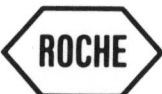

PRESENTED WITH

THE COMPLIMENTS OF

ROCHE LABORATORIES

DIVISION OF

HOFFMANN - LA ROCHE INC.

NUTLEY, N. J.

PRINCIPLES OF

AMBULATORY MEDICINE

THIRD EDITION

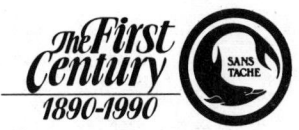

PRINCIPLES OF

AMBULATORY MEDICINE

THIRD EDITION

Edited by

L. Randol Barker, M.D.

Associate Professor of Medicine
The Johns Hopkins University School of Medicine
Co-Director, Division of General Internal Medicine
Francis Scott Key Medical Center
Baltimore, Maryland

John R. Burton, M.D.

Associate Professor of Medicine
Clinical Director, Division of Geriatric Medicine and Gerontology
The Johns Hopkins University School of Medicine
Director, Division of Geriatric Medicine
Francis Scott Key Medical Center
Baltimore, Maryland

Philip D. Zieve, M.D.

Professor of Medicine
The Johns Hopkins University School of Medicine
Chairman, Department of Medicine
Francis Scott Key Medical Center
Baltimore, Maryland

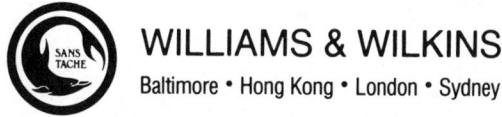

WILLIAMS & WILKINS
Baltimore • Hong Kong • London • Sydney

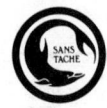

Editor: Michael G. Fisher
Associate Editor: Carol Eckhart
Copy Editor: Susan Vaupel
Designer: Norman W. Och
Illustration Planner: Lorraine Wrzosek
Production Coordinator: Charles E. Zeller

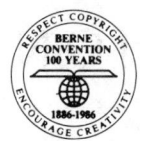

Accurate indications, adverse reactions, and dosage schedules for drugs are provided in this book, but it is possible that they may change. The reader is urged to
review the package information data of the manufacturers of the medications
mentioned.

Printed in the United States of America

First Edition 1982
Second Edition 1986

Library of Congress Cataloging in Publication Data

Principles of ambulatory medicine / edited by L. Randol Barker, John R. Burton,
  Philip D. Zieve. — 3rd ed.
      p.   cm.
    Includes bibliographical references.
    ISBN 0-683-00437-9
    1. Family medicine. 2. Ambulatory medical care. I. Barker, L. Randol (Lee
  Randol), 1939–   . II. Burton, John R. (John Russell), 1937–   . III. Zieve,
  Philip D.,
  1932–   .
    [DNLM: 1. Ambulatory Care. WX 205 P957]
  RC46.P894 1990
  616—dc20
  DNLM/DLC   90-12180
  for Library of Congress   CIP

                                      91 92 93 94
                          1   2   3   4   5   6   7   8   9   10

PREFACE FOR THE THIRD EDITION

The principles stated in the Preface to the First Edition continue to guide the writing of this textbook of ambulatory medicine. Contributors have incorporated into each chapter of the third edition the large amount of new information required to meet the needs of our readers. The recommendations of many practicing physicians have again helped us to achieve this end. The third edition contains one major new chapter, Ambulatory Care for the Patient with HIV Infection.

For this edition, the editors and the publisher have embarked on a new, more efficient book-production process, in conjunction with the Laboratory for Applied Research in Academic Information of the William H. Welch Medical Library of The Johns Hopkins University. The production process utilizes the library's advanced capabilities for electronic information management. The electronic data base for *Principles of Ambulatory Medicine* will make possible two related objectives—continuous updating of the text and on-line access to the text in ambulatory practice settings.

A note on gender pronouns. Readers will note that we have adopted the following approaches to the use of gender pronouns: All text that refers to physicians utilizes language that is inclusive of both genders. Female gender pronouns are employed in all text that refers to conditions that affect women exclusively. Male gender language is often employed for conditions that affect both men and women. This latter approach was elected to avoid awkward phrasing that would occur frequently if inclusive language pronouns were utilized in all references to patients.

PREFACE TO THE SECOND EDITION

Since publication of the first edition of *Principles of Ambulatory Medicine*, the locus of patient care has continued to shift from the hospital bed to the physician's office: hospitalized patients are discharged earlier, and many conditions for which patients were traditionally hospitalized are now managed entirely in the ambulatory setting. These facts, plus the increase in knowledge important in ambulatory care, are the reasons for preparing a second edition of this book. The objectives and the format for the book are identical to those described in the preface to the first edition. This edition is approximately 350 pages longer, due to the addition of several new chapters and to expansion in the scope of many chapters. Every chapter has been revised to incorporate new information. There are a number of new contributors, all with current or previous affiliations with the Francis Scott Key Medical Center (formerly Baltimore City Hospital) and/or the Johns Hopkins University School of Medicine.

New chapters in this edition are Chapter 3: The Doctor-Patient Relationship: Communication and Patient Education; Chapter 31: Ambulatory Care for Selected Subacute Infections: Osteomyelitis, Lung Abscess, and Endocarditis; and Chapter 33: Medical Advice for the International Traveler. In addition, the new version of Chapter 6, Geriatric Patients: Special Considerations, describes in greater depth the practical approach to urinary incontinence, comprehensive evaluation of functional status, and other aspects of this important area of practice; a detailed chapter on Alcoholism, by new contributors, replaces the brief chapter on this subject from the first edition; chapters on a number of other psychiatric and behavioral topics (e.g., evaluation of psychosocial problems, office psychotherapy, psychosomatic syndromes, adjustment disorders, anxiety syndromes, and tobacco abuse) have been revised extensively; the chapter on infectious mononucleosis has been expanded to include a number of other conditions that affect lymphocytes (the acquired immune deficiency syndrome, chronic lymphocytic leukemia, and undiagnosed lymphadenopathy), the chapters on Rheumatoid Arthritis and Plasma Lipids and Hyperlipidemia have been largely rewritten; and the chapters on musculoskeletal problems cover additional conditions and include useful new illustrations and information on the examination of the musculoskeletal system.

To a great extent, the preparation of the second edition of *Principles of Ambulatory Medicine* has been guided by the responses of the book's readers. Uniformly, readers cited the practical details regarding patient management as the feature which set *Principles of Ambulatory Medicine* apart from other textbooks. In addition, they pointed out important conditions that were omitted from the first edition, and these conditions have been included in this edition.

PREFACE TO THE FIRST EDITION

This book is directed primarily to the general physician who cares for ambulatory adult patients. The purposes of the book are (a) to provide an in-depth account of the evaluation, management, and long term course of those common clinical problems which are handled by the generalist in the ambulatory setting, and (b) to provide guidelines for recognizing those problems which require either hospitalization or referral for specialized care and for appreciating the expected course of those problems.

For over 60 years, Baltimore City Hospital has offered education to medical students, residents, fellows, and practicing physicians. During the past decade, the full time professional staff of the hospital has developed major teaching and practice initiatives in ambulatory care. The recognition of the need for a clinical textbook which focused upon the ambulatory patient grew directly out of these initiatives. All of the contributors to this text have a present or recent affiliation with Baltimore City Hospital and/or with The Johns Hopkins University School of Medicine. All have had substantial experience caring for ambulatory patients in their areas of expertise. The editors have worked very closely with all contributors to assure that the material they prepared was focused upon the ambulatory patient.

Three principles have guided the preparation of each chapter.

1. That the physician working in a busy office practice needs to know a great deal about *probabilities* related to his patients' conditions. To address this need, the following types of information are emphasized throughout the book:
   a. Relative frequencies of the conditions which underlie common symptoms.
   b. Distribution of conditions in major subgroups of the population.
   c. The sensitivity, specificity, and predictive value of diagnostic tests and procedures.
   d. The expected course of conditions, in both treated and untreated patients.
   e. The frequency of the complications of treatment.
2. That the patient, in fact, makes most decisions in ambulatory care and that the physician should

emphasize the following aspects of *patient education* to assure that the patient's decisions are appropriate:
   a. Information about the short and long term prognosis of the patient's condition, with special emphasis on the implications of the condition for the patient's usual occupational and recreational activities.
   b. Information about the treatment: *i.e.,* how much the treatment usually helps, the expected duration, the correct schedule for treatment (including options adapted to the patient's life style), common side effects, and cost of the treatment.
   c. Information about the experience the patient will undergo when he is referred for care by a specialist or for diagnostic procedures which require his cooperation.
3. That the physician and the patient should incorporate a *preventive point of view* into all of the actions which they take in dealing with a condition. For example, there should be:
   a. Primary prevention of certain conditions, in all patients.
   b. Risk reduction, in those patients who already have certain risk factors.
   c. Optimum maintenance of the patient's health, after a symptomatic condition has developed.
   d. Anticipation of and prevention of problems associated with an established condition or with the treatment prescribed for that condition.

In planning the scope of the book, we selected those conditions which most office-based general internists and general or family practitioners encounter in caring for adult patients from the general population. It was clear that the book should include all of the common conditions of the major organ systems which have been the focus of internal medicine. It was equally clear that a large group of conditions outside of the traditional scope of internal medicine should be included because of the importance they assume in everyday office practice. For all of the conditions included, we agreed that there is a special body of information needed for care of the ambulatory patient, as defined in the three principles named above.

An introductory chapter, entitled The Distinctive Characteristics of Ambulatory Medicine, defines the domain of ambulatory medicine and delineates the knowledge and the skills which are particularly important in the care of ambulatory patients.

There are a limited number of specific references and a few general references at the end of each chapter. These references are included so that interested readers can pursue in greater depth problems of interest to them. Because we have striven to provide the practical information needed to deal with each of the clinical problems included in this book, readers should be able to make practical decisions for their patients without often having to consult the references.

The book is extensively cross-referenced in order both to avoid redundancy and to facilitate access to useful information contained elsewhere in the book.

In addition, for easy reference, the key topics in each chapter are presented in outline form at the beginning of the chapter.

CONTRIBUTORS

Unless otherwise indicated, hospital appointments are at the Francis Scott Key Medical Center, Baltimore, Maryland, and faculty appointments are at The Johns Hopkins University School of Medicine

Nadim E. Afeiche, M.D.
Staff Physician Orthopedic Surgery
Instructor of Orthopedic Surgery

Richard P. Allen, Ph.D., A.C.P.
Co-Director, Baltimore Regional Sleep
   Disorders Center
Assistant Professor of Neurology

Frank C. Arnett, Jr., M.D.
Professor of Internal Medicine
The University of Texas Health Science
   Center
Houston, Texas

L. Randol Barker, M.D., Sc.M.
Co-Chief, Division of General Internal
   Medicine
Associate Professor of Medicine

Edward Bartlett, B.A., M.P.H., D.R.P.H.
Associate Adjunct Professor
Georgetown University
Department of Community and Family
   Medicine

John G. Bartlett, M.D.
Chief, Division of Infectious Diseases
Johns Hopkins Hospital
Stanhope Bayne-Jones Professor of
   Medicine

Eric B. Bass, M.D.
Staff Physician General Internal Medicine
Johns Hopkins Hospital
Instructor in Medicine

Joan M. Bathon, M.D.
Staff Physician, Rheumatology
Assistant Professor of Medicine

George E. Bigelow, Ph.D.
Director, Behavioral Pharmacology
   Research Unit
Associate Professor of Behavioral Biology
   and Assistant Professor of Psychology

Marc R. Blackman, M.D.
Staff Physician, Endocrinology
Associate Professor of Medicine

Eugene R. Bleecker, M.D.
Professor of Medicine
University of Maryland School of
   Medicine

Margit L. Bleecker, M.D.
Formerly Chairman, Department of
   Neurology and Associate Professor of
   Neurology and Medicine

David G. Borenstein, M.D.
Professor of Medicine
The George Washington University
   School of Medicine

Gary R. Briefel, M.D.
Director of Hemodialysis
Associate Professor of Medicine

E. James Britt, M.D.
Clinical Director, Pulmonary Division
University of Maryland Hospital
Associate Professor of Medicine
University of Maryland School of
   Medicine

John R. Burton, M.D.
Clinical Director, Division of Geriatric
   Medicine and Gerontology
The Johns Hopkins University School of
   Medicine
Director Division of Geriatric Medicine
Associate Professor of Medicine

Ronald P. Byank, M.D.
Chairman Department of Orthopaedic
   Surgery
Assistant Professor of Orthopaedic
   Surgery

Richard E. Chaisson, M.D.
Director AIDS Service
Johns Hopkins Hospital
Assistant Professor of Medicine,
   Epidemiology and International Health

Nisha Chibber Chandra, M.D.
Director, Coronary Care Unit
Associate Professor of Medicine

Lawrence J. Cheskin, M.D.
Staff Physician, Digestive Diseases
Assistant Professor of Medicine

Vanessa E. Cullins, M.D., M.P.H.
Staff Physican, Obstetrics/Gynecology
Fellow in Primary Care Obstetrics/
   Gynecology

Peter E. Dans, M.D.
Director, Office of Medical Practice
   Evaluation
Johns Hopkins Hospital
Associate Professor of Medicine

Mahlon R. DeLong, M.D.
Staff Physician, Neurology
Johns Hopkins Hospital
Professor of Neurology and Professor of
   Neuroscience

Susan J. Denman, M.D.
Medical Director Mason F. Lord Chronic
   Hospital and Nursing Home
Assistant Professor of Medicine

J. Raymond DePaulo, M.D.
Director, Affective Disorders Clinic
Johns Hopkins Hospital
Associate Professor of Psychiatry

Burton D'Lugoff, M.D.
Staff Physician Internal Medicine
Associate Professor of Medicine and
   Associate Professor of Psychiatry

Thomas E. Finucane, M.D.
Staff Physician, Geriatric Medicine
Assistant Professor of Medicine

Robert S. Fisher, M.D.
Staff Physician, Neurology
Johns Hopkins Hospital
Associate Professor of Neurology

Preston Gazaway, M.D.
Staff Physician, OB/GYN
Instructor in Obstetrics/Gynecology

Archie S. Golden, M.D., M.P.H.
Chief, General Pediatrics
Associate Professor of Pediatrics
Associate Professor of International
   Health, School of Hygiene and Public
   Health

Peter J. Golueke, M.D.
Chief of Vascular Surgery
Greater Baltimore Medical Center
Assistant Professor of Surgery

Sheldon H. Gottlieb, M.D.
Clinical Director, Cardiology Division
Associate Professor of Medicine

William B. Greenough, III, M.D.
Staff Physician, Geriatric Medicine and
  Infectious Diseases
Professor of Medicine

Robert I. Gregerman, M.D.
Chief, Endocrinology Division
Professor of Medicine

Diane E. Griffin, M.D., Ph.D.
Johns Hopkins Hospital
Professor of Medicine
Professor of Neurology

Richard J. Gross, M.D., Sc.M.
Assistant Professor of Medicine and
  Public Health

Carol S. Haines, M.D., M.P.H.
Instructor in Medicine

S. Mitchell Harman, M.D.
Staff Physician, Endocrinology
Francis Scott Key Medical Center
Gerontology Research Center, NIA
Associate Professor of Medicine

James Hawthorn, Ph.D.
Director, Southeast Baltimore Drug
  Treatment Program
Assistant Professor of Medical
  Psychology

Janet Horn, M.D.
Director, Ambulatory Infectious Diseases
Sinai Hospital of Baltimore
Assistant Professor of Medicine

George R. Huggins, M.D.
Chairman, Department of Obstetrics and
  Gynecology
Associate Professor of Obstetrics and
  Gynecology

Lorraine F. Josifek, M.D.
Neurologist

Philip O. Katz, M.D.
Deputy Director, Department of Medicine
Assistant Professor of Medicine

James P. Keogh, M.D.
Associate Professor of Medicine
Associate Professor of Epidemiology and
  Preventive Medicine
The University of Maryland School of
  Medicine and Hospital

David E. Kern, M.D.
Co-Director, Division of General Internal
  Medicine
Assistant Professor of Medicine

Dilip S. Kittur, M.D.
Chief, Transplant Surgery
Assistant Professor of Surgery

Joyce Kopicky-Burd, M.D.
Formerly Staff Physician, Rheumatology,
  Instructor in Medicine

Frederick T. Koster, M.D.
Associate Professor
University of New Mexico School of
  Medicine
Department of Medicine
Albuquerque, New Mexico

Edward S. Kraus, M.D.
Staff Physician, Nephrology
Assistant Professor of Medicine

Stanford I. Lamberg, M.D.
Formerly Chairman, Department of
  Dermatology, Associate Professor of
  Dermatology

Bruce S. Lebowitz, D.P.M.
Director, Podiatry Clinic

Mark C. Liu, M.D.
Staff Physician, Pulmonary Medicine
Assistant Professor of Medicine

Douglas K. MacLeod, D.M.D.
Formerly Chief, Department of Dentistry

David F. Martin, M.D.
Assistant Chairman, Department of
  Orthopaedic Surgery
Assistant Professor of Orthopaedic
  Surgery

Theodore L. McLemore, M.D., Ph.D.
Staff Physician, Pulmonary Medicine
Assistant Professor of Medicine

Constance J. Meyd, M.D.
Director of Outpatient Neurology
Instructor in Neurology

Esteban Mezey, M.D.
Professor of Medicine

Hamilton Moses III, M.D.
Deputy Director, Department of
  Neurology
Johns Hopkins Hospital
Associate Professor of Neurology

**Andrew Munster, M.D., F.R.C.S. (Eng. &
  Ed.) F.A.C.S.**
Director, Baltimore Regional Burn Center
Professor of Surgery

David N. Neubauer, M.D.
Staff Physician, Psychiatry
Assistant Professor of Medicine

Nathaniel F. Pierce, M.D.
Professor of Medicine

Thomas J. Preziosi, M.D.
Staff Physician, Neurology
Johns Hopkins Hospital
Associate Professor of Neurology

Michael J. Purtell, M.D.
Staff Physician Hematology-Oncology
Assistant Professor of Medicine

Robert M. Quinlan, M.D.
Chief of Surgery
Medical Center of Central Mass—
  Memorial
Worcester, Massachusetts
Professor of Surgery
University of Massachusetts School of
  Medicine
Worcester, Massachusetts

Peter V. Rabins, M.D.
Department of Psychiatry and Behavioral
  Sciences
Johns Hopkins Hospital
Associate Professor of Psychiatry

Stephen G. Reich, M.D.
Staff Physician, Neurology
Johns Hopkins Hospital
Instructor in Neurology

Robert P. Roca, M.D., M.P.H.
Director, Consultation and Geriatric
  Psychiatry
Assistant Professor of Psychiatry and
  Medicine

Warren Rothman, M.D.
Chief, Otolaryngology-Head and Neck
  Surgery
Assistant Professor of Otolaryngology

R. Bradley Sack, M.D.
Professor of Medicine and International
  Health

Andrew P. Schachat, M.D.
Director, Ocular Oncology Service
Johns Hopkins Hospital
Associate Professor of Medicine

Larry N. Scherzer, M.D., M.P.H.
Northeast Permanente Medical Group
East Hartford, Connecticut
Assistant Professor of Pediatrics
University of Connecticut
Farmington, Connecticut

Chester W. Schmidt, Jr., M.D.
Chairman, Psychiatry
Associate Professor of Psychiatry

Marvin M. Schuster, M.D.
Director, Division of Digestive Diseases
Professor of Medicine and Joint
  Appointment in Psychiatry

Stephen D. Sears, M.D.
Vice President for Medical Affairs
Kennebec Valley Medical Center
Augusta, Maine

Edward P. Shapiro, M.D.
Director, Cardiac Non-Invasive Service
Associate Professor of Medicine

Gardner W. Smith, M.D.
Chairman, Section of Surgical Sciences
Professor of Surgery

Philip L. Smith, M.D.
Co-Director, Baltimore Regional Sleep
  Disorders Center
Associate Professor of Medicine and
  Instructor of Anesthesiology

David A. Spector, M.D.
Director, Division of Nephrology
Associate Professor of Medicine

Robert J. Spence, M.D.
Chief of Plastic Surgery
Assistant Professor of Plastic Surgery

Aaron Spital, M.D.
Associate Physician
University of Maryland Health Center
College Park, Maryland

Kerry J. Stewart, Ed.D.
Director, Cardiac Exercise Program
Assistant Professor of Medicine

Dean J. Storer, M.D.
Staff Physician Psychiatry
Johns Hopkins Hospital
Instructor in Psychiatry and Behavioral
  Science

Ray E. Stutzman, M.D.
Chief, Division of Urology
Associate Professor of Urology

Peter B. Terry, M.D.
Staff Physician, Pulmonary Medicine
Associate Professor of Medicine

Mahmud A. Thamer, M.D.
Director, Cardiac Rehabilitation Program
Assistant Professor of Medicine

Alexander S. Townes, M.D.
Chief of Staff
Veterans Administration Medical Center
Nashville, Tennessee
Professor of Medicine
Vanderbilt University School of Medicine
Nashville, Tennessee

Martin D. Valentine, M.D.
Johns Hopkins Asthma and Allergy
  Center
Professor of Medicine

Larry Waterbury, M.D.
Chief, Division of Hematology-Oncology
Associate Professor of Medicine

Charles L. Whitfield, M.D.
Clinical Associate Professor of Medicine
  and Family Medicine
University of Maryland School of
  Medicine
Baltimore, Maryland

Fredrick M. Wigley, M.D.
Chief, Division of Rheumatology
Associate Professor of Medicine

Elena Yamaguchi, M.D.
Johns Hopkins Hospital
Fellow in Infectious Diseases

Philip D. Zieve, M.D.
Chairman, Department of Medicine,
  Physician-in-Chief
Professor of Medicine

ACKNOWLEDGMENTS

The editors wish to acknowledge the helpful suggestions of many colleagues, both generalists and specialists, who provided feedback on the second edition and who reviewed chapters for this edition. We are greatly appreciative of the excellent help provided by Mrs. Marjorie Gregerman and her staff in the Department of Art as Applied to Medicine. Two persons, Mrs. Carole Messman and Ms. Susan McFeaters, provided excellent administrative and typographic assistance throughout the preparation of all three editions of the book.

CONTENTS

SECTION 1: Issues of General Concern in Ambulatory Care

SECTION 2: Psychiatric and Behavioral Problems

SECTION 3: Allergy and Infectious Diseases

SECTION 4: Gastrointestinal Problems

SECTION 5: Renal and Urological Problems

SECTION 6: Hematological Problems

SECTION 7: Pulmonary Problems

SECTION 8: Cardiovascular Problems

SECTION 9: Musculoskeletal Problems

SECTION 10: Metabolic and Endocrinological Problems

SECTION 11: Neurological Problems

SECTION 12: Selected General Surgical Problems

SECTION 13: Gynecological Problems

SECTION 14: Problems of the Eyes and Ears

SECTION 15: Miscellaneous Problems

Issues of General Concern in Ambulatory Care

Distinctive Characteristics of Ambulatory Medicine

L. RANDOL BARKER, M.D.

The fundamental tenet of this book is that ambulatory medicine has a number of distinctive characteristics that should shape physicians' approaches to their ambulatory patients. This chapter describes the present domain of ambulatory care in the United States and defines the goals and the proficiencies that are central to the practice of ambulatory medicine.

DOMAIN OF AMBULATORY MEDICINE

Who are the physicians providing ambulatory care? Which patients visit physicians in their offices? What are the problems that these patients present to their physicians? What is the ambulatory care provided for these problems? In order to answer these questions, the United States National Ambulatory Medical Care Survey (NAMCS), started in 1973, has collected information periodically from a representative sample of physicians' offices.

Office-Based Physicians

Table 1.1 shows the distribution by physician specialty of the 636 million office visits to physicians in the United States during 1985. Of these visits approximately 30% were to general and family practitioners and 12% were to internists, the two groups of generalists to whom this book is directed primarily.

Table 1.1.
Number and Percentage Distribution of Office Visits by Physician Specialty: United States, 1985[a]

Physician Specialty, Type of Practice, and Professional Identity	Number of Visits in Thousands	Percentage Distribution
All visits	636,386	100.0
Physician specialty		
General and family practice	193,995	30.5
Internal medicine	73,727	11.6
Pediatrics	72,693	11.4
Obstetrics and gynecology	56,642	8.9
Ophthalmology	40,062	6.3
Orthopedic surgery	31,482	4.9
General surgery	29,858	4.7
Dermatology	24,124	3.8
Psychiatry	17,989	2.8
Otorhinolaryngology	16,097	2.5
Urological surgery	11,699	1.8
Cardiovascular disease	10,617	1.7
Neurology	4,992	0.8
All other specialties	52,408	8.2

[a]From National Ambulatory Medical Care Survey, 1985.

Table 1.2.
Percentage Distribution of Visits to General and Family Physicians and to Internists by Age and Sex of Patient: United States, 1985[a]

Age and Sex of Patient	Percentage Distribution	
	General and Family Practice	Internal Medicine
All ages	100.0	100.0
Under 15 years	15.3	3.5
15–24 years	13.6	6.4
25–44 years	28.9	21.7
45–64 years	22.7	29.3
65 years and over	19.6	39.2
Female	60.7	61.1
Male	39.3	38.9

[a]From National Ambulatory Medical Care Survey, 1985.

Ambulatory Patients

The age and sex distribution of the patients who visit these two groups of generalists is shown in Table 1.2. Approximately 60% of visits to all generalists are made by female patients. The principal differences shown in Table 1.2 are that adolescents and young adults account for a larger proportion of visits to general and family physicians than to internists, and that visits by older patients make up a larger proportion of the practice of internists.

The NAMCS definition of an ambulatory patient is "an individual presenting for personal health services who is neither bedridden nor currently admitted to any health care institution." We would add to this definition that an ambulatory or homebound patient (or a member of the household) has most of the responsibility for his or her own care; that is, the patient must administer most or all treatments, must monitor symptoms and functional status, must adapt activity to the constraints imposed by illness, and must decide how to deal with new problems when they arise. These characteristics of an ambulatory patient have important implications for the physician, as discussed below.

Problems of Ambulatory Patients

What types of problems are seen in ambulatory practice? Physicians participating in NAMCS were asked to name the principal diagnoses (using the International Classification of Diseases) for the problems addressed at a large sample of visits. Table 1.3 lists the most common responses given in 1985 by internists and general and family physicians, respectively. For both of these generalist groups of physicians, 25 problems or diagnoses accounted for approximately 50% of total visits.

Ambulatory Care

The NAMCS defined ambulatory care as "health services rendered to individuals under their own cognizance, any time when they are not in a hospital or other health care institution." Table 1.4, from the 1985 NAMCS report, shows the percentage distribution of diagnostic and therapeutic services ordered or provided by internists and general or family physicians for their ambulatory patients. The table also shows the frequency distribution of visit duration and of visit status of patients.

The majority of visits included some type of diagnostic service and the majority included some form of therapy (most commonly a prescription for medicine). At about one in five visits internists and general/family practitioners devoted a significant part of the visit to counseling. These data probably underestimate the amount of time devoted to education of the patient.

At 62% of visits to internists and 53% of visits to general and family practitioners, the patient had been seen before for the same problem, and the patient was seen for the first time at only 14% to 15% of visits.

In addition to office visits, telephone encounters and house calls are important in the care of ambulatory patients. *Telephone encounters* enable physicians and patients to handle many problems efficiently; they constitute approximately 25% of all patient contacts for internists and 19% for family physicians (1). *Home visits* are helpful for providing care to patients who are too frail to make office visits or for learning facts about patients' home conditions that may facilitate management of their problems at future office visits. The roles of house calls and home health services in ambulatory medicine are discussed in Chapters 6 (Geriatric Medicine) and 9 (Selected Special Services).

Self-Care

Before making visits to physicians, patients usually attempt to diagnose and treat their own symptoms. Studies of the domain of self-care have shown that at any one time approximately 30% of persons are taking nonprescribed medications or are engaged in self-care for a problem for which they have not consulted a physician (4). The frequency distribution of conditions managed by self-care has been estimated by Fry (3) on the basis of many years of general practice in a community well known to him: 25% upper respiratory infections, 20% musculoskeletal symptoms, 20% emo-

Table 1.3.
Reasons for Ambulatory Visits to Generalists: United States, January to December 1985[a]

Rank	25 Most Common Reasons (by ICD-9-CM Categories)	
	Internists: Reason for Visit	General and Family Practitioners: Reason for Visit
1	Essential hypertension	Essential hypertension
2	Diabetes mellitus	General medical examination
3	Other forms of chronic ischemic heart disease	Acute upper respiratory infections
4	Acute upper respiratory infections	Diabetes mellitus
5	General medical examination	Normal pregnancy
6	Osteoarthrosis and allied disorders	Suppurative and unspecified otitis media
7	General symptoms	Acute pharyngitis
8	Chronic airway obstruction	Bronchitis
9	Asthma	Chronic sinusitis
10	Bronchitis	Certain adverse effects not elsewhere classif.
11	Neurotic disorders	Health supervision of infant or child
12	Angina pectoris	Sprains and strains
13	Chronic sinusitis	Other disorders of urethra and urinary tract
14	Acute pharyngitis	Obesity and other hyperalimentation
15	Cardiac dysrhythmias	General symptoms
16	Other disorders of soft tissue	Contact dermatitis and other eczema
17	Symptoms involving respiratory system	Neurotic disorders
18	Heart failure	Osteoarthrosis and allied disorders
19	Peripheral enthesopathies	Other and unspecified arthropathies
20	Other and unspecified arthropathies	Other disorders of soft tissues
21	Diseases of esophagus	Other noninfectious gastroenteritis
22	Other noninfectious gastroenteritis	Asthma
23	Other disorders of urethra and urinary tract	Sprains and strains of sacroiliac region
24	Allergic rhinitis	Acute tonsillitis
25	Hypertensive heart disease	Disorders of external ear

[a]From National Ambulatory Medical Care Survey, 1985.

Table 1.4.
Percentage Distribution of Visits to Office-Based Generalists by Selected Diagnostic and Therapeutic Services Ordered or Provided, Duration of Visit, and Visit Status, United States, January–December, 1985[a]

	Percentage of Visits	
	To Internists	To General and Family Practitioners
Selected diagnostic services		
Blood pressure checked	72.1%	52.3%
Breast examination	7.2	4.9
Urinalysis or CBC or chemistries	51.9	32.7
Chest X-ray	7.3	3.1
Electrocardiogram	11.1	3.0
Selected therapeutic services		
Medication prescribed	77.4	72.7
Counseling:		
Diet counseling	10.9	8.9
Psychotherapy	2.2	1.1
Other counseling	11.6	8.0
Physiotherapy	3.8	5.4
Duration of visit		
0 minutes (no face-to-face encounter with physicians)	1.3	3.1
1–5 minutes	4.1	9.0
6–10 minutes	20.2	34.2
11–15 minutes	36.3	31.5
16–30 minutes	29.5	19.7
31–60 minutes	7.5	2.3
Visit status of patient		
New patient	15.2	14.1
Old patient, new problem	22.9	32.6
Old patient, old problem	61.8	53.3

[a]From *The National Ambulatory Medical Care Survey.* Washington, D.C., Department of Health and Human Services, 1985.

tional problems, 10% acute gastrointestinal symptoms, 5% skin rashes, and 20% miscellaneous other symptoms.

The time interval between the onset of a new problem and the decision to go to the physician (i.e., the duration of self-care) is shown for a number of common conditions in Table 1.5, adapted from NAMCS. Not surprisingly, patients with lacerations, symptoms

of acute infections, and new chest pain presented within 1 to 6 days while those with subacute problems (headache or back pain) tended to present after at least 1 week of self-care.

Self-care before professional care is an important way in which the patient, not the physician, makes the decisions in the domain of ambulatory medicine. The patient's primary role in carrying out the plan of care after visiting a physician has already been emphasized in the expanded definition of the ambulatory patient given above. These two features confirm the primacy of the patient's decisions in influencing the course of events in ambulatory medicine.

Temporal Dimension in Ambulatory Medicine

The information from NAMCS contained in Tables 1.1 to 1.5 does not illuminate the longitudinal nature of ambulatory care. Table 1.6 shows the 5-year profile of care for an elderly woman. This patient's story illustrates each of the following important questions for which only the passage of time provided the answers:

1. What is the significance of a recent symptom (e.g., the temporal headache for 1 year reported in 1975, subsequently not a serious problem)?
2. What is the advisability of initiating a referral for a problem (e.g., cataract problem identified but asymptomatic in 1975, evaluated when more symptomatic in 1978 and classified as not mature)?
3. How well will the patient adhere to recommended treatment (e.g., the digoxin for heart failure, taken reliably for 5 years)?
4. What is the impact of treatment upon the patient's health (e.g., adding a diuretic in 1978; heart failure gradually improved during the month after diuretic)?
5. What is the impact of intercurrent medical problems upon the patient's usual activities? (The answer to this question varied over time depending upon intercurrent problems: During the 5 years the patient's ambulation deteriorated greatly; however, other valued activities, such as crocheting and canning, did not.)

Table 1.5.
Percentage Distribution of New Problem Office Visits by Time since Onset of Complaint or Symptom, According to Selected Principal Reasons for Visit: United States, January to December 1977[a]

Principal Reason for Visit	Total	Time since Onset of Complaint or Symptom					
		1 Day	1–6 Days	1–3 Wk	1–3 Mo	>3 Mo	Not Applicable
		%					
All new problem visits	100.0	8.2	37.3	15.6	10.3	13.9	14.8
Symptoms of throat	100.0	6.9	77.9	10.6	2.3	1.9	0.4
Cough	100.0	3.3	73.0	18.6	2.9	2.1	0.2
Head cold, upper respiratory tract infection	100.0	6.2	72.5	16.5	3.0	1.1	0.7
Fever	100.0	17.6	76.4	4.7	0.2	1.0	
Headache	100.0	5.1	35.6	19.0	16.5	19.7	3.2
Back symptoms	100.0	6.5	37.6	26.4	11.8	16.2	1.5
Chest pain	100.0	7.6	45.8	22.6	9.3	13.6	1.2
Laceration, upper extremity	100.0	70.4	15.4	7.8	3.0	2.1	1.3

[a]From *National Ambulatory Medical Care Survey, 1977, Summary.* Hyattsville, MD, National Center for Health Statistics, 1979.

Table 1.6.
Profile of 5 Years in the Care of an Elderly Patient (Each Problem *Italicized*)

Feature	1975	1976	1977	1978	1979
ENCOUNTERS	Initial visit, 4 office visits, many phone calls	3 office visits, many phone calls	5 office visits, 2 hospital admissions, 1 home visit, many phone calls	4 office visits, many phone calls	4 office visits, many phone calls
PRINCIPAL MEDICAL PROBLEMS	*Acute myocardial infarction* (mild congestive heart failure; digitalized; home management by patient's choice)	Stable (digoxin)	Stable (digoxin)	Congestive heart failure (diuretic added)	Stable (digoxin, diuretic)
	Degenerative joint disease (knees for years; cervical spine for years)	Waxes and wanes (aspirin, Motrin)	Same (coated aspirin)	Same (coated aspirin)	Same (coated aspirin)
	Temporal headaches for 1 year (erythrocyte sedimentation rate 30)	Rarely	Rarely	Rarely	Rarely
	Hearing loss (ear, nose, and throat examination: senile high frequency deficit, no prescription)	Stable	Stable	Stable	Stable
	Bilateral cataracts	Stable	Stable	Referred (not mature)	Stable
	Leukoplakia, mouth (biopsy: not malignant)	Stable	Stable	Stable	Referred for change in appearance (biopsy: not malignant)
	Hematocrit 35 (guaiac-negative)	Stable	Stable		Stable
	Constipation (for years)	Waxes and wanes (over-the-counter (OTC) laxative as needed)	Same (OTC laxative as needed)	Same (OTC laxative as needed and stool softener)	Same (OTC laxative as needed and stool softener)
		Leg cramps (quinine at bedtime)	Minimal (quinine at bedtime)	Same (quinine at bedtime)	Same (quinine at bedtime)
		Left cerebral *transient ischemic attack* (TIA)	*Left cerebrovascular accident* (CVA) (hospital, physical therapy)	Stable (right hemiparesis)	Recurrent left CVA (home management)
			Dog bite (cellulitis)	No recurrence	No recurrence
			Rectal bleeding (hospital, negative workup)	No recurrence	No recurrence
			Dysuria (culture negative)	*Family temporarily "exhausted"* (Visiting Nurses Association)	Family doing well
				Painful toe	Persists (codeine)
				Appetite lost temporarily	No recurrence
OVERALL PROFILE	87-year-old widow living with daughter's family, ambulatory and independent in the home, mentally intact, crochets and cans food; weight 166; multiple medical problems identified at initial visit (above)	88 years old, status the same; weight 160; 2 new problems (above)	89 years old, ambulation with walker assistance after CVA; weight 151; 4 new problems (above), hospitalized twice	90 years old, status the same; weight 140; 3 new problems (above)	91 years old; ambulation more impaired after second CVA; mentally intact, crochets and cans food; weight 139; no new problem

GOALS OF AMBULATORY CARE

The Patient's Expectations

The goals of ambulatory care are determined by the fact that the patient is residing at home, not in an institution. Residence at home creates daily expectations that are similar to the expectations of someone who has not in fact become a patient, such as: to play as active a role as possible in the life of one's family and community; to be as capable as possible of taking care of basic needs such as nutrition, clothing, hygiene, travel, etc.; on an average day to be as free as possible of physical and emotional symptoms while engaging in one's usual activities; and to be generally satisfied with one's situation in life. Depending on the severity of their medical problems, ambulatory patients may be greatly, moderately, or not at all constrained from attaining these expectations. But by virtue of living at home, they will be dealing with these expectations daily, in contrast to hospitalized patients for whom these expectations must await return to home.

Implications for Practice

In order to decide how any patient is doing, a physician must know about that person's particular expectations; this usually involves learning about the make-up of the patient's household and the patient's usual role in the household, about the patient's occupation and level of formal education, about valued activities and about short- and long-term plans.

Knowledge of how well a patient is meeting personal expectations is often critical in managing that patient's active medical problems. This point can be illustrated by a common example, namely, that of the head of a household who has had an uncomplicated myocardial infarction. After 3 months, the patient might be assessed as "status postmyocardial infarction—doing well." If he is back at work, then he is indeed "doing well." If he is not back at work, is financially stressed, and his wife reports that he has become irritable, then he is "not doing well" and he needs additional support from his physician.

Awareness of a patient's life circumstances is also important in preventive care (see Chapter 2), in which the patient's degree of "wellness" rather than degree of illness is assessed. Assessing wellness means learning whether a patient is engaging in health-promoting behaviors and determining what health risks the patient has. For example, a 40-year-old mother who is happily married, free of chronic disease, has stopped smoking, has had periodic negative Pap smears and breast examinations, and drinks alcohol only socially would be assessed as very well. If everything were the same but she smoked two packs of cigarettes daily, she would be assessed as only relatively well because of the major risk posed by heavy tobacco exposure. If she were recently divorced, had stopped seeing friends, and was smoking and drinking heavily, she would be assessed as not very well, even though she might not complain of any particular symptoms or have objective evidence of any disease.

KNOWLEDGE AND SKILLS CENTRAL TO AMBULATORY MEDICINE

The picture provided by the National Ambulatory Medical Care Survey and other studies of office practice has clear implications for the knowledge and skills that are most important in the practice of ambulatory medicine. These are a fund of knowledge from clinical epidemiology and clinical pharmacology and proficiency in communication with patients, in record keeping, in coordination of care, and in containing costs.

Clinical Epidemiology

Feinstein has defined clinical epidemiology as follows:

"The territory is the clinicostatistical study of diseased populations. The intellectual activities of this territory include the following: the occurrence rates and geographic distribution of disease; the patterns of natural and post-therapeutic events that constitute varying clinical courses in the diverse spectrum of a disease; and the clinical appraisal of therapeutic agents" (2) and of diagnostic tests (author's addendum).

In patient care, physicians utilize information from clinical epidemiology to (a) make working diagnoses, (b) understand the natural history of conditions and the capacity of treatment to alter them, and (c) make patient care decisions.

Working Diagnosis/Assessment

In ambulatory medicine, the assessment of a patient may range from "healthy without any significant risk factors," to "healthy with risk factors A and B for disease X," to a working diagnosis of "disease X."

In evaluating a patient for the presence of a risk factor or of an established disease, it is critical to be aware of the prevalence (i.e., proportion of the population affected at one particular time) and the incidence (i.e., proportion of the population newly affected during a specified interval of time) of the suspected condition in the general population and in the particular subgroup(s) to which the patient belongs. This information enables a physician to follow a strategy that is particularly important in ambulatory medicine: *focusing upon the probable and not upon the possible.* A familiar example of this strategy is the evaluation of a patient for hypertension. The prevalence of hypertension is 10 to 20% in adults in United States. The prevalence of renovascular hypertension is probably less than 1% in the overall population of hypertensive patients and less than .1% in the population of black hypertensive patients. Based on this information, screening for hypertension is appropriate in all adult patients, but screening for renovascular hypertension is not appropriate in most hypertensive patients, especially those who are black.

Three principal types of clinical data are utilized to reach a working diagnosis:

1. A single diagnostic test, for example, a biopsy that shows a malignant neoplasm.
2. A quantitative deviation in a single physiological function, for example, a fasting blood glucose that satisfies a criterion for diabetes.
3. A cluster of information that may include history of exposures, present or recent symptoms, present signs, and the results of laboratory tests (e.g., the cluster of data that leads one to working diagnosis of transfusion-related non-A, non-B hepatitis).

There are two sets of performance characteristics that describe diagnostic and screening tests and help in assessing the meaning of positive or negative test results (or positive or negative findings from the interview and the physical examination):

1. *The sensitivity and specificity* of the test. The sensitivity of a test is the percentage of affected individuals that will have a positive test (or true positive rate). The sensitivity is determined by utilizing the test on a large group of patients known to have the condition being tested for (see Fig. 1.1). The spec-

ificity of the test is the percentage of non-affected individuals that will have a negative test (or true negative rate). The specificity of a test is determined by utilizing the test on a large group of patients who are known not to have the condition (see Fig. 1.1). Figure 1.2 illustrates two points that are especially important in interpreting sensitivity and specificity values reported from patient studies: that both the cut-point selected for "positive" and the population in which the test is evaluated have major influence on the meaning of a "positive" or "negative" test result.

2. *The predictive value* (or posttest probability) of the test, which means the probability that one's own patient has a suspected condition when the test is positive (positive predictive value) or does not have the suspected condition when the test is negative (negative predictive value). The predictive value of a test is dependent upon the prevalence of that condition in the population to which the patient belongs. The predictive value of a positive test is highest when the prevalence (or prior probability) of a condition is relatively high (≥5%) and the specificity and sensitivity of the test are also relatively high. As shown in Figure 1.1, the predictive value of a test can be calculated when the prevalence of a condition in the population plus the sensitivity

DISEASE

Present   Not Present

TEST

	Present	Not Present
+	True Positive	False Positive
−	False Negative	True Negative

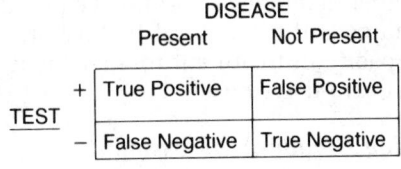

Independent of prevalence of the disease in the population to which a specific patient belongs

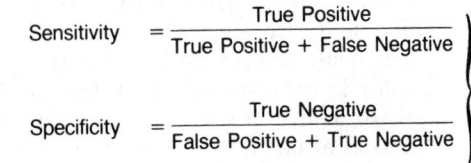

Dependent on prevalence of the disease in population to which the patient belongs

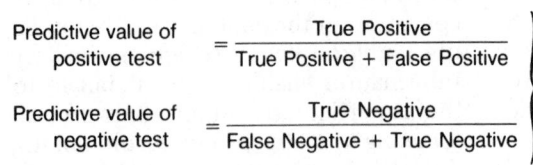

EXAMPLES:

Population to Which Patient Belongs	Prevalence of Condition	Test Characteristics		Predictive Value of a Positive Test	Predictive Value of a Negative Test
		Sensitivity	Specificity		
A	1%	90%	90%	9%	99.9%
B	10%	90%	90%	50%	98.7%

Figure 1.1. Methods for determining sensitivity, specificity, and predictive values of a test. Examples show the influence of disease prevalence upon the predictive values of positive and negative tests.

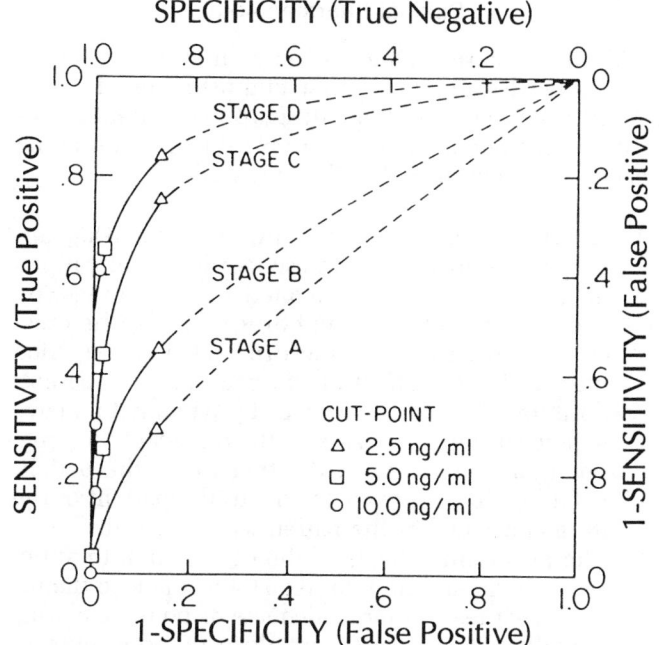

SPECIFICITY (True Negative)

Figure 1.2. The sensitivity/specificity of a test varies with the stage of disease and the cut-point for a "positive" test. ROC (Receiver Operating Characteristic) curve for carcinoembryonic antigen (CEA) as a diagnostic test for colorectal cancer according to stage of disease. From Fletcher R, Fletcher S, Wagner E. *Clinical Epidemiology,* Baltimore, Williams & Wilkins, 1988.

and the specificity of the test are known or can be estimated.

In the examples shown at the bottom of Figure 1.1, it can be seen that only 9% or 9 of 100 patients with positive tests from population A (1% prevalence of condition X) would have the condition and the other 91 with positive tests would not have the condition, whereas 50 of 100 patients with a positive test from population B (10% prevalence) would have the condition.

Natural History and the Impact of Treatment

This information is derived from longitudinal studies and clinical trials.

In order to learn the natural history of a condition (including a risk factor), a group of subjects representative of the universe of patients affected by the condition must be followed longitudinally. Ideally the longitudinal study is conducted prospectively, meaning that the questions to be asked and the data to be collected are chosen before subjects are enrolled. In reality, many of the studies of the natural history of conditions have been performed retrospectively (meaning that the primary data were generated before the study was planned and that the patients selected were those available for review at the time the study was planned). At times, a satisfactory "prospective" study can be reconstructed from events that preceded the planning of the study.

In order to delineate the impact of treatment, the

study design should assure that treated subjects are compared with untreated subjects who are similar in every important characteristic except treatment. Again, ideally, the study is conducted prospectively (a clinical trial); participating subjects are allocated randomly to two groups for concurrent study or the same subjects are allocated randomly to study and comparison treatments for crossover study; the study is double blind, meaning that neither the investigator nor the subjects know who is receiving which treatment; a simulation of treatment in the form of a placebo is utilized in the comparison group; and results include an analysis of all patients who were randomized, whether or not they completed the trial (intention-to-treat analysis). For many of the conditions seen in ambulatory medicine, longitudinal studies of treatment are either inadequate or have not been conducted at all. In these instances, physicians must utilize their own judgment and published evaluations of existing information.

Even the best designed clinical trials rarely address *effectiveness*. The effectiveness of a treatment is a measure of its impact in patients being cared for in the "real world," meaning representative community and practice settings. This concept is different from the familiar concept of the efficacy of a therapy, which is a measure of its impact in patients participating in clinical trials. In recent years, patient compliance—a major determinant of the effectiveness of treatment in ambulatory patients—has been studied in "real world" settings for a variety of conditions (see Chapter 4). Such studies have generally demonstrated that adherence to a prescribed regimen in ambulatory patients is highly variable, and that a number of factors related to patient behavior must be considered if treatment is to be effective for the individual patient.

Patient Care Decisions

To help their patients to select diagnostic and management decisions, physicians combine information from clinical epidemiology, information from their experience and their colleagues' experiences, and special information about the individual patient, in particular the patient's goals and expectations. In recent years, a quantitative method for making decisions (Decision Analysis) has been developed; a decision analysis is usually displayed as a decision tree Fig. 1.3). Formal decision analysis is especially useful for addressing complex decisions for a patient. The steps that are followed in formal decision analysis are similar to the steps used informally in most patient-care decisions. They are:

1. To identify the decision problem. In the example, Figure 1.3, the problem is the patient's already-diagnosed herniated lumbar disc.
2. To identify the principal options that the patient might select to address the problem (choice or *decision nodes*, represented by squares on a decision

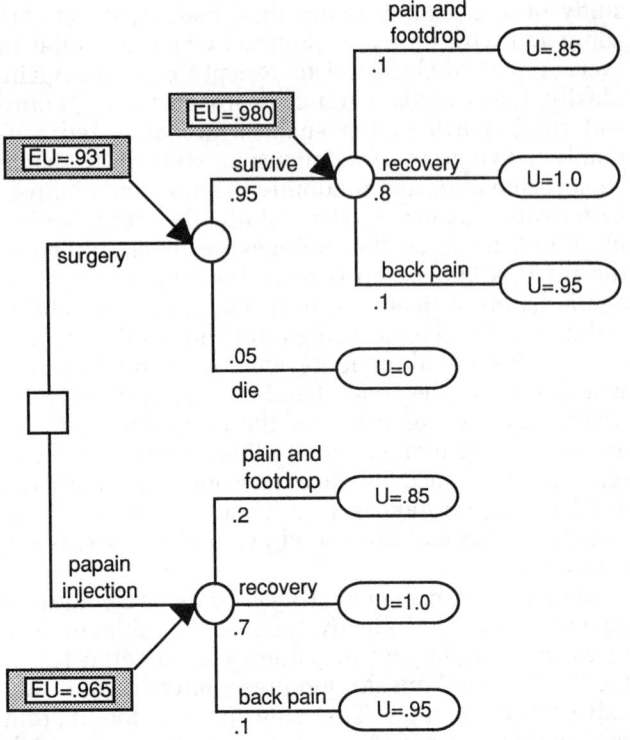

Figure 1.3. This hypothetical decision tree shows utility values (U) selected by the patient for each outcome, probability values for each potential consequence of a decision, and calculated expected utilities (EU) for the chance node associated with each of the two management choices (surgery or papain injection for a herniated lumbar disc). From Sox HC Jr., Blatt MA, Higgins MC, Marton KE (eds.): *Medical Decision Making.* Boston, Butterworths, 1988.

tree). In the example the choices are surgery and papain injection.

3. To identify potential consequences of each decision, quantify the probability of each of these consequences (*chance nodes*, represented by circles on a decision tree), and make this information available to the patient. In the example, one such probability would be the 5% risk of operative mortality.
4. To identify the potential outcomes of care (quality of life and longevity) in terms of the patient's overall health and, based on the patient's input, to assign a quantitative value (*utility value* in the decision tree) to each of these outcomes. One utility value shown in the example is .85, meaning that the probability of surviving the operation and being free from pain and footdrop could be as low as 85% and the patient would accept the operation in lieu of having permanent footdrop.
5. To work backwards from the utility values selected by the patient in order to calculate the value (the *expected utility* in a decision tree) for each of the alternative courses of action. In the example, based on the patient's preferences for the various outcomes shown and the expected utility values, the patient would probably choose papain injection over surgery.

Clinical Pharmacology

Clinical pharmacology is the source for the many details needed for appropriate administration of drugs. Apart from the impact of a drug upon a patient's condition, physicians should be aware of the following aspects of each drug that they prescribe:

1. Practical information about initiating the drug: appropriate starting dose and schedule; modifications in dose and schedule dictated by patient age, by concurrently administered drugs, and by the presence of diseases affecting drug metabolism; time interval for the effect of the drug to be apparent; duration of a course of the drug (when not a maintenance drug); how to assess the impact of the drug; potential interaction with other drugs the patient is taking; the appropriate cost to the patient of the drug and whether the patient can afford it.
2. The major side effects of the drug: when to anticipate them, and how to detect and manage them.
3. The major reasons for inadequate response to a drug: nonadherence, insufficient dose of drug, antagonism of the drug by patient behavior or by concurrent drugs, and primary refractoriness to the drug; and how to recognize and manage each of these problems.

Because administering/prescribing of medications is the single most common action taken by generalists in ambulatory medicine (see Table 1.4), access to these practical types of information is particularly important.

Communication and Patient Education

As stated earlier, the goals of care in ambulatory medicine can be equated with the patient's expectations for activities at home, at work, and in the community. Attaining these goals is an ongoing process, requiring some measure of continuous care for most patients and recognition that the patient has the major responsibility for carrying out the plan of care. Given these characteristics of ambulatory medicine, proficiency in interpersonal communication and in patient education are fundamental to motivating patients to select, concur in, and adhere to appropriate care. In recent years, these proficiencies have been delineated more explicitly, and a growing number of investigations have confirmed the positive impact of specific proficiencies on the outcome of care. This domain is covered in depth in Chapter 3.

Documentation of Care

Clinical records are valuable chiefly for reference at some later time. In ambulatory medicine, the interval between visits is usually weeks or months, so that the physician must rely largely upon recorded facts and not on memory. The various characteristics of ambulatory medicine that have been discussed earlier point to the following information that should be available in the office record if it is to provide useful points of reference for subsequent care:

1. A social profile, including information about family, occupational, educational, and recreational circumstances that determine the patient's expectations (see example, Fig. 1.4).
2. A problem list, that is, a list of all medical problems, with dates, that have been identified in the course of the patient's care (see example, Fig. 1.4).
3. A preventive care profile that provides a record that documents baseline risk factors (see Fig. 1.4) and that documents/promotes periodic preventive care (see example, Fig. 2.3).
4. Concise progress notes that document, by problem, data and thinking (assessment/plan).

To record observations about the course of one or more facets of the patient's condition, separate medication records or flow sheets may also be useful in long-term care (see example, Fig. 2.3). To document patient education, it is helpful to use instruction forms that make a duplicate for mounting in the patient's record (see example, Fig. 3.1). Similar forms are useful to document on-call notes describing telephone encounters.

Coordination of Care

The third general skill that is particularly important in ambulatory medicine is skill in coordinating the patient's care. Coordination of care refers to actions that promote appropriate use of services that the patient may need. During the past 20 years, the number of available laboratory services, support services, and specialty consultative services grew enormously: there are currently more than 200 health-related professions

Department of Medicine
PRIMARY CARE PROFILE

Mrs. Jane Doe

Dates
Initiated: 2/85 Updated:
Provider(s): Dr. Jones

Social Profile

Marital Status Widow (2/83) Highest Education High School Income Source Social Security
Work History/Hazard Exposure: Munitions Plant WWII, Saleslady 1950s – 1976 (Ret.)
Children/Immediate Family: 2 daughters, 6 grandchildren – all live in town
Lives with? Alone Permanent impairments: Hearing Loss (Uses Aid)
Person(s) to contact in event of emergency: Mrs. James Smith Relation: daughter (Phone: 533-0000)
Other (activities, major life events, social support system, etc.): Bowls weekly, Active in church, 2 dogs (walks them daily), several neighbors whom she sees weekly

Allergic/Drug Reactions (Year)

None:
Penicillin (hives 1968)

Family HX (Relation/Age)

ASHD: (N) Y ( )
Colon Ca (N) Y ( )
Breast Ca: N (Y) (Mother)
Other:

Risk Profile

Smoker (N) Y (quit 1980)
Quit Dates: ( )
Etoh N Y✓ ( )
C+A+G+E+ Date: (3/86 → quit)
Drugs (N) Y ( )
Exercise N (Y) (Bowls 3x/week)
Cholesterol: 5/85 186 mg %
Other:

Operations (Year)

None:
Hysterectomy 1968
(R) Carpal tunnel 1982

Problem List

Date of Onset/ Identification	#	Problem & Comments (Key Tests/Consults)
– / –	1	HM (Health Maintenance)
/1976	2	COPD Fvc/FEV-1 1.9/1.3 1979
1950s/1976	3	Smoker – stopped 1977
/1976	4	Pneumonia
/1976	5	Mitral Valve Prolapse Echo 1976
/198	6	Prolonged Grief p̄ husband ↓
1983 /1983	7	Stress incontinence → Learned self control technique
/1984	8	Immature Cataracts → Ophth 1983
3/86	9	Alcoholism → Recovering alcoholic since 6/86
/		
/		
/		
/		
/		
/		
/		

Figure 1.4. Example of form for recording social profile, problem list, and other baseline data in an office record.

and occupations; and the ratio of nonphysician health workers to physicians grew from 10:1 in 1960 to more than 20:1 in 1980. The availability of so many services requires the generalist to be prudent in recommending them and in utilizing the information they provide, and to be aware of the cost of a service to the patient, the nature of the experience the patient will undergo, and the likelihood that the service will be of value to the patient.

The services recommended for patients may involve permanent, temporary, or partial transfer of responsibility for the patient's care, or they may be strictly consultative, meaning that they provide information to be utilized directly by the referring physician (ranging from laboratory test results to a consultant's suggestions).

There are two sets of guidelines that define the role of general physicians in the coordination of services that they recommend for patients:

1. Assure that the patient understands the reason for services that are recommended; arrange to obtain information promptly after a service has been performed; and assure that the patient learns, as soon as is appropriate, the meaning of this information.
2. Whenever referring a patient for a service, assure that proper information is given to the person providing the service. For example, there should be a clear indication of what laboratory test is required or of the facts generally needed by consultants (see Table 1.7).

Patients sometimes obtain services for medical problems without referral by their personal physician. These most often include visits to emergency departments or to specialists such as ophthalmologists. Obtaining information about treatment changes or new diagnoses related to these visits is another way in which the generalists should attempt to coordinate their patients' care.

Containing Costs

This chapter has emphasized that the patient has a dominant role in ambulatory medicine, particularly with regard to carrying out the plan of care recommended by the physician. However, just as in hospital medicine, the office-based physician is largely responsible for describing to the patient those options and recommendations that lead to health care spending. Although the ways in which patients pay for services in ambulatory care vary from prepayment for all

services to paying out of pocket for each service when it is rendered, the decision to purchase these services is influenced greatly by the physician. This is similar to many situations in our society in which the consumer entrusts to a professional or expert recommendations regarding the purchase of a particular service.

Owing to the extraordinary increase in available medical services in the past two decades and because of the parallel increase in the cost and the utilization of these services, the containment of the cost of medical care is generally recognized as a national imperative. The need to contain costs has critical implications for generalist physicians in office practice, for it is they who coordinate much of the medical care provided in our society. Table 1.4 indicates that, in addition to paying for the office visit, the patient, on the recommendation of the physician, purchases one or more discrete services or items at the majority of office visits (diagnostic testing, office procedures, prescribed medications, consultant opinions, etc.). There is little doubt that many of these purchases are not necessary for the health of these patients.

There are important ways in which the generalist physician can limit the costs of care:

- Taking a history carefully and allowing some time to pass before embarking on an extensive diagnostic workup of a new symptom.
- Keeping well informed about the impact on health outcomes of costly diagnostic procedures.
- Avoiding additional tests that will not alter one's decisions.
- Devoting sufficient time to educating patients about their conditions (especially about conditions that often lead to inappropriate and costly doctor shopping by the patient).
- Prescribing only necessary medications and selecting the least expensive preparations.
- Utilizing home health services and other community services to forestall the need for hospital admission, or to shorten length of hospitalization.

Unhappily, third party reimbursement patterns have promoted excessive utilization of procedural services in the United States and have discouraged physicians from engaging in the inquiry, observation, and counseling that might obviate much inappropriate purchasing of health services. It is likely that the federal government and other third party payers will eventually implement payment formulas that reward physicians for those cognitive services that promote the health of patients and reduce the unnecessary use of technical services.

Table 1.7.
Information That Subspecialty Consultants Generally Need from the Referring Physician

The specific reason for the consultation
Relevant current medical problems
Relevant current medications
What the patient has been told about the referral
The patient's attitude about the problem (if relevant)

General References

The National Ambulatory Medical Care Survey. (Periodic publications issued by the Department of Health and Human Services. Washington, D.C.).

Nationwide study of a probability sample of office-based physicians from all medical specialty areas, utilizing physician- and patient-generated information to delineate the ambulatory care activities of physicians and patients, started 1973.

Fletcher RH, Fletcher SW, Wagner EH (eds): *Clinical Epidemiology: The Essentials*. Baltimore, Williams & Wilkins, 1982.
  Lucid book written for clinicians. Uses case examples to illustrate all points.
Fries JF, Vickery DM (eds): *Take Care of Yourself: A Consumer's Guide to Medical Care*. 3rd ed. Reading, MA, Addison-Wesley, 1986.
  Good book to recommend to interested patients; contains sound advice about self-care for most common symptoms.
Fry J: *Common Diseases: Their Nature, Incidence and Care*. 2nd ed. Philadelphia, JB Lippincott, 1979.
  Unique account of the longitudinal course of many common diseases, based upon over 25 years of general practice in a single British community.
Griner PF, Mayewski RJ, Mushlin AI, Greenland P: Selection and interpretation of diagnostic tests and procedures. *Ann Intern Med* 94:553, 1981.
  Lucid guidelines for appropriate use of diagnostic tests (special supplementary issue).
Hsiao W, Brawn P, Dunn D, et al: Special Report. Results and policy implications of the resource-based relative-value scale. *N Engl J Med* 319:881, 1988.
  This paper describes the empiric data that justify increased payment to physicians for cognitive services in office practice.
McCue JD (ed): *The Medical Cost-Containment Crisis: Fears, Opinions, and Facts*. Ann Arbor, Health Administration Press Perspectives, 1989.
  A multiauthor book that covers all facets of the topic.
Mendenhall RC, Tarlov AR, Girard RA, et al: A national study of internal medicine and its specialties. II. Primary care in internal medicine. *Ann Intern Med* 91:275, 1979.
  Nationwide study of a large sample of internists (including subspecialists), utilizing physician-generated information to delineate the primary care activities of internists.
Sox HC Jr., Blatt MA, Higgins MC, Marton KI (eds): *Medical Decision Making*. Boston, Butterworths, 1988.
  Lucid account of the steps involved in quantifying probabilities in order to do formal decision analysis. Appendix contains table with true positive rates (sensitivity) for many tests/clinical situations, with references.

Specific References

1. Curtis P: The practice of medicine on the telephone. *JGIM* 3:294, 1988.
2. Feinstein AR: Clinical epidemiology. I–III. *Ann Intern Med* 69:809, 1968.
3. Fry J: *Common Diseases: Their Nature, Incidence and Care*. Chapter 1, 2nd ed. Philadelphia, JB Lippincott, 1979.
4. Kohn R, White KL (eds): *Health Care*. New York, Oxford University Press, 1976.

C H A P T E R   2

Preventive Medicine in Ambulatory Practice

DAVID E. KERN, M.D.

The practicing physician's tasks in preventive medicine consist of disease prevention, early detection and treatment of presymptomatic disease, and promotion of optimal functioning once disease has become clinically manifest. Two characteristics distinguish preventive from curative care:

1. The physician, not the patient, usually initiates preventive care.
2. Preventive care is designed to protect health *prospectively*; this is true even when "health" may mean, for a chronically ill patient, a sedentary existence in his home instead of hospital admission for preventable worsening of his illness.

A number of considerations underlie the importance of incorporating preventive strategies into routine office practice: (*a*) It has been estimated that 50% of mortality from the 10 leading causes of death in the United States can be traced to alterable behavioral patterns, often termed "life style" (*7*). (*b*) Early detection and treatment of several common disorders—such as hypertension, hypercholesterolemia, breast cancer, and cervical carcinoma in situ—are effective in reducing the morbidity and mortality caused by these conditions. (*c*) Although infectious diseases have been controlled to a large extent in the industrialized nations by public health measures, including immunization, outbreaks continue to occur, particularly in underprotected or unprotected individuals and segments of the population. Influenza, for example, remains a major preventable cause of death. (*d*) The value of a comprehensive approach to prevention is demonstrated by the reduction in maternal and perinatal morbidity and mortality that may be attributable to prenatal care (3, 17). In addition, a comprehensive, preventive approach to care has been shown to reduce mortality, acute hospitalizations, and nursing home placement in high risk elderly patients, while improving their functional status and morale (19, 20). (e) Finally, a significant proportion of iatrogenic illness is probably preventable.

TYPES OF PREVENTIVE CARE

Prevention of disease and disability can be subdivided conceptually into three types according to where in the course of a disease process the preventive intervention occurs (Fig. 2.1).

Primary prevention is any intervention that prevents a pathological process from occurring. Immunization against infectious diseases, for example, neutralizes infectious agents before disease processes can begin. In a similar fashion, identification and control of risk factors (such as cigarette smoking) in healthy individuals can be considered primary prevention, because control or elimination of the risk factors prevents the development of specific diseases.

Secondary prevention occurs when there is intervention after a pathological process has been initiated but before symptoms occur. Secondary prevention is of value when two important conditions exist: (a) the pathological process is detectable during the presymptomatic stage of disease and (b) treatment initi-

ated before symptoms occur is more beneficial than treatment initiated after symptoms occur. The early detection and treatment of breast and cervical cancers are examples of secondary prevention (a) because the former can be detected presymptomatically by periodic physical examination and mammography and the latter by periodic cytological screening of the uterine cervix, and (b) because early treatment reduces morbidity and mortality from these diseases. Behavior modification leading to weight reduction in an obese individual with impaired glucose tolerance would also be considered secondary prevention, because weight loss in such a patient may improve glucose tolerance and forestall or prevent symptomatic diabetes.

Tertiary prevention refers to the prevention of progressive disability or other complications in individuals with established disease. Physical and occupational therapy designed to prevent flexion contractures and to restore independent functioning in a stroke victim is an example of tertiary prevention. Tertiary prevention has also been termed *prevention in clinical medicine* (23).

Although conceptually useful, the distinctions between primary, secondary, and tertiary prevention can become blurred in practice. The early detection and treatment of asymptomatic hypertension, for example, would be considered secondary prevention if one considers hypertension a disease and congestive heart failure, stroke, and renal failure complications of that disease. On the other hand, hypertension can be considered a risk factor for congestive heart failure, stroke, and renal failure, so detection and treatment of hy-

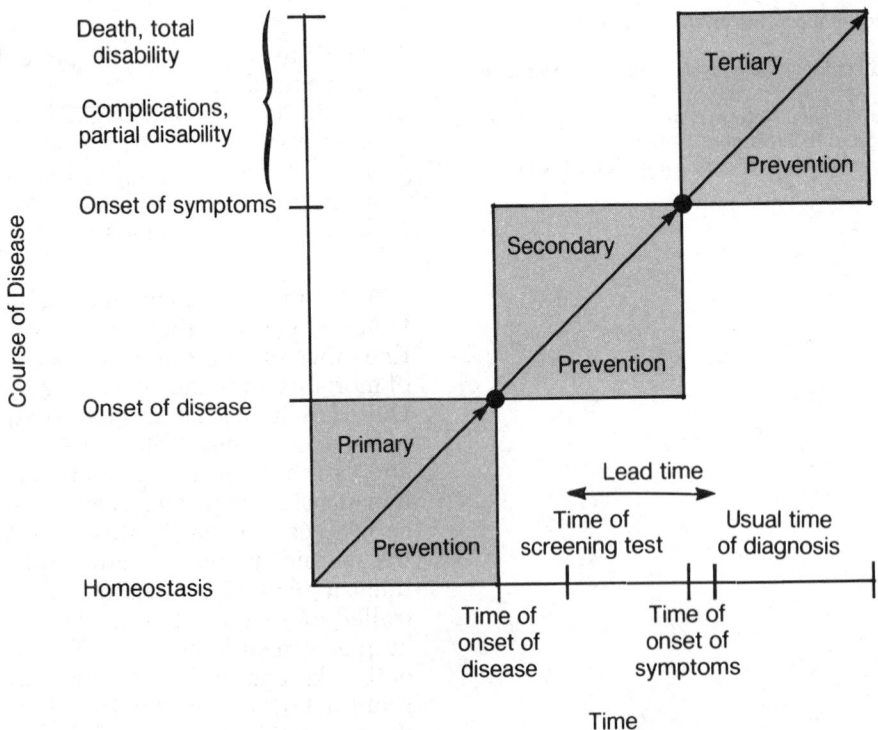

Figure 2.1. Primary, secondary, and tertiary prevention in the spectrum of a disease.

pertension to prevent these diseases from occurring can be considered primary prevention. Smoking cessation, as another example, represents primary prevention in the healthy individual but tertiary prevention in the patient with established coronary artery or chronic obstructive pulmonary disease.

Within the practice of preventive medicine, *screening* is defined as "the process of identifying individuals with one or more remediable asymptomatic diseases or risk factors in a defined population group" (23). When screening tests are applied to large populations, independent of visits to physicians, the process is called *mass screening*. Screening for asymptomatic conditions in office practice is most readily accomplished through a procedure called *case finding*. This is the application of screening tests to patients by their physicians during consultations for unrelated problems.

EVALUATING PREVENTIVE MEASURES FOR USE IN AMBULATORY PRACTICE

The first step in integrating preventive care into office practice is deciding which measures to offer patients routinely. Because the physician usually initiates preventive care, because the patients receiving such care are usually healthy, and because many more patients need to be subjected to preventive care than will benefit from it, there is an ethical obligation for the physician to be quite certain that recommended preventive measures result in more benefit than harm to patients. In deciding which measures to recommend, the physician should consider the importance of each preventable condition, in terms of its prevalence and severity, the efficacy, cost-effectiveness and complications of treatment, the availability of effective screening tests, and the usefulness of each measure in office practice (Table 2.1). Recommendations that are periodically published by organizations such as the United States Preventive Services Task Force, Canadian Task Force on the Periodic Health Examination, the American Cancer Society, the American College of Physicians, the American Medical Association, the Centers for Disease Control, and others can be consulted (see "General References"). For some measures, however, the recommendations are conflicting. The reports of the United States Preventive Services Task Force and the Canadian Task Force are firmly grounded in clinical epidemiology and provide the most scientific, least biased framework to date for evaluating which preventive health measures should be included in periodic health examinations.

In evaluating a given measure, the physician should be aware of certain pitfalls and special considerations. *Lead time* refers to the interval between early detection by a screening test and usual time of diagnosis (Fig. 2.1). In evaluating the efficacy of early detection and treatment, the lead time must be subtracted from the survival times reported for screened patients to avoid *lead time bias*. Otherwise, a preventive measure might be proposed that simply increases the duration of pa-

Table 2.1.
Questions to Ask in Evaluating a Recommended Preventive Measure

IS THE PREVENTABLE CONDITION IMPORTANT?
 What is the prevalence and/or incidence?
 What is the size of the attributable morbidity?
 What is the mortality rate?
IS PREVENTIVE INTERVENTION EFFECTIVE IN RESEARCH SETTINGS?
 Is the intervention efficacious[a] in study groups?
 Are compliance levels in study situations acceptable?
 Are side effects acceptable?
 Is intervention in the asymptomatic stage more beneficial than intervention after symptoms?
DO EFFECTIVE SCREENING TESTS EXIST?
 Do they have acceptable sensitivity, specificity, and predictive value?[b]
 Are they reliable?[b]
 Are they practical and reasonably priced?
 Are the side effects of screening acceptable?
WOULD USE OF THE MEASURE BE EFFECTIVE IN ROUTINE OFFICE PRACTICE?
 Have suitable field trials been conducted?
 Is the measure effective in reducing morbidity and mortality in nonstudy situations?[a]
 Are the compliance levels in nonstudy situations acceptable?
 Are side effects in nonstudy situations acceptable?
 What are the reliability, sensitivity, specificity, and predictive value of screening tests in one's own setting?
 Is the measure cost effective?

[a]A measure is *efficacious* if it results in more benefit than harm to those who are completely compliant. Efficacy is usually established in clinical trials where participants are selected on the basis of their compliance and where special efforts are made to minimize complications from the intervention.
A measure is *effective* if it results in more benefit than harm to those to whom it is offered in practice.
A measure may be extremely efficacious yet minimally effective in practice if patient compliance is lower and/or complications/costs are substantially higher in practice than in controlled study situations.
[b]See Chapter 1 for a discussion of reliability, sensitivity, specificity, and predictive value.

tients' awareness of their disease without reducing morbidity or increasing longevity. *Time-linked biased sampling or length bias* occurs when the same disease (e.g., some malignancies, autoimmune diseases, dementia syndromes) is characterized both by less aggressive forms with long presymptomatic stages and more aggressive forms with presymptomatic stages that are significantly shorter than the screening interval. Hence, individuals with less aggressive forms of disease are more likely to be detected by screening than individuals with more aggressive forms of the disease. Due to this bias, the difference in survival between screened and nonscreened persons will overestimate the efficacy of screening. *Selection bias* occurs when individuals undergoing the preventive measure differ from those with whom they are compared in a manner that affects the likelihood of their developing disease or the natural history of their disease, once acquired. Volunteers, for example, may have healthier lifestyles than those who do not volunteer. In the absence of randomized assignment to preventive care and control groups, these types of biases are difficult to avoid.

The process of screening itself can cause morbidity, independent of any physical complications from the screening test, by falsely labeling some individuals as ill (*false positives*—related to the specificity of the test and the prevalence of the disease*) (2), while inappropriately reassuring other patients that they are healthy (*false negatives*—related to the sensitivity of the test and prevalence of the disease*). Even correctly labeling patients can be associated with morbidity, a risk that has been documented for a number of common conditions (2, 8, 9, 11). In one study, for example, absenteeism rose in screened workers diagnosed as hypertensive, especially if they had previously been unaware of the condition and if they complied poorly with treatment (9). A disadvantage of mass or nonoffice-based screening is that a significant proportion of labeled individuals will not seek recommended follow-up with a physician. Physicians who screen for presymptomatic disease in their own patients may prevent much of the morbidity created by labeling (*a*) by confirming that a problem is present, usually by repeated or additional observations, before presenting a patient with a diagnosis; (*b*) by taking time to explain the meaning of a problem to a patient and to respond to his questions; (*c*) by only screening for conditions for which detection is likely to benefit the patient; and (*d*) by ensuring appropriate follow-up.

Finally, caution must be exercised in adopting recommendations based solely upon proof of efficacy in highly controlled study situations, especially when the proposed measure is expensive or associated with significant complications. Costs and conditions may be different in office practice. Before recommending yearly mammography to all women age 50 and over, the physicians in a large group practice might wish to negotiate the lowest price with local radiologists and obtain some assurance that the sensitivity and specificity of their readings approach published norms. Before recommending routine sigmoidoscopy to all patients aged 45 and over in one's practice (a recommendation based upon less than conclusive evidence in study situations), the costs, availability of diagnostic services, and complication rate in one's own setting must be considered. Although colon perforation rates of less than 1 per 1000 examinations have been reported among trained gastroenterologists, the complication rate for trained and untrained generalists remains to be established.

Despite the precautions listed above, there is sufficiently strong evidence to support the integration of numerous primary and secondary preventive measures into office practice (see below). Failure to do so represents an inadequacy in the provision of primary care.

COMPONENTS OF PREVENTIVE CARE

General Examination and Baseline Data

Most physicians will perform a *baseline general examination* (history, physical, and selected laboratory tests) for some or all of their ambulatory patients. In

addition, some physicians will update all or part of this examination on a periodic basis. In many practices patients complete self-administered history forms. As contrasted to the periodic health examination discussed below, there is no firm scientific evidence linking the general examination to reductions in morbidity and mortality. Most clinicians would agree, however, that knowledge of a patient's past hospitalizations and operations, past and present illnesses, medication and allergic history, diet history, habit history, social history, and family history is indispensable to the provision of effective preventive and curative care for that patient. General examinations may be advantageous in other ways as well. For example:

1. Baseline information may be of value in assessing symptoms that are likely to occur at a later date (e.g., ECG in a patient with a high risk of coronary artery disease or chest X-ray in a patient exposed to asbestos).
2. Occasionally a general approach will detect a treatable asymptomatic condition, such as an abdominal aneurysm, which, because of low prevalence or lack of a highly accurate screening test, cannot justify a directed screening effort.
3. Periodic updates of the medical history may assist the primary care physician in coordinating the patient's care.
4. Comprehensive general examination of individuals upon whom other lives are dependent (e.g., airline pilots) may be of use.
5. A "normal" general examination can provide reassurance, especially to the patient who expressly wants to know if he is in good health.

Periodic Health Examination

Periodic health examinations consist of the periodic provision of selected preventive measures to groups of patients, based upon their age, sex, and risk status. Preventive measures that should be considered for inclusion in the periodic health examination are summarized in Table 2.2. For each measure, the table provides the following information:

1. The required assessment by the physician.
2. Preventable condition(s) for which the assessment is performed.
3. The patient population to which the measure should be applied (age, sex, risk status).
4. Recommended time interval between preventive interventions.
5. Nature of the action to be taken by the generalist.
6. Quality of the evidence regarding the effectiveness of the intervention . . . classified using a rating system (I-III), adapted by the United States Preventive Services Task Force and the Canadian Task Force on the Periodic Health Examination from one originally developed by the Canadian Task Force:
    I. Evidence obtained from at least one properly randomized controlled trial.

---

*See Chapter 1 for a discussion of sensitivity, specificity, and predictive values.

Table 2.2.
Preventive Measures to Consider for the Periodic Health Examination in Nonpregnant Adults

Health Assessment by Generalist	Preventable Condition	Patient Population (Age, Sex, Risk Status)	Time Interval	Nature of Action by Generalist	Quality of Evidence Regarding Effectiveness of Intervention (See Text)	Strength of Recommendation (See Text)	Chapter to See for Details
INFECTION							
Gonococcal culture	Gonorrhea and complications	Sexually active high risk F,M	Discretionary	Antibiotics, report case, counsel regarding prevention	II-1^a, II-3^b	A^{a,b}	27, 94
Risk of hepatitis B	Hepatitis B and complications	High risk M,F of all ages	Once	Hepatitis B vaccine	I^a	A^{a,b}	32, 43
HIV antibody testing	Human Immunodeficiency virus (HIV) infection, AIDS	High risk M,F of all ages	Discretionary	Counseling, notify persons at risk, evaluate for prophylactic therapy	III^a	B^a	34
Risk of influenza	Influenza and complications	High risk and institutionalized M,F of all ages, all M,F ≥65	One year	Influenzal vaccine	I^{a,b,d}, II-3^{a,e}	A^{a,b}	32
Risk of pneumococcal pneumonia	Pneumococcal pneumonia and septicemia	High risk M,F of all ages, all M,F ≥65	Once^f	Pneumococcal vaccine	I^{b,g}, II-1^{a,g}, II-2^{a,h}	A^b, B^a	32
Rubella antibody titer or documented history of rubella vaccination	a) Rubella b) Congenital rubella syndrome	F of childbearing age	Once	Rubella vaccine	a) I^{a,b} b) II-3^c	A^{a,b}	32
Serological test for Syphilis (STS)	Syphilis and complications	High risk M,F	Discretionary	Antibiotics, report case, counsel regarding prevention	II-3^{a,b}	A^b, B^a	27, 94
History of tetanus and diphtheria vaccine within last 10 years	Tetanus, diphtheria	All M,F	Ten years	Tetanus-diphtheria vaccine	I^{a,b}	A^{a,b}	32, 33
Travel to developing countries	Hepatitis, malaria, gastroenteritis, cholera, yellow fever, typhoid fever, poliomyelitis, etc.	All M,F	Varies	Immunization, prophylactic medication, counseling regarding preventive health practices	I^{a,b}	A^{a,b}	32, 33
Tuberculin skin test	Tuberculosis	High risk M,F	Discretionary	Chemoprophylaxis, immunization—depends on age of patient and clinical circumstances	I^{a,b}	A^{a,b}	29
CANCER							
Breast examination by physician and mammography	Breast cancer mortality and morbidity	a) All F 50 to 59 b) All F ≥60 c) High risk F, ≥35	One year^i	Referral	a) I^{a,b} b) II-2^a c) III^c	a) A^{a,b} b) B^{a,b} c) C^c	89
Breast examination by physician	Breast cancer mortality and morbidity	a) All F, 40 to 49 b) All F, <40	1–2 years^i	Mammography, referral	a) III^{a,b} b) III^c	a) C^{a,b} b) C^c	89
Mammography	Breast cancer mortality and morbidity	All F, 35 or 40 to 49	1–2 years^i	Referral	I^c	C^{a,b,c}	89
Teach/encourage breast self-examination	Breast cancer mortality and morbidity	All F ≥20	One month (by patient)	Physician exam, mammography and referral as indicated	III^{a,b}	C^{a,b}	89
Cervical cytology (Pap test)	Cervical cancer morbidity and mortality	a) All F, onset of sexual activity or age 18 (whichever comes later) to age 34 b) All F, 35–60 or 65^j	a) 1 year^k b) 3 years^k, after 2 normal cytologies	Referral	II-2^{a,b}	A^{a,b}	95

Table 2.2. *Continued*

Health Assessment by Generalist	Preventable Condition	Patient Population (Age, Sex, Risk Status)	Time Interval	Nature of Action by Generalist	Quality of Evidence Regarding Effectiveness of Intervention (See Text)	Strength of Recommendation (See Text)	Chapter to See for Details
Stool for occult blood	Colorectal cancer morbidity and mortality	a) All M,F ≥40 to 50 b) High risk <40	One year	Referral for colonoscopy, or air contrast barium enema and sigmoidoscopy	a) III[a] b) I and II-3[b]	C[a], B[b]	38
Sigmoidoscopy	Colorectal cancer morbidity and mortality	a) All M,F ≥40 to 50 b) High risk, M,F	1 year (×2), then 3–5 years	Referral	III[a]	C[a]	38
Rectal exam	Colorectal and prostate cancer morbidity and mortality	All M,F ≥40	1 year (×2), then 3 years	Referral	III[b,c]	C[b,c]	38
Skin inspection	Skin cancer morbidity and mortality	High risk M,F	Discretionary	Counseling regarding reduction of risk factors, referral	II-2[b], III[c]	B[b], C[c]	100
CHRONIC DISEASE							
Blood pressure	Stroke, congestive heart failure, chronic renal failure	All M,F	2 years	Confirm high blood pressure, treat	I[b,c]	A[b,c]	62
Plasma *cholesterol* level (or lipid profile)	Atherosclerotic disease	All M,F	5 years	Confirm abnormal level, treat	I[c]	A[c]	75
Assessment of oral hygiene practices and dental inspection	*Dental caries, periodontal disease,* premature loss of teeth	All M,F	Discretionary	Counseling regarding proper dental hygiene (brush, floss), fluoride, diet, and regular dental visits	I to II[a,l] II-3 to III[a,b,m]	C[n,b,c]	101
Geriatric (medical, psychosocial, accident risk, and functional) *assessment*	Premature morbidity and mortality in high risk geriatric populations	High risk M,F ≥65 to 75	Once	Management of detected disorders	I[c]	A[c]	6
Hearing assessment, assessment of risks for hearing loss	*Hearing impairment*	High risk and elderly M,F	Discretionary	Counseling regarding noise control, hearing protectors, confirm abnormal assessment, treat when possible, selective referral	III[c]	C[c]	96
Visual screening	Decreased function related to *poor vision*	All or elderly M,F	Discretionary	Referral	III[b,c]	C[b,c]	97, 98
Tonometry and Ophthalmoscopy	*Glaucoma*	All M,F ≥40	One year	Referral	III[b,c]	C[b,c]	98
Weight, height	Morbidity and mortality related to *morbid obesity*	All M,F	Discretionary	Counseling regarding diet and exercise, referral	III[c]	C[c]	76
None	Morbidity and mortality from myocardial infarction	High risk M ≥40	Not applicable	*Aspirin prophylaxis*	I[c]	C[c]	59
None	*Osteoporosis, hip and other fractures*	High risk F starting at menopause	Not applicable	a) Radiologic screening b) Estrogen replacement c) Calcium supplements d) Exercise	a) III[b] b) I[b,c,o] II-2[b,c,p] c) I[b,o], II-2[b,p] d) I[a,o], III[a,b,p]	a) D[b] b) C[b,q] c) C[b] d) C[a,b]	74, 77
LIFE STYLE-RELATED DISEASE							
Alcohol abuse	Physical and psychosocial complications of alcoholism	All M,F	1–5 years	Counseling, referral	I[c], III[b]	A[c], C[b]	21
Birth control	Unwanted pregnancy	All M,F childbearing years	1–5 years	Counseling, prescribing, referral	II-2[a,r,u], II-3[a,b,s,u]	A[a,c,t], B[a,b,s,t]	93
Dietary assessment	Cardiovascular, dental, and other health problems	All M,F	1–5 years	Counseling/diet prescription regarding intake of calories, saturated fat, cho-...	I[a,v], II-[a,w,x] III[c,y]	A to C[a,z] A[a,aa], C[c,bb]	62, 75, 76, 101

Topic	Population	Target conditions	Intervention	Frequency	Rating	Rating	References
		carbohydrates, fiber, and sodium	Counseling, referral	1–5 years	I to III[c,cc]	B[c]	22
Drug abuse	All M,F	Physical and psychosocial complications of drug abuse					
Exercise practices	All M,F	Premature mortality, cardiovascular disease, obesity, osteoporosis, some psychosocial problems, unfavorable plasma lipoprotein levels, lack of physical fitness	Counseling, exercise prescription	1–5 years	I[a,dd], II-2[a,ee], III[a,ff]	A[a,gg], B[a,hh], C[a,ii]	58, 75, 76
Seat belt use	All M,F	Morbidity and mortality from automobile accident	Counseling	Discretionary	II[a,jj], III[a,kk]	A[a,jj], C[a,kk], B[a,ll]	—
Sexual history	All M,F	Sexually transmitted disease including AIDS; unwanted pregnancy (v.s.)	Counseling	Discretionary	III[a]	C[a]	18, 34
Smoking, tobacco use	All M,F	Premature morbidity and mortality from cancer, pulmonary, cardiovascular	Smoking tobacco cessation counseling	1–5 years	I[a,mm], II-2[a,nn]	A[a]	20

[a] Rated by the United States Preventive Services Task Force (USTF).
[b] Rated by the Canadian Task Force on the Periodic Health Examination (CTF).
[c] Rated by the author on the basis of USTF, CTF, or other reports.
[d] For efficacy of vaccine.
[e] For efficacy in the elderly.
[f] Patients at highest risk (e.g., splenectomy) who received the 14-valent vaccine (before 1983) should be revaccinated with the 23-valent vaccine. Revaccination should also be considered for those adults at highest risk who received the 23-valent vaccine 6 years or more ago and for those patients shown to have rapid decline in antibody levels (e.g., nephrotic syndrome, renal failure, renal transplants).
[g] For efficacy of vaccine.
[h] For United States population.
[i] Screening at both 1 and 2-year intervals has been demonstrated to reduce breast cancer mortality in women aged 50 and over. The optimal interval for screening has not been established.
[j] Stop at age 60 or 65, after two normal cytologies.
[k] Recommended intervals vary.
[l] For efficacy of interventions.
[m] For efficacy of counseling.
[n] Counseling by the primary care physician.
[o] Prevention of bone loss.
[p] Prevention of fractures.
[q] Estrogen replacement is particularly indicated in patients with symptoms of estrogen deficiency and in patients who have experienced premature surgical/radiological menopause. The use of cyclical estrogen/progestin therapy will abolish the increased risk of endometrial cancer attributable to estrogen therapy, but will result in the return of menses (for further details to Chapter 77).
[r] Effectiveness of, use of birth control methods.
[s] Counseling.
[t] Sexually active adolescents.
[u] Sexually active adults.
[v] Efficacy of counseling in changing patient's dietary habits.
[w] Efficacy of limitations of sweets in preventing dental caries.
[x] Efficacy of low fat, low cholesterol diet in reducing coronary artery disease.
[y] Preventive efficacy for most other preventive interventions.
[z] For dietary fat counseling to limit saturated fat (A), prevent coronary artery disease (B), and prevent cancer (C).
[aa] For counseling patients to limit sweets to prevent dental caries (A).
[bb] For most other preventive dietary counseling.
[cc] Depends on drug.
[dd] To preventive bone loss, obesity, and to improve affect, self-esteem.
[ee] To prevent coronary artery disease and hypertension in men and women, and to increase physical activity by counseling.
[ff] To prevent type II diabetes mellitus, hip fracture in postmenopausal females, bone loss in premenopausal females.
[gg] To prevent coronary artery disease in men, hypertension, postmenopausal bone loss, and obesity.
[hh] To raise self-esteem and to increase physical activity.
[ii] To prevent coronary artery disease in women, type II diabetes mellitus, bone loss in premenopausal women, hip fracture in postmenopausal women, and to improve affect.
[jj] Efficacy of use.
[kk] Efficacy of counseling adult patients.
[ll] Efficacy of counseling patients to use infant care seats.
[mm] To reduce tobacco use.
[nn] To reduce the risk of lung and other cancers, cardiovascular and lung disease, and complications of pregnancy.

II-1. Evidence obtained from well-designed controlled trials without randomization.

II-2. Evidence obtained from well-designed cohort or case-control analytic studies, preferably from more than one center or research group.

II-3. Evidence obtained from multiple time series with or without the intervention. Dramatic results in uncontrolled experiments (such as the results of the introduction of penicillin treatment in the 1940s) could also be regarded as this type of evidence.

III. Opinions of respected authorities, based on clinical experience, descriptive studies, or reports of expert committees.

7. Strength of the recommendation for including or excluding the preventive measure from the periodic health examination . . . classified using a rating system (A-E) developed by the Canadian Task Force on the Periodic Health Examination and adapted by the U.S. Preventive Services Task Force.

A. There is good evidence to support the recommendation that the condition be specifically considered in a periodic health examination.

B. There is fair evidence to support the recommendation that the condition be specifically considered in a periodic health examination.

C. There is poor evidence regarding the inclusion of the condition in a periodic health examination, but recommendations may be made on other grounds.

D. There is fair evidence to support the recommendation that the condition be excluded from consideration in a periodic health examination.

E. There is good evidence to support the recommendation that the condition be excluded from consideration in a periodic health examination.

In determining the strength of recommendation, special emphasis was placed on the strength of the evidence regarding the effectiveness of preventive intervention, but consideration was also given to the burden of suffering caused by the target condition and to the characteristics of the intervention (e.g., cost, invasiveness, complications).

8. Location of additional information elsewhere in this book.

The preventive measures summarized in Table 2.2 pertain to average and high risk adults. Factors that may dictate expanded or more limited surveillance for the individual patient may not be included. A characteristic that should always be considered when planning preventive care, for example, is the expected longevity of an individual patient. Thus, a 55-year-old patient with inoperable lung cancer should receive influenza and pneumococcal vaccines but should not receive most of the other preventive care appropriate for his age and sex. On the other hand, a 50-year-old patient who has survived an uncomplicated myocardial infarction at the age of 48 has a reasonable life expectancy and should be offered all of the preventive care appropriate for an individual in his age group.

Preventive Care for Established Conditions (Tertiary Preventive Care)

Preventive care pertains to the management of a patient's established condition as well as to early detection and treatment for asymptomatic conditions. In an office practice consisting largely of patients with such established conditions as diabetes, congestive heart failure, and degenerative joint disease, physicians may improve the health of their patients as much by preventive care for these conditions as by screening systematically for asymptomatic conditions. Appropriate preventive care for an established disease depends upon the disease, its treatment, and the expectations of the individual patient. Examples of this type of care include periodic monitoring of the serum potassium in patients taking digitalis and diuretics, taking steps to improve compliance and prevent rehospitalization in an elderly poorly compliant patient with congestive heart failure, and short-term counseling for a survivor of a myocardial infarction who is showing early symptoms of depression. The strategies for optimal preventive management of established conditions are discussed in subsequent chapters of this book.

Extending Prevention to the Family and the Community

Physicians should take action to extend preventive care beyond the individual when this is appropriate. In some instances, preventive treatment should be recommended for members of a patient's family and other close contacts. Gamma globulin prophylaxis for the family of a patient with infectious hepatitis and treatment of sexual contacts of patients with sexually transmitted bacterial diseases are classic examples. In other situations, the physician should recommend evaluation of the relatives of patients with certain chronic diseases that show a tendency to occur in families. For example, relatives of patients with familial hypercholesterolemia should have plasma lipid levels determined, and routine screening should be encouraged for at-risk relatives of patients with breast and colon cancers. Prevention should be extended to the community at large when a notifiable communicable disease is diagnosed in an individual patient (see Table 2.3). Similarly, any suspected occupational disease in an individual worker should be reported to local health authorities. Such reporting may be critical in protecting the health of other workers in that environment (see Chapter 7).

PRACTICING PREVENTIVE CARE

Physician Performance

Despite a sound scientific base that supports the routine provision of selected preventive measures,

Table 2.3.
Reportable Diseases and Conditions[a]

Amebiasis[c]	Mycobacteriosis, other than tuberculosis and leprosy
Animal bites	Occupational disease
Anthrax[b,c]	Pertussis[b,c]
Botulism[b,c]	Pertussis vaccine adverse reactions
Brucellosis[b]	Plague[b,c]
Chancroid	Poliomyelitis[b,c]
Cholera[b,c]	Psittacosis[b]
Diphtheria[b,c]	Rabies[b,c]
Encephalitis[b]	Rocky Mountain spotted fever[b]
Gonococcal infection[b]	Rubella (German measles) and congenital rubella syndrome[b,c]
Granuloma inguinale	Salmonellosis
Haemophilus influenzae type b invasive disease[c]	Septicemia in newborns
Hepatitis viral (A,B, non-A/non-B, delta, underdetermined)[b]	Shigellosis
HIV (human immunodeficiency virus) infection (AIDS and all other symptomatic infections)[b]	Syphilis[b]
	Tetanus[b]
Kawasaki syndrome	Trichinosis[b]
Legionellosis[b]	Tuberculosis[b]
Leprosy[b]	Tularemia[b]
Leptospirosis[b]	Typhoid fever (case or carrier, or both, of Salmonella typhi)[b]
Lyme disease	
Lymphogranuloma venereum	
Malaria[b]	
Measles (rubeola)[b,c]	
Meningitis (viral, bacterial, parasitic, and fungal)[b]	An outbreak of disease of known or unknown etiology[c]
Meningococcal disease[b,c]	A single case of a disease, of known or unknown etiology, that may be a danger to the public health
Mumps (infectious parotitis)[b]	An unusual manifestation of a communicable disease

[a]Determined at the state and federal levels. Reportable to local health departments. This list is adapted from Communicable Disease Bulletin, August, 1989, State of Maryland, Department of Health and Mental Hygiene, 201 W. Preston Street, Baltimore, Maryland, 21201.
[b]Notifiable Diseases, United States (reported by state or local health departments to the Center for Disease Control).
[c]Reportable immediately by telephone to the local health department.

studies have shown that physicians in both academic (10, 13, 16, 27) and community (5, 10, 14, 18) practice often fail to provide them. Reported compliance rates for recommended preventive measures range from 75 to 99% for blood pressure determinations, 40 to 80% for breast examinations, 20 to over 100% for Pap examination, 20 to 65% for hemoccult determinations, 10 to 54% for mammography, 5 to 20% for pneumococcal vaccination, 5 to 20% for yearly influenzal vaccination, and 5 to 22% for adult tetanus immunization. Interestingly, in one study (5) the performance of periodic complete physical examinations correlated with improved provision of preventive measures. Favorable physician attitudes toward the preventive measures were even better predictors of performance.

Implementing a Practice Plan for Prevention

It is generally agreed that preventive care must be planned carefully if it is to be offered routinely and effectively to patients in a busy practice. First, a policy must be developed that outlines which measures are to be offered to which patients (see above). This policy can be posted, in abbreviated form, for quick reference in each examining room (Fig. 2.2). Second, a plan must be developed to implement the policy. Including "health maintenance" as a problem at the top of each patient's problem list and including a risk profile on the front sheet in the chart of each patient are means of cueing the physician to provide indicated preven-

tive care (see Fig. 1.2). Maintenance of a preventive care flow sheet (Fig. 2.3) is necessary to determine efficiently which measures are due and which have already been done. Otherwise, much time may be spent trying to retrieve relevant information that has become "buried" in the text of the chart. When an office-based computer is available, it can be programmed to generate flow sheets and produce preventive care reminders for each visit, which are then attached to the front of each patient's chart (15). Nurses (4) or midlevel practitioners can be trained also to monitor or provide preventive care within the office. Audit and timely feedback of individualized performance data and educational messages can result in improvements in physician performance that can be transferred from one setting to another and persist for months to years (10, 12, 26). Whatever the approach, it is essential that it be an organized one.

Although it is desirable to schedule special time for a baseline history and physical examination for patients new to a practice, ongoing preventive care is best incorporated into routine office visits. This is so because few visits to the doctor are purely preventive and because attendance rates are lower for preventive than for problem-based visits (21). The low attendance rates for preventive visits may be explained by low patient motivation and/or by the additional cost and inconvenience of an extra visit for purely preventive care. For otherwise healthy patients who see their physicians infrequently, however, health maintenance visits should be scheduled and appointment reminders sent to increase attendance rates.

FRANCIS SCOTT KEY MEDICAL CENTER

GUIDELINES FOR ROUTINE HEALTH MAINTENANCE OF NONPREGNANT ADULTS

	Interval	Patient Population
Baseline Data		
*Complete history and physical examination	Baseline	All patients
Life-Style History and Counseling		
*Alcohol/drug abuse	Every 1–5 years	All patients
Birth control	Every 1–5 years	M,F childbearing years
Exercise	Every 1–5 years	All patients
Sexual practices	Discretionary	All patients
*Smoking, tobacco use	Every 1–5 years	All patients
Physical Examination		
Blood pressure	At least every 2 years	All patients
*Breast examination	Every 1 year	All F ≥ 40 (high risk F at younger ages)
Laboratory/Procedures		
*Cholesterol	Every 5 years	All patients
Gonococcal culture of cervix	Every 1 year	High risk F
HIV antibody testing	Discretionary	High risk M,F; with informed consent
*Mammogram	Every 1 year	All F, ≥50 (high risk F, ≥35 to 40)
*Pap (cervical cytology)†	Every 1 year	All F, 18–34
	Every 3 years, after 2 normal Paps	All F, 35–65
Rubella antibody titer	Once	F, child bearing age, without documented history of rubella vaccination
Sigmoidoscopy	Every 1 year until 2 successive normal exam, then every 3 to 5 years	High risk M,F
*Stool for occult blood	Every 1 year	All patient ≥45, high risk patients <45
STS (serologic test for syphilis)	Discretionary	High risk M,F
Tuberculin skin test	Discretionary	High risk M,F
Immunizations		
Hepatitis B vaccine	Once	High risk M,F
*Influenzal vaccination	Every 1 year	High risk M,F and all patients ≥65
*Pneumococcal vaccination	Once	High risk M,F and all patients ≥65
Rubella vaccine	Once	Susceptible F of child-bearing age (see above)
*Tetanus/diptheria immunization	Every 10 years	All patients
Health Maintenance Flow Sheet		All patients
Problem List		All patients
Problem-Oriented Flow Sheet	Most patients with chronic active problems	

*Included in chart audits
†Pap examination is not required after hysterectomy, provided the cervix has been removed, unless there is a history of cervical cancer.

Figure 2.2.   Sample of abbreviated preventive care standards posted in each examining room of the Francis Scott Key Medical Center, Baltimore, MD

Motivating Patients

Unfortunately, simply recommending a preventive measure to a patient is not sufficient to ensure compliance. When the preventive measure involves an unpleasant procedure (such as sigmoidoscopy or pelvic examination) or requires active participation (such as collection and return of stool samples or the taking of chronic medication), poor compliance is likely. It is most likely to be a problem when the preventive intervention requires change in behavior on the part of the patient (such as smoking cessation).

Motivating patients to comply with recommendations requires considerable skill on the part of the physician. Important ingredients for success include

establishment of a trusting, friendly, and supportive patient-physician relationship (Chapters 3 and 4), effective patient education (Chapters 3 and 4), involvement of the patient in planning and monitoring his own health maintenance plan (Chapters 3 and 4), use of behavioral strategies to enhance compliance (Chapters 3 and 20), and the promotion of more healthy beliefs, attitudes, values, and self-perceptions in one's patients (Chapter 4). A patient's perceived *self-efficacy* or expectations for success may be the best predictor of whether he will initiate and persist in an activity (1, 25). It should always be remembered that a patient's motivation to comply may be different from the physician's motivation in wanting him to comply. For example, patients tend to be less impressed than

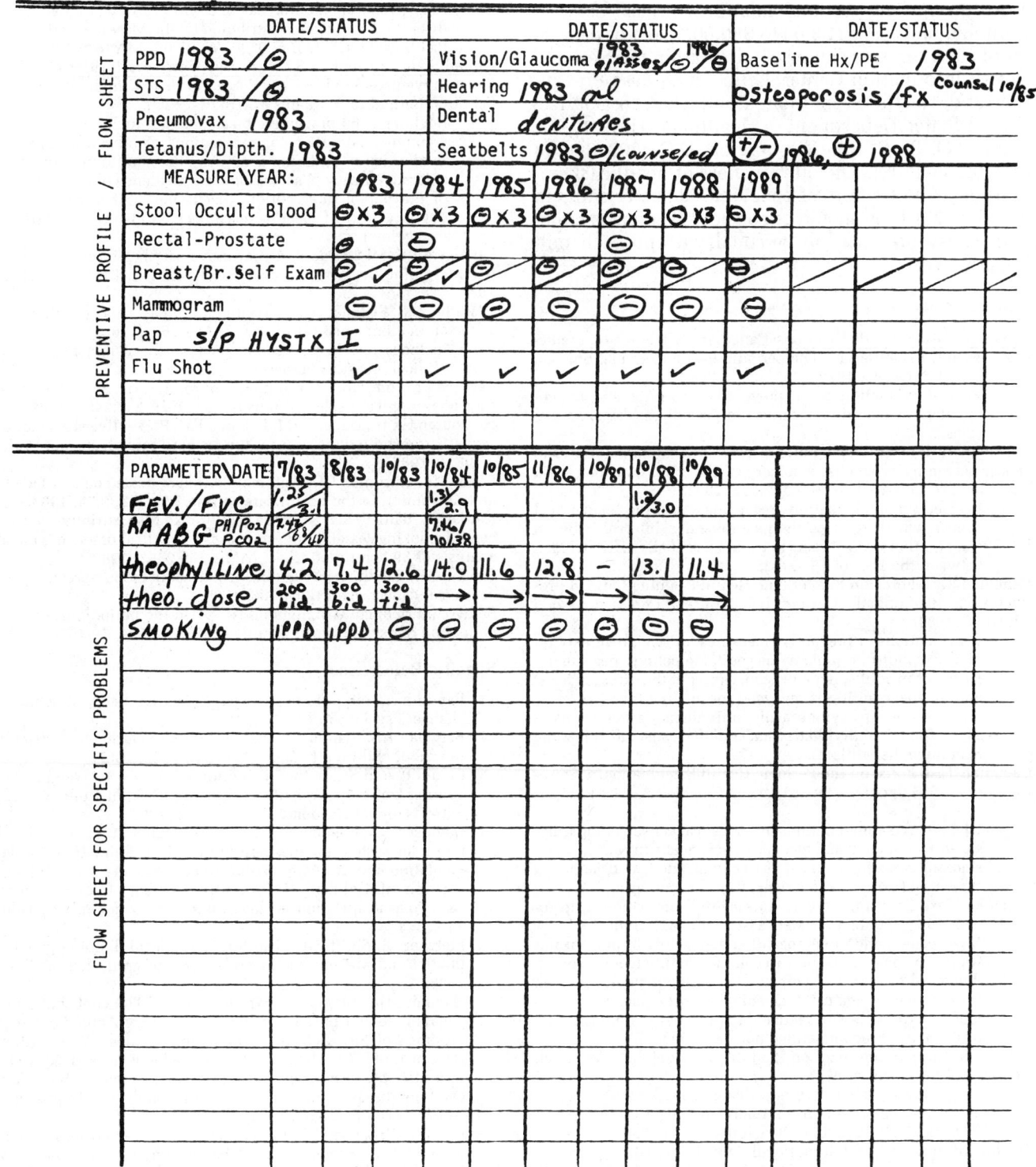

Figure 2.3. Sample preventive care flow sheet. (Department of Medicine, Francis Scott Key Medical Center, Baltimore, Md.)

physicians with long-term and more impressed with short-term benefits. Accordingly, the physician should stress the factors that seem to motivate the patient.

One technologically sophisticated method that is designed to efficiently transmit information to patients about their personal health behaviors and mortality risks is called health risk appraisal (6, 24). After completing a questionnaire that explores numerous health risks, the patient receives a computer-based report that (a) provides him with his risk compared with an average patient's risk of dying within a defined period of time and (b) provides him with an estimate of the amount of reduction in risk that could theoretically be accomplished if he complied with specific health-promoting recommendations. Prices for such printouts range from $3.00 to $30.00. A list of providers of such services can be obtained from the National Health Information Center, Office of Disease Prevention and Health Promotion, Public Health Service, United States Department of Health and Human Services, P.O. Box 1133, Washington, D.C., 20013-1133 (1-800-336-4797). The effectiveness of health risk appraisals as motivators of behavior change remains in question (22).They should be considered adjuncts rather than substitutes for the personalized approach outlined above.

General References

Canadian Task Force Publications: Canadian Task Force on the Periodic Health Examination. The periodic health examination. *Can Med Assoc J* 121:1193, 1979.

Critical evaluation of 78 preventive measures and recommendations regarding their use in periodic health examinations.

Canadian Task Force on the Periodic Health Examination. Cervical cancer screening programs: summary of the 1982 Canadian Task Force Report. *Can Med Assoc J* 127:581, 1982.

Revised recommendations regarding screening for cervical cancer, which reduces the recommended interval between examinations from 3 years to 1 year for sexually active women between the ages of 18 and 35.

Canadian Task Force on the Periodic Health Examination. 1. Introduction. 2. 1984 update. 3. An evolving concept. *Can Med Assoc J* 130:1276, 1984.

Reevaluations of preventive measures for five previously reviewed conditions (chlamydia genital infections, hearing impairment in adults, hypertension, cancer of the skin, scoliosis) and five conditions reviewed for the first time (coronary artery disease in asymptomatic individuals, carotid bruits in asymptomatic individuals, cancer of the testis, infant feeding technique, hepatitis B).

Canadian Task Force on the Periodic Health Examination. 1. Introduction. 2. 1985 update. 2. Breast cancer. *Can Med Assoc J* 134:721, 1986.

Updated recommendations for breast cancer screening (physician examination and mammogram annually in women ≥50), smoking cessation counseling (recommended), and glaucoma screening (neither recommended nor discouraged).

Canadian Task Force on the Periodic Health Examination. 1. Introduction. 2. 1987 update. *Can Med Assoc J* 138:617, 1988.

New recommendations regarding counseling to prevent unwanted teenage pregnancy (recommended), screening for endometrial cancer of asymptomatic postmenopausal women (recommended against), screening for osteoporosis (recommended against), and treatment to prevent osteoporosis/fractures (neither recommended nor discouraged).

Guide for Adult Immunization. 2nd ed. Philadelphia, American College of Physicians, 1989.

Practical and exhaustive paperback manual. Includes references. Can be ordered from American College of Physicians, P.O. Box 7777-RO270, Philadelphia, PA 19175.

Health Information for International Travel. Published yearly by the Centers for Disease Control, United States Department of Health and Human Services.

This monograph provides up-to-date and comprehensive information on immunization requirements and health recommendations for international travelers. For sale by the Superintendent of Documents, United States Government Printing Office, Washington, D.C., 20402, (202) 783-3238.

Morbidity and Mortality Weekly Report. Atlanta, Center for Disease Control, Department of Health and Human Services.

A weekly report containing very current information about communicable disease incidence (for example, regional incidence of influenza), updated recommendations for communicable disease prevention (including immunizations), and

timely reports on outbreaks of a wide variety of preventable diseases. Printed and distributed by the Massachusetts Medical Society, CSPO Box 9120, Waltham, MA 02254-9120.

United States Preventive Services Task Force Publications: United States Preventive Services Task Force. *Guide to Clinical Preventive Services.* Baltimore, Williams & Wilkins, 1989.

Reviews of 60 preventive measures that include Task Force recommendations, recommendations of others, analysis of the burden of suffering caused by the condition being considered, efficacy of screening tests, evidence of effectiveness of preventive intervention, discussion, and references. In-depth reviews of specific measures have also been published (see below).

Lawrence RS, Michelide AD: Preventive services in clinical practice: designing the periodic health examination. *JAMA* 257:2205, 1987.

O'Malley MS, Fletcher SW: Screening for breast cancer with breast self-examination: a critical review. *JAMA* 257:2196, 1987.

Includes Task Force recommendations for mammography and clinical breast examination.

LaForce FM: Immunizations, immunoprophylaxis, and chemoprophylaxis to prevent selected infections. *JAMA* 257:2464, 1987.

Horsburgh CR Jr., Douglas JM, LaForce FM: Preventive strategies in sexually transmitted diseases for the primary care physician. *JAMA* 258:814, 1987.

Polen MR, Friedman GD: Automobile injury—selected risk factors and prevention in the health care setting. *JAMA* 259:76, 1988.

Kottke TE, Battista RN, DeFriese GH, Brekke ML: Attributes of successful smoking cessation interventions in medical practice: a meta-analysis of 39 controlled trials. *JAMA* 259:2882, 1988.

Knight KK, Fielding JE, Battista RN: Occult blood screening for colorectal cancer. *JAMA* 261:586, 1989.

Selby JV, Friedman GD: Sigmoidoscopy in the periodic health examination of asymptomatic adults. *JAMA* 261:594, 1989.

Specific References

1. Bandura A: Self-efficacy; toward a unifying theory of behavior change. *Psychol Bull* 84:191, 1977.
2. Bergman AB, Stamm SJ: The morbidity of cardiac non-disease in school children. *N Engl J Med* 276:1008, 1967.
3. Committee to Study the Prevention of Low Birth Weight. *Preventing Low Birth Weight.* Washington, D.C., Institute of Medicine, National Academy Press, p. 132, 1985.
4. Davidson RA, Fletcher SW, Retchin S, Duh S: A nurse-initiated reminder system for the periodic health examination. Implementation and evaluation. *Arch Intern Med* 144:2167, 1984.
5. Dietrich AJ, Goldberg H: Preventive content of adult primary care: do generalists and subspecialists differ? *Am J Public Health* 74:223, 1984.
6. Fletcher DJ, Smith GL: Health-risk appraisal: helping patients predict and prevent health problems. *Postgrad Med* 80(8):69, 1986.
7. Hamburg DA, Elliott GR, Parron DL (eds): The contribution of behavior to the burden of illness. In: *Health and Behavior, Frontiers of Research in the Behavior Sciences.* Washington, D.C., Institute of Medicine, National Academy Press, p. 33, 1982.
8. Hampton ML, Anderson J, Lavizzo BS, Bergmen AB: Sickle-cell "nondisease": a potentially serious public health problem. *Am J Dis Child* 128:58, 1974.
9. Haynes RB, Sackett DL, Taylor DW, et al: Increased absenteeism from work after detection and labeling of hypertensive patients. *N Engl J Med* 299:741, 1978.
10. Kern DE, Harris WL, Boekeloo BO, et al: Use of an outpatient medical record audit to achieve educational objectives: changes in residents' performance over six years. *J Gen Intern Med* 1990.
11. Knibbs S, Jackson JGL: In: Keen H, Jarrett J (eds): *Complications of Diabetes.* Chicago, Year Book, 1975, p 265.
12. Korn JE, Schossberg LA, Rich EC: Improved preventive care following an intervention during an ambulatory care rotation: carryover to a second setting. *J Gen Intern Med* 3:156, 1988.
13. Kosecoff J, Fink A, Brook RH, et al: General medical care and the education of internists in university hospitals: an evaluation of the Teaching Hospital General Medicine Group Practice Plan. *Ann Intern Med* 102:250, 1985.

14. Lurie N, Manning WG, Peterson C, et al: Preventive care: do we practice what we preach? *Am J Public Health* 77:801, 1987.
15. McDonald CJ, Sui LH, Smith DM, et al: Reminders to physicians from an introspective computer medical record. A two-year randomized trial. *Ann Intern Med* 100:130, 1984.
16. McPhee SJ, Richard RJ, Solkowitz SN: Performance of cancer screening in a university general internal medicine practice: comparison with the 1980 American Cancer Society guidelines. *J Gen Intern Med* 1:275, 1986.
17. Milio N: *Primary Care and the Public's Health.* Lexington, MA, DC Heath, 1983. p 34.
18. Romm FJ, Fletcher SW, Hulka BS: The periodic health examination: comparison of recommendations and internist's performance. *South Med J* 74:265, 1981.
19. Rubenstein LZ: Geriatric assessment: an overview of its impacts. *Clin Geriatr Med* 3(1):1, 1987.
20. Rubenstein LZ, Josephson KR, Wieland GD, et al: Effectiveness of a geriatric evaluation unit. A randomized clinical trial. *N Engl J Med* 311:1664, 1984.
21. Sackett DL, Snow JC: The magnitude of compliance and noncompliance. In: Haynes RB, Taylor DW, Sackett DL (eds): *Compliance in Health Care.* Baltimore, Johns Hopkins University Press, 1979, p 11.
22. Schoenbach VJ, Wagner EH, Beery WL: Health-risk appraisal: review of evidence of effectiveness. *Health Services Research* 22(4):553, 1987.
23. Stokes J, Noren J, Shindell S: Definitions of terms and concepts applicable to clinical preventive medicine. *J Community Health* 8:33, 1982.
24. Werra RJ, Petrakis NL: Prospective medicine. In: Rakel RE (ed): *Textbook of Family Practice.* Philadelphia, WB Saunders, 1984, p 175.
25. Wilson GT: Cognitive factors in life style changes: a social learning perspective. In: Davidson PO, Davidson SM (eds): *Behavioral Medicine: Changing Health Lifestyles.* New York, Brunner/Mazel, 1980.
26. Winickoff RN, Coltin KL, Morgan MM, et al: Improving physician performance through peer comparison feedback. *Med Care* 22:527, 1984.
27. Woo B, Woo B, Cook EF, et al: Screening procedures in the asymptomatic adult. Comparison of physician's recommendations, patients' desires, published guidelines, and actual practice. *JAMA* 254:1480, 1985.

C H A P T E R 3

The Doctor-Patient Relationship: Communication and Patient Education

ARCHIE S. GOLDEN, M.D.
EDWARD BARTLETT, Ph.D.
L. RANDOL BARKER, M.D.

After leaving the hospital, a patient who has emphysema was overheard telling her husband, "You know I don't really feel any better. This going into the hospital for a few days and then not feeling better afterwards hardly seems worth it." When her husband asked, "What do you think the problem is?, " the patient replied, "I think it's the medication. I told the doctor, but he didn't really seem to pay any attention. But I really think it's the medication. If it isn't any better in a few days, I'm going to see another doctor."

The evolution of American medical practice over the last 50 years has witnessed a movement from office practice mixed with house calls to a pattern of practice characterized by a much more rapid pace, a greatly enlarged armamentarium of diagnostic tests and therapeutic regimens, and very few house calls. Thus, there is a tendency to know less about the personal, social, and psychological side of the patient and to rely more on test results to assess a patient. This trend was already noted in 1927 by Francis Peabody when he wrote in the *Journal of the American Medical Association*, "The most common criticism made at present by older practitioners is that young graduates have been taught a great deal about the mechanism of disease, but very little about the practice of medicine—or, to put it more bluntly, they are too 'scientific' and do not know how to take care of patients" (14). He went on to say, "One of the essential qualities of the clinician is interest in humanity, for the secret of the care of the patient is in caring for the patient."

DOCTOR-PATIENT RELATIONSHIP

Our society's concept of the doctor-patient relationship has evolved through the years. Four decades ago, Parsons described the patient's role as essentially passive (13). Later Szasz and Hollender (18) outlined the following three types of interactions between physician and patient: the *active-passive* relationship, in which the physician has all authority (similar to Parson's conceptualization); the *guidance-cooperation* relationship, in which the physician still is somewhat authoritarian and the patient cooperates; *mutual participation*, in which there is active collaboration between patient and physician and the patient assumes more responsibility for his care. The consumer movement of the 1960s and 1970s promoted the mutual participation relationship between doctors and patients (16). This relationship requires physicians to get to know their patients better, restoring a feature essential to good medical practice.

The mutual participation model of Szasz and Hollender is central to the *principles of medical ethics* that have been delineated in the past two decades (1). These principles define a doctor-patient relationship in which the physician respects the sanctity of the individual person and believes that that person's goals should be the basis for medical decisions. In practice, these principles require that physicians learn what their patients' expectations and goals are; and that patients (or their surrogates) participate as fully as possible in each decision about their health care. Such participation requires that several conditions prevail: that the patient is competent to consider a specific decision; that the patient receives sufficient information regarding his options and demonstrates comprehension of that information; and that the patient's decision is voluntary, that is, free from constraints imposed by the interests of other persons. Additional physician actions that are critical in a respectful doctor-patient relationship are truthfulness and protection of confidentiality. Attainment of all of these conditions is not always possible, and although patients generally want to be well informed, many still prefer to have their physicians recommend choices for them (4). Despite these limitations, the relationship delineated by the principles of medical ethics is now widely advocated as the basis for the doctor-patient relationship in American society (5).

Each doctor-patient relationship is established through a person-to-person interaction in which the physician's goals are to (*a*) obtain accurate and critical information from the patient and reach a valid formulation of the patient's problem or status, (*b*) provide information and ensure that the patient comprehends it, (*c*) arrive at plans with which the patient concurs, (*d*) assure patient compliance with the plans, (*e*) attain patient satisfaction with the relationship, and (*f*) facilitate the alleviation or resolution of the patient's illness. The achievement of these goals depends equally upon the physician's knowledge of medicine, respect for the patient's participation in the interaction, and skills in communication and patient education.

COMMUNICATION

Importance of Effective Communication

The importance of effective communication has been confirmed in a variety of studies of the doctor-patient relationship.

Gathering of *valid information* and getting the patient to disclose fully the reasons for a visit are two goals that are achieved better by physicians trained to utilize effective communication skills (8). Satisfaction with the physician correlates well with high interactional skills in the physician (9), and compliance with medical regimens is related strongly to satisfaction (6). In addition, medication errors occur less frequently when the physician utilizes effective techniques to communicate instructions (7). Finally, there is mounting evidence that the incidence of malpractice is related to the communication between the physician and the patient (15).

Although gathering and providing of information may appear to be the primary reason for direct communication with patients, the *therapeutic nature of the interaction* is perhaps the factor that is most important to the health of the patient. If information gathering and giving were the only goals of the interaction, then patients could fill out a questionnaire on their symptoms, and the physician could read the response and provide a treatment plan. This would result in an efficient and cost-effective method of providing medical care but would not produce much satisfaction for the patient or the physician. As summarized by Reiser and Schroder (17):

"Repeatedly, physicians will feel the power of something intangible, yet unmistakable, in the nature of the doctor-patient relationship that helps a sick person to get better. It is hard to overestimate the potency and curative potential of this very unique and special relationship. For all our technical advances, this relationship remains one of medicine's most powerful therapeutic tools."

Or as put by Balint, in describing his classic studies, "by far the most frequently used drug in general practice was the doctor himself" (2).

The skills that establish the therapeutic nature of every medical encounter are described here. Chapter 11 (Psychotherapy in Ambulatory Practice) describes the important phenomenon of transference and additional skills that are useful when the primary purpose of the encounter is to deal with emotional problems.

Fundamental Communication Skills

Recognizing What the Patient Experiences

Effective interaction with a patient always requires that the physician recognize as well as possible the feelings and concerns that the patient brings to the visit.

It is essential for physicians to understand *what it is like for a patient to be seen by a doctor*. Patients come to the office with anxieties concerning what the doctor may find wrong with them. Patients know that their doctor has a busy schedule, and they are reluctant to ask what the doctor may regard as trivial questions. Some social distance often exists between doctor and patient, and the combination of this and the physician's special knowledge gives the physician a great deal of authority. As a result, patients may be reluctant to contradict or correct their physicians' statements; may block or misrepresent their thoughts or feelings in order to provide answers they think the physician wants to hear; and may not ask for clarification despite being confused by medical terminology. Finally, during the physical examination, some patients feel embarrassment at being exposed, and this may further inhibit disclosure of important concerns. Although a long-standing relationship with a physician will diminish these sources of discomfort, it can be expected that most patients possess some degree of uncertainty during an office visit, and it behooves the physician to ask, "If I were this patient, how would I be feeling during this visit?"

The component of communication that most facilitates disclosure of concerns by the patient is the *development and maintenance of rapport*. Rapport is basically a feeling that one has of being with a "friend." Most of the elements in communication described below can facilitate the growth of rapport. Three basic elements of rapport are trust, respect, and understanding—elements that are present when a physician demonstrates genuine interest in the patient and when both the doctor and the patient feel they have been heard. These conditions create a safe atmosphere so that the patient feels comfortable talking about matters that he might otherwise feel reluctant to discuss. The physician's *ability to be empathetic* often determines whether a patient feels that his physician understands his situation. Empathy requires attentive listening and statements that confirm for a patient that one recognizes the patient's feelings. The physician can indicate attentive listening by maintaining eye contact, leaning forward, and using utterances such as "uh-huh" or nodding to encourage the patient to continue. Empathetic statements may either describe a feeling that the patient is showing (e.g., "I can see that this is pretty upsetting for you . . .") or indicate awareness of feelings the patient has recently experienced (e.g., "that made you very angry . . . I can tell from what you have said . . .").

Planning the Interaction

It is important to review critical information about a patient before actually seeing him. This preinteraction planning, accomplished in 1 or 2 minutes, allows the physician to indicate a familiarity with the patient's problems when greeting him and eliminates the need to rummage through the chart in the presence of the patient.

Opening the Interaction

Upon first greeting a patient, one should shake the patient's hand, use the patient's name, and, if it is a first visit, introduce oneself. The first few moments are crucial because the physician and the patient are sizing up one another, and nonverbal behavior will take precedence over what is being said. Both the physician and the patient are paying attention to physical features, type of handshake, voice tone and pitch, age, dress, and overall demeanor. *The seating arrangement* of the office should be conducive to the development of rapport. Where space allows, the patient's and the physician's chairs should be arranged so that the patient and the physician are facing one another without a desk between them. An attentive posture should be maintained by leaning forward slightly.

The eyes are a primary medium of expression and often tell more about an individual's message than words. *Eye contact* is thus an essential element in establishing and maintaining rapport. Looking at one's watch or at the chart while discussing a patient's problem signals to the patient that one is not listening, is not interested, or is too busy to be answering questions that the patient may already be reluctant to ask. Although eye contact is one of the best methods for conveying interest, staring can be uncomfortable and should be avoided.

Gathering Information

For gathering information about a patient's problems, it is pertinent to *begin with an exploratory approach* and move to a more directive approach as needed. An exploratory approach is usually more efficient, aids the physician in detecting underlying problems, and indicates interest in the patient. The most appropriate method for initiating an inquiry is the *use of open-ended or exploratory questions*. Open-ended questions allow patients to discuss symptoms or express concerns in their own words. Asking the patient "How have you been doing since your last appointment?" is an appropriate open-ended question for a follow-up visit. For a new patient visit, or a visit requested by the patient, the physician will want to explore the reason for the visit by asking "Please tell me what brings you in today?" This type of opening provides an opportunity for the patient to describe his reasons for the visit and does not imply that there is a problem. There is a tendency for physicians to ask "What seems to be the problem?" This question implies that a problem exists when the patient may be there for preventive care.

In response to the opening inquiry, a patient might respond "Well, I haven't been doing so well lately. My shoulder has been giving me a problem." Before exploring the first problem mentioned, it is helpful with most patients to ask whether there are any other problems that the patient wants to discuss at the visit.

If one assumes that the patient wishes to discuss only one problem and goes on to ask about the problem, then additional problems may be mentioned whenever the patient finds an opportunity, often when one is preparing to close the visit. By having the patient name each of his concerns at the outset, this dilemma can be avoided. If several issues are mentioned, it is quite appropriate to ask "Which problems seem to be bothering you the most?"

If the patient does not name other problems, one should continue with open-ended questions to explore the main problem. For example, "Tell me about the shoulder pain." The patient will then be able to describe the problem in his own words. One concern with this approach is that it will unnecessarily increase visit time. However, it has been shown that when patients give the history in their own words the length of the interview does not increase (15). Open-ended questions should be curtailed with patients who tend to produce extraneous information.

Exploratory questions can be used throughout the interaction. When one wants to inquire about the patient's life situation, an appropriate question is "Tell me, how have things been going at home?" When the patient produces information that needs clarifying, additional exploratory questions are helpful to establish a common meaning. For example, if the patient complains for the first time of constipation, the physician will want to explore what this means to the patient, e.g., "What do you mean by constipation?" The physician may discover that the patient moves his bowels every other day and yet believes that this means constipation.

The patient rarely provides all of the information needed to evaluate a problem, and one will have to use more direct questions to obtain the additional information. *Direct questions* are those questions that require a specific response. For example: "When did you first notice the pain?" or "What words would you use to describe the pain?" or "Can you show me where the pain is?" When seeking specific information, physicians should avoid asking leading questions, i.e., questions that tend to elicit predetermined answers, usually in the form of a simple "yes" or "no." For example: "You don't have the pain every day, do you?" This leading question gives the message to the patient that the physician does not expect the pain to occur every day. If the patient is somewhat passive, he may agree to whatever his physician suggests even if the answer is not accurate. Once the patient has responded inaccurately, he may become distracted and forget to report important information related to his symptoms.

When a patient is unable to provide needed information, it is sometimes necessary to *give the patient a number of choices* from which to select. For example, if the patient reports chest pain but is unable to provide accurate information about whether the pain radiates, one might ask "Does the pain seem to go anywhere else, such as to your back, one of your arms, your neck, or your legs?" While the physician may have an idea of the likely response, this will not be obvious to the patient since the patient is given several choices. This is contrasted with a question such as "Does the pain move to your left arm?" which is a leading question giving the patient the impression that this is the correct answer.

A patient will at times give a vague, aggregate description of an episodic symptom. In this situation, it is helpful to have the patient *describe in detail a single episode*. For example, "Let's discuss the last time you felt the nausea and crampy pain. . . ."

When asking questions, it is important to *ask only one question at a time* and to phrase each question so that it refers to one piece of information. Thus, when the patient responds one knows what the patient is referring to in his response. For example, to questions such as "Are you having any problems sleeping or eating?" or "Are you constipated or do you have diarrhea?" a positive response may not reveal which is the problem. Conversely, a negative response may only refer to one of these problems, but one may incorrectly assume that the patient is not having either problem.

While responding to questions, the *patient may give verbal cues* related to the discussion or concerning other issues that will need exploration. At times, it is appropriate to pursue a verbal cue when it is mentioned, and at other times it will be more appropriate to pursue it later in the interaction. If a verbal cue is pertinent to the present discussion, it is helpful to repeat the patient's words or to ask an open-ended question to explore what the patient means. For example, in response to a question about pain, a patient may respond "Well, it seems to have gotten worse lately, but maybe its just my nerves." Here, an appropriate response would be an open-ended question such as "Your nerves?" or "What do you mean?" An example of a verbal cue that one would explore at a later time would be a response to a question about sleep disturbance due to pain, such as "Sometimes I wake up in the middle of the night, but it isn't because of the pain." Since one is exploring the pain at this time, it would not be appropriate to pursue the patient's sleep problem then. However, it would be an important problem to pursue later in the interaction.

A patient's *nonverbal cues* may provide important information. One not only needs to pay attention to the content of the message but to the vocal message as well, including the pitch, the tone, and the tempo; each of these may confirm or contradict the content of the patient's verbal message. Nonverbal messages also include what has been called "body language." When interpreting nonverbal messages, the particular situation and person should be taken into account. One needs to distinguish between a patient's usual habits of seating, talking, and gesturing and any nonverbal behavior that is out of character for that patient. For example, although crossing one's legs when seated may be a sign of defensiveness, many people do so out of habit and for comfort. It may be presumptuous to assume that such patients are feeling defensive based on seating alone. Elements of body language that can be observed are the patient's seating position (e.g., sitting on the edge of the chair suggests apprehension, facing away from the physician suggests mental discomfort); head position (e.g., held back in. defiance, anxiety, or fear; or held down in sadness or shame); facial expression (eyes, eyebrows, and forehead show the greatest range of emotions, including surprise, fear, anger, happiness, disgust, sadness); hands (wringing or rubbing of hands can show anxiety, clenched fists or pounding on the table can show anger); arms and legs (crossing of the arms and legs can signify resistance or defensiveness). An astute physician will routinely notice when there is congruity or incongruity between what the patient says and his body language. At times, incongruity in these factors will be the only indicator of an important problem that the patient is hesitant to disclose.

When gathering data, it is important to ensure that one's *judgments* are not visible to nor imposed upon the patient. Judgmental attitudes are often conveyed by one's appearance, e.g., looking dismayed when a patient reports noncompliance with medications. Generally, judgmental statements are conveyed by the way in which one speaks rather than by the content of the message. The inflection and tone of voice can convey judgment on the part of the physician.

The data-gathering phase should always include inquiry about the *patient's life situation*. Awareness of the patient's life situation can be instrumental in developing a diagnosis or management plan, and attention to this information makes the patient aware of the physician's interest in him.

Organizing the Flow of the Interview

The importance of setting a tentative agenda before greeting the patient and then having the patient disclose his own additions to the agenda has been mentioned above. There are a number of other ways in which a visit can be organized to assure optimal effectiveness and efficiency. They are:

1. Keeping the interview focused upon *one problem at a time.*
2. *Delineating the essential features of each problem,* including the meaning of the problem to the patient. The following checklist is useful to keep in mind when assessing new problems: (a) chronology—onset date and time, duration, frequency and time of day of symptoms, duration of symptoms during a typical episode, course over time, remote history of a similar problem; (b) quality—nature and severity of a symptom (in the patient's words), location, radiation; (c) aggravating and alleviating factors; (d) associated factors or symptoms; (e) description of a discrete episode; (f) impact of symptoms on valued activities; (g) patient's explanatory model for what is wrong (patient's own diagnosis, etiological notions, fears, ideas of how to treat the problem and about what will happen, etc.).
3. *Utilizing transitional statements* to assure that the patient understands when the focus of the inter-

view is changing. This is especially important when one wishes to explore a sensitive topic, such as the patient's personal life (e.g., "Since this is your first visit, I would like to find out more about you.").
4. *Summarizing periodically.* This helps by letting the patient know that one has heard what he said and by giving the patient the chance to clarify or expand on important information.
5. *Integrating patient education into the visit in a way that is both efficient and effective.* One should ascertain the patient's educational needs throughout the interview, by hearing or asking what the patient knows or wants to know about a problem. However, the process of providing information and working out a plan should be deferred to the latter part of the visit (see details in "Patient Education" below).
6. *Using vocabulary consistent with the patient's background* and avoiding formulations that may confuse the patient, e.g., telling a patient that his test results are "negative" may convey to the patient that something is wrong.
7. *Taking notes in a fashion that does not diminish rapport* with the patient. It is helpful to point out that one will be making a few notes during the visit; it is equally helpful to suspend the interaction entirely while writing or dictating the complete note for the chart.
8. Communicating appropriately during the *physical examination.* This includes describing what one is doing and avoiding the tendency to give important information (diagnosis and plan) during the physical or when the patient is getting dressed; both are instances when the patient is distracted and cannot be expected to focus upon the physician's message or to formulate his questions as well.

Closing

At the close of a visit, it is important to accomplish a number of rather concrete tasks, i.e., (a) summarize, by problem, the assessment and plan, assuring that the patient comprehends these (see patient education below); (b) ask whether there are any further questions; (c) schedule a follow-up visit at an appropriate interval; (d) instruct the patient explicitly to phone back (or tell the patient that one will phone him) when this is indicated, e.g., when there is a symptom whose course over time is important, when the physician will know the results of a diagnostic test of interest to the patient, etc. At the end of the visit one should use rapport-generating techniques that will reemphasize interest and concern for the patient. Actions such as shaking the patient's hand or touching the patient on the shoulder, using the patient's name, giving him one's professional card, and encouraging him to call for any interval problems will convey to the patient one's interest in him.

Difficult Situations

All physicians have been faced with difficult patients in medical practice. Patients may be difficult to care for because of their style of communicating, because of the nature of their disease(s), because of their failure to adhere to appropriate treatment or behavior, because they present psychosocial distress through somatic symptoms, because they rarely or never respond positively to the physician's efforts, or because they have lifelong maladaptive personalities. Situations that often create difficulty for physicians are covered in Section 2 of this book (Psychiatric and Behavioral Problems) and in chapters describing patients who are noncompliant (Chapter 4), adolescent and geriatric patients (Chapters 5 and 6), and patients who have illnesses that create major psychosocial stress: patients with cancer (Chapter 8), HIV-infected patients (Chapter 34), patients recuperating from myocardial infarction (Chapter 58) and stroke (Chapter 83).

It is common for physicians to react negatively in a variety of ways to difficult patients and situations. Table 3.1 summarizes common negative reactions of physicians and strategies for dealing with these reactions. Most of these strategies require one to take time for self-exploration. Self-exploration can be facilitated by meeting with colleagues to share candidly one's reactions to difficult patients and ways to approach such patients, a process described by Balint many years ago (2).

PATIENT EDUCATION

Introduction

The word doctor means "teacher." Most practicing physicians today would not identify their doctoring as teaching, and most would agree that little of their medical education concerned the acquisition of teaching skills. However, most of the elements of communication during a visit, described in detail above, contribute to the process of patient education, a process that depends as much upon identifying the patient's information needs and upon involving the patient in selecting a plan as it depends upon the giving of information.

Patient education involves three steps:

1. *Establishing rapport and using effective communication skills* (see above).
2. *Providing the information and advice that patients want or need.* Patients wonder about their diagnosis, prognosis, regimen, and how they will be able to cope with the illness. The skills related to this step are discussed below.
3. *Overcoming obstacles to behavior change.* Frequently, it is not adequate to simply inform the patient about the regimen or choice of regimens. It is also necessary to identify and overcome obstacles to the patient following a plan. Skills related to this step are discussed below.

Patient education, then, is defined as a planned learning experience using a combination of methods such as teaching, counseling, and behavior modification techniques that influence patients' knowledge and health behavior. All members of the staff of an office practice may contribute to patient education, including physician, nurse, secretary, and others. For example, the office secretary may explain to the patient how the practice works, while a nurse may learn of special concerns that the patient is hesitant to discuss with the physician.

Clinical experience and research have supported the principle that *knowledge is necessary, but not sufficient, to assure behavior change.* Studies of the impact of patient education upon a number of conditions have confirmed this principle (3, 11, 12). More than information is usually needed when the patient is expected to make a life style change, varying from fitting a medication regimen into his daily routine to altering long-standing pleasurable habits, such as overeating and smoking.

Integrating Patient Education into the Visit

Patient education occurs throughout the three phases of a typical office visit—history taking, physical ex-

Table 3.1.
Common Negative Responses of Physicians to Difficult Patients and Strategies to Cope with These Responses[a]

Physician's Emotional or Behavioral Reaction	Coping Strategies
Avoidance	Analyze why; attempt to understand and master feelings that lead to avoidance; stay with the patient; discuss with colleagues
Identification with patient	Recognize, avoid tendency to deny seriousness of disease or to give way to despair; stay with the patient
Hostility/rejection	Acknowledge and analyze; do not attempt to like the unlikable patient; use behavioral approaches; if situation is intolerable, transfer patient to another physician
Feelings of impotence, inadequacy (*e.g.*, in caring for dying patient)	Discover areas in which help and comfort can be rendered, both physical and emotional; be realistic about limitations of medicine; give the patient time to go through the stages of bereavement
Feelings of loss of control or threatened authority	Acknowledge and analyze; be realistic about personal limitations and actual range of influence and authority; be aware that patient's need for control over his own body may conflict with physician's urge to control the situation
Frustration, confusion, uncertainty about dealing with the patient; coping strategies not effective	Request psychiatric consultation/referral
Anxiety, guilt, and frustration about meeting patient's recognized emotional needs	Allocate time realistically according to need; request consultation/referral

[a] From Gorlin R, Zucker HD: Physicians' reactions to patients. *N Engl J Med* 308:1059, 1983.

amination, and closure of the visit. The process begins when *an educational diagnosis* is made, i.e., the patient's informational and/or behavioral needs are identified. Some degree of educational diagnosis occurs at every visit. The patient may state his needs in the form of specific questions; the physician may note misinformation or information gaps in what the patient says; or the *physician may infer the patient's needs* (e.g., a patient newly diagnosed with chronic lymphocytic leukemia in its asymptomatic stage, or a regular patient in whom the physician suspects noncompliance as the explanation for poorly controlled hypertension). Before inferring the patient's needs, it is helpful always to ask the patient "What do you know about . . .?" At times, a patient's informational needs may be the source of significant psychological distress and the major focus for handling serious emotional problems (see "Meeting Informational Needs" in Chapter 11).

When an educational diagnosis has been made, one has the task of assuring that the patient acquires both the information and the skills (behaviors) that he needs to deal with his medical problem. The case report below illustrates the process of making an educational diagnosis and designing an effective educational intervention.

Guidelines for Providing Information

In most chapters of this book, the patient education content related to specific problems is described. The following general guidelines are important in providing information to patients.

1. *Assure that rapport has been promoted* in the various ways noted earlier and that the patient is able to give his full attention to you (e.g., not getting dressed, not trying to discuss another subject, etc.).

2. When explaining a problem, its treatment, and the expected outcome, *summarize using explicit categorization.* Table 3.2 compares the effectiveness of this approach with a less organized approach for conveying the same information to a patient with a chest infection.

3. *Check for patient comprehension* of the most important information you have just conveyed. Because it has been found that patients tend to recall the diagnosis better than the treatment plan (10), it is especially important to ascertain retention of the essentials of the plan, e.g., for a streptococcal throat infection, that penicillin will be taken for a full 10 days (not the exact dose or schedule, which will be transcribed onto the pill bottle). In order not to offend the patient when checking for comprehension, it is helpful to use a phrase indicating your own interest such as "It would help me if you would tell me what you understand to be the plan . . ." rather than a phrase such as "Now tell me what the plan is."

4. *Whenever appropriate, provide written information* as an adjunct to what you tell the patient. Since it usually requires time to make sense out of information about one's condition (e.g., newly diagnosed hepatitis) and since patients retain only about one-half of the essential information communicated at a visit (10), some written information should be given to the patient at the end of most visits. Written information includes *individual instructions* (e.g., modification in the way a current medication is to be taken, instructions to call back on a certain day, etc.; see example, Fig. 3.1), in addi-

Table 3.2.
The Effect of Explicit Categorization on Recall of Verbal Medical Information Given to a Layperson[a]

Usual Presentation of Information	Explicit Categorization of Information[b]
1. You have a chest infection.	'I am going to tell you: what is wrong with you
2. And your larynx is slightly inflamed.	what tests we are going to carry out;
3. But I think your heart is all right.	what I think will happen to you;
4. We will do some heart tests to make sure.	what treatment you will need; and
5. We will need to take a blood sample.	what you must do to help yourself'.
6. And you will have to have your chest X-rayed.	First, what is wrong with you . . . (statements 1–3)
7. Your cough will disappear in the next 2 days.	Second, what tests we are going to carry out . . . (statements 4–6)
8. You will feel better in a week or so.	Third, what I think will happen to you . . . (statements 7–9)
9. And you will recover completely.	Fourth, what the treatment will be . . . (statements 10–12)
10. We will give you an injection of penicillin.	Finally, what you must do to help yourself . . . (statements 13–15)
11. And some tablets to take	
12. I'll give you an inhaler to use.	
13. You must avoid cold draughts.	
14. You must stay indoors in fog.	
15. And you must take 2 hours' rest each afternoon	

[a]Adapted from Ley P, Bradshaw, PW, Eaves D, Walker CM: A method for increasing patients' recall of information presented by doctors. *Psychol Med* 3:217,1973.
[b] When the information in the left column was explicitly categorized (see right column), recall of information was 50% higher.

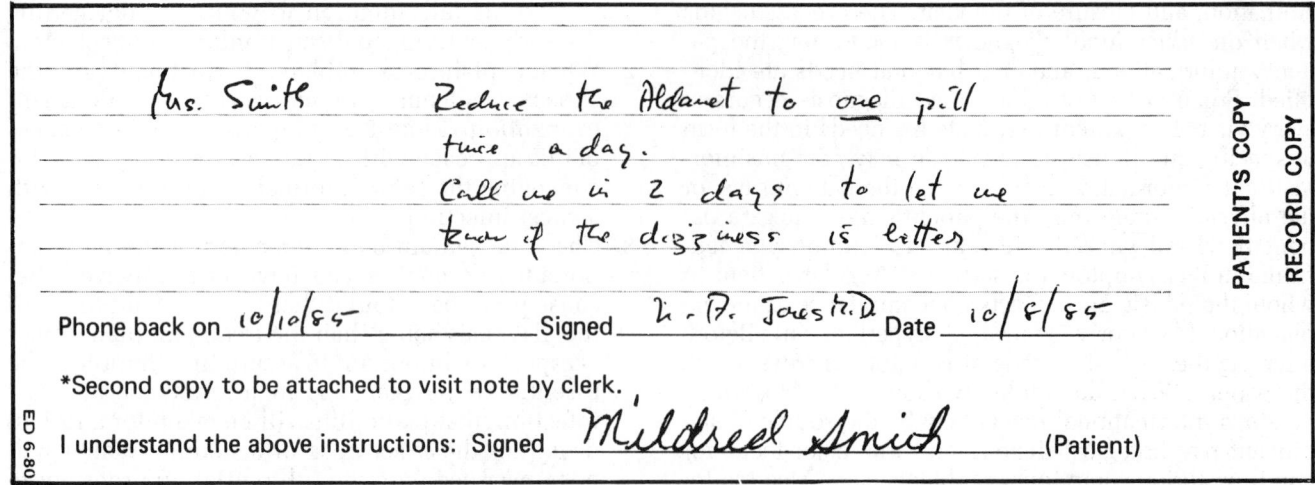

Mrs. Smith

Reduce the Aldomet to one pill twice a day.

Call us in 2 days to let me know if the dizziness is better

Phone back on ___10/10/85___   Signed ___L. B. Jones R.D.___ Date ___10/8/85___

*Second copy to be attached to visit note by clerk.

I understand the above instructions: Signed ___Mildred Smith___ (Patient)

ED 6-80

PATIENT'S COPY   RECORD COPY

Figure 3.1 Examples of written instructions for a patient (form makes a copy for the patient's folder). (Source: Francis Scott Key Medical Center, Baltimore, Md.)

tion to _preprinted patient education materials._ When individual instructions are given in writing, consider having the patient sign those instructions, indicating comprehension or agreement with what is written. When a printed item is given to a patient, it is a good idea to personalize it by underlining important points, writing down additional information that you judge important, and writing the day's date on it. A large collection of printed educational handouts is available in the periodically updated book by Griffith (see "General References"). Condition-specific publications that are widely available (e.g., from the American Heart Association or National Cancer Institute) are cited in many chapters of this book.

Guidelines for Overcoming Obstacles to Behavior Change

There are four steps to overcoming obstacles to behavior change:

1. Assessing the extent of compliance with indicated behavior.
2. Identifying the obstacles to compliance.
3. Using indicated educational intervention(s).
4. Assessing the response to educational interventions.

General strategies for carrying out these four steps are outlined in Chapter 4, Patient Compliance with Medical Advice. Specific strategies are described in chapters covering the many conditions for which behavior change is fundamental to treatment. Table 3.3 lists common problems identified in behavioral diagnosis and educational strategies for addressing them. As noted in the first section of this chapter, a strategy that can be helpful in all aspects of the doctor-patient relationship, especially when the patient needs to modify behavior, is to invite patient in-

volvement in the process. When the patient helps to formulate a plan for behavior change, the likelihood of success is greater.

Case Illustrating Educational Diagnosis and Intervention

The following case example illustrates the process of making an educational diagnosis and designing specific educational interventions.

A 30-year-old black male actor sought care because "his blood pressure was up again." Severe hypertension was diagnosed in this patient 5 years ago and has been treated intermittently since that time. As the patient stated, he had "gotten rid of his high blood pressure several times," only to have it come back again, despite having seen several physicians and having taken "lots of medicine."

Further questioning revealed that, although the patient always tried to do what the doctor said, it was troublesome to remember or to take the time to ingest all 12 pills each day because he worked and had family responsibilities. Moreover, it was hard to keep all of the doctor's appointments and even more difficult to maintain a salt-free diet because he did not do the family cooking. His wife could not understand his illness, since he did not feel or look bad, and thus it was very difficult to ask her to cook separate meals for him. In general, his family found his treatment needs demanding and interfering.

The patient was quite aware of why hypertension needed treatment, and he desired to keep his blood pressure under control. He was willing to come for care in order to control his blood pressure but was "getting tired of not getting anywhere." In brief, he simply wanted a safe, effective, and relatively simple way to control his blood pressure.

From an educational perspective, the following problems of the patient were diagnosed:

1. Lack of family understanding and support.

Table 3.3.
Common Problems Affecting Behavior and Some Strategies for Addressing Them[a]

Finding of Behavioral Diagnosis	Educational-Behavior Strategies
INDIVIDUAL	
1. Lack of awareness or understanding	Teaching, instructional aids, repetition
2. Lack of confidence to control condition	Reassurance, encouragement, attribution, peer group discussions
3. Forgetfulness	Simplifying regimen, cueing pill taking to other activities, providing weekly pill dispenser, involving friend or family member
4. Denial	Supportive exploration of patient's feelings and perceptions, avoiding "sledgehammer" method of sharing diagnosis
5. Inadequate motivation	Pointing out dangers of untreated condition (fear arousal) and benefits of therapy, paradoxical mention, increasing frequency of visits, inviting patient's ideas of how to achieve desired behavior, praise for any positive actions
6. Fear of getting hooked on drugs	Trying nonpharmacological treatment, reassuring patient that drugs will be used as little as possible, explaining known side effects
7. Lack of skills	Demonstration and guided practice
8. Behaviors that are repetitive and unconscious (smoking, diet)	Applying behavior modification techniques (stimulus control, contingency management, recording behavior, contracting, cueing, modeling, etc)
9. Reluctance to accept sick role	Giving patient as much freedom and respect as possible, exploring patient's feelings
10. Psychiatric disturbance	Psychiatric referral, psychotherapy, chemotherapy
11. Skepticism toward provider's statements	Respecting patient's feelings, providing medical textbooks and journals, referring for second opinion
SOCIAL	
12. Lack of support from family, friends, and teachers	Calling significant other on telephone, inviting to accompany patient to next clinic visit, making home visit, asking patient to talk to significant other, using mass media
13. Poor relationships with health provider	Developing provider communication skills, improving accessibility and continuity of care
ENVIRONMENTAL	
14. Inadequate money to purchase medications	Prescribing generic drugs, giving free drug samples, prescribing less expensive drugs, referral to social worker
15. Inadequate money to pay for health care	Providing free care, referral to social worker, community organizing
16. Long clinic waiting time	Using practice management to decrease waiting time, having patient see only nurse at follow-up visit
MEDICAL REGIMEN	
17. Side effects	Taking medications with meals, substituting medications
18. Complex regimen	Simplifying regimen, cueing medication taking with other activities, reducing dosage

[a] From Bartlett EE: Behavioral diagnosis: A practical approach to patient education. *Patient Counseling Health Educ*, 4:29, 1982.

2. Difficulty incorporating the requirements of therapy into his daily life situations.
3. Belief that the problem would "go away."
4. Increasing discouragement regarding his ability to control his high blood pressure.

Thus the approach taken to address these perceived problems included the following educational efforts:

1. Inviting the patient's wife to come to the office to learn first hand what she understood about hypertension, to assure that she understood the reason for treatment, including diet restrictions, and to invite her input regarding how to modify the family's diet.

2. Decreasing the number of medications, and having the patient select ways by which the drug-taking behavior could be cued to other daily behaviors, e.g., taking pills twice daily, with breakfast and dinner.
3. Educating the patient regarding his belief that hypertension could be cured, with the accompanying frustration and discouragement when it was not. Checking his comprehension of and concurrence with the idea that hypertension is a risk factor that requires lifelong treatment.
4. Explicitly describing the behaviors that the patient should follow regarding maintenance of diet, appointment keeping, and medication taking, and obtaining his input on how to achieve these behaviors.

5. Using encouragement and optimism regarding the likely success of the plans that were mutually developed by physician, patient, and spouse.

The effectiveness of the educational efforts was evaluated in the following ways:

1. Self-reports of dietary and medication adherence.
2. Appointment-keeping behavior.
3. Patient's perception of family understanding and support.
4. Patient's reported sense of confidence to control his hypertension.
5. Level of blood pressure.

After 1 year of treatment and educational support, the patient found it much easier to remember to take his pills twice a day and reported that he took his medication about 80% of the time. He also reported that he added salt to his food very infrequently and that he felt more support and cooperation from his family. He was cautiously optimistic about continuing to control his blood pressure in the future. His blood pressures at his last two visits averaged 150/94, as contrasted to readings averaging 200/138 1 year ago.

Integrating Patient Education into an Office Practice

It is possible to enhance the overall patient education effort in an office practice by addressing some practical management issues:

1. Nurses frequently have considerable interest in patient education, and involving them in this effort can save physician time and can enhance the effectiveness of care. Many office practices involve the nurse in educating patients about preventive measures such as breast self-examination, family planning, and the like. In other practices, nurses play a larger role in patient education by working with patients newly diagnosed with such chronic illnesses as diabetes, asthma, or hypertension. In these instances, it is important to delineate in advance which information will be covered by the nurse and which will be covered by the physician.
2. A certain amount of general patient education can be promoted in the waiting room, by setting up a *pamphlet rack* containing 10 to 15 of the most useful printed materials. These might include pamphlets on smoking cessation, weight reduction, low salt diets, exercise, and other topics of interest to patients and their families. Some practices have found it helpful to have a bulletin board with newspaper clippings about current health topics. Finally, removal of ashtrays and a no-smoking policy are important ways in which the waiting room atmosphere can remind smokers of the possibility of discontinuing their habit.
3. One of the most innovative methods of actively

involving patients in their care is the establishment of a *patient advisory group*. This idea has been tried in small and large practices. A patient group can be effective not only in channeling suggestions and complaints but also in helping to promote patient education in the office and to develop community health education programs.

General References

Bartlett EE (ed): *Patient Education and Counseling.* Elsevier Publications.
    Journal of applied patient education research, including current research, literature reviews, collections on special topics, and case studies of innovative programs.
Green LW, Kreuter MW, Deeds SD, Partridge KB: *Health Education Planning, A Diagnostic Approach.* Palo Alto, CA, Mayfield, 1980.
    A valuable book that takes the reader from educational diagnosis to education techniques in patient care.
Griffith HW: *Instructions for Patients,* 4th ed. Philadelphia, WB Saunders, 1988.
    Soft-bound collection of one to two page instructions, which can be reproduced for individual patients, on over 200 conditions. Includes anatomical sketches of most organ systems, useful for instructing patients.
Lipkin M, Putnam SM, Lazare A: *The Medical Interview: A Textbook on Medical Interviewing.* New York, Springer-Verlag, 1990.
    Multiauthored text with extensively referenced chapters on all of the uses of the interview in medical practice.
Novack DH: Therapeutic aspects of the clinical encounter. *J Gen Intern Med* 2:346, 1987.
    Thorough, well-referenced review, focusing largely on ordinary medical encounters.
Quill TE: Recognizing and adjusting to barriers in doctor-patient communication. *Ann Intern Med* 111:51, 1989.
    Delineates the barriers that are common and practical ways to lessen them.
Williams MA (ed): *Patient Education Rx Newsletter.*
    Bi-monthly newsletter that reports on current developments, issues, research, and people in patient education. Available from the International Patient Education Council, 500 N. Washington Street, P.O. Box 1438, Rockville, MD, 20849.

Specific References

1. Arnold R, Forrow L, Barker LR: Medical ethics and doctor-patient communication. In: Lipkin M, Putnam SM, Lazare A (eds): *The Medical Interview: A Textbook on Medical Interviewing.* New York, Springer-Verlag, 1990.
2. Balint M (ed): *His Patient and the Illness.* New York, International University Press, 1972.
3. Bartlett EE: The contributions of consumer health education to primary care practice: a review. *Med Care* 18:862, 1980.
4. Ende J, Kazis L, Ash A, Moskowitz MA: Measuring patient's desire for autonomy. *J Gen Intern Med* 4:23, 1989.
5. Subcommittee on Evaluation of Humanistic Qualities in the Internist, American Board of Internal Medicine. Evaluation of humanistic qualities in the internist. *Ann Intern Med* 99:720, 1983.
6. Hulka BS, Kupper LL, Cassell JC, et al: Medication use and disuse: physician-patient discrepancies. *J Chronic Dis* 28:7, 1975.
7. Hulka BS, Kupper LL, Cassel JC, et al: Doctor-patient communication and outcomes among diabetic patients. *J Community Health* 1:15, 1975.
8. Hutler MJ, Dungy CI, Zakus GE, et al: Interviewing skills: a comprehensive approach to teaching and evaluation. *J Med Educ* 52:328, 1977.
9. Korsch B, Negrete V, et al: Doctor-patient communication. *Sci Am* 227:66, 1972.
10. Ley P: Psychological studies of doctor-patient communication. In: Rachman S (ed): *Contributions to Medical Psychology,* I. Oxford, Pergamon Press, 1977.

11. Mazzuca SA: Does patient education in chronic disease have therapeutic value? *J Chronic Dis* 35:521, 1982.
12. Morisky DE: Five year blood pressure control and mortality following health education for hypertensive patients. *Am J Public Health* 73:153, 1983.
13. Parsons T: *The Social System.* Glencoe, IL, The Free Press, 1951.
14. Peabody FW: The care of the patient. *JAMA* 89:1127, 1927.
15. Putnam SM, Stiles WB, Jacab MC, James SA: Teaching the medical interview, an intervention study. *J Gen Intern Med* 3:38, 1988.
16. Reeder LC: The patient-client as a consumer: some observations on the changing professional-client relationship. *J Health Soc Behav* 13:406, 1972.
17. Reiser DE, Schroder AK: *Patient Interviewing: The Human Dimension.* Baltimore, Williams & Wilkins, 1980.
18. Szasz T, Hollender MH: A contribution to the philosophy of medicine—the basic models of the doctor-patient relationship. *Arch Intern Med* 97:585, 1956.

C H A P T E R   4

Patient Compliance with Medical Advice

DAVID E. KERN, M.D.

The initial sections of this chapter review what is known about patient compliance with medical advice. The short section at the end provides practical guidelines for preventing and managing noncompliance and refers the reader to relevant information contained in the previous sections.

INTRODUCTION

The following case example is representative of a common problem in office-based practice:

Example: Mr. Y is a 45-year-old man who feels dizzy at work. A blood pressure check shows a reading of 180/110. He is told that his "pressure is up" and is referred to a physician. Mr. Y has not seen a doctor in 20 years. After an appropriate physical examination and laboratory work the diagnosis of essential hypertension is confirmed. The physician is happy because he knows that there are efficacious medicines that prevent complications of hypertension such as stroke and congestive heart failure. The patient is given medication, takes it for a couple of weeks, feels better, and then stops taking it.

In this example, the physician might have been more successful if the following questions had been addressed: What is Mr. Y's understanding of hypertension and its management? What is the source of his information? What are his beliefs about the relationship between symptoms and high blood pressure? (A symptom precipitated its detection.) Why has Mr. Y not seen a doctor in 20 years? How does he view himself (in control of his destiny or controlled by forces beyond himself, at risk of or magically protected from disease, etc.)? What is his value system, and where do health promotion and disease prevention fit in?

Before consulting a physician, a patient may already have tried a number of remedies for his symptoms, consulted family, friends, or lay practitioners, and developed half-formed or inaccurate models to explain his illness. His age, sex, race, ethnic background, family, social class, education, past experience, and place in history will have affected his view of the problem and the world. Although he is likely to be more informed about medical care than patients were in the past, he is also more likely to be skeptical of the medical profession. He may have read about successful malpractice suits and medical mistakes, heard about bad experiences in medical care from friends, or had bad experiences himself. He may come from a lower socioeconomic class, be less educated, and have a different value system than the physician. He may have underlying fears and concerns, and certain expectations for the visit, but be reluctant to express them for fear of being thought foolish.

Physicians may be well motivated and highly trained in the diagnosis and treatment of physical disease. They are less likely to have developed their interviewing, communication, and teaching skills to an equivalent degree. Although they may make diagnoses and prescribe effective treatments, they may not detect or allay patients' underlying concerns or meet the patients' expectations for the visit. It is likely they will assume that the patient's value system is similar to their own. It is even more likely they will fail to uncover the patient's beliefs about and understanding of the illness. If a physician has failed to establish rapport and to explain things adequately, the patient may not trust the physician.

Given the difference in perspectives, it is not surprising that noncompliance with medical advice is an extremely prevalent condition. Fortunately, our understanding of this common problem has improved during the past two decades, during which over 4000 articles on the subject have been published. While methodological problems still exist in compliance research, a sufficient number of well-designed studies and a sufficient amount of concordance in results among studies exist to provide clinically useful guidelines. It is true that most studies of factors associated with compliance are cross-sectional, making inferences of causality subject to error. However, an increasing number are prospective. Most studies of compliance have involved hospital-based ambulatory patients, leaving questions about their general applicability; but when private patients have been studied, results tend to be similar. Numerous studies now exist that evaluate the short-term effectiveness of various interventions designed to improve patient compliance. The development and assessment of strategies to maintain such improvements require further research.

DEFINITIONS AND CLASSIFICATION

Patient compliance is defined as the extent to which the patient adheres to medical advice. It encompasses taking medications, keeping appointments, undertaking recommended preventive measures, and, with respect to activities such as dieting, exercising, and ceasing to smoke or take alcohol, changing possibly deep-seated behavioral patterns. Some clinicians favor the term *patient adherence* to *patient compliance*, but the latter is more widely used.

Noncompliance can be caused by a failure to understand instructions, *noncomprehension*, or can exist in the presence of adequate understanding, *volitional noncompliance*.

Noncompliance in medication taking can be classified as *errors of omission* (a prescribed medicine is not taken), *errors of commission* (a nonprescribed medicine is taken), *dosage errors* (the wrong dose is taken), and *scheduling errors* (the medicine is taken according to the wrong schedule, e.g., once instead of twice daily).

Noncompliance should be viewed as a neutral term. It describes one aspect of patient behavior that may be either appropriate or inappropriate to the patient's best interests. For example, it may be appropriate for a patient with mild chronic obstructive pulmonary disease to be noncompliant in taking a regularly prescribed medicine, such as theophylline, if it causes more distress (e.g., nausea) than relief. On the other hand, it would be inappropriate for a patient with severe hypertension to stop taking antihypertensive medication because of denial of his medical problem. In view of the not insignificant frequency of documented prescribing errors and unwise prescribing patterns, patients are justified in critically questioning

their particular regimen (8, 9, 36, 40, 44). That patients may exercise sound judgment is suggested by higher compliance rates for seemingly more important medications, such as cardiac, diabetic, and antihypertensive agents, than for seemingly less important agents, such as sedatives, antacids, and drugs prescribed for symptomatic relief (2, 20–22). Finally, it should be realized that responsibility for noncompliant behavior often rests with the physician. It is not valid, for example, to blame noncompliant patients for failure to understand instructions or to realize the importance of therapy when there has been ineffective communication by the physician (see Chapter 3 on patient education).

IMPORTANCE OF COMPLIANCE

Problems Caused by Noncompliance

Patient noncompliance is potentially important from at least four perspectives: individual patient care, public health efforts, interpretation of the medical literature, and economic consequences.

First, patient noncompliance with efficacious therapeutic regimens may thwart the goals of both physician and patient in reducing suffering, preventing illness, improving functional status, and increasing longevity. If physicians are unaware of their patients noncompliance, they may falsely attribute poor outcomes to inadequate dosage, failure of the regimen itself, or incorrect diagnosis. Any of these conclusions could lead to inappropriate action by the physician. Thus medication might be changed or dosage might be increased, and new diagnoses entertained, so that the patient could be subjected to unnecessary procedures and testing.

Second, noncompliance may increase the cost and reduce the effectiveness of screening, immunization, and disease control programs. For example, a screening program that identifies undiagnosed hypertensives will be less effective and will cost more for each hypertensive complication prevented if the dropout rate after screening is high or compliance with medication is low.

Third, noncompliance may influence the outcome of the therapeutic trials upon which important recommendations are based. Dose-response curves (dose plotted on the abscissa and response on the ordinate) may be shifted to the right by noncompliance, resulting in falsely high estimates for toxic and therapeutic doses. A falsely large response range for a given dose may be reported because of variation in subjects' compliance. In therapeutic trials, noncompliance in the treatment group will reduce the power of the study to detect significant differences between treatment and placebo. Furthermore, differences in compliance among different treatment groups may lead to false conclusions regarding their relative efficacy. Most therapeutic trials now include methods to exclude noncompliers at entry and to motivate and monitor compliance in participants. However, subjects chosen on the basis of proven compliance may not be representative of the population from which they were drawn. Patients with type A (competitive, driving, and independent) personalities, for example, may be less likely to enroll in a coronary prevention program (35) but more likely to have a myocardial infarction. Their under-representation in prevention programs could decrease the overall risk of myocardial infarction for enrollees compared with controls. In the Coronary Drug Project trial of the usefulness of lipid-lowering therapy (4), those subjects who adhered strictly to their regimen of clofibrate had a substantially lower 5-year mortality than those who did not, but so did those control subjects who adhered strictly to their prescribed placebo.

Fourth, noncompliance with indicated medical regimens has been shown to increase medical costs by increasing hospitalization rates for cardiac and other patients, by causing nursing home placement in the elderly, and by increasing utilization of outpatient services (41).

Prevalence of Noncompliance

The high prevalence of noncompliance underlines the importance of the problem. Reported noncompliance rates must be viewed critically and compared with caution, because of differences in definition from study to study. Nevertheless, the results of extensive reports are almost unanimous in identifying noncompliance, variably defined, as an *extremely prevalent* condition. Rates vary from less than 10% to over 90%, depending on the setting. Owing to previous dropouts, cross-sectional studies of patients taking medication chronically tend to underestimate noncompliance, but even then noncompliance is often in the 20 to 70% range. Among newly diagnosed hypertensives, for example, up to 50% fail to follow through with referral advice; over 50% of those who begin treatment drop out by 1 year; and only about two-thirds of those who stay under care consume enough prescribed medications to achieve adequate blood pressure reduction (19).

A review of the literature leads to the following additional conclusions:

1. Noncompliance rates tend to be higher for preventive care than for treatment of established illness.
2. There is a marked increase in noncompliance with duration of therapy.
3. Noncompliance is highest for regimens that require significant behavioral change, such as smoking cessation or weight loss.
4. Missed appointments are more common for provider-initiated than patient-initiated visits. Asymptomatic patients are more likely to miss appointments than are symptomatic patients.
5. Lack of comprehension of a regimen is a common cause of noncompliance. Unfortunately, most studies do not separate noncomprehension from volitional noncompliance, but where studied, noncomprehension has been shown to be responsible for 20 to 70% of objectively measured noncompliance.

MEASUREMENT OF COMPLIANCE

General Considerations

Various methods are available for measuring compliance. Unfortunately, there is no gold standard of validity and each method has strengths and weaknesses. Of general concern are the following issues:

First, it should be recognized that compliance is usually defined arbitrarily. Ideally compliance should be defined in terms of its relationship to therapeutic efficacy. For example, 80% compliance may be required to ensure blood pressure reduction (18), while evidence suggests that consumption of only about one-third of prescribed medicines provides some protection from recurrence of rheumatic fever (31).

Second, compliance reported in terms of percentages does not reflect sequential behavior. For example, omitting medications for 1 week could have an impact on therapeutic efficacy quite different from missing a few doses per week over a much longer period; yet the percentage compliance might be identical.

Third, measuring compliance in populations requires additional considerations. The magnitude of the noncompliance problem will depend upon the particular population at risk (i.e., the denominator), which should be clearly stated. Compliance rates will be higher, for example, for a clinic population studied at a single time than for a clinic population studied longitudinally from the inception of therapy, since only the latter approach adequately accounts for patients who completely drop out from care. The compliance distribution (number of patients versus percent compliance) should also be reported, since its pattern can vary markedly (Fig. 4.1). Reported compliance distribution curves have varied from U-shaped in chil-

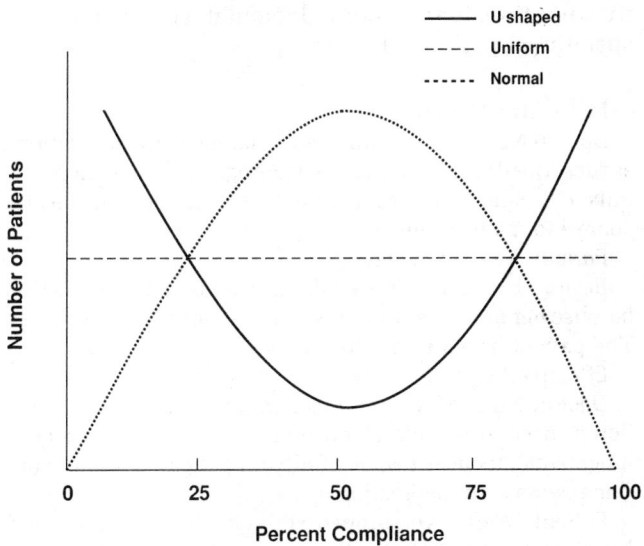

Figure 4.1. Possible compliance distributions.

dren given rheumatic fever prophylaxis (14), to skewed bell-shaped for patients taking chronic antacid therapy (38), to relatively uniform for patients taking antituberculous (24), chronic oral hypoglycemia (10), or psychopharmacological (32) therapy. The shape of the curve may influence the choice of strategies designed to improve compliance. For example, in the case of a U-shaped distribution, attempts to improve compliance might best be directed toward the most noncompliant group of patients, whereas the entire population might be a better target when compliance is normally distributed.

Methods of Measurement

There are several approaches to assessing compliance behavior in patients. Because each method has some limitations, it is *often necessary for the physician to use more than one method* to arrive at a reasonably valid estimate of compliance in the individual patient.

Asking

The simplest and most practical method of assessing compliance behavior is to ask the patient. Self-reports of noncompliance are generally valid, although the degree of noncompliance tends to be underestimated. There is even some evidence that patients who admit to being noncompliant may be more amenable to intervention than those who do not (25).

Because only about 40 to 80% of patients admit their noncompliance, self-reported compliance cannot be relied upon. In studies of various patient populations, reported compliance rates have almost always overestimated true compliance rates.

The *manner of asking* influences the accuracy of patient response. Certain interview methods can provide reasonably valid estimates of patient compliance (43). It is generally agreed that patients should be questioned about compliance in an open-ended, facilitative, nonthreatening, nonjudgmental, yet detailed and specific way. For example:

Ineffective Method:
Doctor: Now, Mrs. Smith, are you taking your medications as prescribed? (judgmental and leading question, which permits a "yes/no" and promotes a "yes" answer; confines response to medications).
Patient: Yes, every day.
Result: The doctor raises dose or adds new medication because her blood pressure is still not adequately controlled. The patient becomes frustrated.
Effective Method:
Doctor: Now, Mrs. Smith, can you tell me what you are doing to control your blood pressure? (open-ended; nonjudgmental; focuses responsibility on patient; does not confine response to medications)
Patient: Well, I've stopped adding salt to my food and have pretty much cut out all salted snacks. I do occasionally

have a frozen dinner when I'm alone. And, of course, I'm taking the medication.
Doctor: Uh, huh. . . . (facilitative)
Patient: Yes, that blue pill.
Doctor: And how are you taking it? (directive, not leading)
Patient: Twice a day.
Doctor: Any other medications? (directive, not leading)
Patient: No. I stopped the fluid pill when we started the blue one.
Doctor: And did you take the blue one this morning? (directive)
Patient: No, I never take my medicine the day I come to the office!
Doctor: What about yesterday? (directive)
Patient: Yes . . . at least in the morning. Yesterday afternoon was so hectic! You know how busy my days are!
Doctor: I guess it's hard to take that afternoon dose? (facilitative, empathetic, nonjudgmental)
Patient: Yes, because my schedule varies so much.
Doctor: What did you decide about starting on an exercise program? (directive, nonjudgmental, focuses responsibility on the patient).
Patient: Thought about it, but haven't done anything yet. Do you really think it's important?
Result: The doctor congratulates (positively reinforces) the patient on salt restriction, tailors a medication regimen to the patient's schedule, explains why she should take her medication on the day of an office visit, provides more information on the value of regular exercise, and provides written instructions/contract to which both agree. The doctor decides not to restart the diuretic because of the patient's compliance with salt restriction and the lack of a blood pressure reading reflecting the effect of the current medication regimen. If the dietary history had been less convincing or the patient had gained weight, the patient might have been asked for a 24-hour diet recall (which is more accurate than general questioning) on this and subsequent visits.

Medication Counting

Medication counting provides a more objective measure of compliance than does simply asking patients, and it has been used to demonstrate the lack of reliability of patient-reported compliance. Results are usually expressed in terms of percentages. The ability to measure sequential behavior depends upon the use of short intervals between counts, which is usually not feasible. Although more accurate than reported compliance, medication counts are still not perfect. If the patient is suspicious of being monitored, he can remove medicines from containers without ingesting them. Overestimates of compliance can also occur if other persons are using medicine from the same container. Compliance may be underestimated if the patient is using more than one medication container but only makes one available for counting. Furthermore, many patients do not bring their medication containers with them to the physician's office, despite reminders. Finally, some patients might take offense at having their medications counted, resulting in deterioration of the physician-patient relationship.

The medication count can be approximated by the more practical and less intrusive method of prescribing quantities of medication that should be consumed within a reasonable interval of time, and then observing the *frequency with which prescription renewals are requested.*

Ingenious medication dispensers have been devised that monitor not only the amount but also the regularity with which medicine is removed (3). They are bulky, however, and are not commercially available.

Assays

Another objective method of estimating compliance behavior involves testing drug levels in blood, urine, breath, or saliva. Drug levels have been shown to correlate with compliance determined by other methods as well as by outcome. Marked variation in drug levels may reflect inconsistencies in medication taking. Monitoring drug levels and relaying results to the patient may also serve as stimuli to improve compliance.

However, there are limitations to the method. Assays can be expensive. For accurate assessment, multiple measurements are required over an extended period. There is the possibility that, if the patient knows he is being monitored, he may take medicine immediately before the collection of specimens but not at other times. More important may be differences in drug absorption, distribution, metabolism, and excretion among individuals, making it impossible in the individual patient to decide whether a low level represents noncompliance or inadequate dosage. The absence of any drug in the specimen suggests noncompliance, assuming the specimen has been collected appropriately. The physician should have a working knowledge of the pharmacokinetics of the medicine being assayed, so that the collection of specimens can be timed correctly. Compliance with short acting drugs, which are rapidly cleared from the blood and excreted, is difficult to monitor by assay techniques because of the difficulty in collecting specimens at appropriate times. Finally, assays are not available for many medications.

Outcome

An even more indirect but objective method of estimating compliance is the monitoring of expected therapeutic or physiological outcomes. For example, blood pressure can be followed in a patient taking antihypertensive medication; weight, in a patient on a weight reduction diet; and pulse rate, in a patient prescribed a β-blocker. Many of the limitations of drug assays also affect assessment of outcome, which can be influenced by variations in drug bioavailability, absorption, distribution, and excretion; multiple measurements are required. Furthermore, other factors can influence outcome. For example, a reduction in stress may lower blood pressure, or the presence of

concomitant heart disease might be responsible for bradycardia.

Supervision

An additional approach to assessing compliance is to compare drug levels or outcome of therapy during supervised versus unsupervised periods of medicine consumption. Depending upon the pharmacokinetics of the drug, supervision may be accomplished either in the office or in the hospital.

Physicians' Ability to Predict Compliance

The need to measure compliance becomes obvious if one considers that studies have shown that physicians are *poor* at predicting compliance behavior in their patients, sometimes performing no better than would be expected by chance. Whether physicians can improve their performance by making determined efforts or by specific training remains to be evaluated.

FACTORS ASSOCIATED WITH COMPLIANCE

There are multiple determinants of compliance behavior, and no single factor or small group of factors seems to account for all of the noncompliance in any study population. Factors associated with noncompliant behavior can be classified as being related to the patient, the environment, the treatment, or the physician-patient relationship. Physicians need to be aware of the most important of these associations in order to improve their ability to predict and manage noncompliance in their own patients.

Patient Characteristics

Patients who are *symptomatic* are more likely to be compliant than those who are not, especially if the symptoms are relieved by treatment recommendations. Surprisingly, such *sociodemographic* variables as age, sex, race, education, occupation, income, and marital status usually do not correlate with compliance behavior. Elderly patients, however, have been shown to have difficulty in opening childproof medication containers, and they may be at increased risk for noncomprehension. *Alcoholism and drug addiction* tend to correlate highly with noncompliance. *Previous compliance or concurrent compliance* with one aspect of treatment usually correlates with adherence to other aspects of the regimen. *Psychological factors,* such as depression, immaturity, impulsivity, paranoia, hostility, fear of dependence, denial, commitment to a bad decision, and type A personality, might be expected to correlate with noncompliance, and in some studies such associations have been demonstrated. *Internal, as opposed to external, locus of control,* or the extent to which an individual perceives events that happen to him as dependent upon his own behavior as opposed to external factors, is usually associated with compliant behavior. Patients with certain *psychiatric illnesses*, such as depression, mania, schizophrenia, antisocial or paranoid personality disorders tend to be less compliant. Factors or illnesses that affect the patient's *ability to comprehend*, or to organize and initiate deliberate behavior, such as a language barrier, dementia, or mental retardation, should be expected to affect compliance adversely. Moreover, some patients who come to physicians are experiencing considerable anxiety, which may interfere with cognitive functioning of which comprehension is one element. Understanding may be further hampered by the tendency of many patients, such as blue-collar workers, to ask few questions of their physicians even when they desire information (16).

Other important patient characteristics that are often overlooked are patients' feelings and beliefs about themselves, their illnesses, their regimen, and their physicians. Patients who believe in their own *self-efficacy*, i.e., their ability to accomplish objectives by exerting control over themselves and their environment, particularly as it relates to the regimen in question, are more likely to be compliant than those who feel unable to exert such control. *Feelings*, such as dislike of taking medication, may also interfere with compliance. Patient's *"health beliefs,"* i.e., their belief about the severity of an illness, their susceptibility to an illness or its complications, the efficacy of treatment, barriers to therapy, their own likelihood of benefiting, and their intent to comply, have usually been found to be associated with compliance. As distinguished from disease, which is an objective entity based upon the presence of independently verifiable findings, a patient's experience of illness is a subjective state that is shaped by personal, interpersonal, and cultural factors. It is the patient's perceptions of disease and treatment that correlate with compliance rather than the objective realities. An extreme example occurs in patients who deny illness. Thus, patients who have had a myocardial infarction, who answer "no" or "maybe" rather than "yes" when asked if they have experienced a heart attack, are less likely to comply with physicians' instructions for decreased activity and reduced cigarette smoking (5).

Patients often have their own *models of disease* and treatment. If this model conflicts with the regimen prescribed for the patient, noncompliance may follow. For example, the not uncommonly held perception of hypertension as an intermittent, symptomatic, stress-related condition encourages an erratic approach to medication taking. Some patients with clearly diagnosable soft tissue injuries may feel that their evaluation was incomplete without an X-ray and therefore mistrust the physician's diagnosis. Ethnic concepts of disease and treatment can also conflict with the physician's approach to diagnosis and management and result in noncompliance. Such concepts are more prevalent among ethnic group members who experience a language barrier, are generationally close to immigration, live in segregated neighborhoods, are lower in education level and socioeconomic class, and

experience barriers to receiving personalized medical care—i.e., those who are least integrated into the mainstream culture. For example, some black patients might change physicians or refuse treatment if they are told they have both "high blood" pressure and a "low blood" count (anemia). According to some folk beliefs these diagnoses are mutually exclusive, so the physician making them may be regarded as ignorant. Among Mexican Americans, lay understanding and management of *caide de la mollera* ("fallen fontenelle") in infants can result in a failure to understand the importance of rehydration therapy in diarrheal disease.

Finally, the patient's *value system* may conflict with that of the physician. An elderly patient, for example, may prefer to accept an increased risk of death rather than endure the inconvenience, impersonalization, and separation from house and family resulting from hospitalization.

Environmental Factors

Patients who have stable *support systems* and stable *family situations* tend to be more compliant. A spouse's concern about a patient's illness can encourage compliance with medication taking, appointment keeping, and prescribed behavior changes (such as diets and smoking cessation). On the other hand, adherence to the *cultural norms* of social class, ethnicity, family, age, and sex are likely to supersede adherence to the norms of the medical profession when the two are in conflict. It should be remembered that a patient's previous experience of *similar disease among his relatives or friends* can profoundly affect his beliefs about his illness. *Advice from friends, family, and lay practitioners* can also be influential. *Nursing and office staff* may promote compliance by demonstrating enthusiasm and positive attitudes regarding patients' adherence to treatment regimen.

Appointment keeping is positively correlated with *appointment scheduling systems* that reduce waiting time, give individual rather than block appointments, minimize the time between scheduling and the actual appointment date, and make referrals to specific doctors rather than to clinics.

Treatment Factors

The *complexity of the medical regimen* correlates inversely with compliance. Compliance decreases as the number of medications or the number of daily doses per medication increases. Unsynchronized schedules (e.g., one drug every 4 hours and another every 6 hours) should also be expected to affect compliance adversely. *Side effects* may cause noncompliance when they cause significant symptoms or interfere with an important function in the individual's life (e.g., impotence secondary to an antihypertensive drug in a young sexually active man). *Medication class* has already been noted to be related to compliance, with seemingly more important drugs (such as cardiac and diabetic agents—over 70% compliance in cross-sectional studies) resulting in higher compliance rates than seemingly less important medicines (such as antacids and drugs prescribed for symptomatic relief—less than 50% compliance). The reason for these differences is unknown and could conceivably be due either to sound patient judgment or to increased physician emphasis, supervision, and teaching. The relationship between independently audited medication need and compliance remains unexplored.

The *duration* of therapy and the requirement for significant *behavioral change* (e.g., weight reduction or smoking cessation) have been previously mentioned as negatively associated with compliance.

Doctor-Patient Relationship

Close supervision of the patient by the physician (or his assistant) has proved a consistent and significant correlate of compliant behavior. In most studies, *continuity* in provider care has also contributed.

Establishment of a good patient-physician relationship is being increasingly recognized as an important determinant of patient compliance. Although *effective communication* is a prerequisite to the establishment of such a relationship, studies show that physicians commonly communicate poorly with their patients (7, 11, 26, 45). However, the necessary skills (see Chapter 3) can be learned (26) and are being taught with increasing frequency in medical schools, residencies, and continuing education courses (26). Among the aspects of the communication process that have a demonstrated relationship to patient compliance are the following:

Effective transfer of information is important (28, 33), since the patient must first understand a regimen before he can be expected to comply with it. To improve retention, instructions need to be clear, concise, explicit, and categorized by subject matter, with important features emphasized and repeated (29). Because patient factors, such as anxiety and reluctance to ask questions, may interfere with understanding, it has been found useful to test the patient for receipt and retention of instructions and to supplement verbal with written instructions. The use of medical jargon needs to be avoided, and use of language should be geared to the educational and cultural backgrounds of the recipient.

It should be remembered that the physician may be the last resource on a long road of self-medication and lay consultation, and that the patient may already have some ideas and concerns about his problem. The physician must, therefore, *justify* or explain the rationale behind a regimen, and in the process detect and correct or accommodate any misconceptions that might interfere with compliance.

Other features of the communication process that correlate with patient compliance include fulfillment of patient expectations (requires detection of and at-

tention to the patient's underlying concerns); physician friendliness; a positive, confident approach on the part of the physician; physician response to patient complaints; encouragement of patient questions; a supportive, nonjudgmental method of eliciting and responding to patient admissions of noncompliance; encouragement of patients to become actively involved in their own care; active patient participation as opposed to physician dominance; negotiation rather than dictation of a treatment plan; identification and resolution of barriers to compliance; congruence between patient and physician in their understanding of a problem and its management; physician effort to motivate the patient; and patient satisfaction (12, 13, 15, 17, 37, 42, 45, 46).

Transference, or the subconscious redirection to one person of feelings and attitudes toward others (e.g., parents or authority figures), may further influence the patient's relationship to his physician. Depending upon its nature, which is based on previous experience, the transference reaction can promote compliance (e.g., the patient who finds it rewarding to please authority figures) or impede it (e.g., the patient who distrusts authority figures). *Countertransference,* the redirection toward the patient of previously developed physician attitudes and feelings, may also be detrimental or beneficial to the patient-physician relationship.

Many of the above features contribute to the development of *patient trust in the physician,* and trust is one of the most important factors in any approach to helping people change. Because a key element of trust is self-disclosure and because self-disclosure exposes the patient to possible rejection, ridicule, shame, or exploitation, the importance of eliciting and responding to admissions of noncompliance in a nonjudgmental manner, in the context of a positive and supportive relationship, is clear.

Some practitioners prefer patients who do not ask too many questions and who simply follow instructions. Although this active-passive relationship may be appropriate for some patients, to be effective with most ambulatory patients the physician must enter into a relationship of *mutual participation* in which he must listen to the patient, educate, and negotiate with him. Such an approach need not be time consuming. It is the quality of the interaction and not the amount of time spent that correlates with compliance and satisfaction (7, 26).

COMPLIANCE-IMPROVING INTERVENTIONS

The techniques designed to improve patient compliance that have been evaluated include organizational or structural, instructional, and behavioral interventions. Successful intervention has increased compliance rates by less than 10% to almost 70%, averaging between 25 and 30% (percentage change = percentage of compliant patients in the experimental group minus percentage of compliant patients in the control group). When studied, compliance-improving interventions have also been shown to have favorable cost-benefit ratios (41).

Appointment Keeping

A number of factors have been shown to improve appointment keeping by patients.

Telephone and mail reminders, in which patients receive messages several days before their scheduled visits informing them of the dates and times of their appointments or messages inviting patients to reschedule after missed appointments, have consistently improved compliance, usually in the range of 10 to 20%. Wording of the message may be influential. In one study of high risk patients (27), postcards with a persuasive educational message resulted in a significantly higher compliance rate for influenza vaccination than those with a "neutral" message simply announcing the availability of the vaccine.

The introduction of *individual rather than block appointment systems and the substitution of a single for multiple providers* have resulted in decreased waiting time and improved appointment keeping. Individual appointment systems give each patient a precise time for his appointment; block systems schedule several or all patients for one time, usually at the beginning of office hours.

If *referral* is required, *educating the patient* about the purpose of referral, *minimizing the elapsed time* between the referral and the referral appointment, secretarial assistance to facilitate scheduling and transportation, and *referral to a specific physician* and not simply to a specialty group or clinic have also been shown to improve appointment keeping for diagnostic studies and/or specialty consultations.

Compliance with Regimens

Structural Strategies

Compliance with therapeutic regimens can be improved by a number of structural interventions. These include *simplification of the treatment regimen*, use of long-acting parenteral therapy, provision for continuity in the physician-patient relationship, use of clearly labeled medication containers, pill calendars (devices on which patients keep track of their medication taking), and special pharmaceutical packaging designed to aid memory.

Long-acting parenteral therapy is especially useful in situations in which compliance is known to be low. For example, the use of a single intramuscular long-acting penicillin rather than 10 days of an oral preparation will improve effectiveness of therapy.

Instructional Strategies

Providing patients with *information* about their illnesses and the rationale for treatment enhances compliance. Information is most effective when it provides an explanatory framework understandable and acceptable to the patient, when it addresses potential barriers to compliance, and when it is targeted to the needs of the patient.

Providing patients with *instructions* about their regimen is, of course, critical. Nevertheless, physicians often communicate poorly both the purpose of a specific regimen and precise directions about how it should be administered (7, 33). *Verbal* instructions should be brief, clear, explicit, categorized by subject matter, with repetition for emphasis and testing for the effectiveness of the communication (29). *Written* instructions further enhance compliance. They provide a remedy for documented forgetfulness and can be reviewed at leisure in the less stressful environment of the patient's home. Interestingly, informing patients of expected drug side effects seems to increase compliance, at least with respect to antidepressant therapy (34).

Behavioral Strategies

Strategies that incorporate various combinations of increased supervision, tailoring of the medical regimen to individual patients' needs or habits, reinforcement, and patient involvement have improved compliance with chronic therapy. Instruction alone tends to be less effective in the setting of chronic diseases, probably because most patients have already learned their regimen and have been taught something about their disease. Verbal and written instructions, however, are still important at the initiation of therapy and whenever the regimen is changed.

Increased supervision includes scheduling of more frequent provider-patient contacts, the use of reminders, the use of drug assays, and the eliciting of family or community support to assist in administering and monitoring treatment. For example, the physician may request more frequent blood pressure values in a hypertensive patient. The blood pressures can be taken either by a nurse at the physician's office, a nurse at work, a family member, or the patient himself.

Tailoring refers to a process whereby the therapeutic regimen is fitted to the patient's characteristics and environment. Effective tailoring requires knowledge of the patient as a person—his beliefs, life style, social and family support systems, and, specifically, any barriers to compliance. Forgetful patients may benefit from linking medication taking or prescribed activities to daily routines, such as eating meals, brushing teeth, getting up in the morning, or going to bed at night. In addition, medication should be kept available where it is taken (e.g., at the breakfast table). If possible, the patient should avoid taking medication during times of the day when his activities are variable or when he is likely to be distracted (e.g., at work). Other examples of tailoring include involving patients who like to be in control in planning and monitoring their own therapy, substituting liquid medication in patients who have difficulties swallowing tablets or capsules, increasing supervision and peer support for patients who are having difficulty on their own following a desired regimen (such as a weight reduction diet), and recommending exercise programs that can be incorporated into the schedules of extremely busy, time-pressured individuals and that eliminate travel, waiting time and the need for special scheduling. The physician needs specifically to search for barriers that interfere with compliance. When cost is a factor, less expensive regimens can be prescribed or financial assistance sought. When a patient's health beliefs or ethnic model of disease interferes, they can sometimes be accommodated. For example, Mexican American or Puerto Rican patients who ascribe to the hot-cold theory of health and disease avoid the use of "hot" substances during pregnancy and, therefore, may refuse to take "hot" medications such as iron and vitamins. Compliance in this situation may be obtained by encouraging the patient to "neutralize" the hot properties of these medications with cool substances such as fruit juices or herb teas.

Reinforcement consists of behavioral feedbacks that can either promote or discourage compliance. It is the physician's task to identify existing reinforcers, support or initiate those that promote, and attempt to eliminate or diminish those that discourage compliance. For example, through *classical (Pavlovian) conditioning* a patient may have learned the habit of eating whenever he watches television, even when he is not hungry. To eliminate this behavior, the physician might try to reach an agreement whereby the patient eats only at the dining room table with the television off. *Operant*, in contrast to classical, conditioning reinforces behavior through its consequences and is more commonly used in clinical medicine. Feeding back to the patient results of drug level assays and therapeutic outcomes (e.g., decrease in blood pressure or weight) are examples of operant conditioning. Because positive feedback is more effective than negative in helping individuals adopt new behaviors, measures and outcomes that indicate compliance should be praised, otherwise rewarded, or viewed by the patient as rewards in themselves. When measures or outcomes suggest noncompliance, the problem should be discussed. Education and use of family and friends may be required to optimize reinforcers at home and in the community. Two common examples for such an intervention are reversal of reinforced psychosocial disability in the physically capable patient after myocardial infarction and maintenance of abstention in the detoxified alcoholic patient.

When a regimen is particularly complex or difficult, compliance may be improved by "*graduated regimen implementation*" or "*shaping*," whereby the patient is initially rewarded for adhering to only part of the regimen. Once the first part is achieved, additional components of the regimen are added in stepwise fashion with rewards being given only when there is compliance with all of the components that have been implemented.

Mechanisms of *enhancing patient involvement* have included various forms of self-monitoring, such as taking blood pressures at home and the signing of contracts between patients and physicians. Therapeutic regimens that have been negotiated with rather than dictated by the physician are more likely to result in patient compliance. By taking active responsibility for their own care, patients may become more motivated to comply with therapy.

Combination strategies that utilize two or more of the above methods are generally much more effective than single interventions. Such a combination strategy utilized to improve behavior in noncompliant postmyocardial infarction patients has been described by Baile and Engel (1). Patient involvement was effected by having patients set their own goals and monitor their own behavior. Frequent contact with the physician allowed reinforcement, modification of goals on a negotiated basis, and discussion of problems with the regimen. Involvement of the spouse also increased supervision.

Direct Supervision of Medication Taking

Direct supervision of drug intake is especially helpful for ensuring compliance in patients with impaired intellectual or psychological functioning, such as those with alcoholism, dementia, and schizophrenia. Examples include the use of intermittent supervised oral antituberculosis therapy and the use of long-acting parenteral drugs in the ambulatory management of schizophrenia.

Maintenance of Compliance/Motivating Patients

Compliance tends to decay toward baseline after cessation of most successful interventions. Hence, there is a need to continue some form of intervention. Unfortunately, there has been little effort to date to study maintenance strategies.

One explanation for the failure of most compliance-improving interventions to have enduring impact is their reliance on actions and supports external to the patient. Based upon reviews of the relevant compliance, psychological, sociological, and behavioral literature, DiMatteo and DiNicola and Meichenbaum and Turk (see "General References") suggest approaches that promote "internalization" of the patient's motivation and ability to comply.

New *beliefs, attitudes, or values* may have to become integrated into the patient's life, and perhaps others may have to be dropped. Because physicians are the major source of health information for most Americans (7), they can assist in this process. They are more likely to succeed if they have earned the patient's trust (see "Doctor-Patient Relationship" above).

The first step for the physician in promoting change in health attitudes is to explore the patient's present knowledge, beliefs, attitudes, and values, as well as his social and cultural norms. Education about his disease and regimen can then be tailored to correct misconceptions, fill in gaps in his knowledge base, provide an explanatory framework understandable and acceptable to the patient, and motivate him in the context of his value system. Simply taking time for discussion will raise the salience in the patient's mind of the issue being discussed. Threat or fear messages can motivate behavioral change but should not be too strong (can cause patient denial or paralysis) or too weak. Furthermore, they should be combined with a positive message about a feasible (for the patient) and effective therapeutic regimen. Because patients are often more present than future-oriented, short-term, as well as long-term, benefits of any regimen should be stressed. Because behavior can influence attitudes, as well as *vice versa*, the practitioner should point out the patient's own behaviors that support the attitude being promoted. One can help integrate the new attitude into the patient's total system of beliefs by noting how it correlates with other beliefs the patient has. One can also note how it adheres to cultural and social norms. Of course, new attitudes and beliefs need positive reinforcement, as previously discussed.

Patients with unhealthy *self-perceptions* may need to be convinced that they can indeed effect a change in their lives. The practitioner can help by emphasizing the patient's past and present behaviors that demonstrated self-control, by enhancing the patient's feelings of responsibility for accomplished changes, by pointing out inaccuracies in the patient's negative self-perceptions, and by having and projecting a positive attitude to the patient about her abilities to change (e.g., "On the one hand you say you have no self-control. On the other, you tell me you stopped smoking for the entire period of your second pregnancy. That demonstrates to me that you can exhibit tremendous self-control." or "Two months ago you told me that you would never be able to manage insulin. Now you are monitoring your own blood sugars and calling me to propose changes in your insulin schedule. What does that tell you about yourself?"). Patients and their physicians often view partial successes as failure (e.g., the patient who has started drinking or smoking after a period of abstinence, the patient who has cut caffeine intake in half). Physicians can promote patients' self-esteem and sense of self-efficacy by reframing these "failures" as "successes," as important steps along the way to the accomplishment of important health goals (e.g., "It's great you were able to stop smoking for a month! That really increases your chances of being able to quit for good. Did you know that most persons who stop smoking require more than one attempt?").

New *skills* can also be taught to patients to enhance their ability, as well as motivation, to initiate and maintain compliance with difficult regimens. They can learn problem solving-skills by analyzing, with the physician, the health problem, treatment alternatives, and the advantages and disadvantages of potential actions. They can participate in the development of overall treatment goals. They can be tutored in developing specific, feasible, and measurable behavioral objectives for themselves, and in breaking down large tasks into several small, manageable steps. When patients have adopted new attitudes, beliefs, or behaviors, they can be taught to anticipate and prepare themselves for likely challenges (e.g., to the recovering alcoholic, "What challenges do you expect to your new sobriety?" and

"How are you going to handle it when people try to get you to drink at your niece's wedding this weekend?"; or to the hypertensive patient who is sensitive to being viewed as ill by others, "How are you going to respond when one of your colleagues at work sees you taking your medication and says 'Oh, you have to take medicine now! What's wrong with you?'"). Patients can also learn to analyze and learn from past failures to enhance the likelihood of future success (e.g., "Why has it been difficult for you to take the second dose?" or "Exactly how did it occur, when you started smoking again?", "What does that tell you?", and "If you could overcome that problem, your chances for success would be really high! Any ideas?").

Efforts to help patients adopt appropriate health-promoting beliefs, attitudes, values, and skills can be integrated into ongoing care and should usually span several office visits. Referral to *supportive groups* that expose patients to others with similar problems (e.g., asthma, postmyocardial infarction, ostomy, and mastectomy groups, Alcoholics Anonymous, Weight Watchers, etc.) is an important adjunct to management.

Example

The following is an example of how structural, information providing, behavioral, and motivational strategies can be integrated into a visit (continuation of example from page 38).

Doctor: Well, Mrs. Smith, your blood pressure is 150/100 today, which is better than when we started but not as low as we'd like it. Do you remember the goal we agreed upon? ("We" implies shared responsibility. Doctor focuses patient upon a specific measurable objective and points out that some progress has been made.)

Patient: I believe it was under 140 on the top and under 90 on the bottom.

Doctor: Right. What do you think you could do to bring it down further? (Doctor further involves and transfers responsibility to the patient.)

Patient: Well, as you said, part of the problem with today's blood pressure could be my not taking the medicine this morning. So I'll be sure to take it from now on, on the days I come to see you.

Also I've been thinking about enrolling at the athletic club. I like dancing. The club has convenient hours and is on my way to work. I'd prefer not to take any more medicines.

Doctor: The athletic club is an excellent idea. Regular exercise not only has a direct effect that lowers blood pressure, but it might also indirectly lower your pressure by helping you to lose weight. (Doctor provides positive reinforcement and notes an added benefit that relates to another goal the patient has for herself.)

Patient: That would be nice.

Doctor: I am concerned though about the difficulty you have getting the second dose of medication into your schedule. Blood pressure pills work best when you can take them almost 100% of the time. (Doctor provides a rationale for this concern.) Would dinner be a good time for you? (Doctor initiates negotiation process)

Patient: My meal times are irregular and I don't always eat at home.

Doctor: How about bedtime?

Patient: Sometimes I'm so exhausted, I just fall to sleep while I'm reading, before I've brushed my teeth or anything. Don't you have a pill that can be taken just once a day?

Doctor: As a matter of fact, that's a possibility. When would you take it?

Patient: With my morning coffee. I never miss that!

Doctor: Fine, I'll give you a prescription for a pill that you can take once a day with your morning coffee . . . 100% of the time, even the mornings you come to my office. Is that a deal?

Patient: Yes! (solution achieved through tailoring and negotiation)

Doctor: The side effects for this medicine are the same as for the other. Since you experienced none with the other, you should tolerate this one well.

Patient: Good.

Doctor: Together with the salt restriction and exercise program, this medicine alone may be enough to control your blood pressure. (Doctor provides further motivation for salt restriction and exercise.) Of course, we'll start with a low dose, so we may have to increase it. Can you come back in 2 weeks?

Patient: How about 2 months?

Doctor: Well, I'd really like to see you more frequently until your blood pressure is controlled. Of course, if you monitored your own blood pressure at home, you could call the results in to me and there would be less need for frequent office visits. (The doctor prefers not to yield on the follow-up interval and uses the opportunity to motivate the patient to become further involved in her own management and to create a new environmental reinforcer.)

Patient: How can I do that?

(Doctor proceeds (a) to explain the process of getting a blood pressure cuff, coming to the office to have it checked, and learning how to use it; (b) to test the patient for her understanding of her responsibilities; (c) to get her verbal commitment; and (d) to write down for her the new management plan.)

Education of Physicians as a Compliance-Improving Strategy

It has been demonstrated in two carefully executed controlled studies (23, 30) but not in another (6) that educating physicians about the importance, recognition, and management of noncompliance can result in improved compliance outcomes in their patients. Additional research is required to identify and refine the components necessary for effective educational intervention.

Ethical Considerations

It has been suggested that the following three conditions be met before attempting to improve compliance: (a) the diagnosis should be correct, (b) the therapy should be proven efficacious and benefits should out-weigh adverse effects, and (c) the patient should be an informed and willing partner in the intervention (39).

Although the first two conditions are probably applicable to interventions directed toward populations, they may be too rigid for application to individual patients. In some circumstances, it may be reasonable to prescribe an efficacious medicine as a therapeutic trial, when the diagnosis is in question. Furthermore, many medicines have not been unequivocally proven to be efficacious, although some evidence supports their usefulness. The physician is justified in encouraging the use of such medications in an attempt to determine whether they relieve symptoms or improve functional status. How else will the physician know whether a given antiarrhythmic or analgesic, for example, is effective for a given patient?

In individual practice, therefore, the first two conditions might be replaced with the following requirements: (a) that the therapy be rational and based upon sound medical knowledge, and (b) that the potential risks of therapy be less than the likely benefits.

The third condition, that of an informed and willing partner in the intervention, is even more difficult to satisfy. In medical practice one may encounter individuals who willfully fail to comply against their own best interest. Is the physician justified in increasing supervision or attempting to elicit familial support in order to improve compliance, without obtaining explicit consent from the patient? On the one hand, the patient has come to the doctor's office and voluntarily entered into the patient-physician relationship, suggesting implicit consent. On the other hand, the patient is willfully noncomplying, suggesting a rejection of this aspect of the relationship. The dilemma may be somewhat artificial since most compliance-improving strategies require participation of the patient and, therefore, implicit consent. Going beyond the patient-physician relationship to enroll family help, however, requires consideration of the patient's feelings with respect to this intervention. Some patients are mentally or psychologically impaired in their ability to understand or make sound decisions regarding their situations. An example might be the symptomatic schizophrenic patient who fails to comply in taking his oral antipsychotic medication, when introduction of long-acting parenteral therapy could reduce symptoms, rate of relapse, and rehospitalization. There are no definitive guidelines in these situations, but the following suggestions may be helpful: (a) The physician should attempt to determine the patient's own best interest, considering not only the disease but also the patient's desires, values, psychological makeup, and social environment, and he should use this information as a guide to action. (b) The physician should weigh the relative benefits versus risks of intervention (self-monitoring of blood pressure in some individuals, for example, might markedly increase their anxiety). (c) The physician should respect the patient's autonomy and legal rights. (d) When the patient is incapable of understanding or making reasonable decisions related to his situation, the physician should consult with the responsible family member or guardian before deciding on a course of action. (See Chapter 10 for determination of mental competence.) (e) In particularly difficult situations, the physician should seek advice from others.

Finally, there is the question of where the patient's responsibilities begin and those of the physician end. Is the physician ethically bound to identify and treat noncompliance when it compromises the health of his patient? Once a patient-physician relationship has been established, it is certainly the physician's responsibility to work with the patient to improve his health status to the best of the physician's ability, taking into consideration the severity of the problem, economic constraints, time constraints, and competing obligations to other patients. To achieve this end a physician should use not only the traditional methods of diagnosis, treatment, and instruction of patients, but when appropriate, interventions for improving compliance as well.

PRACTICAL APPROACH TO NONCOMPLIANCE

In practice, the problem of noncompliance should be handled in the same way as are other clinical problems. Whenever possible it should be prevented. When present, it should be diagnosed and treated by accepted diagnostic approaches and treatment modalities.

Noncompliance with Therapeutic Regimens

Prevention (Table 4.1)

It is usually more efficient to use some strategies that will improve compliance with all patients at the inception of treatment, rather than to attempt to identify the noncompliers at a later time. Minimal preventive strategies for all patients should include (a) *development of rapport and patient trust* (see page

Table 4.1.
Prevention Of Noncompliance

Development of rapport and patient trust
Targeted (limited) education
  Correction of misconceptions
  Provision of explanatory framework for treatment regimen
  Motivation of patient
  Discussion of:
    Likely side effects
    Cost
    Alternative therapies
    Consequences of nontherapy
Use of simplest possible medical regimen
Tailoring of medical regimen
Verbal instructions that are
  Concise
  Clear
  Explicit
  Categorized
  Repeated
Written instructions
Parenteral therapy (when an option)

41); (b) the use of the *simplest possible medical regimen* (page 42); and (c) *brief, clear, explicit, categorized instructions* that include the purpose and duration of therapy, with subsequent repetition and testing for the effectiveness of the communication (page 42). *Written instructions* (in addition to what the pharmacist transcribes onto the medication bottle) should be given when changes are made in the treatment regimen, the regimen is complex, or the instructions are incompletely retained. *Education targeted to correct misconceptions and motivate the patient, and discussion of likely side effects*, what to do in the event of side effects, approximate cost of medications, *alternative therapies, and consequences of nontherapy* may further enhance compliance. Negative transference and countertransference reactions should be recognized and controlled.

Tailoring of care to the individual needs of the patient from the outset may increase his satisfaction and improve the chances for compliance. This requires that the physician routinely answer some of the following questions about most patients: (a) *Who* is this patient? What are his personality traits? Does he need more or less information about and involvement in his own care? (b) *What* are the patient's explanations for and beliefs about his illness? What are his attitudes about care? What perceived barriers to compliance exist? (c) *Where* does the patient come from? What environmental factors, such as family and work hours, might influence his ability to follow a therapeutic regimen? (d) *Why* is the patient here? What are his expectations, motivations, and concerns in seeking care? What triggered today's visit? (e) Does the patient *understand and accept* the physician's explanation and prescription? These answers may then be utilized as described above to tailor a treatment regimen for the patient (page 42). Familiarity with the beliefs and practices of commonly served ethnic groups can also be of assistance (see page 40).

The use of *parenteral therapy* in lieu of more complicated and prolonged oral regimens (e.g., in the treatment of gonococcal urethritis or streptococcal pharyngitis) will reduce noncompliance and thereby increase the effectiveness of therapy.

The use of printed *patient education materials* may be an efficient way to enhance patient understanding of a disease and its management from the outset (see also Chapter 3).

Diagnosis (Table 4.2)

The possibility of noncompliant behavior should be considered in all patients because of its high prevalence and the inability of physicians to predict it intuitively. The failure to see expected therapeutic or side effects should raise suspicions, as should the presence of other factors known to be associated with noncompliance (see discussion above).

The first step in diagnosing noncompliance is to *ask* patients what they are doing to treat their problem in an open-ended, facilitative, nonthreatening, nonjudg-

Table 4.2.
Diagnosis Of Noncompliance

Suspicion
  All patients (special emphasis on patients who fail to achieve expected therapeutic effects or side effects and those with associated risk factors for noncompliance)
Measurement
  Questioning (open-ended, facilitative, nonjudgmental, detailed, and specific) of patient or family (see text)
  Frequency of patient-requested prescription renewals or medication count
  Inspection of all pill bottles
  Drug assays
  Achievement of expected outcomes
  Supervised medication taking (office or hospital)
Cause
  Noncomprehension
  Volitional noncompliance
    Determination of cause of volitional noncompliance

mental, yet detailed and specific manner (see example, page 38). Questioning should continue until the patient has provided information about what medicines he is taking, how frequently he is taking them, how frequently doses are missed, and what nonpharmacological modes of treatment he is using. Patients should be specifically asked about compliance on the day of and the day preceding their visit. (Some diabetic patients, for example, routinely omit all drugs including insulin at the time of a morning visit; 24-hour recalls are more accurate than general reports, which tend to be idealized.) Using such techniques, 50% or more of noncompliers (and all those who do not comply because they do not understand the requirements) will be identified. Sensitivity can be increased by asking family members or housemates.

When the patient appears confused or is unable to provide sufficient information, having him *bring all medication containers to the office* (for both prescribed and over-the-counter medications) may provide invaluable information. For example, it may be discovered that a patient is still taking a discontinued medication or is taking two different preparations of the same drug. Selected patients should be encouraged to bring their medication containers with them at every visit.

If volitional noncompliance is suspected despite denial by the patient, objective measures are required. Medication counts may be instituted but are often impractical as discussed above. Instead observations of the frequency of *actual versus expected prescription renewals* may be substituted for formal pill counts. (A method for keeping track of prescription renewals should be incorporated into the office record, especially when prescriptions are filled by more than one physician.) Review of the longitudinal relationship between medication and *outcome measures* (greatly assisted by the appropriate use of flow sheets) can provide important clues of noncompliant behavior, such as widely varying blood pressures on a constant regimen. The absence of a drug upon *assay* is virtually diagnostic of noncompliance (assuming that the assay is reliable and the samples have been obtained at ap-

propriate times). The failure to achieve therapeutic drug levels or expected outcomes, however, could be secondary either to noncompliance or inadequate therapy. To distinguish between these two alternatives it may sometimes be necessary to observe drug levels or outcome of treatment during a period in which drugs are taken under *direct supervision*. This may require a period of hospitalization. In one common condition, hypertension, hospitalization can be avoided by measuring the patient's blood pressure for several hours after supervised ingestion of medication in the office (for examples, see cases in Chapter 62).

Once the presence of noncompliance has been established, its cause should be determined. Noncomprehension will be detected by simply asking the patient to describe his regimen. If the patient knows his regimen but does not comply, the physician is challenged to discover the reasons for the noncompliance (e.g., inappropriate beliefs about the illness or therapy, presence of side effects, cost of medicines, inconvenience of taking medicines, poor sense of self-efficacy, depression, etc.). The ways in which these factors may affect compliance behavior have been discussed above.

Treatment (Table 4.3)

Once noncompliance has been established and it has been decided to try to treat it (after a review of the ethical considerations previously discussed, see page 45) several methods are possible. If the problem is *noncomprehension*, the use of further verbal and written instructions and/or simplification and tailoring of the medical regimen may be indicated. If the patient is still unable to comprehend, supervision of medication taking by family members or by health personnel, such as visiting nurses, will be required.

Table 4.3.
Treatment Of Noncompliance

Noncomprehension
  Verbal and written instructions
  Simplification and tailoring of treatment regimen
  Supervision of treatment

Volitional noncompliance
  Targeted education to
    Correct misconceptions
    Address barriers
    Motivate the patient
    Boost self-efficacy
    Enhance patient skills
  Patient involvement (goal setting, problem solving, negotiation of regimen, contracts, self-monitoring)
  Simplification of treatment regimen
  Tailoring of treatment regimen
  Use of positive reinforcers
  Family/environmental support
  Increased supervision
  Supervised medication taking
  Long-acting medications

Combined interventions

Development of maintenance strategies, after initial success

When there is *volitional noncompliance*, a strategy designed to improve compliance must be tailored to each individual's needs. Underlying problems, such as depression or alcoholism, should be treated. The use of behavioral methods (see page 42) will often be required, including simplification and tailoring of the regimen, use of special pharmaceutical packaging or drug charts to aid memory, patient self-monitoring, negotiation and involvement of the patient in planning his own care, obtainment of patient verbal commitments and written contracts, increased medical and environmental supervision, monitoring and feedback of blood levels or outcome measures, and alteration of environmental reinforcers. Further education designed to motivate the patient, correct important misconceptions, address barriers to compliance, introduce or alter certain beliefs, attitudes, or values, boost the patient's sense of self-efficacy, and/or enhance his skills and, therefore, ability to comply is usually a necessary concomitant of treatment (see page 42). Long-acting parenteral therapy is occasionally an option. Because compliance tends to decline after the termination of many interventions, effective strategies may have to be continued indefinitely. Attempts to simplify or to discontinue a successful strategy should be done in stepwise fashion while continuing to monitor compliance.

Noncompliance with Appointment Keeping

Techniques to improve appointment-keeping rates in general have been discussed above (page 42). When follow-up is important, the physician can (a) logically *"bridge"* to the next visit by discussing its purpose with the patient (e.g., monitoring for recurrence, review of test results, decision about therapy, etc.); (b) *negotiate a visit interval* that is mutually acceptable; (c) *tailor the appointment time* to the patient's needs; (d) *obtain a verbal agreement* from the patient to comply; and (e) *schedule the appointment* instead of giving the patient instructions to "call for" one. Components (a) and (e) of this strategy have been tested in one successful clinical trial (47). Because *missed appointments* could presage dropouts from treatment, the charts and/or names of these patients should be reviewed daily by the physician. When indicated, the patient can be contacted by telephone, letter, or postcard. When referral is required, the physician should educate the patient about the purpose of the referral, ensure the patient's understanding of and agreement with the referral plan, refer when possible to a specific health care provider rather than to a clinic or specialty group, and arrange for an appointment to be made within a reasonably short period of time.

General References

Bernarde MA, Mayerson EW: Patient-physician negotiation. *JAMA* 239:1417, 1978.
  Practical discussion of some components of patient-provider communication, including negotiation, that can enhance patient compliance.
DiMatteo MR, DiNicola DD: *Achieving Patient Compliance: The Psychology of the Medical Practitioner's Role.* New York, Pergamon Press, 1982.
  Important contribution that describes an in-depth social-psychological approach to the understanding and management of noncompliant behavior.
Harwood A: *Ethnicity and Medical Care.* Cambridge, MA, Harvard University Press, 1981.
  Useful reference on ethnic health beliefs and practices.
Haynes RB, Taylor DW, Sackett DL (eds): *Compliance in Health Care.* Baltimore, Johns Hopkins University Press, 1979.
  Excellent comprehensive reference with annotated bibliography.
Martin AR, Coates TJ: A clinician's guide to helping patients change behavior. *West J Med* 146:751, 1987.
  Short practical "how to" article, with examples, on behavioral methods for improving compliance.
Meichenbaum D, Turk DC (eds): *Facilitating Treatment Adherence: A Practitioner's Guidebook.* New York, Plenum Press, 1987.
  A book, written by two leading clinical researchers in cognitive-behavioral therapy, that provides a useful analysis of the compliance literature. It is clinically oriented and full of suggestions for the health care provider on how to increase patient compliance by enhancement of the doctor-patient relationship and by use of effective patient education, behavioral modification, and motivational strategies.

Specific References

1. Baile WF, Engel BT: A behavioral strategy for the treatment of noncompliance following myocardial infarction. *Psychosom Med* 40:413, 1978.
2. Closson R, Kikuwago C: Noncompliance with drug class. *Hospitals* 49:89, 1975.
3. Cramer JA, Mattson RH, Prevey ML, et al: How often is medication taken as prescribed? A novel assessment technique. *JAMA* 261:3273, 1989.
4. Coronary Drug Project Research Group: Influence of adherence to treatment and response of cholesterol on mortality in the Coronary Drug Project. *N Engl J Med* 30:1038, 1980.
5. Croog SH, Shapiro DS, Levine S: Denial among heart patients. *Psychosom Med* 33:385, 1971.
6. Dickinson JC, Warshaw GA, Gehlbach SH, et al: Improving hypertension control: impact of computer feedback and physician education. *Med Care* 19:843, 1981.
7. DiMatteo MR, DiNicola DD: Practitioner-patient relationships: the communication of information. In: DiMatteo MR, DiNicola DD (eds): *Achieving Patient Compliance, The Psychology of the Medical Practitioner's Role.* New York, Pergamon Press, 1982, pp 29–67.
8. Durbin WA, Lapidas B, Goldman DA: Improved antibiotic usage following introduction of a novel prescription. *JAMA* 246:1796, 1981.
9. Editorial: Need we poison the elderly so often. *Lancet* ii:20, 1988.
10. Eshelman FN: Drug compliance in diabetics. *Br Med J* 1:581, 1978.
11. Fletcher C: Listening and talking to patients. I. The problem. *Br Med J* 281:845, 1980.
12. Francis V, Korsch BM, Morris MJ: Gaps in doctor-patient communication in patients' response to medical advice. *N Engl J Med* 280:535, 1969.
13. Garrity TF: Medical compliance and the clinician-patient relationship: a review. *Soc Sci Med* 15E:215, 1981.
14. Gordis L, Markowitz M, Lillienfeld AM: Studies in the epidemiology and preventability of rheumatic fever. IV. A quantitative determination of compliance in children on oral penicillin prophylaxis. *Pediatrics* 43:173, 1962.
15. Greenfield S, Kaplan SH, Ware JE, et al: Patients' participation in medical care: effects on blood sugar control and quality of life. *J Gen Intern Med* 3:448, 1988.
16. Hackett TP, Cassem NH: White-collar and blue-collar responses to heart attack. *J Psychosom Res* 20:85, 1976.
17. Hall JA, Roter DL, Katz NR: Meta-analysis of provider behavior in medical encounters. *Med Care* 26:657, 1988.
18. Haynes RB: Strategies in improving compliance with referrals,

appointments, and prescribed medical regimens. In: Haynes RB, Taylor DW, Sackett DL (eds): *Compliance in Health Care*. Baltimore, Johns Hopkins University Press, 1979, p 123.

19. Haynes RB, et al: Management of patient compliance in the treatment of hypertension. Report of the NHLBI Working Group. *Hypertension* 4:415, 1982.
20. Hemminki E, Heikkila J: Elderly people's compliance with prescriptions, and quality of medication. *Scand J Soc Med* 3:87, 1975.
21. Hulka B, Kupper L, Cassel J, et al: Medication use and misuse: physician-patient discrepancies. *J Chron Dis* 28:7, 1975.
22. Inui TS, Carter WB, Pecoraro RE, et al: Variations in patient compliance with common long term drugs. *Med Care* 18:986, 1980.
23. Inui TS, Yourtee EL, Williamson JW: Improved outcomes after physician tutorials: a controlled trial. *Ann Intern Med* 84:646, 1976.
24. Ireland HD: Outpatient chemotherapy for tuberculosis. *Am Rev Respir Dis* 82:378, 1960.
25. Johnson AL, Taylor DW, Sackett DL, et al: Self-recording of blood pressure in the management of hypertension. *Can Med Assoc J* 119:1034, 1978.
26. Kern DE, Grayson M, Barker LR, et al: Residency training in interviewing skills and the psychosocial domain of medical practice. *J Gen Intern Med* 4:421, 1989.
27. Larson EB, Bergman J, Heidrich F, et al: Do postcard reminders improve influenza vaccination compliance? A prospective trial of different postcard "cues." *Med Care* 20:639, 1982.
28. Ley P: Cognitive variables and non-compliance. *J Compliance in Health Care* 1:171, 1986.
29. Ley P: Memory for medical information. *Br J Soc Clin Psychol* 18:245, 1979.
30. Maiman LA, Becker MH, Liptak GS, et al: Improving pediatricians' compliance-enhancing practices: a randomized trial. *AJDC* 142:773, 1988.
31. Markowitz M: Eradication of rheumatic fever: an unfilled hope. *Circulation* 41:1077, 1970.
32. Mason AS, Forrest IS, Forrest FM, Butler H: Adherence to maintenance therapy and re-hospitalization. *Dis Nerv Syst* 24:103, 1963.
33. Mazzuca SA: Does patient education in chronic disease have therapeutic value? *J Chron Dis* 35:521, 1982.
34. Meyers ED, Calvert EJ: Knowledge of side effects and perseverance with medications. *Br Med J* 1:1577, 1976.
35. Oldright NB, Wicks JR, Hanley C, et al: Noncompliance in an exercise rehabilitation program for men who have suffered myocardial infarction. *Can Med Assoc J* 118:361, 1978.
36. Ray WA, Federspiel CF, Shaffner W: A study of antipsychotic drug use in nursing homes: epidemiologic evidence suggesting misuse. *Am J Public Health* 70:485, 1980.
37. Rost K, Carter W, Inui T: Introduction of information during the critical medical visit: consequences for patient follow through with physician recommendations for medication. *Soc Sci Med* 28(4):315, 1989.
38. Roth HP: Accuracy of doctors' estimates and patients' statements on adherence to a drug regimen. *Clin Pharmacol Ther* 23:361, 1978.
39. Sackett DL: Introduction. In: Sackett DL, Haynes RB (eds): *Compliance with Therapeutic Regimens*. Baltimore, Johns Hopkins University Press, 1976, p 4.
40. Sheckler WE, Bennett JV: Antibiotic usage in seven community hospitals. *JAMA* 213:264, 1970.
41. Smith M: The cost of noncompliance and the capacity of improved compliance to reduce health care expenditures. In: *Improving Medication Compliance, Proceedings of a Symposium*. National Pharmaceutical Council, 1985, p 35.
42. Steele DJ, Blackwell B, Gutmann MC, Jackson TC: Beyond advocacy: a review of the active patient concept. *Patient Education and Counseling* 10:3, 1987.
43. Steele DJ, Jackson TC, Gutman MC: "Have you been taking your pill?" The adherence monitoring sequence in the medical interview. *J Fam Practice* 30(3):294, 1990.
44. Stolley PD, Lasagna L: Prescribing patterns of physicians. *J Chron Dis* 22:394, 1969.
45. Svarstad BL: Physician-patient communication and patient conformity with medical advice. In: Mechanic D (ed): *The Growth of Bureaucratic Medicine*. New York, John Wiley & Sons, 1976, p 243.
46. Uhlmann RF, Inui TS, Pecoraro RE, Carter WB: Relationship of patient request fulfillment to compliance, glycemic control, and other health care outcomes in insulin-dependent diabetes. *J Gen Intern Med* 3:458, 1988.
47. Waggoner DM, Jackson EB, Kern DE: Physical influence on patient compliance: a clinical trial. *Ann Emerg Med* 10:348, 1981.

CHAPTER 5

Adolescent Patients: Special Considerations

LARRY N. SCHERZER, M.D.

From a developmental perspective, adolescence is a time of dynamic changes, with tremendous physical, sexual, intellectual, and psychological growth. This chapter describes (a) the normal changes and the major problems associated with each of these four spheres of development, and (b) practical approaches to the office care of the adolescent patient.

ADOLESCENT MORTALITY AND MORBIDITY

Adolescence is the healthiest period of life; morbidity and mortality rates are low compared with other age groups; but the absolute number of adolescents who die or suffer from chronic illnesses is considerable. Because the number of productive years at stake for a teenager with a significant illness is large, adolescent health deserves a special priority.

Accidents are by far the leading cause of death among adolescents and young adults. Preventive measures have, by and large, been bypassed by the victims of accidental death; and, in many instances, behavioral problems underlie those deaths. For example, alcohol is implicated in over 50% of automobile accidents, and there may be an element of suicidal intent in many of them.

The second and third leading causes of death in older adolescents (and an important problem in young adolescents) are homicide and suicide, problems that are discussed later in this chapter.

The fourth leading cause of death among adolescents and young adults is neoplasia. The most frequent diagnoses are acute leukemia (both lymphocytic and myelogenous), lymphomas (including non-Hodgkin's lymphoma and Hodgkin's disease), central nervous system tumors (especially supra- and infratentorial gliomas), bone tumors (especially osteogenic sarcomas and Ewing's sarcomas), and solid organ tumors (especially of genital organs).

As medical treatment improves, conditions that were previously fatal in childhood are being seen frequently in adolescents and young adults. It is common for patients with cystic fibrosis, nephritis, congenital heart disease, and leukemia to survive into adolescence and young adulthood.

Most visits to a physician by adolescents are for preventive care or are for problems that are relatively minor (Table 5.1). However, a number of more severe medical problems are either limited chiefly to the adolescent period or are problems of adulthood that begin during adolescence (Table 5.2). The data in Tables 5.1 and 5.2 do not depict the significant distress that many adolescent patients (and their physicians) experience. This distress is often related to the pressures unique to the several chronological stages of adolescence.

The *young teen* (i.e., 11 to 15 years old), with his special concern over physical development, may have anxieties about mutilation and death. Hostility toward an illness may be expressed in a fantasy of invincibility leading to an uncooperative, noncompliant patient. Other young adolescents become greatly depressed by their illnesses and become annoying, complaining, whiny patients, frequently regressing to a child-like dependence on adult caretakers.

The *middle adolescent* (i.e., 14 to 19 years old) who is seriously ill suffers from the loss of valued contact with friends and schools. Important aspirations may be interrupted (and dreams shattered) through illness. Body image is at a critical developmental stage in mid-adolescence, and the teen may be more worried about a cosmetic defect resulting from an illness than about the disease or its therapy. Such fears need to be faced early and dealt with honestly.

Table 5.1.
Number of Office Visits Made by Adolescents and Percentage Distribution by the 20 Most Frequent Principal Diagnoses (By ICD-9-CM Categories), According to Age: United States, 1980–1981[a,b]

Principal Diagnosis[b]	No. of Visits in Thousands	Percentage Distribution	Principal Diagnosis	No. of Visits in Thousands	Percentage Distribution
11–14 years			**15–20 years**		
Total	40,269	100.0	Total	87,172	100.0
General medical examination	2,832	7.0	Normal pregnancy	7,926	9.1
Allergic rhinitis	1,760	4.4	Diseases of sebaceous glands[c]	7,306	8.4
Diseases of sebaceous glands[c]	1,629	4.0	General medical examination	5,457	6.3
Acute pharyngitis	1,297	3.2	Acute pharyngitis	2,439	2.8
Acute upper respiratory infections of multiple or unspecified sites	1,296	3.2	Acute upper respiratory infections of multiple or unspecified sites	2,242	2.6
Suppurative and unspecified otitis media	1,177	2.9	Special investigations and examinations[e]	1,756	2.0
Asthma	1,109	2.8	Disorders of refraction and accommodation	1,525	1.7
Disorders of refraction and accommodation	1,054	2.6	Allergic rhinitis	1,482	1.7
Routine infant or child health check	930	2.3	Other diseases due to viruses and chlamydiae	1,427	1.6
Certain adverse effects not elsewhere classified[d]	808	2.0	Follow-up examination	1,345	1.5
Acute tonsillitis	791	2.0	Acute tonsillitis	1,254	1.4
Other diseases due to viruses and chlamydiae	770	1.9	Contact dermatitis and other eczema	1,146	1.3
Contact dermatitis and other eczema	684	1.7	Suppurative and unspecified otitis media	955	1.1
Fracture of radius and ulna	551	1.4	Contraceptive management	866	1.0
Disorders of external ear	527	1.3	Asthma	851	1.0
Curvature of spine	460	1.1	Disorders of menstruation and other abnormal bleeding from female genital tract	820	0.9
Bronchitis, not specified as acute or chronic	*435	1.1			
Observation and evaluation for suspected conditions	*422	1.0	Bronchitis, not specified as acute or chronic	788	0.9
			Disorders of external ear	731	0.8
Other noninfective gastroenteritis and colitis	*413	1.0	Chronic sinusitis	722	0.8
Follow-up examination	*405	1.0	Neurotic disorders	719	0.8
Residual	...	52.1	Residual	...	52.3

[a] From Cypress BK: *Health Care of Adolescents by Office-Based Physicians: National Ambulatory Medical Care Survey, 1980–1981.* Advance Data from Vital and Health Statistics. No. 99, September 28, 1984.
[b] Based on US Public Health Service and Health Care Financing Administration: *International Classification of Diseases, 9th Revision, Clinical Modification* (ICD-9-CM). Department of Health and Human Services, Publ no. (PHS) 80-1260. Public Health Service. Washington, DC, US Government Printing Office, September 1980.
[c] Chiefly 706.1, acne other than varioliformis.
[d] Chiefly 995.3, allergy unspecified.
[e] Chiefly V72.3, gynecological examination.

Table 5.2.
Selected Medical Problems Limited to Adolescence or Persisting into Adulthood

Limited Chiefly to Adolescence	Chronic Problems That May Begin in Adolescence
Slipped epiphysis	Obesity
Distortion of body image	Hypertension
Delinquency[a]	Diabetes
Anorexia nervosa	Hypercholesterolemia
Primary amenorrhea	Duodenal ulcer
School or learning problems[b]	Inflammatory bowel disease
	Irritable colon
	Dental caries
	Drug abuse
	Alcoholism
	Personality disorders
	Somatization disorder
	Depressive neurosis

[a]May begin earlier.
[b]Often develops earlier.

The *older adolescent* (i.e., 18 to 21 years old) shares many adult concerns. For example, anxiety may be expressed over the cost of an illness and the length of hospitalization, and the burdens these place on the family.

PHYSICAL DEVELOPMENT

Normal Patterns and Concerns

Physical maturation is an important feature of the second decade of life. Although the rate and the timing of maturation may vary, they follow the hormonal changes of puberty in a given individual.

There is a notable *growth spurt* occurring during the adolescent years, with a 20 to 25% increase in height over a period of 2 to 3 years. This spurt usually occurs earlier in the female than in the male (as does sexual maturation).

During puberty, there is an average 2-fold increase in both lean and nonlean body mass. The ratio of lean to nonlean body mass is greater in males than in females. Fat accumulation tends to be greatest at the point that growth ceases and may extend into adulthood.

The *musculoskeletal system* has special characteristics during adolescence. To accommodate growth, the ligaments and tendons become lax and elastic, frequently giving the teen a slouched-over appearance. Similarly, there is an increase in skeletal growth, particularly in long bones; and metaphyseal-epiphyseal junctions remain soft. Thus, the actively growing teen, who may not have developed a muscle mass to correspond to his skeletal growth, may be prone to some special injuries, particularly joint dislocations and fractures along epiphyseal plates.

As with all areas of development, the adolescent may have particular concerns about *growth and weight*. The principal reason for this is that adolescents often base judgment of each other's adequacy and acceptability on size or (for males) on athletic ability; and adult criteria of social status based on other standards (or prejudices) are of less importance.

Children called "squirt" or "runt" are given various types of parental advice; much of it is not helpful. Some children adapt by engaging in an activity where size is unimportant (e.g., debating, chess, fencing, swimming, body building, etc.). Occasionally, normal children with a familial basis for their short stature will require some psychological counseling to promote effective adaptation to their stature. Some individuals who are very sensitive about height and strength limitations may try radical and potentially harmful solutions such as self-injections of purported growth stimulants.

The concern of the adolescent about height may be generalized to many other aspects of appearance, including body habitus, beauty (or lack of beauty), skin condition, etc. It is important to recognize when concern about body image is the patient's primary concern and to provide reassurance that he or she is medically and biologically normal. This reassurance can be greatly facilitated at times by suggesting a book in which the adolescent can learn more about normal growth (see page 61).

Common Problems

Short Stature

This problem is discussed below ("Short Stature and Delayed Sexual Maturation").

Obesity

A practical definition of obesity is a weight of 20% or more over ideal body weight (see also Chapter 76). This can be estimated by determining the weight that corresponds to the growth chart height percentile for the age and sex of the child and dividing this into the actual weight (Fig. 5.1). A result of greater than 1.2 would be suspect. This ratio should be compared with the clinical appearance of the child, since the fat distribution changes at puberty in boys, when extra weight may be transformed into musculature, and in girls, who normally increase their storage of fat. Obesity remains a clinical diagnosis. Adolescent obesity is usually due to overeating. Most estimates place the prevalence between 4 and 10%, with the highest frequency among the lower socioeconomic groups. Frequently, the obesity began in early childhood but becomes a concern in adolescence because of desires to conform to peer standards.

It is recommended that obese teens be screened for other cardiovascular risk factors, such as positive family history, high blood pressure, elevated serum cholesterol or triglyceride, diabetes mellitus, and smoking. If multiple risk factors are present, the patient should be monitored more frequently and risk modification should be encouraged.

In order to treat adolescent obesity successfully, the teen himself must be motivated and must accept the physician's assessments and recommendations. Frequently, the patient has attempted to cope with the problem by himself. Certain fad diets, such as fasting,

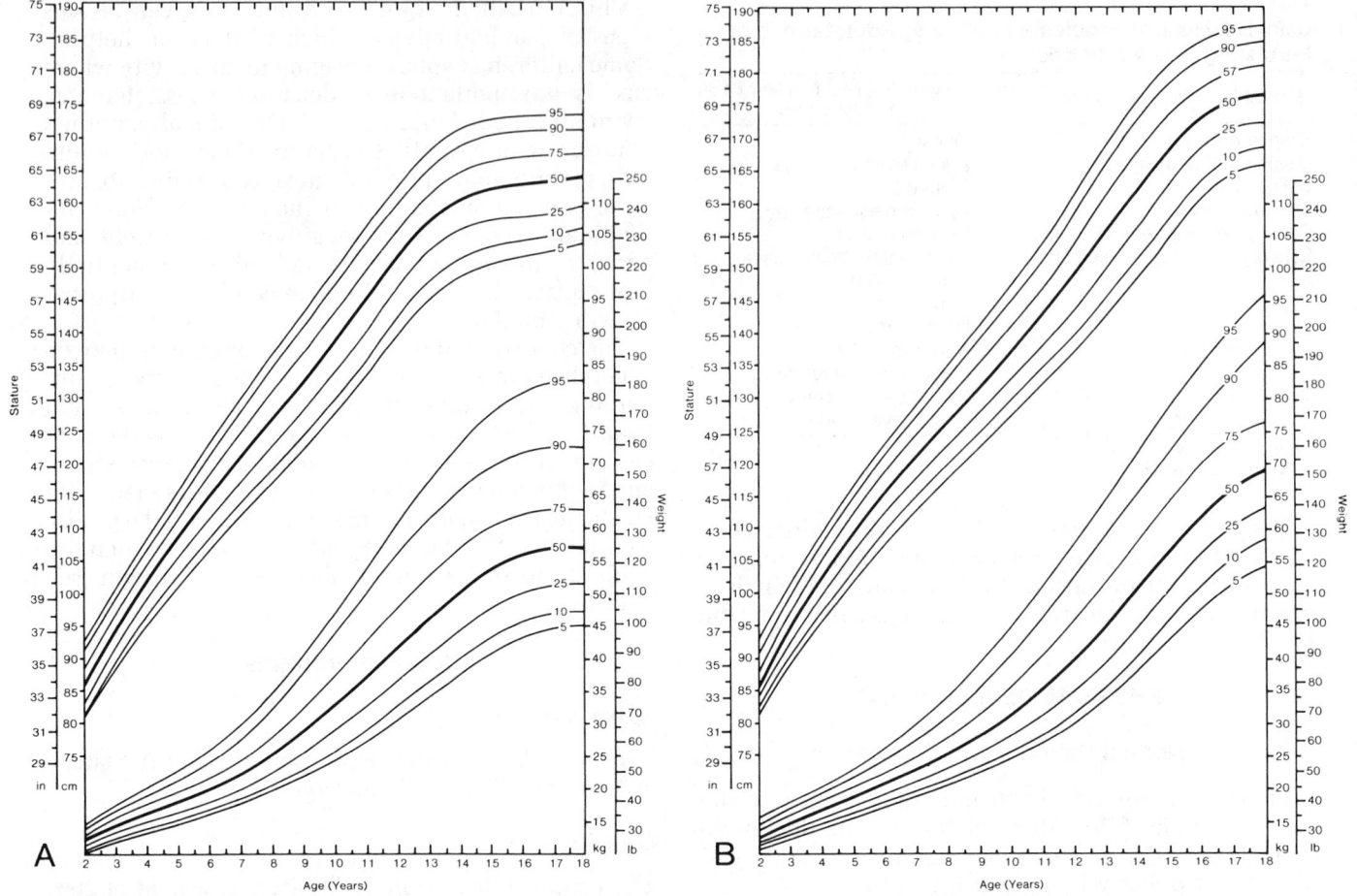

Figure 5.1A. Physical growth in girls. Plot height and weight against and weight against chronological age at each encounter. The curve so obtained should parallel percentile lines within the clear area (growth patterns of 90% of children/adolescents). If the curve deviates from percentile lines, an abnormal growth pattern is likely. The upper series of curves represent the normal range of height at various ages and the lower series of curves, the normal range of weight at various ages. (From National Center for Health Statistics: NCHS Growth Charts, 1976. Monthly Vital Statistics Report. vol 25, no. 3, suppl. (HRA) 76-1120. Rockville, MD, Health Resources Administration, June 1976.) **B.** Physical growth in boys.

water diets, etc., may yield rapid weight loss but will deplete the strength of the child. Generally, since no modification of long-term eating habits is attempted, the weight is regained upon cessation of the diet. Occasionally, serious biological complications are associated with prolonged adherence to highly restrictive diets. Macrobiotic diets have been associated with symptoms of protein and vitamin deficiencies and liquid protein diets have cardiotoxic effects that have resulted in deaths (see details, Chapter 76). Severely calorie-restricted diets will lead to a cessation of linear growth and may cause menstrual irregularities.

Medications have been of no value in weight control. Amphetamines and metamphetamines are contraindicated because of their potential for abuse.

Surgical treatment (e.g., jejunal-ileal bypass or gastric stapling) of obesity is rarely indicated, particularly in the adolescent years.

One is left with methods of dietary control by modification of eating habits and by increasing exercise, together with moderate calorie restriction. These methods, while successful for some, are not successful for all. Frequently, the teen who wants to diet is well motivated, if for personal and emotional reasons rather than for reasons of health. A group meeting of obese teens provides a nucleus of peer support, with an opportunity for mutual discussions of problems of dieting and appetite control that may not be aired in a brief office visit. Such a group may also help to alleviate home pressures. (Parental coercion and control of diet in the context of a normally antagonistic parent-teen relationship may result in an angry, rebellious youngster who is gaining rather than losing weight.)

For overweight young to midadolescents a reasonable goal is to maintain their current body weight, since excess caloric restriction may result in a loss of lean body weight. For the late adolescent, the goal may be weight loss. For all obese patients, one wishes to achieve a change in long-term eating patterns.

Some adolescents overeat because of unresolved psychological difficulties. If there are expressions of problems in peer, school, or parental relationships, these should be explored further. Obesity alone, however, is not an indication of psychopathology.

Anorexia Nervosa and Bulimia

Anorexia nervosa is an infrequent but serious disorder of growth in adolescents. It is marked by extreme loss of appetite and of weight (at least 25% of the baseline weight) that is not attributable to a medical or psychiatric illness ordinarily associated with weight loss (i.e., inflammatory bowel disease or a major affective disorder). Patients characteristically exhibit an intense fear of becoming obese and, even when very thin, have a distorted body image so that they still consider themselves overweight (Table 5.3).

Anorexia nervosa is most commonly a disease of young adolescent girls (about 90% of cases); but occasionally it affects males or older females. Most often, the problem develops in children of upper middle class families. Before their illness, the patients typically have been considered "model children" who have done well in school and have been obedient to their parents.

The cause of the disease is unknown. Although there have been many theories proposed to explain it, none is entirely satisfactory. Frequently there has been some stress in the family (divorce, death, change of location) before the onset of the illness.

There is no simple treatment that can be recommended for patients with anorexia nervosa. Help should be sought from a psychiatrist who has experience with eating disorders. The best results seem to be achieved by involving the patient and her family in an intensive program in which counseling and behavior modification are employed to restructure the patient's eating habits and attitude toward food. Cachectic patients

should be hospitalized so that a proper program of nutrition can be instituted.

Complete remission of anorexia nervosa is unusual, but about 75% of patients achieve an acceptable improvement in both their physical and emotional state. The rest remain chronically undernourished and maladapted, and up to 10% die of complications of the disease.

Bulimia is a second eating disorder seen in adolescents and young adults. The vast majority of bulimic persons are women; bulimic symptoms have been reported by up to 10% of young women interviewed in community surveys (9). Characteristically, a patient with bulimia will periodically gorge herself, only to follow this by self-induced vomiting and by further self-reprisals through abstinence from food (Table 5.3). As the disease progresses, patients may become withdrawn and depressed, leading to further appetite suppression. Amenorrhea is common in these patients, and it may be the presenting complaint. Some patients have a history of both anorexia and bulimia. Management of a patient with severe bulimia requires the help of a professional skilled in the management of eating disorders. Self-help groups such as Overeaters Anonymous may play an important role in the patient's long-term handling of bulimia.

SEXUAL DEVELOPMENT

Normal Patterns and Concerns

A major difference between the child and the adolescent is the conversion of the teen into a sexual being. The onset of puberty is associated with an intensification of sexual feelings and desires that lead to sexual exploration. With the liberalization of sexual mores in recent years, the problems of adolescent pregnancy and venereal diseases have grown to epidemic proportions.

The staging of physical sexual development of adolescents established by Tanner is a widely accepted method of following the physical changes of puberty (Tables 5.4 and 5.5 and Fig. 5.2).

As the adolescent enters puberty, he also assumes a role as a sexual being. He must begin to meet expectations of his society, family, and peer group and is pushed into sexual propriety and conformity. These expectations are transmitted to the teen by multiple messages. However, these messages are often conveyed poorly, and many teens remain ignorant and insecure about sexual issues.

Early adolescence is characterized by a bisexual period, in which close friendships are formed with members of the same sex but heterosexual attitudes develop. One sees young teens developing "best buddy" relationships. The closeness of these relationships may even be on a physical level, but they are not considered characteristic of adult homosexuality. However, the teen (particularly male) may fear that he is a homosexual; and the frequent name calling of this period (in which people are called "gay" or "queer" with

Table 5.3.
DSM-III-R Criteria for Diagnosing Eating Disorders[a]

Anorexia Nervosa	Bulimia
1. Refusal to maintain normal body weight	1. Recurrent episodes of binge eating
2. Loss of more than 25% of original body weight	2. At least three of the following:
3. Disturbance of body image	a. Consumptions of high-caloric, easily ingested foods during a binge
4. Intense fear of being fat	b. Termination of binge by abdominal pain, sleep, or vomiting
5. No known medical illness	c. Inconspicuous eating during a binge
	d. Frequent attempts to lose weight
	e. Frequent weight fluctuations of more than 4.5 kg
	3. Awareness of abnormal eating pattern and fear of not being able to stop voluntarily
	4. Depressed mood after binge
	5. Not due to anorexia nervosa or other physical disorder

[a]From American Psychiatric Association: *Diagnostic and Statistical Manual of Mental Disorders*, 3rd ed, revised. Washington, DC, American Psychiatric Association, 1987.

Table 5.4.
Typical Progression of Female Adolescent Sexual Development (See Also Fig. 5.2).[a]

STAGE 1:
  There is no pubic hair present, and there is no breast enlargement. The ovaries have begun to enlarge. The external genitalia are preadolescent or those of a child.
STAGE 2:
  Breast bud formation usually begins before pubic hair growth. A small mound is formed by the elevation of the breast and papilla. Areolar diameter increases. The adolescent height spurt begins, and there is an acceleration in the deposition of total body fat. The adult female habitus emerges as the breasts enlarge and the hips widen.
STAGE 3:
  There is further spread of pubic hair and further enlargement of breasts and areola with no separation of their contours. The vagina enlarges and the vaginal epithelium, responding to estrogen stimulation from the maturing ovaries, increases in thickness, with considerable deposition of glycogen. The height spurt usually reaches a peak early in stage 3, prior to menarche.
STAGE 4:
  If menarche has not occurred late in stage 3 it should occur during stage 4. Axillary hair appears just before or after menarche, usually in early stage 4. There is a projection of the areola and papilla to form a secondary mound above the level of the breast. The areolar mound may be absent (25% of females). The breasts and pubic hair progress. The ovaries continue to enlarge. Ovulation may occur just after menarche, but it is usually delayed until stage 5.
STAGE 5:
  Pubic hair and breast development resemble that of the adult female; the areola has recessed to the general contour of the breast. Height increase has decelerated since menarche; height may increase from 2 to 4 inches after menarche. By 2 years after menarche regular ovulation may be expected.
STAGE 6:
  In 10% of females there is a further spread of pubic hair.

[a]From Tanner JM: *Growth at Adolescence*: New York, Appleton-Century-Crofts, 1966.

Table 5.5.
Typical Progression of Male Adolescent Sexual Development[a]

STAGE 1:
  The male has no pubic hair or increase in size of the penis.
  This describes the male as a preadolescent or child. However, the testes are beginning to mature. Usually there is considerable acceleration in height and weight gain along with changes in body composition (especially more body fat).
STAGE 2:
  There is early growth of the testes and scrotum before pubic hair appears. The height spurt accelerates; the male physique begins to change as fat and muscle are added; and the areola of the breast increases in size and darkens slightly.
STAGE 3:
  There is further enlargement of the testes and scrotum, enlargement of the penis (mainly in length), and spreading and darkening of the pubic hair. Facial hair first appears at the corners of the upper lip. The height spurt accelerates further; there is broadening of the shoulders relative to the hips and generalized increased moulding of the body, with considerable increase in muscle mass relative to fat. Hair appears in the perineum. Facial expression is significantly altered and appears more adult. The cartilage of the larynx enlarges, and the voice may begin to deepen. There is transient gynecomastia with slight projection of the areola.
STAGE 4:
  Axillary hair first appears. There is continued enlargement of the scrotum, testes, and penis (the last, mainly in breadth). The pubic hair begins to appear adult. Facial hair is still limited to upper lip and chin. The first ejaculation, indicating considerable growth of the prostate gland, occurs early in stage 4. Sebaceous glands are approaching adult size and function. The voice deepens further.
STAGE 5:
  Genital size and pubic hair distribution are adult in appearance. Hairs are present on the sides of the face. Gynecomastia has disappeared. The height spurt has decelerated and the physique is that of the mature male.
STAGE 6:
  Some adolescents have a further spread of pubic hair up the linea alba, which may be described as stage 6. This later development, often not reached until the early twenties, occurs in 80% of males.

[a]From Taner JM: *Growth at Adolescence*. New York, Appleton-Century-Crofts, 1966.

little provocation) may be taken too seriously. Boys who have developed noticeable gynecomastia may be particularly confused about their sexual identity. Such individuals need to be reassured of the normality of these concerns. Masturbation tends to be a frequent practice in this period, and there may be associated guilt that increases as the sex drive stimulates the teen to continue the practice. Again, where appropriate, problems associated with masturbation should be met with reassurance of its normality.

In mid- to late adolescence, dating and heterosexual activities begin in earnest. In the 1980s, the mean age for initiating sexual intercourse was 15.7 for males and 16.2 for females (11). Frequently, teens rush into sexual activity before they fully understand their own feelings about it. It is often part of the dating relationship—a prerequisite to communication, rather than vice versa. It may be part of thrill-seeking behavior for some teens, and others use it to escape from loneliness and depression.

Common Problems

Short Stature and Delayed Sexual Maturation

A frequent problem that comes to the attention of physicians is the teenager with short stature and/or delayed puberty. These two symptoms are often in-

terrelated, and the medical investigation is similar, so they will be discussed together. However, the presence of one does not necessarily indicate a problem with the other.

Most of these patients simply are at one end of the spectrum of normal development (3). Many teenage boys may not appreciate the fact that some individuals fall into the 10th percentile of a normal curve, and they may not accept a cursory dismissal of their concerns about size. Some may be helped by looking at normal growth curves that indicate the predicted ultimate height for persons in their percentile (see Fig. 5.1). Detailed discussion may be necessary for patients to comprehend fully and to cope with normal findings.

Assessment of short stature and delayed puberty by the generalist consists of the following steps:

1. A careful history of the onset of puberty and of the height of siblings, parents, and grandparents should be obtained. In particular, it should be noted if there is a history of several short family members (males under 5'6", females under 5'0").
2. Growth records of the patient should be reviewed.

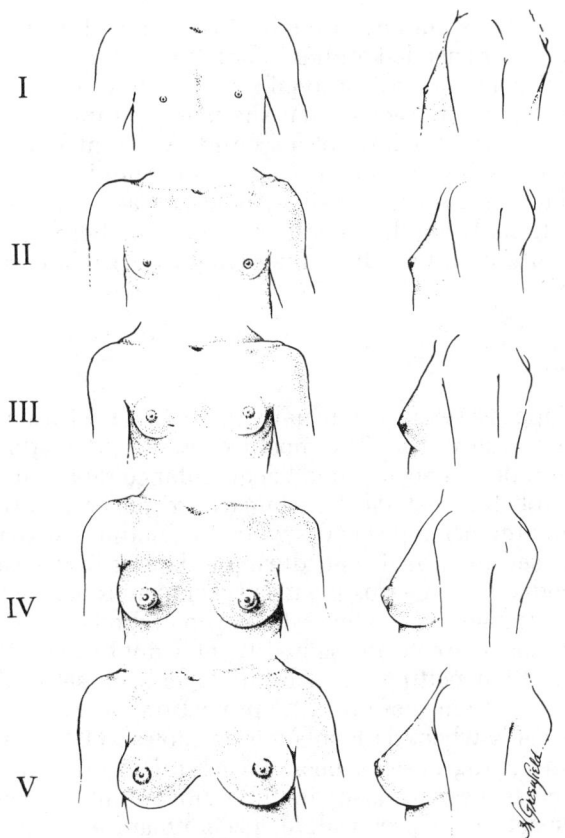

Figure 5.2. Diagrammatic representation of Tanner stages I to V of human breast maturation. (Adapted from Marshall WA, Tanner JM: Variations in pattern of pubertal changes in girls. *Arch Dis Child* 44:291, 1969.)

Heights and weights should be plotted on an appropriate growth curve (see Fig. 5.1). If a child has followed a single curve throughout life, a significant metabolic reason for this short stature is unlikely. If, however, there is a falling away from a growth line, a metabolic problem is more likely.

3. The medical history should be reviewed, including a prenatal and neonatal history. A history of operations, head injuries, or chronic medical conditions that could predispose the individual to failure to thrive should be noted. If the child had a low birth weight, a review of underlying factors may disclose a possible chromosomal abnormality or toxic exposure (e.g., maternal cigarette smoking or alcohol use) that could produce long-term growth delay.
4. A developmental and psychosocial history may indicate possible familial problems and/or emotional neglect that could predispose to constitutional growth delay (so-called psychosocial dwarfism).
5. Inquiries into the teen's general health and daily habits may reveal problems needing investigation, such as poor appetite, frequent infections, drug abuse, chronic abdominal pain, or general fatigue and listlessness.

A physical examination is essential, including an accurate height and weight and Tanner stage assessment (Tables 5.4 and 5.5). If the testes are softening and show enlargement, or if breast budding is present, there usually will be a normal sexual development. Unusual facies or ears, unusual hand creases, clinodactyly (deviation or deflection of the fingers), obesity, or delayed intellectual development may suggest a recognizable hereditary syndrome.

The initial laboratory investigation should include the following: urinalysis; measurement of serum urea nitrogen, creatinine, and electrolytes; hematocrit value and white cell count; as well as X-rays of the hands and wrists to assess skeletal growth.

More specific laboratory investigations may be suggested by the history and physical examination. Examples are: (a) thyroid enlargement (testing for hypothyroidism); (b) normal physical examination and appearance but markedly short stature that is falling away from growth lines (testing for growth hormone deficiency); (c) girls with delayed puberty, heights under the 3rd percentile, associated with a short "webbed" neck, a systolic murmur, or widely spaced nipples (buccal smears performed to rule out Turner's syndrome, i.e., X-O chromosomes); (d) striking pubertal delay without a history of similar delay in other family members (testing for gonadal failure: measurement of serum follicle-stimulating and luteinizing hormones, of estradiol, and of urinary 17-ketosteroids and 17-hydroxysteroids; vaginal smear for maturation index and buccal smear for chromosome analysis).

Definitive diagnosis and planning for adolescents with suspected endocrine, metabolic, genetic, or psychological reasons for maturation delay require referral to an appropriate specialist. Patients with hereditary disorders may benefit from genetic counseling, particularly those who will be unable to bear children—for example, patients with Turner's syndrome.

Sexually Transmitted Disease

Sexually transmitted diseases (STDs) are epidemic in 15- to 19-year-olds. This is partially due to more casual attitudes toward sex, with frequent changes of sex partners. Sex education programs have had little impact on the problem. Fear of infection apparently does not deter some teens, who seem irresponsible, impulsive, emotionally insecure, and who appear to have little respect for others. Frequently parents have failed to provide basic information about sex and the risks of infection and pregnancy that accompany it.

In most states, adolescents have a right to receive treatment for STDs without the parents' knowledge; it is important to be receptive to the teen seeking treatment. Visits for treatment should also be utilized to explain the mechanism of acquiring venereal infection and to explain and encourage the use of condoms to prevent reinfection. The diagnosis and treatment of various STDs are discussed elsewhere in this book (see Chapters 27 and 94).

The high rate of sexual intercourse and adolescent pregnancy in the 1980s, has raised concerns about acquisition of the infection with the human immunodeficiency virus (HIV) in this age group. Given the long incubation period of HIV infection, data showing that 21% of all AIDS cases occur in persons 20 to 25 years of age suggest strongly that adolescence is an important period of acquisition of HIV (2). Other data suggest that a frequent route of spread of the virus in adolescence is by heterosexual transmission, rather than intravenous drug abuse, blood products, or homosexual contacts. Furthermore, many cases of HIV infection in infants may be linked to maternal acquisition of the virus during adolescence. It is imperative that teenagers, especially sexually active teens, be counseled about high risk behaviors that may expose them to HIV infection and about "safe sex" practices. This information and details about the ambulatory care of HIV-infected patients are described in Chapter 34.

Pregnancy

Each year over a million women under the age of 20 become pregnant, half of them out of wedlock. Many of these pregnancies are associated with serious medical risks for the mother and the fetus. Mothers under 14 have particularly high risks of toxemia, anemia, prematurity, infants with low birth weight, prolonged labor, and postpartum complications. Many of these problems can be prevented by good obstetrical care, so that the first goal in adolescent pregnancy should be early diagnosis and entry into a comprehensive treatment program.

There are multiple social and behavioral reasons for the high number of teenage pregnancies. For many adolescents, pregnancy may be part of a maladaptive attempt to solve psychological issues, such as independence from a clinging mother or manipulation of a boyfriend. Such patients may have previously engaged in other maladaptive activites, such as drug abuse or delinquency. There may also be an underlying ignorance about methods and availability of birth control (see Chapter 93).

The teenager herself may be ambivalent about her pregnancy. Often, the manipulations that led to the pregnancy in the sense of achieving a prolonged relationship, etc., have not succeeded and a sense of abandonment is felt. Furthermore, the pregnancy may have resulted in hostility from the family when the teenager is in greatest need of help from her parents.

Clearly the teenager about to make important decisions about herself and her pregnancy requires counseling. It can be provided by her primary physician or by a staff member of a counseling agency such as Planned Parenthood. In either case, the patient's primary physician should be aware of the patient's plan and be available for any problems she may wish to discuss. In most states, adolescents have the right to treatment for pregnancy-related events, including abortion, without parental consent or knowledge. If the teenager decides to continue with the pregnancy, she should be prepared to assume a parenting role. Furthermore, she should be educated about future

pregnancies and given medical assistance for the pediatric care needed for her infant. If possible, day care, vocational, and educational services should be available for the mother so that she may continue her education after the birth of her child. As an integral part of counseling, a stable caring person should be identified (a parent, if possible) who can assist the teen emotionally and financially and who can help her see the future for herself and her baby in a realistic manner.

Rape

Rape is a sexual act, usually intercourse, with a nonconsenting victim. The most frequent type of adolescent rape has been called "acquaintance rape," and it is probable that most instances are never reported. Acquaintance rape occurs when the victim is sexually misused by a boyfriend during a date or by a casual friend, or when a trusting teen accompanies her friends to a strange place where she is gang raped.

Teens, in exploring sexuality, may not have set limits to their petting, or, if limits have been set unilaterally, they may afford little protection for the victim, especially when the assailant is an adolescent for whom limit setting has not been successful in other areas. Some teens may also, in their uncertainty, present themselves in provocative, pseudomature ways, for example, by wearing outrageous and provocative clothing that may be viewed as sexually inviting by male acquaintances.

There is a tendency in dealing with adolescent rape victims to imply that the assault may have been invited by the victim. Regardless of this possibility, rape should be treated as a very serious problem for the victim who reports it.

Initial care for the rape victim should be handled by a physician, with follow-up by a rape counseling service if one exists in the community. Often, a physician who is already acquainted with the patient can provide the best care.

There are several important considerations in caring for the rape victim:

1. Rape is a crime of violence, not a sexual act.
2. Above all else, the adolescent reporting rape has usually had a very frightening experience and needs short-term counseling either by her regular physician (see Chapter 11) or, ideally, through the auspices of a rape victim's support program. She will usually have a number of questions about the physical meaning of her experience, and it is important to assure that she obtains answers to them.
3. She should be examined carefully for evidence of trauma, both to the pelvic organs and to the rest of her body, and the information should be carefully recorded.
4. She must decide whether she wishes to report the rape to the police. In this instance, it is essential to obtain a wet and fixed smear of the vaginal con-

tents as early as possible to confirm the presence of spermatozoa.

5. Most rape victims will need ongoing counseling by their physician and/or a counselor for a number of months to discuss persisting anxieties and questions.

PSYCHOSOCIAL DEVELOPMENT

Normal Patterns and Concerns

The major psychosocial developmental task for the adolescent as he approaches adulthood is to increase independence from his parents and to establish a positive identity congruent with social norms.

In early adolescence, the young teen is faced with the dilemma of seeking independence from parents while at the same time relying on them for emotional and physical support. The conflict over independence is evidenced by contradiction and ambivalence. For example, a teen may refuse to listen to parents' suggestions about study habits, but blame mediocre grades on the fact that the parents did not help with homework assignments.

As the teen enters into middle and late adolescence, he demonstrates a remarkable resourcefulness in coping with anxiety over separation and in learning more mature behavior. Much assistance comes through peer relationships. Teens support each other by experimenting with adult roles that mirror societal expectations of behavior; a sense of moral responsibility begins to take shape. In this period, individual identity tends to be blunted by the seeking of independence from the family. Peers tend to look alike, dress alike, date alike, and experiment with drugs and sex alike. Later, as teens address their concerns about careers, a greater differentiation of personalities takes shape and individual identities emerge.

Normal development also requires the example of secure, healthy parents in an environment in which the teen can feel secure. Thus, parents who are preoccupied with their own psychological problems at work, in their marriage, or with their own families may have difficulties helping and coping with the development of their adolescent offspring. Often such parents have not previously succeeded at their own adolescent tasks and so are unable to proceed with the task of adulthood—they have not developed the ability for intimacy, for close personal feelings, for the sharing of feelings and thoughts with others, and for adhering to reasonable limits.

One clear fact about adolescent development is that its emotional course is variable, even among "normal" adolescents. The idea that adolescence is usually a time of crisis, in which persistent neurotic behavior is essential for development of a personal identity, has not been borne out by longitudinal research. On the other hand, it has been found that at least 20% of college freshmen have psychological problems, usually personality disorders of the compulsive, schizoid, or passive-aggressive type expressed as difficulties in academic, social, and psychosexual functioning (4). A longitudinal study of teenage boys (8) pointed out that achievement of identity is a long-term process. Subjects were first studied when they were high school freshmen and were followed for 7 years. At the end of this interval, most subjects had yet to consolidate their identities to the point where they could develop an intimate relationship, one of the best indicators of progress to adulthood. Despite this, self-satisfaction and parental satisfaction were the norm. For many, adolescence is a crisis but an internalized, noiseless one.

Generally the teen must succeed in the other spheres of development in order to meet tasks in the psychosocial sphere successfully. In retarded, handicapped, or chronically ill children the dependence-independence struggle may persist, impairing the development of self-esteem needed to develop a sense of identity.

Common Problems

Juvenile Delinquency

Juvenile delinquency is a legal term for youthful behavior that violates the law and would be adjudicated and punished if it had been committed by an adult. It is a major social problem and will, at times, be brought to the attention of the practitioner who is asked whether there is an underlying psychological cause for the delinquent behavior. In order to deal with this issue, it is necessary to distinguish between three broad categories of delinquency, described by Weiner (10) as sociological delinquency, characterological delinquency, and neurotic delinquency.

Sociological delinquency refers to illegal acts organized by a subcultural group, i.e., street gang. The delinquent acts are adaptive in that the teen receives the approval of his peers. The following four features of the clinical history suggest sociological delinquency: first, the delinquent acts are performed with valued companions, rather than alone or with strangers; second, these teens see themselves as accepted and integral members of their peer group and rarely exhibit feelings of alienation or inadequacy; third, sociological delinquents give little evidence of neurotic symptom formation or basic character flaws; and fourth, these delinquents frequently have had supportive family relationships during early childhood, although there may have been more recent problems that have led to their current activities. Frequently, involvement in other positive group activities will change the delinquent orientation of these teens.

Characterological delinquents reflect a basically antisocial attitude toward life. Their acts do not evoke in them any guilt or remorse. Such teens are frequently loners who have not established a strong relationship of basic trust in their life. Their past history suggests a series of problems, with a flurry of destructive acts, such as fighting, fire setting, and cruelty to animals, preceding their more destructive delinquent activity.

Such children often require long-term psychiatric treatment. Chapter 14 provides additional details about the course and management of patients with an antisocial personality.

The *neurotic delinquent* commits destructive acts as an atypical (for him) behavior pattern to illustrate and emphasize certain needs. These acts may reflect feelings of being ignored by family or peers, or indicate that the teen is suffering from some form of psychological distress, most frequently depression. The acts are committed in such a way that the teen will be caught in the process or will give himself away soon after; generally, if concealment of illegal acts is repetitive and successful, a neurotic basis of the delinquency is unlikely. There is rarely a history of early behavioral problems, and typically the delinquent has enjoyed a loving relationship with parents and family members. Occasionally, however, some recent family stress may serve as the trigger for the delinquent act. In general, neurotic delinquency may be treated through short-term counseling (see Chapter 11).

Substance Abuse

Although substance abuse, including tobacco use, is a major problem of adult life, it frequently begins during the adolescent years. Because adolescence is a period of experimentation, it is the rare teen who has not had a drink of alcohol, smoked a cigarette, or tried marijuana. Substance abuse may be viewed as a rite of passage bridging the gap between childhood and adulthood or as a condition for belonging to peer groups or organizations. Advertising or exposure to personalities that appear to link the use of cigarettes and alcohol to life successes, popularity, and sex can be important inducements for adolescents to try alcohol or tobacco. A major concern is to identify the adolescent abuser—one whose life is being disrupted by his aberrant activities. It is this teenager who is most likely to continue to abuse alcohol or drugs in adult life.

The routine evaluation of a teen should include skillful questioning about his use of alcohol and of drugs. Substance use should be explored using nonthreatening questions such as those listed in Table 5.6.

Table 5.6.
Sample Questions Concerning Drug Use for Adolescents[a]

I know that many schools have drug problems. Does your school have such a problem?
Do most of your friends drink alcohol or smoke marijuana at parties?
Do any of your friends use drugs other than alcohol or marijuana?
Where do most young people obtain drugs?
Do you smoke cigarettes? How many per day?
Have you ever tried alcohol? Marijuana? Other drugs?
Have you ever been ill as a result of using drugs or drinking?
Have you ever been in trouble with the law as a result of drugs or alcohol?
Do your parents know that you've used alcohol or _____ ?
What would (did) they say?
Have you ever worried about your alcohol or _____ use?
Have you ever been drunk or stoned and driven a car (or motorcycle)?

[a]From Schonberg SK (ed): *Substance Abuse: A Guide for Health Professionals.* American Academy of Pediatrics, Elk Grove, Illinois, 1988.

The presence of drug abuse and/or its impact on a teenager can also be uncovered by asking the parents questions such as those in Table 5.7. If the use of a substance is excessive and hazardous, the physician should explore the factors that might have led to abuse. Drugs and/or alcohol are often abused as a response to some psychosocial problem, and it is only by identifying the problem that the abuse may be stopped. Lecturing on the dangers of alcohol, drugs, or tobacco seems to have little impact on adolescents.

Occasionally, the serious abuser of hazardous substances will develop physiological symptoms that are dramatic enough to come to the physician's attention. Hospitalization for observation is almost always indicated for the teenager presenting with drug intoxication, even if emergency room evaluation indicates that there are no immediate medical risks. The possibility of attempted suicide may be real and must be explored. Even if this is not a factor, there is still concern about the teen's ability to control his own drug abuse behavior.

How to intervene in drug abuse behavior is a difficult question. In part, it is a moral question, and the physician's behavior may be influenced by his own beliefs about the dangers of cigarettes, alcohol, or drugs and about his right to interfere with the actions (albeit dangerous) of an autonomous individual. Current recommendations for physicians' approaches to patients with substance abuse are contained in Chapters 20 (Tobacco Abuse), 21 (Alcoholism), and 22 (Illicit Drugs and Substances).

Depression and Suicide

A behavioral hallmark of adolescents is mood shifts, from the peaks of elation to the depths of despair. Depressive symptoms are normal parts of psychosocial development. The quest for identity is balanced by a sense of loss once independence is achieved. Similarly, rejections by peers (e.g., first loves) may be felt very deeply. It is not unusual, as part of these depressions, for the adolescent to contemplate suicide.

Mattsson (6) describes five depressive states of adolescence. Normal *depressive mood swings* represent transient reactions to personal disappointments or family difficulties. They rarely affect other life functions. *Acute depressive reactions* are more severe states, often lasting weeks or months. They are normal reactions, similar to states of grief (see Chapter 19), often related to separation or to loss of a close friend, relative, or teacher. The adolescent who does not successfully work through his grief, and who becomes increasingly depressed and incapacitated by his loss, suffers from a *depressive neurosis*. Such teens withdraw from their normal functioning, are chronically sad, and begin to entertain suicidal ideation. This is a fairly severe level of depression and demands professional intervention. A fourth form of depression, the *masked depressions of adolescence*, can be viewed as a subgroup of the depressive neuroses. Such teens can-

Table 5.7.
Questions for Interviewing the Parent(s) of the Adolescent Suspected of or Known to be Abusing Drugs and/or Alcohol[a]

1. Does your daughter/son spend many hours alone in his/her bedroom apparently doing nothing?
2. Does your son/daughter resist talking to you or persistently isolate himself/herself from the family?
3. Has your daughter's/son's taste in music had a dramatic change to hard rock music?
4. Has there been a definite change in your son's/daughter's attitude at school? With his/her friends? At home?
5. Has your daughter/son shown recent pronounced mood swings with increased irritability and angry outbursts?
6. Does your son/daughter always seem to be unhappy and less able to cope with frustration than he/she used to be?
7. Has your daughter's/son's personality changed from being a considerate and caring person to being selfish, unfriendly, and unsympathetic?
8. Does your son/daughter always seem to be confused or "spacey"?
9. Have money or valuable articles recently disappeared from your home?
10. Has your daughter/son begun to neglect household chores and homework?
11. Has there been a change in your son's/daughter's friends from age-appropriate friends to older, "unacceptable" associates?
12. Has there been a change in your daughter's/son's appearance (i.e., sloppy dress and poor grooming and hygiene)?
13. Have there been excuses and alibis made, and has there been lying in order to avoid confrontation or not to get caught?
14. Do you feel you have lost control of your son/daughter?
15. Has your daughter/son begun lying in order to cover up sources of money and possessions?
16. Have there been episodes of "ditching" or "skipping" school? Has your son/daughter lied to cover up bad report cards?
17. Have there been stealing, shoplifting, or encounters with the police?
18. Has your daughter/son become a "con artist"?
19. Have you noticed a marked increase in your son's/daughter's interest in drugs, drug literature, and the drug "culture" (i.e., clothing and accouterments, paraphernalia, belt buckles, and tee shirts with a drug theme)?
20. Has your daughter/son recently quit a sport or dropped out of school clubs, social groups, stopped music lessons, quit the band or orchestra, or lost interest in a hobby?
21. Has there been a deterioration of school performance, frequent truancy, or conflict with coaches or teachers?
22. Do you feel your daughter/son has become untrustworthy, insincere, and distrustful ("paranoid")?
23. Has he/she become unpredictable or rebellious?
24. Has your son/daughter been verbally abusive to you or your spouse?
25. Has your daughter/son been physically abusive to you or your spouse?
26. Has your son/daughter tried to introduce any of your other children to drugs or alcohol?
27. Has your daughter/son talked about suicide or running away?
28. Is your son/daughter more argumentative lately? Does he/she tend to blame others for his/her problems?
29. Is there a paranoid flavor to all of your daughter's/son's relationships with adults, siblings, and authority figures?

[a]From Schonberg SK (ed): *Substance Abuse: A Guide for Health Professionals.* American Academy of Pediatrics, Elk Grove, Illinois, 1988.

not tolerate their painful feelings and express them through a variety of somatic or behavioral complaints. They may be frequent visitors to the primary care physician, suffering from ill-defined, atypical symptoms without a clear organic basis. Their behavior may include overeating, delinquent acts, exhibitionist acts resulting in "accidental" self-destruction, drug and alcohol abuse, etc. *Psychotic depressive disorders* are marked by impaired reality testing, thought disorders, paranoia, and suicidal intention, in addition to depressive symptomatology.

The primary care physician is sometimes asked to evaluate the depressed or suicidal adolescent. In taking the history, the physician should try to uncover recent events that may have precipitated the depressive disorder: any long-standing family, school, or peer problems; possibilities of organic brain disease or of drug abuse that may mimic depressive symptoms; symptoms of cognitive or reality disturbances, suggesting a psychosis; and symptoms suggesting a masked depression. The physician should not hesitate to talk about depression with the teen. Indeed, such openness may put the adolescent at ease and let him feel that the physician truly understands what he may be feeling. A physical examination will help the physician rule out physical problems, and communication with the school will give the physician some additional observations about the teen in his daily activities.

Most adolescents with depressive symptoms need

some counseling. If one feels medication is necessary and is unfamiliar with the use of psychoactive drugs in adolescents, conjoint treatment with a psychiatric consultant may prove helpful. Patients with long-standing depressive symptoms, which suggest thought disturbances, and possible suicide attempts should be referred for psychiatric intervention. Additional details about the office management of depression are contained in Chapter 15.

INTELLECTUAL DEVELOPMENT

Normal Patterns and Concerns

In adolescence, a major change occurs with respect to education and intellect. Schools differentiate students, placing them into vocational or academic tracks. The emphasis shifts from the learning of tasks (e.g., basic reading, writing, and arithmetic) to the accumulation of facts and the ability to think abstractly. As teens prepare for college, learning becomes a competitive task. Career choices become limited as an individual's abilities and talents become manifest. Upon entering college, a greater amount of independence and responsibility is expected. Symbolically, the university begins to resemble the workplace both in terms of potential rewards and of potential pressures.

Scholastic Failure

Academic achievement is strongly related to parental aspirations, socioeconomic status, and intellectual ability. Occasionally, the child cannot meet parental expectations, and the resultant crisis may lead to a visit to the physician's office. Failure in school may also be a symptom of a physical impairment, mental retardation, specific learning disabilities, or emotional stress. By making an accurate diagnosis of the underlying problem, a caring practitioner may help such children.

First a history is necessary, to determine the nature of the school difficulties. When did they begin; has educational achievement been a problem throughout a school career, as with a global intellectual deficit, or is it specific to certain subjects or tasks, as with learning disorders? Is there a family history of poor school performance, as is seen with familial dyslexics? How does the teen act with his family and peers? Is there evidence of disturbed behavior outside school as with emotional disorders? Is the family structure stable, or has there been separation, divorce, or death of a parent or grandparent? Is there evidence of substance abuse on the part of the teen or a member of the family? Is there daytime hypersomnolence that suggests a sleep disorder? What has the family done to try to work through problems?

Second, a physical examination, with a careful neurological examination, is indicated, with emphasis on looking for signs of minimal cerebral dysfunction, such as "soft" neurological signs, right-left discrimination or orientation difficulties, or overt signs of cerebral palsy (1). (In such patients, there may be suggestions of a neurological problem in the past medical history; the birth may have been abnormal; or the patient may have shown hyperactivity or attention deficits as a child.) Vision testing and office assessment for slight or moderate hearing loss (see Chapter 96) are also particularly important.

Third, some specific intelligence testing is indicated. Children who are mentally retarded will tend to show low intelligence quotient (I.Q.) scores, and achievement tests will show a delay of several grades in math and reading levels. Children with dyslexia will have a normal I.Q. but will show a wide scatter of scores on subtests, indicating a nonglobal deficit. Achievement tests may also show a difference between abilities in reading and mathematics.

Some learning problems may appear relatively late in a school career (5). The recent criticism of the ability of some college students to write well has given credence to the notion of expressive language disorders, which may not become manifest until adolescence. Some individuals with fine perceptual problems may not reveal difficulties until geometry or drafting is studied in high school.

The Congress, in 1974, passed Federal Law 94-142, assuring a free, appropriate educational placement for all children up to age 21. Thus, adolescents with specific learning problems, retardation, or emotional difficulties are entitled to be placed in a classroom setting where they will learn. If he suspects an unrecognized problem in one of these spheres, the patient's physician may help by referring the patient and his parents for evaluation, usually available through the child's school or the local education system. Unfortunately, problems remain unrecognized for many children, and, out of frustration, they drop out of school.

A SUGGESTED APPROACH TO THE ADOLESCENT PATIENT IN THE OFFICE SETTING

When dealing with adolescents, it is important to be aware of their perspective. Each adolescent approaches the developmental pressures of this period of life with his own particular skills and emotions. From a health perspective, an adolescent can be a responsible partner in maintaining his well-being and complying with medical care; or he can be infantile, dependent, uncommunicative, aggressive, or irresponsible.

Interviewing Strategies

It is important to interview adolescents in private. The adolescent needs to feel that he is the patient and that his problems are being listened to and taken seriously. It is often useful to talk to the parents separately as well.

The Patient

Some adolescent patients are difficult to interview. An uncommunicative patient may have been sent to a physician against his will or may lack verbal skills needed for coherence. One must be verbally active with such patients and watch for any nonverbal cues as wedges to try to get the patient to speak. Examples of nonverbal cues are: a look of interest or initiation of eye contact when a subject is mentioned that the patient would like to discuss; a clenched fist when an anger-provoking subject is raised; frequent position change and fidgeting when the patient is anxious about a specific subject or about the visit to the physician in general. Because adolescents are often reticent about their major concerns, an open-minded invitation to share information ("Is there anything else you wanted to talk about?") should be included in each office contact. The initial comprehensive interview may require several sessions. At the first visit, warmth and interest in the adolescent may open the way to better communication in future sessions.

Many adolescents continue to go to their pediatrician for medical care until they enter college, take a job, or marry. Because of this long-term association, their relationship may be almost like that of a parent and child—warm, intense, and comradely. These feelings cannot be transferred easily to a new physician, and it is unwise to attempt to transfer them.

Physicians can most effectively surmount problems in communicating with adolescents by explaining their *modus operandi* in advance, emphasizing that they will be primarily the adolescent's physician, rather than an agent of the patient's parents as had been the case previously. It is also important to encourage the adolescent to initiate patient-doctor contacts, guard against patriarchal advice giving, and avoid showing disapproval or surprise when the adolescent attempts to impress one with tales of sexual exploits, with the use of vulgar language, etc.

It is wise to establish certain ground rules with adolescents. Patient-doctor confidentiality, for example, can be assured to adolescents only insofar as they do not reveal that they are comtemplating harmful acts, such as running away or committing suicide. However, certain privileged communications should be kept confidential from parents. In particular, adolescent minors have the right to be seen for sexually transmitted or for sex offense-related examinations without the prior consent of a parent. The teen may also wish to keep some health-related or emotional problems, such as drug experimentation, from a parent's knowledge.

The Parents

How does an adolescent's physician communicate with the parent? It is suggested that, whenever possible, a parent should be involved with and concerned about the health of the teen. A separate interview with a parent, immediately before or after the examination, may prove helpful and can emphasize particular concerns downplayed or denied by the patient. The parents of adolescent patients may be useful in providing emotional support and ensuring compliance with therapy; therefore, informing them about the adolescent's problems and needs is important.

Some parents ask physicians to take on the role of health educator or counselor for their adolescent child. Usually, these requests are for anticipatory guidance about birth control or drug usage. At times, the physician is asked to help the child work through an upcoming family crisis, such as divorce, serious illness, or death. Frequently, adolescents welcome the opportunity to discuss these issues in private. Their knowledge in these areas is often found wanting, and the sensitive physician may help the adolescent grasp realities and make intelligent decisions. A number of books on these subjects are directed to an adolescent and young adult audience, and it may be useful to make these titles available:

Ropes E (ed) The Kids Book of Divorce. Louis Publishing Co., 1981.

Bell R (ed) Changing Bodies, Changing Lives. Random House, 1980.

Comfort A, Comfort J (eds) The Facts of Love: Living, Loving, and Growing Up. Crown Publishers, 1980.

C.L. Otis and R. Goldingay: Campus Health Guide. The College Student's Handbook for Healthy Living. College Entrance Examination Board, New York, 1989.

Parents often have questions about specific adolescent behavior. A particular episode or issue may come to the parents' attention, and they may ask the physician whether they should exert control over it. In such instances, the physician should not offer specific advice but should try to discern any moral or behavioral conflicts between the parents and the adolescent. When the parents' behavior is inconsistent with the parents' own stated values, adolescents will often act in opposition to those values. Miller (7) suggests that parents are not helped in this instance by being told how to behave. Advice either increases the parents' uncertainty when faced with later difficulties or implies that the parents' own opinions are inappropriate. Adolescents probably turn out mentally healthier when presented with models of adult behavior with which their parents are comfortable, whether consistent with societal norms or not. Parents must be prepared, however, to make allowances so that their children have freedom to make their own "mistakes." Family counseling is a technique that a general physician can utilize when several members of a household are involved (see Chapter 11).

Health Assessment

The initial interview(s) should be comprehensive enough to ensure that the adolescent is meeting appropriate developmental tasks. Inquiries should be made into teenagers' relationships and functioning with their families, at school, and with peers. It is important to determine whether teenagers are establishing positive personal identities (Have they hobbies? Do they voice their own opinions? Can they choose their own friends or must friends be approved by the parents? Do they have plans for the future?); whether they are accepting their sexuality and adjusting to adult sexual roles (Do they date? Are they sexually active? Do they have a knowledge of contraception? Is contraception used?); whether they are establishing independence from the family (Do they drive? Do they earn money on their own? What sort of hours do they keep?); whether they are working toward a career (What are their plans after high school? What subjects in school do they like? What are their grades? Do they plan to go to college? Are their goals realistic and are they supported by the family?); whether they have established good health habits (What are their views about nutrition? Have they experimented with alcohol, tobacco, or other recreational drugs? What drugs? Have they ever been drugged or high when driving or when attending school?); and whether affective swings are interfering with functioning (Do they often feel down? What makes them happy? Have sad feelings ever made them consider harming themselves?).

As part of the review of systems before examination, a self-administered medical questionnaire may be useful and timesaving. Such a questionnaire should be brief with language simple enough to be understood by teens with poor reading skills. Positive answers often need to be explored further. A physical examination should be performed in the absence of parents. Teenage girls examined by male physicians may be more comfortable with an female adult in the room with them. Some parts of the physical examination occasionally omitted by physicians but essential for adolescent patients include blood pressure measurement, examination of the entire integument, of the spine (for scoliosis), and of the external genitalia (for signs of venereal disease and for assessment of sexual development using Tanner's staging (see Tables 5.4 and 5.5). All sexually active adolescent girls should have a pelvic examination, including gonorrheal cultures and a Pap smear. If the physician is uncomfortable doing this examination, the teen should be referred to a gynecologist who is used to dealing with adolescents.

There are several useful adjuncts to the physical examination of the healthy adolescent. These include testing for myopia and hyperopia (using a Snellen chart) and screening for deafness (by speaking softly). Adolescence is a period marked by noise pollution, in the form of loud music that can cause permanent damage to the eighth nerve (see Chapter 96). Those adolescents who have difficulty in school should be screened for learning disorders. Having a teenager read a newspaper paragraph out loud or do some simple arithmetic may reveal a previously undetected learning disability.

Laboratory screening tests for healthy adolescents should include a full urinalysis, a complete blood count, and tuberculin testing. Screening for hyperlipidemia (Chapter 75) is indicated for all adolescents and is especially important for those with family histories of myocardial infarction or of stroke under the age of 50. Blood chemical screens, chest X-rays, and electrocardiograms are not indicated in healthy adolescents. Specific recommendations regarding periodic health assessment in adolescents and young adults are found in Chapter 2 (Table 2.1).

Examining the Adolescent Athlete

The examination of adolescent athletes requires an evaluation of the individual's health and a consideration of his functional ability, growth, and maturation.

The purpose of the preparticipation health evaluation is to identify medical conditions that might preclude safe and effective athletic participation, including those that might become worse by participation in sports activities. A brief screening questionnaire (Table 5.8) plus information already known to the physician will identify most conditions that may disqualify an adolescent from participation in various types of sports (Table 5.9).

As athletes become more experienced, the most commonly encountered problems are residuals of previous sports injuries, most of them musculoskeletal problems. Common exercise-related musculoskeletal injuries that can be managed in the office are described in Chapter 67.

General References

American College of Physicians Position Paper: Health care needs of the adolescent. *Ann Intern Med* 110:930, 1989.

    Consensus recommendations, with references, for internists.

Committee on Sports Medicine, American Academy of Pediatrics: *Sports Medicine: Health Care for Young Athletes.* Evanston, IL, American Academy of Pediatrics, 1983.

    An updated reference on sports medicine for children and adolescents.

D'Angelo JD, Farrow J: Clinical problems in adolescent medicine. *J Gen Intern Med* 4:64, 1989.

    Brief review of selected problems of adolescents (growth and development, substance abuse, eating disorders, sexual problems, and violence).

Erickson EH: *Identity, Youth and Crisis.* New York, WW Norton, 1968.

    The most widely used theoretical model of adolescent psychosocial development.

Felice ME: Adoelscence: General Considerations. In: Levine MD, Carey WB, Crocker AC, et al (eds): *Developmental-behavioral pediatrics.* Philadelphia, WB Saunders, 1983.

    A brief behavioral prospective on adolescent development.

Gallagher JR, Heald FP, Garell DC (eds): *Medical Care of The Adolescent.* 3rd ed. New York, Appleton-Century-Crofts, 1976.

    An excellent textbook on adolescent medicine. Emphasizes patient-doctor relationship.

Haggerty RJ: In: *Ambulatory Pediatrics.* 2nd ed. Philadelphia, WB Saunders, 1977.

    A brief review of adolescent disorders.

Keniston K: *Youth, Transition to Adulthood.* American Handbook of Psychiatry, Vol. II. 2nd ed. New York, Basic Books, 1974.

Table 5.8
Screening Preparticipation History for the Adolescent Athlete[a]

NAME _____ DATE _____		
PREPARTICIPATION EVALUATION—HISTORY		
Completed by ATHLETE or PARENT	YES	NO
1. Have any members of your family under age 50 had a "heart attack" or "heart problems"?	_____	_____
2. Have you ever been told you have a heart murmur, high blood pressure, extra heart beats, or a heart abnormality?	_____	_____
3. Do you have to stop while running around a (¼ mile) track twice?	_____	_____
4. Are you taking any medications?	_____	_____
5. Have you ever "passed out" or been "knocked out" (concussion)?	_____	_____
6. Have you ever had any illness, condition, or injury that:	_____	_____
a. Required you to go to the hospital either as a patient overnight or in the emergency room or for X-rays?		
b. Required an operation?	_____	_____
c. Lasted longer than a week?	_____	_____
d. Caused you to miss a game or practice?	_____	_____
e. Is related to allergies (hayfever, hives, asthma, or medicine)?	_____	_____

[a]Adapted from Committee on Sports Medicine, American Academy of Pediatrics: *Sports Medicine: Health Care for Young Athletes.* Evanston, IL, American Academy of Pediatrics, 1983.

Table 5.9.
Disqualifying Conditions for Sports Participation by the Adolescent[a]

Conditions	Collision[b]	Contact[c]	Noncontact[d]	Other[e]
General				
Acute infections:				
Respiratory, genitourinary, infectious mononucleosis, hepatitis, active rheumatic fever, active tuberculosis	X	X	X	X
Obvious physical immaturity in comparison with other competitors	X	X		
Hemorrhagic disease:				
Hemophilia, purpura, and other serious bleeding tendencies	X	X	X	
Diabetes, inadequately controlled	X	X	X	X
Diabetes, controlled	f	f	f	f
Jaundice	X	X	X	X
Eyes				
Absence or loss of function of one eye	X	X		
Respiratory				
Tuberculosis (active or symptomatic)	X	X	X	X
Severe pulmonary insufficiency	X	X	X	X
Cardiovascular				
Mitral stenosis, aortic stenosis, aortic insufficiency, coarctation of aorta, cyanotic heart disease, recent carditis of any etiology	X	X	X	X
Hypertension on organic basis	X	X	X	X
Previous heart surgery for congenital or acquired heart disease	g	g	g	g
Liver enlarged	X	X		
Skin				
Boils, impetigo, and herpes simplex gladiatorum	X	X		
Spleen, enlarged	X	X		
Hernia	X	X		
Inguinal or femoral hernia	X	X	X	
Musculoskeletal				
Sumptomatic abnormalities or inflammations	X	X	X	X
Functional inadequacy of the musculoskeletal system, congenital or acquired, incompatible with the contact or skill demands of the sport	X	X	X	
Neurological				
History or symptoms of previous serious head trauma or repeated concussions	X			
Controlled convulsive disorder	h	h	h	h
Convulsive disorder not moderately well controlled by medication	X			
Previous surgery on head	X	X		
Renal				
Absence of one kidney	X	X		
Renal insufficiency	X	X	X	X
Genitalia				
Absence of one testicle	i	i	i	i
Undescended testicle	i	i	i	i

[a]From Committee on Sports Medicine, American Academy of Pediatrics: *Sports Medicine: Health Care for Young Athletes*. Evanston, IL, American Academy of Pediatrics, 1983.
[b]Football, rugby, hockey, lacrosse, and so forth.
[c]Baseball, soccer, basketball, wrestling, and so forth.
[d]Cross country, track, tennis, crew, swimming, and so forth.
[e]Bowling, golf, archery, field events, and so forth.
[f]No exclusions.
[g]Each patient should be judged on an individual basis in conjunction with his cardiologist and surgeon.
[h]Each patient should be judged on an individual basis. All things being equal, it is probably better to encourage a young boy or girl to participate in a noncontact sport rather than a contact sport. However, if a patient has a desire to play a contact sport and this is deemed a major ameliorating factor in his or her adjustment to school, associates, and the seizure disorder, serious consideration should be given to letting him or her participate if the seizures are moderately well controlled or the patient is under good medical management.
[i]The Committee approves the concept of contact sports participation for youths with only one testicle or with an undescended testicle(s), except in specific instances such as an inguinal canal undescended testicle(s), following appropriate medical evaluation to rule out unusual injury risk. However, the athlete, parents, and school authorities should be fully informed that participation in contact sports for youths with only one testicle carries a slight injury risk to the remaining healthy testicle. Fertility may be adversely affected following an injury. But the chances of an injury to a descended testicle are rare, and the injury risk can be further substantially minimized with an athletic supporter and protective device.

Another standard text; the perspective is sociological.

Marks A, Fisher M: Health assessment and screening during adolescence. *Pediatrics* 80(supp):135, 1987.

An excellent discussion of health screening examinations as adolescents.

Neinstein LS (ed): *Adolescent Health Care: A Practical Guide.* Baltimore, Urban and Schwartzenberg, 1984.

A practical approach in outline form emphasizing the diagnosis of diseases and illnesses during adolescence.

Schomberg SK (ed): *Substance Abuse: A Guide for Health Professionals.* American Academy of Pediatrics, 1988.

A comprehensive review of the substance abuse problem in adolescents.

Sorenson RC: *Adolescent Sexuality in Contemporary America.* New York, World, 1973.

A good overview of sexual problems of adolescents and proposed social policy approaches.

Tanner JM: *Growth at Adolescence.* 2nd ed. Springfield, IL, Charles C Thomas, 1962.

A classic system for describing the physiological changes of adolescents.

Specific References

1. Desmond MM, Volderman AL, Fisher ES: Assessment of learning competence during the pediatric examination. *Curr Prob Pediatr* 8:2, 1978.
2. Hein K: Commentary on adolescent acquired immune deficiency syndrome: the next wave of the human immunodeficiency virus epidemic? *J Peds* 114:144, 1989.
3. Kogut MD: Growth and development in adolescents. *Pediatr Clin North Am* 20:789, 1973.
4. Kysar JR, Zaks MS, Schuchman HP, et al: Range of psychological functioning in "normal" late adolescents. *Arch Gen Psychiatry* 21:515, 1969.
5. Levine MD, Zallen BG: The learning disorders of adolescence: organic and non-organic failure to thrive. *Pediatr Clin North Am* 31:345, 1984.
6. Mattsson A: Adolescent depression and suicide. In: Hockelman RA, Blatman S, Bounell PA, et al (eds): *Principles of Pediatrics* New York, McGraw-Hill, 1978.
7. Miller D: Adolescent crisis: challenge for patient, parent, and internist. *Ann Intern Med* 79:435, 1973.
8. Offer D, Marcus D, Offer JL: A longitudinal study of normal adolescent boys. *Am J Psychiatry* 126:917, 1970.
9. Pope HG, Hudson JI, Yurgelun-Todd D: Anorexia nervosa and bulimia among 300 suburban women shoppers. *Am J Psychiat* 141:292, 1984.
10. Weiner IB: Delinquent behavior. In: *Psychological Disturbance in Adolescence.* New York, John Wiley & Sons, 1970.
11. Zelnik M, Kantner J: Sexual activity, contraceptive use and pregnancy among metropolitan-area teenagers. *Fam Plann Perspect* 12:230, 1980.

C H A P T E R   6

Geriatric Medicine: Special Considerations

THOMAS E. FINUCANE, M.D.
JOHN R. BURTON, M.D.

"Geriatrics" is formed from two Greek roots meaning "old age" and "healing or physician." Related words are "gerontology," which refers generally to the study of aging, and "iatrogenic," which literally means "caused by a physician or healer."

Ambulatory adult medicine in the United States is already geriatric medicine to a great extent, and it is likely to become increasingly geriatric in the next several decades. This "demographic imperative" results from two distinct phenomena. First, a large group of postwar baby boomers will turn 70 in the first third of the twenty-first century. Second, at every age life expectancy is increasing. In 1988, a 65-year-old man could expect to live an average of 15 more years and a woman could expect about 19 years (22). This is a 10% increase over corresponding figures from 1974 (23).

The challenge for physicians will be sharpened by two additional effects, the rates of disability and of poverty among the elderly. Projections of disability in the future vary widely. One study based on data from 1974 estimated that 65-year-olds will spend 40% of their remaining life dependent on others for basic Activities of Daily Living (see "Functional Assessment" below) (23). Data from 1987 show that 12% of elderly Americans and 19% of the elderly living alone have incomes below poverty levels. When out-of-pocket medical expenses are considered, 27% of the elderly living alone are below the poverty level (7).

Because of the burgeoning cost of medical care, much of it directed to the frail elderly (Fig. 6.1), geriatrics is closely involved with important aspects of public policy. The elderly are all at risk for prolonged "catastrophic illness," potentially caught in the toils of medical technology. Consequently, ethical issues surrounding limitations of therapy are often a central part of clinical decision making.

The clinical care of the old, and especially the very old (those over 85 years), requires special awareness of the progressive socioeconomic and physiological vulnerability prevalent in old age. More than knowledge of specific disease states, this awareness of the extreme frailty of many of the very old defines clinical geriatrics.

This chapter will briefly discuss public policy debate. The bulk of the chapter will consider specific clinical issues including ethical considerations in limiting therapy. Pertinent clinical issues covered elsewhere in this textbook will be cited.

PUBLIC POLICY

In the wealthiest and most powerful nation in the history of the world, millions of citizens are homeless, hungry, or illiterate. Society's guarantee of a clean, well-lighted place for all of its disadvantaged elderly is ambiguous. In a medical system where some hospitals and physicians advertise openly for patients, millions of people with little or no health insurance have difficulty obtaining medical care. Some patients undergo interventions that are futile and unwanted whereas others cannot afford a home health aide that might permit them to remain in their homes. In the waning days of the Reagan Administration a study of public opinion found that most participants "remained unwilling either to lower their own expectations about what the government should provide, or to pay what is necessary for even a modest level of government-provided coverage . . . while there is a strong support for more government involvement, there is no corresponding inclination to pay for it" (6).

Under considerable pressure, Congress enacted catastrophic illness legislation. When Medicare premiums rose as a result, considerable pressure developed to modify the law. It has now been repealed. Some form of federally sponsored long-term care program is now being considered.

The majority of dependent elderly who require long-term care are not institutionalized. For those remaining in the community, formal sources of care (day care, home health care, etc.) provide less than 15% of the necessary care, with friends and family performing the large majority of the work. These caregivers are predominantly women. Many work outside the home and

a substantial number are caring for their own children as well (34). Medical care for these often home-bound, frail elderly, by physicians and other health professionals, is a very important area of care that is often neglected by physicians.

Although there are exceptions, Medicare is best thought of as an acute illness insurance policy for the elderly. It currently does not, in general, cover preventive services or long-term care. Eligibility is not defined by income. Medicare insures about 95% of all Americans over age 65, without regard for their finances. The program pays for home health services for a (presumably short) period of recovery after acute illness when a skilled care need can be demonstrated. It does not, in the vast majority of cases, pay for long-term nursing home placement. Overall, only about 3% of the Medicare budget is spent on long-term care.

Medicaid pays for acute and long-term services for patients who are poor. In contrast to Medicare, age is unimportant and poverty is necessary (but not sufficient) to obtain Medicaid coverage. If a low-income elderly person requires long-term nursing home placement, he must "spend down" his assets, often by paying nursing home bills, until he is impoverished. He then becomes Medicaid eligible. Of all public funds spent on nursing home care, Medicaid provides 92% (41).

Public policy about medical care of the elderly, and especially the poor and frail elderly, is in flux. Out-of-pocket and government expenses are both rising. Many different legislative initiatives are in various stages of development, and the underlying problems are enormous. Costs are high, rising and likely to accelerate.

CLINICAL ISSUES

General Approach

Several aspects of clinical evaluation deserve emphasis:

Obtain old records before the first visit, where possible, If not, ask for them at the first visit. A patient's prior medical records invariably contain useful information. Patients should routinely bring all of their medications, including over-the-counter medications, to clinic appointments.

Bright, direct light is often uncomfortable for patients with cataracts. Prolonged sitting on a backless examining table or in a chilly room can be uncomfortable. Making a patient comfortable probably improves the quality of the history. For patients with presbycusis, it is more important to face the patient and speak slowly and clearly than it is to speak loudly. Patients with marked kyphosis can lie down comfortably if a rolled-up sheet is placed on the pillow under the occiput.

Some form of minimental status examination should be included in the initial evaluation of every older patient (see Chapter 17). Studies have shown that a

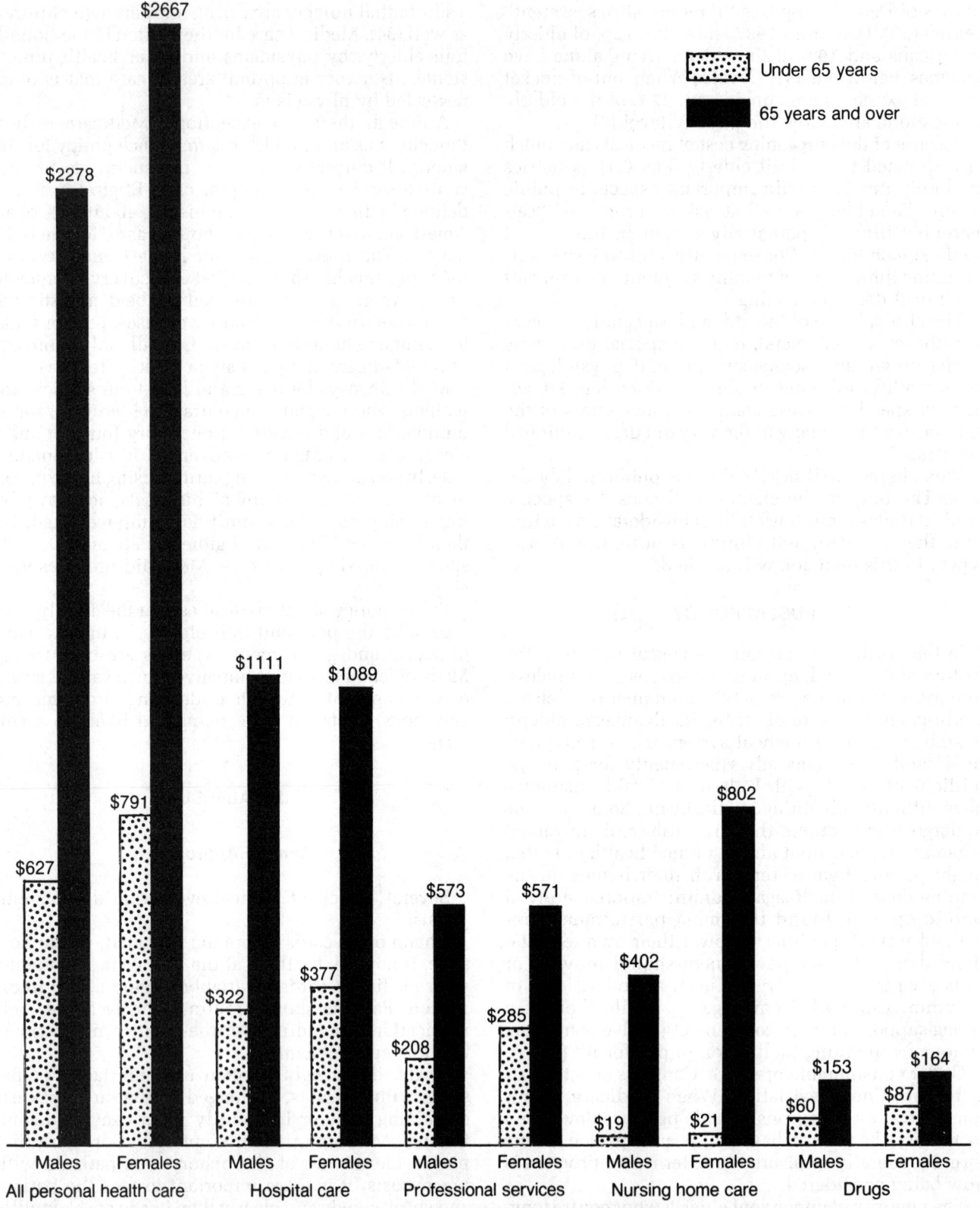

Figure 6.1. *Per capita* personal health care expenditures, according to type of care, age, and sex: United States, 1980. The elderly comprised 11% of the population but consumed disproportionate amounts of health care resources. (Redrawn from Hodgson TA, Kopstein AN: Health care expenditures for major diseases in 1980, National Center for Health Statistics. *Health Care Financing Rev* 5:1, 1984.)

clinician's judgment is insensitive in detecting mild cognitive impairment (27).

It is by now commonplace that symptoms of disease in the elderly may be absent, atypical, or ignored by the physician. Subtle deterioration of cognitive or functional capacity may be the only indication of serious pathology (38).

More time is needed for evaluation of an elderly patient than is usually required for a younger patient. The patient often has multiple problems including sensory and mobility impairments that require a slower tempo of evaluation. Diagnostic testing should be highly selective and stressful tests (which may include X-ray studies for a frail person with a mobility disorder) should have an expected therapeutic implication and should be explained thoroughly to the patient and caregiver. An extensive evaluation may require several visits. Highly streamlined evaluations so characteristic of the practice of modern medicine simply are too stressful for many ill elderly. Empathy and compassion must accompany a visit of low tempo if quality care is to be delivered to the older patient. Several 30- or 60-minute visits may be more easily tolerated than a longer, extensive encounter.

Decisions about Limiting Therapy

Many elderly patients die during acute exacerbation of chronic illness. When patients are critically ill, and if their wishes about aggressive intervention cannot be known, the tendency of the medical care system is to provide treatment. Studies have shown that patients (31) and physicians (2) both believe planning about future illness is a good idea, that physicians are poor predictors of patients' wishes (31), and that planning in advance rarely occurs (2). Offering elderly patients the opportunity to learn about some of the contingencies of severe illness and to express their wishes about aggressive intervention is a very important function of the primary care physician.

"Living Will" laws have been passed in 38 states and the District of Columbia. Although allowing the specification of advance directives, these "living wills" may be rather imprecise and may be valid only in very limited circumstances. In Maryland, for example, the Living Will is only valid when a patient is terminally ill. Finally, large numbers of treatment options may occur in a rapidly evolving clinical context; a single advance directive may be inadequate.

The "durable power of attorney for health care" permits a patient to name a surrogate decision maker who would help the physician plan therapy if the patient were to become incapable of making plans for himself. This form of advance planning permits response to a large number of situations, particularly if the patient has given his surrogate a good idea of his values, wishes, and goals. In practice, informal surrogates are frequently consulted in decisions to limit therapy, even though this practice has very limited legal recognition (14).

Laws about limiting therapy vary from state to state and are evolving continuously. Hospital administrators are generally familiar with pertinent local laws. For the primary physician three general points are worth emphasis:

First, there is no perfect protection from liability. Physicians have been taken to court because they have withdrawn therapy from an incompetent patient at the family's unanimous request. Under almost identical circumstances, physicians have been sued because they have refused to discontinue therapy.

Second, the process of planning with capable patients, in the presence of the family when indicated, is at least as important as the product of the planning session, be it a Do Not Resuscitate order, a Living Will or durable power of attorney. Informed consent, or informed refusal, is as fundamental here as in any other area of medical care.

Third, a unanimous consensus among family and involved health care workers is the surest method of avoiding litigation when making decisions about incapacitated elderly patients.

Elderly outpatients were uniformly pleased when their primary physicians asked them specific questions about their wishes in the event of severe illness (13). For many elderly patients, the prospect of a life of prolonged dependence and discomfort is as dreadful as the prospect of death.

Functional Assessment

Although most elderly people live independently, the prevalence of disability rises steadily with age. Functional assessment is an evaluation in which a patient's degree of independence or disability is the primary focus. In contrast, a standard medical assessment seeks to identify a list of medical diagnoses or problems. If a physician diagnoses stable one-flight angina pectoris in an elderly person, it may be less useful than an assessment of the impact of the problem on the patient's continued independence.

For many patients with mild dementia or gait instability, the precise underlying diagnosis is often less important than the impact of the illness on the patient's function. Dozens of scales have been developed to measure functional disability. The scientific and clinical problems in constructing a valid and useful measure of these behaviors have been carefully described (11). The most commonly used scale is Katz' Activities of Daily Living (ADLs) (Table 6.1).

The six ADLs are feeding, bathing, dressing, transferring, toileting, and continence. Katz has pointed out parallels in child development, and these ADLs may be simply thought of as activities of an average 6-year-old. Inability to perform these ADLs has been an independent predictor of reduced survival (30), nursing home placement, and inadequate recovery after hip fracture (24). To live independently in the community, a higher level of function is necessary. The ability to travel, shop, prepare meals, do housework, and handle finances is called the Instrumental Activities of Daily

Table 6.1.
Areas and Levels of Assessment in the Katz Index of Independence in Activities of Daily Living[a]

Bathing:	____Receives no assistance
	____Receives assistance in bathing only one part
	____Receives assistance in bathing more than one part
Dressing:	____Gets clothes and dresses without assistance
	____Needs assistance in tying shoes only
	____Needs assistance greater than above or stays undressed
Toileting:	____Needs no assistance
	____Needs assistance only in getting to toilet room or in cleaning self
	____Does not go to toilet room
Transferring:	____Needs no assistance from another person
	____Needs assistance with transferring
	____Does not get out of bed
Continence:	____Continent
	____Occasional accident
	____Needs supervision, uses catheter, or is incontinent
Feeding:	____Needs no assistance
	____Needs assistance in cutting meat or buttering bread
	____Needs more assistance or is tube or intravenously fed

[a]From Katz S, Ford AB, Moskowitz RW, et al: Studies of illness in the aged: The index at ADL; standardized measures of biological and psychosocial function. *JAMA* 185:94, 1963.

Living (IADLs) (12). Disability in these IADLs indicates another level of frailty and vulnerability.

Clinicians should inquire specifically about the living situation and functional ability of their frail elderly patients. An evaluation that focuses on pathophysiology and medical therapy may miss a very important dimension of caring for an older person: that person's ability to remain functional and independent.

GERIATRIC ASSESSMENT

Comprehensive geriatric assessment refers to a multidisciplinary, multidimensional assessment of frail elderly patients. Although it has received a great deal of favorable attention (35), geriatric assessment lacks a precise definition and data supporting its usefulness are sketchy. The referral source and initial characteristics of patients, the nature of intervention (for example, whether inpatient, in the office, or in the home, consultation or ongoing therapy), and the measured outcomes vary from study to study.

There is no doubt that certain frail, elderly patients and their companions would benefit from a careful and competent social worker, a nurse who has the time and desire to teach, or perhaps a visit with a pharmacist, nutritionist, or therapist. On the other hand, it is difficult to imagine how this multidisciplinary approach would cause a 50% reduction in mortality in treated subjects compared with randomized controls in 1 year, as reported in a prominent article on inpatient geriatric assessment (40). In contrast, in a randomized outpatient study, no effect on survival

was shown when controls were seen by well-trained internists (10).

Because the concept of the geriatric assessment unit is so amorphous, enthusiasm must be tempered. Clinical care of frail old people requires careful and repeated medical evaluation, sensitivity to social and economic conditions, and attention to drug use, nutrition, and needs for occupational and physical therapies. The central importance of functional ability in the context of the patient's day-to-day environment cannot be overemphasized. Clinicians whose practices include substantial numbers of such patients should have the appropriate resources available.

DRUG USE IN THE ELDERLY

Elderly Americans take large numbers of drugs. Although some drugs are clearly beneficial, many others have little or no evidence of efficacy. A useful clinical strategy is to insist that all medication be brought to each visit and then to consider the justification for each drug.

Studies of drug disposition in the elderly demonstrate wide heterogeneity in several important physiological functions. Although drug absorption is unimpaired in general, distribution within the body compartments may be quite different in older compared with younger subjects. Muscle mass, bone mass, body water, and some serum proteins are lower and body fat higher in older subjects. Hepatic drug clearance, in simplest terms, depends on hepatic blood flow, serum protein binding, and the intrinsic capacity of the hepatocyte mass. The first two of these factors decrease with age resulting in some individuals having impaired drug metabolism. Glomerular filtration rate (GFR) can fall about 30% from the third decade to the eighth (Fig. 6.2). The fall in GFR may not be accompanied by a rise in serum creatinine because muscle mass is falling concomitantly. Due to the variability among subjects, prediction of drug levels from dosage is unreliable (15).

In many cases, very low doses of medication may be effective, for example, 50 mg hydrochlorothiazide per day at most (42), and beginning doses of 0.25 mg of haloperidol or 10 mg of imipramine per day (28). Unless the clinical situation requires otherwise, drugs should be started at low doses in the elderly and titrated carefully upward during frequent early follow-up. Drug levels, when available, are useful in monitoring the patient.

New drugs pose particularly serious risks for the elderly. In general the United States Food and Drug Administration (FDA) approves new drugs after safety has been demonstrated in small trials, usually with healthy young subjects taking no other drugs (25). Once the drugs are released, however, they are frequently used widely in a very different population, the frail elderly. It is often during this phase that serious but uncommon toxicities become apparent especially in this very vulnerable population. In the past few years benoxaprofen (Oraflex), zomepirac (Zomax), suprofen

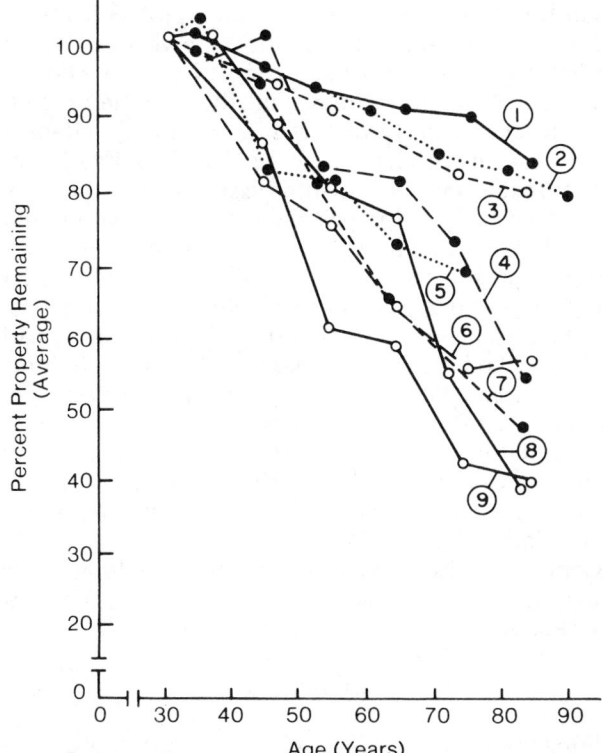

Figure 6.2. Organ system function and aging. *1,* conduction velocity; *2,* basal metabolic rate; *3,* standard cell water; *4,* cardiac index; *5,* standard glomerular filtration rate (inulin); *6,* vital capacity; *7,* standard renal plasma flow (Diodrast); *8,* standard renal plasma flow (para-aminohippurate (PAH)); *9,* maximal breathing capacity. (Adapted from Shoch NN: The physiology of aging. *Sci Am* 206:100, 1962.)

(Suprol), nomifenisine (Merital) and bupropion (Wellbutin) have been heavily promoted and then withdrawn from the market after reports of serious injury or death of patients. Some months after release of the class IC antiarrhythmic agents encainide and flecainide, both of whose advertising campaigns referred specifically to their safety, the National Heart Lung and Blood Institute announced that a clinical trial had demonstrated twice as many deaths in patients taking these drugs rather than placebo for asymptomatic ventricular arrhythmias after myocardial infarction (46).

New drugs should be tried carefully in older patients only after all other more standard drugs have been tried and failed. Older drugs have more well-established safety profiles. Prescribing a new drug means entering a patient into the postmarketing surveillance phase. Promotional statements about the safety or the lack of side effects of newly released drugs should be ignored.

Some specific drugs selected because of their widespread use in the elderly are considered below:

Digoxin. In patients in sinus rhythm and compensated, well-documented congestive heart failure (CHF), digoxin may often be safely withdrawn (33) (see Chapter 61 for a full discussion of the use of digoxin). Patients with compensated CHF who also have an S_3 are

more likely to benefit from continued therapy. Digoxin is a frequent cause of drug toxicity.

Oral hypoglycemic drugs. The FDA requires that all of these drugs, including the new ones, be labeled with a ''Special Warning'' on the possibility of increased risk of cardiovascular mortality. No study has convincingly demonstrated reduction in the microvascular complications of diabetes mellitus as a result of the use of these agents (9). Moderate control of hyperglycemia may result in symptomatic improvement in some patients. Oral hypoglycemic drugs are discussed fully in Chapter 72.

Major tranquilizers. These drugs are associated with increased risk of falls (47), hip fracture (37), and tardive dyskinesia (20). They are sometimes efficacious in treating the behavioral complications of dementia (18). If these drugs are prescribed, evidence of good effect should be sought. If they provide nothing more than sedation, other drugs should be used instead, such as chloral hydrate or short-acting benzodiazepines. The use of psychoactive drugs in the elderly is discussed fully in Chapter 17.

Nonsteroidal anti-inflammatory drugs (NSAIDs). For treatment of inflammatory conditions these are excellent drugs. As analgesia for noninflammatory chronic pain, their considerable toxicities may outweigh their benefit. Current users of NSAIDs are almost five times more likely to have a fatal upper gastrointestinal hemorrhage when compared with former users or subjects who have never used them (16). This study suggests frail, elderly white women are especially at risk. Renal and central nervous system (CNS) toxicities are well known (see Chapter 70 for a full discussion on NSAIDs).

In many cases of pain without underlying inflammation, acetaminophen may have a superior risk/benefit profile, although chronic use of acetaminophen has recently also been associated with renal disease (43).

Cold remedies. There is no cure for the common cold, but there is a multimillion dollar market in remedies. Common treatments bring the risk of antihistaminic or narcotic sedation, sympathomimetic stimulation, or a combination of the two. Many common combinations are irrational, even contradictory.

Clinicians should discourage their elderly patients, who are likely to be susceptible to anticholinergic and sympathomimetic effects, from buying these nostrums, many of which contain a variety of useless ingredients. They will, however, be working against a mammoth advertising campaign as they do so.

NEGLECT AND ABUSE IN THE ELDERLY

Most dependent elderly live in the community and are cared for by relatives. In the vast majority of these cases, excellent, loving care is provided. In some cases, however, there is frank abuse or neglect and in some the situation is ambiguous. The number of older Americans who are abused is likely to increase for a variety of reasons, including the national trend toward smaller families and the rapidly increasing numbers of the very old, who are no longer wage earners and are more likely to be frail and dependent. Clear-cut examples of physical and emotional violence, sexual abuse, and harmful neglect against frail elderly people have been reported.

Definition of abuse can be difficult, in large part because the victims are presumably competent adults who choose to continue the relationship leading to putative abuse. Neglect is also often difficult to define, especially in a relationship in which the caregiver has no legally defined responsibility. Furthermore, some situations offer only tragic options. If a single working mother cares for her demented mother, and if the mother repeatedly wanders or urinates in closets, is it abuse if the daughter uses physical restraints? Suppose neither mother nor daughter will accept a nursing home and employment of professional caregivers is not financially feasible?

Diagnosis is difficult because both abuser and victim may tend to deny or minimize abuse. The diagnosis is often, therefore, inferential. "Treatment" may be problematic in all but extreme cases. Remedies might include an alternative environment that is healthful, supportive, and acceptable to the victim, or the provision of services that can relieve a stressed caregiver. Such "treatment" is often unavailable. Risk factors for abuse are shown in Table 6.2 (8, 21).

Clinicians may be reluctant to become involved in a situation in which there is little reward, poor reimbursement, and potential liability. State statutes vary in defining the physician's liability. The Council on Scientific Affairs of the American Medical Association has published a very useful report on this subject. The report outlines several strategies for prevention and intervention (8). The full report may be obtained by writing to the Council on Scientific Affairs, AMA, 535 N. Dearborn St., Chicago, IL 60610. In severe cases, however, legal advice should be sought and state agencies such as Adult Protective Services, should be involved.

FALLS

Falls are common in the elderly (annual incidence of 35% in persons older than 75) and have serious consequences (9500 deaths per year, in addition to

Table 6.2.
Risk Factors for Elder Abuse

Victim characteristics
  Lives with related relative, not spouse
  Severely demented
  Behavior problem
  Medically ill

Abuser
  Has provided long-term care
  Stressed significantly by care of the victim
  Under severe external stress
  Abused as a child
  Expresses frustration
  Uses drugs, including alcohol

disability, limitation of activity, etc.) (48). A standard history and physical examination are very limited in the identification of the usually multifactorial etiology of falling. Medications may contribute to the problem and, in fact, seem to be a risk factor independent of the illness for which they were prescribed. Evaluation of the patient's environment is essential and the value of a house call in this process cannot be overemphasized. Dangerous throw rugs, poorly lighted areas, inadequate railings, weak or sharp furniture, unsafe bathing or cooking facilities are examples of high risk problems that are easily identified during a house call. Performance-based assessments may provide information unavailable after standard neurological examination (49).

Ambulatory patients with primary degenerative dementia have a higher than average risk of falling and of fractures. Demented patients who wander are at particularly high risk (4).

Commonly implicated drugs include long-acting benzodiazepines, major tranquilizers, tricyclic antidepressants, antihypertensives, and alcohol.

NUTRITION

For a variety of reasons, precise definition of dietary requirements for ambulatory elderly people is difficult. "The elderly" are physiologically and metabolically an extremely diverse group with a variety of illnesses, taking a variety of medicines. Absorptive function in the aging gut is poorly studied. Yet recommended daily allowances (RDAs) for the elderly are extrapolated from data collected in studies of younger people. RDAs based on age alone are imprecise. More complicated calculations will likely replace them (44).

Two general principles have been demonstrated. First, the large majority of elderly Americans who come to see a doctor are not undernourished. Second, desirable body weight may be somewhat heavier than previously thought, based on insurance company tables of mortality and body mass index (BMI). Based on independent analysis of insurance company data, Andres (1) has calculated mortality ratios in various age groups according to BMI. The "best" BMI, the one with the lowest mortality ratio, rises in each age group. At age 50, for example, the BMI (in kilograms/meter^2) associated with the least mortality is about 26. At age 70 the "best" BMI is almost 28. Thus, for a 6-foot-tall 70-year-old person, the "best" weight by these tables can be calculated at 206 pounds. These tables demonstrate that higher weights, per se, are not necessarily harmful. Weight loss is of proven effectiveness in the management of hypertension, hypercholesterolemia, and diabetes mellitus and should be pursued in overweight patients when these illnesses are present.

A variety of psychosocial factors (e.g., isolation, alcoholism, depression, low income) and physiological changes (e.g., diminished taste and smell sensation, dental problems, dementia, dysphagia, acid peptic disease) may contribute to a diminished intake of nutritious meals. Although difficult to demonstrate except in extreme cases, malnutrition may occur in these situations. The benefits of multivitamin supplement are unknown. Although risks are low when vitamins are taken in moderation, costs can be high.

Weight loss can result from a variety of causes, some trivial and some lethal. In general, the known causes of weight loss can be classified as: (a) decreased intake, (b) reduced absorption, and (c) increased utilization. Some cases of weight loss cannot be explained.

In the elderly, decreased intake should be carefully sought. Some potential causes are listed above. Reduced absorption is an area of active investigation. The search for malignancy during a careful history and physical examination and the exclusion of hyperthyroidism with appropriate laboratory investigation are also an important part of the evaluation.

In summary, patients who are eating a reasonably balanced diet and who are not losing weight are unlikely to be malnourished. If either of these conditions is not met, the physician must investigate carefully and intervene judiciously.

URINARY INCONTINENCE

The involuntary loss of urine (urinary incontinence) affects 15 to 20% of ambulatory elderly people and has profound implications, both social and medical. Incontinence is a frequently given reason for admission to a long-term care facility. It is a major reason for social isolation of elderly individuals. When severe it can lead to skin maceration and contribute to pressure sores. In spite of the high prevalence of urinary incontinence in the elderly, especially in women, the problem is not recognized frequently by their physicians. In part this is because patients fail to report urinary incontinence, assuming it to be part of normal aging—"one of the curses of age"—and in part because physicians fail to inquire of their patients about urinary incontinence. General physicians usually have not been involved in the care of the incontinent patient because younger patients with this problem have been managed by urologists and/or gynecologists. In a younger population, most patients are women with urinary incontinence due to sphincter insufficiency (or stress incontinence, see below) and this insufficiency is treated very effectively and often surgically by urologists or gynecologists. In the elderly, however, the general physician must be involved in the care of the incontinent patient for several reasons: The elderly are often resistant to consultation; they often refuse to have an invasive evaluation, a common component of an evaluation by a specialist; frequently the incontinence is multifaceted and the treatment is correspondingly broad-based and not curative; and, in general, surgery is not often as beneficial in elderly as it is in young patients.

Physiology of Micturition

To evaluate and manage patients with urinary incontinence, an understanding of the basic knowledge of the physiology of voiding is necessary. The bladder is innervated by an autonomous spinal reflex arc that can be modulated effectively by the cerebral cortex, permitting the patient, under normal circumstances, to evacuate the urinary bladder in a socially acceptable fashion. Spontaneous contraction of the detrusor muscle usually occurs when the urinary bladder fills to approximately 150 to 250 ml; however, most individuals can suppress this urge to void under normal circumstances. Also, conditioning by chronic high or low volume voiding can change the bladder capacity considerably, in either direction.

Reasons for Urinary Incontinence

It is simplest to classify patterns of urinary continence into four groups: urge, stress, overflow, and functional (Table 6.3).

Urge

Urge incontinence results from an *uninhibited bladder* (or detrusor instability) and occurs when there is an inability by the patient to suppress sensations of bladder fullness; consequently, when a certain bladder volume is achieved, voiding occurs often within moments. (The urge to void is very transient and incompletely suppressible.) This problem is common in patients with dementia or in those who have had a stroke.

Stress

Stress incontinence or *sphincter insufficiency* occurs when there is an inability to increase the resistance in the outflow tract, when an increase in abdominal muscle tone (stress) is transmitted to the urinary bladder. This might occur with increased abdominal tension during lifting, coughing, sneezing, or laughing. In all of these instances increased muscle tone leads to increased intraabdominal pressure. The pressure is transmitted to the urinary bladder, outlet sphincters are unable to resist the increased pressure, and incontinence occurs. This problem is very common in women who have borne children (resulting in perineal trauma) and who are postmenopausal. Tissue relaxation (from estrogen deficiency) results in a malalignment of the bladder and urethra, and the ureterovesical angle is extremely important in maintaining continence. Sphincter insufficiency is frequently present in combination with an uninhibited bladder in elderly women and, occasionally, in men who have had prostate surgery.

Table 6.3.
Classification of Disorders of Urinary Continence

Uninhibited urinary bladder (spastic bladder, urge incontinence)
Sphincter insufficiency (stress incontinence)
Overflow incontinence
Functional incontinence—normally adequate control but imbalance due to drugs (e.g., anticholinergics or diuretics), diminished mobility (arthritis), or environment change (away from home)

Overflow

Overflow incontinence occurs when there is inadequate detrusor function and/or inadequate sensory perception within the bladder wall, or significant outlet obstruction. Overdistension of the bladder results until incontinence occurs from spontaneous bladder contraction at high bladder volumes. This is a typical result of diabetic neuropathy and of obstructive uropathy, as, for example, from prostatic hypertrophy in males.

Functional

Functional incontinence occurs when under ideal circumstances the voiding mechanism is adequate, but because of impaired mobility of the patient or an increase in urinary volume (e.g., from diuretics), the functional reserve is overcome and incontinence results. This pattern is typical in older persons who are in a new environment where they are unable to reach a toilet or when they have been given medications that may alter their voiding, either neurologically (e.g., antidepressant or antiparkinsonian drugs) or volumetrically (e.g., diuretics).

Evaluation of a Patient with Urinary Incontinence

The simultaneous combination of several of these four major patterns is very common in elderly patients.

Reversible Causes

When a patient with urinary incontinence is identified, it is important first to evaluate the patient for the possibility of a functional disorder (see above) and/or an acute reversible cause of urinary incontinence. The most common reversible causes are changes in mental state for any reason, drug effects (especially diuretics, anticholinergics, sedatives, and neuroleptics), fecal impaction, urinary tract infections (rarely), and, in women, atrophic vaginitis. In the latter three of these instances, incontinence results from increased bladder sensory stimulation, which may be incompletely suppressed (because of a marginal decrease in suppressor function). In the case of atrophic vaginitis, there may also be relaxation of the tissues of the urinary bladder outlet, resulting in a pattern of sphincter insufficiency. These problems should be considered routinely and, when identified, treated appropriately. Even so, some patients, especially those with infection, often have persistence of incontinence after eradication of the problem.

History

If reversible causes are not present, it is important to establish the pattern of urinary incontinence by taking a careful history. After first reviewing symptoms with the patient, it is best to ask the patient to record the episodes of incontinence. Figure 6.3 provides examples of *bladder records*. It is best to provide the patient with 7 to 14 copies of a similar form to record the time and to describe any voiding accidents. (Initially, it is not necessary to instruct the patient to void at timed intervals as shown in Figure 6.3, but these same forms may be used later to educate the patient to perform timed voidings.) The physician can review these data with the patient at a follow-up office visit. Usually, in the patient with urge incontinence (*uninhibited bladder*), there are episodes of large volume involuntary losses frequently occurring when the patient simply was not able to suppress the urge to void or could not get to a lavatory in time (Fig. 6.3A). Stress incontinence (*sphincter insufficiency*) is associated with episodes of small volume loss or of dribbling that occurs in association with increased abdominal pressure, e.g., coughing or sneezing (Fig. 6.3B). The physician should also inquire about symptoms that might relate the incontinence to a *neurological cause* (e.g., paresthesia, gait abnormality), a structural cause (e.g., prostatism), or a metabolic disorder (e.g., diabetes mellitus).

Examination

The physical examination seeks to help in the classification of the incontinence and to rule out reversible causes (see above). The bladder should be *carefully palpated* with the patient in the supine position. A palpable bladder is strongly suggestive of overflow incontinence, but a nonpalpable bladder does not rule out this problem. *Neurological examination* should include an assessment of sensation (using fine touch or pin) in the perineal and perianal area and of anal sphincter tone. Also, in men, the bulbocavernosus reflex should be tested (contraction of the bulbous portion of the urethra caused by tapping the penis near the scrotum). Diminished or absent sensation in these areas or lack of sphincter tone suggests a neurological cause of the urinary incontinence. A *rectal examination*, besides assessing sphincter tone, is necessary to evaluate the possibility of fecal impaction and, in men, to assess the prostate for cancer, benign enlargement, or infection. In women, a *pelvic examination* is necessary to evaluate for a relaxation (e.g., cystocele) or for atrophic vaginitis (Chapter 94). It is also necessary to test for urinary sphincter adequacy. This may be accomplished by having the patient, while in the lithotomy position, cough after her bladder is full. If urinary sphincter insufficiency is present, a small urine leak will result. If the patient has a leak after coughing, a Bonney's test may be performed. Incontinence due to a cough is prevented by lifting the urethra and base of the bladder with the tips of two fingers placed just lateral to the urethra in the vagina. Although the test is more likely to be positive in young women, it should be tried in elderly patients as well. Although there is some controversy regarding the predictive value of the test, the correction of the incontinence by this maneuver correlates generally with a good surgical outcome if sphincter insufficiency is the only mechanism of incontinence. If the patient did not have an incontinent episode in the lithotomy position, she should be asked to stand while properly draped, holding an absorbent pad over her urethra, and cough. This maneuver may precipitate an episode of stress incontinence.

After the patient has voided fully, it is important to perform carefully a *catheterization of the urinary bladder.*

Patient experience. Catheterization may be performed simply by obtaining a catheterization kit, which contains all of the materials necessary (cleansing solutions, a catheter, sterile gloves, collection containers, and lubricant). After preparation of the urethral meatus, the sterile catheter is inserted gently into the bladder. In male patients, it is important that the shaft of the penis be extended and lifted in a cephalad direction to align the urethra with the bladder outlet. The urine volume is measured and the catheter removed. When carefully performed, the incidence of infection is less than 1% and only 3 to 4% of patients—usually males—experience mild discomfort, typically a burning sensation. This discomfort may be minimized by careful placement of a well-lubricated catheter and by thoroughly explaining the procedure to the patient prior to its performance.

If the postvoid residual volume is greater than 100 ml of urine, overflow incontinence may be present; this is a special concern with very large residual volumes (over 200 ml). Overflow incontinence (also see Chapter 49) is important to recognize because the patient should be referred to a urologist for further evaluation and treatment, e.g., for relief of obstruction or, in the case of an atonic bladder, for educating the patient in intermittent self-catheterization. The urologist may perform cystometric evaluation and cystoscopy and may consider a trial of bethanecol (Urecholine) if an atonic bladder is confirmed. Analysis of the urine, both microscopically and by dipstick, can be accomplished on the urine specimen obtained by the catheterization and is helpful in evaluating for an infection or in suggesting less common diagnoses. Hematuria may suggest a tumor, for example.

An additional technique useful in the evaluation of selected patients is simple cystometry. This procedure, which requires filling the bladder incrementally with sterile water, can easily be performed by a nurse or physician following the guidelines established by Ouslander and colleagues (36). The procedure is helpful when the patient's history is unclear or suggests a mixed disorder. It also ensures that the tests for stress incontinence and residual volume are performed when the bladder is full thus increasing their validity. Also, involuntary contractions are easily seen using this technique, and when these occur at relatively low volume (e.g., <250 ml) urge incontinence is suggested.

Referral

Younger patients with urinary incontinence should be referred to a urologist or gynecologist. Cystoscopy and cystometrographic studies are often necessary to classify precisely the voiding disorder and to plan for definitive therapy. Frequently, however, this is not possible in frail elderly patients (see above). Further, the value of cystometrographic studies has not been fully validated in elderly patients. When the pattern of incontinence is highly suggestive of urge (large volume accidents often occurring within moments of the first urge to void), for example, there is usually no indication for further evaluation since at present these patients are not surgical candidates. Elderly women who have a pure pattern of stress incontinence may be surgical candidates. The surgical success in correcting this problem is dramatic in younger women. Now with the newer techniques of endoscopic suspension of the bladder neck, a procedure with less operative stress than earlier operations, elderly women with pure stress incontinence may be helped. The physician should refer the patient to a geriatrician with special interest in incontinence or to a urologist or gynecologist when basic therapies (see below) have failed or at any time that there is doubt about the cause of the incontinence or concern about a serious underlying problem (e.g., a bladder tumor or the cauda equina syndrome).

Therapy

It is most important to recognize that small therapeutic gains often are extremely important to an elderly patient. Cure is not accomplished often, but if incontinent episodes can be minimized, the patient and his/her family may express considerable satisfaction.

The bladder record (see above) may provide an important clue to the treatment (as well as the cause) of the incontinence. The physician might advise, for example, avoiding situations that increase the urge to void (the patient who comments that incontinence occurs only when drinking warm milk or listening to running water). The willingness with which the patient uses the bladder record will provide insight as to the likelihood that a program of education (see below) will be successful.

Educational Programs

An *educational program* is an important first step in the therapy of any patient with stress, urge, or both patterns of incontinence who is not significantly demented. The initial focus should be on a thorough explanation of the mechanisms of incontinence and that a great deal can be done by the patient to avoid the problem. Having the patient void at timed intervals permits the beginning of a *behavioral modification program.* The patient learns to empty the bladder by the clock, before a bladder volume is achieved that results in spontaneous detrusor contraction. Occasionally, when asked to void at 2-hour intervals (following the pattern on the Bladder Record, Fig. 6.3), a patient with urge incontinence will become continent. If that happens, the physician can educate the patient to increase the interval between voidings by 30 to 60 minutes every week or so until incontinence recurs.

Bladder Record

Name _____   Date_____

Instructions: 1. In the first column, mark the time every time you void.
2. In the second or third column, mark every time you accidentally leaked urine.
3. Write "dry" if no accident occurred in the 2-hour interval.

Time Interval	Urinated in Toilet	Leaking Accident	or	Large Accident	Reason for Accident
6–8 AM	✓				
8–10 AM					
10–12 AM	✓				
12–2 PM					
2–4 PM	✓	✓			Running water
4–6 PM					
6–8 PM				✓	Waited too long
8–10 PM	✓				
10–12 PM				✓	Running water
Overnight					

Number of pads used today: _____

Comments: _____

Exercises: _____

_____

_____

Total: _____

Figure 6.3A. Bladder record from patient with urinary incontinence: Uninhibited bladder. (Patient data, for *A* and *B*, courtesy of Kathryn L. Burgio, Ph.D., Gerontology Research Center, National Institute on Aging, Baltimore, MD. Bladder record from Whitehead WE, Burgio KL, Engel BT: Behavioral methods in the assessment and treatment of urinary incontinence. In Brocklehurst JC (ed): *Urology in the Elderly.* New York, Churchill Livingstone, 1984, p. 81.)

Then by continuing to void by the clock (at the longest interval without incontinence), acceptable continence often will result.

For patients who are not severely demented and who have a pattern of stress incontinence, the mechanism of sphincter insufficiency should be explained. The patient should learn to avoid increasing abdominal pressure while the bladder is full and to perform exercises that strengthen the sphincter (see below). The patient should be taught to avoid consuming a large volume of fluid 2 to 6 hours prior to being in a situation without easy access to a toilet.

Kegel exercises will help many women with stress incontinence. With the woman in a lithotomy position, the physician places two fingers in the vagina and separates them as much as possible. Then the patient is asked to squeeze the introitus around the fingers. The physician will sense when the musculature has been properly contracted and should instruct the patient to practice repeatedly contracting this mus-

Bladder Record

Name _____ Date _____

Instructions: 1. In the first column, mark the time every time you void.
2. In the second or third column, mark every time you accidentally leaked urine.
3. Write "dry" if no accident occurred in the 2-hour interval.

Time Interval	Urinated in Toilet	Leaking Accident	or	Large Accident	Reason for Accident
6–8 AM	✓	✓			Fast walking
8–10 AM	✓				
10–12 AM	✓				
12–2 PM					
2–4 PM	✓				
4–6 PM		✓			Coughed
6–8 PM	✓				
8–10 PM		✓			Sneezed
10–12 PM	✓				
Overnight					

Number of pads used today: 2 _____

Comments: _____

Exercises: _____

_____

_____

Total: _____

Figure 6.3B. Bladder record from patient with urinary incontinence: sphincter insufficiency.

cle group. Once the patient learns how to do this, she should contract these muscles several times every day. At follow-up visits, the examination should be repeated and the patient advised as to the adequacy of her effort. An alternative to this technique applicable to men and women takes advantage of the fact that the urethral sphincter is innervated almost identically as the anal sphincter and works in parallel with it. During a rectal examination, the examiner asks the patient to squeeze the anal sphincter around the finger. Once the patient understands the importance that such con-

tractions have in controlling the bladder outlet and once contractions can be performed spontaneously, the patient usually is willing to practice the exercise 50 times in succession several times (typically three) a day. This program will strengthen the sphincters considerably. The patient should be taught to perform this exercise occasionally while in various positions, while walking and while voiding. As confidence is gained, the patient should be instructed to contract the sphincters whenever abdominal pressure is increased (e.g., in anticipation of a cough, a sneeze, or a quick movement). This educational program has effectively cured some patients of incontinence (5).

In those with urge incontinence sphincter exercise should be combined with an attempt to have the patient relax at the very first sense of an urge. This will take some effort because patients will have become conditioned to quickly moving toward a lavatory and thus inadvertently increasing abdominal and bladder pressure. The patient, once relaxed, can contract the sphincter muscles and walk slowly to a lavatory to void.

Some elderly patients have difficulty opening their garments to void. Replacing buttons and zippers with Velcro fasteners (easily done by a tailor) will save time and may avoid an accident. Similarly, a lavatory should be conveniently accessible.

Drug Therapy

Although many drugs have been claimed to be effective in the treatment of urinary incontinence, currently only a few have been shown to be effective in the treatment of elderly patients.

Estrogen. For female patients with atrophic vaginitis, estrogen replacement has improved incontinence. Atrophic vaginitis may be diagnosed during the pelvic examination and if there is doubt on inspection, a therapeutic trial still may be beneficial. A course of estrogen therapy should be tried if the patient has no contraindication to this hormone (See Chapter 73). If the patient is willing to try vaginal cream, a topical estrogen such as Premarin may be the best first step. A 1-month trial should be adequate; if there is significant improvement, the physician should discuss with the patient the possibility of long-term estrogen therapy (see Chapter 94 for details). For many patients symptoms can be controlled by applying topical estrogen periodically, e.g., once or twice a week. Topical estrogen therapy does have a systemic effect, and the complications (such as uterine cancer) especially when unopposed by progestins should be considered. Some patients may be unwilling or unable to use vaginal estrogen cream. In that instance a 1-month trial of an oral estrogen (e.g., Premarin, 0.625 mg every day) is appropriate. If successful, long-term administration may be tried. The lowest effective dose of estrogen should be used, and cycling with a progestin (e.g., Provera) should be considered. Such a regimen, described fully in Chapter 77, minimizes or eliminates most risks previously associated with unopposed continuous estrogen therapy.

Oxybutynin. Oxybutynin (Ditropan, 5 mg tablets or liquid) has been shown to be effective when administered in short-term studies in patients with either an uninhibited bladder or sphincter insufficiency. It probably works by increasing sphincter tone and increasing bladder capacity. Oxybutynin is administered orally at a 5-mg-tablet dosage three times a day. In frail elderly patients the drug should be started as a lower dose: 2.5 mg (one half tablet or appropriate volume of the liquid preparation) once or twice a day,

then advanced to a maximum of 5 mg three times per day or until either an acceptable response or a significant side effect is seen. It is effective in approximately 50% of patients, but the side effects of dry mouth, blurred vision, abdominal cramps, urinary retention, or constipation are encountered in nearly 50%; also 20% of patients stop the drug because of intolerance. A trial of this drug for 7 to 10 days may be considered. Long-term studies with this agent are not available. Nevertheless, when symptoms of urgency are present and educational programs (see above) have not been effective, and, in women, when no response to estrogen is seen, a trial of oxybutynin should be considered.

Imipramine. Imipramine (Tofranil, 10-, 25-mg tablets) has been shown to be effective in some elderly patients with either sphincter insufficiency or an uninhibited bladder. It is the only antidepressant carefully studied for this effect. The drug probably works via its anticholinergic activity, by increasing bladder capacity and increasing sphincter tone. It should be begun at 10 to 25 mg orally every night, then increased every third night to a maximum of 150 mg/night or until side effects occur. Drug levels are useful at higher doses in older or smaller patients or those with renal impairment. The most common side effects are postural hypotension, urinary retention, constipation, dizziness, and mucous membrane dryness. Although the drug may be partially effective in 50 to 60% of patients, over half experience some side effects and approximately 20% will discontinue the medication because of intolerance.

Alpha Agonists. Some patients with stress incontinence may benefit from alpha agonists, which are thought to increase the tone of the urethral sphincter. Pseudoephedrine (e.g., Sudafed 30- or 60-mg tablets, available without prescription) may be tried in a dose of 30 to 60 mg twice a day for 1 or 2 weeks. Side effects including palpitation, nervousness, dry mucous membranes, urinary retention, or hypertension limit its use in many older patients.

Other Medications. Many other drugs have been touted as effective in elderly patients with incontinence. Some of these include calcium channel blockers (e.g., Nifedipine), nonsteroidal anti-inflammatory agents (e.g., Indocin), antispasmodics (e.g., Flavoxate). However, none is currently recommended because of unproven efficacy or potential side effects.

Garments and Catheters

Increasingly, comfortable diapers or briefs are available to avoid embarrassing incontinent accidents, e.g., Attends (Proctor and Gamble), Depends (Kimberly-Clarke), Asorb-fil (Sears), or Tranquility (Devilbiss) are available from pharmacies, medical supply stores, or large catalog stores. For men there are also available relatively comfortable (day and night) condom catheter kits (such as United Weimer Urinal, United Medical) drip urinals, or supporters with absorbent liners, generally for under $50 to $75. However, if the patient frequently manipulates the external catheter, urosepsis is a common complication, and in that instance it is probably wise to use a diaper garment. Recently available are external catheter systems for women (e.g., from Hollister). These hold promise but their application requires a large level of dexterity and commitment.

Indwelling urinary catheters have no place in the treatment of urinary incontinence, except in instances in which there is secondary skin maceration or pressure sore development. In those instances, the catheter should be used only temporarily until those complications have been resolved. Intermittent self-catheterization is a useful technique for patients with an atonic bladder and overflow incontinence. However, the patient or his caretaker must be able and willing to perform the procedure several times a day. When this procedure is considered, it is usually best to refer the patient and caretaker to a urologist for education, unless the general physician or a staff member is experienced in educating others in its performance.

Biofeedback techniques are effective in treating elderly men and women with incontinence from sphincter insufficiency or from an uninhibited bladder. Severe dementia precludes this technique, which requires learning skills. Referral to a geriatric center offering this therapy should be considered when educational methods and/or drug therapy (see above) have failed to achieve adequate control.

Surgical techniques of creating artificial urinary bladder sphincters are gaining clinical applicability, but it is still uncertain which candidates will benefit most; a geriatrician with expertise in treating incontinent patients or a urologist should be consulted, initially by telephone, to help determine which patients might be candidates for artificial sphincter surgery.

PREVENTIVE GERIATRICS (ALSO SEE CHAPTER 2)

Rowe and Kahn distinguish "usual" from "successful" aging (39). In a group of "usual" aging Americans, for example, bone and muscle mass fall and glucose tolerance worsens with age. Regular exercise, however, is associated with improved glucose metabolism, increased bone mass, and muscle strength (3) and thus modifies "usual" aging. Exercise may also lower the risk of falling and the risk of coronary artery disease and may alleviate depression in the elderly (3, 29). The risk of initiating an exercise program in a previously sedentary elderly person is real, as prevalence of coronary heart disease is high in this population. As with many other forms of therapy in the elderly, exercise should be begun at low levels and increased slowly under close supervision. Exercise stress testing is indicated in older patients who wish to begin higher levels of training (see Chapter 57). Immunization information is provided in Chapter 32.

Data show that although elderly women visit physicians more frequently, they are less likely to have a pelvic examination and Papanicolaou smear and less likely than younger women to be diagnosed with uterine, ovarian, or cervical cancer in a localized (and potentially curable) stage (17). Prevalence of abnormal Pap smears among elderly women was 13.5 per 1000 in one study, and the death rate from cervical cancer is highest in women over 65 (32). Chapter 95 provides guidelines for gynecological cancer screenings.

Although available data do not permit clear-cut recommendations, most authorities believe that the well elderly should receive periodic testing similar to that of younger patients (see Chapter 2). Elderly patients with marked cognitive impairment or severe chronic disease comprise a separate group of patients for whom the value of screening is particularly uncertain.

Screening for visual loss and for hearing loss are discussed in Chapters 98 and 96, respectively.

In patients at high risk for vertebral compression or hip fracture, and for those with established kyphosis, a careful survey of the house for environmental hazards is recommended; such patients also should not lift heavy objects, specifically grandchildren. Prevention of falls is discussed above.

The benefits of discontinuing cigarette smoking among the elderly are probably substantial. Although several studies of smoking cessation among the elderly have shown little effect on primary prevention of coronary heart disease, in those with established disease, smoking cessation reduces the risk of myocardial infarction and death (19). Cessation is a key step in the primary prevention of lung and other cancers and the primary or secondary prevention of obstructive lung disease, peripheral vascular disease, and peptic ulcer disease. A full discussion of strategies for smoking cessation are discussed in Chapter 20.

The routine use of aspirin (45) and, in women, estrogens (26) in old age is under considerable scrutiny (see Chapters 52 and 77, respectively). Both of these agents may provide valuable benefits to certain elderly people.

PRERETIREMENT COUNSELING AND PLANNING

Several problems of the elderly can be minimized if they are anticipated and planned for well in advance. Books are available to help the older person in planning (see "General References") and large corporations, senior citizen centers, and several colleges offer courses in preretirement counseling and planning. The American Association of Retired Persons (AARP) has a wide range of materials to assist in such planning in their National Gerontology Research Center [1909 K Street, NW, Washington DC 20049; telephone (202) 728-4883]. Important topics for the older person to consider are anticipated economic changes, preparation of wills and estate planning, changes in tempo and nature of activities, the importance of developing hobbies and activities for leisure time, health care resources, and systems of health care and social support. As noted above, advance directives guiding medical therapy in the event of debilitating illness can be extremely valuable. A useful publication on the Medicare insurance program, *Your Medicare Handbook*, is available to patients and physicians. It may be obtained from the Superintendent of Documents, United States Government Printing Office, Washington DC 20402. This concise booklet explains services and provides definitions of terms used by Medicare, e.g., "skilled nursing facility care." An understanding of the Medicare program is important for every elderly citizen. However, Medicare covers only 44% of total health expenditures for the elderly, and therefore the aging patient and his or her family will need sound advice to plan properly for potential health care needs. The physician should encourage utilization of all of these resources by his or her "young" elderly patients before they attain the age at which frailty is more common.

SPECIAL HOUSING

Housing programs primarily for the elderly are increasingly available. States have developed programs where, in the setting of a congregate facility support services such as eating programs or housekeeping, are provided. These programs may be called *sheltered housing* or *elder housing* and are generally available only to individuals who are able to satisfy an economic means test. Information regarding such programs can be obtained through the state or regional office on aging.

Continuing care retirement communities are increasingly available. These require that an elder move (usually while still functionally independent) to a community that provides a variety of resources, and usually includes primary medical care, access to nursing home care and personal care, meal and social programs. Several types of retirement communities exist. Some provide comprehensive services including nursing home and medical service, meals, and programs for an inclusive entrance and monthly fee. Others provide only housing and access to additional services that may be purchased on an a la carte basis. Cost varies tremendously. The physician should advise patients who ask about entering such a community to (a) analyze carefully the services included in the fee, (b) to review the record of the community with the state office on aging, and, (c) review the contract with a lawyer before agreeing to sign it.

Because of the relatively high cost of community care retirement communities, programs are being developed to provide similar support services while patients remain in their own homes. Such programs, typically called social health maintenance organizations or life care at home programs, are still experimental.

OTHER IMPORTANT PROBLEMS OF THE ELDERLY PATIENT

The following problems are discussed in detail elsewhere in this book: constipation (Chapter 39), diverticular disease (Chapter 41), musculoskeletal problems (Section 9), menopause (Chapter 77), osteoporosis (Chapter 77), hearing loss (Chapter 96), skin problems (Chapter 100), dental problems (Chapter 101), disorders of the feet (Chapter 102), hypertension (Chapter 62), cataracts and macular degeneration (Chapter 97), psychiatric illnesses of old age such as dementia (Chapter 17), delirium (Chapter 17), depression (Chapter 15), and bereavement (Chapter 19), and urinary problems such as infection (Chapter 27) and retention.

General References

Action for Independent Maturity: *Looking Ahead: How to Plan Your Successful Retirement.* Washington, DC, American Association of Retired Persons, 1984.
> A 92-page paperback on retirement planning that covers: retirement planning, health and fitness, housing, use of leisure time, and other related topics.

Bowman FJ: *The Complete Retirement Handbook.* New York, Peregee Books, 1983.
> A 249-page paperback covering various aspects of retirement planning.

Cassel CK, Christine K (eds): *Geriatric Medicine,* 2nd ed. New York, Springer-Verlag, 1990.
> A comprehensive two-volume textbook covering all aspects of geriatric medicine.

Downs H: *The Best Years Book.* New York, Delacorte Press, 1981.
> A well known television personality gives his thoughts on retirement.

Hazzard WR, Andres R, Bierman EL, Blass JP (eds): *Principles of Geriatric Medicine and Gerontology,* 2nd ed. New York, McGraw-Hill, 1990.
> A comprehensive textbook of geriatric medicine.

Kane RL, Ouslander JG, Abrass JB: *Essentials of Clinical Geriatrics,* 2nd ed. New York, McGraw-Hill, 1989.
> A short textbook that contains much practical information.

Ouslander JG, Sier HC: Drug therapy for geriatric urinary incontinence. *Clin Geriatric Med* 2:789, 1986.

Resnick NM, Yalla SV: Management of urinary incontinence in the elderly. *N Engl J Med* 313:800, 1985.

Specific References

1. Andres R: Mortality and obesity: the rationale for age-specific height-weight tables. In: Hazzard WR, Andres R, Bierman EL, Blass JP (eds): *Principles of Geriatric Medicine. and Gerontology,* 2nd ed. New York, McGraw-Hill, 1990.
2. Bedell SE, Delbanco TL: Choices about cardiopulmonary resuscitation in the hospital. When do physicians talk with patients? *N Engl J Med* 310:1090, 1984.
3. Blackburn H, Jacobs DR JN: Physical activity and the risk of coronary heart disease. *N Engl J Med* 319:1217, 1988.
4. Buchner DM, Larson EB: Falls and fractures in patients with Alzheimer-type dementia. *JAMA* 257:1492, 1987.
5. Burton JR, Pearce KL, Burgio KL, et al: Behavioral training for urinary incontinence in elderly ambulatory patients. *J Am Geriat Soc* 36:693, 1988.
6. Callahan D: Old age and new policy. *JAMA* 261:905, 1989.
7. Commonwealth Fund Commission on Elderly People Living Alone: *Medicare's Poor.* Baltimore, MD, Commonwealth Fund Commission, 1987.
8. Council on Scientific Affairs—American Medical Association. Elder abuse and neglect. *JAMA* 257:966, 1987.
9. Diabetes Control and Complications Trial. Are continuing studies of metabolic control and microvascular complications in insulin-dependent diabetes mellitus justified? *N Engl J Med* 318:246, 1988.
10. Epstein AM, Hall JA, Besdine R, et al: The emergence of geriatric assessment units: the "new technology of geriatrics." *Ann Intern Med* 106:299, 1987.
11. Feinstein AR, Josephy BR, Wells CK: Scientific and clinical problems in indexes of functional disability. *Ann Intern Med* 105:413, 1986.
12. Fillenbaum GG: Screening the elderly. A brief instrumental activities of daily living measure. *J Am Geriatr Soc* 33:698, 1985.

13. Finucane TE, Shumway JM, Powers RL, D'Alessandri RM: Planning with elderly outpatients for the contingencies of severe illness: a survey and clinical trial. *J Gen Intern Med* 3:322, 1988.

14. Green J: The legal status of consent obtained from families of adult patients to withhold or withdraw treatment. *JAMA* 258:229, 1987.

15. Greenblatt DJ, Sellers EM, Shader RI: Drug disposition in old age. *N Engl J Med* 306:1081, 1982.

16. Griffin MR, Ray WA, Schaffner W: Non-steroidal anti-inflammatory drug use and death from peptic ulcer in elderly persons. *Ann Intern Med* 109:359, 1988.

17. Grover SA, Cook EF, Adam J, et al: Delayed diagnosis of gynecologic tumors in elderly women: relation to national medical practice patterns. *Am J Med* 86:151, 1989.

18. Helms PM: Efficacy of antipsychotics in the treatment of the behavioral complications of dementia: a review of the literature. *J Am Geriatr Soc* 33:206, 1985.

19. Hermanson B, Omenn GS, Kormal RA, Gersh BJ: Beneficial six-year outcome of smoking cessation in older men and women with coronary artery disease: results from the CASS registry. *N Engl J Med* 319:1365, 1988.

20. Jenike MA: Tardive dyskinesia: special risk in the elderly. *J Am Geriatr Soc* 31:71, 1983.

21. Jones J, Dougherty J, Schelble D, Cunningham W: Emergency department protocol for the diagnosis of geriatric abuse. *Ann Emerg Med* 17:1006, 1988.

22. Kasper JD: *Aging Alone: Profiles and Projections*. A report of the Commonwealth Fund Commission on Elderly People Living Alone, Baltimore, MD, 1988.

23. Katz S, Branch LG, Branson MH, et al: Active life expectancy. *N Engl J Med* 309:1218, 1983.

24. Katz S, Stroud MW: Functional assessment in geriatrics. A review of progress and directions. *J Am Geriatr Soc* 37:267, 1987.

25. Kessler DA: The regulation of investigational drugs. *N Engl J Med* 3(20):81, 1989.

26. Kiel DP, Felson DT, Anderson JJ, et al: Hip fracture and the use of estrogens in post-menopausal women. *N Engl J Med* 317:1169, 1987.

27. Klein LE, Tovs RP, McArthur J, et al: Diagnosing dementia: univariate and multivariate analysis of the mental status examination. *J Am Geriatr Soc* 33:483, 1985.

28. Lakshmanan M, Mion LC, Frengley JD: Effective low-dose tricyclic anti-depressant treatment for depressed geriatric rehabilitation patients in a double-blind study. *J Am Geriatr Soc* 34:421, 1986.

29. Larson EB, Bruce RA: Exercise and aging. *Ann Intern Med* 105:783, 1986.

30. Lichtenstein MJ, Federspiel CF, Schaffner W: Factors associated with early demise in nursing home residents: a case-control study. *J Am Geriatr Soc* 33:315, 1985.

31. Lo B, McLeod GA, Saika G: Patient attitudes to discussing life-sustaining treatment. *Arch Intern Med* 146:1613, 1986.

32. Mandelblatt J, Gopaul I, Wistreich M: Gynecologic care of elderly women: another look at Papanicolaou smear testing. *JAMA* 256:367, 1986.

33. Mulrow CD, Feussner JR, Velez R: Re-evaluation of digitalis efficacy: new light on an old leaf. *Ann Intern Med* 101:113, 1984.

34. National Center for Health Services Research. Research Activities. Who takes care of the disabled elderly? 87:1, 1986.

35. National Institutes of Health Consensus Development Conference Statement, 1987. Geriatric assessment methods for clinical decision-making. *Ann Intern Med* 106:299, 1987.

36. Ouslander JG, Leach GE, Staskin DR: Simplified tests of lower urinary tract function in the evaluation of geriatric urinary incontinence. *J Am Geriatr Soc* 37:706, 1989.

37. Ray WA, Griffin MR, Schaffner W, et al: Psychotropic drug use and the risk of hip fracture. *N Engl J Med* 316:363, 1987.

38. Rowe JW: Health care of the elderly. *N Engl J Med* 312:827, 1985.

39. Rowe JW, Kahn RL: Human aging: usual and successful. *Science (Wash DC)* 237:143, 1987.

40. Rubenstein LZ, Josephson KR, et al: Effectiveness of a geriatric evaluation unit. A randomized clinical trial. *N Engl J Med* 311:1664, 1984.

41. Ruchlin HS, Braham RL: Long-term care: a review for the general internist. *J Gen Int Med* 2:428, 1987.

42. Rudd P, Blaschke TF: Antihypertensive agents and the drug therapy of hypertension. In: Goodman AG, Goodman LS, Murad F: *Goodman and Gilman's The Pharmacologic Basic of Therapeutics*. New York, Macmillan, 1985.

43. Sandler DP, Smith JC, Weinberg CR, et al: Analgesic use and chronic renal disease. *N Engl J Med* 320:1238, 1989.

44. Schneider EL, Vining EM, Hadley EC, et al: Recommended daily allowances and the health of the elderly. *N Engl J Med* 314:157, 1986.

45. Steering Committee of the Physician's Health Study Research Group. Final report on the aspirin component of the ongoing physicians' health study. *N Engl J Med* 321:129, 1989.

46. The Medical Letter on Drugs and Therapeutics. Drugs for cardiac arrhythmias: new warning. 31:48, 1989.

47. Tinetti ME, Speechley M, Ginter SF: Risk factors for falls among elderly persons living in the community. *N Engl J Med* 319:1701, 1988.

48. Tinetti ME, Ginter SF: Identifying mobility dysfunctions in elderly patients. *JAMA* 259:1190, 1988.

49. Tinetti ME, Speechley M: Prevention of falls among the elderly. *N Engl J Med* 320:1055, 1989.

C H A P T E R 7

Occupational and Environmental Disease

JAMES P. KEOGH, M.D.

This is an era characterized by widespread proliferation of new and potentially toxic chemicals that are encountered in homes, schools, the general environment, and especially in the workplace. This proliferation has altered our overall environment in ways that affect the health of many individuals. Contamination of air and water from industrial discharges of hazardous waste is reported nearly every day in newspapers all over the country. The extent to which such exposures may be causing unrecognized health problems is a grave concern. In the future, few communities in the United States will escape public scrutiny of the health hazards of pesticide spraying, asbestos in school buildings, contaminated drinking water, or toxic waste disposal.

This chapter provides an overview of how environmental diseases occur and outlines an approach to enable the physician to recognize and deal with them.

Its emphasis on the workplace reflects the fact that clinically diagnosed illness is much more likely to be related to the higher levels of toxic exposure found in this setting. Each year in the United States over 100,000 people die and over 400,000 become ill as a direct result of occupational disease.

VITAL ROLE OF THE PRIMARY PRACTITIONER

Primary practitioners have frequently been the first professionals to recognize the hazards of an occupational exposure, by documenting the link between their patients' illnesses and their patients' work. While the task of following up on such observations involves public health specialists, it is vitally important that primary practitioners take the time to report and follow up suspected occupational diseases. Although theoretically there is a system of surveillance and inspection of workplaces through the Occupational Safety and Health Administration (OSHA), there are, in fact, only enough inspectors to visit every workplace once in about every 200 years. Furthermore, most workers are unaware of their right to request investigation of potential hazards at work, and corporate medical departments and executives usually do not want government inspectors in their plants. Inspectors who do visit workplaces may lack medical training, so that they often focus on safety, rather than on health issues. For these reasons, if a patient has an occupational health problem or is exposed to a dangerous situation at work, physicians and patients need to initiate action to protect the patient and his coworkers.

PATHOGENESIS OF OCCUPATIONAL DISEASE

The pathogenesis of occupational disease is complex and involves not only the interaction between the host and a toxic substance, but a complex set of social interactions as well.

Toxin-Host Interaction

For an occupational disease to occur, there must be a triad consisting of a toxic agent, a host, and an environment in which the host is exposed. The illness that may result depends on the toxic properties of the substance, its route of entry, the dose received by the host, and the susceptibility of the host to the toxin.

Toxic agents can be inhaled, ingested, or absorbed through the skin. With inhalation, the dose received depends on whether the substance is present as a fume or a dust. Deposition of dust in the lungs depends to a great extent on particle size and distribution, since smaller particles can more easily enter the alveoli and become trapped. The concentration of the substance in the air (which is related to room ventilation, temperature, and humidity), the rate at which the worker is exercising and breathing, protective factors such as special clothing or respirator use are other factors that affect the likelihood of illness.

Once the toxic substance is absorbed there may be an instantaneous effect as in the case of carbon monoxide poisoning, a brief latent period as in the case of occupational asthma, or a latent period of years or decades as in the pneumoconioses. A brief, high dose exposure may cause serious illness and death and be relatively easy to recognize. On the other hand, prolonged exposure to a low dose of a toxin may not cause symptoms at the outset, and yet may produce disease years later.

Economic Factors Affecting Pathogenesis

Thousands of new chemicals are introduced into industrial processes every year; few have had testing to detect their potential toxicity. Even when toxicological screening tests are done on a compound, these may not predict human disease. In all too many cases, the hazardousness of a chemical is recognized only after an outbreak of illness.

Economic factors play a major role in determining how safe a workplace is. Industrial hygiene programs to monitor exposure are common only in the largest plants. Important decisions such as improving ventilation or decreasing exposure to noise may involve significant expense. Therefore management must weigh the benefits of protecting employee health against the cost of doing so. A company that consistently chooses health over profits may find itself at a distinct competitive disadvantage.

Workers may be reluctant to complain about working conditions for fear of losing their jobs. This is especially likely during periods of high unemployment, when acceptance of unpleasant and potentially unhealthy working conditions may be the price of having a job. Physicians who fail to recognize this may be perplexed by their patients' unwillingness to take action to secure better conditions at work.

Even when workers are strongly organized, the desire for a safer workplace may be balanced by a concern that increased production costs may result in the decision of a company to relocate its plant to areas where unions are less effective or do not exist.

Despite these factors that tend to make occupational illness more common, progress has been made. Increasingly, American workers and businessmen are both developing the knowledge needed to prevent workplace illness and demonstrating a willingness to place a higher priority on people than on profits. Stringent health and safety regulations with strong enforcement can put competitors on a more equal footing and protect responsible businesses from being undercut by irresponsible ones.

DIAGNOSING WORK-RELATED DISEASE

Although episodes of illness caused or exacerbated by the patient's work are frequently seen in ambulatory practice, they are frequently not recognized as such, and they are not appropriately managed. The consequences of not considering an occupational disease are that the patient does not benefit from correct diagnosis and management, and there is no alteration

in the poor working conditions that may subsequently injure others or even result in death.

Two cases illustrate these points:

Case: A Teenager with Bronchitis

An 18-year-old woman complained to her physician of a severe cough and some wheezing. The physician treated her with erythromycin and fluids and advised her to stay in bed for a few days. She recovered and returned to work feeling well. Several days later she had a severe recurrent cough with wheezing and dyspnea and saw her physician again. The physician again prescribed erythromycin and rest. She remained off work for a week. She felt better and returned to work. After 2 days she became extremely short of breath and was brought to the emergency room. She had severe bronchospasm and was admitted, improving on bronchodilators and corticosteroids after a few days.

History on admission disclosed that her work involved grinding drill bits made of tungsten carbide, a known pulmonary sensitizer. Having been sensitized, each fresh exposure to the dust caused symptoms after a shorter incubation period. Had the first physician considered the diagnosis of extrinsic asthma and inquired about occupational exposures he could have prevented the patient's subsequent deterioration.

Case: A Grouchy Man with a Headache

A 25-year-old man presented to the emergency room of a community hospital with a chief complaint of headache. When seen by the physician he was hostile and complained bitterly about having waited 45 minutes to be seen. He said he had had increasingly severe headaches for several weeks. He initially refused physical examination, pointing out that the pain was only in his head, and insisted "what I really need is something stronger for the pain." Physical examination was negative and he was given an aspirin-narcotic compound.

Seen some weeks later, a coworker warned him that his lead level might be high, and a family member contacted the health department. In addition to the persisting headaches, a history of irritability, abdominal pain, insomnia, and constipation was elicited. The patient worked in an automobile assembly plant where he used a grinding wheel to smooth joints filled with a lead-containing solder. He had actually been under surveillance for lead poisoning, with regular measurement of blood lead level, but the plant physician did not inform workers of their results. His blood lead level had been steadily rising and was 3 times normal. After therapy with a chelating agent he became symptom free. Subsequent investigation revealed that most of his coworkers had high blood lead levels; three of them were subsequently treated for lead poisoning. Questioning the patient about his work could have saved him weeks of discomfort and prevented some of his coworkers from being poisoned.

To avoid the pitfalls these cases demonstrate, the primary practitioner needs to remember only three important principles:

1. Ask every patient about his or her job.
2. Consider the possibility that the patient's illness is related to work or home environment.
3. Follow up on your suspicions. Others may be in danger.

Taking an Occupational History

Inquiring about a patient's job will not only help to identify occupational disease, it will provide other information useful in caring for a patient. Clearly the physical demands of the job are important when advising a patient about a health problem, such as coronary artery disease or diabetes mellitus. Knowing the patient's work schedule is also important since shift work affects medication schedules, diet, and family life. Medications can dramatically affect the patient's comfort or safety at work (e.g., diuretics in an interstate truck driver or antihistamines in an ironworker). Financial and psychological stress may result from layoffs, whereas regular overtime may bring about chronic fatigue and psychological problems of its own. Usually, a brief discussion of the current job, including a brief description of how the patient spends his working day, is sufficient. This rarely takes more than 3 minutes. The major points to cover in this inquiry are summarized in Table 7.1.

When some aspect of the medical or occupational history has raised suspicions of a work-related condition, further questioning will flow naturally. The inquiry should focus upon a temporal relation between symptoms and possible exposure, upon exposure to an agent known to cause disease, or upon a pattern of similar illness among coworkers. Because every patient, every job, and every medical presentation is different, there is no single way of taking a history. If the patient uses jargon or job titles that are unfamiliar, he should be asked for clarification.

Table 7.1.
Components of an Occupational History

Description of the job
  Physical exertion
  Body mechanics
  Pace of work
  Repetitive tasks
  Job stress

Exposure to hazards
  Risk of trauma
  Dusts, fumes, mists
  Contamination of skin and clothing
  Noise and vibration
  Heat and cold
  Ionizing and nonionizing radiation

Protective measures
  Ventilation and respiratory protection
  Protective clothing
  Medical surveillance

Effects of exposure
  Temporal relation of any symptoms to work, e.g., relation to time of day, day of week, change of symptoms on vacation, weekends
  Similar symptoms in coworkers

The screening history will sometimes reveal the need to take a lifelong work history. An account of the previous jobs and exposures is especially important when the patient has a chronic illness or the possibility of work-related neoplasia. In such cases, the following approach is recommended:

1. Begin with parents' jobs and childhood exposures.
2. Review each of the patient's jobs in chronological order.
3. Elicit relevant aspects of each period of employment (see Table 7.1).

Diseases That Are Commonly Related to Work

The occupational diseases that one will encounter depend upon one's location in the United States, the industry in the immediate vicinity, and the demographic makeup of the practice. For example, practitioners near retirement communities may see retired workers with previous exposure in all types of industry. Table 7.2 lists selected examples of clinical problems grouped according to the organ system affected.

Dermatitis and pneumoconiosis are the most frequently reported occupational illnesses. This probably reflects both true incidence (skin and pulmonary epithelium are most in contact with the outside environment) and the greater likelihood of recognition of these disorders as being occupational in origin.

The number of chemicals that are toxic to the *liver and kidney* is so great that a careful exposure history should be taken from all patients with hepatitis and hepatic or renal failure. Many chemicals can affect the gastrointestinal tract and cause functional disturbances that may be misdiagnosed as peptic disease or irritable bowel syndrome.

Low level exposure of the *respiratory organs* to a variety of substances may result in the production of nonspecific upper respiratory syndromes that the patient may describe as an intractable cold or as sinus trouble.

Although occupational diseases periodically present with striking and unusual signs (such as acro-osteolysis in vinyl chloride workers or nasal septal perforation in patients exposed to chromates), more commonly they present with the vague systemic symptoms typical of early intoxication.

There are a few specific clinical situations that deserve to be highlighted:

Any change in personality or behavior. Poisoning due to mercury, lead, pesticides, and a wide variety of other central nervous system toxins may present this way.

New onset of asthma. Owing to the time lapse when an immunological mechanism is involved, wheezing and dyspnea may not be noted until after the workday is over.

Any case of pulmonary fibrosis. A prolonged latent period between exposure and disease onset means that abnormalities that appear on X-ray may result from a job the patient had decades ago.

Table 7.2.
Common Medical Problems with Examples of Environmental Causes

Clinical Problem	Causative Agent	Clinical Problem	Causative Agent
CONSTITUTIONAL		Convulsions	Aldrin
Fever	Heat		2-Aminopyridine
	Radiant heated air		Camphor
	Microwaves		Chlordane
	Metal fumes:		Crag herbicide
	Zinc		DDT
	Copper		Decaborane
	Magnesium		2,4-Dichlorophenoxyacetic acid
	Cadmium		Dieldrin
	Dinitrophenol		1,1-Dimethylhydrazine
	Pentachlorophenol		Endrin
	Dinitro-o-cresol		Heptachlor
	Polymer fume (polytetrafluorethylene)		Hydrazine
SKIN			Lindane
Sweating	Organophosphates		Methoxychlor
	Pentachlorophenol		Methyl bromide
	Dinitro-o-cresol		Methyl chloride
Cyanosis	Methemoglobin formers:		Methyl iodide
	Aniline		Methyl mercaptan
	Anisidine, ortho- and para- isomers		Monomethylhydrazine
	Dimethylaniline		Nicotine
	Dinitrobenzene, all isomers		Nitromethane
	Dinitrotoluene		Oxalic acid
	Monomethylaniline		Pentaborane
	p-Nitroaniline		Phenol
	Nitrobenzene		Rotenone
	p-Nitrocholorobenzene		Sodium Fluoroacetate
	Nitrogen trifluoride		Strychnine
	Nitrotoluene		Tetraethyllead
	Perchloryl fluoride		Tetramethyllead
	n-Propyl nitrate		Tetramethylsuccinoitrile
	Tetranitromethane		Thallium, soluble compounds
	o-Toluidine		Toxaphene
	Xylidine	Headaches	Carbon monoxide
Contact dermatitis	Many chemicals with irritant or sensitizing properties		Nitrites
			Nitrates
Chronic eczematous dermatitis	Solvents		Alcohols
	Detergents		Lead
Folliculitis	Oil exposure		Organic lead compounds
	Grease exposure		Methemoglobin formers (see under cyanosis)
Acne	Polychlorinated biphenyls	Behavioral change	Mercury
	Chlorinated naphthalenes		Lead
	Paraffin		Carbon disulfide
	Coal tar		Carbon monoxide
	Dioxin		Methyl chloride
Photosensitization	Coal tar		Methyl bromide
	Pitch	Ataxia, tremor, spasticity	Manganese
	Asphalt		Organic lead compounds
	Anthracene		Organic tin compounds
	Creosote	Hyperreflexia, micrographia	Mercury
	Fluorescein		DDT
	Phenanthrene	Peripheral neuropathy	Peripheral neurotoxins:
Granulomas	Beryllium		Acrylamide
Corns	Asbestos		Arsenic and compounds
	Fiberglass		Calcium arsenate
Punctate ulcers	Chromic acid		Carbon disulfide
Painful burns	Hydrofluoric acid (deep pain out of proportion to appearance of burn)		n-Hexane
			Lead and inorganic lead compounds
Skin cancer	Soots		Dimethylaminopropionitrile
	Tars		Lucel-7 (2-t-butylazo-2-hydroxy 5-methyl hexane)
	Arsenic		Mercury
	Coke oven emissions		Methyl bromide
	Cutting oils		Methyl butyl ketone
	Sunlight		Thallium, soluble compounds
NERVOUS SYSTEM			2,4,6-Trinitrotoluene
Central Effects			Tri-o-cresyl phosphate
Altered consciousness	Hundreds of chemicals have central nervous system (CNS)-depressant properties and other CNS effects	EYE	
		Conjunctivitis	Ultraviolet radiation (welder's flash)
			Many irritant chemicals

Table 7.2. *Continued*

Clinical Problem	Causative Agent	Clinical Problem	Causative Agent
Corneal irritation or scarring	Acids		Organic mercury
	Alkalies		Phosphorus
	Dimethyl sulfate		Sodium nitrate
	Formaldehyde	Otitis externa	Contamination of earplugs used for noise protection
	Methyl dichloropropionate		
	Osmic acid	Ear pain	Acute shifts in pressure
	Sulfur dioxide	SMELL	
	1-Butanol	Anosmia	Arsenic
	Xylene		Benzine
	Diazomethane		Benzol
	Dichlorobutenes		Cadmium
	Ethylene oxide		Carbon disulfide
	Ethylenimine		Chromium
	Hydrogen sulfide		Ethyl acetate
Corneal edema producing "haloes" around lights	Allyl alcohol		Formaldehyde
	Amines		Hydrazine
	Morpholines		Iodine
	Diethyldigylocolate		Ketone
	Diisopropylamine		Lead
	3-Dimethylamino propylamine		Mercury
	Ethylenediamine		Nickel
	Tetraethylbutanediamine		Osmium tetroxide
	Triethylenediamine		Phosphorus oxychloride
Scarring and discoloration	Benzoquinone		Phthalic anhydride
	Aniline		
Corneal discoloration as a manifestation of systemic intoxication	Arsine	Anosmia (continued)	Potassium iodide
	Nitrobenzene		Selenium
	Siler		Sulfuric acid
Cataracts	Radiant heat		
	Microwave exposure	TASTE	
	Dinitro-o-cresol	Decreased acuity	Bromine
	Dinitrophenol		Caprolactam
	Sunlight	Alterations in taste	Iodine
Lens deposits and discoloration	Copper		Phosgene
	Iron		Antimony
	Mercury		Arsenic
	Phenylmercuric salts		Bismuth
	Silver		Cadmium
Optic neuritis—visual acuity and visual field defects	Carbon dioxide		Copper
	Carbon monoxide		Gallium
	Carbon disulfide		Lead
	Cyanide		Mercury
	Methanol		Nickel
	Methyl mercury		Nitrogen dioxide
	Naphthalene		Selenium
	Thallium		Tellurium
	Lead		Thallium
	Acetylphenylhydrazine		Vanadium
	Benzene		Zinc oxide
	Triethyl tin	RESPIRATORY	
	Phosphorus	Nasal septal perforation	Chromic acid and other chromates
	Ethylene glycol	Laryngeal carcinoma	Asbestos
Nystagmus and extraocular muscle palsy	Carbon disulfide	Laryngitis, bronchitis, tracheitis, pneumonitis	Many irritants including:
	Dieldrin		Ammonia
	Ethanol		Chlorine
	Ethylene Glycol		Oxides of nitrogen
	Lead		Ozone
	Methyl bromide		Phosgene
	Methyl chloride		Sulfur dioxide
	Methyl iodide		Vanadium pentoxide
	Triethyl tin		Mercury
Eye strain—visual fatigue	Visual display terminals		Manganese
			Cadmium dust
HEARING		Bronchiolitis obliterans	Nitrogen dioxide
Decreased acuity and tinnitus	Noise exposure especially above 85 decibels	Allergic alveolitis:	Many different antigens for example:
		Bagassosis	*Thermoactinomyces vulgaris* and *Micropolyspora* sp.
Acoustic neuritis	Aniline		
	Arsenic	Bird-breeder's lung	Avian proteins
	Carbon monoxide	Byssinosis	Cotton, flax, and soft fiber hemps
	Hypoxia	Cheese-washer's lung	*Penicillium caseil*
	Lead	Detergents	*Bacillus subtilis*

Table 7.2. *Continued*

Clinical Problem	Causative Agent	Clinical Problem	Causative Agent
Farmer's lung	*Micropolyspora faeni* and *Thermoactinomyces vulgaris*		Carbon disulfide
			Carbon tetrachloride
Feathers	Feather proteins		Chlorodiphenyl
Furrier's lung	Keratinized particles of hair		Chloroform
Malt-worker's lung	*Aspergillis clavatus*		*p*-Dichlorobenzene
Maple bark-stripper's disease	*Cryptostroma corticale*		Dimethylacetamide
			Dimethylformamide
Paprika-splitter's lung	*Mucor stolinifer*		Dioxane
Bronchospasm	Pulmonary sensitizers:		Ethylene chlorohydrin
	Castor bean pomace		Ethylene dibromide
	Cobalt, metal fume and dust		Ethylene dichloride
	Enzymatic detergents		Hexachloronaphthalene
	Grain dusts		Kepone
	Maleic anhydride		Nitroethane
	Methylene bisphenyl isocyanate		Octachloronaphthalene
	Methyl isocyanate		Pentachloronaphthalene
	Nickel, metal		Picric acid
	p-Phenylenediamine		Tetrachloroethane
	Phthalic anhydride		Tetrachloroethylene
	Platinum salts		Tetrachloronaphthalene
	Polyvinyl chloride (fume from heated film: meat-wrapper's asthma)		Trichloronaphthalene
			2,4,6-Trinitrotoluene
	Toluene 2,4-diisocyanate	Jaundice	Hepatoxins (see above)
	Tungsten carbide		Hemolytic agents:
	Western red cedar		Arsine
	Plicatic acid		Butyl cellosolve
Pulmonary fibrosis	Asbestos		Naphthalene
	Silica		Phenylhydrazine
	Beryllium		Stibine
	Talc	Angiosarcoma of liver	Vinyl chloride
	Coal dust	Abdominal pain	Antimony
	Cobalt		Arsenic
	Hematite		Bromine
	Kaolin		Cadmium
Benign pneumoconiosis deposits in lung without fibrosis	Aluminum powder		Lead
	Barium		Mercury
	Graphite		Nicotine
	Iron oxide		Organophosphates
	Tin		Thallium
	Cerium oxide		Many other chemicals when ingested
	Silver	CARDIOVASCULAR SYSTEM	
	Titanium		
Pleural effusion	Asbestos	Myocardial damage	Antimony
	Paraquat		Arsine
	Talc		Carbon disulfide
GASTROINTESTINAL			Cobalt
Gingivitis and gum pigmentation	Mercury	Ischemic disease	Nitroglycerin
	Lead		Nitrogycol
	Bismuth		Other vasodilating nitrates
Dental erosion	Acetic acid	Hypertension	Noise exposure
	Hydrochloric acid		Aminopyridine
	Lactic acid		Arsenic
	Nitric acid		Barium
	Nitrogen dioxide		Boron hydride
	Sulfuric acid		Carbon disulfide
Tongue paresthesias	Furfural		Cobalt
	Rotenone		Diphenyl
	Cresol		Lead
Green tongue	Vanadium		Mercury
Nausea and vomiting	Many chemicals including:		Thallium
	CNS depressants	Vasospastic disorders "White finger"	Vibrating tools
	Cholinesterase inhibitors		
	Methemoglobin formers	Raynaud's phenomenon	Vinyl chloride
Constipation	Lead	GENITOURINARY	
	Barium sulfate	Renal disease	Nephrotoxins:
	Thalium		4-Aminodiphenyl
	Tellurium		Cadmium
	Vanadium		Carbon disulfide
	Fluorides		Carbon tetrachloride
Hepatomegaly	Hepatoxins:		Chloroform
	Acetylene tetrabromide		

Table 7.2. *Continued*

Clinical Problem	Causative Agent	Clinical Problem	Causative Agent

Renal disease (continued)	Dioxane
	Ethylene chlorohydrin
	Ethylene dibromide
	Lead
	Mercury
	Oxalic acid
	Picric acid
	Tetrachloroethane
	2,4,6-Trinitrotoluene
	Turpentine
	Uranium (natural), soluble and insoluble compounds
		HEMATOLOGICAL PROBLEMS
		Anemia
			Lead
			Hemolytic agents:
			  Arsine
			  Butyl cellosolve
			  Naphthalene
			  Phenylhydrazine
			  Stibine
			Marrow depressants:
			  Benzene
			  Dinitrophenol
			  Tetryl
			  2,4,6-Trinitrotoluene

Renal carcinoma	4-Aminodiphenyl Auramine Benzidine β-Naphthylamine 4-Nitrodiphenyl Magenta	Leukemia	Benzene Radiation Styrene-butadiene Ethylene oxide
Urinary retention Urinary frequency	Dimethylaminopropionitrile Chloroform Fufuryl alcohol Oxalic acid	Splenomegaly	Beryllium Methyl chloride Naphthalene Naphthol Nitrobenzene Phosphorus Resorcinol
REPRODUCTIVE ABNORMALITIES Female sterility Male sterility	 Lead Carbon disulfide Dibromochloropropane (DBCP) Lead Microwaves to testes (radar workers) Stilbestrol	MUSCULOSKELETAL Osteonecrosis Osteomalacia Osteosclerosis Acro-osteolysis	 Phosphorus Cadmium Fluorine Vinyl chloride

Peripheral neuropathy. A toxic neuropathy may be recognizable by an unusual pattern of presentation, but in most cases only careful history taking will reveal the cause.

Hearing loss. Noise-induced hearing loss occurs gradually and usually in older workers, so that it is rarely recognized in time to prevent severe damage.

Inability to conceive. More and more compounds that affect the reproductive system and cause sterility are being identified.

Lung cancer. Exposure to asbestos and cigarette smoke are very common throughout the United States. Other lung carcinogens may be important in certain parts of the country.

Other cancers. Specific carcinogens are identified in Table 7.3.

Determining Work Relatedness

The key to identifying occupational disease is to be sure that a toxic/environmental etiology is at least considered. In addition, the patient should always be asked, *"Do you think this problem could have anything to do with your work?"* and, *"Does anyone else at work have this same problem?"* Very often, if there is a connection, the patient will be able to identify it.

If neither the physician nor the patient knows if a syndrome is occupational in origin, there are resources available that identify (*a*) toxic causes of a given symptom complex, (*b*) toxic exposures of given professions, and (*c*) the potential hazards of exposure to given substances (Table 7.4).

FOLLOW-UP OF OCCUPATIONAL DISEASE

Physician's Role

If there is suspicion that a patient became ill from an occupational exposure, it is the physician's responsibility to follow up. Not only does diagnosing an occupational disease affect therapy and eligibility for compensation for a patient, but it may indicate that the health of others is also in danger. Often physicians overcome their own uneasiness about a patient's job by advising the patient to change jobs. Then, instead of the potentially hazardous job being made safe, another unsuspecting person is brought in to take the risk.

There are some circumstances in which occupational disease is recognized but the original hazard has been eliminated—for example, a patient with asbestosis who worked in a now closed shipyard. Even in these circumstances, former fellow workers need to be informed of the risk resulting from previous exposure.

It is not necessary to wait for absolute proof of etiology before beginning an investigation of a possible workplace hazard. The least severely affected member of a group of workers may be the one who seeks attention. Moreover, for most occupationally induced diseases, proof of a relationship rests on epidemiological data rather than on diagnostic study of the individual patient. Often the most practical way to learn whether a patient's problems are caused or exacerbated by his occupation is to find out whether fellow workers are similarly affected.

Table 7.3.
Cancers Presently Known to Be Caused by Environmental Agents

Site/Cell Type	Toxic Agent	Industry/Occupation
Liver/hemangiosarcoma	Vinyl chloride monomer	Vinyl chloride polymerization industry
	Arsenical pesticides	Vintners
Nose	Hardwood dusts	Woodworkers, cabinet, furniture makers
	Radium	Radium chemists and processors, dial painters
	Chromates	Chromium producers, processors, users
	Nickel	Nickel smelting and refining
	Unknown agent	Boot and shoe industry
Larynx	Asbestos	Asbestos product manufacture, shipbuilding, construction and maintenance work
Lung	Asbestos	Asbestos product manufacture, shipbuilding, construction and maintenance work
	Coke oven emissions	Topside coke oven workers
	Radon daughters	Uranium and fluorspar miners
	Chromates	Chromium producers and processors, users
	Nickel	Nickel smelters, processors, users
	Arsenic	Smelters
	Mustard gas	Mustard gas formulators
	Bis (chloromethyl) ether, chloromethyl methyl ether	Ion exchange resin makers, chemists
Pleura and peritoneum/mesothelioma	Asbestos	Asbestos product manufacture, shipbuilding, construction and maintenance work
Bone	Radium	Dial painters, radium chemists and processors
Scrotum	Mineral/cutting oils	Automatic lathe operators, metalworkers
	Soots and tars, tar distillates	Coke oven workers, petroleum refiners, tar distillers
Bladder	Benzidine, α- and β-naphthylamine, auramine, magenta, 4-aminobiphenyl, 4-nitrophenyl	Rubber and dye workers
Esophagus	Asbestos	Asbestos product manufacture, shipbuilding, construction and maintenance work
Stomach	Asbestos	Asbestos product manufacture, shipbuilding, construction and maintenance work
Colon	Asbestos	Asbestos product manufacture, shipbuilding, construction and maintenance work
Kidney	Coke oven emissions	Coke oven workers
Hematopoietic/lymphoid leukemia, acute	Unknown	Rubber industry
	Ionizing radiation	Radiologists
Myeloid leukemia, acute	Benzene	Refining, chemical, and manufacturing industries
	Ionizing radiation	Radiologists
Erythroleukemia, acute	Benzene	Refining, chemical, and manufacturing industries

Health Department

In many states, there is a health department unit for investigation of occupational disease. Some states require physicians to report all cases of suspected occupational disease. Such laws should and probably will become more widespread. Reporting any suspected occupational disease problem to the local health department can be the first step in follow-up.

Occupational Safety and Health Administration (OSHA)

Although health departments generally have authority to investigate occupational diseases, regulation of workplace conditions is usually the responsibility of a separate state agency or of the local office of the Occupational Safety and Health Administration in the United States Department of Labor (telephone number is listed under United States Government, Labor Department, OSHA). When a state has taken over OSHA enforcement, its regulations are required to be as strict as the federal regulations. In every state, every employer is obligated to report workplace injuries and illness to OSHA.

If other workers may be in imminent danger of being made ill, the physician should communicate this urgently to OSHA to promote an immediate investigation. In most cases OSHA enforcement officers are able to determine relatively easily whether regulations are being violated at a workplace, and they will provide a follow-up report to the referring physician. In some cases, the inspection may suggest that the patient's illness was job related, but that at the time of the inspection no specific OSHA regulation was being violated. If a continuing hazard does exist, OSHA can force changes by invoking the employer's "general duty" to maintain a safe workplace. Especially in these situations the physician may need to be patient but persistent to see that appropriate action is taken.

National Institute of Occupational Safety and Health (NIOSH)

If there is difficulty in clarifying the potential relationship of illness to environment, or if the concerns raised are not addressed by a specific OSHA regulation, it may be helpful to request assistance from the National Institute of Occupational Safety and Health

Table 7.4.
How to Determine the Potential Hazards of an Exposure

1. Characterize the exposure to the extent possible, including the chemical identity of substances; type and wavelength of radiation, light, or noise; likely route of entry; concentration of chemical substance or intensity of energy course; available protection.

2. Look it up in available references:

If you know:	*Then*:
Only a trade or code name	Call the employer to get the chemical identity or at least the name of the manufacturer, then call the manufacturer of the substance to learn the contents;
	or use:
	Gosselin RE, Smith RP, Hodge HC: *Clinical Toxicology of Commercial Products*, 5th ed. Baltimore, Williams & Wilkins, 1984.
The identity of the chemicals or energy	Use the information on the Material Safety Data Sheet only as a guide, confirm health effects from an independent source.
	Look it up in one of the general references listed at the end of this chapter.
	or:
	Use the National Library of Medicine TOXNET (you can access this through Grateful Med on one of many commercial data base). Ask the local librarian for help. Some toxins have separate listing in Toxline and Medline
	or:
	Call your local poison control center for fast help;
Only the general nature of the patient's work	Get an idea of exposures from the patient, the employer or union, or a consultant (see below).

3. Call a consultant:
Your state or local health department may be able to help identify the nature of the problem and even help you get clinical advice. A number of states with "right to know" laws have set up information clearinghouses.
The National Institute of Occupational Safety and Health has a Clearinghouse for Occupational Safety and Health Information. Staff members welcome physicians' inquiries and have rapid access to information and expertise. Telephone 513-533-8326.
The Agency for Toxic Substances and Disease Registries can help with environmental and community exposure issues. Telephone 404-488-4100.

(NIOSH). This institute is that part of the United States Public Health Service (USPHS) Centers for Disease Control that conducts research on occupational disease. An employer, union, or any three employees can request a formal Health Hazard Evaluation (HHE) of a workplace. Furthermore, NIOSH now has Educational Resource Centers (where consultants are available to help physicians, employers, and workers) available in each region of the country. These centers can provide literature searches and information on available publications and current areas of research, and can refer a physician to others who are experts in the field. Access to regional centers can be provided by the central office.

In addition to its investigatory function, NIOSH can provide assistance directly regarding a physician's concern about a patient's exposure. Its clearinghouse responds to practitioners' inquiries with information about the hazards of particular trades and toxic substances. Physicians can contact NIOSH at 513-533-8326.

Consultants

Consultants who are particularly knowledgeable about specific problems are increasingly available to help the practicing physician. Poison centers through their national network of contacts can usually identify an appropriate expert for telephone consultation about an acute problem. The Association of Occupational and Environmental Clinics (AOEC), a national network of primarily university-based clinics, can be contacted at 203-776-8884 to identify resources available in most parts of the country.

WORKER'S COMPENSATION

Every state has a worker's compensation act that provides a system of dispensing funds for medical expenses related to occupational disease and injury and for employee's lost earnings. These laws were passed to provide a "no fault" system of compensating workers injured on the job, and to provide employers with a statutory protection from being sued for negligence by their employees. In almost all states an injured worker or his family may not sue an employer but is entitled to receive prompt compensation for lost earning ability without having to go through a lengthy legal proceeding.

Although this system works well in some situations for on-the-job injuries, it does not respond well to the needs of a worker with an occupational disease. Here the burden of proof that the disease is work related falls on the worker, and the process of obtaining compensation is often slow and difficult. Because most small employers insure themselves with an insurance company, the insurer may delay action on a claim even when the employer himself believes the illness was caused by the job. Usually the worker can obtain legal assistance without having to pay an attorney directly, because provision is made for cases to be taken on a contingency basis (i.e., the attorney receives no fee unless the claim is upheld, and then he receives a fixed percentage). Because illness claims are usually complex, the worker will often need such expert advice.

If a physician concludes or even strongly suspects that a patient has an illness caused or made·worse by his job, the patient should be encouraged to file for worker's compensation (through his employer, the worker's compensation local office, or his lawyer).

There are two reasons for this. First, if a claim is pursued and won (even though it takes time), the patient is usually guaranteed lifetime medical coverage from worker's compensation funds for that illness. Compensation may lift some of the financial burdens from the patient and his family, particularly in cases of chronic or fatal diseases. Second, worker's compensation has the potential to encourage safety and to penalize careless employers.

To a great extent worker's compensation has failed in the area of occupational disease, chiefly because of inadequate physician diagnosis and follow-through. For example, a 1980 Department of Labor survey showed that only 3% of workers disabled by occupational respiratory disease were receiving compensation. The 97% of the disabled workers who were not receiving worker's compensation were living on Social Security or welfare. Their medical bills were being paid by health insurance, Medicare, or state welfare funds. Thus, the economic and social costs of industrial disease are largely borne not by the companies who may have acted irresponsibly but by the victims and the taxpayers, including those businesses that are trying to protect their employees properly.

Physicians are often reticent about involvement with worker's compensation, feeling that a claim may tie them up in court. This is an unsubstantiated fear since the medical record usually provides sufficient medical evidence and the physician does not have to appear at the hearing. If the record does not provide adequate information, the attorneys involved will almost always be willing to take a statement at the physician's convenience.

PART-TIME PLANT PHYSICIAN

A primary practitioner may become involved in a workplace at the invitation of the employer or the union representing the employees. Many small- and medium-sized workplaces need the assistance of part-time physicians to conduct effective programs to detect and prevent occupational disease. The practitioner should welcome the chance to do something to prevent illness but must take special care to meet the ethical obligations such a role requires. Many physicians in occupational medicine regard themselves as responsible to the management of the company that pays them, rather than to the patients they serve. In some instances, physicians have withheld information from patients about work-related diseases. In other cases, physicians modify their therapy for illnesses and injuries to meet the needs of production rather than the needs of the patient. This role of the "com-

pany physician" as servant of management rather than of the patient has had tacit acceptance in the past. In the last decade the American Occupational Medical Association, composed principally of industry-employed physicians, has called for adherence to ethical practice, and many abuses have been ended. Any physicians today who practice as plant physicians differently from the way they practice in their own office may face professional discipline and malpractice suits. In some plants, workers and management are following the Swedish model of jointly selecting a plant physician. Table 7.5 summarizes the principal ethical responsibilities of a plant physician.

HAZARDS AT HOME AND IN THE COMMUNITY

Exposures at Home

The average American home is a Pandora's box of potentially harmful exposures. Between kitchen, bathroom, garage, and garden, family members may have access to caustics, a variety of aerosols, pesticides, solvents, paint removers, adhesives, and electrical equipment. It is important to consider these types of exposure when warning about childproofing for toddlers and when evaluating dermatoses and allergic reactions. Exposures at home may also produce illness in ways that come less readily to mind (see Table 7.6). Case reports have documented poisoning from unwise use of cosmetics and vitamin supplements. Many hob-

Table 7.5.
Responsibilities of the Plant Physician

The primary responsibility of the physician is to the individual patient, no matter who is paying the bill.

The physician may reveal nothing to others, including management, about the patient without his permission. Reports should be limited to a statement about the patient's illness to work and any specific limitations of activity.

The physician must acquire all available information about the workplace that may be relevant to a patient's health.

Everything that the physician learns or may deduce about the safety of the workplace must be explained to those whose health may be affected.

The physician should report occupational disease to the local health department or state OSHA.

The physician should not take sides in any dispute between the management, the workers, or the government, but should only provide accurate information and honest opinion to all concerned.

Table 7.6.
Common Hazards at Home

Heating and air conditioning
Insulation and lack of ventilation
Vitamins and health foods
Cleaning chemicals
Electrical appliances
Water supply
Hobbies
Home repair
Neighborhood pollution sources

bies can involve exposure to chemicals with fewer protections than workers in industry may enjoy. For example, lead poisoning has been documented from ceramics, stained glasswork, and cosmetics; paint strippers containing methylene chloride can produce carbon monoxide poisoning sufficient to aggravate angina and precipitate infarction; and injudicious combinations of cleaning materials can release hazardous fumes.

Homes themselves may have hazards. For example, lead-containing paints are a risk to both children and do-it-yourselfers, and formaldehyde-urea foam insulation can release sensitizing fumes. In cases of illness caused by such exposures, physicians need to take a careful history to recognize the cause.

Heating and ventilation systems deserve special mention. Even up-to-date heating systems can produce carbon monoxide poisoning if flues are blocked or inadequate air for combustion is provided. Because symptoms of early carbon monoxide poisoning are nonspecific and mimic those of stress and depression, a high level of suspicion is critical, especially early in the heating season. With the current emphasis on increased insulation and barriers to air infiltration, houses are often poorly ventilated by fresh air. The increasing use of wood, coal, and kerosene heaters may make matters worse. Use of scrap lumber treated with chemical preservatives is an additional hazard.

Office and commercial buildings are also increasingly "tight," due to recirculation of heated or cooled air. A large number of epidemics of illness caused by chemical or biological agents circulated through the air are being reported. Building-associated illness can be caused by exposure to particulates, to chemical fumes from cleaning materials and office equipment, and from mold spores and other biological antigens. Because symptoms are often nonspecific, diagnosis may depend on recognizing a temporal pattern or symptoms in coworkers. Evaluation of the ventilation system often reveals inadequacies and in many situations improved ventilation may be all the therapy that is needed.

Exposures from Sources in the Community

Physicians are increasingly being asked for advice relating to concerns about contamination of drinking water and air and the cleanup of toxic wastes. Many communities dependent on groundwater have had their supplies threatened by illegal dumping of chemicals or by leakage from licensed landfills.

The discovery of a *chronic source of environmental contamination* is an experience few American communities will escape. There is no substitute in such situations for enlisting the assistance of appropriate experts, and physicians in a community need to take the lead in getting help from state and local agencies. Often there is a continuing role for practitioners to play in facilitating the resolution of problems. In many cases, knowledgeable specialists, have difficulty in

translating what they have to say into language that the lay public can understand. Physicians who spend their entire days translating medical science into advice for their patients in the office, are well suited to serve in this role. At the same time, community members may need someone who can represent their acute personal concerns to the authorities in a reasoned way. The physician may have to serve as the advocate and critical reviewer of the community, making sure that the statements and positions of all of those involved are supported by factual evidence and calling on independent expertise when appropriate. The Agency for Toxic Substances and Diseases Registries (USPHS) has made a commitment to support physicians in communities affected by environmental contamination with information and assistance. Emergency help is available 24 hours a day at 404-488-4100.

Air Pollution

Patients with respiratory disease are especially concerned about the effects of air pollution. There is little evidence to implicate general community air pollution as the primary cause of individual patient illness, except in unusual circumstances. Patients often do develop symptoms of upper respiratory irritation during periods of severe pollution, and patients with cardiac or respiratory disease may suffer exacerbations. Prudent advice is in order in such situations. Advice to move to less polluted areas is rarely a good idea, and such advice should be given only after a great deal of thought about the impact of a move on the patient's entire life. The lack of convincing data linking air pollution with huge excesses in mortality is not a reason

Table 7.7.
Checklist for Physicians Involved in Hazardous Substances Incidents

1. What toxic and hazardous substances have been identified?
   a. What are the concentrations in air, water, and soil?
   b. What are the known health hazards at these concentrations?
   c. What are the potential hazards of fire, explosion, or chemical interactions?
2. How many persons have been exposed and how many are likely to become exposed in the near future?
   a. What groups in the exposed population are likely to be most susceptible to health effects?
   b. How many exposures are resulting in hospital admissions? Outpatient visits?
   c. What clinical findings, if any, are being observed?
3. What technical resources are available on short notice to assist in evaluation and control? Is there a local Hazardous Materials Team?
4. Is the community adequately handling the casualties?
   a. What is the capacity of local hospitals, clinics, and physicians to absorb the additional caseload?
   b. Should hospital disaster plans be mobilized?
   c. Are intensive care or specialty services adequate or available to the degree needed?
   d. Are local physicians experienced and knowledgeable about this kind of problem? If not, what is the best way to obtain expert help quickly?
5. Is this community covered by a control data repository (such as a tumor registry or population-based research study) that could be used to follow the exposed population in the future?

for physicians to be complacent about it in their own communities. Alleviating the immediate discomfort that air pollution causes to nearly everyone and freeing patients with pulmonary disease from imprisonment in their homes during pollution alerts ought to be motivation enough for physicians to join in the battle for clean air. Pollution of indoor air in workplaces and in public facilities from cigarette smoking is an equally important challenge to the medical profession.

Hazardous Materials: Accidents and Disposal

Physicians with no special background in toxicology or public health may be pressed into service in cases of accidental emissions of toxic fumes or accidents involving transport of hazardous materials.

In responding to such emergencies, a practitioner should clarify immediately that the hazard is being contained as effectively as possible, that individuals not needed at the scene are not being allowed to become exposed, and that orderly procedures for the care of casualties are being set up. Many communities have developed a coordinated plan for response to hazardous materials incidents. Usually the local emergency response system (fire department or 911 system) will alert a "HAZMAT" team. A checklist is provided in Table 7.7.

General References

Cullen MR, Cherniack MG, Rosenstock L: Occupational Medicine. *New Engl J Med* 322(9 & 10):594, 1990.
> Up-to-date review emphasizing occupational disorders by body system.

Himmelstein JS, Frumkin H: The right to know about toxic exposures. *N Engl J Med* 312:687, 1985.
> Critical review of facts clinicians should know about the subject.

Levy BS, Wegman DH, David H (eds): *Occupational Health: Recognizing and Preventing Work-Related Disease.* 2nd ed. Boston, Little, Brown, and Co, 1988.
> Excellent introductory text for the practitioner, still very inexpensive.

Merchant JA, Boehlecke BA, Taylor G (eds): *Occupational Respiratory Diseases.* [DHHS (NIOSH) Publication No. 86–102], Washington, D.C., US Government Printing Office, 1986.
> A well-written and illustrated guide published by NIOSH.

Proctor NH, Hughes JP: *Chemical Hazards of the Workplace.* Philadelphia, JB Lippincott, 1978.
> A thorough text on chemical hazards. It includes a section on diagnostic principles.

Rom WN (ed): *Environmental and Occupational Medicine.* Boston, Little, Brown, and Co, 1983.
> An excellent text.

Rosenstock L, Cullen MR: *Clinical Occupational Medicine.* Philadelphia, WB Saunders, 1986.
> A good pocket-sized manual organized both by organ system and by type of hazard.

Zenz C: *Occupational Medicine.* Chicago, Year Book Medical Publishers, 1988.
> A large text, worth the investment for the physician involved in part-time occupational medicine practice.

CHAPTER 8

Primary Care of the Patient with Cancer

LARRY WATERBURY, M.D.
MICHAEL PURTELL, M.D.

The purpose of this chapter is to examine the role of the general physician in the care of patients who have cancer. Common cancers are discussed in other chapters (breast, Chapter 89; lung, Chapter 56; gastrointestinal, Chapter 38; prostate, Chapter 49; gynecological, Chapter 95, skin, Chapter 100). The estimated distribution of newly-diagnosed cancers and of cancer deaths for 1990 is depicted in Figure 8.1.

GENERAL ASPECTS OF CARE

Communicating the Diagnosis

The primary physician is the one who is most likely to evaluate a patient for cancer and to communicate the diagnosis. During these initial steps, the following elements are important: (a) prompt scheduling of tests and notification of results; (b) when the diagnosis is cancer, clear communication (e.g., use of the word "cancer" rather than vague terms such as "a growth") and ample time for the patient to react to this news; (c) prompt explanation of options/recommendations, based upon the type and extent of the cancer.

INITIAL REFERRAL AND TREATMENT

When possible, one should refer patients to oncologists whom one trusts and knows to be helpful, considerate clinicians. Multimodality treatment regimens involving the combined efforts of surgical, medical, and radiation oncologists may result in a bewildered patient without a physician who accepts the primary

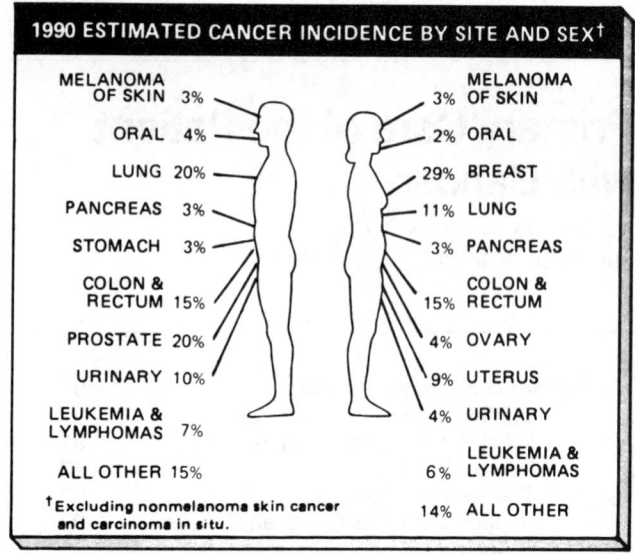

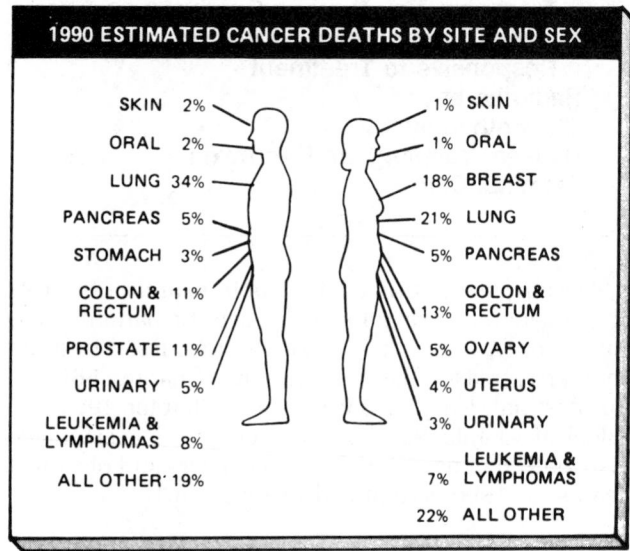

Figure 8.1. Estimates of the American Cancer Society for distribution of newly-diagnosed cancers and cancer deaths, 1990. Source: CA-A Cancer Journal for Clinicians 40:9, 1990.

responsibility for his care; and the patient's personal physician may need to intercede in order to identify who will be the coordinator for the patient's care and who will be accessible to the patient to answer questions, provide support, improve communications, etc. By receiving up-to-date and complete information about the diagnostic and therapeutic plans and about the patient's evolving status, the general physician may be able to assess the overall picture and, as time goes on, to identify when problems resulting from treatment (side effects, expense, family disruption, deteriorating psychological status of patient, etc.) outweigh the likely benefits of continued therapy.

FOLLOW-UP CARE

Many oncologists welcome participation of the patient's personal physician in continuing care. This is particularly important when treatment has been given in an oncology center in a distant city. Some less toxic ambulatory treatment regimens may even be given by the primary physician under the direction of the specialist.

The follow-up of treated patients who may or may not be cured requires knowledge of the common sites and manifestations of tumor recurrence and the appropriate timing of follow-up examinations and tests, as well as a great deal of sensitivity in recognizing the feelings of the individual patient. Some patients function better if scheduled to be seen less frequently, not to be constantly reminded of the possibility of recurrence. Others require the constant reassurance of a negative examination and normal tests and are more comfortable with frequent follow-up visits. Usually there is room for considerable flexibility in a follow-up plan without jeopardizing the care of the patient.

Whenever a cancer patient is seen in follow-up, it is important to explain carefully the meaning of symptoms or physical findings and the rationale for tests. If tests will take several days to return, that should be explained and a time for a phone follow-up arranged.

The Family's Concerns

The crises attending evaluation for possible cancer and the diagnosis and care for cancer profoundly affect the spouses and families of cancer patients. Common dilemmas for family members include emotional strain, physical demands in caring for the patient, altered roles and lifestyles, finances, and uncertainty about prognosis (13). In addition there may be questions about the likelihood of cancer occurring in other members of the family. Each of these dilemmas may require consideration by the patient's primary physician (see for details chapters on specific cancers and Chapters 11, Office Psychotherapy, and 19, Dying, Death, and Bereavement).

Support from The American Cancer Society

The American Cancer Society has chapters in each state and can provide a variety of services to cancer patients and their families. Services vary from state to state but may include loan of supplies (e.g., hospital beds), transportation to treatment facilities, reduced costs for chemotherapy, respite coverage for caregivers, and a wide range of information about support groups and other help available in the patient's community.

NONOPERABLE CANCERS IN WHICH TREATMENT MAY PROLONG SURVIVAL

Table 8.1 lists a number of nonoperable cancers in which survival may be prolonged by modern treatment regimens; patients with such cancers should be referred to cancer specialists. These patients frequently benefit from multimodality treatment. Even within this group of cancers, when specialty help is needed, the general physician will continue to play

Table 8.1.
Some Nonoperable Cancers in Which Treatment Prolongs Survival[a]

Acute leukemia
Hodgkin's disease
Lymphoma
Metastatic testicular cancer
Metastatic ovarian cancer
Small cell carcinoma of the lung
Metastatic breast cancer

[a] Patients with these cancers require specialized treatment, frequently in centers where multimodality therapy is available.

Table 8.2.
Some Cancers in Which Treatment Provides Palliation in Some Patients: Effects on Survival Unproven or Controversial

Non-small cell lung cancer (unresectable)
Metastatic large bowel cancer
Metastatic stomach cancer
Metastatic pancreatic cancer
Metastatic malignant melanoma
Metastatic soft tissue sarcomas
Metastatic cervical cancer
Metastatic endometrial cancer
Metastatic hypernephroma
Metastatic prostate cancer (when patient relapses on hormonal therapy)

an important role, especially if the relationship with the patient or the family has been a lengthy one.

CANCERS UNRESPONSIVE OR POORLY RESPONSIVE TO TREATMENT

Table 8.2 lists a number of cancers less responsive to therapy, when the impact of therapy on survival is unproven or controversial. Diagnosis and initial therapy usually require surgery, but when metastasis is proven, the effect of systemic therapy or radiotherapy or both is at most palliative (21, 22). In such situations, patients often expect their personal physicians to help them select or to actually recommend treatment plans. Several questions will come up at this juncture:

1. *Should palliative therapy be recommended?* Although difficult to generalize, a number of factors must be considered in attempting to help patients and their families decide whether the patient is likely to benefit from palliative therapy. More than age, the functional status of the patient must be considered in such therapeutic decisions. The infirm, ill, poorly functional patient with widely disseminated and rapidly progressive disease may be more harmed by the side effects and discomforts of palliative treatment than benefited, especially if response rates are small and toxicity of treatment is high. Weight loss before therapy correlates remarkably with poor response rates in clinical chemotherapy trials in these less responsive cancers (5). Other patients, even if elderly, in good functional status are much more suitable candidates for attempts at palliation. The patient who feels that any chance of response is worth the price of toxicity, and who cannot feel comfortable unless at-

tempting some therapy, should generally be offered treatment.

2. If some attempt at palliative treatment seems worthwhile, *should it be conventional therapy or experimental protocol therapy?* Every oncology center has current protocols for the metastatic cancers that are listed in Table 8.2. Clinical protocols designed to seek improved methods of treatment are important for advances that may improve the outlook and the comfort of future patients. However, experimental therapy may have undesirable consequences for the individual patient. Frequently, such protocols involve the investigation of treatments with more toxicity than current conventional therapies. They usually require more frequent visits to the physician as well as more frequent diagnostic tests, because of the necessity to document precisely the objective response. They may therefore also involve increased expense to the patient. Patients agreeing to experimental protocol therapy—and their physicians—must be well informed about the side effects and likely benefits of therapy (17). The helpful consultant should describe the currently popular treatment for the patient's disease and should be able to tailor the recommendation to the specific patient. No treatment, conventional low dose palliative chemotherapy or radiotherapy, and experimental therapy are all appropriate choices for individual patients in various clinical situations. Table 8.3 lists the major considerations for patient and physician in selecting among these options.

RADIOTHERAPY

The patient with cancer frequently has misconceptions about and limited knowledge of radiotherapy. It is thus important to explain radiotherapy to the patient in terms of the rationale, experience, and likely benefits of this treatment modality. The initial visit usually includes a focused history and physical examination by the radiotherapist. Further diagnostic tests [X-rays, computerized tomography (CT) scan, etc.] may be obtained. If the therapist agrees that treatment is appropriate, the radiotherapy ports may actually be determined at the first visit; and the patient may receive his first treatment at that time. The patient should be told that skin markings may be placed in order to facilitate the uniformity of subsequent treatments, and that these markings must not be removed. It is im-

Table 8.3.
Factors Affecting Palliative Treatment Recommendations in Patients with Cancer

The natural history of the untreated cancer
The proven effect of treatment on the natural history
 Likely effects on survival
 Likelihood of lessening morbidity
Toxicity of treatment
Functional status of the patient
Ability of the patient to comprehend the implications of treatment
Psychological state and philosophical position of the patient
Emotional strength, and attitudes of immediate family
Financial situation, health coverage status

portant to explain that the therapy machines are bulky and somewhat overwhelming in appearance. Many patients are likely to be frightened by the experience; and if the referring physician appreciates this, it is useful to contact the radiotherapist and to explain the particular fears of the patient ahead of time. Therapists will often give patients and their families a tour of the radiotherapy treatment rooms before starting therapy and will spend extra time answering questions about the treatment and its benefits and complications. The patient should be aware that the treatment itself is not painful. The initial consultation is usually time consuming (several hours), but subsequent treatments are usually scheduled precisely and require only a small amount of time (30 minutes). Treatments are usually given several days a week, and the entire course may take several weeks to complete. The patient usually will not see the radiotherapist at the time of each treatment but will be seen by a radiotherapy nurse or technician. He therefore needs to know precisely with whom to communicate if he has side effects or questions during radiotherapy.

In addition to the timing and types of side effects that the patient may experience, it is important for him to know that the response to treatment is frequently delayed and that sometimes the maximal effect is noted a few weeks after the course of radiotherapy is completed. For example, radiotherapy is useful in the palliation of pain secondary to local bony metastases, but 2 to 3 weeks may elapse before improvement occurs; and improvement may not be maximal until a few weeks after treatment is discontinued. Some responses are more rapid, occurring after only a few days of therapy [e.g., relief of superior vena caval obstruction and neurological deficits from spinal cord obstruction or central nervous system (CNS) metastasis].

Table 8.4 describes important side effects of radiotherapy. The patient will be most concerned by those common side effects that occur during treatment and by those that may remain for a few weeks after treatment is discontinued.

Dermatitis secondary to radiotherapy is less common than it used to be, owing to the use of the modern high energy machines. Severe burning requiring specialized treatment is quite uncommon; however, skin discoloration may occur. The patient should be told that the radiation field should not be exposed to sunlight or extreme cold, and that total, but temporary, hair loss will usually occur in the areas being radiated and that complete return of hair, after high dose radiation, may take many months.

The most troublesome side effects that occur during radiotherapy are gastrointestinal. Patients receiving radiation to the chest or upper back frequently experience symptoms of radiation esophagitis (odynophagia and sometimes reflux symptoms that may respond to elevation of the head of the bed and to antacids). Severe esophagitis is more likely to occur when radiotherapy has been used in patients who have had prior chemotherapy especially with such agents

Table 8.4.
Important Side Effects of Radiotherapy (4, 6, 9, 15, 20, 21ᵃ)

Dermatitis (less common with newer high energy machines; avoid sunlight and extreme cold).
Acute radiation pneumonitis (transient, usually occurring 6–12 weeks after treatment; precipitated by corticosteroid withdrawal, concomitant chemotherapy; clinical manifestations include nonproductive cough, dyspnea, fever, leukocytosis with parenchymal infiltrates on X-ray in the area of the radiation ports; may respond to steroid treatment) (9).
Pulmonary fibrosis (occurs 6–12 months after treatment, not responsive to steroids) (9).
Esophagitis (usually occurs during treatment; particularly severe when radiotherapy and adriamycin are administered together).
Nausea, vomiting, and diarrhea (occur during treatment with most abdominal radiotherapy, usually self-limited).
Enteritis (rare, more likely with very high dose treatment; small bowel more sensitive than large bowel and stomach; occurs weeks to years after radiotherapy; manifestations include obstruction, bleeding, perforation; pelvic irradiation, *e.g.*, in the treatment of bladder or prostate cancer, may cause acute *proctitis* which occasionally becomes chronic sometimes leading to bleeding or stricture formation) (15).
Pericarditis (occurs months to years after radiation, usually resolves, occasionally progresses to constrictive pericarditis or to tamponade requiring pericardiectomy) There is also an increased incidence of coronary artery disease seen after mediastinal irradiation (16).
Neurological side effects (transverse myelitis, very rare; side effects from CNS irradiation in adults are infrequent (5); Lhermitte's sign (the sensation of electric shocks passing down the body when the head is flexed) seen in 10% of patients undergoing mantle irradiation for Hodgkin's disease; after radiotherapy herpes zoster is common).
Hypothyroidism (common in patients treated for Hodgkin's disease with mantle field; may develop years after treatment).
Sterility (usually temporary).
Growth retardation in children (occurs both from direct skeletal effects and from hypopituitarism from CNS irradiation).
Dental side effects (severe dental problems are common after head and neck irradiation because of decrease in saliva formation, increased sensitivity to caries, osteonecrosis) (20).
Cystitis (occurs during treatment with pelvic irradiation; clinical manifestations include urgency dysuria and hematuria occurring usually during the third and fourth weeks of treatment; usually self-limited and treated symptomatically with fluids and phenozopyridine (Pyridium), 200 mg four times a day; chronic bladder fibrosis is a rare late complication manifested usually by painless hematuria).

ᵃ Data used are from sources listed in "Specific References."

as doxorubicin, bleomycin, or cis-platinum. Superinfection of the irritated esophagus with *Candida* is not unusual, especially in patients who are receiving steroids. This usually responds to treatment with oral nystatin (Mycostatin, suspension 100,000 U/ml, 5 ml every 4 hours). Clotrimazole troches (Mycelex troches, one troche dissolved in the mouth five times daily) are also effective and more palatable. Oral ketoconazole (Nizoral) is frequently effective in nystatin failures (200-mg tablets, one daily by mouth). Patients should improve within 1 week of therapy. Occasionally short courses of amphotericin are necessary to cure *Candida* esophagitis, but that treatment is best given in the hospital. Abdominal irradiation may cause diarrhea that may persist to some degree during the entire course of treatment. Other than the importance of replacing fluids and electrolytes, there are some dietary maneuvers that may minimize diarrhea; these are listed in Table 8.5. Nausea and anorexia are the most troublesome side effects of abdominal irradiation and are discussed separately below.

Patients who receive radiotherapy to the head or neck are subject to special dental complications. Before treatment all patients should have a complete den-

Table 8.5.
Dietary Maneuvers for Therapy-Induced Diarrhea

Clear liquids (warm or at room temperature)
Avoid fiber (roughage) in the diet
Take smaller amounts of food more often
Avoid fatty foods
Avoid highly spiced foods
Avoid carbonated drinks, beans, cabbage, broccoli, cauliflower, and corn

Table 8.6.
Common Side Effects of Chemotherapy[a]

Hair loss—alkylating agents, vincristine, vinblastine, adriamycin, mithramycin, daunomycin (7).[b]
Hypercalcemia—estrogens, antiestrogens (tamoxifen).
Fluid retention—estrogens, androgens, steroids.
Skin darkening—adriamycin (nails), 5-FU, bleomycin, busulfan, methotrexate (7).[c]
Dermatitis—methotrexate, 6-MP, 6-thioguanine (7).
Marrow depression—alkylating agents, vinblastine, nitrosoureas, methotrexate, adriamycin, cytosine arabinoside, daunomycin, 5-FU, mithramycin, mitomycin C, cis-platinum, procarbazine, hydroxyurea, 6-MP (10).
Neurological—cis-platinum (deafness), vincristine, vinblastine, methotrexate, hexamethylmelamine, 5-FU, procarbazine (11).
Gastrointestinal ulcerations—methotrexate, 5-FU, bleomycin (mucocutaneous), adriamycin.
Cardiomyopathy—adriamycin, daunorubicin (24).
Pulmonary fibrosis—bleomycin, alkylating agents, mitomycin-C (8).
Renal damage—cis-platinum, methotrexate, streptozotocin, ifosphamide, nitrosoureas (23).
Red urine—adriamycin, daunomycin.
Hepatic toxicity—mithramycin, methotrexate, nitrosoureas, cytosine arabinoside, 6-MP (19).
Sexual and gonadal dysfunction—(3).
Secondary neoplasm—alkylating agents, combination chemotherapy, and especially chemotherapy and radiotherapy (12).

[a] From Perry MC: Chemotherapy, toxicity and the clinician. *Semin Oncol* 9:1, 1982.
[b] Data used are from sources listed in "Specific References."
[c] 5-FU, 5-fluorouracil; 6-MP, 6-mercaptopurine.

tal examination by a dentist experienced in the treatment of patients who have undergone radiotherapy. Damage to the teeth, gums, and bone, plus the xerostomia that results from high dose radiotherapy to the oral mucous membranes and salivary glands, may result in severe problems. Many of these can be prevented by appropriate prophylaxis (aggressive treatment of periodontal disease and of infected teeth before radiation) and an ongoing program during and after radiotherapy, which should be strictly followed. The use of artificial saliva (Saliva Substitute, Roxane Laboratories) may be helpful for patients with xerostomia.

The patient's primary care physician may sometimes be involved with the early treatment of CNS metastases or spinal cord compression, using corticosteroids. Multiple regimens are used. A common regimen consists of dexamethasone (Decadron), 4 to 25 mg four times a day, continued until the patient has received several courses of radiotherapy and then slowly tapered over 2 to 3 weeks. Steroids decrease the local edema that occurs in these situations and help to protect against radiation-induced edema during the first few days of therapy.

An excellent booklet, *Radiation Therapy and You: A Guide to Self-Help During Treatment*, is available free from the National Institutes of Health, to patients undergoing radiotherapy. It is helpful to have copies of this booklet available for patients and families to read when radiotherapy is being considered.

CHEMOTHERAPY

The chemotherapy experience for the patient is so varied (depending on the disease being treated) that it is hard to give a general description. The medical oncologist giving therapy can best explain to the patient the specifics of treatment, including how it is administered, the frequency of treatment, the hoped for response, and the side effects. The most frequent troublesome side effects for the patient are hair loss and nausea and vomiting. The frequency and degree of hair loss vary with the treatment regimen, but it is helpful for the patient to know that hair will regrow once the treatment is discontinued. The treatment of nausea and vomiting is discussed below. Table 8.6 lists other acute and chronic side effects of various chemotherapeutic agents. Knowledge of the long-term side effects of various agents is particularly important for the primary physician who may be responsible for follow-up care of patients with good prognoses after chemotherapy.

There is an excellent free booklet, *Chemotherapy and You: A Guide to Self-Help During Treatment*, on chemotherapy written for patients which is available through the National Institutes of Health (see General References). It is helpful to have this booklet available for patients and families to read when chemotherapy is being considered.

NAUSEA, VOMITING, AND ANOREXIA

Nausea and vomiting are by far the most troublesome and common side effects of both radiotherapy and chemotherapy. Unfortunately the symptomatic treatment of nausea is only moderately effective. However, there are a number of maneuvers that may help to limit the degree of nausea after chemotherapy or radiotherapy. For example, it is frequently helpful for the nauseated patient to be extremely still, lying down in a quiet room without external stimuli. Antiemetics may help but unfortunately may not eliminate the nausea completely, especially that associated with intense chemotherapy regimens. However, for more mild regimens the use of a conventional antiemetic such as prochlorperazine (Compazine) orally or by rectal suppository (e.g., 10-mg capsule orally every 6 hours or 25-mg suppository two to four times daily) may be helpful. Patients in intensive chemotherapy programs, especially with regimens including cis-platinum, are benefited by treatment with high doses of metoclopramide (60 to 120 mg/m² intravenously every 2 hours during cis-platinum infusion), lorazepam (1 to 2 mg intravenously), and corticosteroids (dexamethasone, 10 to 20 mg intravenously) (1, 2, 14).

There are a number of dietary maneuvers that may

be helpful to the patient experiencing nausea and vomiting after therapy (Table 8.7). The patient who experiences severe nausea and vomiting after therapy should probably only drink clear liquids until the symptoms are decreased. In general it is more helpful to take smaller portions of food frequently than to take larger meals less often, to take foods that are low in fat, and to avoid overly sweet foods. Mild nausea, especially that experienced before therapy or in anticipation of therapy, may be helped by taking dry toast or crackers in small quantities. It is recommended that patients do not lie down just after eating. Some patients find also that it is helpful not to drink liquids with their food, (as this may increase their feeling of bloating and subsequent nausea). Many patients become nauseated at the smell of food cooking, and it may be helpful for them to go to another part of the house or to stay out of the house when food is being prepared. Greasy and fried foods seem to be the worst offenders in this regard and are best avoided.

One of the major problems with intensive cancer therapy is general anorexia, which may result in considerable nutritional problems and weight loss. Consultation with a dietitian may be extremely helpful in such a situation.

There is an excellent booklet, *Eating Hints: Recipes and Tips for Better Nutrition During Cancer Treatment*, free and available through the National Institutes of Health (see "General References"). It contains all sorts of dietary advice for cancer patients including many recipes.

TERMINAL CARE

The primary physician who has participated in various phases of the cancer patient's care and who has an ongoing relationship with him and his family is frequently in the best position to help during a patient's terminal illness. The physician who develops some expertise in this regard can find enormous gratification from this role. Chapter 19 deals with many of the issues important in caring for terminal patients including the very important issues of pain control and hospice care. An excellent publication entitled *Coping with Cancer: A Resource for the Health Professional* is available free of charge from the National Institutes of Health (see "General References"). In addition to other useful information, it lists organizations and agencies that provide useful services that may aid the physician in providing support for the dying cancer patient.

Table 8.7.
Dietary Maneuvers for Therapy-Induced Nausea

Smaller portions eaten more slowly
Avoid foods high in fat, and greasy and fried foods
Clear, cool liquids between meals
Crackers or toast
Rest (sitting, not lying) after eating
Avoid food odors (during preparation)

General References

Cancer chemotherapy. *Med Letter* 31:49, 1989.
    Useful review of drugs, toxicities, and indications.
Portlock CS, Goffinet DR (eds): *Manual of Clinical Problems in Oncology.* 2nd ed. Boston, Little, Brown, and Co, 1987.
    Excellent, brief, clinically oriented oncology manual.
Rubin P (ed): *Clinical Oncology: A Multidisciplinary Approach.* 6th ed. New York, American Cancer Society, 1983 (new edition projected for 1990).
    Provided free of charge by the American Cancer Society. Excellent condensed data about all cancers and their treatment.
Booklets from the National Institutes of Health cited in this chapter are available free of charge from The Office of Cancer Communications, Department of Health and Human Services, NIH, Bethesda, Maryland, 20205, telephone: 301-496-4070.

Specific References

1. Aapro MS, Plezia PM, Alberts DS, et al: Double-blind crossover study of the antiemetic efficacy of high-dose dexamethasone versus high-dose metoclopramide. *J Clin Oncol* 2:466, 1984.
2. Cassileth PA, Lusk EJ, Torri S, et al: Antiemetic efficacy of dexamethasone therapy in patients receiving cancer chemotherapy. *Arch Intern Med* 143:1347, 1983.
3. Chapman RM: Effect of cytotoxic therapy on sexuality and gonadal function. *Semin Oncol* 9:84, 1982.
4. Deutsch M, Parsons JA, Mercado R Jr: Radiotherapy for intracranial metastases. *Cancer (Phila)* 34:1607, 1974.
5. Dewys WD: Prognostic effect of weight loss prior to chemotherapy in cancer patients. *Am J Med* 69:491, 1980.
6. Donaldson SS, Lenon RA: Alterations of nutritional status: impact of chemotherapy and radiation therapy. *Cancer (Phila)* 43:2036, 1979.
7. Dunagin WG: Clinical toxicity of chemotherapeutic agents: dermatologic toxicity. *Semin Oncol* 9:14, 1982.
8. Ginsberg SJ, Comis RL: The pulmonary toxicity of antineoplastic agents. *Semin Oncol* 9:34, 1983.
9. Gross NJ: Pulmonary effects of radiation therapy. *Ann Intern Med* 86:81, 1977.
10. Hoagland HC: Hematologic complications of cancer chemotherapy. *Semin Oncol* 9:95, 1982.
11. Kaplan RS, Wiernik PH: Neurotoxicity of antineoplastic drugs. *Semin Oncol* 9:103, 1982.
12. Kyle RA: Second malignancies associated with chemotherapeutic agents. *Semin Oncol* 9:131, 1982.
13. Lewis FM: The impact of cancer on the family: a critical analysis of the research literature. *Patient Educ and Counseling* Elsevier Scientific Publishers Ireland Ltd., 269–289, 1986.
14. Meyer BR, Lewin M, Drayer DE, et al: Optimizing metoclopramide control of cisplatin-induced emesis. *Ann Intern Med* 100:393, 1984.
15. Morgenstern L, Thompson R, Friedman NB: Radiation enteritis. *Am J Surg* 134:166, 1971.
16. Muggia EA, Cassileth PA: Constrictive pericarditis following radiation therapy. *Am J Med* 44:116, 1968.
17. Penman DT, Holland JC, Bakna GF, et al: Informed consent for investigational chemotherapy: patients' and physicians' perceptions. *J Clin Oncol* 2:849, 1984.
18. Perry MC: Chemotherapy, toxicity and the clinician. *Semin Oncol* 9:1, 1982.
19. Perry MC: Hepatotoxicity of chemotherapeutic agents. *Semin Oncol* 9:65, 1982.
20. Regeyi JA, Courtney RM, Kerr DA: Dental management of patients irradiated for oral cancer. *Cancer (Phila)* 38:994, 1976.
21. Richter MP, Coia LR: Palliative radiation therapy. *Semin Oncol* 12:375, 1985.
22. Romond EH, Metcalfe MS, Macdonald JS: Palliative chemotherapy and hormonal therapy. *Semin Oncol* 12:384, 1985.
23. Schilsky RL: Renal and metabolic toxicities of cancer chemotherapy. *Semin Oncol* 9:75, 1982.
24. Van Hoff DD, Rozencwieg M, Piccart M: The cardiotoxicity of anticancer agents. *Semin Oncol* 9:23, 1982.

C H A P T E R 9

Selected Special Services: Disability Insurance, Vocational Rehabilitation, and Home Health Services

L. RANDOL BARKER, M.D.

INTRODUCTION

Maintenance of a patient's overall health often requires efforts beyond those of the physician and the patient. Frequently assistance comes from community-based programs to which physicians may refer their patients. Many of these programs provide services for patients with specific types of illness; the roles of such categorical community services are described in the appropriate chapters in this book. Other services are designed to assist sick persons regardless of their type of illness. This chapter describes two fundamental services of this kind: (a) Social Security income support programs for disabled persons and (b) home health services. The purposes of the chapter are to explain eligibility for these services, the nature of the benefits, and the role of physicians in enabling their patients to receive these services. Chapter 7 provides similar information about another noncategorical program, workmen's compensation, which is designed to provide coverage for health care costs and income support to persons with work-related diseases.

SOCIAL SECURITY PROGRAMS FOR DISABLED PERSONS

Loss or decrease of a person's ability to earn a living accompanies many illnesses. Beginning with 1954 amendments to the Social Security Act, income support for medically disabled persons has been available in the United States. Further modifications since 1954 have led to the program that exists today. Five fundamental benefits are presently available: Disability Insurance (DI), Supplemental Security Income (SSI),

Vocational Rehabilitation (VR), Medicare (for DI recipients), and Medicaid (for SSI recipients). Detailed information about each of these services is available from any local Social Security office.

Definition of Medical Disability

Under Social Security, disability is defined as "inability to engage in any substantial gainful activity by reason of a medically determinable physical or mental impairment that can be expected to result in death or has lasted or can be expected to last for a continuous period of not less than 12 months . . ."

Disability Insurance (DI—Title II)

Eligibility

To be eligible for disability insurance payments, a disabled worker must have paid into the Social Security program for a minimal period of time before becoming disabled; in addition there is a requirement for coverage during 5 of the 10 years before the onset of disability. Today, 9 of 10 workers pay the Social Security tax. For younger workers (up to age 31) there are modified requirements to meet insured status.

The dependents of a fully insured worker who is retired, disabled, or deceased may be eligible for disability insurance payments in two situations: (a) a child who became disabled before age 22 (eligible for disability insurance payments at the time that his parent retires, becomes disabled, or dies; payments may begin as early as age 18 and continue as long as the child's disability lasts); and (b) a widow or widower who is between 50 and 59 years of age and who did not work under Social Security but who became medically disabled before or within 7 years of the death of a fully insured spouse.

Benefits

Disability insurance payments go to disabled workers before the age of 65 (after 65, Social Security Retirement Income replaces disability payments) and to eligible children, widows, or widowers as long as they remain disabled. The first monthly disability insurance check is not paid for the first 5 months after the onset of the worker's disability (for example, if a patient is certified as disabled 6 calendar months after he actually became disabled, he immediately becomes eligible for a check covering the 1 month in excess of the required 5-month wait). Supplemental Security Income (see below) is often awarded to persons who qualify for disability benefits, effective the date they apply for benefits. There is no waiting period. Income from DI for a disabled worker is the same amount as the retirement income the worker would receive if he were 65. The average monthly payment to a disabled worker in 1987 was $508, and to a worker with a wife and dependent children, $918. In that year, 2,786,000 workers and 1,259,000 spouses and children were receiving DI benefits.

In addition to income support, disabled persons under 65 receive Medicare (Social Security Health Insurance) after they have been eligible for disability benefits for 24 months.

Process of Disability Determination

There are three basic steps in the process of determining medical disability.

First Step. The patient completes a detailed application at a local Social Security Office. The patient must not be gainfully employed at the time of application. Most patients will initiate disability claims by themselves, but at times the physician may be helpful in suggesting early application to a patient who may not be aware that his medical condition qualifies him for medical disability.

Second Step. The patient's physician receives a request for medical information and returns this report to the state Disability Determination Office. The report sent by the patient's physician should be succinct and precise, and it should provide objective data regarding the condition for which disability is being claimed. It should be divided into the following subheadings: history, physical, laboratory reports, diagnosis, treatment, and response. The information provided should permit the claims reviewers to determine both the severity and the duration of the patient's condition. If malingering is suspected, the report should describe the circumstances that raise doubts rather than recording this assessment without supporting information. In this report the physician is not expected to rate the ability of the patient to work. The most helpful guide for completing these medical reports is the booklet entitled Disability Evaluation under Social Security (available free from any Social Security Office or the State Disability Determination Office). This manual, which was most recently published in 1986, contains the criteria for medical disability for most common conditions. These criteria are the basis for most allowances made by disability claims reviewers. Table 9.1 through Table 9.6 contain excerpts from this manual illustrating the criteria for several common conditions that may cause medical disability: symptomatic ischemic heart disease, chronic obstructive airways disease, cerebrovascular accident, epilepsy due to major motor seizures, arthritis of a major weight-bearing joint, and rheumatoid arthritis. Since 1980, the Social Security Administration has paid a small fee to physicians for medical reports for the DI program; a small fee has also been paid for SSI reports since the inception of that program in 1974. Previously patients were expected to pay for these reports. In some states, doctors also have access to a free teledictation service for dictating their reports.

Third Step. The information provided by the patient and the physician (the disability claim) is reviewed at the State Disability Determination Office by a team consisting of a disability claims examiner and a physician. If deemed necessary, an independent medical examination is purchased by the Disability Determination Office. In keeping with the 1974 Freedom of Information Act, patients may have access to their disability claims files. If an insured worker has an impairment that does not meet the standard criteria for disability but that nevertheless prevents the individual from doing his usual job, other factors (limitations of age, education, training, work experience) may also be considered by the Disability Determination team in determining whether the individual is unable to perform any gainful work found in the national economy. Most findings of disability are, however, based on the standard Social Security criteria.

Appeal Process

If the initial claim of disability has been denied, the claimant may file for reconsideration within 60 days of receiving a denial notice. The case will then be reevaluated by a different claims examining team. If the claim is denied at this reconsideration, the claimant then has 60 days to file a request for a hearing. Hearings are conducted by administrative law judges. If the claim is again denied, the claimant may make an additional appeal for review by the Appeals Council. After that the case may be taken to the United States District Court.

The patient's personal physician can be instrumental in assuring that the patient gets the fullest consideration throughout the Disability Determination process. If the physician feels that there are aspects of the patient's illness that make it more severe than the criteria indicate, the physician should communicate this information in writing, together with support for this opinion, to the Disability Determination Office.

Return to Work

All claims are reviewed for referral to Vocational Rehabilitation (see below) at the time the disability decision is made. In addition, every person with a permanent impairment is reevaluated every 7 years; and all other persons (i.e., those with impairments that may not be permanent) are reevaluated at least every 3 years to determine whether they are still disabled. Even if the original impairment, on review, is judged not to be severe, payments are continued while the patient enters the vocational rehabilitation program. These two processes and the following conditions are designed to encourage disabled persons to return to work: (a) Disabled beneficiaries may test their ability to work for 9 months while continuing to receive benefits. After this trial work period, a determination is made about whether the work constitutes substantial gainful activity (defined as an activity that yields a monthly income of $300 or greater); if it does, benefits are suspended after an additional 3-month adjustment period. (b) If a person who still has a disabling impairment stops work again within 36 months after Social Security payments have been suspended because of substantial gainful activity, the monthly DI benefits can be resumed, usually without a new application. (c) Medicare coverage generally can continue for 3

Table 9.1.
Impairments Qualifying a Person with *Ischemic Heart Disease* for Medical Disability under Social Security[a]

Ischemic heart disease with chest pain of cardiac origin as described in 4.00E. With:

A. Treadmill exercise test (see 4.00F and G) demonstrating one of the following at an exercise level of 5 METs[b] or less:
  1. Horizontal or downsloping ischemic depression (from the standing control) of the ST segment to 1.0 mm or greater, lasting for at least 0.08 second after the J junction, and clearly discernible in at least two consecutive complexes which are on a level baseline in any lead; *or*
  2. Junctional depression occurring during exercise, remaining depressed (from the standing control) to 2.0 mm or greater for at least 0.08 second after the junction (the so-called slow upsloping ST segment), and clearly discernible in at least two consecutive complexes which are on a level baseline in any lead; *or*
  3. Premature ventricular systoles which are multiform or bidirectional or are sequentially inscribed (3 or more); *or*
  4. ST segment elevation (from the standing control) to 1 mm or greater; *or*
  5. Development of second or third degree heart block; *or*
B. In the absence of a report of an acceptable treadmill exercise test (see 4.00G), one of the following:
  1. Transmural myocardial infarction exhibiting a QS pattern or a Q wave with amplitude at least one-third of R wave and with a duration of 0.04 second or more. (If these are present in leads III and aVF only, the requisite Q wave findings must be shown, by labeled tracing, to persist on deep inspiration); *or*
  2. Resting ECG findings showing ischemic type (see 4.00F1) depression of ST segment to more than 0.5 mm in either (a) leads I and aVL and V_6 or (b) leads II and III and aVF or (c) leads V_3 through V_6; *or*
  3. Resting ECG findings showing an ischemic configuration or current of injury (see 4.00F1) with ST segment elevation to 2 mm or more in either (a) leads I and aVL and V_6 or (b) leads II and III and aVF or (c) leads V_3 through V_6; *or*

4. Resting ECG findings showing symmetrical inversion of T waves to 5.0 mm or more in any two leads except leads III or aVR or V_1 or V_2; *or*
5. Inversion of T wave to 1.0 mm or more in any of leads I, II, aVL, V_2 to V_6 and R wave of 5.0 mm or more in lead aVL and R wave greater than S wave in lead aVF; *or*
6. "Double" Master Two-Step test demonstrating one of the following:
  a. Ischemic depression of ST segment to more than 0.5 mm lasting for at least 0.08 second beyond the J junction and clearly discernible in at least two consecutive complexes which are on a level baseline in any lead; *or*
  b. Development of a second or third degree heart block; *or*
7. Angiographic evidence (see 4.00H) (obtained independent of Social Security disability evaluation) showing one of the following:
  a. 50% or more narrowing of the left main coronary artery; *or*
  b. 70% or more narrowing of a proximal coronary artery (see 4.00H3) (excluding the left main coronary artery); *or*
  c. 50% or more narrowing involving a long (greater than 1 cm) segment of a proximal coronary artery or multiple proximal coronary arteries; *or*
8. Akinetic or hypokinetic myocardial wall or septal motion with left ventricular ejection fraction of 30% or less measured by contrast or radioisotopic ventriculographic methods; *or*
C. Resting ECG findings showing left bundle branch block as evidence by QRS duration of 0.12 second or more in leads I, II, or III and R peak duration of 0.06 second or more in leads I, aVL, V_5, or V_6, unless there is a coronary angiogram of record which is negative (see criteria in 4.04B7).

[a] From *Disability Evaluation under Social Security*, 1986. Number codes refer to additional details in this booklet.
[b] MET, metabolic equivalent.

Table 9.2.
Impairments Qualifying a Person with *Chronic Obstructive Pulmonary Disease* for Medical Disability under Social Security[a]

Chronic obstructive pulmonary disease (due to any cause). With: Both FEV_1[b] and MVV equal to or less than the values specified in table (below) corresponding to the person's height without shoes.

Height without Shoes (Inches)	FEV_1 Equal to or Less Than (liters, BTPS)	and	MVV (MBC) Equal to or Less Than (liters/min, BTPS)
60 or less	1.0		40
61–63	1.1		44
64–65	1.2		48
66–67	1.3		52
68–69	1.4		56
70–71	1.5		60
72 or more	1.6		64

[a] From *Disability Evaluation under Social Security*, 1986.
[b] FEV_1, forced expiratory volume in 1 second; MVV, maximum voluntary ventilation; MBC, maximum breathing capacity.

Table 9.3.
Impairments Qualifying a Person with *Cerebrovascular Accident* for Medical Disability under Social Security[a]

Central nervous system vascular accident. With one of the following more than 3 months postvascular accident:
A. Sensory or motor aphasia resulting in ineffective speech or communication; *or*
B. Significant and persistent disorganization of motor function in two extremities, resulting in sustained disturbance of gross and dexterous movements, or gait and station.

[a] From *Disability Evaluation under Social Security*, 1986.

years after a person's DI benefits stop because of return to substantial gainful activity. If a worker starts receiving DI benefits again within 5 years after the DI was stopped, and if the patient was previously entitled to Medicare, that protection will resume immediately. (d) Work expenses related to the impairment that are paid for by a disabled person may be deducted from the patient's earnings in determining whether these constitute substantial gainful activity. This is true even

Table 9.4.
Impairments Qualifying a Person with *Epilepsy Due to Major Motor Seizures* for Medical Disability under Social Security[a]

Major motor seizures (grand mal or psychomotor), documented by EEG and by detailed description of a typical seizure pattern, including all associated phenomena: occurring more frequently than once a month, in spite of at least 3 months of prescribed treatment.[b] With:

A. Daytime episodes (loss of consciousness and convulsive seizures); or
B. Nocturnal episodes manifesting residuals which interfere significantly with activity during the day.

[a]From *Disability Evaluation under Social Security*, 1986.
[b]Adherence to therapy must be objectively confirmed by measurements of drug levels that are in the therapeutic range.

Table 9.5.
Impairments Qualifying a Person with *Arthritis of a Major Weight-Bearing Joint* for Medical Disability under Social Security[a]

Arthritis of a major weight-bearing joint (due to any cause): With history of persistent joint pain and stiffness with signs of marked limitation of motion or abnormal motion of the affected joint on current physical examination. With:

A. Gross anatomical deformity of hip or knee (*e.g.*, subluxation, contracture, bony or fibrous ankylosis, instability) supported by X-ray evidence of either significant joint space narrowing or significant bony destruction *and* markedly limiting ability to walk or stand; or
B. Reconstructive surgery or surgical arthrodesis of a major weight-bearing joint and return to full weight-bearing status did not occur, or is not expected to occur, within 12 months of onset.

[a]From *Disability Evaluation under Social Security*: 1986.

Table 9.6.
Impairments Qualifying a Person with *Rheumatoid Arthritis* for Medical Disability under Social Security[a]

Active Rheumatoid Arthritis and Other Inflammatory Arthritis. With both A and B:

A. History of persistent joint pain, swelling, and tenderness involving multiple major joints (hip, knee, ankle, shoulder, elbow, or wrist/hand) *and* with signs of joint inflammation (swelling and tenderness) on current physical examination despite prescribed therapy for at least 3 months, resulting in significant restriction of function of the affected joints, and clinical activity expected to last at least 12 months; *and*
B. Corroboration of diagnosis at some point in time by either:
   1. Positive serological test for rheumatoid factor; *or*
   2. Antinuclear antibodies; *or*
   3. Elevated sedimentation rate; *or*
   4. Characteristic histological changes in biopsy of synovial membrane or subcutaneous nodule (obtained independent of Social Security disability evaluation).

[a]From *Disability Evaluation under Social Security*: 1986.

if these expenses also apply to needs for daily living (such as a wheelchair). (e) In addition to disabled workers, persons disabled before the age of 22 and disabled widows and widowers can also have a trial work period.

Supplemental Security Income

Supplemental Security Income is a federal program that was introduced in 1974. It is paid for out of general funds rather than Social Security funds, but it is administered by the same state agencies that administer the Disability Determination program. The application process is similar to that described above for Social Security Disability Insurance. The same criteria are used to evaluate SSI disability claims as are used for DI claims.

The basic differences between SSI and Social Security benefits are as follows: (a) Eligibility: SSI is available for two groups of persons when they are not insured by Social Security: persons under 65 who are medically disabled and all uninsured persons over the age of 65.* In addition to these two groups, persons who have "presumptive disability" (claim for total disability being processed) and disabled persons who are in the 5-month waiting period for their DI payments to begin may be eligible. Eligibility in all of these groups is based on need (total resources below a certain defined level) and the absence of gainful employment (defined as earned monthly income of $300 or more for disability claims). (b) There is no waiting period: A person becomes eligible for the first SSI payment in the month when he files his disability claim. (c) In most states, persons who are approved for SSI are also eligible for Medicaid and other social services provided by their state. (d) All persons receiving SSI are reviewed once each year to determine whether their income and other resources still make them eligible to receive SSI.

The maximal monthly income from SSI in 1989 was $368 for an individual and $532 for a couple. In 1987, there were 4.4 million recipients of SSI, on the basis of disability, blindness, and age (over 65 and without Social Security).

As described above for DI, the physician's report must be received before income support under SSI can be initiated.

Vocational Rehabilitation

State Vocational Rehabilitation agencies existed before the federal Disability Determination program was created in 1954. In many states, these agencies administer the Disability Determination program in addition to providing vocational rehabilitation services.

Eligibility

To be eligible for Vocational Rehabilitation, a person must have a disability that interferes with his capacity to obtain suitable employment or that is a threat to his present career; this does not mean that the person has to meet the criteria for medical disability discussed above. The individual must have a reasonable chance of being able to engage in a suitable occupation after Vocational Rehabilitation services are provided. A "suitable occupation" would include being a housewife provided that Vocational Rehabilitation would enable her to remain in her own home instead of requiring institutional care.

---

*SSI for persons over 65 is similar to Social Security retirement. These claims are not handled by Disability Determination services.

Services

The services provided by Vocational Rehabilitation agencies vary from state to state. However, they usually include the following: (a) A *medical examination*. A complete medical examination is provided to determine the extent of a person's disability. (b) *Counseling* and guidance. A trained rehabilitation counselor is assigned to guide each client through the rehabilitation process. (c) *Physical aids*. Items such as artificial limbs, braces, hearing aids, eyeglasses, and wheelchairs may be provided if needed. (d) *Job training*. Training for the proper job is provided when necessary. This may be given in a vocational school, college or university, rehabilitation facility, or in the home. (e) *Help with living expenses*. Board, room, transportation expenses, and other necessary expenses may be provided if needed. (f) *Equipment and licenses*. Tools, equipment, and licenses necessary for getting started in the right job may be provided. (g) *Job placement*. Placement in the right job is an important part of the rehabilitation process. The abilities of each handicapped individual are carefully matched to job requirements. (h) *Follow-up*. The counselor follows up on each placement to make sure that the client's job is suitable.

Physician's Role

As noted above, all persons applying for Social Security disability benefits are screened for referral to Vocational Rehabilitation. For those persons, the report of the patient's physician (see above) may be utilized by the Vocational Rehabilitation agency. For persons who are not applying for medical disability, the physician will often be asked to provide a general medical report for the Vocational Rehabilitation agency. Perhaps the most important role of the general physician in this regard is to provide encouragement to the patient to apply for Vocational Rehabilitation and to maintain continued interest in the patient's progress. It has been estimated that every $1,000 spent for Vocational Rehabilitation increases by $35,000 the lifetime earnings of those who are rehabilitated. This economic consequence for society, in addition to the benefit to the individual, makes support of Vocational Rehabilitation a particularly important role for the physician.

HOME HEALTH SERVICES

A consequence of illness as distressing to the patient as the loss of the ability to earn an income is the temporary or permanent loss of the ability to remain at home. Most people will require acute hospital care one or more times in their adult life, and a small proportion will also require long-term institutional care. The principal objectives of home health services are to minimize the need for admission to either acute or long-term care facilities and to decrease the length of stay in these facilities. Numerous studies have shown that these objectives are attained when home health services are utilized appropriately; but studies have also shown that home health services are underutilized.

Range of Services

Health services provided to sick persons at home include (a) basic care provided by nonprofessional family members and friends (at times with the help of Red Cross or similar training in basic care technique); (b) home food services available at a nominal cost to the patient ("Meals on Wheels"); (c) care provided by physicians or their associates who make home visits; (d) services provided by the personnel of certified home health agencies, under the supervision of the patient's physician; (e) specimen collection and performance of diagnostic procedures such as X-rays and electrocardiograms, by clinical laboratories; and (f) delivery/rental of equipment such as hospital beds by medical suppliers. Even when professional help is involved, most of the responsibility for carrying out care is given to the patient or to a member of the patient's family; as noted in Chapter 1, it is the assumption of responsibility by patients and their families that most clearly distinguishes ambulatory medicine from in-patient medicine.

Today there are approximately 6000 home health agencies in the United States. Agencies may be part of state and local health departments, nonprofit voluntary agencies, for-profit proprietary agencies, or hospital-based programs. The home care provided by voluntary agencies is coordinated by a visiting nurse. A substantial proportion of the care is often carried out by home health aides, analogous to nursing aides on hospital wards, under the supervision of the nurse. In recent years, nurse practitioners have been added to the staffs of many home health agencies, so that more sophisticated care can be provided. In addition to nursing, the services may include physical, occupational, and speech therapy, nutritional, clinical pharmacology, and social work counseling, and home health aide services. Home health agencies also provide the nursing component of hospice programs (see Chapter 19) in many communities or may have full-fledged hospice programs certified by Medicare for reimbursement.

In recent years, numerous agencies have begun to supply and administer in-home intravenous therapies, ranging from short-term normal saline and electrolyte infusions to courses of antibiotics, cancer chemotherapy, cardiac medications, and total parenteral nutrition. In response to the increase in the AIDS patient population, many home-health agencies have added intravenous and aerosolized administration of a variety of AIDS-related drugs (see details, Chapter 34). These initiatives have emerged in response (a) to efforts to reduce the length of hospitalization and (b) to patients who prefer home care to hospital care for parenteral therapy that may have to be administered during 1 or more weeks. Adequate day-to-day supervision of the overall care of patients receiving in-home parenteral therapy is usually not provided by the company that supplies the equipment; therefore, this responsibility should be delegated to a visiting nurse who knows the physician's comprehensive plan for the patient and is in close contact with the supplier.

The types of clinical problems most frequently referred to home health agencies are listed in Table 9.7.

Third Party Coverage

Any patient (or patient's family) may purchase services from a home health agency. During the past 20 years, patients meeting certain criteria have been eligible for coverage of much of the cost of home care by Medicare, Medicaid, and other third party payers Table 9.8). The minimal criteria are that (a) the patient is under the care of a physician and is largely home

Table 9.7.
Problems Most Commonly Referred for Home Health Services

Postsurgical wound care (teach and/or provide dressing changes)
Orthopaedic problems (Rehabilitation after hospitalization)
Congestive heart failure (provide dietary counseling, assess medication compliance)
Diabetes (supervise insulin technique, provide dietary counseling, teach Puges-stick or urine monitoring of glucose, care of the lower extremities, etc)
Hypertension (supervise and reinforce compliance with medication, check blood pressure response in patient's home)
Incurable cancer and AIDS (provide dietary counseling, intravenous therapies, psychological support, and other aspects of hospice care)
Stroke and other incapacitating neurological problems (provide physical and occupational therapy)
Decubitus and stasis ulcers (teach and/or provide debridement and dressing changes)
Dementia and older person living alone (assess environment for health hazards)
Chronic obstructive pulmonary disease (assess home for oxygen therapy)

Table 9.8.
Criteria for Third Party Reimbursement for Home Health Services

Medicare
Part A pays for all covered services (skilled nursing, home health aide, social work, physical, occupational, and speech therapy). Care must be provided by a certified Home Health Agency and must be medically necessary. There is no limit to the number of visits, as long as the patient's condition meets criteria for services. The following conditions must be met to qualify for reimbursement:
  1. Patient is confined to home.
  2. Need for intermittent skilled nursing, physical therapy, or speech therapy. (One of these three services must be needed to qualify for reimbursement for the other services provided by home health agencies, *i.e.*, social work, occupational therapy, home health aide, and nutrition services.)
  3. Physician must sign renewal of orders every 60 days.
Medicaid
Coverage for home health services varies by state.
Veterans Administration
Home care from hospital-based programs
Blue Cross and other private health insurance.
Coverage for home health services varies by plan.

^aNote that since 1981, Part A Medicare has covered patients even if they have not been recently hospitalized.

bound; and (b) the patient has an active medical problem that requires skilled nursing or other skilled professional service such as physical or occupational therapy. Because of the criterion that the patient must have an active medical problem requiring skilled care, payment for the services of a home health aide is often denied after the active problem becomes stable, even when the home health aide's services are important in maintaining the patient's health.

Physician's Role

All physicians should be well acquainted with the home health services available in their community and with the third party coverage that their patients may have for the services. Although anyone (the patient's family, a nurse, a social worker, etc.) can refer a patient for home health services, orders written by the patient's physician are always needed for third party reimbursement.

The quality of the communication between a patient's physician and the visiting nurse often determines how much the patient will benefit from home health services. When the physician provides clear and thorough initial information, when the physician is accessible to the nurse when needed, and vice versa, patients who would otherwise require in-hospital care can receive excellent care in their homes. Some problems are best managed at home, such as adjustment of insulin and diet in a diabetic patient with an intercurrent illness, adjustment of diuretics and diet in a patient with worsening congestive heart failure, assessment of compliance and the response to medication in a patient whose high blood pressure seems refractory to treatment at office visits, and debridement, dressing, and monitoring of a sacral pressure sore.

General References

Carey TS, Hadler NM: The role of the primary physician in disability determination for social security and worker's compensation. *Ann Intern Med* 104:706–710, 1986.
  Useful review with helpful references.
Disability Evaluation under Social Security: United States Department of Health and Human Services, pub. no. (SSA) 05-10089. February, 1986.
  Gives criteria for impairments that qualify a person for medical disability under Social Security (available free from local Social Security Office and State Disability Determination Service).
Family Health and Home Nursing. Garden City, NY, Doubleday, 1979.
  Inexpensive Red Cross publication for the lay person explaining in detail all aspects of caring for sick persons at home. Available in most bookstores.
Harris MD: *Home Health Administration.* National Health Publishing, 1988.
  Useful reference, reflecting the multifaceted aspects of home health care.
American College of Physicians, Home Health Care. Health and Policy Committee. *Ann Intern Med* 105:454–460, 1986.
  Extensively referenced set of positions on home health care for elderly persons. Focuses on efficacy, reimbursement, quality regulation, physician role.

SECTION

2

Psychiatric and Behavioral Problems

C H A P T E R 10

Evaluation of Psychosocial Problems

L. RANDOL BARKER, M.D.
CHESTER W. SCHMIDT, JR., M.D.

Patients with psychological and social problems often consult their general physicians, usually complaining of not feeling well in some physical sense. The problems these patients present range from temporary distress to rather enduring and disabling conditions.

The *temporary disturbances* that are most often seen by the generalist are anxiety regarding the meaning of a new symptom (e.g., cancer fear), frustrations attending an illness that interrupts valued activities (e.g., recovery phase after myocardial infarction), or dysphoric mood related to recent social stress (e.g., anxiety in the mother of a teenager who has run away from home). Such problems occur frequently in persons with excellent previous mental health. These disturbances usually resolve when the interviewing and counseling skills discussed in Chapters 3 and 11 are utilized in conjunction with management of the patient's medical problem.

Those patients with *more persistent psychosocial problems* are difficult to care for unless one has a knowledge of common psychosocial syndromes and utilizes a systematic approach to the patient. This chapter and the following chapter provide general approaches for the evaluation and management of such patients. Subsequent chapters cover the specific psychosocial syndromes seen by generalists.

The Epidemiologic Catchment Area Survey, conducted in 1980 to 1982, identified the frequency of common psychosocial syndromes in a representative sample of American communities (4). Table 10.1 lists the four most common disorders in major sex and age subgroups. Approximately 12% of adults reported symptoms of a diagnosable mental disorder during the past 6 months, and 25% had had a mental illness at some time in their life. These figures probably underrepresent the true prevalence of mental disorders, since the study instrument did not identify patients with two common syndromes, adjustment disorder and generalized anxiety disorder. Over half of those with mental illness reported that the only health care providers they saw were generalists; and of these persons, the majority had not discussed their mental illness with their health care providers (3). These findings, combined with the finding that at least one-third of patients seen in primary care practice have a significant psychosocial problem (2), point to the importance of evaluating patients for mental illness.

SYNDROMAL DIAGNOSIS

Accurate diagnosis of a psychosocial problem is essential for prognosis and management. The *Diagnostic and Statistical Manual of Mental Disorders (Third Edition Revised) DSM-III-R*, issued in 1987 by the American Psychiatric Association, is a particularly useful resource, as it provides diagnostic criteria, epidemiological information, and prognostic profiles for most of the psychosocial syndromes encountered in office practice. DSM-III-R criteria are stated wherever relevant in the chapters that follow.

Despite the availability of diagnostic criteria, reaching an accurate psychosocial diagnosis in general medical practice can be difficult. There are several reasons for this: (a) When the presenting symptoms are somatic, physical illness must always be considered, even when the patient's presentation suggests a psychosocial problem. (b) Psychosocial symptoms or findings are not often specific for one syndrome. (c) The necessary information is different from that needed to evaluate a physical symptom. The most salient information is obtained by inquiring about or observing thoughts, feelings, behaviors, events, and relationships.

After initial information gathering about mental symptoms, it is usually possible to decide which general phenomenon is the dominant problem, e.g., anxiety, depression, somatization, cognitive impairment, maladaptive behavior, etc. To refine the diagnosis, additional information is needed. For example:

The patient has a depressed mood. With a systematic approach, the diagnosis of "depression" may be more accurately formulated as one of the following:

1. Adjustment disorder with depressed mood
2. Major depression
3. Dysthymic disorder (depressive neurosis)
4. Depression related to a recently prescribed drug
5. Alcoholism presenting as depression.

INFORMATION GATHERING

The order in which information is gathered and the particular information gathered will vary depending upon the style that one has developed with previous patients and the diagnosis being considered. With a minimal amount of prompting, many patients will vol-

Table 10.1.
Four Most Frequent DIS:DSM-III-R Psychiatric Disorders by Sex and Age Based on 6-Month Prevalence Rates[a,b]

Rank	18–24 Yr	25–44 Yr	45–64 Yr	65+ Yr	Total
Men					
1	Alcohol abuse/ dependence	Alcohol abuse/ dependence	Alcohol abuse/ dependence	Severe cognitive impairment	Alcohol abuse/ dependence
2	Drug abuse/ dependence	Phobia	Phobia	Phobia	Phobia
3	Phobia	Drug abuse/ dependence	Dysthymia	Alcohol abuse/ dependence	Drug abuse/ dependence
4	Antisocial personality	Antisocial personality	Major depressive episode without grief	Dysthymia	Dysthymia
Women					
1	Phobia	Phobia	Phobia	Phobia	Phobia
2	Drug abuse/ dependence	Major depressive episode without grief	Dysthymia	Severe cognitive impairment	Major depressive episode without grief
3	Major depressive episode without grief	Dysthymia	Major depressive episode without grief	Dysthymia	Dysthymia
4	Alcohol abuse/ dependence	Obsessive-compulsive disorder	Obsessive-compulsive disorder	Major depressive episode without grief	Obsessive-compulsive disorder

[a] From Myers JK, Weissman MM, Tischler GL, et al: Six-month prevalence of psychiatric disorders in three communities. *Arch Gen Psychiatry* 41:959, 1984.
[b] Dysthmia included. The basis for ranking was the mean 6-month prevalence rates for New Haven, Baltimore, and St. Louis combined. DIS indicates Diagnostic Interview Schedule.

unteer information that would otherwise require systematic questioning. Both the efficiency and the accuracy of the interview are probably enhanced when this occurs. Other interviewing skills useful in eliciting a psychosocial history are described in Chapter 3.

Building upon the patient's initial account, one should assess relevant aspects of the social history, the patient's mental status, the patient's personality and coping styles, the chronology of the patient's problem, and the family history of psychosocial problems. With the patient's permission, additional information should be obtained from family members, other physicians, and previous medical records whenever possible. Current medications should be identified, as psychological disturbances can be caused or worsened by a large number of drugs (1). Tables in other chapters list those drugs that may cause anxiety (Table 13.1), depression (Table 15.1), psychotic symptoms (Table 16.2), delirium (Table 17.5), and sexual dysfunction (Table 18.4).

Social and Developmental History

The history should always include a profile of the patient's current life situation (e.g., marital status, family structure, household makeup, educational level, occupation, recreational activities, and substance use). At times, it is also helpful to know the principal patterns and events that have characterized his development from childhood until the present (e.g., family makeup, interactions, conflicts, losses; relationships in school, the armed services, jobs; and the patient's depiction of the type of person he is and has been). Some of this information will be known already to the patient's personal physician, making the assessment of a new psychosocial problem simpler at times. When

a psychosocial problem seems likely, the presenting symptom should be reexplored in the context of social interactions (e.g., "Tell me just where you were and who was there the last time you noted the nausea and quivering in your stomach"), and the patient should be asked to describe any recent changes in his life situation and to discuss the nature of critical relationships (e.g., with spouse, children, and work associates). If substance abuse is suspected, skillful inquiry will be needed to make a diagnosis (see Chapter 21 on alcoholism and Chapter 22 on illicit drugs).

Much psychosocial illness is related to stresses and maladjustments that will be disclosed by the patient during this inquiry. McWhinney has summarized the social factors most commonly related to psychosocial distress (see Table 10.2). The significance of a report of one of these factors becomes clear when it is integrated into the rest of the history (e.g., an interpersonal conflict may be the stressor causing an adjustment disorder or it may be a *symptom of* alcoholism, depression, or sexual dysfunction).

In addition to providing clues to the diagnosis, the social history will usually disclose important assets and liabilities in the patient's life. This information is always useful in planning management for a psychosocial problem.

Mental Status

In those instances when the patient's behavior is the principal problem and/or when psychological symptoms are causing a great deal of subjective distress (e.g., marked anxiety or depression) or suggest a major psychiatric disorder (e.g., dementia, schizophrenia, or manic-depressive illness), a brief mental status examination should be performed.

Table 10.2.
Common Social Factors Related to Psychological Symptoms[a]

1. *Loss*: (a) Personal loss—loss of a loved one through death or desertion. (b) Loss of things—imposed loss of home, cherished possession, or job.
2. *Conflict*: (a) Interpersonal—conflict within family, with neighbors, or at work, where hostility is recognized. (b) Intrapersonal—role conflict or conflicting demands on the patient (as in a working mother).
3. *Change*: (a) Development—where time of life is the major problem (as in adolescence, menopause, or senescence). (b) Geographic—where a move to an unfamiliar environment is the major problem (as in immigration).
4. *Maladjustment*: (a) Interpersonal—problems between people with no overt conflict (as in failure to achieve a satisfactory sexual relation without hostility between partners). (b) Personal—failure to adjust to the environment (home or job) in the absence of the above-mentioned loss, conflict, or change.
5. *Stress*: (a) Acute—unexpected event not covered under loss, conflict, or change (for example, the sudden illness of self or of a family member or friend). (b) Chronic—long-term situation not included in loss, conflict, or change (for instance, the presence of a handicapped child in the family).
6. *Isolation*—not due to any recent loss, change, or conflict (as in an elderly widow).
7. *Failure or frustrated expectations*—when the patient's goals in life are not fulfilled and when there is no evidence of an intervening event covered by loss, conflict, or change (e.g., failure at school or failure to achieve occupational promotion).

[a] From McWhinney IR: Beyond diagnosis, an approach to the integration of behavioral science and clinical medicine. *N Engl J Med* 287:384, 1972.

The mental status examination is a systematic assessment of the patient's current mental functioning. The elements of the mental status examination most useful for the general physician include:

Appearance: Grooming, attention to dress, motor activity (quiet versus agitated).

General level of consciousness: Alert, sleepy, stuporous, obtunded.

Orientation: The patient knows who he is, where he is, and the date (day, month, and year).

Speech: Ability to use customary syntax. Note slurring, inability to find the right word, pressured speech, flight of ideas, looseness of association, muteness.

Memory: Recent memory—knowledge of recent events, capacity to remember names of current treating physicians. Remote memory—ability to give history and present illness in proper historical sequence.

Attention and concentration: Ability to understand and follow questions or instructions.

Intelligence: Can be estimated from level of schooling achieved, vocational history, use of language.

Mood: A pervasive, sustained emotion described by the patient (depressed, euphoric, neutral).

Affect: An observable and immediately expressed emotion (anger, anxiety, sadness, fear, humor, lability, etc.). Note whether display of affect is consistent with the content of speech, thoughts, and behavior.

Perceptions: Presence of hallucinations (i.e., visual, auditory, or somatic perception occurring in the absence of appropriate external stimuli), delusions, (i.e., fixed beliefs, which are false), paranoid ideas, or persistent phobias (i.e., fears directed toward specific objects or situations).

Suicidal thoughts. Statement or actions that indicate the patient wishes to harm or kill himself.

Homicidal or violent thoughts: Statements or actions that indicate patient wishes to harm or kill others.

Judgment: Capacity to understand the situation in which the patient finds himself and/or to demonstrate appropriate compliance with instructions for care.

Most of the data needed for a brief mental status examination are observable while the patient gives his history. Depending upon the cues the patient provides, he should be questioned more about his mental status and other features of the syndrome(s) suggested by his history. For patients whose mental status suggests focal or global cognitive impairment, a more formal cognitive examination can be administered in a few minutes (see Mini-Mental Status Examination, Table 17.1). For those describing cardinal symptoms of affective, anxiety, or psychotic disorders focused probing is necessary (see Chapter 13, The Anxious Patient; Chapter 15, Affective Disorders; and Chapter 16, Schizophrenia).

Personality and Coping Responses

Personality refers to the relatively enduring attitudes and patterns of behavior that typify an individual. Generally a physician becomes acquainted with a patient's personality, particularly the patient's behavior pattern in the face of illness, through caring for that patient during months or years. Some patients will exhibit the features of a maladaptive personality, and recognition of this may be very helpful in planning the patient's care, as discussed in more detail in Chapter 14.

Coping responses are behaviors that people assume in adapting to life stresses. There are several common coping responses that should be recognized since patients may use them to avoid confronting a problem for which help is needed. When maladaptive coping is recognized, the patient can often be assisted to disclose the primary problem and to reach a healthier adaptation to it.

Denial is a common response by which a distressing problem is avoided. Denial may be relatively silent (i.e., a patient with blood in his stools may keep this information to himself to avoid confronting his fear of cancer) or it may be voiced openly (e.g., a patient who greatly fears sudden death during convalescence from a myocardial infarction may boast of robust health and deny angina or other symptoms he may be experiencing).

Rationalization serves the same function as denial. It is a process in which a patient gives plausible explanations for behavior designed to avoid unpleasant realities (e.g., a relapsing alcoholic explains that his work load increased so much lately that it was impossible to continue to go to Alcoholics Anonymous meetings).

Regression is reversion to dependent behavior typical of childhood. Regressive behavior is a common response to major illness or other circumstances that threaten a person's autonomy (e.g., a man who is recovering slowly from a hip fracture complains excessively about small problems at home, gets upset when his son cannot continue to visit daily, and expects his wife to order for him when they go out to a restaurant on the weekend).

Projection is a process in which an unpleasant aspect of one's self is ascribed to another person (e.g., a teenager who is very angry about limits set by her mother criticizes her older sister for being hostile to their mother).

Displacement is a process in which feelings toward one individual are directed toward another (i.e., a researcher who is furious at a colleague who has beaten him to an important finding becomes very irritable toward his wife for no apparent reason).

Chronology

Accurate information about the chronology of a psychosocial problem is important for diagnosis, prognosis, and management. Therefore, as the interview is closing, one should assure that the patient has provided the following essential information: (*a*) duration of the present episode; (*b*) the time(s) and circumstances during which the current symptoms have either improved or worsened (if temporal relationships are unclear, it is helpful to have the patient *keep a log* of symptoms and events for one or more weeks); (*c*) the patient's optimal level of functioning during the past year (when was it and how long did it last?); (*d*) the time and circumstances of any previous episode of similar symptoms or of previous mental illness.

Family History

In the family of a patient with a chronic psychosocial disorder, occurrence in others of the same disorder or other psychiatric problems is common. Information about psychiatric illness in the family may strengthen one's diagnostic hunches and may help the patient to recognize the nature of his own problem.

OVERALL FORMULATION OF THE PROBLEM

When the essentials of a patient's psychosocial history have been collected, a useful way to formulate the problem is the five-axis approach recommended by the American Psychiatric Association.

Axis I—Psychosocial syndrome(s), plus conditions not attributable to a formal mental disorder that are a focus of attention (e.g., malingering, uncomplicated bereavement, noncompliance with medical treatment, academic or occupational problems, etc.).

Axis II—Personality disorders or styles and specific developmental disorders.

Axis III—Physical disorders and conditions.

Axis IV—Severity of psychosocial stressors: acute events (within past 6 months) and enduring circumstances (lasting longer than 6 months) (see Table 10.3).

Axis V—Global Assessment of Functioning: current and past years (see Table 10.4).

Case example. Mr. J, a 60-year-old married security guard, underwent coronary bypass graft surgery (CABG) in January 1984. His postoperative hospital course was uneventful. Shortly after discharge, he came twice in the same day to the emergency department complaining of severe chest pain and also of cold upper extremities. Evaluation revealed mild tenderness at the location of his sternotomy scar. The next day he returned, this time describing inability to sleep in addition to the previous symptoms. A thorough evaluation, including an exercise stress test, did not disclose a physical basis for his symptoms.

The patient's wife described regressive behavior since the patient returned home (e.g., he wanted her to bring his meals to him in bed, asked her to pick his clothes for him each day, was having occasional urinary incontinence, and had put her in charge of dispensing all of his medicines). He was not sleeping well and awakened his wife whenever he could not sleep. Additional inquiry and observation revealed a somewhat diminished sense of self-worth and some doubts regarding his future. He was worried specifically that he would not return to work, as he had expected to preoperatively, and his calculations suggested that his income would be significantly lower if he applied for Social Security benefits.

The patient eventually disclosed that he was sure that he had been "on the pump too long" and that he feared that his incision would break down (this had happened to a friend after CABG).

Mr. J had always seemed to be a self-reliant man. He had worked as a security guard, on medical therapy for his angina, for several years. The CABG was recommended when his angina worsened in November 1983, making it difficult for him to walk the distances required at his job. He had never developed markedly regressive behavior in the past, although he had depended on his wife to make decisions about almost all purchases they made, had never been separated from her for a full day during their long and tranquil marriage, and often referred to her as "Mother." There was no history of significant psychiatric illness in his family.

Based upon this story and additional inquiry, the formulation of Mr. J's illness was:

Axis I—Adjustment disorder, with depressed mood and physical complaints.

Axis II—No personality disorder; history of dependency that made him vulnerable to the behavior he exhibited after CABG.

Axis III—(a) Coronary artery disease. (b) Status postcoronary artery bypass graft, with good technical result.

Axis IV — Severity of psychosocial stressors: moderate to severe (Code 3-4 in Table 10.3), predominantly acute events, i.e., (a) temporary disability due to major surgery; (b) uncertainty regarding his future financial security.

Table 10.3.
Severity of Psychosocial Stressors Scale: Adults[a]

Code[b]	Term	Examples of stressors	
		Acute events (≤6 months)	Enduring circumstances (>6 months)
1	None	No acute events that may be relevant to the disorder	No enduring circumstances that may be relevant to the disorder
2	Mild	Broke up with boyfriend or girlfriend; started or graduated from school; child left home	Family arguments; job dissatisfaction; residence in high-crime neighborhood
3	Moderate	Marriage; marital separation; loss of job; retirement; miscarriage	Marital discord; serious financial problems; trouble with boss; being a single patient
4	Severe	Divorce; birth of first child	Unemployment; poverty
5	Extreme	Death of spouse; serious physical illness diagnosed; victim of rape	Serious chronic illness in self or child; ongoing physical or sexual abuse
6	Catastrophic	Death of child; suicide of spouse; devastating natural disaster	Captivity as hostage; concentration camp experience
0	Inadequate information, or no change in condition		

Severity of Psychosocial Stressors Scale: Children and Adolescents[a]

Code[b]	Term	Examples of stressors	
		Acute events	Enduring circumstances
1	None	No acute events that may be relevant to the disorder	No enduring circumstances that may be relevant to the disorder
2	Mild	Broke up with boyfriend or girlfriend; change of school	Overcrowded living quarters; family arguments
3	Moderate	Expelled from school; birth of sibling	Chronic disabling illness in parent; chronic parental discord
4	Severe	Divorce of parents; unwanted pregnancy; arrest	Harsh or rejecting parents; chronic life-threatening illness in parent; multiple foster home placements
5	Extreme	Sexual or physical abuse; death of a parent	Recurrent sexual or physical abuse
6	Catastrophic	Death of both parents	Chronic life-threatening illness
0	Inadequate information, or no change in condition		

[a]Adapted from Diagnostic and Statistical Manual of Mental Disorders (3rd edition, revised), Washington, D.C., American Psychiatric Association, 1987.
[b]Code numbers used in DSM-III-R.

Axis V—Global Assessment of Functioning: Current GAF = moderate to serious symptoms and functional impairment (Code 50-60 in Table 10.4). Past year GAF = slight to mild symptoms and functional impairment (Code 70-80 in Table 10.4).

COMORBIDITY IN THE PATIENT'S FAMILY

Psychosocial problems create substantial stress for spouses, children, or other persons with close ties to the affected patient. This is particularly true of chronic problems such as alcoholism, affective disorders, anxiety disorders, and the somatoform disorders. The impact of the patient's illness on others should always be considered in the evaluation of psychosocial problems. As pointed out in other chapters in this section, there are important ways in which the comorbidity of the family can be alleviated as part of the overall approach to these trying problems.

ASSESSMENT OF MENTAL COMPETENCE

A physician assesses the patient's competence implicitly at every medical encounter. At times, assessment of competence must be done explicitly. Common civil issues of mental competence include competence to accept or refuse medical care, commitment to hospitals, contesting of wills, and guardianship decisions.

The usual test of the patient's competence in selecting medical care is the determination of whether the patient understands the nature, benefits, and risks of that care and the consequences of not selecting it. This determination can usually be made by the primary care physician for patients with mental retardation or dementia and for patients with psychological problems short of frank psychosis. Similarly, one can evaluate a patient's cognitive functioning in the office, utilizing a standard test such as the Mini-Mental Status Examination outlined in Table 17.1, in order to

Table 10.4.
Global Assessment of Functioning Scale (GAF Scale)[a]

Consider psychological, social, and occupational functioning on a hypothetical continuum of mental health-illness. Do not include impairment in functioning due to physical (or environmental) limitations. Rate GAF for two time periods: current and past year (highest level of functioning for at least a few months).

Code[b]

90 | 81	**Absent OR minimal symptoms** (e.g., mild anxiety before an exam), **good functioning in all areas, interested and involved in a wide range of activities, socially effective, generally satisfied with life, no more than everyday problems or concerns** (e.g., an occasional argument with family members).
80 | 71	**If symptoms are present, they are transient and expectable reactions to psychosocial stressors** (e.g., difficulty concentrating after family argument); **no more than slight impairment in social, occupational, or school functioning** (e.g., temporarily falling behind in school work).
70 | 61	**Some mild symptoms** (e.g., depressed mood and mild insomnia) **OR some difficulty in social, occupational, or school functioning** (e.g., occasional truancy, or theft within the household), **but generally functioning pretty well, has some meaningful interpersonal relationships.**
60 51	**Moderate symptoms** (e.g., flat affect and circumstantial speech, occasional panic attacks) **OR moderate difficulty in social, occupational, or school functioning** (e.g., few friends, conflicts with co-workers).
50 41	**Serious symptoms** (e.g., suicidal ideation, severe obsessional rituals, frequent shoplifting) **OR any serious impairment in social, occupational, or school functioning** (e.g., no friends, unable to keep a job).
40 | 31	**Some impairment in reality testing or communication** (e.g., speech is at times illogical, obscure, or irrelevant) **OR major impairment in several areas, such as work or school, family relations, judgment, thinking, or mood** (e.g., depressed man avoids friends, neglects family, and is unable to work; child frequently beats up younger children, is defiant at home, and is failing at school).
30 | 21	**Behavior is considerably influenced by delusions or hallucinations OR serious impairment in communication or judgment** (e.g., sometimes incoherent, acts grossly inappropriately, suicidal preoccupation) **OR inability to function in almost all areas** (e.g., stays in bed all day; no job, home, or friends).
20 | 11	**Some danger of hurting self or others** (e.g., suicide attempts without clear expectation of death, frequently violent, manic excitement) **OR occasionally fails to maintain minimal personal hygiene** (e.g., smears feces) **OR gross impairment in communication** (e.g., largely incoherent or mute).
10 1	**Persistent danger of severely hurting self or others** (e.g., recurrent violence) **OR persistent inability to maintain minimal personal hygiene OR serious suicidal act with clear expectation of death.**

[a] Adapted from Diagnostic and Statistical Manual of Mental Disorders (3rd edition, revised), Washington, D.C., American Psychiatric Association, 1987.
[b] Code numbers used in DSM-III-R.

patient's routine financial affairs (e.g., Social Security checks and monthly bills).

In the ambulatory setting, perhaps the commonest problem presented by marginally competent patients is unreliable self-care; here, the assistance of a competent household member or of a visiting nurse is essential.

Commitment laws in most states require examination by a physician and do not specify examination by a psychiatrist. Therefore, the patient's primary physician will occasionally be required to make a commitment determination. A complete psychiatric evaluation, including a complete mental status examination, is necessary to determine whether the patient is dangerous to himself or to others, which is the usual test for commitment.

It is less likely that the primary care physician will be called upon to examine and provide expert testimony in contesting of wills or in determining the need for guardianship for a patient. The ultimate decision in such cases is made by an administrative law judge. These legal proceedings are often adversarial in na-

ture, and familiarity with principles of forensic psychiatry and experience as an expert witness are required of the physician participating.

General References

American Psychiatric Association: *Diagnostic and Statistical Manual of Mental Disorders (Third Edition Revised) DSM-III-R.* Washington, DC, American Psychiatric Association, 1987.
Recently updated diagnostic criteria and epidemiological information for all recognized psychiatric disorders.
Cadoret RJ: In: Cadoret RJ, King LJ (eds): *Psychiatry in Primary Care,* St Louis, CV Mosby, 1983. chap 2.
Chapter that covers in greater depth the approaches to evaluation by the generalist, which are described in this chapter.

Specific References

1. Drugs that cause psychiatric symptoms. *Med Letter* 31:112, 1989.
2. Houpt JL, Orleans CS, George LK, et al (eds): *The Importance of Mental Health Services to General Health Care.* Cambridge, Massachusetts, Ballinger, 1979.
3. Ford DE, Kamerow DB, Thompson JW: Who talks to physicians about mental health and substance abuse problems? *J Gen Intern Med* 3:363, 1988.
4. Myers JK, Weissman MM, Tischler GL, et al: Six-month prevalence of psychiatric disorders in three communities. *Arch Gen Psychiatry* 41:959, 1984.

CHAPTER 11

Psychotherapy in Ambulatory Practice

CHESTER W. SCHMIDT, JR., M.D.
ROBERT ROCA, M.D.

Psychotherapy consists of a number of verbal and behavioral processes that are used in the management of psychosocial problems for the purpose of relieving symptoms and resolving intra- and interpersonal conflicts. Although many different techniques have been described, there are fundamental principles that are common to all. General physicians have many opportunities to use psychotherapy, either formally or informally.

GENERAL PRINCIPLES

Demoralization

Most candidates for office psychotherapy suffer from demoralization, a painful sense of disappointment and personal inadequacy in the face of life circumstances. By the time such patients acknowledge their distress to the doctor, their usual problem-solving methods have failed, and their usual sources of support have been exhausted. Demoralization can usually be formulated as the product of interactions between environmental stressors and personal vulnerabilities. Environmental stressors may be remediable (e.g., temporary unemployment) or irremediable (e.g., conjugal bereavement). Personal vulnerabilities may be "constitutional" (e.g., mental retardation) or "learned" (e.g., excessive dependency or perfectionism). Particular personal vulnerabilities make individuals susceptible

to particular stressors. For example, an exceedingly dependent person may be especially sensitive to the death of a spouse; and rigid, controlling parents may be especially distressed by the rebelliousness of their adolescent children.

Psychotherapy may be viewed as an interactive process intended to restore morale. It involves both cognitive and relational tasks. The primary cognitive task is to develop a working formulation of patients' difficulties as products of environmental stressors and personal vulnerabilities, to appreciate the personal strengths and resources available to patients for problem solving and amelioration of emotional distress, and to help patients apply these strengths and resources to regain a sense of mastery over life problems. Some strategies useful for these purposes are described in subsequent sections of this chapter ("Psychosocial Treatment Techniques" and "Forms of Counseling").

The relational task is to promote in patients what Jerome Frank has termed "expectant trust." This describes an attitude on the part of patients that their physician cares about them, is competent to help, is confident of their recovery, and is committed to remain available until relief is obtained. Expectant trust is an important element in psychotherapeutic success and is enhanced by several of the techniques described below. Its effective mobilization also requires an understanding of the concepts of *transference* and *countertransference*.

Transference

There are potent psychosocial roots to the generally positive initial expectations of the patient as he enters into the relationship with the physician. Each patient brings with him a history of psychosocial development in which pain, fear, and other forms of distress have been repeatedly responded to by parents or by parent surrogates. Through these experiences, individuals both consciously and unconsciously come to expect that new people in their lives will behave with them in ways similar to the ways their parents behaved. These expectations are known as *transference phenomena*. Patients will project onto the patient-physician relationship these conscious and unconscious expectations. In fact, at times patients may react to the physician as if the physician were an important parental figure. To the degree that the transference is *positive*, the physician can exercise powerful supportive and healing psychological forces over the patient. Positive transference may explain placebo responses, and its effect must always be kept in mind when evaluating any therapeutic intervention.

Not all transference reactions are positive. Virtually no one comes through their childhood and adolescence without some psychological scars from disappointments, frustrations, and anger that are the results of unmet expectations and other deprivations experienced during the process of growing up. These psychological scars are the historical-developmental roots of maladaptive and negative personality traits such as dependency, passivity, hostility, obsessive-compulsivity, and sociopathy (see Chapter 14). The conscious and unconscious conflicts associated with these traits can also be projected onto the physician-patient relationship. These *negative* transference reactions often cause troubled physician-patient relationships. The more seriously the patient is deprived of parental affection and support during his childhood, the more likely it is that he will manifest these negative traits as an adult, and therefore the more likely it is that negative transference reactions will develop within the patient-physician relationship.

The significance of the transference phenomenon to psychotherapeutic techniques is that it is a basic tool for bringing about positive attitudinal and behavioral change in the patient. For most ambulatory patients psychological distress results from problems within their current relationships with family, friends, and associates. The transference will recreate, within a controlled setting, modified but reasonably accurate representations of the patient's current and past relationships. As the patient begins to disclose conflicts and to react to the physician as if the physician were one of the individuals with whom he is having difficulty, difficult relationships can be clarified and changes in the patient's attitudes and behavior to improve the relationship can then be considered.

The more intense the therapeutic relationship between patient and physician, the more likely it is that both positive and negative transference reactions will appear and become part of the therapeutic effort. Techniques like short-term counseling (see below) do not produce intense therapeutic relationships and therefore tend to involve chiefly positive transference.

Countertransference

Physicians, like their patients, must go through the trials and tribulations of childhood, adolescence, and maturation, and therefore they are not immune to the development of negative personality traits. However, society and the medical profession assume that physicians will not allow these traits to affect the physician-patient relationship. Physicians are expected to maintain an objectivity in their relationships with their patients, and to be supportive and empathetic.

When practicing psychotherapy, physicians must be aware of their own idiosyncrasies and must keep them under control and out of the therapeutic relationship, i.e., they must avoid countertransference. Chapter 3, The Doctor-Patient Relationship, describes a number of interviewing skills that are helpful in avoiding countertransference.

PSYCHOSOCIAL TREATMENT TECHNIQUES

Because disclosure of distressing information and feelings may in itself be beneficial to the patient, it is artificial to separate evaluation from therapy for psychosocial problems. (General aspects of evaluation for psychosocial problems are described in Chapter 10.)

This section describes the principal techniques utilized in counseling, and the following section describes those forms of counseling useful in office practice.

Establishing a Therapeutic Relationship

As noted above (see "Transference"), the therapeutic relationship recapitulates to some extent the parent-child relationship. Several elements are generic to an effective therapeutic relationship. Above all, the patient must trust his physician. Trust is promoted by being consistent in showing of interest, by accepting sensitive information without being judgmental, by taking the patient's concerns seriously, and by controlling inappropriate reactions to difficult patients (see Table 3.1). In addition to establishing trust, physicians should ensure that their patients understand ways in which there will be access to them during ongoing treatment. When embarking on counseling, it is a good idea to reflect on whether these trust-promoting and condition-setting actions have been accomplished at the outset.

Identifying and Addressing Informational Needs

Much psychosocial distress or harmful behavior is related to misinformation or lack of information. Fear of dread illness, misunderstanding of an established condition, or conviction that one's symptoms must be due to physical illness are common forms of misinformation that patients bring to office visits. Through skillful interviewing, the physician can usually have a patient identify and clarify his informational needs. Providing information, tailored to the patient's needs, and assuring that the patient has received that information is the next step. Clear explanation of normal physiology, disease processes, treatment regimens, etc. is often overlooked as a powerful aid in counseling. Besides imparting knowledge, this effort draws the patient into a collaborative relationship with the physician. Depending upon the problem, other counseling techniques may be as important or more important than this first step, particularly when somatic complaints are due to a psychosocial problem.

Commonly encountered informational needs are the following:

1. Identification/clarification regarding feared or existing physical disorder. For example:

   The son of a recently deceased diabetic patient, who thinks he also has diabetes, receives reassurance and advice after a negative workup for diabetes.

   A woman with mitral valve prolapse who has adopted inappropriate activity limitations receives reassurance regarding the relatively benign course of her condition and assurance that she can resume valued activities that she had curtailed. The American Heart Association booklet entitled Mitral Valve Prolapse is given to her; it reinforces what her physician has said.

2. Identification/clarification regarding a psychophysiological basis for somatic symptoms. For example:

A man with panic disorder obtains partial relief from an explanation of how hyperventilation leads to central nervous system symptoms.

3. Identification/clarification of the role of a psychosocial stressor in producing symptoms. For example:

A man with an adjustment disorder, with anxious mood, recognizes the role of his impending job layoff in precipitating his symptoms; and his and his family's fear that he is "going crazy" is alleviated.

4. Identification of a working diagnosis, the plan, and the likely prognosis. For example:

A woman with the syndrome of major depression develops some hopefulness when she is told the diagnosis, the plan to utilize gradually increasing doses of antidepressants, and the likelihood of significant improvement after a few weeks.

A man with the syndrome of hypochondriasis is not given the name of his syndrome, but he reaches a truce with his physician after being informed that he will probably continue to have some symptoms but that he can engage in valued activities that he has curtailed.

Eliciting and Responding to Feelings

The discomfort of psychosocial illness is often due to the feelings the patient is experiencing. The fundamental ways in which the physician can help the patient to deal with feelings are (a) through empathic listening and (b) having the patient "ventilate" in the office.

Empathic Listening

It is very supportive and reassuring to patients when physicians indicate that they are listening and paying close attention to what the patient is saying. Remembering details of the history, responding with appropriate affect to situations described by the patient, and indicating to the patient that his feelings have been observed are actions that demonstrate to the patient that the physician is concerned and that increase the patient's self-esteem. For example:

A man with generalized anxiety disorder feels better after a visit to his physician at which the physician listens attentively, summarizes what the patient has told him, and tells him that he understands how distressing it must be to have tension headaches and difficulty concentrating on his work when he is plagued by worries.

Legitimizing Feelings

Patients often feel embarrassed or isolated when confronting their reactions to a situation. Legitimization of their reactions, by pointing out that these are reactions that anyone in the patient's situation might experience, can be helpful in alleviating feelings of embarrassment or isolation. For example:

A college professor who is confronting surgery for breast cancer describes constant anger since this problem came up; she was preparing to move to another city when she discovered the lump in her breast. She says that the physician's words helped alot moments after the physician stated, "This anger that upsets you so is very understandable . . . Anyone in your situation would feel the same way. . . ."

Ventilation of Feelings

Patients who keep to themselves strong feelings about past or current experiences usually feel better after releasing their pent-up emotions. An outpouring of emotion can be elicited sometimes by stating that the patient looks tense, angry, or depressed or by commenting that the experience that the patient has just described must have made the patient feel upset. Encouraging the patient to express feelings may loosen his defenses just enough to allow the ventilation to take place. For example:

A middle-aged woman with chronic depressive neurosis (dysthymic disorder) always feels better temporarily when her physician encourages her to ventilate and to cry in the office about her feelings of guilt due to the anger she develops toward members of her family in her week-to-week life.

Problem Solving

In general, the physician who engages in counseling should be an observer-participant and should avoid acting as a powerful, all-knowing figure. An appropriate strategy for problem solving is to help the patient recognize assets (e.g., , supportive people, activities he enjoys) and to make choices that favor resolution of current problems. There are times, however, when the physician may have to be somewhat directive in helping a patient work out plans.

Contingency Planning

The life situations that create stress for patients are often manageable even after slight changes. Distressed patients often cannot see a means of making these changes. Once the particular facts of a patient's dilemma are known, the physician and the patient can engage in creative plans for dealing with specific problems that may arise in the days or weeks ahead. In making contingency plans, it is useful to present hypothetical situations and to have the patient decide how he will try to handle them. For example:

A woman who lives alone is distraught because her only child, a grown daughter who recently moved to another city, has hinted that she may not be able to get home for Christmas. The woman's physician encourages her to make another plan for Christmas rather than face the prospect of being alone. She phones later in the week to say that she still does not know whether her daughter will be able to come for Christmas; she has, however, invited several friends to have Christmas dinner with her and feels much better.

Advice (Persuasion)

The physician is considered by the patient to be an expert and should judiciously exercise that expertise. Concrete recommendations may be very helpful for patients who are upset and temporarily unable to use their own coping skills. The physician's advice provides the patient with something to hang on to until he can make decisions himself. For example:

A middle-aged man with major depression who is beginning to improve is tactfully dissuaded from entering a doctoral program that is known to be particularly demanding. (This example makes the point that stressful life changes should be discouraged during recovery from a major depressive illness.)

Advice may also be used in a confrontational manner, forcing the patient to face up to the fact that he is engaging in dangerous or destructive behavior. The shock value of the confrontation may pierce the complacence and defensiveness of the patient, thereby allowing the physician to persuade the patient to change behavior.

Managing Abnormal Illness Behavior

Abnormal illness behavior is present when the patient's symptoms/impairments are disproportionate to detectable disease. Patients with somatoform disorders (see Chapter 12) express their distress mainly in terms of somatic complaints and/or dreaded conditions; patients with other psychosocial problems also do so at times. The following general strategies are useful in patients whose psychosocial problems present mainly as abnormal illness behavior:

1. *Do not facilitate/reinforce abnormal illness behavior.*
   a. Avoid unnecessary testing.
   b. Avoid unnecessary prescribing.
   c. Avoid unnecessary referral to specialists.
   d. Schedule regular visits (i.e., do not make visits contingent on a new or worsening symptom) and stay within a time frame agreed upon for visits.
2. *Permit the patient to have some symptoms (do not view elimination of symptoms as an essential goal).*
3. *Encourage the patient to talk about his life situation instead of about somatic symptoms.*

Example: A patient with somatization disorder and an unremarkable recent urinalysis states that she plans "to see the urologist who took care of my friend's bladder problem" and is persuaded to come for brief weekly visits to her primary physician instead. At the weekly visits, the physician focuses chiefly on the patient's efforts to keep her teenage daughter in school and commends her for any success that she reports in handling these and other domestic problems.

Involving Family, Friends, and Environment

Two fundamental psychosocial influences external to the patient are family/close friends and the patient's environment. The physician can facilitate optimal involvement of family and the patient's environment in several ways.

1. *Meeting the family's informational needs.* The family and close friends of a patient with a psychosocial syndrome frequently suffer much because of the patient's illness. They often have the same informational needs as the patient (see above). If they are to understand the patient's feelings/behavior and to handle appropriately their own feelings toward the patient, these needs must be addressed. For example:

The grown son of a man with the recent onset of a major depression telephones the patient's physician and says that he is very concerned. He reports that his father has been angrily criticizing his young grandchildren for all kinds of petty reasons and that this is not the way he used to treat the children. Furthermore, the son is worried that his father must have an ulcer because he leaves the table rubbing his stomach and shaking his head after eating a few bites of each meal. The physician empathizes with the patient's son and explains that the behavior change is very typical for a depressed man, that the antidepressant medication that has just been started should lead to some improvement within 1 to 2 weeks, that the history and physical examination did not reveal evidence for anything like an ulcer, and that it is very likely that his father will recover entirely within 2 to 4 months.

2. *Enlisting the family's help.* For some conditions in which the patient demonstrates a failure to make choices favoring improvement, the family may be instrumental in promoting such choices. For example:

The family of an alcoholic patient agrees to participate in a family intervention (see Chapter 21) in order to get the patient to accept treatment.

3. *Facilitating healthy choices regarding the patient's environment.* For example:

A woman with a long-standing depressive neurosis (dysthymic disorder) is encouraged to take a job as a companion and housekeeper for an elderly lady who had a stroke, and her chronic depressive symptoms improve.

Knowing and Utilizing Community Resources

Support groups, recreational opportunities, vocational opportunities, and home health services are among the community resources that may help greatly patients with psychosocial problems. The physician's awareness of and enthusiasm about a community resource can be instrumental in determining its impact on the patient. For example:

The depressed and anxious wife of an alcoholic man experiences marked improvement in the symptoms from this common adjustment disorder after she has been active in Al-Anon, an idea suggested by her physician.

An elderly woman joins a geriatric day center, which provides supervision and activity for her 5 days/week. This idea, which was suggested by her physician, enables the patient's family to continue to have her live with them and alleviates the patient's own negativism and a feeling of guilt toward family members who felt compelled to check on her frequently during the day.

FORMS OF COUNSELING

Short-Term Counseling

This form of intervention is especially useful in a patient who accepts a psychological formulation for symptoms and who wants professional help in resolving a crisis related to those symptoms. It is a *suppressive* form of psychotherapy, meaning that the goals of treatment are to strengthen the defenses of the patient and to relieve symptoms without uncovering, in depth, long-standing intrapsychic conflicts underlying the current problem.

It is usually important at the outset of counseling to establish a "therapeutic contract," specifying the purpose, length, frequency, and cost of the sessions. These details form the boundaries within which the treatment may take place and may become extraordinarily significant during the course of treatment. Patients often react to the boundaries as part of the transference phenomenon by objecting to them, or by attempting to change or violate them. Although there are exceptions, the boundaries should not be modified because of a change in the relationship between the patient and the physician that arises as a result of transference. The contractual agreements should remain stable throughout the course of treatment.

The exigencies of practice usually require that sessions be brief (15 to 20 minutes) and limited in number (5 to 10). The short-term nature of treatment helps limit the emergence of negative transference reactions and inappropriate dependency. Patients are usually seen individually, although occasionally couples and families may be treated together. The aim of such short-term treatment is restoration of morale and relief of emotional distress, not personality change. Treatment should focus on problems that are "conscious" (i.e.,

readily accessible, not repressed) and current; the physician should gently divert patients from repeated recitations of past experiences and injuries. The physician's style should be natural and conversational rather than remote and "analytical" and should be tailored to enhance expectant trust (see above). When appropriate, physicians should tell patients that their emotional states are understandable (i.e., valid) reactions to difficult life circumstances and then, having validated the feelings of distress, express confidence that they will improve. The physician's role is to facilitate problem solving, usually not to "prescribe" solutions. To promote this, physicians should be prepared to help patients identify their strengths and resources, praise their demonstrations of adaptiveness, and help patients explore how they might build on their strengths to solve problems. Patients should be encouraged to try out options for action identified in the sessions by means of "homework assignments" carried out between sessions.

Throughout the course of short-term counseling, it is important to listen for evidence of a complicating major psychiatric syndrome, such as panic disorder or major depression, because in such cases psychotherapy may need to be supplemented by pharmacotherapy (see Chapters 13 and 15) or other methods of treatment.

Example of short-term counseling: A 25-year-old woman came for evaluation because of severe leg pain. She had suffered a severe burn injury one year before and had experienced leg pain intermittently since then. The physician commented that she appeared tired and tense. At this, she became tearful and said that she and her husband had separated and that, although she felt this was for the best, she was extremely anxious and uncertain that she could manage on her own. She had frightened herself during the previous week by thinking that she might be better off dead.

The history revealed that she was not suicidal and did not meet criteria for major depression or panic disorder. The physician viewed the patient as *demoralized* and sought to identify the pertinent personal vulnerabilities and environmental stressors. On the basis of a long relationship, the physician knew the patient to be a quiet, self-conscious woman who depended on attractiveness as a source of self-esteem. She was also ambitious and hard working and had enjoyed considerable occupational success. Her major stressor had been the burn injury. She had been spared facial disfigurement but had considerable scarring on her trunk and lower extremities, which she kept covered at all times. Another stressor was the dissolution of her marriage. She regarded this as a positive development, yet she became tearful when discussing it. When the physician pointed this out, she revealed that she was apprehensive about dating again. She felt certain that the scarring from her burns would make her unattractive to men and that she would therefore remain alone, unable to remarry and have children.

The physician responded that her distress was very understandable in view of the problems she had identified, especially her fears of future loneliness. The physician also told her that these fears might be premature and needed to be examined; and proposed meeting weekly for five visits, 20 minutes each, to talk about her choices and assumptions. She agreed.

During the next session she complained about her dissolving marriage. After five to ten minutes the physician praised her for having stuck with it as long as she had and for managing to hold a demanding job so successfully at the same time. She then spoke of compliments given her by coworkers, one of whom had always paid special attention to her. She was grateful for this now but insisted that no one would take an interest in her if he knew of her injuries. The physician asked her how she knew this, reiterated the position that her assumptions warranted exploration, and asked how she might comfortably undertake this. She considered some options and over the course of several weeks tried several, initially simply discussing her injury with others to assess peoples' responses to the news of her injuries and finally allowing some friends to see her scarring. The physician praised her for her courage as she proceeded with these explorations and empathized with her as she dealt with feelings generated by recalling the accident and risking rejection by testing peoples' responses to her.

By the end of the allotted five weeks, she was no longer convinced that the future was hopeless. Although still anxious about the ongoing separation and her potential need to date again, she was no longer feeling overwhelmed and believed herself capable of overcoming her self-consciousness about the injury. The physician acknowledged her progress and offered future support.

Supportive Therapy

In supportive therapy, the physician utilizes one or more of the psychosocial treatment techniques described earlier. Unlike short-term counseling, the duration of supportive therapy is open ended; and it is often incorporated into the routine management of a chronic disease. Patients should participate in the decision about the frequency of visits and, in so doing, make a contribution at least to that portion of the treatment contract. This form of psychotherapy is useful, for example, in the long-term management of a diabetic patient with a history of poor compliance and multiple family problems. Such a patient is seen once a month for 15 to 30 minutes. The strategies for the sessions are the following:

1. To monitor the patient's diabetic condition;
2. To enhance compliance;
3. To review family problems.

The verbal exchange between the physician and the patient during the visit consists of a review of the therapeutic regimen, an assessment of symptoms, a brief review of what has occurred in the patient's life since the last visit, and a discussion of ways to cope with existing family problems. In this manner, a significant supportive service is provided in the context of management of the patient's organic disease.

Family Counseling

The goals of this form of counseling are (a) to create effective communications among the family members, (b) to bring to their awareness maladaptive patterns of behavior that may be destructive to one or more members of the family, and (c) to have family members change those maladaptive patterns to constructive patterns of behavior. The specific techniques are similar to those used in individual counseling.

Example of family counseling. A couple asked their family physician for help in dealing with their adolescent daughter who was continually misbehaving at school and at home: Evaluation of the problem revealed that the parents had not been consistent in limit setting for their daughter and the family considered the girl to be "the black sheep" of the family. Counseling for the whole family was recommended. During the first session the family members (parents and children) attacked the daughter, blaming her for all of the family's troubles. The physician interrupted the attack by focusing the discussion on the development of a contract between the parents and their daughter designed to define the rules they expected her to follow and the consequences of violating the rules. The next session was a review of the parents' and daughter's adherence to the contract. The parents reported that the daughter broke the contract by misbehaving, but one of the older siblings pointed out the parents were inconsistent in their application of the agreed-upon limit-setting rules. This revelation confronted the family with the fact that the girl's behavior was a shared responsibility within the family. Over the remaining sessions, the physician continued to encourage the family to establish fair rules to which all could adhere consistently. By focusing on the behavior of the entire family, the pressure on the "bad member" was relieved, destructive patterns of interacting were interrupted, and new, constructive patterns were introduced.

General References

Dubovsky SL, Weissberg MP (eds): *Clinical Psychiatry in Primary Care,* 3rd ed. Baltimore, Williams & Wilkins, 1986.
> A practical book that gives excellent examples of good and poor techniques for management of psychosocial problems by the primary care practitioner.

Frank J: *Persuasion and Healing,* revised ed. Baltimore, Johns Hopkins University Press, 1974.
> Presents model of the patient in distress and of the components of practical psychotherapy.

Frank JD: The influence of patients' and therapists' expectations on the outcome of psychotherapy. *Br J Med Psychol* 41:349, 1968.
> A classic paper on the subject of expectations and treatment outcome.

Jacobson GF: In: Arieti S (ed): *American Handbook of Psychiatry,* 2nd ed. New York, Basic Books, 1974.
> A concise review of the subject of crisis theory and technique.

Stuart MR, Lieberman JA: *The Fifteen-Minute Hour. Applied Psychotherapy for the Primary Care Physician.* New York, Praeger Scientific, 1986.
> Provides an overview of rationale for short-term counseling, as well as some helpful techniques.

C H A P T E R   12

Somatization*

ROBERT P. ROCA, M.D., M.P.H.

Persons consulting physicians are expected to have discernible pathological or pathophysiological abnormalities (i.e., disease) accounting for their symptoms. The magnitude of their complaints and the associated disability are expected to be proportional to the disease diagnosed. They are supposed to pursue and cooperate with medical care and to resume normal social functioning as soon as possible. This sequence of responses is called "*normal illness behavior*" (17).

Sometimes there is a discrepancy between diagnosable disease and the magnitude and duration of symptoms and disability. Patients may complain of weakness or pain in the absence of objective findings. They may have "pseudoseizures." They may visit their physicians repeatedly with fears of having AIDS despite several negative HIV serologies and normal physical examinations. Such responses are examples of "*abnormal illness behavior.*"

Patients exhibiting abnormal illness behavior are often manifesting *somatization*, a phenomenon in which unexplained or amplified physical symptoms are linked to psychological factors or conflicts. Somatization is a feature of many formal psychiatric disorders. Its causes are incompletely understood, but factors promoting somatization can often be discovered in individual cases.

WHY PATIENTS SOMATIZE

Explanations of somatization come from at least four distinct perspectives (16): somatization as a symptom of a *disease*, as a manifestation of *personality*, as a modeled or reinforced *behavior*, and as an empathically understandable product of a patient's *life story*. Each perspective calls for different observations and illuminates different aspects of the phenomenon of somatization.

Somatization as a Symptom of Disease

Somatization may occur as a symptom of psychiatric disease, particularly major affective disorder, panic disorder, schizophrenia, and dementia.

Unexplained physical symptoms may also be due to undiagnosed physical disease—even when the symptoms seem to be expressing a psychological conflict or need. Studies of one subset of somatizing patients—those originally diagnosed as "hysterics"—have shown that up to 30% may ultimately be found to have medical or neurological disorders that, in retrospect, explain the presenting "hysterical" symptoms (13).

Somatization as a Manifestation of Personality

The concept of personality implies enduring attitudes and habitual patterns of response. Personality may be viewed dimensionally, as clusters of individual traits (e.g., dependency, assertiveness), or categorically, as approximations of ideal prototypes (e.g., histrionic, or obsessive-compulsive type), as discussed in Chapter 14. Somatization has been associated with personality viewed both ways. Patients with histrionic and obsessive-compulsive personality types may be predisposed to develop somatization disorder and hypochondriasis, respectively (see below). Furthermore, recent empirical work has demonstrated that the tendency to experience and report unexplained physical symptoms correlates with the dimensional traits *introspectiveness* (the tendency to devote diffuse attention to thoughts and feelings about the self) (10), and *neuroticism* (a construct embodying emotional instability, vulnerability to stress, and self-consciousness) (8).

Somatization as Reinforced Behavior

Somatization may be viewed as behavior modeled and/or reinforced by the patient's environment (14). This perspective invites exploration for a past history of similar symptoms in the patient or a close contact and encourages a search for evidence of social benefit associated with the patient's current symptoms.

---

*Walter F. Baile, M.D., contributed to this chapter in previous editions.

Case Example. A 20-year old woman was admitted to the hospital for back pain. Physical examination was unimpressive, and an extensive work-up was unrevealing. Discussions with the family disclosed that the patient's father was about to lose his disability income and that financial hardship was expected. The timing of the patient's symptoms strongly suggested that she was amplifying symptoms in the hope of becoming eligible for disability and thereby helping to ameliorate the family's anticipated financial crisis.

Somatization and the Life Story

Somatization may be viewed as a maladaptive but empathically understandable expression of difficulties originating in early life experiences. Although particular formulations can never be proven, they may help physicians comprehend illness behavior that is otherwise irritating and baffling. For example, patients who suffer parental deprivation and neglect often carry into adulthood potent admixtures of hostility and dependency that may be activated in relationships with physicians. Such patients may develop physical symptoms without diagnosable disease and pursue unrevealing medical evaluations. Often hostile and demanding, they demean the competence and the commitment of their physicians, even as they crave medical attention and insist on even more care. Such behaviors may be seen as expressions of angry disappointment with their earliest caretakers, who did not adequately meet their dependency needs, now displaced onto the physician by means of transference (see Chapter 11). Such a formulation may help one to respond to such patients less defensively and permit the development of a workable doctor-patient relationship. Other common formulations from this point of view have been discussed elsewhere (1, 2).

Reaching A Working Formulation

The development of a working formulation thus requires considering the relative merits of four distinct explanatory points of view in a particular case. The fundamental questions are four: (*a*) Does the patient have a mental illness of which somatization is a symptom? (*b*) Does the patient have personality traits or a personality type associated with somatization? (*c*) Is the patient's abnormal illness behavior modeled and/or reinforced by some aspect of the patient's environment? (*d*) Is this behavior empathically understandable when one considers the patient's unique life history and current predicament? As shown below, the working formulation will often carry specific therapeutic implications.

Somatizing patients frequently fall into defined diagnostic groups. The DSM-III-R disorders associated with somatization are listed in Table 12.1. This chapter describes patients in three groups: those with reactive emotional states, those with primary somatizing disorders (The Somatoform Disorders), and those in whom symptom production is deliberate. Mood dis-

Table 12.1.
DSM-III-R Disorders Associated with Somatization

Mental illnesses
  Mood disorders, especially major depression
  Anxiety disorders, especially panic disorder
  Schizophrenia

Personality disorders, especially histrionic, dependent, and obsessive compulsive

Reactive emotional states
  Adjustment disorder with physical symptoms
  Psychological factors affecting physical illness

Somatoform disorders
  Somatization disorder
  Undifferentiated somatoform disorder
  Hypochondriasis
  Conversion disorder
  Somatoform pain disorder
  Body dysmorphic disorder

Disorders with voluntary symptom production
  Factitious disorder with physical symptoms
  Malingering

orders (Chapter 15), anxiety disorders (Chapter 13), schizophrenia (Chapter 16), and personality disorders (Chapter 14) are discussed in detail elsewhere.

REACTIVE EMOTIONAL STATES (DEMORALIZATION)

Adjustment Disorders

Description

Adjustment disorders are reactive emotional states resulting from difficulty in meeting the demands of the environment (21). Individuals feel overwhelmed by illness, marital discord, or other problems and become demoralized. Their distress may be expressed in somatic terms, both because somatic complaints "legitimate" a visit to the doctor and because emotional distress may cause somatic symptoms such as lightheadedness, fatigue, gastrointestinal problems, cold intolerance, increased frequency of micturition, palpitations, precordial pain, breathlessness, and flushing. When such symptoms arise in response to psychosocial problems, a diagnosis of adjustment disorder with physical complaints may be made (see Table 12.2).

Case Example. A shy 26-year-old parochial school teacher was evaluated for dizziness, abdominal cramps, nausea, excessive urination, and a sensation of fullness in the bladder. When physical examination and laboratory tests revealed no physiological disturbance, a more detailed history was taken. It showed that his symptoms began shortly after a confrontation with his school principal over his attempt to organize a teacher's union and his criticism of several school policies. In his ensuing anger he applied for a job that he did not really want. His symptoms prevented him from taking the scheduled examination for the position.

Individuals such as this patient are often unaware

Table 12.2.
Diagnostic Criteria for Adjustment Disorder[a]

A. Reaction to an identifiable psychosocial stressor (or multiple stressors) that occurs within three months of onset of the stressor(s).

B. The maladaptive nature of the reaction is indicated by either of the following:

(1) impairment in occupational (including school) functioning or in usual social activities or relationships with others

(2) symptoms that are in excess of a normal and expectable reaction to the stressor(s)

C. The disturbance is not merely one instance of a pattern of overreaction to stress or an exacerbation of a mental disorder previously diagnosed.

D. The maladaptive reaction has persisted for no longer than six months.

E. The disturbance does not meet the criteria for any specific mental disorder and does not represent Uncomplicated Bereavement.

Adjustment Disorder with Physical Complaints

This category should be used when the predominant manifestation is physical symptoms, e.g., fatigue, headache, backache, or other aches and pains, that are not diagnosable as a specific physical disorder or condition (recorded on Axis III).

[a]From the American Psychiatric Association: Diagnostic and Statistical Manual of Mental Disorders, 3rd ed, revised. Washington, DC, American Psychiatric Association, 1987.

(or only partially aware) of the relationship between their psychological disturbance and somatic symptoms. Symptoms of an adjustment disorder can mimic almost any disease entity. As illustrated in the following example, diagnosis may be particularly difficult when the symptoms of psychosocial distress resemble those of a patient's established disease process.

Case Example. A 54-year-old widowed white woman recovering from a myocardial infarction complained to her physician on several occasions of fatigue, breathlessness, and pleuritic-like chest pain unrelated to exertion. Her physical examination and ECG had not changed since discharge from the hospital. Questioning revealed that she was forced to leave her job after her heart attack and was barely able to afford the $40/month needed for medication. She tearfully revealed that although her son had offered to help pay for her medication, her daughter-in-law hinted they could really not afford to help. This proud and formerly self-sufficient woman, who was initially reluctant to accept any help, was now made to feel like a "charity case" by her son's wife; and, yes, she reported that the periodic symptoms in her chest invariably occurred while she was thinking about her plight. (Diagnosis: adjustment disorder, with mixed emotional features and physical symptoms)

In this case, emotional distress produced symptoms suggesting cardiac decompensation. The correct diagnosis was made when the appropriate history was elicited.

Three strategies are important in evaluating patients who may have adjustment disorders:

1. *Elicit the relevant history.* Asking the patient openended questions such as "How are things at home

(or at work)?" will generally provide some clue about potential sources of psychosocial distress. It is important to allow the patient to expand on his personal history. Most patients are grateful for a physician's interest, will respect time limits, and, with reassurance and encouragement, will go on to solve the precipitating problem themselves. Even before the physician has taken a psychosocial history, the patient may provide verbal and nonverbal cues suggesting distress (e.g., the comment "things aren't the way they used to be" or hand wringing and looking away when describing a new somatic symptom; a bizarre description of the symptoms, or failure to respond to previous treatment known to work specifically for a somatic disorder) (9).

Patients who are initially reluctant to acknowledge psychosocial distress will often eventually open up in response to gentle, persistent encouragement from a trusted physician.

2. *Rule out major depression.* Patients who attribute their low mood to identifiable psychosocial stressors do not necessarily have an adjustment disorder. Such symptoms as persistently depressed mood, loss of interest in usual activities, poor concentration, reduced energy, diminished appetite, and disturbed sleep suggest a major depressive disorder for which antidepressant medication is usually indicated (see Chapter 15). The presence of an apparent psychosocial precipitant should never deter the physician from pursuing inquiry about these symptoms.

3. *Temper the workup.* The patient should be examined, and appropriate laboratory tests should be ordered. However, extensive workups to exclude improbable diagnoses should be undertaken only after careful consideration because they may imbed the patient in the sick role and prolong his disability.

Management

The identification of a psychosocial basis for a patient's somatic complaints is often sufficient to allow him to begin to marshal his own resources for coping (11). In selected cases, short-term prescription of anxiolytic or hypnotic medications (see details in Chapters 13 and 85) may be helpful. When these measures fail to help, the patient may need goal-focused short-term counseling (see Chapter 11).

There have been only a few reports of the outcome of minor mood disturbances managed by generalists (3, 4, 11, 22). From these studies, the following tentative conclusions can be stated:

1. A large proportion of patients get better *after just one office visit.* Most often, this visit includes empathic listening, a partial physical examination, and reassurance that the patient does not have a serious physical problem.

2. Short-term prescribing of drugs for anxiety or insomnia may not increase the proportion of patients who show significant improvement—about two-

thirds of patients—when they are reevaluated after one month (3). This conclusion derives from a single careful study in which patients with minor mood disturbances were allocated at random to receive brief counseling plus a benzodiazepine drug or just brief counseling.

Several practical considerations regarding longitudinal management are suggested by these findings:

1. It is generally prudent to determine the impact of an initial visit upon a patient's distress—by brief telephone or office follow-up within a week—before prescribing a psychotropic drug for an adjustment disorder.
2. Some patients (approximately one-third) who seem to have an adjustment disorder do not respond to the strategies described above. At follow-up visits, such patients should be interviewed systematically to look for evidence of other syndromes, especially panic disorder (see Chapter 13), major depression (see Chapter 15), alcoholism or another chemical dependency in themselves or in a member of their household (see Chapters 21 and 22), or one of the somatoform disorders (see below). For all of these problems, specific treatment in addition to office psychotherapy is indicated.

Psychological Factors Affecting Physical Condition

Description

Emotional factors or psychological stressors may initiate or exacerbate somatic symptoms due to a physical disorder. The resulting symptoms, which are called "psychophysiological," are usually not accompanied by significant tissue damage. A listing of the most common conditions in which psychophysiological symptoms may occur is found in Table 12.3. When the features listed in Table 12.4 are present, the DSM-III-R diagnosis is "psychological factors affecting physical conditions."

Most of the conditions listed in Table 12.3 may occur either as psychophysiological disorders or as disorders without a significant psychological component. Detailed descriptions of most of these conditions are found elsewhere in this book, as indicated in the table. For a patient's symptoms to be labeled as chiefly psychophysiological, stressful life situations should be present and should have a temporal relationship to the onset of symptoms; in addition symptoms should subside when the stressful situation abates.

Conversion symptoms (see below) are differentiated from psychophysiological symptoms by the absence of pathophysiological condition in the former. Psychophysiological problems are closely related to adjustment disorders, but they are distinguished from them by the fact that the somatic symptoms are due to a recognized pathophysiological condition and the same symptoms may occur in the absence of psychosocial stressors.

Table 12.3.
Common Conditions in Which Psychophysiological Symptoms Are Important

Physiological System	Symptomatic Condition	For Further Information, See Chapter
Cardiovascular	Migraine headache	79
	Vasovagal syndrome (fainting)	81
	Hypertension (usually asymptomatic)	62
	Supraventricular tachycardia	59
	Angina	57
Gastrointestinal	Irritable bowel syndrome	40
	The following symptoms may occur singly or together: anorexia, nausea, vomiting, abdominal cramps, diarrhea, constipation, aerophagia, acid-peptic symptoms	36,37,39
Genitourinary	Menstrual disturbances	77
	Difficulties in micturition: frequency (in both sexes); retention (females); hesitancy (in males)	
	Sexual disorders Dyspareunia Anorgasmia Inhibited sexual excitement; (impotence, frigidity) Delayed ejaculation; premature ejaculation	18
Musculoskeletal	Pain secondary to increased muscle tension: occipital or bitemporal headaches, backaches, myalgia in various muscle groups	65,79
	Fatigue	
	Tremor	82
	Rheumatoid arthritis	70
Respiratory	Hyperventilation syndrome	13
	Bronchospasm	55
	Dyspnea	54
Skin	Hyperhidrosis	100
	Pruritis	100

Table 12.4.
Diagnostic Criteria for Psychological Factors Affecting Physical Condition[a]

A. Psychologically meaningful environmental stimuli are temporally related to the initiation or exacerbation of a specific physical condition or disorder (recorded on Axis III).

B. The physical condition involves either demonstrable organic pathology (e.g., rheumatoid arthritis) or a known pathophysiologic process (e.g., migraine headache).

C. The condition does not meet the criteria for a Somatoform Disorder.

[a]From the American Psychiatric Association: Diagnostic and Statistical Manual of Mental Disorders, 3rd ed, revised. Washington, DC, American Psychiatric Association, 1987.

Management

When initiation or exacerbation of a physical condition is related to environmental stressors, management is the same as that described for adjustment disorder above.

SOMATOFORM DISORDERS

As a group, the somatoform disorders are characterized by the occurrence of physical symptoms lacking an organic basis and linked, by positive evidence or strong presumption, to psychological factors or conflicts. They may be acute or chronic, mild or severely disabling. Because patients with these disorders believe themselves to be physically ill, they are treated primarily by nonpsychiatrists and do not generally accept psychiatric referral.

Somatization Disorder

Description

The best studied disorder in this group is somatization disorder, formerly known as hysteria or Briquet's syndrome. This is a chronic disorder in which the patient seeks treatment for multiple, widely distributed symptoms lacking any known pathological basis or pathophysiological mechanism. To meet DSM-III-R criteria for this disorder, the patient must have at least 13 such symptoms, drawn from a list of 35 (see Table 12.5). The list includes gastrointestinal, cardiopulmonary, neurological, and female reproductive symptoms as well as pain and sexual dysfunction. Accurate diagnosis often requires review of old records and careful history taking to determine that a sufficient number of unexplained symptoms have been presented for evaluation and treatment or have caused the patient to take over-the-counter remedies and/or alter lifestyle. Seven symptoms are especially useful in screening: shortness of breath when not exerting oneself, dysmenorrhea, burning sensations in sexual organs, difficulty swallowing (lump in throat), amnesia, vomiting, and pain in extremities. The presence of three of these symptoms without adequate physical explanation identifies somatization disorder with a sensitivity of 87% and specificity of 95%. A mnemonic has been devised to aid in remembering the seven symptoms: Somatization (shortness of breath) Disorder (dysmenorrhea) Besets (burning sexual organs) Ladies (lump in throat) And (Amnesia) Vexes (vomiting) Physicians (painful extremities) (18). Symptoms are often described in dramatic and colorful terms but details tend to be vague and contradictory.

Somatization disorder occurs in 0.2 to 2.0% of women in the general population, but is much more common in women seen in clinical settings (15). It is rare in men.

Histrionic personality traits may be present. Somatization disorder occurs in 10 to 20% of the female first-degree relatives of women with somatization disorder, whereas antisocial personality disorder and alcoholism are overrepresented among their male relatives.

Common complications include substance abuse and iatrogenic illness. One classic study found that women with "hysteria" undergo more than three times as many operations as control women and lose, by weight, more than three times the mass of organs (5).

The disorder is chronic. In a retrospective study of 49 patients, nearly 70% of women were still symptomatic 15 years after diagnosis (7). However, the mortality of women with somatization disorder is the same as that of normal women (6), and the likelihood of developing another medical or psychiatric disorder explaining the symptoms is only 10% in long-term follow-up (19).

Case example. A 43-year-old married white woman was referred for psychiatric evaluation by her internist who, noting her presentation with "ill-defined symptoms," was requesting help with management. She had presented with complaints of generalized muscle aching and periodic sensations throughout her body described as "what one has when hearing someone scratch his fingers on a blackboard." She also complained of skin lesions on her back and stated that she was hypothyroid and suffered from a chronic urinary tract infection. Her past history included tonsillectomy, groin lymph node biopsy (twice), hysterectomy, bladder suspension (twice), rectocele repair, removal of adhesions, multiple cystoscopies, appendectomy, and removal of a tongue papilloma. The patient stated she suffered from Ménière's disease and episodes of sudden shortness of breath. She also carried a diagnosis of "fibrositis," for which she had taken steroids in the past, and "restless leg syndrome." She had stopped having sexual intercourse with her husband because of pain that "10 gynecologists could not cure." Her current medicines were Clinoril, Valium, and Bellergal. She mentioned that she had "always been ill" and that she "hated men." Her psychosocial history included marriage to an alcoholic who abused her and a positive family history of suicide. In presenting her symptoms, the patient was extremely vague and interjected facts about her emotional life with an inappropriate laugh. She believed that her symptoms were due to "food allergy." She had stopped eating everything and at the time of her initial visit to her internist had ingested only distilled water for four days. Physical examination and laboratory tests were normal.

Management

Because these patients adhere vigorously to the idea that they are physically ill, they usually do not accept psychiatric referral, and their treatment lies largely in the hands of nonpsychiatrists. Guidelines for management include the following:

1. Review all available medical records to determine the range of symptomatic complaints brought to physicians and the adequacy of documented evaluations.
2. Respond to physical symptoms by taking a careful history and doing the appropriate physical examination; avoid hospitalization, specialty consultations, and invasive laboratory tests unless objective indications exist.
3. Review the four explanatory perspectives (see above) for factors that might be promoting the development of somatization: (a) psychiatric disease (especially major depression); (b) personality disorders

Table 12.5.
Diagnostic Criteria for Somatization Disorder[a]

A. A history of many physical complaints or a belief that one is sickly, beginning before the age of 30 and persisting for several years.

B. At least 13 symptoms from the list below. To count a symptom as significant, the following criteria must be met:

   (1) no organic pathology or pathophysiologic mechanism (e.g., a physical disorder or the effects of injury, medication, drugs, or alcohol) to account for the symptom or, when there is related organic pathology, the complaint or resulting social or occupational impairment is grossly in excess of what would be expected from the physical findings.

   (2) has not occurred only during a panic attack

   (3) has caused the person to take medicine (other than over-the-counter pain medication), see a doctor, or alter life-style

Symptom list:

Gastrointestinal symptoms:

(1) vomiting (other than during pregnancy)
(2) abdominal pain (other than when menstruating)
(3) nausea (other than motion sickness)
(4) bloating (gassy)
(5) diarrhea
(6) intolerance of (gets sick from) several different foods

Pain symptoms:

(7) pain in extremities
(8) back pain
(9) joint pain
(10) pain during urination
(11) other pain (excluding headaches)

Cardiopulmonary symptoms:

(12) shortness of breath when not exerting oneself
(13) palpitations
(14) chest pain
(15) dizziness

Conversion or pseudoneurologic symptoms:

(16) amnesia
(17) difficulty swallowing
(18) loss of voice (19) deafness
(20) double vision
(21) blurred vision
(22) blindness
(23) fainting or loss of consciousness
(24) seizure or convulsion
(25) trouble walking
(26) paralysis or muscle weakness
(27) urinary retention or difficulty urinating

Sexual symptoms for the major part of the person's life after opportunities for sexual activity:

(28) burning sensation in sexual organs or rectum (other than during intercourse)
(29) sexual indifference
(30) pain during intercourse
(31) impotence

Female reproductive symptoms judged by the person to occur more frequently or severely than in most women:

(32) painful menstruation
(33) irregular menstrual periods
(34) excessive menstrual bleeding
(35) vomiting throughout pregnancy

Note: The seven items in boldface may be used to screen for the disorder. The presence of two or more of these items suggests a high likelihood of the disorder.

[a]From the American Psychiatric Association: Diagnostic and Statistical Manual of Mental Disorders, 3rd ed, revised. Washington, DC, American Psychiatric Association, 1987.

(especially histrionic type); (c) behavioral models (e.g., sick family members) or environmental reinforcers (increased attention from parents) supporting the sick role; (d) aspects of the patient's life story (e.g., poor attention to early childhood dependency needs) making her symptoms (e.g., end-less recitation of complaints keeping the patient under very close medical scrutiny) empathically understandable. When possible, address the apparently etiological factors in the treatment plan (e.g., treat major depression with antidepressants; counsel family members to give attention for healthy behavior but to refrain from rewarding illness behavior).

4. Do not expect symptoms to remit entirely, and do not promise the patient "cure" or complete resolution of symptoms.
5. Assure the patient of your continuing availability and schedule regular brief visits so that access to medical attention does not require the development of new symptoms.
6. Do not tell the patient that the symptoms are entirely psychological, but point out that emotional factors worsen physical distress and attempt to direct the patient to discuss life problems.
7. Help the family of the patient recognize that, despite the plethora of symptoms, no serious disease has ever been found, and encourage them to support a strategy that deemphasizes expensive and elaborate diagnostic tests and stresses the maintenance of function in the face of symptoms.

The usefulness of measures such as these in the management of somatization disorder has been empirically demonstrated (20).

Undifferentiated Somatoform Disorder (Table 12.6)

This is a residual category designed to accommodate patients who do not fully meet criteria for somatization disorder. Symptoms must be present for at least six months in order for the diagnosis to be made. There need be no identifiable precipitant. Although the disorder has not been well studied, it is believed to be much more common than somatization disorder. The approach to evaluation and management is the same as that described for somatization disorder.

Conversion Disorder Table (12.7)

Description

This is a disorder in which an unexplained loss or alteration of bodily functioning develops in the pres-

Table 12.6.
Diagnostic Criteria for Undifferentiated Somatoform Disorders[a]

A. One or more physical complaints, e.g., fatigue, loss of appetite, gastrointestinal or urinary complaints.

B. Either (1) or (2):
  (1) appropriate evaluation uncovers no organic pathology or pathophysiologic mechanism (e.g., a physical disorder or the effects of injury, medication, drugs, or alcohol) to account for the physical complaints
  (2) when there is related organic pathology, the physical complaints or resulting social or occupational impairment is grossly in excess of what would be expected from the physical findings

C. Duration of the disturbance is at least six months.

D. Occurrence not exclusively during the course of another Somatoform Disorder, a Sexual Dysfunction, a Mood Disorder, an Anxiety Disorder, a Sleep Disorder or a psychotic disorder.

[a]From, American Psychiatric Association: Diagnostic and Statistical Manual of Mental Disorders, 3rd ed, revised. Washington, DC, American Psychiatric Association, 1987.

Table 12.7.
Diagnostic Criteria for Conversion Disorder[a]

A. A loss of, or alteration in, physical functioning suggesting a physical disorder.

B. Psychological factors are judged to be etiologically related to the symptom because of temporal relationship between a psychological stressor that is apparently related to a psychological conflict or need and initiation or exacerbation of the symptom.

C. The person is not conscious of intentionally producing the symptom.

D. The symptom is not a culturally sanctioned response pattern and cannot, after appropriate investigation, be explained by a known physical disorder.

E. The symptom is not limited to pain or to a disturbance in sexual functioning.

Specify: single episode or recurrent.

[a]From, American Psychiatric Association: Diagnostic and Statistical Manual of Mental Disorders, 3rd ed, revised. Washington, DC, American Psychiatric Association, 1987.

ence of evidence that the symptoms express a psychological conflict or need. The symptoms often simulate neurological disease but conform to the patient's notion of bodily function rather than the rules of neuroanatomy, and medical evaluation yields no evidence of diagnosable disease. Amnesia, aphonia, blindness, paralysis, numbness, and seizures are among the most common conversion symptoms. The disorder probably occurs more often in women than men and generally begins in adolescence or early adulthood. Patients may have histrionic or dependent personalities and may exhibit remarkable serenity ("la belle indifference") in the face of their impairments.

Conversion disorder is unique among DSM-III-R somatoform disorders in that the definition not only describes the diagnostic criteria but also proposes psychological "mechanisms" as explanations. A mechanism termed "secondary gain" is invoked when unexplained symptoms allow the patient to avoid onerous tasks or undesirable duties (see "Somatization as Reinforced Behavior").

Case Example. A 15-year-old girl with a history of migraine headache and transient visual field cuts was admitted because of a new visual field cut that had developed without headache over the previous 24 hours. On examination, the visual defect was found to "split the macula." At the time of psychiatric interview she revealed that she expected her visual problems to prevent her from obtaining a driver's license when she turned 16. She went on to say that she was afraid to drive, that no other woman in her family drove, and that she would be called upon by everyone to provide transportation. She was transferred to a child neurology floor, where she received physical therapy and daily psychotherapy. Her field defect resolved prior to discharge.

A second mechanism, "primary gain," is invoked when conversion symptoms appear to resolve an internal conflict created by a feeling, impulse, or wish that the individual may find frightening or morally unacceptable (see "Somatization and the Life Story").

Case example. A 50-year-old man was admitted to the hospital because of amnesia. He spoke normally and was otherwise neurologically intact, although he could not remember his name or any other details of personal history. After about 24 hours he began speaking freely about anger related to the recent dissolution of his marriage. Particularly upsetting had been news that his boss was dating his wife. Immediately before the development of amnesia he had thought that he might be provoked to violence if he discovered them together. His amnesia completely resolved in two days, and he was discharged from the hospital. He briefly participated in outpatient psychotherapy. The working formulation was that the amnesia had served to remove unacceptable violent intentions from his awareness and protect him from acting on them.

Acute conversion symptoms have a good prognosis for recovery, especially if the patient has no other psychiatric disorder.

Management

Guidelines for the management of patients with conversion disorder include:

1. Be certain that the patient has had an adequate medical evaluation since many patients with conversion symptoms have an undiagnosed medical disorder (13).
2. Review the various explanatory perspectives for factors that might be promoting the development of conversion symptoms: (*a*) psychiatric illness (especially major depression); (*b*) personality disorders (especially dependent and histrionic types); (*c*) behavioral models (e.g., sick family members) or environmental reinforcers (increased attention from family members) supporting the sick role; (*d*) aspects of the patient's life story (e.g., violent feelings toward an abusive alcoholic father) making the symptoms (e.g., paralysis of the hand when the patient considered violent revenge against his father) empathically understandable. When possible, address specific interventions to the etiological factors identified (e.g., treat major depression with antidepressants; counsel family members to reward healthy behavior instead of illness behavior; refer the angry child of an alcoholic to Al-Anon).
3. Emphasize the evidence that no serious disease is present, and express optimism about the prospect of full recovery. Consider physical therapy or some other physical rehabilitative intervention to help the patient "save face" as he recovers.
4. Do not bluntly confront the patient with the psychological origins of the symptoms, but stress that emotional factors may exacerbate such problems. Review the patient's current life circumstances and difficulties, and consider undertaking a course of short-term counseling (see Chapter 11).

Hypochondriasis

Description

This is a chronic disorder in which unrealistic interpretation of physical symptoms leads the patient to believe that he has a serious illness in the face of reassurances based on adequate medical evaluation (Table 12.8). Onset is generally in the third decade but may occur later. Both sexes are equally affected. Obsessive compulsive personality traits are often observed. Anxiety, depression, drug dependence, and iatrogenic disease are common complications. The disorder tends to be chronic, with waxing and waning intensity. Symptomatic exacerbations occur in response to psychosocial stress and to stimuli that provoke bodily preoccupation and fear of disease.

Case Example. A 30-year-old accountant had always been self-conscious about his physical appearance, a concern that he attempted to allay by weight lifting. After his father died of a heart attack he became concerned that he might have heart disease and was fearful about the implication of insignificant chest pains. He also worried about his blood pressure, which was transiently elevated at the time of his yearly physical examinations. His most recent examination revealed insignificant liver enzyme elevations, a finding over which he fretted for weeks. Despite these concerns he rarely missed a day's work. He was not sure that he did not have a serious disease but thought he had best trust his physician.

Although patients such as this young man are relatively easy to care for, others present more difficult management problems. Often they will read whatever they can find and will "doctor shop" because of preoccupation with a dreaded illness. Striking features of this disorder are the amount of worry generated by minor symptoms (e.g., a scratchy throat or a cough) and the amount of time invested in seeking a diagnosis. Patients may lose time from work and, in severe cases, become bedridden.

Table 12.8.
Diagnostic Criteria for Hypochondriasis[a]

A. Preoccupation with the fear of having, or the belief that one has, a serious disease, based on the person's interpretation of physical signs or sensations as evidence of physical illness.

B. Appropriate physical evaluation does not support the diagnosis of any physical disorder that can account for the physical signs or sensations or the person's unwarranted interpretation of them, and the symptoms in A are not just symptoms of panic attacks.

C. The fear of having, or belief that one has, a disease persists despite medical reassurance.

D. Duration of the disturbance is at least six months.

E. The belief in A is not of delusional intensity, as in Delusional Disorder, Somatic Type (i.e., the person can acknowledge the possibility that his or her fear of having, or belief that he or she has, a serious disease is unfounded).

[a]From, American Psychiatric Association: Diagnostic and Statistical Manual of Mental Disorders, 3rd ed, revised. Washington, DC, American Psychiatric Association, 1987.

Management

Because patients with hypochondriasis believe that they are physically ill, they rarely accept psychiatric treatment. Guidelines for management by generalists are similar to those for other chronic somatoform disorders and include the following:

1. Respond to physical symptoms by taking a careful history and doing the appropriate physical examination; reassurances cannot be given to the patient if the physical complaints are not investigated. At the same time, avoid hospitalization, specialty consultations, and invasive laboratory tests unless objective indications exist.
2. Review the four explanatory perspectives (see above) for factors that might be promoting hypochondriasis: (a) psychiatric illness (especially major depression and anxiety disorders); (b) personality disorder (especially obsessive compulsive type); (c) behavioral models and/or environmental reinforcers supporting the sick role (e.g., family members who were excessively concerned about patient's childhood health and lavished attention in response to minor ailments); (d) aspects of the patient's life story (e.g., religious upbringing with particular emphasis on sexual morality and punishment of sinners) making the symptoms empathically understandable (e.g., hypochondriacal fear of AIDS in a man with repeatedly negative HIV antibody tests who had a single extramarital encounter five years before). When possible, address specific interventions to etiological factors identified (e.g., treat major depression with antidepressants; counsel family members to give attention for healthy behavior but to refrain from rewarding illness behavior).
3. Do not expect symptoms to remit entirely, and do not promise the patient "cure" or complete resolution of symptoms.
4. Assure the patient of your continuing availability and schedule brief visits so that access to medical attention does not depend upon the development of new symptoms.
5. Do not tell the patient that the symptoms are entirely psychological, but point out that emotional factors worsen physical distress and attempt to direct the patient to discuss life problems.
6. Help the family of the patient recognize that, despite the persistence of symptoms, no serious disease has been found, and encourage them to support a strategy deemphasizing expensive and elaborate diagnostic tests and stressing the maintenance of function in the face of symptoms.
7. Some patients may accept short-term counseling (see Chapter 11). The development of a relationship characterized by expectant trust is crucial if patients are to be persuaded that their worries are excessive and that they should participate more fully in life activities. Kellner describes such a short-

term treatment approach requiring ten sessions over five months (12).

Somatoform Pain Disorder (Table 12.9)

Description

This is a chronic disorder characterized by unexplained or amplified complaints of pain. It usually has its onset in the fourth or fifth decades and is associated with marked functional disability. The diagnosis is most useful when psychological factors can be linked to the onset and maintenance of pain. A typical scenario begins with lower back pain, often developing on the job, initially diagnosed as a sprain. The patient may see his general physician and attempt to return to work. Soon thereafter the pain recurs, sometimes following apparent reinjury. A series of specialty consultations (e.g., orthopaedic, neurosurgical) ensue. Conservative treatments (e.g., physical therapy) are ineffective. Surgery may be performed, perhaps with transient benefit, but soon there is a resurgence of symptoms described as "worse than ever." After six to twelve months of illness the patient is out of work, socially isolated, physically inactive, dependent on narcotic analgesics, angry, and demoralized. He may believe that health professionals and family members do not regard his pain as "real."

Management

Treatment of somatoform pain disorder is similar to the management of other somatoform disorders:

1. Respond to pain complaints with thorough history and physical examination and determine that adequate medical, surgical, and/or neurological evaluations have been done; but avoid procedures and hospitalization in the absence of clear indications.
2. Review the four explanatory perspectives (see above) for factors that might be promoting unexplained or amplified pain complaints, and design a treatment plan that addresses specific etiological factors identified: (a) major psychiatric disease (especially major depression and chemical dependency, both of which are common in patients with somatoform pain); (b) personality traits (especially exaggerated

---

Table 12.9.
Diagnostic Criteria for Somatoform Pain Disorder[a]

A. Preoccupation with pain for at least six months.

B. Either (1) or (2):

    (1) appropriate evaluation uncovers no organic pathology or pathophysiologic mechanism (e.g., a physical disorder or the effects of injury) to account for the pain

    (2) when there is related organic pathology, the complaint of pain or resulting social or occupational impairment is grossly in excess of what would be expected from the physical findings

[a]From, American Psychiatric Association: Diagnostic and Statistical Manual of Mental Disorders, 3rd ed, revised. Washington, DC, American Psychiatric Association, 1987.

dependency); (c) environmental reinforcers (e.g., financial compensation, relief from work responsibility, sympathy of family and friends); (d) aspects of life history making the pain complaints empathically understandable (e.g., , abusive or negligent parenting leading to a yearning to be cared for in a passive-dependent way, often hidden behind a defiant, "pseudoindependent facade").

3. Convey optimism that improvement is likely but do not promise "cure" or complete resolution of symptoms.
4. Assure the patient of your continuing availability and schedule regular, brief visits so that access to medical attention does not require exacerbation of symptoms.
5. Consider topical treatments and physical therapy because of their intrinsic value, safety, and symbolic value as indicators that the physical reality of the patient's pain is understood.
6. Avoid prescribing benzodiazepines and narcotic analgesics and persuade addicted patients to pursue detoxification.
7. Do not tell the patient that the symptoms are entirely psychological, but stress that emotional factors undoubtedly worsen physical distress, and attempt to direct the patient to discuss life problems, especially interpersonal conflicts and disappointments.
8. Enlist the support of the patient's family in an effort to reinforce maintenance of function in the face of symptoms rather than persistence of disability.
9. Consider referral to a center specializing in the multidisciplinary care of patients with chronic pain syndromes.

Body Dysmorphic Disorder (Table 12.10)

Description

This is a disorder characterized by an excessive or completely unfounded preoccupation with a defect in personal appearance. The prevalence of the disorder is not known, but it may be relatively common. Onset typically occurs between adolescence and age 30. Perceived facial imperfections, such as the shape of the nose or jaw, are the most common sources of concern.

Table 12.10.
Diagnostic Criteria for Body Dysmorphic Disorder[a]

A. Preoccupation with some imagined defect in appearance in a normal-appearing person. If a slight physical anomaly is present, the person's concern is grossly excessive.

B. The belief is not of delusional intensity, as in Delusional Disorder, Somatic Type (i.e., the person can acknowledge the possibility that he or she may be exaggerating the extent of the defect or that there may be no defect at all).

C. Occurrence not exclusively during the course of Anorexia Nervosa or Trans-sexualism.

[a]From, American Psychiatric Association: Diagnostic and Statistical Manual of Mental Disorders, 3rd ed, revised. Washington, DC, American Psychiatric Association, 1987.

Case example. A 60-year-old man entered into psychiatric treatment for chronic depression. He reported long-standing attitudes and patterns of behavior suggesting obsessive compulsive and avoidant personality traits. He also reported a preoccupation beginning in adolescence with the shape of his jaw. He had undergone elaborate surgical treatment for this but continued to feel that other people were put off by his appearance, a belief contributing to his social discomfort. The examining psychiatrist found nothing remarkable about the appearance of his face. The patient's preoccupation with this perceived defect was partially ameliorated by antidepressant treatment, but he continued to regard himself as misshapen.

Management

Little is known about the treatment and prognosis of the disorder. Some authors believe it should be regarded as a symptom and not as a distinct condition. In general, patients should be discouraged from pursuing surgical solutions, especially when their concerns are entirely unfounded. Otherwise, many of the management guidelines described above for other chronic somatoform disorders are applicable. In particular, it is useful to review the four explanatory perspectives for factors promoting the development and maintenance of the symptoms and to treat any specific etiological factor identified: (a) an associated major psychiatric illness, usually major depression; (b) personality types or traits predisposing to the disorder, especially obsessive compulsive and avoidant; (c) behavioral models for these concerns (e.g., parents who were dissatisfied with similar physical attributes in themselves); (d) aspects of the life story making the symptoms empathically understandable (e.g., early experiences with critical parents leading patient to feel like a "freak" or "alien").

DISORDERS WITH VOLUNTARY SYMPTOM PRODUCTION

The fundamental feature of these disorders is the *deliberate* simulation of physical symptoms. This characteristic distinguishes these patients from those with chronic somatoform disorders, described above, in whom symptom genesis is not apparently voluntary.

Factitious Disorder with Physical Symptoms

Description

Factitious illness is characterized by the deliberate simulation of physical symptoms with the singular objective of assuming the role of "patient." When this behavior is chronic and leads to multiple hospitalizations, it is known as chronic factitious disorder with physical symptoms (see DSM-III-R criteria, Table 12.11) or Munchausen's syndrome. When there is deliberate simulation of a psychiatric syndrome, it is designated as factitious disorder with psychological symptoms. Almost any physical illness may be simulated. Pa-

Table 12.11.
Diagnostic Criteria for Factitious Disorder with Physical Symptoms[a]

A. Intentional production or feigning of physical (but not psychological) symptoms.

B. A psychological need to assume the sick role, as evidenced by the absence of external incentives for the behavior, such as economic gain, better care, or physical well-being.

C. Occurrence not exclusively during the course of another Axis I disorder, such as Schizophrenia.

[a]From, American Psychiatric Association: Diagnostic and Statistical Manual of Mental Disorders, 3rd ed, revised. Washington, DC, American Psychiatric Association, 1987.

tients may report invented symptoms (e.g., severe right lower quadrant abdominal pain) or deliberately produce physical signs by heating thermometers, tying tourniquets around their legs, or ingesting anticoagulant drugs. The history may be dramatic but vague in medically relevant detail. Onset is usually in early adulthood, often shortly after hospitalization for a bona fide physical illness. Job stability, family life, and other interpersonal relationships suffer profoundly as a result of multiple lengthy hospitalizations.

Management

The main goals of management are to prevent unnecessary hospitalization and to avoid invasive procedures. The management of the hospitalized patient may be facilitated by early psychiatric consultation to assist in diagnosis, to determine whether other treatable psychiatric disorders are present, to help plan tactful confrontation of the patient with the diagnosis, and to attempt to persuade the patient to accept psychiatric hospitalization.

Malingering

Description

Malingering is the deliberate simulation of physical (or psychological) symptoms in order to achieve a specific benefit. It occurs as an important and relatively common problem in settings where sickness is rewarded with certain benefits (e.g., avoidance of military service or court appearances; financial compensation for injuries). Malingering may be of three types (Ford, "General References"):

1. Pure malingering, in which there is deliberate deception by the description and/or production of nonexistent symptoms and/or signs (rare).
2. Partial malingering, which involves the conscious and voluntary exaggeration of symptoms of a real disease.
3. The deliberate attribution of an actual disability to an injury or accident that did not cause it.

The diagnosis of malingering should be suspected whenever symptoms or disability greatly exceeding objective disease are accompanied by obvious social and/or financial benefit. Other observations suggesting the diagnosis include inconsistency of symptoms (e.g., a "blind" person detected reading), unusually vague or markedly exaggerated reports of symptoms, and the expression of indignant anger in response to gentle confrontation.

Malingering must be distinguished from factitious disorders, in which the patient has no goal aside from achieving "patienthood," and from conversion disorders, in which symptom production is not conscious and intentional.

Management

The goal of management is to persuade malingering patients to give up their symptoms. Patients should gradually and tactfully be made aware that malingering is suspected, and the gratifications associated with the sick role should be removed. Reports of symptoms should be given minimal attention. Because serious psychiatric disorders may underlie apparent malingering, psychiatric consultation should be obtained if possible.

General References

American Psychiatric Association. *Diagnostic and Statistical Manual of Mental Disorders-III-Revised.* Washington, DC, American Psychiatric Association, 1987.

Ford CV: *The Somatizing Disorders: Illness as a Way of Life.* New York, Elsevier Biomedical, 1983.
> Practical well-referenced monograph covering all disorders in which somatization is the principal feature.

Kaplan CK, Lipkin M, Gordon GH: Somatization in primary care: patients with unexplained and vexing medical complaints. *J Gen Intern Med* 3:177, 1988.
> Review article focusing upon origins of somatization and upon diagnosis and management by the primary care physician.

Specific References

1. Barsky AJ: Patients who amplify bodily sensations. *Ann Intern Med* 91:63, 1979.
2. Barsky AJ, Klerman GL: Overview: hypochondriasis, bodily complaints, and somatic styles. *Am J Psychiatry* 140:273, 1983.
3. Catalan J, Gath D, Edmonds G, Ennis J: The effects of non-prescribing of anxiolytics in general practice. I. Controlled evaluation of psychiatric and social outcome. *Br J Psychiatry* 144:593, 1984.
4. Catalan J, Gath D, Bond A, Martin P: The effects of non-prescribing of anxiolytics in general practice. II. Factors associated with outcome. *Br J Psychiatry* 144:603, 1984.
5. Cohen ME, Robins E, Purtell JJ, et al: Excessive surgery in hysteria. *JAMA* 151:977, 1953.
6. Coryell W: Diagnosis-specific mortality. Primary depression and Briquet's syndrome (somatization disorder). *Arch Gen Psychiatry* 38:939, 1981.
7. Coryell W, Norten SG: Briquet's syndrome (somatization disorder) and primary depression: comparison of background and outcome. *Compr Psychiatry* 22:249, 1981.
8. Costa PT, McCrae RR: Hypochondriasis, neuroticism, and aging. *Am Psychologist* 40:19, 1985.
9. Drossman DA: The problem patient: evaluation and care of medical patients with psychosocial disturbances. *Ann Intern Med* 88:366, 1978.
10. Hansell S, Mechanic D: Introspectiveness and adolescent symptom reporting. *J Human Stress* 11 (winter):165, 1985.
11. Johnstone A, Goldberg D: Psychiatric screening in general practice. *Lancet* 1:605, 1976.
12. Kellner R: Psychotherapeutic strategies in hypochondriasis: a clinical study. *Am J Psychotherapy* 36:146, 1982.

13. Lazare A: Conversion symptoms. *N Engl J Med* 305:745, 1983.
14. Lipowski ZJ: Somatization: the concept and its clinical application. *Am J Psychiatry* 145:1358, 1988.
15. Manu P, Matthews DA, Lane TJ: The mental health of patients with a chief complaint of chronic fatigue. *Arch Intern Med* 148:2213, 1988.
16. McHugh PR, Slavney PR (eds): *The Perspectives of Psychiatry.* Baltimore, The Johns Hopkins University Press, 1983.
17. Mechanic D: The concept of illness behavior: culture, situation, and personal disposition. *Psychological Medicine* 16:1, 1986.
18. Othmer E, DeSouza C: A screening test in somatization disorder (hysteria). *Am J Psychiatry*142:1146, 1985.
19. Perley MJ, Guze SB: Hysteria: the stability and usefulness of clinical criteria. *N Engl J Med* 266:421, 1962.
20. Smith GR, Monson RA, Ray DC: Psychiatric consultation in somatization disorder: a randomized controlled study. *N Engl J Med* 314:1407, 1986.
21. Stoeckle J, Zola IK, Davison GE: The quantity and significance of psychological distress in medical patients. *J Chronic Dis* 17:959, 1964.
22. Thomas KB: Temporarily dependent patient in general practice. *Br Med J* 1:625, 1974.

C H A P T E R 13

Anxiety*

ROBERT P. ROCA, M.D., M.P.H.

Anxiety is the term applied to a psychophysiological state characterized by worry (apprehensive expectation), muscle tension, autonomic hyperactivity, and hypervigilance. Anxiety may improve performance in response to danger or challenge and thus may serve an adaptive function. However, when excessive or inappropriate in form or context, it leads to subjective distress and impairment in social and occupational functioning.

NORMAL ANXIETY

Patients visiting their physicians or awaiting the results of tests are often anxious. Although such anxiety may be understandable and realistically related to con-

*Walter F. Baile, M.D., contributed to this chapter in previous editions.

cerns about the meaning of symptoms and consequences of disease, it nonetheless requires recognition and management because it may interfere with medical care. Mayou, et al (48) observed that survivors of myocardial infarction and their spouses recollected little of the information given to them during in-hospital convalescence, partly as a result of anxiety. Such findings highlight the importance of detecting normal illness-related anxiety and treating it skillfully. The following approaches are helpful:

1. Assume that patients with new symptoms have concerns about serious illness. It is helpful to ask patients for their ideas about the causes of their symptoms. Frequently, a relative or friend will have had a similar symptom related to a serious disease.
2. Avoid comments or jargon that might sensitize or frighten patients (e.g., commenting, while examining a skin lesion, "It's been a long time since I've seen one like that.").
3. Try to offer a measure of reassurance, even if prognosis is guarded. It is usually possible to find some basis for hopefulness.
4. Prepare the patient for painful procedures with explanations. Assume that any procedure may be frightening to a patient.
5. Assume that any patient recovering from serious illness will be anxious about the future; determine whether any unnecessary disability is due to fear or inadequate education. Hospitalized patients often get incomplete explanations of their illnesses at the time of discharge.

DRUG-RELATED ANXIETY

In evaluating patients with symptoms of anxiety, it is important to identify all medications or substances taken during or just preceding the onset of symptoms of anxiety. Prescribed drugs, over-the-counter preparations, caffeine, alcohol, and other substances can cause symptoms similar to those found in the primary anxiety disorders described below. Common examples of such compounds are listed in Table 13.1.

ANXIETY DISORDERS

The anxiety disorders are a group of conditions in which anxiety is the predominant symptom. Anxiety causes distress and dysfunction because it is excessive (adjustment disorder with anxious mood, generalized anxiety disorder) or inappropriate in form or context (phobia, panic disorder, obsessive-compulsive disorder, posttraumatic stress disorder).

Adjustment Disorder with Anxious Mood

Description

This term is used when excessive and maladaptive anxiety occurs in response to a recent, identifiable stressor. This "reactive" anxiety resolves when the stressor remits or when the patient reaches a new level

Table 13.1.
Drugs and Other Substances That May Exacerbate (or Produce) Anxiety

Toxic Symptoms:
  Anticholinergic drugs
  Marijuana and other drugs that alter perception (see Chapter 22)
  Stimulant drugs of abuse (see Chapter 22)
  Sympathomimetic drugs:
    Decongestants (found in most over-the-counter cold remedies)
    β-2 bronchodilators
    Weight reduction agents
  Thyroid hormone
  Xanthine-containing drugs, foods, and beverages:
    Bronchodilators with theophylline
    Many over-the-counter cold and arthritis remedies
    Caffeine (use and discontinuation)
Withdrawal Symptoms:
  Sedative-hypnotics
  Alcohol
  Caffeine
  Tobacco

Table 13.2.
Adjustment Disorder with Anxious Mood[a]

A. A reaction (characterized by nervousness, worry, jitteriness) to an identifiable psychosocial stressor (or multiple stressors) that occurs within 3 months of onset of the stressor(s).
B. The maladaptive nature of the reaction is indicated by either of the following:
  (1) impairment in occupational (including school) functioning or in usual social activities or relationships with others
  (2) symptoms that are in excess of a normal and expectable reaction to the stressor(s)
C. The disturbance is not merely one instance of a pattern of overreaction to stress or an exacerbation of another mental disorder.
D. The maladaptive reaction has persisted for no longer than 6 months.
E. The disturbance does not meet the criteria for any specific mental disorder and does not represent Uncomplicated Bereavement.

[a] Adapted from, American Psychiatric Association: Diagnostic and Statistical Manual of Mental Disorders, 3rd ed, revised. Washington, DC, American Psychiatric Association, 1987.

of adaptation or "adjustment." DSM-III-R criteria are listed in Table 13.2.

Case example. A 55-year-old married man presented to the office because of nonexertional chest pain, dizziness, and breathlessness. He had suffered a heart attack three months before but had recovered uneventfully. A recent stress test had shown no signs of coronary insufficiency or serious arrhythmia. His wife reported that the patient had not been himself since leaving the hospital and that "every little thing gets on his nerves." Although he had formerly been "on the go all of the time," he was now afraid to go out of the house. Physical examination now showed no evidence of heart failure, and the ECG was unchanged. The physician reviewed the encouraging results of the ECG and treadmill test, reassured the patient about his symptoms, explained that anxiety is common after myocardial infarction, asked the patient to enroll in a cardiac rehabilitation program, to telephone in one week to report on his symptoms, and to return to the office in two weeks for follow-up examination and a review of his progress. The physician also demonstrated some simple relaxation techniques (see below) and

gave the patient a small supply of diazepam to be used on a "prn" basis.

Treatment

By definition, an adjustment disorder with anxious mood is expected to remit within 6 months as the precipitating problems are resolved or as a new level of "adjustment" is reached. Management includes the following steps:

1. Advise the patient to moderate or eliminate use of caffeine and other stimulants.
2. Consider short-term counseling (see Chapter 11) to meet the patient's informational needs, assist in problem solving, and provide encouragement.
3. Offer training in relaxation and other techniques of self-regulation (see below).
4. Consider instituting a short course of anxiolytic medication, usually a benzodiazepine (see below).

Generalized Anxiety Disorder

Description

This is a chronic disorder characterized by persistent and excessive worry accompanied by symptoms of muscle tension, autonomic hyperactivity, and hypervigilance. DSM-III-R criteria are listed in Table 13.3.

Case example. A 63-year-old woman came to her physician complaining of continuous tightness in the chest. She had always been prone to worry and "bad nerves" but had been much more anxious in the year since her husband had died and she had become responsible for managing all aspects of the household. Three of her adult children, one of whom was mentally retarded, lived at home, and she continued to prepare their meals and do their laundry. She admitted that she was "scared of everything," generally tense ("Little things make me jump"), and frequently experienced feelings of shakiness, diaphoresis, and fluttering in the chest, usually in response to contemplating driving by herself or engaging in another activity about which she was apprehensive. She did not describe discrete intense panic episodes (see below) or symptoms of major depression (see Chapter 15). Physical examination, electrocardiogram, and exercise stress test were normal. Although she was reluctant to take medications, she agreed to try alprazolam (Xanax) 0.25 mg three times per day. In addition, she agreed to meet with her physician on a monthly basis for 12 months for counseling. During counseling sessions she learned simple relaxation techniques (see below), helped construct a program of systematic desensitization regarding driving, and developed a plan to request that her children participate more vigorously in the running of the household. At the end of one year she was greatly improved and asked to begin tapering the alprazolam. She was driving regularly to visit friends across town with diminishing apprehension and growing confidence.

Table 13.3.
Diagnostic Criteria for Generalized Anxiety Disorder[a]

A. Unrealistic or excessive anxiety and worry (apprehensive expectation) about two or more life circumstances, e.g., worry about possible misfortune to one's child (who is in no danger) and worry about finances (for no good reason), for a period of six months or longer, during which the person has been bothered more days than not by these concerns. In children and adolescents, this may take the form of anxiety and worry about academic, athletic, and social performance.
B. If another Axis I disorder is present, the focus of the anxiety and worry in A is unrelated to it, e.g., the anxiety or worry is not about having a panic attack (as in Panic Disorder), being embarrassed in public (as in Social Phobia), being contaminated (as in Obsessive Compulsive Disorder), or gaining weight (as in Anorexia Nervosa).
C. The disturbance does not occur only during the course of a Mood Disorder or a psychotic disorder.
D. At least 6 or the following 18 symptoms are often present when anxious (do not include symptoms present only during panic attacks):
Motor tension
  (1) trembling, twitching, or feeling shaky
  (2) muscle tension, aches, or soreness
  (3) restlessness
  (4) easy fatigability
Autonomic hyperactivity
  (5) shortness of breath or smothering sensations
  (6) palpitations or accelerated heart rate (tachycardia)
  (7) sweating, or cold clammy hands
  (8) dry mouth
  (9) dizziness or lightheadedness
  (10) nausea, diarrhea, or other abdominal distress
  (11) flushes (hot flashes) or chills
  (12) frequent urination
  (13) trouble swallowing or "Lump in throat"
Vigilance and scanning
  (14) feeling keyed up or on edge
  (15) exaggerated startle response
  (16) difficulty concentrating or "mind going blank" because of anxiety
  (17) trouble falling or staying asleep
  (18) irritability
E. It cannot be established that an organic factor initiated and maintained the disturbance, e.g., hyperthyroidism, Caffeine Intoxication.

[a] From, American Psychiatric Association: Diagnostic and Statistical Manual of Mental Disorders, 3rd ed, revised. Washington, DC, American Psychiatric Association, 1987.

Epidemiology and Origins

Generalized anxiety disorder (GAD) occurs in 4 to 5% of general medical outpatients (68), usually in the guise of a medical disorder (4). Symptoms usually begin in the teens or twenties (2) during times of stress. Although anxiety is generally persistent thereafter, the severity of symptoms fluctuates markedly as life stresses come and go. Major depressive disorder and alcoholism often complicate the clinical course (2).

The causes of generalized anxiety disorder are not fully understood. There is little evidence for a strong genetic contribution (21, 65). Anxious mothers (69) and traumatic early life experiences, especially the death of a parent (66), may be predisposing factors, although patients with this disorder do not characterize their childhoods as more difficult than nonanxious persons (38). Events in later life—especially unexpected events perceived as important and negative (12)—may also play a role in the emergence of symptoms.

Evaluation and Treatment

A systematic approach to the evaluation and treatment of the patient with GAD includes the following steps:

1. Take a medical history and perform a physical examination to look for evidence of medical disorders (e.g., hyperthyroidism, pheochromocytoma, hypoglycemia) that may present with symptoms of anxiety.
2. Inquire about consumption of alcohol, caffeine-containing beverages, and other drugs (e.g., "diet" pills), and counsel patient to eliminate ingestion of caffeine and other stimulants and to moderate alcohol consumption.
3. Inquire about life stresses and encourage patient to find solutions to problems; anxious patients are often demoralized and benefit from short-term counseling (see Chapter 11) aimed at solving problems and restoring self-esteem.
4. Instruct the patient in self-regulation techniques such as progressive muscle relaxation (see below) and encourage regular practice.
5. If there are prominent symptoms of hypervigilance (especially sleep disturbance), autonomic hyperactivity, and muscle tension, consider a 1 to 2-month course of benzodiazepines to supplement and facilitate short-term counseling; patients should be allowed to use the medications on a "prn" rather than a standing basis if they prefer. Some patients benefit from long-term occasional use of benzodiazepines at times of unusual stress. Long-term continuous use is controversial, but benzodiazepines appear to retain their anxiolytic potency over time and may therefore continue to be of assistance to patients. Antihistamines may be given in place of

benzodiazepines to anxious patients at high risk for drug abuse (see below for discussions of both classes of agents).

6. If there are prominent cognitive symptoms of worry and apprehension, consider use of buspirone or a tricyclic antidepressant (see below for discussions of both kinds of medication). Neither is particularly useful in ameliorating symptoms of tension or hypervigilance. Both must be taken for several weeks before they become effective, and they carry little risk of tolerance or dependence. Effective therapy with these drugs is generally continued for at least six months to one year.

7. Nonresponse to treatment or relapse should lead to reassessment of the diagnosis, examination for medical and psychiatric comorbidity (especially major depression), and possible psychiatric referral.

Phobias

Description

As a group, phobias are enduring fears of harmless objects or situations (phobic stimuli), leading patients to avoid contact with them (phobic avoidance). Patients with *simple phobia* fear discrete objects and situations such as animals, heights, air travel, needles, and visits to the doctor, whereas patients with *social phobia* have specific fears of social humiliation and the scrutiny of others. Persons with *agoraphobia* fear being alone and being in situations from which escape is difficult (literally, fear of the agora or "marketplace"). Although phobic patients generally recognize their fears to be excessive and unreasonable, they nonetheless seek to avoid the phobic stimuli because exposure provokes intense anxiety. The diagnosis of phobia is made only if avoidance of the feared object or situation leads to social or occupational impairment or if the patient experiences great distress as a result of the symptom.

DSM-III-R criteria for simple phobia and social phobia are listed in Tables 13.4 and 13.5, respectively. Because agoraphobia is usually a complication of Panic Disorder, it is described in this chapter under "Panic Disorder".

Case example. A 50-year-old married business executive sought treatment because of addiction to chlordiazepoxide. In his early twenties he had first become aware of his discomfort in large groups, particularly when he was the focus of attention. He discovered that regular use of chlordiazepoxide improved his general level of comfort, and by age 50 he was using 80 mg per day routinely. He avoided parties whenever possible but was frequently obliged to make professional presentations before clients and superiors. In the days preceding a presentation he would experience great "anticipatory anxiety" associated with the fear that he would be unable to recall what he wanted to say or that his "throat would close up," preventing him from articulating his thoughts and causing him great embarrassment. In response

Table 13.4.
Diagnostic Criteria for Simple Phobia[a]

A. A persistent fear of a circumscribed stimulus (object or situation) other than fear of having a panic attack (as in Panic Disorder) or of humiliation or embarrassment in certain social situations (as in Social Phobia).
   Note: Do not include fears that are part of Panic Disorder with Agoraphobia or Agoraphobia without History of Panic Disorder.
B. During some phase of the disturbance, exposure to the specific phobic stimulus (or stimuli) almost invariably provokes an immediate anxiety response.
C. The object or situation is avoided, or endured with intense anxiety.
D. The fear or the avoidant behavior significantly interferes with the person's normal routine or with usual social activities or relationships with others, or there is marked distress about having the fear.
E. The person recognized that his or her fear is excessive or unreasonable.
F. The phobic stimulus is unrelated to the content of the obsessions of Obsessive Compulsive Disorder or the trauma of Post-traumatic Stress Disorder.

---

[a] From, American Psychiatric Association: Diagnostic and Statistical Manual of Mental Disorders, 3rd ed, revised. Washington, DC, American Psychiatric Association, 1987.

to this fear, he would increase his daily chlordiazepoxide dose by 50 to 100%. On the day of the presentation he would take 200 to 300 mg and would perform well. He was dissatisfied with this practice because he now felt depressed and believed that the medication might be playing a role. His diagnosis at the time of evaluation was social phobia and benzodiazepine dependence. A slow chlordiazepoxide taper was undertaken and completed within six months. At the same time he participated actively in a program of in vivo "desensitization" (see below) involving regular attendance at social activities of graded difficulty and the pursuit of opportunities to give group presentations at work without the assistance of benzodiazepines. His social anxiety declined and his confidence grew as he succeeded in attending parties and in giving talks without substantial reliance on medication. Ultimately he continued to use chlordiazepoxide in low doses before stressful gatherings but no longer had a habit of daily use.

Epidemiology and Origins

Simple phobias are among the most common psychiatric disorders in the community, with six-month prevalence rates ranging between 5.4 and 13.4% (51). They occur approximately twice as often among women as men and show a tendency to drop in prevalence after age 65. Phobias beginning in childhood often improve with maturity, whereas those beginning in adulthood rarely resolve without treatment. *Social phobia* has a community prevalence of between 1 and 2%. It is equally common among men and women and declines in prevalence with increasing age (51).

Between 7 and 8% of general medical outpatients may have phobias (68). In this setting, phobias related to medical procedures (e.g., phlebotomy) may interfere with the delivery of medical care, and phobias related to dread diseases (e.g., cancer, AIDS) may prevent patients from undergoing examinations that could disclose evidence of the feared illness.

Table 13.5.
Diagnostic Criteria for Social Phobia[a]

A. A persistent fear of one or more situations (the social phobic situations) in which the person is exposed to possible scrutiny by others and fears that he or she may do something or act in a way that will be humiliating or embarrassing. Examples include: being unable to continue talking while speaking in public, choking on food when eating in front of others, being unable to urinate in a public lavatory, hand-trembling when writing in the presence of others, and saying foolish things or not being able to answer questions in social situations.

B. If an Axis III or another Axis I disorder is present, the fear in A is unrelated to it, e.g., the fear is not of having a panic attack (Panic Disorder), stuttering (Stuttering), trembling (Parkinson's disease), or exhibiting abnormal eating behavior (Anorexia Nervosa or Bulimia Nervosa).

C. During some phase of the disturbance, exposure to the specific phobic stimulus (or stimuli) almost invariably provokes an immediate anxiety response.

D. The phobic situation(s) is avoided, or is endured with intense anxiety.

E. The avoidant behavior interferes with occupational functioning or with usual social activities or relationships with others, or there is marked distress about having the fear.

F. The person recognizes that his or her fear is excessive or unreasonable.

G. If the person is under 18, the disturbance does not meet the criteria for Avoidant Disorder of Childhood or Adolescence.

Specify generalized type if the phobic situation includes most social situations, and also consider the additional diagnosis of Avoidant Personality Disorder.

[a]From, American Psychiatric Association: Diagnostic and Statistical Manual of Mental Disorders, 3rd ed, revised. Washington, DC, American Psychiatric Association, 1987.

Patients with social phobia may become addicted to alcohol or sedative-hypnotics as a result of self-directed efforts to ameliorate their social anxiety. Furthermore, phobias and phobic anxiety may be risk factors for ischemic heart disease and other forms of cardiovascular morbidity. Studies have shown (35) significant associations between measures of phobic anxiety (fears of enclosed spaces, illness, going out alone, heights, and crowds) and the probability of subsequent ischemic cardiac events. Such relationships may be mediated by anxiety-related hyperventilation, which has been shown to cause coronary vasospasm and cardiac ischemia (57), or by anxiety-induced arrhythmia (42).

Treatment

Approaches to treating phobic anxiety are based on the notion that this form of anxiety develops as a product of the pairing of an innocuous stimulus with a threatening one. Phobic avoidance emerges and is maintained by the anxiety-preventing consequences of the avoidance. The treatment of phobias has advanced greatly with the development of behavioral therapies aimed at "extinguishing" phobic anxiety and phobic avoidance. Three commonly used techniques are desensitization, participant modeling, and social skills training.

Systematic desensitization begins with the gradual exposure of the patient to increasingly vivid and anxiety-provoking mental images of the phobic stimulus. As anxiety is generated, the patient induces relaxation by use of a relaxation technique (see below). By exercising a response incompatible with anxiety (i.e., relaxation) in response to the phobic stimulus, the patient gradually "extinguishes" the phobic anxiety. This treatment occurs over a series of sessions until the patient is comfortable enough to encounter the stimulus in vivo. Related to systematic desensitization is *flooding* or *implosion*, in which the imagery is presented suddenly rather than gradually.

In vivo desensitization involves the gradual, stepwise exposure of the patient to the feared stimulus in real life. The patient is often initially accompanied by the therapist or a trained family member. Progress from less to more anxiety-producing tasks is accomplished by mastering anxiety at each level. The basis for the technique is that repeated exposure leads to extinction of phobic anxiety.

Participant modeling is a form of in vivo desensitization in which the therapist models the desired interaction with the feared object. This kind of procedure may be useful with severe needle phobics, whose avoidance of needles is potentially life threatening (e.g., in patients requiring insulin). Therapy may involve the following steps (63):

1. Education aimed at providing realistic information about the feared object.
2. Response modeling in which the therapist handles the feared object.
3. Joint performance in which the patient and therapist are both exposed to the phobic stimulus.
4. Self-directed practice (e.g., inserting a needle into an orange).

Social skills training, especially assertiveness training, is particularly useful in the treatment of social phobics. Its object is to promote the development of comfort in anxiety-provoking social settings (e.g., public speaking; business meetings) by use of modeling and role plays.

Behavioral techniques such as these have been used successfully in treating phobias related to hemodialysis, needles, and return to work after medical illness. They may be carried out by nonphysicians and are usually effective within 15 sessions or less. Among patients treated by these techniques, phobias, hypochondriacal symptoms, and work adjustment often improve within six months; and visits to physicians decrease markedly (45, 46).

Panic Disorder

Description

This condition is characterized by recurrent, discrete attacks of intense fear or discomfort associated with somatic and/or psychic symptoms of anxiety. The attacks generally last for a few minutes and are usually unprecipitated, coming "out of the blue," even waking the person from sleep at night. Persons who experience panic attacks often grow uncomfortable being in places from which escape might be difficult or embarrassing or in which help might not be available in the event of a panic attack; this fear and the associated phobic avoidance are termed *agoraphobia*.

DSM-III-R diagnostic criteria for panic disorder are summarized in Table 13.6.

Case Example. A 27-year-old male business executive was referred because of anxiety. He had no prior psychiatric history, did not abuse drugs or alcohol, and did not consume caffeine excessively. He had recently married and was in the process of buying a house. Immediately prior to the onset of his symptoms, his father had suffered a nonfatal myocardial infarction. Subsequently, the patient began experiencing frequent episodes of chest pain, dyspnea, and palpitations associated with fear of dying and feelings of panic. Medical work-up disclosed no evidence of hyperthyroidism or cardiovascular disease, and he was diagnosed as having panic disorder. He was placed on desipramine and alprazolam and was counseled to eliminate stressors. His panic attacks ceased within a week. He was followed in short-term counseling every three weeks, and after six months his medications were tapered without symptomatic relapse.

Epidemiology and Origins

Less common than simple phobia and generalized anxiety disorder, panic disorder has a prevalence in the community of 1 to 2% and may be more common in women than men (61, 68). The initial attacks usually occur in the second or third decades, are often vividly recalled, and, in about 50% of cases, develop during a time of stress (2). Frequently associated psychiatric conditions include major depression, generalized anxiety disorder, agoraphobia (see below), and obsessive-compulsive disorder (13, 14, 15).

Patients with panic disorder present special differential diagnostic challenges to general physicians and cardiologists. Although panic symptomatology is often difficult to distinguish from angina and may lead to unnecessary cardiac catheterization (8), patients with panic disorder have an increased cardiovascular mortality (22), perhaps as a result of hyperventilation-induced coronary vasospasm (57), and may have a very high prevalence of mitral valve prolapse (47), a controversial finding of uncertain significance. In addition, panic symptoms may be simulated by a number of noncardiac medical disorders, including alcohol and sedative-hypnotic drug withdrawal, marijuana use, pheochromocytoma, hyperthyroidism, hypoglycemia, and temporal lobe epilepsy.

Recent studies have supported the view that panic disorder is primarily a biological disorder, i.e., a disease. Genetic factors have been implicated by family

---

Table 13.6.
Diagnostic Criteria for Panic Disorder[a]

A. At some time during the disturbance, one or more panic attacks (discrete periods of intense fear or discomfort) have occurred that were (1) unexpected, i.e., did not occur immediately before or on exposure to a situation that almost always caused anxiety, and (2) not triggered by situations in which the person was the focus of others' attention.

B. Either four attacks, as defined in criterion A, have occurred within a four-week period, or one or more attacks have been followed by a period of at least a month of persistent fear of having another attack.

C. At least four of the following symptoms developed during at least one of the attacks:
   (1) shortness of breath (dyspnea) or smothering sensations
   (2) dizziness, unsteady feelings, or faintness
   (3) palpitations or accelerated heart rate (tachycardia)
   (4) trembling or shaking
   (5) sweating
   (6) choking
   (7) nausea or abdominal distress
   (8) depersonalization or derealization
   (9) numbness or tingling sensations (paresthesias)
  (10) flushes (hot flashes) or chills
  (11) chest pain or discomfort
  (12) fear of dying
  (13) fear of going crazy or of doing something uncontrolled
Note: Attacks involving four or more symptoms are panic attacks; attacks involving fewer than four symptoms are limited symptom attacks (see Agoraphobia without History of Panic Disorder).

D. During at least some of the attacks, at least four of the C symptoms developed suddenly and increased in intensity within ten minutes of the beginning of the first C symptom noticed in the attack.

E. It cannot be established that an organic factor initiated and maintained the disturbance, e.g., Amphetamine or Caffeine Intoxication, hyperthyroidism.

Note: Mitral valve prolapse may be an associated condition, but does not preclude a diagnosis of panic disorder.

[a]From, American Psychiatric Association: Diagnostic and Statistical Manual of Mental Disorders, 3rd ed, revised. Washington, DC, American Psychiatric Association, 1987.

studies demonstrating a 10-fold increase in panic disorder among first-degree relatives of panic probands (54) and a markedly higher concordance rate for panic disorder among monozygotic than among dizygotic twins (65). Furthermore, lactate infusion (31) and hyperventilation (20) may stimulate panic attacks in individuals with panic disorder, suggesting the existence of specific biological triggers. Finally, pharmacological treatments may by themselves dramatically reduce the frequency of panic episodes (see below). These observations all suggest an important role for biological factors in the etiology of panic disorder.

There are also learning (or conditioning) theories to explain panic disorder. These propose that panic attacks develop when physical sensations occurring at times of stress are interpreted as signs of grave illness, giving rise to panic. The physical sensations of arousal thus become conditioned phobic stimuli, provoking the panic symptomatology (conditioned response) (7). Conditioning models have been particularly persuasive in accounting for the development and maintenance of agoraphobia (30).

Agoraphobia

Agoraphobia is the most disabling psychiatric complication of panic disorder. The first sign is usually the avoidance of selected settings from which escape would be difficult or embarrassing in the event of a panic attack (e.g., traveling in bus, train, or car; being out of the house alone; standing in the check-out line at a store). With the persistence of panic attacks, the inventory of phobic stimuli expands by "generalization," and the patient adopts a variety of behaviors aimed at avoiding contact with a growing number of feared objects and situations (see Table 13.7). Ultimately, this fear of having a panic attack ("anticipatory anxiety") may become incapacitating, and the patient may become "homebound."

Table 13.7.
Frequency of Strategies Adopted by Patients with Agoraphobia to Reduce Anticipatory Anxiety[a]

Strategy	Percentage of Patients
When out, having a way open for a quick return home	91
Being accompanied by husband/wife	85
Sitting near a door in hall, restaurant, etc.	76
Focusing my mind on something else	63
When out for a walk, taking dog, perambulator, etc.	62
Talking problem over with a friend	62
Talking problems over with my doctor	62
Being accompanied by a friend	60
Talking "sense to myself" (reassuring myself)	52
Wearing sunglasses	36

[a] From Burns LE, Thorpe GL: Epidemiology of fears and phobias. *J Int Med Res* 5:1, 1977.

Agoraphobia occasionally occurs in the absence of panic attacks ("agoraphobia without history of panic disorder" in DSM-III-R) but this is apparently very rare, at least in clinical samples (5). Among patients with panic disorder, those most likely to develop agoraphobia are women who have persistent panic attacks (i.e., no history of clinical remissions), a high degree of interpersonal sensitivity, and a history of anxiety or depression in childhood (5).

Evaluation and Treatment

A systematic approach to the evaluation and treatment of panic disorder includes the following steps:

1. Take a history and perform a physical examination looking for evidence of a medical disorder that could simulate panic disorder (e.g., hypoglycemic episodes, temporal lobe seizures, arrhythmias).
2. Inquire about the use of caffeine-containing beverages, stimulant drugs, alcohol, marijuana, and other substances associated with panic symptoms during intoxication or withdrawal.
3. Inquire about life stresses and encourage the patient to solve problems (see Chapter 11). Although this may not eliminate panic attacks, it will help reduce the levels of generalized anxiety that often develops in patients with panic disorder.
4. Use pharmacological means to reduce the frequency and intensity of panic attacks. Tricyclic antidepressants and monoamine oxidase (MAO) inhibitors are effective in the prophylaxis of panic attacks (44), as is the triazolobenzodiazepine, alprazolam (6); other benzodiazepines alleviate anticipatory anxiety but may not *prevent* panic attacks. Several strategies may be used. Alprazolam may be started as a single agent in a dose of .25 mg three times a day and increased to six mg per day in divided doses. Reductions in the frequency of panic attacks and of phobic avoidance may become apparent within the first week of therapy (6). If there is concern about the possibility of abuse of alprazolam (19), an antidepressant may be utilized instead as a single agent. The tricyclic, imipramine, and the MAO inhibitor, phenelzine, are most often used. As a rule, dosages required for prophylaxis of panic attacks approximate those required for antidepressant effects (see Chapter 15). Symptoms may not improve for several weeks and may even intensify at first, especially in patients treated with imipramine, which may produce "hyperstimulatory" reactions in up to one-third of patients treated for panic disorder (44). For these reasons, some physicians combine alprazolam and an antidepressant at the beginning of therapy and taper alprazolam, the more rapidly effective agent, after several weeks. Effective drug treatment is generally continued for at least six to twelve months before tapering is attempted. Relapse is common and may indicate the need for chronic therapy.
5. The conditioned avoidances of agoraphobics may

be reduced by behavioral exposure techniques such as those described above for other phobias.

6. Patients often gain relief from learning that panic disorder is a disease, not a sign of "weakness;" that it is common; and that it is treatable. Such educational efforts supplemented by readily available books written for the lay person (1, 33) may help reduce the patient's sense of isolation and embarrassment and provide practical advice about managing panic symptoms.

Obsessive-Compulsive Disorder

Description

The essential features of obsessive-compulsive disorder (OCD) are recurrent, resisted, troubling thoughts (e.g., objects are contaminated), and repetitive, purposeful, but senseless actions (e.g., washing hands 100 times per day). It is the presence of obsessions and compulsions that distinguishes OCD from obsessive-compulsive *personality* disorder (see Chapter 14), a personality type characterized by meticulousness, perfectionism, and rigidity. The DSM-III-R diagnostic criteria for OCD are listed in Table 13.8.

Case example. An 83-year-old widow was referred for evaluation because of disabling fears of contamination. She was a retired mathematics teacher who liked her subject because "one and one always equal two; I like the certainty." A practicing Catholic, she recalled that during adolescence she had once delayed disposing of a "sanitary napkin" because she had sneezed over it after returning home after Mass and worried that bits of the communion wafer might have lodged in it. She had received psychiatric treatment several times for obsessive-compulsive symptoms but had recently been doing well until she was forced to change apartments. After the move she became preoccupied with worries about contamination with "germs." Especially vexing was deciding when she had adequately washed her hands after def-

ecating; she was consumed by uncertainty about how long she should wash and how she could safely dispose of the towel after drying her hands. Her main fear was that others might be contaminated and become ill as a result of her carelessness. As a result of these ideas, she washed her hands excessively, did not leave her apartment, ate poorly (so she would defecate less), and was unable to engage in normal conversation. Treatment consisted of strict direction to limit hand washing, exhortation about the unreasonableness of her worries, and the use of fluoxetine, an antidepressant with specific antiobsessional properties (see below). Within two weeks she was showing improvement, and by the end of eight weeks she was able to dispel obsessive ideas effortlessly and felt no compulsion to wash excessively.

Epidemiology and Origins

One to two percent of persons in the community (51) and in the general medical clinic (68) meet criteria for OCD. Its prevalence is slightly higher among women and tends to decline with age. Symptoms usually have their onset in adolescence or early adulthood. In one study of patients with OCD (58), the most common obsessions were fear of contamination (55%), of acting aggressively (50%), and of performing unacceptable sexual activities (32%). Somatic obsessions were present in 34% of patients [e.g., a woman who performed breast self-examinations 100 times per day to reassure herself that she had not developed breast cancer (58)], and 36% had obsessive thoughts involving the need for symmetry. The most common compulsions involved checking, cleaning, and counting. In most cases the symptoms were chronic and continuous, with some tendency for symptomatic worsening during times of stress. Associated psychiatric diagnoses included major depression (30%), simple phobia (7%), and panic disorder (5%).

Explanations have been advanced from several perspectives. Psychoanalytic writers have viewed obsessive-compulsive symptoms as products of "reaction

Table 13.8.
Diagnostic Criteria for Obsessive-Compulsive Disorder[a]

A. Either obsessions or compulsions:
Obsessions: (1), (2), (3), and (4):
  (1) recurrent and persistent ideas, thoughts, impulses, or images that are experienced, at least initially, as intrusive and senseless, e.g., a parent's having repeated impulses to kill a loved child, a religious person's having recurrent blasphemous thoughts
  (2) the person attempts to ignore or suppress such thoughts or impulses or to neutralize them with some other thought or action
  (3) the person recognizes that the obsessions are the product of his or her own mind, not imposed from without (as in thought insertion)
  (4) if another Axis I disorder is present, the content of the obsession is unrelated to it, e.g., the ideas, thoughts, impulses, or images are not about food in the presence of an Eating Disorder, about drugs in the presence of a Psychoactive Substance Use Disorder, or guilty thoughts in the presence of a Major Depression
Compulsions: (1), (2), and (3):
  (1) repetitive, purposeful, and intentional behaviors that are performed in response to an obsession, or according to certain rules or in a stereotyped fashion
  (2) the behavior is designed to neutralize or to prevent discomfort or some dreaded event or situation; however, either the activity is not connected in a realistic way with what it is designed to neutralize or prevent, or it is clearly excessive
  (3) The person recognizes that his or her behavior is excessive or unreasonable (this may not be true for young children; it may no longer be true for people whose obsessions have evolved into overvalued ideas)
B. The obsessions or compulsions cause marked distress, are time-consuming (take more than an hour a day), or significantly interfere with the person's normal routine, occupational functioning, or usual social activities or relationships with others.

formation" against unacceptable wishes and impulses, often related to aggression and sexuality. Behavioral theorists and practitioners have stressed the anxiety-reducing effects of compulsive rituals and have proposed that compulsions are maintained precisely because of their positively reinforcing ameliorating effects on conditioned anxiety. The importance of personality traits in the development of OCD is suggested by data showing that preexisting obsessive traits (e.g., meticulousness, perfectionism, indecisiveness) are very common in clinical samples of persons who go on to develop OCD (58) and that persons who are obsessional, anxious, or self-conscious may be especially vulnerable to the emergence of OCD in response to life change (50).

Much recent research suggests that OCD has biologic origins. The importance of genetic factors is supported by studies showing high concordance for OCD among monozygotic twins (17) and increased risk for OCD among first-degree relatives of probands with Gilles de la Tourette's syndrome (55). Brain imaging studies have demonstrated abnormalities of the left orbital frontal gyri (9) and the caudate nuclei (9, 43). Clinical studies linking OCD with head trauma (49) and other neurological disorders (34) add support to the conception that OCD may be a manifestation of brain disease. Of great theoretical and practical importance has been the demonstration that antidepressant medications, especially those inhibiting the reuptake of serotonin (e.g., clomipramine; fluoxetine), may dramatically diminish obsessive-compulsive symptoms, suggesting a role for central serotonergic neuronal systems in the pathophysiology of this disorder (see below).

Evaluation and Treatment

A systematic approach to the evaluation and treatment of OCD involves the following steps:

1. In the history and physical examination, look for evidence of medical conditions, medications, or dietary practices that may simulate or exacerbate symptoms of anxiety.
2. Consider use of antidepressant medications shown to have specific efficacy in obsessive-compulsive disorder. Clomipramine, a tricyclic recently approved for use in the United States, was the first medication noted to be effective in this condition (64). The starting dose is 25 mg per day. Doses as high as 250 mg per day may be required; and maximum improvement may not occur for 6 to 8 weeks. Fluoxetine (Prozac), a nontricyclic antidepressant that selectively inhibits serotonin reuptake, may also be effective (67). Initial dosage is usually 20 mg per day. Clinical response often requires 40 to 60 mg per day, generally given in 2 doses early in the day because fluoxetine may produce insomnia.
3. Consider use of behavioral treatments. This suggestion follows from the view that compulsions are

maintained by their temporary amelioration of conditioned anxiety. Patients are taught to control their obsessive ruminations by commanding themselves to "stop" ruminating when obsessive ideas arise ("thought stopping"), and they are exhorted to resist carrying out their compulsive acts so that they can learn that there are no dire consequences associated with nonexecution of the rituals ("response prevention"). These techniques are often helpful if patients can be persuaded to practice them.
4. Consider short-term, problem-solving counseling (see Chapter 11). Although this may not bring total relief, it is clear that symptomatic exacerbations of this chronic disorder tend to come at times of stress and change, and short-term counseling may help reduce the impact of such influences. On the other hand, insight-oriented, introspective psychotherapies have generally been ineffective in the treatment of OCD.

Post-traumatic Stress Disorder

Description

Persons who have experienced severe physical or emotional trauma may develop a syndrome characterized by intrusive recollections or dreams of the event, avoidance of stimuli provoking memories of the event, and a heightened level of arousal. When this syndrome has been present for at least one month, the diagnosis of post-traumatic stress disorder (PTSD) is made. DSM-III-R criteria are summarized in Table 13.9.

Case example. A 45-year-old mechanic sustained burns on the arms and thorax when an engine exploded during repair. He had no history of psychiatric disorder. His surgical treatment was successful, leaving him with little residual physical disability. However, after discharge he experienced marked sleep disturbance, generalized anxiety, and loss of interest in usual activities. He avoided proximity to fire in any form and could not tolerate listening to reports about fires on the radio. Tricyclic antidepressant treatment aided sleep, improved his mood, and reduced the frequency of his intrusive memories and recurrent dreams, but it did not affect his avoidance behavior: On the anniversary of his injury he would not leave his room because he could not be persuaded it was safe to do so.

Epidemiology and Origins

The prevalence of post-traumatic stress disorder in the community is about 1%. Among men, the full syndrome is usually found among Vietnam veterans who were injured in combat; among women, the most common precipitant is physical assault. Individual post-traumatic stress *symptoms* (particularly nightmares, feelings of "jitteriness," and sleep disturbance) are much more common, occurring in about 15% of the population. Combat, physical assault, seeing someone hurt or die, and experiencing a serious threat or close call

Table 13.9.
Diagnostic Criteria for Post-traumatic Stress Disorder[a]

A. The person has experienced an event that is outside the range of usual human experience and that would be markedly distressing to almost anyone, e.g., serious threat to one's life or physical integrity; serious threat or harm to one's children, spouse, or other close relatives and friends; sudden destruction of one's home or community; or seeing another person who has recently been or is being, seriously injured or killed as the result of an accident or physical violence.

B. The traumatic event is persistently reexperienced in at least one of the following ways:
  (1) recurrent and intrusive distressing recollections of the event (in young children, repetitive play in which themes or aspects of the trauma are expressed)
  (2) recurrent distressing dreams of the event
  (3) sudden acting or feeling as if the traumatic event were recurring (includes a sense of reliving the experience, illusions, hallucinations, and dissociative [flashback] episodes, even those that occur upon awakening or when intoxicated)
  (4) intense psychological distress at exposure to events that symbolize or resemble an aspect of the traumatic event, including anniversaries of the trauma

C. Persistent avoidance of stimuli associated with the trauma or numbing of general responsiveness (not present before the trauma), as indicated by at least three of the following:
  (1) efforts to avoid thoughts or feelings associated with the trauma
  (2) efforts to avoid activities or situations that arouse recollections of the trauma
  (3) inability to recall an important aspect of the trauma (psychogenic amnesia)
  (4) markedly diminished interest in significant activities (in young children, loss of recently acquired developmental skills such as toilet training or language skills)
  (5) feeling of detachment or estrangement from others
  (6) restricted range of affect, e.g., unable to have loving feelings
  (7) sense of a foreshortened future, e.g., does not expect to have a career, marriage, or children, or a long life

D. Persistent symptoms of increased arousal (not present before the trauma), as indicated by at least two of the following:
  (1) difficulty falling or staying asleep
  (2) irritability or outbursts of anger
  (3) difficulty concentrating
  (4) hypervigilance
  (5) exaggerated startle response
  (6) physiologic reactivity upon exposure to events that symbolize or resemble an aspect of the traumatic event (e.g., a woman who was raped in an elevator breaks out in a sweat when entering any elevator)

E. Duration of the disturbance (symptoms in B, C, and D) of at least one month
Specify delayed onset if the onset of symptoms was at least six months after the trauma.

[a] From, American Psychiatric Association: Diagnostic and Statistical Manual of Mental Disorders, 3rd ed, revised. Washington, DC, American Psychiatric Association, 1987.

are the most common traumata associated with such symptoms (36).

PTSD generally develops soon after the traumatic event, although onset was delayed by at least six months among some Vietnam combat veterans. Although symptoms may persist for years after the traumatic event, about half of patients report resolution of symptoms within six months (36).

Persons with PTSD are twice as likely as persons without PTSD to have another psychiatric disorder, particularly obsessive-compulsive disorder, dysthymia, substance abuse, bipolar affective disorder, and antisocial personality. There is also an increased risk of PTSD among persons with a history of childhood behavioral problems, especially lying, stealing, truancy, vandalism, and school expulsion. Among persons with a history of four such behaviors, 6% meet formal criteria for PTSD and 29% report at least one symptom (36).

Explanations of PTSD have been advanced from several perspectives. From the behavioral viewpoint, the post-traumatic symptoms (e.g., hyperarousal, intrusive recollections) are viewed as products of classically conditioned linkages between innocuous stimuli (e.g., a news report about a fire) and the original traumatic event (e.g., painful injury in a fire). The avoidance symptoms are explained in terms of operant conditioning: Avoidance of stimuli reminiscent of the

traumatic event is reinforced by its consequence of protecting the patient from the symptoms of phobic anxiety (i.e., hyperarousal). Biological theorists have proposed explanations involving changes in central adrenergic autonomic arousal (40) and in cerebral mechanisms regulating sleep cycles (62). Important roles for personality traits and early life experience have been suggested by observations of burn patients and other trauma victims demonstrating relationships between maladaptive personality traits, early life behavioral problems, and poor post-traumatic adjustment (3, 36).

Treatment

Pharmacological, psychotherapeutic, and behavioral treatment approaches have all been advocated. Tricyclic antidepressants and monoamine oxidase inhibitors are often effective in ameliorating hyperarousal and recurrent nightmares as well as relieving concurrent major depression. Benzodiazepines are also effective but may be relatively contraindicated in patients at high risk for chemical dependency. Neuroleptic drugs are almost never indicated (24). Behavioral treatments such as desensitization are generally required to help patients overcome the conditioned avoidance of stimuli reminiscent of the traumatic event. Finally, psychotherapy may be needed to assist patients in dealing with guilt about survival and similar themes common among persons with PTSD.

TREATMENT OF ANXIETY DISORDERS: GENERAL CONSIDERATIONS

Nonpharmacological Approaches

A variety of cognitive and behavioral interventions are useful in the treatment of anxiety disorders.

Education and Explanation

Patients with panic attacks, obsessions and compulsions, post-traumatic distress symptoms, and generalized anxiety often feel "different," isolated from others, and confused about the nature of their malady. They often benefit greatly from learning that they have a diagnosable disorder, that they are not alone in their suffering, and that there are effective treatments. Several popular books can be recommended to patients who are interested in reading about anxiety disorders (1, 33).

Self-Regulation Techniques

Many patients benefit from learning specific techniques that reduce motor tension, hyperarousal, and autonomic hyperactivity. These so-called "self-regulation" techniques include muscle relaxation, biofeedback, self-hypnosis, and meditation exercises (29). Interested generalists can develop skills in teaching these techniques to their patients. Alternatively, patients can be referred to behavioral therapists for instruction.

In *progressive muscle relaxation* (see Table 13.10), patients learn to reduce muscle tension and ameliorate anxiety by sequential contraction and relaxation of muscle groups. With regular practice, patients can apply this technique in times of distress and achieve considerable relief. Commercially available audiotapes may help guide patients through the procedure (see "General References"), and *The Relaxation Response* (10), written for the lay person, may also be useful.

In *biofeedback* (25) patients learn to control anxiety with the aid of electromyographic information provided to them in the form of visual or auditory signals. During treatment sessions electrodes are placed in a muscle (e.g., frontalis) or muscle group. Patients then attempt to reduce muscle tension, receive immediate feedback about the effectiveness of their efforts (e.g., a reduction in the amplitude of a tone "fed back" to them through earphones), and learn to alter their technique to achieve more complete electromyographic (and clinical) relaxation.

Self-hypnosis training often begins with office-based sessions during which the therapist uses a standard hypnotic induction technique and then, for example, asks the patient to notice the warm, tingling feeling starting in the legs and feet and spreading slowly throughout the body. Pleasant, peaceful mental images might be suggested. Patients are taught to induce these states on their own and are advised to practice them regularly, reinforced by periodic office visits for reassessment and further practice. Physicians may develop skills in performing hypnosis by attending seminars such as those sponsored by the Society for Clinical and Experimental Hypnosis.

Meditation techniques (e.g., Zen, yoga, transcendental meditation) have been practiced for centuries but have recently become popular treatments for anxiety because they favorably alter anxiety-related physiological variables such as respiratory rate, oxygen consumption, and galvanic skin response, a measure of autonomic activity. Meditation techniques that are effective in ameliorating anxiety include or encourage the following elements (11): (a) A mental device. There should be a constant stimulus such as a sound, word,

Table 13.10.
Essential Steps in (A) Progressive Muscle Relaxation and (B) Rapid Muscle Relaxation Techniques

Muscle	Exercise
(A) Progressive Muscle Relaxation[a]	
Forehead/scalp	Raise the eyebrows high; hold; feel strain; relax.
Forehead	Scowl or frown; bunch eyebrows with nose upward; relax.
Eyes	Squeeze eyes shut; hold; feel strain in temples; relax.
Mouth	Smile broadly until mouth quivers slightly; relax; press lips tightly inward; hold; relax.
Jaw	Grit teeth gently but firmly; hold, relax; part lips slightly.
Neck/arm/shoulder	Press head back against right hand; relax; repeat exercise with left hand.
Neck/arm/shoulder	Press head forward against right hand placed on forehead; relax; repeat with left hand
Back/legs/abdomen	Sitting grip chair sides firmly; raise legs slightly; lift buttocks 1 inch from chair; point toes forward, then backward; relax.
Hands/arm	Make fist; clench tightly; relax.
(B) Rapid Relaxation[b]	
Step 1:	Sit or lie down. The quieter the place, the better.
Step 2:	Take a deep breath through your mouth, hold it for 10 seconds, and exhale slowly.
Step 3:	Mentally repeat the word "relax" 4 times in a calm manner.
Step 4:	Gradually space out repeating "relax" until each repetition takes about 7 seconds.
Step 5:	Keep practicing until you achieve the level of relaxation you desire.

[a]Subject instructed to practice this seated comfortably or reclining.
[b]For immediate relaxation in everyday stressful situation.

or phrase repeated silently or audibly, or fixed gazing at an object. (*b*) Passive attitude. If distracting thoughts occur during the repetition or gazing, they should be disregarded and attention should be redirected to the chosen stimulus. The patient should not worry about the quality of performance. (*c*) Decreased muscle tone. The patient should be in a comfortable position so that minimal muscular work is required. (*d*) Quiet environment. An environment with minimal distractions should be chosen. If visual fixation on an object is not employed, the patient's eyes should generally be closed.

Pharmacological Treatments

Patients with anxiety disorders often benefit from pharmacological treatment. The agents used most frequently are discussed in this section.

Benzodiazepines

Benzodiazepines are prescribed in ambulatory settings primarily for the treatment of anxiety and insomnia. Adverse side effects include oversedation, ataxia, diminished cognitive function, and, rarely, ventilatory depression. The anxiolytic effects of these compounds are believed to result from enhancement of the activity of gamma-amino-butyric acid (GABA), an inhibitory neurotransmitter hypothesized to play a role in the mediation of anxiety. The utilization of these agents in the treatment of specific anxiety disorders is described above in the sections describing the disorders. Their use as hypnotic agents is described in Chapter 85.

Pharmacology. Among the benzodiazepines, alprazolam may be especially effective in the prevention of panic attacks (18). Otherwise, the effects of the various benzodiazepines on the cognitive and somatic symptoms of anxiety are fundamentally similar. These agents do differ, however, in terms of certain clinically important pharmacological properties. These are described below and/or summarized in Table 13.11.

Route of administration. All of the anxiolytic benzodiazepines are well absorbed orally, although the rates of absorption vary widely (see below). Diazepam and lorazepam are available for intravenous use; this is rarely required in the ambulatory treatment of anxiety. Lorazepam is very well absorbed after intramuscular administration. If diazepam must be given by this route, the deltoid muscle should be selected as the injection site. The intramuscular absorption of chlordiazepoxide is particularly slow, even after deltoid injection, and is rarely indicated (32).

Onset of action. The onset of action after oral dosing depends on the rate of absorption from the gastrointestinal tract. The rate of absorption is governed primarily by intrinsic physicochemical properties of the drugs, including lipid solubility. Diazepam and clorazepate are especially rapidly absorbed and produce prompt sedation, relaxation, and even euphoria, a property associated with abuse liability. Prazepam is slowly absorbed and slow in onset. Other benzodiazepines develop their clinical effects at intermediate rates.

Duration of action. The duration of action depends primarily on lipid solubility. Agents with higher lipid solubility (e.g., diazepam) are more rapidly redistributed from their sites of action in the central nervous system to peripheral adipose tissue and, therefore, may produce more short-lived clinical effects after *single* doses than less lipid-soluble drugs (e.g., lorazepam), even those with shorter elimination half-lives. Persistence of drug effect after *multiple* doses depends on elimination half-life.

Rate of elimination. Elimination half-life is affected by several factors, including lipid solubility. The more highly lipid soluble drugs are more completely distributed in body fat relative to blood; therefore, these agents have larger volumes of distribution and are less available to the liver for metabolic transformation and elimination. This is especially important in the elderly, who generally have more body fat than younger persons and are therefore particularly vulnerable to drug accumulation.

The elimination half-life of a benzodiazepine is also influenced by aspects of its hepatic metabolism. Most of the benzodiazepines are metabolized in the liver by microsomal P-450 oxidative pathways (hydroxylation and N-dealkylation) to compounds that retain some pharmacological activity. Several of the drugs are transformed to desmethyldiazepam (half-life >50 hours), a metabolite that accounts for all or most of the activity of clorazepate, prazepam, and halazepam. The elimination half-lives of drugs metabolized to this long-lived intermediary compound are relatively long. All benzodiazepines are finally inactivated in the liver by glucuronide conjugation. Certain agents (oxazepam, lorazepam, temazepam) require only conjugation; they do not undergo oxidation and have no active metabolites. The rates of elimination of drugs requiring oxidation may be affected by aging, liver disease, and concurrent pharmacotherapy (e.g., cimetidine, oral contraceptives). Conjugation is not affected by these factors. For this reason, oxazepam, lorazepam, and temazepam may be less prone to accumulation with multiple dosing in patients who are elderly, have liver disease, or take multiple medications.

Tolerance and Dependence. Tolerance refers to a decline in the effectiveness of a drug at a given dose with continuing usage. Physical dependence describes the development of stereotyped physical signs and symptoms in response to the withdrawal of a substance. Psychological dependence refers to a subjective craving for a drug, usually accompanied by "drug-seeking" efforts.

Although tolerance to the hypnotic effects of benzodiazepines usually develops, it is generally believed (53) that tolerance to their anxiolytic effects is less common. However, both physical and psychological dependence may occur, particularly when high doses are taken for long periods of time, and drug discontinuation may lead to the development of a withdrawal syndrome. Common withdrawal symptoms include

Table 13.11.
Usual Dose and Pharmacokinetics of Anxiolytic Benzodiazepines

Drug (Trade Name) Year Introduced	Onset of Effect after Oral Dose[a]	Available Strengths	Oral Daily Dose Range Divided Two or Three Times a Day	Active Metabolites Present	Elimination Half-life[a]
		mg	*mg*		*hr*
Alprazolam (Xanax) 1981	Intermediate	0.25, 0.5, 1 (scored tablets)	0.25–8	No	8–16
Chlordiazepoxide[b] (Librium) (Libritabs) 1960	Intermediate	5, 10, 25 (capsules) 5, 10, 25 (tablets)	15–150	Yes	5–30
Clorazepate dipotassium (Tranxene) (Tranxene SD) 1972	Rapid	3.75, 7.5, 15 (capsules) 11.25, 22.5 (tablets)	15–60 22.5 (single doses are intended for patients stabilized on 3.75 or 7.5 mg three times a day	Yes Yes	36–200 36–200
Diazepam[b] (Valium) 1961	Rapid	2, 5, 10 (tablets)	4–40	Yes	20–50
Diazepam (Valrelease) 1982	Slow	15 (capsules)	15–30 (single dose is equivalent to 5 mg of Valium three times a day)	Yes	20–50
Halazepam (Paxipam) 1981	Slow to intermediate	20, 40 (tablets)	80–160	Yes	50–100
Lorazepam[b] (Ativan) 1977	Intermediate	0.5, 1, 2 (tablets)	1–6	No	10–20
Oxazepam (Serax) 1963	Slow to intermediate	10, 15, 30 (capsules) 15 (tablets)	30–120 30–120	No	5–10
Prazepam (Centrax) 1977	Slow	5, 10 (capsules)	20–60	Yes	36–200

[a]Drugs with more rapid onset of action are those more rapidly absorbed. Elimination half-life of lipophilic activity.
[b]Generic available.

tension, irritability, sleep disturbance, loss of appetite, pain, tremor, paresthesias, photophobia, and hyperacusis (53). Rarely, seizures or delirium may occur (32). In one study (56), minor withdrawal symptoms occurred in 35% of panic disorder patients slowly tapered off alprazolam after two months of active treatment; seizures and delirium were not observed. It is important to distinguish between withdrawal (development of *new* symptoms that resolve with resumption of medication) and "rebound" (*temporary* return of original symptoms at greater-than-pretreatment frequency or severity), a common, self-limited postdiscontinuation phenomenon (56, 59).

The following measures may be useful in managing the discontinuation of benzodiazepines (53):

1. Although both the dosage and duration of treatment must be ample in order for patients to experience the benefits of therapy, not all patients require high dosages (e.g., alprazolam 6 mg per day) or long-term treatment (e.g., more than one year), both of which make discontinuation more difficult; therefore, dosage and duration of treatment should be minimized.

2. Patients should understand that they may experience rebound or withdrawal symptoms after discontinuation and that these do not indicate the need for long-term treatment.
3. Patients should be seen weekly and be able to reach the physician by phone between visits so that they feel some control over their level of discomfort.
4. Tapering of the drug should occur over 4 to 16 weeks, with 10 to 20% reductions in the daily dose every week. The rate should be closely tailored to the patient's level of discomfort.
5. It may be helpful to switch the patient from a short-acting to a long-acting benzodiazepine [e.g., clonazepam (37)] before beginning the taper; this may reduce fluctuations in medication levels during the day and thereby reduce withdrawal symptoms.
6. It is important to watch for emergence of relapse (as opposed to rebound and withdrawal) during the taper and to be prepared to treat this.

Antidepressants

Tricyclics and MAO inhibitors are useful as antipanic agents and may be effective in ameliorating the "psychic" symptoms associated with generalized anxiety (39) as well as the intrusive memories associated with post-traumatic stress disorders. It is believed that these effects are mediated by effects on central non-adrenergic neurotransmission. Detailed guidelines for their use are found in Chapter 15.

Buspirone (Buspar)

This is the first available *azaspirodecanedione*. Its overall effectiveness as an anxiolytic is comparable to that of benzodiazepines (28), although it may be relatively more effective in treating the cognitive and interpersonal aspects of anxiety than the somatic elements (27, 60). It differs from benzodiazepines in that it has no anticonvulsant or muscle relaxant properties, is nonsedating, does not impair psychomotor function, does not produce euphoria, and does not amplify the effects of alcohol or ameliorate symptoms of alcohol withdrawal. The most common side effects include nervousness, headache, dizziness, lightheadedness, and nausea (52). Tolerance and dependence are not believed to occur, and its abuse liability appears to be low. Its central mechanism of action is unknown; however, it clearly interacts with central monoaminergic, GABAergic, and dopaminergic systems differently than do benzodiazepines (23).

Buspirone is well absorbed orally but is subject to a significant first-pass effect in the liver. Although it is largely protein bound in the circulation, it has not been shown to displace phenytoin, digoxin, propranolol, or warfarin from plasma proteins at therapeutic dosages. It undergoes oxidative metabolism in the liver and is excreted by the kidneys; hence liver and kidney disease may slow its metabolism and clearance. Half-life is usually in the range of 2 to 11 hours and may be prolonged in the elderly (26).

Buspirone is available in 5-mg and 10-mg tablets. The usual starting dose is 5 mg three times per day. Anxiolytic effects generally require two weeks to develop. If there has been only modest response after two weeks, the dose may be increased to ten mg three times per day; further increases rarely improve its effectiveness. Withdrawal and rebound effects are not believed to occur after discontinuation.

β-Adrenergic blockers

Propranolol and the other β-blockers may be more effective than benzodiazepines in reducing the autonomic symptoms (e.g., palpitations) that occur in some anxious individuals (41). β-Blockers may be particularly helpful prophylactically in acutely anxiety-provoking situations such as public speaking and taking examinations; in these situations the cognitive impairment that may be produced by benzodiazepines is undesirable. β-Blockers do not appear useful in preventing panic attacks; however, they may be tried in patients who cannot tolerate the drugs of choice for this disorder (i.e., alprazolam, antidepressants). Details regarding the use of β-blocking drugs are found in Chapter 62.

Antihistamines

Antihistamines may be used to control anxiety as alternatives to benzodiazepines. They appear to be safer for patients with chronic obstructive pulmonary disease in whom benzodiazepines may suppress ventilation, and they are useful in patients who might abuse benzodiazepines. Their major disadvantage is that they are very sedating. Hydroxyzine (Vistaril, Atarax) is most oten used for this purpose and may be prescribed in doses ranging from 10 to 25 mg three times per day.

General References

American Psychiatric Association: *Diagnostic and Statistical Manual of Mental Disorders*. 3rd ed., revised. Washington, DC, 1987.
Relaxation Cassettes.
A variety of audiocassette programs that provide self-instruction in relaxation techniques are available from the following publishers: Guilford Publications, Inc., 72 Spring Street, New York NY 10003; and New Harbinger Publications, 5674 Shattuck Avenue, Oakland, CA 94609.

Specific References

1. Agras MW: *Panic: Facing Fears, Phobias, and Anxiety*. New York, WH Freeman, 1985.
2. Anderson DJ, Noyes R, Crowe RR: A comparison of panic disorder and generalized anxiety disorder. *Am J Psychiatry* 141:572, 1984.
3. Andreasen NJ, Noyes R, Hartford CE: Factors influencing adjustment of burn patients during hospitalization. *Psychosomatic Medicine* 34:517, 1972.
4. Appenheimer T, Noyes R: Generalized anxiety disorder. *Primary Care* 14:635, 1987.
5. Aronson TA, Logue CM: On the longitudinal course of panic disorder: developmental history and prediction of phobic complications. *Comprehensive Psychiatry* 28:344, 1987.
6. Ballenger JC, Burrows GD, DePont RL, et al: Alprazolam in panic disorder and agoraphobia: results from a multicenter trial. *Arch Gen Psychiatry* 45:413, 1988.
7. Barlow DH: Behavioral conception and treatment of panic. *Psychopharmacol Bull* 22:802, 1986.
8. Bass C, Cawley R, Wade C, et al: Unexplained breathlessness and psychiatric morbidity in patients with normal and abnormal coronary arteries. *Lancet* 1:605, 1983.
9. Baxter LR, Phelps ME, Mazziotta JC, et al: Local cerebral glucose metabolic rates in obsessive-compulsive disorder. *Arch Gen Psychiatry* 44:211, 1987.
10. Benson H: *The Relaxation Response*. New York, William Morrow, 1975.
11. Benson H, Beary JF, Carol MP: The relaxation response. *Psychiatry* 37:37, 1974.
12. Blazer D, Hughes D, George LK: Stressful life events and the onset of a generalized anxiety syndrome. *Am J Psychiatry* 144:1178, 1987.
13. Breier A, Charney DS, Heninger GR: Major depression in patients with agoraphobia and panic disorder. *Arch Gen Psychiatry* 41:1129, 1984.
14. Breier A, Charney DS, Heninger GR: Agoraphobia with panic attacks. *Arch Gen Psychiatry* 43:1029, 1986.
15. Breier A, Charney DS, Heninger GR: The diagnostic validity of anxiety disorders and their relationship to depressive illness. *Am J Psychiatry* 142:787, 1985.
16. Burns LE, Thorpe GL: The epidemiology of fears and phobias. *J Int Med Res* 5 (Suppl 5): 1, 1977.
17. Carey G, Gottesman II: Twin and family studies of anxiety, phobic, and obsessive disorders. In: Klein DF, Rabkin JG (eds): *Anxiety: New Research and Changing Concepts*. New York, Raven Press, pages 116-136, 1981.
18. Chouinard G, Annable L, Fontaine R, Solyom L: Alprazolam in the treatment of generalized anxiety and panic disorders: a dou-

ble-blind placebo-controlled study. *Psychopharmacology* 77:229, 1982.

19. Ciraulo DA, Sands BF, Shader RI: Critical review of liability for benzodiazepine abuse among alcoholics. *Am J Psychiatry* 145:1501, 1988.

20. Clark DM, Salkovskis PM, Chalkley AJ: Respiratory control as a treatment for panic attacks. *J Behav Ther Exper Psychiatry* 16:23, 1985.

21. Cloninger CR, Martin RL, Clayton P, Guze SB: A blind follow-up and family study of anxiety neurosis: preliminary analysis of the St. Louis 500. In: Klein DF, Rabkin J (eds): *Anxiety: New Research and Changing Concepts.* New York, Raven Press, 1981.

22. Coryell W, Noyes R, Clancy J: Excess mortality in panic disorder: a comparison with primary unipolar depression. *Arch Gen Psychiatry* 39:701, 1982.

23. Eison AS, Temple DL: Buspirone: review of its pharmacology and current perspectives on its mechanism of action. *Am J Med* 80 (Suppl 3B): 1, 1986.

24. Friedman MJ: Toward a rational pharmacotherapy for posttraumatic stress disorder: an interim report. *Am J Psychiatry* 145:281, 1988.

25. Gaarder KR, Montgomery PS: *Clinical Biofeedback: A Procedural Manual for Behavioral Medicine.* 2nd ed. Baltimore, Williams & Wilkins, 1981.

26. Gammans RE, Mayol FG, Labudde JA: Metabolism and disposition of buspirone. *Am J Med* 80 (Suppl 3B): 41, 1986.

27. Goa KL, Ward A: Buspirone: a preliminary review of its pharmacologic properties and therapeutic efficacy as an anxiolytic. *Drugs* 32:114, 1986.

28. Goldberg HL, Finnerty RJ: The comparative efficacy of buspirone and diazepam in the treatment of anxiety. *Am J Psychiatry* 136:1184, 1979.

29. Goldberg RJ: Anxiety reduction by self-regulation: theory, practice, and evaluation. *Ann Intern Med* 96:483, 1982.

30. Goldstein AJ, Chambless DL: A reanalysis of agoraphobia. *Behavior Therapy* 9:47, 1978.

31. Gorman JM, Dillon D, Fyer AJ, et al: The lactate infusion model. *Psychopharmacol Bull* 21:428, 1985.

32. Greenblatt DJ, Shader RI, Abernethy DR: Current status of benzodiazepines. *N Engl J Med* 309:354, 1983.

33. Greist JF, Ferreroson JW, Marks IM: *Anxiety and Its Treatments: Help is Available.* Washington, D.C., American Psychiatric Press, Inc., 1986.

34. Grimshaw L: Obsessional disorder and neurological illness. *J Neurol Neurosurg Psychiatry* 27:229, 1964.

35. Haines AP, Imeson JD, Meade TW: Phobic anxiety and ischaemic heart disease. *Br Med J* 295:297, 1987.

36. Helzer JE, Robins LN, McEvoy L: Post-traumatic stress disorder in the general population: findings of the Epidemiologic Catchment Area Survey. *N Engl J Med* 317:1630, 1987.

37. Herman JB, Rosenbaum JF, Brotman AN: The alprazolam to clonazepam switch for the treatment of panic disorder. *J Clin Psychopharmacol* 7:175, 1987.

38. Hoehn-Saric R: Characteristics of chronic anxiety patients. In: Klein DF, Rabkin J (eds): *Anxiety: New Research and Changing Concepts.* New York, Raven Press, 1981.

39. Hoehn-Saric R, McLeod DR, Zimmerli WD: Differential effects of alprazolam and imipramine in generalized anxiety disorder: somatic versus psychic symptoms. *J Clin Psychiatry* 49:293, 1988.

40. Kolb LC: A neuropsychological hypothesis explaining posttraumatic stress disorders. *Am J Psychiatry* 144:989, 1987.

41. Lead article: Beta-adrenergic blockade and anxiety. *Lancet* 2:611, 1976.

42. Lown B: Mental stress, arrhythmias, and sudden death. *Am J Med* 72:177, 1982.

43. Luxenberg JS, Swedo SE, Flament MF, et al: Neuroanatomical abnormalities in obsessive-compulsive disorder detected with quantitative x-ray computed tomography. *Am J Psychiatry* 145:1089, 1988.

44. Lydiard RB, Ballenger JC: Antidepressants in panic disorder and agoraphobia. *J Affective Disord* 13:153, 1987.

45. Marks I: *Fears and Phobias.* London, Heinemann, 1969.

46. Marks I: Recent results of behavioral treatments of phobias and obsessions. *J Int Med Res* 5 (Suppl 5): 15, 1977.

47. Matuzas W, Al-Sadir J, Uhlenhuth EH, Glass RM: Mitral valve prolapse and thyroid abnormalities in patients with panic attacks. *Am J Psychiatry* 144:493, 1987.

48. Mayou R, Williamson B, Foster A: Attitudes and advice after myocardial infarction. *Br Med J* 1:1577, 1976.

49. McKeon J, McGuffin P, Robinson P: Obsessive-compulsive neurosis following head injury: a report of four cases. *Brit J Psychiatry* 144:190, 1984.

50. McKeon J, Roa B, Mann A: Life events and personality traits in obsessive-compulsive neurosis. *Br J Psychiatry* 144:185, 1984.

51. Myers JK, Weissman MM, Tischler GL, et al: Six-month prevalence of psychiatric disorders in three communities. *Arch Gen Psychiatry* 41:959, 1984.

52. Newton RE, Marunycz JD, Alderdice MT, Napoliello MJ: Review of the side effect profile of buspirone. *Am J Med* 80: (suppl 3B): 17, 1986.

53. Noyes R, Garvey MJ, Cook BL, Perry PJ: Benzodiazepine withdrawal: a review of the evidence. *J Clin Psychiatry* 49:382, 1988.

54. Pauls DL, Slymen P: A family study of panic disorder. *Arch Gen Psychiatry* 40:1065, 1983.

55. Pauls DL, Towbin KE, Leckman JF, et al: Gilles de la Tourette's syndrome and obsessive-compulsive disorder. *Arch Gen Psychiatry* 43:1180, 1986.

56. Pecknold JC, Swinson RP, Kuch K, Lewis CP: Alprazolam in panic disorder and agoraphobia: results from a multicenter trial. III. Discontinuation effects. *Arch Gen Psychiatry* 45:429, 1988.

57. Rasmussen K, Ravnsbaek J, Funch-Jensen P, Bagger JP: Oesophageal spasm in patients with coronary artery spasm. *Lancet* 1:174, 1986.

58. Rasmussen SA, Tsuang MT: Clinical characteristics and family history in DSM-III Obsessive-Compulsive Disorder. *Am J Psychiatry* 143:317, 1986.

59. Rickels K, Fox IL, Greenblatt DJ, et al: Clorazepate and lorazepam: clinical improvement and rebound anxiety. *Am J Psychiatry* 145:312, 1988.

60. Rickels K, Weisman K, Norstad D: Buspirone and diazepam in anxiety: a controlled study. *J Clin Psychiatry* 43:81, 1982.

61. Robbins LN, Helzer JE, Weissman MM, et al: Lifetime prevalence of specific psychiatric disorders in three sites. *Arch Gen Psychiatry* 41:949, 1984.

62. Ross RJ, Ball WA, Sullivan KA, Caroff SN: Sleep disturbance as the hallmark of posttraumatic stress disorder. *Am J Psychiatry* 146:697, 1988.

63. Taylor CB, Ferguson JM, Wermuth BM: Simple techniques to treat medical phobias. *Postgrad Med J* 53:28, 1977.

64. Thoren P, Asberg M, Cronholm B, et al: Clomipramine treatment of obsessive-compulsive disorder: I. A controlled clinical trial. *Arch Gen Psychiatry* 37:1281, 1980.

65. Torgersen S: Genetic factors in anxiety disorders. *Arch Gen Psychiatry* 40:1085, 1983.

66. Torgersen S: Childhood and family characteristics in panic and generalized anxiety disorders. *Am J Psychiatry* 143:630, 1986.

67. Turner SM, Jacob RG, Beidel DC, et al: Fluoxetine treatment of obsessive-compulsive disorder. *J Clin Psychopharmacol* 5:201, 1985.

68. Von Korff M, Shapiro S, Burke JD, et al: Anxiety and depression in a primary care clinic. *Arch Gen Psychiatry* 44:152, 1987.

69. Windheuser HJ: Anxious mothers as models for coping with anxiety. *Behav Anal Mod* 2:39, 1977.

CHAPTER 14

Maladaptive Personalities

ROBERT P. ROCA, M.D., M.P.H.

CONCEPT OF PERSONALITY

The enduring attitudes, behaviors, and capacities that distinguish individuals from each other are collectively designated the "personality." Personality has been conceptualized in many ways, two of which are in common use. One approach is to specify *categories* of personality and to classify individuals according to the type they most closely resemble. The ancient Greek topology of personality (phlegmatic, melancholic, sanguine, and choleric) was of this sort, and the American Psychiatric Association uses a similar approach in the classification of personality disorders published in the most recent *Diagnostic and Statistical Manual of Mental Disorders* (DSM-III-R) (see below).

Another approach is to view personality as a mosaic of *dimensional* traits, each of which is possessed by individuals in differing degrees (2). "Intelligence," as defined by the intelligence quotient (IQ), serves as a model of such a trait. IQ scores are normally distributed in the population and are highly correlated with academic and occupational achievement. Persons with above-average IQ scores tend to be successful in school and work, while those with below-average IQs often have difficulty meeting the demands of daily life independently. Knowledge of an individual's position on the dimension of intelligence thus illuminates strengths and vulnerabilities and allows one to predict circumstances that the individual might find overwhelming.

Case example. A 30-year-old man was admitted to the hospital for cellulitis of the feet. His physician discovered that he had only completed the 3rd grade and that he was unable to read, write, or calculate. Further investigation disclosed that he had recently lost his job in a laundromat and that he had been observed walking barefoot in a dumpster looking for items he needed. His physician explained to him, carefully and repeatedly, the relationship between his infection and his behavior. A social worker was called to help him apply for financial assistance and other entitlements.

Dimensions can be converted into categories, albeit with some loss of precision. Mental retardation, for example, is said to be present when the IQ is less than 70. While this is a useful categorical definition, it is somewhat misleading since the impairment of someone with an IQ of 68 is essentially the same as that of someone with an IQ of 72 who, by definition, would not be declared mentally retarded. Such a case illustrates that thinking in rigidly categorical terms may obscure areas of vulnerability that a dimensional approach might bring to light.

Other personality traits may be described dimensionally, although none has been studied as thoroughly as intelligence. We use dimensional thinking intuitively when we recognize that some persons are more meticulous, more gregarious, or more ambitious than others. Psychologists use this approach more technically when they administer standardized tests to describe quantitatively how "introverted" or "neurotic" someone is. At some arbitrary point, the meticulous person may be categorized as "obsessional" or the introverted person as "schizoid" and thus be said to have a personality disorder; however, it is useful to recognize that certain patients are more meticulous or introverted than others even when they are not categorically "obsessional" or "schizoid." A dimensional view facilitates the recognition of such important personality traits and thus prepares one to take these attributes into account when dealing with patients.

Development of Personality

Personality evolves out of interactions between constitutional, or in-born, factors and the molding influences of the environment. Constitutional factors include capacities, such as intelligence, and aspects of temperament, such as sociability and emotionality, all of which may have neurobiological correlates and genetic determinants (3). The most important environmental influences are interpersonal relationships, usually with parents. Many theories have been offered to account more specifically for personality development, but none has yet proved adequate, and none will be endorsed in this chapter.

Conceptualization of Personality Disorder

Personality disorders are among the least studied and most controversial conditions in psychiatry. There is no doubt that some people have enduring patterns of maladaptive attitudes and behaviors that interfere with their ability to work effectively and to develop and sustain gratifying interpersonal relationships. It is also clear that such persons are at increased risk for long-term social impairment and for many major psychiatric illnesses (4, 5). The controversy lies in how best to conceptualize and subdivide these disorders. This chapter will refer to three such conceptualizations.

The dominant approach in the United States—that adopted by the American Psychiatric Association in its most current Diagnostic and Statistical Manual (DSM-III-R)—is *prototypic* and *categorical*. In this scheme, the diagnostic criteria for the personality disorders are lists of attitudes and behaviors (e.g., self-dramatization; attention-seeking) that, in combination, evoke an ideal prototype (e.g., the histrionic personality). Only a person exhibiting the requisite number of such attitudes and behaviors (at least four, in the case of histrionic personality disorder) is said to have the condition. Personality disorder is relatively rare when defined in this way.

Maladaptive personalities can also be conceptualized in terms of quantitative deviations from normal along specific personality *dimensions*. Many clinically important personality traits may be viewed dimensionally; persons may be high or low in obsessionality or dependency or self-importance. "Normal" endowments of these and other traits are usually considered "healthy," whereas excesses are likely to produce special vulnerabilities. For example, excessive obsessionality may lead to great distress in circumstances that require flexibility and emotional spontaneity, and poor self-esteem may predispose one to demoralization in response to criticism from a superior. These examples illustrate that dimensional thinking about personality disturbances calls for consideration of the environmental stresses that expose the vulnerability as well as the trait-based vulnerability itself. Since there are many relevant dimensions, and since most people have at least one trait "in excess," a dimensional approach illuminates areas of vulnerability in most patients.

Finally, personality disorders may be viewed as incomplete or atypical expressions of schizophrenia, mood disorders, or other major psychiatric illnesses.

Subtyping of Personality Disorder

As noted above, the American Psychiatric Association adopted a categorical approach to the classification of personality disorders. DSM-III-R describes eleven types of personality disorders and groups them into three *clusters*: the "dramatic" (histrionic, borderline, narcissistic, and antisocial types), the "anxious or fearful" (obsessive-compulsive, dependent, passive-aggressive, and avoidant types), and the "odd or eccentric" (schizoid, schizotypal, and paranoid types) clusters. In the descriptions of the categorical disorders that follow in the remainder of the chapter, it will be clear that many of the disorders may be viewed as manifestations of extreme positions on dimensions of personality such as emotionality, narcissism, trust, sociability, self-esteem, and assertiveness. It will also be seen that the types within each cluster tend to share traits and vulnerabilities and, therefore, implications

for management. A few disorders are linked to major psychiatric illnesses. It is important to emphasize that a patient with clinically obvious disturbances involving dimensions of personality may meet criteria for several DSM-III-R personality disorders or may meet criteria for none.

"DRAMATIC" CLUSTER

Patients with personality disturbances in this cluster tend to occupy extreme positions on the dimensions of emotionality and narcissism. They are intensely emotional, thereby sometimes acting impulsively, aggressively, and/or self-destructively. They are also self-absorbed, lacking in empathy for others, and extreme (unrealistically high or low) in their self-regard. They tend to be demanding of others, and their relationships are unstable, tempestuous, and exploitative, qualities that may characterize their interactions with physicians and complicate the provision of medical care.

Description of "Dramatic" Subtypes

Histrionic Personality

The essence of the *histrionic* type is excessive emotionality, self-dramatization, and attention-seeking. Patients meeting criteria for the categorical disorder are self-centered, unusually eager for approval and praise, overly concerned with physical attractiveness, and often inappropriately sexually seductive or flattering ("Of all the doctors I've had, you are the first to really listen to me"). Their style of speech is dramatic, impressionistic, and factually imprecise, and their expression of emotions is often exaggerated, rapidly shifting, and apparently shallow. They may manifest an unusually warm and sometimes seductive manner with the physician and present to the office with complaints that are dramatically expressed but vague in medically relevant detail. Histrionic patients may be especially inclined to develop somatization disorder (see Chapter 12).

Narcissistic Personality

The *narcissistic* personality type is characterized by an exaggerated sense of self-importance, intolerance of criticism, and insensitivity to the needs of others. These patients also exploit others for their own ends, require constant admiration and attention, believe themselves entitled to special treatment, and envy those who are more successful, attractive, intelligent, or otherwise praiseworthy. Such patients are often difficult to care for because they tend to believe that their problems are unique and can only be solved by remarkable physicians. They may challenge the doctor's knowledge, skill, and judgment and expect that their convenience will be the prime consideration in the scheduling of tests and appointments.

Borderline Personality

Extreme instability—in mood, interpersonal relationships, and self-regard—is the essence of the *borderline* personality, a disorder once alleged to lie on the "border" of schizophrenia. Recent data more strongly support a link with depressive disorders. Substance abuse, sexual impulsiveness, poor self-esteem, self-mutilation, recurrent (often manipulative) suicidal threats, and brief bouts of intense depression and rage superimposed on chronic feelings of emptiness or boredom characterize the long-term functioning of these patients. A shifting tendency to view other people as "all good" or "all bad" and to react to them with extremes of idealization and devaluation creates difficulties in all interpersonal relationships, including those with physicians and other caretakers, who are designated as either "good" or "bad" and are thence pitted against one another ("staff splitting").

Antisocial Personality

The *antisocial* personality type is characterized by a chronic and pervasive pattern of irresponsible and socially unacceptable behavior. Truancy, vandalism, fire setting, lying, and theft in childhood give way to impulsiveness, recklessness, aggressiveness, sexual promiscuity, financial irresponsibility, and outright criminality in adulthood. Often complaining of mistreatment themselves, they shamelessly exploit others in their relationships. In medical settings they may be malingerers (see Chapter 12), consciously feigning disease for obvious gain; and in their dealings with medical staff they may be either demanding and abusive or flattering and ingratiating, depending on what they perceive to be most expedient.

Management of "Dramatic" Subtypes

General Guidelines

Several points are useful to bear in mind when dealing with personality-disordered patients of any subtype:

1. Because the maladaptive trait or traits are of long standing and deeply engrained, it is doubtful that they will change in response to the physician's efforts. The general approach to management is therefore to recognize these sources of vulnerability, take them into account when interacting with the patient, and minimize their adverse impact on the provision of medical care.
2. Patients often become angry or depressed when their maladaptive traits are pointed out to them, and either of these responses defeats the physician's purposes. Yet it is frequently important to call patients' attention to ways in which they are undermining their medical care. When such action is necessary, it is helpful to refer to specific *behaviors* rather than to aspects of personality and to present one's observations plainly but compassionately and with-

out criticism (e.g., "It is difficult for us to provide you with the care you need when you curse at us and criticize every effort we make. I need to ask you to stop behaving in this way.").
3. In general, counseling by the general physician, if undertaken at all, is best symptom-focused and short-term (see Chapter 11). For long-term treatment, persons with seriously disturbed personalities should be referred to a mental health professional.

Cluster-Specific Guidelines

When dealing with dramatic patients one can expect a show of emotional extremes and a pressure to bestow emotional and material favors as well as medical care. It is helpful to maintain equanimity in the face of the patient's emotional excesses, to avoid defensiveness when challenged, and to give special attention to professional boundaries. Socializing or becoming unusually familiar with histrionic or borderline patients is particularly risky. Because patients with these traits lack empathy and exploit others, it is often necessary to spell out—firmly, but nonpunitively—the limits of acceptable behavior with medical staff, nurses, and other members of the health care team; such limit setting is most often needed with narcissistic and antisocial persons.

"ANXIOUS OR FEARFUL" CLUSTER

Persons with these disorders tend to be self-doubting, timid, and tense. Lacking confidence in themselves, they may seek to avoid making decisions or taking on responsibility, preferring to have others decide or perform for them; yet, they are often dissatisfied with and critical of the efforts of others. They tend to be socially unassertive, submitting to the wishes of others and even avoiding friendship in the first place for fear of ultimate rejection. Levels of generalized anxiety are chronically high.

"Anxious" Subtypes

Avoidant Personality

The *avoidant* person craves social contact but avoids it because of intense social discomfort related to expectations of criticism and rejection. These persons often complain of loneliness, but are too "shy" to make the social contacts required to solve the problem unless they are certain of acceptance. Major depression (5) and social phobia commonly occur. Because physicians are generally viewed as accepting of their patients, avoidant persons may feel particularly comfortable in the presence of their doctors and may develop symptoms justifying regular visits to alleviate their loneliness.

Dependent Personality

Dependent persons lack self-confidence and go to great lengths to ensure the availability of others upon whom they can depend for advice and reassurance.

Because they feel uneasy and helpless when alone, they may endure abuse and perform unpleasant or demeaning tasks in order to preserve the dependent relationship. They are exceedingly sensitive to criticism and abandonment. Patients of this type may become quite dependent upon their physicians, particularly when other relationships are unsatisfactory, and may use vague, chronic complaints as a means of remaining in close touch, especially in times of stress. Such patients may also become "ill" prior to a period of planned unavailability on the part of the physician (e.g., a vacation).

Obsessive Compulsive Personality

Persons with *obsessive compulsive* personalities are rigid, parsimonious, morally scrupulous, and emotionally constricted. Exceedingly committed to work, they are reluctant to delegate duties, convinced that no one else can do things correctly; yet they are also indecisive and at times are rendered ineffective by perfectionism or preoccupation with trivial details. They tend to describe upsetting emotional experiences in a cool, detached manner ("isolation of affect"). When ill, they often present their physicians with extremely detailed accounts of their symptoms and request lengthy explanations of their disease and its treatment, including very precise instructions about medication use and likely side effects. They are usually aware of hospital rules and routines and are intolerant of lateness and inefficiency. Persons with obsessive compulsive personalities may be especially prone to developing hypochondriasis (see Chapter 12) and obsessive compulsive *disorder*, a condition characterized by recurrent, resisted thoughts and repetitive, senseless actions (see Chapter 13).

Passive Aggressive Personality

Passive aggressive persons do not want to meet the expectations of others but do not want to be held responsible for this decision. Thus they do not say "no" directly but express hostile resistance in terms of procrastination, intentional inefficiency, and feigned forgetfulness. Usually dependent and lacking in self-confidence, they seek the counsel of others, yet often paradoxically resist following the advice of those whom they consult. In medical settings they insist that they intend to comply with treatment recommendations but then, for example, "forget" to keep a symptom log required to assess the effectiveness of a new treatment or "forget" to make it to the laboratory for an important blood test.

Management of "Anxious" Subtypes

The general guidelines described above are applicable. Because patients with these types of personality traits tend to develop anxious attachment to their physicians, the management of dependency is a central issue. It may be necessary to allow patients to be excessively dependent—within manageable bounds—during times of unusual stress. It may be helpful to give them regular, brief appointments so that they do not need to develop new symptomatic complaints in order to gain access to attention (see Chapter 12), and it may be useful to advise them to call weekly at a specified time to provide updates on their status; this may preempt emergency calls at less convenient times. Such patients also generally benefit from advance notice about vacations and may appreciate meeting the covering physician ahead of time. Treatment for generalized anxiety disorder, phobias, and major depression may be indicated in selected cases (see Chapters 13 and 15).

"ODD OR ECCENTRIC" CLUSTER

Patients with disorders in this group occupy extreme positions on the dimensions of trust and sociability. They tend to be highly suspicious and to isolate themselves from other people due to anxious mistrust, awkwardness, or indifference.

Description of "Eccentric" Subtypes

Paranoid Personality

Patients with *paranoid* personalities tend to perceive threats and insults at every turn. Expecting to be exploited or harmed by others, they hear veiled threats in neutral remarks and readily question the loyalty of friends and the fidelity of spouses. They are guarded, easily slighted, defensive, and unforgiving. Although their suspiciousness does not carry the intensity or conviction of a true delusion, schizophrenia and delusional disorders are overrepresented in their families (3). In medical settings these patients may be reluctant to provide a complete history, especially a social history ("What does this have to do with my medical problem?") and may balk at undergoing laboratory tests ("You doctors are just trying to make money off me.").

Schizotypal Personality

Schizotypal persons exhibit odd behavior, have peculiar beliefs, and suffer social isolation—as a result of their own social anxiety as well as the impact of their beliefs and behavior on others. Their affect is often constricted, their talk vague and digressive, and their appearance unkempt. They tend to be suspicious and superstitious. Persons with this disorder are generally severely impaired, often meeting criteria for other personality disorders simultaneously (5). There are family links with schizophrenia (1), and some have argued that this disorder should be classified as a variant of schizophrenia rather than a personality disorder (3).

Schizotypal patients may be guarded and suspicious in medical settings but may also present to physicians with unusual symptoms (e.g., "feelings of electricity in my scalp") and with idiosyncratic theories of causation ("Could my neighbors be doing this to me?").

Schizoid Personality

The essential features of the *schizoid* personality are indifference to the company of others and constricted emotionality. These persons are "loners" who seldom marry, prefer solitary activities, and appear cold and aloof. Despite its name, this disorder does not appear closely linked to schizophrenia. Schizoid persons tend to shun contact with physicians and may appear very uncomfortable when hospitalization thrusts them into close and constant proximity to others.

Management of "Eccentric" Subtypes

The general guidelines described above apply here as well. The most important specific principle of management is to work gradually toward the establishment of rapport by meticulous honesty, composure in the face of the patient's suspiciousness and reserve, and a consistent demonstration of both sincere concern for the patient's well-being and respect for his privacy.

General References

American Psychiatric Association: *Diagnostic and Statistical Manual of Mental Disorders.* 3rd ed. revised. Washington, DC, American Psychiatric Association, 1987.

Specific References

1. Kendler KS, Gruenberg AM, Strauss JS: An independent analysis of the Danish adoption study of schizophrenia. II. *Arch Gen Psychiatry* 38:982, 1981.
2. McHugh PR, Slavney PR: *The Perspectives of Psychiatry.* Baltimore, The Johns Hopkins University Press, 1983.
3. Rutter M: Temperament, personality, and personality disorder. *Br J Psychiatry* 150:443, 1987.
4. Rutter M, Quinton D: Parental psychiatric disorder: effects on children. *Psychological Med* 14:853, 1984.
5. Zimmerman M, Coryell W: DSM-III personality disorder diagnoses in a nonpatient sample. *Arch Gen Psychiatry* 46:682, 1989.

C H A P T E R 15

Affective Disorders

J. RAYMOND DEPAULO, M.D.

INTRODUCTION

The most common psychological disturbance in the general population is a disturbance of mood characterized by depression with or without anxiety. The prevalence of this type of disturbance ranges from 10% for general populations, to 30% for patients seen in general practice settings, to 50% for general hospital inpatients (3, 4). Implicit in these figures are two powerful arguments for the diagnosis and treatment of many of these patients by general physicians rather than by psychiatrists. First, there are too many patients for psychiatrists alone to provide the primary care, and second, there is a clear association between these mood disturbances and other medical illnesses.

The principal mood disturbances are the following:

1. Dysthymic disorder (synonyms: depressive neurosis, characterological depression, minor depression).
2. Adjustment disorder with depressed mood.
3. Major affective syndromes (major depression, atypical depression, and mania).
4. Organic affective syndromes (mania or depression secondary to medication, Table 15.1) or brain disorders (i.e., dementia, Chapter 17; stroke, Chapter 83).
5. Uncomplicated bereavement (see Chapter 19).

Table 15.1.
Drugs And Substances That May Cause A Mood Disturbance

Depressed Mood
  Alcoholic beverages
  Antihypertensive drugs
    Clonidine
    Methyldopa
    Reserpine
    β-Blockers
  Anxiolytic drugs
  Neuroleptic drugs
  Sedative-hypnotic drugs
Hypomanic Mood
  Antidepressants
  L-Dopa
  Phencyclidine (PCP)

DETECTION OF PATIENTS WITH AFFECTIVE SYMPTOMS

Complaints of loss of energy, poor sleep, poor appetite, weight loss, decreased libido, etc. (i.e., vegetative symptoms) should alert one to the possibility of depression. However, depressed patients may not complain of those symptoms initially. Studies (13) have shown that these patients, in fact, usually present to generalists with three types of more vague complaints: ill-defined somatic symptoms, pains of undetermined etiology at a wide variety of anatomical sites, and nervous complaints such as increased tension and feelings of anxiety. Primary complaints about marital distress or job difficulty are also common.

When they are specifically asked about mood changes and associated symptoms, most depressed patients will acknowledge them. The presence of a mood disturbance should not be taken to explain or to invalidate all physical complaints since coexistence of psychiatric and medical disorders is the rule rather than the exception. Conversely, it is a mistake to conclude that depression (or any other psychiatric illness) is present simply because no objective signs of organic disease can be found in a patient with somatic symptoms. If the patient does suffer from an affective disorder and if appropriate inquiries are made, it is likely that at least some of the classic features of the disorder will be detected.

It is appropriate to ask patients about their mood, their sense of self-esteem and general physical and mental well-being, their sleep, appetite, libido, and their feeling about their future. The diagnostic significance of each of these factors is pointed out in the sections on the principal mood disorders below.

Family members, if available, should be asked to corroborate and augment the information obtained from the patient. With the patient's agreement, the diagnostic assessment, the plans for treatment, and the prognosis should be shared with the patient's family.

Manic symptoms are usually detected by family members or coworkers. They most commonly include rapid, sometimes incoherent speech, hyperactivity, decreased need for sleep, hypersexuality (often recognized as inappropriate for the particular patient),

and irritable aggressive behavior. Manic patients usually feel there is nothing wrong with them and often resist medical attention. If they do go to see a physician, it is because they recognize something wrong in their sleep, because they feel that others are causing them distress, or because they want the doctor to reassure their "nagging" family that there is nothing wrong with them.

DYSTHYMIC DISORDER (DEPRESSIVE NEUROSIS)

Dysthymic disorder is the current name given by the American Psychiatric Association to depressions that lack the severity of major depression (described below) and that are sustained over a 2-year period.

This diagnostic formulation, which is similar to the earlier constructs "depressive neurosis" and "characterological depression," is useful for those patients, many with primary personality disorders, who are chronically troubled people. One important subgroup consists of alcoholic patients who have chronically low moods that would improve with sustained sobriety. It is also apparent that some (perhaps 20%) patients in this grouping have persistent forms of an endogenous depressive disorder. Patients in this subset often have strong family histories for major affective disorders and often respond well to antidepressant medications (1). Dysthymic disorder is separated from adjustment disorder with depressed mood (see below) by the duration of the depressed mood, which is longstanding in dysthymic disorder, and by the additional depressive symptoms that constitute the dysthymic state.

Patients with this disorder outnumber those with major depressive syndromes by approximately 2 to 1. For reasons that are not clear, minor depression is far more common among women than among men. Onset usually occurs around 18 to 30 years, and recurrence during periods of increased stress may characterize the patient's entire adult life. Serious medical illness is likely to precipitate such a depressed mood.

Diagnosis

Most minor depressive disorders are only quantitatively distinct from normal mood responses. The patient's own sense of what is a normal response will often determine why one patient goes to the doctor whereas another attempts to deal with the perceived problem by other means. However, there is no absolute level of severity that distinguishes normal mood from dysthymic disorder or depressive neurosis.

These mood disturbances arise in part from personality traits that make the patient more susceptible to particular stressful events or environmental demands. There is an association between certain personality traits (see Chapter 14) and depressive symptoms, and different environmental stresses lead to depressive responses in people with different personality traits. For example, a dependent person may be more likely to become depressed when a source of security is threatened than would a relatively independent person. The depressive symptoms in such a patient should concern the general physician when the patient asks for help or when the mood change affects the patient's ability to function effectively.

Presenting or complicating problems associated with depressed mood in dysthymic patients include (a) suicide attempts or self-injurious behavior—usually nonfatal but often requiring heroic medical interventions to prevent a fatal outcome, (b) multiple medical complaints and excessive medical care-seeking behavior or "abnormal illness behavior" (see Chapter 12 for additional detail), (c) alcohol and drug abuse (see Chapters 21 and 22), (d) family and marital discord, and (e) job difficulties.

These patients do not usually have the characteristic sustained changes in self-attitude and vital sense (i.e., unwarranted feelings of hopelessness and worthlessness and of bodily deterioration), the psychomotor retardation (i.e., slowed speech and movements), or the characteristic early morning awakening with diurnal mood variation (worse in the morning), that are seen in patients with major depression (see below). However, difficulty in getting to sleep, lack of appetite, mild weight loss, and loss of energy and libido are common, as are anxiety symptoms.

Table 15.2 shows the criteria of the American Psychiatric Association (APA) for making the diagnosis of dysthymic disorder.

Management

Detection of the depressed mood and further interviewing to help delineate the personal antecedents of the depressive symptoms are often therapeutic: The interest shown in the patient's story can help to restore diminished self-esteem. Whereas occasionally some specific guidance and reassurance will help, more often empathic listening and encouraging the patient to outline his own synthesis of the problem and his approach to solving it provide more durable improvement. Weekly or biweekly visits for brief supportive psychotherapy (see Chapter 11) for 3 to 6 weeks will often help during an episode of increased depressive symptoms. Occasionally, adjunctive medication may be helpful in a more severely affected patient. If generalized anxiety symptoms and/or insomnia predominate, a nighttime dose of a benzodiazepine sedative-hypnotic may be helpful for a limited 1- to 2-week time period (see Chapter 85).

Prognosis

In contrast to the major affective syndromes, prognosis in minor depressive disorders cannot be estimated with much confidence. They usually have a limited course even if untreated; the best available data suggest an average duration between 1 and 2 years after diagnosis (10). Although short-term beneficial effects have been shown with the use of tricyclic antidepressants, they are modest at best except in those patients with mild forms of a true depressive syndrome. Various forms of psychotherapy as well as no treatment have been associated with positive outcomes. Poor outcomes are most common in patients with chronic medical disorders, severe social maladjustments, and coexistent personality disorders (see Chapter 14).

Recurrence of minor depression commonly occurs in the setting of later social stress or of medical illness. This is particularly true during the years of peak risk (i.e., 18 to 30 years).

ADJUSTMENT DISORDER WITH DEPRESSED MOOD ("REACTIVE DEPRESSION")

This term is used when depressive symptoms (depressed mood, tearfulness, feelings of hopelessness) occur in response to a recent, identifiable stressor. The criteria of the American Psychiatric Association for this disorder are summarized in Table 15.3. The frequency of adjustment disorders is not known but they are clearly common. Importantly, if a patient's depressive symptoms are profound, a depression that seems to be related to a recent stressor may in fact be a major depressive illness (see below). Stressors that commonly precipitate an adjustment disorder are listed

---

Table 15.2.
American Psychiatric Association Diagnostic Criteria for Dysthymic Disorder (Depressive Neurosis)[a]

A. Depressed mood for at least 2 years.
B. Presence, while depressed, of at least two of the following:
   (1) Poor appetite or overeating
   (2) Insomnia or hypersomnia
   (3) Low energy or fatigue
   (4) Low self-esteem
   (5) Poor concentration
   (6) Feelings of hopelessness
C. During the 2-year period of the disturbance, never without the symptoms for more than 2 months at a time.
D. Not due to drugs, recent major depression, or schizophrenia.

[a]Adapted from American Psychiatric Association: *Diagnostic and Statistical Manual of Mental Disorders*, 3rd ed, revised. Washington, DC, American Psychiatric Association, 1987. Some of the criteria for children have been omitted from this table.

Table 15.3.
Adjustment Disorder with Depressed Mood[a]

A. A reaction (characterized by depressed mood, tearfulness, hopelessness) to an identifiable psychosocial stressor (or multiple stressors) that occurs within 3 months of onset of the stressor(s).
B. The maladaptive nature of the reaction is indicated by either of the following:
   1. Impairment in occupational (including school) functioning or in usual social activities or relationships with others.
   2. Symptoms that are in excess of a normal and expectable reaction to the stressor(s).
C. The disturbance is not merely one instance of a pattern of overreaction to stress or an exacerbation of one of the mental disorders previously described.
D. The maladaptive reaction has persisted for no longer than 6 months.
E. The disturbance does not meet the criteria for any specific mental disorder and does not represent Uncomplicated Bereavement.

[a]Adapted from the American Psychiatric Association: *Diagnostic and Statistical Manual of Mental Disorders*, 3rd ed, revised. Washington, DC, American Psychiatric Association, 1987.

in Table 10.2, and one predictable depressive reaction to a stressor, a normal grief reaction, is described in Chapter 19.

These "reactive" depressions resolve when the stressor remits or when the patient reaches a new level of adaptation or adjustment. The approaches to office psychotherapy described in Chapter 11 facilitate this process for most patients.

MAJOR AFFECTIVE SYNDROMES

Mania and major depression are the two syndromes that give the traditional name manic depressive disorder to this group of disorders. These disorders are characteristically episodic with complete remissions between episodes. Most patients suffer only recurrent depressive episodes (the unipolar group), few suffer only manic episodes (they are grouped with bipolar patients), and the remainder suffer from both manic and depressive episodes (the bipolar group). Based upon a national community survey of mental disorders, the Epidemiologic Catchment Area study, it is estimated that 5 to 10% of women and 2 to 5% of men experience at least one major depressive episode during their adult life; it may occur at any age. Only 0.4 to 1.2% of adults develop a bipolar disorder; it is equally common in men and women; the first manic episode usually occurs before age 30 (9).

Major Depression

Diagnosis

It is important to differentiate major depression from other major disorders, i.e., schizophrenia and dementia (see Chapters 16 and 17), from depressive neurosis (see above) and anxiety neurosis (see Chapter 13), and from adjustment disorder with depressed mood (see above).

The concept of the "endogenous" depression, although flawed, has provided a durable, usable account of major depressive illness. The fully developed syndrome is characterized by a sustained alteration in mood, self-attitude, and vital sense. The sustained lowering of mood is relatively impervious to environmental influence when depression is severe. A major life stress frequently occurs at the onset of symptoms and, thus, is not useful for making or excluding the diagnosis. The change in self-attitude is usually manifested in the development of feelings of guilt, inferiority, uselessness, and hopelessness regarding the future as the mood descends. The changes in vital sense (i.e., the subjective assessment of one's physical and mental functioning) usually include feelings of confusion, poor memory with the inability to concentrate, a lack of energy and easy fatigability, loss of interest in valued activities, and occasionally fears or delusions of dying of cancer, losing one's mind, etc.

Marked psychomotor retardation (i.e., slowed speech and movements), delusions with depressive content, and diurnal mood variation (worst mood in the morning) occur in a minority of patients but are diagnos-

tically useful when present since they are fairly specific to this disorder.

A patient presenting with a history of an episodic disorder and a fully developed symptom cluster as described is not difficult to diagnose. However, many patients with major depressions present either with few of these characteristic "endogenous" symptoms, with a dominant somatic symptom, or with a clear reason to be depressed, guilty, or hopeless. In such patients, recognition of major depression may be delayed, and either the patient may be insufficiently treated or may receive no treatment for this eminently treatable disorder. If the diagnosis is uncertain, the facts should be examined for the specific criteria of the APA for major depressive episode (Table 15.4). These criteria state that patients with five of nine depressive symptoms and functional impairment for 2 weeks and who do not have the characteristic symptoms of schizophrenia should be considered to have a major depressive disorder and treated accordingly. These criteria will result in misclassification of some patients who would be easily classified with more traditional diagnostic concepts. However, these criteria are useful in supporting the working diagnosis for major depression in order to begin therapy. Recent work suggests that the dexamethasone suppression test, described in Chapter 74, may be useful in differentiating a major depressive episode (plasma cortisol not suppressed by dexamethasone) from a minor affective disturbance. However, a sizable number of medical conditions interfere with its interpretation. This and other problems make it more useful in an inpatient psychiatric population than in an ambulatory medical population (5).

So-called atypical depression accounts for some major depressions and a larger number of the dysthymic depressions in which symptoms such as hypersomnia, overeating, and lethargy are seen more frequently than insomnia, anorexia, and psychomotor agitation (11). Such patients usually show the characteristic depressive changes in self-attitude and vital sense, but they may describe their mood changes more in terms of fatigue than sadness. These patients often experience panic-type anxiety symptoms during their depressive episodes (see Chapter 13).

Table 15.4.
American Psychiatric Association Diagnostic Criteria for Major Depressive Episode[a]

A. At least five of the following symptoms have been present during the same 2-week period and represent a change from previous functioning;
  (1) Depressed mood
  (2) Markedly diminished interest or pleasure in almost all activities
  (3) Significant weight loss or weight gain
  (4) Insomnia or hypersomnia
  (5) Psychomotor agitation or retardation
  (6) Fatigue or loss of energy
  (7) Feelings of worthlessness or excessive guilt
  (8) Diminished ability to think or concentrate
  (9) Recurrent thoughts of death or suicide
B. Not due to diagnosable brain injury, bereavement, or schizophrenia

[a]Adapted from American Psychiatric Association: *Diagnostic and Statistical Manual of Mental Disorders*, 3rd ed, revised. Washington, D.C., American Psychiatric Association, 1987. Special criteria for children have been omitted from this table.

Management

Antidepressant Drugs. For the patient with major depression who is in good physical condition and who is neither overwhelmed with depressive delusions nor suicidal, outpatient prescription of antidepressant medication is the appropriate initial treatment. Although very useful, the antidepressant drugs—tricyclic antidepressants (TCA), monoamine oxidase inhibitors (MAOI), and serotonin reuptake inhibitors—are not always effective in eradicating depressive symptoms. About 70% of depressed patients will have a complete remission of symptoms with any antidepressant. For most patients, TCAs are regarded as the drugs of first choice. Among patients with the syndrome of depression, those with delusions, hallucinations, and profound psychomotor retardation tend to be less responsive to drugs than those without these symptoms; referral for psychiatric consultation and consideration for electroconvulsive therapy are appropriate for such patients. Among patients with suicidal intent (see "Suicide Prevention") antidepressant drugs, especially tricyclics, should be dispensed in small amounts (i.e., no more than a 1-week supply) since even a 10-day supply provides enough drug for a lethal overdose.

The mechanism of therapeutic action of antidepressant drugs is unknown. Although much indirect evidence suggests that they exert their therapeutic effects by enhancing catecholaminergic and serotonergic neurotransmission, their clinical use remains empirical. The TCAs can be divided into two groups (see Table 15.5): the secondary amines (e.g., desipramine and nortriptyline), and the tertiary amines (e.g., amitriptyline, doxepin, and imipramine), which have been more widely used but which have more anticholinergic activity and cause more orthostatic hypotension than the secondary amines.

At a 1984 consensus development conference at the National Institute of Mental Health (see "General References"), the secondary amine TCAs were selected as drugs that should be recommended to nonpsychiatrists as effective antidepressants with acceptable toxicity. This approach would suggest beginning with a secondary amine such as nortriptyline or desipramine. Two problems common in the prescribing of TCAs by nonpsychiatrists are (*a*) discontinuing or changing a TCA before the patient has had an adequate trial and (*b*) maintaining a drug for a prolonged period despite no response to it.

Treatment with nortriptyline should begin with 25 to 50 mg per day, and the dose should be increased after a few days to 50 to 75 mg per day. It should be maintained there for 2 weeks; if substantial improvement is noted, then no change should be needed. If improvement is marginal or absent after the first 2 weeks, a plasma tricyclic level should be obtained. The optimal nortriptyline level is 90 to 140 ng/ml. The process of dosage adjustment to produce an effective result is repeated every 2 weeks until the patient is showing definite improvement or 4 weeks of optimal treatment have proven fruitless.

Treatment with most other TCAs should begin at 50 mg (exception: 10 mg for protriptyline) and be increased in 25-mg increments as tolerated to 150 to 300 mg/day, the average effective doses for most of these drugs (exception: 40 mg for protriptyline) (see Table 15.5). Starting doses should be reduced in older patients, especially those with medical illnesses (see Chapter 17 for further details). Giving the total daily dose at bedtime is desirable for most patients. After 8 weeks of a particular antidepressant, an adequate trial will have been completed. Blood levels should be monitored to assure that the patient has gotten an adequate trial, if there is an incomplete response. Because TCAs may interact with a number of commonly prescribed drugs (Table 15.6), simultaneous prescribing of other drugs with TCAs should be avoided; if this is not possible, close monitoring is very important (for example, when a patient is taking antihypertensive drugs and a TCA).

Dosage of MAOIs should begin at 15 mg two times a day for phenelzine or 10 mg two times a day for tranylcypromine or isocarboxazid and be increased by 10 to 15 mg per week to the maximum dose unless therapeutic response or toxicity dictates otherwise (see Table 15.5). The use of MAOIs, particularly tranylcypromine, requires caution with respect to diet and the effects of coadministered drugs, in order to avoid a hypertensive crisis (see Table 15.7).

A number of drugs that are structurally distinct from the MAOIs and TCAs have been marketed in the United States as antidepressants. In addition several others await Food and Drug Administration (FDA) approval.

Three of the *newer antidepressant medications* (fluoxetine, trazodone, and alprazolam) are already frequently prescribed by nonpsychiatrists. Fluoxetine (Prozac), a potent serotonin reuptake inhibitor, is an effective antidepressant that is easy to use. Most responders will be helped by a single 20 mg per day dose and will not need any dosage adjustment during therapy. However, because of the very long half-life of the drug, it may take 6 weeks of therapy before benefits are seen (as noted above, with tricyclics, benefits usually develop 2 to 3 weeks after a therapeutic dose has been attained). If there has been no response after 6 weeks, the dose may be doubled. Common side effects of fluoxetine are mild nausea, insomnia, and transient worsening of anxiety symptoms. Insomnia is less common if fluoxetine is taken in the morning.

Trazodone (Desyrel), a second, less potent, serotonin reuptake inhibitor, is a more sedating medication. Because it is so sedating, it is often given in inadequate amounts to depressed patients. Antidepressant benefit is not regularly seen below 300 mg per day. Trazodone should be given initially as 150 mg at bedtime, and the dose should be increased by 50 mg (tablets are scored so this can be done) every 3 or 4 days until a daily dose of 300 mg has been reached.

The high potency benzodiazepine alprazolam (Xanax) is dramatically and rapidly effective in relieving the most severe anxiety symptoms (such as panic or anxiety attacks) seen in some depressed patients. It is

Table 15.5.
Selected Characteristics of Antidepressant Drugs

						A. TRICYCLICS			
							Side Effects		
Amine Group	Generic Name	Proprietary Name	Strengths of Oral Preparations (mg)	Usual Effective Total Daily Doses in mg (Range)	Therapeutic Plasma Level (ng/ml)	Antihistamine (Sedation)	Antiadrenergic (Orthostatic Hypotension)	Anticholinergic[a]	
Secondary amines	Desipramine	Norpramin, Pertofrane,	25, 50	200 (50–300)	>115[b]	+	+ +	+	
	Nortriptyline	Aventyl, Pamelor	10, 25	100 (50–150)	90–140	+	+	+ +	
	Protriptyline	Vivactil	5, 10	40 (15–60)	70–170	+	+ +	+ +	
Tertiary amines	Amitriptyline	Elavil, Endep	10, 25, 50, 75, 100	150 (50–300)	>120[b]	+ + +	+ + +	+ + +	
	Doxepin	Sinequan, Adapin	10, 25, 50, 100	150 (50–300)	>90[b]	+ + +	+ + +	+ +	
	Imipramine	Tofranil SK-Pramine, Presamine	10, 25, 50	150 (50–300)	>95[b]	+ +	+ + +	+ +	

				B. MONOAMINE OXIDASE INHIBITORS		
					Side Effects	
Generic Name	Proprietary Name	Stengths of Oral Preparations (mg)	Usual Effective Total Daily Doses in mg (Range)	Risk of Hypertensive Crisis	Hypotension	
Tranylcypromine	Parnate	10	30 (20–60)	+ +	+ +	
Phenelzine	Nardil	15	45 (30–90)	+	+ +	
Isocarboxazide	Marplan	10	30 (20–60)	+	+ +	

				C. NEWER ANTIDEPRESSANTS	
Generic Name	Proprietary Name	Strengths of Oral Preparations (mg)	Usual Effective Total Daily Doses in mg (Range)	Major Advantage Over Tricyclics	Major Disadvantage Compared to Tricyclics
Fluoxetine	Prozac	20	20–60	Few anticholinergic effects	Can increase anxiety and insomnia in early phase of treatment.
Trazodone	Desyrel	150, 300	300 (200–600)	Almost no anticholinergic effects	Very sedating (like amitriptyline). Appears to have greater direct cardiotoxicity than TCAs. Priapism requiring surgery reported.
Alprazolam	Xanax	0.25, 0.5, 1	0.75–4	A benzodiazepine without anticholinergic or other tricyclic side effects.	Not established as fully effective in depressions. Some addictive potential. Fairly sedating. Three times a day schedule.
Bupropion	Wellbutrin	75, 100	300–450	Few anticholinergic effects	May be more likely than TCA to induce seizures. Can increase anxiety and insomnia in early phase of treatment. Divided dose needed.

[a]Dry mouth, blurred vision, decreased intestinal motility, decreased bladder tone, tachycardia.
[b]Upper limit not established.

somewhat less effective as an antidepressant and when used for more than a month can lead to unpleasant and protracted withdrawal symptoms if it is stopped abruptly.

Bupropion (Wellbutrin) is another antidepressant that has been used in recent years. Advantages are that it causes few anticholinergic or sedative effects and has not been associated with excess weight gain. It may be associated with seizures, rarely. Agitation has been the most frequent reason for stopping this drug. The recommended starting dose is 100 mg twice daily, with an increase to a full dose, 100 mg three times daily, after three days. To reduce the risk of seizures, it has been recommended that the daily dose should

not exceed 450 mg. The full antidepressant effect of bupropion usually occurs within four weeks.

Combination medications containing TCAs and phenothiazine should not be used in the treatment of depressive disorders, since they carry the risk of side effects from both drugs and they provide no demonstrated advantage over carefully selected TCAs in nondelusional depressed patients.

Drug Side Effects. The antidepressants cause side effects, many of which can be grouped according to probable physiological mechanism (see Table 15.5). Many depressed patients tolerate even mild side effects poorly and need to be reassured that the treatment is safe and likely to be effective in 3 to 8 weeks.

Table 15.6.
Drugs That May Interact with Tricyclic Antidepressants (TCAs)

Drug	Interaction
Anticholinergic antispasmodics	Enhanced anticholinergic side effects
Antihypertensive drugs	Enhanced orthostatic hypotension (Exception: clonidine and guanethidine: TCA may interfere with anti-hypertensive effectiveness)
Antiparkinsonian drugs (L-dopa and anticholinergic drugs)	Enhanced anticholinergic side effects (also decreased L-dopa effect)
Cimetidine	Increased imipramine effect
Dilantin	May block TCA effectiveness
Fluoxetine (Prozac)	Increases TCA plasma levels two-fold or more
Methylphenidate (Ritalin)	May increase TCA plasma levels
Monoamine oxidase inhibitors (MAOIs)	Levels of both TCA and MAOI may be increased, enhanced risk of hypertensive crisis
Sedating drugs (alcohol, antihistamines, anxiolytics, hypnotics, neuroleptics)	Enhanced sedation
Sympathomimetics (decongestants, weight reduction agents, stimulants)	TCA may potentiate blood pressure-raising effects of these drugs

Table 15.7.
Restrictions Needed to Avoid Hypertensive Crisis in Patients Taking Monoamine Oxidase Inhibitors

Items to be avoided[a]	Comments
FOODS	
Cheese	Tyramine content may increase with aging. Sharp cheeses, especially cooked and uncooked cheddar, are highly implicated, but no problem with cream and cottage cheese
Yogurt	
Sour Cream	
Beer	
Wine	Not all wines are implicated equally; the problem is noteworthy with Chianti and sherry in small amounts
Broad beans (fava beans, *Vicia faba*) these beans are an ingredient of pasta fasula	Several reported hypertensive crises
Active yeast preparations	No problem with bread
DRUGS	
Any sympathomimetic drug (decongestants in cold remedies, weight reduction agents, stimulants)	Can lead to hypertensive crisis
Stop monoamine oxidase inhibitors 2 weeks before planned surgery	Hypertensive crisis can occur if sympathomimetic given for vasoconstriction during surgery
Meperidine, fluoxetine, and Buspirone	Hypertension, fever, coma can occur. Fluoxetine should be stopped five weeks before giving MAOI

[a]As little as 6 mg of tyramine may produce a hypertensive reaction in a patient taking a monoamine oxidase inhibitor.

Apart from the specific situations listed in Tables 15.6 and 15.7, there is no useful information for predicting, preventing, or alleviating the side effects of antidepressant drugs. In addition to the side effects named in Table 15.5, TCAs may produce mild paresthesia, increased appetite with weight gain (i.e., in response to treatment, the patient's weight surpasses the weight that was normal for the patient before the onset of depression), granulocytopenia (rarely), anticholinergic delirium (rarely), hypomania, slowed cardiac conduction, and cardiac arrhythmias. Because of the cardiac effects, these drugs should be given cautiously to those patients who have preexisting conduction abnormalities and to those with unstable cardiac conditions, such as a recent myocardial infarction. However, tricyclics are quite safe even in patients with pre-existing stable heart disease (12). The major problem associated with the use of MAOIs is acute hypertension caused by foods containing the sympathomimetic agent, tyramine. Thus, patients taking MAOIs must eliminate certain foods from their diet (Table 15.7).

Duration of Drug Treatment. After recovery from a first or infrequently recurrent depressive syndrome, the medication that induced the remission should be continued usually for 6 months (a period of high risk for relapse); during this interval, dosage should remain at the level that relieved the depression. Occasionally, a lowering of the dose to reduce side effects will be justified. The patient should be told that withdrawal symptoms (nausea, dizziness, headache, increased perspiration, and increased salivation) may occur when tricyclics are discontinued abruptly. For this reason tricyclics that have been given for 2 months or more should be tapered in 25- to 50-mg increments/week prior to discontinuation. After electroconvulsive therapy (see below), maintenance treatment with a tricyclic antidepressant also reduces the risk of relapse. Exceptions to these guidelines include the occurrence of drug toxicity, the appearance of manic symptoms (which can be induced by the antidepressants), and a history of such regular relapses that indefinite maintenance therapy with a tricyclic or lithium is needed (see section below on long-term management).

Office Psychotherapy. For the first 6 to 8 weeks, the patient with major depression should be seen at least every other week for adjustment of medication and for brief supportive psychotherapy as described in Chapter 11. Major life decisions and major shifts in personal relationships should be gently discouraged until the patient returns to his or her premorbid condition. Frank discussion of suicidal feelings, plans, intentions, risk, and alternatives should be a routine part of each visit (see "Suicide Prevention" below). The patient should be checked routinely for side effects of drugs by being asked about them (e.g., dry mouth, tremor, blurred vision, orthostasis, tachycardia, and constipation) and by examining heart rate and rhythm and blood pressure (sitting and standing). The more depressed the patient is, the less tolerant he will be of minor adverse drug effects. The support of the doctor in encouraging persistence with drug therapy can be crucial.

Discussion of prognosis with the patient and his family is extremely important in the management of depression (see page 156, "Prognosis," and page 157, "Counseling the Distressed Family" below).

Referral for Management.   There are four types of patients who should always be referred for the expertise of a psychiatrist: those who have shown no improvement after 8 weeks of treatment with therapeutic doses of antidepressant drugs (about one in three patients); those who cannot or will not take antidepressant medications; those who are overtly suicidal; and those who show delusions, hallucinations, or depressive stupor (the patient becomes mute and unresponsive). In these patients, either hospitalization, intensive psychotherapy, more aggressive drug therapy, or electroconvulsive therapy will usually be suggested by the psychiatric consultant. Some patients will be resistant to the idea of seeing a psychiatrist. Physicians who already have good rapport with their patients can be very persuasive if they explain that additional drug treatments are available, but that their use requires the expertise and experience of the psychiatrist, and that there is an excellent chance of improvement with this.

Electroconvulsive Therapy.   Electroconvulsive therapy (ECT) is an effective and rapid treatment for major depressive disorder. The decision to use ECT should be made by the psychiatrist with the concurrence of the patient and/or the patient's family. This treatment is given only to hospitalized patients; during ECT the patient is anesthetized with a short acting barbiturate anesthetic. There is general agreement that this treatment is not useful for patients with "neurotic" depression (dysthymic disorder). There is even some evidence that among patients with clear-cut major depression those with the more severe symptoms will have a better therapeutic response. Failure of drug therapy, the presence of certain medical illness that make drug therapy excessively dangerous, the need for a prompt response (as in the starving or suicidal patient), and overwhelming severity of the depression are the principal indications for ECT.

The mechanism of action of ECT is unknown, but it appears that the electrical seizure discharge which comes in an all-or-none fashion after the application of current, is required for benefit. There is usually transient memory loss, but therapeutic benefit is not linked to the memory disturbance. Although there are other methods of inducing seizures, electric current is easiest to control and, therefore, safest. The usual risk of general anesthesia is the major hazard associated with ECT.

The adverse effects that follow ECT primarily involve memory. Commonly, retention of new and, occasionally, old memories is mildly defective for weeks to months following a series of ECT treatments. This defect is usually "spotty," that is, it will be apparent for specific domains of memory but will not affect many others. Typically, the patient in whom this effect

becomes clinically apparent (perhaps 40% of treated patients) will have trouble recalling names of recent acquaintances including doctors, nurses, and other patients. Clinically apparent memory defects typically resolve within a month. More detailed formal testing reveals mild defects up to 3 months, but none at 6 months after treatment.

Depressed patients with brain tumors ordinarily should not receive ECT. Patients with dementias from neuropathological causes treated with ECT may have temporary worsening of their cognitive impairments, but not infrequently the removal of depression actually helps overall social functioning. ECT should be avoided, if possible, within 3 months of myocardial infarction, cerebrovascular accident, or perforated viscus repair. Neither anticoagulation therapy nor the presence of a cardiac pacemaker is a contraindication for ECT.

Mania

Diagnosis

The manic syndrome, like major depression, is defined by a sustained change in mood with parallel changes in self-attitude and vital sense. The manic patient's mood may be euphoric or irritable and angry or may alternate between the two. Self-attitude becomes one of overconfidence and of an inflated sense of power, position, and importance. Vital sense reflects a subjective sense of quickened, acutely accurate thinking, unusual ease in decision making, a sense of heightened perception of sounds, colors, tastes, etc. In addition there is usually a sense of increased energy and a decreased need for sleep.

This central triad is often accompanied by parallel psychomotor symptoms. Delusions and hallucinations that are either persecutory or consistent with mood are not uncommon. Occasionally even characteristic symptoms of schizophrenia (see Chapter 16) occur in manic patients, leading to the clinical rule of thumb that so-called "schizophrenic" symptoms are not in themselves diagnostic but should be judged by the company they keep. In the presence of the characteristic manic syndrome and first rank symptoms of schizophrenia some would diagnose "schizoaffective disorder-manic type." Treatment and projected outcomes are similar to those for typical mania. The specific criteria of the American Psychiatric Association for mania are shown in Table 15.8.

Management

Because manic patients are treated with a drug, lithium, that requires supervision by someone familiar with its use, patients with mania should be referred to a psychiatrist. The patient's primary physician often plays a crucial role in recognizing the presence of mania, in persuading a severely manic patient to accept referral, and in sharing care when the patient has a chronic medical problem.

Lithium.   In its milder form (called hypomania), the

Table 15.8.
American Psychiatric Association Diagnostic Criteria for a Manic Episode[a]

A. A distinct period of abnormally and persistently elevated, expansive, or irritable mood.
B. At least three of the following symptoms:
  (1) Inflated self-esteem or grandiosity
  (2) ›Decreased need for sleep
  (3) More talkative than usual
  (4) Flight of ideas or subjective experience that thoughts are racing
  (5) Distractibility
  (6) Increased activity
  (7) Excessive involvement in activities that have a high potential for painful consequences
C. Symptoms sufficiently severe to cause marked impairment in occupational functioning, social activities, or relationships
D. Not due to diagnosable brain injury or schizophrenia
NOTE: A "Manic Syndrome" is defined as including criteria A, B, and C above. A "Hypomanic Syndrome" is defined as including criteria A and B, but not C, i.e., no marked impairment.

[a]Adapted from American Psychiatric Association: *Diagnostic and Statistical Manual of Mental Disorders*; 3rd ed. Washington, DC, American Psychiatric Association, 1980.

Table 15.9.
Important Drug Interactions with Lithium

Drugs that may enhance lithium toxicity:
  Amiloride[a]
  Ethacrynic acid[a]
  Furosemide[a]
  Indomethacin (and probably other nonsteroidal antiinflammatory drugs (NSAIDs)[a]
  Methyldopa[b]
  Phenytoin[b]
  Carbamazepine[b]
  Spectinamycin[a]
  Spironolactone[a]
  Tetracycline[a]
  Thiazide diuretics[a]
  Triamterene[a]
Drugs that may diminish lithium effect:
  Theophylline[c]
  Acetazolamide[c]
Drugs that may aggravate lithium tremor:
  Neuroleptics[b]
  Tricyclic antidepressants[b]

[a]Decreased renal excretion.
[b]Mechanism not established.
[c]Increased renal excretion.

manic syndrome may be successfully treated with a neuroleptic (see Chapter 16 for details on neuroleptics) or lithium alone. Because the neuroleptics reduce manic behavior more rapidly, they are often used in combination with lithium in the early phases of treatment. This combined treatment involves greater risk of adverse effects. For both short- and long-term treatment, lithium carbonate is the most useful drug in the manic patient.

Lithium is given in divided doses. Beginning with 300 to 600 mg on the first day and increasing the dose in small increments every 3 to 4 days to the desired level, and having the patient taken lithium on a full stomach minimizes nausea. The usual maintenance dose is 600 to 1800 mg given in divided doses (three or four times daily with standard preparations and once or twice daily with slow release preparations). Blood levels, which should be measured 12 hours after a dose, should be monitored once or twice/week at first. Even when thoroughly stabilized in a compliant patient, lithium levels should be checked at least six times/year. In addition, because of the possibility of long-term renal effects, maintenance dosage should be aimed at maintaining the lowest therapeutic level (often 0.6 to 0.9 mEq/liter) and not necessarily the level required for acute antimanic activity (0.9 to 1.4 mEq/liter). Lithium should be used cautiously with other medications since there are a number of important drug interactions associated with its use (see Table 15.9).

The *adverse effects* of lithium can be divided into three groups: early (associated with rapidly rising blood levels), maintenance (associated with stable levels within the therapeutic range), and toxic (usually associated with high lithium levels).

The early side effects include nausea and vomiting, diarrhea, mild lassitude, and drowsiness. These effects typically resolve as the serum level stabilizes in the therapeutic range.

The number of possible side effects from the main-

tenance dose is large enough to warrant a medical review of systems to detect them. The three most important ones are hand tremor, thyroid disturbances, and renal toxicity.

1. An accentuated physiological tremor (see Chapter 82) appears in a large percentage of patients (perhaps 60%) but is rarely severe. A family history of benign essential tremor and of concomitant use of other psychotropic drugs is often associated with more severe tremor.
2. In about 3% of patients, lithium therapy causes nontoxic goiter and mild alterations of thyroid function tests (i.e., borderline low thyroxine levels or elevated thyroid-stimulating hormone values). Less frequently, frank hypothyroidism may occur, usually in patients who had subclinical hypothyroidism before receiving lithium. For these reasons thyroid function should be assessed before lithium treatment is begun.
3. Finally long-term lithium therapy is occasionally associated with a renal concentrating defect (partial nephrogenic diabetes insipidus). These abnormalities cause symptoms of polyuria and polydipsia in about 10% of patients. The concentrating defect predisposes the patient to dehydration and, therefore, to frank lithium intoxication. Polyuric patients must be counseled to maintain good hydration even under circumstances that might inhibit their interest in adequate water intake (including depression) or that would increase water loss (e.g., hot weather). They should also be instructed to report the onset of polyuria at any time in the course of lithium treatment. Daily urine volume and glomerular filtration rate (GFR) should be assessed (see Chapter 47) before lithium is started and reassessed yearly thereafter.

The toxic effects of lithium occur uncommonly at normal serum levels but increase in frequency as serum levels rise past 1.5 mEq/liter. Overingestion and inadequate renal excretion (at times, related to one of the drugs listed in Table 15.9) are the only causes of lithium toxicity. Premonitory signs are the recurrence of gastrointestinal side effects and worsening of polyuria and hand tremor, lethargy, and clumsiness. Obvious changes in the level of consciousness are reflected in confusion, delirium, stupor, and finally coma. Focal as well as nonlocalizing neurological signs are often present. Peak levels above 4.0 m Eq/liter are potentially fatal; death in coma complicated by aspiration pneumonitis can occur. The toxic syndrome is not usually relieved rapidly, even though blood levels can be reduced rapidly. A rather prolonged 10- to 14-day resolution of the mental state is usual. Management of suspected lithium intoxication begins with an emergency measurement of serum lithium level and the discontinuation of lithium when the early signs of the disorder appear. If the clinical or laboratory evaluations suggest the likelihood of the toxic syndrome, hospitalization is mandatory.

Treatment of Severe Mania. Severe acute mania requires treatment with both lithium and neuroleptics, which is usually carried out in the hospital. The generalist's role with such patients may include initial diagnosis and then assessment of the acute manic state, persuasion of the manic patient to accept hospitalization voluntarily if needed, assessment of the patient for possible civil commitment (see Chapter 10), and the management of the acutely manic patient at home or in the office. These last three steps are outlined below.

Relating to the acutely manic patient can be very difficult. The euphoric or irritable manic patient often will not be able to accept the notion that his or her behavior is disturbed and requires inpatient therapy. A rationale for treatment that does not call attention to the obviously disordered behavior is usually more palatable to the patient. Consultation with the family about the plan of treatment should be arranged before, not after, confrontation with the patient. The family should be advised to the potential consequences if the patient refuses to follow the physician's recommendation.

Although laws on commitment vary from state to state, all states currently have legal provisions to allow the involuntary hospitalization of patients with mental disorders who are clearly dangerous to themselves or others and for whom no less restrictive alternative is appropriate.

For acute manic agitation the use of parenteral haloperidol (Haldol) is usually quite effective. Modest doses (5 to 10 mg intramuscularly) will calm most patients with little or no depression of blood pressure and little sedation. The sedating phenothiazines such as chlorpromazine (Thorazine) are more apt to produce severe orthostatic hypotension, and repeated doses are often necessary to break the agitated manic state. Within 15 to 20 minutes, intramuscular haloperidol usually brings about a calming effect that lasts for several hours. This period can be used to get the patient admitted to hospital. Even in this short period, however, patients may develop extrapyramidal side effects from haloperidol, most frequently acute dystonic reactions. This condition will be alleviated by 50 mg of intramuscular diphenhydramine (Benadryl).

Prognosis and Long-Term Management of Major Affective Disorders

Because of the fundamental similarities, the prognoses of major depression and mania are discussed together. Before modern treatment, patients with these disorders usually recovered spontaneously within 6 to 18 months. With antidepressants, lithium, and ECT, remissions usually can be achieved much more quickly. However, even with modern treatment, about 20% of patients with severe major depressions may not recover fully in a 2-year period after ending treatment (6). Predictors of poor outcome include severity sufficient to require hospitalization and long duration of major symptoms (1 year) before treatment. It has also been noted that many nonrecovering patients have not been aggressively treated after failure to respond to a trial of antidepressant medications. Although some patients will fail to respond to all treatments, clinical experience teaches that most correctly diagnosed patients who are initially treatment failures will eventually respond to a second, third, or fourth treatment effort.

A hallmark of the course of major affective syndromes is the tendency to relapse. The frequency of relapse is quite variable. However, fewer than 20% of major affective syndromes resolve without relapsing at some point. There is a tendency for relapses to become more frequent later in the life of the patient (or later in the course of the illness). There is some evidence that depressions in later life are more severe and treatment resistant as well. Formerly, this was part of the justification for the now discarded term "involutional melancholia."

The use of lithium and antidepressants has been shown to be beneficial in preventing recurrent affective episodes (8). Depressive relapses that occur in patients taking lithium or tricyclics are usually less severe and of shorter duration. Lithium is the best studied treatment demonstrated to reduce the frequency of manic relapses.

The foundations of long-term care of patients with bipolar or unipolar affective disorders are the following: a trusting doctor-patient relationship; education and counseling of the patient and his family regarding the nature and course of the illness, the early signs of relapse, and the benefits and hazards of treatment; and maintenance on lithium carbonate or a tricyclic antidepressant. Maintenance treatment is usually continued indefinitely for a clearly relapsing disorder. The patient's personal physician can often provide the basic treatment, particularly if that physician is following the patient for chronic medical problems. Brief visits every 2 to 3 months are sufficient when the patient is well. The objectives of these visits are to monitor the mood state, the drug therapy, and the social progress of the patient. If the patient has a well-established trusting and predictable relationship with the doctor, even patients with the most grandiose manic or pessimistic depressive states will be more amenable to accepting necessary additional treatment.

The patient and his family should be educated with respect to the relapsing and remitting course of the illness, which is greatly modified but not usually eradicated by drug therapy. Individual aspects of the illness need to be observed and remembered by the patient, the family members, and the doctor, in particular, (a) the early symptoms of relapse (which differ from patient to patient); (b) certain signs or symptoms that specifically point to the affective syndrome in contrast to other reasons for changed feelings or behavior; and (c) recognized signs for suicidal or other dangerous behavior, as well as ways to relieve the danger.

Counseling the Distressed Family

Family members of patients with serious affective disorders often experience feelings of confusion, hopelessness, guilt, and recrimination toward the patient. These are not only painful feelings; they seriously impede the family's attempts to support or care for their ill relative. Physicians need to address the family needs directly through educational meetings with them. Above all, the family must recognize major affective disorders as diseases and realize that these disorders are not caused by the family, by the patient, or by social predicaments affecting the patient. The family also should know that, although the pathophysiology of affective disorders is unknown, empirical treatments are quite effective and the prognosis for complete recovery from an episode is generally good, although relapses occur frequently. These points will usually require some repetition. The patient education materials provided by the American Psychiatric Association and the National Institute of Mental Health and the recently published book by DePaulo and Ablow can also be recommended to patients and families (see "General References").

It is equally important to reassure families and patients with dysthymic and transiently demoralized mood states that the patients are not suffering from major mental illness.

Evidence from studies of concordance in identical as compared with nonidentical twins suggests a substantial genetic contribution to the etiology of major affective disorders. Because no single pattern of inheritance has been discerned, the evidence for a genetic contribution has been interpreted in several ways: (a) not all cases are genetically transmitted, (b) there is genetic heterogeneity in familial cases, and (c) the condition may be polygenic. Overall, it appears that a sibling or offspring of a patient with a major affective disorder has a 10% chance of developing the disorder. However, in a family in which there is no evidence for a genetic contribution, the risk would not be greater than that in the general population, whereas in some families this risk may be as high as 50%. Counseling patients and their families about the genetic risk must be tailored to the needs and relevant past history in each family. The major themes of counseling should be that most, but not all, cases are genetically influenced, that effective treatment is available, and that treatment is much enhanced by early detection of the disorder.

CYCLOTHYMIC DISORDER

A bipolar affective disorder that is sufficiently mild or so brief that the episodes fail to meet the APA criteria for major depression or mania (Tables 15.4 and 15.8) is categorized as a cyclothymic disorder. These patients must be distinguished from patients with the personality traits of emotional lability and self-dramatization, described in Chapter 14, who will often report rapid but unsustained mood changes. The family histories of cyclothymic patients are similar to those of patients with bipolar affective disorders. The prognosis is also similar to that of bipolar disorders, as 35% of such patients were found to suffer full blown manic, hypomanic, or depressive episodes in a 2- to 3-year period (2).

SUICIDE PREVENTION

The rate of suicide in most countries is low enough (11 per 100,000 in the United States) that accurate prediction of an individual suicide at a given point in time is very unlikely.

Practical strategies in this area are to protect those with relatively high risk in the short term and to reduce the risk in these patients over a longer term. Risk factors for successful suicide include severe depression, older age, male sex, alcoholism, living alone, previous suicide attempt, and refusal to accept referral for psychiatric treatment. Retrospective studies of patient groups with major affective disorders in the era before drugs were available for these disorders suggest that about 15% of the deaths were due to suicide. In addition, clinical observations suggest that the risk of suicide increases when improvement begins (or just after a depressed patient is discharged from the hospital) or when the depressive's ruminations become frankly delusional convictions. Retrospective studies also suggest that there are fewer suicides in depressed patients treated with ECT.

The most crucial activities of physicians in preventing suicides are the recognition, treatment, and prophylaxis of major depressive episodes. When evaluating any patient with depressed mood, direct and open inquiry should be made regarding suicidal ideas, specific plans, and available means that the patient might be inclined to use. This information as well as information about the capability and availability of constant family supervision are essential in determining whether treatment may be attempted safely on an outpatient basis. This evaluation should also be guided by the knowledge that delusional depressed patients have a significantly increased risk of suicide and that patients with prior suicide attempts are more likely than others to attempt it again when depressed. When treating depressed outpatients it should be recalled that a majority of people who commit suicide with medications have obtained the lethal dose in a single prescription at a recent visit to a physician (7). This could represent as little as a 1- to 2-week supply of antidepressant medication. Thus, small prescriptions and, at times, family supervision of medications will be needed. Finally, short-term protection of patients with suicidal intent via hospitalization, including involuntary commitment, is often required.

The majority of patients who present to emergency facilities after overdose of medications do not suffer from major depression but from adjustment disorders and personality disorders, and they usually do not die by suicide. However, they should be methodically evaluated in the same manner as noted above since many such patients are prone to take overdoses again when stressed. These patients may benefit from very brief hospital admissions when social support for them is lacking and suicidal feelings are intense. All should have some outpatient counseling.

General References

American Psychiatric Association: *Diagnostic and Statistical Manual of Mental Disorders*. 3rd ed, revised. Washington, DC, American Psychiatric Association, 1987.
> Recently updated diagnostic criteria and epidemiological information for all recognized psychiatric disorders.

Crowe RR: Electroconvulsive therapy—a current perspective. *N Engl J Med* 311:163, 1984.

DePaulo JR, Ablow KR: *How to Cope with Depression: A Complete Guide for You and Your Family*. New York, McGraw-Hill Publishing Company, 1989.
> A book written for patients, families, and general health professionals.

Gold PW, Goodwin FK, Chrousos GP: Clinical and biomedical manifestations and depression. *N Engl J Med* 319:348 and 413, 1988.

Goldberg RJ: Depression in primary care: DSM-III diagnoses and other depressive syndromes. *J Gen Intern Med* 3:491, 1988.
> Well-referenced review, focusing on what is important regarding depression in primary care practice.

Mood Disorders: Pharmacologic Prevention of Recurrences. Consensus Development Conference, Consensus Statement, United States Department of Health and Human Services, National Institutes of Health, 5 (4), 1984.
> The distilled wisdom of a committee of experts on maintenance treatment for major affective disorders. (Available by request from the National Institutes of Mental Health.)

The following patient education pamphlets are available from the American Psychiatric Association, 1400 K Street, N.W., Washington, DC, 20005:
1. Facts About: Depression.
2. Facts About: Manic-Depressive Disorders.
3. Facts About: Teen Suicide.
4. Facts About: Mental Health of the Elderly.

The following patient education pamphlets are available from the National Institute of Mental Health, 5600 Fishers Lane, Rockville, Maryland, 20857:
1. Depression: What You Need to Know.
2. Helpful Facts About Depressive Disorders.
3. National Educational Program on Depressive Disorders.

Specific References

1. Akiskal HS: Dysthymic disorder: psychopathology of proposed chronic depressive subtypes. *Am J Psychiatry* 140:11, 1983.
2. Akiskal HS, Djenderedjian AH, Rosenthal RH, Khani MK: Cyclothymic disorder: validating criteria for inclusion in the bipolar affective group. *Am J Psychiatry* 134 (1227):177, 1977.
3. DePaulo JR, Folstein MF: Psychiatric disturbance in neurological patients: detection, recognition and hospital course. *Ann Neurol* 4:225, 1978.
4. Goldberg DP, Day C, Thompson L: Psychiatric morbidity in general practice and the community. *Psychol Med* 6:565, 1976.
5. Health and Public Policy Committee, American College of Physicians: The dexamethasone suppression test for the detection, diagnosis, and management of depression. *Ann Intern Med* 100:307, 1984.
6. Keller MB, Klerman GL, Lavori PW, et al: Long-term outcome of episodes of major depression. *JAMA* 252:788, 1984.
7. Murphy GE: The physician's responsibility for suicide. I. An error of commission. II. Errors of omission. *Ann Intern Med* 82:301, 305, 1975.
8. Prien RF, Klett CJ, Caffey Jr. EM: Lithium carbonate and imipramine in prevention of affective episodes: a comparison in recurrent affective illness. *Arch Gen Psychiatry* 29:240, 1973.
9. Robins LN, Helzer JE, Weissman MM, et al: Lifetime prevalence of specific psychiatric disorders in three sites. *Arch Gen Psychiatry* 41:949, 1984.
10. Shepherd M, Gruenberg EM: The age for neuroses. *Milbank Mem Fund Q* 35:258, 1957.
11. Sovner D: The clinical characteristics and treatment of atypical depression. *J Clin Psychiatry* 42:285, 1981.
12. Veith RC, Raskind MA, Caldwell JH, et al: Cardiovascular effects of tricyclic antidepressants in depressed patients with chronic heart disease. *N Engl J Med* 306:954, 1982.
13. Widmer RB, Cadoret RJ, North CS: Depression in primary care—changes in pattern of patients visits and complaints during subsequent developing depressions. *J Fam Pract* 9:1017, 1979.

C H A P T E R 16

Schizophrenia

CHESTER W. SCHMIDT, JR., M.D.

Schizophrenia is a mental disorder or group of disorders of unknown etiology. The American Psychiatric Association lists the essential features of the disorder as the presence of certain psychotic features during the active phase of the disease, characteristic chronic symptoms involving multiple psychological processes, deterioration from a previous level of functioning, onset before the age of 45, and duration of at least 6 months. As noted below, none of these symptoms is pathognomonic for schizophrenia, and each is seen in other psychotic states associated with both functional and organic mental disorders.

Familiarity with schizophrenia is important to the generalist for two principal reasons: (a) in the prodromal stage, the patient frequently presents first to a general physician, and (b) the interested generalist can provide much of the care for a patient with this lifelong disorder.

EPIDEMIOLOGY

Schizophrenia has been found in all societies throughout the world. The distribution is assumed to be similar through all populations. Epidemiological studies in Western societies have found the incidence of schizophrenia to range from 50 to 250 cases/100,000 population/year. Lifetime incidence rates have been reported to range from 0.75 to 2.75%. The recent Epidemiologic Catchment Area survey reported a lifetime prevalence rate of 1.3% for five sites in the United States (5). Studies of incidence and prevalence in Europe using strict and somewhat narrow criteria of schizophrenia have produced case numbers and rates lower than similar studies done in the United States using broader criteria. Currently it is estimated there are 200,000 patients hospitalized in the United States with a diagnosis of schizophrenia. These patients occupy one-half of all of the psychiatric beds in the country. In 1943, Lemkau et al. (4) determined that 15 to 25% of patients with schizophrenia never enter the hospital. Developments in psychopharmacology that occurred in the 1950s and the wide availability of ambulatory treatment resources have expanded that number and have greatly reduced the duration of confinement for those schizophrenics who require hospitalization.

Schizophrenia is found with equal frequency in males and females. Onset is usually during young adulthood, with the first hospitalization generally occurring between the ages of 25 and 34 years. Most schizophrenics are single and are found in lower socioeconomic groups. The proposed reason for the clustering of patients in the lower socioeconomic groups is a downward social drift resulting from deterioration of social and vocational function.

ETIOLOGY

The cause or causes of schizophrenia remain unknown. Numerous theories have been offered: constitutional, genetic, neurological, anatomical, biochemical, nutritional, psychosocial, and psychoanalytical. It is known that people related to schizophrenics are at higher risk for the disorder. The increased risk ranges from 3% for second degree relatives, to 7 to 15% for siblings and children of one schizophrenic parent, to 40% for children of two schizophrenic patients. Concordance rates in dizygotic twins are 10 to 15%, and

in monozygotic twins 45%. This evidence indicates there is a genetic factor, but such a factor has yet to be defined. A more recent clue to the etiology of schizophrenia has emerged from studies of the pharmacological effects of neuroleptic antipsychotic agents on schizophrenia. These antipsychotic agents have been found to antagonize dopamine-mediated neurotransmission, leading to the speculation that excessive activity of the dopamine systems may be part of a biochemical defect in schizophrenics (6).

NATURAL HISTORY OF SCHIZOPHRENIA

Although the first episode of acute psychosis usually occurs in late adolescence or early adulthood, prodromal manifestations of the disease are often present for years before the acute episode. During the prodromal phase, individuals gradually withdraw from social relationships into their own inner psychological world. They become indifferent to their grooming, develop suspicious attitudes about others, and ignore social graces and social rituals. They appear different, peculiar, and sometimes bizarre. Withdrawal often results in a gradual deterioration of scholastic and vocational abilities although some patients who have achieved substantial social skills (including marriage and family), educational skills (college and/or graduate level work), and vocational skills (stable and productive work) show little deterioration of their baseline function. The development of these skills may be a function of the age at onset of the disorder: The older the patient is, the more likely it is that he or she will have developed social, educational, and vocational talents. In other patients the deterioration of social and vocational skills may be so striking that the patient seems to have a changed personality. In many cases of early onset schizophrenia, the patients will have developed only marginal social and vocational skills so that their deterioration appears more insidious.

In one study of the prodromal stage of schizophrenia (8), the majority of patients demonstrated some dysphoria (anxiety or depression) in association with social deterioration; and it is significant that over half of them developed vague somatic complaints for which they sought help from a general practitioner.

Acute psychotic episodes are marked by the presence of a variety of active (or positive) symptoms: delusions (content of thought); hallucinations (perception); blunted, flattened, or inappropriate affect; illogical thinking and loosening of associations (form of thought); preoccupation with fantasies and an inner psychological world (autism); inability to carry out goal-directed behavior because of preoccupation with consequences of alternatives (ambivalence); and stereotyped, bizarre, and sometimes rigid posturing. These episodes are often associated with stressful life events. Before neuroleptics were available, these episodes could last from weeks to years. Currently most episodes are brought under pharmacological control within several weeks to 2 months. After treatment, positive psychotic symptoms subside and in some cases seem to disappear completely. Most patients then display negative symptoms—the withdrawn, distant, odd social manner they manifested before the psychotic episode. Scholastic and vocational ability may slip further. With each subsequent psychotic episode the patients slip further and further into a dependent, regressed state in which they are unable to function and become entirely dependent on family or society. Less than 20% work full time; the majority are financially supported by welfare programs or by federal disability programs. Institutionalization is required in some cases because the patients lose all ability to care for themselves.

Thus, schizophrenia is a lifelong disease consisting of (a) psychotic symptoms that periodically become intense, and (b) an arrest or deterioration of social and vocational functioning probably caused by massive withdrawal of interest in the outside world.

DIAGNOSIS

The diagnosis of schizophrenia, especially during the initial episodes of acute psychosis, is based on clinical judgment and diagnostic criteria that, until recently, were unreliable. There are no pathognomonic symptoms, signs, or laboratory findings that point to the diagnosis. The medical history of the patient does not contribute to the diagnosis and, as discussed above, family history of the disease provides only partial information.

The diagnostic criteria for schizophrenia described in the American Psychiatric Associations' *Diagnostic and Statistical Manual of Mental Disorders DSM-III-R* (third edition revised) are an excellent synthesis of several recognized diagnostic formulations (see Table 16.1). Diagnosis rests upon the findings of the symptoms of psychosis elicited by a mental status examination (see Chapter 10) and a history that documents the prodromal phase.

DIFFERENTIAL DIAGNOSIS

Any kind of psychotic state may resemble acute schizophrenia. However, differences in symptomatology permit differentiation and diagnosis. *Organic mental disorders* (see Chapter 17) are marked by disturbances in consciousness (delirium), by disorientation with respect to time, place, and person, and by impairment in intellectual functions (memory, calculations, etc.). In addition, especially in persons under 50, there is usually evidence from the history, physical examination, and laboratory tests of specific organic findings that are etiologically related to the mental condition. *Single psychotic symptoms*, such as persecutory delusions and auditory hallucinations, may occur de novo in elderly patients either as symptoms of dementia or paraphrenia (see Chapter 17). *Illicit drugs*, especially amphetamine and phencyclidine (see Chapter 22), may mimic the acute phase of schizophrenia. In addition, a number of *prescription drugs*

Table 16.1.
Diagnostic Criteria for Schizophrenia[a]

A. Presence of characteristic psychotic symptoms in the active phase: either (1), (2), or (3) for at least 1 week (unless the symptoms are successfully treated):
   (1) Two of the following:
       (a) Delusions
       (b) Prominent hallucinations (throughout the day for several days or several times a week for several weeks, each hallucinatory experience not being limited to a few brief moments)
       (c) Incoherence or marked loosening of associations
       (d) Catatonic behavior
       (e) Flat or grossly inappropriate affect
   (2) Bizarre delusions (i.e., involving a phenomenon that the person's culture would regard as totally implausible, e.g., thought broadcasting, being controlled by a dead person)
   (3) Prominent hallucinations [as defined in (1) (b) above] of a voice with content having no apparent relation to depression or elation, or a voice keeping up a running commentary on the person's behavior or thoughts, or two or more voices conversing with each other
B. During the course of the disturbance, functioning in such areas as work, social relations, and self-care is markedly below the highest level achieved before onset of the disturbance (or, when the onset is in childhood or adolescence, failure to achieve expected level of social development).
C. Schizoaffective Disorder and Mood Disorder with Psychotic Features have been ruled out, i.e., if a Major Depressive or Manic Syndrome has ever been present during an active phase of the disturbance, the total duration of all episodes of a mood syndrome has been brief relative to the total duration of the active and residual phases of the disturbance.
D. Continuous signs of the disturbance for at least 6 months. The 6-month period must include an active phase (of at least 1 week, or less if symptoms have been successfully treated) during which there were psychotic symptoms characteristic of Schizophrenia (symptoms in A), with or without a prodromal or residual phase, as defined below.
Prodromal phase: A clear deterioration in functioning before the active phase of the disturbance that is not due to a disturbance in mood or to a Psychoactive Substance Use Disorder and that involves at least two of the symptoms listed below.
Residual phase: Following the active phase of the disturbance, persistence of at least two of the symptoms noted below, these not being due to a disturbance in mood or to a psychoactive Substance Use Disorder.
Prodromal or Residual Symptoms:
(1) Marked social isolation or withdrawal.
(2) Marked impairment in role functioning as wage earner, student, or homemaker
(3) Markedly peculiar behavior (e.g., collecting garbage, talking to self in public, hoarding food)
(4) Marked impairment in personal hygiene and grooming
(5) Blunted or inappropriate affect
(6) Digressive, vague, overelaborate, or circumstantial speech, or poverty of speech, or poverty of content of speech
(7) Odd beliefs or magical thinking, influencing behavior and inconsistent with cultural norms, e.g., superstitiousness, belief in clairvoyance, telepathy, "sixth sense," "others can feel my feelings," overvalued ideas, ideas of reference
(8) Unusual perceptual experiences, e.g., recurrent illusions, sensing the presence of a force or person not actually present
(9) Marked lack of initiative, interest, or energy
Examples: Six months of prodromal symptoms with 1 week of symptoms from A; no prodromal symptoms with 6 months of symptoms from A; no prodromal symptoms with 1 week of symptoms from A and 6 months of residual symptoms.
E. It cannot be established that an organic factor initiated and maintained the disturbance.
F. If there is a history of Autistic Disorder, the additional diagnosis of Schizophrenia is made only if prominent delusions or hallucinations are also present.

[a]From American Psychiatric Association: *Diagnostic and Statistical Manual of Mental Disorders*, 3rd ed, revised. Washington, DC, American Psychiatric Association, 1987.

may occasionally produce hallucinations and other manifestations suggesting psychosis (see Table 16.2). History of drug usage and absence of the prodromal phase help to differentiate these conditions from schizophrenia.

The psychotic symptoms of *major affective episodes* (both mania and depression, see Chapter 15) can also be similar to those seen during acute episodes in the course of schizophrenia. Affective disorders differ from schizophrenia in that psychotic symptoms (delusions, hallucinations, etc.) appear after the development of the affective disturbance (depression or mania). In schizophrenia, marked depression or mania may appear, but the affective disturbance occurs after the onset of the psychotic symptoms. These principles of differential diagnosis are far from perfect, and patients with both types of disorder have been mislabeled. Because of the often poor prognosis associated with schizophrenia, mislabeling is not without significant consequence in terms of the physician's attitudes toward the patient and the actual treatment provided.

There are several *other functional psychotic conditions* that have symptoms similar to the acute psychotic phase of schizophrenia. However, these psychoses do not include a prodromal phase of withdrawal and deterioration, and patients return to their baseline level of function after recovery from the psychotic episode and do not experience progressive deterioration of function or recurrence of psychotic episodes.

TREATMENT AND PROGNOSIS

Neuroleptic Antipsychotic Drugs

The primary treatment of the acute and chronic psychotic manifestations of schizophrenia in ambulatory or hospitalized patients is with the "neuroleptic" antipsychotic agents (agents that may produce unwanted symptoms that resemble neurological disease). There are several classes of neuroleptics, with numerous drugs in each class. The common drugs are listed in Table 16.3, together with available strengths and potency equivalents to chlorpromazine.

Although the structures of the various antipsychotics are well known, the pharmacology is not. Dose-response relationships have not yet been worked out for humans. The drugs produce effects within 1 hour after oral administration and within 10 to 15 minutes after intramuscular injection. They are lipid soluble with a high affinity for cell membranes. The drugs and their metabolites are distributed generally throughout the central nervous system with no local or regional accumulation. Metabolites are partially excreted each day with significant portions retained in lipid-rich tissues and connective tissues. As these tissues become saturated, the drugs undergo slow turnover. The drugs are detoxified and inactivated mainly through oxidation by hepatic microsomal enzymes, and they are excreted through both the bile and the urine.

There is no evidence that these agents are addicting,

Table 16.2.
Prescription Drugs That Have Been Reported Occasionally to Cause Hallucinations or Other Manifestations of Psychosis[a]

Acyclovir (Zovirax)
Albuterol (Proventil; Ventolin)
Amiodarone (Cordarone)
Amantadine (Symmetrel)
Amphetamine-like drugs
Anabolic steroids
Anticonvulsants
Antidepressants, tricyclic
Antihistamines
Atropine and anticholinergics
Baclofen (Lioresal)
Benzodiazepines
Beta-adrenergic blockers
Bromocriptine (Parlodel)
Bupropion (Wellbutrin)
Captopril (Capoten)
Chloroquine (Aralen)
Clonidine (Catapres)
Cocaine
Corticosteroids (prednisone, cortisone, ACTH, others)
Cyclobenzaprine (Flexeril)
Cyclosporine (Sandimmune)
Deet (Off)
Digitalis glycosides
Disopyramide (Norpace)
Disulfiram (Antabuse)
Ethchlorvynol (Placidyl)
Fluoxetine (Prozac)
Histamine H_2-receptor antagonists
Isoniazid (INH, others)
Levodopa (Dopar, others)
Methyldopa (Aldomet)
Methylphenidate (Ritalin)
Nalidixic acid (NegGram)
Narcotics
Pantazocine (Talwin)
Nonsteroidal anti-inflammatory drugs
Pergolide (Permax)
Phenelzine (Nardil)
Phenylephrine (Neo-Synephrine)
Prazosin (Minipress)
Procainamide (Pronestyl)
Procaine Penicillin G
Quinacrine (Atabrine)
Quinidine
Salicylates
Thyroid hormones
Trazodone (Desyrel)
Zidovudine (Retrovir)

[a]Adapted from Drugs that cause psychiatric symptoms. Med Lett 31:113, 1989.

although tolerance to some of the side effects (sedation, hypotension, anticholinergic effects, and parkinsonian symptoms) has been reported. The drugs are relatively safe; massive amounts must be taken acutely to produce symptoms of stupor or coma.

The mechanisms of action of the antipsychotics are not fully understood. Although it has been speculated that specific antipsychotic activity may be due to the dopamine-antagonist action of these agents, the drugs have a variety of effects on many metabolic processes.

Treatment of Acute Psychotic Episodes

All of the neuroleptic antipsychotics are equally efficacious for controlling psychotic symptoms associ-

Table 16.3.
Available Strengths and Equivalent Doses of Commonly Used Neuroleptic Antipsychotic Agents[a]

Generic Name	Trade Name	Available Strengths of Oral Preparations	Approximate Equivalent Dose
		mg	*mg*
Phenothiazines			
Aliphatic			
Chlorpromazine	Thorazine (also generic)	10, 25, 50, 100, 200	100
Triflupromazine	Vesprin	10, 25	30
Piperidines			
Mesoridazine	Serentil	10, 25, 100	50
Piperacetazine	Quide	10, 15	12
Thioridazine	Mellaril	10, 15, 25, 50, 100, 150, 200	95
Piperazines			
Fluphenazine[b]	Prolixin, Permitil	1, 2.5, 5, 10	2
Perphenazine	Trilafon	2, 4, 8, 16	10
Trifluoperazine	Stelazine	1, 2, 5, 10	5
Thioxanthenes			
Aliphatic			
Chloroprothixene	Taractan	10, 25, 50, 100	65
Piperazine			
Thiothixene	Navane	1, 2, 5, 10, 25	5
Dibenzazepine			
Loxapine	Loxitane, Daxolin	10, 25, 50	15
Butyrophenone			
Haloperidol[c]	Haldol	0.5, 1, 2, 5, 10	2
Indolone			
Molindone	Moban	5, 10, 25	10

[a] Adapted from Baldessarini RJ: The neuroleptic antipsychotic drugs. *Postgrad Med 65*:108, 1979.
[b] Long acting fluphenazine decanoate or enanthate, for injection once weekly, comes in a concentration of 25 mg/ml.
[c] Haloperidol for injection comes in a concentration of 2 mg/ml.

ated with schizophrenia. The choice of one drug over another depends upon predicted differences in side effects, history of a particular patient's response, and the clinician's familiarity with the agent. The treatment of acute psychotic episodes should begin with the equivalent of 300 to 400 mg of chlorpromazine (Thorazine) a day, in divided doses (usually three times daily). Only one antipsychotic should be given at a time because administration of more than one agent increases the probability of side effects.

Combativeness, hyperactivity, and agitation are usually controlled within 24 to 48 hours after beginning treatment. If these symptoms are not modified within that period of time, the dosage should be increased 100 to 200 mg a day, up to the equivalent of 800 to 1000 mg of chlorpromazine. It may be necessary to administer the drugs intramuscularly during the acute phase of agitation if the patient is unable to take oral medication. The butyrophenone, haloperidol (Haldol), 2 to 5 mg, is a good choice for intramuscular injection because of its minimal effects upon circulatory regulation; an equivalent intramuscular dose of chlorpromazine (25 mg) can also be used, but the likelihood of orthostatic hypotension (occasionally leading to syncope) is greater.

Delusions, hallucinations, associational defects, negativism, and withdrawal begin to subside within 1 to 2 weeks after treatment begins. Continued improvement of these symptoms may take place over an additional 4- to 8-week period. If very high doses of antipsychotic agents were initially required, the dosage should be reduced to the equivalent of 400 to 600 mg of chlorpromazine as soon as possible. This ad-

justment in dosage can usually be made 1 to 2 weeks after reaching the peak dose.

Early Side Effects

Antipsychotic drugs with lower potency per milligram, such as chlorpromazine (see Table 16.3), produce *sedation*, which may be a useful side effect in treating hyperactive or combative patients but a disadvantage in regressed, withdrawn patients. The *anticholinergic* property of all phenothiazines produces annoying symptoms of dry mouth, stuffy nose, blurred vision, and occasional urinary retention in older patients and (with high doses) delirium. These side effects often abate or disappear within 2 to 4 weeks. The most worrisome side effect is *drug-induced Parkinson's syndrome*. It occurs with greatest frequency in association with drugs of higher potency per milligram, such as haloperidol, the piperazine class of phenothiazines, thioxanthene, loxapine, and molindone (see Table 16.3). The syndrome usually appears within 5 to 30 days of the beginning of treatment and includes tremor, rigidity, bradykinesia, fixed facies, drooling, and stooped posture. Because this problem commonly causes patients to discontinue antipsychotic treatment, it should be managed properly (7). Management consists of: (a) reduction of dosage, if possible; (b) change to another drug; or (c) antiparkinsonism medication (for details, see Chapter 82). In most cases reduction of dosage and/or addition of small amounts of an antiparkinsonism agent will control these side effects. The parkinsonian effects of neuroleptic drugs tend to decrease after 1 or 2 months. Therefore withdrawal of antiparkinsonism drugs should be attempted after 6 to 12 weeks. Prophylactic treatment of all patients with antiparkinsonism drugs is generally not a good idea because of the additional anticholinergic effects of these drugs.

Acute dystonias occur in occasional patients, within 1 to 5 days of initiating any neuroleptic; they are most frequently seen with haloperidol and the piperazine class of phenothiazines. The symptoms are the sudden onset of severe, tonic contractions of the musculature of the neck (torticollis), of the neck, back, and heels (opisthotonos), of extraocular muscles (oculogyric crises) of the mouth, and of the tongue. These symptoms remit promptly after parenteral injection of either diphenhydramine (Benadryl, 25 to 50 mg intramuscularly) or benztropine (Cogentin, 2 mg intravenously). Neuroleptic treatment can be continued in these patients; an antiparkinsonism agent should be added for about 1 month to protect against recurrent dystonia. *Akathisia* may also occur early in treatment. This side effect is marked by motor restlessness with pacing, fidgeting, and "restless legs." Treatment is the same as that prescribed for drug-induced parkinsonism. Diazepam (Valium), 5 mg two or three times daily, may also help to control this side effect.

A number of non-neurological side effects can result from administration of the antipsychotics. *Cardiovascular toxicity* is usually limited to orthostatic hypotension; this problem is most commonly seen with the aliphatic and piperazine classes of phenothiazines and with chlorprothixene. Frank syncope may occur, rarely, after intramuscular administration of low potency antipsychotics. Ventricular tachycardia is a very rare side effect; there are no baseline characteristics that help one to recognize persons at risk for this problem. Reversible *cholestatic jaundice* may occur as an allergic response. *Agranulocytosis* is an exceedingly rare side effect.

The *neuroleptic malignant syndrome* is a rare, and occasionally lethal, idiosyncratic complication. It usually occurs at the onset of treatment, when the dose is increased, or when a second drug is introduced. Over 24 to 72 hours, the patient develops muscle rigidity and a high temperature (as high as 42°C). Patients with this syndrome should be hospitalized immediately, in an intensive care unit, since hypoventilation occur as a consequence of the rigidity of the patient's chest wall muscles.

Because older schizophrenics are more prone to the development of the common side effects, dose levels should be lower by the equivalent of 100 to 200 mg of chlorpromazine. The very high dose range described for treatment of combativeness and hyperactivity should be avoided in elderly patients.

Long-Term Drug Treatment of Schizophrenia

The responsibility for the long-term care of schizophrenics can be assumed by interested generalists.

Pharmacotherapy is the principal mode of long-term treatment. Many studies have shown that 60 to 70% of schizophrenics relapse within 1 year if they do not receive medication (3). Most patients require antipsychotics indefinitely, but all patients should be treated for at least 2 years after an acute episode.

The goal of long-term pharmacotherapy is to minimize psychotic symptoms with the lowest dose of antipsychotic possible. Moderate doses appear to be as effective as, and safer than, the larger doses that have been popular in the United States in recent years (1).

For most patients this dose is the equivalent of 100 to 200 mg of chlorpromazine daily. Patients on this dose often continue to have psychotic symptoms but do not seem to be disturbed by them (e.g., "I still hear the voices but they don't seem to bother me").

Some patients temporarily have difficulty maintaining a regular medication schedule because of psychotic disorganization, negativism, or fear of medication (7). Inability to comply with the medication regimen may signal the onset of an acute episode. With the first indication of a disruption in medication schedule, the patient should be evaluated, frequency of visits increased to at least once a week, and medication increased if warranted. If the patient remains unable to comply, a long acting intramuscular agent, fluphenazine (Prolixin), 1 to 2 ml once a week, should be used. The patient can be returned to an oral medication when symptom control is re-established. Long acting intramuscular agents are also useful for new patients for whom no information is available on compliance in aftercare or ambulatory programs.

Late Side Effects of Neuroleptic Antipsychotic Drugs

Side effects are rarely a problem for patients taking maintenance doses of antipsychotics. When an increase in medication is necessary, drug-induced *parkinsonism* may appear. Patients who experience symptoms of parkinsonism over a long period of time should try other antipsychotic medications until one is found that does not produce the side effect. As noted above, long-term use of antiparkinsonism medication is to be avoided if possible (see Chapter 82 for further discussion of drug-induced parkinsonism).

Tardive dyskinesia is an extrapyramidal syndrome that occurs in about 10 to 15% (only 3 to 5% according to some reports) of patients after prolonged (months to years) moderate- to high-dose antipsychotic chemotherapy. The incidence of this disorder increases with age (three times more common over the age of 40 years), and it is more common in women. The disorder has been reported in association with long-term treatment with anticonvulsants. Up to 25% of neuroleptic-treated patients who are evaluated for drug-induced tardive dyskinesia are found to have another disorder causing their dyskinesia. The syndrome consists of involuntary or semivoluntary movements of choreiform, tic-like nature, sometimes associated with a dystonic component that classically involves the tongue, facial, and neck muscles. Early manifestations include fine worm-like movements of the tongue at rest, facial tics, and jaw movements. Later symptoms are bucco-lingual-masticatory movements, chewing motions, lip smacking, puffing of cheeks, blinking of eyes, and choreoathetoid movements of the extremities. Younger patients often have significant involvement of the extremities and trunk. Although the syndrome is painless, it can be socially embarrassing and can interfere with the patient's ability to feed and care for himself. In general, the prognosis is poor, regardless of treatment, and symptoms last for years if not indefinitely. In an occasional patient, the symptoms slowly subside after several years.

There is no satisfactory treatment for tardive dyskinesia. Antiparkinsonism medications usually worsen the symptoms. One short-term effective treatment is the use of more potent antipsychotics to suppress the symptoms, but this usually requires increasing doses of the suppressing agent, and subsequent withdrawal of antipsychotics often leads to worsening of the symptoms for a period of time. The emphasis of treatment should be on prevention of tardive dyskinesia. At the first sign of the disorder, neuroleptics should be gradually lowered and discontinued if possible. Symptoms will gradually disappear over several months in about one-third of patients who can be taken off drugs early. Benzodiazepines, pure lecithin, lithium, and sodium valproate have been reported to be useful in a limited number of cases.

Overall Management of the Patient

The schizophrenic patient is sensitive to change or instability in any aspect of his life. Therefore one practitioner should provide continuity and consistency in his relationship with each of these patients so that the clinician becomes a predictable resource for assisting the patient to develop and maintain his social role in the community. Although few schizophrenics work full time ($\leq 20\%$), the clinician should refer patients for vocational rehabilitation (see Chapter 9) or sheltered workshops when requested. Most patients determine their own level of social activity, and it is fruitless to push them into unwanted activities. The clinician should be available to the patient's family or to foster care providers for periodic review of the patient's progress and expectations. The book *Surviving Schizophrenia* should be recommended to the patient's family (see "General References").

Recreational or social activities are enjoyed by some patients, but many do not care for them. Ideally, residential facilities are available when there is no family for the patient to live with or when the family is a harmful influence. However, in many communities such facilities do not exist. For some patients the clinician and the ambulatory center itself become the source of the few social contacts that the patient has outside his home and his inner psychological world.

Office visits should be scheduled on a regular basis, as frequently as once a month, or as infrequently as twice a year. Frequency of visits should be determined on the basis of the current status of the patient, history of the course of the patient's illness, reliability of the patient in taking medication, and the patient's ability to recognize early signs of onset of acute episodes. Office visits need last only 15 to 20 minutes and should include an interim history, a brief mental status examination, a review of the effectiveness of medications and of significant side effects, and provision of support or advice regarding the ways in which the patient is dealing with day-to-day matters. In other words these office visits may be defined as supportive therapy, which is described in Chapter 11.

In addition to individual office visits a family management approach may be useful for patients who are having difficulties with their families (2). The method involves a two-step process:

Step 1—sessions devoted to educating the patient and family about the nature, course, and treatment of schizophrenia.

Step 2—family sessions aimed at reducing existing family tensions and improving problem-solving skills of the family in coping with causes of stress. (See "Family Counseling" in Chapter 11).

Management is enhanced if the clinician has ready access to social services, emergency mental health services, and psychiatric day care and inpatient services. Social services, especially for financial support (welfare, food stamps, disability payments, etc.) are very important in the management of schizophrenics, because of the usual dependent status of these patients. (Many acute episodes of psychosis are precipitated by threatened or actual withdrawal of welfare and disability payments.)

The generalist caring for a schizophrenic patient may need psychiatric consultation for confirmation of initial diagnosis, for decisions regarding hospitalization, or for treatment recommendations when symptoms respond poorly to antipsychotics or when side effects are intolerable.

Prognosis of the Treated Patient

Schizophrenia is a lifelong disease requiring an open-ended commitment by the clinician. The patient's life is disrupted by periodic psychosis, sometimes necessitating hospitalization, and by an arrest or deterioration of social function. Some patients are able to work and maintain fair levels of interpersonal relationships. Many lead lonely, withdrawn, socially marginal existences. Psychopharmacological treatment is very effective for controlling the symptoms of acute psychosis and for suppressing the intensity of psychotic symptomatology over long periods of time. Suppression of psychosis may permit the patient to use his intellectual and social talents more effectively in developing and maintaining some role in the community; however, the antipsychotics have no direct effect on the deterioration of social function that is so characteristic of schizophrenia.

General References

American Psychiatric Association: *Diagnostic and Statistical Manual of Mental Disorders (Third edition-Revised), DSM-III-R*, Washington, DC, American Psychiatric Association, 1987.
> Recently updated diagnostic criteria and epidemiological information for all recognized psychiatric disorders.

Bleuler E: *Dementia Praecox or the Group of Schizophrenias*. New York, International Universities Press, 1950.
> A classical work on schizophrenia.

Drugs for psychiatric disorders. *Med Letter* 31:13, 1989.
> Concise information on actions and side effects of all currently-used antipsychotic drugs.

Torrey EF: *Surviving Schizophrenia: A Family Manual*.New York, Harper and Row, Publishers, 1983.
> A thorough book that contains invaluable information for families of schizophrenia patients and for generalist practitioners.

Tune LE, McHugh PR, Coyle JT: Management of extrapyramidal side effects induced by neuroleptics. *Johns Hopkins Med J* 148:149, 1981.
> Brief, helpful review of current information.

Specific References

1. Baldessarini RJ, Cohen BM, Teicher MH: Significance of neuroleptic dose and plasma level in the pharmacologic treatment of psychoses. *Arch Gen Psych* 45:79–91, 1988.
2. Falloon IR, Boyd JL, McGill CW, et al: Family management in the prevention of exacerbation of schizophrenia. *N Engl J Med* 306:1437, 1982.
3. Hogarty GE, Goldberg SC, Schooler NR, Ulrich RF: Drug and sociotherapy in the aftercare of schizophrenic patients: two year relapse rates. *Arch Gen Psychiatry* 31:603, 1974.
4. Lemkau PU, Tietze C, Cooper M: Survey of statistical studies on prevalence and incidence of mental disorder in sample population. *Public Health Rep* 58:1909, 1943.
5. Regier DA, Boyd JH, Burke JD, et al: One-month prevalence of mental disorders in the United States. *Arch Gen Psych* 45:977, 1988.
6. Snyder SH: The dopamine hypothesis of schizophrenia: focus on the dopamine receptor. *Am J Psychiatry* 133:197, 1976.
7. Van Putten T: Why do schizophrenic patients refuse to take their drugs? *Arch Gen Psychiatry* 31:67, 1974.
8. Varsamis J, Adamson JD: Early schizophrenia. *Can Psychiatr Assoc J* 16:487, 1971.

C H A P T E R 17

Mental Illness in the Elderly: Principles and Common Problems (Depression, Dementia, Delirium, Psychosis*)

PETER V. RABINS, M.D.
DEAN J. STORER, M.D.

A recent study of over 20,000 Americans found that the elderly are the group least likely to seek help for mental illness. It also demonstrated that the treatment of an elderly patient with mental health problems is most likely to be provided by a primary care provider during a routine medical visit (3).

GENERAL PRINCIPLES

Importance of Diagnosis

Making a correct diagnosis is a crucial first step in determining proper treatment. The most common mistakes made in assessing psychiatric symptoms in older persons are ascribing them to normal aging, confusing symptoms with syndromes and not appreciating the frequent interaction between physical and psychiatric disorders. A significant factor in the recognition of a mental illness is the suspicion that it might be present, that is, including a psychiatric disorder in the differential diagnosis. Asking the appropriate questions and attempting to elicit the classic signs and symptoms should lead to the correct diagnosis even when the presentation is unusual.

---

*John Breitner, M.D., contributed to this chapter in the first and second editions.

Relationship between Physical and Mental States

Physical and psychiatric illnesses commonly co-exist in the elderly. A prudent strategy when facing a patient with both physical and psychiatric complaints is to establish a differential diagnosis for each symptom before assuming that either the physical or the psychiatric disorder is primary. The two types of symptoms may be related in a number of ways:

1. *Mental distress complicating a primary physical illness.* Demoralization, anxiety, grief, irritability, and frustration are especially common in older patients with significant physical illness. These feelings usually begin after the onset of the physical illness, vary over time, and respond to the techniques for psychotherapy described in Chapter 11.
2. *Physical complaints as the primary manifestation of psychiatric disorder.* Particularly in older persons, focused complaints of physical ill health may be the most prominent or only sign of mental illness, especially depression. Although the physical complaint must be appropriately evaluated, a psychiatric etiology should be suspected when the somatic complaint is bizarre, seems to be exaggerated, or has been previously but unsuccessfully evaluated, or when the patient has some symptoms of depression.
3. *Psychiatric disorders arising from specific diseases.* Cancer of the pancreas, hypothyroidism, and several structural brain diseases (stroke, Parkinson's disease, dementia) are commonly accompanied by a depression. Because the rates of depression are higher in these disorders than in arthritic or orthopedic conditions with similar levels of impairment, it is likely that the medical disorder is the cause of the depression or that the medical and psychiatric disorders share a common etiology. These depressions respond well to antidepressant treatment.
4. *Psychiatric syndromes caused by medication and substance abuse.* Psychiatric syndromes can also be precipitated by a variety of medications and by alcohol abuse. Corticosteroids, beta-blockers and other drugs that affect the adrenergic system can induce depressive symptoms. Anticholinergic compounds, dopaminergic agonist compounds, benzodiazepines, and H2 blockers can induce delirium. Patients with dementia are more vulnerable to developing cognitive side effects from these compounds than are cognitively normal elderly. Alcoholism, often hard to recognize in elderly patients, can also cause symptoms of depression and anxiety or cognitive defects (see Chapter 21). Abstinence can lead to resolution of the psychiatric symptoms.

Importance of Psychosocial Factors

Psychosocial factors are important to consider in patients of all ages. They become particularly important in the elderly because reduced physical mobility, isolation from family and friends, and financial limitations are more common and can directly interfere with the treatment of medical and psychiatric disorders. For elderly patients with mental illness, referring the patient to a social service agency or enlisting the help of the patient's family may be especially important in assuring successful treatment and follow-through.

Importance of Cognitive Assessment

Because dementia and delirium are common disorders of the elderly, it is important to be familiar with the assessment of cognitive function. The Mini Mental Status Examination delineated in Table 17.1 is reliable, brief, and standardized.

SPECIFIC PSYCHOGERIATRIC DISORDERS

Psychiatric disorders in older patients may present with the classic symptoms described in other chapters of this book. The following pages focus upon several syndromes that are particularly important in the elderly.

Depression

Depressive Symptoms

Symptoms of depression and sadness become more common in late life even though the syndrome of major depression is less common in the elderly. This dissociation may be due both to the criteria used to make diagnoses and to intrinsic differences between the young and old. The *Diagnostic and Statistical Manual of Mental Disorders, Third Edition Revised (DSM-III-R)* divides mood disorder into several categories (see Chapter 15). The differences among them depend both on symptom clustering and on course. There are a number of ways in which the presentation of these disorders in older persons may differ from the presentation in younger persons.

An *adjustment disorder with depressed mood* is characterized by sad or low mood present for more than 2 weeks but less than 6 months. It should follow, within 3 months, a clearly identifiable stressor or precipitant. In elderly persons, stressors such as those listed above ("Importance of Psychosocial Factors") are particularly common. The approaches to office psychotherapy described in Chapter 11 are fully applicable to elderly patients with adjustment disorders.

A *dysthymic disorder,* conversely, is characterized by the presence of depressive symptoms for more than 2 years. Mood often fluctuates widely but in no discernible pattern. The patient may experience hours, days or weeks of improved mood, mixed with prolonged periods of unhappiness. In the elderly, a dysthymic disorder should be considered when the patient reports chronic depressive symptoms throughout their life and denies the cyclicity and periods of normal mood found in recurrent depressive or bipolar disorder (see Chapter 15). It may require specialty referral because of its chronicity.

Table 17.1.
Mini-Mental Status Examination: Instructions for Administration and Scoring[a]

The test takes 5 to 10 minutes to administer.

ORIENTATION

1. Ask for year, season, date, day, month. Then ask specifically for parts omitted. One point for each correct. (0–5)
2. Ask in turn for name of state, county, town, hospital or place, floor or street. One point for each correct. (0–5)

REGISTRATION

Ask the patient if you may test his memory. Then say the names of three unrelated objects, clearly and slowly, about 1 second for each. After you have said all three, ask him to repeat them. This first repetition determines his score (0–3) but keep saying them until he can repeat all three up to six trials. If he does not eventually learn all three, recall cannot be meaningfully tested.

ATTENTION AND CALCULATION

Ask the patient to begin with 100 and count backward by 7. Stop after five subtractions (93, 86, 79, 72, 65). Score total number of correct answers, one point for each. (0–5)

If the patient cannot or will not perform this task, ask him to spell the word "world" backward. The score is the number of letters in correct order, e.g., dlrow = 5, dlrwo = 3. (0–5)

RECALL

Ask the patient if he can recall the three words you previously asked him to remember. Score 0–3.

LANGUAGE

Naming: Show the patient a wrist watch and ask him what it is. Repeat for pencil. Score 0–2.

Repetition: Ask the patient to repeat this phrase after you: "No ifs, ands, or buts." Allow only one trial. Score 0 or 1.

Three-stage command: "Take a piece of paper in your right hand, fold it in half, and put it on the floor." Give the patient a piece of blank paper and repeat the command. Score 1 point for each part correctly executed. (0–3).

Reading: On a blank piece of paper print the sentence "Close your eyes," in letters large enough for the patient to see clearly. Ask him to read it and do what it says. Score 1 point only if he actualy closes his eyes. (0–1)

Writing: Give the patient a blank piece of paper and ask him to write a sentence for you. Do not dictate a sentence; it is to be written spontaneously. It must contain a subject and verb and be sensible. Correct grammer and punctuation are not necessary. (0–1)

Copying: On a clean piece of paper, draw intersecting pentagons, each side about 1 inch, and ask him to copy it exactly as it is. All 10 angles must be present and 2 must intersect to score 1 point. Tremor and rotation are ignored. (0–1)

Estimate the patient's level of sensorium along a continuum, from alert on the left to coma on the right.

[a] From Folstein MF, Folstein SE, McHugh PR: "Mini-mental state": a practical method for grading the cognitive state of patients for the clinician. *J Psychiatr Res* 12:189, 1975. Total possible score is 30 points. Patients with totals of 20 points or less usually have either dementia, delirium, schizophrenia, or a major affective disorder (pseudodementia).

The diagnostic criteria of the *major affective disorders* and their treatment as described in Chapter 15 are generally applicable to the elderly. Hypochondriacal features, agitation, and suspiciousness or frank paranoia, however, often accompany depression in the elderly and are common sources of diagnostic confusion.

Elderly individuals with a hypochondriacal focus usually deny that their mood is sad but will focus on physical symptoms for which there is minimal or no evidence of abnormality on physical examination or on laboratory assessment. Depressed hypochondriacal patients often have changes in their vital sense ("something is wrong with me") and a negative self-attitude ("I've done something to deserve this or cause this"). Therefore, it is important to ask specifically about these cardinal features of major depression when hypochondriasis is present.

Because suspiciousness and paranoia are common in depressed elderly patients, it is important to seek other evidence for a major depression when these symptoms are present. When paranoia and depression coexist, depression is most commonly the primary disorder.

As in younger individuals, major depression in the elderly requires pharmacotherapy or electroconvulsive therapy (ECT). Practical details about these modes of treatment are found in Chapter 15. It is important to avoid tricyclic antidepressants with the most pronounced anticholinergic properties (e.g., amitriptyline and doxepin). Those tricyclics with the highest likelihood of causing orthostatic hypotension (e.g., amitriptyline and imipramine) should also be avoided, since elderly patients are at higher risk of falls and are more likely to be receiving antihypertensive drugs or other compounds that also can cause orthostasis. Nortriptyline and desipramine are the tricyclic agents that are less likely to cause these side effects. A usual starting dose in the elderly is 25 milligrams at bedtime; however, a dose of 10 milligrams should be prescribed in the frail elderly or in individuals with potential medical complications from the drugs. Fluoxetine (Prozac), a nontricyclic antidepressant, has minimal anticholinergic activity, but it has been only recently introduced, and studies of its use in elderly patients are limited. Its long half life suggests that it should be used in lower dosages in the elderly than in young patients. ECT is sometimes safer than pharmacotherapy for older persons with cardiac disease. It is equally effective in all age groups (see details regarding ECT, Chapter 15, Affective Disorders). Low-dose neuroleptic drugs (see Table 16.3) are indicated when paranoid delusions complicate depression, especially when the suspiciousness is significantly interfering with the patient's function or is life threatening (for example, the patient will not eat because he believes that the food is poisoned) or when it causes distress for the patient or those close to him.

Dementia Syndrome of Depression

Depression in late life can present with a patient believing that he is becoming demented and also with poor performance on routine tests of cognitive function. Previously this condition was called "pseudodementia," but this term has fallen into disfavor because patients with this syndrome perform in the demented range in standardized tests of cognitive function. Furthermore, up to 50% of these patients eventually develop a progressive dementing illness (9). Nonetheless, recognition of the syndrome is important since both the mood disorder and cognitive function can improve with antidepressant treatment. The dementia syndrome of depression should be considered when the onset of cognitive impairment has been subacute (less than 6 months and particularly less than 3 months); when the history of an episode of depression earlier in life is elicited, when a dementia is complicated by hypochondriacal or bizarre delusions (10); when the patient constantly emphasizes his cognitive disability (a behavior that is uncommon in Alzheimer's disease); or when a cognitively impaired patient acknowledges having early morning awakening, lack of energy, self-blame or guilt. At times it is difficult to distinguish whether the patient is suffering from a primary dementing illness with secondary depression or primary depression with reversible dementia. In such cases a therapeutic trial of an antidepressant (e.g., at least four weeks at a therapeutic dose, as described in Chapter 15) may be the best way to determine which disorder is primary.

Depression Coexisting with Brain Disease

Major depression may complicate primarily "organic" disorders of the central nervous system. Stroke, Parkinson's disease, and Alzheimer's disease are three common late life disorders in which major depressive symptoms occur in 20 to 50% of patients. The importance of recognizing these as coexisting disorders is that the physical disorder and the psychiatric disorder may both need to be treated if either problem is to improve. For example, depression has been shown to directly interfere with rehabilitation from stroke (11). Thus, the treatment of depression in stroke patients improves the likelihood of recovery from the stroke; at the same time, gains from rehabilitation improve the stroke patient's morale and mood (see details, Chapter 83.) In Parkinson's disease, depressive symptoms and parkinsonian symptoms (e.g., psychomotor retardation) often overlap, and it can be difficult to determine which disorder is causing specific symptoms. In planning treatment, it is best to focus on the depressive or parkinsonian symptoms separately and to treat first the disorder that is causing the worst impairment in function. The treatment of Parkinson's disease is discussed in Chapter 82. The treatment of depression in patients with Alzheimer's disease or multi-infarct dementia can improve cognitive performance, behavior, and mood although some cognitive impairment will persist.

Age-Associated Memory Impairment

Some older patients complain of memory loss, or members of their families notice a problem, but a history from both the patient and family reveals no social or occupational dysfunction and screening cognitive tests reveal no abnormality. It appears that fewer than 20% of these individuals develop a dementia (1). Those unlikely to have a dementia complain of such things as misplacing keys or having more difficulty remembering names or words than they once did; on questioning they acknowledge that names and words often

come to them minutes later and that they have not forgotten important engagements or events. Patients who complain of memory difficulties and report a decline in function in social, personal, or occupational realms should be referred to a neuropsychologist for better formulation of the problem. Careful attention should be given to the medical status of such individuals since they could be suffering from a subclinical delirium (see below). When no dysfunction is identified and objective testing makes a progressive dementia unlikely, reassurance and an agreement to reassess the patient in 6 months may help to relieve the anxiety associated with this condition.

Paranoia and Suspiciousness

Suspiciousness is more common among the elderly than in younger individuals. This becomes clinically relevant when the suspiciousness interferes with the patient's life. Several types of disorder can present with suspiciousness.

Suspiciousness as an Isolated Symptom

Some elderly individuals become more suspicious as they age but have no accompanying signs or symptoms of other mental illness. It is important to determine whether there is a basis for the patient's suspiciousness, since financial abuse of the elderly is not uncommon and concerns about the environment being unsafe can be appropriate. An understandable reaction to difficult circumstances should not be assumed, however, and a review of symptoms that explore other psychiatric conditions is necessary.

Suspiciousness Complicating Depression

As noted above, suspiciousness occurs in some elderly patients with major depression. Depression should be considered primary if the person feels deserving of persecution or punishment or has changes in vital sense and other manifestations of depression (Chapter 15).

Late Life Schizophrenia or Paraphrenia

Older individuals occasionally develop a syndrome similar to schizophrenia in young people (see Chapter 16). Such patients have delusions (fixed, false, idiosyncratic ideas) or auditory hallucinations, and they lack symptoms of depression or cognitive impairment.

The treatment of late life schizophrenia and paranoia is similar to that of younger individuals (Chapter 16) except that significantly lower doses of neuroleptic drugs are used. Although no single neuroleptic is more efficacious than another, those with high anticholinergic effects such as thioridazine (Mellaril) should be avoided, especially if the patient is taking an antidepressant that also has anticholinergic properties. A starting dose of 1 to 3 mg of haloperidol (Haldol) two to three times daily or trifluoperazine (Stelazine) is recommended. Because old age is a risk factor for developing tardive dyskinesia, it is important to attempt to discontinue neuroleptic treatment after the patient has stabilized. Chapter 16 describes the use of neuroleptic drugs in detail.

Paranoia and Persecutory Delusions as Symptoms of an "Organic" Disease

Paranoia can be symptomatic of a focal brain disease (e.g., *tumor or stroke*), a diffuse brain disease such as Alzheimer's disease (8), a systemic condition such as a metabolic disorder (e.g., hyperthyroidism or hypoparathyroidism), or psychoactive substance abuse. Any patient presenting with a persistent suspicious belief should have a full assessment to rule out these etiologies.

Dementia

Definition and Epidemiology

Dementia is characterized by (*a*) a decline in cognitive abilities from a previous level; (*b*) a decline that is generalized or global and not isolated to one cognitive function such as memory (i.e., amnesia) or language (i.e., aphasia); and (*c*) the presence of clear consciousness. Dementia can have many etiologies, but only 2 to 5% of affected patients have dementia due to a treatable etiology.

Moderate to severe dementia affects about 5% of individuals over 65. Most dementia occurs, however, among the very old: the prevalence is 20% in persons 80 and older, and approximately 30% in persons over 90. These prevalence rates have been found in numerous European, North American, and Japanese prevalence studies (2).

Etiological Evaluation

The assessment of a person presenting with complaints of cognitive decline has two purposes. The first purpose is to identify the probable etiology of the dementia, including the identification of individuals who might suffer from a treatable disorder. The major causes and the approximate percentage distribution of the causes are listed in Table 17.2. The three most common causes of treatable dementia are medication toxicity, depression, and thyroid disease. Commonly used

Table 17.2.
Major Causes and Approximate Frequency Distribution of Progressive Dementias[a]

1. Senile dementia, Alzheimer type	50%
2. Multiinfarct (arteriosclerotic or other vascular cause)	20%
3. Combination of 1 and 2	
4. Communicating hydrocephalus	5%
5. Alcoholic-posttraumatic	5%
6. Huntington's	5%
7. Intracranial mass lesions	5%
8. Uncommon or mixed with above:	10%
Chronic drug use; Creutzfeldt-Jakob; metabolic (thyroid, liver, nutritional); degenerative (spinocerebellar, amyotrophic lateral sclerosis, parkinsonism, multiple sclerosis, Pick's, Wilson's, epilepsy); static dementia	

[a]From Plum F. In: *Cecil Textbook of Medicine*, Wyngaarden JB, Smith Jr, LH (eds), 18th ed, Philadelphia, WB Saunders Co, 1988.

medications that have been found to be associated with global cognitive impairment are the benzodiazepines (most common), methyldopa, neuroleptics, and cimetidine (5). The second purpose of asessment is to identify treatable comorbidity in the patient or family. Because fewer than 5% of patients have a truly reversible dementia, the treatment of medical and behavioral comorbidity is the main focus of both the assessment and the treatment of almost all individuals who present in the ambulatory setting.

The first step in the etiological evaluation of dementia is to search for reversible causes, beginning with the history, physical examination, mental status examination (Table 17.1), and a number of screening tests. The NIA Consensus Conference on the differential diagnosis of dementia suggested the following screening tests for all patients: CBC, serum electrolytes, creatinine, liver function tests, calcium and phosphate concentrations, thyroid function (T4), B12 level and serological tests for syphilis (7). While CT head scanning is listed as optional, most physicians in the United States regard it as a necessary part of the assessment. It is important to emphasize that a CT scan can identify focal lesions such as a tumor, subdural hematoma, or abscess; demonstrate findings compatible with hydrocephalus; or provide confirmatory evidence for vascular etiology of the dementia; but that it is not possible to diagnose Alzheimer's disease from the scan. In the elderly, a magnetic resonance imaging (MRI) scan is not recommended unless there is a high likelihood of a focal lesion such as a tumor (e.g., in a demented patient with recent onset of new focal symptoms).

The second step in the assessment process is to determine whether the dementia is a subcortical or cortical dementia. Most reversible dementias present as subcortical dementias. *Subcortical dementias* are characterized by memory loss, apathy, slowness, and movement disorder with intact language [the patient is able to name objects, repeat a phrase, and follow the 3-step command see (Table 17.1)] and visuospatial function (i.e., the patient is able to copy the diagram on the Mini Mental Status Examination). The common causes of subcortical dementia include Parkinson's disease, multiple sclerosis, Huntington's disease, normal pressure hydrocephalus, the dementia syndrome of depression, and most instances of multi-infarct dementia. The *cortical dementias* are also characterized by memory loss, but impairments in language [making paraphasic errors such as substituting a letter (e.g., "tee" instead of "tie") or saying an incorrect word ("paper" instead of "pencil")], apraxia (inability to perform skilled movements such as showing how to drink with a cup on command) and agnosia (inability to recognize common objects or sensory stimuli) are also present. Alzheimer's disease is the most common cortical dementia, but Pick's disease and rare dementias such as Creutzfeldt-Jakob disease are included in this category.

Alzheimer's disease is diagnosed by inclusion and exclusion criteria. The diagnosis should be made when other specific causes of dementia, including vascular disease, have been excluded, when the condition has been slowly progressive, and when the cognitive disorder includes language impairment, apraxia, or agnosia.

Multi-infarct dementia should be diagnosed when the history suggests distinct episodes of worsening (a so-called stair-step course), when evidence of vascular disease and hypertension are present on examination, and when the neurological examination reveals asymmetries in reflexes, strength, or sensation. A score on the Hachinski scale (Table 17.3) of 7 or more suggests that a multi-infarct or vascular etiology is likely.

Management

The management of the irreversibly demented patient can be divided into six aspects:

1. *The assessment process.* This is the first step in management. The diagnosis has often been suspected by the family or patient, but at times abnormal behavior has been misinterpreted as purposefully irritating. As specific a diagnosis as possible should be made and conveyed to the family. The family may ask about long-term prognosis. The average patient with dementia lives 7 to 10 years after early symptoms, but life span while demented can be as long as 20 years. In general a dementia that has progressed slowly will continue to do so while a history of rapid progression predicts rapid decline. Although the patient has the right to know his diagnosis, many lack the ability to realize they have a deficit. Patients who, when asked, deny they have any problems with their memory usually do not accept that there is a problem when told directly.

The evaluation process should also elicit specific problems in behavior caused by the dementia (see commonly cited problems, Table 17.4). Difficulty in speaking, dressing, and in such potentially dangerous activities as driving, smoking, and cooking

Table 17.3.
Helsinki Ischemic Score
The summation of points produces an *Ischemic Score.* Scores of 4 or less indicate probably Alzheimer's disease and scores of 7 or more indicate multi-infarct dementia.[a]

Feature	Point Value
a) Abrupt Onset	2
b) Stepwise Deterioration	1
c) Fluctuating Course	2
d) Nocturnal Confusion	1
e) Relative Preservation of Personality	1
f) Depression	1
g) Somatic Complaints	1
h) Emotional Incontinence	1
i) History of Hypertension	1
j) History of Strokes	2
k) Evidence of Associated Atherosclerosis	1
l) Focal Neurological Symptoms	2
m) Focal Neurological Signs	1

[a]From Hachinski VC, Lassen NA, Marshall J: Multi-infarct dementia. *Lancet* 2:207, 1974.

Table 17.4.
Behavior Problems of Patients and Problematic Activities of Daily Living Cited by Families of Demented Patients[a]

Behavior	Percentage of Families Reporting Occurrence	Percentage of Families Reporting Behavior to Be a Problem
Memory disturbance[c]	100	93
Catastrophic reactions[b, c]	87	89
Demanding/critical behavior	71	73
Night waking	69	59
Hiding things	69	71
Communication difficulties	68	74
Suspiciousness[c]	63	79
Making accusations[c]	60	82
Meals	60	55
Daytime wandering	59	70
Bathing	53	74
Hallucinations	49	42
Delusions	47	83
Physical violence	47	94
Incontinence[c]	40	86
Cooking	33	44
Hitting[c]	32	81
Driving	20	73
Smoking	11	67
Inappropriate sexual behavior	2	0

[a]Based on an open-ended interview with the primary care-givers of 55 patients with irreversible dementia. Adapted from Rabins PV, Mace NL, Lucas MJ: The impact of dementia on the family. *JAMA* 248:333, 1982.
[b]See example in text.
[c]Cited as most serious problem.

should be inquired about. When present, these problems should be explained as the result of the illness. The family or other caregivers should then try to adapt the environment to the disordered behaviors and should take steps to eliminate dangerous behaviors. Helping the caregivers specifically to identify each problem can enable them to institute common sense solutions they have not otherwise tried. Families needing legal and financial advice should be advised to seek this out early and not wait for a crisis. Guidelines for assessing competence or for obtaining legal guardianship are described in Chapter 10.

2. *Good general medical care.* Congestive heart failure, urinary tract infection, and seemingly minor medical abnormalities can lead to marked deterioration of the demented patient's functioning. Likewise, patients taking drugs that can affect cognition (e.g., cimetidine, beta-blockers, clonidine, methyldopa, digoxin, anticholinergics) should be carefully monitored, and all unnecessary medication should be discontinued. A search for superimposed medical illness should be instituted if there is a sudden deterioration in behavior, cognition, or functional ability. Correction of coexisting medical conditions has been shown to improve functioning in demented patients (4).

3. *Behavioral management and treatment of depression.* Not sleeping at night, suspiciousness, easy irritability, and catastrophic reactions (see below) can be more problematic than cognitive impair-

ment. Nonpharmacological approaches should be tried first. For insomnia these might include keeping the person more active in the daytime (day care centers are a significant help in this regard) and not letting the patient nap during the day. Irritability, suspiciousness, and frustration are often best managed by eliminating tasks that the patient can no longer do or situations that frustrate the patient. When both irritability and sleep disorder are serious enough to necessitate drug treatment, haloperidol (Haldol), .5 mg, up to 2 mg, one hour before bedtime, on a regular basis, is often effective. Patients taking these drugs must be monitored for two common side effects—orthostatic hypotension and extrapyramidal symptoms (see details in Chapter 16). If only insomnia is a problem, chloral hydrate, 500 to 1000 mg, causes the least paradoxical agitation and daytime drowsiness. When daytime irritability is being treated, low doses of haloperidol two to three times daily should be tried. These drugs can worsen cognition and this should be watched for. Suspiciousness sometimes decreases with neuroleptic drugs, but pharmacological treatment should not be instituted for this symptom unless it is causing severe problems.

Depression is present in at least 20% of patients with dementia. When it has the characteristics of an adjustment disorder or demoralized state (see above), it is best managed with supportive therapy (see Chapter 11). However, major depressions with symptoms of early waking, anorexia, notions of guilt, self-blame, worthlessness, nihilistic attitudes, or morbid hypochondriasis also occur. Their treatment is discussed under "organic" depression above.

Demented patients with at least partial insight into their disability may become profoundly distressed when brought into a situation in which they are forced to confront their failing aptitudes. Often an overwhelming sense of frustration, fear, anger, or anxiety ensues. These poorly controlled emotions further impair the patient's already limited functional ability, leading to total decompensation of a previously coping individual.

Example: A 72-year-old woman with a history of several small strokes suffered from moderate forgetfulness and confusion but was generally calm and pleasant. Keeping track of the date with a calendar and making copious notes to herself, she managed to maintain an independent existence at home. At the supermarket check-out counter she could not find her wallet but insisted she had money to pay for her food. The clerk grew impatient, and the patient became increasingly agitated, tearful, and accusatory. When the store manager was called, she picked up grocery items and began throwing them.

These *catastrophic reactions* may have an extremely important impact on both the patient and the patient's family. The explanation of their cause and their prevention through avoidance of provoking circumstances can forestall the need for institutionalization. The use of small doses of the neuroleptic haloperidol (see above) may be beneficial in patients in whom episodes like this recur despite the caretaker's best efforts.

4. *Family support.* Family distress is common. Treating it starts with the assessment and problem-solving approach outlined above. The latter gives families a sense of control and the hope that most problems can be managed in spite of the irreversibility and probable progression of the underlying disorder. Feelings of guilt, anger, discouragement, and demoralization are common. Other common types of distress are concern about loss of friends, hobbies, and leisure time; family conflicts; and worry that the principal caregiver will become ill. Allowing families time to ventilate these feelings and concerns and acknowledging that they are common can be helpful. Participation in a support group for families of demented patients can be helpful. The Alzheimer's Disease and Related Disorder Association can provide information about nearby resources and has a free "800" phone number (1-800-621-0379). It is also helpful to recommend a book such as *The 36-Hour Day* (see "General References"), which explains dementia and provides practical advice for dealing with all of the vexing problems created by a demented family member.

5. *Longitudinal care.* Because the dementing illnesses are progressive (new symptoms appear while old symptoms worsen), expected changes should be described to families. Also it is prudent to discuss the possibility of eventual nursing home placement soon after the diagnosis is made. Although the majority of families report that they do not want to place their loved one in a nursing home, it is important to urge them not to promise this unconditionally since medical issues or behavioral problems may develop to the point where placement is necessary. The family's emotional needs may change over time. Here again, a nonjudgmental, listening approach helps family members feel supported.

6. *Decisions about limiting therapy.* Chapter 6, Geriatric Medicine, describes the processes whereby patients and their families may plan in advance the limitation of therapy (Living Wills and other forms of advance directives) and the delegation of decision making to others. These processes are especially important in planning the care of a demented patient, early in the patient's course of dementia.

Drugs for Dementia

No drug has been shown unequivocally to improve the cognitive impairment of dementia and thereby improve patients' functional abilities. Improvements in behavior have been reported with ergot alkaloids and in memory with cholinomimetic agents, but it is not yet established that quality of life is significantly affected. At present, drug therapy is indicated only for the management of the secondary behavioral symptoms listed in Table 17.4.

Delirium

Definition and Diagnosis

The hallmark of delirium is clouding of consciousness and inattentiveness, with secondary changes in behavior, cognition, or perception. The delirious patient often seems strangely inaccessible or unable to concentrate on his environment or on the task at hand. Bizarre, dream-like hallucinations may occur. The patient commonly suffers illusions, misinterprets his environment, and may fail to recognize persons well known to him. Because of the bizarre, threatening quality of his perceptions, the delirious patient may become wildly agitated. On the other hand, psychomotor underactivity may also dominate the picture. The onset of delirium is acute or subacute, developing over hours or days rather than over weeks or months. The intensity of the disturbance often waxes and wanes through the day and night.

In some patients, the manifestations of delirium may be so subtle that they are not recognized by an examiner who is unfamiliar with the patient's baseline status. At other times the symptoms suggest depression, dementia, or schizophrenia. The elderly are especially prone to delirium as a result of medical illness and drug intoxication (6).

The essential features of delirium are cognitive impairment and difficulty sustaining and shifting attention. Delirious patients may appear drowsy or hyperalert (hypervigilant), trail off in the middle of sentences, fail to answer questions or ask that questions be repeated, or appear perplexed. Perceptual disturbances such as illusions (misinterpretations of real external stimuli) or hallucinations are common. Delirium usually has rapid onset, relatively brief duration, and marked fluctuation throughout the day. Delirium is especially common in patients with dementia. Both demented and delirious patients may experience memory impairment, disorientation, hallucinations, delusions, and disturbed thinking. However, the demented patient is alert while the delirious patient is drowsy, and waxes and wanes over minutes or hours. The abrupt onset of delirium (within hours or days) differs from dementia, which develops over months or years in most instances.

The presence of cognitive impairment and rapid fluctuation distinguishes delirium from schizophrenia or other psychotic disorders. The hallucinations and delusions associated with delirium are often fleeting and poorly systematized in comparison with those of other psychotic disorders in which they are sustained and well organized. The electroencephalogram (EEG) in the delirious patient frequently reveals a generalized slowing of background activity whereas the EEG is generally normal in schizophrenia and depression.

The key to accurate diagnosis of delirium is a high index of suspicion in any elderly patient who presents with a history of recent or sudden change in mental status and behavior. The electroencephalogram shows diffuse slowing in both delirium and dementia. In delirium, the slowing is often marked, even when the cognitive and behavioral impairment is minor; conversely, severe cognitive disorder and a mildly abnormal EEG is most common in dementia.

Etiological Evaluation

Delirium can result from a wide range of organic causes that adversely affect the brain metabolism (Table 17.5). Special attention should be given to medications in the elderly, since they may produce a delirium at "therapeutic" doses. Beta-blockers, H2 blockers, and the many compounds with anticholinergic activity are common causes of delirium. Although electrolyte disturbances are the most common metabolic cause of delirium, any disorder of metabolic homeostasis can cause delirium. Withdrawal from alcohol or sedatives is frequently overlooked in the elderly as a possible cause of delirium. Commonly, multiple etiologies are suspected and no one specific cause is identified in 30 to 50% of cases.

The key to treatment is the identification of the underlying cause (causes) when they can be identified. A thorough physical and neurological examination is important, as is a search for a remediable metabolic abnormality. Attention to nutrition, fluid intake, and electrolyte balance is crucial.

Table 17.5.
Etiological Classification of Delirium[a]

IN A MEDICAL OR SURGICAL ILLNESS (NO FOCAL OR LATERALIZING NEUROLOGICAL SIGNS; CEREBROSPINAL FLUID USUALLY CLEAR):
  Metabolic disorders: hepatic stupor, uremia, hypoxia, hypercapnea, hypoglycemia, prophyria, hyponatremia
  Congestive heart failure
  Pneumonia, septicemia, typhoid fever, other febrile illnesses (especially in elderly)
  Hyperthyroidism and hypothyroidism
  Postoperative and post-traumatic states
IN NEUROLOGICAL DISEASE THAT CAUSES FOCAL OR LATERALIZING SIGNS OR CHANGES IN THE CEREBROSPINAL FLUID:
  Cerebrovascular disease
  Subarachnoid hemorrhage
  Hypertensive encephalopathy
  Cerebral contusion
  Subdural hematoma
  Tumor
  Abscess
  Meningitis
  Encephalitis
  Status epilepticus (by EEG)
  Postconvulsive delirium
THE ABSTINENCE STATES AND EXOGENOUS INTOXICATIONS (SIGNS OF OTHER MEDICAL, SURGICAL, AND NEUROLOGICAL ILLNESSES ABSENT OR COINCIDENTAL):
  Withdrawal of alcohol (delirium tremens), barbiturates, and nonbarbiturate sedative drugs, following chronic intoxication
  Drug intoxication due to benzodiazepines, opiates, neuroleptics, antidepressants, H2-blockers, centrally-acting antihypertensives, anticholinergics, digitalis, illicit drugs (see Chapter 22), etc.
BECLOUDED DEMENTIA:
  Senile or other brain disease in combination with infective fevers, drug reactions, heart failure, or other medical or surgical disease.

[a]Adapted from Adams RD: Delirium and other acute confusional states. In Isselbacher KJ, et al (eds): *Harrison's Principles of Internal Medicine*, 9th ed. New York, McGraw-Hill, 1980.

The treatment of the behavioral and emotional complications of delirium can become as urgent as the identification of the underlying etiology. Frequent reorientation and reassurance, a well-lighted environment, and avoidance of overstimulation are important aspects of treatment. If the agitation, hallucinations, or delusions do not respond to environmental intervention and are overwhelming to the patient or adversely affecting the patient's safety, then a low dose neuroleptic (e.g., haloperidol, .5–1.0 mg every 4 hours) can be ordered.

General References

Clarfield AM: The reversible dementias: do they reverse? *Ann Intern Med* 109:476, 1988.
> A thorough review of clinical relevance.

Mace NL, Rabins PV: *The 36-Hour Day*. New York, Warner Brooks, 1981.
> A book that provides detailed practical information for care providers of persons with dementia.

McGreevey Jr. JF, Franco K: Depression in the elderly: the role of the primary care physician in management. *J Gen Intern Med* 3:498, 1988.
> A well-referenced review article.

Montamat SC, Cusack BJ, Vestal RE: Management of drug therapy in the elderly. *N Engl J Med* 321:303, 1989.
> A readable review of drug treatment.

Moran MG, Thompson TL, Nies AS: Sleep disorders in the elderly. *Am J Psychiatry* 145:1369, 1988.

Specific References

1. Crook T, Bartus RT, Ferris SH, et al: Age-associated memory impairment: proposed diagnostic criteria and measures of clinical change—report of a National Institute of Mental Health Work group. *Developmental Neuropsychol* 2:261, 1986.
2. Gruenberg EM: Epidemiology of senile dementia. *Adv Neurol* 19:437, 1978.
3. Kramer M, German PS, Anthony JC, et al: Patterns of mental disorders among the elderly residents of eastern Baltimore. *JAGS* 33:236, 1985.
4. Larson EB, Reifler BV, Featherstone HJ, English DR: Dementia in elderly outpatients: a prospective study. *Ann Intern Med* 100:417, 1984.
5. Larson EB, Kukull WA, Buchner D, Reifler BV: Adverse drug reactions associated with global cognitive impairment in elderly persons. *Ann Intern Med* 107:169, 1987.
6. Lipowski ZJ: Delirium in the elderly patient. *N Engl J Med* 320:578, 1989.
7. NIA Consensus Conference: Differential diagnosis of dementing diseases. *JAMA* 258:3416, 1987.
8. Psychotic symptoms in Alzheimer's Disease. *Lancet* 2:1193, 1989.
9. Reding MJ, Haycox J, Wigforss K, et al: Follow-up of patients referred to a dementia service. *JAGS* 32:265, 1984.
10. Rabins PV, Merchant A, Nestadt G: Criteria for diagnosing reversible dementia caused by depression: validation by two year follow-up. *Br J Psychiatry* 144:488, 1984.
11. Starkstein SE, Robinson RG, Price TR: Comparison of patients with and without poststroke major depression matched for size and location of lesions. *Arch Gen Psychiatry* 45:247, 1988.

CHAPTER 18

Sexual Disorders

CHESTER W. SCHMIDT, JR., M.D.

The sexual difficulties described by patients to their physicians are evenly divided into sexual problems that accompany physical illness, those that are secondary to side effects of medication or abuse of drugs, and those that are unrelated to physical problems and are purely psychological in origin. Typically the psychologically based sexual problems are related to both psychosocial antecedents and to current stressful life situations, which are often self-limited. Those physically related and stress-related problems that are minor and reversible lend themselves to treatment by counseling techniques that rely heavily on catharsis, reassurance, and education. Although there are limited data to document results of treatment for these types of problems in the ambulatory setting, clinical experience suggests that the outcome for reversible sexual problems is usually good, with improvement rates approaching 75%.

NORMAL SEXUAL RESPONSE CYCLE

In order to assess these disorders rapidly and accurately it is helpful to be familiar with the normal sexual response cycle and the major physiological factors mediating each phase of the cycle. The human sexual response cycle is divided into four phases.

The first phase is one of *desire* and consists of fantasies and wishes to engage in sexual activity. This response is psychic in origin, but the psychic stimulation is mediated, at least in men, by circulating androgens.

The second phase is the *arousal* phase and consists of a number of physiological changes plus the subjective sense of sexual pleasure. In both sexes there is an increase in heart rate, an increase in breathing rate, and development of muscular tension throughout the body, most pronounced in the pelvic area and thighs. For both sexes the major physiological change is the development of vascular congestion in the genital area. For females the manifestations of vasocongestion are vaginal lubrication and swelling of the external genitalia. In males, vasocongestion leads to erection. Vasocongestion may occur via either of two neurological pathways: (*a*) a *local reflex pathway* initiated by tactile stimulation of the penis or clitoris and mediated by sensory fibers entering the dorsal root ganglia at S_2 through S_4 and by parasympathetic fibers from these ganglia to the perivesicular, prostatic, and cavernous plexuses; postganglionic fibers from these plexuses go to the blood vessels of the corpora cavernosa. (*b*) A *cortical pathway* initiated by psychic stimuli and mediated by parasympathetic and sympathetic fibers that originate at the $T_{12}–L_1$ level of the spinal cord. Each of these pathways promotes rapid inflow and retention of blood in the penis and the vulva.

The presence of these two spinal centers governing erection has important clinical implications. Patients with complete cord transections above the sacral center but below the thoracic center may still be capable of psychogenic erections mediated by impulses descending from higher centers and exiting the cord at T_{12}-L_1. With a cord lesion above both spinal centers, psychogenically produced erections are blocked, but the patient may still be capable of reflexogenic erections from direct tactile stimulation of the penis or clitoris even though he or she is unable to experience the sensation.

In addition to neurological pathways, erection in the male depends upon intact arterial blood flow from the right and left internal pudendal arteries.

The third phase is *orgasm*. Subjectively for both sexes orgasm is a peaking of sexual pleasure accompanied by a sense of release from sexual tension. Physiologically in the male, the most obvious manifestation of orgasm is ejaculation. Ejaculation is mediated by the sympathetic nervous system and consists of two processes: emission, resulting from contraction of the vas deferens, prostate, and seminal vesicles; and actual ejaculation, resulting from rhythmic contraction of the muscles of the pelvic floor and from closure of the internal sphincters of the bladder (preventing retrograde ejaculation). In the female, the rhythmic contractions take place within the musculature of the outer third of the vagina and in the perineal muscles. The subjective component of orgasm is a cortical sensory phenomenon, purely psychic in origin; it can occur without ejaculation or bladder neck closure.

The fourth phase is called *resolution*, which subjectively is accompanied by a sense of pleasure, warmth, well-being, and relaxation. Physiologically there is a gradual return of heart rate, breathing rate, and muscle tension to the baseline state. Most males are refractory to entering another cycle of sexual activity for some period of time (minutes in younger men and an hour or longer in middle-aged and older men). Women are not subject to this refractory period and may have multiple orgasms following continued or additional stimulation.

COMMON SEXUAL DISORDERS

The nomenclature and criteria used to classify sexual disorders in this chapter are based upon the American Psychiatric Association *Diagnostic and Statistical Manual of Mental Disorders* (Third Edition-Revised DSM-III-R). The assessment and management of the following common sexual disorders are discussed below: hypoactive sexual desire (loss of libido); inhibited sexual arousal (impotence); inhibited orgasm; dyspareunia; vaginismus; and premature ejaculation.

Organic Etiologies

As is pointed out below in the criteria for each of these disorders, a physical basis must be excluded before the disorder can be attributed to psychological factors. Because sexual functioning involves neural, vascular, and endocrine physiological mechanisms, as well as cellular receptor activity, there are many physical conditions and drugs that can interrupt normal function. To make matters more complicated these pathological conditions can adversely affect one or more phases of the sexual response cycle (see Tables 18.1 to 18.4).

General Characteristics

Incidence

The exact incidence of sexual disorders is not known. Estimates of lifetime incidence have ranged from a high of 75% in marriages and other long-term relationships to a low of 25%. A study involving general internists revealed 53% of new patients evaluated reported sexual dysfunctions (3). In all likelihood, the higher estimates include these disorders in their milder and more transient forms. Each type of sexual dysfunction can be found in both hetero- and homosexual couples. The sex ratio varies for the particular dysfunction. For example, inhibited orgasm is more common in females. By defini-

Table 18.1.
Organic Factors That May Affect Sexual Response in Both Sexes

Organic Factor	Sexual Disorders
Alcoholic neuropathy	Hypoactive arousal, hypoactive orgasm
Angina pectoris or recent myocardial infarction	Hypoactive desire
Any chronic systemic disease	Hypoactive desire, hypoactive arousal
Chronic pain	Hypoactive desire
Degenerative arthritis and disc disease of lumbosacral spine	Hypoactive desire, hypoactive arousal
Diabetes mellitus	Hypoactive arousal, retrograde ejaculation (men) Hypoactive orgasm (women)
Endocrine disorders (thyroid deficiency states, Addison's disease, Cushing's disease, hypopituitarism, hyperprolactinemia)	Hypoactive desire, variable effect on arousal
Multiple sclerosis	Hypoactive desire, hypoactive arousal, hypoactive orgasm
Cord lesions:	
Low lesion	Hypoactive reflex arousal (psychogenic arousal, and reflex ejaculation may be preserved)
High lesion	Hypoactive psychogenic arousal, (reflex arousal, and ejaculation may be preserved)
Radical pelvic surgery	Hypoactive arousal, hypoactive orgasm
Temporal lobe lesions	Hypoactive or increased desire
Vascular disease:	
Large vessel (Leriche syndrome)	Hypoactive arousal
Small vessel (pelvic vascular insufficiency)	Hypoactive arousal

Table 18.2.
Organic Factors That May Affect Sexual Response: Men Only

Organic Factor	Sexual Disorders
Dyspareunia (Genital pain during intercourse):	Hypoactive desire, hypoactive arousal, and hypoactive orgasm are disorders that may occur with any of the organic factors listed at the left.
Disturbed penile anatomy (chordee, Peyrone's disease, traumatic fracture, traumatic amputation)	
Penile skin infections	
Prostatic infections	
Testicular disease (orchitis, epididymitis, tumor, trauma)	
Urethral infections (gonorrhea, nonspecific urethral infections)	
Hypogonadal androgen-deficient states (Klinefelter's syndrome, testicular agenesis, Kallman's syndrome, testicular tumors, orchitis, hyperprolactinemia, castration)	Hypoactive desire, hypoactive arousal, hypoactive orgasm
Mechanical problems (inguinal hernia, hydrocele)	Hypoactive arousal
Surgical procedures:	
Abdominoperineal bowel resection	Hypoactive arousal
Lumbar sympathectomy	Hypoactive orgasm
Radical perineal prostatectomy	Hypoactive arousal

tion, premature ejaculation is confined to men and vaginismus is restricted to women.

Age of Onset of Common Sexual Disorders

Psychological and behavioral antecedents of these disorders can sometimes be found in both adolescent and childhood sexual behaviors and fantasies; however, the common age of onset is early adulthood. Onset can occur at any time during adult life, especially for those dysfunctions that are associated with physical conditions or drugs and for those that are situational or transient.

Predisposing Personality Factors

In general, competent and satisfying sexual function is considered to be associated with a healthy and adaptive personality development. Therefore, defects in personality structure accompanied by maladaptive

personality traits or psychopathology may affect sexual function. However, a study involving 288 patients with a diagnosis of a sexual dysfunction revealed that only 30% of the sample fulfilled criteria for an additional psychiatric disorder (5). *Negative attitudes toward sexuality* due to particular experience, internal psychic conflicts, or adherence to rigid cultural values can predispose individuals to the development of these dysfunctions.

Course and Severity

The course of sexual dysfunctions is variable. They may develop after a period of normal functioning or they may be lifelong. They may be generalized, occurring with all partners, or situational, limited to certain partners. There are differing degrees of impairment from partial to total. Usually, early age of onset and total impairment indicate chronicity and a poor treat-

Table 18.3.
Organic Factors That May Affect Sexual Response: Women Only

Organic Factor	Sexual Disorder

Complications of surgery:
  Ovarian approximation to vagina
Posthysterectomy scarring
Shortened vagina
 	
Dyspareunia (painful intercourse):
  Agenesis or the vagina
  Clitoral phymosis
  Imperforate hymen, rigid hymen, tender hymenal tags
  Infections of external genitalia: herpes genitalis, labial cysts, furuncles, Bartholin cyst infections
  Infections of the vagina: herpes genitalis, *Candida albicans, Trichomonas*
  Injuries due to birth trauma: episiotomy scars, tears, uterine prolapse
  Irritations of the vagina: chemical dermatitis (douches), atrophic vaginitis, intercourse with insufficient lubrication
Miscellaneous pelvic problems
  Cystitis, urethritis, urethral prolapse
  Endometriosis, ectopic pregnancy, pelvic inflammatory disease, ovarian cysts and tumors, pelvic tumors
  Intrauterine device complications
	Hypoactive desire, hypoactive arousal, hypoactive orgasm, and vaginismus are disorders that may occur with any of the organic factors listed at the left.

Table 18.4.
Drugs That May Affect Sexual Response[a]

Drugs	Sexual Disorders
Alcohol and sedatives (high dose)	Hypoactive desire, hypoactive arousal, delayed orgasm
Androgens	Increased desire (women) Hypoactive or increased desire, hypoactive arousal
Antidepressants	Hypoactive or increased desire, hypoactive arousal
Antihypertensives: Centrally acting (β-blockers, clonidine, guanabenz, methyldopa, reserpine)	Hypoactive desire, hypoactive arousal, (?) hypoactive orgasm
Peripherally acting (guanethidine, guanadrel)	Retrograde ejaculation
Antipsychotics	Hypoactive or increased desire, hypoactive arousal, retrograde ejaculation (Mellaril)
Cimetidine	Hypoactive desire, hypoactive arousal
Digoxin	Hypoactive desire, hypoactive arousal
Disopyramide	Hypoactive arousal
Disulfiram	Hypoactive arousal, delayed ejaculation
Diuretics	Hypoactive arousal
Estrogens, progesterone Men	Hypoactive desire, hypoactive arousal, hypoactive orgasm
Women	Hypoactive desire
L-Dopa	Increased desire (elderly men)
Lithium	Hypoactive desire, hypoactive arousal
Marijuana (high dose)	Hypoactive arousal (low dose may produce increased desire in men)
Narcotics	Hypoactive desire, hypoactive arousal, hypoactive orgasm
Stimulants (high dose) (cocaine, amphetamines)	Hypoactive desire, hypoactive arousal, hypoactive orgasm (low dose may produce increased desire)

[a] See also: Drugs that cause sexual dysfunction. *Med Lett* 29:65, 1987, for an exhaustive list, with references.

ment outcome. Conversely, a history of prior adequate sexual function, situational symptoms, and partial impairment indicate a self-limited course and a favorable treatment outcome.

Complications

The major complications are disrupted marital or sexual relationships. In addition, presence of the dys-

function may give rise to a variety of symptoms such as depression, anxiety, guilt, shame, frustration, and anger. These symptoms affect not only the individual but may intrude into most of his or her relationships.

General Approach to the Patient

Because patients often have difficulty discussing sexual activities and problems, it is important to inquire about sexual orientation and function as part of the primary care of each patient. In a study in a general medicine practice, 90% of patients appreciated being asked about sexual function (3). Table 18.5 outlines interviewing approaches that may be useful in this inquiry. In patients who do name a problem, the history of the present problem may be imprecise. Thus it is important to set aside sufficient time with the patient to achieve a clear statement of the problem. Occasionally, more than one scheduled session may be necessary. The setting for the discussion should be private. For those patients whose difficulties involve a partner or a spouse, it is important to have the partner's view of the problem. Sometimes the more functional partner will seek help in order to gain support for bringing the less functional partner into the evaluation.

The evaluation should be organized to obtain information about the onset and duration of the problem, about factors that make the problem better or worse, about concurrent events, such as birth of children, changes in relationships or vocation, onset of physical or emotional illness, and about use of new medications. It is always important to elicit from patients their ideas about the etiology of sexual problems and their expectations of treatment.

Sexual Desire Disorders

Diagnostic Classification

Medical conditions that cause decreased sexual desire should be specifically diagnosed (e.g., angina pectoris). Predominantly psychogenic disorders have been classified as follows in DSM-III-R:

Hypoactive Sexual Desire Disorder (Loss of Libido). Persistently or recurrently deficient or absent sexual fantasies, and desire for sexual activity. The judgment of deficiency or absence is made by the clinician, taking into account factors that affect sexual functioning, such as age, sex, and the context of the person's life.

Sexual Aversion Disorder. Persistent or recurrent extreme aversion to, and avoidance of, all or almost all, genital sexual contact with a sexual partner.

Assessment

As can be seen from Tables 18.1 to 18.4, there are many pathological conditions and drugs that have the potential for inhibiting sexual desire. In practice, most of these conditions will be known or easily diagnosed by the physician. Only a few conditions may present with the initial complaint of decreased or absent desire.

Congenital or acquired *hypogonadism* may be associated with decreased sexual interest in men (14). Because the testosterone level needed to maintain libido is usually lower than that needed for full stimulation of the prostate and seminal vesicles, the patient should also complain of a decrease or absence of emission when loss of sexual desire is due to hypogonadism. Hypogonadism that occurs before puberty results in eunuchoidism (lack of development of secondary sex characteristics). Similar striking physical findings are not present in patients who acquire hypogonadism after puberty; however, subtle physical changes do occur; decrease in beard growth, tendency to female body habitus, and decreased size of testes. An evaluation for hypogonadism should be undertaken in any male with persistent loss of libido (see details in Chapter 77).

In both sexes *prolactin-secreting microadenomas* of the pituitary can cause loss of sexual interest. In men this is partly due to a prolactin-mediated decrease in

Table 18.5.
Suggested Questions Regarding Sexual Practices and Problems

Suggested Opening (Legitimizing Statement)
  "Something that I ask each of my patients about is sexual activity. Is that alright with you?"

Suggested Initial Question(s)
  (Open-ended question) "Can you tell me about your present sexual activity (practices)? . . . . . ".
                                                  Or
  (Closed, somewhat leading question) "Have you noticed any problem in your ability to have and enjoy sexual relations?"
                                                  Or
  (Closed, but facilitative question) "Do you have any problems or questions related to your current sexual activities? . . . . ".

Screening Questions for Sexual Dysfunction (ask for clarification of any positive response)
  (Both sexes) "Have you noticed any loss of interest in having sex?"
  (Men) "Any problems having an erection?"
  (Both sexes) "Any problems having an orgasm?"
  (Both sexes) "Any problems having pain during intercourse?"

Screening Questions Regarding Sexual Orientation
  (Both sexes) "In the past few years about how many partners have you had for sexual relations?"
  (Men) "Do you ever have sex with another man?"
  (Women) "Do you ever have sex with another woman?"

Screening Question for Venereal Disease
  (Both sexes) "Have you ever had any kind of infection that you got from having sex? . . . . ".

Open Question to Obtain Additional Information
  "Is there any other information or any other questions about your sexual activities that you would like to discuss with me? . . . . ".

gonadotropin output, and the testosterone level is low. Hyperprolactinemia causes amenorrhea and galactorrhea in females, but galactorrhea is rare in affected men. Diagnosis can be made in both sexes by measuring serum prolactin levels (normal less than 15 mg/ml). (See additional details in Chapter 77.)

In both sexes *alcohol or other substance abuse* can cause decreased sexual desire. Patients who abuse drugs are usually guarded or untruthful about their habits; therefore, persistence and use of collateral interviews are often necessary in diagnosing the primary problem (see Chapters 21 and 22).

Depression is a common cause of loss of sexual desire. Even mild depressive states may result in decreased sexual desire, but in patients suffering from severe depressions this loss is universally observed. The relationship between loss of sexual desire and the presence of depression may be recognized by noting the patient's mood as well as by obtaining a history of depressive symptoms (see Chapter 15). *Life stresses* (loss of a job, death of a family member or of a friend, birth of a new family member, recent illness such as myocardial infarction, etc.) are common sources of decreased sexual desire related to depression or anxiety.

In married couples decreased sexual desire in one or both partners is often the result of *marital strife*. Arguments between partners create anger that eventually interferes with their sexual relationship. Although spouses may be aware of their anger toward each other, they may fail to draw a connection between loss of sexual interest and their mutual differences. Assessment requires a history taken from the couple together and then separately. Review of their current life situation will usually elicit the precipitating stresses and highlight the conflicts. The uncovering of extramarital relationships during the assessment requires careful handling by the physician. If both partners are aware of the relationship, then it can be discussed openly. If the extramarital relationship is revealed to the physician during the individual interviews, the physician should ask what the partner intends to do about the relationship, and with the "secret" information now shared with the physician. The responsibility for telling the other partner should be left to the patient. In some cases the extramarital relationship is a peripheral issue, and airing it could be destructive to an otherwise salvageable relationship.

Certain patients may give a history of aversion to or avoidance of all forms of genital contact with a sexual partner in contrast to a history of gradual or sudden loss of sexual desire. The complaint is often of long standing but may be of recent onset. The aversion may be so severe as to be associated with panic attacks should the patient find him- or herself confronted with a sexual experience.

Finally, inhibited sexual desire can be caused by the anxiety and frustration of repeated sexual failure associated with one of the other sexual disorders discussed below.

Treatment

Depending upon the etiology, *hypogonadism* in men may be treated by surgery, radiotherapy, hormone replacement, or hormone suppression (in the case of hyperprolactinemia). These treatment modalities are discussed in Chapter 77.

In both sexes, if a *drug* (see Table 18.4) is suspected of interfering with sexual desire, it should be discontinued, if possible, as a diagnostic-therapeutic test. If loss of sexual drive is secondary to alcohol or substance abuse, then treatment should be aimed at controlling the abuse (see Chapters 21 and 22).

Patients with *coronary artery disease*, especially postmyocardial infarction patients, have particular problems associated with sexual function. The management of these patients is discussed as part of the overall approach to rehabilitation after infarction in Chapter 58.

Transient hypoactive sexual desire disorders secondary to *psychological factors* such as stress, anger, or other interpersonal problems can be managed effectively with short-term counseling. When alcoholism, depression, or another psychosocial disorder is the primary problem, specific treatment for that disorder should of course accompany the counseling. The design of a counseling program should include an agreement between the patient or couple and the physician to meet for a specific number of sessions (usually two to five) for approximately 30 minutes/session.

Example. A couple in their midtwenties presents with a history of recent loss of sexual desire on the husband's part, and a decrease in the frequency of their sexual relationships. Assessment reveals a past history of mutually satisfying sexual experiences until 1 month ago when the husband was threatened with a job layoff. Although the husband still has his job, the layoff is still a possibility. The wife reports the husband has become quiet, sullen, and has increased drinking of alcohol. They report fighting frequently over small issues. The assessment is that the husband has an *adjustment disorder* with depressive features (see Chapter 15). During the initial counseling session the physician suggests that a relationship exists between changes in the husband's behavior and the threatened layoff. The wife indicates that the husband has refused to discuss his concerns because "it is unmanly." During the next counseling session the physician assists the couple in sharing their anguish with each other and developing contingency plans to cope with the potential layoff. As they are drawn into the discussions of planning, the couple's anger with each other subsides and a collaborative relationship is reestablished. The third session is utilized to review what contingency plans they have made. As an aside, they report that they have resumed their sexual relationship. During the final session the physician (a) reviews the relationship between stress, anger, and the change in sexual functioning; (b) points out that anger subsided when they worked together and that good sex is difficult to experience when they are angry with each other;

and (c) encourages them to use what they have learned when stresses arise in the future.

Aversion disorders usually require psychotherapy and treatment of associated panic attacks with low dose antidepressant medication (see details regarding panic attacks, Chapter 13).

Patients and their physicians often attempt to treat decreased sexual desire with drugs such as testosterone, alcohol, antianxiety compounds, or stimulants. There is no scientific basis for prescribing drugs for sexual desire disorders, except testosterone for the treatment of confirmed hypogonadism and bromocriptine for treatment of hyperprolactinemia (13), as discussed in Chapter 77.

Sexual Arousal Disorders

Diagnostic Classification

Arousal disorders that are secondary to a medical condition should be diagnosed as a symptom associated with the condition.

Psychogenic disorders have been classified as follows in DSM-III-R:

Female Arousal Disorders. Persistent or recurrent partial or complete failure to attain or maintain the lubrication-swelling or sexual excitement until completion of the sexual activity - OR - Persistent or recurrent lack of a subjective sense of sexual excitement and pleasure in a female during sexual activity.

Male Erectile Disorder (Impotence). Persistent or recurrent partial or complete failure in a male to attain or maintain erection until completion of the sexual activity - OR - Persistent or recurrent lack of a subjective sense of sexual excitement and pleasure in a male during sexual activity.

Assessment

An initial history (including psychosocial evaluation—see Chapter 10) and physical examination will usually lead to a formulation that the problem is either organic (i.e., one of the causes in Tables 18.1 to 18.4) or predominantly psychogenic. The general features in a male patient's history listed in Table 18.6 are helpful in making this important distinction.

Organic Basis. In both sexes, partial or complete failure to begin and maintain genital vasocongestion can be caused by a large number of pathological conditions and drugs. In younger patients, drugs are the commonest organic cause of impotence (Table 18.4). In older men, new impotence is usually organic, mostly due to vascular and/or neurological disease (12). The other conditions that may cause sexual arousal disorders (Tables 18.1 to 18.3) usually present with other manifestations before the patient complains of this problem.

In male patients with diabetes mellitus it is estimated that 25 to 60% will eventually develop impotence (4). Because some patients present with impotence as the initial symptom of diabetes, a fasting blood glucose is indicated for any male patient who presents with a chief complaint of impotence that is not due to an obvious psychosocial stressor or a recently started medication. There is no definitive information at this time about the effect of diabetes on the arousal phase in women; clearly, it can inhibit orgasm in women (10).

There are two conditions in women that may contribute to inhibition of sexual arousal: *vaginitis* and *atrophic vaginal changes* secondary to estrogen deficiency (see Chapter 94). Surprisingly, some women do not associate the presence of vaginitis or atrophic changes with the discomfort or pain these conditions can cause when intercourse is attempted. The history should therefore include questions to determine whether there is pain during intercourse, and the physical examination should include a pelvic examination to look for evidence of atrophy (see Chapter 94).

Occlusive vascular disease causing diminished blood flow to the internal pudendal arteries is more likely to affect men than women. Inhibited sexual arousal has been described with large vessel disease (Leriche's syndrome) as well as with medium and small vessel disease. If it is suspected that there is a vascular basis for impotence, the patient should be referred to a vascular surgeon for evaluation. The diagnostic techniques that may be employed included angiography of the medium size vessels of the corpus cavernosa, comparison of penile systolic pressures to limb systolic pressures, Doppler measurement of penile blood

Table 18.6.
Clinical Features Differentiating Predominantly "Psychogenic" from Predominantly "Organic" Erectile Dysfunction[a]

	Psychogenic	Organic
Onset	Usually abrupt, with temporal relationship to specific stress (marital difficulties, loss of job, bereavement, fatigue, *etc*)	Usually insidious decline from previous competency (90–95% of cases)
Course	Selective, intermittent, episodic, transient	Usually persistent, with progressive deterioration
Degree of impairment	Evidence of potential to respond to erotic stimuli and fantasies, with masturbation, alternate partner	Unable to obtain erection with masturbation, erotic stimuli, other partner
Nocturnal or morning erection	Generally present	Generally absent or reduced in frequency and intensity

[a]From Vliet LW, Meyer JK: Erectile dysfunction: progress in evaluation and treatment. *Johns Hopkins Med J* 151:246, 1982.

flow, and nocturnal penile tumescence studies (NPT) (8).

The *hypogonadal states* that cause hypoactive desire (see above) can also cause inhibited arousal (16), and the approach to diagnosis is the same (see Chapter 77).

Psychogenic Basis. If the assessment for an organic etiology, which will often include a trial off a potentially offending drug, does not yield a convincing diagnosis, a *psychogenic basis* should be assumed, and further inquiry followed by appropriate brief counseling (see below) should be utilized as a diagnostic-therapeutic trial.

Inability to attain and maintain levels of arousal that permit a smooth and trouble-free progression from the beginning of a sexual experience to its completion can be caused by any external or internal psychological events that interfere with the patient's ability to focus on the physical and psychological stimuli that maintain the sexual arousal. A dramatic example of an external event is the ringing of a telephone during the midst of the sexual experience. An internal psychological event might be a recurring thought about how one is performing. The history and assessment should be structured to uncover the presence of external events and the specific content of the psychological events when present. A common finding is a *persistent preoccupation and anxiety about performing successfully.* This problem may be primary or may occur as a secondary response to the frustration associated with organic dysfunction. Worry about a successful performance becomes more and more absorbing during the course of the sexual experience so that the psychological activity crowds out the patient's capacity to focus on the sexual stimuli that create the arousal response. When such patients realize they are losing arousal, they try all the harder, shutting off completely their ability to respond to sexual stimuli. Masters and Johnson have called this process "spectatoring" (see "General References"). The term describes a process whereby the patient, through observation of his performance, psychologically takes himself out of the experience. The mental process is guaranteed to result in loss of sexual arousal. Typically this process may begin after one or two failed experiences secondary to external events or stresses. Once the process begins, it becomes internally reinforcing, leading to further worry and further failure. When this process is suspected, the history should focus on the patient's mental experiences during sexual intercourse. Such information is difficult for most patients to describe, and more than a single interview may be required.

Other common causes of psychologically inhibited sexual arousal are *stressful life situations*. Patients who have recently lost a job, lost a relative, are concerned about retirement, have developed an illness, etc. may not be able to clear their minds of their worries during a sexual experience and therefore cannot respond. Similarly, feelings of anger or resentment directed toward the sexual partner can interfere with the ability to become sexually aroused.

If the patient with suspected psychogenic impotence does not respond to brief counseling (see below), then he should be offered *referral to a sleep laboratory for NPT studies* (8). The diagnostic usefulness of NPT monitoring is based on the assumption that during sleep, the psychological factors impeding erectile function during wakefulness are no longer operative, allowing a demonstration of the integrity of one's physiological capacity. Organic deficits, however, would persist during sleep, and therefore inhibit the number and duration of erectile episodes. Research has tended to confirm this assumption, with two exceptions: first, in certain psychiatric disorders (e.g., endogenous depression) in which rapid eye movement (REM) sleep patterns are also disrupted; and second, in a few men with organically proven erectile failure who occasionally have an episode of full erection during sleep, such as in patients with lower body spasms due to spinal cord injury, patients with a vascular "steal" syndrome, and in a previously unrecognized syndrome of impaired penile tumescence in the presence of sleep apnea, hypoventilation with decreased oxygen saturation, myoclonic jerks, and bradycardia.

Patient experience. This is similar to the experience for evaluation of sleep disorders (see Chapter 85). The patient will usually be scheduled to sleep on three consecutive nights in the sleep laboratory. Parameters monitored include electroencephalography, eye movements (to document the presence of REM sleep), heart rate, blood pressure, changes in penile circumference at the tip (just proximal to the glans) and base using two mercury-filled strain gauges, and an assessment of the degree of penile rigidity during at least one of the erectile episodes. Rigidity is assessed using a specifically designed tonometer that measures the amount of force required to "buckle" the erect penis. The patient is also briefly awakened to observe his erection, and asked to evaluate the quality of this erection, and to estimate its sufficiency for intromission. The technician records his estimate of the degree and rigidity of the erection. A photograph of the erect penis is taken, and later reviewed with the patient. This photograph provides visual evidence of normal erectile capacity to the patient with psychogenic dysfunction; it aids in the interpretation of numerical data obtained; and it reveals or confirms the presence of an anatomical deformity interfering with normal erection and/or intromission.

A do-it-yourself device (the Dacomed Snap-Gauge) for assessing nocturnal erections has been promoted in recent years. Because the role of this potentially cost-saving device has not been validated in careful studies, its place in the evaluation of impotence is not yet clear.

If an NPT study indicates an organic disorder (i.e., no or only partial erections occur during sleep), additional evaluation for vascular or neurological disorders should be carried out. If an NPT study supports psychogenic impotence, psychiatric referral is warranted.

Treatment

The method of treatment of *organically based inhibited sexual arousal disorders in men* will depend on whether the physiological impairment is reversible.

If a disease process, such as an infection, has not caused irreversible anatomical or physiological changes, treatment of the disease is dictated. Similarly, side effects of drugs can be reversed by reduction of dosage or, ideally, discontinuation of the medication. An adequate trial off a drug would be 1 or more weeks. Testosterone replacement for hypogonadism produces improvement in sexual arousal within a few weeks (see Chapter 77 for details). Whenever one is managing a patient with a reversible organic cause, treatment should be accompanied by encouragement and practical advice as discussed below.

When a disease process has caused permanent impairment of neural, vascular, or anatomical function in males, *surgical measures* can be considered. Currently there are two types of penile prosthetic devices that allow the impotent male to engage in intercourse. The Small-Carrion (15) prosthesis is a set of semirigid Silastic rods that are placed in the penis, creating a permanent modest erection. The second prosthesis is a hydraulic device (6) that, when implanted, permits voluntary stiffening of the penis. The commonest indication for penile prosthetic devices has been in impotent diabetics who are otherwise healthy. Counseling of the patient and his spouse or partner is an essential element of a rehabilitative program before and after surgery.

Intracavernosal injection of vasodilating substances such as papaverine hydrochloride (smooth muscle relaxant) or phenoxybenzamine hydrochloride and phentolamine (alpha-adrenergic blockers) has become an important, nonsurgical technique for treating organically caused arousal disorder (7). This technique has not yet been approved by the United States Food and Administration (FDA). Patients can be taught, with supervision, to inject themselves painlessly with 28-gauge needles. The amount of substance (usually a combination of papaverine and phentolamine) necessary to cause erection may vary from patient to patient and must be determined by the physician (usually a consulting urologist) with a challenge injection, which also serves the functioning of initiating instruction of the patient. This method of treatment has been more effective for men with neurogenic impotence than those with vascular or other etiologies for their impotence. Erection occurs 8 to 10 minutes after injection and lasts 2 to 4 hours, with partial detumescence after ejaculation. Priapism has been the major untoward effect of this form of treatment.

In two small studies, *yohimbine, an orally administered alpha-adrenergic blocker* that may effect sympathetic outflow, has been reported to improve sexual function in about 50% of men with either organic (vascular or neurogenic) impotence (11) or psychogenic impotence (13). Yohimbine is available as Yohimex (5-mg tablets) and Yocon (5.4-mg tablets), and the usual dose is one tablet three times a day. Occasional side effects at this dose are nausea, dizziness, or nervousness. The clinical effect may not be seen until the patient has been on medication for 3 weeks. Considering the relative costs of medication versus psychotherapy, a trial of this drug may be indicated for selected patients.

Little is known about the response to treatment in *women* with disease processes that impair the physiological capacity for sexual excitement. As in men, side effects of drugs can be eliminated by adjustment of dosage or discontinuation of the drug, and dyspareunia due to vulvovaginal conditions and atrophic vaginitis can usually be eliminated (see Chapter 94).

The strategy for management of *psychologically based* inhibited sexual arousal in both sexes depends on whether the patient has had the dysfunction for a sustained period of time or whether the dysfunction has appeared recently and there is a prior history of competent sexual functioning. As discussed earlier, transient inhibition of sexual excitement is often secondary to stressful life situations and/or marital discord (adjustment disorders). These clinical situations often respond to brief counseling. The elements of counseling are similar to those described in the example above of the couple with sexual desire disorders. The role of the physician is to help the couple recognize the effect of the stress on their relationship as well as the effect of their feelings (often anger) on their ability to relate sexually. Encouragement of collaborative contingency planning for resolving problems reduces anxiety and anger, often helping the couple to return to their baseline level of sexual function. The same principles and steps are applicable to an individual patient.

When spectatoring is a major factor and does not remit after open discussion, referral to a professional skilled in sex therapy usually brings excellent results. A successful form of treatment is one developed by Masters and Johnson that combines cognitive as well as behavioral techniques to replace spectatoring with appropriate sexual focus and behavior.

The following factors favor a good prognosis after treatment for psychogenic impotence: history of adequate prior sexual functioning, acute versus insidious onset, short duration of sexual impairment, heterosexual orientation, stable social situation, motivation for treatment, presence of sexual desire, willingness of partner to participate in treatment, absence of severe marital conflicts, and absence of significant concurrent psychopathy.

Even in patients for whom excellent function can be expected, the return to normal sexual excitation can be impaired by worry and hesitation. This is especially true when the impaired arousal has been present for more than a few weeks, which is often the case. Such patients should be invited to discuss this situation freely and should be given permission and encouragement to experiment in one or more ways (e.g., masturbation, erotic pictures or movies, new techniques) in order to test or promote their sexual functions. Such advice should, of course, be consistent with the patient's personal beliefs.

Patients who have suffered with inhibited sexual arousal over a long period of time or have never functioned competently may be given a trial of short-term counseling (Chapter 11). If the counseling does not result in reasonable improvement, referral for more expert help should be considered.

Orgasm Disorders

Diagnostic Classification

Orgasm disorders caused by physiological factors should be diagnosed as symptoms associated with the responsible medical conditions. Psychogenic disorders have been classified as follows in DSM-III-R:

Inhibited Female Orgasm. Persistent or recurrent delay in, or absence of, orgasm in a female following a normal sexual arousal phase during sexual activity that the clinician judges to be adequate in focus, intensity, and duration. Some females are able to experience orgasm during noncoital clitoral stimulation, but are unable to experience it during coitus in the absence of manual stimulation. In most of these females, this represents a normal variation of the female sexual response and does not justify the diagnosis of *inhibited female orgasm.* However, in some of these females, this does represent a psychological inhibition that justifies the diagnosis. This difficult judgment is assisted by a thorough sexual evaluation, which may even require a trial of treatment.

Inhibited Male Orgasm. Persistent or recurrent delay in, or absence of, orgasm in a male following a normal sexual arousal phase during sexual activity that the clinician, taking into account the person's age, judges to be adequate in focus, intensity, and duration. This failure to achieve orgasm is usually restricted to an inability to reach orgasm in the vagina, with orgasm possible with other types of stimulation, such as masturbation.

Premature Ejaculation. Persistent or recurrent ejaculation with minimal sexual stimulation or before, upon, or shortly after penetration and before the person wishes it. The clinician must take into account factors that affect duration of the arousal phase, such as age, novelty of the sexual partner or situation, and frequency of sexual activity.

Assessment

The orgasmic response is physiologically governed by the autonomic nervous system in both sexes. The organic conditions that inhibit orgasm are for the most part neurological disorders, drugs that affect the autonomic system, and surgical or traumatic interruption of the involved neural pathways (see Tables 18.1 to 18.4). History-taking and physical examination should focus on these possibilities. In women, diabetic autonomic neuropathy is probably the most common organic cause of inhibited orgasm (10). Men who are experiencing retrograde ejaculation often state they have lost their ability to have orgasms. If history reveals the patient has the subjective sensations of orgasm but has no ejaculate (and the patient is not taking a drug that can cause retrograde ejaculation; see Table 18.4), then the patient should have a urological evaluation of the function of the internal sphincter of the bladder.

Isolated *psychogenic* anorgasmia in men is a rare disorder and is associated with severe personality disturbances. Cases can be divided roughly into two personality types: severe obsessive compulsive character disorder and severe sadomasochistic character disorder.

Premature ejaculation is the most common male orgasmic disorder. There are no known organic causes for premature ejaculation; therefore, the assessment of this dysfunction should focus on psychological issues. Whereas some men recognize that orgasm regularly occurs too soon for their partner to enjoy intercourse fully, others do not; therefore it is necessary to interview both partners in order to make the diagnosis. Typically the couple will report that the male experiences orgasm as he is attempting to penetrate, just as he has penetrated, or within several thrusts after penetration.

Patients usually have had the dysfunction since they became sexually active. Although occasionally patients may report the recent onset of premature ejaculation, these men have invariably experienced this disorder for a sustained period in the past. Another variation is the patient who reports good control with a girlfriend but premature ejaculation with his spouse.

The personality structure of the premature ejaculator is often passive-aggressive (see Chapter 14). Evaluation of the relationship usually reveals an ongoing struggle between the couple. The woman is openly angry about some issue (not necessarily the sexual problem), and the man is complacent, content, and puzzled that his partner is upset. Transient episodes of premature ejaculation may be precipitated by marital conflict. Some men who are sufficiently frustrated by the disorder may develop inhibited sexual arousal (impotence) secondarily.

Psychologically caused inhibited orgasm is a common problem in *women.* Numerous studies estimate that 10% of the female population is anorgasmic to any stimuli and 30 to 50% of all married women are occasionally anorgasmic with intercourse. Assessment should focus on the duration of the problem, a past history of sexual functioning, the status of the relationship with the spouse or partner, and the presence of a stressful situation. A history of recent onset, competent past functioning, and identifiable precipitating stresses predicts a good response to treatment. Patients who have been anorgasmic for many years and are seeking help because of a change in their relationship or life situations are more difficult to treat.

Some women will present with a complaint of anorgasmia but evaluation will reveal the patient is actually experiencing inhibited sexual arousal. Because treatment may differ for these disorders, clarification of the phase in which the dysfunction is operating may be important.

Treatment

Men. It is unusual for men to experience loss of orgasmic capacity due to organic factors while retaining the capacity for erection. In fact it is more usual for men to lose their potency while retaining the capacity for emission and some of the subjective sensations associated with orgasm. Most of the physical conditions, diseases, and drugs listed in Tables 18.1, 18.2, and 18.4 will affect the capacity for erection before orgasmic function is impaired. There may be isolated instances of side effects of drugs in which males report loss of ability to experience orgasm, but retain the capacity for erection. In these instances, it is important to distinguish *retrograde ejaculation* from inhibited orgasm. Retrograde ejaculation can occur with some drugs, including thioridazine (Mellaril) and guanethidine (Ismelin) while the other components of orgasm remain intact.

Men who suffer from inhibited orgasm on a psychogenic basis usually have long-standing personality disorders requiring expert psychotherapy to effect improvement.

There are several behavioral methods of treatment for premature ejaculation that may be adaptable to the ambulatory setting. The key to helping the premature ejaculator is to teach him to become aware of his progression through the sexual response cycle and then, with his partner, to practice one of two control techniques. Patients without regular partners cannot readily use this behavioral method. The techniques are "squeeze technique" and "stop and go." The squeeze technique requires the female partner to place her thumb and first two fingers around the coronal ridge of the penis and press firmly for 10 seconds. The pressure will result in a 10 to 25% loss of erection and a decrease in the subjective sense of arousal. The technique teaches the couple a method of control that can be practiced well before the patient reaches high levels of sexual arousal. The stop and go method accomplishes the same thing by discontinuing all forms of stimulation. The patient and his partner alternately stimulate and practice control with these techniques until they are confident of their ability to exercise control. At this point they progress to coitus, interrupting the experience as necessary with the squeeze or stop and go technique. Additional details can be found in Masters and Johnson's *Human Sexual Inadequacy* (see "General References").

Treatment

Women. Apart from managing local vaginal conditions and discontinuing possible causal drugs, there are no organic therapies for this dysfunction in women. Therefore, in female patients with known neuronal damage, including diabetic neuropathy, the goal of therapy should be to help the patients adjust to the permanent loss of their sexual responsiveness.

Transient forms of anorgasmia caused by psychogenic factors are amenable to treatment with counseling. A history of previous orgasmic response is a good prognostic indicator. The block in orgasmic response is often due to the process of "spectatoring" described above. The interfering process is usually secondary to stressful life situations and/or marital discord. Counseling for married women and women who have a regular sexual partner should include the partner provided that it is agreeable to the patient. Counseling should be aimed primarily at resolving the dominant problems, which are usually life stresses or interpersonal strife. With the single patient, counseling should be directed at helping the patient suppress or remove the psychological events (i.e., spectatoring) that are occurring at a critical time, when the patient has reached a high plateau level of excitement and is prepared for orgasmic release. The interfering psychological events may be removed by having the patient focus to the best of her ability on the physical stimuli that she is experiencing during the excitement phase.

Women with anorgasmia of long duration can be given a trial of counseling. If counseling does not result in substantial improvement, referral for additional evaluation and treatment should be made.

Sexual Pain Disorders

Diagnostic Classification

The diagnosis of psychogenic dyspareunia should be made only after all physical causes have been ruled out. The DSM-III-R diagnostic criteria for *sexual pain disorder* are:

Dyspareunia. Recurrent or persistent genital pain in either a male or female before, during, or after sexual intercourse. The pain is not caused exclusively by lack of lubrication or by vaginismus.

Vaginismus. Recurrent or persistent involuntary spasm of the musculature of the outer third of the vagina that interferes with coitus. The disturbance is not caused exclusively by a physical disorder.

Assessment

The common causes of genital pain during intercourse (dyspareunia) are presented in Tables 18.2 and 18.3. In both sexes the complaint of discomfort or pain during intercourse requires a careful history, physical examination, and laboratory testing. The commonest causes are infections or atrophic vaginitis in women, and urethral or prostatic infection in men. Psychogenic dyspareunia is uncommon, and this diagnosis should be made only after organic causes have been excluded.

Vaginismus is a disorder of women. There are relatively few causes of organic vaginismus, and they are usually secondary to dyspareunia. Diagnosis of functional vaginismus may be made when pelvic examination is attempted and the physician finds it impossible to pass a finger or speculum into the vagina because of contraction of the musculature around the vaginal outlet. Patients may also present with a history of inability to be penetrated during coitus because of tightness of the vaginal outlet caused by muscular spasm.

Treatment

The treatment of dyspareunia caused by organic conditions in both men and women is directed at the condition, usually an infection, causing the pain (see Chapters 27 and 94). Patients with psychogenic dyspareunia will have many of the features described for those with psychogenic inhibited sexual arousal or inhibited orgasm; that is, they will report a prior history of competent sexual function without pain and will have current life stress and/or marital discord. Therefore, the counseling techniques used in the treatment should be very similar to those described for the other two disorders. An important strategy in counseling is to allow the patient a face-saving way of giving up the pain without directly confronting him with the idea that the pain is of psychogenic origin.

A few patients have psychogenic dyspareunia over a sustained period of time. Such patients usually have severe underlying psychiatric conditions and require referral for expert evaluation and treatment.

The treatment of organic vaginismus is the same as the treatment of the organic causes of dyspareunia.

The treatment of functional vaginismus is based upon *desensitizing* the patient to the experience of penetration. Couples are provided with a series of exercises to be performed in the privacy of their home. Following a relaxing bath, the couple engages in general body touching, excluding the genitals. Next, they repeat general touching but include the genitals, avoiding any touching that is frankly stimulating. At following sessions, they repeat the touching but add the passage of graded sized dilators, still avoiding stimulating, touching, or efforts to attain orgasm. When dilators have reached the size approximating the size of the penis, then the penis can be substituted as a dilator. The same process can be applied by having the individual woman dilate herself. One problem with the single patient is the possibility that the experience during the sessions at home will not generally apply to a sexual experience with a partner. Should this occur, treatment may have to be delayed until the patient has a regular partner with whom she has a reasonably good relationship and who can participate in the outlined program.

HOMOSEXUALITY

General Characteristics

Although homosexuality is no longer classified as a sexual disorder, it is the most common sexual deviation that will be seen by the generalist. The diagnostic term *sexual disorder not otherwise specified* may be used for patients who experience persistent and marked distress about their sexual orientation.

Thirty years ago Kinsey et al. (9) estimated that 10% of white American men and 5% of white women were predominantly homosexual. Estimates of the preva-

lence of homosexuality in blacks have not been published.

Predisposing Factors

Various attempts to relate homosexuality to abnormal pituitary and sex hormone function have been unsuccessful. There is no evidence to support the contention that homosexuality is genetically determined. Many theories about the etiology of homosexuality involving psychosocial predisposition have been proposed. However, no studies have clearly demonstrated psychosocial etiological precipitants.

Course

Most individuals who have a homosexual orientation continue that orientation as a lifelong pattern. Some homosexuals are socially open about their life style; others are covert.

Complications

In the past, but to a lesser degree at the present time, the principal complication was the social stigma. Bias against homosexuals leads to occupational and other social problems for some, as summarized in Table 18.7. Recently, criminal penalties for homosexuality have been eliminated for consenting adults. The only legal difficulty currently is for those individuals who are promiscuous and who use public facilities for their sexual activities. Homosexuality *per se* is not a contraindication for developing sustained, affectionate, long-term relationships. There is little evidence to support the contention that homosexual individuals are subject to or manifest greater levels of psychopathology than heterosexual individuals.

Table 18.7.
Influence of Homosexuality on Vocation and Social Life (Results of a Study of 143 Subjects)[a]

	Male Homosexuals N = 86	Female Homosexuals N = 57
	%	%
SOCIAL:		
No negative influence[b]	51	72
Deprived of family life	35	9
Social contacts limited to other homosexuals	14	19
AMBITIONS:		
No negative influence	68	88
Imposed restrictions on choice of work or advancement	32	12
JOB:		
No negative influence	84	88
Reprimanded, fired, or asked to resign because of homosexuality	16	12

[a]From Saghir M, Robins E: *Male and Female Homosexuality—A Developmental, Psychiatric, and Sociological Investigation.* Baltimore, Williams & Wilkins, 1973.
[b]All negative influences listed are those that subjects felt were specifically a result of being identified as a homosexual.

Assessment and Management

Assessment of patients who express concerns about homosexual fantasies or experiences should focus on the frequency of the experiences, on the patients' decisions to continue with homosexual experiences, and on whether they feel comfortable with those decisions. Patients who ultimately choose a homosexual orientation and are comfortable with that choice do not present problems. However, patients who are anxious or depressed about their homosexual inclinations may need therapy. Adolescents or adults who anxiously report isolated episodes of homosexual experiences or fantasies may need brief supportive counseling (see Chapter 11).

Most homosexuals prefer their personal physician to know of their homosexuality and indicate that they are more satisfied with the care they obtain when their physician is aware of their orientation (2).

Homosexuals require special considerations in their *routine medical care*. Those who have multiple partners should always be asked about their knowledge of "safe sex" practices (see Chapter 34) and about symptoms that might be caused by venereal disease, including HIV infection (see Chapter 34); and they should be screened periodically for type B hepatitis (Chapter 43), syphilis (Chapter 30), and gonorrhea (Chapter 27).

SPECIAL CONSIDERATIONS FOR SELECTED AGE GROUPS

Elderly Patients

Aging individuals do not lose their capacity for sexual function on the basis of the aging process alone. It is important to invite questions regarding sexual function in the general care of an older person, as they are often embarrassed to bring up this aspect of their health. Those patients who have any of the sexual disorders discussed above should be evaluated in the same manner as a younger patient. The changes associated with aging are slower arousal phase, increased ability to stay at plateau levels of arousal, and, in men, a longer refractory period.

Children

It is unusual for children to complain of sexual difficulties. However, parents will occasionally ask their own physician questions about the developing sexuality of their children. Parents may express concern about the appearance of sexual behavior in children such as mutual exploration of playmates' genitalia or masturbation. The parents can be assured that the behavior is normal and that the behavior should be discouraged in a nonpunitive fashion. Failure to control the behavior may require further evaluation of both the child and the family.

Occasionally the physician may recognize the presence of *sexual abuse* within a family, either on the basis of physical findings or information disclosed by a child during a medical visit. If the abuse has been committed by someone outside the family, both the child and parents may require supportive counseling to help them vent their fear and anger about the experience. Discovery of sexual abuse within a family needs to be fully evaluated. This should be initiated by reporting the problem to the division of protective services of the local department of social services.

Adolescents

Adolescent sexual difficulties (see Chapter 5) may be brought to the attention of the physician either by the adolescent or by the adolescent's parents. Adolescents who are sexually active may have questions about their sexual function, birth control, venereal disease, or abortion. In most states, the physician may provide service for sex-related problems to the adolescent with or without the parental consent.

Adolescents may request consultation about isolated homosexual experiences and/or homosexual fantasies. In most cases, the physician's role is to reassure the adolescent that these experiences are normal and are not indicative of the development of lifelong homosexuality. Adolescents who have a homosexual orientation or who are in the process of doing so may be brought to the physician by parents disturbed at the discovery of homosexual activities. In these instances, counseling should be given to the parents in order to help them accept the decision of the adolescent. Older adolescents (above 17 years) are unlikely to change their orientation. Younger adolescents (16 years and below) have not consolidated their personality development and should be referred for psychiatric evaluation and possible treatment.

GENDER IDENTITY DISORDERS

Gender identity disorders are divided into (a) transsexualism and (b) gender identity disorders of childhood. The essential feature of both disorders is the incongruence between anatomical sex and gender identity.

Predisposing Factors

No known genetic or biochemical predisposing factors have as yet been elucidated. There is some evidence that these disorders may stem from faulty parent-child relationships in situations in which parents have confused sexual identity, or have a need to raise a child of one sex in the role of the opposite sex.

Prevalence

These disorders are apparently rare. Male cases are more common than female, the reported ratio varying from 8 to 1 to as low as 2 to 1.

Age of Onset

For children the initial expression of the wish to be in the cross-gender role may take place as early as the fourth birthday. For adults, the manifestations of this disorder usually become apparent in early adulthood, although the adults usually state that they had been aware of wishes to be in the cross-gender role since childhood or adolescence.

Course

The course of the disorder for children is as yet unknown. An undetermined number of affected boys and girls may adopt a homosexual orientation during adolescence or as adults. The course in adults is variable. For some it is chronic and unremitting, with a persistent drive toward attaining surgical reassignment. For others, the intensity of the desire for living and functioning in the cross-gender role waxes and wanes, often associated with current life stress and the appearance of psychiatric symptoms, principally depression. Females who are interested in sexual reassignment are a more homogeneous group than the males, in that they are more likely to have a history of homosexuality and by and large have a more stable course with or without treatment.

Complications

The principal complications are those associated with the desire and attempt to live and function socially and occupationally in the cross-gender role. In addition, there is a moderate degree of associated psychopathology, including episodes of depression and of suicide attempts. In rare instances, affected males may attempt to mutilate their genitals.

Assessment

The assessment of these disorders in adults is relatively simple in that most individuals will identify themselves as being unhappy with their anatomical sex and interested in a surgical reassignment. No endocrinological studies are indicated, and physical findings show that the individuals seeking surgical reassignment are genetically normal men or women. However, the generalist may see rare cases of patients who have a congenital intersexed condition and who are confused about their sexual identification.

Treatment

Patients with gender identity disorders should be referred to psychiatrists or to special programs that have the expertise to treat these problems. Transsexuals who are in a cross-gender program and who need continuous administration of cross-gender hormones may be transferred to the generalist. Some physicians may not agree with such treatment, and these patients should select physicians who are comfortable working with these types of problems.

THE PARAPHILIAS

This is a group of disorders in which sexual interests are directed primarily toward objects other than other human beings, toward sexual acts not usually asso-

ciated with coitus, or toward coitus performed under bizarre conditions.

Fetishism

Fetishism is the relatively exclusive displacement of erotic interest in sexual satisfaction to an object, or to a body part other than those usually associated with genital sexuality. Common fetish objects are female undergarments (particularly worn or soiled ones), feet, and shoes. Orgasmic release may be achieved by any of the behavior used by adults in sexual activities.

Zoophilia

Zoophilia is the use of animals as a preferred or exclusive method of achieving sexual excitement. The animal may be the object of intercourse or may be trained to excite the human partner sexually by licking or rubbing. The animal is preferred no matter what other forms of sexual outlet are available.

Pedophilia

Pedophilia is a condition in which adults compulsively involve children in their sexual activities. The sexual behavior that results in orgasmic release may be heterosexual or homosexual and includes any behavior utilized by adults in their sexual activities. In the majority of cases, however, the pedophile is concerned with mutual masturbation or fondling rather than coitus.

Exhibitionism

Exhibitionism is the displaying of the genital organs for the purpose of sexual gratification. This perversion is predominantly a male activity. Orgasmic release is usually achieved through masturbation.

Voyeurism

Voyeurism is a deviation in which sexual stimulation and gratification are obtained from looking at the sexual organs of others or from observing their sexual activities. Orgasmic release is usually achieved by masturbating during, or just following, the period of observation.

Sadism and Masochism

Sadism and masochism are deviations in which sexual arousal and gratification are dependent either upon inflicting pain (sadism) or experiencing it (masochism). There is a broad spectrum of behavior ranging from the dim awareness of cruelty or suffering as part of the sexual experience to overt behavior, including extreme physical injury and murder. Aspects of sadism and masochism are usually found in the same individual, even though one or the other behavior appears dominant.

General Characteristics of the Paraphilias

Predisposing Factors

The etiology is unknown. However, history of physical and/or sexual abuse during childhood appears in a modest number of the cases.

Prevalence

The disorders are rare. The sex ratio is predominantly in favor of males, with the exception of sexual sadism and masochism.

Course

The course of these disorders is usually chronic. Peaks of deviant activity may accompany current life stress or be associated with psychiatric symptomatology, principally depressive episodes. If the deviant behavior brings the individual into conflict with society, the outcome can often include arrest and incarceration. Treatment is difficult because of the egosyntonic nature of the behavior. Anxiety and depression may be associated with the fear of being discovered, arrested, or punished; however, once these dangers have passed, the uncomfortable affect disappears, and the individual has little motivation for treatment.

Complications

Inasmuch as these disorders are often associated with other defects in personality development, the capacity for developing long-term, affectionate relationships may be impaired. The possibility of being involved in criminal violations has already been mentioned. In some instances the behavior may bring the individual into extremely dangerous situations, resulting in severe injury or death.

Assessment

It is not difficult to diagnose a specific paraphilia once the history is obtained. No specific laboratory tests are indicated. The physical examination will usually be normal. Sadistic or masochistic behavior may produce physical injuries. Hypersexuality, including some deviant behavior, has been reported to be associated with temporal lobe epilepsy (1). Thus, in cases in which there is suggestion of a seizure disorder, an electroencephalogram is indicated. Psychiatric disorders, principally depression secondary to loss, may precipitate bursts of deviant behavior in paraphiliacs. Abuse of alcohol or of other substances may also increase the behavior.

Stress, anxiety, organic brain syndrome, and mental retardation may lead to episodic deviant behavior, but these episodes are not diagnosed as paraphilia.

Treatment

Psychotherapy or other psychological treatment designed to control or eliminate paraphiliac behavior is best provided by a psychiatrist. The general physician's role in the care of these patients is in the management of concurrent medical problems. Of major concern are recognition and treatment of venereal disease in those patients whose sexual behavior is promiscuous, and the possibility of child abuse in families that have paraphiliac members. Many individuals who engage in paraphilias were subjected to physical or sexual abuse as children. The pattern is often passed on from generation to generation.

General References

American Psychiatric Association: *Diagnostic and Statistical Manual of Mental Disorders.* DSM-III-R (third edition revised), Washington, DC, American Psychiatric Association, 1987.
   Recently updated diagnostic criteria and epidemiological information for all recognized psychiatric disorders.
Masters WH, Johnson VE: *Human Sexual Inadequacy.* Boston, Little, Brown, and Co, 1970.
   The original and still used descriptive work on the behavioral treatment of common sexual disorders.
Meyer JK, Schmidt CW, Wise TN (eds): *Clinical Management of Sexual Disorders.* Baltimore, Williams & Wilkins, 1983.
   A current textbook that addresses the evaluation, diagnosis, and treatment of a wide variety of sexual disorders.
Segraves RT: Effects of psychotropic drugs on human erection and ejaculation. *Arch Gen Psych* 46:275-284, 1989.
   An excellent current review of the physiology and receptor chemistry associated with male arousal.
Drugs That Cause Sexual Dysfunction. *Med Letter* 29:65, 1987.
   Review article listing drugs that cause sexual dysfunction with excellent reference list.
The Psychiatric Clinics of North America: *Sexuality.* Philadelphia, WB Saunders, 1980.
   A concise review.
Vliet LW, Meyer JK: Erectile dysfunction: progress in evaluation and treatment. *Johns Hopkins Med J* 151:246, 1982.
   An in-depth review article that focuses on impotence but that provides a methodology of evaluation for the practitioner that can be applied to any sexual dysfunction.

Specific References

1. Blumer D: Changes of sexual behavior related to temporal lobe disorders in man. *J Sex Res* 6:173, 1970.
2. Dardick L, Grady KE: Openness between gay persons and health professionals. *Ann Intern Med* 93:115, 1980.
3. Ende J, Rockwell S, Glasgow M: The sexual history in general medicine practice. *Arch Intern Med* 144:558-561, 1984.
4. Ellenberg M: Impotence in diabetes: the neurologic factor. *Ann Intern Med* 75:213, 1971.
5. Fagan P, Schmidt CW, Wise TN, Derogatis R: Sexual dysfunction and dual psychiatric diagnoses. *Compreh Psych* 29 (3): 278–284, 1988.
6. Furlow WL: Surgical treatment of erectile impotence using the inflatable penile prosthesis. *Sex Disabil* 1:299, 1978.
7. Intracavernous injections for impotence. *Med Letter* 29:95, 1987.
8. Karacan I: Diagnosis of impotence in diabetes mellitus: an objective and specific method. *Ann Intern Med* 92:334, 1980.
9. Kinsey AC, Pomeroy WB, Martin CE: *Sexual Behavior in the Human Male.* Philadelphia, WB Saunders, 1948.
10. Kolodny RC: Sexual dysfunction in diabetic females. *Diabetes* 20:557, 1971.
11. Morales A, Surridge DHC, Marshall PG, et al: Non-hormonal pharmacological treatment of organic impotence. *J Urol* 128:45–48, 1982.
12. Mulligan T, Katz G: Why aged men become impotent. *Arch Intern Med* 149:1365, 1989.
13. Reid K, Morales A, Harris C, et al: Double-blind trial of yohimbine in treatment of psychogenic impotence. *Lancet* 421, August, 1987.
14. Schmidt CW: Biochemical treatment of sexual disorders. *Psychiatr Clin North Am* 3:89, 1980.

15. Small MP: The Small-Carrion penile prosthesis: surgical implant for the management of impotence. *Sex Disabil* 1:282, 1978.
16. Spark RF, White RA, Connolly PB: Impotence is not always psychogenic: newer insights into hypothalamic-pituitary-gonadal dysfunction. *JAMA* 243:750, 1980.

C H A P T E R 19

Dying, Death, and Bereavement*

L. RANDOL BARKER, M.D.
MICHAEL PURTELL, M.D.
LARRY WATERBURY, M.D.

Family physicians traditionally took care of their patients from cradle to death, they managed the grief and bereavement of the survivors. This situation has changed dramatically in the last 40 to 50 years, in part because of the mobility of the society, in part because of the increased specialization of physicians. Now 80% of people come to hospitals to receive terminal care, which cannot be given at home either because of the specialized nature of the care or because of lack of family resources. Up until 40 or 50 years ago a dying patient stayed at home or returned home from the hospital to be with his family when death was imminent. Death was not a taboo and was openly discussed with patients and their families. The physician had a major role in managing the moment of death.

During the second half of the 20th century interest in the care of dying patients has steadily grown, stimulated in the last decade by the growth of the hospice movement. It is likely that, because of this interest, the general physician again will be able to manage many dying patients in their own homes.

*Kripa S. Kashyap, M.D., contributed to this chapter in the first and second editions of this book.

SOCIOPSYCHOLOGICAL ISSUES

Fear of Death

Man is the only creature known who buries his dead; this he has done since the very dawn of human culture, possibly as far back as 50,000 B.C. Before the 11th century A.D., life after death was seen as a kind of sleep for an indeterminate period. Death was calmly accepted, without fear. Then the concept of the Last Judgment began to be taken seriously. An awe and fear of death became manifest in art and culture. The image of purgatory, heaven, and hell, which preoccupied the mind of medieval man, continues to exert its influence on a significant sector of society today.

Although aware that death is his ultimate fate, contemporary man is often incapable of facing his own death. In the unconscious, death is always the death of the other. The fear of death is intricately linked with the facing of the finality of one's being and the separation from one's loved ones. Therefore, it is unusual for a person to reflect upon death unless his own life is threatened or unless a close friend or relative is dying.

Fear of Dying

Fear of dying should not be confused with fear of death. Death is the ultimate moment of the cessation of life, and dying is the process whereby that moment is approached. Fear of dying is actually a combination of fear of death and fear of living in dread of death. Whether a man is dying at home or in a hospital, he cannot escape the agony of dying. Writings of doctors who attended many deaths at home give vivid descriptions of patients ravaged by pain and disease to such a point that they were either beyond caring or were a foul-smelling embarrassment to their family and friends. On the other hand, dying in a hospital's impersonal environment surrounded by machines and by unfamiliar staff cannot be glamorized either. The technology that has given us the knowledge and equipment to prolong life is greatly responsible for "the medicalization of death" that we see today. Death is no longer synonymous with the irreversible loss of consciousness. It is a technical phenomenon obtained by cessation of care based upon the decision of the doctor and the family. The management of a dying patient ends with the onset of irreversible coma—and what is left afterward is management of death. Death has been dissected and seen as a phenomenon of several steps—cessation of consciousness, cessation of breathing, and cessation of brain activity, manifested by a flat electroencephalogram. The contemporary fear of dying also involves the dread of such a protracted death.

The fear of dying is further compounded by the following factors: (*a*) helplessness over the hopelessness of the situation; (*b*) self-blame and guilt feelings; (*c*) fear of physical injury, multilation, and crippled existence; and (d) fear of being abandoned.

A dying person continues to hope for a miraculous recovery; but when the hopelessness of the treatment becomes quite evident, a strange sense of helplessness comes over the patient. He starts blaming himself for not having taken good care of himself. He may also feel guilty over his conduct and may see the terminal illness as some kind of punishment. The fear of physical injury and multilation from a drastic investigative procedure, chemo-, radio-, and/or surgical therapy is not to be discounted. Finally, the fear of a crippled existence and of being left alone to die in isolation away from family, friends, and children is present in the back of the mind of every terminal patient.

Emotional Reactions in the Face of Death

Terminally ill patients often go through a series of five stages in accepting the reality of their impending death (3). The duration of these stages and the intensity and sequence with which they are experienced are highly variable from one individual to the next. The stages are:

1. Shock and denial
2. Anger
3. Bargaining
4. Depression
5. Acceptance

During the first stage, when the patient is informed of his diagnosis and poor prognosis, he is usually unable to "hear" it. Some patients may be shocked and surprised temporarily, but a profound sense of disbelief in the physician's pronouncements keeps them calm. They may go from physician to physician to find someone to tell them what they would like to hear—that their condition is not serious. This denial of illness can be best summed up in a phrase—"No, not me." Eventually, all such attempts are deemed to be futile and the patient has to face reality.

During the stage of anger it may be difficult to deal with the patient. He complains about his care and, as a result, he may be avoided by his family, friends, and physicians. This rejection further increases his rage. He is likely to ask "Why me?" He often feels cheated and envious of others. If a person does not feel guilty and lose his self-esteem, he is likely, after this period of anger, to move on to the stage of bargaining. On the other hand, if he feels that he deserves punishment for his past doings as an explanation of his illness, he is likely to become very depressed. From being very "mad" he moves to being very "sad."

During the stage of bargaining the dominant theme is—"Yes, it is me, but. . . ." With the realization of an impending death the patient, in exchange for the prolongation of his life, offers to do things that he did not do before or to live his life differently. A number of patients go through a religious experience, and some

of them believe that they are "born again." Often at this stage the patient will look comfortable and peaceful, but that sense of well-being is short lived. As the illness advances and suffering is compounded, the patient becomes depressed.

During the stage of depression the reality of impending death sinks even deeper. The patient may have already gone through many real (and imagined) losses by this time, e.g., he may have lost a body organ, or he may have missed important events in the life of his family, or he may have lost his job or his savings. Depression at this stage is not so much compounded by anger as it is colored with resignation. The patient begins to separate himself from everyone and everything he loved before. At this time he does not want any false hopes. It is a very private and personal time in his life. He may not want any visitors and may not even say much to his own immediate family members. He wants his family's love, affection, and respect but may not be able to give them anything in return. He may exhaust his caregivers by developing regressive behavior patterns, such as failing to accomplish activities of daily living of which he is capable, making many small demands, and becoming incontinent. This stage is very difficult for the family.

Finally, when the patient has finished his business—experienced anger and experienced grief—he moves to the stage of acceptance. If the patient has the strong support of his family, he will go through all stages to arrive at his final stage of equanimity characterized by tranquility—where the patient is neither happy nor sad. He may simply say "My time is coming close," "It is all right," or "I am ready," etc..

CARE OF A DYING PERSON

The vast majority of patients who experience prolonged but predictable dying are patients with the terminal stage of cancer or, nowadays, AIDS. This discussion focuses on terminal care for such patients, much or all of which can be provided out of hospital. Chapters 8 and 34, respectively, describe the care of the cancer patient and the AIDS patient before the terminal stage.

Throughout the care of a patient with terminal illness, it is important to determine the physical stage of the illness but also the patient's psychological stage of accepting impending death (see above) and the patient's concerns regarding his family or his affairs. Terminally ill patients' needs differ widely, and every effort should be made to provide care that is adapted to these unique needs.

Communication

Communication of Diagnosis, Treatment Plan, and Prognosis

People have different opinions about the need and importance of communication of the diagnosis, treatment plan, and prognosis of terminal patients. A common practice in the past has been to maintain a conspiracy of silence in which the patient's physician in collusion with family members has covered up the diagnosis of a terminal illness in order to "protect" the dying patient from emotional shock. This practice is now recognized usually to be wrong. Honesty and sincerity in dealing with terminally ill patients make effective management possible. Although most patients become temporarily demoralized in the face of this news, they appreciate the truth in the long run. Moreover, it is then easier for their families to relate to them in an open and honest manner. Families participating in a conspiracy of silence have greater emotional difficulties than do families in situations in which truth has prevailed. Occasionally, a patient will indicate that he does not want to know the unpleasant truth; in that case, one should respect the patient's wish. However, invariably these patients come to know the nature of their illness even if it has not been told directly to them.

When the physician is ready to discuss the diagnosis and expected course of the illness with a terminally ill patient, a number of considerations can be very helpful: it is important to sit down with the patient and his family in a private place, to avoid lengthy introductions, to be precise and concise and not hurried, and to pay attention to the emotional reactions of the patient and of the family members, responding with silent pauses, followed by verbal acknowledgement of the patient's emotional reactions, rather than providing details about the patient's disease. It is also important not to use euphemisms (such as swelling, tumor, lump), but to acknowledge the presence of "cancer," or "malignant disease" and to pledge to help to reduce suffering as much as possible, affirming that one will be involved and supportive to the very end. A majority of patients "do not hear" the bad news when it is first delivered and must be told the truth in small doses in the course of several interviews.

Often terminally ill patients receive attention during the early stages of their illness, but that attention wanes as their disease progresses. This occurs largely because of the helplessness that others feel when confronting the patient's plight. The stages of denial, anger, and depression often cause a withdrawal of family, friends, physicians, and other caregivers; and these behaviors establish a vicious cycle, i.e., the more the patient is ignored, the more unmanageable and inaccessible he becomes. For these reasons, a most important principle of the care of a terminal patient is for all parties to maintain a consistency of involvement. The physician should counsel family members in this regard and should plan regular contacts with the patient, either by scheduling office visits or making visits to the home. These physician actions can reduce the patient's anguish, making it easier for him to express feelings and ask questions. Above all, continued and consistent involvement of physician, family, and other caregivers gives dignity to the dying person. The patient continues to feel like a person till the very end.

Advance Directives from the Patient

There is good evidence that patients with terminal illness would welcome early in their clinical course a discussion of the degree and type of support they wish to receive as they become more ill. One recent study (7) revealed that almost 80% of patients with terminal cancer would not want ventilators or other life-support treatment and 50% would want only treatment directed at comfort and pain relief. Ninety percent favored the routine availability of living wills or proxy designation. The majority felt that discussions of these issues should occur early after the diagnosis of a serious illness. Other data suggest that most physicians remain hesitant to initiate discussions of advance directives with patients, especially early in the course of the illness (9). It is important for the physician to help patients and families express their preferences, since patients' preferences frequently are not to have heroic treatment or even continuing supportive care at the end of their terminal illness. These discussions, difficult as they are, will spare the patient inappropriate interventions and help maintain dignity during the dying process. Chapter 6 (Geriatric Medicine: Special Considerations) describes in detail the process of helping patients to delineate advance directives.

The educational organization *Concern for Dying* provides helpful information regarding living wills and other ways to protect the autonomy of a dying person. (Address: 250 West 57th Street, New York, New York, 10107. Telephone: 212-246-6962.)

Communication with the Patient's Family

The emotional problems of the family of the dying person need attention from the physician. Family members go through stages of emotional adjustment and have difficulties in accepting the diagnosis and projected course of a terminal illness, just as the patient does. By encouraging open communication between the patient and his family, the physician can make an important contribution in the care of the dying person. Each family member will react differently to the impending death of a person, depending on their age, personality, role, and relationship with the patient and the rest of the family. To be effective, the physician must be sensitive to these factors and allocate time to meet the needs of individual family members.

The important advice to family members includes the fact that a dying person has a great need to have access to his children and the children have a great need to be close to their dying parent. The physician should encourage these necessary contacts. In addition, the family should be urged to find ways to gratify small needs of the patient. Removing restrictions from food, alcohol, and cigarettes is not only humane but sensible. Considerations such as these are described in an excellent booklet for families, *Taking Time*, available from the National Cancer Institute, Bethesda, Maryland, 20205. It was prepared by terminal cancer patients and their families to help others to deal with many draining and awkward experiences that they will face.

Management of Pain, Anxiety, Depression, Delirium

Pain

A large number of cancer patients have significant pain during the terminal stage of their illness. Therefore, a very basic principle in the care of these patients is to provide adequate relief of pain. This often requires the administration of narcotics. Because of the physician's fear of inducing addiction, patients may receive doses of narcotics that are too small or too infrequent to relieve pain adequately. Physicians should be aware that the risk of addiction, in this setting, is slight and that narcotics should be given on schedule (not "as occasion requires"), including at night, when it is preferable to disturb the patient for his medication and not to wait for pain to waken him.

Another misconception about narcotic use in cancer patients concerns tolerance. Many cancer patients on narcotics do not develop tolerance and are able to remain on the same dose of medication for prolonged periods of time. When tolerance does occur it usually manifests itself as a decrease in the duration of analgesia and can be treated by shortening the dose interval or increasing the dose or both. When the requirement for medication increases, this is frequently caused by disease progression rather than the development of tolerance. Rarely massive doses become necessary (e.g., hydromorphone, 200 mg per hour intravenously). Physical dependence (abstinence syndrome occurring at the time of abrupt withdrawal of narcotics) will develop within two weeks of the initiation of narcotic therapy in most patients.

Important considerations in selecting medication for pain are effectiveness, route of administration (e.g., the cachectic patient may have few sites for injections), available forms for oral administration (e.g., some patients may be able to take only liquids easily; liquid morphine is especially useful for such patients), and duration of pain relief. Table 19.1 summarizes practical information about a number of narcotics that are used in controlling pain.

In order to determine the appropriate dose of a narcotic, pain control should be assessed approximately 1 hour after a dose is given. If the patient reports that he is not getting good relief from pain, the next dose should be higher. In order to determine the appropriate interval between doses, pain control should be assessed at the end of an interval. If the patient reports that pain control regularly abates before the next dose of narcotic, the dosing interval should be reduced.

In evaluating pain control over time, it is helpful to use a visual analogue scale, such as the scale illustrated in Fig. 19.1, providing an ongoing record of the effectiveness of pain treatment (6). Sometimes pain control is inadequate with oral or intramuscular medication. Constant infusion of narcotics may provide more even and satisfactory pain relief. In these instances, morphine or hydromorphone is usually prescribed. If the doses required are not too high, the subcutaneous route may be used (limited by volume requirements and absorption characteristics) and a small portable pump allows mobility. Larger doses require constant intravenous access, which usually (especially if a home disposition is desired) requires a permanent indwelling intravenous catheter. One must be careful not to chose this complicated treatment plan too readily. Appropriate use of oral narcotics will be effective most of the time.

All narcotic analgesics may cause the following *side effects:* sedation, respiratory depression, emesis, suppression of cough, constipation, bladder spasm, or urinary retention. The synthetic narcotics may cause less nausea and constipation than does morphine; however, they may also produce less euphoria than morphine at equivalent analgesic doses.

Nausea and constipation are extremely common side effects of narcotic usage in terminal cancer patients and should be actively treated. Phenothiazines are effective for nausea. Prochlorperazine (Compazine, 10 mg orally or intramuscularly or 25 mg by suppository every 4 to 6 hours) causes less sedation and hypotension than chlorpromazine. The latter is the preferred drug in a bed-bound patient when sedation is desired. Haloperidol (.5 mg to 2 mg orally or subcutaneously every 6 to 8 hours) is useful for nausea in the agitated patient. Metachlopromide (Reglan, 10 to 20 mg orally or intramuscularly every 6 hours) is useful if gastric fullness is a common complaint. Dexamethasone (8 mg every 8 hours) may also be helpful in the nauseated patient and scopolamine (.4 mg to .6 mg subcutaneously every 4 hours) is useful for intractable retching.

Constipation is a universal problem in the terminal cancer patient who is taking narcotics and should be treated prophylactically. Bulk laxatives require an adequate intake of food to be effective and have little use in the terminal patient. A stool softener alone is rarely effective for narcotic-induced constipation. More useful, sequential strategies are the following:

1. Daily use of a preparation that combines a stool softener and a mild laxative such as dioctyl sodium, sulfosuccinite plus casanthranol (Peri-Colace, 1 daily–2 TID) or docusate sodium plus senna (Senikot 1 daily–4 TID).
2. If no success, add bisacodyl (Dulcolax, 5 mg by mouth at bedtime–15 mg TID or Milk of Magnesium, 30–60 cc once or twice daily).
3. If still unsuccessful, add lactulose (Chronulac, 10 grams/15 cc, 30–45 cc HS-BID).
4. If constipation continues, check for impaction. If present with a hard stool, try glycerine suppositories or olive oil retention enemas. If no impaction, add bisacodyl suppositories (Dulcolax, 10 mg) or Fleets enema.

There are other helpful adjunctive measures for the

Table 19.1.
Selected Drugs for Treating Pain

Constituents	Trade Name	Available Preparations	Usual Dose Range[a]	Approximate Equivalent IM Dose of Morphine	Peak Effect (Hr)	Duration (Hr)	Federal Narcotic Schedule
		MODERATELY POTENT					
Codeine phosphate		Tablets 30,60 mg	30–120 mg	2–10 mg	2	3–4	II
		Injectable 10 mg/5 ml					
Codeine-acetaminophen[b]	Tylenol No. 3	Tablets 30 mg codeine	1–2 tablets	2 mg	2	3–4	III
		Tablets 60 mg codeine	1 tablet		2	3–4	
	Tylenol No. 4	Elixir 12 mg codeine/5 ml	15–30 ml				
Oxycodone aspirin-phenacetin-caffeine	Percodan	Tablets 5 mg oxycodone	1–3 tablets	2–4 mg	1	13–4	II
Oxycodone acetaminophen	Tylox[c]	Capsules 5 mg oxycodone	1–3 capsules	2–4 mg	1	3–4	II
	Percocet[b]	Tablets 5 mg oxycodone	1–3 tablets	2–4 mg			
Oxycodone	Roxicodone	Tablets 5 mg	1–3 tablets	2–4 mg	1	3–4	
		Liquid 5 mg/5 ml	5–15 ml	2–4 mg	1	3–4	
		MOST POTENT					
Morphine sulfate[a]		Injectable l0 mg/ml		10 mg	1	3–4	
		Liquid multiple Concentrations	20–200mg	4–40 mg	½	2–3	
		Tablets 30 mg	30–90 mg	5–15 mg	1	3–4	
	MS Contin	Controlled release tablets 30, 60 mg	30–180 mg	5–30 mg	3	8–12	
	RMS suppository	Suppository 5, 10, 20, 30 mg	30–90 mg	5–30 mg	1	3–4	
Methadone[d]	Dolophine	Tablets 5, 10 mg	2.5–20 mg	4–10 mg	2	4–5	II
		Injectable 10 mg/ml		10 mg			
Meperidine	Demerol	Tablets 50, 100 mg	50–300 mg	2–10 mg	2	3–4	II
		Syrup 50 mg/5 ml					
		Injectable 25 mg/ml 50 mg/ml 75 mg/ml 100 mg/ml	50–150 mg	4–10 mg	1	2–4	
Hydromorphone	Dilaudid	Tablets 1, 2, 3, 4 mg	2–8 mg	4–10 mg	1	3–4	II
		Suppository 3 mg					
		Injectable 1 mg/ml 2 mg/ml 3 mg/dl 4 mg/ml	1–2 mg	10 mg	½	3	
Levorphanol[d]	Levo-Dro-moran	Tablets 2 mg	2–4 mg	5–10 mg	2	4–5	II
		Injectable 2 mg/ml	2 mg	10 mg	1	4–5	

[a]Higher doses needed in patients who develop tolerance.
[b]Each tablet contains 300 mg acetaminophen.
[c]Each capsule contains 500 mg acetaminophen.
[d]The plasma half-life of methadone and levorphanol is long (>15 hr), and cumulative effects may occur with continual use of these drugs.

cancer patient with pain. Nonsteroidal anti-inflammatory drugs are frequently helpful for many types of pain, especially bone pain. Tricyclic antidepressants may be helpful for neuropathic pain especially if associated with insomnia or depression. Corticosteroids are useful for spinal cord compression, brain tumors, and other nerve compression syndromes. They also, at least in the short run, increase appetite, mood, and general sense of well-being. Methylphenidate (Ritalin) may be useful to combat the lethargy of analgesics. L-Tryptophan (2 to 4 g per day) has been shown to help

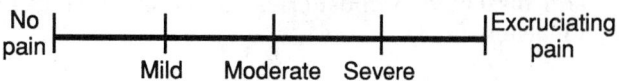

Figure 19.1 Visual analogue scale for rating pain severity.

some patients with neuropathic pain. Transcutaneous nerve stimulation may temporarily be helpful for localized (particularly neuropathic) pain. A number of psychological approaches (hypnosis, relaxation training, distraction techniques) have also been found to be useful for the cancer patient with pain.

Anxiety

The physician's concern and accessibility may be all that are necessary to relieve the anxiety of the dying patient. Anxiolytic drugs also can be of some help in the management of these patients. Commonly prescribed anxiolytic drugs belong to the benzodiazepine group; their use for the control of anxiety is described in detail in Chapter 13. When insomnia is also a major problem, a benzodiazepine hypnotic can be used to induce sleep (see Table 85.6). Hydroxyzine (Atarax, Vistaril), an antihistamine tranquilizer, has a number of properties that may make it more beneficial than one of the benzodiazepines. It has not only sedative but also antispasmodic, antiemetic, and (when given intramuscularly) analgesic effects. In this regard, hydroxyzine has advantages over phenothiazines, which are not analgesic and which may produce hypotension. Hydroxyzine, 25 to 50 mg by mouth three times daily, is often prescribed to patients who have anxiety as the result of prolonged pain.

Depression

Most patients go through the depressive stage without requiring antidepressant medications, although periodically some may require antianxiety medications. The family's and the physician's support is most therapeutic for this kind of depression. Some patients develop severe depression, particularly after a brief stage of anger when they conclude that they are being punished for their sins. Loss of self-esteem, guilt feelings, psychomotor retardation, early morning awakening with a diurnal variation in mood, even suicidal thoughts may appear in this setting. When a number of these and other indicators of a major depression are present, tricyclic antidepressants may bring relief. There is a detailed discussion of the use of these drugs in Chapter 15.

Delirium

Periodic or persistent delirium (inattentiveness, inaccessibility, nonrecognition of loved ones, gross confusion, etc.) is very common in the final days or weeks of terminal disease (4). The cause is almost always an identifiable metabolic derangement, excess analgesic or psychotropic medication, tumor metastasis to the brain, or a combination of these factors. Loss of clear communication due to delirium is very distressing to the patient's family. Management of easily reversible causes is therefore very important except in the patient whose death is imminent. A list of the principal causes of delirium is found in Chapter 17.

Hospice Care

In many communities, patients and their families can be cared for by their physician in cooperation with a hospice, a program devised to provide terminal care, including relief of pain, to the dying patient and to provide support to his family. Services are delivered either in the patient's home or in a hospital or other hospice facility by a multidisciplinary team under the direction of the physician.

In hospice care the primary focus changes from curing to caring, and the overall goal changes from prolongation of life to the enhancement of the quality of life during the patient's final days. Since the introduction of the hospice movement in the United States and founding of the first hospice here in 1974, hospice programs have been developed in virtually every community, and most third party payors now provide hospice benefits. Eligibility criteria for hospice benefits under Medicare are the following: the patient must be terminally ill with a life expectancy of 6 months or less, be unable to benefit from further aggressive (curative) therapy, be able to receive most (80%, by law) care at home, and have a caregiver (relative or friend) who will assume the responsibility for custodial care of the patient and be the decision maker in the event the patient becomes no longer competent to make decisions.

The mushrooming of hospice programs may create an erroneous impression that hospice type care can only be provided in hospices. Comprehensive humanistic treatment for the dying patient and his family can be offered by any physician. Home health agencies can play a pivotal role in this care (see Chapter 9). The essential ingredients of the delivery of hospice-type care at home are physician knowledge and skill in prescribing for symptom relief, willingness and ability to work with a multidisciplinary team, and willingness to spend extra time and effort to foresee and alleviate the problems faced by the dying patient and his family.

Dying patients and their families especially appreciate the assurance that the place of care can be changed at appropriate moments from acute medical services to hospice services or to home, and families appreciate the physician's willingness to pronounce the patient in the home when the patient has voiced a preference for death at home.

A clearinghouse for information on hospice care in the United States is provided by the National Hospice Organization, 1750 Old Meadow Road, McLean, Virginia, 22102.

MANAGEMENT OF GRIEF

If death of a loved one has been unexpected, grief usually begins with an initial stage of shock and disbelief accompanied by a general numbing of all affect. If death has been anticipated, however, this stage is less prominent. There is often a feeling of relief that the dead person's suffering has ended. Soon afterward (within hours to a few days) there is a more demonstrative phase characterized by protest and anguish, often accompanied by tears. These feelings come in waves and may be precipitated by even an indirect reference to the lost person; ordinarily, they do not persist for more than 1 or 2 months. Other symptoms of mourning normally occur throughout the first year after the death of a loved one. During this year, survivors are continuing to grieve while they reorient their lives. As time passes there often is a preoccupation with memories of the lost person. Guilt feelings for not having done enough for the deceased are very common. In some cases, this guilt may be expressed as hostility toward the physician. Bereaved people often have the experience of "seeing" the dead person in a crowd or in some other individual fleetingly, which is then followed by the reality of permanent loss. The bereaved is likely to visit the grave during the first year of loss more frequently than in later years. Sometimes, there is a dramatic change in personality, and the manners and the terminal symptoms of the dying individual are assumed by the bereaved person. This is another way of resolving grief, by attempting to make the lost person a part of the survivor.

Approximately 80% of bereaved people are depressed and have disturbed sleep; and 40% have a poor appetite, weight loss, difficulty in concentrating, and general loss of interest in daily life (1). Depression is especially common in spouses in the middle or later years of their lives. In fact, one-third of this latter group have symptoms that meet the criteria for the diagnosis of a major depression (Chapter 15) (2). Although depression usually lasts for many months, 80% of individuals show improvement within 10 weeks. However, two-thirds of bereaved spouses at the end of the first year of bereavement continue to have some symptoms of apathy, aimlessness, and a disinclination to look to the future. Only a small fraction of these survivors develop complicated and/or atypical mourning.

The *management of normal grief* during the first year of bereavement should be individualized, depending on the patient's personal, family, and social background. All bereaved persons need to be reminded that their grief and its psychophysiological concomitants are normal. This has to be done with special care, acknowledging the irreparable loss while encouraging them to lead a full life without feeling guilty. Bereavement support groups exist in many communities and are usually known to clergy and social workers. Sharing feelings with others who have lost a loved one may be particularly helpful during this lonely time. A physician's encouragement can be important in helping a grieving person decide to seek such support. When severe emotional reactions become prolonged, pastoral counseling or psychotherapy may be necessary.

Bereaved persons may present with new somatic symptoms or amplification of pre-existing symptoms. When evaluation reveals no change in physical status, the management strategies suggested for adjustment disorders are appropriate (see Chapter 12). In time, with the completion of their grieving reaction, those patients will give up their physical symptoms and again become actively engaged in a new life.

Some bereaved persons may need short-term medication for the relief of insomnia and anxiety. A benzodiazepine hypnotic (Chapter 85) at bedtime if needed for sleep, or one of the anxiolytic benzodiazepines with a short half-life (Chapter 13) two or three times a day as needed for anxiety, should be considered for 1 to 2 weeks in the management of normal grief. On the other hand, many patients may feel quite satisfied with an empathetic and supportive physician.

An additional way in which a physician can be supportive early after a patient's death is to telephone or write to the family, acknowledging one's own sense of loss, supporting the family in what they have done to help in the terminal care of the patient, and inviting contacts at a later time. The latter idea is suggested by a finding that over half of bereaved spouses report that they had unanswered questions about their spouse's death 1 year later (8).

During the first year of bereavement special attention should be paid to the patient during holidays, anniversaries, or on other important dates. Some symptoms of acute grief are likely to resurface around these times. Supportive therapy at such times will usually control the symptoms.

The physician is in a good position to detect the early signs of pathological mourning when a person either shows no signs of grieving or shows the exaggerated features of grieving characterized by excessive and/or prolonged (longer than a year) social isolation, unmoderated guilt or anger, panic attacks, and physical symptoms without any clear-cut organic etiology. In such cases, consultation with a psychiatrist is appropriate to help remove obstacles that have inhibited the mourner from undergoing a normal grief reaction (5).

General References

Bowlby J: *Separation*. New York, Basic Books, 1973.
This is the second volume of Bowlby's classic work on attachment and loss, and deals with the issues of anxiety and anger generated in the anticipation of and in the event of separation from a loved one.

Bowlby J: *Loss*. New York, Basic Books, 1980.
This is the third and final volume of Bowlby's work on attachment and loss. This is probably the best book ever written on the subject of bereavement.

Bulkin W, Lukashok MS: Rx for dying: the case of hospice. *N Engl J Med* 318:376–378, 1988.
Editorial-review, contains Medicare hospice guidelines and references to recent literature on the hospice movement in the United States.

Keubler-Ross E: *On Death and Dying*. New York, Macmillan, 1969.
A classic work on the subject of death and dying.

Nelson T: *It's Your Choice, the Practical Guide to Planning a Funeral*. Glenview, IL, Scott, Foresman, and Co., 1982.
A practical paperback on making funeral plans in the face of impending death.

Reuler JB, Girard DA, Nardone DA: The chronic pain syndrome: misconceptions and management. *Ann Intern Med* 93:588, 1980.
Excellent review by general internists that covers both psychogenic and organic aspects of chronic pain, physiology of placebo effect, drug treatment of terminal cancer pain, nondrug modalities (transcutaneous nerve stimulation, acupuncture, neurological block/ablation biofeedback, hypnosis, behavior modification).

Saunders C (ed): *The Management of Terminal Disease*. Chicago, Year Book, 1978.
This book is an excellent guide to any professional involved in the care of a dying patient; it includes a complete discussion of the hospice concept.

Zimmerman JM, et al: *Hospice: Complete Care for the Terminally Ill*. 2nd ed. Baltimore, Urban and Schwarzenberg, 1986.
Well-referenced and practical book that covers all practical aspects of the hospice approach to terminal care.

Specific References

1. Clayton PJ, Halikas JA, Maurice WL: The bereavement of the widowed. *Dis Nerv Syst* 32:597, 1971.
2. Clayton PJ, Halikas JA, Maurice WL: The depression of widowhood. *Br J Psychiatry* 120:71, 1972.

3. Keubler-Ross E: *On Death and Dying.* Chapters 3–7, New York, Macmillan, 1969.
4. Massie MJ, Holland J, Glass E: Delirium in terminally ill cancer patients. *Am J Psychiatry* 140:1048, 1983.
5. Melges FT, DeMaso DR: Grief-resolution therapy: relieving, revising, and revisiting. *Am J Psychother* 34:51, 1980.
6. Partenoy RK: Practical aspects of pain control in the patient with cancer. *Cancer (Phila)* 38:327, 1988.
7. Steinberg MD, et al: Patient preference for treatment options and advance directives in terminal care (abstract). *Pract Am Soc Clin Oncol* 7:268, 1988.
8. Tolle SW, Bascom PB, Hickam DH, Benson Jr. JA: Communication between physicians and surviving spouses following patient deaths. *J Gen Intern Med* 1:309, 1986.
9. Wanzev SH, Federman DO, Adelstein ST, et al: The physician's responsibility toward hopelessly ill patients. *N Engl J Med* 320:844, 1989.

CHAPTER 20

Tobacco Use and Dependence*

GEORGE E. BIGELOW, Ph.D.
CAROL S. HAINES, M.D., M.P.H.

Chronic tobacco use, primarily in the form of cigarette smoking, is the greatest single cause of chronic illness, disability, and death in the United States. The perniciousness of the habit relates largely to a long history of social acceptability and to the reluctance by society to recognize and respond to smoking as a health-damaging behavior.

PREVALENCE OF TOBACCO USE

1987 prevalence data (from the National Health Interview Survey of Cancer Epidemiology and Control) for cigarette smoking are summarized in Table 20.1. Subgroup analysis of these data showed that black men were more likely to smoke (39%) than white men (30.5%) and that smoking rates for black women (26.7%) and white women (28%) were the same. Prevalence data for the use of noncigarette tobacco by men are summarized in Table 20.2 (see "Other Forms of Tobacco Use," below).

ETIOLOGY AND RISK FACTORS

The determinants of tobacco use and dependence are multiple and variable. The smoking habit is so widespread that it defies substantial correlation with discrete environmental, physiological, or psychological factors. Smoking typically begins in the teenage years or in early adulthood. Social influences (e.g., peer pressures, efforts to display independence and to appear mature and self-confident) are major factors in promoting and sustaining initial smoking experiences. The aversive properties of those initial experiences (e.g., coughing, nausea, dysphoria) are described even by individuals who subsequently develop into chronic

Table 20.1.
Percentage of Adults Who Smoke Cigarettes, by Sex and Age—United States, 1987[a]

Age (yrs)	Men	Women	Total
18–24	28.1	26.1	27.1
25–44	35.6	30.8	33.2
45–64	33.5	28.6	30.9
65–74	20.2	18.0	19.0
≥75	11.3	7.5	8.9
Total	**31.2**	**26.5**	**28.8**

[a]From Centers for Disease Control Morbidity and Mortality Weekly Report: 38:685, 1989.

Table 20.2.
Percentage of Men Who Use Noncigarette Tobacco,[a] by Age and Form of Smokeless Tobacco or Alternative Smoking Method—United States, 1987[b]

Age (yrs)	Smokeless Tobacco Form		Alternative Smoking Method	
	Chewing Tobacco	Snuff	Pipes	Cigars
18–24	5.5	6.4	0.8	1.6
25–44	3.2	3.1	2.9	5.8
45–64	3.9	1.6	5.1	7.0
65–74	5.0	1.9	5.0	5.2
≥75	6.1	2.7	4.1	3.9
Total	**4.0**	**3.1**	**3.4**	**5.3**

[a]Prevalence of use among women was ≤0.5%.
[b]From Centers for Disease Control Morbidity and Mortality Weekly Report: 38:685, 1989.

*Maxine L. Stitzer, Ph.D., contributed to this chapter in the first and second editions.

dependent smokers. Nicotine is recognized to be the pharmacological agent responsible for maintaining the habit.

Certain risk factors are associated with an increased likelihood of becoming a chronic cigarette smoker. Chief among these is *family history*. Cigarette smoking runs in families, and this is generally thought to be due to a social modeling process. An individual with parents and siblings who smoke is 4 times as likely to become a smoker as is an individual from a nonsmoking family. Although living with other smokers is often an obstacle to quitting, it can sometimes be used persuasively to motivate parents with young children to stop smoking in an effort to reduce the likelihood that their children will adopt the habit. The possibility of genetic or physiological predisposing factors accounting for this familial aggregation has received little study, but data from twin studies suggest some genetic contribution.

Because smokers almost universally begin the habit during *adolescence or early adulthood*, age is a significant risk factor for initiation of smoking; it is the rare smoker who acquires the habit at an age beyond the early twenties. In the past males were more likely to smoke than females, but this is no longer the case. There is an inverse relationship between smoking prevalence and socioeconomic status that will likely become more pronounced over the rest of this century. There is no personality type that is characteristic of smokers, but on average they tend to be somewhat more extroverted than nonsmokers, to be more adventuresome or risk taking, and to be more likely to deviate from social norms or rules. These latter characteristics may, in adolescence, increase the probability of experimenting with smoking—with a consequent increased risk of chronic dependence.

PRIMARY PREVENTION

Because of the relatively narrow age window when individuals are at risk for experimentation with tobacco products, it is necessary that primary prevention efforts be directed to adolescents and preadolescents. Unfortunately, the age of greatest risk is also the age of greatest resistance to the influence of parents and other authorities. Optimally, formal preventive interventions begin at the fourth to sixth grade and continue for several years. Not to be confused with teaching about the health risks of smoking, these interventions teach specific skills for resisting social pressure. All include explicit instructions and rehearsals with peers in vignettes about resisting offers to use cigarettes, alcohol products, and illegal drugs. Several completed trials of "resistance training" have shown that children who have had such training are either less likely to smoke or initiate smoking later than unexposed children (2, 18).

Primary prevention of smoking occurs in the home, in the classroom, and in the community at large. A major role for physicians is unlikely. As community health leaders, however, physicians should encourage and support families and schools in adopting resistance training. In the community at large physicians should also encourage restrictions on tobacco use in public areas, on sales to minors, and on advertising that glamorizes smoking.

COURSE OF THE HABIT

Until recently, the typical course of the habit was one of relatively unabated chronic smoking from the time of initiation throughout the remainder of the smoker's life. In more recent years, as the health hazards of smoking have become more widely recognized and as the social acceptability of smoking has declined, there has been a growing tendency for smokers to discontinue the habit. Now, in the United States there are nearly as many former smokers (approximately 40 million) as there are current smokers (approximately 50 million).

Most continuing smokers feel considerable ambivalence about their habit. Over one-half of current smokers report having made at least one serious attempt to stop smoking, and about 90% of smokers say they would like to quit if there were an easy method to do so. About 30% of smokers report that they have made an active attempt to stop smoking within the preceding year. As described below, advice from physicians can be a potent force in promoting increased cessation efforts by patients.

Patterns of Quitting and Relapse

Approximately 60 to 80% of smokers who attempt to quit achieve at least a minimal period of abstinence. However, the relapse rate is high, and approximately two-thirds of quitters resume smoking within 3 to 6 months, often within only a few days. Only 15 to 20% of quitters remain cigarette free for 6 months or more.

A cessation attempt should not be considered successful until at least 6 months of abstinence have been sustained. The probability of relapse after 6 months of abstinence is relatively small. About 1% of smokers permanently quit each year, yielding about one-half million new ex-smokers annually.

Smokers express interest in a wide variety of aids for cessation. Most popular are instructional and self-help aids that smokers can use at their own convenience. A substantial proportion of smokers express interest in formal cessation treatment programs; but when such services are offered, even at optimal cost and convenience, fewer than 10% of those expressing interest will actually attend. Because the long-term quit rate upon completion of such programs is about 20 to 30%, their overall public health impact is small.

Approximately 95% of smoking cessation occurs as the result of smokers' self-directed personal efforts, without formal treatment. Abrupt (so-called "cold turkey") cessation is more likely to be successful than are approaches involving gradual reduction. Most quitters require more than one attempt before becoming successful ex-smokers.

Cyclic quitting and relapse are characteristic of the normal, successful cessation process. The risk of relapse is increased (a) when patients are under emotional stress (e.g., anger, frustration, anxiety, depression); (b) when ex-smokers are exposed to cues associated with prior smoking (e.g., after meals, when consuming an alcoholic beverage); and (c) in individuals whose spouse or friends continue to smoke (23). Smokers are vulnerable to interpreting initial relapse as proof of an inability to quit.

HEALTH CONSEQUENCES

Risk of Disease

Although smoking dramatically increases overall population morbidity and mortality, its effects on individual smokers are unpredictable, and some smokers will escape major health consequences. The overall mortality rate for smokers is 70% greater than that for nonsmokers. Life expectancy is significantly shortened by smoking, (e.g., 8.1 years less for the 30-year-old, two-pack-a-day smoker than for a comparable nonsmoker). Risk is dose related in that it increases with increasing number of cigarettes smoked, with increasing number of years smoking, with depth of inhalation, and with increasing yield of tar and nicotine of the cigarettes smoked.

Smoking is associated with increased risk of cancer (especially of the respiratory tract), cardiovascular disease, chronic obstructive pulmonary disease, gastric ulcer, and postmenopausal osteoporosis. Smoking by pregnant women reduces fetal growth, and therefore birth weight, and increases the risk of fetal death; smoking interacts with the use of oral contraceptives by women and increases their risk of myocardial infarction, subarachnoid hemorrhage, and thromboembolic disease.

The risks of cancer and of chronic pulmonary disease in smokers are ten-fold the risks in nonsmokers. The risk of atherosclerotic cardiovascular disease is approximately doubled in smokers. Because of the much greater population prevalence of cardiovascular disease, it is in this area that the greatest overall health benefits of smoking cessation occur.

Benefits of Cessation

The greatest immediate benefit of smoking cessation is the reduction of cardiovascular risk. Within hours of smoking cessation both carbon monoxide and nicotine, the two cigarette products thought to be primarily responsible for cardiovascular disease, are dissipated from the body, with a consequent reduction in cardiac work requirement concurrent with an increase in oxygenation. There is also prompt reduction in the risk for upper respiratory infection. Slower to accrue is a reduction in the rate of pulmonary decline and a reduction in cancer risk; benefits of cessation are measurable in these domains within 3 to 5 years after smoking cessation.

Health benefits of smoking cessation are greater for those smokers who quit before the development of symptoms; however, the benefits of cessation can extend to those individuals who have already experienced symptoms of smoking-related disease. For example, individuals who stop smoking after myocardial infarction have improved survival rates compared with those who continue smoking (3).

Low Yield Cigarettes

Because the risks of smoking are dose related, it is reasonable to advise patients that, even in the absence of total cessation, risks are decreased by reducing the amount of smoke intake. This might be achieved by any of a variety of techniques—reducing the number of cigarettes smoked, taking fewer or smaller puffs per cigarette, inhaling less, or switching to a cigarette with lower tar and nicotine yield. Epidemiological data generally indicate that the overall risks are lower among individuals smoking lower yield cigarettes. However, as a cautionary note, it should be mentioned that these epidemiological data were generally collected at a time when the average tar and nicotine yield of marketed cigarettes was considerably higher than it is today. In the mid-1950s the average yield was 2 to 3 times that of present day cigarettes; the extent to which the earlier data can be extrapolated to the present era is not clear. Several reports have appeared in recent years suggesting that variations in current tobacco yields may have relatively little health impact (14, 25).

When patients switch to lower yield cigarettes, they should be cautioned not to change the pattern of their smoking in a compensatory fashion that could maintain the same biological intake of smoke—e.g., by smoking more cigarettes or inhaling more smoke. Extensive research has documented that such compensatory behavioral changes are common when cigarette yields are changed (11, 26). Cross-sectional studies of smokers have found negligible correlations between the stated yield of the brand smoked and blood levels of nicotine and its major metabolite, cotinine (1). The primary manufacturing technique for producing current low yield cigarettes is to place ventilation holes in the sides of the filter to dilute the smokestream with air. With these low yield brands it is especially likely that biological delivery will significantly exceed assay delivery since the smoker's fingers will tend partially to block these ventilation holes (15). Thus, it appears that biological yield may differ substantially from the yield values published by the Federal Trade Commission.

Abstinence Syndrome and Craving

Upon cessation of smoking, an abstinence syndrome typically occurs (13). The physiological correlates of the tobacco abstinence syndrome are generally inconsequential, consisting of a slight and gradual decline in heart rate and blood pressure. However, the subjective aspects of the syndrome can be very distressing to patients. Symptoms can include irritability, restlessness, sleep disturbances, difficulty in concentrating, anxiety, gastrointestinal disturbances, hunger, weight gain, and, most important, craving for cigarettes. Relatively little is known about the course of the tobacco abstinence syndrome, but most patients feel normal again within approximately 2 weeks of abstinence, except that craving for tobacco may persist for months or years (9, 24).

Recently nicotine chewing gum has been approved as a prescription drug in the United States (see details below). Its primary purpose is to facilitate tobacco abstinence by suppressing the abstinence syndrome. Prior to the availability of nicotine gum there was no specific treatment available for the tobacco abstinence syndrome.

Craving for tobacco is an extraordinarily persistent obstacle to sustained abstinence. More than an occasional ex-smoker reports craving 5 or even 10 years after cessation. The duration of craving is highly variable, but it should be expected to persist for at least 3 to 6 months, with its frequency and urgency diminishing over that interval.

Passive Smoking

Passive smoking—exposure of nonsmokers to air contaminated by the smoking of others—is not only an irritant to many nonsmokers; it has definite adverse health effects. Although the levels of smoke products detected in the blood and urine of passively exposed nonsmokers are low relative to those in smokers, there are significantly increased health risks associated with passive smoking (7). Passive exposure to the smoke of spouses has been associated with impaired pulmonary function, increased lung cancer risk, and increased coronary heart disease risk. Children passively exposed to smoker parents have increased rates of respiratory infections and slower developmental increases in pulmonary function capacity. Maternal smoking contributes to reduced birth weight, and smokers who stop the habit during pregnancy have significantly heavier babies than those who continue smoking (22).

The adverse effects of smoking upon other family members—and especially on young children—might be effectively used in persuading smokers to attempt cessation. Also, as a general practice, physicians should try to protect nonsmokers from cigarette smoke. Smoking (including employee smoking) should be considerately but emphatically prohibited in physicians' offices, and physicians should support similar efforts in all public settings, especially in health care facilities.

RECOGNITION AND DIAGNOSIS

Diagnostic Criteria

Nicotine dependence is now recognized as a diagnosable medical disorder in the American Psychiatric Associations 1987 *Diagnostic and Statistical Manual,* third edition revised (DSM-III-R). The diagnostic criteria are identical to those for other substance use disorders, reflecting the growing recognition of extensive commonalities among alcoholism, drug abuse, and tobacco dependence. The criteria are satisfied by any three of the following (only those items relevant to nicotine dependence are listed): an unsuccessful attempt to or persistent desire to cut down or quit; withdrawal symptoms on cessation; use to avoid or relieve withdrawal symptoms; continued use despite a problem caused or exacerbated by use; giving up important social, occupational, or recreational activities because of use (e.g., not going places where smoking is not permitted); a great deal of time spent in getting or using the addictive substance (e.g., chain smoking); use in larger amounts or for longer durations than intended.

Recording Smoking Status

The greatest impediment to effective professional response to smoking is the widespread failure of health professionals either to recognize and diagnose tobacco dependence or to treat it as an active problem when it is identified. Tobacco use status (i.e., smoker, nonsmoker) is often an item recorded only at initial contact and soon buried in the medical record. However, since prospective guidance is basic to primary care, smoking status should be considered at every visit. Determination of status is most efficiently accomplished at the office reception point. For example, the receptionist can rapidly and routinely identify smokers by asking "Did you smoke at least one cigarette in the past seven days?" Positive responses should initiate action to prompt the physician to follow up. Attaching a questionnaire and/or a smoking cessation booklet (both described below) to the medical record can serve as an effective prompt to the physician. On subsequent visits, recognition of the smoking status and of the actions agreed upon at the previous visit are essential. Rates of follow-up of any previously initiated prevention activity will be disappointingly low with traditional progress note, flow chart, or problem list methods. A simple system of distinctive stickers with shorthand notes can lead to higher levels of provider attention at subsequent visits. This technique is discussed more below.

Objective Assessment

In virtually all patients the assessment of smoking status will be based solely upon patient self-report. However, under some conditions it may be desirable to assess smoking status with an objective biological assay. Three primary indices can be used: (*a*) thiocyanate, a product of the cyanide compounds in tobacco, can be measured in blood, saliva, or urine; (*b*) cotinine, the major metabolite of nicotine, can be measured in blood, saliva, or urine; or (*c*) carbon monoxide, a combustion product, can be measured in blood (as carboxyhemoglobin) or in expired breath. Although none of these is in routine clinical use, all are widely used in clinical research. Assessment of carbon monoxide (CO) concentrations in expired breath is the least intrusive and least expensive procedure and is widely used in smoking cessation programs. Devices for measuring breath CO that would be suitable for routine office use are currently marketed for about $1000. Some experts have suggested that office assessment of expired breath CO should become as routine as the recording of blood pressure. The value of objective assessment of smoking status is indicated by the fact that up to 20 to 30% of self-reported quitters show biological evidence of continuing to smoke.

TREATMENT

A three-step process for integrating smoking cessation advice into an office visit is described in detail below. Factors important in this process (physician communication skill, self-help guides, nicotine gum, dealing with weight gain and relapse) are described first.

Role of the Physician

Physicians can be effective in motivating smoking cessation when they use facilitative techniques. A major reason that patients stop smoking is concern about their health, and smokers cite physicians as the individuals most able to influence their decisions to attempt to quit. The appearance of specific smoking-related symptoms often serves as a stimulus for patients' efforts to break the smoking habit.

The most prevalent error in management of the smoking patient is to do nothing. Fewer than 25% of smokers report ever having any physician advise them to stop smoking.

Most smokers who quit the habit do so on their own, and this is the method that smokers overwhelmingly prefer. Therefore, the optimal physician's role in the treatment of tobacco dependence is to advise all smoking patients to stop and to have them agree to take a number of specific actions to facilitate self-directed quitting. It is a mistake to rely heavily on referral to smoking cessation programs. Results of referral attempts are disappointing when compared with those obtained by devoting equal or less time to a direct advice process, such as the three-step approach described below.

Research indicates that brief advice by a physician can significantly increase rates of smoking cessation (16); and medical economic analyses have shown that smoking cessation advice is as cost-effective as other common interventions, such as treatment of hypercholesterolemia or of mild hypertension (6). Studies have demonstrated a three-fold increase in smoking cessation rates (from 1 to 3%) when physicians simply cautioned each smoker to quit during routine office visits for other problems. Additional efforts beyond the cautionary advice yield even higher quit rates. Physicians who also provide a take-home pamphlet with how-to-quit suggestions have generated quit rates

of 7 to 12% in general practice. Investing a few more moments to negotiate a "quit date" in addition to delivering the cessation message increases the quit rate to 15%. Even higher cessation rates are reported in certain settings. For example, the smoking cessation rate after a first myocardial infarction is as high as 50% for patients given directive smoking cessation advice by their physician, compared with about 35% for patients receiving usual care (3). Similarly high rates of cessation are seen in prenatal care settings— where up to 20 to 30% of smokers may quit during a pregnancy (22).

It is important to recognize at the outset that the achieved rates of cessation are likely always to be frustratingly low. In an individual practice, small changes in smoking cessation rate will be unnoticed. However, in terms of overall health benefit to a patient population, routine smoking cessation advice from physicians can be very worthwhile; even the lowest figures cited above—a change from 1 to 3% cessation rates— would yield an additional 1 million ex-smokers per year in the United States.

There is a small minority of smokers who are so dramatically frustrating that physicians might overestimate the resistance of all smokers to cessation advice. The most extreme cases are those patients who smoke through tracheotomies or while in critical care units where oxygen is used. Discouragement because of these highly resistant patients should be avoided, since it can drain one of desire to assist more responsive and cessation-prone patients.

Communication Techniques

The physician is in a uniquely persuasive position as an authority figure but has limited specific remedies to offer the smoker. Therefore, one must provide advice and utilize motivation of techniques that will maximize the likelihood of patient compliance with a plan to quit. A common tendency in physician communication is excessive reliance upon fear as a motivator; fear is at best a weak motivator of complex behavior change and, at its worst, may stimulate denial and resistance that will actually inhibit behavior change. Patient commitment and confidence are strengthened by enumerating the non-health benefits of smoking cessation—its importance to significant others, the financial savings, the increased self-esteem, and sense of self-control that result.

The smoking advice to patients should be personally relevant, should describe in a positive way the benefits to be gained, and should prescribe a particular course of action. These three objectives can be attained (a) by pointing out the association between smoking and the specific symptoms, illnesses, or health risks of the individual patient; (b) by pointing out that smoking cessation can prevent, reverse, or stop the progression of disease (whichever is appropriate); and (c) by stating clearly, simply, and directively the course of action to be taken—to stop smoking. A general statement that "Smoking is bad for your health and you can kill yourself if you continue" fails on all three of these points. It is not specifically personal; it describes no benefit; and it is not sufficiently directive. Many patients will not perceive this as a medical instruction to stop smoking. More personalized and directive statements can be more persuasive, for example: "I strongly advise you to stop smoking; especially for people like you who use oral contraceptives the risk of heart disease or stroke is very substantially increased as long as you continue to smoke;" or "Both your coughing and your recurring colds and flus are caused in part by your smoking; I want you to try to quit smoking, and then we should see some improvement."

Brochures for Office Use

Self-help smoking cessation brochures can provide useful motivational and skill aids to smokers. A wide variety are available from the offices of the local heart, lung, or cancer societies or the National Institutes of Health. Table 20.3 provides information on several widely available brochures.

Nicotine Substitution

At this time, nicotine substitution treatment, with nicotine chewing gum, is the only recognized specific therapy for tobacco dependence. Clinical trials are in progress to evaluate the efficacy of transdermal nicotine patches, of higher doses of the gum preparation, and of other medications.

Nicotine gum (Nicorette) was approved in 1984 for marketing as a prescription drug in the United States. The gum—a nicotine resin complex—is to be initiated at the time that an individual stops smoking. The purpose of the gum is to reduce symptoms of the abstinence syndrome (see above) and thereby to prevent smoking relapse. The gum has documented therapeutic value when used in this way. *It is important to understand, however, that the gum is not intended for use by continuing smokers who hope that the nicotine substitution will induce either a cessation attempt or a reduction in smoking;* rather, it is to be used as an aid for maintaining smoking cessation once the patient has made the cessation decision and committed to that course. Thus, the prescribing physician must still engage in persuasion and motivation and in the selection/prescription of a quit date (see below).

Available data indicate that use of nicotine chewing gum may approximately double the likelihood of long-term smoking cessation. The absolute rates of cessation depend, of course, upon the context. In organized cessation programs use of the gum has led to cessation success rates of about 45% compared with about 20% in program participants receiving placebo gum (21). In general office practice prescription of nicotine gum in combination with brief directed cessation advice from the physician led to successful cessation in 9% of patients, compared with 4% in control patients receiving the advice without the gum (20). Similar results have been obtained in a family practice trial (27), using a procedure similar to the recommended office procedure discussed below. However, efficacy of nicotine gum in medical practice settings is certainly not universal (12). The gum is thought to be most effective when used in conjunction with other behavioral treatments (8), and effectiveness may depend upon physicians becoming familiar with and instructing patients on how to use the gum properly (5).

It is important to emphasize to patients that the gum is a medication and must be chewed differently than popular sweet chewing gums. The gum should be chewed slowly and intermittently to release the nicotine. Nicotine release can be perceived as a tingling sensation on the tongue and palate. The nicotine is absorbed through the mucous membranes of the mouth. Swallowing the released nicotine can lead to inactivation in the stomach rather than absorption. Too vigorous chewing can lead to an unpleasant excess of nicotine. Patients tend to use too little of the gum and

Table 20.3.
Features of Selected Self-Help Guides to Smoking Cessation

Guide: Name/Source/Cost	Comments
Smart Move! American Cancer Society (all distribution is through local, not state or national, chapter offices—consult phone directory). Usually any reasonable quantity without charge.	Most readable. Effective use of pictures as persuasive testimonials. Devotes nine pages to preparing to stop and seven to maintaining cessation. A "Stop Smoking Contract," which could be used by physicians not using a separate step-wise agreement (see text), is included in the four pages that are devoted to quitting.
Clearing the Air National Cancer institute NIH publication 89-1648 Phone 1-800-4-CANCER and ask for the *Quit for Good* kit.	Dense text totalling 24 pages. Use by smokers with reading level less than grade 11 might be difficult. About seven pages each on preparation, quitting, and maintenance. Fifty guides are packaged in an excellent complete kit that includes agreement forms, chart stickers (Fig. 20.1c), and promotional materials.
Calling it Quits American Heart Association (all distribution from local chapter offices; consult telephone directory). Single copies without charge. Charges for bulk distribution at the discretion of the local chapter.	By offering two separate guides and packaging them together, this product facilitates smoker attention to the distinct requirements of quitting vs. maintaining. The second guide in the packet, *Guide to Becoming an Ex-Smoker*, promotes focused attention on the planning required to avoid relapse.

for too short a period. Most patients should use between 8 and 30 pieces per day, and use (at a tapering frequency) should continue for at least three months.

Nicotine gum is commercially available as Nicorette, in packages of 96 pieces. In 1989 the cost to pharmacists was approximately $20 per package. Each piece of gum contains 2 mg of nicotine—approximately equivalent to the nicotine yield of two cigarettes.

Weight Gain

Weight gain is a frequent, distressing consequence of cessation for smokers. It appears that weight gain results from both dietary changes (increased snacking and selection of high calorie foods) and from release from the metabolic effects of nicotine (17, 19). The magnitude of weight gain of patients remaining abstinent for one year averages 5 to 15 pounds across various studies (though certainly higher for many individual patients). This magnitude of weight gain is medically insignificant relative to the health benefits of smoking cessation. However, the social, cosmetic, and economic (e.g., wardrobe cost) consequences of weight gain may be sufficient to deter some smokers from quitting and to lead others to relapse. Therefore, it is advisable to provide anticipatory guidance concerning weight control to patients for whom this risk is a concern. This would include advice to (a) use daily weighings to attend to weight early, when it is most manageable; (b) keep only low calorie snacks on hand; (c) initiate a moderate, pleasurable exercise program; (d) explicitly accept a priori a "ceiling" weight gain that will be tolerated for several months until smoking abstinence is well established.

Treatment with nicotine gum may significantly reduce weight gain after smoking cessation (10).

Organized Treatment

Physicians often state that they would like to have information concerning formal cessation programs to which they might refer patients. However, as noted above, only a small minority of patients utilize such programs even when they are available. For those patients who desire them, organized programs at little or no cost are often available through local voluntary service organizations such as the Lung Association or Heart Association. Commercial programs may be somewhat more comprehensive, but are also more costly and require greater investment of time by the patient. There is little difference in outcome among organized treatment programs. Most such programs have now incorporated the behavioral principles that have been characteristic of the most successful treatments (self-monitoring, analysis of environmental stimulus factors, and scheduling of rewards).

Relapse Prevention

In a variety of circumstances, the new quitter will be subjected to an urge to smoke again. Anticipation of this temptation and advance planning for ways to cope with it are associated with lower rates of relapse. An excellent resource in this regard is the second in a two-booklet set (*Calling it Quits*) from the American Heart Association (see Table 20.3). This *Guide to Becoming an Ex-Smoker* is devoted entirely to the experience of being a new quitter. There are story-like descriptions of situations other quitters have experienced and one or more coping strategies that helped prevent them from smoking again. Such guides are valuable to the new quitter both for anticipating what temptations may be ahead and in preselecting a coping strategy. The other self-help guides in Table 20.3 have smaller sections devoted to coping strategies.

Maintenance of smoking cessation is a remarkably difficult process. It is to be expected that many attempts will end in relapse. This should not frustrate or discourage either the physician or the patient but should be recognized as a predictable part of the quitting process. Unsuccessful attempts often precede successful cessation; it is important and worthwhile to try again. Relapsed patients will often be disappointed in themselves and fearful of a nagging or humiliating response from the physician. Therefore, it is important that one's response to relapse be understanding and nonjudgmental.

RECOMMENDED OFFICE PROCEDURE

Figs. 20.1a–d presents the components of a three-step procedure for delivering brief, persuasive smoking cessation advice in office practice.

The use of two prompts such as those shown in Fig. 20.1b—a questionnaire that the smoker completes before being seen and an agreement form that the physician completes with the patient while giving the cessation advice—is optimal. The questionnaire provides cues to guide one through the three-step process and makes it possible to tailor smoking cessation advice to the individual patient. Another approach is to use only a self-help guide as a prompt; if this approach is used, it is advisable to select a guide that already contains a contract agreement such as in *Smart Move!* from the American Cancer Society. A supply of *Smart Move!* is available without charge from any local chapter of the American Cancer Society. The three-step procedure should be initiated before the patient sees the physician. Any patient who has answered "yes" to the question "Have you smoked at least one cigarette in the past seven days?" is asked to complete the Smoker's Questionnaire at registration or while being weighed. Copies of the agreement form should be available in the examination rooms along with copies of self-help guides. The National Cancer Institute *Quit for Good* kit contains three of the four materials needed for the three-step procedure in Fig. 20.1: a self-help guide for smokers, (*Clearing the Air*), chart stickers, and an abbreviated agreement form, prepared like a prescription pad. The smoker's questionnaire and a

Step 1: **Personalize and Provide Instructions**: (Questions 1 and 2, Fig. 20.1*b*) Simple facts make a powerful and inarguable beginning. One may feel discomfort about lifestyle advising and may adopt the manner of a scolding parent rather than a concerned professional. A self-check against this common problem is to ensure that one's initial comments to the patient about smoking have a verbal and nonverbal delivery style indistinguishable from "Your hemoglobin is 10.5. That's too low. I must do more lab studies."

Step 2: **Promote Confidence**: (Questions 3–6, Fig. 20.1*b*) It is rare that anyone undertakes a task in order to fail. The remainder of the questionnaire prompts one to promote rather than inadvertently discourage the quit attempt. By acknowledging that quitting is DIFFICULT, one establishes expertise—for this is one truth about smoking of which all smokers are certain. One is then emphatic about the certainty of HEALTH BENEFITS. More valid than risk advising, it also provides easy transition to smoker-identified benefits (Question 5). Because a majority of smokers have made prior quit attempts, these are relabeled as preludes to success. Most successful quitters make multiple attempts before quitting for good.

Step 3: **Contract for Specific Behavior**: Turning to the agreement form, the self-help guide, and the chart sticker, one is now ready to promote action. The smoker is asked to agree to specific actions of increasing difficulty. Asking general questions at this time (Would you like to try to quit?) invites the smoker's self-doubt to dominate. Instead concentrate on a single specific task, give an instruction and elicit a verbal response to each item with "Can you do that?"

Because data point to its efficacy, negotiating a specific quit date is very important. Open-ended questioning here (e.g., "What do you think about a quitting date?") invites self-doubt to dominate. Focusing instead on the usually very different life circumstances a smoker encounters at work (week-days) or home (week-ends) encourages the smoker to consider concrete details of each environment that would promote or undermine a quit attempt. Smokers who truly are not already to make a quit attempt will state this. For others, the physician should suggest the nearest date that matches the smoker's needs. "How about next Monday?"—and readily grant another week if that is too soon. The smoker is given the agreement form after signing it and watches as the physician applies a sticker to the chart. Simple shorthand such as "L/D/Nov 17" on the sticker provides an instant reminder of the agreement to read literature, keep a diary, and quit on November 17.

Figure 20.1A. Components of a Three-Step Procedure for Advising Smokers, Using Prompts Figure.

more complete agreement form can be prepared inexpensively.

It is advisable for the patient's physician or a member of the office staff to telephone the smoker a day or two before the selected quit date. The first purpose of the call is to remind, support, and encourage the smoker. In addition, at this time the smoker will be more concerned about and attentive to information about maintaining cessation. Separating these two types of advice—advice to quit and advice on how to maintain cessation—is more in keeping with the needs of

SMOKER'S QUESTIONNAIRE

1. I smoke ____ packs of cigarettes on average each day.
2. I began smoking when I was ____ years old.
3. Quitting would be difficult for me.
    ____ AGREE ____ DISAGREE.
4. My health would benefit if I quit.
    ____ AGREE ____ DISAGREE.
5. Some concerns of smokers: Circle if a concern for you:

cigarette money is needed for other things	no	maybe	yes
have been short of breath	no	maybe	yes
want to be a better example for children/ grandchildren	no	maybe	yes
cough and cold problems	no	maybe	yes
nagged by others about smoking	no	maybe	yes
chest discomfort or angina	no	maybe	yes
want to be more in control of myself and my life	no	maybe	yes

6. Circle the longest you have gone without cigarettes:

     1 day   1 week   1 month   3 mos   6 mos   1 year

SMOKER'S AGREEMENT

Upon the advice of Dr. John Smith, I, _____, agree that the following will benefit my health and my self-esteem and will receive my full attention and effort:

____ I agree to read *Clearing the Air*
____ I agree to tell someone about my doctor's advice to quit
____ I agree to pay more attention to my smoking habit in these ways:
    ____ Buy packs not cartons, changing brands with each pack
    ____ Move a rubber band from one wrist to the other before each smoke
    ____ Make a written record of where and why before each cigarette
____ I agree that in order to quit I need to have a specific QUIT DATE in mind
____ For me quitting would be easier ____ week-days ____ week-ends

_____ is my QUIT DATE.

_____
Signature

Figure 20.1B. Examples of Two Prompts: Smoker's Questionnaire and Smoker's Agreement

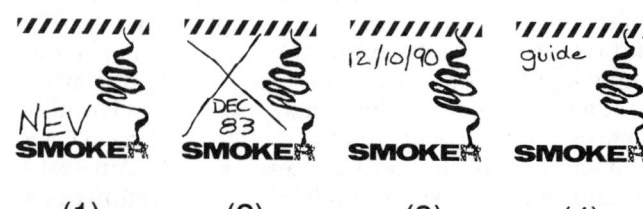

    (1)   (2)   (3)   (4)

Figure 20.1C. Use of labels provided in the *Quit for Good* Kit. Applied to the outside of the chart, these communicate, from left to right, (*1*) a never smoker, (*2*) a person who quit in December of 1983, (*3*) a person who has been advised and selected a quit date of December 10, 1990 and (*4*) a smoker who does not yet have a quit date but has agreed to read a self-help guide.

Mr. Lee, you've smoked 25 cigarettes a day for 15 years. That's a long time. I recommend that you stop smoking. Quitting IS hard; (pause rhetorically) we both know that. But I can assure you that this will benefit your health. We will also find that your blood pressure is easier to control.

. . . And I see here that you would enjoy other benefits, too. You'd feel more in control and be a better example to your grandchildren.

I see that you have quit before for _____ [only if over 1 week]. That gives me a lot of confidence that you will be able to quit for good. I think we can agree on some things you should do to get ready to quit. (Picks up pamphlet)

I recommend this guide (names it and hands it to patient) for you to read. CAN YOU DO THAT?

There are many techniques to make you more aware of your smoking. (Name each and ask CAN YOU DO THAT?)

Now I'd like to tell you how to quit smoking. To quit you must choose a specific date. It must be within 3 weeks or it will be too far away to get ready for.

WOULD IT BE BETTER FOR YOU TO QUIT ON A WEEK-DAY OR A WEEK-END? (Select a date.)

I'll note our agreement on this form for you to sign and keep.

And I'm putting this sticker on the front of your chart to remind me of this important step you have taken.

Figure 20.1D. Illustrative Script for Advising Smokers Using Prompts

the smoker. Quitting is a process, not a single-point event, and continued efforts are necessary.

The follow-up telephone contact can be used to promote successful abstinence by addressing and/or reminding the patient about the use of nicotine gum to suppress withdrawal discomfort, about cautions for avoiding weight gain, and about the use of self-help brochures to anticipate difficulties and to prepare coping strategies.

On the patient's next visit to the office, one must be cautious not to humiliate or discourage the smoker who was not able to quit. If a sticker was used during the initial advising, one can now identify at a glance what level of commitment was agreed upon. If the sticker indicates a quit date, asking "How did it go on (date)?" is useful; the open-ended phrasing assures that the patient will respond with a sentence and will not feel forced to give a simple "yes" or "no." Efforts, whether successful or not, should be praised and encouraged. For those patients who failed or who made no serious effort at all, a repetition of the fact-based cessation instructions, general encouragement, and a repeat request for similar action are most efficient. The currently successful quitter will be best served by a review of his or her coping strategies, use of nicotine gum, and desire for help with weight control or other problems.

OTHER FORMS OF TOBACCO USE

This chapter focuses upon cigarette smoking because it is the most prevalent form of tobacco use and has the greatest health impact. Other forms of tobacco use—cigars, pipes, snuff, chewing tobacco—also have deleterious health effects (4). Prevalence data for the use of these forms of tobacco by men are summarized in Table 20.2. The mortality rates associated with these other forms of tobacco use are intermediate between those of cigarette smokers and nonusers of tobacco. Although the total mortality of cigarette smokers is increased by about 70%, the total mortality of cigar or pipe smokers is about 15 to 20% higher than that of comparable nonsmokers.

Compared with cigarette smoking, cigar and pipe smoking is usually associated with less exposure to carbon monoxide and with less exposure of lung tissue to smoke; some cigar and pipe smokers do, however, inhale. Use of smokeless tobacco (snuff or chewing tobacco) eliminates both of these exposures. However, with all of these tobacco products nicotine is absorbed through the mucous membranes, and there is topical exposure to tobacco or smoke in the oral-nasal cavity and throat. Site-specific cancer rates in these areas are five times as great as in nonusers of tobacco. In addition, there is an increased risk of cardiovascular disease. There is growing concern about the prevalence and adverse health effects of smokeless tobacco use. This form of tobacco dependence is increasing, and among young men in rural areas its prevalence approaches that of smoking.

Treatment approaches for these other varieties of tobacco dependence are the same as those described above for cigarette smoking.

Acknowledgment. Preparation of this chapter was supported in part by Research Scientist Award DA 00050 from the United States Public Health Service.

General References

Benowitz NL: Pharmacologic aspects of cigarette smoking and nicotine addiction. *N Engl J Med* 319:1318, 1988.
An excellent overview.
JAMA 255(8):1986.
JAMA 261(1):1989.
Am J Pub Health 79(2):1989.
The above three journal "special issues" focus on tobacco use and provide convenient access to a broad range of reviews and current research covering the epidemiology, toxicity, prevention, and treatment of tobacco use and dependence.
United States Public Health Service: *Smoking and Health: A Report of the Surgeon General.* DHEW publ. no. (PHS) 79-50066, Washington, DC, United States Government Printing Office, 1979.
The most comprehensive compilation and review of biomedical and behavioral data available. Subsequent volumes have been issued annually (except 1987) and have focused on the special topics of Women, The Changing Cigarette, Cancer, Cardiovascular Disease, Chronic Obstructive Lung Disease, Smoking in the Workplace, Involuntary Smoking, and Nicotine Addiction; all are excellent.

Specific References

1. Benowitz NL, Jacob P: Nicotine and carbon monoxide intake from high- and low-yield cigarettes. *Clin Pharmacol Ther* 36:265, 1984.
2. Botvin GJ, Tortu S: Preventing adolescent substance abuse through life skills training. In: Price RH, Cowen EL, Lorion RP, Ramos-McKay J (eds): *Fourteen Ounces of Prevention: A Casebook for*

Practitioners. Washington, DC, American Psychological Association, 98–110, 1988.

3. Burling TA, Singleton EG, Bigelow GE, et al: Smoking following myocardial infarction: a critical review of the literature. *Health Psychol* 3:83, 1984.
4. Council on Scientific Affairs. Health effects of smokeless tobacco. *JAMA* 255:1038, 1986.
5. Cummings SR, Hansen B, Richard RJ, et al: Internists and nicotine gum. *JAMA* 260:1565, 1988.
6. Cummings SR, Rubin SM, Oster G: The cost-effectiveness of counseling smokers to quit. *JAMA* 261:75, 1989.
7. Fielding JE, Phenow KJ: Health effects of involuntary smoking. *N Engl J Med* 319:1452, 1988.
8. Fortmann SP, Killen JD, Telch MJ, Newman B: Minimal contact treatment for smoking cessation. *JAMA* 260:1575, 1988.
9. Gilbert RM, Pope MA: Early effects of quitting smoking. *Psychopharmacology* 78:121, 1982.
10. Gross J, Stitzer ML, Maldonado J: Nicotine replacement: effects on postcessation weight gain. *J Consulting and Clinical Psychology* 57:87, 1989.
11. Hill P, Haley NJ, Wynder EL: Cigarette smoking: carboxyhemoglobin, plasma nicotine, cotinine, and thiocyanate vs. self-reported smoking data and cardiovascular disease. *J Chronic Dis* 36:439, 1983.
12. Hughes JR, Gust SW, Keenan RM, et al: Nicotine vs. placebo gum in general medical practice. *JAMA* 261:1300, 1989.
13. Hughes JR, Hatsukami D: Signs and symptoms of tobacco withdrawal. *Arch Gen Psych* 43:289, 1986.
14. Kaufman DW, Helmrich SP, Rosenberg L, et al: Nicotine and carbon monoxide content of cigarette smoke and the risk of myocardial infarction in young men. *N Engl J Med* 308:409, 1983.
15. Kozlowski LT, Frecker RC, Khouw V, Pope MA: The misuse of "less-hazardous" cigarettes and its detection: hole-blocking of ventilated filters. *Am J Public Health* 70:1202, 1980.
16. Pederson LL: Compliance with physician advice to quit smoking: a review of the literature. *Prev Med* 11:71, 1982.
17. Perkins KA, Epstein LH, Marks BL, et al: The effect of nicotine on energy expenditure during light physical activity. *N Engl J Med* 320:898, 1989.
18. Perry C, Killen J, Telch M, et al: Modifying smoking behavior of teenagers: a school-based intervention. *Am J Public Health* 70:722, 1980.
19. Rigotti NA: Cigarette smoking and body weight. *N Engl J Med* 320:931, 1989.
20. Russell MAH, Merriman R, Stapleton J, Taylor W: Effect of nicotine chewing gum as an adjunct to general practitioners' advice against smoking. *Br Med J* 287:1782, 1983.
21. Schneider NG, Jarvik ME, Forsythe AB, et al: Nicotine gum in smoking cessation: a placebo-controlled, double-blind trial. *Addict Behav* 8:253, 1983.
22. Sexton M, Hebel JR: A clinical trial of change in maternal smoking and its effect on birth weight. *JAMA* 251:911, 1984.
23. Shiffman S: Relapse following smoking cessation: a situational analysis. *J Consult Clin Psychol* 50:71, 1982.
24. Shiffman SM, Jarvik ME: Smoking withdrawal symptoms in two weeks of abstinence. *Psychopharmacology (Berlin)* 50:35, 1976.
25. Sparrow D, Stefos T, Bosse R, Weiss ST: The relationship of tar content to decline in pulmonary function in cigarette smokers. *Am Rev Respir Dis* 127:56, 1983.
26. Wald NJ, Idle M, Boreham J, Bailey A: Inhaling habits among smokers of different types of cigarette. *Thorax* 35:925, 1980.
27. Wilson DM, Taylor DW, Gilberg JR, et al: A randomized trial of a family physician intervention for smoking cessation. *JAMA* 260:1570, 1988.

C H A P T E R 21

Alcoholism*

L. RANDOL BARKER, M.D.
CHARLES L. WHITFIELD, M.D.

* John E. Davis, Ph.D., contributed to this chapter in the second edition.

Along with cardiovascular disease and cancer, alcoholism ranks among the top three causes of death and disability in the United States. One in three Americans reports that drinking has caused trouble in his or her family (17). The estimated cost of alcoholism to society in 1983 was $117 billion, with an untold additional cost in the suffering of those people who are close to alcoholics (32). It is also estimated that over three-fourths of the alcoholics in the United States do not receive treatment for their alcoholism (7). Many of these persons have early alcoholism and would be likely to recover successfully if diagnosed and treated.

Until recently, alcoholism was widely regarded as a hopeless condition with a poor prognosis for recovery. Yet alcoholism is one of the most treatable of all medical and psychiatric conditions, with a high long-term success rate when a disease model of alcoholism is utilized in diagnosis and treatment.

DEFINITION OF ALCOHOLISM

A useful, broad definition of the disease alcoholism is *recurring trouble associated with drinking alcohol*. The *trouble* may occur in one or more of several domains, including *interpersonal* (e.g., valued relationships, especially within the family), *educational, legal, financial, medical,* or *occupational*. Although there are many exceptions, trouble due to alcoholism usually occurs in that order of progression, so that one's health and job are last to be overtly affected. The trouble often includes the physiological manifestations of dependence or addiction: tolerance (the need for increased amounts of a substance to achieve intoxication or desired effect) and withdrawal symptoms. The drinking that is characteristic of alcoholism includes one or more of the following abnormal patterns: inability to control one's use of alcohol (always present), drinking alone, avoiding situations where alcohol is not available, drinking before going to a party, gulping drinks, drinking of nonbeverage alcohol, continuing to drink alcohol despite occupational, psychosocial, or physical problems caused by drinking.

Alcoholism is classified by the American Psychiatric Association (APA) under the broad rubric *Psychoactive Substance Use Disorders* (2). In its subclassification for these disorders, the APA has generic criteria for *psychoactive substance abuse* (abnormal use, with unwanted consequences) and for *psychoactive substance dependence* (more intensive abuse patterns and/or physiological manifestations of addiction). These criteria are found on page 232. Another widely-used term for these disorders is Chemical Dependence. Many individuals with chemical dependence abuse multiple psychoactive substances (e.g., an alcoholic patient may also abuse cocaine and a benzodiazepine). Chapter 22 describes a number of the other specific psychoactive substance use disorders common in the United States.

ETIOLOGY

The etiology of alcoholism is multifactorial and poorly understood (29, 41, 55). A predisposition to alcoholism appears to be inherited by at least half of all alcoholic patients; and there is some evidence that there are inherited factors associated with inability to control use of alcohol (20, 46). Social conditioning and enabling behavior by others close to the individual (see "Co-Alcoholism" below) and being a child in a dysfunctional family (see below) are important nongenetic factors. For about 10 to 20% of *alcoholic men* another mental disorder (especially antisocial personality disorder, primary abuse of other substances, or an affective disorder) may play an etiological role (47). For *alcoholic women*, there is evidence that pre-existing mental illness, especially a phobic disorder or major depression, may play an etiological role more often (6, 25). In addition, for those elderly alcoholics whose problem began after the age of 50, the losses and isolation that accompany aging are often factors associated with the onset of problem drinking. These factors do not account for all alcoholism. They only add credence to the concept that alcoholism is a complex disease and not the result of moral turpitude.

ALCOHOLIC BEVERAGES: CONTENT AND METABOLISM

Alcoholic beverages can be divided into nondistilled (wine and beer) and distilled varieties. The concentration of alcohol (ethanol) in wine ranges from 10 to 22% by volume and is 12 to 14% in most wines. Beer usually contains 4 to 5% alcohol by volume. The distilled alcoholic beverages are whiskey, brandy, rum, gin, and vodka. Alcoholic fermentation ceases when the concentration of alcohol exceeds 15% by volume, and, therefore, to manufacture more potent beverages distillation is necessary. In the United States, the word "proof" is preceded by a number that is double the percentage of alcohol by volume: thus 90 proof whiskey contains 45% alcohol by volume.

In a 154-pound or 70-kg person, on an empty stomach, one drink of distilled alcohol (usually 1 fluid ounce or 30 ml), which normally contains about 15 ml of absolute ethyl alcohol, produces a peak blood alcohol level (BAL) of about 25 mg/dl within 30 minutes of ingestion. The metabolism of alcohol follows zero-order pharmacokinetics: about 15 mg/dl (or approximately 10 ml) per hour are metabolized, no matter how high the BAL. The alcohol in 120 ml of whiskey (i.e., four drinks each containing about 15 ml of alcohol) or in 1.2 liters of beer would take about 5 to 6 hours to be metabolized. The rate of metabolism is higher—even in the range of from 20 to 25 mg/dl/hour—in the alcoholic who drinks heavily each day for many months. To reach a BAL of 300 mg/dl, which is diagnostic of alcoholism, a 70-kg person generally has to consume between 14 and 20 drinks over the span of a few hours.

EPIDEMIOLOGY

Prevalence

In a recent survey of representative American communities, alcoholism was found to be the commonest psychosocial disorder in American men between the ages of 18 and 65 and the fourth most common in American women in the age range 18 to 24 years (38). For community-dwelling men, the prevalence exceeds 10% for those age 18 to 40 and ranges from 6 to 12% for those 41 to 59, and 2 to 5% for those over 60. For community-dwelling women in these three age groups the prevalence rates are 2 to 3%, 1 to 3%, and .1 to .7%, respectively (28). Studies of teenage students have shown that the rates of problem drinking (heavy drinking or drinking to get drunk) exceed the rates of alcoholism in adults, even though the purchase of alcohol by teenagers is illegal (3).

The apparent annual national consumption of alcohol is 2.7 gallons of pure alcohol or the equivalent of 2.6 drinks a day for every person over the age of 15. Per capita alcohol consumption peaks under the age of 50 and declines with increasing age. Inasmuch as about one-third of the adult population is abstinent, the consumption of alcohol is concentrated in the approximately 94 million drinking Americans. About one-third of that number (30 million) consume approximately 70% of all the alcohol produced. It is this group that uses the health system more frequently, is most at risk of trauma, and has the recurring problems that constitute the disease alcoholism (66).

Alcoholism is common in medical patients. Among general hospital inpatients, alcoholism has been documented in 15 to 42% of men and in 4 to 35% of women (34). Similar percentages have been reported from emergency departments, clinics, and office practices. A conservative estimation would be that at least 1 in 10 ambulatory patients has alcoholism or another form of chemical dependence and that at least another 10 or 20% are suffering from a concomitant condition seen in family members that is now called "co-alcoholism" or co-dependence (see below). Alcoholism

afflicts all ethnic, cultural, and socioeconomic groups, and no single group is immune.

Mortality and Morbidity

Prospective studies have shown that alcoholic patients have 2 to 4 times higher death rates and much higher rates of medical and psychosocial morbidity than matched controls (39, 40). The most common causes of early death in alcoholics are cirrhosis of the liver, cancers of the respiratory and gastrointestinal tracts, accidents, suicide, and ischemic heart disease. Overall, 1 in 10 deaths in the United States is alcohol related (59).

Even recovering alcoholics have considerable excess mortality. This may be because certain diseases initiated during active drinking may be irreversible or because other factors adversely affecting health may have persisted, including surreptitious continued use of alcohol, cigarette smoking, use of other drugs, poor diet, and emotional disturbances.

Utilization of Health Services

Alcoholics who are untreated for their alcoholism tend to be high users of medical care. Overall, it is estimated that 20% of spending for hospital care and 12% of the total expenditure for adult health care is for problems caused by alcoholism (59). A study representing a variety of hospital types showed that alcoholics constituted a major proportion of the high-cost 13% of patients who consumed as many resources as the low-cost 87% (66). The high-cost group was further characterized by having repeated hospitalizations for the same disease and having a 5 times higher incidence of unexpected complications of their illnesses than the low-cost group. Other studies have shown that when alcoholics have been successfully treated, their use of health services decreases to that of the general population (27).

NATURAL HISTORY OF ALCOHOLISM

The natural history of alcoholism in men has been delineated in retrospective and prospective studies. In Jellinek's retrospective study of recovering alcoholic men (29), the majority of subjects identified multiple phases in the progression of their disease: (a) an initial phase, lasting months to years, in which they used alcohol to relieve tension and developed tolerance to alcohol; (b) a phase in which they experienced blackouts (amnesia for drinking-associated events), increasing preoccupation with getting alcohol, and profound loss of control over use of alcohol; (c) a phase in which there were overt psychological and behavioral consequences (rationalization, grandiosity, aggressive behavior, remorse, efforts to abstain); and (d) a stage characterized by chronic intoxication and serious deterioration of health and psychosocial functioning. In Vaillant's prospective study (55), this multiphase course of alcoholism characterized three-quarters of men who became alcoholic. Most of the remaining men exhibited abnormal drinking patterns, usually rituals to constrain the uncontrolled drinking that they themselves recognized as abnormal, and had less alcohol-related trouble with family, job, and health. Importantly, in these and other studies of the course of alcoholism it has been found that periodic abstinence or moderation of use is typical. Although anecdotal information suggests that an occasional individual with what appears to be alcoholism can return to normal drinking, critical studies of this issue have shown that this is very uncommon and not clinically useful (24).

MANIFESTATIONS OF ALCOHOLISM

Alcoholism is a protean disease, and it is probably the most common "great masquerader" today. Table 21.1 lists medical, psychosocial, legal, and other manifestations that are often associated with alcoholism. Manifestations are ranked in the table according to their strength as diagnostic features, ranging from those that are diagnostic of alcoholism to those that should make one at least consider alcoholism. A number of the most important manifestations of alcoholism are discussed here.

Legal Problems

A driving-while-intoxicated (DWI) history or record is highly suggestive of alcoholism. In one study of about 21,000 consecutive people with DWIs (19), about 75% of first time offenders were found to be alcoholic. Of those with two DWI arrests, over 90% were alcoholic, and of those with three, essentially 100% were alcoholic. A prison record is also strongly suggestive, since the majority of prison inmates have a history of alcoholism or other chemical dependence. Child and spouse/partner abuse is also highly associated with alcoholism.

Behavioral, Psychiatric, and Neurological Problems

Miscellaneous

Accidents and trauma are frequently associated with alcoholism; in more than half of patients with severe trauma, alcohol or other psychoactive drug use can be detected (51). Among patients with symptoms of chronic mental illness, especially symptoms of depression and anxiety, alcoholism is common. Usually alcoholism is the primary problem, and treatment of mental symptoms is not successful until the alcoholism is treated.

Alcohol Intoxication

The best known acute consequence of alcoholism is alcohol intoxication, which should usually present no diagnostic problem. Because this condition is so common, diagnostic errors are made when it is forgotten that "drunken behavior"—often with evidence of recent alcohol use—may be caused by a host of conditions, such as infection, metabolic disturbance, neurological disease, or other drug toxicity. Because the alcoholic is especially prone to many disorders

that may be manifested as deranged behavior, he should be examined systematically before a diagnosis of simple drunkenness is made.

Alcohol intoxication may be characterized by one or more of the following: relaxation and sedation, euphoria, impaired coordination, loudness, lowered inhibitions, poor memory and judgment, labile mood, slurred speech, nausea, vomiting, and obtundation (see Table 21.2). An initial period of excitement and euphoria is often followed by depression and sleep, or possibly coma. The duration and magnitude of the intoxication depend on dose, the rapidity with which the alcohol was drunk, and on whether the patient drank on an empty stomach (enhancing the rate of absorption). Tolerance is also a significant factor. As noted above, normal persons metabolize ethanol at a rate of about 15 mg/dl (or 10 ml) per hour, no matter how much is ingested; but an alcoholic may acquire the (reversible) capacity to increase his rate of alcohol metabolism. Moreover, alcoholics characteristically develop substantial central tolerance, so that they appear fairly sober at blood alcohol levels of 150 mg/dl or more. Most nonalcoholic individuals become intoxicated at levels between 100 and 200 mg/dl, and some, at levels as low as 30 mg/dl. Levels over 400 mg/dl may be lethal, death usually resulting from depressed respiration or aspiration of vomitus.

Blackouts

"Blackouts," amnesia for events that occurred during a period of intoxication, are common. However, from 10 to 25% of alcoholics do not have memory blackouts, and some normal drinkers have experienced one to three blackouts after drinking. If they recur more than three times, blackouts are usually an indication of alcoholism.

Alcohol Idiosyncratic Intoxication

Alcohol idiosyncratic intoxication (pathological intoxication) is an uncommon syndrome characterized by an extreme, often aggressive or violent reaction to drinking alcohol, which is frequently followed by amnesia for the episode. The behavior is atypical of the person when not drinking. The duration of this condition is brief (hours), and the person returns to his normal state as the blood alcohol level falls. Temporal lobe epilepsy, sedative-hypnotic use, and malingering should be ruled out (2).

Alcohol Amnestic Disorder (Korsakoff's Psychosis)

Alcohol amnestic disorder is characterized chiefly by short-term memory impairment, associated with some loss of long-term memory, in the absence of clouded consciousness (delirium) or general loss of intellectual abilities (dementia). (For definitions and detailed discussions of delirium and dementia, see Chapter 17.) Patients with less advanced forms of this disorder may be substantially impaired, but they may appear superficially to be normal, particularly as they frequently attempt to minimize their impairment and to confabulate in order to fill in memory gaps.

The amnestic disorder frequently follows an episode of *Wernicke's encephalopathy*, a syndrome of global confusion, ataxia, and impaired eye movement, due to thiamine deficiency, which may occur suddenly or gradually over several days. Parenteral thiamine given during an acute episode of Wernicke's encephalopathy may prevent the amnestic syndrome.

With abstention from alcohol and good nutrition, some patients recover entirely from the alcohol amnes-

Table 21.1.
Medical, Psychiatric, Legal, and Other Findings Suggestive (0 to *) to Highly Suggestive (** to ***) or Diagnostic (****) of Alcoholism and Other Chemical Dependence

Presenting Complaint and History

**** Drinking or drug-related problem, recurring[a]	* Night sweats
*** Blackouts with drinking	* Depression
*** Spouse/other complains of patient's drinking	* Suicide attempt
*** Driving-while-intoxicated (DWI) record	* Sexual dysfunction
*** Prison record	* Legal problem
*** Change in alcohol/drug tolerance	* Noncompliance in treatment
*** Frequent requests for mood-changing drugs	* School learning problem
** Gastrointestinal bleeding, especially upper	* Hypertension
** Automobile accident	Heart trouble
** Traumatic injuries, fracture	Palpitations
** Parent, grandparent, or relative alcoholic	Abdominal pain
** Friends alcoholic or other chemical dependence	Amenorrhea
** Family or other violence	Weight loss
** Child abuse or neglect	Vague complaints
** First seizure in an adult	Seizure
** Job performance problem	Insomnia
* Multiple gastrointestinal complaints	Anxiety or panic attacks
* Untoward responses to a number of medications (see page 262)	Marital discord
* Unexplained syncope	Financial problem
* Frequent infections	Behavior problem

Alcohol or Other Drug Use History

**** Alcohol use recurringly interfering with health, job, or social functioning[a]	*** Word "drinker" said in rounds or report
*** Patient says, "I can stop drinking anytime," or the equivalent; or patient gets evasive or angry, or talks glibly during taking of drinking history	** Heavy alcohol use (more than 3 drinks/day or more than 5 drinks at an occasion for a 154-lb person)
*** Patient states that he has consciously stopped drinking completely for any length of time	** Other drug misuse or dependence
	* Cigarette smoker

Physical Examination

*** Odor of beverage alcohol on breath	* Unexplained arrhythmias, especially chronic borderline tachycardia
*** Parotid gland enlargement, bilateral	* Thin extremities in proportion to trunk
*** Spider nevi or angioma	* Splenomegaly
*** Edematous, "puffy face" (may be subtle); unexplained edema	* Hypertension
*** Tremulousness, hallucinosis, and/or 1 or 2 seizures	Diaphoresis, day or night
** Cigarette stains on fingers	Very neat and clean
** Breath mints odor	Depression
** Many scars or tattoos	Alopecia
** Hepatomegaly	Corneal arcus
** Gynecomastia	Abdominal tenderness
** Small testicles	Cerebellar signs (*e.g.*, nystagmus)
** Unexplained bruises, abrasions, or cuts	Any alteration in consciousness
	Anxiety

Laboratory Abnormalities

**** Blood alcohol level greater than 300 mg/100 ml[a]	** Abnormal liver function tests
*** Blood alcohol level greater than 100 mg/100 ml	** Anemia, macrocytic or megaloblastic
*** High serum osmolality	** Hyperlipoproteinemia-type 4 or 5
*** High serum ammonia	* Positive blood or urine for mood-changing drugs
*** Serum asiaptate transferase elevated on admission, and normal by discharge	* Hyperuricemia (7 to 12 mg/100 ml most often; may be transient)
*** Gamma-glutaryl transpeptidase elevation	* Small intestinal absorption test abnormalities
*** Negative workups for hyperthyroidism	* Hypophosphatemia or hypomagnesemia
** Creatinine phosphokinase elevation	Electrolyte imbalance
** Blood alcohol level positive, any amount	Elevated or low blood glucose
** High amylase	Low white blood cell or platelet count

Table 21.1.—Continued

X-ray Film Findings

***	Pancreatic calcification	*	Hepatomegaly
***	Multiple rib fractures	*	Splenomegaly
**	"Aspiration pneumonia"	*	Nonfilling gallbladder

Diagnosis

****	Hepatitis, alcoholic[a]	**	Attempted suicide
***	Pancreatitis, acute or chronic	**	Gastritis
***	Cirrhosis	**	Refractory hypertension
***	Portal hypertension	**	Cerebellar degeneration
***	Wernicke-Korsakoff syndrome	**	Peripheral neuropathy
***	Frequent automobile or other accidents	**	Aspiration pneumonia
***	Cold injury	*	Cerebral
***	Nose and throat cancer	*	Cardiomyopathy
**	Hepatitis, non-A or B	**	Anxiety
**	Other chemical dependence	**	Any symptom or sign, cause not found, or unknown
**	Drownings	*	Depression
**	Burns, especially third degree	*	Marital discord or family problem
**	Leaves hospital against medical advice	*	Fatty liver

[a]Major criteria of the National Council on Alcoholism for the diagnosis of alcoholism (see "General References").

Table 21.2.
Expected Effects According to Blood Alcohol Level for a Person without Tolerance to Alcohol

Blood Alcohol Level mg/dl	Expected Effect	Approximate Location of Physiological Disturbance
25 to 50	Relaxation, sedation	
50 to 100	Coordination impaired; euphoric; loud conversation; apparent reduction of social inhibitions	Cerebral cortex
100 to 200	Ataxia; depressed fine motor ability, decreased mentation, attention span and memory; poor judgment; labile mood; beginning of slurred speech	Limbic system and cerebellum
200 to 300	Marked ataxia and slurred speech, nausea and vomiting, tremor, irritable	Reticular activating system
300 to 400	Stage 1 anesthesia (unconsciousness) memory lapse	Reticular activating system
above 400	Respiratory failure, coma, death	Medulla oblongata

tic syndrome. Many remain grossly impaired and require institutional care; of these about 20% improve modestly with good long-term institutional support (43).

An amnestic syndrome resembling alcohol amnestic disorder may be caused by bilateral damage to certain diencephalic and medial temporal structures due to head trauma, surgery, hypoxia, or infarction in the territory of the posterior cerebral arteries.

Dementia Associated with Alcoholism

When more generalized intellectual impairment develops after years of heavy drinking, the diagnosis of dementia associated with alcoholism is appropriate. An estimated 70% of actively drinking chronic alcoholics will have cognitive impairments, as measured by psychological testing. Perhaps 10% of these will have dementia that is sufficiently apparent so that it can be noticed without psychological testing. Because

even detoxified alcoholics are likely to show some cognitive impairment for a period of time after cessation of drinking (1), this diagnosis should not be made unless dementia persists for at least 3 weeks after drinking has stopped. Other causes of dementia must be excluded (see Chapter 17).

All alcoholics with any signs of dementia should be treated with high dose thiamine (i.e., 100 mg daily) and multivitamins long term. Some will improve.

Other Medical Complications

Miscellaneous

The various deficiency states involved in a diet composed largely of nutritionally empty alcoholic calories (7 calories/g), as well as the direct toxic actions of alcohol itself, have been implicated in the pathogenesis of many of the medical consequences of alcoholism. These disorders are legion, spare no body system, and most are related to the quantity and duration of alcohol consumed (15). Among the commoner medical complications of alcoholism are gastritis; fatty liver, hepatitis, or cirrhosis; pancreatitis; cerebellar ataxia; peripheral neuropathy; unexplained elevation of serum creatine kinase with or without muscle pain and weakness; hematological abnormalities (elevated mean corpuscular volume of red blood cells, anemia, thrombocytopenia); hypoglycemia, ketoacidosis, electrolyte abnormalities (hyponatremia, hypokalemia); pulmonary infections suggesting aspiration or impaired defenses (tuberculosis and pneumonia); cancers of the liver, respiratory, and gastrointestinal tract; unexplained cardiomyopathy; hypertension; and trauma.

Hypertension is becoming a more frequently recognized manifestation of alcoholism. It is found in about one-third of actively drinking alcoholics. Since it frequently remits within 1 week of discontinuing alcohol, and since the patient usually remains normotensive for the duration of abstinence (45), it may be the most common reversible cause of hypertension (see Chapter 62).

Because it is both serious and preventable, the *fetal alcohol syndrome* deserves special mention (36). It is manifested by morphological abnormalities, low birth weight, and developmental and cognitive impairment. This syndrome is a consequence of alcohol ingestion during pregnancy. The risk of minor abnormalities (e.g., low birth weight) begins with the consumption of one drink per day; this risk increases with increasingly larger amounts of alcohol consumption. Because of this, it is prudent to advise women not to drink during pregnancy.

Medical Consequences: A Summary View

Nearly all of the medical consequences of alcoholism tend to have certain common characteristics:

1. Excessive drinking causes them.
2. A poor diet generally makes most of them worse and makes them occur earlier.
3. Harmful habits, such as cigarette smoking and the misuse of other drugs, also tend to compound the medical consequences.
4. If the patient continues to consume alcohol, damage involving major organs progresses slowly, but relentlessly, over the course of a few years, often ending in organ failure. The organ(s) affected by alcohol and the rate of decline in function of these organs vary greatly among patients. Severity of damage is loosely correlated with dose of alcohol; for one organ, the liver, damage is more common in women at any level of alcohol consumption.

This progression of organic damage will occur no matter what medical or psychological intervention the patient may receive, as long as drinking continues. If the patient stops drinking, many of the pathophysiological processes due to alcohol will reverse rapidly, such as those in the blood and bone marrow (cyto-

penias), those in the small intestine (malabsorption), hypertension, and fluid and electrolyte imbalance. Other processes do not reverse rapidly with sobriety, but they usually do not progress and often improve over weeks and months. Alcoholic hepatitis, chronic pancreatitis, and cognitive deficits are conditions that tend to improve more gradually.

SCREENING FOR AND DIAGNOSING ALCOHOLISM

Overview

Except when a patient presents with overt behavioral or medical evidence for of alcoholism (see diagnostic manifestations, Table 21.1) the diagnosis of alcoholism requires skillful interviewing and careful evaluation of other information about the patient. Such an approach is needed for most alcoholics, whose disease is a private dilemma experienced by themselves and those who are close to them. In addition to unwanted psychosocial and physiological consequences of alcoholism, two cardinal features will inevitably emerge when one is obtaining information from an alcoholic or others who know him: (a) evidence of inability to control the use of alcohol, and (b) denial that a significant problem exists.

Loss of Control

Continuous inability to control the use of alcohol is not always present in alcoholics. Indeed, many can go for periods of a few hours (e.g., at a social gathering) to a few months of apparently "normal" drinking. Therefore, the absence of overt loss of control for a period of time does not rule out alcoholism. In such patients, the loss of control returns eventually. Inability to control one's drinking may be manifested acutely, when the person drinks more than he intended to or is unable to stop drinking and becomes intoxicated; or it may follow a chronic pattern, in which the patient drinks heavily for a few days or most days of each week, often alone, and cannot stop. In addition, some alcoholic patients will describe rituals to constrain their intake because of previous trouble with control (e.g., never having a first drink till after dinner). Normal persons do not describe drinking in these ways, and such information usually indicates that there is a serious problem. Control of alcohol consumption is always an issue for the alcoholic.

Denial

Denial (i.e., the direct or implied message that there is no problem) is present in nearly all actively drinking alcoholics. Denial behavior and responses may be due to one or more of the following mechanisms: (a) conscious lying (one of the least common mechanisms); (b) classic denial (an adaptive coping response to avoid the shame, lowered self-esteem, and distressing inability to overcome the drinking problem that are experienced by most alcoholics); (c) memory blackout due to drinking; (d) euphoric recall (the patient remembers only the good times he had when drinking); (e) the fact that no one points out problems related to drinking; (f) wishful thinking; (g) denial on the part of the family and other close people, including helping professionals; (h) ignorance of what an alcoholic is; (i) toxic effects on information processing and memory; (j) stigma related to the term "alcoholic;" (k) fear of the unknown; and (l) a complex thinking quandary. This last mechanism consists of genuine confusion on the part of the patient; he knows that something is wrong in his life but somehow cannot connect it with drinking alcohol (57).

Some of the ways in which denial presents are (a) as rationalizations (e.g., "I drink because my work is more than any man should try to do"); (b) as glibness and humor (e.g., "That's the way of all flesh doc . . . no problem"); (c) as hostility ("I came to you about my blood pressure and I would appreciate it if we could stay out of my personal life"); (d) as comparison of oneself with a "real" problem drinker ("Now see here, I have a lovely family, a job that I enjoy . . . I have nothing in common with those poor guys who have lost it . . .. those are your alcoholics"); (e) reticence to discuss drinking; and (f) in the assertions by other physicians or family members that the patient has no problem with alcohol. An alcoholic patient's denial responses are usually the result of years of complex adapting to dependence upon alcohol. This helps to explain why these responses may seem to be quite refractory and may cause much frustration during screening/diagnostic interviewing and during efforts to get the patient to accept the diagnosis and agree to treatment (30).

Screening for Alcoholism

Because alcoholism is common and because the evidence for it is usually private information that patients do not volunteer, it is important to screen all patients for this problem. The goal of screening, and of further inquiry when there are positive responses to screening, is to be confident that one has ruled out alcoholism, has detected definite alcoholism, or must continue to consider alcoholism as a possible diagnosis.

There are a number of ways to screen for the cardinal features of alcoholism (23). The approach outlined in Fig. 21.1 incorporates the four so-called "CAGE questions" into the interview. In this approach, exploratory inquiry about the use of alcoholic beverages follows inquiries about less-sensitive habit information; and the inquiry begins with an open-ended question that prompts patients to respond with more than a simple "yes"/"no" or with a quantitative reply (e.g., "a few beers"). In patients who report any current or recent use of alcohol, discomfort, glibness, voluntary reporting of heavy use, or other information suggesting alcoholism (see Table 21.1), including that from the patient's past medical history, increases the likelihood that there is a problem. In the absence of such clues, it is still important for all patients who report alcohol

1. Integrate alcohol use inquiry into interview so that it follows inquiry about less sensitive habits.

   Example: "We have talked about your usual diet and your smoking. Can you tell me how you use alcoholic beverages" (or "How about alcoholic beverages. . .?")

   If the patient says that he has never used alcohol and shows no sign of discomfort, inquire about problem use in others (e.g., "Anyone in your family or other close persons who have a drinking problem?"). This helps to identify a risk factor for alcoholism and to identify patients who may suffer because of the alcoholism of another person.[a]

2. **General Questions**: For patients who report present or past use of alcohol, screen for evidence of alcoholism, with a general question such as the following:

   "Has (Did) your use of alcohol caused (cause) any kinds of problems for you?" or "Have you ever been concerned about your drinking?"

3. **CAGE Questions**:[b] If the patient has not disclosed a problem with drinking, use these four focused questions and probe for clarification of positive or ambivalent responses.

   I'd like to ask you a few more questions about alcohol that I ask all of my patients . . ."

C   "Have you ever felt you ought to CUT DOWN on your drinking (use of _____)?"

A   "Have people ANNOYED you by criticizing your drinking (use of _____)?"

G   "Have you ever felt bad or GUILTY about your drinking (use of _____)?"

E   "Have you ever had a drink first thing in the morning (EYE OPENER) to steady your nerves or get rid of a hangover?" (For other substances: "Have you found that you have to take some _____ most days/some days to feel okay?")

[a]See section on "Co-Alcoholism."
[b]Modifications of questions for substances other than alcohol are shown in parentheses.

Figure 21.1. A recommended approach to the use of interviewing to screen all patients for alcoholism and for problems with alcohol in the family.

use to complete the follow-up questions listed in Fig. 21.1 or other questions that focus upon similar content.

The approach in Fig. 21.1 is designed to uncover specific data that point to the diagnosis of alcoholism. The CAGE questions are derived from the larger Michigan Alcoholism Screening Test (MAST), a standardized instrument that has been used extensively for alcoholism screening (see Table 21.3) (23, 42). Each of the questions in the MAST may be helpful when one is attempting to uncover occult alcoholism. The CAGE questions have the advantage of being simple to incorporate into an office interview, being phrased in a nonthreatening way, and focusing upon several features that are present in most patients with alcoholism, i.e.:

Table 21.3.
Michigan Alcoholism Screening Test (MAST)[a]

	YES	NO
0. Do you enjoy having a drink now and then?	0	
1. Do you feel you are a normal drinker? (By normal we mean you drink less than or as much as most other people and you have not gotten into any recurring trouble while drinking.)		2
2. Have you ever awakened the morning after some drinking the night before and found that you could not remember a part of the evening?	2	
3. Does either of your parents, or any other near relative, or your spouse, or any girlfriend or boyfriend ever worry or complain about your drinking?	1	
4. Can you stop drinking without a struggle after one or two drinks?		2
5. Do you feel guilty about your drinking?	1	
6. Do friends or relatives think you are a normal drinker?		2
7. Are you able to stop drinking when you want to?		2
8. Have you ever attended a meeting of Alcoholics Anonymous (AA)?	5	
9. Have you gotten into physical fights when you have been drinking?	1	
10. Has your drinking ever created problems between you and either of your parents, or another relative, your spouse, or any girlfriend or boyfriend?	2	
11. Has any family member of yours ever gone to anyone for help about your drinking?	2	
12. Have you ever lost friends because of your drinking?	2	
13. Have you ever gotten into trouble at work or at school because of drinking?	2	
14. Have you ever lost a job because of drinking?	2	
15. Have you ever neglected your obligations, your school work, your family, or your job for 2 or more days in a row because you were drinking?	2	
16. Do you drink before noon fairly often?	1	
17. Have you ever been told you have liver trouble? Cirrhosis?	2	
18. After heavy drinking have you ever had severe shaking, or heard voices or seen things that really weren't there?	2(5 DTs)	
19. Have you ever gone to anyone for help about your drinking?	5	
20. Have you ever been in a hospital because of drinking?	5	
21. Have you ever been a patient in a psychiatric hospital or on a psychiatric ward of a general hospital where drinking was part of the problem that resulted in hospitalization?	2	
22. Have you ever been seen at a psychiatric or mental health clinic or gone to any doctor, social worker, or clergy for help with any emotional problem, where drinking was a part of the problem?	2	
23. Have you ever been arrested for drunk driving, driving while intoxicated, or driving under the influence of alcoholic everages or any other drug? (IF YES, How many times? ____)	2 each	
24. Have you ever been arrested, or taken into custody, even for a few hours, because of other drunk behavior, whether due to alcohol or another drug? (IF YES, How many times? ____)	2 each	

[a]Interpretation: *Standard MAST*—0 to 3 points = probable normal drinker; 4 points = borderline score; 5 to 9 points = 80% associated with alcoholism/chemical dependence; 10 or more = 100% associated with alcoholism. The values assigned to each response are shown.

Inability to control one's drinking, which leads to cutting back or quitting attempts (the "C").

Domestic problems caused by one's drinking and that evoke negative responses from other persons ("A"). The phrasing of this question places the blame on the criticizer, so that a positive response is not self-incriminating.

Bad feelings that one has about drinking-related actions ("G"). The phrasing of this question allows the patient to blame the drinking and not himself.

Physiological dependence (the "E"), as denoted by the need to drink to suppress withdrawal symptoms.

Studies of the CAGE questions have shown that they are quite sensitive (70 to 90% of alcoholics respond positively to one or more of the questions; most have at least two positive responses) and specific (80 to 95% of nonalcoholic persons respond negatively to all four questions) (23). These test characteristics of the CAGE questions are superior to laboratory tests—gamma-glutaryl transpeptidase (GGT), other liver function tests, and mean corpuscular volume (MCV)—that are often used to screen for alcoholism (23). Abnormalities in these tests may, however, be helpful in supporting persistent inquiry and in confrontation (see below) in the suspected alcoholic.

Screening questions that focus upon *one common consequence of alcoholism—trauma—*may be quite sensitive, especially the question "Have you ever been injured after drinking?" (51). A positive response to this question, or a history of unexplained repeated trauma or traffic accidents, may be important in patients whose CAGE responses are equivocal or in patients who have few of the social contacts that are implied in the CAGE questions. The latter group includes antisocial younger drinkers, older persons, and others who commonly become isolated.

The approach in Fig. 21.1 does not include direct inquiry about *quantity or frequency of alcohol use.*

Although quantitative inquiry may be helpful for identifying an occasional patient who is ready to discuss problems associated with drinking, its disadvantages are that (a) it does not focus upon inability to control use or upon adverse consequences of drinking; (b) there is no "gold standard" for the cut-off quantity below or above which one can confidently exclude or diagnose alcoholism (23); (c) problem drinkers usually under-report the amount and frequency of their drinking (13) and may become guarded in their response to subsequent questions about patterns of use and consequences.

Diagnosis of Alcoholism

The confident diagnosis of alcoholism requires nonjudgmental exploration of any positive information obtained in screening. This may include asking for clarification (e.g., "Can you tell me more about the last time you decided to cut back a bit . . ." or "Exactly what does she say to annoy you . . .?" or "How do you feel after you take that morning drink on the days that you do take it . . ."), gentle confrontation ("That must have made you feel pretty bad . . . sounds like the drinking had a lot to do with it . . .").

At times, a planned interview with a family member or close friend may be needed to make a confident diagnosis of alcoholism. This means requesting the patient's permission to discuss his drinking with another person; his response to this request may reveal a problem that was denied in response to screening questions (e.g., "No, no, don't talk to her . . . she'll tell you I overdo it every night . . . but that's her problem, not mine . . ."). Questions to another person regarding the patient's drinking patterns and consequences of his drinking (the same kind of information contained in the CAGE and MAST instruments) will usually yield abundant evidence for alcoholism when the problem is present. An exception may be the relatives of an elderly alcoholic who have little contact with him and/or have tacitly agreed to ignore or deny a frustrating, seemingly hopeless situation. In this instance, educating the family about the disease concept of alcoholism may be needed before they are willing to describe the patterns and consequences of the patient's drinking.

In another way, through contact initiated by one or more family members, information will be produced that supports the diagnosis of alcoholism. In these instances, it is important to encourage the family members to tell the patient that they have contacted his doctor to describe these concerns. The ways in which the family can influence the treatment of the patient and can get help for themselves are described below.

In summary, except for the presence of one of the diagnostic manifestations of alcoholism, (Table 21.1), there is no simple way to diagnose alcoholism. When the problem is not overt, skillful interviewing of the patient and evaluation of multiple pieces of information are needed to make this diagnosis. This process

may be accomplished at one or two visits or may span a period of weeks to months.

GENERAL PRINCIPLES OF TREATMENT

Definition of Successful Treatment

Alcoholism is a highly treatable disease. Successful treatment depends largely on the skills of those who motivate the alcoholic patient to accept his diagnosis, to undergo detoxification (see below), and to enter and adhere to a long-term treatment process. Treatment success can be defined as the *achievement of abstinence, or progressively longer periods of abstinence from alcohol (and other drugs), with improved life functioning for the patient and his family.* (A case example is shown in Fig. 21.2.) Using this definition, when treatment is initiated and maintained for about 3 years, at least 70% of alcoholic patients will successfully recover from alcoholism (11, 33, 41, 64). This rate of recovery compares favorably with reported rates of "spontaneous" recovery from alcoholism, which range from 4 to 26%. Factors associated with good and poor outcomes after treatment are summarized below (see "Prognosis with Treatment" below).

The appropriate terms for describing an alcoholic in recovery are "recovered" alcoholic (a public or polite term) or "recovering" alcoholic (a personal or clinical term). The terms "ex-," "reformed," "former," or "cured" alcoholic are inappropriate.

Despite initial reports that some alcoholics can learn "controlled drinking" (53), this goal of treatment has been shown in careful studies to be unrealistic for most alcoholics (24).

Avoiding a Psychoanalytic Approach

It has been repeatedly shown that treating alcoholics as though their abnormal drinking behavior were secondary to underlying psychopathology is usually unsuccessful and often countertherapeutic. Insight-oriented or in-depth psychotherapy early in the treatment of alcoholism is, therefore, contraindicated. By contrast, supportive and directive psychotherapy, using the treatment methods outlined below and focused on the alcoholism as a primary disease, is usually effective in helping the alcoholic patient reach a successful recovery.

Outpatient Treatment: Overview

A trial of outpatient treatment, including detoxification (see below), is appropriate initially for most alcoholics. It is more economical, allows the patient to continue working and to continue daily activities, and promotes recovery in the more realistic environment of the patient's day-to-day life. However, to be successful, outpatient treatment must be *intensive, thorough, and monitored consistently and regularly* over a long period of time. Even with optimal outpatient treatment, many alcoholics also require inpatient treatment (discussed below). Treatment consists

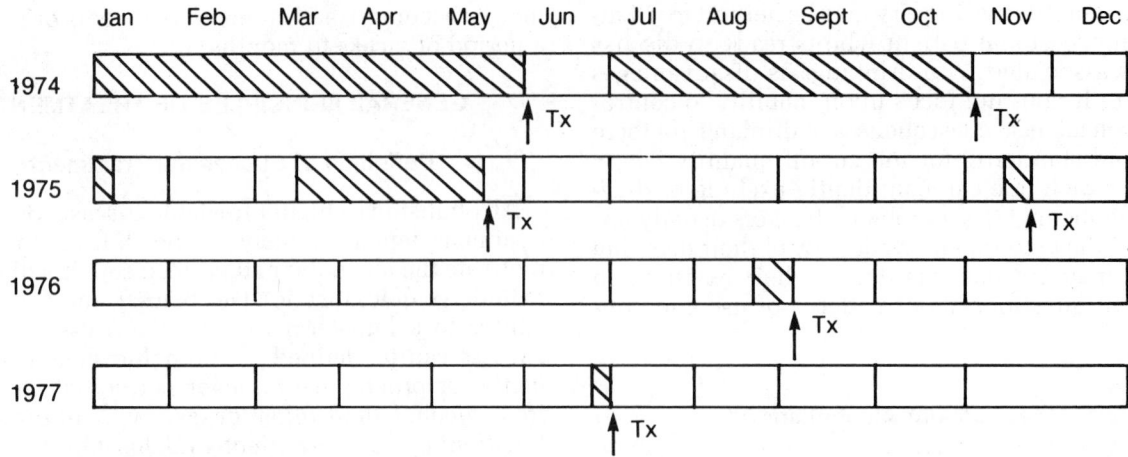

Figure 21.2. Drinking-sober profile of a 53-year-old factory supervisor who had been abusing alcohol for 15 years. The achievement of longer and longer periods of abstinence is typical of the process of recovery from alcoholism. *Hatched areas* = drinking; *clear areas* = abstinence; *Tx* = came in for treatment, after having dropped out of treatment.

of motivating the patient, initiating a treatment plan, and providing regular follow-up.

The clinician who initially motivates an alcoholic to accept treatment may elect not to coordinate his overall treatment but to refer him elsewhere. For this important referral, one should select a specialist or a program with demonstrated expertise in helping alcoholics to recover. The simplest ways to find such expert help are to call the local National Council on Alcoholism, to ask a colleague who has had experience in referring or treating alcoholics, or to refer the patient to an existing community alcoholism treatment program. In selecting skilled help, one should look for several characteristics. The effective alcoholism specialist or program tends to (a) be abstinence oriented; (b) use Alcoholics Anonymous (AA) and/or group therapy as a mainstay of treatment; (c) offer disulfiram to patients; (d) avoid the use of psychoactive drugs in long-term treatment, especially the sedative-hypnotics; (e) refer the spouse to Al-Anon or family therapy; (f) provide close follow-up; and (g) avoid insight-oriented psychotherapy, unless indicated later in the course of recovery. The physician who makes the referral should reinforce participation in the treatment program whenever the patient returns for follow-up.

The importance of being competent in handling alcoholism has been highlighted in legal decisions in recent years in which physicians have lost suits brought by families and patients for (a) failure to diagnose alcoholism; (b) failure to refer alcoholics for treatment; or (c) failure to provide treatment for alcoholism.

Breaking Down Denial and Motivating the Patient

Denial, described above, is the major obstacle to having a patient accept the diagnosis of alcoholism and agree to treatment. Three motivational techniques are fundamental in breaking down denial in patients—and in their family members if necessary: *confrontation, showing empathy, and offering hope.* These techniques are equally important in one-on-one interviews and the other paths to treatment that are described

below. *Confrontation* is telling the person what one observes, including that one has diagnosed the disease alcoholism. The patient will usually deny the diagnosis and may even get angry. However, with persistent and nonjudgmental confrontation, most patients will eventually admit that they have a problem with alcohol. It is important in a confrontation not to argue with the patient but simply to restate the facts.

Statements that convey empathy and offer hope are important in allaying the person's denial, anxiety, anger, and shame. They should be interspersed with confrontational statements. *Empathy* is conveyed by stating that one recognizes the patient's feelings ("I can see that this is upsetting you") and by conveying concern ("I am very concerned about you"). *Offering hope* is crucial. The patient must hear, repeatedly, that there is a "way out" and that there is relief from the misery and bewilderment of his condition. The "way out" is through abstinence from alcohol and other psychoactive drugs—one day at a time—and the liberal and regular use of group treatment, which includes self-help groups and group therapy.

Motivation of the patient is an ongoing process. In follow-up, denial will recur, and it can be dealt with by using the same three techniques. It may be useful to refer to the facts recorded at previous visits and to the patient's Michigan Alcoholism Screening Test results, if available, to help break down the recurring denial.

SPECIFIC ASPECTS OF TREATMENT

After a confident diagnosis of alcoholism has been made, the objectives of care are to have the patient accept the diagnosis and agree to treatment. Specific aspects of this process are described here, beginning with one-on-one confrontation of the patient.

One-on-One Confrontation

Utilizing the motivational techniques described above, one can often persuade an alcoholic patient to accept treatment. Several actions are critical in the one-on-one confrontation of the patient:

— Stating the diagnosis.
— Explaining the disease model.
— Making the model specific to the patient.
— Telling about treatment.
— Getting the patient (and his family) to accept (support) treatment.
— Following through.

Fig. 21.3 summarizes a recommended approach that includes each of these actions. This approach may be incorporated into the interview at a single visit or into interviews at multiple visits. The term "drinking problem" may be used early in the discussion, before the patient's feelings regarding alcoholism are known. Even in the most denying and uncooperative patient, naming the diagnosis is useful, because it "plants a seed" that is likely to grow, given time and motivation. One must be rather directive in confronting a patient with his alcoholism. It is important, however, to include questions that give the patient some sense of control during this rather one-sided interaction (see items 3, 5, 7, and 10 in Fig. 21.3). Because most alcoholic patients will have negative emotional responses, either overt or private, to being told their diagnosis, it should be assumed that they will not register much of what one says and that brevity, repetition, and directness are essential. Repeated statements of concern, optimism, and support for the person are as important as statements of fact about the disease. Such statements will help a patient while he is hearing a diagnosis that inevitably brings shame' despite the message that it is a disease and that it is not his fault.

Telling the patient that *he has a disease*, and that it is not his fault for having it, helps to relieve guilt. To assure that the patient does not conclude that he cannot avoid further drinking because he "has a disease," one should tell him it is his responsibility to seek treatment.

The first goal of treatment is *abstinence from alcohol* and other psychoactive drugs. However, it is never sufficient simply to tell the patient to stop drinking. Early in treatment, the patient must accept help in the difficult process of recovery. This help is *multidimensional*. In addition to regular follow-up by a supportive physician who believes the patient can recover, the most important elements are a plan for detoxification, consideration of disulfiram, family involvement, Alcoholics Anonymous, and group therapy that provides the patient with successful role models. Inpatient treatment in a specialized alcoholism treatment facility will often be needed. It is important to explain each of the possible treatment options to the patient and his family. If one is not familiar with these, one should ask an alcoholism counselor to see the patient to explain them. If the patient is in a crisis and not enough time is available during the first visit, a return appointment should be

STATING THE DIAGNOSIS

1. Tell the patient the diagnosis (e.g., "I think that you have the disease alcoholism . . . and I am very concerned about you").

2. Acknowledge the patient's reaction (e.g., "I can see that this is making you pretty uncomfortable . . .").

EXPLAINING THE DISEASE MODEL

3. Ask the patient to tell you his idea of what alcoholism is. (Patient usually describes stereotype model of a skid-row alcoholic . . . "and that's not me!". . . .)

4. Clarify the patient's model by stating four basic facts:

   a) Alcoholism is a disease ("a disease like other medical diseases . . . for example diabetes").
   b) Like other diseases, alcoholism has an early stage way before what you described.
   c) Like other diseases, alcoholism is not the patient's fault.
   d) Alcoholism can be treated and the chances of recovery are excellent.

MAKING THE MODEL SPECIFIC

5. Ask the patient if he knows why you think he has alcoholism.

6. Tell the patient the evidence that he has alcoholism. (Always restate concern for the patient; if appropriate, stress features of early alcoholism.)

TELLING ABOUT TREATMENT

7. Ask the patient what he knows about the treatment of alcoholism.

8. Tell the patient the basic facts about treatment:

   a) Abstinence
   b) Requires the help of other people

GETTING THE PATIENT (AND FAMILY) TO ACCEPT TREATMENT

9. Offer the patient treatment options that you know of (always include a local program that offers detoxification and Alcoholics Anonymous).

10. Get the patient to select a treatment plan and to make contact promptly (e.g., call available detoxification program, call local AA office and let patient speak with AA representative).

11. With the patient's permission, contact his spouse or other significant person(s) (tell the diagnosis and plan, and initiate plans for family treatment).

FOLLOWING THROUGH

12. Schedule follow-up, appointment in 1 or 2 weeks (consider 1 to 2 days if patient has not agreed to make a treatment decision).

Figure 21.3. A recommended approach for one-on-one confrontation of the patient in whom alcoholism has been diagnosed.

scheduled within a few days, or the patient should be immediately referred to a reliable treatment program.

Formal Intervention

All too frequently, an alcoholic with a concerned family does not respond to efforts to motivate him to accept treatment. In this situation, the family should be told about the option of using a formal intervention (31). This consists of a meeting at which persons closest to the alcoholic (immediate family members, concerned friends, employer, and/or other important people) create a crisis that motivates the alcoholic to accept treatment. An individual with expertise in coordinating formal interventions can usually be identified through the local office of the National Council on Alcoholism. An available film illustrates this technique well (see "General References").

The intervention team is composed of as many persons as possible (up to a dozen) who are emotionally important to the alcoholic. Before the actual intervention this team meets one or more times to talk about the alcoholism, to come together in their thinking, to break down their own denial that this intervention is necessary, and to agree that their purpose is to show the patient in unmistakable terms that there is a problem and that he needs treatment. The process is initiated by having each participant put in writing specific dramatic instances of drinking-related incidents that led to anger, fear, disappointment, sadness, embarrassment, or other distress for the team member. The team then *rehearses* confronting the alcoholic. Each person learns to begin with an expression of concern for the alcoholic, to describe the disturbing event and how it made that person feel, and to name specific measures they will take if the patient does not agree to treatment (e.g., loss of job, no further visits by grandchildren, etc.). As part of a formal intervention, arrangements are made in advance to have the person admitted for alcoholism treatment. Alcoholism treatment centers are familiar with this technique and cooperate. Details of financing of treatment, packing clothes, arranging for absence from work, etc. must all be worked out by the team ahead of time.

After the team has rehearsed, the consequences for not going into treatment are agreed upon, and the details of treatment are worked out, the patient is told that the family wants to meet to talk about some family concerns. The patient is asked by the coordinator to hear the family out and is told that he will be given an opportunity to express his concerns. It is hoped that the intervention will conclude with the patient accepting treatment.

If properly constructed and properly prepared, such an intervention can have enormous power with even an unmotivated alcoholic. Faced with the crisis created by the intervention, the alcoholic will find that there is nowhere left to turn should the entire team pull out its support if treatment is refused. Although an alcoholic may respond angrily to the coercion that drives him into treatment, he will usually eventually be grateful for the help.

Motivating through Employee Assistance Programs

Increasingly employers have recognized the economic and human costs of alcoholism and have developed employee assistance programs to motivate and assist alcoholics into treatment. Employers threaten to terminate employees who have deteriorating job performance due to alcoholism unless they get treatment and remain in treatment. Such programs have demonstrated recovery rates as high as 90% for alcoholics. Cost savings have been estimated to be in the range of $4 to $7 saved for every dollar invested in an employee assistance program. Physicians asked to write work excuses can often work with employee assistance programs to coerce the denying alcoholic to get appropriate treatment for alcoholism. This approach uses the strong motivation to keep a job as leverage for getting treatment and following through to recovery—leverage the physician alone may not have on the patient.

The problem of the impaired professional and the use of measures similar to employee assistance programs are discussed below.

Alcoholics Anonymous and Group Therapy

Alcoholics and other chemical-dependent people seem to recover best in group treatment settings. Groups effectively break down the denial process and heal the associated guilt and shame through a combination of identification, nonjudgmental acceptance, confrontation, and support. Every alcoholic should be strongly encouraged to attend AA regularly. Many physicians who are specialists in alcoholism consider it the single most important aspect of treatment, and studies have shown that regular AA attendance is strongly correlated with long-term recovery and improved functioning (4, 26, 54). Formal alcoholism group therapy is also successful.

Many patients will be reluctant to attend AA or a therapy group. Therefore, when referring a patient it is important to convey that one is familiar with these programs and has confidence in them. Immediate action, taken while the patient is in the office, may consist of (a) telephoning the local AA office and letting the patient request a contact to take him to a convenient AA meeting, or (b) telephoning an alcoholism treatment program and arranging an intake appointment for the patient.

The best way for physicians to learn about these programs is to attend one or more AA and, if available, open group therapy meetings. To locate such meetings, one should call the local AA office or the local National Council on Alcoholism. The AA process is summarized in Table 21.4.

Table 21.4.
The Process of Alcoholics Anonymous

AA was founded in 1935 by two chronic alcoholics, one a stockbroker and one a physician.

Meetings

AA meetings are held frequently in all communities in the United States and in most other countries. Meetings are either open or closed (most are open and most welcome nonalcoholics interested in treating alcoholism). A published directory of meetings, places, times, and information by telephone are available from each local chapter of AA. By contacting AA, an alcoholic can almost always arrange to be taken to a meeting in his community, often on the day he makes the request. Many AA members attend meetings several times a week. Some attend at least one meeting per day. Lifelong activity in AA is the basis for maintaining health for many recovering alcoholics.

Meetings are usually 1 hour in length. Most are held in the evening, although there are many daytime meetings as well. Meetings begin with a recitation by one member of the Twelve Steps and the Twelve Traditions and are devoted to examination and interpretation of these—as illustrated in personal experiences described by a number of members. One member of the group chairs the meeting and calls on speakers. Speakers introduce themselves by their first names (*e.g.,* "I'm Joe—I'm an alcoholic . . . ."). Meetings end with group recitation of the Lord's Prayer or the Serenity Prayer. ('God grant me the Serenity to accept the things I cannot change, Courage to change the things I can, and Wisdom to know the difference.')

AA on the surface can sometimes look insubstantial and unsophisticated, often turning off newcomers. Frequently the spiritual overtones of the program are rejected. The program however is *profound and life changing*. Without an administrative structure, owning no property, and having no dues or fees, it continues to grow because it works and meets human need.

Publications

AA provides printed educational aids in the form of pamphlets (available at meetings) and "the Big Book" (*Alcoholics Anonymous,* a collection of personal stories that illustrate vividly the ways that lives are damaged by alcoholism and the AA path to recovery). One can obtain this book or other literature at meetings, at the local AA office, or by writing AA World Services, Box 459, Grand Central Station, New York, NY 10017.

The 12 Steps and the 12 Traditions

The 12 Steps
1. We admitted we were powerless over alcohol, that our lives had become unmanageable.
2. Came to believe that a Power greater than ourselves could restore us to sanity.
3. Made a decision to turn our will and our lives over to the care of God as *we understood Him.*
4. Made a searching and fearless moral inventory of ourselves.
5. Admitted to God, to ourselves and to another human being the exact nature of our wrongs.
6. Were entirely ready to have God remove all these defects of character.
7. Humbly asked Him to remove our shortcomings.
8. Made a list of all persons we had harmed, and became willing to make amends to them all.
9. Made direct amends to such people wherever possible, except when to do so would injure them or others.
10. Continued to take personal inventory, and when we were wrong promptly admitted it.
11. Sought through prayer and meditation to improve our conscious contact with God, *as we understood Him*, praying only for knowledge of His will for us and the power to carry that out.
12. Having had a spiritual awakening as the result of these Steps, we tried to carry this message to alcoholics, and to practice these principles in all our affairs (*note*: For this step, Altman substitutes "others" for the word "alcoholics").

Boiled down, these steps mean, simply:
  a. Admission of alcoholism.
  b. Personality analysis and catharsis.
  c. Adjustment of personal relations.
  d. Dependence upon some Higher Power.
  e. Working with other alcoholics.

The 12 Traditions of AA
1. Our common welfare should come first; personal recovery depends upon AA unity.
2. For our group purpose there is but one ultimate authority—a loving God as He may express Himself in our group conscience. Our leaders are but trusted servants; they do not govern.
3. The only requirement for AA membership is a desire to stop drinking.
4. Each group should be autonomous except in matters affecting other groups or AA as a whole.
5. Each group has but one primary purpose—to carry out its message to the alcoholic who still suffers.
6. An AA group ought never endorse, finance, or lend the AA name to any related facility or outside enterprise, lest problems of money, property, and prestige divert us from our primary purpose.
7. Every AA group ought to be fully self-supporting, declining outside contributions.
8. Alcoholics Anonymous should remain forever nonprofessional, but our service centers may emply special workers.
9. AA, as such, ought never to be organized; but we may create service boards or committees directly responsible to those they serve.
10. Alcoholics Anonymous has no opinion on outside issues; hence the AA name ought never be drawn into public controversy.
11. Our public relations policy is based on attraction rather than promotion; we need always maintain personal anonymity at the level of press, radio, and films.
12. Anonymity is the spiritual foundation of our Traditions, ever reminding us to place principles before personalities.

Psychotherapy

It is commonly thought that all alcoholic patients have a primary and causative underlying psychological problem. If treatment of this condition is successful, the alcoholism is expected to resolve, since it is considered to be chiefly a manifestation of the underlying psychological problem. Although this approach may seem theoretically valid, experts in treating alcoholism agree that this therapeutic strategy rarely works unless there happens to be a coexisting psychosis. Even in the latter case, the alcoholism must also be treated. After establishing rapport, therefore, the initial effort in psychotherapy should be to work with the patient toward *abstinence and toward regular participation in group treatment*.

For most nonalcoholics in *individual psychotherapy* it is best for the patient to arrive at his own "diagnosis," in order to reinforce insight. This technique works well for patients with emotional problems who do not have chemical dependency, do not have an organic brain syndrome, or are not psychotic. However, active alcoholics by definition have chemical dependency, with a strong denial system, and they often have some degree of cognitive impairment, sometimes severe. Therefore, achieving insight is difficult and often impossible. To circumvent this problem, it is suggested that the therapist utilize confrontive, supportive, and directive approaches, such as those described earlier. Using this approach facilitates the process of having the patient accept and work on his problem.

Ongoing *supportive psychotherapy*, by the patient's personal physician, as described in Chapter 11, is useful for reinforcing the patient's understanding of the disease and the recovery process; for monitoring patient's functioning in important life areas, such as family, job, and interpersonal relations; and for assisting the patient in change and growth.

A year or more after a successful recovery, it is useful to re-examine the need for psychotherapy and recovery from a deeper perspective (see "Adult Children of Dysfunctional Families" below).

Discussions with the Spouse or Closest Family Member(s)

As part of the early management of an alcoholic patient, it is important to discuss the situation with the spouse or person closest to the patient. Through such discussions, which should be conducted without breaking the patient's confidentiality, one can (a) ensure that the family agrees with the goal of abstinence; (b) explore the spouse's own drinking pattern; (c) discern any special problems occurring in any of the close family members, including the children; (d) educate the spouse about the enabling process; (e) refer the spouse to Al-Anon, teenage children to Alateen, or some other available family resource; and (f) schedule a follow-up visit after the spouse has attended several Al-Anon meetings. *If the family does not change and grow, usually through regular attendance at Al-Anon meetings, it will be more difficult for the patient to recover.* Family treatment and the Al-Anon process are described below (Co-Alcoholism).

Disulfiram (Antabuse)

Although controlled studies have not shown unequivocally that it increases duration of sobriety (50), the use of disulfiram to prevent drinking should be considered for some patients. The risks of prescribing disulfiram have probably been overemphasized. Very

few deaths attributed to its interaction with alcohol have been recorded in the medical literature. Most of these occurred early in the drug's history and usually at daily doses exceeding 1000 mg (more than 4 times the present recommended daily dose of 250 mg). Disulfiram is available, as Antabuse, in the form of scored tables containing 250 mg or 500 mg.

Disulfiram-Alcohol Interaction

Alcohol is initially oxidized by the hepatic enzyme alcohol dehydrogenase to acetaldehyde, and disulfiram inhibits acetaldehyde oxidation by interfering with aldehyde dehydrogenase. This effect may persist for up to two weeks after cessation of disulfiram. The symptoms of the alcohol-disulfiram reaction are related to elevated acetaldehyde; they are usually proportional to the amounts of disulfiram and alcohol ingested. Some people will have typical symptoms after drinking as little as 7 ml of alcohol (about half of a drink). A very small percentage of patients seem to be able to drink despite taking disulfiram with no significant symptoms. In these latter patients the dose can be increased up to 500 mg daily but only if the patient seems motivated to abstinence rather than to drinking.

The common symptoms of the alcohol-disulfiram reaction usually begin within 10 minutes of drinking and include flushing, throbbing in the head and neck, headaches, anxiety, general discomfort, sweating, and respiratory difficulty. The reaction typically lasts between 30 minutes and several hours. Less frequently nausea, vomiting, hypotension, thirst, chest pain, palpitation, dyspnea, hyperventilation, tachycardia, syncope, weakness, blurred vision, and confusion can occur. Very rarely, disulfiram may cause an acute exacerbation of a coexisting problem—e.g., respiratory depression, congestive heart failure, convulsions, arrhythmias, angina, or myocardial infarction. These risks must be weighed against the certain risks of continued alcohol drinking.

Treatment for the alcohol-disulfiram reaction, when needed, is usually supportive to restore blood pressure and treat shock. These measures should be instituted in an emergency department.

Side Effects and Contraindications

Disulfiram at recommended doses is tolerated well by most patients. Some patients complain of drowsiness, fatigability, headaches, a garlic-like or metallic aftertaste, and breath odor and acneform eruptions. To avoid the problem with drowsiness, the disulfiram can be taken at bedtime. The other side effects usually subside within a few days or weeks with continued therapy. More rarely confusion (particularly in the elderly), optic neuritis, polyneuritis, and peripheral neuritis may occur.

Contraindications for the use of disulfiram include a history of hypertension, diabetes, emphysema, seizures, liver or renal disease, coronary artery disease, hypothyroidism, pregnancy, or a history of having drunk in the past while taking disulfiram. Disulfiram may impair the metabolism and potentiate the effects of caffeine, warfarin, and phenytoin; and it may interact additively to potentiate the neurological side effects of isoniazid (ataxia, psychosis). It should not be used in conjunction with these drugs or with the following other classes of drugs: beta- or alpha-adrenergic antagonists, vasodilators, sympathomimetic amines, monoamine oxidase inhibitors, tricyclic antidepressants, and neuroleptics. Because bone marrow toxicity and hepatitis may be caused, rarely, by disulfiram, it is recommended that aminotransferase levels be measured at baseline and every two weeks; and that a complete blood cell count be checked at baseline and every 6 months.

Advantages of Disulfiram

There are several advantages to disulfiram: (a) Because the drug is taken daily, it is a constant reminder that one cannot drink safely; (b) it provides evidence of compliance in the treatment program; (c) it is compatible with other forms of treatment of alcoholism; and (d) it can also provide family and employer with reassurance that, as long as it is taken daily, the alcoholic cannot get drunk. There are four additional advantages for the patient to consider. These are (a) the patient has to make the decision not to drink only once a day; (b) because of this, he tends not to worry about whether he can drink or not; (c) not worrying or thinking about drinking saves him considerable energy; and (d) this makes his recovery easier.

Office Prescribing of Disulfiram

Patients who are motivated to succeed in recovery and who have experienced relapse or dread the likelihood of relapse are candidates for disulfiram. Many alcoholism treatment programs utilize disulfiram for some patients, usually under close supervision. Table 21.5 summarizes a practical plan that can be used in office practice. This supervised approach is similar in its demands on patient and physicians to the initiation and management of long-term anticoagulation. A detailed patient education guide accompanies packages of Antabuse.

A decision to stop the drug is best made jointly by the physician, the spouse or other close person, the AA sponsor, and the patient. It should be based on the strength of the person's recovery. Important guidelines in this decision are active AA and/or group therapy participation, coping with crises without recourse to drinking, improved family relationships, dissolution of denial, social ease (diminution in social anxiety), growth in self-esteem, and prolonged abstinence (67).

Alcohol-Drug Interactions

Because of their erratic behavior, alcoholics frequently fail to take prescribed drugs regularly or correctly. In this sense, alcoholism, like other forms of chronic mental illness, adds greatly to the difficulty of treating coexisting medical conditions. In addition to compliance problems, there are a number of drug interactions that must be considered when prescribing to alcoholics and to other persons who use alcoholic beverages (48). Some of the interactions between alcohol and other drugs may provide initial clues to the existence of alcoholism. This may be especially true in elderly persons with unrecognized alcoholism, who are more likely than younger persons to be taking multiple prescribed drugs for chronic physical and mental disorders.

Alcohol-drug interactions may involve (a) antagonism, (b) additive and supra-additive (synergistic) effects, and (c) cross-tolerance or synergism.

Antagonism between drugs and alcohol, such as occurs with disulfiram, can cause specific, deleterious reactions. Some common drugs in this category are: chlorpropamide, tolbutamide, chloramphenicol, griseofulvin, isoniazid, metronidazole, quinacrine, phenylbutazone, and phenacetin.

The additive effects may occur with agents whose pharmacological effects or adverse effects may be aggravated by alcohol. Common drugs in this category are: oral hypoglycemic agents (hypoglycemia), salicylates (gastrointestinal bleeding), antihypertensives, nitroglycerine, and tricyclics (hypotension), warfarin (hemorrhage because prothrombin time increased), sedative-hypnotics, anxiolytic drugs, antidepressant drugs, antihistamines, opiates, metoclopramide [central nervous sytem (CNS) depression], neuroleptic drugs

Table 21.5.
A Suggested Approach to Supervised Use of Disulfiram

1. Satisfy the following indications: the patient is willing to take medication several times a week under supervision, the patient can recall making the decision to take the first drink of a relapse, and the patient is actively involved in an organized outpatient treatment program.
2. Rule out contraindications and ask yourself the following question "Can this patient survive a disulfiram-alcohol reaction?"
3. Ensure sober state prior to the initiation of treatment. Check a CBC and SMA-18.
4. Be sure patient and spouse know how to avoid hidden alcohol in foods, OTC medications, toiletries, ect.
5. Have the patient read, discuss, and sign a consent form prior to initiating treatment.
6. Begin with a dose of one tablet (250 mg) daily.
7. *Keep the medication bottle in the office*, and have the patient come in three times a week to be dispensed two (or three) doses by the office staff. After one month, decrease the visits to twice a week and increase the number of pills dispensed accordingly. After another month, go to weekly visits and continue these for the duration of disulfiram treatment. See the patient at least monthly and repeat laboratory testing every three months.
8. If the patient misses more than one or two appointments in a row, have the office staff contact the people on the consent form, and stop administering the medication.

(CNS depression, hypotension, respiratory depression, impaired hepatic function).

Either *cross-tolerance or synergism* can occur with some drug-alcohol combinations, depending on the time of drug administration. For example, chronic alcoholics may require an unusually large dose of anesthetic because of cross-tolerance, but at the same time would be susceptible to CNS depression with a low dose of anesthetic when a large amount of alcohol has been ingested shortly before the need for emergency surgery and anesthesia (e.g., after major trauma).

Finally, *cimetidine* may inhibit hepatic metabolism of alcohol and/or increase gastrointestinal absorption of alcohol; patients prescribed cimetidine may thus become intoxicated with smaller amounts of alcohol and should be forewarned.

Psychoactive Drug Prescribing

Although many alcoholics present with symptoms that might be helped by sedatives, such as anxiety, insomnia, and tremors, in actuality *these drugs usually interfere with successful recovery.* Anxiolytic drugs may have a role in acute detoxification (see below) and major tranquilizers, antidepressants, and lithium have usefulness in treating, respectively, the schizophrenic, the severe protracted depressive, and the manic-depressive alcoholic (as long as these patients are being treated concomitantly for alcoholism). Apart from these situations, psychoactive drugs should not be prescribed for alcoholics. There are many reasons for this: (a) all of the sedatives are cross-tolerant with alcohol, and thus have a "built-in" escalation factor; (b) combining sedatives with alcohol is often dangerously synergistic; (c) inability to control consumption, a cardinal feature of alcoholism, occurs with prescribed sedative drugs; (d) memory blackouts may also occur with other sedatives and minor tranquilizers; (e) patients may alter the prescription in order to obtain excess quantities of these drugs; (f) prescribing these drugs reinforces psychoactive substance use as a coping mechanism and impairs development of the patient's own coping mechanisms; (g) they interfere with learning to relate to others in a healthy manner; and (h) using these drugs may alienate the patient from perhaps the best treatment he could receive, i.e., Alcoholics Anonymous. Bissell (5) has said "I do think we need to give our patients a substitute for alcohol, but I don't think that substitute can be another sedative. I think it has to be our concern, our time, our caring, and ourselves."

Urine Monitoring in the Alcoholic with other Psychoactive Substance Abuse

For the patient with chemical dependence to one or more drugs other than alcohol, urine monitoring is indicated. This is in part because it can be difficult to recognize that a person is using drugs, especially early in the course of a relapse. Urine monitoring is also therapeutic, in that it gives the patient another type of structure through which to recover. Finally, it is often to the patient's advantage (e.g., to protect his job or to meet court-ordered conditions) to have negative urines documented for a substantial period of time. Low-priced urine screens that check for from 30 to 40 different psychoactive drugs are available in most large communities. For communities that lack these services, specimens can be mailed to a regional laboratory. This should be done by a reliable person other than the patient. The sample should be collected at random and witnessed by a reliable observer. In patients being treated for multidrug dependence, weekly urine monitoring should continue for a minimum of 1 year.

Follow-up: Prevention and Management of Relapse

Next to dealing with denial and motivating the patient, follow-up is the most difficult part of treatment. One reason is that when an alcoholic recovers there may be an early "honeymoon period" during which the patient feels and looks so good that one is lulled into believing that regular follow-up is not necessary. However, because it takes about *2 to 3 years of appropriate treatment* before recovery can be secure, regular follow-up is indicated.

During the first 6 weeks after stopping drinking, the patient needs much support and direction, for this is the time when he is most likely to relapse. Therefore, at least weekly visits are indicated for this time, with a gradually decreasing frequency thereafter. Other high risk times for potential relapse include special days and occasions, such as vacations, holidays, business trips, birthdays, anniversaries; or crises such as separation, divorce, death of a close person, or illness in the family. Other relapse danger times are when a patient stops taking disulfiram or stops going to AA or group therapy meetings.

"Dry drunks" are frequently part of the natural history of recovery. This is the name given by recovering alcoholics to the negative emotions and behaviors reminiscent of those that occurred when the patient was drinking. Dry drunks may last from a few hours to several weeks or even months. Treatment is by recognition, education, and alteration of the diet and other current life habits. Dry drunks are often associated with eating poorly. Regular well-balanced meals should be recommended, and caffeine intake, including coffee, tea, colas, and chocolate, should be markedly decreased or discontinued. Increased attendance at AA and/or group therapy meetings at this time is very important. Moderation in the patient's work and recreational activities and rest should be advised. Beginning to address adult child and co-dependence issues may also be helpful (see below).

The relapse process generally begins long before the person drinks. This process often progresses in the following sequence: (a) reactivation of denial; (b) progressive isolation and defensiveness; (c) building a crisis to justify symptom progression; (d) immobilization; (e) confusion and overreaction; (f) depression;

(g) loss of control over behavior; (h) recognition of loss of control; (i) option reduction; and (j) debilitation—which ends in drinking, using other drugs, or in some other debilitating condition (21).

Although it should not be telegraphed to the patient, relapse is part of the natural history of successful recovery for the majority of alcoholics (21), and one should not become discouraged if it happens (see Fig. 21.3 illustrating the long-term course of a typical recovering alcoholic). Instead, one should *immediately* recruit the patient back into treatment using the same motivational techniques described above. *Relapse is a time for both patient and therapist to learn about their mistakes* and to correct them by strengthening treatment.

OUTPATIENT DETOXIFICATION

It has been shown that about 90% of alcoholics can be detoxified from alcohol by outpatient procedures (18, 22, 62), leaving about 10% that require hospitalization for detoxification. When patients are randomly assigned to outpatient or inpatient detoxification, the principal difference is that more of the inpatients (over 90%) than the outpatients (about 70%) complete a standard detoxification program (22). Although many alcoholics can be detoxified at home, many will also benefit from a community "social setting" detoxification center, described below.

Alcohol Withdrawal Symptoms

The diagnosis of alcohol withdrawal requires (a) a history of recent heavy drinking lasting at least a week followed by reduced intake or cessation of use; (b) the absence of other conditions that could cause symptoms mimicking withdrawal; and (c) one or more of the four major manifestations of alcohol withdrawal: tremors, seizures ("rum fits"), hallucinosis, and delirium tremens. These occur also in other conditions, ranging from withdrawal from other sedative-hypnotic drugs to meningitis (see list of causes of delirium, Table 17.6).

Tremulousness usually begins 8 to 12 hours after the patient's last drink and peaks in 24 to 36 hours. *Withdrawal seizures* occur within 8 to 24 hours. Both of these manifestations can occur before the blood alcohol level has reached zero.

The *alcohol hallucination* is almost never the mythical "pink elephant." Rather, it is usually one of moving insects, small animals, or threatening voices. In a series of 50 consecutive patients, 58% of their hallucinations were purely visual, 16% were purely auditory, and 26% were mixed (56). In certain patients these hallucinations may not be all negative, i.e., the patient becomes used to them and is no longer frightened. Hallucinations may begin up to several days after the patient stops or markedly reduces alcohol (usually in the first 48 hours). Typically, alcoholic hallucinosis lasts from minutes to days (usually less than 1 week) but in a very small percentage of patients

hallucinosis may continue for weeks or months and, rarely, as a continuous symptom.

Delirium tremens is a late manifestation of withdrawal, occurring anytime from 48 hours (most common interval) to 14 days (uncommon) after cessation of drinking. It may begin after the patient has shown signs of improvement from the early manifestations of withdrawal. Any of the symptoms of delirium, described in Chapter 17, may signal the onset of delirium tremens.

At least half of ambulatory alcoholic patients who stop drinking develop *none* of the four major manifestations of withdrawal (62). Additional minor symptoms are common. Anorexia, nausea, and sometimes vomiting are present in varying degrees. Tachycardia, systolic hypertension, and paroxysmal diaphoresis also occur frequently. Generalized weakness may be prominent, and tinnitus, hyperacusis, itching, muscle cramps, mood and sleep disorders are sometimes experienced. The patient is often hyperalert, becomes startled easily, and usually craves alcohol or other drugs to quiet his symptoms. The patient usually experiences varying degrees of disorientation and difficulty concentrating.

Selection of Patients for Outpatient Detoxification

There are a number of indications for referring a withdrawing alcoholic patient to an emergency department Table 21.6), where admission for management of medical problems and/or for detoxification will often be necessary. For the majority of patients, outpatient detoxification, supervised at daily visits to the treatment program or physician's office, is as effective as inpatient detoxification (22). The choice of outpatient versus inpatient detoxification is often based upon what programs are available, upon patient and/or family preference, and upon third party reimbursement policies. The option of undergoing withdrawal without the use of psychoactive drugs, is offered by

Table 21.6.
Some Indications for Referring a Withdrawing Alcoholic to an Emergency Department

1. Vomiting blood
2. A fever greater than 100.5°F (38.1°C)
3. Shortness of breath or respiratory rate >20
4. Sudden onset of chest pain
5. Heart rate >120 in absence of tremulousness or hallucinosis, or as part of withdrawal that does not improve with a talk down
6. A seizure that occurs more than once, or from which the patient does not awaken within 15 minutes, or a localized seizure
7. Shaking chills
8. Severe abdominal pain
9. Protracted vomiting
10. Any trauma other than minor trauma
11. Depression of consciousness where the patient is not arousable
12. History of a recent head injury (within 3 days)
13. Recurring hallucinations
14. Marked agitation that does not respond to talk down
15. Delirium
16. Severe depression or suicidal ideation
17. Uncontrolled violence

many programs and has been shown to be safe and effective (see below).

Using Psychoactive Drugs in Detoxification

Psychoactive drugs may be beneficial in selected patients who are withdrawing from alcohol. The principal reasons for using drugs in the detoxification process are (a) that many detoxification programs have long experience using drugs in the withdrawal process and do not have experience in withdrawal without using drugs and (b) that some patients undergoing withdrawal without drugs require medication to control their symptoms. The time-course of symptom resolution is the same in patients receiving psychoactive drugs and in those receiving placebo treatment (49).

Detoxification using psychoactive drugs appears to be most effective when combined with the nonpharmacological techniques described below and when treatment is given early. The safest and most effective drugs for this purpose are the benzodiazepine sedative-hypnotics. It seems to matter less which sedative-hypnotic drug is used than how it is used. An exception is that oxazepam (Serax) is probably safer in patients with overt liver disease, as it is not metabolized by the liver. What is important is *early recognition of withdrawal, early treatment, frequent monitoring, and continual treatment.* Given the decision to use sedative drugs in the detoxification process, one can choose low or high doses (see Table 21.7). *Low doses* of sedative-hypnotic drugs may be tried first for most patients. The advantage of low dose treatment is that the patient remains more alert, one of the advantages of using nonpharmacological detoxification. *High doses* of these drugs may be indicated when the low dose does not suppress or prevent symptoms in the first few hours.

The aim of drug treatment is to alleviate the most bothersome symptoms and signs of withdrawal. The drug should be given such that withdrawal symptoms are improved but without oversedating the patient. Each day's medication should be dispensed at a brief supervisory visit to the treating program or physician. The total single dose, daily dose, and frequency of administration will vary with the patient's and the staff's needs. Thus the schedule of the drug will usu-

ally be between every 2 to 12 hours "as needed," for a total of 48 to 72 hours. The route of administration of benzodiazepines should be by mouth or, if this is not possible, by slow intravenous push (diazepam or chlordiazepoxide). Hydroxyzine, diphenhydramine, and barbiturates can be given intramuscularly, but not the benzodiazepines, which are inconsistently absorbed.

For the 70-kg patient actively in early delirium tremens (DTs), a slow intravenous push of diazepam, 10 mg, may be the most effective initial treatment, to be repeated every 30 to 60 minutes as needed to lessen the agitation. At times it may be needed more frequently. After diagnosis and initial therapy, patients with DTs should be admitted to the hospital.

Detoxification without Drugs

This technique of detoxification is used in many settings, including the patient's home, "social setting" facilities, and some inpatient alcoholism programs. It is sometimes erroneously called "nonmedical" detoxification. However, medical and nursing supervision are integral features of this approach. Candidates for nonpharmacological outpatient detoxification should be *ambulatory* and, except for their chronic alcoholism and acute withdrawal, should be *otherwise free from serious chronic illness* or acute problems such as those listed in Table 21.6.

The primary aim in nonpharmacological detoxification is to provide a nonthreatening, positive environment for the patient (see Table 21.8). The patient should be kept ambulatory when possible and given a regular diet. Except when asleep or resting comfortably, he should

Table 21.7.
Selected Sedative-Hypnotic Drugs in Low and High Oral Doses as Treatment Aids in Detoxification

Drug	Low Dose[a]	High Dose[a]
	mg	*mg*
Benzodiazepines		
Chlordiazepoxide (Librium)	25	100
Diazepam (Valium)	2–5	10–20
Oxazepam (Serax)	10	30
Antihistamine-Antianxiety		
Hydroxyzine (Vistaril, Atarax)	25–50	100
Diphenhydramine (Benadryl)	25–50	100
Barbiturates		
Phenobarbital	30	100

[a]Every 2 to 12 hours.

Table 21.8.
Environmental Modification in Treating Alcohol and Other Sedative Withdrawal[a]

Sense	Therapeutic	Countertherapeutic
Visual	Lights on, not bright Familiar people, pictures, clock, clothes	Lights off Marked shadows
Sound	Soft music Soft conversation Reassurance and reality Orientation by staff	Loud or abrupt noises
Touch	Reassuring touch by staff (*e.g.,* taking pulse, hand on shoulder) Comfortable chair Low bed Regular clothes	Bed clothes High bed Restraints IVs and tubes
General	Respect Positivity, optimism	Hostility, even if subtle Negativity or pessimism

[a]Modified from Baum R, Iber FL: Initial treatment of the alcoholic patient. In Gitlow SE, Peyser HS (eds): *Alcoholism: A Practical Treatment Guide.* New York, Grune and Stratton, 1980, chap 4, pp 73–87.

be encouraged to perform purposeful activities, such as carrying out small duties or attending introductory group education and therapy sessions.

It is now clear that nonpharmacological therapy can be just as effective and usually is less hazardous than drug therapy in the detoxification of ambulatory and otherwise uncomplicated patients (18, 50, 62).

The advantages of nonpharmacological detoxification without drugs, as compared with traditional detoxification with drugs, are that it may be shorter in duration (usually 2 days); it can be done largely by nonmedical personnel; it is less expensive; it permits earlier diagnosis of psychiatric conditions; it decreases dependence on other drugs; the patient is more likely to remain alert and, therefore, able to participate in treatment; and the patient remembers the withdrawal experience and is thus more likely to realize the damaging consequences of his or her drinking behavior.

The use of all psychoactive drugs should be avoided, and routine medications should not be given unless they are clearly indicated for an ongoing condition. Antimicrobials and antidiabetic and cardiac medications usually should be continued. Antihypertensive drugs should be discontinued during the patient's withdrawal from alcohol. The only routine medication should be vitamins, i.e., 50 to 100 mg of thiamine daily, 1 mg of folate a day, and a potent multivitamin daily. These vitamins should be continued for the first month or more of recovery.

Social setting detoxification: In the past 10 years, many communities have established alcoholism facilities that provide a sheltered, supportive environment to care for alcoholics using a social model for nondrug detoxification. Patients are screened and evaluated to detect any obvious medical problems before or shortly after being admitted. Should complications arise, backup hospital/medical support is available.

The length of stay varies in each program from 3 days to more than 30 days. Most social setting programs use AA extensively, and many of the larger programs use many of the techniques used in other alcoholism treatment centers. These centers can be either day treatment or residential facilities.

Home detoxification: For detoxification at home without the use of drugs, there should be a reliable family member or other person to observe the patient for 2 full days. The physician supervising such detoxification should be in touch with the patient or the family member daily during the 2 to 4 days required for detoxification. The following is a checklist for home detoxification:

1. The patient should be motivated to do it at home.
2. A reliable person should be with the patient or frequently check on him.
3. There should be access to a phone to call the physician or counselor twice or more daily for reassurance and to monitor withdrawal.

4. No active medical problems requiring aggressive treatment, and no high dose chemical dependence to drugs other than alcohol.
5. There should be arrangements to see a supervising physician, nurse, or counselor each day.
6. If sedatives are required, antihistamines should be used (e.g., hydroxyzine 25 to 50 mg orally every 3 to 4 hours).
7. The patient should be as active as possible, attend AA if patient can tolerate, take food and fluid as desired, take multivitamins daily, and avoid caffeinated beverages.
8. Involvement in a strong outpatient program should start upon completion of detoxification.

Prevention of Withdrawal Seizures

It has been shown that phenytoin in a dose of 300 mg daily for 5 days can prevent most withdrawal seizures, even though therapeutic levels are not reached initially (44). This regimen should therefore be included in the outpatient detoxification of any patient with a history of previous withdrawal seizures. Should a withdrawal seizure occur in a patient during outpatient detoxification, the nurses and aides should monitor the patient carefully. If the patient does not recover fairly rapidly after a seizure, he should, of course, be evaluated by a physician.

There is some evidence that a high dose benzodiazepine regimen for withdrawal (Table 21.7) also may prevent seizures (49).

INPATIENT TREATMENT

Although controlled studies have not shown a definite advantage for inpatient treatment over outpatient treatment (35), inpatient treatment for 2 to 6 weeks may be especially helpful for selected patients. It is always planned for in advance when a formal intervention is utilized (see above). Other indications for inpatient treatment are (a) strong denial, especially if it persists in outpatient treatment; (b) unsuccessful or too slow recovery despite adequate outpatient treatment; (c) weak or unavailable support systems; (d) danger to self or others; (e) severe medical, psychiatric, or other problems related to the alcoholism; and (f) patient's desire for inpatient treatment.

Although treatment goals among inpatient treatment programs vary, some of the major goals include (a) breaking down denial; (b) educating about alcoholism/chemical dependence; (c) providing an introduction to group treatment: self-help groups and group therapy; (d) becoming aware of feelings and beginning to learn to handle them; (e) learning how to ask for help; (f) learning how to communicate directly and honestly; (g) learning how to enjoy life while abstinent; (h) beginning family restoration; and (i) developing a specific, appropriate, and structured long-term recovery program.

PROGNOSIS WITH TREATMENT

As stated above, with appropriate and continued treatment for at least 2 years, the prognosis for a successful recovery in alcoholism is about 70%. However, this figure does not apply to every alcoholic. A number of factors, described here, are associated with a good or poor prognosis for recovery. Even factors traditionally thought to be major barriers to treatment success—a "skid row" life style or being an unattached young adult—do not always preclude successful recovery (3, 10, 16).

Factors Associated with a Good Prognosis

The first of these factors is *clinician commitment and patient motivation.* Most patients are only marginally motivated to get well. They can be characterized as being quite ambivalent: a part of them wants to get well, and another part of them wants to continue drinking and stay sick (the patient usually does not know what is wrong with him because no one has told him of the diagnosis in an effective way). Such patients have a good chance of getting into recovery if their physician is committed to the treatment of the patient's alcoholism and consistently utilizes the motivational techniques described above.

The presence of a crisis situation is also a positive prognostic factor *if the crisis is used as a motivational tool.* The crisis may be the threat of a job loss, family separation or divorce, a driving-while-intoxicated charge, a health-related crisis, an organized formal intervention (see above), or some other dramatic event. A physician actually precipitates a crisis whenever the confrontation approach described above (Fig. 21.3) is utilized. As in that approach, it is critical to act promptly if a situational crisis is to be utilized effectively to motivate the patient to accept treatment. If exploitation of this crisis does not work, at least a seed has been planted that may eventually yield results.

A third factor associated with a good prognosis is *appropriate treatment for at least 2 years.* Those people whose alcoholism began before age 25 usually require at least 3 years of treatment. Many alcoholics who begin treatment will either believe they can "do it on their own" or they will return to drinking and drop out of treatment. To recover effectively, most alcoholics need to be with people who are themselves recovering successfully. This favorable environment is found most easily in self-help groups such as Alcoholics Anonymous and in group therapy (see above). Thus, when the patient shows any indication of dropping out of treatment, it is important to promptly persuade him not to do so.

It is very helpful, in keeping the patient motivated to stay in treatment, for him to have a *continued threatened loss for stopping treatment.* However, most clinicians are not trained to use such a therapeutic coercion, and some, especially those trained in the mental health fields, find doing so especially difficult. If the alcoholic patient knows that his physician gen-

uinely cares, he will be more likely to cooperate in treatment that is somewhat coercive. In this regard, the following are helpful ways to obtain participation in treatment: (*a*) using a therapeutic contract between physician and patient, or a patient-employer contract making job security contingent upon continued abstinence and recovery (see "Motivating through Employee Assistance Programs," above), or (*b*) assuring that the family continues to threaten their actions named in a formal intervention (see above).

The prognosis is also better if *family, job, health, and cognitive function are intact.* The status of family, job, health, and cognitive function usually correlates with how far along the alcoholism has advanced. Thus, making a diagnosis early in the course of the alcoholism generally portends a better prognosis, since each of these aspects of the patient's life tends to be more intact early in the illness. Also, in early illness the patient's and family members' denial system and other defense systems tend not to be as strong.

If one or more members of the patient's *family* is receiving treatment for their co-alcoholism (see below), the patient generally has a better prognosis.

Additional factors that increase the likelihood of long-term success are *prompt recognition and intervention when relapse occurs* (see above) and the acceptance by patient and physician of a 3-fold recovery model that views alcoholism as a *physical, mental, and spiritual illness* (60, 61).

Factors Associated with a Poor Prognosis

If the patient has *no perceived threat of loss* from continued drinking, the prognosis for recovery is generally worse.

A second factor that may worsen the prognosis is *one of the following forms of inappropriate treatment:* (*a*) disulfiram alone; (*b*) psychoanalytically oriented psychotherapy in the first year of alcoholism treatment; (*c*) "controlled drinking" treatment; (*d*) use of sedatives in long-term management; (*e*) inpatient or outpatient treatment that does not treat alcoholism as a primary illness; and (*f*) treatment that is too short in duration.

Although many patients who have a *continued self-destructive bent* do not tend to recover, some do. Often, intensive inpatient alcoholism treatment for 2 months or longer can be helpful in such patients.

Cognitive impairment or psychosis often makes treatment difficult. However, the presence of these factors alone does not preclude a full attempt at treatment. With abstinence there is often surprising improvement over time.

Acceptance of a derelict subculture status by the patient makes the prognosis virtually hopeless. However, it can be helpful to screen for a potentially reversible derelict status by looking at prior career and duration of dereliction (16). For example, a person who up until 2 years ago was in a productive profession or trade and is now on skid row has potential for recovery. By contrast, a skid row person who has had no constructive activities for many years generally has little chance for reaching a successful long term recovery.

If the patient has *powerful enablers* (see "Co-Alcoholism" below) to deny, cover up, and protect him from the consequences of his drinking or drug using, it is less likely that he will make a successful recovery.

CO-ALCOHOLISM (CO-DEPENDENCE)

Co-alcoholism can be defined as *ill health or maladaptive, problematic, or dysfunctional behavior that is associated with living with, working with, treating, or otherwise being close to a person with alcoholism.* Co-alcoholism is a specific example of the more general phenomenon *co-dependence*, i.e., suffering or dysfunction associated with or due to focusing upon the needs or behaviors of others (58, 63). The long-term sequelae of one type of co-dependence—growing up in a family dominated by alcoholism or by other unhealthy or dysfunctional abnormal patterns—are described below ("Adult Children of Dysfunctional Families").

Co-alcoholism affects not only individuals and families, but also helping professionals, communities, businesses, other institutions, and even whole societies. Its "signs and symptoms" range from passive acceptance and absence of overt problems to the following range of manifestations:

In Individuals Close to an Alcoholic:

1. Behaviors that protect the alcoholic (enabling).
2. Behavioral or psychological symptoms, such as anxiety disorders, depression, insomnia, hyperactivity, aggression, anorexia nervosa, bulimia, and suicidal gestures.
3. Functional or psychosomatic illness.
4. Family violence or neglect.
5. Alcoholism or another chemical dependence.

In Helping Professionals:

1. Failure to diagnose alcoholism.
2. Failure to treat alcoholism as a primary illness.
3. Treating the alcoholic with sedatives or tranquilizers.
4. Treating the co-alcoholic with sedatives or tranquilizers.

As noted earlier, some of these co-alcoholic behaviors have been the basis for a number of successful suits against physicians in recent years.

In Society at Large:

1. Not confronting relatives, friends, and colleagues who are inappropriately intoxicated or who are chronically abusing alcohol or drugs.
2. Placing a positive social value upon those who drink.
3. Stigmatizing those who are alcoholics or those who do not drink.

Co-Alcoholism in the Individual

The following is a typical case history of co-alcoholism in an individual.

A 38-year-old white, married woman presented with recurring episodes of upper abdominal pain of about 4 years' duration. During that time she had been evaluated by two internists and had been hospitalized once. After extensive evaluations, the working diagnosis was functional abdominal pain. She was treated with antispasmodics and sedatives but there was no substantial improvement. The pain occurred almost every day. On a follow-up visit 6 months later, the patient said that a friend had suggested that she attend the self-help group Al-Anon because her husband's drinking had been bothering her for at least 5 years. The patient reported that after attending 12 Al-Anon meetings over 3 months, her abdominal pain gradually abated. On follow-up 2 years later, she had continued to attend Al-Anon and the symptoms had not recurred. In the meantime, the patient's husband had continued to drink.

This patient illustrates a common manifestation of co-alcoholism, i.e., a psychosomatic illness that resolved after recognizing an alcohol problem in the family and attending Al-Anon regularly.

Recognition and Management of the Co-Alcoholic Individual

When a patient presents with unexplained somatic or psychological symptoms, it is helpful to ask whether the patient has ever been concerned about the drinking (or drug use) of anyone close to him or her. If the answer is yes, the patient should be asked to describe the problem. If the patient is vague or doubtful, one can administer some or all of the questions in the Family Drinking Survey shown in Table 21.9. One can also ask the possible co-alcoholic to answer CAGE questions (see above) or the questions on the Michigan Alcoholism Screening Test (Table 21.3) as though the questions were addressed to, and answered honestly by, the potentially alcoholic person to whom he or she is close (37). A positive score on one of these is a strong indication of co-alcoholism.

Initially, the psychological and behavioral adjustments of the co-alcoholic are normal responses to an abnormal situation. However, these adaptive responses eventually lead to the individual becoming dysfunctional. Co-alcoholism, like alcoholism, is chronic, progressive, and characterized by denial, ill health, or maladaptive behavior and by a lack of knowledge about alcoholism.

The major strategies in treating an individual with co-alcoholism are remarkably similar to those for treating the alcoholic:

1. Have the patient accept the fact that he or she is a co-alcoholic.
2. Motivate the patient to get help (occasionally by

Table 21.9.
Family Drinking Survey

	YES	NO
1. Does someone in your family undergo personality changes when he or she drinks to excess?		
2. Do you feel that drinking is more important to this person than you are?		
3. Do you feel sorry for yourself and frequently indulge in self-pity because of what you feel alcohol is doing to your family?		
4. Has some family member's excessive drinking ruined special occasions?		
5. Do you find yourself covering up for the consequences of someone else's drinking?		
6. Have you ever felt guilty, apologetic, or responsible for the drinking of a member of your family?		
7. Does one of your family member's use of alcohol cause fights and arguments?		
8. Have you ever tried to fight the drinker by joining in the drinking?		
9. Do the drinking habits of some family members make you feel depressed or angry?		
10. Is your family having financial difficulties because of drinking?		
11. Did you ever feel like you had an unhappy home life because of the drinking of some members of your family?		
12. Have you ever tried to control the drinker's behavior by hiding the car keys, pouring liquor down the drain, *etc.*?		
13. Do you find yourself distracted from your responsibilities because of this person's drinking?		
14. Do you often worry about a family member's drinking?		
15. Are holidays more of a nightmare than a celebration because of a family member's drinking behavior?		
16. Are most of your drinking family member's friends heavy drinkers?		
17. Do you find it necessary to lie to employers, relatives, or friends in order to hide your spouse's drinking?		
18. Do you find yourself responding differently to members of your family when they are using alcohol?		
19. Have you ever been embarrassed or felt the need to apologize for the drinker's actions?		
20. Does some family member's use of alcohol make you fear for your own safety or the safety of other members of your family?		
21. Have you ever thought that one of your family members had a drinking problem?		
22. Have you ever lost sleep because of a family member's drinking?		
23. Have you ever encouraged one of your family members to stop or cut down on his or her drinking?		
24. Have you ever threatened to leave home or to leave a family member because of his or her drinking?		
25. Did a family member ever make promises that he or she did not keep because of drinking?		
26. Did you ever wish that you could talk to someone who could understand and help the alcohol-related problems of a family member?		
27. Have you ever felt sick, cried, or had a "knot" in your stomach after worrying about a family member's drinking?		
28. Has a family member ever failed to remember what occurred during a drinking period?		
29. Does your family member avoid social situations where alcoholic beverages will *not* be served?		
30. Does you family member have periods of remorse after drinking occasions and apologize for his or her behavior?		
31. Please write any symptoms or medical or nervous problems that you have experienced since you have known your heavy drinker. (Write on back if more space needed).		

If you answer "YES" to any 2 of the above questions, there is a good possibility that someone in your family may have a drinking problem.

If you answer "YES" to 4 or more of the above questions, there is a definite indication that someone in your family *does* have a drinking problem.

(These survey questions are modified or adapted from validated survey instruments such as the Children of Alcoholics Screening Test (CAST) and the Howard Family Questionnaire, and from the Family Alcohol Quiz from Al-Anon.)

using a coercive intervention, such as the formal intervention described above).

3. Refer the patient to Al-Anon or Alateen (as is true of AA referrals, enthusiasm for and a good understanding of the Al-Anon process on the part of the referring physician are critical to successful referral. The Al-Anon process is described in Table 21.10).

4. Provide supportive psychotherapy at follow-up visits (see description of techniques, Chapter 11) and refer the patient or the family for additional therapy, especially group therapy for co-dependents or adult children of dysfunctional families (see below).

5. Assist in the process of getting the alcoholic(s) who is the source of the problem into treatment. (This is not the responsibility of the co-alcoholic, however.)

Co-Alcoholism in the Helping Professions

Co-alcoholism includes behavior on the part of professionals that "enables" alcoholics to remain en-

Table 21.10.
The Al-Anon Process

Al-Anon began in the 1940s as an AA auxiliary and initially called itself AA Family Groups. In 1952, the wives of the two founders of AA established Al-Anon.

Al-Anon is a fellowship of family members of alcoholics who meet together to share their experience, strengths, and hopes so that they can achieve health and serenity. The organization is modeled after AA and uses the 12 Steps of AA (see Table 21.3) as its principles for individual recovery. Its focus is not on the alcoholic but on the family members, and by so doing it powerfully frees families from their dependence on the alcoholic.

Al-Anon meetings are all open to the public and frequently meet at the same time and location as AA meetings. In most communities, Al-Anon has a telephone listing where meeting information, help, and literature can be obtained. Where there is no local Al-Anon office, the AA office can provide Al-Anon information.

Al-Anon meetings generally last 1 hour and follow the format of AA meetings (see Table 21.3), but they are usually smaller and discussion of topics is often freer than in AA.

Al-Anon is the sponsor of Ala-Teen and Ala-Tots, which are organizations for teenage and young children of alcoholics, respectively. These groups follow the Al-Anon discussion format and in general are not open to the nonalcoholic public, but helping professionals are usually welcome if they request to attend ahead of time. In the last several years in some areas, Al-Anon members have begun groups for adult children of alcoholics. These groups offer help to adults who may no longer live with an alcoholic family member, but whose life continues to be adversely affected by the legacy of growing up in an alcoholic home. These are especially powerful, and many patients whith this background can be profoundly helped.

Al-Anon publishes a number of pamphlets for families that are available at meetings. *Al-Anon Faces Alcoholism*, Al-Anon's "Big Book," describes the family's plight with alcoholism through a variety of stories that graphically describe how families become sick in response to the alcoholic. Its other major book, *Living with an Alcoholic*, offers practical suggestions for recovery.

More information can be had by writing Al-Anon Family Group Headquarters, Box 182, Madison Square Station, New York, NY 10010.

meshed in their disease, as noted above. Enabling behavior often coexists with otherwise excellent clinical skills. The Professional Enablers Screening Test (Table 21.11) is useful for identifying the various ways in which enabling may occur in the context of medical practice. Societal norms (including one's own approach to the use of alcohol or other drugs) plus unawareness of modern approaches to diagnosis, motivation, and management of the alcoholic are probably the major reasons for the co-alcoholism in helping professionals. Several steps are recommended for the professional who wishes to cease being an enabler:

1. Update one's knowledge of alcoholism.
2. Attend a number of AA and Al-Anon meetings.
3. In one's own practice, try using skills such as those described in this chapter. The best "cure" for co-alcoholism in the physician is success in getting a number of alcoholics and their families into the recovery process.

Table 21.11.
Professional Enablers Screening Test[a]

Please check your answer to each question. For medically oriented questions, please check the space to which you would subscribe, even though you may not be a physician.

	Yes	No
1. Do you sometimes avoid raising sensitive issues related to drinking because it might offend your patient, or make him or her angry or feel bad?	(2)	___
2. Do you generally treat the heavy drinking persons' problems without focusing most of the treatment on the drinking behavior?	(5)	___
3. Do you avoid confronting your heavy drinking patient when there is good evidence that he or she has misinformed you about his or her drinking?	(2)	___
4. Do you generally suggest to your alcoholic patients that they cut down on their drinking?	(3)	___
5. Do you believe what your heavy drinking patient tells you about his or her drinking without using other sources such as a spouse, employer, a screening test, blood alcohol level, or other laboratory test?	(5)	___
6. Do you generally prescribe a sedative or minor tranquilizer for the nervous conditions or sleep problems of your alcoholic patients?	(5)	___
7. Do you refer most of your alcoholic patients to attend Alcoholics Anonymous meetings regularly?	___	(5)
8. Do you refer many of your alcoholic patients to an alcoholism therapy group?	___	(3)
9. Do you prescribe disulfiram (Antabuse) to many of your alcoholic patients?	___	(3)
10. When your alcoholic patient has a minor crisis requiring hospitalization, do you routinely hospitalize him or her in a community hospital general ward?	(5)	___
11. Do you refer most of the spouses or family members of your alcoholic patients to attend Al-Anon meetings regularly?	___	(5)
12. Do you subscribe to the theory that most alcoholics have an underlying psychological disorder that is the major cause of their alcoholism?	(5)	___
13. Do you believe that most alcoholics will not respond positively to treatment for their alcoholism?	(5)	___

[a]Numbers in parentheses are the scores recommended for the corresponding responses. A score of 0 to 3 points indicates a probable nonenabler; 4 to 6 points may indicate a possible enabler; 7 points or more indicates a probable enabler.

Summary View of Co-Alcoholism

It is estimated that for each of the 10 to 15 million alcoholics in the United States there are three to five people who are seriously affected by their association with the alcoholic. Better understanding of alcoholism by this enormous segment of the population that, in addition to family members, includes many helping professionals, law enforcement workers, educators, members of the clergy, politicians, employers, and others would probably result in earlier recognition and treatment for numerous alcoholics and effective prevention for many who are otherwise destined to be afflicted with alcoholism.

ADULT CHILDREN OF DYSFUNCTIONAL FAMILIES

In recent years, it has been recognized that many adults in our society grew up in families made dysfunctional by alcoholism or other abnormal behaviors that dominated life at home. The term "Adult Children of Alcoholics" (ACOA) is widely used for those whose childhood is affected by alcoholism or other chemical dependence in one or both parents (65).

A dysfunctional family tends not to support the psychological and spiritual growth of each of its members. Trying to be real, i.e., expressing oneself through one's actual feelings and thoughts, in such a family is generally so painful that the child develops a mask, which can be called a false self or co-dependent self. Living through this false self is survival oriented but not fulfilling. From becoming entrenched in living this way, such individuals come to think that that is all there is to life. When they become adults and leave their family of origin, they generally continue in this stance, unhappy and unfulfilled. Many develop alcoholism or other chemical dependence.

When adult children of dysfunctional families are recognized in adulthood, they usually describe a childhood pattern in which they took on one of several roles: *hero* (overachiever, successful member of a sibship), *scapegoat* (delinquent or "bad" child), *lost child* (quiet, passive one), or *family pet* (mascot, comedian, or little princess) (58). They tend to continue one or a combination of these roles into their adulthood.

Because the ACOA concept has been widely publicized in the lay media, many affected individuals will recognize their situation and seek help from programs in their communities. Some, however, will present their problems in medical visits.

Among the many adult problems that derive from these childhood roles are difficulty in showing feelings and developing intimate relationships, high tolerance for inappropriate behavior in others, difficulty getting one's own needs met, being either very responsible (helping others, never saying no) or irresponsible, and seeking approval of others. Many persons with these patterns enter the helping professions. Although supportive psychotherapy (Chapter 11) can be helpful, these persons tend to have recurring problems unless they enter into a full-recovery program (60, 63).

The major process in a full-recovery program includes identifying and experientially working through one's psychological and spiritual wounding, much of it from one's family of origin. Like recovery from alcoholism and other chemical dependence, a major treatment modality for the adult child syndrome is long-term group therapy in a group that is specific for this condition. Such group therapy has become more widely available in recent years. Also important to full recovery is participation in self-help programs, including Al-Anon groups (described above), ACOA groups (available in many communities, often in association with Al-Anon), or Co-Dependents Anonymous groups (not specific to alcoholism, available in many communities). Individual counseling, keeping a journal or diary, educational experiences, and intensive residential treatment may also be helpful for some individuals (9, 14, 60, 63).

THE TROUBLED PHYSICIAN OR OTHER PROFESSIONAL

The prevalence among physicians of alcoholism and other chemical dependence is probably similar to that for the general population (8). Each year, a substantial number of physicians are lost to the profession because of chemical dependence or other treatable illnesses and many more practice despite being seriously troubled or impaired. Most of these individuals could be successfully treated with early recognition and follow-up. Since the mid-1970s, all state medical societies have developed programs for these physicians. Because of this, each year many troubled physicians are now being rehabilitated and returned to productive practices and better lives. In recent years, numerous other professional organizations have implemented such programs, including organizations of nurses, dentists, pharmacists, psychologists, social workers, lawyers, and others.

Definitions

Impaired professionals may be further defined as those who are troubled by personal difficulties to the extent that (a) they cannot offer reasonable patient care, effectively help others through interpersonal skills, or maintain skills by continuing education or (b) they demonstrate a definite decline from their prior level of functioning, even if they are currently performing adequately. Impairment may be further characterized by denial and ambivalence on the part of the physician, the family, and the community, all of whom may ignore the problem until it is too late. Intervention with appropriate treatment as soon as it is recognized is a major goal of the impaired physician movement.

Impairment may be either transient or chronic and varies along a spectrum of severity of degree and causes. One problem is that presently there is no way to monitor *transient impairment.* For example, any physicians who have been intoxicated have been transiently impaired, since during the period of intoxication they would have provided suboptimal care. Also, physicians can be episodically exposed to extreme personal stresses (e.g., problems in their family, loss of important relationships, or financial disruptions) that render them temporarily impaired. How long impairment should be present to indicate *chronic impairment* is difficult to specify; 6 months might be a reasonable minimum.

Troubled physicians have been described in three major categories: incompetent, due to lack of skill or knowledge; unethical, malicious, or uncaring; and ill, either physically or mentally. The ill physician is by far the most common. The illness may be alcoholism, other chemical dependence, mental illness, cognitive decline, co-dependence related to dysfunctional persons in the family, or another condition.

Recognition and Management

The manifestations, symptoms, or signs of impairment from alcoholism and other chemical dependence among professionals are the same as those seen in nonprofessionals. A checklist of particular clues to assist in the recognition of impairment in helping professionals is shown in Table 21.12. Many of these manifestations are late indicators of impairment, especially those listed under "Manifestations at Hospital." Early manifestations are indicated with an *asterisk*.

When one is concerned about impairment in a colleague, it is advisable to contact one or more close associates of that colleague to confirm the impairment. Likely reasons for the impairment may be uncovered in this discreet inquiry; frequently alcoholism or other chemical dependence will be the underlying problem. Persuasion of an impaired physician to accept the existence of a problem and to agree to rehabilitation can be attempted by a concerned colleague, an approach similar to that for other persons with alcoholism (see Fig. 21.3). Such efforts are likely to be met with intense denial. A second approach is to utilize the state's physician rehabilitation committee. Each state medical society has a committee and maintains telephone access

Table 21.12.
Clues to Impairment in the Physician, Nurse, or Other Helping Professional[a,b]

Home and Family
*Medical use of alcohol or drugs
*Mood swings or inconsistency
*Behavior excused by family and friends
Drinking or substance-using activities more important than other activities
Children neglected, abused, or in trouble
Extreme temper
Fights, arguments, and violent outbursts
Sexual problems
Withdrawal, isolation, and fragmentation of social and family life
Family isolating itself from social supports
Financial problems
Spouse in psychotherapy or taking psychoactive medication
Lack of problem resolution
Separation or divorce

Manifestations at Office
*Overwork
Disorganized schedule
Spasmodic work pace
Unreasonable behavior
Inaccessible to patients and staff
Excessive drug use, prescriptions, and supply
Liberal in prescribing psychoactive drugs to patients
Medical errors
Patient complaints
Frequent absences
Decreased work load and tolerance
Frequent days off for vague reasons
Taking sexual advantage of patients or co-workers

Employment Applications
Frequent job changes or relocations
Unusual medical history
Vague letters of reference
Inappropriate qualifications
Time lapse unexplained in work
Inappropriate job now
Refusal of physical examination or spouse interview

Physical Status
*Insomnia
*Personality and behavior changes
*Amnesias
Multiple physical complaints and illnesses
Many prescriptions for self and family
Frequent emergency room visits and hospitalizations
Inappropriate tremulousness or sweating
Poor hygiene and appearance
Long sleeves in warm weather

Manifestations at Hospital
*Heavy drinking at staff functions
Often late, absent, or ill
Decreased work/chart performance
Inappropriate orders
"Hospital gossip"
Unavailability
Alcohol on breath while in hospital
Drunk when on call, even at home

Friends and Community
*Neglected social commitments
*Embarrassing behavior
Personal isolation
Overreaction to criticism
Exaggerates work accomplishments and finances
Inordinate financial difficulties
Drunk driving arrests
Legal problems
Neglected social commitments
Lessening of ethical values
Unpredictability or unreliability

[a]Modified from Talbott GD, Benson E: Impaired physicians: the dilemma of identification. *Postgrad Med* 68:56, 1980; and Whitfield CL, Bissell L, Wesson DW: Treatment of the professional or "VIP" alcoholic. In Whitfield CL, Liepman MR (eds): *The Patient with Alcoholism and Other Drug Problems*. Baltimore, University of Maryland, 1980. See also Table 21.3.
[b]An *asterisk* indicates early signs.

for confidential reporting of impaired physicians. Subcommittees undertake verification of the problem, followed by confrontation of the troubled physician similar to the formal intervention technique described above. The goal of this process is to rehabilitate the physician, usually through intensive treatment in a residential faculty (52).

The family members of the troubled physician or other professional are often suffering in varying degrees from co-alcoholism or co-dependence or an equivalent debilitating condition. They should be evaluated and appropriately treated.

General References

Alcoholics Anonymous: *The Story of How Many Thousands of Men and Women Have Recovered from Alcoholism ("The Big Book")*. 3rd ed. New York, Alcoholics Anonymous World Services, 1976.

The nature of alcoholism and the recovery process using AA are illustrated in a large number of personal stories.

Barnes HN, Aronson MD, Delbanco TL (eds): *Alcoholism: A Guide for the Primary Care Physician*. New York, Springer-Verlag, 1987.

Bean MH: Alcoholics Anonymous. I. Principles and methods. *Psychiatr Ann* 5:5, 1975.

A psychiatrist's lucid account of the AA process, based on her personal visits to 40 different AA groups.

Bean MH, Zinberg NE (eds): *Dynamic Approaches to the Understanding and Treatment of Alcoholism*. New York, The Free Press, 1981.

Detailed description of the denial process and other psychodynamic aspects of the alcoholics' behavior.

Criteria Committee, National Council on Alcoholism, New York, New York. Criteria for the diagnosis of alcoholism. *Ann Intern Med* 77:249, 1972.

Drews T: *Getting Them Sober: A Guide for Those Who Live with an Alcoholic*. Plainfield, New Jersey, Haven Books, 1980.

Widely available paperback, for families of alcoholics. Quick reading. Advice regarding numerous practical issues ("hide the car keys?"; "don't beg him to stay"; "don't pour out the booze," etc.).

Gorski TT, Miller M: *Staying Sober: A Guide for Relapse Prevention*. Independence, Missouri, Independence Press, 1986.

A book that describes the relapse process and how to deal with it, in detail. For recovering alcoholic patients.

Gravitz H, Bowden J: *Recovery Guide for Adult Children of Alcoholics*. New York, Simon and Schuster, 1986.

For therapists and lay people: a practical and readable map of recovery.

Health and Public Policy Committee, American College of Physicians: Chemical dependence. *Ann Intern Med* 102:405, 1985.

Consensus paper defining the responsibilities of practicing physicians to recognize alcoholism and other forms of chemical dependence and to assure that affected patients get appropriate treatment.

Jellinek EM: *The Disease Concept of Alcoholism*. New Haven, College and University Press, 1960.

Landmark monograph reviewing the history of the disease concept.

Rogers RL, McMillin CS (eds): *Don't Help: A Positive Guide to Working with the Alcoholic*. New York, Bantam Trade, 1989.

Practical account of techniques for group or individual counseling that, in conjunction with Alcoholics Anonymous, are often effective in long-term treatment of alcoholism.

"The Enablers" and *"The Intervention"*: Minneapolis, Johnson Institute, 1978.

Two of the best films ever made on alcoholism. Technique of formal intervention shown.

Turner RC, Lichstein PR, Peden Jr. JG, et al: Alcohol withdrawal syndromes: a review of pathophysiology, clinical presentation, and treatment. *J Gen Intern Med* 4(5):432, 1989.

Vaillant G: *The Natural History of Alcoholism*. Cambridge, MA, Harvard University Press, 1983.

Detailed monograph, much of it based on the author's longitudinal studies.

West LJ, Maxwell DS, Noble EP, Solomon DH: Alcoholism. *Ann Intern Med* 100:405, 1984.

Recent review covering biomedical consequences, alcoholism in older persons, and controversies regarding treatment.

Whitfield CL: *Healing the Child Within: Discovery and Recovery for Adult Children of Dysfunctional Families*. Pompano Beach, Florida, Health Communications, Inc., 1987.

A clinical introduction to the problems of adult children of alcoholic and other dysfunctional families and to successful recovery from these problems.

Whitfield CL: *A Gift to Myself: A Personal Notebook and Guide for Healing My Child Within*. Deerfield Beach, Florida, Health Communications, 1990.

A detailed description of the recovery process for adult children of dysfunctional families.

Specific References

1. Allen RP, Faillace LA, Wagman A: Recovery time for alcoholics after prolonged alcohol intoxication. *Johns Hopkins Med J* 128:158, 1971.
2. American Psychiatric Association: *Diagnostic and Statistical Manual of Mental Disorders. (Third Edition, Revised)* Washington, DC, American Psychiatric Association, 1987.
3. Bean-Bayog M: The adolescent drinker. In: Barnes HN, Aronson MD, Delbanco TL (eds): *Alcoholism: A Guide for the Primary Care Physician*. New York, Springer-Verlag, 1987.
4. Bill C: Probability of continuation of sobriety. *Q J Studies Alcohol* 26:283, 1965.
5. Bissell LC: The treatment of alcoholism: what do we do about long-term sedatives? *Ann NY Acad Sci* 252:396, 1975.
6. Blume SB: Women and alcohol. *JAMA* 256(11):1467, 1986.
7. Bowen OR, Sammons JH: The alcohol-abusing patient: a challenge to the profession. *JAMA* 260(15):2267, 1988.
8. Brewster JM: Prevalence of alcohol and other drug problems among physicians. *JAMA* 255(14):1913, 1986.
9. Brown S: *Treating Adult Children of Alcoholics: A Developmental Perspective*. New York, John Wiley & Sons, 1988.
10. Buckey SF, Edwards D, Berz NH: *Hospitalizations and Discharge Rates of Men Treated at the Navy's Alcohol Centers*. Report No. 75-41, San Diego, Naval Health Research Center, May, 1975.
11. Cahalan D: *Problem Drinkers: A National Survey*. San Francisco, Jossey-Bass, 1970.
12. Criteria Committee, National Council on Alcoholism, New York, New York: Criteria for the diagnosis of alcoholism. *Ann Intern Med* 77:249, 1972.
13. Cyr MG, Wartman SA: The effectiveness of routine screening questions in the detection of alcoholism. *JAMA* 259(1):51, 1988.
14. DeSoto CB, O'Donnell WE, Allred LJ, Lopes CE: Symptomatology in alcoholics at various stages of abstinence. *Alcoholism: Clinical and Experimental Research*, 9:505, 1985.
15. Eckardt MJ, Harford TC, Kaelber CT, et al: Health hazards associated with alcohol consumption. *JAMA* 246:648, 1981.
16. Fagan RW, Mauss AL: Social margin and social reentry: an evaluation of a rehabilitation program for skid row alcoholics. *J Studies on Alcohol* 47(5):413, 1986.
17. Fein R: *Alcohol in America: The Price We Pay*. Newport Beach, California, Care Institute, Page 10, 1984.
18. Feldman DJ, Pattison EM, Sobell LC, et al: Outpatient alcohol detoxification: initial findings on 564 patients. *Am J Psychiatry* 132:407, 1975.
19. Fine E, et al: Philadelphia DWI Study. *US J Alcohol Drug Abuse* 19: March, 1983.
20. Goodwin DW: *Is Alcoholism Hereditary?* New York, Oxford University Press, 1976.
21. Gorski TT: Relapse prevention planning: a new recovery tool. *Alcohol Health and Research World* 6–11, Fall, 1986.
22. Hayashida M, Alterman AI, McLellan T, et al: Comparative effectiveness and costs of inpatient and outpatient detoxification of patients with mild-to-moderate alcohol withdrawal syndrome. *N Engl J Med* 320:358, 1989.

23. Hays JT, Spickard Jr. WA: Alcoholism: early diagnosis and intervention. *J Gen Intern Med* 2:420, 1987.
24. Helzer JE, Robins LN, Taylor JR, et al: The extent of long-term moderate drinking among alcoholics discharged from medical and psychiatric treatment facilities. *N Engl J Med* 312:1678, 1985.
25. Hesselbrock MN, Meyer RE, Kenner JJ: Psychopathology in hospitalized alcoholics. *Arch Gen Psychiatry* 42:1050, 1985.
26. Hoffman NG, Harrison PA, Belille CA: Alcoholics Anonymous after treatment: attendance and abstinence. *Int J Addict* 18:311, 1983.
27. Holden HD, Blose JO: Alcoholism treatment and total health care utilization and costs. A four-year longitudinal analysis of federal emloyees. *JAMA* 256:1456, 1986.
28. Holzer III CE, Robins LN, Myers JK, et al: Antecedents and correlates of alcohol abuse and dependence in the elderly. In: NIAAA, Research Monograph #14, *Nature and Extent of Alcohol Problems Among the Elderly*. U.S. Department of Health and Human Services, DHHS Publication No. (ADM) 84-1321, 1984.
29. Jellinek EM: Phases of alcohol addiction. *Q J Stud Alcohol* 13(4):673, 1952.
30. Johnson B, Clark W: Alcoholism: a challenging physician-patient encounter. *J Gen Intern Med* 4:445, 1989.
31. Johnson VE (ed): *I'll Quit Tomorrow*. New York, Harper and Row, 1980.
32. Kamerow DB, Pincus HA, Macdonald DI: Alcohol abuse, other drug abuse, and mental disorders in medical practice. *JAMA* 255(15):2054, 1986.
33. Kissin B: Theory and practice in the treatment of alcoholism. In: Kissin B, Begleiter H (eds): *The Biology of Alcoholism. Vol 5: Treatment and Rehabilitation of the Chronic Alcoholic*. New York, Plenum Press, 1977, pp 1–51.
34. Lewis DC, Gordon AJ: Alcoholism and the general hospital: the Roger Williams Intervention Program. *Bull NY Acad Med* 59:181, 1983.
35. Miller WR, Hester RK: Inpatient alcoholism treatment: who benefits? *Am Psychologist* 41(7):794, 1986.
36. Mills JL, Graubard BI, Harley EE, et al: Maternal alcohol consumption and birth weight: how much drinking during pregnancy is safe? *JAMA* 252:1875, 1984.
37. Morse RM, Swanson WM: Spouse response to a self-administered alcoholism screening test. *J Stud Alcohol* 36:400, 1975.
38. Myers JK, Weissman MM, Tischler GL, et al: Six-month prevalence of psychiatric disorders in three communities. *Arch Gen Psychiatry* 4:959, 1984.
39. Pell S, D'Alonzo CA: A five-year mortality study of alcoholics. *J Occup Med* 15:120, 1973.
40. Pell S, D'Alonzo CA: The prevalence of chronic disease among problem drinkers. *Arch Environ Health* 16:679, 1968.
41. Polich JM, Armor DJ, Braiker HB: *The Course of Alcoholism: Four Years after Treatment*. R-2433, NIAAA, Santa Monica, Rand Corporation, 1980.
42. Powers JS, Spickard A: Michigan Alcoholism Screening Test to diagnose early alcoholism in a general practice. *South Med J* 77:852, 1984.
43. Reuler JB, Girard DE, Cooney TG: Wernicke's encephalopathy. *N Engl J Med* 312:1035, 1985.
44. Sampliner R, Iber F: Diphenylhydantoin control of alcohol withdrawal seizures. *JAMA* 230:1430, 1974.
45. Saunders JB, Beevers DG, Paton A: Alcohol-induced hypertension. *Lancet* 1:653, 1981.
46. Schuckit MA: Genetics and the risk of alcoholism. *JAMA* 254(18):2614, 1985.
47. Schuckit MA: The clinical implications of primary diagnostic groups among alcoholics. *Arch Gen Psychiatry* 42:1043, 1985.
48. Seixas FA: Alcohol and its drug interactions. *Ann Intern Med* 83:86, 1975.
49. Sellers EM, Naranjo CA, Harrison M, et al: Diazepam loading: simplified treatment of alcohol withdrawal. *Clin Pharmacol Ther* 822, December, 1983.
50. Sellers EM, Naranjo CA, Peachey JE: Drugs to decrease alcohol consumption. *N Engl J Med* 305(21):1255, 1981.
51. Skinner HA, Holt S, Schuller R, et al: Identification of alcohol abuse using laboratory tests and a history of trauma. *Ann Intern Med* 101:847, 1984.
52. Spickard Jr. WA: The impaired physician. In: Barnes HN, Aronson MD, Delbanco TL (eds): *Alcoholism: A Guide for the Primary Care Physician*. New York, Springer-Verlag, 1987.
53. Sobell MB, Sobell LC: Individualized behavior therapy for alcoholics. *Behav Ther* 4:49, 1973.
54. Vaillant G, Clark W, Cyrus C, et al: Prospective study of alcoholism treatment: eight-year follow-up. *Am J Med* 75:455, 1983.
55. Vaillant GE (ed): *The Natural History of Alcoholism*. Cambridge, Massachusetts, Harvard University Press, 1983.
56. Victor M, Hope JM: The phenomenon of auditory hallucinations in chronic alcoholism. *J Nerv Ment Dis* 126:451, 1958.
57. Wallace J: Alcoholism from the inside out: a phenomenological analysis. In: Estes NJ, Heinemann ME (eds): *Alcoholism: Development, Consequences, and Interventions*. St Louis, CV Mosby, 1977.
58. Wegsheider-Cruse S: *Choice-Making*. Pompano Beach, Florida, Health Communications, 1985.
59. West LJ: Maxwell DS, Noble EP, Solomon DH: Alcoholism. *Ann Intern Med* 100:405, 1984.
60. Whitfield CL: Advances in alcoholism and chemical dependence. *Am J Med* 85:465, 1988.
61. Whitfield CL: *Alcoholism, Attachments and Spirituality: Stress Management and Serenity during Recovery*. Baltimore, Perrin and Thegell, 1984.
62. Whitfield CL, et al: Detoxification of 1,024 alcoholics without psychoactive drugs. *JAMA* 239:1409, 1978. and letter response. 241:2597, 1979.
63. Whitfield CL (ed): *Healing the Child Within: Discovery and Recovery for Adult Children of Dysfunctional Families*. Deerfield Beach, Florida, Health Communications, 1987.
64. Whitfield CL: Outpatient management of alcoholism. *Psychiatr Ann* 12:447, 1982.
65. Woititz JG (ed): *Adult Children of Alcoholics*. Pompano Beach, Florida, Health Communications, Inc., 1983.
66. Zook CJ, Moore FD: High-cost users of medical care. *N Engl J Med* 302:996, 1980.
67. Zuska JJ, Pursch JA: Long-term management. In: Gitlow SE, Peyser HS (eds): *Alcoholism: A Practical Treatment Guide*. New York, Grune and Stratton, 1980, pp 131–163.

C H A P T E R   22

Use and Abuse of Illicit Drugs and Substances

BURTON D'LUGOFF, M.D.
JAMES HAWTHORNE, PH.D.

DEFINITIONS

Illicit drugs are drugs that are taken for nonmedical reasons, to modify mood or behavior. The use and abuse of such substances dates back thousands of years. Plant alkaloids, alcohol, and an ever increasing array of newly synthesized chemicals have been used in these endeavors. Patterns of use and the social acceptance of use of these agents have differed from time to time and from place to place. Successive genera-

tions of the same society have held discordant views about which substance to use, at what age, in what amount, and under which circumstances (e.g., attitudes regarding alcohol use in the pre- and post-prohibition eras in the United States). Also, in a single historical epoch, neighboring cultures have differed about the sanctioned use of psychoactive substances. Currently, in 20th century Western society, there are two forms of relatively innocuous use of illicit substances, experimental and social-recreational use, and two defined patterns of abnormal use, substance abuse and substance dependence.

Experimental Use

The experimental use of illicit substances is sporadic; the initial trial and experience usually are associated with youthful rites of passage. These experiments usually have little impact on mental health. They are dangerous to the extent that possible dosage errors and bizarre or unsterile methods of exposure may occur; and because of user behaviors that may endanger himself or other persons when he is intoxicated. Incorrect labeling of such drugs (a common problem) increases the risk of these untoward effects. Experimentation is commonplace. A 1987 national high school survey (14) revealed that 57% of all respondents had engaged in an experimental trial of an illicit drug (primarily marijuana) and 92% had tried alcohol on at least one occasion.

Social-Recreational Use

The social and recreational use of illicit substances suggests that they have been used repetitively but that control has been exerted over the dose and the time of use. The risks due to unintended overdosage, improper exposure, and mislabeling are increased by the frequency of use. To the extent that control of use is effective, enabling one to maintain a high degree of social and behavioral function, recreational use also is not psychologically disabling. Most American use of alcohol and marijuana conforms to this pattern of social-recreational use.

Abuse and Dependence

The 1987 revision of the *Diagnostic and Statistical Manual* of the American Psychiatric Association (DSM III-R) delineates two diagnostic categories for the Psychoactive Substance Use Disorders. (1). The diagnostic criteria are the same for all psychoactive substances including alcohol.

Psychoactive substance abuse refers to a maladaptive pattern of psychoactive substance use indicated by either (a) continued use despite knowledge of having a persistent or recurrent social, occupational, psychological, or physical problem that is caused or exacerbated by use of the psychoactive substance or (b) recurrent use in situations in which use is physically hazardous (e.g., driving while intoxicated).

Psychoactive substance dependence refers to a pattern of use that includes at least three of the following:

1. Substance often taken in larger amounts than the person intended.
2. Persistent desire or one or more unsuccessful efforts to cut down.
3. A great deal of time spent in obtaining or using the substance.
4. Frequent intoxication or withdrawal symptoms when expected to fulfill major role obligations at work, school, or home.
5. Important social, occupational, or recreational activities given up or reduced because of substance use.
6. Continued use in spite of a persistent or recurrent social, psychological, or physical problem that is caused or exacerbated by use.
7. Increased tolerance.
8. Withdrawal symptoms.
9. Substance often taken to relieve withdrawal symptoms.

An important difference between DSM III-R and the preceding edition is that the diagnosis of psychoactive substance dependence no longer requires the presence of tolerance or a withdrawal syndrome. The diagnosis of dependence may now be made solely on the basis of impairment in psychosocial functioning.

Classification by Physiological Effect

Succeeding sections of this chapter describe the manifestations and the principles of management for selected substances of abuse common in the United States today (Chapters 20 and 21 describe tobacco and alcohol abuse/dependence, respectively). A list of all drugs extant today that have abuse potential would be extremely long. It is possible, however, to group the various substances into broad classes, the members of which share common characteristics and are readily distinguishable from other classes (Table 22.1). Psychoactive substances may thus be classified as (*a*) depressants, (*b*) stimulants, and (*c*) drugs that alter perception (including hallucinogens).

SOCIAL AND EPIDEMIOLOGICAL ASPECTS

Social Aspects

Drug abuse has been one of the dominant public concerns of the 1980s. A study commissioned by the National Institute on Drug Abuse showed that the economic cost of drug abuse during fiscal year 1980 was approximately $47 billion (11). A connection between property crime and heroin addiction has been well established (3). Most recently, in the United States, a cause of particularly concern has been the spread of cocaine use and abuse into middle and upper income populations. Media coverage of cocaine abuse by stock brokers, physicians, and lawyers, as well as by prom-

Table 22.1.
Categories of Psychoactive Drugs

DEPRESSANTS
  Narcotics:
    Morphine, hydromorphone (Dilaudid), heroin, meperidine (Demerol), codeine, methadone
  Sedative-hypnotics:
    Alcohol, barbiturates, glutethimide (Doriden), methaqualone (Quaalude)
  Minor tranquilizers:
    Benzodiazepines, meprobamate (Equanil or Miltown)
  Inhalants:
    Nitrous oxide, toluene, volatile hydrocarbons
STIMULANTS
  Cocaine, amphetamine, methylphenidate (Ritalin), Phenmetrazine (Preludin)
DRUGS THAT ALTER PERCEPTION (INCLUDING HALLUCINOGENS)
  Marijuana, lysergic acid diethlamide (LSD), dimethylamine tryptamine (DMT), psylocybin, phencyclidine (PCP), belladonna alkaloids (atropine, scopolamine)

Table 22.2.
Prevalence of Use of Selected Drugs Reported by High School Students, Class of 1988[a]

Drugs	Used One or More Times Last 30 Days	Used Daily for the Last 30 Days
Marijuana/hashish	18.0	2.7
Inhalants	3.0	0.2
LSD	1.8	0.0
PCP	0.3	0.1
Cocaine	3.4	0.2
Heroin	0.2	0.0
Other opiates	1.6	0.1
Stimulants	4.6	0.3
Sedatives	1.4	0.1
Tranquilizers	1.5	0.0
Alcohol	63.9	34.7
Cigarettes	28.7	10.6

[a]Adapted from Johnston LD, O'Malley PM, Backman JG: Drug use, drinking, and smoking: national survey results from high school, college, and young adult populations. Rockville, MD, US Department of Health and Human Services, Public Health Service, Alcohol, Drug Abuse, and Mental Health Association, 1988.

inent entertainment and sports figures, has made it clear that drug abuse, which was previously assumed to be confined to a relatively small segment of society, pervades all segments of society.

Prevalence Trends

Although there is no question that drug abuse continues to be one of the most serious problems faced by public health and law enforcement authorities, survey data suggest that the use of some illicit substances has been declining modestly in important segments of the population. Since 1975, a national survey of high school seniors and young adults has been conducted by the University of Michigan Institute for Social Research (14). The principal measure of use frequency is the 30-day prevalence, meaning the percentage of respondents who admit to use of a particular drug at least one time during the past 30 days. Table 22.2 summarizes these data for selected drugs; the table also summarizes the 30-day prevalence of *daily* use of these drugs by high school seniors. *Trends from these survey data* indicate that use by high school seniors of marijuana, stimulants, tranquilizers, nitrites, sedatives, and most hallucinogens has declined since 1980. The 30-day prevalence of PCP declined from 2.4% in 1979 to .3% in 1988. Marijuana use was down from a peak of 37.5% in 1978 to 18% in 1988. The prevalence of cocaine use, which had increased from 1.9% in 1975 to a high of 6.7% in 1985, declined to 3.4% in 1988. Alcohol use peaked at 72% in 1980 and declined to 63.9% in 1988. Since 1984–85 there have been increases in the use of inhalants and lysergic acid diethylamide (LSD), but less than 2% respondents reported using these substances. A notable finding of the survey is that the decline in use of most drugs has been accompanied by *changes in attitudes.* An increasing number of high school seniors have endorsed the belief that drug use is harmful. The number who say they disapprove of drug use has also increased. In 1975, for example, 43.3% of survey respondents perceived regular marijuana use as harmful. In 1987 the proportion had risen to 75.5%. The percentage of respondents who endorsed the belief that taking cocaine once or twice involved "great risk" rose from 33.5% in 1986 to 47.9% in 1987. These findings suggest that drug education efforts and media representations of the adverse consequences of drug use may be having some effect.

The study of high school seniors has included longitudinal follow-up on representative panels of graduating classes from 1976 through 1988 (14). Data on drug use by each of these panels provide information on a population of young adults between the ages of 19 and 30. These data have revealed essentially the same prevalence trends that were observed in the cross-sectional study of the class of 1987. One of the few differences between the two groups was a sharper decline in cocaine use by the young adults from 1986 to 1987.

The authors note that these studies of high school seniors and high school graduates may somewhat underestimate drug use in the total population since high school dropouts and absentees were not included. However, after applying several approaches in estimating the extent of this bias, they concluded that it would not change prevalence rates by more than 2 or 3% in most cases.

The recent rise in the use of "crack," a potent and relatively cheap formulation of cocaine, is an important exception to the generally favorable trends discussed above. Data from the Drug Abuse Warning Network (DAWN) (20) show a dramatic increase in the frequency with which cocaine is mentioned as a factor in emergency room visits. Between July 1985 and June 1988 there was almost a 300% increase in the frequency with which cocaine was mentioned. The increase in total drug mentions for the same period was 55%, but slightly over half of this increase was attributable to cocaine. The DAWN data show an increase in the frequency of cocaine mentions in 1986 and 1987,

the same period in which high school seniors and young adults were reporting decreased use. This discrepancy may have resulted from a variety of differences between the populations studied. The DAWN population includes a high proportion of inner city residents characterized by lower levels of employment and educational achievement, two of the social factors associated with increased drug use.

ETIOLOGY

Drug abuse as defined above is merely an operational definition. It does not speak to possible etiologies or to legal consequence, nor does it point to possible helpful therapeutic maneuvers. Four models, described here, have been proposed to encompass these concerns.

Moral Failure Model

This view attributes substance abuse to a failure by parents or parental surrogates (religious training, schools, movies, TV, records, etc., loosely grouped as society) to inculcate values and to the absence of an ongoing morality that would prevent the use and abuse of drugs. Paradigms of such societies exist but their relevance to our or any "western" society is dubious. They require a commonly accepted set of central organizing principles, i.e., a religious or political ideology, and a degree of homogeneity in the acceptance and enforcement of coercion for violations of prohibition, that are totally lacking in pluralistic western societies today. The failure of Prohibition in the 1920s to effect a change in American society's view of the consumption of alcohol highlights the irrelevance of the moral failure model for understanding and attenuating our current epidemic of drug abuse.

Legal Model

This view denies a psychological or biological basis for drug abuse. Proponents define behavior as aberrant, and as of consequence to society, only when specific acts violate existing law and then recommend existing legal remedies such as trial, fines, and imprisonment to deal with these infractions. This view neglects and underestimates current research in neurobiology and psychopharmacology that points to a biological basis of mental illness, including drug addiction.

It also ignores the repeated failure of legal sanctions and imprisonment, short of the death penalty, to deter recidivism; and it ignores the inability of victims of drug abuse, when in the throes of their illness, to exert rational control over their acts that would fulfill the specific intent requirement that most humane legal systems require to justify punishment for aberrant acts.

Disease Model

This model hypothesizes a host susceptibility to drugs of abuse that is lifelong, progressive, and incapable of modification and hence can be coped with only by total abstinence. It takes as its substrate only those meeting the definitions of substance abuse or dependence (see above) and does not concern itself with social or experimental use. The disease model encompasses research advances in psychopharmacology that seem to explain the stereotypic behaviors that lead to tolerance and addiction. Positing dependency as a disease—albeit self-induced—it implies a more humane approach than other models.

The disease model of substance abuse is the paradigm for the proponents of methadone maintenance, developed in the 1960s. Chronic narcotic abuse was seen as a biological modification of the brain that required supplementation by a narcotic substitute that does not lead to dysfunction. Methadone, by virtue of being orally ingestible and having a long duration of action, optimally met this criterion. The disease model also offers a nonstigmatizing explanation of substance abuse to organizations such as Alcoholics Anonymous and Narcotics Anonymous. These organizations have helped to unleash a vast movement for self-improvement that is consonant with a yearning for greater personal autonomy and less reliance on narrow technical expertise.

Psychosocial Model

This model sees chemical dependency as the inadvertent effect of repeated self-medication by a vulnerable population intent on relieving overwhelming anxiety and/or psychic pain attendant on loss, hopelessness, boredom, depression, and fear. Drugs of abuse are potent and effective, albeit short-term, chemical alleviators of these symptoms. Vulnerability in this model is not a function of genetic constitution (though this may define an enhanced susceptibility) but of membership in at-risk populations who, because of youthful immaturity, socioeconomic disability, and the lack of responsible familial or peer support systems, have not developed the same repertory of behaviors that the greater part of society uses to cope with the disappointing aspects of the human condition. This model has the virtue of defining an at-risk population from among the young, the drop-outs, and the socially and economically disadvantaged that best fit epidemiologically the majority of abusers in our current epidemic. The model helps explain the potential for endemic abuse by individuals who, although they may be socially and economically advantaged, may also turn to repetitive self-medication in the face of losses or situational anxiety, demoralization, or physical pain. The psychosocial model avoids a simplistic expectation of cure by mere detoxification or by enforced abstinence if release back into the same environment is contemplated without remediation of the conditions of vulnerability. The model also relies on support systems and self-help as a condition of remission and emphasizes a humane approach to treatment as opposed to reliance on ever more punitive but futile efforts at deterrence.

DEPRESSANT DRUGS

Tolerance and Addiction

Central nervous system (CNS) depressants all share the capacity to induce psychoactive tolerance. *Psychoactive tolerance* is the habituation of the CNS that occurs in response to repetitive drug dosages given in a schedule so that there is always a measurable level of the drug in the blood. Tolerance results in a diminution or absence of the expected biological effect of a given dose of the drug. Markedly increased amounts of drug are required to achieve the initially desired effect. Psychoactive tolerance is distinguishable from *"pharmacological" tolerance*, which reflects the induction of catabolic enzymes that metabolize a drug more rapidly on repeated use. Psychoactive tolerance depends upon a change in the neuronal membrane receptors, independent of the rate of metabolism of the drug. Barbiturates induce both pharmacological and psychoactive tolerance. Narcotics produce only psychoactive tolerance.

The time required for the induction of psychoactive tolerance varies from a matter of days after repeated intravenous or intramuscular administration of narcotics, to weeks or months after repeated oral administration of narcotics, barbiturates, alcohol, and other sedatives.

Physiological addiction is defined as the point in the induction of tolerance when abrupt cessation of a drug results in withdrawal symptoms (the abstinence state). Withdrawal symptoms are often the mirror image of the biological effects exerted by the drug in question (Table 22.3). As can be seen in the table, narcotic withdrawal, while uncomfortable, is not life threatening. Sedative withdrawal includes both a minor and relatively innocuous symptom complex that occurs initially in all sedative-tolerant individuals and a major symptom complex, occurring in a small fraction of tolerant individuals, which includes seizures and death. Sedative-tolerant individuals should have a tapering detoxification under medical supervision, similar to that described for alcohol in Chapter 21.

The inhalants, which also are CNS depressants, do not usually induce tolerance because their volatility and short-term use never lead to high blood levels long enough to habituate the neuronal membranes.

Sedative-Hypnotics

Usual Effects

Intoxication with sedatives is similar to intoxication with alcohol. Sufficient amounts are taken to produce a depression of cortical function and to relax social and personal inhibitions. This disinhibition is called

Table 22.3.
Characteristics of Dependence on Depressant Drugs

Drug	Physiological Effect	Withdrawal Symptoms (from 1 to 7 Days after Last Dose)	
Narcotics	Pupillary constriction Analgesia Constipation Respiratory depression	Pupillary dilation Myalgia Diarrhea Stimulation of respiratory centers ("yawning")	
Barbiturate, alcohol, sedative, tranquilizers	Induction of sleep (hypnosis) Sedation Alcohol may increase seizure activity (other sedatives decrease seizure activity)	Insomnia Tremulousness Irritability Hyperpyrexia	Minor symptoms Onset 24–72 hr after last dose Duration 72–96 hr after last dose
		Delirium Seizures Death	Major symptoms Onset 72 hr to 1 week after last dose Duration up to 2 weeks after last dose

"a high," a state of euphoria in which mood is elevated and anxiety is reduced. Depending on dose, route of administration, rate of metabolism, and body size, exact effects of the sedative may vary widely from time to time and from individual to individual.

Acute Adverse Effects

Overshooting the mark may lead to more profound intoxication: slurred speech, impaired judgment, and unsteady gait. Even greater overdose may lead to stupor, coma, respiratory depression, vasomotor collapse, and death. Intoxication from sedatives, as with alcohol intoxication, impairs motor coordination and the ability to make intellectual judgments.

Chronic Adverse Effects

A different population of abusers of sedatives is characterized not by the intent to reach disinhibition (a "high") but by the intent to calm anxiety or induce sleep. Patients often receive prescriptions for sedatives (especially benzodiazepines) without instructions that they should be used only for short-term intermittent treatment. Patients will then use the medications on a regular basis, induce tolerance, and increase the dose (sometimes obtaining prescriptions from multiple physicians) in a misguided effort to control anxiety. The escalating drug use may go undetected until confusion, irritability, slurred speech, and ataxia together are recognized as sedative intoxication. Often the only distinguishing physical features are ecchymoses, which result from the patient being uncoordinated during an intoxicated state. Prescribing and use of individual new sedatives vary widely, almost in a fad-like pattern. Despite assertions to the contrary, all induce tolerance, are dangerous when consumed with alcohol or other CNS depressants, and produce dependency.

Treatment

Sedative overdose is a life-threatening emergency that should be treated in an emergency room.

Because of physiological dependence, patients who use excessive doses of sedative drugs are at risk of serious withdrawal reactions (including life-threatening seizures). Chapter 13, The Anxious Patient,

delineates guidelines for the withdrawal of benzodiazepines in the patient who has developed physiological tolerance.

Heroin and Other Narcotics

The heroin addict will not generally be seen in office practice seeking treatment of his addiction, although a review of medical histories given by patients entering a large methadone maintenance program indicates that these patients do receive treatment for a range of other medical problems. Addicts may also appear in office practice settings attempting to obtain prescription drugs when they experience difficulty in obtaining heroin (diacetylmorphine). Morphine, hydromorphone (Dilaudid), and meperidine (Demerol) are the narcotics most preferred by addicts, but they will readily use the whole range of less potent narcotic and nonnarcotic analgesics if preferred drugs are unavailable. If analgesics are difficult to obtain, addicts will temporarily use virtually any depressant drug but will prefer the barbiturates and other potent sedatives such as methaqualone (Quaalude), glutethimide (Doriden), and ethchlorvynol (Placidyl). Alcohol, the benzodiazepines, and promethazine hydrochloride (Phenergan) are often abused by patients maintained on methadone because of their tendency to potentiate the effects of methadone.

Usual Effects

The acetyl groups on the heroin molecule allow it to penetrate the blood-brain barrier more rapidly than do other narcotics. In the CNS the acetyl moieties are removed, yielding the active compound, morphine. Heroin is usually injected intravenously but can also be injected intramuscularly (skin-popping) or sniffed (snorting). The effects after intravenous injections consist of a brief and intense period of euphoria followed by several hours of a pleasant dreamy state in which the user may slowly nod as if he is falling off to sleep. He may also experience itching of the skin, which leads to characteristic scratching.

Acute Adverse Effects

Narcotic overdose is characterized by depressed consciousness and depressed respiration. Pulmonary edema, a common complication of narcotic overdose, contributes to hypoxia and may cause death, even while the needle is still in the vein. Experimental evidence suggests that a massive sympathetic discharge is responsible for this effect.

Chronic Adverse Effects

The adverse effects of chronic heroin use result from use of dirty needles, the adulterants mixed with the heroin, and the associated life style (poor nutrition and health care) rather than from the drug itself. Heroin generally constitutes only 2 to 5% of the content of a street dose and is usually mixed with milk sugar (lactose) and quinine under nonsterile conditions in which other, more dangerous, adulterants may also be included to mask the dilution of the heroin. Chronic heroin abusers will have needle marks or scars, usually in the antecubital fossae of both arms, on the forearms and wrists, or on the backs of the hands. The presence of abscesses or old abscess scars and of bluish phlebitis scars from past injections also indicates chronic use. Long-time users are usually forced to seek out new injection sites as old sites become unusable because of scarring, and they may exhibit fresh needle marks on the legs and neck. In addition to abscesses, chronic intravenous drug use will result in an increased incidence of cellulitis, endocarditis, and pulmonary hypertension due to microembolization. When needles are shared, there is a high risk of acquiring hepatitis and human immunodeficiency virus (HIV) infection. It has been estimated that at least one-half of all heroin addicts develop chronic liver disease.

Tolerance to heroin develops quickly and can be demonstrated to some degree after only a few days of administration of the drug. The degree of tolerance and the consequent severity of withdrawal symptoms will depend primarily on dosage levels and the frequency and duration of use. However, the severity of a patient's addiction to heroin cannot be defined purely in terms of tolerance or withdrawal symptoms since heroin addiction is as much a function of psychological and social factors as it is a simple consequence of physical tolerance or of withdrawal symptoms.

Narcotic withdrawal is characterized by anxiety, nausea, yawning, diarrhea, sweating, rhinorrhea, dilated pupils, and piloerection ("goose flesh"). In the advanced stages of withdrawal the patient experiences vomiting and muscle spasms that often appear as jerky "kicking" movements of the legs. Acute narcotic withdrawal may be inadvertently induced when a narcotic-tolerant individual is given pentazocine (Talwin) or nalbuphine hydrochloride (Nubain), analgesics that combine agonist and antagonist properties. Although the untreated addict will experience significant anxiety and discomfort during withdrawal, the process itself presents no serious medical risks. Narcotic addicts tend to confuse anxiety with the early symptoms of withdrawal, so that the diagnosis of withdrawal should be made on the basis of observable signs rather than on subjective reports of anxiety and nausea.

Treatment

Narcotic overdose must be treated in an emergency room. Emergency treatment requires cardiorespiratory monitoring and support. A narcotic antagonist (nalorphine, Narcan) is extremely safe and effective in countering the central nervous system depression caused by narcotic overdose.

As a practical matter, any patient who has been abusing heroin or other narcotics and is willing to accept help should be referred for treatment. Few addicts voluntarily seek treatment until the destructive effects of their drug use have made continued use intolerable. Detoxification may be accomplished by substituting methadone for the narcotic previously used by the patient and then gradually reducing the dose over a period of approximately three weeks. The initial dose should be sufficient to suppress withdrawal symptoms without causing sedation. Methadone detoxification is normally done on an ambulatory basis by specially licensed drug treatment programs. Detoxification may also be accomplished using clonidine hydrochloride in conjunction with methocarbamol (Robaxin) to provide symptomatic treatment of withdrawal symptoms (7, 26). As with detoxification from any substance, the patient should be engaged in a program of outpatient chemical dependency counseling during and after detoxification. There appears to be little benefit in hospitalizing patients for narcotic withdrawal since it involves no significant medical risks and since hospitalization does not appear to increase the proportion of patients who achieve abstinence.

Inhalants: Solvent Abuse

The inhalation of solvents is a form of substance abuse that is most commonly found among young people. Because solvents are easily obtainable and inexpensive, they are likely to be preferred by individuals who lack the money or other resources needed to obtain more desirable drugs. A partial list of specific substances subject to this type of abuse includes gasoline, ignition spray, airplane glue, paint thinner, spray paint, lighter fluid, nail polish remover, cleaning fluid, and shoe polish. Inhalation is typically accomplished by saturating a rag with the substance and holding it directly over the face or placing it in a bag that is then placed over the nose and the mouth.

Usual Effects

The effects of solvents are immediate and of short duration, usually dissipating in an hour or less. Acute intoxication is similar to alcohol intoxication except for a shorter duration.

Acute Adverse Effects

A hangover, with symptoms of headache and nausea similar but perhaps milder than the hangover produced by alcohol, has been observed. Some users will experience apparent delirium characterized by tactile hallucinations, spatial distortions, and macropsia or micropsia (body image distortions). Sudden sniffing deaths have been described when inhalants were used during strenuous activity or under conditions in which blood oxygen is reduced. Such deaths apparently occur as a result of cardiac arrhythmias. Other deaths have been caused by suffocation when the user loses consciousness while his nose and mouth are covered by the bag containing the solvent.

Chronic Adverse Effects

Although current information does not permit clear-cut conclusions concerning the extent of organ damage caused by inhalant abuse, there is cause for concern. The effects of solvents on the central nervous system, liver, kidneys, and bone marrow are not known. Numerous studies have demonstrated organ damage from long-term exposure to relatively low concentrations of industrial solvents, but it is not clear to what extent these findings can be generalized to the short-term, high concentration exposures experienced by inhalant abusers. Furthermore, in studies contrasting solvent abusers with control subjects, adverse effects were found in solvent abusers, but the possibility that these were due to factors other than inhalant abuse was not ruled out.

There is evidence that tolerance develops with chronic solvent abuse, but no withdrawal syndrome has been reported, probably because the concentration of the substance in neurons is not sustained.

Treatment

Because the acute effects of solvents are usually of short duration, abusers rarely present for medical treatment. On rare occasions a patient may be brought in for treatment of a solvent-induced delirium. Chronic solvent abuse requires the same type of intense counseling and rehabilitative intervention indicated for other forms of self-destructive substance abuse (see below).

STIMULANT DRUGS

Cocaine and Other Commonly Abused Stimulants

Cocaine, the amphetamines, methylphenidate, and phenmetrazine are the most commonly abused stimulant drugs.

Cocaine is used in several forms. The route for cocaine intake depends upon the form used. As the natural water-soluble powder, cocaine hydrochloride, it is either sniffed ("snorted") and absorbed through the nasal mucosa or it is injected intravenously. Forms of cocaine that can be smoked (using a water pipe or in cigarette form) are produced by extracting or "freeing" the cocaine alkaloid from the hydrochloride salt. When ether is used as the reagent in this process, the resulting product is referred to as freebase. When baking soda and water are used as reagents, the resulting product is "crack," so named because of the crackling sound that is produced when the drug is smoked. Although they may differ in appearance and concentration, freebase and crack are pharmacologically the same.

Cocaine use appears in variable patterns. In the early stages, sessions of cocaine use typically last two to four hours with intervals of days or weeks between sessions. Some individuals are able to maintain this pattern of use without progressing further. Many users, however, follow a pattern of rapidly escalating use in which both the length of sessions and the rate of consumption increase; users of freebase and crack are much more likely to succumb to this pattern than are users who snort cocaine powder.

Chronic abusers typically engage in "runs"—periods of intensive cocaine use that can last anywhere from a few hours to several days. A run is terminated when the user runs out of cocaine or money or is too physically exhausted to continue. A run is followed by a "crash" that may last one or two days. During the crash, the user experiences intense depression, fatigue, anxiety, and irritability, usually accompanied by intense cravings for cocaine.

Amphetamines are swallowed or injected intravenously. Two nonamphetamine stimulants, *methylphenidate* (Ritalin) and *phenmetrazine* (Preludin), which can mimic the effects of naturally occurring stimulants such as cocaine, are taken orally or intravenously.

Abusers of stimulants rapidly develop pharmacological tolerance to the euphoric effects of the drugs but may actually become more sensitive to adverse effects such as irritability, restlessness, hypervigilance, and paranoia. Users report that in any given session of cocaine use the duration and intensity of the euphoric effect seems to recede with successive doses, a phenomenon referred to as "chasing the dragon's tail."

Usual Effects

Central nervous system stimulants produce euphoria, increased confidence and energy, increased heart rate and blood pressure, dilated pupils, constriction of peripheral blood vessels, and increased body temperature and metabolic rate. All of these effects are caused by a massive sympathetic stimulation induced by these drugs acting as agonists on monoaminergic neurons centrally and peripherally. The duration and intensity of effect depends upon the route used for taking in a stimulant. The effect of an oral dose of methylphenidate is muted (less intense but lasts 2 to 4 hours) because of first-pass metabolism of the drug in the liver, whereas the effect of an intravenous dose is rapid in onset (peak effect in about 5 minutes) and lasts about 20 to 40 minutes. Similarly, single oral doses of amphetamines produce effects lasting 2 to 4 hours. The effects of cocaine, when sniffed or used intravenously, are always rapid in onset but relatively short in duration. Smoking freebase or crack produces the most intense but also the shortest duration of effects (i.e., peak effect in 2 to 3 minutes, duration about 10 minutes) due to the fact that smoking is an extremely efficient method of delivering a very concentrated bolus to the brain.

Its capacity to produce an intense euphoria gives cocaine an extremely high abuse potential. In abuse liability studies employing animal subjects, cocaine has displayed a potency that far exceeds that of other drugs of abuse. The temptation to use more cocaine in order to counteract the dysphoria and fatigue that follow the initial euphoria makes the drug particularly seductive. Users often delay entry into treatment until they are physically and emotionally exhausted or are faced with serious financial problems.

When the acute effects of stimulants subside, users often experience lethargy or depression, somnolence, and a voracious appetite. The preference for cocaine over amphetamines and other stimulants is related to its greater potency and hence its greater effect on the dopaminergic neurons in the limbic system associated with the reward and pleasure centers of the brain. Cocaine absorbed in small quantities yields euphoria disproportionate to the dysphoric sympathetic side effects (increased heart rate, blood pressure and temperature, and sensations of irritability and anxiety). These side effects are more commonly associated with higher dosages of cocaine, with intravenous use, and with the use of more potent formulations such as freebase and crack, but they also occur with the longer acting amphetamines.

Acute Adverse Effects

Very large doses of all of the stimulants may cause hyperpyrexia, severe hypertension, and coronary artery vasospasm, leading to myocardial infarction, stroke, convulsion, cardiovascular collapse, and death, even in adolescents and young adults (33). Large amounts of cocaine, in addition, may cause depression of the medullary centers, and death may result from respiratory arrest as well. Death from overdose of CNS stimulants has increased significantly since the introduction of crack.

Chronic Adverse Effects

The chronic abuser of cocaine, amphetamines, and other long acting stimulants is typically hyperactive, jittery, and irritable while using; and he is depressed, exhausted, or lethargic after use. Frequently, however, early signs may take the form of unexplained financial problems or uncharacteristic overnight disappearances. With chronic use there is usually a history of sleep disturbance and weight loss. The patient may be emotionally labile and his periods of irritability, depression, and fatigue may alternate with periods of elation and enthusiasm ("mania"). Physical examination may reveal needle marks, rhinitis, teeth worn from bruxism (grinding of teeth), ulcers on the lips,

tongue, or nose, tremor, flushing, cardiac arrhythmias, and excessive sweating. Although cocaine may initially enhance sexual functioning, chronic use frequently interferes with sexual performance. Extremely heavy users may exhibit rapid, repetitious, and ritualistic body movements, or such movements may be described by companions.

Intravenous use of stimulants can result in the transmission of hepatitis, AIDS, and other infectious diseases and can cause venous sclerosis, cellulitis, and abscesses. Although methylphenidate is water soluble, the tablets contain water-insoluble components, such as talc, which may cause accelerated vascular sclerosis and pulmonary abnormalities (fibrosis, obstructive and restrictive lung disease, and reduced pulmonary diffusing capacity).

Repeated exposure to high doses of stimulants exhausts the supply of preformed monoamine neurotransmitters such as noradrenaline, dopamine, and serotonin. It has been proposed that the release of neurotransmitters in the brain and then their depletion secondary to stimulant use leads to a state of super sensitivity of their receptors and a reversible organic delusional disorder that resembles paranoid schizophrenia (32). This syndrome may occur in normal subjects with no previous psychiatric history (10). Subjects who have taken higher doses of a stimulant (e.g., 10 mg of dextroamphetamine every hour) have developed the disorder within 24 hours, as do high dose cocaine (27) and methylphenidate (24) users.

Treatment

There are no data at present to guide the clinician in distinguishing stimulant-abusing patients who should be hospitalized from those who may succeed as outpatients. Clearly, patients who present a risk of suicide should be hospitalized as should patients who are unable to maintain abstinence long enough to begin a program of outpatient treatment. Although virtually all patients experience a moderate to severe dysphoria after a session of cocaine use, only a small percentage become suicidal. Only a minority of cocaine abusers uses the drug on a daily basis for more than one or two days. In most cases, sessions of continuous cocaine use do not exceed 12 hours, and episodes of use are frequently separated by periods of abstinence lasting several days or more. Abstinence may occur because the user is unable to obtain more cocaine, is too exhausted to continue using, or is making an attempt to stop or control use. In many instances these periods of abstinence last several days or more, long enough for the patient to recover from the worst of the acute dysphoria and lassitude that normally follow a session use. Motivated patients with appropriate external supports can be engaged in outpatient treatment during such breaks in cocaine use provided that treatment involves daily counseling sessions at least five days per week during the first few weeks of abstinence. Necessary external supports would include stable employment, a drug-free home environment, and active involvement in Narcotics Anonymous. For such patients, hospitalization should probably be considered only after an initial attempt at outpatient treatment has failed. A recent, carefully designed study (9) suggests that desipramine is a useful adjunct in helping patients to withdraw from cocaine as outpatients. Patients who received desipramine reported reduced cocaine cravings and were more likely to achieve abstinence than patients who received placebo.

There is no definitive approach for helping patients maintain abstinence over the longer term. The same principles of rehabilitation, described below, that apply to the rehabilitation of abusers of alcohol and other drugs also apply to cocaine abusers.

DRUGS THAT ALTER PERCEPTION

This category encompasses substances that may be CNS stimulants or depressants, but that in their commonly used dose and via their usual route of administration produce exaggerated imaginings, visual hallucinations, altered time perceptions, and subjective feelings of enhancement of sensation.

Marijuana/Hashish

Marijuana consists of the dried leaves of the marijuana (*Cannabis sativa*) plant, which are usually smoked in pipes or cigarettes ("joints"). *Hashish* is a concentrated resin of cannabis and contains approximately 5 to 10 times as much of the psychoactive ingredient, tetrahydrocannabinol (THC) as does marijuana. The discussion that follows applies to both marijuana and hashish, although the effects associated with higher doses are more likely to occur with hashish than with marijuana.

Usual Effects

The effects of marijuana usually last from 3 to 6 hours. The more common effects are elation, relaxation, an increased tendency to laughter and silliness, a sense of sharpened perception and increased insight, increased vividness and appreciation in all sensory modalities, decreased concentration, loosened associations, increased appetite, tachycardia, mild feelings of paranoia, and a sense of detachment or depersonalization. Lower doses tend to produce relaxation and euphoria, whereas higher doses tend to result in increasing visual and auditory perceptual distortions. Doses three to five times higher than those producing relaxation and mild euphoria can result in psychotomimetic effects (depersonalization, auditory and visual hallucinations). Thus, some of the usual effects of marijuana that might be enjoyable to the experienced user can be frightening to the inexperienced user. The setting is also very important in determining the effects of the drug. Marijuana, when smoked in a pleasant and familiar setting, is less likely to produce a negative response than when used in an unfamiliar or threatening setting.

Acute Adverse Effects

Considering the large number of regular users in the United States, it is clear that adverse reactions to marijuana requiring medical treatment are rare. The most frequent adverse response is an acute anxiety reaction that is similar to the panic attacks described in Chapter 13. The *acute anxiety reaction* that is induced by marijuana is different in that it frequently includes paranoid ideation, which is not typically a feature of panic attacks. Acute panic reactions are most likely to occur in novice users or in users who unexpectedly receive a much higher than usual dose. This reaction is characterized by the appearance of many of the usual effects of the drug in an exaggerated form and by mounting anxiety, which often stems from a sense of losing control and which is often expressed as a fear of "going crazy" or, less frequently, of dying. Acute panic reactions can vary in intensity and duration, but most last only the few hours it takes for the effects of the drug to wear off. Some patients experience persistent anxiety for several days after the initial panic subsides. It has been estimated that three intense panic reactions occur per 100, 000 exposures (22).

There have also been reports of *delirium*, in the form of an organic delusional disorder induced by marijuana. A *dysphoric reaction* characterized by disorientation, catatonia-like immobility, acute panic, and heavy sedation has also been reported. As with the anxiety/panic reaction, these conditions tend to remit within 2 to 4 hours as the effects of the marijuana diminish.

Reports of *enduring psychotic reactions* after heavy marijuana use have appeared largely in countries where marijuana is used in much higher doses than in the United States. Reports of confirmed psychotic reactions to marijuana in this country have been rare.

Chronic Adverse Effects

There is substantial evidence that marijuana in dose levels associated with common social usage interferes with intellectual and psychomotor performance. A number of studies indicate that marijuana use will significantly impair driving skills. In the dosage commonly used (10 mg/cigarette), marijuana impairs recent memory, thus interfering with cognition and learning (17).

It is clear that smoking marijuana, even a few cigarettes daily for only a few weeks, adversely affects pulmonary function (30). It has also been reported that marijuana smoke contains 70% more carcinogens, such as benzopyrene, than does tobacco smoke (21). Although there is reason for concern regarding the carcinogenic potential of marijuana smoke, there are no data yet that demonstrate an association of neoplasia with marijuana. There have been conflicting findings concerning possible adverse effects of marijuana on the immune system. Some studies have reported changes in immunological responsiveness, but the clinical implications of these changes are not currently known. There is evidence that marijuana reduces testosterone levels in men, although the average level for users remains within normal limits (15). The clinical implications are unclear, but concern has been expressed over possible effects of even small changes in testosterone levels in adolescent males.

Animal studies involving very high doses of THC have yielded evidence of teratogenicity. However, while there is widespread use of marijuana among women of reproductive age, there have not been reports of a higher level of birth defects among children born to mothers who were regular users of marijuana during pregnancy. Several studies (6, 8, 13) suggest that more subtle effects, such as neurological abnormalities and reductions in birth weight and height, may be associated with maternal use of marijuana.

It should be noted that all reviews of the literature on marijuana include the admonition that the available data simply are not adequate to draw clear conclusions about the effects of chronic use. The current status of marijuana research is quite analogous to the status of research on the effects of smoking some 30 years ago.

Tolerance and Withdrawal. Marijuana is clearly a CNS depressant. It is cross-tolerant with the barbiturate sedatives; high doses induce psychoactive tolerance and physiological dependence, and it is additive with all other depressants (narcotics, sedatives, alcohol) in depressing the function of the central nervous system. Heretofore, because of the low potency of the marijuana used in the United States (1 to 10 mg/cigarette) these effects were not generally appreciated. With greater potency (new plants yielding 20 mg/cigarette) and greater concentration of the active ingredient in hashish or oil of hashish, users ingesting doses as high as 30 to 100 mg report more adverse reactions, greater frequency of hallucinations, and more pronounced CNS depression. In one study (22) volunteers who smoked an average of five marijuana cigarettes a day for 64 days exhibited restlessness, sleep disturbance, loss of appetite, and irritability when they stopped using marijuana.

Treatment of Acute Reactions

Because they must be closely observed and may take several hours to recover, patients suffering from panic reactions are best managed in a setting such as a drug abuse program, mental health center, or emergency room where continuing observation and supportive contact can be provided (29). Generally, these patients require simple reassurance and an explanation that they are experiencing a drug reaction that will dissipate as the drug is eliminated from their bodies.

Delusional or delirious patients should be seen in an emergency room since they present more complicated management problems and may require sedation or hospitalization. Furthermore, other causes of a delirium or an organic delusional disorder such as trauma, infection, or a metabolic disorder should be ruled out. Restraints should only be used when absolutely necessary for the safety of the patient or of others. Drugs

should also not be used unless the patient is extremely agitated and difficult to control. In such cases, diazepam (Valium) is preferred in an initial dose of 20 mg intramuscularly with subsequent doses of 10 mg each hour to a maximum of 60 mg.

Phencyclidine (PCP)

Phencyclidine, a derivative of ketamine, a known barbiturate-like anesthetic, is quite clearly a CNS depressant, capable of inducing psychoactive tolerance. However, PCP exhibits selective action as an anesthetic, appearing to depress sensory tracts, including proprioception, pain, touch, and temperature, to a greater degree than it depresses cortical function. The resultant state of sensory deprivation and relative cortical wakefulness makes for a peculiar sense of detachment, disembodiment, and weightlessness. These sensations are intensely pleasurable for some, whereas for others they induce intense anxiety and even panic. Prolonged sensory deprivation, whether chemically induced or provoked mechanically by shielding out visual, auditory, and tactile stimuli, will predictably induce delusions and hallucinations even in normal subjects.

PCP was developed as an anesthetic but was abandoned for this purpose when it was found to cause disturbing side effects. It continues to be used by veterinarians as an animal tranquilizer or immobilizing agent. Pure PCP is a white powder that dissolves in water. It is usually sprinkled on marijuana, dried parsley flakes, or other organic material and smoked. Less frequently, it is obtained in powder or tablet form and ingested or sniffed ("snorting"). Street names for the drug vary considerably from region to region, but it is most commonly known as angel dust, flakes, crystal, hog, or sheets. An excellent summary of the literature on PCP has been prepared by Luisada (16).

Usual Effects

The effects of PCP tend to be dose related, although there can be marked differences in the response of different individuals to a given dose or in the response of an individual to the same dose at different times. Individuals who take PCP in the relatively low doses normally associated with street use may experience exhilaration, euphoria, a sense of great strength and power, inebriation, tranquilization, and perceptual disturbances. Some unpleasant effects commonly reported include disorientation, hallucinations, anxiety, paranoia, hyperexcitability, and irritability. At usual street dosages, most users reach peak intoxication in 5 to 30 minutes and remain "high" for 4 to 6 hours. It may take 24 hours before the user feels completely normal again.

Acute Adverse Effects

Even in relatively low doses, PCP is capable of occasionally causing severe reactions that may precipitate extreme agitation and *acts of violence* toward the user and to others. With higher doses users are more likely to exhibit *delirium*.

A cardinal symptom of delirium is clouding of consciousness, defined as a reduction in the clarity of awareness of the environment (1). The delirious patient can present a bewildering array of symptoms that can fluctuate markedly over relatively short periods of time. He may be hypervigilant or drowsy, anxious or aggressive, fearful or dauntless. His behavior may fluctuate during the day, alert at times and stuporous at other times. Clouding of consciousness may also appear as impairments in concentration, memory, arithmetical ability, orientation, and complex motor functions, such as in writing a sentence or drawing an abstract design. Thinking may appear fragmented and disorganized or it may be unusually accelerated or slowed. Delirious patients may also experience hallucinations, illusions, and delusions. They frequently show a blank stare, and in some instances they may appear almost catatonic.

There is a difference between the delirium that is seen in acute PCP toxicity and what has been referred to as a *PCP psychosis*, a disorder closely resembling schizophrenia that develops after acute intoxication and persists for 24 hours or more. Such psychoses may develop out of the original intoxication or may occur days after the intoxication has cleared. Approximately one-fourth of the patients who experience a PCP psychosis will go on to develop a schizophrenic psychosis within 2 years, despite abstinence from PCP. It appears that at least half of the patients treated for PCP psychosis use the drug again within 2 weeks of discharge (13).

Ataxia, nystagmus, and ptosis are common features of acute PCP toxicity. Very high doses of PCP, which are normally the result of oral ingestion rather than of smoking, can result in coma, severe respiratory depression, seizures, and death.

Chronic Adverse Effects

Chronic use of PCP may produce persistent changes in personal habits (hygiene or dress), problems with memory or speech, sleep disturbances, mood changes (depression, irritability), paranoid or frankly delusional thinking, and unusual excitability or lethargy. Little is known about long-term physical effects.

Treatment of Acute Reactions

Consistent correlation has been found between the patient's initial level of consciousness and the time course of improvement (4). Patients who present with delirium clear in 3 to 8 hours; patients who remain stuporous or comatose for 1 to 4 hours clear in 5 to 62 hours; and patients whose stupor or coma lasts 6 or more hours clear in 75 to over 200 hours. Therefore, patients who are delirious at presentation can be treated in an emergency room and do not require hospitalization. Repeated mental status examinations should be performed to ensure that the patient is in a state of clear consciousness for at least 4 hours before dis-

charge. Members of the family should be cautioned that the patient should stay in the company of family members or reliable friends for several days. Patients can have the onset of severe depression or a PCP psychosis for several days after the acute effects of the drug have subsided. Patients who remain comatose or stuporous for more than 2 hours or who develop a PCP psychosis require hospitalization.

Lysergic Acid Diethylamide (LSD)

Lysergic acid diethylamide is the prototype of a number of alkaloid substances of such great potency that small doses predictably cause hallucinations. These hallucinogens, including psylocybin, di-methyltryptamine (DMT), and mescaline, are all CNS depressants in higher doses. LSD ("acid") is sold illicitly in the form of powder, tablets, or capsules. Sugar cubes, small squares of gelatin ("window pane"), or paper ("blotter acid") that have been impregnated with the drug are also available. LSD is usually ingested orally and its effects appear within 15 minutes, reaching a peak at about 90 minutes and lasting for approximately 8 to 10 hours.

Usual Effects

LSD usually produces some combination of the following subjective effects: depersonalization, altered time perception, labile mood, profound perceptual distortions (usually visual), body image distortion, and feelings of profound insight. Objective effects include tachycardia, palpitations, anorexia, elevated blood pressure, fever, lack of coordination, and dilated pupils.

Acute Adverse Effects

Inexperienced users may experience an acute panic reaction that occurs because the normal effects of the drug are unfamiliar or unexpected. In more severe reactions, users of LSD may experience hallucinations (usually visual) and delusions that may persist beyond the time when the drug is circulating in the blood.

Flashbacks, spontaneous recurrences of the original LSD experience, have been estimated to occur in 1 of every 20 users (from days to years later). They are more likely to occur in chronic users. There have also been reports of prolonged psychotic reactions after the use of LSD, although these are rare.

Patients with acute LSD toxicity can be differentiated from those with PCP toxicity and from schizophrenia in several ways. LSD causes dilation of the pupils, which is absent in PCP toxicity and in schizophrenia. PCP toxicity usually is characterized by clouding of consciousness, and the patient will often exhibit ataxia, nystagmus, and ptosis, which are not features of LSD toxicity or of schizophrenia.

Chronic Adverse Effects

Some degree of tolerance develops with repeated use of LSD, but no withdrawal syndrome has been observed.

Treatment

Adverse reactions to LSD usually remit in 8 to 24 hours, and hospitalization is usually not necessary. However, the patient should be observed until symptoms clear. Referral to an emergency room or to a drug abuse program that can provide this type of support will usually be necessary. The same supportive measures described earlier for the treatment of adverse reactions to marijuana are appropriate. Extremely agitated patients should be given diazepam (Valium), 20 mg intramuscularly, before being sent to a treatment center.

Belladonna Alkaloids

Belladonna derivatives such as atropine (the active ingredient in Jimson weed) and scopolamine are acetylcholine antagonists that in high doses will also regularly produce hallucinations, delirium, and varying states of excitement, insomnia, and/or amnesia. These effects may be followed by CNS depression and coma. The side effects of these drugs—dryness of the mouth, blurred vision, anhidrosis, and tachycardia—limit their appeal as psychoactive agents. Thus, the rare instances of abuse are mostly by youngsters experimenting with Jimson weed in rural areas or, in the past, by use of over-the-counter soporifics that contained scopolamine until banned by the Food and Drug Administration some years ago. Treatment of toxic overdose is a medical emergency requiring gastric lavage and ingestion of activated charcoal to limit intestinal absorption. Physostigmine, 1 to 4 mg, injected intravenously, intramuscularly, or subcutaneously is a specific antidote that abolishes both the peripheral and CNS effects of these alkaloids. Repeated injection at 1 to 2 hours may be necessary.

REHABILITATION

All forms of drug abuse require both acute and long-term intervention. Acute interventions (see above) include the management of overdose, toxicity, and withdrawal under medical supervision. It is important to recognize, however, that when the immediate physical consequences of drug abuse have been successfully treated, there remains a critical need to identify and treat the underlying conditions that motivated drug misuse in the first place. Most drug abusers will have significant problems of psychological and social adjustment and will require counseling and rehabilitation over extended periods of time before they are capable of sustained abstinence. As described below, the general physician's major role in dealing with long-term rehabilitation is to motivate patients to enter and continue in rehabilitation programs.

Effective rehabilitation programs stress the development of practical social and vocational skills, and the avoidance of social environments conducive to drug use. In recent years, there has been an increasing recognition that families may actually "enable" drug abuse by one or more members. Family therapy has been used successfully with narcotic addicts (28) and would appear to be the treatment of choice with drug-abusing teenagers who are still living with their parents.

Because many drug abusers have important deficits in education and vocational preparation, lack basic social and recreational skills, and are handicapped by problems of poor impulse control and low self-esteem, the process of rehabilitation will often take considerable time. As with alcoholism, relapse is commonplace and recurrent treatment episodes will frequently be required.

There is evidence that existing treatment modalities shorten the course of substance abuse disorders and reduce the amount of injury to both the individual and the community. There is evidence that treatment reduces the economic costs that result from drug abuse and that these cost reductions substantially exceed the actual cost of providing care (26). However, while treatment appears to be cost effective, it must also be acknowledged that definitive treatment methods that result in lasting abstinence from drugs in a significant proportion of patients do not presently exist.

Detoxification

With the exception of patients who enter methadone maintenance treatment, rehabilitation begins with detoxification. Detoxification is the first, and easiest, task for the recovering addict. Patients tend to attach too much significance to the task of physiological withdrawal and too little significance to the more difficult tasks of developing new social and vocational skills and making the life-style changes necessary for continued abstinence.

With proper support, the majority of chemically addicted patients can be detoxified *on an outpatient basis*. Such patients should be seen on a daily basis throughout the detoxification and should be participating concurrently in an intensive program of counseling and education. Medications should be administered on a daily basis so that the patient has only the dosages needed between visits. The other conditions needed for successful outpatient detoxification are described in detail in Chapter 21, Alcoholism.

In general, *inpatient detoxification* is necessary when (a) the patient is unable to discontinue use of illicit substances in spite of appropriate medication and psychological support; (b) the patient has concurrent medical problems that require hospitalization; (c) the patient has developed an extremely high tolerance and has a history of major withdrawal symptoms such as seizures and delirium tremens; (d) the patient presents a clear risk of suicide or, because of chronic intoxication and impaired judgment, is a danger to self or others.

The foregoing restrictions preclude only a minority of patients from outpatient detoxification. Cocaine abusers frequently feel that they are out of control and in need of hospitalization. Careful history taking will reveal, however, that most cocaine use is episodic and that between episodes of use most users experience periods of abstinence in which withdrawal symptoms dissipate. Patients presenting for treatment frequently have been abstinent from cocaine for several days and are not experiencing significant withdrawal symptoms. In many cases, patients press for hospitalization because they are afraid of resuming use. There is little evidence, however, that hospitalizing patients for this purpose produces a better outcome than would be obtained through outpatient detoxification (12).

For most patients, it is not physical dependence that presents the major obstacle to recovery. Rather, it is the patient's willingness and ability to make changes in lifestyle that will determine the success of the patient's efforts to become drug free.

Pharmacological Approaches to the Treatment of Drug Dependence

Methadone Maintenance

Methadone maintenance is the most widely used chemotherapeutic approach to the treatment of narcotic addiction. Methadone is a long acting synthetic narcotic that is effective when taken orally in a single daily dose. Methadone is substituted, at a dose that prevents withdrawal but does not cause sedation or intoxication, for the illicit narcotic previously used by the patient. The methadone dose is gradually increased thereby increasing the patient's tolerance for all narcotics. The patient's tolerance is increased to a level where the patient is unable to experience a significant effect, even from relatively large doses of illicit narcotics. Although this methadone "blockade" can be over-ridden by a sufficiently large dose of another narcotic, the "payoff" for doing so is small in relation to the cost and the use of illicit narcotics. Patients taking methadone are fully tolerant of the effects of the drugs and are thus able to function normally in home and work settings.

Numerous studies have shown methadone maintenance to be a cost-effective approach in treating narcotic addiction (26). Methadone maintenance produces substantial reductions in crime and increases economic productivity of patients in treatment. It has also taken on a new significance in terms of its potential for reducing the spread of AIDS, since needle sharing among addicts is a common mode of transmission. In the late 1980s intravenous drug users have had the highest incidence of AIDS of any identified risk group.

Although demonstrably cost-effective, methadone treatment has several limitations. As with other forms of chemical dependency treatment, there is a high rate of relapse. Patients are required to take methadone under observation at a clinic at least three times a week and this requirement sometimes conflicts with work and family commitments. Although methadone is highly effective in suppressing the use of narcotics, it has no such effect on alcohol or other drugs, and many methadone-maintained patients develop problems with other substances. Methadone-maintained patients become both physically and psychologically dependent on the drug, and many experience considerable difficulty in making the transition from methadone to abstinence. Some treatment professionals believe that narcotic addicts suffer from a biochemical abnormality that is corrected by methadone so that it may be necessary for them to remain on methadone for life. The predominant view, however, is that patients who make appropriate changes in lifestyle and develop good social and emotional support systems should be able to detoxify successfully from methadone.

Naltrexone

Naltrexone is an orally administered narcotic antagonist that is highly effective in blocking the effects of narcotics. It is a long acting drug that can effectively block the use of narcotics when administered three times a week. Candidates for naltrexone treatment must first be detoxified from the narcotic drug to which they are addicted. Unlike methadone, which works by increasing the patient's tolerance for narcotics, naltrexone competes with narcotics at the receptor site. Another important difference between the two drugs is that naltrexone is not addicting, and patients can discontinue use without difficulty. The major disadvantage of naltrexone is that few patients are willing to use the drug and stay on it for an appropriate length of time. Its effectiveness is thus limited to highly motivated patients or patients who can be required to take the drug. Like methadone, naltrexone is not effective in blocking the use of other substances.

The pharmacological equivalents of methadone or naltrexone have not been developed for other drugs such as cocaine, sedatives, or minor tranquilizers. Although a variety of drugs can provide symptomatic relief for patients detoxifying from these drugs, there are no agents presently available that will block their effects (naltrexone) or serve as a substitute (methadone).

Drug-Free Treatment Approaches

Traditional individual psychotherapy alone has not proven effective in treating drug dependence. Most drug-free treatment programs use some form of group rather than individual counseling as a primary component.

Principal Types of Rehabilitation Programs

Residential Treatment Programs

There are two types of residential treatment programs commonly encountered in the United States.

Therapeutic Communities. Therapeutic facilities typically require patients to commit themselves to six months or more of treatment. Patients are subjected to an intense, aggressively confrontational form of group therapy that is intended to facilitate change by stripping away antisocial, drug-oriented beliefs and values and replacing them with socially adaptive beliefs and values. Therapeutic communities tend to have high drop-out rates in the first few weeks of treatment as many patients are not willing to make the commitment required by this form of treatment. Patients who remain for the duration of treatment, however, often achieve an enduring drug-free adjustment.

Intermediate-Term Residential Programs. A more frequently encountered form of residential treatment is the intermediate-term residential program. These programs are typically four weeks in duration and were originally designed to treat alcoholism. Over the last two decades they have evolved into chemical dependence programs that accept patients with a wide range of substance abuse problems. Intermediate-term residential programs utilize a more traditional group therapy approach that is less aggressive than the approach used by therapeutic communities. They also place a strong emphasis on education. In most facilities, patients attend lectures and films designed to increase their understanding of the disease of chemical dependency and the nature of the recovery process. Traditionally, intermediate-term residential programs have been viewed as the treatment of choice for chemical dependency, but in recent years they have come under pressure from a variety of groups concerned about the rising cost of health care benefits. Residential treatment is considerably more expensive than outpatient care, and there is little evidence that the outcomes are different for the majority of patients (18). In response to the demand for most cost-effective treatment approaches, intermediate-term residential facilities have begun to offer flexible lengths of stay rather than admitting all patients for the same 28- or 30-day program.

Intensive Outpatient Treatment Programs

Demands for more cost-effective forms of treatment have led to a greater emphasis on the use of outpatient approaches. Intensive outpatient programs offer a combination of education and group counseling similar to that found in the intermediate-term residential programs, but they provide treatment in the evenings so patients do not have to be absent from home or work. Intensive outpatient programs have patients attend treatment sessions four to six times a week and offer twelve to twenty hours of therapeutic activities each week for a period of four to six weeks.

Self-Help Groups

Self-help groups such as Alcoholics Anonymous (AA) and Narcotics Anonymous (NA) provide another valuable resource for individuals seeking help for a substance abuse problem. These "twelve step" programs provide a clearly defined sequence of steps that the addict must take in order to recover from his or her addiction. They also provide immediate access to the emotional support and encouragement of others who have successfully coped with similar problems. AA and NA both maintain hotlines that are listed in the telephone directories of every major community in the United States and Canada. The NA process is identical to the process of AA, which is described in Table 21.4.

Nar-anon provides support for members of the addict's family using twelve steps modeled on the twelve steps of Al-Anon (see Table 21.10). Even if the patient refuses to accept treatment or try self-help groups, family members (co-dependents) should be referred to Nar-anon. Co-dependents experience a wide range of physical and emotional stresses as a result of another family member's addiction. Co-dependents frequently suffer from guilt, shame, loss of self-esteem, diminished self-confidence, and social isolation. They often believe that they are in some way to blame for the substance abuser's problems, a belief that is frequently fostered by the substance abuser who is more than happy to shift responsibility to others. Co-dependents frequently engage in "enabling" behaviors—actions that are intended to "help" the substance abuser but that in fact only shield the substance abuser from the consequences of his or her behavior and serve therefore to delay serious efforts at recovery. Co-dependents frequently resort to a variety of strategies intended to control or prevent access to drugs by the substance abuser. Such efforts are doomed to failure. Recovery can occur only when the substance abuser feels the need for change and is willing to accept full responsibility for making change occur. Substance abusers who recover are motivated to change in large part by the unpleasant and painful consequences of their drug use. Nar-anon helps family members recognize and discontinue enabling behaviors and helps them cope with the physical and emotional stresses that result from living with a substance abuser.

Twelve step groups do not present themselves as alternatives to treatment although many addicts have successfully recovered in NA without participating in a formal treatment program. Most drug-free treatment programs incorporate the basic tenets of AA and NA into their approach and require or encourage patients to get actively involved with a twelve step program.

Common Obstacles to Recovery

Most authorities believe that a commitment to complete abstinence from mind-altering chemicals is a fundamental requirement of recovery. Although there has been some research support for the belief that alcoholics can be taught to drink in a controlled manner, most experts feel that this approach works primarily with individuals with less severe problems. Total abstinence is a more practical approach for individuals whose problems are serious enough for them to have sought treatment.

Many patients, particularly those in the early stages of addiction, have difficulty accepting the requirement of total abstinence. Although they might not admit it, many patients enter treatment with the unstated agenda of gaining control of their drug use rather than stopping it. They are reluctant to give up the pleasurable effects of drugs or they doubt their ability to cope with emotional distress without the relief afforded by drugs.

They secretly hope to learn how to enjoy the benefits of drugs while avoiding the problems that have accompanied their drug use in the past. Other patients enter treatment believing they have a problem with one type of drug but not with others. Cocaine addicts, for example, often feel that they do not have a problem with alcohol or marijuana and see no reason to give up the use of those drugs. Experience has shown, however, that continued use of "nonproblem" drugs tends to predispose patients to relapse with their problem drug. Furthermore, patients who continue to use other drugs are less likely to make the changes in lifestyle that are important in maintaining recovery over the longer term.

One of the most important tasks for the patient in early recovery is to sever ties with drug users and develop new relationships with nonusers or, at least, with nonabusers. In addition to forming new relationships, the recovering addicts must learn to form a new type of relationship, one that involves a level of trust, honesty, and intimacy that will seem quite alien to most drug users. Such relationships will be fundamental to recovery, however, since they will be the primary source of support for the addict struggling with the physical and emotional demands of recovery. During their addiction, most addicts learn to use drugs as a quick and effective, if ultimately destructive, method of dealing with physical or emotional distress. In recovery, the addict must learn to use supportive relationships instead of drugs as one of the primary methods of coping with distress.

Breaking off relationships with other users is not particularly difficult since these relationships are generally superficial and based on little else than the shared activity of getting high. What is much more difficult is the task of establishing new relationships with nonusers. The active abuse of drugs during adolescence and early adulthood seems to interfere with the development of basic social skills. In addition, addicts are frequently hampered by diminished self-esteem and self-confidence and by the expectation that they will be rejected by "straight" people. Meeting people for the first time and attempting to initiate new relationships generates anxiety for most people under the best of circumstances. When normal social anxiety is compounded by the social and emotional deficits that characterize most addicts in early recovery, the task of forming new relationships can become so intimidating that it may be avoided altogether. The recovering addict who finds himself lonely or isolated will be tempted to resume contact with old friends who are still using.

Another important lifestyle change has to do with the use of leisure time. Drug use is, among other things, a recreational activity. Getting and using drugs provides a daily routine that fills time and provides stimulation and challenge. For some addicts, the enjoyment of certain aspects of the drug-oriented lifestyle is as important as the reinforcing effects of drug use in maintaining drug involvement. For other users, being high makes it possible to tolerate what would otherwise be a tedious daily routine. It is important for the addict in early recovery to identify new activities that will provide a reasonable amount of stimulation and satisfaction. Boredom greatly increases the risk of relapse, and the recovering addict who fails to develop satisfying leisure time activities is in danger of drifting back to people and activities associated with his or her former lifestyle.

Self-help groups are an invaluable resource for people in early recovery. In addition to providing emotional support and guidance they are the best available forum for meeting nonusers and developing new friendships. They also sponsor social and recreational activities and provide opportunities for addicts in early recovery to learn new ways of managing leisure time from individuals who are further along in recovery.

In summary, recovery from chemical dependency requires a multitude of changes in beliefs, relationships, and lifestyle. Some of the required changes are very difficult to accomplish, and the need for them is not immediately apparent to many addicts. In early episodes of treatment, most addicts make some of the needed changes but not enough to avoid relapse over the long term. As a result, relapse rates among patients successfully completing treatment run as high as 80% in the year after treatment. With successive treatment episodes, however, one can hope to see a changing pattern in which periods of abstinence grow longer and periods of active drug use grow shorter. Perhaps it is best to view relapse as an indication that the patient has so far failed to make all of the necessary changes needed to support an enduring recovery. Instead of regarding relapse as an indication that the patient's case is hopeless, the patient's physician can encourage the patient to identify the reasons for the current relapse and to make changes that will help the patient avoid a recurrence.

Urine Testing

Urine testing to establish drug abuse seems a tempting and objective means of cutting through the problems of denial, subjective histories, and the often confusing and less than clear-cut signs and symptoms presented to arrive at a diagnosis. Certainly, in pursuit of other medical diagnoses, laboratory testing is an invaluable tool. In the general physician's office, resorting to testing for drug abuse can, however, prove problematic. Unlike organic illness when the patient is as eager to expeditiously arrive at a diagnoses as the physician, the patient already knows the answer as to whether he is abusing drugs or not. The question is whether he is willing to share that information with family or physician.

The testing requires *informed voluntary consent* of any person 18 years of age or older, except in truly emergent circumstances. Faced with this requirement it does not seem that laboratory testing will yield any more information than the patient is willing to concede voluntarily by history. Testing at the request of an employer or school authority, in particular, is fraught with questions of legality and ethics.

There are major problems of sensitivity and specificity in urine screening tests for drug abusers. False-negatives are frequent (because of deception in collection and insensitive testing); false-positives are reported (because of innocent confounding substances or doubts about the source of the specimen and the normal frequency of testing error); most significantly problems of interpretation of results are seen. Experimental and social and recreational use of illicit substances is so widely practiced that a positive test by no means establishes abuse or dependency.

The testing of minors under the age of 18, which theoretically can be authorized by parents and legal guardians regardless of the wishes of the patient, raises issues of patient trust, ethics, and legality if contested. The scenario of an angry parent hauling a recalcitrant child in for testing should be immediate grounds for referral and consultation to a trained professional, expert in parent-child interactions. Possible drug use can be explored there most productively in the context of the total family relationship without the referring physician appearing to have to take sides, and impeaching the trust required for other medical interventions.

In most instances, testing, like ongoing therapy, should probably be performed by the consulting specialist or treatment program.

THE GENERAL PHYSICIAN'S ROLE

Since the 1920s, with the exception of small numbers of psychiatrists and substance abuse specialists from other disciplines, physicians in the United States have been reluctant to become involved in problems of addiction and substance abuse. This is understandable since, beginning with the passage of the Harrison Narcotic Act in 1914, and until recently, the Federal Government waged an intense battle against the involvement of physicians and health care providers in the treatment of addiction. Over the period of 1920 to 1940, many physicians, nurses, and pharmacists who persisted in regarding narcotic addiction as a medical problem and in prescribing or dispensing narcotics in violation of the Harrison Act were prosecuted and imprisoned. This campaign led to avoidance of the problems of addiction by physicians and other health care providers.

In recent years, substance abuse has been recognized as the major cause of much of the morbidity seen in medical practice—usually a mix of physical, mental, and social consequences—and the responsibility of physicians to care for the patient with substance abuse has been emphasized (19). In light of the complexity of long-term rehabilitation of the patient with substance abuse, the major role of the physician is recognition of the problem, motivation of the patient to accept treatment, referral to a treatment program, ongoing care for the patient's other medical problems, and, importantly, continued motivation to remain in recovery from previous substance abuse.

Discovery of a substance abuse problem starts with a suspicion of the diagnosis if signs, symptoms, and elements of the history suggest the possibility, even in the most unlikely subjects. It is important to remember that people from all walks of life abuse drugs. The stereotype of the drug abuser is of a young, antisocial male of unkempt appearance who uses drugs for their euphoric effect. However, the abuse of illicit drugs such as marijuana and cocaine is now commonplace among middle and upper class Americans, and the misuse and abuse of prescription analgesics and anxiolytics by individuals who are in the mainstream of American society have been recognized for many years. Patients with chronic anxiety, insomnia, or pain are at high risk of abusing medications used to treat those conditions. In most instances, abuse develops not because the patient is seeking drug-induced euphoria or intoxication but because the tolerance that develops during continued use leads the patient to increase the dosage to inappropriate levels. Elderly patients are at particular risk because they are more likely to be given medications and more likely to be receiving multiple prescriptions. Changes in the pharmacokinetics of drugs secondary to the aging process also make the elderly more vulnerable to normally prescribed doses (31) (see also Chapter 6). Furthermore, they often have less recourse to nonpharmacological alternatives in coping with pain, psychological distress, or insomnia.

Behaviors that should arouse suspicion and concern are requests for repetitive prescriptions for tranquilizers, sedative hypnotics, narcotic analgesics, or stimulants such as Ritalin (e.g., a parent who requests this for a "hyperactive" child) without proper indication. A history of unexplained financial reverse, frequent absence from work or school, sudden deterioration in relationships, and requests for medical excuses might suggest abuse and dysfunction in daily living. Unexplained cellulitis, sclerotic veins, skin slough, superficial venous thrombosis, or subacute bacterial endocarditis should raise suspicion of narcotic or cocaine intravenous abuse. The medical side effects of cocaine overdose now seen as a consequence of "crack" use as described above must be kept in mind when unexpected vasospastic episodes, i.e., stroke, myocardial infarction, cardiac arrhythmia, or pulmonary edema, occur in otherwise healthy adolescents or young adults in whom a normal risk factor profile would seem to preclude such events.

Histories of assaultive behavior, unexplained syncope, abrupt onset of mood swings, irritability, anorexia, weight loss, and insomnia are symptoms that should also arouse concern. Slurred speech, multiple ecchymoses (e.g., bruises sustained secondary to sedative abuse and/or ethanolism), nasal mucosal erosion, acute onset of paranoid ideation, or dementia are other signs that might be noted during examination of a patient, leading to further exploration for possible drug abuse.

Interviewing techniques helpful in screening for alcoholism and in motivating the alcoholic to accept treatment are described in Chapter 21. These techniques, including the CAGE questions (Fig. 21.1), can be adapted for the interview of patients who abuse illicit substances.

PRESCRIBING OF CONTROLLED DRUGS

Office-based physicians prescribe large amounts of controlled drugs each year (Table 22.4). When prescribing these drugs, it is important to recognize that chronic pain, anxiety, and insomnia usually cannot be treated with a prescribed daily depressant drug without inducing tolerance and physiological addiction (see above). Intermittent use is required to avoid addiction. Other modalities, i.e., psychotherapy, relaxation techniques, biofeedback, physiotherapy, and exercise regimens, should therefore be utilized also, in order to increase the interval between doses and/or permit intermittent use of depressant drugs. Additional details on prescription of depressant-type drugs for medical conditions are found elsewhere (anxiety—Chapter 13; pain control—Chapter 19; insomnia—Chapter 85). Chapter 12 (somatization) describes somatoform pain disorder, a common condition for which patients frequently seek narcotic analgesics.

Narcotic Analgesics

It has been widely observed that the fear of causing addiction has led physicians to undermedicate in the management of acute pain (2). Conversely, there has been a tendency in managing patients with chronic pain to continue the use of narcotic analgesics when the development of tolerance has rendered them ineffective or even countertherapeutic. Patients who have been taking narcotic analgesics for long periods may experience little pain relief and may, in fact, confuse incipient withdrawal toward the end of a dosing interval with the onset of pain (23). An understanding of the induction of tolerance and of physiological addiction can assure more rational prescribing patterns.

Sedative-Hypnotic Drugs

The change in prescribing patterns, de-emphasizing barbiturates and other potent sedatives in favor of the benzodiazepine anxiolytics, has reduced the potential of serious overdosage. There does not appear to be a very great risk of abuse on the part of nonabusers who are prescribed benzodiazepines for anxiety or sleep disorders (35). Patients should be reminded, however, that benzodiazepines are potentiated by alcohol and other psychoactive substances and must be used with caution. Sedatives and tranquilizers should not be prescribed to individuals known to have had problems of substance abuse or dependence; the risk of abuse is extremely high and the use of these medications

Table 22.4.
Number, Percentage and Therapeutic Use of the 20 Most Prescribed Controlled Drugs, by Frequency of Mention and Control Schedule: United States, 1985[a]

Controlled Drugs Most Frequently Prescribed	Control Schedule	Number of Mentions in Thousands	Percentage	Therapeutic Use
All controlled drug mentions	...	51,877	100.0	...
Tylenol with codeine (acetaminophen, codeine)	III	5,081	9.8	Pain relief
Xanax (alprazolam)	IV	4,071	7.8	Anxiety relief
Valium (diazepam)	IV	3,672	7.1	Anxiety relief
Darvocet-N (Propoxyphene, acetaminophen)	IV	3,610	7.0	Pain relief
Ativan (lorazepam)	IV	2,306	4.4	Anxiety relief
Tranxene (clorazepate)	IV	1,698	3.3	Anxiety relief
Dalmane (flurazepam)	IV	1,478	2.8	Insomnia relief
Halcion (triazolam)	IV	1,271	2.5	Insomnia relief
Librium (chlordiazepoxide)	IV	1,215	2.3	Anxiety relief
Lomotil (diphenoxylate, atropine)	V	1,137	2.2	Antidiarrhea
Restoril (temazepam)	IV	1,103	2.1	Insomnia relief
Phenobarbital	IV	1,096	2.1	Anticonvulsant, insomnia relief
Phenergan expectorant with codeine (promethazine, codeine, phenylephrine)	V	1,062	2.0	Cough relief
Florinal (butalbital, caffeine, aspirin)	III	970	1.9	Migraine relief
Tussi-Organidin (codeine, iodinated glycerol)	V	965	1.9	Cough relief
Percocet-5 (oxycodone, acetaminophen)	II	722	1.5	Pain relief
Fastin (phentermine)	IV	737	1.4	Appetite suppressant
Percodan (oxycodone, aspirin)	II	672	1.3	Pain relief
Demerol (meperidine)	II	631	1.2	Pain relief
Hycomine (hydrocodone, phenylpropanolamine)	III	553	1.1	Cough relief

[a]From Koch H: Utilization of controlled drugs in office-based ambulatory care: National Ambulatory Medical Care Survey, 1985. From Vital and Health Statistics of the National Center for Health Statistics. Advance Data, No. 177, August 29, 1989.

may precipitate a relapse in individuals who have been in recovery for many years.

Addiction to benzodiazepines and the potential for major withdrawal symptoms may occur in as little as two months if doses substantially in excess of therapeutic levels are used. There have also been reports of major withdrawal symptoms (5, 25, 34) in patients taking therapeutic doses daily over long periods of time (six months or more). In the latter cases, the risk of withdrawal can be reduced by simply tapering the dosage. Although chronic use may create the risk of withdrawal symptoms, there is some evidence to suggest that patients may use benzodiazepines on a chronic basis without developing tolerance to the anxiolytic effects of the medication (35). This finding remains somewhat controversial, however.

Stimulants

Prescriptions have been identified as the primary source of methylphenidate (as Ritalin) in a recent study (24) of methylphenidate abusers. The drug was obtained, in every instance, through prescriptions—some forged on stolen prescription blanks but many obtained from primary care physicians ostensibly for the treatment of a child with attention-deficit hyperactivity disorder. The authors suggest that this disorder is often poorly understood by primary care physicians, resulting in diagnostic errors and inappropriate prescribing of methylphenidate.

General References

Brecher EM (ed): *Licit and Illicit Drugs*. Boston, Little, Brown, and Co, 1972.
  Although dated, still an excellent overview of the history of drug abuse in the United States.
Gawin FH, Ellinwood Jr. EH: Cocaine and other stimulants. *N Engl J Med* 318(18):1173, 1988.
  Review covering epidemiology, pathophysiology, treatment for the stimulants discussed in this chapter.
Marlatt AG, Gordon JR (eds): *Relapse Prevention*. New York, The Guilford Press, 1985.
  An excellent review of literature on relapse and relapse prevention.
McLellan AT, Luborsky L, O'Brien CP, et al: Is treatment for substance abuse effective? *JAMA* 247(10):1423, 1982.
  Evidence from multiple programs that current rehabilitation approaches are effective.
Robertson N (ed): *Getting Better: Inside Alcoholics Anonymous*. New York, Fawcett Crest, 1988.
  A description of how Alcoholics Anonymous works. Much of what is said about AA can be generalized to Narcotics Anonymous.
Schuckit MA (ed): *Drug and Alcohol Abuse*. New York, Plenum Medical Book Company, 1989.
  Covers the treatment of withdrawal, overdose, and toxic reactions to commonly abused drugs.

Specific References

1. American Psychiatric Association: *Diagnostic and Statistical Manual of Mental Disorders, III-Revised*. Washington, DC, American Psychiatric Association, 1987.
2. Angell M: The quality of mercy. *N Engl J Med* 306:98, 1982.
3. Ball JC, Nurco DN: Criminality during the life course of heroin addiction. In: *Problems of Drug Dependence 1983*. Rockville, MD, Department of Health and Human Services, 1984.
4. Burns RS, Lerner SE: Perspectives: acute phencyclidine intoxication. *Clin Toxicol* 9:477, 1976.
5. Dysken MW, Chan CH: Diazepam withdrawal psychosis: a case report. *Am J Psychiatry* 134:573, 1977.
6. Finnegan LP: Pulmonary problems encountered by the infant of the drug-dependent mother. *Clin Chest Med* 1:311, 1980.
7. Flemenbaum A, Boza R, Slater VL, Batkis M: Clonidine opiate withdrawal. *Resident and Staff Physician* 35:111, 1989.
8. Fried PA: Marijuana use by pregnant women: neurobehavioral effects in neonates. *Drug Alcohol Dependence* 6:415, 1980.
9. Gawin FH, Kleber HD, Byck R, et al: Desipramine facilitation of initial cocaine abstinence. *Arch Gen Psychiatry* 46:117, 1989.
10. Griffith JD, Cavanaugh JH, Oates JA: Psychosis induced by the administration of d-amphetamine to human volunteers. In: Efron DH (ed): *Psychotomimetic Drugs*. New York, Raven Press, 1970.
11. Harwood HS, Napolitano D, Kristiansen P, Collins J: *Economic Cost to Society of Alcoholism and Drug Abuse and Mental Illness: 1980*. Washington, DC, U.S. Government Printing Office, 1984.
12. Hayashida M, Alterman AI, McLellan T, et al: Comparative effectiveness and costs of inpatient and outpatient detoxification of patients with mild-to-moderate alcohol withdrawal syndrome. *N Engl J Med* 320:358, 1983.
13. Hingson R, Alpert JJ, Day N, et al: Effects of maternal drinking and marijuana use on fetal growth and development. *J Pediatr* 70:539, 1982.
14. Johnston LD, O'Malley PM, Bachman JG:*Drug use, drinking, and smoking: national survey results from high school, college, and young adults populations*. Rockville, MD, United States Department of Health and Human Services, Public Health Service, Alcohol, Drug Abuse, and Mental Health Administration, 1988.
15. Kolodny RC, Lessin PJ, Toro G, et al: Depression of plasma testosterone with acute marijuana administration. In: Braude MC, Szara S (eds): *Pharmacology of Marijuana*. New York, Raven Press, 1976.
16. Luisada PV: Phencyclidine. In: Lowinson JH, Ruiz P (eds): *Substance Abuse: Clinical Problems and Perspectives*. Baltimore, Williams & Wilkins, 1981.
17. Melges FT, Tinklenberg JR, Hollister LE, Gillespie HK: Temporal disintegration and depersonalization during marijuana intoxication. *Arch Gen Psychiatry* 23:204, 1970.
18. Miller WR, Hester RK: Inpatient alcoholism treatment: who benefits? *Amer Psychol* 41:794, 1986.
19. Moore RD, Bone LR, Geller G, et al: Prevalence, detection, and treatment of alcoholism in hospitalized patients. *JAMA* 261:403, 1989.
20. National Institute on Drug Abuse: *Statistical Series G, Trend Data Through January–June 1988*. Washington, DC, United States Government Printing Office, 1988.
21. Novotny M, Lee ML, Bartle KD: A possible chemical basis for the higher mutagenicity of marijuana smoke as compared to tobacco smoke. *Experientia* 32:280, 1976.
22. Nowlan R, Cohen S: Tolerance to marijuana: heart rate and subjective "high". *Clin Pharmacol Ther* 22:550, 1977.
23. O'Brien CP, Weisbrot MM: Behavioral and psychological components of pain management. In: Brown RM, Pinkert TM, Ludford JP (eds): *Contemporary Research in Pain and Analgesia, 1983*. Washington, DC, United States Government Printing Office, 1983.
24. Parran TV, Jasinski DR: Intravenous Ritalin abuse: prescription drug abuse. *Arch Intern Med* 1990.
25. Prevnick JS, Jasinski DR, Haertzen CA: Abrupt withdrawal from therapeutically administered diazepam. *Arch Gen Psychiatry* 35:995, 1978.
26. Rufener BL, Rachal JV, Cruze AM: *Management Effectiveness Measures for NIDA Drug Abuse Treatment Programs*. Vol. 1, Rockville, MD, United States Department of Health, Education and Welfare, 1984.
27. Schuckit MA (ed): *Drug and Alcohol Abuse*. New York, Plenum Medical Book Company, 1989.
28. Stanton MD, Todd TC: *The Family Therapy of Drug Abuse and Addiction*. New York, Guilford Press, 1982.
29. Talbott JA: Emergency management of marijuana psychosis. In: Bourne PC (ed): *Acute Drug Abuse Emergencies*. New York, Academic Press, 1976.

30. Tashkin DP, Sharpiro BJ, Lee YE, Harper CE: Subacute effects of heavy marijuana smoking on pulmonary function in healthy men. *N Engl J Med* 294:125, 1976.

31. Thompson TL, Moran ML, Nies AS: Psychotropic drug use in the elderly. *N Engl J Med* 308:134, 1983.

32. Van Kammen DP: The dopamine hypothesis of schizophrenia revisited. *Psychoneuroendocrinology* 4:37, 1979.

33. Wetli CV, Wright RK: Death caused by recreational cocaine use. *JAMA* 241:2519, 1979.

34. Winokur A, Rickels K, Greenblatt DJ, et al: Withdrawal reaction from long-term, low-dosage administration of diazepam. *Arch Gen Psychiatry* 35:101, 1980.

35. Woods JH, Katz JL, Winger G: Use and abuse of benzodiazepines: issues relevant to prescribing. *JAMA* 260:3476, 1988.

Allergy and
Infectious Diseases

CHAPTER 23

Allergy and Related Conditions

MARTIN D. VALENTINE, M.D.

Allergy is a state of increased immunological reactivity resulting from the synthesis of immunoglobulin E (IgE) antibodies after man is exposed to foreign immunogenic protein. Subsequent allergen-IgE antibody interaction causes release of chemical mediators that cause the symptoms of allergy. Although allergic symptoms are undesirable, the allergen-antibody-mediator sequence may have originally evolved as a host defense mechanism.

It is estimated that 17% of Americans suffer from acute and chronic conditions generally considered to be allergic in origin (see Table 23.1); approximately

Table 23.1.
Estimated Prevalence of Common Allergic Conditions in the General Population[a]

Condition	Prevalence (%)
Allergic rhinitis alone	7
Miscellaneous conditions (eczema, urticaria/ angioedema, food/drug/insect allergy)	6
Asthma	4

[a] From *Asthma and the Other Allergic Diseases*, NIAID Task Force Report. NIH publ no. 79-387, May 1979.

9% of all office visits to physicians are for one of these conditions (1). The majority of visits are for conditions that are known to be mediated by antibodies of the IgE class or for conditions that resemble IgE-mediated allergy. Because the symptoms in these patients result from the release or formation of a limited number of chemical mediators, effective pharmacological treatment may be similar whether or not allergy in the true sense is involved.

It is believed that the ability to synthesize relatively large amounts of IgE with specificity for certain antigens may be inherited. The risk of developing an allergy for a child if one parent is allergic is one chance in three, increasing to two in three if both parents are allergic.

This chapter is concerned with IgE-mediated allergy and similar conditions (with the exception of asthma, which is discussed in Chapter 55). Other immunopathological conditions that are not IgE mediated (drug-induced hepatitis, autoimmune hemolytic anemia, contact dermatitis) are discussed elsewhere in this book.

PATHOPHYSIOLOGY

Antibody

Acute allergic reactions are mediated by IgE antibodies. Never present in large amounts, IgE concentration in serum is greatest between puberty and young adulthood. As indicated in Fig. 23.1, IgE binds to surface receptors on tissue mast cells and blood basophils. The release of histamine and other chemical mediators from these cells is initiated by the bridging of a pair of IgE molecules on cell surface receptors by an antigen molecule of appropriate specificity.

Allergens

Allergens that have clinical relevance are usually proteins with a molecular weight between 10,000 and 40,000. Low molecular weight substances like penicillin can be allergenic if they can combine as haptens with host proteins.

Mediators

The release or formation of biologically significant chemical mediators is a prerequisite to the development of allergic symptoms. In general, mediators affect smooth muscle contractility and vascular tone and permeability. Histamine, released from mast cells and basophils, causes pruritus, flushing, nasal stuffiness, conjunctival injection, bronchoconstriction, uterine contraction, increased permeability of venules, and hypotension. Anaphylatoxin, a substance formed during complement activation, induces histamine release. Bradykinin and similar polypeptides with potent vasodepressor activity may be responsible in part for the shock of anaphylaxis. Members of the leukotriene family have been identified as the slow reacting substances of anaphylaxis (SRS-A), arachidonic acid metabolites with bronchoconstrictor and vasodilator

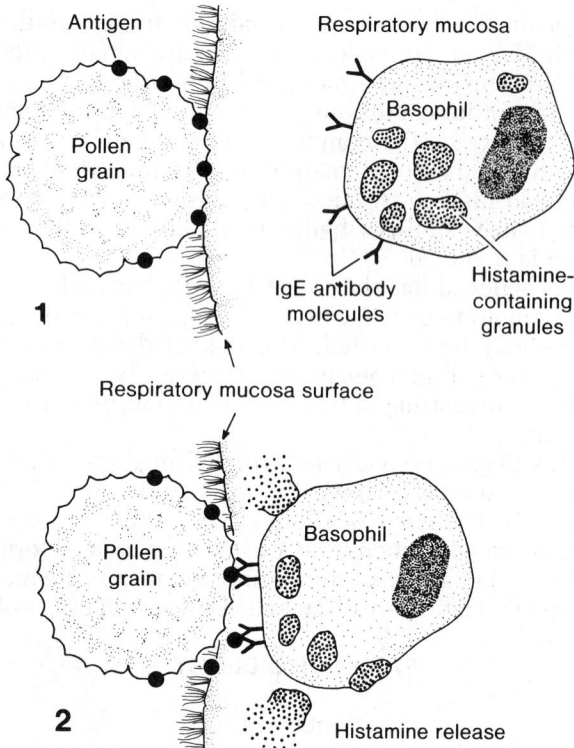

Figure 23.1. Steps in the IgE-mediated response of respiratory mucosa to pollen antigen. *Step 1,* pollen grains containing antigen reach nasal mucosa containing mast cells and basophils with IgE antibodies to antigen. *Step 2,* antigen bridges adjacent IgE molecules, initiating histamine release.

Table 23.2.
Site of Action of "Antiallergic" Drugs

Drug	Action Site	Mode of Action
Cromolyn	Mast cell	Inhibits mediator release
Adrenergics		
α	Postcapillary venules, arterioles	Vasoconstriction
β₂	Mast cell, basophil	Inhibits mediator release (increases cyclic AMP)
	Bronchial muscle	Relaxes bronchial muscle
Methylxanthines	Mast cell, basophil	Inhibits mediator release (increases cyclic AMP)
	Bronchial muscle	Relaxes bronchial muscle
Antihistamines	Histamine receptors	Competitive inhibition
Corticosteroids	Basophil	Inhibits histamine release

activities. These and prostaglandin D_2 (PGD_2) have been found in the nasal secretions of patients with allergic rhinitis challenged intranasally with allergen.

PHYSIOLOGICAL BASIS FOR TREATMENT

Pharmacological

Drugs can favorably influence the outcome of an allergic condition by acting at various sites in the sequence of the allergic reaction (see Table 23.2). Although no drug prevents antigen-antibody interaction, disodium cromoglycate (cromolyn, Intal) prevents mediator release after this interaction has occurred. The formation or release of some mediators is modulated by variation in cellular and tissue levels of cyclic adenosine monophosphate (cAMP), which acts as a "second messenger" for certain energy-requiring metabolic steps. Beta-adrenergic agonists appear to inhibit mediator release and relax bronchial smooth muscle by increasing cAMP. The methylxanthines, such as theophylline, produce similar effects by preventing enzymatic breakdown of cAMP. Conventional (H-1) antihistamines inhibit histamine effects by competing with histamine for H-1 receptor sites. The usefulness of antihistamines is limited by their inability to compete successfully with relatively high tissue concentrations of histamine adjacent to its cellular sites of

origin, and also because nearly all antihistamines are central nervous system (CNS) depressants. Corticosteroids have anti-inflammatory and topical vasoconstrictor effects and inhibit histamine release from basophils but not from mast cells.

Immunological

Immunization of humans with extracts of pollens has been shown to result in the appearance in serum of "blocking" antibody (immunoglobulin G), suppression of specific IgE production, and a reduction in the sensitivity of mediator-containing cells to antigen challenge.

ALLERGIC RHINITIS AND SIMILAR NASAL CONDITIONS

Epidemiology and Natural History

The prevalence of allergic rhinitis in the United States varies from region to region, depending upon the amount and type of airborne allergens present. Onset of symptoms is most common between the ages of 10 and 20. The prevalence is approximately 10% in the age group 16 to 64 and may be as high as 20 to 25% in young adults (1).

During the 10 years after onset, about one-third of young adults get better, and almost one-half get worse (1). Some have a permanent remission of symptoms; in the longitudinal study of the Tecumseh population, typical allergic rhinitis remitted entirely in 8% of subjects during a 4-year interval (2). The severity of symptoms tends to decrease in most subjects after the age of 40. Therefore, it is important to consider other causes for apparent allergic rhinitis that begins after age 40. Whereas it is generally thought that asthma develops in many people with allergic rhinitis, in fact only about 10% develop both conditions (1).

Differential Diagnosis of Noninfectious Rhinitis

Noninfectious rhinitis refers to those conditions in which there is no purulent discharge from the nose; purulent discharge is typical of nasal and paranasal infections such as viral upper respiratory infection and acute and chronic sinusitis (see Chapter 28). Occasionally grossly purulent secretions occur in noninfectious rhinitis; microscopically, large numbers of eosinophils are seen. Subjects with noninfectious rhinitis may belong to one of three categories: typical seasonal allergy, perennial (year-round) allergy, and miscellaneous nonallergic causes for nasal symptoms (see Table 23.3). The classification of an individual patient depends chiefly upon information obtained in the history. Some patients may have elements of more than one of these conditions.

History

Symptoms of noninfectious rhinitis. The symptoms that trouble patients most are obstruction of nasal airflow, dry mouth (from mouth breathing), nasal discharge (usually clear), itching of the nose and the soft palate, and sneezing. In addition, cough and discharge, itching, and puffiness of the eyes may occur, and there may be periodic loss of smell and taste. Occasionally acute sinusitis (see Chapter 28) or serous otitis media (see Chapter 96) may occur as complications. Although these symptoms are not incapacitating, they may interfere significantly with an individual's usual activities and may lead to minor mood disturbance (see Chapter 12) in susceptible individuals. As shown in Fig. 23.2, there is considerable day-to-day variability in the severity of symptoms in patients with typical seasonal allergy. Furthermore, the symptoms may vary substantially from year to year.

Allergic rhinitis. In nasal allergy due to seasonally prevalent allergens, symptoms will recur each year at approximately the same time. Pollen counts are higher in the morning, and outdoor symptoms are apt to be worse at that time. In nonseasonal allergy, symptoms may be induced by exposure to allergens (such as an-

Table 23.3.
Miscellaneous Nonallergic Causes of Noninfectious Rhinitis

RHINITIS MEDICAMENTOSA
  Antihypertensive medication:
    β-Blockers
    Guanethidine
    Methyldopa
    Reserpine
  Aspirin sensitivity (other NSAIDS also)
  Topical decongestant abuse (rebound rhinitis)
ENDOCRINE
  Hypothyroidism
  Pregnancy
  Oral contraceptives
ANATOMICAL
  Nasal polyp
  Deviated nasal septum
  Nasal tumor
VASOMOTOR RHINITIS

imal dander) any time during the day. In vasomotor rhinitis (see below), obstructive symptoms are prominent and, in contrast to allergic rhinitis, irritative symptoms (sneezing and itching) are usually not pronounced.

Environmental Exposures

In seasonal allergy ("hay fever"), the specific source of the patient's trouble can often be identified by a careful history taking. Skin testing and in vitro immunological tests can be utilized to provide definitive evidence; these measures are appropriate when the incrimination of a specific allergen, such as dog dander, will assist in environmental treatment or when immunotherapy is being considered (see below). In patients with year-round allergic symptoms, differentiation from nonallergic rhinitis may be more difficult. Indirect evidence for an allergic etiology for nasal symptoms includes other manifestations of atopy (see Table 23.1) and a history of typical allergic rhinitis in one or both parents. The absence of blood or nasal eosinophilia (<25% eosinophils in Giemsa-stained nasal smear) mitigates against an allergic etiology.

To a certain extent, even a limited knowledge of local flora will assist the physician in history taking. The general rule is that plants capable of causing nasal allergy produce copious quantities of pollen in inconspicuous, unattractive flowers that depend on wind for pollination. Therefore, pollen from attractive, pleasantly scented flowers, such as roses, is not allergenic, since these flowers depend on insects for pollination. So-called "rose fever" is usually due to allergy to grass pollen, which is prevalent during that period of time when roses are in bloom; the pleasant scent of the rose simply aggravates the patient already irritated by the allergic reaction initiated by grass pollen. In those sections of the country where the seasons are well demarcated, tree pollens are found in early spring, followed in late spring by grass pollen (Fig. 23.3). Late summer produces ragweed pollen in the east and midwest and cedar pollen in other sections. Mold spores are also prevalent in the fall, but snow during the winter usually prevents further dissemination of spores.

House dust, a mongrel material of uncertain heritage, can be more of a problem during the heating season in northern climes, since all heating systems, but particularly forced air systems, tend to disperse dust particles. Among important components of urban dust are the following: fragments of cockroach exoskeleton and excreta; the house dust mite, a nonparasitic organism that exists on human skin scales after they are shed; and aerosolized fragments of the saliva and skin of mammalian pets. Animal hair per se, comprising primarily insoluble collagen, is allergenic only by virtue of its burden of dander (shed skin). Symptoms due to animal allergens may be more pronounced in pollen seasons in pollen-sensitive patients and in circumstances when the patient and his pet spend more time indoors, e.g., during the winter months.

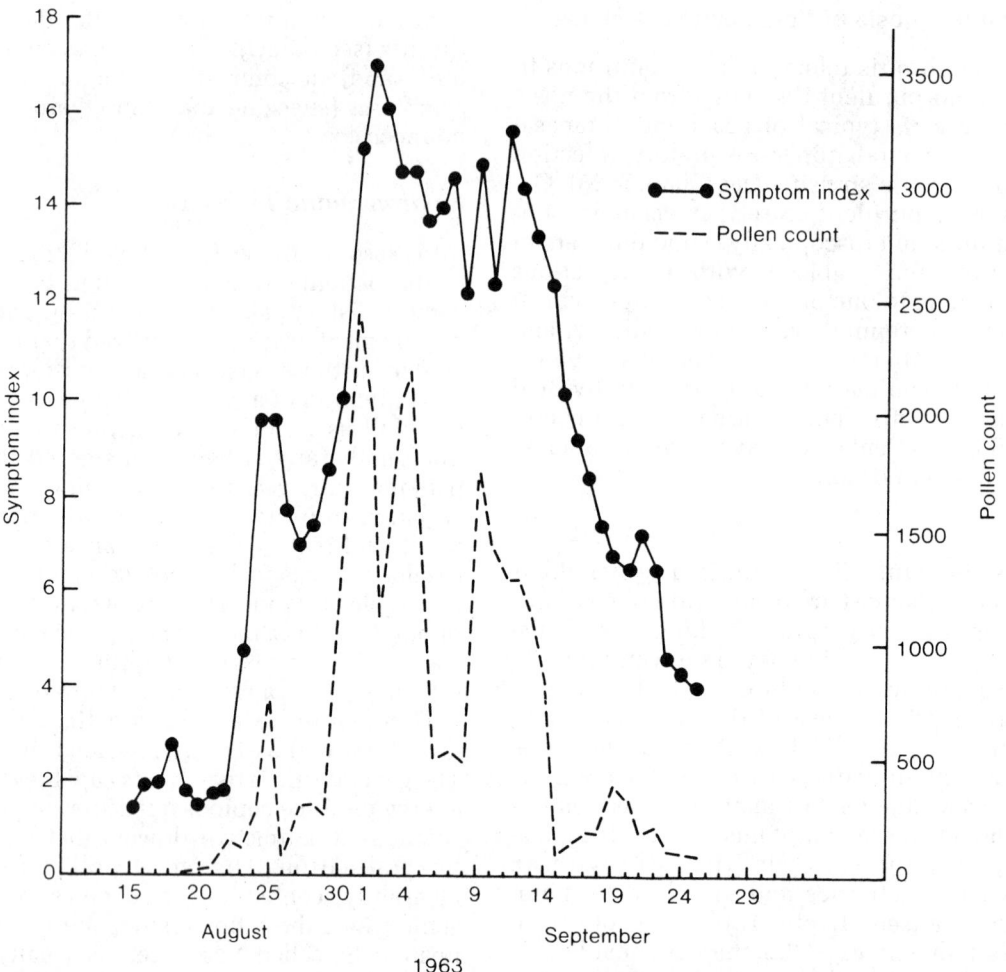

Figure 23.2 Day-to-day variation in self-reported symptoms during the pollen season, in an untreated patient with allergy to ragweed pollen.

Miscellaneous Causes of Nasal Symptoms

As noted above, there are a number of other conditions that may cause symptoms of chronic nasal obstruction. Most of these can be diagnosed or excluded on the basis of the history and physical examination.

Rhinitis medicamentosa refers to symptoms produced by the administration of several sympatholytic drugs (see Table 23.3) or of aspirin [and other nonsteroidal anti-inflammatory drugs (NSAIDs)], and to symptoms associated with abuse of topical decongestant sprays. Individuals susceptible to aspirin-induced symptoms develop profuse rhinorrhea, conjunctival suffusion, and severe bronchospasm minutes to hours after ingestion of aspirin or another NSAID; they may also develop an anaphylactoid reaction (see below). The aspirin rhinitis-bronchospasm reaction, if not fatal, is self-limited and probably does not exist in a subacute or chronic form. Abuse of topical decongestants refers to frequent use, which leads, after 1 to 2 weeks, to tolerance and then to rebound engorgement of submucosal blood vessels as the vasoconstrictive effect of the medication fades. The diagnosis of rhinitis medicamentosa can be made most efficiently by discontinuing the suspected drug. In the case of topical

decongestants, the persistence of symptoms after the drug has been stopped suggests allergic or vasomotor rhinitis.

The nasal symptoms, chiefly obstructive, that may accompany *pregnancy, oral contraceptive use, and hypothyroidism,* are most readily recognized because of their temporal association with one of these conditions and their remission when the inciting condition is no longer present.

The recognition of *anatomical causes* for chronic nasal symptoms depends chiefly upon the physical examination (see below). An uncommon problem such as a tumor may be suspected if there are new and progressive symptoms, especially in older individuals. Polyps or deviated nasal septum may produce chronic obstructive symptoms that are difficult to separate from perennial allergy or vasomotor rhinitis. In patients with the combination of aspirin-induced bronchospasm and nasal symptoms (see below, page 268), polyps are common. Whenever one of these anatomical causes is suspected, the patient should be referred to an otolaryngologist.

In over half of the patients with chronic, nonseasonal nasal symptoms, the clinical evidence will not support the diagnosis of perennial allergy or one of

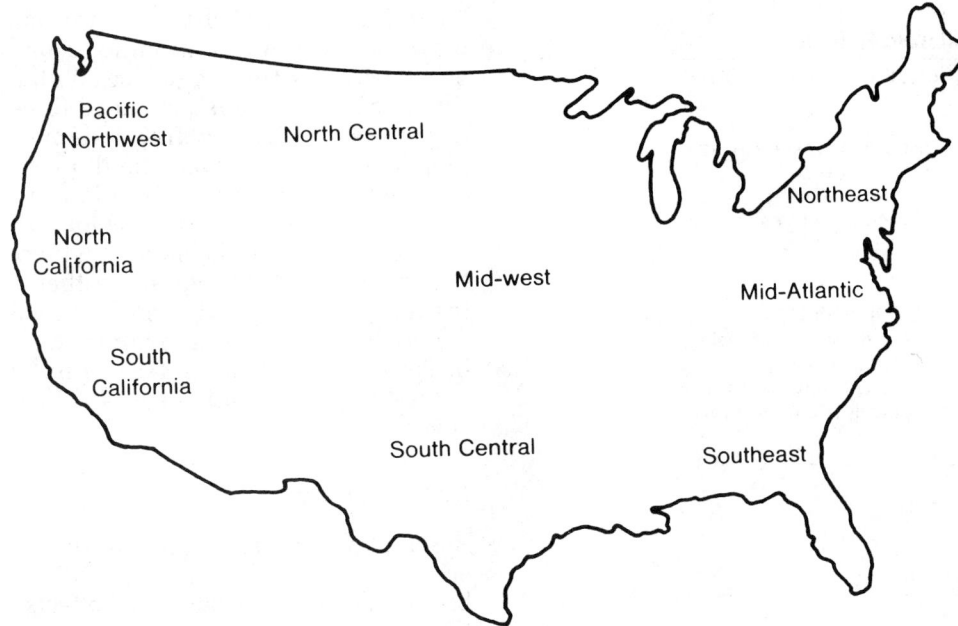

Figure 23.3. Seasonal occurrence of pollens, selected regions:

Pacific Northwest	*North Central*	*Northeast*
Trees: Apr–May	Trees: Mar–May	Trees: Apr–May
Grasses: Apr–Oct	Grasses: May–Aug	Grasses: May–July
Weeds: June–Sept	Ragweed: Aug–Sept	Ragweed: Mid-Aug–Sept
North California	Other weeds: June–Sept	Other weeds: May–Sept
Trees: Feb–May	*MidWest*	*Mid-Atlantic*
Grasses: Apr–Sept	Trees: Mar–May	Trees: Mar–May
Sagebrush: July–Oct	Grasses: May–July	Grasses: May–June
Other weeds: Mar–Oct	Ragweed: Aug–Oct	Ragweed: Mid-Aug–Sept
South California	Other weeds: July–Oct	Other weeds: May–Sept
Trees: Feb–June	*South Central*	*Southeast*
Grasses: Apr–Oct	Mountain Cedar: Dec–Feb	Trees: Feb–May
Sagebrush: July–Oct	Other trees: Feb–Apr	Grasses: May–Oct
Other weeds: June–Oct	Grasses: Feb–Aug	Ragweed: Aug–Oct
	Ragweed: Aug–Oct	Other weeds: May–Oct
	Other weeds: June–Oct	

the miscellaneous causes just described. These patients are thought to have the poorly understood condition known as *vasomotor rhinitis* (10). As is true of allergic rhinitis, symptoms of vasomotor rhinitis are also thought to be provoked by environmental stimuli. The pathophysiology of this condition seems to involve inappropriate heightened reactivity of the nasal membranes to a variety of stimuli. Typically the patient awakes in the morning without symptoms but develops nasal congestion, with or without discharge, and sneezing shortly after getting out of bed; moreover, exposure to a cold bedroom or bathroom, particularly to cold bathroom tiles, is frequently identified by the patient as an inciting stimulus. Pleasant scents (in perfumes or in household products such as soaps and detergents), cooking odors, products of combustion, and emotional stress may all precipitate symptoms.

Physical Examination

Allergic and vasomotor rhinitis, with or without conjunctivitis, usually presents with swollen nasal membranes and enlarged turbinates that are often de-

scribed as "pale" or "blue." The usual healthy pink appearance is absent. It may be difficult to differentiate edematous membranes or turbinates from nasal polyps; the appearance of pearly glistening globules, resembling peeled green grapes, in the nasal cavity suggests polyps and requires the opinion of an otolaryngologist. Polyps usually arise from stalks originating in the ethmoid sinuses. They are usually visible on speculum examination; at times, they may fill the nasal cavity.

Management of Allergic Rhinitis

Table 23.4 outlines the management of the patient with seasonal or perennial allergic rhinitis.

Avoidance and Environmental Control

The treatment of choice is removal of a suspected allergen from the environment. It this is not possible, other environmental manipulations may be carried out. Because the allergic patient is rarely affected by only one allergen, general control of the environment with respect to removal of as many irritants as possible is

Table 23.4.
Management of Allergic Rhinitis

AVOIDANCE AND ENVIRONMENTAL CONTROL
    Control dust
    Isolate furred animals
    Obtain machine-washable polyester pillows
    Seal mattress in zippered cover
    Close windows, use air-conditioning
    Adjust humidity to 30–40% in winter
    Filter air
        Electrostatic
        HEPA
PHARMACOLOGICAL TREATMENT
    Antihistamine alone (for discharge, sneezing, itchy eyes)
    Decongestant alone (for obstruction)
    Antihistamine-decongestant combination
    Topical disordium cromoglycate (cromolyn)
    Topical corticosteroid
    Systemic corticosteroid
IMMUNOTHERAPY
    Rational choice of allergens
        History
        Skin testing
    Adequate dosage essential

often beneficial, even though the irritants play only a contributory role. Thus, the allergic patient will benefit from avoiding smoke in the environment, although smoke is not usually regarded as an antigen-containing substance. Clearly animal-sensitive patients will benefit by removing the animal from the home or attempting to reduce direct contact with it. Improvement of symptoms thereafter is gradual owing to the tendency of microscopic fragments of dander to persist in the environment, even for several months; thorough vacuum cleaning and washing, if feasible, of all fabrics and surfaces are indicated. If it is questionable whether a pet is actually producing allergic symptoms, it is appropriate to send the patient, not the pet, for a short stay away from home. If the symptoms improve when the patient is away but come back when he is at home, this is presumptive evidence of the presence of allergen(s) in the home, usually from an animal or an unsuspected source of mold or related fungal growth, such as a contaminated humidifier reservoir or dust mites.

The quality of the air in closed environments can have a significant impact on symptoms. Regulation of the relative humidity is useful; it should be maintained between 35 and 40% during the winter. Humidifier reservoirs must be kept clean. Reduction of humidity in warm, humid summer weather may also be beneficial, although this is less critical unless the degree of humidity is such that it supports visible mold growth. Air conditioning and dehumidifiers are thus often necessary where the relative humidity is always high. Any heating, humidifying, or air-cooling device that depends upon the delivery of forced air must have an effective air filter. Two types of air filtration devices may be used. One depends on electrostatic precipitation of particulate matter as it is drawn through a charged field by a blower. The second type depends on the trapping of particulate matter in a specially treated cellulose filter (the so-called HEPA

type). Maintenance of the electrostatic filtration devices merely requires cleaning (usually by washing) of the particle-trapping device. With a HEPA type of filter, accessory filters may need to be replaced on a regular basis. These prefilters are necessary for trapping larger particles that would otherwise impair the efficiency of the unit. In addition to air-filtering devices, the following are desirable: floors that are bare or carpeted with washable rugs; windows that are curtained with washable curtains rather than dust-catching venetian blinds; bedrooms furnished with washable materials and containing a minimum of dust-catching books and bric-a-brac; and use of pillows of washable polyester and mattresses encased in zippered plastic covers.

Drug Therapy

Symptomatic drug treatment of allergic rhinitis is empiric and usually involves striking a satisfactory balance between the beneficial effects of the drug and the undesirable side effects. The goal of therapy is reduction of symptoms to a level that enables the patient to function normally, since complete elimination of symptoms is usually not possible (see Fig. 23.4). Antihistamines are the mainstays of empiric therapy. Sympathomimetic decongestants, cromolyn, topical or systemic corticosteroids, and topical ophthalmic agents may be added to antihistamines depending upon the individual patient's needs.

Antihistamines. In many patients, an antihistamine alone may provide adequate relief most of the time. This is particularly true when irritative symptoms (sneezing, itching, discharge) are the major problems. Many antihistamines are available. The older agents produce some sedation and drying of the mucous membranes, and their efficacy in suppressing nasal symptoms generally parallels the degree of these two side effects. As indicated in Table 23.5, there are several chemical classes of antihistamines from which to choose in the treatment of allergic rhinitis. Individual patients may respond more readily to a given class, but within classes, differences in efficacy tend to be slight. Once an effective class has been found for a patient, preference within the class will be determined by relative absence of side effects. There is an enormous cost differential between generic and brand name antihistamines, so that once a patient has found an effective product, he should be encouraged to try an equivalent generic. Subtle manufacturing differences between clinically equivalent products may make a particular one more suitable for a given patient. A useful procedure is to choose one drug from each class as a starting point, beginning with the drug names first in each class in Table 23.5. At first it is better to avoid "sustained-release" preparations; they may be used later as a convenience once the right drug is found.

As shown in Table 23.5, antihistamines are available in a variety of strengths and forms; some are available without prescription. All have their onset of action in 10 to 30 minutes. Sustained-released preparations may

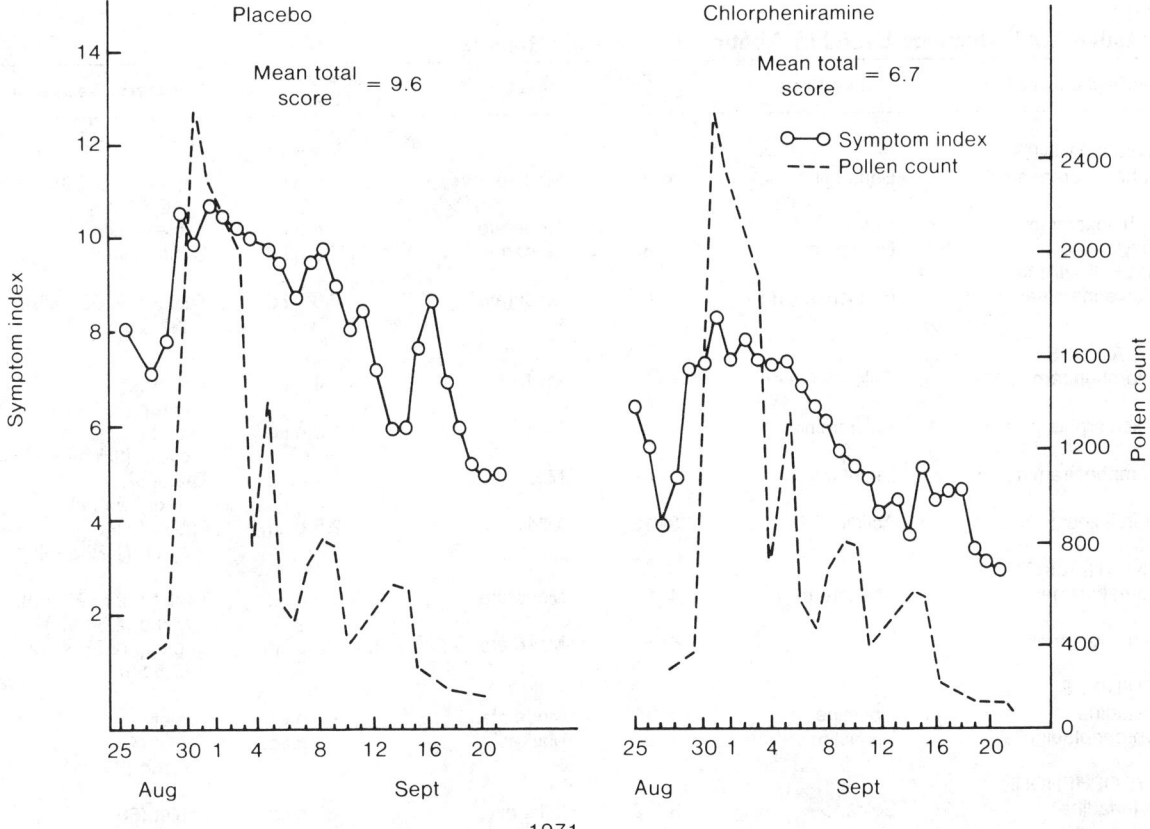

Figure 23.4. Symptom level in patients with allergic rhinitis taking antihistamines. These two sets of data compare the response of carefully matched groups of ragweed-allergic patients either to placebo or to an antihistamine (chlorpheniramine) during the ragweed pollen season. It can be seen that the antihistamine reduces but does not eliminate symptoms (the symptoms recorded by patients were: sneezing, stuffy nose, running nose, red itchy eyes, and cough). (Adapted from Valentine MD, Norman PS, Lichtenstein LM: Evaluation of an antihistamine in ragweed hay fever. In McMahon FG (ed): *Evaluation of Gastrointestinal, Pulmonary, Anti-Inflammatory, and Immunological Agents.* Mount Kisco, NY, Futura, 1974.)

need to be taken every 8 hours for continuous effect. Antihistamines appear to be more effective if dosing is begun in anticipation of symptoms, i.e., before exposure to animals, or before the beginning of the grass or ragweed pollen season.

To obviate sedation some patients omit daytime doses and choose to utilize a sustained-release preparation at bedtime, to help assure a good night's sleep and also to control adequately the irritative symptoms that are so common upon awakening in the morning. Terfenadine (Seldane) and astemizole (Hismanal), recently approved, have little or no sedative or anticholinergic effects. Because of its long half-life, astemizole is used once daily. Loratidine, also nonsedating, awaits approval.

Sympathomimetic decongestants may add significantly to the beneficial effects of antihistamines. They may be particularly effective in patients who have pronounced obstructive symptoms due to nasal mucosal edema; presumably decongestants work by vasoconstriction, which decreases the blood flow to nasal mucosa. A second beneficial property of these agents is that they have a stimulatory effect on the central nervous system, which may counteract antihistamine-induced sedation. Table 23.6 summarizes practical

information about a number of commonly prescribed antihistamine-decongestant combinations (all require written prescription). Extendryl and Histaspan-D incorporate the anticholinergic agent methscopolamine for additional drying effects.

Sympathomimetic decongestants are also available alone in oral preparations and in topical drops and sprays. These forms may be useful in patients with allergic rhinitis whose most troublesome symptom is nasal obstruction or in those who cannot tolerate antihistamines. Decongestant treatment without antihistamine is the treatment of choice in patients with acute sinusitis and serous otitis media, two conditions that may complicate any allergic or nonallergic process producing congestion of the nasal mucosa. Details regarding available decongestant preparations are found in the discussion of serous otitis, Chapter 96.

In therapeutic doses, sympathomimetic decongestants may cause tachycardia and blood pressure elevation (6). Therefore, it is important to determine the individual patient's blood pressure response before prescribing a sympathomimetic for prolonged use; this can be done within 1 to 3 hours of administration of the drug. Patients with allergic rhinitis should be strongly warned against the routine use of nasal de-

Table 23.5.
Representative Antihistamines Useful in Treatment of Allergic Rhinitis

Class and Generic Name	Trade Name	Duration of Action	Sedation	Recommended Adult Dose	Available Preparations
		hr		mg	mg
ETHANOLAMINES					
Diphenhydramine[a,c]	Benadryl	4–6	Marked	25–50 q.i.d.	Capsule (25, 50), elixir (12.5/5 ml)
Carbinoxamine[b]	Clistin	3–4	Moderate	4 q.i.d.	Tablet, elixir
Doxylamine	Decapryn	4–6	Moderate	12.5–25 q.i.d.	Tablet, syrup
ETHYLENEDIAMINES					
Tripelennamine[a,b]	Pyribenzamine	4–6	Moderate	50 q.i.d.	Tablet (25, 50), elixir (37.5/5 ml)
ALKYLAMINES					
Chlorpheniramine[a,b,c,]	Chlor-Trimeton	4–6	Mild	4 q.i.d.	Tablet (4), syrup (2/5 ml)
Dexchlorpheniramine[b]	Polaramine	4–6	Mild	2 q.i.d.	Tablet (2), syrup (2/5 ml)
Brompheniramine[a,b,c]	Dimetane	4–6	Mild	4 q.i.d.	Tablet (4), elixir (2/5 ml)
Triprolidine[a,c]	Actidil	8–12	Mild	2.5 b.i.d.	Tablet (2.5), syrup (1.25/5 ml)
PHENOTHIAZINES					
Promethazine[a]	Phenergan	4–6	Moderate	12.5–25 q.i.d.	Tablet (12.5, 25, 50), syrup (2.5/5 ml)
Trimeprazine[a,b]	Temaril	4–6	Moderate	2.5–7.5 q.i.d.	Capsule (2.5), syrup (2.5/5 ml)
PIPERIDINES					
Azatadine	Optimine	8–12	Moderate	1–2 b.i.d.	Tablet
Cyproheptadine[d]	Periactin	4–6	Marked	4 q.i.d.	Tablet (4), syrup (2/5 ml)
BUTYROPHENONE					
Terfenadine	Seldane	8–12	Little or none	60 b.i.d.	Tablet (60)
MISCELLANEOUS					
Loratidine	Claritin	12–24	Little or none	10 daily	Tablet (10)
Astemizole	Hismanal	up to several weeks	Little or none	10 daily on empty stomach	Tablet (10)
PIPERAZINE					
Hydroxyzine[a,d]	Atarax, Vistaril	6–12	Moderate	10–25 b.i.d., t.i.d.	Capsule (10, 25, 50, 100), suspension (10/5 ml)

[a] Generic available.
[b] Sustained-release preparation available.
[c] Over-the-counter drug.
[d] More useful in urticaria and pruritus.

congestant sprays or drops, as this may lead to rhinitis medicamentosa (see above). Perhaps the best advice for the patient who cannot part with a decongestant spray is that he utilize it only at times when symptom relief is crucial—for example, at bedtime if nasal obstruction makes it difficult to get to sleep (and when the stimulatory effects of oral sympathomimetic decongestants may interfere with sleeping).

For patients whose nasal symptoms are not controlled adequately by antihistamines or decongestants, *topical corticosteroids* may provide excellent relief, at times enabling an almost incapacitated individual to return to normal function. Steroids have a major impact upon obstructive nasal symptoms; simultaneous antihistamine use may, however, be needed to suppress irritative symptoms. Beclomethasone and flunisolide are steroid derivatives with negligible systemic activity that have been extensively tested and shown to be effective when administered intranasally as so-

lutions (Vancenase AQ, Beconase AQ, and Nasalide) or as micronized powder aerosols (Vancenase and Beconase). One or two sprays of any of these agents used on a regular basis twice daily to each nostril is usually effective in relieving the symptoms within 7 to 14 days. With all of these agents the patient should be instructed to sniff more or less synchronously with the administration of the spray so that distribution of the agent within the nasal cavity will be facilitated. The aqueous preparations of beclomethasone are tolerated somewhat better than the other preparations in many patients. Rare side effects include localized Candida infection, epistaxis, mucosal ulceration, and nasal septal perforation. Patients must be told to expect gradual improvement, over the course of days, in contrast to the immediate response to be expected from a topical vasoconstrictor. Dexamethasone as a nasal aerosol has also been available for some time but is rarely indicated because of the increased risk of ad-

Table 23.6.
Representative Antihistamine-Sympathomimetic Combinations Useful in Treating Allergic Rhinitis

Trade Name	Ingredients	Mg. per Tablet or Capsule	Recommended Adult Dosage	Available Preparations[a]
Pyribenzamine with ephedrine	Tripelennamine	25	1 or 2 tablets q.i.d.	Tablet
	Ephedrine	12		
Co-Pyronil	Thenylpyramine	25	1 capsule t.i.d.	Capsule
	Pyrrobutanine	15		Suspension
	Cyclopentamine	12.5		
Omade	Chlorpheniramine	12	1 Spansule b.i.d.	Timed-release spansule
	Phenylpropanolamine	75		
Naldecon[a]	Chlorpheniramine	5	1 tablet t.i.d.	Sustained-action tablet
	Phenyltoloxamine	15		Syrup
	Phenylpropanolamine	40		
	Phenylephrine	10		
Extendryl or Histaspan-D	Chlorpheniramine	8	1 capsule b.i.d.	Timed-action capsule
	Phenylephrine	20		Syrup
	Methscopolamine	2.5		
Isoclor[a,b]	Chlorpheniramine	4	1 tablet q.i.d.	Tablets
	d-Isoephedrine	25		Syrup
				Sustained-release capsule
Dimetapp[a,b]	Brompheniramine	12	1 Extentab b.i.d.	Extended-release tablet
	Phenylpropanolamine	75		Elixir
Actifed[a,b]	Triprolidine	2.5	1 tablet t.i.d.	Tablet
	d-Isoephedrine	60		Syrup
Disophrol	Dexbrompheniramine	6	1 tablet b.i.d.	Chronotab
Drixoral[b]	d-Isoephedrine	120		Extended-release sustained-action tablet
Rondec	Carbinoxamine	2.5	1 tablet q.i.d.	Tablet, syrup
	d-Isoephedrine	60		
Trinalin	Azatadine	1	1 tablet b.i.d.	Extended-action tablet
	d-Isoephedrine	120		

[a] Generic available
[b] Over-the-counter drug.

renal gland suppression that is present with this preparation, when used in maximal dosage. Both flunisolide and beclomethasone can be used safely for prolonged periods. All nasal aerosols occasionally cause transient, mild, local irritation.

Patients who are using intranasal corticosteroids occasionally report symptoms that suggest a new, infectious rhinitis. Although the manufacturers have advised patients to notify their physician in this instance, there is no evidence for a need to discontinue the topical spray. Topical steroids may also be continued while sinusitis is being treated with an appropriate antibiotic.

Systemic corticosteroids are occasionally justified in treating seasonal allergy. For example, in a patient who usually requires topical steroids for obstructive symptoms, a 3- or 4-day course of prednisone (20 mg/day) may be needed to relieve nasal obstruction sufficiently so that the aerosol can effectively reach the nasal mucosa. Only rarely should a longer course of steroids (2 to 3 weeks) be utilized to treat allergic rhinitis. The prednisone can usually be tapered rapidly during the last few days of treatment (see further discussion of steroid use in Chapter 74). Although parenteral, "depot" steroid injections are convenient, they are generally contraindicated because they entail greater risk of adrenal suppression.

A nasal aerosol is available of *cromolyn sodium* (Nasalcrom), an agent that inhibits mediator release in the mast cells of the nasal mucosa (5). Aerosolized crom-

olyn must be administered approximately every 4 hours by metered dose to each nostril in order to prevent symptoms. Mild side effects (chiefly nasal irritation) are common, but they are transient and well tolerated. The disadvantages of this drug are high cost to the patient and the frequent dose schedule. However, for selected patients with unequivocal seasonal allergic symptoms, a trial of cromolyn may be worthwhile because of the absence of antihistamine sedation. In animal-sensitive patients, a trial of cromolyn before exposure is worthwhile; if effective, the drug should be continued every four hours during the period of exposure.

Another type of agent, the *topical anticholinergic,* ipratropium bromide nasal spray (Atrovent), is in clinical trials for use, twice a day, in patients with nonallergic rhinorrhea.

Management of Eye Symptoms

Frequently the nasal symptoms of allergic rhinitis are controlled by one of the above drugs, but the eye symptoms persist. In this situation any of the number of topical preparations containing alpha-adrenergic agents such as Vasocon, Prefrin, Albalon, and Opcon may be effective; two drops should be instilled three to four times daily. The latter two prepartions include "artificial tears" in their formulas. Of these agents, Prefrin can be obtained without prescription. Several are available in the "A" form, denoting inclusion of antihistamine. For the patient who is seriously impaired by conjunctival symptoms despite topical vasoconstrictors, either of two relatively weak topical steroids (HMS Liquifilm or FML Liquifilm) may be tried for brief periods; however, an ophthalmologist should be consulted, at least by telephone, first. Prolonged use of ophthalmic steroids should be avoided unless the patient has periodic slit-lamp examinations by an ophthalmologist, because of the danger of herpetic keratitis. Ophthalmic cromolyn (available as Opticrom) is as effective as corticosteroid preparations for some patients. The dose is one drop in each eye every four hours. Any contact lens wearer should consult an ophthalmologist before using any eye drop, because of the special risks of injury to the cornea by contacts. One complication of contact use, giant papillary conjunctivitis, is often treated with Opticrom.

Referral to an Allergist

If the patient fails to respond to the measures outlined above, he should be referred to an allergist for evaluation, to confirm the diagnosis of allergic rhinitis or to disclose any other cause for nasal symptoms, and to determine whether the patient may be a candidate for immunotherapy.

The *immunological tests* done by an allergist are primarily scratch or intracutaneous tests using solutions of suspected offending allergens. These skin tests are more sensitive, although no more specific, than the in vitro RAST (RadioAllergoSorbent Test) in which the patient's serum level of allergen-specific IgE antibody is measured. Moreover, the skin test is far less expensive than the RAST; therefore, the latter should be reserved for instances when either the skin is not suitable for testing (such as in patients with dermatographism or generalized atopic dermatitis) or when skin reactivity seems to be equivocal when compared with negative and positive controls.

Immunotherapy with sufficient doses of appropriate allergens has been shown to reduce symptoms in 95% of patients with seasonal allergic rhinitis due to ragweed or grass pollens (see Fig. 23.5): however, nearly one-third of patients seem to benefit from a placebo (7). Although there are few controlled studies of animal dander immunotherapy, some allergists try this mode of therapy in selected animal-hypersensitive patients when manipulation of the environment and pharmacological control are ineffective. House dust mites (Dermatophagoides species), commensal occupants of human habitats, are important sources of airborne allergen in some areas. Control is difficult and no practical miticide is available at present. Mite extract is also available for diagnosis and immunotherapy.

Because allergic rhinitis is often present in multiple family members, parents may question their physicians about the value of immunotherapy for their affected children. Immunotherapy is rarely indicated in early childhood. Although it may yield apparently good results in the prepubertal child, it should be borne in mind that puberty may also be accompanied by a diminution in symptoms of allergic rhinitis. Therefore, immunotherapy is indicated chiefly in the postpubertal patient.

Immunotherapy is often arbitrarily recommended for a period of 2 to 3 years. Initially, the patient is given frequent injections of the selected allergen extract in progressively higher doses until a maintenance dose is achieved, after which booster injections are given approximately once or twice per month for the duration of immunotherapy. After 2 or 3 years, a decision must be made whether to continue treatment or to stop it and watch for recurrence of symptoms. Some patients who respond well to several years of immunotherapy may continue to enjoy reduced symptoms even after immunotherapy is stopped. Allergen preparations modified with formalin ("allergoid") or glutaraldehyde are awaiting United States Food and Drug Administration (FDA) approval; this sort of chemical modification allows less frequent dosing and a somewhat reduced risk of systemic reactions to therapy.

The patient's general physician may at times be asked to administer maintenance subcutaneous allergen injections. There are three types of untoward reactions that may occur after allergen injections:

1. An "immediate" local reaction, characterized by formation of a wheal and flare at the site within 15 to 30 minutes of injection. An eruption that is as large as a half dollar is an indication not to increase the dosage of allergen in the subsequent injection. This type of reaction may result from inadvertent administration of the dose too superficially.
2. A delayed local reaction, which begins 2 to 4 hours after the injection of allergen and reaches a peak at 18 to 24 hours. This is most commonly seen when dust and mold spore antigens are included in the extract, and may be due to nonallergens present in the raw material used to make the extract. This type of delayed, large local skin reaction may prevent an increase in the dose of allergen because of local discomfort.
3. Generalized or constitutional reaction. This may be immediate or delayed; the management of generalized urticaria and anaphylaxis is described below.

Management of Rhinitis Due to Topical Decongestant Abuse

Rhinitis medicamentosa of the rebound variety should be suspected whenever there is a history of worsening symptoms of nasal obstruction in association with more than a week of regular (i.e., several times daily) use of a topical decongestant. Management consists of explaining the probable reason for the problem to the patient, discontinuing the topical decongestant, and prescribing a 1- to 2-week course of corticosteroid in aerosol form (see above), which will relieve the symp-

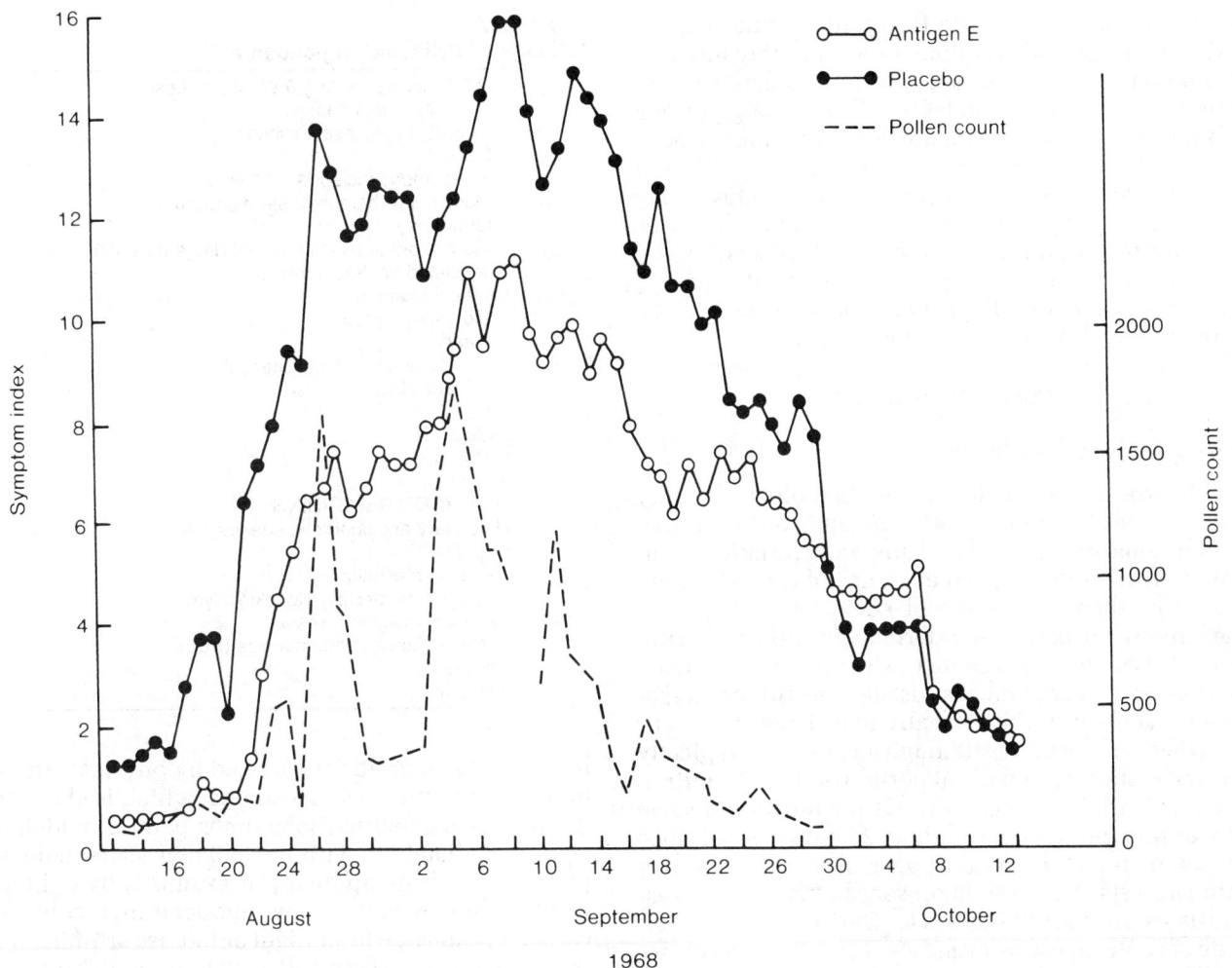

Figure 23.5. Daily symptom scores of patients immunized with a ragweed antigen (Antigen E), compared with matched patients "immunized" with a placebo. (From Lichtenstein LM, Norman PS, Winkenwerder WL: A single year of immunotherapy for ragweed hay fever: immunologic and clinical studies. *Ann Intern Med* 75:663, 1971.)

toms due to rhinitis medicamentosa. In very severe cases, several days of systemic corticosteroids should precede topical steroid use. The patient usually has an underlying chronic nasal condition, and appropriate management will be needed when that condition has been identified.

Management of Intranasal Polyps

Polyps (see description above) may cause symptoms of obstruction to nasal airflow or they may be asymptomatic. They may be seen in association with asthma precipitated by aspirin (see below), and there is often associated chronic or acute sinusitis. They are also often seen in patients with cystic fibrosis. The treatment of symptomatic polyps consists of topical corticosteroids or polypectomy. When polyps are suspected, the patient should be referred to an otolaryngologist to confirm the diagnosis and to plan appropriate management.

Management of Vasomotor Rhinitis (2)

This nonallergic condition (10) shows little or no response to antihistamines, but symptoms may diminish when the patient is treated with oral decongestants alone (see Chapter 96 for details regarding these preparations). Symptoms may respond to intranasal corticosteroids (see above), which can be prescribed for use during troublesome exacerbations. The most important consideration in management for patients with vasomotor rhinitis is ensuring that they understand the chronicity of their condition, the limited symptomatic treatment available, and the importance of avoiding irritants in his environment and of not abusing topical decongestants.

GENERALIZED ALLERGIC AND ALLERGIC-LIKE REACTIONS

There are two categories of generalized reactions that may be seen in ambulatory settings: urticaria/angioedema (usually not life threatening) and anaphylaxis/anaphylactoid reactions (often life threatening). The underlying mechanisms for these generalized reactions are either classic IgE-mediated allergy or one of a number of nonallergic processes in which mediator release and clinical symptoms resemble those in IgE-mediated allergy. These generalized reactions may be precipitated by a wide variety of foreign substances and physical stimuli. At the end of this section, the following five specific causes of generalized reactions are discussed: penicillin, Hymenoptera venom, foods, iodinated contrast materials, and aspirin.

Urticaria/Angioedema

Definition and Incidence

Urticaria and angioedema differ pathologically only with respect to the microscopic depth of the lesion, which consists primarily of the extravascular accumulation of fluid, with no evidence of inflammation. Raised erythematous areas of edema involving only the superficial part of the dermis are urticarial eruptions (hives), whereas edema extending into the deep dermis and subcutaneous tissue constitutes angioedema. These eruptions usually itch. They may occur anywhere on the body, although angioedema typically occurs on the face and distal portion of the extremities. True urticarial eruptions do not remain in the same area of skin for much longer than 24 hours; persistence of lesions for 72 hours or longer in the same area of skin suggests the possible presence of cutaneous vasculitis as an underlying cause. During a typical episode of acute urticaria, evanescent eruptions may arise in different areas for 1 or more days. Urticaria ceases being acute and becomes chronic after eruptions have continued to appear, recur, or persist for 6 weeks or longer.

Urticaria is particularly common in prepubertal females but occurs at some time in approximately one-fifth of the population.

Etiology and Evaluation

A number of etiologies are recognized for urticaria/angioedema (Table 23.7). Both urticaria and angioedema may occur alone or together in each of the conditions listed in the table; the exception to this rule is the rare syndrome hereditary angioedema in which angioedema alone occurs.

The definite (or most likely) cause of *acute urticaria* can often be determined by a history of an exposure preceding the onset of symptoms. The onset of acute urticaria/angioedema may occur from minutes to hours after the exposure to an inciting substance. (Additional discussion of reactions to selected common substances is found in a later section of this chapter.) There are a number of urticaria/angioedema states initiated by physical stimuli. The most common is dermatographism, a linear wheal with flare that occurs at the site of brisk stroking with a firm object; the eruption fades within 30 minutes. There are several

Table 23.7.
Etiology of Urticaria/Angioedema

ACUTE (Episode Lasting 6 Weeks or Less)
Allergy (IgE-mediated):
Foods, drugs, insect stings
Infection:
Virus (mononucleosis, hepatitis)
Bacterial (β-hemolytic streptococcus)
Idiosyncrasy:
Nonsteroid anti-inflammatory drugs (NSAID)
Iodinated contrast material
Physical agents:
Dermatographism
Heat:
Generalized ("cholinergic")
Localized
Cold
Solar
Pressure
Idiopathic
CHRONIC OR RECURRING
Hereditary angioneurotic edema (HAE)
Hepatitis
Parasitic infestation
Neoplasm (especially Hodgkin's lymphoma)
Collagen-vascular disease:
Systemic lupus erythematosus (SLE)
Polyarteritis
Idiopathic

less common conditions induced by physical stimuli: (a) pressure urticaria/angioedema, which is characterized by local swelling, sometimes painful, which occurs immediately or within 4 to 6 hours after constant pressure has been applied (for example, by tight garments); (b) exposure to low temperatures (cold urticaria); (c) exposure to sunlight or intense artificial light (solar urticaria); (d) so-called "cholinergic" urticaria (because it can be reproduced locally in affected subjects by the injection of cholinergic agents), which develops after an increase in core body temperature due to a hot bath, exercise, fever, etc.: and (e) urticaria developing shortly after the local application of heat (heat urticaria).

It is particularly important to consider the rare but potentially life-threatening condition, *hereditary angioedema* (HAE), in any patient with isolated episodes of angioedema, particularly if there is a history of other family members with angioedema. Onset of symptoms usually occurs before age 20. Typically, the patient does not describe itching. Local trauma may precipitate peripheral attacks. Visceral attacks may occur spontaneously, characterized by abdominal pain. Life-threatening oral or laryngeal edema may occur during any attack. HAE is a nonimmunological problem, due to deficiency of the inhibitor of the first component of complement. The diagnosis is suggested by a low level of serum C4 and a normal C3 level. Patients with these findings should be referred to an allergist for definitive evaluation, which involves a functional assay for the inhibitor. An acquired form of C1 inhibitor deficiency has recently been recognized in which the pathophysiology involves consumption of the inhibitor through chronic activation of C1 by circulating immune complexes, the entire syndrome being secondary to lymphoproliferative or other malignant disorders. In both the inherited and the acquired forms, the diagnosis must be confirmed immunologically. Specific therapy with impeded androgens, such as danazol or stanozolol, is indicated in these syndromes but not in other forms of angioedema. Another cause of low values of C4 in urticaria is cutaneous vasculitis; this is usually accompanied by an elevated erythrocyte sedimentation rate.

It is often difficult to determine the etiology for *chronic urticaria*. The diagnostic workup may include complete blood counts with differential, sedimentation rate, urinalysis, stool examination for ova and parasites, and tests for hepatitis antigen (see Chapter 43), cytomegalovirus antibody, heterophile antibody (Mono-spot test, see Chapter 53), cold agglutins, cryoglobulins, C3, C4, or antinuclear antibody. Despite screening tests for underlying conditions, in over 70% of patients with chronic urticaria no etiology is found (so-called idiopathic urticaria).

Management

Many patients with minor episodes of urticaria/angioedema simply tolerate it or learn by trial and error how to eliminate the causative factor(s). Others will seek help from their physician.

The intense itching of acute urticaria usually responds promptly to the subcutaneous administration of epinephrine (for adults: 0.2 to 0.5 ml of a 1:1000 solution of aqueous epinephrine, repeated after 15 minutes if necessary). An antihistamine such as diphenhydramine (50 mg) or chlorpheniramine (4 mg) should be given orally at the same time. If the parenteral route is used, the initial dose should be reduced 50% to avoid marked sedation.

Additional antihistamines are helpful in preventing prolonged symptoms from urticaria. Hydroxyzine (Vistaril or Atarax) appears to be the most effective for controlling itching (8), particularly in chronic urticaria. A low dose (10 mg every 8 hours) should be tried initially, as the usual dose (25 mg every 8 hours) is much more likely to cause significant sedation. If hydroxyzine is ineffective, cyproheptadine (Periactin) may be tried, beginning with 2 mg every 12 hours and increasing to a maximum of 4 mg four times daily. The addition of an H2 antagonist (cimetidine or ranitidine) may enhance the effectiveness of conventional (H1) antihistamines in the management of urticaria. Ephedrine, 25 mg every 4 to 6 hours, may be added to H1 plus H2 regimens with some additional beneficial effect resulting from the alpha-, beta-1, and beta-2 adrenergic effects of this compound.

These measures are useful in most of the allergic and nonallergic urticaria/angioedema states. There are exceptions, however. *Cold urticaria* seems to respond best to cyproheptadine (Periactin), 4 mg every 6 hours. *Pressure urticaria*, when severe enough to require treatment, usually does not respond to antihistamines and may require a short course of corticosteroids. *Solar urticaria* should be managed with a combination of topical sunscreens and hydroxyzine. *Attacks of HAE* may be prevented by long-term treatment with a nonvirilizing androgen derivative (3). This form of treatment should usually be planned in conjunction with a consulting allergist. Life-threatening acute attacks of HAE require hospitalization for observation in an intensive care unit. If C4 levels are less than 50% of normal, any surgical procedure proposed for such patients should not be attempted without pretreatment, because of the risk of precipitating local attacks through trauma. Four mg of stanazol four times a day for three days given preoperatively appears to have sufficient effect to prevent HAE attacks in the intra- and postoperative periods.

When there is a clear indication that certain conditions promote urticaria, it is important to avoid re-exposure, since more severe reactions may result. Acute generalized urticaria/angioedema after exposure to a foreign substance signifies that there is a risk of a life-threatening reaction (see below) on re-exposure. In addition, in patients with a history of solar, cold, or cholinergic urticaria, there is a small risk of vascular collapse on subsequent exposure. These disquieting facts should be made known to affected subjects and their families in order to emphasize the importance of avoiding exposure, of obtaining immediate medical attention if recurrent exposure occurs, and of administering emergency treatment if there is a severe reaction (anaphylaxis, see next section).

Anaphylaxis/Anaphylactoid Reactions

Definition

Life-threatening acute generalized reactions are not uncommon in ambulatory practice. Table 23.8 lists selected therapeutic and diagnostic substances that

Table 23.8.
Selected Therapeutic and Diagnostic Substances Reported to Have Caused Anaphylaxis or Anaphylactoid Reactions[a]

Adriamycin
Antisera (produced in animals)
Aspirin (and other nonsteroidal anti-inflammatory agents)
Barbiturates
Blood and blood products
Bromsulfophthalein (BSP)
Cephalosporins
Cyclophosphamide
Dehydrocholate (Decholin)
Diazepam (and other benzodiazepines)
Insulin (including human insulin)
Iodinated radiopaque contrast agents
Local anesthetics (procaine, lidocaine)
Penicillins
Phenytoin (and other antiepileptics)
Protamine
Streptomycin
Sulfonamides
Tetanus toxoid
Tetracyclines
Various peptide hormones

[a] Modified from *Asthma and the Other Allergic Diseases*, NIAID Task Force Report. NIH publ no. 79-387, May 1979.

have been documented as causes of such reactions; other important causes are insect stings and ingested foods (see below).

Anaphylaxis is an immune response to an agent to which an individual has become hypersensitive by prior exposure. A variety of symptoms may occur. Initially, there may be a diffuse erythema of the skin followed by a sense of warmth and then generalized urticaria. Severe and rapidly progressive respiratory distress due to bronchospasm and/or angioedema involving the larynx may follow. Gastrointestinal symptoms may include vomiting, abdominal cramps, and diarrhea (occasionally bloody). Vascular collapse, with or without other symptoms, can occur (anaphylactic shock). Reactions clinically indistinguishable from anaphylaxis can also occur when no allergic basis can be established for the reaction (idiopathic anaphylaxis or anaphlylactoid reaction).

Management

The recommendations of the National Institutes of Health Task Force on Allergy for the initial management of anaphylaxis and anaphylactoid reactions are summarized in Table 23.9. Because bronchospasm, hypotension, and other hazardous manifestations can recur over a number of hours, the patient should either be hospitalized or kept under close observation during the 12 to 24 hours after anaphylaxis.

Avoidance of the offending substance is, of course, critical in patients with a history of anaphylaxis. The self-treatment kit described below under Hymenop-

Table 23.9.
Treatment of Anaphylaxis[a]

1. When applicable, place tourniquet above site of injection or sting to obstruct venous return or stop the administration of the causative agent. Remove tourniquet temporarily every 10–15 minutes.
2. Place patient in recumbent position and elevate lower extremities.
3. Administer aqueous epinephrine 1:1000. 0.3–0.5 ml subcutaneously or intramuscularly (or if necessary 0.1 in 10 ml of saline solution given intravenously over several minutes) and repeat as necessary or sting.
4. When applicable, inject aqueous epinephrine 1:1000, 0.1–0.3 ml at the site of the injection.
5. Establish and maintain airway, first with oral airway. If necessary, use endotracheal tube.
6. Give oxygen as needed.
7. Monitor vital signs frequently.
8. If patient is not responding, give diphenhydramine hydrochloride (Benadryl), 60–80 mg intravenously over 3 minutes (maximum, 5 mg/kg in 24 hours).
9. If blood pressure cannot be obtained, give normal saline intravenously and maintain blood pressure with levarterenol bitartrate (Levophed), 1 or 2 ampules (8 to 16 mg) in 500 ml of 5% glucose in water. Titrate to maintain blood pressure.
10. If severe asthma without shock give aminophylline, 500 mg intravenously over 10–20 minutes.
11. While corticosteroids will not be helpful for the acute anaphylaxis, they may prevent protracted anaphylaxis.

[a] Modified from *Asthma and the Other Allergic Diseases*, NIAID Task Force Report. NIH publ. no. 79-387, May 1979.

tera sting reaction should be prescribed for subjects who are at risk of recurrent accidental exposures.

Penicillin Allergy

Penicillin allergy is a common concern in ambulatory practice, where short courses of penicillin or one of the semisynthetic penicillins are frequently prescribed. The physician may be confronted with either of two problems.

The commonest problem is the patient who needs penicillin and gives a history of penicillin "allergy." For the infections treated in ambulatory practice, there is almost always a suitable alternative to a penicillin (throughout this volume, the appropriate alternative is named wherever a penicillin is recommended). The most prudent strategy is to select an alternative drug whenever there is a possibility of prior penicillin allergy, even though this will lead to some unnecessary substitution, as almost half of patients giving a history of penicillin allergy do not in fact show allergic reactions when rechallenged with penicillin (11). In an ambulatory patient who has been labeled "allergic to penicillin" on the basis of an atypical "allergic" reaction, genuine penicillin allergy can be confirmed or excluded by skin testing, ideally utilizing both major and minor determinant penicillin antigens (11); this may be particularly desirable in young adults who may be denied access to penicillin throughout their lives on the basis of unsubstantiated "penicillin allergy." When such patients are seen in ambulatory practice, the best plan is to select alternatives to penicillin when antibiotics are needed and to refer them to an allergist for administration and interpretation of these critical skin tests. At present the major determinant is available commercially as Pre-pen from the Kremers Urban Company. The minor determinant mixture is not available yet; until it is available, testing should be carried out with Pre-pen and Penicillin G at a concentration of 10, 000 units per ml. This will detect 90% of penicillin allergic patients.

Approximately half of patients with confirmed penicillin allergy also have positive skin tests to cephalosporin antigens (11). Therefore, cephalosporin antibiotics should not be given to persons allergic to penicillin, and vice versa.

Less commonly, the physician in ambulatory practice will have to manage a first reaction to penicillin. Table 23.10 shows the approximate incidence of each of three types of allergic reactions (immediate, accelerated, late) following either parenteral or oral administration of penicillin. The management of the more common late reactions (usually nonurticarial morbilliform rashes) is reassurance and a short course of an antihistamine if itching is a problem. The acute management of accelerated and immediate reactions is described in the preceding sections on urticaria and anaphylaxis. Long-term management requires assuring that the patient and his immediate family know

Table 23.10.
Estimated Incidence of Allergic Reactions to Penicillin[a]

Type of Reaction	Manifestations	Time of Occurrence after First Dose of Penicillin	Percentage of Treated Patients Showing Reaction
Late reactions	Skin rash	≥72 hr	1.4
Accelerated reactions	Urticaria	1–72 hr	0.3
Immediate reactions	Generalized urticaria	2–30 min	0.3
	Anaphylaxis	2–30 min	0.04
	Anaphylactic deaths[b]		0.001

[a] Modified from *Asthma and the Other Allergic Diseases*, NIAID Task Force Report. NIH publ. no. 79-387, May 1979. Results are based upon 70 to 80 million therapeutic courses of penicillin or semisynthetic penicillin or cephalosporin given per annum in the United States.
[b] From 400 to 800 deaths per year in the United States.

that all forms of penicillin and the related cephalosporin antibiotics should be avoided.

Ampicillin Rash

Ampicillin (and amoxacillin) commonly causes a nonallergic maculopapular rash that is not pruritic. The rash appears 48 to 72 hours after starting ampicillin. It occurs in approximately 9% of all patients given ampicillin and as high as 50% of patients with mononucleosis (1). The risk of developing this type of rash is also higher in patients with lymphatic leukemia and hyperuricemia, and in those taking allopurinol. Rechallenge with ampicillin at a later time often causes no recurrence of the rash or other adverse reactions; therefore, a well-documented history of this kind of ampicillin rash is not a contraindication to subsequent ampicillin (or other penicillin) treatment.

Hymenoptera Venom Allergy

Stings by yellow jackets, hornets, honeybees, and wasps result in generalized allergic reactions of varying severity in approximately 0.4% of the population (1).

IgE-mediated hypersensitivity to these insect venoms may be confirmed by skin testings with suitable dilutions of available venoms; this is most appropriately done by an allergist. Because victims, unless already familiar with the distinguishing features of the various Hymenoptera, are often unable to tell bees from yellow jackets, hornets, or wasps, skin testing with individual venoms is particularly important. After a generalized allergic reaction to an insect sting has been treated (see above), the general physician should immediately initiate a plan to protect the patient's future health. Avoidance of recurrent exposure is critical. In particular, wearing shoes at all times is the single most important safeguard to the patient. However, because of the possibility of unavoidable re-exposure, despite the patient's best efforts, the patient (and ideally a companion whenever the patient is out of doors) should know both the early signs of a generalized reaction and how to administer emergency treatment. An *emergency self-treatment kit* containing a syringe preloaded with epinephrine should be prescribed. An example is the Ana-Kit (Hollister), which contains a two-dose syringe that allows administration

of two measured doses (0.3 ml each) of epinephrine; two 4-mg tablets of chlorpheniramine; two sterile swabs; a tourniquet; and instructions. The Epi-Pen and Epi-Pen, Jr., kits (Center Laboratories) provide a single 0.3- or 0.15-mg dose of epinephrine, respectively, in an automatic injector, which some patients may prefer. General physicians should be familiar with one of these kits, keep one in the office, and review its use with any susceptible patient.

Any adult patient with sensitivity to one of these venoms confirmed by skin test who has had a past history of a potentially life-threatening reaction has a greater than 50% chance of a similar reaction if stung again and should therefore be offered immunotherapy with those venoms to which he is reactive. Such treatment is analogous to that described above for seasonal allergy; it reduces the likelihood of a future severe reaction to less than 5%. Once immunotherapy is instituted for insect venom hypersensitivity, it must be maintained through the use of booster injections at 4- to 6-weekly intervals for a minimum of 5 years. Children through age 16 whose systemic reactions have been confined to the skin (urticaria or angioedema) have a 10 to 20% risk of future systemic reactions of similar or milder type, and a minuscule risk of a more severe reaction. Therefore in this group of patients, immunotherapy may be offered but may be of relatively small benefit.

Even patients who do not have life-threatening reactions (i.e., those who have urticaria/angioedema or other cutaneous symptoms) may be at increased risk of a more severe reaction on re-exposure; therefore, such patients also should be referred to an allergist for skin testing and for a careful explanation of the available methods of protection (immunotherapy or an emergency self-treatment kit). Patients whose reactions have been local (confined to an area contiguous to the site of the sting) are not considered candidates for immunotherapy, even if the reaction is large.

Food Allergy

The gastrointestinal tract is sufficiently permeable to antigens found in food that some individuals experience one or more manifestations of allergy after the ingestion of a food to which they have become sensitive. Clinically apparent food allergy is much more common in young children than in adolescents or adults. In adults food allergy usually manifests as urticaria/angioedema or anaphylaxis. In children (particularly those sensitive to cow's milk), rhinitis, eczema, asthma, and colic may also occur. The most common causes of food allergy are listed in Table 23.11. Allergy to shellfish has nothing to do with susceptibility to the nonimmunological reactions to iodinated contrast materials seen after administration of these materials (see below).

Evidence of sensitization to foods can be detected by skin testing. It has been established, however, that only 50–60% of subjects with positive skin puncture tests will have a reaction on double-blind food challenge. Conversely, virtually no patients with negative skin tests have been found to have positive responses to placebo-controlled, double-blind challenge. Thus, although the puncture test is useful for screening, the placebo-controlled, double-blind food challenge is the definitive test for establishing the diagnosis of food allergy. A blind challenge should not be carried out when an anaphylactic reaction is thought to be due to a particular food, because of the potential danger of the reaction.

There is no good evidence for nonantibody-mediated food hypersensitivity, although many practitioners claim to be able to use various techniques to substantiate food sensitivity. Various symptoms, including hyperactivity, depression, difficulty in concentration, and memory loss, have been blamed on food "allergy." Evidence to support such notions consists of uncontrolled observations by physicians who strongly believe in the existence of such entities.

The management of food allergy is avoidance and, in selected instances, prescription of and education about self-treatment kits (see above). No evidence exists that food sensitivity can be "neutralized" by injections of food extracts or by the administration of food extract drops sublingually.

Reactions to Iodinated Contrast Materials

Patients receiving intravenous iodinated contrast materials may develop one of three reactions that resemble allergic reactions. Neither IgE-mediated allergy nor other immunological mechanisms have been found to explain these reactions, although complement activation may be shown in vitro. The three types of reaction are:

Table 23.11.
Foods That Most Often Cause Allergic Reactions

MOST COMMON:
Seafood
Eggs
Nuts
Seeds
OTHERS:
Milk
Chocolate
Grains (barley, rice, wheat)
Fruits (citrus, melons, bananas, strawberries)
Vegetables (tomatoes, celery, spinach, corn, potatoes, soy bean)

1. Rash. Onset of urticaria/angioedema, usually accompanied by generalized itching.
2. Anaphylactoid. Cough, dyspnea, wheezing, syncope, with or without urticaria/angioedema.
3. Vasomotor. An exaggerated response to dye injection, with more than the usual amount of flushing and nausea, frequently accompanied by a sensation of numbness and tingling of the extremities and transient hypotension of a mild degree.

It is estimated that there is a 1 to 2% risk of developing one of these reactions in the general population and an approximately 35% risk in patients with a prior history of a reaction (1). At the present time, there is no method such as a skin test or a small trial dose to identify prospectively the patient at risk.

Management of the acute reaction is similar to that described for generalized allergic reactions above. The patient should be carefully educated about the risk of recurrence; and repeated studies with iodinated contrast materials should be avoided whenever possible. In the event that a patient with a history of a reaction (either urticaria/angioedema or anaphylactoid) must undergo a later study, the following regimen should be followed: prednisone, 50 mg by mouth 13, 7, and 1 hour before the procedure; diphenhydramine, 50 mg, and ephedrine, 25 mg, by mouth 1 hour before the procedure. This regimen reduces but does not entirely eliminate the risk of a subsequent reaction (4).

Reactions to Aspirin and Other NSAIDs

Aspirin (acetylsalicylic acid) can produce urticaria/angioedema, an anaphylactoid reaction, or severe asthma (in association with acute rhinorrhea, described above) in susceptible subjects. These reactions usually occur in patients with a prior history of some type of allergy. It is estimated that this type of aspirin sensitivity may develop in up to 10% of asthmatics (1); the problem is particularly common in patients with both bronchial asthma and nasal polyps.

IgE-mediated allergy to aspirin has not been demonstrated. Further evidence against an allergic basis is the fact that affected individuals may show similar reactions to other NSAIDs (see description of these drugs in Chapter 70) not related antigenically to aspirin. The yellow food-coloring dye tartrazine (utilized in some foods, beverages, and medications) may also elicit urticaria in NSAID-sensitive patients.

The first generalized reaction to aspirin usually occurs in adulthood, most typically a number of years after the onset of asthma (9). Symptoms may occur immediately after aspirin ingestion or a number of hours later. Because of this delay, the role of aspirin may be overlooked by the patient; therefore, it is important to question any patient with an unexplained generalized reaction about the use of aspirin or one of the other agents known to produce these reactions.

The management of the generalized reactions in these patients is the same as that described earlier for urticaria/angioedema and for anaphylaxis. Avoidance of products containing aspirin (see Table 23.12) and the other agents that may induce these symptoms is essential after the diagnosis has been established. Affected patients should be instructed explicitly to use only acetaminophen (Tylenol or a noncoated generic) when they need a mild analgesic or antipyretic. An

Table 23.12.
Aspirin Preparations and Aspirin-Containing Products

Alka-Seltzer[a]
Anacin[a]
Anahist
Arthritis Pain Formula[a]
Ascodeen-30
Ascriptin[a]
Aspergum[a]
Bayer Aspirin[a]
Bufferin[a]
Cama Inlay-Tabs[a]
Cirin
Congesprin[a]
Cope
Coricidin[a]
Darvon Compound
Dristan[a]
Duradyne DHC Tablets
Duragesic Tablets
Easprin
Ecotrin[a]
Empirin
Emprazil
Equagesic
Excedrin
Fiorinal
Goody's Headache Powders[a]
Measurin
Midol[a]
Momentum Muscular Backache Formula
Pabirin
Panalgesic[a]
Percodan
Persistin
Phenaphen
Quiet World Analgesic/Sleeping Aid[a]
Rhinex
St. Joseph Cold Tablets for Children[a]
Sine-Off Tablets-Aspirin Formula[a]
Stanback[a]
Stero-Darvon
Supac
Synalgos
Triaminicin[a]
Vanquish[a]
Viro-Med[a]
4-Way Cold Tablets

[a] Over-the-counter.

oral "desensitization" regimen using aspirin has been reported to lessen chronic nasal and sinus symptoms in some aspirin-sensitive patients. This regimen should be regarded as experimental and should not be undertaken in the ambulatory patient or in the hospitalized patient without expert consultation.

General References

Lichtenstein LM, Fauci AS: *Current Therapy in Allergy, Immunology, and Rheumatology. 1985–1986.* St Louis, CV Mosby, 1985.
Middleton E, Reed CE, Ellis EF (eds): *Allergy: Principles and Practice.* St Louis, CV Mosby, 1983.
> A two-volume compendium with chapters by many recognized authorities on various topics. It is worthwhile to read about a subject in both this and in Samter (see below), since the discussions are often complementary, and at times contradictory.

Mygind N: *Nasal Allergy.* Oxford, Blackwell Scientific Publications, 1978.
> Recommended for the physician who has more than a superficial interest in nasal problems. One author, one style, clearly written, and reasonably concise.

Samter MD (ed): *Immunological Diseases,* 4th ed. Boston, Little, Brown and Co, 1988.
> Two-volume work containing more detail on treatment of general problems in immunology than in Middleton et al.

Specific References

1. NIAID Task Force Report: *Asthma and the Other Allergic Diseases.* NIH publ no. 79-387, May, 1979.
2. Broder I, Higgins MW, Mathews KP, Keller JB: Epidemiology of asthma and allergic rhinitis in a total community, Tecumseh, Michigan. *J Allergy Clin Immunol* 54:100, 1974.
3. Gelfand JA, Sherins RJ, Alling DW, Frank MM: Treatment of hereditary angioedema with danazol: reversal of clinical and biochemical abnormalities. *N Engl J Med* 295:1444, 1976.
4. Greenberger PA, Patterson R, Radin RC: Two pretreatment regimens for high-risk patients receiving radiographic contrast media. *J Allergy Clin Immunol* 74:540, 1984.
5. Handelman NI, Friday GA, Schwartz HJ, et al: Cromolyn sodium nasal solution in the prophylactic treatment of pollen-induced seasonal allergic rhinitis. *J Allergy Clin Immunol* 59:237, 1977.
6. Horowitz JD, Howes LG, Christophidis N, et al: Hypertensive responses induced by phenylpropanolamine in anorectic and decongestant preparations. *Lancet* 1:60, 1980.
7. Norman PS: Specific therapy in allergy. *Med Clin North Am* 58:111, 1974.
8. Rhoades RB, Leifer KN, Cohan R, Wittig HJ: Suppression of histamine-induced pruritis by three antihistamine drugs. *J Allergy Clin Immunol* 55:180, 1975.
9. Samter M, Beers Jr. RF: Intolerance to aspirin. Clinical studies and consideration of its pathogenesis. *Ann Intern Med* 68:975, 1968.
10. Stewart Jr. TW: Vasomotor rhinitis: neglected cause of nasal congestion. *Postgrad Med* 67:171, 1980.
11. Sullivan TJ, Wedner HJ, Shatz GS, et al: *Skin Testing to Detect Penicillin Allergy.* St Louis, CV Mosby, 1981.

C H A P T E R 24

Undifferentiated Acute Febrile Illness

NATHANIEL F. PIERCE, M.D.

Acute febrile illnesses are encountered frequently in medical practice. Such episodes have many possible causes that range in significance from trivial to life threatening. For those that require treatment, accurate diagnosis is obviously needed to guide the choice of therapy. In most instances, fever is accompanied by localizing complaints or physical findings that suggest specific diagnoses and guide the selection of diagnostic laboratory studies. Such episodes can usually be diagnosed promptly and appropriate management can be readily instituted. Thus, for example, fever plus dysuria suggests the diagnosis of urinary tract infection, indicates the need for a urinalysis and urine culture, and is likely to require antibiotic therapy.

A more difficult problem may be posed, however, when fever occurs as an isolated complaint or is accompanied only by nonspecific constitutional symptoms, such as chills, malaise, anorexia, or modest weight loss. Although such episodes of acute undifferentiated febrile illness may raise the fear of serious illness in the minds of both patient and physician, most are benign and resolve spontaneously in 2 weeks or less, without a specific diagnosis being made. In only a very few instances do undifferentiated febrile illnesses persist and remain unexplained despite continued careful observation of the patient and the performance of routine diagnostic laboratory tests. Only when fever has lasted at least 3 weeks in such patients should it be designated "fever of unknown origin" (FUO). Patients with FUO require more extensive diagnostic evaluation, often in the hospital, whereas unexplained febrile illnesses of shorter duration are usually managed on an ambulatory basis.

The aim of this chapter is to describe a rational approach to the diagnosis and management of acute undifferentiated febrile episodes, emphasizing a balance between cautious observation and active investigation.

NORMAL TEMPERATURE RANGE

In most healthy persons, the normal oral temperature varies between 96.5°F (35.8°C) and 99°F (37.2°C), the lowest value occurring between 2 A.M. and 4 A.M., and the highest between 6 P.M. and 10 P.M. In very hot weather, an individual's temperature may be 0.5°F to 1°F (0.3 to 0.6°C), higher than normal. Very vigorous exercise, such as marathon running, will also cause the temperature to rise temporarily.

ETIOLOGICAL CONSIDERATIONS

Infections

Infection is undoubtedly the most common cause of acute undifferentiated fever. An abrupt onset of fever is especially suggestive of infection; however, other causes are possible. The majority of episodes of undifferentiated fever due to infection are self-limited, eventuate in complete recovery without treatment, and are likely to be of viral etiology. The viral agents that cause these episodes are rarely identified, and attempts to identify causative viruses by cultural or serological methods are not usually warranted.

For certain infections that begin as undifferentiated fever diagnostic signs or symptoms develop after one or several days. These account for only a small portion of the episodes of acute undifferentiated fever but include serious infections that require prompt diagnosis and treatment. Most common among these are viral infections, such as infectious mononucleosis (see Chapter 53), viral hepatitis (see Chapter 43), varicella (chickenpox), rubeola (measles), rubella (German measles), and recent human immunodeficiency virus (HIV) infection (see Chapter 34); rickettsial infections, such as Rocky Mountain spotted fever and Q fever; Lyme disease, a spirochetal infection transmitted by deer ticks (see Chapter 30); a variety of localized bacterial infections, such as those involving the pleura, biliary tract, retroperitoneum, kidney, liver, and spleen; and several bacteremic infections, especially acute bacterial endocarditis and *Salmonella* bacteremia. If there has been recent travel to certain developing countries (see Chapter 33), the list of etiological considerations should include malaria, dengue fever, scrub typhus, and leptospirosis, and the possibility of viral hepatitis and of *Salmonella* bacteremia is increased. Table 24.1 summarizes salient features of important nonbacterial infections that may present with acute undifferentiated fever and that are not discussed elsewhere in this book.

Table 24.1.
Some Acute Nonbacterial Infections for Which Undifferentiated Fever May Be the First Manifestation

Infection	Transmission	Incubation Period	Clinical Features
		days	
Chickenpox (varicella)	Person-to-person *via* respiratory secretions and direct contact; highly contagious	10–21	Malaise and fever precede or occur simultaneously with rash. Rash develops in crops as pruritic maculopapules evolving in hours to vesicles and in days to dried scabs. All stages of rash are seen in the same skin area.
German measles (rubella)	Person-to-person, *via* respiratory secretions and direct contact; highly contagious	14–21	1–7-day prodrome of malaise, headache, fever, mild conjuctivitis followed by maculopapular (occasionally confluent) rash which begins on forehead and spreads to trunk and extremities.
Measles (rubeola)	Person-to-person, *via* respiratory secretions	9–11	3–4-day prodrome with fever, malaise, hacking cough, rhinitis, subsiding 1–2 days following onset of maculopapular rash spreading from face to neck to trunk, to feet (by third day)
Q Fever (*Rickettsia burnetti*)	Spread by airborne rickettsiae in dust contaminated by infected animals (cattle, sheep, goats) or by direct contact with infected animals or their tissue	14–26	Headache, chills, fever, anorexia, myalgias lasting 3 days to 2 weeks. Cough with rales after a few days, persisting after fever remits. Treated with tetracycline or chloramphenicol.
Rocky Mountain spotted fever (*Ricksettsia rickettsiae*)	Bite of infected tick or contamination with tick tissues or feces	3–14	Abrupt onset of severe headache, chills, myalgia, fever. Rash (second to fourth day of fever)—initially *macules* on wrists, ankles, palms, soles, extending in 6–12 hours to buttocks, trunk, face; becomes *maculopapular* by day 2–3 and *petechial* by about day 4, progressing to ecchymoses. Rash may be missed on dark skin. Early treatment with chloramphenicol or tetracycline is lifesaving.

Drugs

A small portion of acute undifferentiated febrile episodes in ambulatory patients is caused by hypersensitivity to drugs. Almost any drug can cause fever, but digitalis preparations, chloramphenicol, insulins, and tetracyclines almost never do. Those most frequently responsible are listed in Table 24.2. Fever may begin promptly after starting the drug or may be delayed by several weeks; however, a drug taken regularly for 3 months or longer is not likely to cause fever. Drug fever may be low grade or may exceed 104°F (40°C). Chills are uncommon with drug fever, but their presence does not exclude this diagnosis. Urticaria, maculo-papular skin rash, and/or eosinophilia occurs in many cases. Rarely, hypersensitivity to some drugs may begin with fever, followed by the syndrome of serum sickness (rash, lymphadenopathy, arthritis, nephritis, edema); these drugs include barbiturates, methyldopa, penicillin, phenytoin, sulfonamides. A lupus-like syndrome characterized by fever, arthralgias, and positive ANA titers may follow the intiation of procainamide. When a drug is the cause of a patient's fever, removal of the offending drug is usually followed by defervescence in 1 to 2 days; however, fever may last several days, or up to 2 to 3 weeks, if the drug is eliminated slowly, e.g., iodides. Readministration of the suspected drug usually causes fever within a few hours, thus confirming its causative role. This approach should only be considered if the drug is important for future therapy and the original febrile episode was not associated with organ damage.

An ambulatory patient may present with drug-induced fever due to several other mechanisms, most of them rare. Temperature elevation due to *altered thermoregulation* can occur because of a direct effect on the central nervous system (amphetamines, cocaine, phenothiazines), decreased heat loss due to decreased sweating, especially in the presence of high ambient temperature (drugs with anticholinergic activity), a state of hypermetabolism (monamine oxidase inhibitors, excessive thyroid hormone, cimetidine). Fever due to the *pharmacological action of a drug* may be seen in the Herxheimer reaction that follows penicillin treatment of syphilis (see details, Chapter 30) and in association with chemotherapy that causes rapid destruction of tumor

Table 24.2.
Drugs That Frequently Cause Fever Due to Hypersensitivity

Allopurinol	Isoniazid
Amphotericin B	Methyldopa
Antihistamines	Nifedipine
Atropine	Nitrofurantoin
Barbiturates	Penicillins
Bleomycin	Phenyolphthalein[b]
Cephalosporins	Phenytoin
Clofibrate	Procainamide
Ethambutol	Quinidine
Hydralazine	Salicylates[c]
Ibuprofen	Sulindac
Iodides[a]	Sulfonamides

[a] Including intravenous contrast media.
[b] Found in many nonprescription laxatives.
[c] When toxic levels occur.

cells. *Administration-related fever* may occur after any intravenous infusion of a drug, either because of contamination with microorganism-induced pyrogens or infusion-induced phlebitis. In addition, repeated intramuscular injections at the same site can cause a sterile abscess that releases endogenous pyrogens.

Other Causes

Other acute processes that may cause undifferentiated fever include vascular occlusive and/or inflammatory events such as deep vein thrombophlebitis, minor pulmonary emboli, and asymptomatic myocardial infarction. Similarly, fever may be the only manifestation of acute hemolytic episodes, such as occur in acute autoimmune hemolytic anemia or hemolytic anemia due to glucose 6-phosphate dehydrogenase (G6PD) deficiency. Recent immunization with certain vaccines (see Chapter 32) may also cause fever. Leukopenia caused by medications such as carbamazepine, captopril, and antithyroid agents may present with undifferentiated fever.

Special Risk Patients

In patients with certain pre-existing conditions, serious infections play an increased role in causing acute undifferentiated fever. Patients with lymphomas or HIV infection and those receiving therapeutic doses of corticosteroids (more than 20 mg daily of hydrocortisone or an equivalent dose of another corticosteroid), especially if combined with other immunosuppressive agents, are at increased risk of developing primary or reactivation tuberculosis, acquiring or reactivating certain fungal infections (e.g., cryptococcosis, histoplasmosis, and coccidioidomycosis), reactivating certain viral infections (e.g., herpes zoster or cytomegalovirus infections), or developing infections due to *Pneumocystis carinii* or *Toxoplasma*; the approach to these problems in patients with HIV infection is described in detail in Chapter 34. Patients with established rheumatic valvular disease, certain types of congenital heart disease (e.g., ventricular septal defect, patent ductus arteriosus, or coarctation of the aorta), or prosthetic heart valves or vascular grafts are at increased risk of bacterial endocarditis (acute or subacute) or other endovascular infection. Patients with multiple myeloma, or surgical splenectomy or autosplenectomy due to sickle cell disease, are at increased risk of serious spontaneous bacteremia, due especially to *Streptococcus pneumoniae*, *Haemophilus influenzae*, or salmonellae. Patients with granulocytopenia (less than 1,000 pmns/mm³) are at increased risk of being bacteremic when febrile. Persons with advanced hepatic cirrhosis, especially when it is accompanied by ascites, may develop spontaneous bacterial peritonitis, often without localizing signs or symptoms. And persons who administer illicit drugs to themselves intravenously are at risk of developing bacterial sepsis due to nonsterile technique.

In other patients, especially elderly people, chronic alcoholics, and those with diabetes mellitus, the usual signs and symptoms of some acute bacterial infections may be diminished or absent. Fever may be the only manifestation of pneumonia, empyema, or localized intra-abdominal infection in such persons; and the febrile response to these infections may be less than usually seen in younger or nondiabetic, nonalcoholic patients.

Chronic Fever

The major causes of unexplained fever lasting more than 3 weeks (FUO) differ appreciably from those described above. The most common causes are (a) chronic infections, especially tuberculosis, subacute bacterial endocarditis, chronic osteomyelitis, cytomegalovirus infections, occult intra-abdominal abscesses, urinary tract infections and HIV infection; (b) collagen-vascular or rheumatic diseases, especially systemic lupus erythematosus, temporal arteritis, rheumatic fever, and rheumatoid arthritis; (c) certain neoplasms, especially lymphoma, acute leukemia, reticulum cell sarcoma, hypernephroma, hepatoma, pancreatic carcinoma, carcinoma of the lung, and malignancies involving bone; and (d) miscellaneous disorders such as granulomatous hepatitis, hyperthyroidism, drug fever, inflammatory bowel disease, sarcoidosis, thyroiditis, and recurrent pulmonary emboli.

Early diagnosis of these disorders is sometimes possible, especially when localizing symptoms or signs are present. Otherwise, these diagnoses are usually considered only when fever has been unexplained for at least 3 weeks despite preliminary diagnostic studies.

DIAGNOSTIC APPROACH

General Objectives

There are two general objectives in managing patients with acute undifferentiated fever; first, early diagnosis in those few instances of serious illness that require specific treatment, and second, the avoidance of unnecessary and expensive diagnostic studies and of "blind therapy" for the majority of patients whose course will prove benign and self-limited. The key to achievement of these objectives is careful, repeated evaluation of the patient's history and physical findings and judicious use of diagnostic tests. A sequential evaluation process, which emphasizes frequent reevaluation combined with increasing diagnostic studies, is summarized in Table 24.3 and described below.

Initial Evaluation

The initial evaluation of most patients with an acute undifferentiated febrile illness requires about 15 minutes. A febrile illness is present if an oral temperature exceeding 99.5°F (37.6°C) is found on examination or by history. The evaluation of such patients should aim to detect signs, symptoms, or historical background

Table 24.3.
Acute Undifferentiated Febrile Illness: Summary of Sequential Evaluation Process

Evaluation Process	Comment
INITIAL EVALUATION	
1. History, physical examination; if negative and not seriously ill, observe 7–10 days; frequent phone contact	Spontaneous defervescence common, benign illness common
2. More thorough evaluation of "special risk" patients, including laboratory studies	Increased risk that fever is caused by serious illness, usually infection
3. If seriously ill: more extensive laboratory studies; may need hospitalization and treatment	
REPEAT EVALUATIONS (AT WEEKLY INTERVALS)	
1. Carefully repeated history and physical examination, expanded laboratory evaluation	Thorough re-evaluation often detects cause of fever
2. Discontinue recent drugs, document fever	
AFTER 3 WEEKS	
1. Begin evaluation for true FUO, often requires hospitalization	Spontaneous defervescence uncommon, fever usually due to serious illness with substantial risk of mortality

that will identify the most likely reason(s) for the fever. A history of similar symptoms among others at home or at work suggests an infectious process. Fever with no other signs or symptoms in a patient recently started on a new drug, especially one known to cause fever (Table 24.2), suggests drug fever. If no localizing signs or symptoms are found and the patients does not seem seriously ill, no further evaluation is needed. The patient should be reassured and instructed to keep a record of morning and evening temperatures at home if the fever persists. A telephone call should be scheduled after 1 or 2 days as a simple means of following the course of the illness, detecting new complaints, and providing reassurance. If undifferentiated fever persists for 7 to 10 days, the patient should return for a thorough re-evaluation.

Exceptions to this pattern of management are patients whose constitutional symptoms are severe, who have those underlying conditions that predispose to serious infections or mask their manifestations (see above), who have been recently hospitalized or have undergone invasive diagnostic studies, or who describe fever of at least 2 weeks' duration when first seen. The initial evaluation of such patients should be expanded to include a thorough history and physical examination, as described below under "Re-evaluation," and the following laboratory studies: chest X-ray with posteroanterior (PA) and lateral views, complete blood count with differential, erythrocyte sedimentation rate, liver function tests, blood cultures (aerobic and anaerobic) from at least two sites, urinalysis, and quantitative urine culture if the urinalysis reveals pyuria or bacteriuria. Positive findings should be used to guide further studies or treatment. Patients with severe constitutional symptoms may require hospitalization and prompt antimicrobial therapy for possible bacteremia, especially if underlying conditions predisposing to bacteremia are present and/or hematological findings suggestive of bacteremia are found (e.g., Döhle bodies or vacuoles in polymorphonuclear neutrophilic leukocytes (PMNs), an increased erythrocyte sedimentation rate, or increased numbers of band-forms with an elevated or depressed total white

count). If not hospitalized, such patients should be reevaluated daily by telephone or at an office visit until severe symptoms subside or the cause of fever is determined.

Re-evaluation

Patients with unexplained fever that has lasted 1 week or more after the initial evaluation should be thoroughly re-evaluated. The history should be carefully reviewed, including recent travel (especially to areas of poor sanitation; see Chapter 33, Medical Advice for the International Traveler), contact with persons with infectious or febrile illnesses (especially hepatitis, mononucleosis, or HIV infection), drug use (including recently prescribed drugs, over-the-counter medications, and illicit drugs), alcohol abuse, homosexual activity, intravenous drug abuse, and familial disorders associated with fever or infection. The past medical and surgical history should be thoroughly explored. The review of systems should be repeated to detect any new complaints or subtle complaints missed at the initial evaluation. Trivial symptoms, such as vague abdominal discomfort, may prove of great value in localizing the cause of fever.

The *physical examination* should be meticulously reperformed. As with the history, subtle findings may prove invaluable. Essential procedures sometimes ignored, but which should be included, are funduscopic examination of the eyes (after dilating the pupils, if necessary), examination for a tender or enlarged temporal artery, search for a new or changing heart murmur, detection of enlargement or tenderness of the thyroid gland, search for pericardial, pleural, or hepatic friction rubs, search for hepatomegaly or splenomegaly, detection of subtle abdominal or hepatic tenderness, examination of the rectum and prostate, pelvic examination, thorough search for lymphadenopathy including epitrochlear nodes, and examination of skin and mucus membranes (including conjunctivae) for petechiae and of nail beds for splinter hemorrhages.

Laboratory studies should also be initiated. A complete blood count, differential white blood cell count, and urinalysis should be performed. Additional studies should include a chest X-ray (PA and lateral views), erythrocyte sedimentation rate, serum alkaline phosphatase, serum aminotransferases, and a test for occult fecal blood. At least two blood cultures (each cultured aerobically and anaerobically) should be obtained. The urine should be cultured if pyuria or bacteriuria is observed. An intermediate strength purified protein derivative (PPD) skin test should be applied unless there is a documented history of a positive PPD or history of tuberculosis. If there has been travel within 6 months to an area where malaria is endemic, appropriate blood smears should be examined. Any medications started during the previous 2 months should be discontinued or, if that is not possible, replaced by chemically unrelated substitutes. This is especially important for those drugs listed in Table 24.2.

Patients should then chart their temperature at least twice daily for another full week. If unexplained fever persists, the history and physical examination should again be reviewed with great care. Additional laboratory studies should include skin tests for cutaneous anergy (if intermediate PPD was negative), an electrocardiogram, serum calcium determination, serum titers of antistreptolysin O, rheumatoid factor, antinuclear antibody, HIV antibody, and a monospot test. The complete blood count, differential white blood cell count, and urinalysis should be repeated.

If fever is still unexplained, temperature should be charted again for a full week. Documentation of temperature recordings by an independent observer is important to rule out factitious fever. Patients remaining febrile for at least 3 weeks after initial evaluation and lacking a recognized cause or provisional diagnosis despite the approach described above should be studied more extensively, usually in hospital.

MANAGEMENT OF FEVER

Fever is not usually harmful and antipyretic therapy is not often needed. Moreover, such treatment may confuse the clinical picture by altering the temperature pattern. In certain circumstances, however, control of fever is desirable. These include (a) persons with severely compromised cardiac function in whom fever-associated tachycardia further stresses the heart, and (b) persons such as alcoholics or those with dementia who develop increasing confusion or delirium when febrile.

Aspirin is usually effective as an antipyretic but may cause an uncomfortable diaphoresis or actually pre-

cipitate shaking chills. These side effects can be minimized by giving the dose of 0.3 to 0.6 g regularly at 3- to 4-hour intervals. Acetaminophen, in similar dosage, may be used in patients allergic to aspirin, in patients with hemorrhagic diatheses, or in patients with a history of gastrointestinal bleeding or with poor tolerance of aspirin. Acetaminophen is preferred in teenaged or younger children when there is a possibility that fever is caused by influenza or varicella infection; use of aspirin during these infections has been linked to the occurrence of Reye's syndrome.

Antimicrobial drugs have no place in the treatment of patients with acute undifferentiated fever, except in those who appear dangerously ill or who have seriously compromised defenses against infection. The premature use of antibiotics serves only to confuse interpretation of the patient's clinical course, add unnecessary expense, and risk the addition of drug toxicity to the patient's complaints. In most instances, antibiotics should be withheld until a diagnosis for which they are indicated is made.

The daily activities of febrile patients need not be severely restricted but should be moderated to provide additional rest, light meals, and the avoidance of strenuous or tiring tasks.

General References

Esposito AL, Gleckman RA: A diagnostic approach to the adult with fever of unknown origin. *Arch Intern Med* 139:575, 1979.
   This article includes initial evaluation of patients with acute undifferentiated fever as well as those with true fever of unknown origin.
Kumar KL, Reuler JB: Drug fever. *West J Med* 144:753, 1986.
   Brief review, especially helpful for description of mechanisms other than hypersensitivity.
Larson EB, Featherstone HJ, Petersdorf RG: Fever of undetermined origin: diagnosis and follow-up of 105 cases, 1970–1980. *Medicine (Baltimore)* 61:269, 1982.
   A follow-up of Petersdorf's original study on fever of unknown origin documenting the changing diagnostic composition of this syndrome.
Lipsky BA, Hirschmann JV: Drug fever. *JAMA* 245:851, 1981.
   A concise review of the problem of drug fever with typical clinical examples and guidelines for management.
Mellors JW, Horwitz RI, Harvey MR, Horwitz SM: A simple index to identify occult bacterial infection in adults with acute unexplained fever. *Arch Intern Med* 147:666, 1987.
   A valuable report on clinical and hematological features that help to identify patients with acute unexplained due to occult bacterial infection.
Petersdorf RG, Beeson PB: Fever of unexplained origin: report on 100 cases. *Medicine (Baltimore)* 40:1, 1961.
   A classic description of true fever of unknown origin.
Vickery DM, Quinnell RK: Fever of unknown origin: an algorithmic approach. *JAMA* 238:2183, 1977.
   A useful example of a systematic approach to evaluation of fever.

C H A P T E R 25

Bacterial Infections of the Skin

NATHANIEL F. PIERCE, M.D.

Skin infections are extremely common. Although most are trivial and can be managed at home without medical assistance, each year about 5% of the population develops skin infections that require medical attention; these are usually caused by *Streptococcus pyogenes* or *Staphylococcus aureus*. The seriousness of these infections depends upon the nature of the infecting organism, especially its array of virulence factors, such as proteolytic enzymes and toxins, and upon the condition of normal host defense mechanisms. Thus, cutaneous infections due to *S. pyogenes* or *S. aureus* in otherwise healthy persons usually cause only modest morbidity and respond rapidly to appropriate treatment. However, the same organisms can cause serious infections in diabetics, in persons with impaired blood supply to, or impaired lymphatic or venous drainage of, the infected site, or in patients with defects in leukocytic or immunological defense mechanisms. Serious infection is also more likely when other bacteria, or combinations of bacteria, are involved (e.g., in bites or in wounds contaminated with fecal material, animal products, or soil).

SUPERFICIAL INFECTIONS CAUSED PREDOMINANTLY BY *STREPTOCOCCUS PYOGENES*

Impetigo, ecthyma, and erysipelas are superficial infections due largely to group A β-hemolytic streptococci (*S. pyogenes*), although *S. aureus* may play a causative role in some instances. These infections arise from breaks in the skin that are often so minor that they are unnoticed.

Impetigo

Impetigo occurs mostly among preschool children, especially in warm humid climates and when personal hygiene is poor. Under these conditions, the disease is highly contagious and distinct outbreaks may occur. Older children and adults are only occasionally affected. Although *S. pyogenes* is usually the causative agent, *S. aureus* is often present and sometimes appears to play a pathogenic role.

Impetigo begins as a pruritic, focal, superficial eruption of small 1- to 2-mm vesicles, often on the face near the nares or on the chin. There is usually no history of preceding trauma. In several days the vesicles change to pustules that break, become crusted, and have an erythematous base. Regional lymphadenopathy is common, but there are no constitutional symptoms. The process may spread due to scratching, or remain localized. Healing occurs without scarring. Streptococcal impetigo may recur if personal hygiene is not improved.

A *bullous form of impetigo* is caused by *S. aureus*. It can cause epidemics among newborns but occurs only sporadically among children; adult cases are uncommon. The process begins as a macular erythematous rash. The characteristic thin-walled, fluid-filled, superficial bullae appear within 1 to 3 days, range from 1 to several centimeters in diameter, and usually involve exposed areas of the body. These rupture, desquamation occurs, and healing without scarring follows in about 7 days. In its most dramatic form, this process causes the "scalded skin" syndrome, a disease of small children in which there is extensive superficial desquamation.

Ecthyma

Ecthyma occurs under the same conditions of poor hygiene that promote streptococcal impetigo. It is characterized by discrete ulcerating lesions (3 to 10 mm diameter) with an adherent necrotic crust and surrounding erythema; a small amount of pus often underlies the crust. The ulcer is sufficiently deep to cause permanent scarring. Lesions are most common on the anterior tibial surface at sites of minor trauma or insect bites. Untreated, the lesions tend to spread distally and there may be associated lymphadenopathy; systemic symptoms, however, are lacking. Cultures of pus may yield both *S. pyogenes* and *S. aureus*, but the former appear to play the major pathogenic role.

Erysipelas

Erysipelas involves progressive, often rapid spread of infection through superficial layers of skin and lymphatics. It may occur after a minor wound in normal skin but is more likely when prior injury or disease has impaired the lymphatic or venous drainage of the skin or left extensive scarring, as for example in a patient with chronic venous insufficiency of the lower extremities or with a radical mastectomy.

The infection is characterized by a rapidly spreading area of marked erythema with warmth, local pain, an elevated sharp margin between involved and uninvolved skin, and firm edema that gives the skin a typical "orange peel" appearance. Fluctuation and dermal necrosis are lacking, although there may be seropurulent drainage at the inoculation site. Erythema frequently extends centrally along superficial draining lymphatics; regional lymph nodes are often enlarged and tender. Systemic toxicity, chills, and fever are common. If untreated, metastatic infection may occur, and there is appreciable mortality. Facial infections are dangerous because of possible intracranial spread via draining lymphatics or veins. Extensive involvement of the trunk causes increased morbidity and a risk of mortality.

Almost all episodes of erysipelas are due to S. pyogenes, although a very few are due to S. aureus and these cannot always be distinguished clinically. Infections resembling erysipelas may also be caused by *Pasteurella multocida* or *Erysipelothrix rhusiopathiae* (see Table 25.4).

Management

Bacterial cultures of the lesions of impetigo, bullous impetigo, and ecthyma are not usually helpful. Impetigo and ecthyma may reveal mixed cultures of S. pyogenes and S. aureus, whereas lesions of bullous impetigo are frequently sterile. Similarly, cultures of early and mild erysipelas are unnecessary. In contrast, blood cultures should be obtained when erysipelas is extensive or associated with marked systemic toxicity [(e.g., temperature greater than 102–161°F (39–61°C)], shaking chills, severe malaise. Should there be seropurulent drainage at the site of inoculation, this should be cultured as well. Placing the culture swab in a transport medium, such as Carey-Blair medium, preserves the specimen until it reaches the diagnostic laboratory. Attempts to isolate the organism by culturing sterile saline injected and withdrawn at the edge of the lesion are usually unrewarding.

Systemic antibiotic therapy is required for all streptococcal and related skin infections (Tables 25.1 and 25.2). In general, an oral penicillin is adequate except in persons with disease likely to be due to S. aureus (e.g., bullous impetigo), with extensive infection associated with systemic toxicity, or with suspected penicillin allergy. Erythromycin is an acceptable substitute in patients who cannot receive penicillin. Tetracycline should not be substituted as many strains of

Table 25.1.
Antibiotic Selection for Skin Infections Due to *Streptococcus pyogenes* or *Staphylococcus aureus*

Infection	Antibiotic[a]	
STREPTOCOCCAL INFECTIONS		
Impetigo	Benzathine penicillin	(i.m.)
	Penicillin V	(oral)
	Erythromycin	(oral)
Ecthyma	As for impetigo	
Erysipelas—mild	Penicillin V	(oral)
	Erythromycin	(oral)
Erysipelas—severe	Penicillin G	(i.v.)
STAPHYLOCOCCAL INFECTIONS		
Folliculitis	None	
Furunculosis, boils	Dicloxacillin	(oral)
	Erythromycin	(oral)
Bullous impetigo	As for furunculosis	
Carbuncle	Dicloxacillin	(oral)
	Nafcillin	(i.v.)
	Vancomycin	(i.v.)
Cellulitis	As for carbuncle	

[a] A single antibiotic is given. Choices are in order of preference and include an alternate choice for patients allergic to penicillin. See the text for duration of therapy and adjunctive treatment. Dosage recommendations are in Table 25.2.

Table 25.2.
Antibiotic Dosage and Schedule for Skin Infections Due to *Streptococcus pyogenes* and *Staphylococcus aureus* in Adults[a]

Antibiotic	Dosage
AMBULATORY TREATMENT: MILD INFECTION	
Benzathine penicillin	1,200,000 units i.m., once
Penicillin V	500 mg p.o. 3 times/day
Erythromycin	250–500 mg p.o. 3 times/day
Dicloxacillin	250 mg p.o. 3 times/day
PARENTERAL TREATMENT: SEVERE INFECTION	
Penicillin G	600,000–2,000,000 units i.v. every 6 hours
Nafcillin	1.0–1.5 g i.v. every 4 hours
Vancomycin	0.25–0.5 g i.v. every 6 hours

[a] Choice of antibiotics for specific infections is described in the text and summarized in Table 25.1. The duration of therapy is described in the text.

S. pyogenes are resistant to it. To eradicate group A streptococci, antibiotic treatment should routinely be given for 10 days, even though marked improvement may occur earlier.

Streptococcal impetigo and ecthyma are treated similarly. Penicillin V given orally is adequate. A single parenteral injection of benzathine penicillin is also effective and assures adequate duration of therapy. Oral erythromycin is a satisfactory alternative. Adjunctive therapy includes careful daily soaking of lesions to remove crusted debris using warm water with an iodophor (a *soap* that releases iodine in a nontoxic, nonstaining form, e.g., Betadine skin cleanser) or with a soap that contains hexachlorophene (e.g., pHisoHex). Topically applied antibiotics are of little value and should not be used. Prevention depends primarily upon improved personal hygiene; the most important preventive measure is careful frequent skin cleansing with soap and water.

Treatment of *bullous impetigo* is directed at penicillin-resistant staphylococci. The same treatment should be used for the small portion of patients with impetigo that does not respond to treatment with penicillin V; in such patients S. aureus appears to play a pathogenic role, and antistaphylococcal therapy is usually effective. Oral dicloxacillin is suitable, with erythromycin as an effective alternative.

Minor episodes of *erysipelas* may be treated with oral penicillin V or erythromycin. Careful local application of moist heat to the affected area appears to hasten clearing of the infection. Serious episodes are those with marked systemic toxicity, extensive lesions, facial lesions, or those occurring in compromised hosts, e.g., diabetics. Such patients usually require hospitalization and more intensive antibiotic treatment (Tables 25.1 and 25.2). Special attention should also be paid to patients with atherosclerotic peripheral vascular disease who have infections of their lower extremities. In such patients, the affected leg should be rested and elevated; sustained pressure on any part of the leg or foot should be avoided.

Persons with pre-existing damage to the veins or lymphatics of an extremity may experience repeated episodes of erysipelas that cause further damage. Patients who have numerous recurrent infections should receive continuous antibiotic prophylaxis with penicillin V (250 mg twice daily), benzathine penicillin (600,000 units intramuscularly monthly), or erythromycin (250 mg twice daily). Reduction of chronic edema by fitted pressure stockings or by diuretics helps to reduce susceptibility to this infection.

Superficial skin infections respond rapidly to appropriate therapy. Systemic toxicity and erythema associated with erysipelas usually abate within 3 or 4 days, and discrete skin lesions show marked healing within 10 days. During this period, activity should be restricted in accord with the extent of morbidity. Minor lesions require no restrictions. Persons with any form of impetigo should avoid contact with infants and small children until lesions heal.

Complications

Streptococcal skin infections do not cause rheumatic fever but may cause acute glomerulonephritis, if the streptococcal strain is nephritogenic. Nephritis is not prevented by antibiotic therapy. The average latency period between initial symptoms of a streptococcal skin infection and the onset of glomerulonephritis is 2 weeks. Therefore, if a nephritogenic strain is known to be present in the community, initial and 14-day follow-up evaluation should include a urinalysis. The majority of patients who develop poststreptococcal glomerulonephritis are asymptomatic; but in some, glomerulonephritis will first be suggested by gross hematuria, acute hypertension, or signs of salt and water retention, such as dependent edema or congestive heart failure.

Bacteremia with metastatic infection may complicate neglected or severe episodes of erysipelas. Metastatic infection should be considered in patients with severe disease who respond poorly to treatment or

develop findings suggestive of distant localized infection. Possible metastatic infections include meningitis, endocarditis, septic arthritis, infection of pre-existing pleural effusions or ascites, or solid organ abscesses, e.g., in the liver or spleen.

PUSTULAR INFECTIONS CAUSED BY *STAPHYLOCOCCUS AUREUS*

These infections include folliculitis, furunculosis, hydradenitis suppurativa, and carbuncles. They represent increasingly severe effects of the infection of hair follicles, sebaceous glands, or sweat glands by S. aureus, the end result being inflammation and abscess formation.

Folliculitis

Folliculitis involves minor inflammation of individual hair follicles, often with formation of small superficial pustules. There is little pain or surrounding erythema. In some persons, lesions may recur for months or even years. A common area of involvement is the bearded part of the face in which minor trauma from shaving may be a contributing factor.

Furunculosis

Deeper infection of follicles or of cutaneous glands leads to formation of pustular furuncles (boils are large furuncles). These lesions range in diameter from about 5 mm to 2 to 3 cm and occur most commonly on hairy areas exposed to friction, trauma, or maceration, e.g., the buttocks, neck, face, axillae, groin, forearms, thighs, and upper back. Furunculosis may also complicate the acne of adolescence. Furuncles begin with pruritus, local tenderness, and erythema, followed by swelling and marked local pain. As pus forms in the center of the lesion, the overlying skin becomes thin, the lesion becomes elevated, pain increases, and spontaneous drainage of pus ultimately occurs, usually with prompt relief of pain and rapid healing. Furunculosis may be a recurrent problem in some persons, especially diabetics and persons who are chronic nasal carriers of S. aureus.

Hydradenitis Suppurativa

This is a particular form of furunculosis due to obstruction of apocrine sweat glands, usually in the axilla, perineum, or groin. The process is chronic, perpetuated in part by the scars, abscesses, and sinus tracts that develop in the involved skin.

Carbuncles

A carbuncle is a coalescent mass of deeply infected follicles or sebaceous glands with multiple interconnecting sinus tracts and cutaneous openings that drain pus ineffectively. Carbuncles usually occur in the thick skin on the back of the neck or the upper back. Once formed, the lesions steadily worsen, with increasing pain, erythema, swelling, purulent drainage, and lateral enlargement; they vary in diameter from 3 to 10 cm or larger. Fever and systemic toxicity are common. Carbuncles occur with increased frequency in diabetics. Once established, they may recur in the damaged area of skin.

Management

Bacterial cultures of typical lesions are usually unnecessary since virtually all are caused by S. aureus and most isolates will prove resistant to penicillin G.

Minimal lesions, such as *folliculitis*, require little therapy. Careful, twice daily cleansing with a mild soap, preferably one containing hexachlorophene, and avoidance of minor trauma and irritants, such as cosmetics or abrasive soaps, are usually sufficient.

Furuncles should be managed initially by application of warm moist heat (either as moist compresses or baths) for about 30 minutes four times a day. Small lesions, i.e., those less than 1 cm in diameter, will often drain spontaneously after 1 to 3 days and require no further treatment. Larger lesions, painful lesions, or lesions that do not drain spontaneously should be drained surgically when they have localized and are fluctuant. This can be done in the office by making a single incision into the abscess with a scalpel, after the incision line has been infiltrated with 0.5 or 1.0% lidocaine for local anesthesia. Lifting the anesthetized skin with a towel clip when the incision is made helps to avoid pain due to downward pressure from the scalpel. Antimicrobial therapy is not required except for more extensive lesions such as multiple furuncles, carbuncles, or lesions associated with marked surrounding inflammation. In such cases oral dicloxacillin or erythromycin (Tables 25.1 and 25.2) should be given until signs of inflammation completely subside, which may take 2 weeks or longer. *Carbuncles* may require extensive surgical drainage, which is best done in a hospital. Patients with severe systemic toxicity, such as diabetics with carbuncles, require parenteral therapy with a penicillinase-resistant penicillin; vancomycin is an effective alternative for those allergic to penicillin.

Recurrent furunculosis may prove a frustrating problem. Management of individual episodes is as described above, but other steps should also be taken to eliminate colonization with staphylococci. The anterior nares should be cultured to determine whether they are the likely source of the reinfecting staphylococci. Patients with positive nasal cultures should be treated by application of bacitracin ointment to the anterior nares three or four times daily for 14 days. Prolonged therapy with bacitracin ointment may be needed if cultures become positive upon cessation of treatment. Bacterial contamination of skin should be meticulously controlled by having the patient bathe and shampoo three times daily with a hexachlorophene soap, and by daily changes of bed and bath linens.

Recurrent furunculosis may occur in certain disorders that impair host defenses. Tests for diabetes mellitus should be made; if positive, control of blood glucose may prove beneficial (see Chapter 72). Defects in polymorphonuclear leukocyte function are a rare cause of recurrent furunculosis but should be considered in patients who show an increased incidence or severity of infections due to staphylococci, Gram-negative bacteria and fungi may be cultured from the furuncles of such patients. If an unusual problem such as a leukocyte defect is suspected, the patient should be referred to a medical center where there may be the capability to investigate such problems.

Hydradenitis suppurativa is an extremely difficult problem that requires prolonged, often lifelong, treatment by multiple methods. These include selective surgical drainage of abscesses; elimination of irritants, such as tight clothing, antiperspirants, and shaving of the axillae; careful frequent cleansing of skin with antiseptic agents; local application of heat; intermittent or chronic systemic antibiotic therapy; and in some cases local irradiation or excisional surgery. Management of such patients is best done by physicians especially skilled in the treatment of skin disorders. (See additional discussion in Chapter 100, Common Problems of the Skin.)

Complications

Staphylococcal skin infections may spread to other sites. This is especially true in patients with extensive inflammation and systemic toxicity, such as those with carbuncles, in whom bacteremia is common. However, even an innocent appearing furuncle may cause metastatic infection, especially in patients with a focus of increased susceptibility, such as a ventricular septal defect, valvular heart disease, or an arthritic joint. Patients at risk of bacteremia who have such preexisting susceptible foci, or whose systemic complaints (fever, focal pain) persist despite antibiotic treatment, should be carefully examined for metastatic infection.

CELLULITIS AND OTHER WOUND INFECTIONS

Any break in the skin may become infected. This includes not only obvious trauma, such as lacerations, burns, abrasions, and animal or human bites, but also minor defects such as scratches and insect bites. The features of the resultant infection vary widely; they depend upon the nature of the wound, the type of infecting organism(s), and the defensive responses of the infected person. In many instances, early appropriate management given on an ambulatory basis is sufficient. In others, recognition of serious infection and prompt hospitalization for vigorous medical and/or surgical treatment are of prime importance. Table 25.3 describes findings that require hospitalization and/or surgical intervention. Table 25.4 lists organisms that may cause life-threatening forms of cellulitis.

Table 25.3.
Wound Infections: Findings That Necessitate Hospitalization and/or Surgical Intervention

Finding	Comment
Extensive cellulitis or erysipelas with systemic toxicity	Needs parenteral antibiotics, close observation
Diminished arterial pulse in cool, swollen, pale, infected extremity	Possible fasciitis, a surgical emergency
Cellulitis with cutaneous necrosis and/or subcutaneous gas	Needs parenteral antibiotics and possible surgical drainage/debridement
Closed space infections of the hand	Needs surgical drainage

Table 25.4.
Causes of Life-Threatening Bacterial Cellulitis

Cause	Important Features
Gram-negative enteric bacilli, especially *Escherichia coli*	Occur in fecally contaminated wounds; gas may be present; surgical drainage required for gas or pus
Mixed anaerobic and enteric aerobic bacteria	Occur in fecally contaminated wounds; gas may be present; symptoms may progress rapidly and may include exquisite pain; surgical drainage required
Bacillus anthracis	Causes anthrax when minor wound is inoculated by spore-contaminated animal products (animal hides and hair, especially from goats); local chancre-like lesion develops followed by systemic toxicity
Erysipelothrix rhusiopathiae	Erysipelas-like lesion with central clearing; due to wound contamination with fish or meat products; treated with penicillin V or tetracycline
Pasteurella multocida	Erysipelas-like lesion which folllows a dog or cat scratch or bite; treated with penicillin V or tetracycline
Marine vibrios	Necrotizing cellulitis after minor wound is contaminated by sea water or contact with shellfish
Aeromonas hydrophilia	Wound contaminated by fresh water swimming

Cellulitis Due to *S. Pyogenes* and *S. Aureus*

Acute cellulitis is a spreading infection of skin and subcutaneous tissues. The involved area, which enlarges steadily, is painful, tender, and intensely erythematous. Chills and fever are common and bacteremia may occur. The lesion differs from erysipelas in that its margin is not as sharply demarcated nor is it elevated. There may be purulent or serous drainage at the inoculation site; in severe cases, patches of involved skin may become necrotic.

The most common causes of acute cellulitis are S. pyogenes and S. aureus. Presence of Gram-positive cocci in drainage from the wound is presumptive evidence that they are causative. Infection due to these agents may progress rapidly, especially when it involves an area of chronic edema. Lower extremity infection in persons with peripheral arterial insufficiency

may precipitate tissue necrosis and secondary infection.

Management of cellulitis should include culture of any wound drainage (as described for erysipelas) and prompt antibiotic therapy. In mild cases, treatment may be given on an ambulatory basis. The treatment selected should be effective for infections due to penicillin-resistant staphylococci, as well as penicillin-sensitive streptococci. Oral dicloxacillin is adequate for infections due to either type of organism; erythromycin is a suitable choice for patients allergic to penicillin (Tables 25.1 and 25.2). Local application of moist heat is a useful adjunct to antibiotic treatment; care should be taken, however, to avoid burns, especially in persons with impaired sensitivity to pain. Improvement is usually apparent in 3 or 4 days; during this period, patients should rest the involved area (with elevation when the cellulitis involves an extremity) and be told to report promptly any worsening of the infection or of constitutional symptoms. Severe infections require hospitalization and parenteral treatment with a penicillinase-resistant penicillin or vancomycin. This includes patients with extensive lesions, lesions of the face, or serious toxicity.

Secondarily Infected Ulcers

Cutaneous ulcers are caused by a wide variety of conditions including peripheral vascular disease, arterial insufficiency, pressure sores, neurological disorders, etc. Management of the ulcer is generally aimed at the underlying cause and seeks to improve blood flow, reduce edema, and avoid pressure and trauma (see Chapter 88). Control of secondary infection is also of considerable importance. Superficial colonization with a variety of bacteria is unavoidable and without consequence; however, infection that is deeper or laterally invasive prevents healing and may interfere with other treatments, such as skin grafting. Infection is best controlled by repeated careful cleaning and local debridement. Systemic antibiotics should be used only when all other methods fail to control surrounding infection. The choice of antibiotic should be based on cultures of the wound or its purulent drainage. Local antibacterials are sometimes helpful. Those effective against a broad spectrum of bacterial agents include polymyxin-bacitracin-neomycin ointment and topical nitrofurazone (Furacin ointment); these should be applied three times daily until healing occurs or until it is apparent they are ineffective. Soaking with 3% acetic acid three to four times daily is helpful in controlling bacterial growth in ulcers colonized with *Pseudomonas aeruginosa*.

Cutaneous Diphtheria

Cutaneous ulcers or other skin lesions may become secondarily infected with *Corynebacterium diphtheriae*, causing cutaneous diphtheria. Although the cutaneous lesion may appear benign, myocarditis or neuropathy develops in about 3% of cases. Outbreaks have occurred in the northwest and southwest parts of the United States, primarily among Native Americans or urban indigents. The presence of cutaneous diphtheria in a community should increase suspicion that skin wounds may harbor this agent. The diagnosis should be suspected when existing wounds develop a gray-yellow or gray-brown covering membrane and surrounding erythema (1). Typically, the membrane can be easily removed to reveal a clean base. Other minor skin lesions may also become infected. Typical organisms can be seen in methylene blue stains of smears from the wound and confirmed by culture on Loeffler's or tellurite agar. Presumptive cases should be reported to public health officials and treated with equine diphtheria antitoxin (20,000 to 40,000 units intramuscularly or intravenously after testing for hypersensitivity to horse serum) and either erythromycin (1.5 g/day, orally) or procaine penicillin (1.2 million units/day, intramuscularly) for 7 to 10 days.

Bites

Bite wounds become infected with the oral, salivary, or dental flora of the biting person or animal and may cause serious local or systemic infections. Initial management before signs of infection appear is of primary importance in preventing certain infections. Appropriate prophylaxis for tetanus is required for all bite wounds (see Chapter 32).

Human bites are contaminated with a complex variety of aerobic and anaerobic oral bacteria. Without treatment, a severe necrotizing cellulitis frequently results. Minor lesions that break the skin should be washed thoroughly and treated with a combination of dicloxacillin (250 mg three times/day) and ampicillin (500 mg three times/day) given orally; oral clindamycin (150 to 300 mg three times/day) is appropriate for patients allergic to penicillin. Antibiotics should be continued for 7 to 10 days. More severe wounds, including wounds of the hands and knuckles, require meticulous debridement and possible tendon repairs. These should be referred for surgical management.

Dog bites carry the risk of local soft tissue infection and raise concern about rabies. Minor abrasions, shallow punctures, or superficial lacerations require no therapy for local infection other than thorough cleansing with soap and water. More extensive or deeper bites require surgical management for debridement and, in some cases, primary closure; ampicillin (500 mg by mouth three times/day for 7 days) should also be given. Rabies precautions should be taken with all dog bites, including bites by domestic pets, even though the risk of rabies from domestic pets—especially when biting was provoked—is very small. The dog should be quarantined for 10 days. If it is a dog whose owner cannot be identified, the local health department should be called to take charge of the dog. If its owner is known, it may be observed at its home. If it remains well, there is no risk of rabies. If the dog develops suspicious symptoms or dies, its brain should be examined immediately; prophylaxis is required if evidence of ra-

bies is found. If the dog escapes after biting, and especially if the bite was unprovoked, rabies prophylaxis with rabies immune globulin and human diploid cell rabies vaccine is usually indicated (see Chapter 32).

Bites by other domestic animals, e.g., cats, should be managed in the same way as dog bites are managed. Bites by *wild animals* carry a greater risk of rabies and are treated similarly, except that rabies prophylaxis is usually required (unless the animal's brain can be examined). Wild animals with the greatest risk of carrying rabies include raccoons, skunks, foxes, coyotes, and bats. The risk of rabies with rodent bites, including squirrel bites, is very small; the local health department should be consulted regarding the need for rabies prophylaxis after a rodent bite (2).

Guidance on the use of rabies prophylaxis, management of the biting animal, and the risk of rabies among various animal species should be sought from local or state health authorities.

Puncture Wounds

Most puncture wounds involve the feet or hands and carry the risk of introduction of infecting bacteria that cannot be removed by washing or debridement. In all instances, patients should receive appropriate prophylaxis for tetanus (see Chapter 32). Low risk wounds, i.e., those not likely to be contaminated by soil or fecal material and in which the wound site is healthy, well-vascularized tissue, need only be thoroughly washed and observed for several days for signs of developing infection. Should infection develop, any wound drainage should be cultured and treatment begun with dicloxacillin (250 mg three times daily) or erythromycin (250 to 500 mg three times daily) for presumptive staphylococcal or streptococcal infection; the wound site should also be soaked in warm soapy water for 30 minutes at least four times a day. Higher risk wounds, i.e., those likely to be contaminated with fecal material, soil, or foreign debris, or occurring in a diabetic or in an extremity with an inadequate blood supply, should be treated with an antibiotic from the outset (adults: ciprofloxacin 750 mg every 12 hours; children below 15 years: one of the antibiotics above), and the wound site should be rested and treated with warm soaks as above. The patient should promptly report any evidence of inflammation, swelling, or persisting pain. If purulent drainage develops, this should be cultured. Antibiotic management will need to be altered if bacteria resistant to the current treatment are isolated. If pus develops, surgical drainage is usually required.

Felon

A felon is an infection of the pulp of the distal phalanx of a finger; it usually follows a recognized local wound. Abscess formation and tissue necrosis are common, and bony or articular involvement may occur. If neglected or inadequately treated, severe damage, including loss of function, may occur. The most common causative agents are *S. aureus* and *S. pyogenes*, although Gram-negative bacilli may occasionally be recovered. Treatment involves surgical drainage, and this should be done by an experienced surgeon. Concurrent antibiotic therapy should be guided by Gram stain and culture of infected material.

Paronychia

A paronychia is an infection, often chronic or recurrent, which involves tissue immediately adjacent to a fingernail. The affected tissue is warm, tensely swollen, erythematous, and painful. When infection is chronic, the nail may become ridged or discolored and may be lost. These infections occur most frequently in persons who bite their nails excessively and in persons whose hands are frequently in water, for example, in mothers of infants or in dishwashers. Diabetics also have an increased risk of this infection. *Candida* species appear to play an etiological role, although a variety of bacteria are also usually present. Management involves keeping hands as dry as possible (e.g., using waterproof gloves for dishwashing) and applying amphotericin B ointment or cream (Fungizone) two to four times a day for several weeks. When localized swelling does not respond to these measures, surgical drainage may be helpful.

The major cause of paronychia of the toe (usually a great toe) is an ingrown toenail. Diagnosis and management of this problem are described in Chapter 102.

Intertriginous Infections

Approaches to diagnosis of infections involving moist intertriginous areas (toe webs, axillae, groin area) are described in Chapter 100.

General References

Koblenzer PJ: Common bacterial infections of the skin in children. *Pediatr Clin North Am* 25:321, 1978.
> A useful review of the subject with excellent pictures of typical lesions.
Musher DM, McKenzie SO: Infections due to *Staphylococcus aureus*. *Medicine (Baltimore)* 56:383, 1977.
> Review article with a section on staphylococcal skin infections, including those that resemble erysipelas.
Peter G, Smith AL: Group A streptococcal infections of the skin and pharynx. *N Engl J Med* 297:311, 1977.
> An excellent, thorough review of basic and clinical features of streptococcal skin infections.
Wannamaker LW: Differences between streptococcal infections of the throat and of the skin. *N Engl J Med* 282:23, 1970.
> A scholarly discussion by an expert on the subject.
Witkowski JA, Parish LL: Bacterial skin infections. Management of common streptococcal and staphylococcal lesions. *Postgrad Med* 72:166, 1982.
> A practical review of the features and treatment of these infections with excellent photographs of typical infections.

Specific References

1. Belsey MA, Sinclair M, Roder MR, LeBlanc DR: *Corynebacterium diphtheriae* skin infections in Alabama and Louisiana: a factor in the epidemiology of diphtheria. *N Engl J Med* 280:135, 1969.
2. Rabies prevention—United States. *MMWR* 33:393, 1984.

C H A P T E R   26

Acute Gastroenteritis and Associated Conditions

R. BRADLEY SACK, M.D. Sc.D.
L. RANDOL BARKER, M.D.

Acute symptoms of gastroenteritis may follow the ingestion of a wide variety of infectious and chemical agents. Ingestion may occur because of direct person-to-person contact or, more commonly, via food or water. With several important exceptions, the acute illnesses caused by these agents are characterized by diarrhea, with or without other gastrointestinal symptoms (nausea, vomiting, abdominal pain), or systemic symptoms (anorexia, fever, malaise, orthostatic hypotension, neurological symptoms).

Diarrhea is defined as an increase in frequency and/or amount of fecal evacuations, which are usually fluid (see Chapter 39). The diarrhea of gastroenteritis usually begins abruptly, sometimes preceded by systemic symptoms, and the hour of onset can usually be documented by the patient. With few exceptions, the illness is self-limited and will terminate within 1 to 5 days.

Tables 26.1 (infectious agents) and 26.2 (chemical agents) summarize the etiological agents, pathophysiology, clinical and epidemiological features, and principles of diagnosis and treatment for those conditions that may occur in the United States.

EPIDEMIOLOGY

The *incidence* of the conditions listed in Tables 26.1 and 26.2 varies from year to year; and the true incidence is never known since a large proportion of cases are not reported to physicians or health authorities. Even when outbreaks of gastroenteritis involving mul-

Table 26.1.
Characteristics of Acute Illness Due to Ingestion of Infectious Agents

Agent	Pathogenesis	Usual Clinical Features	Frequency in USA	Usual pattern[a]	Source (reservoir)	Transmission to Man	Incubation Period	Diagnosis	Specific Therapy
BACTERIA									
Bacillus cereus	Enterotoxin produced in food or in intestine	Vomiting if preformed toxin in food, diarrhea	Not common	CSO	Soil	Foodborne	2–16 hr	Culture suspected food	None
Helicobacter jejuni (3)	Invasion of large and small intestine	Fever, abdominal pain, diarrhea	Relatively common	S or CSO	Animal feces	Foodborne or waterborne[b]	24–48 hr	Culture stool, blood	Erythromycin (see text)
Clostridium botulinum	Neurotoxin produced in food	Vomiting, diarrhea, symmetric motor paralysis: cranial nerves, respiratory paralysis, death	Uncommon	CSO	Animal feces, soil	Foodborne (canned, low pH, anaerobic)	12–36 hr	Culture food, identify toxin in food, blood, stool	Polyvalent antitoxin
Clostridium difficile	Cytotoxic enterotoxin produced in large intestine secondary to overgrowth	Fever, abdominal pain, diarrhea (often bloody) in a patient currently or recently on antibiotics	Uncommon (hospitalized or recently hospitalized patients)	S	Humans (normal intestinal flora) or environment (spores)	Probably not necessary but may occur in hospitals[b]	1–10 days after beginning antibiotics (rarely up to 6 weeks after antibiotics stopped)	Culture stool, identify enterotoxin in stool	Metronidazole or Vancomycin (see text)
Clostridium perfringens	Enterotoxin released during sporulation in large intestine	Diarrhea, occasionally vomiting	Relatively common	CSO	Human feces, animal feces, soil	Foodborne (meats)	12–24 hr	Culture suspected food	None
Escherichia coli (13)									
Enterotoxigenic	Enterotoxin produced in small intestine	Voluminous watery diarrhea without fever (traveler's diarrhea)	Relatively common (travelers)	CSO, S	Human feces	Foodborne	24–48 hr	Culture stool, identify enterotoxin production by bacteria	None
Invasive	Invasion of large intestinal mucosa	Fever, diarrhea (often bloody)	Rare	CSO, S	Human feces	Foodborne (cheeses)	24–48 hr	Culture stool	Same as *Shigella* (see text)
Adherent (4, 20)	Adheres tightly to small bowel mucosa	Acute diarrhea, which may be prolonged	Unknown, probably uncommon	S	Human feces	Probably foodborne	24–48 hrs	Culture stool, small bowel	Antibiotics to which organism is sensitive
Hemorrhagic (16)	Cytotoxin produced in large bowel	Hemorrhagic colitis, may be followed by hemolytic uremic syndrome	Uncommon	CSO	Animal feces	Foodborne	24–48 hrs	Culture stool	None
Salmonella (many species)	Invasion of small and large intestine	Fever and diarrhea (see Table 26.3)	Relatively common	CSO	Animal feces	Foodborne (many foods, see text) person-to-person[b]	12–48 hrs	Culture stool	Ampicillin or Chloramphenicol, in selected cases only (see text)
Salmonella typhi	Invasion of small intestine mucosa, systemic dissemination	Protracted illness: fever, malaise, headache, constipation more often than diarrhea, splenomegaly, occasionally intestinal perforation	Uncommon	S	Human feces	Person-to-person, foodborne[b]	4 days–3 weeks	Culture blood, stool, antibacterial antibodies	Chloramphenicol
Shigella species	Invasion of large intestine	Fever, diarrhea (often bloody) (see Table 26.3)	Relatively common	S	Human feces	Person-to-person[b]	12–48 hr	Culture stool	Trimethoprim-Sulfamethoxazole (see text)

Organism	Mechanism	Clinical features	Frequency		Reservoir	Transmission	Incubation period	Diagnosis	Treatment
Staphylococcus aureus (10)	Enterotoxin produced in food	Vomiting dominates, diarrhea (see Table 26:3)	Very common	CSO	Human skin, nares, mouth	Foodborne (many foods, see text)	2–8 hr	Culture food, and food handlers	None
Streptococcus group A	Invasion of upper respiratory tract	Streptococcal pharyngitis syndrome (see Chapter 28)	Uncommon (by this mode of transmission)	CSO	Human pharynx, skin lesions	Foodborne	1–3 days	Culture throat, food, skin lesions of food handlers	Penicillin (see Chapter 28)
Vibrio cholerae (14)	Enterotoxin produced in small intestine	Voluminous watery diarrhea without fever	Rare	CSO, S	Human feces	Waterborne and food borne	12 hr–5 days	Culture stool, antibacterial and antitoxic antibody	Tetracycline
Vibrio parahaemolyticus	Probably both invasion and enterotoxin production; exact mechanism unknown	Diarrhea, abdominal cramps	Uncommon	CSO, S	Seawater	Foodborne (various types of seafood from estuary and seawater)	15–24 hr	Culture stool	None
Yersinia enterocolitica (19)	Invasion of small and large intestine	Fever, abdominal pain, may suggest appendicitis, diarrhea	Uncommon	CSO, S	Animal feces	Foodborne, person-to-person	Probably 3–7 days	Culture stool	Probably tetracycline or trimethoprim-sulfamethoxazole

VIRUS

Organism	Mechanism	Clinical features	Frequency		Reservoir	Transmission	Incubation period	Diagnosis	Treatment
Parvovirus-like agents (Norwalk agent) (12)	Invasion of small intestine	Vomiting and diarrhea (see Table 26.3)	(may be relatively common)	CSO	Human feces	Food and waterborne, person-to-person (secondary cases)	1–3 days	Rise in antiviral antibody (not generally available)	None
Rotavirus (11, 23)	Invasion of small intestine	Severe gastroenteritis in young children, mild in adults	Relatively common	S	Human feces	Person-to-person (secondary cases)	1–3 days	Virus antigen in stool; Rise in antiviral antibody	None

PROTOZOA AND HELMINTHS

Organism	Mechanism	Clinical features	Frequency		Reservoir	Transmission	Incubation period	Diagnosis	Treatment
Entamoeba histolytica (8)	Invasion of large intestine	Diarrhea, often chronic and bloody	Uncommon (travelers)	CSO, S	Human feces	Food and waterborne, person-to-person[b]	Few days to months	Examine stool for trophozoites	Metronidazole or quinacrine (see text)
Giardia lamblia (18)	Colonization and occasional invasion of small intestine	Diarrhea, flatulence with foul-smelling stools	Uncommon (travelers)	CSO, S	Human feces	Waterborne, person-to-person[b]	1–4 weeks	Examine stool for trophozoites	Metronidazole (see text)
Trichinella spiralis	(a) Encysted trichinae mature, mate, reproduce in small intestine; (b) larvae penetrate intestine, migrate to muscles where they cause inflammation and become encysted	Diarrhea, puffy eyes, muscle aching, fever, occasionally severe heart failure; eosinophilia typical	Uncommon	CSO, S	Animal muscle (swine, many wild animals)	Foodborne	2–28 days	Skin tests, antibody, muscle biopsy	Thiabendazole, occasionally steroids (see text)
Cryptosporidia (5)	Colonization	Diarrhea, acute in children	Chronic in patients with AIDS	S	Human and animal feces	? Probably animal to person[b]	? 2–7 days	Examine stool for trophozoites	None known

[a] CSO, common source outbreak; S, sporadic.
[b] Anal-oral transmission may occur in homosexual men.

Table 26.2.
Characteristics of Acute Illness Due to Ingestion of Chemical Agents[a]

Agent	Pathogenesis	Clinical Features	Epidemiological Features					Diagnosis	Specific Therapy
			Pattern[b]	Source	Transmission to Man	Incubation period	Frequency in USA		
SEAFOOD									
Ciguatoxin	Toxin with character of cholinesterase inhibitor	Vomiting and diarrhea, paresthesia (warmth, extremities), metallic taste, blurred vision, sharp pains in extremities, respiratory paralysis	CSO, S	Food chain of bottom-dwelling fish caught in Florida, Hawaii (red snapper, barracuda)	Foodborne	1–6 hr	Uncommon (Florida)	Clinical and epidemiological features	None (sensory symptoms may last days to months)
Scombrotoxin	Toxin with properties of histamine	Histamine reaction (flushing, headache, dizziness, burning of mouth and throat; urticaria, pruritus, and bronchospasm)	CSO, S	Bacteria acting on fish flesh (tuna, mackerel, bonito, skipjack)	Foodborne	Minutes to 1 hr	Uncommon (Florida, California)	Clinical and epidemiological features	None (lasts few hours–few days)
Paralytic shellfish toxin	Neurotoxin causing motor paralysis	Paresthesia (warmth, extremities), floating sensation, dysphonia, dysphagia, weakness, and respiratory paralysis	CSO, S	Toxic dinoflagellates concentrated in filter feeding bivalves (mussels, clams, oysters, scallops)	Foodborne	<30 min	Uncommon	Clinical and epidemiological features	None (lasts few hours–few days)
MUSHROOMS									
Muscarine	Muscarinic cholinergic response	Colicky abdominal pain, nausea, vomiting, diarrhea, salivation, miosis, blurred vision, bradycardia, hypotension	CSO, S	Amanita muscaria	Foodborne	Few minutes–few hours	Uncommon	Clinical and epidemiological features	Atropine 0.1–0.5 mg s.c. or i.v.
Phalloidin (and other toxins)	Diverse cytotoxic effects, multisystemic	Stage 1: nausea, abdominal pain, vomiting, bloody diarrhea, marked weakness, hypotension (shock) Stage 2: Clinical improvement (day 2 or 3) Stage 3: Severe hepatic failure, delirim frequent fatal outcome	CSO, S	Amanita phalloides and other Amanita species	Foodborne	6–15 hr		Clinical and epidemiological features	None
MISCELLANEOUS									
Heavy metals (antimony, cadmium, copper, iron, tin, zinc)	Upper gastrointestinal irritation	Metallic taste to food, nausea, vomiting, or diarrhea	CSO, S	Containers make of ally which includes a heavy metal	Foodborne (food prepared in, stored in, or eaten from a container from which heavy metal leached)	5 min–8 hr	Uncommon	Clinical and epidemiological features	None
Monosodium glutamate (MSG)	Idiopathic reaction	Burning sensation in chest, neck, abdomen, extremities	S	Foods prepared with large amounts of MSG	Foodborne (Chinese restaurant foods)	3 min–2 hr	Relatively common	Clinical and epidemiological features	None

[a] Data from Gossalin RE, Hodge HC, Smith RP, Gleason MN: *Clinical Toxicology of Commericial Products*, 4th ed. Baltimore, Williams & Wilkins, 1976; and Hughes JM, Merson MH: Current concepts: fish and shellfish poisoning. *N Engl J Med* 295: 1117, 1976.
[b] CSO, common source outbreak, S, sporadic.

tiple persons are fully investigated, the *etiology* can be established with relative certainty only 50 to 75% of the time. Based upon annual surveillance by the United States Centers for Disease Control (CDC), it is known that the majority of reported foodborne outbreaks (and therefore probably the majority of cases) are due to *Staphylococcus aureus*, followed by *Salmonella* species, and *Clostridium perfringens*. The most frequent pathogen isolated in waterborne outbreaks is *Giardia*. Physicians and patients frequently call an illness "viral gastroenteritis," although viral agents probably account for only a modest proportion of acute gastrointestinal illness in adults (21). Studies of outbreaks of viral gastroenteritis in adults have shown that the symptoms it produces overlap with the symptoms produced by several common bacterial pathogens (see Table 26.3). A viral etiology is more likely when secondary cases develop in a household, a pattern that suggests person-to-person spread rather than one-time exposure to a common food.

The *sources and modes of transmission* of the etiological agents causing foodborne illness are summarized in Tables 26.1 and 26.2. These features of the three most common etiological agents illustrate the diverse ways that foodborne disease is acquired:

1. Humans whose skin or nasal mucosa is colonized are almost always the source of *S. aureus*. Contamination of food with small numbers of staphylococci is undoubtedly very common. Staphylococcal food poisoning occurs when contaminated foods are allowed to stand long enough for organisms to multiply and produce enterotoxin. The principal foods in which this occurs are those high in protein (ham, pork, beef, poultry, either cooked or in salads, and cream-filled cakes and pastries) and those with a relatively high salt or sugar content (ham, salads, and custards) (10).
2. Animals are the source of the *Salmonella* serotypes causing most human disease; only *Salmonella typhi* and *Salmonella paratyphi* are carried by humans. Transmission from animal to man occurs chiefly by fecal contamination of equipment and personnel involved in the packaging and preparing of foods—most commonly poultry, red meats, and eggs or their by-products.

3. *C. perfringens* is a ubiquitous organism found in human and animal feces and in soil. Meats are the most frequently contaminated foods; transmission of enough organisms to produce illness occurs typically with inadequately heated or reheated meats (spores may survive at normal cooking temperatures and then germinate and multiply while foods are being held at warm temperatures or being rewarmed at temperatures that do not inhibit bacterial growth).

The vast majority of episodes of foodborne illness follow the ingestion of *normally safe foods*, that have been rendered unsafe due to one or more of the following factors (6): failure to refrigerate foods properly or to heat foods thoroughly, preparing foods a day or more before they are served, allowing foods to remain at warm temperatures, failure to reheat or cook foods at temperatures that kill vegetative bacteria, incorporating raw (contaminated) ingredients into foods that receive no further cooking, failure to clean and disinfect kitchen or processing plant equipment, and contamination by infected food handlers who practice poor personal hygiene.

A small minority of foodborne illnesses are due to the ingestion of *foods that are always unsafe* due to the presence of toxins that cannot be rendered innocuous by cooking or other means, i.e., ciguatoxin, scombratoxin, amanita toxins, paralytic shellfish toxin, mushroom toxin, and heavy metals (7, 9).

The *place of* ingestion of the etiological agent is usually the patient's home or a restaurant, and, less commonly, a social gathering or an institutional eating place.

For many of the conditions listed in Tables 26.1 and 26.2, *individuals are at risk at all ages*, and a single episode may not confer protective immunity against a later episode. However, the vast majority of acute diarrheal episodes occur in children. A particularly high rate of diarrheal illness occurs in people of all ages who travel to developing countries (see Chapter 33).

In the past decade, a wide spectrum of intestinal infections (the *gay bowel syndromes*) has been recognized in homosexual and bisexual men (15). Several factors favor the acquisition and spread of enteric in-

Table 26.3.
Comparison of Symptoms of Viral and Bacterial Gastroenteritis in Adults

Symptom	Percentage with Symptom				
	Viral gastroenteritis		Bacterial gastroenteritis		
	Rotavirus[a]	Norwalk agent[b]	Salmonella[b]	Shigella[b]	Staphylococcus aureus[b]
Nausea	2	85	50	45	62
Vomiting	9	84	23	39	86
Abdominal cramps	26	62	78	60	86
Diarrhea	33	44	73	100	67
Fever	5	32	49	72	10
Headache	NR[c]	37	33	6	8

[a] From Wenman WM, Hinde D, Feltham S, Gurwith M: Rotavirus infection in adults. Results of a prospective family study. *N Engl J Med* 301:303, 1979.
[b] From Adler JL, Zickl R: Winter vomiting disease. *J Infect Dis* 119:668, 1969.
[c] NR = not reported.

fections in this population: (a) oral-genital and genital-anal contact between subjects; (b) exposure to multiple sexual partners; and (c) asymptomatic carriage of enteric pathogens, often more than one. The pathogens transmitted to the gastrointestinal tract by homosexual men include common and uncommon enteric pathogens and also a number of genital pathogens (Table 26.4). The syndromes produced by these infections range from oral ulcerations to gastroenteritis to proctitis. In patients with acquired immune deficiency syndrome (AIDS), a number of agents cause acute and often prolonged diarrhea. *Cryptosporidium* infection, usually a benign self-limited diarrheal illness in children, may cause a prolonged and life-threatening illness in these patients (5). *Isospora belli*, usually not thought of as a diarrheal pathogen, may also cause diarrheal illness in patients with AIDS. Diarrheal illnesses due to *Helicobacter jejuni*, which are usually short illnesses in normal hosts, may be prolonged in AIDS patients (see Chapter 34 for additional discussion of infection in AIDS patients).

PATHOGENESIS

As indicated in Tables 26.1 and 26.2, the majority of the etiological agents produce symptoms due either to inflammation of the gastrointestinal tract or to physiological events related to one or more toxins.

In recent years, the common bacterial diarrheal syndromes have been separated into invasive and enterotoxigenic syndromes (see Table 26.5) (18, 20), an important advance because of the implications for antibiotic treatment. In *invasive disease*, the etiological agent enters the intestinal mucosal cells, often destroying them, and the diarrhea is a result of this destructive process with its accompanying inflammatory response. This usually occurs in the large bowel and produces systemic symptoms (particularly fever), local symptoms (tenesmus, abdominal discomfort), and frequent small amounts of stool that contain pus cells

and often blood. Shigellosis is the prototype of this syndrome. In *enterotoxigenic diarrhea*, the organisms do not invade tissue but colonize and multiply on the small bowel mucosal surface; during this process they produce enterotoxins, which act as chemical mediators and cause hypersecretion of fluid and electrolytes by the small bowel. Little tissue damage is produced, and inflammation of the mucosa is minimal. Symptoms consist of simple watery diarrhea (which may be voluminous), accompanied by minimal systemic signs, unless dehydration becomes significant. The prototypes of this syndrome are diarrheas caused by *Vibrio cholerae* and by enterotoxigenic *Escherichia coli* (13, 14).

More recently, strains of *E. coli* have been characterized that neither invade mucosal cells nor produce enterotoxins, but they tightly adhere to the mucosal surface and produce diarrhea presumably by interfering with normal absorptive processes. These strains produce diarrhea primarily in small children, and many belong to the classical "enteropathogenic" serotypes (4, 20).

A new syndrome of *hemorrhagic colitis* has recently been described that is caused by strains of *E. coli* that produce cytotoxins called verotoxins or Shiga-like toxin, which damage the colonic epithelial surface, resulting in the hemorrhagic symptoms (16). These organisms are transmitted in processed foods, usually meat products, and are responsible for outbreaks of illness from fast food restaurants and in nursing homes. Some persons with this illness, usually children and older adults, develop a hemolytic-uremic syndrome, which may be life threatening.

PATIENT EVALUATION

Historical Information

In addition to a history of the specific symptoms the most useful information will be:

1. A history of *food eaten* within the past 48 hours, particularly noting any deviation from the patient's usual pattern, such as eating an unusual food (e.g., a special fish), eating at a restaurant, attending a picnic or pot-luck dinner, or preparing food in an unconventional container (e.g., in a copper pot).
2. A history of a *similar illness in others* (family members or members of a group who ate with the patient). This will be helpful in suggesting a common source outbreak.
3. The probable *incubation period*. This may be helpful in suggesting the most likely etiology for a patient's illness (see Tables 26.1 and 26.2). For example, the onset of symptoms immediately after ingestion always indicates chemical food poisoning; onset of symptoms within a few hours of eating strongly suggests staphylococcal food poisoning; onset within 24 to 48 hours suggests salmonella infection; and onset of symptoms after 1 or more weeks of ex-

Table 26.4.
Sexually Transmissible Pathogens Resulting in Enteric Infections[a]

Bacteria	Protozoa
Calymmatobacterium granulomatis	*Cryptosporidium* species[b]
Helicobacter species	*Dientamoeba fragilis*
Chlamydia trachomatis	*Entamoeba histolytica*
Haemophilus ducreyi	*Giardia lamblia*
(?) *Mycoplasma hominis*	*Isospora belli*[b]
Neisseria gonorrhoeae	"Nonpathogenic" protozoans
Neisseria meningitidis	
Salmonella species	**Viruses**
Shigella species	Condyloma acuminatum
Treponema pallidum	Cytomegalovirus
(?) *Ureaplasma urealyticum*	Hepatitus A and B
	Herpes simplex

Helminths
Enterobius vermicularis
Strongyloides stercolalis

[a] From Quinn TC: Gay bowel syndrome. *Postgrad Med* 762:197, 1984.
[b] Have been shown to cause enteric disease in homosexual men with acquired immune deficiency syndrome (AIDS), but sexual transmission has not been reported.

Table 26.5.
Characteristics Distinguishing Invasive and Enterotoxigenic Diarrhea

Feature	Invasive Diarrhea	Enterotoxigenic Diarrhea
History	Fever, abdominal pain, tenesmus, may have blood in stool	Watery diarrhea with little or no fever or other systemic symptoms
Physical examination	Fever, abdominal tenderness; proctoscopy may be indicated	May be signs of salt and water depletion
Laboratory studies	Stool culture (may be diagnostic) Fecal leukocytes in large number[a] White count may be elevated	Stool culture usually negative unless special culture techniques available White count usually normal, but may be elevated
Therapy	Oral fluids and electrolytes (usually only small quantities needed) Antimicrobials often indicated[b]	Oral fluids and electrolytes (substantial quantities may be needed) Antimicrobials not indicated
Course	Improvement in 1–2 days, particularly if approppriate antimicrobials used	Duration of 1–2 days usually; may last up to 5 days

[a] Use a drop of methlyene blue stain with liquid stool.
[b] See text for recommendations for specific bacterial pathogens.

posure suggests uncommon problems such as giardiasis.

4. A history of taking antimicrobials (particularly clindamycin, ampicillin, or a cephalosporin), either currently or within the last 2 weeks. This would support the possibility of antibiotic-associated diarrhea that, when severe, is most commonly due to *Clostridium difficile* (2).
5. A history of *neurological symptoms* after ingestion of canned foods should always suggest botulism or one of the other sources of neurotoxins (all rare) listed in Table 26.2.
6. A history suggestive of the *acquired immunodeficiency syndrome* (see Chapter 34) and chronic diarrhea should suggest the possibility of cryptosporidia (5), isospora, or salmonella infection.
7. A history of *homosexuality* in the male should suggest the possibility of the more unusual causes of diarrheal disease (15).

Physical Examination

The physical examination is usually of minimal help in establishing an etiological agent. Probably the most important observation is the temperature: fever or significant abdominal tenderness in association with diarrhea suggests an invasive organism. Poor skin turgor and postural hypotension suggest significant salt and water deficits (relatively uncommon in adults with diarrhea in the United States). Infrequently occurring conditions in which the physical findings may be very helpful are botulism and other neurotoxic forms of food poisoning, and trichinosis (see Tables 26.1 and 26.2).

Laboratory Studies

In the majority of patients with acute gastrointestinal illness, no laboratory studies are indicated. If there is a suggestion of a common source outbreak, however, special cultures and tests for toxins in stools and in food, primarily for epidemiological purposes, should be obtained.

In patients with a combination of diarrhea for more than 24 hours, fever, and blood in the stool or significant dehydration, a minimal number of laboratory studies is indicated (16): (a) stool culture for *Salmonella, Shigella, Helicobacter,* and *Yersinia.* (Unfortunately enterotoxigenic *E. coli,* invasive *E. coli,* vibrios, and most viral agents cannot be identified in routine laboratories because of the special techniques required.) (b) Stool examination for fecal leukocytes. (More than 10 leukocytes per high power field is indicative of an invasive pathogen.) The test is done by mixing a small bit of stool with methylene blue stain on a microscope slide, and placing a coverslip over the mixture. After 2 or 3 minutes, the preparation is examined under the "high dry" objective for the presence of leukocytes. (c) A white blood cell count. (An elevated count and/or shift to younger polymorphonuclear forms supports the diagnosis of invasive diarrheal disease.)

In suspected cases, the laboratory should be asked to culture the stool for *E. coli* that cause hemorrhagic colitis, or to examine the stool for *Giardia lambia, Entamoeba histolytica,* or *Cryptosporidium* (Table 26.1). For optimal identification of trophozoites of these organisms, fresh stools should be examined immediately by an experienced observer. For the diagnosis of giardiasis, stools may need to be examined repeatedly. *E. histolytica* trophozoites are best identified from the mucus taken from the base of ulcerations seen at proctoscopy.

Additional laboratory tests should be ordered for certain conditions (see Tables 26.1 and 26.2). If *C. difficile* enterocolitis is suspected, the laboratory can be asked to identify the cytotoxin in the stool. (Also see Chapter 39 for a discussion of the evaluation of patients with chronic diarrhea.)

MANAGEMENT

In all patients with acute diarrhea, symptomatic treatment is of primary importance. In addition, some patients may require specific therapy (i.e., antibiotics), usually indicated on the basis of the history and physical examination. Most episodes of acute diarrhea are self-limited, lasting 1 to 2 days, but occasionally symptoms last 5 to 10 days. Resolution of illness is thought to be due to the local secretory immune response of the gastrointestinal tract.

Symptomatic Treatment

Fluid Therapy

With the exception of giardiasis, amebiasis, *C. difficile* colitis, and the more severe cases of shigellosis and salmonellosis, practically all acute diarrheal disease seen commonly in the United States can be treated with only symptomatic therapy, the mainstay of which is the replacement of fluids and electrolytes lost in the stool. Because in most patients the disease is mild and the amount of stool is small, replacement is relatively simple. Patients should be encouraged to drink lots of fluids, to avoid spicy foods, and otherwise to eat what they like.

In patients who have a *very large loss of stool* and who experience weakness and a feeling of being "washed out" with or without signs of dehydration, replacement should consist of fluids containing electrolytes and glucose. In many parts of the world, an oral glucose-electrolyte replacement solution is available commercially for this purpose (19). Commerical products available in the United States are Pedialyte and Rehydralyte solutions and Orlyte packets. These products have been developed primarily for treating children but are adequate for adults. Most have sodium concentrations of 50 to 75 mEq/liter and substitute citrate for bicarbonate. A less complete replacement fluid can be made using table salt, sugar, and water (see page 369). Patients should be instructed to replace estimated diarrheal fluid losses roughly on a 1:1 basis (17).

Patients experiencing *severe diarrhea or vomiting* that precludes easy ingestion of oral replacement fluids and those who have evidence of moderate to severe salt and water depletion should be hospitalized for initial intravenous fluid replacement with Ringer's lactate or its equivalent.

Other Symptomatic Measures

Several types of medications are commonly used to treat diarrhea symptomatically. *Diphenoxylate with atropine* (Lomotil) or *loperamide* (Imodium) both cause a decrease in intestinal motility and stool frequency; they may be very useful to the patient at times when frequent defecation would be embarrassing. Because these drugs do not alter the natural course of the disease, however, and are potentially harmful if invasive pathogens such as *Shigella* are causing the diarrhea, they should only be used infrequently. *Kaolin and pectin mixtures* (e.g., Kaopectate) add to the bulk of the stool, and thus the stools become less watery; actual fluid loss, however, is not affected by these agents. *Bismuth subsalicylate* (Pepto-bismol) has been demonstrated to decrease the volume of stools in patients with diarrhea due to enterotoxigenic organisms and may be taken in either liquid or tablet form; the dose

is two tablets or 30 ml every half hour to one hour, as needed, up to a maximum of eight doses per 24 hours.

In patients with the *protracted vomiting,* that may occur with staphylococcal food poisoning, the antiemetic drug prochlorperazine (Compazine) may be very helpful, given as a 25-mg rectal suppository two or three times daily.

Specific Treatment

In patients in whom *shigellosis* is strongly suspected, or from whom the organism has been cultured in the stool, appropriate antibiotic treatment should be given as this will shorten the illness from 3 to 7 days to 1 to 2 days. Trimethoprim-sulfamethoxazole is presently the drug of choice, since most shigella are now resistant to drugs formerly used, such as ampicillin. The dose is one double strength tablet every 12 hours for 3 days; alternative drugs include the newer fluroquinolones (norfloxacin and ciprofloxacin), and there is some data to suggest that a single large dose (800 mg by mouth) of norfloxacin may be adequate (6).

If *Salmonella* is isolated from diarrheal stool, patients should not be given antibiotics unless there is evidence of systemic disease, such as high fever or other signs of toxicity. It has been found that routine treatment of Salmonella gastroenteritis with antibiotics leads to a prolongation of the carrier state in some individuals (1). Even without antibiotic treatment, patients may excrete *Salmonella* in the stool for several weeks to months after their acute illness has terminated. If there is systemic disease, ampicillin or chloramphenicol, 500 mg four times daily for 1 week, is adequate.

Patients infected with *Helicobacter* may benefit from antibiotic therapy, but controlled studies indicate primarily an effect on excretion of the organism rather than a clinical effect. Erythromycin, 500 mg four times a day for 5 days, seems to be the drug of choice; most strains are also sensitive to similar doses of tetracyclines.

In patients who develop *significant diarrhea related to antibiotics,* the antibiotic should be stopped and another substituted if antibiotic therapy must be continued. The majority of cases of significant antibiotic-associated diarrhea in hospitalized or recently hospitalized patients are due to *C. difficile*. Metronidazole (Flagyl), 250 mg by mouth four times a day for 5 days, will shorten the illness in most patients; for those who do not improve after several days of metronidazole, the much more expensive antibiotic vancomycin should be given in an oral dose of 125 to 250 mg four times daily for 7 to 10 days (2).

There is no evidence that antibiotics are useful in patients with *hemorrhagic colitis* due to *E. coli* . Antibiotics are, however, definitely useful in the treatment of traveler's disease, most of which is due to enterotoxigenic *E. coli* (see Chapter 33).

Patients with *giardiasis and amebiasis* definitely require appropriate therapy. For giardiasis, the drug of choice is quinacrine hydrochloride, 100 mg three times a day, for 5 days. Metronidazole (Flagyl), 750 mg three times a day for 5 days, is also effective. For moderate to severe amebic dysentery, metronidazole should be administered, 750 mg three times a day for 10 days, followed by diiodohydroxyquin (Diodoquin), 650 mg three times a day for 3 weeks, to eradicate the cyst forms.

Trichinosis is treated with thiabendazole, 25 mg/kg twice a day for 5 to 7 days. High doses of prednisone (e.g., 30 to 50 mg daily) should be given simultaneously if symptoms are pronounced (see Table 26.1).

Patients with *suspected botulism* should be hospitalized in an intensive care unit immediately and should be given polyvalent antitoxin, which must be obtained through the local health department.

Patients with mushroom poisoning due to *Amanita muscaria* should be treated with atropine (see Table 26.2).

In patients who are thought to have one or more of the gay bowel syndromes, the management for typical enteric infections (e.g., *Salmonella, Shigella, E. histolytica*, etc.) is identical to that for nonsexually transmitted infections. Patients with proctitis or perianal disease (symptoms include constipation, anorectal discomfort, tenesmus, and mucopurulent discharge) should receive empirical treatment for *Neisseria gonorrhoeae* and *Chlamydia trachomatis* (i.e., 4.8 million units of procaine penicillin intramuscularly plus 1 g of probenicid, followed by 500 mg of tetracycline orally four times a day for 7 days). For all patients with a gay bowel syndrome, a serological test for syphilis should be sent, and permission to test for human immunodeficiency virus H(IV)infection should be sought. Chapter 34 describes the selection of antimicrobial therapy for the diarrheal illnesses associated with HIV infection; for one of these, cryptosporidiosis, there is no effective treatment.

The Patient's Role in Therapy

Acute gastroenteritis, like the common cold, is an illness that is often diagnosed and handled by the patient without contacting a physician. In some instances, patients will contact their physician by telephone, and a working diagnosis and plan of therapy can be established without an office visit. This is particularly true for healthy patients with typical symptoms of staphylococcal food poisoning. In all situations, whether the patient is examined or not, it should be stressed that care of gastroenteritis requires taking of sufficient fluids, at times supplemented by an oral electrolyte solution (see above) and by oral antibiotics if prescribed. Patients should be advised to contact their physician if diarrhea becomes worse or if they develop fever or protracted vomiting. There is no need for a follow-up visit unless symptoms persist beyond 2 to 3 days, or unless stool cultures have been taken and reveal that antibiotic therapy is indicated. Limitation of activity should be dictated by how the patient feels and by proximity of toilet facilities.

Course of Illness

The dehydrated patient will feel almost immediate improvement when adequate oral replacement fluids are given. When the patient is given antimicrobial therapy for an invasive pathogen, there should be a noticeable decrease in diarrhea and fever within 24 to 36 hours.

An *atypical course* will occasionally occur after initial diagnosis and treatment. Any patient may develop an increase in diarrhea after being initially seen, which could result in unanticipated significant dehydration. An increase in severity of symptoms could also occur if the patient develops antibiotic-associated enterocolitis. An initial episode of ulcerative colitis could be misdiagnosed as shigellosis, in which case antibiotic therapy would not result in improvement; and the occasional patient with antibiotic-resistant *Shigella* may not respond to initial therapy, indicating the need for an alternative drug.

Rarely, a patient's diarrheal symptoms may not resolve within a few days. In this case, he should return for further evaluation, particularly repeated stool examinations, which may be necessary to confirm the diagnosis of protozoal infections.

PREVENTION

Primary Prevention

Primary prevention of the diseases discussed above can theoretically be accomplished by these measures: (a) reducing the agent's presence in the environment, (b) increasing resistance of the host (by immunization or prophylactic antibiotics), and (c) utilizing environmental measures that block the transmission of the agent (2). Regulations governing sewage treatment, water purification, and food processing, packing, and preparation provide the principal protective barriers to foodborne disease *outside the home*. Unfortunately this is frequently not adequate, as evidenced by the observation that as many as 50% of poultry carcasses sold commercially in super markets are contaminated with *Salmonella* and/or *Helicobacter. In the home*, almost all forms of foodborne disease can be prevented if several measures are followed routinely (see Table 26.6). Many people do not realize that some of the food they prepare each day is contaminated before cooking, and that proper cooking and storing, not absence of contamination, is the way in which most food is rendered safe to eat. Whenever food known to be contaminated is eaten raw, the risk of foodborne disease is present; this is particularly important with respect to shellfish, which concentrate microbial organisms from the waters in which they are grown; routine surveillance of these waters by public health authorities is the major mode of protecting persons who eat raw shellfish (9).

Table 26.6.
Measures to Prevent Foodborne Disease in the Home

1. Refrigerate all foods that are capable of supporting microbial growth (perishable foods).
2. Avoid keeping perishable foods for long periods even in refrigerator.
3. Cook all foods at sufficiently high temperatures before serving (212°F (100°C) or higher for all oven-cooked meats and at least 15 minutes boiling time for all boiled foods. Same procedure when foods are reheated).
4. Avoid preparing perishable foods a day or more before they are to be served.
5. Avoid allowing foods to stand at warm temperatures for several hours before being served.
6. Avoid incorporating raw (contaminated) ingredients into foods that receive no further cooking.
7. Thoroughly clean kitchen equipment after it has been in contact with perishable foods.
8. Avoid using utensils that may contain toxic metals.
9. Avoid foods that are unsafe no matter how they are processed (see text).

Secondary Prevention

After an outbreak of an acute enteric illness, appropriate measures should be taken to prevent additional cases.

In the household, any foods suspected of transmitting illness should be thrown away. (In the event that an epidemiological investigation is warranted, a sample should be submitted to the local health department.) An error in storage or cooking of the suspected food will often be evident; the patient's physician should point out this error and, most important, review the standard precautions as listed in Table 26.6 to prevent repeated episodes of foodborne illness. When a member of a household has an enteric infection that is transmissible from person to person (see Table 26.1), this individual should be instructed to wash his/her hands frequently, especially before preparing food for others. When shigellosis or salmonellosis occurs in a person involved in food handling, it is critical to obtain three negative stool cultures, assuring eradication of the carrier state, before the individual returns to food handling.

When exposure *outside the home* is suspected by the physician, the problem should be reported immediately to the local health department; it is the responsibility of the health department to undertake an epidemiological investigation in order to protect others. Each year, investigations of 400 to 500 outbreaks of foodborne illness are reported to the Centers for Disease Control, and many lead to measures that interrupt potentially widespread outbreaks of diseases, some of them particularly hazardous, such as botulism (3).

Prophylaxis for Travelers to the Developing World

The problem of diarrheal illness and the other problems related to travel are discussed in Chapter 33.

General References

Benenson AS (ed): *Control of Communicable Diseases in Man*. 15th ed. Washington, DC, American Public Health Association, 1990.

A concise summary of epidemiology, management, and prevention of communicable diseases.
Centers for Disease Control: *Foodborne Disease Outbreaks, Annual Summary*. Atlanta, In: *CDC Surveillance Summaries* 35:7ss, 1986.
This report, published annually, provides the most current overview of foodborne disease epidemiology; it includes detailed reports on important new problems each year.
Gorbach SL (ed): *Infectious Diarrhea*. Boston, Blackwell Scientific Publications, 1986.
Tyrrell DAJ, Kapikian AZ (eds): *Virus Infections of the Gastrointestinal Tract*. New York, Marcel Dekker, Inc. 1982. The Medical Letter On Drugs and Therapeutics. *Drugs for Parasitic Infections. The Medical Letter* 30:February, 1988.
Guerrant RL, Shields DS, Thorson SM, et al: Evaluation and diagnosis of acute infectious diarrhea. *Am J Med* 78:91, 1985.

Specific References

1. Aserkoff B, Bennett JV: Effect of antibiotic therapy in acute salmonellosis on the fecal excretion of salmonellae. *N Engl J Med* 281:636, 1969.
2. Bartlett JG: Treatment of *Clostridium difficile* colitis. *Gastroenterology* 89:1192, 1985.
3. Blaser MJ, Wells JG, Feldman RA, et al: *Campylobacter* enteritis in the United States. *Ann Intern Med* 98:360, 1983.
4. Clausen CR, Christie DL: Chronic diarrhea in infants caused by adherent enteropathic *Escherichia coli*. *J Pediatr* 100:358, 1982.
5. Current WL, Reese NC, Ernst JV, et al: Human cryptosporidiosis in immunocompetent and immunodeficient persons. *N Engl J Med* 308:1252, 1983.
6. Gotuzzo E, Oberhelman RA, Maguina C, et al: Comparison of single-dose treatment with norfloxacin and standard 5-day treatment with trimethoprim-sulfamethoxazole for acute shigellosis in adults. *Antimicrobial Agents and Chemotherapy* 33:1101, 1989.
7. Gosselin RE, Hodge HC, Smith RP, Gleason MN: *Clinical Toxicology of Commercial Products*, 4th ed. Baltimore, Williams & Wilkins, 1976.
8. Guerrant RL: The global problem of amebiasis: current status, research needs, and opportunities for progress. Amebiasis: introduction, current status, and research questions. *Reviews of Infectious Diseases* 8(2):218, 1986.
9. Hughes JM, Merson MH: Current concepts: fish and shellfish poisoning. *N Engl J Med* 295:1117, 1976.
10. Holmberg SD, Blake PA: Staphylococcal food poisoning in the United States: new facts and old misconceptions. *JAMA* 251:487, 1984.
11. Kapikian AZ, Chanock RM: Norwalk group of viruses. In: Fields BN, et al (eds): *Virology* New York, Raven Press, 1495, 1985.
12. Kapikian AZ, Chanock RM: In: Fields BN, et al, (eds): *Virology*. New York, Raven Press, 863, 1985.
13. Levine M: *Escherichia coli* that cause diarrhea: enterotoxigenic, enteropathogenic, enteroinvasive, enterohemorrhagic, and enteroadherent. *J Infect Dis* 155:377, 1987.
14. Ouchterlony O, Holmgren J (eds): *Cholera and Related Diarrheas, 43rd Nobel Symposium*. Basel, S. Karger, 1980.
15. Quinn TC, Stamm WE, Goodell SE, et al: The polymicrobial origin of intestinal infections in homosexual men. *N Engl J Med* 309:576, 1983.
16. Riley LW: The epidemiologic, clinical, and microbiological features of hemorrhagic colitis. *Ann Rev Microbiol* 41:383, 1987.
17. Santosham M, Brown KH, Sack RB: Oral rehydration therapy and dietary therapy for acute childhood diarrhea. *Pediatrics in Review* 8(9):273, 1987.
18. Stevens DP: Host-pathogen biology. *Rev Infect Dis* 4:851, 1982.
19. Vantrappen G, Agg HO, Geboes K, et al: *Yersinia* enteritis. *Med Clin North Am* 66:639, 1982.
20. Vial PA, Robins-Browne R, Lior H, et al: Characterization of enteroadherent-aggregative *Escherichia coli*, a putative agent of diarrheal disease. *J Infect Dis* 158:70, 1988.
21. Wenman WM, Hinde D, Feltham S, Gurwith M: Rotovirus infection in adults. Results of a prospective family study. *N Engl J Med* 301:303, 1979.

C H A P T E R 27

Genitourinary Infections*

SUSAN J. DENMAN, M.D.

WILLIAM B. GREENOUGH III, M.D.

Urinary tract infection (UTI) is one of the most common disorders seen by the primary care physician. The majority of these infections respond well to therapy, but complicated urinary infections can cause significant morbidity and mortality. This chapter provides a practical approach to the diagnosis, evaluation, management, and follow-up of patients with urinary tract infections. Sexually transmitted disease and vulvovaginal infections are discussed more extensively in Chapters 30 (syphilis) and 94 (vaginitis), respectively.

---

*Drs. John R. Burton and James K. Smolev contributed to this chapter in the first and second editions of this book.

PATHOGENESIS—GENERAL CONSIDERATIONS

Gram-negative, aerobic bacteria cause the vast majority of urinary tract infections in all age groups with *Escherichia coli*, accounting for approximately 80% of community-acquired infections in women and 30 to 50% of nosocomial urinary tract infections in men and women (23, 34). There are over 100 serotypes of *E. coli*, differentiated by the character of the "O" antigen (a component of the cell wall), but only eight of these commonly cause infection. Other Gram-negative bacteria, such as *Enterobacter*, *Klebsiella*, *Proteus* species, and *Pseudomonas*, and some Gram-positive bacteria, especially *Staphylococcus saprophyticus*, cause urinary tract infections with less frequency than *E. coli*. Viruses, mycobacteria, fungi, and parasites rarely cause urinary infections.

In women, the major cause of UTI is invasion of the urinary tract by bacteria that have ascended the urethra from the introitus. Women who are prone to infection have colonization of the vaginal introitus with the same serotypes of *E. coli* found in the fecal flora. There is evidence that this colonization is favored by a pH of the introitus greater than 4.4, by the absence of the production of cervicovaginal antibody (a surface antibody produced by the local tissues) to colonizing bacteria, and by urethral trauma (e.g., during intercourse).

Risk factors that have been shown to be associated with acute urinary infections in women include increased sexual activity, diaphragm usage, and failure to void after intercourse (47). There is little evidence to support the commonly held views that the direction of wiping after bowel movements, the use of oral contraceptives, or tampons, play a role in the pathogenesis of UTIs in women (15).

Infection of the bladder and kidneys in men is unlikely in an anatomically normal tract (as opposed to its common occurrence in women). The much lower incidence of urinary tract infection in men has been attributed to the long male urethra, to the absence of colonization of bacteria near the meatus, and to an antibacterial factor—prostatic antibacterial factor (PAC)—which is present in the prostatic fluid (and is markedly diminished in some men with recurrent prostatic infection).

The bladder has unique intrinsic defenses against infection. The washout of bacteria by periodic voiding is probably one important defense mechanism. The bladder mucosa also removes surface organisms (perhaps by phagocytosis, the secretion of mucus, surface antibody production, or all of these); this defense mechanism is severely limited if residual urine is regularly present after voiding (6).

Urinary tract infections occur more often and persistently in both men and women who have structural abnormalities of the urinary tract (such as an obstruction) or who have been catheterized or instrumented. Vesicoureteral reflux (the retrograde flow of urine from the bladder to the ureters) may be associated with, but is not necessarily a cause of, ascending infection. Infection in women also occurs more frequently in pregnancy (4 to 6% incidence), especially if they also have sickle cell trait (10 to 15% incidence). Diabetes mellitus does not increase the risk of developing a UTI unless there is an associated disorder of bladder emptying or unless the patient has been instrumented. However, once a UTI has developed in a diabetic patient, it may be more virulent. Sobel and Kay have provided a comprehensive view of host factors in the pathogenesis of UTIs (39). The pathogenesis of other genitourinary infections (vulvovaginitis and sexually transmitted disease) is discussed in Chapters 30 (Syphilis) and 94 (Benign Vulvovaginal Disorders).

GENERAL DIAGNOSTIC EVALUATION

The diagnosis of urinary tract infection is suggested by the history and physical examination (see below) and confirmed by examination of the urine. Sometimes, X-rays and instrumentation of the urinary tract are necessary ancillary procedures.

Urine Examination

The urinalysis is the most important initial study in the evaluation of the patient suspected of having a UTI because a negative urinalysis makes a UTI unlikely and a urinalysis may aid in the localization of an infection within the urinary tract (see below).

Collection

Collection of urine specimens requires careful technique since bacteria and cells on the skin near the urethra may contaminate the urine. However, a carefully instructed patient can usually obtain a satisfactory clean caught midstream specimen.

Men can easily collect an uncontaminated specimen by cleansing the glans of the penis using one or two 4 × 4-inch gauze wipes containing liquid detergent followed by rinsing with gauze soaked in tap water. Uncircumcised males must retract the foreskin. After initially voiding a small amount of urine into the toilet (except when a segmental collection is obtained, (page 293) a midstream specimen is voided into a sterile container.

In women, the procedure is more difficult. While sitting on the toilet with one leg swung fully to the side, the labia are separated and the area around the urethra is cleansed two or three times with a 4 × 4-inch gauze soaked with liquid detergent and rinsed with two or three gauzes soaked with tap water. The initial portion of urine is voided into the toilet and a midstream specimen is then collected in a sterile container. Commercial urine collection kits are available but often are expensive and sometimes contain small cotton balls that may be hard for many patients to use. The "clean caught" procedure may be impossible in women who are very obese or who have other disabilities. If more than an occasional vaginal squamous cell is found in the urine specimen, contamination

has occurred. In this instance, urine must be obtained by bladder catheterization.

Catheterization of the urinary bladder is accomplished by using a no. 14 catheter, inserted through the urethra into the bladder and removed when the specimen has been obtained. This requires careful preparation and cleansing of the urethra (with an aseptic solution such as Betadine) to minimize the risk of introducing an infection.

Urinalysis

If the urine specimen cannot be processed by the laboratory within 10 to 15 minutes of obtaining it, it must be refrigerated (until it reaches the laboratory) or placed on a dip agar transport device (see below). The uncentrifuged specimen can be examined microscopically under a coverslip with use of the oil immersion lens. The finding of bacteria by this method has a 90% correlation with the subsequent culture of over 1 million bacteria/ml of urine. The number of white cells in the uncentrifuged urine can be roughly quantitated microscopically in a counting chamber by the use of the low-powered lens. In women the finding of more than seven white cells/mm^3 is abnormal (although not specific for infection). The finding of seven or fewer white cells/mm^3 suggests that infection is not present (43). In men the finding of any number of white cells should be considered abnormal.

The urine is more easily analyzed, after it is centrifuged: A drop of the sediment is examined by the use of the high dry lens of the microscope. If bacteria are seen, infection is likely. Quantitation of white blood cells after centrifugation is not very reliable; however, it has been estimated that two to five leukocytes/high power field corresponds to > seven/ml in uncentrifuged urine (21); also the identification of white cell casts is diagnostic of pyelonephritis. Red blood cells are often present in urine in association with infection but may reflect a number of other processes as well (see Chapter 45).

The urine may also be analyzed by a multiple reagent dipstick. There may be a nonspecific positive test for blood and/or protein, but the most important measurement is the urinary pH. In an infected patient, a pH greater than 7.0 (if the patient is not a vegetarian) suggests the presence of infection by a urea-splitting organism, usually a *Proteus* species. The recent addition of the nitrite test to the multiple reagent dipstick should not lead to the use of it as a reliable method to rule in or out bacteriuria in a symptomatic patient or in a random urine specimen. The use of the nitrite test for the purpose of detecting infection is most valuable when used in mass screening. Bacteria in the bladder reduce nitrate to nitrite, and the latter can be measured colorimetrically using a dipstick. Because the generation of nitrite from nitrate by bacteria requires time, the test, when it is used for mass screening, is best performed on the first voided morning specimen and is most sensitive when repeated on three different morning specimens.

Culture

When a UTI is suspected, a culture should always be obtained before the initiation of therapy except, for cost/benefit reasons, in certain circumstances: women with first, occasional, or uncomplicated infection (see page 294) or with the urethral syndrome (see page 297)—and in these instances very careful follow-up must be assured. Urine cultures must be performed within a few minutes after collection. Bacteria multiply logarithmically if urine is incubated at room temperature; and, for this reason, the urine should be plated on a dip agar transport device (Uricult, bacteriuria screening test, or Bactercult—available from commercial laboratories) or it should be refrigerated until it reaches the laboratory. (A refrigerator should be in the vehicle transporting the specimen to the laboratory.) Cultures or sensitivity testing should not be done in the office unless a single individual can be dedicated to this task and quality control measures can be maintained.

Traditionally, 10^5 colonies of bacteria/ml have been considered indicative of significant infection; most patients with UTIs have bacterial counts above this level. However, any number of bacteria colonies may be significant if they are present in association with symptoms suggesting an infection. The vast majority of patients with bacterial UTIs have cultured a single species, but occasionally there may be a mixed infection (44). Mixed infections are more likely in patients with anatomical abnormalities such as obstructive uropathy or renal calculi and are frequent in patients with chronic indwelling catheters (16, 28).

When urine specimens are contaminated by surface bacteria, cultures may yield bacterial counts of less than 10^5 organisms/ml, or they may yield multiple species. When contamination is suspected, a carefully collected clean caught urine specimen should be obtained, or, if this is difficult, a specimen should be obtained by catheterization (see above). Not infrequently, a presumptive diagnosis of UTI has been made and antimicrobials have been prescribed by the time the laboratory reports that multiple organisms have been cultured. In this instance, the patient should be contacted by telephone to inquire about symptoms. If improvement has occurred, the antimicrobial course should be completed and a repeat culture obtained at follow-up (see below, page 295). If there has not been a significant response to the prescribed therapy, another urine specimen should be obtained for urinalysis and culture, either by a very careful repeated clean caught collection or preferably by catheterization.

The culture techniques for sexually transmitted diseases are discussed in Chapters 30 (syphilis) and 94 (vaginitis).

LOCALIZING THE SITE OF INFECTION

There are several techniques that may localize infection in selected cases (31). Three of these are available.

The *antibody-coated bacteria* test takes advantage of the host immune response to invasion by bacteria of tissue, such as kidney, bladder wall, or prostate. The bacteria may be identified in the urine by the use of fluorescent antibodies against the immune globulins (generated by the host) that coat the bacteria. The test, although helpful in differentiating bladder bacteriuria from pyelonephritis, is not yet widely reliable when done by commercial laboratories. Furthermore, because it reflects tissue invasion anywhere in the urinary tract, it is not specific for pyelonephritis (33). Currently, its use is limited to the evaluation of patients with frequently recurrent UTIs or to pregnant patients with bacteriuria (see below).

Urinary tract infection may also be localized by the *catheterization* of the ureters by a urologist. In this manner infected urine in the upper tracts can be demonstrated. This technique, however, is only performed if it is necessary to demonstrate that infection is localized to one kidney (e.g., for consideration of removal of a chronically infected nonfunctioning kidney).

A third method of localization, the *bladder washout technique* (12), is too cumbersome for routine office practice.

In the male patient, infection of the prostate and/or bladder can be confirmed by the comparison of quantitative bacterial counts on the first 10 ml of voided urine (urethral specimen—voided bladder specimen 1, VB_1), the midstream urine specimen (bladder specimen—voided bladder specimen 2, VB_2), a drop of expressed prostatic secretion (EPS), and the first 5 to 10 ml of urine voided after prostatic massage (prostatic specimen—voided bladder specimen 3, VB_3) (Fig. 27.1). Prostatic massage is accomplished by firm rolling pressure and working from the superior and lateral margin toward the midline and inferior margin. The seminal vesicles should be stripped also. If no secretions result, stripping the bulbar portion of the urethra may provide several drops of prostatic fluid.

In the performance of this *segmented collection technique*, it is important that the patient have some urine in the bladder at the time of the prostatic massage. Occasionally the prostate gland is too tender to massage, in which case a specimen may be obtained

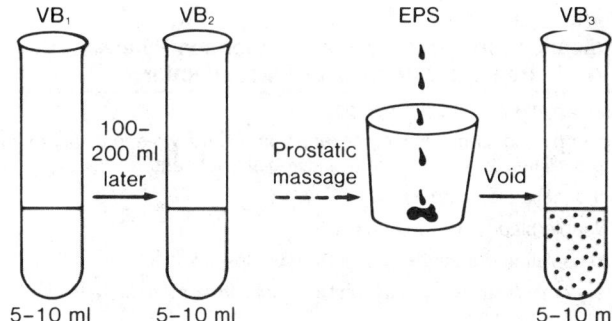

Figure 27.1. Segmented culture of the lower urinary tract in the male patient. VB_1, first voided urine; VB_2, midstream urine; EPS, expressed prostatic secretions; VB_3, first voided urine after massage. (After Stamey TA: *Pathogenesis and Treatment of Urinary Tract Infections*. Baltimore, Williams & Wilkins, 1980.)

by having the patient masturbate and by culturing the ejaculation. The interpretation of the results of this segmented collection is as follows: VB_1 only positive—likely contamination or urethritis alone; VB_2 only positive—UTI; VB_3 or EPS only positive—epididymitis or prostatitis. The VB_1 specimen also may be positive in association with a positive VB_2, EPS, or VB_3.

Radiography

The intravenous pyelogram (IVP) is not necessary in the vast majority of patients with uncomplicated UTI. It may help, however, in the evaluation of certain patients (Table 27.1) who are suspected of having structural abnormalities, the correction of which may prevent recurrence or may even be lifesaving. In addition to identifying problems that predispose to infection (such as reflux, a stone, or obstruction), an IVP will help to identify changes in the upper tract, such as scarring or caliectasis, which represent loss of renal parenchyma as well as abnormalities in the lower tract, such as bladder diverticula (23).

The *voiding cystourethrogram* may show abnormalities of the bladder outlet and urethra and may demonstrate urethral reflux. In adult patients this procedure is rarely necessary, and it is not recommended without a urological consultation.

INFECTIONS IN WOMEN

The Patient with Irritative Symptoms: Diagnostic Approach

Infections in all parts of the female genitourinary system may present with similar symptoms. It is important to localize the source of infection accurately in order to select the most appropriate therapy. Lower urinary tract infections are characterized by symptoms of bladder irritation (frequency, urgency, and dysuria) and occasionally hematuria. Chills and fever almost always indicate pyelonephritis (infection of the renal parenchyma), but the absence of these symptoms does not eliminate that diagnosis (13). Vaginal infections may mimic UTIs (21), underscoring the importance of

Table 27.1.
Indications for Obtaining an Intravenous Pyleogram (IVP) in Patients with Urinary Tract Infections

Acute pyelonephritis in male patients

Acute pyelonephritis in women when symptoms worsen or fail to improve after 2 or 3 days of antimicrobial treatment

Renal colic (see Chapter 47)

Palpable bladder or renal mass

Urea-splitting organism—usual Proteus special

Frequently recurrent urinary tract infections in women (more than three or four per year)

Failure to eradicate infection with appropriate therapy

Patients with newly recognized renal failure [an infusion IVP should be performed in the presence of renal failure; if the renal failure is severe (e.g., serum creatinine > 3–4 mg/dl) alternative imaging techniques should be used—see Chapter 48].

questioning sexually active women about vaginal discharge. A pelvic examination should be performed if the history is suggestive of vulvovaginitis from candidiasis, trichomoniasis, or other infections that may account for the bladder irritative symptoms (see Chapter 94). Chlamydial or gonococcal urethritis should also be considered in sexually active women (see Chapter 94). Chlamydia infection is suggested if the patient has had a sexual partner with recent urethritis, a new sexual partner, the gradual onset of symptoms (onset over days), or if hematuria is present. Chlamydial cervicitis is characterized by mucopurulent cervical discharge with exocervical edema. Gonococcal infection should be suspected in patients with a history of gonorrhea or those whose sexual partners have a urethral discharge. A purulent discharge from the cervicalis should be Gram stained (and cultured on Transgrow).

First Infection, Occasional Infection, or Uncomplicated Infection

The vast majority of women with urinary tract infections experience only one or occasional uncomplicated infections. The diagnosis of a UTI is confirmed by urinalysis and urine culture, as discussed above. Although an uncomplicated infection may clear spontaneously in time, treatment dramatically shortens the symptomatic period and should be given. Forcing fluids, historically a common practice, is not recommended as it may actually dilute significantly the concentration of antimicrobial in the urine.

Treatment

Usually uncomplicated UTIs are sensitive to multiple antimicrobials. Traditionally a 7- to 10-day course of antimicrobials has been given; but a single dose of a parenteral antimicrobial (32) or a single dose or a 3-day course of an oral antimicrobial (1, 11, 14) has been shown to eradicate approximately 90 to 95% of cases of uncomplicated cystitis in young women. There have been several complementary studies that have indicated that the single oral dose now can be recommended in preference to the traditional 7- to 10-day course. The single dose is associated with significantly fewer side effects; the flora of the vagina, periurethral area, and rectum are less likely to be altered; the treatment is less expensive; and compliance is more likely (22, 37).

The following single-dose oral regimens have been shown to be effective: amoxicillin (Amoxil, Polymox, or generic) 3 g (available as 500-mg tablets), sulfisoxazole (Gantrisin or generic) 2 g (available as 500-mg tablets); trimethoprim 160 mg with sulfamethoxazole 800 mg (available in single large tablets, e.g., Bactrim DS, or Septra DS). The trimethoprim/sulfamethoxazole combination is preferred because of somewhat better results (7, 18). The patient should understand that the symptoms may persist for 1 to 2 days, but she should telephone the physician if symptoms persist beyond this time since reassessment is then necessary.

When single-dose therapy is initiated, the patient should return in a few days for a follow-up urinalysis. If the urinalysis is abnormal, a urine culture and sensitivity testing should be done. With this approach the few patients who do experience a relapse, because of a renal infection, can be recognized early and can be given a more prolonged course of therapy (4 to 6 weeks of antimicrobial-specific therapy, see below). Additionally, this follow-up visit provides the opportunity for the physician to reinforce patient education about UTIs (see below, "Follow-up").

Single-dose oral therapy should be reserved only for uncomplicated episodes of cystitis in women. A traditional 7- to 10-day course should be used in all of the following situations: (a) when renal parenchymal infection is suspected (e.g., if fever, chills, or white blood cell casts are present); (b) when more than three or four previous episodes have occurred; (c) if symptoms have been present longer than 2 or 3 days because of the greater likelihood of upper tract infection; (d) if the patient is older than 65 years of age; (e) during pregnancy; (f) if follow-up is uncertain; or (g) if there is any suggestion of an underlying systemic problem (such as diabetes mellitus) or urological problem (such as a history of stones, reflux, or renal failure).

If the single-dose regimen is not used, the well-proven traditional 7- to 10-day course of antimicrobial is a reasonable option. The 3-day or the single parenteral dose regimens do not sufficiently improve upon the single or the 7- to 10-day oral regimens and are therefore not recommended. There is no evidence that treatment beyond 7 to 10 days is beneficial except when tissue infection is present (see below, "Recurrent Infections—Relapse Type in Men and Women"). The selection of an antimicrobial for a 7- to 10-day course should be based on efficacy, cost, and avoidance of any drug to which the patient is allergic. The results of culture sensitivity testing will ultimately guide the choice of therapy for patients with infections with more resistant organisms, but these results often are not available for 48 to 72 hours.

Prompt initiation of therapy is appropriate before the culture report, to control the patient's symptoms (Table 27.2). Sulfonamides are often prescribed except when prior resistance has been noted, in which case trimethoprim/sulfamethoxazole, ampicillin, nitrofurantoin, or tetracycline is a reasonable alternative. There is an increasing pattern of resistance to ampicillin (up to 30% in outpatient-based studies) (34, 42), making trimethoprim, sulfamethoxazole a more appropriate initial therapy. The urinary tract analgesic, phenazopyridine (Pyridium), is generally not required when antimicrobials are prescribed.

The availability of a new class of oral antimicrobial agents, the quinolones, inhibitors of bacterial DNA gyrase, promises to provide greater flexibility in the treatment of UTIs. However, until more data are accumulated, the quinolones should be greeted with cautious enthusiasm. Growing experience in the United States shows norfloxacin and ciprofloxacin to be as effective in treating complicated symptomatic urinary

tract infections as are parenteral agents (8, 35, 36, 38). They are well absorbed from the gastrointestinal tract even in elderly and critically ill patients. Norfloxacin and ciprofloxacin are renally excreted and require dose reduction in azotemic patients. However, the urinary concentrations achieved are high enough to treat most urinary infections, even in patients with renal insufficiency (27).

The quinolones generally are well tolerated. The most common side effect reported is nausea. Animals have developed cataracts after prolonged administration, but no ocular toxicity has been noted in humans. There have been isolated reports of arthralgia, dizziness, headache, restlessness, and depression (27). Most urinary pathogens are sensitive to the quinolones. However, as with all antimicrobials, resistance develops with long-term therapy. There is no evidence currently to support the use of single-dose or 3-day quinolone therapy for UTIs.

A useful way to spare patients given the 7- to 10-day course of treatment the expense of purchasing additional medication, if a change in medication is indicated, is to provide the patient with a 3-day supply of an antimicrobial from the office stock. The patient is instructed to telephone the office (or better, the physician initiates the call) after 3 days, to obtain a prescription to complete the 7- to 10-day course. This practice also provides an efficient follow-up at which time a patient with uncomplicated infection should be nearly symptom free. If the symptoms have not significantly diminished, persistent bacteria may be present, and the patient should be re-evaluated (see below, "Persistent Infection in Men and Women"). Recurrences after the eradication of bacteria and after the patient is no longer taking an antimicrobial are common, however, and follow-up is necessary.

Follow-up

It is usual that the first office visit is taken up in establishing the diagnosis and initiating therapy. As cited above, telephone follow-up will occasionally identify the need for prompt re-evaluation. If the symptoms have cleared, re-evaluation of the patient in the office in 2 to 7 days if single-dose therapy was utilized or in 3 to 4 weeks if a 7- to 10-day course was utilized is recommended, in order to reinforce education about UTIs (Table 27.3) and to reassess the urine. Many patients who have a persisting nidus of infection and who have received only a single-dose regimen or a 7- to 10-day course of antimicrobials will have evidence of a relapse (see page 301) at follow-up (bacteriuria and pyuria), which is frequently asymptomatic.

Recurrent Infection—Reinfection Type

The vast majority of women with recurrent urinary tract infections have reinfection (rather than an exacerbation of a smoldering quiescent infection). Although the infections are symptomatic and occasionally may be associated with pyelonephritis, recurrent rein-

Table 27.2.
Antimicrobial Agents That May Be Used in Uncomplicated Urinary Tract Infections

Agent	Dose
When single-dose therapy is used	
Amoxicillin	6 500-mg capsules at once
Sulfisoxazole (Gantrisin)	4 500-mg tablets at once
Trimethoprim 160 mg and sulfamethoxazole 800 mg (e.g., Bactrim DS or Septra DS)	1 double strength tablet at once
When a traditional 7- to 10-day course of therapy is used	
First Choice	
Ampicillin[a]	250–500 mg 4 times a day
Amoxicillin[a]	250–500 mg every 8 hours
Nitrofurantoin (Furadantin or Macrodantin)	100 mg 4 times a day
Sulfisoxazole (Gantrisin)[a, b]	500 mg 4 times a day
Trimethoprim[c] and sulfamethoxazole[b] (Bactrim or Septra)	2 tablets twice a day or 1 double strength (DS) tablet twice a day
Second Choice	
Cephalosporin (cephalexin)[d]	250–500 mg 4 times a day
Ciprofloxacin (Cipro)[d]	500 mg 2 times a day
Norfloxacin (Noraxin)[d]	400 mg 2 times a day
Tetracycline[c]	250–500 mg 4 times a day

[a]Resistance may occur after frequent episodes of UTI.
[b]Avoid in women who are breast feeding.
[c]Avoid in pregnancy.
[d]Often more costly.

Table 27.3.
Points to Consider in Educating Women Who Have Had an Uncomplicated Infection

Infections are often recurrent. However, the following measures may decrease the recurrence rate:

Avoid a full bladder. This is an especially important reminder during travel.

High fluid intake (1 liter in 2–3 hours) may eradicate an infection that has just become symptomatic.

Irritation to the urethra, as occurs with sexual intercourse, is associated with the movement of bacteria into the bladder. Voiding after intercourse, therefore, helps to prevent recurrent infection.

Diaphragm use is associated with development of urinary tract infection.

Infections in the absence of structural urological disorder are rarely, if ever, associated with the development of chronic renal failure.

Prompt recognition and treatment will help to control symptoms.

Even if recurrent infections are frequent, there is much that can be done to control symptoms (see discussion of prophylaxis under "Recurrent Infection—Reinfection Type").

fection in women with structurally normal urinary tracts rarely, if ever, leads to the development of chronic renal failure.

Treatment

The approach to women with anatomically normal urinary tracts and the syndrome of reinfection has been vastly improved by the understanding of the pathogenesis of UTI in women (41). In the past, the women were often treated with a variety of painful manipulations, such as urethral dilatation, urethral incision, transurethral resection of the bladder neck, installa-

tion of a variety of intravesicle agents, and other inappropriate and ineffective maneuvers. Instead each episode of bacterial infection should be treated as outlined above in the section on first infections. If there are more frequent recurrences, such as three or four or more in a year, prophylactic antimicrobials should be used.

Prophylactic Antimicrobials

After eradicating a recurrent infection a prophylactic antimicrobial may be initiated. A number of studies have confirmed the efficacy of prophylaxis in reducing the number of urinary tract infections in women (40, 45). The agents that have been used are effective when given as a single small dose at bedtime. A dose taken only after sexual intercourse is also effective in patients whose recurrent UTIs are associated with sexual activity: Patient acceptance is good, and side effects are uncommon.

Many agents have been shown to be effective prophylactically, but nitrofurantoin (Furadantin), a 50-mg tablet at bedtime, trimethoprim/sulfamethoxazole 40/200 mg, half a tablet of regular strength Bactrim or Septra at bedtime, and cephalexin (Keflex or generic), a 250-mg capsule at bedtime, are used most commonly and are recommended. Even low doses of nitrofurantoin have been associated with serious adverse effects (50) especially in older women, and this agent is therefore best avoided in women over age 35. Prophylactic therapy should be continued for 6 months. During prophylaxis, the patient should have a urinalysis performed every 3 to 4 months to ensure that there is no pyuria or bacteriuria. If after the cessation of prophylaxis there are still frequent recurrences, prophylaxis for a longer period (such as a year) should be tried (after a course of appropriate eradicative therapy). Prophylactic therapy has improved dramatically the lives of many women with distressingly frequent UTIs.

In addition to the established efficacy of prophylactic therapy for preventing recurrent urinary tract infections in women, a recent study has shown that patient-initiated single-dose antimicrobial therapy may be just as effective and as economically comparable (54). Nevertheless, when symptoms of recurrent cystitis occur, the method of prophylaxis using a small dose of an antimicrobial every night is recommended until more information can be developed regarding the selection of women for the patient-initiated single-dose method.

ASYMPTOMATIC BACTERIURIA

Associated with Pregnancy

Asymptomatic bacteriuria in pregnancy is relatively common, affecting up to 4 to 6% of women in the first trimester. Recognition of this fact is important, since eradication of bacteriuria reduces the high incidence of symptomatic UTI that subsequently occurs during pregnancy and may reduce the risk of immature and premature birth that occurs in women with antibody-coated bacteria in the urine.

Unassociated with Pregnancy

Asymptomatic bacteriuria is more common in women and increases in both sexes with advancing age. Among individuals aged 20 to 50, bacteriuria is present in less than 5% of women and 0.5% of men. In contrast, 3% of men and 20% of women ages 65 to 70 have positive urine cultures. After age 80, 22% of men and 23 to 50% of women have bacteriuria (20).

In addition to advancing age, asymptomatic bacteriuria is also associated with indwelling urinary catheters, urinary incontinence, multiple medical illnesses, impairment in functional status, and impairment of mental status (4, 49).

Several population studies have reported an unexplained increase in mortality in elderly patients with asymptomatic bacteriuria (9, 10, 30). This increase in mortality appears to be secondary to concomitant illnesses rather than to a direct consequence of the bacteriuria. It is not known how frequently nonpregnant patients with asymptomatic bacteriuria develop symptomatic infections. Treatment with antibiotic therapy is frequently unsuccessful in eradicating infection and is associated with the development of more resistant infections (28, 29). Controversy remains about the value of attempting to eradicate bacteriuria with a single course of therapy (5). Screening for asymptomatic bacteriuria in nonpregnant adult women is not recommended, therefore.

CLINICAL SYNDROMES THAT MIMIC URINARY TRACT INFECTIONS

Two syndromes in women that mimic "classic" UTI (i.e., $>10^5$ bacteria/ml of urine) are analogous to prostatodynia in men (see below) and because of their high prevalence deserve special attention. They are the urethral syndrome and interstitial cystitis.

Urethral Syndrome (Dysuria-Pyuria Syndrome)

This syndrome is characterized by bladder irritation, frequency, urgency, and dysuria without "significant" (greater than 10^5) bacterial colonies/ml on culture. With the increased ability to identify bacteria and other infectious agents in the urinary tract (see above), a new understanding of the syndrome has evolved.

Dysuria-pyuria syndrome may be the better term since dysuria is invariable and pyuria (greater than eight white blood cells/mm^3 of clean uncentrifuged urine) has important etiological implications (43). Studies have shown that many women with the syndrome have bacterial infection (43, 44). Patients may have cultures that show fewer than 10^5 colonies of bacteria (especially of *E. coli*, but occasionally of other bacteria) and yet respond to appropriate antimicrobial eradication therapy. Also in many women urine cultured by the usual bacteriological techniques appears sterile, but when the urine is cultured by use of special methods, it will grow infectious agents such as herpes simplex virus, *Chlamydia trachomatis*, and other agents (2). Also, this syndrome may be mimicked by vaginitis or gonococcal urethritis.

When *Chlamydia* infection is suspected (see above, page 294), treatment should be empiric because a culture is relatively expensive; however, commercial laboratories increasingly have available diagnostic methods of detecting *C. trachomatis* in urogenital swab specimens: A fluorescent antibody-staining technique and an enzyme immunoassay are the two methods currently available; both are quite accurate and relatively inexpensive. The laboratory should be consulted about the method of specimen collection and handling. Satisfactory treatment is achieved with doxycycline (Vibramycin or generic), 100 mg twice a day, or tetracycline, 500 mg four times a day for 10 days. Cervicovaginal gonococcal infection may also be eradicated with this regimen, although penicillin is more effective; therefore, if gonococci are identified on Gram stain (or cultured), then procaine penicillin, 4.8 million units intramuscularly plus 1 g of probenecid orally 30 minutes before injection, or either ampicillin, 3.5 g orally, or amoxicillin, 3 g after 1 g of oral probenecid may be used. Spectinomycin, 2.0 g intramuscularly, is recommended for patients allergic to penicillin or for whom penicillin failed to eradicate the gonococcus. Newer cephalosporins may be used to treat penicillin-resistant gonococci also (see Chapter 94). Even when gonorrhea is diagnosed, concomitant therapy to eradicate *Chlamydia* is recommended (see above) since these organisms are present commonly (17).

If a sexually transmitted disease is not suspected and if the urinalysis shows pyuria with some bacteria, then treatment as outlined above for first, occasional, or uncomplicated UTI in women (see above) should be prescribed.

Five to 10% of women who have the urethral syndrome do not have a demonstrable infectious agent even if special culture methods are used; most often these patients do not have pyuria. The cause of the syndrome in these instances is not known. In this group, treatment with reassurance, sitz baths, and the urinary tract analgesic, phenazopyridine (Pyridium), 200 mg three times a day for 5 to 10 days, will provide some relief. The patient should be informed that the medication often causes the urine to appear orange. If symptoms persist, referral to a urologist is indicated for cystoscopic evaluation (3).

Follow-up for patients with this syndrome should be identical to that outlined above or, if there is vaginitis or a sexually transmitted disease present, as outlined in Chapter 94.

Interstitial Cystitis

Interstitial cystitis is an occasionally seen disorder affecting middle-aged women, which early in its course may be confused with the urethral syndrome. Interstitial cystitis causes symptoms of suprapubic discomfort, especially when the bladder is full, and symptoms are relieved by voiding. The patient may experience progressive urinary frequency and eventually patients may have to void four to six times/hour, often throughout the night. The urinalysis is often normal, but hematuria may be present. The urine is sterile. This disease is difficult to diagnose, and therapy is often unsatisfactory. If suspected on the basis of the history, referral to a urologist is indicated. The urologist will perform cystoscopy and often a biopsy of the bladder in order to establish the diagnosis (usually a normal-appearing mucosa with a very small vesicle capacity is identified; tissue histology may show changes consistent with the diagnosis; mucosal hemorrhage may appear with bladder filling). Also, a cystoscopic evaluation will permit the urologist to exclude other causes of the symptoms (bladder tumor, for example). No definitive therapy has yet been developed for treatment of this condition.

VAGINITIS AND CERVICITIS

For discussion, see Chapter 94.

INFECTIONS IN MEN

Bacterial Cystitis

This infection is similar in presentation to that in the female patient and is diagnosed by the same method, but a urine culture should always be obtained. It suggests the presence, however, of an underlying struc-

tural problem, such as prostatic hypertrophy, and a diagnostic workup including a prostatic examination, assessment of renal function by a determination of serum creatinine or creatinine clearance, and an IVP and a urological consultation for consideration of cystoscopy are appropriate.

The treatment of bacterial cystitis should be similar to the traditional 7- to 10-day course described above and in Table 27.2. The treatment course may need to be prolonged further, however, if the workup reveals a structural problem (see below, "Persistent Infection in Men and Women" and "Recurrent Infection—Relapse Type in Men and Women"). A singe dose or a 3-day regimen of an antimicrobial as described for use in female patients with an uncomplicated infection should never be used in men.

Men with bacterial cystitis should be followed carefully even if the initial evaluation was unrevealing, as many will be found to have recurrent infection—relapse type (see below). Many men with relapse infection have bacterial prostatitis; therefore, a follow-up visit in 4 to 6 weeks after the initial infection should include a segmented urine collection (see above).

Prostatitis

Prostatitis is classified as bacterial prostatitis, nonbacterial prostatitis (prostatosis), or the much less common prostatic infections due to a virus, a parasite, tuberculosis, a fungus, or associated with nonspecific granulomatous changes (25).

Acute Bacterial Prostatitis

Acute bacterial prostatitis is characterized often by an abrupt onset of fever, chills, low back pain, and perineal pain with irritative urinary tract symptoms, although on some occasions systemic symptoms are not pronounced. Perineal discomfort may be worsened by defecation. In addition, the patient may have initial, terminal, or occasionally total hematuria (see Chapter 45). Rectal examination usually discloses a tender, swollen, and boggy prostate. The urinalysis as well as expressed prostatic secretions (see above) contain leukocytes, and culture will often grow the responsible bacterial pathogen, which most commonly is *E. coli*. The prostate may be too tender to massage and an EPS or VB_3 specimen may therefore not be obtained. Almost always in this situation the urethral (VB_1) or bladder urine (VB_2) specimen will contain bacteria; and sensitivity testing can be performed on bacteria grown from these specimens. If bacteria are not seen in the urine, material for culture may be obtained by having the patient masturbate as discussed above (page 294).

When the diagnosis is made, the patient may occasionally require hospitalization, although if systemic symptoms are minimal, ambulatory therapy is appropriate. Trimethoprim (Proloprim or Trimpex), 100 mg twice a day, trimethoprim/sulfamethoxazole (Bactrim or Septra), two tablets twice a day, carbenicillin (Geocillin) two tablets four times a day, clindamycin (Cleocin), 150 to 300 mg every 6 hours, or erythromycin, 250 to 500 mg twice a day, achieves a high level of tissue concentration in the prostatic fluid and can be prescribed to an ambulatory patient. Trimethoprim/sulfamethoxazole (Bactrim or Septra) is suggested as initial therapy until culture sensitivity tests are available, and then an adjustment in antimicrobial selection is made if necessary (trimethoprim holds promise as the agent of first choice but further clinical trials are necessary). Treatment with the quinolone norfloxacin has also been proven effective (23, 26). Therapy with antimicrobials for acute prostatitis should be continued for 2 weeks.

Bed rest and sitz baths for 20 to 30 minutes two or three times a day may provide comfort. Occasionally, prostatitis results in acute urinary retention, which requires hospitalization and urgent urological consultation. The palpable irregularity of the prostate gland after acute infection may persist for several months. The acute infection is readily controlled but recurrences may occur, especially in older individuals.

Benign prostatic hyperplasia (BPH) occurs at about age 50; therefore men below this age do not need a urological evaluation if the acute prostatitis responds within several days. Men older than 50 should be referred routinely to a urologist because of the likelihood of associated BPH and the high recurrence rate (see Chapter 49).

Chronic Bacterial Prostatitis

The organisms that cause chronic bacterial prostatitis most often are Gram-negative bacilli, *E. coli* being the most common organism, followed by *Enterococcus*, *Proteus*, and *Klebsiella*. Most patients with chronic bacterial prostatitis present with mild irritative symptoms (frequency, urgency, and dysuria), and occasionally there is a urethral discharge. Fever is absent. Patients may also have painful ejaculation with hematospermia (see Chapter 45). On rectal examination the prostate gland feels somewhat irregular and may be mildly tender, although the examination is often unremarkable.

The diagnosis is confirmed by the presence of greater than 10 to 20 white blood cells/high power field in the prostatic fluid or by the isolation of bacteria from expressed prostatic secretions or from the urine voided after prostatic massage (VB$_3$); at the same time the bladder urine (VB$_2$) is sterile or contains only a few colonies of bacteria and often a small number in the urethral specimen (VB$_1$) (see page 293). Obstructive symptoms are rare. Most often the patients have intermittent symptomatic episodes that have been controlled with short courses of antibiotics. Unfortunately, however, recurrent infection is frequent because of persistence of bacteria within the urinary tract. Chronic prostatitis may also be a reservoir for acute symptomatic cystitis, pyelonephritis, or epididymitis. Therefore, a prolonged course of therapy is indicated when chronic prostatitis is diagnosed.

If the infectious organism is sensitive to trimetho-

prim/sulfamethoxazole (Bactrim or Septra), a 12-week course consisting of two tablets twice a day in patients with chronic prostatitis offers a 30 to 70% chance of a long-term cure (25). Ciprofloxacin has also been shown to be effective in a small group of men with chronic prostatitis (52), but more data are necessary to determine whether quinolone therapy should become a first-line treatment for this chronic infection. For any chance of such a cure, a repeated culture of the expressed prostatic secretions and of the urine voided after prostatic massage should be sterile after 4 weeks of treatment. If the culture at 4 weeks is not sterile, continued therapy will fail and should be stopped. Some patients in whom oral therapy has failed may be cured by the administration of an aminoglycoside antibiotic parenterally for 7 days, but this requires hospitalization and careful monitoring of renal function to avoid renal injury.

If all efforts to eradicate infection fail, symptoms usually can be controlled with very low-dose trimethoprim/sulfamethoxazole, one-half tablet of regular strength Bactrim or Septra nightly indefinitely. The only way to effect a cure is by radical prostatectomy, but the morbidity of this procedure precludes its use for benign disease. Repeated prostatic massage has not been shown to be effective. It is important that patients with refractory chronic bacterial prostatitis be evaluated for the presence of prostatic stones by an X-ray of the kidney, ureters, and bladder; if stones are seen, the patient should be referred to a urologist. Patients with prostatic stones are often infected with a *Pseudomonas* species. On the other hand, patients who are not infected and incidentally are found to have prostatic calculi do not need to be referred to a urologist as the stones are frequently of no significance.

Nonbacterial Prostatitis (Prostatosis)

A certain group of patients have all of the symptoms of chronic bacterial infection of the prostate, but no organism can be demonstrated, i.e., they have nonbacterial prostatitis (prostatosis). This is the most common form of prostatic inflammation. These patients have mild perineal pain and irritative symptoms on urination, as well as white cells on the smear of the expressed prostatic secretions, or in the third voided urine (VB$_3$); yet, no organisms are cultured. Culture of the secretions and urine by special techniques occasionally reveals infectious agents such as mycoplasma, *Gardnerella vaginali*, *Ureaplasma urealyticum*, or *Chlamydia* species; however, the significance of these findings is unknown. Most patients with this condition cannot be cured; nevertheless, they should be given an antimicrobial such as erythromycin, 250 mg four times a day, minocycline (Minocin), 100 mg twice daily, trimethoprim/sulfamethoxazole (Bactrim or Septra), two tablets twice a day, or trimethoprim (Proloprim or Trimpex), 100 mg twice a day for a 2-week course; if there is no response to the therapy or if the syndrome recurs, no subsequent antibiotics should be prescribed. Instead, an antispasmodic agent such as oxybutynin (Ditropan), 5 mg two to three times a day, should be tried. Therapeutic prostatic massage has not been shown to be of value.

Interstitial cystitis and *in situ bladder* cancer may mimic symptoms of nonbacterial prostatitis; both conditions require cystoscopic examination for confirmation. Therefore, if the symptoms of nonbacterial prostatitis recur after a single course of treatment, a urological consultation should be requested to exclude these conditions and to educate the patient about the benign nature of prostatosis.

Prostatodynia. Patients with a syndrome called prostatodynia have symptoms suggesting prostatic inflammation but have no evidence of inflammation on physical examination, have no white blood cells in the urine or expressed prostatic secretions, and have sterile segmented urine cultures. There is some evidence that the syndrome may be due to a neurological disorder and that muscle relaxants or α-sympathetic blocking agents such as phenoxbenzamine (Dibenzyline) are effective in treating it. If this syndrome is suspected, urological consultation is suggested to confirm the diagnosis, to rule out interstitial cystitis and bladder cancer, and to initiate therapy.

Epididymitis

Epididymitis is a common intrascrotal infection that affects adult male patients. Organisms are thought to reach the epididymis through the lumen of the vas deferens from infected urine, the posterior urethra, or seminal vesicles. Epididymitis is manifested as an abrupt swelling of the epididymis that rapidly spreads, presenting often as a generalized inflammation of the entire hemiscrotum and making the differentiation from an acute orchitis impossible. Frequently fever, chills, and irritative bladder symptoms are also present. The differential diagnosis includes torsion of the testicle, acute orchitis, and tumor of the testicle with hemorrhage or hydrocele. Several observations help to differentiate torsion from epididymitis; torsion occurs in young boys and epididymitis occurs after puberty; the urinalysis is normal in torsion but usually shows pyuria and may show inflammatory cells in epididymitis; elevation of the scrotum often relieves the pain of epididymitis but intensifies the discomfort in torsion. Occasionally, however, it is not possible to distinguish torsion from epididymitis, in which case the patient should be referred to a urologist for emergency evaluation.

Epididymitis may be distinguished from orchitis only in its early stages. However, the presence of a urethral discharge or pyuria suggests epididymitis. A tumor of the testis is usually identified by its hardness and insensitivity to pressure. A hydrocele is usually easy to identify as it is painless and transluminates light. Although the gonococcus causes some episodes of epididymitis, *Chlamydia* has been found to be a common cause of epididymitis in men less than 50 years, whereas in older men who have benign prostatic hypertrophy, the coliform organisms are more common. Mumps,

although uncommon in adults, may be associated with epididymo-orchitis. In some instances no infectious agent can be identified. Once the diagnosis of epididymitis is made on clinical grounds, it should be confirmed by culture of the urine and expressed prostatic secretions, which usually demonstrate an infectious agent.

Treatment with ampicillin, 500 mg four times a day, or tetracycline, 500 mg four times a day, in addition to scrotal support, bed rest, and sitz baths will usually control bacterial infection within several days. Treatment should be continued for 14 days, and the patients should be informed that induration and edema in the region of the epididymis may persist for as long as 6 to 8 weeks. In the older patient with acute epididymitis, a search for obstruction at the bladder outlet (see Chapter 49) should be done as soon as the acute symptoms are controlled. On rare occasions, continued pain from chronic epididymitis may occur; if it does, a urologist should be consulted since an epididymectomy may be required.

Urethritis

Urethritis is an acute inflammation of the urethra that may be classified as gonococcal or nongonococcal (19). Nongonococcal urethritis is more common, and the most common cause for it is *Chlamydia* trachomatis. Symptoms of urethritis in the male patient include a discharge from the urethra, dysuria, and a sensation of itching at the distal end of the penis. There is no associated fever. Nearly 25% of men with a *Chlamydia* infection have no symptoms (46). Culture for *C. trachomatis* is quite expensive and is not recommended for routine clinical use; however, commercial laboratories increasingly have available relatively low cost, rapid, and accurate methods of detecting *Chlamydia* in urogenital swab specimens (see above, page 294). These methods, as they become more widely available, will help accurately diagnose *Chlamydia* urethritis. Diagnosis of gonococcal urethritis depends on the examination and culture of the urethral discharge. Material from the male urethra is best obtained using a sterile calcium alginate swab (Calgiswab, Type 1). The Calgiswab is much smaller than the usual cotton swab and, for this reason, is much less irritating to the patient.

A culture of the urethra for gonococci using a calcium alginate swab or a culture of the discharge should always be done by plating the swab on Transgrow, which must be at room temperature. (Because of its low cost, culture for gonococci is recommended whereas the high cost of *Chlamydia* culture precludes its routine use.) Approximately 10% of men with gonorrhea are asymptomatic, and swabbing the urethra for a culture of *Neisseria gonorrhea* is appropriate whenever there is a history of exposure.

Swartz and coworkers (48) have pointed out the usefulness of counting the white blood cells after staining the discharge with Gram stain. A Calgiswab is passed into the urethra, then rolled over a 1 × 2-cm area on a slide, which is stained by Gram stain. Gonococcal urethritis is almost always associated with greater than 50 white blood cells/high power field compared with less than two in normal men and a count of between four and 50/high power field in patients with nongonococcal urethritis.

Gonococcal urethritis is diagnosed by the presence on Gram stain of many white blood cells and of extra- or intracellular Gram-negative diplococci; the treatment is either with parenteral ceftriaxone, or parenteral spectinomycin plus doxycyline or erythromycin because of the likelihood of coexisting chlamydial infection (Table 27.4) (51). In nongonococcal urethritis the discharge continues for a longer period and is more mucoid, and the smear has fewer white blood cells and no stainable bacteria. The treatment is usually effective but recurrences develop commonly (51).

Because all the forms of urethritis must be assumed to be sexually transmitted, the patient's partner or partners should be treated with a regimen appropriate for the urethritis and the patient should use a condom until the infection has been controlled.

When patients continue to have recurrences of nongonococcal urethritis or have persistent symptoms unresponsive to antimicrobial agents, they should have bacteriological studies to evaluate the possibility of a chronic bacterial prostatitis (see above), and they should also undergo urological investigation for evaluation of possible urethral stricture, foreign bodies, or other intraurethral lesions.

Gonorrhea in women is discussed in Chapter 94.

PERSISTENT INFECTION IN MEN AND WOMEN

As noted above, treatment in the male or female patient of infection in a normal urinary tract with an appropriate antimicrobial should result in the sterilization of the urine within 72 hours. By this time, symptoms should have abated or, at least, have markedly diminished. If symptoms continue, a persistent infection may be present, and it should be established by a repeated culture. If any growth of the bacterial species present in the urine before treatment occurs,

further evaluation is necessary. Several causes Table 27.5) should be considered. A test of renal function (determination of a serum creatinine level or of creatinine clearance) and an IVP are suggested if infection persists in a patient who has taken the appropriate antimicrobial therapy. Urinary obstruction is discussed in Chapter 49.

RECURRENT INFECTION—RELAPSE TYPE—IN MEN AND WOMEN

Recurrent infection with the same organism is called relapse infection and implies the persistence of bacteria in tissue within the urinary tract. Relapse infection is, in fact, very similar to persistent infection except that in relapse bacterial sterility has been demonstrated either while the patient is on or has completed antimicrobial therapy, whereas sterility is never demonstrated with persistent infection. Relapse occurs most often within 6 weeks of completion of a course of antimicrobial therapy. An underlying structural problem is often present in both men and women with this problem. In women it is very much less common than reinfection (see above, page 295) but is quite difficult to document because most infections are a result of E. coli, which has many serotypes that cannot be differentiated by routine bacteriological laboratory techniques. Therefore, recurrent UTI due to E. coli may be either relapse (same serotype) or reinfection (different serotype). On the other hand, relapse of infection with organisms other than E. coli may be diagnosed by routine bacteriological culture. In women, if recurrent infection with E. coli occurs three times in a 12-month period, or if relapse infection with other species occurs, evaluation as outlined under "Persistent Infection in Men and Women" to exclude the possibility of structural abnormality is appropriate. If a structural abnormality is identified, it should be corrected if possible; if relapse infection is documented and there is no structural abnormality, a more prolonged course (6 weeks) of an appropriate antimicrobial agent should be prescribed.

If a woman or man has a structural abnormality of the urinary tract that cannot be corrected, sterilization of the urinary tract usually is not possible. However, suppressive therapy may decrease the frequency of symptomatic exacerbations or of episodes of sepsis. Suppressive therapy (as opposed to eradicative or prophylactic therapy) is accomplished for sensitive organisms by the use of sulfisoxazole (Gantrisin), 500 mg twice a day, or trimethoprim/sulfamethoxazole (e.g., Bactrim or Septra), one tablet twice a day. An alter-

Table 27.4.
Management of Urethritis in Men

Treat for gonococcal urethritis plus nongonococcal urethritis simultaneously

Ceftriaxone (Rocephin), 250 mg intramuscularly as single dose
or
Spectinomycin (Trobicin), 2.0 g intramuscularly as a single dose

plus

Doxycycline, 100 mg twice a day for 7 days
or
Erythromycin, 500 mg orally 4 times a day for 7 days

Treat partner(s) appropriately.

Follow-up for recurrence, complications (stricture, prostatitis, epididymitis), or especially in gonococcal urethritis, infection elsewhere (oropharyngeal, arthritis).

Report to local health department as required.

Table 27.5.
Differential Diagnostic Possibilities When Urinary Tract Infection is Not Eradicated by Therapy

Bacterial resistance to prescribed antibiotic
Patient noncompliance with antibiotic therapy
Presence of an underlying structural problem, such as an obstruction, diverticulum, or stone
Renal failure (inadequate urinary concentration of antimicrobial)

native to these agents is methenamine hippurate (Hiprex or Urex), 1 g twice a day, or methenamine mandelate (such as Mendalamine or Thiacide), 1 g four times a day. However, for these latter agents to be maximally active the urine pH must be below 5.5, so that acidifying agents such as ammonium chloride, 300 mg three to four times a day, must be used and the patient must test urine regularly and adjust the dose of ammonium chloride accordingly (often several grams/days are required) to assure the acidification of the urine. Thus these agents are unacceptable for most patients.

ACUTE PYELONEPHRITIS IN MEN AND WOMEN

Pyelonephritis is a bacterial infection of the kidney that most often results from ascending infection. It is suggested by the presence of bladder irritative symptoms, in addition to flank pain, fever, and, frequently, abdominal pain. Bacterial infection of the kidney may also be present without any of these signs or symptoms or with only bladder irritation (13). The urinalysis will show changes as outlined above (page 292), but only the presence of white blood cell casts is diagnostic of pyelonephritis. "Glitter cells" (white blood cells that glitter upon microscopic evaluation because of granules in the cytoplasm) are often touted as diagnostic, but they are not specific (24).

Clinically apparent acute pyelonephritis in men suggests the presence of a structural problem predisposing to infection and is an indication for immediate hospitalization, parenteral antimicrobial therapy, and an urgent IVP. In women, an underlying structural problem is much less likely to be present. Therefore, the decision for hospitalization and evaluation requires careful consideration. The patient can be managed at home if she does not have complicating medical illnesses, is not severely ill, does not exhibit sepsis, is reliable, is able to take antimicrobials by mouth, and if access to the physician is guaranteed should symptoms worsen (34). If a patient is managed at home, follow-up in 24 to 48 hours by phone is necessary. If there has not been significant improvement during that time, the possibility of an undrained infection (due to obstruction or abscess, for example) should be considered, and prompt hospitalization should be arranged for parenteral antibiotics, IVP, and emergency urological consultation.

The initial antimicrobial for the patient who is managed at home can be any of the agents listed in Table 27.2 (except the single dose regimens should not be used) with an appropriate adjustment based on the results of the urine culture and on sensitivity testing (see above). Forcing fluid (once an antimicrobial has been started) is not necessary and may theoretically be detrimental, as the concentration of antimicrobials in the urine and in the renal tissue may be diluted (53). However, intake should be adequate to replace fluid losses, including the additional fluid lost by fever or by vomiting.

If the acute episode of pyelonephritis promptly re-

solves, then follow-up in 3 to 4 weeks is appropriate (see above, page 295). An IVP, unless indicated for evaluation of an unresponsive infection, should not be done until that time. An IVP performed during the acute state sometimes shows a nonspecific diffuse or segmented decrease in the concentration of dye, a delay in the nephogram on the affected side, distortion of the collection system, and mild urethral reflux. Also, the kidneys may be enlarged. These changes will reverse in several weeks as the infection subsides. Therefore, to avoid being misled by these transient changes and thus to avoid repeating studies, an elective IVP should be postponed until several weeks after the acute episode has abated.

General References

Hanno PM, Wein AJ: Interstitial Cystitis. Parts I and II. In: Ball Jr TP (ed): *American Urological Association Update Series*. Vol VI. Houston, American Urological Association, Inc., 1987.

Lipsky BA: Urinary tract infections in Men: Epidemiology, pathophysiology, diagnosis and treatment. *Ann Intern Med* 110(2):138, 1989.

Stamey TA: *Pathogenesis and Treatment of Urinary Tract Infections*. Baltimore, Williams & Wilkins, 1980.

Stamey TA: Recurrent urinary tract infections in female patients: An overview of management and treatment. *Rev Inf Dis* 9(Suppl.12):S195, 1987.

Treatment of sexually transmitted diseases. *The Medical Letter on Drugs and Therapeutics*, 30:5, 1988.

Specific References

1. Bailey RR, Abbott GD: Treatment of urinary tract infection with a single dose of trimethoprim-sulfamethoxazole. *Can Med Assoc J* 118:551, 1978.
2. Berg AC, Heidrich FE, Fihn SD, et al: Establishing the cause of genitourinary symptoms in women in a family practice. *JAMA* 251:620, 1984.
3. Bordner DR: The urethral syndrome. *Urol Clin North Am* 15(4):699, 1988.
4. Boscia JA, Kobasa WD, Knight RA: Epidemiology and bacteriuria in an elderly ambulatory population. *Am J Med* 80:208, 1987.
5. Bosia JA, Kobasa WD, Knight RA, et al: Therapy vs. no therapy for bacteriuria in elderly ambulatory nonhospitalized women. *JAMA* 257:1067, 1987.
6. Brettman LR: Pathogenesis of urinary tract infections: Host susceptibility and bacterial virulence factors. *Urology* 33(3):9, 1988.
7. Carlson KJ, Mulley AG: Management of acute dysuria. *Ann Intern Med* 102:244, 1985.
8. Cox CE, McCabe RE, Grad C: Oral norfloxacin versus parenteral treatment of nosocomial urinary tract infection. *Am J Med* 82(Suppl 6B):59, 1987.
9. Dontas AS, Kasviki-Charvati P, Chem L: Bacteriuria and survival in old age. *N Engl J Med* 304:839, 1981.
10. Evans DA, Kass EH, Hinnekens CH, et al: Bacteriuria and subsequent mortality in women. *Lancet* 1:156, 1982.
11. Fair WR, Crane DB, Peterson LJ, et al: Three-day treatment of urinary tract infections. *J Urol* 123:77, 1980.
12. Fairley KF, Bond AG, Brown RB, et al: Simple test to determine the site of urinary tract infections. *Lancet* 2:7513, 1967.
13. Fairley KF, Carson NE, Gutch RC, et al: Site of infection in acute urinary tract infection in general practice. *Lancet* 2:615, 1971.
14. Fang LST, Tolkoff-Rubin NE, Rubin RH: Efficacy of single dose and conventional amoxicillin therapy in urinary tract infection localized by the antibody-coated bacterial technique. *N Engl J Med* 298:413, 1978.
15. Fihn SD: Behavioral aspects of urinary tract infection. *Urology* 33(4):16, 1988.
16. Garibaldi RA, Brodine S, Matsuriya S: Infections among pa-

tients in nursing homes—policies, prevalence, and problems. *N Engl J Med* 305:731, 1981.

17. Hook EW III, Holmes KK: Gonococcal infections. *Ann Intern Med* 102:229, 1985.
18. Hooton TM, Running K, Stamm WE: Single-dose therapy for cystitis in woman. *JAMA* 253:387, 1985.
19. Jacobs NF, Kraus SJ: Gonococcal and nongonococcal urethritis in men. *Ann Intern Med* 82:7, 1975.
20. Kaye D: Urinary tract infections in the elderly. *Bull NY Acad Med* 57(2):209, 1980.
21. Komaroff AL: Acute dysuria in women. *N Engl J Med* 310:368, 1984.
22. Kunin CM: Duration of treatment of urinary tract infections. *Am J Med* 71:841, 1981.
23. Lipsky BA: Urinary tract infections in Men: Epidemiology, pathophysiology, diagnosis and treatment. *Ann Intern Med* 110(2):138, 1989.
24. McGuckin M, Cohen L, McGregor RR: Significance of pyuria in urinary sediment. *J Urol* 120:452, 1978.
25. Mears Jr EM: Prostatitis. *Kidney Int* 20:289, 1981.
26. Meares Jr EM: Urinary tract infections in the male patient. *Urology* 33(Suppl)(3):19, 1988.
27. Neu HC: A new class of antimicrobial agent with wide potential uses. *Med Clin North Am* 72(3):623, 1988.
28. Nicolle LE, McIntyre M, Zacharias H, et al: Twelve-month surveillance of infections in institutionalized elderly men. *J Am Geriat Soc* 32:513, 1984.
29. Nicolle LE, Mayhew JW, Bryan L: Outcome following antimicrobial therapy for asymptomatic bacteriuria in elderly women residents in an institution. *Age and Aging* 17:187, 1988.
30. Nordenstam GR, Brandberg CA, Oden AS: Bacteriuria and mortality in an elderly population. *N Engl J Med* 314:1152, 1986.
31. Pollock HM: Laboratory techniques for detection of urinary tract infection and assessment of value. *Am J Med* 75:79, 1983.
32. Ronald AR, Boutros P, Mourtada H: Bacteriuria localization and response to single-dose therapy in women. *JAMA* 235:1854, 1976.
33. Rumans LW, Vosti KL: The relationship of antibody-coated bacteria to clinical syndromes. *Arch Intern Med* 138:1077, 1978.
34. Safrin S, Siegel D, Black D: Pyelonephritis in adult women: Inpatient versus outpatient therapy. *Am J Med* 85:793, 1988.
35. Schaeffer AJ: Multiclinic study of norfloxacin for treatment of urinary tract infections. *Am J Med* 82 (Suppl 6B):53, 1987.
36. Schaeffer AJ: Recurrent urinary tract infection in the female patient. *Urology* 33(Suppl 3):12, 1988.
37. Sheehan G, Harding GKM, Roland AR: Advances in the treatment of urinary tract infection. *Am J Med* 76:141, 1984.
38. Scheife RT, Cox CE, McCabe RE, Grad C: Norfloxacin vs. best parenteral therapy in treatment of moderate to serious, multiplyresistant, nosocomial urinary tract infections: a pharmacoeconomic analysis. *Urology* 33(Suppl 3):24, 1988.
39. Sobel JD, Kaye D: Host factors in the pathogenesis of urinary tract infection. *Am J Med* 75:122, 1984.
40. Stamey TA, Cindy M, Mihara G: Prophylactic efficacy of nitrofurantoin macrocrystals and trimethoprim-sulfamethoxazole in urinary tract infections. *N Engl J Med* 296:780, 1977.
41. Stamey TA: Recurrent urinary tract infections in female patients: an overview of management and treatment. *Rev Infect Dis* 9(Suppl 2):S195, 1987.
42. Stamm WE, McKevitt M, Counts GW: Acute renal infection in women: treatment with trimethoprim-sulfamethoxazole or ampicillin for two or six weeks. *Ann Intern Med* 106(3):341, 1987.
43. Stamm WE, Wagner KF, Ansel RL, et al: Causes of the acute urethral syndrome in women. *N Engl J Med* 303:409, 1980.
44. Stamm WE, Counts GW, Running KR, et al: Diagnosis of coliform infection in acutely dysuric women. *N Engl J Med* 307:463, 1982.
45. Stamm WE, Counts GW, Wagner KF, et al: Antimicrobial prophylaxis of recurrent tract infections. *Ann Intern Med* 92:770, 1980.
46. Stamm WE, Koutsky LA, Benedett JK, et al: Chlamydia trachomatis urethral infection in men. *Ann Intern Med* 100:47, 1984.
47. Stom BL, Collins M, West SL, Kreisberg J, Weller S: Sexual activity, contraceptive use, and other risk factors for symptomatic and asymptomatic bacteria. *Ann Intern Med* 107:816, 1987.
48. Swartz SL, Kraus SJ, Hermann KL, et al: Diagnosis and etiology of nongonorrhea urethritis. *J Infect Dis* 138:445, 1978.
49. Turck M, Stamm W: Nosocomial infection of the urinary tract. *Am J Med* 70:651, 1981.
50. Treatment of urinary tract infections. *Med Lett* 23:69, 1981.
51. U.S. Department of Health and Human Services: 1989 Sexually Transmitted Diseases Treatment Guidelines *Morbidity and Mortality Wkly Rpt* 38(5–8):21, 1989.
52. Weidner W, Schiefer HG, Dalhoff A: Treatment of chronic bacterial prostatitis with ciprofloxacin: Results of a one-year follow-up study. *Am J Med* 82(Suppl 4A):280, 1987.
53. Whelton A, Walker WG: An approach to the interpretation of drug concentrations in the kidney. *Johns Hopkins Med J* 142:8, 1978.
54. Wong ES, McKevitt M, Running K, et al: Management of recurrent urinary tract infections with patient-administered single-dose therapy. *Ann Intern Med* 102:302, 1985.

C H A P T E R 28

Respiratory Tract Infections

FREDERICK KOSTER, M.D.

UPPER RESPIRATORY INFECTIONS

Magnitude of the Problem

Upper respiratory infections (URIs) are the most common acute illnesses in the United States and the industrialized world. These infections are the most common causes of absences from school or work. The vast majority of URIs are self-diagnosed and self-treated and do not come to the attention of a physician. (Americans spend $500 to $700 million annually for over-the-counter medications for the relief of upper respiratory symptoms.) However, symptoms of URI rank fourth in order of frequency as for the principal reasons for visits to internists (see Table 1.3).

Principal Syndromes

Common Cold

The common cold is a mild, self-limited syndrome caused by viral infection of the upper respiratory tract mucosa and characterized by one or more of the following symptoms: nasal discharge and obstruction, sneezing, sore throat, cough, and hoarseness.

Epidemiology and Transmission. The common cold syndrome is caused by a variety of viruses that are clinically indistinguishable from each other, yet have distinct seasonal peaks for unknown reasons. Rhinoviruses constitute the etiological agent in 25 to 30% of colds, with seasonal peaks in early fall and mid- to late spring. Coronaviruses account for another 10 to 15% of annual colds, with a seasonal peak in midwinter. Influenza, parainfluenza, respiratory syncytial viruses, and adenovirus are etiological agents for another 10 to 15%, although this group more commonly presents with the typical influenza syndrome (see below). Bacteria associated with pharyngitis (see below) can also cause a common cold syndrome.

The incidence of the common cold syndrome decreases with age. On the average, adults have two to four colds per year; children have six to eight (18). Since person-to-person spread of colds occurs mainly in the home and at school, school children usually serve as carriers for introducing colds into the family. Thus mothers tend to have higher secondary attack rates than do fathers. Transmission of rhinovirus is most efficient by direct physical contact (19). Frequent, unconscious touching of virus-contaminated nasal mucosa contaminates the subject's hands. Infectious material can survive on the hand for as long as 4 hours, during which time hand-to-hand contact with susceptible subjects serves to transmit the virus. Exposure to susceptible subjects across even short distances of air is an inefficient method of transmission of rhinoviruses, although aerosol transmission of particles effectively transmits some viruses (e.g., Coxsackie, influenza, and adenovirus). Thus transmission of colds may be low even in congested offices, theaters, buses, etc. if hand-to-hand contact is avoided.

Clinical Characteristics. The correct diagnosis of the common cold is readily made by the patient. After an incubation period of 48 to 72 hours, the syndrome begins with mild malaise, rhinorrhea, sneezing, scratchy throat, and variable loss of taste and smell. These symptoms increase to maximal severity on the second to fourth day. Viral excretion and communicability are maximal during the period of severest symptoms. Fever is usually not present but, if present, rarely exceeds 1°F (0.5°C) elevation. Cough and hoarseness may begin later, and their severity and duration are increased in cigarette smokers. Conversely, neither cigarette smoking nor exposure to cold appears to increase the attack rate of colds. Colds due to rhinoviruses usually last 1 week but in one-quarter of cases last up to 2 weeks.

Identification of the causative virus by clinical observation is not possible, nor is it necessary for management. The primary challenge for the physician is to identify the cases with complicating secondary bacterial sinusitis (see below) and otitis media (see Chapter 96), for whom antimicrobials will be beneficial. The physical examination should therefore include the pharynx, nasal cavity, ears, and sinuses. The use of X-rays, pneumatic otoscopy, and throat culture is discussed in sections on sinusitis (below), otitis (Chapter 96), and pharyngitis (below), respectively.

Treatment. Most patients with typical URI syndromes can be assessed and managed on the basis of a telephone contact. In view of the absence of specific antiviral therapy for the uncomplicated common cold, symptomatic treatment is the only treatment available. Aspirin is the best drug for relief of fever and myalgias, but it may increase viral excretion, a finding of unknown epidemiological significance (37). Bed rest is not necessary to facilitate recovery. Steam or cool mist helps to liquefy secretions. Sipping hot chicken soup (the only soup studied) increases the clearance of nasal mucus, although it is not clear whether the benefit of this timeless remedy is mediated exclusively through inhaling water vapor or through an additional effect of an aromatic compound (36). There is no symptomatic remedy for hoarseness, which is due to inflammation and edema of the vocal cords; the patient should, however, be advised to rest his voice as this may shorten recovery time.

Nasal congestion is best relieved by *topical decongestants*; sprays rather than drops are preferred for ease of administration. Most over-the-counter short acting (3 to 4 hours) sprays contain 0.5% phenylephrine; some patients prefer the milder effect of 0.25% phenylephrine (sold as Neo-Synephrine). Longer acting topical decongestants (8 to 10 hours) are available—0.1% xylometazoline (Otrivin) or 0.05% oxymetazoline (Afrin); they may occasionally produce a stinging sensation when first used. Patients should be cautioned against using drops or sprays for more than 5 days to avoid the rebound effect, defined as an increase in nasal congestion when decongestant medication is discontinued. In contrast to orally administered decongestants, there has not been a blood pressure-elevating effect reported with topical decongestants. (See additional discussion of topical decongestants in Chapter 23.)

The *oral decongestants* phenylpropanolamine (contained in a large number of over-the-counter products) and pseudoephedrine (Sudafed, 30 mg over-the-counter or 60 mg by prescription; also available as Sudafed S.A., a sustained-action preparation containing 120 mg of pseudoephedrine, taken every 12 hours) are somewhat helpful. When prescribed in the recommended doses, these drugs can be used safely in stable hypertensive patients (27).

Antihistamines have a marginal effect in attenuating cold symptoms (23). The combination of decongestant and antihistamine, although often helpful in allergic rhinitis (see Chapter 23), is a more expensive, less effective alternative to topical decongestants; this is also true of the many cold remedies containing antihistamines, decongestants, analgesics, caffeine, and a variety of other ingredients.

A large number of over-the-counter *cough remedies* are available. These contain various combinations of cough suppressants, expectorants, decongestants, analgesics, and alcohol (33). There is no evidence that any expectorant is effective in URIs, and it is more rational and far less expensive to utilize the other ingredients individually in appropriate doses. (See additional discussion of cough suppressants below.)

Antimicrobials are useless in the uncomplicated cold.

Patient Education. Because transmission of colds occurs chiefly by physical contact, it is reasonable to counsel patients and those around them that transmission can be minimized by handwashing, reduced finger-to-nose contact, and reduced exposure to the cold sufferer. Physicians should be particularly vigilant to avoid contact with the patient's secretions and should wash their hands carefully after examining the infected patient. Although physicians with common colds may examine patients if they wash their hands and avoid sneezing on the patient, physicians with the flu syndrome should avoid patient contact (see below).

Viral upper respiratory infections may be complicated by superimposed bacterial sinusitis, otitis media, or pneumonitis. Therefore, patients should be advised to notify their physician of any symptoms suggesting one of these syndromes, each of which requires antimicrobial treatment.

Prevention. Prophylactic and therapeutic properties of large doses of vitamin C have been examined in a number of trials, and no consistent beneficial effect has been found (9). In those studies suggesting a benefit, the placebo effect could not be excluded since subjects could identify the vitamin C capsule by taste. In doses above 4 g/day, vitamin C may cause diarrhea and has the potential of precipitating urate, oxalate, and cystine stones in susceptible individuals. Other uncommon effects include diminishing the anticoagulant effect of warfarin, and confusing urine glucose tests, causing a false-negative glucose oxidase (Dextrostix, Tes-Tape) or a false-positive copper reduction test (Clinitest tablets).

It is unlikely that vaccines will ever play a role in preventing the common cold, especially since at least 89 different serotypes of rhinoviruses have been confirmed and since infection occurs despite the presence of specific serum antibody.

Flu Syndrome

Although there is considerable overlap in the two syndromes, the flu syndrome is sufficiently distinct from the common cold syndrome, especially in terms of potential complications, that the two are discussed separately. Flu presents as the abrupt onset of malaise, myalgia, headache, and fever; and substantial morbidity (including prostration in severe cases) persists for 1 to 2 weeks. As many as 85% of cases of flu syndrome may be due to the influenza virus during an epidemic (4). Other viruses, especially parainfluenza, respiratory syncytial, and adenovirus, are agents that produce the same clinical syndrome and coinfect patients with influenza (17).

Epidemiology. Epidemic spread of the influenza virus is due to the appearance of new antigenic variations of the virus in nonimmune populations. Antigenic variations occur almost annually in influenza serotype A, whereas variation occurs much less frequently in influenza B. Major variation is called antigenic shift and results in pandemic spread of a new strain, almost always type A, throughout regions of the world where there is little natural immunity. The most recent pandemics were in the winters of 1957 to 1958, 1968 to 1969, and 1977 to 1978, and they varied considerably in severity. In between pandemics, minor antigenic variations occur frequently, resulting in nearly annual epidemics during the winter months. Such interpandemic spread, although less dramatic, occurs frequently and therefore accounts for greater cumulative morbidity and mortality than pandemic spread. In some years there are no influenza epidemics. In recent years, however, epidemic influenza has occurred regularly and has influenced death rates (Fig. 28.1). Although it is often not possible clinically to separate infections due to type A or B, influenza A is responsible for greater excess mortality than type B.

Influenza virus appears to be transmitted by virus-containing small particle aerosols dispersed by sneezing, coughing, or talking. The incubation period is 18 to 72 hours. Viral shedding persists for 5 to 10 days, but virus is present in high titer in secretions for only 48 hours after the onset of clinical illness. In the community, person-to-person transmission is rapid, with spread initially among children, then adults. In local epidemics the incidence of cases reaches a peak in 2 to 3 weeks and persists for only 5 to 6 weeks.

Clinical Characteristics. Uncomplicated influenza, type A or B, has an abrupt onset of systemic symptoms including fever, chills, headache, myalgias, and malaise. The fever, which may rise to 106°F (41°C) in some cases, typically lasts 3 days, although frequently it persists for 5 to 7 days. Headache and myalgias involving the back, arms, legs, and, occasionally, the eyes are the predominant symptoms, persisting as long as the fever. Respiratory symptoms, such as cough, nasal discharge, hoarseness, and sore throat, appear as systemic symptoms wane. Cough and weakness may persist for 2 or more weeks.

Physical findings include general toxicity, flushed face, hot skin, watery red eyes, clear nasal discharge, tender cervical lymph nodes, and, occasionally, localized rales in the chest. The white cell count and differential count usually demonstrate mild neutropenia and relative lymphocytosis, due to absolute granulocytopenia.

Treatment. One antiviral agent, amantadine (Symmetrel), is approved for treatment of type A influenza infections. Amantadine attenuates clinical disease in all patients with influenza A by reducing the fever by 50% and by shortening the duration of illness by 1 or 2 days; these benefits are seen only if the drug is administered within 24 to 48 hours of onset of illness. Side effects, which include insomnia, nervousness, dizziness, and difficulty in concentrating, occur in about 7% of adults, appear a few hours after the first dose, tend to diminish after repeated doses, and disappear upon discontinuation of the drug. The cost of a ther-

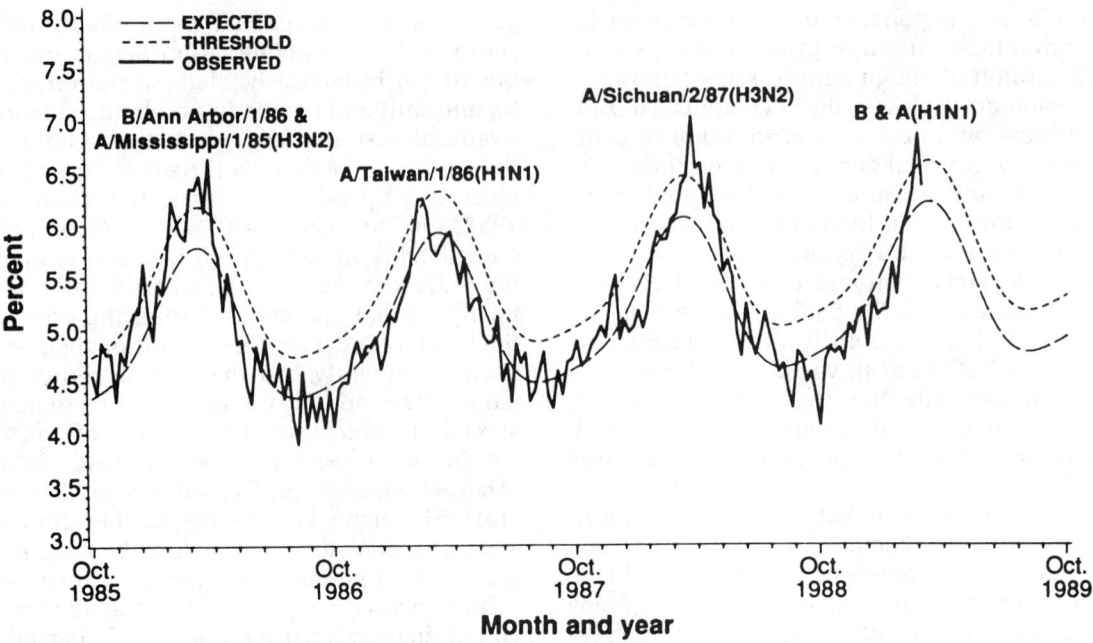

Figure 28.1. Pneumonia and Influenza Deaths as Percentage of Total Deaths—United States, October 1985–February 1989. From Morbidity and Mortality Weekly Report, 38:97, 1989.

apeutic course (200-mg loading dose followed by 100 mg twice a day for 5 days) is approximately $5, in contrast to the more costly prophylactic course (12, 31) discussed in Chapter 32. Treatment with amantadine should be seriously considered for patients at high risk of morbidity and mortality who develop an influenza-like illness in a community where the state or local health department has reported influenza A. Groups at high risk include:

1. Unvaccinated children and adults with chronic diseases including pulmonary, cardiovascular, metabolic neuromuscular, or immunodeficiency diseases;
2. Adults whose activities are vital to community function, including selected hospital personnel;
3. Patients with life-threatening primary influenzal pneumonia, although the efficacy of amantadine in such patients has not been demonstrated.

Because of the side effects, only partial effectiveness, difficulty of identifying influenza A infections in the individual, and difficulty in initiating therapy early in clinical illness, amantadine has not achieved widespread use. Rimantadine, not yet approved for general use, is equally efficacious for prophylaxis and for treatment of uncomplicated influenza and is associated with less insomnia, fever, and central nervous system side effects. Aerosolized ribavirin is also not approved and is not appropriate for outpatient therapy.

Supportive measures are important for symptomatic relief. Bed rest and adequate fluid intake should be advised. Aspirin, 600 to 900 mg every 3 to 4 hours, or acetaminophen if aspirin is contraindicated, reduces headache, fever, and myalgia. Sponging with tepid water is effective in lowering high fever, whereas sponging with isopropyl alcohol only increases the patient's discomfort. Relief of nasal discharge may be obtained by agents discussed in the section above on the common cold. Relief of cough with cough suppressants is discussed in the section below on acute bronchitis.

Complications. Patients should be advised that dyspnea, hemoptysis, wheezing, purulent sputum, fever persisting more than 7 days, and, rarely, dark urine, severe muscle pain, and tenderness, herald complications that demand prompt medical attention and usually hospitalization.

Pulmonary complications exhibit a continuous spectrum of severity, from mild airway hyperreactivity without pulmonary infiltrates, to segmental influenza pneumonia or secondary bacterial pneumonia, to fulminant bilateral influenza pneumonia with the adult respiratory distress syndrome (ARDS).

Airway hyperreactivity is most common after influenza but may occur in less severe form after many viral upper respiratory infections (20). It appears to be caused by destruction of epithelial cells secondary to viral invasion and may result from heightened sensitization of afferent cholinergic irritant receptors in the respiratory mucosa. Exposure to inhaled irritants induces a vagally mediated increase in airway resistance, manifested clinically by bronchospasm, coughing, or both; cough may also be due to direct stimulation of cholinergic irritant receptors as these are the receptors that mediate the cough reflex (for additional details, see Chapter 54). Patients with asthma or chronic bronchitis have even greater bronchoconstrictor responses because of their underlying bronchial smooth muscle hyperreactivity. Airway hyperreactivity can be demonstrated for 3 to 8 weeks after influenza and other viral infections, and occasionally it may last for 4 to 6 months even in nonatopic patients.

The relationship between airway hyperreactivity and persistent symptoms after influenza is not entirely clear; however, it is likely that nonproductive cough, wheezing, and dyspnea on exertion are related to airway hyperreactivity. These postflu symptoms seem to be particularly common in urban areas during periods of high air pollution. Chest roentgenograms are clear. Both cough and wheezing, following an otherwise uncomplicated flu-like infection, may be treated with a trial of a bronchodilator (see Chapter 55) as needed and at bedtime. Patients troubled particularly by nighttime cough will obtain additional relief with 15 to 30 mg of codeine at bedtime.

During influenza epidemics, there is a 2- to 3-fold increase in the *incidence of pneumonia* (4). The incidence of postinfluenzal bronchitis and pneumonia varies with age: low in patients below age 50 and very high in patients over age 70. Mortality from pneumonia during influenza epidemics clearly increases for those with chronic pulmonary disease and congestive heart failure.

Primary influenza viral pneumonia is a rare complication occurring predominantly among persons with cardiovascular disease but occasionally in healthy young adults. After several days of typical influenzal symptoms, fever, cough, and dyspnea rapidly progress to cyanosis and delirium, often developing into adult respiratory distress syndrome. Immediate hospitalization and intensive care are required, but mortality remains high.

Milder influenza pneumonia may be restricted to a single lobe. Patients present with persistent fever, cough and dyspnea, localized rales, normal white blood cell count, and they subsequently experience a benign course.

Secondary bacterial pneumonia and bronchitis complicate up to 10% of influenza A illness, depending on age group and chronic pulmonary or cardiac disease. Pneumonia complications of influenza B are less common but are becoming increasingly recognized (2). The presentation is typically biphasic: The initial influenzal illness is followed by several days of clinical improvement, and then there is an exacerbation of fever with production of purulent or bloody sputum. The predominant bacterial pathogen is *Streptococcus pneumoniae*, but *Haemophilus influenzae* and *Staphylococcus aureus* are also common; the last mentioned has a mortality rate of approximately 50% in this setting. The diagnosis and management of pneumonia are discussed below.

Nonpulmonary complications of influenza are unusual. Myositis, with thigh pain and inability to walk, occurs occasionally in children and adolescents. Severe myositis with myoglobinuria and acute renal failure has been observed in adults after both influenza A and B. Guillain-Barré, syndrome, encephalitis, and transverse myelitis are neurological complications associated with influenza A, and, rarely, B infection, but no firm causal relationship has been established. *Reye's syndrome*, on the other hand, is a rare but severe complication of influenza, usually type B, presenting as a change in mental status and progressing to coma and hepatic failure. The mean age of attack is six years and the incidence has fallen markedly in recent years. The syndrome is very rare in adults, and, unlike the situation in children, there is no known relationship between aspirin and the syndrome in adults. With the exception of mild myositis, all of the nonpulmonary complications of influenza require hospitalization for differential diagnosis and management.

Prevention. The use of influenza vaccine and amantadine prophylaxis in ambulatory practice are discussed in Chapter 32.

Pharyngitis

Sore throat is the fourth most common symptom seen in medical practice (10). The most important task in the evaluation of pharyngitis is to identify and treat group A streptococcal infections in adults, especially those with a history of prior rheumatic fever, and to recognize less common causes of pharyngitis associated with more serious systemic illness.

Pharyngitis in the adult is caused by a variety of bacterial and viral pathogens with no one pathogen predominating (24). Common pathogens include beta-hemolytic streptococci groups A and G, *Mycoplasma pneumoniae*, TWAR strain of *Chlamydia pneumoniae*, *Corynebacterium hemolyticum*, *Neisseria gonorrheae*, respiratory syncytial virus, influenza types A and B, parainfluenza, herpes simplex virus, adenovirus, and Epstein-Barr virus. No pathogens are found in at least one-third of cases.

Accompanying signs and symptoms may suggest the etiology in some cases. *Corynebacterium hemolyticum* is characterized by exudative pharyngitis, a scarlatiniform rash, fever, and adenopathy (30). Infectious mononucleosis (see Chapter 53) is characterized by the clinical triad of sore throat, fever, and lymphadenopathy with or without mild tenderness; it can be distinguished with certainty from streptococcal infection on clinical grounds only when hepatosplenomegaly and a maculopapular skin rash (similar to a drug eruption or rubella) are present. Palatal petechiae may be seen in mononucleosis but may also occur with rubella and streptococcal pharyngitis. Pharyngoconjunctival fever is usually accompanied by influenza-like symptoms and can be distinguished by concurrent conjunctivitis in one-third of cases and a history of swimming pool exposure 1 week prior to onset. Herpes simplex, Coxsackie virus A, herpangina, and aphthous stomatitis are distinguished by the presence of mucosal vesicles or ulcers (see additional details in Chapter 101).

Diagnosis, Management, and Course. Most patients with pharyngitis are not cultured, and the culture technique routinely used in office practice will detect only streptococci. The most common bacterial pathogens are streptococci, *C. hemolyticum, M pneumoniae*, and many experts feel that the drug of choice for the treatment of presumptive bacterial pharyngitis in adults is erythromycin, 500 mg orally twice daily for 10 days. This regimen would cover each of the common pathogens causing pharyngitis.

The failure of initial treatment to relieve symptoms after four days of treatment should prompt an evaluation for one of the five etiologies discussed here, or for a complication such as "Peritonsillar Abscess," pharyngeal abscess or epiglottitis (see page 311).

1. *Group A streptococcal pharyngitis*. The incubation period is 2 to 4 days, followed by the abrupt onset of sore throat, malaise, fever, and headache. The "classic syndrome," including temperature elevation, tender tonsillar lymph nodes (at angle of jaw), and grayish-white exudate on the tonsils occurs in less than 10% of cases of streptococcal pharyngitis (26) and may occur in other types of pharyngitis as well. Importantly cough and rhinorrhea are not usually present in the patient with strep throat. The only clinical feature specific for group A streptococcal infection is a rare scarlatiniform rash (*scarlet fever*), characterized by a diffuse red blush appearing on the trunk early in the disease, spreading centrifugally, blanching with pressure, and acquiring a "sandpaper" texture. One week later the skin desquamates in large sheets, particularly over the palms and soles.

Because clinical findings are not specific, the diagnosis of streptococcal pharyngitis requires a *throat culture*. Office throat culture kits are inexpensive and offer rapid diagnosis and high sensitivity (approximately 95%). To avoid false-negative results, correct plating techniques must be followed. The tonsillar tissue and posterior pharynx are swabbed vigorously enough to induce a gag reflex; the swab is then rubbed on about one-sixth of a blood agar plate and subsequently streaked with a sterile wire loop. The agar is stabbed several times with the loop to enable recognition of subsurface hemolysis. A bacitracin disc is applied and the plate incubated at 37°C for 18 to 24 hours. With a little practice, one can readily recognize beta-hemolytic colonies, estimate the number, and recognize the inhibition of their growth by the bacitracin disc if they belong to group A. Many physicians prefer to send throat swabs in transport media to state or regional laboratories. Rapid diagnosis using Gram stain of pharyngeal swab material yields variable results even with skilled observers and is thus not recommended. Rapid diagnosis using kits to detect streptococcal antigen in throat swab specimens has improved; specificity is adequate, but sensitivity remains less than that of a correctly performed throat culture. If a strep antigen test is used, negative assays must be followed by a standard throat culture. There is no evidence at this time that current strep

antigen tests substantially reduce the number of throat cultures performed (8).

In *deciding whether to culture or treat a patient for strep throat*, the results of a study conducted in multiple primary care settings are helpful (26). In this study, patients complaining of sore throat could be separated into three groups according to clinical features and the results of throat cultures:

—A group with tonsilar exudate, tender anterior cervical adenopathy, and temperature greater than 100°F: 2% of all pharyngitis patients had this constellation of findings and of these 42.1% had positive strep cultures.
—A group with tonsilar exudate or tender adenopathy or a temperature greater than 100°F: 61% had one of these findings and of these 13.5% had positive cultures.
—A group with none of the three clinical findings: 37% were in this category and of these 3.4% had positive cultures.

Based on this study, it would be reasonable to treat patients from the first group with antibiotics before knowing the result of the throat culture, to culture patients from the second group but defer antibiotics until the culture result is known, and to neither culture nor treat patients in the third group. An exception to these guidelines is that all patients with a sore throat who have a *history of rheumatic fever* should be cultured whether or not the above clinical features are present (15). Although some positive cultures will represent asymptomatic carriage, it is best to assume that all positive cultures are significant in these patients and to treat accordingly.

In three types of patients besides those having characteristics of the first group above, antibiotic treatment for streptococcal pharyngitis should be started routinely before throat culture results are known: (*a*) patients with a past history of rheumatic fever not currently on prophylaxis, (*b*) young patients with a strong family history of rheumatic fever, and (*c*) all new cases of pharyngitis in an explosive epidemic of streptococcal disease in semiclosed populations. (Local health authorities should be notified immediately in this situation.)

Symptomatic family contacts of patients with streptococcal pharyngitis should have cultures made and should be treated if the cultures are positive. Routine cultures of asymptomatic family members is not indicated.

In adults over the age of 15 without a prior history of acute rheumatic fever (ARF), first attacks of ARF are extremely rare. Therefore the principal goals of treatment for streptococcal pharyngitis in such adults are the amelioration of symptoms, the prevention of local suppurative complications, and the prevention of spread. Since early therapy (in the first 2 days) is required for symptomatic relief, most physicians do not wait for culture results in patients with severe pharyngitis. In untreated patients, fever, malaise, and sore throat are self-limited, abating in 3 to 5 days; early treatment may reduce modestly the duration and severity of these symptoms. In patients being treated to prevent recurrence of ARF, therapy within 7 days of onset of pharyngitis is sufficient. The mean latent period of ARF is 19 days, with a range of 1 to 5 weeks.

The preferred therapy for streptococcal pharyngitis is parenteral benzathine penicillin, 1.2 million units given once, because it obviates noncompliance. If oral therapy is given, the recommended regimen is penicillin V, 250 mg three times a day for 10 days. For patients allergic to penicillin, erythromycin, 250 mg every 6 hours for 10 days, is recommended. (See practical information about antimicrobials, Table 28.3.) Posttreatment cultures should be done only if there is a history of rheumatic fever in the patient or in a household contact.

2. *Gonococcal pharyngitis.* Gonococcal pharyngitis is diagnosed by throat culture. Special culture techniques should be used to detect gonorrhea in specimens from patients practicing orogenital sex. Gram stain of direct pharyngeal smear is insensitive and nonspecific. Calcium alginate swabs should be used, as ordinary cotton swabs contain inhibitory fatty acids. The swab should be immediately plated on a modified Thayer-Martin medium that is incorporated in a number of inexpensive kits for office culture. For throat cultures, however, *N. gonorrhoeae* must be distinguished from *N. meningitidis* and *N. lactamicus* by carbohydrate fermentation and serology; therefore, cultures should be sent to state or regional laboratories. Effective treatment, based upon the 1989 recommendations of the CDC, is either ceftriaxone, 250 mg as a single intramuscular injection or erythromycin, 500 mg by mouth four times a day for 7 days. The former, newer regimen is highly effective, is comfortable for the patient, and obviates compliance and drug resistance problems. Ampicillin and spectinomycin should not be used, as they are associated with unacceptable failure rates in the treatment of pharyngeal gonorrhea. A follow-up culture 7 days after completion of therapy should be done as a test of cure. Cotreatment for presumed chlamydia should be given (doxycycline 100 mg twice daily for 7 days).

Chapters 27 and 94 discuss in detail sexually transmitted infections in men and women, respectively.

3. *Diphtheria.* This diagnosis should be suspected when there is a grayish membrane in the anterior nares or on the tonsils, uvula, or pharynx. (Infectious mononucleosis and "strep throat" display a creamy white exudate and do not involve the uvula.) Treatment must begin before bacteriological confirmation and requires hospitalization for bed rest, close observation, antitoxin, and peni-

cillin. Management of contacts is discussed in Chapter 32.

4. *Other bacteria.* Throat cultures often grow pneumococci, staphylococci, groups B, C, and G streptococci, and various Gram-negative enterobacteria. These species, which colonize the pharynx, have only rarely been shown to be etiological agents in pharyngitis, and patients who harbor them should not be treated with antimicrobial agents.

5. *Vincents' angina.* This is an anaerobic infection of the pharynx characterized by fever, tender lymphadenitis, a large grayish-brown pseudomembrane in the pharynx, and very foul odor. It is a complication of acute necrotizing ulcerative gingivitis, which is described in Chapter 101. Hospitalization for antimicrobial treatment with penicillin or tetracycline is the appropriate management plan.

Chronic or Relapsing Sore Throat

Some patients will describe a sore throat of several weeks' duration at their first visit. Others will have either a prolonged course after an illness that began as a typical acute pharyngitis syndrome or frequent recurrence of sore throats. The conditions that may cause prolonged and/or recurrent pharyngitis are listed in Table 28.1. Most are discussed in more detail elsewhere in the book as indicated in the table.

One problem, "*chronic tonsillitis,*" often related to recurrent streptococcal pharyngitis, may be alleviated best by tonsillectomy. The clinical diagnosis of chronic tonsillitis is made in patients with recurrent sore throats (several in the same year), very large tonsils, and chronically enlarged, periodically tender lymph nodes (11). Considerable evidence indicates that β-lactamase-producing organisms in the pharynx, including *S. aureus*, *Hemophilus* species, *Bacteroides* species, and *Branhamella catarrhalis*, inactivate the penicillin and protect mucosal streptococci (7); these conditions may underlie some cases of chronic tonsillitis. For recurrent pharyngitis and tonsillitis due to Group A streptococci and aerobic and anaerobic penicillin-resistant pathogens, predictable eradication of streptococci and elimination of recurrent tonsillitis have been achieved with clindamycin or amoxycillin-clavulanic acid (Augmentin).

Table 28.1.
Causes of Chronic or Relapsing Sore Throat

Primary Site of Pain	Condition	See for Details
Pharynx	Chronic tonsillitis	
	Smoking (especially marijuana)	Chapters 20, 22
	Postnasal drip	Chapter 54
	Infectious mononucleosis	Chapter 53
	Chronic Fatigue Syndrome	Chapter 53
	Agranulocytosis	
	Acute leukemia	
	Pemphigus	
Not the Pharynx	Subacute thyroiditis	Chapter 73
	Angina (radiating to neck)	Chapter 57
	Psychogenic	Chapter 12

Acute Sinusitis

This is a bacterial infection of one or more paranasal sinuses, which complicates about 0.5% of viral upper respiratory infections. Sinusitis may also be a complication of noninfectious rhinitis, polyps, foreign bodies, or anatomical nasal obstruction of sinus drainage. Up to 10% of cases of acute sinusitis are an extension of dental abscess. Nursing home or homebound patients with nasogastric tubes occasionally have occult sinusitis as a cause of persistent fever.

Diagnosis. Acute sinusitis in the autumn, winter, and spring usually develops during the course of a viral upper respiratory infection. Sinusitis in the summer often is associated with swimming and diving or with allergic rhinitis (see Chapter 23).

The pain of sinusitis is due to periosteal reaction secondary to an expanding purulent inflammation behind an outlet obstruction. The pain is dull in the early stages but becomes throbbing in later stages. Coughing, dependency, and percussion over the involved sinus exacerbate the pain. Percussion of the teeth is often painful in maxillary sinusitis. The facial pain associated with the noninfectious causes of nasal congestion (see Chapter 23) may resemble the early pain of acute sinusitis, but it is less localized and does not become progressively worse. Other causes of facial pain to be distinguished from sinusitis are dental abscess (Chapter 101), migraine, cluster headache, and trigeminal neuralgia (Chapter 79) (38).

Nontender edema of the eyelids, seen predominantly in children, may occur with uncomplicated ethmoid and maxillary sinusitis. Acute sinusitis may present without pain as in subacute sinusitis (see below), usually in the guise of a cold persisting for more than 2 weeks and accompanied by cough due to postnasal drip, purulent nasal discharge, and headache.

Examination should include the pharynx, nose, ears, and teeth. Transillumination of the sinuses can be attempted, but it is often unreliable.

Radiological examination of the sinuses, comprising four views to visualize all paranasal sinuses, is the most sensitive diagnostic test in acute sinusitis. Fig. 28.2 shows the typical radiological changes seen in acute maxillary sinusitis. X-rays are not necessary in patients with typical signs and symptoms. It is most helpful in the diagnostic workup of headache and in those patients who do not respond to therapy or who are toxic and require accurate diagnosis early.

Most cases of acute sinusitis can be treated without culture. Nasopharyngeal swabs are usually contaminated with normal flora and are of no use. Studies employing antral puncture (14) indicate that S. pneumoniae and unencapsulated H. influenzae are the bacterial agents in 60% of acute infections and probably in most acute exacerbations of chronic sinusitis. Anaerobes, Streptococcus pyogenes, Neisseria catarrhalis, alpha-hemolytic streptococci, Mycoplasma pneumoniae, Chlamydia pneumoniae, and Gram-negative aerobes each cause a small percentage of infec-

tions. S. aureus causes less than 5% and tends to be associated with pansinusitis and general toxicity.

Management and Course. *Antimicrobials.* Ampicillin or amoxicillin provides the best coverage of the most common bacterial pathogens, in a dose of 250 to 500 mg, four times daily for 10 days. In penicillin-allergic patients, trimethoprim-sulfamethoxazole, two tablets twice a day for 10 days, is a good alternative. (See practical information about antimicrobials, Table 28.3.) For patients who respond slowly or relapse, amoxicillin-clavulanic acid (Augmentin) is effective to treat potential β-lactamase-producing pathogens. Effective but more expensive alternatives include cefalor (Ceclor), cefuroxime axetil (Ceftin), and ciprofloxacin (Cipro), the latter being particularly effective for S. aureus.

Symptomatic therapy to improve sinus drainage is important. A decongestant spray, such as Neo-Synephrine 0.25 or 0.5%, is most convenient, administered as an initial squirt to decrease congestion in the membranes of the anterior nares, followed 5 to 10 minutes later by a second squirt delivered deeper to the middle meatus. This is repeated every 4 hours for 2 to 4 days and followed by oral decongestants (see details on the common cold above) for an additional 2 weeks. Steam inhalation is often helpful. Pain relief is important, and codeine may be required. Patients who plan to fly, especially in nonpressurized aircraft, should take an oral decongestant before takeoff, supplemented with topical decongestant spray every 4 hours.

Resolution of facial pain, headache, and fever is expected within several days. If no response occurs by this time, referral to an otolaryngologist for radiography, antral puncture, or surgical drainage is advisable. Toxic patients, especially those with frontoethmoid sinusitis, should be referred at initial presentation for hospitalization, drainage, and definitive parenteral antibiotics. Patients whose symptoms worsen during the first 48 hours of vigorous ambulatory therapy should be referred. Many patients with severe facial pain are benefited by early antral puncture for pain relief.

Complications of acute sinusitis are unusual. They should be regarded as medical emergencies because they represent direct extension of infection to adjacent orbits, bone, blood vessels, and central nervous system. Nontender periorbital edema represents restriction of orbital venous outflow through congested ethmoid veins, is not associated with decreased visual acuity, and is appropriately managed with vigorous medical therapy. However, tender periorbital swelling, associated with proptosis and chemosis, represents orbital cellulitis and requires immediate referral to an otolaryngologist. Subsequent progression of cellulitis to subperiosteal or orbital abscess, associated with ophthalmoplegia and loss of vision, requires emergency surgical drainage. Osteomyelitis is most often a complication of frontal sinusitis. Cavernous sinus thrombosis should be suspected in the patient with signs of orbital complications plus extreme tox-

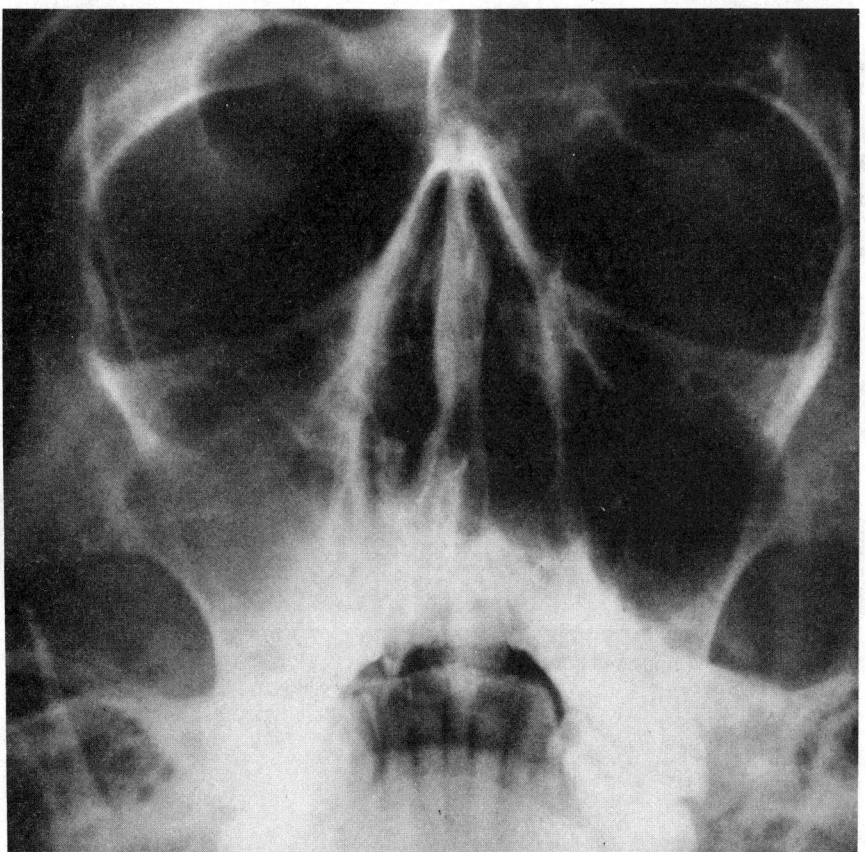

Figure 28.2. Acute infectious maxillary sinusitis. Waters' view shows complete opacity of the right maxillary sinus caused by thickening of the lining mucosa and/or fluid accumulation. The mucoperiosteal line is preserved. The left maxillary sinus is normal in appearance.

icity. Intracranial extension is rare but life threatening, presenting most commonly as meningitis. Abscesses in the brain and epidural and subdural spaces present more insidiously. Frontal lobe abscess may present as mild headache, low grade fever, malaise, and personality change. In poorly controlled diabetics and immunocompromised hosts rhinocerebral mucormycosis begins in the nose and maxillary sinuses and may be recognized by a black eschar on the nasal turbinates.

Subacute and Chronic Sinusitis

When the symptoms of acute sinusitis, especially pain and fever, subside with therapy, but purulent nasal discharge continues, this stage is called *subacute sinusitis*. Despite persistence of radiological changes, this stage usually resolves after an additional 2 to 3 weeks of conservative management, including antibiotics and oral decongestants.

Chronic sinusitis resists accurate definition but appears to result from episodes of prolonged, repeated, or inadequately treated acute sinusitis. This results in the loss of normal ciliated epithelial lining of the sinus cavity, which becomes populated by anaerobic and Gram-negative bacteria. Acute exacerbations occur, due primarily to the common organisms of acute sinusitis (*H. influenzae* and *S. pneumoniae*). Chronic sinusitis

commonly complicates certain systemic diseases, such as sarcoidosis, Wegener's granulomatosis, and allergic rhinitis with asthma. In allergic rhinitis, control of asthma is often facilitated by treatment of the sinusitis.

Diagnosis and Management.   Persistent purulent nasal discharge and postnasal drip, despite adequate medical therapy, are the primary features of chronic sinusitis. Facial pain and tenderness are minimal or absent. The sinuses transilluminate light poorly. Radiological examination usually reveals clouding of the cavities in some patients, thickening (greater than 5 mm) of the mucosal lining, and bony sclerosis (see Fig. 28.3). For this reason sinus films are of limited value in acute exacerbations superimposed on chronic sinusitis.

Referral to an otolaryngologist for appropriate surgical drainage is recommended. Oral penicillin V or ampicillin is the most appropriate antimicrobial, amoxacillin-clavulanate or clindamycin, 300 to 450 mg every eight hours, are appropriate alternates.

Pharyngeal Abscess

Occasionally, after several days of symptoms due to an upper respiratory tract infection, the patient will develop a complicating infection of one of the closed compartments adjacent to the pharynx. The most com-

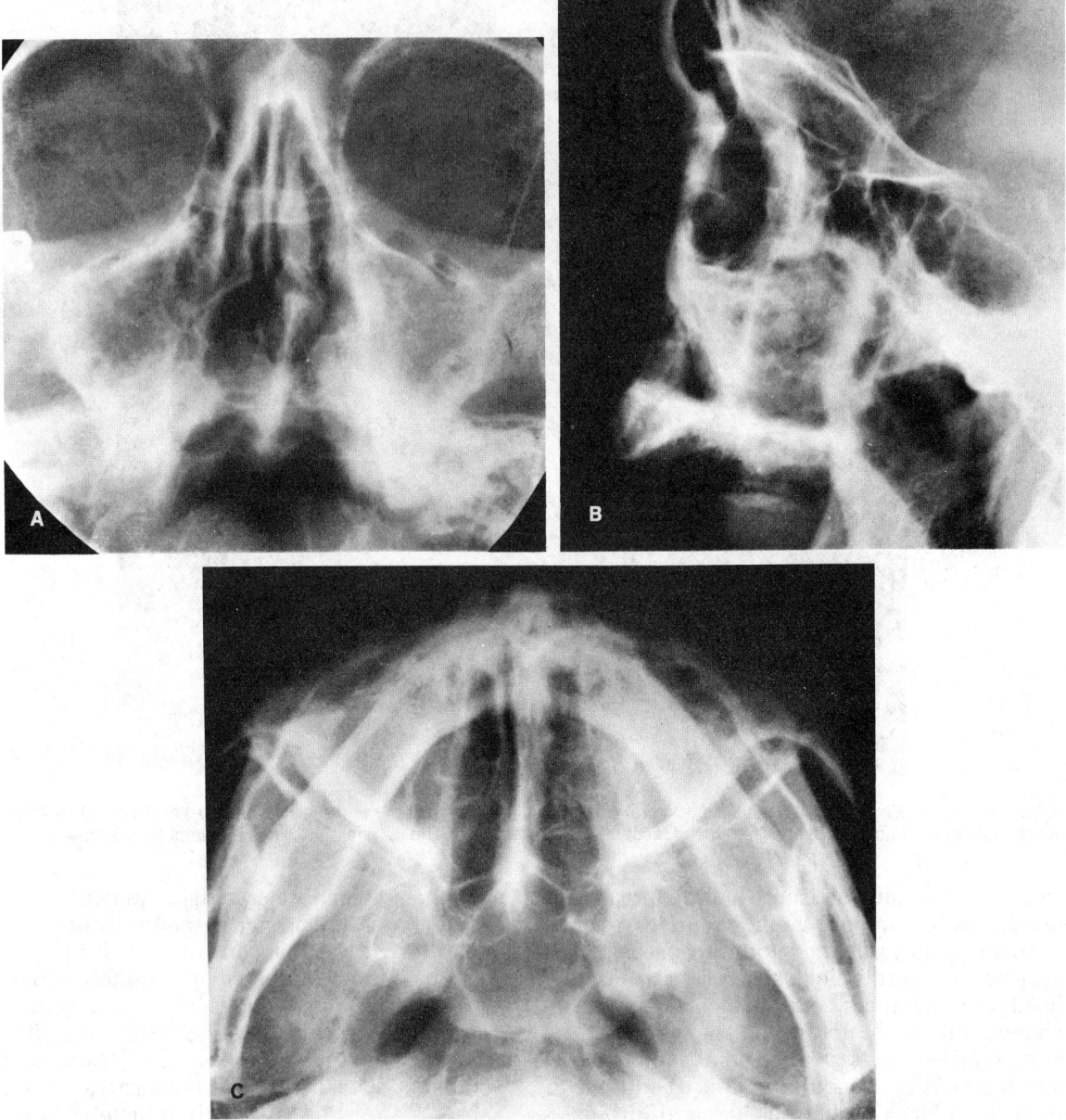

Figure 28.3.   Chronic infectious maxillary sinusitis. *A.* Waters' view: marked opacity of the left maxillary sinus and, to a lesser degree, of the right maxillary sinus, with disappearance of mucoperiosteal lines and sclerosis of the bony walls. *B.* Lateral view: marked bony sclerosis of all of the walls of the maxillary sinuses. *C.* Submentovertical view: marked sclerosis of posterolateral walls of the maxillary sinuses.

mon of these pharyngeal abscesses are peritonsillar abscess and retropharyngeal abscess. When one of these conditions is suspected, the patient should be referred immediately for evaluation and management by an otolaryngologist.

Peritonsillar Abscess. Patients with this condition develop severe odynophagia; they are not only unable to take liquids, but they may be unable to swallow their own saliva, resulting in early dehydration. The voice acquires a muffled quality, and trismus may be present. Fever, malaise, and systemic toxicity are typical. Dramatic relief may occur if the abscess drains spontaneously before the patient seeks medical attention. On physical examination, there is a swelling of

the anterior tonsillar pillar at its superior pole. The involved tonsil itself may or may not be enlarged, but it is displaced medially. This condition is almost always unilateral.

Retropharyngeal Abscess. The symptoms of this condition are similar to those of peritonsillar abscess. In addition, there may be respiratory embarrassment if the process extends inferiorly toward the larynx. Trismus is not common. On examination, a swelling in the posterior oropharynx is readily seen. Lateral soft tissue X-rays of the neck may disclose expansion of the soft tissue density in the posterior pharyngeal space.

Management. Incision and drainage, using either an

18-gauge needle or a surgical blade, is the treatment of choice for both of these conditions. This should be performed by an otolaryngologist or an oral surgeon. Antibiotics and warm saline gargles should follow drainage.

Epiglottitis

Acute epiglottitis is a life-threatening but curable condition. The epiglottis serves as a valve that closes over the proximal portion of the trachea during swallowing, to prevent aspiration. When the epiglottis becomes inflamed, the resultant edema causes it to curl posteriorly and inferiorly, thereby reducing the glottic aperture. Inspiration, which draws the epiglottis down, further reduces the effective airway.

Epiglottitis is a rare complication of upper respiratory infections. Most cases occur in children, although the condition may occur in adults.

The diagnosis of epiglottitis should be suspected in patients presenting with a sore throat, dysphagia, and progressive respiratory distress, all of short duration. On physical examination, stridor may be noted in inspiration. The patients are usually febrile. The oropharynx may be erythematous, but an important clue to the diagnosis is the relatively uninvolved appearance of the oropharynx found in some patients. Soft tissue X-rays of the neck may show edema of the epiglottis and narrowing of the aperture. The diagnosis is confirmed by indirect laryngoscopy, which reveals marked edema of the epiglottis; this procedure must be performed only in circumstances in which emergency intubation could be carried out as it may induce additional obstruction.

Management requires immediate admission to an intensive care unit, where close observation is essential since some patients with acute epiglottitis will require emergency tracheotomy (3).

Telephone Assessment and Self-Care for Upper Respiratory Infection

Most physicians welcome the opportunity to assess URI symptoms initially by phone. The phone assessment should accomplish the following:

1. Differentiate between infectious and allergic problems;
2. Among the patients with acute infections, distinguish those with possible bacterial infections or superinfections who should be examined to decide whether antibiotics should be prescribed;
3. Identify those who may be suffering from complications of a URI that require office evaluation. The following symptoms and signs should be sought: (*a*) symptoms lasting more than 3 weeks; (*b*) fever lasting more than 1 week, or associated with delirium; (*c*) purulent nasal discharge with sinus pain; (*d*) purulent sputum, chest pain, dyspnea, or hemoptysis; (*e*) ear pain or discharge; (*f*) sore throat and a history of rheumatic fever; (*g*) the combination of cough and fever over 102°F (39°C) or fever for more than 4 days; (*h*) hoarseness for more than 1 month; (*i*) pleuritic chest pain; (*j*) marked odynophagia; (*k*) the combination of dysphagia, stridor, and difficulty in breathing.
4. For those patients not needing a visit, provide simple instructions for self-care based upon the measures described earlier.

Increasing numbers of patients will be consulting self-care algorithms (42). The book *Take Care of Yourself* by Vickery and Fries (see "General References") is one of the most widely distributed collections of algorithms. In one evaluation (6), strict adherence to the algorithms for colds, influenza, cough, and sore throat would have increased the number of patient visits to a physician. Thus, this standard set of instructions exhibited sensitivity, missing few people who need to be examined, yet lacked specificity and led to unnecessary visits. This study points to the need to search for symptom complexes that better identify patients likely to be helped by a visit to a physician.

LOWER RESPIRATORY INFECTIONS

Acute Bronchitis

Clinical Characteristics

Acute bronchitis is an inflammatory condition of the tracheobronchial tree that results from respiratory infections with common cold viruses, influenza, adenovirus, *M. pneumoniae*, *Chlamydia pneumoniae*, *B. catarrhalis*, and rarely *Bordetella pertussis*. The role of secondary bacterial invasion by *S. pneumoniae* and *H. influenzae* is not clear. The illness is characterized by cough, with or without sputum production, persisting longer than expected (usually 1 to 2 weeks) after the onset of an acute URI.

Rhinovirus and coronavirus, by virtue of their high prevalence, are common etiological agents for mild bronchitis of short duration and without fever. Influenza, adenovirus, and *M. pneumoniae* cause a more severe bronchitis associated with fever and burning substernal pain. Mucoid sputum production develops in half of all cases and is not helpful in distinguishing etiological agents. Frequency and duration of cough are increased in cigarette smokers.

The patient presenting with a cough as the predominant or only respiratory symptom may have pneumonia, bronchitis, or one of a variety of noninfectious conditions associated with persistent cough. Diagnostic efforts should be directed at identifying those patients with pneumonia and with noninfectious causes of cough, leaving acute bronchitis as a diagnosis of exclusion.

The diagnosis of pneumonia is discussed below. In approaching the patient who has a persistent cough without apparent infectious etiology, it is helpful to consider what is known about the anatomy and physiology of the cough reflex (Chapter 54). Airborne irritants, especially smog containing sulfur dioxide, and allergens cause bronchitic symptoms. Repeated small aspiration of oral and upper airway secretions, especially in the elderly and in the alcoholic with incompetent glottic function, is also associated with nighttime cough.

Identification of the agent in most episodes of acute bronchitis is not possible. Bacterial cultures of sputum are useless, since the contribution of bacteria to acute bronchitis is unclear and sputum is readily contaminated by nasopharyngeal flora. Culture techniques for viral agents and *M. pneumoniae* are not widely available. *M. pneumoniae* may be implicated if bullous myringitis is observed, or suggested if (*a*) the patient is a young adult, (*b*) similar cases are occurring in the family or in the close contacts, and (*c*) the case occurs in the summer or early fall season. The diagnosis can be confirmed by a 4-fold or greater rise in complement fixation titer in convalescent serum.

Pertussis, rare in adults, is characterized by initial nonspecific symptoms of malaise and rhinorrhea followed by 1 to 4 weeks of severe paroxysms of repetitive coughs without inspiration. The paroxysm is terminated by an inspiratory whoop. The clinical symptoms are attenuated in previously immunized adults and children, who act as reservoirs of infection for nonimmune infants. *B. pertussis* is identified by culture of nasopharyngeal swab on special media, or more rapidly by direct immune fluorescent staining of organisms on smear of nasopharyngeal secretions.

Treatment

It is not helpful to treat acute bronchitis with *antibiotics* in patients who are otherwise healthy and free of systemic symptoms. Patients with underlying chronic diseases such as diabetes mellitus or congestive heart failure may benefit from ameliorating symptoms or preventing progression to pneumonia. Whereas randomized trials have supported the use of doxycycline or tetracycline in these patients (35), ampicillin or trimethoprim-sulfamethoxazole have been shown to be modestly effective in several trials. Amoxicillin-clavulanate, cefaclor, cefuroxime axetil, and ciprofloxacin are more expensive alternatives that have been shown to be efficacious in randomized trials. Erythromycin, 500 mg twice daily for 14 days, is an appropriate choice if *M. pneumoniae* is suspected on epidemiological grounds (see below) and since the TWAR strain of *Chlamydia* is commonly encountered. *B. pertussis* infection is treated with erythromycin. (See practical information about antimicrobials, Table 28.3.)

Treatment of acute bronchitis is usually *symptomatic*. Many patients will have tried an over-the-counter cough suppressant containing dextromethorphan without relief. Cough suppression, primarily to get a good night's sleep, is best obtained with preparations containing codeine, although in titrating up to an effective dose, patients should be warned of problems with drowsiness and constipation. (See Chapter 54 for a discussion of narcotic and non-narcotic cough sup-

pressants.) Except in allergic rhinitis with postnasal drip, antihistamines, present in many combination cough remedies, should be avoided because they dry out secretions. There is no consistent evidence that expectorants or glyceryl guaiacolate alter the course of bronchitis. Maintaining hydration with oral fluids is a reasonable approach to preventing mucous plugs. Inhaled steam and cool mist provide symptomatic relief but fail to deliver water droplets into the smaller airways.

Smokers with acute bronchitis should be strongly encouraged to stop smoking at least for the duration of the acute illness. Those smokers with a history of chronic cough before their bronchitis may be more motivated to discontinue smoking permanently in the face of the acute illness. In 50% of those who discontinue smoking, the chronic cough will resolve completely within 1 month. Behavioral approaches to smoking cessation are described in Chapter 20.

Acute Exacerbations of Chronic Bronchitis

Clinical Characteristics

Respiratory infections contribute to the episodic worsening of cough and increased sputum production in the patient with chronic bronchitis, and they are the most common identifiable causes of death in these patients. Evidence that infections in adulthood play an independent role in the deterioration of pulmonary function is lacking, however (39).

The most important indicator of intercurrent infection is the patient's report of a change in color, consistency, and amount of sputum. Patients who consistently produce purulent sputum most of the time may notice increasing cough, dyspnea, and fatigue. Systemic toxicity with fever and chills is generally absent unless pneumonia is present.

The role of bacteria in acute exacerbations of chronic bronchitis is difficult to assess. The bronchial secretions of patients with chronic bronchitis contain pneumococci, unencapsulated *Haemophilus* species, and normal pharyngeal flora, which persist through asymptomatic intervals. The development of purulent sputum is not correlated with the presence of one or more specific bacterial species. These bacteria appear de novo during acute exacerbations in only a small percentage of uncolonized patients. Similarly, the acquisition of a new serotype of either pneumococci or encapsulated *Haemophilus* species is usually not followed by a clinical exacerbation. In summary, a primary role for these bacteria in the pathogenesis of clinical exacerbations remains unclear, and performing Gram stain and a culture of the sputum during acute exacerbations will not provide useful information.

Viruses (influenza, parainfluenza, respiratory syncytial, rhinovirus, and coronavirus) may cause up to 50% of acute infectious exacerbations. *M. pneumoniae* may be the agent in up to 10% of episodes.

Treatment

Acute exacerbations of chronic bronchitis should always be managed with more vigorous applications of routine therapy for chronic symptoms. Clearance of secretions should be promoted with postural drainage and therapeutic doses of bronchodilators (see Chapter 55). Cough suppressants and sedatives should be avoided. Smokers should be strongly counseled to discontinue cigarettes at least until their acute symptoms have resolved. As noted above, chronic cough will resolve completely within 1 month in half of those patients who are motivated by an acute illness to discontinue cigarettes permanently.

Antimicrobial prophylaxis is commonly used in the management of chronic bronchitis, but the efficacy of this practice has not been demonstrated convincingly (39). Many studies have suggested that continuous prophylaxis with tetracycline in low doses reduces the frequency of exacerbations during the winter months. The conclusions of most studies, however, do not stand up to rigorous analysis. In addition, there is considerable concern that widespread use of prophylactic antibiotics without clear effectiveness may promote emergence and dissemination of antibiotic-resistant strains in the community.

Efficacy of *short-term antibiotic therapy* given for acute exacerbations is unclear due to the difficulty in assessing therapeutic benefits and variable results among randomized trials (35). For the individual patient, efficacy appears to be based primarily on the patient's reported response to antibiotics during previous exacerbations. A reasonable approach is to provide reliable patients who have three or more acute exacerbations per year with a prescription for tetracycline, 250 mg four times daily for 7 to 14 days, ampicillin, 250 to 500 mg four times daily, or trimethoprim-sulfamethoxazole, two tablets twice daily. The patient is instructed to begin the antibiotic within 24 hours of the first sign of a "chest cold," since early initiation of therapy may be more effective in alleviating symptoms and preventing lost time from work (39). Those who benefit most from these antibiotics have a triad of symptoms including increased dyspnea, increased sputum, and sputum purulence (1). Oral penicillin V and chloramphenicol are not appropriate alternatives, since penicillin is not effective against the *Haemophilus* species and there are many safer alternatives to chloramphenicol.

Some patients managed at home for acute exacerbations will not improve by any criteria or will deteriorate after self-initiated therapy. The patient should be asked to keep in touch by phone during the acute episode so that symptoms indicating pneumonia will be detected earlier.

Pneumonia

There are over 3,000,000 episodes of pneumonia annually in the United States, responsible for over 30 million days of disability requiring bed rest. With influenza, pneumonia ranks fifth among all diseases as a cause of death and first among infectious diseases (10).

Definition

Distinction from Bronchitis. Bronchitis and pneumonia represent a continuum of lower respiratory infection. Aspirated pathogens including bacteria, mycoplasma, and viruses invade the bronchial epithelium. The extent of involvement of adjacent lung parenchyma determines whether there is an infiltrate on chest roentgenogram. The alveolar inflammation spreads like a grass fire, and the advancing edge of edema and leukocyte infiltration are not radiologically apparent. Patients seen early and those with emphysema and reduced parenchyma may fail to show any infiltrate or may show a patchy infiltrate on their chest film despite the presence of considerable inflammation. Thus the clinical distinction between acute bronchitis and acute pneumonia is often an arbitrary radiological distinction. Early management and the decision for hospitalization must focus on the overall condition of the patient in terms of signs and symptoms of systemic toxicity as well as of localized pulmonary infection.

"Atypical" Versus "Bacterial" Pneumonia. The clinical presentation of pneumonia can be divided into two categories: "bacterial pneumonias" and "atypical pneumonias." "Atypical" historically referred to cold hemagglutinin-positive pneumonias, which have more recently been identified as being due to *M. pneumoniae*. Atypical pneumonias due to a variety of other viral, bacterial, chlamydial, and parasitic agents may be clinically indistinguishable from mycoplasmal pneumonia unless definitive diagnostic studies are done. The usefulness in separating "bacterial" from "atypical" pneumonia lies in predicting outcome and need for hospitalization, at the time of initial presentation in the office. Thus only a small proportion of patients with mycoplasmal and viral pneumonia require hospitalization, whereas a large percentage of patients with bacterial pneumonias are sick enough to require hospitalization. The following discussion is restricted to the recognition of patients requiring hospitalization for pneumonia and to the ambulatory management of patients with pneumonia who do not require hospitalization. Chapter 31 describes the post-hospital management of lung abscess, a complication of pneumonia that may require prolonged antimicrobial treatment.

Pneumonia Syndromes

Bacterial Pneumonia. Bacterial pneumonias comprise half of all adult pneumonias, and 60 to 90% of these are due to S. *pneumoniae*. Pneumococcal pneumonia may occur in a previously healthy adult, or after an upper respiratory infection, usually with the abrupt onset of shaking chills, fever, pleuritic chest pain, and cough productive of purulent or rusty sputum. In the setting of compromised pulmonary clearance of secretions (depressed consciousness, morbid obesity, abdominal surgery, chronic bronchitis, congestive heart failure, and alcoholism) that predisposes to pneumococcal and other bacterial pneumonias, or in the setting of HIV infection, onset of clinical symptoms may be more insidious. Other types of bacterial pneumonias are more common in different clinical settings: staphylococcal and *H. influenzae* after influenza A or B; *Haemophilus*, *Klebsiella*, and anaerobic pneumonias in alcoholics; anaerobic and Gram-negative pneumonias in recently hospitalized patients. In the elderly, particularly those in nursing homes, *S. pneumoniae* continues to be the most common cause of pneumonia, but Gram-negative aerobes, nontypable strains of *H. influenzae*, and mixed pneumococcal-Gram-negative anaerobes are common etiologies. Group B streptococcus, *B. catarrhalis*, and *Legionella pneumophilia* are also occasional etiologies of pneumonia in the elderly (41). *B. catarrhalis* is particularly common in patients with chronic obstructive lung disease (32).

Atypical Pneumonia. The atypical pneumonia syndrome comprises the majority of pneumonias in persons under 40. Atypical pneumonia is distinguished by a prodrome of headache and myaligia before the respiratory symptoms. *M. pneumoniae* is the agent in 60 to 90% of pneumonias in this age group (16). A number of viruses (influenza A and B, respiratory syncytial virus, parainfluenza, adenovirus), *Chlamydia psittaci*, TWAR strain of chlamydia (*C. pneumoniae*), rickettsia (Q fever), and bacteria (tularemia and Legionnaires' disease), and a protozoa (*Pneumocystis carinii*) may present as a pneumonitis that clinically is indistinguishable from mycoplasmal pneumonia (28). The onset is a flu-like illness, with fever, headache, myalgias, and malaise. At onset or several days later a nonproductive hacking cough and substernal chest pain appear, accompanied by dyspnea and respiratory distress in more severe cases. Pleuritic chest pain and hemoptysis are unusual.

Complications of M. pneumoniae are more common in severely ill patients, who probably require hospitalization, but may appear in patients initially managed at home. These complications include sinusitis, otitis media, myringitis (diagnostic if bullae are seen), erythema multiform or erythema nodosum, intravascular hemolysis, meningoencephalitis, toxic psychosis, myocarditis, and pericarditis. Persistent hacking cough, lasting as long as 6 weeks despite therapy, is common and requires symptomatic relief with codeine (see Chapter 54). Relapse of the primary disease occurs in up to 10% of cases, usually 2 to 3 weeks after the initial illness, and is probably related to the fact that mycoplasma persists in bronchial epithelium for up to 14 weeks.

Pneumonia due to *C. pneumoniae* is characterized by fever, cough, and sore throat, and it often presents as a biphasic illness with severe pharyngitis and laryngitis in the first phase (29).

Diarrhea, relative bradycardia, abdominal pain, liver enzyme elevations, and hematuria may occur in Legionnaires' disease but can accompany pneumonia due to viruses or mycoplasma (21). Signs of encephalop-

athy (confusion, delirium, stupor) are clearly more common in Legionnaires' disease.

Since 70% of first opportunistic infections in AIDS are episodes of *P. carinii* pneumonia (PCP), this diagnosis should be entertained particularly if the onset of fever, cough, and dyspnea is insidious over 1 to 4 weeks and the immune status of the host is unknown.

Important clues for the etiological diagnosis may be obtained from a knowledge of seasonal, environmental, and occupational predilections of the different agents that cause atypical pneumonias (see Table 28.2).

Evaluation

Physical Examination. The physical examination does not usually distinguish between bacterial and atypical pneumonia syndromes. Crepitant rales that do not clear with cough are suggestive of pneumonia of either type. Signs of consolidation (bronchial breath sounds, dullness to percussion, and egophony) are more common in bacterial pneumonia. In early stages of pneumonia the examination may be normal, despite an infiltrate on X-ray. On the other hand, rales and rhonchi may indicate pneumonia before the appearance of an infiltrate.

Laboratory Examination. Every patient suspected of having pneumonia should have a chest X-ray, peripheral blood white cell count and differential count, and two blood cultures when possible. A white cell count over 15,000 is usually associated with bacterial pneumonia. Although the X-ray is essential for the firm diagnosis of pneumonia, a normal X-ray does not necessarily rule out pneumonia and X-ray patterns are not specific in terms of the etiology. For example, in one study (40) in which diagnosis was attempted by six radiologists from the chest film alone, mycoplasmal pneumonia was incorrectly identified as bacterial in a significant proportion of patients.

If the chest X-ray or clinical findings indicate pneumonia, a *sputum Gram stain* is often instrumental in directing initial therapy; and cultures of sputum and blood should be obtained. The rapid Gram stain technique requires only 1 to 2 minutes: (*a*) heat fixation; (*b*) 5 seconds crystal violet, water rinse; (*c*) 5 seconds Gram's iodine, water rinse; (*d*) decolorization of the thin part of the smear with 4 to 5 drops of 95% alcohol, water rinse; (*e*) 5 seconds safranine, water rinse; (*f*) blotting dry. The sputum sample is probably of lower respiratory tract origin if there are fewer than 10 squamous epithelial cells and more than 25 polymorphonuclear leukocytes/high dry (100X) field, except in leukopenic patients. The appearance of columnar ciliated epithelial cells assures lower tract origin. Sputum smears positive for pneumococci (Gram-positive, lancet-shaped diplococci) are helpful in directing therapy (34). Sputum, often foul smelling, containing mixed flora with pleomorphic Gram-negative bacilli and tiny or pleomorphic Gram-positive cocci, is consistent with anaerobic aspiration pneumonia. Pneumonia due to *Staphylococcus* or *Haemophilus* organisms usually is accompanied by sputum con-

Table 28.2.
Epidemiological Clues to the Presumptive Diagnosis of Atypical Pneumonia

Organism or Disease	Peak Seasonal Incidence	Incubation Period (days)	Epidemiological Setting
Mycoplasma pneumoniae	Summer, early fall	14–28	Family—3 weeks between onset among individuals
Chlamydia pneumoniae (TWAR strain of Chlamydia)	All year	not known	Community and nosocomial transmission probably person-to-person
Pneumocystis carinii	All year	not known	Patient with known HIV infection or patient from group at high risk of acquiring HIV infection (see Chapter 34)
Respiratory syncytial virus	Late winter and spring	2–8	Bronchiolitis in children <5 years. Mild upper respiratory infection in adult contacts, with mean symptomatic period 9 days. More severe in elderly
Influenza A and B	Winter epidemics	1–3	Adult cases follow school absenteeism
Parainfluenza 1 + 2	Fall	3–8	Croup in children, unusual in adults
Parainfluenza 3	All Year	3–8	Family —mild upper respiratory infection in adults, more severe in elderly
Adenovirus (type 4, 7)	Winter	4–5	Military recruits
Psittacosis	All year	6–15	Occupational or household exposure to birds, especially parrots, turkeys, and pigeons (20% have no bird exposure)
Tularemia (pulmonary)	All year	2–4	Handling infected rodents and rabbits
Q fever	All year	14–28	Contact with sheep, goats, cattle
Legionnaires'	Outbreaks in summer, sporadic through year	2–10	Contact with construction sites and stagnant water in air-cooling apparatus (some reports)

taining abundant large Gram-positive cocci, or small Gram-negative coccobacilli, respectively.

Sputum samples from patients with atypical pneumonia presenting as a flu-like illness characteristically contain few bacteria and only modest numbers of leukocytes. On the other hand, sputum from some mycoplasmal and viral pneumonias contains abundant leukocytes but few bacteria. Many patients produce no sputum, including one-half of patients with *Legionella* pneumonia. If such patients are toxic, they may require hospitalization for more invasive diagnostic studies such as transtracheal aspiration.

Unlike sputum Gram stains, *sputum cultures* have limited utility in the management of ambulatory pneumonias, since sputum samples are often contaminated by oral pneumococci. Moreover, pneumococci fail to grow in 45% of cultures from cases of pneumococcal pneumonia (5). In view of the confusing data, routine sputum cultures are not recommended, with the following important exceptions: patients, such as nursing home residents or those recently discharged from a general hospital, who are at greater risk for nonpneumococcal pneumonia; and patients with sputum Gram stains demonstrating a predominance of a nonpneumococcal bacterial pathogen.

Serological diagnosis. The majority of pneumonias cannot be diagnosed by blood or sputum culture and do not require definitive diagnosis by serology. If, however, the patient fails to respond to 3 to 5 days of therapy and has been ill less than 14 days, an acute serum sample should be obtained and stored. After 3 weeks of illness, a convalescent serum sample should be obtained and both samples submitted to a state or regional health laboratory for diagnostic serology. Guided by epidemiological clues (Table 28.2), complement fixation titers for *M. pneumoniae*, Q fever,

psittacosis, influenza, respiratory syncytial and parainfluenza viruses, and adenovirus may be requested. An indirect immunofluorescent assay on paired sera is available to diagnose Legionnaires' disease. Tularemia is usually diagnosed by an agglutination assay.

The presence of serum cold agglutinins is often used as a rapid diagnostic test for mycoplasmal pneumonia. This test, however, has several drawbacks. The sample must be maintained at close to 37°C for delivery to the laboratory. In addition, the test is not very sensitive; (only about three-quarters of patients with mycoplasmal infection are positive), and not very specific (half of all positive tests are due to other diseases, including pneumococcal and adenovirus pneumonia).

Management: Hospitalization

The need for hospitalization must be individually determined for each patient but in general is based on how sick the patient is and what underlying diseases are present. Patients who are toxic, diaphoretic, dyspneic, cyanotic, fatigued from respiratory effort, have hemoptysis, have difficulty clearing secretions, or cannot be expected to follow a course of oral therapy due either to vomiting or to characteristics predictive of poor compliance (see Chapter 4) should be hospitalized.

Other associated features that should prompt hospital admission are the following:

1. Age over 60 years, obstructive or bronchospastic lung disease, congestive heart failure, diabetes mellitus, renal insufficiency, malignancy, postsplenectomy, HIV infection, sickle cell anemia, alcoholism, drug abuse, or concomitant tuberculosis;
2. Peripheral white cell count <5000, ileus, or abdominal distention;

3. Suspicion of recent major aspiration due to history of head trauma, sedative use, acute alcoholism, seizures, dental anesthesia, loss of consciousness, or esophageal motility disorder;
4. Extrapulmonary complications (large pleural effusion, meningitis, septic arthritis, peritonitis, metastatic abscesses, etc.);
5. Hospitalization within the last 4 weeks or residence in nursing home, two situations that increase the chance of having a Gram-negative or a resistant nosocomial pathogen;
6. Sputum smears showing a predominance of Gram-negative bacteria;
7. Inability to care for self if living alone;
8. Failure to respond to initial therapy.

Management: Ambulatory

Antimicrobial Therapy (Table 28.3). If the clinical presentation supports the diagnosis of pneumococcal pneumonia, the antibiotic of choice is penicillin, 300,000 units of procaine penicillin administered intramuscularly in the office, followed by oral penicillin V, 250 mg every 6 hours for 10 days. If the patient is allergic to penicillin, erythromycin, 250 mg four times daily, is appropriate.

If the clinical presentation is that of the atypical pneumonia syndrome and an adequate sputum smear is nondiagnostic, erythromycin, 250 to 500 mg four times daily for 14 days, is recommended. Patients receiving erythromycin should be advised that crampy

abdominal pain is a frequent benign side effect that often can be ameliorated by taking the medication with meals (without impairing its absorption) or by lowering the dose. Erythromycin can raise blood theophylline levels, occasionally into the toxic range, and doses of the latter drug should be monitored and adjusted.

Many physicians treat all ambulatory patients who have pneumonia with erythromycin. The advantage is coverage for pneumococcal, chlamydial, and mycoplasmal infections, as well as Legionnaires' and many milder anaerobic infections. An alternative is ciprofloxacin, which is efficacious for treating *streptococci, M. pneumoniae, C. trachometis, Legionella, B. catarrhalis* and Gram-negative aerobes. Because up to 10% of pneumococcal isolates are resistant to tetracycline, this drug is reserved for the occasional patient who fails to respond to erythromycin or in whom tularemia or Q fever is suspected epidemiologically. In these situations, a 2- to 3-week course of tetracycline, 500 mg four times daily, is appropriate.

Follow-up

The patient should be advised to keep in close contact by phone, maintain good hydration with oral fluids, use aspirin or acetaminophen to control fever and headache, and avoid cough suppressants and cigarettes. A phone contact with the patient 24 hours after the initial visit provides a check on antibiotic compliance and side effects and on the status of symptoms;

Table 28.3.
Oral Antimicrobial Drugs Used in Ambulatory Treatment of Respiratory Infections

Drug	Available Strengths (mg)	Usual Adult Dose and Schedule	Common Side Effects	Drug (and Food) Instructions
Penicillin V	250, 500	250–500 mg 3 or 4 times daily	Diarrhea nausea, vomiting, vaginitis, skin rash, urticaria	Rash with infectious mononucleosis or concomitant allopurinol, false positive Clinitest (use Clinistix or Testape)
Ampicillin	250, 500	250–500 mg 3 or 4 times daily		
Amoxicillin	250, 500	250–500 mg 3 or 4 times daily		
Amoxicillin-clavulanate	250, 500	250–500 mg every 8 hours		
Erythromycin	250, 500	250–500 mg 3 or 4 times daily	Nausea, vomiting, abdominal pain, diarrhea	False elevation of aminotransferase, raises serum theophylline levels, potentiates warfarin and glucocorticoids
Tetracyline	250, 500	250–500 mg 3 or 4 times daily	Skin photosensitivity, nausea, vomiting, heartburn, diarrhea mucosial candidiasis	Food, milk, antacids, iron interfere with absorption
Doxycycline	100	100 mg twice daily		
Trimethoprim (T) plus Sulfamethoxazole (S)	80 T/400 S (single strength) 160 T/800 S (double strength)	2 single strength or 1 double strength twice daily	Skin rash, gastroinstestinal upset, elevates serum creatinine	Prolongs half-life of warfarin phenytoin, and oral hypoglycemics
Cefuroxime axetil	125, 250, 500	250–500 mg twice daily	Nausea, vomiting, diarrhea	Absorption enhanced with food, false positive Clinitest
Cefaclor	250	250–500 mg every 8 hours		
Ciprofloxacin	250, 500, 750	500 mg twice daily	Nausea, diarrhea, vomiting, restlessness	Prolongs half-life of theophylline. Antacids interfere with absorption. CNS side effects increaseed with caffeine

also it reassures the acutely ill patient that he has access to the physician should his condition worsen or fail to improve.

A follow-up visit to the office 3 to 4 days later will help to assess response to therapy. Symptoms of pneumococcal pneumonia in the uncompromised host abate dramatically within 48 to 72 hours of initiation of penicillin therapy. If substantial clinical response to penicillin has not occurred, either switching to erythromycin or hospitalizing the patient for further diagnostic studies should be contemplated.

Erythromycin will substantially reduce fever and systemic symptoms in most patients with mycoplasmal pneumonia by 3 to 6 days.

Early follow-up chest X-rays are mandatory in patients who fail to show clinical improvement by 5 to 7 days of therapy or who have a later relapse. Because 3% of patients who have a bronchogenic carcinoma initially present with a typical pneumonitis with or without consolidation (13), all patients over 40 and all smokers or former smokers should have a chest X-ray at 4 to 6 weeks, the interval in which radiological clearing is expected for uncomplicated cases of pneumococcal and mycoplasmal pneumonia (25). Old age, chronic obstructive lung disease, and alcoholism may delay radiological clearing for an additional 2 to 6 weeks (25).

Pneumonia in Human Immunodeficiency Virus (HIV)—Infected Patients

HIV-infected individuals are more susceptible to infection with a wide variety of pulmonary pathogens. Because eighty-five percent of all patients with acquired immune deficiency syndrome (AIDS) develop *Pneumocystitis carinii* pneumonia (PCP), the numbers of cases of PCP presenting to physicians will be considerable in the years ahead. As early prophylaxis for PCP becomes widespread, other pathogens will probably account for a larger proportion of the respiratory infections of HIV-infected patients.

PCP presents most frequently with fever, nonproductive cough, and exertional shortness of breath (22). Findings on the chest examination may or may not reveal rales. Examination may reveal other evidence of immunosuppression such as oral thrush, hairy leukoplakia, or cutaneous lesions of Kaposi's sarcoma. The chest radiograph usually reveals a diffuse interstitial infiltrate, although diffuse or focal airspace consolidation can be caused by PCP.

Several antimicrobial agents are effective in treating PCP, and patients with mild PCP can be treated in the ambulatory setting. PCP prophylaxis is also efficacious, both to prevent initial PCP in high-risk patients and to prevent recurrence of PCP. A systematic approach to the HIV-infected patient is described in Chapter 34.

Prevention of Pneumonia

Polyvalent pneumococcal vaccine and influenza vaccines are discussed in detail in Chapter 32. No special precautions need to be taken to isolate the ambulatory patient with pneumonia. Household contacts of these patients need no special surveillance, with the exceptions of pneumonic disease due to tuberculosis (see Chapter 29), tularemia, plague, and meningococci.

Pleurodynia

Pleurodynia is an uncommon acute illness caused by members of the coxsackievirus family. It occurs in summer and early fall. The presenting symptoms may suggest the onset of pneumonia—abrupt onset of severe paroxysmal pain of the thorax or abdomen, worse with cough or breathing. Other manifestations of pleurodynia include fever, headache, cough, anorexia. The physical examination is often normal except that the patient will splint to avoid pain, which is commonly felt in the lower rib cage or under the sternum. The chest X-ray is usually normal. Most patients recover within three days to one week. Rare complications are orchitis, pericarditis, and aseptic meningitis.

General References

Benenson AS (ed): *Control of Communicable Diseases in Man*, 15th ed., Washington, DC, American Public Health Association, 1990.
  A concise summary of epidemiology, prevention, and management of communicable diseases.
Mandell GL, Douglas Jr. RG, Bernett JE (eds): *Principles and Practice of Infectious Diseases*, 3rd ed., New York, John Wiley & Sons, 1989.
  The standard textbook of infectious diseases.
Vickery DM, Fries JF: *Take Care of Yourself: A Consumer's Guide to Medical Care*, 4th ed., Reading, MA, Addison-Wesley, 1990.
  Simple algorithms for self-care of common medical problems.

Specific References

1. Anthonisen NR, Manfreda J, Warren CPW, et al: Antibiotic therapy in exacerbations of chronic obstructive pulmonary disease. *Ann Intern Med* 206:196, 1987.
2. Baine WB, Luby JP, Martin SW: Severe illness with influenza B. *Am J Med* 68:181, 1980.
3. Baker AS, Eavey RD: Adult supraglottitis (epiglottitis). *N Engl J Med* 314:1185, 1986.
4. Barker WH, Mullooly JP: Pneumonia and influenza deaths during epidemics: implications for prevention. *Arch Intern Med* 142:85, 1982.
5. Barrett-Connor E: The nonvalue of sputum culture in the diagnosis of pneumococcal pneumonia. *Am Rev Respir Dis* 103:845, 1971.
6. Berg AO, LoGerfo JP: Potential effect of self-care algorithms on the number of physician visits. *N Engl J Med* 300:535, 1979.
7. Brook I: The role of beta-lactamase-producing bacteria in the persistence of streptococci tonsillar infection. *Rev Infect Dis* 6:601, 1984.
8. Burke P, Bain J, Lowes A, Athersuch R: Rational decisions in managing sore throat. *Br Med J* 296:1646, 1988.
9. Chalmers TC: Effects of ascorbic acid on the common cold: an evaluation of the evidence. *Am J Med* 58:532, 1975.
10. *Current estimates from the Health Interview Survey: United States—1976.* Vital and Health Statistics, series 10, no. 119, DHEW pub no. (PHS) 78-1547, 1977.
11. Davidson TM, Calloway CA: Tonsillectomy and adenoidectomy: its indications and its problems. *West J Med* 133:451, 1980.
12. Delker LL, Moser RH, Nelson JD, et al: Amantadine: does it have a role in the prevention and treatment of influenza? A National Institutes of Health Consensus Development Conference. *Ann Intern Med* 92:256, 1980.
13. Drevvatne T, Frimann-Dahl J: Peripheral bronchial carcinomas: a radiological and pathological study. *Br J Radiol* 34:180, 1961.

14. Evans Jr FO, Sydnor JB, Moore WEC, et al: Sinusitis of the maxillary antrum. *N Engl J Med* 293:735, 1975.

15. Feinstein AR, Spagnuolo M, Wood HF, et al: Rheumatic fever in children and adolescents. *Ann Intern Med* 60:68, 1964.

16. Foy HM, Kenny GE, McMahan R, et al: Mycoplasma pneumoniae pneumonia in an urban area. *JAMA* 214:1666, 1970.

17. Gross PA, Rodstein M, LaMontagne JR, et al: Epidemiology of acute respiratory illness during an influenza outbreak in a nursing home. *Arch Intern Med* 148:559, 1988.

18. Gwaltney Jr. JM, Hendley JO, Simon G, Jordon Jr. WS: Rhinovirus infections in an industrial population. 1. The occurrence of illness. *N Engl J Med* 275:1261, 1966.

19. Gwaltney Jr. JM, Moskalski PB, Hindley JO: Hand to hand transmission of rhinovirus colds. *Ann Intern Med* 88:463, 1978.

20. Hall WJ, Douglas Jr. RG: Pulmonary function during and after common respiratory infections. *Annu Rev Med* 31:233, 1980.

21. Helms CM, Viner JP, Sturm RH, et al: Comparative features of pneumococcal, mycoplasmal, and Legionnaires' disease pneumonias. *Ann Intern Med* 90:543, 1979.

22. Hopewell PC: Pneumocystic carinii Pneumonia: diagnosis. *J Infect Dis* 157:1115, 1988.

23. Howard JC, Kantner TR, Lilienfield LS, et al: Effectiveness of antihistamines in the symptomatic management of the common cold. *JAMA* 242:2414, 1979.

24. Huovinen P, et al: Pharyngitis in adults: the presence and coexistence of viruses and bacterial organisms. *Ann Intern Med* 110:612, 1989.

25. Jay SJ, Johanson Jr. WG, Pierce AK: The radiographic resolution of Streptococcus pneumoniae pneumonia. *N Engl J Med* 293:798, 1975.

26. Komaroff AL, Pass TM, Aronson MD, et al: The prediction of streptococcal pharyngitis in adults. *J Gen Intern Med* 1:1, 1986.

27. Kroenke K, Omori DM, Simmons JO, et al: The safety of phenylpropanolamine in patients with stable hypertension. *Ann Intern Med* 111:1043, 1989.

28. Luby JP: Southwestern Internal Medicine Conference: Pneumonias in adults due to mycoplasma, chlamydiae, and viruses. *Am J Med Sci* 294:45, 1987.

29. Marrie TJ, Grayston JT, Wang S-P, Kuo C-C: Pneumonia associated with the TWAR strain of chlamydia. *Ann Intern Med* 106:507, 1987.

30. Miller RA, Brancato F, Holmes KK: *Corynebacterium hemolyticum* as a cause of pharyngitis and scarlatiniform rash in young adults. *Ann Intern Med* 105:867, 1986.

31. Mostow SR: Prevention, management and control of influenza: role of amantadine. *Am J Med* 82 (suppl 6A):35, 1987.

32. Nicotra B, Rivera M, Luman JL, et al: Branhamella catarrhalis as a lower respiratory tract pathogen in patients with chronic lung disease. *Arch Intern Med* 146:890, 1986.

33. Over-the-counter cough remedies. *Med Lett* 21:103, 1979.

34. Rein MF, Gwaltney JM, O'Brien WM, et al: Accuracy of Gram's stain in identifying pneumococci in sputum. *JAMA* 239:2671, 1978.

35. Rodnick JE, Gude JK: The use of antibiotics in acute bronchitis and acute exacerbation of chronic bronchitis. *West J Med* 149:347, 1988.

36. Sakethoo K, Januszkiewicz A, Sackner MA: Effects of drinking hot water and chicken soup on nasal mucus velocity and nasal airflow resistance. *Chest* 74:408, 1978.

37. Stanley Jackson ED GG, et al: Virus shedding with aspirin treatment of rhinovirus infection. *JAMA* 231:1248, 1975.

38. Strome M: Rhino-sinusitis and midfacial pain in adolescents. *Practitioner* 217:914, 1976.

39. Tager I, Spiezer FE: Role of infection in chronic bronchitis. *N Engl J Med* 292:563, 1975.

40. Tew J, Colenoff L, Berlin BS: Bacterial or nonbacterial pneumonia: accuracy of radiographic diagnosis. *Radiology* 124:607, 1977.

41. Verghese A, Berk SL: Bacterial pneumonia in the elderly. *Medicine (Baltimore)* 62:271, 1983.

42. Wood RW, Tompkins RK, Wolcott BW: An efficient strategy for managing acute respiratory illness in adults. *Ann Intern Med* 93:757, 1980.

C H A P T E R 29

Tuberculosis in the Ambulatory Patient

R. BRADLEY SACK, M.D., Sc.D.
FREDERICK KOSTER, M.D.

DEFINITION OF THE PROBLEM

Epidemiology

The tuberculosis case rate in the United States, which had decreased at a rate of 5.9% per year from 1963 to 1985, began to increase in 1986 when there were 22,768 new cases reported, in contrast to 22,201 in 1985 (3). The increase in cases has occurred mostly among persons in the 25 to 44-year age group; in contrast the numbers of cases in children under 5 years of age continues to decrease. The increase in numbers of cases in large urban centers and in young adults coincided with the epidemic of human immunodeficiency virus (HIV) infections, which is now known to be an important risk factor for developing tuberculosis.

The drop in incidence of tuberculosis prior to 1986 was due entirely to decreases in cases of *pulmonary* tuberculosis; new extrapulmonary tuberculosis continues to appear at a rate of about 4,000 cases/year.

Reactivation and Primary Tuberculosis

The majority of the sporadic new cases of tuberculosis are due to *reactivation* of a remote primary infection; patients in this situation are those who have had untreated or inadequately treated active tuberculosis and those with positive tuberculin reactions who have neither a past history of active tuberculosis nor documented conversion from tuberculin negativity during an interval of 1 year or less. *Primary tuberculosis* means evidence for newly acquired infection (either recent conversion to tuberculin positivity or the onset of active disease shortly after exposure to a patient with known active disease). Persons at highest risk of developing primary tuberculosis are those living with, or having close contact with, a person who has undetected and therefore untreated active disease.

Most patients with tuberculosis are minimally symptomatic or are asymptomatic, which is why public health screening programs are critical for case detection.

Etiology

The etiology of tuberculosis in the United States is almost always *Mycobacterium tuberculosis*. In some parts of the world, or in immunosuppressed patients, other strains (such as bovine and avian strains) may also be important in human disease. Atypical mycobacteria, such as *Mycobacterium kansasii* and *Mycobacterium avium intracellulare*, and certain fungi, such as *Cryptococcus neoformans* and *Histoplasma capsulatum*, may produce disease indistinguishable from tuberculosis and should be considered in the differential diagnosis.

DIAGNOSIS

History

Tuberculosis, when symptomatic, almost always presents with signs and symptoms of weeks' to months' duration. Almost the only time it presents as acute disease is in rare cases of acute meningitis or tuberculous pneumonia. The history should be directed toward both defining the symptom complex and determining possible exposure to known sources of disease.

Because tuberculosis has multiple presentations, one should be suspicious about anyone with chronic unexplained symptoms. Weight loss (documented over a defined period of time), fever (particularly in the late evenings), night sweats (to be differentiated from environmentally induced sweats), decreased appetite, and the loss of a sense of well-being are the most important nonspecific symptoms. Persistent cough (usually with sputum production), hemoptysis, and pleuritic chest pain are more specific findings suggestive of pulmonary involvement.

It is important to know whether the patient has previously had tuberculosis, has previously been skin tested for tuberculosis (and if so, when he was tested and what the results were), and when the patient has had previous chest films (and where they can be obtained).

Possibly significant history also includes any family member or close friend with known tuberculosis, any person in school or at work with known disease, and any recent history of travel to the developing world, where tuberculosis is common.

Because *extrapulmonary tuberculosis* may occur in any organ (in particular, pleura, lymph nodes, endometrium, kidneys, ureters, bones and joints, skin, meninges, small intestine, and peritoneum) or as a disseminated (miliary) form, localized symptoms and signs in any organ must raise the consideration of tuberculosis.

Physical Examination

The physical examination often may be entirely negative, even with obvious evidence of pulmonary disease on the chest film. The following positive findings, when present, may be of considerable help in suggesting the diagnosis: rales localized to the upper posterior chest or auscultatory evidence of pulmonary cavitation (bronchovesicular breathing and whispered pectoriloquy); evidence of pleural effusion; supra- and infraclavicular retraction; lymphadenopathy; evidence of weight loss; and fever. Although rare in the United States, large, matted, nontender cervical lymph nodes (at times with draining sinuses) are almost diagnostic of *scrofula*, a form of tuberculous adenitis (which may also be due to atypical mycobacteria) seen primarily in children.

Tuberculin Skin Tests

If a patient who is being evaluated for TB has previously had a negative skin test or has not had a skin test at all, a test with intermediate strength purified protein derivative (PPD), 5 tuberculin units, Tween-stabilized, should be applied intradermally on the volar skin of the forearm. Ideally, control tests should be placed on the opposite arm, containing ubiquitous antigens (antigens for which most persons have a positive skin test), such as *Candida*, mumps, or tetanus toxoid. The reactions should be read at 48 hours. A practical method for determining the diameter of the indurated area is the ballpoint pen method (13): a line is drawn from a point 1 to 2 cm away from the margin of a positive reaction; when the pen tip reaches the margin of the indurated area, definite resistance is felt; this is repeated on the opposite side, and the diameter of the indurated reaction is measured. The interpretation and significance of tuberculin tests are summarized in Table 29.1. About 80% of patients with reactivation tuberculosis will have positive PPD tests.

A person with a known positive tuberculin skin test does not need to have one repeated; if the test is repeated, there is a small risk of producing a very *strong positive reaction* characterized by tender induration, axillary adenopathy, temperature elevation [as high as 102°F (38.5°C)], and slough of the epidermis after a week. This problem is best treated with a sterile gauze

Table 29.1.
Evaluation of Tuberculin Skin Tests (5 Tuberculin Units)

Reaction[a]	Associated Features	Significance	Therapy[b]
Positive	Unknown duration:		
	Chest film negative	Probably old infection unless recently acquired disease	Consider INH treatment for 1 yr, if under age 35 yr
	Chest film positive (calcified nodes, apical scarring)	Old tuberculous disease, at increased risk for developing reactivation	Consider INH treatment for 1 yr
	Close contact of patients with tuberculosis	May represent recent disease	Consider INH treatment for 1 yr
Positive	Recent development (<1 yr)	Recent acquisition of tuberculosis	INH treatment for 1 yr
Positive	In patient beginning long term course of corticosteroids	Patient at increased risk of developing clinical tuberculosis	Consider INH treatment for duration of steroid course or for 1 yr
Negative	In patient also negative to ubiquitous antigens	Anergic, noninterpretable	Repeat PPD; follow with chest X-ray if necessary
Negative	In patient with recent close contact with tuberculosis patient	Does not rule out early tuberculous infection	Treat with INH; retest in 3 months. If positive continue for 1 yr. If still negative may stop INH
Negative	In patients taking high dose corticosteroids or immunosuppressives	Uninterpretable	Follow with chest X-rays; treat with INH if disease proved or highly suspected

[a] Interpretation of readings:
Negative: 5 mm induration or less. (See the text for a discussion of factors causing a false-negative test and of the booster phenomenon.)
Intermediate: 5–10 mm induration (needs to be repeated; consider atypical mycobacterial disease).
Positive: 10 mm induration or more.
[b] INH, isoniazid; PPD, purified protein derivative.

dressing impregnated with a topical steroid, such as 0.1% triamcinolone.

First strength and second strength tuberculin tests are rarely if ever useful in the diagnosis of tuberculosis. Tine tests are used as screening tests, and positive tests should be confirmed by an intermediate PPD.

M. tuberculosis shares antigens with related mycobacteria, and therefore a positive skin test is not completely specific. However, most cross-reactions will be less than 10 mm in diameter. Skin testing with specific atypical mycobacterial antigens is not possible, since the antigens are not available for general use.

A negative tuberculin skin test does not conclusively rule out the diagnosis of tuberculosis; intercurrent febrile illnesses, skin testing within 30 days of vaccination with a live virus, underlying disease or immunosuppressive drugs that may suppress delayed hypersensitivity reactions, and errors in administration of the test material may explain false-negative reactions.

The *booster phenomenon* may interfere with the interpretation of the tuberculin test (14). Persons with a remote tuberculous or atypical mycobacterial infection who have become skin test negative may, upon repeat annual skin testing, develop a positive response because of the boosting effect of the repeated test. This *boosting effect* can be detected by administering a second tuberculin test 1 week after the first test in persons who initially have a negative response. If the second response is positive, these persons can be said to have had past infection but are not considered to have a recently acquired infection. The booster phenomenon is important in elderly persons, in whom it is common, and in persons such as hospital employees who may be skin tested frequently.

Laboratory Examination

Chest X-Ray

Both postanterior (PA) and lateral views should be obtained. In the patient with strongly suggestive clinical evidence for tuberculosis, an apical lordotic view should also be obtained when the PA and lateral views appear to be normal. The radiological findings typical of tuberculosis (apical scarring, hilar adenopathy with peripheral infiltrate, upper lobe cavitation, miliary infiltrate, etc.) are not specific; however, a negative chest film rules out pulmonary tuberculosis (with the rare exception of early miliary disease), making the chest film a very sensitive test.

Cultures and Smears

Sputum, for smear (rapid screening with an acid-fast fluorescent dye, followed by Ziehl-Nielson staining) and culture, should be obtained at least three times. A positive sputum smear is highly suggestive of tuberculosis (not absolutely diagnostic because of the possibility of atypical infection or of contamination); and a positive culture is diagnostic. If sputum is difficult to obtain, one can obtain morning gastric aspirates, which contain the swallowed sputum. Gastric samples should not be examined by acid-fast stain but should be sent for culture only, since smears of gastric contents frequently show commensal acid-fast organisms.

In a patient with a positive PPD and persistent pyuria without bacteriuria, three urine samples should be obtained for tuberculosis culture (again a positive acid-fast urine smear is only suggestive, since there are commensal acid-fast organisms such as *Mycobacterium smegmatis*, which inhabit the urinary tract; therefore, only cultures are of diagnostic value).

Tuberculosis cultures become positive within 3 to 4 weeks of plating the specimens. The initial positive cultures from any source should be tested for sensitivity to drugs used to treat tuberculosis since resistant organisms may necessitate a change in treatment.

Miscellaneous Laboratory Tests

Complete blood count. The hematocrit value may be normal or low; the anemia due to tuberculosis is normochromic and normocytic, the so-called anemia of chronic disease (see Chapter 50). The white blood cell count and differential count are usually normal; occasionally a monocytosis is seen in persons with severe disease.

Urinalysis. This should be obtained routinely; if sterile pyuria is found, it is suggestive of renal tuberculosis and cultures should be sent as described above.

Liver function tests. Tests of serum aminotransferases, alkaline phosphatase, and bilirubin may be helpful if disseminated disease or liver involvement is suspected.

Other procedures. Other procedures, such as thoracentesis, lumbar puncture, and liver biopsy, are indicated only when specific organ involvement is suspected.

Presumptive Diagnosis

The *presumptive diagnosis of active tuberculosis* can be made when any of the following is found:

1. A typical chest X-ray;
2. A positive sputum smear;
3. A biopsy showing caseating granulomas with or without acid-fast organisms;
4. A recent change (within 1 year) of the tuberculin skin test from negative to positive, associated with other characteristic systemic symptoms/signs.

The diagnosis of active tuberculosis is *confirmed* by a positive culture from any body fluid or biopsy specimen.

All patients with a presumptive or confirmed diagnosis of tuberculosis must be reported promptly to the appropriate state health authority.

COURSE AND MANAGEMENT

Overview

Most persons infected with *M. tuberculosis* are unaware that they have it; only 5 to 10% of infected persons become ill, and a positive PPD or calcified nodes on chest film may be the only indicators of the past disease. Individuals in the latter group are at continual risk of reactivating their disease, however, since it is known that live *M. tuberculosis* may persist in the tissues of an infected individual for a lifetime. Such individuals have a much higher rate of development of clinical disease than do people not previously infected.

When tuberculosis is diagnosed in association with systemic signs or symptoms, there is no question that the patient should be treated. Persons with positive tuberculin reactions as the only manifestation of disease constitute a more difficult problem (see Table 29.2 and "Isoniazid Prophylaxis" below).

Once the diagnosis is strongly suspected or made, the question arises of how best to initiate therapy. Because it may take 4 weeks before cultures of *M. tuberculosis* become positive, therapy must usually be initiated on the basis of presumptive diagnosis (see above). If at 3 months all cultures are negative, therapy may be stopped.

If the patient is well enough to care for himself, can take oral medications regularly, and has no extrapulmonary disease, he can be successfully treated without hospitalization.

Treatment

Chemotherapy

The recommended duration of treatment of tuberculosis has been substantially shortened due to the use of multiple drugs. A single drug should never be used because this increases the risk of the emergence of resistant organisms during therapy.

In 1986, the American Thoracic Society issued its most recent recommendations for the standard treatment of active tuberculosis (1). These recommendations, whch are supported by the outcomes in multiple clinical trials (5A), are summarized here.

Successful treatment of active tuberculosis can be accomplished in as little as *six months with a three-drug regimen* (isoniazid, rifampin, and pyrazinamide), when the organisms are fully susceptible and the patient is fully compliant. A *nine-month two-drug regimen* (isoniazid and rifampin) is also highly successful in such patients. Recommended doses for the drugs, all of which can be taken in a once-a-day schedule, are shown in Table 29.2. When the three-drug six-month regimen is used, pyrazinamide is given only for the first two months, and isoniazid and rifampin for the full six months. Also, in either regimen, isoniazid and rifampin can also be given twice weekly after the first one to two months of daily treatment. The more intensive regimen for treating tuberculosis in HIV-infected patients is described below ("Tuberculosis and HIV Infection").

When isoniazid resistance is suspected, ethambutol should be included in the initial phases of treatment until susceptibility tests have been reported. When isoniazid resistance is documented, rifampin and ethambutol should be given for a minimum of twelve months.

Regimens containing *second line drugs* need to be considered only in patients who have developed adverse reactions to the standard drugs, which is uncommon, or in patients with drug-resistant tuberculosis. This latter group is usually composed of people who have been treated previously for tuberculosis, or who

Table 29.2.
Drugs for the Treatment of Mycobacterial Disease in Adults and Children[a]

Commonly Used Agents	Available Strengths of Oral Tablets or Capsules	Dosage		Most Common Side Effects	Tests for Side Effects	Drug Interactions[b]
		Total Once Daily Dose	Twice Weekly Dosage			
	(mg)					
Isoniazid[c]	100, 300	5 to 10 mg/kg up to 300 mg PO or IM	15 mg/kg PO or IM	Peripheral neuritis, hepatitis, hypersensitivity	Aminotransferases (not as a routine)	Carbamazepine— increased toxicity both drugs Disulfiram— psychosis, ataxia Phenytoin— toxicity increased
Rifampin	600	10 mg/kg up to 600 mg PO	10 mg/kg up to 600 mg PO	Hepatitis, febrile reaction, purpura (rare)	Aminotransferases (not as a routine)	May reduce the effect of the following drugs due to increased hepatic metabolism: oral contraceptives, quinidine, corticosteroids, anticoagulants, disopyramide, diazepam, barbiturates, methadone, digitoxin, digoxin, oral hypoglycemics; p-aminosalicylic acid may interfere with absorption of rifampin
Streptomycin		15 to 20 mg/kg up to 1 g IM	25 to 30 mg/kg	Eighth nerve damage, nephrotoxicity	Vestibular function, audiograms[b]; blood urea nitrogen and creatinine	Neuromuscular blocking agents—may be potentiated to cause prolonged paralysis
Pyrazinamide	500	15 to 30 mg/kg up to 2 g PO	50 to 70 mg/kg	Hyperuricemia, hepatoxicity	Uric acid, aminotransferases	
Ethambutol	100, 400	15 to 25 mg/kg	50 mg/kg PO	Optic neuritis (reversible with discontinuation of drug; very rare at 15 mg/kg), skin rash	Red-green color discrimination and visual acuity[d], difficult to test in a child under 3 years	

[a] Adapted from American Thoracic Society: Treatment of tuberculosis and tuberculosis infection in adults and children. *Am Rev Resp Dis* 134: 355, 1986.
[b] Reference should be made to current literature, particularly on rifampin, because it induces hepatic microenzymes and therefore interacts with many drugs.
[c] With pyridoxine 25 mg daily to prevent peripheral neuropathy
[d] Initial examination should be done at start of treatment.

have acquired tuberculosis in Southeast Asia or in Mexico.

Pregnant women can receive isoniazid, rifampin, or ethambutol, since these regimens are safe for the fetus.

Patients with *impaired renal function* should be treated with isoniazid and rifampin, since ethambutol is excreted mainly by the kidneys, and its dosage would have to be adjusted.

Both pulmonary and extrapulmonary tuberculosis can be treated with identical drug regimens (6).

Symptomatic Therapy

Usually no symptomatic therapy is required, except that patients should be encouraged to eat an adequate diet. If a patient has symptoms that require special management (such as high fever and toxicity for which steroids may be helpful, or a pleural effusion that needs draining), hospitalization may be necessary.

If the patient is eating poorly, pyridoxine (25 mg/day) should be taken with isoniazid to prevent peripheral neuropathy. Pyridoxine should also be taken with isoniazid routinely by pregnant patients and by patients with other diseases that may cause peripheral neuropathy (e.g., alcoholism, diabetes, end-stage renal disease).

Course in Treated Patient

Follow-up Schedule

After treatment has been initiated, the patient should be seen or contacted at least once per month, chiefly to assure drug compliance (see below) and to monitor for drug side effects (see below). Sputum cultures should be obtained monthly for the first 3 months. At 3 months and between 6 months and 1 year chest X-rays should be obtained. Sputum culture should be negative after 3 months of therapy, although occasionally nonculturable acid-fast organisms will be seen on smear for longer periods. A test-of-cure culture should be done on all patients at 5 or 6 months. Resolution of pulmonary infiltrates is often slow; the former practice of monthly chest films is therefore not warranted. Chest films are most helpful in excluding progression of disease and in documenting the patient's status when the tuberculosis is cured.

At the cessation of traditional chemotherapy regimens (9 months) prolonged follow-up is not necessary. After short course, i.e., 6-month, chemotherapy, it is recommended that follow-up be continued for another 12 months to detect relapses by symptoms and sputum cultures.

Usual Response

Patients diagnosed as having tuberculosis who comply with therapy have an excellent prognosis. The only exceptions are the rare patients with organisms resistant to the usual antituberculous drugs or patients who develop adverse effects from the antituberculous therapy. These problems are discussed in more detail below.

The patient should show some symptomatic improvement within 1 week of being started on antituberculous therapy. Improvement is usually indicated by an increased sense of well-being, an increase in appetite, and a decrease in cough, fever, and night sweats; temperature should be normal within 10 days of initiating treatment. The patient is usually back to his usual state of health in 1 to 2 months.

The improvement is due to the antibacterial effects of the drugs, which lead to a decrease in the inflammatory response of the host. After 1 week of therapy, the patient can be considered noninfectious.

Possible Complications

Drug resistance. This problem may occur in 5% of newly diagnosed cases in the United States (4% for isoniazid; 1% for ethambutol or rifampin) (10). The frequency of drug resistance is higher if the disease was acquired abroad, particularly in Southeast Asia (15%) or Mexico. In this case, the patient may show a delayed clinical response during the first few weeks of therapy. Because the laboratory may take 8 to 10 weeks to provide sensitivity data on the original isolates, it may be difficult to detect this problem early. If resistance is strongly suspected (as in a patient with previously treated tuberculosis) or documented, the drug regimen should consist of two antituberculous drugs that the patient has not taken before; ideally these drugs should be selected on the basis of the sensitivity pattern of the organism. It is suggested that consultation be obtained before embarking on a course of therapy with second line, less effective drugs, however.

Drug toxicity. Patients may develop a number of toxicities from antituberculous medications (Table 29.2).

ISONIAZID (7). Hepatic toxicity is the most common adverse reaction; it occurs at a biochemical level in approximately 20% of persons who take the drug; the incidence of toxicity may increase with age and with excessive alcohol intake. Laboratory evidence of mild injury to the liver is not in itself a reason to stop the drug, however, since in most subjects the aminotransferase level returns to normal while the drug is being continued. If the patient develops jaundice or develops fever with elevated liver enzymes, the drug

should, of course, be stopped. The liver injury is usually reversible and will heal without further therapy. In some persons, however (elderly men and particularly those with chronic alcohol-related liver disease), the liver injury may be severe and sometimes fatal. Isoniazid liver toxicity most often occurs early in therapy, so that the first 2 to 3 months are the most critical in the detection of adverse drug reactions. Specific guidelines for monitoring for isoniazid hepatitis are contained in the section on prevention (below). Peripheral neuropathy is an uncommon complication of isoniazid therapy that occurs only in persons on an inadequate diet; it can be prevented by taking 25 mg of pyridoxine every day.

ETHAMBUTOL. The most serious side effect of ethambutol is optic neuritis, resulting in decrease of visual acuity and in inability to distinguish the color green. This problem was seen frequently when the drug was given in a dose of 25 mg/kg. It is extremely uncommon at the recommended daily dose of 15 mg/kg.

RIFAMPIN. Serious allergic complications of rifampin therapy, including thrombocytopenia manifested by purpura, petechiae, and hematuria, acute renal failure, and a "flu syndrome," occur in approximately 1% of patients and necessitate cessation of therapy. There is a modest increase in hepatic toxicity that may be additive to isoniazid toxicity so that patients taking both drugs should be closely supervised. Patients should be warned that rifampin may result in an orange-red color in secretions such as urine, saliva, etc. Rifampin accelerates the metabolism of other drugs (Table 29.2) and may necessitate an increase in the dose of these drugs.

Problems requiring hospitalization. Ambulatory patients started on treatment should not require hospitalization. The few possible exceptions are (a) the development of progressive and debilitating disease, due either to resistant organisms or to poor compliance by the patient, and (b) severe toxic reactions to drugs, particularly isoniazid.

Patient's Role in Therapy

The patient's role is of the utmost importance to the successful treatment of tuberculosis, since he must faithfully administer the drugs daily for a period of 6 or 9 months and return for regular follow-up visits.

Because poor compliance accounts for most therapeutic failures in the treatment of tuberculosis, the most important function of monthly visits is the assessment, reinforcement, and documentation of compliance (see Chapter 4). When therapy is begun, the patient should be thoroughly educated about the course and therapy of his disease, so that the illusion of health when symptoms disappear will not cause premature cessation of therapy. The patient should be asked to devise a strategy to avoid missing daily medication due to forgetfulness. Pill counts at follow-up visits may be helpful. In noncompliant patients, twice weekly regimens (see above) may be particularly useful. If persistent problems with compliance are suspected, the patient should be referred to public health authorities for supervision of long-term care. Such authorities will provide home visits if necessary and will ensure that the patient is not lost to follow-up.

The patient should be advised about the communicable nature of his disease, which is particularly important until he has been on therapy for at least a week. During that first week, he should avoid intimate contact with others and should cough into tissue, which then should be incinerated or disposed of in closed plastic bags. After 1 week, he should be considered not contagious, and his activities can be dictated solely by his sense of well-being. Patients taking isoniazid should be given specific advice and monitored for hepatitis as outlined in the following section.

PREVENTION OF TUBERCULOSIS

Case Detection among Known Contacts

An integral part of initiation of care in any patient with active tuberculosis is case reporting to the local health authority and investigation of contacts. This entails tuberculin testing of all household and intimate "nonhousehold" contacts and retesting of nonreactors in 2 to 3 months. Reactors are examined by chest X-ray and if free of active disease are given chemoprophylaxis with isoniazid for 1 year. With the exception of evaluating family members this type of investigation is usually difficult for a physician to carry out alone and should be done by the local city or county health department. Such departments have trained personnel who are available to visit homes and workplaces in order to detect cases in contacts. In many states, it is required by law that persons with newly diagnosed tuberculosis (or with a strongly suspected diagnosis) be reported to the public health authorities.

Tuberculin Testing in Prevention

(See method above, and interpretation, Table 29.1.)
Ideally the tuberculin skin test status of all individuals should be determined at some time in their early adult life. In almost all school age children, screening for tuberculin positivity is coordinated with school health programs. In adult populations, a number of factors such as urban residence, the presence of chronic disease, a history of residence in underdeveloped countries, and health care occupation increase the importance of periodic tuberculin testing. This is particularly true for those individuals for whom isoniazid would be recommended if the PPD is positive (see the next section).

Because of the increased risk of contact with unrecognized cases of tuberculosis, physicians and hospital personnel have an increased chance of acquiring infection (twice the risk of the general population). Both for personal protection and because of the risk of transmitting tuberculosis to patients, physicians and other health workers should have annual tuberculin testing and should take isoniazid chemoprophylaxis if they convert from negative to positive.

Isoniazid Prophylaxis

Isoniazid prophylaxis (300 mg daily for 6 months to 1 year) has been shown to be very effective in preventing new cases of active tuberculosis among special groups of persons at high risk (9, 12). Because of the recognition of isoniazid-induced hepatitis, however, the indications for the use of isoniazid have narrowed somewhat in recent years. At the present time, isoniazid prophylaxis is recommended for persons in the following groups (1, 5): (a) close contacts of active infectious cases; (b) persons with recent skin test conversion (not those with booster responses, see above); (c) persons with positive skin tests and an abnormal chest X-ray suggestive of old tuberculosis; (d) persons with a known history of old tuberculosis who have never been given antibacterial treatment; (e) persons with positive skin tests who will be given corticosteroid or immunosuppressive therapy, who have silicosis, who have a history of a gastrectomy, or who have conditions such as Hodgkin's disease or HIV infection, which reduces T cell activity; and (f) persons with a positive skin test only, who are under the age of 35 years.

The guidelines recommended by the American Thoracic Society for *monitoring patients taking isoniazid* are the following (1):

Individuals receiving preventive therapy or a responsible adult in a household with children on preventive therapy should be questioned carefully at monthly intervals for (a) symptoms consistent with those of liver damage or of other toxic effects, that is, unexplained anorexia, nausea, or vomiting of greater than 3 days' duration, fatigue or weakness of greater than 3 days' duration, new and persistent paresthesias of the hands and feet; and (b) signs consistent with those of liver damage or of other toxic effects, that is, persistent dark urine, icterus, rash, elevated temperature of greater than 3 days' duration without explanation.

Monitoring by routine laboratory tests (e.g., aminotransferases, serum bilirubin, and alkaline phosphatase) is not always useful in predicting hepatic disease in isoniazid recipients and therefore is not recommended. However, in evaluating signs and symptoms such tests are mandatory. Preventive therapy should be reinstituted only if biochemical studies are normal and signs and symptoms are absent.

Because it has been recognized that this monitoring plan may fail to detect an occasional patient with severe hepatitis (8), periodic measurement of aminotransferase levels is recommended for persons over 35 years of age. This would detect the transient aminotransferase elevation that occurs in approximately 20% of subjects taking isoniazid; a cut-off level, such as a level 3 or 5 times normal, is recommended as the criterion for discontinuing isoniazid. Glassroth et al. (see

"General References") suggest measurement of aminotransferase levels each month in those patients who are in the groups at the highest risk of developing isoniazid hepatitis—i.e., those over 35 years of age, daily "drinkers," patients concomitantly taking other potentially hepatotoxic drugs, and patients with a history of liver disease.

TUBERCULOSIS AND HIV INFECTION

As noted earlier ("Epidemiology"), the recent increase in the incidence of active tuberculosis in the United States is due to the excess number of cases seen in patients with HIV infection. In some urban areas the incidence of tuberculosis among acquired immune deficiency syndrome (AIDS) patients is as high as 10%. In the presence of HIV infection, extrapulmonary tuberculosis, but not pulmonary tuberculosis, is an AIDS-defining illness. Although there is no evidence that HIV infection increases susceptibility to tuberculosis, individuals already infected (indicated by a known positive tuberculin skin test) are at increased risk of developing clinical disease and may present with unusual clinical syndromes (4, 11).

When clinical tuberculosis appears before the development of other AIDS-defining illnesses, presentation occurs in a typical fashion with pulmonary disease predominantly in the apices and often with cavitation. Fever, sweats, cough, anorexia, and wasting are common complaints. The tuberculin skin test is usually positive. It has been recommended that in patients with HIV infection and suspected tuberculosis, a reaction to PPD greater than 5 mm should be considered presumptive evidence for active tuberculosis (4).

When tuberculosis appears after the occurrence of an AIDS-defining opportunistic infection or malignancy, clinical features are often atypical (e.g., more frequent lower lobe disease without cavitation but with intrathoracic adenopathy); and only about half of all AIDS patients with proven tuberculosis will have a positive tuberculin test (10 mm or greater). Extrapulmonary tuberculosis is more common in AIDS patients and involves lymph nodes, liver, brain, meninges, bone marrow, adrenals, and the genitourinary tract. Aspiration or biopsy of the suspected site of infection should be performed for acid-fast stain and culture. When acid-fast bacilli are found, treatment for *M. tuberculosis* should be initiated while awaiting culture results, even though *M. avium intracellulare* is more common.

AIDS patients appear to respond as readily to standard therapy as non-HIV-infected patients, but early reports of relapses led to recommendations of more aggressive therapy in AIDS patients. The recommended regimen for treating tuberculosis in HIV-infected adults is isoniazid, 300 mg/day, rifampin, 600 mg/day; and pyrazinamide, 20 to 30 mg/kg/day (4). Ethambutol may be added if isoniazid resistance is suspected, although resistance is uncommonly encountered. Both ethambutol and pyrazinamide are given

for only 2 months if the isolate is isoniazid susceptible. Isoniazid and rifampin are continued for a total of 6 to 9 months or at least 6 months beyond conversion of sputum cultures to negative. Patients with extrapulmonary disease should be treated with the standard regimen for at least 9 to 12 months. Relapse after completion of therapy has been uncommon, but a few experts recommend lifelong isoniazid therapy.

Because the risk of developing reactivation tuberculosis is significant, preventive therapy with 12 months of daily isoniazid is presently recommended for HIV-infected persons, regardless of age, with a 5 mm or greater reaction to 5 TU of intradermal PPD, or a documented history of a reaction without prior isoniazid prophylaxis. Active infection should first be excluded. Conversely, all individuals in the major HIV risk groups (gay men and intravenous drug abusers) found to have a reactive tuberculin skin test, and all individuals presenting with disseminated or unusually severe tuberculosis, should be considered for HIV serological testing.

Chapter 34 provides a detailed account of the care of HIV-infected patients.

ELIMINATION OF TUBERCULOSIS IN THE UNITED STATES

A strategy has been formulated by the Department of Health and Human Services that calls for elimination of tuberculosis (<1 newly diagnosed case per million population) by the year 2010, and names an interim target of 3.5 incident cases per 100,000 by the year 2000. The present rate is about 8 per 100,000. If tuberculosis is to be eliminated by the year 2010, the percentage of infected persons who are identified and treated for tuberculosis annually must increase substantially beyond the current percentage (about 1%). The national plan of action calls for (a) more effective use of existing prevention and control methods, particularly in high risk populations; (b) the development of new technologies for diagnosis, treatment, and prevention; and (c) rapid transfer of these new technologies into clinical and public health practice (2).

General References

Glassroth MD, Robins AG, Snider Jr. DE: Tuberculosis in the 1980s. *N Engl J Med* 302:1441, 1980.
    Extensively referenced review.
Schlossberg D (ed): *Tuberculosis*, 2nd ed. New York, Springer-Verlag, 1988.

Specific References

1. American Thoracic Society: Treatment of tuberculosis and tuberculosis infection in adults and children. *Am Rev Respir Dis* 134:355, 1986.
2. CDC: *A strategic plan for the elimination of tuberculosis in the United States.* MMWR 38(suppl S-3):269, 1989.
3. CDC: *Tuberculosis, Final Data—United States, 1986.* MMWR 36:817, 1988.
4. Chaisson RE, Sluckin G: Tuberculosis and human immunodeficiency virus infection. *J Infect Dis* 159:96, 1989.
5. Comstock GW, Edwards PQ: The competing risks of tuberculosis and hepatitis for adult tuberculin reactors. *Am Rev Respir Dis* 111:573, 1975.

5A. Davidson PT: Treating tuberculosis: what drugs, for how long? *Ann Intern Med* 112:393, 1990.

6. Dutt AK, Moers D, Stead WW: Short-course chemotherapy for extrapulmonary tuberculosis. Nine years' experience. *Ann Intern Med* 104:7, 1986.

7. Garibaldi RA, Drusin RE, Ferebee SH, Gregg MD: Isoniazid-associated hepatitis: report of an outbreak. *Am Rev Respir Dis* 106:357, 1972.

8. Grosset JH: Present status of chemotherapy for tuberculosis. *Rev Infect Dis* 11(suppl 2):S347, 1989.

9. International Union Against Tuberculosis Committee on Prophylasix. Efficacy of various durations of isoniazid preventive therapy for tuberculosis: five years of follow-up in the IUAT trial. *Bull WHO* 60:555, 1982.

10. Kopanoff DE, Kilburn JO, Glassroth JL, et al: A continuing survey of tuberculosis primary drug resistance in the United States: March 1975 to November 1977. A United States Public Health Service cooperative study. *Am Rev Respir Dis* 118:835, 1978.

11. Selwyn PA, Hartel D, Lewis VA, et al: A prospective study of the risk of tuberculosis among intravenous drug users with human immunodeficiency virus infection. *N Engl J Med* 320:545, 1989.

12. Snider Jr. DE, Caras GJ, Koplan JP: Preventive therapy with isoniazid: cost-effectiveness of different durations of therapy. *JAMA* 255:1579, 1986.

13. Sokal JE: Measurement of delayed skin-test responses. *N Engl J Med* 293:501, 1975.

14. Thompson NJ, Glassroth JL, Snider Jr. DE, Farer LS: The booster phenomenon in serial tuberculin testing. *Am Rev Respir Dis* 119:587, 1979.

C H A P T E R   30

Selected Spirochetal Infections: Syphilis and Lyme Disease

PETER E. DANS, M.D.
DIANE E. GRIFFIN, M.D., Ph.D.

This chapter describes two spirochetal infections, syphilis (caused by *Treponema pallidum*) and Lyme disease (caused by *Borrelia burgdorferi*), each of which has primary, secondary, and tertiary stages.

SYPHILIS

Epidemiology

Syphilis became a major public health menace when a virulent form of the disease swept through Europe in the late 15th and early 16th centuries. It flourished in settings of sexual promiscuity and of heightened mobility, especially during wars. The combination of effective penicillin therapy and contact tracing brought the incidence of new infections in the United States to a low point in the 1950s (Table 30.1).

Beginning with the so-called "sexual revolution" of the 1960s, the frequency of early syphilis rose and then stabilized until the 1980s (Table 30.1). In 1987, the incidence of primary and secondary syphilis was 14.6 cases per 100, 000, the highest rate since 1950. Approximately 57% of all cases were reported from Florida, California, and New York alone. Most cases occurred in large urban centers. For example, rates per 100, 000 persons were 63.5 in New York City compared with 3.4 for the rest of New York state and 41.6 in Philadelphia compared with 2.5 for the rest of Pennsylvania (44). There are major differences in the rates of infectious syphilis by race and sex. The national rates per hundred thousand for primary and secondary syphilis for 1988 were 216 for black males, 135 for black females, 56 for Hispanic males, 24 for Hispanic females, 5.4 for white males, and 3.1 for white females. There has been a marked decline in cases of early syphilis among homosexuals and bisexuals as a result of recent changes in sexual practices, and syphilis is once again a predominantly heterosexual disease.

Several hypotheses have been suggested to explain the increase in early syphilis. These include increased prostitution in which such drugs as "crack" and cocaine are exchanged for sex (29), a decrease in resources available for syphilis control programs as efforts have been directed to acquired immune deficiency syndrome (AIDS) surveillance, and the routine use of spectinomycin for treatment of gonorrhea in some areas. Unlike penicillin, spectinomycin does not cure simultaneously acquired syphilis. The increase in early

Table 30.1.
Annual Reported Cases of Syphilis in the United States for Selected Years[a]

	Infectious (Primary and Secondary) Syphilis	Early Latent <1 year Duration	Late and Late Latent	Total
1943	82,204	149,390	251,958	483,552
1955	6,454	20,054	86,526	113,034
1960	16,145	18,017	81,798	115,960
1965	23,338	17,458	67,317	108,113
1970	21,982	16,311	50,348	88,641
1975	25,561	26,569	27,098	79,228
1980	27,204	20,297	20,979	68,480
1985	27,131	21,689	18,414	67,234
1987	35,594	28,197	22,987	86,778
1988	40,117	35,600	26,987	102,704

[a] From Blount J, Centers for Disease Control, Department of Health and Human Services, Atlanta, Georgia (personal communication), 1989.

syphilis has grave clinical implications, not only for the affected patients but also for others (44).

Stages of the Disease

The acquired form of the disease has different stages (Table 30.2): primary, secondary, early and late latent, and tertiary or late syphilis. The primary and secondary stages may not be clinically apparent, and only a third of untreated patients develop tertiary manifestations.

Primary Syphilis

Primary syphilis is characterized by the development of a "chancre" at the site of intimate sexual contact (genitals, anus, mouth, breast, and occasionally elsewhere). It appears 10 to 90 days (average 21 days) after infection by *T. pallidum*, the etiological organism. It usually starts as a single painless papule that varies in size from a few millimeters to a few centimeters in diameter and progresses to a painless ulcer with indurated edges containing a highly infectious exudate. Multiple lesions occur in about 30% of cases. There is associated painless regional and generalized lymphadenopathy. If secondary infection occurs, the lesions may become painful. Major considerations in the differential diagnosis of a genital ulcer are summarized in Table 30.3. The herpes simplex virus remains the most common cause of chancre-like genital ulcers, but a six-fold increase in chancroid in the United States in the last decade has added further complexity to the differential diagnosis of genital ulcers. Definitive diagnosis is made by microscopic examination of the fluid overlying the ulcer (see "Direct Microscopic Examination"). Serological tests for syphilis (STS) are usually reactive (see "Diagnosis").

Surveillance of the sexual contacts of newly diagnosed patients with infectious (primary or secondary) syphilis has shown active infection in about one-third of those who had such contact in the month preceding the patient's diagnosis (32).

Secondary Syphilis

If untreated during the primary stage, most patients develop secondary syphilis 6 weeks to 6 months after initial contact. When the secondary stage begins, the chancre may still be present. The most characteristic finding is a nonpruritic rash that is usually maculopapular, but not vesicular or bullous. It can involve all areas of the skin, especially the trunk, the palms, and the soles. Scalp and eyelash involvement may lead to alopecia. Mucous patches (gray oral patches on an erythematous base) and lesions in warm, moist areas such as the axillary and genital regions are particularly infectious. Condyloma latum, a flat, wart-like lesion usually found in the genital or anal area, is also highly infectious; it must be distinguished from the more common pointy, fleshy, genital wart (condyloma acuminatum, see Chapter 94). Dark-field or direct fluorescent antibody for *T. pallidum* (DFA-TP) examination of moist skin lesions or the condyloma latum should be positive. In as many as one-half of the patients, skin lesions may not occur or may not be detected.

Constitutional symptoms such as fever, headache,

Table 30.2.
Outline of Clinical Stages of Syphilis[a]

Stage	Characteristic Findings	Usual Onset after Exposure	Duration of Stage in Untreated Patients	Dark Field
Primary	Chancre—may be absent or not visible (*e.g*, in vagina or mouth)	10–90 days (average 21 days)	2–6 weeks	+ (Chancre, lymph nodes)
Secondary	Rash, condyloma latum, lymphadenopathy	6 weeks to 6 months	2–6 weeks; recurrences in 25% over 2-year period	+ (Especially moist lesions)
Acute syphilitic meningitis	Headache, cranial nerve lesions, papilledema	6 weeks to 2 years	Not applicable	+ CSF
Latent			May be lifelong since only ⅓ of untreated patients develop tertiary syphilis	−
Early	None	<1 year after infection		
Late	None	>1 year after infection		
Late (tertiary)				
Benign	Gumma	2–10 years	Indolent	−
Cardiovascular	Aortic aneurysm Aortic insufficiency Coronary artery disease especially of the ostia	10–30 years	Progressive; may be fatal	Aorta may be +
Neurosyphilis		2–35 years	Progressive; may be fatal	Brain may be +
Asymptomatic	None			
Meningovascular	Signs of infection depend on area involved	2–10 years		
Paresis	Minor personality change to frank psychosis	15–35 years		
Tabes dorsalis	Signs of posterior column degeneration	5–30 years		

[a] See details in the text.

Table 30.3.
Differential Diagnosis of a Genital Sore

Primary syphilis (chancre)
   Incubation period 10–90 days (average, 21 days)
   Usually painless (in absence of secondary infection)
   Not vesicular
   Usually single indurated ulcer but multiple lesions are seen in
      30% of cases
   Spirochete on dark field examination
   Nontender inguinal adenopathy
Herpes simplex
   Incubation period 24–48 hours
   Usually painful
   Vesicular
   Usually multiple ulcers
   Multinucleated giant cells on Giemsa stain plus virus on culture
   Tender inguinal adenopathy
Chancroid
   Multiple soft superficial erosions
   Nontender adenopathy. *Haemophilus ducreyi* on Gram stain of
      dried smear (small Gram-negative bacillus)
Granuloma inguinale
   Soft, occasionally raised, granulating lesions in inguinal area:
      Donovan bodies on smear (histiocytes with intracytoplasmic
      encapsulated Gram-negative bacilli)
Other considerations
   Trauma, carcinoma, scabies, lichen planus, psoriasis, fixed drug
      eruption (especially phenolphthalein), fungus infection,
      folliculitis

malaise, and generalized lymphadenopathy are common. Other systemic manifestations occur in 1 to 2% of cases and include hepatitis, immune complex nephropathy, and frank meningitis. The latter is characterized by headache, stiff neck, seizures, and cranial nerve signs including papilledema and involvement of the 3rd, 6th, 7th, and 8th nerves. Associated with involvement of the latter, there is tinnitus, followed by deafness that can be reversed by treatment (1). Cerebrospinal fluid (CSF) contains increased mononuclear cells and protein; there may also be a decrease in CSF glucose. The CSF-VDRL (see below) is positive in about 90% of cases of active meningitis (5). There is continuing controversy about the utility of the CSF-FTA-ABS, but it has been shown to be uniformly positive in such cases when the test is performed at the Centers for Disease Control (CDC) (5, 22). Spirochetes may also be detected on dark-field or DFA-TP examination of the CSF. Even in the absence of positive laboratory findings, clinical signs may warrant treatment; in such cases, a therapeutic response may be the only way to verify the diagnosis.

Serological tests for syphilis are reactive in virtually 100% of patients at this stage (see "Serological Tests in Diagnosis" below).

Untreated, secondary syphilis lasts 2 to 6 weeks and may relapse in about 25% at some time during the first 4 years after infection; 90% of all relapses occur within a year. Although relapses are usually identical to initial episodes, condyloma latum may be more common in the relapse episode than in the initial episode. The major considerations in differential diagnosis are drug reactions, psoriasis, and pityriasis rosea (see descriptions of these conditions, Chapter 100).

Latent Syphilis

Latent syphilis is, as the name implies, the period after infection with *T. pallidum* when there are no clinical manifestations. The division between early and late latent infection has been set at 1 year because following up of contacts of patients with syphilis of more than 1 year's duration rarely turns up infectious cases; this therefore becomes a useful demarcation for reporting purposes.

The majority of patients with latent disease come to diagnosis through routine serological testing (see "Diagnosis"). Detection early in this stage is important not only for epidemiological purposes but also to prevent further complications in the one-third of untreated patients who go on to develop late manifestations of syphilis.

Tertiary (Late) Syphilis

Tertiary or late disease is divided into three principal forms: late benign syphilis, cardiovascular syphilis, and neurosyphilis. Since the advent of penicillin therapy, all forms of tertiary syphilis have become uncommon although there appears to be an increase in human immunodeficiency virus (HIV) positive individuals (see "HIV Infection and Syphilis" below). In addition, the late manifestations have become milder and more subtle (18).

Late benign syphilis is characterized by the development of a gumma, a lesion that may grow to several centimeters in size. The gumma is thought to be a hypersensitivity reaction because viable organisms are rarely seen. Gummas usually occur within 2 to 10 years of infection, most commonly on the skin (ulcerative or nodular-ulcerative), in bone, or in the liver, and are especially destructive when in the brain, liver, or heart. Diagnosis is made on the basis of typical pathological findings and of dramatic healing of visible gummas after treatment.

Cardiovascular syphilis, which is very uncommon today, was reported in 13.6% of untreated men and 7.6% of untreated women from 5 to 30 years after acquisition of the disease. However, recent reports of syphilitic aortitis confirm previous studies that revealed unsuspected tertiary syphilis in a significant number of patients autopsied in areas where the prevalence of syphilis was thought to be low (45). Syphilitic aortitis occurs when the organism destroys the elastic tissue of the media of the aorta and produces an endarteritis of the vasa vasorum. Clinical manifestations include aneurysm of the ascending aorta and progressive dilatation of the aortic ring, resulting in aortic insufficiency and heart failure. When the coronary ostia are involved, angina pectoris may result. Linear calcification of the ascending aorta is a common radiological finding in syphilitic aortitis; it may precede clinical symptoms and signs of aortic involvement.

Asymptomatic neurosyphilis is defined by the occurrence of a reactive Venereal Disease Research Laboratory (VDRL) test for syphilis in the spinal fluid of a patient who has no neurological or psychiatric signs or symptoms. A pleocytosis and an elevated protein concentration may be present in the fluid. Asymptomatic neurosyphilis occurred in 10% of all untreated patients in the preantibiotic era. The current rate of occùrrence in untreated persons is unknown. The diagnosis of asymptomatic neurosyphilis and its significance are the subject of controversy (5, 22). The following facts are important to know: First, dissemination of *T. pallidum* to the central nervous system is very common at all stages, even primary syphilis. Second, in the preantibiotic era only about 10% of patients developed clinical neurosyphilis. Third, after the widespread use of intramuscular penicillin, even in doses that did not produce spirochetocidal levels in the central nervous system, the incidence of clinical neurosyphilis fell to virtually zero. Consequently, the regimens recommended for the routine treatment of primary, secondary, and early latent syphilis have not been substantially altered in the most recent CDC guidelines (33). However, interest in this issue has been rekindled because patients infected with HIV seem to develop neurosyphilis more frequently despite treatment with intramuscular penicillin, possibly because of their immunocompromised state (17). HIV-infected patients with neuropsychiatric manifestations can present difficult diagnostic problems because of limitations in the diagnostic tests for neurosyphilis (see below) and the lack of specific markers for HIV infection of the central nervous system. Diagnosing asymptomatic neurosyphilis and defining its natural history in HIV-infected patients are even more difficult. However, because of concerns about the sufficiency of current treatment schedules, this issue is receiving considerable attention (see "HIV Infection and Syphilis" below).

Symptomatic neurosyphilis, which is also uncommon, occurred in 9.4% of men and 5% of women with untreated syphilis in the Oslo study of the natural history of untreated syphilis (see "General References"). The risk of developing symptomatic neurosyphilis after a primary infection is greater in whites than in blacks. Symptomatic neurosyphilis is divided into various types depending upon the site of major involvement.

1. *Meningovascular syphilis* usually occurs within 2 to 10 years after untreated primary infection. Common manifestations include headache, irritability, and personality changes. Vasculitis involving small end arteries results in focal neurological signs. The severity of the patient's disability depends upon the extent and location of the accompanying cerebrovascular inflammation and occlusion.
2. *Tabes dorsalis* usually occurs 5 to 30 years after infection. It is characterized by symptoms and signs of posterior column degeneration (ataxia, areflexia, broad-based gait, incontinence, impotence, abdominal pain crises, and paresthesias or "lightning" pains in the extremities). Characteristic findings also include trophic joint changes (Charcot's joints),

the Argyll Robertson pupil (small, irregular pupil that accommodates but does not react to light), and optic atrophy (in about 10% of patients).
3. The syndrome of *general paresis* usually occurs 15 to 35 years after infection. It is due to destruction of the parenchyma of the cerebral cortex. It consists of personality changes, irritability, poor judgment, insomnia, and memory loss. The progressive dementia in these patients may be characterized by periodic euphoria and delusions of grandeur.

A definitive diagnosis of neurosyphilis is based upon spinal fluid findings: elevated protein concentration and an increased number of mononuclear cells, as well as a reactive serological test for syphilis (see "Diagnosis").

Serology for Diagnosis and Follow-up

Direct Microscopic Examination

As syphilis decreased in prevalence, both the availability of dark-field microscopy and the competency of those performing it declined. Some reference laboratories now perform direct fluorescent microscopy using specific antisera (DFA-TP) to identify the organism. Large medical centers with special sexually transmitted disease (STD) clinics and larger health departments ordinarily provide reliable testing. One should call ahead to assure that a working microscope and a knowledgeable reader are available. To obtain material, one should (*a*) abrade the lesion gently with gauze so as to produce a nonbloody, serous exudate; (*b*) after wiping the surface, squeeze the lesion between gloved thumb and forefinger; (*c*) collect the exudate in a capillary tube or a microscope slide; and (*d*) finally, give it to someone who knows how to do the test. Microscopic examination should be performed on 3 consecutive days in highly suspect patients before being called definitively negative. This is especially so if antibiotic ointments have been used. Dark-field examination should not be done on material obtained from oral lesions because of the potential for confusion with *Treponema microdentium*, a common mouth inhabitant. The DFA-TP test is more specific and can be performed on oral smears.

Serological Tests in Diagnosis

Serological tests are of two basic types; nontreponemal and treponemal. *Nontreponemal tests* detect reagin, a nonspecific antibody to cardiolipin, a normal component of many tissues. Wassermann in 1906 was the first to use this reaction to detect patients with syphilis. Since then about 100 different forms of the original Wassermann test have been developed. Of the five flocculation tests in common use today, the Venereal Disease Research Laboratory (VDRL) and the rapid plasma reagin (RPR) tests are most frequently used.

The *treponemal tests* include the fluorescent treponemal antibody-absorption test (FTA-ABS) and microhemagglutination test for *T. pallidum* (MHATP or HATTS). Both tests detect specific antibodies to *T. pallidum*. Fig. 30.1 shows the pattern of reactivity of various serological tests during the course of untreated syphilis.

The *sensitivity* (the percentage of syphilitic patients with a reactive test) varies at each stage of the disease and for different tests (see Table 30.4). The RPR is slightly more sensitive than the VDRL; the FTA-ABS tests and hemagglutination procedures are more sensitive than the VDRL and RPR. The range of values for sensitivity is accounted for by differences in case definition in different studies. Where case definition is more rigorous (e.g., using a positive dark-field or DFA-TP to assure the diagnosis of primary syphilis rather than simply clinical criteria), the sensitivity is higher.

STS *specificity* (the percentage of nonsyphilitic patients with a negative test) is also shown in Table 30.4. There are two major reasons for the variance in specificity given for each test. First, study populations have differed in the proportion of patients with conditions that cause false-positive test results. For example, studies of the specificity of the VDRL or the FTA-ABS in a group of nuns or other healthy volunteer populations have revealed very few false-positives. On the other hand, studies in sexually transmitted disease clinic populations, facilities serving drug addicts, or arthritis clinic populations with many patients with systemic lupus have yielded higher rates of false-positives and consequently lower estimates of specificity. Second, test performance can vary in different laboratories with devastating effects on both the specificity and sensitivity of such vulnerable tests as the FTA-ABS (6). Table 30.4 gives consensus sensitivity and specificity figures for serological tests done on serum from patients in an STD clinic population and performed at the Centers for Disease Control (CDC) reference laboratory (21). As with any other test, one must determine how applicable they are to tests done in one's patient population and at one's reference laboratory. Most of the discussion of treponemal tests will be confined to the FTA-ABS test, which is used more extensively than the MHATP. However, some laboratories are substituting the hemagglutination tests as the treponemal test of choice because they are less subject to technical error.

When a nontreponemal test is reactive and the FTA-ABS or the hemagglutination test is consistently non-reactive, the patient is considered to have a *biological false-positive test result*. "Acute" biological false-positive VDRL and RPR tests are defined as those lasting less than 6 months. They have been reported in patients with viral and bacterial pneumonia, hepatitis, pregnancy, mononucleosis, measles, malaria, and after smallpox vaccination. "Chronic" false-positive nontreponemal test reactions (those lasting more than 6 months) occur in diseases of disordered immunity, such as systemic lupus erythematosus, rheumatoid arthritis, and Waldenström's macroglobulinemia, as well as in chronic liver disease, and in intravenous drug addicts, elderly persons (approximately 1% of persons over 70 and 10% of persons over 80), and occasional patients on a hereditary basis. Biological false-positive VDRL or RPR titers are usually 1:8 or lower but occasionally can be higher, especially in hereditary cases. A false-positive nontreponemal test result should not be dismissed but should be used as a clue to the diagnosis of the conditions listed above. However, in as

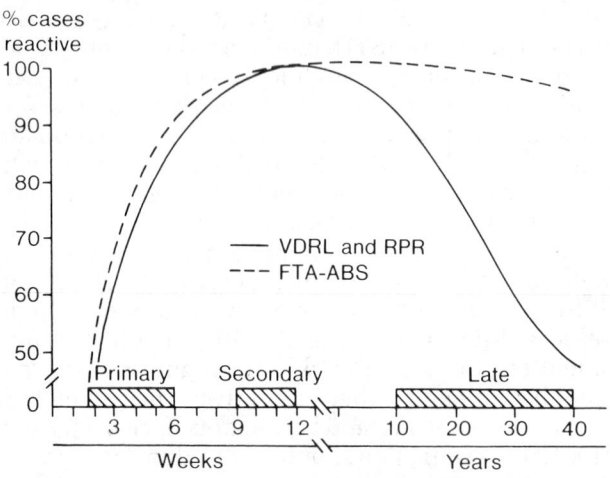

Figure 30.1. Serology of untreated syphilis. (Adapted from Wallace AL, Norins LC: Syphilis serology today. *Prog Clin Pathol* 2:198, 1969.)

Table 30.4.
Sensitivity and Specificity of Serological Tests for Syphilis[a] at Different Stages

Stage of Syphilis	Percentage of Sensitivity (Sens.) and Specificity (Spec.)							
	VDRL[b]		RPR[b]		FTA-ABS[b]		MHA-TP[b]	
	Sens.	Spec.	Sens.	Spec.	Sens.	Spec.	Sens.	Spec.
Primary	80 (59–87)	98 (80–99)	86 (81–100)	98 (80–99)	98 (93–100)	98 (84–99)	82 (64–90)	99 (98–100)
Secondary	100 (99–100)	98	100 (99–100)	98	100 (99–100)	98	100 (96–100)	99
Latent	96 (73–100)	98	99	98	100 (96–100)	98	100 (96–100)	99
Tertiary (Late)	71	98	73	98	96	98	94	99

[a] The consensus figures for the sensitivity and specificity are for tests done in the Centers for Disease Control Reference Laboratory (10) on samples derived from a well run STD clinic. The figures in parentheses demonstrate the variability in published reports. Responsible factors include (a) study of populations with different prevalences of syphilis and other confounding illnesses, (b) variable performance by the laboratory, and (c) different clinical criteria for the diagnosis of syphilis (see the text).

[b] See text for fuller discussion of these tests.

many as 50% of cases, no explanation can be found and the patient remains symptom free. Whatever the case, a patient should be informed of his or her test status in order to prevent inappropriate labeling and treatment for syphilis.

When properly performed, the FTA-ABS tests have a specificity of 98%. A positive FTA-ABS test is essentially a "true" positive in patients with related treponemal conditions such as yaws, pinta, and behel. These must be considered where those diseases are endemic, e.g., parts of Africa, and Central and South America. False-positive reactions occur in patients with lupus erythematosus, rheumatoid arthritis, chronic liver disease, some infections, and in other patients for unexplained reasons. Because small errors in laboratory technique can affect the results of the FTA-ABS tests more than the results of the nontreponemal tests, the FTA-ABS should be utilized selectively (6), i.e., only when nontreponemal tests are reactive. Exception should be made when either primary or tertiary syphilis is highly suspect, when there are neurological or psychiatric signs suggestive of tabes or paresis, or if signs of aortic insufficiency and aneurysm of the ascending aorta are present. In these situations, the treponemal test may occasionally be the only reactive test (Table 30.4).

In diagnosing *latent syphilis*, a single reactive nontreponemal test, even if confirmed by a treponemal test result, should not be relied upon as the only datum, especially if there is no other reason to suspect syphilis. The test should be repeated to assure that there was not a mix-up of blood specimens. The clinical, psychological, and social implications of this diagnosis are too serious to rely on a single datum.

The sensitivity *of the CSF-VDRL* for the detection of neurosyphilis ranges from 10 to 89%. It is highest for meningitis, meningovascular, and paretic forms and lowest for asymptomatic neurosyphilis and tabes dorsalis. Although virtually 100% specific for neurosyphilis, instances of false-positive CSF-VDRL have been reported after traumatic lumbar puncture and in a case of meningeal tumor. Recent evidence suggests that the CSF FTA-ABS has an excellent sensitivity and specificity when performed at the CDC reference laboratory. However, because of vulnerability to performance error, its use should be restricted to the CDC or a carefully monitored laboratory and only in highly suspect cases. Thus, the CSF-VDRL, with all of its limitations, remains the test of choice in the workup for neurosyphilis in selected patients (5).

Serological Tests in Screening

A nontreponemal serological test for syphilis should be used as a screening test in patients who are sexually active with multiple partners and who are thereby at increased risk for acquisition of syphilis (3). Patients found to have another STD, such as gonorrhea, should also have a screening STS because their pattern of sexual activity puts them at higher risk for having acquired syphilis in the past. The occasional patient who acquires syphilis and gonorrhea simultaneously will have a negative serology when the gonorrhea becomes manifest, since the latent periods for the development of these two diseases differ so widely. This is of concern for contact tracing, and when therapy for gonorrhea is other than penicillin (e.g., spectinomycin), since penicillin treatment for gonorrhea during the incubation period aborts the development of syphilis (32). In most office settings, an STS should be done routinely on a sexually active patient's first visit. In subsequent visits, a repeated STS should be done only in those patients deemed to have been at risk for acquiring a new infection during the interval.

Pattern of Serological Tests after Treatment (Fig. 30.2)

The nontreponemal test reverts to nonreactive in more than 90% of patients adequately treated for primary or secondary syphilis, but the FTA-ABS rarely does so except when patients are treated very early in the course of their disease (31). The FTA-ABS should be repeated once, 6 to 12 months after syphilis is diagnosed and treated. If it remains reactive, it should not be repeated. In later serological testing of patients who have had syphilis, the nontreponemal test titer becomes the most useful tool (see "Follow-up") (31). In patients treated for early latent syphilis, nontreponemal tests become nonreactive within 5 years of treatment in approximately 75%, whereas only about 25% of patients with treated late latent syphilis will be seronegative in 5 years (10). Many middle-aged and older persons with a titer of 1:4 or lower reactivity in the nontreponemal test will fall into the category of adequately treated serofast syphilis; differentiation from late latent syphilis can usually be made through careful history.

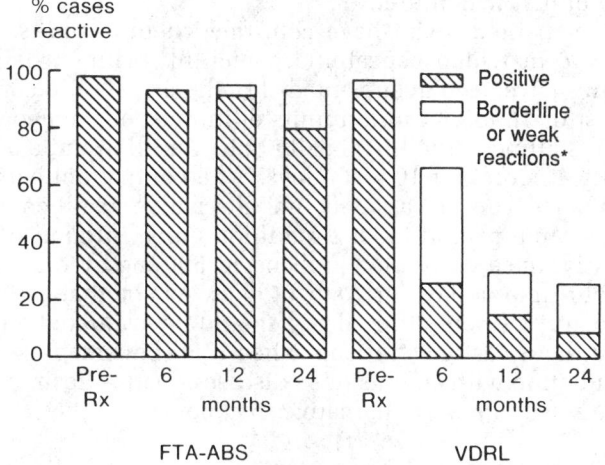

Figure 30.2. Serological reactivity of 80 patients treated for dark-field positive primary or secondary syphilis and observed for 2 years, with use of FTA-ABS and VDRL tests. (Adapted from Schroeter AL, et al.: Treatment for early syphilis and reactivity of serologic tests. *JAMA* 221:471, 1972.) *These reactions are now classified as nonreactive.

Treatment

Regimens

The treatment of choice for *primary, secondary, and early latent syphilis*, as well as for known contacts of a patient with infectious syphilis, is 2.4 million units of benzathine penicillin G (LA Bicillin) intramuscularly (33). Some advocate administering a repeated dose 1 week later (10). An alternative for persons allergic to penicillin is a total dose of 30 g of oral tetracycline (2 g a day for 2 weeks) or 3 g of doxycycline (200 mg a day for 2 weeks). In penicillin-allergic patients who cannot tolerate tetracycline or doxycycline, erythromycin (2 g a day for 2 weeks) or possibly ceftriaxone (250 mg intramuscularly daily for 10 days) may be used. While follow-up is essential with any regimen, it is especially important when alternatives to penicillin are used. As previously noted, penicillin, but not spectinomycin, regimens for gonorrhea therapy are also effective against incubating syphilis, acquired simultaneously (32).

The treatment of choice for *late latent syphilis, gummas, and cardiovascular syphilis* is 2.4 million units of benzathine penicillin G intramuscularly (LA Bicillin) weekly for 3 weeks. For patients who are allergic to penicillin, alternative drugs can be used; however, the CDC suggests that a CSF examination be done first to exclude neurosyphilis. It is best to validate a history of penicillin allergy by careful history and, where possible, by skin testing, using the major and minor penicillin determinants if available (see Chapter 23). Alternative regimens are tetracycline (2 g a day for 4 weeks) or doxycycline (200 mg a day for 4 weeks). Erythromycin is no longer advocated because of the lack of studies demonstrating efficacy in late latent and late syphilis as well as concerns about the association of congenital syphilis with treatment failure (53). It is also worth noting that some would treat cardiovascular syphilis with the regimen for neurosyphilis, which follows.

In patients who have *confirmed neurosyphilis*, a stage in which benzathine penicillin treatment failures have been documented (11), therapy should consist of 12 to 24 million units of intravenous aqueous crystalline penicillin G daily (2 to 4 million units every 4 hours) for 10 to 14 days. When outpatient compliance can be assured, an alternative regimen is procaine penicillin G: 2.4 million units, intramuscularly, once daily plus probenecid 500 mg by mouth, four times a day, for 10 to 14 days. As noted above, a history of penicillin allergy should be evaluated and in the occasional patients when it is confirmed, consultation with an infectious disease expert is desirable to select the best alternative treatment.

Effectiveness

The effectiveness of treatment varies depending on the stage of syphilis treated. In one study of patients with primary and secondary syphilis, retreatment was required in 5% of patients after the usual doses of benzathine penicillin G, and in 10% of patients after the usual doses of tetracycline (31). The criteria for retreatment in this study were recurrence or persistence of clinical manifestations or failure of the VDRL titer to decrease 4-fold within 1 year.

The effectiveness of treatment in patients with latent syphilis is difficult to assess because of the absence of any markers to follow. However, in one follow-up study, all 469 patients with late latent syphilis treated at various centers with the recommended doses of penicillin were symptom free 12 years later (19).

The effectiveness of treatment of cardiovascular syphilis has been debated (7). Most investigators believe that treatment may arrest the disease but not reverse it. Because of the weakening of the media of the aorta, aneurysms may continue to enlarge even after adequate treatment.

The results of treatment for neurosyphilis vary directly with the extent of the disease and inversely with its duration. Thus, treatment often reverses the signs and symptoms of acute meningovascular syphilis and stabilizes tabes dorsalis, but is less effective in reversing the signs of general paresis, especially if given late in its course (52). In addition to the reversal of clinical signs, the return of any CSF reactivity to normal is an index of effective therapy. If the initial CSF examination reveals a pleocytosis, the lumbar puncture should be repeated every 6 months until the cell count is normal. If the examination shows no improvement in 6 months or is not normal by 2 years, retreatment is probably indicated.

Jarisch-Herxheimer Reaction

The Jarisch-Herxheimer reaction is characterized by a mild temperature elevation within 6 to 8 hours of administration of the first injection of penicillin (25, 46). It appears to be caused by microbial lysis and the release of endotoxin. The reaction resolves after several hours and does not occur after subsequent injections. A Jarisch-Herxheimer reaction is estimated to occur in 50% of patients with primary syphilis, 75 to 90% of patients with secondary syphilis, and 30% of patients with late disease. When it occurs during treatment of secondary syphilis, skin lesions become more prominent. Because the Jarisch-Herxheimer reaction is common, patients should be told that the reaction usually is mild and lasts only a few hours and that it can be treated with mild analgesics. Uncommonly the reaction may be quite severe and consist of high fever, chills, headache, muscle and joint pains, sore throat, and transient hypotension. It may produce significant exacerbation of neurological signs in a small percentage of patients treated for neurosyphilis. For this reason, corticosteroid therapy has been used both before and after treatment, but its efficacy is not established (46).

Practical Approach to the Patient

Sexually active patients in whom syphilis is a consideration usually present to their physicians because of (a) a "sore" or rash, (b) referral as a known contact of a patient with syphilis, (c) worry about a recent sexual liaison, or (d) a positive serological test in routine premarital, blood donor, or health screening. The diagnosis of syphilis must be made carefully, as it can have a major impact on the relationships of patients with their contacts and on how they view themselves. A systematic approach to diagnosis and management is outlined here.

Evaluation

The *history* should include a description of any sore or rash, determination of a previous history of STD especially syphilis, review of the results of previous serological tests for syphilis, an inquiry into the patient's type of sexual practices to guide the physical examination, and information about recent partners and their disease status.

The *physical examination* should include a careful search for typical lesions in all areas of sexual contact. Special care should be taken in examining the anogenital area and the mouth. Other features to look for include regional and generalized lymphadenopathy, enlarged liver, and neurological, psychiatric, and cardiovascular signs when late disease is a concern.

Laboratory data should include direct microscopy of the exudate from any suspicious lesions and serological testing for syphilis (see "Diagnosis"). CSF examination is mandatory in patients with psychiatric or neurological signs or symptoms. In asymptomatic patients who have had syphilis for more than 1 year, the CDC recommends a lumbar puncture to exclude asymptomatic neurosyphilis. However, the CSF examination is virtually always negative in such patients. Furthermore, in the most comprehensive study of the subject, only 1 of 765 patients with asymptomatic neurosyphilis treated with penicillin in doses equivalent to the 3 weekly benzathine penicillin G injections developed clinical neurosyphilis (12). Thus, for asymptomatic patients who have low serum nontreponemal test titers (1:16 or less), who are not positive for HIV antibody, and who do not have a confirmed penicillin allergy, it is reasonable to administer the recommended regimen for late latent syphilis (see above) without performing a lumbar puncture (5, 51). These patients should be followed to assure that they remain asymptomatic. Other clinical approaches have been recommended (20, 22).

In *patients who were treated for syphilis with heavy metals* before the penicillin era, the question sometimes arises about the need for further treatment. Most experts do not recommend retreating such patients, if there are no suspicious signs or symptoms and there is no history of exposure to infectious syphilis in the interim.

Special difficulty is presented by *patients who are pregnant* and who are found to have an abnormal serological result when a routine STS is performed either at their initial visit or, in areas of high prevalence, when it is repeated during the third trimester and at

delivery. Because pregnancy has been reported to be a cause of a biological false-positive nontreponemal test, the treponemal test is an essential confirmatory test. If the treponemal test is nonreactive and there is no clinical evidence of syphilis, nontreponemal and treponemal tests should be repeated monthly for 3 months. If the treponemal tests remain negative, this can be considered to be a biological false-positive reaction. If there is clinical or serological confirmation of syphilis, the staging is similar to that for nonpregnant patients. The only difference in therapy is that in penicillin-allergic patients, tetracycline and doxycycline are contraindicated. Current CDC treatment guidelines suggest that pregnant patients who give a history of penicillin allergy should be skin tested for penicillin with major and minor determinants and, if positive, desensitized (Chapter 23). Because women treated in the second half of pregnancy are at high risk for premature labor and/or fetal distress if their treatment precipitates a Jarisch-Herxheimer reaction (see above), treatment should be coordinated with the obstetrician. Nontreponemal tests should be performed at monthly intervals to determine therapeutic response and to detect any reinfection. Infants born even to adequately treated mothers will be seropositive at birth because of passive transfer of IgG across the placenta. If the baby appears healthy, no further treatment is indicated, but the baby should be followed carefully over the next 6 to 12 months to assure that no signs develop and that the serological reactivity disappears (33).

Management

The management plan is contingent upon making the appropriate diagnosis. The diagnosis rests on positive results of direct microscopy or on the combination of a reactive nontreponemal and treponemal test. When the diagnosis is made, the disease should be staged appropriately, as outlined above.

The most common errors in the diagnosis of syphilis are: (a) failing to take proper note of an abnormal serology and missing the diagnosis entirely, or (b) noting the serological change but inadequately staging the disease (e.g., "positive VDRL, treat with penicillin.") Treatment of syphilis at a given stage is indicated, not treatment of a reactive VDRL. Appropriate antibiotic regimens are listed above for each stage of syphilis.

Follow-up. In following up the patient, the nontreponemal test titer remains the most useful index of the effectiveness of treatment. A high titer is more likely to occur in early syphilis or in active late disease. When a 1:4 titer or greater is present, a nontreponemal test should be performed every 3 months for a year to see if the patient has a 4-fold or greater fall in titer (for example, a 1:32 titer that falls to 1:2). If the expected fall in titer does not occur within 9 to 12 months, the patient should be retreated. It is important to use the same nontreponemal test on all serial specimens because of the differences in their sensitivity, i.e., the RPR titer will often be at least one dilution higher than a VDRL done on the same specimen.

Patients with persistently high titers after 1 year may represent either treatment failures or undetected reinfections and should be retreated. A spinal fluid examination to rule out neurosyphilis is indicated in such patients especially if one has not been done. Patients who have a 4-fold or greater rise in titer during follow-up should be considered to be reinfected and staged and treated accordingly. In patients with very low titers, as is usually the case in the late latent stage, there is no practical way of assessing the adequacy of therapy.

Contact Tracing. In most jurisdictions, physicians are obligated by law to report the patient's name and the stage of the disease to the health department for both statistical purposes and for contact tracing by specially trained investigators. Because of rapport with the patient, a physician may choose to coordinate contact tracing. In this era of freer discussion of human sexuality, this poses less of a problem; however, the physician may encounter a situation in which the patient does not wish to be straightforward with partners about outside liaisons. This presents a conflict between patient confidentiality and the binding legal requirement to report the patient. Health department investigators make every effort to keep the patient's name from being divulged; however, when there is a spouse involved, this may be impossible without resorting to deception, which is not recommended. When the patient balks at informing a spouse or steady partner, it must be impressed upon the patient that the relationship may well benefit from frank and honest discussion of the situation. In any case, not to do so would put the partner at risk and this cannot be condoned.

All identified contacts of patients with infectious syphilis should be thoroughly evaluated for signs of syphilis. When the contact has signs of syphilis, the disease should be staged and treated accordingly and their contacts should be located. Even if there are no signs or serological evidence of active disease, contacts of patients with syphilis should receive prompt treatment for primary syphilis without waiting for clinical manifestations or a positive serology (14).

Education. Education should focus on prevention. If patients have sexual relations with multiple partners, they should be counseled about the risk this entails for contracting syphilis and other STDs. At the time that a patient is treated for infectious syphilis, he or she should be told to abstain from sex until the sore or rash disappears or for at least 1 week, whichever is longer. If the patient plans to continue to be promiscuous, he should be cautioned to use a condom as a protection against venereal disease transmission and acquisition. To be effective, condoms must be used during foreplay, be properly worn, and remain intact (7); detailed instructions for condom use are summarized in Table 34.3. Condoms cannot prevent infection if lesions are outside of the area covered. Contraceptive vaginal creams and jellies may provide some prophylaxis as well. Nonetheless, patients who continue to be promiscuous should have checkups for gonorrhea, HIV, and syphilis whenever they suspect they may have acquired one of these diseases or on a 6-month or yearly basis.

HIV INFECTION AND SYPHILIS

The biological, clinical, psychological, social, political, and economic consequences of HIV infection are as far reaching as those that were associated with syphilis from the 15th to the middle of the 20th century. Studies in Africa and the United States have shown that patients who have had syphilis are at increased risk of being infected with HIV. This results in part from common exposure, through prostitution and intravenous drug use (29), but also because of the facilitation of HIV transmission through genital ulcerations. Safer sexual behaviors that decrease the risk of infection with one disease also decrease the risk for the other.

Because of the strong association of these two diseases, patients suspected of having syphilis should be encouraged to be tested simultaneously for HIV infection (26). Although most patients infected with HIV have normal serological and clinical responses to *T. pallidum*, immunocompromised patients may develop altered seroreactivity, and possibly, even altered clinical manifestations of syphilis. There is some evidence that HIV-infected patients are more prone to develop clinical neurosyphilis and to fail to respond to standard treatment for syphilis. This issue is under intense study. At the present time, standard treatment for syphilis (see above) is still recommended for HIV-infected patients, but VDRL tests, at monthly intervals for 6 months rather than at 3-month intervals, are recommended, to search for evidence of treatment failure (stable or rising titer) (17). Treatment failures should be retreated in conjunction with an infectious disease consultant. Chapter 34 provides a comprehensive account of the ambulatory care of the HIV-infected patient.

LYME DISEASE

Epidemiology

Lyme disease is a tick-borne spirochetal disease that is endemic in several areas of the United States, Russia, and central Europe. The agent, *B. burgdorferi*, is transmitted by ixodid ticks that have mice and deer as important hosts. The pinhead-sized nymphal ticks are the ticks most likely to bite humans. Areas of the United States that are endemic for Lyme disease are the northeast, upper midwest, and northern California (see Fig. 30.3). However, cases are seen by physicians throughout the United States because of summertime vacation travel and, infrequently, transmission in nonendemic areas. Trans-

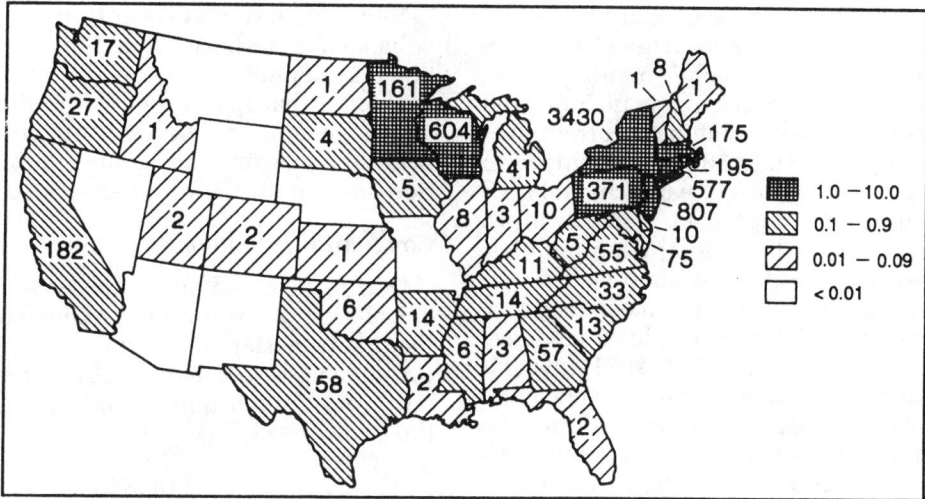

Figure 30.3. Number and average annual incidence rates of reported Lyme disease cases, per 100,000 population—United States, 1987–1988. Data for Oregon and California are for 1987 only. From: Centers for Disease Control *MMWR* 38:669, 1989.

mission and onset of illness occur most frequently when the nymphal ticks are most abundant and active. However, since the adult tick can also transmit Lyme disease, infection can occur at nearly any time of the year. Onset of illness is most common in the northeastern and north central states in May through August and in the northwestern states in January through May. The incidence of Lyme disease has been steadily increasing since its recognition in the township of Lyme, Connecticut, in 1975 (42). In some areas virtually 100% of the ixodid ticks are infected. Lyme disease is currently the most common arthropod-borne disease in the United States.

Stages of the Disease

Primary Lyme Disease

The organism is introduced into the skin of a susceptible host by the tick bite. The period between tick bite and onset of illness (incubation period) varies from 3 to 32 days. The most common manifestation of primary disease, occurring in 60 to 80% of cases, is an expanding lesion appearing within days to weeks at the site of the bite, usually the thigh, buttock, axilla, or trunk. The lesion starts as a red macule or papule. The later appearance of the lesion is characteristic with an erythematous border and clearing center that may expand to become very large (e.g., 6 to 16 cm in diameter). This typical lesion of *erythema chronicum migrans* (ECM) may continue to increase for many days, is usually warm but not particularly painful or pruritic, and is the best clinical marker for the disease (41, 42). The primary stage of the disease is often accompanied by flu-like symptoms including fever (low-grade and intermittent), chills, malaise, stiff neck, arthralgias, and headache. In addition to ECM, regional and/or generalized lymphadenopathy is often present. Even without treatment these early signs and symptoms, including the ECM eruption, resolve within 3

to 4 weeks without treatment (35, 40, 41). Despite the neurological complaints, CSF examination is almost always normal when a lumbar puncture is performed to look for meningitis.

Secondary Lyme Disease

The secondary stage of the disease is due to systemic spread of the organism and usually occurs within one to six months after exposure. It most often presents with multiple ECM lesions (35, 40), carditis (36), or neurological disease (28), but hepatitis, ophthalmitis, pneumonitis, orchitis, and nephritis have been reported.

Dermatological Manifestations. Dissemination to form multiple secondary annular skin lesions is usually accompanied by more intense systemic manifestations with severe lethargy, encephalopathy, myalgias, generalized lymphadenopathy, and splenomegaly (35, 40). A second type of skin eruption called *lymphocytoma* or *lymphadenosis benigna cutis* may be seen during secondary Lyme disease. This condition consists of a solitary red or violaceous lesion most commonly located on the ear lobe in children or on the nipple in adults. It may be accompanied by regional lymphadenopathy as well as by other manifestations of late Lyme disease (arthritis, nerve palsies, etc.) (49).

Cardiac Manifestations. Carditis occurs in approximately 8% of untreated infected individuals and presents with palpitations associated with atrioventricular conduction abnormalities and occasionally S-T segment and T wave changes. These signs and symptoms usually resolve within 6 weeks (36).

Neurological Manifestations. Neurological complications occur in 10 to 15% of patients and include meningitis, meningoencephalitis, cranial nerve palsies, and radiculitis (28). Systemic symptoms may be present, but ECM and lymphadenopathy have usually resolved.

Meningitis is present in 80% of those patients with

neurological disease during the secondary stage and is often combined with other neurological manifestations (24). Intermittent headache, meningismus, nausea, vomiting, malaise, and fatigue in untreated patients may last several weeks and be recurrent over several months. Approximately 50% of patients with meningitis have some symptoms of parenchymal CNS involvement—most often depressed consciousness, impaired concentration, or behavioral abnormalities. A subset of patients has additional abnormalities including seizures, ataxia, paresis, or movement disorders. Cerebrospinal fluid usually shows a mild to moderate mononuclear pleocytosis (usually < 500 cells) and moderately elevated protein and normal glucose concentrations. Plasma cells are often present and IgG may be increased, with oligoclonal bands of electrophoretic examination (16). The electroencephalogram (EEG) usually shows diffuse slowing or increased sharp wave activity. The head computed tomography (CT) scan is often normal but may show focal areas of increased attenuation with contrast enhancement (27, 28).

The most characteristic neurological abnormalities are *cranial and peripheral neuropathies.* Approximately 50% of patients with neurological involvement during secondary Lyme disease have cranial nerve palsies, and 39 to 50% have peripheral nerve palsies. Bell's palsy, often bilateral, is the most common cranial neuropathy, but any cranial nerve or combination of cranial nerves may be involved. The most characteristic peripheral manifestation is asymmetrical radicular pain accompanied by decreased sensation, weakness, and loss of reflexes (24, 28). Electrophysiological testing has shown evidence for both axonal injury and demyelination. Chapter 84, Peripheral Neuropathy, describes these patterns.

Tertiary Lyme Disease

The later stages of Lyme disease occur weeks to months or even years after the primary infection.

Rheumatological Manifestations. The most common late manifestation is arthritis, which may be monoarticular or oligoarticular, is asymmetrical and occurs in approximately 60% of patients who are not treated (37). Large joints, particularly the knees, are most frequently affected, but occasionally there is involvement in small joints as well. The arthritic attacks last weeks to months and may become recurrent over years. Joint destruction with erosion of cartilage or bone is infrequent and occurs in only a subset of patients with HLA DR2 or DR4 who appear to be predisposed to a more severe, possibly immunologically mediated, form of the disease.

Dermatological Manifestations. Tertiary Lyme disease also has a characteristic skin eruption, *acrodermatitis chronica atrophicans,* which is more commonly seen in Europe. This chronic skin disease begins insidiously on the distal portions of the extremities with redness and swelling followed by atrophy and ultimately by loss of fingers and toes. It is often accompanied by joint deformities (30%) or polyneuropathy (40%) (49).

Neurological Manifestations. Neurological involvement in tertiary Lyme disease is not well defined but may include a chronic progressive meningoencephalitis that may resemble multiple sclerosis (27) and a generalized polyneuropathy (13). These illnesses may begin many years after the primary infection and are difficult to diagnose conclusively.

Congenital Infection

During the blood-borne phase of infection the Lyme borrelia can be transmitted to the fetus at least during the first trimester (30). In one study 5 of 19 monitored pregnancies associated with Lyme disease had adverse outcomes though none could be definitely linked to the Lyme disease agent (23).

Diagnosis

The diagnosis of Lyme disease is currently based on clinical presentation and may or may not be aided by serology (34, 40). The history of tick exposure is often helpful, though, because of its small size, the tick may be overlooked by the patient. Therefore, history of living or vacationing in a known endemic area in a season when ticks are active is also important information. The ECM rash is characteristic and sufficient for the diagnosis of primary disease. Antibody to *B. burgdorferi* appears weeks or months after infection and is often not present early in the disease. The clinical features of the secondary stage, especially the combination of meningitis and cranial or peripheral neuropathy, should suggest Lyme disease as the leading diagnosis (24). In untreated patients with secondary or tertiary manifestations of the disease, antibody to the organism, as measured by enzyme-linked immunosorbent assay (ELISA) or solid phase fluorescence assay, is usually present. In neurological disease antibody is usually also present in CSF. The CDC, most state laboratories and many private and hospital laboratories, can test for antibody to the Lyme disease agent, but considerable variability from one laboratory to another has been documented (15). False-positive reactions may occur in individuals with other spirochetal infections (e.g., syphilis, leptospirosis, relapsing fever) and at lower titers in patients with rheumatoid factor or antinuclear antibody. Early treatment of the primary disease may reduce or abort the antibody response to the organism but not eliminate the late manifestations of infection (9). Immune response may be detectable by lymphotyte proliferation or Western blot assay, but these tests are not widely available. Therefore, serological diagnosis may be unreliable, leaving only the history and physical examination on which to base a diagnosis (2).

Treatment

Primary Lyme Disease

The generally accepted treatment for primary disease is orally administered tetracycline in adults and amoxicillin in children under 8 years of age. The organism is also sensitive to erythromycin, penicillin, imipenam, and ceftriaxone. Nonpregnant women, other adults, and children more than 8 years old should be treated with oral doxycycline (100 mg two times daily) for 10 to 21 days, depending on the rapidity of the clinical response, or amoxicillin, 250 mg three times daily or 20/mg/kg/day in 3 doses for 10 to 21 days. Amoxicillin is the preferred treatment for pregnant or lactating women and children under the age of 8 years. Erythromycin, 250 mg four times daily or 30 mg/kg/day can be used as alternative therapy in patients allergic to tetracycline or penicillin (47). A Jarisch-Herxheimer reaction (see above, page 334) has occurred in some patients (39). Early treatment both shortens the course of ECM and reduces the incidence of later arthritis, carditis, and neurological disease. Nearly 50% of treated patients will have minor late symptoms such as headache, musculoskeletal pain, facial palsy, or lethargy, and major late complications will occur in less than 10% (39). Because early treatment often blunts the immune response, reinfection can occur (50).

Secondary and Tertiary Lyme Disease

Patients with acrodermatitis, minor cardiac (e.g., first degree A-V block with P-R interval less than .30) or neurological (e.g., Bell's palsy alone) involvement without other significant symptoms should be treated with the regimens outlined above for early disease, but for patient's with Bell's palsy therapy should be continued for one month. Those with more severe cardiac conduction abnormalities or neurological disease (meningitis, other cranial and peripheral neuropathies) or with arthritis should be treated with intravenous penicillin (20 million units/day) or with intravenous ceftriaxone (2 g/day) for 14 days (8, 38, 43). A one-month course of oral doxycycline (100 mg two times daily) or amoxicillin (500 mg three times daily) may also be effective in patients with established arthritis (47). Responses of patients with tertiary neurological disease or arthritis is often slower, with approximately 50% showing improvement (8, 38).

Prevention

The best preventive measure is to avoid exposure to ticks by use of protective clothing and insect repellent. Daily inspection for ticks is also important since early removal can prevent transmission. Prophylactic antibiotic therapy for tick bites has been suggested but is not recommended since in at least one study the risk of acquiring Lyme disease was approximately equal to the risk of an adverse reaction to the drug (4). There is no available vaccine.

General References

Syphilis:
Clark EG, Danbolt N: The Oslo study of the natural course of untreated syphilis. Med Clin North Am 48:613, 1964.
    Long-term study of the natural history of syphilis in 1404 subjects.
Fiumara NJ, Shinberg JD, Byrne EM, Fountaine J: An outbreak of gonorrhea and early syphilis in Massachusetts. N Engl J Med 256:982, 1957.
    Detailed account of the spread of syphilis and of contact tracing in a local outbreak.
Holmes KK, Mardh PA, Sparling PF, Weisner P (eds): Sexually Transmitted Diseases. New York, McGraw-Hill, 1990 (in press).
    Detailed accounts of syphilis and other STDs by leading experts.
Jones JH: Bad Blood. New York, Free Press, 1981.
    A popular account of the Tuskegee study of untreated syphilis in black male subjects.
Rosebury T: Microbes and Morals. New York, Vebany Press, 1971.
    Fascinating account of the history of sexually transmitted disease.

Lyme Disease:
Benach J, Bosler EM (eds): Lyme Disease and Related Disorders. Vol. 539. Ann NY Academy Science, 1988.
    Multiauthored monograph with individual chapters on many aspects of Lyme disease.
Steere AC: Lyme disease. N Engl J Med 321:586, 1989.
    General review of all aspects of Lyme disease by the person who first described and has extensively studied the disease.

Specific References

1. Balkany TJ, Dans PE: Reversible sudden deafness in early acquired syphilis. Arch Otolaryngol 104:66, 1978.
2. Barbour AG: The diagnosis of Lyme disease: rewards and perils. Ann Intern Med 110:501, 1989.
3. Brown ST, Zaidi A, Larsen SA, Reynolds GH: Serological response to syphilis treatment. JAMA 253:1296, 1985.
4. Costello CM, Steere AC, Pinkerton RE, Feder, Jr. HM: A prospective study of tick bites in an endemic area for Lyme disease. J Infect Dis 159:136, 1989.
5. Dans PE, Cafferly I, Oller SE, Johnson RT: Inappropriate use of the cerebrospinal fluid venereal disease research laboratory (CSF-VDRL) test to exclude neurosyphilis. Correspondence, Ann Intern Med 104:86, 1986. 104:724, 1986.
6. Dans PE, Judson FN, Larsen SA, Lantz MA: The FTA-ABS test. A diagnostic help or hindrance? South Med J 70:312, 1977.
7. Darrow WW: Condom use and use-effectiveness in high-risk populations. Sex Transm Dis 16:43, 1989.
8. Dattwyler RJ, Halperin JJ, Volkman DJ, Luft BJ: Treatment of late Lyme borreliosis: randomised comparison of ceftriaxone and penicillin. Lancet 1:1191, 1988.
9. Dattwyler RJ, Volkman DJ, Luft BJ, et al: Seronegative Lyme disease: dissociation of specific T and B lymphocyte responses to Borrelia burgdorferi. N Engl J Med 319:1441, 1988.
10. Fiumara NJ: Serologic responses to treatment of 128 patients with late latent syphilis. J Am Vener Dis Assoc 6:243, 1979.
11. Greene BM, Miller NR, Bynum TE: Failure of penicillin G benzathine in the treatment of neurosyphilis. Arch Intern Med 140:1117, 1980.
12. Hahn RD, Cutler JC, Curtis AC, et al: Penicillin treatment of asymptomatic central nervous system syphilis. I. Probability of progression to symptomatic neurosyphilis. Arch Dermatol 74:355, 1956.
13. Halperin JJ, Little BW, Coyle PK, Dattwyler RJ: Lyme disease: course of a treatable peripheral neuropathy. Neurology 37:1700, 1987.
14. Hart G: Epidemiologic treatment for syphilis and gonorrhea. Sex Transm Dis 7:149, 1980.
15. Hedberg CW, Osterholm MT, MacDonald KL, White KE: An interlaboratory study of antibody to Borrelia burgdorferi. J Infect Dis 157:790, 1988.
16. Henriksson A, Link H, Cruz M, Stiernstedt G: Immunoglobulin abnormalities in cerebrospinal fluid and blood over the course of lymphocytic meningoradiculitis (Bannworth's syndrome). Ann Neurol 20:337, 1986.
17. Hook EW: Syphilis and HIV infection. J Infect Dis 160(3):530, 1989.
18. Hooshmand H, Escobar MR, Kopf SW: Neurosyphilis, a study of 241 patients. JAMA 219:726, 1972.
19. Idsoe O, Guthe T, Willcox RR: Penicillin in the treatment of syphilis. The experience of three decades. Bull WHO 474 ([Suppl]): 1972.

20. Jaffe HW, Kabins SA: Examination of cerebrospinal fluid in patients with syphilis. *Rev Infect Dis* 4 (Suppl): S842, 1982.

21. Larsen SA, Hunter EF, McGrew BE: Syphilis. In: Wentworth B, Judson FN (eds): *Laboratory Methods for the Diagnosis of Sexually Transmitted Diseases.* Washington, DC, American Public Health Association, 1984.

22. Lukehart SA, Hook EW, Baker-Zander SA, et al: Invasion of the central nervous system by *Treponema palidum:* implications for diagnosis and treatment. *Ann Intern Med* 110:855, 1988. Correspondence. 110:6, 7, 494, 574–575, 1989.

23. Markowitz LE, Steere AC, Benach JL, et al: Lyme disease during pregnancy. *JAMA* 255:3394, 1986.

24. Pachner AR, Steere AC: The triad of neurologic manifestations of Lyme disease: meningitis, cranial neuritis, and radioculoneuritis. *Neurology* 35:47, 1985.

25. Putkonen T, Salo OP, Mustakallio KK: Febrile Herxheimer reaction in different phases of primary and secondary syphilis. *Br J Vener Dis* 42:181, 1966.

26. Recommendations for diagnosing and treating syphilis in HIV-infected patients. *MMWR* 37:39, 1988.

27. Reik L, Smith L, Khan A, Nelson W: Demyelinating encephalopathy in Lyme disease. *Neurology* 32:1302, 1985.

28. Reik L, Steere AC, Bartenhagen NH, et al: Neurologic abnormalities of Lyme disease. *Medicine (Baltimore)* 58:281, 1979.

29. Relationship of syphilis to drug use and prostitution—Connecticut and Philadelphia, Pennsylvania. *MMWR* 37:755, 1988.

30. Schlesinger PA, Duray PH, Burke BA, et al: Maternal-fetal transmission of the Lyme disease spirochete, *Borrelia burgdorferi. Ann Intern Med* 103:67, 1985.

31. Schroeter AL, Lucas JB, Price EV, Falcone VH: Treatment for early syphilis and reactivity of serologic tests. *JAMA* 221:471, 1972.

32. Schroeter AL, Turner RH, Lucas JB, Brown WJ: Therapy for incubating syphilis. Effectiveness of gonorrhea treatment. *JAMA* 218:711, 1971.

33. Sexually Transmitted Diseases, Treatment Guidelines. *MMWR* 38: No. 5–8, 1989.

34. Shrestha M, Grodzicki RL, Steere AC: Diagnosing early Lyme disease. *Am J Med* 78:235, 1985.

35. Steere AC, Bartenhagen NH, Craft JE, et al: The early clinical manifestations of Lyme disease. *Ann Intern Med* 99:76, 1983.

36. Steere AC, Batsford WP, Weinberg M, et al: Lyme carditis: cardiac abnormalities of Lyme disease. *Ann Intern Med* 93:8, 1980.

37. Steere AC, Gibofsky A, Patarroyo ME, et al: Chronic Lyme disease: clinical and immunogenetic differentiation from rheumatoid arthritis. *Ann Intern Med* 90:896, 1979.

38. Steere AC, Green J, Schoen RT, et al: Successful parenteral penicillin therapy of established Lyme arthritis. *N Engl J Med* 312:869, 1985.

39. Steere AC, Hutchinson GJ, Rahn DW, et al: Treatment of the early manifestations of Lyme disease. *Ann Intern Med* 99:22, 1983.

40. Steere AC, Malawista SE, Bartenhagen NH, et al: The clinical spectrum and treatment of Lyme disease. *Yale J Biol Med* 57:453, 1984.

41. Steere AC, Malawista SE, Hardin JA, et al: Erythema chronicum migrans and Lyme arthritis: the enlarging clinical spectrum. *Ann Intern Med* 86:685, 1977.

42. Steere AC, Malawista SE, Syndman DR, et al: An epidemic of oligoarticular arthritis in children and adults in three Connecticut communities. *Arthritis Rheum* 20:7, 1977.

43. Steere AC, Pachner AR, Malawista SE: Neurologic abnormalities of Lyme disease: successful treatment with high dose intravenous penicillin. *Ann Intern Med* 99:767, 1983.

44. Syphilis and congenital syphilis—United States, 1985–1988. *MMWR* 37:32, 1987.

45. Tertiary syphilis deaths—South Florida. *MMWR* 36:29, 1987.

46. The Jarisch-Herxheimer reaction. *Lancet* 1:340, 1977.

47. Treatment of Lyme disease. *Med Lett* 31:57, 1989.

48. Vlay SC: Complete heart block due to Lyme disease. *N Engl J Med* 315:1418, 1986.

49. Weber K, Schierz G, Wilske B, Preac-Mursic V: European erythema migrans disease and related disorders. *Yale J Biol Med* 57:463, 1984.

50. Weber K, Schierz G, Wilske B, et al: Reinfection with erythema migrans disease. *Infection* 14:32, 1986.

51. Wiesel J, Rose DN, Silver AL, et al: Lumbar puncture in asymptomatic late syphilis. An analysis of the benefits and risks. *Arch Intern Med* 145:465, 1985.

52. Wilner G, Brody JA: Prognosis of general paresis after treatment. *Lancet* 2:1370, 1968.

53. Zenker P: Background paper for syphilis treatment guidelines. *Reviews of Infectious Diseases* 1989 (in press).

C H A P T E R 31

Ambulatory Care for Selected Subacute Infections: Osteomyelitis, Lung Abscess, and Endocarditis

JOHN G. BARTLETT, M.D.

The three types of infections reviewed in this chapter are initially managed with intravenous antibiotics administered in the hospital. Patients with these infections are often seen first in an office setting and the relatively long courses of antibiotics used to treat them are usually completed after discharge from hospital. These infections involve diverse bacteria and different anatomical sites but share the propensity for relapse due to persistent bacteria at the infected site. This explains the requirement for prolonged courses of antimicrobial treatment. Antibiotics may be administered by two different routes out of hospital: the oral route, to complete a course initiated parenterally during hospitalization, and the intravenous route, utilizing the same regimen provided for inpatients. This latter form of treatment is gaining popularity due to concerns regarding hospital costs, and it is also attractive to patients who would prefer to receive their antibiotics at home, particularly when other hospital resources are not required. Details about the use of home health services are found in Chapter 9.

OSTEOMYELITIS

Definition

Osteomyelitis is an infection of bone. There are three major categories: osteomyelitis following hematogenous spread of infection, osteomyelitis secondary to a contiguous focus of infection, and osteomyelitis associated with vascular insufficiency. There are major differences between these three categories according to age of occurrence, bones involved, predisposing conditions, usual bacterial pathogens, and presentation (Table 31.1).

Clinical Presentation and Bacteriology

Hematogenous

Hematogenous osteomyelitis is classically described as a disease of children, usually under 16 years of age and usually due to *Staphylococcus aureus*. The tendency for this infection to occur during active growth reflects the enhanced susceptibility of the vascular network of the metaphysis, especially of the femur or tibia. About one-third of patients have a history of preceding nonpenetrating trauma in the area that is subsequently involved. The infection begins in the metaphyseal sinusoidal veins; it is contained by the epiphyseal growth plate and tends to spread laterally with perforation of the cortex and lifting of the loose periosteum. Hematogenous osteomyelitis of the long bones in adults is rare, different in presentation and bacteriologically distinct. In these individuals, the growth cartilage has been resorbed so the subarticular space is more vulnerable; and the periosteum is firmly attached so that subperiosteal abscess formation is uncommon. The most frequent form of hematogenous osteomyelitis in adults involves the vertebrae (see Fig. 31.1) and the most common pathogens are Gram-negative bacilli as well as *S. aureus*. The initial site of infection is the richly vascularized bone adjacent to cartilage;

there is subsequent involvement of adjacent bone plates and of the intervertebral disc. The infection may extend longitudinally to involve adjacent vertebrae, anteriorly to produce a paraspinal abscess, or posteriorly to form an epidural abscess.

Acute hematogenous osteomyelitis usually presents with precipitous onset of pain, swelling, chills, and fever. With vertebral osteomyelitis there is fever with back pain, stiffness, and often point tenderness over the infected vertebra. Many patients have a more subacute presentation, with vague symptoms of 1 to 2 months' duration prior to presentation with few constitutional complaints. One well-described variant is "Brodie's abscess" (also referred to as a "cold abscess")—subacute staphylococcal osteomyelitis located in the metaphysis of a long bone, which presents with local pain and fever. Patients with recurrent or chronic osteomyelitis often simply note increased or persistent drainage and pain after a prior episode involving the same anatomical location.

Contiguous Infection

Osteomyelitis secondary to contiguous foci of infection accounts for at least half of all cases. The most frequent precipitating factor is previous surgery, usually involving the lower extremities, such as open reduction of fractures of the femur or tibia. Next in frequency is a soft tissue infection involving the digits of the hand or feet. These infections usually become apparent within 1 month of a precipitating event, although many patients have chronic or recurrent infections that occur intermittently for years or decades. A variant in this category that is being seen with increasing frequency is infection associated with prosthetic devices. This complication is noted in 0.5 to 2% of patients with total hip replacement. Infections in the early postoperative period usually result from contamination at the time of surgery. Late infections presumably reflect either persistent perioperative sepsis, hematogenous spread

Table 31.1.
Types of Osteomyelitis

	Hematogenous	Secondary to Contiguous infection	Complication of Vascular Insufficiency
Approximate proportion of all cases	20%	50%	30%
Commonest age group(s)	1–16 years >50 years	Any age	>50 years
Bones involved	Long bones (children) Vertebrae (adults)	Hip, femur, tibia, digits	Feet
Predisposing causes	Trauma Bacteremia	Surgery Soft tissue infection	Diabetes mellitus Vascular insufficiency
Usual bacteria	*S. aureus* Gram-negative bacilli	Often polymicrobial: Gram-negative bacilli, *S. aureus*	Usually polymicrobial: Gram-negative bacilli, anaerobes, streptococci, *S. aureus*
Presentation: Initial episode	Fever, local pain swelling, tenderness, limited movement	Fever, local pain swelling, tenderness, limited movement	Ulceration drainage ± pain
Recurrent eposode	Sinus drainage ± pain	Sinus drainage ± pain	Drainage ± pain

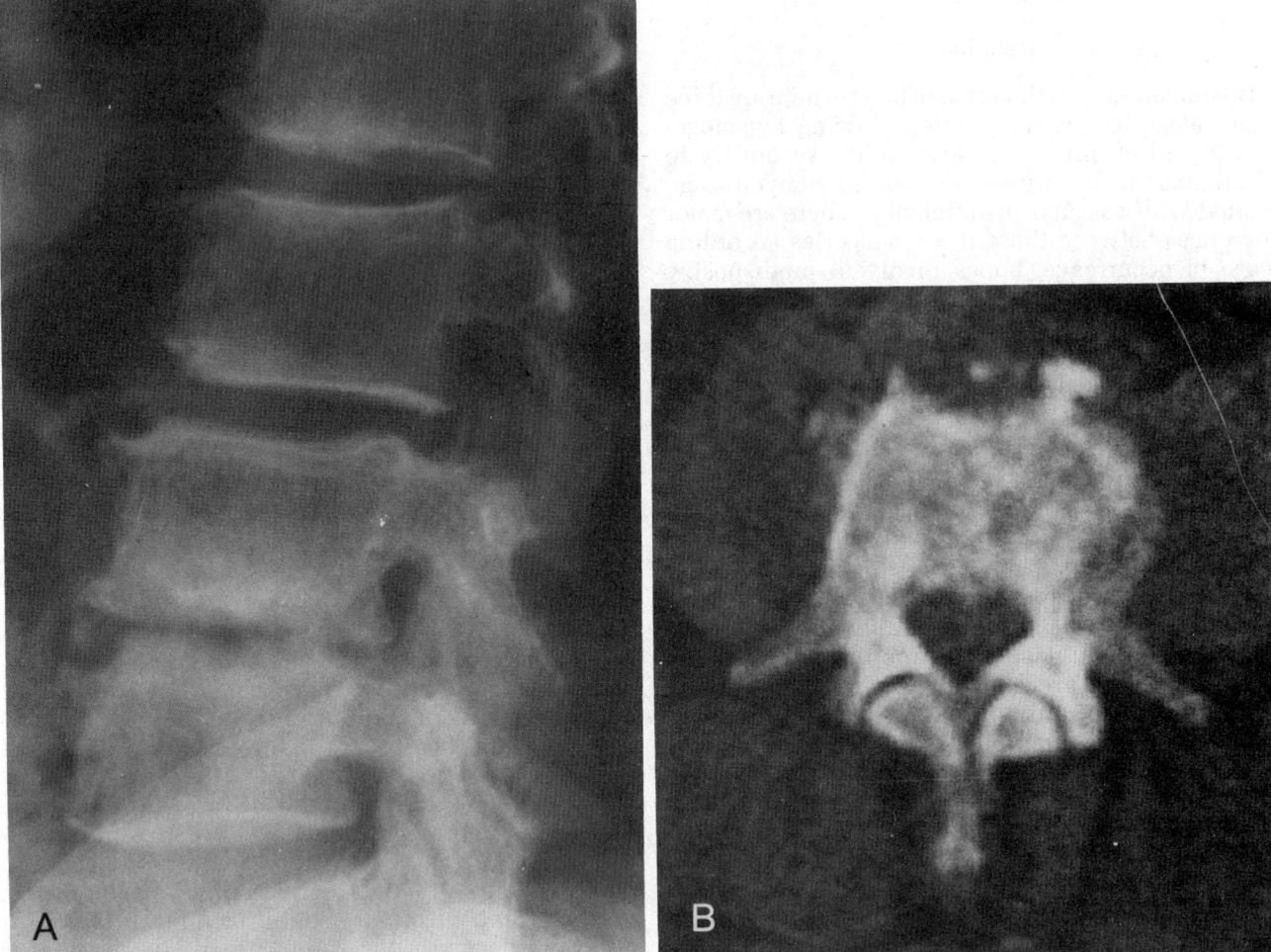

Figure 31.1. *A.* L3-4 staphylococcal osteomyelitis of 3 months' duration with disc narrowing and sclerosis seen on plain film. *B.* Computed tomographic scan in same patient showing small soft tissue abscess and minimal bone destruction. Hazy bone outline. (From Post MJD (ed): *Computed Tomography of the Spine*. Baltimore, Williams & Wilkins, 1984, p 740.)

from another infection, or seeding from transient bacteremia in a fashion analogous to the situation in endocarditis. The major pathogens are S. *aureus* and *Staphylococcus epidermidis*, although multiple different bacteria, including many relatively non-pathogenic organisms, may be involved.

Vascular Insufficiency

Osteomyelitis associated with vascular insufficiency is most frequent in patients with diabetes mellitus and/or severe atherosclerosis. The most common sites of infection are the toes or small bones of the feet, usually with overlying soft tissue infections (see Fig. 31.2). These infections are often detected with the routine X-rays performed to evaluate chronic draining sinuses or skin ulcers that are so common in the patients at risk. Both the adjacent soft tissue infection and the osteomyelitis usually involve a polymicrobial flora that may include anaerobic bacteria, coliforms, pseudomonads, streptococci, and S. *aureus*.

Laboratory Evaluation

Diagnostic studies include X-rays or radionucleotide studies to demonstrate typical bone changes and cultures to identify the etiological organism.

The earliest changes on plain X-rays are lytic lesions; other findings may include soft tissue swelling, periosteal reaction, cortical irregularity, demineralization, and sequestrum formation. However, typical changes are not visible on plain films until 30 to 50% of the bone has been resorbed, and this usually requires 10 to 14 days. Therefore, in a patient with a normal plain film but suspected osteomyelitis, a bone scan should be obtained. The bone scan is a radionuclide examination that employs Tc99 as a marker bound to diphosphonate that concentrates in bone due to incorporation at sites of osteoblastic activity. This scan is positive in nearly all patients with osteomyelitis within 1 to 3 days after the onset of symptoms. Problems with this test are (a) that a "positive" scan may reflect increased blood flow associated with soft tissue infections or with osteoblastic activity due to

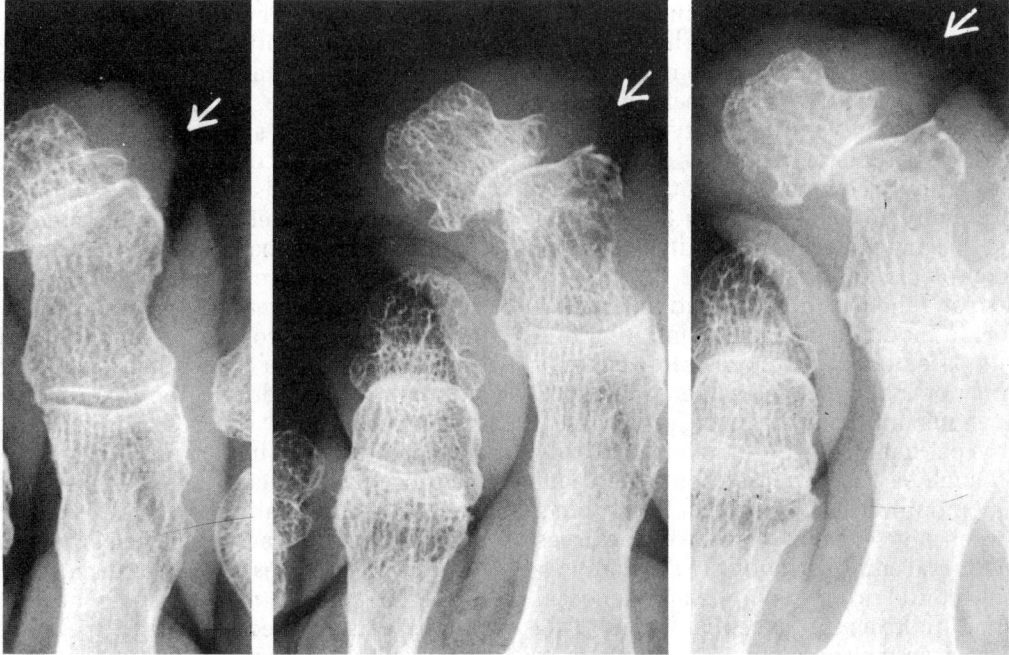

Figure 31.2.   Infected soft corn, sinus tract, and osteomyelitis distal interphalangeal joint. As destruction increases, the joint becomes dislocated (From Gamble, FO, Yale I: *Clinical Foot Roentgenology*. Baltimore, Williams & Wilkins, 1966.)

other processes, such as degenerative joint disease; and (b) that it may show increased uptake for extended periods after eradication of infection due to continuing osteoblastic activity. Thus, the bone scan is sensitive but is nonspecific in detecting osteomyelitis and is not particularly useful for following the course of infection. These problems may be partially overcome with three-phase imaging that increases specificity (12). Gallium uptake is not as dependent on bone blood flow and more accurately reflects inflammation than it does osteoblastic activity. Thus, a Ga-67 citrate scan may complement a positive bone scan and is more useful in following the course of an infection.

Because antimicrobial treatment, often prolonged, is the mainstay of management, accurate bacteriological data are imperative for making the diagnosis and for planning treatment. The list of possible organisms is legion, and sensitivity patterns for these organisms show considerable variation, making empirical selection of antimicrobials hazardous. These considerations justify an aggressive attempt to identify the responsible organism. Conclusive bacteriological studies require isolation of the pathogen from either the bone or blood cultures.

When osteomyelitis is suspected, an orthopaedist should perform a needle aspiration over the involved bone, either in an ambulatory setting (when the presentation is not acute) or in the hospital. If subperiosteal pus is obtained, surgical drainage is mandatory. If no pus is obtained, the needle is inserted into bone to obtain a specimen. The diagnostic yield with a needle aspirate of bone is approximately 60%, and for a surgical biopsy it is about 90% (5). Cultures from draining sinus tracts tend to show a poor correlation

with cultures obtained directly from bone (11); this experience supports the need for bone biopsy or possibly deep aspiration in patients with chronic osteomyelitis. Care must be exercised in the interpretation of culture results, even of bone aspirates since these are often contaminated, especially if the specimen is obtained by traversing soft tissue infections (15). Organisms recovered in relatively small concentrations, especially those growing only in the broth culture, must be viewed with skepticism. Common skin contaminants include *S. epidermidis*, diphtheroids, and proprionibacteria. These organisms tend to cause osteomyelitis only in the presence of prosthetic devices. Gram stain of exudate or tissue aspirate should verify the culture results and represents an important correlate in deciding upon the etiological organism.

Treatment

General Principles

Immobilization was commonly advocated in the treatment of osteomyelitis in the preantibiotic era. However, this appears to be less important at the present time, and most authorities conclude that strict immobilization is not necessary.

Antimicrobial Treatment: Acute Osteomyelitis

For newly diagnosed or acute osteomyelitis, optimal management is a 3- to 6-week course of parenteral antibiotics. This recommendation is based on several studies, but particularly the work of Dich and colleagues, who noted that 19% of patients developed recurrent or chronic disease when treatment was less than 21 days compared with only 2% in those who received more prolonged courses (5). The preferred regimen for acute staphylococcal osteomyelitis is a pencillinase-resistant penicillin such as nafcillin given intravenously in a dose of 1.5 to 2 g every 6 hours for adults. Alternative parenteral regimens are cephalothin (2 g every 6 hours), vancomycin (500 mg every 6 hours), or clindamycin (600 mg every 8 hours). In stable patients, these regimens can be initiated in the hospital and completed at home.

To decrease cost, length of hospitalization, and patient discomfort, a modified regimen, consisting of a short course of parenteral antibiotics followed by a prolonged course of oral agents, has been developed (7). The intravenous antibiotic is given for at least 3 days, or until the patient is afebrile, or for an arbitrarily defined period such as 1 to 2 weeks. The same agent is then taken by mouth, usually at home, to complete a total 3- to 6-week course, usually 4 weeks. The drugs recommended for oral administration are clindamycin (300 mg every 6 hours) or an oral antistaphylococcal penicillin such as dicloxacillin or cephalexin (500 mg every 6 hours). It should be noted that this therapeutic approach has been tested successfully in children but that comparable studies have not been done to establish efficacy in adults.

Antimicrobial choice for osteomyelitis involving *Enterobacteriaceae* or *Pseudomonas aeruginosa* should be based on in vitro sensitivity tests. The importance of bactericidal activity and the relative merits of drugs for bone penetration as factors in drug selection are debated issues that remain unresolved.

Antimicrobial Treatment: Chronic Osteomyelitis

Therapeutic guidelines are less precise for chronic osteomyelitis. Because necrotic bone may serve as a nidus for sequestered bacteria, surgical excision of dead tissue and adequate debridement are often essential components of treatment. Antibiotic selection should be based on bacteriological diagnosis using deep aspirates or, preferably, cultures obtained from bone. The route of administration and duration of treatment are arbitrary, but most authorities recommend prolonged courses. The initial treatment may be parenteral antibiotics for 1 to 3 months in the hospital or in the home, followed by oral agents for several months (17). An alternative approach is the use of oral agents exclusively for extended periods, such as 6 months or longer (2). In view of the difficulty of obtaining adequate antibiotic levels in avascular bone, there has been an attempt to deliver higher concentrations locally using regional perfusion of the wound after surgery with antibacterial solutions (8). There are no controlled trials to document superiority of this approach, and there is a potential problem of selection for antimicrobial-resistant bacteria.

Late Complications

The major complication of osteomyelitis is recurrence that may occur months, years, or decades after the initial event. The patient should be warned of this potential complication. The clinical features of recurrences are fever, draining sinuses, local pain, elevated sedimentation rate, and the typical changes noted on X-rays or scans as summarized above. Chronic osteomyelitis may be complicated by secondary amyloidosis, although this has become extremely rare since the advent of antibiotics. Another complication is epidermoid carcinoma arising in a draining sinus of osteomyelitis that occurs in 0.2 to 1.5% of cases, with a mean delay of 34 years (18). Patients with orthopaedic devices such as prosthetic joints are at risk for infection after transient bacteremia. However, unlike the situation with endocarditis, there are no guidelines from authoritative sources to direct treatment. It is reasonable to administer prophylactic antibiotics for the procedures that are considered a risk by the American Heart Association for patients susceptible to endocarditis. However, the major pathogens for infected orthopaedic devices are *S. aureus*, *S. epidermidis*, and to a lesser extent *Streptococcus*, whereas endocarditis prophylaxis is directed primarily against *Streptococcus*. For this reason a regimen that employs vancomycin is preferable in this situation (see endocarditis section below).

LUNG ABSCESS

Definition

Lung abscess refers to pulmonary suppuration with parenchymal necrosis caused by bacterial infection. The lesions are traditionally classified on the basis of clinical and bacteriological observations. Lung abscesses are considered acute or chronic depending on the duration of symptoms at the time of initial presentation, with the usual dividing line being 4 to 6 weeks. Clinically, lung abscesses are often grouped as (a) "putrid lung abscess," in reference to the foul odor of sputum that is regarded as diagnostic of anaerobic infection; or (b) "nonspecific lung abscess," indicating that aerobic sputum cultures have not grown out a pathogen. Anaerobic bacteria are the presumed pathogens in these cases also. Lung abscesses may also be classified clinically as "primary" or "secondary" depending on predisposing conditions. Primary lung abscesses are those that occur in patients who are prone to aspiration or in previously healthy individuals. Secondary abscesses represent complications of a local lesion such as a pulmonary malignancy or of a systemic disease that compromises immunological defenses. Approximately 80% of lung abscesses are primary; 60% are putrid, and 40% are nonspecific (probably mostly anaerobic). Patients with lung abscess frequently present in the ambulatory care setting due to the chronicity of these infections. Most patients are hospitalized for diagnostic studies and initial treatment with intravenous antibiotics. The hospital course is usually followed by prolonged courses of antibiotics and follow-up chest X-rays.

Clinical Presentation and Bacteriology

Many bacteria are potential pulmonary pathogens, but the number of organisms likely to cause parenchymal necrosis is relatively modest. The most common pathogens are anaerobic bacteria that comprise the normal flora of the gingival crevice and are aspirated during periods of altered consciousness. The usual pathogens in such cases are *Bacteroides melaninogenicus*, anaerobic streptococci, and *Fusobacterium nucleatum* (1). The most frequent aerobic bacteria that cause suppurative pulmonary infections are S. aureus and *Klebsiella pneumoniae*; less frequent causal pathogens are *Streptococcus pyogenes, Streptococcus pneumoniae, Haemophilus influenzae, P. aeruginosa, Legionella, Nocardia,* and enteric Gram-negative bacilli other than *K. pneumoniae.*

Patients with *anaerobic lung abscesses* usually present with indolent complaints that date for weeks or even months. Common symptoms include fever, malaise, cough, and sputum production. Pleuritic pain and hemoptysis are relatively common and may be the factors that persuade a chronically ill patient to seek medical attention. Chills are occasionally noted, but true rigors are rare. The frequent observation of anemia and weight loss reflects the chronicity of many of these infections. The sputum is usually purulent, and putrid odor is noted in about 60% of bacteriologically confirmed anaerobic lung abscesses. The usual sites of involvement are the anatomical segments of the lung where passive aspiration is most likely to occur in the recumbent position. These are the superior segments of the lower lobes and the posterior segments of the upper lobes. Less frequent abscess sites are the basilar segments of the lower lobes, which are dependent in the upright or semiupright position.

Lung *abscesses due to aerobic bacteria* are usually found in specific clinical settings. Staphylococcal pulmonary infections with abscess formation are particularly common in young children and in adults with influenza or with hospital-acquired pneumonia. *Klebsiella* is often suspected as a cause of lung abscess in alcoholic patients, but even in these patients anaerobic organisms are the commonest pathogens. The immunologically compromised patient may have pulmonary suppuration due to a variety of both bacterial and nonbacterial organisms, but anaerobes appear to be distinctly unusual in this population.

Laboratory Examination

The initial evaluations in patients with the symptoms of lung abscess are those recommended for patients with suspected pulmonary infections in general. These include a chest X-ray, a complete blood count, blood cultures, and an examination of expectorated sputum. The lung abscess is generally readily apparent with the chest X-ray (see Fig. 31.3), although other causes of a pulmonary cavity must be considered in the differential diagnosis. Alternative considerations include a cavitating neoplasm, cavitating pulmonary

infarction, tuberculosis, fungal infection, an infected pulmonary cyst or bulla, a loculated empyema (i.e., pleural space infection) with an air-fluid level due to a bronchopleural fistula, gas-producing organisms, or Wegener's granulomatosis.

When a cavitary lesion appears to be due to bacterial infection, there is controversy about the approach to identifying the likely pathogen. Sputum should be examined using Gram stain and Ziehl-Neelson stain in order to determine from the outset whether an anaerobic pathogen or *Mycobacterium tuberculosis* is the likely cause of the abscess.

Expectorated sputum is easily obtained from most patients, and standard cultures will usually show a predominance of an aerobic organism when it is the etiological pathogen. The problem with these specimens is that they are not appropriate for anaerobic culture, and the results with aerobic cultures are frequently misleading due to contamination by bacteria that reside in the upper airway. To confirm by sputum culture the presence of anaerobic bacteria, the ideal specimen for patients without an empyema is a *transtracheal aspirate*. However, this procedure is not necessary in most patients who have a typical presentation. This particularly applies to patients with an associated condition that predisposes to aspiration, to infection involving a typical pulmonary segment, and to patients with putrid sputum. Such individuals may be treated with antibiotics selected empirically.

Bronchoscopy is generally not useful for microbiological studies except for mycobacterial and nonbacterial pathogens; a possible exception is when specimens are obtained with a specialized double catheter and are cultured quantitatively (19).

Antimicrobial Treatment (Table 31.2)

Antimicrobials are the mainstay of treatment for lung abscess. The best studied regimens are those for anaerobic lung abscesses since these account for the majority of cases. Nevertheless, there is considerable controversy regarding the selection of agents and the duration of treatment.

Anaerobic Infections

With regard to drug selection, the initial antimicrobial recommended by some authorities for anaerobic lung abscess is penicillin G, 5 to 10 million units daily, given intravenously until fever resolves and there is definite clinical improvement. Successful treatment has been reported, however, using oral penicillin G from the start, in relatively high doses (750 mg four times daily) (16). The argument favoring high dose parenteral penicillin initially is that this provides a definitive conclusion regarding response to penicillin, thus obviating subsequent changes to a higher dose of penicillin if the patient fails to respond.

The major alternative drug for anaerobic lung abscesses is clindamycin, which is active against most anaerobic bacteria. In approximately 25% of patients anaerobic organisms resistant to penicillin are present,

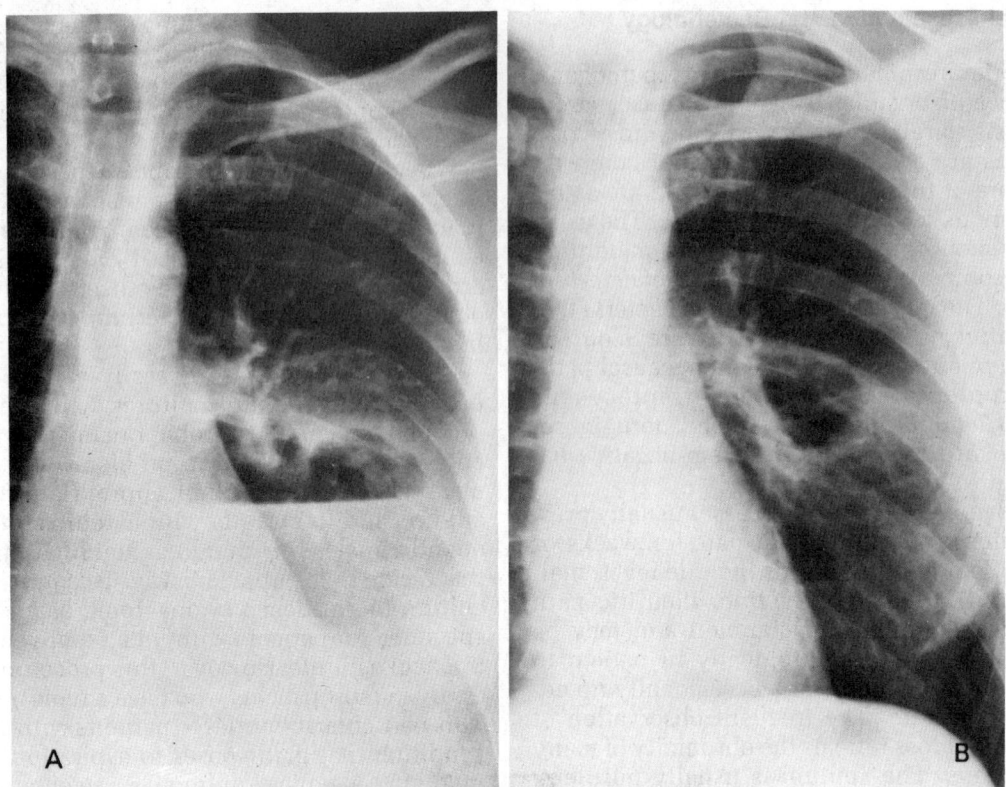

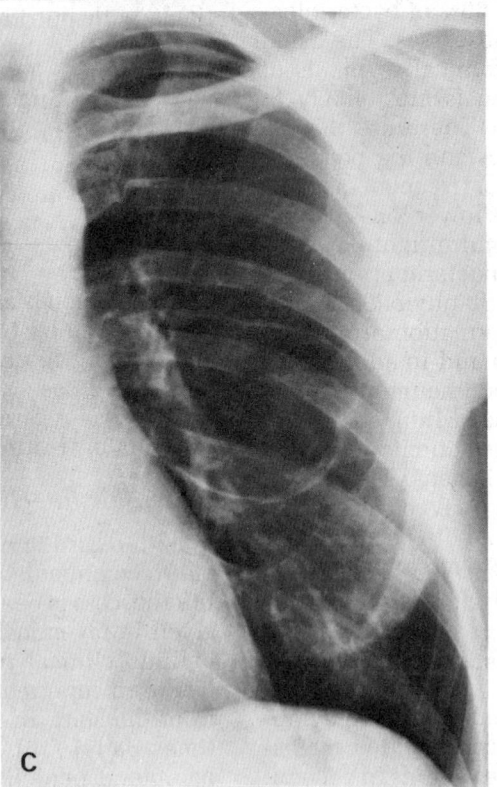

Figure 31.3.   Putrid lung abscess. *A*. July 6, 1976. The patient developed fever and coughed up foul sputum after an epileptic attack. The huge cavity with an air-fluid level in the left lower lobe suggests a pyopneumothorax. However, the irregularity of the cavity wall indicates that it lies within the lung rather than in the pleura. *B*. August 3, 1976. On antibiotic therapy, the cavity has become much smaller and there is no longer an air-fluid level. *C*. September 20, 1976. Although the patient was clinically well, the cavity has increased in size. Its wall is thin and smooth and there are no infiltrations in the lung around the cavity. The ballooning of the cavity was noted after an attack of asthma. The increase in size was due entirely to air trapping because of the bronchospasm and does not indicate reactivation of the infection. (From Rabin CB, Baron MG: *Radiology of the Chest*, ed 2. Baltimore, Williams & Wilkins, 1980, p 340.)

Table 31.2.
Antimicrobial Regimens for Primary Lung Abscess

Intravenous[a]	Oral[a]	Comments
Aqueous penicillin G 5–10 million units/day	Penicillin G or V 500–750 mg four times a day *or* Amoxicillin 500 mg four times a day	Regarded as standard *Advantages*: inexpensive and well tolerated *Disadvantage*: About 20% fail to respond and additional patients have delayed response
Clindamycin 600 mg every 6–8 hours	Clindamycin 300 mg four times a day	*Advantages*: Optimal response rates *Disadvantages*: Expensive; side effects include 10–20% with diarrhea and occasional patients with pseudomembranous colitis

[a] Intravenous treatment until patient is afebrile and clinically improved; oral treatment is given either to complete an arbitrary total course of 3 to 6 weeks of treatment or until chest X-rays show clearance or a small stable residual lesion.

and nearly all of these organisms are highly sensitive to clindamycin. Not surprisingly, a comparative trial showed that clindamycin was superior to penicillin in terms of the primary response rates and the duration of fever after the institution of treatment (10), two factors that may allow earlier hospital discharge. The advantage of penicillin for initial treatment is that this makes one more confident in prescribing oral penicillin for posthospital treatment. This is desirable because the high cost of clindamycin may lead some patients to discontinue treatment or "spread out" their supply of medicine after discharge.

With either penicillin or clindamycin, initial treatment is usually given parenterally until the patient is afebrile and there is subjective improvement. This generally requires 3 to 7 days but may be considerably longer in patients with very large lung abscesses, patients with prolonged symptoms prior to treatment, and patients with pleural complications (primary empyema).

Aerobic Infections

Guidelines for antimicrobial selection are less precise for lung abscesses involving other organisms. In these cases, the antibiotic is selected on the basis of in vitro sensitivity tests. Abscesses involving *S. aureus* or Gram-negative bacilli are regarded as more serious infections, and intravenous antibiotics should be given for a more prolonged period; in selected stable patients, the intravenous regimen can be completed at home.

Duration of Treatment

Rigorous studies to determine the optimal duration of antimicrobial treatment for lung abscesses have not been done. Most authorities recommend at least 3 to 6 weeks. It is reasonable to base the duration of treatment also upon observations on serial chest X-rays (weekly or less frequently). Antibiotics are given until

the chest X-ray either is clear or shows only a small stable residual lesion (see Fig. 31.3). These recommendations are based on experiences in which patients have had relapses despite treatment for at least 1 month; in these patients the infiltrate was still resolving when drugs were discontinued, and the patients were subsequently readmitted for recurrent abscesses in the same pulmonary segment.

For abscesses due to anaerobes, one of the following oral regimens should be used: penicillin G or penicillin V (500 to 750 mg four times daily), amoxicillin (500 mg three times daily), or clindamycin (300 mg four times daily).

Regardless of the total duration of treatment, adequate follow-up is necessary to assure resolution with serial X-rays. These should be obtained at 2- to 3-week intervals, or earlier if there is clinical deterioration. Most patients with lung abscess treated with antibiotics improve clinically before there is demonstrable improvement in the chest X-ray; cavities gradually close, but 20 to 30% persist beyond 6 weeks, and the roentgenographic criteria for cure as defined above may require several months (9).

Inadequate Response to Treatment

If the patient is taking oral penicillin at home and does not show continued improvement, a change to clindamycin is appropriate. An alternative regimen, which has been used in Europe with considerable success, is the combination of oral metronidazole (Flagyl), 500 mg four times daily, combined with a penicillin in the doses noted above. It is necessary to use penicillin with metronidazole due to the frequent presence of microaerophilic and aerobic streptococci that are resistant to metronidazole. The anticipated outcome is either a clear X-ray, a small stable residual scar, or a thin-walled cyst. Failure to show progressive improvement, especially if accompanied by clinical symptoms, necessitates a change in medical therapy, bronchoscopy (to rule out obstruction), or, on rare occasions, surgery. The major indications for surgery are an abscess that is totally refractory to antibiotic treatment, life-threatening or persistent hemorrhage, and abscesses occurring in association with an obstructed bronchus (6).

ENDOCARDITIS

Definition

Endocarditis refers to infections involving heart valves, usually due to bacteria, but occasionally due to other microbes such as *Rickettsia* or fungi. There is a spectrum of clinical findings, but patients with the subacute form of the disease may present with symptoms that are notably vague and nonspecific. The principal criteria for making the diagnosis are documented fever, heart murmur, and positive blood cultures. A unique feature of the disease is that most patients have continuous bacteremia so that blood cultures are positive in 90% of patients, regardless of the temporal relationship between blood samplings and temperature profile. All patients with endocarditis should be hospitalized for complete diagnostic evaluation, supportive care, and initiation of treatment with antibiotics given intravenously. This discussion addresses the management of these patients in the ambulatory care setting following hospitalization.

Treatment

Antimicrobial Treatment Out of Hospital

Antibiotics are selected for patients with endocarditis according to in vitro sensitivity tests, with emphasis on bactericidal activity. Most patients are treated with specific regimens according to guidelines from authoritative sources. The duration of treatment is usually 4 to 6 weeks of intravenous antibiotics. Some authorities now endorse a 2-week regimen of penicillin and streptomycin for infections due to penicillin-sensitive strains of viridans streptococci and *Streptococcus bovis* (3); and most recommend prolonged courses for patients with prosthetic valve endocarditis (14). When intravenous antibiotics are planned for several weeks, part of the parenteral course can be administered at home, to expedite hospital discharge.

Abbreviated courses of intravenous antibiotics have been suggested also for *staphylococcal endocarditis as a complication of intravenous drug abuse* (13). The advantage of this plan is that it limits the period when an intravenous access is available for the patient to use, surreptitiously, to continue his habit. This occurs frequently and adds the risk of superinfection involving antibiotic-resistant organisms, such as Gram-negative bacilli and *Candida* species. Furthermore, these patients often leave the hospital against medical advice, before a long course of intravenous treatment has been completed. One plan is to restrict the intravenous route to 2 weeks or less and then continue oral treatment on an outpatient basis using cephalexin or dicloxicillin (2 to 8 g/day, usually 1 g every 6 hours) to complete a 6-week course of treatment. Another option is to simply discontinue treatment after two weeks (4). Either of these approaches can be endorsed only in patients who are clinically stable at the time intravenous therapy is discontinued, and when the blood culture isolate is highly sensitive to the drug used orally.

Patients with *prosthetic valve endocarditis* have infections that have proven particularly difficult to cure without intervening surgery. Nevertheless, intravenous antibiotics are given in the hopes of avoiding reoperation; this is a realistic goal with antibiotic-sensitive organisms. The most common pathogen in these cases is *S. epidermidis*, which is treated for at least 6 weeks with intravenous drugs selected on the basis of in vitro sensitivity tests. The usual regimen is a penicillinase-resistant penicillin (nafcillin or oxacillin, 2 g every 4 hours) or vancomycin (30 mg/kg/day) for at least six weeks combined with gentamicin (1 mg/kg every 8 hours) for the first two weeks (3). For methicillin-resistant strains the regimen is vancomycin and rifampin (300 mg orally every 8 hours) for at least six weeks and gentamicin for two weeks. Many authorities recommend prolonged courses of oral antibiotics, after the initial intravenous regimen, such as dicloxicillin or cephalexin in a divided dose of 2 g per day. Because these patients are often stable, it is reasonable to complete a course of dicloxacillin or cephalexin combined with rifampin, 600 to 900 mg per day, out of hospital. This oral regimen is continued for arbitrarily defined periods that range from several weeks to 6 months or longer (14).

Long-Term Follow-up and Prognosis

Patients with endocarditis treated medically or surgically should be followed carefully after discontinuation of antibiotics. Major complications during this recovery phase include congestive heart failure, relapse, mycotic aneurysms, and recurrences involving new organisms.

Blood cultures are commonly recommended after discontinuation of antibiotic treatment, usually 2 to 3 days later. Patients who have had an inadequate course of therapy will usually relapse within this time frame. Patients most likely to relapse are those with prosthetic valve endocarditis and endocarditis involving organisms resistant to antibiotics. The presence of positive blood cultures without a clearly identifiable portal of entry in the recovery phase is presumptive evidence of relapse. The usual recommendation is another course of antibiotics or surgery for a refractory infection. The choice between these two approaches is made on the basis of the extent of the initial treatment course, underlying valve disease, and the in vitro sensitivity of the organism, with particular attention to bactericidal activity. The patient should also be forewarned of the possibility of relapse and should be instructed to monitor temperature with attention to measurements in the evening when elevations are most likely to be noted.

The status of cardiac function should be followed carefully. Valve replacement is a rather common practice during active infection, especially in the 6 to 20% of patients who satisfy certain, often somewhat arbitrary, criteria. It should be noted, however, that the mortality rate of surgery performed during active infection is substantially higher than surgery performed on an elective basis. When possible, it is preferred that valve replacement be conducted 6 weeks or longer after antibiotics have been discontinued. The major indication is congestive heart failure that proves difficult to control with medical management.

Mycotic aneurysms may become apparent at any time during the course of endocarditis, but most become clinically apparent several months or even years after treatment. These lesions usually occur at arterial bifurcations and have been reported in up to 15% of cases. The most frequent vessels involved are intracranial; next in frequency are chest and abdominal arteries. The diagnostic evaluation usually consists of computed tomography, when the central nervous system is involved, and arteriography for lesions suspected there or in other locations. Surgical correction is almost always indicated.

Anticoagulation is usually avoided during active endocarditis due to the danger of bleeding from unrecognized aneurysms or emboli. However, patients who are receiving anticoagulants for prosthetic valves should have anticoagulation continued in the absence of a bleeding complication.

Antibiotic Prophylaxis.   It must be remembered that any patient with endocarditis is at risk for another infection. These patients should be warned about this potential complication with endoscopy, surgery, and dental procedures. It is good practice to supply all patients who are at risk for endocarditis with a wallet-sized card that contains the current antibiotic recommendations for prophylaxis with various procedures (see Table 86.12). This serves the dual role of emphasizing the importance of prophylaxis to the patient and assuring that specific guidelines will be available to those health professionals who may be performing procedures on the patient that can cause bacteremia.

General References

Osteomyelitis:
Waldvogel FA, Medoff G, Swartz M: Osteomyelitis: a review of clinical features, therapeutic considerations and unusual aspects. I, II, and III. *N Engl J Med* 282:198, 260, 316, 1970.
    A thorough, well-referenced review.
Waldvogel FA, Vasey H: Osteomyelitis: the past decade. *N Engl J Med* 303:360, 1980.
    An update of the 1970 review by the same author.

Lung Abscess:
Bartlett JG: Lung abscess. *Johns Hopkins Med J* 150:141, 1982.
Bartlett G, Gorbach SL: Penicillin or clindamycin for primary lung abscess? *Ann Intern Med* 98:546, 1983.
Gopalakrishna KV, Lerner PI: Primary lung abscess. *Clev Clin Q* 42:3, 1975.
Perlman LV, Lerner E, D'sops N: Classification and analysis of 97 cases of lung abscess. *Am Rev Respir Dis* 99:390, 1969.

Endocarditis:
Bayliss R, Clark C, Oakley CM, et al: The teeth and infective endocarditis. *Br Heart J* 50:506, 1983.
Bayliss R, Clark C, Oakley CM, et al: The microbiology and pathogenesis of infective endocarditis. *Br Heart J* 50:513, 1983.

Specific References

1. Bartlett JG, Anaerobic bacterial infections of the lung. *Chest* 91:901, 1987.
2. Bell S: Further observations on the value of oral penicillins in chronic staphylococcal osteomyelitis. *Med J Aust* 2:591, 1976.
3. Bisno AL, Dismukes WE, Durak DT, et al: Antimicrobial treatment of infective endocarditis due to viridans streptococci, enterococci, and staphylococci. *JAMA* 261:1471, 1989.
4. Chambers HF, Miller RT, Newman MD: Right-sided *Staphylococcus aureus* endocarditis in intravenous drug abusers: two-week combination therapy. *Ann Intern Med* 109:619, 1988.
5. Dich V, Nelson J, Haltalin K: Osteomyelitis in infants and children. *Am J Dis Child* 129:1273, 1975.
6. Hagan JL, Hardy JD: Lung abscess revisited. A survey of 184 cases. *Am Surg* 197:755, 1983.
7. Kaplan SL, Mason EO, Feigin RD: Clindamycin versus nafcillin or methicillin in the treatment of Staphylococcus aureus osteomyelitis in children. *South Med J* 75:138, 1975.
8. Kelly P, Wilkowske C, Washington II J: Comparison of Gram-negative bacillary and staphylococcal osteomyelitis of femur and tibia. *Clin Ortho* 96:70, 1973.
9. Landay MJ, Christensen EE, Bynum LJ, Goodman C: Anaerobic pleural and pulmonary infection. *AJR* 134:233, 1980.
10. Levison ME, Mangura CT, Lorber B, et al: Clindamycin compared with penicillin for the treatment of anaerobic lung abscess. *Ann Intern Med* 98:466, 1983.
11. Mackowiak POA, Jones SR, Smith JW: Diagnostic value of sinustract cultures in chronic osteomyelitis. *JAMA* 239:2772, 1978.
12. Maurer AH, Chen DCP, Camargo EE, et al: Utility of three-phase skeletal scintigraphy in suspected osteomyelitis: concise communication. *J Nucl Med* 22:941, 1981.
13. Parker RH, Fossieck BE: Intravenous followed by oral antimicrobial therapy for staphylococcal endocarditis. *Ann Intern Med* 93:832, 1980.
14. Sande MA, Scheld WM: Combination antibiotic therapy of bacterial endocarditis. *Ann Intern Med* 92:390, 1980.
15. Sugarman B, Hawes S, Musher DM, et al: Osteomyelitis beneath pressure sores. *Arch Intern Med* 143:683, 1983.
16. Weiss W, Cherniack NS: Acute nonspecific lung abscess: a controlled study comparing orally and parenterally administered penicillin G. *Chest* 66:349, 1980.
17. Wagner DK, Collier BC, Rytel MW: Long-term intravenous antibiotic therapy in chronic osteomyelitis. *Arch Intern Med* 145:1073, 1985.
18. West WF, Kelly P, Martin WJ: Chronic osteomyelitis. I. Factors affecting the results of treatment in 186 patients. *JAMA* 213:1837, 1970.
19. Winberly N, Faling J, Bartlett JG: A fiberoptic bronchoscopy technique to obtain uncontaminated lower airway secretions for bacterial culture. *Am Rev Respir Dis* 110:337, 1979.

C H A P T E R   32

Immunization to Prevent Infectious Disease

R. BRADLEY SACK, M.D., Sc.D.
L. RANDOL BARKER, M.D.

Protection against infectious diseases can be conferred by active immunization with vaccines and by passive immunization with immune globulin preparations. As newly purified antigens become available, and as the mechanisms of the immune response become better understood, there will continue to be new vaccines and revised recommendations for protection against important infectious diseases. This chapter describes available vaccines and immune globulin preparations utilized in the United States, focusing upon the two critical questions commonly considered in practice: (a) Who should receive immunization? and (b) When should they receive it? Chapter 33 provides similar information on immunization for travelers to developing countries.

PATIENT ASSESSMENT

History

There are a number of questions that should be asked whenever immunization is contemplated.

The history of *previous immunizations* should be determined. In young adults, this may be readily known; in older persons, this information is often hard to obtain. Patients may or may not keep personal records that can be of use. For example, persons who have served in the military will have received a large number of immunizations. They and persons who frequently travel abroad may have this information recorded on their International Vaccination Card. Immunization history is particularly important in determining (a) whether to give tetanus toxoid or antitoxin after an injury, (b) whether diphtheria should be seriously considered in the diagnosis of acute pharyngitis (see Chapter 28), and (c) what immunizations to give to patients traveling outside the United States (see Chapter 33).

A history of *prior allergic reactions or of other untoward reactions* to vaccines or their components should always be excluded before giving an immunization. Most vaccines are now highly purified, and allergic reactions after their use are rare. However, persons with a history of an allergic reaction after eating eggs, for instance, should not receive vaccines made in eggs (e.g., influenza, measles, mumps, and yellow fever vaccines). Some persons experience unusually severe reactions to bacterial vaccines such as typhoid and cholera vaccines. A history of a previous severe response to a vaccine is a contraindication to its use. Some antiviral vaccines contain trace amounts of antibiotics (used often in tissue culture preparations) to which the patient may be hypersensitive; this information should be determined from the package insert before administration of vaccine to susceptible patients.

The following conditions are those for which use of a *live virus is generally contraindicated*: patients with either a known immunodeficiency disease or recent treatment with an immunosuppressive drug, and pregnant women, in whom the live virus vaccine might pose a risk to the developing fetus. Persons known to be infected with the Human Immunodeficiency Virus (HIV) may be at some risk when receiving live vaccines, although adverse effects have not been well documented. Guidelines for use of vaccines in these persons are still being formulated (see Chapter 34).

A *recent injection of gamma globulin* (within 3 months) requires that the use of some live virus vaccines be postponed, since there may be interference with the antibody response. For the same reason, gamma globulin should not be administered earlier than 2 weeks after live virus vaccine. However, yellow fever and oral polio vaccines can be given without regard to gamma globulin administration, since interference does not occur.

Finally, a patient with an *acute febrile illness* should generally not be immunized until after the illness has resolved, because any side effects might add to the patient's morbidity, and because the effectiveness of the vaccination may be diminished. However, a minor illness (e.g., upper respiratory infection with or without a low-grade fever) is not a contraindication to give a necessary immunization.

Physical Examination

When immunization is contemplated, the physical examination usually adds little to the assessment of the patient. Pregnancy or an active infection (see above) may be confirmed on examination.

Immunological Testing

Immunological tests may be useful in deciding about immunization in two situations: (a) in considering the use of hyperimmune globulin preparations or hepatitis B vaccine for protection against hepatitis B; if the exposed person already has antibody to hepatitis B surface antigen, additional protection is unnecessary; and (b) when considering the use of rubella vaccine for a woman of childbearing age; if she already has antibodies to rubella, further immunization is unnecessary.

IMMUNIZATION PROCEDURES

It is important to be familiar with the information contained in the package insert when giving a vaccine. This information includes dose, route of administration, common and uncommon side effects, contraindications, whether there is contamination with antibiotics, interval between immunizations, and additional detail.

All gamma globulin preparations made in the United States have been shown to be free of any possibility of transferring human immunodeficiency virus (HIV) infection, although antibodies to HIV may be present in the preparation. This could lead to a "false-positive" HIV antibody test if it were done within a month or two of receiving the globulin preparation.

Many of the widely used vaccines can be given simultaneously. The Centers for Disease Control list the following guidelines for simultaneous vaccine administration: (a) Inactivated vaccines can be administered simultaneously at separate sites (at the same site in the case of widely used combination vaccines such as tetanus and diphtheria toxoids). However, when vaccines commonly associated with side effects are given together (e.g., cholera, typhoid, plague) the side effects may be accentuated; and consideration should be given to vaccinating on separate occasions (see also Chapter 33). (b) An inactivated vaccine and a live, attenuated virus vaccine can be administered simultaneously at separate sites. Some vaccines are routinely given together. Measles, mumps, and rubella (MMR vaccine) is a combined live virus vaccine that can be given to any age group. Tetanus and diphtheria (Td) are most effectively given together in the combined vaccine.

Patients should be told at the time of immunization that they may experience some local soreness and possibly fever and malaise during the following 24 to 48 hours. They can be instructed to take aspirin or acetaminophen if these symptoms are bothersome. Because of the rare possibility of anaphylactic reactions, persons receiving any immunization should wait in the office where they can be observed for about 15 minutes. Finally, patients should be clearly informed of the name of the immunizations they have received and be encouraged to keep a written record of them. Official immunizations cards are available in every state for this purpose.

Physicians and health care providers must now legally maintain permanent records of immunization and report certain adverse effects after immunization to the United States Department of Health and Human Services. These recording requirements became effective March 1988 (5).

CURRENT RECOMMENDATIONS FOR VACCINES AND IMMUNE GLOBULINS

Table 32.1 summarizes information on the major available vaccines and immune globulin preparations. The following sections provide practical information on infections for which immune protection for adults is most likely to be given in ambulatory practice.

PROTECTION AGAINST SELECTED INFECTIONS

Hepatitis

Hepatitis A

At present, only passive immunization with preparations of gamma globulin is available for prevention of hepatitis A. Pooled human gamma globulin (immune serum globulin, ISG) is 80 to 90% effective in preventing hepatitis A in exposed persons. It should be given to the following: (a) close contacts of persons with known hepatitis A (family members or intimate friends, but not schoolmates or fellow workers unless some unusually high possibility of fecal-oral transmission is suspected); ISG should be given as soon as possible after the known exposure, certainly within 1 week; the usual adult dose is 0.02 ml/kg intramuscularly; (b) persons traveling to the developing world where risk of exposure is known to be high (see Chapter 33 for doses and schedules) (11).

Vaccines are being developed for prevention of hep-

atitis A, using both killed and attenuated viruses, and should be available within the next several years.

Hepatitis B

Although pooled gamma globulin (ISG) in relatively large doses (0.06 ml/kg intramuscularly in two doses 4 weeks apart) may also be useful in preventing hepatitis B, a globulin preparation of high titer (hepatitis B immune globulin, HBIG) is preferred and is approximately 75% effective in preventing hepatitis in those persons known to have direct exposure to hepatitis B virus. When HBIG is given at the same time as hepatitis B vaccine (see below), this protection is considerably higher (16). Exposed persons who are known to have antibody to the surface antigen (HBsAg) do not need postexposure prophylaxis.

There are presently two vaccines for prevention of Hepatitis B; one is plasma derived (Heptavax-B), and the other is a recombinant DNA vaccine (Recombivax HB, Eugerix-B) made in yeast. Both have shown similar immunogenicity and their efficacy is also similar, about 90%. The vaccines are given intramuscularly at 0, 1, and 6 months. Booster doses are not routinely recommended at this time (7, 11). The arm should be used as the hepatitis vaccination site for adults since suboptimal responses to the vaccine have occurred when the vaccine was injected into the buttock. The only side effect of the vaccine is occasional soreness and redness at the injection site. The protection after the completed immunization schedule is about 80 to 95% for at least 5 to 7 years.

Table 32.2 summarizes the 1990 recommendations of the Centers for Disease Control (CDC) for *postexposure HBIG and vaccine prophylaxis* for persons in the following groups: (a) newborns with perinatal exposure to a mother who has acute hepatitis B or is HBsAg positive; it is now recommended that all pregnant women be routinely tested for HbsAg during an early prenatal visit; (b) sexual contacts of persons who have active hepatitis B or are HBsAg carriers. Table 32.3 summarizes recommendations for postexposure prophylaxis for (a) persons who have had percutaneous, ocular, or mucous membrane exposure to blood from patients who have active hepatitis B or are HBsAg carriers; (b) persons who receive a human bite that penetrates the skin from a patient who has active hepatitis B or is a carrier of HBsAg; (c) persons with similar exposures to patients whose HBsAg status is unknown.

Hepatitis B vaccine for *primary prevention of hepatitis B* is recommended for persons who are at high risk of exposure: (a) health care professionals exposed frequently to blood or blood products (e.g., laboratory and blood bank personnel, operating room staff, surgeons, dentists, endoscopists, pathologists, and the staff in oncology, dialysis, and emergency room units); (b) homosexually active men; (c) family members or partners, in particular sexual partners, of chronic HBsAg carriers; (d) patients who frequently receive transfusions of blood or blood products; (e) patients in he-

Table 32.1.
Identity, Characteristics, and Administration of Available Vaccines and Immune Globulin Preparations

Vaccine or Immune Globulin (References)	Type of Preparation	Population to Be Immunized	Age at Which Immunization Usually Done	Immunization Schedule[a]	Possible Adverse Reactions
Beginning in Childhood (All Children)					
Diphtheria vaccine (8)	Killed bacteria and toxoid	All	Child or adult	Series of three primary injections with boosters (day 0, 1 month, 6–12 months) every 10 yr[b]	Local pain and swelling
Tetanus toxoid (8)	Toxoid	All	Child or adult	Series of three injections (day 0, 1 month, 6–12 months) with boosters every 10 yr[b]	Local pain and swelling
Tetanus immune globulin	Human antiserum	Unimmunized person with dirty wound		Single injection	Not significant
Pertussis vaccine (8)	Killed bacteria	All children	Child only	Series of three injections (day 0, 1 month, 6–12 months) with boosters to age 6	Fever, occasionally severe neurological reactions
Polio vaccine					
Oral	Live attenuated virus	All	Child	Primary series of three oral preparations	Not significant, rare clinical disease
Parenteral	Killed virus	All	Child	Primary series of four injections	Not significant
Measles vaccine (9)	Live attenuated virus	All children	Child ≥15 months of age	Two injections (age ≥15 months and 4–6 years)[c]	Fever
Rubella vaccine	Live attenuated virus	All children and unimmunized women	Child ≥15 months females through childbearing age	Single injection[c]	Arthralgias, fever in young women
Mumps vaccine	Live attenuated virus	All children and young adults without history of mumps	Child ≥15 months	Single injection[c]	Not significant
Hemophilus influenza	Conjugate purified polysaccharides	All children	Children ≥18 months	Single injection	Not significant
Usually Beginning in Adulthood (Selected Populations)					
Influenza vaccine (10, 15)	Killed virus (whole virus and "split virus" preparations) preparations of virus change yearly	Persons at risk, chronic illness	Child or adult	Adults: Single injection (whole virus) repeated yearly. Children under 13: split virus preparation, two doses	Mild fever, allergic reactions, Guillain-Barré syndrome rarely
Hepatitis B vaccine (7, 11, 12, 16)	Inactivated viral constituents from infected humans and recombinant virus in yeasts	Health workers and others at increased risk	Usually adults	Three injections (0 time, 1 month, 6 months)	Not significant
Hepatitis globulin (11, 16)					
Pooled (ISG) (11)	Pooled human γ-globulin	Persons exposed to hepatitis A (and B)	Usually adults	Hepatitis A: 0.02 ml/kg, once. Hepatitis B: 0.06 ml/kg, twice	Not significant
High titred	Hepatitis B immune globulin (HBIG)	Persons exposed to hepatitis B only	Usually adults	0.06 ml/kg at time of exposure and again 1 month later	Not significant
Meningococcal vaccine (6)	Purified polysaccharide (serogroups A, C, Y, W135)	Only during epidemic disease. Persons with high risks (military)	All ages; young adult military	Single injection	Erythema at injection site; not significant
Rabies vaccine (2, 4)	Killed virus (human diploid vaccine)	Persons bitten by possible rabid animal or at high risk of exposure	All ages—postexposure and pre-exposure	Postexposure: multiple does of vaccine intramuscularly (days 0, 3, 7, 14, 30)	Pain, rare neurologic reactions

Table 32.1.—Continued

Vaccine or Immune Globulin (References)	Type of Preparation	Population to Be Immunized	Age at Which Immunization Usually Done	Immunization Schedule[a]	Possible Adverse Reactions
				Pre exposure: 3 doses of rabies vaccine, intradermally (days 0, 7, 28)	
Rabies immune globulin	Human rabies immune globulin (HRIG)	Unimmunized persons with suspicious animal bite	Any age	Single injection	Not significant
Pneumococcal vaccine (17)	Polyvalent purified polysaccharides (23 serotypes)	Persons with asplenia or splenic dysfunction; persons with chronic illness	Any age (over 2 yr)	Single injection, not repeated	Erythema at injection site
Bacillus Calmette and Guérin (BCG) vaccine (14)	Live attenuated bacteria	Used to immunize newborns in developing countries and persons with excessively high risk of developing tuberculosis.	Infants and children	Single injection, intradermal	Prolonged granuloma or ulcer at injection site, lymphadenitis

[a] All injections are intramuscular unless otherwise specified.
[b] Boosters of diphtheria and tetanus are particularly important for those traveling to underdeveloped countries. Diptheria and tetanus vaccines should be given in combined (Td) preparation.
[c] Given as the combination mumps, measles, rubella (MMR).

Table 32.2.
Recommendations for Hepatitis B Prophylaxis After Perinatal or Sexual Exposure

Exposure	HBIG		Vaccine	
	Dose	Recommended Timing	Dose	Recommended Timing
Perinatal	0.5 ml IM	Within 12 hours of birth	0.5 ml IM	Within 12 hours of birth[a]
Sexual	0.06 ml/kg IM	Single dose within 14 days of last sexual contact	1.0 ml IM	First dose at time of HBIG treatment[a]

[a] The first dose can be given the same times as the HBIG dose but at a separate site; subsequent doses should be given as recommended for specific vaccine. From *Morbidity and Mortality Weekly Report*, vol 39, no. RR-2, 1990.

Table 32.3.
Recommendations for Hepatitis B Prophylaxis After Percutaneous or Permucossal Exposure

Exposed Person	Treatment When Source Is Found To Be:		
	HBsAg-positive	HBsAg-negative	Source not tested or Unknown
Unvaccinated	HBIG × 1[a] and initiate HB vaccine[b]	Initiate HB vaccine[b]	Initiate HB vaccine[b]
Previously vaccinated Known responder	Test exposed for anti-HBs 1. If adequate,[c] no treatment 2. If inadequate, HB vaccine booster dose	No treatment	No treatment
Known nonresponder	HBIG × 2 or HBIG × 1 plus 1 dose HB vaccine	No treatment	If known high-risk source, may treat as if source were HBsAg-positive
Response unknown	Test exposed for anti-HBs 1. If inadequate,[c] HBIG × 1 plus HB vaccine booster dose 2. If adequate, no treatment	No treatment	Test exposed for anti-HBs 1. If inadequate,[c] HB vaccine booster dose 2. If adequate, no treatment

[a] HBIG dose, 0.06 ml/kg IM.
[b] Adult dose, 1.0 ml IM.
[c] Adequate anti-HBs is ≥ 10 SRU by RIA or positive by EIA. (From *Morbidity and Mortality Weekly Report* Vol 39, No RR-2, 1990.)

modialysis units; (f) inmates and staff of institutions for the mentally retarded; (g) users of illicit injectable drugs; (h) selected international travelers (see Chapter 33); (i) members of a family that adopts a child from an area where hepatitis B is endemic—if the child is HBsAg positive. The vaccine is not routinely recommended for individuals who come in contact with HBsAg carriers at work or in school. Screening for antibodies to hepatitis B virus prior to immunization is not routinely done, except in high risk populations where the prevalence is high (such as intravenous drug abusers), and thus the testing is cost effective. Vaccination of individuals who have anti-HBs from previous infection does not cause adverse effects.

The patterns of appearance of antigens and antibodies in hepatitis B infection are illustrated in Figure 43.1.

Non-A, Non-B Hepatitis

There is no immune globulin preparation known to be protective against non-A, non-B hepatitis, which is now the most frequent cause of post-transfusion hepatitis.

Hepatitis in ambulatory patients is discussed in Chapter 43.

Tetanus

Currently, about 50 cases of tetanus are reported each year in the United States (8). There is no known subclinical "natural" immunity to tetanus, so that every person is susceptible unless he has been actively immunized. The majority of cases in the United States occur in persons over 60 years old, a population containing many persons who have never been immunized. Tetanus usually follows penetrating wounds due to accidents and animal bites (see Chapter 25). The incubation period is 4 to 21 days with an average of 10 days. In persons who have been actively immunized at any time in their life, injection of toxoid once every 10 years is necessary to boost their antitoxin titers to protective levels. If a person at risk of developing tetanus from a wound has received a toxoid booster in the last 10 years, no additional toxoid is required; if such a person has never received toxoid immunization, has not received a toxoid booster within the past 10 years, or is unsure about it, passive immunization with tetanus antitoxin (250 units intramuscularly) should be given. This preparation is made from human serum, and therefore hypersensitivity reactions are not a problem. Persons who require tetanus antitoxin should at the same time (but at a different site) be given their first dose of toxoid, followed by repeated doses of toxoid 1 month and 6 to 12 months later. Combined diphtheria-tetanus (Td) toxoids are preferred in order to produce immunity to both diseases.

Diphtheria

Currently, about 1 to 5 cases of diphtheria are reported each year in the United States (8). Although

subclinical infection may occur and confer immunity in unimmunized persons, it is recommended that persons who have never been given diphtheria toxoid should receive it if their occupation places them at increased risk of exposure to diphtheria (i.e., physicians, nurses, other hospital personnel, teachers, and staff and patients of institutions for the mentally handicapped) or if they plan travel in developing countries (see Chapter 33). For unimmunized school-aged children and adults, adult type (Td), tetanus and diphtheria toxoids are used. This preparation contains only about 25% of the diphtheria toxoid contained in the DPT (diphtheria-pertussis-tetanus) combined vaccine utilized in infants; this minimizes the risk of severe reactions in adults, previously a significant problem. Primary immunization consists of an initial dose, a 1-month dose, and a third dose at the 6th to 12th month; a booster (Td) is recommended every 10 years to assure protection. In adults, there is a high incidence (25 to 50%) of local soreness, swelling, and itching after Td injections; fever occurs in less than 10% and urticaria in approximately 2% of individuals. Serious reactions (massive swelling of the whole arm, or anaphylaxis) occur rarely.

For asymptomatic unimmunized contacts of patients with diphtheria, management includes: (a) prophylactic antibiotics (600,000 units of benzathine penicillin intramuscularly or a 7-day course of erythromycin, 250 mg four times daily); (b) primary vaccination as outlined above; and (c) daily surveillance for 7 days for clinical evidence of diphtheria (see Chapter 28).

Mumps

In the interval 1972 to 1987, the number of cases of mumps reported annually in the United States fell from approximately 70,000 to approximately 10,000. This decline is probably in part due to the use of mumps vaccine during this interval.

Live attenuated virus mumps vaccine is now recommended routinely for children and for those young adults with no history of mumps; most people born before 1957, however, can be considered immune. Because in adults the mumps virus can cause severe symptoms (orchitis, meningitis, or pancreatitis), there is good reason to provide this protection to younger adults who may be susceptible. Unimmunized persons may have had an immunizing subclinical infection, since only one of every three cases of mumps in childhood is symptomatic.

Measles

Measles is a moderately severe illness in most persons and has a case fatality rate of 1:1,000. Since 1963, measles vaccines have been available (initially, killed virus vaccines, and since 1968, attenuated live virus vaccines). In the interval 1960 to 1980, when measles vaccination of children was introduced generally in the United States, the number of cases reported annually fell from over 400,000 to less than 15,000. In 1983, only 1,497 cases were reported, but subsequently the annual rate began to rise. In 1989, more than 14, 000 cases were reported (9). This increase in measles incidence occurred despite a strategy announced in 1978 for the eradication of measles.

Investigation of the recent increase in measles incidence has shown that vaccination before the age of 15 months (i.e., between 12 and 14 months) may be ineffective in some children because of persisting maternal antibody and that single-dose vaccination at ≥15 months of age does not confer lifelong immunity in some individuals. In response to these problems, a two-dose vaccine schedule was recommended, as of 1990, in place of the previous one-dose schedule. Table 32.4 summarizes this new policy. Table 34.5 summarizes recommendations for control of a measles outbreak in each of the following situations: in preschool aged children, in institutions (day centers, schools, colleges, etc.), and in medical facilities.

Rubella

In the interval 1970 to 1988, the number of cases of rubella reported annually in the United States fell from approximately 55, 000 to less than 300. The number of reported cases of congenital rubella syndrome remained unchanged during the decade 1970 to 1980 (50 to 60 cases) but fell dramatically in 1982 (13 cases reported) and 1988 (1 case reported).

Since about 1970, immunization against rubella, using an attenuated live virus vaccine, has been administered routinely to children between ages 1 and 2. The major rationale for this vaccine is to prevent the spread of rubella to pregnant women and thereby to reduce the incidence of the congenital rubella syndrome.

Adolescent females and women in the childbearing age group should be offered immunization also, if not previously immunized or known to have had the disease. Although immunological testing can be done to prevent unnecessary immunization of women with preexisting titers, this is not necessary. Before the vaccine is given, a woman should be cautioned against becoming pregnant (see Chapter 93, Birth Control) for the 3 months immediately after the immunization since there is the possibility of fetal damage by the live virus. However, such an occurrence has not actually been documented and the risk is estimated to be extremely low.

Influenza

Killed virus vaccines have been available for the prevention of influenza for many years. Earlier preparations contained nonspecific protein that frequently led to fever and malaise after the vaccine had been administered. Preparations now available are highly purified, and reaction rates are very low. Each year's vaccine is polyvalent, containing antigenic material from the type A and type B strains that are expected to prevail in a given year.

Influenza vaccine is recommended annually for those persons in whom influenza causes the highest morbidity and mortality: individuals over 60 years old and individuals of all ages with significant heart, lung, or chronic debilitating disease (10). The vaccine is also recommended for those involved in critical jobs where their absence may be highly detrimental (e.g., firemen, policemen, selected hospital personnel).

Influenza vaccine is about 70% protective, as determined in a number of experimental trials involving healthy adults and in retrospective studies involving young and elderly individuals (15). The antigens in

Table 32.4.
1989 Recommendations for Measles Vaccination (Column on Right Lists Criteria for Adequate Protection)

Routine childhood schedule, United States	
Most areas	Two doses[a, b] —first dose at 15 months —second dose at 4–6 years (entry to kindergarten or first grade)[c]
High risk areas[d]	Two doses[a, b] —first dose at 12 months —second dose at 4–6 years (entry to kindergarten or first grade)[c]
Colleges and other educational institutions post-high school	Documentation of receipt of two doses of measles vaccine after the first birthday[b] or other evidence of measles immunity[e]
Medical personnel beginning employment	Documentation of receipt of two doses of measles vaccine after the first birthday[b] or other evidence of measles immunity[e]

[a] Both doses should preferably be given as combined measles, mumps, rubella vaccine (MMR).
[b] No less than 1 month apart. If no documentation of any dose of vaccine, first dose of vaccine should be given at the time of school entry or employment and second dose no less than 1 month later.
[c] Some areas may elect to administer the second dose at an older age or to multiple age groups.
[d] A county with more than five cases among preschool-aged children during each of at least 5 years, a county with a recent outbreak among unvaccinated preschool-aged children, or a county with a large inner-city urban population. These recommendations may be applied to an entire county or to identified risk areas within a county.
[e] Prior physician-diagnosed measles disease, laboratory evidence of measles immunity, or birth before 1957.
(From *Morbidity and Mortality Weekly Report*, Vol 38, No.S-9, 1989.)

Table 32.5.
Recommendations for Measles Outbreak Control[a]

Outbreaks in preschool-aged children	Lower age for vaccination to as low as 6 months of age in outbreak area if cases are occurring in children <1 year of age[b].
Outbreaks in institutions: day-care centers, K-12th grades, colleges, and other institutions	Revaccination of all students and their siblings and of school personnel born in or after 1957 who do not have documentation of immunity to measles[c].
Outbreaks in medical facilities	Revaccination of all medical workers born in or after 1957 who have direct patient contact and who do not have proof of immunity to measles[c]. Susceptible personnel who have been exposed should be relieved from direct patient contact from the 5th to 21st day after exposure (regardless of whether they received measles vaccine or IG) or—if they become ill—for 7 days after they develop rash.

[a] Mass revaccination of entire populations is not necessary. Revaccination should be limited to populations at risk, such as students attending institutions where cases occur.
[b] Children initially vacinated before the first birthday should be revaccinated at 15 months of age. A second dose should be administered at the time of school entry or according to local policy.
[c] Documentation of physician-diagnosed measles disease, serologic evidence of immunity to measles, or documentation of receipt of two doses of measles vaccine on or after the first birthday.
(From *Morbidity and Mortality Weekly Report*, Vol 38, No. S-9, 1989.)

the vaccine must, of course, be appropriate for the prevailing influenza virus strain. The vaccine should be given in the fall, before the influenza season, which usually occurs between December and April.

Amantidine Prophylactics. During confirmed local outbreaks of influenza A, the antiviral drug amantadine (Symmetrel) can be utilized prophylactically as well as therapeutically (see Chapter 28 for a discussion of therapeutic use) (1, 3). Amantadine prevents clinical disease due to influenza A viruses in approximately 70% of subjects. The prophylactic use of this drug has been recommended for the following groups of subjects:

1. Unvaccinated children and adults at high risk of serious morbidity and mortality because of underlying diseases, which include pulmonary, cardiovascular, metabolic, neuromuscular, or immunodeficiency diseases;
2. Adults whose activities are vital to community function and who have not been vaccinated with an appropriate contemporary influenza vaccine—for example, policemen, firemen, selected hospital personnel. Such persons are in frequent contact with others who may have influenza and should be considered at higher risk of contracting influenza than the general population.
3. Persons in semiclosed institutional environments, especially older persons, who have not received the current influenza vaccine.

The drug should be taken once daily (100 mg) during the local outbreak and at the same time influenza immunization should be given. The drug can be stopped after two weeks, at which time protective antibodies will have developed. Subjects should be warned of the following transient central nervous system side effects, which may occur during the first few days in 5 to 10% of subjects: insomnia, lightheadedness, nervousness, drowsiness, difficulty in concentrating.

Influenza in ambulatory patients is discussed in Chapter 28.

Pneumococcal Disease

A purified polyvalent polysaccharide vaccine is available for the prevention of pneumococcal disease in persons at high risk, including persons who have had a splenectomy, those with sickle cell anemia, and adults with chronic lung disease. The vaccine is about 80% protective against the pneumococcal serotypes that it contains (23 serotypes that are responsible for approximately 90% of pneumococcal disease in the United States) (17). The vaccine produces very few untoward effects and can be given as a single injection. Because of a high incidence of adverse local reactions to reinjection of pneumococcal vaccine, second or "booster" doses should not be given.

Pneumococcal pneumonia in ambulatory practice is discussed in Chapter 28.

Tuberculosis

Efforts to control tuberculosis in the United States are based upon early identification of active disease and upon isoniazid prophylaxis of the contacts of tuberculous patients and other groups at increased risk (see Chapter 29). Because the incidence of new tuberculosis is relatively low in this country (approximately 25, 000 cases/year) and because most new cases are due to reactivation of disease in older individuals who acquired their infection in an era when the risk of infection was much higher, the indications for immunization with bacillus of Calmette and Guérin (BCG) vaccine are very limited. The 1988 recommendations of the United States Public Health Service (14) are as follows:

1. BCG vaccination should be seriously considered for infants and children who are tuberculin skin test negative and who have repeated exposure to persistently untreated or ineffectively treated, sputum-positive pulmonary tuberculosis.
2. BCG vaccination should be considered for tuberculin-negative infants and children in groups in

which an excessive rate of new infections can be demonstrated (1% per year) and the usual surveillance and treatment programs have failed or have been shown not to be applicable. Such groups might exist among the socially disaffiliated and those without a regular source of health care. BCG is not recommended for health care workers, who should have periodic tuberculin skin testing.

The recommended route of administration for the BCG strain utilized in this country is intradermal or subcutaneous, depending on the specific vaccine given. Contraindications to BCG vaccine are compromised immunity due to malignancy or immunosuppressive therapy and pregnancy. After BCG immunization, it is not possible to distinguish between a positive tuberculin skin test resulting from infection with virulent M. tuberculosis and one resulting from the BCG vaccine. Because the protective efficacy of BCG vaccine is not absolute, tuberculosis should be included in the differential diagnosis of any tuberculosis-like illness occurring in vaccinated individuals.

Rabies

In the past 10 years, zero to four cases of human rabies have been reported each year in the United States. Theoretically all of these cases are preventable if protective treatment is given promptly after exposure. The incubation period is usually 2 to 8 weeks, but it may be as short as 10 days or as long as a year or more.

Since 1980, killed virus rabies vaccine produced in human diploid cells has been in use in the United States. This vaccine is given intramuscularly.

For *postexposure prophylaxis* following an animal bite (see Chapter 25), the recommended treatment schedule is as follows: on day 1, simultaneous administration of antirabies globulin (as human rabies immune globulin, HRIG), and the first dose of rabies vaccine, given intramuscularly, not subcutaneously; vaccine is repeated on days 3, 7, 14, and 30. The effectiveness of this vaccine in stimulating antibody and in protecting patients from rabies has been well established (4). Adverse reactions (urticaria, anaphylaxis, transient headache, and fever) occur in less than 0.5% of persons receiving this vaccine (2). The vaccine and antiglobulin are available from local health departments.

Pre-exposure Prophylaxis.   For persons working in areas where rabies exposure may be high, the vaccine should be given before exposure. In this situation, it can be given intradermally in small doses (0.1 ml), on days 0, 7, and 28 (see Chapter 33 for details regarding frequency of vaccine for those living in endemic areas). Pre-exposure immunization does not mean that postexposure immunization is not necessary; but it obviates the need for immune globulin and decreases the number of immunizations required.

General References

ACP Task Force on Adult Immunization and Infectious Diseases Society of American, 2nd ed., Philadelphia, American College of Physicians, 1990.

Contains all standard recommendations in a single source, with critical discussion of effectiveness, indications, administration, adverse consequences of individual vaccines and immune globulin preparations.

Benenson, AS (ed): *Control of Communicable Diseases in Man*, 15th ed., Washington, DC, American Public Health Association, 1990.

A concise summary of epidemiology and management of communicable diseases.

Recommendations of the Immunization Practices Advisory Committees. *Morbidity and Mortality Weekly Report* 38:205, 1989.

Summary recommendations, updated periodically; also published periodically in the *Annals of Internal Medicine* and *The Medical Letter*.

Morbidity and Mortality Weekly Report, Annual Summary. United States Department of Health and Human Services, Centers for Disease Control.

This annual report summarizes the incidence of reportable diseases for the current year and for previous years and decades (beginning with 1940).

Specific References

1. Arden NH, Patriarca PA, Fasano MB, et al: The roles of vaccination and amantadine prophylaxis in controlling an outbreak of Influenza A (H3N2) in a nursing home. *Arch Intern Med* 148(4):865, 1988.
2. Bernard KW, Roberts MA, et al: Human diploid cell rabies vaccine: effectiveness of immunization with small intradermal or subcutaneous doses. *JAMA* 247:1138, 1982.
3. Douglas Jr. RG: Influenza prevention and treatment. The primary care physician's role. *Postgrad Med* 83(5):207, 1988.
4. Fishbein DB, Arcangeli S: Rabies prevention in primary care. A four-step approach. *Postgrad Med* 82(3):83, 93, 1987.
5. Food and Drug Administration. New reporting requirements for vaccine adverse events. *FDA Drug Bull* 18(2):16, 1988.
6. Frasch CS: Prospects for the prevention of meningococcal disease: special reference to Group B. *Vaccine* 5(1):3–, 1987.
7. Krugman S, Davidson M: Hepatitis B vaccine: prospects for duration of immunity. *Yale J Biol Med* 60(4):333, 1987.
8. Recommendations of the Immunization Practices Advisory Committee (ACIP). Diphtheria, tetanus, and pertussis: guidelines for vaccine prophylaxis and other preventive measures. *MMWR* 34(27):405, 1985.
9. Recommendations of the Immunization Practices Advisory Committee (ACIP). Measles prevention. *MMWR* 38(1):11, 1989.
10. Recommendations of the Immunization Practices Advisory Committee (ACIP). Prevention and control of influenza: Part I, vaccines. *MMWR* 38 (No. 5–9), 1989.
11. Recommendations of the Immunization Practices Advisory Committee (ACIP). Protection against viral hepatitis. *MMWR* 39(S2), 1990.
12. Recommendations of the Immunization Practices Advisory Committee (ACIP). Update on hepatitis B prevention. *MMWR* 36(23):353, 1987.
13. Recommendations of the Immunization Practices Advisory Committee (ACIP). Update: prevention of Haemophilus influenza Type B disease. *MMWR* 37(2):13, 1988.
14. Recommendations of the Immunization Practices Advisory Committee (ACIP). Use of BC vaccines in the control of tuberculosis: a joint statement of the ACIP and the Advisory Committee for elimination of tuberculosis. *MMWR* 37(43):663, 1988.
15. Ruben FL: Prevention and control of influenza. *Am J Med* 82(6A):31, 1987.
16. Stevens CE, Taylor PE, Tong MJ, et al: Yeast-recombinant hepatitis B vaccine. Efficacy with hepatitis B immune globulin in prevention of perinatal hepatitis B virus transmission. *JAMA* 257(19):2612, 1987.
17. Williams WW, Hickson MA, Kane MA, et al: Immunization policies and vaccine coverage among adults. The risk for missed opportunities. *Ann Intern Med* 108(4):616, 1988.

C H A P T E R   33

Medical Advice for the International Traveler

STEPHEN D. SEARS, M.D., M.P.H.
R. BRADLEY SACK, M.D., Sc.D.

SCOPE OF THE PROBLEM

Approximately 25 million Americans travel by air to foreign countries each year. This does not include the many who take boats, cruises, or go by car to Canada and Mexico. Of these 25 million, it is estimated that between 3 and 5 million journey to developing areas of the world where infectious diseases are commonly encountered. Malaria, schistosomiasis, yellow fever, polio, typhoid fever, and amebiasis are just a few of the diseases that are more prevalent in tropical developing countries. Many travelers make little, if any, provision for the prevention of illness while traveling. This is unfortunate because the overall attack rate for several infectious diseases is much higher in international travelers than it is in comparable populations that remain at home. This fact is well illustrated by the results of a study of Swiss travelers that found that three quarters had at least one symptom of infectious illness while traveling; and of the 16,500 travelers surveyed in this study, greater than 30% had at least one episode of a diarrheal illness (15). In a follow-up study, travelers not only were found to have illnesses while traveling, but almost one-third became ill within a month of returning home (16). Another study of 2,000 travelers returning to the United Kingdom found that 43% became ill during or shortly after their journeys (12).

The previously cited studies offer a small glimpse into the medical problems of travelers. Even so, we do not have any reliable measurement of the amount or severity of disease encountered by the traveler. Only a portion of the most dramatic cases of illness in travelers such as malaria, lassa fever, or African trypanosomiasis are ever reported to public health authorities. At present, there is no mechanism for obtaining accurate surveillance data on either the incidence or prevalence of illness in American travelers, nor are there data on significant risk factors for acquiring infectious diseases. This lack of data hampers scientific investigation of interventional strategies in travelers. Even so, significant progress has been made in the prevention of malaria, travelers' diarrhea, and diseases for which immunizations exist.

Factors such as the low cost of air travel and being accustomed to safe water, safe food, and unrestricted access to swimming place large numbers of Americans at risk of contracting diseases in the tropics and presenting to their physicians at home: e.g., a college student on a safari in Kenya can be bitten by an Anopheles mosquito carrying sporozoites of *Plasmodium falciparum* and 2 weeks later be back at college when the fever and chills begin.

To prevent unnecessary illness, it is imperative that travelers undertake appropriate pretrip health planning. When approached by a person about to embark upon an international journey, it is important to ascertain several key aspects of the proposed trip. "Where are you going?," "Where will you stay?," "What is the purpose of your trip?," "Where will you be eating? In restaurants or in private homes?" are all questions that need to be asked. After the traveler has answered these questions, one can categorize the traveler as either high or low risk. The *low risk traveler* is exemplified by the businessman staying for a short period of time in a first class hotel in a large city in a developed country. This traveler is rarely if ever at any greater risk than that associated with traveling in the United States. However, such travelers to developing countries should not be complacent about food and water (see below) because they plan to stay at first class hotels. At the other end of the spectrum is the *high risk traveler*, such as the college student who will be living at the village level in multiple developing countries. This traveler is at significant risk and should receive complete pretrip health planning. Most travelers fit somewhere between these two extremes. In addition to the risks associated with the itinerary, the traveler's present health status, history of chronic diseases, use of medications, allergies, and immunization record are important in planning for a safe trip.

Immunizations, malaria prevention, food and water safety, diarrhea, schistosomiasis, and a number of general health hazards are topics that may need to be discussed with the traveler. Two useful resources that are updated yearly provide practical information on these issues: "Health Information for International Travel" published by the United States Public Health Service (available from the Centers for Disease Control, Atlanta, GA 30333) and "Vaccination Certificate Requirements for International Travel and Health Advice to Travelers" published by the World Health Organization (available from WHO Publication Center, USA, 49 Sheridan Avenue, Albany, NY 12210).

IMMUNIZATIONS

Vaccines are now available against a number of the major viral and bacterial diseases encountered in developing areas (see Table 33.1). Immunizations can be broadly separated into those that are legally required and those that are recommended. Legally required vaccinations are public health measures that certain countries demand prior to entry, to benefit the country as a whole, whereas recommended immunizations are designed only to benefit the individual. In order to enter or return to the United States, there are no legally required vaccines. Many countries, however, do have strict entry requirements, and travelers who arrive without proper vaccination certificates may be denied entry, quarantined, or possibly vaccinated at the point of entry. Therefore, it is important to determine what vaccines are required before beginning a journey.

Presently, the only legally required vaccinations are those for cholera and yellow fever, and each country has its own requirements for them. In the past, smallpox vaccination was required by many countries, but in 1980 the World Health Organization declared the global eradication of smallpox and on January 1, 1982, smallpox was deleted from the list of diseases subject to regulation.

Yellow Fever

Yellow fever vaccine, containing a live attenuated strain of the yellow fever virus, is one of the most important and effective vaccines. It is required by some countries before travelers are allowed entrance, particularly when areas to be visited are endemic for yellow fever. If yellow fever exists in the country of destination, the traveler should be vaccinated regardless of the regulations of the country (Figs. 33.1 and 33.2). The vaccine is relatively nontoxic and induces long lasting immunity. Reactions, which are generally mild, occur in 1 to 5% of vaccinees. These include mild headache, myalgia, low grade fever, or other minor symptoms 5 to 10 days after inoculation. Because yellow fever vaccine is a live attenuated virus, it poses a theoretical risk to the pregnant woman, although teratogenicity has not been encountered. Pregnant women who must travel to yellow fever endemic areas should be vaccinated. It is presumed that the unknown but small risk to the fetus is less than the risk to the mother. If at all possible, the trip should be postponed until after delivery. The vaccine is contraindicated in immunocompromised patients. Because the vaccine strain is grown in chick embryo culture, it should not be given to travelers with known hypersensitivity to eggs. Yellow fever immunization is also not recommended in children less than 9 months of age. Yellow fever vaccine is available only through official yellow fever vaccine centers; locations of these centers can be obtained by calling the local health department. The dose of vaccine is 0.5 ml subcutaneously, and it must be given within 1 hour of reconstitution. The vaccine should be stored at 5°C until it is reconstituted. The vaccine gives solid immunity for at least 10 years. If it is contraindicated for a traveler to receive yellow fever vaccine for any of the above reasons, a detailed letter explaining the contraindications should be provided to the traveler.

Cholera

In 1973, the World Health Assembly recommended discontinuing required vaccination against cholera. Even so, vaccination against cholera is still required for entry into a few countries. Presently, no country requires cholera vaccination for travelers coming directly from the United States, but several countries do require proof of cholera vaccination for those travelers coming from areas where cholera is endemic. Unless the vaccine is legally required, it is not recommended because, although cholera is widespread around the world, infection in travelers is extremely rare; and the vaccine, a killed vaccine, is of limited effectiveness (14). For travelers following usual tourist routes and using standard precautions in countries endemic for cholera, the estimated attack rate is less than one in a million trips (11). Therefore, rather than recommend immunization, one should emphatically instruct travelers to cholera endemic areas not to eat uncooked vegetables and to always drink boiled water or bottled beverages.

If a traveler requires vaccination, one injection will satisfy entry requirements. The vaccine can be given both intradermally or subcutaneously, but intradermal injection may cause fewer reactions. The intradermal

Table 33.1.
Vaccines and Immune Globulins for International Travel

Vaccine/Immune Globulin	Patient	Route	Dose	Booster	Comments
Yellow Fever	>9 mos	SC[a]	0.5 ml	0.5 ml Q 10 yrs	May be required
Cholera	6 mos–4 yrs	SC	0.2 ml	0.2 ml Q 6 mos	May be required
	5–10 yrs	or	0.3 ml	0.3 ml Q 6 mos	Limited efficacy
	>10 yrs	IM[b]	0.5 ml	0.5 ml Q 6 mos	
Typhoid	<10 yrs	SC	0.25 ml	0.25 ml Q 3 yrs	Local reactions common
	>10 yrs		0.50 ml	0.5 ml Q 3 yrs	
Poliomyelitis					
OPV	all ages	Oral	3 doses	1 dose pretravel	IPV is preferable for adults
IPV	all ages	IM	4 doses	1 dose Q 10 yrs	
Japanese Encephalitis	<3 yrs	SC	0.5 ml	unclear	Not available in the United States
	>3 yrs		1.0 ml		
Immune Serum Globulin	<23 kg	IM	0.5 ml	—	Immune globulin is used
(short term <3 mos)	23–45 kg		1.0 ml	—	for prophylaxis of
	>45 kg		2.0 ml	—	hepatitis A
(long term >3 mos)	<23 kg	IM	1.0 ml	1.0 ml Q 6 mos	
	23–45 kg		2.5 ml	2.5 ml Q 6 mos	
	>45 kg		5.0 ml	5.0 ml Q 6 mos	
Tetanus-diphtheria	>7 yrs	IM	3 doses	1 dose Q 10 yrs	Always use combined vaccine
Meningitis A, C, Y, W135	>2 yrs	IM	0.5 ml	Unclear	For specific areas of travel
Rabies	All ages	IM	1.0 ml	1 dose Q 2 yrs	Still required postexpo-
		ID[c]	0.1 ml (3 doses)	1 dose Q 2 yrs	sure treatment
Hepatitis B	all ages	IM	1.0 ml 3 doses	unclear	Protection lasts 5–7 yrs

[a] Subcutaneous.
[b] Intramuscular.
[c] Intradermal.

dose is 0.2 ml for those 5 years and older. For intramuscular or subcutaneous dosing, see Table 33.1. Chlorea vaccination is not recommended for infants under 6 months old. The vaccine certificate is valid for 6 months.

Typhoid Fever

The Centers for Disease Control (CDC) has analyzed all cases of typhoid fever in American citizens from 1970 to 1979. Over 900 cases were reported; 62% of those occurred in travelers. In addition, many areas of the world are reporting multiple antibiotic resistance in *Salmonella typhi*, the organism that causes typhoid fever.

Typhoid vaccination, though not legally required, is recommended for certain high risk travelers because typhoid fever is endemic in most areas of the developing world (17). *S. typhi* is transmitted by the ingestion of contaminated food and water. If such travelers are likely to stray off the usual tourist route, stay in small villages, and eat local food, they should be immunized because of the increased risk.

The currently available killed typhoid vaccine provides approximately 70 to 90% protection depending in part on the degree of subsequent exposure. The acetone-dried typhoid vaccine should be used without the paratyphoid component. Paratyphoid antigen offers little protection and is responsible for many of

the side effects common with typhoid immunization. Even so, the typhoid vaccine frequently causes pain at the injection site, fever, headache, and malaise for 1 to 3 days. If the traveler has never been vaccinated before, the primary sequence is two inoculations 1 month apart (see Table 33.1 for doses). Booster doses should be given every 3 years.

A new live oral attenuated typhoid vaccine as well as a Vi capsular polysaccharide vaccine have been recently studied and show promise, but these are not yet available for routine use.

Polio

Status of protection against poliomyelitis should be considered in any traveler visiting developing areas because poliomyelitis remains endemic in most parts of the developing world. Travelers who have previously completed primary series with either the Sabin (oral, live) or Salk (parental, inactivated) vaccine should have a booster dose if the last immunization was given more than 10 years previously. A history of at least three doses of oral polio vaccine (OPV, Sabin) or four doses of inactivated polio vaccine (IPV, Salk) with IPV boosters each 5 years until age 18 is evidence of adequate primary immunization. Such fully immunized people need only one dose of polio vaccine before traveling to high risk areas. If a traveler is only partially immunized, he should complete the primary series.

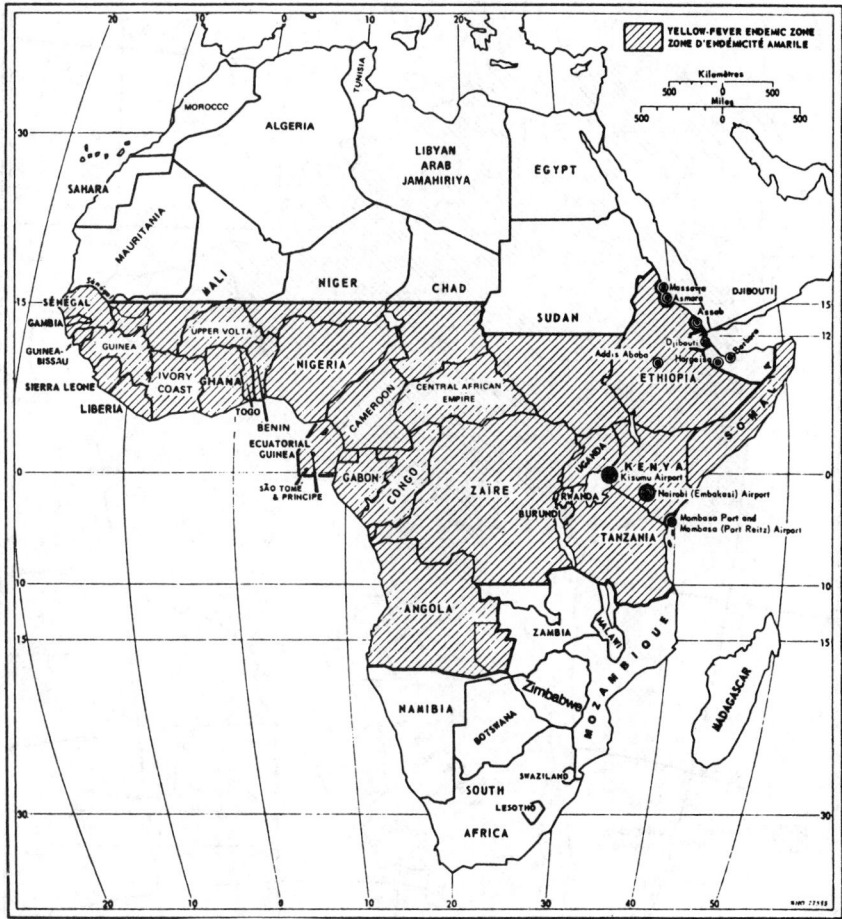

Figure 33.1. Yellow fever endemic zone in Africa. (From *Health Information International Travel, 1983.* Supplement to *Morbidity and Mortality Weekly Report*, vol 32, August, 1983. US Department of Health and Human Services, HHS Publication no. (CDC) 83-8280.)

Adults who require a primary series should receive IPV. IPV is preferred in adults because the risk of OPV-associated paralysis is somewhat higher in adults than in children. If children are not already vaccinated, they should receive a primary series with OPV, which is the preferred vaccine for individuals younger than 18. If an unimmunized adult traveler does not have time to complete a primary IPV series prior to departure, a single dose of OPV may offer reasonable protection. On return, he should be primarily immunized with IPV. Live (OPV) vaccine should not be given routinely to women known to be pregnant, although teratogenicity has not been shown. If the risk of polio is significant and the pregnant woman is unimmunized, primary vaccination with IPV would be prudent. Because OPV is a live virus, immunocompromised patients and their families should not receive OPV; instead they should be immunized with IPV. Table 33.1 summarizes information regarding doses for polio vaccines.

Tetanus and Diphtheria

Tetanus occurs worldwide but is slightly more common in the tropics. Thus, tetanus immunization should be kept up to date in travelers. Boosters need to be given every 10 years regardless of age. Travelers, if they injure themselves, are less likely to seek medical help so that adequate pretravel immunization becomes more important. Diphtheria is endemic in many developing countries, and most cases occur in unimmunized or partially immunized individuals. Therefore, routine immunization with tetanus-diphtheria (Td) should be given rather than tetanus toxoid alone. For primary immunization, persons older than 7 years should receive three doses of Td. (Before age 7, the primary immunizing agent is the diphtheria, pertussis, tetanus combination or DPT.) The first doses are 1 to 2 months apart and the third 6 to 12 months later. Local reactions may occur within 12 to 48 hours after vaccination. Severe local reactions can occur in adults if the booster is given within a short time of the previous vaccine. Therefore, routine boosters should not be given more often than every 10 years. The only contraindication to Td is a history of hypersensitivity reactions after prior immunization.

Hepatitis A

Hepatitis A continues to be an important risk for travelers to many areas of the developing world. Although the risk is small for individuals who travel on

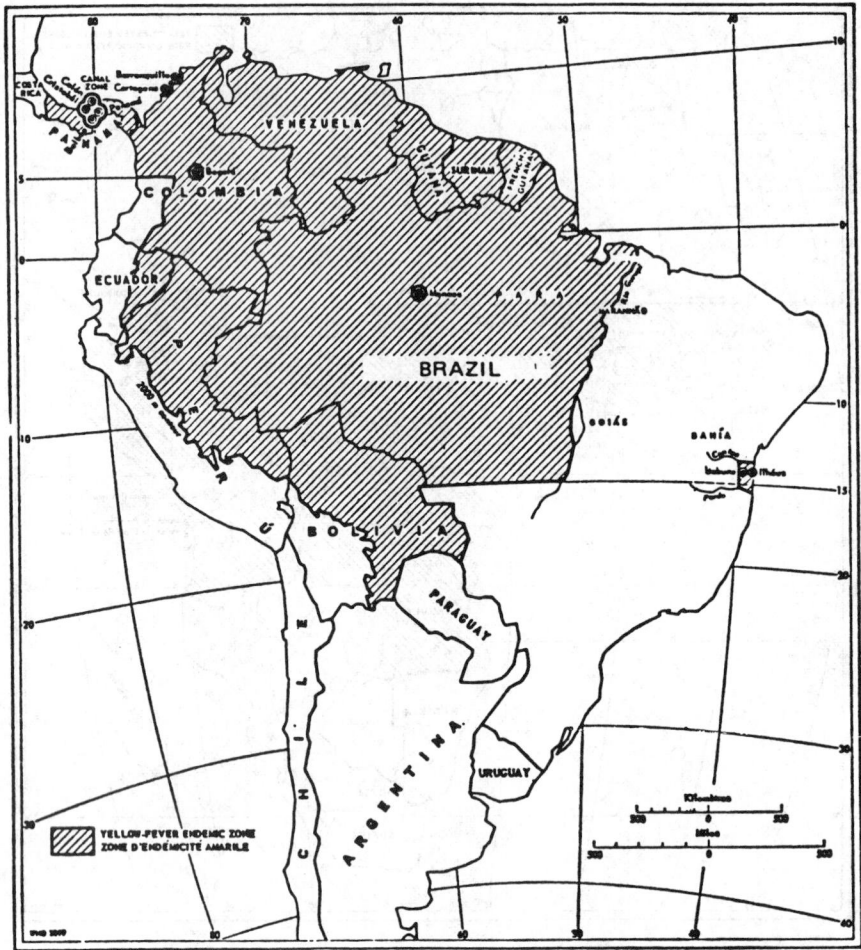

Figure 33.2.   Yellow fever endemic zone in the Americas. (From *Health Information for International Travel, 1983*. Supplement to *Morbidity and Mortality Weekly Report*, vol 32, August, 1983. US Department of Health and Human Services, HHS Publication no. (CDC) 83-8280.)

ordinary tourist routes and stay for short periods of time, it may be considerable for those individuals who bypass the tourist routes and stay for extended periods of time. Immune globulin provides passive protection against hepatitis A and should be strongly advised for high risk travelers. The dose of immune globulin given may be based on weight, but in practice, for adults, injection of 2 ml for stays of less than 3 months, and 5 ml for stays of 3 to 6 months, is usually given. Travelers who will be staying for an extended period of time should have repeated immune globulin, in the same doses, every 6 months. Immune globulin should be given very near to the date of departure to ensure longer efficacy. The only side effects are muscle soreness at the injection site. Immune globulins prepared in the United States carry no risk of transmission of human immunodeficiency virus (HIV) or other infectious agents. Pregnancy is not a contraindication to immune globulin.

Hepatitis B

The risk of hepatitis B is generally low for the routine traveler. Health care workers who are likely to have contact with blood or secretions from patients in areas endemic for hepatitis B should receive hepatitis B vaccine. The prevalence of hepatitis B virus carriers is 5 to 15% in sub-Saharan Africa and Southeast Asia including China and Indonesia, and between 1 and 5% in North Africa, South Central Asia, and Southern Europe. Because hepatitis B can be transmitted through sexual contact, travelers should be counseled appropriately when going to endemic areas. Vaccination or hepatitis B immune globulin (HBIG) prophylaxis may be appropriate for individuals who are likely to have sexual contacts. Primary adult vaccination consists of three intramuscular doses of 1 ml of vaccine. The first two doses are given 1 month apart and the third dose should be given 6 months later (see additional details in Chapters 32 and 43).

Rabies

Rabies remains an important public health problem in many areas of the developing world and has occurred in travelers. Rabies transmission occurs when rabies virus is introduced into open cuts or wounds, usually through the bite of an infected animal. Pre-exposure rabies prophylaxis, which consists of three inoculations of human diploid cell killed-virus vaccine (1 ml intramuscularly on days 0, 7, and 21 or 28) is appropriate for long-term travelers who will live in endemic areas. Individuals who anticipate animal exposure such as veterinarians, animal handlers, and laboratory workers should also be vaccinated. Persons with continued risk of rabies exposure should receive a booster dose of vaccine (1 ml) every 2 years. Children are especially at risk because of the increased likelihood of contact with stray dogs. The human diploid cell vaccine is more immunogenic and causes fewer reactions than the old duck embryo vaccine. Occasional local reactions and rare systemic reactions such as headaches, myalgias, and dizziness may occur.

The human diploid cell vaccine (HDCV) may be also administered to travelers by the intradermal route (0.1 ml on days 0. 7, and 21 or 28) if the three-dose series is completed 30 days or more before departure. Intradermal rabies vaccine is as immunogenic as intramuscular vaccine, but since the dose is one-tenth of the intramuscular dose, it is less costly. The HDCV should not be administered by the intradermal route when chloroquine or other drugs that may interfere with the immune response are being used.

Pregnancy is not a contraindication to pre-exposure prophylaxis. If the previously vaccinated traveler is exposed to rabies, he or she should still seek medical help for postexposure immunization, described in Chapter 32. Any animal bite should be thoroughly cleansed with soap and water to help reduce the rabies risk.

Tuberculosis

Tuberculosis continues to be a worldwide health problem, but the risk to the short-term traveler is small. *Mycobacterium tuberculosis* is primarily a respiratory pathogen contracted by inhaling droplet nuclei, but unpasteurized milk products can also spread the disease. Travelers who will be spending extended periods of time in tuberculosis endemic areas should have a tuberculin skin test prior to departure. Calmette-Guérin bacillus (BCG) vaccine use is controversial and most United States experts do not recommend it. Periodic skin tests in long-term travelers are recommended to detect subclinical infections.

Measles, Mumps, Rubella, Influenza

In most developing and developed countries other than the United States, measles, mumps, and rubella remain uncontrolled. Therefore, prior to travel children should have received routine immunizations against these diseases. Adolescents and adults who have neither had these diseases nor been immunized against them are at risk of becoming infected while traveling. These diseases may be much more serious in adults, and vaccination should be strongly considered. Rubella vaccine is indicated for females of childbearing age without serological evidence of prior rubella infection.

Certain travelers may benefit from pretrip vaccination with influenza vaccine. Influenza causes morbidity and mortality throughout the world and poses risk to unvaccinated travelers. The same criteria for selecting candidates for influenza vaccine in the United States should be used.

Chapter 32 contains details regarding doses and schedules for these vaccines.

Japanese Encephalitis

Japanese encephalitis (JE) is a mosquito-borne viral encephalitis that occurs in epidemics in much of Asia including China and endemically in the tropical areas of Southeast Asia. The risk to short-term travelers and persons who confine their travel to urban centers is low. Persons at greatest risk are those living for prolonged periods of time in endemic or epidemic areas. No vaccine for JE is licensed for use in the United States. The Biken vaccine, manufactured in Japan, appears to be immunogenic, efficacious, and safe and has been used to vaccinate millions of people. Vaccination with this vaccine should be considered for persons planning long-term residence in endemic areas, and for those travelers visiting rural farming areas or sleeping in unscreened rooms in endemic or epidemic areas. Travelers may inquire about the availability of the vaccine at American embassies in countries where JE is endemic. The agency that has been involved with this vaccine on an experimental basis in this country is the Center for Disease Control, Fort Collins, Colorado (303-221-6429).

Miscellaneous Vaccines: Typhus, Plague, Meningococcal

Typhus vaccine is no longer available, and the disease poses little risk except for those working with louse-infected refugees. No typhus has been reported in an American traveler since 1950.

Plague exists in certain rural areas in Africa, Asia, and South America. Vaccination is not recommended for most travelers, but if the traveler will have direct contact with wild rodents in plague-enzootic areas, vaccination should be considered. Local and systemic reactions after plague vaccine occur frequently.

Meningococcal meningitis occurs throughout the developing world, often in devastating epidemics. Although cases in American travelers are rare, vaccine may be indicated in travelers going to countries with known epidemics. Most recently, pretravel immunization has been recommended by the CDC for travelers to (a) New Delhi and Northern India, (b) the meningitis belt of Sahel (subSaharan Africa), (c) Saudi Arabia after outbreaks in pilgrims returning from Mecca, and (d) Nepal, especially in mountain travelers. Currently the only vaccine available for use in the United States is the A, C, Y, W-135 Quadrivalent vaccine (Menomune, Connaught). The dose of vaccine is 0.5 ml given subcutaneously.

Timing of Vaccines

Many travelers go to see their physician just before their departure. In this situation, all active immunizations can be given concurrently. There is, however, some evidence that cholera vaccine may decrease slightly the efficacy of yellow fever vaccine if the two vaccines are given within 3 weeks of each other. Otherwise, simultaneous administration of multiple vaccines produces good antibody responses to all the antigens. However, when it is possible, multiple vaccinations should be spread out over time, and all should be completed by 1 week before arrival in a developing country to decrease the likelihood of reactions and to assure that adequate antibody levels have been attained. When vaccines are administered concurrently, they should be given with separate syringes at different body sites. Killed vaccines can be given at the same time as immune globulin. With certain live attenuated vaccines (especially measles, mumps, rubella), passively acquired antibody may interfere with replication of the vaccine virus and decrease the efficacy of the vaccine. Therefore, if possible, live virus vaccines should be given at least 14 days *before* the administration of immune globulin and probably 3 months *after* administration. Immune globulin does not interfere with either yellow fever or oral polio vaccines, both of which are live.

MALARIA PROPHYLAXIS

Malaria is a potentially fatal parasitic disease caused by infection of red blood cells with plasmodia species. It is usually transmitted by *Anopheles* mosquitoes but can be acquired from transfused blood and intravenous drug use. Malaria tends to be more severe in immunologically "virgin" travelers than in residents of endemic areas. The disease is characterized by high fevers, chills, sweats, myalgias, and headache with no obvious focal signs or symptoms of infection. Malaria exists worldwide (Fig. 33.3). The risk of contracting malaria varies from country to country and from season to season depending upon local conditions such as rainfall, altitude, and mosquito density. Because malaria is almost a totally preventable disease in travelers, there should be no deaths in travelers due to malaria. Each year, though, American travelers still die because of inadequate protection against malaria. Prevention of malaria requires a 2-fold approach: (a) to minimize mosquito contact and (b) to take appropriate prophylactic medicine.

To avoid mosquito exposure, travelers should sleep in screened rooms and under mosquito nets. *Anopheles* mosquitoes feed predominantly from dusk to dawn. Therefore, travelers who must be out during this time should try to cover exposed body parts with clothing or insect repellent. Long-sleeved shirts, long-legged trousers, and occasionally a face net should be worn if at all possible. Mosquito repellent containing N, N-diethyl-meta-toluamide (deet) should be applied to ex-

posed skin. Outdoor nighttime activity should be avoided whenever possible.

Even with appropriate mosquito protection, travelers may get bitten by malarious mosquitoes. It is therefore necessary when traveling to a malarious area to take an appropriate chemoprophylactic drug (Table 33.2). Malaria chemoprophylaxis should preferably begin 1 to 2 weeks prior to travel and should continue for 4 weeks after leaving the malarious areas. Regardless of the chemoprophylaxis employed, it is still possible to contract malaria. Symptoms of malaria can develop as early as 1 week after initial exposure and as late as several months after departure from a malarious area. Before deciding on a chemoprophylactic regimen, it is important to obtain recent information regarding country-specific malaria risk. The Centers for Disease Control maintains up-to-date information that is available by calling (404-639-1610).

In selecting the appropriate chemoprophylactic agent(s) several factors need to be taken into consideration. The most important consideration is whether the traveler will be at risk of acquiring chloroquine-resistant *Plasmodium falciparum* (CFPF) malaria (see below).

For travel to malarious areas where CRPF has not been reported or is at a very low level, once weekly chloroquine phosphate, 500 mg of the phosphate salt (300 mg base), should be taken. Chloroquine is usually well tolerated, but a few people may experience mild side effects including itching, nausea, and disorientation. Side effects can be minimized by taking the drug with meals or in divided twice weekly doses. As an alternative, the related compound hydroxychloroquine may be better tolerated. Amodiaquine, another related compound (not available in the United States), should not be used because of associated hepatotoxicity and marrow depression. When chloroquine is used for prolonged periods of time in high doses as in the therapy of rheumatoid arthritis, it may be associated with a severe retinopathy. This serious side effect is very rare when chloroquine is used at the relatively low doses for malaria chemoprophylaxis. The risk of retinopathy appears to increase after a cumulative dose of 100 g of base, and periodic retinal examinations should be considered in persons who have taken this much chloroquine. Chloroquine is believed to be safe in pregnant and lactating women and should be recommended to pregnant women traveling to malaria endemic zones.

Routine chemoprophylaxis with chloroquine has been complicated by the emergence of chloroquine resistance in *P. falciparum*. Travelers to areas with known chloroquine resistance, including South East Asia, parts of Africa, Indonesia, and Oceania, as well as the Amazonian basin (Fig. 33.4), are at risk of contracting chloroquine-resistant malaria if chloroquine alone is used for chemoprophylaxis. Until recently, it was recommended that travelers to these areas take Fansidar (pyrimethamine, 25 mg, and sulfadoxine, 500 mg) in addition to chloroquine. Because of the risk of adverse reactions to Fansidar, which include blood

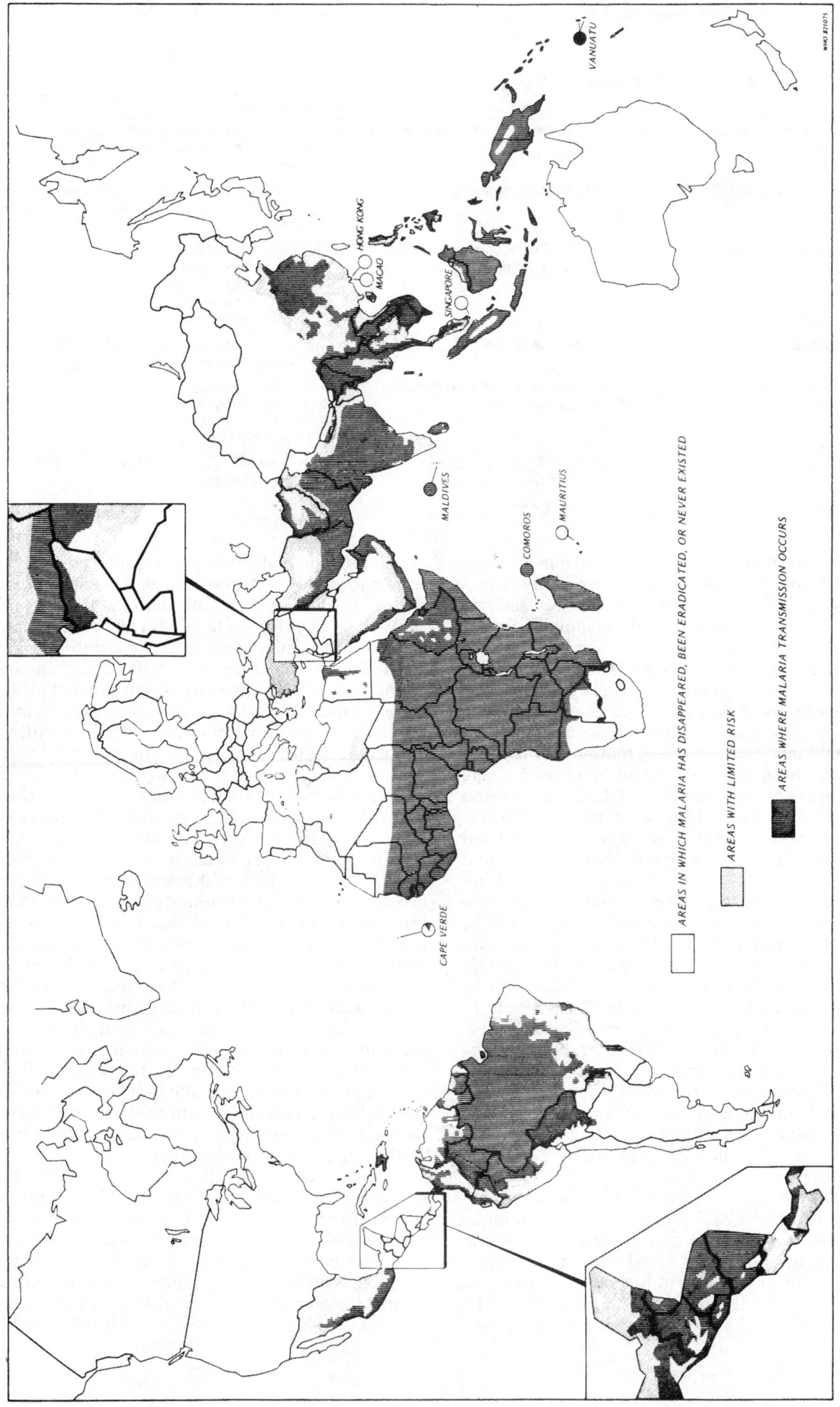

Figure 33.3. Epidemiological assessment of status of malaria, 1982. (From *Vaccination Certificate Requirements for International Travel and Health Advice to Travelers.* Geneva, World Health Organization, 1984.)

AREAS IN WHICH MALARIA HAS DISAPPEARED, BEEN ERADICATED, OR NEVER EXISTED

AREAS WITH LIMITED RISK

AREAS WHERE MALARIA TRANSMISSION OCCURS

VANUATU

HONG KONG

MACAO

SINGAPORE

MALDIVES

COMOROS

MAURITIUS

CAPE VERDE

WHO 871075

Table 33.2.
Drugs Used In The Prophylaxis of Malaria

Drugs	Adult Dose	Pediatric Dose
Choloroquine phosphate (Aralen)	300 mg base (500 mg salt) orally, once/week	5 mg/kg base (8.3 mg/kg salt) orally, once/week, up to a maximal dose of 300 mg base
Hydroxychloroquine sulfate (Plaquenil)	310 mg base (400 mg salt) orally, once/week	5 mg/kg base (6.5 mg/kg salt) orally, once/week, up to maximal adult dose of 310 mg base
Pyrimethamine-sulfadoxine (Fansidar)	1 tablet (25 mg pyrimethamine and 500 mg sulfadoxine) once/weekly	2–11 mos: ⅛ tablet/week 1–3 yrs: ¼ tablet/week 4–8 yrs: ½ tablet/week 9–14 yrs: ¾ tablet/week >14 yrs: 1 tablet/week
Doxycycline	100 mg orally, once/day	>8 years of age: 2 mg/kg of body weight orally/day, up to adult dose of 100 mg/day
Proguanil (not available in United States	200 mg orally, once/day in combination with weekly chloroquine	<2 yrs: 500 mg/day 2–6 yrs: 100 mg/day 7–10 yrs: 150 mg/day >10 yrs: 200 m g/day
Primaquine	15 mg base (26.3 mg salt) orally, once/day for 14 days	0.3 mg/kg base (0.5 mg/kg salt) orally once/day for 14 days
Mefloquine	250 mgm once/week	

dyscrasias, erythema multiforme, Stevens-Johnson syndrome, and toxic epidermal necrolysis, these recommendations have been altered (6). The revised recommendations place increased responsibility on individual travelers and their physicians. *Short-term travelers (less than 3 weeks)* to areas with a high level of transmission of chloroquine-resistant *P. falciparum* malaria, including East Africa and Oceania (Papua, New Guinea, Solomon Islands, Vanuatua, and Irian Jaya), should take chloroquine as routine prophylaxis. In addition, these travelers should be given a single treatment dose of Fansidar (three tablets) to be taken if they develop a febrile illness compatible with malaria and they are unable to get prompt professional medical care. This is a temporary measure only, and travelers still should be advised to seek medical follow-up as soon as possible. *For travelers staying more than 3 weeks in* these areas, consideration should be given to using Fansidar, one tablet weekly, in combination with chloroquine. If weekly use of Fansidar is prescribed, the traveler should be advised to discontinue it immediately if any side effects occur. In laboratory animals, pyrimethamine has been shown to be teratogenic and therefore Fansidar should not be prescribed to women who are pregnant or may become pregnant. Travel to chloroquine-resistant areas should be avoided if at all possible, and, if necessary, extreme precaution should be used to avoid mosquitoes. Chloroquine can be made into a liquid form for children (dose is 5 mg/kg).

There are a number of *alternative chemoprophylactic regimens for CRPF.* There is now preliminary evidence that doxycycline may be effective as a suppressive agent, and it may be taken as a chemoprophylactic agent for short-term travelers to areas with CRPF. It is especially useful for those with a sulfa allergy. Travelers who use doxycycline must be alert to potential side effects including sun sensitivity and gastrointestinal tract intolerance. The dose of doxycycline is 100 mg by mouth daily, and it should be started one to two days before travel to the malarious areas and for four weeks after departure. Proguanil (Paludrine) has been used both alone and in combination with other antimalarials, but it is not available in the United States. The British use proguanil as their prophylactic agent of choice. Proguanil is a dihydrofolate reductase inhibitor and some resistance to it has been reported. Limited data suggest that it is effective in Kenya, but not in Thailand and Papua New Guinea. If travelers use proguanil, it should be taken as a daily 200-mg dose in combination with chloroquine. Mefloquine, a new antimalarial that is similar to quinine, is very effective against CRPF, although resistance to it is also beginning to be reported. It has only recently been licensed in the United States, and general guidelines for its use are being developed. Mefloquine should be used in areas where there is a high risk of transmission of CRPF or where CRPF and Fansidar resistance exists. The adult prophylactic dose is 250 mg once weekly. Minor side effects include dizziness and gastrointestinal disturbances, which tend to be transient and self-limited. Mafloquine has occasionally been associated with asymptomatic bradycardia and a prolonged QT interval and should not be used by travelers taking beta blockers, calcium channel blockers, or other cardiac drugs that alter conduction.

Routine malaria prophylaxis with either chloroquine or Fansidar does not prevent delayed attacks of malaria from *Plasmodium vivax* or *Plasmodium ovale* because these species have an extra-erythrocytic chronic liver phase not eradicated by these two agents. Primaquine is an 8-aminoquinolone drug that is effective against the chronic liver forms of vivax and ovale malaria. For travelers with minimal mosquito exposure

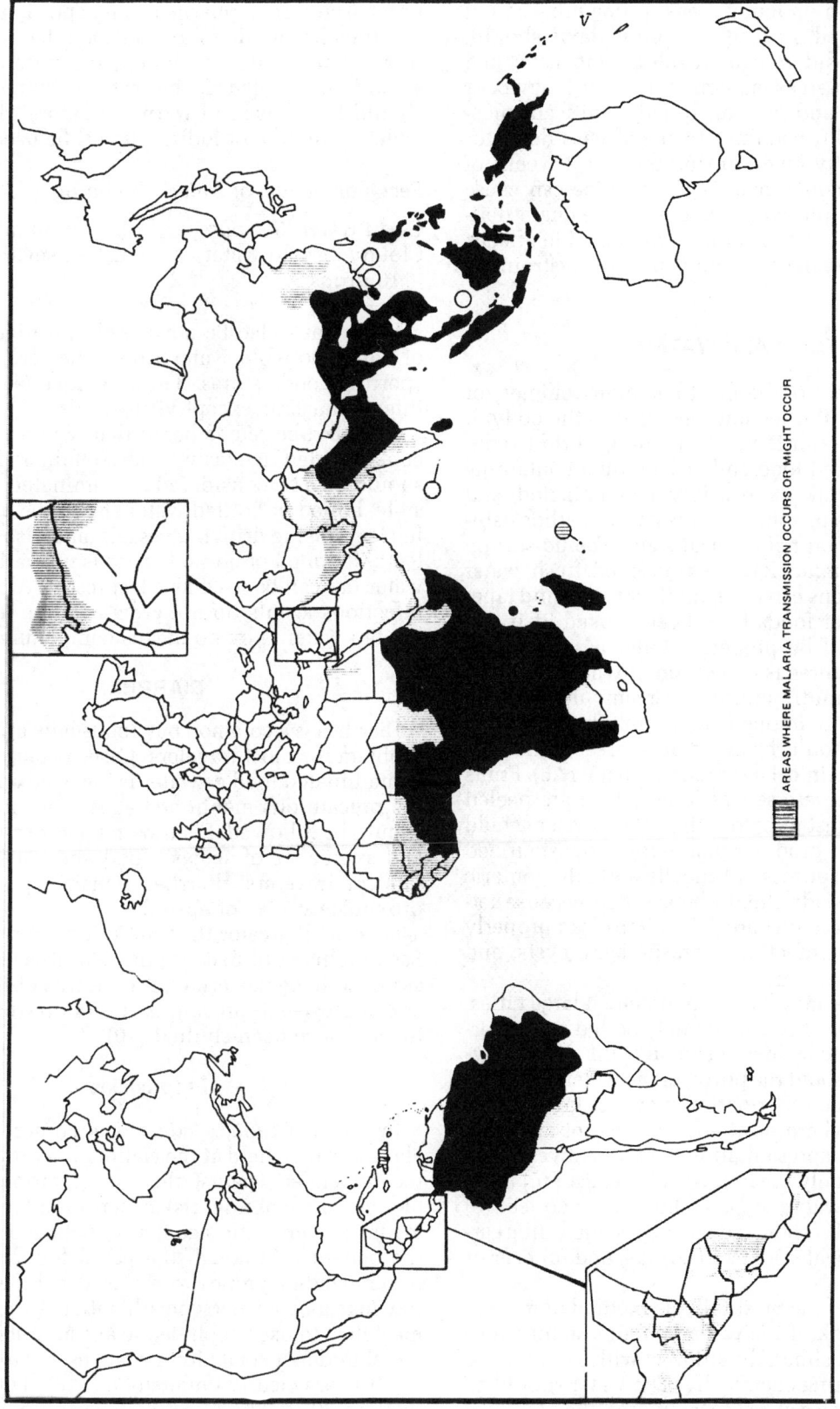

Figure 33.4. Areas with chloroquine-resistant *Plasmodium falciparum*, 1988. (From Malaria Branch, Centers for Disease Control, Atlanta, Georgia.)

AREAS WHERE MALARIA TRANSMISSION OCCURS OR MIGHT OCCUR

and short stays in endemic areas, primaquine is not routinely indicated. Primaquine prophylaxis should, however, be considered in travelers who have had extended stays in areas endemic for either *P. vivax* or *P. ovale* malaria and who have had significant mosquito exposure. Primaquine, 15 mg of base daily for 14 days, is usually given during the last 2 weeks of chloroquine chemoprophylaxis. Primaquine can cause hemolysis in people with glucose 6-phosphate deficiency, and it has several other potential side effects, such as headache, nausea, vomiting, and gastrointestinal distress.

FOOD AND WATER

Food and water are the most common vehicles for the introduction of infectious agents into the body. It is best for the traveler to the developing world to consider any uncooked food and any product containing unpasteurized milk as possibly contaminated and therefore not safe to consume. Meats can harbor pathogens such as *Trichinella spiralis* and *Taenia solium* and *Taenia saginata*. Raw or uncooked fresh water fish and crustaceans can transmit liver flukes and tapeworms. Even after foods have been cooked, it is imperative that food be properly stored. Food held at ambient temperatures is a medium in which bacterial pathogens can rapidly multiply. Creamy desserts are often vehicles for *Salmonella* and staphylococcal food poisoning and should be avoided in areas with poor refrigeration (see clinical description, Chapter 26). Fruits that can be peeled are safe as long as they are peeled by the consumer just prior to eating. The traveler should be wary of cheese products made from unpasteurized milk as possible sources of brucella and other enteric pathogens (2). Salads should be avoided because lettuce and leafy vegetables are difficult to clean properly and often harbor infectious parasite eggs, cysts, and bacteria.

Although water may be safe in hotels in large cities, only water that has been adequately boiled and chlorinated should be considered safe to drink. If the traveler is uncertain about the purity of the water, it should be boiled. Routine chlorination may not kill all parasites. In areas where purified water is not available or where hygiene and sanitation are poor, travelers are advised to drink only the following beverages: (*a*) those that use boiled water, such as hot tea or coffee; (*b*) canned or bottled carbonated beverages, including carbonated bottled water and soft drinks; and (*c*) beer or wine.

Boiling is by far the most reliable method of making water safe to drink. If the water contains sediment or floating matter, it should be strained with a cloth prior to boiling or treating chemically. The water should be boiled vigorously for at least 10 minutes, then allowed to cool to room temperature. If boiling is not possible, water can be chemically disinfected with tincture of iodine or tetraglycine hydroperiodide tablets. Cloudy water should always be strained to remove sediment before adding iodine. The purification tablets can be purchased from a pharmacy or a sporting goods store. The traveler should follow the manufacturer's instructions. If the water is cloudy, the number of tablets should be doubled. If the water is extremely cold, it should be allowed to warm up before dissolving the tablets. Tincture of iodine should be used as follows:

Per Quart or Liter of Water	Timing
Clean water, 5 drops	Let sit 30 minutes
Cloudy or cold water, 10 drops	Let sit several hours

Water may also be adequately purified by the use of small portable water filters that are available in sporting goods stores. These remove all water-borne infection agents except viruses.

It should be remembered that where water may be contaminated, ice (as well as containers for drinking) should also be considered contaminated. If at all possible, boiled or bottled water should be used for making ice, rinsing drinking vessels, and also for brushing teeth. If boiled or bottled water is unavailable, the hot water tap can be used as a last resort. Although many infectious agents do not grow at these temperatures, hot tap water is by no means completely safe.

DIARRHEA

Diarrhea is a common but not usually a serious health problem for most travelers. Cases occur when fecally contaminated food or water is ingested and, therefore, the precautions mentioned above for food and water should be followed. Even with good personal hygiene and avoidance of suspect food and water, the attack rate for travelers' diarrhea remains quite high. Approximately 75% of episodes are caused by bacterial agents, with greater than 50% due to enterotoxigenic *Escherichia coli*. Because the causative agents can be assumed to be bacterial three-fourths of the time, several strategies to prevent bacterial diarrhea or to treat it early have been studied (10).

Prophylaxis

In January 1985, a consensus conference on traveler's diarrhea held at the National Institutes of Health recommended against the use of prophylactic antibiotics. The potential risk of serious adverse reactions to the prophylactic agent was believed to outweigh the benefits. Although the panel found no basis for recommending prophylaxis, they concluded that "some travelers may wish to consult with their physician and may elect to use prophylactic antimicrobial agents for travel under special circumstances, once the risks and benefits are clearly understood" (18). Two antibiotics that are 80 to 90% effective for prophylaxis are doxycycline (100 mg) and trimethoprim-sulfamethoxazole (one double-strength tablet), taken once daily (13). Limited studies have also shown that norfloxacin (Noroxin), 400 mg daily, is also effective. The usual traveler should not be subjected to the risk of antimicrobials, but if antimicrobials are used they should be limited to those persons traveling to developing countries for less than 3 weeks, especially persons with medical conditions that could be worsened by diarrhea.

Treatment

Most cases of diarrhea are self-limited and may only require rest and *replacement of fluids and salts*. This can usually be accomplished with fruit drinks or carbonated beverages. When traveler's diarrhea is severe, the traveler should be advised to take a few packets of oral rehydration salts (ORT), such as Orlyte, to be mixed with clean water (see above) when needed. Severe diarrhea can cause dehydration and can possibly result in significant morbidity. Drinking the oral rehydration solution prevents the dehydration and increases the sense of well-being even though it does not stop the diarrhea. Commercial ORT products are available in most countries. Commercial products designed to replace losses through perspiration (e.g., Gatoraid) are not equivalent to ORT preparations. If no packets are available, a similar solution can be prepared by placing 1 level teaspoon of salt plus 4 level teaspoons of table sugar in a liter of water. The packet is preferable, however, because it provides a more "complete" formula. Any solution remaining after 24 hours should be discarded as it may become contaminated with bacteria.

Early antimicrobial treatment with either doxycycline (100 mg every 12 hours) or trimethoprim-sulfamethoxazole (Bactrim or Septra, one double-strength tablet every 12 hours) will limit the length of an episode of traveler's diarrhea to less than 36 hours; both of these antimicrobials are available in generic forms. Generally, these antimicrobials should be started soon after the diarrhea starts and continued for 3 to 5 days. Potential side effects, although uncommon, consist of (a) for trimethoprim-sulfamethoxazole, allergic reactions, skins rashes, and Stevens-Johnson syndrome; (b) for doxycycline, photosensitivity, expressed as exaggerated sunburn, and *Candida* vaginitis in women. These small risks and inconveniences may be justified in a traveler who has a limited amount of time and cannot afford 3 to 5 days of a typical traveler's diarrhea. Other therapies for traveler's diarrhea have been recently studied: the fluorinated quinolone, ciprofloxacine (Cipro tablets), has been found to be effective (5) as has symptomatic therapy of nondysenteric traveler's diarrhea with either loperamide (Imodium) or bismuth subsalicylate (Pepto-Bismol) (9).

The choice of modalities to use in treating acute traveler's diarrhea should be based on the patient's symptoms. Fluid replacement should be encouraged for any episode of diarrhea but is all that is necessary in mild cases. For diarrhea of moderate severity (2 to 3 unformed stools per day, no fever, no symptoms of frank dysentery, i.e., severe crampy pain and/or bloody stools), nonspecific symptomatic therapy may be all that is needed. Either bismuth subsalicylate or loperamide is useful. Antimicrobial agents should be used only for moderately severe to severe illness (greater than four unformed stools, mild fever, dysentery). After antimicrobial agents have been started, symptomatic treatment with an antimotility agent such as loperamide may be considered.

Drugs that inhibit bowel motility such as diphenyoxylate/atropine (Lomotil) or loperimide (Imodium) may provide temporary relief when diarrhea is especially inconvenient (such as during an 8-hour country bus trip). They provide brief relief of symptoms but may be contraindicated in diarrhea caused by invasive organisms. Loperimide, which does not cause atropine-like side effects, should be taken after each voluminous stool in a dose of two 2-mg capsules or 5 to 10 ml (1 to 2 mg) of the liquid preparation.

Liquid *bismuth subsalicylate* (Pepto-Bismol) may also be helpful, but very large amounts are needed to significantly reduce diarrhea. Also, its use is not without possible complications due to the salicylates it contains. A recent study of the tablet formulation of Pepto-Bismol has found it to be almost as effective as the liquid preparation (4). Pepto-Bismol will bind the antibiotic doxycycline and negate its effectiveness, so these two drugs should not be taken together. The dose of Pepto-Bismol is two tablets or 30 ml every half hour to one hour, as needed, up to a maximum of eight doses per 24 hours.

Kaopectate is not effective in reducing the frequency and volume of diarrhea. At best, it may cause the stool to be somewhat less liquid.

For diarrhea that is very severe, is associated with repeated vomiting, or does not improve after several days, the traveler should be advised to consult a physician rather than attempt self-treatment. He should also see a doctor if (a) there is blood in the stool; (b) there is a fever higher than 101°F, especially if accompanied by shaking chills; or (c) antimicrobial therapy does not provide rapid improvement. Finally, in preparation for possible diarrhea, the traveler should be reminded that toilet tissue is difficult to find in many developing countries and that it is prudent to take a supply.

Additional information regarding the pathogenesis, epidemiology, and treatment of diarrheal illnesses is contained in Chapter 26.

SCHISTOSOMIASIS

Schistosomiasis is one of the world's major public health problems. Three predominant species exist (*Schistosoma mansoni*, *Schistosoma japonicum*, *Schistosoma haematobium*) and are found worldwide (see maps, Figs. 33.5–33.7). Although few travelers are aware of schistosomiasis, it is a relatively common disease in much of the developing world. After infection, the disease may lie dormant, until it causes problems later in life. People contract schistosomiasis by wading or swimming in fresh or estuary water that harbors the snail vector of this trematode parasite. The cercariae (larval stage) can penetrate the skin and pass into the bloodstream without causing any symptoms

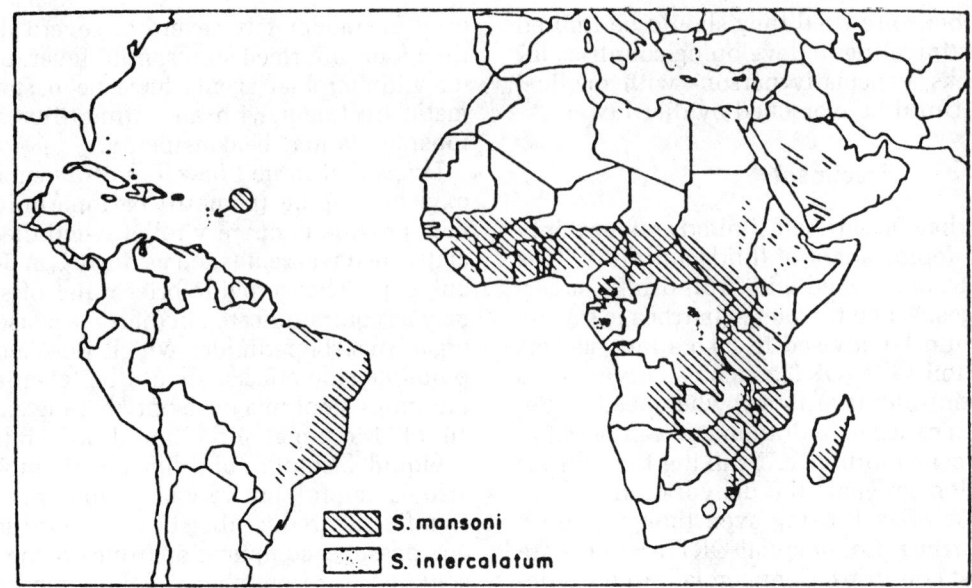

Figure 33.5. Geographic distribution of *S. mansoni* and *S. intercalatum*. (From Warren KS, Mahmoud AAF (eds): *Tropical and Geographical Medicine*. New York, McGraw-Hill, 1983.)

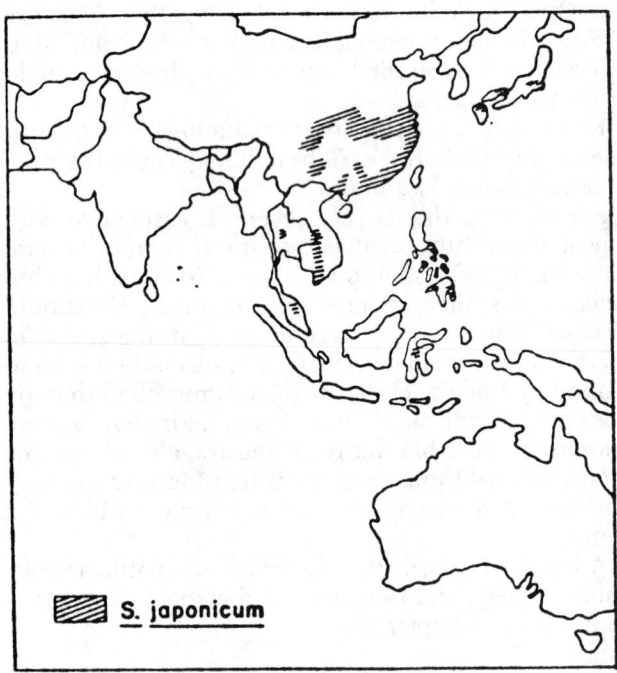

Figure 33.6. Geographical distribution of *S. japonicum*. On the mainland of Indochina, *S. mekongi* is probably the predominant species. (From Warren KS, Mahmoud AAF (eds): *Tropical and Geographical Medicine*. New York, McGraw-Hill, 1983.)

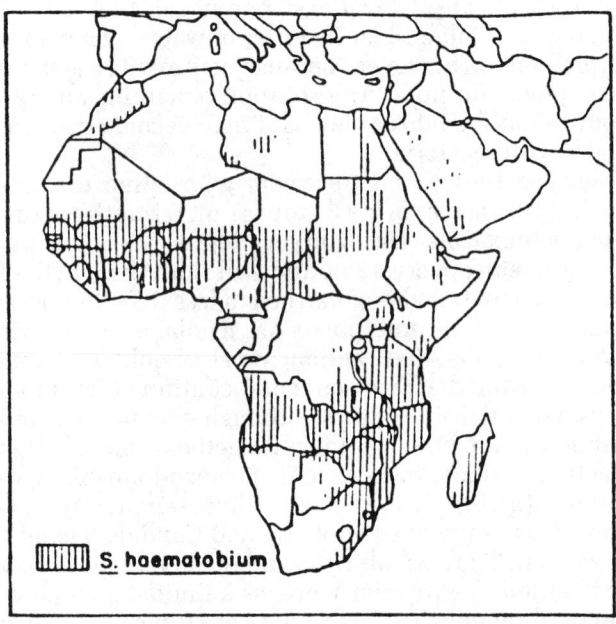

Figure 33.7. Geographical distribution of *S. haematobium*. (From Warren KS, Mahmoud AAF (eds): *Tropical and Geographical Medicine*. New York, McGraw-Hill, 1983.)

at the time. Symptoms that may occur with schistosomiasis depend on the stage of the infection. Sometimes, there may be a rash at the site where the cercariae invaded, but this is not common. About 4 or 5 weeks after infection, an episode of fever, cough, and general malaise may occur. Still later (6 months to several years), more severe complications may occur, usually related to liver or urinary tract disease.

In recent years, severe cases of schistosomiasis have occurred in Americans after river rafting in Ethiopia (8) and after swimming in fresh water in Kenya (1). Although treatment has improved with the advent of praziquantel, it is better to advise travelers to avoid fresh water contact in endemic areas and thereby prevent disease acquisition. For a returning traveler who has been exposed to fresh water in a schistosome-endemic area, screening tests including a complete blood count and specific serology may be useful. This is particularly important in a patient with unexplained systemic symptoms. Eosinophilia in the peripheral blood may be present during the initial stages of the parasitic infection, although it is not a constant finding in late chronic infections. Positive serology indicates likely exposure, especially in the nonimmune traveler. If serology is positive, a further laboratory evaluation including urinalysis and stool examination for ova should be undertaken, recognizing that the acute syndrome described above may occur before there is detectable egg excretion. Proven, or strongly suspected, acute schistosomal infection requires treatment with praziquantel (Biltricide), which is very effective in early schistosomal infection. This drug is supplied in 600-mg tablets, scored so that they can be broken into four 150-mg units. Treatment is accomplished in one day by giving three doses four to six hours apart. Each dose should approximate 20 mg/kg.

MISCELLANEOUS HEALTH CONCERNS

Jet Lag

Jet lag seems to be nearly universal for travelers traversing several time zones (see Fig. 33.8), though some seem to be more affected than others. More than simple travel fatigue, jet lag occurs when the body's physiological clock has not yet adjusted to the new time zone. Symptoms include sleepiness during the daytime, lying awake and hungry at night, and often a feeling that one's thinking processes are not quite normal. Several days to a week are usually needed to recover completely from jet lag.

Although time is the only cure, a few suggestions seem to help. Patients should be advised to avoid overeating and excess alcohol ingestion during air travel and to keep a light snack handy for middle-of-the-night hunger. Also they should be advised to try to

schedule a day of rest after passing six or more time zones before proceeding with their business or vacation. Taking a mild sleeping medication before bed for 2 or 3 days may also help them to get back on schedule (see also Chapter 85, Sleep Disorders).

Accidents

The major cause of serious morbidity and leading cause of mortality in travelers to the developing world is from accidents, especially involving motor vehicles. Other major accidents include drowning, electric shocks, and trauma associated with dangerous sports (hand gliding, white water rafting). Defensive driving is a must. In developing areas, roads are generally not as well engineered as in developed areas, and road hazards are common. Compounding the problems of accidental trauma is the usual lack of a developed emergency medicine infrastructure. Many countries have no formal emergency transport system, and hospital supplies are often lacking. Blood is often not available and/or not carefully screened, and quality control is not available. For serious trauma, it is often best to arrange transport to a medical facility in or operated by a developed nation.

Injectable Medications and Blood Transfusions

Travelers should be advised to avoid, if possible, receiving any injectable medication or blood transfusions when traveling in the developing world. Both hepatitis B and HIV can be readily transmitted by this route, since needles and syringes may not always be sterilized properly. In addition, blood in most developing countries is not routinely screened for HIV (and may also not be screened for hepatitis B).

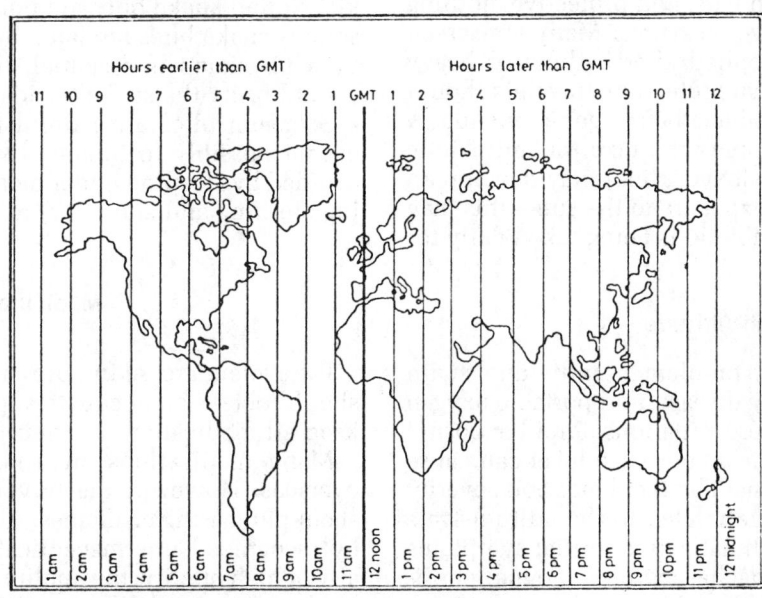

Figure 33.8. Time zones ("jet lag" typically occurs when five or more time zones are crossed). (*GMT*, Greenwich Meridian Time.) (From Walker E, Williams G: ABC of healthy travel: during travel and acclimatization. *Br Med J* 286:865, 1983.)

Motion Sickness

Travelers with a history of motion or sea sickness can attempt to avoid these symptoms by taking one of the antihistamines useful for this problem or trans-dermal scopolamine. Further details are found in Chapter 81.

Swimming and Bathing

Swimming in contaminated water may result in eye, ear, skin, and some intestinal infections. Wading, washing, and swimming should be avoided in water that is likely to be infested with the snail hosts of schistosomiasis (see above) or with human sewage or with animal urine that may contain *Leptospira*. Generally, only chlorinated pools should be considered safe places to swim in developing countries. Ocean beaches may be safe, if not contaminated by sewage, but bathers should be advised to wear light shoes to protect against exposure to coral and other contact hazards.

Insects

The bites, stings, and contact of some insects cause unpleasant reactions. Many insects, such as mosquitoes, can bite and transmit disease without the traveler being aware of the bite. Insect repellents, protective clothing, and mosquito netting, which prevent the bite of insects, are the best prevention for some communicable disease, particularly malaria (see above). Travelers therefore should take a supply of insect repellent cream, lotion, or spray.

Sunburn

Sunburn is a particular hazard in tropical and high glare environments. Sunshades, sunscreens (see Chapter 100), broad-brimmed hats, and protective clothing are important preventive measures. Many sunscreen lotions need to be reapplied after bathing or heavy perspiration. For maximal protection, travelers should apply all sunscreen products before going outside. A small percentage of people who take the antiobiotic tetracycline (including doxycycline) may develop an exaggerated burn after exposure to the sun—this may be important if this antibiotic is being taken daily for diarrhea prevention.

High Altitude

High altitudes can be a problem for individuals with preexisting heart or lung disease, and portable oxygen may be advisable for these situations. Rapid exposure to altitudes over 8,000 feet above sea level can cause serious medical problems. The incidence and severity of mountain sickness are related to the altitude, rate of ascent, and prior acclimatization. Initial symptoms include dizziness, headache, extreme fatigue, chilliness, nausea, and vomiting. More severe symptoms may also occur, most commonly difficulty in concentrating, extreme shortness of breath, and more severe headache. In most individuals, symptoms are mild and clear within 24 to 48 hours. If symptoms persist or are severe, a return to lower altitude may be required. Administration of oxygen generally relieves acute symptoms. Preventive measures include adequate rest before travel, avoidance of alcohol and tobacco, and decreased physical activity at high altitude.

The carbonic anhydrase inhibitor acetazolamide (Diamox) has been shown to reduce the time needed for acclimatization to high altitudes by 24 to 48 hours, in both simulated and actual climbing situations. The United States Food and Drug Administration (FDA) has approved this drug for use in the prevention of altitude sickness (7). The recommended dosage for travelers is 250 mg every 8 to 12 hours, with medication initiated 24 to 48 hours before and continued for 48 hours after ascent. Although its mechanism of action is poorly understood, acetazolamide is known to promote excretion of bicarbonate by the kidneys. This bicarbonate excretion compensates for the respiratory alkalosis seen at high altitudes and this property may contribute to the beneficial effects of the drug on acclimatization. Recent studies suggest that dexamethasone (4 mg every 6 or 8 hours for 48 hours before and 48 hours after ascent to high altitude) may also be useful in preventing altitude sickness; acetazolamide is still regarded as the agent of choice because of the more extensive use of it for this purpose (7).

Snakes and Scorpions

Poisonous snakes live in many developing countries, although most travelers will never see them unless they visit a zoo. If travelers will be walking through brush or jungle, or will be walking at night, they should wear good quality leather boots that go above the ankle. Not all snake bites are poisonous and not all poisonous snake bites are fatal, but immediate treatment by a physician is essential. If possible, the traveler should bring the snake for identification.

Scorpion bites are painful but seldom dangerous, except possibly to infants. Exposure to bites can be avoided by sleeping under mosquito netting and shaking clothing and shoes before putting them on.

Medicines

If travelers are taking prescribed medications, they should obtain an adequate supply before leaving and keep all medications in their luggage.

Many medications are sold without prescription overseas. However, the traveler should be cautious about purchasing medicines. Although medicines made by recognized pharmaceutical companies are generally of high quality, the quality of other medicines may not be guaranteed. The traveler should be advised not to self-medicate, as many medicines have serious side effects.

Women and Children

Some medications used commonly in travelers should not be given to pregnant women, in particular doxycycline (impairs tooth development in the infant) and Fansidar (see "Malaria" above) (3). Travel late in pregnancy may precipitate labor. In fact, many airlines will not allow air travel during the final month. Immunizations recommended for children are, in general, the same as those recommended for adults (see Table 33.1) except that yellow fever vaccine is not usually required under 1 year of age. Routine "baby shots" are even more important for children traveling to developing countries since diphtheria, whooping cough, polio, and measles are relatively common. The dosages of medicines have to be adjusted for children. This is especially important for malaria medications. Because children may be restless on long airline trips, some parents are tempted to sedate their children. This is not recommended, however, because children may react adversely to sedatives.

Sexually Transmitted Diseases

The risk of contracting sexually transmitted diseases is very high in some parts of the world. Very importantly, HIV infection has become a global health problem. In addition to the risk of HIV infection, sexually transmitted pathogens such as penicillinase-producing *Neisseria gonorrhoeae* are becoming increasingly common. Likewise less common pathogens such as chancroid and *Lymphogranuloma venereum* and hepatitis B are more commonplace in certain areas. To reduce the risk of sexually transmitted infections, travelers need to be discriminating in sexual relations and avoid multiple partners, anonymous partners, prostitutes, and persons who have had multiple sexual partners. If a traveler chooses to have sexual relations, then during intercourse condoms should always be used.

Miscellaneous Infections

Many people experience a "traveler's cold" during a trip. These are thought to be due to infection with respiratory viruses to which the traveler has no immunity. Travelers should bring their favorite cold remedy and an extra box of tissues with them. Fungal infections, especially "jock itch" and athlete's feet, may also be more common, especially in hot humid environments. Travelers should wear clean dry socks, or sandals when possible, and use antifungal powders and ointments as needed.

In recent years the incidence of *dengue fever* has increased dramatically in most of the countries in the Caribbean. Dengue fever is a mosquito-borne viral illness found in parts of tropical Asia, Africa, and the Pacific and is characterized by sudden onset of high fever, severe headache, joint and muscle pain, and rash. There is no vaccine and no specific therapy. Travelers to areas where dengue is endemic need to take precautions to avoid mosquito bites (see "Malaria" above).

Long-Term Travelers

Recommendations for long-term travelers are generally the same regarding food and water, immunizations, malaria prophylaxis, etc. In addition, gamma globulin should be given every 6 months and immunizations for typhoid (every 3 years) and yellow fever (every 10 years) should be kept up to date. If the traveler hires people to work in the house, these people should be examined medically before starting work. The employee will benefit from this, and it will minimize the possibility of infections being transmitted to the traveler's family.

Medical Emergencies

If the traveler becomes seriously ill or injured while traveling, the United States consulate can provide advice on where to go for help.

INTERNATIONAL TRAVELERS HEALTH KIT

The following is a suggested first aid and health kit that represents the minimal necessary equipment for the traveler to the developing world:

1. *International Immunization Card* with documentation of vaccines received
2. Appropriate medication for *malaria prophylaxis*
3. *Mosquito repellent*
4. *Water purification tablets or tincture of iodine,* and/or water filters
5. *Oral rehydration salt packets*
6. *Antimicrobial medication for treatment or prevention of diarrhea* as arranged with the traveler's physician
7. *Imodium or Lomotil*
8. *Sunscreen*
9. *Bandaids* (for blisters)
10. A spare pair of glasses or at least the lens prescription
11. Any prescription medication the traveler takes regularly
12. The traveler's favorite "cold" remedy
13. Fever thermometer
14. Aspirin or acetaminophen (paracetamol in most other countries)
15. Astringent or antiseptic
16. Antifungal powder
17. Toilet paper

POST-TRAVEL SCREENING

Most persons who acquire viral, bacterial, or parasitic infections in developing countries will become ill within 6 weeks after returning, but certain infectious diseases, such as malaria and schistosomiasis, may not manifest themselves until later. The traveler should be advised to seek medical help for any unexplained symptoms during the 12 months after the end of his trip. When an unexplained late illness occurs, it is necessary to identify all of the developing countries that the traveler visited in order to know which infectious disease risks the travel encountered.

For travelers who stay for relatively long periods in the developing world, it is prudent to provide routine screening on arrival home. This should include a complete blood count, liver function tests, tuberculosis skin test, stool examination for occult blood, urinalysis, and stool examination for ova and parasites. If these tests all are normal, the traveler has probably not acquired a serious unrecognized infectious disease, but post-trip surveillance for another 6 months is still warranted.

General References

Gorbach SL, Edelman R: Travelers diarrhea: National Institutes of Health Consensus Development Conference. *Rev Inf Dis* 8(suppl 2):S109, 1986.
A thorough review of traveler's diarrhea.
Health Information for International Travel. Supplement to Morbidity and Mortality Weekly Report, DHHS publ no. (CDC) 88-8280, Atlanta, Centers for Disease Control,
A practical manual, updated yearly, available free of charge.
Jong EC (ed): *The Travel and Tropical Medicine Manual.* Philadelphia, WB Saunders Company, 1987.
A manual written for the clinician that is relevant and contains a list of travel clinics.
Schroeder D (ed): *Staying Healthy in Asia, Africa, and Latin America.* Stanford, Volunteers in Asia Press, 1988.
A handbook that contains the nuts and bolts of health maintenance while traveling in the developing regions of the world.
Wolfe M: Diseases of travelers. *CIBA Clin Symp* 32:2, 1984.
Well-illustrated publication, with practical recommendations concerning common infectious disease problems.

Specific References

1. Acute schistosomiasis with transverse myelitis in American students returning from Kenya. *MMWR* 33:445, 1984.
2. Arrow PM, Smaron M, Ormiste V: Brucellosis in a group of travelers to Spain. *JAMA* 251:505, 1984.
3. Barry M, Bia F: Pregnancy and travel. *JAMA* 261:728, 1989.
4. DuPont HC, Ericsson CD, Johnson PC, et al: Prevention of travelers diarrhea by the tablet formulation of Bismuth Subsalicylate. *JAMA* 257:1347, 1987.
5. Ericsson CD, Johnson PC, DuPont HC, et al: Ciprofloxacin or trimethoprin-sulfamethoxasole as initial therapy for travelers diarrhea. *Ann Intern Med* 106:216, 1987.
6. Herwaldt BC, Krogstad DS, Schlesinger PH: Antimalarial agents: specific chemoprophylaxis regimens. *Antimicrob Agents Chemo* 32:953, 1988.
7. High altitude sickness. *Med Lett* 30:89, 1988.
8. Istrie GR, et al: Acute schistosomiasis among Americans rafting the Omo River, Ethiopia. *JAMA* 251:508, 1984.
9. Johnson PC, Ericsson CD, DuPont HC, et al: Comparison of Loperamide with Bismuth Subsalicylate for the treatment of acute travelers diarrhea. *JAMA* 255:757, 1986.
10. Kean BH: Travelers diarrhea: an overview. *Rev Infect Dis* 2(S):S111, 1986.
11. Monger H, Steffe R, Schar M: Epidemiology of cholera in travelers, and conclusions for vaccination recommendations. *Br Med J* 286:184, 1982.
12. Reid D, Dewar RD, Fallon RJ, et al: Infection and travel: the experience of package tourists and other travelers. *J Infect* 2:65, 1980.
13. Sack DA, et al: Prophylactic doxycycline for traveler's diarrhea: results of a prospective double-blind study in Peace Corps volunteers in Kenya. *N Engl J Med* 298:758, 1978.
14. Snyder JD, Blake PA: Is cholera a problem for United States travelers? *JAMA* 247:2268, 1982.
15. Steffen R, van der Linde F, Gyr K, Schar M: Epidemiology of diarrhea in travelers. *JAMA* 249:1176, 1983.
16. Steffen R, Rickenbach M, Wilhelm U, et al: Health problems after travel to developing countries. *J Infect Dis* 156:84, 1987.
17. Taylor P, Polland R, Blake P: Typhoid in the United States and the risk to the international traveler. *J Invest Dermatol* 148:599, 1983.
18. Consensus Conference: Travelers' diarrhea. *JAMA* 253:2700, 1985.

C H A P T E R 34

Ambulatory Care For the HIV-Infected Patient

JANET HORN, M.D.
ELENA YAMAGUCHI, M.D.
RICHARD E. CHAISSON, M.D.

Since its recognition in 1981, infection caused by the human immunodeficiency virus (HIV) has rapidly become one of the major health problems of this century. As HIV infection and its uniformly fatal sequel—the acquired immune deficiency syndrome (AIDS)—become more widespread, physicians will be called upon with increasing frequency to care for patients who are infected with this virus. A major proportion of the care for these patients, including those with extensive opportunistic infections and those in the terminal stages of illness, is now provided in ambulatory settings or in hospice programs.

GENERAL CONSIDERATIONS

Etiology

The human immunodeficiency virus or HIV 1 was isolated and found to be the etiological agent of AIDS in 1983 (2). Because of the confusion caused by several different names for the same virus—e.g., lymphadenopathy-associated virus (LAV), human T cell lymphotropic virus, type III (HTLV III), and AIDS-associated retrovirus (ARV)—an international committee on taxonomy of viruses recommended the current term in 1986. Since that time, at least one additional human immunodeficiency virus, designated HIV 2, has been discovered (12). Other related human retroviruses include HTLV I and HTLV II, which cause syndromes such as T-cell leukemia, and progressive spastic paraparesis, that are quite distinct from AIDS.

HIV is a member of the lentivirus subfamily of human retroviruses. These viruses code for an enzyme known as reverse transcriptase, which permits transcription of viral RNA into proviral DNA and subsequent integration into the host's cellular genome, leading to a persistent and latent infection. The retroviruses are associated with diseases of long incubation period, involvement with the hematopoietic and central nervous systems, and immune suppression.

Epidemiology

In 1989, the Centers for Disease Control (CDC) estimated that between 1 and 1.5 million Americans were infected with HIV (4). Because HIV seropositivity is not a reported condition, these figures are derived from numerous data regarding high-risk behaviors and the numbers of people who engage in these behaviors. By 1988, AIDS, a reportable condition, had been diagnosed in over 100,000 Americans; and the CDC estimated that the cumulative number of cases will reach 365,000 by 1992 (4).

The major *distribution characteristics* of the AIDS epidemic in adults in the United States are as follows:

1. AIDS has been diagnosed in all fifty states. The case incidence is especially high in large cities in the states with high incidence rates (see Fig. 34.1).
2. AIDS occurs in adults belonging to the major risk groups for HIV infection. These risk groups and the distribution of AIDS cases among them are shown in Table 34.1, based on cumulative experience in the United States up to 1988. In the late 1980s, the proportion of AIDS diagnoses in homosexual and bisexual men began to decline and that in intra-

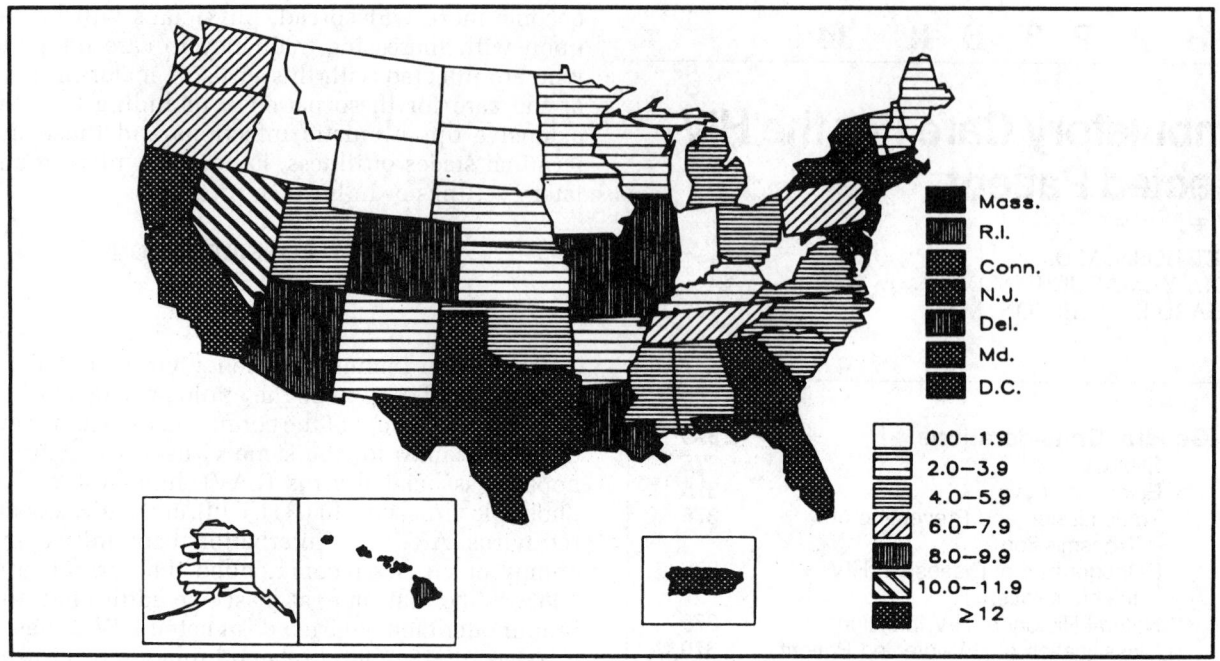

Figure 34.1. AIDS incidence rates per 100,000 population, United States, 1988(4). From *Morbidity and Mortality* 38(14):231, 1989.

venous drug users increased; and heterosexual transmission, the major mode of transmission in developing countries, became increasingly important in the United States and Europe.

3. AIDS onset is most frequent in the age range 20 to 50, with the peak incidence between 30 and 39. Because primary HIV infection precedes AIDS by a number of years (see below), a substantial proportion of infection occurs in adolescents and young adults.

4. About 10% of AIDS cases in adults diagnosed in 1988 were in women, an increase from 7% in 1984. In women of all races, intravenous drug use has been the commonest mode of transmission, followed by heterosexual contact with men from high risk groups.

5. The ratio of AIDS case incidence is 3.2 to 1 for blacks and 2.8 to 1 for Hispanics compared with whites.

Transmission and Prevention of Transmission

To date, only blood and semen have been shown conclusively to transmit HIV infection. These are the two body fluids in which the virus occurs in high concentration. It is also detectable, in lower concentrations, in cervical and vaginal secretions; and it is present in very low concentration in saliva, tears, breast milk, and amniotic fluid. It appears that HIV is transmitted by only three modes: sexual intercourse, exposure to infected blood or blood products, and in utero from infected mother to fetus (14). The behaviors and conditions most commonly associated with these modes of transmission are those listed in Table 34.1,

respectively, for adult males, adult females, and pediatric-age children.

Sexual Transmission

HIV infection can be transmitted during sexual intercourse between men and between men and women. The following patterns, practices, and situations greatly increase an individual's risk of infection:

1. Relations with multiple partners, especially partners from groups in which HIV infection is most common.

2. Receptive anal intercourse. The mucosa of the rectum is delicate and tears easily during intercourse. Tearing of tissues, allowing semen to contact the blood stream, can also occur during vaginal intercourse.

3. The presence of a sexually transmitted disease in either partner, especially a disease causing genital ulcers such as syphilis, chancroid, and genital herpes. Genital ulcers can act as conduits for infected blood *from* or for infected semen, blood, or vaginal secretions *into* the person with the ulcer.

The prevention of sexual transmission of HIV requires that sexually active persons choose sexual practices that minimize or eliminate the high-risk situations listed above. In the care of every patient who is sexually active, and in public education messages, the fundamentals of safe and unsafe sex should be clearly communicated. The fundamentals include information about those forms of sexual intimacy that are safe, possibly safe, and definitely unsafe (Table 34.2). Spe-

Table 34.1.
Distribution Percentage of AIDS Cases by Transmission Category and Year of Report, United States, 1981–1988[a]

Category	AIDS cases (%)				
	Before 1985	1985	1986	1987	1988
Adult Male (≥13 years)					
Homosexual/bisexual only	69	72	71	70	63
IV-drug user	15	15	15	14	20
Homosexual and IV-drug user	10	8	8	8	7
Hemophilic	1	1	1	1	1
Heterosexual					
Heterosexual contact	<1	<1	1	1	1
Born in Pattern II country[b]	3	1	1	1	1
Transfusion	1	1	2	2	2
Undetermined	2	2	2	3	4[c]
Total	**100**	**100**	**100**	**100**	**100**
Adult Female (≥13 years)					
IV-drug user	58	53	49	49	53
Coagulation disorder	<1	1	<1	<1	<1
Heterosexual					
Heterosexual contact	16	21	28	27	26
Born in Pattern II country[b]	8	6	6	4	3
Transfusion	8	11	10	13	10
Undetermined	10	9	6	6	8[c]
Total	**100**	**100**	**100**	**100**	**100**
Pediatric (<13 years)					
Coagulation disorder	4	6	6	7	7
Transfusion	11	14	13	14	11
Mother with/at risk for AIDS, HIV infection					
IV-drug user	45	47	44	41	40
Sex with person at risk	11	17	24	21	21
Born in Pattern II country[b]	22	14	6	7	7
Other	0	2	5	8	9
Undetermined	6	0	2	3	6[c]
Total	**100**	**100**	**100**	**100**	**100**

[a]From the Centers for Disease Control: AIDS and human immunodeficiency virus infection in the United States: 1988 update. *Morbidity and Mortality Weekly Report* 38(S-4), May 1989.
[b]Pattern II countries are WHO-designated countries with predominatly heterosexual transmission of HIV.
[c]Of patients initially reported with an undetermined transmission category, 75% are reclassified into known risk categories following investigation. Increases in the proportion of cases with undetermined risk in more recent reporting periods reflect a higher proportion of patients who have not been investigated.

cific instructions for the most effective use of condoms Table 34.3) is particularly important.

Transmission through Transfusion of Blood and Blood Products

This mode of transmission accounts for about 10% of the women and children and 1 to 2% of the men who have developed AIDS in the past decade (Table 34.1). HIV can be transmitted only by whole blood, blood cellular components, plasma, and clotting factors. No other blood products (e.g., immune globulin preparations, albumin, plasma protein fraction, hepatitis B vaccine) have been implicated.

Since recognition of the problem, transmission of HIV infection by blood transfusion has been almost eliminated. This has been achieved by blood donor education programs (to eliminate donors who belong to high-risk groups), uniform blood product screening since April 1985, HIV-inactivating treatment of clot-

Table 34.2.
Safe Sex Guidelines

Safe Sex Practices
- Massage
- Hugging
- Mutual masturbation
- Social kissing (dry)
- Body-to-body rubbing
- Voyeurism, exhibitionism, fantasy

Possibly Safe Sex Practices
- French Kissing (wet)
- Anal intercourse WITH CONDOM[a]
- Vaginal intercourse WITH CONDOM[a]
- Limiting the number of partners with whom one has sex

Unsafe Sex Practices
- Semen, vaginal fluid, menstrual blood, or urine in mouth or in contact with the skin where there is an open cut or sore
- Anal intercourse WITHOUT CONDOM[a]
- Vaginal intercourse WITHOUT CONDOM[a]
- Rimming (oral-anal contact)
- Fisting (possible percutaneous inoculation with blood from trauma caused by inserting fist into anus)
- Having sex when you or your partner has an open genital sore

[a]See Instructions for Condom Users in Table 34.3.

Table 34.3.
Instructions for Condom Users[a]

- Use a condom every time you have intercourse.
- Always put the condom on the penis before intercourse begins.
- Put the condom on when the penis is erect.
- Do not pull the condom tightly against the tip of the penis. Leave a small empty space—about 1 or 2 cm—at the end of the condom to hold semen. Some condoms have a nipple tip that will hold semen.
- Unroll the condom all the way to the bottom of the penis.
- If the condom breaks during intercourse, withdraw the penis immediately and put on a new condom.
- After ejaculation withdraw the penis while it is still erect. Hold onto the rim of the condom as you withdraw so that the condom does not slip off.
- Use a new condom each time you have intercourse. Throw used condoms away.
- If a lubricant is desired, use water-based lubricants such as contraceptive jelly. Lubricants made with petroleum jelly may damage condoms. Do not use saliva because it may contain virus.
- Store condoms in a cool, dry place if possible.
- Condoms that are sticky or brittle or otherwise damaged should not be used.

[a]Adapted from *Population Reports* XIV No. 3, 1986.

ting-factor concentrates, the use of autologous blood transfusions for elective surgery, and efforts to avoid all nonessential transfusions. The estimated risk of HIV infection is now about 1 in 100,000 to 1 in 1,000,000 transfusions (14).

Needle Transmission

This mode of transmission explains the large proportion of AIDS patients in the United States in whom the only identified risk factor is the sharing of needles for intravenous drug injection. HIV-infected individuals in this group pose a threat both to needle partners and to sexual partners. In developing countries this mode of transmission may also occur because of reuse of improperly-cleaned needles and syringes for the injections of medicines.

Definitive interruption of transmission by this mode

requires that the user discontinue the practice, as part of a recovery program (see Chapter 22, Use and Abuse of Illicit Drugs and Substances). The interruption of transmission by those who continue intravenous drug use requires that they either avoid needle sharing or cleanse their shared needles with bleach after assuring that the syringe does not contain blood. These protective behaviors have been very difficult to promote in this subset of individuals, who engage in a variety of high-risk behaviors.

Perinatal Transmission

Several modes may account for perinatal transmission from an HIV-infected woman to her infant: intrauterine transmission by cord blood, during delivery due to inoculation or ingestion of maternal blood or fluids, and postnatal due to breast feeding. Only the first mode has been documented conclusively (14). It is estimated that 30 to 50% of infants born to HIV-infected mothers become infected. Prevention of this form of transmission requires a combination of primary prevention through safe-sex practices and secondary prevention through HIV testing and subsequent counseling, of HIV-infected women, about the risks of pregnancy.

Casual Contact and the Risk of HIV Transmission

It is presently believed that casual transmission of HIV does not occur (6). Thus, household contacts of HIV-infected patients who are not sexual partners are not at risk during ordinary circumstances. Although the virus has been isolated in urine and saliva, there have been no documented cases of transmission through kissing or through exposure to urine, stool, or saliva. It is generally recommended, however, that the same precautions taken to prevent transmission of hepatitis B in the household setting be observed by HIV-infected persons (see Chapter 43). Precautions for avoiding transmission to health care workers and caretakers are described at the end of this chapter.

Knowledge and Attitudes about Transmission

The 1989 National Health Interview Survey (22), a periodic survey of persons 18 years of age and older, showed the following crude levels of knowledge and attitudes regarding transmission of the AIDS virus:

1. Over 75% of persons knew of the three principal modes of transmission.
2. More than 80% felt that condoms and a monogamous relationship between two uninfected persons were methods that were at least somewhat effective in preventing transmission of the AIDS virus.
3. Over half thought that kissing with exchange of saliva can definitely transmit the AIDS virus. About one in four persons perceived that transmission can occur by other modes that are not known to transmit HIV, e.g., being coughed or sneezed on, sharing eating utensils with an HIV-infected person, or by mosquito or other insect bites. Eleven percent or

less felt that more indirect contacts (e.g., school and work setting) could transmit the virus.
4. 12% of adults reported knowing someone with AIDS or HIV infection; and of these, half reported knowing the person very well or fairly well.

Practicing physicians are responsible for disseminating accurate information in a dispassionate manner, not only to all of their patients and families, but to the public at large. This is especially important in a hospital setting, as lack of accurate information about modes of transmission of HIV can lead to unnecessary fears by health care workers.

Pathogenesis of Disease in HIV-Infected Patients

The human immunodeficiency virus causes illness by impairing important components of the patient's immune system, making the patient susceptible to a wide variety of infections. This virus also causes illness by its direct effect upon other body systems, especially the nervous system (15).

HIV preferentially infects human T lymphocytes of the helper/inducer subset (also referred to as T4 or CD4 cells), resulting in both quantitative and qualitative defects in helper-cell function. Because helper T lymphocytes are crucial in *cell-mediated immunity*, HIV infection impairs this type of immunity, making the patient susceptible to a number of opportunistic infections. Uninfected individuals usually have more than 800 CD4 cells/mm^3 of blood, whereas HIV-infected patients with opportunistic infections usually have less than 200 CD4 cells/mm^3. Thus, monitoring the CD4 cell count has become useful for predicting the degree of suppression of a patient's cell-mediated immunity and for deciding when to initiate antiretroviral treatment and prophylaxis for opportunistic infection (see below).

Other abnormalities of immune function are also found in HIV-infected persons. HIV can infect, and impair the function of, macrophages and monocytes as well as of CD4 lymphocytes. HIV infection may also result in B lymphocyte activation and nonspecific hypergammaglobulinemia, which may impair de novo antibody response to some antigens; this may place the patient at increased risk for infection with encapsulated bacteria. Additionally, some studies suggest that HIV infection may cause derangements in polymorphonuclear neutrophil phagocytosis and intracellular killing.

Although most of the illnesses in patients with HIV infection are due to impaired resistance to infection, a number of clinical manifestations are *direct consequences of HIV infection*. There is good evidence that the virus plays an etiological role in some neurological syndromes; these include a subacute encephalitis syndrome, the AIDS dementia syndrome, and other abnormalities of the central nervous system, where the virus predictably infects monocytes and macrophages. Other tissues in which HIV infection seems to play a direct role in producing symptoms are the gastrointestinal tract, the heart, and the kidneys.

Natural History of HIV Infection

Fig. 34.2 depicts the time course of HIV infection from initial infection to symptomatic disease. Because the virus may remain latent with no demonstrable signs of immunodeficiency or symptoms for many years (1, 21), asymptomatic patients play a major role in transmitting the virus. Patients with HIV infection may be asymptomatic; they may have symptoms that do not meet the diagnostic criteria for AIDS; or they may have AIDS. This progression reflects the variable severity of the underlying immunodeficiency. Studies indicate that virtually all individuals with longstanding HIV infection have laboratory evidence of cellular immunodeficiency and that at least 50% of infected persons will progress to AIDS. The median time from HIV infection to AIDS, without treatment, is estimated to range from 2 to 10 years.

For the two principal subgroups of HIV-infected patients that are seen in ambulatory settings, longitudinal studies in the 1980s provided information about the chance of developing AIDS (13). Patients who were *asymptomatic or had only persistent generalized lymphadenopathy* had a 10 to 15% chance of developing AIDS within two to three years of identification; this figure increased to 36% in 88 months. Patients having *constitutional symptoms, oral thrush, herpes zoster, or a low CD 4 count* had a 40% chance of developing AIDS within 36 months of identification.

Survival after the diagnosis of AIDS depends upon the natural history of the disease and upon the efficacy of treatment for opportunistic infections and for HIV infection. There is as yet no evidence that any treatment cures AIDS, and the impact of evolving treatments on the course of AIDS remains to be learned. Fig. 34.3 shows the survival experience for a cohort observed before anteretroviral drugs were available for general use. In this cohort, two subgroups with quite different survival curves were black women who were intravenous drug users and had pneumocystis pneumonia at the time of diagnosis (worst survival) and white men who were homosexual and had Kaposi's sarcoma at the time of diagnosis (best survival).

Classification of HIV-Infected Patients and Case Definition for AIDS

In the late 1980s, the Centers for Disease Control published a four-category *classification that encompasses all patients with HIV infection* (Table 34.4); this system utilizes the principal type(s) of clinical manifestation(s) that a patient has at any point in time. The CDC has also published criteria for *case definition of AIDS*, updated most recently in 1987 (Table 34.5). Importantly, the diagnosis of AIDS by these criteria makes a patient eligible automatically for Social Security Disability and other social service benefits (see "Social and Economic Issues" below).

In previous years the term *AIDS-related complex (ARC)* was used for symptomatic HIV-infected patients, who did not meet criteria for AIDS. The term ARC is no longer used because it generated more confusion than clarity and did not help to separate patients into prognostic groups to to guide treatment decisions.

As described below ("Early Drug Treatment"), classification of HIV-infected patients according to their CD4 counts has become a major determinant of treatment decisions.

SEROLOGICAL DIAGNOSIS AND ASSOCIATED COUNSELING

Serological Tests

Antibody to HIV usually appears between four and twenty four weeks after infection (see Fig. 34.2). The body's immune response to HIV does not, however, lead to elimination of the virus from host tissues. As described above, a persistent carrier (and persistent seropositive) state follows infection with this type of virus. The diagnosis of HIV infection is based on detection of anti-HIV antibodies by the enzyme-linked immunosorbent assay (ELISA), confirmed by the more specific Western blot method (WB). In the Western blot method several individual HIV proteins are transferred onto nitrocellulose paper and reacted against the patient's serum and known positive and negative sera; HIV antibody is detected by an antihuman immunoglobulin antibody coated with an enzyme that,

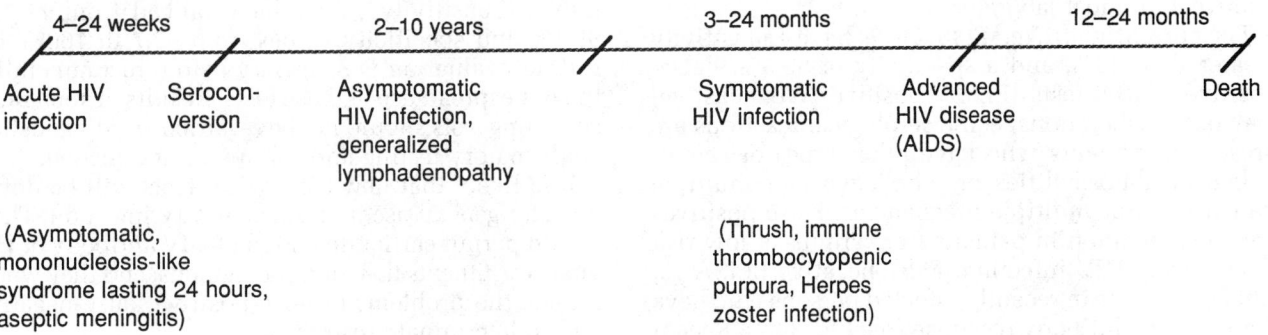

Figure 34.2. Natural history of HIV infection (without treatment).

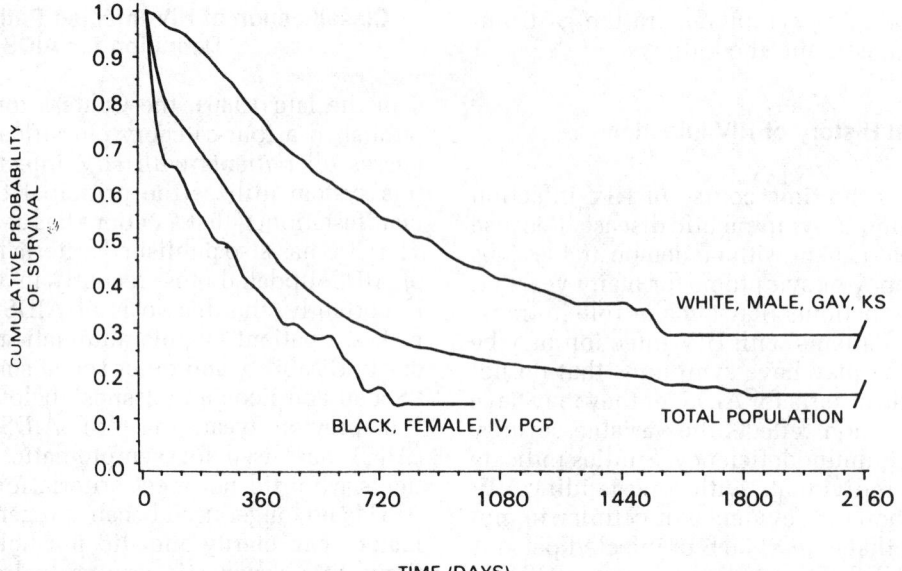

Figure 34.3. Survival in a cohort of 5833 patients with AIDS (diagnosed in New York City through December 1985) and in two subgroups. From Rothenberg R, et al: Survival with the acquired immunodeficiency syndrome. N Engl J Med 317(21): 1299, 1987. KS = Kaposis sarcoma, IV = intravenous drug use, PCP = *Pneumocystis carinii* pneumonia.

Table 34.4.
CDC Classification System for Patients with HIV Infection

I. Acute Retroviral Syndrome
II. Asymptomatic
III. Persistent Generalized Lymphadenopathy
IV. Other Disease
    A. Constitutional disease
    B. Neurologic Disease
    C. Secondary Infections
    D. Secondary Malignancies
    E. Other

in the presence of substrate, produces a colored band. A positive WB test (the presence of one of several combinations of colored bands) indicates that the individual has been infected with HIV.

ELISA tests are reported as positive or negative. WB tests are reported as positive, negative, or indeterminate. The routine processing of a specimen that is positive on initial ELISA testing always includes rerun of the ELISA, to confirm the result, followed by the WB test. Turn around time from obtaining the patient's initial specimen to reporting of the WB result is about one week in most laboratories.

The *currently utilized ELISA tests* have a sensitivity greater than 99%, and a specificity of 99.5%. False-positive ELISA tests (ELISA positive, WB negative) may occur when nonspecific serological reactions are present in patients who have other types of immunological abnormalities or who have had multiple transfusions or multiple pregnancies. False-positives are most common in patients from groups at low risk of acquiring HIV infection. False-negative ELISA results may occur in recently infected persons who have not made an antibody response (see Fig. 34.2). Recent

findings suggest that a subset of infected persons may be ELISA negative for periods much longer than the 4 to 24 week interval shown in the figure (27); the size of this subset is not yet known.

Patients whose Western blot tests are reported as *indeterminate* are those whose sera yield at least one positive color band but do not yield one of the color-band patterns defined as WB positive. This result may signify that a person is in the process of converting to WB positive or it may not signify HIV infection. The CDC recommends retesting of such patients every 8 to 12 weeks for at least 6 months (7). If the WB pattern remains indeterminate for at least 6 months—in the absence of any known risk factors or clinical findings to suggest HIV infection—the test may be considered negative. Patients having risk factors or findings compatible with HIV-induced disease should have continued evaluation.

Several *rapid serological screening tests for HIV* have been evaluated in research and field conditions. The need for proficiency in performance and expertise in test interpretation, as well as quality control measures, raises concern about the possibility that such test methods may become available for use by the general public. Sensitivity values have ranged from 71.4 to 99.1% and specificity values from 92.7 to 100%, but further evaluation is necessary before recommending the widespread use of these tests. Results of such rapid screening tests should not be regarded as "diagnostic"; confirmatory testing and follow-up are needed.

It is likely that new serological tests will be developed for general use in diagnosing HIV infection. These would permit earlier detection of HIV antibody or HIV viral constituents than current methods; and they would reduce the problems of false-positive, false-negative, and indeterminate results.

Table 34.5.
Centers for Disease Control Case Definition of AIDS for Surveillance Purposes[a]

The presence of reliably diagnosed disease that is at least moderately indicative of underlying cellular immunodeficiency, in a person WITH NO KNOWN CAUSE of immunodeficiency other than HIV infection.[b]

DISEASES DIAGNOSTIC OF AIDS

BACTERIAL
- Extrapulmonary *Mycobacterium tuberculosis*[c]
- Disseminated *Mycobacterium avium-intracellulare*
- Recurrent *Salmonella* septicemia[c]

FUNGAL
- *Candida* esophagitis
- *Cryptococcus neoformans* meningitis or other extrapulmonary form
- Disseminated *coccidioidomycosis*[c]
- Disseminated *histoplasmosis*[c]

VIRAL
- *Cytomegalovirus* infection of an organ other than liver, spleen, lymph nodes in a patient >1 month of age
- Chronic mucocutaneous *herpes simplex* (lasting >1 month)
- *Herpes simplex* causing bronchitis, pneumonitis, or esophagitis in a patient >1 month of age
- Progressive multifocal encephalopathy (*papovavirus*)
- HIV "wasting syndrome"[c] (large-volume diarrhea with >10% weight loss)
- HIV encephalopathy[c] (also called AIDS dementia)

PROTOZOA
- *Pneumocytis carinii* pneumonia
- *Toxoplasma gondii* infection of brain in patient >1 month of age
- *Cryptosporidiosis* (diarrhea lasting >1 month)
- *Isospora belli* diarrhea (>1 month)[c]

MALIGNANT
Kaposi's sarcoma in a patient <60 years of age
Primary lymphoma of the brain in a patient <60 years of age
Non-Hodgkin's lymphoma[c]

[a]Adapted from *Morbidity and Mortality Weekly Report Supplement* 36: No. 1S, 1987.
[b]1. High dose corticosteroid therapy or other immunosuppressive/cytotoxic therapy ≤3 months *before* onset of indicator disease
2. Any of the following diagnosed ≤3 months *after* diagnosis of indicator disease: Hodgkins or non-Hodgkins lymphoma, lymphocytic leukemia, multiple myeloma, other malignancy of lymphoreticular or histocytic tissue
3. A genetic or congenital immunodeficiency syndrome or an acquired immunodeficiency syndrome other than HIV infection, such as hypogammaglobulinemia
[c]With positive HIV serology (regardless of the presence of other causes of immunodeficiency).

Indications for Serological Testing

Serological testing is indicated both to confirm suspected HIV infection or AIDS and to identify asymptomatic HIV carriers. At the present time, mandatory HIV testing is done on members of many military and prison populations and on all new participants in residential training programs of the Job Corps (4). Prenatal screening may become mandatory in some settings. Patients for whom HIV testing should be part of the diagnostic evaluation include those who have asymptomatic lymphadenopathy, any unexplained symptoms that could be due to HIV infection, or any of the AIDS-defining illnesses listed in Table 34.5.

Pre- and Post-Test Counseling

The most important aspect of HIV testing is *pre- and post-test counseling*. Because of the ominous meaning of HIV infection, it is important to assure privacy and to allow sufficient time to respond to the patient's feelings and questions. Many settings require the patient's written informed consent as part of pretest counseling. Recommended points of discussion during counseling are shown in Table 34.6. Information about behaviors associated with the risk of acquiring HIV infection is important in both stages of counseling.

Information about available printed materials useful in post-test counseling and about regional programs for HIV-infected persons can be obtained by contacting The National AIDS Information Clearing House, P.O. Box 6003, Rockville, Maryland, 20850 (telephone 1-800-458-5231).

EARLY EVALUATION AND MANAGEMENT OF THE HIV-INFECTED PATIENT

Baseline History, Physical Examination, and Laboratory Studies

The apparently asymptomatic patient with HIV infection requires an initial evaluation and ongoing psychological support and medical assessment. Important manifestations to be sought in initial and/or subsequent evaluations of HIV-positive patients are summarized by organ system in Table 34.7. Detailed

Table 34.6.
HIV Pre- and Post-test Counseling: Points for Discussion

Pretest Counseling
1. Meaning of positive test:
   - Positive test means HIV infection
   - Positive test does NOT mean AIDS
   - Positive test means individual is an HIV carrier
   - Not every HIV-infected person will develop AIDS (it is estimated that 50% will develop AIDS in 5–7 years, that the remaining 50% may not)
2. Confidentiality of test results and medical information
3. Availability of anonymous and confidential counseling and testing sites
4. Potential adverse psychosocial consequences if information becomes known, e.g., possible adverse effects on employment, housing, insurance status
5. Sources of additional AIDS/HIV-related information[a]
6. Means for reducing risk of HIV transmission or exposure (depends on patient's current or likely high-risk behaviors)
   - "Safe Sex" practices (See Tables 34.2 and 34.3)
   - Sterilization of IV drug equipment
   - Treatment for drug addiction
   - Discontinuation of sharing IV needles

Post-Test Counseling
1. Interpretation of HIV antibody test results
2. Information about long-term chances of developing symptoms
3. Planning for medical follow-up
4. Referral to psychosocial support services
5. Reinforcement of recommendations for prevention of HIV transmission/exposure
6. Discussion of notification of sexual partner(s) or needle-sharing partner(s)
7. Reproductive issues in women

[a]A single source for information is The National AIDS Information Clearing House, P.O. Box 6003, Rockville, Maryland, 20850 (1-800-458-5231).

Table 34.7.
Significant History and Physical Manifestations in Initial and Follow-Up Evaluation of HIV-Infected Patients

HISTORY
General: Weight loss, fevers, night sweats
Skin: New Rashes or pigmented lesions
Lymphoid System: Localized or generalized lymph node enlargement

HEENT: Change in vision, unusual headaches, sinus problems, oral lesions
Respiratory: Cough, shortness of breath, decrease in exercise tolerance
Gastrointestinal: Painful swallowing, diarrhea (chronic), tenesmus
Neuropsychiatric: Difficulty thinking, depression, paresthesias or weakness

PHYSICAL FINDINGS
Oral: Oral hairy leukoplakia, thrush, Kaposi's sarcoma
Eyes: Cytomegalovirus retinitis, other abnormal funduscopic findings
Skin: Kaposi's sarcoma, petecchiae (immune thrombocytopenic purpura), nodules (fungal, *Mycobacterium avium*-intracellulare)
Lymph nodes: Adenopathy—Particularly noting distribution
Abdominal: Hepatosplenomegaly
Anorectal and Genital: Ulcers or other evidence of sexually transmitted disease
Neuropsychiatric: Ataxia, hypesthesia, hypo- or hyperreflexia, psychomotor slowing, cognitive impairment, depression

descriptions of symptomatic manifestations are found in the next section ("The Symptomatic HIV-Infected Patient").

When asked, at least half of all HIV-positive patients may report a history of *acute HIV infection*, which presents clinically as a mild to severe mononucleosis-like illness lasting one to two weeks (fevers, diaphoresis, malaise, myalgias, arthralgias, pharyngitis, retro-orbital headaches, and in some patients lymphadenopathy), or an aseptic meningitis (16). Less common manifestations of acute HIV infection include polyneuropathy, brachial neuritis, and odynophagia with esophageal ulcers. The incubation period (time from exposure to onset of illness) for the acute syndromes may range from 5 days to 3 months, usually 2 to 4 weeks. Knowledge of when a patient's acute HIV illness occurred may be helpful with prognosis (Fig. 34.2).

In addition to *a baseline history* focused upon the target organ systems named in Table 34.7, seropositive patients should be asked about a history of sexually transmitted diseases; tuberculosis or a positive PPD; exposure to or history of hepatitis B; and immunosuppressive therapy (e.g., an asthmatic patient who intermittently requires corticosteroids). Important information to obtain in the social history includes current sexual practices (type and number of sexual partners), types of contraception used, and past or present intravenous drug use.

The *baseline physical examination* should cover each of the systems most likely to be affected by either HIV infection or the opportunistic infections associated with HIV infection.

Initial laboratory evaluation should establish a data base that will be useful for identifying already-present abnormalities and for comparison when abnormalities

are identified at a later time in the care of the patient. This data base should include a complete blood count (including a differential and platelet count), SMA-12, urinalysis, hepatitis B surface antigen, syphilis serology, CD4 lymphocyte count, and a chest X-ray. Baseline serological tests for antibody to toxoplasma and cytomegalovirus are not usually useful because of the high prevalence of positive tests in the normal population. Unless the patient has a history of a positive PPD skin test or tuberculosis, the patient should have a PPD. To establish whether the patient's delayed immune response is intact at baseline, he should have skin tests for ubiquitous antigens (separate tests using antigens from at least two ubiquitous organisms, such as mumps and *Candida*, or a commercially available anergy-panel kit that includes these and other antigens).

Many patients who complain of no symptoms at baseline will have one or more abnormalities found on physical examination or laboratory evaluation, most commonly generalized lymphadenopathy (see definition below), reduced CD4 count (less than 700/mm^3), or mild suppression of the elements of the bone marrow (19). If a history of constitutional symptoms (weight loss, fevers, night sweats) is elicited, this should be evaluated further as discussed in the next section. Findings in the oral cavity that may not cause symptoms but suggest some degree of immunodeficiency include oral hairy leukoplakia or early *Candida* infection (see descriptions below). A finding of an isolated low platelet count may be indicative of immune thrombocytopenic purpura, which may also be predictive of progression of disease. Laboratory abnormalities (e.g., hypochromic anemia) should be evaluated in the same manner as in a non-HIV infected patient.

Follow-up Care

Depending on results of the initial evaluation, medical follow-up is recommended every three to six months and should include a brief history and physical examination, as well as a laboratory evaluation consisting of a CBC and CD4 count (CD4 count every 3 months if baseline count is 500 to 600/mm^3 and every 6 months if baseline count is >600/mm^3). CD4 counts are performed reliably by all licensed clinical laboratories. The cost per test varies from $50 to $100; for patients without means to pay for these tests, it is worthwhile to check for local health department clinics that may perform CD 4 counts without charging the patient.

HIV-positive patients are as likely as HIV-negative patients to have common acute or chronic diseases, and the two groups should be approached in the same way.

Many HIV-infected patients will describe minor problems—such as fatigue, night sweats, mild chronic diarrhea, pruritus, and low-grade temperature elevation—for which specific infection etiologies cannot be identified. It is likely that many of these problems are manifestations of chronic HIV infection per se. In addition, for some patients a focus upon somatic concerns will be the way in which they present their mental distress (see Chapter 12 for a detailed discussion of somatization). When an identifiable opportunistic infection has been excluded (see below) and there is no evidence for a conventional infection, simple palliative measures should be recommended (e.g., increased rest, the use of acetaminophen or aspirin as needed, skin lubricants). Importantly, patients should be encouraged to bring up their mental distress as well as being queried and advised about physical symptoms.

Preventive care for all HIV-infected persons should include pneumococcal and influenza vaccination and should follow guidelines for other patients for non-live vaccines and other preventive measures, according to age, symptoms, and risk factors (Chapters 2 and 32). Although their response to hepatitis B vaccine is often suboptimal, HIV-infected persons who are hepatitis B antigen and antibody negative should receive this vaccine because they are at high risk of acquiring hepatitis B infection and of becoming chronic carriers. It is currently recommended that HIV-infected persons should not receive live vaccines (25).

Early Drug Treatment

The CD4 count has proven to be the most useful laboratory test in following disease progression and in making early decisions regarding drug treatment. Early initiation of antiretroviral treatment (zidovudine, AZT) and prophylaxis for *Pneumocystis carinii* pneumonia are now recommended, as there is evidence that this approach delays the occurrence of major opportunistic infections. Table 34.8 summarizes guidelines for initiating these therapies, based upon the CD4 count and the presence of AIDS-defining opportunistic infection (see Table 34.5). It was estimated in 1990 that up to 500,000 individuals may have asymptomatic HIV infections and CD4 counts below 500/mm^3, making them candidates for early treatment with AZT. Details regarding early AZT treatment and pneumocystis prophylaxis are found below (pages 387 and 394).

Psychosocial and Ethical Aspects

Dealing with the psychosocial issues accompanying the diagnosis of asymptomatic HIV infection is usually much more difficult than the medical management of

Table 34.8.
Treatment and Prophylaxis Guidelines for HIV Seropositive Patients[a]

Category	Zidovudine (AZT)	Pneumocystis Prophylaxis
CD4 > 500/mm^3	No	No
CD4 200–500/mm^{3b}	Yes	No
CD4 < 200/mm^3	Yes	Yes
Opportunistic infection[c]	Yes	Yes

[a]From Unpublished data, September 1989, from NIAID AIDS Clinical Trial Group; "Recommendations for Zidovudine: Early Infection" JAMA 263:1606, 1990; and "Guidelines for Prevention of PCP in patients with HIV infection." *Morbidity and Mortality Weekly Report* 38:5, 1989. Additional data from clinical trials may result in important changes in these guidelines.
[b]Two CD4 counts below 500 should be obtained at least 1 week apart before initiation of therapy.
[c]See Table 34.5.

the patient. Patients who have learned that they have a high likelihood of developing a fatal disease, which may have been acquired sexually and which is stigmatizing for a variety of reasons, will usually feel extremely isolated and despondent. Because the patient's emotional response may impair the ability to process information, it is important to reiterate those points covered in the post-test counseling session (Table 34.6) and to respond to the feelings and questions that these points will evoke. The patient must understand how the virus is and is not transmitted, the usual course of the disease, and therapeutic interventions that are available.

The HIV-infected patient has an intense need for hope and support. In addition to assuring the patient of one's ongoing support and utilizing counseling techniques that are helpful for a patient in crisis (see Chapter 11), it is appropriate to offer psychological or psychiatric consultation after the diagnosis of HIV positivity. Among the major psychosocial consequences of this diagnosis are the uncovering of homosexuality in men whose gay orientation has been confidential; the threatened loss of family, social, and occupational relationships; the release of irresponsible promiscuity in antisocial individuals (especially intravenous drug users); and a greatly increased risk of suicide. These are the kinds of problems that particularly require expert counseling.

HIV-positive patients should be assured of confidentiality about their condition but at the same time be instructed to inform others who may have been infected by them. Although asymptomatic HIV infection is not reportable in most jurisdictions, the patient's physician may have a responsibility for informing others who may be infected if the patient will not do so. This raises the difficult conflict between the patient's right to confidentiality and the rights of other persons to protect their health. Laws governing physicians' actions and obligations and ethical aspects of caring for an HIV infected patient are discussed further in a later section (Public Health and Legal Responsibilities of the Physician).

THE SYMPTOMATIC HIV-INFECTED PATIENT

General Principles

The most important aspect of the primary care of the symptomatic HIV-infected patient is knowing the patient well. Many newly diagnosed HIV positive patients are young and have been previously healthy; symptoms and illness are often new to them. They may either overreact to each symptom or deny symptoms entirely. Good rapport with patients is thus essential to having them disclose information and to distinguishing the significance of new symptoms.

The CD4 lymphocyte count is the most useful marker for the progress of immunodeficiency in HIV-infected patients and for deciding on early treatment of these patients (see Table 34.8). When a patient's CD4 count is less than 500/mm^3, new symptoms should lead to a careful search for an opportunistic infection; when a patient's CD4 count is normal (800/mm³ or higher), the symptoms are more likely to be due to conventional infections or other noninfectious illnesses.

The less severe opportunistic infections of HIV-infected patients can be diagnosed and treated in ambulatory settings. Most patients will also require repeated hospital admissions for rapid evaluation and initial treatment of new, worrisome symptoms; but for acute problems diagnosed in the hospital, the completion of the course of antimicrobial treatment, and maintenance antimicrobial treatment, will be accomplished after discharge from the hospital (see "Duration and Location of Treatment for Opportunistic Infections," below).

Constitutional Manifestations and Lymphadenopathy

Fevers, night sweats, or weight loss may be the presenting manifestations of one of the opportunistic infections described below or of a malignancy; or they may be due to HIV infection itself. When one or more of these symptoms are present, a careful evaluation for a treatable problem is mandatory.

The laboratory evaluation of fever, chills, or night sweats should include a CBC with differential, liver function tests, chest X-ray, serum cryptococcal antigen test, blood and urine cultures, and sputum cultures if sputum is available. If the history, physical examination, and these screening laboratory data do not reveal an explanation for fever, a more extensive workup should be performed. Considerations should be given to blood, bone marrow, and stool cultures for *Mycobacterium avium intracellulare (MAI)*, and to specialized imaging techniques [computed tomography (CT) or gallium scans] to look for an occult infection. MAI is now the most common mycobacterial species isolated from AIDS patients. Infection with this organism, which is not curable, typically causes systemic symptoms as well as wasting and persistent diarrhea. This species of *Mycobacterium* is not communicable.

Lymphadenopathy is always a troublesome finding, as it may represent reaction to HIV, infection with another agent, or a malignancy. Prospective studies of a large cohort of homosexuals have shown about a 30% frequency of persistent generalized lymphadenopathy—defined as nodes 1 cm or greater in diameter in two or more noncontiguous extrainguinal sites—during the first six months after diagnosis of HIV positivity (19).

Nodes most often enlarged are anterior and posterior cervical, axillary, submental, and femoral nodes; preauricular and epitrochlear nodes are rarely enlarged. Patients with generalized lymphadenopathy will often have one or more other abnormalities in the history, physical examination, or laboratory evaluation; but no single abnormality coexists predictably with adenopathy. Lymphadenopathy per se has not been found to be predictive of the patient's future experience (23).

Young, sexually active patients with HIV infection are at risk for other diseases causing diffuse adenopathy such as secondary syphilis, hepatitis B, toxoplasmosis, and infectious mononucleosis. These can usually be diagnosed or excluded by utilizing specifical serologic studies and referring to the baseline results of such studies (see baseline evaluation of asymptomatic patients above). If a patient's lymphadenopathy is most pronounced in the inguinal region, with or without an active genital lesion or a history of a lesion, other sexually transmitted diseases, such as chancroid or lymphogranuloma venereum should be considered. If lymphadenopathy is localized in one area, progressively enlarging, associated with constitutional symptoms, or of a different texture (very firm or irregular), consideration should be given to biopsy to exclude malignancy. Chapter 53 provides additional details regarding the causes of lymphadenopathy and when to consider a lymph node biopsy.

Clinical Manifestations by Organ System

The commonest opportunistic infections and other manifestations of HIV infection are described here according to the ways in which they present and the organ systems involved. Tables 34.9 and 34.10 summarize the principal features, diagnostic approaches, and the acute and maintenance antimicrobial treatments for the opportunistic infections of HIV-infected patients. Practical details regarding antiretroviral treatment are found below (page 394).

Respiratory System

The lung is the organ most frequently involved in HIV-related opportunistic infections. In approximately 60% of AIDS patients, the diagnosis of AIDS is made on the basis of *P. carinii* pneumonia (PCP), and an additional 20% of patients experience at least one episode in the course of their disease (5, 17). Despite the frequency of this pathogen as the etiological agent for pneumonia in AIDS patients, other opportunistic and conventional agents may cause pneumonia, either as the sole agent or simultaneously. For this reason, a systematic diagnostic approach to lower respiratory tract symptoms is very important in HIV-infected patients with pneumonia. Moreover, as chemoprophylaxis for pneumocystis becomes more widely used for patients with HIV infection, other causes for respiratory infection will probably become more prevalent.

P. Carinii Pneumonia. Symptoms of PCP are similar to those of other pneumonias, but the symptoms may be less acute in onset. Common complaints include fever, night sweats, dyspnea, and nonproductive cough. The duration of respiratory symptoms is usually 1 to 3 weeks, although the systemic symptoms may have been present for several months. Because many of these patients have been previously healthy, their clinical presentation may be subtle. For example, it is not unusual for a patient with PCP to have had no more than a mild dry cough and a modest decrease in exercise tolerance. Thrush or hairy leukoplakia (see

Table 34.9.
Principal Features of Common Opportunistic Infections in HIV-Infected Patients

Organ System/Organism	Mode of Transmission/Isolation Procedures	Major Clinical Features	Definitive Diagnosis: Method/Source	Antimicrobial Agents[a]
RESPIRATORY SYSTEM				
Pneumocystis Carinii[b,c]	—Not human-to-human —Patient with PCP not contagious to others —No respiratory isolation	Dry cough, mild SOB, subacute presentation, may have no findings on P.E.	Cytologic stain: bronchial lavage or lung tissue	1. Trimethoprim-sulfa (TMP/TMX) or 2. Pentamidine or 3. Dapsone-trimethoprim
Mycobacterium tuberculosis	—Aerosolized droplets —Human-to-human —Respiratory isolation	Productive cough, SOB, fever; usually with findings on P.E.	Smear or culture: bonchial lavage	Isoniazid, Rifampin and 3rd anti-TB drug (ethambutol, pyrazinamide, etc.)[d]
NEUROLOGIC SYSTEM				
Cryptococcus neoformans[b,c] (meningitis)	—Not human-to-human —Patient not contagious —No isolation	Headache, fever, change in mental status; often no findings on P.E.	Positive India ink or cryptococcal antigen or culture: CSF	1. Amphotericin B (Flucytosine is added only in severe cases) or 2. Fluconazole
Toxplasma gondii[b,c] (cerebritis or abscess)	—Not human-to-human —Patient not contagious —No isolation	Headache, seizures, focal neurologic deficit, ± fever	1. Head CT with contrast 2. Toxoplasma serology not helpful 3. Definitive dx: brain biopsy 4. Dx often made by response to empiric Rx	1. Pyramethamine and Sulfadiazine and Folinic Acid or 2. Clindamycin as alternative to sulfa
Herpes simplex or *Varicella zoster* (encephalitis)	—Human-to-human —Wound and skin precautions if peripheral lesions present	Headache, seizures, change in mental status, ± fever	1. Heat CT—cerebritis or WNL 2. LP—pleocytosis 3. EEG—focal temporal slowing 4. Brain biopsy—culture: definitive 5. Empiric Rx often tried	Acyclovir
Progressive multifocal leukoencephalopathy[b] (*papovavirus*)	? mode of transmission —No isolation	Change in mental status	1. Head CT with contrast or MRI: distinctive pattern 2. Brain biopsy—definitive	None
ORAL CAVITY AND GASTROINTESTINAL SYSTEM				
Thrush (*Candia albicans*)[c]	—Not human-to-human —No isolation	Typical white placques in mouth	Potassium hydroxide microscopy or culture: Scraping of plaque	1. Nystatin or 2. Clotrimazole or 3. Ketaconazole or 4. Fluconazole
Candida esophagitis[b,c]	Same as above	Dysphagia/odynophagia ± thrush	Biopsy of esophagus for pathology	1. Ketaconazole or 2. Amphotericin B or 3. Fluconazole
Herpes Simplex esophagitis[b,c]	—Human-to-human transmission —Contact of mucous membrane/open skin wound with lesion —Wound and skin precautions if peripheral lesions present	Dysphagia/odynophagia ± oral mucocutaneous HSV infections	1. Biopsy of esophagus for pathology, culture 2. May be assumed with definite oral herpes and esophageal symptoms	Acyclovir
Cytomegalovirus[b,c] esophagitis/ ileocolitis	—Human-to-human —Sexual, intravenous, vertical, breast milk, ? other —No isolation (? pregnant caretakers)	Esophagitis: same as above Ileocolitis: cramping abdominal pain ± fever ± diarrhea	Biopsy of site for pathology, culture	Ganciclovir

(continued)

Table 34.9.—Continued

Organ System/Organism	Mode of Transmission/Isolation Procedures	Major Clinical Features	Definitive Diagnosis: Method/Source	Antimicrobial Agents[a]
Salmonella sp.[c]	—Fecal-oral transmission —Enteric precautions	Diarrhea, fever, systemic toxicity	Stool culture	1. Amoxicillin or 2. TMP/TMX or 3. Quinolones
Cryptosporidia[b]	—No human-to-human —No isolation	Chronic, profuse diarrhea	1. Stool O and P exam 2. Biopsy	?
Isospora Belli	—No human-to-human —No isolation	Chronic, profuse diarrhea	1. Stool O and P exam 2. Biopsy	TMP/TMX

OTHER ORGAN SYSTEMS
SKIN:
  Mucocutaneous
  Herpes Simplex
  virus (HSV)[c]
	—Human-to-human
	—Contact of mucous membrane or open skin with active lesion
	—Skin and wound precautions until lesion crusted
		Classic vesicular lesion and distribution	Smear (Tzanck prep) or culture	Acyclovir

Varicella-zoster (shingles)	Same as HSV	Same as HSV in dermatomal distribution	Same as above: Only culture differentiates from HSV	Acyclovir

EYE:
  Cytomegalovirus[b]
  (retinitis)
	Same as for cytomegalovirus under GI above	Asymptomatic—or loss of vision	1. Ophthalmologist-diagnosed classical retinal lesion
			2. Positive CMV urine or blood cultures
				Ganciclovir

DISSEMINATED INFECTIONS *Mycobacterium avium-intracellulare*[b]	—No human-to-human —No isolation	"Wasting" syndrome, diarrhea/abd pain, fever of unknown origin	1. Blood cultures 2. Stool cultures 3. Tissue biopsy (bone marrow, liver, colon)	Requires multiple agents if treated: Suggested: Rifampin +, Ethambutol +, Ciprofloxacin +, Clofazimine
Histoplasmosis[b]	—No human-to-human —No isolation	Nonspecific: FUO, weight loss Pulmonary SX	1. Bone marrow biopsy and culture 2. Blood culture 3. Biopsy of lymph node, liver, lungs	Amphotericin B (ketaconazole—maintenance)
Coccidioidomycosis[b]	—No human-to-human —No isolation	Same as above plus CNS: meningoencephalitis cutaneous: nodules, ulcers	1. Sputum/tissue pathology 2. Cultures: Bone marrow, blood, lymph node, liver, urine 3. ± Serology	Amphotericin B (ketaconazole-maintenance)

[a]For details regarding treatment, see Table 34.10 and text section entitled, "Duration and Location of Treatment."
[b]AIDS-defining illness.
[c]Requires maintenance or prophylaxis after initial treatment.
[d]See Chapter 29 for details.

below) may be present, or may have occurred in the past, as indicators of immunosuppression. The physical examination is often not specific. Fever, tachycardia, and tachypnea may be present and, if so, are indicative of more severe disease. Auscultation of the chest is frequently normal.

HIV-infected patients with only a history of respiratory symptoms should undergo a *stepwise laboratory evaluation* that is designed to rule in or out PCP and other pulmonary infections (Fig. 34.4 on page 390). In patients with abnormal chest X-rays, the pattern of infiltrates is very helpful in determining the next step. The timing of onset of symptoms is also very helpful. A lobar infiltrate on radiograph and a history of acute onset of symptoms is most consistent with a community-acquired pneumonia, either typical (e.g., pneumococcal) or atypical (e.g., mycoplasma). A lobar infiltrate in the presence of subacute or chronic symptoms is more consistent with mycobacterial or fungal disease. A diffuse interstitial pattern is present in 60 to 80% of patients with PCP; some have only focal infiltrates, however, and up to 10% initially have normal chest X-rays. Therefore, since PCP is so common in this group of patients, a normal radiograph in the presence of even minimal lower respiratory tract symptoms should be followed by screening tests such as arterial blood gases, pulmonary function tests, or gallium lung scanning. In the presence of any objective findings of pulmonary infection (radiographic infiltrates, hypoxia, abnormal diffusing capacity, or pulmonary uptake of gallium), one should attempt to make a specific diagnosis by inducing the production of sputum; this is done by having the patient inhale an aerosol of hypertonic saline, produced by an ultrasonic nebulizer. *P. carinii* is diagnosed by microscopic examination of sputum; there is no technique for culturing this organism. Examination of induced sputum for *P. carinii* has a sensitivity of approximately 80% in selected patients, although its negative predictive value is low (17). Therefore, if a specific diagnosis is not made on induced sputum, the patient should undergo fiberoptic bronchoscopy with bronchoalveolar lavage. Sputum can also be stained and cultured for mycobacteria, fungi, and viruses. Patients with no diagnosis even after bronchoalveolar lavage should have transbronchial biopsy. Hospital admission for open lung biopsy may be indicated in selected cases. Importantly, when PCP is suspected, one can initiate antimicrobial treatment since this will not alter the chance of identifying the organism, even in specimens obtained after a week of treatment.

Details of treatment for PCP are summarized in Tables 34.9 and 34.10. First-line agents for the treatment of PCP include TMP-SMX, dapsone-TMP, and pentamidine isothionate. Although extremely effective in treating PCP, those agents may cause serious adverse reactions in 25 to 50% of patients treated for two or more weeks. A number of investigational agents are available for patients who are unable to tolerate first-line agents. Improvement may be very slow. Therefore, patients should not be considered to have failed treatment until at least 5 to 7 days of therapy have elapsed. At this time, discontinuation of the initial therapy and substitution of an alternative drug is warranted. Patients who require a change in drug because of toxicity usually do well, whereas those requiring a change because of treatment failure often do poorly. Seventy to eighty percent of patients with first episodes of PCP recover. Higher mortality rates are seen in patients who are sick enough to require hospital admission and who have, or develop in the hospital, severe hypoxemia, elevated lactate dehydrogenase levels, and severe lung damage (3). The use of corticosteroids in patients with PCP has been advocated by some investigators, but proof of benefit in clinical trials is lacking at the present time.

PCP Prophylaxis. Recurrences of PCP are very common after successful therapy; 50 to 60% of patients surviving one year from an initial episode will relapse without preventive therapy. Prophylactic (maintenance) therapy is therefore recommended for all patients after a first episode of PCP. PCP prophylaxis is also indicated for all patients with CD4 counts of under 200/mm^3 who have not had an initial episode of PCP (see Table 34.8). Several agents have been effective for prophylaxis (5, 18, 28): aerosolized pentamidine (300 mg monthly) and oral TMP-SMX (5 mg TMP/kg per day). The less toxic and more convenient monthly aerolized pentamidine regimen is the prophylactic regimen of choice (see details, Table 34.10). The aerosolized dose of pentamidine is administered over about 20 to 25 minutes, with a jet nebulizer (Respigard no. 2). Side effects are cough and/or brochospasm, most often seen in smokers or patients with preexisting asthma. Pretreatment with a metered-dose bronchodilator will often prevent this problem. Oral TMP-SMX is much less expensive than aerosolized pentamidine and may be more effective in suppressing disease, particularly extrapulmonary pneumocystis. Adverse reactions, however, are more common than with aerosolized pentamidine, especially bone marrow toxicity, hepatotoxicity, and cutaneous reaction.

Tuberculosis (TB). Mycobacterial infections are well recognized complications of immunosuppression. The incidence of *Mycobacterium tuberculosis*, which is highly communicable, is increasing in AIDS patients, and TB may be the presenting illness in some HIV-infected patients. Because TB is one of the few respiratory diseases occurring in HIV-positive individuals that is transmissible, curable, and preventable, special care should be taken to exclude it as a cause of pulmonary symptoms; and all HIV-infected patients with positive tuberculin tests should be treated prophylactically with isoniazid (11). Chapter 29 (Tuberculosis in the Ambulatory Patient) has a detailed account of the approach to TB in the HIV-infected patient.

Other Respiratory Tract Infections. If the chest radiograph of an HIV-infected patient shows a lobar infiltrate, sputum should be obtained and processed for a Gram stain and routine culture, mycobacterial and fungal stains and culture, and diagnostic tests (immunofluorescent staining of sputum and serological tests) for *Legionella* and mycoplasma as described in Chapter 28. Treatment should be based on the results.

HIV-infected patients may also have a simple bronchitis or sinusitis presenting with cough and a negative chest radiograph. Though it would be reasonable to treat for one of these entities if the patient is not acutely ill, a high index of suspicion for PCP should be maintained if the patient does not respond.

Neurological Manifestations

The nervous system is frequently involved in patients with HIV infection. More than 10% of patients with AIDS present with an initial AIDS-defining neurologic disease (see Table 34.5), and more than two-thirds are found to have neurological involvement at autopsy (20). Involvement of the nervous system may be categorized as disease secondary to HIV infection itself or disease secondary to opportunistic pathogens or neoplasms. Manifestations may be due to diseases of the central nervous system (CNS) or the peripheral nervous system, as shown in Table 34.11. Table 34.9 and 34.10 summarize features and treatment of the principal opportunistic CNS infections of AIDS patients.

Global CNS Disorders Caused by HIV. In a small proportion of patients, *acute HIV CNS infection* may occur, manifested as a focal or diffuse encephalitis, or aseptic meningitis; there may be associated cranial neuropathies, myelopathy, or peripheral neuropathy.

Table 34.10.
Practical Information about Antimicrobial Agents Used for the Treatment of the Opportunistic Infections Listed in Table 34.9

Antimicrobial Agent	Organism(s) and Syndromes	Dosage/Schedule/Route	Duration/Maintenance	Common Adverse Effects	Drug Interactions	Dosage Change with Renal/Hepatic Failure	Available Strengths, Preparations
ANTIFUNGAL							
Nystatin	• *Candida:* Thrush	Suspension 100,000 Units TID P.O. or Troches (lozenge) 200,000 Units five times/d P.O.	1–2 weeks ± Maintenance or prn	1. Transient nausea, vomiting (N and V) 2. Unpleasant taste	None	None	100,000 u-per 5 ml of suspension 200,000 u per troche
Clotrimazole	Same as nystatin	Troches 10 mg five times/ d P.O.	1–2 weeks ± Maintenance or prn	1. GI side effects 2. ↑ LFTs–reversible	None	None	10 mg per troche
Fluconazole	• *Candida* sp.: Esophagitis • *Cryptococcus neoformans:* Meningitis	200 mg/d P.O. 100 mg/d P.O. 400 mg/d P.O. 200 mg/d P.O.	First day ≥4 weeks First day 10–12 weeks then Maintenance of 200 mg per day	1. GI side effects 2. Headache 3. ↑ LFTs	1. Warfarin: potentiated 2. Phenytoin: increased levels 3. Hypoglycemics: increased levels	↓ with renal failure	Tablets: 50 mg, 100 mg, 200 mg
Ketaconazole	• *Candida:* 1. Thrush 2. Esophagitis • *Histoplasmosis* • *Coccidioidomycosis*	200 mg/d P.O. 200–400 mg/d P.O. 200–400 mg/d P.O. 200–400 mg/d P.O.	2 weeks or until Sx resolve + Maintenance RX Maintenance only Maintenance only	1. N and V 2. Mild ↑ LFTs 3. Severe hepatitis (1/15,000) 4. Adrenal insufficiency	1. H₂ blockers, antacids: prevent absorption of ketaconazole 2. Warfarin: anticoagulant effect enhanced. 3. Hypoglycemics: severe ↓ glucose 4. Rifampin: causes ↓ levels of ketaconazole 5. Phenytoin: may alter concentration of either	Renal—none Precaution with hepatic failure	200 mg capsule
Amphotericin Bª	• *Candida:* Esophagitis Other organs • *Crytococcus neoformans:* meningitis (Synergistic with Amphotericin)	0.6–1.0 mg/kg/d IV 0.5–1.0 mg/kg/d IV	1. Up to 500 mg *total* 2. 1.5–2.0 gms total To total of 1.0 g, then maintenance of at least 100 mg per week	1. ↓ renal function 2. Anemia, thrombocytonia (leukopenia-rare) 3. Reactions assoc. with infusion: fever, chills, H/A 4. Thrombophlebitis 5. Anaphylaxis, hepatoxicity-rare	May cause additive nephrotoxicity with aminoglycosides	When creatine >3.5, ↓ daily dose by ½ or use same dose qod	
	• *Histoplasmosis:* Disseminated • *Coccidiodomycosis:* Disseminated	0.5–1.0 mg/kg/d IV 0.5–1.0 mg/kg/d IV	Total = 2.0–2.5 g Total = 2.0–2.5 g				
5-Flucytosine (usage limited due to bone marrow suppression)	• *Crytococcus neoformans:* meningitis	150–200 mg/kg/day in four divided doses P.O. (IV available on request) can ↓ Amphotericin dose	Only to be used with Amphotericin × 6 weeks	1. N,V, diarrhea 2. Bone marrow suppression 3. Hepatoxicity	Should avoid when using other marrow suppressive drugs	1. ↓ in renal failure 2. Caution in hepatic failure	Capsules: 250 mg, 500 mg
ANTIPROTOZOAN							
Trimethoprim (TMP) Sulfa methoxazole (SMX)	• *Pneumocystis carinii:* pneumonia	5 mg/kg of TMP component IV q 6 hrs or equivalent (2 DS tabs quid) P.O.	21 days	1. Nausea, vomiting 2. Rash; drug fever 3. Hematologic: bone marrow ↓ 4. Reversible renal impairment	1. ? potentiation of warfarin phenytoin 2. Avoid when using other drugs	1. Renal—"use cautiously"	DS tablets: 160 mg TMP component, 800 mg sulfa component

Drug	Indication	Dosage	Duration	Toxicity / Side effects	Drug interactions	Dose adjustment	How supplied
Dapsone-TMP	• Pneumocystis carinii pneumonia	150 mg TMP/1600 mg TMX BID or BID 2 days a week P.O.	Maintenance	Same as TMP/SMX	Same as TMP/SMX	Same as TMP/SMX	100 mg tablet (Dapsone)
	• Pneumocystis carinii pneumonia	100 mg P.O. Dapsone 320 mg TMP bid P.O.	Maintenance	Same as TMP/SMX	Same as TMP/SMX	Same as TMP/SMX	Tablets: 25 mg Pyrimethamine 500 mg sulfadoxine
Pyrimethamine-sulfadoxine	• Pneumocystis carinii pneumonia	25 mg pyrimethamine/500 mg sulfa a week or 50 mg pyrimethamine 1000 mg sulfa q 2 weeks	Maintenance				
Pentamidine	• Pneumocystic carinii pneumonia	4 mg/kg/day IV slowly (im causes sterile abscesses)	21 days	1. Rapid infusion: tachycardia, orthostatic hypotension 2. Renal insuff. 3. Hypo/hyperglycemia 4. Bone marrow → Bronchospasm	None	No guidelines available	300 mg (for IV use)
		300 mg aerosolized q month	Maintenance			None	
Pyramethamine	• Toxoplasma gondii cerebritis/abscess (used in conjunction with sulfadiazine or clindamycin)	100–200 mg loading dose → 75–100 mg/d P.O. (must supplement with Folinic Acid → 10–50 mg/d)	x ≥6 weeks	1. Hematologic: ↓ bone marrow (↓ WBC, → platelets, megaloblastic anemia)	Avoid other bone marrow toxic drugs	No guidelines available	25mg tablet
Sulfadiazine	• Toxoplasma gondii (with pyrimethamine, folinic acid)	25–50 mg/day P.O.	Maintenance	Same as TMP-SMX	Same as TMP-SMX	Same as TMP-SMX	500 mg tablet
		6–8 g/day in 4 divided doses P.O.	≥6 weeks				
Clindamycin	• Toxoplasma gondii (alternative to sulfa)	2–4 g/day in 4 divided doses	Maintenance	1. Nausea, vomiting, diarrhea 2. Pseudo-membranous colitis 3. Mild transaminitis 4. Hypersensitivity	1. Enhanced action of curare-like drugs 2. Worsened colitis	1. None 2. Avoid with hepatic dysfunction	Capsules: 75 mg 150 mg 300 mg
		900–1200 mg q 6–8 hrs. IV	≥6 weeks				
		300–450 mg q 6–8 hrs. P.O.	Maintenance				
ANTIVIRAL Acyclovir	• Herpes simplex infections: 1. Shingles 2. Esophagitis 3. Encephalitis	5 mg/kg IV q8 hr 10 mg/kg IV q8 hrs Mucocut: 200–400 mg BID-TID P.O.	7–10 days or until lesions crusted or symptoms gone Maintenance	1. Nausea, vomiting, lightheaded 2. Renal insufficiency with rapid infusion 3. Neurotoxicity 4. Hematologic unusual	1. Possible additive nephrotoxicity with aminoglycosides	1. ↓ with renal failure	200 mg capsule
	• Varicella-zoster infections: 1. Shingles	10 mg/kg IV q8hrs or 600–800 mg 5×/day P.O.	7–10 days or until lesions crusted				
	2. Encephalitis	10 mg/kg IV q8 hrs					
Ganciclovir	• Cytomegalovirus infection: 1. Retinitis 2. Colitis 3. Other disseminated	5 mg/kg IV q 12 hrs induction then 5 mg/kg IV q day	2–3 weeks Maintenance (dose not clearly est.)	1. Neutropenia, thrombocytopenia 2. Neurotoxicity—confusion 3. GI—nausea, vomiting		↓ with renal failure	

[a] Dosage based on cumulative, not daily, dose.

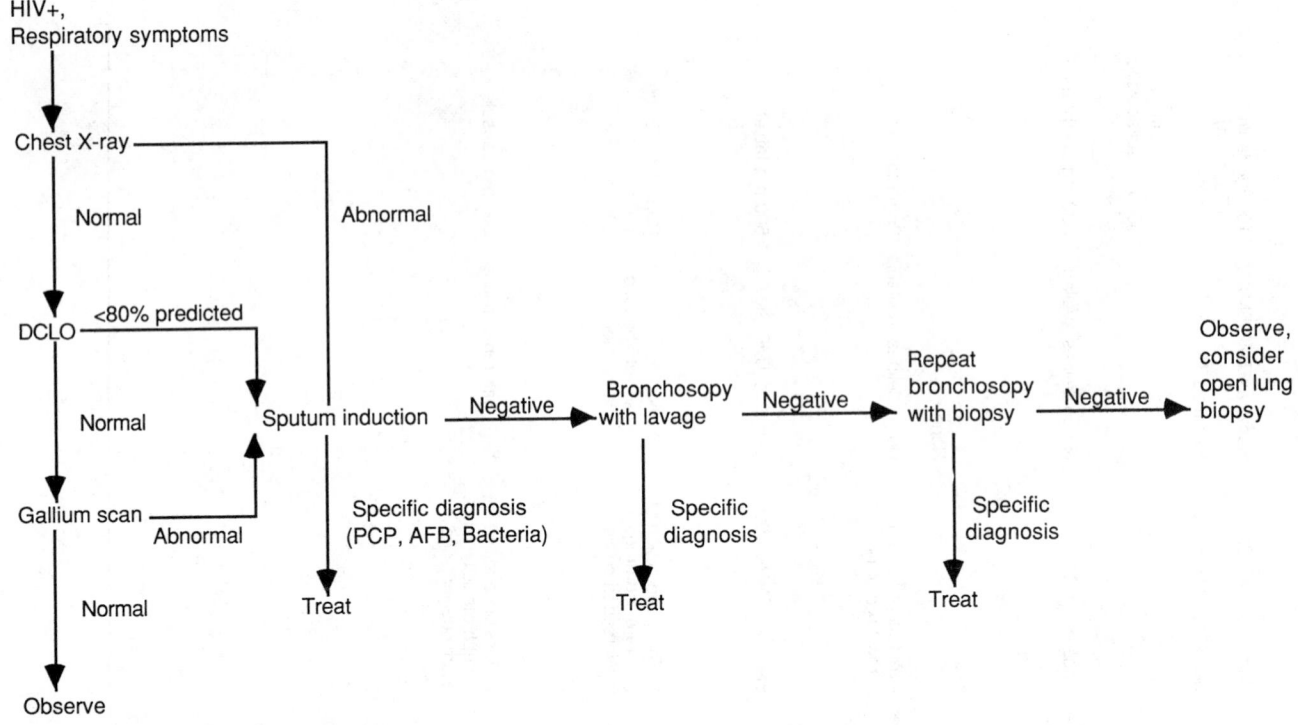

DLCO = Diffusing capacity for carbon monoxide
PCP = Pneumocystis carinii pneumonia
AFB = Acid fast bacilli

Figure 34.4. Step-wise laboratory evaluation of HIV-infected patient with new respiratory tract symptoms.

Several of these manifestations may occur simultaneously. Typically these acute CNS manifestations resolve within 1 to 4 weeks.

In later stages of HIV infection, many patients develop the *AIDS dementia complex,* a disorder characterized by cognitive, motor, and behavioral dysfunctions. Dementia is the most common CNS complication of AIDS, found eventually in up to 65% of patients. This disorder is included in the CDC case definition of AIDS (Table 34.5). Diagnostic features include positive HIV serology; history of cognitive/behavioral changes (especially impaired concentration and attention, apathy, memory loss); and associated neurological findings including hyperreflexia, hypertonia, signs of myelopathy (spastic paraparesis or ataxia), and, frontal release signs. In early stages of HIV infection of the CNS, the mental status and neurological examinations can be completely normal. Cerebrospinal fluid findings are nonspecific: normal or slightly elevated protein concentration, normal glucose concentration, a slight mononuclear pleocytosis, negative cryptococcal antigen, and nonreactive VDRL. CT scan of the brain or magnetic resonance imaging (MRI) of the brain may show atrophy with changes in white matter. Before making a working diagnosis of AIDS dementia, it is important to exclude metabolic or toxic encephalopathies, opportunistic infections, neoplasms, and neurosyphilis. The Mini-Mental Status Examination is helpful for identifying most significant cognitive abnormalities in a brief office interview (see Table 17.1). In a patient whose Mini-Mental Examination is normal, neuropsychological testing may be useful in assessing suspected early AIDS dementia, and in following the course of the disease; this may be especially important in assessing patients whose work requires a high level of cognitive function. Characteristic abnormalities include difficulty with complex sequencing, impairment of fine and rapid motor movements, and slowed verbal fluency. In rare instances, brain biopsy may be indicated to exclude other metabolic, neoplastic, or infection causes. The efficacy of antiviral treatment of AIDS dementia is still unproven, but there are preliminary reports of improved cognitive function after several weeks of zidovudine (AZT) treatment.

Opportunistic CNS Infections. Opportunistic infections of the CNS occur in many HIV-infected patients. *Cryptococcus neoformans* is the most common pathogen causing meningitis in AIDS patients; this meningitis usually presents as a nonfulminant process. Focal CNS disease is most often caused by *Toxoplasma gondii,* though primary CNS lymphoma, tuberculoma, or cryptococcoma may present in the same way. *Progressive multifocal leukoencephalopathy* (PML) may also present as a focal CNS disease. This is a progressive demyelinating disorder, caused

Table 34.11.
Neurological Syndromes in HIV-Infected Patients

Diffuse Brain Disease
  Encephalitis (toxoplasmosis, herpes simplex, cytomegalovirus, acute HIV)
  AIDS dementia complex

Meningitis
  Aseptic (acute HIV infection)
  Cryptococcal
  Tuberculous
  Lymphomatous

Focal Brain Disease
  Toxoplasmosis
  Primary CNS lymphoma
  Progressive multifocal leukoencephalopathy (papovavirus)
  Tuberculoma
  Cryptococcoma
  Herpes simplex/varicella-zoster virus encephalitis

Peripheral Neuropathies/Radiculopathies/Myelopathies
  Neuropathies/Radiculopathies
    Mononeuritides (brachial plexopathy)
    Guillain-Barré syndrome
    Sensorimotor polyneuropathy
    CMV polyradiculopathy
    Varicella-zoster (may involve multiple dermatomes)

  Myelopathies
    Transverse myelitis (varicella-zoster virus, cytomegalovirus, lymphoma)
    HIV vacuolar myelopathy

by reactivation of a papovavirus in immunosuppressed individuals, including AIDS patients. It presents as a subacute disease, progressing over several weeks, with focal neurological deficits without alteration of consciousness until its terminal stages. There is no specific treatment for this condition.

The clinical presentation of opportunistic CNS infections in HIV patients may be subtle. Headache and fever are the most common presenting symptoms of CNS infections, although fever may not be present. Focal neurological findings and meningismus are found in less than half of patients with CNS infection. Therefore, a high index of suspicion must be maintained in any HIV-positive patient with new onset of severe headache, a change in a usual headache pattern, or persistent headache. As sinusitis may present with fever and a headache, this diagnosis should be considered as well.

Laboratory evaluation. Because the physical examination usually is not diagnostic, a thorough laboratory evaluation is important in any patient with new neurological symptoms. The evaluation should begin with plain and contrast-enhanced computed tomographic (CT) scan of the head to exclude mass lesions. The presence of a ring-enhancing lesion is fairly characteristic for toxoplasmosis, although lymphoma and other etiologies cannot be excluded. Because toxoplasmosis is the most common cause of such a lesion and because definitive diagnosis requires a brain biopsy, it is reasonable to begin empirical treatment for toxoplasma on the basis of the CT scan. If

after 10 to 14 days of therapy the patient has not clinically improved or the CT scan shows no improvement, further diagnostic measures should be considered. Unless the CT scan shows a mass lesion that might lead to herniation, lumbar puncture should also be performed in evaluating new CNS symptoms. Cerebrospinal fluid (CSF) should be sent for cell count, protein and glucose concentrations (with a simultaneous serum glucose), Gram stain, India ink preparation, culture for bacteria, mycobacterial and fungal stains and cultures, cryptococcal antigen, and a VDRL. Cryptococcal meningitis may be present even with few or no cells in the CSF; in most cases, cryptococcal antigen is present in both the CSF and the serum. A working diagnosis of neurosyphilis should be considered in the presence of a positive serum VDRL, CSF pleocytosis, and negative cultures and stains for other organisms, even if the CSF VDRL is negative. If the CT scan, CSF examination and culture, and serological studies do not reveal a cause for the patient's symptoms, an MRI scan should be obtained. Once opportunistic infections and neoplasms are excluded, especially in a patient in whom mental status changes are pronounced, the AIDS dementia complex should be the working diagnosis.

Peripheral Neuropathy. Peripheral neuropathies may occur at all stages of HIV infection, including demyelinating neuropathies such as the Guillain-Barré; syndrome in early HIV infection, a painful sensory neuropathy of the feet, and infectious radiculopathies caused by varicella-zoster virus or cytomegalovirus. There is some evidence that zidovudine, when given for indications in Table 34.8, may improve some symptoms of peripheral neuropathy. Chapter 84 (Peripheral Neuropathy) provides additional information about these syndromes in HIV-infected patients.

Psychiatric Manifestations

Psychiatric disorders may predate the acquisition of HIV infection in some patients; and management of patients with a preexisting psychiatric illness and HIV infection may be extremely challenging. Virtually all HIV-infected patients will have gone through a very stressful experience upon initially learning that they are infected (see above). In the months to years that follow diagnosis of HIV infection, these patients may require supportive counseling and the assistance of professional social workers and social service agencies to deal with psychosocial dilemmas. Some patients will develop major psychiatric disorders, symptoms of which may be difficult to distinguish from the symptoms of organic CNS disease or drug toxicity (24). For example, apathy and mental slowing are often prominent in the presentation of major depression in HIV-infected patients; and paranoid thoughts or other symptoms of functional psychosis may accompany symptoms that suggest delirium or cognitive impairment. When organic etiologies have been excluded, or when there is a strong possibility that both organic and functional CNS syndromes coexist in a patient, psychotropic medications should be prescribed.

For depression, either a tricyclic antidepressant with minimal anticholinergic effects or a nontricyclic antidepressant should be selected, as these patients seem to be quite prone to the anticholinergic effects of the tricyclics (including delirium). The doses of all antidepressants should be lower than the usual recommended doses since HIV-infected patients seem to be more sensitive to all of the effects of these drugs. (See Chapter 15, Affective Disorders, for practical information about antidepressants.) Early experience suggests that psychostimulant drugs (e.g., methylphenidate and dextroamphetamine) may be particularly helpful in alleviating the apathy in depressed HIV-infected patients (24); advice regarding the use of these drugs should be sought from a psychiatrist who has used them to treat depression.

For patients who develop psychotic symptoms, the high-potency neuroleptic haloperidol is recommended, as it has few anticholinergic side effects. Psychotic symptoms in HIV-infected patients respond to rather low doses of haloperidol (e.g., 1 to 5 mg one to three times a day). Details regarding the use of neuroleptic drugs are found in Chapter 16, Schizophrenia.

Oral Cavity and Gastrointestinal System

The oral and gastrointestinal manifestations of HIV infection may be due to opportunistic pathogens or, in the case of some patients with diarrhea, to non-opportunistic pathogens. Tables 34.9 and 34.10 summarize the features and treatment of the opportunistic oral and gastrointestinal infections most common in HIV-infected patients.

Oral Lesions. Oral lesions are common in HIV-positive individuals, and they are frequently the first symptoms of immunodeficiency. The commonest oral problem is *thrush, or candidiasis,* which occurs most typically as whitish coating of the oral mucosa or tongue (see Fig. 101.6), in 5 to 10% of patients within the first six months of known seropositivity (24) and probably occurs in one-third to one-half of patients at some point in their disease. Other manifestations of oral *Candida* infection are angular cheilosis and erythema without coating. As noted earlier ("Natural History of HIV Infection") the presence of thrush increases the likelihood of development of AIDS. The topical regimens listed in Table 34.10 usually control symptoms of thrush; if they fail, systemic ketoconazole usually works.

Other oral manifestations include oral hairy leukoplakia (OHL), Kaposi's sarcoma, mass lesions secondary to neoplasms and opportunistic infections, and difficult-to-control periodontal disease. *Oral hairy leukoplakia* is particularly important to recognize since, like herpes zoster infection (shingles) and thrush, it is a manifestation of immunodeficiency. It presents as symptomless hypopigmented shaggy lesions, histologically showing hyperparakeratosis of the mucosa, on the lateral aspects of the tongue. It may be confused with thrush from which it may be distinguished by

scraping the lesion and examining the scrapings microscopically after application of potassium hydroxide. The absence of typical fungal forms generally excludes thrush. A distinct *HIV-gingivitis* that may lead to severe periodontitis and occasionally acute necrotizing gingivitis (ANUG) may occur despite good oral hygiene. Management of periodontal disease may include topical treatment (e.g., povidone-iodine, or chlorhexidate) or systemic antibiotics. Management of these problems requires coordination of care with a dentist. *Oral Kaposi's sarcoma* appears as bluish, black, or red flat lesions, usually on the hard palate. Biopsy of suspicious lesions establishes the diagnosis.

Esophagitis. Esophagitis should be considered when the patient complains of odynophagia, dysphagia, or retrosternal chest pain. The most common cause of esophagitis in HIV-positive patients is *Candida albicans;* the majority of patients have oral thrush concomitant with or preceding esophagitis. Invasive *Candida* esophagitis is an AIDS-defining illness, whereas oral thrush alone is not. Esophagitis may also be due to herpes simplex virus or cytomegalovirus. Rarely, Kaposi's sarcoma, primary lymphoma, and esophageal squamous cell carcinoma have been found as the cause of esophageal symptoms. In a patient with thrush and severe odynophagia, the clinical diagnosis of *Candida* esophagitis can be made. Odynophagia without thrush should be evaluated with endoscopy or a barium swallow. Definitive diagnosis of *Candida* esophagitis or malignancy requires endoscopic biopsy of the involved portion of the esophagus. Barium contrast radiographs may be useful for evaluating suspected esophageal disease before endoscopy; when there is extensive esophagitis, the mucosal contour is typically ragged in appearance.

Gastric and Hepatobiliary Diseases. The stomach is the most frequent gastrointestinal location for visceral Kaposi's sarcoma (KS); lesions are commonly found by endoscope in patients with cutaneous KS. Gastric lymphomas may also be found. Acalculous cholecystitis, rare in younger persons, occurs occasionally in HIV-infected patients; the majority of these patients have cytomegalovirus (CMV) or cryptosporidium found in tissue specimens.

Hepatic parenchymal disease is also common in HIV-infected patients. They commonly have elevated concentrations of serum alkaline phosphatase and serum aminotransferases. The underlying pathology includes, most often, fatty infiltration, portal inflammation, and noncaseating granulomata. Serological evidence of past hepatitis B infection is almost universal. Frequently liver abnormalities are due to an already-diagnosed disseminated infection. When this is not likely, admission for liver biopsy is appropriate. MAI is the most common opportunistic pathogen isolated. KS is also found frequently.

Diarrhea. Diarrhea occurs in about 50% of patients during the course of HIV infection; when careful evaluation does not yield an etiology (about one-third of the time), diarrhea can be ascribed to HIV infection. *Large volume diarrhea,* indicative of small bowel disease, often with associated crampy abdominal pain and weight loss, is common. The opportunistic and conventional enteric pathogens that may cause small bowel disease, include *Isospora belli*, microsporidia and cryptosporidium, CMV, MAI, *Giardia lamblia*, *Salmonella*, *Shigella*, and *Helicobacter*. Multiple stool specimens for culture and microscopic examination for ova and parasites are necessary to diagnose each of these entities; special cultures must be requested for CMV and MAI. In some cases, small bowel biopsy may also be necessary. HIV itself may be associated with abnormal small bowel mucosa. Chapter 26 contains details regarding the diagnosis and management of gastroenteritis due to conventional pathogens.

It has been pointed out that the rate of control of chronic diarrhea (about 75% of patients) is no better, but more costly, when an extensive investigation is conducted than when the initial approach is limited to stool cultures, specific treatment when a pathogen is identified, and diphenoxylate hydrochloride for symptom control if no treatable pathogen is identified. When this strategy is followed, more extensive evaluation would be reserved for those patients (about 25%) whose stool frequency is still abnormal after 1 month (18a).

Diarrhea indicative of colorectal disease is also common in HIV-infected patients. This presents as frequent small-volume stools, tenesmus, and proctalgia. Laboratory examination and culture of stool specimens are helpful for establishing a diagnosis, and in some cases sigmoidoscopy or colonoscopy with biopsy may be utilized. In patients who practice receptive anal intercourse, perianal herpetic ulcerations may account for proctalgia and tenesmus, as may a number of other sexually transmitted infections (e.g., syphilis, gonorrhea, chlamydia).

The diagnosis of *HIV wasting syndrome*, an AIDS-defining illness (Table 34.5), is made in patients with the combination of pronounced weight loss (>10% from baseline) plus either chronic diarrhea (at least two loose stools per day for ≥30 days) or chronic weakness and fever (intermittent or constant for ≥30 days) in the absence of other opportunistic infection or malignancy that could explain the findings.

Cutaneous Manifestations

A wide variety of skin lesions may occur in HIV-positive patients. Probably the best known is *Kaposi's sarcoma* (KS), which occurs more frequently in homosexual men than in patients from other risk groups. KS is thought to arise from lymphatic endothelial cells. It presents as painless, violaceous papules, usually .5 to 2 cm in diameter, often multiple, occurring most commonly on the face, on the extremities, and in the oral cavity. The lesions are bluish in light-skinned persons and may appear nearly black in dark-skinned persons. Kaposi's sarcoma requires a biopsy for definitive diagnosis. This is especially important as it is an AIDS-defining illness (Table 34.5). KS may also involve the lungs, oral cavity, and the gastrointestinal tract.

Seborrheic dermatitis and exacerbations of *psoriasis* are also commonly seen in HIV-infected individuals.

Diagnosis and management of these two conditions are described in Chapter 100 (Common Problems of the Skin).

A number of the invasive opportunistic infections of HIV-infected patients, such as cryptococcosis and histoplasmosis, may present with cutaneous lesions that are rather insignificant in appearance. In the presence of symptoms of systemic disease, one should have a high index of suspicion and consider biopsy of new skin lesions.

Mucocutaneous herpes simplex virus infection, described in Chapter 100, is another syndrome frequently seen in HIV-infected patients, and if persistent for more than a month, is also an AIDS-defining illness. *Shingles*, or reactivation of latent varicella-zoster infection, is also common in HIV-infected patients and may involve multiple dermatomes; it may be the harbinger of the onset of AIDS when it occurs in an otherwise asymptomatic individual. Diagnosis is based on a cytological examination of the vesicle fluid (the Tzanck smear), and viral cultures (see details in Chapter 100). The mucocutaneous erosions caused by these viruses also predispose the individual to local and disseminated bacterial superinfection.

Diagnosis and treatment for cutaneous infections are summarized in Tables 34.9 and 34.10. The treatment of Kaposi's sarcoma may vary from expectant observation to a variety of antineoplastic regimens. The consultation of an oncologist should be obtained in deciding on the management of this tumor.

Other Organ Systems: Ophthalmological, Hematological, Renal, Cardiac, and Gynecological

Other organ systems are involved in HIV-infected patients, though not as frequently as those mentioned above.

The predominant *ophthalmological disease* is CMV retinitis, which may be completely asymptomatic but, if left untreated, progresses to blindness. Cytomegalovirus (CMV) retinitis occurs in approximately 20% of patients with AIDS. Routine fundoscopic examination, especially in patients with proven CMV disease in the past, is crucial. Diagnosis is confirmed by an ophthalmologist, as the lesions, which are hemorrhagic and exudative, are specific for this entity.

Hematological disease is usually secondary to involvement of the bone marrow by one of the opportunistic infections, such as tuberculosis, MAI, or histoplasmosis, or secondary to adverse effects of medications used to treat these patients, especially zidovudine (see below) and TMP-SMX. Bone marrow aspirate and biopsy are frequently indicated to ascertain the etiology of the abnormality.

Both reversible and irreversible *renal abnormalities* are encountered in persons with HIV infection. Although some of these abnormalities may be caused by HIV infection, many will be due to identifiable causes, especially drug toxicity.

The diagnostic approach to *cardiac disease* in HIV-infected individuals should also focus upon identifiable causes other than HIV infection. Although a distinct HIV cardiomyopathy has been described, it has not been well defined. One relatively common cardiac disease is the infective endocarditis seen in intravenous drug users, which is unrelated to their HIV seropositivity.

With the increase in the numbers of HIV-positive women, involvement of the *reproductive tract* has been recognized. Women with HIV infection will frequently present with chronic vulvovaginal candidiasis or herpes, unresponsive to therapy, as the first manifestation of underlying immunodeficiency. Immunosuppressed women may also be at more risk for the progression to malignancy of cervical papillomavirus infection, and such patients should be followed with Papanicolaou smears every six to twelve months.

Duration and Location of Treatment for Opportunistic Infections

Duration of therapy is an important consideration for each of the opportunistic agents that cause AIDS-defining infections. For each specific treatment shown in Table 34.10, the recommended length of treatment is listed. In the absence of a fully functional immune system, most opportunistic infections are never completely cured despite apparently successful therapy; therefore, for many of these infections some form of maintenance therapy is recommended as prophylaxis against recurrent infection. This is especially true of PCP, cryptococcal meningitis, cerebral toxoplasmosis, thrush, esophageal candidiasis, mucocutaneous herpetic infections, and CMV retinitis. Maintenance regimens for these infections are also shown in Table 34.10.

Because of the need for prolonged therapy, *home administration of intravenous (IV) antibiotics and fluids* is used with increasing frequency. Home treatment often follows a brief hospital admission when the patient is evaluated, specific treatment is initiated, and a Hickman catheter is placed for long-term use. Even medications as difficult to administer as amphotericin B and intravenous pentamidine are now being given in the patient's home by nurses trained to monitor the patient during drug infusion. In patients with chronic intractable diarrhea, intermittent home IV fluid replacement may be needed; and patients with reversible causes of weight loss can receive total parenteral nutrition at home.

Antiretroviral Treatment

As of 1990, the only United States Food and Drug Administration (FDA)-approved and readily available antiviral drug for treatment and prophylaxis for HIV-infected patients was *zidovudine* or *AZT* (3'-azido, 3'-deoxy-thymidine). AZT is a dideoxynucleoside analogue of thymidine and acts as an antiviral compound by inhibiting viral reverse transcriptase and/or by terminating viral DNA chain elongation. AZT inhibits replication of HIV in vitro and in controlled clinical trials has been shown to prolong survival in HIV-

seropositive patients. Nevertheless, this drug does not cure HIV infection and it has important toxicity.

The 1990 indications for continuous treatment with AZT are summarized in Table 34.8 (page 383). For *asymptomatic patients*, the benefit of AZT prophylaxis accrued to about 4% of patients in the first controlled trial of prophylaxis (i.e., progression to symptomatic disease was reduced from 7.6 to 3.6 per hundred persons years (26). For *patients with AIDS or ARC*, the benefit of AZT treatment accrued to about 20% of patients in the first controlled trial of treatment (i.e., probability of developing an opportunistic infection the 24-week study period fell from .43 to .23) (13A). The principal benefits that have been found in clinical trials of AZT have been the forestalling of the onset of opportunistic infections, reducing the frequency and severity of infections that do occur, improvement in patients' overall functional status, and weight gain in a significant proportion of treated patients. Subjective improvement is often apparent within the first few weeks of initiating AZT; and the risk of developing opportunistic infections is reduced after six weeks of treatment. The duration of these benefits varies, but within months there is often failure to maintain improvement or inability to tolerate AZT.

AZT is available (as Retrovir) in 100-mg capsules and as an elixir (50 mg/5 ml); it is not available for parenteral administration. Once AZT has been initiated, it should be taken continuously unless it must be temporarily stopped due to toxicity or because the patient cannot take medicine by mouth. The usual dose for both asymptomatic and symptomatic patients is 100 mg 5 times a day by mouth (every 4 hours while awake), taken indefinitely. The previously recommended regimen was 200 mg every 4 hours, but the 1989 analysis of results of a multicenter randomized trial by the NIAID AIDS Clinical Trials Group have shown that 100 mg 5 times daily is as efficacious as, and more convenient and less toxic than, the larger dose; these findings are based on studies of patients with previous PCP infection. AZT 100 mg 5 times daily was also as effective but less toxic than 200 mg 5 times daily in preventing asymptomatic HIV-seropositive patients from developing systemic disease in a placebo-controlled trial (26).

Zidovudine is eliminated from the body primarily by renal excretion after metabolism in the liver.

Toxicity of AZT is mostly hematological, primarily anemia and neutropenia. Both are more frequent in patients with advanced AIDS and in patients who are taking other drugs with bone marrow toxicity (e.g., TMP-SMX, pentamidine, sulfas, pyrimethamine, ganciclovir). Common adverse reactions to AZT include nausea, insomnia, headaches, agitation, mild confusion, and myalgias. These adverse reactions occur in many patients taking AZT and often subside with time.

Once AZT is initiated, the patient's complete blood count (CBC) should be monitored every 2 weeks for two months and then, if stable, once every 4 to 6 weeks; Table 34.12 summarizes dose adjustments and other actions related to bone marrow toxicity. Renal and

Table 34.12.
Dose Adjustment of AZT in Patients with AZT Bone Marrow Toxicity

Toxicity	Options
Hgb 6.5–7.9 g/dl	Transfuse and/or dose reduction[a] until >9.5 gm/dl or entry level; discontinue if transfusion requirement exceeds 2–3 units/2 weeks
<6.5	Transfuse and discontinue[a] until >9.5 mg/dl or entry level
WBC 1000–1500/cmm	Dose reduction[a]
<1000	Discontinue until >2600/cmm or entry
Granulocytes 500–750/cmm <500/cmm	Dose reduction[a] until >1300/cmm or entry level
	Discontinue until >1300/cmm or entry level
Platelets 25,000–50,000/cmm	Dose reduction until >75,000/cmm or entry level
<25,000	Discontinue until >75,000/cmm or entry level

[a]Dose reduction may be reduction to half dose or discontinuation of the drug. When discontinued and restarted, use half dose.

hepatic function should be monitored monthly. For patients with hepatocellular disease or renal insufficiency (creatinine greater than 2 mg per deciliter), the dose of AZT should be reduced to 100 mg every 6 hours.

Two other inhibitors of reverse transcriptase, which are under investigation, are 2'3" dideoxyinosine (DDI) and dideoxycytidine (DDC). In preliminary trials, DDI appears to be as effective as AZT but to have less bone marrow toxicity. As of early 1990, DDI was only available for investigational use in patients who could not tolerate AZT or had failed treatment with AZT; and DDC was available for investigational use in those who had failed or became intolerant of AZT and DDI.

SPECIAL CONSIDERATIONS

Problems Unique to Specific Patient Populations

Intravenous Drug Users

These patients have very difficult medical and social problems, even in the absence of HIV disease. Hospital admission for complications related to drug use, including endocarditis, thrombophlebitis, and cellulitis, is common. In some cases, the intravenous drug user uses multiple substances, including alcohol with its related medical complications. Thus, when an intravenous drug user is infected with HIV, the care becomes even more challenging. Although coinfection must always be considered in such patients when they present with signs of an acute illness (tremors, tachycardia, fever, prostration, changes in sensorium), they should also be evaluated for drug toxicity or withdrawal.

Lack of intravenous access is a common and frustrating problem in these patients. Frequently, placement of a central line expedites therapy and prevents much of the frustration experienced in looking for peripheral vascular access. Unfortunately, a central line also provides the active drug user with a site for injecting himself, while being treated in the hospital or at home.

In addition to their medical problems, drug abusers also present many behavioral problems. Often noncompliant with medication and manipulative, and at times callous about the risks they pose to others, these patients require much patience and expertise. Effective treatment for their substance abuse is critical to having them follow appropriate care for their HIV infection. Information regarding treatment of substance abuse is found in Chapter 22 (Use and Abuse of Illicit Drugs and Substances).

Women

HIV-infected women generally fall into one of two categories, based on age. A minority are older female patients who have acquired their infection through transfusion of blood products and who have an underlying medical condition. The majority are younger patients who have histories of intravenous drug use and/or multiple sexual partners from an early age; thus they are at risk not only for other diseases transmitted by needle sharing and sexual promiscuity, but also for unplanned pregnancy. As the diagnosis of HIV seropositivity may come as a surprise, these young women will frequently deny the diagnosis and will not return for medical follow-up.

Women capable of childbearing should be counseled about the risk of transmission of HIV infection to their newborn should they become pregnant; the risk of transmission to the fetus is currently estimated as between 30 and 50%. Barrier contraception (condom use by the partner) is of paramount importance not only to prevent pregnancy but also transmission of HIV (For details, see "Sexual Transmission" above).

Social and Economic Issues

As noted above ("Early Evaluation and Follow-up of the HIV-Infected Patient"), the diagnosis of HIV seropositivity or AIDS can be devastating to the individual. Not only are AIDS patients faced with coping with a fatal disease, which is sexually transmissible, but also with the social stigmata attached to the disease. These individuals must confront the need to inform their sexual partner(s) (for the partners' own protection) and also the risk of losing close friends. They must face the risk of employment, housing, or insurance discrimination. Women must face the effect of this disease on their childbearing future, as well as the effect on children they are already rearing. Because many individuals who are seropositive were in dire financial straits prior to their illness, the disease may create an unbearable financial burden. In addition to the medical complications of AIDS, these social and economic dilemmas will come to the attention of the patient's physician(s), who must repeatedly present unpleasant facts to the patient and help the patient come to terms with them.

The patient's financial stress may be ameliorated somewhat by the fact that AIDS (and some HIV-related illnesses that do not meet diagnostic criteria for AIDS) qualifies a patient for Social Security Disability. This means that the patient receives Social Security income immediately but must wait 24 months before receiving Medicare health insurance. An AIDS patient who meets the needs criteria for Supplemental Security Income (SSI) can obtain health insurance through Medicaid immediately (see Chapter 9 for further information). The cost of AZT alone (more than $1.00 per capsule) gives some indication of the size of the health care cost of AIDS, even for the ambulatory patient.

In addressing the social aspects of the patient's disease, the patient's right to privacy and confidentiality should be assured at the outset, and the patient should be asked to specify those persons to whom he plans to disclose the nature of his illness. Intensive psychological counseling is of paramount importance in helping AIDS patients to cope with these decisions and the many changes in their lives caused by their disease. A team approach to the management of all aspects of AIDS is crucial. In addition to the physician's input, the supportive counseling of a social worker and help from community-based support groups and health department AIDS services should be enlisted.

Death and Dying

As AIDS is at present a uniformly fatal disease, dealing with the issues of death and dying is extremely important. It is probably not appropriate to begin such discussions when an individual first learns of seropositivity, other than to answer questions about the prognosis frankly. It should be emphasized that HIV infection has a long latency period (see Fig. 34.2), and that it is not known that all HIV-positive individuals will develop AIDS. In these circumstances, hope is extremely powerful in maintaining one's psychological and physical well-being.

The more appropriate time to explore the issues of death and dying is when the individual develops signs and symptoms related to progressive immunodeficiency. Open discussions should be initiated about financial planning and about advance directives regarding resuscitation and other aspects of care when one may not be competent. It is specially important that these discussions take place early in the course of AIDS while the individual is still fully competent. Again, the team approach is very important here, as the individual needs as much support as possible. Issues of death, dying, and bereavement are discussed in further detail in Chapter 19, and Chapter 6 describes legal considerations in specifying and documenting advance directives.

Public Health and Legal Responsibilities of the Physician

No disease in recent times has emphasized to a greater extent the confrontation between the defense of in-

dividual privacy and the protection of public health. Clearly, this remains a major challenge to health care professionals dealing with HIV infection. The physician's primary responsibility is to the patient. The unique trust inherent in the physician-patient relationship allows the physician to guide the patient to protect those who may be at risk because of intimate exposure. The physician has the responsibility of emphasizing to the patient, on multiple occasions if necessary, the importance of informing sexual and/or needle-sharing partners of seropositivity. Guidelines governing the physician's responsibility when the patient refuses to inform others are included in many state laws, and advice regarding these guidelines should be sought from public health authorities in one's state.

Physicians are required by law to report all newly diagnosed cases of AIDS, using confidential morbidity report forms. Some states now require reporting of most symptomatic HIV-associated disease.

Information/Support for Household Members

Persons who live with and/or care for HIV-infected patients at home have special needs.

First, they need clear information about the transmission of HIV infection—both about the safety of nonintimate contact with the patient and the risks and precautions related to intimate contact. Household caretakers should be advised to follow the precautions recommended to health care workers for the care of all patients, the so-called "universal precautions" described in the next section. Guidelines for social interaction in the household should be based on information described above ("Transmission and Prevention of Transmission").

Second, persons close to patients with HIV infection and AIDS invariably have a variety of intense emotional reactions and must also confront distressing social implications of the patient's illness. Thus, taking the time to share information and, more important, to respond to the questions and feelings of the patient's caretaker(s) is a critical part of being the physician(s) for HIV-infected and AIDS patients.

Precautions for Health Care Workers

The possibility of transmission of the human immunodeficiency virus to health care workers and caretakers in the patient's household has been of concern since the identification of HIV as the cause of AIDS. The cumulative results of several studies of health care workers have shown that health care workers are at an extremely low but finite risk of occupational infection with the virus (8). The predominant occupational risk for infection is through accidental needlestick exposure; however, the risk of infection after exposure to HIV-infected blood through a needlestick is less than 0.5% (9).

It has been shown that accidental infection is preventable by conscientious use of the *universal precautions* summarized in Table 34.13. The word "universal" refers to the fact that these precautions

Table 34.13.
Health Care Workers' Universal Precautions That Should Be Used in the Care of ALL Patients

1. Wear gloves for touching blood and body fluids, mucous membranes, or nonintact skin of the patient.
2. Wash hands immediately before and after patient care.
3. Wear gowns, mask, and goggles if aerosolization or splattering of blood or body fluids is likely.
4. Handle sharp instruments with great care and discard them immediately in containers designed for this purpose. Used venipuncture needles MUST NOT be recapped.
5. Clean blood spills promptly with disinfectant such as 1:10 dilution of bleach.
6. Refrain from direct patient care if you have exudative skin lesions.

should be followed in the direct care of *all* patients and in handling the body fluids of *all* patients (8).

If a health care worker has a parenteral (needlestick or cut) or mucous membrane (splash in eye or mouth) exposure to blood or other body fluids, the source patient should be assessed clinically and should be queried about risk factors for HIV infection by the patient's physician, to determine the likelihood of HIV infection. If that assessment suggests that infection with HIV may exist, the patient should be informed of the incident and asked to consent to serological testing (see pretest counseling, Table 34.6). If the source patient has clinical evidence suggesting HIV infection, declines testing, has a known positive test, or if the source is unknown, the exposed worker should be advised to have a baseline HIV antibody test and repeated tests at 3 and 6 months. Because the risk of transmission of hepatitis B virus (HBV) is much greater than that for HIV, the approach for exposure to possible HBV, outlined in Table 32.3 also should be followed in caring for the exposed health care worker.

General References

Centers for Disease Control: *Update: AIDS-United States, 1981–1988.* MMWR 38:229–236, 1989.
  A summary of the epidemiological aspects of AIDS in the United States between 1981 and 1988.
Cohen PT, Sande MA, Volberding PA (eds): *The AIDS Knowledge Base.* Waltham, Massachusetts, The Medical Publishing Group, 1990.
  Ten years' experience, fifty experts, 1100 pages of text.
Institute of Medicine, National Academy of Sciences: *Confronting AIDS: Directions for Public Health, Health Care, and Research.* Washington, DC, National Academy Press, 1986.
  An excellent review and discussion of policy issues relating to AIDS.
Kucers A, Bennett NM: *The Use of Antibiotics.* Philadelphia, JB Lippincott Company, 1987.
  A comprehensive review of the pharmacology, actions, interactions, and indications of the antibiotics most commonly used in the treatment of infections associated with AIDS.
Makadon HJ, Williamson P, Pisaneschi JI (eds): *AIDS and the Primary Care Provider.* New York, The American Foundation for AIDS Research, 1989.
  Multi-author book focusing on both psychosocial and medical aspects of primary care for the AIDS patient.
McArthur JC: Neurologic manifestations. *Medicine (Baltimore)* 66:407, 1987.
  An excellent, comprehensive review of the wide range of neurological manifestations associated with AIDS.
Acquired Immunodeficiency Syndrome. In: Mandell GL, Douglas RG, Bennett JE (eds): *Principles and Practice of Infectious Diseases.* New York, John Wiley & Sons, pp 1029–1123, 1989.
  An overview of the pathophysiology, clinical manifestations, and treatment of the disorders associated with AIDS.

Turner CF, Miller HG, Moses LE (eds): *AIDS: Sexual Behavior and Intravenous Drug Use.* Washington, DC, National Academy Press, 1989.
  Exhaustive multicontributor resource on behavioral aspects of prevention, acquisition, and management of HIV infection.

Specific References

1. Allain JP, Laurian Y, Paul DA, et al: Long term evaluation of HIV antigen and antibodies to p24 and gp41 in patients with hemophilia: potential clinical importance. N Engl J Med 317:1114, 1987.
2. Barrácute;-Sinoussi F, Chermann JC, Rey F, et al: Isolation of a T-lymphotropic retrovirus from a patient at risk for acquired immune deficiency syndrome (AIDS). Science (Washington, DC) 220:868, 1983.
3. Brenner M, Ognibene FP, Lack EE, et al: Objective clinical and histological prognostic factors for patients with Pneumocystis carinii pneumonia and acquired immunodeficiency syndrome. Am Rev Resp Dis 136:1199, 1987.
4. Centers for Disease Control: AIDS and human immunodeficiency virus infection in the United States: 1988 update. MMWR 38(S-4), May 1989.
5. Centers for Disease Control: Guidelines for prophylaxis against Pneumocystis carinii pneumonia for persons infected with human immunodeficiency virus. MMWR 38:5, 1989.
6. Centers for Disease Control: Human immunodeficiency virus in the United States. A review of current knowledge. MMWR 36:5, 15, 1988.
7. Centers for Disease Control: Interpretation and use of the Western blot assay for serodiagnosis of human immunodeficiency virus type I infections. JAMA 262(24):3395, 1989.
8. Centers for Disease Control: Recommendations for prevention of HIV transmission in health care settings. MMWR 36 (suppl 2):1S, 1987.
9. Centers for Disease Control: Update: acquired immunodeficiency virus infection among health care workers. MMWR 37:229, 1988.
10. Centers for Disease Control: Update: universal precautions for prevention of transmission of human immunodeficiency virus, hepatitis B virus, and other bloodborne pathogens in health care settings. MMWR 37:377, 1988.
11. Chaisson RE, Schecter GF, Thever CP, et al: Tuberculosis in patients with acquired immunodeficiency syndrome: clinical features, response to therapy and survival. Am Rev Resp Dis 136:S70, 1987.
12. Clavel F, Mansinho K, Charmaret S, et al: Human immunodeficiency virus type 2 infection associated with AIDS in West Africa. N Engl J Med 316:1180, 1987.
13. Cooper GS, Jeffers DJ: The clinical prognosis of HIV-1 infection: a review of 32 follow-up studies. J Gen Intern Med 3:525, 1988.
13a. Fischl MA, Richman DD, Grieco MH, et al: The efficacy of azidothymidine (AZT) in the treatment of patients with AIDS and AIDS-related complex; a double-blind, placebo-controlled trial. N Engl J Med 317:185, 1987.
14. Friedland GH, Klein RS: Transmission of the human immunodeficiency virus. N Engl J Med 317:1125, 1987.
15. Ho DD, Pomerantz RJ, Kaplan JC: Pathogenesis of infection with human immunodeficiency virus. N Engl J Med 317:278, 1987.
16. Ho DD, Sarngadharan MG, Resnick L, et al: Primary human T-lymphotropic virus type III infection. Ann Intern Med 103:880, 1985.
17. Hopewell PC: Diagnosis of Pneumocystic carinii pneumonia. In: Sande MA, Volberding PA (eds): Medical Management of AIDS. Inf Dis Clin North Am 2(2):409, 1988.
18. Hughes WT, Kuhn S, Chaudhary S, et al: Successful chemoprophylaxis for Pneumocystic carinii pneumonitis. N Engl J Med 297:1419, 1977.
18a. Johanson JF, Sonnenberg A: Efficient management of diarrhea in the acquired immunodeficiency syndrome (AIDS). Ann Intern Med 112:942, 1990.
19. Kaslow RA, Phair JP, Friedman HB, et al: Infection with the human immunodeficiency virus: clinical manifestations and their relationship to immune deficiency. Ann Intern Med 107:474, 1987.
20. Levy RM, Bredesen DE, Rosenblum ML: Neurological manifes-

tations of the acquired immunodeficiency syndrome (AIDS): experience of UCSF and review of the literature. *J Neurosurg* 62:75, 1985.

21. Moss AR, Bachetti P: Natural history of HIV infection. *AIDS* 39(2):55, 1989.
22. Hardy AM: Vital and Health Statistics of the National Center for Health Statistics: *AIDS knowledge and attitudes for April–June 1989. Advance Data*, United States Department of Health and Human Services, 179, November 1, 1989.
23. Osmond P, Chaisson RE, Moss AR, et al: Lymphadenopathy in asymptomatic patients seropositive for HIV. *N Engl J Med* 317:246, 1987.
24. Ostrow D, Grant I, Atkinson H: Assessment and Management of the AIDS Patient with Neuropsychiatric Disturbances. *J Clin Psychiatry* 49(5, Supple):14, 1988.
25. Poland GA, Love KR, Hughes CE: Routine immunization of the HIV-positive asymptomatic patient. *J Gen Intern Med* 5:147, 1990.
26. Volberding PA, Lagakos SW, Koch MA, et al: Zidovudine in asymptomatic human immunodeficiency virus infection. *N Engl J Med* 322:941, 1990.
27. Wolinsky SM, Rinaldo CR, Kwok S, et al: Human immunodeficiency virus type 1 (HIV-1) infection a median of 18 months before a diagnostic Western blot. *Ann Intern Med* 111:961, 1989.
28. Young FE, Nightingale SL, Cooper EC, Trapnell CB: Aerosolized pentamidine: approved for HIV-infected individuals at high risk for Pneumocystis carinii pneumonia. *Arch Intern Med* 149:2412, 1989.

Gastrointestinal Problems

Disorders of the Esophagus: Dysphagia, Noncardiac Chest Pain, and Gastroesophageal Reflux*

PHILIP O. KATZ, M.D.

PHYSIOLOGY OF SWALLOWING

Normal swallowing requires the coordination of the skeletal muscles of the pharynx, the cricopharyngeus muscle (the upper esophageal sphincter), and the proximal one-third of the esophagus, with the smooth muscle of the distal body of the esophagus and the lower esophageal sphincter. Thus, the initiation of swallowing is voluntary, but involuntary processes subsequently propel the swallowed bolus through the esophagus into the stomach. The following sequence of events occurs during normal swallowing: relaxation of the upper esophageal sphincter to permit entry of the bolus into the esophagus; closure of the sphincter to prevent esophageal-pharyngeal regurgitation and aspiration; propulsion of the bolus distally by esophageal peristalsis; relaxation of the lower esophageal sphincter (LES), to allow easy entrance of the bolus into the stomach; and prompt closure of the LES to prevent reflux of gastric contents.

DYSPHAGIA

Dysphagia, difficulty in swallowing, may occur from a disturbance of any of the anatomical structures or of the physiological events involved in normal swallow-

---

*Dr. Harold Tucker contributed to this chapter in the first two editions of this book.

ing. It is an extremely specific symptom and should never be dismissed as an "emotional" problem or as a symptom of "globus hystericus" (see page 409). The patient frequently says that food is sticking in his chest, often pinpointing the precise area. Occasionally, dysphagia may be accompanied by pain on swallowing, *odynophagia*, but the two symptoms are quite distinct and may occur independently. There are two types of dysphagia: oropharyngeal dysphagia (the inability to initiate the act of swallowing) and esophageal dysphagia (difficulty in transport of material down the esophagus).

Clinical Evaluation

History

Because of the complexity of the swallowing mechanism, the causes of dysphagia are quite varied. Certain aspects of the history are very helpful in elucidating the underlying disorder. Difficulty in swallowing solids strongly suggests an anatomical obstruction such as carcinoma, stricture, or esophageal ring, whereas difficulty in swallowing solids and liquids suggests a motility disturbance such as achalasia, scleroderma, or diffuse esophageal spasm.

The history may also be useful in identifying the region of abnormal function as either *oropharyngeal* or *esophageal*. Symptoms suggestive of oropharyngeal dysphagia include regurgitation of liquid through the nose, aspiration with swallowing, and an inability to propel a bolus of food into the pharynx. Patients with esophageal dysphagia complain of retrosternal fullness after swallowing and of the feeling that food is stuck at a certain point in the esophagus—often relieved by regurgitation. Esophageal dysphagia is most commonly caused by structural abnormalities (ring, stricture, tumor) but may be due to reflux esophagitis or to a primary motility disorder. The most common causes of dysphagia are illustrated in Table 35.1.

Mild weight loss may be described by patients with any type of chronic dysphagia due to voluntary decrease in intake of food that often accompanies their symptoms. More severe weight loss, plus anorexia, suggests carcinoma or achalasia.

Special Studies

To delineate the cause of dysphagia, one or more of the following procedures should be employed: radiological studies, esophagoscopy, and esophageal motility studies. The workup can establish a diagnosis in 95% of cases. Consultation with a gastroenterologist is recommended for most patients with dysphagia, both for evaluation of the clinical problem and for the performance of esophagoscopy and motility studies.

Radiology. The initial study in most patients with dysphagia should be a *barium swallow*, a procedure that can identify motility disturbances as well as anatomical deformities, and is the easiest procedure for the patient to tolerate (it takes only 15 to 20 minutes and is associated with essentially no discomfort). As

Table 35.1.
Types of Dysphagia

		Symptoms		Causes
Oropharyngeal		Nasal regurgitation, cough, aspiration with swallowing, difficulty initiating swallow	CNS:	CVA, Parkinson's disease, brainstem tumors
			Muscle:	Myasthenia, polymyositis, thyroid disease, systemic lupus erythematosus
			Structural:	Web, Zenker's diverticulum, extrinsic compression
Esophageal		Dysphagia for solids Continuous Intermittent		Carcinoma, stricture, ring, diverticulum
		Dysphagia for solids and liquids		Motility disorder (see text), severe narrowing from tumor, stricture

with all radiological studies, the radiologist should be informed about the specific disorders that are most suspected. Without this communication, the radiologist may perform a routine barium swallow looking for only carcinoma, stricture, or reflux. Special techniques need to be applied to identify esophageal rings and diverticula. Careful fluoroscopic control is required to evaluate motility. In addition, to observe the rapid activity of pharyngeal contractions and to detect abnormal esophageal contractions, the barium swallow should be recorded on videotape or cine film if oropharyngeal dysphagia is suspected. A double contrast study should be performed to identify mucosal abnormalities associated with gastroesophageal reflux. In this way, barium studies often can detect both organic and functional abnormalities that have led to dysphagia. However, a negative study does not exclude either anatomical or motor disorders of the esophagus and a positive study seldom permits a specific diagnosis to be made; therefore, a barium swallow should always be followed by endoscopy or esophageal manometry.

Endoscopy. *Esophagoscopy* is an essential part of the evaluation of dysphagia. Because of the insensitivity of the barium swallow, endoscopy should be performed in all patients with persistent dysphagia, particularly in those with persistent difficulty in swallowing solid food. Esophagoscopy is complementary to the radiographic examination. The procedure is well tolerated and can generally be performed on an ambulatory basis. When a lesion is detected by radiography, endoscopy provides the most direct approach to establish the nature of the lesion, whether inflammatory or neoplastic. Biopsies and brushings for cytological evaluation can be obtained under visual guidance. Further, the instrument may disrupt esophageal webs or rings that are causing the dysphagia and thus may be both a diagnostic and a therapeutic tool. Inability to pass the endoscope through the esophagus into the stomach confirms an anatomical cause of the dysphagia and rules out a primary motor disturbance (e.g., achalasia). The patient's experience with upper gastrointestinal endoscopy is described in Chapter 36.

Recording of Esophageal Motility. *Esophageal manometry* is the best procedure for the evaluation of esophageal motor function (Table 35.2). This study measures the strength, function, and coordination of both the upper and lower esophageal sphincters and of the body of the esophagus in response to a swallow (Fig. 35.1A). The procedure is well tolerated, takes only about 30 minutes and involves the passage of a narrow catheter through either the nose or the mouth into the stomach. Recordings are made of the amplitude and coordination of contractions within the pharynx and esophagus. Various motility disturbances can be diagnosed by use of this technique (see below). Esophageal manometry should be performed in all patients for whom a structural cause for the dysphagia cannot be found.

Specific Causes of Dysphagia

Carcinoma of the Esophagus

Cancer of the esophagus should always be suspected as the cause of dysphagia in a patient over the age of 40. The incidence of esophageal carcinoma in the United States is approximately 9300 cases/year. Men, especially black men, are more likely to develop esophageal cancer than are women. Predisposing factors include cigarette smoking, heavy alcohol use, lye strictures, achalasia, Plummer-Vinson syndrome (see below, page 408), and Barrett's mucosa.

In the vast majority of cases, esophageal cancer is of the squamous cell type. These tumors are most common in the middle third of the esophagus. Adenocarcinoma is more likely to be seen when the normal squamous cells of the esophagogastric junction are destroyed by reflux (see below) and are replaced by columnar cells (Barrett's mucosa). Carcinoma of the cardia of the stomach may directly extend into the lower esophagus and obstruct the esophageal lumen.

Diagnosis. The diagnosis of esophageal cancer is generally made only after symptoms have developed, by which time the lesion is already advanced, with involvement of regional lymph nodes. In patients with predisposing conditions, such as achalasia or Barrett's mucosa, earlier detection of the cancer may be achieved by annual esophagoscopy with cytological brushings of the entire esophagus. Most patients present with

Table 35.2.
Esophageal Motility Disorders

Disorder	Manometry: Esophageal Body	Manometry: LES	Primary Symptoms
Primary			
Achalasia	Absent peristalsis, low amplitude	High pressure, normal, incomplete relaxation	Dysphagia, regurgitation, chest pain
Diffuse esophageal spasm	Simultaneous contractions mixed with normal peristalsis	Normal pressure, ⅓ with incomplete relaxation	Chest pain, dysphagia
Nutcracker esophagus	High amplitude, normal peristalsis	Normal pressure	Chest pain
Hypertensive LES	Normal amplitude	High pressure, normal relaxation	Chest pain
Nonspecific motility disorder	Nontransmitted, low amplitude with normal peristalsis	Normal pressure	Dysphagia, chest pain
Secondary			
Reflux esophagitis	Low amplitude, poor peristalsis	Low pressure	Heartburn, dysphagia
Scleroderma	Aperistalsis (smooth muscle) low amplitude	Low to absent pressure	Dysphagia, heartburn
Polymyositis	Proximal muscle disorder (low amplitude disordered peristalsis)	Normal pressure	Regurgitation, oropharyngeal dysphagia

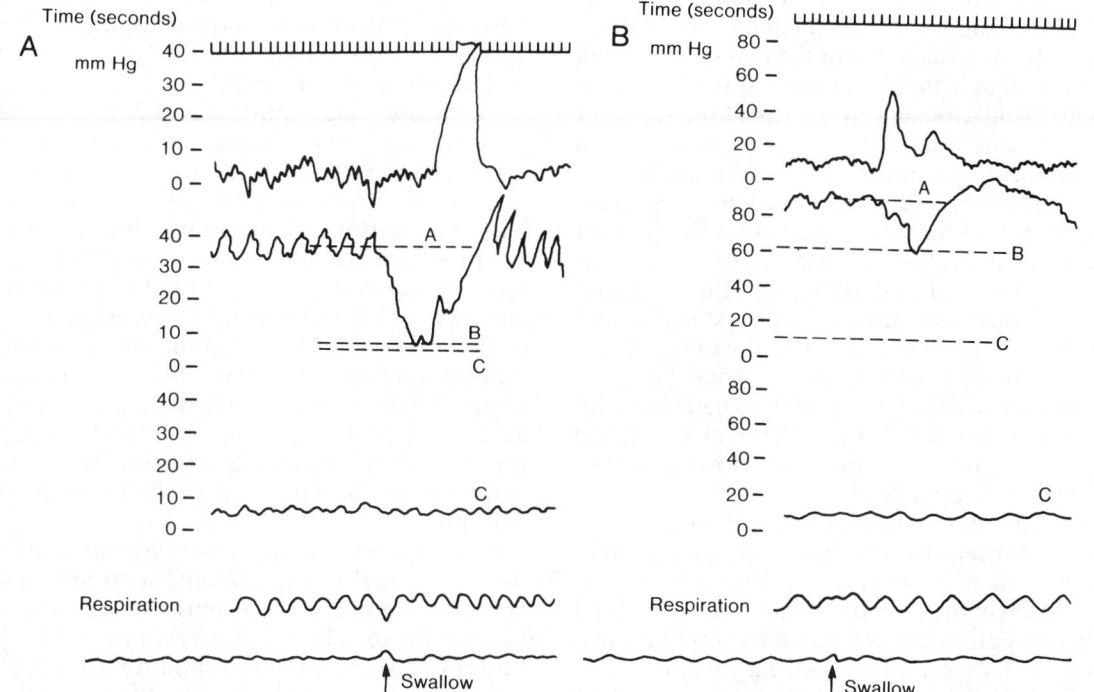

Figure 35.1. *A.* Esophageal manometry tracing in a normal subject demonstrating the esophageal response during a single swallow. Pressure recordings are obtained at 5-cm intervals from the esophagus, lower esophagus, lower esophageal sphincter (LES), and stomach. Before the swallow, the LES maintains a high pressure (*A*) compared with intragastric pressure (*C*). With a swallow, there is prompt relaxation of the LES (*B*) toward gastric pressure (*C*). An esophageal contraction occurs in the esophageal body in response to a swallow (primary peristalsis). The LES returns to its basal level as the esoph-ageal contraction reaches the LES. *B.* Esophageal manometry tracing in a patient with achalasia. The basal LES pressure (*A*) is abnormally high (>80 in tracing). With a swallow, there is incomplete relaxation of the LES (*B*), leaving a residual high pressure compared with gastric pressure (*C*). In the esophageal body, nonperistaltic, repetitive contractions may be found, but there is no normal peristalsis. (Adapted from Cohen S, Lipshutz W: Lower esophageal sphincter dysfunction in achalasia. *Gastrointerology* 61:814, 1971.)

dysphagia for solid food for several months that progresses to dysphagia for solids and liquids, usually with progressive weight loss. Odynophagia (pain on swallowing) may accompany the dysphagia. Occult blood loss is common but hematemesis is unusual.

The diagnostic workup in all patients includes both a barium swallow and upper endoscopy. If the X-ray is negative, the endoscope may still reveal mucosal lesions. When the tumor is already defined by X-ray, endoscopy is necessary to establish a histologic diagnosis, which is important in deciding whether surgery or radiation is indicated. Multiple biopsies and directed brush cytologies obtained via the endoscope provide a positive tissue diagnosis in over 95% of cases of esophageal cancer. However, radiological evaluation remains important as it provides useful information concerning the degree of esophageal obstruction, the length of the tumor, and the appearance of the fundus of the stomach. With the combined use of these two techniques, differentiation can be made between cancer of the esophagus and other esophageal lesions—such as peptic stricture of the esophagus, achalasia, severe esophagitis, and esophageal varices.

After the diagnosis is confirmed, a computed tomography (CT) scan of the chest should be performed to evaluate the possibility of extraesophageal extension, and, if CT is negative, liver function should be assessed to screen for hepatic metastases.

Therapy. Therapy for esophageal cancer is generally *surgery* (6) or *radiation*. The choice between these two forms of therapy depends on the cell type and the location of the neoplasm. Adenocarcinoma is less radiosensitive, usually occurs in the distal one-third of the esophagus, and therefore, is better suited for a surgical approach. Squamous cell carcinoma is relatively radiosensitive, and numerous studies suggest that radiation of lesions in the distal and middle third of the esophagus is as effective as is surgery (see Chapter 8 for a discussion of radiotherapy in the treatment of cancer). Surgical resection is more extensive and less well tolerated, the more proximal the tumor. Combination radiotherapy and resection have been reported to improve survival, but greater experience with this approach is needed. With either approach, the prognosis is very poor: 75% are dead within 1 year of diagnosis, and 95% by 5 years.

Palliation, i.e., maintenance of an open esophagus so that the patient can swallow food and saliva, should be the major aim of therapy if the tumor is not resectable. Dilation of the lumen with mercury-weighted rubber dilators, guidewire-assisted polyvinyl dilators, or with various balloon dilators all may achieve successful palliation. Treatment with thermal coagulating dilators or laser therapy may occasionally be helpful. Celestin tubes (esophageal protheses) have been used in palliation of tracheoesophageal fistulas. Chemotherapy or surgical palliation should also be considered in selected cases. Unfortunately no well-designed clinical trials that compare different modalities are available. The choice of palliation therefore must be

individualized after consultation with a surgeon, an oncologist, and/or a gastroenterologist.

Achalasia

Achalasia is characterized by the complete absence of esophageal peristalsis and by failure of lower esophageal sphincter (LES) relaxation. The condition occurs in all age groups, with a peak incidence in the fourth and fifth decades. The incidence of this disorder is about 1/100,000 population/year. Men and women are equally susceptible to the disease. Patients present most commonly with progressive dysphagia for both solids and liquids and, frequently, with regurgitation of ingested material. Pulmonary symptoms such as nocturnal coughing and even aspiration pneumonia may be the initial mode of presentation. Occasionally, substernal chest pain is associated with the dysphagia.

Pathogenesis. The pathogenesis of achalasia is not known. There have been several studies that have described abnormalities in the myenteric ganglion cells in the distal esophagus (LES zone) and in the body of the esophagus, as well as abnormalities in the vagal nucleus and its peripheral fibers. However, these findings have not been consistent. Pharmacological studies have further supported the concept of denervation of the esophagus. There is an exaggerated response of the LES and of the body of the esophagus to cholinergic stimulation (e.g., in the Mecholyl test) and to the hormone gastrin, consistent with the concept of denervation hypersensitivity. The cause for the neuropathic injury is unknown.

Diagnosis. The routine chest X-ray frequently suggests the diagnosis. The normal gastric air bubble is absent, and an air-fluid level in the dilated esophagus is sometimes seen behind the heart. With a very dilated and tortuous esophagus, the mediastinum appears widened. The typical features on barium esophagogram (Fig. 35.2) include (a) smooth tapered narrowing of the distal end of the esophagus that fails to open properly, (b) retention of barium and secretions in the more proximal esophagus, and (c) absence of peristalsis. The distal narrowing is often described as a "bird beak" or "pen quill" deformity. It is important that the patient be examined while upright, to demonstrate the height of the retained barium-filled column.

Esophageal manometry has demonstrated three distinct abnormalities in patients with achalasia: (a) absence of peristalsis of the entire esophagus, (b) failure of the LES to relax after a swallow, and (c) elevated LES pressure. Manometry should be done, if possible, in every patient with the disease to confirm the diagnosis. In achalasia, the basal LES pressure is usually elevated, at times to very high levels, and the degree of relaxation is incomplete, generally less than 50% (Fig. 35.1B). Thus, there is a constant high pressure zone that impedes the passage of the esophageal contents. Peristalsis is also absent, further impairing the propulsion of the bolus distally. Manometry may dem-

the patient in the upright position will confirm delayed emptying and the abnormal LES (4).

Differential Diagnosis. Achalasia must be differentiated from other disorders that lead to obstruction of the passage of food into the stomach. *Esophageal strictures*, both peptic and neoplastic, and *carcinomas* at the esophagogastric (EG) junction may result in symptoms and even in a radiographic and manometric picture similar to that of achalasia (12). Thus, it is important that all such patients be evaluated with endoscopy. Failure to pass the endoscope into the stomach indicates an anatomical obstruction. *Scleroderma* (see below) with its associated esophageal motility disturbance may result in dysphagia with diminished peristalsis seen on X-ray. If stricture has not occurred, the patient will demonstrate a wide open sphincter through which barium passes easily. By the time patients with esophageal scleroderma develop stricture and dilation of the esophagus that may mimic achalasia, they usually have other obvious stigmata of scleroderma (particularly tight skin of the face and hands or Raynaud's phenomenon). Further, on esophageal manometry the LES pressure in scleroderma is low rather than high as it is in achalasia, and the disorder of motility is confined to the smooth muscle portion (distal two-thirds) of the esophagus, with a normally functioning proximal segment. In patients from South America, *Chagas' disease* may result in a megaesophagus and present with manometric patterns identical to that of achalasia. Patients with *idiopathic intestinal pseudo-obstruction* have a manometric pattern similar to that of achalasia (10); esophageal manometry may be used to help confirm the diagnosis.

Therapy. There are two types of therapy for achalasia: pneumatic dilation and surgery. Both forms of therapy are aimed at reducing the pressure gradient between the esophagus and the stomach, thus decreasing the severity of the dysphagia. The aperistalsis and impaired sphincter relaxation persist after therapy. *Pneumatic dilation* is performed by a gastroenterologist in the hospital. The esophagus is aspirated completely before the dilation. After premedication with analgesics and sedatives, a bag dilator is passed into the stomach. The dilator is a weighted tube, the distal portion of which includes an inflatable balloon. Under fluoroscopic guidance, the balloon portion is positioned across the area of the LES. It is then inflated for 30 seconds to 2 minutes, causing a forceful disruption of the LES muscle. The dilator is then removed and can be expected to be blood streaked. The patient usually experiences chest pain during the procedure. The major risk of the procedure is esophageal perforation, which occurs in 1 to 5% of dilations. Satisfactory results, i.e., improvement in dysphagia, weight gain, and decrease in retention of barium, can be expected in about 75% of cases. In successful cases, there is immediate relief of symptoms. The patient is then observed overnight and is discharged the following day. Dilation can be repeated if symptoms of dysphagia recur or worsen, but most patients have only

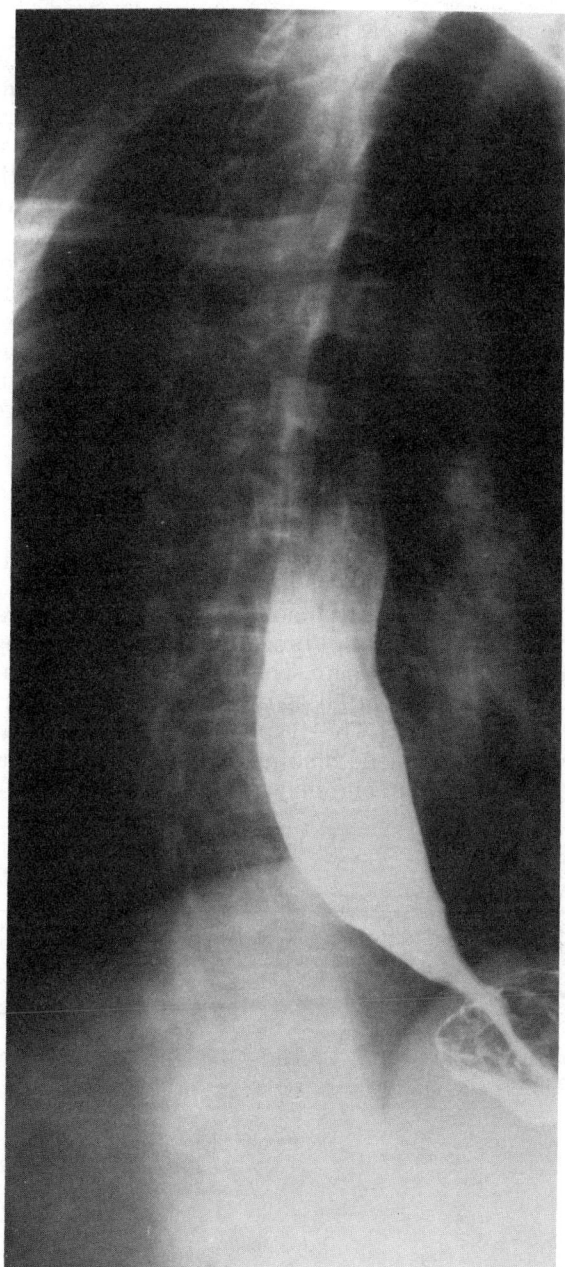

Figure 35.2. Barium swallow in a patient with achalasia. The esophagus is dilated, and the tapered distal segment never opens normally. Under fluoroscopy, no peristalsis is seen, but simultaneous contractions are noted.

onstrate high-amplitude, simultaneous, repetitive contractions that are not peristaltic. These patients are classified as having vigorous achalasia and often have severe chest pain (1).

Patients who present early in the course of disease with mild symptoms and minimal esophageal dilation may, at manometry, appear to have normal LES relaxation (due to a manometric artifact) and normal sphincter pressure and yet have true achalasia. In such cases, utilizing technetium-labeled food studies with

minimal symptoms for many years after therapy. Repeat esophageal manometry is not necessary if symptoms have been relieved.

Surgical therapy involves a thoracotomy with transection of the circular muscle of the LES zone to the level of the mucosa, the Heller myotomy. This surgical approach provides similar satisfactory results, with a success rate of 75 to 80%. The procedure may cause significant reflux esophagitis in 10 to 25% of patients. As a result of this complication, some have advocated combining a fundoplication with the myotomy. Because of the ease to the patients of pneumatic dilation compared with a thoracotomy, and because of the high incidence of reflux after surgery, pneumatic dilation is generally the initial procedure of choice. Surgery should be reserved for (*a*) failure of repeated dilations to provide symptomatic relief, (*b*) esophageal perforation secondary to pneumatic dilation, (*c*) inability to perform dilation because of the shape of the esophagus or the presence of an epiphrenic diverticulum, and (*d*) inability to exclude carcinoma.

Medical therapy with nitrates, calcium channel blockers (see Table 35.3), and even mercury bougienage may offer transient improvement in some patients. Pharmacologic therapy should be reserved for patients in whom pneumatic dilation or myotomy is contraindicated or patients with very mild disease.

Complications. Many studies suggest that patients with achalasia are at increased risk of esophageal cancer. The incidence of this complication ranges from 6 to 29% in various series (2). The development of cancer in patients with achalasia should not be confused with cancer of the esophagogastric junction presenting with an achalasia-like picture. The cancer that develops in patients with primary achalasia usually occurs many years after the diagnosis of achalasia has been established, is of the squamous cell type, and generally occurs in the midportion of the esophagus. There is no evidence that successful therapy of achalasia prevents the development of cancer. Thus, all such patients should have periodic endoscopy with esophageal cytology every 3 to 5 years after diagnosis.

Diffuse Esophageal Spasm

Clinical Presentation. Symptomatic diffuse esophageal spasm (DES) (9) is a disorder characterized by nonperistaltic (simultaneous) esophageal contractions, often of high amplitude, that result in dysphagia and substernal chest pain. The disorder is seen equally in both sexes and at all ages (although it appears to be rare in children). The dysphagia is intermittent and is experienced for both solids and liquids. The pain also is intermittent and may, at times, be provoked by

Table 35.3.
Therapy for Esophageal Motility Disorders Associated with Chest Pain

Treatment Modality	Dose	Mode of Administration	Major Complications
Reassurance			
Nitrates[a]			
Nitroglycerin	0.4 mg s.l.	Usually before meals and prn	Headache
Isosorbide	10–30 mg orally	30 min before meals	
Anticholinergics			
Dicyclomine (Bentyl)	10–20 mg orally	4 times a day	Dry mouth, blurred vision
Sedatives/Antidepressants			
Diazepam (Valium)	2–5 mg orally	4 times a day	Drowsiness
Trazodone (Desyrel)	50–100 mg orally	4 times a day	Drowsiness, impotence
Doxepin (Sinequan)	50 mg orally	At bedtime	Drowsiness
Calcium Channel Blockers[a]			
Nifedipine (Procardia)	10–30 mg	4 times a day	Dizziness, nausea, dyspepsia
Diltiazem (Cardizem)	90 mg	4 times a day	Headache, edema, nausea
Smooth Muscle Relaxant[a]			
Hydralazine	25–50 mg orally	3 times a day	Headache, lupus-like syndrome
Static Dilatation	50 French	Repeat as needed	None
Pneumatic Dilatation[b]			Perforation (5–10%)
Esophagomyotomy[c]			Thoracotomy required; GE reflux (20%)

[a]Orthostatic hypotension is a common complication of this class of drugs.
[b]May be indicated if dysphagia is a prominent symptom.
[c]Rarely indicated (intractability).

certain foods, particularly hot and cold beverages. At other times, the pain occurs spontaneously and may even awaken the patient at night. The pain is highly variable in quality and is sometimes described as knife-like, sometimes as dull and crushing; it may radiate to the neck, back, or arms. It may be brief, or it may last for hours. Because of its location, radiation, and "crushing" quality, it is frequently confused with the pain of ischemic heart disease. When no cardiac disease is found, many of these patients are believed to have a psychogenic disturbance. Thus, this condition is often undiagnosed and is easily confused with other conditions.

Diagnosis. The procedures for the diagnosis of this condition include radiographic studies and esophageal manometry. The *barium swallow*, or preferably the *cine-esophagogram*, may demonstrate nonperistaltic, spontaneous, and simultaneous contractions (tertiary waves) of the body of the esophagus. These abnormal contractions are frequently encountered during routine barium swallow, especially in the elderly, and by themselves do not make a diagnosis of esophageal spasm without the appropriate clinical history. Further, as DES is an intermittent condition, the barium swallow may be normal or may be too insensitive to detect the motility disturbance. Since the barium study is not specific, patients with suspected DES should have esophageal motility studies to confirm the diagnosis. *Esophageal motility* studies are more specific. Provocative agents (edrophonium) can be employed during the motility studies to identify more clearly those patients who develop chest pain associated with abnormal esophageal contractions (see below) (3).

Therapy. Therapy for DES and other motility disorders that cause chest pain is discussed in greater detail later in this chapter (see page 410) and is outlined in Table 35.3.

Other Primary Motility Disorders

In addition to achalasia and diffuse esophageal spasm two other distinct primary motility abnormalities of the esophagus have been described that rarely are associated with dysphagia. The *nutcracker esophagus* and the *hypertensive lower esophageal sphincter* (excessively high LES pressures with normal esophageal peristalsis) are two abnormalities associated primarily with chest pain and, rarely, with dysphagia, and they will be discussed later in this chapter. A large number of patients referred with dysphagia for esophageal motility testing will have contraction abnormalities outside the range of normal and yet do not fit neatly into one of the four disorders classified above. These patients are classified currently as having *nonspecific esophageal motility disorders* and are briefly discussed in the section below on esophageal chest pain.

Secondary Motility Disorders

Chronic reflux esophagitis (see below) may result in scarring of the distal esophagus with resultant de-

creased force of esophageal contractions and/or ineffective esophageal peristalsis that lead to dysphagia. There is ample evidence against the concept that acute acid reflux induces esophageal spasm, but chronic reflux may cause symptoms and motility abnormalities radiographically and monometrically similar to those of diffuse esophageal spasm. Treatment is aggressive antireflux therapy (see below). Improvement in dysphagia and in contraction abnormalities is variable but the pain of chronic reflux usually does diminish with treatment.

Abnormalities of esophageal contractions associated with dysphagia may be seen in patients with hyper- or hypothyroidism, amyloidosis, and myotonic dystrophy. Diabetes mellitus has been associated with multiple radiographic and manometric abnormalities, but patients are seldom symptomatic. Collagen vascular disease (see below), particularly scleroderma, may affect the esophagus as well. Chronic idiopathic intestinal pseudo-obstruction may produce manometric abnormalities indistinguishable from those of achalasia. Many authorities have used esophageal manometry to help make this diagnosis. The use of the term presbyesophagus should be abandoned. Aging itself does not produce significant alteration of esophageal motility.

Scleroderma of the Esophagus

The esophagus is involved in as many as 80% of patients with scleroderma. At times the esophageal symptoms are the presenting complaints that lead to the diagnosis. Indeed, the esophagus may demonstrate the characteristic abnormalities even before skin changes occur. The main symptoms of esophageal scleroderma are heartburn and dysphagia. The cause for these symptoms can readily be appreciated by examining the changes in esophageal motility. In esophageal scleroderma the LES pressure is very low, resulting in free gastroesophageal reflux. In addition, the peristaltic waves initially are of reduced amplitude, progressing later to complete aperistalsis in the smooth muscle portion of the esophagus, sparing the skeletal muscle portion. As peristalsis is impaired, the refluxed acid remains abnormally long in the esophagus, perhaps accounting for the frequent development of an esophageal stricture in this disorder. Thus, the dysphagia may be due to the primary motor abnormality or may signify the development of a peptic stricture.

The pathogenesis of scleroderma is unknown. In the esophagus, the disorder is not simply secondary to replacement of muscle fibers with collagen, since the motility dysfunction can be demonstrated in the absence of histopathological changes. Several studies have suggested a neural defect rather than a primary myogenic disorder.

Scleroderma is a chronically progressive disease for which no specific treatment exists. Therapy of esophageal manifestations is directed at symptomatic relief and prevention of strictures.

Patients with scleroderma, whether they have dysphagia or heartburn, should be referred to a gastroenterologist for evaluation of esophageal motility, and to rule out reflux esophagitis and stricture formation. If reflux is present, the patient should be treated intensively with antireflux therapy (Table 35.4) (see page 411) to try to prevent stricture formation. Strictures should be dilated by bougienage. Stimulation of the smooth muscle by bethanechol (Urecholine) or metoclopramide (Reglan) to enhance LES tone and improve peristaltic contractions may be useful (see below, page 411). If muscle atrophy is already present, however, these agents may not be helpful and therapy with omeprazole (Losec), a $H+ -K+$ ATP inhibitor, a more potent inhibitor of acid secretion than H_2 antagonists, may be useful. Antireflux surgery should be avoided if at all possible because the motility disorder may lead to significant dysphagia after fundoplication.

Esophageal Webs and Rings

Dysphagia for solid foods may be caused by esophageal webs or rings. An *esophageal web* is a mucosal structure that protrudes into the lumen, most commonly in the proximal esophagus. The association of an iron deficiency anemia with a proximal esophageal web constitutes the *Plummer-Vinson syndrome*. *Esophageal rings* are located in the distal esophagus and may be either mucosal or muscular; rings can be demonstrated in up to 10% of the population, but rarely cause symptoms.

The ring that occurs at the gastroesophageal junction is referred to as *Schatzki's ring*. The origin of these lesions is unclear, though they are probably acquired. They are often found in asymptomatic individuals. There is no evidence that gastroesophageal reflux is associated with the development of the Schatzki ring, even in the presence of a hiatal hernia.

Symptoms arise when the ring narrows the esophageal lumen to less than 13 mm in diameter and are rare if the ring is >20 mm in diameter. A typical presenting symptom of a patient with an esophageal ring is intermittent dysphagia for solid foods. The patient may point to the area of the ring. At times a bolus of food may become impacted; the patient then regurgitates and subsequently may be able to resume eating without further difficulty. The intermittency of the dysphagia, the chronicity of the condition, and the difficulty in making the diagnosis unless specifically suspected often results in misdiagnosis and inappropriate therapy.

The diagnosis of esophageal ring is best made by barium swallow. The lower esophageal ring is best detected when the lower segment of the esophagus is distended as it is during a Valsalva maneuver. Endoscopy is sometimes helpful to differentiate rings from annular strictures secondary to either reflux esophagitis or carcinoma. Cervical webs are frequently missed on conventional radiography but may be detected with cine studies. The webs are usually detected on the anterior surface of the esophagus, and

Table 35.4.
Treatment of Gastroesophageal Reflux

Intervention	Specific Change	Mechanism of Improvement
Phase I		
Elevate head of bed (wedge)		Decreases acid contact time
Avoid drugs that decrease LES pressure	Theophylline, nitrates, calcium channel blockers, benzodiazepines	Avoids decrease of lower sphincter pressure
Avoid irritants	Citrus, coffee	Avoids direct mucosal damage
Stop smoking		Removes inhibition of H2 blockers, increases lower sphincter pressure
Avoid eating before sleep	3 hours	Avoids gastric distention
Antacids	As needed	Decreases gastric acid
Alginic acid (Gaviscon)	As needed	Barrier protectant
Phase II		
H_2 Antagonists[a]		
Cimetidine (Tagamet)	400 mg 2 times a day, 300 mg 4 times a day	Decreases acid secretion
Ranitidine (Zantac)	150 mg 2 times a day	
Famotidine (Pepcid)	20 mg 2 times a day	
Metoclopramide (Reglan)	5–10 mg 4 times a day	Increases lower esophageal sphincter pressure, increases esophageal clearance, accelerates gastric emptying
Bethanechol (Urecholine)	25 mg 4 times a day	Increases lower sphincter pressure, accelerates esophageal clearance
Sucralfate (Carafate)	1 g 4 times a day	Mucosal protection
Omeprazole (Losec)	20 mg a day	Decreases acid secretion
Phase III		
Surgery	Nissen fundoplication Belsey Mark IV repair Hill procedure	Creates intraabdominal esophagus and increased lower sphincter pressure

[a]Nocturnal H_2 antagonists are insufficient antireflux therapy.

lateral and oblique films are needed to demonstrate these lesions. Endoscopy frequently fails to visualize cervical webs but may disrupt the lesion during blind passage of the instrument into the esophagus. The endoscope may demonstrate an esophageal ring during air sufflation of the distal esophagus.

Therapy generally involves reassurance with recommendation to chew food well and slowly, as well as mechanical disruption of the ring or web. If the webs are associated with iron deficiency, the treatment of the anemia is believed to cause rapid regression of the web. Bougienage with a large caliber dilator frequently disrupts the lower esophageal ring with complete relief of the dysphagia. The procedure causes transient discomfort but much less pain than does pneumatic dilation. It is ordinarily done by a gastroenterologist in his office. Rarely symptoms may persist after bougienage, and pneumatic dilation (see above) or even surgery may be necessary.

Globus Hystericus

Globus hystericus is a diagnosis frequently made in patients with dysphagia who have no demonstrable organic disease. However, this condition does not produce dysphagia and should not be used to explain away the symptom of dysphagia. Patients with globus describe the sensation of a "lump" in the throat, but they do not actually have difficulty swallowing. At times, these symptoms may be more pronounced with eating. However, when specifically questioned, patients will deny dysphagia or food "sticking" or being "held up" in this region and they will state that the symptom is present even when they are not eating. The pathogenesis of this condition is unknown, but hypertonicity of the upper esophageal sphincter, as a primary disorder or as a consequence of esophageal reflux, has been suggested. Gastroesophageal reflux should be ruled out (see below) before a psychological disturbance (see Chapter 12) is diagnosed. If reflux cannot be ruled out, a trial of antireflux therapy (Table 35.4) for a month is reasonable. Reassurance and an explanation of the problem form the basis for treatment. Mild sedation may be helpful. The significance of this disorder is mainly its differentiation from other conditions that produce true dysphagia.

ESOPHAGEAL CHEST PAIN

Chest pain (7) is a common and difficult diagnostic challenge. It is now well accepted that esophageal disease can be implicated as a cause of recurrent "anginal" chest pain. The prevalence of esophageal chest pain is unknown. However, over 600,000 new patients have cardiac catheterizations each year and 10 to 30% are normal. An estimated 50% of these patients will have identifiable esophageal abnormalities to account for their pain; thus at least 100,000 new cases are seen each year. It is important to be aware that 50% of patients with normal coronary arteries continue to be disabled by chest pain, despite being told they do not have heart disease. These patients still receive cardiac drugs, continue to have approximately two physician visits a year for chest pain, and are hospitalized about once a year for continuing evaluation, at significant cost.

Etiology and Pathogenesis

Esophageal chest pain has been attributed to stimulation of esophageal chemoreceptors by acid or bile reflux or of mechanoreceptors by smooth muscle spasm or esophageal distention. Cold or hot liquids may cause severe chest pain suggesting there may also be alteration in temperature receptors in the esophagus. Transient myoischemia may be a cause of pain in patients with spastic motility disorders. Such patients have an increased frequency of psychiatric disorders and have personality profiles similar to those of patients with the irritable bowel syndrome (Chapter 40), suggesting that chronic stress may play a role in the pathogenesis of chest pain.

Two major abnormalities have been associated with esophageal chest pain, esophageal motility disorders and gastroesophageal reflux (see Diagnosis p. 410).

Approximately 30% of patients with esophageal chest pain will have a demonstrable motility disorder and, of this group, the most common disorder is the *nutcracker esophagus* (hypertensive esophagus, "supersqueezer"). This manometric abnormality is characterized by normal peristaltic contractions in the distal esophagus with contraction amplitude greater than 2 standard deviations above normal (>180 mmHg) associated with chest pain (Table 35.2). Many of these patients will have prolonged duration of contractions as well. *Diffuse esophageal spasm* (DES) (see above) is the motility disorder usually considered as the principal cause of esophageal chest pain; however, recent studies have found it to be uncommon, representing only 10% of esophageal motility abnormalities in patients with noncardiac chest pain. Other disorders, such as an *isolated elevated LES pressure* (hypertensive LES) and *achalasia* have been rarely associated with noncardiac chest pain. A large number of patients (approximately 35%) will have contraction abnormalities that do not fit into one of the four categories defined above. These patients are grouped under the general category of nonspecific esophageal motility disorders (NEMDs).

Evaluation requires consultation with a gastroenterologist. Few patients will have spontaneous chest pain during stationary esophageal motility testing (even if esophageal motility is abnormal) but will have their typical chest pain reproduced when the esophagus is stimulated with intravenous edrophonium (Tensilon). This cholinergic agonist will reproduce chest pain accompanied by high amplitude esophageal contractions in 20 to 30% of patients with chest pain and normal coronary arteries. Edrophonium does not cause narrowing of the coronary arteries nor does it cause chest pain in normal individuals or in patients with irritable bowel syndrome. A positive test indicates the chest pain is of esophageal origin.

Diagnosis

Unfortunately the history is not reliable in differentiating esophageal from cardiac pain nor in differentiating the various esophageal causes of chest pain. Location, exertional onset, and radiation do not distinguish the two entities. Heartburn, dysphagia, or odynophagia suggest an esophageal etiology, but overlap does exist. Pain lasting greater than an hour is more likely to be esophageal but is occasionally seen with cardiac disease. Therapeutic trials with antacids or nitrates will not distinguish between the two diseases. It is important to be aware that intraesophageal acid perfusion can cause pain and STT wave changes indistinguishable from coronary artery disease, so cardiac disease must always be ruled out before the esophagus can be implicated. Musculoskeletal etiology should be sought by careful examination of the chest wall and the costochondral joints. Peptic ulcer disease or esophageal mucosal disease should be excluded by either esophagoscopy or barium radiographs and biliary tract disease, by ultrasound. If these studies are normal, gastroesophageal reflux should be excluded with a short (3- to 4-week) therapeutic trial of antireflux therapy (see below). If this is unsuccessful, the patient should be referred, if possible, to a gastroenterologist who has equipment to perform 24-hour ambulatory esophageal pH monitoring. With this latter method the frequency of reflux can be assessed, episodes of pain can be correlated with episodes of reflux, and esophageal pH can be monitored during exercise. If this study is negative, esophageal manometry with provocative testing with edrophonium should be performed. Using this systematic approach an esophageal etiology can be established in approximately 50 to 60% of patients with noncardiac chest pain.

Treatment

If gastroesophageal reflux is diagnosed, treatment should proceed in a stepwise fashion as outlined later in this chapter. Treatment of esophageal motility disorders of patients with only positive provocative tests is more difficult and controversial (see Table 35.3). Reassurance should be given to all patients, specifically indicating that the esophagus is the cause of their pain and that the heart is normal. Many will experience a decrease in pain with this single intervention. Patients with spastic disorders or with nutcracker esophagus may respond to nitrate or to a calcium channel blocker. Hydralazine may be tried in patients with symptomatic esophageal spasm if calcium blockers are not successful. Trazadone HCl (Desyrel), an antidepressant, has been used successfully to relieve chest pain in these patients and is particularly useful in patients with other symptoms suggestive of depression. Tranquilizers or anticholinergics have been used successfully in some patients. Patients with symptomatology unresponsive to these measures may respond to biofeedback or to other psychological interventions.

Surgery with a long esophageal myotomy is occasionally required in patients with severe pain in whom pharmacologic therapy has failed. Many patients with esophageal chest pain, whatever the cause, will continue to have intermittent symptoms despite therapeutic intervention.

GASTROESOPHAGEAL REFLUX

Gastroesophageal reflux disease (GERD) (8) is a common problem in the United States. Approximately 10% of Americans will suffer daily heartburn and up to 33% will have symptoms monthly. Most patients complain of burning substernal pain that radiates upward, often aggravated by meals and by lying down and relieved by sitting up. Approximately 10% of people will present with chest pain as the sole manifestation of reflux. An unknown number of people will have GERD manifested as hoarseness, cough, or wheezing. In most cases the diagnosis and treatment can be managed successfully by the primary care provider; however, 10 to 15% of patients will develop complications and will require referral to a gastroenterologist.

Etiology and Pathogenesis

The etiology of GERD is unknown. Several defects contribute to the development and progression of the disease. By far the most significant is an abnormal antireflux barrier—the lower esophageal sphincter (LES). Two major abnormalities of the LES are associated with an increased frequency of reflux: *a low basal LES pressure* or *transient inappropriate LES relaxation* unassociated with a swallow. The latter abnormality is the most common cause of an episode of reflux. Abnormal esophageal epithelial resistance (increased permeability to hydrogen ions), abnormalities of gastric emptying, gastric distention, and the nature of the gastric refluxate (acid, pepsin, and bile) all contribute to the development of GERD.

Diagnosis

Several diagnostic tests are readily available to establish the clinical diagnosis. No single test provides complete information about the cause and consequences of reflux, so careful selection among the available modalities is required. In patients with mild heartburn a therapeutic trail of phase I therapy including antacids (see below) is an effective diagnostic approach. If successful, no further workup may be needed. Patients who have dysphagia and chest pain who have other atypical symptoms or who fail to respond to phase I measures should have a diagnosis established by one of the tests described below.

A *barium swallow* is the simplest, least expensive procedure used to diagnose GERD. A double contrast study should always be performed to evaluate for mucosal irregularities associated with esophagitis. Several points are important in interpreting the barium study. Hiatal hernia is present in 40 to 60% of the general population. Mild "free reflux" may be seen in

30% of normal individuals. These findings, together or alone, should not be used to make a diagnosis of reflux disease. The presence of mucosal irregularities, stricture, or esophageal ulcer suggests a high likelihood (85 to 95%) that GERD is present. A normal barium swallow may be seen in 40 to 60% of patients with symptomatic GERD and does not rule out significant disease. It is most useful as a screening study to rule out complications and to evaluate patients with dysphagia.

Endoscopy (esophagoscopy) is the best study for the diagnosis and evaluation of reflux esophagitis or of other complications of GERD such as stricture or Barrett's epithelium. If esophagitis is present at endoscopy, the diagnosis is established with 95% certainty, and no further work up is required. If a stricture is encountered, it should be biopsied to rule out carcinoma (dilation may be done at the same sitting in some patients). If Barrett's mucosa (see below) is observed, biopsies can be taken to confirm the diagnosis and to rule out dysplasia or in situ carcinoma. Though more sensitive than a barium swallow, endoscopy may be normal in 40% of patients in whom reflux is subsequently verified by prolonged intraesophageal pH monitoring.

Intraesophageal acid perfusion (the Bernstein test) provides objective evidence that the esophagus is sensitive to acid and is particularly useful when atypical symptoms such as noncardiac chest pain or dyspepsia are the presenting complaint. The acid perfusion test can be performed in the office by a primary physician. A nasogastric tube is placed 30 to 35 cm from the tip of the nares. Saline is infused at 7 to 8 ml/min for 3 to 5 minutes followed by 0.1 N HCl at the same rate for up to 30 minutes. Reproduction of the patient's presenting complaint during acid perfusion, with relief by saline, suggests that the symptoms are due to acid. The overall sensitivity of this test is about 80%. False positives may be seen in patients with cholelithiasis and rarely with coronary artery disease (see Esophageal Chest Pain above).

The diagnosis of GERD will be established in most patients by the combination of barium studies, endoscopy or intraesophageal acid perfusion test. However, if the diagnosis is still in doubt, 24-hour ambulatory pH monitoring should be performed. This newly developed technology, available in many medical centers, has added much to our understanding of this common condition. The test is performed by placing a 2-mm flexible antimony probe transnasally 5 cm above the LES. The probe is connected to a recording box similar to a Holter monitor and worn about the waist. The patient can then be observed in his home environment eating a normal diet. Ambulatory monitoring is extremely useful in patients with noncardiac chest pain, chronic pulmonary or otolaryngologic symptoms suggestive of reflux, or in patients with typical symptoms when a diagnosis is illusive. All patients who are being considered for surgery should have pH monitoring to confirm the diagnosis before the operation. The study is extremely reproducible

and is currently the most sensitive and specific diagnostic test for the presence of abnormal acid reflux. A suggested approach to the diagnosis of GERD is outlined in Figure 35.3.

Treatment

Treatment is divided into three phases (Table 35.4). *Phase I therapy* is predominantly aimed at modification of lifestyle. This includes elevation of the head of the bed on 6 to 8 inch blocks or asking the patient to buy a wedge designed to be placed in bed under the shoulders and upper back. The patient should avoid sleeping on more pillows as this might actually increase abdominal pressure and contribute to more reflux. Certain foods such as coffee, citrus juice, and spices are direct esophageal irritants and should be avoided. The patient should be instructed not to lie down after a meal as this promotes greater reflux. Avoidance of food 3 hours before going to bed has also been shown to decrease episodes of reflux. Drugs that decrease LES pressure, such as calcium channel blockers, nitrates, sedatives, and theophyline, should be avoided. The use of antacids is part of phase I therapy and should be used as needed to relieve daytime symptoms. Phase I therapy is successful for the majority of patients with symptoms who have minimal esophagitis. If symptomatic improvement is not seen in 2 to 3 weeks, phase II therapy should be started.

Phase II therapy is primarily pharmacologic and is aimed at decreasing gastric acid secretion (H_2 antagonists), augmenting LES pressure, and improving esophageal clearance with prokinetic agents (metoclopramide or bethanecol) or enhancing mucosal protection (Sucralfate). Each agent has similar healing rates when compared to placebo in acute studies, though the largest and most consistent experience is with the H_2 antagonists ranitidine and cimetidine. Trials with other H_2 antagonists are currently in progress. Treatment should be begun with an H_2 antagonist in twice daily dosage. Treatment is continued for 8 to 12 weeks and, if successful, is discontinued. If symptoms do not resolve, a second drug should be added. Metoclopramide has been used successfully in combination with cimetidine in one study (5). Extrapyramidal side effects are common and make this agent difficult to use in the elderly. A starting dose of 5 mg three times a day may be useful in limiting side effects. Bethanecoll (Urecholine) has a lower incidence of side effects and is a useful drug if a prokinetic agent is desired. If the patient is elderly or taking multiple medications, sucralfate (Carafate), 1 g four times a day, may be added as second line therapy instead of a prokinetic agent. This drug is not systemically absorbed, acts as a mucosal protectant, and is remarkably free of side effects. Constipation, a problem in the elderly, is seen in 2 to 3% of patients taking this agent. Second line therapy is continued for an additional 8 to 12 weeks. If therapy is not successful at this time, referral to a gastroenterologist should be considered for experimental therapy with higher doses of H_2 blockers, or with newer

Approach to Patients with Gastroesophageal Reflux

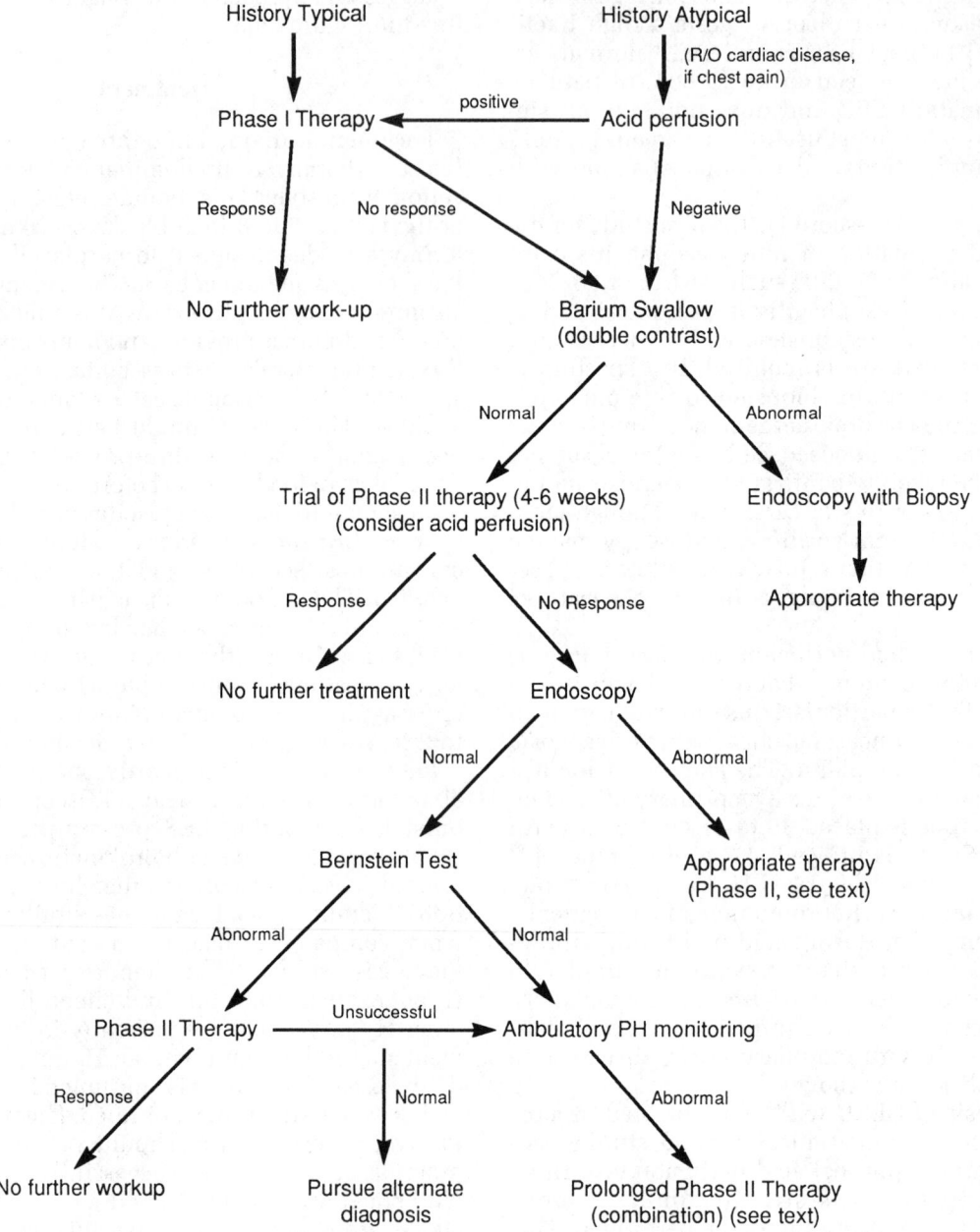

Figure 35.3.

agents such as omeprazole (Losec, a H+ K+ ATPase inhibitor) or cisapride (a prokinetic agent).

Surgery (phase III) is indicated in 5 to 10% of patients with reflux disease. Indications are strictures unresponsive to medical therapy, hemorrhage secondary to erosive esophagitis, esophageal ulcers unresponsive to medical therapy, aspiration pneumonia secondary to reflux, reflux-induced hoarseness, as well as symptoms refractory to medical management as discussed above. Barrett's esophagus (see below) is considered by some authorities to be an indication for surgery. Most would, however, attempt to treat such patients with aggressive medical therapy before surgery, as there is no indication that surgery alters the risk for esophageal cancer. Before surgery all patients should have esophageal manometry to evaluate LES pressure and esophageal peristalsis. As mentioned previously ambulatory pH monitoring must be done to confirm the diagnosis of abnormal acid exposure before surgery. Operations incorporating a fundoplication around the distal esophagus provide symptomatic improvement in about 90% of patients. Simple repair of hiatus hernia, if present, has not been equally effective nor have the benefits been as long lasting. Fundoplication provides an effective barrier to reflux. Several variations of the operation are available and local surgical expertise generally dictates the specific operation that is performed. Complications include dysphagia, which is usually transient, and the "gasbloat" syndrome from inability to belch. Antireflux surgery for patients with scleroderma should be avoided at all costs as it may markedly exacerbate dysphagia. Vagotomy is not indicated in the treatment of gastroesophageal reflux disease.

There is no evidence that nocturnal, single-dose H_2 antagonists are effective in the acute treatment or in the maintenance therapy of esophagitis associated with GERD. A therapeutic approach to reflux is outlined in Table 35.4.

Complications

The complications of reflux include hemorrhage, ulcerations, stricture formation, and development of Barrett's epithelium (11). Esophagitis is the cause of 5 to 10% of all cases of upper gastrointestinal hemorrhages. Peptic ulcers and strictures must be differentiated from malignancy and caustic ingestion. The presence of a midesophageal ulcer or stricture should raise the suspicion of Barrett's epithelium (columnar-type mucosa that replaces the squamous mucosa of the tubular esophagus). This type of columnar mucosa contains several different cell types, including parietal cells capable of secreting acid. Of further significance is that this mucosa is a metaplastic response to inflammation and is a premalignant condition. Patients with this type of mucosa should therefore be under regular endoscopic surveillance for the development of cancer.

HIATUS HERNIA

Herniation of a part of the stomach through the diaphragm through the normal esophageal hiatus into the thorax is called a hiatus hernia. The defect is quite common, but the precise prevalence is very much influenced by the zeal of the radiologist during the performance of an upper gastrointestinal series. Estimates of prevalence therefore have ranged from 30 to 60% overall. The defect is twice as common in women as in men and is extremely common in elderly people, affecting perhaps 70 to 80% of the population who are older than age 60. Many physicians still erroneously correlate hiatus hernia with reflux esophagitis, but certainly a hernia may exist without producing symptomatic reflux and reflux may occur without hernia. If a patient has clear-cut reflux esophagitis, the treatment of it (see page 411) should not be influenced by the presence of a hiatus hernia. If a patient who does not have reflux is inadvertently discovered to have a hiatus hernia, no treatment is indicated. (In the past needless surgery has been done to reduce a hiatus hernia in patients whose symptoms were not clearly attributable to the defect.)

A *paraesophageal hernia*, the hernia of part of the stomach through the diaphragm adjacent to the gastroesophageal junction, is potentially dangerous because about one-third of the time the hernia incarcerates and produces acute obstruction, a surgical emergency.

General References

Katz PO, Castell DO: Esophageal motility disorders. *Am J Med Sci* 290:61, 1985.
    Review of classification and treatment of esophageal motility disorders.
Richter JE, Castell DO: Gastroesophageal reflux: pathogenesis, diagnosis, and therapy. *Ann Intern Med* 97:93, 1982.
    Concise review of approach to diagnosis and therapy.
Richter JE, Bradley LA, Castell DO: Esophageal chest pain: current controversies in pathogenesis, diagnosis and therapy. *Ann Intern Med* 110:66, 1989.
    Comprehensive review of the subject.

Specific References

1. Bondi JL, Goodwin DH, Garrett JM: "Vigorous" achalasia: its clinical interpretation and significance. *Am J Gastroenterol* 58:145, 1972.
2. Just-Viera J, Haight C: Achalasia and carcinoma of the esophagus. *Surg Gynecol Obstet* 128:1081, 1969.
3. Katz PO, Dalton CB, Richter JE, et al: Esophageal testing of patients with non cardiac chest pain or dysphagia. Results of three years experience with 1161 patients. *Ann Intern Med* 106:593, 1987.
4. Katz PO, Richter JE, Cowan R, Castell, DO: Apparent complete lower esophageal sphincter relaxation in achalasia. *Gastroenterology* 90:978, 1986.
5. Lieberman DA, Keefe EB: Treatment of severe reflux esophagitis with cimetidine and metoclopramide. *Ann Intern Med* 104:21, 1986.
6. Parker EF, Moertel CG: Carcinoma of the esophagus: is there a role for surgery? *Am J Dig Dis* 23:730, 1978.
7. Richter JE, Bradley LA, Castell DO: Esophageal chest pain: current controversies in pathogenesis, diagnosis and therapy. *Ann Intern Med* 110:66, 1989.
8. Richter JE, Castell DO: Gastroesophageal reflux: pathogenesis, diagnosis, and therapy. *Ann Intern Med* 97:93, 1982.

9. Richter JE, Castell DO: Diffuse esophageal spasm: a reappraisal. *Ann Intern Med* 100:242, 1984.
10. Schuffler MD, Pope CE II: Esophageal motor function in idiopathic intestinal pseudo-obstruction. *Gastroenterology* 70:677, 1976.
11. Spechler SJ, Goyal RJ: Barrett's esophagus. *N Engl J Med* 315:362, 1986.
12. Tucker H, Snape Jr WJ, Cohen S: Achalasia secondary to carcinoma: manometric and clinical features. *Ann Intern Med* 89:315, 1978.

C H A P T E R   36

Abdominal Pain

MARVIN M. SCHUSTER, M.D.

Abdominal pain is one of the most common presenting complaints of ambulatory patients to their physicians. Many patients complain of having chronic pain that is constant or recurrent; and in this population it is important to consider functional as well as organic causes for the symptom. Acute abdominal pain (onset within 24 hours before the patient seeks help) almost always reflects an organic process. In any case, whether chronic or acute, abdominal pain due to an organic cause is more often a symptom of gastrointestinal disease than nongastrointestinal disease.

The physician's response to the patient with abdominal pain will be influenced by its rapidity of onset, its apparent severity, its location, and by accompanying signs and symptoms (fever, gastrointestinal bleeding, diarrhea, etc.) that may suggest a specific process. Although there is no information about the relative frequency of the various causes of abdominal pain, experience suggests that, most often, acute pain is self-limited (abates within hours) and the pain is usually attributed (without proof) to viral gastroenteritis or to dietary indiscretion. Chronic pain, if associated with an organic process, is most often due to

peptic, gallbladder, or diverticular disease, to chronic relapsing pancreatitis (primarily in alcoholics), or to carcinoma (most commonly pancreatic or colonic). The symptoms and signs that accompany these processes are discussed in a general way in this chapter and more specifically in the chapters devoted to these conditions. Chronic pain, not associated with a demonstrable organic process, is most often due to the irritable bowel syndrome (see Chapter 40).

The significance of pain is determined by two major factors—the characteristics of the pain and the characteristics of the patient. The relative significance of pain to the patient depends on its severity and frequency, the degree to which it interferes with his daily life or sleep patterns, and its meaning to him, both implied and symbolic. Even severe pain can be tolerated for brief periods if it appears infrequently, whereas less severe pain may be less tolerable if it interrupts important activities or disturbs sleep. Pain that has no anticipated end is generally less well tolerated than pain that, even though intense, has a predictable span. The threshold of pain tolerance varies considerably from one individual to another, because of both neurological and psychological factors. When pain suggests to the patient a serious underlying disorder, such as cancer, this concern itself may decrease his tolerance for pain. Also, pain that is primarily organic may be reinforced by the secondary psychosocial gains that it provides.

Elderly patients with abdominal pain require special attention. Even serious underlying conditions may be manifested by minimal subjective complaints and minimal objective signs. For example, the diagnosis of appendicitis and of ruptured appendix is easily missed because pain may not be severe and fever and leukocytosis may be minimal or absent. Therefore careful follow-up of abdominal pain in the elderly warrants repeated abdominal and rectal examination and serial determinations of temperature and laboratory tests (such as white blood cell and differential counts).

Management of any type of pain can be significantly improved by consideration of certain general principles. For example, reassurance that pain can be relieved by medication or surgery can significantly raise the threshold of tolerance. On the other hand, the existence of severe pain sensitizes patients to additional, less intense pain (such as lumbar puncture or venipuncture), and the patient's "overreaction" to the second pain should not be taken to imply that the primary pain is psychogenic. Another common misconception is that alleviation of pain by placebo implies psychogenc origin; in fact, organic pain may be more readily relieved by placebo than is psychogenic pain. A post hoc rationalization that accounts for this phenomenon views the patient with organic pain as a person who wants desperately to get rid of his pain, whereas the person with psychogenic pain may be unwilling "to give it up" because of secondary gain.

TYPES OF ABDOMINAL PAIN

A few general concepts concerning abdominal pain are reviewed here, since understanding them can be quite helpful diagnostically. Pain involving the digestive system can be visceral, parietal, referred, neurogenic, or psychogenic. Pain caused by metabolic disease (see below) is ordinarily visceral or neurogenic.

Visceral Pain

Visceral pain can result from spasm or stretch of the muscle wall of a hollow viscus, from distension of the capsule of a solid organ such as the liver, or from inflammation and ischemia of a visceral structure. Tenderness associated with visceral pain (sometimes including rebound tenderness) is often felt directly over the part of the digestive system that is involved, although (except for the terminal ileum) small bowel tenderness is usually not well localized. Abdominal viscera are insensitive to cutting, tearing, crushing, and burning.

Parietal Pain

The parietal peritoneum, mesentery, and posterior peritoneal covering are sensitive to forces similar to those that affect the viscera, but the omentum and anterior abdominal wall are less sensitive. Parietal tenderness is more localized than visceral tenderness, and rebound tenderness is experienced over the involved area. Parietal pain that is the result of generalized inflammation (peritonitis) encompasses a large area of the peritoneum. A rigid abdomen, associated with pain, usually means that the inflammation is severe.

Referred Pain

Both visceral and parietal pain may be referred to a remote site along shared nerve pathways (dermatomes). Gallbladder pain, for example, typically radiates to the infrascapular area, and right diaphragmatic pain to the right shoulder. Esophageal pain can be confused with the pain of myocardial ischemia because the sites to which the pain radiates may be identical (e.g., neck, left arm, etc.). The more severe the visceral pain, the more likely it is to be referred to the back, as for example with esophageal spasm or with cholecystitis. The skin overlying the dermatome to which the pain is referred may be hypersensitive. Deep palpation of the primary site of the painful organ may intensify the pain, not only locally, but at its referred site, whereas the reverse is not true; deep palpation over the referred site does not usually enhance pain over the primary site.

Abdominal Pain Caused by Metabolic Disease

Metabolic disease may produce intestinal pain by a direct effect on the alimentary tract as, for example, when intestinal spasm is induced by porphyria, lead poisoning, or familial Mediterranean fever. In hered-

itary angioneurotic edema, C-1 esterase deficiency may produce intestinal swelling, which can result in pain due to partial obstruction or to intestinal spasm. On the other hand, metabolic disorders may secondarily produce gastrointestinal pain; for example, hyperparathyroidism may produce a painful peptic ulcer or pancreatitis. Hyperlipidemia also may cause pancreatitis but may be associated with abdominal pain in the absence of this entity.

Neurogenic Pain

Neurogenic abdominal pain (causalgia) is experienced by the patient as a burning sensation along the route of distribution of the nerve and is sometimes associated with hyperesthesia. Usually the spinal root is involved by herpes zoster, carcinoma, arthritis, etc., but peripheral neuropathies due to operative trauma or to diabetes mellitus may also produce neurogenic abdominal pain. There is no relationship of neurogenic pain to digestive function (e.g., eating or defecating).

Psychogenic Pain

Psychogenic pain may represent a conversion reaction that results in the perception of pain when no organic dysfunction exists; or it may result from psychophysiological reactions characterized by pathological or physiological responses to psychological stress (see Chapter 12). For example, emotional stress can lead to painful intestinal spasm in patients with irritable bowel syndrome (Chapter 40). This spasm is a measurable physiological event. Similarly, stress may lead to peptic symptoms due to gastric hypersecretion, which also can be quantitated. Pain or tenderness that represents a conversion reaction (emotions converted into somatic complaints) may disappear during periods of distraction. Such pain may be inconsistent and incompatible with known neuroanatomy and neurophysiology.

HISTORICAL CLUES TO DIAGNOSIS

Although the successful diagnosis of conditions that present with abdominal pain depends on meticulous pursuit of leads that are provided by history and physical examination, familiarity with standard questions and examination techniques assists in ensuring completeness. Questions relating to local features include the nature and quality of pain, its location, radiation, intensity, timing, duration, and course, and the factors that precipitate, aggravate, and alleviate it. Associated symptoms and signs include tenderness, fever and chills, anorexia, nausea and vomiting, diarrhea and constipation, obstruction, borborygmus, rectal bleeding, passing of mucus, jaundice, and genitourinary symptoms. Although aggravation of pain by emotional tension is seen with functional disorders such as irritable bowel syndrome, the pain of many organic disorders can also be accentuated by stress.

Rapidity of Onset of Pain

The temporal development of abdominal pain is an important factor that guides the physician in the urgency and direction of the evaluation. In particular, pain that develops abruptly or within minutes and becomes rapidly severe is very ominous (Table 36.1).

In addition, situations in which a silent period follows the initial symptoms are notoriously deceptive problems. For example, a perforated viscus or an intestinal infarction may be characterized by resolution of the intense initial pain hours after perforation or infarction first occurs and by a recurrence of pain several hours later when peritonitis and volume depletion are well established.

Almost always, therefore, if the patient complains of an abrupt onset of severe abdominal pain on the day that he visits the physician, even if the pain has resolved and the abdominal examination is unrevealing, a complete blood count, urinalysis, chest X-ray, plain and upright films of the abdomen, and close surveillance over several hours are imperative and are usually best accomplished in an emergency room.

Table 36.1.
Causes of Acute Abdominal Pain According to Rapidity of Onset[a]

Intestinal Causes	Extraintestinal Causes
Abrupt onset (instantaneous)	
Perforated ulcer	Ruptured or dissecting
Ruptured abscess or hematoma	aneurysm
Intestinal infarct	Ruptured ectopic preg-
Ruptured esophagus	nancy
	Pneumothorax
	Myocardial infarct
	Pulmonary infarct
Rapid onset (minutes)	
Perforated viscus	Ureteral colic
Strangulated viscus	Renal colic
Volvulus	Ectopic pregnancy
Pancreatitis	
Biliary colic	
Mesenteric infarct	
Diverticulitis	
Penetrating peptic ulcer	
High intestinal obstruction	
Appendicitis (gradual onset more common)	
Gradual onset (hours)	
Appendicitis	Cystitis
Strangulated hernia	Pyelitis
Low small intestinal obstruction	Salpingitis
Cholecystitis	Prostatitis
Pancreatitis	Threatened abortion
Gastritis	Urinary retention
Peptic ulcer	Pneumonitis
Colonic diverticulitis	
Meckel's diverticulitis	
Crohn's disease	
Ulcerative colitis	
Mesenteric lymphadenitis	
Abscess	
Intestinal infarct	
Mesenteric cyst	

[a]Adapted from Way LW: Abdominal pain. In Sleisenger MH, Fordtran JS (eds): *Gastrointestinal Disease, ed. 4.* Philadelphia, WB Saunders, 1989, p 247.

When the onset of pain is more gradual, there are many more possible causes, and considerable judgment is necessary in deciding about the urgency and direction of the evaluation. The physician will need particularly to be guided by the patient's history, the nature and location of the pain (see below), and by the examination (see below). In all cases follow-up examination is warranted. Newly experienced abdominal pain should never be dismissed, even if it is felt to be innocuous, without follow-up, at least by phone, within a few days. In this way, any important new symptoms will not be missed. It is best for the physician to initiate this follow-up since it will obviate the need for the patient to decide whether a change in symptoms is important enough to trouble the physician.

Nature and Location of Pain (Tables 36.2 and 36.3)

Esophageal pain is generally described as pressing, constricting, or burning. It is usually located in the substernal area and, when severe, radiates through to the back. The location of the pain is a good clue to the location of the underlying disease. Although pain from the lower esophageal region may be referred higher, lesions high in the esophagus do not refer to the lower part of the esophagus (see also Chapter 35).

Gastric pain is usually experienced in the subxiphoid area or the left upper quadrant. Although gastritis is perceived as a true pain (often burning or cramping in quality), the distress caused by both duodenal and gastric ulcer is experienced as a gnawing discomfort or as a hunger sensation rather than as pain. The discomfort caused by peptic ulcer is felt on an empty stomach and is relieved by eating. Thus nocturnal pain of peptic ulcer usually awakens the patient between 1 and 3 A.M. In contrast, pain of gastritis may be aggravated by eating or relieved only momentarily and then subsequently intensified over a period of 10 to 15 minutes. A change from ulcer distress to a burning, boring, or knife-like pain (especially when there is radiation through to the back) is an indication of a complication of ulcer—namely penetration. Pain that is precipitated by meals also suggests gastric outlet obstruction (often due to pyloric channel ulcer) or high intestinal obstruction (see also Chapter 37).

Duodenal pain is felt also in the epigastric area or slightly to the right of it, and it, too, may radiate through to the back. When perforation of an ulcer occurs, the pain appears abruptly in the epigastric region and later settles into the right lower quadrant as gastric contents are spilled into the right gutter.

Small intestinal pain is generally diffuse and poorly localized. It is experienced in the periumbilical area and, when severe, radiates through to the back. Pain deriving from the terminal ileum may be localized to the right lower quadrant. Uncommonly it may radiate down the leg. Small intestinal pain is generally crampy, sharp, or aching. Bloating, distension, and dull ache are terms that frequently are associated with prolonged mechanical obstruction or reflex ileus, whereas

Table 36.2.
Nature and Location of Gastrointestinal Pain

Organ Involved	Nature of Pain	Location of Pain
Esophagus	Burning, constricting	Upper lesions → high substernal
		Lower lesions → low substernal or referred upward Severe → back
Stomach	Gnawing discomfort, pain	Epigastric Left upper quadrant
Duodenum	Gnawing discomfort, hunger, pain	Epigastric
Small intestine	Ache, cramp, bloating, sharp	Diffuse Periumbilical Terminal ileum → right lower quadrant
Colon	As above	Lower abdomen Sigmoid → left lower quadrant Rectum → midline and sacrum
Pancreas	Excruciating, constant	Upper abdomen radiating to back
Gallbladder	Severe, later dull ache	Right upper quadrant Radiates to right scapula or interscapular area
Liver	Ache, occasionally sharp	Right lower rib cage Right upper quadrant if liver is enlarged

more acute forms may be manifested by sharp steady pain. Associated fever and chills suggest inflammatory bowel disease.

Colonic pain is better localized, often to the lower abdomen. Sigmoid pain is felt in the left lower quadrant, and rectal pain is often described by the patient as being located over the rectum, usually in the midline. Gas pocketed in the splenic flexure of the colon (seen most commonly in patients with the irritable bowel syndrome) produces left upper quadrant or left chest pain that may be confused with the pain of myocardial ischemia. Temporary relief is obtained by passing gas (see also Chapter 40). Colonic pain generally is crampy or of an aching quality unless perforation occurs, and then it is frequently severe and constant. Associated fever and chills suggest diverticulitis, diverticular abscess, or ulcerative colitis.

Pancreatic pain is excruciating and constant and usually located in the upper abdomen with radiation through to the back, but it may be felt in almost any area of the abdomen. Chronic pancreatic pain (due to inflammation, pseudocyst, or carcinoma) is similar in nature and location to acute pancreatic pain but may be less severe. Pancreatitis is almost invariably associated with vomiting. If vomiting is not present, other diagnoses such as pancreatic carcinoma, should be considered.

Appendicitis often begins as diffuse abdominal pain that intensifies over a period of hours as it settles in the right lower quadrant. The pain of appendicitis is frequently aggravated by extension of the right leg.

Gallbladder pain generally begins in the right upper quadrant or epigastrium and radiates to the interscapular area or to the right infrascapular area. It is excruciatingly severe, may be aggravated by deep inspiration, and is replaced by a dull, aching sensation that persists for hours after the severe pain subsides. Tenderness can often be elicited by deep palpation under the rib

in the area of the gallbladder, especially during deep inspiration. Gallbladder pain often appears several hours after a heavy dinner. Associated fever and chills suggest ascending cholangitis (see also Chapter 90).

Hepatic pain localizes over the liver, and a tender liver can be demonstrated by palpating the edge during deep inspiration or by fist percussion over the lower right rib cage anteriorly (or over the right upper quadrant if the liver is enlarged).

PHYSICAL EXAMINATION

The patient's general appearance provides clues concerning the severity, the duration, and frequently the cause of the underlying condition. The cold, sweat, and pallor of shock along with the marble skin (superficial vessels seen over blanched skin) indicating vasoconstriction are signs of significant hemorrhage. Tachycardia and perspiration are seen in both shock and sepsis, but the skin in shock is cold and clammy whereas in sepsis it is warm and moist. Signs of sepsis suggest bacterial enteritis, inflammatory bowel disease, intra-abdominal abscess, cholangitis, pancreatitis, peritonitis, or pyelonephritis.

The position assumed by the patient may be characteristic of a particular disorder. A position of truncal flexure often typifies patients with pancreatitis, whereas patients with gallbladder colic tend to pace or writhe about and appear restless in their unsuccessful attempt to find a comfortable position. This is in sharp contrast to the immobile position assumed by patients with peritonitis who attempt to avoid even the slightest jarring movement.

Inspection of the abdomen is facilitated by using incident lighting to visualize abdominal asymmetry and to outline masses and pulsations. In thin patients with partial obstruction peristaltic intestinal movement may be seen through the abdominal wall, and churning peristalsis may coincide with reports of

Table 36.3.
Differential Diagnosis of Abdominal Pain Due to Gastrointestinal Disorders[a]

A. Character, Location, Production or Relief

Disorder	Character	Location	Produced or Relieved by
Peptic ulcer	Gnawing hunger discomfort, occasionally burning, gastric—within minutes after meals; duodenal—usually several hours after meals	Subxiphoid, may radiate to back	Produced by empty stomach, relieved by food, antacids or H_2 receptor blockers
Penetrating ulcer	Severe boring constant pain	Subxiphoid radiating to back	May awaken patient in early morning hours, may be relieved by antacids or H_2 receptor blockers
Perforated ulcer	Abrupt, severe pain followed within 6 hours by deceptive refractory period with diminishing of pain	Initially epigastric—then right lower quadrant (right gutter)	Initial pain spontaneous, peritonitis aggravated by movement
Small bowel obstruction	Crampy severe pain with partial obstruction, constant pain develops with complete obstruction or strangulation	Generalized periumbilical or localized over strangulation	Relieved by intubation decompression
Large bowel obstruction	Crampy pain initially, constant pain with subsequent distension or strangulation, onset less sudden than upper intestinal obstruction	May be localized or generalized	Occasionally relieved by intubation decompression
Intestinal infarct	Severe, excruciating, abrupt onset	Generalized	Relieved only by surgery
Intussusception	Sudden onset severe crampy pain	Periumbilical	Temporary relief may occur with emesis
Appendicitis	Initially colic then continuous with varying intensity	Initial colic in periumbilical area, subsequently continuous in right lower quadrant, occasional testicular radiation	Aggravated by extension of right leg
Pancreatitis	Severe constant pain	Epigastric, radiation to back or lower abdomen	Often initiated by alcoholic binge or eating after binge, by common duct obstruction, penetrating ulcer, or blunt trauma
Cholecystitis	Constant, severe pain preceding nausea and vomiting; subsidence of pain followed by aching	Right upper quadrant radiating to infrascapular region	Precipitated by heavy meal and aggravated by deep inspiration
Biliary colic	Crampy, severe pain	Epigastrium, radiating to right upper quadrant and subscapular region	Precipitated by heavy meal within 1–3 hours
Diverticulitis	Crampy or continuous pain	Left lower quadrant, may radiate to back	Relieved by anticholinergics and antibiotics
Crohn's disease	Crampy with partial obstruction and continuous pain with inflammatory mass	Periumbilical or right lower quadrant, may radiate to back	May be precipitated by milk. Relieved by defecation or intubation decompression
Ulcerative colitis	Crampy pain usually, may be constant with toxic dilation	Often left lower quadrant or any area of colon, generalized with toxic megacolon or perforation	Precipitated by emotional stress or infection; toxic megacolon by opiates or enemas; relieved temporarily by defecation

B. Abnormal Physical Findings, Associated Signs, and Laboratory Features

Disorder	Abnormal Physical Findings	Associated Signs and Symptoms	Laboratory Features
Peptic ulcer	Subxiphoid tenderness	Nausea, vomiting, retrosternal burning; weight gain with duodenal ulcer; weight stable or loss with gastric ulcer	Endoscopic or X-ray demonstration of ulcer, possible occult blood in stool or melena and iron deficiency anemia
Penetrating ulcer	Marked subxiphoid tenderness	Writhing, clutching abdomen	Amylase may be elevated
Perforated ulcer	Initially rigid with rebound, during refractory stage tenderness disappears to return later, absence of liver dullness with intraperitoneal air	Patient lies rigidly still, pale perspiring; emesis may be present	Upright film shows free air under diaphragm, leukocytosis

Condition	Physical Examination	Symptoms / History	Laboratory and X-ray Findings
Small bowel obstruction	Borborygmus, high pitched sound with rushes initially; later quiet abdomen; tenderness may be mild or rebound tenderness may be present	Emesis (may be feculent with lower obstruction), obstipation, may be weak with shock-like appearance	Plain film of abdomen showing air-fluid levels, may show stepladder pattern.
Large bowel obstruction	Initially hyperperistalsis with high pitched rushes, subsequently distension and decrease in bowel signs	Nausea but less vomiting than with high obstruction, obstipation or marked constipation	Large bowel distension with air-fluid levels and no air demonstrated distal to obstruction
Intestinal infarct	Quiet bowel sounds, tenderness present but not commensurate with pain, later rebound tenderness	Shock, bloody diarrhea, melena, vomiting; history of intestinal angina	Leukocytosis, hemoconcentration; bloody fluid on paracentesis; plain film of abdomen may reveal normal gas pattern or no gas pattern due to fluid-filled loops
Intussusception	Tender mass in abdomen, high pitched peristaltic rushes	Initially normal stool after onset, then blood mucus and constipation; vomiting is late; fever after strangulation	Barium enema demonstrates coiled spring appearance of invagination; with ileocecal intussusception, small bowel loop is in colon
Appendicitis	Localized rebound tenderness, hyperesthesia over area	Initially diarrhea, then constipation; nausea, vomiting may be present; fever, tachycardia; rectal tenderness in right perirectal area	Leukocytosis
Pancreatitis	Marked epigastric tenderness, guarding and upper abdominal distension; the pain of chronic pancreatic disease may be less pronounced	Emesis almost invariable, fever, with hemorrhagic pancreatitis purple color in flank or periumbilical region; emesis is less common in patients with chronic pancreatic disease	Marked leukocytosis, hyperamylasemia; serum calcium depression on days 2 and 4, toxic psychosis on days 2 and 4; X-ray may show calcification, localized ileus, or colon cut-off sign; upper gastrointestinal series demonstrates pancreatic enlargement and spicules in C loop of duodenum; may have left pleural effusion
Cholecystitis	Tenderness over gallbladder area especially on deep inspiration; Murphy's sign may be positive	More common in obese women 40 years or older or after pregnancy; high incidence among some American Indian populations	Leukocytosis; plain film may show calcified stone; oral cholecystogram nonvisualized during attacks, TcHIDA nonvisualized; cholangiograms may show radiopaque stones
Biliary colic	As above	As above; jaundice may be present	Radiopaque stones may be seen on plain film; nonvisualization on cholecystogram during colic: subsequently may show radiolucent stones; i.v. cholangiogram may show dilated duct; bilirubin, alkaline phosphatase increase; may have hyperamylasemia
Diverticulitis	Guarding and tenderness in left lower quadrant	Constipation, fever, tachycardia; rectal tenderness on left; may have urinary frequency or dysuria from periocolonic involvement	Leukocytosis, barium enema shows diverticula but may not visualize during acute episode, may show partial obstruction
Crohn's disease	Tender mass in right lower quadrant, borborygmus	Nausea, vomiting, diarrhea, fever; may have perirectal fistula; tender mass in right rectal area, occasional clubbing	Anemia, elevated sedimentation rate; small bowel series shows cobble-stone appearance or string sign
Ulcerative colitis	Tender over involved area, distended especially over transverse colon with toxic megacolon	Frequent passage of small amounts of bloody liquid stool; tenesmus with rectal involvement; fever, tachycardia, arthralgia, erythema nodosa; proctoscopy reveals bleeding and friability	Anemia; elevated sedimentation rate; barium enema demonstrates ulcerations, shortening, effacement of colon

ᵃModified from *Handbook of Differential Diagnosis*, vol 2, part 1: *The Abdomen*. Nutley, NJ. Rocom Press. 1974.

crampy abdominal pain. Flank discoloration (Gray-Turner sign) or periumbilical discoloration (Cullen sign) results from retroperitoneal or intraperitoneal hemorrhage dissecting into the subcutaneous tissues and may indicate hemorrhagic pancreatitis. A strangulated hernia may protrude visibly from ventral defects, the inguinal area, or into the scrotum where peristaltic contractions may occasionally be appreciated. Patients with subphrenic abscess or gallbladder disease may have inspiratory pain that results in splinting and in avoidance of deep inspiration.

Auscultation should always be performed before palpation so that abdominal sounds may be evaluated before they are altered by palpation. At times borborygmus will be audible without the stethoscope. Specifically one should search for hyper- or hypoperistaltic sounds, for the high tinkles of obstruction, and for bruits suggesting vascular distortion from aneurysms, compression of blood vessels, or invasion of blood vessels (as, for example, invasion of the splenic artery in advanced pancreatic carcinoma). Although a silent abdomen implies reflex ileus, bowel sounds may also be quiet or markedly diminished late in the course of mechanical obstruction. Whenever obstruction (especially gastric outlet obstruction) is considered, the physician should try to elicit a succussion splash. This is done by placing the stethoscope over the area (e.g., the stomach) and shaking the patient gently but abruptly. A sloshing sound indicates the presence of air and fluid. This finding in the stomach 3 or more hours after eating or drinking indicates delayed gastric emptying or, rarely, marked hypersecretion.

Gentle percussion should precede palpation and is an excellent means for detecting rebound tenderness, masses, and tympany (either generalized or localized) over an area of ileus or obstruction. Because air will rise to the area between the liver and the abdominal wall, absence of liver dullness with the patient in a recumbent position is an important finding indicating the presence of free air in the abdominal cavity.

Before palpation, it is wise to ask the patient to point to the site of maximum pain. Gentle palpation should at first avoid that site to minimize the chances that muscle guarding will interfere with the examination. Preferably the patient should be lying perfectly flat on his back with knees flexed to facilitate relaxation of abdominal muscles. Guarding may be localized over specific lesions (often inflammatory), or there may be marked rigidity if pain is severe, as in perforation or penetration. Subxiphoid tenderness suggests an active ulcer. Tenderness over the liver, especially when the liver edge is brought down against the examining finger by deep inspiration, suggests inflammation in this organ. With gallbladder disease tenderness is localized to the region of the gallbladder, and with cystic or common duct obstruction a distended viscus can sometimes be felt as well. Right lower quadrant tenderness is found with appendicitis as well as with Crohn's disease involving the ileum or the ileocecal area. A left lower quadrant tender sigmoid cord is felt most commonly with irritable bowel syndrome but can also indicate diverticular disease. A distinct tender mass in the right lower quadrant suggests inflammation (usually Crohn's disease) extending beyond the bowel; a similar finding in the left lower quadrant is suggestive of diverticulitis. Board-like rigidity indicates an intra-abdominal catastrophe such as perforation or infarction. Pulsatile masses should be differentiated from laterally expansile masses since the former can represent a mass overlying an artery, whereas the latter implies aneurysmal dilation. When localized perforation has occurred, rebound tenderness may be localized over the area. Hyperesthesia may exist over the segmental distribution of the spinal nerve that innervates the particular area of the viscus. This finding is detected by gently rubbing the fingers over the skin of the involved dermatome.

Rectal examination can be extremely helpful in localizing areas of tenderness as well as in palpating masses through the rectum. Periappendiceal abscesses can sometimes be identified in this manner, as can a perforated diverticulum. On digital examination the finger should circumscribe a complete circle examining the entire perirectal area.

Genital and pelvic examination, like the rectal examination, should be performed in all patients with abdominal pain since it can detect hernias as well as genitourinary and other pelvic problems.

If analgesic drugs have been administered, it is useful to re-examine the patient after pain has been relieved to identify masses or localized tenderness that may have been obscured by guarding and rigidity.

LABORATORY TESTS

A complete blood count, urinalysis, and test for occult blood in the stool are required in every person with serious acute abdominal pain (see above), as are a chest X-ray and plain and upright films of the abdomen. Other laboratory tests should be ordered as indicated by the specific findings.

A low hematocrit value or hemoglobin concentration can call attention to intraperitoneal or retroperitoneal bleeding, whereas hemoconcentration raises consideration of mesenteric vascular occlusion. High white count and high erythrocyte sedimentation rate suggest inflammation or infection. Blood in the urine points to kidney disease as a possible source of pain, and white cells point to infection. Glycosuria may arouse suspicion of a diabetic crisis.

The presence of occult blood in the stool reinforces concern about the gastrointestinal tract as a source of painful symptoms and may be an early sign of vascular ischemia or intussusception, or a sign of more common lesions such as peptic ulcer, polyp, or inflammatory bowel disease.

RADIOLOGY

Plain and upright films of the abdomen are helpful in delineating gas patterns, which may demonstrate displacement of intestine by intra-abdominal masses or may show localized loops of ileus such as one sees with pancreatitis or pyelonephritis. Air is distributed more widely in the small bowel in reflex ileus and in intestinal obstruction. In the latter the typical stepladder pattern is often encountered, with slight separation of the loops due to edema of the wall of the small bowel; an upright film demonstrates air-fluid levels in the dilated loops. Absence of air distal to a specific point suggests obstruction at that point. Volvulus can be diagnosed on the plain film, which demonstrates a sausage-shaped air- or air-fluid-filled viscus coming to an apex. In gastric volvulus the greater curvature is seen above the lesser curve; and a double air-fluid level is a classic finding, one level being in the lesser curvature of the fundus and the other in the antrum (because of the inverted U-shaped stomach under these conditions). Free air under the diaphragm on the upright film indicates a perforated viscus unless the patient has had recent surgery (at which time air was introduced) or has *pneumatosis cystoides intestinalis,* in which case a large amount of air may appear subdiaphragmatically from ruptured pseudocysts. The important clue to pneumatosis cystoides intestinalis is the presence of free air in the absence of signs or symptoms of perforation or peritonitis. Radiopaque gallbladder or kidney stones or pancreatic calcification seen on plain film may help to corroborate a suspected diagnosis or point attention toward one of these organs.

Contrast studies are performed for specific indications. For example, an upper gastrointestinal series (see Patient Experience, page 426) can be performed instead of upper endoscopy (see below) when the history is typical of peptic ulcer and not suggestive of esophagitis, gastritis, or duodenitis (diagnoses that are not well demonstrated by X-ray examination). An upper gastrointestinal series is also helpful when pancreatitis or pancreatic pseudocyst is thought to be the basis of the pain, since the compression on the C loop of the duodenum may suggest these diagnoses. Barium enema (see Patient Experience, page 437) can be useful not only in demonstrating a low site of obstruction but also in reducing an intussusception. When pain is thought to result from gallbladder disease (see Chapter 90) and opaque stones are not visible on plain abdominal film, ultrasonography is an excellent means of demonstrating stones in the gallbladder but is not reliable in detecting ductal stones. An oral cholecystogram may demonstrate radiolucent stones; if the gallbladder fails to be visualized with reinforced dosage, a diseased gallbladder is quite likely. A *TcHIDA or PipHIDA radioisotopic study* may demonstrate obstruction of the common or cystic duct. This technique requires injection of isotope and serial views for 1 hour while the appearance of isotope in the gallbladder is examined. (A sonogram is usually performed beforehand to localize the gallbladder.)

Ultrasonography is also useful in showing pancreatic edema or pseudocysts, in evaluating a suspected abdominal aortic aneurysm, and in evaluating a patient who is difficult to examine for an intra-ab-

dominal mass; this technique has the advantage of avoiding irradiation. Sonography is often unsatisfactory in obese persons and in persons with metal abdominal sutures because adipose tissue and metal reflect sound.

Computed tomography (CT) is a sensitive means of demonstrating masses, infarcted tissue, and cysts but is expensive and exposes the patient to irradiation. Table 36.4 compares the ultrasound and CT technique and the patient experience.

Selective mesenteric angiography should be performed in patients suspected of having mesenteric vascular ischemia (particularly in elderly persons with postprandial abdominal pain) or mesenteric vascular occlusion (e.g., in women taking contraceptive medication). This is particularly helpful in older patients since normal arteriographic findings rule out mesenteric vascular disease; on the other hand, occlusion even of two of the three major aortic branches (celiac, superior mesenteric, and inferior mesenteric arteries) may occur without symptoms of mesenteric vascular disease. It may be prudent to hospitalize the patient for this procedure. The patient experience is similar to that described for renal arteriography (Chapter 62).

ENDOSCOPY

Upper gastrointestinal endoscopy requires referral to a gastroenterologist (see below). It should be con-

Table 36.4.
Ultrasound and Computerized Tomography (CT) Scanning: Comparison of the Technique and the Patient Experience[a]

Characteristic	Ultrasound	CT
Basis of tissue attenuation	Tissue elasticity, acoustic impedance	Electron density; linear attenuation coefficient
Radiation dose or toxic effect	None known at diagnostic energy levels	8–10 R (skin exposure)
Morphological detail	Good	Excellent
Contrast medium useful	None	Iodinated intravascular and oral agents; diatrizoate meglumine (Gastrografin)
Time for examination	½–1 hour	½–1 hour
Operator skill	Substantial	Minimal
Ease of interpretation	Complex—many artifacts	Straightforward
Preparation	Nothing by mouth after midnight (for pelvis, three glasses of water 1 hour before study and do not void)	Evacuate barium from recent gastrointestinal studies (or wait 1 week)
Cooperation	Lie still, supine	Lie still, supine

[a]Adapted from Ferrucci JT Jr: Body ultrasonography (first of two parts). *N Engl J Med* 300:538, 1979.

sidered as an ambulatory procedure to clarify or confirm findings in upper gastrointestinal series or to obtain a biopsy for diagnosis (e.g., when cancer is suspected). Endoscopy should be one of the first diagnostic procedures performed when abdominal pain is associated with upper gastrointestinal bleeding (see Chapter 38), but these patients should be hospitalized (see below).

Proctoscopy should be performed in any patient with abdominal pain and rectal bleeding or a change in bowel habits or in any patient in whom inflammatory bowel disease (proctitis, ulcerative colitis, Crohn's disease) is suspected. Moreover, anal lesions such as hemorrhoids and fissures are best demonstrated by proctoscopy. The procedure routinely should precede roentgenographic examination of the lower bowel since the barium enema does not visualize the lower rectum.

Colonoscopy, like upper endoscopy, requires referral to a gastroenterologist (see below). It should be considered in patients with abdominal pain who have occult rectal bleeding (see Chapter 38), in those with suspected diffuse colonic inflammatory disease (ulcerative colitis, Crohn's disease) or suspected ischemic colitis, and in patients with polypoid lesions on barium enema who require biopsy or, often, resection of the lesion. Colonoscopy cannot be performed within a day or 2 of a barium X-ray of the lower or upper gastrointestinal tract.

Patient Experience. In addition to concerns about facts relating to endoscopy, many patients have specific apprehensions and misconceptions that can only be managed appropriately if the patient is encouraged to express them. The most common questions concern the indication for the procedure, its anticipated benefits, and technical details about the procedure itself, including prior preparation, side effects, and risks. Much of the patient's anxiety can be allayed if the referring physician can answer these questions appropriately. The physician may find it helpful to emphasize that the fiberoptic instruments can be passed with relatively little discomfort and that photographs can be taken for detailed study, as well as brushings for cytology and biopsy for histology.

Upper Endoscopy (Esophagoscopy, Gastroscopy, Duodenoscopy). Preparation varies, but usually the patient will be asked to fast for 8 hours before the procedure and will be given a topical anesthetic by gargle or atomizer spray and also an intravenous or intramuscular sedative or tranquilizer. It is often helpful to reassure patients that the procedure can be and in fact often is performed without any premedication, as, for example, in patients with massive bleeding. Moreover, although the swallowing of tubes sounds like an awesome task, the knowledge that endoscopy is performed in patients of all ages and that children as well as elderly people tolerate the procedure well is also reassuring. The instrument is about the diameter of the fifth finger and introduction produces discomfort rather than pain. The entire procedure seldom lasts more than 20 minutes. Instillation of air, which

is necessary to distend the organ so that it can be well visualized, tends to produce a sensation of bloating. This air can be aspirated at the end of the procedure.

The discomfort from upper endoscopy is usually much less than that from a barium enema, and biopsies are painless. A topical anesthetic is administered initially to minimize gagging. During the procedure, the patient experiences the sensation of having something in his throat that he cannot swallow. Bleeding and perforation, the most serious complications, are extremely rare. The procedure is usually performed on an outpatient basis, and since sedation is generally employed, the patient should be accompanied by someone who will be able to take him home after the procedure.

Proctosigmoidoscopy. Whether prior preparation is appropriate depends on the suspected pathology. If proctoscopy is performed to detect or biopsy a mass lesion, a laxative is used the day before and a cleansing enema is given on the morning of the procedure. On the other hand, mucosal lesions (such as inflammatory bowel disease) are best demonstrated without preparation (other than a natural bowel movement the morning of the procedure). Most enema preparations tend to produce some mucosal edema that may obscure mucosal lesions. Proctosigmoidoscopy is not painful, but there is an uncomfortable sensation produced by the distention of the rectosigmoid region by the instrument and by air.

Fiberoptic sigmoidoscopy and colonoscopy. Fiberoptic sigmoidoscopy can generally be performed if a laxative is administered the day before the procedure and if an enema is given on the morning of the procedure. Colonoscopy requires further cleaning, usually necessitating a liquid diet 2 to 3 days before the procedure in addition to laxatives and an enema. Good cleansing is especially important if polypectomy is contemplated. However, the patient should be warned that the ensuing 12 to 16 hours of cramps and watery diarrhea may be quite uncomfortable. For colonoscopy premedication similar to that used in upper endoscopy (see above) is appropriate, as well as an intravenous analgesic such as Demerol to minimize the discomfort and crampy pain commonly associated with insufflation of air and negotiation of curves. The procedure may take from 30 minutes to over 1 hour. Polypectomy adds additional time as well as additional risk (perforation and bleeding) but generally does not increase discomfort nor involve the additional recovery time that would be required after an abdominal operation to remove polyps.

TREATMENT

The treatment of patients with abdominal pain depends on the severity of the pain, its rapidity of onset, and the nature of the underlying condition, if known. Severe pain with an abrupt or rapid onset frequently reflects a gastrointestinal disorder that will require surgical intervention (see Table 36.1). Hospitalization and consultation with a gastroenterologist and a surgeon should be requested immediately in almost all cases. Less severe pain (pain that does not prevent the patient from ambulating, talking normally, thinking coherently, etc.) should not be treated aggressively with analgesic drugs until an attempt has been made to establish a diagnosis, since the pain will often abate spontaneously within minutes or hours and will not recur. In such circumstances, no further evaluation is indicated. If the pain recurs or persists and the cause is not obvious, the screening tests described on page 420 should be done. If these tests do not provide a diagnosis, referral to a gastroenterologist is indicated.

As a general rule, analgesic drugs may be prescribed to patients with persistent pain, but opiates should be avoided if possible because they may aggravate the underlying condition. (For example, morphine may aggravate pancreatitis by producing duodenal and ampullary spasm, thus enhancing pancreatic duct obstruction; and opiates or anticholinergics may produce toxic megacolon in patients with active ulcerative colitis. Furthermore, there is a risk of narcotic addiction in any patient whose pain is likely to be of prolonged duration.)

General References

Ferrucci Jr JT: Body ultrasonography (first of two parts). *N Engl J Med* 300:538, 1979.
  Good review of the clinical uses of sonography, with useful comparison of computerized tomography scanning.
Handbook of Differential Diagnosis, vol 2. part I, The Abdomen. Nutley, NJ, Rocom Press, 1974.
  Excellent illustrations by M. F. Netter and good tables.
Hendrix TR, Bulkley GB, Schuster MM: Abdominal Pain. In: Harvey AM, Johns RJ, McKusick VA, et al (eds): *Principles and Practice of Medicine*, ed 22. East Norwalk, Appleton and Lange, 1988. p. 787.
  Describes the physiological and clinical aspects of abdominal pain.
Way LW: Abdominal Pain. In: Sleisenger MH, Fordtran JS (eds): *Gastrointestinal Disease*, ed 4. Philadelphia, WB Saunders, 1989.
  Very good discussion organized along classical rather than problem-oriented lines; written by an experienced surgeon.

C H A P T E R   37

Peptic Ulcer Disease*

PHILIP O. KATZ, M.D.

NORMAL GASTRIC FUNCTION

The two primary functions of the stomach are the secretion of various substances that are important in digestion and absorption and the movement of gastric contents downstream into the small intestine. There are four primary classes of secretory cells: mucus-secreting cells of the cardia, hydrochloric acid-secreting parietal cells of the body (which also secrete intrinsic factor—see Chapter 50), pepsinogen-secreting chief cells of the body, and gastrin-secreting G cells of the antrum. Gastric function is regulated by neural and hormonal influences that determine the rate and amount that the various cells secrete and the rate at which the stomach empties its contents into the duodenum. During the *cephalic phase* of gastric activity, the anticipation of eating initiates cholinergic impulses that, via the vagus nerve, stimulate parietal cell secretion of acid and G cell secretion of gastrin (which then also stimulates acid secretion). During the *gastric phase*, distention of the stomach by food causes local

---

*Dr. Harold J. Tucker contributed to this chapter in the first and second editions of this book.

nerve endings to stimulate acid and gastrin secretion further—the G cells are also directly stimulated by protein and protein breakdown products and inhibited by acid. During the *intestinal phase* of gastric activity, intestinal hormones (secretin, cholecystokinin, and probably others), the secretion of which is stimulated directly by gastric acid, inhibit the action of gastrin on the parietal cells.

EPIDEMIOLOGY—NATURAL HISTORY

Peptic ulcer disease is a common clinical problem. It is estimated to have a lifetime incidence of 10%. Between 1 and 2% of the population has an ulcer at any point in time and approximately 200,000 to 400,000 new cases are seen each year. The rate of hospital admissions for uncomplicated duodenal ulcer has decreased significantly in the last 30 years; but gastric ulcer and complications of ulcer disease—bleeding and perforation—have not diminished, suggesting that the treatment of peptic disease has become primarily an ambulatory function. Duodenal ulcer is twice as common in men, as it is in women and 1.5 times as common as gastric ulcer. The peak incidence for duodenal ulcer is in the fifth decade in men and in the 6th decade and older in women. Gastric ulcer is slightly more common in men and in both sexes is more common in the elderly.

Ulcers are usually less than 1 cm in diameter, though giant ulcers (>2.5 cm) occasionally occur. Duodenal ulcers are almost always located in the duodenal bulb or immediately postbulbar, within 3 cm of the pyloric duodenal junction. Ulcers distal to the duodenal bulb should raise the suspicion of the Zollinger-Ellison syndrome (see below) or of Crohn's disease of the duodenum. Gastric ulcers are most commonly located on the lesser curvature, at the junction of the body and antrum of the stomach. There is no risk of cancer in a duodenal ulcer; but 1 to 3% of gastric ulcers occur in carcinomas.

Duodenal ulcer disease is a chronic disease. Estimates are that 60 to 80% of patients will have a recurrence within 1 year of diagnosis. Many recurrences will be asymptomatic. Recurrences are thought to decrease over 10 to 20 years, but symptomatic duodenal ulcer is seen with some frequency in the elderly. The recurrence rate of gastric ulcers has not been as extensively studied but appears to be not as frequent. Both duodenal and gastric ulcers tend to recur in the same place as the index ulcer. Long-term studies suggest that bleeding or perforation will occur at a rate of 1 to 3% a year with a lifetime incidence of about 20%. Recurrent hemorrhage occurs in about 50% of patients who have had a prior bleed. A few studies suggest that the complication rate may be reduced by maintenance therapy (see below) (2). The major risk of death from ulcer disease is in the first 1 to 2 years after diagnosis (4).

RISK FACTORS

Certain factors are associated with an increased risk of developing peptic ulcer disease (Table 37.1). Ge-

Table 37.1.
Risk Factors for Peptic Ulcer Disease

Male sex
First degree relative with duodenal ulcer
Genetic markers:
  Elevated levels of pepsinogen I
  Presence of HLA-B5 antigen
  Decreased red blood cell acetylcholinesterase
Stress
Cigarette smoking
Zollinger-Ellison syndrome
Chronic renal failure—for duodenal ulcer disease only
Chronic obstructive pulmonary disease—for duodenal ulcer disease only
Alcoholic cirrhosis—for duodenal ulcer disease only
Drugs: aspirin, nonsteroidal antiinflammatory drugs
Helicobacter pylori?

netic factors appear to play an important role. Men (see above) are more prone to both duodenal and gastric ulcers than are women. Duodenal ulcer is three times more common in first degree relatives of a patient with a duodenal ulcer than in the general population. Furthermore, certain genetic markers, such as pepsinogen I, HLA-B5 and red blood cell acetylcholinesterase, can identify groups at increased risk. With the aid of such markers, peptic ulcer disease has been shown to be genetically heterogeneous. In certain families there appears to be an autosomal dominant mode of inheritance, whereas in others no discernible pattern is found.

The role of *stress* in the pathogenesis of peptic ulcer disease is well recognized but difficult to quantitate. Nevertheless, it is clear that threats to the psychological or physical well-being of some people appear to predispose them to peptic ulceration. Why some people react to stress by developing peptic disease and others by developing another disease (e.g., asthma or hypertension) is unknown (see Chapter 12 for a discussion of psychosomatic illness).

Cigarette smoking has been repeatedly demonstrated to be associated with an increased frequency of duodenal ulcer disease with frequencies ranging between 33 and 100% above that of nonsmokers (14). In addition, there is evidence that cigarette smoking may delay the healing rate of both gastric and duodenal ulcers and increase the frequency of their recurrence. There is no epidemiological evidence that alcohol is ulcerogenic, although it is a known cause of acute gastritis. Coffee, both caffeinated and decaffeinated, is a mild stimulant of gastric acid secretion. Symptoms may be exacerbated by coffee, but a definite causal relationship with ulcer disease has not been demonstrated.

Certain disease states have been associated with an increased risk of peptic ulcer disease. Evidence for such associations must be carefully evaluated in light of the high prevalence of ulcer disease in the general population and the frequent use of ulcerogenic drugs. There is, however, good evidence linking duodenal (but not gastric) ulcer disease with chronic obstructive pulmonary disease, alcoholic cirrhosis, chronic renal failure, and hyperparathyroidism.

Conditions that lead to increased gastric acid secretion also predispose to ulcer disease. The Zollinger-Ellison syndrome, or gastrinoma (see below), is the best example of such a condition. Extensive small bowel resection may also lead to hyperplasia of antral gastrin-containing cells and result in ulcer disease. Retained antrum after gastric surgery is yet another example of a situation in which there is uninhibited acid production associated with recurrent ulcerations.

Many drugs are reputed to be ulcerogenic, although the evidence is not well established for most of them. Aspirin is one drug that does cause gastric and, possibly, duodenal ulcers. Experimentally, aspirin disrupts the gastric mucosa both physiologically and anatomically, leading to ulcer formation. The risk of gastric ulcer increases 6-fold when patients use more than three aspirin a day (1). Aspirin use also increases the risk of bleeding from peptic lesions (see Chapter 52). Enteric coated or buffered aspirin has no advantage over regular aspirin with respect to these untoward effects.

There is good evidence that all nonsteroidal antiinflammatory drugs (NSAIDs) cause gastric ulcers. As with aspirin, the association with duodenal ulcer is less certain. The greatest risk of NSAID-induced gastric or duodenal bleeding appears to be in patients over 60 years of age (8). The risk of NSAID complications in patients with a history of ulcers is uncertain. Corticosteroids have frequently been linked to the formation of ulcers and to the complications of hemorrhage and perforation. Prospective and retrospective studies have concluded that chronic use of corticosteroids does not increase the risk of peptic ulcer disease or of its complications (15).

PATHOPHYSIOLOGY

The pathophysiology of duodenal ulcer disease differs from that of gastric ulcer disease.

Duodenal Ulcer

Duodenal ulcer disease can be viewed as the result of an imbalance between the normal duodenal defense mechanisms and the amount of acid delivered to the duodenum from the stomach. Multiple abnormalities have been identified that result in this imbalance: (a) increased parietal cell mass, (b) increased capacity of parietal cells to secrete acid, (c) increased vagal "drive" to secrete acid, (d) defective inhibition of gastrin release and of gastric secretion after gastric acidification or after a meal (these first four abnormalities result in a considerably increased acid production compared with normal), (e) abnormally rapid gastric emptying, and (f) altered duodenal defense mechanisms.

Duodenal defense mechanisms include neutralization of acid by pancreatic bicarbonate and absorption of acid by duodenal contents. Bicarbonate secretion is lower in patients with duodenal ulcer than in normal subjects. There are some data, also, to suggest that pancreatic bicarbonate secretion is decreased by nicotine. This observation may provide an explanation for the association between smoking and ulcer disease, but its true significance is still uncertain. Other key elements in mucosal defense that may break down include vascular epithelial integrity, endogenous prostaglandin formation, and mucus production.

Helicobacter Pylori (3)

Since its identification in 1983 the role of *H. pylori* (formerly *Campylobacter pylori*) in the pathogenesis of duodenal ulcer disease has received a great deal of attention. This Gram-negative bacillus is believed by most authorities to be the causative agent for chronic nonerosive antral gastritis (see below page 435), an associated finding in 80% of patients with duodenal ulcer disease. *H. pylori* has been demonstrated in 85% of patients with duodenal ulcers, usually in the gastric antrum or in areas of duodenum exhibiting gastric metaplasia (but in only approximately 5% of controls). *H. pylori* antibodies are found in high titers in most patients with duodenal ulcers. However, at present it can be said only that *H. pylori* has a strong association with duodenal ulcer and may play a role in relapse. Current evidence does not support this agent as etiologic. No change should be contemplated in the approach to treatment of duodenal ulcer because of the presence or absence of this organism, and, in fact, routine cultures of gastric and duodenal contents of patients with peptic disease are not warranted.

Gastric Ulcer

The current understanding of the pathogenesis of gastric ulceration is less clear. It is generally believed that the basic defect in gastric ulcer formation is the disruption of the gastric mucosal barrier. It has been shown that this barrier can be broken by such irritants as bile, alcohol, and aspirin. These experimental observations help explain the epidemiological data associating alcohol with acute gastritis, and aspirin with gastric ulcers and erosions. Furthermore, in patients with gastric ulcers, radiological and manometric studies have suggested that there is an increased duodenal gastric reflux. This reflux of bile across an incompetent pyloric sphincter results in the disruption of the mucosal barrier. Once the barrier is broken, hydrogen ion may diffuse back into the gastric cells, leading to ulceration via local histamine release, vasodilation, and tissue damage. Thus, according to this concept, gastric ulcer formation requires injury to the gastric mucosal barrier and the presence of some, but not necessarily an excessive amount of, acid.

Another factor that may be involved in the formation of some gastric ulcers is pyloric stenosis, which most commonly occurs secondary to a chronic duodenal ulcer that antedates the formation of a gastric ulcer. With pyloric deformity there may be poor gastric emptying, resulting in stasis and antral distension. This distension leads to increased gastrin release and increased gastric acid production. This hypothesis is supported by the frequent association radiographically of both duodenal and gastric ulcerations. In the Veterans Administration (VA) Cooperative Study of gastric ulcer, over 40% of patients had radiographic evidence of concurrent duodenal ulcer disease (9). Furthermore, patients with gastric ulcers just proximal to the pylorus are frequently found to produce increased amounts of acid, just as patients with duodenal ulcers do.

DIAGNOSIS

History

The most common symptom of peptic ulcer disease is epigastric distress—vague discomfort or a feeling of gnawing hunger—usually in the midline. If actual pain occurs, it is typically aching or burning.

Classically, the distress of duodenal ulcers occurs 1 to 3 hours after a meal and may awaken the patient from sleep, usually between 1:00 and 2:00 A.M.; it is relieved within minutes by food, antacids, or vomiting. Pain is minimal before breakfast. In patients with gastric ulcers, the history is more variable. In some, a similar distress-food-relief pattern exists, whereas in others there is no relationship with food. Occasionally, the distress is actually exacerbated by food.

Other less frequent symptoms of ulcer disease include nausea, vomiting, and heartburn. However, in some patients with ulcers one or more of these symptoms may occur in the absence of typical ulcer pain. Weight loss occurs in up to 50% of patients with a benign gastric ulcer (and is therefore not a helpful feature in distinguishing a benign from a malignant ulcer). Patients with duodenal ulcer often gain weight because they eat more in an attempt to control their pain.

The history may also suggest certain complications. Pyloric obstruction presents first with early satiety and then with persistent vomiting, frequently of undigested food. A change in the quality of the pain or radiation of the pain to the back or shoulder suggests penetration of the ulcer. A history of melena suggests bleeding. Occasionally, one of these complications is the first clinical manifestation of peptic ulceration.

Physical Examination

The physical examination may provide supportive, although nonspecific, information. Localized epigastric tenderness is common. The presence of a succussion splash 4 hours or more postprandially is evidence of gastric outlet obstruction. Rectal examination should be included in the initial physical examination to obtain a stool specimen for testing for occult blood.

Radiological Studies

Confirmation of the presence of peptic ulcer disease can be made with barium studies or with endoscopy.

Patient experience. The patient should be told that the upper gastrointestinal series requires him to have a series of X-rays taken after he swallows a bolus of barium, that peristalsis is monitored fluoroscopically during the procedure, and that to coat as much of the stomach and duodenum as possible, he will be X-rayed while he is prone. The entire procedure takes about 20 to 25 minutes.

Endoscopically demonstrable duodenal or gastric ulcers are visible by barium X-ray in up to 80% of cases.

Duodenal Ulcer

The radiographic diagnosis of duodenal ulcer disease depends upon the detection of an ulcer crater. Associated findings include edema and radiation of the duodenal folds adjacent to the ulcer, deformity of the bulb, and spasm. Occasionally the ulcer crater may not be detected because of overhanging edematous folds that prevent filling of the crater with barium, shallowness of the ulcer crater, or an inadequate technique. Overall, the sensitivity of X-ray in detection of duodenal ulcer is 40 to 80%, with the greatest sensitivity achieved with double contrast radiographs. Ulcers less than 0.5 cm are often missed radiographically. Ulcers larger than 2.5 cm are classified as giant duodenal ulcers. Duodenal ulcers do not carry the risk of malignancy that gastric ulcers do, and therefore follow-up X-rays to confirm healing are generally not needed. In patients with chronic ulcer disease with severe deformity of the bulb, distinction radiographically between old scarring with deformity and new active ulcerations is often very difficult. Comparison with previous films and correlation with the clinical state are needed in these cases.

In the postoperative patient, barium studies are often difficult to evaluate. With conventional studies, anastomotic ulcers are detected in only 50% of cases. The air contrast technique may be of more value in this situation. Distinction between surgical deformity and recurrent ulcerations is often difficult without a previous postoperative study for comparison.

Gastric Ulcer

A well-performed double contrast X-ray can detect approximately 65 to 80% of gastric ulcers seen at endoscopy; of greater importance is its ability to differentiate benign from malignant ulcers. The radiographic features characteristic of a benign gastric ulcer include (a) penetration of the ulcer crater beyond the expected course of the gastric lumen; (b) radiating gastric folds converging on the ulcer reaching right up to the ulcer margin; (c) smooth appearance of surrounding mucosa; (d) central location of the ulcer, surrounded by a smooth mound of edematous mucosa; and (e) smooth and round or oval margins of the ulcer crater. The radiation of the gastric folds up to the thin overhanging margin of the ulcer is probably the most reliable sign of benignity. Appreciation of the surrounding gastric mucosa and the radiation of the folds is best achieved with good air contrast technique (Fig. 37.1). (The air contrast study causes distension of the stomach but no real pain.) The size of the ulcer is not helpful as a differential point in an individual case, except that the incidence of malignancy in gastric ulcers increases with increasing size of the ulcer crater. Similarly, location of the ulcer is not of predictive value. Coexistent duodenal ulcer disease (seen in 40% of gastric ulcer patients) considerably decreases the likelihood that a gastric ulcer is malignant but does not rule it out. Multiple ulcers need to be evaluated and followed individually.

In evaluating a gastric ulcer, the radiologist generally describes it as benign, malignant, or indeterminant. As many as 10% of gastric ulcers may be classified in this last category. Although the radiographic impression of a benign or malignant ulcer is generally very accurate, discrepancies still occur. The prevalence of malignancy in an ulcer diagnosed radiographically as benign ranges from 3 to 7% with higher frequencies when "indeterminant" lesions are included. Air contrast techniques may decrease this error rate. Furthermore, barium studies may miss lesions, particularly when multiple ulcers are present. Even carefully performed radiography will miss up to 20% of ulcers seen by endoscopy. Thus, while a barium study is frequently the initial procedure of choice for gastric ulcers, it must be recognized that its sensitivity is less than that of endoscopy and that it is associated occasionally with erroneous results.

Endoscopy

Comparison studies clearly indicate increased sensitivity and specificity of endoscopy over radiography. Experienced endoscopists will diagnose 85 to 95% of gastroduodenal ulcers when the initial 5 to 15% failure

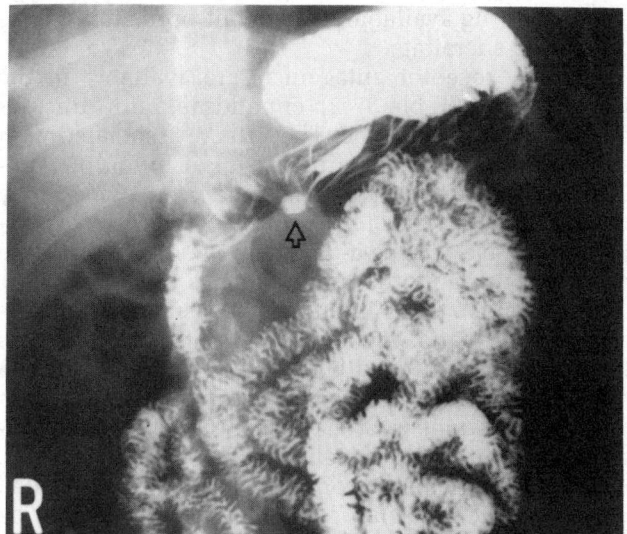

Figure 37.1. X-ray study in a patient with a benign gastric ulcer. The presence of gastric folds radiating to the edge of the ulcer, with no distortion of the surrounding mucosa, is characteristic of a benign gastric ulcer.

rate is documented by a second endoscopy, surgery or radiography (6). When both ulcers and erosions (duodenitis) are considered as diagnostic criteria, the sensitivity of radiography in the detection of both duodenal and gastric lesions is 54% compared with 90% for endoscopy (12). The question of the primary diagnostic procedure of choice for diagnosis of ulcers remains to be settled. Clearly this must be based on the clinical presentation as well as the overall condition of the patient. Guidelines for endoscopy in peptic ulcer disease can only be suggested. In patients with typical symptoms of duodenal ulcer (see above) a diagnosis can be strongly suggested by response to a therapeutic trial of medical therapy. Patients with longstanding abdominal pain refractory to medical treatment or with negative X-rays should have endoscopy. Other indications for endoscopy include suspected outlet obstruction, active or suspected gastrointestinal bleeding, and the need to evaluate equivocal or indeterminant findings on upper gastrointestinal series. There is a higher diagnostic yield of endoscopy in patients over the age of 65 (7). No follow-up endoscopic evaluation of an uncomplicated duodenal ulcer is required since the risk for malignancy is nil.

Another controversial issue is the indication for endoscopy when a gastric ulcer is diagnosed by X-ray. The argument for endoscopy in all patients with gastric ulcer is that 3 to 7% of radiographically benign ulcers will be found subsequently to be malignant. It has been "documented" that malignant ulcers do heal radiographically. The argument against routine endoscopy is that most endoscopies will only confirm the radiographic impression so the patient will incur unnecessary discomfort, risk, and cost. Unfortunately no data are available to help, nor are any likely to be forthcoming because of the number of patients required to do conclusive study. It is the opinion of the American Society for Gastrointestinal Endoscopy (5) that all patients with gastric ulcers that appear benign should have endoscopy with biopsy at some point in the therapy (after 8 weeks of therapy, for example). It is reasonable to do early endoscopy in all patients with ulcers that are not clearly radiographically benign or that are large (2.5 cm). Biopsies can be obtained at that point and all parties can be reassured. The ulcers should then be followed until they have healed, as confirmed by endoscopy.

Gastric Analysis

Gastric secretory studies have enhanced the understanding of the pathophysiology of ulcer disease but are of limited clinical usefulness. Although many patients with duodenal ulcer disease can be shown to hypersecrete acid, over one-half of such patients actually have normal levels of acid production. The presence of hypersecretion, furthermore, does not predict the development of ulcer disease in an individual patient. Dyspepsia with a negative X-ray is not an indication for gastric analysis.

In patients with gastric ulcers, gastric analysis is not helpful. No reliable criteria exist to differentiate benign from malignant gastric ulcer.

The main indications for gastric analysis are for preoperative evaluation of patients with suspected Zollinger-Ellison syndrome (see below) or in the postgastrectomy patient with recurrent ulcer disease. However, gastric analysis is not useful as an indicator of the type of surgery needed—more acid production does not necessarily require more gastric resection (13).

Serum Gastrin Measurements

Measurements of the level of gastrin in the blood are readily available and are of use in the evaluation of selected patients with peptic ulcer disease. The fasting basal serum gastrin level is normal (i.e., <150 pg/ml) in patients with duodenal and gastric ulcer disease but is elevated, often to very high levels (usually 1000 pg/ml or more), in patients with the Zollinger-Ellison syndrome (see below). Therefore, fasting gastrin determinations are very useful in screening for this condition. In patients with frequently recurrent ulcers and in patients refractory to conventional therapy—features suggestive of the syndrome—two or three fasting serum gastrin determinations should be made to rule out this condition since the levels may fluctuate. Also, in all patients undergoing elective ulcer surgery, a preoperative gastrin level should be measured (see page 432 for a discussion of hypergastrinemia).

MEDICAL THERAPY

The treatment of peptic ulcer disease revolves around two issues: healing of the ulcer and prevention of its recurrence. Acute treatment involves dietary manipulation, a change in lifestyle, and relief of pain with pharmacologic agents. Occasionally, a patient will be refractory to medical treatment or will have complications and will require surgery.

Nonpharmacological Therapy

There is no evidence that dietary modification affects the treatment of peptic ulcer disease. Frequent feedings, bland diets, increased milk consumption, decreased consumption of spices and fruit juices have never been demonstrated to effect healing. Although alcohol and caffeine increase acid secretion, no evidence exists that discontinuing either of these substances enhances healing. Dietary restrictions should be limited to those substances that cause symptoms; otherwise patients should be allowed to eat as they wish.

The most important nonpharmacologic intervention is to discontinue cigarette smoking. Cigarette smoking both increases the risk and delays the healing of duodenal ulcers. Impaired healing of duodenal ulcers in smokers compared with nonsmokers has been repeatedly demonstrated in controlled trials with H_2 antagonists. The impact of smoking is more dramatic when recurrence of ulcers is examined. Nontreated non-

smokers have a yearly recurrence rate of approximately 20% (equal to smokers treated with maintenance therapy) compared with a recurrence rate of about 70% in nontreated smokers. Several studies have demonstrated that patients who smoke fewer than 10 cigarettes a day have healing rates similar to nonsmokers. Healing rates are dramatically lower in patients who smoke greater than 20 cigarettes a day (14, 16). In this group recurrence approaches 100% in the first 3 months after therapy is discontinued. Smoking may predispose to perforation and bleeding. The effect of smoking on gastric ulceration appears to be similar to that in duodenal ulceration, though not as extensively studied.

Aspirin and other nonsteroidal anti-inflammatory drugs are well-known risk factors for gastric erosions and ulcers. There is a trend toward an increased risk of duodenal ulcers and erosions as well. All such agents should be discontinued when a patient has a peptic ulcer.

Pharmacological Therapy

In general, pharmacological agents will heal 75 to 80% of acute duodenal ulcers in 4 to 6 weeks and 85 to 90% will heal in an additional 2 weeks. Pain relief usually occurs in the first week to 10 days. If significant pain continues for greater than 2 weeks, the diagnosis should be reconsidered. Gastric ulcers require longer therapy—usually 8 to 12 weeks and pain relief may be slower. Gastric ulcers usually heal at a rate of 2 to 3 mm per week (also see below, page 431).

Ulcers can be treated either by inhibiting secretion of or neutralizing gastric acid or by augmenting protection of the mucosa. Inhibition of acid can be accomplished by five classes of drugs: H_2 receptor antagonists, antacids, proton pump (H+, K+, ATPase) inhibitors, anticholinergics, and prostaglandins. The only drug available to augment protection of the mucosa is sucralfate.

Four H_2 receptor antagonists are available in the United States (Table 37.2): cimetidine, ranitidine, famotidine, and nizatidine. They all are associated with similar healing rates in clinical trials. Cimetidine, ranitidine, and famotidine all may be used twice a day or in single doses before bedtime. Nizatidine is approved for use as once-a-day therapy only. Cimetidine has been available the longest and is extremely safe. Common side effects include gynecosmastia (approximately 0.2%) and impotence. Both of these problems have been reported with ranitidine therapy, though rarely. The major side effect of cimetidine is inhibition of the cytochrome P450 pathway, thereby causing interference with drug metabolism of benzodiazepines, warfarin, phenytoin, propranolol, and theophylline. Ranitidine, famotidine, and nizatidine appear to be free of this interaction. Other side effects such as confusion, dizziness, and somnolence—especially important problems in elderly patients and in patients with hepatic or renal dysfunction—appear to be more common with cimetidine but do occur with ranitidine

Table 37.2.
Drugs Approved for Treatment of Peptic Ulcer Disease

	Available Strengths	Initial Dose[a, b]	Maintenance Dose	Principal Side Effects
Cimetidine (Tagamet)[c]	200 mg 300 mg 400 mg 800 mg	300 mg four times a day 400 mg twice a day 800 mg at bedtime	400 mg at bedtime	Gynecomastia, confusion, impotence, blood dyscrasia, drug interaction (text)
Ranitidine (Zantac)	150 mg 300 mg	150 mg twice a day 300 mg at bedtime	150 mg at bedtime	Gynecomastia, impotence, hepatitis (rare)
Famotidine (Pepcid)[c]	20 mg 40 mg	20 mg twice a day 40 mg at bedtime	20 mg at bedtime	Headache, decreased libido, depression, mild increase in aminotransferase
Nizatidine (Axid)	150 mg 300 mg	150 mg twice a day[d] 300 mg at bedtime	150 mg at bedtime	Sweating, urticaria (<1%), somnolence, elevated liver enzymes
Sucralfate (Carafate)[c]	1 g	1 g four times a day[d] 2 g twice a day	1 g twice a day[e] 2 g at bedtime	Constipation

[a]Duodenal ulcer, 4–6 weeks.
[b]Gastric ulcer, 8–12 weeks (document healing).
[c]Available in liquid suspension.
[d]Not approved for gastric ulcer by FDA.
[e]Not approved for maintenance by FDA.

as well. It is unknown, because of relatively little use compared with the other H_2 blockers, whether these problems occur with famotidine and/or nizatidine. Other rare but important reactions to H_2 blockers include bradycardia, headache, and rarely hepatitis. The hepatitis is reversible on withdrawal of the drug.

Healing rates for duodenal ulcers for all dosage regimens are equal (75 to 90% at 4 to 8 weeks). Healing rates for gastric ulcers (65 to 90% at 8 to 12 weeks) are also equal among H_2 antagonists.

Cimetidine is the least expensive H_2 blocker, and ranitidine (based on length of use) appears to be the safest (side effects of famotidine and nizatidine appear to be similar to those of ranitidine but experience is limited). Actually there is little upon which to base a choice between the four available H_2 blockers. Although there is some relationship, especially at lower doses, between dosage of an H_2 blocker and ulcer healing, ordinarily there is little to be gained by exceeding the dosages listed in Table 37.2.

Antacids (Table 37.3), the backbone of pain relief for symptomatic peptic ulcers, are rarely used as the sole pharmacologic agents for healing. Though a 70 to 80% healing rate has been demonstrated with full dose antacid therapy, there is no advantage in cost or side effect profile compared with H_2 antagonists or to mucosal protective agents. Liquid antacids must be given seven times a day to give consistent healing. Side effects include hypermagnesemia, particularly in patients with renal disease, and phosphate depletion from aluminum hydroxide antacids. Prolonged therapy with aluminum-containing antacids may produce osteoporosis or osteomalacia and, in patients with severe chronic renal falure, neurologic dysfunction and anemia. Sodium overload may be a problem in patients with congestive heart failure. Hypercalcemia, alkalosis, renal impairment, and milk alkali syndrome have all been reported with calcium-containing antacids.

Table 37.3.
Comparison of Various Antacids[a]

Brand Name	Contents			One Dose[b]		Cost (¢)
	Al	Mg	Ca	Vol (ml)	Na (mg)	
Mylanta-II[c,d]	+	+		30	47.9	20
Maalox	+	+		48	53.8	25
Mylanta[d]	+	+		52	40.6	23
Riopan	+	+		56	7.9	22
Amphojel	+			64	77.0	28
Gelusil	+	+		93	132.7	37
Camalox	+	+	+	35	17.8	16

[a]From Ippoliti A, Peterson W: The pharmacology of peptic ulcer disease. *Clin Gastroenterol* 8:54, 1979.
[b]Dose defined as volume of antacid with neutralizing capability equivalent to 30 ml (1 ounce) of Mylanta-II.
[c]Mylanta-II has twice as much aluminum hydroxide and magnesium hydroxide per unit volume as Mylanta.
[d]Contains simethicone.

Inhibition of absorption of antibiotics, digoxin, anticonvulsants, anti-inflammatory agents, cimetidine, and warfarin also have been reported. The side effects, coupled with the fact that compliance with full dose antacid regimens is difficult, have largely eliminated antacids from a major primary therapeutic role in peptic ulcer disease. It is current practice to use antacids on an as needed basis for relief of pain early in the course of treatment.

Omeprazole, a hydrogen potassium ATPase (proton pump) inhibitor, is the most potent antisecretory agent currently available for treatment of ulcer disease but as of this writing has not been approved by the United States Food and Drug Administration (FDA). This agent blocks the terminal step in acid secretion. A single dose of 40 to 60 mg a day will reduce acid secretion to zero for 24 hours. Single doses of 20 or 40 mg per day results in 90 to 100% duodenal ulcer healing at 4 weeks, and 95% healing of gastric ulcer at 8 weeks (19). The side effect profile in acute studies is low, mild elevation of liver enzymes being the principal side effect. Long-term side effects from such profound inhibitions of secretion of gastric acid are unknown at present. This agent, if approved, should be especially valuable in the treatment of refractory ulcers and of reflux esophagitis.

Anticholinergic agents are mild inhibitors of basal and food-stimulated acid secretion. These drugs have limited usefulness because of significant side effects— dry mouth, blurred vision, tachycardia, ileus, and urinary retention. Pirenzepine, a selective anticholinergic that inhibits acid secretion by blocking the M2 receptor on the parietal cell, results in 70 to 80% healing at 6 weeks and does so with few anticholinergic side effects, but the drug is not yet available in the United States.

Prostaglandins have two major therapeutic effects: acid inhibition and mucosal protection. The only available agent is misoprostil (Cytotec), a prostaglandin E1 analogue. In doses of 200 mg four times a day or twice a day, duodenal ulcers heal at a frequency equal to that of H_2 antagonists. Unfortunately this regimen produces significant abdominal cramps and diarrhea (13 to 33%). In addition at this dose uterine contractions are stimulated. Doses below 100 mg four times a day, so called mucosal (or cyto) protective dosages, cause few side effects but fail to heal ulcers with greater frequency than do placebos. Thus there is little to recommend prostaglandins in the treatment of peptic ulcer disease.

Sucralfate (Carafate) is an aluminum hydroxide salt of sucrose octasulfate and is the only available agent in the United States that promotes effective treatment of peptic ulcer disease without inhibition of gastric acid secretion. It appears to have a multifactorial node of action. It binds to ulcerated mucosa to form a protective barrier on the ulcer base and thus prevents further damage. It appears to inhibit peptic activity by binding to pepsin substrate. It is "cytoprotective" to the gastric mucosa, either by augmenting prostaglandin secretion or gastric mucus production. In addition it binds bile salts, which can be irritative to the gastric mucosa. There is little to no systemic absorption and it is only a weak antacid. The single major side effect is constipation, in 2 to 4%. An occasional patient will complain of headache, dizziness, or dry mouth. The basis for these latter side effects is unknown. The approved dosage regimen (a 1-g tablet four times a day between meals) gives healing rates comparable to H_2 blockers, with fewer side effects. Duodenal ulcer healing with 2 g twice a day before breakfast and at bedtime is equal to the four times a day dose but has not yet been approved for use in the United States. A recent study has suggested that sucralfate may be particularly advantageous in smokers (11). In this study smokers had similar healing rates to nonsmokers, a result different from that of H_2 blocker therapy.

Colloidal bismuth, another gastric mucosal protectant, appears to decrease peptic activity, increase mucous secretion, and bind to mucosal proteins of the ulcer base. Bismuth compounds either in liquid or tablet form appear to be as effective as H_2 blockers in acute treatment of duodenal ulcer disease. Of greater importance is that these drugs appear to delay the onset of ulcer recurrence, perhaps related to inhibition of *H. pylori*. Colloidal bismuth is not available in the United States.

General Recommendations

The current available pharmacologic agents are equally efficacious in promoting healing of acute peptic ulcers. The choice of initial therapy should be based on local pharmacy costs, physician and patient preference, side effects, and drug interactions. There is no evidence that addition of a second drug—e.g., sucralfate plus an H_2 antagonist—is more effective than a single agent.

Patients whose ulcers fail to heal in 6 to 8 weeks should be treated an additional 2 to 4 weeks with the same agent. If the Zollinger-Ellison syndrome is not suggested (see below) and nonpharmacologic therapy (see above) has been maximized, another class of drug should be tried. Switching from one H_2 antagonist to another rarely results in significant improvement in the rate of healing.

Maintenance Therapy

It is now well known that the acute treatment of uncomplicated ulcer disease is not difficult. Unfortunately recurrences are common. Maintenance therapy, although effective and remarkably free of side effects, is expensive. It is therefore important to develop a rational strategy. Patients over the age of 60; men; patients with chronic obstructive lung disease, coronary artery disease, or renal failure; patients with a history of complications such as bleeding or perforation, a history of refractory symptoms, or the need for nonsteroidal anti-inflammatory drugs are at high risk for recurrence and are candidates for maintenance therapy. Perhaps the greatest risk for recurrence is cigarette smoking. As mentioned above, patients who are nonsmokers have recurrence rates when treated with placebo equal to the recurrence rate with active drug therapy in smokers, suggesting that simply the elimination of cigarette smoking will obviate the need for maintenance therapy in many patients.

Patients who do not fall in high risk categories should be treated on an individual basis. Less than 20% of this population will have a recurrence within 1 year. There is little reason to treat these people with continuous maintenance therapy. Intermittent therapy for infrequent recurrences is logical in this group. However, if a patient has two or more recurrences in a year after diagnosis, continuous maintenance therapy is indicated.

Patients who are given maintenance therapy are usually treated for 1 year. Treatment in a single dose at bedtime with H_2 blockers (cimetidine, 400 mg; ranitidine, 150 mg; famotidine, 20 mg) is effective for maintenance of "remission" of duodenal ulcers. In these dosages the recurrence rate is reduced to 20%

at 1 year. A recent 2-year study with ranitidine suggested that these rates can be maintained over time (18). A 4-year experience with cimetidine in European trials has suggested that maintenance of remission can be maintained with few side effects over this extended period, if necessary. Sucralfate appears to prevent recurrence at a dose of 1 g twice a day. In a single trial 2 g at bedtime appeared to be effective also, but this drug has not received approval for maintenance therapy in the United States. The available data do not allow separation among the available therapeutic modalities. The decision must be based on cost and the profile of side effects for the individual patient.

A small body of evidence is emerging that the choice of initial therapy may have an effect on ulcer recurrence. Several trials have shown lower recurrence rates after initial therapy with colloidal bismuth (currently not available in the United States) or sucralfate compared with H_2 blockers (11). Recurrence rate at 1 year appears to be slightly lower when these modalities are used for initial healing. The reason for these results is unknown but may relate to elimination of H. pylori or the prevention of rebound acid secretion that may occur after stopping a course of antisecretory therapy. The numbers are small and require confirmation.

In summary, immediate maintenance therapy can be recommended if patients are at risk for recurrence. Low risk patients can be watched and maintenance therapy can be given based on the frequency of recurrence. Nonsmokers and smokers who quit can be expected to have a low rate of recurrence. H_2 blockers in half doses are effective and reduce recurrence to 20% at 2 years. Sucralfate, 1 g twice daily, appears equally effective. It is current practice to attempt stopping maintenance therapy after 1 to 2 years; however, the optimum length of therapy is not known and must be individualized.

Gastric Ulcers

In general the same drugs available to treat duodenal ulcers are effective in the treatment of gastric ulcer. A few differences in approach to acute treatment deserve comment. Limited experience is available using single dose (bedtime) H_2 antagonists in gastric ulcer. Though single doses are probably as effective as multiple doses, the current recommendation is for therapy two or four times a day. Sucralfate is as effective as cimetidine but has not been approved for maintenance therapy of gastric ulcer. If used it should be given 1 g four times a day. Omeprazole is probably the most effective drug for gastric ulcer but is not yet approved for treatment of this condition.

In general treatment should be for at least 8 weeks and healing must be documented, preferably by endoscopy. No dietary restriction affects healing, and hospitalization (in the absence of complications) is not necessary. Nonsteroidal anti-inflammatory drugs (NSAIDs), including aspirin, should be discontinued, though a few studies suggest that healing may occur even if the NSAID is continued. Smoking cessation

should be strongly recommended. Maintenance therapy should be prescribed according to the guidelines for duodenal ulcer (see above).

SURGICAL THERAPY

Surgery is effective therapy for the relief of ulcer symptoms and for the prevention of ulcer recurrence. Although certain postoperative problems are common, the vast majority of patients feel significantly better after surgery. Thus, in the appropriate setting, surgery should be considered as a good and effective alternative form of therapy, rather than as a punishment for failure to respond to medical therapy.

Indications

The indications for ulcer surgery are perforation, uncontrolled hemorrhage, gastric outlet obstruction, and intractability. At times surgery is performed as an emergency, but often it is performed after a prolonged period of symptomatic ulcer disease. Intractability is probably the weakest indication for ulcer surgery, although it may be the one most commonly used. It should be recognized that intractability may be due to the disease itself, to the patient's noncompliance with an appropriate medical regimen, or to insufficient medical therapy provided by the clinician. Thorough review with the patient of maximal medical therapy as outlined above will help to delineate the cause for the refractoriness of medical therapy (see Chapter 3).

Before surgery, except for emergency situations, some preoperative assessment should be made to rule out Zollinger-Ellison syndrome (see below) and hypercalcemia.

Types of Operations

Various operations are available for the treatment of ulcer disease. The physician should discuss with the surgeon the various alternatives and reach an agreement about which operation may be best suited for the individual patient. Of course, the final decision is generally made in the operating room after the surgeon has evaluated the gastroduodenal area. The patient should also be educated about the rationale for the planned surgical approach and the expected outcome.

Duodenal Ulcer

Three major operations are currently employed for duodenal ulcer: vagotomy with pyloroplasty, vagotomy with antrectomy, and parietal cell (or highly selective) vagotomy. The first two procedures involve a selective vagotomy (gastric vagal fibers only) plus a drainage procedure to facilitate gastric emptying postoperatively. The third procedure involves cutting vagal fibers to the body (acid-secreting cells) of the stomach, preserving antral innervation, and eliminating the need for a drainage procedure. Vagotomy with pyloroplasty has the lowest mortality, shortest operation time, and a recurrence rate of 6 to 8%. Vagotomy with antrectomy is technically more difficult and may predispose to more postoperative morbidity (because an anastomosis to the remaining stomach is required) but has the lowest recurrence rate (<2%) (10). Postoperative complications are significantly more frequent with either procedure compared with parietal cell vagotomy (see Table 37.3). A parietal cell vagotomy has a recurrence rate of 10% at 10 years (10), approximately 4 to 5 times that of vagotomy with antrectomy. Long-term complications (of dumping syndrome and diarrhea) are less than 60% that of vagotomy and antrectomy. In the hands of experienced surgeons a parietal cell vagotomy is the operation of choice. The higher recurrence rate (which can be managed medically in 80%) is an acceptable tradeoff for the decreased complication rate.

Gastric Ulcer

For gastric ulcers the type of surgery is less certain since our understanding of the condition is less clear. In contrast to duodenal ulcer disease a vagotomy may not be indicated in all patients with a gastric ulcer who undergo surgery. However, in patients who have evidence of concomitant duodenal ulcer disease (approximately 10 to 40% of patients with gastric ulcers) and in patients who have pyloric ulcers, which generally behave as duodenal ulcers, a vagotomy is clearly indicated. If the ulcer is within the antrum, an antrectomy or hemigastrectomy that includes the ulcer is frequently the preferred operation. When the ulcer cannot be included in the gastric resection, a full thickness biopsy of the ulcer should be taken for frozen section to rule out malignancy. The recurrence rate for gastric ulcers after these types of operation is very low (1 to 2%).

After antrectomy or hemigastrectomy, the stomach may be anastomosed to the duodenum (Bilroth I anastomosis) or to the jejunum (Bilroth II). The type of anastomosis is determined by the surgeon based on the degree of duodenal deformity and on technical considerations.

Postgastrectomy Syndromes

A wide variety of problems develop in the postgastrectomy state (Table 37.4). In 10% of patients, the postgastrectomy complications are severe. Many of these conditions result from the altered physiology created by the surgery.

ZOLLINGER-ELLISON SYNDROME

The Zollinger-Ellison syndrome represents dramatically the relationship between gastrin, acid secretion, and ulcer formation. The syndrome results from a non-β islet cell tumor of the pancreas that autonomously secretes gastrin and is therefore called a *gastrinoma*. In the majority of cases there are multiple tumors, most commonly found in the head of the pancreas. They vary considerably in size from several millimeters, often undetectable at surgery, to huge masses that may even be palpable through the abdominal wall. Approximately two-thirds of gastrinomas are malignant in their biological behavior and histological appearance; they can metastasize and be a cause of death, although generally they are slow growing.

With the introduction of readily available measurement of gastrin, the concept of the clinical features of the Zollinger-Ellison syndrome has begun to change. The original description of the syndrome focused on the virulent nature of the ulcer diathesis and on the atypical location for the ulcers. It is now recognized, however, that 75% of ulcers in patients with Zollinger-Ellison syndrome occur in the duodenal bulb and appear as routine single duodenal ulcers. The finding, however, of postbulbar and jejunal ulcerations should alert the physician to the possibility of the syndrome. Over one-quarter of patients undergo ulcer surgery before the diagnosis of the syndrome, which is usually made only when anastomotic ulcers develop. Diarrhea is another frequent symptom, occurring in more than one-third of patients, and may precede the formation of ulcers by several years; however, 7% of patients have diarrhea and never develop an ulcer. (The diarrhea is due principally to the increased secretion of gastric acid, which, when it enters the duodenum, lowers the pH of the normally alkaline duodenal fluid and thereby interferes with absorption of water and electrolytes.)

Diagnosis

The diagnosis of Zollinger-Ellison syndrome should be considered under the following conditions: (a) failure of medical therapy, resulting in the need for ulcer surgery; (b) giant ulcer; (c) multiple ulcers; (d) postbulbar or jejunal ulcers; (e) anastomotic ulcer; (f) ulcer disease in association with diarrhea (but not diarrhea secondary to drugs); and (g) radiographic or secretory evidence of gastric hypersecretion.

The diagnosis of Zollinger-Ellison syndrome is usually based on the fasting serum gastrin concentration, normally less than 150 pg/ml. Elevations greater than 1000 pg/ml in association with the typical clinical picture are nearly diagnostic of a gastrinoma.

However, in patients with mild elevations of the serum gastrin concentration (i.e., between 150 and 300 pg/ml) and in postoperative patients, differentiation between Zollinger-Ellison syndrome and other causes for hypergastrinemia is important. Consultation with a gastroenterologist is advisable. Other conditions that may lead to hypergastrinemia include (a) retained antrum, (b) G-cell hyperplasia, (c) postvagotomy plus pyloroplasty, (d) small portion of the population with routine duodenal ulcer disease, and (e) pernicious anemia. Also, H_2 receptor blockers cause a slight increase in the serum gastrin concentration so that these drugs should be stopped 12 hours before blood is drawn for the measurement.

Differentiation of these disorders from the Zollinger-Ellison syndrome requires the use of provocative tests, the secretin and calcium infusion tests, generally per-

Table 37.4.
Postgastrectomy Syndromes

Syndrome	Clinical Features	Pathophysiology	Diagnosis/Treatment
Early			
Stomal dysfunction	Vomiting, gastric retention	Edema, inflammation, hypokalemia	Electrolyte repletion, time, no suction
Duodenal stump dehiscence	Pain, fever, signs of abscess, sepsis, death	Bilroth II anastomosis: tension and poor closure; adjacent pancreatitis; excessive inflammation in area of surgery.	Reoperation
Afferent loop syndrome	Pain, vomiting bile without food, may occur acutely or chronically	Bilroth II anastomosis: afferent loop too long, kinked, twisted, herniated, etc. Loop fills, then empties	Reoperation
Vagotomy complications Transient dysphagia	Dysphagia	Lower esophageal sphincter dysfunction	Usually transient, disappears in 1–2 weeks
Diarrhea	Diarrhea transient or slight, 20–40% of patients; troublesome, 5%. Occurs mainly with selective vagotomy and drainage procedure	Most common after truncal vagotomy; appears to be related to increased output of dihydroxy bile salts, the cause of which is uncertain	Cholestyramine, Amphogel
Late or persistent			
Dumping syndrome	Early phase: with or shortly after meals—nausea, abdominal fullness or pain, cramping, palpations, dizziness, sweating	Distention of gastric pouch and upper jejunum from rapid emptying; peripheral intravascular volume depletion from rapid entry of fluid into jejunum due to osmotic changes in jejunum; vasomotor symptoms related to release of vasoactive substances into circulation, such as serotonin and bradykinin	Small frequent meals, high protein, low carbohydrate. Small volume of liquids only
	Late phase: symptoms of hypoglycemia	Early hyperglycemia → insulin production → late hypoglycemia	
Gastric cancer	Increased incidence of 3–5% in gastric stump 15–20 years after surgery	Possibly related to chronic gastritis developing after gastrectomy	Endoscopy for diagnosis, surgical resection
Diarrhea	Chronic diarrhea	Rapid gastric emptying, lactose intolerance unmasked by vagotomy, malabsorption, ZE syndrome, bile acid output increased, bacterial overgrowth	Lactose free diet; if no response, malabsorption work-up (Chapter 39)
Stomal or recurrent ulcer	Recurrent ulcer symptoms; hemorrhage in approximately 50%	Hyperacidity due to inadequate resection, incomplete vagotomy, retained antrum, unrecognized Zollinger-Ellison syndrome (gastrinoma)	Endoscopy; H2 antagonists, (successful in 80%), reoperation
Anemia	Iron deficiency	Chronic blood loss; impaired iron absorption	Repletion of deficient nutrient
	Nutritional anemia	Defective vitamin B_{12} absorption due to decreased intrinsic factor production (resection and gastritis); possible blind loop bacterial overgrowth; folate deficiency	
Osteomalacia	Bone pain	Diminished calcium intake, poor vitamin D absorption; duodenal bypass	Calcium or vitamin D

formed by a gastroenterologist. The secretin test is preferred because it is more reliable and is safer. In both tests, the response of the serum gastrin level to the infusion of a stimulating substance is monitored. In the secretin test, the serum gastrin level rises, usually within the first ½ hour, after the injection of secretin in patients with Zollinger-Ellison syndrome, whereas in all other disorders the gastrin level falls or is unchanged.

In the calcium infusion test, serum gastrin deter-

minations are made immediately before and then repeatedly for 4 hours after the intravenous administration of calcium. In all conditions, the gastrin level increases. However, in the Zollinger-Ellison syndrome, the response is exaggerated with a greater than 50% rise over basal levels.

Gastric analysis may provide further supportive data. Marked hypersecretion is found in both the basal state and after pentagastrin stimulation. Because the stomach is being influenced by an autonomous tumor, further stimulation with exogenous pentagastrin provides little additional stimulation to secretion. Thus, the basal acid output (BAO):maximal acid output (MAO) ratio is 0.6 or greater in this syndrome. However, there is considerable overlap with normal values so that the gastric secretory data alone cannot be used to make the diagnosis.

Various attempts have been made to localize the gastrinoma in the hope that excision of an isolated tumor would be curative. Unfortunately, such efforts have not been successful since multiple tumors are frequently present; small lesions are undetectable by surgical inspection of the pancreas; and these tumors frequently have metastasized by the time surgical exploration is performed. The use of selective pancreatic venography with measurements of gastrin levels from each venous site may provide an improved method to localize the gastrinoma.

Therapy

Because the tumor mass is rarely localized and therefore curable by local resection, therapy has been directed at the end organ. Total gastrectomy historically has been the procedure of choice. Although there is little evidence to suggest that gastrectomy alters the biological behavior of the gastrinoma, it does prevent the consequences of the hypersecretion of acid. In the past, patients died from this condition most often because of the virulent nature of the ulcer diathesis, including frequent recurrences, diarrhea, and even malabsorption, as well as multiple operations. Complete removal of the end organ prevents these complications. In some patients a parietal cell vagotomy may be an alternative procedure to gastrectomy.

In recent years it has become clear that medical therapy is often successful in controlling the ulcer disease and the diarrhea and that surgery may not be necessary. Even if surgery is performed, medical therapy can provide time to stabilize the patient, to correct nutritional deficiencies, and to allow the surgery to be performed on an elective basis. The H_2 receptor antagonists (see page 428) have been used successfully to control acid secretion, though large doses are often needed. The $H+ K+$ ATPase inhibitor, omeprazole (see page 429), also is extremely successful in decreasing acid secretion in these patients.

NONULCER DYSPEPSIA (17)

Dyspepsia is a symptom of persistent epigastric discomfort, occasionally related to meals and sometimes associated with nausea, belching or bloating. It is estimated to be present in 7% of the United States population, most of whom rarely seek medical treatment. When patients with dyspepsia are evaluated with endoscopy, only ⅓ will have demonstrable peptic ulcer disease or gastric cancer. The remaining group—termed nonulcer dyspepsia—present a diagnostic and therapeutic dilemma.

If large groups of patients with nonulcer dyspepsia are evaluated, four major diseases are found to be as-sociated—irritable bowel syndrome (IBS), cholelithiasis, gastroesophageal reflux, and chronic pancreatic disease. In IBS (see Chapter 40) the dyspepsia is associated with diffuse abdominal pain and altered bowel habits. Patients with gastroesophageal reflux disease will have associated heartburn. Chronic pancreatic disease is less common but usually is associated with more severe pain and steatorrhea. The most difficult diagnostic dilemma, due to the high prevalence of gallstones in the general population, is distinguishing patients with symptomatic gallstones from patients with dyspepsia and asymptomatic (incidental) gallstones (see Chapter 90). It is now well established that patients with dyspepsia fail to respond to cholecystectomy unless they have had an identifiable attack of acute cholecystitis or a good history of biliary colic. The absence of either should suggest that gallstones are not the cause of dyspepsia.

Patients without one of these identifiable conditions are said to have *essential dyspepsia*. The etiology of this condition is unknown. A small subset of patients has been described with delayed gastric emptying of solids; however, correlation of improvement of symptoms with treatment has been poor. About 50% of patients will have *H. pylori* gastritis (see page 435). Again symptomatic response to treatment for this infection has been inconsistent. It is clear that patients with essential dyspepsia do *not* have increased basal acid secretion nor has a definite association with stress been documented.

The approach to the patient can be difficult. As mentioned above the yield of diagnostic procedures is low and, particularly with cholelithiasis, may be confusing. Response to empiric therapy with H_2 blockers has been disappointing and may be misleading and lead to inappropriate long-term therapy.

At the present time—until more controlled trials are available—patients below age 40, with a short history and with no evidence of organic disease by physical examination and by appropriate laboratory tests require no investigation, may be treated with reassurance and some modification of their diet or avoidance of caffeine, alcohol, and tobacco. Drugs with a low incidence of side effects—such as H_2 blockers, sucralfate and antacids—may be used, if necessary, in short courses of 3 to 4 weeks. If no response occurs in 2 to 4 weeks and no evidence of reflux disease or IBS is present, endoscopy should be performed. If endoscopy is negative, the other diagnoses discussed above should be pursued. Patients over age 60 are candidates for early investigation (within 1 to 2 weeks), particularly if symptoms are severe and have occurred for the first time. In this group the diagnostic yield for endoscopy is 60% (6, 17).

The long-term prognosis is good with or without treatment in patients in whom endoscopy is negative.

GASTRITIS

Gastritis—inflammation of the stomach mucosa—is a nonspecific diagnosis that is made by endoscopic biopsy. It may be variably associated with dyspepsia though cause and effect have not been documented. Several types of "gastritis" are seen in clinical practice.

Acute erosive or hemorrhagic gastritis is seen most commonly in seriously ill hospitalized patients, patients taking NSAIDs including aspirin, after heavy alcohol ingestion, and rarely in patients prescribed potassium chloride or iron supplements. Symptoms are variable but usually include nausea and/or vomiting and gastrointestinal bleeding that requires hospitalization.

Nonerosive or chronic antral gastritis is a histologic entity, common in the general population, particularly the elderly. This entity has attracted intense attention recently because of its association with *H. pylori* (see above, page 425), a Gram-negative bacillus found in gastric biopsies in 75 to 95% of patients with nonerosive, superficial, chronic active gastritis. Studies in two individuals have demonstrated a syndrome of severe nausea, vomiting, and epigastric pain associated with hypochlorhydria after ingestion of large numbers of the organism (3). Gastric biopsies demonstrated antral gastritis and the presence of the organism. Resolution of symptoms and of the histologic lesion was associated with disappearance of the organism. Unfortunately there is no good evidence that infection with the organism is responsible for any acute or chronic clinical syndrome. No clinical correlation between resolution of gastritis, eradication of *H. pylori* and dyspepsia, bloating, etc. has been adequately demonstrated. The organism can be easily identified by biopsy, noninvasive "urea-breath" tests or serology and can be eradicated by combination therapy of metronidizole, ampicillin, or tetracycline with bismuth compounds (Pepto-bismol), but specific treatment for patients infected with this organism should be resisted until it is established to be efficacious. Symptomatic treatment of patients with nonerosive gastritis is the same as it is for patients with nonulcer dyspepsia (see above).

General References

McGuigan JE: The Zollinger-Ellison Syndrome. In: Sleisenger MH, Fordtran JS (eds), *Gastrointestinal Disease: Pathophysiology, diagnosis, management*. Philadelphia, W.B. Saunders, Co., 1989, p. 909.

Soll AH: Duodenal ulcer and drug threapy. In: Sleisenger MH, Fordtran JS (eds):*Gastrointestinal Disease: Pathophysiology, diagnosis, management*. Philadelphia, W.B. Saunders, Co., 1989, p. 814.

Specific References

1. Aspirin Myocardial Infarction Study Research Group: A randomized, controlled trial of aspirin in persons recovered from myocardial infarction. *JAMA* 243:661, 1980.
2. Bardhan KD, Hinchliffe RCF, Bose K: Low dose maintenance treatment with cimetidine in duodenal ulcer: intermediate-term results. *Postgrad Med J* 62:347, 1986.
3. Blaser MJ: Gastric campylobacter-like organisms, gastritis, and peptic ulcer disease. *Gastroenterology* 93:371, 1987.
4. Bonnevie O: Survival in peptic ulcer. *Gastroenterology* 75:1055, 1978.
5. Committee on Endoscopic Utilization: *Appropriate use of Gastrointestinal endoscopy*. American Society for Gastrointestinal Endoscopy. Manchester, Massachusetts June, 1986. p. 6.
6. Dooley CP, Larson AW, Stace NH, et al: Double contrast barium meal and upper gastrointestinal endoscopy: a comparative study. *Ann Intern Med* 101:538, 1984.
7. Fjosne U, Kleveland PK, Waldum H, et al: The clinical benefit of routine upper gastrointestinal endoscopy. *Scan J. Gastroenterol* 21:433, 1986.
8. Fries JF, Miller SR, Spitz PW, et al: Toward an epidemiology of gastropathy associated with nonsteroidal anti-inflammatory drug use. *Gastroenterology* 96:647, 1989.
9. Hanscom D, Buchman E: The follow-up period (V.A. Cooperative Study on Gastric Ulcer). *Gastroenterology* 61:585, 1971.
10. Jordan PH, Thornby J: Should it be parietal cell vagotomy or selective vagotomy—antrectomy for treatment of duodenal ulcer. A progress report. *Ann Surg* 205:572, 1987.
11. Lam SK, Hui WM, Lau WY, et al: Sucralfate overcomes the adverse effect of cigarette smoking on duodenal ulcer healing and prolongs subsequent remission. *Gastroenterology* 92:1193, 1987.
12. Martin TR, Vennes JA, Silvis SE, Ansel H: A comparison of upper gastrointestinal endoscopy and radiography. *J Clin Gastroenterol* 2:21, 1980.
13. McCarthy D: The place of surgery in the Zollinger-Ellison Syndrome. *N Engl J Med* 302:1344, 1980.
14. McCarthy DM: Smoking and ulcers—time to quit (editorial). *N Engl J Med* 311:726, 1984.
15. Messer J, Reitman D, Sacks HS, et al: Association of adrenocorticosteroid therapy and peptic-ulcer disease. *N Engl J Med* 309:21, 1983.
16. Sontag S, Graham DY, Belsito A, et al: Cimetidine, cigarette smoking, and recurrence of duodenal ulcer. *N Engl J Med* 311:689, 1984.
17. Talley NJ, Phillips SF: Non-ulcer dyspepsia: potential causes and pathophysiology. *Ann Intern Med* 108:865, 1988.
18. VanDeventer GM, Elashoff JD, Reedy TJ, et al: A randomized study of maintenance therapy with ranitidine to prevent recurrence of duodenal ulcer. *N Engl J Med* 320:1113, 1989.
19. Walan AW, Bader JP, Classen M, et al: Effect of omeprazole and ranitidine on ulcer healing and relapse rates in patients with benign gastric ulcer. *N Engl J Med* 320:69, 1989.

C H A P T E R   38

Gastrointestinal Bleeding*

LAWRENCE J. CHESKIN, M.D.

The presence of blood in the stool or in the upper gastrointestinal tract is always a significant finding that requires thorough investigation. Gastrointestinal bleeding may present as (*a*) occult blood, (*b*) melena (black stool) or intermittent hematochezia (the passage of overtly bloody stool), and (*c*) hematemesis. Massive hemorrhage requires immediate hospitalization and, often, emergency diagnostic procedures. (The vomiting of blood, also, almost always dictates immediate hospitalization.) Otherwise, the evaluation of gastrointestinal bleeding often can be performed in an ambulatory setting. Table 38.1 shows the common conditions associated with gastrointestinal bleeding.

TESTS FOR DETECTION OF BLOOD IN STOOL

In "normal" subjects, the hemoglobin concentration of the stool is less than 2 mg of hemoglobin/g of stool as measured by tagged red cell assay. A variety of tests are available to detect abnormal amounts of blood in the stool. These tests differ in sensitivity and specificity and therefore differ in their value as indicators of disease. The most commonly used test for fecal occult blood is the modified guaiac slide test (Hemoccult). This test depends on the peroxidase activity of hemoglobin and reflects the concentration of hemoglobin in the stool. The false-positive rate is as low as 2% (2). If multiple slides (three pairs) are evaluated, the false-negative rate for Hemoccult is 15 to 20%. Therefore, a positive test for occult blood with the Hemoccult slide test is highly specific for significant bleeding although only moderately sensitive. Because colonic cancers and polyps may bleed intermittently, multiple stool specimens should be evaluated. In patients over the age of 40 with at least one positive slide test, about 10% have carcinoma, and another 20 to

Table 38.1.
Common Causes of Gastrointestinal Bleeding

Occult Bleeding
  Colonic polyps
  Colonic cancer
  Peptic ulcer disease
  Gastric cancer
  Gastritis

Melena
  Duodenal ulcer
  Gastric ulcer
  Gastritis
  Gastric carcinoma
  Esophagitis

Hematochezia
  Rectal outlet disorders (hemorrhoids, cryptitis, fissures)
  Colonic polyps
  Colonic cancer
  Diverticulosis
  Inflammatory bowel disease
  Angiodysplasia

Hematemesis
  Esophageal varices
  Mallory-Weiss tear
  Peptic ulcer disease
  Gastric cancer
  Gastritis

40% have polyps greater than 5 mm in diameter (2). Left-sided lesions are detected more often than are right-sided ones. In asymptomatic patients with a positive slide test who have carcinoma, over 80% have lesions limited to the bowel. Thus, a positive Hemoccult test for occult blood in the stool requires further investigation and may favorably influence the patient's prognosis. More reliable methods for detecting fecal blood are under investigation.

Laxatives increase both the number of true-positive and false-positive results of the Hemoccult test (probably by an irritant effect on the normal colonic mucosa and on colonic lesions—such as cancer). For this reason, many screening programs have recommended a high bulk diet for several days before the stool is tested in the hope of maximizing the discovery of occult lesions. False-negative results are more likely in patients taking high doses of vitamin C. False-positive tests may result from peroxidase-rich foods (rare red meat and uncooked vegetables like broccoli, turnips, and cauliflower) and from iron compounds. Salicylates and nonsteroidal anti-inflammatory agents may cause occult gastrointestinal bleeding, either because of a direct irritant effect on the stomach or duodenum or because of unmasking of an underlying lesion. Rehydration of the fecal material also increases the false-positive rate and is not recommended.

The optimal number and the timing of the collection of stool samples have not yet been determined. The object is to detect bleeding from lesions that are known to bleed sporadically. Because compliance is a major factor in this screening test, convenience for the patient is important. Therefore, the recommendation is to obtain two different samples from three different stools over a 3-day period once a year. Patients should

---

*Dr. Harold J. Tucker contributed to this chapter in the first and second editions of this book.

avoid raw red meat, high doses of vitamin C and aspirin, and other nonsteroidal anti-inflammatory agents for 3 days before and during the period of testing. The stool slides can be stored up to 6 days if necessary without a decrease in the sensitivity of the test.

EVALUATION OF PATIENTS WHO HAVE GASTROINTESTINAL BLEEDING

Choosing Appropriate Tests

The history and physical examination direct the sequence of the various tests used to investigate a patient with gastrointestinal bleeding. The patient's age, the nature of associated symptoms, and the severity of bleeding are all important factors. For example, patients with peptic symptoms or with risk factors such as the use of nonsteroidal anti-inflammatory medications (Chapter 37) require an initial evaluation of their stomach and duodenum, whereas patients with a change in bowel habits require an initial evaluation of their colon. In general, patients under the age of 40 are less likely to have a colonic lesion than are patients over 40. Peptic disease and benign rectal lesions are more evenly distributed in adults of all ages.

In asymptomatic patients with occult fecal blood or in patients with hematochezia but with no other symptoms, the lower bowel should be investigated first. In patients with melena but with no other symptoms, the upper gastrointestinal tract should be investigated first. One reasonable approach to the evaluation of lower and upper gastrointestinal bleeding is described below.

Lower Gastrointestinal Tract

Flexible or rigid proctosigmoidoscopy is almost always the first test done in the evaluation of the lower bowel; it should be followed by an air contrast barium enema or a colonoscopy. In patients over the age of 40, colonoscopy should be performed, even if a previous barium enema was negative.

The finding of hemorrhoids, polyps, or even a rectal cancer on proctosigmoidoscopy does not obviate the need for examination of the rest of the colon. However, if the pattern of bleeding is consistent with rectal disease (see Chapter 91), if a rectal lesion is seen during proctosigmoidoscopy, and if the colonic mucosa is well visualized by barium enema and is normal, colonoscopy is not necessary. Also, diverticulosis (see Chapter 41), found on barium enema, should not be considered the cause of intermittent mild hematochezia until colonoscopy has failed to provide another explanation.

Proctosigmoidoscopy

Anorectal lesions are poorly visualized by barium enema. Cryptitis, bleeding hemorrhoids, fissures, and proctitis can only be seen by rigid proctoscopy; and rectal polyps or cancer are much better seen by proctoscopy than by a barium enema. The preparation of the patient for this procedure and the patient's experience during the procedure are described in Chapter 36.

Flexible sigmoidoscopy is used to evaluate the rectum and descending colon. It is better tolerated and identifies more lesions than does rigid proctosigmoidoscopy. It is most useful in screening asymptomatic individuals for colorectal adenoma or carcinoma. It has limited value, however, in patients with gastrointestinal bleeding, as colonoscopy is still required to evaluate the possibility of more proximal colonic lesions.

Radiological Studies

The barium enema is a valuable test in the detection of colonic lesions. Even in patients with suspected anorectal disease, a colonoscopy or barium enema is indicated to rule out other lesions, particularly in patients at high risk for polyps and cancer. The barium enema may also detect diverticula, inflammatory bowel disease, strictures, extraluminal masses, or intramural filling defects from endometriosis or from metastatic tumor.

The double (air) contrast barium technique is preferred in the search for a colonic source of bleeding. This technique has the advantage over the conventional single contrast barium enema in providing much better detail of the mucosa. Early changes of inflammatory bowel disease are also detectable by this technique though not with as high a sensitivity as colonoscopy. However, because of the risk of perforation, the double contrast barium enema should not be requested in patients suspected of having an obstructing lesion or diverticulitis.

Patient experience. The patient's colon must be cleaned before the study can be performed satisfactorily. A reasonable regimen is the ingestion of 2 to 3 liters of liquids as well as a low residue diet (see Table 39.2, Chapter 39) the day before the examination and administration of a laxative, such as 2 to 4 tablespoons of milk of magnesia at night; on the morning of the examination, a sodium phosphate enema (Fleet) is self-administered. This preparation will be effective in about 90% of patients. Patients who are chronically constipated may need 2 days of preparation.

The patient should be told that the barium will be introduced into his rectum, through a lubricated plastic enema tip, while he lies on his left side on a hard table. Often a balloon is then inflated around the tip to seal the rectal ampulla. He will then be told to lie on his back while the barium is allowed to flow in, intermittently, under fluoroscopic observation. Frequently, cramping is experienced during this process. After the colon is filled, several films will be taken, with the patient in various positions. The barium will then be evacuated. The films will be developed and an additional film will be taken after evacuation. The entire procedure takes 45 to 60 minutes.

The air contrast barium enema differs from the standard technique in that a smaller amount of very dense barium is introduced followed by insufflation of air. All patients experience cramping during this procedure (usually more than is experienced during the standard barium enema), and atropine may be given to inhibit cramping. The patient will be flatulent for several hours after the procedure.

Colonoscopy

Colonoscopy is indicated in patients with gastrointestinal bleeding of suspected colonic origin in whom proctosigmoidoscopy and barium enema have not provided an unequivocal diagnosis. Most gastroenterologists may do colonoscopy instead of a barium enema because of its higher positive predictive value in the evaluation of rectal bleeding (4). Also, in patients with polyps, colonoscopy provides a way in which the polyps can be removed without major surgery (see below). An experienced endoscopist can reach the cecum in over 90% of cases. The complications from the procedure are mainly perforation and hemorrhage; the overall complication rate for diagnostic colonoscopy is 0.3 to 0.4%, with a mortality rate of 0.02%. If polypectomy is performed, the morbidity rate increases to 1 to 2%, but the mortality rate remains the same (6).

The sensitivity of colonoscopy in experienced hands is much higher than that of even an air contrast barium enema (see above): only 2% of polyps are not diagnosed. In anemic patients with occult bleeding Tedesco et al. (7) showed that colonoscopy revealed polyps (greater than 5 mm) or cancer in 15% of patients with negative barium enema examinations and that, in patients with rectal bleeding, 34% had a significant lesion (including 11% with cancer) when the barium enema was reported as negative or simply as showing diverticulosis.

Patient experience. Preparation for colonoscopy usually includes a liquid diet for 2 or 3 days and laxatives and enemas (prescribed by the consultant gastroenterologist). A newly available alternative procedure is to drink 4 liters of a nonabsorbed isosmolar salt solution the night before the procedure (GoLYTELY). Before the procedure, the patient is sedated intravenously (usually with Demerol and Valium or Versed). During the procedure, the patient may experience discomfort when the bowel is distended with air for inspection and as the colonoscope is maneuvered through the bowel lumen. The duration of the procedure is variable, depending on the tortuosity of the colon, the presence of disease, and on the skill of the endoscopist; but, the average is 30 to 60 minutes.

Upper Gastrointestinal Tract

The sequence of tests performed in evaluating the upper gastrointestinal tract depends on the severity of the bleeding and on the diagnosis that is suspected. An *upper gastrointestinal series* is often done first in patients with suspected peptic disease or carcinoma when the bleeding is slow and chronic or is occult. On the other hand, if an inflammatory process is suspected (esophagitis or gastritis), endoscopy should be done, since contrast radiography is less sensitive in detecting mucosal lesions that are not severe. Also, in acute bleeding, endoscopy is preferred over an upper GI series because actively bleeding lesions can often be treated at the time of the procedure—by endoscopic sclerotherapy in the case of bleeding esophageal varices or by electrocautery in the case of bleeding ulcers or angiodysplasias. If the patient has melena and an upper gastrointestinal series is negative or reveals a gastric ulcer (Chapter 37) or a tumor, endoscopy should be the next routine procedure. If the upper and lower gastrointestinal tract have been evaluated in a patient with gastrointestinal bleeding, and the studies have been negative, *a small bowel series* should be considered to investigate the possibility of Crohn's disease and other disorders that affect mainly the small intestine.

Radiological Studies

The *upper gastrointestinal series* is valuable in the detection of mass lesions in the esophagus and stomach and in identifying gastric and duodenal ulcerations. It is well tolerated, serves as a permanent guide for follow-up evaluation, and is relatively inexpensive. The patient's experience during the performance of an upper gastrointestinal series is described in Chapter 37.

The conventional *small bowel series* is very poor at detecting small lesions of the intestine (such as cancer or a leiomyoma). Disorders like Crohn's disease or lymphoma are more likely to be revealed by X-ray (although a definitive diagnosis will only be made by biopsy). These sources of bleeding are relatively uncommon and should be suspected only when the more frequent conditions (peptic ulcer disease, colonic polyps) have been excluded. The patient should be warned that the small bowel series will require him to spend 1 to 5 hours in the radiology waiting room during which time films will be taken every 30 minutes.

Endoscopy

Upper endoscopy is now a widely used and readily available means of investigating gastrointestinal blood loss. This technique not only is more sensitive than are X-rays but also provides a direct means of obtaining specimens for histological examination. Because of the increased sensitivity, endoscopy is indicated even if barium studies have been negative in the evaluation of a suspected upper gastrointestinal source of bleeding.

Patient experience. Upper endoscopy is an outpatient procedure that usually takes less than 15 minutes. The patient fasts overnight before the procedure. He is sedated with intravenous medication [Valium or Versed (midazolam) and Demerol] and his throat is anesthetized with a topical anesthetic. Some gagging is common during passage of the endoscope into the esophagus. Under direct vision, biopsies and cytological brushings can be obtained from suspicious lesions and for histological confirmation. Complications include perforation and bleeding but are extremely uncommon. Newer, smaller caliber endoscopes have greatly improved patient tolerance of the procedure.

SELECTED LESIONS THAT BLEED

The commonest cause of upper gastrointestinal bleeding—peptic disease—is discussed in Chapter 37. Several common causes of lower gastrointestinal bleeding are discussed in other chapters: benign anorectal disorders (Chapter 92), inflammatory bowel disease (Chapter 39), and diverticulosis (Chapter 41).

Colonic Polyps

Colonic polyps or colonic cancer should be suspected in any patient over 40 years of age who has gastrointestinal bleeding or a change in bowel habits. Bleeding may be occult or may occur as intermittent hematochezia. The patient is often totally asymptomatic but may complain of a change in bowel habits, abdominal pain, or of passing mucus per rectum. It is believed that all cancers of the colon (excluding those associated with ulcerative colitis; see Chapter 39) arise from these benign epithelial tumors, though only a small percentage of premalignant polyps will grow into invasive cancers. It has been estimated that it takes a minimum of 5 years for an early polyp to become an invasive cancer. Thus the removal of polyps before they become malignant has the potential of preventing the occurrence of colonic cancer in predisposed individuals. Although polyps are most common in the rectosigmoid region, they may be found anywhere in the colon. The detection of a polyp on proctoscopy or on barium enema is an indication for referral to a gastroenterologist.

The risk of polyps becoming malignant is related to their histological type and size. *Hyperplastic polyps*, the most common type in adults, are thought to have no malignant potential. *Villous and tubular adenomas*, however, carry a definite risk of malignant transformation that increases as they increase in size. The risk that a villous adenoma over 2 cm is cancerous is over 50% (5) (Table 38.2). Fortunately, if the cancer remains confined to the mucosa of the polyp (*carcinoma in situ*), colonoscopic polypectomy is curative. Once the cancer has infiltrated the stalk of the polyp, surgery is indicated. Because the cancerous change in the polyp may be focal, single biopsies of a polyp are not sufficient to exclude the presence of a malignancy; the entire polyp must be excised.

Once a polyp has been detected, surveillance for additional polyps is indicated. In 30% of patients more than one polyp is present at the time of initial investigation and the risk of recurrence rises with the number of polyps that are initially discovered. Subsequent development of new polyps occurs in at least 10% of patients. The patient should continue to be tested yearly for occult blood in the stool. The finding of a single positive test is an indication for a repeated evaluation. Even when the stools are negative for blood, periodic evaluation of the colon is still recommended. Colonoscopy or air contrast barium enema should be repeated in a year, then every 3 to 5 years if subsequent examinations reveal no further polyps.

Multiple polyposis syndromes are rare inherited abnormalities that are significant for their malignant potential. *Familial polyposis, Gardner's syndrome,* and *Turcot syndrome* all are associated with multiple adenomatous polyps of the colon (Fig. 38.1) and therefore carry a high risk of the development of carcinoma. Gardner's syndrome includes osteomas and soft tissue tumors, and Turcot syndrome includes tumors of the central nervous system. Familial polyposis and Gardner's syndrome are inherited as an autosomal dominant defect, Turcot syndrome, as an autosomal recessive. The diagnosis of a polyposis syndrome is usually made when the patient is in his twenties, with cancer developing some 20 years later. There is considerable controversy about the therapy of these conditions. Colonic resection is indicated but its extent

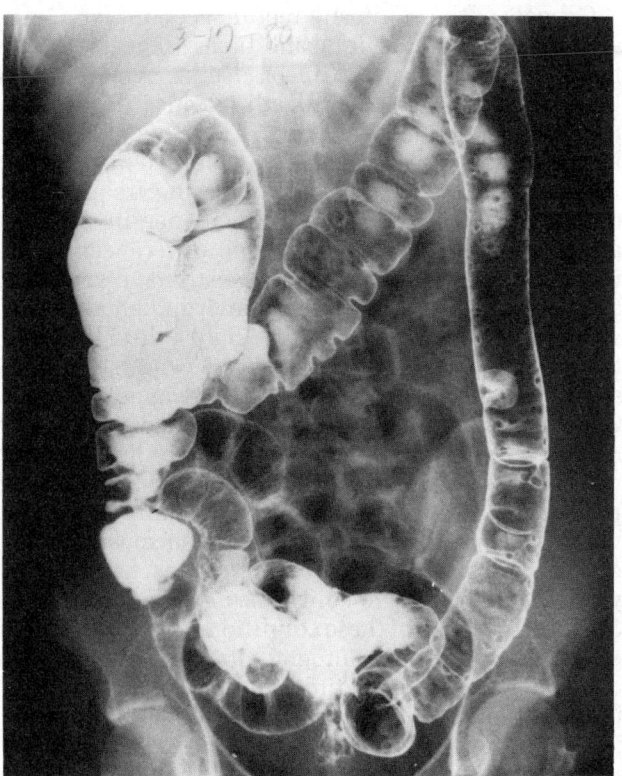

Figure 38.1. Double (air) contrast barium enema performed in a patient with familial polyposis. With this technique, numerous polyps of varying sizes may be seen throughout the colon.

Table 38.2.
Polyps: Relationship of Size, Histological Type, and Risk of Carcinoma

Histological Type	Size		
	Under 1 cm (%)	1–2 cm (%)	Over 2 cm (%)
Tubular adenoma	1.0	10.2	34.7
Intermediate type	3.9	7.4	45.8
Villous adenoma	9.5	10.3	52.9

and timing are not uniformly agreed upon. Ideally, when rectal polyps are present, a proctocolectomy should be performed to eliminate the risk of cancer. However, as the patients are generally quite young, the prospect of an ileostomy (see Chapter 42) and of potential sexual dysfunction is often overwhelming to them. Newer operations involving ileorectal pull-through procedures are now available and early results are encouraging. Consultation with a gastroenterologist and gastrointestinal surgeon is recommended as soon as the diagnosis is made.

Colonic polyposis syndromes should be distinguished from conditions associated with juvenile polyps or hamartomas that are of low malignant potential. The *Peutz-Jeghers syndrome* consists of multiple hamartomas, predominantly of the small intestine, associated with buccal and cutaneous pigmentation. Although the malignant potential of the hamartomas is low, duodenal and ovarian carcinomas have been reported in 2 to 5% of patients. Rarely juvenile polyps may occur throughout the gastrointestinal tract. In the absence of associated extracolonic manifestations, this syndrome is called generalized juvenile polyposis; when accompanied by alopecia, nail bed changes, hyperpigmentation, and malabsorption, it is called the *Cronkhite-Canada syndrome*.

Colorectal Cancer

Epidemiology and Etiology

Cancers of the colon and rectum account for 15% of all cancers and, after lung and breast cancers, are the third leading cause of cancer deaths overall in the United States, the second leading cause in men and the first in women over age 75. There is about a 6% lifetime chance of developing a colorectal cancer.

Colon cancer occurs with increasing frequency in older age groups, with a peak incidence in the sixth and seventh decades. Geographic differences in the mortality rates due to this neoplasm have suggested an etiologic role for dietary and environmental factors. The proportion of cancers in the right side of the colon has been increasing in recent years with a commensurate drop in the proportion of rectosigmoid lesions. Currently, about one-third of colon cancers are within reach of the rigid sigmoidoscope, two-thirds within reach of the flexible sigmoidoscope, and one-third proximal to the splenic flexure and only accessible with a colonoscope. The three main predisposing causes of large bowel cancer are colonic polyps, familial polyposis, and ulcerative colitis (see above and Chapter 39). The presence of these conditions dictates the need for a strict surveillance program in patients with these conditions and even, at times, prophylactic surgery to prevent the development of large bowel cancer. (See page 454 for risk of cancer in ulcerative colitis.) Though it is accepted that a family history of colorectal cancer predisposes one to polyps and to colorectal cancer, there is some evidence that the risk does not rise significantly above that of the general population unless more than one first-degree relative has had colorectal cancer (3).

Screening Tests

Because of the high incidence of colon cancer and its precursor, the colonic polyp, screening tests should be performed routinely in all patients over 40 years old. However, there are currently no definitive studies that demonstrate that early detection of colon cancer improves survival; studies to examine this question are in progress. The most comprehensive screening program would involve periodic colonoscopy, but its cost and complications make this impractical for patients who are at average risk. One reasonable compromise of cost and efficacy is the guidelines offered by the American Cancer Society, which are that six stools should be tested consecutively for occult blood annually by use of the guaiac-slide test (see above). These slides or cards are convenient for the patient because they can be mailed to the physician's office without a significant loss in sensitivity. In one study, 80% of patients ultimately found to have colonic cancer after detection of occult blood in their stool in a screening program had disease limited to the bowel (and therefore had a good prognosis).

In addition to tests for occult blood, a yearly rectal examination should also be performed in patients over the age of 40 to 50. Proctosigmoidoscopy, preferably by use of a flexible sigmoidoscope, should also be performed in 2 consecutive years to ensure a normal rectal and rectosigmoid area. Subsequently, proctoscopy can be performed every 3 to 5 years in the asymptomatic patient who has negative tests for fecal blood.

Diagnosis

History. Unfortunately, most patients with adenocarcinoma of the colon are diagnosed only after symptoms have developed. Less than 5% are asymptomatic at time of diagnosis, and it is in this group that the highest chance for cure exists. The major presenting symptoms are abdominal pain (25 to 75%) and a change in bowel habits (20 to 50%), either constipation or diarrhea. Abdominal pain is least common in patients with cancer of the rectum, where even large lesions can be accommodated without producing symptoms. Gross blood in the stool is another common complaint, occurring in 75% of patients with rectal cancer and in 30 to 40% of patients with colonic cancer above the rectum. Unfortunately, this hematochezia is frequently mistakenly attributed to hemorrhoids.

Physical Examination. The findings on physical examination vary according to the location and extent of the lesion. The primary tumor may be palpable as an abdominal mass, particularly in lesions of the right colon where lesions can remain "asymptomatic" for long periods of time. Metastatic disease may be suggested by the presence of a large, hard nodular liver, ascites, peripheral adenopathy, or by palpating a mass in the cul-de-sac on rectal examination. Signs of anemia may be present, particularly in lesions of the cecum and ascending colon that may bleed occultly for months or even years before the diagnosis is made. Most patients will have a positive test for occult blood (at least one) sometime during their course of illness.

Radiological Studies. The diagnosis of colon cancer is often made by barium enema. Findings may include a polypoid mass, stenosis, either as a stricture or with an "apple-core" appearance, distortion of the mucosa, and localized rigidity of the bowel wall. At times, distortion or fixation of adjacent structures may be seen. The development of a gastrocolic fistula, best seen on barium enema, is also suggestive of a primary colonic neoplasm.

The accuracy of the radiographic diagnosis of colon cancer is excellent, except at opposite ends of the large bowel. The cecum is often difficult to evaluate because of the inability to cleanse the region completely and, at times, to distinguish a "prominent" ileocecal valve or sphincter from a mass. The rectum is also difficult to visualize optimally, as frequently it is obscured by the balloon through which the barium is administered. Thus, proctoscopy is essential in any patient suspected of having a colorectal carcinoma.

Endoscopy. The role of endoscopy varies depending on the nature of the initial evaluation. If a very suspicious lesion is detected on barium enema, it may be most efficient to proceed directly to a search for metastases (see below), followed by surgery. However, it should be recognized that spasm, benign strictures, and even stool can be confused with cancer on radiographic examination and that some polypoid lesions, even if large or sessile, can be removed via the colonoscope, avoiding surgery in many cases.

In addition, colonoscopy has an important role in the evaluation for other colonic lesions (see page 438). The prevalence of coexistent polyps in patients with colon cancer is high, ranging from 10 to 30%. These residual polyps may develop later into carcinoma, accounting for the incidence of a second colon cancer in 5 to 10% of patients with cancer of the colon who have been followed for up to 25 years (5). In addition, synchronous colon carcinomas occur in 3 to 5% of patients. Thus, colonoscopy is helpful in ensuring that the rest of the colon is free of neoplastic lesions. Optimally, colonoscopy should be performed preoperatively; otherwise, it should be done within the first year postoperatively.

Carcinoembryonic Antigen

Carcinoembryonic antigen (CEA) is a normal fetal antigen that is found in the blood of many patients with carcinoma of the colon (from 30% of patients with local disease to 83% of patients with metastatic disease). It also is found sometimes in the blood of patients with other malignancies or with a variety of benign conditions, including cigarette smoking, peptic ulcer, pancreatitis, diverticulitis, and inflammatory bowel disease. Therefore, CEA titers are not useful screening tests for the presence of colon cancer.

The assay is helpful, however, in the postoperative management of patients who have CEA in their blood at the time of diagnosis. Persistently elevated CEA levels postoperatively suggest metastatic disease; falling levels that then rise on follow-up evaluation suggest the re-emergence of the malignant tumor, usually at a remote site.

Therapy

Surgery is the most effective therapy for colon carcinoma. Inoperable low rectal and anal lesions may be palliated with radiation or electrocoagulation. For inoperable colon or rectal tumors, 15 to 20% of patients will have a temporary response to 5-fluorouracil, but there is no proven benefit for chemotherapy or radiation as an adjuvant to surgery.

Preoperative Evaluation

Before surgery, most patients should undergo evaluation for metastatic disease. Liver function tests should be performed routinely. The role of routine computed tomography or ultrasound of the liver in the diagnosis of hepatic metastasis remains to be determined. In patients with bowel obstruction or bleeding, surgery may still be needed as palliation, despite the presence of liver metastases. In patients asymptomatic from their bowel lesions, the presence of hepatic metastases should deter surgical intervention. However, abnormal liver function tests alone should not be considered absolute evidence of metastatic disease. A histological diagnosis should be made, if possible. Needle liver biopsy is a simple way to obtain tissue and may be guided by ultrasound or computerized tomography. A preoperative CEA level should also be determined as a baseline (see above).

For patients requiring an ostomy, preoperative evaluation by an enterostomal therapist is very helpful, not only to discuss with the patient problems and concerns about the ostomy, but also to mark the proper location of the ostomy preoperatively (see Chapter 42).

Prognosis

The prognosis for colon carcinoma is based on several variables. The major variable is the extent of the tumor, in terms of its invasion through the bowel wall and of its lymph node involvement (Table 38.3). Vessel invasion and the degree of differentiation of the tumor histologically also affect survival. The pathol-

Table 38.3.
Colon Carcinoma

Classification[a]	Staging and 5-Year Survival	
	Microscopic Findings	Percentage of 5-Year Survival
A	Disease limited to mucosa	95
B	Tumor extends to serosa	60–70
C	Tumor extends to serosa and nodes involved	<40
D	Distant metastases	<5

[a]Modification of the Dukes' classification.

ogist's interpretation of the resected specimen is much more meaningful than the surgeon's estimation of "curable."

Follow-up Care

Most patients undergoing resection of colon cancer do well in the early postoperative period. Diarrhea may be present early, but it is usually transient and is easily controlled with antidiarrheal medication if needed. The patient with a colostomy needs continued follow-up care by the surgeon and the enterostomal therapist to ensure proper functioning and handling of the ostomy (see Chapter 39).

The long-term follow-up is aimed at detection of recurrence or spread of the cancer and at continued surveillance for new colonic lesions. Most commonly, metastases occur in adjacent nodes with spread to the liver. Physical examinations should be done and liver function tests and CEA levels should be measured every 2 to 6 months for 3 to 5 years.

To evaluate for new colonic lesions, or for the infrequent occurrence of tumor at the anastomosis, colonoscopy should be performed within the first 6 to 12 months, postoperatively. If no lesions are found, colonoscopy should be repeated a year later. The interval may then be increased to once every 3 years if no recurrence or polyps are detected. Yearly evaluation for occult fecal blood loss should be performed with three to six Hemoccult slides. Should any of these slide tests be positive, colonoscopy should be repeated.

Arteriovenous Malformations of Colon

Arteriovenous malformations of the colon are a common source of gastrointestinal bleeding, most often in the elderly and in patients with chronic renal failure. A variety of terms have been used to describe these abnormalities including angiodysplasia, hemangioma, and vascular ectasia. The etiology of the disorder is unknown. Although the lesions may occur throughout the gastrointestinal tract, they are found most commonly in the mucosa of the cecum and ascending colon where multiple lesions are often found, ranging in size from 1 mm to over 1 cm. An association of angiodysplasia of the colon with aortic stenosis has been observed repeatedly (1).

The prevalence of angiodysplasias and the frequency with which they cause bleeding are still uncertain. With increasing utilization of endoscopy and selective angiography, the disorder is being recognized more frequently. In one study of patients over the age of 60 without a history of gastrointestinal bleeding, submucosal vascular ectasis was detected in 53% and mucosal lesions in 27% (1). Angiodysplasias may be the most common cause of bleeding from the right colon, and they are the most common cause of major lower intestinal bleeding in the elderly.

These lesions, when they bleed, usually produce hematochezia. The bleeding is often brisk, and may be massive, but occult blood loss also may occur. Bleeding often stops spontaneously but commonly recurs. The lesions cannot be detected by barium enema, are not recognizable from the serosal surface by the surgeon, and are often overlooked by the pathologist. The diagnosis is best made by selective arteriography (by which a malformation can be visualized even when the bleeding has stopped) or by colonoscopy. It should be recognized, though, that like diverticula, the mere presence of angiodysplasias does not incriminate them as the source of bleeding per rectum, and other potential sources of bleeding should be sought. Lesions that have bled should be excised, preferably by surgical resection in the involved colon. However, colonoscopic removal or cauterization of discrete mucosal lesions can be performed by an experienced gastroenterologist.

The generalist should be aware of this disorder, especially in elderly patients who present to him with gastrointestinal bleeding in whom initial evaluation (see above) is unrevealing; but the diagnosis will be made only after consultation with a gastroenterologist and a radiologist.

General References

Cheung PSY, Wong SKC, Boey J, Lai CK: Frank rectal bleeding: a prospective study of causes in patients over the age of 40. *Postgrad Med J* 64:364, 1988.
Ehrinpreis MN, Kinzie JL, Jaszewski R, Peleman RL: Management of the malignant polyp. *Gastroenterol Clin North Am* 17(4):837, 1988.
Fleischer DE, Goldberg SB, Browning TH, et al: Detection and surveillance of colorectal cancer. *JAMA* 261:580, 1989.
> Guidelines from a study section of the American Gastroenterological Association and the American Society for Gastrointestinal Endoscopy.
Fletcher RH, Carcinoembryonic antigen. *Ann Intern Med* 104:66, 1986.
> Good review.
Ho SB, Toribara NW, Bresalier RS, Kim YS: Biochemical and other markers of colon cancer. *Gastroenterol Clin North Am* 17(4):811, 1988.
Potter GD, Sellin JH: Lower gastrointestinal bleeding. *Gastroenterol Clin North Am* 17(2):341, 1988.

Specific References

1. Boley SJ, Sammartano R, Adams A, et al: Nature and etiology of vascular ectasias of the colon. *Gastroenterology* 72:650, 1977.
2. Fleischer DE, Goldberg SB, Browning TH, et al: Detection and surveillance of colorectal cancer. *JAMA* 261:580, 1989.
3. Grossman S, Milos ML: Colonoscopic screening of persons with suspected risk factors for colon cancer. I. Family history. *Gastroenterology* 94:395, 1988.
4. Irvine EJ, O'Connor J, Frost RA, et al: Prospective comparison of double contrast barium enema plus flexible signoidoscopy v. colonoscopy in rectal bleeding. *Gut* 29:1188, 1988.
5. Muto T, Bussey HJ, Morson BL: The evolution of cancer of the colon and rectum. *Cancer* (Phila) 36:2251, 1975.
6. Silvis SE, Nebel O, Rogers G, et al: Results of the 1974 American Society for Gastrointestinal Endoscopy Survey. *JAMA* 235:928, 1976.
7. Tedesco F, Wayne J, Raskin J, et al: Colonoscopic evaluation of rectal bleeding—a study of 304 patients. *Ann Intern Med* 89:907, 1978.

C H A P T E R 39

Constipation and Diarrhea*

LAWRENCE J. CHESKIN, M.D.

CONSTIPATION

Definition

Constipation is often defined as the infrequent, difficult passage of stool. However, it may mean different things to different people: that the stools are too infrequent, too difficult to expel, too hard, too small, or that there is a sensation of incomplete evacuation. Of these, frequency of bowel movements is the most readily measured aspect. Several studies have identified that there is a wide variation in the frequency of bowel movements among normal subjects of both sexes and of all ages, ranging from three per day to three per week. Therefore, someone who has fewer than three bowel movements per week is constipated, by definition. On the other hand, a change in frequency of movements from, say, two per day to three per week may also signify constipation. It is probably not necessary, however, to work up or to treat people merely because they report fewer than three bowel movements per week. Even one movement per week is acceptable if it does not represent a recent change in bowel frequency and is not associated with symptoms such as pain on defecation or bloating.

Almost always, constipation is due to a delay in transit within the colon. A wide variety of conditions may affect colonic transit (Table 39.1). There may be structural abnormalities that obstruct the passage of intraluminal contents, or there may be conditions that alter colonic motility. Evaluation of patients with constipation must therefore include consideration of a wide variety of possible etiologies. Although it is difficult to be precise about the relative frequencies of these etiologies, chronic constipation (months or longer)

---

*Dr. Harold J. Tucker contributed to this chapter in the first and second editions of this book.

Table 39.1.
Various Causes of Constipation

IDIOPATHIC (POSSIBLE MECHANISMS):
 Dietary factors—low residue
 Motility disturbances—colonic inertia or spasm (irritable bowel syndrome)
 Sedentary living

STRUCTURAL ABNORMALITIES:
 Anorectal disorders—fissures, thrombosed hemorrhoids
 Strictures
 Tumors

ENDOCRINE/METABOLIC:
 Hypercalcemia
 Hypokalemia
 Hypothyroidism
 Pregnancy

NEUROGENIC:
 Cerebrovascular events
 Hirschsprung's disease
 Spinal cord tumors
 Trauma

SMOOTH MUSCLE/CONNECTIVE TISSUE DISORDERS:
 Amyloidosis
 Scleroderma

DRUGS:
 Antacids—aluminum, and calcium-containing compounds
 Anticholinergics
 Antidepressants
 Calcium channel blockers (especially verapamil)
 Cholestyramine
 Narcotics
 Sympathomimetics—pseudoephedrine

PSYCHOGENIC (especially depression)

---

is most commonly due to a motility disorder (such as in sedentary people eating a low fiber diet or in patients with the irritable bowel syndrome), to the use of constipating drugs, and to local anorectal problems (fissures, hemorrhoids, and tumors).

Evaluation

History

The history provides the most useful information about the etiology of constipation. It may reveal a gross misconception about normal bowel habits or a neurotic preoccupation with bowel function. Reassurance that there is a broad range of normal bowel frequency may be all of the treatment that is needed in many cases of self-defined constipation. It is important to determine whether there is a history of, or suggestion of, a systemic process (e.g., hypothyroidism, hyperparathyroidism, or scleroderma), a neurological disorder (e.g., cerebrovascular disease or Parkinson's disease), or the taking of drugs (e.g., anticholinergics, opiates, antidepressants), all of which are known to impair colonic motility. Most systemic or neurological diseases are almost certain to affect organs outside the gastrointestinal tract so that, in addition to constipation, patients have symptoms that reflect extraintestinal dysfunction. On the other hand, local processes (e.g., strictures or tumors) often produce other gastrointestinal symptoms in addition to constipation, such as abdominal pain or rectal bleeding. Thus, rectal bleeding should always be thoroughly evaluated (see Chapter 38) even though, in constipated patients, it frequently is caused by perianal disease (fissures, hemorrhoids, cryptitis). Abdominal pain, with constipation, is also a prominent feature of the irritable bowel syndrome (see Chapter 40). Most patients with "idiopathic" diet-related, or drug-induced constipation are otherwise asymptomatic, although a complaint of a "bloated" sensation is common if constipation is prolonged.

Physical Examination

The physical examination should be focused on the identification of underlying causes of constipation. Rectal examination should be done routinely to look for fissures, hemorrhoids, and inflammation as well as anal stenosis or stricture, secondary to previous surgery or inflammation. The anal sphincter normally is closed. A gaping anal opening or asymmetry of the anal opening may indicate a neurological disorder (spinal cord trauma, peripheral neuropathy) that impairs sphincteric function. After inspection, a careful digital examination should be performed to evaluate the strength of the anal sphincters, the presence of masses, the consistency of the stool, and the presence of any painful or tender areas.

Endoscopy

Anoscopy and proctosigmoidoscopy should be performed routinely in newly constipated patients in whom the cause is not obvious. Because it is much more comfortable to the patient, visualizes more of the colon, and is easier to manipulate, flexible sigmoidoscopy (see Chapter 36) is now to be preferred over rigid sigmoidoscopy. Proctosigmoidoscopy can be performed in the office, often without a prior enema. In fact, when the appearance of the mucosa is important (as it is in patients with suspected ulcerative colitis), an enema should be avoided. In contrast, if exophytic bleeding lesions (i.e., polyps) are suspected, a cleansing enema (e.g., Fleet enema) is desirable and is usually administered by the patient at home before the office visit. Anoscopy may be needed to search properly for hemorrhoids or fissures (see Chapter 92). Proctosigmoidoscopy can be performed with the patient in the knee-chest position on a routine examining table, or in the left lateral position. Sigmoidoscopy should be performed to the highest level possible, with limitations imposed by the patient's tolerance of the procedure, the presence of stool, and the length of the instrument (a rigid scope extends to 25 cm whereas a flexible instrument can be passed to 60 cm). It is important to recognize that even a good air contrast barium enema is not a substitute for sigmoidoscopy because subtle mucosal abnormalities cannot be detected and the most distal 15 to 20 cm of the colon are difficult to evaluate radiographically. The patient's experience during proctosigmoidoscopy is described in Chapter 36.

Inflamed hemorrhoids and fissures found during sigmoidoscopy may be caused by constipation, but may also cause pain on defecation, and thus may promote constipation. These are also common causes of bleeding in the chronically constipated patient. A spotty or diffuse brown pigmentation, *melanosis coli*, is indicative of chronic laxative abuse, particularly of the anthraquinone family (e.g., cascara, senna, and aloe). A lesion, such as a carcinoma or polyp, may also be identified by proctosigmoidoscopy.

A *rectal biopsy* may diagnose amyloidosis, ulcerative colitis, or Crohn's disease, and a deeper, suction biopsy of a rectal valve may diagnose Hirschsprung's disease. Biopsies of the rectal mucosa can be taken safely below the peritoneal reflection (about 12 cm proximal to the anus in men, 8 cm in women). Punch biopsies can be performed by a general physician who has had appropriate training and experience. Suction biopsies should be performed only by a surgeon or gastroenterologist. Rectal biopsy should be painless unless a tender inflamed lesion is biopsied, and, if done properly, the risk of bleeding and perforation, the major complications, is very low.

Radiographic Studies

Radiographic examination is primarily helpful in the detection of obstructing lesions and should be performed in all adult patients who complain of constipation of relatively recent onset (within the preceding 6 months). The plain film of the abdomen may occasionally diagnose an obstructing carcinoma before a barium study has been done. The presence of a megacolon or a volvulus, either of the sigmoid or cecum, also may be easily diagnosed by a plain film. The more recent the onset of constipation, the more likely it is that the barium enema (see patient experience, Chapter 38) will yield positive results. Obstructing neoplasms and strictures can be identified by barium studies. Sometimes, patients with Hirschsprung's disease reach adolescence or adulthood without the diagnosis having been made. A narrowed rectal segment on X-ray is a clue to the diagnosis in such cases; it can be best seen when the patient is in the lateral oblique position and the X-ray is taken just as the barium is being instilled. The radiologist may also comment on the motility of the colon, particularly if there is significant spasm or if haustral markings are absent, as seen in patients who use laxatives chronically or who have an atonic megacolon. Repeated barium studies are rarely helpful unless some aspect of the history or physical examination suggests a new development.

Other Studies

Colonic motility tests and transit studies are additional procedures that may provide insight into the pathophysiology of constipation. These studies are generally available only in selected centers where there is specific interest in this problem. They should be performed in the few patients who are severely impaired by constipation and who are refractory to conventional therapy.

Colonic motility studies are generally performed by placing catheters, which monitor intracolonic pressures, in the rectal and sigmoid regions. The study can identify various patterns of colonic activity in patients with constipation. In some, high amplitude phasic contractions are seen spontaneously as well as in response to stimulation. This type of segmental activity is sometimes associated with pain and is believed to cause constipation by impeding the distal flow of luminal contents. In other patients an atonic pattern is found, characterized by a decreased response to stimulation and a loss of resistance to distension (4).

Colonic transit time can be measured by plotting the expulsion of radiopaque markers after daily ingestion of a capsule containing 24 markers. Once a steady state is reached, the number of markers entering the gastrointestinal tract must equal the number being excreted and the transit time in hours is equal to the number of markers still in the colon on plain film (5). Moreover, the distribution of these markers may have a relationship to the underlying motility disturbance.

Treatment

The treatment for constipation should, if possible, be based on correction of the underlying abnormality—for example, if there is a systemic disease that can be treated (e.g., hypothyroidism) or a constipating drug that can be stopped. The simple use of laxatives as a reflex response to complaints of constipation should be discouraged. Successful therapy must include discussion with the patient about the broad limits of normal bowel function and about the patient's own concepts of normal bowel activity.

Bowel Retraining

Bowel retraining is an important initial aspect of therapy for those patients whose constipation does not have an identifiable and remediable cause. The patient should be encouraged to have a regular daily routine with time set aside for having a bowel movement, preferably within 5 to 10 minutes after a meal, to take advantage of the strong stimulus of the gastrocolic reflex. This behavior modification program allows the patient to become more aware of and responsive to the normal urges to defecate. Patients should be advised always to respond to such urges. In the severely constipated patient, a bowel retraining program may be initiated with the use of enemas or suppositories to enhance bowel activity at the desired time. For enemas, lukewarm tap water should be used since all other solutions may be irritating if used repetitively. The enema should be given within an hour of eating a meal to take advantage of the gastrocolic reflex. For suppositories, glycerin or bisacodyl (Dulcolax) should be used, again just after eating; however, they should not be used for more than a few days because they may eventually be irritating.

Diet

Diet is an important factor in bowel function. There is epidemiological evidence that greater amounts of crude dietary fiber are associated with a lesser prevalence of constipation as well as of other gastrointestinal disorders, including diverticular disease and colorectal cancer. The mechanism for the effect on constipation is unclear. Studies in which fiber is added to the diet have demonstrated an increase in stool weight but a variable effect on whole gut transit time. Some studies have showed a speeding of transit when baseline transit was slow but no change or slowing when the baseline transit was rapid (3, 7). Several mechanisms may account for these observations: (a) fiber may act as a bulk-forming agent; (b) fiber may increase the concentration of fecal bile salts, which have a pronounced cathartic effect; and (c) fiber, metabolized by colonic bacteria to nonabsorbable volatile fatty acids, may act as an osmotic cathartic. The low fiber diet generally consumed in this country along with other variables such as sedentary lifestyle may account for the large number of patients who complain of constipation. As an initial step in treatment, the patient should be placed on a diet rich in fiber content. As listed in Table 39.2 there are a variety of foods high in fiber that are suitable for the patient's daily diet.

Table 39.2.
Fiber Content of Various Foods

Type of food	Dietary Fiber per Average Serving
	g
Vegetables	
Beans (navy, lima, kidney, baked)	8.5–10.0
Beans (string)	2.0
Broccoli	3.2
Brussel sprouts	2.3
Cabbage	2.0
Carrots	2.0
Celery	1.0
Corn	2.6
Corn on the cob	5.9
Lettuce	1.0
Potato (baked with skin)	3.0
Potato (french fried)	1.6
Peas, canned	6.0
Rice	0.8
Fruit	
Apple with peel	2.0
Apple juice	0.0
Banana	1.5
Grapefruit (fresh)	0.6
Orange	2.0
Peach	2.0
Raspberries	4.6
Strawberries	1.8
Breads	
Whole wheat	1.3
White, rye, French	0.7
Cereal	
All-Bran (100%)	8.4
Corn Flakes	2.6
Wheaties	2.6
Meats, chicken, liver, fish, lamb	0.0
Cheese, milk, yogurt	0.0

As a practical matter, it may be reasonable to add a commercial fiber preparation (see below) to a high fiber diet.

Laxatives

Despite numerous warnings, laxatives are still popular in the treatment of constipation. The presence of an estimated 700 or more commercially available laxatives and enema preparations attests to the widespread use of these agents. The mechanism of action for most laxatives is poorly understood, and the potential for toxicity is often underestimated (Table 39.3). Few data are available for comparison among the various laxatives, and the decision to use a particular laxative often is determined by individual preference rather than by objective evidence of efficacy or safety.

There are a number of different mechanisms by which a laxative effect may be achieved. *Bulk-forming agents* are natural or synthetic polysaccharides or cellulose derivatives that exert their laxative effect by absorbing water and increasing fecal mass. Methylcellulose, psyllium seed, and bran are examples of such laxatives. In addition to their hydrophilic properties, these agents are metabolized by colonic bacteria, resulting in accumulation of osmotically active metabolites. These laxatives are effective in increasing the frequency and in softening the consistency of stool. There have been isolated reports of obstruction secondary to hydrophilic agents in patients with esophageal or small bowel strictures. In the majority of cases, however, this type of laxative is highly effective and the potential for adverse effects appears to be low. However, in patients with an atonic form of constipation, particularly with megacolon, these agents are often ineffective and produce an uncomfortable sensation of bloating and gaseousness at high doses. Bloating is common in all patients when they begin to take bulk agents, but it is generally transient and can be minimized by increasing the dosage gradually over a period of weeks.

Dioctyl sodium sulfosuccinate (Colace) is frequently labeled as a *stool softener* or a wetting agent. It works by lowering surface tension, allowing water to enter the stool more easily.

The *saline laxatives* are magnesium or sodium salts (e.g., milk of magnesia and sodium phosphate), which

Table 39.3.
Laxatives

Classification and Active Ingredient	Examples	Dose	Average Onset of Action	Potential Adverse Effects
BULK				
Psyllium seed	Konsyl Effersylliuum Perdiem (with senna)	1 tsp to 2 tbsp/day	12–24 hours or more	Increased gas and bloating sensation; bowel obstruction if stricture present
Plus dextrose	Metamucil			
Bran		4+ tbsp/day		
EMOLLIENT (SOFTENERS)				
Dioctyl sodium (or calcium) sulfosuccinate	Colace, Pericolace (with casanthranol) Surfak	1–3 caps/day	24–48 hours	Electrolyte imbalance
STIMULANT				
Phenolphthalein	Correctol, Ex-Lax	1–2 tablets (100–200 mg)	6–8 hours	Dermatitis; electrolyte imbalance, melanosis coli
Bisacodyl	Dulcolax	2–3 tabs (10–15 mg)		Senna
Senokot, Perdiem (with psyllium)	1-4 tsp or 2-4 tabs			
Cascara (Casanthranol)	Pericolace (with dioctyl sodium)	1–2 tabs		
CO_2	Ceo-two suppositories	1–2	10–30 minutes	
OSMOTIC				
Ricinoleic acid	Castor oil	1–2 tsp		
Lactulose[a]	Cephulac, Chronulac	1–2 tbsp/day		Excessive gas production
Magnesium salts	Milk of Magnesia, magnesium citrate	2–4 tbsp	3–6 hours or less	Hypermagnesemia, hypocalcemia, hyperphosphatemia in chronic renal failure
Sodium salts	Phospho-Soda	2 tbsp in ½ glass of H_2O		
	Fleet enema	120 ml	2–5 minutes	Dehydration; hyperphosphatemia in chronic renal failure

[a]Requires a prescription.

are poorly absorbed and therefore act as hyperosmolar solutions. They may also release cholecystokinin, a hormone that stimulates colonic motility. Complications include hypermagnesemia in patients with renal failure and hypocalcemia from phosphate overdoses.

Stimulant laxatives, such as anthraquinone derivatives (senna, aloe, cascara) and diphenylmethane compounds (phenolphthalein, bisacodyl), exert their effects primarily by altering electrolyte transport by the intestinal mucosa and thereby increasing intestinal motor activity. The effect of these agents is claimed to be more specific on the colon. Phenolphthalein, an ingredient found in many over-the-counter preparations, has been associated with severe allergic dermatitis and the Stevens-Johnson syndrome. The chronic use of the anthraquinone derivatives has been reported to induce damage to the myenteric plexus, and thus actually to worsen bowel motility. Agents such as these that affect electrolyte transport may result in significant hypokalemia, factitious diarrhea, protein-losing enteropathy, and salt overload. Although these agents are undoubtedly effective, their chronic use may lead to significant side effects, and they should be avoided when possible.

Castor oil, previously thought to be a stimulant laxative, is now understood to exert its cathartic effect by alteration of intestinal fluid and electrolyte secretion. Ricinoleic acid, the active ingredient of castor oil, has effects on the small and large intestine similar to that of bile acids: It inhibits absorption of sodium and glucose and stimulates fluid and electrolyte secretion by increasing cellular cyclic adenosine monophosphate (AMP) and by inhibiting sodium-potassium adenosine triphosphatase (ATPase). This increase in intraluminal fluid content may then secondarily affect intestinal motility.

Lactulose (Cephulac or Chronulac syrup) is a semisynthetic disaccharide that is not metabolized by the intestinal enzymes. As a result, water and electrolytes are retained within the intestinal lumen by the osmotic effect of this undigested sugar. In addition, this agent is converted by colonic bacteria to organic acids, which may further alter electrolyte transport and/or affect colonic motility. Lactulose is commonly used in patients with hepatic encephalopathy (see Chapter 43). It has also been shown to be an effective laxative in patients with chronic constipation. There is little current information on the relative merits of lactulose versus bulk laxatives except that lactulose is relatively expensive and requires 24 to 48 hours to achieve its effect.

Surgery is rarely necessary in the treatment of constipated patients. It is, however, required for resection of an obstructing lesion, and myectomy may be needed for treatment of Hirschsprung's disease. Various procedures have been recommended for patients with megacolon who suffer from recurrent volvulus, ranging from simple tacking down of the loose mesentery to resection of bowel. Finally, in severe cases of intractable constipation, extensive surgery has been advocated, varying from resection of redundant sigmoid loops to subtotal colectomy with ileal proctostomy. The exact role and precise indication for this type of surgery remain to be more clearly defined.

General Recommendations

Therapy of constipation should always be directed first at identifying and treating any underlying disorder (Table 39.1). If the constipation is drug induced, the drug should be discontinued (if possible) or an alternative that is less constipating should be substituted. When constipation is "idiopathic" or is due to an irreversible, underlying disorder (e.g., diabetes), or is secondary to a necessary drug, then dietary changes and some form of laxative therapy may be necessary.

In practically all patients with constipation, a high fiber diet or a bulk laxative will be helpful. The amount of dietary fiber and/or bulk laxative that is needed varies from patient to patient and must be titrated individually. As the only significant side effect from this form of therapy is "excessive" gas and a bloated sensation, the dose can be gradually increased until either the constipation is resolved or the side effects become too uncomfortable. For the vast majority of patients, this form of therapy will be successful and appears to be very safe on a chronic basis. No other laxatives need be used.

However, in patients with partial bowel obstruction (as recognized on X-ray), or in those with an atonic form of constipation (e.g., institutional megacolon), the high fiber-bulk laxative approach is not usually effective. A patient with constipation due to partial obstruction must be treated surgically. A patient with an atonic colon may need a stimulant laxative. Senna compounds, bisacodyl (either as a tablet or a suppository), or enemas are most effective in such cases. Combinations of a stimulant laxative with a bulk agent (e.g., Perdiem) or with a softener (e.g., Pericolace) are reasonable and effective forms of therapy. Bulk agents alone in such cases simply distend the already distended bowel further without improving bowel function.

Special consideration must be given to the bedridden or chair-bound patient. In such patients laxatives may result in incontinence, as the patient may not be able to recognize or respond quickly enough to the sudden urge to defecate. In these circumstances, bulk agents are useful to keep the stool soft, but suppositories or enemas should be used (simple tap water enemas are usually sufficient; also see Table 39.3), with the patient already positioned on the commode. In this fashion, the embarrassment and soilage of fecal incontinence can be avoided, and fecal impactions can be prevented. These enemas or suppositories should be used regularly (daily to every third day) to prevent fecal impactions and "overflow" diarrhea and incontinence.

DIARRHEA

Diarrhea is a troublesome problem that almost everyone has experienced. In the vast majority of cases, the diarrheal illness begins abruptly, lasts only a day or 2, and resolves without serious sequelae (see Chapter 26). Only occasionally does the illness continue for more than a week or do symptoms recur after the initial attack. The task facing the clinician is to identify the few patients with a significant underlying disorder who may require a specific therapeutic approach.

Definition

Patients complaining of diarrhea generally have an increase in the frequency and fluid volume of the bowel movement. Stool weight is the best objective measurement of diarrhea, with mean weights in this country ranging normally between 100 and 200 g/day. In the patient with chronic diarrhea, objective documentation of daily fecal output is sometimes necessary (see below). Most cases of significant diarrhea will have in excess of 250 g of stool/day. There is a subset of patients with diarrhea who present with the frequent passage of small volumes of liquid stool. Patients with inflammatory conditions or space-occupying lesions of the rectum may present in this fashion. Patients with the irritable bowel syndrome have stool volumes either within or slightly above the normal range. Patients with secretory forms of diarrhea, or small bowel disorders with malabsorption, frequently pass large volumes of stool, often in the range of 500 to 1000 (or greater) g/day.

Pathophysiology

There are four basic mechanisms of diarrhea: (a) osmotic load within the intestine resulting in retention of water within the lumen, (b) excessive secretion of electrolytes and water into the intestinal lumen, (c) exudation of protein and fluid from the intestinal mucosa, and (d) altered intestinal motility resulting in rapid transit through the colon.

Osmotic diarrhea occurs when poorly absorbable material retains fluid within the intestinal lumen. This mechanism operates in patients with malabsorption or with lactose intolerance in which poorly absorbed sugars accumulate within the intestinal lumen and exert a considerable osmotic load. Magnesium-containing laxatives and some magnesium-containing antacids (e.g., Maalox) probably produce diarrhea through a similar mechanism.

Secretory diarrhea occurs when the intestinal mucosa secretes increased amounts of water and electrolytes under the stimulation of a variety of substances. Cholera toxin is the prototype, and some enterotoxigenic *Escherichia coli* produce diarrhea in the same way (see Chapter 26). Other substances that induce secretory diarrhea include bile acids and long chain fatty acids (postileal resection, Crohn's disease, or a malabsorption syndrome), certain gastrointestinal hormones, and anthraquinone laxatives. Many of these stimulating agents have been shown to increase intracellular cyclic AMP and to inhibit sodium potassium

ATPase. The increase in cyclic AMP leads to increased secretion.

Exudative diarrhea results from the outpouring of protein, blood, or mucus from an inflamed or ulcerated mucosa. Ulcerative colitis, Crohn's disease, invasive infections, and infiltrative disorders like Whipple's disease and lymphoma are examples of this mechanism.

Motility disorders may lead to diarrhea, although the exact correlation between the abnormal motility and the diarrhea is not completely understood. The *irritable bowel syndrome* (see Chapter 40) is generally believed to be a motor disorder that causes abdominal pain and altered bowel habits, with diarrhea predominating in many patients. Diabetes mellitus may also lead to diarrhea due to neurogenic dysfunction. Other conditions, like scleroderma, can lead to stasis of the bowel with resultant bacterial overgrowth, steatorrhea, and diarrhea.

It is not always possible to identify one particular mechanism to account for diarrhea in a given patient; sometimes more than one mechanism is operative. However, an appreciation of pathophysiology enables the physician to understand better the clinical features of a diarrheal illness and to select appropriate therapy.

Evaluation of Acute Diarrhea

(Acute diarrhea due to infectious agents is discussed in greater detail in Chapter 26). The vast majority of patients who present to the physician with a sudden onset of diarrhea have a benign, self-limited illness. These patients do not require extensive evaluation and can be simply reassured. It is important, however, to recognize that a small percentage of such patients may actually have a significant underlying illness for which specific therapy is needed.

If diarrhea persists for more than 72 hours or if there is gross blood in the stool, an evaluation is indicated. In any case, the patient should always be evaluated before medicine is prescribed, since in certain situations even nonspecific antidiarrheal therapy may actually be harmful. In particular, it has been shown that antidiarrheal drugs such as diphenoxylate (e.g., Lomotil) may prolong the course of acute infectious diarrhea by hindering the natural mechanism of clearing the body of the organism (1).

History

The history reveals whether the illness is acute or chronic and also provides clues to the underlying cause. The sudden onset of loose watery stool is most commonly due to an infectious process, and much less often due to ingestion of drugs or poisons. Infectious diarrhea is likely to affect more than one person. Frequently, no specific bacterial agent is identified and the syndrome is labeled "viral gastroenteritis." Bacteria may cause diarrhea by a direct effect on the bowel or by elaboration of a toxin that produces intestinal dysfunction. Toxin-induced diarrhea, often associated with vomiting, begins within 6 hours of ingestion of contaminated food, whereas bacteria-induced diarrhea does not begin for 12 to 24 hours. Bloody diarrhea should never be ascribed to "viral" or to toxin-mediated diarrhea; it is more likely to be due to bacterial infection (*Shigella, Helicobacter, Yersinia,* and *Salmonella*), to ulcerative colitis, or to ischemic bowel disease. Information about recent travel should include not only trips out of the country but also camping or fishing trips. Giardiasis, for example, may be carried by beavers who contaminate water supplies and cause both epidemic outbreaks as well as individual cases of acute diarrhea among campers and hikers. Recent use of drugs is a common cause of new onset diarrhea (Table 39.4) that is often overlooked by both the physician and the patient. Some antihypertensives (e.g., methyldopa, hydralazine, reserpine, and guanethidine), magnesium-containing antacids, broad spectrum antimicrobials, and quinidine are commonly used drugs that can lead to diarrhea.

A number of human immunodeficiency virus (HIV)-associated intestinal disorders cause diarrhea so that appropriate questions should be asked to identify patients who are at risk of having HIV infection (see Chapter 34).

Physical Examination

The physical examination in acute diarrhea is generally unremarkable. The patient's state of hydration should be estimated, as it is an important measure of the severity of the diarrhea and of the need for hospitalization. Abdominal examination may reveal mild diffuse tenderness. The bowel sounds are clearly active or hyperactive. Rectal examination is essential since diarrhea may be the initial manifestation of obstructing rectal carcinoma; furthermore in the geriatric population, fecal impactions may result in "overflow" diarrhea so that constipating agents may be mistakenly recommended.

Table 39.4.
Common Drugs That May Induce Diarrhea

ANTIBIOTICS:[a]
  Clindamycin
  Ampicillin
  Cephalosporins
ANTACIDS: Magnesium-containing
ANTIHYPERTENSIVE AGENTS:
  Guanethidine
  Hydralazine
  Methyldopa
  Propranolol
  Reserpine
CARDIOVASCULAR AGENTS:
  Digitalis
  Quinidine
ANTIMETABOLITES: Colchicine
ALCOHOL
NUTRITIONAL SUPPLEMENTS: Hyperosmolar solutions (enteral feedings)
POTENT DIURETICS:
  Furosemide
  Ethacrynic acid

[a]All antibiotics can induce pseudomembranous colitis (see Chapter 26).

Stool Examination

If diarrhea has continued for more than 3 to 4 days, the stool should be examined for the presence of blood, fecal leukocytes, and enteric pathogens. Blood in the stool suggests mucosal disruption and is not a feature of osmotic, secretory, or motor diarrhea. Inflammatory conditions like ulcerative colitis and pseudomembranous colitis (see below, page 455, and Chapter 26) frequently present with bloody diarrhea.

Fecal leukocytes are best seen by microscopic examination of the liquid portion of the stool after staining with methylene blue or Gram's stain. They are not seen in infectious processes that do not invade the mucosa such as "viral enteritis," toxin-mediated diarrhea, cholera, or infection with noninvasive E. coli (see Chapter 26). *Salmonella, Shigella, Amoeba,* and *Helicobacter,* which are invasive organisms, typically lead to exudation of fecal leukocytes, as does chronic inflammatory bowel disease. In these conditions, in which the mucosal barrier is broken, the course of the diarrheal illness is unpredictable and may even become life threatening. The absence of fecal leukocytes or blood is, therefore, very reassuring and, in these cases, the disease is usually transient.

Stool cultures for bacterial pathogens should be obtained in all patients who have fecal leukocytes. Specific isolation techniques are needed to diagnose *Yersinia* and *Helicobacter,* common causes of acute diarrhea, and should be requested. Acute infectious diarrhea secondary to *Salmonella* or *Shigella* or other invasive organisms is impossible to differentiate from acute inflammatory bowel disease, especially without a stool culture. In the absence of fecal leukocytes, stool cultures are generally negative. Gram stain of the stool is not helpful except in cases of suspected staphylococcal enterocolitis or gonococcal proctitis.

Examination of the stool for parasites such as *Entamoeba histolytica* and *Giardia lamblia* is very important even in the absence of a history of travel since the organism may be passed by contact with a carrier. Microscopic examination of the inflammatory exudate of a patient with acute amoebic colitis will almost always demonstrate motile trophozoites, but only if the slide is prewarmed (e.g., over a light bulb) and then examined immediately. Slides sent to a laboratory for processing are unlikely to reveal amoeba. Rectal biopsy may identify the organisms in the exudate. Amoebic serology can be useful but does not distinguish recent from distant infection. Measuring acute and convalescent titers is more specific for recent infection but gives the diagnosis only in retrospect. *Giardia* can be detected on examination of fresh stool in only about 50% of patients. Duodenal aspiration or biopsy is more sensitive in diagnosing giardiasis.

Endoscopy

Proctosigmoidoscopy is important in patients with acute diarrhea associated with fecal leukocytes or bloody diarrhea. The examination should be performed without a prior enema, as enemas may alter the appearance of the mucosa and reduce the chance of detecting intestinal pathogens like amebae. The marginal diagnostic return in examining the entire colon is quite small, so flexible or rigid proctosigmoidoscopy is preferable to colonoscopy in evaluation of acute diarrheal illness.

Many acute diarrheal illnesses produce a similar abnormal but nonspecific mucosal appearance on proctoscopy. Certain findings, however, are suggestive of specific diseases. In viral enteritis, giardiasis, toxin-mediated diarrhea, drug-induced diarrhea, and other conditions not accompanied by fecal leukocytes or blood loss, the proctoscopy is normal. In ulcerative colitis the rectal mucosa is involved in at least 95% of cases, and the mucosa is uniformly abnormal with bleeding and a granular, friable appearance. Uncommonly, Crohn's disease affects the rectum and causes discrete aphthoid ulcers with normal intervening mucosa. Amebiasis occasionally produces classical flask-shaped ulcers that may be single or multiple, with normal intervening mucosa; more often, however, it produces a pattern very similar to ulcerative colitis. In shigellosis, multiple small superficial ulcers may be seen, but the appearance may also be indistinguishable from that of ulcerative colitis. Pseudomembranous colitis is identified by the presence of numerous raised yellow plaques covering an inflamed mucosa. Occasionally a carcinoma or large villous adenoma may be detected by sigmoidoscopy. Proctoscopy also provides an opportune time to obtain samples of stool and exudate for culture and microscopic examination. The patient's experience with proctosigmoidoscopy is described in Chapter 36.

Radiographic Studies

Radiography is of very limited value in the evaluation of acute diarrhea and may, in fact, be confusing. In patients suspected of having inflammatory bowel disease or ischemic colitis, plain films of the abdomen may demonstrate an irregular appearance to the bowel wall secondary to mucosal edema, often described as "thumbprinting." In the gravely ill patient with fulminant colitis, the X-ray may confirm the presence of "toxic megacolon." In the vast majority of cases of acute diarrhea, a plain film is not needed. Barium studies during the acute phase of the diarrhea are likewise not needed and in certain conditions may even be hazardous, as in patients with severe colitis or ischemic bowel disease. Similarly, a small bowel series during acute "viral enteritis" may be frighteningly abnormal, resembling sprue, and yet may rapidly return to normal after resolution of the acute illness.

Evaluation of Chronic Diarrhea

The approach to patients with either acute diarrhea that lasts longer than 3 to 4 days or chronic diarrhea (lasting longer than 2 weeks) is very much the same. Although the physician may be reassured, knowing that the majority of such patients do not suffer from any serious progressive or disabling disease, the patient requires a specific diagnosis and effective therapy. The differential diagnosis is so varied, and the available tests are so numerous, that the diagnostic workup of chronic diarrhea poses a difficult problem. The following discussion provides a practical approach to this problem.

History

The history is often very helpful in differentiating organic from "functional" diarrhea—i.e., irritable bowel syndrome (see Chapter 40). If organic diarrhea is suspected, the physician must determine whether the pathogenic mechanism is osmotic, secretory, motor, or exudative (see above).

In patients with so-called "functional diarrhea," the history of diarrhea often dates back many months or years, although occasionally it can be traced to a specific acute diarrheal illness. Despite the chronicity, no sequelae, such as weight loss, anemia, or hypoalbuminemia, have occurred. The patient typically complains of several watery, at times explosive, bowel movements early in the morning, and then no subsequent movements the rest of the day. Nocturnal bowel movements are rare. The total stool output is usually small, however—often less than 200 g/day and rarely, if ever, greater than 500 g/day. Mucus is present frequently. There is no blood in the stool unless secondary conditions, such as anal fissures, have developed. Postprandial pain is a feature of irritable bowel syndrome but is absent in many patients. The condition frequently waxes and wanes in severity, and stress often exacerbates the symptoms.

The most common cause of chronic secretory diarrhea is *laxative abuse*. It should be suspected in apparently healthy patients with large volume diarrhea, especially if they have *melanosis coli* on proctoscopic examination (see above, page 444). Although such patients may have emotional problems with which the physician must deal (see Chapter 12), often the abuse simply reflects an individual's misconception about how often he should have a bowel movement and his attempt to adhere to that standard.

In patients with organic disease, the history may indicate the part of the intestinal tract that is involved. The passage of a large volume of frothy, malodorous stools without blood suggests small bowel diarrhea, often secondary to malabsorption. The frequent passage of small volumes of poorly formed bloody stools suggests inflammatory, exudative disorders of the colon like ulcerative colitis. The presence of recognizable fat droplets (oil) suggests malabsorption, frequently secondary to pancreatic insufficiency. (Floating stools and undigested food in the stools are not helpful observations as they may be seen in both organic and functional diarrheal states.) The association of diarrhea with the ingestion of certain dietary products (milk, hyperosmolar solutions) may not be recognized by the patient unless he is specifically asked. A detailed drug history is also important since many drugs may cause diarrhea.

Other symptoms may help the physician to arrive at a specific diagnosis. *Arthritis* and *arthralgias* may suggest the presence of one of several uncommon bowel diseases, e.g., inflammatory bowel disease and Whipple's disease; conversely, diarrhea may be an important feature of Reiter's syndrome (Chapter 71). *Weight loss*, in the absence of anorexia, should suggest malabsorption, hyperthyroidism, or a malignant tumor. *Abdominal pain* may reflect the irritable bowel syndrome (Chapter 40), in which case it is generally in the left lower quadrant or in the suprapubic region, or a disease of the small bowel (e.g., Crohn's disease) in which case it is periumbilical or in the right lower quadrant, or a gastrinoma (Zollinger-Ellison syndrome) with accompanying peptic ulcers.

Physical Examination

The physical examination may reveal additional information about the etiology of the diarrhea. Patients with malabsorption may have evidence of weight loss, peripheral neuropathy (secondary to vitamin B deficiency), and carpopedal spasm (secondary to hypocalcemia). Erythema nodosum and pyoderma gangrenosum may be seen in some cases of inflammatory bowel disease. Hyperpigmentation is a feature of Whipple's disease and Addison's disease. Diabetic diarrhea is frequently associated with other evidence of autonomic dysfunction, such as postural hypotension. Nondeforming arthritis is a feature of Whipple's disease and inflammatory bowel disease. Hepatosplenomegaly and lymphadenopathy suggest lymphoma or Whipple's disease. The abdominal examination may reveal an arterial bruit or an aortic aneurysm, which suggests ischemic bowel disease. A rectal examination may disclose perianal disease (e.g., abscesses or fistulas, secondary to Crohn's disease), a rectal tumor, or a fecal impaction.

Endoscopy

Proctoscopy should be performed during the initial visit without a prior cleansing enema. Proctoscopic examination of the rectal mucosa and a rectal biopsy (see pages 444 and 450) may suggest specific etiologies—ulcerative colitis, Crohn's disease, amebiasis, pseudomembranous colitis, Whipple's disease, or amyloidosis. The finding of melanosis coli (spotty or diffuse brownish mucosal pigmentation) in a patient complaining of diarrhea indicates laxative abuse. At the time of proctoscopy, stool specimens are obtained for microscopic evaluation and culture. Gonococcal proctitis appears similar to ulcerative proctitis (see below) and requires direct plating on a warm special culture medium (Thayer-Martin) with prompt incubation. Routine stool cultures should be taken as well. The stool should be examined for leukocytes, blood, fat (Sudan stain), and parasites (see page 449).

After this initial evaluation, the etiology of the chronic diarrhea in most patients is either evident or strongly suspected. It is usually possible to distinguish functional from organic diarrhea, to detect evidence of inflammatory or infiltrative disease, to suspect the presence of malabsorption; to characterize the diarrhea as "small bowel" or "large bowel," and even to suggest the underlying pathophysiology. Further evaluation is then dictated by the results of this initial workup.

Laboratory Studies

Laboratory studies should be selected to support the clinical impression but rarely are able to make or exclude a specific diagnosis. For example, the erythrocyte sedimentation rate (ESR) may be elevated in a variety of inflammatory diseases that cause diarrhea, but a normal ESR does not exclude inflammatory bowel disease or a connective tissue disorder.

Radiological Studies

A plain film of the abdomen may reveal pancreatic calcifications (indicative of chronic pancreatitis), a dilated small bowel, or an abnormal bowel contour (such as in inflammatory bowel disease or lymphoma).

In the patient over 40 years old with chronic or recurrent diarrhea, a *barium enema* or *colonoscopy* is indicated during the initial evaluation. In younger patients, barium studies are unlikely to be useful unless a specific disorder is suspected. The presence of blood in the stool, at any age, is a clear indication for a colonoscopy or barium enema, regardless of the presence of hemorrhoids or fissures. Neoplastic and inflammatory conditions may be diagnosed in this way, and ulcerative colitis and Crohn's disease of the colon can be differentiated in most cases. When inflammatory bowel disease is suspected, during the barium enema an attempt should be made to reflux contrast material into the terminal ileum to rule out Crohn's disease of the ileum.

The timing of the barium enema is important. Barium will interfere with the collection of stool for measurement of volume and fat and with the detection of parasites. A barium enema should be delayed for 1 week following a rectal biopsy to prevent colonic perforation. The patient's experience with the barium enema is discussed in Chapter 38.

A *small bowel series* (see Chapter 38 for a discussion of the patient's experience with this procedure) is helpful in distinguishing mucosal disease (celiac sprue), inflammatory conditions (Crohn's disease), and infiltrative processes (Whipple's disease or amyloidosis). In addition, a small bowel series is indicated in postsurgical patients to clarify the anatomy (e.g., a blind loop or fistulas) and to detect localized areas of dilation and stasis.

Other Studies

A quantitative 72-hour stool collection, although regarded as unpleasant by both the patient and laboratory personnel, is a very informative test. It should be employed early in the evaluation of patients in whom the initial routine workup does not suggest a diagnosis. The test can be performed in the ambulatory setting by having the patient collect all of his stool in a preweighed container, supplied by the clinical laboratory. (He can also defecate into a bedpan or into a special stool collection trap, placed inside a commode, and then transfer the stool to a preweighed container.) The test should be performed before barium studies or other invasive tests in these patients. As mentioned previously, the normal stool weight is less than 250 g/day (or less than 250 ml/day). Most patients with the irritable bowel syndrome will have stool volumes within this range. A stool volume of greater than 1000 ml/day suggests a secretory diarrhea.

Fecal fat should also be measured during this collection. Normally less than 7% of ingested fat is secreted in the stool per day (6 to 7 g on an average American diet containing 70 to 100 g of fat). The presence of steatorrhea dictates a different approach to the remainder of the workup (see below). In the absence of excessive fat excretion, or of evidence of an exudative process (e.g., inflammatory bowel disease), high volume diarrhea suggests a secretory process. The *osmolality* and *electrolyte* concentration of the specimen can also be measured. In osmotic diarrhea, the measured fecal osmolality is greater than twice the sum of the concentration of fecal sodium and potassium. In secretory diarrhea, the calculated and measured osmolality are the same.

In patients suspected of having a secretory diarrhea, further evaluation will generally require hospitalization and consultation with a gastroenterologist. In secretory diarrhea, having the patient ingest nothing by mouth for 48 hours will not alter the volume of diarrhea, whereas in osmotic diarrhea the stool volume will significantly decrease. Causes of chronic secretory diarrhea include hormone-secreting tumors and surreptitious laxative abuse. Evaluation of such patients frequently requires availability of various hormone assays.

Evaluation of Malabsorption

When the quantitative fecal collection demonstrates steatorrhea, the evaluation of the diarrhea should be focused on the cause of malabsorption. Malabsorption can result from small intestinal disease, pancreatic disease, hepatobiliary disease, and gastric disease. A series of diagnostic studies is utilized initially to define the organ involved and then to diagnose the specific disease. Consultation with a gastroenterologist is generally recommended to help perform and analyze these various tests.

The *d-xylose test* measures the absorptive capacity of the proximal small bowel and is useful in distinguishing malabsorption from maldigestion. This sugar does not require the intraabdominal pancreatic stage of digestion in order to be absorbed by the intact small intestinal mucosa. After absorption it enters the blood and is excreted in the urine. The test is performed in the same manner as an oral glucose tolerance test and can be performed in the ambulatory setting by most clinical laboratories. A 25-g oral dose of xylose is given,

and the patient's urine is collected over the next 5 hours. A blood sample is collected at 1 hour after ingestion. In disorders of the intestinal mucosa (e.g., sprue, Whipple's disease) xylose is poorly absorbed and low levels are found in the serum and urine. Uncommonly, massive bacterial overgrowth may also produce an abnormal d-xylose test that reverts to normal with treatment. Because an abnormal xylose test suggests mucosal disease, a small bowel biopsy should be performed next. Dehydration, renal insufficiency, third spacing of fluid, vomiting, and hypothyroidism may spuriously decrease urine, but not serum, levels of d-xylose.

If the d-xylose test is normal, maldigestion, usually due to *pancreatic insufficiency*, is the most likely cause of steatorrhea. In this chronic pancreatitis, pancreatic calcifications may be seen on an abdominal plain film, and diabetes mellitus is frequently present. Pancreatic insufficiency can be confirmed by measuring pancreatic secretions or by measuring intraluminal contents after a test meal. These tests, performed usually in the gastroenterology laboratory of a medical center, involve intubation of the duodenum, with collection of intraluminal contents. Newer methods do not require intubation but simply a prolonged urine collection, e.g., the Bentiromide test, which utilizes a nonabsorbable synthetic peptide that is cleaved by pancreatic enzymes, then becomes absorbable and is measured when it is excreted in the urine. Often, however, if a presumptive diagnosis of pancreatic insufficiency is made, the patient is treated empirically with pancreatic enzymes (e.g., Viokase, three to six tablets with meals or Pancrease, two to three tablets with meals); diagnostic and therapeutic decisions should be made in consultation with a gastroenterologist.

Suction biopsy of the small intestine is often useful in the detection of various disorders that may cause malabsorption and/or diarrhea. The procedure can be performed by a gastroenterologist in an ambulatory setting. The biopsy instrument, a small caliber weighted tube, is passed by mouth through the stomach and positioned fluoroscopically at the duodenal-jejunal junction. The patient may be given prior mild sedation (Valium intravenously) and a topical anesthetic is sprayed onto the back of the pharynx. The procedure may last from 15 minutes to 2 or 3 hours depending on the ease of passage of the tube (usually the tube can be passed rapidly). Complications (including perforation and bleeding) are extremely rare. Disorders that may be diagnosed by small bowel biopsy include sprue, Whipple's disease, intestinal lymphoma, amyloidosis, lymphangiectasia, and eosinophilic gastroenteritis. Giardiasis also can be diagnosed by examination of the intestinal mucosa and of the intestinal mucus or fluid by the pathologist or the consulting gastroenterologist.

Disorders of the terminal ileum (Crohn's disease, ileal resection) may also lead to diarrhea and malabsorption. Evaluation should include a *Schilling test* or a *bile salt breath test*. The Schilling test measures vitamin B_{12} absorption, which is abnormal in disorders of the terminal ileum, the site of B_{12} absorption. Absorption is impaired despite the presence of intrinsic factor (see Chapter 50) or the administration of antibiotics.

Similarly, the bile salt breath test measures bile acid absorption, which is also abnormal in disorders of the terminal ileum, the site of bile salt absorption. The patient is given orally a radiolabeled (^{14}C) bile salt. In the presence of terminal ileal disease, the bile salt is malabsorbed and excess acid reaches the colon, where bacteria deconjugate it and release $^{14}CO_2$, which diffuses across the colon and is excreted in the breath. Therefore, in ileal disease, the level of $^{14}CO_2$ in the patient's expired air is abnormally high. The same abnormality can be seen when there is bacterial overgrowth in the small bowel, so that the bile acid is deconjugated and metabolized there instead of in the colon. Bile acid malabsorption due to bacterial overgrowth is reversed when the patient is given antibiotics. Both the Schilling test and the bile salt breath test are performed by nuclear medicine specialists.

Specific Causes of Chronic Diarrhea

Lactose Intolerance (See Also Chapter 40, Page 460)

Lactose is by far the most commonly malabsorbed carbohydrate. Lactose intolerance results from a deficiency or total absence of the enzyme lactase in the brush border of the intestinal mucosa, which causes maldigestion and therefore malabsorption of lactose. The unabsorbed carbohydrate exerts an osmotic effect that draws water into the intestinal lumen. In the colon, the lactose is metabolized by bacteria to organic acid, CO_2, and hydrogen. The acid contributes to the diarrhea by both an osmotic effect and an irritatant effect on the colonic mucosa. Thus, the unabsorbed carbohydrate, if present in sufficient quantities (the critical amount varies widely), may cause diarrhea, gaseousness, bloating, and abdominal cramps.

Lactose intolerance may be present either as an inherited condition or one that is acquired because of damage to the intestinal epithelium (e.g., due to infectious enteritis or sprue). Even in patients with a genetic disorder, the onset of the disease is unpredictable and may not occur until adult life. The secondary cases are usually, but not always, reversible if the underlying disease is successfully treated. The severity of the clinical symptoms is highly variable.

In some patients even small amounts of lactose produce severe symptoms, whereas in others large quantities may be consumed with no or only minimal symptoms. Isolated lactase deficiency is most common in blacks (50 to 80% prevalence) and in Asians (75 to 100%) but may also be found in 10 to 20% of the white population in this country (2). The condition is more pronounced in certain clinical settings: when superimposed on another diarrheal disorder, most commonly irritable bowel syndrome; after gastric surgery, which permits rapid delivery of lactose to the small bowel; and when a patient consumes extra amounts of milk as part of (misguided) therapy for ulcer disease.

The diagnosis of lactose intolerance is suggested by the history and by the response to a lactose-free diet. Nearly a third of patients with symptomatic lactose intolerance, however, may not have made the correlation between the dietary intake and the resulting symptoms, as a wide variety of foods, ranging from bread to instant coffee, contain lactose (see Table 40.2).

Specific tests for the diagnosis of lactose intolerance include the lactose tolerance test and the hydrogen breath test. The *lactose tolerance test* measures changes in the concentration of serum glucose at 1 and 2 hours after ingestion of 50 g of lactose. A rise in glucose of 20 mg/100 ml above fasting is normal. The test has about a 30% false-positive rate, and its validity depends on a variety of factors besides simply the presence of the lactase enzyme. The *hydrogen breath test* is easier to perform and is more accurate. Unabsorbed lactose is fermented by colonic bacteria, and the resultant hydrogen is absorbed and expired in the breath. In normal subjects after a lactose load, there is only a trace amount of hydrogen in the expired air, whereas in lactose-deficient patients substantial levels are recorded. This test is widely available; it is usually performed by a nuclear medicine specialist or in a gastrointestinal laboratory and requires 2 to 4 hours of the patient's time.

Ordinarily, a 3-week trial of a diet that is free of milk and milk products is a satisfactory therapeutic trial to test the diagnosis of lactose intolerance. The other tests are indicated only in equivocal cases or when the patient's nutritional status would be compromised by eliminating milk products unnecessarily.

Fecal Impaction

Although it is the result of chronic constipation, fecal impaction (8) commonly causes diarrhea. The adults most at risk for impaction are elderly sedentary people—often bedridden. The feces are usually impacted in the rectum or in the rectosigmoid region but occasionally may extend high up into the colon (rarely, even to the cecum). The leaking of colonic fluid around the impaction, resulting in the passage of frequent, small volume, watery bowel movements, accounts for the diarrhea. Other symptoms are common but are usually nonspecific: a sense of fullness in the rectum, vague lower abdominal pain, nausea, and headache. On physical examination, the firm stool is palpable in the left lower quadrant of the abdomen, which is best examined bimanually (a finger of one hand in the rectum and the other hand on the abdomen). The impaction is best removed manually if it is low enough, or through the sigmoidoscope if it is not. Repeated enemas (e.g., phosphosoda) may be helpful once some of the very hard stool is removed. Complications of impaction include recurrent urinary tract infection (because of compression of the ureters—more common in women), urinary incontinence, intestinal obstruction, perforation of the colon, and local ulceration.

Ulcerative Colitis

Ulcerative colitis is a chronic inflammatory disorder of colonic mucosa; its cause is unknown. It is recommended that patients with this condition be followed by the general physician in consultation with a gastroenterologist. The disorder may affect patients of any age with a peak incidence in the third decade and a second peak in the seventh decade.

The clinical picture of ulcerative colitis is highly variable. The disorder may be limited to the rectum (ulcerative proctitis) or may involve the entire colon. Symptoms may range from occasional rectal bleeding, even without diarrhea, to profuse purulent and bloody diarrhea. The severity of the initial presentation and the extent of the disease at the time of the initial attack have been shown to be useful predictors of the eventual course of the disease. Most patients (about 60%) have mild disease, i.e., fewer than four bowel movements a day without fever, weight loss, or hypoalbuminemia. The vast majority of these patients will have colitis limited to the rectosigmoid region or to the descending colon. About 10 to 15% of patients with ulcerative colitis develop severe pancolitis with accompanying deterioration in their general health. Another 25% have moderate disease with more troublesome diarrhea, often containing blood, accompanied by crampy lower abdominal pain. Patients with moderate or severe disease may also have systemic symptoms of fever, fatigue, and weight loss. The clinical course is characterized by periodic exacerbations that in general respond well to adjustments in medical therapy. The smallest group of patients with ulcerative colitis consists of those with severe disease. This group includes the 1% of patients who present initially with fulminant colitis. In patients with severe colitis, symptoms may suddenly worsen, with profuse diarrhea, rectal bleeding, and high fevers. Plain films of the abdomen may demonstrate a dilated bowel ("toxic megacolon"). Mortality is high in this group of patients.

As there is no specific test for or histopathology of ulcerative colitis, the diagnosis depends on the constellation of symptoms, on the appropriate endoscopic and histological appearance of the colonic mucosa, on the exclusion of other inflammatory conditions, and on the natural history of the disorder. Patients with acute presentations, depending on the circumstances, must be differentiated from patients with bacterial diarrheas (see Chapter 26), amebiasis (see above page 449), Crohn's disease (see below), and ischemic colitis (ischemic colitis presents with acute abdominal pain and the passage of bloody stool; this is a disease of middle-aged or older people who usually have evidence of generalized atherosclerosis).

Treatment. Medical therapy for ulcerative colitis is determined by the severity of the attack. Mild attacks may respond to sulfasalazine (Azulfidine), whereas moderate or severe attacks require treatment with oral or intravenous steroids. Steroids are very useful for acute exacerbations but are not helpful in preventing relapses. Conversely, sulfasalazine is of limited value in the treatment of acute attacks but has been shown to reduce the frequency of exacerbations and may allow reduction of the dosage of steroids. A minority of patients with ulcerative colitis need continuous steroid therapy. Other drugs, such as cytotoxic agents, require further evaluation before they can be recommended.

Surgery in ulcerative colitis is curative, and patients should be counseled early in their course about the role of surgery in the treatment of this disorder. Patients should be informed about the indications for surgery and the types of operations that are available. Early attention to this issue will enable the patient to accept an operation more readily if it is needed. Surgery for ulcerative colitis (see Chapter 42) involves a proctocolectomy with an ileostomy to which a stomal appliance is attached to assure continence. Construction of a continent ileostomy (Kock pouch) avoids the need for a stomal appliance, but the procedure is technically difficult and often requires revision. Another alternative is construction of an internal pouch from a loop of small bowel anastomosed to the anus (Park's procedure). These last two procedures are most successful in highly motivated young patients undergoing elective colectomy.

Cancer of the Colon. The risk of cancer of the colon is increased 5 to 10 times in patients with ulcerative colitis. The major risk factors are (a) duration of disease—risk increases significantly after 8 to 10 years of disease; (b) extent of colonic involvement—pancolitis carries the highest risk, whereas the risk in patients with ulcerative proctitis is similar to that of the general population; and (c) age of onset of disease—patients under the age of 25 at the time of onset have the highest risk, independent of the extent of disease. The cancer may be found anywhere in the colon, although most commonly it is within the rectum or rectosigmoid. It may be multicentric. It is important that the patient know about the risk of cancer since it may influence his decision to undergo colectomy. After they have had the disease for 8 to 10 years, high risk patients should have yearly evaluations of the colon by colonoscopy. In addition, since dysplastic changes of the colonic mucosa have been identified as "precancer" and have been shown to correlate closely with the development of cancer elsewhere in the colon, serial colonic and rectal biopsies should be obtained during yearly colonoscopy in high risk patients.

Crohn's Disease

Crohn's disease or regional enteritis is a chronic inflammatory condition of unknown cause involving all layers of the intestine as opposed to just the mucosa as in ulcerative colitis. The condition most commonly affects the terminal ileum, but any area from the esophagus to the anus can be involved. The onset of the disease most commonly is in adolescence and young adulthood. The incidence of Crohn's disease has been rising in recent years, particularly Crohn's disease of the colon.

Presentation. Crohn's disease may be localized initially to the small bowel, involve small bowel and colon, or be confined to the colon only. The inflammatory process often remains confined to the initial site of involvement unless surgery is performed. Recurrence is the rule after surgery, and the condition may then involve additional segments of bowel. Spontaneous progression of the disease tends to be in a proximal (orad) direction. As the inflammatory process persists, the bowel wall becomes thickened and stenotic, leading to bowel obstruction. Fistula formation is characteristic and may involve any contiguous structure. As a result, abscess formation and infection may complicate the clinical course. Diarrhea, abdominal pain, and weight loss are the most common symptoms. Unlike ulcerative colitis, rectal bleeding is not a prominent feature unless the colon is the major site of involvement.

The *differential diagnosis* includes disorders of both the small and large bowel. Occasionally the patient presents with fever and acute right lower quadrant pain resembling acute appendicitis. When there is terminal ileal involvement, Crohn's disease must be distinguished from lymphoma and tuberculosis. Colonic involvement may suggest ulcerative colitis (see above), ischemic colitis, or carcinoma (see Chapter 38). Involvement of the distal small bowel and the right colon, the presence of characteristic skip areas, stricturing of the bowel, perianal disease, and fistula formation are helpful diagnostic features that suggest Crohn's disease.

Treatment. Therapy for Crohn's disease is similar to that for ulcerative colitis, depending heavily on corticosteroids and sulfasalazine (Azulfidine). These agents may be effective in treating the recurrent attacks that characterize Crohn's disease, but neither agent has been shown to be effective in preventing relapses. In addition, sulfasalazine has not been shown to be useful in disease limited to the small bowel. Metronidazole (Flagyl) seems to be effective for perianal fistulas. Immunosuppressants, like 6-mercaptopurine and azathioprine (Imuran), have produced variable results, and their use in this condition is still controversial.

Surgery is sometimes necessary in Crohn's disease for (a) resection of fibrotic obstructing lesions, (b) drainage of abscesses, and (c) resection of complicated fistulas. Occasionally the disease is refractory to medical therapy, and the diseased bowel must be resected. It must be recognized that surgery is not intended to be curative, so that removal of normal bowel to achieve wide "disease-free" margins is generally not indicated. In the rare patient whose disease is extensive and unresponsive to medical and surgical intervention, or in whom a short bowel syndrome has developed secondary to the disease and to repeated surgery, long-term home parenteral hyperalimentation can be beneficial in providing good nutritional support and in ameliorating symptoms.

Course. Despite its chronicity and tendency for recurrence, Crohn's disease takes a highly variable course. Prolonged relatively asymptomatic periods occur, even after years of disease activity and after multiple operations. There is a poor correlation between the clinical severity and the radiological appearance of the disease. Mortality from the disease is low though morbidity is high. Since the natural history is so variable, the physician should approach the patient with Crohn's disease in a positive and hopeful fashion, yet be aware of the potential for significant morbidity. All patients should be followed in close consultation with a gastroenterologist.

Drug-Induced Diarrhea

A variety of commonly used medications may cause diarrhea (Table 39.4). The diarrhea may be a direct result of the pharmacological activity of the drug (e.g., magnesium-containing antacids or colchicine); or the mechanism for the induction of diarrhea may be unknown (e.g., hydralazine or propranolol). The diarrhea may also signify drug toxicity (e.g., digitalis). Certain drugs have repeatedly been associated with diarrhea (antibiotics, antacids, quinidine, digitalis, alcohol), whereas in other cases (hydralazine, propranolol) the relationship is rare and not well defined.

Diarrhea associated with antibiotics may range from a mild increase in the frequency and volume of stools to a toxic, life-threatening condition. Diarrhea may develop during the course of antibiotic therapy, after either parenteral or oral use, but may also occur up to 3 weeks after discontinuation of the drugs. The antibiotics most commonly associated with diarrhea are ampicillin, tetracycline, clindamycin, and the cephalosporins.

In the more severe forms of antibiotic-associated diarrhea the diarrhea is bloody and is accompanied by abdominal cramps and fever. Endoscopy may reveal pseudomembranes which appear as raised plaques on edematous friable mucosa. Histologically these pseudomembranes, are collections of fibrin, mucin, and leukocytes. Pseudomembranous colitis is due to proliferation of *Clostridium difficile* and the elaboration of its toxin. This organism accounts for the vast majority of cases of pseudomembranous colitis and for 20 to 30% of antibiotic-associated diarrhea in general. The toxin elaborated by *C. difficile* can be assayed in stool. The organism can also be cultured but is difficult to grow. Because culture is less sensitive than the toxin titer and does not correlate as well with symptoms, it is not recommended.

Therapy involves discontinuation of the antibiotics and, in cases of pseudomembranous colitis, administration of metronidazole (Flagyl), 500 mg four times a day for 7 days (see Chapter 26). This antibiotic is effective against clostridial organisms, and the response is fairly rapid. Relapses after discontinuation of metronidazole have been reported. In such cases, vancomycin, a much more expensive drug, should be prescribed, 125 to 500 mg four times a day for 7 days.

Oral cholestyramine has also been used effectively to bind the toxin. Antidiarrheal medications are contraindicated as they may actually prolong the duration of the disease. It is probably not necessary to treat patients who are found to have *C. difficile* toxin-positive stools, as is common in nursing homes, unless there are accompanying symptoms. Relapses are common and when they occur, a course of vancomycin for at least 10 days is appropriate (even if metronidazole was prescribed initially).

Postsurgical Diarrhea

A variety of surgical procedures may result in diarrhea. Obviously, *extensive small bowel resections*, e.g., for mesenteric vascular occlusions, result in severe diarrhea and steatorrhea. Management of such patients requires careful attention to nutritional factors and often requires narcotics for control of the diarrhea. Long-term home hyperalimentation has allowed patients to overcome the severe malabsorption that would accompany massive small bowel resection.

Resection of the ileum is less well tolerated than is resection of the jejunum since the ileum serves as the only site for absorption of bile acids. When the ileal resection is limited (less than 100 cm), the total bile acid pool remains sufficient to prevent significant steatorrhea. However, there is still an excessive loading of bile salts into the colon where they stimulate mucosal secretion and result in diarrhea. Therapy for this form of diarrhea is aimed at binding the fecal bile acids with an agent such as cholestyramine. The dose is 4 g given before meals and at bedtime. When ileal resection is more extensive (greater than 100 cm), the total bile acid pool becomes diminished below the critical level needed for proper digestion and absorption of fat, and steatorrhea develops. The use of cholestyramine in this situation only further depletes the bile acid pool and worsens the steatorrhea and diarrhea. Therefore, dietary fat should be supplied in the form of medium chain triglycerides, which do not require bile salts for absorption. Commercial preparations are available (e.g., Portagen), and consultation with a nutritionist as well as a gastroenterologist is recommended.

Diarrhea may also follow *gastric surgery*. At times the vagotomy causes diarrhea by altering intestinal motility and, for unclear reasons, by increasing the concentration of fecal bile salts. Therapy with cholestyramine has been successful in this postvagotomy syndrome. Gastric surgery may also unmask a latent lactase deficiency or, rarely, a latent celiac sprue. The blind loop syndrome with resultant bacterial overgrowth, dumping syndrome, inadvertent gastroileal anastomosis, and gastrocolic fistula are all complications that may result in diarrhea in patients after gastrectomy (see Chapter 37).

Diarrhea occurs rarely after routine cholecystectomy, associated with an increased concentration of fecal bile salts. Therapy with cholestyramine is effective. Subtotal colectomy, with an ileal-rectal anasto-mosis (e.g., for multiple polyposis), frequently results in diarrhea that is usually easily controlled by antidiarrheal medication (see below) and diminishes with time. Segmental colonic resection usually does not result in diarrhea.

Symptomatic Antidiarrheal Therapy

Diarrhea is merely a symptom, and therapy, if possible, should be directed at the primary underlying process. However, a wide variety of agents are available for symptomatic control of diarrhea. The efficacy of these agents is highly variable, and the mechanism of action of many is poorly understood. Symptomatic treatment should be avoided in patients with acute infectious diarrhea (except in minimal doses to prevent marked discomfort), since early suppression of bowel movements in these conditions prolongs the diarrhea.

Hydrophilic bulk-forming agents, like psyllium (Metamucil, Konsyl), have been shown to improve the consistency of ileostomy and colostomy effluent (see Chapter 42). These agents, which paradoxically are also used in treating constipation (see page 446), are particularly useful in patients with irritable bowel syndrome (Chapter 40).

Another group of antidiarrheal medications consists of those classified as *adsorbents* on the premise that these agents adsorb factors within the intestinal lumen that cause diarrhea. Medications of this group include kaolin and pectin (Kaopectate), bismuth salts (Pepto-Bismol), aluminum hydroxide (Amphojel), and cholestyramine (Questran). Most of these agents are available over the counter, but their value is not well established. Pepto-Bismol has been shown, however, to be effective in controlling the symptoms of traveler's diarrhea (see Chapter 26). Cholestyramine, as previously mentioned, is effective in treating bile acid-induced diarrhea, as occurs in patients after ileal resection, vagotomy, or cholecystectomy. This drug also may bind other compounds, like digoxin and warfarin, and thereby decrease their absorption.

Opiate and opioid derivatives are probably the most effective antidiarrheal medications. Opiate drugs delay the transit of intraluminal contents through the small and large intestine. A possible central effect cannot be excluded. In patients with extensive small bowel resection, tincture of opium or codeine may be the only effective form of therapy. The synthetic agents, diphenoxylate-atropine (Lomotil) and loperamide (Imodium) are effective also and generally are very well tolerated. The atropine in Lomotil contributes little to its antidiarrheal effect and may cause significant toxicity. Imodium has the theoretical advantages of a more favorable ratio of gastrointestinal effects to central nervous system effects and a longer duration of action. Imodium has the practical disadvantage of being relatively expensive. The development of megacolon, prolongation of symptoms, and worsening of pseudomembranous colitis have all been linked to the injudicious use of these agents in patients with bacterial diarrhea. The potential risk for abuse is theoretically less for Imodium.

Another class of drugs that is under investigation is classified as "antisecretory." Some of these drugs inhibit the synthesis of prostaglandins, which increase intestinal secretion by stimulating adenylate cyclase activity within intestinal cells. (Adenylate cyclase is the enzyme that catalyzes the formation of cyclic AMP, the concentration of which influences certain transport systems in cell membranes.) Other drugs of this class inhibit adenylate cyclase directly. For example, indomethacin (Indocin) inhibits prostaglandin synthesis and has been shown experimentally to inhibit the effect of enterotoxin; and propranolol, an inhibitor of adenylate cyclase, suppresses bile acid-induced fluid accumulation in intestinal loops. Certain diuretics, like ethacrynic acid, which act on electrolyte transport, also have been shown to be effective enterotoxin antagonists. Endorphin-like peptides are also under study as antidiarrheal agents. Although these antisecretory agents are not now recommended for use in antidiarrheal therapy, investigation into their mechanism of action may lead to the development of new effective forms of therapy against diarrhea.

Because there are few data to allow an objective comparison of the various antidiarrheal medications, the choice of drug must be based on efficacy, safety, and cost. For acute self-limited illnesses, drugs like kaolin-pectate and bismuth salts are often tried by patients, even before a physician is consulted. For such patients, diphenoxylate-atropine or loperamide is highly effective. Patients should be instructed to use medication after a diarrheal movement, not to exceed 8 tablets/day. Loperamide may provide longer diarrhea-free intervals with fewer side effects (6).

For patients with chronic diarrhea, the choice of medication is based on the severity of the diarrhea and on its cause. In patients with the diarrhea-predominant form of the irritable bowel syndrome (Chapter 40), hydrophilic agents may be useful. The dose should be titrated to the desired bowel habits, with doses ranging from 1 teaspoon to 2 tablespoons/day mixed in 8 ounces of juice or water. In patients with diarrhea from other causes diphenoxylate-atropine or loperamide should be tried. These medications can be given in divided doses throughout the day. Diarrhea can also be prevented by taking one or two tablets before engaging in an event associated with diarrhea (meals, examinations, etc).

In more severe cases of diarrhea, narcotics are necessary. Tincture of opium is convenient because it can easily be titrated (by the drop) to control diarrhea at the lowest possible dose. A recommended starting dose is six drops every 4 to 6 hours, to be adjusted by one or two drops per dose depending on the patient's response. Codeine, at a dose of 15 to 30 mg, may also be used with the same dosage schedule.

General References

Cranston D, McWhinnie D, Collin J: Dietary fibre and gastrointestinal disease. Br J Surg 75:508, 1988.

Review of relationship of fiber to constipation, diverticular disease, and colorectal cancer.

Gerding DN: Disease associated with *Clostridium difficile* infection. Ann Intern Med 110:255, 1989.

A good review of the clinical spectrum from asymptomatic carriers to fulminant disease.

Sawer MK, Gehlbach SH: Bacterial disease of the colon. *Prim Care* 15:125, 1988.

Good review. Emphasizes selection of patients with self-limited disease and discusses oral rehydration as primary treatment in these patients.

Smith PD, Janoff EN: Infectious diarrhea in HIV infection. *Gastroenterol Clin North Am* 17:587, 1988.

Specific References

1. Dupont HL, Hornick RB: Adverse effects of Lomotil therapy in shigellosis. JAMA 226:1525, 1973.
2. Erickson RA: Disaccharidase insufficiency and other disorders of carbohydrate digestion. In: Gitnick G (ed): *Principles and Practice of Gastroenterology and Hepatology.* New York, Elsevier, 1988. p. 405.
3. Harvey RF, Pomare EW, Heaton KW: Effects of increased dietary fibre on intestinal transit. Lancet 1:1278, 1983.
4. Kaufman N, Schuster M: Colonic motility studies differentiate three types of constipation. Gastroenterology 76:1166, 1979.
5. Metcalf AM, Phillips SF, Zinsmeister AR, et al: Simplified assessment of segmental colonic transit. Gastroenterology 92:40, 1987.
6. Palmer KR, Corbett CL, Holdsworth CD: Double blind cross-over study comparing loperamide, codeine, and diphenoxylate in the treatment of chronic diarrhea. Gastroenterology 79:1272, 1980.
7. Payler DK, Pomare EWJ, Heaton KW, et al: The effect of wheat bran on intestinal transit. Gut 16:209, 1975.
8. Wrenn K: Current concepts: fecal impaction. N Engl J Med 321:658, 1989.

C H A P T E R 40

Irritable Bowel Syndrome

MARVIN M. SCHUSTER, M.D.

DEFINITION AND EPIDEMIOLOGY

Irritable bowel syndrome (IBS) is the most common gastrointestinal condition encountered in medical practice. The syndrome is diagnosed on the basis of (a) abdominal pain, (b) altered bowel habits, and (c) the absence of detectable organic pathology. A related condition, painless (or "nervous") diarrhea, should be considered either as a separate entity, or at best a variant of IBS, because it affects persons with different personality profiles, is more directly and immediately related to emotional stress, and has a different course and prognosis. Symptoms of IBS generally appear during late teenage years or in the early twenties and more commonly afflict women than men, the disorder having a female to male predominance of 2:1. The symptoms rarely appear for the first time after the age of 50, and therefore this diagnosis should be made extremely reluctantly in the older patient who has had a recent onset of symptoms. There is some question about whether recurrent abdominal pain of childhood is a form of IBS or leads to IBS in later life.

There are many other terms by which irritable bowel syndrome is known. These include mucus colitis, nervous colitis, spastic colon, nervous colon, irritated colon, and unstable colon. The term "colitis" is especially inappropriate since no inflammation is present and since it is frightening to the patient, who easily confuses it with ulcerative colitis. This misconception imposes unnecessary stress on patients whose condition is readily aggravated by stress. The term irritable bowel syndrome is more appropriate than other terms because it refers to general gastrointestinal irritability, indicating that areas other than the colon may be involved, and it also emphasizes that this is a syndrome and not a specific disease.

PATHOPHYSIOLOGY

The signs and symptoms of irritable bowel syndrome appear related predominantly to exaggeration of normal intestinal motility patterns. In normal subjects the dominant type of motor activity is that of segmenting contractions, which tend to retard the forward movement of intraluminal contents. This impeding activity represents about 90% or more of the wave types recorded in normal individuals. When this type of activity is excessive, constipation ensues. In diarrheal states this activity is markedly diminished or abolished and is replaced by infrequent mass propulsive movements (which may occur five or six times a day during episodes of diarrhea). The symptoms of irritable bowel syndrome (abdominal pain, constipation, diarrhea) are related to excessively strong, spastic contractions either of the segmenting (impeding) or of the propulsive type. The motility pattern of IBS has been described as the paradoxical motility of constipation and diarrhea, but the paradox is a spurious one, if these basic principles are understood.

Motility can be influenced by a number of factors such as meals, emotionally stressful situations, anxiety, and various drugs (e.g., opiates). In IBS, exacerbation of symptoms by meals (i.e., pain, distension, and occasional diarrhea) is thought to be related to an exaggeration of the normal biphasic postprandial response—the gastroileocolic response, which consists of an early neurogenic (reflex) component during the first 15 to 30 minutes postprandially, and hormonally stimulated contractions that appear after 40 minutes. The hormonal phase may be initiated by gastrointestinal hormones released during feeding. For example cholecystokinin, which is released as food enters the duodenum, can reproduce postprandial symptoms in some patients with IBS, and these symptoms are associated with increased motility. Whether this or other hormones of this type are clinically important is unknown.

DIAGNOSIS

History

Most patients with IBS come to medical attention after their symptoms have been present for months or years. Major complaints are those of pain and altered bowel habits. Which of these two components is emphasized depends on which is the more disturbing to the patient. This, in turn, is determined by the intensity of each symptom, by the patient's reaction to it, and by the disruptive effects of the symptom on the patient's function and activities. For example, some patients are less bothered by abdominal pain, which can be hidden from others, but are perturbed by urgent diarrhea, which interferes with their job or social functions. The pattern of symptoms varies considerably from person to person but remains fairly consistent for a given individual, with changes for an individual occurring predominantly in intensity or frequency of occurrence. Typically, symptoms are intermittent with symptom-free periods lasting days, weeks, or, rarely, months. An occasional patient will have symptoms every day.

Pain

The quality of pain may be described by one patient as crampy, by another as sharp or burning. For most, the pain is relieved temporarily by a bowel movement. One of the most important features that differentiates functional from organic pain is that the pain does not awaken the patient from sleep. It is important that the question concerning this feature is carefully phrased, since there is an important distinction between awakening with pain and being awakened by pain. Patients with IBS who are depressed have early morning awakening, and, after awakening, experience pain; but close questioning can determine that the patient was not awakened by the pain. The location of pain may vary from person to person but is fairly consistent for a given person. Pain may be localized to any quadrant, although it is more common in the lower abdomen than anywhere else and in the left lower quadrant more common than in the right. Although the pain usually does not radiate, some patients describe transmission into the lower back or down the legs. The distribution of the pain is generally over a wide enough area so that the patient, when asked to point to the location of the pain, does so with the flat of his hand rather than with a finger, and often makes a circular motion covering a broad area. More often than not, the onset of pain does not appear to correlate with any known precipitating stressful event; instead, periods of illness may correlate with general periods of stress over months or years. It is important to determine what life experiences or interpersonal relationships constitute stress for a particular person so that this can be taken into account when establishing a treatment program.

Altered Bowel Habits

The altered pattern of defecation in patients with irritable bowel syndrome may consist of constipation, diarrhea, or, more commonly, alternating constipation and diarrhea, with one of the two predominating. (Chapter 39 discusses these symptoms in detail.) As with pain, the altered pattern of defecation, though variable from person to person, is fairly consistent for a given individual, changing only in periodicity and intensity.

Not infrequently the major disordered bowel function occurs in the morning, with the first stool being normal in consistency followed in rapid succession by increasingly loose stools, sometimes associated with flatulence and sometimes also precipitated by meals. The bowel movements are accompanied by a great deal of urgency and are preceded by cramps that are relieved by defecation. Formed stools are often compressed and of narrow pencil-sized diameter because of the molding effect of rectosigmoid spasm. In other instances spasm of the colon results in the passage of scybalous stools described by the patient as dehydrated pellets. Mucus may cover the stools or be passed separately. Stools may mistakenly be referred to as diarrheal when they consist of frequently passed small quantities of soft fragments that are narrow in caliber. Explosive defecation may result from evacuation of gas along with the stool.

Painless Diarrhea. Patients who present with diarrhea but do not have abdominal pain generally are thought to have a disorder that is different from irritable bowel syndrome, although sometimes painless diarrhea is classified as a variant of the irritable bowel syndrome. Compared with patients with IBS their symptoms are more directly related to a stressful event, follow more immediately upon that stress, and respond more readily and dramatically to alleviation of stress. Also the prognosis is generally better than it is in classical IBS.

Relationship of Symptoms to Meals

Some, but not all, patients with IBS experience exacerbation of their symptoms postprandially (see above). They appear to be a special subset of patients. Some patients report intolerance of specific foods, most commonly milk, caffeine, fried foods, and red wine.

Gas

Intestinal gas derives either from swallowing of air, from bacterial breakdown of poorly digested foods, or from diminished absorption of gas (which may occur during the rapid transit that accompanies diarrhea). Aerophagia is aggravated by frequent swallowing while chewing gum and during nervous states and is induced by a dry throat or by the excessive intake of carbonated beverages, including beer. Increased gas production follows eating of legumes (beans, for example) that contain stachyose and raffinose, substances that can only be digested by colonic flora, resulting in release of large amounts of hydrogen in the colon. If patients have milk intolerance because of lactase deficiency, undigested lactose enters into the colon where it is broken down by colonic bacteria, also resulting in gaseous distension.

Although gaseous distension is a frequent complaint, actual measurements have demonstrated that patients with IBS have no more gas than do normal subjects. Instead, they have a decreased tolerance to distension from normal amounts of gas, a factor that may be related to hypermotility of their bowel and to the lowered threshold for distension-induced spasm. Gas, because it tends to rise, usually forms pockets under the splenic flexure, which is the highest portion of the colon in the upright position. This entrapment of air is further facilitated by distal rectosigmoid spasm that impedes its passage. The *splenic flexure syndrome* that ensues is experienced as chest pain, which may mimic the pain of myocardial ischemia. A similar hepatic flexure syndrome can accompany gas trapped on the right side and may mimic the pain of cholecystitis. Relief often occurs with passage of gas.

Studies in which air has been instilled into the small bowel have demonstrated that patients with IBS tend to reflux gas more readily into the stomach than do normal subjects, which may explain their complaint of increased belching. This complaint also seems to result from abnormal intestinal motility.

Upper Gastrointestinal Symptoms

One-fourth to one-half of patients with IBS complain of dyspeptic symptoms such as heartburn, "indigestion," pain, and nausea (but rarely vomiting). These upper gastrointestinal symptoms reinforce the concept that the motor abnormality is not restricted to the colon alone.

Significance of Weight Loss and Bleeding

Irritable bowel syndrome per se is not associated with either weight loss or gastrointestinal bleeding, and the appearance of either of these two symptoms in patients with IBS should alert the physician to another disorder. However, significant depression accompanying irritable bowel syndrome may explain substantial weight loss, just as anal fissures or hemorrhoids resulting from the altered bowel habits of the syndrome may explain bright red rectal bleeding. Nevertheless, either of these two symptoms warrants a meticulous search for other disorders, including cancer. A sudden change in symptom pattern after a period of many years also warrants a search for a new disorder.

Psychological Factors

Seventy percent of patients with IBS have abnormal scores on psychological testing (see Table 40.1). The psychological disturbances that most commonly accompany irritable bowel syndrome are somatoform disorder, anxiety, depression, and cancerphobia. Of these, anxiety

Table 40.1.
Psychological Features of Irritable Bowel Syndrome[a]

Psychopathology	Diagnostic Features	Treatment
Depression	Sad, tearful, hopeless, fatigue, loss of interest, early morning awakening	Antidepressant medication, environmental manipulation
Anxiety	Symptoms increased by stress	Relaxation training; environmental manipulation; learn coping techniques
Gratification from illness behavior	Symptoms often interfere with work or socializing	Treat as a physical deformity; encourage maximal activity; discourage talking to others about illness; recognize chronic nature of disorder
Cancer phobia	Patient or family reports fear; patient describes similarity of his symptoms with a known cancer victim	Adequate early workup, then limit further investigation; discuss openly with patient

[a] After Whitehead WE, Schuster MM: Psychological management of irritable bowel syndrome. *Prac Gastroenterol* 3:32, 1979.

is the most readily detected and perhaps the easiest to treat by pharmacological means, by psychological approaches, or by environmental manipulation. Depression is generally masked and is commonly overlooked by patient and physician alike (see Chapter 15). This is in part because somatization, a common manifestation of depression, results in a focus upon complaints that may misdirect the physician's attention from underlying psychological factors. Depression should be suspected in patients who appear preoccupied or sad or who by their report or the report of family members have lost interest in matters that formerly interested them.

Community studies comparing people with IBS who do not seek medical attention with those who do demonstrate that patients who seek medical attention have more psychological distress then those who do not (3). Cancerphobia may be suggested when the patient compares his symptoms with those of a relative or friend who has had cancer. In addition to determining whether the patient has an unwarranted and excessive fear of cancer, an attempt should be made to elicit from him and from other informants any other fears or concerns that the patient has with respect to himself and his illness.

Physical Examination

Except for an anxious demeanor, patients with IBS usually look remarkably healthy, and physical examination is correspondingly normal with the frequent exception of mildly increased tympany to percussion over one or more areas of the colon and a tender cord-like sigmoid palpable in the left lower quadrant. A palpable sigmoid itself is not an unusual finding, even in normal people, because firm stool may be present in this area, but tenderness is significant. Tenderness may be present in other areas also, particularly in the right lower quadrant, where a squishy cecum may be palpated.

Digital rectal examination is usually unremarkable but may reveal excessive tenderness. Proctoscopic examination should demonstrate no structural abnormality but often does reveal rectal and rectosigmoid spasm and excessive tenderness that precludes advance beyond 12 or 13 cm. At times excessive mucus is encountered.

In patients with symptoms of IBS, the physician should look for signs of hyperthyroidism, masses, ad-

enopathy, and partial intestinal obstruction as well as for abdominal bruits, which might signal ischemic intestinal angina in the elderly.

Laboratory Tests

Basic laboratory tests should be carried out to demonstrate the absence of anemia, a normal white blood cell count and sedimentation rate, the absence of blood, ova, and parasites on three stool examinations, a negative sigmoidoscopy, and (when symptoms are severe enough or prolonged enough to warrant the study) a barium enema negative except for spastic contractions. Effacement of haustra may be seen in the barium enema if there has been prolonged laxative abuse (see Chapter 39). Occasionally a small bowel series will be necessary to rule out Crohn's disease, especially when diarrhea predominates or when there is associated weight loss. Painful splenic flexure symptoms sometimes require studies to rule out coronary artery disease (see Chapter 57).

The basic principle in the selection and timing of laboratory tests is to perform as early as possible those tests that are necessary to convince both the physician and the patient that organic disease has been ruled out. It is generally imprudent to postpone some tests for a later date or to repeat tests continually, since this behavior arouses the suspicion that the diagnosis is uncertain, that the disease might be progressive, or that a new and more dire consequence such as cancer or colitis, may be developing.

Differential Diagnosis

Many of the symptoms of irritable bowel syndrome are nonspecific and can be produced by other disorders. A careful travel history should be obtained relative to possible bacterial infection or parasitic infestation, including giardiasis and amoebiasis.

Because patients with lactose intolerance often do not associate their symptoms with milk, the failure to find a direct relationship between milk intake and diarrhea should not dissuade the physician from testing for milk tolerance. Lactose intolerance is best ruled out by a therapeutic trial on a lactose-free diet (see sample lactose-free diet, Table 40.2) for 3 weeks, eliminating all milk and milk products, including butter,

Table 40.2.
Lactose-Free Diet[a]

Type of Food	Food Allowed	Food to be Avoided
Milk and milk products	Nutramigen and soya bean milk used in place of milk. Nondairy "milk" that does not contain lactose. Lactaid milk.	All milk or any species and all products containing milk as skim, dried, evaporated, condensed yogurt, cheese,[b] ice cream, malted milk, sherberts.
Meat, fish, fowl	Plain beef, chicken, fish, turkey, veal, pork, ham, liver, or other organ meats.	*Creamed* or *breaded* meat, fish, or fowl; sausage products such as weiners, liver sausage; cold cuts that contain milk.
Eggs	All	None
Vegetables	All	Creamed, breaded, or buttered vegetables. Any vegetables to which lactose has been added during processing.
Potatoes and substitutes	White potatoes, sweet potatoes, yams, macaroni, noodles, rice, spaghetti.	Any creamed, breaded, or buttered potatoes or starch and instant potatoes if lactose has been added during processing.
Breads and cereals	Any that do not contain milk or milk products.	Prepared mixes as muffins, biscuits, waffles, pancakes, dry cereals with added skim milk powder. Instant cream of wheat and other instant hot cereals. Read labels carefully.
Fats	Margarines that do not contain milk or milk products. Salad dressings that do not contain milk or milk products. Bacon, salad oils, shortening.	Margarines and dressings containing milk or milk products; butter, cream cheese.
Soups	All except those listed under foods excluded.	Cream soups, chowders, commercially prepared soups which contain lactose.
Desserts	Water and fruit ices; Jello, angel food cake; homemade cakes, pies, cookies made without milk from acceptable ingredients; Ice cream made with nondairy mix.	Commercial cakes and cookies and mixes; custard, puddings, ice cream made with milk; any containing chocolate.
Fruits	All fresh, canned, or frozen that are not processed with lactose.	Any canned or frozen that are processed with lactose.
Miscellaneous	Nuts and nut butter, unbuttered popcorn, olives, pure sugar candy, jelly or marmalade, sugar, Karo, chewing gum.	Gravy, white sauce, coffee, powdered drink, carmels, molasses, molasses candies, instant coffee (Folger's instant coffee and Tang are lactose free).

[a]In all instances labels should be carefully read and any product that contains milk, lactose, dry milk solids, or curds should be omitted. Avoid also whey and sugar substitutes with lactose. For milk products use Coffeemate, soy milk baby formulas, or Lactaid milk.
[b] Swiss, Jarlsberg, Edom, and *sharp* cheddar are the only cheeses allowed.

cottage cheese, yogurt, and soft cheeses. Aged cheeses, such as Swiss and Jarlsberg, are permissible since most of the lactose in them has been eliminated. Yogurt contains little lactose and may be reintroduced later as tolerated. Acidophilus milk (cultured with *Lactobacillus acidophilus*), contrary to popular misconception, contains the same amount of lactose as does regular milk. However, the amount of lactose in milk can be virtually eliminated by adding 12 drops of lactase (Lactaid, obtained over-the-counter) to a quart of milk, which is then permitted to remain overnight in the refrigerator; this procedure reduces, but does not eliminate entirely, the symptoms of lactose intolerance (2). Also, Lactaid tablets or Lactrase capsules taken just before ingestion of milk products will reduce the lactose load substantially. Otherwise, nondairy (lactose-free) substitutes such as Coffeemate, Cremora, or Mocha Mix, may be used. Margarine may be substituted for butter. If all symptoms disappear on a lactose-free diet, then the diagnosis is lactose intolerance. Partial improvement implies that, in addition to irritable bowel syndrome, the patient has lactose intolerance and that some of the symptoms (usually those of gaseous bloating and diarrhea) are due to the intolerance. The therapeutic dietary trial is more useful than a lactose tolerance test, which simply tests the patient's response to a given amount of lactose in a single dose at a particular time (see also Chapter 39, page 453).

Among the other disorders that can mimic symptoms of diarrhea-predominant irritable bowel syndrome are hyperthyroidism, nontropical sprue, carcinoid, Zollinger-Ellison syndrome, medullary carcinoma of the thyroid, diabetic autonomic neuropathy, Addison's disease, Whipple's disease, and HIV-associated diarrhea (see Chapter 34). Constipation-predominant IBS may be mimicked by hypothyroidism, hyperparathyroidism, diverticular disease, intestinal obstruction, and colon cancer. Suspicion of any of these disorders justifies the appropriate tests to rule them out. Further evaluation of patients with atypical symptoms of irritable bowel syndrome should be done in consultation with a gastroenterologist.

NATURAL HISTORY

There is evidence that approximately 15% of the general adult population have the irritable bowel syndrome but have not sought medical attention for it (4). Patients who seek medical attention have more psychopathology than those who do not and may give a false impression of an increased incidence of psychopathology in IBS. Approximately one-fourth of patients who seek medical treatment for IBS ultimately have a permanent remission. It is unclear whether this represents the natural course of the disease or a response to early treatment of mild disease. The patient who is referred for gastroenterological consultation often has correspondingly more severe and chronic symptoms and generally experiences a more prolonged course.

Although there is little information concerning patients with IBS who present to the primary care physician, it has been shown that the course of patients seen by gastroenterologists follows a fairly consistent pattern that is characteristic for the given individual. In fact, the pattern is so consistent that any significant change should be accepted as a warning of a new superimposed problem warranting further investigation.

THERAPY

General Principles

Because the underlying etiology of IBS is unknown, treatment is symptomatic and relies on education, reassurance, diet, supportive and behavioral therapy, and pharmacotherapy aimed at both the underlying motor disorder and its psychological concomitants. Successful management requires an interest in the patient and his disorder, an understanding on the part of both patient and physician of what is known about IBS, and, above all, a recognition of the chronic nature of the disorder, which implies acceptance of a prolonged cooperative therapeutic endeavor.

Education and Reassurance

Treatment begins with the first interview and physical examination, which should be designed to begin to establish a relationship of mutual interest and confidence and which should be thorough enough to demonstrate to the patient that the physician has taken seriously the complaints and is performing all necessary maneuvers to rule out organic causes. At the same time attention to the details of all contributing factors, including diet, emotional reactions, interpersonal relationships, social interactions, and the patient's fears and concerns, provides ample evidence to the patient that these are important factors for him to consider and with which he must deal. The worst mistake that a physician can make is to downplay the symptoms on the grounds that they exist only in the patient's mind. This is incorrect physiologically and therapeutically; a definite motor disorder exists and can be demonstrated by both myoelectric and motility recordings.

It is important to take the time to explain to the patient the present understanding of the disordered motility (see page 458) and the factors influencing it to emphasize that, although the disorder is chronic, it can be managed by appropriate cooperation between patient and physician. The demonstrated ability of the physician to predict the course promotes confidence. Furthermore, if the patient knows what to anticipate and understands that treatment can be expected to ameliorate rather than eliminate the disorder, he is better prepared to face recurrence, which otherwise might be disappointing and frightening. Labeling and understanding the abnormal motor activity can be reassuring to the patient and may provide him with the patience required to wait for gradual improvement. At the same time the positive implications of the diagnosis should be underscored, emphasizing that IBS, though often persistent, does not lead to cancer, colitis, or ileitis and does not alter life expectancy.

Diet

Even when the patient keeps a meticulous daily log relating onset of symptoms to life events (including activities, interpersonal relations, and food intake), it is often difficult to make direct associations with any degree of specificity. It is best to explain to those individuals who have postprandial distress that, although some foods may be bothersome, it is usually the act of eating (rather than a specific food) that aggravates the symptoms. Because a lactose-free diet can provide dramatic relief for patients who are lactose intolerant, it is worthwhile trying such a diet in every patient (as stated above). (Those patients who improve on a 3-week lactose-free trial may then add small amounts of lactose-containing foods until symptoms appear. This will establish the level of lactose that can be tolerated by that person.) Otherwise the most that can be said about food intolerance is that some people react badly to coffee, carbonated beverages, and spicy sauces, although no convincing evidence exists in this regard. Therefore patients may wish to abstain from these foods for a period, noting whether symptoms recur on at least two occasions when each substance is reintroduced. Any food that is definitely associated with precipitation of symptoms should obviously be avoided, but one should be careful not to create a dietary cripple.

Some patients with constipation-predominant IBS derive benefit from a diet that includes a large amount of bran. This can be administered as 2 tablespoons of miller's unprocessed bran three times daily. Bran can be obtained from a health food store. Because it looks and tastes like sawdust, it can be camouflaged in cereal, baked in cookies, or taken with a beverage. Studies in another disorder, diverticular disease, show that the effect of bran on transit and motility appears to be specific and is not common to all fibers (1). Therefore lettuce, celery, and fruits may not produce similar results. Bran has been shown to increase the size of stool and the frequency of its passage. Patients should be warned that there might be some increase in flatulence when bran is first administered but that it will wear off by the end of 3 weeks in 80% of patients. However, 15 or 20% of people find these side effects intolerable even after 3 weeks. Dosage should be titrated for each patient, weighing the beneficial effects against the annoying side effects.

The hydrophilic colloids (bulk agents such as Metamucil, Konsyl, or L.A. Formula containing psyllium seed) may be especially useful in those patients who have alternating constipation and diarrhea. Because of their hydrophilic qualities they tend to bind water and therefore decrease the fluidity of diarrheal stools, while preventing excess dehydration in constipated patients. Initially, 1 to 2 tablespoons of hydrophilic powder are prescribed in conjunction with a meal two to three times a day, and the dose is gradually diminished to once a day (adjusting to the patient's response). It is better to prescribe the agent before or after a meal rather than at bedtime, so that it becomes mixed with the meal as it traverses the gastrointestinal tract. When taken at night the medication can result in the passage of rock-hard stool followed by a gelatinous mass. Patients who are thin should take the bulk agent after meals, since it tends to suppress appetite, whereas obese patients may derive benefit from taking it before meals, thus achieving satiation without caloric content.

Drugs

Although there are ample theoretical grounds for prescribing antispasmodic medication, clinical experience with spasmolytic agents has been disappointing. Nevertheless, some patients improve with antispasmodic drugs, particularly those whose symptoms are induced by meals and those who complain of tenesmus. Well-controlled studies are needed to determine whether anticholinergic medication has more than a placebo effect. When used for those whose symptoms are related to meals, anticholinergics should be prescribed 30 to 45 minutes before meals so that the major benefit of the drug will be available at the time of anticipated symptoms. Patients with tenesmus should take the drug on a regular basis, timing the dose so that it is given as close as possible to 1 hour before anticipated symptoms. There is no evidence that one anticholinergic is better than another, but it seems logical to use drugs that have the highest ratio of antispasmodic to antisecretory effect, so that a large dose can be administered to suppress spasm without producing undesirable side effects such as dry mouth. Mebeverine, a spasmolytic agent with little or no antisecretory effect, is available in most countries outside the United States and is prescribed in doses of 100 to 200 mg four times a day (½ hour before meals if symptoms are meal related). In this country dicyclomine hydrochloride (Bentyl) is given in dosages of 20 to 40 mg, four times a day, as tolerated. The major side effects are tachycardia and orthostatic hypotension. Thus, baseline and follow-up recordings of pulse rate and blood pressure with the patient seated and standing are very important. Dicyclomine should be prescribed in small quantities to elderly people who are susceptible to orthostatic changes; for example, 10-mg doses on a divided basis, gradually increasing to reach the desired effect as tolerated. If improvement ensues, long-term medication for months or years is warranted. Tolerance usually does not develop, but change to a different anticholinergic may be helpful if benefit decreases. A therapeutic trial should be carried out for at least 3 weeks to test the efficacy of the drug.

Significant diarrhea may respond to diphenoxylate-atropine (Lomotil), 1 to 2 tablets every 6 hours while diarrhea persists. The related drug, loperamide (Imodium) has a longer duration of action, and 1 to 2 tablets every 8 hours may be given. Care should be taken to discontinue medication as soon as the diarrhea is controlled in order to avoid inducing constipation, especially in those patients who are prone to have alternating diarrhea and constipation. Patients who have strongly diarrhea-predominant IBS and who do not respond to the above medications may benefit from codeine, 30 to 60 mg every 6 hours, especially if pain is disabling. Because of its potentially addicting qualities, codeine should be prescribed with caution, although addiction is rare when codeine is taken for diarrhea. This is partially because intestinal tolerance to the drug does not develop. The same dose that controls diarrhea at one stage continues to control it subsequently, and escalating doses are not required as they are in patients who have developed central nervous system addiction.

Analgesic medication should be avoided if possible and when needed should be prescribed in the mildest form and lowest dose possible. Aspirin and acetaminophen, however, are rarely effective. Pentazocine (Talwin), 50 to 100 mg, can be given every 6 hours as needed for severe pain, but the number of tablets taken should be monitored. Morphine and codeine (see above) generally should be avoided, especially when constipation exists, because they tend to aggravate spasm; and Demerol should be reserved for extreme pain on unusual occasions.

Gas Control

Most medications designed to alleviate gaseous distension have proven disappointing. However, simethicone (Mylicon), 2 to 4 tablets with meals, or activated charcoal, 4 tablets with meals and at bedtime, can be prescribed as a therapeutic trial. Phazyme 95 or 125, 1 to 2 tablets with meals and at bedtime, or similar enzymes such as Ilozyme, Pancrease, Viokase, Cotazym, etc., can also be tried, although their efficacy has not been documented.

Psychological Management

Psychological management begins with the recognition of depression, anxiety, and somatization of affect (see Table 40.1). Symptoms of IBS often are anxiety provoking and frequently are perpetuated by social reinforcement (secondary gain). Psychological evaluation and management usually can be effectively performed by the interested physician without the need for psychiatric referral. The condition itself is not an indication for psychiatric consultation. Referral should be reserved for those patients who would need expert psychotherapy whether or not they have irritable bowel syndrome.

Psychological management is dictated by answers to the following questions:

1. Is there evidence of anxiety, and are the symptoms aggravated by stress? If so, what are the specific stresses? Stress-induced anxiety can be handled by avoiding or modifying situational factors, and by teaching relaxation techniques (using audio-tapes).* Occasionally mild tranquilizing agents are indicated (see Chapter 13).
2. Is the patient depressed? As with anxiety, attempts should be made to determine specific depressing situations, especially to determine whether simple maneuvers can alter them. If not, the patient sometimes can learn new ways of handling situations that cannot be avoided. Tricyclic antidepressants (see Chapter 15) may prove helpful in depression.
3. Does gratification from illness behavior (see Chapter 12) reinforce the illness? Evidence that this is so derives from the history that the illness keeps the patient from job-related or social discomfort and stress. The spouse, family, or friends respond sympathetically to the patient's symptoms, providing further reinforcement. The patient's motivation is generally unconscious, and it is a strategic error to accuse a patient of trying to derive benefit from the illness. Treatment is designed to reduce the amount of gratification that illness behavior evokes. The patient is asked not to discuss his illness with family members, but instead to reserve his complaints for the physician. In return family members are instructed to help the patient by discouraging excessive discussion of his illness and by avoiding overly sympathetic responses. The patient is instructed to view the illness as he would a physical disability that he would like to overcome by pushing his performance to maximal capacity.
4. What misconceptions does the patient have about his illness? The answer to this question can be obtained from questions directed to the patient as well as to his family members who may provide information that the patient is reluctant to give. A rational explanation of the patient's disorder is necessary, but the physician should also listen attentively to the patient's irrational fears (of cancer, for example) and should deal with them as well. Patience is required since these issues may need to be worked through repetitively. A steady, supportive approach is most desirable, as well as a clear demonstration that the physician is acquainted with and sensitive to the patient, his disorder, and his needs. Regular (although not necessarily frequent) follow-up visits supply reassurance to the patient while "p.r.n." (as the need arises) visits are often viewed as abandonment or as an indication of impotence on the part of a physician who feels incapable of providing further help. Furthermore, "as

needed" visits lend themselves to greater abuse by the patient who is seeking secondary gains (see Chapter 12 for a discussion of the management of abnormal illness-behavior).

PROGNOSIS

Whether treatment alters the prognosis or simply affects the patient's ability to accept or deal with his symptoms has not been established. It is difficult to determine the impact of a specific form of treatment on the natural course of irritable bowel syndrome for a number of reasons. First, each patient is different: some have milder symptoms, some more severe; some have frequent recurrences, some infrequent. Second, patients with painless diarrhea (see page 457) have been included in some of the studies and excluded from others. Prognosis for this group is better than that of IBS patients with pain; and the number of such patients included in any given study markedly influences the results of a particular treatment program. Third, the more serious the associated psychological factors, the more prolonged the course of IBS, no matter what the underlying precipitating factors and presentation. Fourth, physicians are different in their training, interest, background, and approaches. Fifth, various treatment programs have been fashionable from time to time and none has undergone systematic, long-term evaluation in a manner that provides useful scientific data. All of these factors underscore the need for organized, individualized, multifaceted management by a physician who is interested, educated, skillful, and compassionate.

General References

Read NW (ed): *Irritable Bowel Syndrome.* London, Grune & Stratton, Ltd, 1985.
   An authorative anthology by international experts on specific aspects of IBS and its management.
Schuster MM: Irritable Bowel Syndrome. In: Sleisenger MH, Fordtran JS, (eds): *Gastrointestinal Diseases.* 4th ed, Philadelphia, W.B. Saunders, Co, 1989, p. 238.
   Comprehensive review of pathophysiology, clinical features and treatment of IBS.
Schuster MM, (ed): Irritable bowel syndrome. *Pract Gastroenterol* 3(3, 4, 5, 6): (May-Dec) 1979.
   In-depth and still up-to-date symposium consisting of 15 articles by leading experts, each focusing on a specific clinical aspect of irritable bowel syndrome.
Thompson WG: *The Irritable Gut.* Baltimore, University Park Press, 1979.
   A delightfully written overview of functional disorders of the gut including irritable bowel syndrome.

Specific References

1. Eastwood MA, Smith AN, Brydon WG, Pritchard J: Comparison of bran, ispaghula and lactulose on colon function in diverticular disease. Gut 19:1144, 1978.
2. Reasoner J, Maculan TP, Rand AG, Thayer WR: Clinical studies with low-lactose milk. Am J Clin Nutr 34:54, 1981.
3. Whitehead WE, Bosmajian L, Zonderman AB, et al: Symptoms of psychologic distress associated with irritable bowel syndrome. Comparison of community and medical clinic samples. Gastroenterology 95:709, 1988.
4. Whitehead WE, Winget C, Fedoravicius A, et al: Learned illness behavior in patients with irritable bowel syndrome and peptic ulcer. Dig Dis Sci 27:202, 1982.

*An excellent program was developed by Brudzinski and is sold by BMA Audio Cassettes, 200 Park Ave. South, New York, NY 10003.

C H A P T E R   41

Diverticular Disease of the Colon*

LAWRENCE J. CHESKIN, M.D.

DEFINITIONS

The terminology for conditions subsumed under the phrase "diverticular disease" is widely misunderstood. The phrase refers to a variety of clinical states that may differ in their etiology and prognosis. The nomenclature of diverticular disease of the colon is listed in Table 41.1. As can be seen from this classification, *diverticulosis* refers simply to the presence of colonic diverticula , without presuming that there are accompanying signs and symptoms. *Symptomatic diverticular disease* refers to diverticulosis associated with pain and/or altered bowel habits in the absence of evidence of diverticular inflammation. *Diverticulitis* is inflammation of one or more diverticula, generally implying perforation of a diverticulum and is almost always symptomatic. The *prediverticular state* is characterized by the radiographic, pathological, and often clinical features of diverticulosis without the

Table 41.1.
Nomenclature of Diverticular Disease of Colon[a]

Diverticulosis (presence of multiple diverticula)
  Asymptomatic
  Symptomatic (pain, altered bowel habit)
  Complicated by hemorrhage
Diverticulitis (necrotizing inflammation in one or more diverticula)
  With microperforation (local inflammation)
  With macroperforation, manfested by abscess, fistula, peritonitis, obstruction, or hemorrhage
Prediverticular state: Muscular thickening and shortening of colonic wall without recognizable diverticula

[a]Adapted from Almy T, Howell D: Diverticular disease of the colon. *N Engl J Med* 302:324, 1980.

*Dr. Harold Tucker contributed to this chapter in the first two editions of this book.

formation of diverticula. The distinction between these entities is more than semantic, as the pathophysiology and natural history of each of these conditions probably vary.

EPIDEMIOLOGY AND PATHOGENESIS

The prevalence of diverticular disease in the United States is strongly correlated with advancing age: about 20% of men and women over 40, and 50% over 60, have diverticulosis of the colon. These figures reflect a striking rise in the frequency of the condition over the last 70 years (5% of people over 60 were affected in the early years of this century), coincident with the advent of milling, which removes 2/3 of the fiber content of flour. It is known, in addition, that vegetarians have a much lower prevalence of diverticular disease than nonvegetarians. In animals, a life-long low fiber diet is associated with the formation of diverticula, whereas a high fiber diet is not. This evidence has led to the hypothesis that a low fiber diet increases intraluminal pressure and that the increased pressure leads to herniation of the mucosa through weakened or porous parts of the colonic muscle. In support of this hypothesis is the demonstration in some cases of diverticular disease of higher resting pressures in the colon and of exaggerated contractile activity in response to meals and cholinergic stimulation. Thus, both a low fiber diet and disordered colonic motility have been implicated in the pathogenesis of diverticulosis.

Another aspect in the pathogenesis of this condition is the weakness in the colonic wall through which the mucosa herniates to form the diverticulum. The site of herniation occurs at areas of least resistance, most often at points of penetration of intramural vessels through the circular muscle layer. The association of colonic diverticula with scleroderma and with Marfan's and Ehlers-Danlos syndromes suggests that loss of muscle mass or defects in collagen may be important factors. Changes in collagen synthesis are known to occur with aging and may explain the increased prevalence of diverticular disease in elderly people. Thus, the formation of diverticula may also involve a degenerative process of the colonic muscle with a change in tensile strength of the wall of the colon.

ASYMPTOMATIC DIVERTICULOSIS

The majority of patients with diverticulosis detected on barium enema are entirely asymptomatic. The diverticula may be localized to the rectosigmoid junction or may involve the entire colon diffusely. The sigmoid colon is involved almost always (95% of the time). This colonic segment accounts for 75% of all diverticula. It is believed that this predilection is explained by the narrow caliber of the sigmoid colon, resulting in higher intraluminal pressures and hence a greater risk of herniation. The more proximal the position in the colon, relative to the sigmoid, the higher the incidence of diverticula. Rectal and appendiceal diverticula rarely occur.

The natural history of diverticulosis is variable. A large majority of patients never present clinically, either because their diverticulosis is asymptomatic or because the symptoms are not severe enough to cause them to seek medical attention. Symptomatic diverticular disease presents either as painful diverticular disease (75%) or as diverticulitis or hemorrhage (25%). In most cases, diverticula precede the onset of symptoms by several years. In a minority of cases, however, typical symptoms precede anatomic disease (the prediverticular state).

There is little evidence that therapy for asymptomatic diverticulosis is of any value. If the development of diverticulosis is really related to low fiber intake with resultant increased intraluminal pressure during segmental activity, then a high fiber diet may be beneficial. However, there is currently no evidence that such therapy prevents or even delays the occurrence of symptomatic diverticular disease or of such complications as diverticulitis or hemorrhage. Maintenance of regular bowel habits without the use of laxatives is probably the best advice for these patients. It is also prudent to alert them to the manifestations of symptomatic diverticular disease (see below) and to urge them to seek medical care promptly should such symptoms develop.

PAINFUL DIVERTICULAR DISEASE

Diagnosis

Diverticular disease may at times cause abdominal pain and an alteration in bowel habits. The pain may be colicky or steady, is generally in the left lower quadrant, and is usually made worse by meals (presumably due to gastrocolic reflex) and at least partially relieved by having a bowel movement or by passing flatus. Bowel habits, usually during the painful episodes, become irregular in 46 to 63% of cases, with development of constipation, diarrhea, or both in an alternating fashion. Constipation is more common than the other alterations in bowel habit. These attacks are usually episodic rather than continuous.

Physical examination may reveal tenderness, at times marked, in the left lower quadrant of the abdomen. A tender sigmoid loop, which feels like a sausage, may be palpable, but there is no other palpable mass and the entire abdominal examination is often unremarkable. The stool should be negative for occult blood, but rectal bleeding may be found due to coincidental rectal outlet disorders such as fissures or hemorrhoids. The presence of fever, leukocytosis, or peritoneal signs points towards the more serious diagnosis of diverticulitis.

Proctosigmoidoscopy, if performed during an attack, will show a normal colonic mucosa. However, considerable pain and spasm may be caused by the procedure.

The *barium enema* (see Chapter 38, "Patient Experience") is essential both for the diagnosis of diverticulosis and for excluding other reasons for symptoms.

Spasm may be a feature of diverticular disease, but fistulas or a mass suggests diverticulitis, carcinoma, or Crohn's disease.

Therapy

The therapy for symptomatic diverticular disease is based on the assumption that low fiber diets and increased colonic pressure are important pathogenetic factors. Diets high in fiber (see Table 39.2, Chapter 39) are prescribed and have been shown to be effective in improving bowel transit and in relieving symptoms. Commercial preparations of hydrophilic colloids made from vegetable fiber are available and convenient but are expensive compared to dietary sources (see Table 39.3, Chapter 39). Thus, patients should be instructed about high fiber diets, and, if necessary, should be given fiber supplements at a dose of 4 to 6 g (1 tablespoon 1 to 3 times/day in a glass of water or juice).

In addition to dietary maneuvers, anticholinergic drugs or antispasmodic drugs may also be helpful for the relief of abdominal pain. Although these agents are not of proven value for this condition, some patients do respond. Dicyclomine (Bentyl), at a dose of 10 to 20 mg before meals and at bedtime, is an often used initial drug. Other more potent anticholinergics may produce adverse side effects and may aggravate the constipation.

The patient should be told that the course of the disease is unpredictable and that attacks will probably be experienced at irregular intervals (months to years) for the rest of his life. There is no benefit in continuing to take medication for the condition between attacks, but maintenance of a high fiber diet is prudent.

DIVERTICULITIS

Diverticulitis results from perforation of one or more diverticula. Perforation may result from persistently high colonic pressures or from an inflammatory process that weakens the wall of the diverticulum. The perforation may be grossly evident, with fistulization and abscess formation, or it may be only microscopic and well confined. Diverticulitis increases in incidence with lengthening duration of the underlying diverticulosis, and is more common in patients with the largest number of diverticula. Fistulas may form to bladder, vagina (especially after hysterectomy), small bowel, or skin.

Diagnosis

The cardinal symptoms of acute diverticulitis are abdominal pain and fever. In classic cases, the pain is severe, abrupt in onset, and persistent, worsening with time and localizing to the left lower quadrant. The pain is often accompanied by anorexia, nausea, and vomiting. Altered bowel habits, especially constipation, is common. Urinary tract symptoms and purulent vaginal discharge may occur because of fistula formation or because of inflammation of contiguous structures.

Abdominal tenderness and fever are found on physical examination. Localized peritonitis may be noted by the marked direct and rebound tenderness over the involved area, generally most pronounced in the left lower quadrant. The abdomen is often distended and tympanitic to percussion and the bowel sounds diminished. A mass may be felt at the site of inflammation in the left lower quadrant, or on pelvic or rectal examination. Rectal bleeding occurs in about 25% of patients and is usually occult.

Leukocytosis is almost always present. Pyuria and/or hematuria may be found when there is involvement of the bladder or ureter.

The *differential diagnosis* includes painful diverticular disease, carcinoma of the colon, and inflammatory or ischemic bowel disease. The presence of peritonitis, fever, and leukocytosis rules out simple symptomatic diverticular disease. The other conditions are distinguished from diverticulitis by their clinical course and by proctoscopy and barium enema.

The diagnosis of acute diverticulitis is made largely on clinical grounds, but some testing may be useful in confirming the clinical impression. Plain abdominal radiographs (flat and upright or decubitus) may show signs of ileus and the location of the inflammatory mass, or air in the bladder in some cases of colovesical fistula. Plain films are also important in detecting free air due to perforation, a surgical emergency. A limited flexible sigmoidoscopy is indicated in many cases when the diagnosis is in doubt, both to rule out other processes and to see whether there are indeed diverticula in the sigmoid colon. Once the presence is verified, the procedure is terminated to avoid worsening or to avoid causing perforation. Weeks later, after successful medical therapy, it is safe to complete the examination of the rest of the colon, either by colonoscopy or barium enema. This is not so much to make the diagnosis of diverticulitis but to exclude other conditions, such as carcinoma or Crohn's disease.

The diagnosis of diverticulitis is based on the finding of a mass effect on the contour of the bowel or the extravasation of the barium outside a diverticulum. The presence of spasm or thickening of the bowel wall are not, by themselves, radiographic evidence of diverticulitis.

Therapy

Most patients with diverticulitis should be hospitalized, placed on bowel and bed rest, and given analgesics, intravenous hydration, and antimicrobial drugs (such as ampicillin and metronidazole or gentamicin, to treat both aerobic and anaerobic infection). Selected patients, with mild tenderness and low grade fever, may be treated on an ambulatory basis with oral broad spectrum antibiotics (e.g., tetracycline, 250 mg four times a day).

Although more than 75% of patients will respond to conservative medical management, it is wise to obtain surgical consultation early in the hospital course to facilitate operative intervention should it prove necessary. The patient's clinical condition usually improves markedly in 3 to 10 days if medical therapy is going to prove successful. For those patients who respond to conservative management, a recurrence rate of 25%, mostly in the first 5 years, can be expected.

Failure to resolve the acute inflammatory process, recurrent attacks of diverticulitis, and obstructive stricture formation are indications for surgical intervention. It seems reasonable that patients be placed on a high fiber diet after recovery from an acute episode of diverticulitis.

DIVERTICULAR BLEEDING

Diverticulosis is the most common cause of massive lower gastrointestinal bleeding in adults, followed by bleeding from angiodysplasias. Both diverticulosis and angiodysplasia are common in the older population, and both frequently are found in the proximal colon. Diverticular bleeds, in contrast to diverticulitis, occur in the right colon in two-thirds of cases (even though the evidence of diverticula is higher in the left colon). The exact mechanism for initiating diverticular bleeding is uncertain. There is no evidence that dietary therapy reduces the risk of hemorrhage. Most instances of bleeding occur in patients who are otherwise asymptomatic.

Massive hemorrhage is a common mode of presentation for diverticular bleeding though in many cases the bleeding is occult and chronic. It should be appreciated that massive lower gastrointestinal bleeding in a patient known to have diverticula is not automatically diverticular in origin. In 30% of cases, colonoscopy detects a second lesion (cancer, angiodysplasia) equally capable of causing bleeding. Occult bleeding, also, should be ascribed to diverticulosis only after other causes have been excluded by a thorough evaluation (see Chapter 38).

Patients with diverticular hemorrhage require hospitalization for hemodynamic stabilization, diagnosis, and therapy. About 80% of patients will stop bleeding spontaneously. The recurrence rate is 20 to 25% and increases with each subsequent episode of bleeding.

General References

Almy T, Howell D: Diverticular disease of the colon. *N Engl J Med* 302:324, 1980.
    A good review of pathophysiology and classification of diverticular disease. Well referenced.
Levien DH, Mazier WP, Surrell JA, Raiman PJ: Safe resection for diverticular disease of the colon. *Dis Colon Rectum* 32:30, 1989.
Pohlman T: Diverticulitis. *Gastroenterol Clin North Am* 17:357, 1988.
Tedesco F, Waye J, Raskin J, et al: Colonoscopic evaluation of rectal bleeding—a study of 304 patients. *Ann Intern Med* 89:907, 1978.
Trotman IF, Misiewicz WP: Sigmoid motility in diverticular disease and the irritable bowel syndrome. *Gut* 29:218, 1988.
Woods RJ, Lavery IC, Fazio VW, et al: Internal fistulas in diverticular disease. *Dis Colon Rectum* 31:591, 1988.
    The five articles above are good reviews of specific aspects of diverticular disease.

C H A P T E R 42

Care of Patients with Colostomy or Ileostomy

MARVIN M. SCHUSTER, M.D.

Ostomies are openings of a portion of the gastrointestinal tract—usually the ileum or the colon—that have been surgically diverted to the abdominal wall. It is estimated that there are in excess of 1 million ostomates (the preferred term for people with ostomies) in North America. Unfortunately the amount of time devoted in medical curriculum and postgraduate training to the care of ostomies is not commensurate with these impressive numbers, and therefore few physicians have the necessary background to be appropriately helpful to the ostomate. This is particularly unfortunate in light of the fact that the partial or total colectomy that results in an ileostomy or colostomy often cures the underlying condition, leaving a healthy patient who is capable of normal function, assuming that he receives appropriate preoperative preparation and postoperative ostomy care.

Ninety percent of ileostomies are performed for ulcerative colitis. Less often, other conditions, such as Crohn's disease of the colon or familial polyposis, require this operation. Most of the patients are young, 75% or more being between the age of 20 and 45 years of age.

In contrast, colostomies are usually performed for cancer of the rectum, and, less often, for diverticulitis or for neurological impairment or gunshot wounds that have led to incontinence. Both children and young adults with congenital disorders, such as imperforate anus, may have colostomies, but 80% of patients who have colostomy surgery are over the age of 50.

Appropriate management of the stoma begins before surgery and continues for a short period after successful surgery and for a longer period when old problems persist or new ones arise.

PREOPERATIVE CARE

Ostomy management should begin as soon as ostomy surgery is seriously considered. For preparation of the patient to be most effective, family members should be included, since the approach is best tailored to meet the needs of the patient and the family. Preparation should encompass a brief description of the surgery, emphasizing the benefits to be derived, and of the stoma, stressing the fact that the stoma itself need not interfere with any aspect of future life except for vigorous body contact sports. Emphasis is placed on the fact that modern developments in appliances permit normal functioning and that there is no way that anyone will be able to tell that the clad patient has an ostomy. After these brief introductory comments the patient and family should be given an opportunity to voice their concerns and to ask questions, both during this first discussion and later, when the initial shock has worn off.

Many resources are available during the preoperative stage: the informed physician or surgeon, specially trained stoma nurses or enterostomal therapists (most of whom are nurses who have had specialized training at one of the schools of enterostomal therapy), and members of the visiting committee of the local chapter of the United Ostomy Association. The latter are usually lay ostomates trained as members of the visiting committee, who are specifically selected whenever possible to match the patient in age and sex (and frequently in socioeconomic status), so that the patient can identify readily with the visitor. The benefits to be derived from the visiting team cannot be overemphasized; for even the most comforting of professionals cannot be as reassuring to the patient as some kindred soul who has undergone similar surgery, has adjusted to it, and is leading a healthy, productive, and joyful life.

Pamphlets, available through the local ostomy chapters, can assist the patient's acceptance of the procedure, provide an optimistic projection for the future, and educate him in the use of ostomy appliances and in colostomy irrigation. In addition, films on preoperative preparation are available; these can be shown in portable projectors so that they can be viewed in the doctor's office, hospital clinic, or the patient's home.* These films are particularly useful when viewed by the patient after the first discussion of the topic, because they not only depict healthy ostomates who discuss their initial and subsequent adjustment but also provide minimal basic anatomical information and information concerning appliances. Such infor-

---

*One such film is Ostomy: A New Beginning. Available from Milner Fenwick, 2125 Greenspring Dr., Timonium, MD 21093. $250.00.

mation not only allays fears and misconceptions but also provides the basis for logical questions.

What to Tell the Patient about Conventional Ileostomy

Conventional ileostomies require that the patient continuously wear a pouch, which is applied to the body using a skin barrier (a wafer-like adhesive) to provide a watertight seal. In this manner the intestinal contents (a better term than stool or waste material) discharge into the pouch, which can be emptied into the toilet simply by unclipping the end of the pouch four or five times a day. The contents are liquid and usually odorless. The pouch is flat and cannot be detected through the clothing or even in a bathing suit. The seal is tight enough so that persons can swim, dive, and participate in dancing and in sports such as skiing or baseball. Modern materials are so effective that the pouch can be worn for a week at a time without being removed.

What to Tell the Patient about a Kock or Internal Pouch

The Kock or internal pouch (sometimes called "continent ileostomy") consists of several loops of small intestine sutured to each other and opened so that they form a reservoir pouch (artificial rectum) within the abdomen. This reservoir is connected to the abdominal wall with a short segment of ileum and opens into the abdominal wall much as a conventional ileostomy does, except that it can be placed much lower on the abdomen since it will not require a pouch if it performs well. Between the pouch and the short ileal conduit, a nipple valve is constructed by inverting the ileum into the pouch in such a manner that it prevents leakage and therefore provides continence. In order to evacuate the contents of the pouch the patient inserts a Silastic catheter into it through the ileostomy and the nipple valve. The ileal contents then drain through the catheter into the toilet bowl. Although frequent drainage is necessary initially, eventually most patients drain three or four times a day. Because it does not require an external appliance the stoma can be placed near the groin, permitting the wearing of brief attire, such as a bikini.

This type of surgery is not recommended for patients who have Crohn's disease involving the ileum. Moreover, one-third of the operations are not initially successful in providing total continence and therefore require revision, and in some instances more than one revision. These factors need to be taken into consideration when deciding the appropriate form of surgery for the specific patient, especially when patients with conventional ileostomies ask about the advisability of converting their conventional, well-functioning ileostomy to the "continent ileostomy." This operation is also not appropriate for people who have neurological disorders that impair manual dexterity and interfere with insertion of the Silastic catheter. For these reasons the Kock procedure has been largely replaced by the endorectal pull-through operation (see below).

What to Tell the Patient about Sphincter-Saving Operations

The operation that has largely replaced the Kock pouch as a "continent" procedure is the endorectal pull-through with ileal pouch (1). Like the Kock procedure, the endorectal pull-through involves the construction of a reservoir pouch formed by suturing several adjacent loops of small bowel to each other and opening up the contiguous walls to form a reservoir. The distal (efferent) limb is then brought through the rectal stump, which has been denuded of its mucosa; and the distal ileum is sutured to the distal rectal wall from inside. The denuded rectum then adheres to the serosal surface of the efferent ileal limb. Thus the anal sphincters are spared and nerve damage from anterior dissection is avoided. This approach can be utilized when rectal involvement from ulcerative colitis is not so severe that it prevents lifting the mucosa off the submucosal surface and removing it. Generally this procedure is contraindicated in Crohn's disease because of the risk of local inflammation around the intestinal surface and anastomosis and because of the danger of fistula formation. When successful, this sphincter-forming surgery can preserve continence. The construction of an adequate reservoir and the appropriate placement of the efferent limb is technically quite difficult. Therefore, this procedure should only be performed by surgeons who have had substantial experience with the operation.

What to Tell the Patient about Colostomy

There are basically four different types of colostomies: the dry colostomy, the wet colostomy, the loop colostomy, and the continent colostomy utilizing the magnetic cap. Most permanent colostomies are *dry sigmoid colostomies*, which result from rectal resection, usually for cancer of the rectum. Because only the rectum has been removed, there is no alteration of the usual stool consistency. This is an important feature since it means that patients who have frequent and erratic bowel habits, e.g., the irritable bowel syndrome, will continue to have these bowel habits and therefore will have unpredictable evacuation. They will most likely have to wear an appliance. Patients who have more regular bowel habits can often develop controlled evacuations by use of irrigation (enemas) that they initially administer daily for proper control and later in most instances every 2 days. Some colostomates simply wear a small adhesive Band-Aid or gauze pad, although most prefer to wear a small appliance (stoma cap) to protect them against incontinence during those few days a year when they develop the same episodes of diarrhea that affect the general population. Patients who suffer from irritable bowel syndrome (see Chapter 40) or nervous diarrhea before surgery will continue to have similar symptoms after surgery and therefore may not achieve continence during intervals between irrigations.

The *wet colostomy* refers to loose stool that occurs when a colostomy is situated proximal to the splenic flexure. This type of colostomy is usually performed as a temporary bypass and is generally less desirable, since evacuations are more frequent and cannot be controlled by irrigation, and since the contents are malodorous because of colonic bacterial action. A permanent ileostomy is generally preferable to a permanent wet colostomy. The wet colostomy requires an appliance large enough to contain the colonic evacuations.

Loop colostomies and double barrel colostomies are performed as (usually temporary) diverting procedures in the proximal colon. The loop is brought over a glass or plastic rod, and the resultant irregular oblong shape may make a watertight appliance fit difficult.

Research is currently under way toward perfecting a magnetic cap that covers the colostomy in order to provide continence. It is held in place by a magnetic ring sutured around the stoma. The cap is removed when evacuation is desired. At present the procedure is available only at selected centers since there are many complications, and the success rate is less than 50%.

Informed consent for colostomy requires that the patient be made aware of possible postoperative impotence. If impotence does occur, psychological adjustment to it is improved with preoperative counseling. Impotence is uncommon among ileostomates, but some degree of sexual impairment occurs in 80% of colostomates, 50% of whom are totally impotent after surgery. This is due to the wide resection that is necessary for rectal cancer surgery, the major indication for a colostomy, as well as to the advanced age of the colostomate compared to the ileostomate. Patients may be reassured that sexual counseling is available if problems arise and that many couples have found alternative satisfactory means of sexual gratification. In selected patients, it may be appropriate to offer the possibility of penile implants (see Chapter 18). Obviously these concerns are less significant for the female ostomate who does not suffer from impaired performance, although impaired gratification may still be an important factor.

POSTOPERATIVE MANAGEMENT

Only late postoperative problems will be discussed here since the early problems will be managed in the hospital. Four major categories of problems are (*a*) psychological adjustment, (*b*) sexual adjustment, (*c*) appliance management, and (*d*) local and physiological problems. Again, all can be minimized by appropriate preoperative preparation and counseling of the patient and the patient's family by an informed physician working with the appropriate members of the health team.

Psychological Adjustment

A concerted effort should be made postoperatively by the medical team as well as by the family, and particularly the spouse, to restore self-esteem and foster independence. During the early postoperative months men tend to depend on their wives for nursing care, but women seem to prefer help from other women (daughters, mothers, sisters) rather than from husbands. This is explained by the fact that wives express more concern about being physically unacceptable to the husband than vice versa. On the other hand, one-fifth of wives have been reported to react by vomiting, fainting, or showing frank expressions of disgust when first exposed to their husband's stoma. This obviously engenders a sense of rejection, degradation, and loss of self-esteem. All too often little consideration is given by the physician to the possibility of such exaggerated responses or to their consequences. Attendance at meetings of local ostomy chapters is a good way of preparing the family during the postoperative period. Formal psychotherapy may be needed when depression is severe, when suicidal inclinations appear prominent, or when behavior is bizarre.

Sexual Adjustment

When debilitating illnesses, such as inflammatory bowel disease, have led to decreased libido and impaired sexual function, ileostomy may lead to improved postoperative sexual function and more satisfactory sexual relations. This is less often true when colostomies, performed with proctectomy and radical pelvic dissection, lead to neurological impairment of potency. Even in these circumstances psychological factors may play a major role, as demonstrated by a survey (2) that reported that all men who had had extramarital affairs before surgery terminated these relationships postoperatively, feeling that only their wives would accept them. Also, cessation of relationships involving a female colostomate was invariably initiated by the female and was never reported to be a result of rejection by the husband.

In general, impaired sexual relationships may result from neurological impairment, depression with loss of libido, inhibitions due to a sense of humiliation and embarrassment, or, in some unfortunate instances, from rejection by the spouse. An awareness of these possibilities will prepare the physician to assist with preventive or corrective measures. Frank discussions with the male patient may in some instances indicate the advisability of urological referral for prosthesis. Sexual counseling by the attending physician or specially trained counselors may assist in adjustment to alternate forms of sexual gratification.

Appliance Management

Modern improvements have impressively decreased the number of problems that are directly attributable to the appliance.

Skin Problems

Skin breakdown, a problem which used to plague 50% of ileostomates, is now uncommon because of effective skin barriers that have replaced the old cement adhesives. Hypersensitivity to adhesives or to the pouch can be diagnosed when the contour of skin reaction conforms to that of the adhesive or the pouch. If hypersensitivity is suspected, a patch test utilizing the arm or trunk distant from the stoma may confirm the suspicion. Skin problems are more common among ileostomates than colostomates because ileostomy effluent contains digestive enzymes. Skin that has been excoriated by ileal leakage should be treated with a cortisone spray, such as Kenalog, and an antifungal powder, such as Mycostatin, neither of which interferes with adherence of the appliance. Patients with more serious skin problems should be referred to gastroenterologists and to enterostomal therapists experienced with ostomy care. Skin complications for proximal colostomies may be similar to those of ileostomies.

Odor

Odor problems are more commonly encountered by colostomates than ileostomates because of putrefactive bacteria present in the colon. Some bacterial colonization of the ileum takes place after colectomy, but odor problems occur only occasionally in 50% of ileostomates and more often in about a third. Sudden increase in gas and odor may signify partial intestinal obstruction. Dietary factors such as oils, fat-soluble vitamins, eggs, and onions may be associated with offensive odors and may be diagnosed by careful dietary history or by use of elimination diets. Odors may also be due to malabsorption resulting from small bowel disease or resection. A number of deodorants are available that can be placed into the pouch (Nilodor, Banish, Aspirin, and Ostoban powder), and additionally oral bismuth subcarbonate may be helpful.

Leakage

Under ordinary circumstances leakage is rarely seen with new appliances, but may become a problem if pregnancy or postoperative weight gain (as, for example, when a patient has been emaciated from inflammatory bowel disease) may change body contour requiring refitting of the appliance. The stoma may shrink during the first 6 to 8 weeks after surgery, and good follow-up care is vital for at least the first postoperative year. Minimal bleeding at the stoma may occur occasionally and is no cause for alarm. A soft wet cloth should be used to clean the stoma, since dry materials may stick to the surface and cause bleeding. Skin excoriation can occur as a result of perspiration under the pouch, particularly in hot weather. This can be prevented by wearing a cover over the pouch and also by powdering the skin liberally.

Equipment Update

Stoma nurses and enterostomal therapists are usually familiar with state-of-the-art supplies and equipment. Some new products include the following: (a) Sur-Fit flexible flange, which allows removal and replacement of the pouch without disturbing the skin barrier, helps avoid discomfort and skin irritation and allows easy repositioning for supine bedside drainage without removal of the pouch; (b) Stomahesive paste and Stomahesive protective powder can be used to fill in skin irregularities around the stoma; (c) The Guardian two-piece system has the only drainable pouch with replaceable filters; (d) First Choice drainable pouch with convex barrier is a one-piece unit that provides excellent skin protection for flush, recessed, or retracted stomas; (e) Closed pouch styles and closed minipouches are interchangeable with the two-piece units for patients who have colostomies; (f) Stoma caps provide a convenient stomal covering for discharge that is controlled by irrigation. The caps contain carbon cloth filter to absorb the odorous components of flatus.

Local and Physiological Complications

Ileostomates are much more likely to experience complications of this type than are colostomates, and most of these complications appear within the first year after surgery. Obstruction due to volvulus, herniation, or adhesions is the most commonly encountered problem, whereas prolapse, retraction, and fistula formation are seen less frequently. These problems usually require consultation with a surgeon or gastroenterologist and often need surgical correction. Crampy abdominal pains, abdominal distension, vomiting, and excessive diarrheal discharge suggest the presence of obstruction. Gastroenteritis may mimic some of these symptoms but persists only for several days.

Because of the absence of normal colonic absorptive function, ileostomates may be susceptible to dehydration or electrolyte imbalance (particularly salt depletion), especially in hot weather because of sweating and increased incidence of infectious diarrhea. For this reason ileostomates should be encouraged to increase water and salt intake during the summer unless there are medical contraindications. Antidiarrheal agents such as deodorized tincture of opium, Lomotil, or Imodium may be needed during these periods and also should be available during travel to foreign countries where traveler's diarrhea may be a problem.

With these minimal precautions neither ileostomy nor colostomy imposes any dietary restrictions, except that ileostomates should avoid excessive quantities of peanuts or fibrous foods such as bean sprouts, which have been reported to be associated with obstruction. Taken in moderation, however, these foods usually present no problem.

Effects Of Colectomy On Handling Of Medications

For the most part colectomy does not influence drug absorption, since most drugs are absorbed in the small bowel. A major exception is sulfasalazine (Azulfidine), one of the drugs most commonly used for inflammatory bowel disease. The inactive form of this drug is broken down by colonic bacteria into an active constituent that is reabsorbed into the blood stream and secreted in connective tissue of the gut. Colectomy obviously can seriously impair this process. On the other hand because sulfasalazine is most effective for colonic involvement in inflammatory bowel disease, it is not often required after colectomy.

When resection of parts of the small bowel is performed for the treatment of inflammatory bowel disease, the patient is left with decreased absorptive surface and often intestinal hurry. This rapid transit may lead to poor absorption of medication as well as of foodstuffs. Particularly, enteric and sustained release preparations should be avoided under these circumstances. Patients with short bowel syndrome are especially prone to have problems and may benefit from medications prescribed in liquid rather than tablet form, since liquid is more rapidly absorbed.

Residual inflammatory disease as well as bacterial overgrowth in the terminal ileum of ostomy patients may result in poor absorption of vitamin B12, and the need for B12 replacement.

Colostomy Irrigation

Although a few colostomates (having distal colostomy) find that they can have controlled bowel movements by careful dietary manipulations, the vast majority use irrigation to control evacuation. This simply involves the instillation of 1 liter of warm tap water through the colostomy. The replacement of the old irrigating catheter with the blunt cone (which is placed against the stoma to prevent backflow) has virtually eliminated the problems of perforation. Although tepid water is preferred in order to avoid cramping, some patients find cold water more effective. It is normal for patients to have an initial evacuation followed within ½ hour by further excretion; for this reason the patient should be advised to continue wearing the irrigation sleeve (long pouch) with the end closed for ½ hour after irrigation. Cramps experienced during the irrigation may be due to rapid instillation of water, air distension of the bowel resulting from failure to expel the air from the irrigating tip, or from obstruction. Constipation and diarrhea should be handled in the same way as with patients who have intact colons (see Chapter 39), relying on dietary manipulations as much as possible (prunes and bran for constipation and hard cheeses and rice for diarrhea).

General References

Kretschmer KP: The intestinal stoma. *Major Probl Clin Surg* 24:1975.
       Valuable for both physicians and patients.
Schuster MM, Bengel JR: In: Spittell Jr J (ed): *Clinical Medicine.* New York, Harper & Row, 1982. vol 10, Chap 523.

       A comprehensive review directed primarily at physicians.
Sparberg M: *Ileostomy Care.* Springfield, IL, Charles C Thomas, 1971.
Walter FC: *Modern Stoma Care.* New York, Churchill Livingstone, 1976.
       The two references above are useful texts for both physicians and patients.

Specific References

1. Coran AG, Sarahan TM, Dent TL, et al: The endorectal pull-through for the management of ulcerative colitis in children and adults. *Ann Surg* 197:99, 1983.
2. Dyk RB, Sutherland AM: Adaptation of spouse and other family members to the ostomy patients. *Cancer* 9:123, 1956.

C H A P T E R   43

Diseases of the Liver

ESTEBAN MEZEY, M.D.

HEPATITIS

Hepatitis is an inflammatory condition that may be localized in the liver or may be part of a generalized systemic process. Acute hepatitis is usually a self-limited disease. The principal causes of acute hepatitis are viruses, drugs, and alcohol. Chronic hepatitis refers to unresolved hepatitis that has persisted for a period longer than 6 months. Cirrhosis is often the principal consequence of chronic hepatitis.

Acute Hepatitis

Viral Hepatitis

Viral hepatitis is a systemic infection whose principal manifestations are hepatic. The two types of viral hepatitis that are well-defined separate entities are type A and type B. Delta (δ) hepatitis (hepatitis D virus) refers to infection by a defective virus-like particle that is dependent on persisting or concomitant infection with type B virus. The term non-A, non-B hepatitis has been used to refer to those cases that cannot be identified as either hepatitis A or B and are not caused by other viruses (such as cytomegalic virus or Epstein-Barr virus). Most cases of non-A, non-B hepatitis that are acquired by transfusion (see below) appear to be due to a specific virus, now termed hepatitis C virus (7).

The characteristic features of type A, B, and non-A, non-B hepatitis are shown in Table 43.1. Type A hepatitis, previously known as infectious hepatitis, is more common than the other types. It is usually transmitted by the fecal-oral route and has a particularly high incidence wherever persons come in close contact under poor hygienic conditions. A number of epidemics have been described after fecal contamination of the water or food supply. Ingestion of contaminated shellfish has been associated with sporadic cases as well as with epidemics.

Type B hepatitis, previously named serum hepatitis, is usually transmitted by the parenteral route from blood, blood products, or contaminated needles. However, it has also been shown to be transmitted by the ingestion of contaminated blood, by sexual contact, and from the mother to the fetus. The δ agent is transmitted by the same routes as type B hepatitis (23). Its incubation period ranges from 3 to 13 weeks. Infection with δ agent may become manifest as a biphasic pattern of hepatitis when there is simultaneous infection with hepatitis B virus, or as a clinical exacerbation of hepatitis in patients who are carriers of hepatitis B virus with or without chronic liver disease. The δ agent has been implicated in cases of fulminant hepatitis and in worsening of chronic liver disease with more rapid progression to cirrhosis. The incidence of δ hepatitis, however, is unknown.

In the United States 5–10% of all cases of non-A, non-B hepatitis are acquired by transfusion, 40% by parenteral use of illicit drugs, 10% by sexual exposure, and less than 5% by occupational exposure to infected blood; the source of infection of the remaining 35–40% of the cases is unknown (3). It now appears that about 60% of cases of non-A, non-B hepatitis are due to infection with hepatitis C virus (17). At least one other virus causes non-A, non-B hepatitis, usually in epidemics in developing countries or sporadically in developed countries; this virus appears to be transmitted by the fecal-oral route (2).

Clinical Presentation. The clinical symptoms of the various types of hepatitis are similar. However, viral hepatitis, type B and type non-A, non-B, is usually more severe and is associated with a higher incidence of morbidity and mortality and late sequelae. The majority of cases of hepatitis are anicteric; patients have a few nonspecific symptoms such as fatigue and nausea; and the disease is often misdiagnosed as a flu-like illness. The correct diagnosis, if suspected, is made by demonstrating bilirubin in the urine and an increase in serum aminotransferases. In icteric disease the symptoms that usually precede jaundice are anorexia, fatigue, abdominal discomfort, and nausea. Erythematous skin rashes, urticaria, arthralgias, and low-grade fever may also appear. These initial symptoms are followed within 10 days by the appearance of dark urine, often pruritus, and jaundice. It is at this stage that most patients seek medical attention. On physical examination a tender palpable liver is found in about 70% of the patients. Posterior cervical lymphadenopathy and splenomegaly may also be present. Jaundice usually increases in intensity in the first few days and then begins to decrease, disappearing completely by 2 to 8 weeks after onset.

Laboratory Features. A mild degree of transient anemia, granulocytopenia, lymphocytosis with the appearance of atypical lymphocytes, and mild hemolytic anemia, with an increase in the reticulocyte count, are commonly found in patients with viral hepatitis. Both direct and total fraction of serum bilirubin rise, the height reached by the total bilirubin being an indication of the severity of the disease. However, total

Table 43.1.
Comparison of Characteristics of Various Types of Viral Hepatitis

Characteristic	Type A	Type B	Type Non-A, Non-B (Type C)
Hepatitis A antibody	Appearance or increase in titer	Absent No change in titer	Absent No change in titer
Hepatitis B surface antigen	Absent	Present in early stage of illness	Absent
Hepatitis C antibody	Absent	Absent	Appears 4–32 weeks after onset of hepatitis
Incubation period	15–50 days	50–160 days	15–160 days
Route of infection	Oral and parenteral	Usually parenteral, also oral or sexual	Usually parenteral, also oral or sexual
Age preference	Children	Any age	Any age
Seasonal incidence	Autumn-winter, epidemic outbreaks	All year	All year
Severity	Usually mild	Often severe	Often severe
Mortality	0.1%	1.0%	1.0%
Prophylactic value of gammaglobulin	Good	Good with hyperimmune hepatitis B globulin	Unclear
Hepatitis B vaccine		90% efficacy	

serum bilirubin levels greater than 30 mg/dl are almost invariably due to complicating hemolysis. The serum aminotransferases generally rise before the onset of detectable jaundice, may reach levels as high as several thousand units, and may remain elevated for several weeks. The height reached by the aminotransferases in the serum provides only a rough estimate of the degree of hepatocellular injury and is of no prognostic value. However, a rapid fall in aminotransferases from a high peak value to normal in less than 1 week may be an indication of fulminant hepatitis with massive necrosis and collapse of liver parenchyma. The serum alkaline phosphatase usually rises in the early, cholestatic phase of hepatitis, remains elevated throughout the illness, and is often the last serum enzyme to return to normal levels after clinical recovery. The concentration of serum albumin is normal in acute hepatitis. Serum gammaglobulins are frequently transiently elevated. The prothrombin time is usually normal and, if prolonged, is usually responsive to the administration of vitamin K. Prolongation of the prothrombin time with no response to vitamin K administration suggests severe hepatitis; and if the prolongation increases, it is indicative of fulminant hepatitis.

Immunological Features. A marked advance in the diagnosis of hepatitis occurred with the discovery in 1964 of an antigenic substance in the blood that was later documented to be associated only with type B hepatitis. This antigen, initially named Australian antigen because it was first detected in the serum of an Australian aborigine, is now designated hepatitis B surface antigen (HB_sAg). In 1973 the hepatitis A antigen was discovered, and the determination of serum antibodies to this antigen began to be used for the identification of type A hepatitis. Delta agent, which is associated with HB_sAg, was discovered in 1977. Recently an antibody to hepatitis C was developed as a diagnostic test for the identification of parenterally transmitted non-A, non-B hepatitis (17).

In acute type A hepatitis fecal excretion of hepatitis A antigen (HA Ag) can be demonstrated a few days before the increase in serum aminotransferases, rising to a peak during maximal serum aminotransferase elevation, and then falling as jaundice appears. Antibody to hepatitis (anti-HA, predominantly IgM) appears in the serum as HA Ag disappears from the stool and rises rapidly to high levels. Afterwards antibody titers (predominantly IgG) remain detectable for at least 10 years, indicative of immunity against reinfection. Because hepatitis A infection is very common, many healthy individuals have detectable anti-HA in the serum. The prevalence of positive anti-HA is about 30% in the United States and as high as 90% in certain areas of Latin America and Asia (30). Hence, identification of an acute episode of hepatitis as type A requires a high titer of anti-HA of the IgM class or the appearance of or a rise in anti-HA titer in the serum collected during the convalescent as compared with the acute stage of hepatitis.

The hepatitis B virus by electron microscopy appears as a double-shelled 42-nm spherical particle originally called the Dane particle. The outer shell of this particle is HB_sAg, and the inner core contains an antigen that has been designated the hepatitis B core antigen (HB_cAg). The inner core also contains double-stranded DNA and DNA polymerase activity. In acute type B viral hepatitis HB_sAg first appears in the blood 1 to 2 weeks before, and usually disappears by 2 months after, the onset of clinical symptoms (Fig. 43.1). Radioimmunoassay and reverse passive hemagglutination are the only reliable procedures for detection of HB_sAg. (The hemagglutination technique is slightly less sensitive than the radioimmunoassay.) Antibody to hepatitis B core antigen (anti-HB_c) appears in the serum at the onset of clinical symptoms, reaches a peak soon after the maximal level of serum aminotransferase is reached, and then falls gradually, becoming undetectable 1 to 2 years after the infection. Antibody to the hepatitis B surface antigen (anti-HB_s) usually appears during the convalescence when HB_sAg is no longer detectable and then persists for many years. The presence of HB_sAg, IgM anti-HB_c, or a rise in anti-HB_s titer during the acute illness is evidence that the hepatitis is due to the hepatitis B virus (16). Persistence of HB_sAg in the serum beyond 3 months after the infection suggests that the patient has become a chronic carrier of the hepatitis B virus (24). High titers of anti-HB_c but absent anti-HB_s are usually found in association with HB_sAg in the carrier state. The presence of anti-HB_s indicates that the patient has had a prior infection with type B hepatitis and now is immune to reinfection. In 1972 a new antigen termed e antigen was discovered in HB_sAg-positive sera. The e antigen (HB_eAg), although associated only with type B hepatitis, is immunologically distinct from HB_sAg and HB_cAg. HB_eAg appears transiently in the serum during the early phase of acute type B hepatitis. In chronic carriers of HB_sAg the presence of HB_eAg is a marker of active virus replication and correlates with

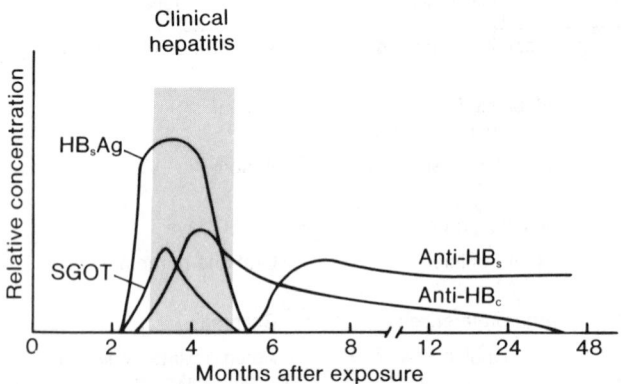

Figure 43.1. Pattern of appearance of hepatitis B surface antigen (HB_sAg) and antibodies to hepatitis B surface antigen (anti-HB_s) and to hepatitis B core antigen (anti-HB_c) in acute hepatitis B infection. (From Mezey E: Specific liver diseases. In Halsted JA, Halsted CH (eds): *The Laboratory in Clinical Medicine*, ed 2. Philadelphia, WB Saunders, 1981.) SGOT is now properly called serum aspartate aminotransferase.

infectivity of the carrier (11). Some studies suggest that the presence of HB_eAg in the chronic carrier is an indicator of progression of acute hepatitis B to chronic hepatitis or cirrhosis.

Delta agent is a defective virus-like particle that is composed of a small RNA genome surrounded by δ antigen and a coat of HB_sAg. Acute δ hepatitis agent infection (23) is associated with a brief rise in δ antigen lasting approximately 10 days followed by the appearance of δ antibody (anti-δ). Initially the antibody is of IgM type, lasting 10 to 20 days, followed by the appearance of IgG anti-δ. A characteristic of δ infection is a lowering of HB_sAg titers; probably hepatitis D virus requires hepatitis B virus for its replication.

Hepatitis non-A, non-B has been transmitted to chimpanzees by serum derived from patients with acute and chronic non-A, non-B hepatitis, suggesting that patients can become carriers of the agent responsible for this type of hepatitis. A portion of the genome of a virus (C) responsible for parenterally transmitted non-A, non-B hepatitis has been cloned and a test for antibody has been developed. Anti-HCV becomes detectable in about 60% of patients with acute and in over 80% of patients with chronic non-A, non-B hepatitis acquired by transfusion (17, 1). The antibody appears a mean of 15 weeks (4–32 weeks) after the onset of the clinical illness. It clears from the blood when acute hepatitis resolves, but persists in most patients with chronic hepatitis (1).

At present the practical diagnostic usefulness of the immunological markers for hepatitis is as follows: Hepatitis A infection is confirmed by the demonstration of a rise in anti-HA titer in the serum collected during convalescence as compared with the acute stage of hepatitis, or preferably the presence of anti-HA of the IgM class. Infection with hepatitis B is usually confirmed by the presence of HB_sAg; but if the antigen is absent and it is clinically indicated, the diagnosis can be confirmed by demonstrating IgM anti-HB_c. The determination of anti-HB_s is useful to find out whether a person is immune to hepatitis B and is a candidate for prophylaxis, a subject that is discussed later in this chapter (page 476). Acute δ infection is diagnosed by the presence of δ antigen or IgM anti-δ. Parenterally transmitted chronic non-A, non-B (C) hepatitis is diagnosed by the appearance of anti-HCV 4–6 months after the onset of the illness.

Management. Acute viral hepatitis usually resolves completely in 1 to 3 months. There is no specific therapy. Bed rest is indicated initially in the symptomatic patient because it often alleviates the symptoms, although there is no evidence that it changes the overall course of the illness (22). As the patient's symptoms improve, a gradual increase in activity is allowed as tolerated by the patient. Intake of a normal calorie, high protein diet should be encouraged, although it is often difficult for the patient to eat because of nausea and anorexia. However, these symptoms are usually minimal in the morning and, hence, the patient should be encouraged to eat a large breakfast. Strict isolation of the patient to his own room and

bathroom is often impractical and probably unnecessary. General hygienic measures, such as washing the hands after contact with the patient and careful handling of stool and blood samples, are mandatory.

Hospitalization is indicated in patients in whom the diagnosis is uncertain and in those who have severe symptoms of nausea and vomiting, changes in mental status, or a prothrombin time that is prolonged more than 4 seconds above the control value. In addition, it is advisable to admit to the hospital patients who do not have somebody at home who can observe and help them.

Nausea can be controlled with oral Benadryl, 25 mg three times a day, or by Compazine, 10 mg two to four times a day, without danger of central nervous system depression. No sedatives or tranquilizers should be given because they may precipitate hepatic encephalopathy. Corticosteriods are of no value in the treatment of acute viral hepatitis.

Patients should be followed at intervals varying from 1 to 3 weeks and should not be discharged from ambulatory care until all symptoms have disappeared and all laboratory tests have returned to normal. Patients are advised not to ingest alcoholic beverages until 1 month after all laboratory tests have returned to normal.

An informative booklet for patients, entitled Viral Hepatitis, Everybody's Problem, is available from the American Liver Foundation (Cedar Grove, NJ 07009).

Liver Biopsy. Liver biopsies are only indicated if the diagnosis is uncertain or if the clinical course of the disease is prolonged beyond 6 months. A specialist in liver disease should be consulted to evaluate the patient and to perform the liver biopsy.

For liver biopsy the patient is admitted to the hospital. Before admission for this procedure the patient should be demonstrated to have a history of normal hemostasis, a prothrombin time less than 4 seconds above control, and a platelet count greater than 80,000/mm³. A liver biopsy is contraindicated if there is an infiltrate in the right lower lung or a right-sided pleural effusion, absent hepatic dullness to percussion, suspected liver hemangioma or abscess, massive ascites, extrahepatic obstruction, or severe anemia (hemoglobin less than 10 g/dl). After application of local anesthesia, the liver biopsy is performed by the intercostal right subcutaneous route using suction with a needle 1.6 mm in diameter. It entails minimal risk when done by a skilled operator. The most common complication is pleuritic pain lasting a few hours after the biopsy, which is noted in about 5% of the cases. The most serious complications are bleeding and bile peritonitis, which occur in less than 1% of cases. The incidence of mortality from liver biopsy is 0.2%.

Prognosis. The majority of patients with acute viral hepatitis recover from their illness without any sequelae. The mortality rate from all types of hepatitis is less than 0.1%. The principal cause of death is the development of fulminant hepatitis, which is more common in type B hepatitis. Fulminant hepatitis, which is rare, usually overcomes the patient within 10 days of the onset of the symptoms of hepatitis. Older patients and patients with other medical illnesses, such as diabetes mellitus, are more likely to have a prolonged course and higher mortality. Type non-A, non-B hepatitis, transmitted by the fecal-oral route, results in a high mortality in pregnant women. Indications of a poor prognosis are changes in mental status, a nonpalpable liver that is also small on hepatic scan, a liver that decreases rapidly in size, or a prothrombin time that is prolonged more than 4 seconds above normal.

Chronic hepatitis and cirrhosis occur in 3 to 5% of patients with type B and in 10 to 20% of patients with parenterally transmitted non-A, non-B (C) hepatitis (2). They do not occur after type A hepatitis. These complications should be suspected in patients who continue to have clinical and laboratory evidence of liver disease 6 months after the onset of acute hepatitis (14). Most patients clear the HB_sAg from their serum within 3 months of the onset of the illness. About 10% of patients with type B hepatitis become chronic carriers of HB_sAg. Chronic carriers of HB_sAg with abnormal levels of serum aminotransferases should be evaluated for the development of chronic active hepatitis by liver biopsy. An increased incidence of hepatocellular carcinoma has been found in carriers of HB_sAg.

Differential Diagnosis. A number of other viruses have been reported to cause hepatitis. *Cytomegalic inclusion infection*, usually clinically inapparent in the adult, can present with manifestations of hepatitis in patients being administered immunosuppressive therapy, who have diseases that are characterized by immunosuppression (see Chapter 34), or after blood transfusions in healthy subjects; the diagnosis can be made promptly by examination of biopsy specimens for intranuclear inclusions and detection of the virus in tissue with specific antibodies. Alternatively, the diagnosis can be made by showing a rise of specific IgM antibody to the virus or by culture of the urine. *Mononucleosis* (caused by the Epstein-Barr virus) frequently is associated with hepatocellular dysfunction with mild transient jaundice in 5 to 10% of patients. The presence of a heterophil antibody, that is not absorbed by guinea pig kidney, or a positive mononucleosis spot test confirms the diagnosis (see Chapter 53).

Hepatitis due to *leptospirosis* should be suspected in patients who have been in close contact with rodents; the diagnosis is established by recovery of leptospiras in culture of the blood or by a rise in antibodies in the course of the disease. *Drug hepatitis* (page 477) presents with clinical features that are indistinguishable from viral hepatitis, and a history of drug intake is a most important clue in suspecting the diagnosis. *Alcoholic hepatitis* (page 478) usually develops after recent heavy alcohol ingestion; the serum aminotransferases are rarely elevated more than 10 times above normal and the elevation is primarily in the serum aspartate aminotransferase (AST). In patients with marked cholestasis, as evidenced by persistent elevation of the bilirubin, high serum alkaline phospha-

tase, and pruritus in association with persistent dark urine and light stools, the diagnosis of *extrahepatic biliary obstruction* should be entertained. An abnormal sonogram may provide a clue to extrahepatic obstruction if the biliary ducts are found to be dilated, and the patient should then be referred to a specialist in liver diseases for further evaluation.

Prevention and prophylaxis of viral hepatitis. General hygienic measures, such as washing the hands after contact with the patient, are the most effective means of preventing the spread of hepatitis from patients to other persons. The patient's dishes and eating utensils can be shared by other persons only if cleaned by heating above 120°C for 15 to 20 minutes in a dishwasher after the patient has used them. Assignment of the patient to a separate bathroom is ideal but often impractical. The viruses are present in feces, blood, and other body fluids of the patients. The handling of all of these materials should be done with care. Because the virus appears in the stool during the prodromal period of hepatitis, the precautions mentioned should be taken routinely in environments where there is a high risk of development of hepatitis, such as in institutions for the mentally retarded. The screening of blood for HB_sAg before transfusion has virtually eliminated the development of type B hepatitis after blood transfusions. Hence 90% of post-transfusion hepatitis at present is type non-A, non-B (C). The development of post-transfusion hepatitis can be reduced further by using voluntary rather than commercial blood donors. Other sources of type B and non-A, non-B (C) that can easily be controlled are contaminated needles, pins used to test sensation, and dental and surgical instruments. All used needles or pins should be discarded in specially labeled bottles containing 40% formalin, which is known to inactivate the hepatitis virus. The preferred method for cleaning surgical and dental instruments is by heat sterilization. The risk that most health workers who are HB_sAg positive pose to their patients is minimal if high standards of hygiene are maintained (18). The exceptions are dentists and surgeons who often develop cuts on their hands while operating. Dentists are urged to wear gloves regardless of whether they are HB_sAg positive to protect themselves and their patients. Patients who have had hepatitis B or hepatitis non-A, non-B and have recovered (clinically and, in the case of hepatitis B, serologically) may be infectious for many years and therefore should not be allowed to donate blood. Spouses of patients with hepatitis B should receive hepatitis B vaccine. Unvaccinated sexual partners of patients who have recovered from hepatitis B may be at risk. Sexual partners of patients who have recovered from non-A, non-B hepatitis may also be at risk.

Standard immune serum globulin (ISG) is known to prevent the clinical manifestations of hepatitis A in 80 to 90% of persons when administered early after exposure. However, it does not prevent subclinical infection. It is indicated for close personal contacts of patients with known hepatitis A, inmates of institutions during an epidemic of hepatitis A, and travelers to areas where hepatitis is endemic. It is not indicated for casual acquaintances or coworkers of the patient or for persons who are known to have anti-HA antibody in their serum. The recommended dose of standard immune globulin is 0.02 ml/kg. For continuous protection of persons in hepatitis-endemic areas repeated doses of standard immune serum globulin, 0.06 ml/kg, should be given every 6 months.

The role of standard immune serum globulin in the prevention of type B hepatitis is uncertain. Hepatitis B immune globulin (containing a high titer of anti-HB$_s$) prevents approximately 75% of cases of type B hepatitis in people who have been stuck with needles contaminated by HB$_s$Ag-positive patients, in sexual partners of HB$_s$Ag-positive individuals, in newborns of HB$_s$Ag-positive mothers, and in the staff of dialysis units (25). It is not indicated for casual or work contacts of patients with type B hepatitis or for persons who have been demonstrated to have anti-HB$_s$. Testing for anti-HB$_s$ should be done routinely before administration of hepatitis B immune globulin provided that the results of the tests can be obtained within 1 week of exposure to the virus.

Hepatitis B vaccine currently is available in two forms, a suspension of highly purified formalin-inactivated HB$_s$Ag particles obtained from chronic HB$_s$Ag carriers and a recombinant DNA vaccine (Recombiax HB).

Chapter 32 contains details regarding indications, doses, and schedules for (*a*) primary prevention of hepatitis B with hepatitis B vaccine, (*b*) postexposure prophylaxis for adults and newborn infants exposed to persons who either have active hepatitis B or are known HB$_s$Ag carriers, and (*c*) postexposure prophylaxis for adults exposed to persons whose HB$_s$Ag status is not known.

There have been insufficient studies to know whether the incidence of post-transfusion non-A, non-B (C) hepatitis is decreased by the administration of standard immune serum globulin. Avoiding the use of commercial blood donors has been a more practical way of preventing post-tranfusion hepatitis but screening of blood donors for anti-HVC will virtually eliminate the problem.

Drug-Induced Hepatitis

The liver is the principal organ concerned with drug metabolism; hence, it is not surprising that it is also a principal target for drug toxicity. Every drug has the potential for producing hepatocellular damage. Drug-induced hepatitis results either from direct hepatotoxicity or from an idiosyncratic reaction (host hypersensitivity). Hepatotoxic reactions caused by direct toxins such as carbon tetrachloride and inorganic phosphorus are dose dependent and reproducible with a brief interval after exposure to the drug. Idiosyncratic reactions are the more common response to drugs. Characteristically, they are not dose dependent, occur in only a small number of individuals who are ex-

posed, and are preceded by a sensitizing period of 1 to 4 weeks of exposure or a history of prior exposure. Drug reactions may be cholestatic, simulate viral hepatitis, or combine features of both processes.

Cholestatic Reactions. Cholestasis is due to a direct dose-related effect of the administration of anabolic steroids and oral contraceptives. Cholestasis occurs in 1 to 2% of patients receiving anabolic steroids but occurs less frequently after the ingestion of oral contraceptive drugs. Jaundice and pruritus are prominent symptoms. The elevated serum bilirubin is composed principally of the direct fraction. Serum alkaline phosphatase and cholesterol are elevated, whereas serum aminotransferases are normal or only slightly elevated. Cholestasis disappears soon after withdrawal of the offending drug.

A much larger number of drugs cause cholestasis due to hypersensitivity. Examples are phenothiazine derivatives such as chlorpromazine, antibiotics such as erythromycin, antithyroid drugs such as propylthiouracil and methimazole, hypoglycemic agents such as tolbutamide and chlorpropamide, and cytotoxic drugs such as chlorambucil. Common clinical features of these drug reactions are fever, right upper quadrant abdominal pain, pruritus, skin rash, and eosinophilia. Serum aminotransferases are moderately elevated (less than 10 times above normal). The clinical and laboratory abnormalities usually subside between 2 and 4 weeks after discontinuation of the drug, although on occasion cholestasis persists for months to years. Severe pruritus is treated with cholestyramine (Questran) given in a dose of 4 g three times a day before meals. Relief of pruritus is obtained in 4 to 7 days after starting this medication. Patients with cholestasis should be hospitalized whenever the jaundice persists unchanged or increases 2 to 4 weeks after discontinuation of the drug to investigate the possibility of other causes of cholestasis (see Chapter 90).

Hepatocellular reactions. Most agents that produce direct hepatocellular damage are toxins rather than drugs. Acetaminophen, however, is a drug that produces hepatic necrosis in all individuals if ingested in a large dose (greater than 10 g), usually in a suicide attempt. Alcoholics and patients taking drugs such as phenobarbital, which are inducers of microsomal enzymes, are at risk of developing hepatic necrosis after the ingestion of lower doses of acetaminophen. Shortly after ingestion the patient develops nausea and vomiting, but evidence of hepatocellular damage often does not become apparent until 48 hours later when serum aminotransferases rise and the prothrombin time becomes prolonged. The patient's condition then deteriorates; jaundice appears and central nervous system depression may occur. The mortality rate of patients who took an overdose of acetaminophen was found to be 3.5% in one large study (5). Thus patients who are known or are suspected of ingesting toxic amounts of acetaminophen should be hospitalized.

Idiosyncratic hepatocellular reactions have been reported after the administration of a number of drugs, the most common of which are isoniazid, α-methyldopa, phenylbutazone, 6-mercaptopurine, and halothane. Asymptomatic increases in serum aminotransferases, which subside despite continued administration of the drug, have been reported in 5 to 10% of patients taking isoniazid or α-methyldopa (31). Because of the frequent transient nature of the serum aminotransferase elevations, there is no need to monitor this test in asymptomatic patients. However, the development of symptoms of fatigue and anorexia or of nausea and general malaise is an indication for determination of serum aminotransferases; if aminotransferase activity is increased, the drug should be discontinued immediately because this often heralds the onset of severe hepatocellular damage. The incidence of acute hepatitis in patients taking the drugs listed above is 0.1 to 0.3%. Women and older patients are more likely to be affected. The onset of the reaction is between 1 and 10 weeks after the start of therapy. The symptoms, laboratory tests, and findings on liver biopsy are indistinguishable from those of viral hepatitis (see page 472). The hepatitis usually resolves within a few weeks after the drug is discontinued. However, a mortality rate as high as 12% has been reported for severe hepatitis due to isoniazid. Moreover, chronic active liver disease can develop if the drug responsible for the hepatitis is continued. Administration of corticosteriods is not indicated in drug-induced hepatitis.

Alcoholic Hepatitis

This condition is seen most frequently after prolonged heavy alcohol intake. Women are more susceptible to alcoholic liver disease than men and it usually does not develop in men who drink less than 80 g of ethanol/day or in women who drink half this amount (equivalent to 8 and 4 ounces of 86 proof whiskey, respectively). Many of the presenting clinical characteristics of patients with alcoholic hepatitis (such as anorexia, marked fatigue, jaundice, and tender hepatomegaly) are indistinguishable from those of viral hepatitis (see pages 472 to 473). However, patients with alcoholic hepatitis are more likely to have fever and leukocytosis. The elevation of the serum aminotransferases is rarely 10 times above normal, and frequently there is a prolongation of the prothrombin time. The elevation of AST is characteristically higher than that of ALT. Patients with alcoholic hepatitis should be admitted to the hospital and a definite diagnosis established by liver biopsy, if not contraindicated by abnormal hemostatic function. Liver biopsy differentiates alcoholic hepatitis from drug-induced hepatitis and viral hepatitis and gives an indication of any underlying chronic liver disease. The illness is often more severe than in patients with viral hepatitis, and decompensation with hepatic encephalopathy and death can occur. About one-third of patients with alcoholic hepatitis have been shown to progress to cirrhosis, often in a short period of 6 months (21). However, if patients are able to abstain from further drinking of alcohol (see Chapter 21), about half of

them will recover completely, both clinically and histologically, usually within a month.

Chronic Hepatitis

Chronic hepatitis refers to chronic inflammation of the liver detected by abnormal liver tests or by abnormal liver histology that has persisted for longer than 6 months. The spectrum of chronic hepatitis varies from a benign reversible process to an unrelenting process that often progresses to cirrhosis. Liver histology is essential both for the diagnosis and to establish the severity of the disease and the need for treatment. Two types of chronic hepatitis are recognized by the examination of tissue obtained on liver biopsy: chronic persistent hepatitis, which is a self-limited disease and does not require therapy, and chronic active hepatitis, which is a progressive process associated with increased morbidity and mortality and which often improves with therapy. In chronic persistent hepatitis, liver biopsy reveals portal inflammation, often with expansion of the portal areas, and focal parenchymal necrosis with preservation of the lobular architecture and slight or absent fibrosis, whereas in chronic active hepatitis there is extension of inflammation and necrosis from the portal area to the hepatocytes adjacent to it (piecemeal necrosis), disruption of the lobular architecture, and increased fibrosis with the formation of intralobular septa of fibrous tissue (bridging) (6).

The principal causes of chronic hepatitis are infection with hepatitis viruses, both type B and type non-A, non-B (not type A), idiopathic (formerly called lupoid hepatitis), and drugs such as isoniazid, α-methyldopa, nitrofurantoin, and oxyphenacetin. In addition, Wilson's disease, α_1-antitrypsin deficiency, and primary biliary cirrhosis may present with clinical and histological features of chronic hepatitis.

Chronic Persistent Hepatitis

Patients with chronic persistent hepatitis are either asymptomatic or have mild nonspecific symptoms such as fatigue. On physical examination there are no peripheral manifestations of chronic liver disease, but there may be mild hepatomegaly. Laboratory tests show mild elevation of serum aminotransferases (2 to 5 times normal), but the remainder of the liver tests are usually normal. Forty percent of the patients have detectable HB$_s$Ag in the serum. The diagnosis is established by liver biopsy and the patient is then reassured about the benign course of his condition. If symptoms and elevation of the aminotransferases persist, a liver biopsy is indicated after 2 to 3 years to rule out a sampling error on the initial liver biopsy. Patients with persistent hepatitis have been shown to have elevated serum aminotransferases for over 10 years without any evidence of progression of the disease.

Chronic Active Hepatitis

The onset of chronic active hepatitis is usually insidious. The patient may be asymptomatic and liver disease may be detected by aminotransferase elevations done on routine testing, or he may present symptoms of general malaise, fatigue, abdominal discomfort, anorexia, and jaundice. In about a third of the patients the disease evolves from a clinically overt episode of acute hepatitis. Physical examination in patients with chronic active hepatitis reveals hepatomegaly and often peripheral manifestations of chronic liver disease, such as spider angiomas, palmar erythema, and gynecomastia. Elevations of serum bilirubin, aminotransferases, and globulins are the most sensitive indicators of the activity of the hepatocellular damage, whereas decreases in serum albumin and prolongation of the prothrombin time reflect loss of hepatocellular function and a poor prognosis. Older male patients are more likely to have HB_sAg in the serum and to present with an acute onset of illness. On the other hand, HB_sAg-negative patients are more likely to be women and to present with systemic symptoms of acne, amenorrhea, arthralgia and arthritis, pleurisy, or intermittent fever. In addition, they may have associated thyroiditis, Sjögren's syndrome, ulcerative colitis, glomerulonephritis, or hemolytic anemia. Laboratory tests on these patients show evidence of immunological hyperactivity: serum γ-globulin is often markedly elevated; lupus erythematosus (LE) cells are present; and there is an increased prevalence of elevation of the titer of antinuclear antibodies and smooth muscle antibodies. In addition, antimitochondrial antibodies are found in 15% of these patients.

The clinical course of patients with chronic active hepatitis is quite variable. Patients can be asymptomatic for a long time, have periods of intermittent worsening and remission, or have a progressive course to cirrhosis and death if untreated (26). Delta agent is associated with clinical exacerbation of chronic hepatitis and more rapid progression to cirrhosis (23).

Differential Diagnosis. The diagnosis of *Wilson's disease* (about 1 in 1 million people are affected) should be considered in all patients, particularly those under 25 years who present with clinical and laboratory features of chronic hepatitis (28). Wilson's disease is discussed in more detail in the section on cirrhosis (page 480). The diagnosis of chronic hepatitis due to α_1-antitrypsin deficiency (1 in 1000 people are affected) is suggested by the finding of an absent or low α_1-globulin on serum protein electrophoresis (10). The diagnosis is established by demonstrating a low value of α_1-antitrypsin in the serum by quantitative measurement and by protease inhibitor (Pi) typing (10). The common allele is PiM, whereas liver disease occurs in about 20% of individuals who are homozygous for the allele PiZ. Liver biopsy reveals PAS-positive cytoplasmic inclusions that are resistant to diastase in both homozygous and heterozygous individuals for the allele PiZ. There is no known therapy for this deficiency, which is transmitted by codominant inheritance. The diagnostic characteristics of *primary biliary cirrhosis* are discussed in the section on cirrhosis (page 480). The diagnosis of *drug-induced chronic hepatitis* (page 477) is dependent on a careful

history and on the demonstration of improvement of the patient after discontinuation of drugs that are known to produce this illness. In most cases chronic active hepatitis due to drugs will revert to normal after discontinuation of the offending drug (31).

Therapy. Corticosteroids have been shown to be beneficial in symptomatic patients with chronic active hepatitis who are HB_sAg negative. Clinical, biochemical, and histological improvement and even remission have been observed; and mortality rates have been reduced after therapy with corticosteroids (27). Prednisone or prednisolone, 40 to 60 mg, is given initially to suppress the activity of the disease and then tapered slowly, usually over a period of 1 to 3 months, to a maintenance dose of 15 to 20 mg. Symptomatic improvement followed by a fall in serum aminotransferases occurs in the first few weeks. Histological transformation to a lesion of persistent hepatitis will occur in some patients within a 2-year period. Treatment with corticosteroids is discontinued in patients who attain remission. In the remainder of the patients it is not continued beyond 4 years because the prospect of remission diminishes whereas the risk of side effects increases (8). Asymptomatic patients with chronic active hepatitis who are HB_sAg negative are usually only treated if they have marked elevations of serum aminotransferases (greater than 10 times above normal) and histological evidence of severe liver disease (marked multilobular necrosis and bridging). Administration of corticosteroids to patients with chronic type B hepatitis is contraindicated because it appears to favor replication of hepatitis B virus, resulting in a higher morbidity and mortality (19). Alpha interferon has shown some promise in controlling the activity of chronic type B, and type C hepatitis (13). However, relapse after discontinuation of treatment is very common (9).

UNEXPLAINED ELEVATIONS OF LIVER ENZYMES IN SERUM

Elevations of serum aminotransferases and alkaline phosphatase are occasionally found in normal subjects or in patients not suspected of having liver disease. In such a situation the abnormality should first be confirmed by repeated testing. Next, it is important to remember that elevated serum aminotransferases and alkaline phosphatase do not necessarily originate from the liver. For example, elevated serum aminotransferases can be due to injury to the heart and striated muscle; if the source of the serum aminotransferases is muscle, the more specific creatine kinase will also be elevated. An isolated increase of serum alkaline phosphatase can originate from liver or bone. The hepatic origin of alkaline phosphatase can be confirmed by demonstration of an elevated 5'-nucleotidase, which, unlike alkaline phosphatase, is present only in the liver and in the epithelium of the bile ducts. By contrast, an elevated serum alkaline phosphatase accompanied by a normal serum 5'-nucleotidase is almost invariably due to bone disease; a very common cause of such an occurrence is a recent bone fracture. Any persistent elevation of serum aminotransferases for longer than 6 months that remains unexplained is an indication for liver biopsy to rule out chronic hepatitis. A persistent elevation of serum alkaline phosphatase in the absence of an elevated serum bilirubin can occur in patients with fatty liver, which is common in the diabetic and obese patient or can be the result of space-occupying lesions, such as granulomas or metastatic carcinoma. A liver scan is recommended in these cases to rule out metastatic carcinoma, but a liver biopsy is indicated only if the scan shows a space-occupying lesion or if there is clinical suspicion of diseases such as tuberculosis and sarcoidosis that may result in hepatic granulomas.

ALCOHOLIC FATTY LIVER

Fatty liver is due to alterations of lipid metabolism caused by alcohol and therefore occurs in all persons ingesting alcohol in excessive amounts. It is manifested mainly by a feeling of abdominal fullness due to hepatomegaly and mild elevation of the serum aminotransferases (rarely more than two times above normal). On occasion marked fatty infiltration is associated with symptoms of malaise, weakness, anorexia, tender hepatomegaly, and even jaundice. These symptomatic patients require admission to the hospital and a liver biopsy to distinguish fatty liver from alcoholic hepatitis and cirrhosis. The treatment of fatty liver consists of abstinence from alcohol. With abstinence the abnormal accumulation of fat will disappear in a period of 4 to 6 weeks. As the patient improves, the liver decreases in size and becomes nontender. Serum bilirubin and aminotransferases promptly return to normal. Recurrent episodes of symptomatic fatty liver are common after heavy alcohol ingestion, but there is no evidence that this lesion in itself leads to cirrhosis.

CIRRHOSIS

Cirrhosis is a chronic diffuse liver disease characterized by widespread hepatic fibrosis and nodule formation. The fibrosis is the result of extensive destruction of liver cells, and the nodularity represents regeneration. For clinical purposes cirrhosis can be classified into the following major categories: alcoholic (micronodular), postnecrotic (macronodular), cardiac, biliary, Wilson's disease, hemochromatosis, and schistosomiasis. The two major types of cirrhosis are alcoholic, which is characterized by regular small nodules, and postnecrotic, in which there is extensive scarring of the liver and the presence of irregular nodules of various sizes (29). On occasion cirrhosis of the alcoholic is of the macronodular type; this is more common in chronic alcoholics who no longer drink alcohol. The onset of cirrhosis is usually insidious and associated with nonspecific symptoms such as fatigue, anorexia, weight loss, nausea, and abdominal discomfort. As the disease progresses, signs of hepatocellular failure become prominent: jaundice, edema, ascites, electrolyte abnormalities, bleeding tendencies, spider

angiomas, palmar erythema, gynecomastia, impotence, and loss of axillary and pubic hair. Hepatomegaly and portal hypertension resulting in splenomegaly and a venous collateral circulation are common. The most severe complications of cirrhosis are hepatic encephalopathy, bleeding from esophageal varices, and infection. Patients with alcoholic cirrhosis often present with recurring episodes of hepatocellular failure, precipitated by hepatocellular necrosis and fatty infiltration induced by alcohol ingestion, which is reversible with clinical improvement after abstinence from alcohol, and after bed rest, and optimal nutrition. By contrast, patients with postnecrotic cirrhosis are more likely to present insidiously with evidence of portal hypertension. When hepatocellular failure occurs in these patients, it is usually a terminal event because it is the result of excessive fibrosis and reduced hepatic parenchymal mass rather than of reversible lesions such as necrosis and fatty infiltration found in alcoholic cirrhosis. Rapid deterioration of patients with cirrhosis should raise the suspicion of a complicating hepatocellular carcinoma. Common laboratory findings in patients with cirrhosis include anemia, a normal or slightly decreased white blood cell count, and moderate thrombocytopenia. The most frequent abnormal liver tests are hyperbilirubinemia, a depressed serum albumin, elevated serum globulins, and a prolonged prothrombin time. Liver biopsy is indicated to establish a firm diagnosis in all cases in which hemostatic function allows this procedure to be done (see page 475).

Differential Diagnosis

The diagnostic characteristics of some of the other types of cirrhosis are as follows: (a) *Cardiac cirrhosis* develops only after prolonged and severe cardiac failure, usually due to valvular disease, particularly in patients with tricuspid incompetence or in patients with constrictive pericarditis. Jaundice, hepatomegaly, and ascites are prominent features, but the diagnosis can only be established with certainty by liver biopsy. Treatment of cardiac failure, in particular of constrictive pericarditis by pericardiectomy, results in improvement of liver function. (b) *Primary biliary cirrhosis* (15) is a chronic disease of unknown cause which is characterized by progressive intrahepatic cholestasis and is most frequently seen in middle-aged women. The principal manifestations are jaundice with pruritus, hepatomegaly, hypercholesterolemia with the formation of xanthoma and xanthelasma, and steatorrhea due to the decreased delivery of bile acids to the intestine. Antimitochondrial antibodies are found in 95% of these patients, and their presence is virtually diagnostic. Liver biopsy in the early stages reveals injury to the septal and large intralobular bile ducts with surrounding accumulation of the inflammatory plasma cells and lymphocytes and with granuloma formation. In the end stages of the disease cirrhosis develops that is nearly indistinguishable from postnecrotic (macronodular) cirrhosis. (c) *Wilson's disease* is a rare disorder of copper metabolism that is inherited as an autosomal recessive disorder (28). Its symptoms are due to hepatic and neurological dysfunction. In children the principal symptoms are due to liver involvement, whereas in adults neurological symptoms tend to predominate. The diagnosis should be suspected in all children or young adults who develop cirrhosis since treatment with copper-chelating agents can arrest the disease and alleviate all symptoms. A characteristic finding that is virtually diagnostic is the presence of Kayser-Fleischer rings, which are greenish-brown rings found in the posterior surface and periphery of the cornea. Because these rings cannot often be seen by the naked eye, it is important to refer all suspected patients to the ophthalmologist for slit-lamp examination of the cornea. Serum ceruloplasmin, the copper-binding protein, is reduced in most but not all cases. Histological examination of a liver biopsy is not diagnostic. However, quantitative determination of copper with a finding of more than 250 μg/g of dry liver weight or the urinary excretion of more than 50 μg/24 hours is diagnostic. Hospitalization is not required for treatment of Wilson's disease with d-penicillamine. (d) *Hemochromatosis* is an inherited disorder of iron metabolism, resulting in excessive body iron; it is principally characterized by cirrhosis, diabetes mellitus, and grayish pigmentation of the skin. Other symptoms are cardiac failure and arrhythmias, peripheral neuritis, arthritis, and testicular atrophy. The iron overload appears to be due to an increased absorption of dietary iron, and the mode of inheritance is autosomal recessive. The disease usually appears in persons over 40 years of age and develops earlier in men, probably because of the menstrual loss of iron in women. The diagnosis is made by demonstrating a high serum iron (greater than 150 μg/dl), a high saturation of iron-binding protein (greater than 50%), and increased serum ferritin, usually in a patient with a family history of the disease (4). Therapy consists of removal of excess iron by repeated phlebotomy (1 to 2 units weekly). (e) *Hepatic schistosomiasis* may occur in persons from tropical areas who have been infected by schistosome cercariae while swimming or walking in infested water. The liver disease is due to the deposition of ova of *Schistosoma mansoni* in the portal areas, with the development of an inflammatory reaction, often with granuloma formation and periportal fibrosis. Jaundice is uncommon in these patients on presentation. The most common laboratory abnormalities are increases in serum alkaline phosphatase and mild elevations of serum bilirubin and aminotransferases. The diagnosis of active infection is made by demonstrating mobile *Schistosoma* ova on fresh examination of rectal biopsy, and the diagnosis of liver involvement is made by showing the presence of ova capsules on liver biopsy.

Management

The treatment of uncomplicated cirrhosis consists of voluntary restriction of activity if the patient has weakness and fatigue, a diet high in protein but low in salt, and abstinence from alcohol (see Chapter 21).

This regimen almost invariably results in improvement of hepatocellular function in patients with alcoholic cirrhosis and occasionally in patients with postnecrotic cirrhosis. Tranquilizers and sedatives should be avoided. Infection and gastrointestinal bleeding, which in addition to alcohol ingestion are frequent precipitating factors of decompensation, should be searched for and treated. Vitamin K, 15 mg parenterally, may improve prolongation of the prothrombin time. Multivitamins and folic acid, 1 mg/day, may be given if the patient's dietary intake does not appear to be adequate or if there is evidence of vitamin deficiencies. Potassium deficiency is frequent and may contribute to the precipitation of hepatic encephalopathy, but its extent is difficult to assess because serum potassium concentration is a poor reflection of the total body potassium. However, when serum potassium falls below 3.5 mEq/liter, the deficit of body potassium is approximately 300 to 500 mEq. This can be replaced over a period of a few days with oral solutions of 10% potassium chloride, which provides 40 mEq of potassium/30 ml. Fluid retention is treated with sodium restriction (500 mg of sodium chloride/day) and diuretics. The induced diuresis should be slow and should result in a loss of no more than 2.27 kg (5 lb) of weight per week because of the danger of precipitating electrolyte depletion and hypokalemia. Diuresis can be initiated by spironolactone, 25 mg orally three times a day. Thiazide diuretics or furosemide can be added to the regimen in gradually increasing doses if diuresis is inadequate. The development of acute hepatic encephalopathy manifested by asterixis or by changes in mental status is an indication that the patient should be hospitalized for evaluation and treatment. Acute and chronic gastrointestinal bleeding is also an indication for hospitalization.

Protein can be restricted in stable cirrhotic patients to 45 g/day without development of a negative nitrogen balance as long as a minimum of 400 g of carbohydrate are ingested a day. A change from animal protein to a vegetable protein diet may also improve hepatic encephalopathy. The exact mechanism whereby vegetable protein is better tolerated is unknown. However, vegetable protein contains smaller amounts of ammonia, methionine, and aromatic acids and also results in alterations of small intestinal and colonic bacterial flora (12). Lactulose is a nonabsorbable synthetic disaccharide that when administered in doses of 20 to 30 g (30 to 45 ml) three to four times a day reduces blood ammonia and improves encephalopathy in over 80% of patients. Lactulose usually is effective only when it also increases the frequency of bowel movements. Other than producing mild abdominal cramps and flatulence, lactulose is devoid of side effects. The mechanism of its action is not well defined, but its effectiveness is related to its ability to trap nitrogen in the stool and decrease ammonia production. Some of the decrease in ammonia production may be due to a decrease in contact time of the stool with colonic bacteria. The beneficial effects of a vegetable protein diet and lactulose on hepatic encephalopathy are additive. Chronic hepatic encephalopathy can be treated with protein restriction and lactulose on an ambulatory basis. Patients with decompensated cirrhosis who are not responding to therapy should be considered for liver transplantation (20) and should be referred to a hepatologist for evaluation.

General References

Hoyumpa Jr AM, Greene HL, Dunn GD, Schenker S: Fatty liver: biochemical and clinical considerations. *Am J Dig Dis* 20:1142, 1975.
> Discusses various causes, clinical presentation, and management of fatty liver.

Leevy CM, Popper H, Sherlock S: *Diseases of the liver and biliary tract. Standardization of nomenclature, diagnostic criteria and diagnostic methodology.* DHEW Publication No. (NIH) 76-725, Fogarty International Center Proceedings No. 22, 1976.

Lemon SM: Type A viral hepatitis. New developments in an old disease. *N Engl J Med* 313:1659, 1985.
> Excellent review of all aspects of hepatitis A, including epidemiology, clinical characteristics of hepatitis A, and prophylaxis.

Perillo RP, Aach RD: The clinical course and chronic sequelae of hepatitis B virus infection. *Sem Liver Dis* 1:15, 1981.
> A review of the characteristics of the hepatitis B virus and of clinical characteristics of hepatitis B virus infection.

Zimmerman HJ: *Hepatotoxicity: The Adverse Effects of Drugs and Other Chemicals on the Liver.* New York, Appleton-Century-Crofts, 1978.
> A comprehensive source of information on drug hepatotoxicity.

Specific References

1. Alter HJ, Purcell RH, Shih JW, et al: Detection of antibody to hepatitis C virus in prospectively followed transfusion recipients with acute and chronic non-A, non-B hepatitis. *N Engl J Med* 321:1494, 1989.
2. Alter MJ: Non-A, Non-B hepatitis: sorting through a diagnosis of exclusion. *Ann Intern Med* 110:583, 1989.
3. Alter MJ, Sampliner RE: Hepatitis C. And miles to go before we sleep. *N Engl J Med* 321:1538, 1989.
4. Bassett ML, Halliday JW, Ferris RA, et al: Diagnosis of hemochromatosis in young subjects: predictive accuracy of biochemical screening tests. *Gastroenterology* 87:628, 1984.
5. Black M: Acetaminophen hepatotoxicity. *Ann Rev Med* 35:577, 1984.
6. Boyer JL: Chronic hepatitis—a perspective on classification and determinants of prognosis. *Gastroenterology* 70:1161, 1976.
7. Choo Q-L, Kuo G, Weiner AJ, et al: Isolation of a cDNA clone derived from a blood-borne non-A, non-B viral hepatitis genome. *Science* 244:359, 1989.
8. Davis GL, Czaja AJ: Prolonged steroid therapy for severe chronic active liver disease (CALD): a diminishing return? *Gastroenterology* 78:1153, 1980.
9. DiBisceglie AM, Martin P, Kassianides C, et al: Recombinant interferon alfa therapy for chronic hepatitis C. A randomized, double blind, placebo-controlled trial. *N Engl J Med* 321:1506, 1989.
10. Fagerhol MK, Laurell CB: The polymorphism of "prealbumins" and α_1-antitrypsin in human sera. *Clin Chim Acta* 16:199, 1967.
11. Grady GF, and the U.S. National Heart and Lung Institute Collaborative Study Group: relation of e antigen to infectivity of HB$_s$Ag-positive inoculations among medical personnel. *Lancet* 2:492, 1976.
12. Greenberger NJ, Carley J, Schenker S, et al: Effect of vegetable and animal protein diets in chronic hepatic encephalopathy. *Am J Dig Dis* 22:845, 1977.
13. Hoofnagle JH, Mullen KD, Jones DB, et al: Treatment of chronic non A, non B, hepatitis with recombinant human alpha interferon. *N Engl J Med* 315:1575, 1986.
14. Hoofnagle JH, Shafritz DA, Popper H: Chronic type B hepatitis and the "healthy" HB$_s$AG carrier state. *Hepatology* 7:758, 1987.
15. Kaplan MM: Primary biliary cirrhosis. *N Engl J Med* 316:521, 1987.
16. Krugman S, Overby LR, Mushahwar IK, et al: Viral hepatitis, type B. Studies on natural history and prevention re-examined. *N Engl J Med* 300:101, 1979.
17. Kuo G, Choo Q-L, Alter HJ, et al: An assay for circulating antibodies to a major etiologic virus of human non-A, non-B hepatitis. *Science* (Wash DC) 244:362, 1989.
18. LaBrecque DR, Freeman R: Risk of transmitting hepatitis B from staff to patient in a renal dialysis unit. *Gastroenterology* 75:972, 1978.
19. Lam KC, Lai CL, Trepo C, Wu PC: Deleterious effect of prednisolone in HB$_s$Ag-positive chronic active hepatitis. *N Engl J Med* 304:380, 1981.
20. Maddrey WC, Van Thiel DH: Liver transplantation: An overview. *Hepatology* 8:948, 1988.
21. Mezey E: Alcoholic liver disease. *Prog Liver Dis* 7:555, 1982.
22. Repsher LH, Freebern RK: Effects of early and vigorous exercise on recovery from infectious hepatitis. *N Engl J Med* 281:1393, 1969.
23. Rizzetto M, Verme G, Gerin JL, Purcell RH: Hepatitis δ virus disease. *Prog Liver Dis* 8:417, 1986.
24. Sampliner RE, Hamilton FA, Iseri OA, et al: The liver histology and frequency of clearance of the hepatitis B surface antigen (HB$_s$Ag) in chronic carriers. *Am J Med Sci* 277:17, 1979.
25. Seeff LB, Koff RS: Passive and active immunoprophylaxis of hepatitis B. *Gastroenterology* 86:958, 1984.
26. Sherlock S: Chronic hepatitis. *Gut* 15:581, 1974.
27. Soloway RD, Summerskill WHJ, Baggenstoss AH, et al: Clinical, biochemical, and histological remission of severe chronic active liver disease: a controlled study of treatments and early prognosis. *Gastroenterology* 63:820, 1972.
28. Sternlieb I, Scheinberg IH: Chronic hepatitis as a first manifestation of Wilson's disease. *Ann Intern Med* 76:59, 1972.
29. Summerskill WHJ, Davidson CS, Dible JH, et al: Cirrhosis of the liver. A study of alcoholic and non-alcoholic patients in Boston and London. *N Engl J Med* 262:1, 1960.
30. Szmuness W, Dienstag JC, Purcell RH, et al: Distribution of antibody to hepatitis A antigen in urban adult populations. *N Engl J Med* 295:755, 1976.
31. Zimmerman HJ: Drug-induced liver disease: an overview. *Sem Liver Dis* 1:93, 1981.

Renal and Urological Problems

C H A P T E R   44

Proteinuria*

EDWARD S. KRAUS, M.D.

Normally less than 150 mg of protein per 24 hours are present in urine although values may be as high as 300 mg/24 hours in adolescents. Sixty percent of this urinary protein is plasma protein (two-thirds of this being albumin) that has been filtered by glomeruli and only partially reabsorbed by renal tubules. The remaining 40% of urinary protein is synthesized and secreted into the urine by the renal tubules as well as by the more distal portions of the urogenital tract.

Increased urinary protein excretion (proteinuria) is frequently encountered in ambulatory practice. Proteinuria may be due to renal disease, either glomerular dysfunction that allows more protein to be filtered and/or changes in the renal tubules so that there is decreased reabsorption of filtered proteins. Alternatively, increased urinary protein excretion may reflect increased extrarenal generation of protein. In many instances proteinuria may simply be an abnormal laboratory finding in an asymptomatic individual with no significant impact upon his present or future health, but it may signify a serious underlying disorder. This chapter will discuss the methods of detection of protein in the urine and describe an approach to the evaluation and management of patients with proteinuria.

---

*Dr. John Burton contributed to this chapter in the first and second editions of this book.

METHODS FOR DETECTING PROTEINURIA

Office screening for proteinuria is easily accomplished by several accessible and inexpensive semiquantitative methods described in detail below. All methods are sensitive (dipstick detects 20 to 30 mg of protein/dl, sulfosalicylic acid and heat and acetic acid, 5 to 10 mg/dl) so that positive results may be obtained when testing concentrated urine, even though 24-hour urinary protein excretion is normal. With all of these methods, false-positive and negative results may occur (Table 44.1).

Dipstick

This is the most practical and easiest test for semiquantitation of urinary proteins. When moistened with urine, the stick becomes yellow when protein is absent. As protein concentration increases, interference with the dye-buffer combination results in an increasingly green color. Although simple and inexpensive, the technique has several limitations: (a) Because the color reaction is pH dependent, false-positive reactions may be observed if the urine is alkaline (pH greater than 7.5). This error can be avoided by adding a drop of strong acid (e.g., 1 N HCl) before testing to assure that the pH in the urine is less than 7.0. (b) The dipstick method is primarily sensitive to albumin. Therefore, globulins or parts of globulins (heavy or light chains—Bence Jones protein) may be missed. Because of these last two limitations, an alternative method of screening for proteinuria should be available in the physician's office. Either of the methods described below is satisfactory.

Sulfosalicylic Acid

Another relatively easy and inexpensive semiquantitative test for proteinuria is protein precipitation with a 3 to 10% solution of sulfosalicylic acid (SSA). SSA is available from some pharmacies or from hospital laboratories. It is also marketed as Ames Micro-Bumintest by the Miles Company and is available through physician or surgical supply stores. When urine and then water are placed on the tablet, a distinctive reaction occurs in the presence of protein.

SSA is used most frequently to detect globulins or light chains, since the dipstick is insensitive to these proteins. False-positive test results occur, however, if the urine is already turbid. In this situation the urine must be filtered before it is tested. False-positive results also occur when the test is done within 3 days of the administration of iodinated radiographic contrast media or after the administration of some drugs (Table 44.1). In addition, the SSA test will detect proteins of prostatic and vaginal origin. The physician should take care to avoid these contaminants by not palpating the prostate before collecting urine from men and by obtaining a clean voided urine specimen from women, which should show no or only a few vaginal cells microscopically.

Table 44.1.
Urinary Constituents That Alter the Results of Protein Screening Tests[a]

Urinary Constituents	Dipstick	Sulfosalicyclic Acid	Heat and Acetic Acid
Radiographic contrast media	No effect	False-positive	False-positive
Drugs and drug metabolites[b]	No effect	False-positive	False-positive
Bence Jones Protein	False-negative	No effect	False-negative[c]
Highly alkaline urine	False-positive	False-negative	False-negative
Urine turbidity	No effect	False-positive	False-positive
Vaginal or prostatic secretion	No effect	False-positive	False-positive

[a]Modified from Bradley M, Schumann GB, Ward PCJ: Examination of urine. In Henry JB (ed): *Todd-Sanford-Davidsohn Clinical Diagnosis and Management by Laboratory Methods*, 16th ed. Philadelphia, WB Saunders, 1979.
[b]Tolbutamide, tolmetin, chlorpromazine, sulfisoxazole, and high doses of cephalosporins and penicillin.
[c]Precipitated protein may disappear rapidly and be missed with continued heating.

Heat and Acetic Acid

This method is more time consuming and is recommended as a second method of urine protein testing only when SSA is not available. Glacial acetic acid may be purchased at a photography store and must be diluted for accurate results. The diluted solution, one volume of glacial acetic acid to two volumes of water, may be stored and used as necessary. The test is performed by heating the top of a test tube containing approximately 10 ml of urine. After the top of the urine begins to boil rapidly, three or four drops of the diluted acetic acid are added. Reheating to boiling causes a white precipitate to form if protein (either globulin or albumin) is present in the urine specimen. False-positive results occur if the specimen is contaminated with prostatic or vaginal secretions or in the presence of certain drugs or radiographic contrast media (Table 44.1). Further, the rapid boiling may mask the visualization of a transient precipitation of Bence Jones protein.

OFFICE ASSESSMENT OF PATIENTS WITH PROTEINURIA

When proteinuria is suggested by a screening test, further data can be obtained in the office to determine diagnosis, prognosis, and the need for additional consultation. Screening tests should be repeated two or three times. Transient, nonrecurrent mild proteinuria may be seen in association with changes in systemic hemodynamics due to the stress of fever, exercise, or decompensated congestive heart failure.

Persistent or recurrent proteinuria requires additional evaluation. Historically, the chronicity of proteinuria may be become apparent, when the patient is asked about urinalysis performed as a part of previous insurance, school, military or employment examinations. Patients may be aware of prior renal or urological problems but may not associate them with proteinuria. Therefore, a detailed urological history should be obtained, including past history of infection and/or stones, prior radiological evaluations, and family history of renal insufficiency. Because drugs such as gold, penicillamine, captopril, and nonsteroidal anti-inflammatory agents can cause proteinuria, medications should be thoroughly reviewed. Proteinuria may represent only one facet of a systemic illness, suggested by dermatological, rheumatological, infectious, and cardiovascular review of systems. The date of onset of edema, nocturia, or hypertension may help determine the duration of a disease associated with proteinuria. Occasionally, the patient may have noticed a foaming of urine upon voiding if proteinuria has been massive.

Physical examination should be reviewed for the presence of signs that may be associated with the cause of renal disease (such as diabetic retinopathy, abdominal masses suggestive of polycystic kidneys, or rashes, murmurs, or arthropathy indicative of systemic illness) or that may result from renal disease (such as edema) or both (such as hypertension).

Laboratory evaluation should include several studies. First, a microscopic urinalysis should be performed. The presence of other abnormalities, such as hematuria, casts, and/or inflammatory cells, will suggest specific patterns of renal disease of which proteinuria may just be a part. Second, serum creatinine or creatinine clearance should be measured to identify whether renal filtration function is impaired (see Chapter 48, Chronic Renal Insufficiency). Third, proteinuria should be quantitated by either examining a 24-hour urine sample or by determining the protein:creatinine ratio in a single voided sample. This will help classify the disorder (see below) and will assist in the development of the differential diagnosis.

Twenty-Four-Hour Urine Collection for Protein

A clean container without preservatives, usually a gallon jug, is given to the patient with instructions about the collection process. The 24-hour collection is best done on a day when the patient will be using one toilet; and it is helpful for the patient to place a note on the toilet on the day of collection to remind him to collect all required specimens. On the day of collection the first voided morning specimen is discarded; and then all urine in the next 24 hours, including the next morning's first voided specimen, is collected in the container. Once collected, it is not critical when protein determination is done. When delays in analysis are prolonged, however, bacterial growth can falsely raise protein concentrations. Therefore, it is advisable to refrigerate the urine until it is brought to the laboratory if the specimen is not brought in on the day the collection is completed. Alternatively, where refrigeration is not possible, 1 to 2 g boric acid should be added to the container. Other preservatives (e.g., strong acids, thymol) must be avoided since they will interfere with the protein assay.

Quantitation of urine protein is a precise measurement in a well-controlled laboratory, and any value greater than 200 mg/day is considered abnormal. Proteinuria is classified as non-nephrotic if the excretion is between 200 mg and 3500 mg in 24 hours and classified as nephrotic (definitely indicative of glomerular disease) when the excretion is greater than 3500 mg in 24 hours, regardless of the presence or absence of other manifestations of the nephrotic syndrome (low serum albumin, edema, high serum cholesterol). The simultaneous measurement of urinary creatinine is helpful as an index of the adequacy of collection. Most individuals who are not wasted and are of average body mass produce between 800 and 1500 mg of creatinine/day (21 to 26 mg/kg/day in adult men; 16 to 22 mg/kg/day in adult women).

Protein:Creatinine Ratio

An excellent correlation exists between 24-hour urinary protein excretion and the protein:creatinine concentration ratio, mg/dl of protein ÷ mg/dl of creatinine, determined in a random sample of urine obtained during normal daytime activity (1). A ratio of greater than 0.2 is considered abnormal. A ratio greater than 3.5 represents nephrotic range proteinuria. The ratio may overestimate 24-hour urinary protein excretion in certain circumstances, most notably when urine is collected from diabetic patients after strenuous exercise and from individuals whose daily urinary creatinine excretion is considerably less than 1 g, e.g., frail adults. Conversely, determination of this ratio from a first morning urine specimen may underestimate daily urinary protein losses (see below). The urinary protein:creatinine ratio is especially useful, whenever a 24-hour collection is difficult to obtain or there is doubt about the completeness of the sample.

NON-NEPHROTIC PROTEINURIA

A variety of primary renal and systemic diseases may be associated with non-nephrotic range proteinuria. Also most, if not all, patients with nephrotic range proteinuria (see below) may have, at some time, had non-nephrotic range protein excretion. Evaluation is best defined by considering separately patients who have normal physical examinations and laboratory profiles (isolated proteinuria) from patients with other stigmata of disease, e.g., active urinary sediment, hypertension (nonisolated proteinuria).

Isolated Proteinuria in Apparently Healthy Persons

If the initial evaluation is negative except for the presence of isolated proteinuria, the proteinuria may be further classified as persistent (25 to 30% of patients) or intermittent (70 to 75% of patients) (8). The physician can determine which pattern is present by obtaining five or six specimens for semiquantitative analysis over several months. Also, the 24-hour urine protein excretion is almost always less than 1 g in patients with isolated proteinuria. If the total protein excretion is greater than 2 g/24 hours, the chance of significant occult kidney disease is high and further investigation as described below for nonisolated proteinuria should be considered.

Intermittent Proteinuria

A study of individuals with intermittent isolated proteinuria (protein in less than 80% of specimens) revealed definite abnormalities by light microscopy in the renal tissue of approximately 60% of patients, and approximately 40% had a normal or nearly normal biopsy (7). The significance of these findings is unclear, however, in light of another study that retrospectively analyzed the prognostic significance of proteinuria in male college students and found there was no excess mortality 37 to 45 years later. Morbidity was not studied (6). More recently, the Framingham study reported that overall mortality and cardiovascular mortality rates in men were slightly, but significantly, increased (approximately three-fold) in association with proteinuria, in some cases intermittent (2).

In any case, patients who are found to have asymptomatic intermittent proteinuria and who have no evidence of systemic or renal disease can be given an optimistic prognosis. It is not necessary to perform kidney biopsy in these individuals, but it would be prudent to follow them yearly with measurement of urine protein excretion, a urinalysis, and determination of serum creatinine. Should deterioration in renal function, significant increase in protein excretion, or new abnormalities occur, then reassessment and possibly a renal biopsy are necessary.

Persistent Proteinuria

Patients with protein in greater than 80% of urine specimens are defined as having persistent proteinuria. The disorder may be further classified by evaluating the effect of posture. *Orthostatic persistent proteinuria* is present when the patient is in the upright position only. *Constant persistent proteinuria* is not influenced by the position of the patient.

Orthostatic Proteinuria

A simple method of determining the presence of this phenomenon is to have the patient collect two urine specimens. The patient rests quietly for 2 hours and then voids just before retiring in the evening to ensure an empty bladder on assuming the recumbent posture. The patient then does not get out of bed for 8 hours. Upon arising he voids completely into a container labeled "recumbent urine" (Specimen 1). The patient then stays up but is not vigorously active and collects all subsequent urine over the next 8 hours. This specimen is labeled "ambulatory urine" (Specimen 2). The protein concentrations in the urine specimens are then compared. This protocol may be simplified if the patient does not drink during the night. In the morning after overnight fluid deprivation, two or more urine specimens are collected consecutively. The first specimen is marked "recumbent" and should be collected immediately upon arising. The following specimen(s) should be labeled "ambulatory." A semiquantitative test (dipstick or SSA) and a measurement of urine concentration to confirm antidiuresis are performed on each sample (8). In patients with orthostatic proteinuria the "recumbent" protein excretion is negligible, whereas proteinuria is found when the patient assumes the upright posture.

A renal biopsy is not necessary in the evaluation of a patient with this problem; but, when done as part of a research protocol, minor abnormalities have been defined in approximately half of the individuals and the others have had a biopsy that appeared normal on light microscopy (studies utilizing electron and/or immunofluorescent microscopy have not been done) (8). It would, however, be prudent to follow the patient by measuring urinary protein excretion and serum creatinine or creatinine clearance on a yearly basis even after the proteinuria has cleared (see below).

If orthostatic persistent proteinuria is documented, the prognosis seems to be excellent. Military recruits with this problem have been followed for 20 years (10). None developed renal failure, and approximately 80% were no longer proteinuric. Not all patients who were free of protein in the urine at 10-year follow-up remained protein free after 20 years, although none of those patients showed significant deterioration in renal function. Also, a small number of patients re-evaluated 42 to 50 years after the establishment of the diagnosis of postural proteinuria manifest good health (9).

Constant Proteinuria

In most patients with constant proteinuria, diverse morphological changes are identified in kidney biopsy specimens. Few long-term studies of these patients have been made, but their course is likely to be indolent. Renal failure develops very rarely, although most patients develop abnormal urine sediment, and 50% develop hypertension (4). It is not necessary to perform renal biopsy when there are no other findings, but yearly re-evaluation is appropriate and should include blood pressure measurement, urinalysis, and determination of 24-hour protein excretion and of serum creatinine and creatinine clearance. If proteinuria exceeds 2 g/day, additional evaluation including sonogram or intravenous pyelogram and collagen vascular screens may be appropriate.

Nonisolated Proteinuria

If an abnormality related to proteinuria is discovered during initial evaluation (e.g., hypertension, he-maturia, casts in the urine, or renal failure), further investigation may be necessary. The direction and extent of the investigation depend on the nature of the abnormality. Renal biopsy may be indicated, especially if there is hematuria, red blood cell casts, mild renal failure, or evidence of systemic disease [e.g., systemic lupus erythematosus (SLE)]. Table 44.2 lists some additional investigations that may be indicated to evaluate abnormalities associated with proteinuria. A telephone consultation with a nephrologist may be helpful in deciding the need for further evaluation.

NEPHROTIC PROTEINURIA

When a 24-hour protein quantitation reveals greater than 3.5 g of protein or the protein:creatinine ratio is greater than 3.5, nephrotic range proteinuria is established by definition and is indicative of glomerular disease. Once nephrotic range proteinuria has been identified, consultation with a nephrologist is appropriate to help decide the extent of the workup, as well as to provide suggestions for treatment (3). There are many causes of nephrotic syndrome, but there are relatively few conditions that are seen with significant frequency in a general medical practice (Table 44.3). Clinical and laboratory screens for systemic illness should be performed first in an effort to establish the etiology of the nephrotic syndrome (e.g., detection of Bence Jones proteinuria or collagen vascular screens for systemic lupus). Table 44.2 lists some of the laboratory evaluations that may be helpful in determining the cause of renal disease. When nephrotic range proteinuria develops in a patient who has been diabetic for over 10 to 15 years, the renal lesion is almost always diabetic glomerulosclerosis, particularly if the patient also has diabetic microaneurysms in the retina.

Table 44.2.
Selected Investigations That May Be Appropriate in the Diagnosis of Proteinuria That is Not Isolated or That is Nephrotic

Antinuclear antibody, if systemic lupus erythematosus (SLE) is suspected
Antistreptolysin (ASO) titer, if there is a possibility of post-streptococcal glomerulonephritis
Complement (C_3, C_4), if glomerulonephritis is suspected
Complete blood count, to provide a baseline evaluation for subsequent use and to provide a clue to a systemic illness (such as leukemia)
Erythrocyte sedimentation rate, if collagen vascular disease is suspected
Fasting blood sugar, to consider the possibility of diabetes mellitus
Hepatitus B surface antigen, if hepatitis-associated vasculitis may be present
Intravenous pyelogram, to provide evidence for structural renal disease (such as papillary necrosis)
Lupus erythematosus (LE) prep, if SLE is suspected
Serum albumin, if nephrotic range proteinuria is present
Serum electrolytes (Na^+, K^+, Cl^-, HCO_3^-, Ca^{2+}, PO_4^{2-}), to provide a screen for abnormalities subsequent to renal disease
Serum and urine protein electrophoresis, if multiple myeloma is suspected
Uric acid, to screen for urate-related renal disease
Urine culture, if pyuria is present
X-ray of chest, to provide evidence for a systemic disease—for example, sarcoidosis

Table 44.3.
Cause of Nephrotic Syndrome in Adults[a]

MOST COMMON
  Diabetes mellitus
  Idiopathic membranous glomerulopathy
  Idiopathic lipoid nephrosis—(including minimal change disease, mesangial proliferative glomerulonephritis, focal segmental glomerulosclerosis)

LESS COMMON
  Proliferative glomerulonephritis—(crescenteric glomerulonephritis)
  Membranoproliferative glomerulonephritis
  Collagen vascular disease
  Amyloidosis

[a]An extensive list of potential causes of nephrotic syndrome can be found in Glassock RJ: Syndrome of glomerular diseases, In Massry SG, Glassock RJ (eds): *Textbook of Nephrology*, Baltimore, Williams & Wilkins, 1983.

In this setting, a renal biopsy is usually not necessary. On the other hand, a biopsy is usually necessary to diagnose a specific primary renal disease if a diagnosis cannot be made by other tests (e.g., detection of Bence Jones proteinuria or rectal biopsy for amyloid), or it may be needed to guide therapy or to help determine prognosis (e.g., SLE).

Renal Biopsy

Patient experience. Renal biopsy requires hospitalization for 24 to 48 hours. Generally, in patients without renal failure and normal hemostasis, percutaneous biopsy is performed under local anesthesia with fluoroscopic or sonographic guidance. This technique permits the nephrologist to sample the lower portion of the kidney, thus avoiding the hilar vessels and the renal collecting system. With percutaneous biopsy the patient usually experiences minimal discomfort and is able to be out of bed in 12 hours.

The biopsy core is approximately 1 mm in diameter and approximately 10 to 20 mm in length. Usually two such tissue cores are obtained. The risk associated with percutaneous renal biopsy is small if performed by an experienced physician.

Microscopic hematuria is almost inevitable, and usually there is a small hematoma at the biopsy site on the surface of the kidney. However, it is usually of no clinical consequence. Gross hematuria occurs in approximately 5 to 10% of patients, but less than 5% require a transfusion to replace blood loss. Fewer than one in 1000 patients requires nephrectomy because of continued massive bleeding, and death from biopsy is very rare. A renal arteriovenous fistula may develop after biopsy, but it usually closes spontaneously. Rarely this complication may require treatment if bleeding continues or if hypertension develops (5). Even more rarely, there may be perforation of another viscus.

When percutaneous biopsy is not feasible, open biopsy can be obtained; some surgeons perform this procedure under local anesthesia in selected patients. Regardless of the technique of obtaining the biopsy, the evaluation of tissue by the pathologist should include light, immunofluorescent, and electron microscopy, and it should be done by a pathologist experienced in preparation and interpretation of renal biopsy material.

The physician who has referred to a nephrologist a patient in whom a renal biopsy has been performed should expect communication of the following: the probable diagnosis, based upon all aspects of the microscopic assessment; whether specific therapy for the condition is indicated; and what prognostic judgment can be made.

MANAGEMENT OF PATIENTS WITH PROTEINURIA

Non-nephrotic proteinuria requires no special treatment. The physician's major effort is directed at diagnosis, education, surveillance, and treatment of any underlying disease. However, if the proteinuria is felt to be caused by a drug, it should be discontinued. Proteinuria from drugs may take several months to resolve and occasionally it is permanent.

Some patients with nephrotic range proteinuria are asymptomatic and require no therapy unless the results of the renal biopsy dictate that treatment be given. When either edema or hypoalbuminemia is present, special therapy may be indicated. In the absence of renal failure, albumin synthesis is either increased or normal in patients with the nephrotic syndrome. Until recently, treatment included provision of a high protein diet (2 to 3 g of protein/kg dry weight, i.e., estimated or actual weight before edema developed). Nutritional recommendations are currently being re-evaluated, especially for patients whose proteinuria is associated with renal insufficiency. Currently, mild to moderate protein restriction rather than protein supplementation is advised. At present, appropriate standards for protein intake in this setting remain controversial and are a subject of intense research.

In the presence of edema, salt restriction to a tolerable level such as a no added salt diet (approximately 2 to 3 g of Na, see Table 62.12) is appropriate. If the edema is more severe and is unresponsive to sodium chloride restriction, cautious use of diuretics may be helpful, beginning with thiazides and then substituting a loop diuretic (furosemide or bumetanide) if necessary. There should not be an attempt to rid the patient entirely of edema, which could risk contraction of the circulating volume with serious consequences. The patient may benefit from alternate-day diuretics, which will diminish the risk of inducing serious volume contraction. Potassium-sparing diuretics (spironolactone, triamterene, or amiloride) may be added if renal failure is absent and if loop diuretics have not been entirely adequate. If acceptable control is still not achieved, consultation with a nephrologist is appropriate.

Numerous extrarenal complications are associated with nephrotic syndrome. These include alterations in cellular immunity leading to increased infections, hyperlipidemia, and changes in calcium and bone metabolism. A life-threatening complication, *renal vein thrombosis*, occurs in a number of patients with certain histological patterns of idiopathic nephrotic syndrome (especially membranous glomerulopathy). Clues to the development of this complication include pulmonary embolism, sudden deterioration in renal function, marked increase in the level of proteinuria, or the development of hematuria. Suspicion of this complication requires hospitalization of the patient for urgent evaluation.

Prediction of the course and selection of specific therapy in patients with nephrotic range proteinuria depend on the pathological pattern that is identified in the biopsy. Patients with nephrotic range proteinuria will need regularly scheduled office visits at 1- to 4-month intervals. Usually this follow-up is done by the primary physician and the patient will see the nephrologist only once a year. The office visit provides an opportunity to review the patient's symptoms and to perform a limited physical examination (which, at a minimum, should include weight, volume assessment, and blood pressure) as well as to evaluate the 24-hour urine protein excretion, or a protein:creatinine ratio, the renal function (creatinine or creatinine clearance), and the serum electrolytes if diuretics are being used. Less frequently an assessment of the serum albumin may be necessary.

General References

Abuelo JG: Proteinuria: diagnostic principles and procedures. *Ann Intern Med* 98:186, 1983.
Brenner BM, Stein JH (eds): *Nephrotic Syndrome.* Vol 9, Contemporary Issues in Nephrology. New York, Churchill Livingstone, 1982.
Dennis VS, Robinson RR: Clinical proteinuria. *Adv Intern Med* 31:243, 1986.
Striegel J, Michael AF, Chavers BM: Asymptomatic proteinuria: benign disorder or harbinger of disease? *Postgrad Med* 83:287, 1988.

Specific References

1. Ginsberg JM, Chang BS, Matarese RA, Garella S: Use of single voided urine samples to estimate quantitative proteinuria. *N Engl J Med* 309:1543, 1983.
2. Kannel WB, Stampfer MJ, Castelli WP, Verter J: The prognostic significance of proteinuria: the Framingham study. *Am Heart J* 108:1347, 1984.
3. Kassirer JP: Is renal biopsy necessary for optimal management of the idiopathic nephrotic syndrome? *Kidney Int* 24:561, 1983.
4. King SE: Diastolic hypertension and chronic proteinuria. *Am J Cardiol* 9:669, 1962.
5. Leiter E, Gribetz D, Cohen S: Arteriovenous fistula after percutaneous needle biopsy—surgical repair with preservation of renal function. *N Engl J Med* 287:971, 1972.
6. Levitt JI: The prognostic significance of proteinuria in young college students. *Ann Intern Med* 66:685, 1967.
7. Muth RG: Asymptomatic mild intermittent proteinuria. A percutaneous renal biopsy study. *Arch Intern Med* 115:569, 1965.
8. Robinson RR: Isolated proteinuria in asymptomatic patients. *Kidney Int* 18:399, 1980.
9. Rytand DA, Spreiter S: Prognosis in postural (orthostatic) proteinuria. Forty- to fifty-year follow-up of six patients after diagnosis by Thomas Addis. *N Engl J Med* 305:618, 1981.
10. Springberg PD, Garrett LE, Thompson Jr AL, et al: Fixed reproducible orthostatic proteinuria: results of a 20-year follow-up study. *Ann Intern Med* 97:516, 1982.

C H A P T E R   45

HEMATURIA*

DAVID A. SPECTOR, M.D.
JOHN R. BURTON, M.D.

Normal individuals excrete up to 2 million red blood cells (RBCs) into the urine daily. This rate extrapolates to as many as one to three red blood cells per high power microscopic field (HPF) using standard urinalysis techniques. The finding of greater numbers of RBC/HPF constitutes abnormal hematuria, although the exact level separating normal from abnormal is arbitrary. Benzidine or orthotolidine-impregnated, hemoglobin-sensitive dipsticks, widely used as screening tests for hematuria, are less sensitive than microscopy but are usually positive in urine containing more than three to five RBCs/HPF. However, there are certain limits to their use (Table 45.1).

Microscopic hematuria may or may not be indicative of serious genitourinary tract disease (2, 9, 12). The constellation of symptoms, signs, and laboratory findings associated with hematuria and the clinical sitting in which it occurs help considerably in predicting the seriousness of the finding. For example, hematuria associated with proteinuria or pyuria or gross hematuria is highly predictive of a significant disease. Conversely, asymptomatic microhematuria in a young adult has little predictive value.

PSEUDOHEMATURIA

A large number of substances can impart a color to urine that may be mistaken for hematuria (16). *Exogenous sources* of some of these substances are listed in Table 45.2. *Endogenous substances* capable of producing a reddish hue include porphyrins, myoglobin,

---

*James K. Smolev, M.D., contributed to the chapter in the first and second editions of the book.

Table 45.1.
Limits of Dipstick Method for Detection of Blood in the Urine

REASONS FOR A POSITIVE TEST
Hematuria—greater than approximately 5–10 red blood cells/high power field
Hematuria with red blood cells lysis
From hypotonic urine (specific gravity less than 1.008)
From highly alkaline urine (pH greater than 6.5–7.0)
Hemoglobinuria—from intravascular hemolysis
Myoglobinuria—from muscle injury
False positive reactions
From hypochlorite (bleach) contamination of container
From peroxidase (from heavy growth of bacteria)
REASONS FOR A FALSE NEGATIVE TEST
Vitamin C—ingestion by the patient of large amounts vitamin C (>200 mg/day) results in diminished oxidation potential of the test material. The dipstick test may miss trace quantities of blood, although usually there is a quantitative decrease in the estimate of blood (such as 3+ to 2+). (This is of concern only if red blood cells are observed but the dipstick test is negative.)
Formaldehyde—ingestion of bacterial suppressant agents (such as Mandelamine or Hiprex) which produce formaldehyde in acid urine or contamination of the container with formaldehyde will diminish the oxidizing potential of the reagent strips. This results in a quantitative estimate error or, if hematuria is minimal, false negative results.

Table 45.2.
Exogenous Substances That May Cause Pseudohematuria[a]

Medications

Analgesics:	Phenacetin
	Phenazopyridine (e.g., Pyridium)
Antibiotics:	Nitrofurantoin
	Rifampin
	Sulfonamides
Antimalarials:	
	Chloroquine
	Primaquine
Laxatives:	Anthraquinones: Cascara, Senna, danthron (e.g., Modane or Dorbane)
Anticancer Agents:	Doxorubicin, daunoribicin
Others:	Deferoxamine (an iron-chelating agent)
	Dimethylsulfoxide (DMSO)
	Levodopa
	Phenothiozines
	Methyldopa (rare)

Vegetable Dyes

Anthrocyanins:	beets, blackberries
Paprika	
Rhubarb	
Fuscin (a reddish dye used in topical agents)	

Other

Antiseptics:	mercurochrome, phenols, cresols, povidine isodine (Betadine)
pHisoHex	
Urate crystals (in acid urine)	

[a]Some of these agents cause hemoglobinuria.

and hemoglobin. Myoglobin and hemoglobin also cause positive reactions in tests for red blood cells (e.g., Labstix or Multistix). Therefore when the dipstick is positive in urine and the microscopy is negative for red blood cells, myoglobinuria or hemoglobinuria should be suspected. The dipstick reaction, however, may not detect hemoglobin (or red blood cells) or myoglobin when these substances are present if there is heavy hypochlorite (bleach, chlorine) or peroxidase (from bacteria) contamination of the urine specimen or its container. Conversely, a false-negative dipstick test may occur when formaldehyde (e.g., present as a breakdown product of mandelamine) or large amounts of vitamin C are in the urine, since both substances decrease the sensitivity of the test reagent.

INNOCENT HEMATURIA

Microscopic hematuria is often identified after a genitourinary tract examination such as a pelvic or prostate examination, cystoscopy or bladder catheterization, or biopsy of prostate, bladder, or kidney. Occasionally gross hematuria may be seen in this setting. Gross or microscopic hematuria, also, is present sometimes after vigorous exercise such as swimming, lacrosse, boxing, football, or running. This finding has been most frequently reported in long-distance runners, and in one study 18% of athletes were found to have hematuria after the completion of a marathon (14). Hematuria in all such settings subsides in 24 to 48 hours. It does not signify underlying genitourinary pathology when it resolves quickly and does not recur spontaneously. In exercisers (especially runners), proteinuria and/or cast formation sometimes accompanies the hematuria, and the red cells have been found to be dysmorphic (see below), suggesting the bleeding site is the glomerulus.

SYMPTOMATIC HEMATURIA

Hematuria with Pyuria

If a patient is found to have hematuria associated with pyuria (with or without irritative symptoms—frequency, urgency, or dysuria), an infectious cause is most likely and bacterial cultures should be obtained. If a specific organism is identified, appropriate antimicrobial therapy should be given (see Chapter 27). After treatment the patient should be followed carefully (including the performance of a urinalysis) for 4 to 6 weeks to ensure that the hematuria has been eradicated and does not recur. If irritative symptoms suggesting infection have been present and the routine culture is sterile, *a sexually transmitted disease* (especially *Chlamydia* infection or gonorrhea), a viral infection or, rarely, tuberculosis should be suspected. *Chlamydia trachomatis infection* (see Chapters 27 and 94), especially, may be manifested by hematuria and pyuria with minimal irritative symptoms. When a sexually transmitted infection is suspected, but cannot be proven, a therapeutic trial of an antimicrobial may be given (see Chapters 27 and 94). *Viral cystitis* is a fairly common infection of young women. It has a short-lived (2 to 3 days) natural course, and it is nonrecurrent. Suspicion of *tuberculosis of the urinary tract* requires several weeks to confirm by culture (an acid-fast stain of the urine is not a reliable indicator because of the regular presence of acid-fast material from smegma bacilli). Because noninfectious disorders of the bladder (including malignancies) may also present with irritative symptoms (see Chapter 49), one should ensure that symptoms, especially in patients over age 50, have abated and that the patient's urinalysis is normal on two or three occasions in the following 4 to 6 weeks.

Hematuria with Proteinuria, Red Blood Cell Casts, or Dysmorphic Red Blood Cells

Hematuria associated with proteinuria reflects either glomerulonephritis or interstitial nephritis. When proteinuria is greater than 3.5 gm/24 hours (i.e., nephrotic range) and/or red cell casts are present, the diagnosis is most likely glomerulonephritis (see Chapter 44). The morphological appearance on microscopy of the RBCs may help to differentiate glomerular from nonglomerular bleeding (5). This observation takes advantage of the deformation of cytoplasmic content of RBCs after their passage into Bowman's space. If greater than 80% of at least 100 (counted) red cells appear dysmorphic (abnormal size, shape, and cytoplasmic staining) using Wright's stain (or phase contrast microscopy, if available) of urinary sediment, glomerular bleeding is very likely. If glomerulonephritis is suspected, estimation of glomerular filtration rate, quantitative 24-hour urine protein, and serological survey (ANA, antistreptococcal antibodies, serum complement, etc.) are indicated (see Chapter 44). Although any form of glomerulonephritis may be present, IgA nephropathy (Berger's disease) (8) and Alport's syndrome (hereditary nephritis often associated with deafness) are especially likely in situations in which the hematuria has been an incidental finding. Both of these diseases are characterized by recurrent episodes of hematuria (microscopic or gross), fluctuating proteinuria, and a variable course. A nephrologist should be consulted when these or other forms of glomerulonephritis are suspected. Often the nephrologist will perform a renal biopsy (see Chapter 44 for patient experience) to establish the diagnosis, to estimate the prognosis, and to determine treatment.

ASYMPTOMATIC ISOLATED MICROHEMATURIA

The prevalence of isolated microscopic hematuria is quite high. Twelve percent of adult men and postmenopausal women in one study were found to have asymptomatic hematuria (12, 13). On the other hand studies that have used more stringent definitions of hematuria in a variety of populations have demonstrated a 2 to 5% prevalence of microscopic hematuria (Table 45.3). Neoplasia is more frequent in series derived from an older population of patients referred to urologists, and it is rare in series of nonreferred young individuals.

In all series, no specific diagnosis was made for many patients because the evaluations were not always complete and most often did not include a renal biopsy, which may have revealed subtle glomerular or interstitial disease. For example, in one study 20 of 29 adult patients with hematuria with minimal or no proteinuria and with a negative urologic work-up had a specific diagnosis established only after the performance of a renal biopsy (6, 15).

Patients with isolated hematuria should have the concentration of calcium and uric acid in a 24-hour urine specimen measured. Hypercalciuria (>300 mg/24 hours) and/or hyperuricosuria (>750 mg/24 hours in women; >800 mg/24 hours in men) has been shown to be a cause of hematuria (presumably due to irritation of the tubules by microcrystals), and it has been shown that thiazide therapy (which reduces calciuria) and/or allopurinol stops the bleeding (1).

EVALUATION OF PATIENTS WITH HEMATURIA

Pseudohematuria as discussed above and drug-induced hematuria (Table 45.4) should be ruled out. The evaluation then depends on associated symptoms, on whether the bleeding is gross or microscopic, and on the results of the complete urinalysis (see above). Localization of the site of the bleeding in the genitourinary tract is the first priority. The associated symptoms and the history of temporal events often provide a diagnostic clue. For example, colicky flank pain suggests that the hematuria is emanating from the ureter whereas dysuria and frequency suggest that the bleeding is from the bladder. All patients should be asked about the temporal relationship of the hematuria to exercise and to ingestion of medications or food. The urinalysis is helpful also if there are findings suggestive of glomerular disease or infection (see above). The number of red cells/HPF is, however, not predictive of the seriousness of the problem.

A history and physical examination should be performed to evaluate the patient for clues to illnesses with which hematuria is associated (for example, a nodular prostate suggestive of prostate cancer or cutaneous or other abnormalities suggestive of a collagen vascular disease). When the history and physical examination plus selected laboratory tests (for example, urine culture) and treatment (for example, antimicrobials) do not support a working diagnosis, a basic laboratory data set should be obtained. This information should include a complete blood count, an estimate of glomerular function (e.g., serum creatinine), a sickle cell preparation (if the patient is black), a 24-hour urine specimen for determination of the concentration of calcium and uric acid (see above), and an intravenous pyelogram with tomography (if the creatinine is not significantly elevated and if the patient gives no history of dye allergy). In patients suspected of having a bleeding disorder, a platelet count and the measurement of the prothrombin, partial thromboplastin, and bleeding times should be done. If an underlying bleeding diathesis is identified, the search for a pathological process in the genitourinary tract should continue since one will usually be identified (see Chapter 51). If symptoms or signs of infection are present, appropriate cultures should be obtained (see above). In

Table 45.3.
Distribution (%) of Selected Urological Findings in Asymptomatic Patients with Microhematuria Reference

Reference No. of Patients Type Population	11 500 Urology Referral	3 200 Urology Referral	10 246 Urology Referral	9 636 Young Israeli Men[a]	13 781 Rochester MN Population[a]	2 177 Young Women Urology Referral
Neoplasia	2.2	13.0	9.3	0.2	1.0	0
Other disorders						
Renal Calculi	2.6	14.0	0	0.6	3.3	1.6
Ureteral Calculi	0.4	1.5	1.0	0	0.9	0.6
Nephritis/Renal Insufficiency	0	3.5	2.0	0.1	14.4	0
Benign Prostatic Hypertrophy	23.6	20.0	8.0	0	37.7	---
Urinary Tract Infection	3.6	10.5	2.0	0	0.5	b
Urethrotrignitis/Prostatitis	24.6	18.0	18.0	0.1	1.8	26.6
Any finding[c]	56.0	81.0	47.6	b	62.5	63.0

[a]Complete urological workup not performed on all patients.
[b]Unable to determine from data.
[c]Includes those listed above, in addition to other findings that may or may not have been related to the hematuria. These include: hydronephrosis, renal cysts, polycystic kidney disease, vesicoureteral reflux, intersitial and radiation cystitis, diverticuli, ureteropelvic junction obstruction, ureterocele, cystocele, neurogenic bladder, atrophic vagina, scarred kidney, cystitis cystica, polyps, papillary necrosis, calcified renal mass, trabeculated bladder. Some patients in all series had more than one disorder.

Table 45.4.
Examples of Drugs Causing Hematuria

Antibiotics
Penicillin analogues[a]
Cephalosporin analogues[a]
Sulfa analogues[a]
Polymycin[a]
Rifampin[a]

Analgesics and Anti-inflammatory Agents
Aspirin[b]
Penacetin[b]
Aminosalicylic acid[b]
Non-steroidal anti-inflammatory agents[a]

Diuretics
Furosemide[a]
Ethacrynic Acida Thiazides[a]

Anticoagulants
Warfarin (Coumadin)[c]

Other
Cyclophosphamide[d]
Ifosfamide (Isex—an antineoplastic agent)[d]
Danazold[a]

[a]Infrequent bleeding due to interstitial nephritis, usually occurring within days to weeks of taking drugs; usually reversible.
[b]Infrequent bleeding due to medullary/papillary necrosis, usually following many months or years of combination analgesic preparations; partially reversible.
[c]An underlying cause of hematuria is often found and a work-up should be considered (7).
[d]Bleeding due to hemorrhagic cystitis in 10-20% of patients; dose-related and usually reversible.

older patients (e.g., >40 to 50 years) two or three morning urine specimens should be evaluated by a cytology laboratory for the presence of tumor cells. The sensitivity of cytology in this setting is 30% when an upper tract tumor is present and 50 to 90% when a bladder tumor is present. (The higher rates of detection are in situations in which a higher grade of cancer is present.)

When neoplasia is a consideration [those patients over 40 to 50 years of age or those who are younger but have a risk factor for bladder cancer (see below)], a urologist should be consulted and the patient should undergo cystoscopy (see Chapter 49 for patient experience) (4). Risk factors for bladder cancer include a heavy occupational exposure [e.g., to aromatic amines, dyes, benzidine and paint ingredients (see Chapter 7)], prolonged daily use of analgesics (phenacetin, acetominophen, and aspirin combinations have been reported), or heavy smoking. When neoplasia is a strong consideration, the urologist might also suggest the evaluation of the patient by computed tomography (CT) scanning, magnetic resonance imaging, or renal angiography.

When neoplasia is not strongly considered, and persistent hematuria is present or recurrent, the patient should be referred to a nephrologist for consideration of the performance of a renal biopsy (see Chapter 44 for patient experience).

Gross Hematuria

When gross hematuria is present, the evaluation should initially proceed in the same manner as in the patient with microscopic hematuria, but there are several caveats: Blood clots in the urine suggest that bleeding is from the bladder. However, clots may result occasionally from upper tract bleeding and in that situation ureteral colic may occur. Another caution is important when gross hematuria develops: Plasma protein may be lost into the urine (and detected by qualitative or quantitative test) in relatively large quantities, yet not reflect a glomerular disease. However, the concentration of urinary protein rarely exceeds a daily excretion of 1 g when it occurs from gross bleeding. The "*three glass test*" is sometimes useful in determining the site of gross bleeding. This test is performed by having the patient void into containers in a sequence: the *initial* 10 ml of urine represents the urethral specimen, the *middle* portion of urine voided is nondiagnostic of a specific location, and blood in the *terminal* portion (the last few drops of urine) suggests that the site is likely to be the prostate, bladder neck, or proximal urethra. Blood present in all three specimens is not specific for the site of origin.

In patients with persistent gross hematuria a urologist should always be consulted promptly as the most opportune time to establish the site is when the bleeding is active.

The surveillance of a patient found to have gross hematuria will depend on the cause (Table 45.5). If no cause is found, close surveillance (every 6 months for several years) is indicated since some of these individuals will have a serious underlying disorder, such as a tumor or glomerulonephritis. This surveillance should include reviewing the history, performing a physical examination, obtaining a urinalysis and the urea nitrogen and creatinine concentration, and, in situations in which a tumor is considered, obtaining a urine specimen for cytological examination and referring the patient to a urologist for a cystoscopic examination.

HEMATOSPERMIA

The presence of blood in the ejaculate of males is an alarming but usually innocuous symptom. This problem occurs most often in men over 40, and most often the episodes recur over several weeks or months. When it occurs in an otherwise asymptomatic man who has a normal physical examination (including rectal examination of the prostate and seminal vesicles) and a normal urinalysis, the patient should be reassured that it is innocuous and that no further workup is necessary. If there is any abnormality, further evaluation for benign prostatic hypertrophy or cancer of the prostate, seminal vesicles, bladder, or urethra should be considered and a urologist should be consulted.

Table 45.5.
Diagnosis Established in 1000 Cases of Gross Hematuria[a]

Diagnosis		% Patients
Kidney	15.2	
Tumor		3.5
Pyelonephritis		3.0
Calculus		2.7
Trauma		2.0
Hydronephrosis		1.5
Polycystic disease		0.6
Chronic glomerulonephritis		0.6
Other		1.3
Ureter	6.5	
Calculus		5.3
Tumor		0.7
Other		0.5
Bladder	39.5	
Cystitis		22.0
Tumor		14.9
Calculus		1.2
Other		1.4
Prostate	23.8	
Benign hyperplasia		12.5
Chronic prostatitis		9.0
Carcinoma		2.1
Urethra	4.3	
Stricture		1.7
Calculus		1.3
Gonorrhea		0.4
Tumor		0.3
Other		1.8
Other Causes	1.2	
Urinary tuberculosis		0.7
Hemophilia		0.2
Uremic syndrome		0.1
Thrombocytopenia		0.1
Dicumarol poisoning		0.1
"Essential" hematuria	8.5	
TOTAL		100.0

[a] Adapted from Lee LW, and Davis E. Gross urinary hemorrhage: A symptom, not a disease. *JAMA* 153:782, 1953.

General References

Abuelo JG: Evaluation of hematuria. *Urology* 21:215, 1983.
Copley JB: Isolated asymptomatic hematuria in the adult. *Am J Med Sci* 291:101, 1986.
Leary FJ, Aguilo JJ: Clinical significance of hematospermia. *Mayo Clin Proc* 49:815, 1974.

Specific References

1. Andres A, Praga M, Bello I, et al: Hematuria due to hypercalciuria and hyperuricosuria in adult patients. *Kid Int* 36:96, 1989.
2. Bard RH: The significance of asymptomatic microhematuria in women and its economic implications. *Arch Intern Med* 148:2629, 1988.
3. Carson III CC, Segura JW, Greene LF: Clinical importance of microhematuria. *JAMA* 241:140, 1979.
4. Carter III WC, Rous SN: Gross hematuria in 110 adult urologic hospital patients. *Urology* 18:342, 1981.
5. Chang BS: Red cell morphology as a diagnostic aid in hematuria. *JAMA* 252:1747, 1984.
6. Copley JB, Hasbargen JA: Idiopathic hematuria. A prospective evaluation. *Arch Intern Med* 147:434, 1987.
7. Cuttino Jr JT, Clark RL, Feaster SH, Zwicke DL: The evaluation of gross hematuria in anticoagulated patients: efficacy of IV urography and cystoscopy. *AJR* 149:527, 1987.
8. D'Amico G: Clinical features and natural history in adults with IgA nephropathy. *Am J Kid Dis* 12:353, 1988.
9. Froom P, Ribak J, Benbassat J: Significance of microhematuria in young adults. *Br Med J* 288:20, 1984.
10. Golin AL, Howard RS: Asymptomatic microscopic hematuria. *J Urol* 124:389, 1980.
11. Greene LF, O'Shaughnessy Jr EJ, Hendricks ED: Study of five hundred patients with asymptomatic microhematuria. *JAMA* 161:610, 1956.
12. Mohr DN, Offord KP, Owen RA, Melton III J: Asymptomatic microhematuria and urologic disease. A population-based study. *JAMA* 256:224, 1986.
13. Mohn DN, Offord KP, Melton III LJ: Isolated asymptomatic microhematuria. *J Gen Int Med* 2:318, 1987.
14. Siegel AJ, Hennikens CH, Solomon HS, Von Boeckel B: Exercise-related hematuria. Findings in a group of marathon runners. *JAMA* 241:391, 1987.
15. Tiebosch ATMG, Frederik PM, van Breda Vriesman PJC, et al: Thin-basement-membrane nephropathy in adults with persistent hematuria. *N Engl J Med* 320:14, 1989.
16. Young DS, Pestoner LC, Gibberman V: Effects of drugs on clinical laboratory tests. *Clin Chem* 21:1D, 1975.

Hypokalemia*

AARON SPITAL, M.D.

Hypokalemia, defined as a serum potassium concentration less than 3.5 mEq/liter, is frequently encountered in ambulatory practice. Although the consequences are often trivial, rarely they may be life threatening. Loss of potassium through the gastrointestinal tract or the kidneys accounts for the majority of patients with hypokalemia seen in ambulatory practice; occasionally, other less common causes will be encountered. This chapter will review the physiology of potassium homeostasis, outline the clinical consequences of potassium depletion, develop an approach to differential diagnosis, and discuss the management of patients with hypokalemia.

PHYSIOLOGICAL BACKGROUND

The serum potassium concentration depends upon two factors: (a) the total body potassium content and (b) the distribution of potassium between the intracellular and extracellular spaces (15). Total body potassium, normally about 50 mEq/kg, is determined by external potassium balance (the difference between intake and excretion); in health, excretion matches intake and total body potassium remains essentially constant (Fig. 46.1). The distribution of potassium between the intracellular and extracellular spaces is referred to as internal potassium balance, which may vary in the absence of changes in external balance (15).

External Potassium Balance

The average intake of potassium is about 60 to 100 mEq/day (17). Normally, about 90% is absorbed and then excreted in the urine; the remainder is eliminated in the stool (Fig. 46.1). However, in diarrheal states, large amounts of potassium may be lost in the stool.

---

*John R. Burton, M.D., contributed to this chapter in the first and second editions of this book.

Furthermore, in severe renal failure the amount of potassium eliminated by the gastrointestinal tract increases so that about 1/3 of potassium intake may be excreted by this route. Only trivial amounts of potassium are lost through the skin (<5 mEq/day) unless sweating becomes profuse.

By adjusting the rate of urinary potassium excretion in proportion to intake, the kidney acts as the major regulator of external potassium balance. Because potassium is freely filtered by the glomerulus and nearly completely reabsorbed in the proximal parts of the nephron, urinary potassium excretion is largely a function of distal tubular secretion. Factors affecting the rate of potassium secretion (and excretion) include (Fig. 46.2) (3): (a) the serum potassium concentration, (b) the luminal flow rate, (c) distal sodium and chloride delivery, (d) the plasma aldosterone concentration, (e) distal transepithelial voltage, (f) acid-base balance, (g) antidiuretic hormone concentration, and (h) dietary potassium intake. Any factor that increases the urinary flow rate, distal sodium delivery, aldosterone secretion, and transepithelial voltage that decreases distal chloride delivery, or that causes metabolic alkalosis, will stimulate potassium secretion and predispose to the development of potassium depletion. Dietary potassium deficiency also predisposes to mild potassium depletion since the ability of the kidney to conserve potassium is not as efficient as is the ability to conserve sodium.

Internal Potassium Balance

Most of body potassium is located intracellularly; maintained by membrane bound Na-K-ATPase, the ratio of intracellular to extracellular potassium concentration normally is about 30:1 (15). Indeed, of total body potassium, less than 2% (50 to 60 mEq) resides in the extracellular space (Fig. 46.1). Therefore, relatively small transcellular potassium shifts can have marked effects on the serum potassium concentration, even in the absence of changes in total body potassium. Factors known to stimulate cellular potassium uptake and thereby predispose to hypokalemia include (16): (a) β_2 adrenergic stimulation, (b) insulin (independent of its effect on glucose transport), (c) high pH and bicarbonate levels, (d) anabolism, and (e) possibly aldosterone.

Because transcellular potassium shifts are not infrequent, and because potassium is not lost proportionally from the extracellular and intracellular spaces, it is not surprising that the serum potassium does not always accurately reflect total body stores. Nevertheless, in the absence of major alterations in internal potassium balance, there is a roughly linear inverse relationship between the decrement in the serum potassium concentration and the magnitude of the potassium deficit. The serum potassium falls about 0.27 mEq/liter for each 100 mEq of potassium depletion (Fig. 46.3) (15). This relationship is valid for deficits up to about 500 mEq; with larger deficits, the serum

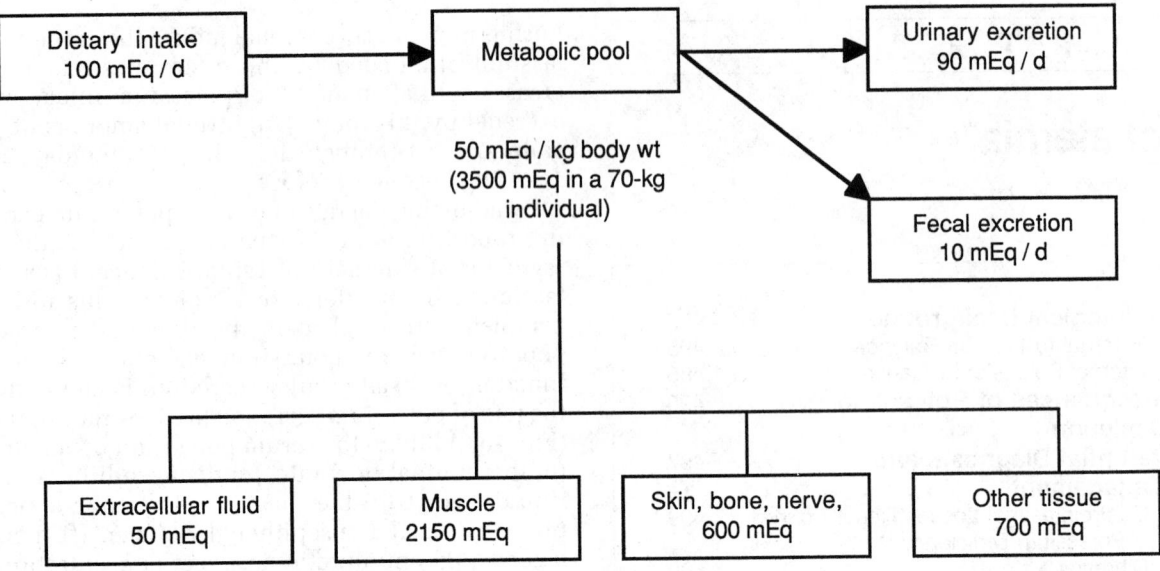

Figure 46.1. Balance of potassium. (Adapted from Kliger AS, and Hayslett JP: Disorders of potassium. In Brenner BM, Stein JH (eds): *Acid-Base and Potassium Hemostatis*. New York, Churchill Livingstone, 1978.)

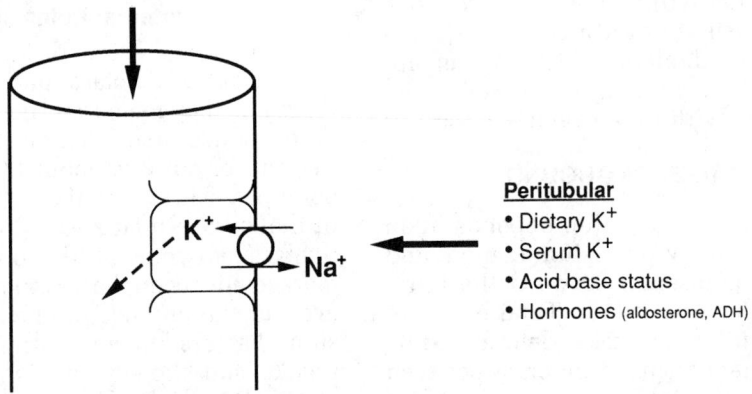

Figure 46.2. Factors influencing potassium secretion by the distal tubule modified from Giebisch G: Physiology of Potassium Metabolism. In: Whelton PK, Whelton A, Walker WG (eds), *Potassium in Cardiovascular and Renal Medicine*. New York, Marcel Dekker, Inc, 1986.

potassium falls less for every 100 mEq of potassium lost.

CONSEQUENCES OF POTASSIUM DEPLETION

Most often the practitioner detects mild hypokalemia on a set of electrolytes in an asymptomatic individual. Almost as often, the symptoms of the problems that have led to potassium depletion are prominent, for example, vomiting or diarrhea. However, severe potassium depletion may occasionally have serious consequences (Table 46.1) (17). Many of these con-

sequences are the result of changes in cell membrane potential that affect the function of excitable tissue, primarily nerve and muscle.

Of greatest concern is the effect of hypokalemia on the heart. Although some have claimed that severe potassium depletion can cause myocardial necrosis, it is difficult to exclude other etiological factors in these reports. On the other hand, changes in potassium balance can clearly affect cardiac conduction and rhythm; during hypokalemia (as with hyperkalemia), characteristic electrocardiographic changes may be seen (Fig. 46.4).

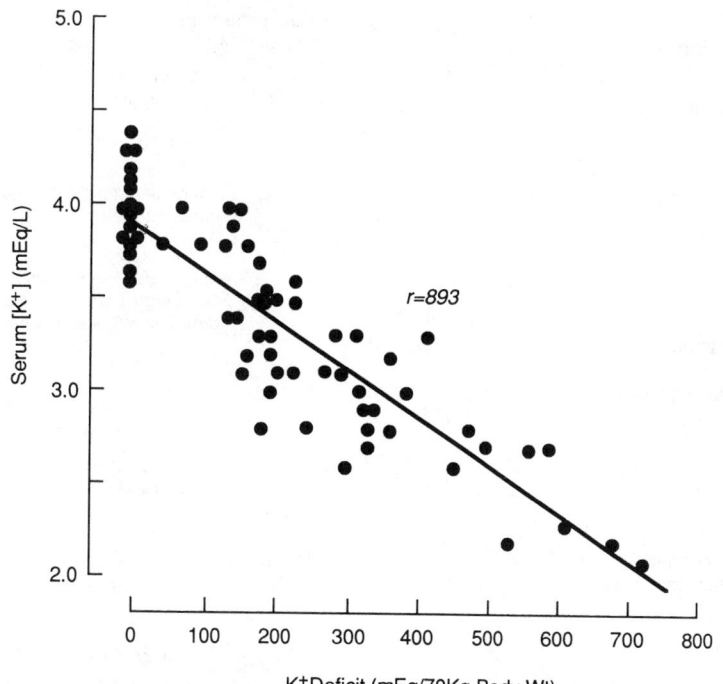

Figure 46.3. Effect of uncomplicated potassium depletion on the plasma potassium concentration. The fall in serum potassium concentration equals 0.27 mEq/L per 100 mEq potassium deficit (r = 0.893). Taken with permission from Sterns RH, Cox M, Feig PU, Singer I: Internal potassium balance and the control of the plasma potassium concentration. *Medicine* (Baltimore) 60:339, 1981.

Hypokalemia has also long been known to predispose to digitalis intoxication manifested by a variety of rhythm disturbances. However, whether mild to moderate hypokalemia per se is a cause of dangerous ventricular ectopy is presently a matter of controversy. Although some investigators found increased ventricular ectopy in hypertensive subjects after diuretic-induced hypokalemia, others have been unable to confirm these findings (11). It may be that hypokalemia is arrhythmogenic only in certain individuals; thus in a small group of patients, diuretic-induced hypokalemia led to increased ventricular ectopy only in those subjects with underlying heart disease (1). It has also been suggested that hypokalemia may be particularly arrhythmogenic during acute myocardial infarction; but even in this setting the studies are not all in agreement (11). It is possible that during a myocardial infarction, hypokalemia is merely a marker of high catecholamine levels with the latter being responsible for both the induction of arrhythmias and hypokalemia (via an intracellular shift of potassium secondary to stimulation of β_2 receptors).

Both smooth and skeletal muscle function may be altered by potassium depletion. Severe hypokalemia can cause decreased gastrointestinal tract motility resulting in ileus, as well as proximal muscle weakness that can progress to paralysis. On occasion, the respiratory muscles may be involved resulting in respiratory failure. Hypokalemia may also predispose to rhabdomyolysis after vigorous exercise, at least in part by interfering with exercise-induced vasodilation. On the other hand, postural hypotension and a decrease in systemic vascular resistance have been re-

ported in potassium-depleted patients. Rarely tetany may be seen even in the absence of changes in pH or serum calcium.

Potassium depletion has several effects upon the kidney. The most characteristic alteration in renal function is an impaired ability to concentrate the urine; however, the severity of the defect is generally mild and the polyuria sometimes seen may be in large part due to direct stimulation of thirst. With prolonged severe potassium depletion, the glomerular filtration rate and renal blood flow may be reduced. This is usually reversible with potassium repletion, although rarely permanent renal injury can occur. Potassium depletion also predisposes to the development of metabolic alkalosis through renal and extrarenal mechanisms.

The state of potassium balance also affects a variety of hormones. Thus, hypokalemia inhibits the synthesis of aldosterone, increases plasma renin activity, and decreases insulin secretion. The latter may precipitate or worsen diabetes mellitus. Despite much investigation, the effects of hypokalemia on prostaglandin metabolism and the resulting clinical consequences remain unclear.

Finally, by stimulating renal ammonia production, potassium depletion may precipitate hepatic encephalopathy in patients with severe liver failure.

DIFFERENTIAL DIAGNOSIS AND MANAGEMENT

Three fundamental mechanisms, alone or in combination, may lead to hypokalemia (Table 46.2): (*a*) a shift of potassium into the cells, (*b*) reduced potassium

Table 46.1.
Clinical Sequelae of Hypokalemia*[a]*

Cardiovascular
Predisposition to digitalis intoxication
Abnormal electrocardiogram
Ventricular ectopic rhythms
Cardiac necrosis
Decreased peripheral vascular resistance
Decreased blood pressure

Neuromuscular
Gastrointestinal: Constipation
                   Ileus
Skeletal muscle: Weakness, cramps
                   Tetany
                   Paralysis (including respiratory)
                   Rhabdomyolysis

Renal
Decreased renal blood flow
Decreased GFR
Renal hypertrophy
Pathologic alterations (interstitial nephritis)
Predisposition to urinary tract infection

Fluid and Electrolyte
Polyuria and polydipsia
   Renal concentrating defect
   Stimulation of thirst center
   ADH release (?)
Increased renal ammonia production
   Predisposition to hepatic coma
   Altered urinary acidification
Renal chloride wasting
Metabolic alkalosis
Sodium retention
Hyponatremia (with concomitant diuretic therapy)

Endocrine
Decrease in aldosterone
Increase in renin
Altered prostaglandin metabolism
Decrease in insulin secretion
   (Carbohydrate intolerance)

[a]Modified from Tannen RL. Potassium Disorders. In Kokko JP, Tannen RL (eds): Fluids and Electrolytes. Philadelphia, WB Saunders Co, 1986.

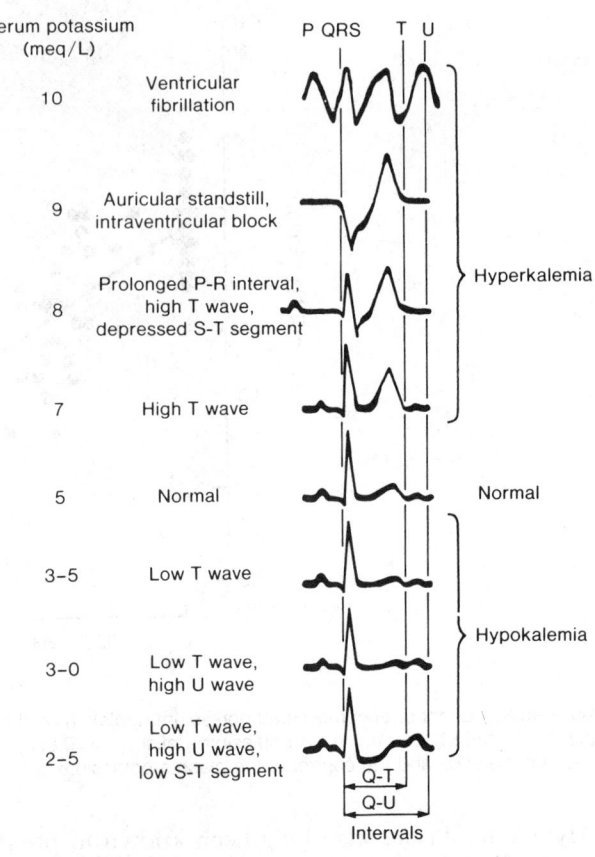

Figure 46.4. Electrocardiogram in assessment of potassium. (Adapted from Burch GE, Winsor T: *A Primer of Electrocardiography*, 6th ed. Philadelphia, Lea & Febiger, 1972, p. 128.)

Table 46.2.
Basic Mechanisms of Hypokalemia

1. Intracellular shift of potassium
2. Decreased intake of potassium
3. Increased loss of potassium
   a) Renal source
   b) Extrarenal source

intake, and (c) excessive potassium loss. The latter category may be subdivided according to whether potassium losses are renal or extrarenal (primarily gastrointestinal).

The first step in evaluating the hypokalemic patient is a careful history, asking specifically about diet, medications [especially diuretics, laxatives, and β_2 agonists (e.g., salbutamol)], vomiting, diarrhea, urine output, hypertension, diabetes mellitus, and family history. The physical examination should be directed toward a careful assessment of volume status, including measurement of blood pressure in the supine and upright positions. Laboratory data should always include a set of electrolytes, glucose concentration, and a measure of renal function, best reflected by the serum creatinine. At this point, the etiology of hypokalemia may be obvious, and if the patient responds to therapy as expected, further evaluation is not necessary.

If the cause of hypokalemia remains unclear, the following approach is recommended (Fig. 46.5) (10). First decide whether there is any reason to suspect an intracellular shift of potassium; for example, is the patient using a β_2 agonist for asthma or is the blood pH elevated? If not, the patient is likely to be potassium depleted. In this case, the next step is to determine where the potassium was lost—was it via a renal or extrarenal route? This usually can be achieved by measuring the urinary potassium. If renal potassium excretion is high (>20 mEq/liter on a spot urine specimen or >20 mEq in a 24-hour collection) despite hypokalemia, excessive renal potassium losses are, at least in part, responsible for potassium depletion. On the other hand, if renal potassium excretion is appropriately low, this suggests an extrarenal loss of potassium. However, on occasion potassium may have been lost through the kidneys even though the present urinary potassium excretion is low; this occurs when the stimulus to excessive renal potassium excretion is only temporary—as with diuretics that have been discontinued.

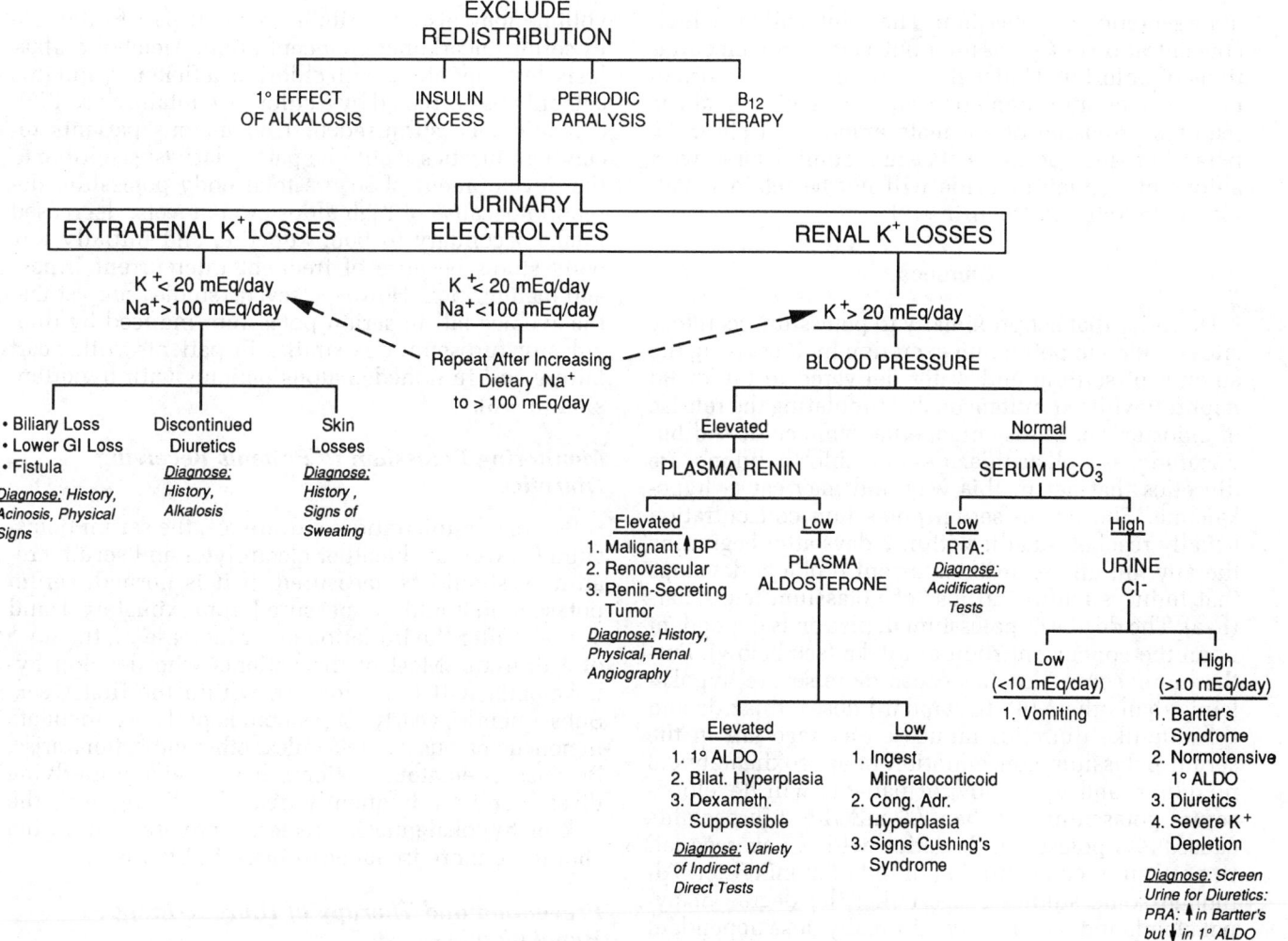

Figure 46.5. Diagnostic approach to hypokalemia. Taken with permission from Narins RG, Jones ER, Stom MC, et al: Diagnostic strategies in disorders of fluid, electrolyte and acid-base homeostasis. *Am J Med* 72, 496, 1982.

As shown in Figure 46.5, further studies depend on whether potassium has been lost through a renal or extrarenal route. The acid-base status and blood pressure provide useful clues. It is also important to remember that magnesium depletion and potassium depletion often go hand in hand, and that magnesium depletion can cause renal potassium wasting. Therefore, the serum magnesium level should be checked in any patient with severe or refractory hypokalemia.

Gastrointestinal Losses Resulting in Potassium Deficiency

Diarrhea

Because potassium and bicarbonate are normally present in the stool in high concentrations, diarrhea is a common cause of hypokalemia that is frequently associated with metabolic acidosis. Occasionally, hypokalemia may be a clue to the presence of a villous adenoma of the colon or surreptitious laxative abuse; in these conditions, the acid-base status is variable. Diarrheal states in general are usually associated with

clinical contraction of the extracellular fluid volume, detected on physical examination by weight loss, low jugular venous pressure, poor skin turgor, tachycardia, and orthostatic hypotension. Urinary potassium excretion should be low when potassium deficiency results from gastrointestinal losses, since in this setting the kidney conserves potassium maximally.

Loss of Gastric Fluid

Hypokalemia is well known to accompany vomiting or gastric drainage. Yet, although gastric fluid is rich in hydrochloric acid, it contains only small amounts of potassium (about 5 to 10 mEq/liter). Therefore, most of the potassium lost from the body during removal of gastric fluid is not lost from the stomach; indeed, the major route of potassium loss in this setting is the urine (14). The loss of gastric contents induces metabolic alkalosis, chloride deficiency, extracellular volume depletion, and secondary hyperaldosteronism. The increased filtered load and increased distal delivery of bicarbonate, decreased distal delivery of chloride, and high levels of aldosterone all act together to stimulate secretion of potassium. The urine will have high concentrations of potassium but very low concentrations of chloride. Under these circumstances, correction of potassium depletion and metabolic alkalosis requires provision of adequate amounts of chloride, potassium and sodium. Potassium administered with anions other than chloride will not be retained but, rather, excreted in the urine (5).

Diuretics

Diuretics that act proximally to potassium secretory sites accelerate potassium excretion by increasing the amount of sodium and water delivered to the distal nephron while simultaneously stimulating the release of aldosterone. Furosemide, ethacrynic acid, and bumetanide, as well as thiazides and chlorthalidone, are diuretics that act in this way and may cause hypokalemia. The fall in serum potassium concentration usually reaches a nadir within 7 days after beginning therapy (8), unless an intercurrent problem develops that induces additional loss of potassium (e.g., diarrhea). The degree of potassium depletion is dependent upon the concurrent sodium intake (see below). Furthermore, some diuretics cause more severe hypokalemia than others (8): In standard doses, thiazide and thiazide-like diuretics induce an average fall in the serum potassium concentration of approximately 0.6 mEq/liter, and up to 50% of patients will develop a serum potassium less than 3.5 mEq/liter; furosemide causes less potassium depletion with an average fall in potassium concentration of only 0.3 mEq/liter. Although some studies suggest that the degree of hypokalemia induced is only minimally dose dependent (8), the use of multiple (non-potassium-sparing) diuretics acting at different nephron sites (e.g., furosemide and thiazide) is likely to cause significant hypokalemia.

Patients who take diuretics but who are not edematous (for example, patients with mild hypertension being treated with thiazides) do not usually become severely depleted of potassium. Less than 7% of such individuals develop a serum potassium concentration less than 3.0 mEq/liter (8). Levels below 3.0 mEq/liter should suggest two additional explanations (18): (a) *Excessive sodium intake.* A high intake of sodium chloride in a patient taking potassium-wasting diuretics will increase the amount of sodium and water delivered to the distal nephron, thereby accelerating potassium secretion and exacerbating potassium depletion. (b) *An unrecognized potassium-wasting state.* Both primary and secondary aldosteronism should be suspected when marked hypokalemia develops after the introduction of potassium-wasting diuretics, particularly if the potassium level before treatment was low.

Metabolic alkalosis frequently accompanies hypokalemia in patients taking diuretics. Many potassium-wasting diuretics stimulate renal hydrogen ion secretion and induce a net loss of acid, causing a rise in serum bicarbonate. Contraction of the extracellular

volume may also contribute in small part to the rise in serum bicarbonate concentration. Metabolic alkalosis develops along with chloride deficiency, and this can only be corrected by a chloride containing salt (5).

It might be surmised that edematous patients receiving diuretics would be particularly susceptible to the development of severe total body potassium depletion because of high aldosterone levels, decreased intake secondary to poor appetite, and initially low body stores because of frequent intercurrent illness and malnutrition. However, several studies suggest that the average fall in serum potassium induced by thiazides or furosemide is similar in patients with heart failure and in nonedematous patients with hypertension (8, 18).

Monitoring Potassium in Patients Receiving Diuretics

Before administration of diuretics, the serum potassium (as well as the other electrolytes and serum creatinine) should be measured. If it is normal, serum potassium should be measured approximately 1 and 4 weeks after the initiation of, or increase in, the dose of a diuretic. Most of the patients who develop hypokalemia will have done so within the first week. Subsequently, yearly assessment is probably adequate in nonedematous patients unless other indications arise. Because edematous patients have major underlying disease and are frequently treated with digitalis, the risk of hypokalemia is greater; therefore monitoring should be more frequent in these individuals.

Prevention and Therapy of Diuretic-Induced Hypokalemia

As previously outlined, whether mild diuretic-induced hypokalemia per se is dangerous remains controversial (11). Nonetheless, when a diuretic is indicated, it seems reasonable to employ simple measures that can minimize this problem (6). These include using the lowest effective dose of an agent with an intermediate duration of action (e.g., hydrochlorothiazide) and prescribing a moderate restriction of dietary sodium (75 to 100 mEq or ≥2 g per day) (see Tables 62.12 and 62.13). Although an increase in dietary potassium seems logical, much of the potassium in food is accompanied by anions other than chloride; because only potassium chloride can correct potassium depletion in this setting, a high potassium diet is unlikely to be effective.

Even with preventive measures, about 30% of diuretic treated patients become hypokalemic (6). The physician must then decide whether normalization of serum potassium is indicated. Because it is likely that only certain patients will benefit from correction, and potassium therapy is costly, inconvenient, and not without risks (4), the management of diuretic-induced hypokalemia should be individualized. It is important to maintain a normal serum potassium in groups of patients listed in Table 46.3 (18). Potassium may also be prescribed as a therapeutic trial for patients with

Table 46.3.
Indications for Potassium Maintenance Therapy[a]

1. Digitalis therapy
2. Predisposition to hepatic coma
3. Serum potassium < 3.0 mEq/liter
4. Development of glucose intolerance
5. Underlying cardiac disease
6. Symptoms attributable to hypokalemia

[a]Taken with permission from Tannen, RL. Diuretic induced hypokalemia. *Kid Int* 28:988, 1985.

Table 46.4.
Commonly Available Potassium Salts

Source	Potassium Concentration
Solutions	
Potassium chloride	
5% (generic)	10 mEq/15 ml
10% (generic, Kaochlor 10%, Kaon Cl-10, Klor-10%, Klorvess 10%)	20 mEq/15 ml
20% (generic, Kaon Cl-20)	40 mEq/15 ml
Potassium citrate (Polycitra-K)	30 mEq/15 ml
Potassium gluconate (generic, Kaon Elixir)	20 mEq/15 ml
Effervescent Granules or Tablets	
Potassium chloride (Klorvess)	20 mEq/packet
Tablets	
Potassium chloride (K-Tab, Kaor-Cl, Slow-K, Micro-K, Extencaps)	6, 7, 8 and 10 mEq/tablet
Potassium gluconate (Kaor)	5 mEq/tablet

*Available with or without sugar and in different flavors. Taste generally improved by chilling.

mild diuretic-induced hypokalemia who develop nonspecific complaints such as fatigue and muscular aches; if there is no improvement, potassium should be discontinued.

When normalization of the serum potassium is indicated and the diuretic must be continued, the physician must then decide whether to use potassium supplements or potassium-sparing diuretics (see Table 62.9 for detailed discussion). Although a variety of potassium supplements are available (Table 46.4), just as with the loss of gastric contents, *only potassium chloride* will correct diuretic-induced hypokalemia associated with metabolic alkalosis (5). However, liquid preparations have a bad taste that limits compliance. Wax matrix tablets (Slow-K) or the newer microencapsulated preparations (Micro-K Extentabs) avoid this problem, but they are expensive and contain only small amounts of potassium, thereby requiring frequent dosing. Salt substitutes are composed mostly of potassium chloride (about 50 to 65 mmol/teaspoon) and have been suggested as a cheap and effective alternative. However, diuretic-induced hypokalemia may be relatively refractory even to large doses of potassium chloride because the renal clearance of potassium remains high during continued diuretic therapy (2, 12); in one study, potassium chloride in doses up to 96 mmol/day normalized the serum potassium in only eight of 16 hypertensive patients with diuretic-induced hypokalemia (12).

When compared with potassium supplements, po-

tassium-sparing diuretics (including spironolactone, triamterene, and amiloride) offer several advantages (6): (a) by reducing urinary potassium losses, they act to correct the underlying pathophysiology; (b) they minimize the development of metabolic alkalosis by reducing acid excretion; (c) they limit renal magnesium wasting; and (d) they are frequently accepted better by the patient. For these reasons, potassium-sparing diuretics are often preferable to potassium supplements when maintenance of a normal serum potassium is deemed appropriate. In one study, conversion from hydrochlorothiazide (with or without potassium supplements) to Moduretic (hydrochlorothiazide plus amiloride) once daily or two capsules of Dyazide (hydrochlorothiazide plus triamterene) without potassium supplements, increased the serum potassium by about 0.5 to 0.7 mEq/liter and brought it into the midnormal range (13). Spironolactone can also be used but has the disadvantage of sometimes causing gynecomastia in men. Triamterene can cause nephrolithiasis and in combination with indomethacin can markedly decrease the glomerular filtration rate.

The major risk of attempts to raise the serum potassium is hyperkalemia. To avoid this potentially life-threatening complication, all patients beginning therapy with potassium supplements or potassium-sparing agents should be assessed for risk factors for hyperkalemia. These include renal insufficiency, diabetes mellitus, old age, and the ingestion of other agents known to interfere with potassium homeostasis (e.g., converting-enzyme inhibitors, nonsteroidal anti-inflammatory drugs, cyclosporine, and heparin). Rarely even patients without apparent risk factors may develop hyperkalemia when treated with potassium-sparing agents. Therefore, all patients beginning potassium therapy should have their serum potassium measured after 1 and 4 weeks and then every 6 to 12 months. If a hypokalemic patient is found to have renal insufficiency or other risk factors for hyperkalemia, potassium supplements and potassium-sparing diuretics are generally contraindicated and should not be used without consultation from a nephrologist; if raising the serum potassium is deemed necessary in these patients, more frequent measures of the serum potassium are mandatory. Even in the patient with normal renal function, potassium supplements and potassium-sparing diuretics generally should not be given together or along with other drugs that interfere with potassium homeostasis.

Less Common Causes of Hypokalemia

Less common causes of hypokalemia seen in ambulatory practice are dietary deficiency, excessive urinary potassium loss due to several causes, and an altered distribution of potassium across the cell membrane. The approach to diagnosing these problems is based on the history, physical examination, urinary electrolyte levels, acid-base status, and occasionally the measurement of plasma renin activity and aldosterone levels. An unexpectedly low serum potassium value should always be confirmed by repeated testing before initiating an extensive workup.

Deficient Potassium Intake

Potassium is widely distributed in many foods. Therefore, inadequate potassium intake is an unusual cause of hypokalemia unless the patient fails to eat for prolonged periods. Alcoholics and patients with terminal illnesses may become mildly hypokalemic in this manner. More severe hypokalemia may develop if insufficient potassium is provided during anabolism as cells take up potassium; examples include refeeding malnourished patients and treating megaloblastic anemia (16). Dietary deficiency of potassium, particularly in the elderly, may also exacerbate diuretic-induced hypokalemia. Dietary deficiency is established by history, clinical evidence of malnutrition, the absence of other causes of hypokalemia, and correction with potassium replacement. In such patients, the urinary potassium excretion should be less than 10 to 20 mEq/day while they are hypokalemic.

Excessive Urinary Potassium Losses

In the presence of chronic hypokalemia, an unexplained excessive loss of potassium in the urine (>20 mEq/liter or >20 mEq/day) is diagnostic of renal potassium wasting. The differential diagnosis in this setting is complex, but it can be simplified by assessing the acid-base status and blood pressure of the patient (Fig. 46.5) (10).

Renal Potassium Wasting

When hypokalemia secondary to renal potassium wasting is accompanied by an elevated blood pressure, mineralocorticoid (or glucocorticoid) excess is suggested. There are several causes that must be considered (Table 46.5). The evaluation of such a patient is complex. However, certain basic diagnoses may be made in an office, which may minimize the need for referral to a center experienced in the evaluation of these syndromes.

Unless the cause is readily apparent (e.g., a patient with essential hypertension treated with diuretics), the first step in the evaluation of renal potassium wasting in a hypertensive patient is the determination of plasma renin activity (Fig. 46.5); if elevated, this suggests a primary renin excess state, such as renovascular, accelerated, or malignant hypertension (see Chapter 62), or rarely a renin-producing tumor. On the other hand, if the renin level is low, the plasma renin activity should be remeasured along with a plasma aldosterone level. If both levels are low, the presence of excessive amounts of endogenous or exogenous steroids, other than aldosterone, is likely; licorice, chewing tobacco, carbenoxolone, and steroid-containing nasal sprays are rare exogenous causes of this syndrome. Finally, if the renin level is low but the simultaneous aldosterone level is high, primary aldosteronism is strongly suggested. The sensitivity

Table 46.5.
Causes of Hypertension with Associated Renal Potassium Wasting[a]

Hyperreninemic forms
  Renovascular
  Renin tumor
  Malignant or accelerated essential hypertension

Hyporeninemic steroid-dependent forms
  Mineralocorticoid
    Exogenous
      Licorice, desoxycorticosterone,
      Fluodrocortisone, chewing tobacco,
      Carbenoxalone
    Endogenous
      Adrenal adenoma
      Adrenal glomerulosa hyperplasia
      Enzyme deficiency: 17-OHase; 11-OHase
      Liddle syndrome
  Glucocorticoid
    Endogenous
      Cushing syndrome, pituitary, ectopic
      ACTH, adrenal cortical
    Exogenous

[a]Taken with permission from Narins RG, Jones ER, Stom MC, et al: Diagnostic strategies in disorders of fluid, electrolyte and acid-base homeostasis. *Am J Med* 72:496, 1982.

and specificity of this screening test may be increased by determining the aldosterone:renin ratio 2 hours after 25 mg of captopril; in primary aldosteronism the ratio remains high but is suppressed in patients with essential hypertension (7).

Primary Hyperaldosteronism

Most patients with primary aldosteronism are asymptomatic (19). Clinical manifestations, in addition to hypertension, are related to potassium depletion and occur only when such depletion is severe. These include weakness, paralysis, tetany, arrhythmias, polyuria, and polydipsia. Edema is rare. Patients with primary aldosteronism usually have spontaneous hypokalemia, but as many as 25% have serum potassium levels above 3.5 mEq/liter. However, many of these patients manifest hypokalemia if challenged with potassium-wasting diuretics or large intakes of sodium chloride [200 mmol/day (about 4 to 5 g sodium)]; both interventions result in increased delivery of sodium and water to the distal nephron where, under the influence of excessive aldosterone, sodium is reabsorbed whereas potassium and hydrogen ions are secreted—hypokalemia and metabolic alkalosis ensue. Indeed, the development of severe hypokalemia after the initiation of thiazide therapy is a clue to a hypermineralocorticoid state. On the other hand, a serum potassium greater than 4.0 mEq/liter on a high sodium diet (documented by a 24-hour urinary sodium excretion of about 200 mEq/day) virtually excludes the diagnosis (19).

When the combination of hypokalemia, suppressed plasma renin activity, and elevated aldosterone levels appears likely, the patient should be referred to an endocrinologist or nephrologist with expertise in this area. Localization procedures will then be undertaken by the consultant to distinguish adenomas from bilateral adrenal hyperplasia. The techniques used usually are computed tomography (CT) followed, if negative, by adrenal scintography using an isotope or cholesterol (this latter technique seems superior especially for small tumors). The treatment of adenomas is primarily surgical, and excision has frequently led to the cure of hypertension and hypokalemia. If bilateral hyperplasia is found, surgery is not indicated since it is seldom curative. A trial of spironolactone may be useful in all patients. Large doses (up to 400 mg daily) are usually necessary, and the full effects may not be seen for several weeks. Failure of spironolactone to normalize the blood pressure while normalizing hypokalemia strongly suggests that—regardless of the anatomical basis for the aldosterone excess—surgery would not correct the hypertension. Although spironolactone has been the mainstay of medical therapy for primary aldosteronism, amiloride (up to 40 mgm/day) is also effective and may be the drug of choice for sexually active men and for patients intolerant of spironolactone (19).

Normotensive Renal Potassium Wasting

When renal potassium wasting is discovered in a normotensive patient, the acid-base status is the next parameter to be evaluated (Fig. 46.5). If metabolic acidosis is present, renal tubular acidosis or diabetic ketoacidosis is suggested. If metabolic alkalosis is present, the urinary chloride provides an important clue to the underlying process. If the urinary chloride concentration is low, vomiting is the likely cause; if the urinary chloride is high, the most likely cause is diuretics, but other less common etiologies are possible. It should be emphasized that diuretic abuse and self-induced vomiting are common concealed causes of hypokalemia and metabolic alkalosis in women concerned about their weight.

Bartter's Syndrome

This rare disorder presents with hypokalemic metabolic alkalosis and excessive urinary potassium losses; blood pressure is normal and edema is absent. Plasma renin activity and aldosterone levels are markedly elevated. This presentation is mimicked by diuretic abuse, from which Bartter's syndrome must be differentiated. Urine screens for diuretics can be helpful.

Bartter's syndrome may be due to reduced solute reabsorption in the diluting segment of the nephron. Hypokalemia is usually refractory to potassium supplementation but may be ameliorated by prostaglandin synthesis inhibitors or by amiloride (17).

Disordered Internal Potassium Balance

It has been well shown that β_2 adrenergic agonists lower the serum potassium concentration by stimulating cellular potassium uptake (16). Thus it is not surprising that a reduction in serum potassium is seen commonly when β_2 agonists are used in the treatment of asthma or premature labor; though the decrease in serum potassium is usually mild, significant hypokalemia can occur, which usually resolves within hours after the drug is discontinued. Similarly, *high levels of endogenous catecholamines* released during stress may explain transient reductions in serum potassium (that resolve with or without potassium supplementation) sometimes seen during acute hospital admissions (9), before delirium tremens, and during acute myocardial infarction (16).

Metabolic and respiratory alkalosis are associated with small shifts of potassium from the extracellular to the intracellular space. This may sensitize the individual to digitalis, even in the absence of total body potassium depletion.

Insulin stimulates cellular potassium uptake in liver and skeletal muscle, independent of its effects on glucose transport. This dose-dependent action forms the basis for using insulin in the treatment of severe hyperkalemia. When insulin is used to correct hyperglycemia and the initial serum potassium is normal, hypokalemia may ensue.

Hypokalemic periodic paralysis is a rare familial disorder characterized by spontaneous episodes of paralysis that may be precipitated by a variety of stimuli including insulin, glucose, and a high carbohydrate meal. A similar syndrome may also be seen in hyperthyroidism, especially in oriental men. Although a fall in the serum potassium is regularly demonstrated during paralysis, there is a dramatic decrease in urinary potassium excretion, signifying an intracellular shift of potassium. In the thyrotoxic form, beta-blocking agents may be effective in preventing attacks.

Vitamin B$_{12}$, when administered in the therapy of megaloblastic anemia, may cause large intracellular shifts of potassium as metabolic activity is increased in hematopoietic cells. Provision of adequate quantities of potassium and careful monitoring will avoid this complication.

Finally, *ingestion of soluble barium salts* may cause profound hypokalemia by competitively blocking cellular potassium channels and inhibiting potassium exit from the cells. Severe muscle weakness, paralysis, and respiratory failure may result. Though sporadic barium poisoning is rare, epidemics have occurred secondary to contamination of table salt with barium chloride. Provision of potassium improves paralysis, most likely by competing with barium for potassium channels.

General References

Nader PC, Thompson JR, Alpern RJ: Complications of diuretic use. *Semin Nephrol* 8:365, 1988.

Papademetriou V: Diuretics, hypokalemia, and cardiac arrhythmias: a critical analysis. *Am Heart J* 111:1217, 1986.
    A review of the controversy about the cardiac risks of diuretic-induced hypokalemia.

Sterns RH, Cox M, Feig PU, et al: Internal potassium balance and the control of the plasma potassium concentration. *Medicine* (Baltimore) 60:339, 1981.

Tannen RL: Diuretic-induced hypokalemia. *Kidney Int* 28:988, 1985.

Tannen RL: Potassium disorders. In: Kokko JP, Tannen RL (eds): *Fluids and Electrolytes.* Philadelphia, WB Saunders, 1986.

Young WF, Klee GG: Primary aldosteronism: diagnostic evaluation. *Endocrinol Met Clin North Am* 17:367, 1988.

An excellent review of primary aldosteronism with emphasis on diagnosis and differentiation of subtypes.

Specific References

1. Caralis PV, Materson BJ, Perez-Stable E: Potassium and diuretic-induced ventricular arrhythmias in ambulatory hypertensive patients. *Min Electrolyte Metab* 10:148, 1984.
2. Down PF, Polak A, Rao R: Fate of potassium supplements in six outpatients receiving long-term diuretics foroedematous disease. *Lancet* 2:721, 1972.
3. Giebish G: Physiology of potassium metabolism. In: Wheaton PK, Whelton A, Walker GW (eds): *Potassium in Cardiovascular and Renal Medicine.* New York, Marcel Dekker, 1986.
4. Harrington JT, Isner JM, Kassirer JP: Our national obsession with potassium. *Am J Med* 73:155, 1982.
5. Kassirer JP, Berkman PM, Lawrenz DR, et al: The critical role of chloride in the correction of hypokalemic alkalosis in man. *Am J Med* 38:172, 1965.
6. Krishna GG, Shulman MD, Narins RG: Clinical use of the potassium-sparing diuretics. *Semin Nephrol* 8:354, 1988.
7. Lyons DF, Kem DC, Brown RD, et al: Single dose captopril as a diagnostic test for primary aldosteronism. *J Clin Endocrinol Metab* 57:892, 1988.
8. Morgan DB, Davidson C: Hypokalemia and diuretics: an analysis of publications. *Br Med J* 280:905, 1980.
9. Morgan DB, Young RM: Acute transient hypokalemia: new interpretation of a common event. *Lancet* 2:751, 1982.
10. Narins RG, Jones ER, Stom MC, et al: Diagnostic strategies in disorders of fluid, electrolyte and acid-base homeostasis. *Am J Med* 72:496, 1982.
11. Papademetriou V,: Diuretics, hypokalemia, and cardiac arrhythmias: a critical analysis. *Am Heart J* 111:1217, 1986.
12. Papademetriou V, Burris J, Kukich S, et al: Effectiveness of potassium chloride or triamterene in thiazide hypokalemia. *Arch Intern Med* 145:1986, 1985.
13. Ridgeway NA, Ginn DR, Alley K: Outpatient conversion of treatment to potassium-sparing diuretics. *Am J Med* 80:785, 1986.
14. Stein JH: Hypokalemia: common and uncommon causes. *Hosp Prac* 23:55, 1988.
15. Sterns RH, Cox M, Feig PU: Internal potassium balance and the control of the plasma potassium concentration. *Medicine* 60:339, 1981.
16. Sterns RH, Spital A: Disorder of internal potassium balance. *Semin Nephrol* 7:206, 1987.
17. Tannen RL: Potassium disorders. In: Kokko JP, Tannen RL (eds): *Fluids and Electrolytes.* Philadelphia, W.B. Saunders, 1986.
18. Tannen RL: Diuretic-induced hypokalemia. *Kidney Int* 28:988, 1985.
19. Young WF Jr, Klee GG: Primary aldosteronism: diagnostic evaluation. *Endocrinol Metab Clin North Am* 17:367, 1988.

C H A P T E R 47

Urinary Stones*

DAVID A. SPECTOR, M.D.

Urinary stones are very common in the United States. In an office practice such patients will be encountered frequently and one will therefore need to be familiar with the evaluation and management of this common problem. Although urological intervention or nephrological consultation may occasionally be required, the vast majority of patients with stones can be evaluated, treated, and followed by the primary care physician. This chapter will review the various manifestations of stone disease; the types of urinary stones; the evaluation of patients with stones; the acute and chronic management of patients with urinary stones, and, finally, when to obtain consultation for these patients.

*Drs. John R. Burton and James K. Smolev contributed to this chapter in the first and second editions of this book.

PRESENTATION OF URINARY STONE DISEASE

Physicians will encounter patients who have urinary stone disease in one of five clinical settings: (a) a patient with acute colic, (b) a patient with persistent or recurrent urinary tract infection, (c) a patient with isolated hematuria, (d) a patient with no symptoms in whom a stone is discovered incidentally on an X-ray taken for other purposes, or (e) a patient who gives a history of having had a stone.

Acute Colic

Presentation

Most patients with urinary stones will have at some time an acute episode of colic. The stone, if obstructing, causes ureteral spasm, resulting in severe intermittent pain. The location of the pain depends on the location of the stone in the ureter but is most often felt in the flank; and then as the stone moves distally, pain radiates in a characteristic pattern around the groin and into the testicles in the male or into the labia majora in the female. Nausea, vomiting, paralytic ileus, and other gastrointestinal symptoms that often suggest a primary gastrointestinal problem may be associated with pain. Examination reveals an uncomfortable, restless patient. There may be costovertebral tenderness as well as deep tenderness in the abdomen. More importantly, there are no signs of peritoneal irritation present (guarding, rebound, or rigidity). Fever is not present unless urinary tract infection has developed in the obstructed urinary tract.

Urinalysis almost always demonstrates microscopic (or gross) hematuria. The presence of pyuria is important since chronic bacterial infection may be associated with the development of urinary stones; however, pyuria may be absent even if infection is present during complete ureteral obstruction.

Diagnosis and Management

The aim of management of a patient with colic should be (a) relief of discomfort, (b) surveillance for infection, and (c) determination of whether stones will pass spontaneously or will require surgical removal. The abdominal X-ray is useful in monitoring the site and progression of the stone. Approximately 90% of renal stones are radiodense and will be seen on a good quality X-ray. The size and position of the stone will help to decide the urgency of subsequent studies, such as an intravenous pyelogram (IVP). In general, stones that are smaller than 5 mm will pass spontaneously; those between 5 and 10 mm have a 50% chance of passing spontaneously; and those larger than 10 mm usually require surgical removal. The common sites where stones become lodged are (a) the renal calyx, (b) the ureteropelvic junction, (c) in the ureter at the pelvic brim where the ureter begins to pass over the iliac vessels, (d) in the lower third of the ureter, and (e) at the ureterovesical junction. If there is doubt about whether calcification seen on the plain X-ray is within the urinary tract, an oblique view may help. It is also important to review old abdominal films taken for any reason to see whether a stone was present at that time. An intravenous pyelogram should also be obtained as soon as possible in the patient with colic, as it will help to establish the diagnosis, especially in patients with radiolucent stones, and it will provide certain important information (see below) that will aid in management.

Several factors will help one decide whether to hospitalize a patient with renal colic, to obtain urgent urological consultation, or to manage the patient at home. First, the patient with nausea and vomiting cannot be assured of an adequate fluid intake or of adequate oral analgesia and should be admitted to a hospital. Second, fever suggests infection proximal to an obstructing stone, and urgent urological consultation should be obtained. Third, if an IVP reveals any of the following findings, urgent urological consultation should be obtained: (a) a nonfunctioning kidney (completely obstructed ureter), (b) a partially obstructed ureter from a solitary kidney, and (c) urine extravasation. Fourth, if the stone is larger than 10 mm, spontaneous passage is very unlikely and urological consultation should be obtained. Eighty percent of all stones that become symptomatic are ureteral, and 85 to 90% of these will pass spontaneously. Thus only 10 to 15% will require interventional treatment (2).

Most patients can be managed at home. Forced hydration of 2 to 3 liters of fluid/24 hours is necessary to maintain a good urinary flow and to help in moving the stone. When the patient is voiding, all of the urine voided during the period of intermittent colic should be collected and strained through an old stocking, a fine knit screen, or a filter paper so that the passed stone may be saved and analyzed. It is important to prescribe analgesic medication such as meperidene (Demerol), 100 to 150 mg every 3 to 6 hours, to control the discomfort. A phenothiazine (e.g., Phenergan, 25 mg) given with the Demerol will provide additional relief by controlling any associated nausea. Some prostaglandin synthesis inhibitors such as indomethacin (Indocin or generic), 50 mg three to four times per day, have been shown to give effective analgesia in renal colic. This effect is possibly due to reductions in ureteric wall muscle tension, to reduced renal pelvic pressure due to decreased glomerular filtration rate, and to a reduction of ureteral edema. Indomethacin may be tried in combination with traditional analgesics when symptoms of colic are prolonged. The patient should be hospitalized if fever, pain, or vomiting develop (see above). The patient should have a weekly X-ray of the abdomen to determine the progression of the stone. If by 6 weeks the stone has not passed, it is unlikely that spontaneous passage will occur, and urological consultation should be obtained. Because of the demands of their occupation or for social reasons, some patients will want to consider surgical removal of the stone earlier and therefore will ask their physician to request urological consultation sooner.

Stones that pass from the ureter into the bladder generally pass with ease through the urethra. In the event of a bladder outlet obstruction, a stone may be retained in the bladder (*bladder stone*) where it may grow and in time become an *infection stone* (see below).

An occasional patient who has acute ureteral colic will give a history of allergy to radiological dye. In this instance, an ultrasonic study of the collecting system of the kidney may help in deciding about the presence of obstruction or the presence of a solitary kidney. If ultrasonography is unavailable, then urological consultation should be obtained so that either an antegrade (i.e., via a catheter passed percutaneously into the renal pelvis) or retrograde pyelogram can be considered. These methods are safe for individuals who have given a history of allergy to IVP dye.

It is important to recognize that occasionally a patient with a history strongly suggestive of renal colic may have another cause for the pain. A dissection of the aorta, acute back strain or lumbar disc disease, the passage of blood clots in the ureters as in sickle cell disease or renal infarct, as well as malingering should be considered. A malingerer is often difficult to identify but usually will give a classic history of acute renal colic to a physician whom he is seeing for the first time and may also relate a history of allergy to IVP dye. Often these patients will have blood (obtained from a fingerstick or oral injury) in the urine specimen they give to the physician.

Patient Requiring Urological Referral. When a patient is referred to a urologist for *stone removal*, there are several options. Lower ureteral stones may be removed using a basket that is inserted through a cystoscope or ureteroscope. This procedure is very similar to cystoscopic examination but requires general or spinal anesthesia and hospitalization (see Chapter 49 for details). This procedure has a success rate greater than 95% and a low rate of complications. Until the early 1980s, stones located more proximally required removal by open ureterolithotomy, open pyelolithotomy, or, in the case of a staghorn calculus, nephrolithotomy.

However, in recent years two new techniques, percutaneous *nephrostolithotomy (PCNL)* and *extracorporeal shock wave lithotripsy (ESWL)*, have supplanted traditional open stone removal operations. Both techniques give results similar to operative stone removal but are associated with less convalescent time and less morbidity.

PCNL requires that the patient be sedated and an intravenous pyelogram performed to localize the kidney and the stone. Under fluoroscopy, a percutaneous nephrostomy tube is placed near the posterior axillary line. Subsequently, the tract is dilated and various nephroscopes, buckets, and forceps are utilized to extract the calculi. For struvite (triple phosphate, or "infection") calculi (see below), *Hemiacidrin (Renacidin)* irrigation sometimes is useful to dissolve residual

stones. Antegrade X-rays are performed to confirm stone removal and ureteral patency. Successful removal occurs in over 95% of renal stones, and 88% of ureteral stones, with a complication rate of less than 1% (13, 14). Typically, a 4- to 5-day hospitalization is needed for a patient to undergo PCNL.

The number of centers providing extracorporeal shock wave lithotripsy (ESWL) has multiplied rapidly in recent years. ESWL also requires that the patient have anesthesia (spinal or general), after which the patient is lowered into a water bath and the stone is located fluoroscopically. A shock wave, generated by an underwater electrode similar to a spark plug, is focused by the lithotripser for a precise impact on the stone (Fig. 47.1). When the shock wave encounters materials (calculus) with different acoustical properties from surrounding tissue, a tensile force is produced which shatters that material. This treatment takes an average of 45 to 60 minutes. ESWL usually is done in outpatients but often a short postprocedure hospital stay is part of the routine. (When the lithotripser is not in a hospital the patient is transported to a hospital by ambulance after a short recovery period at the site.) Following ESWL, fragments of stone generally pass in the urine for a few days and usually cause colic. Retreatment is occasionally needed in a few patients, and macroscopic hematuria occurs transiently in most.

The selection of treatment modalities for a given patient depends in large part on local resources and expertise. Where all modalities are available, ESWL used alone is the treatment of choice in 70% of patients. Individuals suitable for treatment using ESWL are those with single or multiple renal stones of less than 2.5 cm diameter, some smaller staghorn stones (those in which the pelvis is not dilated), and some stones located in the upper third of the ureter. Larger calculi, most staghorn calculi, and calculi composed of cysteine (see below) are usually treated by percutaneous nephrolithotomy in combination with ESWL, or by open operation alone.

Results of ESWL are excellent. Ninety percent of patients with stones less than 1 cm in size located in the kidney or ureter become stone free or are left with small asymptomatic residual fragments. Convalescence from ESWL requires several days. Most patients experience some flank discomfort from the trauma to the kidney. This discomfort frequently requires analgesics for a few days. Immediate complications of ESWL are infrequent, but renal or perirenal tissue injury has been demonstrated in experimental studies and suggested by magnetic resonance imaging and tissue enzyme release in up to 85% of patients. Approximately 8% of patients developed new hypertension or experienced exacerbation of pre-existing hypertension within a year after treatment (7).

Other Patterns of Stone Presentation

Urinary stones usually produce symptoms that suggest acute colic, at least at some time in their course. When stones are discovered in patients who do not

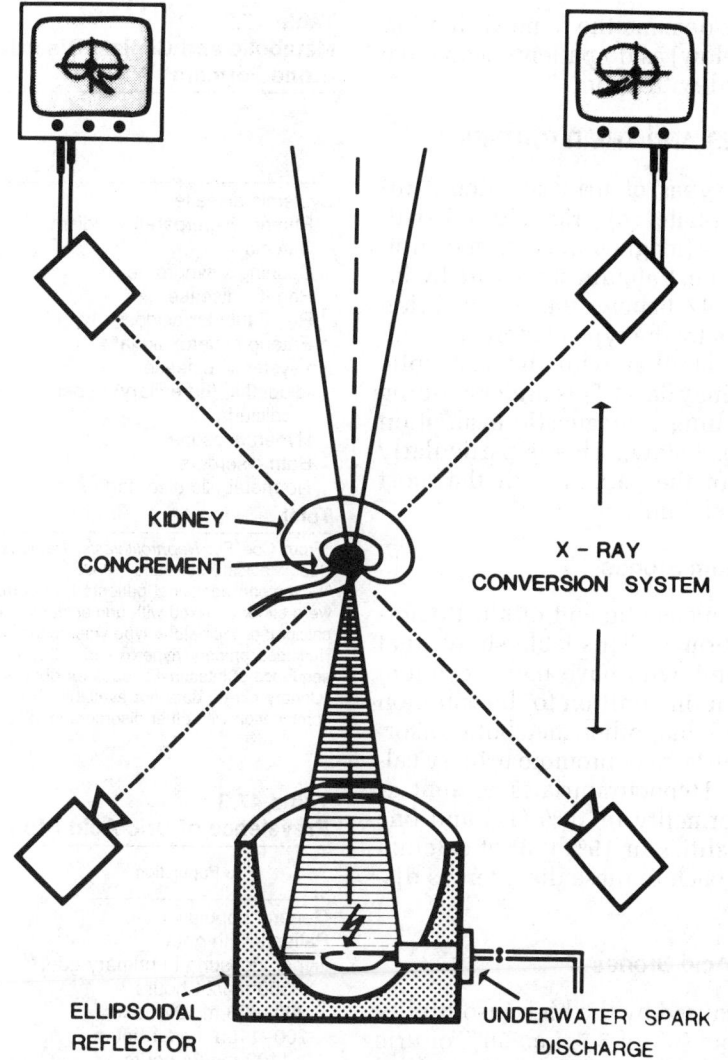

KIDNEY

CONCREMENT

X - RAY
CONVERSION SYSTEM

ELLIPSOIDAL
REFLECTOR

UNDERWATER SPARK
DISCHARGE

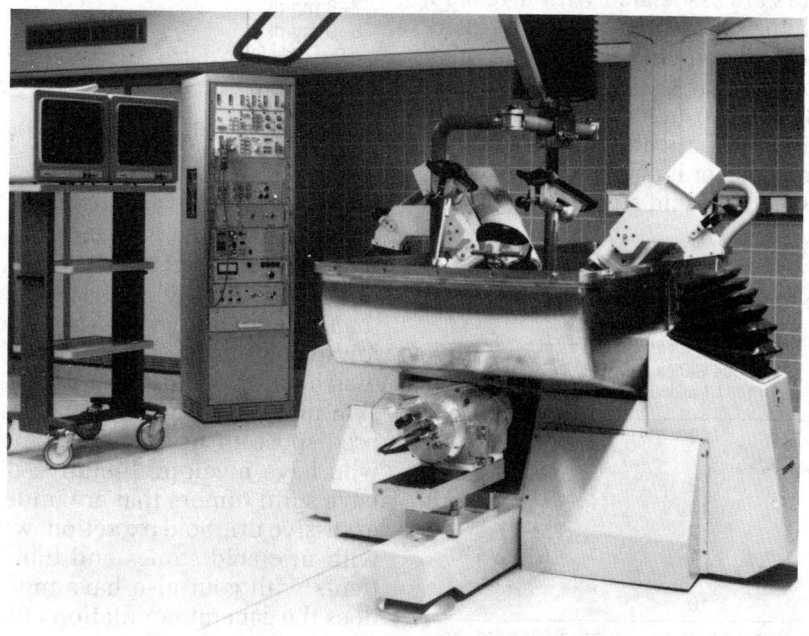

Figure 47.1. Schematic drawing of the technical arrangement (*top*) and photograph of the actual apparatus (*bottom*) for extracorporeal shock wave lithotripsy. (From Chaussey C, Schmidt E, Jocham D: Nonsurgical treatment or renal calculi with shock waves. In Roth RA, Finlayson BF (eds): *Stones: Clinical Management of Urolithiasis*. Baltimore, Williams & Wilkins, 1983.)

have colic, these patients demand the same evaluation and management (see below) as do patients who have passed a stone associated with colic.

TYPES OF STONES AND THEIR CAUSES

There are four main types of urinary calculi: (a) calcium oxalate or phosphate, (b) uric acid, (c) struvite—triple phosphate—(magnesium, ammonium phosphate), and (d) cystine. Calcium stones are by far the most common. Table 47.1 shows the classification of stone-forming patients by the type of stone passed.

It is important to be familiar with the metabolic disorders these patients may have. This understanding will be helpful in planning a diagnostic evaluation and specific therapy (see below). This is particularly true in the evaluation of the patient with the most prevalent stone type—calcium.

Calcium Stones

Table 47.2 shows the metabolic and clinical disorders in calcium stone formers. This table shows that in almost 80% of patients who have had a calcium stone the cause is known. In addition to the common disorders shown in the table, other metabolic disorders, such as hypocitraturia, may promote urinary calcium salt precipitation. Hypocitraturia is present as the sole metabolic abnormality in 10% (12) and one of two or three abnormalities in 19% (16) of calcium stone formers. The approach to these disorders is discussed below.

Uric Acid Stones

Uric acid stones are caused by the high insolubility of undissociated uric acid (pK of 5.7, i.e., 50% of uric acid is undissociated at pH 5.7, 90% is undissociated at pH 4.7). Three factors are associated with uric acid stone formation: (a) hyperuricosuria, (b) highly acid urine, and (c) low urinary volume. The lifetime incidence of uric acid stones in the general population is very low (Table 47.3). On the other hand, uric acid stones are very prevalent in patients who have gout, asymptomatic hyperuricemia, or hyperuricosuria. Many patients will have passed uric acid stones long before

Table 47.1.
Classification of Stone-Forming Patients by Type of Stone Passed[a]

	Coe Series 1431 Patients	Series Combined Other 1870 Patients
Calcium oxalate (with or without phosphate)	69[b]	63.2[b]
Calcium phosphate	2	7.4
Calcium and uric acid	10	
Uric Acid	2	5.4
Cystine	1	2.5
Struvite	7	21.5
Unknown	10	

[a]From Coe FL: *Nephrolithiasis: Pathogenesis and Treatment.* Chicago, Year Book Medical Publishers, 1988.
[b]All values expressed as percentages of patients in each category.

Table 47.2.
Metabolic and Clinical Disorders in 989 Calcium Oxalate Stone Formers[a]

	No. of Patients	
	Men	Women
Systemic disease	%	
Primary hyperparathyroidism[b]	26 (4)	24 (10)
Sarcoid	6 (1)	1 (1)
Cushing's syndrome	5 (1)	1 (0.4)
Paget's disease	1 (0.1)	1 (0.4)
Renal tubular acidosis, type I	7 (1)	4 (2)
Enteric hyperoxaluria[c]	39 (5)	13 (5)
No systemic disease		
Idiopathic (hereditary) hyper-calciuria	213 (29)	121 (49)
Hyperuricosuria	126 (17)	9 (4)
Both disorders	120 (16)	22 (9)
No metabolic disorder[d]	186 (26)	52 (11)
Total	**729**	**249**

[a]From Coe FL: *Nephrolithiasis: Pathogenesis and Treatment.* Chicago, Year Book Medical Publishers, 1988.
[b]Seventeen additional patients had primary hyperparathyroidism; their stones were either admixed with uric acid, struvite, or cystine; they had stones with no calcium; or their stone type was unknown.
[c]Includes primary hyperoxaluria (three patients) and hyperoxaluria as a consequence of intestinal bypass for obesity.
[d]Urinary citrate data not available. Hypocitraturia has been found alone or in combination with other disorders in 19% of hypercalciurias (13).

Table 47.3.
Prevalence of Uric Acid Stones in Various Populations

Population	Lifetime Incidence (%)
General population	0.01
Patients with gout	22
Hyperuricosuria in primary gout[a]:	
<300 mg/24 hours	11
300–699 mg/24 hours	21
700–1100 mg/24 hours	35
>1100 mg/24 hours	50
Hyperuricemia in men[b]:	
7–8 mg/dl	12.7
8–9 mg/dl	22
>9 mg/dl	40

[a]From Yüu T, Gutman AB: Uric acid nephrolithiasis in gout. *Ann Intern Med* 67:1133, 1967.
[b]From Hall AP, Barry PE, Dawber TR, McNamarea PM: Epidemiology of gout and hyperuricemia. *Am J Med* 42:27, 1967.

a gouty attack has occurred. It is known that many patients with gout produce an abnormally high fraction of their daily acid load as titratable acid rather than as ammonium and therefore have an unusually low average urinary pH. Further, patients with chronic diarrhea or patients with excessive fluid loss from the skin may have highly concentrated urine, which will predispose to uric acid calculus formation. Patients who have myeloproliferative disease and those who have solid tumors that are undergoing lysis may have excessive uric acid excretion, which may be associated with uric acid stones and tubular plugs of urate. Patients with gout also have more calcium stones than does the general population (19). The association may result from crystallization of uric acid, which then forms a nidus for calcium deposition.

Struvite Stones (Infection Stones)

It is generally believed that infection stones form primarily as a consequence of the hydrolysis of urea and the production of ammonium by the bacterial enzyme urease. The production of ammonia leads to a highly alkaline urine, which promotes the precipitation of magnesium, ammonium, and phosphate. These are the components of the infection-induced or struvite stone. The majority of urea-splitting organisms are *Proteus* species; however, *Pseudomonas, Klebsiella, Staphylococcus,* and some *Escherichia coli* strains are capable of producing urease. Struvite stones do not form de novo but almost always are a complication of another primary stone disease in which infection has become superimposed, and they are especially likely to grow into staghorn calculi (large stones that cannot pass the ureteropelvic junction and that form a cast of all or a portion of the pelvicalyceal system).

Cystine Stones

Cystine stones are rare and most likely will be seen in young patients, as the onset is usually in childhood. The stone forms because of crystallization of cystine when the urine is supersaturated with this substance, which occurs when there is a defect in renal tubular resorption of filtered cystine. This is a particularly virulent form of stone disease and may be associated with staghorn calculi. In addition to cystinuria, there is usually urinary loss of other basic amino acids, including ornithine, lysine, and arginine. The disorder is an inherited autosomal recessive trait, although some heterozygous patients have excess cystine excretion, as is shown in Table 47.4. Cystine is much less soluble in acid urine than it is in alkaline urine, and cystine stones generally, therefore, will form when urine is acid and cystine excretion is greater than 400 mg/24 hours.

NATURAL HISTORY OF URINARY STONE DISEASE

Urinary calculus disease is a chronic illness. Once a stone has formed there is a tendency for recurrence, and management (see below) should be tailored to the stone activity, to the type of stone, and to any associated metabolic abnormality.

Stone activity—the number of stones formed and the change in size of existing stones—is an important, although at times difficult, determination to be made. It requires a yearly review of stones passed and removed, as well as an evaluation by abdominal X-ray of increase in size of known stones or the appearance of new stones. The activity of urinary calculi depends on a number of factors: stone type, associated meta-

bolic abnormality, treatment received (both specific and nonspecific), and age. Precise rates of recurrence, therefore, cannot be given with real accuracy.

Because calcium stone formers make up the largest population of patients with stones, there is more information about recurrences in this group. In solitary calcium stone formers (history of passing a single stone) there is a recurrence in half of the patients by 5 years and in two-thirds of the patients by 9 years, with a peak recurrence at about 2 years and a second smaller peak at 8 years after passage of the initial stone (Fig. 47.2).

Because of this high recurrence rate it is suggested that evaluation for associated metabolic abnormalities be undertaken in every patient who has formed a calcium stone. This is also reasonable in patients who have passed uric acid, struvite, or cystine stones since recurrence is also likely. Because multiple metabolic defects may be responsible for stone formation, it is wise to evaluate each stone former comprehensively, as discussed below.

DIAGNOSTIC WORKUP OF PATIENTS WITH URINARY STONE DISEASE

Evaluation of patients with stone disease can be accomplished entirely in an ambulatory setting. This evaluation depends on history, physical examination, and certain laboratory measurements.

History

A history is important in determining the activity of stone disease (see above) as well as in providing clues to the nature of the stone. The number of passed stones, the frequency of attacks of colic and/or hematuria, and the history of infection should be obtained. Previous abdominal X-rays and, most important, chemical analysis of prior stones should be obtained, if possible. *Family history* may provide a clue to cystine stones, uric acid stones (gout), and some calcium stones (e.g., those associated with renal tubular aci-

Table 47.4.
Urinary Cystine Excretion

Normal individuals	<100 mg
Heterozygotes for cystinuria	150–300 mg
Homozygotes for cystinuria	>600 mg

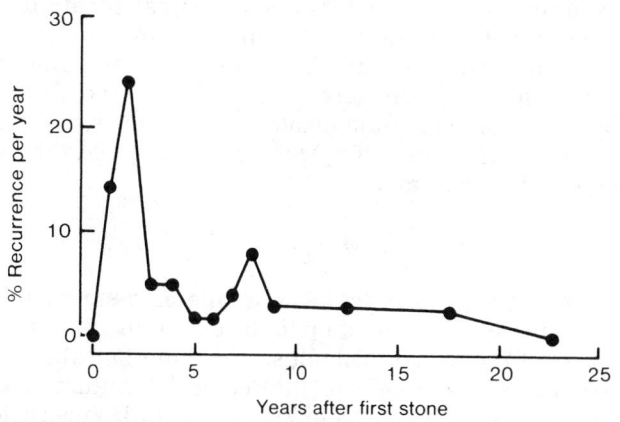

Figure 47.2. Rate of stone recurrence in patients who have formed a single calcium stone. (From Coe FL: *Nephrolithiasis: Pathogenesis and Treatment.* Chicago, Year Book Publishers, 1978.)

dosis). *Dietary history* may reveal excessive intake of calcium, purine, and/or oxalate (see below). The *eating habits* are important. For example, if a patient takes only one large meal a day, there may be a sudden surge of uric acid that requires excretion in a highly acid urine, resulting in predisposition to uric acid calculi. High protein meat diets may be associated with excess ingestion and excretion of acid and thereby may be connected with stone disease. An approximate daily fluid intake is also an important part of the history. Some individuals may ingest as little as 500 to 700 ml/day and thus have concentrated urine most of the day. *Medication history* is important. For example, aspirin in high doses (more than 5 g/day, especially if the urine is also alkaline) and probenecid are associated with increased uric acid excretion and may cause a predisposition to uric acid calculi. Further, calcium-containing antacids (e.g., Camalox, Bisodol, Titralac, Tempo, or Tums) as well as vitamin D may be associated with hypercalciuria and calcium stone formation. Acetazolamide (Diamox) may be associated with development of chronically alkaline urine and a higher incidence of calcium calculi. Triamterene and its metabolites have been found as the nidus in urinary calculi (and occasionally it may be the only ingredient). For this reason, a history of the use of triamterene preparations (Dyazide or Dyrenium) should be sought (6) and use of these medications discontinued in patients with a history of urinary calculus. Moreover, certain medications, such as thiazides or allopurinol, will decrease calcium and uric acid excretion, respectively, and interfere with results of testing in a patient who is being evaluated for renal stone disease. *Occupational history* is important in that the environmental temperature (and therefore fluid losses) and/or the accessibility to fluids are factors influencing stone formation by promoting decreased output of highly concentrated urine.

Physical Examination

Physical examination (when there is no colic) occasionally will give clues to specific problems. For example, band keratopathy (stippled calcification of the perimeter of the cornea, which may require a slit-lamp for visualization) may be seen in hyperparathyroidism; or there may be signs of sarcoidosis, hyperthyroidism, inflammatory bowel disease, neoplasia, or gouty arthritis. Most often, however, the examination is normal.

Urinalysis

The urinalysis provides a simple assessment that may give specific direction to the determination of the cause of the urinary calculus. It is important that the urinalysis is complete, including the determination of pH. The pH is usually acid in patients with a uric acid or a cystine stone and is invariably alkaline in patients with struvite stones. Also, the pH may suggest the presence of renal tubular acidosis: The first voided morning urine is usually acid, so that finding a urine pH > 6.0 in this specimen suggests the possibility of renal tubular acidosis. The microscopic analysis may show hematuria (although this is often absent in the intercritical period), crystals, or evidence of infection. Crystals of cystine have the appearance of a benzene ring and are highly suggestive of cystinuria. Other crystals are more variable and are not diagnostic. Oxalate crystals appear in urine normally, and their identification should not suggest a disorder.

Stone Analysis

If a stone is available it should be analyzed because the stone type will determine the approach to evaluation and treatment. Stones can be analyzed inexpensively at commercial laboratories, and stones may be mailed without preservative for this purpose.

Laboratory Assessment (Table 47.5)

A thorough laboratory analysis is important even in patients in whom a stone has been available for analysis. This evaluation is necessary because it is increasingly recognized that many patients have more than one metabolic disorder that has led to stone formation: For example, struvite stones often start as some other primary stone type—most often calcium; and patients with pure uric acid or cystine stones occasionally may have other types of stones as well. Patients will usually comply with the testing necessary for proper evaluation of a metabolic disorder if they understand the relative ease with which it can be accomplished, the high rate of recurrent calculi, and the effectiveness of

Table 47.5.
Laboratory Assessment of Patients with Urinary Calculi[a]

Measure	Day of Testing		
	1	2	3
24-hour urinary volume	✓	✓	✓
24-hour urinary calcium[b]	✓	✓	✓
24-hour urinary uric acid[c]		✓	✓
24-hour urinary creatinine	✓	✓	✓
24-hour urinary oxalate	✓	✓	
24-hour urinary citrate	✓	✓	
24-hour urinary sodium	✓	✓	
Urinalysis	✓		
Urine cystine screen (cyanide-nitroprusside test)	✓		
Urine culture (if pyuria)	✓		
Urine pH (taken on first voided morning specimen collected under mineral oil)	✓		
Serum calcium	✓	✓	✓
Serum phosphorus	✓		
Serum uric acid	✓		
Serum chloride	✓		
Serum bicarbonate	✓		
Serum creatinine	✓		
Serum urea nitrogen	✓		

[a]During evaluation patients should follow their usual diet and life habits except on day 3 when a 1-g calcium intake should be ensured (see page 511).
[b]The 24-hour urine container should contain 15 ml of concentrated HCl (with warning to avoid contact).
[c]The 24-hour urine container should contain a few crystals of thymol to retard bacterial overgrowth.

specific therapy for different metabolic problems (see below).

Laboratory assessment of patients who have formed urinary calculi is relatively simple and noninvasive and can be easily performed in the office. It is important that this initial evaluation be accomplished without the patient modifying his diet or habits so that an underlying process associated with urinary calculus disease will not be masked. The reason for obtaining most studies listed in Table 47.5 is self evident. Urinary creatinine is measured to monitor completeness of collections and to estimate glomerular filtration rate. Urinary sodium (reflecting dietary intake) is measured because increased urinary sodium excretion promotes hypercalciuria. Serum calcium should be repeated at least once and ionized calcium determined, if possible, since the latter is a more accurate index of hypercalcemia. Urinary citrate should be measured in patients with calcium stones. Citrate combines with calcium to form a soluble complex, thus reducing the availability of calcium for crystallizing with oxalate or phosphate.

An *intravenous pyelogram*, if not done previously as part of the evaluation of an episode of acute colic, should be done in an attempt to search for underlying structural disease (such as anatomical abnormality of the lower tract or medullary sponge kidney).

In addition to the laboratory assessment outlined in Table 47.5, *parathyroid hormone* should be measured if hypercalcemia and hypercalciuria are documented and if other causes of hypercalcemia are ruled out (see Chapter 74). Urinary *oxalate* should also be determined when hyperoxaluria is expected clinically (Table 47.6), although oxalate determination is not always a reliable analysis and hyperoxaluria is uncommon; therefore, it is not a routinely performed measurement.

Hypercalciuria

Although calcium excretion varies somewhat with intake of calcium and of protein, generally the upper limits of calcium excretion for individuals eating a normal diet are 250 mg/24 hours for women and 300 mg/24 hours for men. Patients with hypercalciuria without hypercalcemia deserve special attention because they are seen quite commonly and because of the variable pathogenesis of their stones. Table 47.7 lists the causes of hypercalciuria that may be unassociated with hypercalcemia.

Most patients will have idiopathic hypercalciuria

Table 47.6.
Situations in Which Hyperoxaluria May Be Expected

Hereditary overproduction—usually virulent stone disease with frequent recurrences and nephrocalcinosis often occurring before age 12 years
Methoxyflurane anesthesia—immediately after
Ethylene glycol ingestion—immediately after
Chronic inflammatory bowel disease affecting the ileum, ileal resection, or small bowel bypass
Cellulose phosphate ingestion—during entire period of ingestion
Oxalate gluttony (tea, spinach, rhubarb)

Table 47.7.
Causes of Hypercalciuria That May Not Be Associated with Hypercalcemia

Idiopathic hypercalciuria
Administration of loop diuretics (furosemide, ethacrynic acid, or bumetanide)
Excessive salt ingestion
Exogenous adrenal corticosteroids
Cushing's syndrome
Paget's disease of bone
Immobilization
Progressive bone disease
Malignant tumors
Hyperthyroidism
Sarcoidosis
Renal tubular acidosis
Other causes of metabolic acidosis
Medullary sponge kidney
Severe phosphate deprivation

either from a *renal leak* (renal hypercalciuria) or from *excessive gastrointestinal absorption* of calcium (absorptive hypercalciuria). In the latter, which occurs much more commonly, there is excess gastrointestinal absorption (and then excretion) of calcium after the ingestion of calcium. The differentiation of renal from absorptive hypercalciuria requires the use of an *oral calcium tolerance test* (1, 9), which is not routinely recommended in a general medical office practice. However, it is important to be aware that some patients with absorptive hypercalciuria may have normal calcium excretion if they inadvertently restrict their calcium intake on the day of the urine collection. Therefore, it is advantageous to ensure that the patient has at least a 1-g intake of calcium on the days that the calcium concentration will be determined, as noted in Table 47.5. This calcium intake may be ensured by having the patient drink 1 quart of milk (approximately 250 mg of calcium/8 ounces) or, if milk is not tolerated or not desired, calcium glubionate (Neo-Calglucon Syrup, available from a pharmacy without a prescription), 1 tablespoon three times a day (345 mg of calcium/tablespoon). It is easiest if the physician dispenses this from office stock because the test requires that the patient ingest a relatively small amount. Some patients with hypercalciuria, especially the absorptive type, will benefit by restriction of calcium in the diet (see below).

PREVENTIVE TREATMENT OF URINARY CALCULUS DISEASE

General Measures

It is important to educate patients who have formed stones about the nature of urinary calculi, their natural history, the importance of regular surveillance, and the effectiveness of therapy. Increasing fluid intake and eliminating dietary excesses or deficiencies will control stone formation in about 60% of patients.

Diet

Diet can play a role in most conditions in which stones form. Because obtaining a detailed diet history is often not practical in the office, it is usually helpful to have a dietician or nutritionist evaluate the patient both to determine dietary excesses or deficiencies and to begin to plan dietary therapy depending on the results of the evaluation for metabolic abnormalities. Specific diet restriction is discussed under the various stone types (see below).

Fluid Intake

A low urine volume, reflecting low fluid intake, is common in many stone formers. Regardless of the type of stone that has been formed, a patient should maintain a high intake of fluids to ensure a urinary output of 3 to 4 liters/day. This high urinary output prevents supersaturation, and the high flow rate may wash out small crystalline formations before they produce any obstructive symptoms.

Patients with recurrent stone disease require a high fluid intake throughout the day and night (10). This can be accomplished by having the individual drink 3 liters through the day and then take one or two glasses of water before retiring. This should result in a nocturnal diuresis necessitating voiding 3 to 4 hours later, at which time a further ingestion of one or two glasses of water will continue the diuresis until morning. Although annoying to the patient, once the habit is formed it is a small nuisance compared with the benefit of preventing subsequent stone formation. Continuing to encourage patients is critical to the success of the treatment program.

Avoidance of Dehydration

Patients should be counseled to avoid dehydration and, consequently, concentrated urine when participating in sports, during travel, or work.

Specific Therapy for Calcium Stone Formers

Calcium is present in the vast majority of urinary calculi, and hypercalciuria is the most frequent disorder uncovered during the evaluation of patients with urinary calculus disease. In addition to the general measures described above, there are several specific therapies.

The decision, however, to use specific therapy (especially pharmacological therapy) must be made on an individual basis. The rate of stone recurrence for a large population of patients may not apply to an individual patient. It is prudent to use only general therapeutic measures until there is an increase in stone activity reflected by the passage of gravel or a stone or an increase in size or number of stones on X-ray. At this time a decision should be made about adding such specific therapy as might be appropriate from the workup.

Restricted Calcium Diet

Excesses of dietary calcium should be considered in every patient with hypercalciuria. Modest restriction of dietary calcium should be attempted in patients with "absorptive" hypercalciuria, but not "renal leak" hypercalciuria, because of the induction of chronic negative calcium balance and the potential for subsequent bone disease (a seriously calcium restricted diet is generally not indicated for the same reason). Generally a calcium-restricted diet is obtained by limiting intake of milk and milk products (including cheese), in which case the calcium intake may fall from 1500 to 2000 mg to 400 to 700 mg/day.

Thiazide Diuretics

Thiazide administration has been shown to result within a day or two in a fall in urinary calcium excretion by as much as 50 to 60%. It also increases (by action on the tubular transport mechanism) magnesium, zinc, and oxalate excretion, which may be important in the inhibition of calcium crystallization. Thiazides are an ideal theoretical choice in the treatment of renal hypercalciuria, but thiazides also seem to be effective in other metabolic disorders associated with renal stones. Many studies attest to as much as 60 to 90% efficacy in reducing the frequency of stones using thiazides in all types of stone formers. Although there are serious methodological concerns about some of these studies (3), the vast majority of experts consider thiazide the drug of choice in hypercalciurics. However, they should be avoided in patients with hypercalcemia (e.g., those with hyperparathyroidism or sarcoidosis).

Any thiazide diuretic is usable, but trichlormethazide (2 to 4 mg) or hydrochlorothiazide (25 to 50 mg) twice daily, or chlorthalidone (25 to 50 mg) once daily are most commonly prescribed. The exact dose of thiazide to be used for the prevention of urinary calculi is uncertain. The incidence of side effects was nearly 35% in one early study (18) utilizing a dose of hydrochlorothiazide of 50 mg twice a day, the regimen that usually resulted in maximal hypocalciuria. Most side effects were seen soon after initiation of the drug. Intolerance of thiazides can be limited to less than 10% of patients by gradually increasing the dose, and reducing the dose if side effects develop. Although thiazides elevate the plasma uric acid level (see Chapter 69), this is not detrimental to patients with urate stones. Chapter 45 provides a discussion of the management of the hypokalemic complications of thiazides. If a potassium-sparing diuretic is used, amiloride, 5 to 10 mg daily, is the drug of choice. Triamterene should not be given because of the association of this agent with the formation of urinary calculi (see above). A good choice for prevention or treatment of thiazide-induced hypokalemia would be the addition of oral potassium citrate (e.g., Urocit-K, Polycitra-K) in a dose of 0.5 to 2 mEq/kg/day in two to four divided doses daily. This provides both potassium and base. The latter increases tubular secretion of citrate, which may be reduced as a consequence of thiazide therapy (8). Citrate therapy has also been useful in hypercalciuric patients who continue to form stones in spite of thiazide therapy, presumably by increasing urinary citrate concentration (see below) (11).

Citrate

Citrate (sodium, potassium, or both, e.g., Polycitra) is useful in many metabolic conditions associated with renal stones. Its usefulness is due to the alkalinizing effect on the urine (for calcium stones associated with renal tubular acidosis, hyperuricosuria, and diarrheal syndromes, and for uric acid and cystine stones, see below), as well as to the increase in urinary citrate, a natural inhibitor of stone formation (for calcium stones associated with hypocitraturia). Although provision of base as sodium bicarbonate is theoretically just as efficacious, sodium bicarbonate is often not well tolerated, in contrast to citrate therapy.

The object of treatment is to provide enough base to increase urinary pH to between 6.0 and 7.0, and to restore normal urinary citrate excretion (greater than 320 mg/day and as close as possible to the normal mean of 640 mg/day). Twenty-four-hour urinary citrate and/or urinary pH measurement should be obtained to determine the adequacy of the initial dose. Once an acceptable level is achieved it should be confirmed every 6 to 12 months.

Orthophosphate (Inorganic Phosphate)

The administration of neutral (not acidic) inorganic phosphate results in the complete cessation of new urinary calculi formation in 90% of patients (15). However, because of the large doses required and the high incidence of side effects, the use of inorganic phosphate is still controversial. Although some clinical trials suggest efficacy, others do not, and there is no randomized control study available. Its method of action may be to decrease calcium absorption directly by forming unabsorbable complexes in the gastrointestinal tract (therefore making it theoretically ideal for treatment of patients with absorptive hypercalciuria), but also to some extent by increasing plasma phosphate and by increasing the excretion of urinary stone inhibitors. This, in turn, leads to a fall in the ionized calcium concentration, resulting in increased parathyroid hormone production, a subsequent fall in the glomerular filtration rate, and an increase in renal tubular calcium absorption.

There are risks associated with using orthophosphates. The excess stimulation of parathyroid hormone could result in bone disease, and many patients have had intolerable diarrhea, nausea, or vomiting.

The inorganic phosphate salts are prescribed primarily as a mixture of sodium and potassium phosphate (e.g., K-Phos), 1 g four times a day. Its use is probably best restricted to patients in whom thiazides and oral citrates are contraindicated or not tolerated. The administration of inorganic phosphate is not recommended without at least a telephone consultation with a nephrologist or urologist.

Cellulose Phosphate

This is an ion exchange resin (Calcibind). Taken with meals, the resin binds calcium so it is not absorbed. Urine calcium falls but urine oxalate rises. There are no controlled studies of its efficacy, and the value of treatment is uncertain. Its use is especially promulgated for the treatment of absorptive hypercalciuria. This agent may result in chronic negative calcium balance and subsequent bone disease. Cellulose phosphate also binds magnesium, and hypomagnesemia may develop but can be corrected with magnesium supplementation. Its use, because of the quantity required, may be unacceptable to many patients, and it frequently causes unacceptable diarrhea and/or occasional offensive stools. For these reasons its use is not recommended without consultation with a nephrologist or urologist.

Patients with Calcium or Uric Acid Stones Who Are Found to Have Hyperuricosuria

Patients with calcium stones who have hyperuricosuria or those who have mixed calcium and uric acid stones should be treated in the same way as if they had pure uric acid stones.

If purine gluttony is present hyperuricosuria can be modified by dietary restriction of purine-rich food, such as liver, kidney, and fish roe. Gluttony, however, is not often the problem, and other means are necessary.

Uric acid stone formation can be markedly modified by increasing the urinary pH; increasing the pH of the urine from 4.5 to 5.5 or 6.5 increases uric acid dissociation from 15 to 40% and 80%, respectively. Alkalinization can be accomplished by the administration of sodium bicarbonate several times a day. However, because sodium bicarbonate frequently causes gas and gastrointestinal discomfort, citrate salts (Polycitra solution containing 2 mEq base/ml) are more palatable and therefore preferable. Most patients require 10 ml three times/day, but the dose should be adjusted as necessary based on the results of regular urine pH testing. The metabolism of citrate results in the generation of bicarbonate. During the initial week of treatment and periodically thereafter, the patient should be taught to measure his urinary pH several times a day to ensure proper alkalinization (urine pH > 6.5).

Should these agents not be effective in controlling recurrence of uric acid stones, if the urine pH cannot be kept above 6.5, or if uric acid excretion is above 650 mg, allopurinol (which decreases uric acid production) may be used and is very effective in reducing stone recurrence. Allopurinol (Zyloprim, available in 100- and 300-mg tablets) should be initiated at a dose of 200 mg once a day and raised to a level that controls uric acid excretion to below 500 or 600 mg/24 hours (doses greater than 300 mg are divided in two daily doses). Complications from allopurinol are usually minor (minor skin rash, drug fever, or precipitation of an acute gouty attack); the drug should be discontinued whenever a skin rash or fever occurs because diffuse fatal systemic vasculitis has been reported. Allopurinol also has been reported to be associated, although rarely, with the acceleration of cataract formation, with cholestatic hepatitis, and with leukopenia. The use of allopurinol is especially important as a preventive measure in patients who have excess uric acid excretion because of a myeloproliferative disease or in anticipation of tumor lysis. Also, when allopurinol is not entirely satisfactory, a thiazide (see above) alone or in combination with allopurinol is beneficial in reducing the frequency of recurrence.

Hyperoxaluria

In this group of patients the aim is lower oxalate excretion. Treatment depends to some extent on the cause of hyperoxaluria, and frequently a telephone consultation with a nephrologist may be helpful in managing a patient with this complex problem. The consultant may consider the use of cholestyramine in a dose of 8 to 16 g/day, in addition to increased calcium supplementation and a low oxalate, low fat diet. In patients who have had ileal resection or a disease that has caused malabsorption, pyridoxine deficiency may develop. This deficiency results in the reduction of the transamination of glyoxylate to glycine, and hyperoxaluria results. In this situation the use of pyridoxine (150 to 400 mg every 24 hours) may be beneficial. In addition providing additional intake of oral fluids, electrolytes (sodium, potassium, and magnesium), and base may correct deficiencies that result from malabsorption and that promote stone formation.

Cystinuria

This group of stone formers generally have particularly virulent disease and are best managed in consultation with a nephrologist. Generally it is necessary to raise urinary pH in a manner similar to the method used in patients with uric acid stones (see above) and, if stone activity continues, to use D-penicillamine, which forms complexes with cystine and prevents its precipitation.

Struvite or Infection Stones

Infection stones are particularly virulent. Untreated patients with infected staghorn calculi frequently develop sepsis and require urgent nephrectomy. Further, when the disease is bilateral there is an associated 25% mortality rate in 5 years (17). In view of this morbidity and with the recent advance in techniques for controlling infection stones, early urological referral is suggested. The goal of surgery in such patients is to remove the stone totally. This may be done by a variety of approaches. The mortality for these procedures in skilled hands is less than 1%. Application of hypothermia combined with a technique permitting the kidney to be bivalved has permitted great success in total stone removal with preservation of renal function. There is, however, still a relatively high recurrence rate. Also, percutaneous nephrostolithotomy may be used for smaller stones. This procedure usually requires that the stone be broken up by a shock wave probe (ultrasonic lithotripsy) (see page 506). In another treatment the stone may be perfused and dissolved by an acid solution—hemiacidrin (Renacidin)—using a percutaneous catheter placed antegrade into the pelvis of the kidney (5).

In addition to the surgical treatment of stone disease, medical therapy is an important adjunct. Associated metabolic abnormalities should be sought and treated. Specific antimicrobial therapy is necessary in conjunction with surgery, and, where stones cannot be removed surgically, suppressive therapy with antimicrobials may decrease the incidence of septicemia. The use of oral agents that prevent infecting bacteria from splitting urea (urease inhibitors) has been shown to decrease recurrence of some struvite stones by preventing the formation of highly alkaline urine caused by the ammonium produced by urea-splitting organisms. Acetohydroxamic acid (Lithostat) may be used as an adjunct to antimicrobial therapy and surgery in patients with struvite stones. Acetohydroxamic acid, 250 mg, three to four times a day or a total dose of 10 to 15 mg/kg/day (but never more than 1.5 g/day) should be used only when the patient is infected with urea-splitting organisms as evidenced by a high urinary pH. Because of its teratogenic effects, it is contraindicated in women who are pregnant. Also it is not effective in the presence of moderate renal failure (creatinine ≥ 2.5 or creatinine clearance < 20 ml/minute). Side effects occur in nearly 30% of patients and some are serious, such as thrombophlebitis and hemolysis. Experience with the drug is still limited, and the general physician should prescribe it only after consultation with a urologist.

Urinary Calculi in Patients without an Identifiable Metabolic Disorder

Approximately 10 to 15% of stone formers found after evaluation not to have a metabolic disorder may respond to thiazides and/or allopurinol as outlined above (4).

General References

Coe FL, Parks JH: *Nephrolithiasis Pathogenesis and Treatment*, 5th ed. Chicago, Year Book Medical Publishers, Inc, 1988.
    This is a review monograph covering all aspects of urinary stone disease and provides an extensive documentation of the literature.
Lingeman JE, Smith LH, Woods JR, Newman DM: *Urinary Calculi: ESWK, Endourology, and Medical Therapy.* Philadelphia, Lea & Farber, 1989.
    A well-referenced monograph that covers all aspects of stone disease, including the newer treatments utilizing shock waves and surgery.
Narins RG (ed): *Controversies in Nephrology and Hypertension.* New York, Churchill Livingstone, 1984.
    Contains a thorough and well-referenced discussion on the extent of the workup for hypercalciuric patients with stone disease.

National Institutes of Health, Concensus Development Conference on Prevention and treatment of Kidney Stones. *J Urol* 141:705, 1989.
Uribarri J, Oh MS, Carroll HS: The first kidney stone. *Ann Intern Med* lll:1006, 1989.

A literature review analyzing the approach to the work-up of a patient passing their first calcium-containing kidney stone.

Specific References

1. Broadus AE, Dominguez M, Bartter FC: Patholphysiological studies in idiopathic hypercalciuria: use of an oral calcium tolerance test to characterize distinctive hyperalciuria subgroups. *J Clin Endocrinol Metab* 47:751, 1978.
2. Chaussy CG, Fuchs GJ: Current state and future developments of noninvasive treatment of human urinary stones with extracorporeal shock wave lithotripsy. *J Urol*141:782, 1989.
3. Churchill DN: Medical treatment to prevent recurrent calcium urolithiasis: A guide to critical appraisal. *Min Electrolyte Metab* 13:294, 1987.
4. Coe FL: Treated and untreated recurrent calcium nephrolithiasis in patients with idiopathic hypercalciuria, hyperuricosuria, or no metabolic disorder. *Ann Intern Med* 87:404, 1977.
5. Dretler SP, Pfister RC, Newhouse JH: Renal stone dissolution via percutaneous nephrostomy. *N Engl J Med* 300:341, 1979.
6. Ettinger B, Oldroyd NO, Surgel F: Triamterene nephrolithiasis. *JAMA*244:2443, 1980.
7. Lingerman JE, Woods J, Toth PD, et al: The role of lithotripsy and its side effects. *J Urol* 141:793, 1989.
8. Nicor MJ, Peterson R, Sakhaee K, et al: Use of potassium citrate as potassium supplement during thiazide therapy of calcium nephrolithiasis. *J Urol* 131:430, 1984.
9. Pak CYV, Kaplan RA, Bone H, et al: A simple test for the diagnosis of absorptive, resorptive and renal hypercalciurias. *N Engl J Med* 292:497, 1975.
10. Pak CY, Sakhaee K, Crowther C, Krinkley L: Evidence justifying a high fluid intake in treatment of nephrolithiasis. *Ann Intern Med* 93:36, 1980.
11. Pak CYC, Peterson R, Sakhaee K, et al: Correction of hypocitraturia and prevention of stone formation by combined thiazide and potassium citrate therapy in thiazide-unresponsive hypercalciuric nephrolithiasis. *Am J Med* 79:284, 1985.
12. Preminger GM: The metabolic evaluation of patients with recurrent nephrolithiasis: a review of comprehensive and simplified approaches. *J Urol* 141:760, 1989.
13. Segura JW, Patterson DE, DeRoy AJ, et al: Percutaneous removal of kidney stones: review of 1000 cases. *J Urol* 134:1077, 1985.
14. Segura JW: The role of percutaneous surgery in renal and ureteral stone removal. *J Urol* 141:780, 1989.
15. Thomas Jr WC: Use of phosphates in patients with calcureous renal calculi. *Kidney Int* 13:390, 1978.
16. Wilson DM: Clinical and laboratory approaches for evaluation of nephrolithiasis. *J. Urol* 141:780, 1989.
17. Wojewski A, Zajaczkowski T: The treatment of bilateral staghorn calculi of the kidneys. *Int Urol Nephrol* 5:249, 1974.
18. Yendt ER: Medical management of calcium stones. In: Roth RA, Finlayson B (eds):*Stones: Clinical Management of Urolithiasis.* Baltimore, Williams & Wilkins, 1983, pp 187–209.
19. Yeu T, Butman AB: Uric acid nephrolithiasis in gout. Predisposing factors. *Ann Intern Med* 67:1133, 1967.

CHAPTER 48

Chronic Renal Insufficiency

GARY R. BRIEFEL, M.D.

Renal insufficiency, presenting either as a primary event or complicating another illness, is a common clinical problem that will have to be managed by the general physician. This chapter reviews the epidemiology, evaluation, manifestations, clinical course, and management of patients with renal insufficiency. In addition, the chapter provides guidelines describing when consultation with a nephrologist is necessary; it also contains a discussion about dialysis and renal transplantation.

The healthy kidney performs a wide variety of functions that contribute to the maintenance of the internal environment of the body. In addition to its role in maintaining the balance of water and electrolytes, the kidney has important endocrine and metabolic functions. It produces hormones responsible for normal bone formation (1, 25-dihydroxyvitamin D_3), red blood cell production (erythropoietin), and blood pressure control (renin, prostaglandins). The kidney is responsible for degrading a number of polypeptide hormones, including parathyroid hormone, insulin, gastrin, and prolactin among others. Also, the kidney serves as a major excretory route for many toxic metabolic wastes and a wide variety of drugs or their breakdown products.

In parallel with the progressive destruction of renal mass that occurs with many chronic kidney diseases, patients pass through a sequence of clinical stages before reaching *end-stage renal failure* (the point when dialysis is required). The divisions between these stages are somewhat arbitrary and may vary between individuals; nevertheless, these distinctions are useful in predicting the kinds of abnormalities that are to be expected for any given degree of renal dysfunction. Frequent reference to the glomerular filtration rate (GFR) throughout this chapter should not be misinterpreted to mean that the physicians know the precise value of this measurement in order to manage the patient. Prior to end-stage renal disease the blood urea nitrogen (BUN) and serum creatinine concentrations are often within the normal range, despite a fall of the glomerular filtration rate to as low as 50 ml/minute. Signs and symptoms, if present during this stage, are usually attributable to the underlying disease (e.g., diabetes, hypertension). As renal function declines further (GFR 20 to 50 ml/minute), the BUN and serum creatinine levels become noticeably increased and some metabolic abnormalities appear (e.g., metabolic acidosis, carbohydrate intolerance, reduced synthesis of 1, 25-dihydroxyvitamin D_3). Also at this point, the kidney's ability to respond to acute changes in body fluid and electrolyte composition is reduced. In this stage of renal insufficiency, although the BUN and serum creatinine concentration are increased (azotemia), symptoms attributable to the retention of nitrogenous wastes are absent. However, the patient may begin to experience symptoms related to anemia (fatigue), loss of urine-concentrating ability (polyuria), or volume expansion (dyspnea and/or edema). When the GFR falls below 20 ml/minute (serum creatinine concentration usually > than 5 mg/dl), the patient enters the stage of renal failure. This stage is associated with a further reduction in the ability of the kidney to maintain homeostasis and is characterized by multiple biochemical abnormalities (e.g., hypocalcemia, hyperphosphatemia, metabolic acidosis, fluid overload). The term uremia is employed to describe the entire set of signs, symptoms, and metabolic disturbances that occur in advanced kidney failure (GFR <10 ml/minute, serum creatinine concentration usually > than 8 mg/dl), and that may affect virtually all organ systems. Examples of some uremic manifestations include nausea, vomiting, anorexia (gastrointestinal tract), lassitude, reversal of the sleep cycle (nervous system), heart failure, hypertension (cardiovascular system), pruritis (skin), and infertility (endocrine system).

EPIDEMIOLOGY OF CHRONIC RENAL INSUFFICIENCY

There are currently over 90,000 patients on dialysis in the United States and many more living with successful kidney transplants. Since 1974, the year Medicare coverage was extended to patients with chronic renal failure who needed dialysis, the incidence of end-stage renal failure in patients who enter dialysis programs has increased from 71/million/year to over 100/million/year in 1983 (8). In actual numbers, 20,000 new patients require dialysis each year. The incidence of end-stage renal disease requiring dialysis has been noted to be 30 to 40% higher in males than in females and to peak between the ages of 65 and 74 years. The rate has also been estimated to be from three to four times greater in nonwhites than in whites due either to higher prevalence of hypertension or a greater end organ sensitivity to its effects in nonwhites (Fig. 48.1).

The reported distribution of patients entering the End-Stage Renal Disease Program (the Medicare-managed program that provides coverage for virtually all patients in the United States needing dialysis) by primary diagnosis is as follows: primary hypertensive disease, 23.4%; diabetic nephropathy, 21.8%; glomerulonephritis, 19.7%; interstitial nephritis, 6.4%; polycystic kidney disease, 5.9%; etiology unknown, 8.8%; miscellaneous, 14% (8).

CLASSIFICATION

Kidney diseases are often classified according to whether they produce acute or chronic renal failure. Acute renal failure is defined as a deterioration of glomerular filtration that occurs over days or weeks, whereas the course of chronic renal failure often runs from months to years. Many of the diseases that cause acute renal failure are reversible, and recovery is often complete (e.g., aminoglycoside nephrotoxicity). Recovery from those diseases that produce chronic renal failure is less common. It should be emphasized that some illnesses producing acute renal failure may not be entirely reversible and can progress to end-stage renal disease (e.g., Goodpasture's syndrome, acute cortical necrosis). Conversely, some of the chronic forms of renal disease can improve spontaneously or with therapy and may, therefore, never progress to the point of requiring dialysis treatments (e.g., membranous glomerulonephritis or the nephropathy of systemic lupus erythematosus).

The causes of kidney failure may be further subdivided into those with prerenal, renal, or postrenal components. *Prerenal azotemia* is caused by factors that produce a decrease in renal perfusion. Diminished perfusion may result from anatomical lesions such as might occur with renal artery stenosis, but

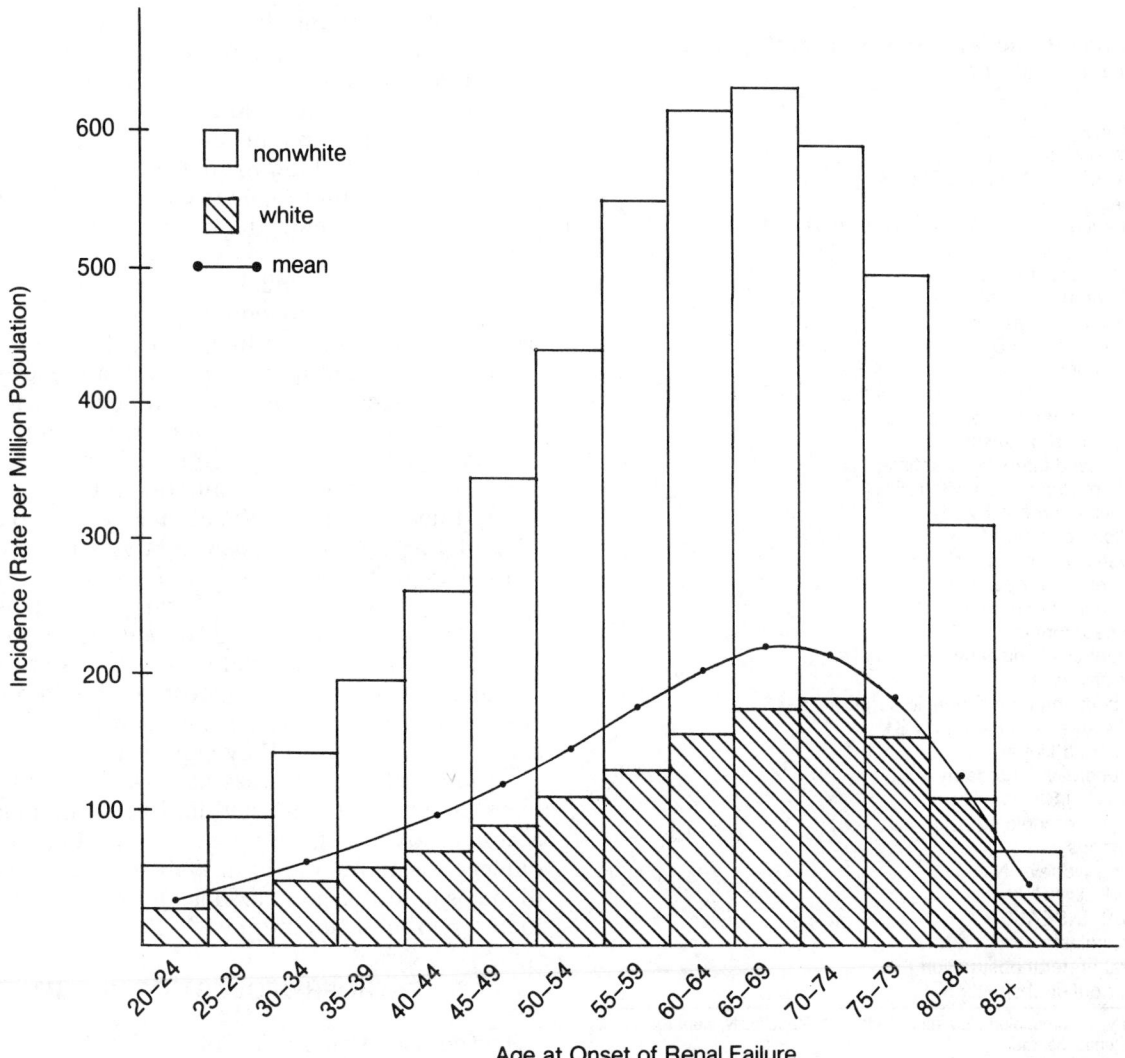

Figure 48.1. Curves show the incidence (rate/million) of patients entering the End-Stage Renal Disease Program (starting dialysis) for whites, nonwhites, and the population as a whole. (Adapted and redrawn from Eggers PW, Connerton R, McMullan M: The Medicare experience with end stage renal disease: trends in incidence, prevalence, and survival. Working Paper series. Department of Health and Human Services, Health Care Financing Ad ministration, Office of Research and Demonstrations, May 1983.)

more commonly it is related to pathological states of decreased cardiac output (heart failure), vasodilatation (septic shock), or volume depletion (vomiting or excessive diuretic use). Prerenal azotemia due to volume depletion, for example, may often be superimposed on existing chronic renal failure due to other causes. *Postrenal azotemia* is caused by lesions that occur distal to the kidney parenchyma involving the renal pelvis, ureters, bladder, or urethra. Common examples of such lesions would include prostatic enlargement, nephrolithiasis, or retroperitoneal cancers.

Most of the diseases that cause chronic renal failure directly involve the kidney parenchyma and are classified according to the anatomical region that is primarily affected (Table 48.1). *Glomerular lesions* can be due to proliferation of endothelial or mesangial cells (e.g., postinfectious glomerulonephritis), thickening of the basement membrane (e.g., membranous glomerulopathy, diabetic nephropathy), glomerulo-

sclerosis (e.g., focal sclerosis), or combinations of the three (e.g., membranoproliferative glomerulonephritis). Any of the diseases that cause glomerular lesions, if sustained, can lead to what is termed chronic glomerulonephritis. Clinically, glomerular diseases are often associated with hypertension, edema, renal insufficiency, hematuria, and significant (greater than 1 g/day) proteinuria.

Diseases that primarily affect the tubulointerstitial areas of the kidney are characterized morphologically by interstitial inflammation, fibrosis, and tubular atrophy. In the past these lesions were often equated with bacterial infections of the kidney (pyelonephritis), but most are thought currently to be due to toxins (e.g., analgesics, heavy metals), metabolic derangements (e.g., hyperuricemia, hypercalcemia), or immunological disorders (e.g., methicillin interstitial nephritis). The glomeruli are only secondarily involved in the tubulointerstitial diseases. *Polycystic and medullary cystic*

Table 48.1.
Classification of Kidney Diseases That May Result in Chronic Renal Failure[a]

PRERENAL DISEASES
    Renal artery stenosis   S
    Hepatorenal syndrome   S
RENAL PARENCHYMAL DISEASES
   Glomerular diseases
    Membranous glomerulonephritis (GN)   I
    Membranoproliferative GN   I
    Focal glomerulosclerosis   I
    Rapidly progressive GN   I
    Goodpasture's syndrome   I,S
    Lupus nephritis   I,S
    IgA nephropathy   I
    Alport's syndrome—hereditary nephritis   H,S
    Diabetic glomerulosclerosis   M,S
   Tubulointerstitial diseases
    Drug-induced interstitial nephritis   N[b]
    Chronic pyelonephritis with reflux
    Analgesic nephropathy   N
    Radiation nephritis   N
    Polycystic kidney disease   H,S
    Sickle cell nephropathy   S
    Heavy metal nephropathy   N
    Gouty nephropathy   M,S
    Medullary cystic disease   H
   Vascular diseases
    Thrombotic thrombocytopenic purpura   S
    Hemolyic-uremic syndrome   S
    Scleroderma kidney   S
    Hypertensive nephropathy   S
    Vasculitis   I,S
    Wegener's granulomatosis   I,S
   Miscellaneous
    Myeloma kidney   N,S
    Amyloidosis   S
POSTRENAL DISEASES
    Nephrolithiasis
    Bilateral ureteral obstruction
    Bladder outlet obstruction

[a]H, hereditary; I, immunologically mediated; M, metabolic; N, nephrotoxic; S, part of a systemic disorder.
[b]See Table 48.3.

kidney diseases represent a subgroup of the tubulointerstitial nephropathies and are characterized histologically by the presence of a multitude of thin-walled cysts derived from tubular epithelium. Patients with interstitial forms of kidney disease are not usually hypertensive or edematous, and they often produce large volumes of urine with high sodium contents. Typically, glycosuria, non-nephrotic range proteinuria (<3 g/day), sterile pyuria, and hyperchloremic metabolic acidosis are present.

Lesions of the renal vessels may be located in the main renal arteries (e.g., atherosclerosis, fibromuscular dysplasia), medium-sized arteries or arterioles (e.g., polyarteritis nodosa, scleroderma), or the renal veins (e.g., renal vein thrombosis). Renal insufficiency is a result of a reduction in blood flow to the glomeruli. Involvement of the renal vessels is often a part of a systemic illness that also affects vessels in other areas of the body. The clinical features of the renal vasculitides are very similar to those of glomerulonephritis (see above) except that nephrotic range proteinuria (>3 g/day) is uncommon.

A number of renal diseases can variably affect one or more of the kidney's anatomical regions. For instance, renal involvement in *multiple myeloma* may take the form of a diffuse thickening of the glomerular basement membrane, or more frequently it causes a tubulointerstitial nephropathy. *Systemic lupus erythematosus* is another example of a disease that can produce either glomerular or tubulointerstitial damage.

One can further subclassify renal diseases as to whether they are congenital, part of a systemic disorder, primary to the kidney, or by the mechanism of injury. The congenital or hereditary diseases most often encountered are polycystic kidney disease and Alport's form of hereditary nephritis. Diabetes mellitus and hypertension are the two most common systemic disorders producing chronic renal failure, and together they are listed as the etiology of approximately 45% of the patients entering dialysis programs. Immunological injury to the kidney can be in the form of glomerular immune complex deposition, as in systemic lupus erythematosus, or antiglomerular basement membrane antibody disease, best exemplified by Goodpasture's syndrome. Most of the immunologically mediated diseases predominantly affect the vessels or glomeruli, but they can also cause damage to the tubulointerstitial areas as in a drug-induced interstitial nephritis (e.g., methicillin). Drugs (e.g., phenacetin) or toxins (e.g., heavy metals) most often produce damage to the interstitium. Metabolic disorders (e.g., diabetes mellitus, gout, oxalosis) can result in damage to any region of the kidney.

PATHOPHYSIOLOGY OF UREMIA

The course of many chronic kidney diseases is characterized by the progressive loss of functioning nephrons. The kidney undergoes a number of adaptive changes that allow most patients with chronic renal failure to have few signs or symptoms until 80% of the original number of nephrons is lost.

Once a certain level of renal impairment has been attained, further deterioration seems to be inevitable, even when the original insult is transient and when other causes of additional damage have been excluded. An example of this phenomenon is the course of renal disease after ureteral reimplantation in patients with vesicoureteral reflux and mild renal insufficiency. Even in the absence of continuing reflux or infection some of these patients will, in time, develop proteinuria and progressive renal insufficiency. Renal biopsies in these patients have revealed the lesion of glomerulosclerosis.

The mechanism that has been postulated to explain the progressive nature of renal disease is related to the "adaptive" injury (6). According to this hypothesis, after a reduction in nephron mass, renal vasodilatation occurs and leads to hyperperfusion of the remaining glomeruli. These changes are considered to be adaptive because they result in increased glomerular filtration rates. However, experiments have shown that this state of *glomerular hypertension,* if sustained, can in itself be harmful Fig. 48.2). Glomeruli of nephrons exposed to prolonged hyperperfusion begin to leak protein, become sclerotic, and eventually are destroyed. As more and more nephrons are lost, the stimulus for hyperperfusion of the residual nephrons is increased and the process becomes self-perpetuating. Evidence is gathering that many diseases that produce limited kidney damage (e.g., patchy cortical necrosis, analgesic nephropathy, radiation nephritis) may progress to end-stage disease by this mechanism.

The ability of the impaired kidney to maintain the concentrations of individual components of the body's fluids within normal limits is variable. The concentrations of substances that are simply filtered and neither secreted nor resorbed by the tubule, such as urea and creatinine, begin to rise relatively early in the course of renal impairment (GFR 50% of normal). In contrast, the serum concentration of phosphorus, which is under the influence of parathyroid hormone (PTH), is kept within the normal range until more than 80% of renal function is lost. This is because in renal failure increased PTH activity progressively reduces the amount of phosphorus resorbed by the tubule (normally 80% of filtered phosphorus is resorbed) in parallel with the reduction in renal mass. Once the GFR falls below 20% of normal, this mechanism can no longer keep pace, and the serum phosphorus level begins to rise. Other solutes, such as sodium and potassium, are even better regulated, and their concentrations are maintained within the normal range until the GFR is less than 5 ml/minute.

Eventually the reserve capacity of the kidney is overwhelmed, and a number of signs, symptoms, and metabolic abnormalities appear that are characteristic of uremia (Table 48.2). Uremia is a complex syndrome that results from the failure of the kidney to fulfill its excretory, endocrine, and metabolic functions. In the patient with end-stage renal disease virtually every organ system is affected to some degree. The mechanisms for only some of the abnormalities that appear in uremia are well understood. Efforts to explain the metabolic consequences of renal failure by the retention of toxic wastes are only partially satisfying. Because urea is easily measured, it is the putative toxin that has been most thoroughly examined. Other nitrogenous waste products (e.g., ammonia, guanadinosuccinic acid), "middle molecules" (polypeptides of intermediate molecular weight), and a variety of organic and inorganic compounds have been implicated in the pathogenesis of uremia. Each of these toxins, individually or together, potentially could interfere with a specific cellular metabolic function and give rise to a manifestation of uremia.

It is clear that not all of the manifestations of uremia can be attributed to the retention of metabolic waste products. There are a number of well-described endocrine and metabolic derangements of equal significance in the pathogenesis of uremia. A deficiency of certain hormones results when the failing kidney is no longer able to produce them in adequate quantities (e.g., erythropoietin, 1, 25-dihydroxyvitamin D_3). Other hormones, normally degraded or metabolized by the kidney may be present in excess (e.g., parathyroid hor-

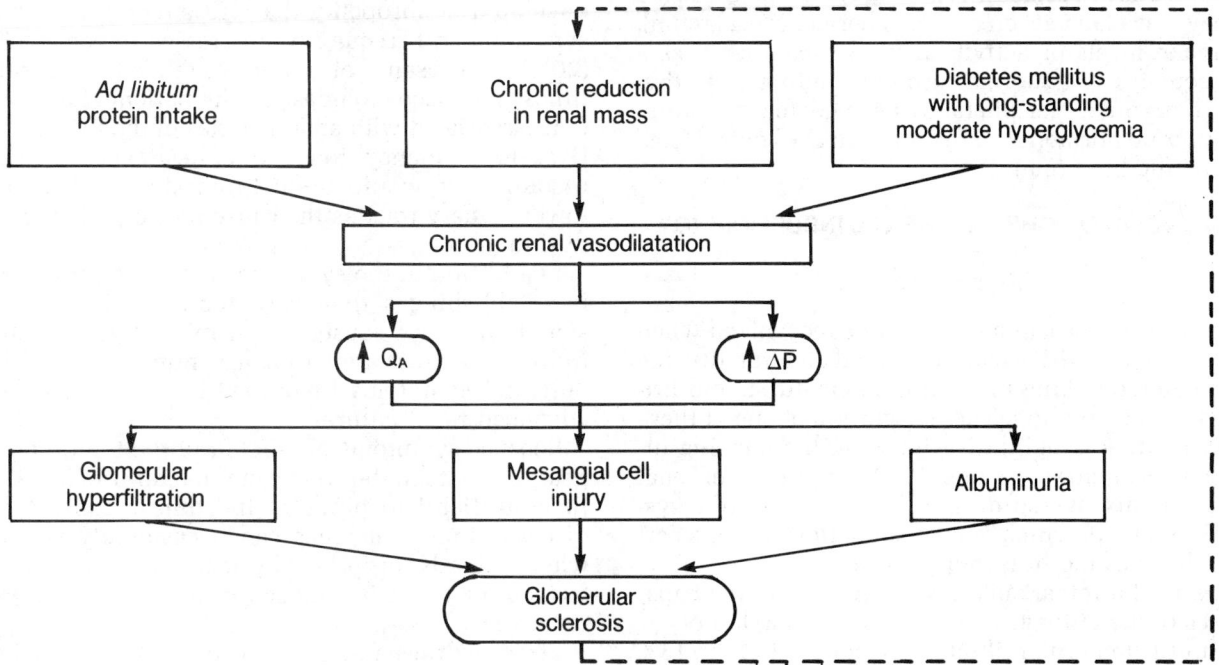

Figure 48.2. Proposed sequence of events whereby a chronic reduction in kidney mass and the consequent increase in glomerular pressures and flows leads to progressive renal damage. Q_A, blood flow; $\overline{\Delta P}$, transcapillary hydraulic pressure. (Redrawn from Brenner BM, Meyer TW, Hostetter TH: Dietary protein intake and the progressive nature of kidney disease: the role of hemodynamically mediated glomerular injury in the pathogenesis of progressive glomerular sclerosis, aging, renal ablation, and intrinsic renal disease. *N Engl J Med* 307:652, 1982.)

Table 48.2.
Major Physiological and Clinical Abnormalities of Uremia

Fluid and electrolyte abnormalities
   Volume expansion
   Hyperkalemia
   Hypocalcemia
   Hyperphosphatemia
   Metabolic acidosis
Endocrine-metabolic abnormalities
   Vitamin D deficiency
   Hyperparathyroidism
   Carbohydrate intolerance
   Impotence and infertility
   Hypertriglyceridemia
Hematological-immunological abnormalities
   Impaired platelet function
   Abnormal T and B cell function
   Anemia
Cardiovascular abnormalities
   Hypertension
   Accelerated atherosclerosis
   Pericarditis
Dermatological abnormalities
   Pruritis
   Increased pigmentation
   Acne
Gastrointestinal abnormalities
   Nausea and vomiting
   Anorexia
   Pancreatitis
Neuromuscular abnormalities
   Peripheral neuropathy
   Seizures
   Coma
   Asterixis
   Myoclonus

mone, insulin, prolactin). Alternatively, the damaged kidney may elaborate an excess of hormone (e.g., renin). Hormone levels or activity may also be altered as a consequence of abnormal protein binding (e.g., thyroid hormone), peripheral resistance (e.g., insulin, parathyroid hormone), or loss of feedback control (e.g., luteinizing hormone).

DIAGNOSIS OF CHRONIC RENAL INSUFFICIENCY

Presentation

Kidney disease can most easily be recognized when it is associated with a clearly defined abnormality, the most common being proteinuria, hematuria, and urinary tract obstruction. The recognition of one of these abnormalities is helpful in focusing the ensuing diagnostic evaluation. Frequently, the presence of renal disease is discovered during the evaluation of a systemic disease of which renal dysfunction is only a part (e.g., diabetes mellitus, hypertension).

Due to the remarkable reserve and adaptive capabilities of the kidney, symptoms of uremia do not appear until glomerular filtration is reduced to 10 to 15% of normal. Therefore, unless clearly overt signs of renal involvement are present (e.g., gross hematuria), many patients will progress to advanced renal failure asymptomatically. In other patients whose renal insufficiency is detected early in its course by routine blood

tests, specific findings on history and physical examination may also be absent. Special laboratory testing in these patients frequently permits establishment of a definitive diagnosis. The complete evaluation may vary from brief, in the patient with advanced renal failure and markedly shrunken kidneys, to extensive, in the patient who may have potentially reversible disease of recent onset. Most of the evaluation can be performed on an ambulatory basis.

History and Physical Examination

Findings in the history and physical examination can provide useful information that helps to establish the nature of the kidney disease, estimate its duration, and determine its effect on the patient. One of the major goals in evaluating the patient with recently identified renal failure is to distinguish those patients with primary kidney diseases from those whose renal failure is due to familial, congenital, or systemic illnesses.

First the family history should be reviewed for the presence of polycystic kidney disease, Alport's syndrome, medullary sponge kidney, hypertension, diabetes mellitus, or renal failure. The presence of an hereditary form of renal disease in the family should help to establish the etiology of the patient's kidney problem. Next, there should be a careful review of the past medical history with a particular emphasis on discovering the presence of a systemic illness that can cause renal failure (e.g., hypertension, diabetes mellitus, collagen vascular disorders). Patients with acquired immune deficiency syndrome (AIDS) may develop a nephropathy that presents with nephrotic syndrome and frequently progresses to renal failure (20). In the absence of symptoms related to a systemic illness one needs to question the patient about symptoms associated with abnormalities of the urinary tract. Dysuria, frequency, renal colic, hesitancy, or urinary incontinence would point to an abnormality of the lower urinary tract as the cause of the patient's renal dysfunction.

In addition to the symptoms that may prove useful in establishing a diagnosis, there are a number of symptoms (e.g., nausea, vomiting, fatigue, nocturia, itching, restless leg) that are nonspecific. These "uremic" symptoms are present in most patients with advanced renal failure.

Because symptoms of renal failure often do not appear until late in the course of renal failure, it is sometimes difficult to pinpoint the time of onset of the disease. Important clues can occasionally be found when records of past physical examinations performed for work, insurance, or military purposes are reviewed.

Because drugs may either be the cause of renal dysfunction (e.g., heroin, analgesics, aminoglycosides) or may aggravate pre-existing renal insufficiency (e.g., diuretics, nonsteroidal anti-inflammatory drugs) (Table 48.3), there should be a complete inventory of past and current drug use.

Table 48.3.
Some Commonly Used Drugs That May Adversely Affect Renal Function[a]

ANTIBIOTICS
　Aminoglycosides (ATN)
　Penicillins (IN)
　Tetracyclines (increased azotemia and acidosis)
ANALGESICS
　Aspirin (PN and reduction in RBF)
　Phenacetin (PN and IN)
　Nonsteroidal analgesics (IN, nephrotic syndrome, and reduced RBF)
DIURETICS
　Thiazides (volume depletion and IN)
　Furosemide (volume depletion and IN)
MISCELLANEOUS
　Radiocontrast materials (ATN)
　Methysergide (retroperitoneal fibrosis causing obstructive uropathy)
　Penicillamine (NS)
　Gold (NS)
　H_2 receptor antagonists (interfere with secretion of creatinine and produce false elevations of the serum creatinine concentration)
　ACE inhibitors (precipitates renal failure in patients with renovascular disease)

[a]ATN, acute tubular necrosis; PN, papillary necrosis; IN, interstitial nephritis; NS, nephrotic syndrome; RBF, renal blood flow.

The physical examination should be focused on a search for signs of systemic illnesses and for genitourinary structural abnormalities. These might include high blood pressure, hypertensive or diabetic retinopathy, vascular bruits, vasculitic skin rashes, gouty tophi, or ocular abnormalities (e.g., band keratopathy of hypercalcemia). Enlarged kidneys to palpation may be found in patients with polycystic disease or hydronephrosis. A pelvic or rectal examination should be performed to evaluate causes of lower urinary tract obstruction, such as prostatic or cervical cancer. When obstruction or neurogenic bladder is suspected, the bladder should be catheterized after the patient voids in order to measure a residual volume (see Chapter 6 for technique). A residual volume that is larger than approximately 100 ml should raise concern for bladder outlet obstruction (see Chapter 49) or neuropathic bladder (most commonly seen in diabetics). Signs of heart failure, pericarditis, or neuropathy are most often related to the stage of renal failure and are not helpful in establishing an etiology.

Laboratory Investigation

Laboratory testing of patients with chronic renal insufficiency serves to establish the severity and etiology of the kidney disease, as well as to determine the presence of complicating abnormalities.

Diagnostically, the *urinalysis* can often provide important information. Red blood cells (RBCs), particularly when associated with RBC casts, are most indicative of a glomerular or vascular lesion. White blood cells, with or without casts, are found in the interstitial nephropathies including, but not limited to, bacterial pyelonephritis. Hyaline or granular casts are not indicative of a specific pathological process.

The urine dipstick is only a rough guide to the amount of proteinuria (see Chapter 44). Most dipsticks are designed to detect only albumin and may therefore miss the presence of other proteins, such as light chains. The dipstick only measures the concentration of protein and therefore the reading must be interpreted in conjunction with the urine specific gravity. When quantification of proteinuria is desired, a 24-hour urine specimen should be obtained and can also be used to calculate the creatinine clearance (see below). Alternatively a protein:creatinine ratio may be determined in a specimen of urine as described in Chapter 44. The finding of nephrotic range proteinuria (greater than 3 g/day) usually indicates a glomerular lesion, whereas lesser amounts are seen in some glomerular or vascular disorders and in most interstitial forms of nephritis (Chapter 44). In patients over the age of 40 with unexplained renal insufficiency, regardless of the amount of urinary protein by dipstick, a serum and urine electrophoresis should be obtained to exclude the possibility of multiple myeloma.

The following tests should be ordered when an immunological disease is suspected: measurement of the serum complement levels (C3 and C4), screening for the presence of antistreptococcal antibodies, antinuclear antibodies, rheumatoid factor, and cryoglobulins. A test for human immunodeficiency virus (HIV) antibodies (see Chapter 34 for guidance before ordering) should be performed in patients with nephrotic syndrome or renal failure who are at risk for AIDS. Hepatitis B surface antigen (see Chapter 43) can be demonstrated in the blood of some patients with membranous glomerulopathy and in some forms of vasculitic renal disease. This antigen should also be screened for in any patient being referred for chronic dialysis or transplantation, since precautions to prevent the spread of hepatitis will need to be taken, if the test is positive.

The severity of anemia roughly parallels the blood urea nitrogen, as shown in Figure 48.3. The absence of anemia in patients with renal insufficiency should suggest either recent onset, the presence of polycystic

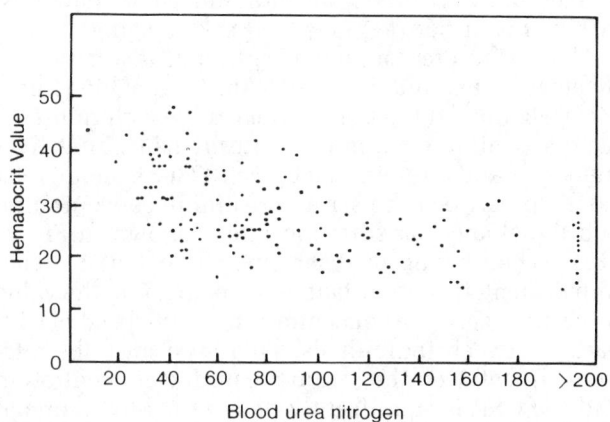

Figure 48.3. Relationship of blood urea nitrogen concentration to the hematocrit value in patients with chronic renal failure (From Erslev AJ: Erythrocyte function of the kidney. In Wesson LG (ed): *Physiology of the Human Kidney*. New York, Grune & Stratton, 1969, p. 521.)

kidney disease, or hydronephrosis. Both polycystic kidney disease and hydronephrosis can be associated with normal or elevated hematocrit values. The peripheral blood smear should be examined carefully for abnormalities associated with diseases that can produce renal failure. Rouleaux formation may be present in multiple myeloma, and leukopenia may be associated with collagen vascular diseases. A microangiopathic hemolytic anemia can be seen in patients with thrombotic thrombocytopenic purpura, the hemolytic-uremic syndrome, postpartum renal failure, accelerated hypertension, or scleroderma.

Measurements of the concentration of blood glucose, serum electrolytes (Na, K, Cl, HCO_3, Ca, PO_4), and uric acid are helpful in monitoring the patient. The presence of hypercalcemia may suggest a tumor or hyperparathyroidism. The uric acid level is usually elevated in patients with renal insufficiency, but a level greater than 12 mg/dl may indicate the presence of primary hyperuricemia or of a myeloproliferative disorder.

The physician will need some measure of overall kidney function in order to determine the degree of impairment, monitor the progression of disease, assess the effects of therapy, and adjust the dosage of drugs that are excreted by the kidney. The glomerular filtration rate is the standard means of expressing the level of renal function. In clinical practice, the GFR may be estimated from (a) the serum creatinine concentration; (b) the endogenous creatinine clearance; or (c) formulae that incorporate the patient's serum creatinine level, age, and weight (see below).

The normal GFR is approximately 100 to 140 ml/min in men and 85 to 115 ml/min in women. A gradual deterioration of GFR with age has been well documented and occurs even in the absence of overt renal disease in some individuals (21). The following equation may be used for estimating the "expected" creatinine clearance in healthy men.

GFR(ml/min) = 133 − 0.64 × age (years)

The clearance for women aged 50 or greater is approximately 5 to 10 ml/min less than for men. Thus, at age 70, for example, an individual may have lost 30% of his or her previous GFR due to aging.

The serum creatinine concentration is a better indicator of renal function than is the level of blood urea nitrogen since the latter is affected by such nonrenal factors as volume status, diet, intestinal bleeding, liver function, and protein catabolism. The general relationship between the serum creatinine concentration and the glomerular filtration rate is shown in Figure 48.4. When trying to determine the extent of renal impairment, it is important to remember that the value of serum creatinine concentration for any level of GFR varies between individuals. This is because the relationship between the serum creatinine concentration and the GFR is significantly determined by nonrenal factors such as the patient's muscle mass and age. Creatinine is produced by muscle, and its production rate parallels directly the muscle mass. The amount of creatinine produced per day also falls with age. As

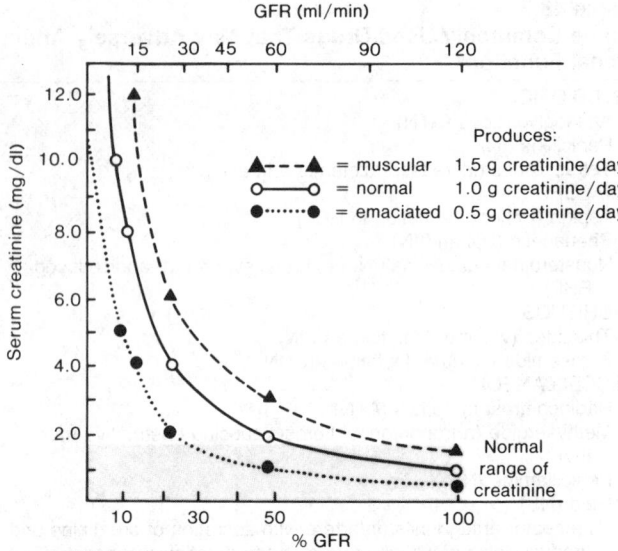

Figure 48.4. Relationship of the serum creatinine concentration to glomerular filtration rate in serum creatinine concentration (*l*/[*Scr*]) over time in a patient patients with different muscle mass.

can be seen in Figure 48.4, a small or elderly patient may have a doubling of the serum creatinine concentration, from 0.8 to 1.6 mg/dl, and still have a level within the "normal" range. Also, a young muscular patient who produces 1.5 g of creatinine per day will have a GFR of 30 ml/min when his serum creatinine concentration is 5 mg/dl, whereas an elderly, thin patient who produces only 0.5 g of creatinine per day will have a creatinine clearance of only 10 ml/min at the same level of serum creatinine. Once the factors affecting the level of serum creatinine concentration are understood the physician should have a clinically useful measure of overall renal function.

Because of the difficulties in interpreting the level of renal function from the serum creatinine concentration alone, the physician should be familiar with alternative methods for estimating the GFR. These methods are generally employed when adjusting dosages of drugs that are excreted by the kidney or when assessing renal function in elderly or small patients.

The endogenous creatinine clearance is a reasonable approximation of GFR in patients with normal or modestly reduced function but overestimates the GFR in advanced renal failure. The formula used for calculating clearance is UV/P divided by 1440, where U is the urine creatinine in mg/dl, V is urine volume in ml/day, P is the plasma creatinine concentration in mg/dl, and 1440 is the number of minutes in 24 hours. The result is expressed in milliliters per minute. A correction can be made for body surface area, but in adults this is not needed for usual clinical purposes. A 24-hour urine collection is used to determine daily creatinine production (UV). To confirm the adequacy of this collection the expected daily creatinine production may be estimated by multiplying body weight by (28 − 0.2 age) for men and (23.8 − 0.17 age) for women. For example, the expected daily creatinine production in a 50-year-old male patient weighing 70 kg would be 70 × [28 − (0.2 × 50)] = 1260 mg. In collecting the 24-hour urine, the patient should be instructed to choose a convenient time to begin the collection—usually upon rising in the morning. At this time the patient voids and discards the urine but collects all subsequent urine until the same time the following day when the patient again voids and adds that specimen to the collection. The blood sample for measurement of creatinine is generally obtained at the end of the collection period but may be drawn at any time during the collection. The estimation of the GFR by measuring creatinine clearance is often inaccurate, mainly due to collection errors. Although radionuclide measurements of GFR that do not require urine collection are available, there is rarely a need for such accuracy in office practice, and these tests are largely reserved for research purposes.

An alternative to calculating the creatinine clearance that avoids the difficulties entailed in collecting urine samples and that can be performed in the office is based on a formula that takes into account the patient's body weight and age:

$$(140 - age) \times body\ weight\ in\ kg \div 72\ (serum\ creatinine\ concentration)$$

(The value should be multiplied by 0.85 in the case of a small woman.) It should be recognized that the value of GFR determined by the above formula or measured by creatinine clearance may vary significantly from the more accurate determination of GFR by inulin clearance. These differences however, for clinical purposes, are generally considered insignificant.

When monitoring the course of kidney disease, it should be recalled that the serum creatinine concentration increases in a nonlinear fashion as renal function declines. In the early stages of renal insufficiency, when the GFR falls by 50%, the absolute increase in the serum creatinine concentration is small. Therefore, most of the loss of functioning nephrons occurs at levels of serum creatinine that would be considered to be only modestly elevated. Once the GFR is reduced to 20 to 30% of normal, the curve expressing the relationship between serum creatinine and GFR rises steeply. Absolute changes in the serum creatinine concentration when there is end-stage renal disease are therefore relatively less significant, when related to losses of GFR, than those seen in early renal insufficiency.

Alternative methods of monitoring the progression of renal disease have been devised in order to overcome the limitations of using the serum creatinine concentration alone and because measuring sequential creatinine clearances is often impractical or improperly done. Because the daily urinary creatinine excretion rate (UV, the numerator in the creatinine clearance calculation) remains essentially constant for a given individual, a plot of the *reciprocal of the serum creatinine concentration versus time* (Fig. 48.5) should

produce a function that parallels the rate of decline in GFR. In many, but not all, patients the plot will be linear with the slope reflecting the rate of progression and the x axis intercept the estimated time of end-stage renal failure. It has been suggested that the slope is constant for an individual and that any deviation reflects the effects of therapy or the presence of a superimposed process. Mathematical formulations such as this may be useful but must be interpreted only in conjunction with the remainder of the clinical and laboratory information. It is also important to understand that changes in GFR (reflected by an increasing serum creatinine concentration or a falling creatinine clearance) are not necessarily related to permanent changes in intrinsic kidney function and may be due to other factors (see below page 527).

Renal Imaging Techniques

Anatomical and functional evaluation of the kidney can be obtained through a variety of tests, all of which need not be performed on any individual patient. Renal imaging techniques in chronic renal failure should be used to (a) establish renal size, (b) detect remediable lesions, and (c) determine etiology.

Renal sonography is a reliable means of estimating kidney size and will usually detect the presence of significant hydronephrosis. Because of the risk of radiocontrast dye toxicity in patients with renal impairment (see below), the sonogram should be used in place of the intravenous pyelogram (IVP) as the initial imaging technique in most instances. Normal kidney length as measured by sonography is from 9 to 10 cm, with the left kidney being 0.5 cm larger than the right. An abdominal X-ray to include kidneys, ureters, and bladder (KUB), with tomograms if necessary, is the simplest and least expensive test for estimating renal size but will not detect the presence of hydronephrosis. Normal kidney length as measured by X-ray is approximately 12 to 13 cm or roughly the same as three to four lumbar vertebrae and discs. The kidneys appear longer when measured by X-ray due to a projection effect. Small kidneys by either technique usually indicate advanced chronic renal disease. However, normal or large kidneys may be seen in chronic renal failure (e.g., diabetes mellitus, amyloidosis).

Hydronephrosis, due to obstruction, should be ruled out in every patient with chronic renal insufficiency. If the screening sonogram reveals the presence of hydronephrosis, subsequent evaluation of the obstructed kidney may include an IVP, retrograde pyelogram, computerized tomographic (CT) scan, or a sonographically guided percutaneous antegrade pyelogram. The advantage of the latter technique is that it allows for the placement of a simultaneous percutaneous nephrostomy tube for drainage. Occasional cases of nondilated hydronephrosis have been described and further evaluation is indicated, even when the sonogram is normal, when the suspicion of obstruction is high.

The IVP is most useful in determining the etiology of renal failure in those diseases that produce gross

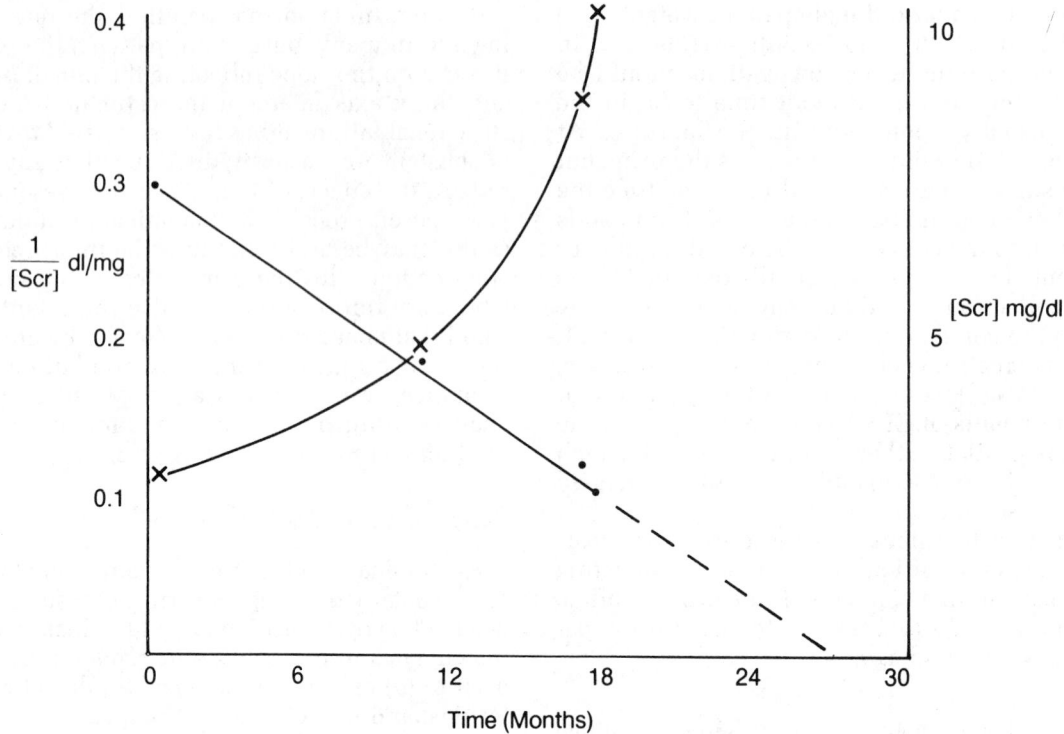

Figure 48.5.   Relationship between serum creatinine concentration ([*Scr*]) and the reciprocal of during an 18-month period. The linear relationship between the reciprocal of serum creatinine concentration over time suggests that nephrons are being lost at a constant rate. This kind of plot can also be used to monitor the course of renal failure. By extending the line derived from observed data it is possible to make a rough estimate (– – –) as to when dialysis will be necessary.

$$[Scr] = \times - \times; \frac{1}{[Scr]} = \cdot - \cdot.$$

anatomical abnormalities such as chronic pyelonephritis, nephrolithiasis, polycystic kidneys, obstruction of papillary necrosis. The IVP is not useful in patients with parenchymal disorders that are not associated with gross anatomical defects. CT scans are not routinely used in the evaluation of patients with chronic renal disease to localize the site of obstruction.

Nuclear medicine imaging techniques, useful in the evaluation of patients with hypertension due to unilateral renal artery stenosis, have been found to be less reliable in detecting bilateral renovascular disease (RVD). Bilateral atheromatous RVD, an often overlooked cause of renal failure (15), is more difficult to diagnose with radionuclide studies because the standard renal scan relies on asymmetrical blood flow as a diagnostic criterion. When blood flow is reduced to both kidneys, it is difficult to distinguish bilateral renal artery stenosis from parenchymal diseases. Even captopril renography, which depends on captopril-induced hemodynamic alterations, is of limited value in patients with renal insufficiency and bilateral RVD (11). Because none of the "noninvasive" tests is of proven efficacy in diagnosing patients with presumed bilateral RVD, an arteriogram should be obtained when the index of suspicion is high. The guidelines in Table 48.4 can be used as an aid in judging which patients should be considered for further evaluation. The most difficult decisions arise in patients with probable type II diabetic nephropathy who often have significant pe-

Table 48.4.
Clinical Presentations of Atheromatous Renal Disease[a]

1. Acute renal failure following reduction in blood pressure (particularly with ACE inhibitors).
2. Progressive azotemia in a patient with known renovascular disease.
3. Azotemia associated with new onset hypertension or a change in severity of hypertension.
4. Unexplained azotemia in an elderly patient with peripheral vascular disease.
5. Progressive renal failure with evidence of cholesterol embolization.

[a]Adapted from Jacobson: *Kid Int* 34:729, 1988.

ripheral vascular disease. The decision to perform angiography is usually based on the clinical judgment that the course deviates from what is generally seen in diabetes, or when the vascular component seems prominent (severe hypertension, claudication, bruits).

It is advisable to discuss these patients with a nephrologist and a vascular surgeon before performing the angiogram. Because arteriography is associated with significant risks (ATN, atheromatous embolization), one must first be absolutely sure that the patient is a suitable candidate for therapy (angioplasty or bypass). Furthermore, because these patients often have multiple sites of atheromatous involvement, additional radiological information beyond the renal arteries (views of the splenic or mesenteric arteries) may be required. Although the quality of the image of the intra-arterial digital subtraction angiogram is less than that of the standard renal arteriogram, the smaller volume of dye that is usually administered may reduce the risk of contrast-induced acute renal failure (ARF).

The incidence of radiocontrast-induced ARF seems highest in patients with renal insufficiency (serum creatinine concentration >2 mg/dl), diabetics, or the elderly; however, some argue that the only significant risk factor is pre-existing renal disease. Although incidence rates of ARF as high as 50% have been reported, the majority of these cases have been clinically insignificant and reversible. More recent reviews of ARF in "high risk" patients have found lower rates of ARF (9 to 16%), and it has been suggested that a greater awareness of the role of pre- and post-test hydration may be proving of benefit (18). The use of nonionic contrast materials has offered no advantage in the prevention of ARF, and the efficacy of mannitol infusions prophylactically is still unsettled. In summary, although transient increases in the level of serum creatinine concentration can be seen after the use of radiocontrast materials, few patients require dialytic therapy. Therefore, the presence of renal insufficiency should not be considered as an absolute contraindication to the performance of intravascular dye studies, particularly when the needed information cannot be obtained by alternative means (e.g., coronary angiography). Finally, because the decline in renal function from radiocontrast materials appears to be particularly preventable by avoiding volume depletion, patients should be instructed to maintain salt and fluid intake both before and after the examination.

Renal Biopsy

Once the baseline data have been accumulated, a nephrologist should be consulted, at least by telephone, to help in interpreting the information and to decide whether a renal biopsy is indicated. The renal biopsy provides histological information and for many disease entities is the most specific diagnostic test available. The biopsy should be considered when the diagnosis is uncertain, to estimate prognosis and to help demonstrate renal involvement of a systemic illness. Most renal biopsies can be performed percutaneously, under local anesthesia, but do involve a brief hospitalization (see Chapter 44). If the kidneys are very small or if renal failure is advanced, a biopsy is usually not done.

MONITORING THE PATIENT WITH RENAL INSUFFICIENCY

The interval between visits is determined by the stage of renal insufficiency, the rate of progression, and the presence of complicating disorders. Early in the course, patients should have office visits scheduled every 3 to 6 months for monitoring of their symptoms, signs (e.g., weight, blood pressure, edema, etc.), and laboratory data (e.g., serum creatinine concentration, BUN, electrolytes, complete blood counts, urinalysis, and possibly creatinine clearance). As renal failure progresses, visits will have to be spaced more

closely, usually at 1-month intervals until dialysis becomes necessary. Once the GFR falls below 10 ml/minute, clinical decisions are based more on the presence of symptoms or specific electrolyte abnormalities, such as hyperkalemia or acidosis, than on further changes in the serum creatinine clearance or the creatinine clearance. Drug dosages should be reviewed at each visit and adjusted according to the degree of renal dysfunction (see below). When the creatinine clearance falls below 5 ml/minute, many patients develop potentially serious electrolyte imbalances and usually require weekly visits for careful monitoring.

COURSE AND PROGNOSIS

The underlying renal disease largely determines prognosis. Many renal diseases have characteristic rates of progression. For example, patients with polycystic kidney disease typically have very indolent courses and some never progress to end-stage renal failure. More aggressive courses, with advanced renal failure developing within months to a year, are more likely to occur in patients with diseases such as rapidly progressive glomerulonephritis, systemic sclerosis, or malignant hypertension. However, most renal diseases fall into an intermediate group, with end-stage renal failure developing within 1 to 5 years after the initial diagnosis.

Therapy

Goals

The goals of therapy fall into four major categories. The first is to treat the underlying renal disease, if possible (e.g., corticosteroids for membranous nephropathy). The second is to slow the progression of renal deterioration by modifying the known or suspected factors that are thought to aggravate the primary process (e.g., treatment of hypertension) and to avoid factors that may aggravate existing renal failure (e.g., avoiding nonsteroidal anti-inflammatory drugs). The third goal is to treat the specific complications of renal disease (e.g., acidosis), as they occur, and also attempt to prevent the long-term complications of uremia before they can become fully established (e.g., secondary hyperparathyroidism). Finally the patient should be referred to a dialysis and transplantation center before the need for dialysis (see below).

Specific Treatments

Once a diagnosis is established, a nephrologist should be consulted, in order to decide whether effective therapy is available for the patient's renal disease. In general, the earlier in the course a treatment is started, the more likely it is to be successful in halting or reversing the disease. When the patient's renal disease is advanced or the effectiveness of the treatment is not well established, it is often advisable to forego potentially toxic therapies, as the hazards often outweigh the benefits.

Many of the immunologically mediated renal diseases (e.g., membranous nephropathy, Wegener's disease, Goodpasture's syndrome, lupus nephritis) may respond to treatment with corticosteroids, cytotoxic agents, or plasmapheresis. For others, there is no proven effective therapy (e.g., IgA nephropathy). Those patients with immunologically mediated renal diseases who require therapy should be under the care of a rheumatologist or nephrologist.

When the renal disease is associated with a metabolic disorder such as occurs in gout or diabetes mellitus, it is reasonable to treat the underlying abnormality (e.g., hyperuricemia, hyperglycemia). Treatment directed at metabolic control may slow the course of renal deterioration but is not likely to result in significant reversal of established disease. In fact, the cause and effect relationship between hyperuricemia and renal failure in patients with gout is debatable (22) as is the efficacy of strict metabolic control on the natural history of diabetic nephropathy.

When a drug (e.g., methicillin, indomethacin) or other toxic substances (e.g., heavy metal) is identified as the cause of renal failure, the offending agent should be withheld or avoided. A trial of corticosteroids may be given to patients with drug-induced interstitial nephritis, but this treatment is still controversial and the decision should be made in conjunction with a nephrologist.

It has been demonstrated that the vascular lesions in the kidney due to malignant hypertension may resolve slowly and usually only partially with control of blood pressure. In some patients this will correlate with significant improvement in the GFR. Patients with renal failure secondary to bilateral RVD may have significant improvement in their renal function after successful angioplasty or bypass surgery.

Obstructing lesions of the urinary tract may require surgical excision (e.g., benign prostatic hypertrophy) or urinary diversion (e.g., retroperitoneal fibrosis) in order to preserve or improve renal function. Other patients can be managed more conservatively (e.g., intermittent straight catheterization of the bladder) if the lesion is not amenable to surgical therapy (e.g., neurogenic bladder).

Nonspecific Treatments

There is currently considerable interest among nephrologists about the use of *protein-restricted diets* to retard the progression of renal disease in order to delay or even obviate the need for dialysis (5). The glomerular filtration rate in healthy animals and humans varies directly with protein intake. Protein restriction has been shown in animal experiments to reduce the degree of compensatory hypertrophy after renal injury and to forestall the development of glomerular sclerosis, proteinuria, and progressive renal failure. Several studies have been published describing the effects of various protein-restricted diets, with or without concomitant phosphorus restriction, on the course of patients with renal insufficiency (serum creatinine

concentration between 2 and 6 mg/dl) (14, 16). The results of these studies lend support to the hypothesis that protein restriction can, in fact, slow the rate of renal deterioration ordinarily expected in this group of patients (Fig. 48.6). Further studies are in progress that should clarify the exact indications, the time of initiation, the composition, and the potential long-term benefits/complications of protein-restricted diets. At this time, it seems reasonable, in the absence of more specific therapy, to advise patients with moderate renal insufficiency (serum creatinine between 2 and 6 mg/dl) to reduce their protein intake to about 40 g/day (14).

Hypertension, present in many patients with renal insufficiency, may also aggravate pre-existing kidney failure. Long-term control of hypertension appears to slow the progression of renal insufficiency (see Chapter 62). This has been most convincingly demonstrated in diabetics in whom the rate of decline in renal function was reduced when blood pressure was treated (17).

Epidemiological and retrospective studies also support the proposition that treatment of hypertension can attenuate the rate of progression of a variety of established kidney diseases. Although angiotensin-converting enzyme (ACE) inhibitors and calcium channel blockers have shown some advantage in protecting the kidneys in animal models of renal failure, it is not yet known whether there is a particular superiority of any specific antihypertensive regimen in patients. The degree of blood pressure reduction that is optimal has also not been established, but systolic pressures of <140 mm Hg and diastolics of <90 mm Hg have been recommended.

Antihypertensive therapy in patients with mild to moderate renal insufficiency is similar to that of patients with normal renal function and hypertension. A salt-restricted diet (e.g., 2 g/day) may be attempted as a first step. Loop diuretics such as furosemide or bumetanide can be added when salt restriction is insufficient or when nondiuretic drugs (e.g., hydralazine, captopril) lead to secondary salt retention. Thiazides are generally avoided in patients with GFRs below 30 ml/minute because they often lose their diuretic effect. Potassium-sparing diuretics (spironolactone, triamterene, amiloride) should not be used in patients with significant renal impairment due to the increased risk of developing hyperkalemia.

Methyldopa, hydralazine, prazosin, clonidine, calcium channel blockers, ACE inhibitors, and beta blockers all are useful in patients with chronic renal insufficiency (see Chapter 62). Many vasodilating drugs induce a state of fluid and salt retention and must be used in conjunction with a diuretic in order to be effective. As renal function deteriorates, the use of larger doses of diuretics will often be necessary to control hypertension. There is often a fine line between effective blood pressure control and hypotension when potent diuretics and antihypertensives are being used; therefore, careful monitoring of blood pressure (both supine and upright) and of serum cre-

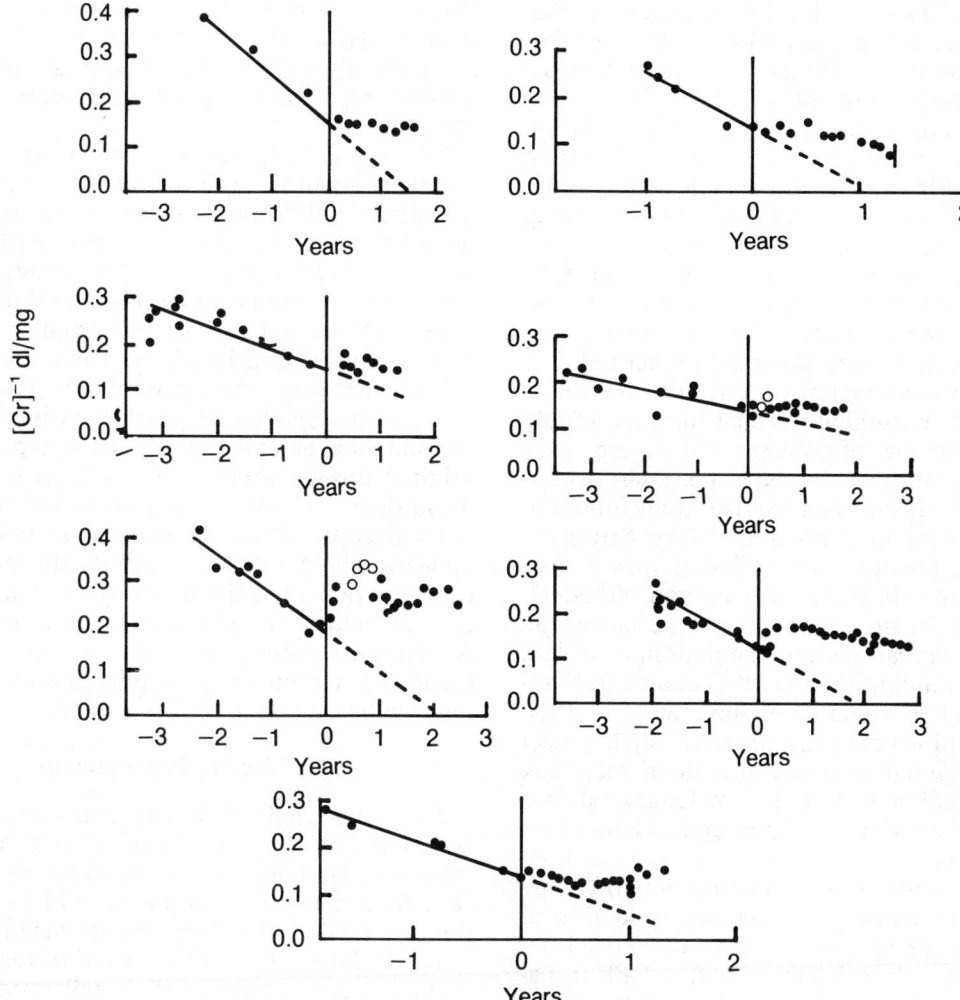

Figure 48.6. Data showing how the rate of progression of renal failure, as determined by a plot of the reciprocal of serum creatinine concentration over time, in seven different patients, was affected by the institution at time 0 of a low phosphorus, low protein diet. A decrease in the slope reflects stabilization of renal function. The *dashed line* indicates the projected course. (Data redrawn from Mitch WM, Walser M, Steinman TI, *et al*: Effect of a keto acid-amino acid supplement to a restricted diet on the progression of chronic renal failure. *N Engl J Med* 311:623, 1984.)

atinine concentration are necessary. Renal insufficiency is not a contraindication to using ACE inhibitors, though some side effects, particularly hyperkalemia, may be more common. With the use of potent drugs such as minoxidil (for detailed discussions of these drugs see Chapter 62) bilateral nephrectomy (which results in a severe anemia and the requirement for dialysis) for the treatment of refractory cases of hypertension can generally be avoided. Long-term control of hypertension may be important in reducing the risk of atherosclerosis in patients on dialysis.

Treating Reversible Causes of Deterioration of Renal Function

Before any change in serum creatinine concentration is attributed to the natural progression of the underlying renal disease, several alternative possibilities should be considered (Table 48.5).

Extracellular volume depletion is probably the most

Table 48.5.
Causes of Renal Functional Deterioration

Volume depletion (salt and water depletion)
Congestive heart failure
Drug nephrotoxicity
Ureteral or urethral obstruction
Orthostatic hypotension
Microcrystal deposition (*e.g.*, acute hyperuricemia)
Hyperphosphatemia-hypercalcemia
Hypertension
Radiocontrast materials (oral and parenteral)
Glomerular hyperperfusion

common cause for a fall in GFR. It may be related to an intercurrent illness associated with anorexia, fever, gastrointestinal losses of sodium and water, overexcessive salt restriction, or diuretic use. The usual clinical signs of volume depletion (e.g., low jugular venous pressure, orthostatic hypotension, tachycardia, decreased skin turgor, and weight loss) may be absent, and a therapeutic trial of salt administration may be required to establish the diagnosis. Weight loss between office visits is usually the most important diagnostic clue to the presence of volume depletion. The urinary sodium concentration or urine osmolality, usually helpful in establishing the diagnosis of volume depletion, is of little value in the patient with chronic renal failure since concentrating and salt-conserving ability in these patients is often impaired.

Patients with decompensated *congestive heart failure* may also present with superimposed prerenal azotemia. Optimal treatment of heart failure may improve renal function in these patients (see Chapter 61).

Drugs given for treatment of various other disorders can be related to worsening of renal function (Table 48.3). A careful review of both prescribed and over-the-counter medications is therefore necessary whenever assessing unexpected changes in kidney function. Of the drugs prescribed in the ambulatory setting diuretics and nonsteroidal anti-inflammatory agents (NSAIDs) are probably the most common offenders. Diuretics can aggravate pre-existing renal failure by inducing intravascular volume depletion, and less commonly by producing an interstitial nephritis. Careful monitoring of the blood pressure, weight, BUN, and serum creatinine concentration will help to detect early signs of prerenal azotemia in patients receiving diuretics. Withholding diuretic therapy for several days usually allows intravascular volume and GFR to return to baseline values.

The NSAIDs can also cause a deterioration in kidney function either by causing a reversible reduction of renal blood flow, or by producing an interstitial nephritis. NSAIDs are most likely to reduce GFR in patients with prerenal states, such as volume depletion, congestive heart failure (CHF), or nephrosis. At this time it cannot be said that one nonsteroidal compound is safer to use in the patient with renal insufficiency than another. It is therefore best to avoid them altogether once the GFR is less than 50 ml/minute. It should be noted that ibuprofen (e.g., Advil or Nuprin) is available without a prescription.

There have been numerous reports of reversible renal dysfunction when ACE inhibitors have been administered to patients with bilateral RVD or stenosis of a solitary kidney. Such patients should be considered for further diagnostic evaluation of their vascular disease (see below).

Obstruction, because of its reversibility, should always be considered in patients with a fall in the GFR. This is particularly true in elderly men predisposed to prostatic hypertrophy or in diabetics who may have autonomic neuropathy affecting bladder emptying. Drugs that reduce bladder tone (e.g., antidepressants, antispasmodics, and antiparkinsonian drugs with anticholinergic properties) should always be considered as causes of obstruction. If obstruction is a possibility, the patient should have a measurement of a postvoid residual volume (see Chapter 6 for technique).

Orthostatic hypotension, due to drugs or autonomic neuropathy, can cause a worsening of renal failure.

Drugs and other causes of this problem are summarized in Table 81.7. Orthostatic hypotension should be managed by adjusting or stopping the drugs and/or prescribing the practical measures summarized in Table 81.8.

Microcrystal deposition in the kidney has been suggested by some as a cause of progressive deterioration in patients with azotemia. Serum uric acid concentrations are often elevated in patients with renal insufficiency. There is no evidence, however, that reducing the serum uric acid concentration will prevent further deterioration when the original kidney disease was not due to gout. Allopurinol is not used, therefore, unless it is needed to control symptomatic gout.

Calcium phosphate deposits have been found in the parenchyma of end-stage kidneys regardless of the original disease process. It has been postulated that these deposits have some role in the progression of renal disease. Although dietary phosphorus restriction appears to help reduce the rate of deterioration of renal function in both animal and human kidney failure, the mechanism by which this occurs is still unclear. Nevertheless, many nephrologists currently recommend that patients reduce phosphorus intake to 800 mg (see below) once GFR falls below 50 ml/minute.

Dietary Management

The major goals of dietary management in the patient with chronic renal insufficiency are to optimize intravascular volume, correct electrolyte abnormalities, relieve uremic symptoms, and prevent or slow the progression of kidney disease (Table 48.6).

The volume of the intravascular space is directly related to salt balance, which is in turn regulated by the kidney. As renal function declines, the ability of the kidney to maintain salt balance in response to changes in sodium intake becomes limited, especially when the changes occur abruptly. The intravascular volume may be depleted if the intake of salt is reduced

Table 48.6.
Dietary Management of Renal Failure

Therapy	Goals
Salt 4–6 g/day	Maintain intravascular volume
Fluid 1–3 liters/day	Avoid dehydration
Potassium if [K] > 5.5 mEq/liter restrict intake to 2–2.4 g/day	Prevent hyperkalemia
Protein Restrict intake to 0.55–0.6 g/kg/day (50% rich in essential amino acids)	Relieve uremic symptoms Retard progression of renal failure
Calories provide 35–45 kcal/kg/day	Maintain nutrition
Calcium provide 1–1.5 g/day	Maintain [Ca] = 9–10 mg/dl
Vitamins multivitamin + folate	Replace vitamins lacking in protein-restricted diet
Phosphorus restrict intake to 600–900 mg/day	Prevent secondary hyperparathyroidism

(e.g., excessive salt restriction, anorexia) or if there are losses of salt (e.g., vomiting, diarrhea, diuretics). A reduction in intravascular volume can lead to a further increase in the BUN and serum creatinine concentrations above the baseline values (prerenal azotemia). Conversely, the intravascular volume will increase if the intake of salt is suddenly augmented (dietary indiscretion), and the patient can develop hypertension, edema, and/or heart failure.

Most patients with chronic renal insufficiency maintain sodium balance on a 4- to 6-g salt intake. Patients with congestive heart failure or hypertension may need further limitation of salt intake (2 g of salt), whereas the rare patient with severe "salt-wasting" nephropathy may require salt supplements to prevent volume depletion. Most of these latter patients have some form of interstitial renal disease.

Salt intake should be adjusted to maintain intravascular volume at the level that maximizes the GFR for any given degree of renal failure. Assessing the state of the intravascular volume can be aided by obtaining serial body weights (rapid changes in weight are usually due to fluid gains or losses), by the physical examination (e.g., orthostatic change of pulse and blood pressure, jugular venous pressure, skin turgor, edema), and by measuring changes in the BUN and serum creatinine concentrations (increases in the level of BUN are proportionately greater than that of the serum creatinine concentration in states of volume depletion). It is often useful to establish an "ideal" weight. This is the weight at which the patient has optimal renal function without overt signs of volume overload. For some patients, those with congestive heart failure or nephrotic syndrome, for example, a small amount of edema is acceptable, since worsening of azotemia may develop when further diuresis is attempted. Whenever there is a significant change in the GFR, the intravascular volume and the ideal weight should be re-evaluated.

When the glomerular filtration rate falls as a result of volume depletion, it is necessary to restore the intravascular volume. This can be accomplished either by adding salt to the diet or by prescribing sodium chloride (600 mg four times a day) or sodium bicarbonate tablets (600 mg four times a day) until the patient's weight and GFR return to baseline values. If oral replacement is not practical (e.g., persistent vomiting), the patient should be hospitalized for intravenous therapy.

If volume overload develops or persists despite salt restriction, diuretics can be used to increase salt excretion (Table 48.7). Because the thiazide diuretics, with the exception of metalazone (Zaroxalyn), lose their effectiveness when the GFR falls below 30 ml/minute, it is often necessary to use a loop diuretic, such as furosemide (Lasix) or bumetanide (Bumex). Another loop diuretic, ethacrynic acid (Edecrin), has been associated with an unacceptable level of ototoxicity and should not be used in patients with renal insufficiency. The potassium-sparing diuretics, spironolactone (Aldactone), triamterene (Dyrenium), and amiloride (Moduretic) are also best avoided in patients with significant renal failure due to the risk of inducing serious hyperkalemia.

Potassium restriction is usually unnecessary until the late stages of renal failure (GFR <15 ml/minute), except in the small number of patients with the syndrome of hyporeninemic-hypoaldosteronism (see below), but careful monitoring of serum potassium levels is indicated nonetheless. If hyperkalemia develops, potassium restriction to between 2 and 2.4 g/day (40 to 50 mEq) is necessary. A dietitian should be consulted to help plan a potassium-restricted diet. Foods with high potassium contents include: dairy products, many greens, beans, potatoes, tomatoes, bananas, dates, prunes, raisins, and citrus fruits. Patients who are on sodium-restricted diets must also be informed that many salt substitutes are unacceptable because they are often composed of potassium salts.

The association of hyperkalemia and hyperchloremic metabolic acidosis in patients with mild to moderate renal insufficiency (GFR > 25 ml/minute) should lead one to consider the presence of the *hyporenin-hypoaldosterone syndrome* (19). This syndrome occurs most frequently in azotemic patients with hypertension, diabetes mellitus, or interstitial nephritis. This disorder probably has many causes, but it is due in part to a suppression of the renin-aldosterone axis. The diagnosis is usually made on clinical grounds, after excluding other reasons for hyperkalemia (e.g., high potassium intake or drugs that reduce the renal excretion of potassium), but it can be more firmly established by the demonstration of a low plasma renin concentration that fails to rise after stimulating the patient with furosemide (Lasix), 40 mg orally, and upright posture for 2 hours. The patient should also have no evidence of glucocorticoid deficiency (random cortisol concentration of 15 to 25 μg/ml; see also Chapter 74). Because, in the absence of aldosterone, potassium excretion by the kidney is dependent on an adequate urine flow rate (1.5 to 2 liters/day), patients with this syndrome are at risk for developing severe hyperkalemia during periods of salt restriction or of volume depletion. Normotensive patients may be treated with a mineralocorticoid (fluorohydrocortisone (Florinef), 0.1-mg tablets, ½ to 1 tablet/day). Alternatively, if hypertension is present or develops after the administration of the mineralocorticoid, the patient may be treated with a combination of furosemide (Lasix) (40 to 80 mg twice a day) plus sodium bicarbonate (600 mg four times a day). The furosemide is used to promote a good urine flow rate, whereas the sodium bicarbonate helps to prevent salt depletion and also is of use in correcting the associated metabolic acidosis. The goal of therapy is to keep the serum potassium concentration within the normal range. Because therapy is frequently complicated, these patients are best managed in conjunction with a nephrologist or endocrinologist.

Although *diluting and concentrating abilities* are impaired in renal failure, most patients are able to ingest 1 to 3 liters of fluid/day without developing

Table 48.7.
Diuretics in Renal Failure

Drug	Available Strengths (mgs)	Dose	Route of Excretion	Comments
Thiazides (Hydrochlorthiazide)	25, 50	50–200 mg/day	Renal	May induce volume depletion and hyperuricemia. Loses effectiveness if GFR < 30 ml/minute but may be used in combination with loop diuretics in advanced renal failure.
Metalozone (Zaroxalyn)	2.5, 5, 10	5–20 mg/day	Renal	May induce volume depletion and hyperuricemia. Effective when GFR > 10.
Furosemide (Lasix)	20, 40, 80	20–400 mg/day	Renal	May induce volume depletion and hyperuricemia. Effective when GFR > 5. May produce ototoxicity and rarely interstitial nephritis. May increase nephrotoxicity of antibiotics.
Bumetanide (Bumex)	.5, 1, 2	1–10 mg/day	Renal	May induce volume depletion and hyperuricemia. Side effects include ototoxicity and muscle pains and may also increase the risk of antibiotic nephrotoxicity.
Ethacrynic acid (Edecrin)		Avoid	Hepatic	Usually avoided in renal failure since the risk of ototoxicity is significantly higher than with furosemide or bumetanide.
Spironolactone (Aldactone) Triamterene (Dyrenium) Amiloride (Moduretic)		Avoid	Hepatic	Avoid when GFR < 50 ml/minute due to the risk of inducing serious hyperkalemia.

hyponatremia. If hyponatremia occurs, fluids should be limited to less than 1.5 liters/day in order to prevent water intoxication.

Protein-restricted diets, in addition to their use in reducing the rate of decline in kidney function (see above), are indicated for patients with advanced renal failure (GFR < 15 ml/minute) who develop nausea, vomiting, or other symptoms attributable to uremia. Because many of the end products of protein metabolism have been implicated in the causation of the uremic syndrome, therapy consists of reducing protein intake to about 0.6 g/kg of body weight/day (approximately 40 g of protein/day in a 70-kg individual). Normal protein intake in the United States exceeds 70 g/day. Half of the protein intake should be in the form of meats, fish, eggs, or milk, since these foods are rich in essential amino acids. In order for the patient on a protein-restricted diet to maintain adequate nutritional balance, total caloric intake must be adjusted to provide 35 to 45 kcal/kg/day. This can be accomplished by increasing the intake of fats and carbohydrates.

Because protein-restricted diets are often deficient in vitamins, calcium, and phosphorus, patients should receive a daily vitamin supplement and 1 to 1.5 g of elemental calcium/day (a single 600-mg calcium carbonate tablet provides 250 mg of elemental calcium). The reduction in dietary phosphorus is desirable (see below), and therefore phosphorus supplements are not given.

If symptoms such as nausea and vomiting related to uremia persist or the creatinine clearance falls below 5 ml/minute, the patient should be started on dialysis. Further restriction of protein intake is possible but should only be attempted for limited periods and under the direct supervision of a nephrologist. With the present availability of dialysis, little is to be gained by trying to maintain a very symptomatic patient on a highly restricted diet. Proper planning for patients with progressive renal disease should prevent referral of debilitated, malnourished, and neuropathic patients to a dialysis center (see below).

Considering the complexity of such diets and the need for individualization of salt, mineral, protein, and potassium intake, consultation with a dietician or a nephrologist proficient in prescribing renal diets is suggested. Constant encouragement and supervision of dietary therapy are needed. The success of dietary treatment often depends on the involvement of family members as well as an enthusiastic dietician.

Calcium and Phosphorus

Renal osteodystrophy is a general term that encompasses osteitis fibrosa, osteomalacia, and a variety of other bone lesions that occur in patients with kidney failure. The pathophysiological factors that lead to osteodystrophy originate in the early stages of renal failure, although clinical manifestations generally do not develop until the patient is on dialysis.

The pathophysiology of renal osteodystrophy is complex but can be briefly summarized as follows: Parathyroid hormone (PTH) secretion increases during the early stages of renal failure (GFR > 30 ml/minute) for two major reasons. The first is to keep the serum phosphorus concentration within normal limits. PTH acts to increase the rate of phosphorus excretion by the remaining nephrons and thereby prevents the rise in serum phosphorus concentration that would otherwise occur during the course of renal failure. The second is to maintain a normal serum calcium concentration. Small, but significant, decreases in serum ionized calcium concentrations can result from equally small increases in the serum phosphorus level as well as from diminished gastrointestinal absorption of calcium. Decreased calcium absorption in renal failure is predominantly a consequence of an intestinal defect (related to vitamin D deficiency) but may in part be due to diminished intake because of anorexia or protein restriction. PTH serves to maintain serum calcium concentrations in the normal range largely by mobilizing calcium from the bones.

The increased rate of PTH secretion is successful at keeping serum calcium and phosphorus levels within the normal range until the GFR is less than 30 ml/minute. In more advanced renal failure hypocalcemia and hyperphosphatemia develop. The most important consequence of prolonged *secondary hyperparathyroidism* is the development of bone disease (osteitis fibrosa cystica).

Osteomalacia, in renal insufficiency, is due partly to the failure of the diseased kidney to convert 25-hydroxyvitamin D_3 to its more active form, 1, 25-dihydroxyvitamin D_3. The active form of vitamin D is necessary for normal bone mineralization. Although the serum levels of vitamin D can be normal in patients with GFRs above 30 ml/minute (since this level is not elevated), such levels may still represent a relative deficiency of the hormone. Absolute deficiencies of vitamin D are found once the GFR falls below 30 ml/minute. Abnormal collagen synthesis, the titration of bone buffers, and the accumulation of aluminum in the bone matrix have also been implicated in the pathogenesis of osteomalacia.

Patients with renal insufficiency should have periodic (see above for frequency) measurements of calcium, phosphorus, magnesium, and alkaline phosphatase. Routine measurements of PTH levels are not indicated unless the patient is hypercalcemic, since virtually all patients with renal insufficiency will have increased levels. Levels of PTH, when measured by the carboxy-terminal assay, will be uniformly high, since the kidney is responsible for the elimination of that fragment. Therefore, determination of PTH levels, when necessary, should be by an assay that measures the intact or N-terminal hormone. Bone X-rays or biopsies are not routinely obtained in the patient not yet on dialysis, unless the patient has symptomatic bone disease.

The clinical features of deranged calcium and phosphorus metabolism, including bone pain, fractures, and proximal myopathy, are not often seen until after the patient is on dialysis. Nevertheless, therapy to correct these abnormalities should begin during the early stages of renal failure (Table 48.8).

Based on a knowledge of calcium, phosphorus, and vitamin D alterations in early renal insufficiency, described above, it is possible to outline a plan of therapy directed at reducing the incidence and severity of osteodystrophy in late renal insufficiency. The goals of therapy are to limit the rise in PTH secretion that usually accompanies renal failure and to prevent the development of osteomalacia. These goals can be achieved by maintaining a positive calcium balance, by providing vitamin D, and by reducing phosphorus intake.

Because *calcium* absorption is diminished in patients with renal insufficiency, the first step in treatment is to assure an adequate intake of calcium. This is particularly important if the patient is on a protein-restricted diet that often contains only 300 to 400 mg of calcium (normal calcium intake is 800 to 1000 mg/day). Supplements in the form of calcium carbonate (generic), 600 mg four times per day, will provide 1000 mg of elemental calcium per day. Calcium lactate (generic), 300 mg (two tablets four times/day), can be substituted if the carbonate is not tolerated because of constipation or bloating.

Until recently, the use of vitamin D therapy, in the predialysis patient, to prevent the development of renal osteodystrophy, was based on limited and uncontrolled data. It has now been shown, in a prospective, controlled trial, that low doses of orally administered vitamin D (Rocaltrol) given to patients with GFRs between 60 and 20 ml/minute can improve the biochemical and histological markers of osteodystrophy (2). Whether initiating therapy early, rather than waiting for the patient to start dialysis, is better in terms of preventing the long-term complications of deranged calcium-phosphorus metabolism has not been proven. If, after consultation with a nephrologist, it is decided to treat early, one should start at the lowest dose of the vitamin D preparation selected and raise the dose every 4 weeks until the serum calcium is in the upper range of normal. It appears, from experience, that most patients with renal insufficiency will not tolerate a Rocaltrol dose of >0.5 μ/day without developing hypercalcemia. Hypercalcemia may be associated with increases in the serum creatinine concentration, which should be reversible once the dose of vitamin D is reduced and calcium levels return to the normal range. Therefore, due to the frequency of hypercalcemia and its potential effects on renal function, it is crucial that serum calcium levels be monitored weekly, after a change in dosage, until the serum calcium concentration stabilizes, and monthly thereafter. At this time there does not appear to be any value to monitoring the levels of vitamin D metabolites during therapy. In general, one expects to see a fall in the levels of alkaline phosphatase and PTH, but as yet there are no treatment guidelines based on these values.

Table 48.8.
Steps in the Management of Calcium and Phosphorus Balance in Patients with Renal Failure

Therapy	Goals
GFR 50–30 ml/minute	
Calcium supplements (1–1.5 g/day) (see text)	Maintain serum calcium concentration at 9–10 mg/dl
Vitamin D (Rocaltrol 0.25–0.5 mcg/day, available in 0.25 mcg tablets)	Maintain serum calcium concentration at 9–10 mg/dl
GFR < 30 ml/minute	
Restrict phosphorus intake (600 mg/day)	Maintain serum phosphorus concentration at 4.0–6.0 mg/dl
Phosphorus-binding antacids (calcium carbonate, aluminum carbonate or aluminum hydroxide taken with meals)	Maintain serum phosphorus concentration at 4.0–6.0 mg/dl

Vitamin D therapy should not be initiated when serum calcium or phosphorus levels are greater than 10.5 and 6 mg/dl, respectively, because of the possibility of inducing metastatic calcification or renal dysfunction. If the serum phosphorus level is elevated, as is common in patients whose GFR is below 30 ml/minute, it is necessary to first reduce the level of phosphorus to normal before starting vitamin D therapy (see below).

The serum phosphorus concentration may rise following institution of vitamin D therapy because both calcium and phosphorus absorption are increased. If dietary phosphate restriction (600 to 900 mg/day) is not sufficient to maintain serum phosphorus levels within the normal range, phosphate binders must be used (see below).

The form of *vitamin D* used is important since preparations (e.g., vitamin D_2 or D_3) that require final activation by the kidney have proven to be ineffective in the usual doses. The most commonly used vitamin D preparations that do not require renal activation are 1, 25-dihydroxyvitamin D_3 (Rocaltrol) and dihydrotachysterol (DHT). When given orally both Rocaltrol (0.25 to 1.0 μ/day) and DHT (0.125 to 0.5 mg/day) are effective in improving calcium absorption and raising serum calcium levels in azotemic patients. Studies comparing the effectiveness of DHT and Rocaltrol have not been performed, although the latter, because it is the native hormone, has possible advantages. Both can produce hypercalcemia, but due to its shorter half-life the hypercalcemia induced by 1, 25-dihydroxyvitamin D_3 tends to be of shorter duration.

Restriction of dietary phosphorus to 600 to 900 mg/day (normal intake is 1 to 1.8 g/day) should be initiated when the serum phosphorus level first becomes elevated. This degree of phosphorus restriction can be achieved by restricting the intake of protein to 50 g/day (foods such as eggs, meat, and fish contain 15 mg of phosphorus/g of protein) and dairy products (20 to 30 mg/g). Despite restriction of phosphorus intake, the serum phosphorus level often becomes elevated when the GFR falls below 30 ml/minute. At this juncture it is necessary to start treatment with phosphate binders. Calcium carbonate and oral antacids containing aluminum hydroxide (Alternajel or Amphojel) or aluminum carbonate (Basaljel) bind phosphate in the intestine and thereby reduce phosphate absorption. These binders are available in liquid, tablet, and capsule forms. Liquids are the most effective but the least well tolerated preparation (they may produce nausea, bloating, and/or constipation). Stool softeners may be used to counter the constipation, but occasionally osmotic laxatives such as lactulose or sorbitol may be required (see Chapter 39). Other medications (Table 48.9) should not be given simultaneously with phosphate binders since their absorption may be increased or decreased. The initial dose of antacid should be 1 or 2 tablespoons or tablets/capsules given with meals; the dose should be increased (at 2-week intervals) until the serum phosphorus concentration is reduced to between 4 and 6 mg/dl. Serum phosphorus concen-

Table 48.9.
Drugs Whose Bioavailability Is Altered by Phosphate Binders

DECREASED
Digoxin
Oral anticoagulants
Tetracycline
Anticholinergics
Aspirin
Chlorpromazine
INCREASED
Penicillin
Pseudoephedrine

tration should be monitored every 1 to 2 months to avoid the syndrome of phosphate depletion (low serum phosphorus), which may result in muscle weakness, osteomalacia, and fractures.

Aluminum-containing antacids should also be used for the treatment of gastritis or ulcers since magnesium toxicity can occur in patients with chronic renal failure who regularly take magnesium-containing antacids, such as Maalox or Mylanta (see also Chapter 37). However, it has been demonstrated that aluminum from the antacids is absorbed and can accumulate in the brain and bones of patients with renal failure. This aluminum accumulation has been implicated in the pathogenesis of the *dialysis dementia syndrome* (myoclonus, seizures, and dementia), anemia (see Chapter 50), and a particular form of osteomalacia that develops in some patients with end-stage renal failure. Therefore, many nephrologists now recommend that calcium carbonate be used as the initial agent for binding phosphorus, with the addition of aluminum-containing compounds only in refractory cases of hyperphosphatemia.

Acidosis

A mild hyperchloremic (normal anion gap) metabolic acidosis develops commonly in patients with early renal insufficiency (Fig. 48.7). This occurs because production of ammonia by the failing kidney results in the retention of hydrogen and chloride ions. However, the acidosis in moderate renal insufficiency is generally not severe enough (serum bicarbonate > 18 mEq/liter) to warrant therapy. It should be realized that the hypochloremic (with an abnormal anion gap) acidosis commonly associated with renal failure does not generally appear until the GFR has fallen below 20 ml/minute.

A patient whose level of serum bicarbonate has fallen below 18 mEq/liter has a seriously reduced buffer reserve and runs the risk of severe acidosis during periods of stress (e.g., from infection or volume depletion). If protein restriction (see above, page 530), which reduces exogenous acid load, is insufficient to restore buffering capacity, base in the form of sodium bicarbonate, 600 mg four times a day, may be given, provided edema is not a problem. Should sodium bicarbonate not be tolerated because of gastrointestinal complaints (belching and bloatedness), sodium

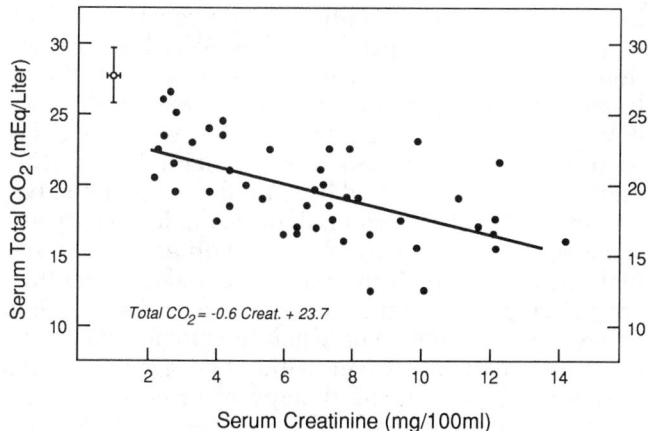

Figure 48.7. Relationship between the serum bicarbonate and serum creatinine concentrations in patients with chronic renal insufficiency. (From Widmer B, et al: Serum electrolyte and acid-base composition. The influence of graded degrees of chronic renal failure. *Arch Int Med* 139:1099, 1979.)

citrate liquid (1 ml liquid = 1 mEq bicarbonate) can be substituted. An attempt should be made to maintain the serum bicarbonate level above 18 mEq/liter.

Anemia

A normochromic, normocytic anemia develops in patients with chronic renal failure, and its severity is proportional to the degree of renal insufficiency (Fig. 48.2). The hematocrit value will generally fall to between 15 and 25% in a patient with advanced renal failure. The anemia of renal failure results mainly from shortened red blood cell survival and an inability of the bone marrow to compensate because of decreased erythropoietin production and/or effect. Other causes of anemia (e.g., iron deficiency) must also be considered.

All patients should be placed on a multivitamin regimen that includes folate, to replace the vitamins lacking in the restrictive diets. Blood transfusion, when necessary, should not be withheld for fear of sensitizing a potential transplant recipient. Patients who have received multiple blood transfusions have higher rates of retention of functioning transplanted kidneys than do those who have not received transfusions. Iron deficiency is almost universal in patients on hemodialysis but may also occur in the predialysis patient, particularly if multiple blood samples have been taken or if there is bleeding. Iron deficiency is best diagnosed in patients with chronic renal failure by measuring the level of serum ferritin. The serum iron and iron-binding capacity are often low in patients with renal failure and are not reliable in establishing the state of iron stores. The values of serum ferritin that are associated with normal iron stores are higher in patients with renal failure than they are in those without kidney disease. Therefore, the laboratory should be consulted in order to interpret serum ferritin levels properly in the uremic individual. The treatment of iron defi-

ciency is the same in azotemic patients as it is in any other patient (see Chapter 50).

Early trials using human erythropoietin (50 to 150 U/kg intravenously three times a week), produced by recombinant DNA techniques, have shown promising results with normalization of serum hemoglobin levels and improvement in the quality of life (9). Although blood pressure control becomes more difficult for some patients, there is no evidence that the progression of renal failure is accelerated. The cost of human erythropoietin is quite high, but at least for dialysis patients Medicare will pay. It is likely that most patients with renal insufficiency whose hematocrit values fall below 30% will be treated with erythropoietin.

DRUG USE IN RENAL FAILURE

The incidence of adverse drug effects is increased in patients with renal failure, a fact that is largely attributable to the alterations in pharmacokinetics that occur as renal function declines. Adverse drug effects, in this group of patients, can be divided into those that are due to abnormal drug metabolism (e.g., increased incidence of digitalis toxicity) and those that are due to an effect on renal function that is part of the anticipated pharmacological action of the drug (e.g., reduction in GFR with thiazides or nonsteroidal anti-inflammatory drugs) (4). In renal failure, drug bioavailability, volume of distribution, and protein binding may be abnormal; however, the most significant derangement is the prolongation of half-life of many drugs or their metabolites. Therefore, it is necessary to have a basic understanding of how a drug's administration should be modified when renal failure is present. This information is available from several sources (1, 3).

Because even over-the-counter preparations (aspirin, ibuprofen, magnesium-containing antacids) have the potential for causing toxicity, patients should be reminded to telephone their physician before using nonprescription drugs. Whenever possible, drugs that require no modification of dosage or that do not affect kidney function adversely should be substituted for those with a greater potential for inducing toxicity. The avoidance of drugs with marginal efficacy will help to reduce the frequency of adverse effects.

A complete review of the topic of drug usage in renal failure may be found elsewhere (1). Guidelines are provided below for the drugs most commonly prescribed in ambulatory practice (see Tables 48.10 and 48.11).

Before initiating therapy with a drug that requires dose modification in renal failure, it is necessary to have an accurate estimation of GFR. Predicting the GFR from the serum creatinine level alone is not recommended; rather one should either measure the creatinine clearance directly or use one of the formulas for estimating GFR (see page 522).

Depending on what modifications are required for a particular drug, an appropriate loading and maintenance dose can be chosen. A loading dose must be

Table 48.10.
**Some Commonly Used Drugs That Require Dosage
Reduction in Renal Failure (GFR < 30 ml/minute)**

Cardiovascular drugs
  Digoxin (Lanoxin)
  Nadolol (Corgard)
  Atenolol (Tenormin)
  Procainamide (Pronestyl)
  Disopyramide (Norpace)
Antihypertensive drugs
  Captopril (Capoten)
  Clonidine (Catapres)
  Guanethidine (Ismelin)
H_2 receptor antagonists
  Cimetidine (Tagamet)
  Ranitidine (Zantac)
Hypoglycemic drugs
  Insulin
Drugs used in the treatment of gout
  Allopurinol (Zyloprim)

Table 48.11.
**Some Commonly Used Drugs That Should Be Avoided
in Patients with Renal Failure (GFR < 30 ml/minute)**

Antimicrobials
  Cephaloridine (Loridine)
  Tetracyclines
  Nitrofurantoin (Macrodantin)
  Nalidixic acid (Negram)
Analgesics
  Aspirin
  Nonsteroidal antiinflammatory agents (Motrin, Nalfon, *etc*)
  Meperidine (Demerol)
Diuretics
  Potassium-sparing diuretics (Aldactone, Moduretic, Dyrenium)
  Ethacrynic acid (Edecrin)
  Thiazides (Diuril, *etc*)
Antacids
  Magnesium-containing antacids (Maalox, Mylanta, *etc*)
Hypoglycemic drugs
  Acetohexamide (Dymelor)
  Chlorpropamide (Diabinase)
Drugs used in the treatment of gout
  Phenylbutazone (Butazolidine)
  Sulfinpyrazone (Anturane)
  Probenecid (Benemid)

given whenever rapid achievement of therapeutic drug levels is desired. Maintenance doses are adjusted either by lengthening the interval between administrations or by reducing the size of each dose. The use of nomograms or tables does not guarantee that adverse drug effects will not occur. The monitoring of serum drug levels is therefore often helpful, particularly when using drugs with low toxic/therapeutic ratios. Finally, the list of drugs should be reviewed periodically and the patient questioned specifically about side effects.

Antimicrobials

When renal impairment is not advanced (GFR > 30 ml/minute), no change is necessary for most of the commonly used antimicrobials in the dosages employed in ambulatory practice (e.g., penicillins, cephalosporins, erythromycin, metronidazole, chloramphenicol). The administration of tetracyclines,

however, with the exception of doxycycline, is not recommended in the patient with impaired renal function as these drugs tend to aggravate uremia. When treating urinary tract infections in patients with GFRs below 50 ml/minute the urinary antiseptic drugs, such as nitrofurantoin (Macrodantin) or naladixic acid (Negram), should not be used because they are ineffective and there is an increased risk of systemic toxicity associated with the retention of metabolites. Antimicrobials such as ampicillin and the cephalosporins that are secreted by the renal tubular cells achieve a high urine concentration, even when the glomerular filtration rate is very low. Given without dosage reduction, they are effective in the therapy of urinary tract infections in patients with advanced renal failure. Trimethoprim-sulfamethoxazole in usual doses is also effective in patients with impaired renal function.

Analgesics

The dosages of acetaminophen, codeine, oxycodone (Tylox) and pentazocine (Talwin) require no dosage modification in renal failure. Further, none of these drugs adversely affects kidney function in patients with chronic renal insufficiency. There is some epidemiological evidence that the regular, heavy use of acetaminophen is associated with an increased risk of developing renal damage. The use of meperidine (Demerol) for more than two to three doses is hazardous due to the accumulation of its metabolites, which may induce seizures.

The use of NSAIDs, including aspirin, is generally not recommended in patients with renal insufficiency since they predictably result in a 25 to 50% decrease in glomerular filtration rate (7). The effects of NSAIDs on GFR are due to changes in renal blood flow consequent to inhibition of renal prostaglandin synthesis and appear greatest in patients who have diminished effective circulatory volume (patient on diuretics or with CHF). The reduction in GFR is generally reversible, once the NSAID is discontinued, but the return to baseline may take up to 1 month. It is not clear whether the reduction in GFR associated with NSAIDs results in any permanent harm to the kidney.

There are several possible approaches to the patient with renal insufficiency for whom it is believed important to use a NSAID. Sulindac (Clinoril) appears not to affect renal prostaglandin synthesis to the same extent as the other NSAIDs and at least in one study did not appear to have any adverse effects on GFR in a group of patients with mild renal insufficiency. The nonacetylated salicylates are only weak inhibitors of prostaglandin synthesis and theoretically should not affect renal function. Currently, however, there are no data on the safety of nonacetylated salicylates in patients with renal insufficiency. In any event, when NSAIDs are given to patients with renal failure it is necessary to monitor kidney function carefully, and it is probably prudent to discontinue their use if more than a minimal change in renal function is seen.

Patients with renal insufficiency are predisposed to

developing salt retention, hyponatremia, and hyperkalemia when given NSAIDs. The latter is more common when NSAIDs are given in conjunction with potassium-sparing diuretics or ACE inhibitors. Finally, there have been numerous case reports of patients with previously normal renal function developing acute renal failure with nephrotic syndrome, as an idiosyncratic reaction, after having been given NSAIDs. When biopsied, these patients generally are found to have an interstitial form of nephritis.

Sedatives, Hypnotics, and Tranquilizers

In the patient with renal failure, no alteration in dosage is necessary for the benzodiazepines (e.g., Valium, Librium, Dalmane), short-acting barbiturates (e.g., Seconol, Nembutal), neuroleptics (e.g., Haldol), phenothiazines (e.g., Thorazine), and tricyclic antidepressants (e.g., Elavil), since all are chiefly metabolized by the liver. However, the phenothiazines and tricyclics must be used with caution since they have significant anticholinergic properties and, accordingly, may cause urinary retention. All of the psychoactive drugs are capable of causing excessive sedation in patients with advanced renal failure. Lithium, which is renally excreted, should be used with great caution once the GFR falls below 50 ml/minute. Levels must be monitored frequently (for details see Chapter 15).

Antacids and H₂ Receptor Antagonists (See Also Chapter 37)

Many of the commonly prescribed or over-the-counter antacids contain magnesium compounds as a major constituent, and magnesium absorption with toxicity may occur when the GFR falls below 30 ml/minute. Therefore, the patient should be instructed to use antacids that are based on aluminum (as opposed to magnesium). Because there is concern that, with prolonged ingestion, significant amounts of aluminum will be absorbed and accumulate in the tissues of patients with renal failure, they should only be prescribed for periods less than 1 month. Sucrafate, although containing aluminum, may be used since the compound is minimally absorbed compared with other aluminum-containing compounds.

The dosage of the H₂ receptor antagonists, cimetidine and ranitidine, must be reduced to 75% and then 50% as the creatinine clearance falls below 50 and 30 ml/minute, respectively. Both can cause an increase in serum creatinine levels, probably due to inhibition of the tubular secretion of creatinine.

Cardiovascular Drugs (See Also Chapters 59 and 61)

Both the loading and maintenance doses of digoxin must be reduced once the GFR falls below 50 ml/minute (12). The loading dose of digoxin should be reduced by 75% and the maintenance dose by 50% once the GFR falls below 50 ml/minute. Despite the use of nomograms and the monitoring of drug levels, digoxin

toxicity remains a problem in the uremic patient. Therefore, whenever feasible, other treatments for heart failure should be tried before resorting to digoxin.

There are now available to the physician a large variety of beta-blocking agents, each with slightly different pharmacological or pharmacokinetic properties. The most important consideration in patients with renal failure is the route of excretion. The dosages of propranolol (Inderal), metoprolol (Lopressor), labetalol (Normodyne), and penbutalol (Levetol), which are all metabolized by the liver, are unchanged even in advanced renal failure. Atenolol (Tenormin), nadolol (Corgard), pindolol (Visken), carteolol (Cartrol), timolol (Blockadren), and the metabolites of acebutolol (Sectral) are excreted largely by the kidney and require dosage reduction. All beta-blocking agents should be used with caution in patients with impaired renal function as they reduce cardiac output and may thereby aggravate azotemia.

The dosage interval should be increased by 2- to 4-fold to avoid toxicity when giving procainamide (Pronestyl) and disopyramide (Norpace) in patients with renal failure. Monitoring blood levels of the drug, and in the case of procainamide, its active metabolite (N-acetylprocainamide), is important in guiding therapy. Once the GFR falls below 10 ml/minute the dosages of flecainide and tocainide should be halved. Quinidine and encainide do not require dosage modification, even in advanced renal failure.

The use of antihypertensive drugs in patients with renal failure is discussed in Chapter 62.

Hypoglycemic Agents (See Also Chapter 80)

The half-life of insulin is prolonged in renal failure, and therefore attention to dosage is required in the diabetic with developing renal insufficiency in order to avoid hypoglycemia. The oral hypoglycemic agents acetohexamide and chlorpropamide have active metabolites that accumulate in renal failure and may produce prolonged hypoglycemia. Therefore, non-insulin-dependent diabetic patients taking oral hypoglycemic agents should be converted to tolbutamide (Orinase), glipizide (Glucotrol), or glyburide (Micronase, Diabeta) once the GFR falls below 50 ml/minute.

Anticonvulsants

The dose of phenytoin (Dilantin) is essentially unchanged in renal failure since an increased volume of distribution and a shortened half-life are offset by reduced protein binding. Because the unbound fraction of phenytoin is increased, the therapeutic and toxic effects of Dilantin occur at lower measured total serum levels in patients with renal failure than they do in patients without kidney disease (Fig. 48.8).

Drugs Used in the Treatment of Gout

Colchicine may be used for the prophylactic treatment of symptomatic gout in usual dosages (0.6 to 1.2 mg/day). The incidence of colchicine myopathy ap-

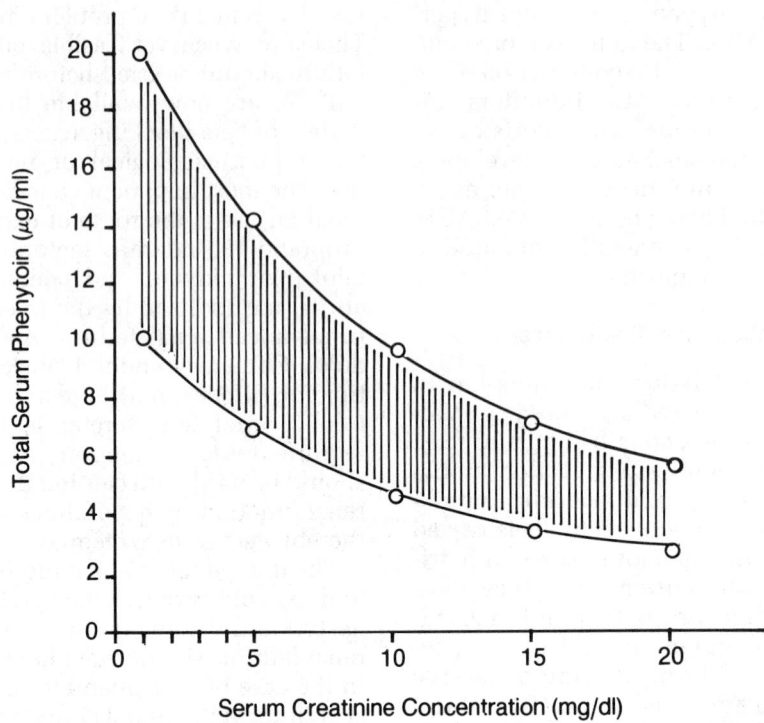

Figure 48.8. Range of total serum phenytoin concentrations in patients with varying degrees of renal failure that provide therapeutic levels of free drug. (Redrawn from Reidenberg NM, Affrime M: Influence of disease on binding of drugs to plasma proteins. *Ann NY Acad Sci* 226:115, 1973.)

pears to be increased in patients with kidney impairment, and when prescribed the patient should be monitored closely for this complication by measuring creatinine phosphokinase concentration and muscle strength. The dose of allopurinol must be reduced to 200 mg/day in patients with GFRs below 50 ml/minute and to 100 mg/day when the GFR is below 30 ml/minute. The uricosuric agents probenecid (Benemid) and sulfinpyrazone (Anturane) are ineffective when the GFR falls below 50 ml/minute and should therefore not be used. Phenylbutazone (Butazolidin) should not be used in patients whose GFRs are below 50 ml/minute since it can cause sodium retention and also because many of its active metabolites depend on renal excretion. Indomethacin (Indocin) is almost entirely metabolized by the liver, and therefore it does not accumulate in patients with even advanced renal failure. However, patients who receive indomethacin for the treatment of acute gout must have their BUN and serum creatinine concentrations monitored carefully, as indomethacin can cause a transient worsening of renal function.

CHRONIC RENAL FAILURE AND COEXISTING DISORDERS

Nonrenal diseases often occur in patients with uremia. In some, such as patients with systemic lupus erythematosus or diabetes mellitus, the renal disease is part of a generalized illness that affects many other organ systems. Others may have diseases unrelated to the kidneys, such as coronary artery disease, chronic obstructive pulmonary disease, or malignancy. The coexistence of multiple disorders often complicates management. For example, angina in patients with coronary artery disease may be aggravated by the anemia of chronic renal failure.

Diabetes Mellitus

Up to 50% of insulin-dependent diabetics and a substantial portion of non-insulin-dependent diabetics develop chronic renal failure, and patients with diabetes account for up to 30% of many dialysis populations with the majority being type II. The mechanism whereby diabetes affects the kidney is predominantly through a microvasculopathy-producing nodular glomerulosclerosis. In humans a relationship between poor glucose control and the development and progression of renal disease is suspected but has not been unequivocally established (Chapter 72). It has been suggested that the increased GFR and renal blood flow seen during the early stages of diabetic nephropathy may have pathophysiological significance (Fig. 48.5). This state of renal hyperperfusion, in part, can be reversed with strict glucose control. Control of systemic hypertension in the later stages of diabetic nephropathy has also been shown to reduce the rate of renal deterioration. The onset of renal disease (in type I diabetes) usually develops after 10 to 15 years of diabetes and is initially manifest by proteinuria. Renal insufficiency soon follows, and there is usually a rapid decline in kidney function leading to end-stage renal failure within another 1 to 2 years. The natural history for patients with type II diabetes has not been as well defined.

Renal disease may reduce the requirement for insulin, an effect related at least in part to decreased hormone degradation in the renal tubules as nephrons are progressively lost. Some oral hypoglycemic agents, notably chlorpropamide and acetohexamide, also have prolonged half-lives in uremic patients. As a consequence of these pharmacological abnormalities, the first overt manifestation of renal disease in some diabetics is the occurrence of hypoglycemia. Therefore, the dose of insulin or oral hypoglycemic drugs should be regularly assessed in the patient with renal impairment.

Diabetes, per se, is not a contraindication to performing dialysis or transplantation, although the course of diabetics is more complicated than that of patients with isolated renal failure. The form of therapy best suited for these patients with end-stage renal failure is uncertain. Hemodialysis, peritoneal dialysis, and transplantation each have proponents. The diabetic patient should be reminded that dialysis and transplantation are supportive therapies for renal dysfunction and will not improve their diabetes. The referring physician should also remember that the course of these patients is less favorable than that of patients with kidney disease without diabetes (see below, "Dialysis and Transplantation"). The microvasculopathy that destroys the kidney also affects the retinal and peripheral vessels. Because blindness and peripheral vascular disease are important causes of morbidity and mortality in the dialysis and transplant population, it is critical for these patients to have appropriate attention to eye (see Chapter 72) and foot (see Chapter 102) (10).

Heart Disease

Patients with congestive heart failure and/or angina often require more frequent monitoring as renal function declines. Diuretics may lose their effectiveness, or as anemia worsens patients with ischemic heart disease may become more symptomatic. In this situation transfusions are necessary if there has been an inadequate response to antianginal therapy, although erythropoietin may be useful in improving the anemia.

Patients with renal failure have been noted to have an accelerated rate of atherogenesis. This may be explained by the presence of hypertension, glucose intolerance, hypertriglyceridemia, and reduced levels of high density lipoproteins in this group of patients.

AIDS (See Also Chapter 34)

A chronic, progressive nephropathy characterized by proteinuria and renal failure can be seen in patients with AIDS. Most of these patients have a history of intravenous drug abuse, but AIDS nephropathy has

also been found in homosexuals and in children. The prognosis of these patients is grim and many die of infections, complications, or inanition before they reach the point of needing dialysis. Similarly only a small percentage of the patients who start on a dialysis program live more than 6 months (20). The experience is somewhat better for patients who are HIV positive but have unrelated renal failure. However, once clinical AIDS develops, life expectancy is measured in months. Given the grim prognosis for AIDS patients with chronic renal failure, some have questioned the advisability of initiating dialysis therapy.

Malignancy

Renal failure as a result of hypercalcemia, sepsis, or drug nephrotoxicity is not an uncommon occurrence in patients dying with a malignancy. In many of these patients it would be inappropriate to prolong their lives by initiating dialysis. However, patients with multiple myeloma or other neoplasms that may have a relatively long survival might benefit from dialysis. Dialyzing patients with neoplastic diseases should be recommended, therefore, only after careful discussion with the patient, his family, an oncologist, and a nephrologist.

SYMPTOMATIC THERAPY OF ADVANCED RENAL INSUFFICIENCY

Patients with advanced renal failure (GFR < 10 ml/minute) invariably develop a variety of uremic symptoms. Gastrointestinal disturbances, such as nausea, anorexia, and vomiting, are frequent. Treatment involves further restriction of protein (see above), and/or antiemetics (e.g., Compazine). Itching is often a bothersome problem of unknown etiology. Reduction of serum phosphorus to normal levels, skin lubricants (see Chapter 100), and antihistamines (e.g., Benadryl, 25 to 50 mg four times/day) are all worth 1- to 3-week trial periods. Ultraviolet light therapy may also be helpful, but this requires consultation with a dermatologist performing this form of therapy. Fatigue, dyspnea, and chest pain may be due to worsening anemia or volume overload and should respond to blood transfusions or diuretics. Neuromuscular symptoms, such as myoclonus, restless legs, and disturbed sleep, are signs of advanced uremia and should serve as warnings that more severe abnormalities (e.g., seizures, coma) may soon develop. The persistence of these symptoms despite the best conservative medical management is an indication for dialysis regardless of the BUN or serum creatinine concentration. Although there are no absolute laboratory criteria defining the time at which dialysis should be initiated, a serum creatinine concentration of greater than 10 to 12 mg/dl or a creatinine clearance of less than 5 ml/minute is commonly accepted as an indication. Many nephrologists believe that diabetics develop uremic symptoms at lower levels of BUN and creatinine concentrations than do nondiabetics. Delay in starting dialysis can lead to patients developing severe peripheral neuropathy, malnutrition, and/or pericarditis from which complete recovery might not be possible.

DIALYSIS AND TRANSPLANTATION

In 1989 over 90,000 patients were being maintained on dialysis in the United States. Most facilities provide hemodialysis, peritoneal dialysis, and transplantation (or referral to a transplant center) for patients with end-stage renal failure (Table 48.12). Either form of dialysis therapy can be performed at a center or at the patient's home. Some patients will choose dialysis as a permanent form of treatment, whereas others will undergo dialysis temporarily until they receive a kidney transplant. Although dialysis does not correct all of the metabolic abnormalities of chronic renal failure, it has enabled thousands of patients to lead productive lives.

Hemodialysis

The hemodialysis procedure involves circulating the patient's blood through a machine that corrects electrolyte abnormalities and has the capability of removing excess fluid and toxic metabolic wastes. In the case of slowly progressive renal failure, provisions for dialysis should be made months in advance of need. The goal of dialysis therapy is to maintain health at a level consistent with a relatively normal life-style. Therefore, it is not advisable to wait for signs and symptoms of far advanced uremia (e.g., pericarditis, seizures, coma, or bleeding) to appear before initiating dialysis. The patient should be referred to a nephrologist associated with a dialysis center when the creatinine clearance approaches 20 ml/minute. In this way the patient may be familiarized with the various forms of therapy offered at that facility and become acquainted with the staff.

Before actually starting dialysis, it is necessary to provide some kind of vascular access to allow for the repeated venipunctures required for this form of therapy. The preferred access is the arteriovenous fistula, which is usually created at the wrist of the nondominant arm. The creation of a fistula can be performed, in most instances, under local anesthesia and often in an outpatient surgical unit. Because there is often a 1- to 2-month maturation period necessary before the fistula can be used, arrangements for the creation of the

Table 48.12.
Treatments for End-Stage Renal Failure

Hemodialysis
  Home
  Hospital based
  Satellite or self-care (*e.g.*, those not situated in a hospital)
Peritoneal dialysis
  Continuous ambulatory peritoneal dialysis (CAPD)
  Intermittent peritoneal dialysis (PD)
Renal transplantation
  Living donor transplant
  Cadaveric transplant

fistula should be made early, and always before the GFR falls to less than 10 to 15 ml/minute. If the patient's vessels are inadequate to support the creation of an arteriovenous fistula, an alternative would be to insert a synthetic (Dacron, Gortex) graft under the skin of the forearm. The synthetic graft can generally be used within 3 weeks of placement. The most common complications after placement of a fistula or graft are clotting and infection.

Hemodialysis is performed in most centers three times/week, and each session lasts about 3 to 4 hours. Except for needle insertion, the procedure, per se, is not painful; but some patients do experience muscle cramps, headaches, nausea, or syncope during or just after dialysis. Hospital-based dialysis should be reserved for those patients who require intensive monitoring. Home dialysis is encouraged for those patients with good home situations who have willing and able partners. Home dialysis patients have the advantage of more flexible schedules and a greater sense of control than do hospital-based patients and, therefore, have the greatest chance of maintaining their previous life style. The remainder of the patients can be treated at outpatient dialysis centers.

As a group, hemodialysis patients have an 80% survival rate for the first year, and at 5 years the survival rate falls to about 55%. The development of the long-term complications of chronic renal failure, including progressive neuropathy, osteodystrophy, cardiovascular disease, and an array of endocrine disturbances, reflects the fact that dialysis does not correct all of the metabolic disturbances of uremia.

Peritoneal Dialysis

Peritoneal dialysis procedures involve the instillation of dialysis fluid through a catheter into the abdominal cavity. Fluid and toxic solutes are transferred across the mesenteric capillary bed into the dialysis fluid, which is then removed through the catheter. Recent improvements in the techniques of peritoneal dialysis have increased its popularity among patients. In the past peritoneal dialysis required 12- to 16-hour periods of being connected to an automatic cycling machine, two to three times/week (*intermittent peritoneal dialysis*, IPD). Even then, its simplicity and freedom from hemodynamic complications made this form of therapy attractive, particularly to the elderly or to those with heart disease. Currently, *continuous ambulatory peritoneal dialysis* (CAPD) has nearly replaced the older machine-based therapy. In this technique the patient constantly carries 2 liters of dialysis solution in his abdomen (13). The fluid is exchanged four times a day, every day. However, because fluid movement is determined by gravity, and no machine is necessary, the patient is able to perform dialysis at home, at work, or virtually anywhere. This degree of freedom is one of the most attractive aspects of CAPD. Its other attributes, at least theoretically, are the greater removal of larger molecular weight substances than that provided by hemodialysis, and the continuous nature of the dialysis that eliminates the large swings in the concentration of electrolytes, creatinine, etc. that occur with the more intermittent forms of therapy. Also the abdominal catheter for CAPD can be placed at the time of the first dialysis and does not require a maturation period. The major difficulty associated with peritoneal dialysis is the development of peritonitis. The incidence in the typical patient is about one infection every 9 to 12 months, but these infections generally respond to antimicrobials and continued peritoneal dialysis; often treatment of peritonitis does not require hospitalization. However, the peritoneal dialysis catheter may need periodic replacement.

Comparative survival statistics between hemodialysis and peritoneal dialysis are difficult to interpret due to significant population selection biases. Whether hemodialysis or peritoneal dialysis is used depends on the center to which the patient is referred and on patient preference. At most dialysis facilities the patient will have a choice and may change dialysis modes if the outcome of one is unsatisfactory.

Renal Transplantation

Of all available therapies, a successful renal transplant provides for the most complete correction of the uremic syndrome. Unfortunately, many transplanted kidneys are lost because of immunological rejection. Innovations in antirejection therapy, such as the use of the potent immunosuppressant drug, cyclosporine, or of monoclonal antibodies, has improved the rate of graft survival.

The success of renal transplantation depends greatly on the antigenic similarity between donor and recipient. Except in the cases of identical twins (in which rejection does not occur) the best results are found in living related donor, HLA antigen identical, sibling transplants (Fig. 48.9). In this instance, kidney survival is greater than 90% at 2 years. More commonly performed are two HLA antigen matched, sibling to sibling, or parent to child organ transplants with a success rate of 88% at 1 year and 83% at 2 years. Patient survival for non-HLA identical living related donor transplants is over 90% at both the 1- and 2-year intervals. The majority of patients do not have the potential for living related donors (less than 25% of patients are able to receive living related donor transplants) and must await a cadaveric transplant, which, despite the best tissue typing, has a significantly lower success rate of 72% at 1 year and 61% at 2 years. Patient survival rates for cadaveric transplants are 90% at 1 year and 88% at 2 years. Comparison of survival statistics between cadaveric transplants and dialysis patients is complicated because of selection bias. Transplant patients tend to be younger, have better myocardial function, and have fewer coexisting illnesses than their dialysis counterparts. If these factors are taken into account, then no significant difference in the survival rate can be found between patients receiving cadaveric kidney transplants and those being treated by dialysis.

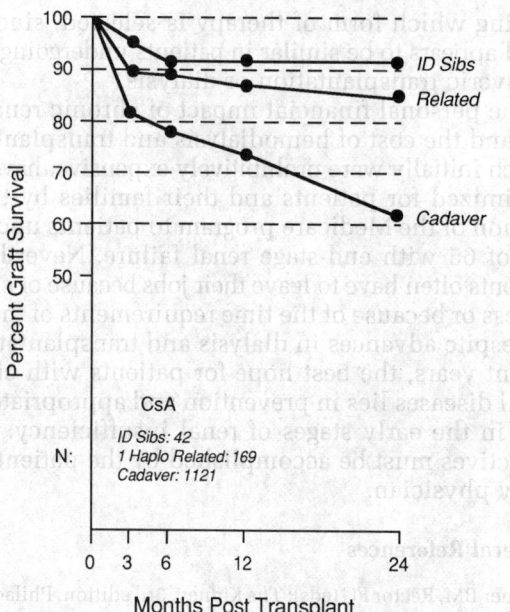

Figure 48.9. Two year kidney graft survival according to donor source in patients treated with cyclosporine. (From Cats S. The effect of cyclosporine-A in kidney transplantation. In *Kidney Transplants 1985*. Terasaki P (ed.) UCLA Tissue Typing Laboratory, Los Angeles, 1985.)

Patients with uncomplicated renal transplants usually require a 10- to 21-day hospitalization. After transplantation (except for those performed between identical twins), the patient requires lifelong immunosuppression, usually with a combination of cyclosporine, prednisone, and azathioprine (Imuran). The patient must understand that there is always the risk of rejection and the possibility of graft failure with a return to dialysis. Although there is no doubt that a successfully functioning transplant restores health better than any other therapy, patients on immunosuppressive therapy have considerable risks—corticosteroid complications, malignancies, or serious infections.

Because the primary physician is most familiar with the patient, he can be of great value in advising which forms of therapy might coincide best with the patient's expectations. Frequently, patients will have a better understanding of their choices if they visit a dialysis or transplant unit and talk with patients or staff. The decision to suggest a renal transplant is most clear-cut in adolescents or young adults who wish to pursue an active, vigorous life, to have a job, and to have intact sexual functions. This is particularly so if a well-matched living donor is available. Elderly patients or those with extensive multisystem disease may not be able to tolerate the rigors of transplantation. For others, a period of dialysis and assessment of the patient's adjustment to this therapy will often help in determining whether to continue dialysis or to consider transplantation. The patient who adjusts well to dialysis can often be fully rehabilitated and can maintain a job as efficiently as the patient with a successful renal transplant. At the present time it appears that quality of life is the most important criterion determining which form of therapy is selected, since survival appears to be similar in patients undergoing either cadaveric transplantation or dialysis.

The personal financial impact of chronic renal failure and the cost of hemodialysis and transplantation, which initially were prohibitively expensive, have been minimized for patients and their families by the extension of the Medicare program to patients under the age of 65 with end-stage renal failure. Nevertheless, patients often have to leave their jobs because of chronic illness or because of the time requirements of therapy.

Despite advances in dialysis and transplantation in recent years, the best hope for patients with chronic renal diseases lies in prevention and appropriate therapy in the early stages of renal insufficiency. These objectives must be accomplished by the patient's primary physician.

General References

Brenner BM, Rector FC (eds): *The Kidney*, 3rd edition. Philadelphia, WB Saunders, 1989.
> General reference for nephrology.

Campbell JD, Campbell AR: The social and economic costs of end-stage renal disease. *N Engl J Med* 299:386, 1978.
> A patient's view of the effects of living with renal failure.

Fine LG: Preventing the progression of human renal disease: have rational therapeutic principles emerged? *Kid Int* 33:116, 1988.
> Critical review of the therapies directed at slowing the course of progressive renal failure.

Jacobson HR: Ischemic renal disease: an overlooked entity? *Kid Int* 34:729, 1988.
> Comprehensive review of atheromatous renovascular disease as a cause of chronic renal failure.

Waltzer WC: Procurement of cadaveric kidneys for transplantation. *Ann Intern Med* 98:536, 1983.
> Discussion of issues related to obtaining kidneys for transplantation.

Specific References

1. Anderson RJ, Schrier RW (eds): *Clinical Use of Drugs in Patients with Kidney and Liver Disease*. Philadelphia, WB Saunders, 1981.
2. Baker LRI, Louise Abrams SM, Roe C, et al: 1, 25(OH)$_2$ D$_3$ administration in moderate renal failure: a prospective double blind trial. *Kid Int* 35:661, 1989.
3. American College of Physicians: *Drug prescribing in renal failure. Dosing guidelines for adults*. Philadelphia, 1987.
4. Bennett WM, Plamp C, Porter GA: Drug related syndromes in clinical nephrology. *Ann Intern Med* 87:582, 1977.
5. Bergstrom J: Discovery and rediscovery of low protein diets. *Clin Nephrol* 21:29, 1984.
6. Brenner BM, Meyer TW, Hostetter TH: Dietary protein intake and the progressive nature of kidney disease: the role of hemodynamically mediated glomerular injury in the pathogenesis of progressive glomerular sclerosis, aging, renal ablation, and intrinsic renal disease. *N Engl J Med* 307:652, 1982.
7. Clive DM, Stoff JS: Renal syndromes associated with nonsteroidal antiinflammatory drugs. *N Engl J Med* 310:563, 1984.
8. Eggers PW, Connerton R, McMullan M: *The Medicare experience with end stage renal disease: trends in incidence, prevalence, and survival*. Working Paper Series, Department of Health and Human Services, Health Care Financing Administration, Office of Research and Demonstrations, May, 1983.
9. Eschbach JW, Egrie JC, Dowing MR, et al: Correction of the anemia of end-stage renal disease with recombinant human erythropoietin. Results of a combined phase I and II clinical trial. *N Engl J Med* 316:73, 1987.
10. Friedman EA, L'Esperance JR (eds): Clinical management of

diabetes mellitus. In: *The Diabetic-Renal-Retinal Syndrome*. New York, Grune and Stratton, 1980.
11. Geyskes GG, Dei HY, Puylaert CB, et al: Renovascular hypertension identified by captopril-induced changes in the renogram. *Hypertension* 9:451, 1987.
12. Jelliffe RW, Brooker G: A nonogram for digoxin therapy. *Am J Med* 57:63, 1974.
13. Levey AS, Harrington JT: Continuous peritoneal dialysis for chronic renal failure. *Medicine* (Baltimore)61:330, 1982.
14. Maschio G, Oldrizzi L, Tessitore N, et al: Effects of dietary protein and phosphorus restriction on the progression of early failure. *Kidney Int* 22:371, 1982.
15. Meyrier A, Buchet P, Simon P, et al: Atheromatous renal disease. *Am J Med* 85:139, 1988.
16. Mitch WM, Walser M, Steinman TI, et al: Effect of a keto acid-amino acid supplement to a restricted diet on the progression of chronic renal failure. *N Engl J Med* 311:623, 1984.
17. Mogenson CE: Long-term antihypertensive treatment inhibiting progression of diabetic nephropathy. *Br Med J* 285:695, 1982.
18. Parfrey PS, Griffitch SM, Steinman TI, et al: Contrast material-induced renal failure in patients with diabetes mellitus, renal insufficiency or both. A prospective controlled study. *N Engl J Med* 320:1, 1989.
19. Phelps KR, Lieberman RL, Oh MS, Carroll HJ: Pathophysiology of the syndrome of hyporeninemic hypoaldosteronism. *Metabolism* 29:186, 1980.
20. Rao TKS, Friedman EA, Nicastri AD: The types of renal disease in the acquired immunodeficiency syndrome. *N Engl J Med* 316:1062, 1987.
21. Rowe JW, Andres R, Tobin JD: et al: Age-adjusted standards for creatinine clearance. *Ann Intern Med* 84:567, 1976.
22. Yu T, Berger L, Dorph DJ, Smith H: Renal function in gout. Factors influencing the renal hemodynamics. *Am J Med* 67:766, 1979.

C H A P T E R   49

Bladder Outlet Obstruction*

RAY E. STUTZMAN, M.D.

The bladder, bladder outlet, prostate, and urethra may be affected by a wide variety of conditions that result in symptoms of urinary obstruction or bladder irritability. These disorders are common, especially in older men.

---

*Dr. James Smolev contributed to this chapter in the first and second editions of this book.

Benign prostatic hyperplasia (BPH) is the most common cause of bladder outlet obstruction in men over 50 years of age. Autopsy studies have shown that 50 to 60% of men over 50 have significant enlargement of the prostate due to BPH and the prevalence increases with age. A number of other conditions may also cause symptoms of bladder outlet obstruction in the male: urethral stricture, carcinoma of the prostate, neurogenic bladder, bladder calculus, prostatitis, bladder neck contracture, and carcinoma of the bladder. Functional obstruction, seen in both women and men, may result from chronic bladder distention, debilitating disease, psychogenic retention, or medications.

HISTORY

Bladder outlet obstruction is characterized by symptoms of urinary hesitancy, diminished force and caliber of the stream, and postvoid dribbling. The symptoms of urinary frequency, urgency, and nocturia result from a diminished functional bladder capacity, bladder muscle hypertrophy, and often bladder instability. The hypertrophy results in increased intravesical pressure during voiding, thereby providing compensation for the obstruction. In time, however, the bladder will decompensate, and this may lead to residual urine, infection, hematuria, hydronephrosis, and renal failure.

Patients with urethral stricture usually have a history of prior urethral trauma, instrumentation (most commonly, indwelling Foley catheter), or urethritis and, in association with symptoms of bladder outlet obstruction, may notice a split stream. Carcinoma of the prostate may present with obstructive symptoms that are often of a shorter duration than those seen in patients with BPH, in whom symptoms of outlet obstruction usually progress over several years. Recent onset of back or bone pain, anorexia, or weight loss suggests malignancy. *Neurogenic bladder* should be suspected when other symptoms of neurological disease are present, when disorders of bowel or sexual function coexist with bladder outlet obstruction, or when a systemic disease that causes neurological bladder dysfunction (such as diabetes mellitus) exists.

A review of current and recently used medications (Table 49.1) is mandatory in the evaluation of the patient with symptoms of bladder outlet obstruction (16). Anticholinergic agents, antispasmodic and antiparkinsonian drugs, as well as many antidepressant drugs depress bladder muscle contractility; sympathomimetic agents (such as ephedrine) increase bladder outlet resistance. Diuresis (such as from a diuretic, glucosuria, or a large, brisk fluid intake) may overstretch a partially decompensated detrusor muscle and cause acute urinary retention.

It is important to distinguish *bladder outlet obstructive* symptoms—hesitancy, decreased stream, postvoid dribbling—from *irritative bladder symptoms*—frequency, urgency, nocturia. Although anatomical or functional obstruction may produce both types of

Table 49.1.
Pharmacological Agents with Known Influence on Bladder Function

DRUGS THAT INCREASE BLADDER TONE AND CONTRACTILITY
  Bethanecol (Urecholine)
DRUGS THAT DECREASE BLADDER CONTRACTILITY
  Anticholinergic drugs (e.g., Pro-Banthine, Donnatal, Ditropan)
  Calcium antagonists (verapamil, nifedipine, diltiazam)
  Prostaglandin inhibitors (e.g., ibuprofen)
  Tricyclic antidepressants (e.g., imipramine, nortriptyline)
  Beta adrenergic agonists (e.g., terbutaline)
DRUGS THAT INCREASE BLADDER OUTLET RESISTANCE
  Sympathomimetic drugs (e.g., ephedrine, Sudafed, Ornade)
  Antiparkinsonian drugs (e.g., levodopa, Sinemet)
  Beta adrenergic antagonists (e.g., propranolol)
  Estrogens
DRUGS THAT DECREASE OUTLET RESISTANCE
  Antispasticity drugs (e.g., diazapan, Baclofen)
  Alpha-adrenergic antagonists (e.g., prazosin, phenoxybenzamine, terazosin)
DRUGS THAT INCREASE URINARY VOLUME
  Diuretics

symptoms, only irritative symptoms are seen with cystitis, prostatitis, bladder stones, and bladder carcinoma. Finally, the differentiation of polyuria from urinary frequency, and nocturia from enuresis (involuntary bedwetting) can be made by appropriate questioning.

PHYSICAL EXAMINATION

The physical examination of the patient with symptoms of bladder outlet obstruction should be thorough, with special emphasis on the urinary tract.

The *abdominal examination* may reveal several findings: a distended bladder from retention, renal tenderness (infection or hydronephrosis) or a renal mass (hydronephrosis, neoplasm, or cystic disease), and inguinal hernia from straining at urination when outlet obstruction is present. In the male patient, the *examination of the penis* may reveal phimosis or urethral meatal stenosis that could cause obstruction. The *examination of the epididymides* may show evidence of acute or chronic infection, which may be a complication of bladder outlet obstruction and concomitant prostatitis. A brief *neurological examination*, particularly of the anal sphincter tone, genital and perineal sensation, and motor, sensory, and reflex activity of the lower extremities may disclose abnormalities that suggest a neurogenic bladder as the cause of the patient's symptoms.

A careful *rectal examination* of the prostate is important in evaluating the patient with suspected BPH or prostatic carcinoma. Even though there are certain limits, rectal palpation permits examination of the lateral lobes of the prostate and the posterior lobe, adjacent to the apex. The anterior lobe cannot be felt, and very rarely is the median lobe palpable unless it is markedly enlarged. BPH most commonly involves the lateral and median lobes; moreover, the size of the prostate gland as estimated by rectal examination is not directly related to the degree of urinary obstruction.

The most important information obtained from the rectal examination is the *consistency of the prostate gland*. In patients with prostate enlargement, BPH can be differentiated from prostatic carcinoma with over 75% certainty based on the rectal examination. The patient may be examined when he is in the decubitus, knee-chest, or standing-bending position. The patient should void as fully as possible before the examination since a full bladder will distort the size of the prostate. The patient should be told that he may feel the urge to void when the prostate is examined. To prevent anal sphincter spasm, appropriate time should be used to explain the procedure to the patient. Using ample lubricant, the anal sphincter should be slowly and gently dilated by gradual insertion of the finger through the anus, asking the patient to bear down slightly. This examination will permit the determination of shape, size, and consistency of the prostate, the presence of tenderness, any other rectal masses, and the adequacy of anal sphincter tone.

The normal prostate is palpable 2 to 5 cm from the anal verge through the anterior rectal wall. The examining finger can normally reach over the top (base) of the prostate, as well as over each lateral border. A median sulcus is appreciated in the midline. The palpable prostate can be compared in size, configuration, and consistency with the tip of the nose.

BPH often results not only in obliteration of the median sulcus but also in a failure of the examining finger to reach the base of the gland. The consistency of the gland in BPH is smooth and rubbery—very similar to the thenar eminence of the hand. The gland is not tender unless prostatitis is present. BPH may be characterized by symmetrical or asymmetrical enlargement and can be nodular. The clinical differentiation between carcinoma and asymmetric or nodular BPH is usually based on the degree of induration or hardness of the gland.

Classically, prostatic carcinoma is characterized by a rock hard nodule or mass involving one or both posterior lobes. The zygomatic arch of the face has a similar consistency to that of prostatic carcinoma. However, not all hard nodules will be found on biopsy to be cancer nor are all cancerous nodules hard. Granulomatous prostatitis, prostatic calculi, spheroids of BPH, or nodularity resulting from transurethral prostatic resection may present as prostatic nodules and induration. Only 30 to 40% of prostatic nodules biopsied as suspicious for carcinoma will be positive on histological examination.

If there is suspicion of prostatic carcinoma, it is important to determine the extent of the local lesion—single nodule, diffuse involvement, or extension outside the capsule—and to refer the patient to a urologist.

PRELIMINARY LABORATORY ASSESSMENT

If the patient is thought to have bladder outlet obstruction due to BPH, one must determine the need

and urgency for urological consultation. A urinalysis and the determination of the urinary flow rate, the performance of a urine culture (if pyuria is present), and measurement of serum creatinine or creatinine clearance will provide the information that will aid in making this decision.

The *urinary flow rate* is easily obtained by measuring the volume of urine voided during a timed 5-second period (3). Normal men will have 5-second volumes exceeding 75 ml, whereas men with urinary obstruction have flows less than 50 ml in 5 seconds.

If the patient does not have hematuria, urinary tract infection, or renal failure and if the diagnosis of BPH is likely, further evaluation will depend on whether the patient is a candidate for surgery (Table 49.2). If there is no indication for surgery, then no further evaluation is necessary at this juncture.

UROLOGICAL INVESTIGATION

When surgery is a consideration and a patient is referred to a urologist, several further assessments are frequently made.

Radiology

Intravenous pyelography (IVP) is usually performed to determine whether there is hydronephrosis or other structural disease of the urinary tract. Besides assessing the upper tract, this study may demonstrate bladder trabeculations, significant residual urine, or a bladder stone. Elevation of the floor of the bladder by an enlarged prostate may be seen as well as "J-ing" or fish hooking of the distal ureters. The pelvic and vertebral bones can also be evaluated and may provide a clue to the presence of metastatic prostatic cancer.

If a patient has a history of an allergic reaction to intravenous contrast material, there are several alternative methods for studying the urinary tract. *Renal ultrasound* is useful in the detection of significant obstruction and other renal disorders such as masses or stones. Depending on the agent used, a *renal scan* may be used to evaluate renal blood flow or delayed excretion suggestive of obstruction. A *retrograde pyelogram* done in conjunction with cystoscopy (see below) will provide visualization of dilated ureters. The contrast medium used during this procedure is not absorbed and can be used safely in patients allergic to it.

If the history suggests a urethral stricture, a retro-

Table 49.2.

Indications for Surgery in Patients with Benign Prostatic Hyperplasia and Bladder Outlet Obstruction

Urinary retention
Intractable symptoms due to obstruction
Recurrent or persistent urinary tract infection
Recurrent prostatic bleeding
Significant postvoid residual urine
Changes of the kidneys, ureters, or bladder caused by prostatic obstruction
Abnormally low urinary flow rate
Bladder calculi

grade urethrogram may be performed. This procedure requires instillation of contrast material into the urethra with appropriate X-rays. There is no need for anesthesia during this procedure, and there is only minimal discomfort during injection per urethra.

If an IVP is felt to be mandatory in a patient with a history of previous mild to moderate reaction, there is approximately a 35% chance of reaction. Newer agents may be used with a much lower risk of reaction. A decision to perform a study in this instance must be made on an individual basis and in consultation with the radiologist and urologist.

Instrumentation

A urologist will gain considerable information in the evaluation of a patient with symptoms of bladder outlet obstruction by performing several invasive procedures. Because these procedures may be associated with the development of infection, they should not be done casually.

Bladder Catheterization for Postvoid Volume (see also Chapter 6)

Inserting a urethral catheter immediately after a patient has voided will determine the amount of residual urine (greater than 100 ml is abnormal), as well as help to determine if there is a urethral stricture. There is a risk of urosepsis if infection is present; also hematuria or urinary retention may result from the instrumentation. Ultrasound of the lower abdomen and pelvis may accurately estimate postvoid residual urine without an invasive procedure such as catheterization.

Cystometrogram

If a neurogenic bladder is suspected, the patient should be referred to a urologist for a consultation and the performance of a cystometrogram and possibly a cystourethroscopy. A cystometrogram is easily performed by a urologist in his office. The procedure is similar to a catheterization for residual urine. After the catheter is placed, a sterile solution is used to fill the bladder and to record and classify the detrusor response to the increasing volume.

Cystourethroscopy

Patient experience. Cystourethroscopy is a procedure permitting visualization of the entire urethra, the prostate, and the bladder. It usually is done in a urologist's office or outpatient clinic using topical anesthesia without premedication. A lighted instrument, typically 6 mm in diameter, is used. The patient will often perceive a feeling of suprapubic pressure as the bladder is being filled with the irrigating fluid, but the degree of discomfort is usually slight. The examination takes just a few minutes. However, if a retrograde ureteropyelogram is performed, another 15 minutes may be required. After cystoscopy, patients will often experience dysuria. The patient should have been advised about this and informed that it may be relieved by voiding while sitting in a bathtub filled with warm water or by taking

phenazopyridine (Pyridium), 100 mg three times a day for one or two days. Hematuria after cystoscopy is also common and may persist for 2 or 3 days. The patient should be informed of this possibility, reassured that it is not uncommon, and advised to force fluids (2 to 3 liters/day). Infection in the urinary tract occurs only rarely after cystoscopy. Occasionally, acute urinary retention occurs from edema of the prostate subsequent to instrumentation. If this complication occurs, the insertion of an indwelling catheter and possible hospitalization are necessary. An uncommon long-term complication of cystoscopy is urethral stricture. The use of smaller instruments and new flexible cystoscopes is likely to eliminate this complication.

The urologist learns a great deal from the cystoscopic examination. The entire urethra is seen. The size of the prostate, the degree of occlusiveness, trabeculation in the bladder, the presence of a bladder stone and diverticula are all directly visualized. This information is most important in helping the urologist decide the need for and the type of surgery.

TREATMENT OF BLADDER OUTLET OBSTRUCTION

Benign Prostatic Hyperplasia

The current treatment for BPH is prostatectomy. Because of operative risk, the urologist may not be able to perform surgery, and urinary retention may have to be treated with long-term indwelling catheterization or clean intermittent catheterization if this is possible. A suprapubic cystostomy may occasionally be necessary when the patient is intolerant of a urethral catheter.

Nonoperative Management

The nonoperative management of benign prostatic hyperplasia is becoming more popular and may be applicable in selected patients (10, 11). Balloon dilation of the prostatic urethra and bladder neck is currently under investigation, but it is too early to recommend its use. Alpha-adrenergic blockade (e.g., prazosin, terazosin), which relaxes the bladder neck, has been used with some success. Its use is primarily in younger patients (e.g., < 55 years) with mild outlet obstructive symptoms and is best discussed by at least a telephone conversation with a urologist. Androgen deprivation (e.g., castration or estrogens) results in impotence and loss of libido and currently has no place as a treatment of BPH. A recent, potent, safe 5-alpha reductase inhibitor that produces regression of benign prostatic hyperplasia without loss of libido and potency is currently under evaluation in phase three clinical trials. It appears that it may be effective in only 30% of patients with outlet obstructive symptoms secondary to BPH. More studies will be necessary to identify which patients will benefit from this drug.

Operative Management

Obstructing prostatic tissue may be surgically removed either transurethrally (TURP) or by one of the open operative approaches (suprapubic, retropubic, or perineal). The particular approach used will depend on the condition of the patient, the size and configuration of the prostate gland, and the urologist's experience. In general, glands that are very large are removed by open prostatectomy and smaller glands by TURP.

Transurethral Resection of the Prostate. TURP is the most commonly used procedure in the treatment of BPH; over 90% of prostatectomies for benign disease are performed this way. It requires hospitalization for 3 to 5 days; general or spinal anesthesia is used.

Complications have been minimized by the use of smaller more efficient instruments, by improved lighting, and by isotonic irrigating fluids. Nevertheless, bleeding, infection, and plasma hypo-osmolality (from absorption of irrigation fluid) may occur. Long-term complications of TURP include urethral stricture, bladder neck contracture, and incontinence.

A frequent consequence of TURP is *retrograde ejaculation*, a situation characterized by the ejaculation of semen into the bladder rather than externally through the urethra. This phenomenon occurs because the bladder neck is opened as part of the TURP and cannot subsequently contract as is necessary to produce antegrade ejaculation. Retrograde ejaculation results in sterility but does not usually affect orgasm. This consequence should be discussed with sexually active patients and their partners before prostatectomy. TURP should not produce organic erectile impotence; however, psychogenic impotence may follow genitourinary surgery. The management of psychogenic impotence is described in Chapter 18.

Most patients can resume normal physical and sexual activity in approximately 4 weeks after TURP. Complete healing of the prostatic fossa, however, usually takes 2 to 3 months, and during this period a urinalysis may reveal white and red blood cells.

Open Prostatectomy. Open prostatectomy requires a slightly longer hospitalization and recovery period. This approach is used when, in addition to having a large prostate, the patient has a coincidental bladder condition that can be repaired at the same time (e.g., bladder diverticulum or bladder stone). Organic erectile impotence occurs occasionally, especially when the perineal approach has been used. If this complication occurs, an evaluation should be performed before attributing the impotence to the surgery and presuming it to be irreversible.

It is very important for a patient undergoing any form of prostatectomy for BPH to understand that the entire prostate gland is not removed. Because of the presence of residual prostate tissue, these patients have a risk equal to that of the general population of developing prostatic carcinoma. Rectal examinations should be done every 12 months to detect changes that may suggest malignancy. Because residual prostatic tissue remains, recurrent symptoms or complications from prostatic hypertrophy may develop later. The frequency of recurrence depends primarily on the extent of the initial surgery and is highly variable.

Urethral Stricture

A urethral stricture may be treated with urethral dilation, transurethral incision of the stricture, or open urethral surgery. The method selected depends on the length and location of the stricture, the patient's overall health, and the urologist's experience.

Prostatic Carcinoma

Prostatic carcinoma may present with bladder outlet obstruction although this is less common than with BPH. The most frequent sign leading to the diagnosis of adenocarcinoma of the prostate is that of a prostatic nodule or induration discovered on a routine rectal examination of the prostate. Either finding should lead to a urological consultation and to a biopsy of the prostate. Approximately 30 to 40% of prostatic nodules or induration in the prostate will be adenocarcinomas. The prevalence of unsuspected or incidental carcinoma of the prostate found at transurethral resection of the prostate (TURP) ranges from 4% in the 4th decade to 80% in the 9th decade of life. The prevalence at autopsy is even higher as many cancers begin in the outer periphery of the prostate gland and are missed by incomplete transurethral resection.

The therapy of prostatic carcinoma is somewhat controversial but may be approached on the basis of the stage of disease (Table 49.3). If the neoplasm is limited to the prostate (no evidence of local spread or metastatic disease) and the patient is under 75 years of age, has an anticipated 10-year survival, and has no contraindicating medical diseases, he is a candidate for a curative treatment. Radiation therapy and radical prostatectomy are primary considerations. Radical prostatectomy appears to provide slightly less morbidity and longer survival. In the hands of a urologist experienced in this type of surgery, the complications are minimal and less than 2% of patients develop incontinence. A modification of the traditional radical prostatectomy permits the removal of all cancerous tissue, yet spares the pelvic nerves that control erection; there is preservation of pre-existing potency in greater than 90% of patients (6, 15).

Stage A prostatic carcinoma is disease unsuspected on rectal examination of the prostate, but discovered at the time of prostatectomy for obstructive symptoms

Table 49.3.
Staging of Prostatic Carcinoma

Stage		Description
A		Clinically undetectable; found on pathological examination after prostatectomy
	A1	Focal and well differentiated
	A2	Diffuse (>5%) or poorly differentiated
B		Limited to prostate on rectal examination
	B1	Solitary nodule; < 1.5 cm; one lobe
	B2	One whole lobe or both lobes
C		Locally extending outside of prostatic capsule or into seminal vesicles
D		Metastatic disease
	D1	Pelvic lymph node metastases
	D2	Distant metastases, usually bone

thought to be secondary to benign hyperplasia (12). If carcinoma is reported, the percentage or volume of neoplasm to the total amount of tissue removed and the histological grade of the neoplasm should be noted (8). This information will aid in the management and determination of prognosis of the patient. Stage A is further subdivided into *stage A1* disease, well-differentiated carcinoma in less than 5% of resected tissue. All other incidentally discovered carcinomas are *stage A2* and are considered potentially more aggressive. The urologist will initiate a metastatic evaluation by determining the concentration of the serum acid phosphatase and by evaluating the bones with a nuclear scan. Prostatic specific antigen (PSA), a tumor marker, will be measured (14). Although not specific, its clinical usefulness lies in the fact that it may reflect tumor mass, and therefore it is of value in following a patient after surgery.

If there is no evidence of local or distant metastatic disease, the management in stage A disease is controversial. In a younger (< 65 yr) individual with A1 disease who is at a higher risk for recurrence because of his expected longevity, radical prostatectomy is recommended (7). For the older patient (> 65 yrs), observation is usually recommended. The patient with A2 disease is at considerable risk for developing metastases, and radical prostatectomy is recommended.

Stage B carcinoma is defined as disease limited to the prostate gland that is detected clinically either as a nodule or as diffuse hardness with no extension or fixation. If the neoplasm is limited to the prostate and the patient is under 75 years of age, has an anticipated 10-year survival, and has no contraindicating medical diseases, he is a candidate for curative radical prostatectomy (see above) (13).

More extensive localized prostatic cancer, *stage C*, is best treated by definitive radiotherapy (6). If significant bladder outlet obstruction is present, the patient may also need a TURP; this combination of treatment results in an increased risk of urinary incontinence.

Studies have shown that the obturator and iliac nodes are usually the first site of metastases, and these structures will be positive in 5 to 50% of patients with prostatic cancers. However, current imaging techniques are unfortunately not reliable in picking up early lymph node metastases.

Metastatic or *stage D prostatic cancer* is best managed by hormonal therapy (i.e., androgen deprivation) via surgical (castration) or pharmacological methods. Studies have shown that hormonal therapy initiated at the time of diagnosis does not prolong survival but may delay the onset of symptomatic metastases compared with hormonal therapy initiated only in response to symptoms (e.g., bone pain) (2, 4). Nevertheless, its use before the development of symptomatic metastasis remains controversial, and, since life expectancy is unchanged, many urologists ordinarily would wait until symptomatic disease develops before initiating hormonal therapy. Diethylstilbestrol (3 mg/day) and orchiectomy give similar results, pro-

ducing an 85 to 90% partial symptomatic response rate in previously untreated patients. The duration of response is 18 months on the average, although prolonged remissions have been documented. There is no advantage of combining orchiectomy and estrogen therapy. Generally, estrogen therapy, which causes salt and water retention, should be avoided in patients who also have an edema-forming illness (such as severe congestive heart failure or nephrotic syndrome) not controlled by diuretics. With newer medications, diethylstilbestrol is not as commonly used. Leuteinizing hormone/releasing hormone (LH/RH) analogues (Luprolide, Zoladex) have proven to be just as effective as surgical or estrogen castration with fewer side effects (9). These analogues in combination with a potent antiandrogen (flutamide) provides total androgen blockade and appears to be more effective than either alone. There have been a number of investigational trials utilizing cytotoxic chemotherapy in all stages of prostatic carcinoma, but none is as effective as androgen deprivation, which is only partially effective in patients who fail hormonal therapy or who have extensive metastatic disease (1).

Much of the controversy in the diagnosis and treatment of prostatic cancer results from the inability to assess accurately the influence of prostatic cancer on longevity (5). Prostatic cancer occurs in older men who often have coexisting diseases that influence longevity. Also, the natural history of the disease is not well understood. The best estimates for survival with various stages of prostatic cancer with the treatments discussed above are listed in Table 49.4.

URINARY INCONTINENCE

Urinary incontinence is a common problem of the elderly and of younger women. It may be a manifestation of urinary outlet obstruction. The evaluation of incontinence is described in Chapter 6. In general, younger patients with incontinence are best referred to a urologist or gynecologist for evaluation and definitive treatment, which is usually surgical. Elderly patients with urinary incontinence are usually managed by the general physician; their treatment is described extensively in Chapter 6, Geriatric Medicine—Special Considerations.

General References

Resnick MI, Kursh E (eds): *Current Therapy in Genitourinary Surgery*. Philadelphia, BC Decker, Inc, 1987.
Walsh PC: Benign prostate hyperplasia. In: Walsh PC, Perlmutter

Table 49.4.
Survival with Appropriately Managed Prostatic Carcinoma

Stage	% of Survival		
	5 yr	10 yr	15 yr
A1	Normal life expectancy		
A2	50–80	40–70	15–35
B	50–90	40–70	15–40
C	15–70	5–60	0–30
D	5–30	3–10	0–3

AD, Gittes RF, Stamey TA (eds): *Campbell's Urology*. Philadelphia, WB Saunders, 1986.

Specific References

1. Anderson T: Chemotherapy of urologic cancer—principles and practice. In: Javadpour N (ed): *Principles and Management of Urologic Cancer*, 2nd ed. Baltimore, Williams & Wilkins, 1983.
2. Bailar JC, Byar DP: Estrogen treatment for cancer of the prostate: early results with three doses of diethylstilbestrol and placebo. *Cancer (Phila)* 26:257, 1970.
3. Bloom DA, Foster WD, McLeod DG, et al: Cost-effective uroflowmetry in men. *J Urol* 133:421, 1985.
4. Byar DP: The Veterans Administration Cooperative Urologic Research Group's studies of cancer of the prostate. *Cancer (Phila)* 32:1126, 1973.
5. Catalona WJ, Miller DR, Kavoussi LR: Intermediate-term survival in clinically understaged prostate cancer patients following radical prostatectomy. *J Urol* 140:540, 1988.
6. Catalona WJ, Scott WW: Carcinoma of the prostate: a review. *J Urol* 119:1, 1978.
7. Epstein JI, Oesterling JE, Walsh PC: The volume and anatomical location of residual tumor in radical prostatectomy specimens removed for stage A1 prostate cancer. *J Urol* 139:975, 1988.
8. Epstein JI, Oesterling JE, Walsh PC: Tumor volume versus percentage of specimen involved by tumor correlated with progression in stage A prostatic cancer. *J Urol* 139:980, 1988.
9. The Leuprolide Study Group: Leuprolide versus diethylstilbestrol for metastatic prostatic cancer. *N Engl J Med* 311:1281, 1984.
10. Kadow C, Feneley RCL, Abrams PH: Prostatectomy or conservative management in the treatment of benign prostatic hypertrophy. *Br J Urol* 61:432, 1988.
11. Lepor H: Nonoperative management of benign prostatic hyperplasia. *J Urol* 141:1283, 1989.
12. McNeal JE, Price HM, Redwine EA, et al: Stage A versus stage B adenocarcinoma of the prostate: morphological comparison and biological significance. *J Urol* 139:61, 1988.
13. Middleton AW: Radical prostatectomy for carcinoma in men more than 69 years old. *J Urol* 138:1185, 1987.
14. Oesterling JE, Chan DW, Epstein JI, et al: Prostate specific antigen in the preoperative and postoperative evaluation of localized prostatic cancer treated with radical prostatectomy. *J Urol* 139:766, 1988.
15. Walsh PC, Lepor H, Eggleston JC: Radical prostatectomy with preservation of sexual function: anatomical and pathological considerations. *Prostate* 4:473, 1983.
16. Wein AJ: Drug treatment of voiding dysfunction, Part I-II. *AUA Update Series* 7:14, 1988.

Hematological Problems

C H A P T E R 50

Anemia

LARRY WATERBURY, M.D.

GENERAL CONSIDERATIONS

Anemia, a reduction of the proportion of red cells or of hemoglobin in the blood, is a condition, like hypoxia or jaundice, which always reflects a primary underlying disease. Although there are sometimes symptoms (e.g., shortness of breath on exertion) or signs (e.g., pallor) that are associated with anemia, the diagnosis of the condition is essentially dependent on one or more laboratory measurements—such as the hematocrit value (the amount of red cells in a volume of blood) or the hemoglobin concentration. In general, anemia is defined in a man as a condition in which the hematocrit value is less than 42% or the hemoglobin concentration less than 14 g/100 ml and in a woman as a hematocrit value less than 37% or a hemoglobin concentration less than 12 g/100 ml. When anemia is diagnosed, other measurements, described below, are important in establishing the cause of the process and in selecting appropriate therapy.

Most of the routine complete blood counts (CBCs)

obtained in clinical practice in this country are determined by automated counting methods (Table 50.1). The CBC usually reports the hemoglobin (Hgb) concentration, hematocrit (Hct) value, red blood cell count (RBC), white cell count, mean corpuscular volume (MCV), mean corpuscular hemoglobin (MCH), and mean corpuscular hemoglobin concentration (MCHC). One commonly used automated system (Coulter) measures the hemoglobin, RBC, and MCV and from these variables calculates the hematocrit value, MCH, and MCHC. With the use of the automated counters the indices (MCH, MCHC, MCV), especially the MCV, are precise, accurate measurements that can be utilized in approaching the diagnostic workup of anemia. The calculated Hct value is slightly lower than that obtained by centrifugation (packed cells trap plasma, distorting the ratio of red cells to plasma).

APPROACH TO EVALUATION OF ANEMIA

The routine data base that should be obtained for every anemic patient includes the hematocrit value, hemoglobin concentration, MCV, MCHC, and reticulocyte count (Table 50.2). A smear of the peripheral blood should be obtained by fingerstick or from unanticoagulated blood on the tip of a venipuncture needle. (Anticoagulants may distort the morphology of the blood cells.) The smear may be stained in the physician's office or transported to an outside laboratory to be stained and interpreted. On the basis of all of these data, and a complete history and physical examination, the physician can progress a long way toward an etiological diagnosis of the anemia. Three questions should be asked:

1. *What is the MCV?* With the use of the automated counters the MCV is a direct measurement of red cell size. The normal range varies with individual laboratories but is approximately 82 to 98 femtoliters (fl). Actually it is helpful to use a broader

Table 50.1.
Representative Normal Values (Coulter S)

	Men	Women
Hemoglobin, g/dl of blood	14–18	12–16
Hematocrit value, %	42–54	37–47
Mean corpuscular volume, MCV, fl	82–98	82–98
Mean corpuscular hemoglobin, MCH, pg	27–32	27–32
Mean corpuscular hemoglobin concentration, MCHC, g/dl of red blood cells	31.5–36	31.5–36

Table 50.2.
Routine Data Base for Anemic Patients

Hematocrit value
Hemoglobin concentration
Mean corpuscular volume
Mean corpuscular hemoglobin concentration
Reticulocytic count (and calculation of reticulocytic index)
Evaluation of a peripheral blood smear (fingerstick)

normal range of 80 to 100 fl to classify the anemia as microcytic (MCV less than 80 fl), normocytic (MCV 80 to 100 fl), or macrocytic (MCV greater than 100 fl). Microcytic and macrocytic anemias have very limited differential diagnoses, and therefore by simply noting the MCV the physician's diagnostic approach can be limited greatly when the anemia is microcytic or macrocytic.

2. *What is the basic mechanism of the anemia?* There are only three ways patients become anemic: (*a*) decreased effective production of red cells by bone marrow, (*b*) bleeding, or (*c*) hemolysis. The most helpful laboratory measurement in defining the mechanism of anemia is the reticulocyte count. The *reticulocyte count* is used to assess the appropriateness of the response of the bone marrow to anemia. The normal reticulocyte count is approximately 1%, representing the 1% of new cells that are released into the circulation from the bone marrow daily (the ordinary red cell life span being in the range of 100 days). Under the stimulus of erythropoietin, in the anemic patient the bone marrow should be able to triple acutely its output of new cells; when anemia is chronic and severe, the bone marrow may be able to increase its output of cells to 8 to 10 times normal. This increased bone marrow activity is reflected in an appropriately elevated reticulocyte count. The reticulocyte count must be adjusted for the level of anemia to obtain a value known as the *reticulocyte index* (Table 50.3), a more accurate reflection of erythropoiesis. In patients with bleeding or hemolysis the reticulocyte index should be at least 3%, whereas in patients with anemia due to decreased production of red cells the reticulocyte index is less than 3%, and frequently less than 1.5%.

In addition to the reticulocyte index serial hematocrit values over a few days or weeks may provide clues to the mechanism of the anemia. Total shutdown of production in the marrow in the absence of bleeding or hemolysis will result in a fall in the hematocrit value of only 3 or 4 percentage points/week. If the value has fallen more rapidly, bleeding or hemolysis must have taken place. Anemia with an appropriate reticulocyte response in the absence of bleeding usually means hemolysis.

3. *Does the patient have another problem that is commonly associated with anemia?* Table 50.4 lists anemias commonly associated with various clinical characteristics and diseases. For this purpose race and sex are also taken into consideration. Women are more frequently iron deficient than are men, and black patients are more likely than are

Table 50.3.
Reticulocyte Index

Reticulocyte index = reticulocyte count $\times \dfrac{\text{patient Hct}}{\text{normal Hct}}$

Example: reticulocyte count 6%, hematocrit 15%

Reticulocyte index $= 6 \times \dfrac{15}{45} = 2\%$

Table 50.4.
Anemias Associated with Various Clinical Settings

Female:
  Iron deficiency
Blacks:
  Glucose 6-phosphate dehydrogenase (G-6-PD) deficiency, hemoglobinopathies, thalassemia
Mediterranean origin:
  G-6-PD deficiency, thalassemia
Far East origin:
  Hemoglobinopathies, thalassemia
Viral infections:
  Immune hemolysis
  Decreased production
Bacterial infection:
  Anemia of inflammation
  Microangiopathic hemolysis
  Oxidative hemolysis (G-6-PD deficiency)
  Other hemolytic mechanisms
Malignancy:
  Microangiopathic hemolysis
  Immune hemolysis
  Decreased production
Alcoholic liver disease:
  Bleeding
  Hypersplenism
  Folate deficiency
  Decreased production
  Sideroblastic anemia
  Iron deficiency
  Hemolysis
Hyper-hypothyroidism:
  Decreased production
  Pernicious anemia
  Iron deficiency
Renal Failure:
  Decreased production
  Hemolysis
  Bleeding
Aortic valve replacement:
  Microangiopathic hemolysis
Malignant hypertension:
  Microangiopathic hemolysis
Rheumatoid syndromes:
  Anemia of inflammation
  Iron deficiency
  Immune hemolysis
Collagen vascular disease:
  Immune hemolysis
  Anemia of inflammation
Drugs:
  α-Methyldopa: Immune hemolysis
  Quinine/quinidine: Immune hemolysis
  Penicillin: Immune hemolysis (rare)
  Butazolidin/chloramphenicol: Dose-related marrow depression; idiosyncratic aplastic anemia
  Gold: Aplastic anemia
  Antituberculosis drugs: Sideroblastic anemia
  Phenytoin: Megaloblastic anemia (folate); pure red cell aplasia
  Sulfa/sulfones: G-6-PD hemolysis
  Methotrexate: Megaloblastosis
  Amphotericin, cisplatinum, zidovudine: production defect

whites to have hemoglobinopathies or glucose 6-phosphate dehydrogenase deficiency.

In summary, the initial data base should enable the physician to classify the anemia on the basis of the MCV, to categorize the basic mechanism of the anemia, and to consider possible causes based upon the patient's problem list. This initial assessment should then suggest the appropriate further diagnostic workup.

ANEMIA WITH A LOW MCV

Table 50.5 lists those anemias commonly associated with a low MCV. For the most part the diagnosis rests between iron deficiency anemia and thalassemia. Occasionally the anemia of chronic inflammation and, even more rarely, sideroblastic anemia are microcytic, although more often they are normocytic or, in the case of sideroblastic anemia, frequently macrocytic.

Iron Deficiency Anemia

Although dietary iron deficiency does occur in the infant and during the rapid growth phase of adolescence, in this country iron deficiency generally occurs only as a result of bleeding. Iron deficiency from menstruation and from pregnancy is extremely common in women; but iron deficiency in a man or in a postmenopausal woman should be considered to be due to gastrointestinal bleeding until proven otherwise.

Diagnosis

The history and physical examination may yield information that suggests the presence of iron deficiency (8). Such information includes a history of multiple past pregnancies in a woman; strange dietary habits such as the eating of ice, starch, or clay (pica); any past history of gastrointestinal bleeding, a sore tongue, brittle and ridged fingernails, spoon nails, and cheilosis. The physical findings are seen only in patients with long-standing and severe iron deficiency.

Most of the body's iron is incorporated in hemoglobin, but approximately one-third of it is stored in reticuloendothelial sites, primarily in the spleen, liver, and bone marrow. In patients with slow continued bleeding the reticuloendothelial iron stores supply the requirement of the bone marrow for iron until the stores are depleted. It is at this point that iron deficiency anemia begins to develop. In iron deficiency cell size (MCV) correlates with the degree of anemia, so that very mild iron deficiency anemia may be associated with normal sized cells (11). The MCV progressively decreases as the anemia becomes more severe, but the MCHC usually remains normal until the hematocrit value falls below 30%. As the anemia becomes more marked, the red cells also become progressively more distorted (poikilocytosis). Table 50.6 illustrates the relationship between the hematocrit value, the MCV, and the degree of red cell distortion (poikilocytosis)

Table 50.5.
Causes of Anemia with Low Mean Corpuscular Volume

Iron deficiency
Thalassemia
Anemia of chronic inflammation (occasionally)
Sideroblastic anemia (rarely)
Aluminum toxicity

seen in iron deficiency anemia of varying degrees of severity.

Often the diagnosis of iron deficiency is obvious after the initial history, physical examination, and standard laboratory evaluation. If not, a number of other tests may be useful; the *reticulocyte index* is inappropriately low for the degree of anemia. The *serum iron concentration* (SI) is low but is usually low also in patients with acute and chronic inflammation and malignancy. Furthermore, an acute infectious process such as pneumococcal pneumonia will cause an immediate drop in the serum iron even though the patient is not iron deficient. Classically, the *total iron-binding capacity* (TIBC) is elevated. It is a measure of the serum transferrin, the iron transport protein that supplies bone marrow reticulocytes with iron. However, many iron-deficient patients have a normal TIBC, and it may be low in cases of chronic inflammation or of malignancy whether or not iron deficiency is present. The *bone marrow iron stain* is the most definitive way to prove a diagnosis of iron deficiency, since iron stores are depleted when iron deficiency anemia is present and are normal or elevated in patients with microcytic anemia due to other causes.

Serum ferritin may be helpful in the assessment of body iron stores (14). Ferritin is a water-soluble complex of iron and a binding protein, apoferritin. The serum ferritin concentration reflects the status of the reticuloendothelial stores and, in general, is a more specific test than the serum iron and iron-binding capacity in the diagnosis of iron deficiency. A low serum ferritin concentration almost always reflects iron deficiency. A very elevated serum ferritin concentration usually signifies iron overload, as in the patient who has received multiple transfusions. There are, however, a number of clinical situations in which the serum ferritin may be spuriously normal or even elevated in the presence of iron deficiency anemia (Table 50.7). In these situations it may be difficult to make a definitive diagnosis of iron deficiency without a bone marrow iron stain.

Treatment

After institution of oral iron therapy, the reticulocyte response is maximal at around 7 to 10 days. The hematocrit value begins to rise after about 1 week, and in the uncomplicated case a normal hematocrit value is reached in a few weeks. However, it takes many months of therapy for patients to replete their iron stores. In the menstruating woman with iron deficiency anemia, treatment for a year may be necessary; and in the man with iron deficiency anemia, treatment for 6 months is frequently indicated. Iron deficiency is very common in menstruating women, especially in those with heavy menstrual periods and a history of multiple pregnancies. Some may require constant iron therapy to maintain a normal hematocrit value. Standard treatment with oral iron consists of 1 tablet of iron (e.g., ferrous sulfate, 300 mg, which contains 60 mg of elemental iron) three times daily on an empty

Table 50.6.
Representative Data Base at Various Stages in the Slow Development of Severe Iron Deficiency Anemia[a]

Hct	42	42	35	27	19
MCV (82–98 fl)	92	88	82	75	68
MCHC (32–36 g/dl)	33	33	33	31	29
SI (65–175 μg/dl)	70	60	35	20	20
TIBC (250–375 μg/dl)	300	300	300	400	450
Serum ferritin (10–200 μg/ml)	60	30	5	3	1
Peripheral smear	Normal	Normal	Normal	1+ poikilocytosis 1+ hypochromia	4+ poikilocytosis 4+ hypochromia
Bone marrow iron stores	Present	Absent	Absent	Absent	Absent

[a]Hct, hematocit value; MCV, mean corpuscular volume; MCHC, mean corpuscular hemoglobin concentration; SI, serum iron; TIBC, total iron-binding capacity. Numbers in parentheses are the range of normal values.

Table 50.7.
Inappropriately Normal or Elevated Serum Ferritin Levels

Acute liver disease
Cirrhosis
Hodgkin's disease
Acute leukemias
Solid tumors (occasionally)
Fever
Acute inflammation
Renal dialysis patients
Recent treatment with iron

stomach (1 hour before meals). If it is difficult for patients to take the noontime dose, it is reasonable to omit it. There are numerous preparations of iron other than ferrous sulfate, but there is usually no justification for recommending any of them unless a reduction in the dose of elemental iron is required (see below). Generally time-release spansules and enteric coated preparations are to be avoided. They are costly, and absorption is variable. Preparations containing iron, including ferrous sulfate, can be obtained without prescription. The most vigorously promoted iron preparation, Geritol, costs the patient approximately 5 times as much as ferrous sulfate for an equivalent dosage of elemental iron. The addition of ascorbic acid to iron preparations to increase absorption is not worth the cost.

Side effects. Approximately 15% of patients have gastrointestinal side effects from oral iron, most commonly constipation, but abdominal cramping and diarrhea are also seen. When such side effects develop, the physician may elect to administer iron only once a day, or may instruct the patient to take iron with meals instead of on an empty stomach. Taking iron with food will decrease iron absorption by approximately 50%, but absorption will still be sufficient to replenish the body's iron if treatment is continued long enough. If symptoms still continue after these alterations in dose and schedule, it is helpful to decrease the individual dose of oral iron. If the dose is decreased to less than 40 mg of elemental iron, symptoms will frequently abate. This can be done by using pediatric liquid preparations, which are usually well tolerated. If these adjustments in the dosage and schedule of oral iron administration are made, parenteral iron is rarely indicated. Parenteral therapy is

indicated, however, in patients with small and large bowel inflammation, rapid gastrointestinal transit, or malabsorption, and when the patient has severe iron deficiency and noncompliance has been repetitively proven. Iron dextran is the most commonly used form of parenteral iron and is usually given in 2.0-ml (100-mg) doses intramuscularly or intravenously. If the intravenous route is chosen, it must be given slowly (no more rapidly than 1.0 ml/minute). Guidelines for the dosage of parenteral iron are provided in the Physicians' Desk Reference but may be grossly calculated by age and hemoglobin concentration (Table 50.8). Injections may be given daily until the calculated required dose has been administered. Side effects from parenteral iron include pain and rash at the injection site, staining of the skin, fever, and rare anaphylactoid reactions.

Thalassemia

In the normal adult there are three hemoglobins present in mature red cells: A, the major component, and two minor components, A_2 and F (fetal). Each hemoglobin molecule consists of four heme groups and four globin chains; the globin chains in each molecule are of two different types. All three hemoglobins have two α-globin chains but differ in the second set (β, δ, γ) of globin chains (Table 50.9). Anemia is due to a combination of decreased hemoglobin production and, usually, mild hemolysis.

Thalassemia is an inherited defect in globin chain production. β-Thalassemia (23) is seen in the United States primarily in black patients, patients from Southeast Asia, or those of Mediterranean (Greek and Italian) origin. The genetics of α-thalassemia are complicated, and the disorder appears to have a wider racial dis-

Table 50.8.
Representative Total Body Iron Deficits (mg) at Various Body Weights and Hemoglobin Concentrations

Patient Weight	Iron Deficit at Various Hemoglobin Levels			
	4 g/dl	6 g/dl	8 g/dl	10 g/dl
lb				
100	2250	1750	1400	1000
120	2650	2100	1650	1150
140	3050	2500	1950	1350
160	3550	2850	2200	1550
180	3950	3200	2500	1750

Table 50.9.
Globin Chain Composition of Normal Adult Hemoglobins

		Percentage of Total in Normal Adults
Hgb A	$\alpha_2\beta_2$	97
Hgb A$_2$	$\alpha_2\delta_2$	2
Hgb F	$\alpha_2\gamma_2$	1

Table 50.10.
Heterozygous Thalassemia: Typical Data Base[a]

Hct	37%
MCV	69 fl
MCH	20 pg
MCHC	32 g/dl
Reticulocyte count	2.5%
Red blood cell morphology	Microcytosis, poikilocytosis, stippling
Ferritin	Normal or increased

[a]Abbreviations are as in Table 50.6.

tribution than does β-thalassemia, but it is especially common in American blacks (21). Most patients have inherited only one defective gene (heterozygotes) and are clinically asymptomatic but may have red cell microcytosis. The diagnosis is important as the entity is frequently confused with iron deficiency anemia resulting in lifelong repetitive workups for gastrointestinal bleeding and inappropriate treatment with iron. Microcytosis in black patients living in the United States is more likely due to α-thalassemia than to iron deficiency.

Diagnosis

Table 50.10 lists the typical data base for the patient with heterozygous α- or β-thalassemia. The combination of a low MCV and a mild anemia should alert the physician to the diagnosis, since in iron deficiency the degree of microcytosis parallels the severity of the anemia (see above). This discrepancy between the MCV and the Hct value, plus the frequent presence of coarsely stippled red cells on peripheral smear, should result in the presumptive diagnosis of heterozygous thalassemia.

In the forms of β-thalassemia most commonly seen in the United States there is a decreased production of β chains with a compensatory increase in the production of δ chains, resulting in a decreased production of hemoglobin A and an increased production of hemoglobin A$_2$. This increase can be assessed by electrophoresis of the hemoglobin and is a definitive diagnostic test for β-thalassemia. Less commonly, in this country, increases in hemoglobin F may be seen in patients with β-thalassemia. Hemoglobin F must be assayed by a separate special technique (alkali denaturation test).

The α-thalassemias are more difficult to diagnose since a decreased production of α chains will affect the relative concentrations of all of the normal adult hemoglobins. A definitive diagnosis of one of the α-thalassemia syndromes may be quite difficult and may require family studies or techniques available only in

research laboratories. However, the diagnosis of presumptive α-thalassemia in the setting of an appropriate data base (hematological values consistent with the diagnosis in the absence of iron deficiency and of β-thalassemia) is reasonable even in the absence of laboratory confirmation.

Patient Education

It is important to explain to patients with heterozygous thalassemia that the clinical features of their condition mimic iron deficiency. The patient should be put on guard against repetitive diagnostic workups for iron deficiency. The physician should emphasize the benign nature of the illness and that the anemia, being mild, usually does not cause any symptoms. He should caution the patient against taking oral iron since thalassemic patients actually have an increase in iron stores. Genetic counseling is important; a couple, both heterozygous for β-thalassemia, have a 25% chance of having a child with homozygous β-thalassemia. Furthermore, the genetic defect for thalassemia and those for hemoglobin S and C are alleles. Hemoglobin S-β-thalassemia is a clinically significant disease.

Miscellaneous

The *anemia of chronic disease* and the *anemia of malignancy* may be associated with a low MCV (although the MCV is usually normal). These entities are discussed below in the section dealing with normocytic anemia (page 561). *Sideroblastic anemias* (characterized by increased iron stores and by ringed sideroblasts in the bone marrow) are occasionally microcytic, and some hemoglobinopathies are associated with a low MCV (hemoglobin E). The former are best treated in consultation with a hematologist; the latter are rare in this country. Aluminum toxicity in patients with chronic renal failure (the result of the use of aluminum-containing antacids and, in some centers, an increased concentration of aluminum in the dialysate) sometimes causes microcytosis (16).

ANEMIA WITH A HIGH MCV

An MCV greater than 100 fl is abnormal and an attempt should be made to explain the abnormality. Table 50.11 lists conditions associated with an elevated MCV (10). For the most part, the diseases associated with an elevated MCV are liver disease, the

Table 50.11.
Differential Diagnosis of Mean Corpuscular Volume Greater Than 100 fl

Spurious
Reticulocytosis (marked)
Liver disease
Alcoholism
Myelodysplastic syndromes
Myelophthisis
Drugs
Megaloblastic anemias
Normal variant

megaloblastic anemias (including drug-induced megaloblastosis), and the refractory anemias with hypercellular bone marrows (preleukemia, sideroblastic anemia). Occasionally an elevated MCV measured by the automatic counter is spurious, caused by red cell antibodies or by marked rouleaux formation in patients with a very high erythrocyte sedimentation rate. Because young red cells are large, patients with a marked reticulocytosis may have an elevated MCV.

Liver Disease

Chronic hepatocellular and obstructive liver disease results in loading of cholesterol in the lipid portion of the red cell membrane so that the cell increases in size. Thus the MCV is frequently elevated but is usually not greater than 115 fl. On smears, cells appear to be round and centrally targeted, without significant variation in shape. This morphological abnormality is not a cause for anemia. However, patients with liver disease frequently have other reasons to be anemic (bleeding, hemolysis, folic acid deficiency). The severe alcoholic often has an elevated MCV even in the absence of overt liver disease or of marked megaloblastosis (7). Presumably the elevated MCV results from either periodic episodes of alcoholic liver disease, or from folic acid deficiency, or both. Owing to poor diet, the alcoholic frequently becomes folic acid depleted. In addition, alcohol interferes with folic acid metabolism.

Megaloblastic Anemia (18)

Table 50.12 lists the various etiologies of megaloblastic anemia related to vitamin B_{12} or folic acid deficiency. The body's stores of B_{12} are such that a diet without B_{12} (one in which animal protein was completely excluded) would not result in megaloblastosis

Table 50.12.
Causes of Megaloblastosis Due to Vitamin B_{12} and Folic Acid Deficiency

B_{12}
  Pernicious anemia (acquired and congenital)
  Gastrectomy
  Ileal resection
  Crohn's disease and tropical sprue
  Fish tapeworm infestation
  Blind loop syndrome
  Nutritional deficiency (vegans diet, rare)
  Familial selective malabsorption (Imerslund's syndrome)
Folic Acid
  Dietary (old age, the alcoholic, chronic disease)
  Malabsorption (sprue)
  Hemodialysis
  Severe exfoliative skin disease (*e.g.*, psoriasis)
  Drugs:
    Interference with absorption or utilization (Phenytoin, alcohol)
    Dihydrofolate reductase inhibitors (methotrexate, trimethoprim)
  Increased requirements:
    Pregnancy
    Infancy
    Hemolysis (*e.g.*, sickle cell anemia)

due to B_{12} deficiency for several years; therefore, dietary B_{12} deficiency is extremely rare. By far, the most common etiology of B_{12} deficiency is pernicious anemia, an acquired defect of the gastric mucosa resulting in deficient formation of intrinsic factor, a substance that binds ingested B_{12} and allows its absorption in the terminal ileum. Patients with pernicious anemia are usually elderly and complain of sore mouth, indigestion, and constipation or diarrhea. Neurological problems, including peripheral neuropathy, dorsal column dysfunction (loss of vibratory and position sense in the lower extremities), and changes in affect, are common. If the deficiency is not corrected, lateral column dysfunction (weakness and spasticity) also occurs. The anemia develops so slowly that patients frequently present with very low hematocrit values and yet remarkably good cardiovascular compensation for their anemia. Such patients usually have an expanded total blood volume and are prone to develop heart failure if given transfusions. B_{12} deficiency from other causes (Table 50.12) is less common. Patients who have had total gastrectomy or ileal resection or who have ileal disease (Crohn's disease, tropical sprue) are likely to develop B_{12} deficiency and should receive prophylactic B_{12}. B_{12} deficiency after partial gastrectomy is much less frequent. There is growing evidence that subtle B_{12} malabsorption may occur and lead to neuropsychiatric sequelae secondary to vitamin B_{12} deficiency. These patients may have normal hematologic values and normal Schilling tests (see below). Their vitamin B_{12} levels are usually low, although frequently not as low as those seen in pernicious anemia. Diagnosis requires more sensitive tests of B_{12} metabolism, which are not readily available, such as serum or urine methylmalonic acid and homocysteine (19). The mechanism of B_{12} deficiency in such patients is unclear, although it may be due, at least in some patients, to an inability to absorb food-bound B_{12}, even though they secrete normal amounts of intrinsic factor (4).

In contrast to B_{12} the body's stores of folic acid are depleted rapidly when patients eat a diet deficient in folate. (The main sources of folate in the diet are leafy vegetables, fruits, nuts, and liver.) Folic acid deficiency, therefore, is most often dietary. For example, pregnant women have an increased need for folate and without prenatal supplementation may develop folate deficiency, as may patients whose dietary intake is severely restricted because of chronic disease or multiple surgical procedures. Intestinal malabsorption due to any cause is also a common cause of folate deficiency. Finally, a number of drugs may be associated with folate deficiency: Phenytoin (Dilantin) interferes with folate absorption; alcohol interferes with folate utilization; and methotrexate and trimethoprim-sulfamethoxazole (Bactrim, Septra) interfere with folate metabolism. Also some chemotherapeutic agents used in the treatment of cancer and to induce immunosuppression in patients with a variety of disorders (e.g., psoriasis, systemic lupus) cause megaloblastosis (e.g., hydroxyurea, cytosine arabinoside, methotrexate, Imuran) by inhibiting DNA synthesis.

Diagnosis

The morphology of the peripheral blood and bone marrow is the same in patients with folic acid and B_{12} deficiencies. With a severe megaloblastic anemia the MCV is frequently markedly elevated. An MCV of greater than 120 fl is almost always due to a megaloblastic anemia. The red cells in the peripheral blood are characterized by marked variation in size and shape. The common cell is a macro-ovalocyte (large egg-shaped cell). One may also see Howell-Jolly bodies (nuclear fragments), Pappenheimer bodies (iron granules), and nucleated red blood cells. The nuclei of the neutrophils are frequently hypersegmented, and commonly there is a neutropenia and thrombocytopenia. The bone marrow is typically markedly cellular, revealing characteristic megaloblastic changes of all cell lines. The bone marrow iron stain usually reveals increased numbers of iron-containing nucleated red cells (sideroblasts).

Folic acid and B_{12} assay. Classically in B_{12} deficiency (pernicious anemia), the serum B_{12} level is quite low (less than 100 pg/ml) and the serum folate level is high. Spuriously normal B_{12} levels may occasionally be seen in B_{12} deficiency, and spuriously low levels may be seen without B_{12} deficiency in some patients with folic acid deficiency (see Table 50.13). The serum folate assay has little clinical usefulness in the workup of a megaloblastic anemia secondary to folic acid deficiency. The red cell folate concentration does reflect chronic folate deficiency, although it may be falsely low in some patients with B_{12} deficiency (Table 50.13).

The Schilling Test. The Schilling test is a measure of B_{12} absorption and requires the measurement of total radioactivity excreted during a 24-hour period after the ingestion of radioactive B_{12}. This test is primarily useful in cases where the data are confusing and/or in patients already treated with B_{12}, when the serum levels are no longer helpful. The Schilling test requires a cooperative patient who is able to collect a 24-hour urine sample. The test includes the following steps: After voiding, the patient takes 0.5 μCi of ^{60}Co or ^{57}Co cyanocobalamine by mouth. A 24-hour urine

collection is initiated; at 2 hours 1 mg of B_{12} is given by injection (the flushing dose) and the percentage of the radioactive B_{12} excreted in 24 hours is determined. Normally 7% or more of the dose is excreted in 24 hours. Incomplete collection will result in a spuriously low Schilling test and a false diagnosis of B_{12} malabsorption. In addition, if there is severe megaloblastic anemia, there are changes in the gastrointestinal mucosa that will affect B_{12} absorption. For example, the Schilling test may be abnormal in folic acid deficiency until the megaloblastic process is treated for a week or 2 (see Table 50.14).

Table 50.15 outlines a stepwise approach to the use of the laboratory in differentiating between folic acid and B_{12} deficiency in a patient with a megaloblastic anemia.

Other laboratory features. Megaloblastic anemias are essentially hemolytic in that there is marked destruction of abnormally formed cells within the marrow (ineffective erythropoiesis), which frequently results in indirect hyperbilirubinemia and an elevated serum lactate dehydrogenase. The serum iron is usually elevated, and the reticulocyte index is inappropriately low.

Gastric achlorhydria is present in pernicious anemia, and antibodies to gastric mucosal cells and to intrinsic factor are frequently present, as are other autoantibodies, especially antithyroid and antiadrenal antibodies. The most useful of these tests is the assay of anti-intrinsic factor antibody in serum, which is reasonably specific for pernicious anemia and is present in approximately 70% of cases. There is an increased prevalence of thyroid disease (hypo- and hyperthyroidism and euthyroid goiter) in patients with pernicious anemia.

Treatment

The usual treatment for B_{12} deficiency is monthly intramuscular administration of 100 μg of B_{12} for the rest of the patient's life. Many physicians will treat patients daily while they are in the hospital, particularly if they have neurological signs; however, there is little evidence that this practice is efficacious.

One to 5 mg of folic acid daily is adequate treatment for patients with folic acid deficiency. Treatment should be given at least until a normal hematocrit level is reached and should be continued if the patient is not eating an adequate diet or if the underlying disease persists (e.g., malabsorption). Patients with a chronic

Table 50.13.
B_{12} and Folate Concentrations

Serum B_{12} Concentration
  1. Spuriously low in some patients with folate deficiency.
  2. Spuriously low in some pregnant patients.
  3. May be elevated for weeks after one injection of B_{12}.
  4. Increased in myeloproliferative syndromes.
RBC Folate Concentration
  1. Reflects chronic folate deficiency.
  2. Falsely low in some patients with B_{12} deficiency.
  3. Falsely high in patients with reticulocytosis.
Serum Folate Concentration
  1. A measure of recent dietary intake of folate.
  2. May be low, normal, or elevated in B_{12} deficiency.

Table 50.14.
Causes, Other Than Pernicious Anemia, of a Positive Schilling Test

1. Incomplete urine collection
2. Renal failure
3. Some patients with megaloblastic anemia before treatment
4. Gastric antibodies to intrinsic factor
5. Defective intrinsic factor
6. Drugs (alcohol, colchicine, neomycin, cholestryamine)
7. Pancreatic insufficiency

Table 50.15.
Differentiating between Folate and B$_{12}$ Megaloblastosis

Etiology by History	RBC Folate	Serum B$_{12}$	Interpretation	Further Testing
Suggests folate	↓	Nl or ↑	Folate deficiency	None
Suggests folate	↓	Sl ↓	Folate deficiency	Recheck B$_{12}$ after folate Rx for 1 week
Suggests B$_{12}$	Nl or ↑	↓	B$_{12}$ deficiency	None
Suggests B$_{12}$	↓ (serum folate usually ↑)	↓	B$_{12}$ deficiency	May confirm with Schilling test
All other combinations → Schilling test.				

hemolytic state, such as sickle cell anemia, patients on hemodialysis (folic acid is dialyzable), and pregnant patients, should receive prophylactic treatment. Whether patients are hospitalized depends on the severity of their symptoms and signs, the severity of their anemia, and, in the case of folate deficiency, the nature of their underlying disease.

With appropriate treatment of megaloblastic anemia there is a rapid reticulocytosis, which reaches a peak at about 7 to 10 days; the hematocrit value begins to rise in about 1 week; in uncomplicated cases it will rise at a rate of 4 to 5 percentage points/week. The leukopenia and thrombocytopenia respond dramatically, and white blood cell and platelet counts may return to normal in a day or 2. There is a variable response of the neurological complications of B$_{12}$ deficiency. "Megaloblastic madness" usually abates dramatically. Dorsal column problems and peripheral neuropathies will usually improve, but more slowly. Cortical spinal tract signs are usually refractory to treatment.

The Myelodysplastic Syndromes

These syndromes (17) are acquired disorders of bone marrow stem cells, seen in elderly patients, that at presentation may mimic a megaloblastic anemia. However, the morphological features of the bone marrow, and usually the peripheral smear, are different (Table 50.16). White cell and platelet morphology may

be abnormal, the serum B$_{12}$ and folic acid levels are high, and the patients do not respond to folic acid or B$_{12}$. In the bone marrow ringed sideroblasts (red cell precursors containing granules of iron that form a ring around the nuclei) are common, as are megaloblastoid changes. Approximately 25% of patients develop acute nonlymphocytic leukemia, usually within a year, but sometimes only after several years.

ANEMIAS WITH NORMAL MCV AND APPROPRIATE RETICULOCYTE INDEX (HEMOLYSIS AND BLEEDING)

Anemias due to bleeding and hemolysis are associated with an appropriate bone marrow response manifested by an appropriate reticulocyte index. The MCV is usually normal; however, if the reticulocyte count is high, the MCV may be slightly elevated. The diagnosis of hemolysis is suggested by an anemia with a reticulocyte index of at least 3% in the absence of overt bleeding. It should be remembered that bleeding is far more common than hemolysis and that bleeding in certain body sites (e.g., retroperitoneal bleeding in patients taking anticoagulants or bleeding into the site of a hip fracture) may be associated with a marked drop in hematocrit value and a high reticulocyte count, without external evidence of blood loss. Furthermore, the correction of anemias that are due to decreased bone marrow production may also give a data base that mimics hemolysis (e.g., patients with an appro-

Table 50.16.
Laboratory Features in Three Conditions Associated with an Elevated Mean Corpuscular Volume

	Liver Disease	Megaloblastic Anemia	Myelodysplastic Syndrome
MCV	Usually <115 fl	Frequently >115 fl	Usually <115 fl
White blood cell count (WBCs)	Variable	Frequently decreased	Frequently decreased
Platelet count	Variable	Frequently decreased	Frequently decreased
Red blood cell (RBC) morphology	Targets, no poikilocytosis	Marked anisocytosis and poikilocytosis, macro-ovalocytes	Marked anisocytosis and poikilocytosis, may mimic megaloblastic anemia
Nucleated RBCs	Not common	Common	Common
WBC morphology	Normal	Hypersegmented nuclei of neutrophils	May have abnormal mononuclear cells, no nuclear hypersegmentation of neutrophils
Platelet morphology	Normal	Normal	May be large and degranulated
RBC folate	Depends on diet	Decreased in folate deficiency, normal or slightly decreased in B$_{12}$ deficiency	Normal or elevated
Serum B$_{12}$	Normal	Decreased in B$_{12}$ deficiency, may be slightly decreased in folate deficiency	Normal or elevated

priate reticulocyte response after being treated with iron, folic acid, or B$_{12}$, or after alcohol withdrawal).

Approach to Hemolysis (25)

It is appropriate to attempt to prove that hemolysis is occurring before obtaining diagnostic tests in a search for specific etiologies. The diagnostic approach to hemolysis varies, depending upon whether hemolysis is primarily intravascular or extravascular.

Intravascular Hemolysis

Table 50.17 lists hemolytic mechanisms associated with intravascular destruction of red cells. Almost all of them require that the patient be hospitalized and that, if possible, diagnostic testing and treatment be planned in consultation with a hematologist. In intravascular hemolysis red cell lysis occurs within the vascular space, resulting in hemoglobinemia. The plasma becomes visibly red or brown (methemoglobinemia) at a low concentration of hemoglobin (approximately 30 mg/100 ml). Free hemoglobin initially binds to haptoglobin (a binding protein produced in the liver). Once haptoglobin is saturated, free hemoglobin passes through the glomerulus and hemoglobinuria occurs. Some of the hemoglobin in the renal tubules is absorbed by the renal tubular cells, which slough into the urine several days later and stain positively for iron (urine hemosiderin). The latter test, therefore, is helpful in documenting the presence of intravascular hemolysis several days after it has occurred. Table 50.18 suggests an appropriate data base when hemolysis is suspected in those clinical states associated with intravascular hemolysis.

Extravascular Hemolysis

Most hemolysis occurs extravascularly within cells of the reticuloendothelial system. A diagnosis of extravascular hemolysis is more difficult to prove than

that of intravascular hemolysis. There is no hemoglobinemia, hemoglobinuria, or hemosiderinuria. Haptoglobin is only partially saturated because there is a slight leakage of free hemoglobin into the circulation. There may be indirect hyperbilirubinemia, but this is an extremely insensitive sign of hemolysis. There is an increase in fecal and urine urobilinogen, but these substances are also difficult to quantitate. Other tests of hemolysis, such as red cell survival, are difficult, and the results are not known for several days. The physician must frequently be satisfied with only a presumptive diagnosis of extravascular hemolysis. Therefore, when extravascular hemolysis is suspected, it may be appropriate to obtain tests diagnostic of specific disease states based on a knowledge of the patient's other problems and on the baseline data base (Table 50.19).

Information from the peripheral smear. In hemolytic states the peripheral smear frequently reveals only evidence of the response of the bone marrow to hemolysis (large polychromatophilic or finely stippled red cells). It does not, as many physicians believe, always reveal fragmented red cells. Occasionally, however, the smear may give further clues about the specific etiology of the hemolysis as indicated below.

Spherocytes. Spherocytes are seen in small numbers in many hemolytic states. When present in large numbers they suggest either hereditary spherocytosis, autoimmune hemolysis, or one of the hemoglobin C hemoglobinopathies.

Elliptocytes. In large numbers these suggest a diagnosis of hereditary elliptocytosis.

Fragmented cells (schistocytes). Sharply pointed fragmented cells (helmet cells, spiculated cells, triangle cells) are seen in microangiopathic states (see page 559).

Spiculated cells. Sometimes these cells are seen in patients with severe liver disease and hemolysis (usually in a terminal stage of liver disease). Spiculated cells are also one type of schistocyte found in the blood of patients with microangiopathic hemolysis.

"Bite" cells (blister cells). Such cells are sometimes seen in patients with oxidative hemolysis (e.g., glucose 6-phosphate dehydrogenase deficiency). In "bite" cells all of the hemoglobin appears to be pushed to one side of the cell.

Poikilocytosis and the hemoglobinopathies. In patients with sickle cell disease and in the various other sickle cell syndromes the peripheral smear is frequently diagnostic (see below).

Table 50.17.
Clinical States Associated with Intravascular Hemolysis

Acute hemolytic transfusion reactions
Severe and extensive burns
Physical trauma (*e.g.*, march hemoglobinuria)
Severe microangiopathic hemolysis (*e.g.*, aortic value prosthesis)
Glucose 6-phosphate dehydrogenase deficiency
Paroxysmal nocturnal hemoglobinuria
Clostridial sepsis

Table 50.18.
Appropriate Further Data Base When Intravascular Hemolysis Is Suspected

Observation of the color of the serum/plasma
Observation of the color of the urine
Measurement of free plasma hemoglobin
Heme pigment test of the urine if there are no red cells in the urine sediment
Measurement of serum haptoglobin
Iron stain of urine sediment for hemosiderin several days after a presumed hemolytic event

Table 50.19.
Most Common Causes of Extravascular Hemolysis

Autoimmune hemolysis
Delayed hemolytic transfusion reactions
Hemoglobinopathies
Hereditary spherocytic and nonspherocytic anemia
Hypersplenism
Hemolysis with liver disease

Hemolysis with a Positive Coombs' Test (22)

Once the physician suspects hemolysis, the diagnostic testing should be guided by the patient's problem list. Because of the relatively common occurrence of immune hemolysis and the important therapeutic implications of such a diagnosis, it is desirable to obtain a Coombs' test at this stage in the workup.

Positive Direct Coombs' Test

The direct Coombs' test is done by mixing the patients cells with Coombs' antiserum containing antibody to IgG and to complement. If the test is positive, the physician should first ascertain from the laboratory personnel that the positive result is attributable to antibody and/or complement on the red cell surface. If this is the case, it is important to determine whether the antibody is an *alloantibody* or an *autoantibody*.

Alloantibodies are antibodies induced by prior transfusion or, in a woman, by placental transfer of fetal red cells. The antibodies are directed against specific minor red cell antigens, and it is important to identify them in the event that future transfusions are necessary. Ordinarily the antibody is primarily present in the patient's plasma and is identified by an antibody screen (indirect Coombs' test). However, a direct Coombs' test would also be positive due to the presence of alloantibodies if the patient had recently been transfused with cells that were still circulating and sensitized by the antibody.

In a patient with hemolysis, if there has not been a recent transfusion, a positive direct Coombs' test generally implies the presence of an autoantibody. In this situation the antibody may be present in the serum as well as on the surface of the red cells. Table 50.20 describes the differences between allo- and autoantibodies. Autoantibodies are classified as either *warm antibodies* or *cold antibodies*. Warm antibodies are usually IgG and cannot be identified by direct agglutination of red cells, but require a Coombs' test. Cold antibodies, however, are usually IgM, cause direct agglutination of red cells in the cold, and result in a positive Coombs' test because of fixation of complement to the red cell, which is identified by nonspecific Coombs' antiserum.

Hemolysis Due to Warm Antibodies

Table 50.21 lists the conditions commonly associated with autoimmune hemolysis resulting from a warm antibody. Patients may develop such antibodies secondary to one of a number of conditions, including infections (particularly viral), collagen vascular disease [systemic lupus erythematosus (SLE)], lymphoproliferative diseases, other malignancies, and secondary also to the effect of drugs. The most common drug causing a positive Coombs' test is α-methyldopa (Aldomet) (26). A positive Coombs' test is not usually observed unless the patient has been taking high doses of Aldomet for a long period of time; in such circumstances a positive Coombs' test is not uncommon, but hemolysis is rare.

Autoimmune hemolysis is a relatively infrequent condition; sometimes it precedes the development of SLE or lymphoma. Patients usually present with anemia, which may be severe. On physical examination the spleen is slightly enlarged in 50% of patients, and mild jaundice and fever are not uncommon. The peripheral smear shows a marked polychromatophilia, spherocytosis, and, frequently, a markedly elevated reticulocyte count. Autoimmune hemolysis that is temporary, e.g., caused by drug administration or by viral infections, usually requires no treatment (although if a drug is implicated, it should be discontinued). The process gradually remits over the course of 3 to 4 weeks. Patients receiving Aldomet, who do not have hemolysis but do have a positive Coombs' test, need not discontinue use of the drug. Patients with chronic primary autoimmune hemolysis should be referred to a hematologist, who usually prescribes corticosteroids, which are usually effective if first given in reasonably high doses and slowly tapered as the anemia improves. Occasionally splenectomy is required for refractory cases. In patients with secondary chronic autoimmune hemolysis treatment of the underlying disease is the most important therapy. Autoimmune hemolysis may sometimes present as a fulminant life-threatening anemia, sometimes associated with reticulocytopenia. In such cases patients should be hospitalized immediately and transfused in spite of the incompatible cross-match.

Cold Agglutinin Hemolysis

The most common etiology of autoimmune hemolysis due to a cold antibody is a viral illness or mycoplasma pneumonia (15). Severe hemolysis is rare. Chronic cold agglutinin hemolysis secondary to a collagen vascular disorder or to a lymphoproliferative disease is frequently more refractory to treatment with steroids and splenectomy than is the case with warm antibody hemolysis. Transfusion therapy may be a problem in such cases since the antibody is a panagglutinin and reacts with all blood types; therefore, a

Table 50.20.
Compairson of Alloantibody and Autoantibody

	Alloantibody	Autoantibody
Direct Coombs' test	Frequently negative; may be positive if sensitized foreign red cells are still circulating	Positive
Indirect Coombs' test	Positive	Positive or negative
Antibody screen (panel)	Specificity is seen	Panagglutination, no specificity seen

Table 50.21.
Autoimmune Hemolysis Due to a "Warm Antibody":
Differential Diagnosis

Idiopathic
Secondary
  Infection (particularly viral)
  Drugs
    α-Methyldopa
    Penicillin
    Quinine/quinidine
  Collagen vascular disease (systemic lupus erythematosus)
  Lymphoproliferative disorders
  Miscellaneous (thyroid disease, malignancy, *etc*)

Table 50.22.
Hemolysis with Fragmented Red Cells on Peripheral
Smear: Differential Diagnosis

Aortic value prosthesis
Arteritis (malignant hypertension, polyarteritis, *etc*)
Disseminated intravascular coagulation
Thrombotic thrombocytopenic purpura
Hemolytic uremic syndrome
Malignancy
Giant hemangiomas
Renal transplant rejection
Eclampsia

compatible cross-match may be impossible to obtain. Ordinarily the IgM antibody in cold agglutinin hemolysis is not significantly hemolytic, and transfusions with warmed washed red cells may be attempted when absolutely necessary (24).

Hemolysis with Fragmented Red Cells on Peripheral Smear (3)

Table 50.22 lists those conditions associated with hemolysis and the presence of fragmented red cells on peripheral smear. The peripheral blood is characterized by the presence of sharply pointed poikilocytes (schistocytes). Such cells are quite characteristic and are clearly differentiated from abnormally shaped red cells seen in other conditions. The hemolysis may be severe and in such cases is usually intravascular, resulting in hemoglobinemia, hemoglobinuria, haptoglobin saturation, and, subsequently, hemosiderinuria (page 557). Red cell fragmentation may occur after insertion of a prosthetic aortic valve. Rarely this may be associated with clinically significant hemolysis. More frequently red cell fragmentation is due to arteriolar lesions (fibrin, inflammation, etc.) that cause damage to red cells as they pass through the damaged vessel. When fragmented red cells are accompanied by thrombocytopenia, one should consider the possibility of *disseminated intravascular coagulation* (Chapter 51) and of *thrombotic thrombocytopenic purpura*. This latter syndrome is usually accompanied by fever and neurological deficits, which characteristically fluctuate. Patients suspected of suffering from this condition should be hospitalized immediately and treated in consultation with a hematologist. The hemolytic uremic syndrome is a related (perhaps identical) syndrome, more common in children, characterized

by the prominence of renal failure over other organ dysfunction.

Hemolysis with Enlarged Spleen (Hypersplenism) (9)

It is important to remember that not all large spleens cause "cytopenias" and that the degree of cytopenia does not necessarily correlate with the size of the spleen. Thrombocytopenia and leukopenia are more common than is anemia. Splenomegaly, from almost any cause, may result in hypersplenism, but the syndrome is seen most often in patients who have chronic liver disease and congestive splenomegaly. Splenomegaly is sometimes seen in patients with hemolysis from other mechanisms, such as autoimmune hemolysis or hereditary spherocytosis. Rarely, splenectomy is necessary because of severe cytopenias resulting from hypersplenism. Occasional patients with Felty's syndrome (see Chapter 70) are benefited by splenectomy, as are some patients with chronic leukemia or lymphoma.

Glucose 6-Phosphate Dehydrogenase Deficiency

Glucose 6-phosphate dehydrogenase (G-6-PD) deficiency (2) is seen primarily in black patients in the United States. Inheritance is sex linked. Ten percent of black males are affected (hemizygotes), as are 20% of black females (heterozygotes). In the affected black patients hemolysis due to G-6-PD deficiency is an acute intravascular hemolytic event usually precipitated either by infection or by an oxidant drug. Drugs known to precipitate hemolysis include sulfonamides, nitrofurantoin, and primaquine. Caucasian-type G-6-PD deficiency is seen primarily in patients from Mediterranean countries and usually is more severe than the African type, sometimes causing chronic persisting, partially compensated, hemolysis.

Diagnosis after a hemolytic event may be difficult, especially in the female heterozygotes. Screening tests for G-6-PD deficiency (available from most commercial and hospital laboratories) may be normal at this time, and even the affected hemizygote black male may have a normal screening test for several weeks after hemolysis (young cells have more G-6-PD activity). Occasionally a characteristic cell ("bite cell") is seen in the peripheral blood during a hemolytic event.

Although the frequency of the genetic defect is high, the incidence of severe hemolysis with provocation (infection, drugs) is low. Ordinarily routine screening before treatment with a known oxidant drug (e.g., sulfonamide) is not advocated. Affected patients should be given a list of drugs to avoid (2), including over-the-counter medications such as phenacetin.

Sickle Cell Disorders (1)

Approximately 8% of the black population in the United States carry the sickle cell gene. The gene is also present to a lesser extent in Greeks, Italians, Arabians, and persons from India. Hemoglobin S results from a mutation in the β-globin chain in hemoglobin that, when oxygen tension is reduced, causes the formation of rigid elongated tactoids that distort red cell shape and increase red cell rigidity. The clumping together of sickled cells leads to tissue ischemia and infarction. A number of common inherited disorders involving hemoglobin S are listed below.

Sickle Cell Trait

Most people who are heterozygous for hemoglobin S (sickle cell trait) are completely well and are not anemic. The peripheral smear appears normal, although sickling is seen if the blood is deoxygenated. Hemoglobin electrophoresis reveals approximately 40% hemoglobin S and 60% hemoglobin A, whereas hemoglobins A_2 and F are present in normal concentration.

Most patients with sickle trait lead a normal life. However, rare clinical events attributable to the presence of sickle cell hemoglobin do occur. For example, splenic infarction at high altitudes (>10,000 feet) has been reported. (Oxygen pressures in commercial aircraft are high enough that individuals with sickle cell trait may fly safely.) Occasionally infarctions occur in other more vital organs during vigorous exercise. All individuals with sickle cell trait have renal tubular dysfunction resulting in hyposthenuria; and on occasion severe hematuria may occur due to hypertonicity in the renal medulla, resulting in sickling and leading to ischemia and tubular infarction. Persons with sickle cell trait have a higher incidence of renal infections, especially during pregnancy.

It is important to identify patients with sickle cell trait so that they may be given genetic counseling. A couple, both heterozygous for hemoglobin S, should be informed that they have a 25% chance of having a child with sickle cell anemia. Prenatal diagnosis of sickle cell anemia by amniocentesis is now possible.

Sickle Cell Anemia (Hemoglobin SS) (1, 6)

Sickle cell anemia exists in approximately 0.15% of the black population in the United States. The disease is usually severe, resulting in significant morbidity as well as in a shortened life expectancy. One of the most disturbing clinical features of the illness is the occurrence of painful ("thrombotic") crises, recurrent episodes of severe pain, usually in the limbs and the abdomen, due to sickling-induced ischemia. Patients have a lifelong, often severe, anemia, with hematocrit values that range from the high teens to the low thirties (average—midtwenties). The primary mechanism of the anemia is extravascular hemolysis, so that there is a chronic reticulocytosis and a chronic indirect hyperbilirubinemia. The patients usually have a leukocytosis, the white count rising occasionally as high as 30,000 to 40,000/ml during a painful crisis. A mild thrombocytosis is also common. The peripheral smear shows markedly distorted red cells including characteristically sickled cells. Upon electrophoresis only

hemoglobin S with a variable amount of hemoglobin F (no hemoglobin A) is detected.

The multiple and repetitive episodes of organ ischemia due to sickling result in a host of abnormalities. The bones characteristically appear abnormal on X-ray, revealing areas of old infarction that mimic the changes of osteomyelitis. The medullary spaces are usually widened due to the marked compensatory expansion of bone marrow. The spine frequently takes on a distorted appearance, and aseptic necrosis of the femoral (and, rarely, humeral) head is common, sometimes requiring joint replacement. Puberty is frequently delayed. Splenomegaly usually disappears by age 8 due to repeated infarctions of the spleen. An adult with sickle cell anemia is essentially autosplenectomized. This lack of splenic function contributes to the propensity for infections, related especially to a decreased ability to resist pneumococcal infections. *Gallstones* (pigment stones) are common, and sicklers do develop cholecystitis, which may be extremely difficult to differentiate clinically from a syndrome of intrahepatic cholestasis secondary to sickling in the hepatic sinusoids. There is some hazard to *surgery*, but patients with recurrent abdominal pain consistent with cholecystitis, who have gallstones, should probably have elective cholecystectomy (see Chapter 90). *Pregnancy* in women with SS disease is complicated by an increased risk of pyelonephritis, pulmonary infarction, antepartum hemorrhage, prematurity, and fetal death. With time, patients develop cardiomegaly and chronic myocardial disease related to repetitive microinfarctions of the heart. Murmurs are frequent and may suggest rheumatic or congenital heart disease. Patients with sickle cell anemia develop venous thromboses and pulmonary embolism. They also develop thromboses in situ in the lungs followed, after many years, by chronic scarring and fibrosis. Pulmonary thrombosis/embolism may lead to pulmonary hypertension and heart failure. Cerebral vascular accidents are common, including infarction and intracerebral and subarachnoid hemorrhage. Seizures are frequent as well. Up to 75% of patients with sickle cell anemia develop *leg ulcerations* that may be chronic and extremely difficult to heal. Sickle cell patients are very prone to serious *retinopathy*, which rarely may lead to blindness, due to plugging of small retinal capillaries and subsequent neovascularization. It is important for these patients to be examined yearly by an ophthalmologist, because some of the problems can be prevented by photocoagulation of abnormal new retinal vessels.

SC Disease

The genes that code for hemoglobin S and hemoglobin C are alleles. The C hemoglobin mutation is relatively common in blacks (about 2% prevalence), and patients doubly heterozygous for S and C constitute approximately 0.15% of that population. The syndrome is very similar to that of SS disease but is usually somewhat more mild. In contrast to sickle cell anemia, the spleen is palpable in 50% of adult patients.

S-Thalassemia

Patients doubly heterozygous for hemoglobin S and β-thalassemia trait have a syndrome similar to sickle cell anemia but usually much more mild. Characteristically the MCV is low. The spleen may be palpable, and the hemoglobin electrophoresis reveals 70 to 80% hemoglobin S and smaller amounts of hemoglobin A and F (the reverse of the pattern in sickle cell trait).

Treatment

Painful "thrombotic" crisis. Painful crises are frequently severe and may last for a few hours to several days and occasionally for several weeks. They may be associated with high fever and with neutrophilia, which makes it difficult but important to differentiate crises from infection. There is no specific therapy. The patient is usually treated with narcotics and with hydration. Because patients can become addicted to narcotics because of the repetitive episodes of severe pain, it is important to limit strictly the amount of narcotics given them in ambulatory practice. When pain is severe and persistent, hospitalization is indicated.

Infection. As mentioned above, patients with sickle cell anemia are prone to infections, especially with the pneumococcus. Patients with sickle cell anemia should receive pneumococcal vaccine (see Chapter 32) and should be encouraged to seek medical help at the first evidence of infection or fever.

Hemolytic and aplastic crises. Acceleration of hemolysis is quite unusual. If hematocrit values drop significantly below baseline, it is most likely to be because of decreased marrow production, associated with infection. Such episodes are much more common in children. If they occur, hospitalization and transfusion are often necessary. Patients with chronic severe hemolysis have an increased requirement for folic acid, and folic acid deficiency may occur, resulting in reticulocytopenia and more severe anemia. Therefore, daily folic acid therapy (1 mg) is reasonable for all patients with sickle cell anemia.

Thrombosis/embolization. When patients with sickle cell disease develop deep vein thrombosis or pulmonary embolism, they should be treated with anticoagulants as would any patient with such problems (see Chapter 52). However, venography should be avoided because of the danger of the development of leg ulcers in any patient with SS hemoglobin whose lower extremities are traumatized. It is frequently difficult to distinguish pulmonary thrombotic/embolic problems from pneumonia.

Leg ulcers. Leg ulcers are often large and are particularly refractory to treatment. Skin grafting is usually only temporarily helpful and frequently does not seem to be worth the time and discomfort involved. It is important to keep the ulcers clean, to elevate the legs

frequently, and to use surgical stockings and elastic wraps (see Chapter 88).

Hematuria. Patients with sickle cell trait, sickle cell anemia, SC disease, and sickle cell-thalassemia all are prone to bouts of severe hematuria related to sickling and to medullary ischemia precipitated by the hypertonicity of the renal medulla. Bleeding can occur for days or even weeks. Maintenance of a high urine flow is important in order to prevent clots from causing obstruction, and usually the hematuria stops spontaneously.

Priapism. Priapism is common in SS and SC disease and usually results in permanent impotence once it has resolved. If urological intervention is to be attempted, it must be done within a few hours of the onset of the priapism. It is frequently only temporarily helpful. Once impotence has occurred, penile protheses are frequently quite helpful.

Recommendations for Preventive Care

1. *General.* It is important to remember that patients with sickle cell disorders have a lifelong chronic illness and will require frequent and recurrent use of the health care system. The patient needs one general physician who is familiar with him. The availability of emergency care 24 hours a day is also exceedingly important.
2. *Infection.* There should be rapid evaluation of fever, chills, or other signs of infection. The patient should be immunized with the pneumococcal vaccine (see Chapter 32). Because heart murmurs and cardiomegaly are common, it is often difficult to know whether a patient with sickle cell anemia has valvular heart disease. If there is any doubt, it is reasonable to prescribe prophylactic antibiotics before dental procedures, etc. (see Chapter 86).
3. *Narcotic abuse.* As mentioned above, analgesics should be given in doses sufficient to relieve pain during a thrombotic crisis. However, the use of narcotics on an ambulatory basis should be avoided if at all possible, since addiction can occur. Easy access to the physician should obviate the need to give the patient a supply of narcotics to take in case of pain.
4. *Folic acid.* Patients should receive 1 mg of folic acid daily.

ANEMIAS WITH NORMAL MCV AND AN INAPPROPRIATELY LOW RETICULOCYTE INDEX

Mild normocytic anemias without appropriate reticulocyte responses are among the most common problems seen in clinical practice. Before considering possible etiologies and embarking on a diagnostic workup, it is important to be sure that the hematocrit value/hemoglobin concentration is reproducibly low. Moreover, the normal values for the laboratory should be known. For example, in some laboratories a hematocrit value of 35% in a woman is normal. One should also consider the variation in normal values related to age, sex, pregnancy, etc. Finally one should be sure that volume overload is not the etiology. Marked volume shifts may result in swings in hematocrit value of 6 or 8 percentage points. Table 50.23 lists the differential diagnosis of a normocytic anemia with an inappropriately low reticulocyte count.

Anemia of Renal Failure (12)

Patients with uremia are anemic primarily because of decreased production of erythropoietin. The red cell morphology on smear is usually normal, but occasionally spiculated cells (burr cells) may be seen. An occasional patient may have a microangiopathic peripheral smear (see page 559). There may be a mild thrombocytopenia, and the nuclei of the neutrophils may be hypersegmented even in the absence of folic acid deficiency. The hematocrit value depends on the degree of renal failure (see Fig. 48.3, Chapter 48). Anemia is unusual if the creatinine is less than 3 mg/100 ml. The hematocrit value seen in patients with renal failure on dialysis is extremely variable (from the low teens, requiring transfusion, up to the midthirties). Recombinant human erythropoietin has been released for the treatment of anemia of renal failure. Responses appear to be dramatic, and although the preparation is expensive, side effects are few (e.g., hypertension in some patients) (13). It is important to remember that patients in renal failure may also be anemic because of iron deficiency (secondary to blood loss) or because of folate deficiency (since folic acid is dialyzable). Some patients with glomerulonephritis or arteritis may have a microangiopathic hemolytic anemia.

Anemia of Chronic Disease (5)

Any chronic inflammatory disease (e.g., rheumatoid arthritis) or malignant neoplastic disease may cause mild to moderate anemia, unrelated to blood loss or hemolysis. (If the hematocrit value is less than 25%, another explanation should be sought.) Red cell morphology is usually normal but occasionally the MCV may be less than 80 fl, requiring differentiation of the process from other causes of a microcytic anemia (see page 551). The serum iron and the total iron-binding capacity are low; the percentage of saturation may be just as low as it is in iron deficiency ($</=10\%$). The

serum ferritin is normal or elevated, and bone marrow iron stores are normal or increased.

In addition to chronic infections, an acute infection or inflammation will cause a decrease in serum iron, reticulocytopenia, and bone marrow red cell production. If present for 1 week or more, therefore, an acute inflammatory process may result in a fall in the hematocrit value of several percentage points.

Mild Early Iron Deficiency

Although severe iron deficiency results in microcytic anemia (see pages 551–553), in the early stages mild iron deficiency may result in anemia with a normal peripheral smear and a normal MCV. Diagnosis can usually be made by measurement of serum ferritin or by a bone marrow iron stain. In addition, a patient with severe iron deficiency, when it accompanies a macrocytic anemia such as a megaloblastic anemia (as in an alcoholic patient with iron deficiency and folic acid deficiency) may have a severe anemia that is normocytic. The reticulocyte count is inappropriately low until alcohol is withdrawn and iron and folate are administered.

Anemia in the Elderly (20)

Old age per se is not an explanation for a significant normocytic anemia. Hematocrit values in healthy patients in their seventies are only slightly lower than they are in the normal adult range (Table 50.1). However, it is in elderly patients that frustrating, mild, unexplained, normocytic anemias occur. In such patients the following possible explanations should be considered: (a) fluid overload, (b) blood loss from phlebotomy if the patient has been hospitalized recently, and (c) any recent inflammatory disease (viral or bacterial infection, inflammatory joint problem) that may depress bone marrow production and, if present for several days, may result in a drop in hematocrit value. If none of the above explanations seems appropriate and there is no reason to suspect an underlying problem to explain the hematocrit value, it is reasonable simply to follow the hematocrit value without further diagnostic workup. If it is known that the anemia is relatively recent (e.g., if there is a record of a normal hematocrit value 3 months previously), then other efforts should be made to explain it. For example, the possibility of occult gastrointestinal bleeding with early iron deficiency and of the anemia of chronic disease (has there been a recent weight loss, fever, etc?) should be entertained.

Table 50.23.
Anemia with a Normal Mean Corpuscular Volume and Low Reticulocyte Index: Differential Diagnosis

Renal failure
Anemia of chronic disease (inflammatory disease and malignancy)
Anemia of hypoendocrine states (hypothyroidism, *etc*)
Mild (early) iron deficiency
Combined iron deficiency and megaloblastic anemia
Sideroblastic anemia
Aplastic anemia
Bone marrow infiltration (myelophthisis)
Bleeding or hemolysis plus one of the above

General References

Williams WJ, Beutler E, Erslev AJ, Lichtman MA (eds): *Hematology*, 4th ed. New York, McGraw-Hill, 1990.
    The currently standard text.

Specific References

1. Abramson H, Bertles JF, Wethers DL (eds): *Sickle Cell Disease*. St Louis, CV Mosby, 1973.
2. Beutler E: Glucose-6-phosphate dehydrogenase deficiency: di-

agnosis; clinical and genetic implications. *Am J Clin Pathol* 47:303, 1967.

3. Brain MC: Microangiopathic hemolytic anemia. *N Engl J Med* 281:833, 1969.

4. Carmel R, Sinow RM, Siegel ME, Samloff IM: Food cobalamin malabsorption occurs frequently in patients with unexplained low serum cobalamin levels. *Arch Intern Med* 148:1715, 1988.

5. Cartwright GE: The anemia of chronic disorders. *Semin Hematol* 3:351, 1966.

6. Charache S: Treatment of sickle cell anemia. *Ann Rev Med* 32:195, 1981.

7. Colman N, Herbert J: Hematologic complications of alcoholism: overview. *Semin Hematol* 17:164, 1980.

8. Cook JD: Clinical evaluation of iron deficiency. *Semin Hematol* 19:6, 1982.

9. Dameshek W: Hypersplenism. *Bull NY Acad Med* 31:113, 1955.

10. Davidson RJL, Hamilton PJ: High mean red cell volume: its incidence and significance in routine hematology. *J Clin Pathol* 31:493, 1978.

11. England JM, Ward S, Down MC: Microcytosis, anisocytosis and the red cell indices in iron deficiency. *Br J Haematol* 34:589, 1976.

12. Erslev AJ: Management of anemia of chronic renal failure. *Clin Nephrol* 2:174, 1974.

13. Eschbach JW, Eqrie JC, Downing MR, et al: Correction of the anemia of end-stage renal disease with recombinant human erythropoietin. Results of a combined phase I and II clinical trial. *N Engl J Med* 316:73, 1987.

14. Halliday JW, Powell LW: Serum ferritin and isoferritins in clinical medicine. *Prog Hematol* 11:229, 1979.

15. Jacobson LB, Longstreth GF, Edgington TS: Clinical and immunologic features of transient cold agglutinin hemolytic anemia. *Am J Med* 54:514, 1973.

16. Kaiser L, Schwartz KA: Aluminum induced anemia. *Am J Kid Dis* 5:348, 1985.

17. Koeffler HP, Golde DW: Human preleukemia. *Ann Intern Med* 93:347, 1980.

18. Lindenbaum J: Status of laboratory testing in the diagnosis of megaloblastic anemia. *Blood* 61:624, 1983.

19. Lindenbaum J, Healton EB, Savage DG, et al: Neuropsychiatric disorders caused by cobalamin deficiency in the absence of anemia or macrocytosis. *N Engl J Med* 318:1720, 1988.

20. Lipschitz DA, Udupa KB, Milton KY, Thompson CO: Effects of age on hematopoiesis in man. *Blood* 63:502, 1984.

21. Pierce HI, Kurachi S, Sofroniadou K, Stamatoyamopoulos G: Frequencies of thalassemia in American blacks. *Blood* 49:981, 1977.

22. Pirofsky G: Clinical aspects of autoimmune hemolytic anemia. *Semin Hematol* 13:251, 1976.

23. Rawley PT: The diagnosis of β-thalassemia trait: a review. *Am J Hematol* 1:129, 1976.

24. Rosenfield RE, Jagathambal : Transfusion therapy for autoimmune hemolytic anemia. *Semin Hematol* 13:311, 1976.

25. Waterbury L: *Hematology for the House Officer*, 3rd ed. Baltimore, Williams & Wilkins, 1988, p.31.

26. Worrledge SM: Immune drug-induced hemolytic anemias. *Semin Hematol* 10:327, 1973.

C H A P T E R   51

Disorders of Hemostasis

PHILIP D. ZIEVE, M.D.

In healthy man a number of different processes interact to ensure that blood is maintained in a fluid state until the integrity of a blood vessel wall is compromised; at that point, a plug is rapidly formed to prevent exsanguination. Three major systems are involved in this regard: the vasculature itself, the blood platelets, and the coagulation system.

EVALUATION OF PATIENTS

The history is the most important aid in determining whether a patient has a hemorrhagic diathesis. Patients with either congenital disorders of hemostasis or acquired disorders of long standing will almost certainly have had unexpectedly excessive bleeding in response to minor trauma or to surgery. The clinician should ask specifically whether the patient has required transfusion after an operative procedure or a seemingly minor trauma.

Bleeding due to trauma to the vasculature is overwhelmingly more common than bleeding due to defective hemostasis. Therefore, patients who present, for example, with gastrointestinal or genitourinary hemorrhage are more likely to have a lesion, such as a peptic ulcer, a carcinoma, a diverticulum, or a tumor of the kidney or of the bladder that has bled than a disorder of hemostasis. Similarly, nose bleeds, bleeding gums, or excessive menstrual flow most likely reflect local (usually benign) problems. Furthermore, even if patients have hemostatic dysfunction, they are likely to bleed from local lesions, the propensity to bleed of which has been accentuated by the hemostatic abnormality.

Specific disorders of hemostasis may be suspected strongly on the basis of the patient's history and because of characteristic findings on physical examination (see Fig. 51.1 and below), but in almost all instances laboratory tests are required before a specific diagnosis can be made. Screening tests, procedures that are extremely sensitive to alterations in hemostasis, are ordinarily relied upon first in a patient with a suspected hemorrhagic diathesis (Table 51.1). If any of these tests is abnormal or if it is strongly suspected that a disorder of hemostasis exists, even if the tests are not abnormal, more specific tests are indicated; these are best performed in consultation with a hematologist. A number of years ago, the bleeding time and the clotting time were the most common tests performed to screen patients for possible disorders of hemostasis. Although both of these have lost favor because of their lack of sensitivity, the bleeding time, as mentioned below, despite its limitations is still the only readily performed procedure to detect qualitative abnormalities of blood platelets (see page 569).

DISORDERS OF BLOOD VESSELS

Vascular disease (Table 51.2) is diagnosed uncommonly as a cause of a hemorrhagic diathesis, in part because, except for trauma, disorders of the vasculature that result in untoward bleeding are relatively rare (2) and in part because there is no reliable screening test to detect generalized vascular dysfunction. The primary hemorrhagic manifestation of vascular disease is purpura, a confluent purplish discoloration of the skin due to extravasation of blood from cutaneous and subcutaneous blood vessels. Although patients with an abnormal vasculature may occasionally experience bleeding from relatively large blood vessels, most commonly they bleed into the skin or mucous membranes. Because purpura is a common response to minor trauma, it cannot in itself be taken as evidence of an underlying hemorrhagic diathesis.

Cutaneous Lesions

Unexplained bruises, especially on the lower extremities, are common and usually are not associated with an underlying disease process. A history of "easy bruisability" therefore is not likely, in itself, to lead to a diagnosis of a disorder of hemostasis. Similarly, *senile purpura*, which occurs characteristically on the dorsum of the hand and the extensor surfaces of the forearms, does not represent a generalized hemorrhagic diathesis but results from the loss of connective tissue support to intracutaneous blood vessels, which then are easily traumatized and bleed within the substance of the skin. Identical lesions are seen sometimes in patients with Cushing's syndrome or in patients who have received corticosteroid therapy.

Allergic purpura (Henoch-Schönlein purpura) (4) represents a hypersensitivity reaction to an antigenic stimulus that usually cannot be identified (although occasionally a drug or a bacterial infection can be incriminated as a provocative agent). Characteristically patients develop a symmetrical petechial rash, most prominent on the extremities. The lesions are slightly raised, distinguishing them from the petechiae of thrombocytopenia. No hemostatic dysfunction is associated with this condition; the cutaneous manifestations of the disorder are part of a widespread vasculitis, the manifestations of which also may include arthralgias (sometimes with evidence of joint effusions), fever, malaise, abdominal pain, gastrointestinal bleeding, and renal disease due to a focal glomerulonephritis that occasionally may progress to chronic renal failure. There is no specific treatment for this condition, although if the patient is taking a drug that is suspected to be a sensitizing agent, it should be discontinued. Most patients recover spontaneously within 3 or 4 weeks, but sometimes signs and symptoms of the disease continue for up to a year. Patients should be reassured while they are symptomatic that unless they have evidence of progressive renal disease, they will ultimately recover.

Autoerythrocyte sensitization (17) is a disorder characterized by apparently spontaneous painful ecchymoses, usually on the lower extremities and anterior trunk. The disorder is named as it is because of a belief at one time that it arose as the result of a hypersensitivity response to the patients' red cells or red cell stroma, and in fact the lesions can sometimes

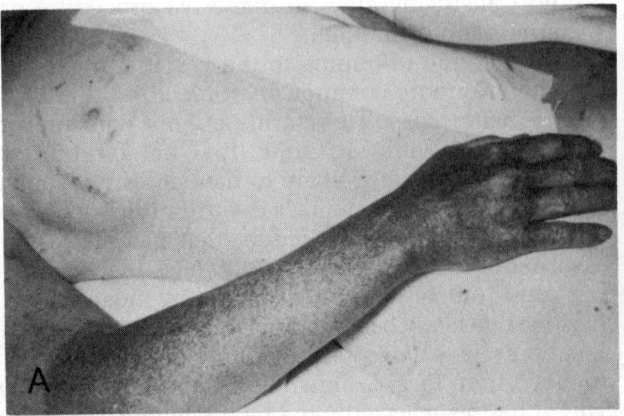
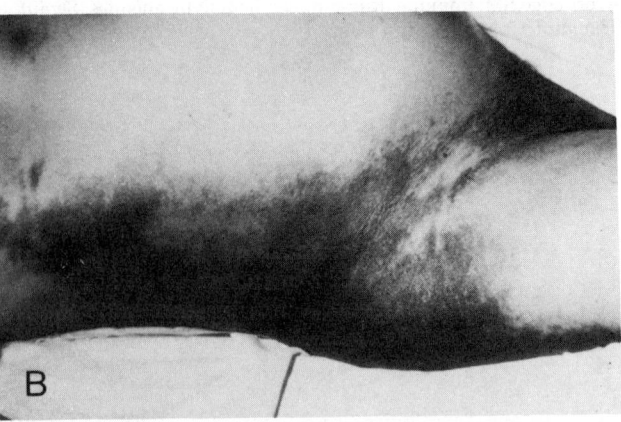

Figure 51.1. Bleeding due to thrombocytopenia compared with bleeding due to abnormal coagulation. *A.* Immune thrombocytopenic purpura. *B.* Hemophilia A. (From Zieve PD, Levin J: *Disorders of Hemostasis.* Philadelphia, WB Saunders, 1976.)

Table 51.1.
Laboratory Evaluation of Hemostatic Function

System	Screening Tests	Specific Tests
Blood vessels	None	Depends on suspected underlying disorder (see the text)
Platelets— quantitative	Scanning of a stained smear of the peripheral blood	Platelet count
Platelets— qualitative	Bleeding time	Platelet aggregation
Coagulation	Partial thromboplastin time, prothrombin time, thrombin time	Factor assays

Table 51.2.
Bleeding Due to Vascular Disease

Cutaneous	Muccutaneous
Senile purpura	Amyloidosis
Steroid purpura	Myeloma
Autoerythrocyte sensitization	Macroglobulinemia
Cryoglobulinemia	Vitamin C deficiency
Hyperglobulinemia of Waldenström	Hereditary hemorrhagic telangiectasia

be produced by injection of autologous red cells into the skin of these patients. It has become apparent, however, that virtually all patients with the disorder, most of whom are women, are severely psychoneurotic and in some instances frankly psychotic; and many people believe now that the lesions are self-inflicted.

Cryoglobulinemia (8, 9) as a primary abnormality or as a special feature of an underlying disease such as dysproteinemia (see below), lymphoma, or collagen vascular disease may also cause purpuric bleeding, especially on the lower extremities. The cryoglobulins may be isolated monoclonal proteins or may be immune complexes of either monoclonal IgG or IgM and polyclonal IgG or of mixed polyclonal immunoglobulins. There is often an associated glomerulonephritis and, in the patient with immune complex formation, sometimes evidence of hepatitis B infection (8).

The diagnosis of cryoglobulinemia may be made by placing a sample of the patient's serum in a refrigerator overnight and then inspecting the serum to see whether a white gel or precipitate has formed that disappears when the specimen is warmed. The blood for this test should be drawn in a warm syringe, and then it should be allowed to clot and retract in a 37°C water bath. Primary cryoglobulinemia is poorly responsive to treatment; secondary cryoglobulinemia may respond to treatment of the underlying disease.

Hyperglobulinemic purpura of Waldenström (11) is a rare poorly defined condition characterized by purpura, especially of the lower extremities, an elevated erythrocyte sedimentation rate, mild anemia, and a polyclonal increase in the blood of a mixture of IgG and anti-IgG immunoglobulins. The disease is more common in women and, particularly after the age of 40, may be associated with an underlying collagen

vascular disorder. The primary condition is untreatable but is generally benign.

Mucocutaneous Lesions

Some patients with vascular disease are prone to bleed from the oral, nasal, or gastrointestinal mucosa, as well as from the skin. Such patients may present to their physicians, not only with cutaneous hemorrhage, but with bleeding gums, epistaxis, hematemesis, or melena.

Amyloidosis (7, 12). Mucocutaneous bleeding may be a symptom of amyloidosis because of the deposition of amyloid within the walls of blood vessels. Periorbital bleeding and bleeding in skin folds are especially common. The skin in the areas of hemorrhage sometimes appears thickened because of palpable amyloid deposits within it. Patients suspected of having this disorder should have skin biopsies with appropriate staining as well as serum and urine electrophoresis in an attempt to make a specific diagnosis.

Dysproteinemia (16). Either myeloma or macroglobulinemia may be associated with untoward bleeding, either because of increased viscosity of the blood or because the coating of blood vessels and platelets with the abnormal protein interferes with normal hemostatic function. Abnormal coagulation is also common in patients with these disorders. Patients suspected of having dysproteinemia should have samples of their serum and urine examined by electrophoresis in an attempt to demonstrate a monoclonal protein. If the diagnosis of dysproteinemia seems likely on the basis of this test and of the clinical presentation, consultation with a hematologist or oncologist is appropriate.

Vitamin C deficiency (10). There are three situations in which symptomatic vitamin C deficiency (scurvy) might be seen in this country: in chronic alcoholics, in food faddists, and in chronically ill or debilitated patients. Because humans, unlike most animals, are unable to synthesize vitamin C, they are dependent upon exogenous sources such as fruits or leafy vegetables. People who cannot or will not eat an adequate diet of foods that contain the vitamin are subject to the manifestations of scurvy. The signs and symptoms of scurvy are largely attributable to the formation of defective connective tissue, because of the human body's absolute dependence on vitamin C for the synthesis of normal collagen. Mucocutaneous bleeding is common in patients with vitamin C deficiency who present characteristically with large ecchymoses on their extremities, with bleeding gums, and, very suggestive of this disorder, with perifollicular hemorrhages that appear commonly on the lower extremities and anterior trunk. Sometimes patients with vitamin C deficiency develop hemarthroses similar to those seen in patients with severe coagulation disorders. All of the manifestations of scurvy are readily reversed by administration of vitamin C, so that although the disorder is uncommon it should be considered in patients with compatible signs and symptoms. Vitamin C deficiency can be confirmed by assay of the blood, but this is usually unnecessary since, if the diagnosis is suspected, a therapeutic trial of vitamin C (250 mg once a day) is innocuous.

Hereditary hemorrhagic telangiectasia (15). This is an inherited abnormality of blood vessels (an autosomal dominant condition) in which there is dilation of abnormally thin-walled venules and capillaries. The dilations result in characteristic telangiectases, which are small, flat, red, or purple lesions that blanch on pressure. They occur throughout the body but can be seen externally most commonly on the lips, the tongue, the mucous membranes of the nose, and the hands. Lesions of larger blood vessels also occur in this disease, most commonly pulmonary arteriovenous fistulas, which develop in up to one-third of patients and which may cause "high output" heart failure. Vascular malformations of the liver or the brain also may occur. The mucocutaneous lesions may bleed excessively when traumatized. Recurrent epistaxis is the most common symptom of patients with the disorder, but the most troublesome problem is recurrent gastrointestinal bleeding, which is notoriously difficult to manage. Accessible lesions can ordinarily be treated by local compression. There is no pharmacological agent that will alter the course of the condition, but symptoms are quite variable; many patients experience relatively little difficulty during the course of their life.

DISORDERS OF PLATELETS

Platelets provide a cellular defense against the loss of blood from traumatized vessels, especially where blood flow is relatively rapid, as it is on the arterial side of the circulation and in the left heart. Platelets are particularly effective in sealing leaks from small arterioles and capillaries; when platelets are abnormal, either quantitatively or qualitatively, it is these vessels that bleed most prominently. The platelet plug is initiated by the exposure of platelets to subendothelial collagen, which is exposed by injury to the vascular intima. The absorption of a protein, von Willebrand factor (VWF—see page 570), to specific receptor sites on the platelet surface is important in the mediation of this process. Thereafter, aggregating agents such as thrombin and adenosine diphosphate cause the accretion of platelets at that site, eventually forming an adhesive plug that within minutes prevents the further flow of blood. Eventually the plug is replaced by fibrin laid down by the activation of the coagulation mechanism, which occurs simultaneously with the initiation of platelet plug formation.

Thrombocytopenia is one of the most common acquired disorders of hemostasis. The normal platelet count is between 150,000 and 350 to 400,000/mm³, but the platelet count ordinarily must be reduced below 50,000/mm³ before untoward bleeding is observed, and even then bleeding usually does not occur unless the patient is traumatized. So-called spontaneous bleeding is unlikely unless the platelet count is reduced below 20,000/mm³. The characteristic lesion of thrombocytopenia is the petechia, a small purpuric

hemorrhage occurring on the skin or mucous membranes, especially at sites of elevated capillary pressure, such as the lower extremities, the forearm after inflation of a blood pressure cuff, or the face after prolonged crying or coughing. In fact, if capillary pressure is raised high enough, or if capillaries are damaged after sunburn, for example, petechiae may be seen in otherwise normal people. Although cutaneous bleeding may be the first clue to the diagnosis of thrombocytopenia, morbidity from the disorder is more likely to result from gastrointestinal or genitourinary hemorrhage. As previously mentioned (see page 563), if bleeding from these sites occurs, the patient should be examined at an appropriate time to determine whether an organic lesion, such as a carcinoma of the colon or of the kidney, has bled in association with defective hemostasis. The most feared complication of thrombocytopenia is intracerebral bleeding that, although it occurs infrequently, is still one of the major causes of death in patients with the disorder.

Evaluation of the Thrombocytopenic Patient

The best screening test for the evaluation of the numbers of platelets in the blood is observation of a stained smear of the peripheral blood. With relatively little experience it is easy to determine whether the platelet count is unusually low or high. In unanticoagulated blood (e.g., from a fingerstick,) at least one clump of platelets should be seen, on the average, in every oil immersion field. In anticoagulated blood, one platelet should be seen for every 10 to 20 red cells. If a quantitative abnormality is suspected, a precise platelet count can be obtained. Such tests as the bleeding time and the measurement of clot retraction are much less useful as screening tests for detecting quantitative abnormalities of platelets. However, the bleeding time, despite its limitations, is still the best screening test to evaluate qualitative abnormalities of platelet function (see page 569).

Patient experience. The bleeding time should be done by use of a commercially available, spring-loaded, disposable device (Simplate), which makes a small incision in the forearm. The examiner should puncture the skin with a disposable lancet. A blood pressure cuff should be inflated to 40 mm Hg above the elbow during the test. The time between the instant the puncture is made and the point at which blood from the wound can no longer be adsorbed onto a piece of filter paper is the bleeding time (normally 3 to 7 minutes). The patient should be warned of the very transient sharp pain that he will experience when the wound is made and of the small scar, usually inapparent, that may form when the wound heals.

Patients with an immune thrombocytopenia (see below) characteristically have increased amounts of gammaglobulin adsorbed to their platelets. Serologic tests to detach these proteins are widely available but have proved to be relatively nonspecific and therefore of little value in establishing a precise diagnosis.

In ambulatory practice patients will most often be encountered with platelet counts lower than normal in whom the precise pathophysiology of thrombocytopenia is not clear.

Many patients are found to have thrombocytopenia during the course of routine hematological studies performed to obtain baseline data, or as part of an evaluation of an apparently unrelated condition. If the platelet count is over 50,000/mm^3 in such circumstances, and the history, physical examination, and other hematological evaluation do not suggest that an underlying disease is present that urgently requires diagnosis and treatment, it is probably justifiable to simply follow the patient with serial platelet counts (performed monthly until it is determined how stable the counts are). If the counts do not decrease further, and if no other evidence of a disease process emerges, there is no need to stress the patient with further diagnostic procedures.

Symptomatic thrombocytopenia due to decreased production of platelets is usually observed in conjunction with processes such as aplastic anemia, leukemia, disseminated tuberculosis, or metastatic carcinoma that affect other hematological cell lines. In contrast, severe thrombocytopenia due to increased destruction of platelets does not necessarily indicate the presence of a disease process that is affecting parts or systems of the body other than the blood platelets or their precursors. In order to be reasonably certain about the pathophysiology of thrombocytopenia, however, it is necessary to perform an aspiration of the bone marrow and to evaluate the numbers of megakaryocytes on a properly stained smear. That requires referral to a hematologist. Patients who have thrombocytopenia because of diseases involving the bone marrow will, except in cases of megaloblastic anemia, have reduced numbers of megakaryocytes; if the underlying disease process is severe, it is likely that abnormalities of production of, or qualitative changes in, other cell lines also will be noted. On the other hand if the patient is thrombocytopenic because of increased destruction of platelets, the numbers of megakaryocytes will be increased and the marrow will otherwise appear normal (although increased erythroid activity might be seen in those patients who are bleeding). If it is decided that a bone marrow aspirate is indicated because of the severity of the thrombocytopenia (ordinarily less than 20,000 to 30,000 platelets/mm^3), because of evidence of a hemorrhagic diathesis at higher platelet counts or because of a suspicion of a generalized underlying disease affecting the bone marrow, referral to a consultant in hematology is warranted. Depending on the nature of the underlying disease, it would then be appropriate for the hematologist to initiate and maintain therapy, or to refer the patient back to the primary physician.

Decreased Production of Platelets

Decreased production of platelets is a common mechanism for thrombocytopenia in ambulatory pa-

tients (Table 51.3). Apparent suppression of thrombopoiesis is often associated with viral infections such as benign upper respiratory infections, infectious mononucleosis, and childhood exanthems. In most cases, bone marrow aspirates show megakaryocytes in normal or reduced numbers, although they sometimes appear morphologically abnormal. At other times increased numbers of megakaryocytes are seen, suggestive of a destructive process (perhaps immunological) to which the marrow has responded with increased production of platelets. In general, patients with benign viral infections are not likely to have severe thrombocytopenia and so are not at major risk of bleeding. The process ordinarily dissipates as the infection resolves.

Certain drugs predictably produce thrombocytopenia by affecting thrombopoiesis. Among these, cytotoxic agents are unlikely to be administered by the general internist. Chloramphenicol suppresses hematopoiesis and if given for a long period of time (usually more than a few weeks) may produce pancytopenia. It is unlikely that the practitioner would prescribe chloramphenicol for long periods in ambulatory practice, but if he does, he should be aware that the process is reversible when the drug is discontinued, in contrast to the much rarer cases of aplastic anemia caused by chloramphenicol, which do not appear to be dose related and are probably not reversible.

Although thiazide diuretics have been reported to produce mild to moderate thrombocytopenia commonly, in fact a clear-cut cause and effect relationship has not been demonstrated unequivocally. In the reported studies platelet counts have fallen several weeks after the beginning of therapy, sometimes associated with morphologically abnormal megakaryocytes. Rarely, however, thiazides have been clearly implicated in immunologically induced destructive thrombocytopenia (see below). Thiazide diuretics also are a common cause of allergic purpura (see page 564), but patients with this condition have normal platelet counts.

A large number of drugs have been implicated, on occasion, in the production of thrombocytopenia by the suppression of thrombopoiesis. Therefore, if patients are symptomatic from thrombocytopenia or have

Table 51.3.
Thrombocytopenia Due to Decreased Production of Platelets

GENERALIZED DISORDERS OF HEMATOPOIESIS
 Aplastic anemia[a]
 Invasive processes: leukemia, metastatic carcinoma, disseminated infection (e.g., tuberculosis)[a]
 Folate or vitamin B$_{12}$ deficiency[a]
 Drugs: cytotoxic agents, choloramphenicol, alcohol
SPECIFIC DISORDERS OF THROMBOPOIESIS
 Certain infections (usually viral)[b]
 Certain drugs (in most cases, cause and effect have not been demonstrated)

[a] Not discussed in the text.
[b] Processes most likely to be seen in ambulatory practice.

counts below 50,000/mm^3 and the cause of thrombocytopenia is not known, it would be reasonable to discontinue administration of all drugs that are not considered absolutely essential.

Management

Unless thrombocytopenia is severe or unless patients have demonstrated a hemorrhagic diathesis, treatment is not necessary. Clearly, if drugs are incriminated in the process, they should be discontinued, if possible. If it is expected that thrombocytopenia will be transient (as, for example, in patients being treated with cytotoxic therapy for an underlying malignancy), treatment with platelet transfusions sometimes is indicated. Also, some patients with chronic diseases of the bone marrow, such as aplastic anemia, may require more regular platelet transfusion. In any event, patients who are considered candidates for platelet transfusions should be followed by hematologists or oncologists as well as by the primary physician.

Increased Destruction of Platelets (Table 51.4)

Destruction of platelets as a cause of thrombocytopenia is infrequently seen in ambulatory practice but, when seen, is most likely to have an immunological basis. *Autoimmune thrombocytopenia* (3), the most common of the antibody-induced disorders associated with a low platelet count, is a diagnosis made in a practitioner's office by exclusion. Such patients characteristically present with petechial bleeding. Physical examination reveals no other evidence of disease; in particular, the spleen is usually not palpable. An acute disease, often preceded by benign viral infection, is seen more commonly in children and, by definition, lasts less than 6 months. The chronic illness (formerly called ITP, idiopathic thrombocytopenic purpura) lasts longer than 6 months and is seen more often in women than men (ratio of 3 or 4 to 1). It

Table 51.4.
Thrombocytopenia Due to Increased Destruction of Platelets

Immunological
  Autoimmune[a]
    Primary
    Secondary to an underlying disease, *e.g.*, systemic lupus, lymphoma, viral infections such as EB or HIV infection
  Isoimmune
    Neonatal
    Post-transfusion[b]
  Drug-induced
    Quindine
    Quinine
    Gold
    Heroin
  Nonimmunological
    Infections[b]
    Drug-induced: alcohol[a]
    Mechanical injury[b]

[a] Processes most likely to be seen in ambulatory practice.
[b] Not discussed in the text.

sometimes is associated with an underlying lymphoproliferative disorder, a collagen vascular disease, especially systemic lupus erythematosus, and, more rarely, with autoimmune hemolytic anemia. There is an increased incidence of immune thrombocytopenia in association with HIV infection (14, 18) (see Chapter 34). Autoimmune thrombocytopenia has been shown to be due to an antibody adsorbed to the surface of circulating platelets that results in their premature destruction by the reticuloendothelial system. [Recently, it has been demonstrated that the disorder is characterized by ineffective production of platelets as well (6).]

A large number of drugs (13) have been associated with thrombocytopenia on an immunological basis. The most common are quinidine and quinine, but even these agents are implicated rarely. However, if a patient presents to the practitioner with severe thrombocytopenia due to increased destruction of circulating platelets, it is important to ask what drugs the patient is taking and to consider stopping them if there is any question of the drugs being involved in the process. Occasional patients with rheumatoid arthritis treated with gold salts will develop thrombocytopenia that has an immunological basis; in fact, this process appears to be much more common than the generalized suppression of hematopoiesis occasionally associated with the administration of gold. In addition, several cases have been reported in which heroin addicts have thrombocytopenia of an immune type, apparently produced by heroin (or an adulterant used with it).

It is not unusual for *alcoholics* to develop thrombocytopenia, usually to a moderate degree, after a binge. Alcohol appears to damage platelet membranes, causing their premature destruction, and also to inhibit compensatory increase in platelet production by marrow megakaryocytes. Once the binge is over, the platelet count returns to normal (or transiently higher than normal) in 4 to 5 days. Alcoholics of long standing who have developed cirrhosis of the liver and portal hypertension may have chronic thrombocytopenia because of increased sequestration of platelets in their spleens.

Management

Patients who are thrombocytopenic because of increased destruction of platelets also should be treated in consultation with a hematologist. If the patient presents with untoward bleeding, or if platelet counts are lower than 20,000/mm^3 and immediate consultation is not available, it is justifiable to begin treatment with the equivalent of 60 mg of prednisone a day and to hospitalize the patient while awaiting expert advice. Modification of the steroid dose and decisions about splenectomy or other kinds of therapy should be made in conjunction with an experienced hematologist. Treatment of immune thrombocytopenia in patients with HIV infection is the same as it is for patients who do not have HIV infection (18).

After treatment, approximately 80 to 90% of patients

with chronic autoimmune thrombocytopenia ultimately have a permanent remission to the point where their platelet counts are high enough to support normal hemostasis without continued therapy. The rest require the continuing care of a hematologist.

Increased Sequestration of Platelets

Patients with large spleens often have thrombocytopenia because of redistribution of platelets within a larger splenic pool, most commonly because of congestive splenomegaly associated with portal hypertension. Splenectomy reverses thrombocytopenia but should only be considered if there is a clear-cut hemorrhagic diathesis and if the underlying disease responsible for the enlarged spleen permits an operation to be performed.

Increased Utilization of Platelets

Patients with disseminated intravascular coagulation (5) characteristically have thrombocytopenia almost always in association with multiple defects in coagulation. Such patients often present acutely ill because of the underlying disease that has incited the hemostatic disorder. For example, in patients with various complications of pregnancy, with disseminated carcinoma, or in some patients with septicemia, hemostatic mechanisms have been activated because of exposure of the circulating blood to thromboplastic material. The hemorrhagic diathesis is manifest most commonly by widespread bruising, petechiae, and mucous membrane bleeding, occasionally, but not often, associated clinically with evidence of venous or arterial thrombosis. In addition to thrombocytopenia, patients present with disordered coagulation, which can be identified by measuring the prothrombin time, the partial thromboplastin time, and the concentration of fibrinogen in the plasma, and by the demonstration of increased titers of fibrinogen and fibrin degradation products in the plasma or serum. These products are formed by the lysis of fibrinogen and of fibrin by plasmin, the major proteolytic enzyme of the blood. Patients who are strongly suspected of having disseminated intravascular coagulation or in whom the diagnosis has been made should be hospitalized for further treatment and to identify and treat the underlying disease.

Qualitative Disorders of Platelets (1)

A number of inherited abnormalities of platelets have been identified that result in impaired hemostasis even though platelet counts are often within normal limits. In general the hemorrhagic diathesis associated with these conditions is milder than it is in patients with severe thrombocytopenia. Practitioners are unlikely to see these patients in their practice, but in patients who have unexplained bleeding, such as frequent epistaxis or recurrent gastrointestinal hemorrhage, with apparently normal coagulation and normal or slightly reduced platelet counts, it is reasonable to perform a

bleeding time (see above), which is almost always abnormal in patients with qualitatively abnormal platelets. Similar abnormalities may be acquired in patients with various disease states, most commonly uremia; in fact, patients with chronic renal failure who have a tendency to bleed often improve after hemodialysis. Perhaps the most common acquired qualitative disorder of blood platelets occurs after the ingestion of *small doses of aspirin*, which regularly prolongs the bleeding time and irreversibly interferes with platelet aggregation and with the release of certain intracellular platelet constituents. Although untoward bleeding is unusual in patients who have taken aspirin, the drug may intensify a pre-existing tendency to bleed. Other nonsteroidal anti-inflammatory drugs (NSAIDs) also may impair platelet function but, unlike aspirin, the effect is less predictable and is reversible when the drug is stopped.

Thrombocytosis

Platelet counts above 350 to 400,000, unless associated with a myeloproliferative disorder such as polycythemia vera, myeloid metaplasia, or chronic granulocytic leukemia are not in themselves associated with an increased risk of morbidity from excessive bleeding or clotting. They may, however, signify the presence of an underlying disease that requires attention. If on a routine evaluation there are a large number of platelets on the patient's peripheral blood smear, a platelet count should be obtained. If thrombocytosis exists, the most common causes are inflammatory disease and solid tumor malignancies. Because there are, however, a large number of conditions that have at least on occasion been associated with an elevated platelet count, there is no reason for the practitioner to perform more than the usual comprehensive history and physical examination and any laboratory tests suggested by these examinations in an attempt to explain the thrombocytosis.

Patients with myeloproliferative disorders, if they have thrombocytosis, almost always also have large distorted platelets on smear and other hematological abnormalities typical of the particular disease. The great majority of those patients will also have splenomegaly. The treatment of thrombocytosis associated with myeloproliferative disease should be planned in consultation with a hematologist.

COAGULATION DISORDERS

The generation of a solid fibrin clot from circulating soluble fibrinogen is the body's major defense against the loss of blood from the vasculature, especially from blood vessels larger than the capillary, arteriole, and venule. Coagulation is initiated by the exposure of proteins to an altered blood vessel surface, most commonly after trauma, and to thromboplastic substances to which the blood is exposed normally also when blood vessels are injured. Thereafter a series of enzymatic reactions occurs that results in the conversion

Table 51.5.
Advise to Give to Patients with a Disorder of Hemostasis

Take only medicine prescribed by your doctor. Do not take aspirin or cold remedies. You may take Tylenol instead of aspirin for pain, colds, etc.

Do not drink any alcoholic beverage.

Avoid any activity that might expose you unnecessary to trauma— e.g., contact sports.

Wear a bracelet (prescribed by the phyician), identifying you as a "bleeder" and giving the name of your disorder.

Call your physician:
Whenever you experience any abnormal bleeding (including excessive menstrual bleeding);
Before you visit your dentist;
Before seeing any other physician;
If you are hospitalized for any reason, without your physician's knowledge.

of fibrinogen by the proteolytic enzyme, thrombin, to fibrin. There are two converging pathways of coagulation that are important in this mechanism: the first, the so-called intrinsic pathway, which begins with surface activation of coagulation proteins, and the second, the so-called extrinsic pathway, which begins with the exposure of the blood to tissue thromboplastin. The best screening tests to detect abnormalities of clotting are the partial thromboplastin time, which tests the intrinsic and the final common pathway, and the prothrombin time, which tests the extrinsic and the final common pathway. Both of these tests are reliably performed by hematology laboratories. The clotting time is an insensitive test and should not be relied upon as a screening procedure to detect abnormalities in this system.

There are enzymatic mechanisms that oppose coagulation and that prevent unwarranted widespread clotting of the blood when a blood vessel is injured. These mechanisms, although clearly important physiologically, are rarely recognized clinically; but a few cases have been reported of patients with an increased tendency to thrombosis and low levels of activity of one of the various protease inhibitors that normally circulate in the blood and regulate coagulation. The best characterized of these inhibitors is antithrombin III, which inhibits the activity of a number of coagulant proteins as well as that of thrombin, and protein C, a vitamin K-dependent protein that catalyzes the proteolysis of activated factors V and VIII (see also page 571). The fibrinolytic system generates the proteolytic enzyme, plasmin, which adsorbs to the clots and results in their ultimate dissolution. Bleeding as the result of increased endogenous fibrinolytic activity is essentially unheard of. There has been interest in recent years in stimulating fibrinolysis by the infusion of activating enzymes in the treatment of thrombotic disease, but the therapy, which may result in bleeding, requires hospitalization.

Patients who have a deficiency of one or more of the coagulation proteins are more likely to have extensive soft tissue bleeding or major hemorrhage in response to trauma than are patients with disorders of the vasculature or of blood platelets [petechiae (see page 566) are never a sign of abnormal coagulation]. Congenital disorders of coagulation are relatively rare; the most common of them is hemophilia A (factor VIII deficiency), an X-linked disorder that affects only 1 of 10,000 males in the population. Congenital disorders are ordinarily readily diagnosed because of the history of lifelong bleeding and because, in the case of hemophilia, of a history of characteristic hemorrhage into joints and soft tissues. Patients who have a severe hemorrhagic diathesis because of a congenital abnormality of clotting almost always have markedly low levels of the deficient coagulation protein. Therefore, screening tests such as the partial thromboplastin time are almost always abnormal and provide clues to the presence of the disorder. It is unlikely that the practitioner will encounter such patients since most of them are diagnosed in childhood and are treated by experienced hematologists thereafter. If such a patient is encountered, however, who is suspected of having a congenital disorder of coagulation but who has not previously been diagnosed, referral to an appropriate center would be warranted.

Von Willebrand's disease (19) is an inherited abnormality of hemostasis (autosomal dominant) in which there is a reduction in the concentration and/or the structure of a protein, the von Willebrand factor (VWF), which ordinarily binds to platelets and mediates their adhesion to subendothelial collagen in the course of platelet plug formation (see page 566). Normally VWF forms a complex with antihemophilic globulin (factor VIII:C), the protein that is deficient in the blood of patients with classic hemophilia. It seems likely that VWF acts as a carrier of factor VIII so that patients with von Willebrand's disease often have reduced levels of factor VIII.

The qualitative disorder of platelets is reflected in a prolonged bleeding time and decreased platelet adhesiveness. The platelets of these patients characteristically do not aggregate in vitro when exposed to the obsolete antibiotic ristocetin. The course of the disease as well as the extent of the laboratory abnormalities are quite variable from one patient to another, but in general the hemorrhagic diathesis is milder than it is in hemophilia A. Patients bleed most commonly from their gastrointestinal tract; it is not unusual that symptoms of the disease are not apparent until the patient is an adult. The bleeding time and the partial thromboplastin time are useful screening tests, but any patient suspected of having the disorder should have plasma factor VIII assayed as well. The diagnosis and treatment of patients with von Willebrand's disease require the ongoing participation of a qualified hematologist.

Acquired disorders of coagulation are more common than congenital ones. By their nature they are more likely to be associated with multiple defects in hemostasis such as are seen in patients with disseminated intravascular coagulation (see page 569) or in patients taking anticoagulant drugs (see Chapter 52). The diagnosis and management of these problems are discussed on those pages.

ADVICE TO PATIENTS WHO HAVE A DISORDER OF HEMOSTASIS

Table 51.5 lists some rules to give patients who have hemostatic dysfunction (also see Table 52.2 Chapter 52). It is also important that the patient knows the name of his disease and its clinical manifestations.

General References

Colman RW, Hirsh J, Marder VJ, Salzman EW (eds): *Hemostasis and Thrombosis: Basic Principles and Clinical Practice*, 2nd ed. Philadelphia, JB Lippincott, Co, 1987.
An authoritative, exhaustively referenced text.
Kitchens CS (ed): *Semin Thromb Hemostasis* 10:173, 1984.
A review of purpura due to vascular disease.
Ratnoff OD, Forbes CD (eds): *Disorders of Hemostasis*. New York, Grune & Stratton, 1989.
A well-edited review.

Specific References

1. Bellucci S, Tobelem G, Caen JP: Inherited platelet disorders. In: Brown EB (ed): *Progress in Hematology*. New York, Grune & Stratton, 1983, vol 13, p. 223.
2. Bick RL: Vascular disorders associated with thrombohemorrhagic phenomena. *Semin Thromb Hemostasis* 5 (3): 167, 1979.
3. Burns TR, Saleem A: Idiopathic thrombocytopenic purpura. *Am J Med* 75:1001, 1983.
4. Cream JJ, Gumpel JM, Peachey RDG: Schönlein-Henoch purpura in the adult. A study of 77 adults with anaphylactoid or Schönlein-Henoch purpura. *Q J Med* 39:461, 1970.
5. Deykin D: The clinical challenge of disseminated intravascular coagulation. *N Engl J Med* 283:686, 1970.
6. Gernsheimer T, Stratton J, Ballem PJ, Slichter SJ: Mechanisms of response to treatment in autoimmune thrombocytopenic purpura. *N Engl J Med* 320:974, 1989.
7. Glenner GG: Amyloid deposits and amyloidosis. *N Engl J Med* 302:1283, 1333, 1980.
8. Gorevic PD, Kassab HJ, Levo Y, et al: Mixed cryoglobulinemia: clinical aspects and long-term follow-up of 40 patients. *Am J Med* 69:287, 1980.
9. Grey HM, Kohler PF: Cryoimmunoglobulins. *Semin Hematol* 10:87, 1973.
10. Hodges RE, Hood J, Canham JE, et al: Clinical manifestations of ascorbic acid deficiency in man. *Am J Clin Nutr* 24:432, 1971.
11. Kyle RA, Gleich GJ, Bayrid ED, Vaughan JH: Benign hypergammaglobulinemic purpura of Waldenström. *Medicine* (Baltimore) 50:113, 1971.
12. Kyle RA, Greipp RR: Amyloidosis (AL): clinical and laboratory features in 229 cases. *Mayo Clin Proc* 58:665, 1983.
13. Miescher PA: Drug-induced thrombocytopenia. *Semin Hematol* 10:311, 1973.
14. Morris L, Distenfeld A, Amorosi E, Karpatkin S: Autoimmune thrombocytopenic purpura in homosexual men. *Ann Intern Med* 96:714, 1982.
15. Perry WH: Clinical spectrum of hereditary hemorrhagic telangectases. (Osler-Weber-Rendu disease). *Am J Med* 82:989, 1987.
16. Perkins HA, MacKenzie MR, Fudenberg HH: Hemostatic defects in dysproteinemias. *Blood* 35:695, 1970.
17. Ratnoff OD: The psychogenic purpuras: a review of auto-erythrocyte sensitization, autosensitization to DNA, "hysterical" and factitial bleeding, and the religious stigmata. *Semin Hematol* 17:192, 1980.
18. Walsh C, Krigel R, Lennette E, Karpatkin S: Thrombocytopenia in homosexual patients. Prognosis, response to therapy, and prevalence of antibody to the retrovirus associated with acquired immunodeficiency syndrome. *Ann Intern Med* 103:542, 1985.
19. Zimmerman TS, Ruggeri ZM, Fulcher CA: Factor VIII/von Willebrand factor. In: Brown EB (ed): *Progress in Hematology*. New York, Grune & Stratton, 1983, p. 279.

C H A P T E R 52

Thromboembolic Disease

PHILIP D. ZIEVE, M.D.
LARRY WATERBURY, M.D.

Patients with acute vascular occlusions, whether they be venous or arterial, almost always require hospitalization for initial diagnosis and treatment. The responsibility of the clinician in the office, therefore, is to recognize the problem, to arrange for hospitalization in an appropriate facility, and ultimately to manage the patient after discharge from the hospital.

VENOUS THROMBOEMBOLISM

Risk Factors

The majority of patients who present to the physician with venous occlusion have formed clots in the veins of the lower extremities. The primary pathological process is stasis of blood (such as might be seen in people who are chronically ill, obese, or for other reasons lead sedentary lives or who have sustained trauma to their lower limbs).

There is a strong association between the use of oral contraceptive agents and venous thromboembolism (an increased risk historically of 5- to 10-fold). The risk only exists during the time the contraceptive is being used but does not increase with duration of use (48). Because oral contraceptives currently contain less estrogen than they once did, the risk appears to have diminished (48).

Occasionally, an *underlying malignancy*, not always apparent, is associated with venous (and/or arterial) thromboembolic disease (20, 43). More rarely, an *inherited deficiency of a naturally occurring anticoagulant* [e.g., *protein C*, an inhibitor of activated coagulation factors V and VIII (8); *protein S*, a cofactor in reactions that involve protein C (8, 15); or *antithrombin III*, an inhibitor of thrombin as well as of several other activated coagulation factors (11)] is implicated in the genesis of recurrent thrombosis. Also, rarely, an inherited or acquired abnormality of fibrinogen (a *dysfibrinogenemia*) revealed usually by a prolonged thrombin time (see Chapter 51), may be associated with thromboembolic disease. Some patients develop *antibodies to phospholipids* that, for reasons that are not clear, may potentiate both venous and/or arterial thrombosis (22). Some antiphospholipid antibodies, directed against a complex of activated clotting factors and phospholipid, have been called "lupus anticoagulants" (a misnomer). These latter antibodies paradoxically prolong the partial thromboplastin time, the recalcified plasma clotting time, and, less often, the prothrombin time (see Chapter 51). Other antiphospholipid antibodies are directed against cardiolipin and cause a false-positive serologic test for syphilis (see Chapter 30). The antibodies characteristically persist for months or years and may recur. When patients with antiphospholipid antibodies develop venous or arterial thrombosis, they should be anticoagulated (see below) for as long as the antibodies are detectable in their blood.

Presentation and Evaluation

Superficial thrombophlebitis is readily recognized as inflammation of a visible tender, often palpably thrombosed, vein. There is no risk of embolism from such clots, unless the deep veins are also involved. In one study superficial thrombophlebitis was much more likely to be associated with deep vein thrombosis (DVT) if the superficial veins were not varicose (3) (see Chapter 88). Otherwise, treatment does not require administration of anticoagulant drugs (see below) and is confined to nonsteroidal anti-inflammatory drugs, elevation of the extremity, local moist heat, and, if there is concomitant infection, antibiotics. If deep vein thrombosis is suspected in a patient with superficial phlebitis, impedance plethysmography (see below) should be performed.

Signs and symptoms of pulmonary embolism (see Chapter 54) may be the sole manifestation of venous thrombosis in the deep veins of the lower extremities. More frequently, patients present with swelling, pain, and tenderness of the affected extremity, although swelling alone may be the presenting symptom. In any case the prevention of pulmonary embolism is the primary reason why diagnosis and treatment of venous thrombosis are urgent. On the basis of history and physical examination alone, however, it is virtually impossible to distinguish DVT from other processes. At least half of the time other diagnoses (especially musculoskeletal injury) prove to be responsible for these signs and symptoms (29). Therefore, patients suspected of having thrombosis of the deep veins or of having had pulmonary embolism without clinical evidence of peripheral thrombosis must undergo specific diagnostic studies so that appropriate therapy for venous thromboembolism may be instituted. The test of reference (the "gold standard") is contrast venog-

raphy. If characteristic filling defects are seen in radiographs of the veins after injection of contrast material, the diagnosis is established (Fig. 52.1). Some medical centers employ radionuclide blood-pool venography (38) in patients in whom contrast venography is technically difficult or is medically contraindicated. The procedure involves injection in an antecubital vein of technetium-labeled red cells and then scanning over the symptomatic extremity. Sensitivity and specificity of the test in the diagnosis of deep vein thrombosis of both the calf and thigh are approximately 85 to 90%.

There are two noninvasive tests used in the diagnosis of DVT: impedance plethysmography (IPG) and Doppler ultrasonography. The Doppler technique is very dependent on the skill of the technician who performs the test and of the interpreter who evaluates it and so is much less preferable than plethysmography, which is far simpler to perform and to evaluate. Plethysmography is highly sensitive in detecting thrombosis in deep veins of the thigh but is relatively insensitive in detecting thrombosis in deep veins of the calf. However, calf vein thrombi are very unlikely to embolize unless they first propagate into the thigh (39, 42). A reasonable protocol then is to do IPG in a patient with a suspected DVT and, if it is positive, to admit the patient to the hospital for treatment. If it is

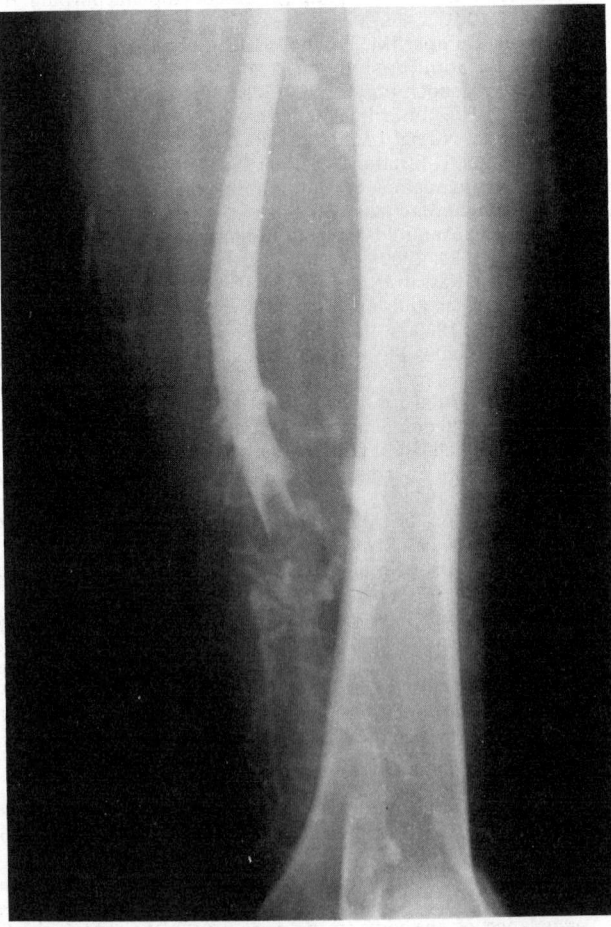

Figure 52.1. Venogram showing clots of deep veins of thigh.

negative or if thrombosis, on clinical grounds, is thought to be limited to the calf, serial IPGs should be done (e.g., days 2 and 7) to ensure that detectable thrombosis has not occurred in a deep vein of the thigh (26, 30). Patients with calf vein thrombosis alone need not be given anticoagulant drugs (see below); they can be treated in the same way as are patients with superficial thrombophlebitis. If IPG is not available, however, patients with venographically demonstrable calf vein thrombosis should be anticoagulated.

Once a definite diagnosis of deep venous thrombosis is made, the patient must be hospitalized for treatment.

Patient experience. Contrast venography is performed after injection of the contrast medium into a dorsal vein of the foot. The patient should be warned that the procedure commonly is associated with unpleasant burning or cramping in the lower extremity while the dye is being injected. In addition, up to one-quarter of patients develop a painful swelling of the leg and ankle that begins 2 to 12 hours after the study, intensifies for 12 to 24 hours, and then begins to subside. The pathogenesis of this delayed reaction is unclear; no specific therapy, therefore, is indicated. There is a risk that venography itself will cause thrombosis; the incidence of deep vein thrombosis, proved by repeated venography, is probably in the range of 3 to 13%, and of superficial thrombosis, 6 to 25% (4).

Impedance plethysmography is performed by inflating a pneumatic cuff at the midthigh to occlude venous return and then rapidly deflating it. The changes in blood volume are measured by changes in electrical resistance detected by a pair of electrodes attached to the cuff. There is no discomfort associated with this procedure other than the mild transient sensation of increased pressure during the few seconds of inflation.

If patients present with signs and symptoms of pulmonary embolism (see Chapter 54), the first diagnostic procedure should be a ventilation/perfusion scan of their lungs. If the scan is negative or read as "low probability" and the patient has signs and symptoms of venous occlusion of the lower extremities, further diagnostic studies should be done, as described above, to establish that diagnosis. If the lung scan is interpreted as indeterminate or high probability, the patient should be hospitalized—in the first instance for pulmonary angiography and in the second for treatment. In many instances, however, the clinician will elect to admit the patient to the hospital on the basis of the clinical presentation and then obtain all necessary diagnostic procedures.

Treatment

The most important therapy for patients with deep vein thrombosis in the lower extremities is anticoagulation, instituted to prevent extension of the clot. The larger the clot, the more likely it is to break off and become an embolus. Anticoagulation is usually instituted in the hospital with heparin, which is administered on the average for 10 days, the approximate time for clots to become adherent to the vessel wall. Heparin is utilized because its onset of action is immediate and because of an unsubstantiated impression that it is a more effective anticoagulant than are coumarin compounds, the other major class of available anticoagulant drugs.

Coumarin Compounds

Coumarin compounds are the drugs commonly used in the anticoagulation of ambulatory patients. Warfarin and dicumerol are the two available coumarins and, of these, warfarin is the preferred drug because response to it is more predictable. *Coumadin* is the brand-name product that is commonly prescribed; other products, including generic products, are reliable but are not interchangeable, because of variation in bioavailability. Ordinarily patients who have been hospitalized for diagnosis and initial treatment of venous thromboembolic disease are given warfarin while heparin is being administered so that by the time that drug is discontinued, the full effect of the coumarin has become established. Coumarins interfere with the synthesis of vitamin K-dependent clotting factors (factors II, VII, IX, and X) by the liver. Their effect is not fully realized, therefore, until they have been given for approximately 5 days. The administration of warfarin, the commonly used coumarin, usually is initiated in doses of 10 mg/day (2-, 2.5-, 5-, 7.5- and 10-mg tablets are available) and then adjusted depending upon the therapeutic response, which is monitored by use of the prothrombin time, a reproducible, dependable test performed reliably by most clinical laboratories.

There is now an internationally accepted uniform system for reporting the prothrombin time (34). The system dictates that all results be related to those obtained by use of a standardized thromboplastin, the critical reagent used in the performance of the test. The relationship is expressed as an International Normalized Ratio (INR), and laboratories doing prothrombin times should report their results in terms of the INR [the INR is the ratio of the patient's prothrombin time to the normal standard prothrombin time of the testing laboratory, raised by an exponent, the International Sensitivity Index (ISI)], supplied by the manufacturer of the thromboplastin.

In most circumstances, the goal of anticoagulant therapy with warfarin is to maintain the INR between 2.0 and 3.0 since it is within this range that a reasonable therapeutic effect is achieved and the risk of untoward bleeding is relatively small. The ratio of the patient's prothrombin time to that of the control will vary, depending on the ISI of the thromboplastin that is used. It should be noted that these recommendations result in significantly lower prothrombin times than have been thought appropriate in the past. During the first several weeks of administration of warfarin, the prothrombin time should be measured at least every few days until it is determined that the proper dosage schedule has been achieved. Thereafter it is appropriate to measure the anticoagulant response monthly. At the same time it is prudent to examine the patient's urine and stool for occult blood and to assess his hematocrit value or hemoglobin concentration.

During the course of anticoagulation with coumarin compounds, patients should be instructed to avoid predictable trauma such as might be expected from playing contact sports or from working in an environment associated with a high risk of injury. The physician should not give intramuscular injections to the anticoagulated patient; subcutaneous injections, done properly, are safe. Venipunctures are also safe, but the wound should be compressed for 10 to 15 minutes after the needle is withdrawn. Arterial punctures are contraindicated as outpatient procedures, for which prolonged compression and observation of the puncture site are impractical.

Factors Affecting Response. Ordinarily, patients taking a given dose of warfarin maintain a consistent hypoprothrombinemic response, once a steady-state is reached. However, there are a number of factors that might alter the patient's responsiveness to warfarin after a period of stability (Table 52.1). Rarely the amount of vitamin K ingested in the patient's diet might be altered drastically, increasing the potency of warfarin if less vitamin K is ingested and decreasing it if considerably more is ingested. Significantly decreased ingestion of vitamin K is almost always associated with a markedly decreased intake of food, e.g., in patients who are anorexic because of illness or who have instituted severe dietary restrictions in an attempt to lose weight. The effect of reduction in intake of vitamin K will be most pronounced in those patients who are concomitantly receiving antibiotics, which will inhibit the synthesis of vitamin K by normal flora of the intestinal tract. Because the vitamin K-dependent clotting factors are synthesized in the liver and because coumarins are metabolized by the liver, patients who develop intercurrent hepatic illness (e.g., hepatitis) should be watched carefully for enhanced effective anticoagulation. In such a circumstance, the clinician would be wise to measure prothrombin times more

Table 52.1.
Some Factors That May Affect a Patient's Response to Warfarin

Enhanced Response	Reduced Response
Vitamin K. Deficiency	Barbiturates
Liver Disease	Cholestyramine
Drugs	Glutethimide (Doriden)
Anabolic steroids	Griseofulvin
Cimetidine	Rifampin
Clofibrate	Spironolactone
Disulfiram (Antabuse)	Foods[a]
Heparin	Fish
Metronidazole (Flagyl)	Broccoli
Phenylbutazone	Spinach
Quinidine	Cabbage
Tamoxifen	Kale
	Cauliflower

[a]Rich in vitamin K.

frequently but would not be required to discontinue warfarin unless bleeding ensued or the prothrombin time became significantly prolonged over the baseline therapeutic control.

One of the major problems confronting the clinician in dealing with a patient taking coumarin anticoagulants is the possibility of drug interaction. A number of pharmacological agents will potentiate the anticoagulant effect of coumarins and a few will inhibit it. The major drugs implicated are listed in Table 52.1. The clinician should be cautious, however, when initiating any new forms of therapy or discontinuing old ones in a patient who is receiving coumarin anticoagulants. Prothrombin times should be checked more frequently for several weeks to be sure that the pharmacological response to coumarin has not been altered. In general, the likelihood of a potentiated response is much higher than that of an inhibitory one, so that there is greater risk of an increased susceptibility to bleeding than of an inhibition of anticoagulation. The clinician should also be careful about the use of drugs, such as aspirin that have an effect on hemostasis that might be enhanced by warfarin or that may produce bleeding by injuring the gastric mucosa. Other nonsteroidal anti-inflammatory agents (see Chapter 70) may be safer than aspirin, but all of them have at least a potential for compromising hemostasis (few data are available) and should be used cautiously.

Complications. By far the major complication experienced by patients taking coumarin anticoagulants is hemorrhage (10, 12, 40). Minor episodes, such as small bruises and bleeding gums after brushing of the teeth, are relatively common but ordinarily do not require a change in the dose schedule of the anticoagulant. Occult rectal bleeding, minor bleeding from hemorrhoids, microscopic hematuria, and menorrhagia will be encountered in less than 10% of patients. When bleeding of this kind is observed, it is essential to make every attempt to establish the site of bleeding by the use of appropriate diagnostic studies. If prothrombin times have been maintained within the therapeutic range, the rapidity and extent of bleeding will dictate to the clinician whether the anticoagulant drug should be discontinued, at least temporarily. Major genitourinary or gastrointestinal bleeding sufficient to lower the hematocrit value or hemoglobin concentration, or bleeding of any degree in the central nervous system, dictates prompt discontinuation of the anticoagulant and immediate hospitalization for further diagnosis and treatment. It is prudent to administer 25 to 50 mg of vitamin K_1 (AquaMephyton) intravenously at a rate no greater than 5 mg/minute while arranging for hospitalization. (The prothrombin time will begin to shorten in 4 to 6 hours and, in most patients, will be in a safe range in 12 to 24 hours.) Bleeding is often associated with an independent organic process, such as a peptic ulcer or a carcinoma of the colon; bleeding of this kind is likely to occur even when the prothrombin time is in the so-called therapeutic range (31).

There is a major risk in the use of coumarin compounds in pregnant patients (21, 36). Major hemor-rhagic complications occur in the fetus as well as teratogenic effects unrelated to the anticoagulant action. It is recommended, therefore, that pregnancy be avoided in women who are being treated with coumarin drugs since a normal infant can be expected only about two-thirds of the time. The risk of heparin in pregnancy is less clear cut; an increased incidence of fetal wastage has been reported (21) but also has been disputed; in any case, if anticoagulation is necessary, heparin is clearly safer than coumarins (see below) (19, 36).

Advice for management of patients who are taking a coumarin compound and who are to undergo a surgical procedure is provided in Chapter 86.

Rarely, patients administered a coumarin anticoagulant will develop, within 10 days, hemorrhagic infarcts in their skin (often in women's breasts) with eventual sloughing of necrotic tissue. Under such circumstances, the drug must be stopped immediately.

Table 52.2 provides information useful for patients at the onset of anticoagulation or at the time that the patient is discharged from hospital. Selection of patients who are able to follow these rules will diminish considerably the incidence of hemorrhagic complications in patients taking anticoagulant drugs (also see Table 51.5, Chapter 51).

Heparin

Because heparin must be administered parenterally, it is not a drug that can be conveniently used by outpatients. If, however, because of unacceptable side effects unrelated to its anticoagulant effect, a coumarin cannot be used, the practitioner should instruct the patient or his family in the use of subcutaneous heparin, administered every 12 hours in doses designed to maintain the partial thromboplastin time (PTT, like

Table 52.2.
Advice to Be Given Patients Taking a Coumarin Anticoagulant

Take *only* medicines prescribed by your doctor. DO NOT take mineral oil, laxatives, aspirin (or any product such as a cold remedy, that contains aspirin), or another proprietary anti-inflammatory agent (currently only ibuprofen—Advil or Nuprin—is available), or any multivitamin preparation that contains vitamin K. You may take acetaminophen (*e.g.*, Tylenol) instead of aspirin for pain.

Take your coumarin at the same time each day.

Avoid wide variation in the kinds and amounts of food you eat, especially fish, broccoli, spinach, cabbage, kale, or cauliflower.

Do not drink more than 1 or 2 glasses of beer or wine or the equivalent of more than 1 ounce (1 "shot") of whiskey/day.

Avoid any activity that might expose you unnecessarily to trauma—for example, contact sports.

Call your doctor immediately whenever:
 You experience any abnormal bleeding;
 Before you visit your dentist;
 Before seeing any other physician;
 If you cannot keep your scheduled appointment;
 Before leaving on a trip;
 If you are hospitalized, for any reason, without his knowing it.

the prothrombin time, a reliable, easily obtained test) at 1.5 to 2 times control (27). Once a dosage regimen is established (usually in the range of 10,000 to 12,000 units twice a day), it probably is not necessary to measure the PTT again unless the patient develops bleeding or recurrent thrombosis. It has been demonstrated that prevention of recurrent thromboembolism is comparable to that achieved by the use of warfarin (27). So-called low dose heparin (5000 units twice a day) is probably inadequate treatment for patients with established thrombosis (28).

In recent years it has been recognized that heparin—especially bovine heparin—causes thrombocytopenia in 5 to 10% of patients to whom it is administered (32). The mechanism of this phenomenon is unclear, although an immunological process may be involved. The onset is usually within a week or 2 of initiation of therapy, and therefore the problem is likely to be recognized in hospital. A small proportion of these thrombocytopenic patients develop, paradoxically, arterial thrombosis. Platelet counts under 40,000 to 50,000/mm^3, thrombocytopenic bleeding, or arterial thrombosis dictate that the heparin be discontinued and that an alternative form of therapy for venous thromboembolic disease be sought. Heparinized ambulatory patients who exhibit untoward bleeding or clotting should be hospitalized, and a platelet count should be done as part of their evaluation. However, routine platelet counts are probably not cost effective in the follow-up of patients receiving heparin.

Prolonged use of heparin (4 months or more) in doses in excess of 10,000 units/day has been reported to cause osteoporosis; spontaneous spinal and rib fractures have been observed. The risk of this complication developing is unknown; until more data are accumulated, treatment with heparin for longer than 3 months is at least relatively contraindicated.

Heparin (especially the bovine preparation) also commonly causes reversible elevation of aminotransferase activity, without other evidence of hepatic dysfunction (13). No pathological correlation with this reaction has been identified.

Aspirin

Although aspirin (see below) has been recommended in the prophylaxis of venous thromboembolism, there is no consensus that it is useful; and there is no justification for prescribing it as treatment of venous thrombosis.

Course

Patients who are being treated with coumarin anticoagulants have a recurrence rate of venous thromboembolism of 10 to 40 episodes/1000 patient months (9). One month after discharge from the hospital, the rate stabilizes at approximately 10 episodes/1000 patient months and remains in that range or slightly lower thereafter. The beneficial effect of anticoagulant therapy in such patients is most pronounced during the first month after discharge from hospital; after 1 to 2 months the recurrence rate is the same whether the patient is anticoagulated or not. It has been the standard of practice to discontinue therapy after 3 months in patients who are not at continued high risk (9). There is good evidence, however, that anticoagulation can be safely discontinued even earlier (4 to 6 weeks) in such patients (24, 40). Patients who maintain risk factors for thromboembolic disease [chronic venous stasis for whatever reason or an abnormality of their coagulation mechanism (see above, page 571)] may, barring complications of drugs, be considered for more prolonged periods of treatment. Although there is no reliable information in this regard, it is reasonable to continue therapy for high risk patients indefinitely unless a contraindication—such as major bleeding—develops.

Patients who have sustained thromboses of the deep veins of the lower extremities should be advised to avoid prolonged sitting or standing in one position, should be encouraged to elevate their legs for two to three periods of 30 minutes each day, and to wear elastic stockings to promote venous return. Although the effectiveness of these maneuvers has not been established, there is little or no risk associated with any of them, and they may be of some value. At such time when a decision is made to discontinue anticoagulation therapy, it may be terminated abruptly without fear of an increased risk of early recurrence of venous thrombosis; the so-called "rebound phenomenon" has never been demonstrated.

Recurrent DVT may be difficult to diagnose (35). Many patients who have had a documented acute DVT develop recurrent pain and swelling of the same extremity. Even contrast venography may be equivocal in such patients because of persistent occlusion of a vein by a previous clot. In such circumstances, IPG is probably the most reliable test, if it has been demonstrated to have become normal after treatment of an acute thrombotic event [normalization occurs in 70% of patients by 3 months and in 90% by 9 months (25)]. If IPG has not become normal and if a contrast venogram is not interpretable, or if recurrent thrombosis has been definitively diagnosed, anticoagulation for a year is probably reasonable.

The Postphlebitic Syndrome

Some patients, after repeated attacks of thrombosis of the veins of the lower extremities, will develop chronic changes in those veins with loss of competence of the valves and hemorrhage of small tributary veins leading to chronic edema and discoloration of the legs and ankles (44). Sometimes painful stasis ulcers also will develop that make it very difficult for the patient to move about. The treatment of this postphlebitic syndrome is the promotion of venous return from the lower extremities by the use of support stockings during the day and by elevation of the lower extremities for several hours each day. In those patients who have developed ulcers, bed rest with persistent elevation of the extremity above the level of the heart is recommended and, if necessary, administration of appropriate antibiotics. On such a regimen, the ulcers will invariably heal, although they may recur if the patients are not careful to continue to follow prescribed conservative therapy (see Chapter 88). It should be noted that signs and symptoms of chronic venous insufficiency are often manifest in patients who have no history or evidence of DVT (14).

ARTERIAL THROMBOEMBOLISM (See also Chapters 59 and 87)

Unlike clots that form in the venous circulation, arterial thrombosis is primarily initiated by platelet plug formation, begun by the adherence of ambient platelets to altered surfaces in arterial vessels or in the left heart. Symptoms and signs of thromboembolism appear more abruptly than do those of venous occlusion and commonly are associated with necrosis of tissue that had been fed by the now obstructed vessel. Heparin and coumarin anticoagulants, both experimentally and clinically, are of little use in preventing the formation of such clots or in preventing their propagation. There is a great deal of interest, therefore, in the use of drugs that interfere with platelet plug formation and that might be useful in the prophylaxis of arterial thromboembolism. Although a number of agents have been tested and others are being actively evaluated, of the currently approved drugs, only aspirin, in some circumstances (see below), has been shown to be efficacious. Dipyridamole (Persantine), a very commonly prescribed drug, has never been shown clearly to be useful (16). Ticlopidine, an inhibitor of platelet aggregation and adhesion, in a multi-center study (18) was shown to be effective in reducing the incidence of vascular events in patients who had recently had a thromboembolic stroke, but the drug is not yet approved for use and more information is needed before it can be recommended.

Aspirin

This drug, the most commonly used therapeutic agent in the world, has for some years been recognized to interfere with platelet function and therefore to inhibit platelet plug formation. Aspirin interferes with the formation of a very potent aggregating and vasoconstricting substance, thromboxane A_2, formed in platelets by the metabolism of prostaglandins. Aspirin inhibits the rate-limiting enzyme in this reaction, cyclo-oxygenase; as a result, the aggregation of platelets by collagen or connective tissue is inhibited and the release of substances, which themselves stimulate platelet aggregation, is impaired. Presumably as a result of the impairment, the bleeding time in patients taking even a single tablet of aspirin a day is prolonged.

Aspirin inhibits not only prostaglandin synthesis in platelets but also the formation by vascular endothelium of prostacyclin, a potent inhibitor of platelet aggregation. Although there is not precise information on the proper dose of aspirin to be administered to achieve an optimum effect (presumably at the point where there is maximum inhibition of thromboxane A_2 synthesis and minimum inhibition of prostacyclin synthesis) (17), there is no evidence that aspirin at any dose is thrombogenic.

Unless aspirin is administered to patients with an underlying hemostatic disorder (including the administration of an anticoagulant drug—see above), a hemorrhagic diathesis is unusual. However, it has been well established that aspirin has a toxic effect on the mucosa of the gastrointestinal tract that may result in bleeding or may increase the likelihood of hemorrhage from pre-existent peptic ulcerations.

There have been a number of studies performed to assess the efficacy of aspirin as a prophylactic agent in patients with cardiovascular and cerebrovascular disease. A recent meta-analysis (a statistical evaluation of the sum of all published interpretable trials) of 29,000 patients with a history of transient ischemic attacks, occlusive strokes, unstable angina, or myocardial infarction reported that allocation to "antiplatelet treatment" (essentially aspirin) reduced vascular mortality by 15% and nonfatal vascular events by 30% (1). There was no significant difference between patients with cardiovascular disease and those with cerebrovascular disease, and no significant difference in effect between different doses of aspirin or aspirin combinations. Individual, relatively small studies have indicated that aspirin is effective as a prophylactic agent in patients with a history of transient ischemic attacks (5, 45, 46) or of unstable angina (6, 37). In these populations it is prudent to recommend aspirin, 325 mg a day. There is little risk of hemorrhagic side effects at this dose. In patients with other manifestations of atherosclerotic disease, the physician must make his recommendations, in consultation with his patient, on a case-by-case basis. There is no convincing evidence in individual studies that aspirin is of benefit to patients who have had a myocardial infarction (2).

It has become a routine in most centers to administer dipyridamole (75 mg three times a day) and aspirin (325 to 975 mg every day) indefinitely to patients who have undergone coronary artery bypass surgery, largely as the result of one well-controlled study that showed a significant reduction for at least a year or more postoperatively of vein-graft occlusion (7). Whether dipyridamole is important to this regimen (see above) is unknown.

There have also been two recent studies (one American and one British) of aspirin in the primary prevention of atherosclerotic disease (given prophylactically to apparently healthy people (41, 47). Despite some difference in design and in results the combined studies showed a significant, 1/3 reduction in the number of nonfatal myocardial infarctions (23). There was no reduction in overall vascular mortality (the studies did not have sufficient power to do so) or in the number of strokes. In fact there was a significant increase in the number of hemorrhagic strokes, al-

though the numbers were small. Based on these results physicians may consider advising their patients to take aspirin (325 mg every other day in the American study) but other factors (such as hypertension, increasing the risk of hemorrhagic stroke) must be taken into account.

Fish Oil

There has been a great deal of interest in exploring the value of fish oil as an agent in the prevention of atherosclerotic disease. Eicosopentanoic acid, the major ingredient in fish oil, competes with arachidonic acid for cyclo-oxygenase and reduces thereby the formation of thromboxane A_2 (see above). Supportive studies have been primarily epidemiologic; showing that populations that eat a great deal of fish have a lower incidence of occlusive vascular disease. However, the effect of fish oil on platelet function is more palatably achieved by administration of aspirin (33), and its use cannot therefore be recommended, on the basis of current evidence.

General References

American College of Chest Physicians and the National Heart, Lung, and Blood Institute. National Conference on Antithrombotic Therapy. *Chest* 89:15, 1986.
    A consensus on the use of antithrombotic therapy, as of 1986.
Deykin D: Current status of anticoagulant therapy. *Am J Med* 72:659, 1982.
    A concise, sensible review.
Oates JA, Fitzgerald GA, Branch RA, et al: Clinical implications of prostaglandin and thromboxane A_2 formation. *N Engl J Med* 319:761, 1988.
    A well-referenced detailed review.

Specific References

1. Antiplatelet trialists' collaboration: Secondary prevention of vascular disease by prolonged antiplatelet treatment. *Br Med J* 296:320, 1988.
2. Aspirin Myocardial Infarction Study Research Group: A randomized, controlled trial of aspirin in persons recovered from myocardial infarction. *JAMA* 243:661, 1980.
3. Bergquist D, Jaroszewski H: Deep vein thrombosis in patients with superficial thrombophlebitis of the leg. *Br Med J* 292:658, 1986.
4. Bettmann MA, Paulin S: Leg phlebography: the incidence, nature, and modification of undesirable side effects. *Diagn Radiol* 122:101, 1977.
5. Bousser MG, Eschwege E, Haguenau M, et al: "AICLA" controlled trial of aspirin and dipyridamole in the secondary prevention of athero-thrombotic cerebral ischemia. *Stroke* 14:5, 1983.
6. Cairns JA, Gent M, Singer J, et al: Aspirin, sulfinpyrazone, or both in unstable angina. Results of a Canadian multicenter trial. *N Engl J Med* 313:1370, 1985.
7. Chesbro JH, Fuster V, Elveback LR, et al: Effect of dipyridamole and aspirin on late vein-graft patency after coronary bypass operation. *N Engl J Med* 310:209, 1984.
8. Clouse LH, Comp PC: The regulation of hemostasis: the protein C system. *N Engl J Med* 314:1298, 1986.
9. Coon WW, Willis PW III: Recurrence of venous thromboembolism. *Surgery* 73:823, 1973.
10. Coon WW, Willis PW III: Hemorrhagic complications of anticoagulant therapy. *Arch Intern Med* 133:386, 1974.
11. Cosgriff TM, Bishop DT, Hershgold EJ, et al: Familial antithrombin III deficiency: its natural history, genetics, diagnosis and treatment. *Medicine* (Baltimore) 62:209, 1983.

12. Davis FB, Estruch MT, Samson-Corvera EB, et al: Management of anticoagulation in outpatients. *Arch Intern Med* 137:197, 1977.
13. Dukes GE, Sanders SW, Russo J Jr, et al: Transaminase elevations in patients receiving bovine or porcine heparin. *Ann Intern Med* 100:646, 1984.
14. Editorial Post-thrombotic venous disorders. *Lancet* 1:1488, 1985.
15. Engesser L, Brockmans AW, Briet E, et al: Hereditary protein S deficiency: clinical manifestations. *Ann Intern Med* 106:677, 1987.
16. Fitzgerald GA: Dipyridamole. *N Engl J Med* 316:1247, 1987.
17. Fitzgerald GA, Oates JA, Hawiger J, et al: Endogenous biosynthesis of prostacyclin and thomboxane and platelet function during chronic administration of aspirin in man. *J Clin Invest* 71:676, 1983.
18. Gent M, Blakely JA, Easton JD, et al: The Canadian American ticlopidine study (CATS) in thromboembolic stroke. *Lancet* 1:1215, 1989.
19. Ginsberg JS, Hirsh J, Turner DC, et al: Risk to the fetus of anticoagulant therapy during pregnancy. *Thrombosis and Haemostasis* 61:197, 1989.
20. Goldberg RJ, Serreff M, Gore JM, et al: Occult malignant neoplasm in patients with deep venous thrombosis. *Arch Intern Med* 147:251, 1987.
21. Hall JG, Pauli RM, Wilson KM: Maternal and fetal sequelae of anticoagulation during pregnancy. *Am J Med* 68:122, 1980.
22. Harris EN, Asherson RA, Hughes GRV: Antiphospholipid antibodies—autoantibodies with a difference. *Ann Rev Med* 39:261, 1988.
23. Hennekens CH, Peto R, Hutchison GB, Doll R: (letter) An overview of the British and American aspirin studies. *N Engl J Med* 318:923, 1988.
24. Holmgren K, Andersson G, Fagrell B, et al: One-month versus six-month therapy with oral anticoagulants after symptomatic deep vein thrombosis. *Acta Med Scand* 218:279, 1985.
25. Huisman MV, Buller HR, ten Cate JW, et al: Utility of impedance plethysmography in the diagnosis of recurrent deep-vein thrombosis. *Arch Intern Med* 148:681, 1988.
26. Huisman MV, Buller HR, ten Cate JW, et al: Management of clinically suspected acute venous thrombosis in outpatients with serial impedance plethysmography in a community hospital setting. *Arch Intern Med* 149:511, 1989.
27. Hull R, Delmore T, Carter C, et al: Adjusted subcutaneous heparin versus warfarin sodium in the long-term treatment of venous thrombosis. *N Engl J Med* 306:189, 1982.
28. Hull R, Delmore T, Genton E, et al: Warfarin sodium versus low-dose heparin in the long-term treatment of venous thrombosis. *N Engl J Med* 301:855, 1979.
29. Hull R, Hirsh J: Advances and controversies in the diagnosis, prevention, and treatment of venous thromboembolism. In: Brown EB (ed): *Progress in Hematology*. New York, Grune & Stratton, 1981, vol 12, p. 73.
30. Hull RD, Hirsh J, Carter CJ, et al: Diagnostic efficacy of impedance plethysmography for clinically suspected deep-vein thrombosis. *Ann Intern Med* 102:21, 1985.
31. Jaffin BW, Bliss CM, Lamont JT: Significance of occult gastrointestinal bleeding during anticoagulation therapy. *Am J Med* 83:269, 1987.
32. King DJ, Kelton JG: Heparin-associated thrombocytopenia. *Ann Intern Med* 100:535, 1984.
33. Knapp HR, Reilly AG, Alessandrini P, FitzGerald GA: In vivo indexes of platelet and vascular function during fish-oil administration in patients with atherosclerosis. *N Engl J Med* 314:937, 1986.
34. Koepke JA, Triplett DA: Standardization of the prothrombin time—finally. *Arch Pathol Lab Med* 109:800, 1985.
35. Leclerc JR, Jay RM, Hull RD, Hirsh J: Recurrent leg symptoms following deep vein thrombosis. A diagnostic challenge. *Arch Intern Med* 145:1867, 1985.
36. Letsky EA, de Swiet M: Thromboembolism in pregnancy and its management. *Br J Haematol* 57:543, 1984.
37. Lewis HD Jr, Davis JW, Archibald DG, et al: Protective effects of aspirin against acute myocardial infarction and death in men with unstable angina. *N Engl J Med* 309:396, 1983.
38. Lisbona R: Radionuclide blood-pool imaging in the diagnosis of deep-vein thrombosis of the leg. In: Freeman LM, Weissman HS (eds): *Nuc Med Ann* 1986, p. 161.
39. Moser KM, LeMoine JR: Is embolic risk conditioned by location of deep venous thrombosis? *Ann Intern Med* 94:439, 1981.
40. Petitti DB, Strom BL, Melmon KL: Duration of warfarin anticoagulant therapy and the probabilities of recurrent thromboembolism and hemorrhage. *Am J Med* 81:255, 1986.
41. Peto R, Gray R, Collins R: Randomized trial of prophylactic daily aspirin in British male doctors. *Br Med J* 296:313, 1988.
42. Philbrick JT, Becker DM: Calf deep venous thrombosis. A wolf in sheep's clothing. *Arch Intern Med* 148:2131, 1988.
43. Sack GH, Levin J, Bell WR: Trousseau's syndrome and other manifestations of chronic disseminated coagulopathy in patients with neoplasms: clinical, pathophysiologic, and therapeutic features. *Medicine* (Baltimore) 56:1, 1977.
44. Strandness DE, Langlois Y, Cramer M, et al: Long term sequelae of acute venous thrombosis. *JAMA* 250:1289, 1983.
45. The Canadian Cooperative Study Group: A randomized trial of aspirin and sulfinpyrazone in threatened stroke. *N Engl J Med* 299:53, 1978.
46. The Dutch TIA Study Group: The Dutch TIA trial: protective effects of low-dose aspirin and atenolol in patients with transient ischemic attacks or nondisabling stroke. *Stroke* 19:512, 1988.
47. The steering committee of the physicians' health study research group: Final report on the aspirin component of the ongoing physicians' health study. *N Engl J Med* 321:129, 1989.
48. Vessey M, Mant D, Smith A, Yeates D: Oral contraceptives and venous thromboembolism: findings in a large prospective study. *Br Med J* 292:526, 1986.

C H A P T E R 53

Selected Illnesses Affecting Lymphocytes: Mononucleosis, Chronic Lymphocytic Leukemia, and the Undiagnosed Patient with Lymphadenopathy

LARRY WATERBURY, M.D.
PHILIP D. ZIEVE, M.D.

A number of illnesses affect the lymphoreticular system, some of them benign (such as most cases due to viral infection), some of them malignant (e.g., lymphoma). The diagnosis is sometimes readily apparent from the clinical presentation, but at other times extensive studies are necessary before a precise diagnosis can be made. This chapter reviews two conditions that affect lymphatic organs and lymphocytes: the mononucleosis syndrome and chronic lymphocytic leukemia. Both of these are conditions in which the general physician will be involved in the diagnosis and treatment of the patient.

INFECTIOUS MONONUCLEOSIS

There are four infectious diseases caused by herpes viruses that affect humans: infectious mononucleosis [Epstein-Barr virus (EBV)], cytomegalovirus (CMV) infections, herpes simplex infections (Chapters 94 and 100), and varicella/zoster infections (Chapter 100).

Epidemiology and Pathogenesis

The EBV is the cause of infectious mononucleosis (3), an acute febrile illness that primarily affects teenagers and young adults (the age group between 15 and 25 years). Infection with the virus is extremely common; for example, over 50% of college students of both sexes have antibodies to it; and each year 12 to 13% of college students who do not have antibodies to EBV develop them (most of them in the course of clinical mononucleosis) (16). Because of the ubiquity of exposure relatively early in life, infectious mononucleosis is rare in people over the age of 30 and, when it does occur, may present atypically (see below). The virus seems to be spread by oral contact, first infecting the throat, then B lymphocytes that generate a T cell response that results in the atypical lymphocytosis that is a hallmark of the disease.

EBV has also been cultured from tumor cells of patients with Burkitt's lymphoma and with nasopharyngeal carcinoma, and such patients also have antibodies to the virus in their blood. It seems likely, therefore, that EBV has a role in the development of these neoplasms.

Signs and Symptoms

Clinical illness usually begins after a 1- to 2-month incubation period. Classically patients present with pharyngitis, lymphadenopathy, splenomegaly, and marked atypical lymphocytosis. Table 53.1 lists the relative frequency of the characteristic signs and symptoms associated with the illness. Pharyngitis can be extremely severe and is frequently accompanied by an exudate, which may be foul smelling. Rarely it may be so severe that it leads to respiratory obstruction. Of the relatively few patients who do not present with pharyngitis (especially children), most simply have a nonspecific febrile illness associated with malaise. Other patients present with mild jaundice and a syndrome that mimics infectious hepatitis. Posterior cervical adenopathy is characteristic of almost all patients, and there is frequently generalized lymph node enlargement as well; approximately 60% have an enlarged spleen. Some patients may experience a protracted course with nonspecific symptoms, slight to moderately tender lymphadenopathy, and splenomegaly that persist for weeks. Most patients are significantly improved by the end of 3 weeks.

Patients usually present to the physician at the end of the first week of a nonspecific illness characterized by malaise and perhaps by anorexia, mild headache, and fever (up to 104°). Adenopathy, splenomegaly, and pharyngitis usually appear at about this time and slowly resolve over the following weeks. However, as noted below, the classical laboratory features of the illness may not be present until the 2nd or 3rd week of the clinical illness. Patients over 40 years of age tend to have more prolonged fever and less adenopathy than do young adults (9).

Table 53.1.
Signs and Symptoms of Infectious Mononucleosis

Common Symptoms	%	Common Signs	%	Less Common Signs and Symptoms	%
Malaise	100	Adenopathy	100	Jaundice	10
Sore throat	85	Fever	90	Arthralgia	5
Warmth, chilliness	70	Pharyngitis	85	Skin rash	5
Anorexia	70	Splenomegaly	60	Diarrhea	5
Headache	50	Bradycardia	40	Photophobia	5
Cough	40	Periorbital edema	25		
Myalgia	25	Palatal enanthem	25		

Laboratory Features

The hematocrit value is usually normal, although occasionally mild hemolysis and, rarely, a severe autoimmune hemolytic anemia are seen. The peripheral white cell count is usually elevated, reaching its height during the 2nd and 3rd weeks of the clinical illness. Early in the course there may be a severe absolute neutropenia, and occasionally the absolute neutrophil count is less than 500/μl. The differential count of the white cells is characterized by an absolute lymphocytosis with large numbers (over 10% of the total white cell population) of atypical lymphocytes (large lobulated or indented nuclei and vacuolated and/or bluish cytoplasm). The platelet count is normal to slightly decreased in the majority of patients; severe thrombocytopenia may occur rarely. Slight increases in the activity of hepatic enzymes are common but never reach the height seen in viral hepatitis; older patients, however, tend to have more marked hepatic dysfunction, and in this group jaundice is common (9).

Serological Features

Diagnosis is based upon the presence of typical clinical features and characteristic serological tests. A number of different EB virus antibodies have been identified (7). They are summarized in Table 53.2. *Immunoglobulin M antibody to viral capsid antigen* (IgM anti-VCA) appears within 1 to 6 weeks after onset of infection and disappears within 3 to 6 months; a rising titer during the first few weeks of clinical illness is the most useful, generally most easily available serological evidence of recent primary infection. Antibodies to the early antigen (EA) complex of EBV of the diffuse (D) type (known as anti-D antibodies) also appear early in primary infection and disappear by 2

Table 53.2.
Serological Evidence of Epstein-Barr Virus (EBV) Infection (3)

1. IgM antibody to viral capsid antigen (IgM anti-VCA). Appears early in primary infection and disappears within 3 to 6 months.
2. IgG antibody to viral capsid antigen (IgG anti-VCA). Appears slightly later than IgM anti-VCA and remains detectable for life.
3. Antibodies to the early antigen (EA) complex of EBV of the diffuse (D) type (anti-D). Anti-D antibodies appear early in primary infection and disappear by 2 to 3 months.
4. Antibodies to EB nuclear antigen (anti-EBNA). Anti-EBNA appears very late (months) after primary infection and is detectable for life.

to 3 months, but anti-D antibody testing is much less available than IgM anti-VCA testing (8). *Heterophil antibodies* are elevated in most patients; the highest titers are reached during the first week of clinical illness. Differential absorption studies are necessary to identify the presence of those heterophil antibodies that are specific for infectious mononucleosis (the antibodies are absorbed by bovine red cells but not by guinea pig kidney). A number of rapid macroagglutination slide tests are commercially available (14). Most utilize horse red cells, which are more sensitive than sheep red cells in the detection of heterophil antibodies. Some kits utilize differential absorption techniques as well. In general, the slide kits are quite sensitive to the detection of heterophil antibodies but may yield positive results also in other conditions associated with such antibodies (serum sickness, viral hepatitis, cytomegalovirus infections, other viral illnesses, leukemia).

In patients with classic symptoms of infectious mononucleosis a positive mononucleosis slide test is sufficient serological confirmation for the diagnosis for clinical purposes. Some 5 to 10% of patients with clinical infectious mononucleosis and serological evidence of recent primary EBV infection are heterophil antibody negative. Another 5 to 10% of patients with clinical features of infectious mononucleosis have another illness (cytomegalovirus infection, toxoplasmosis, etc.).

Complications

Severe complications of infectious mononucleosis are rare but do occur (2). They include neurological problems (encephalitis, meningitis, peripheral neuropathy, Guillain-Barré syndrome), bacterial superinfection, and splenic rupture. The latter has accounted for a number of deaths, especially since the diagnosis is easily missed. The diagnosis should be suspected if there is a recent history of sudden, brief, sharp abdominal pain. Occasional deaths have been seen also with severe pharyngitis and airway obstruction. All of these complications are even more rare when the mononucleosis syndrome is caused by an infectious agent other than the EB virus (see below). The pharyngitis in infectious mononucleosis may closely resemble that of exudative streptococcal pharyngitis, and all patients should have throat cultures to rule out bacterial infection.

Treatment

There is no specific treatment for infectious mononucleosis, and all that is usually necessary is patient education and supportive care. There is no evidence that prolonged bed rest is helpful. It is reasonable for patients to avoid strenuous activities until they feel strong enough to participate. Contact sports should be avoided if the spleen is tender or significantly enlarged. Since splenomegaly may persist for months, however, it seems unreasonable to avoid contact sports until the spleen is no longer palpable. Although contacts do occasionally develop infectious mononucleosis, there is no evidence that the disease is highly infective and patients should not be rigidly restricted from interpersonal contacts. (However, the patient continues to shed the virus for several months after onset of the illness).

Surgery, of course, is indicated for splenic rupture (15). Corticosteroids are usually reserved for patients with severe pharyngitis and impending airway obstruction, in which situation they are usually dramatically effective. Ordinarily a high dose (such as 40 to 60 mg of prednisone daily) is given initially, with rapid tapering of treatment by 1 week to 10 days.

Other Causes of the Mononucleosis Syndrome

Cytomegalovirus Infection

Although CMV infections may cause devastating clinical illness in the newborn (in utero) and in the immunocompromised host, infection in the noncompromised adult causes a clinical syndrome essentially indistinguishable from infectious mononucleosis except that exudative pharyngitis is very unusual in CMV infection. Unlike exposure to EBV, which has occurred in most adults in the United States by age 25, primary CMV infections usually occur at an older age, making CMV mononucleosis the most common cause of the mononucleosis syndrome in patients over 25 to 30 years of age. Up to 50% of people over the age of 40 have antibodies to CMV, although most do not have a history of infection. Diagnosis usually depends on the demonstration of at least a 4-fold rise in CMV complement-fixing antibodies over a 4- to 6-week period. When available, the demonstration of IgM antibodies to CMV antigens or the demonstration of cytolytic antibodies to CMV antigens is more useful in proving recent primary infection (Table 53.3).

Toxoplasmosis

Acute toxoplasmosis may also cause a clinical syndrome that resembles infectious mononucleosis, but pharyngitis does not occur and splenomegaly and lymphadenopathy are usually not as prominent. Diagnosis usually depends on a constellation of serological findings indicative of recent primary infection (see Table 53.3).

Other Infections

Other infections may mimic infectious mononucleosis. These include hepatitis A, hepatitis B, non-A-, non-B hepatitis, rubella, and adenovirus infection. Sometimes an etiological agent cannot be identified even after extensive serological testing. Table 53.4 suggests a stepwise plan for the serological evaluation of patients with the mononucleosis syndrome.

The Chronic Fatigue Syndrome

Since 1985 there has been an epidemic in this country, predominantly in young women, of an illness characterized universally by debilitating fatigue and by a host of other symptoms (Table 53.5), many of them suggestive of EBV infection. Initially people who complained of these symptoms were thought to have

Table 53.3.
Etiologies Other Than EBV for the Mononucleosis Syndrome—Serological Diagnosis of Recent Infection

CMV	Four to 8-fold rise in complement fixation titer. Elevated IgM or cytolytic antibodies to CMV antigen, if available, are more helpful.
Toxoplasmosis	Dye Test (DT) or immunofluorescent antibody (IFA) titers of > 1:1000 plus an IgM-IFA titer of > 1:64.
Hepatitis A	Elevated titer of IgM antibody to hepatitis A antigen (IgM anti-HAAg). (See Chapter 42.)
Hepatitis B	Elevated hepatitis B surface antigen (HBSAg). Chronic carrier state identification will require follow-up measurement of HBSAg, HBeAg, and lack of rise of anti-HBS. (See Chapter 42.)
Rubella	The hemagglutination inhibition antibody (HIA) titer is the most widely used. The antibody is first detected after onset of the rash, and the titer rises rapidly for 1 to 2 weeks thereafter. If one does not catch this rise with acute and convalescent sera, the titer usually remains high for several months, so a single high titer is not meaningful. However, a low titer (<1:16) 2 weeks after the rash is strongly against the diagnosis.

Table 53.4.
Stepwise Serological Testing in the Diagnosis of the Etiology of the "Mononucleosis Syndrome"

1. Typical clinical features with a positive heterophil slide test. This essentially establishes a diagnosis of infectious mononucleosis, usually due to EBV. *Recommendation:* No further testing is needed.
2. Typical clinical features with a negative heterophil slide test at the time the patient first presents to the physician. *Recommendation:* Draw acute serum samples (save frozen in two containers) for pertinent serological testing for EBV, toxoplasmosis, CMV, hepatitis A, hepatitis B, and rubella (see Table 53.3). Repeat heterophil slide test during the third week of clinical illness. If positive, no further testing is necessary. If negative, repeat EBV serology (at least 2 weeks post acute sample) and send with one of the acute serological samples for EBV IgM anti-VCA testing (and anti-D testing if available). If the EBV serologies are diagnostic of recent infection, no further testing is necessary.
3. Typical clinical features, negative slide test at week 3 of clinical illness, and negative EBV serology (IgM anti-VCA or anti-D). *Recommendation:* Draw convalescent sera for testing for toxoplasmosis, CMV, hepatitis A, hepatitis B, and rubella and send with acute sera for appropriate serological testing (Table 53.3).
4. Typical or atypical clinical features with negative serologies for all of the above. Consider other etiologies (leukemia, lymphoproliferative disease, granulomatous disease, collagen vascular disease, *etc.*) *Recommendation:* Consider lymph node biopsy and other tests (*e.g.*, bone marrow aspiration and biopsy).

Table 53.5.
Common Symptoms in Patients with The Chronic Fatigue Syndrome[a]

Easy fatigueability
Difficulty concentrating
Headache
Sore throat
Tender lymph nodes
Muscle aches
Joint aches
Fever
Difficulty sleeping
Psychiatric problems

[a] Adapted from Straus SE: The chronic mononucleosis syndrome. *J Infect Dis* 157:405, 1988.

Table 53.6.
Chronic Fatigue Syndrome[a]

Major Criteria
Persistent or relapsing fatigue of new onset that reduces average daily activity by 50%,
Identifiable conditions that may produce similar symptoms must be excluded.

Minor Criteria
Mild fever · sore throat · adenopathy · weakness · myalgia · headache · prolonged post-exercise fatigue · migratory arthralgia neuropsychologic complaints · sleep disturbance · relatively rapid onset

[a] Adapted from Holmes GP, Kaplan JE, Gantz NM: Chronic fatigue syndrome: a working case definition. *Ann Intern Med* 108:387, 1988. The diagnosis of the syndrome requires that the major criteria and 8 of the minor symptom criteria be met. For other nuances of the "working definition" of the syndrome see the reference.

chronic mononucleosis, because of the demonstration of antibodies to EBV in their blood (10, 21). It soon became evident, however, that antibody titers to a number of viruses (CMV, herpes simplex, measles) were elevated in the blood of these patients (7), casting doubt on the role of EBV as an etiologic agent of the illness. Therefore, the illness was renamed the Chronic Fatigue Syndrome, and criteria were formulated for its diagnosis (Table 53.6) (6). It has become obvious that the prevalence of psychiatric illness (depression, somatoform disorder, anxiety, etc.) is increased considerably in patients with the syndrome (20) so that it is tempting to think that all of the symptoms reflect underlying psychopathology. However, it has been shown that, in addition to the elevated viral antibody titers, a variety of immunologic perturbations, both cellular and humoral, also occur in the syndrome (20). Although it is possible that immunologic dysfunction may be caused by psychiatric illness (19), whether the Chronic Fatigue Syndrome has a psychiatric cause is still not clear. Affected patients are likely to remain symptomatic indefinitely; they need the understanding and support of their families and their physicians and specific attention to psychiatric problems, when they are manifest (see Chapters 12, 13, and 15).

CHRONIC LYMPHOCYTIC LEUKEMIA

Chronic lymphocytic leukemia (CLL) is a disease characterized by the monoclonal proliferation of lymphocytes (usually B cells) that, unlike normal lymphocytes, often are unable to synthesize immunoglobulin.

Clinical Features

CLL is the most common type of leukemia that is encountered in the United States. It is primarily a disease of older men (17) in that two-thirds of patients are 60 or older and 2 to 3 times as many men are afflicted as are women. A mild tendency for the disease to segregate in families suggests that genetic factors may play a role in its acquisition (1).

Many patients are asymptomatic when diagnosed (see below), but complaints of malaise and of increased fatigability are common. Ultimately most patients develop generalized lymphadenopathy and splenomegaly.

A persistent absolute lymphocytosis (greater than 10,000/μl for 3 months or longer) is the hallmark of the disease; lymphocyte counts as high as 200,000 to 300,000/μl may be seen occasionally. Other tests (bone marrow aspiration, lymph node biopsy) are ordinarily not necessary to establish the diagnosis.

As the disease progresses, hypogammaglobulinemia, anemia, granulocytopenia, and thrombocytopenia may develop. Autoimmune disorders (autoimmune hemolytic anemia and thrombocytopenia and pure red cell aplasia) develop in 10 to 15% of patients.

Treatment and Course (4)

The survival of patients with CLL correlates best with the stage of their disease at diagnosis (13). For example, asymptomatic patients with only an absolute lymphocytosis have an essentially normal life expectancy. Patients with lymphadenopathy alone have a median survival of 6 to 8 years, and patients with anemia or thrombocytopenia have a median survival of 2 to 3 years.

Treatment does not influence survival but can be very helpful in decreasing the severity of signs and symptoms in the later stages of the disease. Thus, stable, asymptomatic patients with or without lymphadenopathy and/or splenomegaly do not require treatment. On the other hand, patients with marked constitutional symptoms (weight loss, severe malaise) or with symptomatic anemia or thrombocytopenia should be treated, usually with an oral alkylating agent (chlorambucil or cyclophosphamide) and with prednisone. Various treatment schedules are utilized, dependent primarily on the preference of the therapist. However, side effects may be minimized if therapy is given in short courses (an alkylating agent on day 1, prednisone on days 1 to 4) every 2 to 3 weeks. Patients with autoimmune hemolysis and thrombocytopenia require more aggressive treatment with corticosteroids, and splenectomy is sometimes necessary in severely anemic or thrombocytopenic patients who are unresponsive to corticosteroids. A hematologist or medical oncologist should be consulted at the time of diagnosis of CLL and should be involved in the care of patients who require treatment.

Differential Diagnosis

A number of neoplastic conditions other than CLL may be associated with a chronic lymphocytosis; macroglobulinemia, B and T cell lymphomas, hairy cell leukemia, prolymphocytic leukemia, and adult T cell leukemia. The morphology of the cells and/or other manifestations of the disease usually lead to the correct diagnosis. These conditions should be managed in close consultation with an oncologist.

In the last 15 years a new syndrome has been recognized (12), most often in older people, characterized by a clonal proliferation of large granular T lymphocytes (up to 10,000 per cumm) and, usually, chronic neutropenia. Anemia (rarely, red cell aplasia) and thrombocytopenia are relatively uncommon. Lymphocytic infiltration of the bone marrow and spleen (with splenomegaly) is characteristic; lymph node involvement is rare. Some patients have coexistant seropositive rheumatoid arthritis; and the majority of patients, with or without arthritis, have serologic abnormalities (e.g., in addition to increased titers of rheumatoid factor, antinuclear antibodies, polyclonal hypergammaglobulinemia, and circulating immune complexes). The major morbidity from the disease is due to recurrent bacterial infections; otherwise, most patients require no treatment and their mortality rate is low.

THE UNDIAGNOSED PATIENT WITH LYMPHADENOPATHY: WHEN TO RECOMMEND LYMPH NODE BIOPSY

Lymphadenopathy is a common physical finding that is associated with multiple disease processes (11). The decision about when to biopsy an enlarged lymph node is one of the more difficult in clinical medicine (5). The problem most often arises in younger patients. Older patients with localized lymphadenopathy, unexplained by infection or inflammation, should be assumed to have cancer until proven otherwise, and the biopsy decision, therefore, is usually an easy one. However, lymphadenopathy in children and in young adults is usually due to inflammation, and biopsy is usually not diagnostic. The clinician is often concerned in such circumstances about the possible harm from a delay in the diagnosis of a malignancy (Hodgkin's disease or non-Hodgkin's lymphoma most commonly) or a granulomatous condition (tuberculosis, sarcoid, etc.) for which specific treatment is indicated. However, considerable harm may result from unnecessary biopsy. There is, for the patient, both psychological and physical discomfort from the procedure, and most important of all there is frequently uncertainty about the interpretation of the biopsy of a "reactive" node. The histology of reactive nodes, especially those encountered in the mononucleosis syndrome, can be difficult to interpret. Reed-Sternberg cells (ordinarily pathognomonic of Hodgkin's disease) can be seen in the nodes of patients with infectious mononucleosis, and reactive nodes can sometimes look like and be interpreted as diagnostic of Hodgkin's disease or of non-Hodgkin's lymphoma. Because of these problems, the physician should avoid, if possible, performing a biopsy of a lymph node in a patient with the mononucleosis syndrome. However, since patients with systemic lymphoma, Hodgkin's disease, miliary tuberculosis, etc. may have symptoms suggestive of the infectious mononucleosis syndrome (fever, anorexia, weight loss, malaise, etc.), one of the main reasons to pursue, by serological studies (see above, page 581), a specific etiology for the syndrome is to attempt to make a diagnosis without having to do a biopsy.

If a specific diagnosis cannot be made on the basis of serological studies, there are relatively few criteria upon which the clinician can rely in order to decide whether a biopsy is indicated. However, one helpful retrospective study reported that in the age range of 9 to 25 years three variables were important in determining whether a lymph node biopsy might be diagnostic of an illness requiring specific treatment (18): (a) the size of the node to be tested by biopsy, (b) the presence or absence of ear-nose-throat symptoms, and (c) the presence or absence of an abnormality on chest X-ray. Nodes greater than 2 cm in diameter were more likely to contain important histological information than were smaller nodes. An abnormal chest X-ray (adenopathy, infiltrate) in a patient with peripheral adenopathy correlated with useful biopsy information. Patients with cervical lymphadenopathy but without any ear-nose-throat symptoms were more likely to have a diagnostic lymph node biopsy. Table 53.7 summarizes some of the features that can be utilized by the physician, especially in the young patient, to help decide about the advisability and timing of a lymph node biopsy.

Table 53.7.
When to Recommend Lymph Node Biopsy in the Teenager and Young Adult

Features against early biopsy
1. Mononucleosis syndrome, especially when proven serologically.
2. Ear-nose-throat symptoms (earache, sore throat, coryza, tonsillar, or dental infection).
3. Lymph nodes less than 2 cm in diameter.
4. Normal chest X-ray, especially when associated with one of the above.

Features for early biopsy
1. Systemic illness with atypical features of the mononucleosis syndrome and without serological proof of a cause of the mononucleosis syndrome (see Table 53.4).
2. Lymph nodes greater than 2 cm in diameter and an abnormal chest X-ray, absence of ear-nose-throat symptoms, or no proof of a typical mononucleosis syndrome.
3. Localized supraclavicular lymphadenopathy. This may be seen in the mononucleosis syndrome but in its absence is suggestive of mediastinal (right supraclavicular) or abdominal (left supraclavicular) granulomatous or neoplastic disease.

General References

Niederman JC: In: Hoeprich PD (ed):*Infectious Disease*, 3rd ed. Philadelphia, Harper and Row, 1983.
>A concise authoritative review.

Rundles RW: In: Williams WJ, Beutler E, Erslev AJ, Lichtman MA (eds): *Hematology*, 3rd ed. New York, McGraw-Hill, 1983.
>A detailed, well-referenced review.

Specific References

1. Conley CL, Misiti J, Laster AJ: Genetic factors predisposing to chronic lymphocytic leukemia. *Medicine* (Baltimore) 59:323, 1980.
2. Dorman JM, Glick TH, Shannon DC, et al: Complications of infectious mononucleosis. *Am J Dis Child* 128:239, 1974.
3. Evans AS, Niederman JC, McCollum RW: Seroepidemiologic studies of infectious mononucleosis with EB virus. *N Engl J Med* 279:1121, 1968.
4. Gale RP, Foon KA: Chronic lymphocytic leukemia. Recent advances in biology and treatment. *Ann Intern Med* 103:101, 1985.
5. Greenfield S, Jordan MC: The clinical investigation of lymphadenopathy in primary care practice. *JAMA* 240:1388, 1978.
6. Holmes GP, Kaplan JE, Gantz NM et al: Chronic fatigue syndrome: a working case definition. *Ann Intern Med* 108:387, 1988.
7. Holmes GP, Kaplan JE, Stewart JA, et al: A cluster of patients with a chronic mononucleosis-like syndrome. Is Epstein-Barr virus the cause? *JAMA* 257:2297, 1987.
8. Horwitz CA, Henle W, Henle G, et al: Heterophile-negative infectious mononucleosis and mononucleosis-like illness. *Am J Med* 63:947, 1977.
9. Horwitz CA, Henle W, Henle G, et al: Infectious mononucleosis in patients aged 40 to 72 years: report of 27 cases, including 3 without heterophil-antibody responses. *Medicine* (Baltimore) 62:256, 1983.
10. Jones JF, Ray CG, Minnich LL: Evidence for active Epstein-Barr virus infection in patients with persistent, unexplained illnesses: Elevated anti-early antigen antibodies. *Ann Intern Med* 102:1, 1985.
11. Libman H: Generalized lymphadenopathy. *J Gen Int Med* 2:48, 1987.
12. Loughran TP, Starkebaum G: Large granular lymphocyte leukemia. Report of 38 cases and review of the literature. *Medicine* (Baltimore) 66:397, 1987.
13. Rai KR, Sawitsky A, Cronkite EP, et al: Clinical staging of chronic lymphocytic leukemia. *Blood* 46:219, 1975.
14. Rippey JH, Bowman HE: Infectious mononucleosis test performance on CAP survey specimens. *Am J Clin Pathol* 72:363, 1979.
15. Rutkow IM: Rupture of the spleen in infectious mononucleosis. *Arch Surg* 113:718, 1978.
16. Sawyer RN, Evans AS, Niederman JC, McCollum RN: Prospective studies of a group of Yale University freshmen. I. Occurrence of infectious mononucleosis. *J Infect Dis* 123:263, 1971.
17. Skinnider LF, Tan L, Schmidt J, Armitage G: Chronic lymphocytic leukemia. A review of 745 cases and assessment of clinical staging. *Cancer* (Phila) 50:2951, 1982.
18. Slap GB, Brooks SJ, Schwartz JS: When to perform biopsies of enlarged peripheral lymph nodes in young patients. *JAMA* 252:1321, 1984.
19. Stein M, Keller SE, Schleifer SJ: Stress and immunomodulation: the role of depression and neuroendocrine function. *J Immunol* 135:827s, 1985.
20. Straus SE: The chronic mononucleosis syndrome. *J Infect Dis* 157:405, 1988.
21. Straus SE, Tosato G, Armstrong G, et al: Persisting illness and fatigue in adults with evidence of Epstein-Barr virus infection. *Ann Intern Med* 102:7, 1985.

SECTION

7

Pulmonary Problems

Common Pulmonary Problems: Cough, Hemoptysis, Dyspnea, Chest Pain, and the Abnormal Chest X-Ray

PHILIP L. SMITH, M.D.
E. JAMES BRITT, M.D.
PETER B. TERRY, M.D.

Patients who develop acute respiratory problems usually present with symptoms that result in the rapid diagnosis and treatment of the underlying disorder. On the other hand, chronic diseases of the lung that cause slowly progressive symptoms may go undetected unless incidentally discovered as part of a general medical evaluation that includes routine chest roentgenogram and screening pulmonary function tests. This chapter will discuss common pulmonary problems with which the general physician is often confronted: cough, hemoptysis, dyspnea, noncardiac chest pain, and the abnormal chest X-ray.

COUGH

Cough is an important defense mechanism that clears the airways of both secretions and inhaled particles (7). Although it is often associated with other respi-ratory symptoms, cough may be the major symptom that prompts a patient to seek medical advice. A cough is composed of three phases: a deep inspiration, closure of the glottis accompanied by a rapid increase in pleural pressure, and a final opening of the glottis with an explosive release of pressure.

Mucosal neural receptors that initiate a cough reflex are located throughout the nasopharynx, larynx, trachea, and bronchi down to the level of the terminal bronchioles. Stimulation of these receptors in the nasopharynx may cause sneezing, whereas stimulation of tracheal and bronchial receptors may also cause bronchospasm. After activation of the receptors, impulses are conducted along afferent pathways in the 9th and 10th cranial nerves to the cough center in the medulla. The reflex is completed through efferent pathways that cause forceful contraction of the diaphragm and other expiratory muscles. Although many different stimuli activate these receptors, all essentially initiate cough by some form of mechanical or chemical irritation. Additional factors, such as acute inflammation of the airways, may disrupt the bronchial mucosa, increase its permeability, and expose the receptors. The accompanying increases in respiratory secretions will lead to cough. Environmental pollutants, such as cigarette smoke, can directly stimulate the receptors without necessarily provoking an inflammatory reaction. Finally, although stimulation of irritant receptors may cause reflex bronchoconstriction, the bronchospasm itself, through reflex pathways, induces cough.

Acute Cough Syndromes

Table 54.1 shows the common and uncommon causes of cough. Generally cough that occurs as a symptom of acute inflammatory disease, such as *tracheitis* or *bronchitis*, is limited by the length of the illness. In contrast, cough that is triggered by mild bronchospasm may persist for weeks to months after a viral upper

Table 54.1.
Causes of Cough

Causes	Examples
COMMON CAUSES	
Acute	
Inflammation	Tracheitis, bronchitis, pneumonia
Irritation	Environmental pollutants
Bronchospasm	Infection
Chronic	
Inflammation	Bronchitis, pollution, cigarettes, bronchiectasis, aspired foreign body
Irritation	Cigarettes, cancer, postnasal drip
Bronchospasm	Asthma, heart failure
LESS COMMON CAUSES	
Irritation	Aortic aneurysm, chronic aspiration, auditory canal stimulation (cerumen, hair)
Inflammation	Sarcoid, alveolitis
Psychogenic	

respiratory tract infection (see below). Usually viral infections and atypical pneumonias are associated with nonproductive coughs, and bacterial infections are associated with significant sputum production. Younger patients tend to have a more productive cough associated with *pneumonia*, whereas older individuals, especially those with chronic obstructive pulmonary disease, may retain secretions because of impaired clearance. When a productive cough follows a typical viral syndrome, it may signal the development of a superimposed bacterial bronchitis or pneumonia. High concentrations of *industrial pollutants, such as insoluble gases (for example, SO_3 or NO_2),* which are not removed in the upper airway, can cause either a nonproductive or a productive cough secondary to chemical irritation.

Chronic Cough Syndromes

Coughing that is persistent is more bothersome than the acute cough syndrome described above. Clearly the most common cause of coughing is *cigarette smoking*. Such coughing is usually dry and hacking and is worse in the morning. The number of cigarettes smoked bears little relationship to the development of cough except when three to four or more packs of cigarettes a day are consumed. Perhaps because they inhale more deeply, smokers of marijuana may complain of a persistent cough after smoking only one to two cigarettes daily. By definition, all patients with bronchitis have productive coughs that may interfere with their sleep (14). As opposed to patients with *bronchogenic and mediastinal tumors,* who often complain of coughing, patients with metastatic tumors or with nodules that arise peripherally outside the airways or beyond irritant receptors seldom present with cough. In nonsmokers, the most common cause of chronic cough is *postnasal drip* resulting from chronic sinusitis or allergic rhinitis (6, 13). It is important to recognize that *lower airways obstruction* (bronchospasm) in smokers as well as nonsmokers can be associated with a chronic dry cough. This, in fact, may be the only manifestation of early asthma and need not be associated with dyspnea, wheezing, or changes in baseline pulmonary function. A dry hacking cough, associated with dyspnea, is common in patients in *heart failure* (see Chapter 61).

Other less common causes of chronic cough include any process that stimulates the neural receptors in the pleura and pericardium (7). Even *impacted cerumen* in the external auditory canal can elicit a chronic cough. If a history and physical examination have revealed no positive findings, it is often tempting to attribute chronic cough to a psychogenic etiology; however, this is an extremely rare cause of coughing, most often reported in children. Characteristically, *psychogenic cough* is not productive, it subsides during sleep, and it is clearly related to emotional stress (10).

Evaluation

Evaluation of the acute and chronic cough syndromes is similar. Usually a history and physical examination will yield a presumptive diagnosis. Information should be obtained about the circumstances surrounding the development and duration of the cough, environmental exposure, smoking history, and any past history of obstructive airways disease. A history of constant swallowing or of throat clearing is associated with postnasal drip, even though the patient may deny many other symptoms associated with sinusitis.

Although the physical examination seldom provides a specific diagnosis, it may provide important clues. Careful examination of the ears, nose, throat, and lungs may yield relevant clues to a diagnosis. Cobblestoning in the oropharynx represents lymphoid hyperplasia and is commonly seen in patients with chronic sinusitis. Examination of the chest may reveal rhonchi caused by the loose secretions that result from acute or chronic infection. A localized wheeze suggests a bronchogenic tumor, whereas wheezing at end expiration suggests the diagnosis of obstructive airways disease. Finally, the physical examination allows the quality and severity of the cough to be observed. A harsh cough associated with loose secretions is characteristic of tracheobronchitis resulting from viral upper respiratory infection. When little or no coughing occurs in the course of the visit, the patient should be asked to cough to determine whether the cough is productive or is associated with wheezing. This is also useful since some patients, especially women, refuse to admit to expectoration of sputum and often unconsciously swallow their secretions.

If a diagnosis is not obvious after a history and physical examination, a chest X-ray is indicated. It may reveal a tumor, a major infection, or another chronic inflammatory process involving the parenchyma of the lungs. The X-ray also may demonstrate atelectasis associated with a bronchogenic tumor or with an aspirated foreign body. Patients with coughing due to viral and bacterial tracheobronchitis, asthma, or cigarette smoking will usually have a normal chest X-ray.

In patients with a normal roentgenogram, examination of the sputum may be useful, especially in individuals who are suspected of having asthma. Frequently purulent-appearing sputum will have eosinophils that can be distinguished on a microscopic examination of a "wet prep" of sputum. Spirometry can be routinely employed in the office to screen for evidence of early obstructive airways disease. However, a normal spirogram does not necessarily exclude the diagnosis (see Chapter 55).

If no specific diagnosis has been made after this evaluation, the patient should be seen periodically for 1 to 2 months before other invasive diagnostic procedures are attempted. When the chest X-ray is normal, bronchoscopy seldom provides additional useful information. Although a proximal bronchogenic tumor can be hidden on a chest X-ray by the mediastinal shadows, patients with these tumors often have associated hemoptysis (see below) (22).

Confirmation that bronchospasm or hyper-reactive airways are the causes of persistent coughing can be obtained in some pulmonary function laboratories by bronchoprovocation tests with pharmacological agents, such as histamine or methacholine (see Chapter 55).

Therapy

The specific therapy of the various acute inflammatory and irritating processes likely to cause coughing is discussed in detail in individual chapters dealing with these topics.

In general, viral tracheobronchitis requires only symptomatic therapy since coughing will usually spontaneously subside in 2 to 4 weeks. Patients with persistent coughing and a history compatible with bronchospasm secondary to allergic airways disease, intermittent chronic obstructive airways disease, or with bronchospasm and coughing after a viral upper respiratory tract infection may benefit significantly from bronchodilators. Treatment should begin with an inhaled long-acting specific β_2-sympathomimetic agonist (metaproterenol, terbutaline, fenoterol), and later, if necessary, an oral methylxanthine can be added. A detailed therapeutic approach to the pharmacological treatment of bronchospasm is presented in Chapter 55.

Cessation of cigarette smoking and avoidance of a polluted environment may be the most important aspects of the therapy of both acute and chronic cough. In one study of 200 patients with a chronic cough, 50% had relief within 1 month of cessation of cigarette smoking while eventually 77% of these patients had complete resolution of their cough (21). Thus, the patient who continues to smoke and to complain of cough is particularly frustrating since it is often difficult to convey the notion that as few as one or two cigarettes/day cause airway irritation and inflammation.

Removal of impacted cerumen in the auditory canal provides immediate relief (see Chapter 96). The treatment of postnasal drip is dealt with in Chapter 28.

After specific therapy has been initiated, the use of antitussives should be considered. In spite of the enormous demands made for *antitussives*, there are few situations in which these preparations are absolutely necessary. Moreover, the expectoration of sputum is a major goal in the therapy of patients with chronic obstructive airways disease. Therefore, when antitussives are needed in patients with productive coughs, it is usually better to attempt cough reduction (not total suppression), primarily to allow patients to sleep. In the United States there are several hundred cough and decongestant preparations usually sold as combination products. Many of them combine so-called expectorants with antitussives and should be avoided since, insofar as they have an effect, they work at cross purposes.

Antitussives act on the cough reflex either by anesthetizing the peripheral irritant receptors or by increasing the threshold of the cough center. Probably the two most effective "non-narcotic" antitussives are dextromethorphan and benzonatate (Table 54.2). Dextromethorphan is chemically derived from the opiates; however, it is classified as non-narcotic because at prescribed doses it has no sedative or analgesic effects and, therefore, has little potential for abuse. Dextro-

methorphan suppresses cough centrally. Occasionally, the drug will cause nausea or dizziness, and overdosages of more than 200 mg may lead to central nervous system depression. Benzonatate is a peripherally acting anesthetic similar to tetracaine. Its only side effects are mild dizziness, vertigo, and occasional nausea. If the drug is accidentally chewed, both unpleasant taste and prolonged oral anesthesia will occur. Overdosage has been associated with central nervous system stimulation resulting in tremors followed by profound central nervous system depression. It is reasonable to treat patients initially with dextromethorphan and, if intolerable cough persists, to substitute benzonatate.

If non-narcotic antitussives are ineffective, then codeine can be tried. Many clinicians will prescribe codeine preferentially to patients with persistent cough because it is a more potent cough suppressant than the non-narcotic agents. Codeine is effective in doses of 20 to 30 mg administered every 3 to 6 hours. The common side effects—nausea, vomiting, constipation, dry mouth, and sedation—are usually not experienced at these lower doses.

Topical oral anesthetics can be used as cough suppressants, but they are weak, usually ineffective, and may cause hypersensitivity reactions. If abused or used in excessive doses, the gag reflex will be abolished and the risk of pulmonary aspiration will be increased. The use of expectorants and humidification of the airways in patients with respiratory disease is discussed in Chapter 55.

HEMOPTYSIS

Hemoptysis is defined as the expectoration of blood. It can range from the coughing of minimal amounts of blood-tinged sputum to the coughing of large amounts of blood with clots. Distinguishing between hemoptysis and hematemesis can be difficult. Expectorated blood usually is bright red, frothy, has an alkaline pH, and is usually mixed with sputum containing macrophages and white blood cells. Frequently, patients with hemoptysis will complain of a tickling or bothersome irritation in their chest. On the other hand, hematemesis is characterized by blood that is darker brown, has an acid pH, and is mixed with food particles. Sometimes blood from a lesion in the sinuses or in the upper airway will be aspirated and later expectorated, making it appear that the bleeding occurred in the lower respiratory tract. A careful history and physical examination must be performed to avoid inappropriate treatment. The patient should be instructed to collect and save his bloody sputum so that the hemoptysis can be quantified. Nevertheless, a history of hemoptysis should not be ignored if a patient cannot produce a specimen on command since the symptom can be intermittent.

The various pulmonary causes of hemoptysis are summarized in Table 54.3.

In the typical ambulatory practice, blood streaking of the sputum is caused by bronchitis or bronchiectasis 30 to 60% of the time, and by lung cancer 20 to 30%

Table 54.2.
Non-Narcotic Antitussives

Drug	Brand Name	Usual Dose	Site of Action	Comment
Dextromethorphan	Many preparations	15–30 mg four times a day	Central	Considered most effective central agent
Benzonatate	Tessalon	100–200 mg four times a day	Peripheral	Considered most effective peripheral agent

Table 54.3.
Pulmonary Causes of Hemoptysis

COMMON	
Inflammatory	Bronchitis, bronchiectasis, tuberculosis, pneumonia, lung abscess
Neoplasm	Lung cancer
Vascular	Pulmonary embolus/infarction
LESS COMMON	
Inflammatory/ immunological	Goodpasture's syndrome, idiopathic pulmonary hemosiderosis, cavitary disease (with a "fungus ball"), parasites, broncholithiasis, cystic fibrosis
Neoplasm	Bronchial adenoma, metastatic cancer
Vascular	Arteriovenous malformation, sequestration, mitral stenosis, anticoagulation
Chest trauma	

of the time. *Bronchiectasis* is less common today than it once was, principally because of the successful treatment of many serious childhood pulmonary infections. Active cavitary *tuberculosis* also is now a less common cause of hemoptysis than it once was, but residual upper lobe bronchiectasis, the result of old tuberculous infection, is still frequently found. *Bronchogenic carcinoma* presents with hemoptysis at two stages: blood streaked sputum may be a brief manifestation of a small irritative mucosal lesion; the symptom may resolve only to be replaced at a later date by major hemoptysis from a large endobronchial tumor that is friable or necrotic or is eroding central vessels. Usually blood from *pneumonia* or a *lung abscess* is mixed with "pus," and the sputum appears red-brown or red-green. Hemoptysis from *pulmonary emboli* occurs in approximately 30% of cases of documented emboli associated with an infarction of the lung (2). Interestingly, even with the advent of the fiberoptic bronchoscope, the cause of hemoptysis remains undiagnosed 5 to 15% of the time (22).

Less common causes of hemoptysis are also listed in Table 54.3, but this ranking reflects to some extent the location of a practice since mycetomas within fungus cavities (9) and parasitic diseases that cause hemoptysis, for example, will be much more frequently seen in areas of the country where those problems are endemic. Although the more common presentation of bronchial adenomas is atelectasis with cough and fever, these vascular tumors do cause hemoptysis. Metastatic tumors tend to enlarge within the lung parenchyma; thus bleeding as the initial presentation is exceedingly rare. Patients with *mitral stenosis* and

pulmonary vascular congestion are prone to hemoptysis with any source of lung irritation. Although certainly less frequent today, this valvular abnormality is often silent and the history of rheumatic fever forgotten. Patients being *anticoagulated* with warfarin or heparin may develop hemoptysis. Whether this symptom is a clue to a specific bronchial lesion is not clear insofar as no substantial experience with this problem has yet been published. Any inflammation of the airways in an anticoagulated patient may be complicated by hemoptysis. Occasionally *blunt chest trauma* will produce hemoptysis in an otherwise healthy individual.

Evaluation

The diagnostic evaluation of hemoptysis is aimed at determining the cause, localizing the site, and quantifying the amount of bleeding. The history and physical examination are directed at uncovering clues to the causes outlined in Table 54.3. An attempt should be made to quantitate the amount of hemoptysis by history and by repeated examination of the sputum since patients who have expectorated more than 25 to 50 ml of bright red blood during a 24-hour period require hospitalization in case bleeding becomes massive. Massive hemoptysis, defined as more than 600 ml of blood during a 24-hour period, represents a medical emergency, and survival of the patient is dependent on rapid diagnosis and, often, on surgical therapy (15).

During the physical examination, extrathoracic sources of bleeding from structures such as the nasal passages, sinuses, and pharynx should be sought. The significance of localized wheezing or rales must be interpreted with caution insofar as the sounds may be produced by aspired blood or secretions.

Evaluation of the chest X-ray is essential since all acute inflammatory diseases, such as active tuberculosis, pneumonia, and lung abscess, will produce obvious pulmonary infiltrates. In addition, 85% of neoplasms and most pulmonary emboli with an associated infarction will also show localized pulmonary lesions. However, localization of the bleeding source is frequently precluded by bilateral aspiration of blood or by the presence of bilateral pulmonary disease on chest roentgenogram. Patients with bronchitis or bronchiectasis often have normal films. If the bronchiectasis is a result of old tuberculosis, however, apical scarring may suggest the diagnosis; otherwise, there may be increased lower lobe markings or infiltrates if there is recurrent infection. Bronchitis is a clinical diagnosis made in patients with a productive cough, although differentiation of bronchitis from bronchiectasis is difficult by history and chest roentgenogram alone. Bronchography can be used to distinguish these entities, but the complications of this procedure do not warrant its diagnostic use unless bleeding is recurrent and severe, and unless surgical resection is being considered. Furthermore, the medical management of both bronchitis and bronchiectasis is the same.

When the chest X-ray is normal, endobronchial malignancy is the principal disease to exclude. However, bronchitis and bronchiectasis are the most likely diagnoses. Individuals under 40 years old, including smokers, with hemoptysis that has lasted less than 1 week are unlikely to have cancer (16). In such patients, the evaluation can be limited to analysis of the sputum for tuberculosis as well as to cytologic examination of three sputum samples for malignant cells. Sputum collection should include an overnight sample and an early morning sample, freshly delivered to the laboratory as one complete specimen.

Persistent or recurrent hemoptysis mandates a more thorough evaluation that includes bronchoscopy. In individuals who smoke, who are over 40 years of age, and who have hemoptysis with a normal chest roentgenogram, one in six to seven patients will have lung cancer (22). Sputum cytology will provide the diagnosis in half of these patients, but bronchoscopy will be required to characterize or to locate the site of malignancy and plan for therapy in all patients. A few patients with positive sputum cytology under these conditions will be found to have a head and neck malignancy.

Therapy

Patients who expectorate more than 25 to 50 ml of blood a day should be hospitalized (see above) for diagnosis and treatment. Patients with lesser amounts of hemoptysis should also be hospitalized if they have an abnormal chest X-ray or if subsequent evaluation (sputum cytology or bronchoscopy) reveals a tumor. Patients with the diagnosis of bronchitis or of bronchiectasis can usually be treated on an ambulatory basis with antibiotics, such as tetracycline or ampicillin, 1 to 2 g/day for 10 days. Blood streaking of the sputum usually resolves within 2 to 3 days, but a full course of antibiotic therapy should be completed. In the case of cryptogenic hemoptysis, the prognosis is good in patients with a normal chest X-ray and a nondiagnostic fiberoptic bronchoscopy (1).

Blood is very irritating to the tracheobronchial tree and triggers constant cough, which by itself is traumatic. Mild cough suppression will help. Heavy sedation is undesirable. The patient must maintain the ability to expectorate blood as it accumulates.

DYSPNEA

Breathing is an unconscious act that usually occurs effortlessly; yet even a normal person becomes aware of his breathing during deep sighs or during moderate to severe exercise. Dyspnea, the abnormal, uncomfortable sensation of breathlessness, is difficult to define since patients often cannot accurately perceive or quantitate the feeling. Similar to an individual's threshold for the recognition of pain, the complaint of dyspnea is dependent both on the individual's limit for discomfort and on the specific circumstances that provoke shortness of breath. Thus, dyspnea must be defined in terms of what is abnormal for a particular individual in the context of his level of fitness and of the amount of activity that is associated with breathlessness. Some patients become dyspneic with relatively small measurable alterations in ventilation, whereas others, such as patients who are hyperventilating with Kussmaul breathing, may not complain of dyspnea. Fortunately, a reasonable correlation exists between the degree of dyspnea and objective measurements of physiological dysfunction.

Often the actual complaint of dyspnea may not be expressed as such, and it may vary depending on the type of precipitating illness as well as on whether it developed abruptly or over a longer period of time. Thus, the asthmatic may complain of acute shortness of breath or of a "tightness" in his chest, whereas the patient with an acute pulmonary embolism may state that his breath has suddenly been taken away, and he cannot "get enough air" even though he ventilates easily. In contrast, the patient with emphysema who has modified his life style may dismiss the sensation of breathlessness as part of his advancing age.

Normal Ventilation

There is no single mechanism responsible for dyspnea. Because dyspnea is the result of a variety of diverse influences acting alone or together, a brief discussion of the control of ventilation may help the practicing physician understand the complexity of dyspnea and the reason why this sensation often does not immediately respond to correction of obvious physiological abnormalities. Normally ventilation is coupled to the individual's metabolic demands as reflected in the oxygen consumption and carbon dioxide elimination necessary to meet a given level of activity. These needs are sensed by peripheral (carotid and aortic bodies) and central (medullary) chemical chemoreceptors that respond to the O_2, CO_2, and pH of blood and cerebral spinal fluid. The acute stimulation of these receptors provokes changes in minute ventilation. In addition, the control and regulation of the rate and pattern of breathing are influenced by the reflex effects of activation of neural receptors that lie in the lung parenchyma, airways, blood vessels, respiratory muscles, and chest wall. For example, receptors in the chest wall and diaphragm will respond to increased stiffness (decreased compliance) in the lung that occurs with fluid accumulation or with interstitial fibrosis. In addition, interstitial edema may activate "C" fibers located in the alveolar interstitium and may reflexly cause dyspnea in patients with pulmonary edema. Other receptors located in the airway epithelium cause rapid shallow breathing, coughing, and bronchospasm when irritating substances are inhaled. Finally, the central nervous system alone can cause large alterations in breathing that lead to hyperventilation in association with anxiety attacks (see Chapter 13). This discussion should help in understanding, for example, why the correction of arterial hypoxemia alone in a patient with an asthmatic attack usually does not relieve the sensation of breathlessness. In this situation, dyspnea results from the complex interaction of both chemical and neural stimuli to breathe, coupled with an individual's response to these signals. Correction of only one of these problems, therefore, is not sufficient to abolish dyspnea.

Evaluation

The causes of dyspnea are diverse and include essentially all diseases that result in significant functional impairment of either the respiratory system (gas exchange and/or pulmonary mechanics) or the cardiovascular system (circulatory and/or cardiac function) as well as any hematological abnormality that impairs oxygen delivery. Table 54.4 summarizes the general disease categories that are likely to cause abnormal breathlessness.

In ambulatory practice the major causes of dyspnea are obstructive airways disease and arteriosclerotic and hypertensive heart disease, either alone or in combination. The prevalence of symptomatic lung disease in a specific geographic region or socioeconomic group is further modified by the prevalence of cigarette consumption, urban pollution, and occupational exposure to inhaled toxic substances. Furthermore, the clinical circumstances and sequence of events in which dyspnea occurs will aid in its evaluation.

One of the first steps in evaluating a patient who complains of dyspnea is deciding whether the symptoms reflect an acute or chronic event since the more serious causes of dyspnea tend to present abruptly. In general, dyspnea of sudden onset is easier to evaluate, but the workup must proceed quickly to determine whether the patient should be admitted to the hospital for more intensive evaluation and therapy. On the other hand, the evaluation of chronic dyspnea can usually be accomplished more slowly in an ambulatory setting.

Acute Dyspnea

The history, physical examination, and chest X-ray form the focal point of the evaluation of a patient with acute dyspnea. In a young patient, the medical history and physical examination alone will often suggest the presumptive diagnosis. Where necessary, additional distinction of primary cardiac from pulmonary disorders will be aided by the chest X-ray, spirogram, and electrocardiogram (ECG). *Acute tracheobronchitis* should be considered in the middle-aged smoker with cough, dyspnea, and purulent sputum in association with a clear chest X-ray. When wheezing and rhonchi are present, the term "asthmatic bronchitis" is often used.

Spontaneous pneumothorax (see also below, page 602) presents with sudden sharp chest pain and dyspnea. A small significant pneumothorax on chest X-ray can be easily missed, and diagnostic accuracy will be improved with an expiratory film. Previously undiagnosed *interstitial lung disease, bullous lung disease,* and *cystic fibrosis* may also present with spontaneous pneumothoraces. In these cases, the chest film should demonstrate characteristic abnormalities.

Acute dyspnea in association with fever, cough, and purulent sputum with localized infiltrates suggests *pneumonia,* usually bacterial (see Chapter 28). Diffuse infiltrates and nonproductive cough suggest atypical pneumonia (see Chapter 28).

The patient with acute dyspnea and known *heart failure* will present with usual cardiac symptoms and signs including paroxysmal nocturnal dyspnea, rales, cardiomegaly, and a relatively symmetrical interstitial pattern with or without pleural effusions suggest heart failure. *Psychogenic dyspnea* or the hyperventilation syndrome has a rapid onset and is usually found in

Table 54.4.
Causes of Dyspnea

Dyspnea	Acute	Chronic
COMMON		
Pulmonary		
Obstructive airways disease	Asthma, bronchitis	COPD
Restrictive lung disease	Pneumothorax	Pleural effusions, cancer, diffuse interstitial lung disease
Inflammatory	Pneumonia	
Vascular	Pulmonary embolism	
Cardiac	Heart Failure (ischemic)	Heart failure (myopathic)
Other	Psychogenic	Obesity, anemia
LESS COMMON		
Pulmonary		
Upper airway obstruction	Epiglottis, aspiration (foreign body)	Goiter
Restrictive Lung Disease		Diaphragm paralyses, kyphoscoliosis
Vascular		Pulmonary hypertension
Cardiac		Heart failure (pericardial disease)
Other	CO intoxication	

emotionally disturbed or anxious patients (see Chapter 13).

Less common but important causes of acute dyspnea include acute *foreign body aspiration*, usually evident from the history of aspiration, and a physical examination that demonstrates decreased breath sounds over that part of the lung supplied by the occluded bronchus. During the heating season or in certain industrial settings, *carbon monoxide intoxication* should be considered as a cause of headaches and dyspnea. Diagnosis requires a high degree of suspicion and awareness of the problem. Confirmation requires measurement of carboxy hemoglobin with a co-oximeter. The partial pressure of oxygen measured in the arterial blood gas sample will remain normal.

Pulmonary Embolism

Pulmonary embolism is a major life-threatening cause of acute dyspnea, but the diagnosis can be difficult. Its evaluation requires a systematic approach with a logical sequence of diagnostic testing.

The incidence of pulmonary embolism is high in patients with a recent history of peripheral venous disease, prolonged immobilization, chronic obstructive lung disease, or congestive heart failure. In a multicenter study (2) 60% of patients with pulmonary embolism were men, and, of the women under age 45 who had pulmonary emboli, 75% were found to be using oral contraceptives (see Chapter 93). In this same study, the most frequent symptoms present at the time of diagnosis were dyspnea and chest pain, which were found in over 80% of patients. Hemoptysis, cough, and apprehension were seen less frequently. The physical examination is usually not helpful in the diagnosis, especially since many of the patients have underlying respiratory and cardiovascular diseases that may, in themselves, produce abnormal physical findings: tachycardia, tachypnea, an accentuated second pulmonic heart sound, etc.

Most laboratory tests are not useful in the diagnosis of pulmonary embolism (17). Chest roentgenograms are frequently abnormal, but the findings are nonspecific (localized infiltrates, atelectasis, an elevated hemidiaphragm, or a pleural effusion). The arterial gas tensions are also often abnormal (reduced PaO_2 and $PaCO_2$) but are not helpful diagnostically, in part because of considerable variation and in part because of the high prevalence of cardiopulmonary diseases that alter both the PaO_2 and $PaCO_2$.

The most useful procedure in the screening of patients for pulmonary embolism is a ventilation/perfusion (V/Q) scan of the lungs. (A perfusion scan alone will not always permit the probabilities of embolism to be established accurately.) Whether the patient is hospitalized before having the scan depends on the severity of the presentation.

Patient experience. There is little discomfort associated with a lung scan. The patient should be instructed that he will inhale an oxygen and xenon mixture for 3 to 4 minutes, followed by a venous injection of radioactive-labeled technetium. Several different projections are then recorded on a scanner while the patient is lying on a table.

The V/Q scan is 100% sensitive, but it can be nonspecific depending on the configuration, location, and number of perfusion defects seen (12). If the V/Q scan is normal, the diagnosis of an acute pulmonary embolus is excluded. In general, 5 to 7% of patients with a low probability scan, 20 to 30% of patients with a moderate probability scan, and 80 to 90% of patients with a high probability scan have a pulmonary embolism. However, it must be emphasized that the use of these probabilities is dependent on strict adherence to accepted published criteria for interpreting lung scans (3) and on the experience of the individual nuclear medicine laboratory. Patients with low, moderate, or high probability scans should be hospitalized for further diagnostic studies (angiography) and/or anticoagulation with heparin (see Chapter 51). Patients with acute dyspnea and simultaneous symptoms and signs of peripheral venous thrombosis (less than 40% of patients with pulmonary emboli) should undergo venography to confirm the diagnosis (see Chapter 51). If venography is positive, the patient should be hospitalized for initiation of anticoagulant therapy.

The resolution of pulmonary emboli varies and can occur as early as 1 to 2 weeks in patients who have had small emboli. With larger emboli and in those patients with underlying cardiopulmonary disease, there may be angiographic evidence of emboli that persist for 2 or 3 months (4). If chest pain occurs after discharge, a repeated lung scan (and perhaps, depending on the results, angiography) is necessary to determine whether embolization has recurred.

Evaluation of Chronic or Progressive Dyspnea

In contrast to acute dyspnea, chronic dyspnea usually is more difficult to diagnose and often requires more extensive diagnostic procedures; therefore, the evaluation should proceed in a logical sequence to avoid initially expensive and invasive laboratory testing. The first step is a careful history. Because shortness of breath is appropriate to certain levels of activity depending on the fitness of the individual, the physician must decide whether the patient's symptoms are abnormal and over what period of time they have developed. Many patients with chronic cardiopulmonary disease adapt to the insidious onset of dyspnea by subconsciously changing daily habits and avoiding physical activity. The degree of dyspnea should be determined by comparing the patient's abilities to perform work with an appropriate peer group and with his baseline performance. Thus, the complaint of dyspnea in a 35-year-old who normally runs 5 miles and now becomes short of breath after running only 2 miles should not be ignored.

The most useful initial laboratory test is the chest X-ray, which is often abnormal and therefore directs subsequent evaluation. Patients with *chronic obstruc-*

tive pulmonary disease associated with emphysema have hyperinflation, decreased lung markings, and usually evidence of bullous formation (see Chapter 55). Large *pleural effusions, lung cancer,* or *heart disease* associated with dyspnea will result in obvious changes in the chest roentgenogram with evidence of fluid occupying at least half of one hemithorax, large mass lesions, or cardiomegaly, respectively. *Interstitial lung disease* that has led to fibrosis is revealed by chest X-ray, although the precise cause often requires intensive investigation (see below).

Patients with dyspnea and a normal or nonspecific chest X-ray usually represent the most difficult group to diagnose. Most of these patients have obstructive lung disease. In general, *obesity* is not associated with dyspnea unless body weight is markedly increased (50 to 100% or more or 100 pounds or more over ideal weight). *Primary pulmonary hypertension* may be associated with subtle dilation of the pulmonary arteries on chest X-ray and is most commonly seen in young asthenic women. Upper airway obstruction due, for example, to *goiter* often is not apparent on a routine posterior-anterior and lateral chest roentgenogram.

A spirogram is useful to screen for occult lung disease since a normal spirogram virtually excludes significant parenchymal or airways disease. Although patients with exercise-induced asthma may have a normal spirogram during symptom-free periods, more commonly there is evidence of slight reduction in the baseline forced expiratory volume, as a percentage of forced vital capacity. Additional specialized procedures that aid in the diagnosis of exercise-induced asthma are discussed in Chapter 55. Finally, initial laboratory testing should include a hemoglobin determination or hematocrit value to determine whether a patient is severely anemic or polycythemic.

If an obvious cause of dyspnea is not found after these initial investigations, additional more specialized tests may be necessary. They can usually be obtained by referral of patients to pulmonary function or cardiac diagnostic laboratories.

1. *Complete pulmonary function tests.* In addition to baseline spirometry (see Chapter 55) other pulmonary function tests include the measurement of total lung capacity and functional residual capacity, which quantitate the degree of hyperinflation or restriction. Categorization of a disorder as obstructive or restrictive will direct the physician to a narrowed list of causes. The diffusion capacity measures the amount of alveolar capillary surface area available for gas exchange. Thus, the diffusion capacity is reduced in patients with pulmonary emboli and other vascular occlusive diseases as well as in patients with emphysema. In contrast, an elevated diffusion capacity is found in conditions that elevate the pulmonary blood volume—for example, erythrocytosis or early congestive heart failure. These additional tests should only be considered if spirometry is abnormal. Measurement of inspiratory and expiratory pressures helps characterize

neuromuscular problems. Flow-volume loops will help identify upper airway sources of obstruction. The experience of the patient during the performance of these tests is described in Chapter 55.

2. *Arterial blood gas analysis.* An arterial blood gas determination should be performed to document the presence of hypoxemia or hypercapnia and to characterize the acid-base status. Several general points require emphasis: First, a normal resting arterial blood gas does not exclude significant pulmonary disease. In fact, many patients with severe chronic obstructive lung disease may have normal resting arterial $PaCO_2$ and pH with only slight reductions in PaO_2. Therefore, during an evaluation of dyspnea, a blood gas should be obtained in conjunction with other assessments of pulmonary function. Second, arterial blood gases should be drawn during exercise in a dyspneic patient since abnormalities in gas exchange that occur during exercise usually reverse immediately. Third, measurement of blood gases should not be used as a definitive screening procedure to exclude the diagnosis of pulmonary embolism since normal values may be obtained even with large pulmonary emboli.

3. *Cardiovascular testing.* The use of specialized noninvasive cardiovascular evaluation, including echocardiograms and gated heartpool nuclear scanning to assess right and left ventricular function or the presence of valvular heart disease, is discussed in Chapters 60 and 61.

4. *Exercise testing.* If a patient is dyspneic on exertion and baseline testing of cardiopulmonary function, as described above, is normal or only mildly abnormal, exercise testing should be considered.

In general, there are two types of exercise tests available. The first is a standard *cardiac stress test* during which the patient is exercised and is observed for the development of chest pain and for electrocardiographic ischemic changes (Chapter 57). The cardiac stress test can be modified to permit functional evaluation of cardiac performance during exercise by using radioisotope scanning techniques with thallium (Chapter 57). The second type of exercise testing is a *cardiopulmonary stress test* in which cardiac function, pulmonary gas exchange, ventilation, and physical fitness are quantitated at specific work loads. The two types of tests are similar, but the patient should be told that the cardiopulmonary test requires continuous exercise while breathing into a mouthpiece, measurement of oxygenation is made either by an oximeter or by means of an indwelling arterial line. Such complicated cardiopulmonary stress testing is justified and useful in order to determine whether dyspnea is due to (a) cardiac disease, (b) pulmonary disease including exercise-induced asthma or occult pulmonary vascular disease, or (c) poor physical fitness. This type of testing is particularly useful in evaluating patients for disability compensation, since static pulmonary function and noninvasive cardiac testing may not accurately predict the functional state of a given patient during actual working conditions. It is usually possible for the referring physician to determine presumptively the most likely etiology for dyspnea and to make the appropriate referral for the specific exercise test. In large hospital centers with combined cardiopulmonary laboratories, simultaneous consultation and exercise testing by cardiologists and pulmonologists may be available.

This approach to the evaluation of dyspnea will almost always answer the questions necessary for diagnosis of the underlying condition and for establishment of a therapeutic regimen in patients with dyspnea. At times, a patient with circulatory abnormalities may need a brief hospital admission for additional invasive cardiac catheterization studies to assess the state of the pulmonary vasculature or the degree of cardiac dysfunction. For example, it may be necessary to insert a Swan-Ganz catheter into the pulmonary circulation and to measure directly pulmonary arterial pressures and pulmonary capillary wedge pressures to learn whether a patient with severe obstructive lung disease and cor pulmonale also has significant functional left ventricular failure that requires treatment.

Therapy

Treatment of dyspnea is primarily aimed at therapy of the underlying cardiac, pulmonary, or hematological disorders that cause abnormal breathlessness. In certain patients with underlying irreversible lung disease, specific measures that improve respiratory muscle function may alleviate symptomatic dyspnea. Training programs that increase both muscle strength and endurance are available in selected hospital or community rehabilitation centers and have resulted in decreased shortness of breath in some patients. In addition, there is recent evidence that patients with chronically fatigued respiratory muscles may benefit from total rest by use of outpatient noninvasive mechanical ventilation. Finally, since anxiety or depression is commonly associated with the development of chronic cardiopulmonary disorders associated with dyspnea, appropriate anxiolytics or antidepressants may be useful (see Chapter 13). Benzodiazepines and tricyclic antidepressants in the usual recommended dosages do not cause significant respiratory depression and are generally recommended in combination with good supportive psychological counseling (19). Although codeine has been suggested as potentially useful (20), there is more recent evidence that worsening respiratory failure may occur in patients treated with codeine.

NONCARDIAC CHEST PAIN

Chest pain is a particularly frightening symptom because of the widespread knowledge and concern about heart disease; however, nonspecific musculoskeletal pain is more common than angina, especially in patients less than 40 years old (5). Most patients with chest pain can be evaluated and treated in an ambulatory setting; a few patients require referral to a specialist. The common noncardiac cause of chest pain will be discussed in this section, which should be read in conjunction with Chapter 57.

Afferent neural impulses responsible for thoracic pain are carried by the sympathetic chain, vagus, and phrenic nerves. Visceral structures, which include the lung, diaphragm, heart, and esophagus, all lie within the thoracic cage and have overlapping innervation. Chest pain arising from these different organs will often have similar referral patterns; therefore, irritation of the diaphragmatic pleura, diaphragm, or pericardium, due to either thoracic or abdominal disease, causes chest pain that radiates to the shoulder. In addition, patients may have difficulty localizing pain from the deeper anatomical structures within the chest, whereas diseases involving the superficial structures, muscles, and ribs will be more easily localized. Because there is no sensory innervation of the lung parenchyma, alveolar or interstitial disease does not cause chest pain unless the pulmonary vasculature, bronchi, or pleura are involved.

Table 54.5 lists selected common and less common causes of chest pain. Fleeting, sharp, or lance-like chest pain is the most common complaint in patients who do not have evidence of organic heart disease. Smokers complain more frequently than nonsmokers of both angina-like and nonangina-like chest pain. This has resulted in use of the term "tobacco angina" to describe two distinct types of chest pain in smokers (5). There are smokers with pre-existing angina whose pains clearly are precipitated by smoking. There is also a second, larger group of smokers who have normal or diseased hearts and who complain of intermittent atypical chest pain that is not necessarily associated with smoking a cigarette. This chest pain is not relieved by nitroglycerin or provoked by exercise. It gradually disappears within weeks to months, some-

Table 54.5.
Causes of Chest Pain

COMMON CAUSES	
Chest wall (musculoskeletal)	Nonspecific (smokers, nonsmokers with increased exertion) Costochondritis (Tietze's syndrome)
Cardiac	Angina
Pulmonary	Tracheitis, cough, pleuritis, pneumonia
Neurological	Radicular pain of cervical spine disease
LESS COMMON CAUSES	
Chest wall (musculoskeletal)	Thoracic outlet syndrome, herpes zoster, fractured rib, tumor
Cardiac	Aneurysm, pericarditis
Pulmonary	Pneumothorax, pulmonary embolus, pulmonary hypertension, cancer
Gastrointestinal	Stomach disease, duodenal ulcer, abdominal infection, peritonitis, esophageal reflux

times years after the cessation of smoking; and it is assumed that it is not due to myocardial ischemia.

Musculoskeletal pain is very common in young individuals who increase their exercise abruptly (including the patient who acutely hyperventilates as part of an anxiety state—see Chapter 13). A history of unusual exertion with increased breathing plus tenderness of intercostal muscles usually suffices to make this diagnosis.

Pain caused by *tracheitis* or *tracheobronchitis* is a distinctive substernal burning sensation that is precipitated by coughing and is most often associated with viral respiratory infections. This is in contrast to the sharp, stabbing, pleuritic chest pain that is experienced with pneumonia. The latter is clearly localized to the chest wall and arises from stretching the inflamed parietal pleura during breathing or coughing.

Other causes of chest pain include *costochondritis* (Tietze's syndrome), which is an anterior localized pain associated with tenderness over one or more costochondral junctions; *herpes zoster*, which commonly causes unilateral aching and/or itching, limited to one dermatome, which may precede by several days the eruption of vesicles; *rib fracture* or *bone metastases*, which are more chronic and pleuritic in nature; and *cervical spine disease* with referred pain to the chest (see Chapter 64). Acute stabbing chest pain can occur with a *spontaneous pneumothorax*, which occurs primarily in young men or in older patients with obstructive pulmonary disease. Frequently, a small (< 20%) pneumothorax is not accompanied by significant dyspnea in otherwise healthy individuals. Pleuritic chest pain associated with *pulmonary emboli* results from infarction of parenchymal lung tissue with irritation of the parietal pleura and almost always is associated with dyspnea; and in most patients, the chest roentgenogram will show an infiltrate. The pain associated with *pulmonary hypertension* is heavy and aching and often similar to that of cardiac ischemia (see Chapter 57). *Gastrointestinal disorders*, such as reflux esophagitis or gastric or duodenal ulcer, are usually distinguished from cardiopulmonary chest pain by their association with eating and by their relief by antacids (Chapters 35 and 37).

Evaluation

Many of the common causes of noncardiac chest pain can be diagnosed by a thorough history and physical examination. Because discrete anatomical structures must be involved in order to cause noncardiac chest pain, the physical examination is more useful in the diagnosis of noncardiac chest pain than it is in the diagnosis of dyspnea and hemoptysis. Inspection of the chest wall may reveal the characteristic unilateral eruption of herpes zoster along a dermatome. Light palpation over the chest wall will elicit pain and crepitus from fractured ribs. Mild pressure over the costochondral junctions anteriorly will reproduce the pain of Tietze's syndrome. (In general, cardiac pain is not worsened by pressure over the chest wall.) In pneu-

monia or pulmonary infarction a distinct friction rub can be heard directly over the specific area of chest pain. With pericardial involvement a friction rub that varies with respiration or with the cardiac cycle is usually present. A thorough abdominal examination is important because diseases involving the abdominal visceral organs can cause referred chest pain that is indistinguishable from that produced by involvement of the thoracic structures. Often laboratory studies and a chest roentgenogram will not be necessary for the diagnosis of these common causes of chest pain.

Therapy

The treatment of chest pain requires therapy of the underlying disease process, as well as analgesic drugs for the pain itself. Nonspecific chest pain found in normal people requires reassurance; however, angina-like pain in smokers ideally requires, first, diagnostic testing to exclude ischemic heart disease, followed by discontinuing cigarette smoking for both diagnosis and therapy. Tracheal irritation is limited to the duration of the viral illness but can be treated by cough suppression and bronchodilators (see under "Cough"). Tietze's syndrome is treated with standard anti-inflammatory agents and heat. Although the pain of herpes zoster is often severe, it may be controlled with mild narcotics such as codeine, 30 to 60 mg every 4 to 6 hours. The chest pain experienced in pulmonary hypertension often does not respond to treatment with non-narcotic analgesics, and narcotics may be required if the hypertension does not improve with treatment.

Pleuritic pain in patients with pneumonia or pulmonary embolus responds to specific therapy of the inflammatory process. Nevertheless, narcotics may be needed to reduce splinting of the chest wall and thereby to prevent atelectasis. Codeine (60 mg) is usually adequate therapy. In situations in which pain is extreme an intercostal block may be useful. This is performed by local infiltration of the inferior surface of the rib near the spine with 5 to 10 ml of lidocaine (1 to 2%). Although this therapy only lasts from 4 to 6 hours, local block in combination with the administration of narcotics often provides more long-term control of pleuritic chest pain.

THE ABNORMAL CHEST ROENTGENOGRAM

It is essential that a chest X-ray always be compared with any previous available film since changes may have been present for many years and therefore not require further evaluation. Also, depending on the appearance of the abnormality, it is often most appropriate simply to plan follow-up serial films.

Specific Patterns Indicative of an Abnormal Chest Roentgenogram

This section will review common abnormalities that indicate the presence of pulmonary disease that requires further evaluation.

Air Bronchogram (Fig. 54.1)

Normally, bronchi beyond the mainstem division cannot be seen; however, when lung tissue surrounding a bronchus is devoid of air because of either collapse or consolidation, an air bronchogram can be seen. The presence of an air bronchogram distinguishes a collapsed or consolidated part of the lung from an extrapulmonary density such as a pleural effusion. However, an air bronchogram is not present in every collapsed or consolidated lung because bronchi may fill with secretions or exudate. Therefore, its absence is less significant than its presence.

Silhouette Sign (Fig. 54.2)

The obliteration on a chest roentgenogram of the margin of a normally opaque structure in the chest by an abnormal pulmonary density is called the silhouette sign. If the physician has knowledge of thoracic anatomy and of spatial relations, he can use the silhouette sign to localize abnormalities within the lung parenchyma. Edges of organs that are in contact with parenchymal infiltrates will be obliterated because the normal air interface is eliminated. On the other hand, intrathoracic lesions that are not anatomically contiguous will not interfere with the outlines of nearby structures. For example, obliteration of the cardiac border localizes an abnormality to the right middle lobe or the lingular segment of the left upper lobe (Fig. 54.2). In contrast, an infiltrate that overlaps but does not obliterate the cardiac border is posterior and represents a lower lobe lesion. Lower lobe abnormalities obliterate diaphragmatic borders whereas obliteration of the left border of the aortic knob, a posterior structure, occurs with lesions of the apical posterior segment of the left upper lobe.

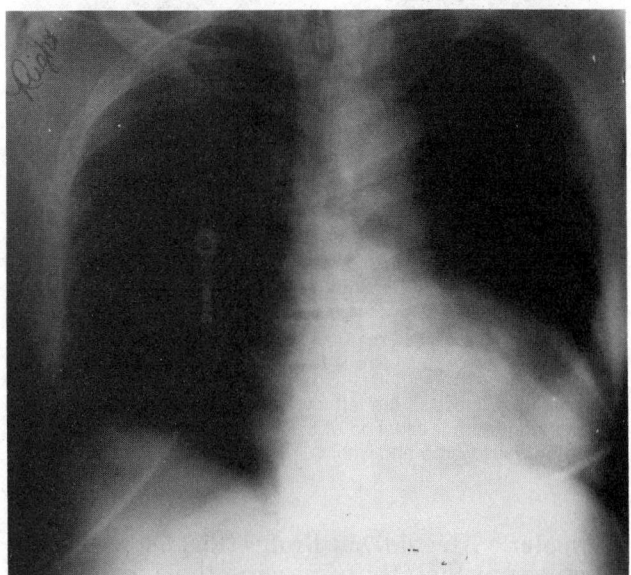

Figure 54.1. Air bronchogram. Patient presented with fever and sputum production; the initial roentgenogram demonstrates a branching air bronchogram seen behind the heart on the left, which is consistent with a lower lobe infiltrate.

Collapse (Fig. 54.3)

The collapse or diminution in volume of the whole lung, a lobe, or a segment of one of the lobes can be an important clue to the presence of asymptomatic pulmonary disease, such as bronchial carcinoma, or it may be the cause of a symptom, such as dyspnea in an asthmatic patient with mucous plugging. The primary mechanisms that cause pulmonary collapse are (a) bronchial obstruction either due to an intrinsic bronchial mass or to an extrinsic or intrinsic stenosis of the bronchus, (b) compression of the lungs from a large pleural effusion or from a pneumothorax, (c) peripheral bronchial plugging with subsequent pulmonary collapse, and (d) contraction of the lung secondary to chronic inflammatory disease. The signs of collapse are related to anatomical landmarks within the lung and are manifest by displacement of the fissure in the lung, loss of aeration within the pulmonary parenchyma, and crowding of the vascular and bronchial lung markings. Other signs that are suggestive of collapse reflect the secondary effects of loss of lung volume such as elevation of the diaphragm, shift of the mediastinal structures toward the collapsed area, diminution in the size of a hemithorax, compensatory hyperinflation, hilar displacement, and tracheal deviation. These latter signs are much more difficult to interpret in patients with underlying lung disease in whom many of these signs may exist in the absence of collapse.

Septal Markings

Normally lung markings reflect vascular patterns within the pulmonary parenchyma and are rarely due to the bronchi or the lymphatics. There are three types of linear shadows that represent septal markings within the lung: Kerley A lines, thin nonbranching lines several inches long radiating from the hilum; Kerley B lines (Fig. 54.4), up to 1 inch in length found at the lateral lung bases, radiating from the pleura; and Kerley C lines, fine interlacing structures throughout the lung parenchyma that produce a spiderweb appearance. The most common cause of these lines is interstitial edema due to congestive heart failure.

Common Problems in Patients with Abnormal Chest X-rays

In this section three general disease categories will be discussed in which the chest roentgenogram provides the basis for diagnosis and further evaluation. A general approach will be outlined including the initial evaluation that should be completed by the physician before referral to a pulmonary specialist or a thoracic surgeon. Frequently, this diagnostic evaluation can be completed in an ambulatory setting, with or without consultation.

Infiltrates

Infiltrates represent alveolar and/or interstitial lung disease and seldom show sharp borders except at pleural surfaces. They may be radiographically separated into

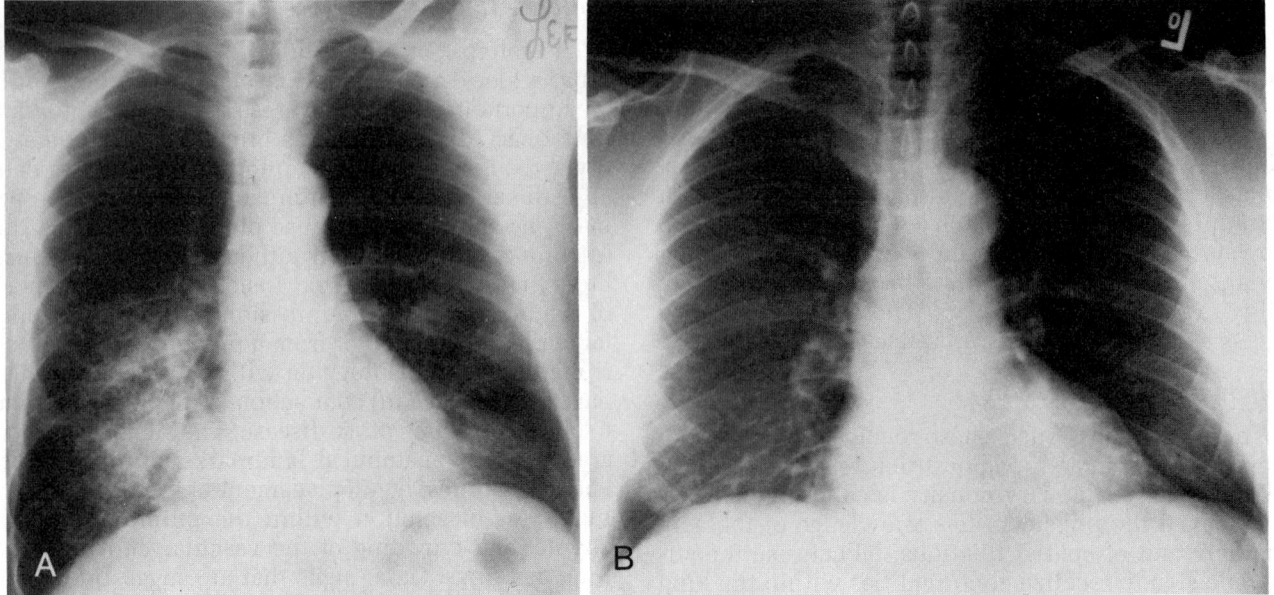

Figure 54.2. Silhouette sign. In this figure, a middle lobe infiltrate obscures the border of the heart (*A*). A previous X-ray is shown for comparison (*B*).

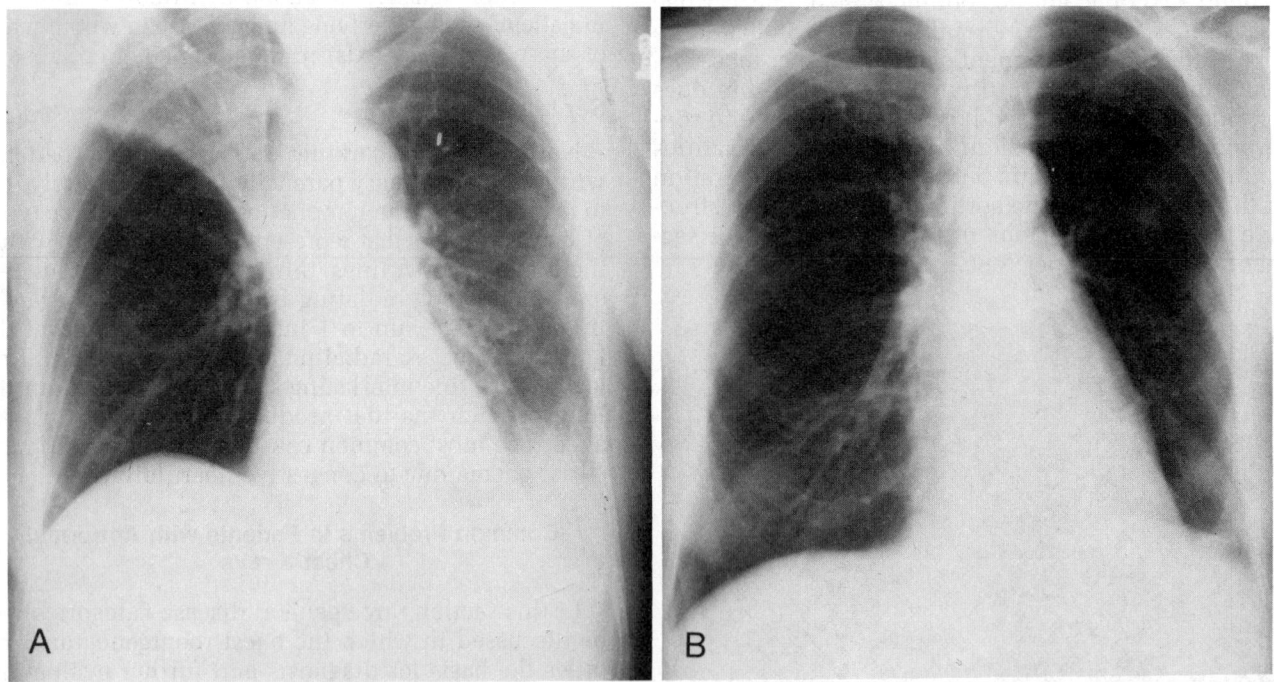

Figure 54.3. Collapse. This demonstrates collapse of the right upper lobe and partial collapse of the left lower lobe in a patient complaining of cough and increased sputum (*A*). The middle lobe fissure is displaced upwards and there is blunting of the left hemidiaphragm. Note that there is no air bronchogram in either collapsed segment. Aggressive physical therapy was initated and within 24 hours there is resolution of the collapse on the right and almost complete resolution on the left (*B*).

diffuse and localized infiltrates. "Diffuse" implies bilaterality and generalized involvement, if not of the entire lungs, then at least the majority of both lung fields. "Localized" implies discrete lesions that may or may not be bilateral but that have intervening normal lung tissue between the localized lesions.

Alveolar. *Alveolar infiltrates* (Fig. 54.5*A*) can be recognized by their fluffy margins, their coalescence into "rosette" formations, their occasional "butterfly" configuration involving hilar and central lung zones, and the presence of air bronchograms or air alveolograms.

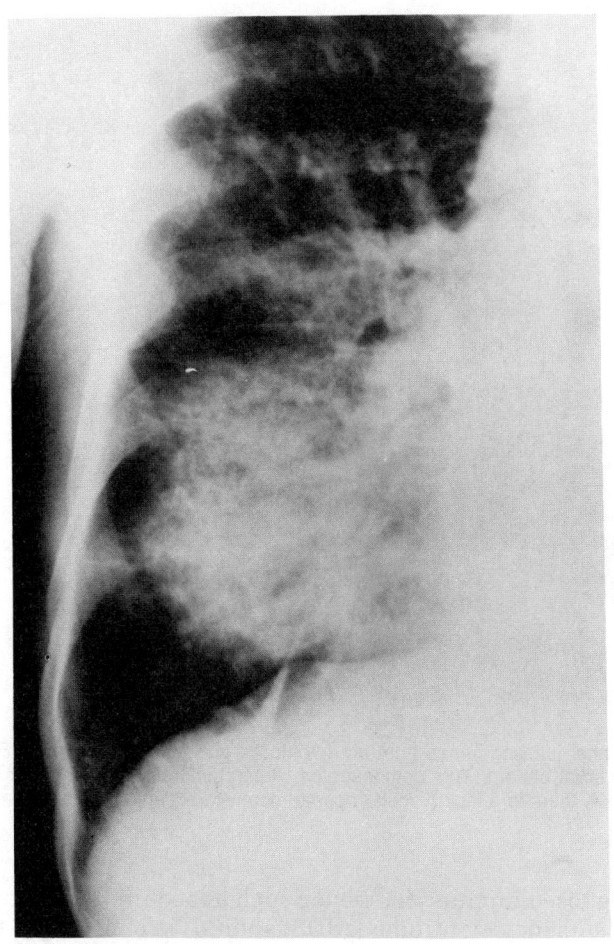

Figure 54.4. Kerley B lines. A close view of the right lower lung in a patient with congestive heart failure demonstrates horizontal linear lines that run to the edge of the lung.

Although there are numerous causes of diffuse interstitial pulmonary disease, there are few causes of diffuse alveolar lung disease. Therefore, the distinction between an alveolar and an interstitial process is important. Unfortunately, it is not always possible to distinguish between the two entities and there may be a mixture of both. Moreover, a disorder that begins as an interstitial process can often merge into an alveolar process, such as early congestive heart failure progressing to severe pulmonary edema.

The causes of diffuse *alveolar filling disease* of the lung are shown in Table 54.6. The three most frequent causes are infection, edema, and hemorrhage, and they are characterized by rapid progression and regression. In contrast, diffuse interstitial lung disease develops more slowly. Therefore, the time course for the development of pulmonary symptoms and roentgenographic abnormalities is an important aspect in the differential diagnosis of diffuse lung disease.

Interstitial. An *interstitial pattern* may be primarily linear or reticular and often consists of multiple, discrete, noncoalescent round nodules, 1 to 5 mm in diameter (Fig. 54.5*B*). Although there can be a summation effect, these small nodular densities retain a distinct identity as compared to the larger, fluffier infiltrates characteristic of alveolar disease. In certain disease processes, such as tuberculosis, histoplasmosis, or healed viral pneumonia, these nodules may calcify and thus appear more dense. The presence of honeycombing is pathognomonic of interstitial disease and pulmonary fibrosis. It can be identified on a chest roentgenogram as round or oval, irregular air spaces that have a reasonably uniform diameter of 1 to 10 mm and are arranged in grape-like bunches, thus giving the impression of a beehive.

Although *interstitial* lung disease (Table 54.7) can be idiopathic, the primary goal in the evaluation is to determine whether a treatable disease is present. The initial medical history, physical examination, and laboratory testing should be oriented toward evaluating the patient for the presence of a pneumoconiosis secondary to occupational exposure, pulmonary involvement associated with collagen vascular disease, sarcoidosis, and granulomatous (tuberculous) infections of the lung.

Bilateral interstitial infiltrates in the lower lung fields are a commonly seen radiographic pattern. The vast majority of patients with this pattern have one of the following diseases: bronchiectasis, aspiration, collagen vascular diseases, asbestosis, sarcoidosis, or idiopathic pulmonary fibrosis. Localized interstitial processes often represent residue of prior pulmonary infections. If new, they may represent acute processes like mycoplasma pneumonia or lymphangitic spread of carcinoma.

Once the more common causes of interstitial lung disease are excluded, the less common causes must be considered before the diagnosis of idiopathic pulmonary fibrosis is made. Specialized pulmonary function testing, including lung volume determination, diffusion capacities, and cardiopulmonary exercise testing, is necessary in addition to routine spirometry. In many of these patients transbronchial biopsy using a fiberoptic bronchoscope may be recommended. The findings in lung biopsy are often useful in guiding therapy in patients with collagen vascular pulmonary diseases, sarcoidosis, idiopathic pulmonary fibrosis, and infectious disease. If the tissue obtained with transbronchial biopsy is inadequate for diagnosis, consultation with a thoracic surgeon for open thoracotomy and pulmonary biopsy may be indicated.

Slowly Resolving or Recurrent Infiltrates. Obstructing pulmonary carcinoma must be considered in any patient who has a slowly resolving pneumonia. Most patients with bacterial pneumonia respond rapidly to antibiotic therapy, and their chest roentgenogram will return to normal over 3 to 6 weeks (see Chapter 28). Patients with chronic obstructive lung disease (Chapter 55) who have difficulty mobilizing their bronchial secretions and patients with superimposed congestive heart failure or with necrotizing pneumonia may have significant pulmonary infiltrates that persist for 8 to 12 weeks (8). If the patient shows symptomatic improvement with a decrease in both the amount and purulence of sputum, a decrease in fever,

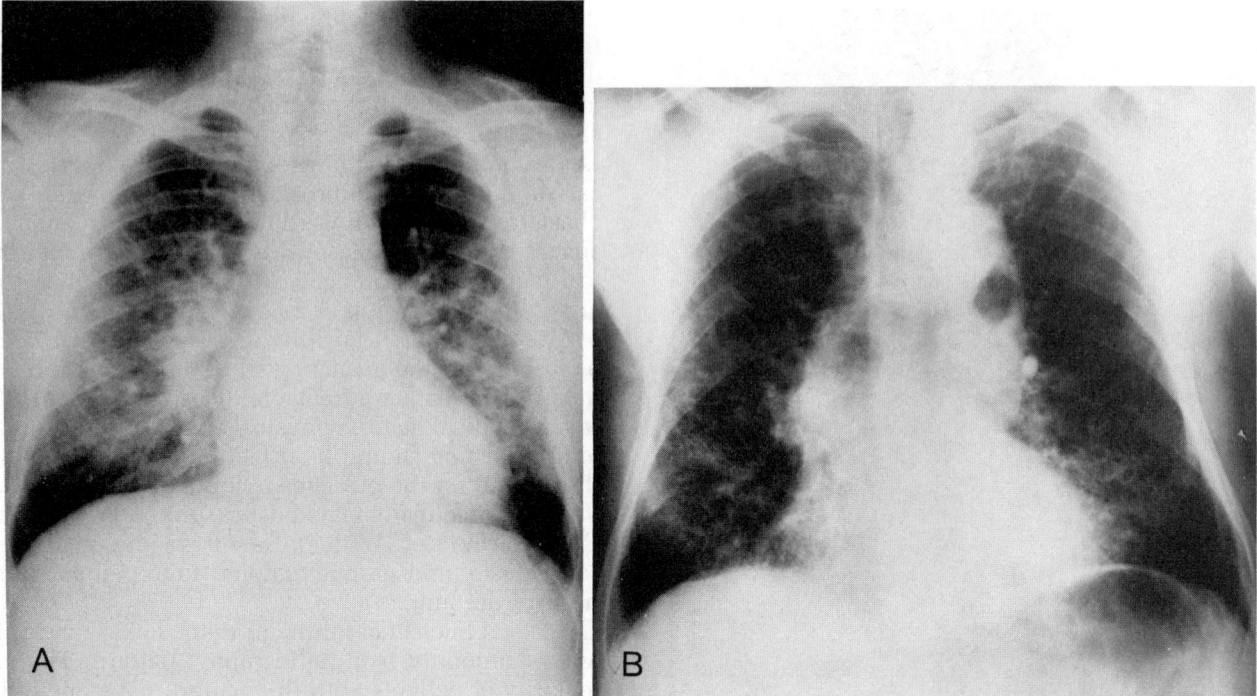

Figure 54.5. *A.* Alveolar patterns. This patient has progressive dyspnea after inhaling fumes from an automobile accident. Compared to *B*, little air is visible in the infiltrate because fluid is filling the alveoli. *B.* Interstitial pattern. This demonstrates bilateral interstitial infiltrates in a patient with progressive dyspnea and with fibrosis on biopsy. Compared to *A*, there is a lacy reticular appearance with accentuation of the air spaces by the fibrosis.

Table 54.6.
Causes of Diffuse Alveolar Pulmonary Disease

Disorder	Common	Uncommon
Infection (pus)	Pneumonia	
Edema (fluid)	Cardiac and noncardiac pulmonary edema	
Hemorrhage (blood)		Anticoagulation
		Trauma
		Hemoptysis with aspiration
		Goodpasture's syndrome
		Idiopathic pulmonary siderosis
Cells	Sarcoidosis	Bronchoalveolar cell cancer
		"Eosinophilic" infiltrative disorders
Foreign material		Lipoid pneumonia
		Contrast media
		Alveolar proteinosis

and slow but progressive roentgenographic clearing, further evaluation during this period is usually not warranted. If roentgenographic abnormalities persist and if there is other evidence of poor response to therapy or if the pneumonic infiltrate is found in an asymptomatic individual, further evaluation to exclude pulmonary carcinoma is warranted (see Chapter 56). In contrast to an older patient, a younger patient with recurrent pneumonia should be suspected of having an altered pulmonary defense such as cystic fibrosis, which may escape detection until late adolescence or early adulthood. In addition, undiagnosed immunodeficiency such as acquired immune deficiency syndrome (AIDS) should be considered if antimicrobial therapy is not effective for a "routine" pneumonia (Chapter 34).

Older patients with recurrent pneumonias (18) should also be evaluated for the possibility of lung cancer. More frequently, these patients have associated chronic diseases such as underlying airways disease, congestive heart failure, diabetes mellitus, or bronchiectasis. In evaluating patients with recurrent pneumonia, it is essential to review previous chest roentgenograms to document the anatomical location and the characteristics of the recurrent pneumonic infiltrate. In general, if a pneumonia recurs in multiple lobes or in pulmonary segments that are unrelated anatomically, the likelihood of bronchogenic carcinoma is small. For example, a recurrent pneumonia that initially involves the right upper lobe and subsequently the lower lobe is unlikely to be the result of a single obstructive carcinoma. In addition to the anatomical location, it is important to consider the time during which recurrent pneumonias have occurred. If the interval is more than 3 years, the possibility of an underlying obstructing lung cancer is unlikely.

Apical. Frequently roentgenographic patterns that range from increased pulmonary markings or minor scarring to cystic or cavitary disease in the upper lobes will be interpreted by a radiologist as showing old granulomatous lung disease with possible active tuberculous infection. The evaluation of these patients includes questioning about previous tuberculous lung

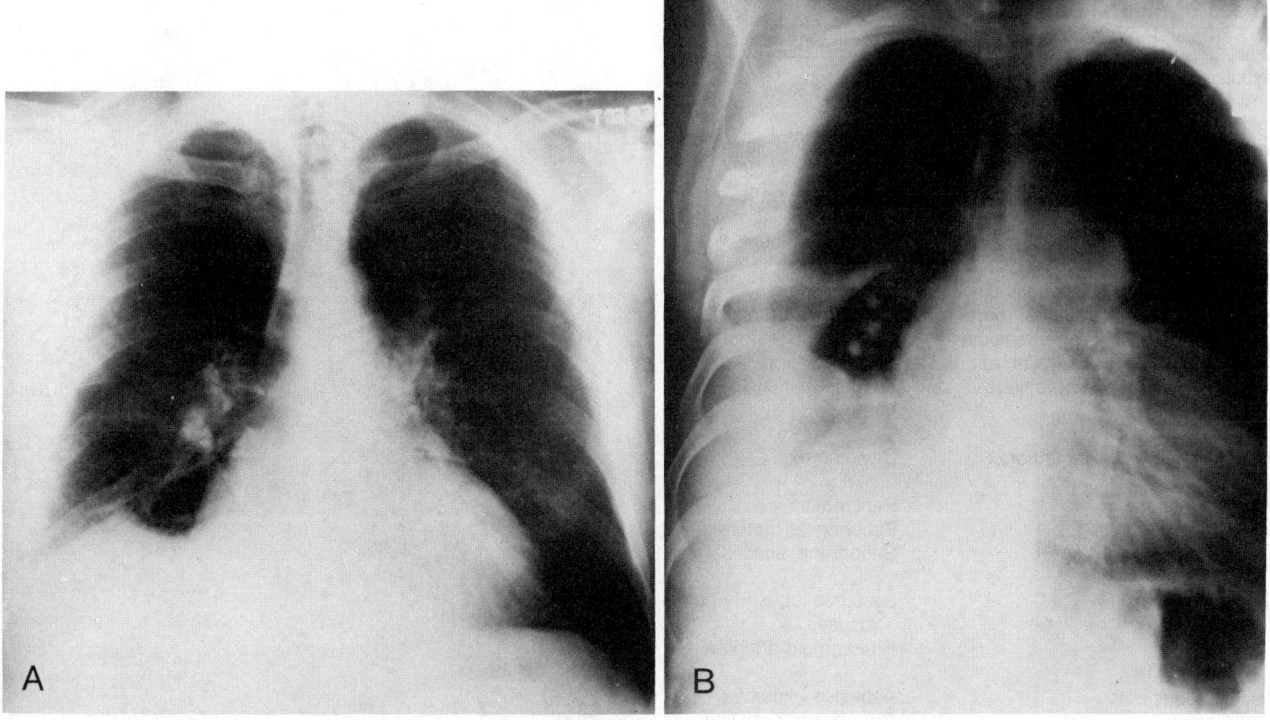

Figure 54.6. Subpulmonic effusion. The diaphragm appears to be elevated on the right (*A*). This represents subpulmonic fluid; when the patient is placed in the right lateral decubitis position (*B*), fluid layers on the right and tracks in the minor fissure and along the apex and diaphragm.

Table 54.7.
Causes of Diffuse Interstitial Pulmonary Disease

Disorder	Common	Uncommon
KNOWN CAUSES		
Infection		Miliary tuberculosis
		Fungal
		Viral and atypical pneumonia
		Pneumocystis infection
Collagen vascular disease	Scleroderma	
	Rheumatoid arthritis	
	Systemic lupus erythematosus	
Occupational (pneumoconiosis)	Asbestosis	
	Silicosis	
	Coal miner's pneumoconiosis	
Hypersensitivity and drug reactions	Extrinsic allergic alveolitis	Nitrofurantoin
		Cytotoxic drugs
Physical agents		Radiation
Vascular	Early heart failure	
Neoplastic		Lymphoma
		Lymphatic metastasis
UNKNOWN CAUSES		
Idiopathic pulmonary fibrosis	Sarcoidosis	Eosinophilic granuloma

disease (including the type and duration of antituberculous therapy) and an assessment of the reactivity of the tuberculin skin test. Comparison with chest roentgenograms is useful because the activity of an infiltrate cannot be determined from an isolated chest roentgenogram. Frequently, old chest roentgenograms demonstrate that no change has occurred. The evaluation and treatment of patients with tuberculosis are discussed in Chapter 29.

Superior sulcus tumors, usually adenocarcinomas, form in the apex of the lung and may be difficult to distinguish initially from pleural thickening or old granulomatous disease; later in the course, roentgenograms may reveal erosion by tumors of adjacent ribs (see also Chapter 56, page 638).

Pleural Effusion (Fig. 54.6)

Small amounts of free fluid within the pleural space will obliterate the costophrenic or costocardiac angles. Because the density of pleural fluid is greater than the density of the lung, a subpulmonic collection will displace laterally the crest of the diaphragm. An increased density between the stomach gas bubble and pulmonary tissue may also indicate the presence of fluid within the pleural space. The diagnosis of a large pleural effusion is not difficult because fluid within the pleural space on an upright chest roentgenogram will form a concave density across the chest cavity; decubitus roentgenograms will demonstrate free pleural fluid in the dependent hemithorax. If the patient is

Table 54.8.
Causes of Pleural Effusion

Effusion	Common	Uncommon
Vascular	Congestive heart failure[a] Pulmonary infarction	
Metabolic		Hypoproteinemia[a] Cirrhosis[a] Nephrotic syndrome[a] Glomerulonephritis[a]
Malignancy	Metastatic disease	Mesothelioma
Infection	Bacterial (parapneumonic and empyema)	Mycoplasma (and other atypical pneumonias)
	Tuberculous	Fungal Viral
Trauma	Hemothorax	Chylothorax
Gastrointestinal		Pancreatitis Esophageal rupture Subphrenic abscess
Collagen vascular disease		Systemic lupus erythematosus Rheumatoid arthritis
Miscellaneous		Asbestos exposure Drug hypersensitivity Postmyocardial infarction syndrome Meig's syndrome[a] Lymphoma and lymphatic abnormalities

[a] Usually transudative pleural effusion.

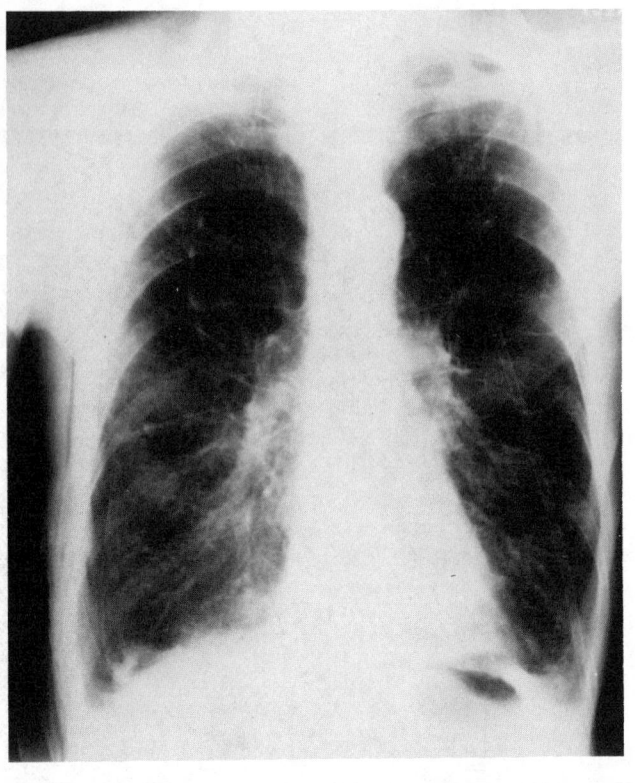

Figure 54.7. Pneumothorax. If the roentgenogram is not carefully examined, the pneumothorax in the right lower lung can be easily missed. Note the widespread bullae throughout the lung.

recumbent, the pleural fluid will layer over the entire hemithorax, causing the lung to appear opaque.

In general, when a pleural effusion is seen on a chest roentgenogram, it is important to examine the fluid. The major exception to this rule is the patient who develops acute pulmonary edema associated with a rapidly developing pleural effusion that resolves with therapy for congestive heart failure (see Chapter 61). The physician should perform a thoracentesis in order to determine the etiology of the effusion (Table 54.8). The fluid should be collected in both a heparinized and a nonheparinized tube so that cytological examination can be performed, if necessary. Most pleural effusions are clear and straw colored, and deviations from this norm are useful diagnostically. For example, a bloody effusion suggests pulmonary infarction or tumor, a lime-green effusion suggests tuberculosis, and a viscous fluid with feculent odor strongly suggests an anaerobic empyema.

Pleural fluids can either be classified as transudates or exudates (11). An exudate is characterized by a pleural fluid protein concentration that is greater than 50% of the concentration of serum protein. Because of their high protein content, exudative pleural effusions usually have a specific gravity of more than 1.015 or a protein concentration of greater than 3 g/100 ml. A cell count and pleural fluid cytology should be performed since polymorphonuclear leukocytes in pleural fluid suggest acute inflammation and infection, whereas a predominance of lymphocytes suggests tuberculosis or malignancy. The presence of more than 5% pleural mesothelial cells usually excludes the diagnosis of tuberculosis. Low pleural fluid glucose concentrations occur in infections as well as in rheumatoid arthritis. If pleural effusion is bloody or appears infected, the patient should be hospitalized for further diagnostic studies and for therapy (pleural fluid pH, pleural biopsy, etc.).

Pneumothorax (Fig. 54.7)

There are three major types of pneumothorax: (a) spontaneous, (b) iatrogenic, and (c) traumatic. Of these, the general physician is most commonly faced with a spontaneous pneumothorax either in a young healthy individual or in the older patient with underlying pulmonary disease. In the former, a subpleural apical bleb ruptures into the pleural space, causing varying amounts of air to collect. This is most commonly seen in 20- to 30-year-old men and is usually unrelated to activity, although 20% may admit to severe coughing at the time. In the older patient, emphysema with concomitant bullous disease is frequently associated with pneumothoraces. Pleuritic chest pain is a major manifestation of small pneumothoraces (10 to 20%), whereas dyspnea predominates in patients with larger collections of air.

After the diagnosis of pneumothorax is made, the patient may need observation (ambulatory or inpatient) or insertion of a chest tube. Needle aspiration to expand the lung is discouraged since further laceration can occur. In general, patients with underlying lung disease should be hospitalized and have a chest tube inserted since the leak seldom seals immediately. On the other hand, a young patient who is not in distress may remain at home and be followed with repeated roentgenograms as long as the pneumothorax does not enlarge. There should be obvious shrinking of the space within 3 to 5 days, and eventually the lung should totally re-expand.

Solitary Nodule

This radiological finding always requires evaluation. A detailed discussion of the problem is to be found in Chapter 56, Lung Cancer.

General References

Felson B: The chest roentgenologic workup—what and why? Convenient methods. Published by the American Thoracic Society, *Basics of RD* 8 (5): 1980.
> A concise selective review.

Hyers TM (ed): Pulmonary embolism and hypertension. *Clin Chest Med* 5 (no 3): 1984.
> Excellent monograph on epidemiology, pathophysiology, diagnosis, and treatment.

Jones NL, Campbell EJ: *Clinical Exercise Testing*, 2nd ed. Philadelphia, WB Saunders, 1982.
> The standard text on this subject.

McLoud TC (ed): Chest radiology. *Clin Chest Med* 5 (4): 1984.
> Excellent monograph on old and new techniques used in the diagnosis of thoracic disease.

Murray JF, Nadel JA (eds):*Textbook of Respiratory Medicine*. Philadelphia, WB Saunders, 1988.
> A comprehensive pulmonary textbook.

Ziment I: *Respiratory Pharmacology and Therapeutics*. Philadelphia, WB Saunders, 1978.
> An exhaustive review of this subject.

Specific References

1. Adelman M, Haponik EF, Bleecker ER, Britt EJ: Cryptogenic hemoptysis: Clinical features, bronchoscopic findings, and natural history in 67 patients. *Ann Intern Med* 102:829, 1985.
2. Bell WR, Simon TL, DeMets DL: The clinical features of submassive and massive pulmonary emboli. *Am J Med* 62:355, 1977.
3. Biello DR, Mattar AG, McKnight RC, Siegel BA: Ventilation-perfusion studies in suspected pulmonary embolism. *AJR* 133:1033, 1979.
4. Dalen JE, Banas Jr JS, Brooks HL, et al: Resolution rate of acute pulmonary embolism in man. *N Engl J Med* 280:1194, 1969.
5. Friedman GD, Siegelaub AB, Dales LG: Cigarette smoking and chest pain. *Ann Intern Med* 83:1, 1975.
6. Irwin RS, Pratter MR, Holland PS, et al: Postnasal drip causes cough and is associated with reversible upper airway obstructions. *Chest* 85:346, 1984.
7. Irwin RS, Rosen MJ, Braman SS: Cough: a comprehensive review. *Arch Intern Med* 137:1186, 1977.
8. Jay SJ, Johanson Jr WG, Pierce AK: The radiologic resolution of Streptococcus pneumoniae pneumonia. *N Engl J Med* 293:798, 1975.
9. Kaplan J, Johns CJ: Mycetomas in pulmonary sarcoidosis: nonsurgical management. *Johns Hopkins Med J* 145:157, 1979.
10. Kravitz H Gomberg RM, Burnstine RC, et al: Psychogenic cough tic in children and adolescents. *Clin Pediatr* 8:580, 1969.
11. Light RW, MacGregor I, Luchsinger PC, Ball WF: Pleural effusions: the diagnostic separation of transudates and exudates. *Ann Intern Med* 77:507, 1972.
12. McNeil BJ, Hessel SJ, Branch WT, et al: Measures of clinical efficacy. III. The value of the lung scan in the evaluation of young patients with pleuritic chest pain. *Nucl Med* 17:163, 1976.
13. Poe RH, Harder RV, Israel RH, Kallay MC: Chronic persistent cough. Experience in diagnosis and outcome using an anatomic diagnostic protocol. *Chest* 95:723, 1989.
14. Power JT, Stewart IC, Connaughton JJ, et al: Nocturnal cough in patients with chronic bronchitis and emphysema. *Am Rev Respir Dis* 130:399, 1984.
15. Rogers RM, Bedrossian C, Coalson JJ, et al: The management of massive hemoptysis in a patient with pulmonary tuberculosis. *Chest* 70:519, 1976.
16. Snider GL: When not to use the bronchoscopy for hemoptysis. *Chest* 76:1, 1979.
17. Szucs Jr MM, Brooks HL, Grossman W, et al: Diagnostic sensitivity of laboratory findings in acute pulmonary embolism. *Ann Intern Med* 74:161, 1971.
18. Winterbauer RH, Bedon GA, Ball Jr WC: Recurrent pneumonia. Predisposing illness and clinical patterns in 158 patients. *Ann Intern Med* 70:689, 1969.
19. Woodcock AA, Gross ER, Geddes DM: Drug treatment of breathlessness: contrasting effects of diazepam and promethazine in pink buffers. *Br Med J* 283:343, 1981.
20. Woodcock AA, Gross ER, Gellert A, et al: Effects of dihydrocodeine, alcohol, and caffeine on breathlessness and exercise tolerance in patients with chronic obstructive lung disease and normal blood gases. *N Engl J Med* 305:1611, 1981.
21. Wynder EL, Kaufman PL, Lesser RL: A short-term follow-up study on ex-cigarette smokers. *Am Rev Respir Dis* 96:645, 1967.
22. Zavala DC: Diagnostic fiberoptic bronchoscopy: techniques and results of biopsy in 600 patients. *Chest* 68:12, 1975.

C H A P T E R   55

Obstructive Airways Disease

EUGENE R. BLEECKER, M.D.
MARK C. LIU, M.D.

Obstructive diseases of the airways are the most common forms of pulmonary disease encountered in ambulatory practice. They include asthma (intermittent episodic bronchospasm), chronic obstructive bronchitis (bronchitis complicated by progressive airways obstruction), and emphysema (destruction of pulmonary parenchyma with associated obstructive lung disease). Although these diseases may differ in their clinical presentation, etiology, and prognosis, they all share the common feature of reduced expiratory airflow. Usually, patients with obstructive lung dis-

ease present with acute intermittent dyspnea or with the insidious onset of progressive dyspnea during exercise. On the other hand, the diagnosis of early obstructive airways disease can only be made in asymptomatic patients by demonstrating a decrease in forced expiration that is objectively measured with a spirometer (Fig. 55.1) (43). Furthermore, since the severity of airways obstruction often does not correlate with clinical symptoms such as wheezing and dyspnea, objective tests of pulmonary function are needed both to establish the initial diagnosis as well as to follow the clinical course of these diseases (Table 55.1). To understand the pathophysiological disturbances found in these patients and to assess the severity and prognosis in an individual patient, a review of some basic principles of pulmonary physiology is important.

PATHOPHYSIOLOGICAL ABNORMALITIES IN OBSTRUCTIVE LUNG DISEASE

To quantitate the amount of air leaving the lungs over a period of time, a forced expiration is performed by having the patient exhale maximally into a spirometer. This apparatus records the volume and speed of expiration. The factors that determine the speed and volume of a forced expiration are schematically represented in Figure 55.2. The lung is an elastic structure enclosed by the rigid chest wall with a potential cavity, the pleural space, located between. During normal respiration, the inspiratory muscles contract, and both pleural and alveolar pressures become negative, causing air to flow into the lungs. With expiration, air leaves the lungs as a result of their tendency to deflate when the respiratory muscles relax. Normally, as expiratory effort is increased, pleural pressure, which surrounds the intrathoracic airways, rises and compresses them (Fig. 55.2). This tendency for airways to collapse is opposed by the elastic properties of the lung that stabilize the bronchi and keep the airways open. Although slight airway compression occurs in normal subjects during a maximal expiratory effort, there is a marked tendency for airways to collapse in patients with emphysema in whom the structural components of the lung are destroyed (38).

Figure 55.3 diagrammatically illustrates airway morphology and the supporting elastic structures in the lung and shows how asthma, chronic bronchitis, and emphysema produce decreased expiratory airflow. In these diseases, forced expiration is limited by several factors (Table 55.2). In asthma, there is bronchospasm often followed by mucosal edema and retained secretions. During an acute asthmatic attack, bronchial smooth muscle may narrow and even close the airways, causing air trapping and subsequent hyperinflation. In bronchitis, the onset of airflow obstruction may be insidious with initial mucous gland hyperplasia and retained bronchial secretions, especially in the peripheral airways (< 2 mm). In addition, the presence of bronchial infection and airflow obstruction may lead to airway hyper-responsiveness to

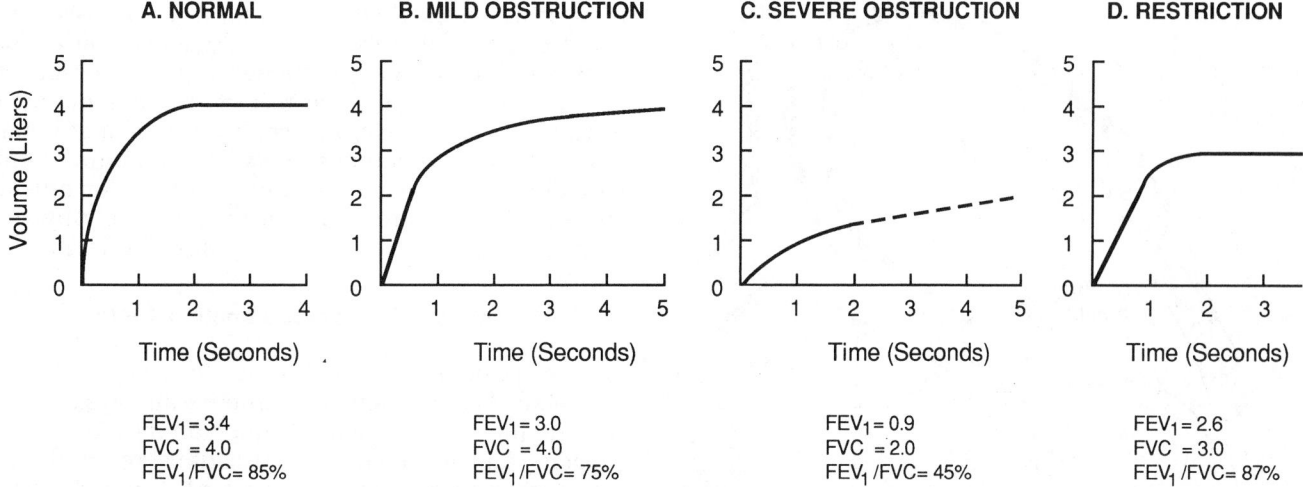

Figure 55.1. Spirographic tracings of forced expiration. Exhaled volume is plotted against time. The forced vital capacity (FVC) is represented by the total volume expired. One-second forced expiratory volume (FEV$_1$) is the volume of air expired during the first second. *A*. Normal spirogram. *B*. Spirogram from a patient with mild obstructive airways disease. *C*. Spirogram from a patient with severe obstructive defect.

If the spirogram were incorrectly terminated after 2 seconds, the FVC would be artificially reduced (see the text). When it is performed correctly (*dotted lines*) it is obvious that there is airway obstruction and that there is no restrictive disease. *D*. Spirogram showing restrictive pulmonary disease (FEV$_1$/FVC is normal but FVC is reduced).

Table 55.1.
Indications for Pulmonary Function Testing in Obstructive Airways Disease

To establish the presence and severity of airway obstructon
To evaluate objectively the reversibility of airways obstruction and the results of therapy
To assist in the differentiation between emphysema and other forms of airways obstruction
To serve as a basis to predict the course and prognosis of chronic obstructive disease
To evaluate work potential (see Chapter 9) or operative risks (see Chapter 86)

Table 55.2.
Mechanisms of Airway Obstruction

Smooth muscle spasm
Bronchial inflammation and edema
Mucous gland hyperplasia
Increased bronchial secretions
Airways collapse
Airways hyperreactivity to inhaled substances (cigarette smoke, dust, histamine)

various inhaled agents (10, 11, 32), causing additional bronchospasm. Finally, in emphysema, airways may collapse even during normal tidal breathing because of destruction of structural elements in the lungs (64).

PULMONARY FUNCTION TESTING IN OBSTRUCTIVE AIRWAYS DISEASE

Spirometry

Spirometry (Fig. 55.1) is the most useful pulmonary function test to assess airflow limitation in asthma and obstructive pulmonary disease (38). This test is performed in all pulmonary testing facilities, and relatively inexpensive spirometers are readily available

(1, 29). Physicians who treat a significant number of patients with chronic obstructive airways disease should have a spirometer in their offices. Ideally, a spirometer should provide a graphic record of the patient's forced expiration, which should be maintained for at least 4 to 5 seconds in order to measure both forced expiratory volume during the first second (FEV$_1$), and the forced vital capacity (FVC, the total volume that can be exhaled after a maximal inspiration). An electronic spirometer is less desirable, but if one is used, a graphic record is still necessary to evaluate the quality and reproducibility of the patient's effort. In addition, with either mechanical or electronic spirometers calibration must be performed frequently with a calibrating syringe to document that the measurements made are accurate (63). The American Thoracic Society has published guidelines for the use of spirometers (1). Three reproducible tracings should be obtained and the FEV$_1$ or another measurement of expiratory flow (maximal or midmaximal expiratory flow rates) should be calculated. Airway obstruction can be quantitated in three ways: measurement of absolute FEV$_1$, the FEV$_1$ as a percentage of predicted, using readily available nomograms, and the ratio of FEV$_1$:FVC. Severe obstruction is usually present when the FEV$_1$ is less than 1.0 liter, less than 25% predicted, or less than 25 to 40% of the FVC. The ratio of the FEV$_1$ to FVC is used to evaluate airways obstruction since pure restrictive ventilatory defects cause an equal reduction in the FEV$_1$ and the vital capacity; and the FEV$_1$:FVC ratio will be normal (Fig. 55.1D). A reduction of the FEV$_1$:FVC ratio below 75% indicates the presence of airflow obstruction. Because patients with obstructive lung disease empty air from their lungs slowly (Fig. 55.1, *B* and *C*), their spirograms do not show a normal plateau. Therefore, if expiration is not prolonged, the FVC will be artificially reduced and the diagnosis of

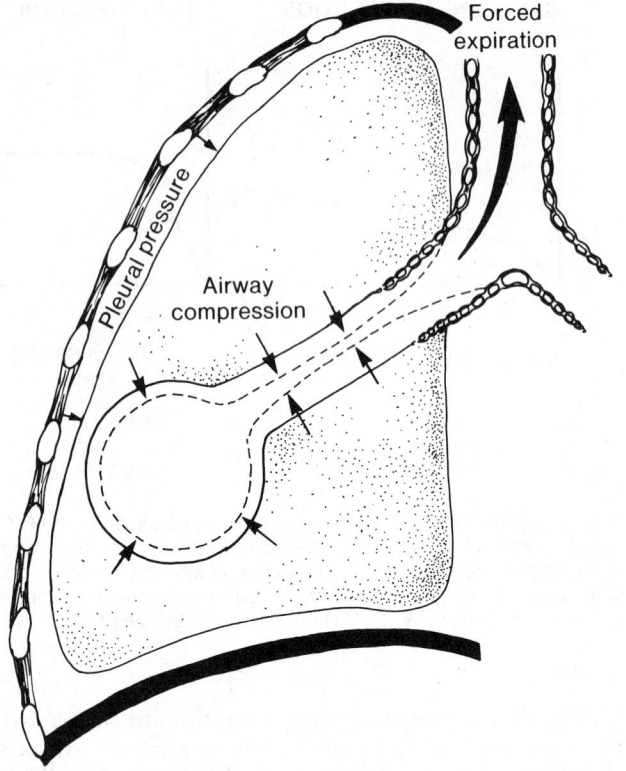

Figure 55.2. Schematic representation of the lungs and chest wall during a forced expiration. With maximal forced expiration, pleural pressure increases and becomes positive. At the point where pleural pressure exceeds intraluminal airway pressure, the airways are compressed. The structural components of the lung stabilize the airways, hold them open, and oppose their tendency to collapse during expiration (see the text).

airflow obstruction may be overlooked. For example, if a patient with obstructive airways disease exhales for only 2 seconds, the spirogram will be artificially truncated (Fig. 55.1 C). If it were stopped at 2 seconds, the FCV would be recorded as 1.1 liters, the FEV_1 as 0.9 liter, and the FEV_1:FVC as 82%. When it is correctly performed and expiration is prolonged for 4 to 6 seconds (Fig. 55.1 C, *dotted line*), the actual FVC is measured as 2.0 liters and the FEV_1:FVC ratio (0.9:2.0) is 45%. Therefore, if the spirogram were not examined, an erroneous diagnosis of restrictive, rather than severe obstructive, lung disease would be made.

Patient experience. There is little discomfort associated with spirometry in normal individuals or in patients with mild to moderate obstructive airways disease. After a nose clip is applied, the patient is instructed to take a deep inspiration, immediately followed by a forceful expiration that should continue for 6 seconds. Forced expiration can occasionally result in coughing and, extremely rarely, cyanosis and hypoxemia in patients with severe airways disease and resting hypoxemia.

The peak expiratory flow rate can be measured in patients with obstructive lung disease by use of an inexpensive peak flow meter (20) (e.g., Mini-Wright or Assess, available from medical supply houses for between $20 and $60). Although a peak flow meter does not provide a printed record or a measurement of vital capacity, it can be used by a patient at home to monitor lung function serially. Thus, improvement with therapy or worsening pulmonary function during an exacerbation can be measured objectively by the patient and the results reported to his physician.

Complete Pulmonary Function Tests

Other pulmonary function tests that are useful in the detailed assessment of obstructive airways disease include the measurement of lung volumes, diffusion capacity, and arterial blood gases both at rest and during exercise (see Chapter 54, under "Dyspnea"). The measurement of *lung volumes* quantitates the degree of hyperinflation that may be found either in patients with long-standing airway obstruction or in patients with acute asthma. Occasionally, initial clinical and symptomatic improvement in airways obstruction during recovery from an asthmatic attack will be reflected by a decrease in the degree of hyperinflation (71). Lung volume measurements are also useful in the evaluation of patients with restrictive pulmonary diseases. The single breath diffusion capacity for carbon monoxide reflects the amount of functional alveolar capillary surface area available for gas exchange. Diffusion capacity is reduced not only in pulmonary fibrosis and congestive heart failure but also in emphysema. The findings of expiratory airflow limitation, hyperinflation, and a reduced diffusion capacity often correlate with the pathological diagnosis of anatomical emphysema (30, 64) (Fig. 55.8, below).

Patient experience. There is no discomfort or risk during the measurement of lung volumes, but it is necessary that a patient be able to remain seated for 6 to 8 minutes, breathing a mixture of air and helium. Severely obstructed patients whose vital capacity is less than 1 liter cannot perform a single breath diffusion capacity since they must inspire and hold at least a 1-liter inspiratory volume for 10 seconds.

Other pulmonary function tests, such as the measurement of pulmonary compliance or airway resistance using a body plethysmograph, are sophisticated tests that are not usually helpful in the routine management of patients with obstructive airways disease. Flow volume curves provide similar information to routine spirometry; however, the apparatus for this test is more complicated, is often more difficult to calibrate accurately, and is expensive. Nevertheless, many testing facilities use flow volume curves rather than spirometry. Flow volume curves are specifically useful in the evaluation of extrathoracic airway obstruction. Some examples of inspiratory and expiratory flow volume curves obtained in upper and lower airway obstruction are illustrated in Figure 55.4 (33).

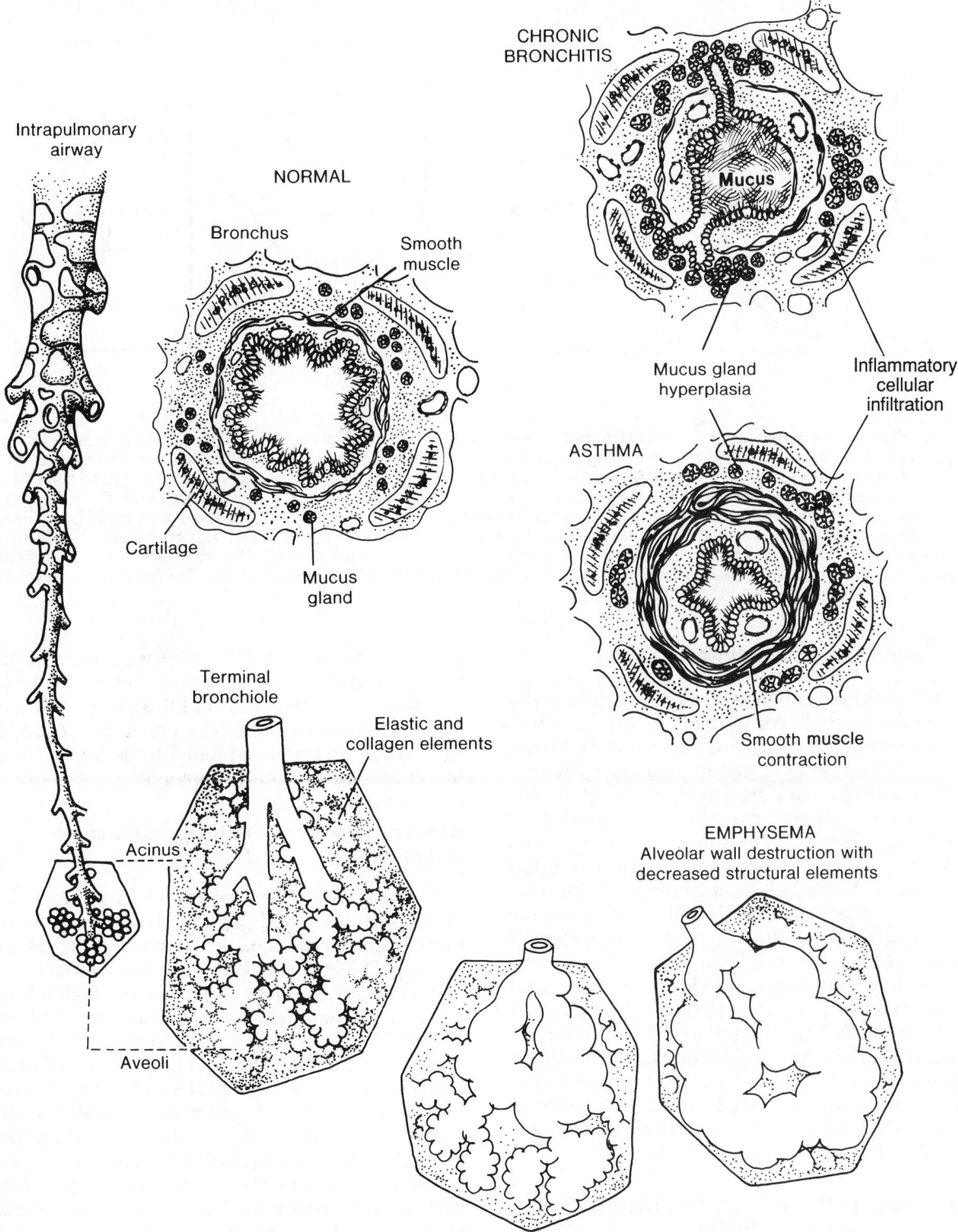

Figure 55.3. Schematic representation of the morphology of normal airways and lung parenchyma and the changes produced in these structures by asthma, chronic bronchitis, and emphysema (see the text).

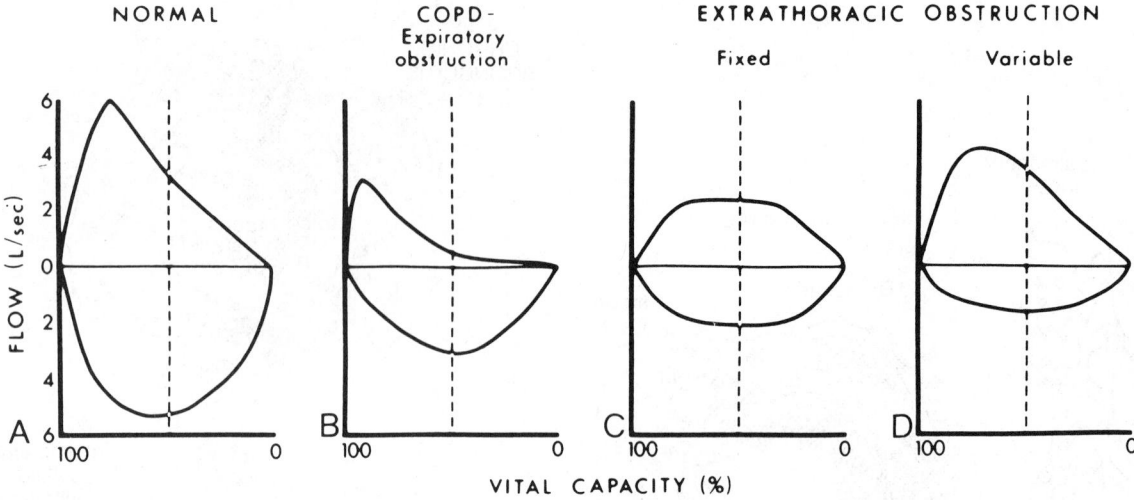

Figure 55.4. Flow volume curves (loops) of maximal forced expiration (*upper*) and maximal inspiration (*lower*). Expiratory and inspiratory flow is plotted against lung volume expressed as a percentage of vital capacity. The *dotted line* can be used to compare flow rates at 50% of the vital capacity where inspiratory flow rates normally exceed expiratory flow rates. *A.* Normal flow volume curves. *B.* Flow volume curves illustrating expiratory airflow obstruction showing decreased flow rates at all points in lung volume throughout maximal expiration. *C.* Fixed extrathoracic airway obstruction (cancer or fracture of the larynx) produces a pattern where there is a decrease and flattening of both inspiratory and expiratory flow volume curves. Inspiratory flow rate at 50% of the vital capacity is equal to similar expiratory flow rate. *D.* Variable extrathoracic obstruction (vocal cord paralysis) produces a pattern where there is a decrease and flattening of maximal inspiratory flow volume curves. Inspiratory flow rates at 50% of the vital capacity are less than similar expiratory flow. (Modified from Hyatt RE, Black LF: The flow-volume curve: a current perspective. *Am Rev Respir Dis* 107:191, 1973.)

Early Detection of Airways Disease

The early diagnosis of chronic obstructive lung disease depends on sensitive pulmonary function tests that correlate with the presence of peripheral airway obstruction (airways of < 2 mm in diameter). Anatomically, these airways lack significant cartilage, have a smooth muscle wall that contains large numbers of mucus-secreting goblet cells, and rely entirely on the surrounding lung parenchyma for structural support. Correlations of the pathological findings in the lungs of patients with early bronchitis and emphysema (30, 64, 66) show abnormalities in these peripheral airways. Early obstructive peripheral airways disease may be predicted by a spirogram in which the FEV_1 is relatively normal (80% of predicted) and the FEV_1:FVC ratio is 70 to 75% but in which the FVC does not reach a plateau within 4 seconds, thereby indicating slowly emptying parts of the lungs (38). This can be further shown by measuring the forced expiratory volume after 3 seconds, the FEV_3, which is normally 98 to 100% of the FVC (FEV_3:FVC ratio: Fig. 55.1).

ASTHMA (INTERMITTENT OBSTRUCTIVE AIRWAYS DISEASE)

Definition

Asthma is difficult to define; for many physicians it simply implies wheezing from any cause. More specifically, asthma is a disease that is characterized by variable airflow obstruction and airway hyper-reactivity that cause intermittent dyspnea and wheezing. Unlike other causes of airflow obstruction, the key features in asthma are reversibility of airway obstruction with relatively symptom-free periods between attacks and increased responsiveness of the airways to a wide variety of inhaled stimuli. The prevalence of asthma in the United States is estimated to be 3% of the population or almost 9 million people.

Airways Hyper-reactivity and Bronchial Inflammation

A characteristic feature found in all asthmatics is airways hyper-reactivity, an exaggerated degree of bronchospasm induced by various inhaled agents (10, 11, 32). These agents include immunological mediators, such as histamine and some prostaglandins; cholinergic agents, such as methacholine; and various irritants, such as dust, cigarette smoke, and cold air (exercise-induced asthma). The presence of increased nonspecific airways reactivity is thought to correlate with the severity of asthmatic symptoms such as coughing and intermittent wheezing. Many patients with chronic obstructive lung disease also show increased airways reactivity (51). Some patients have symptoms consisting primarily of airways irritability such as persistent coughing (see Chapter 54, under "Cough"). They have airways hyper-reactivity to inhaled agents (methacholine), and their symptoms improve after treatment with bronchodilators (40).

Neural reflex mechanisms may be partially responsible for bronchospasm induced by inhaled irritants. These substances activate irritant receptors whose afferent pathways travel in the vagus nerves. Subsequent reflex bronchoconstriction is caused by activation of efferent vagal pathways. These same parasympathetic mechanisms mediate the cough reflex and control bronchial secretions. Although these neural reflex mechanisms may play a role in the development of airways hyper-reactivity, there is increasing evidence that bronchial inflammation is the major factor responsible for airways hyper-responsiveness (3, 10, 32). Various biochemical, cellular, and morphologic changes appear to be present in the airways of asymptomatic asthmatics. These inflammatory events could cause all of the pathophysiologic changes that are found in asthma, including alterations in epithelial integrity, abnormalities in the autonomic neural control of airway tone, changes in mucociliary function, and increased responsiveness of bronchial smooth muscle (3). An important therapeutic implication is that asthma is a chronic inflammatory airway disease (32). Thus treatment with bronchodilators alone may improve symptoms but will not alter the underlying inflammatory processes (6, 32, 35).

Types of Asthma

The definition of asthma above describes only the clinical characteristics of this heterogeneous disease. Asthma can also be classified according to precipitating factors, namely, the presence or absence of an allergic etiology. On the basis of clinical findings, more than half of an asthmatic population can be assigned to one of the five types that are listed in Table 55.3, although even these, as well as the rest of the asthmatic population, show considerable overlap in the clinical features of their disease.

Nonallergic Intrinsic Asthma

The most common type of asthma is not due to allergy but to poorly defined intrinsic factors. These asthmatics have persistent hyper-reactivity of the airways to multiple nonallergic stimuli (see below). Although some intrinsic asthmatics have allergies that occasionally trigger an acute asthmatic attack, the usual clinical course of their disease does not correlate with their allergic hypersensitivities. Instead, asthmatic attacks may be related to infection, exercise, inhaled irritants, or psychological stimuli. Intrinsic asthmatics may have findings that are similar to those of allergic asthmatics such as significant eosinophilia in their blood and sputum and elevated total serum IgE levels. Asthmatic symptoms may begin at any age but often start during adulthood. Commonly, patients may date the onset of asthma to an acute upper respiratory tract infection. Although intrinsic asthmatics may improve with appropriate therapy after their first attack, they subsequently develop chronic symptomatic asthma.

Table 55.3.
Types of Asthma

Nonallergic intrinsic asthma
Allergic extrinsic asthma
Nonallergic extrinsic asthma
Asthma associated with chronic obstructive lung disease
Exercise-induced asthma

Frequently the clinical manifestations of their disease are severe and have a tendency to persist throughout the year, showing variations in severity rather than complete symptomatic remissions. Some of these patients have chronic bronchitis that either complicates or precipitates asthmatic attacks (see below).

Allergic Extrinsic Asthma

In 5 to 10% of asthmatics, clinical asthma is primarily caused by specific allergic factors. These stimuli include seasonal exposure to the pollens of grasses, ragweed, and trees or to other specific allergens, such as animal dander, dust, or some occupational agents. Allergic asthmatics frequently note the onset of recognizable symptoms early in life and relate a family or personal history of asthma or of other allergic diseases (allergic rhinitis, eczema, and urticaria). Many allergic extrinsic asthmatics also have attacks triggered by multiple nonallergic causes.

In these allergic patients, the intradermal injection of a specific allergen causes a wheal and flare reaction; inhalation of this same antigen causes airways obstruction. When a susceptible individual is exposed to an allergen, specific IgE or reaginic antibody is produced. This antibody sensitizes mast cells and basophils (3) and re-exposure to that allergen initiates a sequence of biochemical reactions within these sensitized target cells (type I immunological reaction) (see Chapter 23, Fig. 23.1). These reactions cause the formation, release, and synthesis of histamine and other vasoactive substances that cause contraction of bronchial smooth muscle, alter vascular permeability, and attract inflammatory cells to the reaction site (3).

The release of these mediators is inhibited by increases in cellular cyclic AMP (adenosine 3′:5′-monophosphate) and facilitated by increases in cyclic GMP (guanosine 3′:5′-monophosphate). β-sympathomimetic agonists (such as isoproterenol) directly increase cyclic AMP. Cholinergic stimulation, on the other hand, may enhance the release of mediators by increasing levels of cyclic GMP. These interactions are the basis for the pharmacological treatment of allergic asthma. Theophylline preparations (such as aminophyllin) were until recently thought to inhibit the activity of phosphodiesterase, an enzyme that catalizes the breakdown of cyclic AMP, but at the concentrations achieved *in vivo* that inhibition is weak so that the mechanism of action of theophylline preparations is not really known (19).

Nonallergic Extrinsic Asthma Due to Specific Agents

In some patients, exposure to inhaled or ingested agents causes asthma that does not seem to be caused by the irritant effects of the inhaled substances, nor is it mediated by classic immunological reactions. However, studies have shown that some of these substances [toluene-2, 4-diisocyanate (TDI) or phthalic acid anhydride] may cause their effects through immunological mechanisms. They may act as haptens and combine with serum albumin to form a complete antigen that provokes an IgE-mediated asthma attack (37). When the exposure to these agents occurs in industrial settings, the reversible bronchospasm they produce is called "occupational asthma." Examples of these agents include metal fumes and salts (chromium, nickel, ammonium), wood (oak and western red cedar), vegetable, grain, and coffee bean dusts (flour—baker's asthma), industrial chemicals used in manufacturing processes of plastics, polyurethane foams (TDI, phthalic acid anhydride, epoxy resins, soldering fluxes), pyrolysis products of plastics (meat wrapper's asthma), enzymes (*Bacillus subtilis* detergents), as well as exposures during the manufacture of pharmaceutical agents (penicillin, pancreatic enzymes) (13) (see Chapter 7 and General References under "Asthma").

Aspirin and Other Drug Sensitivity. Other agents such as aspirin, nonsteroidal anti-inflammatory drugs (e.g., indomethacin and phenylbutazone), and tartrazine (yellow dye no. 5), a common coloring agent used in many foods and drugs, precipitate bronchospasm in 5 to 10% of all asthmatics (62) and urticaria in susceptible individuals (Chapter 23). Although the precise mechanisms through which these ingested substances trigger asthma are unknown, it is believed that they are probably not initiated through classic IgE-mediated immunological reactions. Asthmatics with aspirin sensitivity are more commonly female and have associated nasal polyps and sinusitis. Bronchospasm occurs within 2 hours of the aspirin ingestion, and severe reactions may culminate in vascular shock and, rarely, death. Therefore, asthmatics should avoid taking these substances, and challenges with these agents should be performed with extreme care. Table 23.12, Chapter 23, lists both prescription and nonprescription compounds that contain aspirin.

Asthma Associated with Chronic Obstructive Lung Disease

There are patients with chronic obstructive airways disease (chronic obstructive bronchitis or emphysema) whose disease is characterized by intermittent "asthmatic" attacks. A small number of these patients give a history of typical childhood asthma or of other allergic diseases (51). The importance of this somewhat artificial grouping is to emphasize that, although the prognosis in these patients is determined by their chronic obstructive lung disease (see below), the pathophysiology and treatment of an acute exacerbation of bronchospasm are similar to those of typical asthma.

Exercise-Induced Asthma (Cold Air)

Most asthmatics, regardless of etiology, develop wheezing and dyspnea after moderate to severe exercise, especially in cold environments (9). Some forms of exercise, such as running or bicycle riding, are more asthmogenic than others, such as swimming, where ambient air is usually warm and humid. It has been shown that the production of postexertional asthma is directly related to increased heat and water loss from the pulmonary airways during exercise-induced hyperventilation. The mechanisms by which these stimuli trigger bronchospasm are not completely understood, but they may act directly on airway smooth muscle or may produce bronchoconstriction by altering the osmolarity of respiratory secretions. Thus, in experimental situations, exercise-induced bronchospasm can be prevented by having an asthmatic breathe air that is humidified and heated to body temperature (42). The response to exercise or breathing of cold air represents another instance of airways hyper-reactivity in asthma (17). In some mild asthmatics, attacks of exercise-induced bronchospasm represent the primary clinical manifestation of their disease. Also, an elderly intrinsic asthmatic complaining of dyspnea on exertion outdoors on a cold winter day may actually be experiencing exercise-induced asthma rather than cardiac or pulmonary decompensation.

Clinical Presentation of Asthma

Usually asthmatic attacks are episodic, lasting hours to several days, separated by symptom-free periods during which airflow obstruction is absent or mild. Although the patient notes wheezing and coughing productive of white mucoid sputum during a mild asthmatic attack, he can perform ordinary tasks without difficulty. During more severe asthmatic attacks, however, he will experience exertional dyspnea that persists even at rest. Frequent coughing reflects airway hyperirritability. Status asthmaticus refers to a very severe and persistent asthmatic state that does not substantially improve despite intensive therapy.

Evaluation of Mild or Asymptomatic Asthma

History

A complete medical history is essential in the initial evaluation of patients with bronchial asthma to determine the overall severity, the specific factors that precipitate or aggravate symptoms, and the therapeutic modalities that are effective in an individual patient. The medical history should also establish the frequency and severity of asthmatic attacks as well as a description of exercise tolerance during symptom-free periods. If the asthmatic attacks are associated with bronchitis, the frequency, quantity, and duration of sputum production should be documented. The occurrence of seasonal exacerbations should alert the physician to the possibility of environmental factors such as ragweed or grass allergy (see Chapter 23, Fig. 23.3). A history of cough and wheezing precipitated by exposure to cigarette smoke suggests the presence of nonspecific airways reactivity. On the other hand, a personal history of cigarette smoking is unusual in asthma. The severity of exercise-induced bronchospasm should be elicited, especially in adolescents and young adults, in whom the presence of postexercise asthma may interfere with normal social and physical development (9).

Physical Examination

Tachypnea, tachycardia, and a pulsus paradoxus (a drop in systolic blood pressure of greater than 15 mm Hg with inspiration) should be looked for (55). The upper airways should be examined for the presence of sinusitis, nasal polyps, or evidence of allergic rhinitis (boggy, pale nasal mucosa, conjunctivitis). During the rest of the physical examination particular emphasis should be placed on breathing pattern, the use of accessory muscles of ventilation, and the presence of rhonchi and rales during auscultation of the chest. If wheezing is not heard during quiet breathing, a maximal timed forced expiratory maneuver should be performed by asking the patient to blow out all of the air in his lungs as fast as possible after a maximal inspiration. This will frequently induce wheezing not present during quiet breathing; and by timing the forced expiration, a simple index of airways obstruction is obtained. Normal subjects are able to perform a forced expiration in less than 4 seconds, but with airflow obstruction the duration of expiration is greater than 5 or 6 seconds.

Laboratory Testing

In mild asthmatics spirometry is useful to document baseline normal pulmonary function during a symptom-free period. In those patients with more severe asthma, spirometry provides an objective measure of severity and serves as a guide for therapy. Measurement of peak expiratory flow rates provides an objective means of assessing variability of airflow obstruction in asthma. Every asthmatic, even those with mild disease, should own and be taught to use a peak flow meter as well as how to monitor responses to therapy. For a transient time after the initial improvement from an acute attack, significant residual abnormalities in airways function often persist (43). Depending on the individual asthmatic, these residual abnormalities in airways function either resolve or persist with varying severity. It is possible that this subclinical airways obstruction can serve as a focus for future recurrent asthmatic attacks. In asthmatics without superimposed chronic obstructive airways disease, blood gas analysis is indicated only to assess severe asthmatic episodes (see below). In older patients (> 40 years), especially those with evidence of persistent airways obstruction or associated cardiovascular disease, baseline spirometry, an electrocardiogram, and a chest roentgenogram should always be obtained.

A complete blood count (CBC) with differential and sputum examination should be performed in asthmatics who have clinical findings of an acute infectious process. Eosinophils can make sputum appear grossly purulent; therefore, microscopic examination of the sputum in an asthmatic is necessary in order to avoid inappropriate use of antibiotics. Besides eosinophils, sputum may also contain Charcot-Leyden crystals (pointed elongated eosinophilic crystals) and Curschmann's spirals (mucous casts of small bronchioles) (24). If parenchymal pulmonary infection is suspected because of the presence of fever, purulent sputum, and physical findings such as rales and consolidation, a chest roentgenogram and sputum culture are indicated.

Skin testing (Chapter 23) is indicated when a specific allergen is suspected and confirmation of that suspicion is necessary for proper management (see below, page 613). Common allergens that cause allergic asthma include ragweed pollens, various grasses, extracts of trees, molds indigenous to specific localities, and animal danders (cat, dog). Skin testing is most easily obtained by referral to an allergist. Total serum IgE is usually only moderately elevated in patients with allergic asthma, and its measurement is not indicated in the routine clinical management of this disease. Specific serum IgE, measured by the radioallergosorbent test (RAST), provides information similar to that provided by allergy skin testing. Therefore, the RAST is helpful only when skin testing cannot be performed (36).

Bronchial Challenge Procedures

Diagnostic testing with exercise or inhalation challenge with pharmacological agents is occasionally useful to confirm the presence of hyper-reactive airways in patients with questionable symptoms. These tests involve inhaling gradually increasing concentrations of either histamine or methacholine and observing spirometric changes in airflow obstruction (16, 17). Similarly, an exercise challenge can be performed and pulmonary function can be quantitated during the first 30 minutes after maximal exercise. When positive, these tests can cause some mild to moderate distress in an asymptomatic asthmatic since a 20 to 30% reduction in FEV_1 is used as an end point for the diagnosis of hyper-reactive airways. For example, an exercise challenge might help to confirm the diagnostic impression of exercise asthma in a young patient who complains of excessive coughing and dyspnea after physical exertion (17). These challenges require referral to a pulmonary function laboratory that is able to perform provocative testing. Inhalation challenge with specific antigen is almost never indicated since it does not distinguish allergic nonasthmatic patients (grass and ragweed hay fever) from asthmatics with these specific allergies (11). An exception is inhalation challenge in suspected occupational exposure when it may be important to establish the relationship between symptoms and a specific incriminating substance.

Acute Asthma

In order to understand fully the basis for the symptoms, signs, and laboratory findings that correlate with severe asthma, a review of the pathophysiology of acute bronchospasm is indicated.

Pathophysiology of Acute Asthma

Obstruction to expiratory airflow is caused by a combination of bronchial smooth muscle spasm, bronchial wall edema, and inflammatory cell infiltration. During acute asthma these abnormalities may worsen, and mucous plugging of the airways may occur. With progressively more severe asthma ($FEV_1 < 1.5$ liters), the asthmatic is forced to compensate for airway obstruction in order to permit gas exchange to take place. He does this by breathing at high lung volumes since, as the lungs enlarge to total lung capacity, the airways are mechanically opened. Unfortunately, breathing in a hyperinflated state requires a marked increase in the inspiratory muscle forces and results in varying degrees of dyspnea and fatigue. A reduction in vital capacity correlates with the degree of hyperinflation, and, in very severe attacks, the vital capacity may be only slightly larger than the asthmatic's tidal volume. Therefore, the severity of the asthmatic attack is highly correlated with the two simple measures of forced expiration, the FEV_1 and the FVC (Fig. 55.1) (43, 55).

Another major physiological change that occurs during a severe asthmatic attack is the development of pulmonary hypertension due to the direct effects of hypoxia and the mechanical effects of hyperinflation on the pulmonary vasculature. These changes are manifested by electrocardiographic abnormalities such as acute right axis deviation, "p" pulmonale, and right ventricular strain. In addition, during breathing in acute asthma the marked swings in pleural pressure are associated with hyperinflation that affects left ventricular function and accounts for the development of pulsus paradoxus. A summary of these pathophysiological changes is listed in Table 55.4.

Evaluation of an Acute Asthmatic Attack

Unfortunately, subjective symptoms such as dyspnea and wheezing do not correlate with severity of asthma (43), and the physician must rely on objective physical findings and laboratory tests to evaluate an acute asthmatic attack (Table 55.5). During the physical examination, the findings of a pulsus paradoxus and the use of accessory muscles of ventilation with sternocleidomastoid contractions correlate with the development of severe airflow obstruction, hyperinflation, and a marked reduction in FEV_1 ($< 40\%$ predicted or 1.25 liters) (43, 55).

When physical findings are present that suggest severe asthma, objective pulmonary function measurements should be performed in every asthmatic who is

Table 55.4.
Pathophysiological Changes in Acute Bronchial Asthma

Expiratory airflow obstruction (FEV_1 and expiratory airflow are reduced)
Breathing at high lung volumes to prevent airway closure at resting lung volumes (vital capacity is reduced)
Pulmonary hypertension (P pulmonale and right ventricular strain on ECG)
Large fluctuations in pleural pressure with respiration (pulsus paradoxus)
Ventilation-perfusion mismatch (arterial blood gases show hypoxemia always, hypocapnea (low $PaCO_2$) usually, and hypercapnea (high $PaCO_2$) only in very severe asthma)

Table 55.5.
Objective Evaluation of Acute Asthma

Vital signs: tachycardia and pulsus paradoxus
Physical examination: use of accessory muscles of respiration with sternocleidomastoid contractions
Spirometry: reduced FEV_1 and increase in FEV_1 after administration of a bronchodilator
Chest X-ray: hyperinflation
ECG: acute cor pulmonale
Arterial blood gases (low PaO_2, low or high $PaCO_2$)
Sputum smear and culture: eosinophils or evidence of infection

Table 55.6.
Indications of Severe Asthma Necessitating Immediate Hospitalization (Acute Respiratory Failure)

$FEV_1 < 1.0$ Liters, FVC < 1.4 Liters (absent bronchodilator response)
$PaO_2 < 50$ mm Hg, $PaCO_2 > 40$ mm Hg
Disturbance of consciousness, obvious exhaustion
Silent chest
Pulsus paradoxus > 15 mm
Pneumothorax or pneumomediastinum

old enough to cooperate. Objective assessment should consist of either spirometry with measurement of FEV_1 and FVC or peak expiratory airflow measurements. An FEV_1 less than 1.25 liters or 40% of predicted correlates with severe hypoxemia ($PaO_2 < 60$ mm Hg) (46) while peak flow rates less than 100 liters/minute indicate severe airflow obstruction (20). Spirometry or peak flow measurements can then be used to monitor the course of the asthmatic attack as well as the response to bronchodilator treatment. An absent bronchodilator response suggests status asthmaticus. When there is evidence of severe asthma, the patient should be treated in a hospital emergency room or a similar setting where aerosol and parenteral drug therapy is available; O_2 can be administered; and there is the capability to treat acute respiratory failure. The findings listed in Table 55.6 indicate severe respiratory failure in status asthmaticus; such patients require immediate hospitalization.

A chest roentgenogram is indicated in those patients with acute asthma who do not improve readily with initial treatment or in those in whom pulmonary infection is suspected. The chest roentgenogram should be inspected for atelectasis due to mucous plugging of the airways, for pulmonary infiltrates due to infectious processes that could precipitate or complicate an asthmatic attack, and for a pneumothorax or a pneumomediastinum. Furthermore, the presence of acute hyperinflation on a chest roentgenogram indicates a severe asthmatic attack (Fig. 55.5). The significance of electrocardiographic abnormalities consistent with acute cor pulmonale and pulmonary hypertension has been discussed. The measurement of arterial blood gases should be performed when physical findings and spirometry ($FEV_1 < 1.25$ liters or 40% predicted) suggest a severe asthmatic attack. Arterial hypoxemia develops during acute episodes of bronchial asthma (46), and in the very severe attack ($FEV_1 < 1.0$ liter or 25% predicted) hypoxemia can be life threatening. Usually in mild to moderately severe asthmatic attacks

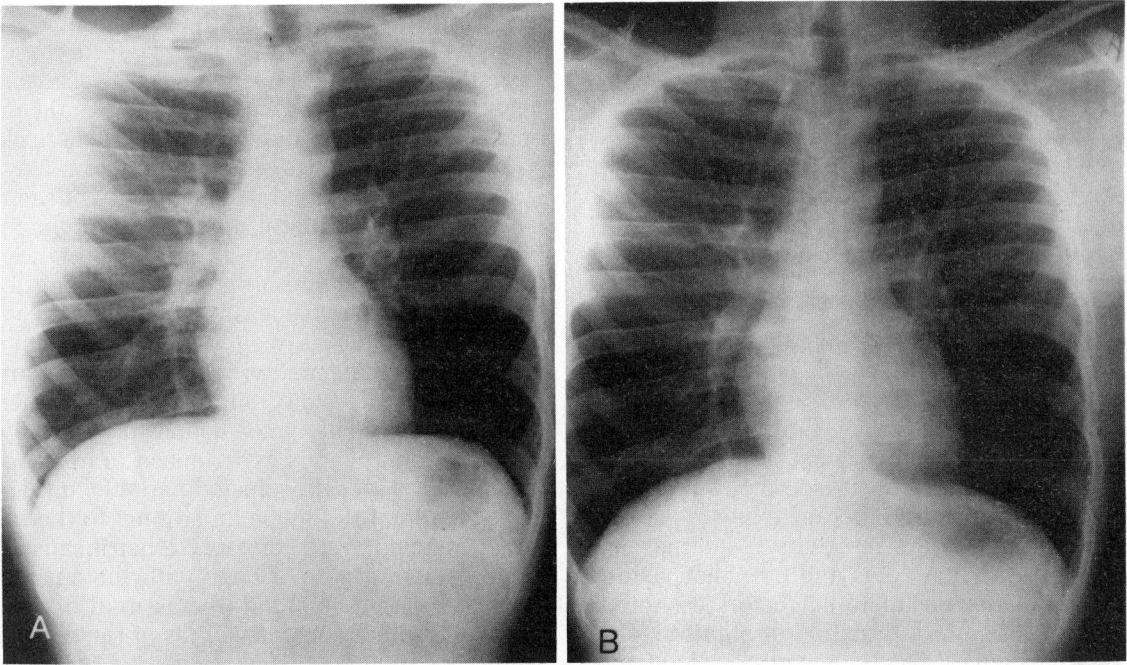

Figure 55.5. Acute hyperinflation in severe asthma. *A.* Normal chest roentgenogram in an asthmatic. *B.* Acute hyperinflation (lowered flattened diaphragms and widened intercostal spaces) in the same patient during a severe asthmatic attack. Pulmonary function tests showed a marked reduction in FEV$_1$ (0.8 liter, 18% predicted) and FVC (2.1 liters, 38% predicted) and an elevated total lung capacity (7.3 liters, 112% predicted).

alveolar hyperventilation is maintained and arterial CO_2 tensions are reduced. In asthma an arterial CO_2 tension that rises into the normal range or becomes elevated predicts imminent respiratory failure.

Differential Diagnosis

Because of its characteristic clinical presentation, acute bronchial asthma is easily differentiated from the other cardiopulmonary diseases that present with cough, wheezing, and dyspnea. In middle-aged and elderly patients one must consider acute left ventricular failure with "cardiac asthma," pulmonary embolism, or an exacerbation of chronic obstructive pulmonary disease. Occasionally patients only complain of persistent coughing and deny wheezing or dyspnea. These patients often have pulmonary function tests that reveal mild obstruction, have bronchial hyper-reactivity, and may improve with bronchodilator treatment (43).

Airflow limitation produced by obstruction in the upper airways (larynx, trachea) caused by a foreign body, tumor, secretions, edema, inflammation, or tracheal malacia can sometimes be confused with lower airway obstruction. In upper airway obstruction, there may be a history of goiter, hoarseness, or prior endotracheal intubation. Physical examination usually reveals inspiratory stridor (wheezing during inspiration). Inspiratory flow volume curves (33), performed in a pulmonary function laboratory, show a reduction in inspiratory flows and a specific diagnostic pattern (Fig. 55.4). Direct or indirect laryngoscopy may visualize an anatomical abnormality.

Treatment of Asthma

Since asthma has multiple etiologies, its management requires a combined therapeutic approach that should attempt to maintain pulmonary function in a nearly normal state as well as to prevent recurrent asthmatic attacks (Table 55.7). Precipitating factors in an individual asthmatic must be identified and avoided. Clinical manifestations, including bronchospasm and pulmonary infections, must be effectively treated, and medical complications should be prevented.

Table 55.7.
Treatment of Asthma

GENERAL MEASURES
  Control of environmental factors:
    Cigarette smoke, air pollutants
    Occupational exposures
    Control of environmental temperature and humidity
  Control of allergy to specific inhaled or ingested agents
  Control of emotional and psychological factors
  Control of respiratory infections
  Avoidance of aspirin and other non-steroidal antiinflammatory agents
SPECIFIC TREATMENT
  Pharmacological
    Smooth muscle spasm—bronchodilators: local/systemic inflammation (corticosteroids)
  Mechanical airways obstruction—mucus:
    Hydration—local/systemic
    Physical therapy
    Mucolytic agents: to be avoided
  Infection: appropriate antibiotics
  Hypoxemia: humidified oxygen
  Sedation: to be avoided

Avoidance of Precipitating Factors

As indicated above, numerous, often apparently unrelated, factors precipitate or worsen clinical asthma. Some of these stimuli are easily defined and controlled, whereas in other asthmatics the exact precipitating factors are difficult to determine with certainty. Knowledge of the triggers of asthma is of prime importance in its evaluation and treatment.

Environment. Asthmatics should avoid exposure to irritating dusts, sprays, or aerosols, both at home and at work. For example, passive exposure of asthmatics to cigarette smoke, especially in enclosed spaces such as cars, airplanes, or poorly ventilated rooms, will cause worsening of airway function. The exact role of air pollutants in provoking asthma is still not completely known. However, it is known that ozone, sulfur dioxide, and nitrogen dioxide exposure can increase nonspecific airways reactivity in normal subjects and can cause symptoms and bronchospasm in asthmatics (11). Often occupational factors are not immediately obvious since asthmatic symptoms may occur several hours after leaving the workplace (coughing and dyspnea awakening the patient from sleep). Because direct challenge with suspected provoking agents is not always practical and is often dangerous, the etiology of an asthmatic's symptoms may be indirectly ascertained by systematically avoiding specific, potentially provoking factors. At home, the control of environmental temperature and humidity is accomplished with an air conditioner that will also help to filter pollens and air pollutants. The filter should be changed regularly to avoid the accumulation of sensitizing airborne molds and fungi. In rare circumstances, removal to a more favorable climate may be indicated to control chronic asthma (see page 631).

Allergy. Desensitization consists of injections of increasing concentrations of an antigen to which the asthmatic is sensitive, thereby inducing blocking antibody (IgG antibody that interferes with the antigen-antibody reaction). It is indicated when there are a limited number of allergens, demonstrated by skin testing, that appear to be etiologically related to an individual's asthma (36). Desensitization therapy is expensive, time consuming, and not always effective. Therefore, before it is started, every attempt should be made to eliminate or reduce specific allergen exposure. At times, only a reduction in exposure to a known allergen can be effected. For example, if it is not possible to remove a household pet from the home of an allergic asthmatic patient, the pet should be excluded from the patient's bedroom. Down-filled pillows and shag rugs that accumulate dust should not be used.

Emotion. Asthmatic attacks can be produced and reversed in some patients by appropriate verbal suggestion (45). For example, less bronchodilation is produced by isoproterenol if the asthmatic is told he is being treated with a bronchoconstrictor rather than a bronchodilator. Therefore, the expectations of the asthmatic patient as well as of those treating him have a significant influence on the therapeutic efficacy of any given therapeutic regimen. Despite these considerations, all asthmatic patients must receive adequate medical treatment, and symptoms should not be ignored because they may have psychogenic etiologies.

In some asthmatics, emotional factors play a much greater role in modulating the course of their disease and often cause difficult therapeutic problems. In addition, asthma can be a chronic, debilitating disease that in itself will stress the asthmatic and his family. Usually supportive measures initiated by a sympathetic physician, as well as by the patient's family members and friends, will avoid the need for psychiatric care. Occasionally, supportive psychotherapy will be useful, especially when counseling is available from a professional who is experienced in treating psychosomatic illnesses. In selected patients, mild sedatives (see Chapter 13) may be an adjunct to the total treatment regimen, but preferably other means should be used to help a patient cope with the anxiety caused by his disease. He should be assured of the concern of those around him, as well as of the constant availability of adequate emergency care. Sedation is specifically contraindicated in severe (Table 55.6) asthmatic attacks since sedating a severely ill, exhausted asthmatic can result in acute respiratory failure (46) and even death.

An important adjunct to the psychosocial management of childhood asthma is the encouragement of a general exercise program. Asthma should not be an automatic excuse preventing participation in physical education and sports. With appropriate premedication, asthmatics can participate in most activities. Some activities may be less asthmogenic than others (see "Exercise-Induced Asthma" above) (9). It is important not to isolate the asthmatic from his peers by unnecessary restrictive measures.

Infections. Upper respiratory tract infections can cause transient increases in nonspecific airways reactivity with persistent coughing and occasional bronchospasm in nonasthmatics (see Chapter 28, Respiratory Infections, and Chapter 54, under "Cough"). In fact, these reactions may be so severe and persistent that these "nonasthmatics" require treatment with bronchodilators. Therefore, it is not surprising that most asthmatics have attacks triggered by respiratory infections.

If there is clinical evidence of an acute bacterial respiratory infection associated with an asthmatic attack, antibiotic therapy should be initiated. Usually, the initial drug of choice is either tetracycline or ampicillin, administered for 7 to 10 days, unless the sputum smear or culture dictates the use of a different antibiotic regimen.

Pharmacological Treatment

Pharmacological therapy is the primary therapeutic modality used to treat reversible bronchospasm and to reduce bronchial inflammation in asthma and in chronic obstructive lung disease (41, 57). The five major drug categories generally available include (a) sympathomimetics, (b) theophylline preparations, (c) antiallergic drugs, (d) anticholinergics, and (e) corticosteroids. Detailed knowledge of the mechanism of action and side effects of these drugs is important for every physician who takes care of patients with reversible airways disease. The selection of an appropriate drug regimen is complicated by the many preparations available for most of these agents. Specific combinations, dosage, and route of delivery will often be determined by whether these drugs are used for preventive therapy in stable asthmatics or for the emergency treatment of acute asthma.

Sympathomimetic Agents. This group of drugs may be functionally divided into agents that have α- and β-sympathomimetic activities. More recently, β-agonists have been further divided into those with β_1 and β_2 selective actions (Table 55.8). The undesirable side effects of beta agonists are due to their β_1 actions, which stimulate the cardiovascular system, causing tachycardia and, possibly, arrhythmias. The β_2 actions of these drugs increase cyclic AMP levels in mast cells and bronchial smooth muscle, thereby inhibiting mediator release and directly dilating the airways smooth muscle.

Epinephrine has both α- and β-adrenergic effects, while isoproterenol is a potent β_1- and β_2-sympathomimetic agent. Besides lack of specificity, these older sympathomimetics have a shorter duration of action because they are rapidly metabolized by catechol-ortho-methyltransferase (COMT), an enzyme present in high concentrations in the gut. Therefore, these drugs can only be administered by an aerosol or parenteral route, and their duration of action is shorter. Two proprietary medications, Bronchaid and Primatine Mist, are metered dose inhalers that deliver 0.23 and 0.20 mg of epinephrine, respectively. Newer β_2-sympathomimetic agonists (metaproterenol, terbutaline, bitolterol, pirbuterol, albuterol) are not metabolized by

COMT and thus have a longer duration of action than isoproterenol. These agents have progressively greater β_2 selectivity and potency as shown in Table 55.8. Improved effectiveness of the newer β-sympathomimetic aerosol preparations has made them an integral part of the treatment of reversible airways obstruction. Unfortunately, these agents still retain some β_1 cardiac side effects, and, furthermore, when administered systemically, all cause skeletal muscle tremor, a specific β_2 side effect. This annoying symptom may occur even when oral treatment with terbutaline or metaproterenol is begun at reduced doses, but it frequently improves with continued therapy (2 weeks). *Ephedrine* has been widely used because it is well absorbed orally, but its side effects include stimulation of the cardiac and central systems, thereby limiting its usefulness. The need to counteract these side effects has led to fixed dose combination tablets that contain ephedrine, a sedative, and a theophylline preparation. These drug combinations, although convenient and popular, do not meet the specific needs of an individual and usually do not deliver an adequate therapeutic dose of any of its components. Because newer β_2 agonists are well absorbed orally, they should replace ephedrine.

For the ambulatory treatment of asthma, the new β_2-sympathomimetic agonists can be used as aerosols to prevent asthmatic attacks caused by known trigger factors, such as exercise, cold air exposure, or inhaled irritants. When therapy with an inhaled agent is begun, all patients should be shown how to use a metered dose inhaler, and thereafter their technique should be checked periodically (48). Illustrations showing the correct technique are usually included in the package insert. This process is described in detail on page 618. In patients who require continuous treatment for either short periods during an exacerbation or chronically because of persistent bronchospasm, two inhalations are taken every 6 to 8 hours. Some physicians prescribe the use of inhaled sympathomimetics at more frequent intervals (every 4 to 6 hours).

Table 55.8.
β-Sympathomimetic Agonists

Generic Name	Trade Name	β_2 Selectivity		Onset of Action	Inhalation Peak Effect	Duration of Effect	Dosage Form
				min.	min.	hours	
Isoetharine	Bronkosol Bronkometer	$\beta_2 >$	$\beta1$	5	5–15	2–3	Metered dose inhaler, 340 µg/puff Nebulized solution, 1%
Metaproterenol[a]	Alupent	$\beta_2 >>>$	β_1	1–5	30–60	2–5	Metered dose inhaler, 0.65 µg/puff Nebulized solution, 5% Tablets 10 and 20 mg
Terbutaline	Brethine Bricanyl Brethaire	$\beta2 >>>$	β_1	1–5	30–60	2–5	Metered dose inhaler, 200 µg/puff Injection, 1 mg/ml Tablets 2.5 and 5 mg
Bitolterol	Tomalate	$\beta_2 >>>$	β_1	3–5	30–60	4–8	Metered dose inhaler, 370 5µ/puff
Pirbuterol	Maxair	$\beta_2 >>>$	β_1	5	30–60	4–5	Metered dose inhaler, 0.2 mg/puff
Albuterol	Proventyl Ventolin	$\beta_2 >>>>$	β_1	5–15	60–90	3–6	Metered dose inhaler, 90 µg/puff Tablets 2.4 and 4.8 mg
Fenoterol[b]	Berotec	$\beta_2 >>>>$	β_1	1–5	60	4–8	Metered dose inhaler, 200 µg/puff

[a] Available as an over-the-counter product.
[b] Not available in the United States.

Although this treatment may be safe, it should not be used in patients with cardiac disease (49). In addition, prolonged therapy with β_2-sympathomimetics may be associated with tachyphylaxis and a diminished response to these agents (56, 65).

Often acute asthmatic attacks are initially treated in the physician's office, but when they are severe (Tables 55.5 and 55.6), treatment should be started in the office and the patient should then be sent to an emergency room. In an acute asthmatic attack, subcutaneous epinephrine (0.1 to 0.3 ml of 1:1000) or inhaled isoproterenol (two inhalations of 131 μg/metered dose/breath) are effective therapeutic regimens (25, 41, 59). These medications can be repeated three times at 30-minute intervals in young patients without heart disease. However, since both of these drugs have significant cardiac side effects, there is a trend to replace them with one of the specific β_2-sympathomimetic agonists, all of which are available for aerosol administration (Table 55.8) (41). Terbutaline is currently available for parenteral administration and may be preferred to parenteral epinephrine because of its sustained action. However, repeated administration of parenteral terbutaline should be performed cautiously since this drug has a long duration of action and unwanted cardiac side effects may occur.

Theophylline Preparations. Numerous theophylline preparations are available for the treatment of reversible airways disease. The physician should become familiar with two of these compounds, choosing an inexpensive short-acting agent (such as generic aminophylline) and a long-acting preparation (such as LaBid, Phyllacintin, Somophyllin-CRT, Sustaire, or Theo-Dur) (52, 57). Theophylline preparations with a longer duration of action (24 hours) are also available and may improve patient compliance because of a once daily dosing schedule, but further experience is necessary before they can be recommended routinely. The toxic side effects of theophylline include stimulation of the central nervous system, nausea, vomiting, and inotropic and chronotropic cardiac actions. Toxic levels of these drugs cause grand mal seizures, cardiac arrhythmias, and even death (68). For the most part, gastrointestinal side effects are related to serum levels of theophylline and not to the direct effects of oral theophylline on the gut mucosa. Absorption from the gastrointestinal tract and metabolism of theophylline in the liver vary and may require adjustment of dosage in different individuals. The dose of theophylline should be reduced in patients with liver disease, congestive heart failure, or a history of seizures. Several drugs (e.g., cimetidine, propranolol, and erythromycin) depress the metabolism of theophylline. Adolescents and heavy smokers often metabolize this drug more rapidly and may require increased doses. Most clinicians attempt to maintain peak plasma theophylline levels between 10 and 20 μg/ml although most of the bronchodilator effects of theophylline are produced at plasma levels of 5 to 15 μg/ml (57). At higher plasma levels, there is an increase in serious side effects, such as central nervous system irritability and

cardiac tachyarrhythmias. In many ambulatory patients, the measurement of serum theophylline levels is usually not indicated, especially when there is a good therapeutic response and no evidence of side effects. However, in patients with altered theophylline clearance (liver or cardiac disease) or in those in whom high doses are required to achieve therapeutic effects, monitoring the serum theophylline level is important. Blood should be sampled 1 to 2 hours after a drug dose to establish the peak serum level.

Initial therapy with oral aminophylline should start with 200 mg administered three or four times/day; however, some patients may require ultimately as much as 1200 to 1600 mg daily. The dose can be increased every 2 to 5 days while the patient is observed for therapeutic and toxic effects. The long-acting theophylline preparations, although more expensive, appear to be useful because patient compliance is improved since these preparations are usually taken only once or twice a day. However, more frequent dosing may be required in individuals who metabolize theophylline rapidly. In addition, the absorption of many of these long-acting theophylline preparations may be affected by the relationship to food intake and to the fat content of the meal. Because these effects vary for each drug preparation, the prescribing physician must know the specific pharmokinetics of the preparation he prescribes. Frequently, therapeutic levels are achieved with lower doses. Treatment should begin with 200 mg twice a day, and the dose should be increased by a 100-mg increment/day every 2 to 3 days. Many patients complain of nervousness, mild gastric distress, and headache when any of the theophylline preparations are started. These distressing side effects usually resolve during continued therapy (2 to 4 weeks).

Antiallergic Drugs. Cromolyn (Intal) is a drug that does not act as a bronchodilator, and although its exact mechanism of action is unknown, it may stabilize mast cells, preventing immunological release of mediators (8), or may improve nonspecific airways reactivity. It is available for administration in the following preparations: capsules for use with a spinhaler, a nebulized solution, and as a metered dose inhaler. Usually it is administered three to four times a day. It occasionally causes coughing and mild bronchospasm in some asthmatics and because of these irritant properties, it should not be used in acute asthmatic attacks, and it may be necessary to administer a nebulized sympathomimetic bronchodilator before cromolyn during routine use.

Cromolyn is an effective prophylactic agent in some allergic and nonallergic asthmatic patients and is specifically useful in patients with significant exercise-induced asthma. Acute administration before exercise may prevent exericise-induced bronchospasm. It is usually used chronically in allergic asthmatics with known factors that specifically trigger asthma such as animal dander. Its effectiveness in patients with other forms of reversible obstructive airways disease is difficult to predict, but when effective, some severe asthmatics may be able to reduce systemic steroid requirements (see below). Some physicians use cromolyn for the initial therapy of chronic allergic asthma. Initially it should be administered for a trial period of 2 to 4 weeks. Symptoms and objective pulmonary function tests (spirometry or peak expiratory flow rates) should be used to assess its efficacy. Patients for whom cromolyn is prescribed should understand that its effect is to prevent but not to treat an asthma attack. This is important because many patients associate the use of inhaled medications with the symptomatic treatment of acute asthma. New oral or inhaled antiallergic agents are undergoing clinical testing in the United States (6).

Pretreatment with *antihistamines* does not prevent or reduce bronchospasm produced by inhaled specific antigen. Therefore, antihistamines should not be used to treat airways obstruction in allergic asthmatics. However, these drugs can be used to control allergic or vasomotor rhinitis (Chapter 23) in patients who also have asthma.

Anticholinergic Agents. One of the first forms of treatment for asthma was inhalation of anticholinergic agents. A rationale for the use of these drugs is that airway tone is maintained by the parasympathetic nervous system; inhaled anticholinergic agents block postganglionic efferent vagal neural control of airway tone and cause bronchodilation. Another reason is that anticholinergic agents also block reflex bronchospasm (see "Airways Hyper-reactivity and Bronchial Inflammation," page 608). Use of these agents was abandoned until recently because of unwanted side effects such as drying of respiratory secretions, reduced bronchial mucociliary transport, blurred vision, urinary retention, and cardiac and central nervous system stimulation. Atropine is the most potent anticholinergic agent, but when inhaled some of it is absorbed systemically. Although atropine is frequently used to treat bronchospasm, it is not officially approved for use as a bronchodilator by the Food and Drug Administration. When atropine is used, a total dose of 0.8 to 1.6 mg (atropine sulfate parenteral solution) is inhaled from a nebulizer every 4 to 8 hours. Some asthmatics, and many patients with chronic obstructive bronchitis, improve airways function with atropine treatment, and it may be tried in combination with or as an alternative to inhaled sympathomimetic agents (13, 54, 65). Ipratropium (Atrovent), a quaternary ammonium compound, has been approved for the treatment of bronchospasm. Its major advantage is that it is not absorbed systemically during inhalation therapy (14, 31). It appears to be a very effective bronchodilator in patients with chronic airflow obstruction (65). Although a less potent bronchodilator than inhaled sympathomimetics, approximately 50% of asthmatics will show at least a 15% improvement in pulmonary function after treatment with ipratropium (two inhalations, 36 μg, four times a day). However, its precise role in the therapy of asthma requires further investigation.

Corticosteroids. Corticosteroids are effective agents for treating reversible obstructive airways disease, but their exact mechanism of action is unknown. They cause bronchodilation and reduction in bronchial inflammation and improve the response to β-sympathomimetic agents. The onset of their therapeutic effects is delayed and does not begin for 6 to 12 hours (26, 44). Steroids may be administered as "burst" therapy in which high doses (40 to 80 mg of prednisone) are started and tapered rapidly (10 to 20 mg a day) over a 7- to 10-day period. "Burst" therapy is used to treat severe asthma attacks or acute severe exacerbations of bronchospasm in patients with reversible chronic obstructive lung disease. The major side effects from "burst" therapy are steroid-induced abnormalities in glucose metabolism. However, when corticosteroids are used to treat severe obstructive airways disease for prolonged periods, they may produce many other unwanted systemic side effects (Cushing's syndrome, adrenal pituitary suppression, osteoporosis, etc.). In addition, the patient's ability to deal normally with infectious processes is impaired. Because reactivation of tuberculosis can occur during chronic corticosteroid treatment, any patient with a positive purified protein derivative (PPD) skin test should receive simultaneous INH (isoniazid) prophylaxis. Acute adrenal insufficiency may occur during stressful medical or surgical illnesses (Chapter 74). Whenever chronic steroid therapy is begun in an ambulatory setting, objective pulmonary function tests are required to evaluate its therapeutic effectiveness since some patients will feel better due to the euphoria produced by steroids but have unchanged pulmonary function. The lowest effective dose should be employed, and, if possible, alternate-day steroid therapy should be attempted. This should be done by decreasing the dose of prednisone by 5 mg every 2 to 3 days and measuring the FEV_1 periodically (weekly). When symptoms of bronchospasm worsen, the tapering process should be slowed. If bronchospasm improves after prolonged treatment, then further reduction or elimination of prednisone therapy may be possible. Aerosolized steroids or cromolyn may be useful to help reduce or even eliminate the need for systemic steroids in some patients.

Nonabsorbable corticosteroid aerosols (beclomethasone, dexamethasone, flunisolide, triamcinolone) are available. The technique for inhaler use described on page 615 should be reviewed with the patient who is beginning to use an aerosolized steroid. The use of these agents often permits a reduction or, if the patient is taking 20 mg of prednisone or less a day, even the elimination of oral steroid therapy. Treatment may also be initiated with these inhaled agents.

Because of the recognition of bronchial inflammation in the pathogenesis of asthma, some physicians advocate early or initial treatment with inhaled corticosteroids (32, 61). Although this approach may reduce asthmatic symptoms and airways hyper-reactivity (6, 23, 35), it may make some mild asthmatics dependent on inhaled corticosteroids. Further studies are needed to evaluate the efficacy and side effects of this therapy.

Side effects from aerosolized steroid preparations are negligible but include the development of oral candidiasis, which is prevented by rinsing the mouth with water immediately after inhaling the steroids or treated by gargling with small doses of an antifungal agent, e.g., mycostatin. Particle deposition in the mouth and the development of oral candidiasis can also be reduced by administering these agents with a spacer or chamber (see below, Metered Dose Inhalers). The usual dose of these preparations is two breaths inhaled three to four times a day; the maximal dose, in severe asthmatics, is 20 inhalations a day. Whenever inhaled steroid therapy is used to reduce systemic corticosteroid dependence, the dose of oral steroids should be decreased slowly (5 to 10 mg weekly) in patients who have been treated with systemic corticosteroids for long periods of time. If patients being treated with inhaled corticosteroids have an acute exacerbation of asthma, treatment with oral prednisone should be reinstituted.

General Approach to Pharmacological Therapy of Reversible Airways Disease

The purpose of this section is to integrate some of the principles of the pharmacological treatment of bronchospasm that have been discussed separately under specific drug categories (41, 67).

Metered Dose Inhalers

Most of the medications for the treatment of asthma are currently available in the form of metered dose inhalers (MDIs) and nearly all patients with obstructive airways disease use this form of drug administration. The obvious advantage to delivering drugs directly into the airways is that high concentrations can be delivered to the primary site of disease and systemic toxicity can be avoided. The major disadvantage is that a degree of skill is required to coordinate activation of the nebulizer and breathing. Unlike oral medications, patients usually require individualized training and observation to learn these techniques (41, 48).

The following technique for MDI use is suggested: After shaking the canister to suspend the medication, the MDI is positioned two finger breadths in front of the open mouth (an exception to this rule is with anticholinergic agents that should be administered directly into the closed mouth to avoid contamination of the eyes). At the end of a normal exhalation (i.e., at functional residual capacity) a slow inhalation is started, taking 5 seconds to reach total lung capacity. The MDI is discharged at the beginning of this slow inspiration. The breath should be held for 5 or more seconds to allow particles that have penetrated into the smaller airways to settle by gravity. Further inhalations of medications can be taken immediately, or in the case of bronchodilators, the patient can wait 15 minutes before the second dose. This waiting period allows bronchodilation to occur and permits deeper penetration of the second aerosol administration into the lungs. Despite intensive instruction, some patients

cannot use a MDI properly. In such cases, there are devices (e.g., InspirEase, Aerochamber, Breathancer) that allow discharge of the MDI into a chamber creating a suspension of particles that can be inhaled without the need for precise coordination of inhalation and the MDI discharge. Thus, with the drug particles held in suspension, the patient has a short time period (3 to 5 seconds) to inhale the drug more effectively. Chambers should be used by patients who are unable to use a MDI correctly. These devices also eliminate the rapid initial particle velocity and reduce the irritant properties of the aerosol and the tendency to cough. They also reduce aerosol deposition in the mouth and oropharynx, decreasing the frequency of oral candida infections when they are used with inhaled corticosteroids (48).

Occasional Symptomatic Use of Bronchodilators

During remission or in patients with very mild asthma ($FEV_1 > 70\%$ predicted), the occasional symptomatic use of aerosolized specific β_2-sympathomimetic agonists usually controls intermittent episodes of bronchospasm (Fig. 55.6). Administration of a sympathomimetic before exercise or an anticipated allergen exposure is usually effective in preventing an asthmatic attack. Alternatives to aerosol therapy are the use of theophylline derivatives or oral preparations of β_2-sympathomimetic agonists. Such occasional use of bronchodilators can control intermittent episodes of bronchospasm and prevent bronchospasm from specific known stimuli (exercise, cold air, irritants). Also cromolyn can be used intermittently to treat exercise-induced asthma.

Chronic Bronchodilator Therapy

There are two choices for initial continuous therapy in patients with reversible obstructive airways disease who cannot be managed with occasional intermittent bronchodilators. One choice is to treat these patients with aerosolized β_2-sympathomimetic agents. Ordinarily these drugs are effective and have fewer systemic side effects than theophylline preparations (41, 48, 59). However, many physicians use theophylline as the drug of choice for chronic bronchodilator therapy. Those patients whose bronchospasm is not controlled with a single bronchodilator require combination therapy. Questions have arisen about potential unwanted cardiac side effects during combination therapy with theophylline and oral β_2-sympathomimetics in patients with cardiovascular disease (49). In patients with known cardiac disease, oral theophylline preparations should be combined with inhaled specific β_2-sympathomimetics (54, 70). There is increasing evidence that anticholinergic agents are more effective in patients with chronic bronchitis and airflow obstruction than in asthmatics (31). However, anticholinergics can produce significant and prolonged bronchodilitation in some asthmatics. Thus, a therapeutic trial with objective pulmonary function assessment may be used in asthmatics who require

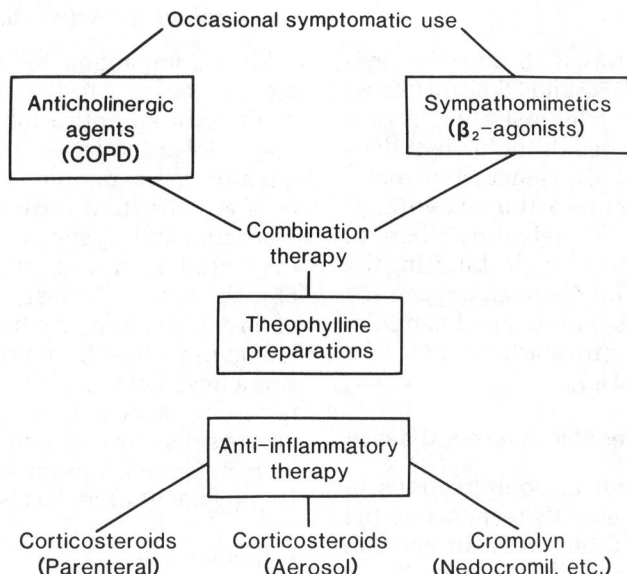

Figure 55.6. Approach to the pharmacological treatment of reversible airways disease (see the text).

combination bronchodilator therapy to control their symptoms.

Because bronchial inflammation appears to be an important mechanism for airway hyper-reactivity and asthmatic symptoms, anti-inflammatory therapy is gaining acceptance. Inhaled corticosteroids can reduce symptoms and oral corticosteroid dependence in many asthmatics. Some physicians are using these agents in the initial treatment of chronic asthma, whereas others will prescribe inhaled corticosteroids when symptoms are not controlled with standard bronchodilators (sympathomimetics and theophylline) (23, 32). Cromolyn also provides effective prophylactic treatment for allergic and exercise-induced asthma. In allergic patients, this drug must be used continuously. Systemic corticosteroids should be reserved for status asthmaticus and for severe chronic asthma that does not respond to conventional therapy.

Acute Asthmatic Attacks

Less severe acute asthmatic attacks can be treated either with aerosolized β_2-sympathomimetics or oral theophylline preparations. If there are objective signs of severe asthma (Tables 55.5 and 55.6), regimens such as subcutaneous injections of epinephrine or inhaled sympathomimetics are more effective than theophylline preparations (59). The addition of theophylline is indicated in the treatment of severe acute asthma (FEV_1 < 1.0 liter) (25). More recently, systemic therapy with subcutaneous injections of terbutaline is being substituted for epinephrine. Also, the new selective β_2-sympathomimetic agents may be preferable to inhaled isoproterenol. Corticosteroids should be administered when there is no objective improvement after 4 hours of therapy in patients with severe asthma (26).

Depending on individual reliability, patients with reversible airways obstruction should be instructed what medications (usually a sympathomimetic aerosol or an oral theophylline compound) they can use for self-treatment before they must contact the physician (39). For example, an intelligent young adult asthmatic should know that he can use an inhaled β-sympathomimetic agonist more frequently (every 2 to 4 hours) and can take an extra dose of aminophylline to self-treat a mild asthma attack. The severity of asthma should be monitored by the patient with measurement of peak expiratory flow rates (see page 606). Peak expiratory flow rates that have fallen more than 40% below an asthmatic's usual range or are less than 120 liters/minute indicate a severe attack that requires treatment by a physician (20). If the asthmatic does not improve after a 2-hour period, he should call his physician or go directly to a hospital emergency room for care.

Other Specific Therapeutic Measures in Asthma

Respiratory Therapy

During acute asthmatic attacks, there is increased water loss from the respiratory tract and a tendency, especially in young children, for patients to become dehydrated. Usually oral rehydration is adequate. During the winter months when ambient room air is dry, a home humidifier will effectively increase the water content of the air. Care should be taken to clean these humidifiers to prevent the accumulation of molds or fungi. Rarely dehydration is so severe that parenteral or nebulized humidification becomes necessary. Ultrasonic aerosols irritate the airways and produce bronchospasm and coughing. Therefore, these forms of respiratory therapy should be avoided. Finally, there is no scientific basis for the use of intermittent positive pressure breathing ventilators (IPPB) either as a form of respiratory therapy or as a means of delivering bronchodilators (47).

Oxygen

In rare cases when asthmatics with objective evidence of severe asthma (Tables 55.5 and 55.6) are treated in the physician's office, the administration of humidified oxygen may be indicated. If the patient does not improve, he should be sent to an emergency room. In the usual uncomplicated young asthmatic without chronic hypoventilation and CO_2 retention, there is little risk of causing respiratory failure by blunting the hypoxic ventilatory control. Only enough oxygen (28 to 35% venturi mask or 2 liters/minute nasal cannula) should be administered to improve arterial PO_2 into a normal range (65 to 80 mm Hg).

Medical Complications of Reversible Airways Disease

There are a number of medical complications of asthma that may impair the patient's response to the usual therapeutic regimens (Table 55.9). In general, these complications should be sought if there is not an appropriate therapeutic response.

Complications of Pharmacological Treatment

In severe asthma, bronchodilators may cause a paradoxical fall in arterial oxygenation by altering the pulmonary homeostatic mechanisms that match ventilation and perfusion in the lungs. These falls in arterial oxygenation are small (5 to 10 mm Hg) and are easily treated with supplemental oxygen. Although this paradoxical hypoxemia is an indication for oxygen administration, it is not an indication to withdraw bronchodilator therapy.

Very rarely, the propellants used to aerosolize sympathomimetics and corticosteroids may provoke paradoxical bronchospasm. If an asthmatic complains of coughing and wheezing after using one of these aerosols, a different preparation should be employed.

Sympathomimetics and theophylline preparations stimulate cardiac activity and may cause arrhythmias, especially when used in high therapeutic doses, in the presence of moderate hypoxemia or in elderly patients with pre-existing cardiac disease (49). However, arrhythmias can also be triggered by bronchospasm and hypoxemia during acute airways obstruction. In these situations, reversal of bronchospasm and improvement in gas exchange often improve the arrhythmias.

Table 55.9.
Medical Complications of Reversible Airways Disease

COMPLICATIONS OF BRONCHODILATORS
  Paradoxical fall in arterial oxygenation
  Paradoxical bronchospasm
  Cardiac arrhythmias
ATELECTASIS
PULMONARY INFECTIONS
  Bronchitis
  Pneumonia
AIR IN EXTRAPULMONARY SPACES
  Penumothorax (tension)
  Pneumomediastinum
ALLERGIC BRONCHOPULMONARY ASPERGILLOSIS

Mechanical Airways Obstruction

Mucus impaction in the airways may lead to microatelectasis or to the collapse of a pulmonary segment or of an entire lobe of the lung. Patients with major lobar collapse should be hospitalized. Frequently, the symptoms and physical signs of atelectasis are obscured during acute asthmatic attacks by wheezing and dyspnea. Therefore, atelectasis is best diagnosed with a chest roentgenogram (see Chapter 55). Usually, atelectasis will improve after treatment of bronchospasm, hydration, and physical therapy (coughing, chest percussion, and postural drainage). Bronchoscopy to remove an obstructing mucous plug is rarely needed. In fact, in a patient with reactive airways disease and acute bronchospasm, it may even worsen bronchospasm and provide only temporary improvement of atelectasis.

Infection

Whereas pulmonary infections often precipitate asthmatic attacks, bronchitis and pneumonia (see Chapter 28) may develop as a complication of asthma. Development of purulent sputum during the course of a prolonged or persistent asthmatic attack requires re-evaluation for superimposed infection, with a sputum smear followed by appropriate antibiotic therapy.

Extrapulmonary Air

Rarely, air can accumulate abnormally in the extrapulmonary spaces. The presence of a pneumomediastinum is best detected by a chest roentgenogram, but it is frequently associated with subcutaneous air in the neck, thorax, and groin (palpable crepitus). Although no specific therapy is indicated, the patient should be hospitalized for careful observation because air may dissect into the pleural space. A pneumothorax can only be detected effectively by a chest roentgenogram, and if a pneumothorax develops during an acute attack, regardless of its size, the patient should be hospitalized since the subsequent development of a tension pneumothorax can be life threatening.

Allergic Bronchopulmonary Aspergillosis

Rarely, allergic bronchopulmonary aspergillosis complicates chronic asthma (60). These patients have airways obstruction that does not improve with usual therapeutic measures; they have febrile episodes associated with a cough productive of purulent sputum containing dark brown plugs, and a chest roentgenogram that shows central bronchiectasis and mucous impaction. They often have pulmonary infiltrates that change location during serial roentgenographic studies. These patients usually have blood eosinophilia, markedly elevated total serum IgE levels, and serum precipitins as well as immediate and delayed skin reactions to Aspergillus antigen. Early treatment with corticosteroids may improve bronchospasm, and it prevents progression to irreversible bronchiectasis. If this diagnosis is suspected, consultation with a pulmonologist or an allergist is advisable.

Course and Prognosis of Asthma

The course and prognosis of pure bronchial asthma are not well understood. Traditionally, it is thought that uncomplicated asthma developing during childhood or early adult life is not a risk factor for progressive fixed obstructive pulmonary disease. However, there is also evidence that airways hyper-reactivity and allergy are found more frequently in patients with severe obstructive pulmonary disease, so that these factors may be risks for the development of chronic airways obstruction. These asthmatic characteristics (allergy and airway hyper-responsiveness) may combine with exposures to cigarette smoke and environmental pollutants to promote bronchial inflammation and facilitate the development of chronic airflow obstruction (10). Further epidemiological studies are necessary to define these relationships (5, 9, 38, 51).

In general, when bronchial asthma begins at an early age, it usually improves, although the estimation of the rate of remission from childhood asthma varies in different studies from 30 to 70% (34, 51). After a spontaneous remission, some childhood asthmatics will experience a recurrence of symptomatic asthma during adulthood. These latter patients, as well as patients with adult onset intrinsic asthma, often have asthma that is persistent and severe. Other patients who had a history of bronchial asthma during childhood, which seemed to resolve spontaneously, develop chronic progressive airways obstruction later in life. Additional risk factors, such as chronic cigarette smoking and exposure to urban and industrial air pollution, complicate their disease making the distinction between asthma and chronic airflow obstruction difficult (see page 610).

Although death from asthma, or one of its complications, is rare, it does occur with a recorded incidence in the United States of one in 100,000 or approximately 2,000 deaths during the course of a year. A recent trend toward an increase in deaths from asthma has caused concern (7). Some of these changes in mortality rate may be due to better recognition and reporting and to increases in mortality rate in the elderly due to the survival of more individuals to old age. Of greater concern is that this shift in mortality is due to adverse reactions to bronchodilators and the complications of severe airflow obstruction. These developments may be complicated by the inability of an individual to recognize severe asthma and access appropriate medical treatment. Inadequate or delayed treatment may occur not only in rural areas but also in urban environments where access of the poor to appropriate health care can be limited.

Deaths in young asthmatics are usually preventable since they are caused by one of the medical or therapeutic complications that have been discussed. For example, in England in the early 1970s, increased mortality from bronchial asthma coincided with the marketing of high dose isoproterenol inhalers. It was postulated that these patients developed cardiovascular toxicity and arrhythmias from isoproterenol overdosage by the repeated use of these inhalers. Often acute respiratory failure and death in status asthmaticus are attributable to sedation of seemingly anxious patients whose respiratory drive is easily depressed because of fatigue and exhaustion. All asthmatics should be taught to assess the severity of their asthma using peak flow measurements. Those asthmatics who manifest the objective signs of severe asthma (Tables 55.5 and 55.6) should receive rapid emergency treatment and should be hospitalized if they do not improve rapidly. Asthma can worsen as quickly as it can improve with appropriate therapy.

Management of the Pregnant Asthmatic

Most studies suggest that pregnancy has an unpredictable effect on asthma, with most patients experiencing no change in their disease and a small percentage either improving or experiencing deterioration. However, asthma may affect the outcome of pregnancy with a reported 2-fold increase in perinatal mortality and a small increase in the risk of infant prematurity. Although the incidence of these complications is slight, prolonged asthmatic attacks produce hypoxemia and acid-base disturbances that can cause serious fetal complications. Therefore, prompt treatment of severe asthmatic attacks is important, and this may require the use of drugs that, at least theoretically, may produce some adverse effects on maternal and fetal function.

In general, management of the pregnant asthmatic is the same as is the treatment of the nonpregnant asthmatic (69). Theophylline and sympathomimetic agents are generally safe for the fetus but may cause uterine smooth muscle dilatation and may, thereby, inhibit labor. Although the newer inhaled specific β_2-sympathomimetic drugs are not officially approved for use during pregnancy, there are no reports of adverse fetal effects caused by any of these agents. In contrast, drugs such as epinephrine, which have α-adrenergic properties, can reduce uterine and placental blood flow due to vasoconstriction and, at least theoretically, may impair fetal circulation. Although cromolyn also has not been approved for use during pregnancy, animal studies have not documented adverse effects in the fetus. Commonly used corticosteroid preparations, such as prednisone and prednisolone, cross the placenta poorly, and therefore fetal adrenal steroid production is not compromised when the mother receives these drugs. However, systemic corticosteroids do suppress maternal adrenal function, and supplemental steroids are frequently required to treat maternal stress during labor. Inhaled steroids have not been officially approved for treatment of pregnant asthmatics, but it would appear, because of their reduced systemic absorption, that their potential for affecting the fetus is negligible.

CHRONIC AIRWAYS OBSTRUCTION: CHRONIC OBSTRUCTIVE BRONCHITIS AND EMPHYSEMA

Patients with advanced chronic airways obstruction have a clinical course characterized by progressive loss of pulmonary function that eventually leads to respiratory failure and death. Usually management of these patients focuses upon the treatment of exacerbations of airways obstruction and pulmonary infection, basically providing palliative support for the complications of this disease. However, before the development of irreversible progressive air flow obstruction, there is a period when functional impairment and pathological abnormalities are potentially reversible. Therefore, this discussion will emphasize not only the therapy of symptomatic obstructive lung disease but also the identification of susceptible individuals at a time when the development of irreversible airways disease is preventable (38).

Chronic progressive airways obstruction is most commonly caused by chronic obstructive bronchitis and emphysema (64). Chronic bronchitis is defined in clinical terms but has certain pathological correlates. In contrast, emphysema, a specific morphological diagnosis, has associated clinical correlates, pulmonary function abnormalities, and characteristic roentgenographic patterns. In their pure forms, these two diseases represent distinct processes with different pathological features and clinical manifestations. However, clinically they usually coexist (66).

It is very difficult to estimate the prevalence of chronic bronchitis and emphysema in the United States since there is often an insidious onset of respiratory symptoms and many patients are not diagnosed until relatively late in the course of their disease. However, approximately 15 to 25% of the adult population who smoke cigarettes will develop symptomatic airways obstruction. There is a greater incidence of chronic bronchitis since not all bronchitics develop chronic airflow obstruction. At present, chronic obstructive lung disease is the fifth leading cause of death in the United States. This mortality rate is increasing despite an overall reduction in cigarette smoking. This may reflect increased survival of the population to older age and the fact that this disease primarily affects the elderly.

Definitions

Chronic Bronchitis

Chronic bronchitis is defined as a clinical syndrome characterized by cough and sputum production that occurs on most days for at least a 3-month period during 2 consecutive years. Most often these symptoms are due to chronic bronchial irritation that is precipitated by agents such as cigarette smoke and air pollution. This results in inflammatory changes in the airways, in hyperplasia of goblet cells and mucus-secreting glands, and in chronic mucus hypersecretion. By definition this excessive production of mucus is not due to specific diseases such as bronchiectasis, tuberculosis, or heart disease. Morphological changes that correlate with the clinical diagnosis of chronic bronchitis are initially found in small airways (< 2 mm) and later progress to involve other parts of the tracheal bronchial tree (Fig. 55.3). The hypertrophied mucous glands occupy a greater proportion of the bronchial wall, which is inflamed, edematous, and eventually fibrotic. The lumina of peripheral airways are frequently filled with mucopurulent secretions (64, 66).

Simple Chronic Bronchitis. A large proportion of patients who smoke develop chronic bronchitis. Most of these patients cough up a small quantity of mucoid sputum each morning. They either ignore this chronic cough or willingly accept it as a minor complication of cigarette smoking. Some of these patients will have intermittent episodes of purulent sputum production and occasional mild wheezing associated with upper respiratory tract infections. Many of these patients do not have a demonstrable impairment of expiratory airflow or an increased rate of decline in pulmonary function.

Chronic Obstructive Bronchitis. At the other end of the spectrum is a disease characterized by progressive airflow obstruction and chronic mucopurulent sputum production. The bronchi, normally sterile, are chronically infected. The factors that protect certain individuals and place others at risk for the development of airflow obstruction are not completely understood (see below). It is known that those who are susceptible to the effects of cigarette smoking and chronic bronchopulmonary infection have a progressive course, with accelerated loss of lung function that leads to pulmonary disability and eventual respiratory failure (Fig. 55.7).

Emphysema

Pulmonary emphysema is defined in anatomical terms and is a diagnosis that is made with certainty only by a pathologist (30, 66). It is morphologically defined as permanent abnormal dilation and destruction of the alveolar ducts and air spaces distal to the terminal bronchioles (see Fig. 55.3). Each component of this definition is important. The enlargement must be permanent; therefore, the temporary overdistension of the lung that occurs in asthma cannot be regarded as emphysema. The enlargement must be abnormal; thus the changes that occur with normal aging cannot be considered to be true emphysema. Perhaps the most important concept is that there should be accompanying disruption of alveolar walls. Because the pathological definition of emphysema is nonspecific, it is necessary to classify emphysema into anatomical subtypes. The most important, clinically, are centrilobular and panlobular emphysema (66).

Centrilobular Emphysema. This form is generally considered to represent the commonest type of emphysema. In centrilobular emphysema there is mainly destruction of the respiratory bronchioles and alveolar ducts, which become confluent to form emphysema-

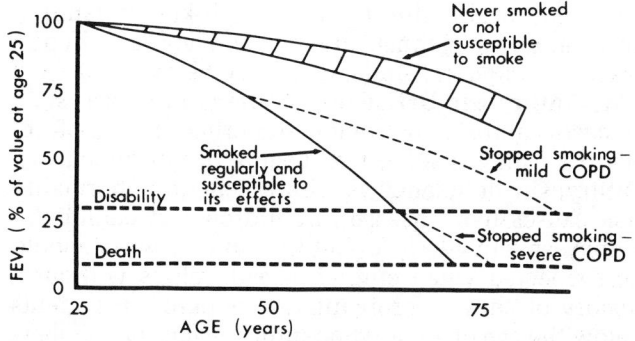

Figure 55.7. Effect of risk factors from smoking on the loss of lung function (FEV_1). The *upper curves* are derived from subjects who do not smoke or are not susceptible to the effects of smoking. They lose lung function gradually throughout adult life (15 to 30 ml/year). *Lower curves* show accelerated loss of lung function in subjects who are susceptible to the effects of cigarette smoke. At age 65 there is respiratory disability since FEV_1 has decreased to 25 to 30% of predicted (1 to 1.2 liters) and further functional deterioration will eventually cause death due to complications of respiratory insufficiency. If that subject stops smoking, life may be prolonged but a respiratory death will still eventually result. If intervention is initiated earlier in life (40 to 50 years) when there is mild COPD, accelerated loss of lung function is reversible and a respiratory death will be avoided. Although this figure illustrates theoretical loss of FEV_1 for an adult cigarette smoker, susceptible smokers will lose lung function at different rates, thereby becoming disabled at different ages. (Modified from Fletcher C, Peto R: The natural history of chronic airflow obstruction. *Br Med J* 1:1645, 1977.)

tous spaces. Deposits of carbonaceous material are found in these areas. The distal alveolar sacs are often spared. The emphysematous lesions are located in the proximal acinar space at the center of the lobules between the conducting airways and the alveolar sacs. The major clinical association of centrilobular emphysema is chronic obstructive bronchitis due to cigarette smoking in which pathological abnormalities in the peripheral airways are the rule. Early disease with patchy pulmonary involvement does not cause roentgenographic abnormalities. But when it is far advanced, pathological and roentgenographic examination shows that centrilobular emphysema is primarily located in the upper lung fields.

Panlobular Emphysema. This less common form of emphysema is characterized by uniform involvement of the pulmonary lobule with morphological destruction of the distal structures and alveolar capillary membrane. Panlobular emphysema is less commonly associated with chronic bronchitis and cigarette smoking, tends to occur in the lower lung fields, is more frequently associated with the formation of cysts and bullae, and is found in patients with hereditary α_1-antitrypsin deficiency (see below) and with bronchiolar obliteration. Frequently the two major forms of emphysema occur in combination, with centrilobular emphysema in the upper lung zones and panlobular in the lower. However, pathological distinction is difficult to make when severe disease exists.

Other forms of emphysema include paraseptal emphysema, which is associated with spontaneous pneumothorax, and irregular emphysema, which is found in patients with diffuse pulmonary fibrosis.

Etiology

There are many risk factors and proposed etiologies associated with the development of chronic obstructive airways disease. They are listed in order of relative importance in Table 55.10. Knowledge of these factors is important in understanding those measures that may alter the progression and thus prevent the development of irreversible chronic airways obstruction (27, 51).

Age

The average nonsmoking adult shows a yearly decline of 15 to 30 ml in FEV_1 with increasing age. Thus an FEV_1 of 4 liters in a 25-year-old would be expected to fall to almost 3 liters by age 65 (Fig. 55.7) (27). However, this normal loss of lung function is not associated with pulmonary disease. Additional risk factors add to the effects of this loss of pulmonary function and act synergistically to cause clinical airways obstruction (18, 38).

Inhaled Irritant and Noxious Agents

The common factor that exists in the great majority of patients with chronic airways obstruction is exposure to inhaled irritant and noxious agents.

Cigarette Smoking. Cigarette smoke represents the most obvious and widespread pulmonary contaminant. Since 1940 when cigarette consumption in the United States increased to present high levels (10 lb of cigarettes per capita), there has been a progressive rise in the incidence and death rate from obstructive pulmonary disease and lung cancer. Various studies have shown that there is pathological evidence of either chronic bronchitis or emphysema in all patients with more than a 40-pack year history of smoking (defined as number of years smoking times the number of packs of cigarettes/day). Approximately 15 to 25% of cigarette smokers will develop symptomatic chronic airflow obstruction.

The deleterious effects of cigarette smoke may be specific or may be due to nonspecific effects of inhaled irritants on the tracheal bronchial tree. For example, stimulation of mucous secretion may result in the loss of normal mucociliary clearance mechanisms. If infection develops, inflammatory cells release proteolytic enzymes that may cause destruction of the

Table 55.10.
Risk Factors and Airways Obstruction (Approximate Order of Relative Importance)

AGE
INHALED IRRITANT AND NOXIOUS AGENTS
Smoking
Urban and industrial air pollution
HEREDITY
Familial incidence
α_1-Antitrypsin deficiency
SEX (MALE > FEMALE)
SOCIOECONOMIC STATUS
AIRWAYS HYPERREACTIVITY

pulmonary parenchyma by overwhelming the protective defenses of the lungs. Moreover, smoking also depresses the phagocytic function of the alveolar macrophage, increasing the tendency for respiratory infections (4).

Specifically, cigarette smoking and individual host susceptibility seem to have a significant effect on pulmonary function, resulting in a more rapid loss in function over time. For example, FEV_1 may decrease by an average of 40 to 60 ml/year. A patient whose FEV_1 was 4 liters at age 25 would have an FEV_1 of 2 liters by the age of 65 (Fig. 55.7) (27). Unfortunately, some smokers lose lung function even more rapidly and approach a loss in FEV_1 of 60 to 80 ml/year. Nevertheless, it is possible that individuals who stop smoking may resume the normal 30 ml/year rate of decline within 1 year after the cessation of cigarette smoking. The mechanisms by which some patients are more sensitive to the effects of cigarette smoke are unknown and is the subject of active investigation. In susceptible patients who continue to smoke, the rapid decline in lung function causes clinical obstructive pulmonary disease (Fig. 55.7) (18, 38).

Urban and Industrial Air Pollution. The effects of air pollution from exposure to urban or industrial environments on the development of chronic obstructive airways disease are unknown. Photochemical oxidant air pollutants include ozone and nitrogen dioxides, which are formed by the effect of solar radiation on automobile and truck emissions. Low concentrations of sulfur dioxide and other particulate matter from the burning of fossil fuels are also present in an urban environment where there are also trace amounts of miscellaneous substances (arsenic, asbestos, cadmium, hydrogen sulfide, lead, and mercury). Periods of atmospheric inversions with increased environmental levels of air pollutants have been associated with exacerbations and even death in patients with cardiopulmonary disease. The sequelae of high exposures to these agents are airways inflammation, pulmonary parenchymal damage, and obstructive pulmonary disease. Furthermore, studies of low level exposures to these agents demonstrate that they cause transient airways hyper-reactivity in normal subjects and an exacerbation of respiratory symptoms in asthmatics (11). Therefore, it is probable that air pollution and cigarette smoking act synergistically to trigger symptomatic exacerbations and pulmonary function abnormalities in patients with chronic obstructive pulmonary disease. However, it is not known to what extent exposure to low levels of urban and industrial air pollutants contributes to the etiology and progression of pulmonary disease.

Heredity

Familial incidence. First degree relatives of patients with chronic obstructive airways disease have abnormal lung function and an increased rate of decline of their FEV_1. This relationship holds even when other risk factors, such as smoking, are controlled. The relationship of this finding to the well-known familial aggregation of asthma, allergy, and airways hyper-reactivity is poorly understood (see below) (18).

α_1 **Antitrypsin Deficiency.** Whereas diseases such as cystic fibrosis are obvious inherited causes of obstructive lung disease that begins in childhood, α_1-antitrypsin deficiency is a rare genetic abnormality that causes liver disease in children and panlobular emphysema in adults. α_1-antitrypsin deficiency should be suspected when emphysema develops without a history of chronic bronchitis or smoking in patients below the age of 45 or when multiple family members develop obstructive lung disease at an early age. Serum antiproteolytic activity is determined by a pair of genes at the Pi locus. Normal individuals have two M genes (MM), whereas patients with α_1-antitrypsin deficiency have two Z genes (ZZ). Homozygous α_1-antitrypsin deficiency is found in only one in 4000 people, but at least 60% of ZZ homozygotes will develop severe emphysema during adulthood. These individuals also have a high incidence of cirrhosis, and the combination of lung and liver disease with an onset in early to middle adult life may indicate the presence of this syndrome. It is postulated that a deficiency of α_1-antitrypsin activity makes the lung vulnerable to damage by the endogenous proteolytic enzymes released by inflammatory cells. Inheritance is codominant so that the heterozygote, MZ, as well as several other mixed genotypes have intermediate levels of circulating antitrypsin. Partial deficiency (heterozygote) is not a risk for the development of obstructive lung disease even when other factors such as smoking are present. The diagnosis of this condition is discussed below (page 628).

Sex

Male sex seems to be an important predisposing factor for the development of obstructive airways disease. Even in nonsmoking young men, there is still accelerated loss of lung function compared with nonsmoking premenopausal women. After menopause, women appear to have a more rapid decline in FEV_1 than similarly age-matched male controls (18, 38). In addition, the acute and chronic physiological effects of cigarette smoking are different in men. In young men, cigarette smoking causes changes in peripheral airways function, whereas similar changes are not produced by cigarettes in premenopausal women. This is especially interesting since the earliest pathological abnormalities of chronic bronchitis are in the peripheral airways. The reasons for these sex differences are unknown, but they may relate either to the protective effects of female sex hormones or to the deleterious effects of androgens.

Socioeconomic Status

People from lower socioeconomic groups seem to decrease FEV_1 at a faster rate than those from higher economic groups. Although the risk factor is still found after controlling for the effects of smoking, sex, and age, it may well relate to increased exposure of the respiratory tract to airborne pollutants in urban environments or to industrial exposures to noxious agents (18).

Airways Hyper-reactivity

Studies of first degree relatives of patients with obstructive lung disease show that those with hyperirritable airways lose lung function at accelerated rates (12, 51) as do patients with significant chronic airways obstruction who are hyper-reactive to inhaled agents (methacholine) (5, 51). It is not known whether this airways hyperirritability develops as a consequence of obstructive lung disease or is a risk factor per se. Allergy may also influence this relationship since allergic factors are associated with hyper-reactivity and have been found with increased frequency in patients with far advanced obstructive lung diseases (38).

Clinical Presentation

History

Usually, patients with emphysema present with dyspnea and those with chronic obstructive bronchitis, with cough and sputum production. These two diseases are so interrelated that most patients have manifestations of both. It is useful, however, to recognize the characteristic features of these syndromes (Table 55.11). Although these two types represent extremes of a clinical spectrum, occasional patients are seen who qualify as having relatively pure emphysema (type A) or bronchitis (type B).

The usual patient with chronic airways obstruction has a long history of a chronic cough with mucopurulent sputum production. The onset of dyspnea is insidious but progressive. Frequently, these patients attribute their poor exercise tolerance to the effects of age or sedentary life style and their chronic cough to the effects of smoking. Often they develop clinically apparent airflow obstruction (wheezing) during upper respiratory tract infections, and the recovery period from these respiratory infections is prolonged. Eventually, dyspnea becomes so severe that it interferes with routine activities and medical attention is sought. In other patients, a respiratory tract infection triggers airway obstruction and acute respiratory failure. Milder forms of obstructive airway diseases are often diagnosed as incidental findings during a routine physical examination, a preoperative evaluation, or a medical evaluation for an unrelated disease. Occasionally, patients with chronic airways obstruction (emphysematous type) will be seen because of progressive weight loss that may initially suggest the presence of an occult malignancy.

When the diagnosis of advanced obstructive airways is well established, its course is relentlessly progressive. In patients with bronchitis, daily cough and sputum production usually increase, becoming more purulent and tenacious during infectious exacerbations. Some patients have difficulty clearing respiratory secretions during attacks of airflow obstruction. In these patients, the production of scant, viscous, purulent sputum may precede the development of respiratory failure. Wheezing and dyspnea are often persistent features of severe disease. Chronic hypoxemia causes cor pulmonale, and the patient will note peripheral edema and weight gain. Some patients will experience asthmatic episodes that periodically worsen their baseline airways obstruction. Usually, these are associated with respiratory infections, but they may be triggered by any of the stimuli that precipitate an acute asthmatic attack.

Physical Examination

In individual patients, physical findings depend on the severity and type of chronic obstructive airways disease (Table 55.11). Vital signs may be normal or show tachypnea and a pulsus paradoxus (see page 612) during severe bronchospasm. In milder forms of obstructive lung disease ($FEV_1 > 1.2$ liters), auscultation of the chest may be unremarkable or may reveal either rhonchi due to mucus within the airways or wheezing if bronchospasm is prominent. Breath sounds may be distant in patients with severe emphysema. Frequently, the diagnosis of airways obstruction is best made during the physical examination by performing a timed FVC. After inspiring to total lung capacity, the patient should perform a complete maximal expiration through an open mouth. This maneuver usually produces audible wheezing in patients with chronic obstructive bronchitis, whereas in patients with severe emphysema whose airways collapse, faint wheezing may be all that is heard. In everyone with significant expiratory airflow obstruction, the timed FVC will be prolonged beyond 4 to 5 seconds. Many other respiratory findings occur with progressively severe disease and primarily reflect pulmonary hyperinflation. These include an increased anteroposterior diameter of the chest, widened intercostal spaces, hyper-resonance, a decreased area of cardiac dullness, and low diaphragms. The same signs of severity found in patients with asthma, such as use of accessory muscles of respiration, occur in individuals with chronic airways obstruction during acute attacks of bronchospasm (Tables 55.5 and 55.6).

When cor pulmonale develops there is often cyanosis, a right ventricular heave, a holosystolic murmur along the left sternal border, an S_3 gallop, and varying degrees of hepatomegaly and peripheral edema. Neck veins will be distended and a large V wave with a Y descent is visible as pulmonary hypertension worsens, causing tricuspid valve dilation and insufficiency.

Laboratory Testing

Pulmonary Function Testing. The most characteristic functional defect in patients with chronic obstructive bronchitis and emphysema is decreased forced expiratory flow. This obstructive defect is best measured with a spirogram, which should be employed in

Table 55.11.
Findings in Emphysematous and Bronchitic Varieties of Chronic Airways Obstruction

Findings	Type A (Emphysema)	Type B (Bronchitis)
CLINICAL PRESENTATION:		
Dyspnea	Early onset, severe progressive	Insidious onset, intermittent during infection
Cough	Onset after dyspnea	Precedes onset of dyspnea
Sputum	Scant and mucoid	Copious and purulent
Respiratory infection	Rare	Frequent
Body weight	Thin, weight loss	Normal or overweight
Respiratory insufficiency	Late manifestation	Frequent episodes
PHYSICAL EXAMINATION:		
Cyanosis	Absent	Often present
Plethora	Present	Absent
Chest percussion	Hyperresonant	Normal
Chest auscultation	Distant breath sounds, end expiratory wheezing	Rales, rhonchi, wheezes
Cor pulmonale	Often terminal	Common
LABORATORY EVALUATION:		
Hematocrit value	Normal	Occasional erythrocytosis
Chest roentgenogram	Hyperinflation with increased anteroposterior diameter and flat diaphragms. Attenuated vascular markings, bullous changes, small vertical heart	Increased bronchovascular markings with normal to enlarged heart and evidence of old inflammatory disease
PHYSIOLOGICAL EVALUATION:		
Spirometry	Irreversible expiratory obstruction, airway closure	Expiratory obstruction, reversible component
Total lung capacity and residual volume	Marked increase	Mild increase
Lung elastic recoil	Marked reduction	Near normal
Diffusion capacity	Marked decrease	Normal or slight reduction
PaO_2		
Rest	Slightly decreased (65–75 mm Hg)	Marked decrease (45–65 mm Hg)
Exercise	Often falls	Variable (decrease to increase)
$PaCO_2$	Normal or low (35–40 mm Hg)	Normal or elevated (40–60 mm Hg)
Pulmonary hypertension	None to mild, worsens during exercise	Moderate to severe variable exercise response
PATHOLOGY	Widespread emphysema, may be panlobular	Chronic bronchitis with or without mild centrilobular emphysema

the diagnosis and assessment of severity in chronic obstructive airways disease as well as for the evaluation of specific therapeutic regimens (see page 606 for the patient experience during this procedure). It is also useful in predicting the prognosis, course, operative risk (see Chapter 86), and work potential Tables (55.1 and 9.2, Chapter 9) (15, 22, 44). In general, it is unusual for patients with a FEV_1 of approximately 2 liters, or 60% of predicted, to experience significant dyspnea during normal physical activities. On the other hand, reduction of the FEV_1 below 1.2 liters or 40% of predicted is associated with dyspnea on mild exertion and significant disability. The severity of hyperinflation will be reflected by a reduction in vital capacity as well as by increases in lung volumes (71). Residual volume is usually elevated and, in emphysematous patients, total lung capacity is increased. When emphysema is present, the diffusion capacity of the lung is reduced, reflecting the loss of functional alveolar capillary membrane available for gas exchange. The presence of significant airways obstruction, hyperinflation, and a reduced diffusion capacity for carbon monoxide correlates with the pathological finding of emphysema (Fig. 55.8) (30, 66).

Arterial Blood Gas Analysis. In evaluating and treating patients with significant chronic obstructive airways disease (FEV_1 < 1.2 liters), baseline arterial blood gas analysis is necessary to measure the level of oxygenation and adequacy of alveolar ventilation. When the FEV_1 is greater than 1.2 liters, resting arterial blood gases are usually normal or show only mild hypoxemia. With more severe airways obstruction (FEV_1 < 1.0 liter), the degree of hypoxemia and hypercapnea will depend on the ventilation-perfusion abnormalities and pulmonary homeostatic mechanisms. Because hypoxemia correlates only roughly with the severity of airways obstruction as reflected by spirometry, arterial blood gases must be measured to evaluate the degree of resting hypoxemia in order to guide the treatment of cor pulmonale (see below). In addition to hypoxemia, it is important to know whether the patient has a chronically elevated arterial $PaCO_2$ indicating alveolar hypoventilation. The diagnosis of acute respiratory failure in patients with severe obstructive lung disease is usually made by finding either an acute fall in arterial oxygenation (absolute PaO_2 < 55 mm Hg) and/or an acute increase in $PaCO_2$ tension of more than 10 mm Hg with associated acute respiratory acidosis.

A

	Actual	Predicted	% Predicted	Post BD[a]	Post/Pre BD[a]
SPIROMETRY					
FVC	2.32 liters (L)	3.99 L	58	2.50	107
FEV$_1$	0.98 L	3.17 L	30	1.15	117
FEV$_1$/FVC %	42	79.4		46	
LUNG VOLUMES					
(He dilution)					
TLC	7.82 L	6.29 L	124		
VC	2.86 L	3.99 L	71.7		
FRC	5.64 L	3.72 L	152		
RV	4.96 L	2.30 L	215		
DIFFUSING CAPACITY					
(single breath)					
DLCO[c] ml	11.6	24.4	47.5		
ARTERIAL BLOOD GASSES[b]					
PaO$_2$	56 mm Hg				
PaCO$_2$	48 mm Hg				
PH units	7.38				

[a] Bronchodilator.
[b] At rest, sitting, breathing room air.
[c] Diffusion capacity for carbon monoxide.

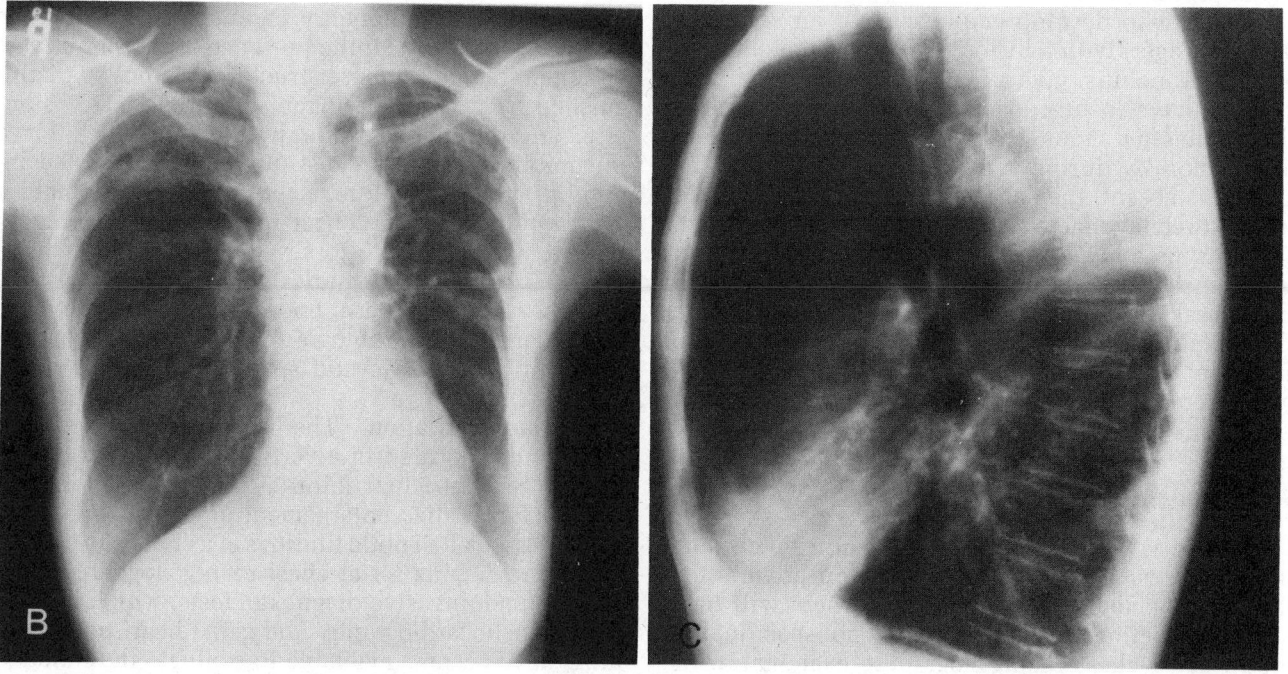

Figure 55.8. *A.* Typical pulmonary function test results in a patient (male, 60 years old, 161 lb, 69 inches tall) with severe chronic obstructive pulmonary disease and probable emphysema. Forced expiration demonstrates a severe obstructive ventilatory defect with an immediate response to aerosolized bronchodilators. Spirograms do not reach a plateau, indicating slowly emptying areas of lungs. Lung volumes show an elevated total lung capacity (*TLC*) and residual volume (*RV*) indicating hyperinflation consistent with obstruction, suggesting early airway closure. Single breath CO diffusion capacity is reduced, indicating loss of effective alveolar capillary surface area for gas exchange. Reduced diffusion capacity and airway obstruction are consistent with the presence of emphysema. Arterial blood gases show an elevated carbon dioxide tension indicating hypoventilation, a mild compensated respiratory acidosis, and low oxygen tension with desaturation. This patient with chronic airflow obstruction is hyperinflated, has a reduced diffusion capacity suggesting emphysema, and has hypoxemia associated with chronic CO$_2$ retention. His chest roentgenogram (*B* and *C*) is compatible with emphysema and shows hyperinflation and bullous changes with loss of vascular lung markings (see the text). *VC*, vital capacity; *FRC*, functional residual capacity.

Such acute changes usually require hospitalization and intensive treatment (21).

Other Laboratory Tests. Normally, the mucopurulent sputum produced by patients with chronic obstructive bronchitis is infected with a mixed bacterial flora including *Streptococcus pneumoniae* and *Haemophilus influenzae*. Other pathogens may be present, depending on the frequency and type of broad spectrum antibiotic treatment. Sputum culture is usually indicated only when there is parenchymal pulmonary infection (pneumonia), and specific treatment will depend on the predominant organism seen on Gram stain and cultured from the sputum. A complete blood count may reveal erythrocytosis, which indicates chronic hypoxemia, and eosinophilia, which suggests allergic or asthmatic etiologies. A white blood count and differential count are helpful in the evaluation of pulmonary infection in a patient with increased sputum production and chronic airflow obstruction. An electrocardiogram may show arrhythmias, atrial hypertrophy (P pulmonale), and evidence of pulmonary hypertension (persistent S waves in the lateral precordial leads).

Patients who develop emphysema at an early age (45 or younger) with a history of cigarette smoking or chronic bronchitis, give a familial history of emphysema, or have roentgenographic evidence of panlobular emphysema should be screened with serum protein electrophoresis during symptom-free periods. If the α_1-peak is absent, then an α_1-antitrypsin level should be measured (available from a commercial laboratory). α_1-Antitrypsin is an acute phase reactant and should not be measured during periods of infection. If both the α_1-peak and antitrypsin level are low, then genetic phenotyping should be obtained if possible. This is important for prognosis and genetic counseling. However, phenotyping is only done in a few medical centers in this country.

Roentgenographic Findings

As many as 50% of patients with significant chronic airways obstruction will have normal or nearly normal chest roentgenograms. In the others, there will be a variety of findings that are relatively nonspecific. Despite this, a chest roentgenographic examination is important both in the diagnosis and in the overall management of patients with airways obstruction. Specifically it is useful as a baseline study for the future evaluation of radiological abnormalities as well as to exclude other associated pulmonary diseases, such as pneumonia, atelectasis, or a pneumothorax.

Bronchitis. In patients with chronic obstructive bronchitis, there may be increased tubular markings, especially at the lung bases, that suggest thickening and disease of the bronchi. These patients may have increased vascular markings, evidence of pulmonary hypertension, and right heart enlargement, but their roentgenograms usually do not show marked hyperinflation or cystic or bullous changes.

Emphysema. The diagnosis of emphysema can of-

ten be made from a chest roentgenogram when severe morphological changes in the lung result in obvious roentgenographic findings (Fig. 55.8). In milder cases of emphysema, it is difficult to make a specific diagnosis. Many of the findings that are associated with emphysema only reflect hyperinflation, which also occurs in asthma or during a bronchospastic exacerbation in patients with chronic obstructive bronchitis. The changes characteristic of hyperinflation include an increased radiolucency of the lungs, an increase in the anteroposterior diameter of the thorax, an enlarged retrosternal air space, and a low and flat diaphragm that makes a greater than 90° angle with the sternum on the lateral views (Fig. 55.8). Changes in vascular markings in the lung fields are often subtle and difficult to detect, especially when there is congestion of the pulmonary veins or parenchymal infection. Regional or generalized loss of vascularity in the peripheral lung fields with rapid tapering of the proximal branches of the pulmonary artery occurs more frequently in panlobular emphysema, especially in the lower lung fields. Centrilobular disease tends to show increased bronchovascular markings, especially in the lung bases. The pulmonary parenchyma needs to be examined carefully for the presence of cysts or bullae, although frequently these structures cannot be distinguished from the hyperlucent lung fields. Occasionally, an upper lobe bulla will be mistaken for a pneumothorax, and a chest tube will be inserted inappropriately. Therefore, it is necessary to obtain a good quality baseline chest roentgenogram of every patient with moderate to severe obstructive airways disease. Although not indicated in the routine diagnosis of bullous disease, both chest tomography and computerized axial tomographic (CT) scanning of the lung will visualize cystic spaces in the pulmonary parenchyma.

Cardiac Evaluation. The heart frequently appears small and is located in a vertical position. In the diagnosis of ventricular failure, the usual radiological criteria for cardiac enlargement are not valid. Often one must look for subtle findings of a change in cardiac size by reviewing serial chest roentgenograms. More recently, noninvasive diagnostic tests, which include biplane echocardiography and gated heart pool scanning, have become available to evaluate the function of both the left and the right ventricles (see Chapter 60).

MANAGEMENT OF THE AMBULATORY PATIENT

General Measures

The primary goal in managing the ambulatory patient with obstructive airways disease is to prevent progression of the disease. When there is severe fixed airflow obstruction, therapeutic goals include improving symptoms and decreasing pulmonary disability by treating any reversible components of bronchospasm, heart failure, and infection. It is clear that prevention and prompt treatment of exacerbations in chronic airways obstruction will improve the quality and duration of life.

The successful management of this chronic disease requires a comprehensive approach either by the physician or by a medical team that includes a respiratory therapist, vocational counselor, and nurse clinician as well as active participation by the physician. Studies have shown that patients consider their physician to be very influential. Whatever preventive and therapeutic measures are selected, they will be more effective if the physician actively coordinates and supports them. For example, it seems that physicians advise their patients to stop smoking only when there are findings consistent with overt lung disease such as objective evidence of abnormal chest roentgenograms, pulmonary function tests, or evidence of respiratory infection. Furthermore, in smoking cessation programs only 25% of participants said their physician actively participated, and on further questioning most indicated that their physician would have been influential in affecting the outcome of the program (see Chapter 20).

If possible, the nurse, respiratory therapist, and physician should work together as a team, instructing the patient and his spouse. Ideally, general instruction should include information about pulmonary anatomy and physiology as well as basic information about the etiology and prognosis of chronic airways obstruction. This instruction can be given in individual as well as in group sessions and should be supplemented with visual aids and booklets that are published by the American Thoracic Society and available for distribution through the local (state) and national lung associations.

Even if therapeutic interventions do not markedly improve respiratory function, appropriate adaptation of a patient's life style and recreational activities is worthwhile. For example, although exercise programs do not improve pulmonary function, they physically condition sedentary patients, making them able to participate in a wider range of activities (see below). In patients with severe disease resulting in curtailment of their usual recreational activities, counseling on alternative hobbies and activities may help to prevent depression and maintain useful family interactions. Although sexual dysfunction is extremely common in these patients, this important aspect is rarely discussed with the physician. Sexual activity is often made easier by the use of supplemental oxygen or pretreatment with a bronchodilator. Alternatives include making the nondyspneic person the more active partner or the use of different positions (see Petty in "General References"). If the patient's disease precludes ambulation, then follow-up patient care is often best performed by home visits. The respiratory nurse clinician with the aid of the patient's spouse can facilitate this type of care. When the disease becomes terminal, the nurse and the physician can counsel the patient and his family about the possibility of dying at home (see Chapter 19). The physician should allay the patient's fears of suffocation and struggling since

death is often peaceful, with the patient eventually dying in a coma secondary to CO_2 retention. Furthermore, one needs to discuss with the patient and his family whether resuscitative attempts such as intubation and prolonged mechanical ventilation in an intensive care unit are appropriate and desirable. During this period, support from the physician, family, and clergy is vital. The patient may often be made comfortable with therapeutic modalities that include fluids, oxygen (see below), and sedation, if necessary.

Preventive Management

The *early diagnosis* of very mild peripheral airways disease is made with sophisticated pulmonary function testing that is not generally available. Furthermore, it is questionable whether physicians can motivate patients with subclinical asymptomatic disease to modify their life style. However, there is a period when mild to moderate airways obstruction is easily diagnosed using a spirogram (Fig. 55.1) and modification of the patient's habits, and treatment with bronchodilators, if indicated, may prevent the development of irreversible obstructive lung disease (Fig. 55.7). The routine screening with spirometry of patients at risk (greater than 35 years of age who have a significant smoking history or chronic bronchitis) will identify many patients with significant obstructive lung disease. For example, the National Institutes of Health are sponsoring a large clinical trial in which the long-term effects of smoking cessation and bronchodilator therapy will be evaluated in 6000 subjects with early obstructive lung disease. Initial results show that screening cigarette smokers using spirometry will identify individuals with asymptomatic airflow obstruction. Prevention of the development of irreversible airways obstruction may well depend on behavior modification in such patients. Smoking cessation and the avoidance of industrial irritants will be better accepted by the patient when he knows the results of objective testing and the prognostic significance of these abnormalities. It is probable that the course of obstructive lung disease can be favorably altered by a systematic program (smoking cessation and bronchodilator therapy) (38).

Important to any preventive regimen is complete *cessation of cigarette smoking*. This is especially true in any patient with homozygous PiZZ (α_1-antitrypsin deficiency). There are many smoking cessation programs and regimens that have been used with varying success rates. In evaluating the results of these programs, objective methods to assess their efficacy must be used (blood carboxyhemoglobin levels, sputum thiocyanate levels). Furthermore, the follow-up period must be long enough to judge that their effectiveness was not transient. At present, objective evaluation of these programs shows that only approximately 15 to 20% of subjects are able to abstain from smoking for 1 year. Strategies and methods for the physician to utilize in counseling patients about smoking cessation are described in Chapter 20.

Although pulmonary infections cannot be specifically linked to the progression of obstructive airways disease, the effective treatment of bacterial exacerbations is important since acute respiratory failure can be precipitated if exacerbations are not promptly treated. Furthermore, vaccination with anti-influenza and antipneumococcal vaccines may be useful in preventing pneumonia, which can be devastating in patients with severe obstructive lung disease (see Chapter 32).

Reduction of Secretions

Removal of Secretions

In patients with chronic airways obstruction and mucous hypersecretion, therapeutic interventions are aimed at the reduction and removal of respiratory secretions. Pulmonary secretions are normally cleared from the lung by mucociliary clearance and coughing. In obstructive airways disease, both of these mechanisms are impaired (see Chapter 54, under "Cough"). Often coughing is not effective because of airway collapse during forced expiration. *Postural drainage* and *chest percussion* can remove mucous secretions from the airways, and these measures should be used by the ambulatory patient whenever there is persistent hypersecretion. Patient instruction in postural drainage and chest percussion can be obtained by referral to a respiratory therapy department, or the physician can learn these principles by referring to the literature such as is given under "General References" (Respiratory Therapy). In addition, the mobilization of secretions is aided by pretreatment with two breaths of an aerosolized bronchodilator (β_2-sympathomimetic, see page 615). Often the best times for this type of respiratory therapy are before retiring at night and after arising in the morning. Thus the patient may be able to sleep more restfully and also may be aided in clearing secretions that have accumulated during the night. If significant pulmonary hypersecretion is not present, these measures are not indicated (28).

Avoidance of Irritants

Respiratory secretions will be stimulated both directly and reflexly by inhaled irritants. Furthermore, these substances cause bronchospasm, which prevents mobilization of secretions. Therefore, smoking, urban and industrial pollutants, and other irritating inhaled substances must be avoided. This includes avoiding "passive smoking" by inhaling ambient air that is contaminated with tobacco smoke since this has been shown to increase airways obstruction in asthmatics.

Alteration of Sputum Character

It has never been effectively proven that oral hydration will thin respiratory secretions and improve pulmonary function in obstructive lung disease (see "General References"—Conference on Scientific Basis of Respiratory Therapy). Nevertheless, most physicians still recommend that patients without significant heart failure should drink approximately 1 liter of fluid daily.

Mucolytic agents are irritating substances that may cause direct and reflex bronchospasm. Furthermore, liquefaction of bronchial secretions in patients who are unable to mobilize them adequately with effective coughing may be deleterious.

Even if bronchial secretions are thick and viscous, treatment with a bland aerosol (normal saline) has not been shown to be effective. For example, patients with cystic fibrosis with thick bronchial secretions do not show improvement in clinical status after bland aerosol treatment (58).

Treatment of Infection

Most patients with chronic bronchitis have a course that is characterized by intermittent infection with mucopurulent sputum. Treatment of these acute infectious exacerbations with a broad spectrum antibiotic that is active against S. pneumoniae, H. influenzae, and other common pathogens is indicated. Usually, a 7- to 10-day course of either ampicillin, tetracycline, or trimethoprim-sulfa-methoxazole is administered. In intelligent, cooperative patients, antibiotic therapy may be initiated by the patient when he notes a change in sputum character or color. In general, continuous antibiotic therapy should be avoided unless there is evidence of persistent chronic infection or bronchiectasis.

Physical Therapy and Rehabilitation

Intermittent Positive Pressure Breathing (IPPB)

Historically, IPPB machines have been used for both physical therapy and the delivery of bronchodilators. However, there is no scientific basis for the use of IPPB machines. In fact, IPPB may induce transient pulmonary overdistension that is harmful in these patients who are already hyperinflated (28, 47). IPPB may be useful in the delivery of medications to patients who are so severely obstructed that they are unable to take a deep breath from a freon-powered metered dose inhaler or hand bulb nebulizer (DeVilbiss). This circumstance is rare in ambulatory practice. Many patients who already have IPPB machines at home are so psychologically dependent on this form of physical therapy that the physician may decide that the use of such a machine should be continued. The administration of oxygen through any IPPB machine is contraindicated, because the oxygen mixture setting that supposedly delivers 40% oxygen usually administers much higher concentrations.

Breathing Exercises

There is evidence that pursed lip breathing may help an emphysematous patient maintain airways stability during expiration (see Petty, "General References"). Diaphragmatic exercises may give the patient a sense of well-being and may improve diaphragmatic muscle function. These breathing exercises are usually taught by a respiratory therapist. Specific details about them are available in the medical literature (28).

Exercise Rehabilitation

Exercise retraining programs do not improve pulmonary function, but they do seem to improve exercise tolerance and skeletal muscle function. Probably this is due to the nonspecific effects of training in sedentary poorly conditioned patients. Furthermore, after exercise training the patient may be able to perform a given level of exercise at a lower oxygen consumption and a lower minute ventilation. Community-based exercise training programs are more frequently available for cardiac rehabilitation (see Chapter 58). Occasionally, these may be adapted to the needs of patients with chronic obstructive pulmonary disease. If no organized programs are available, the physician should consider instructing patients in an informal program of graded increases in physical activity (see Ref. 28 and "General References").

Change in Environment

In selected circumstances environmental change may be important. Some patients seem to improve when they move from cold winter climates to either warm humid or warm dry climates. There is no evidence that the course of obstructive lung disease is altered by such environmental changes. Perhaps some of these patients improve by escaping from urban industrialized areas with air pollution. When such a move is contemplated, its social and economic effects must be carefully weighed by the patient and his family. Environmental changes are more important in patients with hypoxemia who live at altitudes above 4000 feet where atmospheric oxygen tensions are less than 120 mm Hg compared to 150 mm Hg at sea level. A move to a low altitude may improve hypoxemia and decrease pulmonary hypertension. Because the adverse psychological consequences of such a move may outweigh its medical benefits, those patients may do as well remaining at high altitude by using treatment with low flow oxygen (see below). Travel in an airplane or vacationing in high altitude areas may be contraindicated in patients with severe hypoxemia. Because airplane cabins are maintained at a pressure equivalent of 5000 to 8000 feet, low flow supplemental oxygen should be administered throughout flight to patients with arterial PaO_2 under 55 mm Hg. Also, vacations in high altitude locations (above 4000 feet) should be avoided in patients with severe chronic hypoxemia (PaO_2 less than 55 mm Hg).

Treatment of Bronchospasm

Initial and maintenance therapy of bronchospasm is outlined in detail in the discussion of asthma in this chapter. In patients with chronic reversible airways disease, the principles of pharmacological treatment are similar to those used in asthma; however, the response of patients to bronchodilators is usually not as marked. Some patients (Fig. 55.8) increase their FEV_1 only by 10 to 15%, but this improvement of only a few hundred milliliters may increase exercise tolerance. A poor response to inhaled bronchodilators during laboratory testing does not preclude improvement after chronic therapy with pharmacological agents. Such patients should have an assessment of their lung function repeated after a period of 1 to 2 months. Initial bronchodilator therapy should begin with either an inhaled sympathomimetic agent or inhaled ipratropium. Recent studies suggest that anticholinergic agents are more effective bronchodilators in patients with chronic airflow obstruction and that prolonged therapy is not associated with tachyphylaxis, a problem that may occur after long-term use of sympathomimetics (31, 65). Theophylline may not be as potent a bronchodilator, but it does seem to produce additional dilation when added to either of these inhaled bronchodilators. Theophylline may also improve diaphragmatic function in some patients with chronic airflow obstruction. If there is no response to high doses of bronchodilators, patients with severe bronchospasm ($FEV_1 < 1.2$ liters) should be given a therapeutic trial with corticosteroids (see below). When there is no objective or symptomatic improvement, bronchodilators may be discontinued, although some physicians recommend continued maintenance therapy to prevent bronchospastic exacerbations. There is increasing evidence that patients who do not respond to inhaled β-sympathomimetic agonists may improve airways function with inhaled anticholinergic agents (see page 617). Also, combinations of these two agents have been used successfully to treat patients with chronic bronchitis and obstructive lung disease (41, 46, 65). Very rarely, patients with a history of allergy or childhood asthma may improve with cromolyn (8).

If exercise tolerance is severely impaired by dyspnea, or if there is a poor or absent response to standard bronchodilators, a trial with corticosteroids is indicated (see page 617). A favorable response to steroids occurs more frequently in patients with reversible airways disease when there is blood or sputum eosinophilia or when there is a previous history of allergy or asthma. Usually, a trial of systemic corticosteroids such as prednisone (40 mg/day) is maintained for 3 to 6 weeks. Before, during, and after therapy, objective evaluation of lung function with spirometry is mandatory. Systemic steroids are used in these trials because they are more effective than aerosolized preparations. If there is improvement, the steroid dose should be reduced while the patient is monitored with serial spirometry. Alternatively treatment with aerosolized corticosteroid agents can be used to supplement standard bronchodilators. Although aerosolized corticosteroids are less effective in chronic obstructive lung disease than in asthma, there are individuals who will demonstrate objective improvement in pulmonary function. Aerosolized steroids can be used with systemic steroid therapy or may even be substituted if the effective dose of oral prednisone is less than 20 mg/day. Prednisone doses of 5 mg/day or less are not therapeutic and should be discontinued, or aerosolized steroid agents should be substituted.

Treatment of Heart Failure

Cor Pulmonale

In severe chronic airways obstruction ($FEV_1 < 1.0$ liter) pulmonary hypertension and cor pulmonale (Table 55.12) are caused by chronic hypoxemia ($PaO_2 < 50$ mm Hg) (21). This severe hypoxemia also causes erythrocytosis, renal function abnormalities, impaired cognitive function, emotional instability, and dyspnea at rest and during exercise. Chronic low flow oxygen therapy is indicated when severe oxygen desaturation persists despite appropriate treatment (Table 55.13) (2, 27, 50). Other supplementary measures include the use of diuretics, salt restriction, and phlebotomy when the hematocrit value exceeds 60. When oxygen therapy is effective, erythrocytosis and peripheral edema usually improve. Because chronic therapy with oxygen is costly (approximately $3000 to $4000/year for 2 liters of O_2 per minute for 24 hours), it should be used judiciously. Furthermore, when high concentrations of oxygen are administered to severely hypoxemic patients with elevated levels of arterial $PaCO_2$,

Table 55.12.
Treatment of Heart Failure

COR PULMONALE
  Oxygen
  Salt restriction, diuretics, KCl
  Phlebotomy
PULMONARY VASCULAR CONGESTION (LEFT VENTRICULAR FAILURE)
  Salt restriction, diuretics, KCl
  Digitalis (?) (increased sensitivity to digitalis in cor pulmonale)

Table 55.13.
Low Flow Oxygen Therapy in Obstructive Airways Disease

INDICATIONS
  Pulmonary hypertension and cor pulmonale
  Erythrocytosis
  Neuropsychological impairment
  Exercise intolerance
COMPLICATIONS
  Cost
  Respiratory depression
METHODS OF DELIVERY
  Source of oxygen (compressed air tank, O_2 generator, portable O_2 source)
  Nasal cannula/Venturi mask/Transtracheal cannula
DURATION OF THERAPY
  Intermittent—low flow oxygen when resting $PaO_2 > 55$ to 60 mm Hg with:
    Exercise-induced dyspnea and hypoxia; relieved by oxygen: documentation by exercise testing
    Nocturnal-dyspnea, restlessness, or insomnia: documented and relieved by oxygen
  Continuous—$PaO_2 < 55$ to 60 mm Hg after treatment
    Cor pulmonale and congestive heart failure
    Diminished cognitive function
    Persistent erythrocytosis

there may be depression of the respiratory drive, causing acute hypercapneic respiratory failure. Only enough oxygen to raise the resting arterial PaO_2 above 60 to 65 mm Hg is required.

The source of oxygen will be determined by the duration of daily therapy, the flow of oxygen required, and the mobility of the individual patient. For example, oxygen from a large compressed air tank or from an oxygen generator can be delivered to a sedentary patient who does not leave home. If tanks are used, one can be placed in the bedroom and the other in the area of the living quarters where the patient spends most of the day. The use of a costly portable oxygen apparatus is not indicated for a sedentary patient. On the other hand, a patient with exercise-induced hypoxemia who wants to continue to remain active may require a portable oxygen apparatus. Oxygen may be administered through a nasal cannula, a Venturi mask, or directly by a transtracheal cannula. Although the mask will deliver a complete range of specific oxygen concentrations (24 to 35%), nasal cannulas are usually preferred because they can be used during meals and do not interfere with coughing. A 1-liter flow rate through a nasal cannula delivers approximately 24 to 26% inspired oxygen concentrations, and a 2-liter flow rate delivers approximately 28 to 30%.

The duration of oxygen therapy must be individualized for each patient. If the resting arterial PaO_2 is greater than 55 to 60 mm Hg, intermittent oxygen therapy should be considered for exercise-induced dyspnea or at night when there is evidence of restlessness or insomnia. In these situations, the effect of exercise (see Chapter 54, under "Dyspnea") or sleep (see Chapter 85, Sleep Disorders) on arterial oxygenation must be documented. One cannot predict whether these moderate degrees of resting hypoxemia will worsen, stay the same, or improve during exercise. The clinical implications of arterial oxygen desaturation during sleep are not fully understood. Many patients with obstructive lung disease and moderate hypoxemia ($PaO_2 < 55$ mm Hg) have worse hypoxemia during sleep. If these changes are documented, low flow oxygen should be employed to prevent the development of cor pulmonale. Continuous therapy with low flow oxygen is indicated when the arterial PaO_2 is less than 55 to 60 mm Hg. In these situations, oxygen administration for at least 12 to 15 hours/day improves survival and reverses pulmonary hypertension (2, 27, 50). Usually erythrocytosis will improve and repeated phlebotomies are not necessary.

Left Heart Failure

The diagnosis of left ventricular failure in patients with severe chronic obstructive lung disease is often difficult. Noninvasive cardiac testing may help to diagnose the presence of left ventricular dysfunction (see "Laboratory Testing" above). The treatment of left heart failure should begin with diuretics and salt restriction. Frequently slight pulmonary vascular congestion is sufficient to cause respiratory decompensation in these patients. The role of digitalis is very controversial, and it should be used as a last resort (see Chapter 60). Many patients with end-stage cor pulmonale have cardiac arrhythmias, especially multifocal atrial tachycardia, which are worsened by digitalis. Therefore, throughout the course of digitalis treatment, careful evaluation for toxic side effects is necessary.

Course and Prognosis of Chronic Airways Obstruction

It has been emphasized that lung function deteriorates with advancing age, and risk factors, especially cigarette smoking, accelerate this loss of pulmonary function (Fig. 55.7) (27). Some subjects are more susceptible to these risk factors and lose lung function more rapidly. When the FEV_1 falls below 50% of predicted, its decline seems to be accelerated, and unless progression is prevented, irreversible obstructive lung disease results. Severe pulmonary disability occurs when the FEV_1 is between 1 and 1.6 liters or about 30 to 40% of predicted (see Chapter 9, Table 9.2).

Once obstructive airways disease is established, there is a tendency for the disease to worsen. In a general way, the prognosis of patients with airways obstruction can be estimated from their FEV_1 (15, 23). In moderate obstructive airways disease when the FEV_1 is more than 1.25 liters, the 5-year survival is similar to that determined by the patient's age and sex. If the FEV_1 remains above 1.25 liters, these patients continue to have nearly normal expected survival (15, 22). If there is evidence of cardiac disease, resting tachycardia, or if the FEV_1 is between 0.75 and 1.25 liters, 5-year survival decreases to approximately 66% of normal. This figure is further reduced to 33% if the FEV_1 is less than 0.75 liter or there is evidence of cardiac disease, tachycardia at rest, hypercapnea, or a very low pulmonary diffusion capacity for carbon monoxide (emphysema). There are obvious exceptions to these general estimates of prognosis (53) since the short- and long-term response to bronchodilator therapy may alter the progression of airways obstruction. However, it is very useful to have a general understanding of the prognosis for different levels of airways obstruction based on objective measurement of pulmonary function.

The progressive course of obstructive pulmonary disease should not justify withholding treatment from these patients. There is little doubt that symptoms as well as the quality of life can be markedly improved and life can be prolonged. Figure 55.9 illustrates the response to treatment and subsequent loss of pulmonary function in two patients with severe obstructive airways disease. In patient A, initial therapy increased FEV_1 by 300 ml (25%), but after this response, lung function deteriorated progressively, leading to eventual respiratory failure and death. The second patient was lost to follow-up for 1 year and his FEV_1 deteriorated during this period. However, with therapy, there

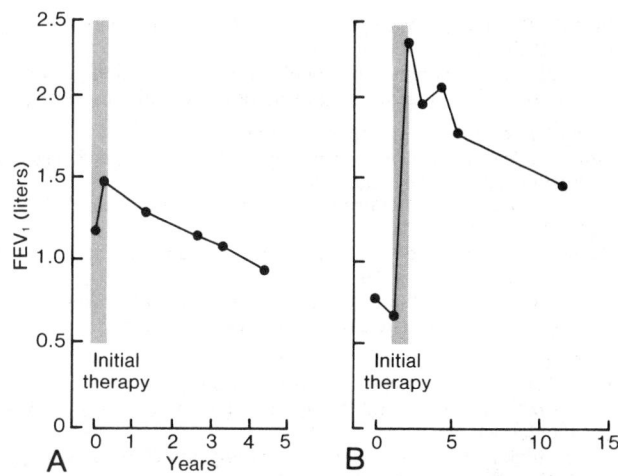

Figure 55.9. Response to treatment and subsequent loss of pulmonary function in two patients with severe chronic airways obstruction. *A.* In this patient, initial therapy increased FEV_1 by 300 ml. However, from this improved FEV_1, there is still progressive deterioration of pulmonary function leading to an eventual respiratory death. *B.* This patient was lost to follow-up for 1 year and FEV_1 deteriorated during that period. He had a better therapeutic response with marked improvement in pulmonary function. Although there was still progressive loss of lung function, from the new baseline FEV_1, respiratory disability was prevented during the 15-year follow-up period. (Modified from Burrows B: *Lung Biology in Health and Disease* (Petty TL, ed). New York, Marcel Dekker, 1978, vol 9.)

was marked improvement in pulmonary function. Although after treatment there was still progressive loss of lung function, respiratory disability was prevented during a 15-year follow-up period.

Expiratory airflow obstruction seems to be the major cause of disability and increased mortality in patients with chronic obstructive bronchitis and emphysema. There is considerable evidence that early changes in lung function can be detected and diagnosed with a spirogram (Fig. 55.1*B*). Serial measurements, perhaps at yearly intervals, in subjects who are at high risk for the development of chronic obstructive lung disease (cigarette smoking, chronic bronchitis, α_1-antitrypsin deficiency, air pollution, etc.) would objectively demonstrate an abnormal rate of deterioration and provide the physician with essential diagnostic information. The effectiveness of preventive treatment of early obstructive lung disease would obviously depend on the physician's ability to modify those factors that are important in the etiology of airways disease in an individual patient. Therefore, a screening spirogram with measurements of FEV_1 and FVC is an important initial step in preventing the development of progressive irreversible airflow obstruction.

General References

Normal and Abnormal Physiology
Murray JF: *The Normal Lung.* Philadelphia, WB Saunders, 1976.
    This very readable textbook provides a more extensive discussion of pulmonary mechanics, circulatory physiology, and acid-base balance.
West JB: *Respiratory Physiology: The Essentials,* 2nd ed. Baltimore, Williams & Wilkins, 1979.

West JB: *Pulmonary Pathophysiology: The Essentials*, 2nd ed. Baltimore, Williams & Wilkins, 1981.

These two concise handbooks are excellent reviews of the essentials of pulmonary physiology and pathophysiology.

General Textbooks of Pulmonary Disease

Baum GL, Wolinsky E (eds): *Textbook of Pulmonary Diseases*, 4th ed. Boston, Little Brown Co, 1989.

Fishman AP (ed): *Pulmonary Diseases and Disorders*, 2nd ed. New York, McGraw-Hill, 1988.

Murray JF, Nadel JA (eds): *Textbook of Respiratory Medicine*. Philadelphia, WB Saunders, 1988.

These three textbooks of pulmonary disease provide excellent extensive discussion of obstructive pulmonary disease.

Asthma

Bailey WC (ed): Asthma. *Clin Chest Med* 5 (4): 1984.

Comprehensive multiauthored review of all aspects of bronchial asthma.

Bienenstock J (ed): *Immunology of the Lung and Upper Respiratory Tract*. New York, McGraw-Hill, 1984.

This book reviews the immunological basis of lung disease.

Brooks SM, Lockey JE, Harber P (eds): Occupational lung diseases. I. *Clin Chest Med* 2 (2): 1981.

Brooks SM, Lockey JE, Harber P (eds): Occupational lung diseases. II. *Clin Chest Med.* 2 (3): 1981.

Morgan WKC, Seaton A (eds): *Occupational Lung Diseases*. 2nd ed. Philadelphia, WB Saunders, 1984.

These three textbooks form a comprehensive review of occupational asthma and lung disease, providing a basis to approach the diagnosis and therapy of disease related to industrial and environmental factors.

National Asthma Education Programs Expert Panel. *Guidelines for the management of asthma*. The National Heart, Lung and Blood Institute, Bethesda, Maryland 20892.

Patterson R (Chairman), Sogn DD (Executive Secretary) (eds): *Asthma and the Other Allergic Diseases*. NIAID Task Force Report, NIH Publication no. 79-387, Washington, DC, US Government Printing Office, May 1979.

This task force report by the National Institute of Allergy and Infectious Diseases provides an extensive discussion of asthma and allergic diseases.

Chronic Obstructive Airways Disease

Hugh-Jones P, Whimster W: The etiology and management of disabling emphysema. *Am Rev Respir Dis* 117:343, 1978.

State-of-the-art review about the etiology and management of emphysema.

Petty TL, (ed): Chronic obstructive pulmonary disease. In: *Lung Biology in Health and Disease*. New York, Marcel Dekker, 1978, vol 9.

This textbook is a comprehensive multiauthored review of all aspects of the diagnosis and the management (including respiratory therapy) of obstructive pulmonary diseases.

Snider GL, (ed): Emphysema. *Clin Chest Med.* 4: (3): 1983.

Epidemiology and Course of Chronic Obstructive Airways Disease

Epidemiology of Respiratory Diseases Task Force Report. NIH #81-2019, Bethesda, MD, National Institutes of Health, October 980.

National Institutes of Health publication that reviews the epidemiology and etiology of chronic respiratory diseases.

Fletcher C, Peto R, Tinker C, Speizer FE (eds): *The Natural History of Chronic Bronchitis and Emphysema*. New York, Oxford University Press, 1976.

Macklem PT, Permutt S: *The lung in the transition between health and disease*. In: *Lung Biology in Health and Disease*. New York, Marcel Dekker, 1979, vol 12.

Rom WN (ed): *Environmental and Occupational Medicine*. Boston, Little, Brown, and Co, 1983.

Extensive theoretical and practical multiauthored review of the epidemiology, etiology, and course of chronic obstructive lung disease.

Respiratory Therapy and Pharmacological Treatment

Lertzman MM, Cherniack RM: *Rehabilitation of patients with chronic obstructive pulmonary disease*. In: *Lung Disease—State of the Art 1976 to 1977*. New York, American Lung Association, 1978.

State-of-the-art review discussing respiratory therapy and rehabilitation.

Proceedings of the Conference on the Scientific Basis of Respiratory Therapy, Temple University Conference Center at Sugarloaf. Philadelphia, May 2 to 4, 1974. *Am Rev Respir Dis* 110:193, 1974.

Excellent critical review of the scientific basis of oxygen, aerosol, physical, and intermittent positive pressure breathing therapy.

Shapiro BA, Harrison RA, Trout CA: *Clinical Application of Respiratory Care*. 2nd ed. Chicago, Year Book Medical Publishers, 1979.

Textbook with discussion of specific modes of respiratory therapy.

Ziment I: *Respiratory Pharmacology and Therapeutics*. Philadelphia, WB Saunders, 1978.

Extensive review of pharmacological treatment of obstructive lung diseases.

Specific References

1. American Thoracic Society: Standardization of Spirometry—1987 update. *Am Rev Respir Dis* 136:1285, 1987.
2. Anthonisen NR: Long-term oxygen therapy. *Ann Intern Med* 99:519, 1983.
3. Austen KF, Orange RP: Bronchial asthma: the possible role of the chemical mediators of immediate hypersensitivity in the pathogenesis of subacute chronic disease. *Am Rev Respir Dis* 112:423, 1975.
4. Ayres SM: *Cigarette Smoking and Lung Diseases: An Update*. vol 3, no 5. New York, American Thoracic Society, 1975.
5. Barter CE, Campbell AH: Relationship of constitutional factors and cigarette smoking to decrease in 1-second forced expiratory volume. *Am Rev Respir Dis* 113:305, 1976.
6. Bel EH, Timmers MC, Hermans J, et al: Long-term treatment with nedocromil sodium or beclomethasone dipropionate attenuates bronchial hyperresponsiveness in non-atopic asthma. *Am Rev Resp Dis* 139:A431, 1989.
7. Benatar Sr MB: Fatal Asthma. *N Engl J Med* 314:423, 1986.
8. Bernstein IL, Johnson CL, Ted CS: Therapy with cromolyn sodium. *Ann Intern Med* 89:228, 1978.
9. Bleecker ER: Exercise-induced asthma. Physiologic and clinical considerations. *Clin Chest Med* 5:109, 1984.
10. Bleecker ER: Airways reactivity and asthma: significance and treatment. *J Allergy Clin Immunol* 75:21, 1984.
11. Boushey HA, Holtzman MJ, Sheller JA: Bronchial hyperreactivity. *Am Rev Respir Dis* 121:389, 1980.
12. Britt EV, Cohen B, Menkes H, et al: Airways reactivity and functional deterioration in relatives of COPD patients. *Chest* 77:260, 1980.
13. Brooks SM: Bronchial asthma of occupational origin. *Scand J Works Environ Health* 3:53, 1977.
14. Brown IG, Chan CS, Kelly CA, et al: Assessment of the clinical usefulness of nebulized ipratropium bromide in patients with chronic airflow limitation. *Thorax* 39:272, 1984.
15. Burrows B, Earle RH: Course and prognosis of chronic obstructive lung disease: a prospective study of 200 patients. *N Engl J Med* 280:396, 1969.
16. Chatham M, Bleecker ER, Norman P, et al: A screening test for airways reactivity. An abbreviated methacholine inhalation challenge. *Chest* 82:15, 1982.
17. Chatham M, Bleecker ER, Smith PL, et al: A comparison of histamine, methacholine, and exercise airway reactivity in normal and asthmatic subjects. *Am Rev Respir Dis* 126:235, 1982.
18. Cohen BH, Menkes HA, Bias WB, et al: Multiple factors in airways obstruction. *Chest* 77S:257, 1980.
19. Cushley MJ, Tattersfield AE, Holgate ST: Adenosine antagonism as an alternative mechanism of action of methylzartines in asthma. *Agents Action* 13:109, 1983.
20. Delroth E, Hargreave FE, Ramsdale EH: Do physicians need objective measurements to diagnose asthma? *Am Rev Respir Dis* 134:704, 1986.
21. Derenne JP, Fleury B, Pariente R: Acute respiratory failure of chronic obstructive pulmonary disease. *Am Rev Respir Dis* 138:1006, 1988.
22. Diener CF, Burrows B: Further observations on the course and

prognosis of chronic obstructive lung disease. *Am Rev Respir Dis* 111:719, 1975.

23. Dutoit JI, Salome CM, Woolcock AJ: Inhaled corticosteroids reduced the severity of bronchial hyperresponsiveness in asthma but oral theophylline does not. *Am Rev Respir Dis* 136:1174, 1987.

24. Epstein RL: Constituents of sputum: a simple method. *Ann Intern Med* 77:259, 1972.

25. Fanta CH, Rossing TH, McFadden Jr ER: Emergency room treatment of asthma. *Am J Med* 72:416, 1984.

26. Fanta CH, Rossing TH, McFadden ER: Glucocorticoids in acute asthma. *Am J Med* 74:845, 1983.

27. Fletcher C, Peto R: The natural history of chronic airflow obstruction. *Br Med J* 1:1645, 1977.

28. Fox MJ, Snider GL: Respiratory therapy: current practice in ambulatory patients with chronic airflow obstruction. *JAMA* 241:937, 1979.

29. Gardner RM, Hankinson JL, West BJ: Evaluating commercially available spirometers. *Am Rev Respir Dis* 121:73, 1980.

30. Gelb F, Gold WM, Wright RR, et al: Physiologic diagnosis of subclinical emphysema. *Am Rev Respir Dis* 107:50, 1973.

31. Gross NJ: Ipratropium bromide. *N Engl J Med* 319:486, 1988.

32. Hogate ST, Beasley R, Twentyman OP: The pathogenesis and significance of bronchial hyperresponsiveness in airway disease. *Clin Sci* 73:561, 1987.

33. Hyatt RE, Black LF: The flow-volume curve: a current perspective. *Am Rev Respir Dis* 107:191, 1973.

34. Johnstone DE: A study of the natural history of bronchial asthma in children. *Am J Dis Child* 115:212, 1968.

35. Kerrebijn KF, van Essen-Zandvliet EEM, Neijens HJ: Effect of long-term treatment with inhaled corticosteroids and beta-agonists on the bronchial responsiveness in children with asthma. *J All Clin Immunol* 79:653, 1987.

36. Lichtenstein LM: An evaluation of the role of immunotherapy in asthma. *Am Rev Respir Dis* 117:191, 1978.

37. Maccia CA, Bernstein IL, Emmett EA, Brooks SM: In vitro demonstration of specific IgE in phthalic anhydride hypersensitivity. *Am Rev Respir Dis* 113:701, 1976.

38. Macklem PT, Permutt S: *The Lung in the Transition between Health and Disease.* New York, Marcel Dekker, 1979.

39. Maiman LA, Green LW, Gibson G, MacKenzie EJ: Education for self-treatment by adult asthmatics. *JAMA* 241:1919, 1979.

40. McFadden ER: Exertional dyspnea and cough as preludes to acute attacks of bronchial asthma. *N Engl J Med* 292:555, 1975.

41. McFadden ER: Aerosolized bronchodilators and steroids in the treatment of airway obstruction in adults. *Am Rev Respir Dis* 122:89, 1980.

42. McFadden ER, Ingram RH: Exercise-induced asthma. Observations on the initiating stimulus. Seminars in Medicine of the Beth Israel Hospital, Boston. *N Engl J Med* 301:763, 1979.

43. McFadden ER, Kiser R, DeGroot WJ: Acute bronchial asthma: relations between clinical and physiologic manifestations. *N Engl J Med* 288:221, 1973.

44. McFadden ER, Kiser R, deGroot WJ, et al: A controlled study of the effects of single doses of hydrocortisone on the resolution of acute attacks of asthma. *Am J Med* 60:52, 1976.

45. McFadden ER, Luparello T, Lyons HA, Bleecker ER: The mechanism of action of suggestion in the induction of acute asthma attacks. *Psychosom Med* 31:134, 1969.

46. McFadden ER, Lyons HA: Arterial-blood gas tension in asthma. *N Engl J Med* 278:1027, 1968.

47. Murray JF: Review of the state of the art in intermittent positive pressure breathing therapy. *Am Rev Respir Dis* 110:193, 1974.

48. Newhouse MT, Dolovich MB: Control of asthma by aerosols. *N Engl J Med* 315:870, 1986.

49. Nicklas RA, Whitehurst VE, Donohoe RF, Balacz T: Concomitant use of beta adrenergic agonists and methylxanthines. *J Allergy Clin Immunol* 73:20, 1984.

50. Nocturnal Oxygen Therapy Trial Group: Continuous or noctural oxygen therapy in hypoxemic chronic obstructive lung disease. A clinical trial. *Ann Intern Med* 93:391, 1980.

51. O'Connor GT, Sparrow D, Weiss ST: The role of allergy and nonspecific airway hyperresponsiveness in the pathogenesis of chronic obstructive pulmonary disease. *Am Rev Respir Dis* 140:225, 1989.

52. Piafsky KM, Ogilvie RI: Dosage of theophylline in bronchial asthma. *N Engl J Med* 292:1218, 1975.

53. Postma DS, Burema J, Gimeno F, et al: Prognosis in severe chronic obstructive pulmonary disease. *Am Rev Respir Dis* 119:357, 1979.

54. Rebuck AS, Gent M, Chapman KR: Anticholinergic and sympathomimetic combination therapy of asthma. *J Allergy Clin Immunol* 71:317, 1983.

55. Rebuck AS, Read J: Assessment and management of severe asthma. *Am J Med* 51:788, 1971.

56. Repsher LH, Anderson JA, Bush RK, et al: Assessment of tachyphylaxis following prolonged therapy of asthma with inhaled albuterol aerosol. *Chest* 85:34, 1984.

57. Rogers R: The pendulum swings again towards rational use of theophylline. *Chest* 87:280, 1985.

58. Rosenbluth M, Chernick V: Influence of mist tent therapy on sputum viscosity and water content in cystic fibrosis. *Arch Dis Childhood* 49:606, 1974.

59. Rossing TH, Fanta CH, Goldstein DH, et al: Emergency therapy of asthma: comparison of the acute effects of parenteral and inhaled sympathomimetics and infused aminophylline. *Am Rev Respir Dis* 122:365, 1980.

60. Safirstein BH, D'Souza MF, Simon G, et al: Five-year follow-up of allergic bronchopulmonary aspergillosis. *Am Rev Respir Dis* 108:450, 1973.

61. Salmeron S, Guerin JC, Godard P, et al: High doses of inhaled corticosteroids in unstable chronic asthma. *Am Rev Respir Dis* 140:167, 1989.

62. Samter M, Beers RF: Intolerance to aspirin. *Ann Intern Med* 68:975, 1968.

63. Shigeoka JW, Gardner RM, Barkman HW: A portable volume/flow calibrating syringe. *Chest* 82:598, 1982.

64. Snider GL, Kleinerman J, Thurlbeck WM, Bengali ZH: The definition of emphysema. Report of a National Heart, Lung, and Blood Institute, Division of Lung Diseases workshop. *Am Rev Respir Dis* 132:182, 1985.

65. Tashkin K, Bleecker ER, Britt EJ, et al: Comparison of the anticholinergic bronchodilator ipratropium bromide with metaproterenol in chronic obstructive pulmonary disease. *Am J Med* 81:81, 1986.

66. Thurlbeck WM: Aspects of chronic airflow obstruction. *Chest* 72:341, 1977.

67. Webb-Johnson DC, Andrews JL: Bronchodilator therapy (two parts). *N Engl J Med* 297:476, 1977.

68. Weinberger M, Hendeles L, Bighley L: The relation of product formulation to absorption of oral theophylline. *N Engl J Med* 299:852, 1978.

69. Weinberger SE, Weiss ST, Cohen WR, et al: State of the art. Pregnancy and the lung. *Am Rev Respir Dis* 121:559, 1980.

70. Wolfe JD, Tashkin P, Calvarese B, Simmons M: Bronchodilator effects of terbutaline and aminophylline alone and in combination in asthmatic patients. *N Engl J Med* 298:363, 1978.

71. Woolcock A, Read J: Lung volumes in exacerbations of asthma. *Am J Med* 41:259, 1966.

C H A P T E R   56

Lung Cancer

THEODORE L. MCLEMORE, M.D, PH.D.
PHILIP L. SMITH, M.D.

EPIDEMIOLOGY/ETIOLOGY

Currently in the United States, lung cancer is the leading cause of cancer-related deaths for both men and women. The most recent statistics reveal approximately 72 male deaths per year per 100,000 population and approximately 27 female deaths per 100,000 per year directly related to primary pulmonary carcinomas (6, 12, 17, 24) (Fig. 56.1). Generally, worldwide there is an increasing rate of lung cancer, and lung cancer mortality correlates well with the use of cigarettes. Furthermore, the risk for developing lung cancer is directly proportional to the number of cigarettes smoked per day (i.e., pack years history of smoking), the degree of deep inhalation of the smoker, and the tar content of the tobacco consumed.

To a lesser extent, lung cancer is linked with exposure to other environmental carcinogens and cocarcinogens including asbestos, arsenic, beryllium, polycyclic aromatic hydrocarbons, ionizing radiation (including radon gas exposure), and vinyl chloride (6). For the most part, these exposures occur in occupationally related environments. In addition, asbestos, in combination with other agents such as cigarette smoke, appears to act synergistically (6, 10). The exact mechanisms for this synergism are unclear, but the relationship between different carcinogens, cocarcinogens, and promoting substances may explain, in part, the differential lung cancer rate among individuals exposed to similar levels of carcinogens (i.e., cigarette smoke).

EARLY DETECTION

Despite the alarming lung cancer rates and the growing awareness of the association between cigarette smoking and other environmental agents with an increased risk for development of lung cancer, there has been little advancement in either the diagnosis or the treatment of this disease in the past 40 years (17).

Because lung cancer is presumed to take years before it advances to a clinically detectable stage, it would seem plausible that screening programs could detect nascent cancer. However, early detection with subsequent surgical intervention, although intuitively appealing, has not proved effective in reducing long-term mortality from lung cancer in high-risk populations. A prospective study of more than 30,000 male heavy smokers over the age of 45 initiated in the early 1970s by three centers in the United States screened individuals by chest X-rays and sputum cytology for the early detection of primary lung tumors. The results have been very discouraging. Even when lung tumors were detected by positive sputum cytologies before they were apparent on chest X-ray, immediate aggressive treatment did not result in any significant increase in 5-year survival rates (Early Lung Cancer Detection—"General References"). Therefore, at present, it seems reasonable to screen with an annual chest roentgenogram and sputum cytology only high risk patients who are concerned about the risk of developing lung cancer.

HISTOLOGIC CLASSIFICATION OF HUMAN LUNG TUMORS

The current histologic classification of lung cancer is subdivided into two major groups (26): small cell carcinomas of the lung (SCCL) and non-small cell carcinomas of the lung (NSCCL) (Table 56.1). The majority of the common lung cancer cell types are classified as NSCCL. Squamous cell carcinoma remains the most common cell type—32% of all lung cancers; adenocarcinoma is second—29%; and large-cell carcinoma is third—8%. SCCL comprises only 16% of total lung cancer cell types. Another 5% are made up of rare tumor types including carcinoids, cylindrinomas, sarcomas, papillary tumors, carcinosarcomas, melanomas, embryonal carcinomas, and mesotheliomas. The remaining 10% of lung tumors cannot be histologically classified (22, 26). For unclear reasons, one type of adenocarcinoma, bronchioloalveolar cell carcinoma, has increased approximately 6-fold in incidence al-

Age-Adjusted Death Rates* For Selected Sites,
Females, United States, 1930-1985

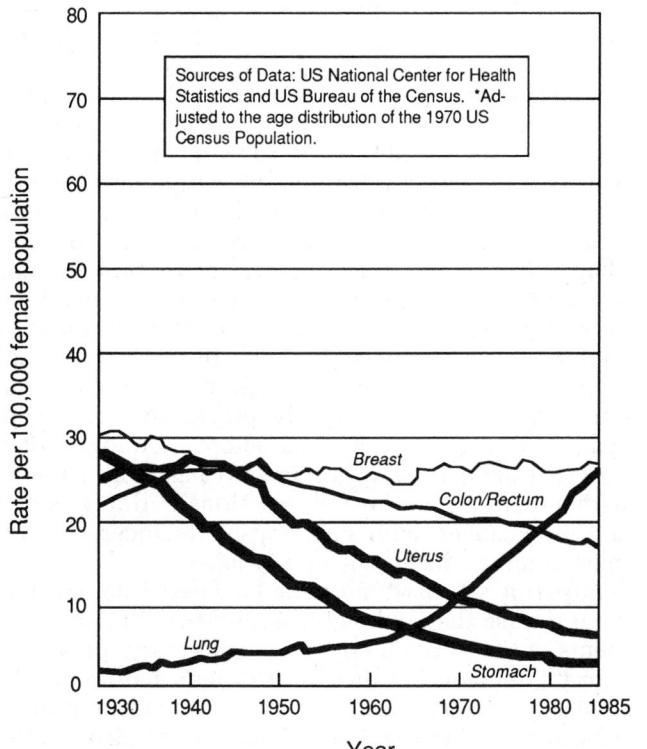

Age-Adjusted Death Rates* For Selected Sites,
Males, United States, 1930-1985

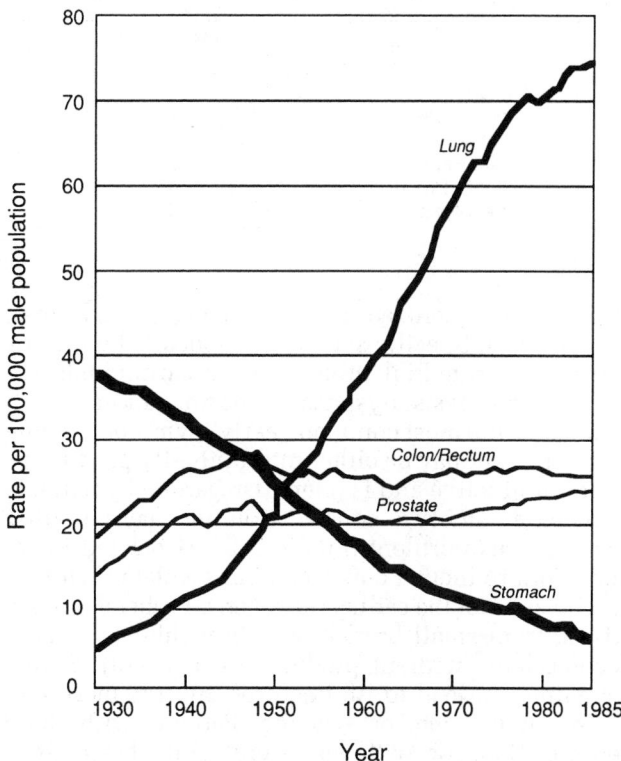

Figure 56.1.

Table 56.1.
Histological Classification of Lung Cancer

CLASS	Approximate Percentage
Non-small cell	
Squamous cell	30
Adenocarcinoma	30
Large cell carcinoma	10
Small cell	15
Rare	5
Unclassified	10

though it is a rare type of adenocarcinoma (approximately 2 to 3% of all cases).

HISTORY

Clinical Presentation of Lung Cancer

Primary lung carcinoma is most often diagnosed by the development of a new or increasing symptom in the patient or by an abnormality on the chest roentgenogram. The signs and symptoms detected at the time of diagnosis depend on the location and size of the primary tumor, the location and size of the metastases, the degree of invasion of nodes or distant organs, and rarely on the occurrence of paraneoplastic syndromes. These patterns of tumor spread also vary to some extent with the histologic subtype of the lung cancer. In general, patients who are symptomatic at presentation have a poorer prognosis, and those who present with pain have the worst prognosis. Nevertheless, patients who are symptomatic for a longer time before their clinical presentation have a better prognosis than those who present with rapid onset of local and systemic symptoms, regardless of tumor type (5). Selected symptoms or signs are sometimes important for assessing prognosis or for determining treatment options, whereas others may represent oncologic emergencies in which recognition and early intervention are important.

Common Symptoms

With the exception of those patients with lung cancer identified by early screening programs, the vast majority of patients present with symptomatic disease. In a large study of patients who had bronchogenic carcinoma, 27% had symptoms related to their primary tumor, 32% had symptoms related to metastatic disease, 34% had systemic symptoms that suggested cancer, such as anorexia, weight loss, or fatigue, and only 6% were asymptomatic (2).

Symptoms due to the primary tumor usually develop gradually in patients and are often attributed to a smoker's cough or a "cold"-like illness. Thus, it is common for the patient to delay seeking medical advice for weeks to months after onset of mild symptoms. Although there is not a hard and fast set of signs or symptoms for the diagnosis of lung cancer, some are observed more frequently than others (Table 56.2). The

Table 56.2.
Common Presenting Symptoms of Patients with Lung Cancer

Symptom	Approximate Percentage
Cough	75
Weight Loss	70
Dyspnea	60
Chest Pain	60
Sputum Production	45
Hemoptysis	30

three most frequent symptoms are cough, weight loss, and dyspnea. Specific symptoms associated with primary endobronchial bronchogenic carcinomas are cough, hemoptysis, dyspnea, wheezing, and fever.

Cough is the most common "early" symptom of lung cancer (13). It may be either intermittently productive or nonproductive and is often disregarded by patients as being a "smokers cough." Sputum may be either clear or mucopurulent if there is an associated infection. Nonproductive cough can be associated with tumor invasion of the carina. However, peripheral tumors, arising from small bronchi and bronchioles, usually become large without producing cough (13). Severe coughing can lead to rib fractures, rupture of an emphysematous bleb, or syncope. Patients with these complications or with any significant change in a smoker's cough should be evaluated for bronchial carcinoma.

Dyspnea is often an early symptom (13). Central lung cancers cause dyspnea by obstruction of a major bronchus in association with postobstructive pneumonitis, and peripheral tumors cause dyspnea by restriction of the lung, associated with pain, fixation, or pleural effusions. Dyspnea may not be directly related to physical exertion but can be positional in nature. Occasional patients complain of dyspnea when lying on the unaffected side (trepopnea) or when assuming an upright position (platypnea) (8, 18).

Chest pain is another common symptom that is observed frequently when the tumor extends beyond the lung parenchyma either into the adjacent medastium or into the thorax. Pain from a superior sulcus tumor (Pancoast tumor) is often misdiagnosed as arthritis, and as a result, the patient may complain of shoulder pain for months before the correct diagnosis is made.

In the majority of the large studies, bronchogenic carcinoma is responsible for about 20% of all cases of *hemoptysis*. Thus, hemoptysis, even in smokers who have another likely etiology, should be considered possibly to be due to lung cancer until radiographic and bronchoscopic evaluation proves otherwise (27). Hemoptysis is rarely due to cancers metastatic to the lung.

METASTATIC COMPLICATIONS

Patients commonly present with evidence of extrathoracic metastatic disease (most often to the liver, brain, bone, kidneys, and adrenal glands). Spread of the tumor to hilar or mediastinal structures is seen in 30% of patients at diagnosis, with chest wall involvement in 14% and involvement of phrenic nerve (dyspnea), recurrent laryngeal nerve (hoarseness), and superior vena cava in 6% (4, 13).

Superior vena cava syndrome. The diagnosis of superior vena cava obstruction, an oncologic emergency, is strongly suggested by cervical veins that are dilated when the patient is sitting and by symptoms that may include headache, dizziness, drowsiness, vertigo, blurred vision, dyspnea, chest pain, cough, or dysphagia. Associated upper airway obstruction or signs of cerebral edema are very poor prognostic signs. However, superior vena cava syndrome by itself does not confer a poor prognosis and can in some cases call attention to a small tumor (21). Furthermore, only patients with the most rapidly progressive or severe symptoms require treatment before histologic diagnosis is established. Approximately half of all patients with superior vena cava obstructions will have small cell lung cancer, with squamous cell cancer the next most common histologic cell type.

Superior sulcus tumors (or Pancoast tumors) may compromise the sixth cervical and first thoracic segments of the sympathetic nerve trunks and plexus by direct extension, resulting in *Horner's syndrome*. Patients classically present with unilateral enophthalmos, ptosis, meiosis, and ipsilateral anhidrosis (13). Horner's syndrome also commonly presents with radiographic evidence of destruction of the first and second ribs.

PARANEOPLASTIC SYNDROMES

Paraneoplastic syndromes are clinically important manifestations of primary lung cancers that occur in a significant fraction of patients, particularly those with small cell carcinomas of the lung (Table 56.3). Approximately 15% of patients present with a paraneoplastic syndrome before any other symptoms of lung cancer. A paraneoplastic syndrome is defined as a distinct effect of a neoplasm that is not directly associated with actual dissemination of tumor cells. A subgroup

Table 56.3.
Paraneoplastic Syndromes Associated with Lung Cancer

Endocrine-metabolic
  Inappropriate antidiuretic hormone (IADH) syndrome
  Cushings syndrome
  Hypercalcemia
  Hyperthyroidism

Neuromuscular syndromes
  Encephalopathy
  Myelopathy
  Neuropathy—sensory, sensory motor
  Myopathy—myasthenia, Eaton-Lambert

Vascular/hematological
  Thrombophlebitis
  Purpura/anemia

Other
  Hypertrophic osteoarthropathy

of paraneoplastic syndromes in patients with lung cancer causes specific endocrine paraneoplastic effects. The most common include Cushing's syndrome, hyperthyroidism, syndrome of inappropriate antidiuretic hormone (SIADH), and hypercalcemia unrelated to bony metastases. Another subgroup of paraneoplastic syndromes is related specifically to neurologic paraneoplastic syndromes and may be associated with effects on the central nervous system, peripheral nerves, or muscle.

One of the most common distant effects of primary pulmonary carcinomas is the development of *hypertrophic osteoarthropathy,* which is observed in approximately 5% of patients with lung cancer and is particularly common in patients with adenocarcinoma (12%) (9). Hypertrophic osteoarthropathy may precede the diagnosis of tumor by as much as 1 year and may respond promptly to surgical removal of the cancer (15). The dominant clinical findings are clubbing of the fingers and toes and bone pain associated with roentgenographic proliferating periostitis of the distal ends of long bones. Bone roentgenograms show an ossifying periostitis, and the bone scan is positive in affected bones, reflecting ongoing deposition of osteoid and new bone formation along the inner aspect of the periosteum (7). It should be noted that hypertrophic osteoarthropathy is not solely associated with lung cancer and is observed in patients with chronic lung diseases such as abscesses and bronchiectasis, as well as in patients with benign chest tumors or with cancers metastatic to the chest.

PHYSICAL EXAMINATION

The physical examination of the lungs is often unrevealing in patients with lung cancer unless obstruction of a major bronchus has occurred leading to wheezing or stridor associated with sudden dyspnea. Wheezing is seen in only 2% of patients with lung cancer at diagnosis and is most significant when it is unilateral or of recent origin (13). When palpable, scalene nodes are positive in about 85% of all cases. The most common sites of visible or palpable lymph nodes are in the supraclavicular fossae, which may be involved in about 15 to 20% of patients with lung cancer (3).

DIAGNOSTIC PROCEDURES

Chest Roentgenogram

The laboratory diagnosis of cancer begins with an examination of the chest roentgenogram. Although a roentgenogram does not diagnose the lesion, it serves as a focal point for subsequent procedures and for the sequence in which they will be performed. Centrally located lesions associated with atelectasis or pneumonia are most commonly squamous cell carcinomas. Adenocarcinomas and large cell carcinomas tend to arise as peripheral nodules and, therefore, are not associated with atelectasis or pneumonia. On the other hand, small cell tumors most commonly present with hilar adenopathy, often with no primary tumor visible on roentgenogram. Squamous cell carcinoma is the most frequently cavitating tumor, but even with this tumor, cavitation is uncommon. Cavitation represents either tumor necrosis, usually with lesions larger than 2 cm, or infection that develops into a lung abscess distal to the tumor. The solitary pulmonary nodule is discussed in detail below (pages 642–643).

Approximately 15% of patients with lung cancer will present with a negative chest roentgenogram (27). This will occur predominantly in patients with hemoptysis from squamous cell carcinoma that arises proximally but is obscured by mediastinal tissues. Therefore, patients with their first episode of hemoptysis and a negative chest roentgenogram should be referred to a chest physician for further evaluation and for possible bronchoscopy (see Chapter 54).

Computer Tomography

Computer tomography (CT) scanning should not be routinely performed in the evaluation of lung cancer. It is most useful in directing the bronchoscopist/surgeon in primary diagnosis of specific lesions or of specific regional lymph nodes. Documentation of extensive intrathoracic metastatic disease by CT is useful in determining surgical resectability. However, the CT scan should not be used for staging of mediastinal lymph nodes without histologic confirmation.

Cytology

The frequency of diagnosis of lung cancer from cytology submitted from spontaneously expectorated sputum or from bronchoscopy is dependent on the cell type and the location of the tumor. Squamous cell tumors shed cells into the airways, and cytologies are positive approximately 80% of the time, whereas patients with a peripheral adenocarcinoma will have positive cytologies less than half of the time. Screening sputum cytologies should be done before hospital admission. However, the completion of the diagnostic evaluation during hospitalization should not be delayed in situations in which sputum cytological examination is not readily available. In general, spontaneously expectorated sputum is the material most often submitted for cytological examination. Patients should be instructed to produce a deep sputum sample by inhaling to total lung capacity in order to produce a forceful cough. Three to five early morning specimens should be collected in a tightly fitting container, and if they cannot be submitted daily to the laboratory within 2 to 3 hours of collection, a fixative should be added so the specimens can be pooled and submitted together. Saccomanno's solution, which contains 50% alcohol and approximately 7% carbowax, is one of the best fixatives; it can be prepared by the laboratory (14) and stored by the physician for later use. More than five samples does not increase the likelihood of a positive diagnosis of cancer. If the patient is not producing sputum, induction by the inhalation of an aerosolized solution of saline can be helpful. The patient inhales, for 15 to 30 minutes, normal saline or a balanced salt solution (Hanks' BSS) that is aerosolized by an ultrasonic nebulizer (DeVilbiss 3583). In general, sputum induction is not a routine office procedure and should be done by experienced personnel. In addition to the sputum collected immediately after induction, there is good material produced on the following morning. The addition of chest vibration or percussion does not improve the yield from sputum cytology. In cases in which there is obstruction of the bronchus as evidenced by the physical examination or the chest roentgenogram, it is reasonable to start collecting sputum after therapy, including antibiotics and perhaps bronchodilators, which may re-establish airway patency and allow sputum to be produced.

Bronchoscopy

Bronchoscopy will generally be necessary either to diagnose patients suspected of having cancer or to determine resectability in those patients with positive sputum. Patients deemed inoperable may not need bronchoscopy. The fiberoptic bronchoscope has greatly aided in the diagnosis of lung cancer since smaller lesions can now be approached even though the lesion may not be visualized through the bronchoscope. Those lesions seen at bronchoscopy yield a diagnosis by biopsy and brushing in greater than 90% of cases. Fluoroscopy will be necessary to guide the biopsy forceps and brush in those patients whose cancers present as peripheral nodules beyond the vision of the bronchoscope. Depending on the experience of the operator and the size and location of the tumor, a positive diagnosis will be made on 30 to 70% of peripheral lesions. With recent advances in technique it is now also possible to obtain transbronchial needle aspirates of paratracheal, subcarinal, and peribroncheal lymph nodes, thus establishing a diagnosis as well as a staging of the tumor. Using this approach, even tumors located near the apex of the lung or near the pleura may be successfully examined by biopsy and staged (11).

Patient experience. In order to reduce expense, bronchoscopy may be performed on an ambulatory basis by a pulmonologist or a thoracic surgeon. The patient is told that he will have to fast (including liquids) 12 hours before bronchoscopy and that he will not be able to eat for approximately 4 hours after its completion when the effects of topical anesthesia wear off. The only discomfort the patient will experience is coughing caused by irritation of the trachea and main bronchi. There is usually no pain associated with this procedure. Risks include bleeding and pneumothorax in 5 to 15% of patients in whom transbronchial biopsy is attempted. However, death is rare and almost always is associated with a transbronchial biopsy that has caused significant bleeding.

Needle Biopsy

If a diagnosis of a lesion still has not been made, transpulmonary needle biopsy of the lung can be performed. This technique is most useful when a mass or a nodule is located peripherally near the pleura or in the apex of the lung. It is especially helpful in the diagnosis of metastatic carcinoma since these tumors are difficult to diagnose by bronchoscopy, particularly when they are less than 2 cm in size. The technique and experience of the operator are of paramount importance in the success of the procedure. When the pathology report indicates nonspecific inflammatory changes on two separate attempts, there is less than 5% chance of malignancy, and under these circumstances certain types of lesions should be followed by chest roentgenograms every few months and further diagnostic procedures should not be done unless the lesions enlarge or cavitate. Needle biopsy does not ordinarily require hospitalization.

Contraindications to the procedure include large blebs that are in the direct path of the needle, a patient with an uncontrollable cough, in which case general anesthesia may be necessary, and contralateral pneumonectomy, in which case the production of a pneumothorax would be devastating. In addition, there is a relative contraindication to needle biopsy in patients with pulmonary hypertension since they have an increased risk of bleeding. However, biopsies can be performed in patients with emphysema, although they have a greater risk of pneumothorax.

Patient experience. The patient should be informed that he will feel a mild pressure with the introduction of the needle. Otherwise, there is no significant pain. Bleeding and pneumothorax occur in 30% of patients in whom biopsies are performed, but only 10% of these patients require insertion of a chest tube. Most patients can resume normal activity within 24 hours.

Mediastinoscopy

Rarely, mediastinoscopy will be necessary to make the diagnosis of lung cancer. More commonly, the procedure is performed to stage the tumor (see below). In either case, the patient must be hospitalized for the procedure. An anterior cervical or parasternal incision is made under general anesthesia, and biopsies are taken of any palpable lymph nodes. There is less than a 1% mortality and approximately a 5 to 10% complication rate that includes infection, pneumothorax, and bleeding.

Recently the technique of transbronchial (see above) needle aspiration has been developed. It has allowed the fiberoptic bronchoscopist to sample lymph nodes in the mediastinum for the simultaneous diagnosis and staging of lung cancer. The procedure can be done during fiberoptic bronchoscopy under local anesthesia; therefore, hospitalization may not be required. This technique has eliminated the need for mediastinoscopy in many circumstances.

STAGING

Regardless of the diagnostic sequence chosen for an individual patient, the process should lead to an accurate histological diagnosis and to accurate clinical staging. This information is essential for planning treatment and for understanding the prognosis, as discussed below. Tables 56.4 and 56.5 summarize the criteria for the clinical stages proposed by the international staging protocol (19). By employing the protocol, a better separation of patients according to stage of disease will be possible (19) (Fig. 56.2). At the time of initial diagnosis, approximately 30% of patients will have evidence of metastatic disease (1). Adenocarcinoma and small cell carcinoma tend to metastasize earlier in their course than does squanous cell cancer. For non-small cell tumors, extensive evaluations for metastatic liver, brain, and bone disease are discouraged unless there is clinical evidence of metastases. In the case of small cell carcinoma, an extensive metastatic evaluation is always prudent, even in the absence of symptoms, since this type of tumor metastasizes early and is only responsive to chemotherapy or irradiation.

Table 56.4.
New International Staging System for Lung Cancer: TNM Classification[a]

Primary tumor (T)

TX	Tumor proven by the presence of malignant cells in bronchopulmonary secretions but not visualized roentgenographically or bronchoscopically
TO	No evidence of primary tumor
Tis	Carcinoma in situ
T1	A tumor that is 3.0 cm or less in greatest dimension, and no evidence of invasion proximal to a lobar bronchus
T2	A tumor more than 3.0 cm in greatest diameter or a tumor of any size that either invades the visceral pleura or has associated atelectasis or obstructive pneumonitis extending to the hilar region
T3	A tumor of any size with direct extension into the chest wall (including superior sulcus tumors), diaphragm, or the mediastinal pleura or pericardium without involving the heart, great vessels, trachea, esophagus, or vertebral body, or a tumor in the main bronchus within 2.0 cm of the carina without involving the carina
T4	A tumor of any size with invasion of the mediastinum or involving heart, great vessels, trachea, esophagus, vertebral body, or carina or presence of malignant pleural effusion

Nodal involvement (N)

NO	No demonstrable metastasis to regional lymph nodes
N1	Metastasis to lymph nodes in the peribronchial or the ipsilateral hilar region
N2	Metastasis to ipsilateral mediastinal lymph nodes and subcarinal lymph nodes
N3	Metastasis to contralateral mediastinal lymph nodes, contralateral hilar lymph nodes, and ipsilateral or contralateral scalene or supraclavicular lymph nodes

Distant metastasis (M)

MO	No (known) distant metastasis
M1	Distant metastasis present. Specify site(s).

[a] From Mountain CF: A new international staging system for lung cancer. *Chest* 89 (suppl):225S-233S, 1986.

Table 56.5.
New International Staging System for Lung Cancer; Stage Grouping[a]

TX NO MO	An occult carcinoma with broncopulmonary secretions containing malignant cells, but without evidence of primary or metastatic tumor
Stage O	Tis No Mo Carcinoma in situ
Stage I	T1 NO MO, T2 NO MO A tumor that can be classified T1 or T2 without metastasis
Stage II	T1 N1 MO, T2 N1 MO Any tumor classified as T1 or T2 with metastasis or peribronchial or ipsilateral hilar lymph nodes only
Stage IIIA	T3 NO MO, T3 N1 MO, T1 N2 Mo, T2 N2 MO, T3 N2 MO A tumor that can be classified as T3 without nodal metastasis or with metastasis limited to the peribronchial mediastinal lymph nodes
Stage IIIB	Any T, N3 MO, T4 any N, MO Any tumor more extensive than T3 or any tumor with supraclavicular or contralateral mediastinal lymph node involvement or any tumor with a malignant pleural effusion, but without evidence of distant metastasis
Stage 1V	Any T, any N, M1 Any tumor with distant metastatic spread

[a] From Mountain CF: A new international staging system for lung cancer. *Chest* 89(suppl) 225S-233S, 1986.

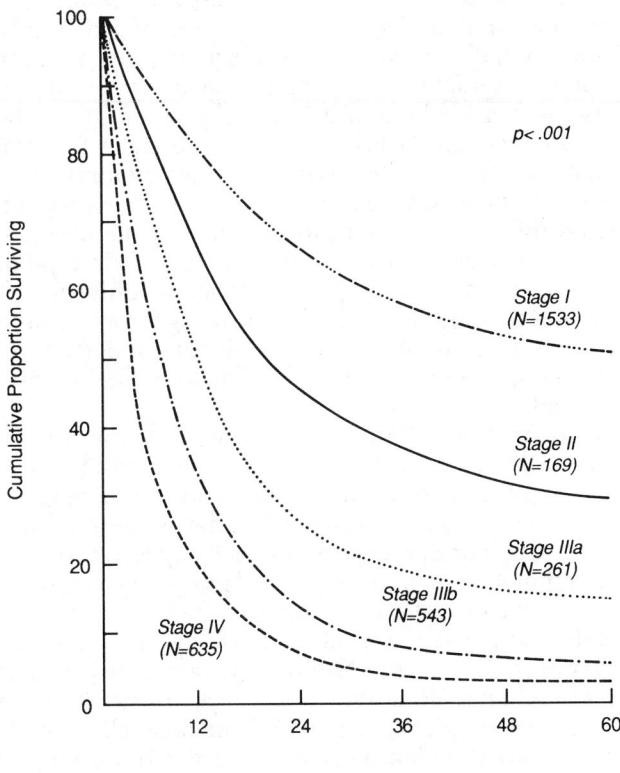

Figure 56.2. Cumulative proportion of patients surviving 5 years by clinical stage of disease based on New International Staging System. From Mountain CF: A new international staging system for lung cancer. *Chest* 89 (Suppl):225S-233S, 1986.

SOLITARY NODULES

Definition

As opposed to patients with mass lesions on chest roentgenogram, those who present with solitary nodules are usually asymptomatic. Solitary pulmonary nodules or "coin" lesions have been variously described as circumscribed densities ranging in size to 6 cm. Because lesions of 6 cm can hardly be classified as coin lesions, the term solitary pulmonary nodule is more appropriate to denote a lesion less than 6 cm in diameter. Until recently, most small pulmonary nodules were resected. Predictably, many benign lesions were removed; therefore, major efforts have been made to improve preoperative diagnostic accuracy.

Diagnostic Procedures

Chest Roentgenogram

When evaluating an asymptomatic patient with a solitary pulmonary nodule, one should begin with a careful examination of the chest roentgenogram. The obvious first question facing the clinician is whether the nodule is benign or malignant since the diagnosis of a benign lesion will allow unnecessary and extensive evaluations to be avoided. There are specific roentgenographic features that will permit the patient to be followed with a reasonable assurance that a lesion is benign.

Growth. At one time, if old chest roentgenograms were available and a lesion had not changed in size for 2 years, it was assumed to be benign (20). It is now appreciated that such lesions can be malignant; therefore, further evaluation is necessary unless it can be documented that a lesion has not grown in 5 years. Prospectively, a doubling time (double in volume) less than 500 days suggests that the lesion is malignant, while doubling times of longer than 18 months are usually associated with benign lesions. This type of measurement is not simple, and when no old films (at least 5 years old) are available, waiting for a lesion to grow may result in spread of the tumor. Therefore, observing a new lesion for growth is not recommended.

Calcification. Calcification represents one of the most reliable signs that a nodule is benign. The following patterns of calcification indicate a benign lesion: (a) a central dense calcified nidus; (b) a diffuse or irregular nodular deposit (i.e., the popcorn-type calcification that occurs in hamartomas); (c) calcifications scattered throughout the lesion; and (d) a laminated pattern of calcium deposited in concentric layers throughout the lesion, a pattern that is found in granulomas. Finally, a few specks of calcium are not a reliable sign that a lesion is benign. Small amounts of eccentrically placed calcium visualized in a nodule can occur with scar carcinoma.

The roentgenographic diagnosis of calcification is often arbitrary and depends on interpretation. Siegelman et al. (23) have reported the use of the CT scan

to assess density and to distinguish benign from malignant lesions by grading the density of the nodule. More dense tissue has higher absorption and, therefore, higher CT density attenuation. Thus, although calcium diffusely spread throughout a lesion may go undetected on a standard chest roentgenogram, it results in a CT scan with a high attenuation number that allows separation of benign from malignant lesions. This method may prove useful in the ambulatory assessment of the solitary pulmonary nodule.

Shape/Size. The shape and configuration of a lesion do not provide help in deciding whether the nodule is benign or malignant. Although malignant lesions tend to have poorly defined, fuzzy borders, are often lobulated, and sometimes notched, none of these signs is diagnostic of a malignant growth. For that matter, a discretely circumscribed, round, sharply defined nodule is not always benign. Although size itself offers little aid in deciding whether a lesion is benign or malignant, larger nodules are more frequently malignant and offer a poor prognosis (Table 56.6). However, even small nodules of less than 1 cm can be malignant and require appropriate evaluation and follow-up.

Age. Although malignant solitary nodules can occur at any age, they are almost never seen (0.5%) in patients less than 30 years of age; therefore, lesions in this age group can simply be observed. However, a semiannual chest roentgenogram should be obtained for at least the first 2 years of follow-up.

Metastasis to Lung

Approximately 7% of solitary pulmonary nodules represent metastatic disease (1, 16). Those patients presenting with a solitary pulmonary nodule due to metastatic disease will almost always have a prior history of cancer. Only 20% of metastatic nodules occur in patients with occult disease. Furthermore, there is no evidence that extensive metastatic workups will uncover these occult tumors (16). Based on these data,

Table 56.6.
Comparison of Nodule Size and Malignancy

	No. of Tumors		
	Study A[a]		% Malignant
Centimeters	Benign	Malignant	
> 4	0	5	100
3–4	0	6	100
2–3	4	13	70
1–2	18	28	50
0–1	11	6	47
Study B[b]			
> 4	9	56	87
3–4	20	59	75
2–3	91	105	50
1–2	225	78	34
0–1	104	8	5

[a] Adapted from Siegelman SS, Zerhouni EA, Leo FP, et al: CT of the solitary pulmonary nodule. AJR 135:1, 1980.
[b] Adapted from Steele JD: The solitary pulmonary nodule. Report of a cooperative study of resected asymptomatic solitary pulmonary nodules in males. J Thorac Cardiovasc Surg 46:21, 1963.

it is unwise to look for an extrapulmonary primary tumor before precise diagnosis of the solitary nodule is undertaken. A complete medical history, physical examination, and laboratory evaluation, including urinalysis, liver function tests, and screening for occult blood from the gastrointestinal and genitourinary tract, will be adequate to uncover most metastatic disease to the lung. If any of these tests is positive, the possibility of a primary extrapulmonary neoplasm should be investigated further.

Evaluation

The actual sequence in evaluating a solitary pulmonary nodule is similar to that already outlined for bronchogenic carcinoma. Cytology will be positive in less than 20 to 30% of patients who present with peripheral nodules. Bronchoscopy will increase the yield if the lesion is greater than 1 cm. Transbronchial needle biopsy is being used more frequently in the evaluation of the solitary pulmonary nodule in an effort to obtain tissue before thoracotomy. Using transbronchial forceps biopsy combined with transbronchial needle aspiration, it is now possible to diagnose and stage lesions before thoracotomy (25). In situations in which reliable transbronchial or transpulmonary needle biopsy is not available, physicians will need to proceed directly to mediastinoscopy and/or thoracotomy for diagnosis. Based on the survival curves from the new international staging system (Fig. 56.2), all patients with solitary nodules should undergo complete staging of their mediastinal lymph nodes to assign an appropriate prognosis and to decide upon appropriate treatment.

COURSE/MANAGEMENT

Prognosis

Even with treatment, the prognosis and course of lung cancer are dismal. The present overall 5-year survival for treated and untreated cancer of the lung is 5 to 10%. Seventy-five percent of tumors are unresectable based on clinical evidence of far advanced disease at the time of presentation. Furthermore, less than 50% of those considered clinically resectable (see below) can have their tumor removed when staging procedures are completed. However, even with earlier diagnosis and increased resectability, the overall prognosis appears little altered (see "General References," Early Lung Cancer Detection). Thus, of 100 patients with lung cancer, only 25 will undergo complete staging. Of these, 11 will be resectable and only 8 to 10 will be alive in 5 years. In general, if the tumor is unresectable, the median survival is 2 to 3 months. However, even in patients with unresectable cancer, the 2-year survival is 4% for cancer limited to one hemithorax (2, 3, 6). As with other cancers, survival is correlated with the histological type of tumor and the stage at the time of presentation (19). Squamous cell carcinoma and adenocarcinoma are associated with the best prognosis, and small cell carcinoma is associated with the poorest. Within the respective cellular groupings, those with more undifferentiated cell types tend to have the worst prognosis. Except for small cell carcinoma, tumor type becomes relatively unimportant if the carcinoma presents as a small nodule less than 1 cm. Frequently tumors contain more than one cellular element, and depending on the amount of tissue available and the number of specimens examined histologically, disagreement among pathologists frequently occurs. In addition, even the same pathologist, after reviewing different microscopic slides from the same tumor, may reclassify the tumor.

Treatment

Surgical resection remains the only potentially curative therapy for non-small cell carcinoma. Irradiation of larger tumors is considered appropriate for the palliation of atelectasis associated with bronchial obstruction and for relief of symptoms associated with paraneoplastic syndromes. In certain instances irradiation is recommended to patients who have stage I or II disease but who are considered inoperable (see below). Chemotherapy for small cell carcinomas often improves the quality and duration of life. However, chemotherapy of lung cancer is in constant evolution and thus patients with such tumors should be referred to an oncologist for definitive therapy (see Chapter 8).

Operability and Resectability

Before proceeding to lung resection, two questions face the clinician: (*a*) operability: is the patient able to withstand an operation and resection? and (*b*) resectability: can the tumor be resected? The determination of resectability should be made in consultation with a pulmonary physician and a thoracic surgeon. Whether a tumor can be removed is determined from information derived from bronchoscopy, mediastinoscopy, and, finally, visualization of the tumor at thoracotomy. Unfortunately, only a small number of tumors are resectable at the time of presentation.

The determination of whether a patient is operable should begin as soon as the patient is suspected of having cancer since an inoperable patient can be spared an extensive workup that includes staging procedures. Factors such as age, coexistent medical conditions, and nutritional status are discussed in detail elsewhere (Chapter 86). Although there are relatively few absolute criteria that preclude resection of the lung, patients with an FEV_1 less than 1 liter and a pCO_2 greater than 50 mm Hg are poor candidates for any kind of resection. By using both the ventilation/perfusion lung scan and the spirogram, one can predict the amount of functional lung remaining after pneumonectomy, although this prediction is more difficult in patients undergoing lobectomy or segmentectomy. If the predicted postoperative FEV_1 is greater than 800 ml, resection can be performed on patients who otherwise might not have been considered operable candidates. It is important to realize that a normal blood gas concentration does not exclude significant pulmonary disease since patients with emphysema and advanced obstructive lung disease can maintain relatively normal arterial blood gases (see Chapter 55). This underscores the need for obtaining the FEV_1 early in the evaluation, but a word of caution is necessary. Frequently, the initial evaluation reveals pulmonary function that precludes operation; however, after aggressive therapy, including bronchodilators for bronchospasm, antibiotics for infection, percussion and drainage for excessive secretions, and discontinuation of cigarette smoking, a marked improvement may be achieved so that a resection can be attempted.

Operable Patients

The course of lung carcinoma after curative resection is variable depending on the functional lung remaining. Often immediately after the operation there is a significant amount of bronchospasm, which improves with conventional treatment. Most patients with postoperative bronchospasm have underlying bronchitis with preoperative evidence of bronchospasm on spirogram; therefore, routine spirometry, before lung resection, is recommended. In addition spirometry postoperatively will aid in assessing whether there has been worsening of bronchoconstriction. After resection there appears to be some chronic compensatory hyperinflation of any remaining lung parenchyma; therefore, in time, pulmonary function can improve 20 to 30% over the immediate postoperative function and is often associated with improved exercise capability. Normal activities can be resumed within several weeks of surgery, depending on pulmonary reserve. Routine follow-up at least every 3 to 4 months for the first 2 years after resection is advised in order to detect metastasis, local recurrence, or a second primary tumor. Yearly sputum cytology and chest X-ray are recommended in patients who continue to smoke (see page 636).

Inoperable Patients

If the patient is inoperable or the tumor is unresectable, and significant tumor remains or recurs, ambulatory treatment is directed at symptomatic relief. Dyspnea resulting from recurring pleural effusions can be effectively relieved in an ambulatory setting by repeated thoracentesis; chest tube drainage and sclerosing of the pleura can be employed (on referral to an oncologist or pulmonary physician) for more chronic resolution. Bone pain from metastasis often responds to local irradiation better than it does to narcotic sedation. Chest wall pain is the most difficult symptom to treat, but local intercostal blocks add to the analgesic effects of narcotics. Pneumonia often occurs when bronchogenic tumors obstruct major bronchi, and therapy with antibiotics alone is usually insufficient. In this situation, palliative irradiation may reduce the tumor size and temporarily allow drainage of the bronchus. Hemoptysis and the superior vena cava syndrome also may respond to radiotherapy. Consultation with an oncologist is useful for the primary physician when a patient has a residual tumor and is difficult to manage. Additional discussion of the care of the patient with incurable cancer is found in Chapter 8, Primary Care of the Patient with Cancer and Chapter 19; Dying, Death, and Bereavement.

General References

DeVita VT, Vincent T, Hellman S, et al. (eds): *Cancer: Principles and Practice of Oncology.* Philadelphia, JB Lippincott, 1985.
Johns Hopkins Medical Institutions, Mayo Foundation, Memorial Sloan-Kettering Cancer Center, University of Cincinnati Medical Center, and the National Cancer Institute: Early lung cancer detection: summary and conclusions. *Am Rev Respir Dis* 130:549, 1984.
Roth JA, Ruckdeschel JC, Weisenburger TH (eds): *Thoracic Oncology.* Philadelphia, WB Saunders Co., 1989.
United States Department of Health, Education, and Welfare: *Smoking and Health: A report of the Surgeon General.* Washington, DC, 1979.
United States Department of Health, Education, and Welfare: *The Health Consequences of Smoking. Cancer. A Report of The Surgeon General.* Washington, DC, 1982.

Specific References

1. Boucot KR, Cooper DA, Weiss W, Carnahan WJ: The natural history of lung cancer. *Am Rev Respir Dis* 89:519, 1964.
2. Carbone PP, Frost JK, Feinstein AR, et al: Lung cancer: perspective and prospects. *Ann Intern Med* 73:1024, 1970.
3. Cohen MH: Signs and symptoms of bronchogenic carcinoma. *Semin Oncol* 1:183, 1974.
4. Cromartie RS, Parker EF, May JE, et al: Carcinoma of the lung: a clinical review. *Ann Thorac Surg* 30:30, 1980.
5. Feinstein AR, Wells CK: Lung cancer staging. A critical evaluation. *Clin Chest Med* 3:291, 1982.
6. Frank AL: Epidemiology of Lung Cancer. In: Roth JA, Ruckdeschel JC, Weisenburger TH (eds): *Thoracic Oncology.* Philadelphia, WB Saunders Co., 1989.
7. Freeman MH, Tonkin AK: Manifestations of hypertrophic pulmonary osteoarthropathy in patients with carcinoma of the lung. *Radiology* 120:363, 1976.
8. Gacad G, Akhtar N, Cohn JN: Ortostatic hypotension in a patient with lung carcinoma. *Arch Intern Med* 134:1113, 1974.
9. Green N, Kurohara SS, George FW, et al: The biologic behavior of lung cancer according to histologic type. *Radiol Clin Biol* 41:160, 1972.
10. Hammond EC, Selikoff IJ: Relations of cigarette smoking to risk of death of asbestos-associated disease among insulation workers in the United States (Biological Effects of Asbestos. Lyons, France.) *IARC Sci Pub* 8:312, 1973.
11. Haponik EF, Summer W, Terry PB, Wang KP: Clinical decision-making with transbronchial lung biopsies: the value of nonspecific histology. *Am Rev Respir Dis* 125:524, 1982.
12. Horm JW, Asire AJ, Young JL, Pollack ES: *SEER Program: Cancer Incidence and Mortality in the United States. 1973–81.* NIH Publication No. 85-1837. Bethesda, MD, Department of Health and Human Services, 1984.
13. Hyde L, Hyde CI: Clinical manifestations of lung cancer. *Chest* 65:299, 1974.
14. Koss LG: *Diagnostic Cytology and Its Histopathologic Bases.* vol 2, 2nd ed. Philadelphia, Lippincott/Harper, 1979.
15. Knowles JH, Smith LH: Extrapulmonary manifestations of bronchogenic carcinoma. *N Engl J Med* 263:506, 1968.
16. Lawhorne Jr TW, Baker RR, Carter D: Adenocarcinoma of the lung presenting as a solitary pulmonary nodule. *Johns Hopkins Med J* 133:82, 1973.
17. Loeb LA, Ernster VL, Warner KE, et al: Smoking and lung cancer: an overview. *Cancer Res* 44:5940, 1984.
18. Mahler DA, Snyder PE, Virgilto JA, et al: Positional dyspnea and oxygen desaturation related to carcinoma of the lung. *Chest* 83:826, 1983.
19. Mountain CF: A new international staging system for lung cancer. *Chest* 89(suppl):225s, 1986.

20. Nathan J: Management of solitary pulmonary nodules. An organized approach based on growth rate and statistics. *JAMA* 227:1141, 1974.
21. Nogeire C, Mincer F, Botstein C: Long survival in patients with bronchogenic carcinoma complicated by superior vena caval obstruction. *Chest* 75:325, 1979.
22. Percy C, Sobin L: Surveillance, epidemiology, and end results lung cancer data applied to the World Health Organizations classifications of lung tumors. *JNCI* 70:663, 1983.
23. Siegelman SS, Zerhouni EA, Leo FP, et al: CT of the solitary pulmonary nodule. *AJR* 135:1, 1980.

24. Silverberg E, Lubera A: Cancer statistics, 1989. *Cancer J Clin* 39:3, 1989.
25. Wang K, Brower R, Haponik E, Siegelman S: Flexible transbronchial needle aspiration for staging of bronchogenic carcinoma. *Chest* 84:571, 1983.
26. World Health Organization: The World Health Organization Histologic Typing of Lung Tumors. *Am J Clin Pathol* 77:123, 1982.
27. Zavala DC: Diagnostic fiberoptic bronchoscopy. *Chest* 68:12, 1975.

Cardiovascular Problems

C H A P T E R   57

Angina Pectoris

NISHA CHIBBER CHANDRA, M.D.

Chest pain is one of the most frequent complaints of patients in an ambulatory practice. The major early objective in the diagnosis of such patients is the separation of noncardiac from cardiac pain. Chapters 35 and 53 describe the various causes of noncardiac pain and their distinguishing characteristics. This chapter describes the diagnosis and treatment of the commonest cause of cardiac pain, transient myocardial ischemia. Chapter 58 describes the posthospital medical care and rehabilitation of patients who have had a myocardial infarction.

Ischemic heart disease due to atherosclerosis is one of the most prevalent ailments in the Western world; in the United States, it remains the leading nontraumatic cause of disability and death, even though, due to increased public awareness and health education, the mortality from ischemic heart disease has declined over 20% in the last 20 years. Most lay people recognize that chest pain may be an important symptom of ischemic heart disease and may be a prodrome of myocardial infarction (a "heart attack") and sudden death. Hence patients with chest pain will often seek prompt medical attention. It is essential that physicians know how to respond to these people in order to make appropriate diagnostic and therapeutic decisions.

In the approach to the patient with chest pain, a detailed history and physical examination must not be replaced by sophisticated noninvasive or invasive cardiovascular procedures. Such procedures are often painful, risky, usually expensive, and often overutilized. A detailed history and physical examination permit the physician to tailor these studies to meet more specifically the needs of the patient, thereby increasing the efficiency and yield of such procedures.

PATHOPHYSIOLOGY

Normally, the myocardium produces most of its energy by means of aerobic metabolism. When totally deprived of oxygen, the heart stops beating within a few minutes. Oxygen demands (Table 57.1) are a function of the amount of work that cardiac muscle is called upon to perform. That work, in turn, is a function of the heart rate, the systolic blood pressure, the duration of systole, the tension of the walls of the left ventricle, and the contractility of the myocardium (55). Tension (T), described by the Laplace relationship ($T = P \cdot r \div 2h$), is directly proportionate to the ventricular blood pressure (P) and volume (r = radius of the ventricular cavity) and is inversely proportionate to the thickness (h) of the ventricular wall. Contractility essentially is the amount of work that the myocardium can do under a given load and, in the normal heart, is influenced primarily by the peripheral vascular tone (generated by the sympathetic nervous system) and by the intra- and extracellular electrolyte concentration of cardiac muscle. These interrelationships, which affect the heart's ability to do work, are also important in the pathophysiology of heart failure (see Chapter 61).

In practical terms these concepts reveal why the heart is more prone to ischemia when its rate is increased (e.g., by exertion or emotional stress), when left ventricular tension is increased (e.g., by increased blood pressure or by ventricular dilation), or when myocardial contractility is increased (e.g., by the sympathetic discharge that accompanies exertion or emotional stress).

Oxygen supply (Table 57.1) is dependent on the oxygen content of the blood and on the volume of blood flowing through the coronary arteries per unit of time. Normally, the myocardium extracts as much oxygen as it can from coronary blood; this is reflected in a low coronary sinus blood oxygen saturation (approximately 30%) and a wide arteriovenous oxygen

Table 57.1.
Some Factors That Influence Myocardial Metabolism

Oxygen Demand	Oxygen Supply
Heart rate	Oxygen content of the blood
Tension (T) of the wall of the left ventricle[a]	Volume of blood flowing through the coronary arteries per unit of time
Ventricular blood pressure (P)	
Radius (r) of the ventricular cavity	
Thickness (h) of the wall	
Contractility of the myocardium	

[a] $T = P \cdot r \div 2h$ (see the text).

649

concentration difference across the coronary circulation. Therefore, an increased demand for myocardial oxygen can only be met by an increase in coronary blood flow. This flow occurs primarily during diastole (since during systole the coronary arteries are squeezed and deliver much less blood to the myocardium) and is determined by two major factors: coronary perfusion pressure and coronary vascular resistance. However, there is little change in total coronary flow over a wide range of coronary perfusion pressures because of flow autoregulation (35). Hence, changes in coronary blood flow occur primarily as a result of changes in coronary vascular resistance. Coronary vascular resistance, in turn, is determined by the degree of collateralization and the patency of the coronary blood vessels; when the vessels are narrowed by spasm or by an atherosclerotic plaque, coronary resistance increases and oxygen demands may not be satisfied. Normal resting coronary blood flow is 0.7 to 0.9 ml/g of left ventricular muscle mass per minute; with exercise it may need to increase as much as four to five times above resting levels.

If the myocardium receives insufficient oxygen to satisfy its metabolic demands, the resultant ischemia usually results in pain, arrhythmia, or left ventricular dysfunction. Transient myocardial ischemia causes transient chest pain—angina pectoris; prolonged ischemia causes more prolonged chest pain, most commonly because of myocardial infarction. The character of the pain is the same in both situations. Also, when ischemic, the heart is much more susceptible to arrhythmias, which can, in themselves, produce symptoms. The treatment of ischemia is directed at reducing myocardial oxygen demand and at increasing coronary blood flow.

RISK FACTORS

Both genetic and environmental factors influence the development of atherosclerotic heart disease. Recent research has been targeted at defining the role of these factors in the premature development of cardiovascular disease. The recognition of these risk factors is especially important insofar as they may be modified to prevent disease. In this regard, it is noteworthy that the Lipid Research Primary Preventional Trial has conclusively shown that a reduction in plasma cholesterol lowers the incidence of coronary artery disease (37). A pamphlet entitled Risk Factors and Coronary Disease: A Statement for Physicians is available from the American Heart Association (2); it summarizes the various risk factors that have been identified and makes recommendations for dealing with them (Tables 57.2 and 57.3).

It is difficult to assign a specific risk to a particular factor because often the risk is proportionate to the degree of exposure (e.g., the number of cigarettes smoked a day or the concentration of cholesterol in the blood) and because the various factors interact in a complicated way to compound the risk of disease in a given patient. However, an active attempt should be made to attenuate the risk associated with those factors that can be modified. *The importance of abstinence from tobacco and control of blood pressure and plasma lipids in high risk patients cannot be overemphasized.* Table 57.3 lists the proposals of the American Heart Association in this regard and indicates also those actions that are most likely to be effective in the primary prevention of coronary artery disease.

Although it is not a risk factor per se, recent myocardial infarction is a powerful predictor of new angina; almost 50% of patients with no prior history of angina will develop typical angina in the first year after myocardial infarction.

DIAGNOSIS

History

Onset of Ischemic Pain

Many patients with ischemic cardiac pain can document the circumstances and sometimes the date and time of their first pain. This is not as true in patients with pain of neuromuscular or gastrointestinal origin unless trauma or some catastrophe such as a bowel perforation has occurred. The ability of the patient to describe the first experience with chest pain is useful, therefore, in differential diagnosis.

Character and Location of the Ischemic Pain

The discomfort of myocardial ischemia is variously described; some describe it as squeezing, crushing, burning, or smothering, whereas others describe it as a shortness of breath or simply a feeling of heaviness. A sharp pain is unlikely to be of cardiac origin, but the patient should be asked to characterize it further, if possible, since "sharp" to some patients means "severe" rather than knife-like or piercing. Ischemic pain begins and ends gradually, is usually steady in character, but occasionally may wax and wane. Patients with angina frequently press a clenched fist against their midchest when asked to describe their pain (Levine's sign)—a suggestive sign, when present, of myocardial ischemia.

Typically, the discomfort is midline and substernal; it often radiates to the shoulder, arm, hand, or fingers—usually to the left. Radiation down the inside of the arm into the fingers supplied by the ulnar nerve is classic. Pain may radiate also into the neck, the lower jaw, or the intrascapular region. Occasionally, the patient may have pain only in a referred location and experience no chest discomfort at all. The atypical pain may be such that the patient may actually consult his dentist because he ascribes pain in the lower jaw that is due to myocardial ischemia to a toothache. In addition, the pain of myocardial ischemia is diffuse and cannot be easily localized: rarely is the patient able to point with one finger to the location of the pain; when pain can be localized in this way, it is likely to be noncardiac in origin (see Chapter 53).

Table 57.2.
Risk Factors for Coronary Artery Disease

Factor	Comment	Documentation
Blood pressure (Chapter 62)	Risk is directly proportionate to increase of systolic or diastolic blood pressure	Excellent
Blood lipids (Chapter 75)	Risk is directly proportionate to increase in concentration of total cholesterol and of low density lipoprotein (LDL) and inversely proportionate to concentration of high density lipoprotein (HDL)	Excellent
Diabetes mellitus (Chapter 72)	Risk is 2 times control in diabetic men, 3 times control in diabetic women	Excellent
Cigarette smoking (Chapter 20)	Proportionate to number of cigarettes smoked per day (3 times control at a pack or more per day)	Excellent
Oral contraceptives (Chapter 93)	Risk is much greater in women over age 35	Excellent
Personality type	A competitive, driving person (so-called type A personality) is more prone to coronary artery disease	Good
Sedentary living	Individuals who do not exercise regularly may have a greater risk of myocardial infarction than do individuals who exercise regularly	Fair
Diet[a] (Chapter 75)	High lipid content of diet may potentiate coronary artery disease	Good in humans Excellent in animals

[a] Alcohol and caffeine—though claimed by some in the past to be independent risk factors—have not been established to be so. However, obesity, by increasing the severity of hypertension, hyperlipidemia, and diabetes mellitus, may have an important influence on the development of coronary artery disease.

Table 57.3.
Primary Prevention of Coronary Artery Disease: Recommended Actions[a]

Demonstrated risk factors that can be modified
  Discontinue cigarette smoking
  Control hypertension
  Control blood lipids
  Monitor use of oral contraception
Demonstrated risk factors that cannot or probably cannot be modified
  Identify ECG abnormalities
  Identify type A behavior
  Identify diabetes mellitus and gout
Factors that are not established risks
  Encourage regular physical activity
  Monitor intake of alcohol and coffee

[a] Modified from American Heart Association: Risk factors and coronary disease: a statement for physicians. *Circulation* 62:449A, 1980.

Initiation of Ischemic Pain

The single most important diagnostic feature of the discomfort of myocardial ischemia is its predictable relationship to exertion, to emotional stress, or to other situations that may either increase myocardial oxygen demand or decrease myocardial oxygen supply. The cause of atypical pain, pain in an unusual location or of an unusual character, may be clarified by this relationship. Pain that is experienced at rest, if it is due to cardiac ischemia, suggests unstable angina (page 667), variant angina (page 667), or myocardial infarction.

Anxiety is an important and often overlooked provoking factor in many patients. Myocardial oxygen demand may be increased by anxiety to an extent and duration greater than that produced by exercise, resulting in prolonged pain. This is important in understanding environmental factors in a patient with angina. The common cycle of anxiety producing chest pain and the pain in turn producing more anxiety should be recognized as an important mechanism of prolonged pain.

Angina is more likely to occur during cold or windy weather because of increased peripheral vascular resistance and consequently increased myocardial work and perhaps because of cold-activated reflexes that produce a decrease in coronary flow. In some patients a specific diurnal pain pattern may be evident with angina occurring only with an early daily activity, such as an early morning shower or a walk from a car to a place of work. It is important to recognize this pattern because it has specific therapeutic implications. Sometimes ischemic discomfort will follow a heavy meal, perhaps because of the shunting of blood to abdominal viscera and because of increased sympathetic tone.

Nocturnal angina may be a consequence of left ventricular failure or may represent unstable angina. Similarly, patients who describe breathlessness and chest pain with exertion may have angina as a consequence of transient left ventricular failure (53).

Increase in carboxyhemoglobin level is an important though seldom recognized cause of angina in some persons. Commonly this may occur through exposure to high carbon monoxide (CO) levels in heavy traffic or through inhalation of CO in tobacco smoke. Recent studies have confirmed that patients with stable angina may have pain at much lower work loads than usual if exposed to levels of carbon monoxide that are commonly encountered in congested city traffic or in traffic tunnels (22).

Relief of Ischemic Pain

Because angina is due to a discrepancy between oxygen supply and demand, relief of pain is achieved by increasing coronary blood flow or by decreasing oxygen demand. Cessation of effort or relief of anxiety decreases oxygen demand, and angina begins to disappear within minutes thereafter. So-called "walk through angina" is uncommon. Most people must stop or at least slow the activity responsible for precipitating the pain before it is relieved. A history of relief of pain by sublingual nitroglycerin is also useful. However, the patient must be told that the use of nitroglycerin in this way is a diagnostic trial and that the prescription of nitroglycerin does not necessarily mean coronary artery disease. The physician and the patient both need to know that the relief of chest pain by nitroglycerin is not specific for myocardial ischemia. For example, the pain of esophageal spasm is commonly relieved by nitroglycerin (see Chapter 35). A placebo effect may relieve chest discomfort due to other causes as well.

Duration of Ischemic Pain

Angina pectoris responds promptly to measures directed at reducing myocardial oxygen demand (cessation of effort usually) or possibly at increasing coronary blood flow. Pain is usually relieved within 5 minutes; if it persists beyond 20 minutes, a myocardial infarction is likely and the patient should be hospitalized.

Physical Examination

The examination of a patient who complains of possible ischemic cardiac pain should be done with particular attention to uncovering circumstantial evidence that would support a diagnosis of cardiovascular disease: high blood pressure, evidence of abnormal lipid metabolism such as xanthomas (Chapter 75), funduscopic changes reflecting long-standing hypertension or diabetes mellitus, or evidence of peripheral vascular disease (Chapter 87).

Several physical findings suggest ischemic heart disease. A systolic bulge may be felt at the apex of the heart, especially when the patient lies in the left lateral decubitus position. A third or fourth heart sound (S_3 or S_4) may be heard transiently during an episode of ischemia. There may be a paradoxic split of the second heart sound caused by a delay in aortic valve closure because of a decrease in contractility of the left ventricle.

The opportunity to examine a patient during an episode of chest pain should not be missed. The examination should be done promptly, while someone else connects the electrocardiograph machine, before the pain resolves. Physical findings (e.g., S_4, paradoxical splitting of S_2, or a murmur of mitral insufficiency—see Chapter 60) may be present transiently during an episode of chest pain; in such instances, they provide stronger evidence of ischemic heart disease than they would if found incidentally, when the patient was asymptomatic. The blood pressure should also be recorded if the patient is examined while he is experiencing chest pain; transient hypertension during an ischemic attack is seen commonly. Hypotension detected during myocardial ischemia is an ominous sign and likely indicates global ischemia produced by left main coronary artery disease or severe triple vessel disease. This is important to recognize because early

arteriography and bypass surgery should be considered in such patients.

Electrocardiogram

A 12-lead standard electrocardiogram (ECG) should be obtained in any patient with suspected ischemic cardiac pain.

The most reliable ECG sign of chronic ischemic heart disease is a Q wave (9), recorded by those leads of the ECG that are measuring electrical activity of a part of the myocardium that has been infarcted (Fig. 57.1A). Nonspecific ST-T wave changes, abnormalities of conduction (except for left bundle branch block—see below), and arrhythmias do not help to establish the diagnosis of myocardial ischemia. ST depression with a flat or down-sloping ST segment, however, is indicative of subendocardial ischemia (Fig. 57.1B). It is seldom present in the ECGs of patients with ischemic heart disease unless they are experiencing angina at the time the tracing is being recorded. On the other hand, these "ischemic" changes are seen commonly when a patient with ischemic heart disease is exercised to a point where he develops chest pain. Such ECG changes, appearing with exercise or pain and resolving with rest or with the resolution of pain, are strongly indicative of myocardial ischemia. *Hence the necessity of repeating the ECG at rest or after the chest pain has been resolved cannot be overemphasized.* ST elevation at rest (Fig. 57.1C) during an episode of chest pain suggests variant angina (see below) or myocardial infarction and allows localization of the diseased coronary artery. T wave inversion in an ECG taken at rest is a nonspecific finding but can also be seen after infarction or as a specific transient finding in a patient experiencing angina. Thus, ECG changes noted during episodes of chest pain not only confirm the diagnosis of myocardial ischemia but also indicate to some degree the extent and location of the ischemic myocardium. As a general rule, the more widespread the changes the more myocardium is involved.

Listed below are some important general guidelines in regard to using the ECG for evaluating chest pain. It is important to caution that some exceptions to these guidelines do exist.

1. A patient who has not had a previous myocardial infarction and who has had angina pectoris for less than a year will usually have a normal ECG, if the ECG is done at a time when the patient is not experiencing chest pain. The finding of a normal resting ECG in such a patient is not good evidence against the diagnosis of coronary artery disease. Fifty percent of all patients with known coronary artery disease will have a normal resting ECG (40).
2. A patient with a normal resting ECG will usually have ischemic ECG changes during an episode of angina. Also such patients will usually have a positive exercise stress test (see below). The absence of changes in such circumstances suggests that the pain may not be cardiac.

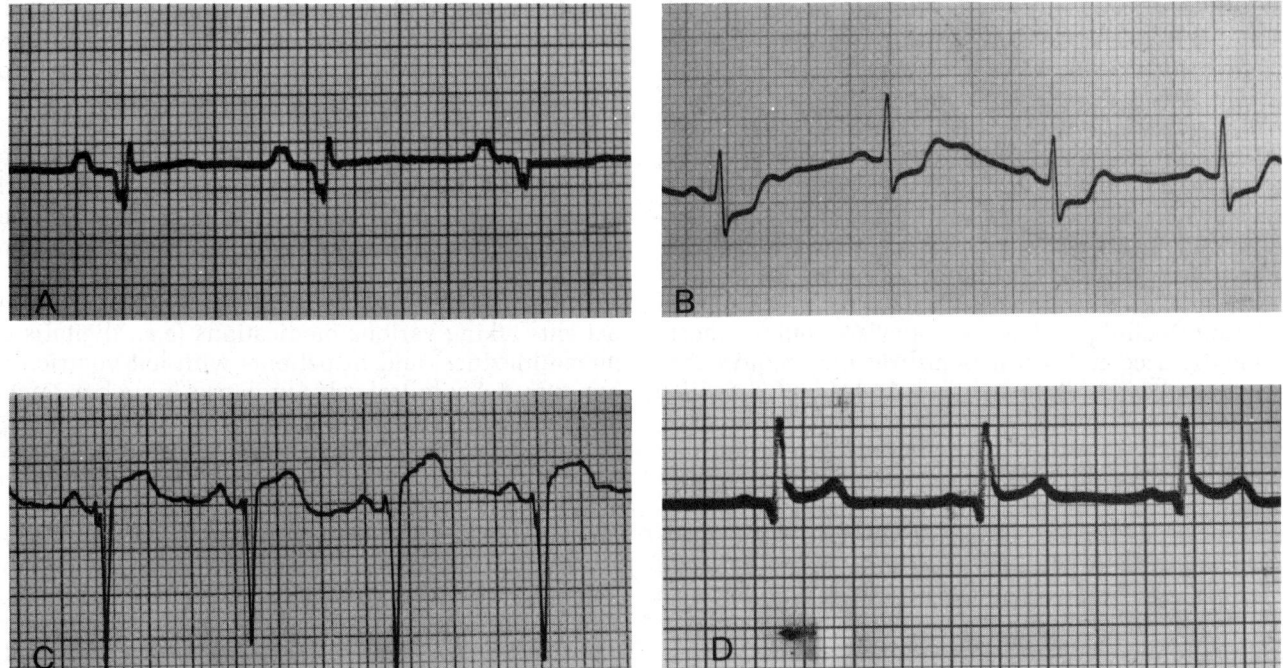

Figure 57.1. Electrocardiographic strips of patients with suspected ischemic heart disease. *A.* Q waves suggestive of chronic myocardial disease. *B.* ST depression developing after exertion. *C.* ST elevation during coronary artery spasm (variant angina). *D.* early repolarization (a normal variant).

3. A patient with a baseline abnormal resting ECG, due to previous infarction, left ventricular hypertrophy, bundle branch block, etc., may develop only minor ECG changes during an attack of angina, making confirmation of the diagnosis difficult. However, a careful review of the ECG in such patients may unmask subtle findings (such as "pseudonormalization" of downsloping ST waves and of inverted T waves in V_4-V_6 in patients with left bundle branch block) that strongly suggest ischemia.

4. An abnormal resting ECG, in the absence of other evidence, does not justify a diagnosis of ischemia or of coronary artery disease. Although there is a high degree of statistical correlation between an abnormal ECG and coronary artery disease, the vast majority of people in whom this correlation exists have other evidence of coronary artery disease, such as clinically documented infarction, typical angina pectoris, heart failure, cardiac enlargement, or arteriographically proven disease. When one sees a patient with a negative cardiac history, a normal cardiovascular examination, and an abnormal ECG, it is likely that the ECG abnormalities are due to some form of cardiac abnormality other than coronary artery disease or that there is no cardiac disease. The QRS abnormalities of infarction are conduction abnormalities that may have many causes (21), although the most common is infarction. Thus, a pattern suggesting old infarction can be seen in patients without coronary artery disease and may be due to healed myocarditis, to an infiltrative disease such as amyloidosis or sarcoidosis, or to Wolff-Parkinson-White syndrome (see Chap-

ter 59). Similarly ST segment elevation suggesting acute infarction may be seen in the resting ECG of healthy persons with so-called "early repolarization." This pattern (see Fig. 57.1*D*) is found most often in young adult men, usually in the midleft chest leads but also in right chest leads and in limb leads. The ST elevation may reach 4 mm, but there is no ST depression in reciprocal leads and the ST elevation usually normalizes during exercise. The presence of nonspecific ST-T abnormalities in an otherwise well person should not be regarded as evidence of heart disease in the absence of other confirmatory findings. Nonspecific ST-T abnormalities per se are rarely diagnostic of anything and that is why they are called "nonspecific."

5. There is a high degree of correlation between left bundle branch block and organic heart disease (see Chapter 59), especially coronary artery disease. Right bundle branch block, on the other hand, especially in younger patients, is seen commonly in the absence of other cardiac abnormalities. It is presumed that right bundle branch block in the absence of other evidence of cardiac disease is congenital; in many instances it is a totally benign finding.

Exercise Stress Tests

The exercise stress test is not only a means of establishing the diagnosis of myocardial ischemia, but it can also be used to assess the efficacy of antianginal therapy and the extent of myocardium at risk, to identify patients likely to have more severe coronary artery disease, and to assess serially the degree of conditioning or exercise capacity in patients of all age groups.

The rationale behind exercise stress testing is that by increasing the work performed by the patient, cardiac work is increased. This increase in work results in an increase in myocardial oxygen utilization, which demands an increase in coronary blood flow. If narrowed or obstructed coronary arteries prevent the required increase in coronary blood flow, ischemia may occur and be manifest as chest pain and/or ECG changes.

Various techniques have been devised, but the most frequently used and best standardized ones require the patient to be monitored with a 12-lead ECG while walking on a treadmill at workloads that can be progressively increased by increasing the speed and inclination of the device. A bicycle ergometer may be substituted for a treadmill, permitting the patient to exercise with his arms instead of his legs. This is particularly useful in patients who cannot use the treadmill, because of claudication, arthritis, or amputation, and also in the evaluation of patients who have chest pain predominantly or exclusively with work that involves the arms and shoulders.

The stress test should be performed in a facility that has equipment and staff trained to deal with arrhythmias and other cardiac emergencies. With properly selected patients and with an appropriately equipped laboratory and a trained staff, an exercise stress test is a safe procedure with reported mortality rates in the range of 0.01% (52).

Ordinarily a patient exercises until a predetermined heart rate is attained. This is usually 80 to 90% of the maximal heart rate predicted on the basis of the patient's age (see Table 58.7, Chapter 58). This goal can be modified according to the pre-exercise evaluation of the patient, keeping in mind the needs of the patient and of his physician. For example, in a young person in whom there is a low probability of ischemic heart disease, attempting to reach the maximal heart rate or exercising the patient to the point of exhaustion is reasonable and adds to the sensitivity of the study. A negative study under such circumstances is yet stronger evidence against myocardial ischemia. On the other hand, in an older patient a negative study (no chest pain and no ischemic ECG changes) may be clinically meaningful at a lesser work load if the work load approximates that patient's normal daily activity.

Criteria

The electrocardiographic criterion for a positive stress test is generally considered to be downsloping or horizontal ST depression of more than 1 mm (Fig 57.1B). Correlation of significant angiographic (usually defined as > 50% luminal narrowing) and electrocardiographic results shows a 65% sensitivity of the test (49). This means that only 65% of patients with documented significant coronary artery disease will have an abnormal exercise ECG and 35% will have a false-negative result. However, the specificity of the exercise ECG is 90%, which means that 90% of people without coronary artery disease will have a normal exercise ECG and 10% will have a false-positive response. If stricter criteria for a positive stress test are used, e.g., 2 mm ST depression for the diagnosis of ischemia, the sensitivity decreases and the specificity increases. It is important to note, however, that with more extensive coronary disease (e.g., severe three-vessel or left main disease), false-negative studies are rare.

False-positive stress tests are often encountered in patients taking various medications (e.g., digitalis or phenothiazines) and in patients with left ventricular hypertrophy or mitral valve prolapse. In such patients, or in patients with baseline ST segment abnormality (LBBB, RBBB, etc.), the sensitivity of the exercise stress test can be enhanced by concurrent radioisotopic imaging (see below).

Occasionally, especially in patients after transmural myocardial infarction, ST segment elevation may be noted during exercise. Recent studies have shown that this finding does not indicate ischemia but rather relates to the size of the underlying infarct and likely suggests left ventricular dysfunction.

In evaluating the results of exercise stress testing it is important to keep in mind Bayes' theorem: the predictive accuracy (number of subjects with true positive tests divided by the number of positive tests) of any diagnostic test is directly related to the sensitivity of the test (the percentage of patients with the disease in whom the test is positive), the specificity of the test (the percentage of patients without the disease in whom the test is negative), and the prevalence of the disease in the population studied. This relationship exists whenever the specificity of any test is less than 100%. In populations that have a high prevalence of disease, the predictive accuracy will be very high even when sensitivity and specificity are low. Conversely, the predictive accuracy will be very low in groups of patients with a low prevalence of disease even when the procedure has high specificity and high sensitivity. Therefore, the predictive accuracy of an exercise stress test is dependent upon the characteristics of the population studied. In men with classic angina pectoris or previous myocardial infarction, a positive exercise stress test will accurately predict the presence of occlusive coronary artery disease about 85% of the time (59).

Occasionally an otherwise asymptomatic patient will be found to have a positive exercise test on routine evaluation. In such patients, a "false-positive" result must be ruled out, and the diagnosis confirmed, if necessary, by stress-thallium testing. The MRFIT study (42) shows that such people have a significantly higher incidence of cardiac events over 7 years compared with patients who do not have a positive stress test. Aggressive modification of risk factors and antianginal therapy can effectively improve outcome in such patients. Hence, if the diagnosis of ischemia is confirmed, even in the asymptomatic patient, antianginal therapy is warranted.

Indications for Exercise Stress Testing

In general, exercise stress testing is used for diagnostic or prognostic purposes or to assess the effectiveness of therapy:

1. *To clarify the etiology of chest pain.* This is probably the most common reason for recommending an exercise stress test in an ambulatory population. In some practices exercise stress tests will be recommended for many patients in order to provide reassurance that chest pain is not due to cardiac ischemia. In such cases factors influencing sensitivity, specificity, and predictive accuracy of the test must be kept in mind.
2. *To assess prognosis* in patients with known ischemic heart disease and after myocardial infarction (58). A positive stress test after minimal exertion likely indicates severe triple vessel disease or left main coronary artery disease. Similarly a positive submaximal stress test in patients after myocardial infarction identifies a high risk population (see Chapter 58). Serial stress tests, at 6-month or 1-year intervals, can also be used to follow patients with stable angina. A deterioration in performance (angina or ischemic changes on the ECG at a lower work load) strongly suggests worsening coronary artery disease. Occasionally, the physiological significance of an anatomical lesion (e.g., 30 to 50% left anterior descending coronary artery stenosis) noted at coronary arteriography may be questionable. In such a patient a positive stress test in the appropriate ECG leads (i.e., V_1 to V_4 in this example) or a reperfusion defect on a thallium scan (see below) would clearly define the critical nature of the anatomical lesion.
3. *To ascertain the effects of medical or surgical management of coronary artery disease,* particularly when baseline studies have been performed. The exercise stress test documents objectively whether a patient has improved, and, if so, to what extent. The documentation of improvement with a stress test is often reassuring to the patient. On the other hand, patients with worsening coronary artery disease can also be identified, and in such patients more aggressive evaluation, e.g., coronary arteriography, may be indicated.
4. *To identify patients in whom early coronary arteriography is indicated.* Patients with positive stress tests after minimal exertion, or those who develop a hypotensive response to exercise, should undergo early coronary arteriography. The referring physician might decide, for example, that a patient with good exercise tolerance who has chest pain associated with 1-mm ST depression in leads II, III, and AVF after maximal exercise will be treated medically, whereas the patient who has chest pain associated with several millimeters of ST depression in many leads after relatively minimal exercise should undergo coronary arteriography.
5. *To evaluate functional capacity of patients* in order to recommend appropriate activities and to assess the ability of the patient to return safely to work. It may be helpful to know how much activity is necessary to produce evidence of ischemia in a given patient so that the patient can be advised about specific limitations in activities. The patient should be asked whether he has already done "stress tests" on himself—i.e., trials of various activities to determine which produce angina (most patients have done this). This information, together with the results of the stress test, should then be used for making specific recommendations about exercise and activity.

Some physicians feel that an exercise stress test is advisable in an apparently healthy middle-aged person who wishes to undertake a new physically stressful activity. For example, a preliminary exercise stress test is considered an appropriate part of the evaluation of a person who wishes to begin mountain climbing or serious running, especially if that person has previously led a largely sedentary life style or has coronary risk factors; the caveats regarding predictive accuracy should be recalled when interpreting stress tests in such persons. Table 58.5 in Chapter 58 lists the metabolic equivalents (METs) of a number of common activities. Stress test data reported in terms of METs achieved before symptoms appear are useful in counseling the patient regarding safe levels of exercise.
6. To document the response of a patient with a cardiac arrhythmia to exercise and to document the response of the arrhythmia to therapy (see Chapter 59).

Contraindications to Exercise Stress Testing

There are a number of contraindications to stress testing:

1. *The recent onset of unstable angina pectoris* (see below) or an acute myocardial infarction is a relative contraindication to exercise stress testing. Most of these patients should not be subjected to maximal exercise stress tests. However, modified submaximal stress tests can be performed with a reasonable degree of safety in selected patients as early as day 7 to 10 after myocardial infarction (58). The information thus obtained may be invaluable for making recommendations about physical activity and further therapy.
2. *Uncontrolled hypertension* is a relative contraindication and depends upon the level of blood pressure and upon the degree of end organ impairment.
3. *Exercise stress testing should not be performed* in patients with severe uncontrolled congestive heart failure because of the risk of acute pulmonary edema, of hypotension due to low cardiac output, and of serious arrhythmias.
4. *Significant ventricular arrhythmias* are a relative contraindication to exercise stress testing. However, it may be difficult to know before the test

whether a given ventricular arrhythmia is significant, since patients with frequent multifocal premature ventricular contractions may show a decrease or an increase in ectopic activity when stressed. If ventricular ectopy increases with exercise, the test should be terminated.

5. *Suspected severe valvular disease,* particularly obstructive valvular disease such as mitral stenosis, aortic stenosis, or subvalvular aortic outflow obstruction, may impose serious risks to patients who are exercised. This is because the heart may be unable to increase cardiac output in response to an increased demand. In such patients the usual increase in blood pressure with exercise significantly increases ventricular afterload and thus reduces perfusion. Again, however, modified stress tests can probably be performed with a reasonable degree of safety in appropriately selected patients.

6. *Exercise stress testing should be performed* with caution in a variety of other conditions. Exercise testing is contraindicated in patients with myocarditis, acute pericarditis, severe pulmonary hypertension, recent pulmonary embolism, atrial fibrillation with an uncontrolled ventricular response, intercurrent acute systemic illness, or significant infection. Patients with a high degree of atrioventricular block should be exercised cautiously since they may not be able to increase their heart rate appropriately. Patients with severe chronic pulmonary disease may have difficulty when exercised, such as increased bronchospasm, increased hypoxemia, or cardiac arrhythmias. However, exercise stress tests in such patients, with concomitant pulmonary function studies and blood gas analyses, can provide useful information (see Chapter 55).

7. *Neurological or orthopaedic disease* may make it difficult for the patient to engage in an exercise stress test. Modifications of stress testing, by use of a bicycle ergometer, for example, can sometimes circumvent these problems.

Patient Experience. The patient should be told that he will spend a total of 1 to 1½ hours at the stress test laboratory; that he should not eat for at least 2 hours before the test; that the preceding meal should be light and should not contain butter, cream, coffee, tea, or alcohol; and that he should wear clothes and shoes that are comfortable to walk in. He should also be told which of his regular medicines he should take on the day of the test (if he has not been told at the time the appointment was made, he should be instructed to telephone the stress test laboratory to inquire about his medications several days in advance). Before testing, ECG leads are applied to the chest and a blood pressure cuff is applied to one arm. The test consists of walking on a treadmill; the speed and the slope of the treadmill are increased during the test. Alternatively, the test may consist of pedaling on a bicycle ergometer. The patient should be told that he will be asked to exercise to a point where he finds it uncomfortable; but that if he experiences chest pain, shortness of breath, claudication, or lightheadedness, the

test will be terminated. He should be told that he will not be asked to exercise to a degree inconsistent with his age and physical condition. The duration of the test will be determined by the time it takes to reach an age-predicted maximal heart rate (usually no more than 10 to 15 minutes).

If radioactive scanning is included in the stress test, the patient will receive an intravenous injection containing thallium-201 at the time of maximal exercise and will have cardiac scanning immediately after exercise and again 3 hours later.

Radioisotopic Imaging

Thallium-201 is the isotope most used for clinically assessing myocardial regional blood flow. The rationale for using thallium is based on its ability to substitute biologically for ionic potassium; healthy myocardial cells rapidly extract thallium-201 shortly after it is injected; uptake is proportionate to regional perfusion. Low energy emissions permit recording of the myocardial pattern of radioactivity. Areas of infarcted myocardium have no thallium uptake and hence show diminished or absent activity, so-called "cold spots." Perfusion defects are also seen in transiently ischemic myocardium, however, these defects disappear or "fill in" as the ischemic episode resolves, i.e., during the reperfusion scan (28).

Thallium-201 scans are commonly performed as part of an exercise stress test. Thallium is injected intravenously at the time of peak exercise, and scintigraphic images obtained shortly thereafter depict regional myocardial perfusion at the time of peak stress. Scintigraphic images taken 3 hours later show redistribution of isotope. A "filling in" of a cold spot defined on the stress images is likely indicative of transient ischemia. On the other hand, a persisting cold spot, or one with only partial redistribution, is likely due to infarction.

Thallium scanning with exercise stress testing is more sensitive and more specific for detection of occlusive coronary artery disease than exercise stress testing alone (51). A carefully done normal maximal stress-thallium study rules out significant coronary artery occlusions with a 90% confidence. It is not reasonable, however, to recommend that all patients undergoing exercise testing should incur the additional expense of a thallium scan. The use of thallium with exercise stress testing is of particular value in those conditions that render ECG interpretation difficult or impossible. It has been shown to be particularly useful in patients after transmural myocardial infarction (20).

Besides its value in evaluating selected patients for exercise-related ischemia, thallium-201 scanning is also useful for detecting evidence of a recent or remote myocardial infarction (e.g., in patients with nonspecific ECG changes and a history of a clinical event too remote to be evaluated by measurement of cardiac enzymes) and for identifying viable myocardium in an area of previous infarction. A resting defect on a thallium-201 scan is more sensitive than an ECG Q wave for identifying an old infarction. Patients who are unable to exercise can be evaluated by thallium-201 imaging after the oral or intravenous administration of dipyridamole. This agent dilates the normal coronary arteries, thus creating an intracoronary "steal syndrome" with reduced blood flow to areas of myocardium supplied by vessels with fixed stenosis. The sensitivity and specificity of this test approximates that of stress-thallium imaging (36).

Ambulatory Electrocardiography

The ambulatory ECG ("Holter monitor") may also be useful in detecting myocardial ischemia, especially in patients suspected of having variant angina (39, 40). It is not a good tool, however, for screening patients to make the diagnosis of coronary artery disease. In patients with coronary artery disease who are symptomatic during ambulatory ECG monitoring, ST segment elevation or depression can be observed during episodes of pain (38, 39) and at other times as well ("silent ischemia"; see below). In patients with silent ischemia the ambulatory ECG is particularly useful in quantitating the degree and frequency of ischemia and in assessing the efficacy of therapy.

Coronary Arteriography

Figure 57.2 shows diagrammatically the coronary arteries and their branches as they appear on coronary arteriography. This technique provides direct information about the presence of coronary artery disease and defines the distribution and severity of obstructive coronary lesions. Coronary arteriography is usually performed in conjunction with detailed intracardiac hemodynamic monitoring and a left ventriculogram. The addition of the latter two procedures allows for the detailed evaluation of valvular lesions and of overall left ventricular function. Coronary angiography has greatly expanded our understanding of the prognosis of coronary artery disease and it has become a major tool for decision making in the individual patient.

Indications

Our expanding clinical experience together with the changing spectrum of therapeutic options make it difficult to define firm guidelines for the use of coronary arteriography. There are certain indications for coronary arteriography that are generally accepted. However, some physicians believe that coronary arteriography should be performed in all (or almost all) patients with angina or myocardial infarction and others who believe that it should only be used as a last resort. It is essential that referring physicians not abdicate their responsibility to a patient through the process of referral for catheterization and arteriography. In addition, the morbidity and mortality of the procedure in the chosen laboratory should also be known. Ideally, each laboratory should systematically and periodically analyze its performance so that its results and risks are known to referring physicians.

The principal indications for coronary arteriography are:

1. To determine the *suitability for revascularization* of patients who have failed maximal medical therapy (see below). This indication is clear-cut since revascularization offers an excellent chance for clinical improvement. In patients with good left ventricular function there is about an 80% chance of operability and a > 90% likelihood of a significant reduction in angina after surgery.
2. To detect *left main* or *severe three-vessel coronary artery disease*. Patients with these lesions can often be clinically identified on the basis of the history

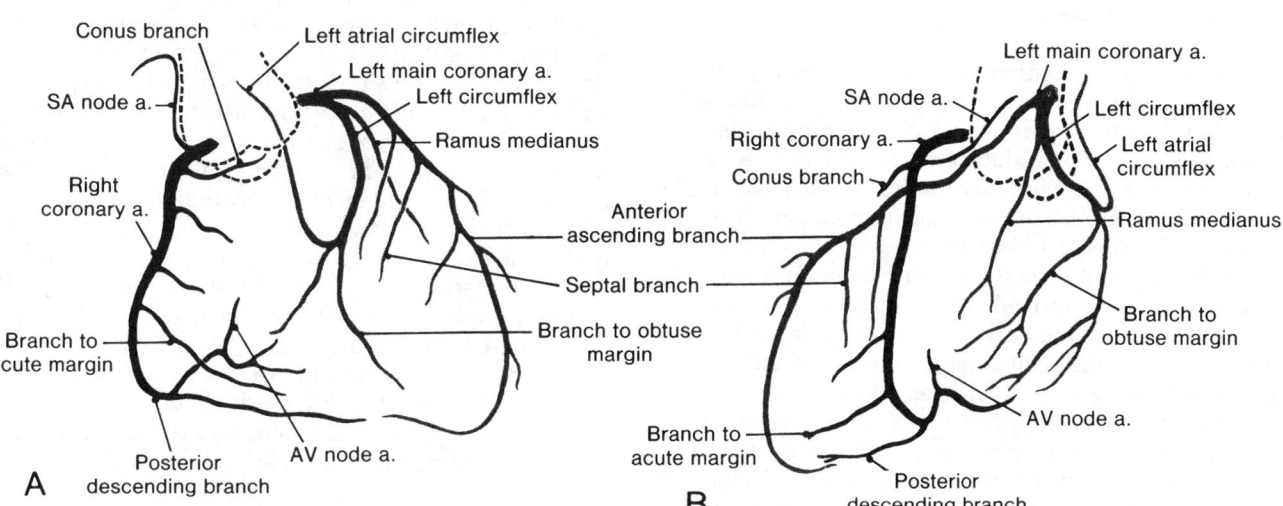

Figure 57.2. Anatomical representation of the coronary arteries. These vessels are represented as they would be seen on the angiogram. No attempt to convey the third dimension has been made. Careful study of the changes in position of the various branches with rotation of the heart is essential to intelligent interpretation of arteriograms. *A.* Anteroposterior. *B.* Lateral. (From Abrams HL, Adams DF: The coronary arteriogram. First of two parts. Structural and functional aspects. *N Engl J Med* 281:1276, 1969.)

and/or stress test performance (see above). In addition, patients who are postmyocardial infarction, with a positive early submaximal exercise stress test, represent a high risk population that is likely to have severe triple vessel disease. Both of these patient populations have a high 1-year mortality and should undergo early arteriography. Demonstration of left main or severe triple vessel disease in such patients is an indication for early coronary bypass surgery. Recent data suggest that patients with a subendocardial infarction are at high risk for further ischemic events (30). In such patients coronary arteriography is generally recommended.

3. To permit decisions concerning *management in young patients* with coronary artery disease who desire to continue an active or stressful life style; ideal recommendations regarding therapy and prognosis can only be made with knowledge of coronary anatomy. This is particularly true if exercise stress testing or radioisotope imaging suggests that there is a large amount of myocardium at risk for infarction.

4. To evaluate patients with chest pain suggestive of angina in whom the diagnosis remains unclear despite other tests (e.g., thallium imaging) and in whom it is important to know whether coronary artery disease exists (e.g., airline pilots). This becomes particularly important in patients with atypical chest pain and a fear of death or of a heart attack. In such patients, the knowledge that the coronary arteries are anatomically normal may be essential to prevent the patient becoming a "cardiac cripple."

Inherent in the recommendation for coronary arteriography is the assumption that the patient is a potential candidate for coronary revascularization. If the patient's general medical condition or other medical problems preclude revascularization, or if the patient refuses to consider revascularization, irrespective of catheterization results, arteriography is ill advised.

Technique and patient experience. Usually the patient is hospitalized the night before or the morning of the catheterization. In some centers, stable patients are not hospitalized overnight.The procedure is not painful and the patient remains awake throughout the study. One hour before the procedure he is given a sedative, usually diazepam (Valium), 10 mg orally. What happens next depends upon the technique that is used. There are two commonly used techniques; both are performed under fluoroscopic control.

By the Sones technique, an incision is made, under local anesthesia, over the right brachial artery, and the catheter is threaded through a small incision into the artery and then via the subclavian and brachiocephalic arteries into the aorta near the coronary sinuses. By the Judkins technique, a special catheter is inserted percutaneously into the femoral artery and then threaded up the aorta to the coronary sinuses. The tip of the catheter is moved into either the right or left sinus; contrast medium is injected; and then, under direct fluoroscopic visualization, the orifices of the right and left coronary arteries are injected sequentially with contrast me-

dium. The patient is asked to hold his breath during the few seconds of the injection. The catheter used in the Judkins technique is designed to enter easily either the right or left artery, so that after one arterial system is visualized adequately, the catheter must be withdrawn and the complementary catheter inserted.

After the coronary circulation has been visualized, ventricular pressures are measured and dye is injected directly into the left ventricular cavity to observe ventricular contraction. During ventriculography, aneurysms and valvular lesions, such as mitral regurgitation, can also be assessed. (Another special catheter is introduced in the Judkins technique for this phase of the study.) Ejection fraction (the ratio of stroke volume to end-diastolic volume) is measured, then the catheter is withdrawn, and (if the Sones technique has been used) the incisions are sutured.

During this procedure the patient feels slightly woozy from the sedation: there is no pain except for occasional mild midsternal burning or a sensation of hot flushing when the dye is injected. The patient is usually discharged from the hospital the following day. (See also Heart Catheterization, an illustrated brochure published for patients by the American Heart Association.)

Complications of Coronary Arteriography

The major complications of coronary arteriography are myocardial infarction, stroke, and death. The minor complications include false aneurysms, arterial thrombosis, bleeding, transient impairment of renal function, allergy to contrast material (see Chapter 23), arrhythmias, and hypotension.

The risks of complications after coronary arteriography are related to the experience of the laboratory performing the studies and to the types of patients being studied. Risks tend to be lower in young, otherwise healthy patients and higher in older patients with poor left ventricular function, particularly those with associated peripheral vascular disease. The incidence of side effects, especially impairment of renal function, is also higher in diabetics. Risks are lower in those laboratories doing a large number of procedures, and the low risk is related to the experience and proficiency of the team performing the study. In laboratories doing six or more procedures a week the overall mortality and the risk of myocardial infarction and of stroke should be of the order of 0.1(%). Another way of evaluating the skill and proficiency of a laboratory is to look at the incidence of studies that have to be repeated because of inconclusive results after the original study. It should not be necessary to repeat more than 1 to 2% of studies. A newly established facility may take some time to reach a critical volume of coronary arteriographic studies before which there may be a higher risk of major and minor complications as well as an increased incidence of repeated studies.

Interpretation of Coronary Arteriography

There is often considerable variation among observers in the interpretation of coronary arteriograms. If there is 70% or more obstruction of a coronary artery, a significant impairment of coronary blood flow, even at rest, may be expected. A 50% narrowing may produce no significant decrease in flow at rest but may produce serious physiological impairment when there is an increase in myocardial oxygen demand. Sometimes the consulting cardiologist will utilize the combined results of stress testing or thallium stress testing and arteriography to decide whether a given coronary occlusion may be significant enough to consider bypassing. For example, marked anterior ST depression and chest pain and an anterior thallium reperfusion defect during an exercise stress test may indicate that there is a severe decrease in flow through a left anterior descending coronary artery even when the arteriogram demonstrates a lesion that obstructs 50% or less of the lumen.

PROGNOSIS

Mortality

The crude annual mortality rate after the onset of angina in persons without known infarction is about 5% (33). In contrast, the crude first year mortality rate ranges between 10 and 30% for patients with unstable angina (see below), 10% for patients surviving 30 days after myocardial infarction, and 5 to 10% for patients with stable angina of 2½ years' duration (3, 33, 44).

Stress testing (see above) helps to detect those patients with angina who have relatively good or relatively poor prognoses and complements the predictive value of arteriography. Patients with typical symptoms of ischemia who have positive exercise stress tests have an annual incidence of subsequent events and mortality that is higher than patients who have negative stress tests (15). Symptomatic patients with equivocal tests will have intermediate risks. The prognosis is worse when ST depression is more down sloping, when the ST depression occurs earlier during exercise, when the degree to which the ST segments are depressed increases, when the ST depression persists longer after termination of exercise, or if left ventricular function is reduced. This information may be helpful in selecting patients for further studies such as coronary arteriography.

The two most important determinants of mortality in patients with coronary artery disease are the location and extent of coronary artery occlusion and the left ventricular ejection fraction. Coronary arteriography (see above) identifies with considerable precision those subsets of patients with relatively poor or relatively good prognoses, regardless of clinical manifestations of their coronary artery disease. Studies of patients with stable angina indicate that medical therapy is associated with a 4-year mortality of approximately 35% for left main disease, 27% for three-vessel disease, 12% for two-vessel disease, and 2% for one-vessel disease (5, 47). In patients with reduced left ventricular ejection fraction (ejection fraction <35 to 40%), these figures are considerably higher (48). Data from the Coronary Artery Surgery Study (CASS) reg-

istry of over 14,000 patients indicate that the annual mortality rate for patients with one-vessel disease is 2%, for two-vessel disease 4%, and for three-vessel disease 8% (41).

In terms of assessing the effect of therapy, The Veterans Administration Study has demonstrated significantly better survival with surgery than with medical therapy in patients with left main coronary artery disease, and in patients with three-vessel disease and impaired left ventricular function (57). The European Cooperative Coronary Surgical Study Group data, support these findings but also show a benefit for surgery (over medical therapy) in patients with >75% lesions in two vessels, one of which was the proximal left anterior descending (16). The CASS randomized study compared medical and surgical therapy in patients with mild angina and found no significant difference in 5-year survival among patients with one-, two- or three-vessel disease with normal left ventricular function (6).

Chapter 58 provides additional information about prognosis for subsets of patients with unstable angina or recent myocardial infarction.

Morbidity

Although angina may spontaneously remit after it has been present for a long interval (either as a consequence of myocardial infarction or of collateral circulation), the usual course is one of periodic symptoms and, for many patients, progressive disease (gradually worsening angina, unstable angina, myocardial infarction, congestive heart failure, arrhythmias, or sudden death) (33). Within 5 years of the onset of angina, about one in four men and one in eight women will have had a myocardial infarction (33).

The impact of angina upon a patient's functional capacity depends upon the nature of his usual activities and upon the status of his disease. As described below, pharmacological and nonpharmacological measures can have an important impact upon changing these limitations of activity, even though such measures usually have no impact upon the overall mortality. Many patients with angina can continue to engage in most if not all of their usual activities after therapy. (Table 9.1 lists the criteria that qualify a person with ischemic heart disease for Social Security benefits.)

TREATMENT OF ANGINA PECTORIS

A useful booklet, Living with Angina, can be obtained from the American Heart Association. It will help the patient better understand his illness and the rationale behind its treatment.

General Therapeutic Considerations

In evaluating and treating patients with angina, it is of paramount importance to identify and treat underlying potential causes.

Hypertension is often present in patients with angina. There is a linear relationship between left ventricular work and myocardial oxygen demand. Left ventricular systolic pressure increases in response to an increase in peripheral vascular resistance. Both systolic and diastolic hypertension can increase myocardial oxygen demand. An attempt should always be made to reduce resting blood pressure to normal in patients with chronic hypertension, including those with isolated systolic hypertension. A reduction in blood pressure from 160/100 to 130/85 mm Hg may achieve a reduction of 15 or 20% in myocardial oxygen demand. This can be of crucial importance in reducing the frequency and severity of angina pectoris in the hypertensive patient. Although any sympatholytic antihypertensive agent is reasonable in the hypertensive patient with angina (see Chapter 62), β-blockers are an excellent choice in such patients since they have other antianginal properties and may also control hypertension without diuretics in some patients. Agents such as hydralazine and minoxidil that cause a reflex tachycardia may be less desirable.

It is important to achieve a maximal level of pulmonary compensation in patients with angina and coexisting lung disease (see Chapter 55). Chronic hypoxemia and acidosis and the increased work of breathing in patients with pulmonary disease increase myocardial oxygen demand and decrease myocardial oxygen delivery, or both. Abstinence from cigarettes, avoidance of environmental pollutants, and the judicious use of bronchodilators are also important in the overall management of such patients. In heavy smokers without clinical lung disease, a decrease in smoking may also decrease susceptibility to angina by eliminating the inhalation of carbon monoxide in tobacco smoke (see Chapter 20). Carbon monoxide exposure in heavy traffic should also be avoided in patients whose angina is precipitated in this setting.

The possibility of *hyperthyroidism* (Chapter 73) in patients with angina should never be overlooked, particularly in older patients or in patients with increasing angina. Often, particularly in the older patient, other obvious signs of hyperthyroidism may not be present. For example, hyperthyroidism may be manifest only by an increased frequency or severity of angina, an increase in heart rate in people with atrial fibrillation, or by increasing heart failure.

Anemia also requires serious consideration, particularly when the hemoglobin concentration falls below 7 g/dl. This is the point at which cardiac output must increase to maintain peripheral oxygen delivery at rest.

Heart failure (see Chapter 61) in patients with angina should always be treated. The real possibility that latent heart failure exists in patients with angina decubitus or nocturnal angina should be considered. Diuretics or the use of digitalis may be effective in such patients and may reduce the frequency and severity of angina or eliminate angina altogether. Nifedipine and diltiazem are often ideal therapeutic agents for such patients since their reduction of preload and afterload helps to decrease left ventricular end-diastolic pressure, lower peripheral vascular resistance, and thus improve left ventricular function.

In the management of patients with angina, vigorous *modification of risk factors* is essential (see page 650). This is discussed in detail elsewhere in this text; however, it is important to note that the recent Multiple Risk Factor Intervention Trial (MRFIT) demonstrated a significant reduction in coronary deaths among men with abnormal exercise ECGs who underwent closely supervised risk factor modification (42).

Physical conditioning can also improve the exercise tolerance of patients with stable angina (34). For interested patients, referral to a physician-supervised exercise program is the best plan. In recent years, most large communities have developed such programs for patients with coronary artery disease. Chapter 58 describes the physiological basis of physical conditioning and describes a supervised exercise program for cardiac patients. The booklet, entitled Exercise Testing and Training of Individuals with Heart Disease or at High Risk for Its Development; A Handbook for Physicians, available from the American Heart Association, provides additional information on this subject.

In addition to recommending exercise programs for selected patients, the physician should counsel patients with angina about physical activities that may increase their symptoms and should always ask them to raise any matters of concern about their regular activities. The energy requirements for a broad range of activities are summarized in Table 58.5 in the following chapter.

Medical Treatment

The basic objective in treating patients with angina pectoris is to relieve or prevent pain by improving the relationship between myocardial oxygen demand and supply. This objective can be attained by increasing coronary blood flow and/or by decreasing myocardial oxygen demand. Angina that occurs with exercise is due usually to an increase in myocardial oxygen demand that cannot be met because of fixed arterial obstruction. A decrease in or cessation of the work that produced angina usually results in a prompt reduction in myocardial oxygen demand. Thus, rest or a decrease in the level of activity may relieve angina in 1 to 2 minutes. When anxiety is a contributing or provoking factor, it may take longer for myocardial work to decrease and the episode of angina may be prolonged.

The major advance in the medical management of angina in recent years has been the demonstration that long-acting nitrates, β-blocking agents, and calcium channel blockers can decrease the frequency of anginal attacks and can increase the exercise tolerance and work capacity of many people who suffer from angina. In general, the duration or intensity of exercise before angina is doubled when these drugs are used optimally. Table 57.4 lists practical information about the drugs used most often in the treatment of angina.

Nitrates

Traditionally, nitroglycerin and related compounds have been the mainstay of treatment of patients with angina pectoris. Initially these agents were thought to increase coronary blood flow by producing coronary artery dilation. Although nitrates may increase coronary blood flow in patients with spasm or may increase collateral flow to obstructed vessels, evidence suggests strongly that the mechanism of action of nitrates in most patients is due not to an increase in blood flow but to a decrease in myocardial oxygen demand. These compounds produce dilatation of the venous circulation, which in turn reduces venous return and decreases ventricular volume. The decrease in ventricular volume improves the efficiency of the heart and decreases wall tension. These effects ultimately reduce myocardial oxygen demand. Nitrates also produce, to a lesser degree, arterial dilatation, and thereby reduce the resistance to ventricular ejection. This effect further decreases myocardial oxygen demand by reducing left ventricular work. Thus, the beneficial antianginal effect of nitrates is due primarily to peripheral vasodilatation.

Sublingual nitroglycerin is still the drug of choice for the relief and prevention of discrete episodes of angina pectoris in most patients. In many patients with mild or infrequent angina, nitroglycerin is often the only medication required for the prevention or relief of pain. The initial dose should be small (0.4 mg) in order to minimize unpleasant side effects (flushing, headache, lightheadedness) in those patients in whom higher doses may be unnecessary.

Patients should be taught that it is important that their pain be relieved as soon as possible and they should be instructed to take nitroglycerin whenever such symptoms appear. Use of nitroglycerin in this way may do more than simply prevent ischemic pain. Angina often produces some anxiety, which may increase heart rate, left ventricular contractility, and hence myocardial oxygen demand. Thus, ischemia may be increased and the severity and the duration of pain may be prolonged. Additionally, some patients, during periods of ischemia, develop serious arrhythmias, hypotension, or incipient heart failure, which the prompt administration of nitroglycerin may abort (53). If pain is not relieved by 2 to 3 tablets of nitroglycerin (the patient should wait for 3 minutes before taking another tablet) or if tablets must be taken more often than every 30 to 60 minutes, the patient should be instructed to call his physician or to go to an emergency facility immediately, because of the danger of impending myocardial infarction. Because nitroglycerin may lose potency on storage, the physician should advise patients not to keep tablets longer then 3 to 4 months after opening the bottle, and if pain is not relieved and usual side effects are also not experienced, the problem may be due to a change in the drug rather than to a change in cardiac status. Prophylactic use of nitroglycerin is of particular value in patients who have mild or moderate angina in response to specific and reproducible stress. For example, the patient who develops angina after walking from a car to a place of work can be taught to take nitroglycerin after the car is parked, to wait a few minutes, and then to walk to work, thereby preventing pain altogether. The use of prophylactic nitroglycerin before sexual intercourse may also prevent angina and may alleviate the anxiety that is naturally associated with sexual activity when angina is anticipated.

It is important to teach the patient to use sublingual nitroglycerin correctly. The patient should take it while he is sitting to maximize the vasodilating effect (reduced in the supine position) and to avoid the possible untoward effects of hypotension (increased in the standing position). When initiating treatment with sublingual nitroglycerin, it is advisable to administer the first dose in the office so that the patient can experience the side effects and receive reassurance from a physician or nurse that this is an expected response. Patients who start taking nitroglycerin at home may otherwise become so frightened by side effects that they may delay taking it or may avoid its use altogether. The most common side effects are flushing and headache; both may diminish with increasing usage of the drug. Recently a nitroglycerine oral spray has been developed that is designed to deliver 0.4 mg of nitroglycerine sublingually with each compression of the nebulizer. Some patients find this preparation more acceptable and reliable than the tablet.

Long-acting nitrates. As shown in Table 57.4, long-acting nitrates are available in a variety of preparations. Careful studies have confirmed the clinical efficacy of both nitroglycerin ointment and isosorbide tablets (11, 50). Both of these preparations produce about a 50% increase in the exercise time before symptoms appear. These effects last from 4 to 6 hours after drug administration. Patients restudied on an average of 6 months after beginning isosorbide tablets maintained the same increase in exercise tolerance (11). The dose of nitrate needed to improve symptoms may be relatively high; fortunately, available preparations permit a great deal of flexibility in dose adjustment, as shown in Table 57.4.

In selecting among available preparations, the major considerations should be the known efficacy and convenience of a particular nitrate for the patient. Using these criteria, isosorbide is probably the best choice for ambulatory patients. The disadvantages of nitroglycerin ointment are that it is messy to apply, that it is difficult to apply similar amounts evenly each time, and that irritation of the skin may occur after prolonged use. Its major advantage is that it can be removed promptly if a patient develops a significant side effect (e.g., severe hypotension) shortly after application. Many patients are treated in the hospital with nitroglycerin ointment; if its disadvantages become apparent after discharge, substitution of isosorbide is the best plan.

A topical nitrate preparation for once a day use also

Table 57.4.
Selected Drugs Used in the Treatment of Angina[a]

Class	Brand Name	Available Strengths	Usual Starting Dose	Usual Maximum Dose	Onset	Duration
Nitrates						
Nitroglycerin Sublingual[b]	Nitrostat and others	0.15-, 0.30-, 0.40-, 0.60-mg tablets, sublingual	1 tablet (0.4 mg) at time of, or in anticipation of pain	2–3 tablets at time of pain	30 sec	3–5 min
Topical						
Ointment	Nitro-Bid, Nitrol	2% ointment	½ inch every 4–6 hr as needed	4–5 inches every 3–4 hr	30–60 min	3–6 hr
Patch[c]	Transderm Nitro, Nitro-Dur and Nitrodisc	2.5-, 5-, 10-, 15-, mg/24 hr rated release	5 mg	2–3 patches that deliver 15 mg/24 hr	30 min	24 hr
Long-acting						
Erythrityl[b] tetranitrate	Cardilate	5-, 10-, 15-mg tablets oral or sublingual; 10-mg tablets, chewable	5 mg sublingually in anticipation of pain or 10 mg orally or chewed three times a day	100 mg a day in divided doses	5 min (sublingual and chewed)	4 hr
Isosorbide[b] dinitrate	Isordil, Sorbitrate and others	5-, 10-, 20-mg tablets, oral; 40-mg tablets or capsules, oral	10 mg every 4–6 hr	60–80 mg every 4 hr	15–30 min	4–6 hr
β-Adrenergic Blockers[b]						
Propranolol[b]	Inderal	10-, 20-, 40-, 80-mg tablets, oral	10-20 mg three or four times a day	320 mg a day in divided doses	1.1.5 hr	4–6 hr
Nadolol	Corgard	40-, 80-, 120-mg tablets, oral	40 mg once a day	240 mg	1–2 hr	24 hr
Tenormin	Atenolol	50-, 100-mg tablets, oral	50 mg once a day	100–150 mg	1–2 hr	24 hr
Calcium Channel Blockers						
Nifedipine	Procardia	10-mg capsule	10 mg three or four times a day; 10 mg at time of pain if sublingual	40 mg every 6 hr	20–30 min	8 hr
Verapamil	Calan, Isoptin	80-, 120-mg tablets	80 mg three or four times a day	120 mg four times a day	30–45 min	6–8 hr
Diltiazem	Cardiazem	30-, 60-mg tablets	30 mg four times a day	60 mg every 6 hr	30–45 min	6–8 hr
Nicardipine	Cardene	20-, 30-mg capsules	20 mg three times a day	40 mg three times a day	30–120 min	8 hr

[a] Other drugs, other doses of the drugs listed, and combinations of different drugs are marketed. The drugs and dosages shown are the ones most often used.
[b] Generic available. Table 59.3 (page ##724) provides information on the pharmacology of all six of the currently available β-blockers.
[c] The brand name of these preparations is followed by a number (5, 10, 15, 20). It is important to know whether that number refers to milligrams per 24 hours (Transderm-Nitro or Nitrodisc) or to square centimeters of the patch (Nitro-Dur).

is available. It provides controlled release of 5, 10, 15, or 20 mg/day of nitroglycerin through a semipermeable membrane applied to the skin by means of an adhesive tape. It has two advantages compared with nitroglycerin ointment: It is not messy to use and it delivers a standardized dose. However, constant serum levels of nitrate predispose to the development of tolerance. A tachyphylactic effect has been conclusively demonstrated in patients with heart failure treated with the nitroglycerin patch (1, 54), and a similar effect occurs in patients with angina treated with frequent oral doses (e.g., every 4 hours) of nitrates, intravenous nitroglycerine, or the topical patch (1, 14). It appears that a "nitrate-free interval" is needed for the drug to exercise its maximal effect. Hence patients who develop increasing angina while using the topical patch may benefit from being changed to an oral nitrate regimen or from having the patch removed at night.

The side effects of all long-acting nitrates are similar to those produced by sublingual nitrates. Many patients will have already experienced the headache produced by sublingual nitroglycerin before being treated with a long-acting preparation.

Because of persistent headache, some patients are unable to take long-acting nitrates, although in most patients this is not a problem. Because long-acting nitrates can produce orthostatic hypotension, and occasionally syncope, it is very important to check a patient's orthostatic blood pressure response before and after initiating treatment with or increasing the dose of a long-acting nitrate. Two relative contraindications to long-acting nitrates are a history of migraine or cluster headache and demonstrated orthostatic hypotension before initiation of treatment.

β-Blocking Agents

The introduction of β-blockers heralded a new era in the medical treatment of angina. Seven β-blockers are currently available in the United States. Though all are approved by the Food and Drug Administration for use in hypertension, only timolol and propranolol are approved for use after myocardial infarction, and only propranolol and nadolol are approved for use in angina. The others (atenolol, pindolol, metoprolol, acebutolol, and timolol), though used to treat angina in England and Europe, are under evaluation for use in patients with angina in the United States. These agents vary in their cardioselectivity, their metabolism, and, to some degree, their side effects (see below and Chapters 59 and 62).

In many respects β-blockade is an ideal approach to the treatment of angina. It decreases heart rate, contractility, and in many patients systemic blood pressure. These effects alone or in combination significantly reduce myocardial oxygen consumption and thus prevent the frequency and/or severity of angina in most patients.

An added benefit for patients with ischemic heart disease is that β-blockade often effectively prevents arrhythmias (see Chapter 59). It may decrease or eliminate premature ventricular contractions (PVCs), and the ventricular rate in patients with atrial fibrillation may also be decreased. Control of PVCs is beneficial to patients with ischemic heart disease because such patients are at increased risk for ventricular tachycardia or ventricular fibrillation, particularly during an episode of ischemia (7). Furthermore, when PVCs are frequent, the number of hemodynamically effective ventricular contractions is diminished, which in turn decreases coronary as well as peripheral perfusion. In patients who are in atrial fibrillation, decreasing the ventricular response improves left ventricular dynamics by decreasing heart rate, increasing diastolic filling period, and decreasing myocardial oxygen consumption.

The dose of a β-blocker can be rapidly increased over hours or days until the desired effect is obtained. The heart rate is the best guide to maximal treatment; sinus bradycardia at a rate at rest between 50 and 60 beats/minute is a reasonable goal. However, it must be noted that the ideal dose is one that not only results in sinus bradycardia at rest but also "blocks" an increase in heart rate with exercise. It should be recognized that the dose necessary to produce this effect and that necessary to relieve angina pectoris may vary considerably.

Because β-blocking agents decrease myocardial contractility, they must be used cautiously in patients with heart failure. If failure increases (sometimes expressed first as decreased exercise tolerance), reducing the dose of the β-blocker and/or adding digitalis (10) may improve cardiac compensation and at the same time reduce the severity or frequency of anginal attacks. If it is approved for the treatment of patients with angina, pindolol may be the β-blocker of choice in such circumstances. It is the only available β-blocker with intrinsic sympathomimetic activity and has, therefore, less negative inotropic effect than the other β-blockers. Often, it can be safely used in patients with reduced left ventricular function.

Extreme caution must be exercised while using all β-blockers in patients with second or third degree block (Chapter 59) since life-threatening bradycardia can be precipitated in such patients.

The nonselective β-blockers (propranolol, nadolol, pindolol, timolol) are contraindicated in patients with intrinsic asthma. A history of allergic asthma or of bronchospasm during pulmonary infections should therefore be sought in all patients for whom β-blockers are being considered. Furthermore, patients with chronic obstructive lung disease may develop increased bronchospasm from β-blockers even if they have no history of allergic or intrinsic asthma; therefore, in such patients a selective β-blocker with minimal β_2-blocking effects should be used. Metoprolol and atenolol are both relatively cardioselective and can often be safely used in such patients and in patients with peripheral arterial disease, particularly Raynaud's disease, in whom nonselective β-blockers may exacerbate symptoms. However, even these agents have β_2-blocking effects at moderate and high doses and should be used cautiously in these situations.

Impotence, though it occurs in 1% or less of the susceptible population, is perhaps the major reason that the use of β-blockers is limited in middle-aged men. It can sometimes be overcome by prescribing a β-blocker with poor lipid solubility and thus less penetration of the nervous system, e.g., atenolol instead of propranolol. Atenolol also is less likely to cause depression or to alter sleep patterns, occasional side effects of other β-blockers.

Several of the newer β-blockers can be administered once or twice a day, a feature that significantly promotes patient compliance. They have been shown to be effective at this schedule and in comparison studies nadolol (administered once a day) and propranolol (administered four times a day) have been shown to be equivalent for control of angina. Because some of the β-blockers are excreted entirely by the kidneys, the interval between doses should be increased in patients with renal insufficiency who are taking those preparations (see Table 59.3). Also, after the abrupt cessation of therapy with certain β-blocking agents, exacerbation of angina and sometimes myocardial infarction have been reported. Hence patients should be instructed never to stop therapy abruptly; all β-blockers should be gradually tapered over several days if therapy is to be discontinued.

Calcium Channel Blockers

Calcium channel blockers have added a new dimension to the treatment of angina. These drugs reduce the influx of calcium into the slow channels of the myocardium and smooth muscle (see Chapter 59) and thereby cause several important hemodynamic effects (56): (a) dilatation of coronary arteries and prevention of coronary vasospasm and (b) production of systemic vasodilation, thus effectively reducing preload and afterload. They have been shown to be effective in the treatment of both stable and unstable angina (19, 45). Four calcium channel blockers are currently available in the United States (Table 57.4). Although all are effective in the treatment of angina, knowledge of their specific effects permits selection of the most appropriate drug.

Nifedipine is the one most often prescribed for patients with angina. It is a potent coronary and systemic vasodilator and therefore reduces the need of the myocardium for oxygen. It is usually given by mouth but for a rapid effect in patients unresponsive to nitroglycerin, a 10-mg capsule can be punctured and the contents taken sublingually. The common side effects of nifedipine are dizziness, flushing, headache, nausea, diarrhea, and, because of systemic vasodilatation, peripheral edema. The major adverse effect is severe hypotension, which, in association with a reflex tachycardia, can actually intensify myocardial ischemia in an occasional patient. All side effects can usually be controlled by a reduction in dosage of the

drug. Nifedipine (and other calcium channel blockers) should be used cautiously in patients taking digoxin since excretion of digoxin may be inhibited and digitoxicity may be induced. At higher doses in patients with reduced left ventricular function, negative inotropy may be observed with nifedipine. It is also an effective antihypertensive, especially in older patients.

Verapamil is most often prescribed for the treatment of arrhythmias but it too is an effective antianginal agent. However, it has a more potent negative inotropic effect than does nifedipine and, unlike nifedipine, significantly retards atrioventricular conduction. Therefore, it should not be used in patients with compromised left ventricular function or with sinus bradycardia, sick sinus syndrome, or atrioventricular block (see Chapter 59). In these situations, nifedipine is a safer choice. Verapamil might reasonably be prescribed to a patient with a supraventricular arrhythmia who also has angina.

Diltiazem also significantly retards atrioventricular conduction, but it has less of a negative inotropic effect than does verapamil and, in contrast to nifedipine, is unlikely to cause hypotension or other side effects of vasodilation (flushing, headache, edema, etc.). Therefore, some cardiologists prefer it to nifedipine in the treatment of patients who do not have an abnormal atrioventricular conducting system, and in older patients.

Nicardipine has recently been released and is similar to nifedipine. Its major advantage is that it reportedly has minimal negative inotropic effects.

Caution must be exercised when treating older patients with calcium blockers, especially if used in conjunction with a β-blocker or other agents that slow atrioventricular conduction (e.g., digitalis) or if used in patients with pre-existing conduction system disease. In such patients, significant heart block and bradycardia can be precipitated that will usually resolve after stopping administration of the calcium blocker and/or the administration of calcium intravenously. This effect, though most commonly seen with verapamil and diltiazem, may occur with all calcium blockers.

Initiating and Adjusting Long-Acting Drugs for Angina

The choice of an antianginal agent should be made on evaluation of the patient's age, angina frequency, lifestyle, and possible mechanism of angina. In addition, the patient's financial resources should also be considered in advising therapy since many of the newer agents, though effective, are expensive and not available as generic substitutes. In patients with stable angina either a nitrate preparation or a β-blocker can be tried initially (Table 57.4). If the patient fails to improve, the dose can be increased weekly until a response is achieved. If the type of treatment selected initially fails to help at a maximally tolerated dose, the other agent can be added or substituted. Because nitrates and β-blockers decrease myocardial oxygen demand by different mechanisms, the continued use of the two types of therapy is quite reasonable.

A number of relative contraindications to either long-acting nitrates or β-blockers have been mentioned above; these contraindications are important in selecting the initial treatment in some patients.

A good argument can be made for administering a β-blocker to most patients with angina, especially younger patients desirous of an active life style unless there is a specific contraindication. In patients who have infrequent or mild episodes of angina relieved promptly by rest or by sublingual nitroglycerin, however, a β-blocker may add little benefit. In patients with more frequent or more severe episodes of angina, it is reasonable to initiate treatment with a β-blocker and to prescribe sublingual nitroglycerin for the relief of discrete episodes of pain. If a β-blocker is effective in reducing or eliminating angina pectoris, additional preparations may be unnecessary. In patients with maximal effects from β-blockade who continue to have pain, addition of a long-acting nitrate preparation or a calcium channel blocker may bring symptoms under better control.

Because of the possible risk of precipitating worsening angina when a β-blocker is abruptly discontinued and because of indirect evidence for a similar problem when long-acting nitrates are abruptly discontinued, these drugs should be tapered over several days when they are being stopped. [However, if a patient is taking a β-blocker and a calcium blocker, the former can be rapidly withdrawn, with no ill effect (25).] It is important to warn all patients of this problem so that they do not casually stop and start these drugs; a corollary to this is the importance of explaining that these drugs are being prescribed chiefly to prevent symptoms, so that patients whose symptoms remit do not conclude that they can try stopping medication themselves.

The potency of β-blockers and of calcium channel blockers in the treatment of angina is about the same. In general, β-blockers are prescribed first to patients with predictable angina (chest pain reproducible after a given effort) who are likely to have fixed obstruction of their coronary arteries—unless there is a specific contraindication, such as chronic obstructive lung disease. A calcium channel blocker is prescribed to patients who have variable chest pain, in whom coronary artery spasm (see "Variant Angina," below) may be playing a role, or to those intolerant of β-blockers.

Because patients who fail to improve after maximal medical management for angina pectoris are considered candidates for coronary arteriography and possible revascularization, it is important to define maximal medical therapy. In practical terms, administration of a β-blocker in increasing doses, until side effects militate against further increase, in conjunction with a dose of long-acting nitrates increased to the point where side effects begin to become intolerable, together with maximal doses of calcium channel blockers, would be considered to constitute maximal medical manage-

ment in most patients. If a β-blocker and a calcium channel blocker are used together, the dose of both may have to be lower than if either is used alone, because of an additive adverse effect on left ventricular function. Similarly, if a nitrate and nifedipine are used together, severe hypotension is more likely and the doses may have to be reduced. If side effects limit the addition of the third drug, the combination of a β-blocker and calcium channel blocker is likely to be more effective than a β-blocker and a long-acting nitrate.

Role of Anticoagulants and of Drugs That Interfere with Platelet Plug Formation

Despite their occasional use, there are no data to support the use of anticoagulants or dipyridamole in patients with angina. The role of aspirin in the treatment of patients with atherosclerotic heart disease is discussed on page 577. In essence, aspirin, 325 mg a day, is probably beneficial to patients with unstable angina (q.v.), but there are no convincing data to support its use in patients with stable angina.

Percutaneous Transluminal Coronary Angioplasty

Percutaneous transluminal coronary angioplasty (PTCA) (26) has introduced an important option for the treatment of coronary artery disease that cannot be controlled by the administration of drugs. This technique has the ability to restore nearly normal coronary flow in diseased native coronary arteries, without the cost and morbidity of bypass surgery. It involves the compression of a critical coronary lesion against the wall of the affected coronary artery by means of an inflatable balloon mounted on a special catheter. Patients are identified as candidates for PTCA after cardiac catheterization has clearly delineated coronary anatomy and after it has been determined that bypass surgery would otherwise be indicated. PTCA was initially used to treat patients with single vessel, proximal, discrete, noncalcific coronary lesions. However, in skilled hands, triple vessel coronary lesions, if they do not straddle branch vessels, can be successfully dilated also (13). Though there are no absolute contraindications to the procedure, patients with arterial dissection or with eccentric and long stenotic lesions are poor candidates and have a higher risk of complications during PTCA. These patients are best treated with surgery.

Patients who are appropriate candidates for PTCA undergo the procedure either immediately after cardiac catheterization or at a subsequent time, depending on the clinical situation and on the needs of the particular patient. The catheter is usually introduced through a femoral artery under local anesthesia. A brachial approach can also be used but requires a cutdown. The coronary orifice is reached with a pre-shaped guiding catheter through which the balloon catheter with the balloon decompressed is inserted. The balloon is positioned halfway across the lesion, and translesional pressure gradients are measured.

(Most significant coronary lesions cause a significant pressure drop across the lesion.) Under fluoroscopic control the balloon is dilated with increasing pressures until there is no more indentation of the balloon or until the previously recorded pressure gradient is essentially abolished and dye injections through the guiding catheter show normal flow and a sufficiently patent coronary artery. Steerable catheters have recently been designed and have significantly widened the spectrum of lesions that can be successfully treated by PTCA. The dilatation results in an actual intimal tear and occasionally a coronary dissection may occur. Therefore, a cardiac surgical team is ordinarily on standby during the procedure. Barring complications, the patient's experience during PTCA and the time of the procedure are the same as they are for coronary angiography (see above). The incidence of major side effects (including dissection, myocardial infarction, and sudden death) is related to the skill and experience of the operator and can be as low as 2 to 4% (4). Overall, the procedure is successful 60 to 80% of the time. After successful angioplasty, patients are maintained on aspirin (see Chapter 52) along with a calcium channel blocker. The calcium channel blocker is ordinarily continued for 2 months after PTCA. However, if there is evidence of ischemia on stress testing or if there is angina, it is appropriate to continue administering the drug. Patients can usually be discharged on the second hospital day and it is advised that they undergo regular stress tests at 3-, 6-, and 12-month intervals. The long-term results of coronary angioplasty are favorable. Though the recurrence rate of stenotic lesions in most centers is about 30%, most recurrences can be successfully treated a second time by the same procedure (27). The vast majority of recurrences occur within the first 8 months after PTCA. Therefore, a lack of symptoms at 8 to 9 months usually indicates an excellent long-term prognosis. Recent European data have shown that the insertion of "stents" into the coronary artery at the site of dilatation reduces the incidence of recurrence. The technique however is still experimental in the United States.

PTCA is an especially attractive therapeutic option in younger patients (40 to 50 years of age) in whom coronary bypass grafts, given the current state of the art, could be expected to remain patent for only 10 to 12 years. Also the comparative cost and morbidity of PTCA versus bypass surgery make the former more attractive if the therapeutic benefit is likely to be the same. Patients can often return to gainful employment 1 week after PTCA versus 3 to 6 months after bypass surgery (31, 32).

Surgical Management

Coronary artery bypass surgery is one of the most common surgical procedures performed in this country today. It is accepted generally that patients with incapacitating angina pectoris who have good left ventricular function and who have failed maximal medical therapy should be considered as candidates for coronary arteriography and subsequent surgery. It has been demonstrated that patients with left main coronary artery disease or its equivalent benefit symptomatically and have increased longevity after surgical intervention designed to increase coronary blood flow (57). Recommendations and results regarding surgery for patients with other lesions are discussed above.

The two surgical methods used today consist of saphenous vein bypass graft or implantation of an internal mammary artery into the native coronary artery circulation. The technique that is used is often based on the surgeon's preference and experience. A well-illustrated brochure, Coronary Artery Bypass Surgery, which explains the procedure and the patient's experience, is available from the American Heart Association.

Patients with good left ventricular function have a 1 to 2% mortality rate from surgery and 5 to 10% of patients will develop evidence of myocardial infarction during the perioperative period. The risk of complications from myocardial infarction in these patients, however, is small since the infarct occurs at a time when myocardial oxygen need is diminished because of cardiopulmonary bypass. Also, the infarct occurs in a setting where complications such as arrhythmias are recognized and treated promptly. Nevertheless, it does represent a risk of loss of functioning myocardium. Perioperative infarction is more likely to occur in older patients and in patients with severe disease distal to a proximal obstruction.

About 60% of properly selected patients initially will have complete (or nearly complete) relief of angina pectoris, and another 20% will have a significant decrease in angina (43). There will be a demonstrable increase in exercise tolerance after surgery in about 60 to 80% of such patients.

Historically, up to 50% of patients have developed recurrent angina within 5 years of bypass surgery (18). The diagnosis of recurrent angina should be confirmed by exercise stress testing. Initial treatment is the same as it is for patients who have not had bypass surgery: nitrates, β-blockers, or calcium channel blockers. Patients who prove to be unresponsive to medical treatment should undergo coronary angiography in an effort to delineate new lesions that possibly could be amenable either to percutaneous angioplasty or to repeat bypass surgery. In an attempt to prevent formation of such lesions it is now common practice to administer aspirin and persantine to patients after bypass (see page 577) and to treat hyperlipidemia aggressively (see Chapter 75).

The postpericardiotomy syndrome develops in approximately 30% of patients after bypass surgery, usually within 2 to 4 weeks (but sometimes as early as a few days or as late as 6 months after the operation.) The syndrome is characterized by fever, pleuritic chest pain, and, often, by pleural and pericardial effusions. Large effusions may require drainage, but most patients respond to diuretics and to a nonsteroidal anti-inflammatory agent (e.g., indomethacin, 25 to 50 mg three times a day for 1 to 2 weeks). Patients who are refractory to such treatment usually respond to prednisone, initially 60 mg a day for 2 to 3 days with tapering of the dose over 7 to 10 days. Recently, it has been suggested that graft occlusion is more likely in patients with postbypass pericarditis. Constrictive pericarditis is a late rare complication of the postpericardiotomy syndrome; when it occurs, pericardial stripping is often necessary.

Dysesthesia, swelling, and itching are not uncommon in the leg from which the vein was harvested and can persist for several months. The swelling usually responds to the use of support hose or to elevation of the legs periodically during the day. If the itching is severe and if there is no evidence of local infection, topical corticosteroid ointments are often very effective.

Bypass surgery has been shown to prolong life in several patient subsets (see above). In addition 60% of patients who either were working just before bypass surgery or discontinued work because of cardiac symptoms return to work after surgery. Early ambulation is advisable and the role of cardiac rehabilitation, as early as 6 to 8 weeks postoperatively, cannot be overemphasized (see detailed discussion, Chapter 58).

UNSTABLE ANGINA

Unstable angina is a term used to describe pain due to cardiac ischemia that is becoming more intense, is occurring more frequently—often provoked by diminishing effort (perhaps even at rest)—and is being relieved less readily by nitroglycerin. The syndrome has also been called crescendo angina and preinfarction angina. Sometimes unstable angina will develop in a patient with previously stable, reasonably controlled angina; at other times, it will develop in a patient with recent onset of ischemic symptoms. During the episode, the ECG shows ST elevation or depression and/or T wave inversion that revert to normal when the pain has abated. Because of the increased risks of myocardial infarction and of sudden death and because of the need for aggressive medical therapy, patients with unstable angina should be hospitalized (17, 19, 45). Aggressive medical treatment with heparin, β-blockers, calcium channel blockers, and intravenous nitroglycerin is usually implemented. Coronary arteriography is indicated as soon as possible in all patients, especially those in whom pain is not controlled by medical therapy, to determine their suitability for coronary bypass surgery or PTCA (see above).

The prognosis of these patients after hospital discharge is described in Chapter 58.

VARIANT ANGINA

Variant angina (Prinzmetal's angina) is, in a sense, unstable in that it occurs usually at rest but, unlike typical angina, does not occur on exertion or in response to emotional stress. Attacks of pain are experienced often at the same time each day, frequently awakening the patient early in the morning. During the attacks, there is ST segment elevation that reverts to baseline when the attack is over; there are also, in about one-third of the patients, transient atrioventricular blocks and/or arrhythmias (including ventricular tachycardia or fibrillation). Unlike unstable angina, pain is usually promptly relieved by sublingual nitroglycerin.

It is now clear that coronary artery spasm (29) often plays a major role in the pathogenesis of variant angina. Two groups of patients have been identified. By far the larger group (85% of patients) have fixed, often proximal, obstruction of a major coronary artery; angina in this group frequently is associated with spasm of the artery near the site of obstruction. The variant syndrome in this group of patients commonly follows months or years of stable typical angina pectoris or follows a myocardial infarction.

The smaller group with variant angina (15% of patients) have normal coronary arteries but have spasm of one of the arteries, thereby reducing blood supply to the myocardium, resulting in ischemic pain. These patients are usually younger and are predominantly women. There is usually no history of typical angina or of myocardial infarction in these patients, and infrequently a history of a systemic arteritis syndrome may be obtained. The ST elevation observed during the anginal attack is a manifestation of coronary artery spasm. It can often be confirmed by arteriography, either by the spontaneous occurrence of arterial spasm and chest pain during the procedure or by induction of arterial spasm by the administration of ergonovine. It is important to perform arteriography in such patients since those with normal coronary arteries are obviously not candidates for bypass surgery or PTCA and most respond favorably to treatment with calcium channel blockers. Calcium channel blockers are the drugs of choice in such patients. If used without calcium channel blockers, β-blockers may potentiate coronary artery spasm because of unopposed α-adrenergic vasoconstriction. However a double blind study of patients with rest angina showed that β-blockers, when added to nifedipine and nitrates, significantly reduced the number of episodes of angina in treated patients as compared with a control group on treatment with nifedipine and nitrates alone (25).

ANGINA WITH NORMAL CORONARY ARTERIES

Recently several investigators have reported large series of patients with typical angina, angiographically normal coronary arteries, and no obvious myocardial abnormality (46). Such patients may have ischemic exercise ECG responses. There are several possible etiologies for this condition. Accumulating evidence implicates coronary spasm (see above) in several patients; therefore it is important during angiography to confirm the diagnosis if possible by infusing ergonovine. The symptoms may also be due to abnormal coronary reserve (e.g., in patients with hypertension, aortic stenosis and regurgitation, and hypertropic cardiomyopathy). Abnormalities of platelet function, small vessel disease, and mitral valve prolapse have been found in some patients. The prognosis of such patients is generally favorable with survival being comparable to age- and sex-matched controls with normal coronaries. In the treatment of such patients nitrates, calcium channel blockers, and β-blockers are often effective. Such patients must be distinguished from the occasional patient who uses chest pain for secondary gain and who likely fails to respond to all therapy.

SILENT ISCHEMIA

Recent studies have demonstrated that many episodes of myocardial ischemia are in fact painless. Such "silent" ischemic episodes may be detected either during exercise treadmill testing (ETT) or by continuous electrocardiographic (ECG) monitoring. Asymptomatic ischemic ST segment changes on ECG monitoring are common in patients with coronary artery disease and have been correlated with transient abnormalities in myocardial perfusion and function (12).

Recent studies have focused on the prognostic value of silent ischemia as detected by ECG monitoring in patients with various manifestations of coronary artery disease. Studies in patients with stable angina have shown that there are many asymptomatic episodes of ischemia noted in ambulatory patients that often occur at low heart rates during activities of every day life, without an apparent significant increase in myocardial oxygen demand; and such episodes may even be precipitated by mental stress (12). Studies in patients with unstable angina or in the early postinfarction phase have identified silent ischemia to be a powerful predictor of poor outcome (23, 24). Patients with unstable angina who also have silent ischemia have a significantly greater frequency of bypass surgery, angioplasty, or recurrent symptomatic angina as compared with patients without silent ischemia (23). In high risk patients after myocardial infarction (patients with ejection fraction < 40% and/or Lown Class IV arrhythmias) silent ischemia detected on predischarge ECG monitoring has been shown to be the single most powerful predictor of poor outcome (24). The presence of silent ischemia within the first 3 days of myocardial infarction has also been shown to be associated with a greater frequency of recurrent ischemic events. Though several studies have identified silent ischemia to be a poor prognostic factor for patients with coronary artery disease (8), it is unknown whether treatment in such patients affects prognosis favorably. Studies to address this issue are ongoing.

General References

Diamond GA, Forrester JS: Analysis of probability as an aid in the clinical diagnosis of coronary-artery disease. *N Engl J Med* 300:1350, 1979.

A review of the application of Bayes' theorem to this problem. Heberden W: *Commentaries on the history and cure of diseases.* New York, Hofner, 1962.

Available from the New York Academy of Science.

Rutherford J, Braunwald E, Cohn PF: Chronic ischemic heart disease. In: Braunwald E (ed): *Heart Disease.* Philadelphia, WB Saunders, 1988, p. 1314.

A complete discussion of the diagnosis and management of angina pectoris.

Specific References

1. Abrams J, Gerety B, Schroeder K, Raizada V: Lack of hemodynamic effects of transdermal nitroglycerin discs. *Circulation* 70 (suppl II): 188, 1984.
2. American Heart Association: Risk factors and coronary disease: a statement for physicians. *Circulation* 62:449A, 1980.
3. Block Jr WJ, Grumpacher EL, Dry TJ, Gage RP: Prognosis of angina pectoris. *JAMA* 150:259, 1952.
4. Bredlau CE, Gruentzig AR, Douglas JS, King SB: Acute complications of percutaneous transluminal coronary angioplasty (PTCA)-initial experience in 3000 consecutive patient attempts. *Circulation* 70 (suppl II): 106, 1984.
5. Bruschke AVC, Proudfit WL, Sones Jr FM: Progress study of 590 consecutive nonsurgical cases of coronary disease followed 5-9 years: arteriographic correlations. *Circulation* 47:1147, 1973.
6. CASS Principal Investigators and Their Associates. Coronary artery surgery study (CASS): a randomized trial of coronary artery bypass surgery. *Circulation* 68:939, 1983.
7. Chiang BN, Perlman LV, Ostrander LD: Relationship of premature systoles to coronary heart disease and sudden death in the Tecumseh epidemiologic study. *Ann Intern Med* 70:1159, 1969.
8. Cohn PF: When is concern about silent myocardial ischemia justified? *Ann Intern Med* 100:597, 1984.
9. Cohn PF, Gorlin R, Vokonas PS, et al: A quantitative clinical index for the diagnosis of symptomatic coronary-artery disease. *N Engl J Med* 286:901, 1972.
10. Crawford MH, LeWinter MM, O'Rourke RA, et al: Combined propranolol and digoxin therapy in angina pectoris. *Ann Intern Med* 83:449, 1975.
11. Danahy DT, Aronow WS: Hemodynamics and antianginal effects of high dose oral isosorbide dinitrate after chronic use. *Circulation* 56:205, 1977.
12. Deanfield JE, Shea M, Ribiero P, de Landsheere CM, et al: Transient ST-segment depression as a marker of myocardial ischemia during daily life. *Am J Cardiol* 54:1195, 1984.
13. Dorros G, Singh S, Janke LM: Coronary angioplasty in multivessel coronary disease. *Circulation* 70 (suppl II): 107, 1984.
14. Elkayam U, Kulick D, McIntosh N, et al: Incidence of early tolerance to hemodynamic effects of continuous infusion of nitroglycerin in patients with coronary artery disease and heart failure. *Circulation* 76:577, 1987.
15. Ellstad MH, Wan MKC: Predictive implications of stress testing: follow-up of 2700 subjects after maximum treadmill stress testing. *Circulation* 51:363, 1975.
16. European Coronary Surgery Study Group: Prospective randomised study of coronary artery bypass surgery in stable angina pectoris: second interim report. *Lancet* 2:491, 1980.
17. Gazes PC, Mobley Jr EM, Faris Jr HM, et al: Preinfarction (unstable) angina—a prospective study. Ten years followup. Prognostic significance of electrocardiographic changes. *Circulation* 48:331, 1973.
18. Gersh BJ, Kronmal RA, Schaff HV, et al: Long-term (5 year) results of coronary bypass surgery in patients 65 years or older: a report from the coronary artery surgery study. *Circulation* 68 (suppl II): 190, 1983.
19. Gerstenblith G, Ouyang P, Achuff SC, et al: Nifedipine in unstable angina: a double-blind randomized trial. *N Engl J Med* 306:885, 1982.
20. Gibson RS, Watson DD, Craddock GB, et al: Prediction of cardiac events after uncomplicated myocardial infarction; a prospective study comparing predischarge exercise thallium-201 scintigraphy and coronary angiography. *Circulation* 68:321, 1983.
21. Goldberger AL: Recognition of ECG pseudo-infarct patterns. *Mod Concepts of Cardiovasc Dis* 49:13 (March), 1980.
22. Gottlieb SO, Allred EN, Bleecker ER, et al: "Urban Angina"— Low levels of carbon monoxide exacerbate myocardial is-

chemia: a multicenter, randomized controlled trial. *Circulation*78 (Supp II):II-257, 1988.

23. Gottlieb SO, Weisfeldt ML, Ouyang P, et al: Silent ischemia as a marker for early unfavorable outcomes in patients with unstable angina. *N Engl J Med* 314:1214, 1986.
24. Gottlieb SO, Gottlieb SH, Achuff SC, et al: Silent ischemia on Holter monitoring predicts mortality in high-risk post-infarction patients. *JAMA* 259:1030, 1988.
25. Gottlieb SO, Weisfeldt ML, Ouyang P, et al: Propranolol for unstable angina in the era of calcium antagonists: a double blind randomized trial. *Circulation* 70 (suppl II): 48, 1984.
26. Gruentzig A: Transluminal dilatation of coronary artery stenosis. *Lancet* 1:263, 1978.
27. Hall DP, Gruentzig AR: Recurrence rate after double-vessel dilatation. *Circulation* 70 (suppl II): 107, 1984.
28. Hamilton GW: Myocardial imaging with thallium-201: the controversy over its clinical usefulness in ischemic heart disease. *J Nucl Med* 20:1201, 1979.
29. Hilles LD, Braunwald E: Coronary-artery spasm. *N Engl J Med* 299:695, 1978.
30. Hutter Jr AM, DeSantis RW, Flynn T, et al: Nontransmural myocardial infarction: a comparison of hospital and late clinical course of patients with that of matched patients with transmural anterior and transmural inferior myocardial infarction. *Am J Cardiol*48:595, 1981.
31. Jang GC, Block PC, Cowley MJ, et al: Comparative cost analysis of coronary angioplasty and coronary bypass surgery: results from a national co-operative study. *Circulation*66 (suppl II): 124, 1982.
32. Jang GC, Gruentzig AR, Block PC, et al: Work profile of patients following coronary angioplasty or coronary bypass surgery: results from a national cooperative study. *Circulation* 66 (suppl II): 123, 1982.
33. Kannel WB, Feinleib M: Natural history of angina pectoris in the Framingham study: prognosis and survival. *Am J Cardiol* 29:154, 1972.
34. Kennedy CC, Spiekerman RE, Lindsay Jr MI, et al: One-year graduated exercise program for men with angina pectoris. *Mayo Clin Proc* 51:232, 1976.
35. Kirk ES, Factor SM: Pathophysiology of myocardial ischemia. In: Hurst JW (ed): *The Heart*. 6th ed. New York, McGraw-Hill, p. 856, 1986.
36. Leppo J, Boucher CA, Okada RD, et al: Serial thallium-201 myocardial imaging after dipyridamole infusion: diagnostic utility in detecting coronary stenoses and relationship to regional wall motion. *Circulation* 66:649, 1982.
37. Lipid Research Clinics Program: The lipid research clinics coronary primary prevention trial results. II. The relationship of reduction in incidence of coronary heart disease to cholesterol lowering. *JAMA* 251:365, 1984.
38. Maseri A, Chierchia S: Coronary artery spasm: demonstration, definition, diagnosis, and consequences. *Prog Cardiovasc Dis* 25:169, 1982.
39. Maseri A, Severi S, De Nes M, et al: "Variant" angina. One aspect of a continuous spectrum of vasospastic myocardial ischemia. Pathogenetic mechanisms, estimated incidence and clinical and coronary arteriographic findings in 138 patients. *Am J Cardiol* 42:1019, 1978.
40. Mattingly TW, Robb GP, Marks HH: Stress tests in the detection of coronary disease. *Postgrad Med* 24:4, 1958.

41. Mock MB, Ringqvist I, Fisher LD, et al: Survival of medically treated patients in the Coronary Artery Surgery Study (CASS) registry. *Circulation* 66:562, 1982.
42. Multiple Risk Factor Intervention Trial Research Group: Baseline rest electrocardiographic abnormalities, antihypertensive treatment, and mortality in the Multiple Risk Factor Intervention Trial. *Am J Cardiol* 55:1, 1985.
43. Mundth ED, Austen WG: Surgical measures for coronary heart disease. *N Engl J Med* 293:13, 75 and 124, 1975.
44. Norris RM, Caughey DE, Mercer CJ, Scott PJ: Prognosis after myocardial infarction. Six-year follow-up. *Br Heart J* 36:786, 1974.
45. Ouyang P, Brinker JA, Mellits ED, et al: Variables predictive of successful medical therapy in patients with unstable angina: selection by multivariate analysis from clinical, electrocardiographic, and angiographic evaluations. *Circulation* 70:367, 1984.
46. Pasternak RC, Thibault GT, Savoia M, et al: Chest pain with angiographically insignificant coronary arterial obstruction. Clinical presentation and long-term follow-up. *Am J Med* 68:813, 1980.
47. Read RC, Murphy ML, Hultgren HN, et al: Survival of men treated for chronic stable angina pectoris. A cooperative randomized study. *J Thorac Cardiovasc Surg* 75:1, 1978.
48. Passamani E, Davis KB, Gillespie MJ, Killip T: A randomized trial of coronary artery bypass surgery. Survival of patients with a low ejection fraction. *N Engl J Med* 312:1665, 1985.
49. Redwood DR, Borer JS, Epstein SE: Whither the ST segment during exercise? (Editorial) *Circulation* 54:703, 1976 .
50. Reicheck N, Goldstein RE, Redwood DR, Epstein ST: Sustained effects of nitroglycerin ointment in patients with angina pectoris. *Circulation* 50:348, 1974.
51. Ritchie JL, Zaret BL, Strauss HW, et al: Myocardial imaging with thallium-201: a multicenter study in patients with angina pectoris or acute myocardial infarction. *Am J Cardiol* 42:345, 1978.
52. Rochmis P, Blackburn H: Exercise tests: a survey of procedures, safety, and litigation experience in approximately 170,000 tests. *JAMA* 217:1061, 1971.
53. Sharma, B, Taylor SH: Reversible left-ventricular failure in angina pectoris. *Lancet* 2:902, 1970.
54. Silber S, Krause KH, Theisen K: Nitrate-tolerance: dependence on dosage intervals? *Circulation* 70 (suppl II): 189, 1984.
55. Sonnenblick EH, Strobeck JE: Derived indexes of ventricular and myocardial function. *N Engl J Med* 296:978, 1977.
56. Stone PH, Antman EM, Muller JE, Braunwald E: Calcium channel blocking agents in the treatment of cardiovascular disorders. II. Hemodynamic effects and clinical applications. *Ann Intern Med* 93:886, 1980.
57. Takaro T, Hultgren HW, Lipton MJ, et al: The V.A. cooperative randomized study of surgery for coronary arterial occlusive disease. II. Subgroup with significant left main lesions. *Circulation* 54 (suppl III): 107, 1976.
58. Theroux P, Waters DD, Halphen C, et al: Prognostic value of exercise testing soon after myocardial infarction. *N Engl J Med* 301:341, 1979.
59. Weiner DA, Ryan TJ, McCabe CH, et al: Exercise stress testing. Correlations among history of angina, ST-segment response and prevalence of coronary-artery disease in the coronary surgery study (CASS). *N Engl J Med* 301:230, 1979.

C H A P T E R   58

Postmyocardial Infarction Care, Cardiac Rehabilitation, and Physical Conditioning

MAHMUD A. THAMER, M.D.
KERRY J. STEWART, Ed.D.
L. RANDOL BARKER, M.D.

The average hospital stay for acute myocardial infarction (MI) in the United States decreased from over three weeks in the 1960s to about two weeks in the 1970s and is now approximately one week. This decrease in the length of hospital care of MI patients has added greater weight to the ambulatory care of these patients.

EPIDEMIOLOGY OF MYOCARDIAL INFARCTION

Care of the patient who has survived a myocardial infarction is common in ambulatory practice. There are roughly 7 million survivors of myocardial infarction in the United States at any time. Each year, approximately 1 million persons are added to this group, and about 1 million die (4). About two-thirds of the

survivors have had uncomplicated MIs and, therefore, have relatively good long-term prognoses.

The majority of persons who have MIs are under the age of 60. It is estimated that in the United States one man in five will have an MI before the age of 60 and that one in 10 to 15 men in this age group will die of atherosclerotic heart disease. These risks are 2 to 3 times lower in age-matched women (37). The higher male mortality rates from coronary artery disease (CAD) are particularly striking among young white males. In 1979, the male to female ratios of mortality from CAD in the United States were 5.2:1 at ages 35 to 44 and 2.4:1 at ages 65 to 74; among nonwhites, the respective ratios were 2.8:1 and 1.6:1 (22). However, these findings appear to be related to the higher incidence and prevalence of CAD in white males. For patients hospitalized with an acute MI, females, particularly black women, have higher mortality during hospitalization and in the 48 months after discharge (44).

Two epidemiological observations underscore the importance of ambulatory care in reducing mortality due to CAD.

1. About three-quarters of all deaths from CAD occur outside the hospital.
2. In the past two decades, the number of people dying of CAD in the United States has decreased significantly; this decrease seems to be due largely to changes that have occurred outside the hospital (i.e., reduction in CAD risk factors and prehospital and postdischarge management of acute MI).

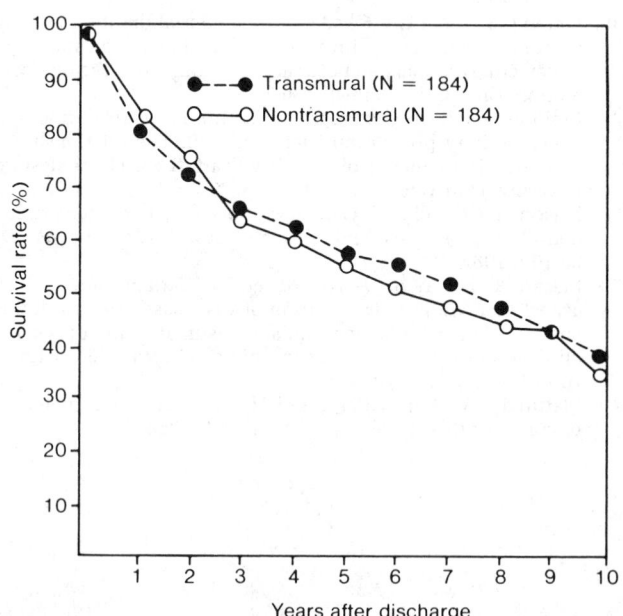

Figure 58.1. Survival rates in matched samples of transmural and nontransmural myocardial infarction patients discharged alive in metropolitan Baltimore, 7/1/66 to 6/30/67 and 1/1/71 to 12/31/71. (From Szklo M, *et al*: Nontransmural MI: prognostic implications, *Primary Cardiology* 6:76, 1980.)

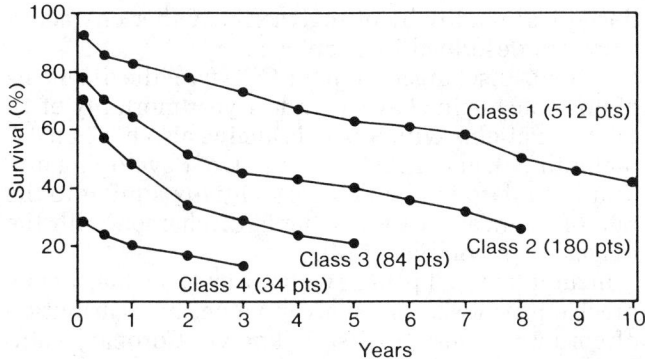

Figure 58.2. Survival after acute myocardial infarction based upon Killip classification (810 patients admitted to the Duke Medical Center Coronary Care Unit from 1967 to 1978). (From: Rosati RA, Harris PJ): In Fries J, Ehrlich GE (eds): *Prognosis; Contemporary Outcomes of Disease.* Bowie MD, The Charles Press Publishers, 1981.)

Table 58.1.

Characteristics Associated with Increase in Mortality after Discharge of Patients Who Have Had Myocardial Infarction (MI)[a]

ADMISSION CHARACTERISTICS
   History of a previous MI
   Congestive heart failure (chest X-ray or Killip classification)
   History of hypertension
   Extent of left ventricular ischemia (radionuclide scintigraphy, cardiac enzymes)
CHARACTERISTICS AT DISCHARGE
   Early (within 10 days) post-MI angina, with transient ST-T changes[b]
   Ejection fraction ≤ 40% (radionuclide ventriculography, arteriography)
   Complex ventricular arrhythmia[c] (Holter monitor)
   Left main proximal, left anterior descending, or three-vessel CAD (arteriography)
   Positive limited early post-MI ECG stress test (within 2–3 weeks after MI)
   Ventricular aneurysm developing in acute stage of MI (28)
CHARACTERISTICS FOLLOWING DISCHARGE
   ECG abnormalities, especially S-T segment depression, ≥ 3 months after MI
   Cigarette smoking

[a] Numbers in parentheses are references.
[b] Mortality risk highest when ECG shows "ischemia at a distance," i.e., transient ischemic S-T changes in myocardial location that is different from the location of the patient's MI.
[c] Multifocal premature ventricular contractions (PVCs), runs of two or more sequential ectopic ventricular beats, or PVCs with R on T pattern.

PROGNOSIS OF PATIENTS DISCHARGED FROM CORONARY CARE UNITS

Patients discharged after hospitalization in coronary care units (CCUs) may be divided into three broad categories: those who have had a confirmed MI, those who have had unstable angina, and those who have had cardiac arrest without a confirmed MI. The different prognoses for patients in these three categories have been delineated in the past two decades.

Survivors of Myocardial Infarction

Mortality

The overall first year mortality for hospital survivors of an MI is about 5 to 10%. Thereafter, the annual mortality remains between 3 and 5% for the next 15 years. These figures are the same for patients surviving transmural or subendocardial MIs (Fig. 58.1). Most of the deaths in the first year occur during the 3 months after discharge, and they occur chiefly in patients with one or more of the high risk characteristics listed in Table 58.1.

The classification of acute MI developed by Killip according to the presence and severity of congestive heart failure (CHF) on admission to the CCU is one of the most useful prognostic indices. Class I patients have no evidence of CHF on admission; class II patients have mild CHF; class III patients present with pulmonary edema; and class IV patients present with shock. Figure 58.2 shows the strikingly different survival rates among persons in these four classes, ranging from a 2-year survival rate of about 80% in class I to less than 20% in class IV (33).

Of the other characteristics listed in Table 58.1, the most powerful predictors of mortality during the first year following an MI are one or more of the following: a history of a previous MI; the development of early (within 10 days) post-MI angina accompanied by transient ST segment or T wave changes; an ejection fraction of 40% or less, late hospital phase (predischarge), complex ventricular arrhythmia, proximal left main, left anterior descending, or three-vessel coronary artery occlusive disease; and a positive submaximal stress test within the first month after an MI. The incidence of sudden death in patients discharged from hospital with *both* left ventricular (LV) dysfunction (ejection fraction <40%) and frequent premature ventricular contractions (PVCs) (>10/hour) is 11 times that of otherwise similar patients with neither of these findings. On reclassification of survivors 6 months after MI with regard to the presence or absence of frequent PVCs and LV dysfunction, these factors are no longer associated with increased risk of sudden coronary death over a further follow-up period of up to 18 months (28). Left ventricular aneurysm developing within two days of the acute MI also brings a high risk of death during the first year, independent of LV function (27).

Morbidity

Postinfarction angina occurs during the year after an MI in approximately 75% of persons who had angina before their MI, and in about 50% of those who did not have it before their MI (46). In patients who are free of angina or other cardiac symptoms in the hospital, limited (target heart rate of 130 beats/minute or limiting symptoms or ischemic signs) electrocardiogram (ECG) stress testing before discharge increases the ability to predict whether or not a patient will develop angina. Angina during the years after an

MI occurs in 86% of patients with positive stress tests (96% of patients with both a positive early post-MI stress test and a previous history of angina) and in 36% of those with negative stress tests (only in 26% of patients with both a negative stress test and no previous history of angina) (46). Additionally, cardiac patients whose limited, early post-MI stress testing shows ischemic ST changes (≥0.1 mV exercise-induced ST depression) and/or limited work capacity (≤5 METs) have two or more times the risk of recurrent myocardial infarction and of death over the ensuing year (41).

Other medical complications include congestive heart failure, life-threatening arrhythmias, systemic emboli, and post-MI syndrome.

The psychological and social sequelae during the year after an MI depend both upon the severity of the patient's MI and upon his premorbid psychosocial situation. Of survivors of MIs, 10 to 20% are never able to return to their former occupational and recreational activities, whereas the other 80 to 90% are able to do so within 2 to 6 months. Based upon extensive observations, Cassem and Hackett have developed a hypothetical profile of emotional and behavioral reactions to an MI (Fig. 58.3); in this scheme, depression or maladaptive behavior related to preexisting personality traits will be present in 10% or more of patients during the period after discharge from the hospital. Persistent denial, anxiety, depression, and dependency after an MI are associated with a decrease in the rate of return to work and usual social activities, regardless of the patient's physiological status.

Patients with Unstable Angina

Unstable angina is defined as pain due to cardiac ischemia that is becoming more intense, meaning that it is occurring more frequently—often provoked by less effort (even occurring at rest)—and is being relieved less readily by nitroglycerine. Other characteristics are described in Chapter 57.

Patients discharged from the CCU with the diagnosis of unstable angina have a crude 1-year mortality of 10 to 30%. Patients with unstable angina also have an 8% 6-month risk and a 12% 1-year risk of developing myocardial infarction, which is essentially similar to the rate of recurrent MI for patients discharged with the diagnosis of completed MI.

In an individual patient with unstable angina, a more precise prognosis can be given when the distribution of coronary artery disease is known. Coronary catheterization has shown that left main coronary artery disease is more common in patients discharged with the diagnosis of unstable angina than in those discharged with the diagnosis of completed MI (15 *versus* 5%, respectively). Another 10% have diffuse coronary artery disease, 10% have normal coronary arteries (and are presumed to have coronary artery spasm or small vessel disease as the etiology of their chest pain), and the remaining 65% are more or less equally divided between single, double, and triple coronary vessel disease (31). This information is of clinical importance because of the demonstrated superiority of surgical over medical treatment of left main coronary artery disease. The prognoses associated with each of the above patterns and the management of unstable angina are described below and in Chapter 57.

Survivors of Cardiac Arrests Who Have Not Had a Myocardial Infarction

The first year mortality of all survivors of out-of-hospital cardiac arrest who have not had an MI is about 25%, with about three-quarters of deaths occurring within the first 6 months after hospital discharge. This is approximately 3 times the mortality rate of survivors of out-of-hospital cardiac arrest who subsequently show completed MIs. In a study of over 200 survivors of out-of-hospital cardiac arrest, followed for over 4 years, the rate of recurrence of ventricular fibrillation or of sudden death in patients without an acute MI was 31% compared with 5% for out-of-hospital survivors of cardiac arrest who subsequently evolved electrocardiographic changes of acute MI. The median time to recurrent circulatory arrest was 20 weeks. More than 70% of the episodes of ventricular fibrillation were unexpected, occurring during sleep or during the usual activities of daily living (35).

Therefore, the survivors of non-MI ventricular fibrillation constitute a highly unstable group of patients who require aggressive and highly individualized management. The multiplicity of recent advances in electrophysiology, antiarrhythmics, automatic implantable defibrillators, and the many innovative surgical approaches to the medically intractable but symptomatic ventricular dysrhythmia dictate prompt referral of such high risk patients to a consulting cardiologist.

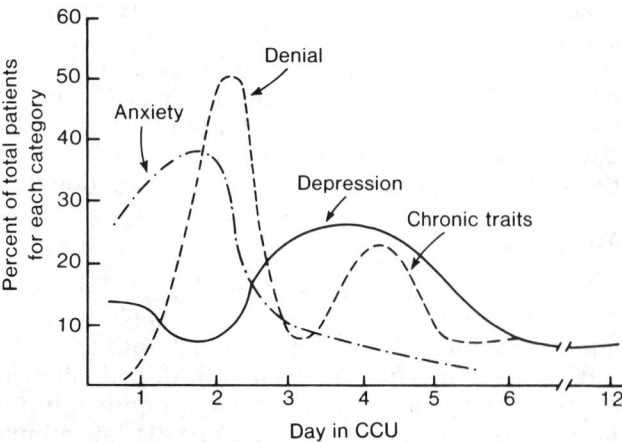

Figure 58.3. Hypothetical patterns and frequencies of emotional and behavioral reactions of coronary care unit (CCU) patients. (Adapted from Cassem NH, Hackett TP: Psychiatric consultation in a coronary care unit. *Ann Intern Med* 75:9, 1971.)

Table 58.2.
Plan of Care for Survivors of Myocardial Infarction after Hospital Discharge

PATIENT EDUCATION (OBJECTIVES FOR ALL PATIENTS)[a]
  Understands disease process (damage to the heart which heals in a few months, leaves a scar)
  Understands likely prognosis
  Understands and follows progressive activity schedule[b]
  Understands approximate timetable for return to work[b]
  Understands importance of controlling major risk factors (smoking, hypercholesterolemia, hypertension) and takes action to control them
  Knows how to recognize principal cardiac symptoms (angina, tachycardia, heart failure, hypotension) and understands how to use sublingual nitroglycerine
  Participates in group classes after discharge[c]
  Gets answers to questions specific to his/her lifestyle
MEDICAL MANAGEMENT
  All patients
    Review in-hospital course for prognostic characteristics (see Table 58.1) and for medications prescribed at discharge
    Assess and reinforce above patient education
    Check periodically for complications of infarction (see Table 58.6)
    Check for behavioral-psychiatric complications
    Check ECG 2–3 months after discharge
  Selected patients
    β-Blocker, calcium antagonists, and/or aspirin treatment (when not contraindicated)
    Referral for physical conditioning[c]

[a] Essential to include the patient's spouse in all aspects of education.
[b] Serial exercise stress tests may be utilized to plan progressive activity (see the text).
[c] If programs are available in the community.

REHABILITATION AND MANAGEMENT AFTER MYOCARDIAL INFARCTION

The majority of patients discharged after MI can expect to return to most of their usual activities within 6 weeks to 6 months. For a smaller number of patients, complications of their MI make this outcome impossible. In either situation, an organized plan for care should be followed (Table 58.2). This plan should include the education of the patient and his family, so that they can participate effectively in the rehabilitation process, and should assure optimal monitoring and medical treatment of the patient by the physician and cardiac rehabilitation specialists.

Patient Education

Most hospitals initiate education about myocardial infarction as soon as the patient is clinically stable. The educational program is often the responsibility of a cardiac rehabilitation nurse. Patient education should cover the following: the nature of coronary heart disease; cardiac symptoms; cardiac drugs; modification of major risk factors (smoking, hypertension, and hyperlipidemia); and guidelines for resumption of physical activities (includes sexual activity) and return to work. It should be emphasized that myocardial infarction is a manifestation of a disease process that has been going on for many years. Many patients will attribute their MI to what they were doing at the moment it actually occurred. The patient must under-

stand that the MI would have occurred regardless of what he was doing that particular day and that the likelihood of a recurrence may best be diminished by following prescribed medical therapy and making lifestyle changes. These matters may be discussed in a general sense, usually in a group setting.

Individualized information should be provided in a *predischarge conference* at which the patient and his spouse are encouraged to ask questions. The conference should include review of any adverse prognostic features identified before discharge (Table 58.1); the medications prescribed at discharge; discussion of specific plans for cardiac rehabilitation, diet, and smoking modification; a chance for ventilation about emotional stress-laden issues; and realistic appraisal of expectations of return to work. Because of the high frequency of postinfarction angina (see above), it is especially important to describe this symptom to patients who have never had it and to point out to all patients that it may occur with the increased activity recommended for the coming weeks. Every patient should be given sublingual nitroglycerin, and the correct use of this drug should be reviewed (see Chapter 57).

Because patients may not retain the information they hear in the hospital, it is important to *provide this information in writing* and to assess and reinforce patient understanding of it after discharge. The patient education booklet *After a Heart Attack* (available from the American Heart Association) gives a useful general account of the disease process, prognosis, coronary risk factors, and rehabilitation process. Risk factor modification is discussed in detail in Chapter 20 (practical approaches to smoking cessation), Chapter 62 (treatment of hypertension), and Chapter 75 (low cholesterol diet).

Many community hospitals have developed *group classes* for survivors of MIs and their spouses. Typically, patients and their spouses are invited to participate in a number of weekly meetings during the first or second month after discharge. Sessions are usually led by a nurse, a social worker, or a cardiologist with the objective of having participants raise questions about the recovery period so that they provide mutual support by sharing experiences with each other. Additional resources available in many communities are patient-run "heart clubs" and physician or allied health professionally-supervised physical conditioning programs (see "Physical Conditioning" below). There are also several nationally distributed newsletters for patients with coronary artery disease (e.g., "The Coronary Club Bulletin", 9500 Euclid Avenue, Cleveland, Ohio, 44195, telephone: 216-444-3690).

Postdischarge Appointments

In general, each patient who has had an MI should be encouraged to telephone his physician at least once during the first week at home, to discuss any questions that arise, and an office visit should be scheduled within

Table 58.3.
Recommendations According to Stress-Test Risk Stratification 3 to 6 Weeks after Myocardial Infarction[a]

LOW RISK PATIENTS
These patients have a peak workload of 5 METs[b] or more in the absence of exercise-induced angina pectoris or ST-segment depression.
Recommendations
Further diagnostic testing is unlikely to identify patients at an even lower risk and is, therefore, not indicated. The effect, if any, of medical or surgical therapy on the prognosis of these patients is difficult to demonstrate because of their very low risk. Treatment should emphasize the reduction of risk factors, especially the control of hypertension, cessation of smoking, and modification of diet.
MODERATE RISK PATIENTS
These patients have a peak workload of less than 5 METs, a peak systolic pressure of less than 110 mm Hg, or severe myocardial ischemia, defined as angina or ischemic ST-segment depression of 0.2 mV or more appearing at a heart rate of 130 to 140 beats per minute or less.
Indication for Coronary Arteriography
In patients at moderate risk, coronary arteriography is indicated.

[a] From Evaluation of Patients after Recent Acute Myocardial Infarction. (Position paper, American College of Physicians. *Ann Intern Med* 110:485, 1989.)
[b] MET (metabolic equivalent) is the energy requirement for a certain level of activity. One MET is the energy requirement at rest.

2 to 3 weeks. Before this visit, it is important to review the patient's hospital summary to determine whether adverse prognostic features were present (see Table 58.1) and to identify the medications prescribed at discharge. The visit should be divided between an assessment of the patient's progress in his rehabilitation (physical activity level, diet and smoking modifications, emotional status, understanding of the overall plan of care, expectation about return to work) and an assessment of his medical status (manifestations of ischemia and heart failure, blood pressure status, and review of current medications). Two or more additional office visits, similar to the first visit, should be scheduled during the 3 months after an MI, and the patient should be encouraged to telephone at any time about symptoms or questions.

At about 4 to 6 weeks post-MI, a maximal exercise stress should be considered, as this can provide helpful therapeutic and prognostic information regarding the patient's disease. Table 58.3 summarizes the recent criteria and recommendations of the American College of Physicians, based on stratification into low-risk and moderate-risk findings in this stress test. The stress test is also used to assess functional capacity and is very helpful in guiding the return to work process (see below). At about 3 months, an ECG should be obtained; it will constitute the patient's new "baseline" ECG with which future tracings should be compared.

Activity Schedule

Table 58.4 contains a practical summary (for use by the patient) of symptom recognition and of a schedule of progressive physical activities for the first 2 to 3 months after MI. Table 58.5 lists a broad array of activities corresponding to the recommended energy levels during the recuperation period and thereafter.

Resumption of activities with different energy requirements should be gradual; in particular, the duration of certain activities should be brief at first, with gradual increase, according to how the individual patient feels. The schedule in Table 58.4 can be given to most patients. A more aggressive plan can be tailored for the individual patient if an early physical conditioning program, guided by early stress testing, is available. Similarly, stress test-guided conditioning can also be planned for patients after the first 1 to 2 months of convalescence from an MI. Programs that enroll patients 2 months after MI are widely available. Local affiliates of the American Heart Association commonly maintain lists of local exercise programs. A comprehensive discussion of exercise conditioning for cardiac patients can be found later in this chapter (see "Physical Conditioning," below).

Return to Work

Because the majority of patients have their first MI during their active working years, they are commonly concerned about returning to work. Patients who do not return to work within 6 months of myocardial infarction are unlikely even to return to work (34), and this is often due to psychological not physical factors (see "Psychological Problems" below). Telling the patient, soon after discharge that he should expect to return to work is important in preventing disability due to psychological factors. Obviously, the type of work is also an important consideration. Patients whose occupations involve mental stress and hectic schedules should be advised to return to work on a part time basis at first, leaving plenty of time for rest and relaxation. For patients whose work involves significant physical exertion, the timing of return to work can be based upon the information contained in Tables 58.4 and 58.5 and guided by the results of exercise stress testing and monitored responses during a supervised rehabilitation program. From Table 58.5, it is evident that most occupations require an energy level of 6 metabolic equivalents (METs) or less. Occupational activities classified as heavy work, such as digging ditches, require energy expenditure of 7 or more METs. Certain activities may produce an increased work load on the heart because of psychological stress (e.g., driving a vehicle) or because they entail significant isometric exercise (e.g., carpentry, plumbing, shoveling, operating pneumatic tools, or carrying objects heavier than 30 lb).

Patients with myocardial infarctions complicated by poorly controlled angina, CHF, or arrhythmias should be evaluated in conjunction with a consulting cardiologist (see "Medical Complications," below) before a plan for return to work and other activities is recommended. Some of these patients will qualify for permanent medical disability (see criteria for disability due to coronary artery disease, Table 9.1) or for job retraining through vocational rehabilitation (see Chapter 9). The fundamental difference between impairment and disability due to

Table 58.4.
Activity Schedule and Symptom Recognition for Patients Convalescing from Myocardial Infarction

GENERAL POINTS

All activities, including sitting and lying down, require energy. The amount of energy required to perform a specific activity is expressed as METs. One MET is your resting energy requirement. As activities become more strenuous, the amount of energy required (METs) also increases, as does the work load imposed on your heart.

The schedule recommended in this program is based on the number of METs needed for various activities. Some specific recommendations are given for each of the first 3 months following your return to home. Table 58.4 gives the energy requirements for a wide variety of additional activities. If the table omits your favorite activities, ask your doctor about them.

Warnings: Generally the following activities impose an added strain on your heart and should be avoided, especially during the first 3 months after a heart attack:

1. Taking very hot or cold showers or baths.
2. Holding your breath while exercising, lifting or straining.
3. Working in a bent or stooped position or with arms held above your head.
4. Work that requires continuous tensing of your muscles.
5. Working or exercising during very hot, cold, humid, or windy weather (in bad weather, plan your regular exercise at a nearby shopping mall).
6. Working or exercising during the first hour after a meal or after consuming alcohol.
7. Consuming excessive amounts of alcohol (e.g., more than 1–2 ounces of whiskey, 2–3 beers, 1–2 glasses of wine).
8. Walking or exercising on a hill or an inclined surface.
9. Any activity which creates emotional stress or worry for you.

A. RECOMMENDED ACTIVITY SCHEDULE[a]

First Month (1–3 METs)

From Discharge to 1 Week

Regular exercise: walk 5 minutes at a leisurely pace once/day on a level surface.

Some specific advice: this week, primarily get used to being at home. Occupy yourself with sit-down activities such as watching television, playing cards, sewing, painting, sketching, *etc.* Avoid lifting objects heavier than 5 lb or doing activities which require reaching above your head. You may go up and down the stairs. However, take your time and limit the number of times you need to climb them. Do all of the things you were doing in the hospital. Get up and get dressed each day. You may be surprised at how tired and weak you feel. This is natural. Be sure to take rest periods when you need them, particularly after meals, before you exercise or climb the stairs.

Week 2

Regular exercise: walk 5 minutes at a leisurely pace twice/day.

Some specific advice: continue all of your previous activities, and add others, such as taking rides in the car (however, no driving yet), cooking a meal, washing clothes in a machine (have someone else remove them), making your bed, attending a relaxing movie, going out to dinner, going shopping with your family (let others lift things from the shelves to the basket and carry the groceries), shooting pool, playing shuffle board, throwing a softball underhand, playing a piano or organ.

Weeks 3 and 4

Regular exercise: advance gradually to walking 10 minutes at leisurely pace twice/day during 2 weeks.

Some specific advice: continue your previous activities and others, such as going to church, sweeping floors, polishing furniture, driving the car (beginning with short drives, avoiding heavy traffic).

Second Month (3–5 METs)

Regular physical exercise: progressively increase leisurely walking from 15 minutes once a day at a slightly faster pace to 30 minutes once or twice a day.

Some specific advice: the attached table of activities lists the approximate energy requirements of each. You may gradually increase your activities, by adding additional activities and spending more time at them; consult the attached table for activities requiring 5 METs or less (or more).

RECOGNIZING HEART SYMPTOMS

Your heart will give you warning signs if it is not ready for increased activity. Here are some guidelines to use:

Pulse: Locate your pulse and count the number of times it beats for 15 seconds and multiply that number by 4. This is your heart rate for 1 minute. Take your pulse before you begin your walk or any new activity and at the end of the activity. Contact your doctor before resuming exercise if:
  1. There is an increase of 20 heart beats or more/minute in postexercise pulse over pre-exercise pulse.
  2. If your heart rate exceeds 120/min.[b]
  3. If you detect abnormal heart action: pulse becoming irregular, fluttering or jumping in chest or throat, very slow pulse rate, sudden burst of rapid heartbeats.

Chest Pain: Contact your doctor before resuming exercise if you experience pain or pressure in the chest, arm, or throat precipitated by exercise or following exercise. Remember to take your nitroglycerine and rest if you do experience pain.

Dizziness: Contact your doctor before resuming exercise if you become dizzy, light-headed, or faint during exercise.

Breathing difficulty: Contact your doctor before resuming exercise if you become short of breath during or after a new exercise, or if you awaken from sleep short of breath.

---

[a] Pace of these activities may be scaled up or down by results of early post-MI stess test when available.
[b] These figures may be markedly modified by results of early stress test and/or medication.

coronary artery disease is underscored in the recent Bethesda Conference on "Insurability and Employability of the Patient with Ischemic Heart Disease" (8). Impairment is a medically defined disorder and is an important component of disability, but it is just one of several factors that determine the overall ability of a person to perform meaningful work. Addi-

tional factors include other medical disorders, age, sex, education, training, and psychosocial support. The main points in the report include: (*a*) most MI patients can return to work; (*b*) prognosis can be estimated by clinical examination and noninvasive studies that evaluate left ventricular function (echocardiogram), myocardial jeopardy (thallium stress

Table 58.5.
Energy Requirements of Certain Activities[a]

Activity Level	Self-Care or Home	Occupational	Recreational	Physical Conditioning
Very light (3 METs or less)	Washing, shaving, dressing Desk work, writing, washing dishes Driving auto[b]	Sitting (clerical, assembling) Standing (store clerk, bartender) Driving truck[b] Crane operator[b]	Shuffleboard Horseshoes Bait casting Billiards Archery[b] Golf (cart)	Walking (level at 2 mph) Stationary bike (very low resistance) Very light calisthenics
Light to moderate (3–5 METs)	Clean windows Raking leaves Weeding Power lawn mowing Waxing floors (slowly) Painting Carrying objects 15–30 lb[c]	Stocking shelves (light objects)[c] Light welding Light carpentry[c] Machine assembly Auto repair Paper hanging[c]	Dancing Golf (walking) Sailing Horseback riding Volleyball Tennis (doubles) Sexual intercourse[b] (see details in the text)	Walking (3–4 mph) Level bicycling (6–8 mph) Light calisthenics
Moderate (5–7 METs)	Easy digging in garden Level hand lawn moving Climbing stairs (slowly) Carrying objects 30–60 lb[c]	Carpenty (exterior home building)[c] Shoveling dirt[c] Pneumatic tools[c]	Badminton (competitive) Tennis (singles) Snow skiing (downhill) Light backpacking Basketball Football Skating (ice and roller) Horseback riding (gallop)	Swimming (breast stoke)
Heavy (7–9 METs)	Sawing wood[c] Heavy shoveling[c] Climbing stairs (moderate speed) Carrying objects 60–90 lb[c]	Tending furnace[c] Digging ditches[c] Pick and shovel[c]	Canoeing[c] Mountain climbing[c] Fencing Paddleball Touch football	Jogging (5 mph) Swimming (crawl stroke) Rowing machine Heavy calisthenics Bicycling (12 mph)
Very heavy (9 METs)	Carrying loads upstairs[c] Carrying objects 90 lb or more Climbing stairs (quickly) Shoveling heavy snow[c] Shoveling 10/minute (16 lb)	Lumber jack[c] Heavy laborer[c]	Handball Squash Ski touring over hills[c] Vigorous basketball	Running (6 mph) Bicycling (13 mph or steep hill) Rope jumping

[a]From Haskell WL: Design and implementation of cardiac conditioning programs. In Hellerstein HK (ed): *Rehabilitation of the Coronary Patient*. New York, John Wiley & Sons, 1978, p. 203.
[b]May cause added psychological stress that will increase load on the heart.
[c]May produce disproportionate myocardial demands because of use of arms or isometric exercise.

test), and electrical instability (Holter); (c) cardiac catheterization is not routinely required; (d) special assessment may be needed for jobs requiring sudden or sustained high effort or heat exposure (e.g., fire-fighters) or for those in which sudden disability may endanger others (e.g., pilots); (e) a trial period of progressively increasing part-time work may be necessary for smooth transition from total disability to full time work; (f) maximal functional capacity should be evaluated as soon as stability is present; this is usually 3 to 5 weeks after uncomplicated MI, seven weeks after coronary bypass surgery, and one week after coronary angioplasty.

Sexual Activity

It is safe for patients who are symptom free during usual activities of daily living to resume sexual intercourse within 4 to 6 weeks of their MI. Available data suggest that the energy requirement approximates 3 METs during foreplay and afterplay and 5 METs at climax (18). These are equivalent to the oxygen demands of a brisk walk around the block or of climbing one flight of stairs. In a study of patients after MI, coitus accounted for less than 1% of sudden deaths. These usually occurred during extramarital affairs in

which the men were considerably older than their companions and frequently were inebriated at the time of intercourse (45).

When counseling patients about resumption of sexual activity, one should give specific advice and should also encourage questions. The pamphlet *Sex and Heart Disease*, available from the American Heart Association, is a helpful adjunct to counseling. Frequency of sexual intercourse can be similar to the frequency before the patient's MI. Sexual foreplay without completion of intercourse can be recommended to patients who wish to resume sex cautiously. In general, sexual activity can be resumed in the position that was most gratifying before the MI; however, the patient should avoid positions in which he supports his weight on his arms, as this requires an isometric type of work (see "Physical Conditioning," below) and may put extra stress on the heart. Sexual activity should be engaged in when both partners are relaxed. It is best to abstain from intercourse for 2 or 3 hours after eating a large meal since eating increases the work of the heart.

Inability to return to a previous pattern of sexual activity may be due to angina precipitated by intercourse, to new medications, or to psychological stress associated with the recent MI. If an otherwise stable patient develops angina during intercourse, he should be advised to take sublingual nitroglycerin just before sexual activity. The evaluation and management of drug-induced and psychological sexual dysfunction, both of which may occur in the post-MI patient, are discussed in Chapter 18.

Psychological Problems

It is normal for patients to experience *anxiety and depression* during the first few weeks after discharge from the CCU. Some of these symptoms are due to misconceptions about the nature and prognosis of myocardial infarction, and they respond to clarification of the facts. Most patients do well when encouraged to ventilate their concerns and when reassured that their response is normal. A small supply of a minor tranquilizer (see Chapter 13) can be prescribed to be used if needed. As noted earlier ("Patient Education"), participation in group classes and group exercise programs can also help patients adjust to changes in their lives after myocardial infarction.

Another common psychological complication of MI is an *inappropriate fear of physical activity* of any kind, i.e., the so-called cardiac cripple. Early participation in supervised physical activity including the treadmill test and exercise conditioning have been shown to enhance the patients's self-confidence and ability to perform physical tasks (12). Having the spouse observe the early treadmill test establishes confidence in the spouse that his/her partner is not a cripple. In some medical centers, spouses are offered an opportunity to walk on the treadmill as well. This serves to establish a reference point for estimating ability to engage in activity. Engaging in a wide range of activities in the months after an MI is important since self-confidence is task specific (11, 12). Most cardiac exercise programs (see below) emphasize activities using the legs, such as walking and jogging. Although this increases self-confidence in tasks requiring leg work, it does little for arm self-confidence. To increase arm self-confidence, patients must practice arm exercises as well (11, 15). This is especially important for patients who plan to return to work that requires upper body and arm efforts.

Another common problem is *denial of illness* persisting beyond the first few days in hospital. The behavior associated with persistent denial may create substantial risks. This is especially true of patients who are extremely competitive and are used to controlling most of the circumstances of their lives (2). They are typically determined to return to work as soon as possible and will refuse cardiac rehabilitation on the basis that they can do it better on their own. This behavior arouses anxiety, fear, and concern in the spouse and family and may lead to significant marital conflict. An open discussion with patient and spouse, with each acknowledging the other's concerns, can often lead to resolution of these conflicts and more appropriate behavior from each partner.

At times it is useful to teach patients to use *various*

forms of feedback to guide their activities. Specifically, patients are taught to (a) use a target heart rate based on an exercise stress test; (b) observe themselves and how they feel, with the basic instruction to rest if fatigue or any cardiac symptoms occur during exercise, and to call the physician if symptoms persist after using nitroglycerin; and (c) view the spouse as a source of feedback. In most cases, the spouse's observation of how the patient looks is remarkably accurate. If she says he looks tired or does not look right, she is probably right. By having the patient agree to consider her comments as well meaning and for his benefit, he will usually comply with her advice. Thereafter, the number of reminding behaviors from the spouse is reduced progressively, and the rehabilitation process can proceed with greater enthusiasm from both partners. With more difficult patients, or where there is preexisting marital strife, the consultation of a psychiatrist or psychologist may be helpful in managing adjustment problems.

Some patients have relatively *severe psychological and behavioral problems* after MI that may interfere with their rehabilitation. The most common problem is *persistent depression*, which may have characteristics of a major or minor depressive illness or may present as an adjustment disorder characterized by anxiety, depression, somatization, or a mixture of these responses (36). The diagnosis and management of these problems are discussed in Chapters 12 (somatization), 13 (anxiety), and 15 (depression).

More recent studies of the possibly coronary prone behavior, the so-called *Type A behavior*, suggest that its basic components are not only time urgency, but also free floating hostility. On the other hand, long working hours, sustained drive, reasonable competitiveness, and enthusiasm do not necessarily connote coronary prone behavior. Apparently, type A behavior can be modified by proper counseling. Such modification has been associated with significant decrease in mortality and morbidity (13).

Medical Prophylaxis

For many years, smoking cessation (47) and treatment with β-blocking agents (14) have been known to improve the prognosis after MI. More recently, aspirin, afterload reducers, and calcium antagonists have also been shown to affect significant reduction in morbidity and mortality in certain subsets of post-CCU patients.

The benefits from *β-blockers* appears to be related to the general class action of β-blockers and do not seem to be related to any cardioselectively, membrane stabilization activity, or intrinsic sympathomimetic activity. The benefits are seen in all ages and in all types of MI although older patients (>60 years) and patients with complicated MI (as long as the complications do not constitute contraindications to the use of β-blockers) seem to show greater benefits than low risk patients as defined in Table 58.3. The overall magnitude of benefit from the use of β-blockers seems to be about one-third reduction in mortality and about the same magnitude of reduction in reinfarction. The contraindications to the use of β-blockers include congestive heart failure, asthma, and bradycardia. The recommended dose of β-blocker is the amount required to produce significant attenuation of heart rate and blood pressure response to exercise without producing significant side effects (14). Characteristics of the available β-blocking drugs are summarized in Table 62.11.

A 1988 meta-analysis of randomized trials of *antiplatelet therapy* for secondary prevention of vascular disease demonstrated that prolonged treatment with aspirin had no effect on nonvascular mortality but reduced vascular mortality by about 15% and nonfatal vascular events (stroke or myocardial infarction) by about 30% in patients with cardiac and cerebral occlusive vascular diseases (1). Benefits for post-MI patients were similar to those in post-stroke and post-TIA patients. There was no difference in the degree of protection afforded by aspirin alone at a dose of 325 mg a day and that afforded by higher aspirin doses or by other antiplatelet agents. In a recent randomized placebo-control study of patients with unstable angina, aspirin (325 mg twice daily during the first 6 days after hospital admission) decreased the incidence of acute myocardial infarction from 12 to 3% (42). Aspirin, 100 mg daily, has also been shown to improve aortic coronary bypass graft patency at 4 months (90% of grafts patent versus 68% in the placebo group) (24) and to decrease significantly the frequency of restenosis after percutaneous transluminal coronary angioplasty (PTCA) (43) and thrombolysis (32).

In chronic ischemic congestive cardiopathy, the use of *prophylactic vasodilator therapy*, such as the angiotensin convertor enzyme (ACE) inhibitors (e.g., captopril or enalapril), is associated with significantly improved survival (5). The impact of these agents on survival in patients with postinfarction left ventricular dysfunction is being evaluated in large-scale clinical trials. ACE inhibitors should be started in small doses

with gradual increases guided by blood pressure response and renal function monitor. Characteristics of these drugs are summarized in Table 62.11.

In patients with *non-Q wave myocardial infarction*, prophylactic use of the calcium antagonist diltiazem (Cardizem), 90 mg every 6 hours for two weeks, was associated with a 50% reduction in the rates of early reinfarction and refractory angina (16). This may be related to the high propensity for coronary artery spasm in this subset.

There have been no trials of *cholesterol-lowering drugs* in post-MI patients, but it is prudent to advise all post-MI patients to follow a low-cholesterol diet, and patients with hypercholesterolemia may benefit from cholesterol lowering drugs. Controlled trials have shown that cholesterol-lowering drugs (cholestyramine and gemfribrizol) reduce the incidence of new coronary artery disease in hypercholesterolemic men (23, 25). Other trials have shown either reversal or delayed progression of atherosclerotic plagues in patients whose cholesterol was reduced (3, 21, 30). Additional information regarding cholesterol and atherosclerotic disease is found in Chapter 75.

Medical Complications

Table 58.6 lists the principal medical complications of MI, the procedures that may be useful in diagnosing or evaluating them, and potential therapies. In general, the use of sophisticated and costly procedures to evaluate these complications should be coordinated by a consulting cardiologist.

Postinfarction Angina

As pointed out in the discussion of prognosis above, this is a very common problem in survivors of MIs. The medical management of angina is described in detail in Chapter 57. Because protection of the heart from transient ischemia may be especially important during recovery from an MI, the prescription of long-acting nitrates or β-blockers and calcium blockers to

Table 58.6.
Medical Complications of Myocardial Infarction

Complications	Diagnostic Procedures for Selected Patients[a]	Management Approaches
Angina or other evidence of reversible ischemia	ECG stress testing; radionuclide stress testing; Holter monitor for silent ischemia; coronary arteriography	Standard antianginal therapy (see Chapter 57); coronary artery bypass or Percutaneous Transluminal Coronary Angioplasty (PTCA) for selected patients; physical conditioning
Congestive heart failure	Radionuclide ventriculography and/or echocardiography (ejection fraction, segmental dysfunction, rupture, ventricular aneurysm)	Afterload reduction and ? standard therapy for hear failure (see Chapter 61); surgery in a few selected patients
Arrhythmias	Holter monitor; ECG stress testing, electrophysiological study in selected patients	Standard antiarrhythmic therapy (see Chapter 59); surgery or implanted defibrillator in selected patients
Postmyocardial infarction syndrome (Dressler's)	Echocardiography (pericardial effusion)	Aspirin or other anti-inflammatory agents
Systemic emboli	Echocardiography (intracardiac thrombus)	Anticoagulant therapy (see Chapter 52); surgery in selected patients

[a]Should be coordinated and intepreted by consulting cardiologist.

prevent angina is advisable in most patients who develop angina within the first 3 months after MI. Careful clinical observations, serial stress testing, and ambulatory ECG monitoring are useful in adjusting the dose, the combination, and the duration of the antianginal therapy. Because of the poor prognosis associated with angina occurring very early after an MI, patients with this problem should be referred to a cardiologist for consideration of coronary catheterization and possible coronary angioplasty or bypass surgery.

Postinfarction Congestive Heart Failure

A small proportion of patients develop chronic congestive heart failure (CHF) after MI. This complication usually develops before discharge from the hospital. Nowadays, many patients have their left ventricular ejection fraction measured as part of their evaluation before discharge, so that those at increased risk of developing new CHF after discharge are known. The regimens described in Chapter 61 should be utilized in treating the CHF of patients after MI. As mentioned above, the use of afterload reduction (with ACE inhibitors) in chronic CHF seems to be associated with improved survival. A small proportion of patients with persistent CHF may have segmental or global left ventricular dysfunction, or significant mitral regurgitation that may improve significantly after cardiac surgery.

Postinfarction Arrhythmias

A substantial number of survivors of MIs are found to have complex ventricular arrhythmias (see Table 58.1) on 24-hour ambulatory ECG monitoring, which is performed routinely after the first week of hospitalization in many hospitals. It has never been shown convincingly that antiarrhythmic therapy improves the prognosis of patients with asymptomatic ventricular arrhythmias; however, some patients will be discharged from the hospital on antiarrhythmic drugs. The drugs utilized to control arrhythmias are discussed in detail in Chapter 59. Once medical control of arrhythmias has been established, the patient should be treated for 3 to 6 months. If ECG monitoring shows no arrhythmia after this period, antiarrhythmic treatment can be stopped and the patient can be checked 1 week later for recurrent arrhythmia. Ventricular irritability and left ventricular dysfunction seem to be independent risk factors for the occurrence of sudden cardiac deaths during the first 6 months after MI (see above); the combination of both of these risk factors is particularly ominous, resulting in an incidence of sudden death that is 11 times that of patients with neither of these risk factors (28).

The use of antiarrhythmic agents in the posthospital management of patients with the combination of complex ventricular arrhythmias and low ejection fractions documented at the end of their stay in the hospital seems prudent, although efficacy has not been established and proarrhythmic complications are particularly ominous in this setting.

Postmyocardial Infarction (Dressler's) Syndrome

It is estimated that 3 to 4% of patients develop this complication, usually within 1 to 6 weeks after a myocardial infarction. The syndrome is characterized by the pain of pericarditis (substernal pain, relieved by leaning forward and increased with inspiration); presence of a friction rub; fever; a pericardial effusion (which can best be demonstrated by echocardiography) and often a unilateral or bilateral pleural effusion.

The principal considerations in the differential diagnosis are pulmonary embolism and recurrence or extension of the recent MI.

When a patient develops the symptoms of Dressler's syndrome, he should be hospitalized immediately, and serial ECGs, cardiac enzymes, and a lung scan should be obtained. If these tests do not show pulmonary embolism, a new MI, or another explanation of the symptoms, the clinical diagnosis of Dressler's syndrome can be made. Echocardiographic evidence of a pericardial effusion and an elevated erythrocyte sedimentation rate may also be present.

Dressler's syndrome usually responds to salicylates or to indomethacin; in patients who do not respond to these drugs, prednisone gives prompt relief of symptoms. Once the diagnosis is secure and symptoms are controlled, the patient can be discharged. The anti-inflammatory drug chosen in the hospital should be administered for 1 to 2 months. Prednisone should be tapered according to the schedule described in Chapter 74. Patients who have recurrent symptoms when anti-inflammatory treatment is discontinued should resume treatment for another month or longer.

Arterial Embolization

This complication occurs in 5 to 10% of post-MI patients. The emboli seem to originate from mural thrombi that are typically seen in the left ventricular apex adjacent to akinetic or dyskinetic wall segments. About 30 to 40% of hearts with akinetic or dyskinetic left ventricular apices show mural thrombi on the echocardiogram. Anticoagulation (see Chapter 52) in patients demonstrating mural thrombi seems prudent, although its effect on reducing subsequent morbidity and mortality has not been established.

Shoulder-Hand Syndrome (Reflex Sympathetic Dystrophy)

This syndrome, characterized by pain and stiffness of the shoulder and pain and swelling of the hand, may occur during the first 1 to 2 months after an MI. It usually affects the left side. This syndrome rarely occurs when patients are mobilized early after an MI. Management of the shoulder-hand syndrome is described in Chapter 83, Cerebrovascular Disease.

Referral for Cardiology Consultation

Selected patients who have had an MI, especially persons under the age of 60, and patients with uncontrolled angina refractory to medical therapy, with a markedly positive exercise stress test, with a ventricular aneurysm, with CHF refractory to medical therapy, with evidence for "ischemia at a distance" (see footnote to Table 58.1 for definition), or with mechanical complications such as ventricular septal defect (suggested by holosystolic murmur and thrill at the left sternal border) or papillary muscle rupture (suggested by refractory CHF and holosystolic apical murmur), may benefit from coronary angioplasty or cardiac surgery, either by having their symptoms reduced or their prognosis improved. Such patients should be referred promptly to a cardiologist, to assure optimal medical therapy and to obtain an opinion about the advisability and the timing of invasive procedures. Post-MI patients presenting with CHF and severe diffuse left ventricular dysfunction should probably continue to be treated conservatively because the coronary artery bypass grafting has not been helpful for these patients. Cardiac transplantation offers a glimmer of hope to a very small, highly selected subset of such patients.

Noncardiac Surgery

Noncardiac surgery carries a very high risk during the first 3 to 6 months after an MI (see Chapter 86 for details).

HOME CARE FOR ACUTE MYOCARDIAL INFARCTION

A controlled trial in Great Britain has shown that for patients with uncomplicated acute MIs the outcome is similar whether the patient is cared for in the home or in an intensive care unit (26). The authors concluded that home care was ethically acceptable for such patients. Because hospital care is the norm for an acute MI in the United States, it is unlikely that home care will gain significant acceptance here. However, for an occasional older person who presents with a stable acute MI and objects to hospitalization, or for a person who consults his physician several days after an infarct, management at home may be appropriate. The scheme for rehabilitation after MI described in this chapter can be adapted to these situations.

MANAGEMENT OF UNSTABLE ANGINA AFTER DISCHARGE FROM HOSPITAL

Of patients admitted to a hospital with unstable angina, 15 to 30% will continue to have pain despite vigorous medical management. Patients in this subgroup have a 25 to 45% 1-year mortality rate. Therefore, most are evaluated for and referred for coronary angioplasty or coronary artery bypass surgery. These interventions relieve or eliminate symptoms in the majority and improve the prognosis for those with left main coronary artery disease, triple vessel disease, and two vessel disease with left ventricular dysfunction.

To date, the rehabilitation of the medically managed patient with unstable angina has not been studied as systematically as the rehabilitation of the patient after MI. These patients should receive education similar to that recommended for patients after MI regarding the nature of coronary artery disease, the recognition of symptoms, and the control of risk factors (see above). Because these patients do not have an ischemic injury that may take 2 or more months to heal, they can usually be permitted to return to their usual activities more rapidly than patients who have had an MI. This is true particularly if their angina is well controlled and a stress test shows minimal or no changes due to ischemia.

Additional information regarding the medical management of unstable angina is found in Chapter 57.

PHYSICAL CONDITIONING

Regular exercise, with the goal of attaining the physiological adaptation known as the conditioning effect, is safe and beneficial for most patients after MI, just as it is for healthy persons. The basic principles of exercise training are applicable to persons with and without heart disease. In addition to the cardiovascular principles related to exercise, principles regarding the musculoskeletal system are important (see Chapter 67).

General Principles

Muscular and Cardiovascular Effects

The body will respond and adapt to the kind and amount of physical demands placed upon it. The response is *specific*, meaning that the greatest changes are observed only in those areas upon which demands are placed. For exercise to bring about an improvement in physical fitness, it must *overload* the muscles or organ system involved in the exercise. To overload is to exercise at a greater intensity than the intensity to which one is accustomed. The overload must be applied gradually, in stages, for maximal effectiveness and safety. This is known as *progressive resistance*. *Threshold of training* refers to the amount of exercise that must be done to produce fitness improvements. The factors that must be considered when establishing the right amount of exercise are:

1. *Type of activity*. As stated, the effects of exercise are specific to the type of activity engaged in and the particular body function it exercises. Thus, if

Table 58.7.
Target Heart Rates for Healthy Persons, by Age (Approximately 80% Maximal Predicted Heart Rate)[a]

Age	Heart Rate
20–29	170
30–39	160
40–49	150
50–59	140
60–69	130

[a]From Parmely JF, Jr, Blair S, Gazes PC, *et al* (eds): Proceedings of the National Workshop on Exercise in the Prevention, Evaluation, and Treatment of Heart Disease. *J South Carolina Med Assoc* 65 (suppl 1):December, 1969.

the objective is to improve cardiovascular endurance, then exercise that increases heart rate and peripheral oxygen consumption is required. If the objective is to improve strength, then exercise with increasing amounts of resistance is required. There is little carryover of the effects of an exercise from one component of fitness to another. Activities for cardiovascular fitness entail rhythmic repetitive movements of large muscles groups against relatively small resistance. Such activities are of low intensity and can be performed for a long time. They include walking, jogging, swimming, cycling, rowing, jumping rope, skating, running, and cross-country skiing. These activities increase the demand for oxygen and the muscles adapt by enhanced extraction of oxygen, which is the reason they are called "aerobic" activities. They are also referred to as dynamic activities. On the other hand, sustained, slow-movement activity, frequently involving relatively small muscle groups, against high resistance is known as static activity. Examples are weight lifting, push-ups, sit-ups, isometrics, carrying heavy packages, and hand grip. Most activities requiring lifting and straining, such as shoveling, have a large static component. In such activities there is increased peripheral vascular resistance with subsequent increase in blood pressure but relatively little increase in heart rate or cardiac output. Such exercises do not bring about enhancement in oxygen extraction; hence they are generally not aerobic. There are inadequate data to suggest that brief episodes of moderate resistive exercise are dangerous. In fact, cardiac patients who were required to carry or lift weights or to perform isometric exercise after myocardial infarction had less ischemic electrocardiographic changes and arrhythmias during resistive exercise rather than during aerobic exercises (9, 40). Gradual involvement in activities such as weight lifting may be beneficial and desirable, especially in blue collar workers since their jobs require static efforts.

2. *Intensity.* Exercise intensity is set at a level that requires more effort than normal activity. This level is usually set at 70% of predicted maximal oxygen uptake, a level that is attained when the heart rate reaches approximately 80% of the age-predicted maximal rate. Optimal conditioning occurs when a person sustains this rate during an aerobic activity. Table 58.7 lists target heart rates for healthy persons in various age groups. Lower levels of aerobic exercise also produce a partial conditioning effect. Exercise prescription for patients with heart disease will be discussed later in this chapter.

3. *Duration.* Exercise must be performed for a sufficient amount of time to be effective. Duration can be varied in several ways: (a) increase repetitions while maintaining the same rate, such as in weight training; (b) increase the distance covered at the same rate, such as in walking or jogging; (c) reduce the number of rest periods between different ex-

ercises; or, (d) reduce the rest time during a rest period. Studies in exercise physiology have suggested that the total work done during an exercise session (i.e., duration X intensity) may be more important in eliciting improvements than intensity or duration alone. Therefore, a long, low-intensity workout may be equivalent to a short, high-intensity workout if the total work is the same. A long, low-intensity workout may be more suitable for beginners and for middle or older aged individuals since it would reduce the risk of injury. For cardiovascular fitness, duration should be at least 20 minutes at the target heart rate.

4. *Frequency.* This factor refers to the number of times per week exercise is to be done. Exercise must be performed regularly, and for most types of exercise three to five times/week are desirable. However, two to three times/week are probably more sensible for the beginner since many musculoskeletal injuries occur at the start of a program due to overuse. This can increase to three to five times/week as adaptation takes place.

The *principal hemodynamic adaptation* to aerobic exercise in patients with heart disease takes place in the peripheral vascular and muscular systems. Trained muscles can extract more oxygen from a given blood flow and there is a better distribution of the cardiac output. Heart rate and blood pressure are lower at rest and at a given submaximal work load. As a result, the patient can do more work with less cardiac effort, i.e., less myocardial oxygen demand. This is extremely beneficial to cardiac patients who have limited blood supply through the coronary arteries. Angina may occur at the same threshold, i.e., the same double product (heart rate X systolic blood pressure), but it is at a higher level of body work or MET level. Metabolic equivalents (METs) are used to rate the energy requirement of different physical activities. One MET is 3.5 ml of O_2/kg of body weight/minute and is equivalent to oxygen requirement at rest; 2 METs are twice the resting requirements, etc. (See Table 58.4 for the METS required for a broad range of activities.) The higher the MET level attained during exercise testing, the more fit the individual is considered to be. In patients with coronary artery disease, the increase in angina-free exercise capacity achieved with regular exercise is similar to that achieved with medications such as the β-blockers and nitrates. In healthy people who practice aerobic exercise there are also changes in the heart itself, including increase in diastolic volume, increase in ejection fraction at rest and to a greater extent during exercise, and enhancement of contractility. Few studies have shown any of this central effect in cardiac patients. However, there is evidence suggesting that cardiac patients may achieve these changes if they train hard and long enough (10). Improvement in coronary collateral circulation or myocardial perfusion as a result of training has not been demonstrated in cardiac patients.

Hormonal and Metabolic Effects

In addition to the effect of training on the muscular and cardiovascular systems, aerobic exercise is associated with beneficial changes in a number of other systems: there is increased vagal tone, lowering of catecholamines, decrease in serum triglycerides, increase in the ratio of high to low density lipoprotein, reduction in adipose tissue, and augmentation in plasma fibrinolytic activity.

Conditioning in Healthy Persons

Healthy individuals can develop their own physical conditioning programs, utilizing a self-instruction programs (6, 48). The objective of conditioning programs is to reach an exercise level at which the body is achieving about 70% of maximal predicted oxygen uptake, a level that is attained when the heart rate reaches approximately 80% of the maximal predicted rate (Table 58.7). As stated previously, optimal conditioning in healthy persons occurs with aerobic activity at the target heart rate for 20 minutes, at least three times/week. Lower levels of aerobic exercise also produce a partial conditioning effect in healthy persons.

Selected individuals should consult their physicians before beginning a conditioning program. In general, persons over the age of 35 and those with major risk factors for atherosclerosis should have a physical

Table 58.8.
Individuals for Whom Stress Testing Should Be Considered When Beginning Exercise Programs

Status	Test or Training Mode
Healthy, under 35	No special test
Healthy, over 35	Stress test[a]
Coronary prone, all ages	Stress test
Coronary stricken, all ages	Stress test

[a]Tests performed by paramedical personnel to assess baseline exercise capacity.

Table 58.9.
Rating of Perceived Exertion (RPE) Scale Perceived Exertion[a]

6	
7	Very, very light
8	
9	Very light
10	
11	Fairly light
12	
13	Somewhat hard
14	
15	Hard
16	
17	Very hard
18	
19	Very, very hard
20	

[a]The rating of perceived exertion scale (RPE) developed by Borg. (From Borg G: Subjective effort in relation to physical performance and working capacity. In Pick HL (ed): *Psychology: From Research to Practice.* New York, Plenum, 1978, p. 333.

examination and a resting ECG. Exercise stress tests should be considered for individuals in a number of categories, as summarized in Table 58.8. Nondiagnostic fitness tests for apparently healthy individuals are usually available at health clubs, YMCAs, wellness centers, and community colleges. When supervised and interpreted by qualified allied health professionals, these tests can provide the basis for the exercise prescription. Fees are usually nominal and are included in the overall package for exercise sessions.

Physical Conditioning in Patients after Myocardial Infarction

Benefits of Conditioning

Cardiac patients who exercise regularly and who have become conditioned show better control of angina and enhancement of physical working capacity.

Because of the peripheral cardiovascular adaptations described earlier, angina pectoris occurs at higher exercise levels. This increased anginal threshold allows the patient to do more work; and at any given level of work, the patient feels more comfortable since the work represents a lower percentage of a now higher maximal capacity. Rating of perceived exertion (RPE) is a scale that measures how hard any given level of work feels. The scale is shown in Table 58.9. The RPE is administered during exercise testing. The patient is asked to rate the work at each stage of the test. After conditioning, the RPE is lower at any given stage and is associated with a lower heart rate and blood pressure at that stage (17). RPE is also a useful way to prescribe exercise. This approach focuses on how the patient actually feels and correlates closely with the target heart rate and/or desired MET level. For most cardiac patients, a prescription at 13 to 14 on the RPE scale is both safe and effective for cardiovascular conditioning.

The effect of exercise training on longevity in patients after MI has been recently established. Meta analysis on the combined results of ten randomized clinical trials has demonstrated a 25% reduction in cardiovascular mortality although not in nonfatal reinfarction for patients in rehabilitation programs (29). Benefits of exercise conditioning on the psychometric profile do not seem to be firmly established (see Greenland and Chu in "General References").

Risks of Conditioning

With proper selection, supervision, monitoring, and precautions, physical conditioning for cardiac patients has proven to be remarkably safe. Cumulative data from over 1.5 million man-hours of exercise, done predominantly 3 months after MI, show that the risks of ventricular fibrillation, acute MI, and death are 1/10,000 to 1/32,000, 1/253,000, and 1/100,000 to 1/212,000 man-hours of exercise, respectively (7). There is no comparable large series in the literature on exercise conditioning earlier than 3 months after MI. In the authors' experience with exercise programs beginning an average of 10 days after hospital discharge, there have been no untoward events during exercise over a 4-year period. These patients exercise three times/week, for an average of 6 to 8 weeks at a conditioning heart rate of about 80% of what they safely achieved on a previous post-MI stress test, usually performed before hospital discharge.

Cardiovascular Medications and Conditioning

Many patients enrolling in exercise programs are taking one or more medications. Many of these medications alter the cardiovascular response to exercise. Patients enrolled in a conditioning program should always be stress tested (see below) while taking their regular medications, and the effects of their drugs must be considered in interpreting test results. For example, β-blockers attenuate the heart rate response to exercise. Thus, heart rate is less useful as an end point for stress testing or as a parameter for the patient to monitor during exercise conditioning. In a patient on β-blockers, symptoms, ECG changes, fatigue, and RPE are used as end points during stress testing. These parameters are also useful for establishing the exercise prescription in patients on certain medications. Table 58.10 summarizes the effects of a number of commonly prescribed cardiac drugs on the hemodynamic response to exercise.

Persons taking a variety of drugs have been evaluated and have participated safely in physical conditioning programs. There is some controversy regarding the effect of β-blockers on the response to training. It has been suggested that β-blockers may attenuate the beneficial effects of training. A recent clinical trial to establish whether β-blockers or calcium channel blockers limit exercise capacity and training showed that neither drug interfered with muscle strength whereas propranolol, a β-blocker, reduced aerobic capacity by 20% (19).

Table 58.10.
Effect of Various Classes of Medications on Hemodynamic Status during Exercise[a,b]

Drug	Peak Heart Rate	Peak Systolic Blood Pressure
ANTIHYPERTENSIVES		
Ace inhibitors	=	↓
Hydralazine	↑	↓
Minoxidil	↑	↓
Clonidine	↓	↓
Guanethidine	↓	↓↓
Methyldopa	↓	↓
Prazosin	↑	↓
NITRATES	↑	↓
ANTIARRHYTHMICS	=	↓
β-BLOCKERS	↓	↓
DIGITALIS[c]	=	↑
CALCIUM BLOCKERS		
Nifedipine	↑	↓
Diltiazem	=	↓
Verapamil	↓	↓

[a]Expanded from Powles ACP: The effect of drugs on the cardiovascular response to exercise. *Med Sci Sports Exercise* 13:252, 1981.
[b]↓, decreased; ↑, increased; =, no discernible effect.
[c]Patients with congestive heart failure.

Referral for Conditioning

The decision to refer a patient for physical conditioning after MI depends on the patient's clinical status, his motivation, and the availability of well-supervised and staffed programs designed for such patients. Medically supervised programs, offering ECG monitoring and the immediate availability of emergency care, often accept patients within 2 weeks of hospital discharge. If such a program is not available, guidelines such as those shown in Table 58.3 are appropriate. After 2 months, when there is no supervised program available, patients with uncomplicated MI can be advised to increase their exercise level gradually, using the results of a stress test to establish target heart rates or RPE.

Before beginning a conditioning program, the patient should have an ECG stress test (see Chapter 57 for a description of the patient's experience), the results of which are used in planning the exercise program. In general, the conditioning target heart rate is 70 to 85% of the maximal heart rate safely achieved on the stress test. Figure 58.4 shows the results of such a stress test, performed 3 weeks after an MI in a patient who was evaluated just prior to enrollment in a supervised exercise program.

Contraindications

A patient should not be enrolled or should be discontinued from a conditioning program if the following problems are present: poorly controlled angina, severe dyspnea at low work loads, moderate to severe uncontrolled hypertension (diastolic >110 mm Hg), complex arrhythmias, atrial fibrillation with a rapid ventricular response, second or third degree heart block, significant valvular or congenital heart disease, significant orthopaedic or pulmonary limitations, chronic alcoholism, or recent acute physical or mental illness.

Exercise Programs

Exercise sessions should be supervised by personnel trained in exercise physiology and cardiopulmonary resuscitation, with immediate availability of monitoring and resuscitative equipment. Programs that accept patients 2 to 3 weeks post-MI should have equipment for continuous ECG monitoring. Sessions are usually held three times a week on nonconsecutive days. The total duration of an average session is about 45 minutes. The pattern for a workout is illustrated in Figure 58.5. During the stimulus phase, the patient exercises at an intensity that elicits a heart rate or rating of perceived exertion (RPE, see above) that falls within the prescribed target zone. Figure 58.6 shows recommendations for exercise intensity based on heart rate response during an exercise stress test. Exercising near the 70% level, for 20 to 30 minutes, will promote fitness, and beginners should be instructed to maintain intensity near this level. Experienced exercisers can advance to the 85% level if a more intense workout is desired. The stimulus, or period at the target heart rate, is preceded by 5 to 10 minutes of warm-up and

```
PATIENT: J T  ID#: 00 00 00   DATE:  6 / 6 / 81
REFERRING PHYSICIAN: CCU


************************PATIENT DATA************************


AGE: 34   SEX: MALE   HGT: 68   WGT: 162  INDICATION: EARLY S/P MI
PRESENT SYMPTOMS: NONE
CCU ADMISSION DATE:  5 / 12 / 81    DX: INFERIOR MI
PRIOR EST:  4 / 14 / 75     RESULTS: NEGATIVE EXERCISE STRESS TEST
MEDS: NITROPASTE
RISK FACTORS: SMOKING FAMILY HX


********************PRE-EXERCISE SCREENING********************


SUPINE: HR: 62  BP: 114 / 78      STANDING: HR: 66  BP: 112 / 80
RESTING EKG:AXIS/PATTERNS:    INFERIOR MI
RESTING EKG:RHYTHM:           NORMAL SINUS RHYTHM
POST-HYPERVENTILATION:        NO SIGNIFICANT CHANGES


**************************EXERCISE RESULTS**************************


REASON FOR STOPPING TEST: TARGET HEART RATE ATTAINED
EXERCISE PROTOCOL: MODIFIED NAUGHTON     TOTAL TIME: 14 MIN, 30 SEC
PEAK SPEED: 3 MPH  ELEVATION: 10 % GRADE   METS: 7  NYHA CLASS: 1
PHYSIOLOGICAL DATA: PREDICTED MAX HR:  186   90% MAX HR:  167
PEAK HR:  132      THIS WAS ADEQUATE FOR THE WORK PERFORMED
PEAK BP:  150/120    THIS WAS ADEQUATE FOR THE WORK PERFORMED
THE RATE-PRESSURE PRODUCT WAS:  19800


     EXERCISE EKG:ST-T CHANGES:
THERE WERE NO SIGNIFICANT CHANGES NOTED.


     EXERCISE EKG:RHYTHM:
THERE WERE NO ARRHYTHMIAS NOTED.


     SYMPTOMS:
THERE WERE NO SYMPTOMS REPORTED.


     CONCLUSIONS:
1.   ADEQUATE, NEGATIVE EARLY POST MI STRESS TEST.
2.   ACCELERATED DIASTOLIC BLOOD PRESSURE RESPONSE TO EXERCISE.
     RECOMMENDATIONS:
A.   MAY START MONITORED EXERCISE PROGRAM.
B.   CONSIDER BETA BLOCKADE IN VIEW OF #2 ABOVE.
```

Figure 58.4. *A.* Example of a formal report of an exercise stress test useful for planning rehabilitation, conducted 3 weeks after myocardial infarction (see data Fig. 58.4*B*).

is followed by 5 to 10 minutes of cool-down (Fig. 58.5). Warm-up and cool-down should include stretching and range of motion calisthenic exercises (see illustration in Chapter 67). Warm-up provides for gradual acceleration of the heart and circulation; it is beneficial to joints and muscles and helps to prevent musculoskeletal injuries. Cool-down provides for gradual deceleration of the cardiovascular system and prevents pooling of blood in the muscles when exercise stops abruptly. Pooling can lead to a precipitous drop in venous return and, consequently, postexercise hypotension.

As discussed earlier, training is specific to the muscles used in a particular exercise. Therefore, a training session should consist of a variety of activities designed to provide a well-rounded workout. Exercises for both the legs and arms should be incorporated into the session. Aerobic training of the legs can be achieved through bicycling, walking, jogging, and aerobic dance. The arms can be trained with shoulder wheels, rowing machines, and arm ergometers. Swimming, cross-country ski machines, and combination arm-leg cycles are excellent for exercising both lower and upper extremities at the same time.

For selected cardiac patients, *circuit weight training* can be used to improve both aerobic capacity and upper and lower body strength (20, 38). Three-year experience with this type of training indicates increased muscle strength and self-efficacy, enhanced compliance to the exercise program, and no cardiac or orthopaedic complications (39). In circuit weight training, the patient moves from weight machine to weight machine, performing for 30 seconds at 40% of maximal capacity, with 30 seconds of rest between each exercise, for a total of 20 minutes. This type of exercise

Protocol

Stage	Bruce Treadmill	Mets	Mod. Naughton Treadmill	Mets	BP	HR	Comments
1	1.7/0*	2	2/0	2	140/100	87	NO SYMPTOMS; NO EKG CHANGES
2	1.7/10	5	2/3.5	3	145/105	92	NO SYMPTOMS; NO EKG CHANGES
3	2.5/12	7	2/7	4	140/115	98	NO SYMPTOMS; NO EKG CHANGES
4	3.4/14	10	2/10.5	5	140/110	108	NO SYMPTOMS; NO EKG CHANGES
5	4.2/16	13	2/14	6	150/120	128	NO SYMPTOMS; NO EKG CHANGES
6			3/10	7	145/95	132	FATIGUE; NO EKG CHANGES
7			3/12.5	8			
8			3/15	9			
9			3/17.5	10			
10							

*Miles per hr/percent elevation

Recovery

Min	BP	HR	Comments
0	145/95	132	NO SYMPTOMS; NO EKG CHANGES
2	114/85	94	NO SYMPTOMS; NO EKG CHANGES
4	112/80	88	NO SYMPTOMS; NO EKG CHANGES
6	112/84	75	NO SYMPTOMS; NO EKG CHANGES
8	112/84	78	NO SYMPTOMS; NO EKG CHANGES
10	110/82	84	NO SYMPTOMS; NO EKG CHANGES

Target Heart Rate____130____

Figure 58.4. *B*. Data from stress test reported in Figure 58.6*A*.

combines elements of dynamic and static forms of exercise. Patients selected for this type of exercise should be preconditioned in a traditional program of walking and jogging for at least 3 months, and achieve at least 6 METs on a treadmill test without symptoms or ischemic electrocardiographic changes.

Termination of Supervised Training

Criteria for terminating supervised exercise training and transfer to nonsupervised maintenance programs are not clearly established. ECG monitoring for 6 to 8 weeks, and longer, during early exercise programs is generally recommended. Clinical stability and functional capacity above 7 to 8 METs (Table 58.4) are generally accepted exit criteria.

After a few months of supervised exercise, repeated stress testing is useful for measuring the change in physical working capacity and for adjusting more accurately the optimal exercise training intensity.

Long-Term Compliance

Long-term compliance with formal exercise programs is often poor. Patients must understand that it is necessary to exercise regularly, at the proper inten-

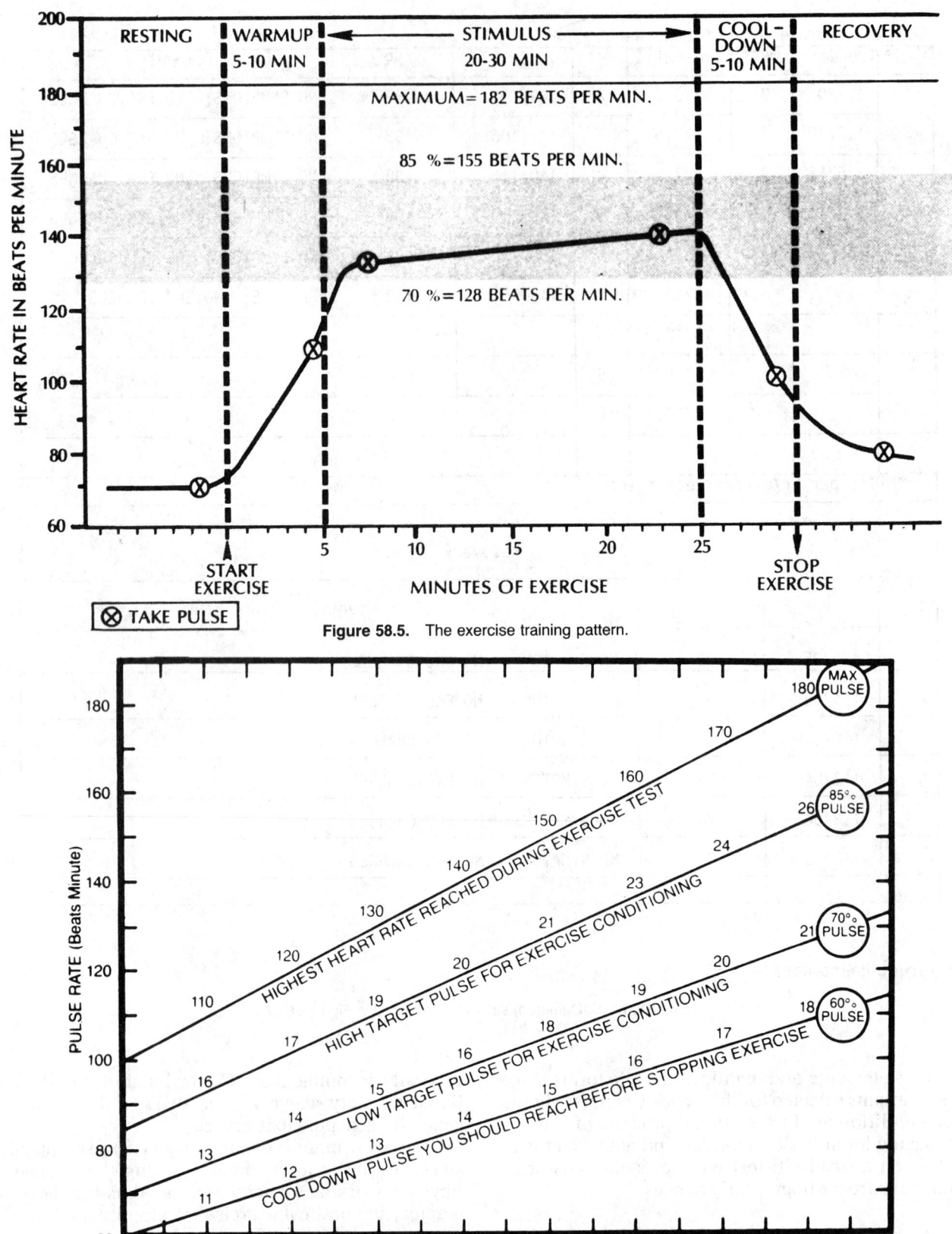

Figure 58.5.   The exercise training pattern.

Figure 58.6.   Target pulse rates for 10-second counts that should be measured the first 10 seconds after exercise. To convert the count to beats per minute, multiply by 6. To determine a patient's target pulse rate range, identify the highest rate safely achieved during the most recent exercise test on the top line (maximum pulse line); then locate the corresponding values on the 85 and 70% lines directly below. These two values represent the limits of target rate range for exercise conditioning (From Haskell WL: Design and implementation of cardiac conditioning programs. In Wenger NK, Hellerstein HK (eds): *Rehabilitation of the Coronary Patient*. New York, John Wiley & Sons, 1978, p 209.)

sity, frequency, and duration if physical fitness is to be maintained. Measurable deterioration in the conditioning effect occurs after missing only a few weeks. The time required to retrieve lost ground seems to be directly related to the length of time without exercise and to the degree of physical fitness achieved before cessation of exercise. Exercise must become a part of the patient's weekly routine, and not something that is done only during the recovery from MI.

General References

American College of Physicians: Evaluation of patients after recent acute myocardial infarction. Position paper. *Ann Intern Med* 110:485, 1989.

DeBusk RF: Specialized testing after recent acute myocardial infarction. *Ann Intern Med* 110:470, 1989.

Greenland P, Chu JS: Efficacy of cardiac rehabilitation services with emphasis on patients after myocardial infarction. Review paper. *Ann Intern Med* 109:650, 1988.

Moss AJ, Benhorin J: Prognosis and management after a first myocardial infarction. *N Engl J Med* 322 (11):743, 1990.

> Review that focuses on survivors of a first infarction, the largest subgroup of postinfarction patients (60 to 80% of all postinfarction patients).

Specific References

1. Antiplatelet Trialists' Collaboration: Secondary prevention of vascular disease by prolonged antiplatelet treatment. *Br Med J* 296:320, 1988.
2. Baile WF, Engel BT: A behavioral strategy for promoting treatment compliance following myocardial infarction. *Psychosom Med* 40:412, 1978.
3. Blakenhorn DH, Nessim SA, Johnson RL, et al: Beneficial effects of combined cholestipol–niacin therapy on coronary atherosclerosis and coronary venous bypass grafts. *JAMA* 257:3233, 1987.
4. Braunwald E: Treatment of the patient after myocardial infarction. *N Engl J Med* 302:290, 1980.
5. The Consensus Trial Study Group: Effect of enalapril on mortality in severe congestive heart failure. Results of the Cooperative North Scandinavian Enalapril Survival Study. *N Engl J Med* 316:1429, 1987.
6. Cooper KH (ed): *The New Aerobics.* New York, Bantam Books, 1970.
7. Council on Scientific Affairs, American Medical Association: Physician-supervised exercise programs in rehabilitation of patients with coronary heart disease. *JAMA* 245:1463, 1981.
8. DeBusk RF: *Report of the twentieth Bethesda Conference. Insurability and employability of the patient with ischemic heart disease.* 38th Annual Scientific Session. Anaheim, California, American College of Cardiology, March, 1989.
9. DeBusk RF, Valdez R, Houston N, Haskell W: Cardiovascular responses to dynamic and status efforts soon after myocardial infarction. *Circulation* 58:368, 1978.
10. Ehsani AA, Heath GH, Hagberg JM, et al: Effects of 12 months of intense exercise training on ischemic ST-depression in patients with coronary artery disease. *Circulation* 64:1116, 1981.
11. Ewart CK, Stewart KJ, Kelemen MH, et al: Self-efficacy mediates strength gains during circuit weight training in men with coronary artery disease. *Med Sci Sports Exerc* 18(5):531, 1986.
12. Ewart CK, Taylor CB, Reese LB, DeBusk RF: Effects of early postmyocardial infarction exercise testing on self-perception and subsequent physical activity. *Am J Cardiol* 51:1076, 1983.
13. Friedman M: Diagnosis and treatment of Type A Behavior as a medical disorder. *Prim Cardiol* 15:68, 1989.
14. Furberg CD, Friedwald WT, Eberlein KA: Proceedings of the workshop on the implications of recent Beta-Blocker trials for postmyocardial infarction patients. *Circulation* 67:1, 1983.
15. Gillilan RE, Chopra AK, Kelemen MH, et al: Prediction of compliance to target heart rate during walk-job exercise in cardiac
16. Gibson RS, Boden WE, Theroux P and Diltiazem Reinfarction Study Group: Diltiazem and reinfarction in patients with non-Q wave myocardial infarction. Results of a double blind, randomized multi-center trial. *N Engl J Med* 315:423, 1986.
17. Gutmann MC, Squires RW, Pollack ML, et al: Perceived exertion-heart rate relationship during exercise testing and training in cardiac patients. *J Cardiovasc Rehabil* 1:52, 1981.
18. Hellerstein HK, Friedman EH: Sexual activity in the post-coronary patient. *Arch Intern Med* 125:987, 1970.
19. Kelemen ME, Effron MB, Valenti SA, Stewart KJ: Exercise training versus exercise training with diltiazem or propranolol: effects on maximal oxygen uptake and exercise duration in men with mild hypertension (abstract). *J Am Coll Cardiol* 13:241A, 1989.
20. Kelemen MH, Stewart KJ, Gillilan RE, et al: Circuit weight training in cardiac patients. *J Am Coll Cardiol* 7:38, 1986.
21. Levy RI, Brensike JF, Epstein SE, et al: The influence of changes in lipid values induced by cholestyramine and diet on progression of coronary artery disease: results of the NHLBI Type II coronary intervention study. *Circulation* 69:325, 1984.
22. Levy RI, Feinlab M: Risk factors for coronary artery disease and their management. In: Braunwald E (ed): *Heart Disease: A Textbook for Cardiovascular Medicine.* Philadelphia, WB Saunders, 1984.
23. The Lipid Research Clinics Coronary Primary Prevention Trial Results. I: Reduction in incidence of coronary heart disease. *JAMA* 251:351, 1984.
24. Lorenz RL, et al: Improved aortocoronary bypass patency by low-dose aspirin (100 mg daily): effects on platelet aggregation and thromboxane formation. *Lancet* 1:1261, 1984.
25. Manninen V, Elo O, Heikki F, et al: Lipid alterations and decline in incidence of coronary heart disease in the Helsinki Heart Study. *JAMA* 260:641, 1988.
26. Mather HG, Pearson NG, Read KLQ, et al: Acute myocardial infarction: home and hospital treatment. *Br Med J* 1:334, 1971.
27. Meizlish JL, Berger HJ, Plankey M, et al: Functional left ventricular aneurysm after acute myocardial infarction. *N Engl J Med* 16:1001, 1984.
28. Mukharji J, Rude RE, Poole WK, et al and The MILIS Study Group: Risk factors for sudden death after acute myocardial infarction: two-year follow-up. *Am J Cardiol* 54:31, 1984.
29. Oldridge NB, Gyuatt GH, Fischer ME, et al: Cardiac rehabilitation after myocardial infarction: combined experience of randomized clinical trials. *JAMA* 260:945, 1988.
30. Ornish DM, Scherwitz LW, Brown SC: Can lifestyle changes reverse atherosclerosis? (abstract) *Circulation* 78:II-11, 1988.
31. Plotnick GD: Approach to the management of unstable angina. *Am Heart J* 98:243, 1979.
32. Randomized trial of intravenous streptokinase, oral aspirin, both or neither among 17, 187 cases of suspected acute myocardial infarction: ISIS-2. *Lancet* 2:349, 1988.
33. Rosati RA, Harris PJ: Acute myocardial infarction. In: Fries JF, Ehrlich GE (eds): *Prognosis: Contemporary Outcomes of Disease.* Bowie, MD, Charles Press Publishers, 1981.
34. Russell Jr. RO, Abi-Mansour P, Wenger NK, et al: Return to work after coronary artery bypass surgery and percutaneous transluminal angioplasty: issues and potential solutions. *Cardiology* 73:306, 1986.
35. Schaffer WA, Cobb LA: Recurrent ventricular fibrillation and modes of death in survivors of out-of-hospital ventricular fibrillation. *N Engl J Med* 293:259, 1975.
36. Schleifer SJ, Macari-Hinson MM, Coyle DA, et al: The nature and course of depression following myocardial infarction. *Arch Intern Med* 149:1785, 1989.
37. Stamler J: Acute myocardial infarction-progress in primary prevention. *Br Heart J* 33:145, 1971.
38. Stewart KJ, Effron MB, Valenti SA, Kelemen MH: Circuit weight training with diltiazem or propranolol: effects on muscle strength in men with mild hypertension. (Abstract) *Med Sci Sports Exercise* 21(2):S107, 1989.
39. Stewart KJ, Mason M, Kelemen MH: Three year participation

in circuit weight training improves muscular strength and self-efficacy in cardiac patients. *J Cardiopul Rehab* 8:292, 1988.

40. Taylor JL, Copeland RB, Cousin AL, et al: The effect of isometric exercise on the graded exercise test in patients with stable angina. *J Cardiopul Rehabil* 1:450, 1981.
41. Theroux P, Marpole DGF, Bourassa MG: Exercise stress testing in the postmyocardial infarction patient. *Am J Cardiol* 52:664, 1983.
42. Theroux P, Ovimet H, McCans J, et al: Aspirin, heparin, or both to treat acute unstable angina. *N Engl J Med* 319:1105, 1988.
43. Thornton MA, Greventzig AR, Hollman J, et al: Coumadin and aspirin in prevention of recurrence after transluminal coronary angioplasty: a randomized study. *Circulation* 69:72, 1984.
44. Toffler GH, Stone PH, Muller JC, et al: Effect of gender and race in prognosis after MI: adverse prognosis for women, particularly black women. *J Am Coll Cardiol* 9:473, 1987.
45. Ueno M: The so-called coitus death. *Jpn J Legal Med* 17:330, 1963.
46. Waters DD, Theroux P, Halphen C, Mizgala HF: Clinical predictors of angina following myocardial infarction. *Am J Med* 66:991, 1979.
47. Wilhelmsson C, Vedin JA, Elmfeldt D, et al: Smoking and myocardial infarction. *Lancet* 1:415, 1975.
48. Zohman LR: *Beyond Diet: Exercise Your Way to Fitness and Heart Health.* Englewood Cliffs, NJ, Mazola Products, Best Food, 1974.

C H A P T E R 59

Arrhythmias

SHELDON H. GOTTLIEB, M.D.

Contraction of the heart is normally the result of a well-orchestrated electromechanical system. The orderly function of the system is maintained by the domination of the heart rate by a single pulse generator known as the pacemaker, by the relatively fast and uniform conduction of the electrical signal via specialized conduction pathways, and by the relatively long and uniform duration of the electrical signal relative to its velocity of conduction through these pathways, thereby assuring uniform electrical excitation and contraction of the heart. An arrhythmia is any disturbance in the normal sequence of impulse generation and conduction in the heart.

Arrhythmias may occur in the absence of heart disease or may be symptoms of severe disease. They must be evaluated in the context of the clinical situation in which they occur. A precise etiological diagnosis and an understanding of the pharmacology of the medications used are necessary to treat arrhythmias effectively.

PHYSIOLOGY OF IMPULSE GENERATION AND CONDUCTION

The Action Potential

Muscle contraction is stimulated by an electrical impulse, the action potential. In skeletal muscle, the action potential is transient, and the electrical activity is essentially dissipated before the beginning of contraction. In cardiac muscle, however, the action potential is sustained and lasts almost as long as the contraction itself (Fig. 59.1). In this way, the action potential not only stimulates contraction of the heart but also determines the duration and intensity of contraction. Furthermore, as long as the action potential is maintained, the heart cannot be stimulated to contract again.

The action potential is generated by depolarization and repolarization of the muscle cell (Fig. 59.2). In the resting state the intracellular concentration of potassium is high and that of sodium is low compared with the extracellular fluid. These gradients are maintained by metabolic activity within the cell membrane. The resting membrane potential is strongly negative (i.e., there is an electrochemical gradient across the membrane so that the inside of the membrane is negatively charged compared with the outside of the membrane). If an electrical stimulus is applied, the membrane becomes very permeable to sodium ions, which rapidly leak into the cell (phase 0). The membrane is thus depolarized (loses its negative charge) and, in fact, is transiently positively charged (overshoot). Repolarization occurs relatively slowly as first chloride (phase 1), calcium ions (phase 2), and then potassium ions (phase 3) move back into the cell and thereby restore the resting potential (phase 4).

Relationship to the Electrocardiogram

In the heart the phases of rapid depolarization and overshoot correspond to the QRS complex of the electrocardiogram (ECG); phase 2 corresponds to the ST segment; and phase 3, to the T wave (Fig. 59.2). During phase 2 the membrane is absolutely and in phase 3 relatively refractory to propagation of another electrical impulse.

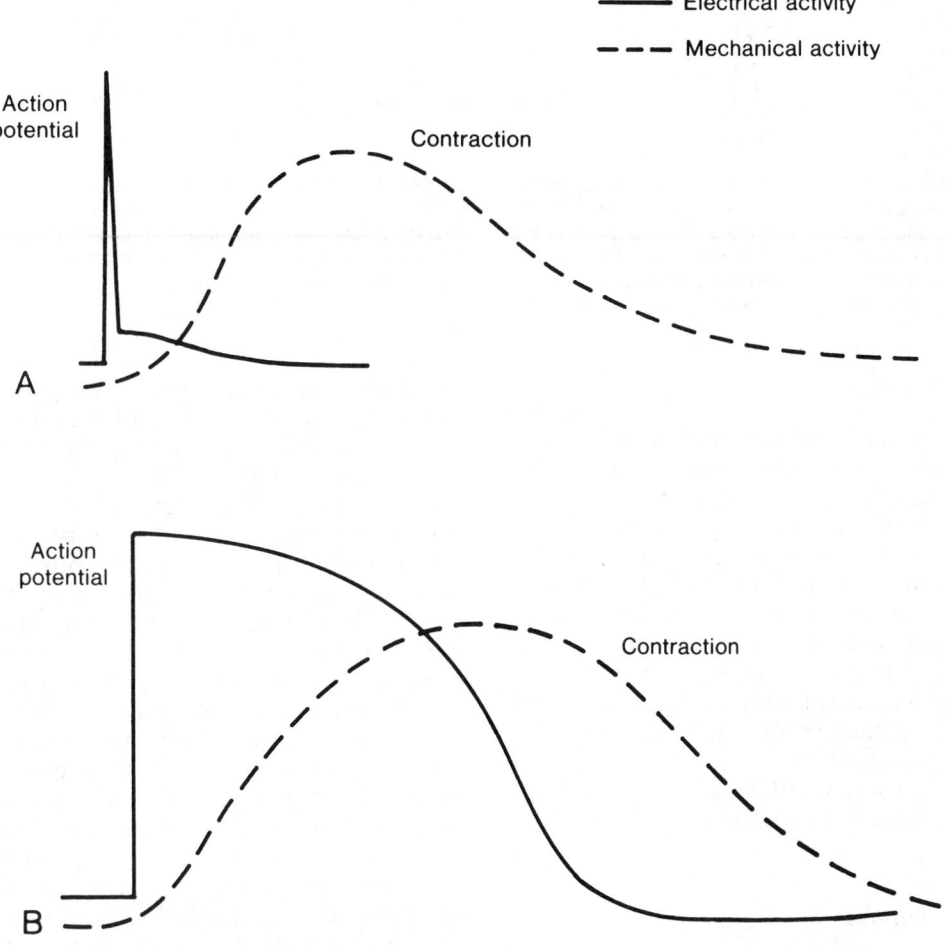

Figure 59.1. Comparison between relative time scales of electrical (*continuous curve*) and mechanical (*interrupted curve*) activity in skeletal (*A*) and cardiac (*B*) muscle. (From Noble D: *The Initiation of the Heart Beat.* Oxford, Clarendon Press, 1975 (17).)

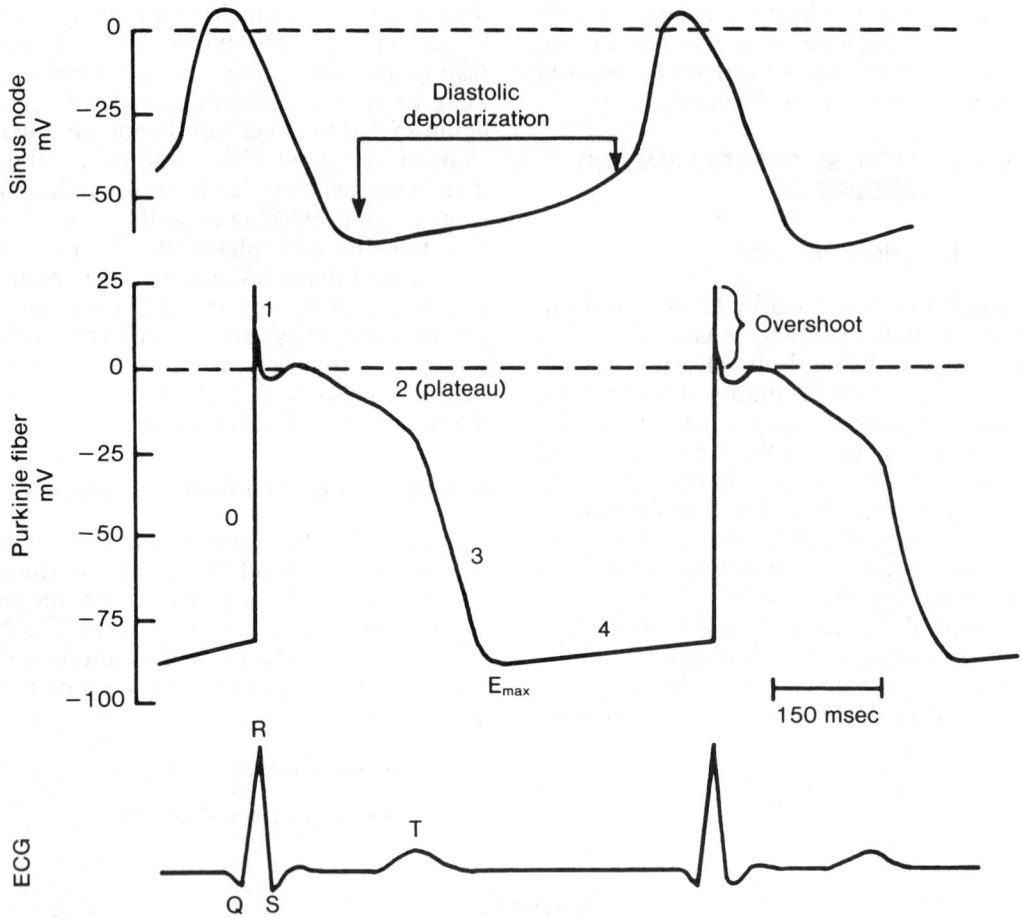

Figure 59.2. Transmembrane potentials from the sinus node and a Purkinje fiber. Note the spontaneous diastolic depolarization in the upper panel, characteristic of pacemaker fibers. The numbers in the *middle panel* are explained in the text. The *lower panel* shows the correlation of the time sequence of changes in the action potential and that of the surface electrocardiogram. Alterations in depolarization will be reflected in changes in the QRS duration of the surface record; those in repolarization will be associated with alterations in the Q-T interval. (From Singh BN, Collett JT, Chew CYC: New perspectives in the pharmacologic therapy of cardiac arrhythmias. *Prog Cardiovasc Dis* 22:243, 1980 (23).)

Fast and Slow Currents

Although in most cardiac tissue, excitation is propagated by the rapidly depolarizing sodium current (so that the action potential is conducted rapidly), excitation of the sinoatrial node and the proximal part of the atrioventricular node is propagated by a slowly depolarizing current generated by the influx of calcium ions into the cell. Also, in diseased cardiac muscle, the sodium current may be inhibited and depolarization may occur entirely via the slow calcium current; therefore the action potential may be conducted very slowly. This difference in conduction velocity between cells depolarized by the sodium versus the calcium current has important implications in both the generation and the treatment of arrhythmias (see below).

Pacemaker Generation

In most cardiac cells, an action potential will not be generated until an electrical stimulus is applied.

In pacemaker cells, slow spontaneous depolarization occurs until a threshold is reached whereupon phase 0 rapidly ensues (Fig. 59.2); this process is called automaticity. In the absence of heart block, the heart rate will be controlled by the pacemaker cells that depolarize most rapidly, because then the action potential is conducted rapidly throughout the heart and initiates rapid depolarization of other cells, even if they already have begun spontaneous slow depolarization. Automaticity is affected by the rate of slow spontaneous depolarization and by the threshold potential. Automaticity is enhanced by increased sympathetic tone, decreased vagal tone, increased catecholamine concentration in the blood, thyroid hormone, and digitalis. It is suppressed by decreased sympathetic tone, increased vagal tone, decreased thyroid hormone concentration, and various drugs (e.g., the drugs used in the treatment of arrhythmias). Antiarrhythmic drugs may also *increase* automaticity under some conditions; this phenomenon is known as proarrhythmagenesis and is discussed below.

Impulse Generation and Conduction (Fig. 59.3)

Sinoauricular Node

The sinoauricular (SA) node is composed of pacemaker cells and is located at the junction of the right atrium and the superior vena cava. The cells of the SA node spontaneously depolarize more rapidly than any other cells within the heart and thereby control the heart rate.

Atrial Fibers

The action potential generated by the SA node traverses the atrium rapidly along discrete bundles of specialized conduction tissue known as internodal fibers. A specialized bundle of tissue connects the right and left atrium and the contractions of the atria are therefore nearly synchronous.

Atrioventricular Node

The internodal fibers terminate in the atrioventricular (AV) node cells, which lie at the junction of the right atrium and the interventricular septum just above the tricuspid valve and through which the action potential is conducted slowly. Electrical delay in the AV node allows the mechanical activity of the atria (which

is slower than their electrical activity) to be synchronized with the mechanical activity of the ventricles. The AV node serves as a protective "gate" and will not respond to extremely rapid impulses generated in the atria, thereby protecting the ventricles from too rapid stimulation. The AV node may function as a subsidiary pacemaker if the SA node fails to pace.

Bundle of His

When the action potential leaves the AV node, it enters the specialized conducting fibers known as the bundle of His. The main bundle of His divides into three branches: the right bundle branch, which runs along the right ventricular surface of the septum, the anterior superior branch, which runs along the left ventricular surface of the septum, and the posterior inferior branch, which runs along the posterior wall of the left ventricle. The action potential is conducted through the bundle branches and into the myocardium by a widespread network of smaller fibers known as Purkinje fibers.

MECHANISM OF CARDIAC ARRHYTHMIAS

There are three basic causes of disturbance in the rhythm of the heart: suppression or enhancement of

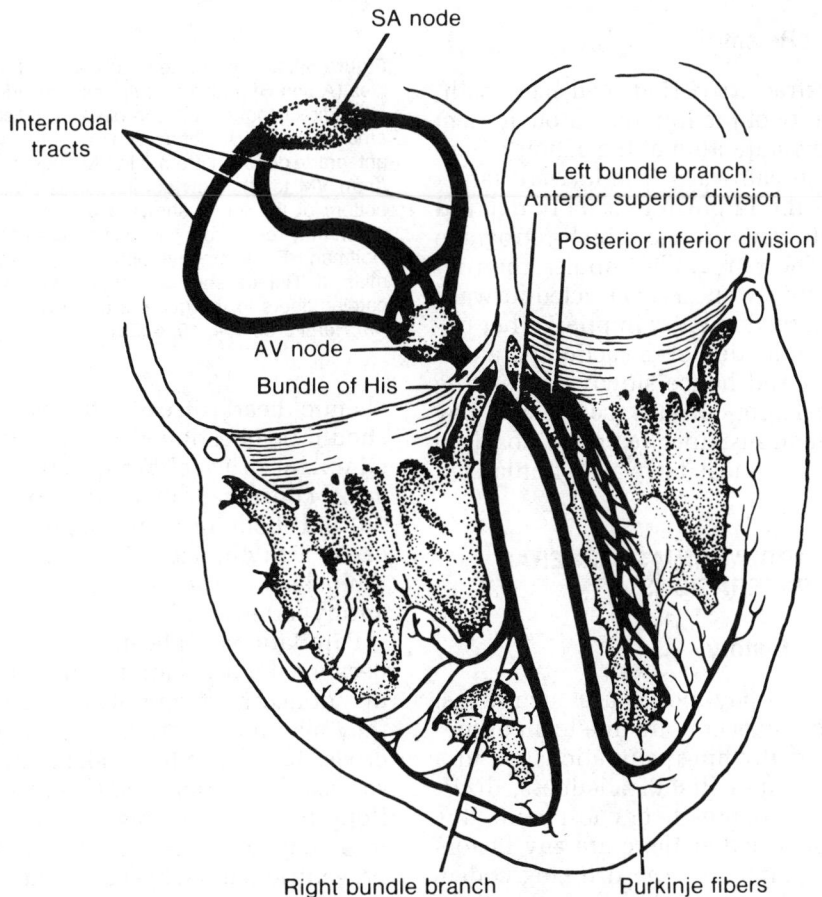

Figure 59.3. Anatomy of impulse conduction. *SA*, sinoatrial; *AV*, atrioventricular. (From Greene HL, Humphries JO: Cardiac arrhythmias. In Harvey AM, Johns RJ, McKusick VA, *et al* (eds): *Principles and Practice of Medicine*. New York, Appleton-Century-Crofts, 1980.)

initiation or propagation of the action potential, ectopic pacemaker activity, and re-entry of the action potential into a pathway through which it has already passed. More than one of these mechanisms may be operative in producing a particular arrhythmia, e.g., ectopic supraventricular tachycardia in a patient with sinus node dysfunction.

Suppression of Initiation or Propagation of Action Potential

A disease process that interferes with pacemaker activity within the SA node or with the movement of the electrical impulse through the normal conduction pathways of the heart results either in abnormal slowing of the heart rate (bradyarrhythmia) and/or in one of the various forms of heart block.

Ectopic Pacemaker Activity

Enhanced automaticity of a part of the cardiac conduction system may result in the initiation of an impulse more rapidly than is normally generated by the SA node. If that happens episodically, occasional premature contractions will occur, the nature of which will depend on the location of the ectopic pacemaker. On the other hand, if there is rapid sustained firing of the ectopic focus, a tachyarrhythmia will be produced.

Re-entry

Alterations in the refractory period of adjacent pathways and of the velocity of the impulse through them may allow retrograde conduction of the action potential through one of the pathways. The forward (antegrade) conduction of the impulse is usually delayed or blocked in the pathway through which retrograde conduction occurs. The retrograde impulse then re-enters an adjacent pathway and is conducted forward again (Fig. 59.4). Sustained re-entry implies either unusual pathways for conduction of the action potential or poorly functioning and hence slowly conducting myocardium. Slow calcium currents (see above) may play an important role in sustained re-entry. Most premature contractions and most tachyarrhythmias are re-entrant rhythms.

DIAGNOSIS OF ARRHYTHMIAS: GENERAL CONSIDERATIONS

History

Arrhythmias may or may not cause symptoms. Symptoms, when they do occur, are due to an appreciation of the irregular rhythm (palpitations) or to a reduction in cardiac output (lightheadedness, dizziness, syncope, shortness of breath, or chest pain). It is important to establish whether there are any factors that seem to trigger symptoms (e.g., drinking coffee, smoking, exercise, emotional stress) and whether there are symptoms of an underlying disease that may be associated with arrhythmia (e.g., heart failure, is-

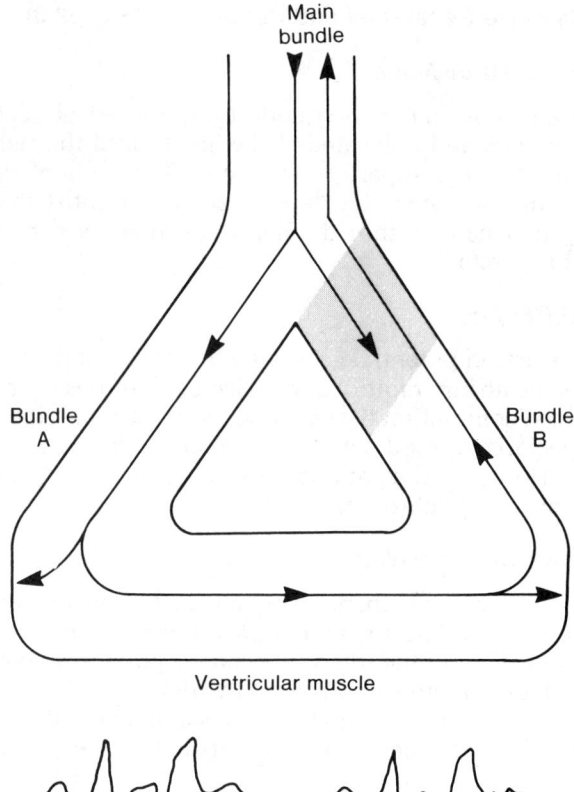

Figure 59.4. Sequence of activation of a loop of Purkinje fiber bundles (A and B) and ventricular muscle (VM) during re-entry. A region of unidirectional conduction block is indicated by the *darkly shaded area* in branch B. Conduction cannot occur through this area in the antegrade direction (from B to VM), but only in the retrograde direction (from VM to B). Slow conduction is present through the loop. The bottom of the figure shows a possible electrocardiographic pattern which may result from this type of re-entry. (From Wit AL, Rosen MR, Hoffman BF: Electrophysiology and pharmacology of cardiac arrhythmias. II. Relationship of normal and abnormal electrical activity of cardiac fibers to the genesis of arrhythmias. B. Re-entry, Section I. *Am Heart J* 88:664, 1974 (29).)

chemic heart disease, thyrotoxicosis). The patient should be questioned specifically about the taking of stimulant drugs either illicitly (see Chapter 22) or as an ill-conceived attempt to lose weight (see Chapter 76) and about the taking of prescription drugs that may cause arrhythmias (digitalis, theophylline, diuretics, β-blockers, β agonists, tricyclic antidepressants, and antihypertensives).

Palpitations are heartbeats that are sensed—usually because the beats are fast or irregular. However, they do not necessarily imply a significant arrhythmia and they may represent only sinus tachycardia in an otherwise healthy individual. Palpitations are usually described by patients as sensations of beating, flip-flopping, or throbbing in the chest. They are often localized to the area of the apex beat, but rapid supraventricular tachycardias are commonly felt substernally or in the neck. Some people seem to sense the compensatory pause (see below) after an extra heart beat, but some may sense the extra beat itself. Often the contraction after an extra beat is more powerful than a normal beat (so-called postextrasystolic potentiation), and this stronger beat may be the one that is felt. Supraventricular beats are more commonly sensed as palpitations than are ventricular beats; and in fact potentially dangerous runs of ventricular tachycardia are commonly asymptomatic.

Light-headedness, dizziness, and syncope are common symptoms of significant arrhythmias. These symptoms and the conditions associated with them are discussed in detail in Chapter 81.

Physical Examination

An arrhythmia is best revealed on physical examination by inspection of the jugular pulse, palpation of the arterial pulse, and auscultation of the heart.

Conditions associated with arrhythmia—e.g., heart failure (Chapter 61), chronic obstructive lung disease (Chapter 55), or valvular heart disease (Chapter 60)—can often be recognized by characteristic physical findings.

Inspection of the jugular venous pulse reveals atrial activity. If there is atrioventricular dissociation or complete heart block, so-called cannon waves may be seen intermittently in the jugular veins; they are due to ejection of blood back into the veins when the right atrium contracts against a closed tricuspid valve. Cannon waves that coincide with the arterial pulse may reflect supraventricular tachycardia. If there is atrial fibrillation, there are no atrial waves visible in the jugular pulse.

Palpation of the arterial pulse establishes the ventricular rate—at least of conducted beats—and rhythm. In conjunction with the jugular pulse, it may provide more specific information as well about the nature of an arrythmia.

Auscultation of the heart also establishes the ventricular rate and rhythm and the intensity of S_1, the most useful heart sound in the evaluation of arrhythmia. For example, variation in the intensity of S_1 during a regular tachycardia suggests AV dissociation; variation during a regular bradycardia suggests second or third degree heart block. The intensity of S_1 is also a function of the P-R interval. A loud S_1 suggests a short P-R interval and is also heard in patients with mitral valve prolapse; a soft S_1 suggests a long P-R interval, due, for example, to digitalis toxicity or to electrolyte abnormalities.

Use of the ECG

It is essential to obtain an ECG when evaluating a patient who has an arrhythmia. Without it, with few exceptions, a specific diagnosis is impossible. Usually a surface resting ECG is all that is needed. Occasionally, ambulatory (Holter) monitoring or an exercise ECG is indicated to detect a sporadic arrhythmia or an arrhythmia that is induced by stress. Even less commonly, a complex arrhythmia cannot be diagnosed accurately by standard ECG, and an intracavity elec-

trophysiological study must be obtained by catheterization in order to make a precise diagnosis.

Surface Resting ECG

There are a number of features of the standard ECG that must be assessed:

Atrial activity. Atrial activity is best assessed in leads 2, 3, aVf, and in V_1. The presence of P waves must be identified. If P waves are present, their configuration and their relationship to QRS complexes must be established. Normally the P-R interval is between 0.12 and 0.20 second, and each QRS complex is preceded by a P wave. If P waves are not present, other evidence of atrial activity (fibrillation or flutter waves) should be sought.

Ventricular activity. The duration of the QRS complexes (normally less than 0.10 second) should be measured and the regularity of ventricular activity should be assessed. A basically regular rhythm may be interrupted by so-called premature beats—QRS complexes that appear before the next regular beat is expected. If premature beats are present, it should be noted whether they have a fixed relationship to the preceding normal beat and whether their configuration is the same as the regularly occurring complexes.

Ambulatory ECG

The ambulatory (Holter) ECG (22) records on magnetic tape the electrical activity of the heart—usually for a 24-hour period. The recording device is small and does not interfere with virtually any of the patient's activities (except bathing and swimming). The technique is useful in the following circumstances:

1. Assessing whether suspicious symptoms—e.g., palpitation, light-headedness, dizziness, or syncope—in a patient with a normal resting ECG are due to an episodic arrhythmia;
2. Assessing whether episodic, but potentially life-threatening, arrhythmias are occurring in a patient with known heart disease (e.g., iscshemic heart disease or congestive heart failure);
3. Assessing the efficacy of antiarrhythmic therapy or the function of a cardiac pacemaker.

The majority of episodic arrhythmias are detected during 24 hours of Holter monitoring. If symptoms are infrequent, however, it may be necessary to record the ambulatory ECG for 48 to 72 hours. It is important to ask the patient to keep a record of symptoms during the time that he is being monitored in order to determine whether those symptoms are, in fact, attributable to arrhythmia.

Exercise ECG

This technique is described in detail in Chapter 57. It is a useful test in the evaluation of patients who have symptoms suggestive of an arrhythmia during or after exercise or those with premature ventricular contractions—to determine whether they become more or less frequent during or after exercise (see page 708).

GENERAL PRINCIPLES IN MANAGEMENT OF ARRHYTHMIAS

Once it has been established that a patient has a particular arrhythmia, the physician must decide whether treatment is necessary. That decision will be influenced by the effect of the arrhythmia on cardiac output, the potential for thromboembolic complications, the potential for degeneration of the arrhythmia into a more dangerous rhythm, and the relative risk of the treatment versus the relative risk of the arrhythmia to the patient's well-being and survival. It must also be determined whether the arrhythmia is constant or intermittent and whether it is secondary to a noncardiac process (e.g., hypoxia, electrolyte imbalance, fever) or a cardiac process (e.g., heart failure, ischemia, pericarditis, digitalis intoxication), the correction of which will restore a normal cardiac rhythm.

If the physician determines that specific therapy is indicated, he must decide which of the various possible regimens is appropriate: one or more of the antiarrhythmic drugs, a cardiac pacemaker, electrical conversion of the arrhythmia, or a combination of these regimens.

Pharmacology of Antiarrhythmic Drugs

There are four classes of antiarrhythmic drugs (10, 28). *Class I drugs*, whose prototype is quinidine, interfere with the fast inward sodium current. *Class II drugs*, whose prototype is propranolol, affect sympathetically mediated excitability. *Class III drugs*, whose prototype is amiodarone, prolong the duration of the action potential by decreasing the late inward (phase 3) potassium current. *Class IV drugs*, whose prototype is verapamil, block calcium-mediated slow channel currents in the myocardium.

Table 59.1 shows some of the characteristics of the orally administered antiarrhythmic drugs that can be used to treat an ambulatory patient.

Most antiarrhythmic drugs have a low toxic:therapeutic ratio and some are exceedingly toxic (Table 59.2). In addition to direct toxic effects, antiarrhythmic drugs may paradoxically induce arrhythmias. These so-called proarrhythmic effects may include virtually any arrhythmia but frequently are seen as an increase in the frequency of PVCs or the sudden onset of ventricular tachycardia or fibrillation. Proarrhythmic effects are usually seen within several days after an antiarrhythmic drug is started or the dose is changed, and they usually are seen in patients with severe heart disease, with an ejection fraction below 40% (11). The safe and effective use of antiarrhythmic drugs depends on a careful assessment of the etiology and physiology of an arrhythmia and a knowledge of the pharmacology of the drugs that are used. Doses must, therefore, be individualized, and drug levels

should be checked periodically (at first, after a steady state has been reached—see Table 59.1—and then one to three times a year, depending on the patient's response). Levels should be obtained approximately 4 hours after an oral dose of a drug that is taken every 6 to 8 hours, and approximately 8 to 12 hours after an oral dose of a drug that is taken once a day.

Digitalis, the other major drug used in the treatment of arrhythmias, is not, strictly speaking, an antiarrhythmic drug in that it does not have a direct effect on membrane function. It acts indirectly as an antiarrhythmic agent by increasing vagal activity, thereby increasing the refractory period of the specialized conduction tissue of the atria and slowing the velocity of the action potential through the AV node. General considerations in the use of digitalis including dosages, choice of a preparation, and recognition and treatment of toxicity are discussed in Chapter 61.

Class I Drugs

All Class I drugs block the fast sodium channel (see pages 690) but the effect on the duration of the action potential and on repolarization varies depending on the kinetics of the blockage (10). This has practical application in the choice of drugs for treatment of specific arrhythmias and in the use of a combination of drugs, although it would be advisable to combine these drugs only after consultation with a cardiologist.

Class I drugs have been subdivided into 3 classes, IA, IB, IC (see Table 59.1).

Class IA Drugs. Class IA drugs prolong the duration of the action potential and so prolong the QRS and QT interval. These drugs include quinidine, procainamide, and disopyramide.

QUINIDINE. In addition to its direct effects on the heart, quinidine blocks parasympathetic stimulation by the vagus nerve and may enhance AV conduction (and the ventricular rate) in some patients. For this reason patients with supraventricular tachyarrhythmias should be digitalized to suppress AV conduction before they are given quinidine. Quinidine also is a moderately potent inhibitor of α-adrenergic activity.

Several preparations of quinidine are available; quinidine sulfate is the recommended preparation on the basis of cost, but quinidine gluconate has fewer gastrointestinal side effects. A sustained release preparation containing gluconate (Quinaglute, Duraquin) may be preferred in some patients because it can be given every 8 to 12 hours.

Table 59.1 shows the time necessary to reach a steady state after administration of usual doses of quinidine. If a faster effect is desired, loading doses may be given (e.g., 300 mg every 3 hours for three doses); in this circumstance hospitalization is advisable, both to monitor the effect of the drug and because the arrhythmia presumably is more dangerous.

Quinidine is used most often to prevent recurrence of supraventricular and ventricular tachyarrhythmias. It is also moderately effective but is no longer the first

Table 59.1.
Characteristics of Antiarrhythmic Drugs

Drug	Common Brand Name	Effects on ECG	Half-life	Time to Steady State (day)	Available Strength (mg)	Usual Oral Dose	Maximal Daily Dose (mg)	Therapeutic Plasma Levels
Class IA								
Quinidine	Generic	Prolongs QRS, Q-and (±) P-R	6	1–2	200 (sulfate) 342 (gluconate)	200–600 mg every 6–8 hr	2400	3–7 μg/ml
Procainamide	Pronestyl	Prolongs QRS Q-T, and (±) P-R	3–4	1	250, 500 500, 750 (sustained release)	500–1000 mg every 3–4 hr or every 6 hr (sustained release)	8000	3–8 μg/ml[a]
Disopyramide	Norpace	Prolongs QRS Q-T, and (±) P-R	6–9	1–2	100, 500	150 mg 4 times daily	1200	2–4 μg/ml
Class IB								
Tocainide	Tonocard	Shortens Q-T	15	1.5–3	400, 600	400–600 mg every 8 hr or 600 mg every 12 hr	3200	4–10 μg of base/ml
Mexiletine	Mexitil	Shortens Q-T	10–12	2–3	200, 250	200–300 mg every 8 hr	1200	0.5–2 μg/ml
Phenytoin (diphenyl-hydantoin)	Dilantin	Shortens Q-T	24–36	3–5	100	300–400 mg a day	800	10–20 μg/ml
Class IC								
Encainide	Enkaid	Prolongs P-R QRS	1–2 for drug 3–12 for active metabolite	3–5	25, 35, 50	35 mg 3 times a day	200	N/A
Flecainide	Tambocor	Prolongs P-R, QRS, QT, bradycardia	12–27	2–3	100	200 mg every day	600	.2–1–.0 μg/ml
Class II								
Propranolol	Inderal	Prolongs (±) P-R, shortens Q-T	6	1	10, 20, 40, 60, 80	10–40 mg every 6 hr	640	50–100 ng/ml
Class III								
Amiodarone	Cordarone	Prolongs P-R, QRS	53	8 days after loading dose	200	200–600 mg once daily	800	Not useful
Class IV								
Verapamil	Calan, Isoptin	Prolongs P-R	4.5–12	1–2	80, 120	80–120 mg every 8 hr	480	125–400 ng/ml
Diltiazem	Cardizem	Prolongs P-R	3.5	1	30, 60, 90, 120	30–120 mg 3–4 times daily	480	Not useful

[a] It may also be important to measure, especially in patients in cardiac or renal failure, the level of the active metabolite of procainamide, N-acetylprocainamide (NAPA).

Table 59.2.
Adverse Effects of Antiarrhythmic Drugs

Drug	Cardiac — Common	Cardiac — Uncommon	Noncardiac — Common	Noncardiac — Uncommon
Class IA				
Quinidine	Decreased digoxin excretion (may precipitate digitoxicity)	Ventricular arrhythmias, myocardial depression, hypotension	Nausea, diarrhea, tinnitus, vertigo, rash, fever	Hepatic dysfunction, thrombocytopenia, hemolytic anemia
Procainamide	None	Myocardial depression	Nausea, vomiting	Agranulocytosis, lupus-like syndrome
Disopyramide	Myocardial depression (should be used with caution in patients with severe or poorly compensated congestive heart failure)	Severe hypotension in absence of known heart disease	Anticholinergic effects—especially urinary retention, dry mouth, blurred vision, constipation, aggravation of narrow angle glaucoma	Acute psychoses, cholestasis
Class IB				
Tocainide	None	Ventricular arrhythmias	Dizziness, paresthesias tremor, nausea, vomiting and sweating	Rashes, convulsions
Mexiletine	None	Increased frequency of ventricular arrhythmias	Nausea, vomiting, indigestion, dizziness, tremor	Sleep disturbances, fatigue
Phenytoin (diphenylhydantoin)	None	Heart Block	Cerebellar-vestibular effects, especially ataxia, nystagmus, vertigo: nausea, lethargy, seizures, rashes	Pseudolymphoma, megaloblastic anemia peripheral neuropathy
Class IC				
Encainide	Increased frequency of ventricular arrhythmias	Congestive heart failure	Dizziness, nausea, blurred vision, headache	Ataxia, gait abnormalities, rash
Flecainide	Increased frequency of ventricular arrhythmias, myocardial depression—use with caution in patients with ejection fraction < 40%	New supraventricular arrhythmias	Dizziness, visual disturbances, dyspnea, nausea, tremor	Constipation, edema, abdominal pain
Class II				
Propranolol[a]	Bradycardia, myocardial depression	Anginal syndrome may worsen if drug suddenly discontinued	Fatigue, nausea, vomiting, depression, impotence, potentiates bronchospasm in patients with asthma	Peripheral vascular insufficiency, hyperglycemia, alopecia
Class III				
Amiodorone	Bradycardia, increased heart block, increased digoxin concentration	Ventricular arrhythmias	Nausea, corneal microcrystalization, thyroid function abnormalities, decreased pulmonary diffusing capacity	Blue tint of exposed skin, pulmonary fibrosis
Class IV				
Verapamil	Bradycardia, prolongation of P-R interval, peripheral edema, increased digoxin level	Precipitation of congestive heart failure or pulmonary edema, severe hypotension, heart block	Dizziness, headache, constipation, nausea	Confusion, sleep disorders
Diltiazem	Bradycardia, prolongation of P-R interval	Heart block, increased digoxin level	Dizziness, headache, constipation	Rash, itching

[a]Other β-blocking agents have the same adverse effects, although bronchospasm and peripheral vascular insufficiency may be less likely with use of β-specific agents (see Table 59.3).

approach in the conversion of atrial flutter or fibrillation to normal sinus rhythm. The uses of the drug in specific situations are discussed below.

Toxicity. There are a number of possible toxic effects of quinidine. The most common are gastrointestinal, especially diarrhea, and occur often within hours of administering the drug. Cinchonism (tinnitus, headache, visual disturbances) occurs occasionally. Hypersensitivity reactions (e.g., rash, arthralgias, immune thrombocytopenia, or hemolytic anemia) are rare. These reactions often necessitate substitution of another antiarrhythmic drug.

Cardiac toxicity is usually dose related, often signaled by a prolongation of the Q-T interval; Q-T prolongation of 50% or more beyond baseline is an indication for reduction of the dose of quinidine. Serious toxicity is manifest by a high degree of AV block, ventricular tachycardia, or fibrillation—all emergency situations that may require cardiorespiratory support and warrant immediate hospitalization. Occasionally, patients taking quinidine die suddenly, sometimes with relatively low plasma levels of the drug. Patients with prolonged Q-T intervals before institution of therapy with quinidine may be more prone to sudden death and therefore probably should not be given the drug.

If patients taking quinidine are asymptomatic, ECGs need be recorded no more frequently than once a year; if they are symptomatic (e.g., complain of exertional chest pain, light-headedness, shortness of breath, etc.), more frequent tracings should be obtained (perhaps every 3 or 4 months).

Drug interactions. Because patients prescribed quinidine are commonly being treated with digitalis as well, it is especially important to recognize that digoxin levels may increase significantly in patients given quinidine. Quinidine decreases the excretion of digoxin by the kidneys, and therefore it is important to monitor serum digoxin concentrations when quinidine is first prescribed and to alter the dose of digoxin to prevent digitoxicity.

Quinidine is an α-adrenergic blocker and, if it is prescribed with vasodilators (e.g., nitrates, nifedipine, hydralazine, prazosin) or with potent diuretics (e.g., furosemide) may cause symptomatic (especially postural) hypotension.

Drugs that are metabolized by hepatic microsomal enzymes may alter the pharmacokinetics of quinidine, and conversely, quinidine may alter the kinetics of one of these drugs. For example, phenytoin may accelerate the metabolism of quinidine, shortening its effect, and quinidine may inhibit the metabolism of warfarin, prolonging its effect.

PROCAINAMIDE. The suppressive effects of procainamide on the electrical activity of the heart are the same as those of quinidine; but, unlike quinidine, procainamide has very little effect on vagal or on α-adrenergic activity.

The drug has been thought to be most useful in preventing recurrence of ventricular arrhythmias, although in somewhat higher doses (4 to 8 g/day instead of the more usual 2 to 6 g/day) it is as effective as quinidine in preventing the recurrence of atrial arrhythmias and in converting atrial flutter or fibrillation to normal sinus rhythm.

Toxicity. The noncardiac toxicity of procainamide is different from that of quinidine. Gastrointestinal symptoms occur less often; and when they do, nausea and vomiting are more common than is diarrhea. Fever or granulocytopenia occurs occasionally.

Fifty percent of people taking procainamide develop antinuclear antibodies (ANAs) within 3 months and 90% within 12 months (4). Twenty to 30% of patients with ANAs develop a lupus-like syndrome characterized by serositis (pleuritis, pericarditis, synovitis), fever, hepatomegaly, and a positive lupus erythematosus preparation. Unlike classical systemic lupus erythematosus, vasculitis is not a manifestation of drug-induced lupus, so that renal disease, for example, does not occur; and, most important, the syndrome abates, usually within months, when the drug is discontinued. The major threat of the syndrome is hemorrhagic pericarditis, and one must watch for signs and symptoms of pericardial tamponade.

DISOPYRAMIDE. Disopyramide has direct membrane effects very much like quinidine and, like quinidine, blocks parasympathetic activity. It is licensed for the treatment of specific ventricular arrhythmias: unifocal or multifocal premature ventricular contractions and ventricular tachycardia. Disopyramide is used in ambulatory practice primarily for patients with one of these ventricular arrhythmias who cannot tolerate quinidine or procainamide.

The noncardiac toxicity of disopyramide is due mainly to its anticholinergic effects; these include dry mouth, blurred vision, urinary hesitancy, and constipation. Nausea, vomiting, and diarrhea are less common than they are after administration of quinidine or procainamide. The cardiac toxicity of the drug is, in part, similar to that of quinidine in that it can prolong the Q-T interval and produce ventricular tachycardia. Disopyramide may also cause or intensify heart failure or cause profound hypotension in patients who have compromised left ventricular function; it should be administered cautiously to such patients and stopped immediately if adverse reactions occur.

Class IB Drugs. Class IB drugs shorten repolarization and the QT interval and have little effect on the duration of the QRS complex. This class includes phenytoin, tocainide, and mexiletine. Class IB drugs are generally not effective for supraventricular arrhythmias.

PHENYTOIN. Phenytoin decreases automaticity and the duration of the action potential in the Purkinje fibers of the myocardium. Its use is limited in the treatment of arrhythmias. Its primary value is in the treatment of complex arrhythmias associated with digitoxicity, and therefore it is seldom prescribed as an antiarrhythmic agent in ambulatory practice. Occasionally, patients will be discharged from the hospital and will be taking phenytoin for control of a ventricular arrhythmia that has proved resistant to other drugs (or that has only been controlled by lidocaine, a drug that cannot be used on an ambulatory basis). Such patients are best followed in conjunction with a cardiologist.

Phenytoin toxicity is discussed in detail in Chapter 80.

TOCAINIDE. Tocainide is an analogue of lidocaine but can be given orally and has high bioavailability. It is used to suppress ventricular ectopy, and in the approximately 60% of patients who respond to it, the number of premature ventricular contractions is reduced by 90% (18). In this regard it is no more effective than are quinidine, procainamide, or disopyramide. Adverse effects include a high incidence of nausea, tremulousness, dizziness, and anxiety. Bone marrow depression is occasionally seen.

MEXILETINE. Mexiletine has electrophysiologic effects similar to those of tocainide and also has similar adverse effects. It may be very useful in combination with a class IA or class III drug (see below), but consultation with a cardiologist is advised before using it in combination.

Class IC Drugs. Class IC drugs slow conduction and widen the QRS complex but cause only small changes in refractoriness or in the QT interval. The class IC drugs currently available, flecainide and encainide, are both highly effective against serious ventricular arrhythmias and may be particularly useful in treatment of supraventricular arrhythmias, especially those associated with pre-excitation (see below). However, both of these drugs have recently been shown to be associated with a high incidence of sudden death (more than three times that among patients treated with placebo) when used in patients after myocardial infarction, and the FDA has approved these drugs for use only in patients with life-threatening ventricular arrhythmias. Noncardiac side effects are largely nausea and epigastric pain. These are largely controlled by dosing with meals in order to reduce peak drug levels. Flecainide is associated with significant myocardial depression and should be used with caution in patients with an ejection fraction below 40% and probably not at all in patients with an ejection fraction below 30%. Encainide is less likely to cause myocardial depression but should nevertheless be used with caution in patients with an ejection fraction below 30%. Until further studies are completed, both drugs should be used only in consultation with a cardiologist.

Class II Drugs (Sympathetic Blocking Agents)

These drugs block the effects of catecholamines (which may potentiate the development of arrhythmias) and slow conduction in the atria, AV node, and myocardium.

β-Blockers are used primarily to lower the ventricular response in patients with atrial tachyarrhythmia; occasionally, in the process, they will convert paroxysmal atrial tachycardia, atrial flutter, or fibrillation to normal sinus rhythm. In addition, ventricular arrhythmias initiated by exercise or ischemia (see Chap-

ter 57) or associated with the prolonged Q-T syndrome (see below) may be prevented by these drugs. β-Blockers appear to be synergistic with digoxin, and relatively low doses of propranolol and digoxin, for example, may be very effective in controlling heart rate in patients with atrial fibrillation, or in maintaining normal sinus rhythm in patients who have been cardioverted.

Toxicity. β-Blockers sometimes, by blocking sympthetic tone, precipitate heart failure in patients with poor ventricular function (an effect that can be overcome by digitalis), and they are contraindicated in patients with bronchial asthma. Gastrointestinal side effects (primarily nausea and diarrhea) occur occasionally. Most β-blockers may cause hair thinning in occasional patients; this effect appears to be reversible when the dose is reduced or the drug is discontinued. Peripheral vascular disease is occasionally exacerbated by nonselective β-blockers, in which case a relatively cardioselective β-blocker such as metoprolol or atenolol, should be used.

The properties of the currently available β-blocking agents are listed in Table 59.3. Propranolol is the preparation prescribed most commonly. However, it crosses the blood-brain barrier and may cause such side effects as depression and sleep disturbances. Atenolol is long acting, does not cross the blood-brain barrier, and is relatively cardioselective. It appears to have fewer side effects than propranolol. It is not yet clear whether any of the other available β-blockers offers significant advantages over these preparations. There is no current clear-cut cost advantage in choosing one of these drugs over another.

Class III Drugs (Potassium Current Blockers)

Amiodarone. Amiodarone (15), the only class III agent available, is a very potent drug that effectively suppresses both supraventricular and ventricular arrhythmias. Especially in high doses, it is associated with a number of troublesome side effects, including photosensitivity, corneal microdeposits, hypothyroidism, pulmonary interstitial firbosis, hepatotoxicity, a variety of neurologic complaints, and exacerbation of arrhythmias. Amiodarone also interacts with many other drugs and, for example, may potentiate the toxic effects of digoxin and of β-blocking agents. Because of these problems it has been recommended that the drug be prescribed only for patients with life-threatening recurrent ventricular arrhythmias that have not responded to other antiarrhythmic drugs or for patients with recurrent hemodynamically unstable ventricular tachycardia. However, amiodarone is so effective an antiarrhythmic agent that it should be considered in patients with less severe arrhythmias (such as paroxysmal supraventricular tachycardia) that are refractory to other membrane-active drugs. In such circumstances, amiodarone usually can be prescribed in lower doses that are less likely to produce side effects. The drug should be administered initially in the hospital, and a cardiologist, familiar with the drug, should

Table 59.3.
Currently Available β-Blockers[a]

	Acebutolol (Sectral)	Labetalol (Normodyne Trandate)	Atenolol (Tenormin)	Metoprolol (Lopressor)	Nadolol (Corgard)	Pindolol (Visken)	Propranolol (Inderal)	Timolol (Blocadren)
β-Blocking plasma levels	0.2–2.0 μg/ml	0.7–3.0 μg/ml	200–500 ng/ml	50–100 ng/ml	50–100 ng/ml	50–100 ng/ml	50–100 ng/ml	5–10 ng/ml
Eliminating half-life (hr)	3–4	5–6	6–9	3–4	14–24	3–4	3.5–6	4
Active metabolites	Yes	No	No	No	No	No	Yes	No
Predominant route of elimination[b]	HM	HM	RE (mostly unchanged)	HM	RE	RE (40% unchanged and HM)	HM	RE (20% unchanged and HM)
β_1-blockade potency ratio (propranolol = 1.0)	0.3	0.3	1.0	1.0	1.0	6.0	1.0	6.0
Relative β_1 selectivity	+	0	+	+	0	0	0	0
Available strengths (mg)	200, 400	100, 200, 300	50, 100	50, 100	40, 80, 120, 160	5, 10	10, 20, 40, 60, 80	10
Usual maintenance dose	200 to 600 mg twice daily	100 to 600 mg twice daily	50 to 100 mg every day	50 to 100 mg twice daily	40 to 50 mg every day	5 to 20 mg 3 times daily	40 to 80 mg 4 times daily	20 mgm twice daily

[a] Modified from Frishman WH: Beta-adrenoceptor antagonists: new drugs and new indications. N Engl J Med 305:550, 1981.
[b] RE:, renal excretion; HM, hepatic metabolism.

be closely involved in the patient's care. Because of a long mean half-life of nearly 2 months, the effects may persist for weeks after the drug is discontinued.

Class IV Drugs (Calcium Channel Blockers)

Calcium channel blockers (5, 24) (see page 690) are effective and useful drugs for controlling supraventricular arrhythmias. Conduction through the AV node is dependent on calcium-mediated currents. By blocking these currents, calcium channel blockers may control the ventricular response in atrial fibrillation and may convert to sinus rhythm supraventricular arrhythmias dependent on conduction through the AV node. *Verapamil* is the only calcium channel blocker approved for control of supraventricular arrhythmias, although diltiazem also is effective. Verapamil may be useful in an ambulatory setting for the conversion of paroxysmal atrial tachycardia (PAT) to sinus rhythm. Doses of 80 to 120 mg orally may be used safely in patients known to have PAT; conversion to sinus rhythm usually occurs in 1/2 to 1 hour; alternatively, a dose of 5 to 10 mg intravenously may convert PAT in minutes. If the drug is not effective, referral to a hospital emergency room should be considered. Oral verapamil in doses of 80 to 120 mg every 8 hours may be used for prophylaxis against supraventricular arrhythmias. Verapamil may also be used in doses of 80 to 120 mg every 8 hours for control of heart rate in patients with atrial fibrillation. Diltiazem in doses of 30 to 60 mg every 6 hours may also be effective (14). These drugs are not effective for control of ventricular arrhythmias. Verapamil is metabolized by the liver and should be used with caution in patients with impaired liver function.

Toxicity. The most common side effects of calcium channel blockers are headache, light-headedness, dizziness, hypotension, and constipation. Both verapamil and diltiazem interfere with renal clearance of digoxin and may precipitate digitoxicity. All calcium channel blockers are myocardial depressants, and both verapamil and diltiazem may suppress the SA node, decrease heart rate, and prolong the P-R interval. Verapamil should be used with caution in patients with cardiomyopathy although diltiazem may be used even in patients with heart failure and a decreased ejection fraction.

Pacemaker Therapy

Implantable electrical pulse generators (pacemakers) are the treatment of choice for patients with symptomatic bradyarrhythmias and heart block. In addition, specialized types of pacemakers may be used to terminate tachyarrhythmias by generating a current pulse that interferes with re-entrant tachycardias (so-called overdrive pacing). The decision to implant a pacemaker and the type of unit to use must be determined in consultation with a cardiologist. In general, patients in atrial fibrillation will require ventricular demand pacemakers. Most patients in sinus rhythm will be best served by a multiprogrammable atrio-ventricular sequential unit. The modest increase in cost and complexity of the atrioventricular sequential units appear in practice to be more than offset by the improved physiological response of patients over long-term follow-up. Pacemakers are less than 1 cm thick, weigh less than 70 g, and may function for 10 to 15 years. Pacemaker leads are easily implantable via a percutaneous transvenous technique and rarely become dislodged even during vigorous activity. Symptoms are relieved in a majority of patients who are symptomatic due to bradyarrhythmias and conduction block (see below).

Patient experience. The units are implanted subcutaneously under local anesthesia in the pectoral area, and the pacemaker lead is inserted via the cephalic vein or directly with the use of a special introducer into the subclavian vein and lodged in the apex of the right ventricle. The procedure takes about 1 1/2 hours; the patient experiences some discomfort when the anesthetic is injected and, often, an unpleasant sensation when the tissues are manipulated to create a pocket for the pacemaker unit.

After the procedure, patients, depending on their age and condition, are discharged from the hospital within 3 to 7 days. Patients with sedentary jobs may return to work approximately 2 weeks after pacemaker insertion, but patients with more active jobs should be kept off work for approximately 6 weeks to allow the wound to heal completely. After that, there is little or no discomfort and the unit feels like part of the chest wall. Patients may exercise if they wish but should avoid extreme exertion (for example, doubles tennis rather than singles; jogging rather than hard running).

Patients with implanted pacemakers require careful, long-term follow-up. They must be seen approximately every 3 months, and the function of the pacemaker must be assessed with a 12-lead ECG yearly and a rhythm strip at each visit. The ECG documents that the complexes have not changed, implying that the pacemaker lead has not shifted position; and the sensing and pacing functions of the pacemaker are determined with the rhythm strip. Long-term follow-up is usually done in conjunction with a cardiologist.

It is important that the make of the pacemaker, its registration number, and its rate be entered into the patient's record and that the patient keep the registration card for the pacemaker on his person in the event of malfunction of the instrument or of an emergency intercurrent problem.

Cardioversion

The electrical conversion of atrial or ventricular tachyarrhythmias is done by the application of a short burst of direct current to the chest wall. The shock is synchronized with the QRS complex of the ECG to avoid applying it during the vulnerable period of the cardiac cycle when ventricular tachycardia or fibrillation might be induced.

Cardioversion is a more reliable technique for the

conversion of tachyarrhythmias than is the administration of antiarrhythmic drugs. It may be required on an emergency basis if a patient has developed severe heart failure, hypotension, or ischemia as a result of an arrhythmia. Otherwise the procedure should be planned with the cardiologist who will attempt the conversion.

Digitalis should be withheld for 1 day before the procedure to ensure that an excess amount of drug is not circulating, and quinidine, 400 mg every 6 hours, should be given for 1 day before the procedure to minimize the development of arrhythmia at the time of the conversion. (Some patients will convert to sinus rhythm after administration of quinidine.) It is not clear whether patients to be subjected to cardioversion should be treated with anticoagulants. It seems reasonable, however, to give anticoagulants to patients in chronic heart failure who have a history of prior embolism or who have mitral stenosis. Anticoagulation (see Chapter 52) in these circumstances should be maintained for 2 weeks before and 2 weeks after the procedure; many cardiologists maintain anticoagulation indefinitely in these patients.

Patient experience. Cardioversion is done in a hospital with an anesthesiologist in attendance and with resuscitation equipment available. The patient is sedated, usually with 1 to 3 mg of intravenous midazolam or with intravenous Surital (thiamylal, a very short acting barbiturate), given to effect. Normally the patient cannot recall afterward the details of the procedure. For atrial fibrillation, cardioversion is attempted at 100 watt-seconds; the energy level is doubled repetitively and other shocks are administered until there is conversion or until a level of 400 watt-seconds is reached, after which the procedure must be terminated. Complications—embolism or a new arrhythmia—are unusual. After cardioversion, the patient is observed for a day or 2 while his rhythm is monitored and then is discharged. Quinidine is usually administered chronically in an attempt to prevent recurrence of the arrhythmia.

When to Refer a Patient for an Invasive Electrophysiological Study

The development of electrophysiological (EP) testing has created a sub-subspecialty whose science and art remain obscure to many practicing cardiologists, and for which the indications remain controversial. EP testing cannot yet reliably identify which patients who are at high risk of sudden death after myocardial infarction by clinical criteria (i.e., poor left ventricular function, persistent ischemia) may benefit by therapy with antiarrhythmic medications or with implantable defibrillators, which themselves carry great risks of morbidity. Several categories of patients appear to be candidates for referral to an EP laboratory. Most of these patients will already be under the care of a cardiologist. These patients include (a) patients who have survived an episode of cardiac arrest with documented ventricular fibrillation in the absence of acute myocardial infarction; (b) patients who have recurrent sustained ventricular tachycardia despite (or perhaps because of) treatment with adequate doses of antiarrhythmic agents; (c) patients with frequent episodes of supraventricular tachycardia, thought to be due to preexcitation (see below), who have not responded to conventional drug therapy. Some of these patients may be candidates for treatment with amiodarone plus a Class I agent, or with an automatic implantable cardiac defibrillator (AICD) (16).

The AICD has prolonged the lives of patients who would have previously been unresponsive to medical therapy, but many of them develop psychological problems that may be responsive to supportive care from a general internist or a family physician.

SPECIFIC ARRHYTHMIAS

Sinus Tachycardia

Definition and Etiology

In adults the normal sinus rate is 60 to 100 beats/minute. Sinus tachycardia, a sinus rhythm at a rate greater than 100 beats/minute, is usually a physiologic rhythm in that the rate is ordinarily appropriate to the physiological state of the patient—a state that requires an increased cardiac output to meet increased metabolic demands. The maximal sinus heart rate that can be attained varies with age but usually does not exceed 140 beats/minute unless demands are excessive (vigorous exercise, for example). The common factors that stimulate an increase in the rate of sinus rhythm, other than exercise, are fever (an increase of approximately 10 beats/minute for each Fahrenheit degree rise in body temperature), emotional stress, heart failure, and a variety of drugs that affect the autonomic nervous system (e.g., caffeine, aminophylline, amphetamine, alcohol, antidepressants, phenothiazines, etc.).

Physical Findings

A regular rapid pulse and heart rate are detected, although there may be a slight variation in rate—so-called sinus arrhythmia. S_1 is normal and the jugular pulsations are normal.

Electrocardiogram

A P wave precedes each QRS complex; the P-R interval is normal for the rate (0.16 to 0.17 at rates over 130/minute); and the P wave vector is normal (upright P waves in II, III, and aVf).

Treatment

In most cases persistent sinus tachycardia need not be treated; it is the underlying condition that requires therapy. Digitalis, especially, should not be used to treat a patient with sinus tachycardia unless he is in heart failure.

In the occasional patient with an unexplained sinus tachycardia in whom a thorough evaluation fails to reveal an underlying cause, and in whom tachycardia is symptomatic, the use of small doses of propranolol may be justified. Treatment should be initiated with 10 mg, two or three times a day. Recent experience has documented that low dose propranolol may also be helpful in treating the anxiety and tachycardia associated with anticipated stressful situations. Used only as necessary, doses of 20 to 40 mg of propranolol an hour before a public speaking engagement, for example, may help to relieve the associated anxiety and tachycardia experienced by some people.

Sinus Bradycardia

Definition and Etiology

Sinus bradycardia is a heart rate below 60 beats/minute. Impulse generation in the sinus node is often slow in well-conditioned people (e.g., long distance runners, heavy laborers). Inappropriately low sinus rates are commonly due to increased vagal tone such as is seen in association with pain, vomiting, or vasovagal syncope. A hypersensitive carotid sinus, more common in elderly people, may also result in marked bradycardia when the sinus is compressed by a tight collar or by the patient's tensing his neck. Parasympathomimetic drugs such as neostigmine, tranquilizers, phenothiazines, and digitalis, and sympatholytic drugs such as reserpine, methyldopa, clonidine and all β-blockers, also may produce sinus bradycardia. Vagally induced bradycardia may be severe and result in asystole (and loss of consciousness) when the stimulus is marked or prolonged or occurs in a hypoxic patient.

Physical Findings

A regular slow pulse and heart rate are detected. S_1 is normal and the jugular pulsations are normal.

Electrocardiogram

A P wave precedes each QRS complex; the P-R interval is normal for the rate (0.20 to 0.21) and the P wave vector is normal (upright P waves in II, III, and aVf).

Treatment

Asymptomatic sinus bradycardia discovered as an incidental finding does not require treatment. However, patients who present with symptoms of lightheadedness or syncope and are found to have sinus bradycardia may have underlying sinus node disease or may be subject to paroxysms of tachycardia and bradycardia, the so-called "sick sinus syndrome" (see below). Patients with sinus bradycardia and symptoms should be evaluated with an ambulatory ECG to determine whether they are suffering from this condition. In any case, patients with symptomatic sinus bradycardia, not due to a drug, are best treated with permanent pacemaker implantation.

Sick Sinus Syndrome

Definition and Etiology

The term sick sinus syndrome refers to a heterogeneous group of arrhythmias involving defective impulse generation by the sinus node and/or abnormal impulse conduction in the atria and AV node. The syndrome is characterized by periods of inappropriate sinus bradycardia (often severe with rates between 25 and 40/minute) that may precede or follow supraventricular tachyarrhythmias and by varying degrees of sinoatrial block including, sometimes, sinus arrest. The rubrics "bradycardia-tachycardia syndrome" or "tachycardia-bradycardia syndrome" are sometimes used, depending upon whether bradycardia precedes or follows a tachyarrhythmia.

The sick sinus syndrome is caused by degenerative fibrotic changes within the sinus node. It is often associated with similar abnormalities in other parts of the cardiac conduction system that result in varying degrees of atrioventricular and intraventricular block. These pathological changes are much more common in patients over the age of 60; although their precise cause is unknown, they are often associated with hypertensive or ischemic heart disease.

Symptoms and Signs

Many patients are asymptomatic. When symptoms do occur, they are produced either by spontaneous sinus arrest or by the tachyarrhythmia itself (palpitations). If there is coexistent left ventricular dysfunction or coronary artery disease, symptoms of heart failure or ischemia may occur.

The physical examination is often normal unless the patient is examined during an episode of brady- or tachyarrhythmia in which case the findings will depend on the type of arrhythmia that is present (see below). Sometimes light carotid sinus massage will produce symptomatic bradyarrhythmia in a patient with sick sinus syndrome who is in normal sinus rhythm.

Electrocardiogram

The ECG may be normal or may simply reveal sinus bradycardia. Often, there are varying degrees of sinoatrial block, characterized by varying P-P intervals on the ECG. Sometimes sinus arrest occurs, manifest by absent P waves and associated, usually, with a junctional escape rhythm. Some patients have slow atrial fibrillation reflecting a concomitant AV conduction abnormality (see above). The ECG changes of the various atrial tachyarrhythmias are described below in the discussions of these entities.

If there is a history of unexplained syncope or palpitations and the resting ECG is normal, ambulatory ECG monitoring is indicated (see page 693).

Treatment and Course

The treatment of choice for patients with the sick sinus syndrome who are symptomatic from bradyarrhythmias is permanent pacemaker implantation (see page 700). Otherwise symptoms are often progressive. Patients with relatively minor symptoms (e.g., light-headedness or dizziness) often will find that they feel significantly better after pacemaker therapy. Vagolytic drugs (atropine, for example) or β-adrenergic agonists (e.g., isoproterenol) are only of transient benefit.

Tachyarrhythmias associated with the syndrome are often not prevented by electrical pacing. However, pacing does allow the use of such drugs as digitalis and propranolol that depress the sinus node and increase the likelihood of sinus arrest or of asystole. It is reasonable, after a pacemaker is implanted, to administer propranolol, 10 mg four times a day, and to increase the dose to 40 mg four times a day in an attempt to prevent tachyarrhythmias. If propranolol is not effective, digoxin should be administered as well. If tachyarrhythmias continue, consideration should be given, in conjunction with the consulting cardiologist, to the use of an antiarrhythmic drug (see above).

Patients with sick sinus syndrome have an incidence, unaffected by pacemaker therapy, of arterial embolization of approximately 10%/year. However, except in patients with recurrent or chronic atrial fibrillation (see below), there is no evidence to support the use of anticoagulants in this condition.

A high mortality rate is associated with the sick sinus syndrome in elderly people, usually because of coexistent atherosclerotic vascular disease (1, 30). Nearly half of patients over the age of 60 die within 2 years of pacemaker implantation (30).

Premature Atrial and Junctional Contractions

Definition and Etiology

Premature atrial and junctional contractions (PACs and PJCs) are commonly seen in patients who are otherwise well. They often are induced by the same stimuli that produce sinus tachycardia, especially caffeine or nicotine. However, in patients with congestive heart failure or chronic pulmonary disease PACs or PJCs may progress to atrial fibrillation or flutter.

Symptoms and Signs

Usually patients are unaware of premature atrial or junctional contractions. Occasionally they will note the PAC or PJC as a palpitation; and the physician, on listening to the heart or palpating the arterial pulse, will be aware of a slight irregularity in the cardiac rhythm.

Electrocardiogram

Premature atrial contractions are reflected in the ECG by a premature morphologically abnormal P wave followed by a premature morphologically normal QRS complex. Often these impulses are not conducted (Fig. 59.5) in which case, if the P wave is buried in the preceding T wave, a false diagnosis of sinus arrest may be made. At other times the premature impulse may be aberrantly conducted, the result of relative refractoriness of one of the bundle branches (usually a right bundle branch pattern is seen after the premature atrial beat).

Premature junctional contractions are reflected in the ECG by a retrograde P wave (negatively deflected in leads II, III, and aVf) that may follow, be hidden in, or precede a morphologically normal but premature QRS complex.

Treatment

Patients with premature contractions who are otherwise well do not require treatment.

Rarely, it may be necessary to prescribe digoxin or propranolol to reduce the frequency of PACs or to prevent their conduction to the ventricles in patients who have annoyingly frequent palpitations. In patients with underlying cardiac or pulmonary disease, digitalization may prevent the progression of PACs to atrial fibrillation. Quinidine or procainamide is also effective in the control of PACs, but the risk associated with the use of these drugs usually is not warranted (see page 697).

Paroxysmal Supraventricular Tachycardia

Definition and Etiology

Supraventricular tachycardias (SVTs) are rapid heart rates (120 to 220 beats/minute) triggered by a premature impulse generated anywhere between the sinus node and the AV junction. Most of these arrhythmias are due to re-entry (see page 692)—usually in the AV node, occasionally through an accessory pathway or in the atria. Less often they are initiated by an ectopic atrial pacemaker.

About half of the time, patients with SVTs have an otherwise normal heart (3). The common forms of heart disease associated with SVT are the pre-excitation syndrome (see page 714), mitral valve prolapse (see Chapter 60), and atrial septal defect (see Chapter 60). Nonparoxysmal atrial tachycardia with block (due to gradually accelerated automaticity of an ectopic atrial focus) is a common manifestation of digitalis toxicity.

Symptoms and Signs

Patients are almost always aware of a suddenly rapid heart rate; usually there are no other symptoms, but if there is coexistent heart disease, patients may complain of shortness of breath or ischemic chest pain. Often the patient will be able to terminate the arrhythmia abruptly by a Valsalva maneuver or by coughing. Frequently, polyuria will be experienced for as long as the arrhythmia lasts.

Attacks often occur spontaneously but may be precipitated by physical or emotional stress, caffeine, or nicotine. They may be as short as a few seconds and as long as several weeks. The frequency of the attacks is also quite variable: some people have attacks every day; some, only a few times during their entire life.

On examination, the physician will note a rapid

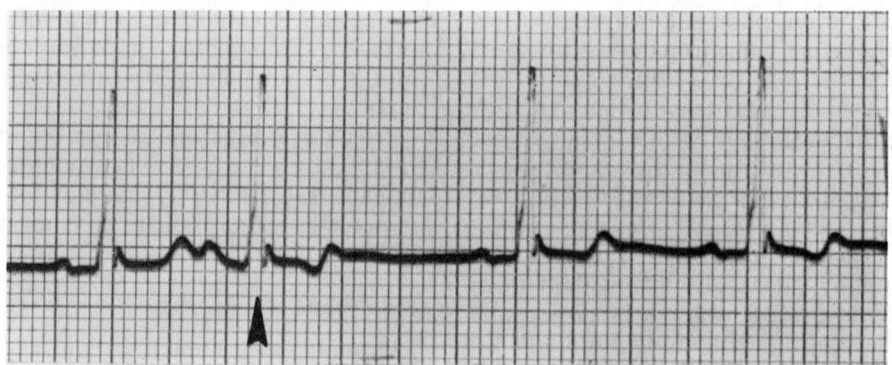

Figure 59.5. A premature atrial contraction (*arrow*). Note the normal configuration of the premature QRS complex.

regular arterial pulse and heart rate—often faster than that measured in patients with sinus tachycardia and usually not associated with the same stimuli. When the atria and ventricles contract simultaneously, cannon waves will be seen in the jugular veins.

Electrocardiogram

Paroxysmal SVT is characterized by a rapid regular heart rate. There is a fixed relationship of the P wave to the QRS complex. If the impulse is generated in the AV node, the P wave may be buried in the QRS complex, but the process can be identified by the normal appearance of the QRS complex and the regularity of the rate. When the P wave is visible, it may follow the QRS complex (some nodal re-entry rhythms, all accessory pathway re-entry rhythms) and will be inverted in leads II, III, and aVf. It may also precede the QRS complex and may appear morphologically normal (atrial re-entry or ectopic rhythm), in which case the diagnosis can only be made (by ECG) if the rate is high enough to make sinus tachycardia unlikely. The P wave also may be hidden in the T wave; but, again, the regularity of the rate and the usually normal duration of the QRS complex establish the diagnosis.

If SVT occurs in association with an AV conduction abnormality, the ventricular rate will be slower than the atrial rate. The arrhythmia can be diagnosed by the rapid regular atrial rate. Various degrees of block may occur (see below)—for example, 2:1 AV block in which the atrial rate is twice the ventricular rate (Fig. 59.6).

Sometimes in patients with SVT there are coexistent bundle branch or intraventricular conduction abnormalities, and prolonged abnormal QRS complexes may occur. If P waves are not visible, the only way to distinguish this arrhythmia from ventricular tachycardia is by comparison with an ECG taken when the rate was slow (in which the abnormal QRS complexes will still be seen) and by the regularity and rate (ventricular rates greater than 160 beats/minute are unlikely to represent ventricular tachycardia). If SVT occurs in a patient with an accessory AV conduction pathway (see below), conduction may be aberrant and it may not be possible with a surface ECG to distinguish the ar-

rhythmia from ventricular tachycardia. If there is any question about which of these diagnoses is correct, urgent consultation with a cardiologist is in order.

Treatment and Course

Therapy of paroxysmal SVT always starts with attempts to increase vagal tone. As mentioned above (see "Symptoms and Signs") the patient often has learned to do this himself. If the arrhythmia persists despite the patient's efforts, the physician should first apply carotid sinus massage. This must be done after auscultation of the carotid arteries to ensure that there are no bruits; if there are, carotid sinus massage is contraindicated. The carotid sinus is at the point of maximal impulse of the carotid artery in the neck. The right sinus should be massaged first for up to 20 seconds; if that has no effect, the left sinus should be massaged; the two sinuses should never be massaged simultaneously. During massage, the patient's ECG should be monitored continuously, and resuscitation equipment should be available.

If carotid sinus massage fails, pharmacological therapy is indicated. This is best done in an emergency room or in a similar facility. If that is not logistically possible, the drug of choice is verapamil, 5 to 10 mg intravenously; it usually converts the arrhythmia to normal sinus rhythm within 5 minutes. If, after administration of verapamil, SVT persists, propranolol (1 mg intravenously every 5 minutes until conversion occurs or until 0.1 mg/kg has been given), digoxin (0.5 mg intravenously), or phenylephrine (0.5 to 1.5 mg intravenously) may be given. One of these drugs is usually successful; rarely electrical cardioversion is necessary.

Chronic administration of digoxin, often in conjunction with an antiarrhythmic agent (see above), is indicated for prevention of recurrent attacks of SVT in patients with frequent symptomatic episodes. Digoxin is probably the drug of choice in otherwise healthy individuals (because it need be taken only once a day and is inexpensive) and in patients with heart failure. Verapamil or β-blockers may be useful in patients with hypertension or with hypertrophic cardiomyopathy. If the attacks recur despite prophylaxis, cardiology

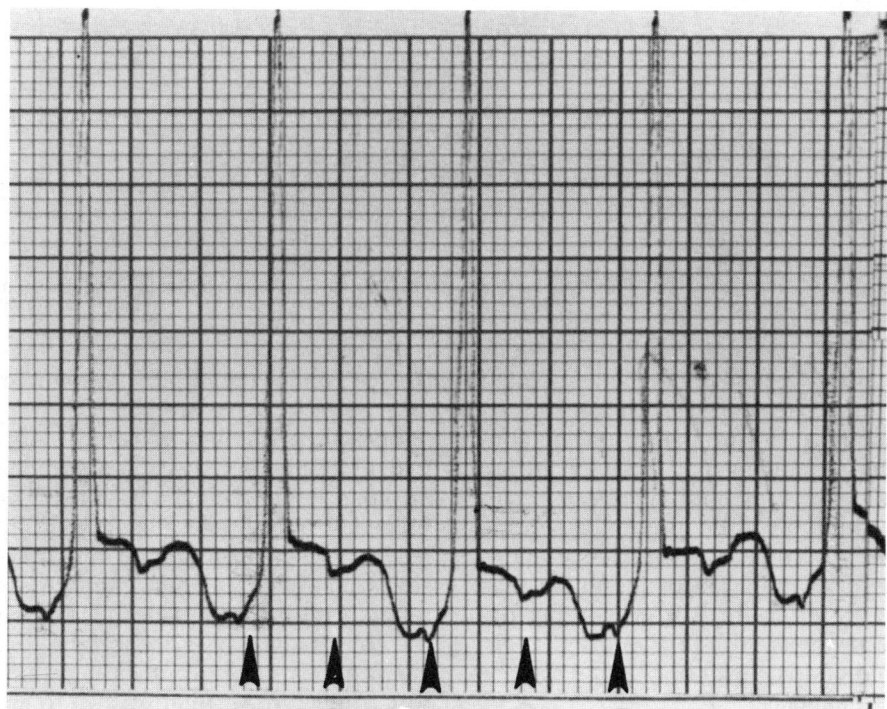

Figure 59.6. Supraventricular tachycardia with 2:1 AV block. The *arrows* point to consecutive P waves.

consultation is again indicated for advice about the use of antiarrhythmic agents and for possible electrophysiologic studies to determine the precise nature of the arrhythmia and the regimen most likely to prevent it.

The course of patients with SVT is dependent on its cause. If the arrhythmia occurs in patients who are otherwise healthy, there is no morbidity between attacks and essentially no effect on survival. If it occurs in patients with underlying cardiac or pulmonary disease, there is a real but undefined risk of heart failure, myocardial ischemia, or sudden death during an episode. Otherwise, survival is dependent on the nature and severity of the underlying disease.

If SVT occurs in association with an AV conduction abnormality (commonly 2:1 block), and the patient is taking digitalis, the drug should be withheld and serum potassium concentration should be measured. If the patient is hypokalemic, potassium repletion is, of course, in order; usually this can be accomplished by administration of oral potassium salts (i.e., 20 mEq three times a day—see Chapter 46). Patients with refractory digitoxic arrhythmias with block should be hospitalized for more aggressive treatment. If SVT with atrioventricular block is not due to digitoxicity, it should be treated in the same way as SVT without block.

Multifocal Atrial Tachycardia

Multifocal atrial tachycardia (MAT) is a chaotic supraventricular arrhythmia characterized electrocardiographically by varying morphology of the P waves, varying P-R intervals, and a rapid heart rate, usually 100 to 200 beats/minute; QRS morphology is normal and every QRS complex is preceded by a P wave (Fig. 59.7). The arrhythmia is usually seen in patients with serious underlying disease, especially decompensated chronic obstructive pulmonary disease, and is better treated by, for example, improving ventilatory function than by attempting directly to suppress the rhythm. Digitalis will not alter this arrhythmia (which is usually well tolerated) and therefore should not be administered. Both verapamil and diltiazem may be used to control the heart rate in patients with MAT. Oral doses of 40 to 80 mg three to four times a day of verapamil or 30 to 60 mg three to four times a day of diltiazem should be tried.

Atrial Fibrillation

Definition and Etiology

Atrial fibrillation is defined electrophysiologically as rapid uncoordinated generation of electrical impulses by the atria. It is usually triggered by a premature atrial contraction (see above) that, by re-entry, generates multifocal impulses at a rate of 300 to 500/minute. These impulses enter the AV node randomly; and, because of the slower rate of conduction of the AV node, not all of them are conducted. Therefore, the ventricular rate is slower than the atrial rate and is irregular. In untreated patients with normal AV conduction the ventricular rate is between 150 and 200 beats/minute.

Atrial fibrillation may occur paroxysmally in people, even in young adults, who have no other evidence

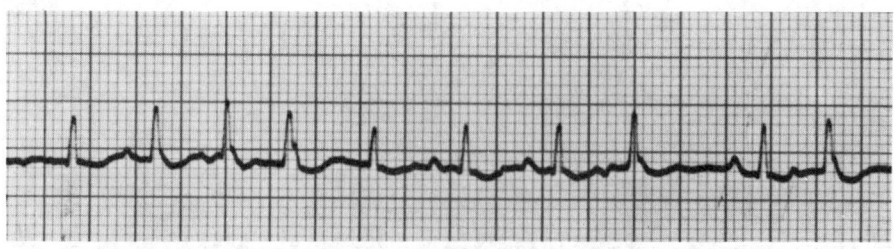

Figure 59.7.   Multifocal atrial tachycardia. Note the variation in the morphology of the P waves and in the duration of the P-R intervals.

of heart disease. In such cases it often is associated with the same stimuli that produce other atrial arrhythmias (sinus tachycardia, premature atrial contractions, paroxysmal supraventricular tachycardia): physical or emotional stress, alcohol, nicotine, or caffeine. Soaking in a "hot tub" while inbibing alcoholic beverages has recently become a recognized precipitating cause of atrial fibrillation. The major noncardiac illness associated with atrial fibrillation is hyperthyroidism; and in the presence of a fast ventricular response refractory to digitalis, atrial fibrillation may be the first clue to the diagnosis.

There are many forms of heart disease that predispose to the development of atrial fibrillation; the commonest are hypertensive, atherosclerotic, and rheumatic (especially when it involves the mitral valve), but almost every kind of myocardial disorder has been associated with it. Also, the tachyarrhythmic component of the sick sinus syndrome (see above) may be atrial fibrillation.

Symptoms and Signs

The most common symptoms of atrial fibrillation are palpitations and fatigue. If the ventricular response is fast (as it often is at onset of arrhythmia), patients often complain of feeling "strange," weak, or faint as well. Because atrial contraction normally provides approximately 20% of the total cardiac output, patients with incipient heart failure, ischemic heart disease, or valvular heart disease may develop symptoms (and signs) of those disorders (especially on exertion) when cardiac output is reduced as the result of atrial fibrillation.

Atrial fibrillation is characterized by an irregularly irregular heartbeat and pulse with variation in intensity of the sounds (including murmurs) on both auscultation and palpation. It is prudent to look for signs of diseases known to be associated with atrial fibrillation (e.g., hypertension, mitral stenosis, and hyperthyroidism)—especially since those signs may be subtle or may be altered by the arrhythmia.

Electrocardiogram

The ECG shows rapid irregular fibrillatory atrial activity at rates between 300 and 500/minute; no P waves are present. The ventricular rhythm is irregularly irregular, at rates that at onset are usually between 150 and 200/minute—unless there is coexistent disease in the AV node, in which case slower rates are likely (Fig. 59.8).

The QRS complex is usually morphologically normal. Occasionally there is aberrant conduction of an impulse in the ventricles, after a beat that has been preceded by a long pause. The aberrant beat usually has a right bundle branch block configuration. This so-called *Ashman phenomenon* is due to prolonged refractoriness of the (usually) right bundle branch after the long pause. It is important to distinguish these aberrant beats from ventricular premature beats. Apart from their typical relationship to a preceding long R-R interval, aberrant beats are often triphasic (RSR') in lead V_1 and their initial vector is the same as that of the normally conducted beats; neither of these features is characteristic of ventricular premature beats.

Treatment and Course

The approach to the treatment of atrial fibrillation should always include a search for underlying or precipitating factors. Treatment of the arrhythmia has two objectives: to slow the ventricular rate if it is fast and to convert the patient to sinus rhythm if possible.

Paroxysmal atrial fibrillation in a patient who does not have underlying heart disease often will revert to normal sinus rhythm once precipitating factors (e.g., stress, alcohol, nicotine) are removed. Specific treatment is indicated in the following circumstances: a rapid ventricular response associated with symptoms (e.g., extreme fatigue, syncope, angina, or shortness of breath); the presence of known underlying severe heart disease (e.g., aortic stenosis, severe mitral stenosis, ischemic heart disease, chronic congestive failure)—these patients are unlikely to revert to normal sinus rhythm spontaneously; persistent atrial fibrillation—especially if the resting ventricular rate is greater than 110 beats/minute or if the rate after moderate exercise (climbing a flight of stairs, for example) is greater than 150 beats/minute.

Symptomatic patients and patients with underlying severe heart disease are best admitted immediately after onset of the arrhythmia to the hospital for cardioversion or for pharmacotherapy. Patients with persistent atrial fibrillation of less than 6 months' duration, particularly if there is no left atrial enlargement, should be hospitalized for elective cardioversion. Patients with atrial fibrillation that has lasted longer than 6 months or patients with large left atria are likely to be refrac-

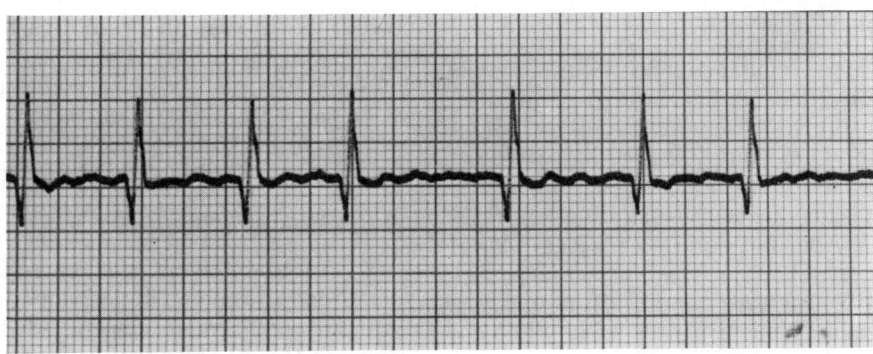

Figure 59.8. Atrial fibrillation. The ventricular rate is 90 to 100 beats/minute, indicative (since digitalis had not been administered) of an associated disorder of atrioventricular conduction.

tory to cardioversion. In general, cardioversion restores normal sinus rhythm in approximately 90% of patients, but the relapse rate is high—50% in 1 year and 90% in 3 years (12)—unless the underlying disorder can be corrected or atrial fibrillation has been of short duration.

Asymptomatic or mildly symptomatic patients who have a rapid ventricular response should be treated with digitalis with a goal of a resting ventricular rate between 70 and 100 beats/minute and a rate after modest exercise of below 150 beats/minute. A loading dose by mouth of 0.75 to 1.0 mg of digoxin followed by 0.25 mg a day is ordinarily sufficient. If rapid digitalization is desired, it is best to hospitalize the patient and administer intravenous digoxin. Approximately 20% of patients will convert to normal sinus rhythm after receiving digitalis.

If digitalization slows the rate but the ventricular response is still too high, verapamil (80 mg three to four times a day), diltiazem (30 to 60 mg three to four times a day), or small doses of propranolol (10 to 20 mg four times a day) will often lower the rate further (see pages 698 to 700 for a general discussion of the use of these drugs).

Patients who cannot or will not be electrically cardioverted may be given an antiarrhythmic drug after they are digitalized (quinidine is ordinarily the first choice and will cause a return to normal sinus rhythm in about one-third of patients).

A slow ventricular response to atrial fibrillation in untreated patients suggests an associated disorder of AV conduction. Such patients do not require specific therapy for the arrhythmia unless they are hemodynamically compromised (i.e., in refractory heart failure) and their heart rate is under 60 to 70 beats/minute, in which case implantation of a pacemaker may be indicated.

Patients with atrial fibrillation are at increased risk of arterial embolization. For example, the Framingham study reported that, over a 24-year period, patients with chronic atrial fibrillation with and without rheumatic heart disease had a 17- and 5-fold increase, respectively, in the incidence of stroke (31). Overall the incidence of arterial embolization in patients with chronic atrial fibrillation is about 10% a year (19). It is the practice to give all patients the anticoagulant warfarin before elective cardioversion (see page 700 and Chapter 51), and, although there are no prospective, randomized, trials to support it, many physicians routinely treat with anticoagulants any patient with chronic atrial fibrillation if there are no contraindications. It seems reasonable to recommend anticoagulation for all patients who have had even one episode of arterial embolization as well as for patients with mitral stenosis or those who have paroxysmal atrial fibrillation as part of the sick sinus syndrome (see page 702).

Apart from the morbidity and mortality associated with atrial embolization, the prognosis of patients with atrial fibrillation depends on whether there is underlying heart disease and, if there is, what the nature of it is.

Atrial Flutter

Definition and Etiology

Atrial flutter is a relatively coordinated rapid atrial activity due to re-entry of premature atrial impulses. Atrial beats are generated at about 300/minute. Usually there is a 2:1 AV conduction block so that the ventricular response is abut 150/minute and, unlike atrial fibrillation, both atrial and ventricular responses are regular. Atrial flutter is almost always seen in patients who have underlying disease: ischemic heart disease, rheumatic heart disease, congestive cardiomyopathy, atrial septal defect, mitral valve disease, chronic obstructive pulmonary disease, and thyrotoxicosis—the same diseases often associated with atrial fibrillation. In contrast to atrial fibrillation, however, atrial flutter is not often seen in patients who are otherwise healthy.

Symptoms and Signs

Patients are usually aware of a rapid heart rate; whether other symptoms develop depends on the severity and nature of the underlying heart disease.

A regular rapid heart rate and atrial pulse are detected. Sometimes the flutter waves are visible in the jugular pulse. An S_4 is occasionally audible (in contrast to atrial fibrillation).

Electrocardiogram

The ECG shows rapid regular sawtooth flutter waves at about 300/minute (Fig. 59.9); P waves are absent. The ventricular response is regular, usually at about 150/minute, and the QRS complex is ordinarily morphologically normal. If the AV node is diseased, higher degrees of AV block may be seen—usually a multiple of 2 (4:1, 8:1, etc.). Aberrant conduction (see "Atrial Fibrillation") is unusual.

If the diagnosis is unclear, carotid sinus massage may help to distinguish atrial flutter from other paroxysmal supraventricular tachyarrhythmias. It usually causes an abrupt temporary slowing of the rate; and flutter waves, which may have been difficult to detect at a higher rate, will be visible in the electrocardiogram, most commonly in leads II, III, aVf, and V_1.

Treatment and Course

Atrial flutter is an unstable rhythm and usually converts spontaneously to normal sinus rhythm or to atrial fibrillation. Because the rhythm is unstable and patients usually have underlying heart disease, they are best hospitalized for observation and treatment. Unlike the situation in patients with atrial fibrillation, it is often difficult to lower the ventricular rate with digitalis. Nevertheless, digitalization is reasonable—especially if hospitalization must be delayed—since some patients will convert to normal sinus rhythm after administration of digoxin alone.

If there is no contraindication, however, electrical cardioversion is the treatment of choice if atrial flutter persists, even if there is a high degree of AV block. Almost every patient can be converted to normal sinus rhythm, usually after application of a much lower current than is necessary to convert atrial fibrillation.

Digitalis (i.e., digoxin, 0.25 mg a day) should be administered to prevent recurrences of atrial flutter. If digitalis is not effective alone, propranolol, 20 to 40 mg every 6 hours, or quinidine, 200 to 300 mg every 6 hours, should also be prescribed. All of these drugs are much more effective in preventing recurrence of flutter than they are in converting it to normal sinus rhythm. Patients who have recurrent symptomatic atrial flutter or fibrillation despite treatment with digitalis and a Class I antiarrhythmic agent should be considered for treatment with amiodarone, but only in consultation with a cardiologist.

Ventricular Premature Beats

Definition and Etiology

Ventricular premature beats (VPBs) are impulses generated in the ventricles, usually as the result of reentry of an impulse conducted down from the atria through the AV node, but sometimes as the result of the firing of an ectopic (parasystolic) focus.

Occasional VPBs occur in many healthy people sporadically during their life, more frequently in older people. However, often VPBs are associated with underlying organic heart disease, e.g., ischemic heart disease, cardiomyopathy, or mitral valve prolapse. The frequency of VPBs may be increased in people both with and without heart disease by caffeine, alcohol, sympathomimetic drugs, tricyclic antidepressants, phenothiazines, hypokalemia, hypoxia, and excitement. VPBs are a common manifestation of digitoxicity. Exercise usually abolishes VPBs activity in normal people; an increase in the number of VPBs after exertion is highly suggestive of underlying heart disease.

Symptoms and Signs

Patients may not be aware that they have had a VPB, but often they experience a palpitation—either sensing the premature beat itself or the more forceful normal beat that follows it after a compensatory pause.

Electrocardiogram

The ECG shows a premature ventricular response with a morphologically abnormal, often bizarre, wide QRS complex (27). No P wave precedes a VPB but, by retrograde conduction, a P wave sometimes follows it. The ST segment and the T wave have an opposite vector from the QRS complex. Typically, a VPB is followed by a compensatory pause, i.e., the R-R interval between two normal beats separated by a VPB is the same as that between two normal beats separated by another normal beat (Fig. 59.10), due to retrograde

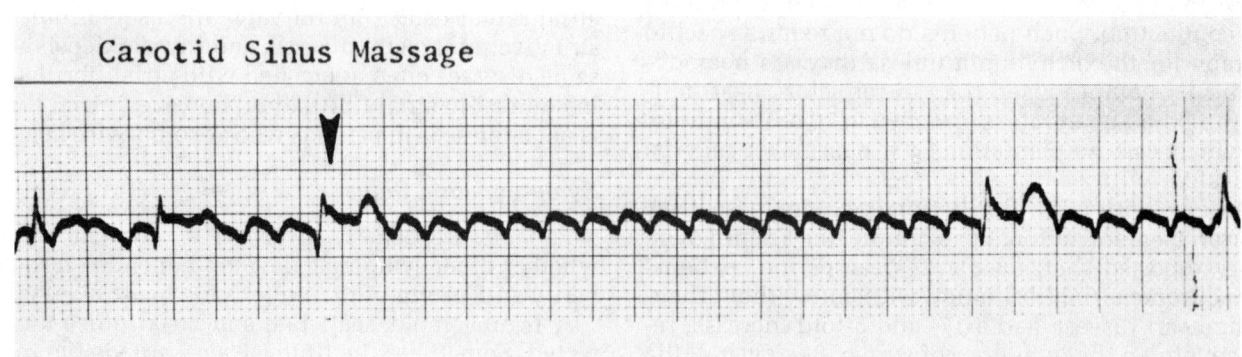

Figure 59.9. Atrial flutter. The flutter waves are clearly revealed after carotid sinus massage (*arrow*).

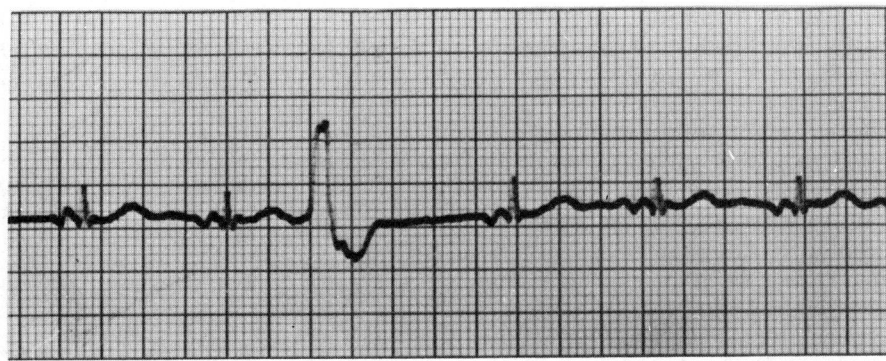

Figure 59.10.   Premature ventricular beat. Note that the R-R interval between the two normal beats separated by the PVB is the same as that between two normal beats separated by another normal beat.

conduction of the premature beat to the AV node, thereby blocking the succeeding sinus beat.

When VPBs are due to re-entry, they have a fixed temporal ("coupled") relationship to the preceding normal beats. When they are due to the firing of an ectopic (parasystolic) focus, they have no fixed relationship to the preceding normal beats but do have a regular pattern (i.e., the ectopic intervals are constant or are multiples of a constant). Ectopic beats may occasionally fuse with normal beats, producing a complex that is intermediate between the two (Fig. 59.11).

Treatment and Course

Ventricular premature beats in patients with otherwise normal hearts are not harmful. However, there is an increased incidence of sudden death and of myocardial infarction in patients with VPBs who have underlying ischemic heart disease (25). It has not been demonstrated that suppression of VPBs in these latter patients alters their course (25). Because all antiarrhyhmic agents have potentially serious side effects (see page 696), the physician must consider for each patient the relative risks of treating or not treating VPBs. The following generalizations may be useful:

1. Apparently healthy young people with asymptomatic ventricular premature beats probably do not need treatment.
2. Apparently healthy young people with ventricular premature beats causing symptomatic palpitations also probably do not need to be treated. If symptoms interfere with normal life style in spite of

reassurance, a trial of low dose propranolol beginning with 10 mg four times a day and increasing if needed to 40 to 80 mg four times a day may abolish VPBs and relieve symptoms. Propranolol commonly produces a sensation of sluggishness in young people, and often they will not continue the medication. In that case, a long acting β-blocker—e.g., atenolol (Tenormin), 50 mg every morning—will often give symptomatic relief with good compliance. β-Blockers should be discontinued after several weeks. Often VPBs will not recur and no further treatment will be necessary.

3. Patients with known ischemic heart disease and symptomatic ventricular arrhythmias, especially symptomatic multiformed premature ventricular beats, should probably be treated. Quinidine remains the drug of choice in initial doses of 200 mg four times a day. The dose should be titrated to serum levels of 3 to 7 μg/ml just before the next dose (the level should be measured every 3 or 4 days until the desired concentration is attained). In patients who do not tolerate quinidine, sustained-release procainamide (Procan-SR), 500 to 750 mg every 6 hours, should be tried. The efficacy of the antiarrhythmic therapy should be assessed by an ambulatory ECG (see page 693).

4. When ventricular arrhythmias occur in the setting of congestive heart failure, an attempt should be made to achieve a maximal state of cardiac compensation before instituting antiarrhythmic therapy. Hemodynamic compensation may decrease or eliminate ventricular premature beats so that specific antiarrhythmic therapy is not needed. Diso-

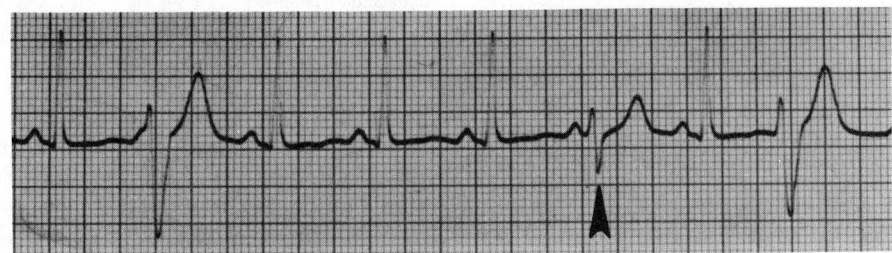

Figure 59.11.   Premature ventricular beats due to the firing of an ectopic focus. The *arrow* points to a fusion beat.

pyramide and flecainide are myocardial depressants and are specifically contraindicated in patients whose hearts are enlarged and hypocontractile. Furthermore, patients in severe chronic heart failure, many of whom are taking diuretics, are more likely to experience problems such as hypokalemia, hypomagnesemia, alkalosis, hypoxemia, and digitalis toxicity, thus increasing the risk of serious side effects from antiarrhythmic agents. Such patients are best treated in consultation with a cardiologist.

5. Patients with recurrent symptomatic VPBs, recurrent ventricular tachycardia, or ventricular fibrillation may be best managed with a drug regimen that is selected using intracardiac electrophysiological techniques to assess the response to the drugs. This approach requires hospitalization and consultation with a cardiologist.

6. If VPBs have been suppressed for a year and the patient is asymptomatic, it is reasonable to discontinue antiarrhythmic therapy and to obtain an ambulatory ECG 1 week later. If the arrhythmia does not recur, the therapy need not be reinstituted. However, this issue is controversial and consultation with a cardiologist may be advisable before stopping the therapy.

7. The possibility that a patient may experience a proarrhythmic effect from an antiarrhythmia agent must always be kept in mind (see page 694).

Heart Block

Heart block, a delay or failure of conduction of the cardiac impulse, is categorized electrocardiographically.

Right Bundle Branch Block

A delay or block of conduction through the right bundle branch (RBBB) (Fig. 59.12) causes a modest prolongation of the QRS complex (> 0.12 second). The initial QRS vector is unaffected since this is accounted for normally by initial left ventricular depolarization. The right ventricle is activated by a spread of the action potential from the left ventricle, which is seen best in leads I and V6 where the S waves are wide and slurred and in V_1 where there is a double peak (R-R') of the R wave. RBBB is sometimes seen in the ECGs of patients who have otherwise normal hearts. More often it is associated with an underlying congenital or acquired disorder, e.g., interatrial septal defect and hypertensive or ischemic heart disease. Patients with newly acquired RBBB have an increased risk of cardiovascular morbidity and death from cardiovascular disease (20).

Left Bundle Branch Block

A delay or block of conduction through the left bundle branch (LBBB) (Fig. 59.13) causes a marked prolongation of the QRS complex (0.14 to 0.16 second). The entire

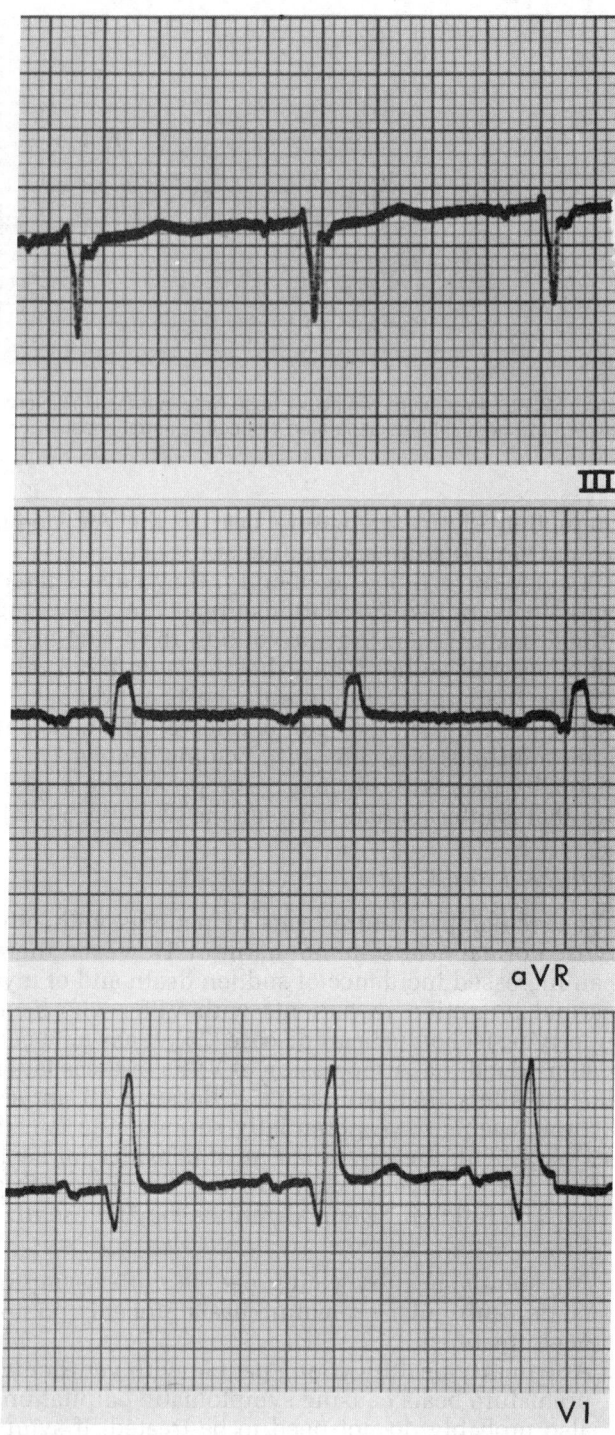

Figure 59.12. Right bundle branch block and left anterior hemiblock (bifascicular block).

sequence of ventricular depolarization is affected so that the QRS complex is widened and the QRS axis is directed to the left and posteriorly. Abnormal repolarization is reflected in the T wave, which is always in the opposite direction of the QRS complex.

LBBB almost always signifies heart disease—usually ischemic heart disease or cardiomyopathy.

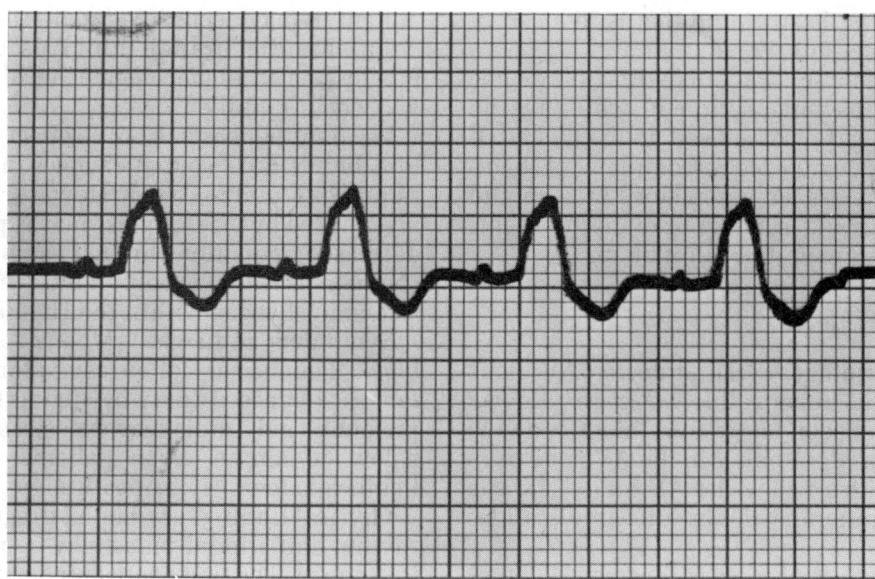

Figure 59.13. Left bundle branch block.

Hemiblocks

Left anterior hemiblock (LAH). When there is delay or block of the cardiac impulse in the anterior-superior portion of the left bundle branch, the anterior-superior wall of the left ventricle is activated late, resulting in marked left axis deviation on the ECG (Fig. 59.12). The duration of the QRS complex is usually normal or slightly prolonged (< 0.10 second). The causes of left anterior hemiblock are the same as those of LBBB. LAH is occasionally seen in patients with no discernible heart disease. Whatever the cause, LAH is not in itself a poor prognostic sign and, at least in an ambulatory setting, requires no specific therapy.

Left posterior hemiblock (LPH). When there is delay or block of the cardiac impulse in the posterior portion of the left bundle branch, the posterior wall of the left ventricle is activated late. The ECG pattern of LPH is characterized by marked right axis deviation (> +110°). The causes of LPH are the same as those of LAH and LBBB. Because the posterior portion of the left bundle branch is larger and better perfused than is the anterior-superior portion, LPH is less common than is LAH and usually indicates more extensive left ventricular disease.

Bifascicular Block

Right bundle branch block with LAH (manifest by a RBBB pattern and left axis deviation—Fig. 59.12) or RBBB with LPH (manifest by a RBBB pattern and right axis deviation) indicates that only one pathway remains to maintain passage of the cardiac impulse from the atria to the ventricles. If bifascicular block is detected in an ambulatory setting, especially if there is a history of syncope or of light-headedness, a cardiologist should be asked to advise whether electrophysiological studies (page 693) and/or pacemaker implantation is indicated. The risk that unselected patients with bifascicular block will develop complete heart block is 5 to 6% a year (13). There is conflicting evidence, however, about the course of patients, generally, with bifascicular block: some report no increased morbidity (13); others, a considerably shortened survival (7, 8). Although there is not a consensus about how to deal with the problem, the prognosis seems to be related to the extent of the underlying disease.

First Degree Heart Block

Definition and etiology. The P-R interval normally varies with heart rate but should not exceed 0.21 second in people in normal sinus rhythm. First degree AV block is defined as a prolonged P-R interval. The block may be due to a prolongation of conduction in any of the structures between the SA node and the bundle of His. Most commonly, when the QRS duration is normal, a long P-R interval is due to a delay in conduction in the AV node. When first degree block coincides with left bundle branch block, it is likely that there is a delay in conduction in the His bundle. A prolonged P-R interval with right bundle branch block may be due to a block in the AV node or in the bundle of His.

A prolongation of the P-R interval is usually due to degenerative, ischemic, or inflammatory changes in the AV conduction systems. It is commonly seen in older people without other evidence of heart disease, in patients who have had an inferior wall myocardial infarction, or in association with myocarditis (including acute rheumatic fever). Drugs such as digitalis, which affect vagal activity, and sympatholytic drugs also may produce a first degree AV block.

Symptoms and signs. First degree AV block in itself does not produce symptoms or abnormal physical findings except a first heart sound that is reduced in intensity (see Chapter 60).

Treatment and Course. Patients with first degree AV block who are asymptomatic and who have no other evidence of heart disease need not be treated. If patients with first degree block complain of lightheadedness or dizziness, an ambulatory ECG should be obtained (see page 693) since some of these patients may have episodic higher degrees of block.

Second Degree AV Block

Definition and etiology. Second degree AV block is present when some but not all P waves are followed by QRS complexes. Second degree AV block is due to conduction delay or block either in the AV node or in the conduction system below the AV node. The site of the block has important therapeutic implications (see below).

Mobitz-I or Wenckebach second degree AV block (Fig. 59.14). Second degree AV block within the AV node results in the Wenckebach phenomenon, characterized by progressive lengthening of the P-R interval for several cycles until the P wave is blocked completely; and the sequence begins again, often with a normal P-R interval in the beat that follows the blocked P wave. In the absence of disease elsewhere in the conducting system, the QRS complex is normal. The "degree of Wenckebach" is characterized by the ratio of the number of P waves to the number of QRS complexes in each cycle of block. In other words, if block occurs after every third P wave, it is called 3:2 Wenckebach.

Because conduction through the AV node is influenced by vagal tone, type I—second degree AV block—may be precipitated by anything that increases vagal tone. It therefore is sometimes seen as a transient phenomenon in people with no other evidence of heart disease. Otherwise, it is produced by the same processes that are associated with first degree AV block.

Mobitz-II second degree AV block (Fig. 59.15). Mobitz-II block is defined as intermittent failure to conduct a P wave due to block below the level of the AV node. The P-R interval of the conducted beat before a blocked P wave is usually normal. The block may be inter-

mittent or may occur in a fixed 2:1 or 3:1 ratio. Coexistent bundle branch block is commonly seen. Progression to higher degrees of block or to asystole may occur rapidly.

Vagal influences have little effect on conduction below the AV node so that changes in vagal tone do not influence Mobitz-II block. However, the block may be precipitated by medications such as propranolol, which decrease conduction through the bundle of His. The common causes of Mobitz-II block are degenerative or ischemic changes within the His-Purkinje system.

Symptoms and signs. *Mobitz-I second degree AV block.* Patients are often asymptomatic but if vagal tone is increased (e.g., by digitalis or propranolol), profound bradycardia may ensue, sometimes with rates below 30/minute. Such patients may complain of lightheadedness, syncope, or extreme fatigue.

Physical findings are subtle; irregularity of the heart rhythm and arterial pulse may be noted when a beat is dropped. The first heart sound of the last beat before the dropped beat will be softer than that of the first beat after the pause (because of the variation in P-R interval—see Chapter 60).

Mobitz-II second degree AV block. Symptoms and physical findings are similar to those of patients with Mobitz-I block except that they are not influenced by changes in vagal activity and the intensity of the first heart sound is constant.

Treatment and course. *Mobitz-I second degree AV block.* Asymptomatic patients need not be treated since the risk of rapid progression of the block and of asystole is slight. Symptomatic patients usually have pronounced bradycardia. If so, medications such as digitalis or propranolol, which may be increasing the block, should be discontinued. If such medications are essential to the patient's management, a cardiac pacemaker should be implanted (see page 700).

Mobitz-II second degree AV block. Because of the risk of rapid progression of the block and of asystole, all patients, even if asymptomatic, should be treated with a permanent cardiac pacemaker.

Patients with a history of light-headedness or dizziness who have new bundle branch block should be suspected of having had Mobitz-II block. This suspicion often can be confirmed with the use of an am-

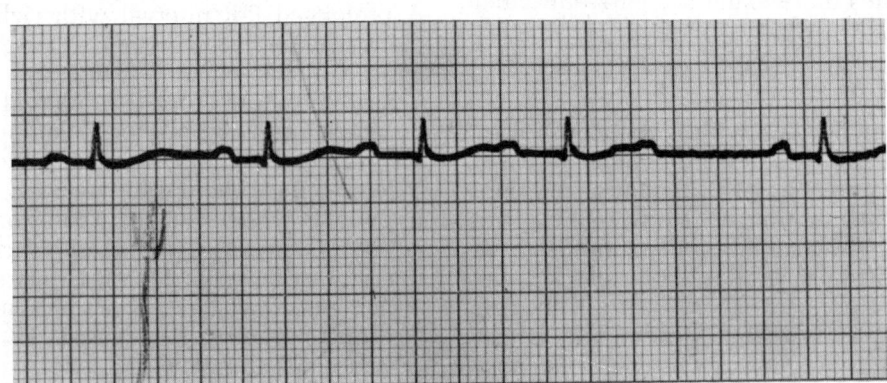

Figure 59.14. Mobitz-I or Wenckebach second degree atrioventricular block.

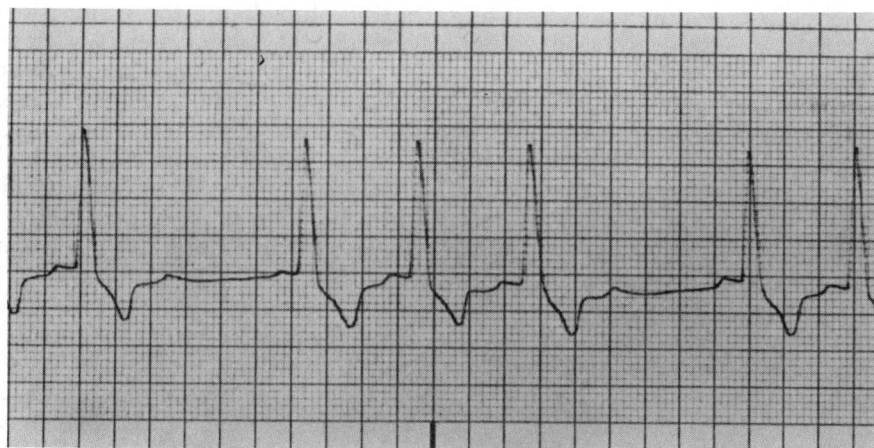

Figure 59.15. Mobitz-II second degree atrioventricular block.

bulatory ECG (page 693). An intracardiac ECG (page 693), if necessary, may also show prolonged conduction through the His bundle. Patients with a known history of coronary artery disease and with new or increased bundle branch blocks who have a clear-cut history of syncope must be thought to have had Mobitz- II block or complete heart block until proven otherwise.

Third Degree (Complete) Heart Block

Definition and etiology. Complete heart block occurs when there is total failure of conduction of impulses from the atria through the AV junction to the bundle of His (or, more rarely, if all three fascicles below the His bundle are diseased). The life of the patient then depends upon the escape of a ventricular pacemaker. A rhythm generated in the upper portion of the His bundle may have a QRS configuration nearly identical to that of normally conducted impulses and will have a rate between 40 and 60 beats/minute (Fig. 59.16). It is more likely to be a stable rhythm than is a rhythm generated by a lower pacemaker. If the pacemaker is located more distally in the conducting system, the ventricular rate decreases; the QRS morphology becomes wider and more bizarre; and the risk of asystole increases. In children or young adults, complete heart block may occur due to congenital defects in development of the AV cushion or of the conduction system itself; escape rhythms are, in such cases, usu-

ally generated relatively high in the bundle of His. In older people complete heart block is most commonly due to degenerative and fibrotic changes in the conduction system (6). It is also seen sometimes in association with infiltrative disease of the myocardium (e.g., sarcoid or amyloid), inflammatory processes (e.g., rheumatoid arthritis), and myocardial infections (tuberculosis, syphilis, etc.) or ischemic heart disease. Occasionally digitalis toxicity may produce complete heart block as may excessive doses of β-blockers, α-methyldopa, and clonidine.

Complete heart block is a sub-category of *atrioventricular (AV) dissociation*, a situation in which the atria and ventricles are depolarized independently. In instances of AV dissociation, other than complete heart block, the ventricles may be paced independently because of enhancement of the rate of discharge of a latent ventricular pacemaker (e.g., ventricular tachycardia) or because of marked slowing of the rate of discharge of the ordinarily dominant atrial pacemaker. In these instances, the ventricular rate is usually greater than the atrial rate and is also greater usually than it is in patients with complete heart block.

Symptoms and signs. A major symptom of complete heart block is sudden loss of consciousness (a Stokes-Adams attack), the result of asystole or of tachyarrhythmia (ventricular tachycardia or fibrillation). The asystole is due to failure of the ventricular pacemaker; the tachyarrhythmia, to escape of another focus when the idioventricular rate falls too low (a variant

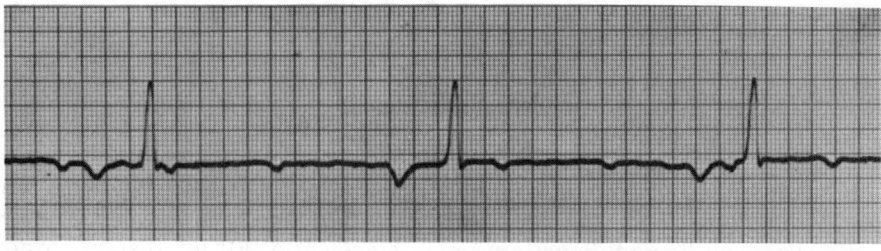

Figure 59.16. Third degree heart block.

of the bradycardia-tachycardia syndrome—see page 702). If the heart begins to pump effectively again within seconds—as it usually does—the patient promptly regains consciousness and is alert and oriented. If perfusion of vital organs is delayed, seizure-like activity (ordinarily not generalized) and even death may ensue. If they are unconscious for more than a few minutes, patients may not become fully alert for some hours.

Complete heart block in patients with underlying myocardial disease may cause symptoms of heart failure (see Chapter 61) primarily because of further reduction in cardiac output as the result of bradycardia.

Physical findings of heart block are all attributable to the dissociation between atrial and ventricular contraction: variation in the intensity of the first heart sound, variation in systolic blood pressure, variation in the intensity of heart murmurs and of third and fourth heart sounds, and the appearance of cannon waves in the jugular pulse. The heart rate, of course, is slow.

Treatment and course.   The treatment of complete heart block is permanent pacemaker implantation. The life expectancy of treated patients with complete heart block who have no other evidence of cardiac or systemic disease is excellent and approaches that of their age-matched cohort. Patients with complete heart block due to coronary disease have a prognosis that is determined by the extent of their underlying coronary artery disease and by their myocardial function.

Pre-excitation Syndrome

Definition and Etiology

The atria and ventricles are electrically isolated from each other by the AV groove, and the electrical signal from the atria is conducted to the ventricle via the AV node and conducting system. If the AV groove is short circuited by muscle fibers, if muscle fibers from the atria enter the His bundle below the AV node, or if muscle fibers from the His bundle bypass the bundle branches, a variable portion of the right or left ventricle will be depolarized early. These short circuiting fibers are known as accessory atrioventricular, nodoventricular, and fasciculoventricular pathways—the atriofascicular bypass tract and the intranodal bypass tract, depending on their location (Fig. 59.17).

The classic example of pre-excitation is the *Wolff-Parkinson-White (WPW) syndrome*, which is due to accessory atrioventricular connections. This syndrome is characterized electrocardiographically by a short P-R interval followed by a wide QRS complex, which is a fusion beat between the area of the ventricle that is pre-excited and the area of the ventricle excited via normal conduction pathways (Fig. 59.18). The portion of the complex due to pre-excitation is called the δ wave because of its resemblance to the Greek capital letter δ. If the accessory bundle connects the atria with the left ventricle, the electrocardiographic pattern resembles right bundle branch block (type A WPW). If,

on the other hand, the connection is with the right ventricle, the pattern resembles left bundle branch block (type B WPW); the negative δ wave in lead II in this situation may be taken for a Q wave, and the mistaken diagnosis of remote myocardial infarction may be made.

If the atrial fibers insert into the bundle of His and short circuit the AV node, the P-R interval is short, but no δ wave is seen since below the AV node conduction occurs along the usual pathways. This syndrome is known as the *Lown-Ganong-Levine (LGL) syndrome*. A number of other variants of pre-excitation have been described but are much rarer than these two relatively common disorders (26).

The ECG manifestations of pre-excitation may vary from time to time within a given individual since, if conduction occurs through the normal anatomical pathways rather than through accessory fibers, no pre-excitation will be seen on the ECG. When pre-excitation is facilitated because of disease in the AV node or because of drugs that suppress conduction through the AV node (e.g., digitalis or propranolol), abnormalities on the ECG will be seen.

Re-entrant supraventricular arrhythmias are common in patients with pre-excitation syndromes [estimates vary from 13 to 60%—usually paroxysmal supraventricular tachycardia, but atrial fibrillation and flutter also occur (2)]. The morphology of the QRS complex during the tachyarrhythmia will depend on the direction in which the re-entrant tachycardia occurs. If re-entry occurs antegrade through the AV conducting system and retrograde through an accessory pathway, then the QRS duration during the tachyarrhythmia may be normal since the ventricle is depolarized in a normal direction through its normal specialized conducting tissue. If the circuit is established in the opposite direction, the QRS complex will be wide, with a bundle branch block pattern, because most or all of the ventricle will be depolarized by way of the accessory pathway, and the arrhythmia easily can be confused with ventricular tachycardia.

Symptoms and Signs

The pre-excitation syndrome may be an incidental finding on an ECG or it may come to the attention of the physician because of symptoms. Other symptoms of tachyarrhythmia will depend on the nature of the arrhythmia and on the presence or absence of underlying heart disease.

There are no physical findings due to pre-excitation other than occasionally a loud S$_1$, except during periods of tachyarrhythmia; and then the findings depend on the type of arrhythmia that is present.

Prevalence

Pre-excitation syndromes are not rare. The prevalence of pre-excitation is between 1 and 30/1000 people (26). Accurate prevalence rates are difficult to obtain since short P-R intervals with normal QRS durations are commonly seen in people without arrhythmias so

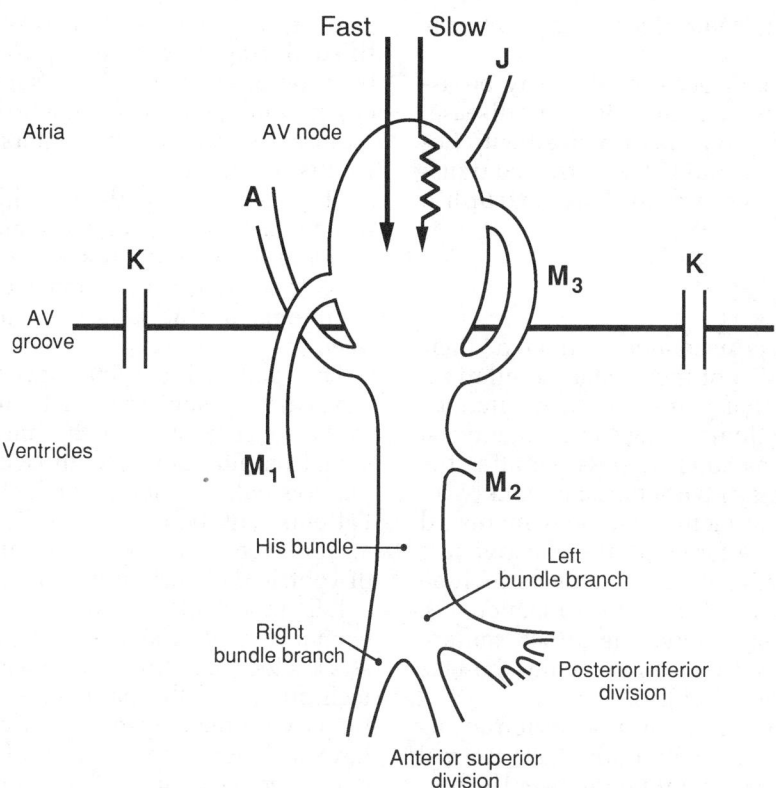

Figure 59.17. Schematic diagram of possible accessory conduction pathways. (Old eponymic nomenclature in parentheses.) *A* indicates atriofascicular (atrio-Hisian) bundles, *K* indicates accessory atrioventricular (Kent) bundles, J indicates intranodal bypass (James) tracts. *M* (Mahaim) fibers: M_1 indicates accessory nodoventricular, M_2 accessory fasciculoventricular; M_3 nodofascicular fibers. Dual AV node pathways are represented by the fast and slow symbols. Adapted from Wellens HJJ, Brugada P, Penn OC: The management of preexcitation syndromes. JAMA 257:2325, 1987.

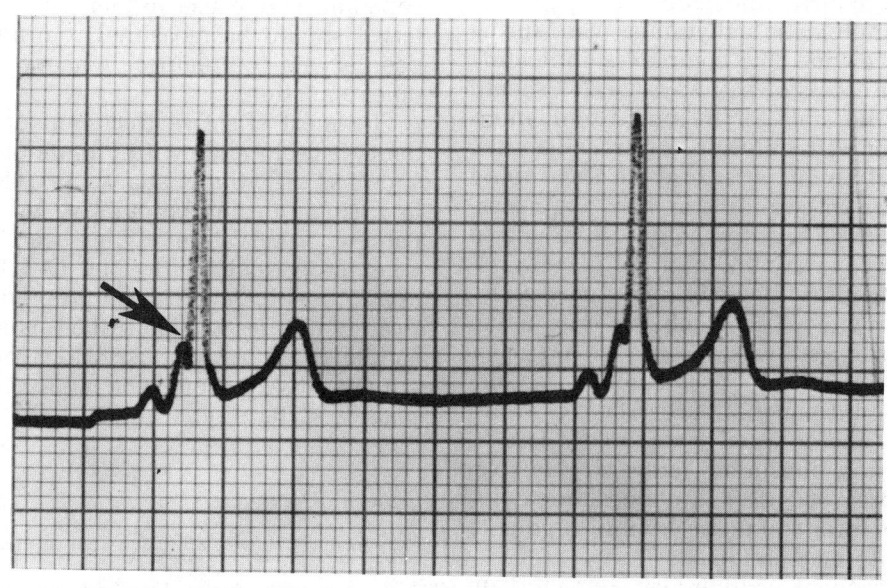

Figure 59.18. The Wolff-Parkinson-White syndrome. Note delta wave (δ).

that no studies are done to determine whether a bypass tract exists.

Pre-excitation syndromes occasionally may be associated with certain forms of congenital heart disease. Pre-excitation of the WPW type is associated with Ebstein's anomaly of the tricuspid valve, corrected transposition of the great vessels, and hypertrophic cardiomyopathies.

Treatment and Course

Asymptomatic patients need not be treated; their survival is the same as that of the normal population.

Patients with occasional symptoms can often be taught to break the arrhythmia using vagal maneuvers. These should be tried as soon as possible after the onset of tachycardia, as sympathetic tone quickly increases after the onset of tachycardia and increased sympathetic tone will interfere with the effectiveness of the maneuvers. Effective vagal maneuvers include straining against a closed glottus (Valsava maneuver), gagging by sticking a finger down the throat, self-applied carotid sinus massage, and immersing the face in cold water (the diving reflex).

Patients with symptomatic supraventricular arrhythmias who, during the arrhythmia, have normal QRS complexes—indicating conduction over the normal pathways—are best treated with propranolol, 10 to 40 mg four times a day. If that approach fails, digitalis is a reasonable alternative (0.25 mg of digoxin/day). Occasionally it will be necessary to administer quinidine or procainamide. If these drugs fail, then amiodarone in modest doses (100 to 200 mg/day) is usually effective. The use of these drugs is discussed on pages 694 and 697. Verapamil is not a useful drug for patients with pre-excitation syndromes. It does not directly affect refractoriness of accessory pathways and may reflexly increase conduction through the accessory pathway, thereby increasing the ventricular response in patients in atrial fibrillation.

Patients with symptomatic arrhythmias who, during the arrhythmia have wide QRS complexes, indicating conduction over the accessory pathways (26, 27), should be hospitalized if possible for treatment with intravenous lidocaine or with quinidine or procainamide. Suppression of arrhythmic attacks thereafter should be attempted first with quinidine and then, if necessary, with procainamide or propranolol. It is important that the physician be aware that digitalis is contraindicated in this situation. By increasing the refractoriness of the AV junction, it may enhance conduction through the accessory pathway and induce a dangerously rapid ventricular response. Amiodarone decreases conduction through both accessory pathways and the AV node and is usually effective. Class IC drugs (flecainide and encainide), are also effective, often in modest doses (50 to 100 mg of flecainide twice a day). All of these three should be administered only in consultation with a cardiologist.

Patients with frequent arrhythmias, refractory to treatment and to suppression, may be candidates for

an operation to transect the accessory pathway—identified during surgery by epicardial mapping. It has been reported that 90% of such operations are successful in preventing further arrhythmia (26); this will require referral to a few centers that have specialized in this technique.

The course of patients with pre-excitation syndromes is unpredictable—some have no or very infrequent arrhythmic attacks; others, despite therapy, have them frequently. Some patients have minimal symptoms during attacks, and others are incapacitated.

The long-term survival of patients with pre-excitation who are subject to arrhythmic attacks is related to the severity of the arrhythmia. Patients with occasional palpitations or with easily controlled bouts of paroxysmal ventricular tachycardia are at low risk. Patients with bouts of atrial flutter or fibrillation and a rapid ventricular response are at considerable risk of ventricular fibrillation and of sudden death.

It is important that asymptomatic patients with pre-excitation who wish to engage in strenuous work have stress electrocardiography (Chapter 57 describes the technique and the patient's experience with it). Patients who develop tachyarrhythmias on exercise or have a documented history of tachyarrhythmias despite treatment should not undertake strenuous exertion.

Long Q-T Interval Syndrome

An inherited syndrome has been described in which delayed repolarization is expressed as a long Q-T interval (>0.45 second when corrected for heart rate). In some families the inheritance is autosomal recessive and is associated with nerve deafness; in others, the inheritance is autosomal dominant and hearing is normal. The long Q-T interval predisposes to re-entry ventricular tachyarrhythmias, which often cause syncope and may cause sudden death (21). The Q-T interval should be measured routinely in the ECG of people who complain of syncope for which there is no explanation.

The most effective treatment of symptomatic patients is β-blockade with propranolol; if this does not suppress arrhythmic attacks, excision of the left stellate ganglion may be curative by interrupting sympathetic innervation of the heart. It is not known whether patients with long Q-T intervals who are asymptomatic benefit from propranolol, but certainly treatment is reasonable if there is a family history of sudden death. An exercise ECG is indicated in patients with negative personal and family histories of arrhythmias to determine whether arrhythmias can be induced by exertion.

General References

Schamroth L: How to approach an arrhythmia. *Circulation* 47:420, 1973.

A practical approach to the analysis of arrhythmias. Treatment of cardiac arrhythmias. *Med Lett* 31:35, 1989.

A brief synopsis of the treatment of the most common arrhythmias.

Zipes DP: Genesis of cardiac arrhythmias, management of cardiac arrhythmias, and specific arrhythmias. In: Braunwald E (ed): *Heart Disease. A Textbook of Cardiovascular Medicine*. Philadelphia, WB Saunders, 1988. pp. 518, 621, 658.

A comprehensive description, exhaustively referenced.

Constant J:*Learning Electrocardiography*. Boston, Little, Brown and Co., 1981.

The one ECG textbook to buy when you're buying only one.

Specific References

1. Aroestz JM, Cohen SI, Markin E: Bradycardia-tachycardia syndrome; results in twenty-eight patients treated by combined pharmacologic therapy and pacemaker implantation. *Chest*66:257, 1974.
2. Berkman NL, Lamb LE: The Wolff-Parkinson-White electrocardiogram: a follow-up study of five to twenty-eight years. *N Engl J Med* 278:492, 1968.
3. Bigger Jr JT: Supraventricular tachycardia. *Hospital Practi* 15:8, 1980.
4. Blomgren SE, Condemi JJ, Bignall MC, Vaughn JH: Antinuclear antibody induced by procainamide. A prospective study. *N Engl J Med* 281:64, 1969.
5. Braunwald E: Mechanism of action of calcium-channel-blocking agents. *N Engl J Med* 307:1618, 1982.
6. Davies M, Harris A: Pathological basis of primary heart block. *Br Heart J* 31:219, 1969.
7. Denes P, Dhringra RC, Wu D, et al: Sudden death in patients with chronic bifascicular block. *Arch Intern Med* 137:1005, 1977.
8. Dhingra RC, Denes P, Wu D, et al: Prospective observations in patients with chronic bundle branch block and marked H-V prolongation. *Circulation* 53:600, 1976.
9. Guarneri T, Griffith LSC: Cardiac Arrhythmias. In: Harvey AM, Johns RJ, McKusick VA, et al (eds): *The Principles and Practice of Medicine*. New York, Appleton and Lange, 1988.
10. Harrison C: Antiarrhythmic drug classification: new Science and practical applications. *Am J Cardiol* 56:185, 1985.
11. Horowitz LN: Proarrhythmia—taking the bad with the good. *N Engl J Med* 319:304, 1988.
12. Jensen JB, Humphries JO, Kouwenhoven WB, Jude JR: Electroshock for atrial flutter and atrial fibrillation: follow-up studies on 50 patients. *JAMA* 194:1181, 1965.
13. Kulbertus HE, deLeval-Rutten F, Duboir M, et al: Prognostic significance of left anterior hemiblock with right bundle branch block in mass screening. *Am J Cardiol* 41:385, 1978.
14. Maragno I, Santostasi G, Gaion RM, et al: Low- and medium-dose diltiazem in chronic atrial fibrillation: comparison with digoxin and correlation with drug plasma levels. *Am J Med* 116:385, 1988.
15. Mason JW: Amiodarone. *N Engl J Med* 316:455, 1987.
16. Mirowski M, Reid PR, Winkle RA, et al: Mortality in patients with implanted automatic defibrillators. *Ann Intern Med* 98:585, 1983.
17. Noble D: *The Initiation of the Heart Beat*. Oxford, Clarendon Press, 1975.
18. Pottage A: Clinical profiles of newer class I antiarrhythmic agents—tocainide, mexiletine, encainide, flecainide and lorcainide. *Am J Cardiol* 52:24C, 1983.
19. Roy D, Marchand E, Gagne P, et al: Usefulness of anticoagulant therapy in the prevention of embolic complications of atrial fibrillation. *Am Heart J* 112:1039, 1986.
20. Schneider JF, Thomas HE, Kreger BE, et al: Newly acquired right bundle branch block. The Framingham study. *Ann Intern Med* 92:37, 1980.
21. Schwartz PJ, Periti M, Malliani A: The long Q-T syndrome. *Am Heart J* 89:378, 1975.
22. Sheffield LT, Berson A, Bragg-Remschel D, et al: Recommendation for standards of instrumentation and practice in the use of ambulatory electrocardiography. *Circulation* 71:626A, 1985.
23. Singh BN, Collett JT, Chew CYC: New perspectives in the pharmacologic therapy of cardiac arrhythmias. *Prog Cardiovasc Dis* 22:243, 1980.
24. Stone PH, Antman EM, Muller JE, Braunwald E: Calcium channel blocking agents in the treatment of cardiovascular disorders; II. Hemodynamic effects and clinical applications. *Ann Intern Med* 93:886, 1980.
25. Surawicz B: Prognosis of ventricular arrhythmias in relation to sudden cardiac death: therapeutic implications. *J Am Coll Cardiol* 10:435, 1987.
26. Wellens HJJ, Brugada P, Penn OC: The management of preexcitation syndromes. *JAMA* 257:2325, 1987.
27. Wellens HJJ, Bär FWHM, Lie KI: The value of the electrocardiogram in the differential diagnosis of a tachycardia with a widened QRS complex. *Am J Med* 64:27, 1978.
28. Williams EM: A classification of antiarrhythmic actions reassessed after a decade of new drugs. *J Clin Pharm* 24:129, 1984.
29. Wit AL, Rosen MR, Hoffman BF: Electrophysiology and pharmacology of cardiac arrhythmias. II. Relationship of normal and abnormal electrical activity of cardiac fibers to the genesis of arrhythmias. B. Re-entry, Section I. *Am Heart J* 88:664, 1974.
30. Wohl AJ, Laborde NJ, Atkins JM, et al: Prognosis of patients permanently paced for sick sinus syndrome. *Arch Intern Med* 136:406, 1976.
31. Wolf PA, Kannel WB, McGee DC, et al: Duration of atrial fibrillation and imminence of stroke: The Framingham Study. *Stroke* 14:664, 1983.

C H A P T E R   60

Common Cardiac Disorders Revealed by Auscultation of the Heart*

EDWARD P. SHAPIRO, M.D.

HEART SOUNDS

First Heart Sound (S₁)

The first heart sound is a high frequency ("clicky") sound produced by closure of the atrioventricular (AV)

---

*Drs. Barbara B. Bell and Philip D. Zieve contributed to this chapter in the first and second editions of this book.

valves, i.e., M_1 (mitral valve closure) followed by T_1 (tricuspid valve closure). Mitral valve closure is louder than tricuspid valve closure.

Abnormally wide splitting of the first heart sound is produced by delays in closure of the tricuspid valve as in patients with right bundle branch block, ventricular ectopic beats, idioventricular rhythm, or left ventricular pacing. In mitral stenosis, mitral valve closure may be so delayed that tricuspid valve closure may actually precede mitral valve closure.

Increased intensity of the first heart sound is associated with a rapid increase in ventricular pressure, which occurs when the ventricles are presented with an increased volume (e.g., ventricular septal defect and atrial septal defect) or with a wide open AV valve at the end of diastole, which occurs when there is shortening of the AV filling time (e.g., atrial tachycardia and conditions associated with a short P-R interval) and when AV filling time is prolonged (e.g., mitral stenosis).

Reduced intensity of the first heart sound may indicate an immobile valve (e.g., severe mitral regurgitation or stenosis) or a long P-R interval.

Second Heart Sound (S_2)

The second heart sound is produced by closure of the semilunar valves, i.e., A_2 (aortic valve closure) followed by P_2 (pulmonic valve closure). Normal splitting of the second heart sound occurs at the height of inspiration, when the splitting may be as wide as 0.10 second and is due to the increase in stroke volume in the right heart with the increase in venous return with inspiration. The two components of the second heart sound are synchronous and virtually single during expiration.

Abnormally wide splitting of S_2 without change in expiration is characteristic of an atrial septal defect or of anomalous pulmonary venous return. S_2 is widely split but variable in patients with pulmonary stenosis. In the presence of severe aortic stenosis, A_2 is delayed beyond P_2, resulting in wide splitting during expiration with no splitting during inspiration (reversed or paradoxical splitting). Paradoxical splitting of the second heart sound also occurs in the presence of a left bundle branch block, severe hypertension, or severe left ventricular failure.

Increased intensities of A_2 and P_2 are features of aortic and pulmonary hypertension, respectively. *Decreased intensities* of A_2 or P_2 are features of an immobile or severely thickened aortic or pulmonic valve.

Gallops

The identification of a gallop sound affords valuable information concerning diagnosis, prognosis, and treatment. Gallops are diastolic sounds and appear to be related to the two periods of filling of the ventricles: the rapid filling phase (the S_3 or ventricular diastolic gallop) and the presystolic filling phase (related to atrial systole S_4 or atrial gallop).

The *atrial gallop sound* or S_4 is a low frequency presystolic sound and is found in patients with primary myocardial disease, coronary artery disease, systemic or pulmonary hypertension, or severe aortic or pulmonic stenosis. The atrial gallop is an indication of severity of the underlying disorder and, as the patient's condition improves, the sound may become fainter or disappear. With ventricular hypertrophy an S_4 is a fixed finding of no prognostic significance.

The *ventricular gallop sound* or S_3 is a low frequency sound. It occurs with the same timing as the normal physiological third sound, approximately 0.14 to 0.16 second after the second heart sound. The third sound is a normal finding in children and young adults up to the age of 30. An S_3 gallop is a feature of severe cardiac decompensation, whatever the underlying cause (hypertension, coronary artery disease, rheumatic heart disease, etc.) and is an indication of a relatively poor prognosis.

Ejection Sounds ("Clicks")

Ejection sounds are produced at the time of ejection of blood from the left ventricle into the aorta or from the right ventricle into the pulmonary artery. The sound may originate in a thickened valve or in a dilated great vessel. The aortic ejection sound is located in the area of aortic auscultation—namely, from the second right intercostal space in a straight line to the cardiac apex—and occurs 0.05 second after M_1. It is a high frequency sound, often called a click. In the presence of systemic hypertension, the aortic ejection sound is an indication of severity. It disappears as hypertension improves. Aortic ejection clicks may also be heard in patients with aortic stenosis, aneurysm of the ascending aorta, and aortic insufficiency.

Pulmonic ejection sounds (or clicks) are frequently localized to the second left intercostal space and may increase in intensity with expiration. They occur immediately after M_1. Pulmonic clicks are a feature of valvular pulmonic stenosis and also of pulmonary hypertension.

A *midsystolic clicking* sound, with or without a late systolic murmur, may indicate mitral valve prolapse (see below).

Opening Snaps

An opening snap occurs because of a stenotic, but still mobile, mitral or tricuspid valve. The mitral opening snap is best heard between the pulmonic area and the cardiac apex. It occurs 0.04 to 0.12 second after S_2 in early diastole. It is heard in patients with a thickened mitral valve. The earlier the snap, the more severe the stenosis. The tricuspid opening snap is best heard at the lower left or right sternal border and occurs immediately after S_2 in early diastole.

Murmurs

Evaluation of a heart murmur is one of the most common tasks that confronts a physician conducting a physical examination. Virtually all normal people have a systolic murmur during some period of their lives. On the other hand, a murmur may be a sign of serious underlying cardiac or noncardiac disease. It is important to be able to distinguish the innocent murmur from those that reflect an underlying disorder and to be able to select appropriately the tests that will lead to the precise diagnosis and to proper management.

General Characteristics of Murmurs

A murmur is a series of audible vibrations produced by turbulence in the circulation. These vibrations can be characterized by intensity, pitch, shape, quality, and timing in the cardiac cycle, precordial location of maximal intensity, and radiation.

The intensity or loudness of a murmur is, by convention, graded on a scale of 1 to 6. A grade 1 murmur is audible only after concentrated auscultation. A grade 2 murmur is faint but readily audible. A grade 3 murmur is prominent but not loud. Grade 4 murmurs are loud and are frequently, but not always, associated with a palpable thrill. A grade 5 murmur is very loud. A grade 6 murmur is heard with the stethoscope held 1 cm above, but not actually touching, the chest wall.

The pitch of a murmur refers to the frequency of the sound—from high to low. High frequency murmurs usually reflect high velocity and/or high pressure.

The shape of a murmur refers to the change in intensity throughout the duration of the sound: for example, crescendo (increasing in intensity), decrescendo (decreasing in intensity), or constant.

The quality of a murmur refers to the nature of the sound: harsh, blowing, musical, cooing, rumbling, etc. Although these terms are not precise, they are useful in identifying various benign and significant conditions, as will be described below.

The timing of a murmur is particularly important in establishing the cause of the sound—first, whether the murmur is systolic, diastolic, or continuous, and second, whether it is heard in early, middle, or late systole or diastole. Murmurs that last throughout systole are called holosystolic. Late diastolic murmurs are sometimes called presystolic.

The location of a murmur refers to that site on the chest wall where the sound is loudest. The direction of radiation refers to the other sites where the murmur, though less intense, can still be heard; those sites may be outside the chest (the back or neck, for example). Aortic murmurs may be heard anywhere in a straight line from the second right interspace to the apex. Pulmonic murmurs are heard best at the second left intercostal space; tricuspid murmurs, at the lower left sternal border; and mitral murmurs, at the cardiac apex radiating into the axilla.

There are two kinds of systolic murmurs—ejection and regurgitant murmurs. The ejection systolic murmur may be an innocent flow murmur or it may reflect organic heart disease. The regurgitant murmur may be due to dilation of the annulus of the valve in an otherwise normal heart or may represent organic heart disease.

The ejection murmur is a crescendo/decrescendo (or "diamond-shaped") murmur caused by the turbulence of blood flowing through either the aortic or pulmonic valve. The murmur is most commonly midsystolic and ends before the second or closing sound (S_2) of the valve from which the murmur was generated; that is, aortic ejection murmurs end before A_2 and pulmonic ejection murmurs end before P_2. The loudness of the murmur depends in part on the pressure gradient across the valve and in part on other factors, such as thickness of the chest, the cardiac output, etc.; the shape depends on the acceleration and deceleration of blood flow across the valve as systole proceeds. When diastole is prolonged, for example, by premature ventricular contraction or by atrial fibrillation, ejection murmurs become louder because of the passage of a large volume of blood through the valve. In general, the larger the cardiac output, the louder the murmur. Increases in cardiac output due to hypermetabolic states, such as anemia, fever, or thyrotoxicosis, will increase the loudness of the murmur. Decreases in cardiac output, such as congestive heart failure, will decrease the loudness of the murmur.

Regurgitant murmurs are murmurs produced by backward flow of blood from a high pressure chamber to a compartment of lower pressure. Intensity may be constant as in mitral regurgitation, tricuspid regurgitation, or ventricular septal defect or may be decrescendo as in aortic and pulmonary regurgitation.

A number of maneuvers can be performed that alter the intensity of a systolic murmur and help to determine its origin. For example, the Valsalva maneuver reduces intrathoracic venous return and softens the murmur of aortic stenosis while intensifying that of hypertrophic cardiomyopathy. Squatting, which increases venous return, has the opposite effect. Isometric handgrip, which increases blood pressure and therefore reduces forward flow, softens the murmur of aortic stenosis and intensifies that of mitral regurgitation.

Innocent Murmurs

Innocent murmurs are a series of vibrations that are produced in the absence of significant abnormalities of cardiac anatomy or function (Table 60.1).

The innocent murmur can usually be distinguished from significant murmurs by the absence of other physical, radiological, or electrocardiographic evidence of disease. Also, innocent murmurs are usually in early or midsystole, are grade 1 or 2 in intensity, and vary with respiration and/or position. Occasionally, echocardiography (see below) is done to clarify

Table 60.1.
Benign or Innocent Systolic Murmurs

Vibratory ejection systolic murmur
Continuous murmur of venous hum
Pulmonic ejection systolic murmur
Aortic ejection systolic murmur
Murmur associated with pregnancy

the etiology of a murmur, but more elaborate studies, such as stress tests, radionuclide studies, and cardiac catheterization, are employed only after it has been decided that a murmur is not innocent and that a more precise diagnosis is necessary.

The most common innocent *systolic murmur of childhood* and young adulthood that is clearly recognizable as benign based on the characteristics of the murmur alone is the musical or vibratory midsystolic murmur (best heard at the lower left sternal border) that is caused by the vibration of the leaflets of the pulmonary valve.

The *venous hum* is a continuous murmur, loudest in the neck, caused by altered flow through the jugular veins. It can be eliminated by turning the patient's head, compressing the internal jugular vein on the side where the murmur is heard, or placing the patient in the supine position.

The *pulmonic ejection systolic murmur* is a systolic crescendo/decrescendo murmur generated by the flow of blood through the pulmonary valve. It is loudest in the left second intercostal space or at the midleft sternal border.

Similarly, the *aortic ejection systolic murmur* is an early systolic murmur generated by the flow of blood through the aortic valve. It is loudest in the right second intercostal space or at the apex of the heart. This innocent or flow murmur, due to sclerosis of the aorta and/or aortic valve, is the most common benign systolic murmur in the middle-aged or elderly patient and may have a cooing quality. An electrocardiogram (ECG) and an echocardiogram may be necessary to rule out left ventricular hypertrophy and aortic stenosis.

Benign flow murmurs commonly are heard in *pregnant women*. Because of the normally increased stroke volume at 28 to 30 weeks of gestation, diastolic filling sounds and systolic ejection murmurs of turbulent flow are common. In pregnant patients also, an S_3 may be prominent enough to be confused with the middiastolic murmur of mitral stenosis. The S_3 of pregnancy may be distinguished from the murmur of mitral stenosis, however, by the absence of an opening snap and by the accompanying hyperdynamic apical movement. An echocardiogram is indicated in some patients to make a precise diagnosis.

In the pregnant patient it is critical to compare the femoral and brachial pulses and the blood pressures in the presence of a heart murmur, since coarctation of the aorta may present with a soft heart murmur and, if left undiagnosed, rarely may result in aortic dissection or rupture.

Clinical Applications of Echocardiography

Echocardiography is a valuable adjunct to the clinical assessment in patients suspected of cardiovascular disease (25). This technique utilizes high frequency pulsed sound waves to record echoes of cardiac structures as they move within a beam of sound directed into the chest. Sometimes the cardiologist will use phonocardiography in combination with ech-

ocardiography to time the various normal and abnormal heart sounds more precisely.

A piezoelectric crystal is used to transmit a short pulse of ultrahigh frequency sound (1 to 8 mHz) into the tissues of the chest. To record an M-mode electrocardiogram, the pulse transducer is placed at one point on the chest wall and rocked to inscribe an arc that will encompass several areas of the heart sequentially. It serves as a source of the sound beam and as a receiver of the echoes. A two-dimensional echocardiogram is recorded using a pulse transducer that is automatically rocked across an arc (mechanical two-dimensional echocardiography) or one that contains multiple piezoelectric crystals directed along the arc (phased array two-dimensional echocardiography). These techniques provide a simultaneous view of the cardiac structures, which is recorded on videotape. These procedures are of no discomfort to the patient; however, he must be able to lie flat for 20 minutes for performance of the test.

Echo spikes arise from the chest wall, right ventricular wall, interventricular septum, mitral leaflets, posterior left ventricular wall, aorta, and left atrium (Fig. 60.1). The size and function of these structures are analyzed and patterns of specific diseases may be recognized.

Two-dimensional (2-D) echocardiography provides a simultaneous view of these structures and, therefore, reveals their function more precisely than does M-mode or one-dimensional echocardiography. Where possible, both modes should be used for optimal visualization of the heart (25). Two-dimensional echocardiography is particularly helpful in assessing left ventricular function in patients with ischemic heart disease where regional structure and function are most important. The noninvasive nature of the test and its ease of performance make two-dimensional echocardiography extremely useful for assessing patients with acute cardiac decompensation. One-dimensional echocardiography is most useful in situations where visualization of rapidly moving structures is important (e.g., mitral leaflet flutter as the result of aortic regurgitation) and in situations where repeated measurements of dimensions of cardiac structures are important.

The echocardiogram is diagnostic in cases of pericardial effusion, idiopathic subaortic stenosis, mitral valve stenosis or prolapse, aortic regurgitation, intracardiac masses, cardiomyopathy, and Ebstein's anomaly of the tricuspid valve. The technique is helpful in cases of aortic stenosis, infectious endocarditis, cardiac tamponade, atrial septal defect, other forms of congenital heart disease such as ventricular septal defect, tetralogy of Fallot and bicuspid aortic valve, and any other structural abnormality of the heart.

During the last several years, *Doppler echocardiography* has developed into an extremely useful tool for the detection and quantification of severity of valvular heart disease. High frequency sound is directed at a column of moving red blood cells, and the reflected sound is analyzed for changes in frequency, which indicate the direction and velocity of flow. Newer

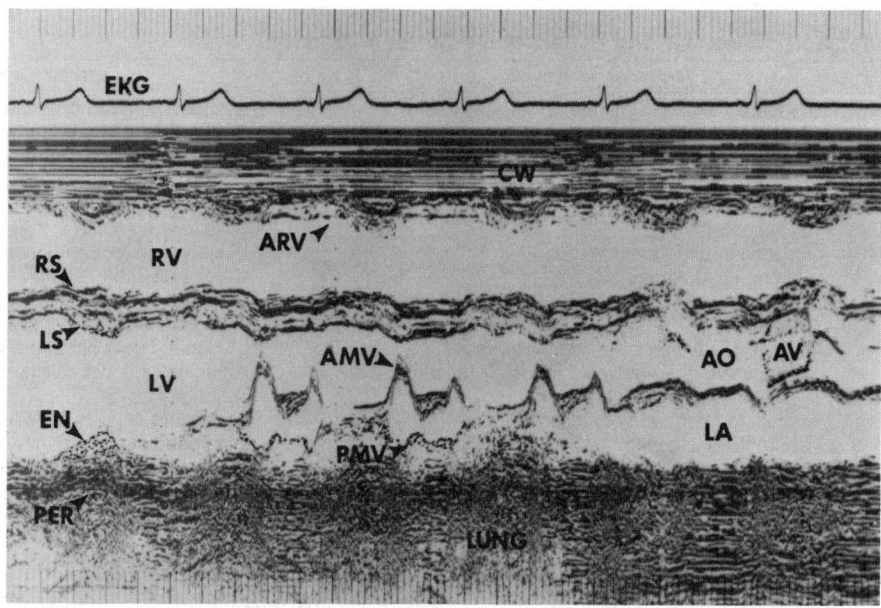

Figure 60.1. Normal one-dimensional echocardiogram. The tracing was taken as the transducer was scanned from the apex to the base of the heart. *AO*, aorta; *AMV*, anterior leaflet of the mitral valve; *ARV*, anterior wall of the right ventricle; *AV*, aortic valve opening; *CW*, chest wall; *EN*, posterior left ventricular endocardium; *LA*, left atrium; *LS*, left ventricular septum; *LV*, left ventricle; *PER*, pericardium; *PMV*, posterior mitral valve leaflet; *RS*, right ventricular septum; *RV*, right ventricle.

instruments allow flow velocity information to be color coded and superimposed on the 2-D echocardiographic image, providing visual representation of blood flow through the heart and great vessels.

In valvular stenosis a high velocity jet of blood is detected distal to the stenosis; the higher the transvalvular gradient, the higher the velocity of the jet. The pressure gradient across a valve and the area of the aortic (34) and mitral (11) valves can also be calculated, providing precise quantification of the severity of aortic and mitral stenosis.

Valvular regurgitation can be detected by reverse flow and its severity estimated, usually by measuring the extent to which the regurgitant jet is detectable in the chamber proximal to the leaking valve. For example, mitral regurgitation is considered severe on a color Doppler study if the regurgitant jet occupies more than 40% of the area of the left atrium during systole (12). It should be noted that a small degree of regurgitation of the tricuspid valve is commonly seen in normal subjects and does not represent disease. The presence of tricuspid regurgitation allows the estimation of right ventricular systolic pressure, which is equal to the pulmonary artery systolic pressure. This is useful in the detection and follow-up of patients with pulmonary hypertension of any etiology.

SELECTED DISORDERS ASSOCIATED WITH ABNORMAL HEART SOUNDS

Aortic Stenosis

Stenosis of the aortic valve obstructs the flow of blood into the aorta and therefore raises the left ventricular pressure above the aortic pressure. The pressure gradient across the valve reflects the severity of the stenosis. The elevated pressure results in a concentric hypertrophy of the left ventricle. Symptoms develop when the left ventricle can no longer compensate for the pressure load; the heart fails and the cardiac output declines.

Aortic stenosis may occur at any one of several levels. The most common obstruction (75% of patients) is at the aortic valve, although patients with subvalvular and supravalvular aortic stenosis may present with symptoms and signs of severity similar to those of valvular disease. It is particularly important to differentiate fixed aortic outflow obstruction from idiopathic hypertrophic disease, which is a functional disorder (Table 60.2 and below).

Etiology and Epidemiology (27)

In patients below the age of 30, aortic stenosis is most likely to be due to a congenitally stenotic unicuspid valve. Between the ages of 30 and 65, a bicuspid aortic valve, which has become calcified and gradually more rigid over the years, is the most common cause of aortic stenosis. (One or 2% of the general population have a bicuspid aortic valve, and 50% of these valves have calcified by age 50). Rheumatic valvular disease accounts for only 6 to 27% of cases of isolated aortic stenosis in patients between the ages of 30 and 70 years. Over the age of 65, degeneration and sclerosis of the valve account for most cases of aortic stenosis. Except in the elderly, in whom the prevalence is the same in both sexes, isolated aortic stenosis is three to four times more common in men.

Table 60.2.
Comparison of Valvular Aortic Stenosis and Hypertrophic Cardiomyopathy

	Valvular Aortic Stenosis	Hypertrophic Cardiomyopathy
Symptoms	Dyspnea, angina, syncope, or near syncope	Dyspnea, angina, syncope, or near syncope
Signs	Systolic ejection murmur loudest at aortic area or at apex; louder if patient squats	Systolic ejection murmur loudest at left lower sternal border; louder if patient stands or performs a Valsalva maneuver
	A_2 may not be audible	A_2 is usually audible
	S_4 is common	S_4 is very common
	Ejection sounds are common	Ejection sounds are uncommon
	Carotid upstroke is delayed	Carotid upstroke is brisk
ECG	Left ventricular hypertrophy (LVH) and strain pattern	LVH and strain pattern; Q waves in inferior and lateral leads are common
Chest X-ray	LVH is a late sign	LVH may occur but unpredictably
	Aortic valve is always calcified (may be seen only on fluoroscopy)	Aortic valve is not calcified
	Ascending aorta may be dilated	Ascending aorta is not dilated
Echocardiogram	Characteristic echos of valvular calcification and of valvular stenosis	Disproportionate septal hypertrophy, systolic anterior displacement of mitral valve

Natural History and Symptoms

Patients with aortic stenosis are usually asymptomatic until relatively late in the course of their disease. Mild to moderate obstruction does not compromise left ventricular function greatly, and even patients with severe stenosis may compensate for years before they develop symptoms. Symptoms ordinarily develop late in the sixth decade after which, if the lesion is not corrected, the average patient dies in about 4 years.

The earliest symptoms are easy fatigability and excessive dyspnea after unusual exercise. Syncope or near syncope with effort (see Chapter 81), angina (see Chapter 57), and dyspnea on unusual exercise (see Chapter 53) are indicative of severe valvular obstruction. Patients with heart failure survive less long (2 years) as a rule than do patients with syncope (3 years) or with angina (5 years) (28). Sudden death occurs in about 15% of symptomatic patients and, particularly worrisome, in about 5% of asymptomatic patients (28).

Physical Findings

Patients with aortic stenosis usually have a loud (grade 3 to 4) systolic ejection murmur. The maximal intensity of the murmur is at the second right intercostal space and/or at the cardiac apex. At the apex the murmur often has a musical cooing quality. There is usually a thrill in the suprasternal notch or in the second right intercostal space. However, the loudness of the murmur may not correlate with the severity of stenosis. Also, if cardiac output is reduced, as in congestive heart failure, or if the diameter of the chest is increased, the intensity of the murmur may be less than it otherwise would be. A late peak to the murmur does suggest severe obstruction, but this is difficult to appreciate with a stethoscope, and absence of the peak does not mean that obstruction is not severe. Augmentation of the murmur when the patient suddenly squats and diminution of the murmur when the patient stands or performs a Valsalva maneuver are characteristic of aortic stenosis.

The systolic murmur, although it may not be loud, is an invariable sign of aortic stenosis; other cardiac sounds are dependent on the nature of the stenotic lesion. An early systolic ejection click is commonly heard when the valve is still mobile. The second aortic sound (A_2) is often not audible when the valve is rigid so that S_2 has only one component (P_2). Paradoxical splitting of the second heart sound, in the absence of left bundle branch block, is a sign of severity. A small pulse pressure (< 30 mm Hg) also indicates severe obstruction (in elderly people, the pulse pressure may be normal despite severe stenosis). A slowly rising pulse—best assessed by palpation of a carotid artery—is characteristic. Under the age of 40, an S_4 is another sign of severe obstruction; over the age of 40, S_4 is common because of the high prevalence of hypertensive and ischemic heart disease and does not correlate with severity of stenosis.

The regurgitant early diastolic murmur of aortic insufficiency is heard in 30 to 40% of patients with aortic valve stenosis.

Laboratory Evaluation

An ECG, a chest X-ray, and an echocardiogram should be obtained routinely in a patient suspected of having aortic stenosis.

Electrocardiogram. The ECG is usually normal until stenosis becomes severe, at which point left ventricular hypertrophy Table 60.3 and (Fig. 60.2) and nonspecific ST depression and T wave inversion are common—but not invariable. In older patients particularly, an abnormal ECG cannot be relied upon to reflect severity since there are often other reasons why it might be abnormal.

Chest X-ray. Calcification of the aortic valve is always present in patients with aortic stenosis who are older than 35 to 40; but often fluoroscopy is necessary to reveal it. Poststenotic dilation of the ascending aorta is also commonly seen. The heart size and configuration are usually normal until the disease is far advanced.

Echocardiogram. Echocardiography reveals multiple diastolic echoes of aortic valve leaflets, due to valvular calcification and, sometimes, an eccentric di-

Table 60.3.
Principal Electrocardiographic Features of Left Ventricular Hypertrophy[a]

Electrocardiographic Criteria	Point System for Diagnosis[b]
Negative components of P in $V_1 \geq 1$ mm and ≥ 0.4 second	3 points
QRS	
Largest limb lead R or S ≥ 20 mm or largest chest lead S before transition or R after transition ≥ 30 mm	3 points
OR	
Largest S before transition plus largest R after transition = 45 mm:	
Frontal plane axis $\geq -30°$	2 points
Duration in extremity lead ≥ 0.09 second	1 point
Intrinsicoid deflection ≥ 0.05 second	1 point
ST-T	
In general, opposite QRS:	
Without digitalis	3 points
With digitalis	1 point

[a] Modified from Horan LG, Flowers NC: Electrocardiography and vectorcardiography. In Braunwald E (ed): *Heart Disease: A Textbook of Cardiovascular Medicine.* Philadelphia, WB Saunders, 1980, p. 229 (14).
[b] Interpretation of point score: 6 points, left ventricular hypertrophy; 5 points, probable left ventricular hypertrophy; 4 points, possible left ventricular hypertrophy. If only voltage criteria are met, ECG may be designated as borderline, and the statement should be made that "left ventricular hypertrophy is suggested only by voltage and should be excluded by other clinical means."

astolic closure line. An increase in ventricular wall thickness on echocardiography implies severe obstruction, if there is no other cause for hypertrophy. Doppler echocardiography (see page 720) can provide an estimate of the transaortic gradient and the aortic valve area. Doppler echocardiography is very helpful in distinguishing aortic stenosis from aortic valve sclerosis, in which no gradient is present.

Management

Asymptomatic patients should be reassessed every 12 months so that signs of progressive disease can be detected promptly. Reassessment should include interval history, pertinent physical examination, ECG, chest X-ray, and echocardiogram.

Patients should be cautioned to avoid undue exertion since acute heart failure, arrhythmia, and sudden death are more likely under such circumstances.

The risk of subacute bacterial endocarditis is increased in patients with aortic stenosis and is unrelated to the severity of the stenosis (the risk is unchanged after aortic valve surgery—see below) (21). Therefore, antibiotic prophylaxis (see Chapter 86) is necessary before dental and surgical procedures.

Atrial arrhythmias are uncommon; if they occur, they must be treated aggressively (see Chapter 59) because they are more likely to cause angina, heart failure, or syncope than in a patient without aortic stenosis. β-Blocking agents are probably best avoided because they may compromise left ventricular function further. If heart failure develops, it should be treated with digitalis and diuretics (see Chapter 61), but great care must be taken to avoid volume depletion, which may reduce cardiac output to a point where serious underperfusion of vital organs occurs.

Table 60.4 lists the indications for referral of a patient with aortic stenosis to a cardiologist. In general,

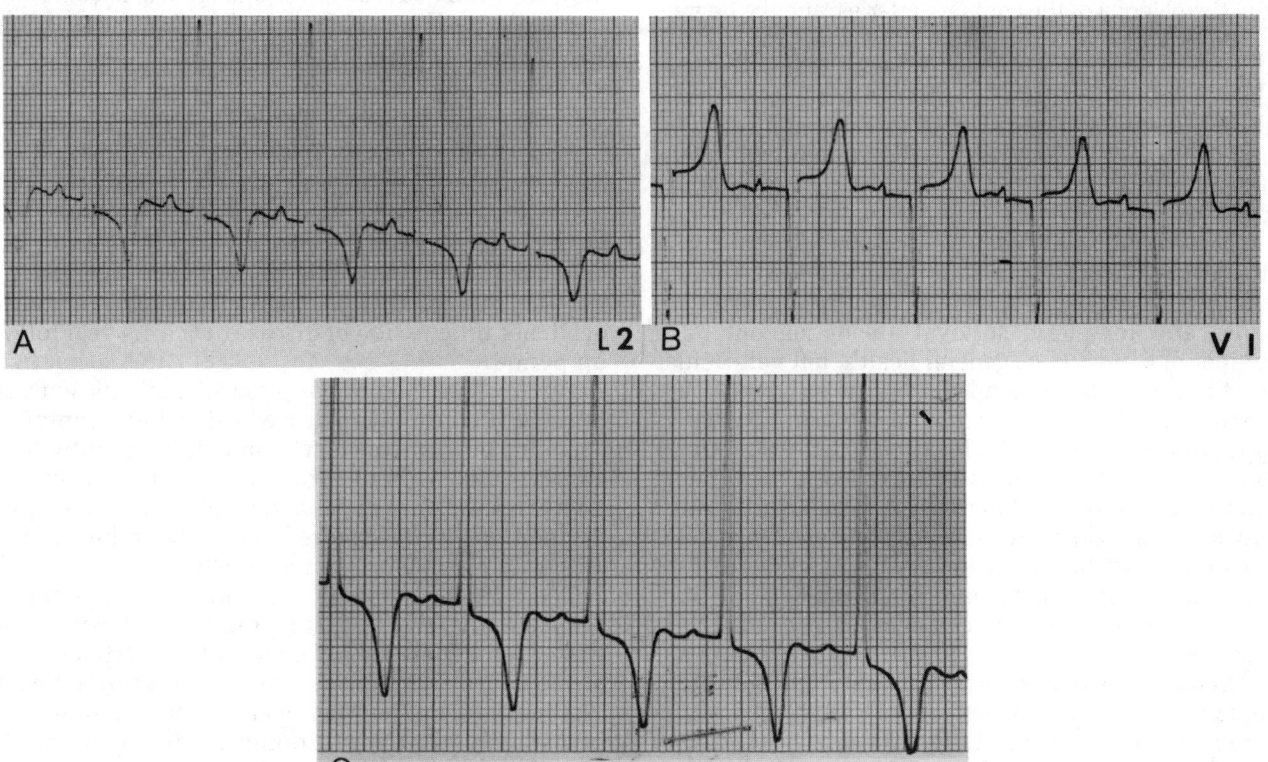

Figure 60.2. ECG of a patient with left ventricular hypertrophy (see Table 60.3).

Table 60.4.
Indications for Referral of Patients with Aortic Stenosis

If there is a question about the diagnosis
If the patient is symptomatic
If the asymptomatic patient has signs of severe obstruction:
   Physical signs:
      Small pulse pressure (< 30 mm Hg)
      Late peak to systolic murmur
      Diminished A_2
      Paradoxical splitting of A_2
   ECG
      Left ventricular hypertrophy
      ST depression, T wave inversion
   Chest X-ray: Concentric left ventricular hypertrophy
   Echocardiogram:
      Concentric left ventricular hypertrophy
      Calcification of aortic valve in patients under 60

referral is indicated if the diagnosis is unclear, the patient is symptomatic, or an asymptomatic patient has evidence of severe obstruction. Cardiac catheterization (see Chapter 57) is the definitive technique for assessing the severity and site of aortic stenosis. It should be performed in all symptomatic patients and in asymptomatic patients who have signs of severe disease. Hemodynamically significant stenosis is usually associated with a gradient of 50 mm Hg or greater (unless cardiac output is reduced, in which case the gradient may be much lower even if there is severe stenosis). The effective aortic valve orifice in patients with severe obstruction is usually less than 0.5 cm/m² of body surface area (compared to 1.6 to 2.6 cm in normal people). At the time of catheterization, angiography is also done to assess left ventricular function, the patency of the coronary arteries, and the degree, if any, of aortic and mitral regurgitation.

The cardiologist is likely to recommend replacement of the stenotic aortic valve with a prosthesis in all symptomatic patients and in asymptomatic patients with signs of severe obstruction who are found to have a large gradient or evidence, on angiography, of left ventricular dysfunction.

Operative mortality in patients without left ventricular failure is 5 to 10%; in patients with left ventricular failure it is 10 to 25%. The patient's postoperative health and long-term survival are dependent on a number of factors (age, general health, left ventricular function, etc.), but overall the 5-year survival is approximately 80 to 85%, and the 10-year survival is approximately 70 to 75%. Most patients experience a considerable improvement in their sense of well-being and in their exercise tolerance (21). When patients die, however, their death is usually due to a cardiac complication (heart failure, myocardial infarction, or sudden death). (For further details regarding the long-term course/management of the patient with a prosthetic valve see page 733.)

Percutaneous balloon valvuloplasty is a new technique in which one or more balloons are placed across a stenotic aortic valve and then inflated in an attempt to reduce the severity of stenosis. This method has been applied mainly to very elderly patients or to those who are poor surgical candidates for other reasons. Although the transaortic gradient is usually reduced and initial clinical improvement is achieved, overall results to date have not been encouraging, since high rates of death (24%) and recurrences of severe symptoms of aortic stenosis (47%) have been reported within 6 months of the procedure (22). However, a subset of patients does experience sustained improvement from the procedure. At present, aortic valvuloplasty can only be recommended for severely symptomatic patients who would be at very high risk were they to undergo aortic valve replacement.

Hypertrophic Cardiomyopathy

Hypertrophic cardiomyopathy is a disease of cardiac muscle in which the ventricular septum is thickened disproportionately compared with the free wall of the left ventricle (asymmetric septal hypertrophy). The left ventricle is hypercontractile and during systole ejects essentially all of its blood, leaving a "clenched fist" with very high wall stress. The asymmetric hypertrophy distinguishes this condition from those, such as hypertension and aortic stenosis, that cause secondary hypertrophy of the heart muscle (Table 60.2). A common, but not invariable, feature of the disease is obstruction to the left ventricular outflow tract.

Etiology and Epidemiology

The etiology of hypertrophic cardiomyopathy is unknown, although there is evidence that it is usually inherited. Some patients become symptomatic when they are young adults, but the diagnosis is sometimes not made until much later in life. Men and women are equally likely to be affected.

Natural History and Symptoms

As echocardiography has become more widely utilized for the evaluation of patients with heart murmurs, it has become clear that most patients with hypertrophic cardiomyopathy are asymptomatic or have only mild symptoms. The prognosis in this group is excellent; one study (35) of 25 patients showed neither death nor progression of disease over a 4.4 year follow-up period.

The most common symptom of patients with hypertrophic cardiomyopathy who develop symptoms is dyspnea, but patients also complain frequently of angina (with or without evidence of occlusive coronary artery disease) and of syncope or near syncope. These symptoms are much more likely to be induced by exertion than to occur spontaneously.

Once marked symptoms develop, some patients become rapidly worse, with progressive heart failure, angina, or arrhythmias. The most troublesome feature of the illness is its propensity to cause sudden death. The incidence of sudden death is about 3 to 4%/year in patients with hypertrophic cardiomyopathy, but some families have a particularly high incidence. Unfortunately, there is no way to identify in any given patient an increased risk of sudden death; in fact, death may be the first manifestation of the disease.

Physical Findings

The characteristic signs of the disease are a sustained left ventricular apical impulse, a loud S$_4$, and a harsh systolic ejection murmur, loudest at the left lower border of the sternum and often accompanied by a thrill. The location of the murmur helps to distinguish the condition from valvular aortic stenosis. Other distinguishing features are as follows: the second heart sound (A$_2$) is usually audible; a diastolic murmur is rare; the pulse pressure is normal; ejection sounds are uncommon; and, most important, the upstroke of the carotid pulse is brisk. In addition, the murmur of hypertrophic cardiomyopathy is augmented when the patient stands or performs a Valsalva maneuver and is diminished when the patient squats—the opposite of the findings in patients with aortic stenosis.

Laboratory Evaluation

An ECG, chest X-ray, and echocardiogram should be obtained routinely in patients suspected of having hypertrophic cardiomyopathy.

Electrocardiogram. The ECG is abnormal in the majority of patients and is always abnormal in patients with obstruction. Typically, there is evidence of left ventricular hypertrophy (Fig. 60.2 and Table 60.3) and there is nonspecific ST depression and T wave inversion. Q waves are often seen in the inferior and lateral leads, reflecting septal hypertrophy.

Chest X-ray. The left ventricle is sometimes enlarged, but unpredictably so. In contrast to aortic valvular stenosis, the aortic valve is not calcified and the ascending aorta is not dilated.

Echocardiogram. Echocardiography is diagnostic; it demonstrates a thickened ventricular septum, hypertrophied out of proportion to the posterior wall of the left ventricle. Also, the mitral valve apparatus is displaced anteriorly during systole, and the aortic leaflets may close suddenly in early systole and reopen as systole continues. (These abnormalities of the aortic valve may only be present after the patient is administered amyl nitrate.)

Management

The goal of therapy is to reduce the hypercontractile state of the left ventricle. Currently this is best done by means of the calcium channel blocker, verapamil, (80 to 120 mg four times a day) unless the patient has signs or symptoms of heart failure. Alternatively, a β-blocker may be prescribed (e.g., propranolol, 10 to 80 mg four times a day). Angina, especially, is often relieved by treatment, but dyspnea also may be decreased as a result of a slower heart rate and of more time for the ventricle to fill. Although it is not clear that the risk of sudden death is reduced by therapy, most patients are symptomatically improved or at least stabilized by treatment.

Drugs that increase ventricular contractility or decrease ventricular volume are best avoided if possible—digitalis, vasodilators, β-adrenergic stimulants, and diuretics. Patients, even if asymptomatic, should avoid undue exertion (e.g., running).

There is an increased risk of endocarditis in patients with hypertrophic cardiomyopathy and they should therefore receive antibiotic prophylaxis before dental and surgical procedures (see Chapter 86).

Surgical removal of a portion of the hypertrophied septum should be considered in severely symptomatic patients. Such a decision should be made in consultation with a cardiologist and a cardiac surgeon. Although the operative mortality is relatively high (5 to 10%), symptoms are usually relieved in patients who survive and postoperative annual mortality is only 1.5 to 2%. In one series the incidence of sudden death appeared to be reduced after operation (32).

Symptomatic patients should limit their activities to those that do not require heavy exertion. It is not clear whether asymptomatic patients should limit their activity.

Atrial Septal Defect

Atrial septal defect of the ostium secundum type (in the midportion of the septum) is one of the most common congenital cardiac diseases that is diagnosed in adults. It causes, until late in the course (see below), a left to right atrial shunt with a volume overload of the right ventricle and overperfusion of the lungs.

Etiology and Epidemiology

The defect is more common in females; the reported female to male ratio ranges from 1.5 to 3.5:1. Occasionally the defect is associated with other cardiac abnormalities. For example, 10 to 20% of patients with an atrial septal defect have mitral valve prolapse (15).

Natural History and Symptoms

Patients with atrial septal defect are usually asymptomatic until their third or fourth decade. Thereafter, symptoms invariably develop—usually dyspnea on exertion, fatigue, and palpitations—the result of heart failure and of supraventricular arrhythmias. Less commonly, symptoms of pulmonary embolism (Chapter 53) or paradoxical embolism (e.g., a stroke) occur. Virtually all patients are symptomatic by age 60. In fact, three-quarters of untreated patients are dead by age 50 and 90% by age 60. Increased pulmonary blood flow eventually produces pulmonary vascular disease and, consequently, pulmonary hypertension in about 15% of patients (5). When this happens, the left to right shunt first decreases and then reverses; it is at that point that cyanosis develops. Coexistent atherosclerotic or hypertensive cardiovascular disease may complicate the course of older patients with atrial septal defect and may make diagnosis and treatment more difficult.

Physical Findings

Atrial septal defect usually causes a wide fixed split of the second heart sound, the result of late closure of the pulmonic valve, and a soft blowing systolic pulmonic ejection murmur. A low-medium frequency middiastolic flow murmur across the tricuspid valve is common. The precordium may be hyperdynamic with a palpable S_3. If pulmonary hypertension has developed (see below), clubbing and cyanosis may be observed, and P_2 will be accentuated. Signs of right ventricular failure (edema, distended neck veins, hepatomegaly) are common late in the disease.

Laboratory Evaluation

An ECG, a chest X-ray, and an echocardiogram should be obtained routinely in a patient suspected of having an atrial septal defect.

Electrocardiogram. The ECG displays an incomplete right bundle branch block or rSR^1 in lead V_1 90 to 95% of the time with a vertical frontal plane axis or right axis deviation. Atrial fibrillation occurs commonly in symptomatic patients; atrial flutter and paroxysmal atrial tachycardia occur less often.

Chest X-ray (Fig. 60.3). The chest X-ray in this disease is almost invariably abnormal and shows increased pulmonary vascularity with a prominent main pulmonary artery and increased heart size. The right pulmonary artery is usually more prominent than the left because of differential flow due to the jet effect.

Echocardiogram. The echocardiogram demon-

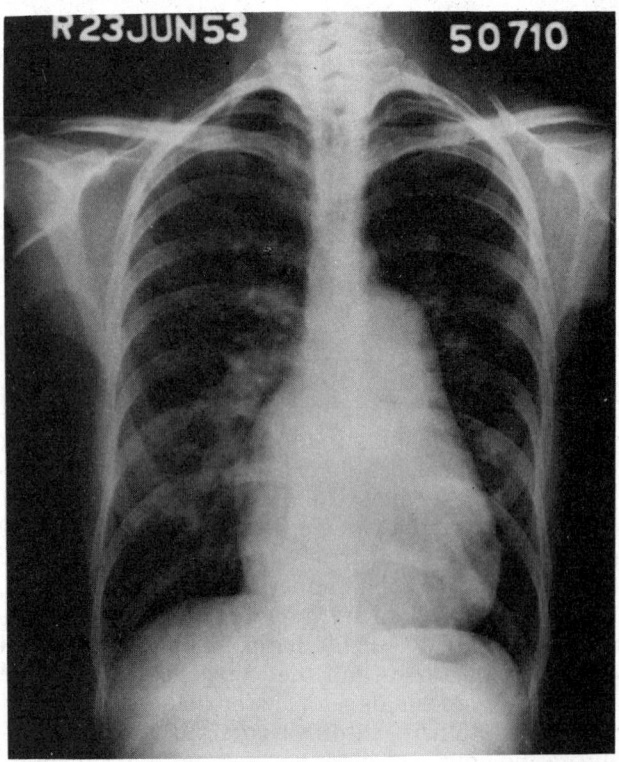

Figure 60.3. Chest X-ray of a patient with atrial septal defect (see the text).

strates right ventricular enlargement and paradoxical motion of the ventricular septum with respect to the posterior wall of the left ventricle. These findings are also seen with other lesions that cause volume overload of the right ventricle, such as tricuspid and pulmonic regurgitation, and partial anomalous pulmonary venous return. Flow across the atrial septum can often be visualized using color Doppler echocardiography.

Management

Patients suspected of having an atrial septal defect should be referred to a cardiologist for definitive diagnosis. The cardiologist will usually perform cardiac catheterization (see Chapter 57 for a description of the patient experience). All patients, even if they are asymptomatic, should have their defect repaired if pulmonary blood flow is more than 1 1/2 times systemic blood flow. The operative mortality is less than 2%, although some degree of persistent right or left ventricular dysfunction is common in adults. If severe pulmonary hypertension has developed (pulmonary pressure equal to or greater than the systemic pressure), corrective surgery is contraindicated, but patients with lesser degrees of pulmonary hypertension may still benefit from repair of the defect. Survival after corrective surgery is influenced by the age of the patient and the degree of persistent cardiac dysfunction. Patients with otherwise normal hearts have normal survival rates after successful repair of the atrial defect and usually can resume normal activity.

Endocarditis prophylaxis is unnecessary for patients with atrial septal defect.

Mitral Regurgitation

Mitral regurgitation (3) may develop because of an abnormality of any part of the mitral valve apparatus: the valve leaflets, the chordae tendineae, the papillary muscles, or the annulus. Such abnormality may result in either acute or chronic signs and symptoms, depending on the nature of the lesion.

An incompetent mitral valve allows regurgitation into the left atrium of blood from the left ventricle. The reduced load on the ventricle reduces the tension in the ventricular muscle and allows it to utilize more energy in contraction. Therefore, in patients with chronic mitral regurgitation, cardiac output remains normal for years until, because of age or intercurrent disease, the ventricle no longer can compensate and heart failure ensues. In patients with acute mitral regurgitation, ventricular compensation is inadequate and heart failure develops abruptly.

Chronic Mitral Regurgitation

Etiology and Epidemiology. Chronic mitral incompetence in adults may occur in association with a great variety of disorders. Rheumatic fever is the cause of only 5 to 15% of cases—usually in association with some degree of mitral dysfunction. Otherwise, chronic mitral regurgitation is most often due to papillary muscle necrosis—the result of ischemic heart disease, to an inherited (e.g., Marfan's syndrome or mitral prolapse—see below) or an acquired (e.g., systemic lupus erythematosus) disorder of connective tissue, to idiopathic calcification of the valve—primarily a disorder of the elderly—or to congenital maldevelopment of the mitral apparatus.

Natural History and Symptoms. Patients with chronic mitral regurgitation may remain asymptomatic for many years, even, if the regurgitation is not severe, for their entire lives. Characteristically, when symptoms do develop, they appear gradually over years as the left ventricle slowly loses its ability to compensate for the loss of more than half of its stroke volume back into the left atrium. Dyspnea and fatigue are the usual symptoms of left ventricular failure. Supraventricular arrhythmias, especially atrial fibrillation, are likely to develop if left atrial enlargement becomes marked, compromising somewhat the ability of the heart to compensate. Acute pulmonary edema occasionally occurs but is uncommon. Sometimes severe pulmonary hypertension develops without much enlargement of the left atrium. Early surgical correction of the lesion in patients with pulmonary hypertension and signs of right ventricular hypertrophy is important.

In a series of patients with mitral regurgitation, 80% treated medically survived 5 years, and 60% survived 10 years (26). Moderately to severely symptomatic patients do less well; in one report 46% of patients with chronic rheumatic mitral insufficiency survived 5 years (21).

Physical Findings. A high pitched holosystolic murmur, loudest at the apex, is characteristic of chronic mitral regurgitation (patients with mild regurgitation may have only a late systolic murmur). The holosystolic murmur is constant in intensity and radiates always to the axilla and sometimes to the back and to the base of the heart. It is best heard when the patient is in the left lateral decubitus position. The murmur is diminished when the patient stands or performs a Valsalva maneuver and is intensified when he squats. If regurgitation is severe, the precordium is usually hyperdynamic and there is an S$_3$ gallop. S$_1$ is soft. If pulmonary hypertension has developed, an S$_4$ gallop, a loud P$_2$, and a right ventricular heave may be appreciated. Signs of right ventricular failure—edema, hepatomegaly, distended neck veins, hepatojugular reflux—may also be seen late in the course of this disease.

Laboratory Evaluation. An ECG, a chest X-ray, and an echocardiogram should be obtained routinely if a patient is suspected of having mitral regurgitation.

Electrocardiogram. The ECG shows evidence of left atrial enlargement (Fig. 60.4 and Table 60.5) and, if present, of atrial fibrillation. The pattern of left ventricular hypertrophy (Fig. 60.2 and Table 60.3) is often seen as well, primarily in patients with severe disease. A pattern of right ventricular hypertrophy (Table 60.6) indicating pulmonary hypertension is less common and, when seen, is cause for great concern.

Chest X-ray. Left ventricular and left atrial enlargement are common. On a posteroanterior (PA) film, elevation of the left bronchus and prominence of the left atrial appendage are the earliest signs of left atrial enlargement; a double density is seen posteriorly when the left atrium is grossly enlarged (Fig. 60.5).

Echocardiogram. Echocardiography demonstrates left atrial and left ventricular enlargement and hyperdynamic motion of the left ventricle, especially the septum. Two-dimensional echocardiography usually can define the etiology of the valvular disease, i.e., rheumatic, prolapsing, ischemic, etc. However, in contrast to mitral stenosis, aortic stenosis, or aortic regurgitation, there are no specific echocardiographic signs of mitral regurgitation. Therefore, even if there is clear auscultatory evidence of mitral regurgitation, the echocardiogram may show only the left atrial enlargement. Doppler echocardiography (see page 720) is sensitive in detecting mitral regurgitation and can estimate its severity.

Management. Patients who do not have severe disease can be managed medically. Antibiotic prophylaxis against bacterial endocarditis should be administered before all dental and surgical procedures (Chapter 86). If atrial fibrillation is present, restoration of sinus rhythm should be attempted unless the left atrium is greatly enlarged or mitral regurgitation has been present for many years. (A detailed discussion of the treatment of atrial fibrillation is in Chapter 59). If heart failure develops, it should be treated by use of the measures described in Chapter 61. Afterload reduction by use of an arteriolar vasodilator may be particularly useful in this condition; by lowering peripheral resistance, ejection of blood into the aorta, rather than back into the left atrium, is favored.

When, despite therapy, patients become more than mildly symptomatic or if the diagnosis is unclear, referral to a cardiologist is indicated (Table 60.7). It is likely that cardiac catheterization and angiography (see Chapter 57) will be done to confirm the diagnosis, establish the severity of the lesion, evaluate the function of the left ventricle and, often, the patency of the coronary arteries. At this point a decision will be made about the value of operative repair of the lesion. Unless the patient has severe noncardiac disease or left ventricular function is so severely reduced that the patient would not tolerate an operation, replacement of the defective valve with a prosthesis is very likely to be recommended. The operative mortality reported from various centers is 3 to 10%.

The health and survival of patients who have undergone successful valve replacement depends on a number of factors (also see page 733). Advanced age, the presence of concomitant mitral stenosis, poor left ventricular function (ejection fraction under 50%), and severity of symptoms preoperatively (New York Heart Association class III or IV—see Chapter 61) are adverse factors that reduce long-term postoperative survival. In general, patients with mitral regurgitation on the basis of ischemic heart disease do less well than do patients with rheumatic heart disease. Nevertheless,

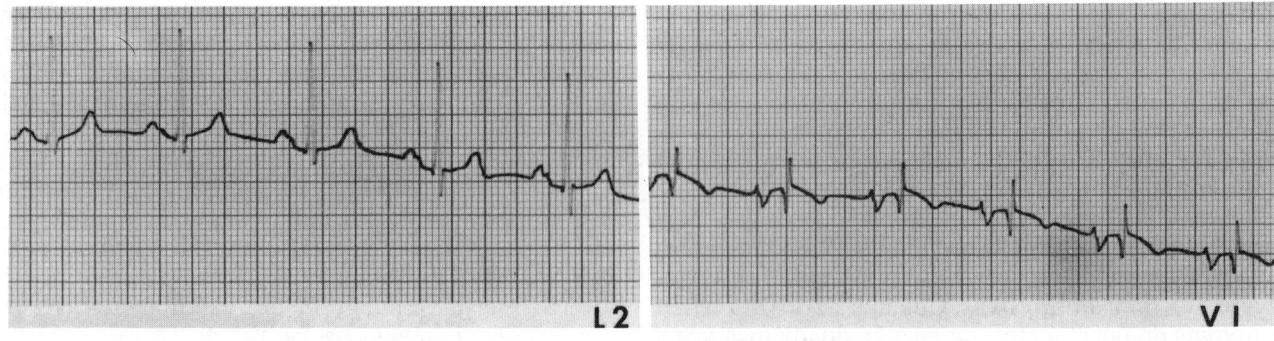

Figure 60.4. ECG of a patient with left atrial hypertrophy (see Table 60.5).

Table 60.5.
Principal Electrocardiographic Features of Left Atrial Hypertrophy[a]

P wave:	
Axis	$+45°$ to $-30°$
Amplitude (II, III, aVf) duration	> 0.11 second (broad)
Component (V_1)	
Early	Positive but inside normal
Late	Negative, ≥ 0.04 area units[b]

[a] Modified from Horan LG, Flowers NC: Electrocardiography and vectorcardiography. In Braunwald E (ed): *Heart Disease: A Textbook of Cardiovascular Medicine.* Philadelphia, WB Saunders, 1980, p. 223 (14).
[b] Area units = mm-seconds. One small block on standard ECG paper = 0.04 mm-second.

Table 60.6
Electrocardiographic Criteria of Right Ventricular Hypertrophy in Adults without Conduction Defects Known NOT to Have Infarction[a]

Sign	Points[b]
Ratio reversal (R/S V_5:R/S $V_1 \leq 0.4$)	5
qR in V_1	5
R/S ratio in $V_1 > 1$	4
S in $V_1 < 2$ mm	4
R in V_1 + S in V_5 or $V_6 > 10.5$ mm	4
Right axis deviation $> 110°$	4
S in V_5 or $V_6 \geq 7$ mm and each ≥ 2 mm	3
R/S in V_5 or $V_6 \leq 1$	3
R in $V_1 \geq 7$ mm	3
S_1, S_2, and S_3 each ≥ 1 mm	2
S_1 and Q_3 each ≥ 1 mm	2
R' in V_1 earlier than 0.08 second and ≥ 2 mm	2
R peak in V_1 or V_2 between 0.04 and 0.07 second	1
S in V_5 or $V_6 \geq 2$ mm but < 7 mm	1
Reduction in V lead R/S ratio between V_1 and V_4	1
R in V_5 or $V_6 < 5$ mm	1

[a] Modified from Horan LG, Flowers NC: Electrocardiography and vectorcardiography. In Braunwald E (ed): *Heart Disease: A Textbook of Cardiovascular Medicine.* Philadelphia, WB Saunders, 1980, p. 226 (14).
[b] Interpretation of point score: 10 points, right ventricular hypertrophy; 7 to 9 points, probable right ventricular hypertrophy or hemodynamic overload; 5 to 6 points, possible right ventricular hypertrophy or hemodynamic overload. These criteria do not take into account serial ECG comparisons. Such additional data may alter the interpreter's impression of the likelihood of fixed enlargement or dynamic overload.

even patients with one or more adverse risk factors live longer, on the average, with a prosthetic valve than they would without one (10), and most patients are able to be more active than they were before surgery. The overall 10-year survival for patients who have undergone successful mitral surgery is approx-

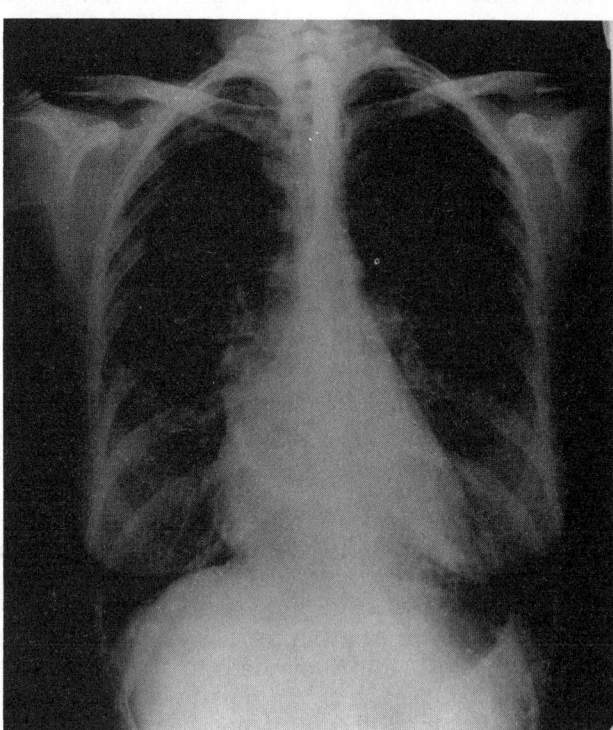

Figure 60.5. Chest X-ray of a patient with left atrial enlargement. Note the straight left heart border and the calcification of the wall of the left atrium.

Table 60.7.
Indications for Referral of Patients with Mitral Regurgitation

Progressive dyspnea or fatigue
Development of supraventricular arrhythmia
A mildly symptomatic or an asymptomatic patient with progressive cardiac enlargement
Uncertainty about the diagnosis
Acute mitral regurgitation
Patients with mitral valve prolapse who have symptomatic arrhythmias, symptomatic mitral regurgitaion, infectious endocarditis, or transient ischemic attacks

imately 70% (10). Postoperatively, anticoagulation with warfarin is used routinely to prevent thromboembolic complications (see Chapter 52).

Surgical reconstruction of the incompetent mitral valve has recently been shown to be an excellent alternative to mitral valve replacement, particularly for valves leaking due to myxomatous degeneration (see mitral valve prolapse, below). Repaired valves usually maintain their competency (92%), seem not to be susceptible to infectious endocarditis, and do not require chronic anticoagulation (7). The decision of whether to recommend valve repair or replacement is dependent on the availability of a surgeon who is skilled at this relatively new procedure and is usually made in consultation with the cardiologist and the cardiac surgeon.

Acute Mitral Regurgitation

Etiology and Epidemiology. Acute mitral incompetence is most often due to rupture of the chordae tendineae, the cords that connect the valve cusps to the papillary muscles of the left ventricle. Most of the time the cause of the rupture is myxomatous degeneration of the valve (see "Mitral Valve Prolapse," below), although occasionally rheumatic fever or acute left ventricular dilation can be incriminated. Much less commonly, acute mitral regurgitation will be caused by papillary muscle rupture or dysfunction (complications of myocardial infarction) or by perforation of a mitral cusp as the result of bacterial endocarditis. The disorder is primarily encountered in middle-aged and elderly patients.

Natural History and Symptoms. Because the left atrium is suddenly presented with a volume load to which it cannot rapidly accommodate, acute pulmonary edema is much more common in patients with acute, compared with chronic, mitral regurgitation. The primary symptom of pulmonary edema is severe dyspnea at rest.

Physical Findings. A harsh holosystolic murmur of constant intensity, loudest at the apex, is characteristic; if a posterior cord has ruptured, the murmur may radiate to the base of the heart and may mimic the murmur of aortic stenosis. Sometimes an early or midsystolic, or even a crescendo-decrescendo, murmur is heard. An S_3 gallop is almost always heard and an S_4 gallop is common. Unlike the situation in patients with chronic mitral regurgitation, S_1 is normal or even loud. Signs of left-sided heart failure (rales) and of right-sided failure (edema, distended neck veins, etc.) are also common.

Laboratory Findings. *Chest X-ray.* The chest X-ray shows marked pulmonary congestion. The left atrium and the left ventricle are minimally enlarged. These findings are the opposite of those found in patients with chronic mitral regurgitation.

Echocardiogram. Chamber enlargement is usually not seen, but increased systolic motion of the valve is common. If the chordae have ruptured, the flailing chordae or marked prolapse of the leaflets into the left atrium may be visualized by two-dimensional echocardiography. Doppler echocardiography allows detection of the lesion, but Doppler criteria for estimating the severity of *acute* mitral regurgitation are not yet established.

Management. Patients suspected of having suffered acute mitral regurgitation should be hospitalized immediately for diagnosis, for treatment of acute heart failure, and for consideration for early operative repair.

Mitral Valve Prolapse (6)

Etiology and Epidemiology. Systolic prolapse of a leaflet of the mitral valve into the left atrium has proved to be a very common phenomenon, affecting over 5% of the population (17). Women are more likely to be affected than are men, although reported sex ratios vary considerably. The exact nature of this abnormality is not entirely clear, but in most cases the condition appears to be inherited (autosomal dominant), with reduced penetrance in men and in children. Histological study of prolapsing valves removed at operation shows "myxomatous degeneration," a proliferation of the spongiosa layer of mucopolysaccharides into the fibrosa layer of collagen, resulting in a weakness in the supporting structure of the valve. This abnormality is also seen in a number of known disorders of connective tissue, including Marfan's syndrome and Ehlers-Danlos syndrome. However, echocardiographic prolapse is also frequently reported in patients with documented coronary artery disease, asymmetric septal hypertrophy, and atrial septal defect, and these cases may represent "secondary prolapse" in which the valve is normal but changes in ventricular geometry cause prolapsing of the leaflets. In these "secondary" cases the click and associated symptoms (see below) are usually not present.

Natural History and Symptoms. Most patients are asymptomatic and the condition is identified during a routine physical examination. Less often, patients complain of palpitations, chest pain, or dyspnea. The palpitations reflect arrhythmias (see below) or, more commonly, just an awareness of sinus tachycardia. The chest pain sometimes mimics angina (or, in fact, is angina if there is concomitant ischemic heart disease) but more often is sharp lancinating pain in the left chest, unrelated to exertion, and the cause of it is unknown.

In the great majority of patients the syndrome is benign. However, in about 15% of patients (20) significant mitral regurgitation occurs, and patients may complain of dyspnea, due to left ventricular failure.

It is now recognized that patients with mitral valve prolapse are at risk for embolic strokes. In one study 40% of patients under 45 who had had a stroke had mitral valve prolapse compared with 6.8% of matched controls (1). The risk of infective endocarditis in patients with mitral valve prolapse is approximately five times that of the general population. This risk is highest in patients with mitral regurgitation.

The most feared complication of mitral valve prolapse, sudden death, is quite rare. The risk is higher in patients with a family history of sudden death or in patients with a prolonged Q-T interval on their ECG (see below).

The hemodynamic and infectious complications appear to be more common in men than in women, and in patients who have mitral regurgitation at the time of presentation. The echocardiographic findings of thickening and redundancy of the mitral leaflet also identify patients with mitral valve prolapse who are at higher risk (18). These findings allow targeting of prophylactic antibiotic therapy and frequent follow-up of specific groups.

Physical Findings. The characteristic finding in patients with mitral prolapse is a midsystolic click, best heard at the lower left sternal border, due to sudden tensing of the prolapsed valve. It occurs later than the systolic ejection sound heard commonly in association with systemic hypertension (see page 718). Very often the click is followed immediately by a crescendo late systolic murmur that continues until A_2.

The physical findings may vary from time to time in any given patient and may also vary with the position of the patient. In those relatively rare instances in which chronic mitral regurgitation has developed, the typical physical findings—including the holosystolic murmur—of this condition will be encountered (see above).

The mitral valve prolapse syndrome is commonly associated with skeletal abnormalities, such as scoliosis and pectus excavatum, suggesting that valve prolapse may be only one component of a generalized disease of connective tissue.

Laboratory Findings. *Electrocardiogram.* The ECG is usually normal, especially in asymptomatic patients. Symptomatic patients may show nonspecific ST-T wave changes, usually in the inferior leads, and, sometimes prolongation of the Q-T interval.

A variety of arrhythmias may occur in patients with mitral valve prolapse. The commonest are premature ventricular contractions (PVCs) and paroxysmal supraventricular tachycardia. When patients are exercised, it has been reported that many of them develop frequent PVCs and that up to 40% develop atrial arrhythmias (9).

Echocardiogram. The M-mode echocardiogram is usually diagnostic in this condition. It shows late systolic or holosystolic prolapse of one or both leaflets of the mitral valve. Sometimes, however, the M-mode echocardiogram shows no abnormalities despite the typical cardiac findings. These patients probably have minor degrees of prolapse. Mitral regurgitation, if present, can be detected by Doppler echocardiography.

Management. Asymptomatic patients need no treatment but should be reassessed by interval history, physical examination, and echocardiogram every few years. Care should be taken to ensure that the diagnosis does not provide unwarrented anxiety in these people. Those patients who have a systolic murmur or have echocardiographic evidence of thickening or

redundancy of the mitral leaflet should receive prophylaxis against bacterial endocarditis before dental or surgical procedures (see Chapter 86). Other patients probably do not need prophylaxis.

Patients with palpitations should have ambulatory electrocardiographic monitoring to determine the severity of their arrhythmia, and therapy should be prescribed on the basis of the type of arrhythmia that is present (see Chapter 59). A β-blocking agent is often a drug of choice in the treatment of these patients and also in those with mitral prolapse who complain of chest pain (e.g., propranolol, usual dose 10 to 40 mg, four times a day or atenolol, usual dose 25 to 50 mg a day). The mechanism of action of the drug in the relief of pain is unknown but possibly may be explained by the fact that many untreated patients have been shown to have increased blood levels of norepinephrine and to have increased sympathetic (and vagal) tone.

Patients with symptomatic mitral regurgitation should be treated as described above (page 727).

Referral to a cardiologist is recommended at any time patients become symptomatic from arrhythmia, chronic mitral regurgitation, or thromboembolism.

Mitral Stenosis

Stenosis of the mitral valve obstructs the flow of blood out of the left atrium and therefore raises the left atrial pressure above the left ventricular diastolic pressure. The pressure gradient across the valve is a measure of the severity of the stenosis. Because of the increase in left atrial pressure, there is an increase in pressure in the pulmonary blood vessels. The pulmonary congestion accounts for most of the symptoms of the disease.

Etiology and Epidemiology

By far the most common cause of mitral stenosis in adults is rheumatic fever (although a history of rheumatic fever can be elicited in only 50% of patients with pure mitral stenosis). Pure mitral stenosis occurs in 40% of all patients with rheumatic heart disease. The rest of the time there is associated mitral regurgitation, aortic valve disease, and, uncommonly, tricuspid valve disease. Two-thirds of patients with rheumatic mitral stenosis are women.

Natural History and Symptoms

On the average, there is a latent period of nearly 20 years between an attack of acute rheumatic fever and the development of symptomatic mitral stenosis (31). Thus, symptoms usually do not develop before the fourth decade. The severity of symptoms is quite variable: some people, in fact, are never symptomatic; some are mildly symptomatic indefinitely; and some develop progressively severe cardiopulmonary decompensation. Of the patients with progressive disease, it has been estimated that an average of 7 years elapses between the onset of symptoms and the development of total disability (class IV cardiac status—see Chapter 61). In one series the 5-year survival from that point in patients treated medically was only 15% (24).

Pulmonary congestion causes many of the symptoms of mitral stenosis: dyspnea, orthopnea, and paroxysmal nocturnal dyspnea. If left atrial pressure rises acutely because of a sudden stress, frank pulmonary edema may occur. Hemoptysis due to rupture of small bronchial veins or to pulmonary edema is not unusual.

As the disease progresses, pulmonary hypertension develops followed by symptoms of right heart failure: edema, distended neck veins, a tender liver, and ascites. At this point, the flow of blood into the left heart is limited, and the pulmonary arterioles hypertrophy, diminishing the risk of pulmonary edema. Low cardiac output is responsible for the fatigue that is a common complaint of patients at this stage.

Atrial fibrillation (Chapter 59) complicates the course of 40 to 50% of patients with mitral stenosis. The 20% reduction in blood flow across the mitral valve by the loss of left atrial contraction may intensify symptoms of heart failure and fatigue.

At some time in their course, 20% of patients with mitral stenosis experience symptomatic thromboembolism—most often to the brain; 80% of these patients are in atrial fibrillation.

Physical Findings

A middiastolic rumbling murmur with presystolic accentuation is characteristic of mitral stenosis. It is best heard at, and is often limited to, the cardiac apex. To hear it, it may be necessary to turn the patient to the left lateral position and to have him expire fully. Sometimes the patient must be exercised before the murmur is audible. The murmur is best heard with the bell of the stethoscope pressed lightly against the chest. A loud first heart sound S_1 and opening snap (see page 718) usually accompany the murmur when the valve is mobile.

Late in the course, signs of pulmonary hypertension (a loud P_2 and a right ventricular heave) and of right heart failure may be found.

Laboratory Findings

Electrocardiogram. The ECG shows left atrial enlargement (Fig. 60.4 and Table 60.5) in 90% of patients who are in sinus rhythm. With the development of pulmonary hypertension, signs of right ventricular hypertrophy appear (Table 60.6).

Chest X-ray. Left atrial enlargement (see page 727 and Fig. 60.5) is seen in virtually all patients with symptomatic mitral stenosis, but the size of the left atrium does not correlate with the severity of stenosis. Late in the course right ventricular and right atrial hypertrophy will be seen as well. Symptomatic patients are also likely to show radiological signs of pulmonary congestion, the severity of which will determine the findings that are seen (Chapter 61).

Calcification of the mitral valve is not unusual in patients with long-standing mitral stenosis, but this is better visualized by fluoroscopy than by a plain X-ray.

Echocardiogram. Mitral stenosis can be easily diagnosed by echocardiography. Mitral valve thickening can be seen; there is reduced excursion of the anterior leaflet of the valve and abnormal anterior motion of the posterior leaflet during diastole (it normally moves posteriorly). The severity of the stenosis can be accurately assessed by two-dimensional and Doppler echocardiography (see page 720).

Management

Asymptomatic patients need no treatment except prophylaxis for bacterial endocarditis when they are to undergo dental or surgical procedures (Chapter 86). Newly diagnosed adult patients with mitral stenosis do not ordinarily require prophylaxis for β-hemolytic streptococcal infection unless they have had an attack of rheumatic fever within the last 5 to 10 years or are in a population where β-hemolytic streptococcal infection is more prevalent (e.g., military personnel or hospital workers). Patients who have received prophylaxis throughout childhood should continue to receive it indefinitely. When prophylaxis is necessary, the best regimen is 1 to 2 million units of benzathine penicillin G intramuscularly once a month.

Mildly symptomatic patients should be treated with diuretics and sodium restriction (see Chapter 61 for a detailed discussion of the treatment of heart failure). Digitalis, since it does not affect the hemodynamic abnormality, is not useful in this situation unless rapid atrial fibrillation or flutter develops. The treatment of atrial fibrillation is discussed in detail in Chapter 59, but it should be recognized that there is a 1 to 2% incidence of systemic thromboembolism at the time of conversion of atrial fibrillation to normal sinus rhythm in patients with mitral stenosis. The conversion, whether pharmacological or electrical, should be done in the hospital.

Warfarin anticoagulants should be administered to patients with mild mitral stenosis who have had one or more episodes of systemic or pulmonary thromboembolism (see Chapter 52), who are in atrial fibrillation, or who have echocardiographic evidence of left atrial enlargement. All patients with moderate or severe mitral stenosis should be anticoagulated.

Table 60.8 lists the reasons to refer patients with

Table 60.8.
Indications for Referral of Patients with Mitral Stenosis[a]

Progressive dyspnea or recurrent attacks of pulmonary edema
Symptomatic disease of the aortic and/or tricuspid valve
Women, whether symptomatic or not, who wish to become pregnant
Patients whose symptoms have developed recently who have no history of rheumatic fever (to rule out an atrial myxoma)
Patients with chronic obstructive lung disease
Patients with angina pectoris
Patients with evidence of pulmonary hypertension (including right ventricular hypertrophy)
Patients with new onset of atrial fibrillation

[a]Modified from Brandenburg RO, Fuster V, Guiliani ER: Valvular heart disease. When should the patient be referred? *Practical Cardiol* 5:50, 1979 (2).

mitral stenosis to a cardiologist. In general referral is indicated to confirm the diagnosis, assess the severity of the process, and consider whether to recommend operative repair or replacement of the mitral valve. The cardiologist is likely to perform a cardiac catheterization to measure the size of the mitral orifice and to decide whether to recommend surgery for a patient with moderate or severe stenosis. However, the age of the patient, the presence of severe noncardiac disease, and the presence of other cardiac lesions (e.g., severe ischemic heart disease) will influence the recommendation. Patients with pulmonary hypertension or evidence of right ventricular hypertrophy should be referred even if asymptomatic.

The relatively poor prognosis of medically treated patients with progressive disease (see "Natural History and Symptoms" above) dictates that such patients, unless there are specific contraindications, should be offered surgery. The preferred procedure will depend on the anatomy of the valve at the time of operation. If possible a mitral commissurotomy will be performed. The operative mortality of this procedure is low (1 to 3%), and the long-term results are excellent for a number of years. However, after commissurotomy, 10% of patients within 5 years and 60% within 10 years require reoperation because of restenosis or because of the development of symptomatic mitral regurgitation or of symptomatic aortic stenosis (13). If a prosthetic valve is implanted, the operative mortality is 3 to 10%; the course of patients who survive surgery depends on a number of factors (see page 733) but certainly is better than that of symptomatic patients treated medically.

Nonsurgical mitral valvulotomy can now be achieved using a balloon catheter passed percutaneously through the venous system and then across the atrial septum to the mitral valve. The relative merits of this approach have not yet been defined.

Aortic Regurgitation

An incompetent aortic valve allows regurgitation into the left ventricle of blood ejected into the aorta (8). In order to compensate for the increased volume load, the left ventricle dilates and hypertrophies so that the effective stroke volume may for a long time be normal. Eventually, however, the left ventricle cannot maintain the work load, and clinical signs and symptoms of heart failure ensue.

Etiology and Epidemiology

Aortic regurgitation may be due to disease of the aortic valve cusps and/or to dilation of the aortic root.

Rheumatic fever now accounts for 29% of cases of chronic aortic valvular incompetence (23), many fewer cases than it did 20 to 30 years ago. Congenital aortic valvular incompetence due to a bicuspid valve accounts for 12% of cases. Bacterial endocarditis is the most common cause of acute aortic valvular incompetence. Traumatic rupture of a cusp of the aortic valve is relatively uncommon.

Chronic aortic regurgitation is due to dilation of the aortic root in 12% of cases, most commonly idiopathic. Relatively rare causes include rheumatoid arthritis, ankylosing spondylitis, Reiter's syndrome, congenital disorders of connective tissue (Marfan's syndrome, Ehlers-Danlos syndrome, and osteogenesis imperfecta), and syphilitic aortitis. Acute aortic regurgitation due to dilation of the aortic root is most commonly due to a dissecting aneurysm—usually associated with medial necrosis of the aorta. Dissection is associated with systemic hypertension in approximately 50% of cases. Occasionally a primary disorder of connective tissue, such as Marfan's syndrome, can be incriminated.

Aortic regurgitation in general is more common in men than women, but there are specific exceptions (rheumatoid arthritis, for example).

Natural History and Symptoms

Patients with chronic aortic regurgitation remain asymptomatic sometimes for up to 20 years or have only mild dyspnea on exertion. When symptoms do develop (progressively more severe dyspnea, orthopnea, paroxysmal nocturnal dyspnea, and, less often, angina), they reflect an ominous deterioration in the condition.

Patients with acute aortic regurgitation develop fulminant pulmonary edema because of the inability of the left ventricle to compensate for the sudden volume load and for the abrupt rise in left ventricular end-diastolic pressure. Marked dyspnea and weakness may be experienced virtually overnight and in most cases within 2 or 3 months. Other symptoms depend on the underlying cause: fever, for example, if it is endocarditis; severe pain in the chest or back, if it is a dissecting aneurysm.

Physical Findings

Patients with chronic aortic regurgitation have a characteristic high frequency early diastolic decrescendo murmur, best heard at the aortic area and at the left sternal border. The duration (but not the intensity) of the murmur correlates with the severity of the lesion so that the murmur is holodiastolic in patients with severe aortic regurgitation. Often there is an accompanying harsh systolic ejection murmur as well, heard at the base of the heart. Severe aortic regurgitation may also cause a loud apical diastolic murmur (the Austin Flint murmur), simulating the murmur of mitral stenosis. Unlike the situation in true mitral stenosis, however, S_1 in patients with aortic regurgitation is sometimes soft, the result of premature closure of the mitral valve, and there is no opening snap. If aortic regurgitation is moderate or severe, the pulse pressure is ordinarily wide, reflecting peripheral vasodilation. The combination of an increased systolic pressure and a reduced diastolic pressure (sometimes as low as 30 mm Hg) produces characteristic changes in the peripheral pulse (waterhammer pulse, "pistol-shot" sounds heard over the femoral artery, etc.) and a typical bobbing of the head with each heartbeat.

Patients with acute aortic regurgitation often show signs of left- and right-sided heart failure. The regurgitant diastolic murmur is lower pitched and shorter than it is in patients with chronic aortic incompetence; S_1 is often absent and S_3, uncommon with chronic regurgitation, is usually present. The pulse pressure is normal—the result of intense peripheral vasoconstriction.

Laboratory Findings

Electrocardiogram. The ECG also reflects the severity and duration of aortic regurgitation. Patients with chronic disease show the ECG pattern of left ventricular hypertrophy (Fig. 60.2 and Table 60.3), whereas patients with acute disease do not (although they commonly do show nonspecific ST-T wave changes).

Chest X-ray. The size of the heart in patients with aortic regurgitation depends on the duration and severity of the disease. Patients with chronic severe disease have very large left ventricles, but patients with acute regurgitation may have no cardiac enlargement at all.

Echocardiogram. Echocardiography is useful in the assessment of left ventricular function, the degree of hypertrophy of the left ventricle, and of the degree of dilation of the aortic root. Fluttering of the anterior leaflet of the mitral valve during diastole is characteristic of moderate to severe aortic regurgitation and also indicates mobility of the mitral valve (a useful sign in ruling out significant mitral stenosis). Premature mitral valve closure is helpful in confirming very severe aortic regurgitation. The severity of aortic regurgitation also can be estimated by Doppler echocardiography using a number of described criteria.

Management

Asymptomatic patients need not be treated but should be assessed once or twice a year by interval history, physical examination, and chest X-ray. Yearly ECGs and echocardiograms should also be obtained. Prophylaxis for bacterial endocarditis is indicated when patients are to undergo dental or surgical procedures (Chapter 86).

If symptoms of heart failure develop, digitalis and diuretics should be prescribed. Also afterload-reducing agents are usually effective in otherwise unresponsive patients (see Chapter 61).

Table 60.9 lists the reasons to refer patients with aortic regurgitation to a cardiologist. In general, referral is indicated in patients with chronic disease to confirm the diagnosis and to consider whether to recommend aortic valve replacement for symptomatic patients and for asymptomatic patients with physical findings of severe disease (widened pulse pressure, holodiastolic murmur, increasing left ventricular enlargement). All patients with suspected acute aortic regurgitation should be seen by a cardiologist as soon as possible. The cardiologist is likely to perform car-

Table 60.9.
Indications for Referral of Patients with Aortic Regurgitation[a]

Uncertainty about the diagnosis
Symptomatic chronic aortic incompetence (dyspnea, fatigue, angina)
Acute aortic incompetence
Asymptomatic patients with evidence of severe chronic aortic incompetence: widened pulse pressure, holodiastolic murmur, left ventricular hypertrophy, progressive cardiac enlargement

[a]Modified from Brandenburg RO, Fuster V, Vuiliani ER: Valvular heart disease. When should the patient be referred? *Practical Cardiol* 5:50, 1979 (2).

diac catheterization (see Chapter 57) to assess the severity of the lesion, the presence of other valvular disease, and the function of the left ventricle. Recently radionuclide angiography and echocardiography have provided the cardiologist with a convenient noninvasive technique for making these measurements easily (see Chapter 61). Patients with marked left ventricular diastolic and systolic enlargement and ejection fractions of less than 50% are at high risk of requiring aortic valve replacement for symptoms of deteriorating left ventricular function within 3 years (33).

Patients with chronic aortic regurgitation do well until they become symptomatic. Thereafter, 50% of patients are dead within 2 years (19). Thus, valve replacement is warranted in all symptomatic patients, preferably before severe left ventricular dysfunction develops. The operative mortality is 3 to 10%, but of the patients who survive surgery, 50% live 10 years or more (30) and their quality of life is usually significantly improved (see below).

The possibility that long-term vasodilation (Chapter 61) therapy may alter the clinical course of high risk patients, with or without symptoms, has been raised. However, to date there is no evidence that this therapy will delay or prevent the need for valve replacement.

The Patient with a Prosthetic Valve

Although patients usually demonstrate clear improvement in symptoms and prognosis after valve replacement, they should not be considered cured. Despite refinements in design, no valve currently available is free of potential serious complications, which, since they may occur many years after surgery, dictate careful long-term follow-up of all patients who have prosthetic valves.

Many varieties of mechanical and tissue valves have been developed. The most commonly used mechanical valves are the Starr Edwards ball-in-cage series, the Bjork-Shiley tilting disk valve, and the St. Jude valve, which has two semicircular tilting leaflets. The most common tissue valves are the Hancock and Carpentier-Edwards valves, which are constructed of porcine aortic valve leaflets that have been fixed in glutaraldehyde.

Potential Complications

Thromboembolic phenomena are perhaps the most frequent life-threatening complications of prosthetic valves and may present as sudden stroke, myocardial infarction, or peripheral arterial occlusion. Alternatively, thrombus may accumulate around the valve ring and prevent proper valve motion, resulting in gradual or sudden obstruction of flow and the development of severe congestive heart failure. Thomboembolic events have been more common with prosthetic valves in the mitral than in the aortic position, and they are much more frequent with the mechanical valves than with the tissue valves (4). Despite treatment with full anticoagulation, the incidence of thromboembolic complications with most mechanical valves is about 1 to 2%/year. The incidence is lower with the St. Jude valve.

Perivalvular leakage resulting in regurgitation occasionally develops in the postoperative period and may require reoperation.

Prosthetic valve endocarditis develops in 2 to 3% of patients (36) and may present as a febrile illness, a new murmur of valvular regurgitation or stenosis, hemodynamic deterioration, or embolization. Because the infection is at the site of a foreign body, the prognosis for recovery with standard antibiotic therapy is worse than in native valve endocarditis. Recurrence after one trial of medical therapy is generally an indication for replacement of the valve. Prognosis is worse in infections that develop within 60 days of surgery (72% mortality), in which contamination may have occurred at operation, than in those that develop later (45% mortality), when transient bacteremia may be the source of infection.

As long-term follow-up data accumulate, late valvular degeneration may become a significant problem after tissue valve implantation. Histological studies have revealed fibrin deposition, tears in the leaflets, and calcification that commonly results in some degree of valvular stenosis (16) and/or regurgitation 5 to 10 years after operation. In some cases in which clinical deterioration occurs, reoperation is required. This process is greatly accelerated in children but also occurs commonly in young adults (younger than 35).

Physical and Laboratory Findings

Auscultatory findings after valve replacement are variable. In general, the ball-in-cage valves produce loud opening and closing clicks. In the aortic position, therefore, there is a prominent systolic "ejection" click, and S_2 is loud and metallic. In the mitral position, S_1 is loud and there is a prominent systolic opening click after S_2, which is similar in timing to the opening snap of mitral stenosis. With the Bjork-Shiley valve the closing sounds are loud but the opening sounds are variable. Porcine valves are the most physiological, and like a native valve, the closing sounds are audible but opening sounds are rare. All valves in either position produce systolic ejection murmurs. Diastolic flow murmurs are common with the Bjork-Shiley valve in the mitral position.

It is important to document the baseline physical examination repeatedly so that the significance of any changes that occur in association with new symptoms can be assessed. The most reliable sign of prosthetic valve dysfunction is the loss or muffling of the opening and closing clicks. New regurgitant murmurs may occur. Congestive heart failure may develop.

The two-dimensional echocardiogram may show abnormal, delayed, or intermittent leaflet motion. Changes from previous studies are helpful, so all patients should have a baseline echocardiogram after valve replacement. Tissue valves are well visualized and can be readily assessed by echocardiography. However, mechanical valves are usually not well seen, and most of the signs of mechanical valve dysfunction are neither sensitive nor specific. The technique of Doppler echocardiography (see pages 720 to 721) is extremely helpful (37) in accurately detecting and quantifying new valve gradients and regurgitation.

Management

Management of the patient with a prosthetic valve should begin before the valve is implanted; the selection of the proper type of valve for the individual patient is crucial. A tissue valve is most appropriate for the patient who is likely to be noncompliant with anticoagulation or who is at high risk for bleeding complications. This includes alcoholics; patients with psychiatric problems, unexplained syncope, or previous gastrointestinal bleeds; the elderly; and patients whose occupations put them at high risk of injury. Women of childbearing age who desire future pregnancies should receive tissue valves (see below), but they should be made aware that valve replacement may have to be repeated in 8 to 10 years. Young men, or women who do not anticipate pregnancy and who will tolerate anticoagulation, may be better off with the more durable mechanical valves so that reoperation may not be necessary (the ball-in-cage valves, the oldest type in current use, have lasted up to 20 years). These decisions are usually made by the cardiac surgeon after discussing the options with the patient, but it is important that the practitioner communicate his opinions to the surgeon well in advance.

All patients with mechanical valves in the aortic or mitral position must be fully anticoagulated with Coumadin indefinitely (see Chapter 52). Antiplatelet agents (see Chapter 52) are not adequate to prevent thromboembolic complications. If an elective surgical procedure is planned, Coumadin may be safely discontinued 3 days before surgery and resumed afterward. Reversal of anticoagulation with vitamin K is not recommended.

Patients with tissue valves in the aortic position should be anticoagulated for 6 weeks after operation only, so that endothelialization of the valve may occur. Coumadin should then be discontinued. There is controversy over whether tissue valves in the mitral position require long-term anticoagulation. Most cardiologists would not anticoagulate indefinitely unless atrial fibrillation were present, left atrial enlargement were detected on echocardiogram (a common finding in mitral valve disease), or a previous thromboembolic episode had occurred. Strict antibiotic prophylaxis against endocarditis is indicated. Table 86.9 lists regimens recommended by the American Heart Association before and after various procedures. Note, however, that parenteral rather than oral regimens should always be used in patients with prosthetic valves, and that streptomycin or another aminoglycoside should be added for procedures involving the mouth or respiratory tract.

Prosthetic valve dysfunction is an indication for referral to a cardiologist, who will usually recommend cardiac catheterization (see Table 60.10 for all of the reasons to refer a patient with a prosthetic valve to a cardiologist).

Pregnancy in a patient with a prosthetic valve.

Pregnancy poses a serious problem in patients with mechanical prosthetic valves. The ingestion of Coumadin during pregnancy results in a definite increase in the incidence of fetal death and birth defects (see Chapter 52). The spontaneous abortion rate is approximately 30%, probably because Coumadin crosses the placenta barrier and predisposes the fetus to intrauterine hemorrhage. Between 8 and 16% of the liveborn infants will have various birth defects, most commonly nasal hypoplasia with stippled epiphysis (a specific Coumadin embryopathy), but including optic atrophy, microcephaly, and mental retardation.

On the other hand, the risk of thromboembolism is greater during pregnancy, and discontinuation of anticoagulation greatly increases the danger of systemic embolism. In one study (29) systemic embolism was seen in 31% of such patients despite antiplatelet therapy. Most of the patients had Starr-Edwards valves.

There is no consensus regarding the management of early pregnancy when a prosthetic valve is in place. Some authors have recommended substituting full dose heparin, which does not cross the placenta, for Coumadin during the first trimester of pregnancy. However, such therapy requires prolonged hospitalization and the incidence of fetal death appears to be high with this regimen as well (see Chapter 52). Many pregnant patients with prosthetic valves are treated with low dose subcutaneous heparin, which the patient learns to administer herself. The safety and efficacy of this regimen are not clearly established (see Chapter 52). Many clinicians strongly counsel patients with prosthetic valves to avoid pregnancy. Patients with prosthetic valves, especially the mechanical valves,

should be well aware of the risks if pregnancy is contemplated.

The proper management of anticoagulation at the end of pregnancy is more clearly defined. If Coumadin has been given, it should be replaced by heparin 2 weeks before delivery is expected. Heparin can then be stopped at the onset of labor, to prevent peripartum hemorrhage. The best approach to these problems is to urge the surgeon to place a tissue valve rather than a mechanical valve in every patient in whom future pregnancy is possible.

General References

Braunwald E (ed):*Heart Disease: A Textbook of Cardiovascular Medicine*, 3rd ed. Philadelphia, WB Saunders, 1988.
    Encyclopedic review of cardiac physical examination, heart sounds, and cardiac graphic techniques.
Constant J: *Bedside Cardiology*. Boston, Little, Brown, 1976.
    The best teaching text for understanding the physiological basis of heart sounds and how to hear and describe them.
Tavel ME: The systolic murmur—innocent or guilty? *Am J Cardiol* 39:757, 1977.
    Concise characterization of the most commonly heard murmur in an ambulatory practice.

Specific References

1. Barnett JHM, Boughner DR, Taylor DW, et al: Further evidence relating mitral valve prolapse to cerebral ischemic events. *N Engl J Med* 302:139, 1980.
2. Brandenburg RO, Fuster V, Guiliani ER: Valvular heart disease. When should the patient be referred? *Practical Cardiol*5:50, 1979.
3. Braunwald E: Mitral regurgitation: physiologic, clinical, and surgical considerations. *N Engl J Med* 281:425, 1969.
4. Cohn LH, Koster GK, Mee RBB, Collins Jr JJ: Long term followup of the Hancock Bioprosthetic Heart Valve. A six-year review. *Circulation* 60 (suppl 2): 93, 1979.
5. Craig RJ, Selzer A: Natural history and prognosis of atrial septal defect. *Circulation* 37:805, 1968.
6. Devereux RB, Perloff JK, Reichels N, Josephson ME: Mitral valve prolapse. *Circulation* 54:3, 1976.
7. Galloway AC, Colvin SB, Baumann FG, et al: Long-term results of mitral valve reconstruction with Capentier techniques in 148 patients with mitral insufficiency. *Circulation* 78 (suppl I):97, 1988.
8. Goldschlager N, Pfeifer J, Cohn K, et al: The natural history of aortic regurgitation. A clinical and hemodynamic study. *Am J Med* 54:577, 1973.
9. Gooch AS, Vicencio F, Markanlov V, Goldberg H: Arrhythmias and left ventricular asynergy in the prolapsing mitral leaflet syndrome. *Am J Cardiol* 29:611, 1972.
10. Hammermeister KE, Fisher L, Kennedy JW, et al: Prediction of late survival in patients with mitral valve disease from clinical, hemodynamic, and quantitative angiographic variables. *Circulation*57:341, 1978.
11. Hatle L, Angelsen B: *Doppler Ultrasound in Cardiology, Physical Principles and Clinical Applications*. Philadelphia, Lea and Febiger, 1985.
12. Helmcke F, Nanda NC, Hsiung MC, et al: Color Doppler assessment of mitral regurgitation with orthogonal planes. *Circulation* 75:175, 1987.
13. Heger JJ, Wann LS, Weyman AE, et al: Long-term changes in mitral valve area after successful mitral commissurotomy. *Circulation* 59:443, 1979.
14. Horan LG, Flowers NC: Electrocardiography and vectorcardiography. In: Braunwald E (ed): *Heart Disease: A Textbook of Cardiovascular Medicine*. Philadelphia, WB Saunders, 1980.
15. Leachman RD, Cokkinos DV, Cooley DA: Association of ostium secundum atrial septal defects with mitral valve prolapse. *Am J Cardiol* 38:167, 1976.
16. Lipson LC, Kent KM, Rosing DR, et al: Long term hemodynamic

Table 60.10.
Indications for Referral of Patients with Prosthetic Valves

Progressive symptoms of congestive heart failure
Progressive cardiac enlargement
Change in prosthetic heart sounds
Pregnancy, or the desire to become pregnant
Embolization
Endocarditis

assessment of the porcine heterograft in the mitral position. Late development of valvular stenosis. *Circulation* 64:397, 1981.

17. Markiewicz W, Stoner J, London E, et al: Mitral valve prolapse in one hundred presumably healthy young females. *Circulation* 53:464, 1976.

18. Marks AR, Choong CY, Sanfilippo AJ, et al: Identification of high-risk and low-risk subgroups of patients with mitral-valve prolapse. *N Engl J Med* 320:1031, 1989.

19. Massell BF, Ameccua FJ, Czohiczer G: Prognosis of patients with pure or predominant aortic regurgitation in the absence of surgery. *Circulation* 34 (suppl 2): 164, 1966.

20. Mills P, Rose J, Hollingsworth J, et al: Long-term prognosis of mitral-valve prolapse. *N Engl J Med* 297:13, 1977.

21. Munoz S, Gallardo J, Diaz-Gorrin JR, Medina O: Influence of surgery on the natural history of rheumatic mitral and aortic valve disease. *Am J Cardiol* 35:234, 1975.

22. Nishimura RA, Holmes Jr DR, Reeder GS, et al: Doppler evaluation of results of percutaneous aortic balloon valvuloplasty in calcific aortic stenosis. *Circulation* 78:791, 1988.

23. Olson LJ, Subramanian R, Edwards WD: Surgical pathology of pure aortic insufficiency: a study of 225 cases. *Mayo Clin Proc* 59:835, 1984.

24. Oleson KH: The natural history of 271 patients with mitral stenosis under medical treatment. *Br Heart J* 24:349, 1962.

25. Popp RL, Rubenson DS, Tucker LR, French JW: Echocardiography: M mode and two-dimensional methods. *Ann Intern Med* 93:844, 1980.

26. Rapaport E: Natural history of aortic and mitral valve disease. *Am J Cardiol* 35:221, 1981.

27. Roberts WC: Anatomically isolated aortic valve disease: a case against its being of rheumatic etiology. *Am J Med* 49:151, 1970.

28. Ross Jr J, Braunwald E: Aortic stenosis. *Circulation* 38 (suppl 5): 61, 1968.

29. Salazar E, Zajarias A, Gutierrez N, Iturbe I: The problems of cardiac valve prostheses, anticoagulants and pregnancy. *Circulation* 70 (suppl 1): 169, 1984.

30. Samuels DA, Curfman GD, Friedlich AL, et al: Valve replacement for aortic regurgitation: long-term follow-up with factors influencing the results. *Circulation* 60:647, 1979.

31. Selzer A, Cohn K: Natural history of mitral stenosis: a review. *Circulation* 45:878, 1972.

32. Shah PM, Adelman AG, Wigle ED, et al: The natural (and unnatural) history of hypertrophic obstructive cardiomyopathy. *Circ Res* 34 (suppl 2): 179, 1974.

33. Siemienczuk D, Greenberg B, Morris C, et al: Chronic aortic insufficiency: factors associated with progression to aortic valve replacement. *Ann Int Med* 110:587, 1989.

34. Skjaerpe T, Hegrenaes L, Hatle L: Noninvasive estimation of valve area in patients with aortic stenosis by Doppler ultrasound and two-dimentional echocardiography. *Circulation* 72:810, 1985.

35. Spirito P, Chiarella F, Carratino L, et al: Clinical course and prognosis of hypertrophic cardiomyopathy in an outpatient population. *New Engl J Med* 320:749, 1989.

36. Watanakunakorn C: Prosthetic valve endocarditis. *Prog Cardiovasc Dis* 22:181, 1979.

37. Weinstein IR, Marbarger JP, Peerez JE: Ultrasonic assessment of the St. Jude prosthetic valve: M-mode, two dimensional, and Doppler echocardiography. *Circulation* 68:897, 1983.

C H A P T E R   61

Heart Failure

SHELDON H. GOTTLIEB, M.D.

DEFINITION

The amount of blood that the heart pumps per minute (the cardiac output) is normally precisely adjusted to the metabolic needs of the body. The cardiac output may increase by two or three times as an individual goes from sleep to exercise. An increase in cardiac output may occur within the space of one heartbeat by a sudden decrease in vagal tone, which causes an increase in heart rate. After several seconds of exercise, sympathetic tone increases, which causes a further increase in cardiac output by increasing the heart rate and the amount of blood pumped per heart beat (the stroke volume). The increased cardiac output soon brings about an increase in the amount of blood returning to the right side of the heart (the venous return); also the heart further increases its output in response to the stretch in the heart muscle resulting from the increased volume of venous return (the Frank-Starling principle). If the heart is not able to pump enough blood to meet the metabolic needs of the body, compensatory mechanisms are brought into play by the heart, kidney, lung, and peripheral vascular system. These adjustments cause symptoms and signs recognized as the syndrome of heart failure. Acute heart failure, manifest usually by pulmonary edema (recognized by the abrupt onset of extreme breathlessness and evidence of alveolar edema by physical and radiological examination), warrants immediate hospitalization for diagnosis of the underlying and/or precipitating cause and for treatment. However, chronic heart failure is usually a problem that can be managed in an ambulatory setting.

EPIDEMIOLOGY OF HEART FAILURE

The incidence of heart failure is approximately 0.3/1000/year below age 45, remains constant at approximately 3/1000/year in the middle-age groups, and increases to 10/1000 in patients above the age of 65 (8, 9). The incidence among men is slightly higher than among women in the 45 to 84 year range but is higher among women in the 85 to 94 year range (8).

The prevalence of heart failure increases greatly in patients above 60 years old (Fig. 61.1). Above the age of 70, women with congestive heart failure outnumber men. This is true in spite of the higher incidence in men and probably reflects the earlier mortality among men from coronary artery disease.

PHYSIOLOGY OF HEART FAILURE

The Heart as a Pump

Length Tension Relation: Frank-Starling Mechanism and Preload

As heart muscle is stretched, it develops increased tension. The relationship of length to tension defines the compliance of heart muscle; the inverse of compliance is *stiffness*. If the ventricle is distended with blood, pressure is developed within the cavity. A higher pressure is needed to distend the ventricle to a given volume in a less compliant, i.e., stiffer, ventricle. The pressure needed to stretch the ventricle to a given end-diastolic volume is called the preload, or left ventricular end-diastolic pressure (LVEDP). The relationship between the volume of the ventricle just before contraction and the force developed during contraction defines the Frank-Starling law of the heart. If the LVEDP is plotted against stroke work (the stroke volume times the mean blood pressure), a ventricular function curve is defined (Fig. 61.2). It can be seen from this relationship that the normal ventricle is compliant and will develop an adequate amount of force during contraction with a relatively low preload. However, the failing ventricle requires a high preload in order to increase its stroke work (Fig. 61.2). The implications of this relationship are discussed below.

Afterload

Afterload is the dynamic resistance against which the heart contracts. It determines the degree of stress within the myocardium. Systolic blood pressure closely approximates and is clinically the most useful indicator of afterload. Afterload determines the ease or speed of ventricular contraction and hence the ejec-

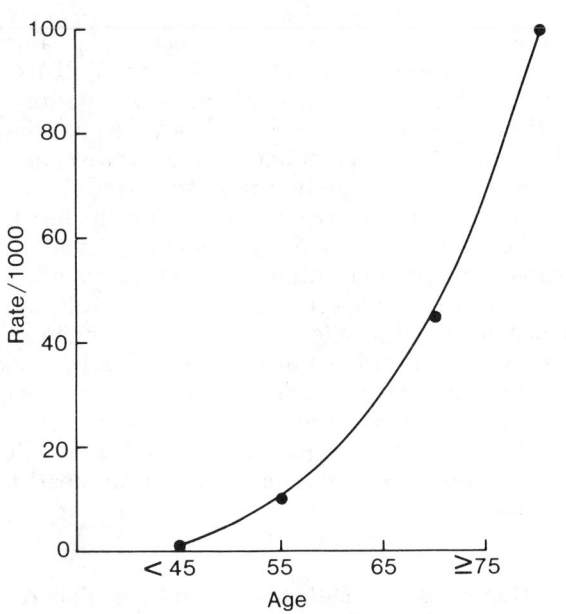

Figure 61.1. The prevalence of heart failure reported from physicians' offices as a function of patient age. Note the marked increase in the sixth and seventh decades. Between 10 and 20% of patients older than age 60 followed regularly by a physician will have a history of heart failure. (From McKee P, Castelli W, McNamara P, Kannel W: The natural history of congestive heart failure: the Framingham study. *N Engl J Med* 285:1441, 1971.)

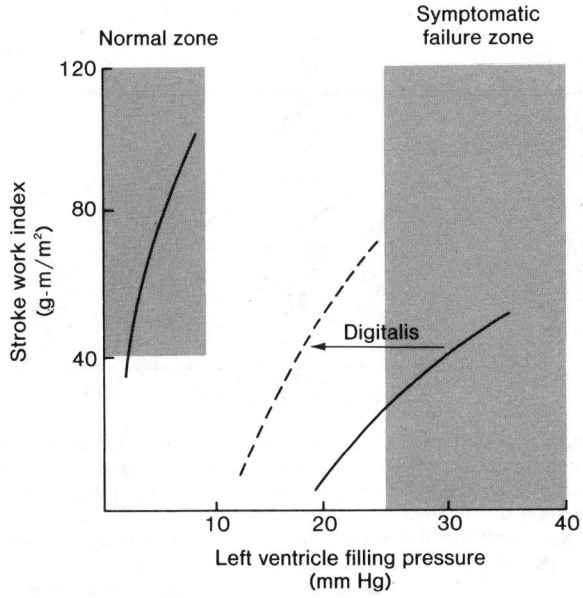

Figure 61.2. Ventricular function curves showing the relationship between left ventricular filling pressures and stroke work. The relative position of the curve defines the *inotropic state* of the heart. Note that for a given curve, *i.e.*, a given inotropic state, the *function* of the heart, or the amount of work the heart is capable of performing, varies with the left ventricular filling pressure. (Adapted from Weisfeldt ML: Congestive heart failure: pathophysiology and the evaluation of ventricular function. In Harvey AM, Johns RJ, McKusick VA, *et al* (eds): *The Principles and Practice of Medicine.* New York, Appleton-Century-Crofts, 1984.)

tion fraction (that portion of the ventricular volume that is ejected with each beat) (Fig. 61.3).

Contractility and Inotropic State

The relationship of preload to stroke work defines the functional state of cardiac muscle (see above). The relative position of the curve defines the inotropic state of the muscle (see Fig. 61.2). For example, infusing the heart with an inotropic substance such as digitalis causes the ventricular function curve to shift to the left, to perform a higher stroke work at a given preload. In other words, the contractility of the heart is increased.

Inter-relationship between Preload, Afterload, and Inotropic State

The inter-relationship between the preload, afterload, and inotropic state is summarized in Fig. 61.3. If preload is kept constant, an increase in afterload will cause a depression in ventricular function. Thus, if afterload or blood pressure increases, ventricular function or ejection fraction decreases. That causes the ventricular end-diastolic volume, or preload, to increase, restoring the ventricular function to baseline. A further increase in afterload leads to a further depression in ventricular function, which again may be restored by increasing preload, i.e., by increasing left ventricular end-diastolic pressure. Eventually, a limit is reached beyond which preload cannot be increased, as noted in the figure. This is the left ventricular filling pressure, the preload reserve, above

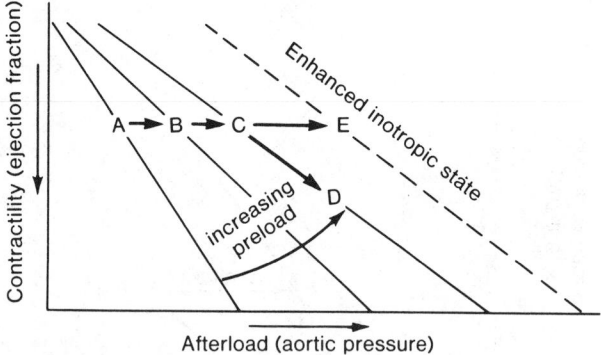

Figure 61.3. The interrelationship between preload, afterload, and inotropic state. The three *solid lines* are a family of curves at different levels of preload but with inotropic state kept constant. Taken together, they represent *ventricular function* as a function of both *preload* and *afterload*. Note that if preload is kept constant, an increase in afterload will cause a decrease in *contractility* as measured by the *ejection fraction*, but that when afterload is decreased to 0, the curves converge, because the *inotropic state* of the muscle is unchanged. As afterload increases, contractility may be maintained by increasing preload (shifting from *point A* to *B* to *C*). When preload reaches the point (*C*) at which an increase will cause pulmonary congestion (the *preload reserve*), any further increase in afterload will decrease contractility (*point C* to *D*). Contractility may then be increased only by measures, such as digitalization, which enhance the inotropic state (*point D* to *E*). Patients are most sensitive to changes in afterload when their filling pressures are at the preload reserve. (Adapted from Ross J Jr: Afterload mismatch and preload reserve: a conceptual framework for the analysis of ventricular function. *Prog Cardiovasc Dis* 18:255, 1976.)

which the pulmonary capillary oncotic pressure is exceeded, fluid passes into the alveoli, and pulmonary congestion occurs. Any increase in afterload that occurs when the preload reserve is reached will cause a decrease in ventricular function. The preload reserve varies with the compliance of the ventricle. If heart muscle is made stiffer or less compliant by a chronic disease process such as hypertension or aortic stenosis, or by an acute process such as ischemia, a higher filling pressure will be necessary to set the level of ventricular function by means of the Frank-Starling principle; and the preload reserve will be reached sooner. The only way to improve ventricular function when the preload reserve is reached is either to decrease the afterload or to change the inotropic state, or contractility, of the muscle. The clinical significance of these inter-relationships will be discussed at greater length under "Management."

Biochemical Basis for Altered Contractility in the Failing Heart

The contractile unit of heart muscle is the sarcomere, which consists of fibers of protein called actin and myosin. *Actin* and *myosin* interact with each other by interlocking protein cross bridges called troponin. The interlocking mechanism is facilitated by adenosine triphosphate (ATP) and magnesium. An inhibitory protein, *tropomyosin*, is present on the myosin fibers. Tropomyosin inhibits the interaction between actin and myosin and allows the muscle to relax. Calcium inhibits the tropomyosin complex, frees the troponin cross-bridges, and allows actin and myosin to interact and to develop tension. Calcium is therefore necessary for myocardial contraction to take place. Large amounts of calcium are stored within the heart in a distinctive network of *sarcoplasmic reticulum*. Excitation contraction coupling takes place in heart muscle when an action potential, via mechanisms not yet understood, causes a release of calcium from the sarcoplasmic reticulum, thereby initiating contraction. In heart failure, there appears to be decreased energy available for cardiac contraction leading to *decreased systolic function* and slow transport of calcium back into the sarcoplasmic reticulum after contraction, leading to a delay in relaxation of cardiac muscle. Clinically this is noted as an increase in resistance to filling or, in other words, the *diastolic compliance of the myocardium* is reduced in heart failure (6). Abnormalities in calcium transport may also predispose the failing heart to *arrhythmias*.

Compensatory Mechanisms in Heart Failure

Heart Rate

If stroke volume remains constant, an increase in heart rate will cause a proportionate increase in cardiac output in patients in heart failure.

Hypertrophy and Dilation

Left ventricular hypertrophy and dilation may allow compensation to be achieved for many years. The stress in the wall of the heart varies with the radius of the ventricular cavity. If the heart is subjected to a volume load, it dilates in order to accommodate the load and to increase its ability to eject the load (the Frank-Starling principle—see above). However, ventricular dilation causes an increase in ventricular wall stress, which serves as a stimulus to ventricular hypertrophy. The hypertrophy is eccentric, so-called because it causes the left heart border to move laterally. Eventually the heart becomes both dilated and hypertrophied, and the ratio of wall thickness to cavity size returns to normal, which returns wall stress to normal; therefore a state of compensated ventricular dilation is achieved. The response to a pressure overload is different. An increase in wall stress in the absence of volume overload leads to concentric hypertrophy; wall stress per unit area returns to normal, but the cavity size is unchanged.

Redistribution of Cardiac Output in Heart Failure

There is a marked increase in peripheral vascular resistance in heart failure, and that causes a redistribution of cardiac output. In less severe failure, when the resting cardiac output is normal, redistribution occurs only during exercise. In severe heart failure, when the resting cardiac output is significantly decreased, redistribution occurs at rest. The decrease in blood flow is most marked in the kidneys and the skin. Decreased renal blood flow causes a release of renin from the juxtaglomerular apparatus, and therefore plasma angiotensin activity is increased. Angiotensin is a potent vasoconstrictor and acts both directly on smooth muscle and indirectly by increasing release of norepinephrine from vascular nerve endings. The increase in angiotensin activity leads to an increase in aldosterone production, which causes an increase in sodium resorption from the distal tubule of the nephron, thereby increasing plasma volume. The renal resorption of sodium is also facilitated by the decrease in cardiac output and in glomerular filtration rate, which causes an increase in the fraction of sodium resorbed in the proximal tubule of the nephron.

DIAGNOSTIC PROCESS

There is no one symptom, sign, or laboratory test that is pathognomonic of heart failure. Diagnosis must therefore be based on a process of clinical inference. The significance of symptoms and signs must be evaluated with regard to the patient's overall condition and to where the patient appears to be in the natural history of his disease. In ambulatory practice, a patient will often present to a new physician with the diagnosis of "heart failure" and will be taking medicine for this condition. In this situation, the diagnosis of heart failure should be verified before it is accepted and before treatment is maintained.

Diagnostic Classification of Heart Failure

Etiology of Heart Failure

When the diagnosis of heart failure is made, it is essential to decide upon the most likely etiology, since the prognosis and the treatment of heart failure vary greatly depending upon its cause.

Heart failure is due to one of three basic mechanisms: an increased work load to which the heart cannot accommodate; a disorder of the myocardium so that it is unable to accommodate normal work loads; or a restriction of ventricular filling so that an adequate stroke volume cannot be achieved. Table 61.1 lists selected examples of these conditions. In this country the most common condition associated with heart failure is ischemic heart disease, followed by systemic hypertension (8). Among the elderly hypertension aortic stenosis and ischemic heart disease are the most common causes of heart failure.

The most common precipitating causes of heart failure (Table 61.2) are noncompliance with medication or diet in a patient with previously compensated heart failure, acute myocardial infarction pneumonia, and uncontrolled hypertension. In patients for whom the precipitating cause is not obvious, it is important to consider arrhythmia (Chapter 59) and pulmonary embolism (Chapter 53). In addition, it is important to inquire about psychosocial stress, which has been shown to precede the onset of symptoms in as many as 50% of patients hospitalized for heart failure (15).

Functional Classification of Heart Failure

The amount of exercise that a patient can perform without symptoms of heart failure determines his

Table 61.1.
Causes of Heart Failure[a]

INCREASED WORK LOAD TO WHICH THE HEART CANNOT ACCOMMODATE
  High output states:
    Hyperthyroidism[b]
    Anemia[b]
    Systemic arteriovenous fistulas[b]
    Certain dermatological disorders (*e.g.*, psoriasis, erythroderma)[b]
    Valvular regurgitation or left to right shunts[b]
  Increased impedance to ejection:
    Systemic hypertension[b]
    Pulmonary hypertension
    Pulmonic or aortic stenosis[b]
DISORDER OF MYOCARDIUM SO THAT THE HEART IS UNABLE TO ACCOMMODATE NORMAL WORK LOADS
  Cardiomyopathies
  Myocardial infarction
RESTRICTION OF VENTRICULAR FILLING
  Pericardial constriction or effusion[b]
  Mitral and tricuspid valvular stenosis[b]
  Increased ventricular stiffness:
    Infiltrative myocardial disease (*e.g.*, amyloid)
    Ventricular hypertrophy
    Hypertrophic cardiomyopathy

[a]Adapted from Weisfeldt ML: Congestive heart failure: pathophysiology and the evaluation of ventricular function. In Harvey AM, Johns RJ, McKusick VA, *et al* (eds): *The Principles and Practice of Medicine.* New York, Appleton-Century-Crofts, 1984.
[b]Indicates causes of heart failure that are potentially treatable by specific therapy.

Table 61.2.
Precipitating Causes of Heart Failure

FACTORS DECREASING MYOCARDIAL EFFICIENCY
  Myocardial infarction
  Ischemia
  Arrhythmia
  Hypoxia
  Alcohol and other toxic substances
  Recent initiation of a β-blocking drug
  Discontinuation of a cardiac glycoside
  Myocardial depressant drugs (*e.g.*, verapamil, disopyramide (Norpace), adriamycin)
  Pericardial tamponade
  Myocardial infections (*e.g.*, bacterial endocarditis, myocarditis, parasitic infection)
  Vasculitis
FACTORS INCREASING CARDIAC LOAD
  Noncompliance with low salt diet
  Uncontrolled systemic hypertension
  Pneumonia
  Psychological stress
  Exercise, especially in extremes of heat or humidity
  Discontinuing diuretics, antihypertensive drugs, or afterload reducing agents
  Drugs which retain or contain sodium
  Infection
  Anemia
  Pulmonary embolism
  Thyrotoxicosis
  Acute valvular dysfunction

functional class. Several classification schemes that are useful in categorizing patients in this regard are presented in Table 61.3. Correctable disease may be present despite severe symptoms so that the functional classification provides useful prognostic information only within selected subsets of patients. Functional class is best determined by questioning the patient regarding his performance during daily activities. For example, a patient may be asked how many stairs he can climb before he has to stop and rest, or how heavy a load he can carry, and what work activities have had to be modified.

History

The most common symptom of heart failure is *dyspnea*. Dyspnea means uncomfortable breathing. It is not the shortness of breath experienced by normal people when they exercise or by anxious people when they hyperventilate (see also Chapters 13 and 53). Dyspnea in heart failure is a symptom of increased LVEDP leading to pulmonary venous and capillary congestion. The increase in pulmonary congestion causes an increased stiffness of the lungs and a decrease in the vital capacity. The work of breathing increases and breathing becomes rapid, shallow, and forced.

Orthopnea is dyspnea in the recumbent position. It is frequently experienced by patients with heart failure, although it may also be a symptom of patients with obstructive lung disease or with obesity. Blood normally pools in the lower extremities when a person is upright. When the patient who is in heart failure lies down, there is an increase in venous return to the heart that leads to an increase in pulmonary congestion because of the inability of the compromised left ventricle to accept and to pump the increased load. The severity of orthopnea is assessed by the number of pillows the patient must use to be able to breath comfortably in the recumbent position.

Patients in heart failure with dyspnea and orthopnea often have a dry hacking cough; at times this is the patient's most troublesome symptom. The cough usually improves concomitantly with improvement in other symptoms. A dry hacking cough also develops in 2 to 10% of patients treated with angiotension-converting enzyme (ACE) inhibitors (11, 12). This symptom may respond to reducing the dose of the drug, but in many

Table 61.3A.
Assessment of Functional Capacity

	New York Heart Association Classification[a]	Severity of Symptoms[b]	Max Oxygen Uptake ml/mm/kg[b]	Goldman's Specific Activity Scale, METs[c, d]
I	Patients with cardiac disease but without resulting limitations of physical activity. Ordinary physical activity does not cause undue fatigue, palpitations, dyspnea or anginal pain.	None to Mild	>20	10 METs
II	Patients with cardiac disease resulting in slight limitation of physical activity. They are comfortable at rest. Ordinary physical activity results in fatigue, palpitations, dyspnea or angina pain.	Mild to Moderate	16–20	5–6 METs
III	Patients with cardiac disease that results in marked limitation of physical activity and causes fatigue, palpitations, dyspnea or anginal pain.	Moderate to Severe	10–16	3.6–4.2 METs
IV	Patients with cardiac disease that results in inability to carry on any physical activity without discomfort. Symptoms of cardiac insufficiency or of the anginal syndrome may be present even at rest. If any physical activity is undertaken, discomfort is increased.	Severe	<10	2–2.3 METs

[a] The Criteria Committee of the New York Heart Association, Inc. *Diseases of the Heart and Blood Vessels, Nomenclature and Criteria for Diagnosis.* 6th ed, Boston, Little & Brown, 1964.
[b] Adapted from Weber KT, and Janiski JS: *Cardiopulmonary Exercise Testing.* Philadelphia, WB Saunders Co., 1986.
[c] Adapted from Goldman L, Hashimoto B, Cook EF, Loscalzo A: Comparative reproducibility and validity of systems for assessing cardiovascular functional class: Advantages of new specific activity scale. Circulation 64:1227, 1981.
[d] METs = metabiolic equivalents of activity, where 1 MET = 3.5 mg O2/Kg/min at rest.

Table 61.3B.
Goldman's Specific Activity Scale

	Any yes	No
1. Can you walk down a flight of steps without stopping? (4.5-5.2 mets[a])	Go to #2	Go to #4

2. Can you carry anything up a flight of 8 steps without stopping (5-5.5 mets) or can you:
  (a) have sexual intercourse without stopping (5-5.5 mets)
  (b) garden, rake, weed (5.6 mets)
  (c) roller skate, dance foxtrot (5-6 mets)
  (d) walk at a 4 mile-per-hour rate on level ground (5-6 mets)
	Go to #3	Class III

3. Can you carry at least 24 pounds up 8 steps (10 mets) or can you:
  (a) carry objects that are at least 80 pounds (8 mets)
  (b) do outdoor work—shovel snow, spade soil (7 mets)
  (c) Do recreational activities such as skiing, basketball, touch football, squash, handball (7-10 mets)
  (d) Jog/walk 5 miles per hour (9 mets)
	Class I	Class II

4. Can you shower without stopping (3.6-4.2 mets) or can you:
  (a) strip and make bed (3.9-5 mets)
  (b) mop floors (4.2 mets)
  (c) hang washed clothes (4.4 mets)
  (d) clean windows (3.7 mets)
  (e) walk 2.5 miles per hour (3-3.5 mets)
  (f) bowl (3-4.4 mets)
  (g) play golf (walk and carry clubs) (4.5 mets)
  (h) push power lawn mower (4 mets)
	Class III	Go to #5

5. Can you dress without stopping because of symptoms? (2-2.3 mets)	Class III	Class IV

[a] Mets = metabolic equivalents of activity, where 1 met = oxygen consumption at rest = 3.5 ml O_2/Kg/min.

cases the drug may have to be discontinued (see below).

Paroxysmal nocturnal dyspnea is characteristic of poorly compensated chronic heart failure. Patients commonly complain of paroxysmal dyspnea approximately 2 hours after falling asleep. It is often associated with bad dreams or nightmares and is relieved by sitting up or by getting out of bed and sitting in a chair. Because the dyspnea often is associated with wheezing, it must be distinguished from the nocturnal shortness of breath sometimes experienced by people with obstructive lung disease (see Chapter 55).

Fatigue is a common complaint of patients in heart failure. It is frequently described as a general sense of weakness or of lassitude. Some patients may complain of fatigue rather than of dyspnea. In this setting fatigue is a symptom of low cardiac output, often due to overdiuresis after the aggressive use of potent diuretics.

A history of *edema* and/or *weight gain* (from retention of salt and water) is often elicited from patients in heart failure. Many will also give a history of having taken digitalis in the past for a "heart problem."

Chest pain due to myocardial ischemia is common in patients in heart failure (see Chapter 57). Patients with pre-existing poor left ventricular function may rapidly develop marked left ventricular dysfunction when their hearts become ischemic, or they may develop paroxysmal mitral regurgitation due to acute papillary muscle dysfunction. This may happen in association with exercise in patients with stable ischemic heart disease or may occur paroxysmally and at rest in patients with unstable ischemic heart disease or in patients who may be experiencing spasm of the coronary arteries (see Chapter 57). Paroxysmal dyspnea associated with exercise-induced ischemia is sometimes referred to as an "anginal equivalent." The symptomatic response to nitroglycerin does not by itself differentiate between dyspnea due to ischemia and dyspnea due to chronic congestive heart failure; sublingual nitroglycerin rapidly relieves congestion due to either condition (see below).

Nocturia, a common symptom of heart failure, often occurs early in the illness. It is due to the redistribution in cardiac output that occurs in the recumbent position, restoring in part blood flow to the kidney that, in the upright position, has been diverted to other organs (see above).

Decreased cardiac output by itself or in association with cerebrovascular disease may lead to *impairment in mental function*, ranging from mild confusion to overt psychosis. The most common neuropsychiatric complaints, however, are mild chronic anxiety and depression; these may be the presenting complaints, especially in elderly patients with previously undiagnosed heart failure.

Symptoms of *congestion of the gastrointestinal system* are common in patients with chronic, poorly compensated heart failure. Chronically increased right heart pressures cause passive congestion of the liver with swelling and discomfort in the right upper quadrant of the abdomen. In extreme cases there will be marked anorexia and weight loss due to gastrointestinal congestion.

Physical Findings in Heart Failure

The physical findings in heart failure depend upon which compensatory mechanisms are utilized to adjust the cardiac output to the metabolic needs of the body. Findings vary depending upon whether the heart failure is compensated or uncompensated.

Uncompensated Heart Failure

In chronic uncompensated or poorly compensated heart failure there will be signs of an attempt at cardiac compensation (increased heart size and heart rate) and signs of increased renin, angiotensin, and aldosterone activity (vascular redistribution and evidence of cardiac, pulmonary, and peripheral congestion). Congestion is manifest by a ventricular gallop sound (S_3), rales, jugular venous distention, hepatojugular reflux, and peripheral pitting edema.

Increased heart size may be recognized by inspection, palpation, and percussion of the precordium. The precordium should be palpated with the patient in the supine and in the left lateral position. The location, quality, and size of the point of maximal impulse (PMI) should be noted. The PMI of an eccentrically enlarged heart is displaced laterally and caudally and is heaving and diffuse. The PMI of a concentrically enlarged heart is not displaced but may be thrusting or sustained. The heart border should be percussed, and its position relative to the PMI should be noted.

Sinus tachycardia, defined as a resting heart rate in an adult greater than 100 beats/minute, is a relatively sensitive but nonspecific sign of heart failure; it is a compensatory mechanism to increase cardiac output (see below). *Pulsus alternans*, a regular rhythm in which contractions are successively strong and weak, is most common in patients with increased resistance to left ventricular ejection (e.g., systemic hypertension) and is due to repetitive changes in stroke volume because of incomplete recovery of contractility by the failing heart.

The second pulmonic sound (P_2) is often accentuated in patients in left ventricular failure, because of increased pulmonary artery pressure. Paradoxic splitting of the second heart sound, an indication of prolonged left ventricular ejection time, may be heard in patients with chronic heart failure and is often associated with a left bundle branch block.

The *ventricular* or S_3 gallop sound is the most specific sign of heart failure (7). The S_3 gallop sound is heard shortly after the second heart sound (S_2) and is due to sudden restriction of filling in a relatively noncompliant left ventricle. It is usually heard directly over the PMI and may be audible only when the patient is in the left lateral position. The sound is low pitched and often may be sensed by the cadence of the heart sounds rather than specifically heard. The cadence closely approximates the word "Kentucky," pronounced KYN-TUC'-KY. The middle syllable is accentuated to represent the loud second heart sound due to increased pulmonary artery pressure in patients in heart failure. The timing of the last syllable closely approximates the timing of the third heart sound when the word is repeated 100 times/minute.

Rales are high pitched sounds (similar to the sound of a clump of hair rubbed between the fingers) produced by the sudden filling with air of fluid-filled alveoli. They are a sign of moderately to severely decompensated left heart failure.

Neck vein distention and hepatojugular reflux are relatively insensitive but specific findings of heart failure (4). In chronic heart failure, right ventricular filling pressures will usually increase as the LVEDP increases. With time the right ventricle becomes increasingly more stiff and unable to accept a sudden volume load.

Neck vein distention is assessed while the patient is semirecumbent with the head turned slightly away from the examiner. Ideally the internal, rather than the external, jugular vein is inspected since the latter contains valves and may not reflect accurately the right heart pressure. Internal jugular venous distention is seen as a broad-based filling in the anterior cervical triangle. However, since the external jugular venous

system is often more easily identified, it may be used as an index of the pressure in the superior vena cava if the physician examines the neck properly. If the external jugular is compressed in the supraclavicular fossa, and the examining finger then strips the vein cephalad, blood will rise in the more proximal portion of the vein and the height of this volume of blood reflects the central venous pressure. An arbitrary reference point may be chosen (such as 10 cm anterior to the posterior axillary line at the sternal angle—this approximates in many the level of the right atrium), and the column of blood above this point may be measured without regard for the angle of elevation of the thorax. The value of this observation is that accurate serial assessments are possible, permitting the physician to confirm worsening failure (increasing jugular venous pressure) or to recognize a too vigorous diuretic response (abnormally low jugular venous pressure).

Hepatojugular reflux is assessed by having the patient lie supine and semirecumbent at 45°. The patient is asked to breathe normally and is warned that the examiner will apply pressure over the right upper quadrant of the abdomen. Patients so warned will comply and will not hold their breath or perform a Valsalva maneuver that will make the sign impossible to elicit. The sudden increase in venous return causes right ventricular end-diastolic pressure and right atrial pressure to rise and to remain elevated; and this will be seen as jugular venous distention (4).

Peripheral pitting edema is a relatively common, although not a specific, sign of heart failure. It occurs in the dependent portions of the body, which in ambulatory patients means the feet and lower legs. Edema in heart failure is due to increased resorption of salt and water by the kidney. Because pitting edema in the lower extremities becomes detectable only when the leg volume increases by about 10%, an increase in weight may precede pitting edema as an early objective manifestation of decompensated heart failure in ambulatory patients.

Because of low cardiac output and vascular redistribution, patients may have a slightly cyanotic cast to their skin and a drawn colorless look to their face. Their extremities may be cool and their nailbeds may be cyanotic. Delayed capillary filling in the skin of the abdomen may be apparent when the examiner's hand is removed after assessing hepatojugular reflux.

Compensated Heart Failure

In contrast to the findings in patients with acute or chronic uncompensated heart failure, there may be few or no specific physical findings in compensated patients at rest other than signs of increased heart size. A presystolic gallop or fourth heart sound (S_4) can be heard in most patients with long-standing high blood pressure or ischemic heart disease who are in normal sinus rhythm. The fourth heart sound is thought to be due to atrial contraction into a stiff ventricle. A soft systolic murmur, approximately grade 1 to 2, is commonly heard at the PMI in patients with chronic compensated heart failure. This murmur usually represents minor degrees of mitral or tricuspid insufficiency. In well-compensated patients the signs and symptoms of heart failure may only be present during exercise, and these patients should be examined immediately after exercising.

Laboratory Diagnosis

Chest X-ray in Heart Failure

The chest X-ray is a useful diagnostic procedure for the evaluation of suspected heart failure (7). The radiological signs of heart failure are cardiac enlargement and pulmonary congestion.

There are a number of factors that influence heart size on the chest X-ray. These include body build, the depth of inspiration when the film is taken, and the chambers that are enlarged. Nevertheless, determination of the ratio of the transverse diameter of the heart to the greatest diameter of the chest, the cardiothoracic ratio, is a reliable and valid measurement of heart size and should be part of the data base of every patient who is thought to have or to have had heart failure. The normal *cardiothoracic ratio* is less than 0.5.

The pulmonary vasculature should be examined, and signs of vascular redistribution, caused by pulmonary venous hypertension, and of enlarged hilar vessels, caused by acute or chronic pulmonary hypertension, should be noted.

Normally, the lower lobes of the lungs are better perfused than the upper lobes. The earliest radiological sign of pulmonary congestion is reduction of blood flow to the lower lobes due to compression of vessels by extravascular fluid that has gravitated to the lung bases. In early heart failure, there is simply an equalization of the size of the vessels to the upper and lower lobes; but as congestion increases, the vessels to the upper lobes become more prominent, the so-called "cephalization" of flow. More severe failure is manifest by signs of interstitial edema and ultimately by alveolar edema and pleural effusion (Chapter 54).

Electrocardiogram

There are no ECG changes that are diagnostic of heart failure. The ECG may, however, reflect an underlying disease (e.g., left ventricular hypertrophy due to hypertension; Q waves or ST-T wave changes due to infarction) or the presence of an unstable rhythm (such as rapid atrial fibrillation) that has caused heart failure.

Patients with well-compensated concentric or eccentric hypertrophy of the heart may show only relatively minor nonspecific ST-T wave changes. Grossly abnormal changes are seen in patients who have both dilation and hypertrophy of the left ventricle. The most common manifestations of left ventricular hypertrophy are left axis deviation, increased QRS voltage and QRS duration, and ST-T wave changes. Although there are numerous ECG criteria for left ventricular hypertrophy (LVH), a clinically useful criterion is the index of Lewis: Net positivity in lead 1 plus net negativity in lead 3 equals 2.0 mV or more (see also Table 60.3, Chapter 60). Also, an R wave greater than 11 mm in aVL is highly specific for LVH. However, LHV should not be diagnosed on the basis of voltage changes alone; ST-T wave changes should be present in order to make the diagnosis.

Conduction abnormalities are common in patients in heart failure, especially left bundle branch block. Left bundle branch block may be an early sign of congestive cardiomyopathy, especially when it occurs in young patients. It is nearly always a sign of organic heart disease.

Left atrial enlargement is diagnosed by the presence of a negative P wave with an area of greater than 1 mm^2 in lead V$_1$. It commonly is seen in the ECG of a patient with acute heart failure and may disappear as the patient is treated and the volume of the heart decreases.

Right ventricular hypertrophy is most reliably diagnosed in adults by a shift of the QRS axis toward the right greater than 90° (see also Table 60.6, Chapter 60). The QRS axis normally shifts toward the left with age.

Certain ECG changes suggest a decreased ejection fraction, especially in patients with heart failure due to ischemic heart disease. These include (a) Q waves in leads 1, aVL, and V$_1$ through V$_4$ with persistently upward coving of the ST segments in the precordial leads (seen in patients with extensive anterior wall infarctions with aneurysms); and (b) deep Q waves in both inferior and precordial leads with QRS duration greater than 0.1 second (suggesting ischemic cardiomyopathy).

Low voltage (less than 10 mm in all leads) is commonly due to pericardial effusion, hypothyroidism, or infiltrative disease of the heart (e.g., amyloid) but also may be seen in patients with severe emphysema or marked obesity.

Echocardiogram

The two-dimensional echocardiogram is a reliable technique for determining ventricular size and thickness, the presence of valvular and other structural abnormalities, and the presence or absence of pericardial effusion. Echocardiography should be considered for patients with suspected valvular or pericardial disease or for patients in whom the cause of heart failure is unclear. (The use of echocardiography in the diagnosis of valvular heart disease is discussed more fully in Chapter 60.)

Ejection fraction can be estimated by two-dimensional echochardiography. The echocardiogram is highly operator dependent, and in only about 80% of patients will the ejection fraction be able to be estimated accurately. The primary physician should attempt to review the echocardiogram with the echocardiographer before major therapeutic decisions are made. Two-dimensional echocardiography with color flow Doppler is useful in the evaluation of the degree of valvular stenosis or regurgitation; pulmonary artery pressures may be estimated accurately and noninvasively only in patients who have tricuspid regurgitation.

Radionuclide Angiography

Radionuclide angiography ("gated blood pool scan") is a technique for visualizing the cardiac chambers throughout the cardiac cycle. As most commonly performed, pyrophosphate is injected to bind with the patient's red blood cells. One-half hour later technetium-99m is injected intravenously to bind with the red blood cell-pyrophosphate complex. The intracardiac blood pool is scanned in multiple images with a scintillation camera that is synchronized (gated) with the ECG. A computer interfaces with the image from the scintillation camera, divides the cardiac cycle commonly into 32 equal segments, and displays on a television screen in a continuous loop the images obtained sequentially so that a moving image of the heart is seen. The technique is painless and exposes the patient to approximately the same amount of radiation as three plain films of the chest. The cost of radionuclide angiography is approximately 10 times that of an ECG.

The major advantages of this technique over echocardiography is that good images may be obtained even in patients who are obese or who have severe chronic lung disease, and the ejection fraction may be determined precisely.

Radionuclide angiography is an effective tool to differentiate between dyspnea due to cardiac and pulmonary causes, to evaluate left ventricular wall motion abnormalities including ventricular aneurysm, to evaluate left ventricular function reflected in the ejection fraction, and to confirm the clinical diagnosis of cardiomyopathy.

The general physician will not ordinarily consider radionuclide angiography without the advice of a cardiologist. However, the technique is an accurate way to complement the clinical assessment of myocardial function in a patient with heart failure.

Cardiac Catheterization and Myocardial Biopsy

Cardiac catheterization (see Chapter 57) should be considered in any patient in chronic heart failure in whom an etiological and anatomical diagnosis has not been made by noninvasive techniques. Cardiac catheterization may be the only way to diagnose occult valvular or pericardial disease or septal defects (see Chapter 60); myocardial biopsy may be useful in young patients, suspected of having a cardiomyopathy, who have the sudden onset of heart failure of uncertain etiology. Consultation with a cardiologist should be obtained before cardiac catheterization or biopsy is recommended.

Exercise Testing

It is often difficult to determine the functional status of patients claiming Social Security disability or workmen's compensation, and functional limitation is frequently over- or underestimated. Studies have shown that the most precise determination of functional classification is given by exercise testing with assessment of oxygen consumption (13). The protocol used should be one in which the level of exercise is increased in small increments (see Chapter 57). The test should be obtained in consultation with a cardiologist or a pulmonologist and only if functional classification cannot be satisfactorily determined by clinical means.

MANAGEMENT

The goal of therapy is not merely to control symptoms but to treat specifically the underlying causes of heart failure if possible (see Table 61.1). If the underlying disease cannot be effectively treated, an attempt should be made to increase the capacity of the heart to do work and/or to decrease the amount of work that the heart has to do. Table 61.4 shows the various measures that can be utilized to accomplish these goals in ambulatory patients. These measures are discussed in detail below.

General Principles

Life Style

It is not always possible to improve the function of the failing heart, but it usually is possible to decrease the metabolic needs of the body by encouraging a patient to stop smoking, to avoid emotionally stressful situations and people, and to get an adequate amount of rest. A thorough understanding of the patient's work environment and the relationship of the patient to his spouse and family is important. The patient is more likely to change his life style and priorities if the practitioner discusses the recommended therapy with both the patient and his family. The ambulatory patient should be encouraged to exercise, but to take care to avoid exertion to the point of causing further symptomatic cardiac decompensation. Sometimes this simply means performing the same activities more slowly.

There is a decreased stimulus to renin, angiotensin, and aldosterone production during supine rest, and

---

Table 61.4.

Measures Used in Ambulatory Treatment of Heart Failure

INCREASING CAPACITY OF HEART TO DO WORK
  Digitalis
  Antiarrhythmic drugs (Chapter 59)
  Pacemaker (Chapter 59)
DECREASING AMOUNT OF WORK THAT HEART HAS TO DO
  Rest
  Low sodium diet
  Diuretics
  Vasodilator drugs
  Home oxygen

even severely disabled patients may be able to lead socially useful and satisfying lives if they take a nap in the afternoon and in the early evening or before social or business engagements. Strict bed rest is rarely necessary.

It is important that the temperature and humidity of the patient's home and work environment be controlled as much as possible. Patients should be encouraged to have air conditioners for the summer months to reduce the extra demand placed on the heart by hot humid weather.

Diet

There is surprisingly little experimental evidence that a severely salt-restricted diet is of benefit in the long term in controlling heart failure in patients who respond well to moderate doses of diuretics. It is commonly observed, however, that sudden increases in salt intake may precipitate acute heart failure in patients who have moderately well-compensated but relatively severe heart failure. Holiday seasons are particularly dangerous in this regard, probably also because of the increased activity and emotional stress during these times. The physician must be aware of the various types of food that the patient is likely to eat. Most ethnic groups have certain foods that are prepared during festive occasions and many of these foods have a high salt content. Examples include "down-home cooking" among Blacks, which is characterized by use of fatback or salt pork, and many foods prepared by traditional Jewish, Italian, or Polish cooks. Many patients attempt to substitute condiments in place of salt and are not aware that ketchup, hot sauce, etc. have high salt concentrations. A no-added-salt diet, which contains approximately 2 to 4 g of sodium, will suffice for most patients in compensated heart failure. Patients with poorly compensated heart failure may require a diet that contains 500 mg to 1 g of sodium. The physician must take the time to discuss diet sympathetically and meticulously with the patient or should refer the patient to a dietician. Guidelines for planning these diets and a list of foods to be avoided by patients being treated for heart failure are given in Table 62.9 of Chapter 62.

Patients with heart failure may wish to know whether they can continue to drink *alcoholic beverages*. In any patient with a cardiomyopathy apparently related to prolonged heavy alcohol use, total abstinence from alcohol may be essential to the management of heart failure. In other patients moderate alcohol use (e.g., wine with meals or a cocktail before dinner) is reasonable.

Drugs That Promote Positive Sodium Balance

A number of drugs can promote a positive sodium balance: (a) Renal sodium retention may be caused by corticosteroids, estrogens, and nonsteroidal anti-inflammatory agents other than aspirin; and (b) some antacid preparations contain a significant amount of sodium (see Table 37.3, Chapter 37). Patients with

heart failure should not receive these drugs, or, if the drugs are necessary, the patients should be monitored for and treated for increased symptoms of heart failure.

Drug Therapy (Table 61.5)

Heart failure is the result of mismatch between preload, afterload, and inotropic state; each of these interrelated factors may be adjusted by use of appropriate measures. Preload may be adjusted by the use of diuretic therapy, salt restriction, and venodilator therapy. Afterload may be adjusted by the control of hypertension and by the use of arteriolar dilating drugs. The inotropic state of the heart may be adjusted by the use of digitalis or by other oral inotropic agents (see page 748).

There are important differences in the approach to treatment of patients whose heart failure is due primarily to systolic dysfunction (dilated left ventricle with decreased ejection fraction) as opposed to those patients whose heart failure is due primarily to diastolic dysfunction (hypertrophied heart and normal or increased ejection fraction, often with a loud S_4) (6, 20). For example, a young patient with failure due to viral myocarditis (primarily systolic failure) will be treated with diuretics, digitalis and/or an angiotensin-converting enzyme inhibitor. A middle-aged patient with ischemic cardiomyopathy is likely to have both systolic dysfunction and variable degrees of diastolic dysfunction; treatment may include diuretics and one or another of an angiotensin-converting enzyme inhibitor, a calcium channel blocker, a long-acting nitrate, and digitalis. Elderly patients with long-standing hypertension occasionally present with congestive failure due to hypertrophic cardiomyopathy with hypercontractility. Vasodilators and digitalis (except for control of supraventricular arrhythmias) are contraindicated in these patients, who respond best to verapamil or diltiazem, β-blockers, and diuretics (20).

Diuretic Drugs

Diuretic drugs are used when it is not possible to treat the underlying cause of heart failure or when signs and symptoms of heart failure persist despite treatment of the underlying condition (19). Diuretics reduce symptoms of circulatory congestion by increasing sodium and water excretion. If the contractility of the heart is depressed, the ventricular function curve is relatively flat and preload may be reduced with little change in ventricular function unless the reduction is excessive (Fig. 61.2). The goal of diuretic therapy is to reach the patient's dry weight. Physiologically, this is the weight at which signs of peripheral congestion are substantially relieved and at which the left ventricular filling pressure remains at the preload reserve (i.e., function is optimized via the Frank-Starling principle). Clinically, this is the weight at which peripheral edema is substantially resolved, and a significant increase in diuretic dose is necessary to achieve further weight loss. If the heart has dilated because of fluid overload, the decrease in ventricular wall stress

Table 61.5.
Characteristics of Selected Diuretic Drugs[a]

Generic Name	Brand Name	Available Preparations	Usual Daily Dose (mg)	Frequency of Dose/Day	Onset of Effect	Peak Effect	Duration
Chlorothiazide	Diuril	500-mg tablet	500–1000	1–2	1 hour	4 hours	6–12 hours
Hydrochloro-thiazide	Generic, Hydro-Diuril, Esidrix	25/50/100-mg tablet	25–100	1–2	2 hours	4 hours	12 hours or more
Chlorthalidone	Generic, Hygroton	50/100-mg tablet	50–100	1	2 hours	6 hours	24 hours
Metolazone	Diulo, Zaroxolyn	2.5/5/10 mg tablet	2.5–10	1	1 hour	2 hours	12–24 hours
Furosemide	Lasix	20/40/80 mg tablet	20–160	1–2	1 hour	1–2 hours	6 hours
Ethacrynic acid	Edecrin	50-mg tablet	50–100	1–2	30 minutes	2 hours	6–8 hours
Bumetanide	Bumex	0.5/1 mg tablet	0.5–2	1	30 minutes to 1 hour	1–2 hours	4 hours
Triamterene	Dyrenium	100-mg capsule	100–300	1–2	2 hours	6–8 hours	12–16 hours
Spironolactone	Aldactone	25 mg tablet	50–400	1–2	Gradual onset	2–3 days after initiation of therapy	2–3 days after cessation of therapy
Amiloride	Midamor	5-mg tablet	5–10	1	2 hours	6–10 hours	24 hours

[a]Modified from Frazier H, Yager H: The clinical use of diuretics. *N Engl J Med* 288:246, 455, 1973.

(i.e., afterload) and the improvement in ventricular contraction pattern brought about by a decrease in heart size after diuresis often lead to a prompt improvement in ventricular function.

There are three classes of diuretics in common use: thiazides (hydrochlorothiazide) and thiazide-like agents (metolazone), the so-called loop diuretics (ethacrynic acid, furosemide, and bumetanide), and the potassium-sparing diuretics (spironolactone, triamterene, and amiloride) (Table 61.5) (see also Chapter 46).

The thiazides act on the distal convoluted tubule (diluting segment) of the nephron; although their mechanism of action is unknown, they inhibit sodium transport and they cause a moderate increase in the excretion of sodium, chloride, and water. Potassium and hydrogen losses are accentuated because of the increased delivery of solute to the even more distal portion of the nephron where potassium secretion occurs and is modulated by aldosterone. Thiazide-like agents such as metolazone may act on both the diluting segment and the more distal segments of the nephron and may be particularly effective in patients with very low renal blood flow. The loop diuretics inhibit tubular resorption of chloride and sodium in the thick ascending limb of the loop of Henle. These diuretics are potent and result in a substantial increase in the excretion of sodium, chloride, and water. Like thiazides, the loop diuretics increase the delivery of solute to the more distal portion of the nephron where potassium and hydrogen secretion is accentuated.

Potassium-sparing diuretics by themselves are only weak diuretics. However, they may be especially useful in combination with a thiazide or loop diuretic in preventing hypokalemia or when a patient becomes refractory to the more potent diuretics. The effect of thiazides and loop diuretics may be dampened by the resorption of sodium in the distal segment since they act proximal to the portion of the distal nephron where aldosterone influences sodium resorption. Spironolactone is structurally similar to aldosterone and competitively inhibits aldosterone binding to cellular receptors. Triamterene and amiloride block sodium resorption and potassium excretion but do not compete with aldosterone or even depend on its presence to be effective. These diuretics may cause life-threatening increases in the serum potassium level. Patients must not receive potassium supplementation while taking them. Also, patients with renal failure are at increased risk for developing hyperkalemia if given these diuretics. In any patient serum potassium must be monitored carefully when these agents are used.

Use of diuretic drugs. Diuretic therapy should start with the lowest effective dose of a thiazide compound. Generic hydrochlorothiazide is the drug of choice. It is inexpensive, effective, and the tablet is small and easy to swallow. Many patients with mild heart failure may effectively control symptoms by use of the drug every other day or three times a week. Patients with progressive disease may become resistant gradually to the effect of thiazides and may require doses of 100 mg of hydrochlorothiazide a day for control of edema and dyspnea. Patients become resistant to thiazides when there is significant renal failure (such as when the serum creatinine is > 2 to 4 mg/dl) or when renal blood flow is decreased markedly, as it may be in severe heart failure. There is no evidence that if one thiazide has failed, another will be effective. Metolazone, however, may be effective in such circumstances, even in patients with very low renal blood flow.

When a patient becomes resistant to thiazide or has complications of thiazide therapy (see below), the loop diuretics—furosemide, ethacrynic acid, or bumetanide—should be prescribed. These drugs are often effective in relatively low doses. Furosemide is the most popular of the three drugs because gastrointestinal and ototoxic side effects are more common with ethacrynic acid, especially in higher doses, and because bumetanide is more expensive (bumetanide is, however, the least ototoxic of the loop diuretics). Furosemide should be started at a dose of 20 mg daily and increased as necessary for control of symptoms. A single dose should be administered each day, usually in the morning, although patients in severe failure may sleep better at night if the dose is given in the late afternoon.

Doses of furosemide higher than 160 to 240 mg/day are rarely required and may cause ototoxicity. When more than 160 to 240 mg/day are required, however, the patient becomes at risk for ototoxicity and the physician should reconsider whether the etiology of heart failure has been accurately determined and whether correctable causes of heart failure have been dealt with. If so, it is at this point (if not previously prescribed for potassium control) that a potassium-sparing diuretic—spironolactone or triamterene—should be added to the drug regimen. The addition of a thiazide diuretic in modest doses (25 to 50 mg of hydrochlorothiazide or 2.5 to 5 mg of metolazone) may markedly potentiate the effect of loop diuretics, leading to a rapid mobilization of fluid and thereby allowing these patients to be managed in an ambulatory setting. Careful monitoring of electrolyte levels is essential, and the diuretic dose should be reduced when the desired effect is achieved (14).

Side Effects of Diuretics

Hypokalemia (see Chapter 46). The thiazide and loop diuretics have marked kaliuretic effects and, especially in edematous patients, hypokalemia is a common complication of the use of diuretic therapy. Hypokalemia may lead to fatigue/depression and muscle cramps and frequently precipitates digitalis toxicity. A high sodium diet will often lead to hypokalemia in patients taking loop diuretics because of sodium-potassium exchange in the distal tubule and the collecting duct of the nephron. Patients with persistent hypokalemia should be encouraged to adhere to a low sodium diet. If hypokalemia persists despite a low sodium diet, then a potassium-sparing diuretic such as spironolactone or triamterene should be added, or the patient should be treated with an angiotensin-converting enzyme inhibitor (see below). Triamterene is probably the drug of choice since it has a more rapid onset of action and may be less expensive than spironolactone if more than three tablets/day of spironolactone are required. Because these medications will ordinarily be used in patients who have received potassium supplementation (although such supplementation should be discontinued before the administration of a potassium-sparing diuretic) and who may have renal failure, the patient's electrolyte concentration must be carefully monitored when these medications are started, when the dose is adjusted, or when there is a change in the severity of the heart failure. Potassium supplementation should be stopped when the drugs are prescribed, and the level of serum potassium should be measured again 1 week later. The usual dose of triamterene is 100 mg, one to three times a day; and of spironolactone, 25 to 100 mg, once or twice daily. The indication for and use of potassium salts in patients taking diuretics is fully discussed in Chapter 46.

Contraction of the Extracellular Volume. Diuretics are therapeutically effective by causing a net loss of sodium, chloride, and water. If the response is excessive, depletion of the extracellular fluid compartment (the maintenance of which depends on sodium and chloride) will occur. This may have catastrophic consequences such as hypotension (or postural hypotension) with precipitation of ischemia due to changes in cerebral, coronary, or renal blood flow. This complication is especially common when loop diuretics are used but may occur after the use of thiazides or of combination diuretics. The patient should be monitored carefully, therefore, for evidence of excessive contraction of extracellular volume by assessment of weight, the presence or absence of edema, the degree of fullness of the neck veins, and by assessment of the blood pressure and pulse. Not infrequently a dose of a diuretic that initiated diuresis will need to be reduced once cardiac compensation has improved.

Acid-Base Disturbance. By their different actions on the nephron, diuretics have an effect on acid-base balance. The thiazides and the loop diuretics are often associated with the generation and maintenance of a metabolic alkalosis. This usually requires no therapy. To correct the alkalosis, the associated volume and potassium deficiency would have to be corrected. If the volume were replenished, the effect of the diuretic would be negated. Therefore usually only potassium chloride supplements are given (see Chapter 46). If the alkalosis is thought to be detrimental, for example in patients with respiratory failure, then the diuretic should be discontinued.

Potassium-sparing diuretics may be associated with diminished hydrogen ion excretion and therefore with a mild metabolic acidosis. This is usually of no consequence and requires no treatment.

Hyponatremia. The loop diuretics and the thiazides may be occasionally associated with hyponatremia by impairing free water clearance, and therefore caution is especially appropriate in patients who tend to consume relatively large quantities of fluid. These diuretics also may be associated with hyponatremia when the extracellular volume has become contracted (a potent stimulus to the release of antidiuretic hormone) and fluid intake has not been restricted. In both of these instances, water restriction is mandatory. Usually this hyponatremia may be corrected by restricting water intake to less than 1 liter/day, but occasionally more severe restriction is necessary. Finally, the thiazides may be rarely associated with hyponatremia in euvolemic patients who also are severely potassium depleted. This situation resembles clinically the syndrome of inappropriate secretion of antidiuretic hormone, although the exact mechanism of this complication is not fully known. The drug must be withdrawn should this complication develop.

Hyperuricemia. Thiazides, loop diuretics, and triamterene commonly elevate the concentration of serum urate by blocking urate secretion by the proximal renal tubules and/or by enhancing resorption through contraction of extracellular volume. Symptomatic gout, however, is not usual, nor is the elevation of uric acid likely to cause renal injury or stone formation. Therefore, unless gout does occur, treatment is not necessary.

Hyperglycemia. Thiazides and, less commonly, loop diuretics may cause glucose intolerance. Hypoglycemic therapy may be required (or changed, in diabetics already receiving a hypoglycemic agent) if the diuretic is to be continued (see Chapter 72).

Ototoxicity. Loop diuretics may impair hearing, usually reversibly, especially if large doses are taken or if the patient has renal insufficiency.

Other Effects. Thiazides are occasionally associated with a hypersensitivity-induced small vessel vasculitis (Chapter 51), with thrombocytopenia (Chapter 51), and with hypercalcemia (Chapter 74) and may be associated with impotence. Furosemide in high doses has been associated with the development of interstitial nephritis and renal failure, especially in patients with marked proteinuria. Spironolactone, a weak androgen antagonist, commonly causes gynecomastia and may reduce libido or even cause impotence; these side effects resolve within a few months of discontinuing the drug.

When diuretics have not adequately controlled the signs and symptoms of congestive heart failure, additional medication should be considered.

Inotropic Agents: Digitalis

Inotropic drugs may help to restore cardiac compensation by increasing the inotropic state, or contractility of cardiac muscle, thereby increasing the ejection fraction at a given preload and afterload, as described above (see page 738). The only inotropic drugs currently available for oral use are the digitalis glycosides.

The digitalis drugs appear to improve contractility by increasing the delivery of calcium to the contractile apparatus of the heart. Digitalis inhibits sodium-potassium ATPase, and it is postulated that this results in an increase of influx of both calcium and sodium into the myocardial cell (17).

Indications for the use of digitalis drugs. Despite more than 200 years of clinical experience with digitalis preparations, the indications for digitalis therapy remain controversial, and there are conflicting reports regarding the utility of digitalis preparations in acute and chronic heart failure. Digitalis preparations may improve ventricular performance by moderating the heart rate of patients in atrial fibrillation or atrial flutter and by increasing ventricular contractility in some patients who are in heart failure. However, the degree to which digitalis preparations increase ventricular contractility is modest; the toxic to therapeutic ratio is small, and the drug must be pushed to near toxic limits in many cases before significant clinical effect is seen. Furthermore, the indiscriminate use of digitalis as a first line medication for control of heart failure has led to its use in many patients in whom heart

failure is not due primarily to a decrease in the inotropic state of myocardial muscle. These include patients whose heart failure is due to valvular heart disease or to systemic hypertension, patients in whom heart failure is due to restrictions to ventricular filling (e.g., hypertrophic cardiomyopathy or pericardial tamponade), and patients in whom symptoms of fatigue are due to a decreased cardiac output induced by excessive diuresis.

Recommendations for use of digitalis compounds :

1. Digitalis glycosides should be prescribed only for patients in congestive heart failure with dilated hearts (a cardiothoracic ratio > 0.5 suggests dilation; echocardiography, however, is the most precise way of demonstrating cardiac chamber size and thickness) and in whom the symptoms of heart failure appear to be due to a decreased inotropic state of heart muscle (usually reflected by an ejection fraction of less than 40 to 45% or the presence of an S_3 gallop). It is also a useful drug for certain types of arrhythmias (see Chapter 59).

2. The practitioner should become familiar with the purified glycoside, digoxin, and should use it exclusively. It is well absorbed, can be used parenterally if necessary, and has an intermediate duration of action (half-life of 36 to 48 hours). The Burroughs Wellcome preparation of digoxin, Lanoxin, is the preferred digoxin preparation, because of variable absorption of many other brands. Digitalis elixir in capsules, Lanoxicaps (0.05-, 0.10-, and 0.20-mg capsules) may be even more dependably absorbed and may be useful when careful titration of the dose is important. Digitalization is best accomplished in an ambulatory patient by daily administration of the drug at the maintenance dosage (see below). Within four or five half-lives of the drug (approximately 7 days) full digitalization is ordinarily achieved.

3. The effect of digitalis on the patient's condition should be monitored and reassessed periodically. If there is no objective decrease in heart size within 1 or 2 months or increase in exercise capacity after a trial of digitalis therapy, the drug should probably be discontinued. Before doing that, however, serum digoxin concentration (see below) should be measured to be certain that adequate blood levels are being attained. Digitalis should be used cautiously in older patients and in any patient known to have impaired renal function. There is no evidence that elderly patients are intrinsically more sensitive to digitalis compounds, but they have a smaller body mass, often have impaired renal excretion of the drug, and have higher serum levels for a given oral dose of the drug.

4. The average dose of digoxin is 0.25 mg/day (of Lanoxicaps, 0.20 mg/day). In patients older than 65 years or in patients with known impairments of renal function, doses of 0.125 mg/day of digoxin (0.1 mg of Lanoxicap) should be prescribed.

5. Digitalis may interact with other medications, and

because of its low therapeutic ratio, the possibility of an interaction should be considered when any medication is added to the regimen of a patient already taking digoxin (1). The administration of quinidine causes a decrease in excretion of digoxin, which may lead to digitalis toxicity; similar effects have been seen when digitalis is prescribed along with either of the calcium channel blockers, verapamil or diltiazem (but not with nifedipine). The use of thiazides and the loop diuretics may lead to digitalis toxicity either because of increased retention of these drugs secondary to decreased renal blood flow or (and) because of increased sensitivity to digitalis as the result of hypokalemia. Cholestyramine and neomycin and some antacids impair digoxin absorption and may result in a subtherapeutic effect.

Recognition and treatment of digitalis toxicity. Digitalis toxicity commonly is caused by administration of too much digitalis or by overdiuresis (often with associated hypokalemia), by intercurrent development of renal insufficiency, or by administration of drugs that interfere with digitalis excretion. Digitalis toxicity is especially common in older patients in an ambulatory practice. Approximately 10% of patients in the 7th and 8th decades being seen regularly by a physician will be taking digitalis (17).

The manifestations of digitalis toxicity are protean and may be difficult to recognize in older patients and in patients whose normal baseline level of function is not familiar to the practitioner. They include changes in the cardiovascular system, the gastrointestinal tract, and the central nervous system. The most frequent cardiac manifestations of digitalis toxicity are progressive slowing and regularization of the heart rate (i.e., development of a nodal rhythm) of patients in atrial fibrillation, and frequent premature ventricular contractions (PVCs). Digitalis toxicity should be suspected in any older patient who is taking digitalis and has PVCs or any patient in atrial fibrillation whose heart rate falls below approximately 60 and becomes regular. Because digitalis both increases automaticity and decreases conduction through the AV node, paroxysmal atrial tachycardia (PAT) with block may be seen. The peripheral pulse in PAT with block is usually 100 to 120 beats/minute (see Chapter 59). Cardiac toxicity may occur in the absence of other signs or symptoms of digitalis overdose.

Gastrointestinal side effects are common manifestations of digitoxicity. They include anorexia, mild nausea, and occasionally vomiting and diarrhea.

Digitalis may cause changes in the sensorium ranging from mild confusional states to frank delirium and psychosis. In an older patient it may be difficult to determine, without stopping the drug, whether these symptoms are due to primary cerebral disease or to digitalis excess.

The diagnosis of digitalis toxicity is based on clinical and laboratory findings. If symptoms compatible with digitalis toxicity are present, especially in an elderly patient who is also taking a diuretic, the drug should be stopped immediately. The patient should be examined in approximately 3 days and the symptoms should be reassessed. If symptoms have abated, a presumptive diagnosis of digitoxicity is warranted.

At the time of presentation, it is reasonable to measure the serum digoxin concentration. That is done in many commercial and hospital laboratories by use of a radioimmunoassay. It is important that the quality control of the laboratory be known, to ensure reliability of the procedure. An adequately digitalized patient will have a serum digoxin concentration of approximately 0.7 to 1.4 ng/ml; most toxic patients have concentrations above 2.0 ng/ml. However, if a patient has symptoms compatible with digitalis toxicity and his serum digoxin level is within the normal range, toxicity has not been ruled out since at therapeutic levels hypokalemic (or hypercalcemic) patients may become digitoxic. Most patients with digitoxicity can be managed by temporary withdrawal of the medication and by reinstitution of it at a lower dose. Often, diuretic therapy must also be modified and/or potassium supplements administered. However, patients with symptomatic arrhythmias are best hospitalized for a few days so that they can be monitored closely.

Any patient who has become digitalis-toxic should have the indications for digitalis therapy carefully reviewed. In many cases the drug may be stopped without any apparent change in the patient's condition.

Vasodilator Therapy

A major advance in the treatment of heart failure in the past 10 years has been the introduction into clinical practice of vasodilator therapy. In ambulatory practice, vasodilator drugs should be considered for patients whose heart failure cannot be controlled by diuretics and digitalis.

Physiological rationale for vasodilator therapy. The syndrome of heart failure is not due to left ventricular dysfunction per se, but to the compensatory responses triggered by the inadequate response of the left ventricle to stress (see above, page 738). The net result is an increase in both left ventricular preload and afterload. These compensatory mechanisms probably developed in the course of evolution to protect against circulatory collapse due to blood loss. In the setting of left ventricular dysfunction, however, these potentially lifesaving compensatory mechanisms lead to a further deterioration of cardiac function (Fig. 61.4). The judicious use of vasodilator agents may promptly optimize cardiac function and may improve the functional state of patients with chronic heart failure.

The hemodynamic effects of *venodilator drugs* and diuretics are essentially the same. Both classes of drugs cause a decrease in preload, thereby relieving symptoms of vascular congestion (see Fig. 61.2). Venodilators are most useful in patients with severe heart failure in whom preload reserve is exceeded during exercise, leading to an increase in LVEDP and to pulmonary vascular congestion. This may occur in as-

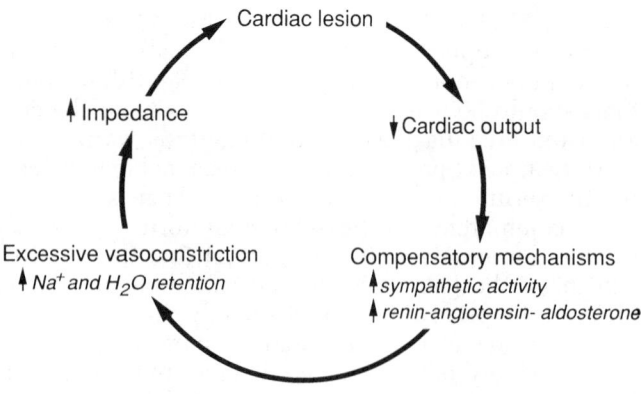

Vicious circle in congestive heart failure

Figure 61.4. From Wester PO, Dyckner T: Intracellular electrolytes in cardiac failure. *Acta Med Scand* 219(Suppl 707):33, 1986.

sociation with ischemia in patients with ischemic heart disease or in association with advanced disease in patients with cardiomyopathy or with valvular heart disease. These drugs should not be used in patients with heart failure due to restriction to ventricular filling (e.g., hypertrophic cardiomyopathy) and should be used with caution in patients with aortic stenosis in whom a reduction in preload may lead to a marked decrease in cardiac output.

Arteriolar vasodilators increase cardiac output by decreasing afterload (i.e., decreasing ventricular wall stress during contraction), thereby allowing the myocardium to contract more efficiently and increasing the ejection fraction and cardiac output (see Fig. 61.3). These medications are most effective in patients with severe peripheral and central congestion, who have signs of peripheral hypoperfusion, such as cool hands and peripheral cyanosis. It is important to note that arteriolar vasodilators increase cardiac output only if preload remains near the preload reserve (see Fig. 61.3). With afterload reduction the left ventricle unloads more efficiently, and volume shifts from the central to the peripheral venous circulation, thereby lowering preload. If preload drops significantly, cardiac output cannot be maintained, and the blood pressure falls. Thus, in an ambulatory setting, vasodilators must be used with caution, and often with a concomitant adjustment of diuretic dosage.

Four classes of vasodilators are available: drugs that act directly on smooth muscle, drugs that act by blocking the α-adrenergic system, drugs that act by blocking calcium channels, and drugs that block angiotensin-converting enzyme (Table 61.6). The choice of an appropriate agent and the effective use of that agent depends upon an understanding of the physiological properties of these drugs.

Smooth muscle dilators. Nitroglycerin in various formulations is an effective venodilator at the low end of the dose range and a mixed veno- and arteriolar dilator at higher doses. The practitioner should be familiar with the use of nitrates in four forms (see also Chapter 57): a short-acting sublingual nitrate, long-acting nitrates taken orally, nitroglycerin in a petrolatum base, and nitroglycerin dermal patches. *Sublingual nitroglycerin* is generally used in a dose of 0.4 mg. The medication is sensitive to body heat, light, and moisture and must be kept in a sealed brown glass or plastic container. Patients should be encouraged to purchase new sublingual nitroglycerin every 6 months to be sure that the medication is active. Sublingual nitroglycerin may be used liberally to control symptoms of pulmonary congestion during normal physical activity such as walking up stairs, shopping, and so forth. Small bottles of 25 tablets may be prescribed and should be kept in strategic locations about the patient's home, car, and workplace. An effective long-acting medication is isosorbide dinitrate (generic, Isordil, Sorbitrate) in doses of at least 20 mg orally, four times a day. If symptoms have not improved within a few days, the dosage should be increased. Doses as high as 40 to 60 mg orally, four times a day, may be used safely depending upon the patient's blood pressure response. Before and after each increase in the dose, the patient should be checked for orthostatic hypotension. If there is a drop of more than 15 to 20 mm Hg systolic blood pressure 3 minutes after going from the supine to standing position, the dosage should be decreased slightly. *Nitroglycerin,* 2% in a petrolatum base, gives effective long-acting venodilation but is messy and may be difficult for some patients to apply. It is best used under an occlusive polyethylene wrapping. The usual dose is 1 to 4 inches, four times daily. Again, titration of the dose depends on whether or not heart failure is improved and on whether orthostasis develops. *Nitroglycerin dermal patches* give sustained high blood levels of nitrate over 24 hours. Tolerance to the effect of sustained levels of nitroglycerin develops after 7 to 10 days of continuous use of nitroglycerin patches, and patients should be advised to remove the patch at bedtime and reapply a fresh patch upon awakening. The usual dose is a 5 to 10 mg/24-hour patch, applied to the skin of the chest. The patient need not be concerned about having the patch in contact with water during bathing or swimming; if it does fall off, however, a new one should be applied at a different site. (The patient will receive an instruction booklet with the patch).

The most common side effects of nitrate therapy are headache and nausea. Skin irritation is occasionally seen with the use of nitrol paste or dermal patches. Headache can usually be controlled by aspirin or acetaminophen, and it usually abates after several days of nitrate therapy. Gastrointestinal side effects can occasionally be eliminated by switching to a different preparation of long-acting nitroglycerin or switching to nitroglycerin patches. Rubbing alcohol should be used to remove nitroglycerine dermal patches. If skin irritation develops, a different brand of patch should be tried (16).

Hydralazine is an effective direct arteriolar vasodilator. In properly selected patients and when used in effective doses, hydralazine may increase the car-

Table 61.6.
Vasodilators Useful in Treating Heart Failure

Site of Action	Drugs	Venodilation/Ar-teriolar Dilation	Available Tablet Strength	Usual Dose	Effectiveness after 1 year
Smooth Muscle	Isosorbide dinitrate (Isordil)	+ + +/+	10, 20, 40 mg	20–60 mg every 6 hours	?
	Topical nitroglycerine[a]			2% paste, 1–4 inches every 6 hours	
				Dermal patches, 10–30 cm²/day	
	Hydralazine (Apresoline)	0/+ + +	10, 25, 50, 100 mg	25–50 mg every 6 hours	?
	Hydralazine plus long acting nitrate	+ + +/+ + +		As above, in combination	+ + +
α-Adrenergic blockade	Prazosin (Minipress)	+ +/+ +	1, 2, 5 mg	3–5 mg every 6 hours	+
Calcium channel blockers	Nifedipine (Procardia)	+/+ + +	10, 20 mg	10–30 mg every 6 hours	?
	Diltiazem (Cardizem)	+/+ +	30, 60 mg	30–60 mg every 6 to 8 hours	?
	Verapamil (Calan, Is-optin)	+/+ +	40, 80, 120 mg	80–120 mg every 8 hours	?
Angiotensin converting enzyme inhibitors	Captopril (Capoten)	+ +/+ + +	12.5, 25, 50 mg	6.25–50 mg every 6 hours	+ + +
	Enalapril (Vasotec)	+ +/+ + +	2.5, 5, 10, 20 mg	5–20 mg every 24 hours	+ + +
	Lisinopril (Zestril, Prinivil)	+ +/+ + +	5, 10, 20 mg	5–20 mg every 24 hours	?

[a] In order to avoid development of tolerance, an 8- to 12-hr period without topical nitrates should be scheduled daily. Usually, this means applying nitroglycerine patches upon awakening and removing them at bedtime.

diac output as much as 2-fold. This improved cardiac output may persist chronically in patients who respond initially.

Hydralazine for afterload reduction must be used cautiously in ambulatory patients. Doses of hydralazine less than 200 mg/day are rarely effective. If the patient's preload is not near maximum, hydralazine may cause a marked fall in blood pressure. In an ambulatory setting it is safest to start hydralazine in a dose of 10 mg and to observe the patient in the office for approximately 2 hours for signs of orthostatic hypotension. The patient can then be given a dose of 25 mg every 6 hours and observed the following day. If orthostatic hypotension or tachycardia is not observed, the dose is increased to 50 mg every 6 hours. At an effective dose the patient's handshake, previously cool, becomes warm and firm, and the patient experiences a general sense of increased well-being and of decreased fatigue. The increased cardiac output may lead to an increase in renal blood flow, and diuretics often become more effective. If signs of peripheral vasodilation are not achieved, the dose of hydralazine should be increased to as high as 100 mg, four times a day. The major complication of hydralazine is a reversible lupus-like syndrome. However, this syndrome usually does not become apparent until 18 to 24 months of treatment with hydralazine in doses above 200 mg/day. Because of the severity of their heart disease, most patients who require such large doses of hydralazine for afterload treatment of congestive heart failure will not live long enough to develop a lupus-like syndrome. Additional information about the properties of hydralazine and other vasodilators is provided in Chapter 62.

Hydralazine is now used chiefly in patients who are unable to tolerate any of the angiotensin-converting enzyme inhibitors (see below) or in whom the relatively modest cost advantage of generic hydralazine is an important consideration.

In severe heart failure it may be desirable to achieve both venous and arteriolar dilation simultaneously. This may be done by the use of hydralazine and a long-acting nitrate such as isosorbide dinitrate, in doses as described above. The combination of hydralazine and long-acting nitroglycerin has been shown to prolong survival in patients with severe heart failure treated concomitantly with diuretics and digitalis. Their use has been largely superseded by the angiotensin-converting enzyme inhibitors (see below).

Sympathetic blockers. Prazosin (Minipress) is an α-sympathetic blocker with both veno- and arteriodilatory actions and may be useful as a single agent with both preload and afterload reducing properties. The usual dose of prazosin is 2 to 5 mg every 6 hours, although some patients may require larger doses for effective afterload reduction. The effect of prazosin is often only apparent during exercise, and many patients appear to develop tachyphylaxis to the drug. Additional information about prazosin is found in Chapter 62.

Calcium channel blockers. These drugs interfere with contractility of smooth muscle by blocking the entry of calcium into muscle cells, resulting in vasodilation, especially of the arterioles. All of the currently available calcium channel blockers also cause cardiac depression. *Nifedipine*, 10 to 30 mg every 6 to 8 hours, may be the most effective of this class of drugs in patients with ischemic cardiomyopathy, due to its anti-ischemic and vasodilatory properties. In this situation afterload reduction is predominant, and because the negative inotropic effect is relatively slight, it may be used even in patients with severe left ventricular (LV) dysfunction [ejection fraction (EF) less than 30%]. *Verapamil* is an arteriolar vasodilator that has a significant antihypertensive effect. It may be particularly useful, in doses of 80 to 120 mg three times a day, in patients with heart failure due to a restriction to cardiac filling caused by hypertrophic cardiomyopathy with hypercontractility, but it should not be used, because of its negative inotropic effect, in patients with congestive cardiomyopathy and an ejection fraction less than 40%. Common side effects of calcium channel blockers include headache, hypotension, nausea, and fluid retention. Often *diltiazem* may be safely used in patients with ischemic cardiomyopathy and relatively mild impairment of LV function (EF from 30 to 40%) and in patients with hypertrophic cardiomyopathy.

Angiotensin-converting enzyme (ACE) inhibitors. As discussed above (page 739), the syndrome of heart failure is due in large part to the stimulation of the renin-angiotensin-aldosterone system by the kidney. ACE inhibitors block the conversion of angiotensin I to angiotensin II, a potent vasoconstrictor and a regulator of renin and aldosterone production. ACE inhibitors cause a marked decrease in angiotensin II levels approximately 30 minutes after administration. They are thus effective vasodilators and also block aldosterone-mediated salt and water retention. ACE inhibitors appear to be the most effective vasodilators currently available and they retain their effectiveness after long-term use (10).

The currently available ACE inhibitors and their dose ranges are described in Table 61.6. Captopril is most useful for initiating ACE inhibitor therapy because of its relatively short half-life and wide dosage range. In patients with obvious signs of circulatory congestion a dose of 12.5 mg of captopril should be given and the blood pressure checked in 1 hour. The usual effective dose of captopril for heart failure is 12.5 to 50 mg three to four times a day. Patients who are hyponatremic or at their dry weight should be started at 6.25 mg (one-half of a 12.5-mg cross-scored tablet) and their diuretic dose adjusted (because the danger of symptomatic hypotension is greater in such situations). Patients who are stable and have relatively mild heart failure (EF, 30 to 40%; creatinine, less than 2.0) may respond well to enalapril, 5 to 10 mg/day, or lisinopril, 10 mg/day in one dose. Because of their antialdosterone effect, potassium supplementation may need to be decreased, and potassium levels should be monitored a week or 2 after initiation of ACE inhibitor therapy.

Side effects. The most common side effect of all ACE inhibitors is cough. A persistent dry hacking cough is seen in 2 to 10% of patients treated with ACE inhibitors. Decreasing the dose of ACE inhibitor will occasionally decrease the severity of the cough. Switching to a different ACE inhibitor is only occasionally helpful. The pathophysiological basis for the cough is not well understood although it has been suggested that the increased levels of bradykinin produced by ACE

inhibitors may irritate the larynx and cause the cough. Patients who have had significant symptomatic relief of heart failure after ACE inhibitor therapy may wish to try continuing the drug at a lower dose. In some cases, the drug must be discontinued, in which case therapy with hydralazine and long-acting nitrates should be considered (see above). Other side effects are uncommon. The ones most often seen are skin rash in patients taking an ACE inhibitor with a sulphydral group (captopril) and angioedema in patients taking long-acting ACE inhibitors (enalapril, lisinopril). Taste alteration and neutropenia are rarely seen. Proteinuria and worsening renal failure are occasionally seen in patients with significant pre-existing renal disease who have a significant blood pressure drop after starting ACE inhibitors (11).

General recommendations for use of afterload reduction therapy in an ambulatory setting:

1. Select patients whose heart failure is due to decreased left ventricular function, with evidence of both central and peripheral congestion.
2. ACE inhibitors appear to be the most effective agents for long-term use in an ambulatory setting. When medication cost is an important issue, hydralazine plus a long-acting nitrate (isosorbide dinitrate, nitroglycerin ointment or patch) may be used at approximately one-half the cost of full dose of an ACE inhibitor.
3. Patient weight should be measured and signs of circulatory congestion (jugular venous distention and hepatojugular reflux) should be assessed *each time* the physician sees the patient. Symptomatic postural hypotension is a frequent complication of vasodilator therapy in patients in whom diuresis has been excessive.

β-Blocker Therapy

β-Blockade may be useful in the treatment of heart failure due to the following conditions: thyrotoxicosis, severe hypertension responsive to β-blockade therapy, hypertrophic cardiomyopathy, and in patients with failure due to recurrent ischemia. The combination of β-blockade therapy with nitrate therapy may be effective in patients with ischemic cardiomyopathy and chest pain. In these cases, β-blockade therapy is given until the resting heart rate falls below 70 beats/minute and does not show a significant increase with mild to moderate exercise. This usually requires relatively high doses of propranolol (e.g., 160 mg daily in divided doses). Lower doses may be effective in patients with depressed hepatic blood flow or function due to congestive heart failure. β-Blockade therapy should not be used in patients with uncompensated or poorly compensated heart failure and should be used with caution, if at all, in patients with bronchospasm. Small doses of β-blocker (15 mg of metoprolol) have been shown in some studies to be of benefit in patients with congestive cardiomyopathy, but this use is experimental.

Importance of Control of Hypertension in Patients in Heart Failure

Hypertension increases ventricular wall stress, and therefore the afterload on the heart, and reduces the cardiac output, especially as the heart begins to fail. It is essential, therefore, that hypertension be controlled in patients in heart failure. This subject is discussed in detail in Chapter 62.

Home Oxygen Therapy

Patients with severe end-stage heart failure and arterial oxygen desaturation at rest due to low cardiac output or to concomitant pulmonary disease may often feel more comfortable with the use of home oxygen. Patients who require home oxygen therapy because of congestive heart failure rarely survive for more than 6 months to a year. The most efficient way to administer oxygen therapy at home is by means of tanks delivered to the house. This form of therapy is paid for in part by Medicare, Medicaid, and most private insurance plans. The physician should obtain an arterial blood gas determination to confirm the hypoxia before oxygen is prescribed.

Anticoagulation Therapy

Patients in severe chronic congestive heart failure are at great risk for pulmonary and peripheral emboli. The incidence of peripheral arterial embolization in these patients may be as high as 10%/year. A patient with a markedly dilated left ventricular cavity or a patient with a left ventricular aneurysm, especially if in atrial fibrillation, should be considered for treatment with coumarin anticoagulants (see Chapter 52). However, such therapy may be hazardous in patients in severe heart failure who have wide swings in prothrombin time due to liver dysfunction. In such circumstances, the prothrombin time should be checked more frequently, perhaps every few weeks.

Control of Arrhythmias in Heart Failure

Patients with persistent bradycardia due to sick sinus syndrome or complete heart block and patients with persistent tachyarrhythmias may develop heart failure. More than 50% of patients with chronic heart failure die suddenly, presumably of ventricular tachyarrhythmias. Patients with an ejection fraction below 30 to 40% are at an increased risk of sudden death, and frequent PVCs or ventricular tachycardia should be aggressively treated in these patients. The treatment of these problems is discussed in Chapter 59.

Operative Correction of Mechanical Problems Causing Heart Failure

The most commonly encountered surgically correctable problems in patients with chronic congestive failure include valvular heart disease, atrial septal defect (Chapter 60), and ischemic heart disease with ventricular aneurysm. Any patient who is in heart failure due to a surgically correctable cause of myocardial dysfunction should be considered for operative correction, and consultation with a cardiologist should be obtained.

The possibility of a ventricular aneurysm should be considered in any patient with known ischemic heart disease and heart failure. Patients with known ventricular aneurysm who are uncomfortable performing their usual daily tasks should be referred for cardiological consultation and consideration of coronary artery bypass graft surgery with aneurysmectomy. As noted above, radionuclide angiography and two-dimensional echocardiography are the best methods currently available for the noninvasive detection of ventricular aneurysms.

Coronary Artery Bypass Graft Surgery and Congestive Heart Failure

Patients with chronic congestive heart failure and angina pectoris (Chapter 57) should be sent for cardiological consultation. Some of these patients will benefit from coronary artery bypass graft surgery, an aneurysmectomy, or an infarctectomy.

Community Health Services

Many community health services are available to help the physician deal with the patient and the patient deal with his illness (5).

Home Visits

In two situations, home visits by the patient's physician or by a visiting nurse should be considered in the management of a patient in heart failure: (a) when the patient has repeatedly returned to the office with heart failure due to dietary neglect or to failure to use his medications correctly and (b) when the homebound patient's symptoms are so severe (NYHA class IV, Table 61.3) that he is unable to come for an office visit without becoming exhausted.

Information Booklets

The American Heart Association has useful free booklets describing low salt diets and has other booklets describing the management of congestive heart failure to the patient and his family. These booklets may be obtained from a local office of the American Heart Association.

Exercise Programs (Chapter 58)

Graduated regular exercise may increase the exercise tolerance and help to relieve feelings of depression in some patients with heart failure even in patients with severe LV dysfunction (18). However, there is no evidence that myocardial function can be improved by exercise. Isometric exercise should be prescribed with caution in patients in heart failure because of the extra afterload this form of exercise imposes on the heart. Exercise may be contraindicated entirely in left heart failure due to valvular heart disease and in most patients with functional class III or IV congestive heart failure.

PROGNOSIS

The prognosis in heart failure is related to the etiology of the heart failure, the left ventricular ejection fraction, the functional status of the patient, the initial response to treatment, the compliance of the patient, and the patient's age. Most patients in chronic congestive heart failure die suddenly, presumably from ventricular arrhythmia (8) or from complications of cerebral and peripheral emboli.

In the Framingham study, which included heart failure from all causes, the probability of dying within 5 years of onset of heart failure was 62% for men and 42% for women. The etiology of heart failure in most of these patients was hypertension and ischemic heart disease. The mortality from ischemic heart disease complicated by congestive heart failure is related to ventricular function; patients with an ejection fraction of less than 40% have a particularly poor prognosis and may have a mortality rate of 10 to 20%/year (2, 8). Patients with heart failure due to regurgitant valvular lesions have a mortality in the same range. Heart failure complicating uncorrected aortic stenosis is a particularly ominous sign, and the majority of these patients die also within 3 years (Chapter 60).

In general, prognosis is related to the age of the patient and to his functional class (page 739), although there are few studies available in which functional class was accurately determined and prognosis was calculated on a stratified sample. Patients who are functional class II have an annual mortality of approximately 8%. Patients who are functional class III have a slightly higher annual mortality. Patients who are functional class IV rarely live longer than 18 months to 2 years. It is important that the practitioner not venture a prognosis to the patient and family until an optimal level of response to therapy has been achieved.

Prognosis of congestive heart failure has been shown to be improved slightly by the use of vasodilating drugs, including the combination of hydralazine and isosorbide (2) and an ACE inhibitor (3). Whether these drugs are effective beyond a 1- to 2-year follow-up remains to be seen, however. Although vasodilator drugs enable patients with chronic heart failure to be more comfortable in their final years of life, the mortality remains very high (2, 8).

General References

Braunwald E (ed):*Heart Disease: A Textbook of Cardiovascular Medicine*, 3rd ed. Philadelphia, WB Saunders, 1988.
    The current standard text. Exhaustively referenced.
Dollery CT, Corr L: Drug treatment of heart failure. *Br Heart J* 54:234, 1985.

The William Withering Lecture of the Royal College of Physicians, 1985. A clinically useful and very readable summary.
Packer CT (ed): Symposium on therapeutic challenges in the management of congestive heart failure. *J Am Coll Cardiol* 12:, Part I, 262; Part II, 546, 1988.
    Excellent review of controversies regarding major issues in congestive heart failure: use of digoxin, treatment of asymptomatic arrhythmia, the role of neurohormonal activation, and of positive inotropic agents in improving the prognosis of patients with heart failure.
Perloff J, Lindgren K, Groves B: Uncommon or commonly unrecognized causes of heart failure. *Prog Cardiovasc Dis* 12:409, 1970.
    Exhaustive but readable review of commonly unrecognized causes of heart failure.
Ross Jr J: The failing heart and the circulation. *Hosp Prac* 18:151, 1983.

Specific References

1. Bussey HI: Update on the influence of quinidine and other agents on digitalis glycosides. *Am Heart J* 107:143, 1984.
2. Cohn JN, Archibald DG, Ziesche S, et al: Effect of vasodilator therapy on mortality in chronic congestive heart failure. Results of a Veterans Administration Cooperative Study. *N Engl J Med* 314:1547, 1986.
3. The Consensus Trial Study Group: Effects of enalapril on mortality in severe congestive heart failure. *N Engl J Med* 316:1429, 1987.
4. Ducas J, Magder S, McGregor M: Validity of the hepatojugular reflux as a clinical test for congestive heart failure. *Am J Cardiol* 52:1299, 1983.
5. Gibson TC: Community health services in the management of congestive heart failure. *J Chron Dis* 19:133, 1966.
6. Harizi RC, Bianco JA, Alpert J: Diastolic function of the heart in clinical cardiology. *Arch Intern Med* 148:99, 1988.
7. Harlan W, Oberman A, Grimm R, Rosati R: Chronic congestive heart failure in coronary artery disease: clinical criteria. *Ann Intern Med* 86:133, 1977.
8. Kannel WB, Plehn JF, Cupples LA: Cardiac failure and sudden death in the Framingham study. *Am Heart J* 115:869, 1988.
9. Klainer L, Gibson T, White K: The epidemiology of cardiac failure. *J Chron Dis* 18:797, 1965.
10. Kostis JB: Angiotensin-converting enzyme inhibitors. I. Pharmacology *Am Heart J* 116:1580, 1988.
11. Kostis JB: Angiotensin-converting enzyme inhibitors. II. Clinical Use. *Am Heart J* 116:1591, 1988.
12. Likoff MJ, Chandler SL, Kay HR: Clinical determinants of mortality in chronic congestive heart failure secondary to idiopathic dilated or to ischemic cardiomyopathy. *Am J Cardiol* 59:634, 1987.
13. Neuberg GW, Friedman SH, Weiss MB, Herman MV: Cardiopulmonary exercise testing. *Arch Intern Med* 148:2221, 1988.
14. Oster JR, Epstein M, Smoller S: Combined therapy with thiazide-type and loop diuretic agents for resistant sodium retention. *Ann Intern Med* 99:405, 1983.
15. Perlman L, Ferguson S, Bergum K, et al: Precipitation of congestive heart failure: social and emotional factors. *Ann Intern Med* 75:1, 1971.
16. Sharpe N, Coxon R, Webster M, et al: Hemodynamic effects of intermittent transdermal nitroglycerin in chronic congestive heart failure. *Am J Cardiol* 59:895, 1987.
17. Smith TW: Digitalis. Mechanisms of action and clinical use. *N Engl J Med* 318:358, 1988.
18. Squires RW, Lavie CJ, Brandt TR, et al: Cardiac rehabilitation in patients with severe ischemic left ventricular dysfunction. *Mayo Clin Proc* 62:997, 1987.
19. Thier SO: Diuretic mechanisms as a guide to therapy. *Hosp Prac* 22:81, 1987.
20. Topol EJ, Traill TA, Fortuin NJ: Hypertensive hypertrophic cardiomyopathy of the elderly. *N Engl J Med* 312:277, 1985.

C H A P T E R   62

Hypertension

L. RANDOL BARKER, M.D.

In the National Ambulatory Medical Care Survey, hypertension was named as the most common "principal problem" at office visits to internists and general practitioners (see Table 1.3). The ambulatory management of this important condition is a longitudinal process requiring skill in enlisting the patient's cooperation and in selecting, monitoring, and adjusting treatment.

EPIDEMIOLOGY

Hypertension has been studied extensively by epidemiologists and clinicians in recent years. The findings from these studies provide the rationale for the care of the individual patient. Because the patient with high blood pressure is usually asymptomatic, an understanding of the risks attending the condition and of the benefits of treatment is especially important.

Prevalence

As shown in the data from the Health and Nutritional Examination Survey (Fig. 62.1), the prevalence of hypertension, defined as a systolic blood pressure of ≥160 mm Hg or a diastolic blood pressure of ≥95 mm Hg, increases with age, and hypertension is more common in black subjects at all ages. These crude data, based on blood pressure screening on a single occasion, probably overestimate the prevalence of sustained hypertension. Depending upon the patient's age group, on repeat examination 10 to 30% of people who are hypertensive on initial screening will have a nor-

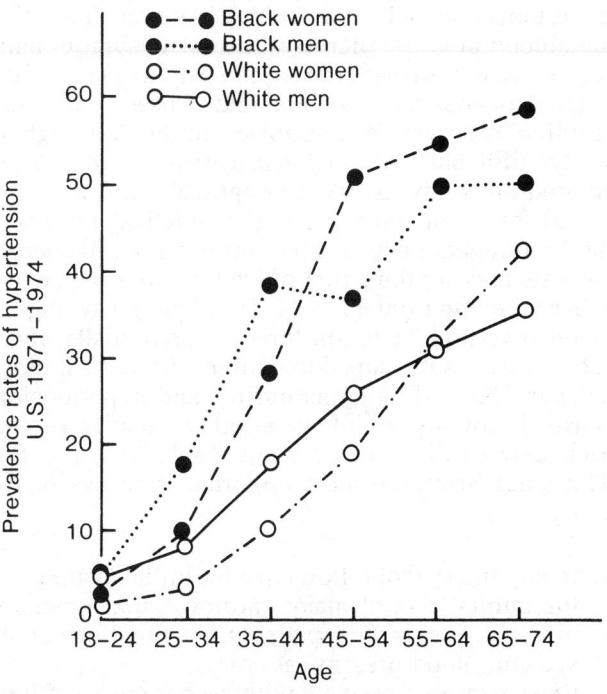

Figure 62.1. The prevalence of hypertension in the United States, defined as a systolic blood pressure of at least 160 mm Hg or a diastolic blood pressure of at least 95 mm Hg. Data from the Health and Nutrition Examination Survey, 1971 to 1974. (From *Advance Data*, Vital and Health Statistics of the National Center for Health Statistics, no. 1, October 18, 1976.)

mal blood pressure, defined as <140 mm Hg over <90 mm Hg (12).

For clinical purposes, it is generally accepted that sustained hypertension is present when the average of two or more diastolic blood pressure readings on two or more occasions are ≥90 mm Hg (32). Of those individuals with hypertension, approximately 75% have *mild hypertension* (diastolic 90 to 104 mm Hg), 15 to 20% have *moderate hypertension* (diastolic 105 to 114 mm Hg), and only 5 to 10% have *severe hypertension* (diastolic ≥115 mm Hg). These prevalence data indicate that in a typical practice decisions must be made more often for patients with mild hypertension than for those with moderate or severe hypertension. The data also explain why the absolute number of morbid events attributable to untreated hypertension in any community is greater in the population of patients with mild hypertension, although the risk of morbid events is much lower in this group than in the other two groups.

The following additional categories for adults 18 years and older have been recognized since 1984 by the Joint National Committee (JNC) on Detection, Evaluation, and Treatment of High Blood Pressure (32): *high normal blood pressure* (diastolic 85 to 89), *borderline isolated systolic hypertension* (systolic 140 to 159, diastolic <90), and *isolated systolic hypertension* (systolic ≥160, diastolic <90). The prevalence of these patterns has not been established, but each is common.

Risks

For the patient and the physician, the single most important concept in approaching hypertension is that high blood pressure increases the risk of symptomatic cardiovascular disease during the patient's entire life.

This concept has been elucidated best by the longitudinal observations on subjects in the Framingham study. Adult subjects ranging in age from 45 to 74 years entered the study in 1951 through 1953 and were followed for 18 or more years. For practical purposes, the Framingham subjects (at entry) can be likened to patients making their first office visit to a physician, at ages ranging from 45 to 74. Based on the average of blood pressures taken on three separate visits, these subjects were subgrouped into those with normal blood pressure, borderline hypertension, and hypertension. During follow-up, an intense effort was made to detect each new cardiovascular event. Table 62.1 and Fig. 62.2 summarize the most important findings of the study:

1. In any interval of follow-up after initial evaluation, the annual risk of major cardiovascular events is much higher for older patients, as a function of both age and blood pressure at entry.
2. Risks rise progressively with each increase of both systolic and diastolic blood pressure.
3. At all ages and blood pressures, the annual incidence of events is somewhat higher for men than for women, although the gradient of risk according

Table 62.1.
Risk of Cardiovascular Events According to Blood Pressure Status, Men and Women, 45 to 74 (Framingham Study: 18-Year Follow-up)[a]

| Age | Average Annual Incidence/1000 Population | | | | | |
| | Men | | | Women | | |
	Normal[b]	BHBP[c]	HBP[d]	Normal[b]	BHBP[c]	HBP[d]
45–54	8.3	14.6	23.4	2.4	5.0	8.9
55–64	15.5	29.3	44.4	6.2	14.2	22.7
65–74	16.4	31.9	52.3	8.3	24.9	33.2
45–74[e]	12.4	21.1	35.3	5.7	10.4	18.8

[a] Adapted from Kannel WB: Hypertension in Framingham. In Paul O (ed): *Epidemiology and Control of Hypertension.* Miami, Symposia Specialists, 1975.
[b] Normal, ≤ 140/90.
[c] Borderline, 141/91 to 159/94.
[d] High, ≥ 160/95.
[e] Age-adjusted rates.

Table 62.2.
Placebo-Treated Subjects, Veterans Administration Trial: Impact of Blood Pressure, Age, and Cardiovascular Abnormalities on Attack Rate[a]

Risk Factor at Entry	Number Randomized	Attack Rate[b]
CARDIOVASCULAR AND RENAL ABNORMALITIES[c] AND DIASTOLIC BLOOD PRESSURE (mm Hg):		
Without abnormality		
90–104	36	0.145
105–114	51	0.173
With abnormality		
90–104	48	0.352
105–114	50	0.426
AGE AND DIASTOLIC BLOOD PRESSURE (mm Hg):		
<50 years		
90–104	43	0.121
105–114	56	0.413
50+ years		
90–104	41	0.413
104–114	54	0.459

[a] Adapted from Veterans Administration Cooperative Study Group on Antihypertensive Agents: Effects of treatment on morbidity in hypertension. III. Influence of age, diastolic pressure, and prior cardiovascular disease; further analysis of side effects. *Circulation* 45:991, 1972.
[b] Rate observed during 3 years.
[c] Presence of any of the following: grade 2 or greater hypertensive retinopathy, cardiomegaly on chest X-ray, left ventricular hypertrophy on ECG, evidence of renal damage, myocardial infarction, congestive heart failure, cerebrovascular accident.

to blood pressure is identical for both sexes at all ages.

By consulting the Framingham data, one can appreciate the degree of risk for an individual patient. For example, for a man 55 to 64 years old with a blood pressure ≥160/95, the risk that a stroke, myocardial infarction, or congestive heart failure will occur during the ensuing 18 years is approximately 80%.

Findings in the placebo-treated subjects in the Veterans Administration (VA) Therapeutic Trial and other placebo trials (described below) have added to the Framingham findings more concrete information about the risks attending untreated diastolic hypertension, albeit in subjects selected for a study. Table 62.2, for example, summarizes the attack rates in the VA trial for placebo-treated patients with entry diastolic pres-

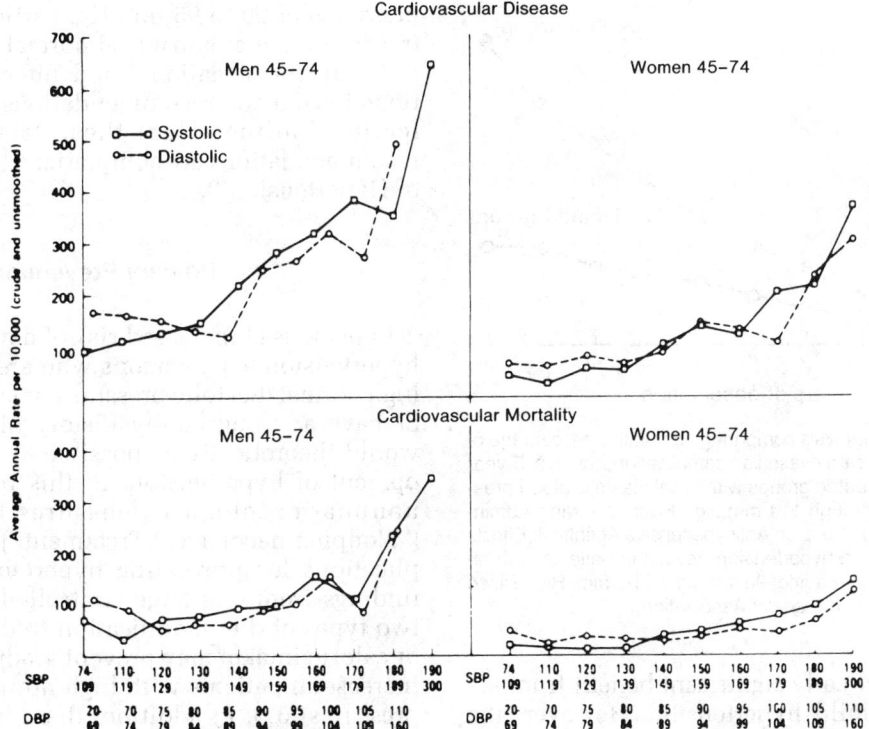

Figure 62.2. The incidence of cardiovascular morbidity (*top*) and mortality (*bottom*) during 18 years' follow-up of the Framingham cohort, plotted according to systolic and diastolic blood pressure at the time of entry for men and women ages 45 to 74. (From Kannel WB, Sorlie P: Hypertension in Framingham. In Paul O (ed): *Epidemiology and Control of Hypertension*. Miami Symposia Specialists, 1975.)

sures in two ranges (90 to 104 mm Hg and 105 to 114 mm Hg) and shows the impact of two associated characteristics (age and presence/absence of established cardiovascular or renal morbidity at entry) upon these risks. Based on these data, for example, the 3-year risk of major morbidity in an untreated man with left ventricular hypertrophy on electrocardiogram and a usual diastolic blood pressure of 100 mm Hg would be approximately 35%.

Although hypertension, especially severe hypertension, almost always alarms physicians and patients, it is important to recognize that *other treatable risk factors can be just as important.* This is illustrated by the fact that the following two hypothetical male patients, one with mild and the other with severe hypertension, have similar long-term risks:

Age	Cigarettes Per Day	Total Cholesterol	Diastolic Blood Pressure
50	0	220 mg/100 ml	125 mm Hg
50	30	220 mg/100 ml	96 mm Hg

Risk Reduction with Drug Treatment

For diastolic hypertension, a number of major clinical trials (active drug versus placebo) have been completed; they are summarized here. For isolated systolic hypertension, clinical trials are still in progress, as described in a later section ("Hypertension in the Elderly").

Veterans Administration Trials

The Veterans Administration controlled trials established the benefit of treatment in patients with severe and moderate hypertension and in some groups with mild hypertension (see below). Treatment reduced by more than 90% the morbidity in patients with entry diastolic pressures of 115 to 129 mm Hg (severe hypertension) (59) and by 50% or more the morbidity in both the subgroup with diastolic blood pressure of 105 to 114 mm Hg (moderate hypertension) and in those subgroups with diastolic pressure of 90 to 104 mm Hg (mild hypertension) who either were over 50 or had one or more cardiovascular-renal abnormalities at entry to the study (Fig. 62.3) (60). Specifically, the risk of congestive heart failure, cerebrovascular accident, or accelerated hypertension (i.e., new retinal hemorrhages or progressive renal insufficiency) was almost entirely eliminated although there was no significant reduction in the risk of myocardial infarction.

Mild Hypertension

The impact of treatment upon mild hypertension in middle-aged adults has been studied in five controlled trials (25, 30, 38, 58, 60), summarized in Table 62.3. A sixth controlled trial of treatment for mild to moderate hypertension in elderly patients (the European Working Party on Hypertension in the Elderly, EWPHE) is described in a later section ("Hypertension in the Elderly"). On balance, these studies have confirmed

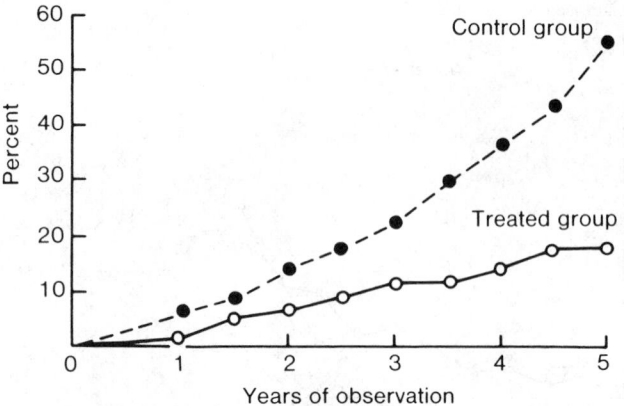

Figure 62.3. Life table analysis comparing cumulative percentage of patients who developed cardiovascular complications over a 5-year period in control *versus* treated groups with initial diastolic blood pressure in the range of 90 through 114 mm Hg. (From Veterans Administration Cooperative Study Group on Antihypertensive Agents: II. Effects of treatment on morbidity in hypertension: results in patients with diastolic blood pressures averaging 90 through 114 mm Hg. *JAMA* 213:1143, 1970. © American Medical Association.)

that there is a statistically significant benefit from active treatment for mild hypertension. However, the benefit for individual subjects who were treated in these trials was small, since the majority of both control and treatment subjects had no assessable events during 3 to 9 years. In addition to the modest size of the benefit of treatment found in these trials, there is evidence from another study, Multiple Risk Factor Intervention Trial (MRFIT), suggesting that treatment of mild hypertension with diuretics may actually increase mortality in those subjects with entry diastolic

pressures of 90 to 95 mm Hg, particularly if the electrocardiogram at entry is abnormal (43).

A number of national and international organizations have made recommendations based on the collective findings from these trials (32, 39). The recommendations are summarized below ("Treatment of Hypertension").

Primary Prevention

In persons at increased risk of developing sustained hypertension (e.g., persons who are overweight, have high normal diastolic pressures or labile hypertension, or have a strong family history of hypertension), it would theoretically be possible to prevent the development of hypertension. In this regard, each of the nonpharmacological measures discussed below ("Nonpharmacological Treatment") has important implications for preventing hypertension. Preliminary findings from one large controlled trial suggest that two types of diet modification (reduced sodium and/or caloric intake) may prevent gradual blood pressure increase in patients with high normal diastolic blood pressures (31). In addition, there is abundant epidemiological evidence that suggests that avoiding weight gain, avoiding excessive salt and alcohol intake, maintaining physical fitness, avoiding excessive stress, and engaging in relaxation techniques may forestall or prevent blood pressure increase. Measures such as these and other measures known to protect cardiovascular health (e.g., not smoking, avoiding a diet high in saturated fats) should be recommended to anyone who is motivated to follow a healthy life style and espe-

Table 62.3.
Characteristics of Completed Controlled Trials of Treatment for Mild Hypertension

Study (Report Year)	No. of Patients Randomized	% Male	Entry Diastolic BP Range	Design		Drugs for Active[a] (Step No.)	Duration (years)	% Reduction in Complications	No Assessable Events	
				Control	Active				Control	Active
Veterans Administration, 1970[b]	170	100	90–104	Placebo	Fixed dose	TZ, R, H	3.8	35	21	14
USPHS Study[c]	389	80	90–104	Placebo	Single fixed-dose regimen	TZ and R	6.5–9.0		89	37
Hypertension and Detection Follow-up Program 1979[c]	7,825	54	90–104	Referred care	Step care	TZ, K-S (1) R, M (2) H (3) G (4) OTH (5)	5	20	287	231
Australian, 1980[b]	3,427	63	95–109	Placebo	Step care	TZ (1) BB, M (2) H, C (3)	3	30	127	91
Oslo, 1980[b]	785	100	90–109	No therapy	Step care	TZ (1) BB, M (2)	5.5	25	37	28
British Medical Research Council, 1985[b]	17,354	52	90–109	Placebo	Step care	TZ (1) BB, M (2) or BB (1) TZ or G (2)	5	19	352	286

[a] TZ, thiazide or thiazide-like diuretic; R, reserpine; H, hydralazine; K-S, potassium-sparing diuretic; M, methyldopa; BB, β-blocker; C, clonidine; G, guanethidine; OTH, other drugs.
[b] Principal end points: cardiovascular morbidity and mortality.
[c] Endpoints: stroke, heart failure, new ECG abnormalities, cardiomegaly, retinopathy, renal insufficiency.
[d] Principal end points: all-cause mortality.

cially to those who have a family history of hypertension or have high normal blood pressures.

PATHOPHYSIOLOGY AND NATURAL HISTORY OF ESSENTIAL HYPERTENSION

It is estimated that 95 to 99% of hypertensives do not have an identifiable etiology for their hypertension. Their problem has, therefore, been designated "essential hypertension." Nevertheless, a number of abnormal physiological characteristics have been demonstrated in essential hypertension; these provide a conceptual basis for understanding the clinical consequences of hypertension and the mechanisms of action of antihypertensive drugs.

As indicated in Figure 62.4, the patient with established essential hypertension has an increase in peripheral arterial resistance; this is hypothesized to be the final consequence of either or both of two mechanisms: inappropriate renal retention of salt and water or increased endogenous pressor activity. Serial studies on small numbers of subjects have suggested that a stage of increased cardiac output may precede the stage of increased peripheral resistance (7). This earlier stage may be manifest in some young hypertensives as a high resting heart rate. In general, however, the evaluation of the individual patient with essential hypertension will not yield much information about the dominant mechanism contributing to that patient's hypertension.

The major complications of untreated hypertension are named in Figure 62.4. These complications can be seen as the clinical manifestations of two pathophysiological processes that are operating during the many "silent years" of increased peripheral resistance: (a) trauma to the vessels in the arterial circulation, leading to accelerated atherosclerosis in large vessels and to obliterative changes (see Fig. 62.5) or thinning and rupture (see Fig. 62.6) in small vessels; and (b) increase

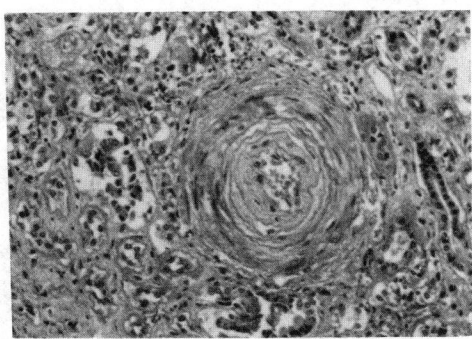

Figure 62.5. Hyperplastic arteriosclerosis in renal tissue from a patient with essential hypertension.

in the work load of the heart, leading to congestive heart failure and/or angina pectoris.

As noted above, blood pressure reduction diminishes the risk of the vascular complications due to hypertension. Although this benefit has only been assessed for drug treatment of hypertension, it is reasonable to assume that nonpharmacological measures that reduce blood pressure are at least as effective.

EVALUATION OF THE PATIENT

In this discussion, hypertension is defined as a diastolic pressure of 90 mm Hg or greater, and the approaches recommended are based upon the general guidelines of the 1988 Report of the Joint National Committee on Detection, Evaluation, and Treatment of High Blood Pressure (32).

Measuring the Blood Pressure

In measuring a patient's blood pressures, the following standard practices should be followed (21):

1. *Select an appropriate-sized cuff*: Ideally, the rubber bladder in the cuff should be about 20% wider than the diameter of the arm, and bladder length should be at least 80% of arm circumference. When bladder dimensions are too small for the patient's arm, the indirect blood pressure obtained may be higher than the actual blood pressure. The dimensions of the bladders in available cuffs are: 13 × 24 cm (standard), 17 × 32 cm (large adult), 20 × 42 cm (thigh cuff).
2. Take the *initial blood pressure after the patient has sat quietly* for a few minutes in the sitting position. Measure the pressure in each arm, with the arm held across the chest or resting on a table so that the stethoscope head is placed over the brachial artery at the level of the heart (about the level of the junction of the fourth intercostal space with the lower left sternal border). If a difference between arms is noted and confirmed on repeated measurement, take all subsequent blood pressures in the arm with the higher pressure.
3. Use the *first Korotkoff sound* for systolic pressure. The cuff pressure should be high enough to

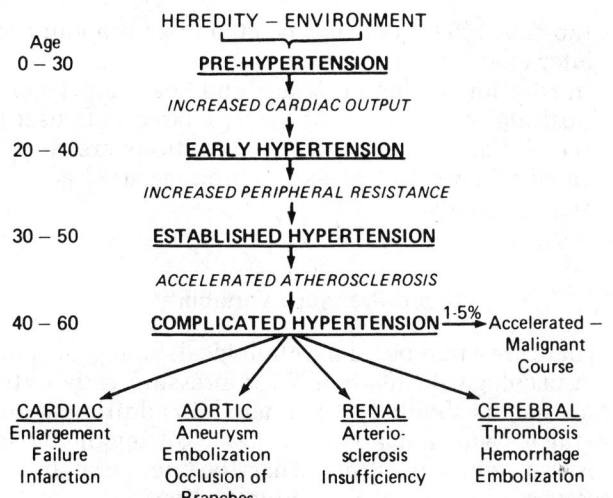

HEREDITY – ENVIRONMENT

Age	
0 – 30	**PRE-HYPERTENSION**
	INCREASED CARDIAC OUTPUT
20 – 40	**EARLY HYPERTENSION**
	INCREASED PERIPHERAL RESISTANCE
30 – 50	**ESTABLISHED HYPERTENSION**
	ACCELERATED ATHEROSCLEROSIS
40 – 60	**COMPLICATED HYPERTENSION** — 1-5% → Accelerated – Malignant Course

CARDIAC	AORTIC	RENAL	CEREBRAL
Enlargement	Aneurysm	Arterio-	Thrombosis
Failure	Embolization	sclerosis	Hemorrhage
Infarction	Occlusion of	Insufficiency	Embolization
	Branches		

Figure 62.4. A representation of the natural history of untreated essential hypertension. (From Kaplan N: *Clinical Hypertension*. Baltimore, Williams & Wilkins, 1978.)

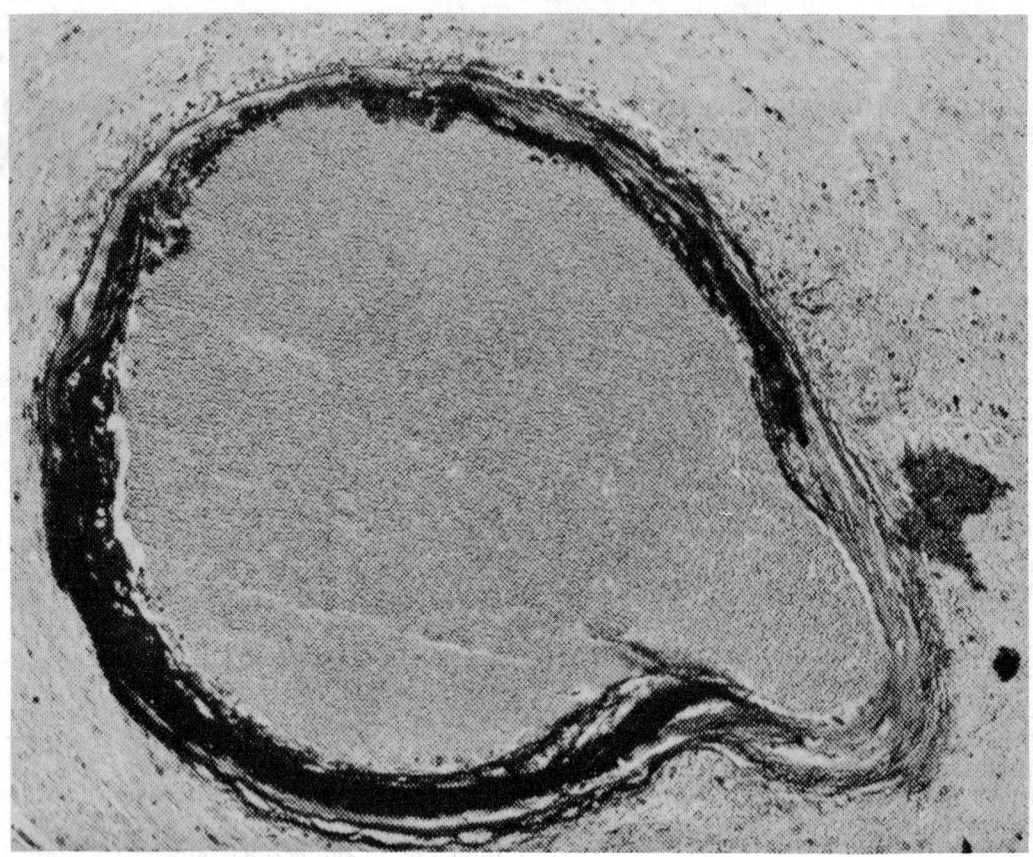

Figure 62.6. A cross-section of a microaneurysm in a small intracerebral artery from a hypertensive patient. (From Russell RW: How does blood pressure cause stroke? *Lancet* 2:1283, 1975.)

obliterate the radial pulse; by assuring that this occurs, one will avoid reading a falsely low systolic pressure due to the silent "auscultatory gap" that occasionally occurs between the first and second Korotkoff sounds.

4. Use the *fifth Korotkoff sound* (disappearance) for *diastolic pressure.*
5. *Wait 1 to 2 minutes before repeating* measurement in the same arm, to permit the return of blood trapped in the veins distal to the cuff.
6. Before initiating antihypertensive treatment, take the blood pressure *when the patient is standing* in order to detect significant baseline orthostatic hypotension.
7. *After starting or increasing antihypertensive drugs,* again check the blood pressure with the patient resting and with the patient standing, preferably after a standard exercise (e.g., 10 steps on a footstool or walking a fixed distance), because the or-

thostatic effects of drugs is often most pronounced after exercise.
8. In addition to blood pressure and heart rate, *record position, arm, and cuff size* (if large cuff used), thereby assuring that these conditions are duplicated when blood pressures are measured at subsequent visits.

Blood Pressure Variability

There are a number of psychological, biological, and pharmacological causes of blood pressure variability. These factors should be considered, in addition to following a systematic approach to measuring the blood pressure, when deciding what the measured blood pressure means in an individual patient.

In a 24-hour period, the average person's resting blood pressures fluctuate (systolic, 20 to 40 mm Hg;

diastolic, 10 to 20 mm Hg). These ranges occur in patients with normal blood pressure and in hypertensive persons who are or are not taking antihypertensive drugs. During and after vigorous exercise, normotensive and hypertensive persons who are not taking antihypertensive drugs show systolic increases of as much as 60 mm Hg and sometimes a modest decrease in their diastolic pressures.

Common causes of transient or short-term blood pressure elevation are (a) physicians taking blood pressures ("white-coat" hypertension), especially if the patient has not had time to relax; (b) mental stress, both intellectual and psychological; (c) self-medication with large amounts of nonprescription sympathomimetic decongestants (44); (d) nicotine use (20); (e) caffeine use (20); and (f) alcohol or sedative-hypnotic withdrawal.

Common causes of a short-term decrease in a patient's blood pressure are (a) intercurrent illness causing volume contraction due to fluid losses or reduced intake, (b) bed rest for several days, and (c) hospitalization with or without strict bed rest (26).

Clinical Classification

Evaluating hypertension in an individual patient consists of (a) deciding which of four clinical presentations describes the patient (labile, chronic, accelerated, or emergency hypertension); (b) for the patient with sustained hypertension, determining in which JNC category the patient belongs (Table 62.4); and (c) completing a baseline evaluation (see below). The classification of the patient should be accomplished carefully, for it leads to a label (and notions) that will have a significant effect on the patient's and the physician's future behavior. Two findings underline this point. First, a sizable proportion of people who are found to be hypertensive in screening programs do

Table 62.4.
Classification of BP in Adults Aged 18 years or Older[a]

BP Range, mm Hg	Category[b]
DBP	
<85	Normal BP
85–89	High-normal BP
90–104	Mild hypertension
105–114	Moderate hypertension
≥115	Severe hypertension
SBP, when DBP <90 mm Hg	
<140	Normal BP
140–159	Borderline isolated systolic hypertension
≥160	Isolated systolic hypertension

[a] From The Joint National Committee on Detection, Evaluation, and Treatment of High Blood Pressure. *Arch Intern Med* 148:1023, 1988.
   Classification based on the average of two or more readings on two or more occasions. BP indicates blood pressure; DBP, diastolic blood pressure; and SBP, systolic blood pressure.
[b] A classification of borderline isolated systolic hypertension (SBP, 140–159 mm Hg) or isolated systolic hypertension (SBP, ≥ 160 mm Hg) takes precedence over high-normal BP (DBP, 85–89 mm Hg) when both occur in the same person. High-normal BP (DBP, 85–89 mm Hg) takes precedence over a classification of normal BP (SBP, <140 mm Hg) when both occur in the same person.

not have sustained hypertension (12). Second, being labeled hypertensive may have significant "side effects, " such as increased sick days, increased life insurance premiums, or certain employment restrictions (24).

On their initial visits, many patients will state that they have hypertension. For some of these, recorded blood pressures from other sources will be available. Some will be taking antihypertensive drugs, presumably for sustained hypertension. Based upon this information, upon blood pressure recordings made at the initial and follow-up visits, and upon clinical and laboratory data regarding end-organs, the patient's hypertension can usually be classified with confidence.

Labile Hypertension

By definition, labile hypertension is present in any individual who has a recorded diastolic blood pressure of 90 mm Hg or above but has a usual diastolic pressure of less than 90 mm Hg. A labile rise in blood pressure can be produced in almost anyone by stresses (including visits to physicians) that provoke increased sympathetic nervous system activity. A high prevalence of labile hypertension has been found in community blood pressure screening programs, especially in young adults (12).

In practice, patients found to have a diastolic pressure of ≥90 mm Hg should have their blood pressure remeasured within 2 weeks to determine whether they have labile or sustained (i.e., chronic) hypertension. If the diastolic pressure at the first visit is relatively high (e.g., ≥115 mm Hg), the repeated blood pressures should be obtained within 1 week; even single diastolic pressures in this range may represent labile hypertension.

It is estimated that 10 to 25% of labile hypertension progresses to chronic hypertension. Therefore, patients with labile hypertension should have their blood pressures checked carefully once each year. It is important to assure that such patients understand that they do not have sustained hypertension. In addition, they should be advised to avoid excess salt and to follow other practices that reduce the likelihood of their developing hypertension (see "Nonpharmacological Aspects of Treatment" below).

Chronic Hypertension

By definition, hypertension is chronic if the diastolic pressure is consistently 90 mm Hg or greater. In some patients, especially those with high initial pressures, electrocardiographic or X-ray evidence of left ventricular hypertrophy is adequate to confirm the suspicion of chronic hypertension at the first visit. Eye ground findings indicative of arteriolosclerosis (grade 1, narrowing of arteriolar lumen; grade 2, arteriovenous crossing changes) are less reliable and less specific indicators of chronic hypertension and should not be substituted for blood pressure measurements on separate occasions.

The prognosis of untreated chronic hypertension and the benefits of treatment are summarized above.

Accelerated Hypertension

By definition, hypertension is in the accelerated or malignant stage if the diastolic pressure is relatively high (usually ≥115 mm Hg) and there is clinical evidence of severe arteriolosclerosis, meaning either grade 3 or 4 hypertensive retinopathy (grade 3, hemorrhages and/or fresh exudates; grade 4, papilledema); both are shown in (Fig. 62.7) or renal insufficiency for which there is no apparent cause except the hypertension.

The prognosis in untreated accelerated hypertension is poor: approximately 95% of subjects die of cardiac, renal, or central nervous system complications within 5 years of initial evaluation. Control of blood pressure, and (for those with end stage renal disease) dialysis, have dramatically improved the prognosis in these individuals.

Hypertensive Emergency

By definition, a hypertensive emergency exists when severe elevation of the blood pressure will predictably cause a catastrophic outcome within hours or days. Patients with two types of hypertensive emergency—hypertensive encephalopathy and dissecting aneurysm of the thoracic aorta—may present initially in an office setting. When either of these diagnoses is suspected, the patient should be transported immediately to a hospital emergency room for evaluation and treatment.

Hypertensive encephalopathy is the result of cerebral edema that develops gradually over 1 or more days in a patient with severe diastolic hypertension. In such a patient, global cerebral symptoms, such as headache, confusion, and irritability, have usually been present and progressive for hours or days. Papilledema may be present. Hypertensive encephalopathy should be diagnosed when intracerebral mass or hemorrhage, which may also present with hypertension, have been excluded by computed tomography scanning. Diffuse or focal white matter edema in the supratentorial compartment will usually be seen on the scan (61).

Thoracic aortic dissection results from an expanding hematoma in the wall of the aorta; in the patient who is dissecting, hypertension may promote perforation of the intima overlying the softened wall of the aorta. The patient with acute dissection will usually have a history of known hypertension and will present with a story of sudden "ripping" pain in the back. Computed tomography (CT), magnetic resonance imaging (MRI), and contrast aortography are all very sensitive and specific diagnostic tests for dissection. By definition, a proximal dissection involves the aorta

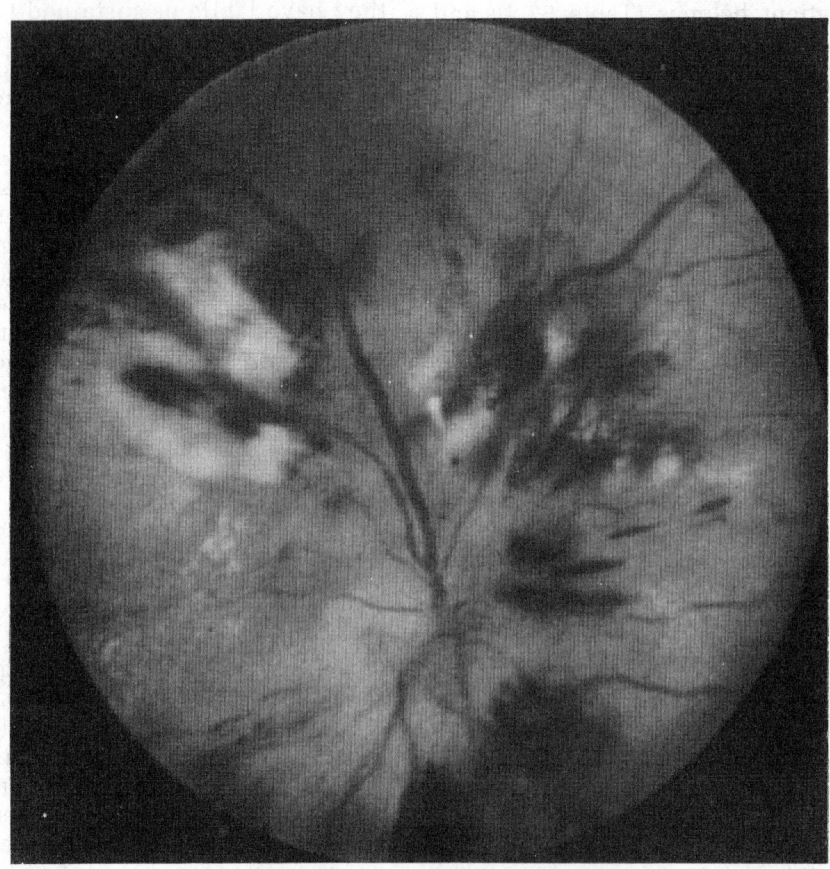

Figure 62.7. Grade 4 Keith-Wagener retinopathy.

between the aortic root and the left subclavian artery (pulses may be absent or decreased in the right arm and neck; there may be a murmur of aortic regurgitation) and a distal dissection involves only that part of the aorta distal to the left subclavian artery.

The prognosis in encephalopathy and aortic dissection, when either condition is diagnosed before there has been irreversible damage, depends upon prompt hospitalization for antihypertensive treatment and, for some patients with dissection, surgery. Despite the overwhelming threat to life without treatment, good outcomes can be achieved with appropriate intervention.

In the past decade, the term *hypertensive urgency* has been used to categorize patients with severe hypertension (diastolic greater than 115 mm Hg) who are asymptomatic; and rapid lowering of the blood pressure, using hourly doses of oral medication, has been advocated for these patients. There is no evidence for benefit—and there is anecdotal evidence for harm—to asymptomatic patients who are treated hourly till their "urgent" hypertension responds. As discussed below ("Treatment"), using currently available drugs it is usually possible to control severe hypertension within one to two weeks.

Baseline Evaluation: Overview

The baseline evaluation of the patient with sustained hypertension should accomplish five objectives:

1. Indicate the status of end organs affected by hypertension;
2. Identify clues to the presence of a treatable etiology for the hypertension;
3. Guide the selection of initial treatment;
4. Establish the pretreatment status of parameters commonly affected by antihypertensive drugs;
5. Detect the presence of additional cardiovascular risk factors.

Table 62.5 lists by source the information that should be obtained in the baseline evaluation to accomplish these five objectives.

End Organ Status

At baseline evaluation, most patients with sustained hypertension, including those with accelerated hypertension, have no symptoms attributable to their hypertension. In the past, it was thought that headache, tinnitus, epistaxis, and dizziness were common symptoms of hypertension, but community-based studies have demonstrated that these symptoms are not more prevalent in hypertensives than in normotensives (63). A minority of patients do have genuine hypertensive headaches, that are occipital in location, are worse in the morning, and resolve with lowering of the blood pressure.

The major morbidity of hypertension is due to cardiac, renal, and cerebral disease. Because the control of hypertension does not eliminate entirely the increased risks of disease, it is important both in baseline and in follow-up care to monitor the status of the end-organs affected by hypertension.

Heart

A history of symptoms due to congestive heart failure or to coronary artery disease will occasionally be obtained at baseline evaluation. Auscultation of the heart commonly reveals accentuation of the aortic second sound and a systolic ejection murmur. Infrequent auscultatory findings include a systolic ejection sound at the base of the heart, paradoxical splitting of the second heart sound, or a short high pitched diastolic murmur at the base. Objective evidence of cardiac hypertrophy is frequently found at baseline evaluation, either on physical examination (left ventricular heave or fourth heart sound) or on the electrocardiogram. Evidence of left atrial abnormality is the earliest change on the electrocardiogram, reflecting atrial contraction against a left ventricle with decreased compliance. The electrocardiographic criteria for left ventricular hypertrophy (LVH) are summarized elsewhere (Table 60.3). The concentric hypertrophy typical of hypertension causes only a modest increase in the left ventricular silhouette on the chest X-ray, and the plain film of the chest is much less sensitive than the electrocardiogram in identifying changes due to LVH.

The functional derangements associated with LVH have been the subject of intense study in recent years. In some asymptomatic patients, the resting ejection fraction (measured by echocardiogram) is normal but the ejection fraction shows a subnormal increase during exercise. In hypertensive patients with symptoms of left ventricular failure, echocardiographic studies have revealed that some have global left ventricular dysfunction; some have functional subaortic stenosis; some have a hyperkinetic left ventricle with a normal or high ejection fraction and with diminished relaxation during diastole; and some in the latter group (usually older patients) have "cavity obliteration" during diastole (50). Because appropriate drug therapy for patients in these groups differs in important ways (see below), it is recommended that hypertensive patients with signs and symptoms of heart failure should have echocardiograms to assure that the drugs prescribed for them improve rather than worsen the heart failure.

Most symptoms of coronary artery disease in hypertensive patients are related to occlusive disease of the coronary arteries. There is also evidence that some hypertensive patients who describe angina and who have normal coronary arteriograms may have ischemia caused by increased resistance of the microvasculature of the myocardium (10).

Kidney

Simple tests of kidney status (urinalysis and serum creatinine concentration) are normal in the majority of hypertensives at baseline. In the patient with a

Table 62.5.
Baseline Evaluation of the Patient with Sustained Hypertension

Information	End Organ Status	Etiology Screening	Selecting Treatment	Factors Modified by Treatment	Additional Cardiovascular Risk Factors
INTERVIEW, OLD RECORDS					
Age and race		X	X		
Blood pressure levels		X	X	X	
Hypertension treatment, results		X	X		
Family history		X	X		X
Congestive heart failure	X		X		
Angina	X		X		
Transient ischemic attack or cerebrovascular accident	X				
Renal disease	X	X	X		
Comprehension of hypertension			X	X	
Diet (Na, K, fats)		X	X	X	X
Exercise habits			X		X
Current drugs[a]		X	X	X	X
Alcohol use		X	X		
Tobacco use					X
Current life stresses		X	X		X
Coexisting conditions[b]		X	X		
Periordic sympathetic symptoms		X			
PHYSICAL EXAMINATION					
Weight		X	X	X	
Blood pressure (right, left, resting, standing)		X	X	X	
Heart rate		X	X	X	
Eye grounds	X		X		
Peripheral pulses	X	X	X		
Heart	X				
Lungs			X		
Abdomen (mass, bruit)		X			
Neurological	X				
LABORATORY					
Complete blood count				X	
Calcium		X		X	
Creatinine	X	X	X	X	
Potassium		X	X	X	
Sodium			X		
Fasting glucose			X	X	
Cholesterol (total, high density lipoprotein)				X	X
Uric acid			X	X	
Urinalysis		X		X	
ECG	X				

[a]Identify drugs that may cause hypertension or may interfere with antihypertensive drugs (e.g., oral contraceptives, tricyclic antidepressants, sympathomimetic decongestants, appetite suppressants, corticosteroids, nonsteroidal anti-inflammatory drugs, cyclosporine, monoamine oxidose inhibitors).
[b]See Table 62.7.

high diastolic pressure, either an elevated creatinine concentration, proteinuria (sometimes more than 1 g/24 hours), or microscopic hematuria may be found as evidence for accelerated hypertension; other forms of urogenital disease should be excluded in such patients before these findings are attributed to hypertension.

Central Nervous System

A history of stroke—lacunar or major vessel syndromes—or transient ischemic attacks (see Chapter 83), an asymptomatic carotid bruit, or neurological findings of a remote stroke may be present at baseline evaluation, but the majority of patients will have no evidence of cerebrovascular disease when first evaluated.

Eye

Ophthalmic symptoms attributed to hypertension (decreased acuity due to retinal hemorrhages or retinal detachment) are uncommon. However, examination of the retina has been emphasized in the evaluation of hypertensive patients because it offers direct inspection of blood vessels affected by hypertension. Most patients with chronic hypertension have evidence of arteriolosclerosis (grades 1 and 2 hypertensive retinopathy), but these findings have little practical value as they are not specific for hypertension, and there is significant interobserver and intraobserver variability in detecting them. On the other hand, grades 3 or 4 retinopathy (see Fig. 62.8) should be sought in any patient with a high diastolic pressure, for these changes are quite specific for accelerated hypertension.

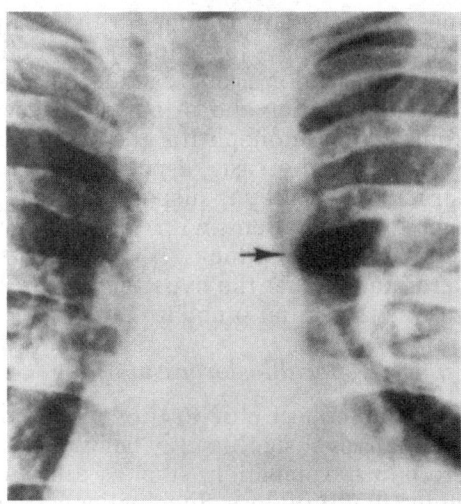 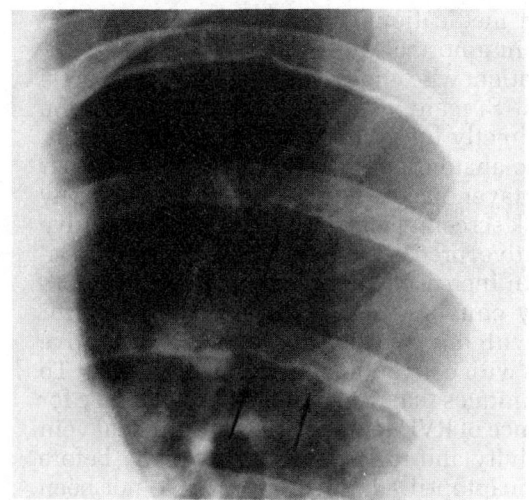

Figure 62.8. Chest X-ray features of coarctation. *Left.* The "3 sign" at the left parasternal border of the descending aorta. *Right.* Notching of the ribs from enlarged collateral vessels. (From Smith PT, Edwards JE: Pseudocoarctation, kinking, or bucking of the aorta. *Circulation* 46:1027, 1972. By permission of the American Heart Association, Inc.)

Evaluation for Secondary Hypertension

Information obtained at baseline evaluation or during follow-up will identify those patients who may have hypertension secondary to a treatable condition. The *rarity of surgically curable hypertension* is indicated by the reports from referral centers in which only 1 to 3% of referred (i.e., selected) patients have had these forms of hypertension (56).

Current Use of an Oral Contraceptive

This cause of hypertension should be considered in any patient currently using an oral contraceptive hormone. To confirm this etiology, there should be evidence for a normal blood pressure before oral contraceptive use; and the patient's blood pressure should become normal within 6 months of discontinuing oral contraceptives (see additional details below).

Chronic Alcoholism

In some individuals, heavy, chronic alcohol use causes sustained hypertension. For patients found to have both hypertension and alcoholism at the baseline evaluation, blood pressure control should be attempted initially through detoxification and treatment of the alcoholism (see Chapter 21). The blood pressure becomes normal in those with alcohol-induced hypertension within about 1 week of alcohol cessation.

Renovascular Hypertension (RVH)

It is estimated that.5% of hypertensive patients have renovascular hypertension (hypertension caused by unilateral stenosis of the main or of a segmental renal artery) (17). RVH is very uncommon in blacks.

A number of findings in the baseline evaluation increase the prior probability that the patient has RVH: the presence of an abdominal bruit radiating to the flank (especially if both systolic and diastolic components are audible); well-documented recent (span of 1 or 2 years) change from normal blood pressure to moderate or severe hypertension; hypertension that is refractory to maximal tolerated doses of multiple antihypertensive drugs; refractoriness to previously effective drugs that is unexplained (see below), a very high baseline diastolic pressure (e.g., ≥115 mm Hg) in a person under 30 years of age; or evidence of accelerated hypertension (i.e., grade 3 or 4 hypertensive retinopathy or renal insufficiency due to hypertension) in any patient.

If a patient has one or more of these findings and is a candidate for surgery, the following choices can be presented to the patient:

1. *Attempt to control the hypertension with drugs*, including drugs not previously tried in those patient who seem to be refractory to maximal doses of multiple drugs. This choice is supported by the findings that RVH generally responds to medical therapy and that many patients with RVH due to atherosclerosis (the commonest cause of RVH) need to resume drug treatment within 1 or more years of surgery (17).
2. *Look for renal artery stenosis (RAS), which may be the cause of the patient's hypertension.* The patient should declare an interest in accepting angioplasty or surgery before undergoing testing for RAS and should understand that if RAS is found the only way to establish whether *renovascular hypertension* is present is to undergo angioplasty or vascular surgery, then await the blood pressure response to the procedure. The generally accepted criteria for confirmed RVH are stable postangioplasty/surgery "cure" (blood pressure of 140/90 or less off medicine) or "significant improvement" (systolic or diastolic pressure reduced by at least 15% without a

change in medication; or less medication needed to maintain a normal pressure) (17).

For a patient who chooses evaluation for the presence of RAS, many experts advocate referring the patient directly for an imaging study that demonstrates the anatomy of the renal arteries, i.e either (a) for intravenous digital subtraction angiography (a low-risk screening study that has a high positive and negative predictive value when used in patients with increased chances of having RVH), followed by conventional renal arteriography for patients with positive findings; or (b) for definitive diagnosis with conventional arteriography only. To date, techniques that detect functional evidence for the presence of RVH (e.g., peripheral and renal vein renin activity and radioisotope renography before and after captopril administration) have not been found to have the same usefulness for screening as intravenous digital subtraction angiography (54). However, because it is simple to perform in the office and inexpensive, the measurement of plasma renin activity (PRA) after two hours of ambulation has been recommended to help guide the decision for or against expensive imaging studies (18). Depending upon the cut-level selected, PRA can be very sensitive and not very specific or quite insensitive but very specific in screening for RVH.

If unilateral renal artery stenosis is found and the patient has fibromuscular hyperplasia, percutaneous transluminal angioplasty (PTA) may yield results equal to those of surgical correction of the RVH. Neither PTA nor surgery has produced very satisfactory long-term results if RVH due to atherosclerosis is present. However, in some patients with the combination of hypertension resistant to medical therapy, renal insufficiency, and arteriosclerosis causing either bilateral renal artery stenosis or renal artery stenosis in a single functioning kidney, surgery or PTA may control the hypertension and stabilize or improve the renal function (66).

Patient experience. The patient can expect the following experience when undergoing radiological evaluation for RVH:
Intravenous Digital Subtraction Angiography. For this study, dye is injected intravenously and multiple images are made while the patient is supine. This method obviates the additional discomfort and risks that accompany arteriography, but the visualization of the main renal arteries is less precise and stenotic lesions in sequential branches may not be visualized.
Renal Arteriography. The patient experience is similar to that described for cerebral arteriography in Chapter 78. For both studies femoral artery catheterization is utilized, and if a very small catheter is used the patient does not need hospital admission.

Kidney Disease

This should be suspected as a possible cause of hypertension in patients with a history of hematuria, stones, or recurrent pyelonephritis; or in patients in whom large kidneys (e.g., due to obstruction or to polycystic disease) or a large bladder (after voiding) are palpated; or when the urinalysis suggests acute or chronic glomerulonephritis (i.e., significant proteinuria and/or many casts, especially red cell casts). If obstructive uropathy is suspected, a sonogram should be obtained. In patients with established chronic renal failure and small kidneys, it is usually impossible to determine whether the hypertension or the renal disease was the initial problem.

Primary Hyperaldosteronism

The commonest clue to this etiology is a baseline potassium level significantly below normal for which there is no explanation, such as diuretic use or gastrointestinal fluid loss. Such patients should be asked about excess consumption of licorice, which contains glycyrrhetinic acid, a moiety with mineralocorticoid-like activity; there are case reports of hypertension that abated when the patient discontinued consuming large amounts of licorice. The ambulatory evaluation of the patient with suspected primary hyperaldosteronism is discussed in detail in Chapter 45, Hypokalemia.

Pheochromocytoma

Clues to the presence of pheochromocytoma are a history of a hypermetabolic state (which may resemble hyperthyroidism) and/or of periodic clusters of symptoms of sympathetic nervous system hyperactivity including tachycardia, palpitations, diaphoresis, with associated headaches and symptoms of orthostatic hypotension (in patients who intermittently have predominant beta-2 sympathetic activity, causing vasodilation). These symptoms are especially important when there is no evidence for the more common causes for them, i.e., hyperthyroidism (see Chapter 73), reactive hypoglycemia (see Chapter 74), or panic attacks and other anxiety disorders (see Chapter 13). The absence of such symptom clusters virtually excludes the presence of pheochromocytoma. Additional findings that raise the prior probability of pheochromocytoma are (a) a marked change in blood pressure or heart rate in response to minor injury, parturition, or general anesthesia; (b) a neurocutaneous syndrome (von Recklinghausen's disease or von Hippel-Lindau syndrome); (c) a blood relative with a pheochromocytoma; (d) possible type II multiple endocrine neoplasia (medullary carcinoma of the thyroid or parathyroid adenoma, or both, with symptoms suggesting pheochromocytoma).

Because pheochromocytoma is very uncommon, and all screening tests will yield between 2 and 5% false-positive results, the best practice is to screen only those patients in whom clinical suspicion is relatively high. Measurement of 24-hour urinary excretion of markers for increased pressor synthesis is widely available and has a 70 to 80% sensitivity; screening techniques with better performance characteristics, such as the clonidine suppression test (9), may be available for general use in the future. For the 24-hour urine tests, the patient is given a plastic container that contains a fixed amount of a strong acid and is instructed to collect a 24-hour specimen. One specimen can be used to screen for catecholamines, metanephrines, and vanillylmandelic acid. With modern assay techniques, no foodstuffs and only a small number of drugs interfere with test results (catecholamines may be increased by methyldopa, L-dopa, theophylline, hypoglycemia, isoproterenol, prochlorperazine; metanephrines may be increased by monamine oxidase inhibitors, clonidine withdrawal, occasionally methyldopa; vanillylmandelic acid may be decreased by monoamine oxidase inhibitors and clofibrate, increased by nalidixic acid). In the rare patient who has a normal blood pressure between paroxysms of hypertension, the urine specimen should be taken when the patient is hypertensive. Patients with positive screening tests, ideally on more than one occasion, should undergo definitive diagnostic testing to localize the purported tumor. This process has been improved by the availability of radioisotope scanning using labeled iodobenzylguanidine, followed by CT or MRI scanning of the site that takes up this substance (51). Almost all pheochromocytomas are located in the adrenal glands; 1 to 3% may be located in the posterior mediastinum.

Coarctation of the Aorta

Clues to the presence of this condition are hypertension in a relatively young patient (most will be recognized in the pediatric age group); decreased blood pressure in the lower extremities, suggested by diminished or absent femoral pulses and corroborated by auscultation over the popliteal artery blood pressures, using a large cuff; and evidence of poststenotic dilatation of the aorta (Fig. 62.8) or collateral arterial vessels either on inspection of the trunk or on the plain chest X-ray (Fig. 62.8). In a minority of patients, the coarctation occurs proximal to the left subclavian artery, and the blood pressure will be high only in the right arm. To confirm the presence of a coarctation, the patient must be hospitalized for aortography.

Baseline Status of Factors Modified by Treatment

Table 62.5 lists a number of factors that should be documented at the baseline evaluation because they may be modified as part of the treatment plan or as an unwanted consequence of treatment. These include information obtained in the history (baseline understanding of hypertension, usual diet, alcohol consumption, current medications), in the physical examination (weight, blood pressure, heart rate and rhythm, edema), and in the laboratory examination (creatinine, electrolytes, fasting glucose, complete blood count, uric acid, cholesterol, and urinalysis).

Other Cardiovascular Risk Factors

At least one other cardiovascular risk factor is present in the majority of patients found to have hypertension (32). Therefore, the baseline evaluation of a hypertensive patient should include checking for other risk factors (Table 62.5), and these factors should be considered in planning the overall management of the patient. These include family history of premature cardiovascular disease, high cholesterol diet, sedentary living, tobacco use, stressful life style, overweight, diabetes mellitus, and hypercholesterolemia.

TREATMENT

Goals of Treatment

When sustained hypertension has been diagnosed, the initial goal of treatment is a normal blood pressure, defined as a diastolic pressure under 90 mm Hg. Although some data have suggested that increased risks of myocardial infarction may attend drug-induced lowering of the diastolic pressure to less than 85 mm Hg, this finding has not been reported in analyses from the major controlled trials and it therefore awaits further study (27). Partial reduction of blood pressure is an acceptable goal for patients with moderate to severe hypertension in whom it is not possible to achieve a diastolic pressure of <90 mm Hg (55).

In patients with mild hypertension who choose a nonpharmacological regimen (see below), a trial of this regimen for a number of months is usually needed to evaluate its impact on the blood pressure. When drug treatment is selected, a goal of satisfactory blood pressure control without significant drug side effects can usually be achieved within 1 to 3 months.

As part of the treatment of any hypertensive patient, the control of other treatable cardiovascular risk factors should be a second goal that is discussed and addressed with the patient.

Recommendations Regarding Initial Treatment Modality

Based on the controlled trial of antihypertensive treatment summarized above, the Joint National Committee (JNC) recommends initiating pharmacological treatment for all patients with sustained *moderate* or *severe* diastolic hypertension (32).

For *mild hypertension*, initial treatment with an antihypertensive drug is advocated for most patients with diastolic pressures of ≥95 mm Hg by the JNC (32) and ≥100 mm Hg by the World Health Organization (39). Both expert groups suggest individualized treatment decisions for patients below these cut-off levels. The presence of other cardiovascular risk factors (smoking, hypercholesterolemia, overweight, diabetes), a strong family history of cardiovascular morbidity, end organ effects of hypertension (left ventricular hypertrophy on the electrocardiogram, renal insufficiency, history of cerebrovascular disease), and coexisting high systolic pressures are characteristics that favor drug treatment for such patients if nonpharmacological treatment (see below) does not control the blood pressure within a few months. For patients with blood pressure below the above cut-off levels who do not have these associated risk factors, nonpharmacological treatment is advocated as the principal approach.

Practical approaches to the treatment of *isolated systolic hypertension* and to hypertension in *young* and *elderly* subjects are discussed in subsequent sections of this chapter.

Nonpharmacological Aspects of Treatment

A number of nonpharmacological modalities may promote lowering of blood pressure. Those for which the evidence for effectiveness is best include sodium restriction, weight reduction, physical exercise, various techniques combining psychological and physical relaxation, and limiting alcohol intake (32). Each of these has been shown to lower blood pressure without the use of antihypertensive drugs in some patients and to add to the blood pressure lowering effect in patients who are taking antihypertensive drugs. There is accumulating evidence that nonpharmacological control of hypertension favorably influences cardiac status after a number of years (52).

Because nonpharmacological measures require significant changes in life-style, it is generally more difficult to achieve long-term adherence to them than to drug treatment. Nevertheless, for motivated patients with mild hypertension, one or more of these can be tried as primary treatment; and they should be recommended, whenever they are pertinent, to all patients who also are beginning treatment with antihypertensive drugs.

Weight Reduction and Sodium Restriction

In 1979, the National High Blood Pressure Coordinating Committee published the following practical recommendations for weight reduction and sodium restriction in the care of and prevention of hypertension. These recommendations, with modifications made in the 1988 JNC report (32), are as follows:

Weight Reduction

1. Weight reduction should be recommended routinely in the treatment of all overweight persons with borderline or sustained hypertension. The goal should be a body weight within 15% of desirable weight (see Chapter 76).
2. If blood pressure is reduced to and maintained at normal levels by weight reduction, maintenance of weight reduction should be regarded as definitive treatment for the patient.
3. For overweight patients who experience significant side effects from drugs, weight reduction should be considered as adjunctive therapy to help reduce drug dosages.
4. Persons with a family history of hypertension should avoid excessive weight gain and should reduce if overweight.
5. Prevention or control of obesity in the young should be regarded as having positive health benefits and as a possible preventive step for hypertension.

Chapter 76 contains a full discussion of obesity and its treatment.

Sodium Restriction

1. Moderate sodium restriction (70 to 90 mEq daily, 1.5 to 2 g of elemental sodium or 4 to 6 g of salt) should be routinely prescribed, and if blood pressure is reduced to and maintained at normal levels, it should be used as definitive therapy.
2. For patients who experience significant side effects from drugs, sodium restriction should be considered as adjunctive therapy to help reduce drug dosages or increase drug efficacy.
3. Persons with a family history of hypertension should be encouraged to restrict sodium intake even though they may not be hypertensive.
4. Practitioners recommending sodium restriction should indicate specific diets appropriate to each patient's condition and life-style and should ensure that the diet is explained satisfactorily.

Tables 62.6 and 62.7, which can be copied for distribution to patients, summarize what the patient should know in order to follow a low salt diet. When giving this information to the patient, it is important to point out (a) that the majority of one's daily intake of salt usually comes in prepared foods ("What not to eat" column, Table 62.7) and (b) that there are many ways to make food tasty without adding salt (see Table 62.6).

As pointed out below, when a patient continues to ingest a large amount of salt while taking diuretics, potassium wasting is increased. Therefore, salt restriction may both prevent excessive potassium loss and facilitate blood pressure reduction in patients taking diuretics.

Muscle Relaxation and Biofeedback

The 1988 JNC report (32) points out that muscle relaxation and biofeedback techniques have been shown to produce sustained modest blood pressure reduction, both in patients who are poorly controlled on drug therapy and in patients who are not on drug therapy. These techniques can therefore be recommended to motivated patients. Muscle relaxation techniques are described in Chapter 13. Biofeedback techniques and "doses" vary and require the involvement of therapists experienced with the method (6).

Physical Exercise

The 1988 JNC report (32) strongly recommends advising motivated patients to engage in conditioning level isotonic exercises. There is suggestive evidence that such exercise may produce sustained blood pressure reduction and/or a need for less antihypertensive medication to control blood pressure. Chapter 58 provides details regarding the level of exercise needed to achieve cardiovascular conditioning.

Although physical conditioning may be recommended as part of the initial treatment for selected

Table 62.6.
Information for Patients Who Are Advised to Follow a 2-g Sodium Diet[a]

Americans eat about **20 times more sodium** than they need, most of which comes from salt, which is one source of sodium.

Sodium is:

found naturally in foods, even those that do not taste salty.

added to food by manufacturers in food processing.

added in cooking in the form of salt, baking powder, baking soda, or seasonings such as monosodium glutamate (MSG).

added as salt to food at the table.

ADD NEW FLAVORS TO YOUR FOOD!

☐ Herbs and spices can give new zest to your unsalted cooking.

☐ A little herb goes a long way. If you are making your own substitution without the benefit of a recipe, try ¼ teaspoon of dried herb or spice to:

a recipe for 4 servings,

a pound of meat, poultry, fish, or vegetable or 2 cups of sauce.

If you are using red pepper or garlic powder start with only ⅛ teaspoon. Taste and add a little more depending on your preference.

☐ If you use fresh herbs use 4 times the amount of dried herb. Instead of ¼ teaspoon of dried herb use 1 full teaspoon of fresh herb.

☐ Add dried herbs to soups and stews during the last hour of cooking.

☐ Use whole spices in slow cooking dishes and add them at the beginning of the cooking period.

BEWARE OF HIDDEN SODIUM!
Processed Foods

Salt is added to many packaged, convenience, "fast," and canned foods. Examples are: packaged dinners (such as macaroni and cheese), packaged coatings and "helpers," combination dinners (such as frozen meals and casserole dishes), canned soups, dried soups, canned vegetables, and frozen vegetables with sauces.

"Fast Foods"

Generally, meals served at "fast food" places are high in sodium. A typical meal of a hamburger, french fries, and a vanilla shake can total over 1000 mg of sodium—more than half of your total daily allowance. Remember pizza, hot dogs, burgers, fried chicken, fried fish, omelettes, and tacos served at "fast food" places are usually high in sodium. Just one whole dill pickle contains 1900 mg of sodium, almost the total allowed in this diet.

Read labels carefully. Foods which list salt or sodium as ingredients should be avoided. Compare different brands of the same product. It's unnecesary to purchase special dietetic foods. Many dietetic foods contain sodium or salt, **so read the labels carefully.**

SOME TIPS ON EATING OUT!

☐ Select restaurants that offer à la carte service.

☐ For breakfast, order from the allowed cereals. Poaches or boiled eggs with toast may be ordered at most restaurants.

☐ For lunch, try fruit or tossed salads; roast beef, sliced chicken or turkey breast sandwich; and fruit for dessert.

☐ At dinner, try fruit (fresh, canned, or forzen), fruit juice, or fruit cup as an appetizer.

☐ If you select broiled meats, fresh fish, or chicken, you may request that no salt or other condiments like garlic salt or onion salt be added before or after broiling.

☐ Inside cuts of roast beef, lamb, pork, veal, chicken and turkey have less sodium than outside cuts. Trim off the edges that would have been salted. Ask that it be served without gravy or sauce.

In the body, sodium acts like a sponge to hold water in the body tissues. Sometimes the body cannot get rid of enough of the sodium. High blood pressure may result. If not controlled, high blood pressure leads to stroke, kidney failure and heart disease.

Using no salt in cooking or at the table and eliminating highly salted food cuts down the sodium level of the food you eat to about **2000 mg a day.**

☐ When using ground spices add them 15 minutes beore the end of the cooking period. If adding them to uncooked dishes, add them several hours before serving. As a start, try one or a combination of the following popular herbs:

Basil	Rosemary
Celery seed	Sage
Marjoram	Savory
Mint	Thyme

Additives

Sodium may be added to food as a preservative; for quick cooking; to soften or loosen skins of fruits and vegetables; to cure meats, fish, sausage; to stop growth of molds. Additives which contain sodium include:

Monosodium glutamate (MSG)

Baking soda

Disodium phosphate

Sodium alginate

Sodium benzoate

Sodium hydroxide

Sodium nitrate

Sodium propionate

Sodium sulfite

☐ In ordering rice, ask if it has been cooked in salted water. Some restaurants cook rice without salt. Rice pilaf is usually prepared with salt.

☐ You can count on baked potato. For toppings use butter, margarine, or sour cream.

☐ If in doubt about cooked vegetables, order sliced tomatoes or a salad such as tossed salad, lettuce wedge or fruit salad. Try lemon or oil and vinegar for the dressing. Ask the waiter to leave off the croutons!

☐ Help yourself to the bread basket, but avoid salted breadsticks and crackers with salted tops.

☐ For dessert select fruit, sherbet, ice cream, or plain yogurt.

☐ Most airlines provide "special meals." A low sodium meal may be ordered at no extra cost when you make your flight reservation.

☐ "Fast food" menu items (except for the salad bar where you can select low sodium items) have usually been salted. If food can be prepared to order, request that no salted seasonings be added.

Table 62.6. Continued

TO SUM IT UP!

☐ Using less salt is advisable for almost everyone, even children, so let the whole family join in.
☐ Avoid shaking salt on your food. Substitute a blend of herbs for your salt shaker.
☐ Cook without salt. Try leaving it out of recipes.
☐ Experiment with new flavors by using herbs and spices. Fine restaurants rely on herbs, spices, and the natural flavor of food, *not salt*, for good taste.
☐ Avoid "fast foods" and other processed foods high in sodium.
☐ Read the labels of foods and medicines to find "hidden" sodium. Look for the symbol: Na⁺;
  the words: salt, sodium, soda, brine.
☐ Become familiar with foods high in sodium.

☐ Low sodium salt, such as "Lite Salt," is a combination of sodium and potassium. Do not be misled that it is free of sodium. It has about half the sodium content of regular salt.
Use of low sodium salt and salt substitutes can be dangerous because of the very high potassium content. It is essential that you ask your doctor if you may use them. Also ask how much you may use each day.

*ᵃ*From "Health Is In—Salt is Out," courtesy of The Maryland High Blood Pressure Coordinating Council.

patients, all patients should be informed about the implications of hypertension and antihypertensive drug therapy for ordinary physical activity. Subjects with untreated hypertension have the same patterns of blood pressure fluctuation during exercise as normotensive subjects, only at higher pressures: with vigorous exercise, the systolic pressure rises (as much as 60 mm Hg) while the diastolic pressure may rise or fall slightly. Similar patterns are found in patients treated with antihypertensive drugs. The impact of a number of antihypertensives and other cardiovascular drugs on blood pressure during exercise is summarized in Table 58.9. Overall, it is reasonable to inform patients that their hypertension does not make them "different" and to reassure them that they can engage in all of their usual activities after beginning treatment for hypertension.

Other Nonpharmacological Measures

A number of other measures may promote blood pressure reduction and should be recommended to hypertensive patients. These are:

1. Limiting alcohol intake to 2 ounces/day in social drinkers and treating alcoholism as a primary mode of treatment for hypertension in alcoholics (see Chapter 21);
2. Consuming a diet with substantial potassium content. This often occurs as a consequence of changing to a low sodium diet, which tends to contain more potassium-rich natural foods in place of processed food.
3. Reducing dietary saturated fats.

Recently, there has been enthusiasm for supplementing the diet of hypertensive patients with calcium and magnesium. To date, there is insufficient evidence to suggest this as part of the nonpharmacological approach to hypertension.

Pharmacological Treatment: Step-Care Method

To date, objective methods for selecting the most appropriate antihypertensive drug for an individual

patient have not been developed. Therefore, drug treatment for most patients should be initiated and modified using the step-care strategies recommended in 1988 by the Joint National Committee (see Fig. 62.9). As discussed below, there are a number of considerations in individual patients that may be helpful when selecting drugs in step-care.

In the JNC strategy, either a diuretic, a beta-blocker, an angiotensin-converting enzyme (ACE) inhibitor, or a calcium antagonist (calcium channel blocker) is recommended for initial monotherapy; previously, only a diuretic or a beta-blocker was recommended. Initial and maximal doses of drugs in each class are delineated below.

For most patients, it is reasonable to initiate monotherapy and assess the response after 1 to 3 weeks. More than 50% of patients will respond to low-dose monotherapy alone. Increasing the dose of the initial drug, substituting another drug, or adding a drug or drugs from another class are strategies that will lead to control in most patients who do not respond to or tolerate the initial regimen.

In general, the level of a patient's baseline blood pressure is not a reliable predictor of the amount or kind of drug the patient will need. Patients with severe hypertension (diastolic greater than 114 mm Hg) should be evaluated frequently until there is evidence that the blood pressure is responding to the drug(s) and/or dose(s) prescribed. This is feasible since the major antihypertensive effect of most nondiuretic drugs is apparent within 1 to 2 days (see below).

Most nondiuretic antihypertensive drugs may promote renal sodium retention as a response to blood pressure lowering, attenuating the antihypertensive effect. Therefore, in a patient who cannot be easily controlled with nondiuretic drugs, the addition of a diuretic should be considered, especially if the patient gains weight or develops edema despite instructions to restrict salt intake. Large doses of loop diuretics and/or the addition of potassium-conserving diuretics may be needed to accomplish this in some patients, as discussed below.

Two or more of some antihypertensive drugs are available in fixed-dose combination tablets, and more will probably be available in the future. The appropriate combination may provide additional convenience at no additional cost.

Promoting Compliance with Pharmacological Treatment

Compliance with treatment as a generic feature of ambulatory care is discussed in detail in Chapter 4. Because poor compliance is so common in hypertensive patients, the problem has been studied extensively in recent years (35). A number of strategies in patient care have been shown to improve compliance with antihypertensive treatment, and several of these should be employed routinely. More intensive strategies should be used for those patients who appear to be especially noncompliant.

The following strategies should be employed routinely from the outset of treatment:

1. Assuring that the patient knows several critical facts about hypertension: that it increases the risk of disabling illness (stroke, heart disease, kidney failure) or premature death; that it is usually asymptomatic when initially found; that treatment greatly reduces the risk of illness or premature death; and that treatment is continuous for life. This information is covered well in patient information pamphlets available from the American Heart Association and from a number of companies that manufacture antihypertensive drugs. One of these pamphlets should be given to each hypertensive patient as an adjunct to a verbal summary of this information by the physician or nurse, and the patient's comprehension of the fundamentals of hypertension should be ascertained periodically. (For further information on techniques for effective patient education, see Chapter 3.)
2. Prescribing drugs that can be taken once or twice per day (see Tables 62.9 and 62.10 below);
3. Having the patient state how he is taking his medication at each visit (including what he has taken "today" and, for drugs with a duration of action under 12 hours, when the last dose was taken). Patients taking multiple drugs should be encouraged to bring their bottles of medicine to every visit.
4. Assuring that supervision is provided frequently enough. During the first year of treatment, this should probably be at least every 2 to 3 months, at scheduled visits.
5. Assuring that the practice is planned to maximize convenience for the patient, meaning that waiting time is brief, that telephone access to the practice is easy, that requests for appointment changes are accommodated, and that prescription renewals are easy to obtain.

For patients who admit poor compliance, the reason should be explored and addressed (see practical approaches, Chapter 4).

For patients with uncontrolled hypertension in whom poor compliance is suspected but not admitted, the following strategies have been shown to help:

1. Having the adult with whom the patient has the most contact (usually the spouse) become an active participant in promoting compliance. This other adult should know in detail the treatment regimen and should be asked to provide specific reinforcement for medication taking. Sometimes it is helpful to have a visiting nurse provide initial education and check blood pressures in the patient's home.
2. Having the patient or another person take blood pressures at home and bring the record to office visits. When this is done, the home measuring technique should be observed periodically, using the equipment that is used at home.
3. Observing the patient's blood pressure response when his prescribed medications are given under supervision in the office (see case example in Fig. 62.9).
4. Having the patient participate in group meetings with other hypertensive patients, coordinated by someone skilled in promoting group support mechanisms.

The following general findings from studies of compliance in hypertension may also be helpful in developing strategies for use in the office:

1. Compliance-promoting strategies are additive.
2. Compliance decays in many patients who initially do well and in those noncompliers who improve after short-term intensive interventions, such as home visits. Because of the problem of compliance decay, it is important to maintain some compliance-promoting strategies continuously in the long-term care of hypertensive patients.
3. The cost of drugs and side effects from drugs explain only a modest proportion of noncompliance in the treatment of hypertension.

Individualizing Drug Selection

There are a variety of diuretic regimens and more than 20 drugs from the four major classes of nondiuretic antihypertensives: adrenergic inhibitors, ACE inhibitors, calcium channel blockers, and vasodilators. In addition to the step-care strategy of the JNC, a number of factors may be helpful in choosing drugs for individual patients.

The baseline evaluation (see Table 62.5) often discloses useful information. The patient's previous experience with specific drugs may be important (e.g., a history of side effects, nonresponse, or good response). The patient's race and age should be considered. In general, black subjects respond less often than whites to beta-blockers and more often than whites to monotherapy with diuretics; and older patients respond best to diuretics or calcium antago-

Table 62.7.
Food List for Patients Who Are Advised To Follow a 2-g Sodium Diet (Shows What to Eat and What Not to Eat)[a,b]

Vegetables

What to Eat	What Not to Eat
Fresh and most frozen vegetables	
Artichoke	Canned vegetables
Asparagus	Canned tomato juice
Avocado	Canned vegetable juice
Bamboo shoots	Frozen peas
Bean sprouts	Frozen lima beans
Beets	Frozen vegetables with seasoned sauce
Broccoli	Olives
Brussels sprouts	Pickled vegetables
Cabbage	Pickles
Carrots	Sauerkraut
Cauliflower	Seaweed
Celery	
Chicory	
Collards	
Corn	
Cucumber	
Dried beans	
Dried peas	
Eggplant	
Endive	
Escarole	
Green beans	
Kale	
Kohlrabi	
Leeks	
Lettuce	
Lima beans	
Mixed vegetables	
Mushrooms	
Mustard greens	
Okra	
Onion	
Parsley	
Parsnips	
Peas	
Peppers	
Potato, sweet white	
Pumpkin	
Radishes	
Rutabaga	
Scallions	
Soybeans	
Spinach	
Squash, summer acorn winter	
Tomato	
Tomato juice, low sodium	
Turnip	
V-8 Juice, low sodium	
Water chestnuts	
Watercress	
Wax beans	
Yams	

Note: Low sodium canned vegetables may be used.

What to Eat	What Not to Eat
Breads	Danish pastries
Cracked wheat	Muffins
French	Pancakes
Hamburger roll	Pizza
Hot dog roll	Spoonbread
Italian	Stuffing mix
Raisin	Sweet rolls
Rye	Waffles
Vienna	
White, enriched	**Crackers/Snack foods***
Whole wheat	Crackers with salted tops
Matzoh	Pretzels
Melba toast	Soda crackers
Rusk	*Consider crackers, chips, pretzels to be high in sodium unless labeled as "unsalted"
Rye Krisp	
Zwieback	**Cereals**
Cereals	Dry cereals, except those listed under "What to Eat"
Barley	Instant grits
Cream of Wheat, regular	Instant hot cereals
Cornmeal	Salted popcorn
Granola	**Pastas**
Grits, regular	Chow mein noodles
Oatmeal, regular	Prepackaged meals, such as macaroni, noodle, or spaghetti dinners
Petijohns	
Popcorn, unsalted	
Puffed Rice	
Puffed Wheat	
Ralston	
Rice	
Shredded Wheat	
Special K	
Tapioca	
Wheatena	
Pastas, Cooked without Salt	
Macaroni	
Noodles	
Spaghetti	

Protein Foods

What to Eat	What Not to Eat
Lean fresh meat	Bacon
Beef	Canned meats
Lamb	Corned beef
Liver	Dried chipped beef
Pork	Ham, cured or "low salt"
Veal	Hot dogs
	Luncheon meats
	Salt pork
	Sausage
	Scrapple
	Smoked meats
	Salted or pickled meats
	Mean extenders and "helpers"
	TV and frozen meat dinners
	"Fast food" meats

Fruits

What to Eat	What Not to Eat
Fresh, frozen, canned or dried fruit	Dried fruits that contain sodium preservative
Apple	
Apple juice	
Applesauce	
Apricots	
Banana	
Berries	
*Cantaloupe	
Cherries	
Cranberries	
Dates	
Figs	
*Grapefruit	
*Grapefruit juice	
*Lemon	
Nectarine	
*Orange	
*Orange juice	
Peach	
Pear	
Pineapple	
Pineapple juice	
Plums	
Prunes	
Prune juice	
Raisins	
Raspberries	
Rhubarb	

Food group	Recommended	Avoid / Restricted
Fresh fish	Bass, Bluefish, Carp, Cod, Flounder, Hake, Haddock, Halibut, Ocean perch, Pike, Pollack, Pompano, Porgy, Red snapper, Rockfish, Salmon, Shad, Sole, Swordfish, Trout, Tuna, Whitefish	Anchovy, Canned fish, Commercially frozen fish, "Fast food" fish, Herring, Salted fish, Sardines, Smoked or pickled fish, TV and frozen fish dinners
Fresh Shellfish	Crab, Crab, Lobster, Oysters*, Shrimp	Crabs, prepared with salty seasoning, Mussels, Scallops
Peanut butter		
Dried beans, cooked without salt, salt pork, or ham		Canned beans
Lean fresh poultry	Capon, Chicken, Cornish hen, Duck, Goose, Turkey	Canned chicken, Canned turkey, Commercial fried chicken, TV dinners, Turkey roll, Frozen turkey or chicken casseroles/pies, Frozen omelet, Frozen quiche, Frozen souffle
Desserts	Grapes, Grape juice, Honeydew, *Strawberries, *Tangerine, Watermelon, Custard, homemade, Fruit, Fruit cake, Fruit cobbler, Gelatin desserts, all flavors, Ice cream, Ice milk, Lady fingers, Sherbert, Sponge cake, homemade, Yogurt, plain	**Commercially prepared:** Cake, Cookies, Donuts, Pie, Pudding mixes, Sweet rolls
Seasonings	Garlic, fresh or powdered, Herbs and spices, Horseradish, fresh or prepared, Lemon, juice and peel, Onion, fresh, powered, flaked, Pepper, Tabasco sauce, Vanilla extract, Vinegar, Wine, Worcestershire sauce (used sparingly)	Barbeque sauce, Catsup, Celery salt, Chili sauce, Cooking wine (has salt added), Garlic salt, Lemon pepper seasoning, Meat tenderizers, Monosodium glutamate (MSG), Onion salt, Pickle relish, Prepared mustard, Salt, seasoned or plain, Sea salt, Soy sauce, Steak sauce
Dairy Products	Skim, Dry, Evaporated, Yogurt, plain, Brie, Chedder, Colby, Cottage, Gruyere, Monterey, Mozzarella, Muenster, Natural swiss, Neufchatel, Port du Salut, Ricotta, Cheese labeled "low sodium" or "unsalted"	Buttermilk (commercial), Condensed milk, "Fast food" shakes, Blue, Camembert, Cheezola, Edam, Feta, Gouda, Limburger, Parmesan, Processed Cheese, American and Swiss, Processed cheese foods, Processed cheese spreads, Provolone, Roquefort, Romano, Slim Line cheese, Tilsit
Beverages	Alcoholic beverages, in moderation, Club soda, Cocoa, Coffee—ground, instant, decaffeinated, Soft drinks, Sugar-free beverages, in moderation, Tea—loose, teabags, instant, Tonic water, Wine	
Breads, Crackers, Cereals, Grains	**Breads** Cinnamon, Corn and molasses **Crackers** Any crackers with unsalted tops	**Breads** Biscuits, Cornbread, Croutons, packaged

* If from saltwater bed, rinse saltwater out with fresh water.

[a] Adapted from "Health Is In—Salt Is Out," courtesy of The Maryland High Blood Pressure Coordinating Council.
[b] Useful conversions: 100 mg of sodium = 4.35 mEq of sodium.
100 mg of sodium = 250 mg of salt.
1 teaspoon of salt = 6 g of sodium.

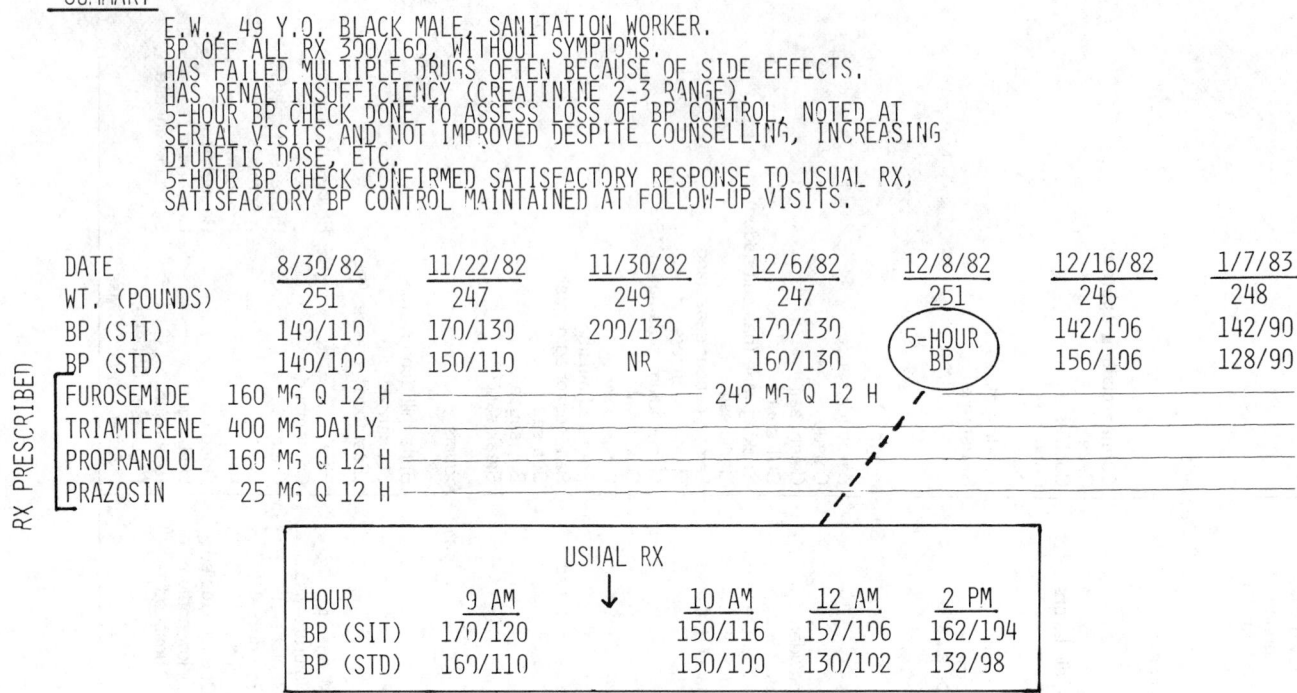

SUMMARY

E.W., 49 Y.O. BLACK MALE, SANITATION WORKER.
BP OFF ALL RX 300/160, WITHOUT SYMPTOMS.
HAS FAILED MULTIPLE DRUGS OFTEN BECAUSE OF SIDE EFFECTS.
HAS RENAL INSUFFICIENCY (CREATININE 2-3 RANGE)
5-HOUR BP CHECK DONE TO ASSESS LOSS OF BP CONTROL, NOTED AT
SERIAL VISITS AND NOT IMPROVED DESPITE COUNSELLING, INCREASING
DIURETIC DOSE, ETC.
5-HOUR BP CHECK CONFIRMED SATISFACTORY RESPONSE TO USUAL RX,
SATISFACTORY BP CONTROL MAINTAINED AT FOLLOW-UP VISITS.

DATE	8/30/82	11/22/82	11/30/82	12/6/82	12/8/82	12/16/82	1/7/83
WT. (POUNDS)	251	247	249	247	251	246	248
BP (SIT)	140/110	170/130	200/130	170/130	5-HOUR BP	142/106	142/90
BP (STD)	140/100	150/110	NR	160/130		156/106	128/90

RX PRESCRIBED

FUROSEMIDE	160 MG Q 12 H	— 240 MG Q 12 H
TRIAMTERENE	400 MG DAILY	
PROPRANOLOL	160 MG Q 12 H	
PRAZOSIN	25 MG Q 12 H	

USUAL RX

HOUR	9 AM	↓	10 AM	12 AM	2 PM
BP (SIT)	170/120		150/116	157/106	162/104
BP (STD)	160/110		150/100	130/102	132/98

Figure 62.9. Five-hour office observation of response to usual antihypertensive regimen to determine whether "loss of response" is due to tolerance, noncompliance, or secondarily resistant hypertension. From Barker LR: HBP Commentary. *Maryland Med J*, Feb. 1986, p. 94.

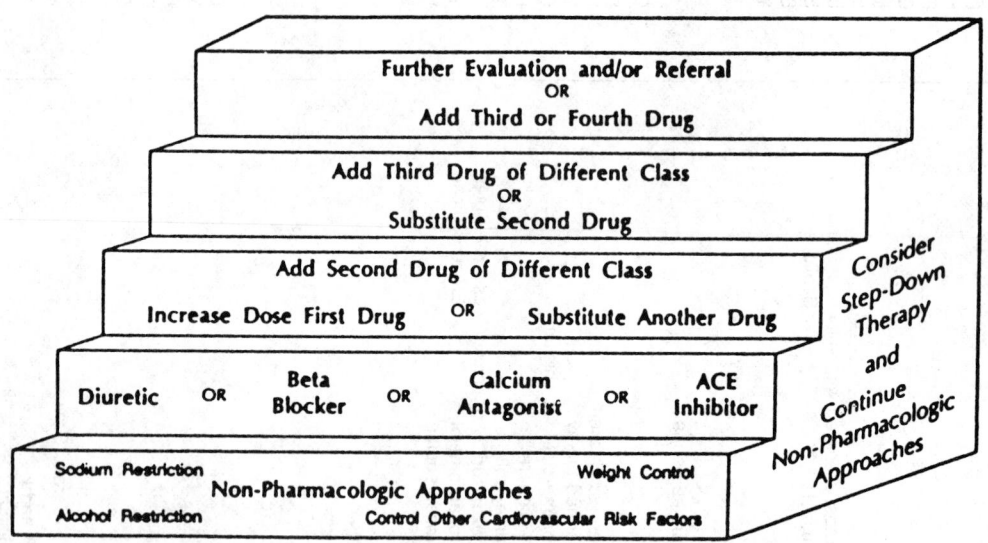

Figure 62.10. Step-care as recommended by JNC. (From The Joint National Committee on Detection, Evaluation, and Treatment of High Blood Pressure. *Arch Intern Med* 148:1023, 1988.)

nists. Additional considerations in managing young and elderly hypertensives are discussed in later sections of this chapter.

Coexisting medical conditions should always be considered in selecting antihypertensive drugs. Table 62.8 summarizes considerations in patients with a number of conditions. Selected antihypertensives may either exacerbate coexisting conditions (e.g., beta-blockers and obstructive airways disease) or favorably influence coexisting conditions (e.g., beta-blockers and

angina pectoris). New illness occurring during longitudinal care of hypertension may also affect management (see "Co-morbidity," below).

Drug Side Effects: Overview

Modification of the regimen may be needed when drugs control the hypertension but cause troublesome side effects. After any drug has been initiated, the patient should be encouraged to discuss any drug-as-

Table 62.8.
Considerations for Selecting Antihypertensive Drugs in Patients with Coexisting Medical Conditions

Coexisting Condition	Drugs That May Be Contraindicated or Disadvantageous	Drugs That May have Special Advantages
Obstructive airways disease	β-Blockers	None
Peripheral arterial insufficiency or Raynaud's phenomenon	β-Blockers	Calcium channel blockers
Congestive heart failure		
Dilated hypokenetic heart	β-Blockers diltiazem, verapamil	ACE inhibitors Vasodilators
Hyperkinetic heart with diminished diastolic relaxation	Vasodilators Diuretics	β-Blockers Calcium Channel Blockers
Angina pectoris	Vasodilators	β-Blockers Calcium channel blockers
Atrioventricular nodal disease	β-Blockers Verapamil, diltiazem	None
Sinus bradycardia	β-Blockers	None
Supraventricular arrhythmia	None	Verapamil
Migraine or cluster headaches	Vasodilators	β-Blockers Calcium channel blockers
Possible bilateral renal artery stenosis (abdominal bruits, widespread atherosclerosis)	ACE inhibitors	None
Diabetes		
On Insulin	β-Blockers	ACE inhibitors
Diet controlled	Thiazide and loop diuretics β-Blockers	ACE inhibitors
Depressed mood	Central adrenergic inhibitors Reserpine	None
Chronic liver disease[a]	Methyldopa	None
Chronic renal disease[a]	None	High dose loop diuretics
Chronic constipation	Verapamil	None
Chronic diarrhea (e.g., irritable bowel syndrome)	Methyldopa, guanethidine, hydralazine	Verapamil
Allergic or perennial rhinitis	Reserpine	None

[a] See Table 62.11 for principal routes of excretion for nondiuretic antihypertensives.

sociated disturbances, such as reduced mental alertness, mood change, or impairment in physical exercise or sexual activity. It should be remembered that from 5 to 15% of subjects discontinue therapy in the trials of most antihypertensive drugs because of such side effects and that many more subjects notice minor side effects as long as they are taking antihypertensive drugs. On the other hand, learning that one has hypertension may cause some apparent "side effects." This point is illustrated in Table 62.9, which displays the frequency of a number of side effects reported by subjects taking a diuretic, a beta-blocker, or a placebo in the British Medical Research Council Trial.

In recent years, *quality of life indices* have been developed to better measure the impact of antihypertensive drugs on patients (14). In general, thiazide diuretics, the ACE inhibitors, and calcium channel blockers have caused the least interference in quality of life as measured by these instruments.

Because *orthostatic exaggeration of the hypotensive effect* can occur with any antihypertensive drug, patients should be asked about orthostatic symptoms and should have a standing blood pressure measured after every change in the regimen. For those with a fall in systolic pressure of more than 15 mm Hg, a standing blood pressure should also be measured after exercise (e.g., 10 steps on a footstool or walking a fixed distance), as exercise may exacerbate drug-induced orthostatic hypotension. For patients reporting transient orthostatic symptoms shortly after taking their daily medication, direct observation of their blood pressure response may be useful (see example case in Fig. 62.11).

Cost of Antihypertensive Drugs

The cost for treating hypertension, a symptomatic risk factor, is substantial. Prescribing should take into account the cost as well as the other properties of antihypertensive drugs. The cost for a one-month supply of most brand-name nondiuretic antihypertensive drugs is between $25 and $75. When generic preparations are available, the cost is substantially lower. The least expensive regimens (less than $10 per month) are monotherapy with a generic preparation of propranolol or a diuretic. When combination therapy is needed, a combination of drugs available in generic forms may still be relatively inexpensive (e.g., the combination of hydrochlorothiazide, propranolol, hydralazine, and KCl supplement may cost less than $25 per month, whereas the same combination in brand-name preparations may cost up to $75 per month).

Properties of Individual Drugs: Overview

The diuretics used for hypertension are listed by class in Table 69.10, which also lists available strengths and recommended dose ranges. For each nondiuretic antihypertensive, the following properties are summarized in Table 62.11: generic and proprietary names, available strengths, recommended dose range, sched-

Table 62.9.
Prevalence of Symptoms at 12 Weeks and at 2 Years after Entry, British Medical Research Council Trial[a]

	Men—percentage of affirmative answers (N = 1130)						Women—percentage of affirmative answers (N = 958)					
Complaint[b]	Bendrofluazide		Propranolol		Placebos		Bendrofluazide		Propranolol		Placebos	
	12 Wk	2 Yr	12 Wk	2 Yr	12 Wk	2 Yr	12 Wk	2 Yr	12 Wk	2 Yr	12 Wk	2 Yr
Dizziness	13.7[c]	9.3	6.9	9.0	5.9	8.4	25.3[d]	19.4	18.1	17.8	16.8	16.1
Muscle pain	13.5	22.2	15.7	14.1	14.6	16.8	25.2	14.6[d]	21.6	17.2	22.5	26.8
Slowed walking	2.6	9.9	7.9	11.0	6.6	7.6	10.0	7.1	12.6[d]	10.6	6.2	6.9
Exertional dyspnea	16.1	23.8	19.4	27.9[d]	14.0	16.4	20.9	25.8	18.4	26.1	21.0	21.1
Headaches	19.6	16.5	21.9	19.7	27.1	26.2	31.9[d]	36.0	33.1	29.8	42.4	37.8
Cold/numb digits	8.4	15.8	14.2	12.6	11.5	10.7	18.8	16.1	18.3	29.3[d]	16.3	15.6
Paresthesias	11.6	14.9	14.7	14.3	14.7	11.2	28.9[d]	28.9	19.7	25.0	18.4	17.5
Dry mouth	13.7	12.4	11.2	7.5	7.7	7.7	26.6	28.1[d]	18.8	18.2	21.3	13.6
Blocked or runny nose	13.7	14.7	23.2[c]	26.8	12.5	18.2	11.5	18.3	20.1	22.6	19.2	12.9
Vomiting/nausea	3.9	5.0	7.9[c]	3.7	3.2	4.5	13.4	5.1	6.3	4.3	8.2	10.3
Impotence	16.2[d]	22.6[d]	13.8	13.2	8.9	10.1						

[a]From Report of Medical Research Council Working Party on Mild to Moderate Hypertension: Adverse reactions to bendrofluazide and propranol for the treatment of mild hypertension. *Lancet* 1:8246, 1981.
[b]Reported in questionnaire.
[c]$p < 0.01$.
[d]$p < 0.05$. Significance levels refer to prevalence rates for each active drug separately compared with those for all control patients. The figures do not indicate comparisons between the two active drugs.

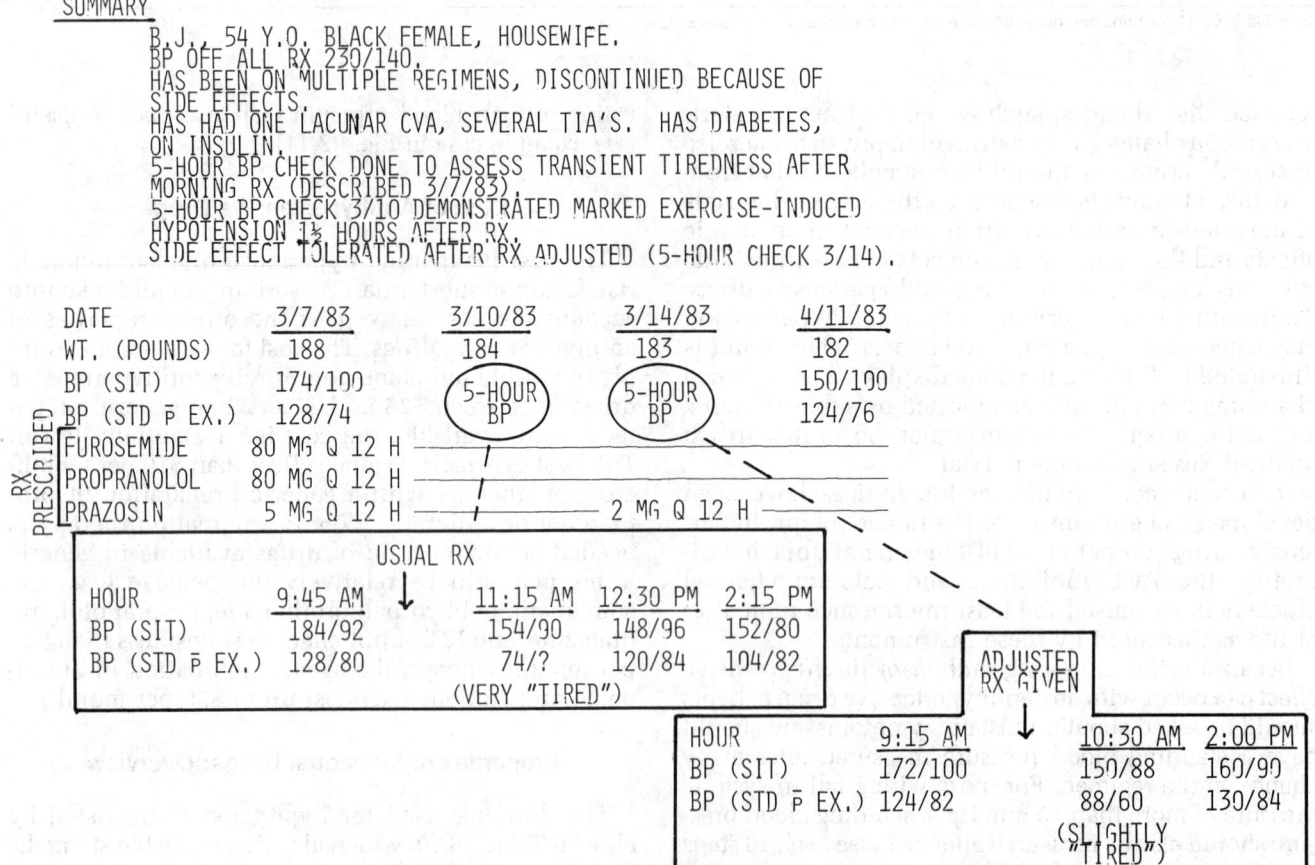

SUMMARY
B.J., 54 Y.O. BLACK FEMALE, HOUSEWIFE.
BP OFF ALL RX 230/140.
HAS BEEN ON MULTIPLE REGIMENS, DISCONTINUED BECAUSE OF SIDE EFFECTS.
HAS HAD ONE LACUNAR CVA, SEVERAL TIA'S. HAS DIABETES, ON INSULIN.
5-HOUR BP CHECK DONE TO ASSESS TRANSIENT TIREDNESS AFTER MORNING RX (DESCRIBED 3/7/83).
5-HOUR BP CHECK 3/10 DEMONSTRATED MARKED EXERCISE-INDUCED HYPOTENSION 1½ HOURS AFTER RX.
SIDE EFFECT TOLERATED AFTER RX ADJUSTED (5-HOUR CHECK 3/14).

Figure 62.11.   Five-hour observation of response to usual medication in a patient who described transient symptoms after medication every day but had satisfactory pressures at office visits. (From Barker LR: HBP commentary. *Maryland Med J,* Feb. 1986.)

Table 62.10.
Diuretic Drugs Utilized for Hypertension

Class/Name of Drugs[a]	Available Strengths (mg)	Dose Range for Hypertension (mg/day)
THIAZIDES AND RELATED SULFONAMIDE DIURETICS		
Bendroflumethiazide (Naturetin)	2.5, 5, 10	2.5–5
Benzthiazide	25, 50	25–50
Chlorothiazide sodium (Diuril)[b]	250, 500	250–500
Chlorthalidone (Hygroton)[b]	25, 50, 100	25–50
Cyclothiazide (Anhydron, Fluidil)	2	1–2
Hydrochlorothiazide[b]	25, 50	25–50
Hydroflumethiazide (Diucardin, Saluron)[b]	50	25–50
Indapamide (Lozol)	2.5	2.5–5
Methyclothiazide[b]	5	2.5–5
Metolazone (Diulo, Zaroxolyn)	2.5, 5, 10	2.5–5
Polythiazide (Renese)	1, 2, 4	2–4
Quinethazone (Hydromox)	50	50–100
Trichlormethiazide (Metahydrin, Naqua)[b]	2, 4	2–4
LOOP DIURETICS		
Bumetanide (Bumex)	0.5, 1	0.5–10
Ethacrynic acid (Edecrin)	50	50–200
Furosemide (Lasix)[b]	20, 40, 80	20–480
POTASSIUM-SPARING DIURETICS		
Amiloride hydrochloride (Midamor)[c]	5	5–10
Spironolactone (Aldactone)[b,d]	25, 50, 100	50–100
Triamterene (Dyrenium)[e]	50, 100	50–100

[a]If more than two proprietary formulations are available, names are not listed.
[b]Generic is available.
[c]Combination form (Moduretic): Amiloride/hydrochlorothiazide 5 mg/50 mg.
[d]Combination forms (Aldactazide and generic): spironolactone/hydrochlorothiazide 25 mg/25 mg and 50 mg/50 mg.
[e]Combination forms (Dyazide: triamterene/hydrochlorothiazide 50 mg/25 mg, Maxide: triamterene/hydrochlorothiazide 75 mg/50 mg, Maxide-25, which contains 37.5/25 mg, and generic).

ule (and alternate schedule for some), onset time and duration of principal action, and principal route(s) of metabolism and elimination.

Diuretics

Mechanism

Diuretics probably lower blood pressure by decreasing modestly the circulating volume and by decreasing peripheral resistance. A chronic increase in plasma renin activity has been demonstrated in diuretic-treated patients; this provides indirect evidence that the decrease in circulating volume persists as long as the patient is taking the diuretic.

Thiazide and Loop Diuretics

Doses and schedules. For monotherapy or combined diuretic-nondiuretic therapy, a once daily schedule, using the dose ranges listed in Table 69.10, is satisfactory, and the patient can select the time of day that is most convenient (e.g., after rather than before work because of the modest diuresis). Recommended starting and maximal doses for diuretics are the equivalent of 12.5 to 25 mg and 50 mg of hydrochlorothiazide; in most patients, the principal antihypertensive effect of diuretics is realized at these doses, and higher doses increase the likelihood of unwanted metabolic consequences of diuretics. The major antihypertensive response is seen within 1 to 2 weeks of initiating or increasing a diuretic. Full reversal of antihypertensive effect occurs within 1 week of discontinuing the drug.

Relatively high doses of loop diuretics (furosemide,

bumetanide) may be necessary in an occasional patient who requires large doses of one or more nondiuretic drugs. These more potent diuretics may also be needed to control hypertension in patients who will not restrict salt use and have edema that does not respond to thiazides; the serum potassium concentration should be monitored closely in such patients (e.g., within 1 or 2 weeks of adding or increasing a loop diuretic) since precipitous potassium depletion may occur.

Precautions. Mild side effects, such as increased urination and transient orthostatic symptoms, are common when diuretics are initiated. Sexual impotence is an important, though infrequent, side effect of diuretics (see Table 62.9). Of the other side effects, those seen most commonly are the following, due to metabolic effects of diuretics: hypokalemia, gout related to hyperuricemia, impaired glucose tolerance, and an increase in low density lipoprotein cholesterol and triglyceride levels (thiazides and chlorthalidone). A modest reduction in total body potassium occurs in most patients, and frank hypokalemia (less than 3.5 mEq/liter) in some. In nonedematous patients taking thiazide diuretics, restriction of sodium intake (see above) and the use of the equivalent of 50 mg of hydrochlorothiazide or less will prevent most hypokalemia. Because ventricular ectopy may be precipitated by hypokalemia, patients should be monitored for hypokalemia (at 3 to 4 weeks; if greater than 3.5 mEq/liter, twice yearly) and the hypokalemia should be treated whenever it is detected. In nonedematous patients with hypokalemia, potassium supplements do not restore a normal potassium level as reliably as potassium-sparing diuretics (see the next section). If

Table 62.11.
Pharmacological Characteristics of Nondiuretic Antihypertensive Drugs

Class/Name of Drug	Available Strengths (mg)	Dose Range (mg/day)	Schedule (Alternative)	Major Action Onset/Duration (Hours)	Metabolism and Elimination[a]
ADRENERGIC INHIBITORS					
β-Blockers					
Acebutolol (Sectral)[b, c]	200, 400	200–1200	Once daily (twice daily)	3–8/24[e]	L, K
Atenolol (Tenormin)[b]	50, 100	25–100	Once daily	2–4/24-48[e]	K
Carteolol (Cartrol)	2.5, 5	2.5–10	Once daily	?/?	K
Metoprolol (Lopressor)[b]	50, 100	50–300	Once daily (twice daily)	2–4/24-48[e]	L
Nadolol (Corgard)	40, 80, 120	20–120	Once daily	2–4/24-48[e]	K
Penbutolol (Levatol)[c]	20	20–80	Once daily	1–3/20-24	L
Pindolol (Visken)[c]	5, 10	20–60	Twice daily	?	L
Propranolol (Inderal)[d]	10, 20, 40, 60, 80	40–≥480	Twice daily	2-4/24-48[e]	L
Propranolol long acting (Inderal LA)	80, 120, 160	80–>480	Once daily	?	L
Timolol (Blocadren)	5, 10, 20	20–60	Twice daily	?	L
Central acting sympatholytics					
Clonidine (Catapres)	0.1, 0.2, 0.3	0.2–2.4	Twice daily	1-2/8-12	K
Catapres TTS	0.1, 0.2, 0.3	0.1–0.3	Once daily	3 days/7 days	K
Guanabenz (Wytensin)	4, 8	8–32	Twice daily	2–4/12	L, K
Guanfacine (Tenex)	1	1–3	Once or twice daily	?/24	K
Methyldopa (Aldomet)[d]	250, 500	250–3000	Twice daily (once at bedtime)	4–6/24-48	K
α-Blockers					
Prazosin (Minipress)	1, 2, 5	2–320	Twice daily (3 times daily)	1-2/12-24	L
Terazosin (Hytrin)	1, 2, 5	1–20	Once daily	2–3/24	L
α-β Blocker					
Labetalol (Trandate, Normodyne)	200, 300	200–≥1200	Twice daily (3 times daily)	1–3/8-24	L, K
Peripheral acting sympatholytics					
Guanadrel (Hylorel)	10, 25	20–75	Twice daily	2–6/?	K
Guanethidine (Ismelin)	10, 25	10–200	Every day	3–5 days/31 wk	K
Reserpine[d]	0.1, 0.25	0.1–0.25	Once daily	1–2 wk/31 wk	K
ANGIOTENSEN-CONVERTING ENZYME INHIBITORS					
Captopril (Capoten)	12.5, 25, 50, 100	19.5–450	3 times daily	1–3/8-12	K
Enalapril (Vasotec)	5, 10	10–40	Once daily	3–4/24	K
Lisinopril (Prinivil, Zestril)	5, 10, 20	5–40	Once daily	2–4/24	K
CALCIUM CHANNEL BLOCKERS					
Diltiazem (Cardizem)[f]	30, 60, 90	120–240	3 times daily	1–3/8-12	L, K
Nicardipine (Cardene)	20, 30	60–120	3 times daily	1–3/8-12	L
Nifedipine (Procardia, Adalat)[f]	10, 20	30–180	3 times daily	1–3/8-12	K
Verapamil (Calan, Isoptin)[f]		240–480	3 times daily	1–3/8/12	L, K
VASODILATORS					
Hydralazine (Apresoline)[d]	10, 25, 75, 100	20–3300	Twice daily (3 times daily)	1–4/12-24	K
Minoxidil (Loniten)	2.5, 10	5–340	Once daily (twice daily)	1–3/24-48	

[a] L, Liver; K, kidney.
[b] Cardioselective β-blockade.
[c] Has intrinsic sympathomimetic activity (ISA)
[d] Generic is available.
[e] Refers to cardioinhibitory action (principal antihypertensive effect may be delayed 1 to 7 days).
[f] Available in slow-release preparation (see details in text).

diabetes mellitus is found at the baseline evaluation or if new diabetes develops in the course of long-term diuretic therapy, strict calorie and sodium restriction should be prescribed instead of diuretic therapy, and nondiuretic antihypertensives should be utilized if dietary modification fails to control the blood pressure. With these measures, glucose tolerance does not deteriorate (or returns to normal) in many patients. Diuretic-induced increases in plasma lipid levels may not persist during long-term treatment; and they can be prevented by adherence to a diet low in saturated fat and cholesterol; therefore, it is appropriate to rec-

ommend this diet to all patients when diuretic treatment is started.

The metabolic abnormalities that may be associated with diuretics are discussed in detail in Chapters 45 (hypokalemia), 69 (gout), 72 (diabetes mellitus), and 75 (hyperlipidemia).

Apart from allergy and a number of uncommon coexisting conditions (e.g., psychogenic polydipsia, hypercalcemia, history of hyponatremia due to inappropriate antidiuretic hormone excretion), there are no absolute contraindications for diuretics in hypertension. Because thiazides can cause an increase in renal reabsorption of lithium, it is advisable to select an alternative drug for hypertension in patients who are taking lithium. Because thiazide-treated patients with abnormal electrocardiograms in the MRFIT trial had an increased mortality rate (43), some authorities caution against the use of thiazides as initial treatment in such patients.

Potassium-Sparing Diuretics

The potassium-sparing diuretics (amiloride, spironolactone, and triamterene) have modest antihypertensive effects when used alone in some patients with essential hypertension. They are useful in combination with other diuretics, chiefly to avoid or reverse hypokalemia (see Chapter 45). One preparation (triamterene-hydrochlorothiazide) is the diuretic that is most frequently prescribed for hypertension in the United States, presumably because of its potassium-sparing property. The diuretics in this group may also be used to enhance diuretic action in the occasional patient who remains edematous while taking thiazide or loop diuretics and potent nondiuretic antihypertensives, especially the vasodilator minoxidil. In such patients blood pressure control may improve dramatically when a potassium-conserving drug is added.

Precautions. To avoid iatrogenic hyperkalemia, potassium-sparing diuretics should not be given concurrently with potassium supplements or with ACE inhibitors (see below) and should be used with caution in diabetic patients because some diabetics have an increased risk of developing hyperkalemia when they take these diuretics. Spironolactone has a number of undesirable endocrine side effects (especially gynecomastia and, occasionally, impotence). Therefore, amiloride or triamterene is preferable to spironolactone in male subjects. The compositions of the principal thiazide/potassium-sparing combinations are listed in the footnotes of Table 62.10.

Adrenergic Inhibitors

Beta-Blocking Drugs

The beta-blocking drugs available in the United States are listed in Table 62.11.

Mechanism. One or more of the following mechanisms probably accounts for the major antihypertensive effect in patients who respond to beta-blocking agents: blockade of cardiac beta-receptors causing decreased cardiac output, blockade of renal beta-receptors causing inhibition of renin release, blockade of central nervous system beta-receptors causing decreased sympathetic outflow, or blockade of presynaptic beta-receptors causing decreased release of catecholamines. Evidence of some cardiac beta-receptor blockade (heart rate of 64 beats or less per minute at rest and less than 80 per minute after brief exercise in the office) is present in many but not all patients whose hypertension responds to these drugs. However, there is no clinically useful way to determine which blocking mechanism is dominant in responders.

Selected Properties. Carteolol, penbutolol, pindolol, propranolol, nadolol, and timolol are *nonselective* beta-blockers, whereas acebutal, atenolol, and metaprolol are *cardioselective*. The major theoretical advantage of a cardioselective beta-blocker is the relative lack of beta 2-receptor blockade. Beta 2-receptors mediate bronchodilation, dilation of resistance vessels, and the sympathetic response to hypoglycemia (tachycardia, sweating). Three beta-blockers—acebutal, penbutolol, and pindolol—have *intrinsic sympathomimetic activity* (ISA), which may be reflected clinically by less tendency to produce bradycardia or to precipitate bronchospasm or heart failure in patients whose baseline respiratory or cardiac function is partly dependent on beta-sympathetic stimulation.

Atenolol, carteolol, and nadolol are *less lipid soluble* and more water soluble than other beta-blockers. This has two consequences that may affect clinical decisions: (*a*) These drugs are dependent on renal excretion and dose intervals may be longer in patients with kidney disease; (*b*) they enter brain tissue less readily than do other beta-blockers and may cause fewer central nervous system side effects (e.g., depression, insomnia, nightmares).

Most beta-blockers may be useful over a broad dose range (see Table 62.11). Atenolol, however, produces little or no additional blood pressure reduction when the daily dose exceeds 100 mg.

For all of the beta-blocking drugs (except for those drugs with ISA), slowing of heart rate and some blood pressure response occur within 2 to 4 hours of taking an initial dose, but the full antihypertensive effect may not be seen until the patient has taken the drug for 1 week. The principal antihypertensive effect of these drugs resolves within 1 to 2 days of discontinuing the drug.

For the subset of hypertensive patients who have symptoms of left ventricular heart failure, good left ventricular function, and a small left ventricular cavity due to poor diastolic phase relaxation, beta-blockers, like calcium channel blockers (see below), may reverse the diastolic stiffness and lower the blood pressure (50). This form of hypertensive cardiomyopathy has been described chiefly in older hypertensive patients.

Precautions. Whenever a beta-blocking agent is being discontinued after prolonged use, it should be tapered over 1 to 2 weeks rather than abruptly stopped, because of the possibility of precipitating angina, acute rebound to pretreatment blood pressure levels, or a number of other withdrawal symptoms (e.g., anxiety, tachycardia, palpitations, tremor, perspiration, or increase in headaches in patients with migraine).

The most common side effects are nausea, abdominal cramps, diarrhea, mild sedation, fatigue, nightmares, cool extremities, and asymptomatic bradycardia. Sexual impotence has been reported occasionally. Of note is the fact that hypertensive athletes tolerate beta-blocking agents well.

With certain coexisting conditions, the beta-blocking properties of these drugs may cause serious side effects. Absolute contraindications to the use of beta-blockers are baseline-marked bradycardia (heart rate less than 50), impaired left ventricular function due to dilated cardiomyopathy, high degree heart block, symptomatic asthma or chronic obstructive pulmonary disease, and severe peripheral vascular disease (e.g., gangrene, skin necrosis, severe or worsening claudication). For patients with mild asthma or chronic obstructive pulmonary disease, stable peripheral vascular disease, or stable insulin-requiring diabetes, it would be reasonable to try a low dose of a cardioselective beta-blocker or a beta-blocker with ISA if other antihypertensive regimens have been unsuccessful. It is recommended that a selective beta 2-bronchodilator (see Chapter 55) be used concurrently whenever a beta-blocking agent must be prescribed for a patient with asthma or chronic obstructive pulmonary disease.

Modest decreases in glucose tolerance may accompany long-term use of propranolol; and those beta-blockers that do not have ISA cause small increases in serum triglyceride and decreases in high density lipoprotein concentrations in some patients. The significance of these changes has not been established.

Drug Interactions. In diabetic patients taking insulin or sulfonylureas, beta-blockers may potentiate acute hypoglycemia and may mask the peripheral signs of hypoglycemia. In combination with digitalis, beta-blockers may produce additional suppression of atrioventricular nodal conduction; they may also partly blunt the inotropic effect of digitalis. Cimetidine, because it decreases hepatic blood flow, may decrease the first pass extraction of the lipid-soluble beta-blockers (i.e., all beta-blockers except atenolol, carteolol, and nadolol), thereby enhancing their antihypertensive and other effects. Beta-blockers should also be used cautiously if at all with the calcium channel blockers that have cardiodepressive effects (verapamil and diltiazem).

Combination with Other Antihypertensives. The addition of a diuretic usually enhances the antihypertensive effect of beta-blocker therapy. The addition of a vasodilator or the calcium channel blockers nicardipine and nifedipine is usually very effective in patients not controlled with a beta-blocker; the beta-blocker prevents the reflex tachycardia that may be provoked by vasodilators and by nicardipine and nifedipine. Any other adrenergic inhibitor or an ACE inhibitor may also be synergistic with a beta-blocker.

Central Acting Alpha-Adrenergic Agonists: Clonidine, Guanabenz, and Guanfacine

Mechanism. These drugs are alpha-adrenergic agonists. Their locus of action is thought to be the medulla oblongata where, through a feedback effect, sympathetic outflow to the peripheral vasculature is reduced. In addition, these drugs suppress renin release, but a relationship between this property and the antihypertensive effect of the central alpha-agonists has not been established.

Selected Properties. Clonidine has been used extensively since it was introduced in 1975. The major antihypertensive response to clonidine occurs within 1 hour and remits after 8 to 16 hours. Because of its rapid onset of action, oral clonidine can be given hourly in doses of 0.1 or 0.2 mg in order to determine rapidly the dose needed to treat an individual patient. This property has been exploited to lower the blood pressure over several hours in symptom-free patients with very high pressures (so-called hypertensive "urgencies"). However, apart from hypertensive emergencies requiring hospitalization and parenteral treatment (see above), there are no indications for such rapid lowering of the blood pressure.

Clonidine is also available in a *sustained-release clonidine patch* (the Catapres Transdermal Therapeutic System, TTS), which lasts 7 days. In addition to the advantage of once a week application, the TTS delivers a smaller dose of the drug and may therefore cause fewer side effects; also blood levels subside slowly at the end of a week, eliminating the risk of rebound hypertension due to abrupt termination of clonidine. The patch is available in three sizes, delivering, respectively, 0.1, 0.2, and 0.3 mg per day. The major antihypertensive effect is not seen until the third day after applying the initial TTS or after applying a new patch containing a higher dose. About two-thirds of patients with mild hypertension have been well controlled; however, up to 20% of patients have had to discontinue the clonidine TTS because of a rash. The role of the TTS in managing a broad spectrum of hypertensive patients has not yet been established.

Guanabenz may lower total serum cholesterol modestly, a unique property among antihypertensive drugs.

Guanfacine, introduced in 1987, has a longer duration of action than oral clonidine and guanabenz, so that it can be taken once per day. Patients should be instructed to take quanficine at bedtime to minimize problems due to the sedating effect of the drug.

Precautions. Rebound to pretreatment, or higher-than-pretreatment, blood pressure, with accompanying symptoms of increased sympathetic nervous system activity (tachycardia, perspiration, headache, palpitations) may follow within one to two days the abrupt discontinuation of oral clonidine, guanabenz, or guanfacine. Treatment for this problem is reinstitution of the drug. As there is no way to recognize prospectively the patients at risk of developing this problem, all patients must be regarded as at risk. In selecting antihypertensive drugs, patients known to be erratic in taking medication should thus not receive these drugs, and all patients for whom they are prescribed should be warned explicitly of the risk of discontinuing the drug.

The most common side effects are sedation, dry mouth, constipation, and orthostatic symptoms. Impotence has been reported. There are no absolute contraindications to the use of these agents.

Drug Interactions. Tricyclic antidepressants may diminish the blood pressure lowering effect of these drugs. Excessive sedation may occur when clonidine, guanabenz, or guanfacine is taken concurrently with any drug having central nervous system depressant effects, including alcohol.

Combination with Other Antihypertensive Drugs. Clonidine has been used with hydralazine to prevent the reflex sympathetic response to hydralazine (see below). This combination is useful in patients needing a vasodilator who cannot take the more widely studied combination of beta-blocking drugs and hydralazine, such as patients with a history of bronchospasm. Synergy between clonidine and prazosin has also been demonstrated.

Other Central Acting Adrenergic Inhibitors: Methyldopa

Mechanism. There is evidence that the derivative of methyldopa, methylnorepinephrine, displaces norepinephrine in the central nervous system and that the hypotensive effect of methyldopa is related to this effect. Methyldopa also suppresses renin release from the kidney, but a relationship of this property to its antihypertensive action has not been clearly established.

Selected Properties. Although 250 to 3000 mg is the daily dose range publicized frequently, an additional hypotensive response is rarely attained with doses greater than 2000 mg. Over long intervals of continuous treatment (e.g., 10 years), most patients require a gradual increase in their daily dose of methyldopa to maintain satisfactory blood pressure control.

In studies of small numbers of patients, it has been shown that hypertension is controlled for 24 hours regardless of whether the same total daily dose is given on a four times daily, three times daily, twice daily, or once daily schedule. For patients who comply poorly or who experience sedation after daytime doses of methyldopa, a single dose at bedtime can be tried in place of the usual twice daily schedule. The major antihypertensive effect of methyldopa occurs within 4 to 6 hours of oral administration, and the hypotensive response remits within 1 to 2 days.

Precautions. Rapid rebound to pretreatment pressures, with or without symptoms, has been reported in a few patients after abrupt discontinuation of methyldopa. The most common side effects are orthostatic symptoms, sedation, mood alteration, impotence, and diarrhea (soft stools, two to four times daily). After 6 to 12 months, about 10% of patients taking methyldopa develop a positive direct Coombs' test, and rarely there is associated hemolysis. Because methyldopa may cause hepatitis, it is contraindicated in patients with active liver disease.

Drug Interactions. Tricyclic antidepressants may diminish the blood pressure lowering effect of methyldopa; chronically coadministered phenobarbital may reduce the effect of methyldopa due to induction of hepatic microsomal enzymes. When methyldopa is given with L-dopa, the hypotensive effect of the former may be potentiated and the antiparkinsonian effect of

the latter may be reduced. Finally toxicity from lithium and from neuroleptic drugs may be increased when methyldopa is taken concurrently.

Combination with Other Antihypertensive Drugs. The combination of methyldopa and a beta-blocker is more effective than either drug alone. In patients who show a partial response to one of these drugs, adding a small amount of the other may at times be more practical than starting a different drug. Synergy with prazosin and with hydralazine has also been demonstrated.

Alpha-Adrenergic Blockers: Prazosin and Terazosin

Mechanism. These drugs block postsynaptic alpha-receptors in arterioles and venules, presumably decreasing blood pressure by impairing sympathetic tone at both sites. They do not block presynaptic alpha-receptors. This may explain why they do not predictably cause tachycardia and renin release, as both of these adaptive responses to blood pressure lowering are inhibited by activation of the presynaptic alpha-receptors.

Selected Properties. Although the recommended maximal dose of prazosin is 20 mg/day, an additional antihypertensive effect may be attained at higher doses; in the patient with hypertension refractory to other drugs, a trial of high dose prazosin is therefore reasonable. Because of the broad range of doses that may be needed to control blood pressure in different patients, prazosin may require more dosage changes than other antihypertensive drugs in patients who do not respond to an initial low dose.

The usual schedule for prazosin is twice daily. Studies have shown that some patients may have to follow a three times daily schedule, whereas others may be able to take prazosin once a day. It is helpful to check the blood pressure just before the next scheduled dose in order to determine the most appropriate schedule for prazosin. The major antihypertensive response to a dose of prazosin occurs within 1 to 2 hours and remits entirely after 24 hours.

Terazosin was introduced in 1988. Its properties and effectiveness are identical to those of prazosin except that it has a longer duration of action, meaning that it can be taken once per day.

Prazosin and terazosin have the effect of lowering slightly the serum concentration of low density lipoprotein-cholesterol; when added to diuretics or beta-blockers, it may counterbalance the unfavorable effects of these drugs on serum lipids.

Precautions. The most common side effects from these two drugs are postural hypotension, headache, drowsiness, dry mouth, and palpitations. Sexual impotence is uncommon. Postural hypotension, usually without tachycardia and at times asymptomatic, occurs as a transient problem in up to half of patients during the first few days they take prazosin. Syncope occurring within ½ hour after the initial dose is a very rare, but severe, side effect. It may occur after taking a 1-mg dose. Clearly, warning and reassurance about postural symptoms (for the first few days) are important whenever this drug is prescribed. In addition, patients should either take their first dose, 1 mg for either drug, in the office (and be observed for about 1 hour) or they should be instructed to take it at bedtime, so that they will be recumbent during the initial adjustment to the drug.

There are no absolute contraindications to the use of prazosin or terazosin.

Drug Interactions. Apart from the risk of additive orthostatic hypotension when they are given with drugs that can cause this problem, there are no important interactions with drugs that might be administered with prazosin or terazosin.

Combination with Other Antihypertensive Drugs. The combination of prazosin or terazosin and a beta-blocker is frequently effective in patients with moderate or severe hypertension that does not respond to either drug alone. Synergism has also been reported with clonidine, methyldopa, and hydralazine.

The use of prazosin in the ambulatory management of congestive heart failure is discussed in Chapter 61.

Alpha-Beta-Blocker: Labetalol

Mechanism. Labetalol combines nonselective beta-blockade and intrinsic sympathomimetic activity (ISA) with postsynaptic alpha-blockade. These two properties exist on separate molecules, making labetalol a fixed-dose combination and not a single drug. During labetalol treatment, control of hypertension is usually accompanied by a modest reduction in resting and postexercise heart rate. The cardiac index and peripheral resistance are reduced during the first year of treatment, but after several years cardiac index returns to normal whereas total peripheral resistance remains lower.

Selected Properties. Labetalol is effective as monotherapy in somewhat more than 50% of patients with mild or moderate hypertension and in about one-third of patients with severe hypertension. It seems to be equally effective in black and white subjects.

The dose range is large (200 to ≥1200 mg per day). Because the full impact of a dose occurs within 1 to 3 hours, the dose can be titrated up rapidly. Most responders are controlled with daily doses of 400 to 800 mg. Abrupt discontinuation does not appear to cause a withdrawal state similar to that observed occasionally with the beta-blockers.

Precautions. The most frequent side effects seen with labetalol are fatigue, nausea, dyspepsia, dizziness, nasal stuffiness, and pruritic rash. Impotence has been the commonest reason for early termination of labetalol.

Because of its ISA, labetalol may be somewhat safer than pure beta-blockers in patients with obstructive airways disease; however, it has been associated with a modest fall in 1-second forced expiratory volume when given chronically to patients with mild obstruc-

tive airways disease. Labetalol is contraindicated in patients with greater than first degree heart block.

Drug Interactions. Apart from an enhancement of the bioavailability and action of labetalol when it is taken concurrently with cimetidine, interactions with commonly prescribed drugs have not been described.

Combination with Other Antihypertensive Drugs. As is true of all antihypertensives, diuretics may enhance the effect of labetalol on blood pressure.

Peripheral Acting Sympatholytics: Guanadrel and Guanethidine

Mechanism. These drugs prevent release of and deplete stores of norepinephrine in peripheral tissues but not in the central nervous system. Their hypotensive action is ascribed to the loss of sympathetic regulation of vessel tone in the venous and arterial circulation. Because their hypotensive effect depends predominantly upon impaired venous tone, the effects of guanethidine and guanadrel are always more pronounced when patients are standing, particularly after exercise.

Selected Properties. With large enough doses, these drugs will lower the blood pressure in most patients. For this reason, guanethidine (the older of the two) was previously recommended for the treatment of hypertension resistant to other drugs. The major antihypertensive effect of guanadrel occurs within 4 to 6 hours of the first dose and lasts 12 to 24 hours. The major effect of guanethidine is seen after 3 to 5 days of initiating treatment and remits within 1 to 2 weeks of discontinuing the drug.

Precautions. Orthostatic exaggeration of the hypotensive response severely limits the usefulness of these drugs. Most patients show one of two unsatisfactory patterns: a normal resting pressure and an unacceptably low pressure after exercise, or a high resting pressure and a normal pressure after exercise. In addition, sexual dysfunction in male patients (impairment of erection and/or ejaculation) and diarrhea are quite common. Because of the frequency of orthostatic hypotension and because of the availability of better tolerated, potent drugs (e.g., minoxidil, the ACE inhibitors, and the calcium channel blockers nifedipine and nicardipine), the initiation of guanethidine or guanadrel can almost always be avoided in the management of hypertension. Patients who currently take either of these drugs should be monitored carefully, and an alternative regimen should be considered whenever there is any suggestion that the exaggerated orthostasis is producing symptoms.

Drug Interactions. Tricyclic antidepressants and sympathomimetic decongestants may reverse the antihypertensive effect of guanethidine. Presumably the same may occur with guanadrel.

Combinations and Interactions. Guanethidine has been used effectively as a sympatholytic drug in conjunction with hydralazine. Because of its undesirable side effects, it provides no advantage over the other sympatholytic drugs that have been tested with hydralazine (beta-blockers, clonidine, reserpine).

Peripheral/Central Sympatholytic: Reserpine

Mechanism. Chronic administration of reserpine depletes the stores of catecholamines in many tissues, probably by impairing the uptake of essential precursors. The antihypertensive effect is attributed to impaired uptake centrally and peripherally of dopamine, a precursor for the intracellular synthesis of norepinephrine.

Selected Properties. The major antihypertensive effect occurs 1 to 2 weeks after initiating treatment and remits within 1 to 2 weeks of stopping the drug. The principal advantages of reserpine are the once a day schedule and low cost.

Precautions. Frank depression occurs in some patients, and slight decrease in mental alertness is common. Both are dose related and occur chiefly at doses higher than the recommended range (0.1 to 0.25 mg) (23). Nasal and gastric hypersecretion occurs at therapeutic doses and may produce nasal stuffiness or dyspepsia. Because of side effects and the availability of other drugs, reserpine has not been recommended prominently in recent years. Two definite contraindications are active peptic ulcer and a history of depression.

Drug Interactions. Reserpine may interact unfavorably with a number of drugs. Because it releases stored norepinephrine, a hypertensive crisis may occur if it is given with a monoamine oxidase inhibitor. Reserpine plus digitalis may cause cardiac arrhythmias (ventricular ectopy and atrial arrhythmias, similar to those caused by digitalis toxicity). Tricyclic antidepressants can reduce the blood pressure lowering effect of reserpine. The central nervous system depressant effects of many drugs may be increased by reserpine. Finally reserpine antagonizes the antiparkinsonian effect of L-dopa.

Combination with Other Drugs. In the Veterans Administration controlled trial (see above), the combination of reserpine, hydralazine, and hydrochlorothiazide was shown to be highly effective. These three drugs are available in a fixed-dose combination tablet (Ser-Ap-Es or generic) that contains small amounts of each drug, i.e., 0.10 mg of reserpine, 25 mg of hydralazine, and 15 mg of hydrochlorothiazide.

Vasodilators

Hydralazine

Mechanism. Hydralazine directly relaxes smooth muscle in resistance vessels (arterioles and small arteries); it has a similar but lesser effect on capacitance vessels (venules and small veins). Secondary effects are stimulation of renin release and reflex increase in activity of the sympathetic nervous system that may cause tachycardia, palpitations, headache, or increased angina. Because of this latter effect, hydrala-zine is not recommended for monotherapy but should be used in combination with an adrenergic inhibitor.

Selected Properties. The daily dose range is 20 to 400 mg. An upper limit of 200 mg is sometimes recommended because of the increased risk of hydralazine-induced lupus at higher doses. However, 400 mg or more may be effective and appropriate in patients with severe hypertension who are difficult to control and who do not tolerate other drugs.

Hydralazine can be taken twice daily. The major antihypertensive response occurs within 2 to 4 hours and remits within 12 to 24 hours. If there is evidence that an individual patient's response does not persist for 12 hours, a three times daily schedule may be required. Hydralazine should be taken with meals, as absorption is maximal with food and blood pressure response may be erratic if the drug is taken irregularly.

Precautions. The most common side effects (headache, palpitations, tachycardia) occur when hydralazine is given without an adrenergic inhibitor. The uncommon but widely publicized lupus-like hydralazine syndrome has the following features in most affected subjects: occurs after 6 or more months of exposure to 200 mg or more daily, begins as new arthritis or arthralgia, rarely affects the kidneys, stimulates the production of antinuclear antibodies, and remits entirely within 6 months of discontinuing hydralazine (a few patients have had persistence of rheumatological symptoms or antinuclear antibodies long after discontinuation of hydralazine). Another uncommon, reversible side effect is peripheral sensory neuropathy presenting as paresthesias and numbness and responding to pyridoxine, 50 mg daily, or to discontinuation of the drug.

Except for a history of systemic lupus erythematosus, there are no absolute contraindications to hydralazine when used in combination with an adrenergic inhibitor.

Interactions with Other Drugs. There are no significant unwanted interactions between hydralazine and other commonly used drugs.

Combination with Other Drugs. When hydralazine is added to any adrenergic inhibitor, the hypertension responds well in the majority of patients who are not controlled with the adrenergic inhibitor alone. The addition of hydralazine to a beta-blocking agent is widely practiced, both because of the effectiveness of this combination and the protection against reflex sympathetic activity that the beta-blockers provide.

Minoxidil

Mechanism. Minoxidil is a very potent peripheral arteriolar vasodilator. Like hydralazine, it stimulates renin release and induces reflex hyperactivity of the sympathetic nervous system. Therefore, the patient should always be taking an adequate dose of an adrenergic inhibitor (usually a beta-blocker) before minoxidil is initiated.

Selected Properties. The daily dose range is 5 to

100 mg. Because of its extraordinary potency, minoxidil should be initiated at a trial dose of 2.5 mg; dose increases can be made daily until a response occurs. The major antihypertensive effect occurs within 1 to 3 hours and remits within 1 to 2 days.

Minoxidil can be given once or twice daily. When minoxidil is being substituted for another drug (hydralazine, for example), this drug should be continued until response to minoxidil occurs; then the other drug should be gradually discontinued while the minoxidil dose is increased if necessary.

Precautions. Fluid retention, often marked, occurs in most patients as a consequence of the hypotensive action of the drug; and furosemide or another potent loop diuretic should be given in a dose adequate to eliminate the problem. Most patients also develop hirsutism within 1 month of starting minoxidil. In addition, darkening of facial pigment and thickening of facial features may occur (so-called "leonine" facies). These effects limit severely the acceptance of this drug by women. There are no other common side effects. A minority of patients (estimated at 3% of those not on dialysis) develop a pericardial effusion (transudate) after prolonged use of minoxidil; rarely cardiac tamponade occurs. The effusion usually resolves or decreases with added diuretic treatment; it resolves entirely if minoxidil is discontinued. The development of anasarca, which remits when the drug is stopped, has been seen in an occasional patient taking minoxidil.

Interactions with Other Drugs. There are no significant interactions between minoxidil and other commonly used drugs.

Combination with Other Drugs. Minoxidil should always be used in conjunction with a diuretic and an adrenergic inhibitor. All minoxidil studies to date have utilized beta-blockers. Presumably the other sympatholytics are also effective with minoxidil. The addition of an ACE inhibitor to a minoxidil beta-blocker diuretic regimen has been shown to control refractory hypertension.

For patients with severe hypertension, a once daily regimen of minoxidil, a long acting beta-blocker, and a diuretic is highly effective and increases the likelihood that the patient will not forget a dose.

Angiotensin-Converting Enzyme Inhibitors: Captopril, Enalapril, Lisinopril

Mechanism

Angiotensin I is the product of the interaction between the proteolytic enzyme renin and an alpha-2 globulin, renin substrate. The ACE inhibitors block the enzymatic conversion of angiotensin I to the potent vasoconstrictor angiotensin II; their antihypertensive effect has been attributed to this action. Because ACE inhibitors lower the blood pressure in patients with low and normal peripheral renin activity as well as those with high peripheral renin activity, and because they also may inhibit the enzymatic degradation of the potent vasodilator bradykinin, there is controversy regarding their mechanism of action. These drugs do not cross the blood-brain barrier, and their antihypertensive action is therefore strictly peripheral.

Selected Properties. When an ACE inhibitor is being substituted for another drug, especially a drug that stimulates renin release (diuretics and vasodilators), the first drug should either be discontinued or gradually tapered, in order to avoid hypotension, while the ACE inhibitor is being introduced. Because a profound fall in blood pressure (and occasional syncope) may follow the first dose of captopril, this dose should be given; and sitting and standing blood pressure should be measured for 1 to 2 hours in the office whenever possible.

Patients should be instructed to take captopril at least 1 hour before meals since absorption is impaired when the drug is taken with meals. This problem does not occur with enalapril and lisinopril.

The major antihypertensive effect of captopril occurs within a few hours of a dose and remits within 12 hours. The full impact of a dose is seen after 1 to 2 weeks at that dose. After prolonged use of captopril, the antihypertensive effect may diminish in occasional patients with severe hypertension, and a larger dose may be required. Black individuals seem to be less responsive to captopril monotherapy than are white.

Enalapril and lisinopril are similar to captopril except that the onset of antihypertensive action of enalapril does not occur for 3 to 4 hours, and the duration of action of both drugs is longer than that of captopril. Both have been found to be effective for 24 hours in most patients, meaning that a once a day schedule can be used.

ACE inhibitors may be of special value in treating hypertensive diabetic patients, both because they may slow the progress of diabetic nephropathy and may improve glucose tolerance.

Precautions. Side effects that may be seen with all of the ACE inhibitors are maculopapular rash, dysgeusia (decreased, totally lost, or altered taste), and nonproductive cough (65). These effects occur within the first 1 to 2 months of use and they remit with either a temporary decrease in dose or discontinuation of the drug. Serious, although rare, adverse reactions are proteinuria, neutropenia, and angioedema. All occur within the first 1 to 2 months of treatment and all are reversible. Angioedema, which may be life threatening if it affects the upper airway, usually occurs after the first dose or within the first few weeks of treatment.

Because renal function may depend upon the action of angiotensin upon postglomerular arterioles in patients with bilateral renal artery stenosis, renal artery stenosis in a solitary kidney, or in renal transplant patients with stenosis of the transplanted renal artery, the ACE inhibitors may cause acute renal failure in patients with these conditions. The type of patients most likely to have the former two problems are those with widespread atherosclerosis, manifested by multiple bruits and diminished peripheral pulses. The renal deterioration, which occurs within one or two days of initiating treatment, remits promptly after the ACE inhibitor is discontinued. In patients who do not have stenotic renal arteries, ACE inhibitors do not cause renal insufficiency, even though transient reduction in renal function may occur in patients with pre-existing renal disease (34).

Drug Interactions. In some patients, nonsteroidal anti-inflammatory drugs reduce the antihypertensive action of ACE inhibitors. This property may be related to the inhibition of the synthesis of vasodilating prostaglandins, which may mediate the response to ACE inhibitors in some patients. Other unwanted drug interactions are those with other drugs used in managing hypertension, especially potassium-sparing diuretics and potassium supplements (discussed in the next paragraph).

Combination with Other Drugs. The action of ACE inhibitors is enhanced by adding a diuretic. A low dose diuretic, low dose ACE inhibitor regimen may be effective and well tolerated in patients who do not respond to monotherapy with either drug, especially black patients on diuretic monotherapy. The prevention of secondary hyperaldosteronism, which is dependent upon the action of angiotensin II upon the adrenal glands, has two important implications regarding diuretics: (a) the development of diuretic-induced hypokalemia, a problem due in part to secondary hyperaldosteronism, is less likely during concurrent treatment with thiazide or loop diuretics, and potassium supplements should be given only for well-documented hypokalemia, with careful monitoring to avoid hyperkalemia; and (b) potassium-sparing diuretics should not be utilized in conjunction with ACE inhibitors, as this combination increases the risk of hyperkalemia.

Combination of an ACE inhibitor with a calcium channel blocker is a second strategy that has been found to be very useful in patients who fail to respond to monotherapy. A disadvantage is the relatively high cost of drugs from both classes.

ACE inhibitors should be used cautiously with agents that affect sympathetic activity, as the sympathetic nervous system may be especially important in supporting the blood pressure in the event of acute hypotension. Despite this concern, beta-blockers have been used in conjunction with captopril in patients whose blood pressure did not respond to captopril alone.

Calcium Channel Blockers: Diltiazem, Nicardipine, Nifedipine, Verapamil

Mechanism

Calcium channel blockers (also referred to as calcium antagonists and calcium entry blockers) are very effective antihypertensives (33). They block or alter cell membrane calcium flux, thereby reducing blood pressure through one or more of the following mechanisms: decreased vascular smooth muscle contractibility in both the arterial and venous circulation,

negative inotropic and chronotropic effects (slows atrioventricular nodal conduction) on the heart, and inhibition of secretion of catecholamines. Nifedipine and nicardipine lower blood pressure chiefly via arteriolar and venous vasodilation. Verapamil and diltiazem probably lower blood pressure via combined peripheral vasodilation and a negative inotropic effect. These differences in mechanism may be important in drug selection.

Selected Properties. Each of the calcium channel blockers has been shown to be effective for monotherapy. The short acting preparations of all of these drugs must be taken three times daily. Long acting preparations are now available for once daily use (nifedipine as Procardia XL in 30-, 60-, and 90-mg strengths and verapamil as Calan SR or Isoptin SR in 240-mg strength) or twice daily use (diltiazem as Cardizem SR in 60-, 90-, and 120-mg strengths). Because the full impact of a dose of the short acting preparations occurs within 1 to 2 hours, the response to a calcium channel blocking agent can be evaluated rapidly.

Like ACE inhibitors, calcium channel blockers may slow the progress of diabetic nephropathy, possibly because they reduce the resistance in the efferent arterioles of the glomeruli.

There is evidence that verapamil reduces left ventricular mass in elderly patients who have hypertension and mild left ventricular hypertrophy (49). It is not known whether this effect adds to the reduction in risk that accompanies blood pressure lowering.

Nicardipine may cause a mild natriuresis, obviating the need for a diuretic.

When the liquid contents of a 10-mg nifedipine capsule are given sublingually, the patient's blood pressure may drop within minutes. This property has been exploited to lower the blood pressure over several hours in symptom-free patients with very high pressures (so-called hypertensive "urgencies"). However, apart from hypertensive emergencies requiring hospitalization and parenteral treatment (see above), there are no indications for such rapid lowering of the blood pressure.

Precautions. Side effects commonly reported with nicardipine and nifedipine are nausea, flushing, headache, and tachycardia. Vasodilator effects (flushing and headache) are less common with verapamil and diltiazem. All of these drugs may cause orthostatic symptoms, ankle edema (not due to salt retention), and palpitations. Verapamil causes constipation, especially when large doses are used, and nifedipine occasionally causes diarrhea.

Because of their effects on the heart, diltiazem and verapamil are contraindicated in patients with bradycardia, atrioventricular conduction disturbances, or uncontrolled heart failure. Because the cardiodepressive effects of these two drugs may be additive to the cardiodepressor effects of beta-blocking drugs, such combinations should be avoided. Although their cardiodepressor actions are much less pronounced, nicardipine and nifedipine should also be used with caution in patients with underlying dilated cardiomyopathy. On the other hand, nifedipine may be useful in treating left ventricular failure in that subgroup of patients with severe hypertension and well-preserved cardiac function, whose heart failure is due to the diastolic stiffness associated with left ventricular hypertrophy (50).

Drug Interactions. The serum digoxin level increases after nifedipine or verapamil, and the potassium level may fall during nifedipine treatment. Because of the latter property, a potassium-sparing agent should be considered when nifedipine is used with a thiazide or loop diuretic.

Combinations with Other Drugs. The combination of nifedipine or nicardipine and a beta-blocker has been shown to be an effective combination regimen in patients with severe hypertension. In addition to its synergy, the beta-blocker blunts the reflex tachycardia that is common with nifedipine monotherapy. Nifedipine has also been shown to be additive when combined with methyldopa.

Problems in the Course of Treatment

Four problems that occur during the long-term treatment of many patients with hypertension are (a) the need for adjustment of the antihypertensive regimen, (b) instability in blood pressure control, (c) orthostatic symptoms, and (d) intercurrent or concurrent morbidity.

Medication Adjustment

Within 2 to 3 months of initiating treatment, most patients should have satisfactory blood pressure control without significant medication side effects. In the ensuing months and years, minor or major changes in the medical regimen will be needed for some patients. Each medication change requires the patient to learn a new habit and brings the possibility for medication error. Therefore, whenever a medication adjustment is contemplated, the reason should be well established. Whenever medication adjustments affect one or more of the medications that the patient is already taking, it is critical to write down the new instructions for the patient.

Instability in Blood Pressure Control

Most patients in whom satisfactory control has been achieved will have inadequate blood pressure control at an occasional follow-up visit. At those visits, one can usually identify the probable cause and design a plan to restore control. A prompt follow-up visit should always be part of this plan. In assessing loss of blood pressure control for which the cause is not clear, it is always useful to look at the information recorded at the most recent visit when the blood pressure was controlled and ask: "What is different today?" The differential diagnosis of instability in blood pressure control is summarized in Table 62.12, divided into common and uncommon causes.

Home monitoring of the blood pressure, either by the patient or by someone else, can be very useful in

Table 62.12.
Differential Diagnosis of Instability in Blood Pressure Control

COMMON CAUSES:
Noncompliance
Increased salt consumption
Weight gain
Psychological stress
Withdrawal from ethanol
UNCOMMON CAUSES:
Concurrent medications[a]
Tolerance
Refractory hypertension

[a]See Table 62.13.

assessing apparent nonresponse to antihypertensive drugs. If this strategy is used, it is important to have the patient obtain and document the following information: blood pressure, arm, position, heart rate, time since last dose of each medication. The currently marketed home monitoring devices range from inexpensive devices that require skill in auscultation and to more expensive electronic devices that give digital readouts. Almost all have been found to give accurate information (8, 29). However, if one plans to rely on data from home monitoring, it is advisable to have the patient (or family member) bring the device to the office periodically to check technique and accuracy.

Noncompliance. Noncompliance can often be identified by nonjudgmental inquiry, as described in Chapter 4. If a patient has deliberately discontinued a medication, he will often explain his reasons.

At certain times, patients will simply omit their medication(s) on the day of the visit. On the other hand, they may be taking medication(s) faithfully but incorrectly. Because this may be due to an error in dispensing of medication, patients who report that they are complying should be asked to telephone the office and read the information on their medication bottles or to bring their medication bottles to the next visit.

If patients with uncontrolled blood pressures report taking their medication correctly, this can be further evaluated by having them take their medicine under supervision in the office and then measuring the blood pressure response for several hours (see example case above, Fig. 62.9).

Increased Salt Consumption and/or Weight Gain. A significant increase in salt consumption may lead to a positive sodium balance, which can blunt the effects of antihypertensive drugs. This problem is not uncommon in the summer months. It should be expected whenever loss of blood pressure control is associated with a weight gain of 2 to 3 lb (1 kg) or more, with or without edema. Brief review of the patient's current diet will often help to support this hypothesis. Management consists of having the patient resume moderate sodium restriction or substituting more potent diuretic treatment. Temporary use of furosemide (e.g., 40 to 80 mg daily for a week) to eliminate excess sodium is often useful in this situation. For patients in whom sodium overload is a recurrent problem, furosemide in doses adjusted to maintain a stable weight is very effective (42).

If the patient's weight gain is associated with increased calorie intake, reduced caloric intake, leading to weight reduction, may restore response to antihypertensive medications.

Psychological Stress. In the patient who is adhering faithfully to treatment, psychological stress may explain failure to respond as usual to antihypertensive drugs. This is probably because increase in sympathetic nervous system activity is often present during psychological stress.

Stress may be associated only with visits to a physician's office ("white coat hypertension"), especially if the patient is being seen by a new physician, and the rise in blood pressure may be strictly transient. This problem can be minimized by assuring that the patient is at ease before taking the blood pressure and by repeating the measurement later in the visit if the initial pressure is high. When stress is suspected as the reason for erratic office blood pressures, home blood pressure measurements may provide better information for judging the effectiveness of treatment and may spare patients from inappropriate increases in antihypertensive drugs and the associated side effects.

Psychological stress may also be due to serious job- or family-related crisis. Brief inquiry may reveal additional stress-related symptoms, such as headache, dyspepsia, sleeplessness, irritability, etc. In such patients, management consists of supportive counseling (see Chapter 11) and, if deemed appropriate, short-term prescription of an anxiolytic medication (see Chapter 13).

Withdrawal from Alcohol. Because hypertension may occur as a manifestation of alcohol withdrawal, it is important to check for alcoholism in a patient who has previously had controlled hypertension. This cause of unstable blood pressure control is probably most common in alcoholic patients whose medical appointments occur after a weekend.

Concurrent Medications. A number of prescribed and over-the-counter (OTC) medications (Table 62.13) may attenuate the response to antihypertensive drugs.

Table 62.13.
Medications That May Attenuate Response to Antihypertensive Drugs

PROMOTES POSITIVE SODIUM BALANCE:
  Nonsteroidal anti-inflammatory drugs
  Corticosteroids
  Estrogens
  Sodium-containing antacids
SYMPATHOMIMETIC:
  Decongestants (oral)
  Amphetamine
  Bronchodilators
MECHANISM NOT ESTABLISHED
  Tricyclic antidepressants
  Phenothiazines
  Monoamine oxidase inhibitors
  Nonsteroidal anti-inflammatory drugs
  Oral contraceptives
  Cyclosporine

The significance of this problem has been assessed for two common classes of drugs: (*a*) OTC preparations containing phenylpropanolamine, which may raise the blood pressure if taken in excessive amounts but do not impair the response to a variety of antihypertensives when no more than the recommended OTC dose is taken (36); and (*b*) nonsteroidal anti-inflammatory drugs, some of which (especially indomethacin) have been shown to interfere with the response to antihypertensives (45).

Because of the potential for this problem, awareness of or inquiry about concurrent, especially recently started, medications is always important in assessing unstable blood pressure control. Hypertensive patients should be told which common drugs are contraindicated and that chronic use of such drugs as nonsteroidal anti-inflammatory agents and over-the-counter decongestants (e.g., for seasonal allergy) requires careful supervision of blood pressure.

Tolerance. Whenever a patient appears to become "tolerant" to a drug that worked well initially, other causes of unstable blood pressure control should be sought. In those with no alternative cause, a larger dose of their current drug will often restore blood pressure control. This finding may signify the development of true tolerance, or it may signify progressive hypertension. In evaluating apparent tolerance to a previously effective drug or combination of drugs, office observation of a patient's response to his usual regimen can be quite helpful (see case example above, Fig. 62.9).

Refractory Hypertension. Rarely, a patient's blood pressure may become refractory to previously effective drugs, and none of the above causes will be found. In such patients, two questions must be answered:

1. *Is the hypertension really refractory to the patient's usual medication?* This question can be answered best by supervision of medication taking and blood pressure response in the office, or at home, by a nurse. It is usually found that the patient was not taking his medication correctly (see Fig. 62.9) and that, under supervision, he responds appropriately. Some patients, however, do not respond at all to previously effective drugs.
2. *What is the reason?* This question is especially important for the occasional patient whose refractory hypertension is confirmed and who does not respond to other antihypertensive drugs. Such persistently refractory hypertension in a previously responding patient is unusual (1) and suggests that one of the causes of secondary hypertension may be present, especially new renovascular hypertension (RVH). Evaluation for RVH is appropriate at this juncture (see above).

"Primary" Refractory Hypertension. Occasionally, a newly diagnosed patient fails to respond to a variety of drugs and doses. This apparent primary refractoriness to antihypertensive drugs, also called resistant

hypertension (22), can be assessed, and potent new drugs can be tried, most efficiently by office supervision, as illustrated in Fig. 62.12.

Regimens that may be particularly effective in controlling refractory hypertension, each of which can be given in forms that allow only once-a-day dosing, are:

1. Minoxidil or nifedipine with a beta-blocker;
2. An ACE inhibitor in conjunction with a calcium channel blocker or in combination with a minoxidil beta-blocker regimen;
3. High dose furosemide in conjunction with potent nondiuretic drugs;
4. High dose prazosin or terazosin.

Orthostatic Symptoms

Many patients describe occasional brief orthostatic dizziness of faintness, particularly when they first stand up in the morning. Either (a) advice to sit for a few minutes before standing or (b) a modest reduction in drug dose will usually alleviate the problem.

At times a patient who has satisfactory blood pressures at office visits will describe orthostatic symptoms lasting an hour or more after taking medicine. In this situation, it is important to reduce or discontinue the medication promptly. If such a patient has severe hypertension off medicine, it is important to evaluate objectively the orthostatic symptoms before reducing medications (see case example, Fig. 62.11).

Occasionally a patient, usually an older person, will describe orthostatic symptoms related to medications even when the standing blood pressure is normal. In patients with known atherosclerosis (e.g., carotid bruits), this may be due to *positional cerebral ischemia* (41). In other patients the problem may be due to *pseudohypertension*, a measurement artifact caused by a difficult-to-compress calcified brachial artery. Pseudohypertension can be tentatively diagnosed by the finding that the (presumably calcified) radial artery does not collapse when the pulse is obliterated during blood pressure measurement (40); definitive diagnosis requires arterial catheterization in order to directly measure the blood pressure, which is then compared with the cuff pressure. When either positional cerebral ischemia or pseudohypertension is suspected, a trial of less (or no) antihypertensive drugs is appropriate; if the patient's symptoms improve, it is reasonable to withhold antihypertensive drugs or to prescribe doses that do not cause the symptoms.

Co-morbidity

During long-term treatment, most hypertensive patients will develop acute or chronic conditions that require adjustment of their antihypertensive drugs. One of the commonest situations in which less medication may be needed to control hypertension is hospitalization for any reason (26). For patients with selected chronic conditions, one or more antihypertensive drugs may be inappropriate, as summarized in Table 62.8.

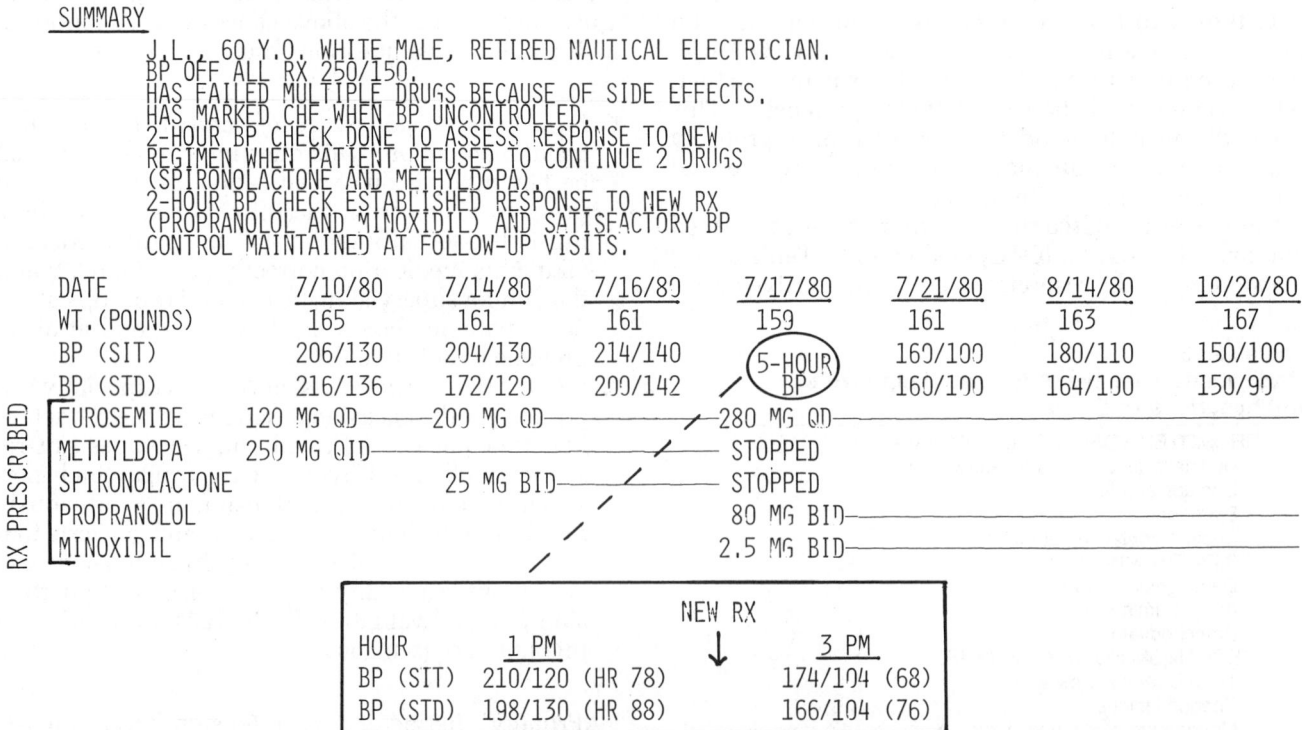

Figure 62.12. Two-hour office observation of response to new regimen in a patient being changed to a more potent antihypertensive drug (minoxidil) because of apparent "primary" refractory hypertension. (From Barker LR: HBP commentary. *Maryland Med J,* Feb. 1986.)

A number of common conditions, discussed here, require extra caution with any antihypertensive drug regimen.

Acute Illness. All patients with hypertension will have intercurrent acute illnesses. The following factors, which increase a person's sensitivity to antihypertensive drugs, may accompany some of those intercurrent illnesses:

1. Reduced intake of food, including salt;
2. Bed rest. In previously healthy individuals, bed rest for more than a few days produces a modest reduction in recumbent blood pressures and may cause a marked reduction in standing blood pressure;
3. Vomiting or diarrhea, leading to fluid and electrolyte deficits;
4. Hypotension, presumably due to vasodilation, during febrile illnesses.

If lower blood pressures are documented or if the patient describes orthostatic symptoms, short-term decrease or withholding of antihypertensive drugs will protect such patients from the additional morbidity brought by hypotension or electrolyte depletion. The patient's usual antihypertensive regimen should be resumed gradually as the blood pressure returns to hypertensive levels. In some situations, for example, after major surgery, the previous regimen may not be needed for 1 or more months.

Concurrent Chronic Illness. *Cerebrovascular disease.* Hypertensive patients with suspected or known cerebral atherosclerosis should have their blood pressure lowered carefully to avoid hypoperfusion of an already compromised vascular network. Patients who develop typical orthostatic symptoms despite standing blood pressures in the "normal" range should have a trial of lower dose treatment or no treatment to determine whether positional cerebral ischemia is present (41).

In patients with completed strokes, controlled studies of antihypertensive treatment have shown both a reduction or no reduction in the occurrence of second strokes; these studies have not reported the impact of treatment on other morbidity from hypertension in poststroke patients, particularly congestive heart failure, a problem that should be prevented by antihypertensive treatment. Patients who remain hypertensive after their neurological status has stabilized should be treated continuously.

Coronary artery disease. In the hypertensive patient with angina pectoris, management of the angina always includes adequate blood pressure control.

The hypertensive patient who has had a recent myocardial infarction may have a normal blood pressure or less severe hypertension during convalescence. Because this may be transient, the blood pressure should be evaluated at least monthly in the first 3 to 4 months after discharge.

Diabetes mellitus. In the patient with coexisting diabetes, consistent control of hyperglycemia will pre-

vent erratic responses to antihypertensive drugs; the diabetic patient who periodically develops volume deficits from osmotic diuresis risks symptomatic hypotension. In the sizable subgroup of diabetics who have postural hypotension due to diabetic neuropathy, the risk of exaggerated hypotension accompanies any antihypertensive regimen; therefore, the orthostatic pressure and not the recumbent pressure should be monitored to determine the response to therapy in these patients and in other patients with baseline orthostasis.

Asthma. In the hypertensive patient with coexisting asthma, blood pressure elevation may accompany episodes of increased bronchospasm. This may occur in untreated hypertensives as well as in those whose blood pressures are usually controlled on antihypertensive drugs. In patients who are already taking antihypertensive drugs, restoration of blood pressure control depends upon improvement in the asthma and not upon increased antihypertensive medications. As noted in Table 62.8, hypertensive patients with a history of bronchospasm should not receive beta-adrenergic blocking agents.

Preplanned Surgery (See Chapter 86)

HYPERTENSION IN ADOLESCENTS AND YOUNG ADULTS

Adolescents and young adults have not been included in the major studies of the epidemiology and treatment of hypertension. However, on the basis of available information about the natural history of hypertension in this age group recommendations for evaluation and management have been published and updated periodically (48).

Epidemiology

Information from the longitudinal Evans County, Georgia, study has provided important information about the prevalence of hypertension and the incidence of new hypertension in adolescents and young adults (57). The study utilized a probability sample of the population between the ages of 15 and 24 at entry. Hypertension was defined as an average of three diastolic blood pressure readings of 90 mm Hg or greater. At entry in 1960, the overall prevalence of hypertension was 14.6% (3.0% for subjects 15 through 19 years of age and 20.6% for subjects 20 through 24 years of age). The follow-up study in 1976, when all subjects were in their third or fourth decade, showed an overall prevalence of hypertension of 26.4%; during 16 years there was a 26% incidence of new hypertension for those 15 to 19 years old at entry and a 12% incidence for those 20 to 24 years old at entry. Overweight status and the development of obesity correlated highly with prevalence and incidence of hypertension, respectively. A small percentage of those hypertensive at entry had a normal blood pressure at follow-up; presumably they had labile hypertension when first examined.

In addition to prevalence and incidence rates, this study has yielded preliminary data on long-term morbidity in the young adult with hypertension. During the first 10 years of follow-up (before the publication of the Veterans Administration study results) none of the hypertensive subjects in this study was treated. An interim study in 1968 disclosed that a number of those who were hypertensive at entry had developed cardiovascular events attributable to hypertension. The 16-year follow-up in 1976 disclosed a much higher incidence of electrocardiographic abnormalities in those hypertensive at entry compared with those normotensive at entry.

Other epidemiological studies of hypertension in young adults have indicated that labile hypertension may be more common than sustained hypertension in teenagers; that there is a striking incidence of sustained new hypertension between the ages of 15 and 25; and that most young adults with sustained hypertension have essential hypertension. The guidelines for baseline evaluation and for suspecting secondary hypertension are therefore the same as those summarized earlier. Oral contraceptive treatment, discussed below, is a particularly important etiology to consider in the baseline evaluation of young women with hypertension.

Recommendations

In 1987, the United States Task Force on Blood Pressure Control in Children (48) published the following recommendations for the care of adolescents with systolic or diastolic blood pressure levels above the 90th percentile (Fig. 62.13):

1. Periodic blood pressure determination;
2. Advice on weight reduction, if needed;
3. Avoidance of excess salt intake (see details above);
4. Encouragement to be physically active;
5. Encouragement to discontinue smoking cigarettes (nonsmokers should be discouraged from starting the habit);
6. Examination for other risk factors (e.g., serum lipids, glucose, etc.).

The Task Force named the following indications for considering the initiation of antihypertensive drug treatment: all patients with significant sustained diastolic hypertension, defined as above the 95th percentile (≥86 mm Hg for ages 13 to 15 and ≥92 mm Hg for ages 16 to 18) and/or evidence of target organ injury attributable to hypertension.

The 1988 report of the Joint National Committee on Detection, Evaluation, and Treatment of Hypertension differs in that it recommends initial use of nonpharmacological modalities, for at least a year, in adolescents unless their diastolic pressure is persistently above the 99th percentile (≥92 mm Hg for ages 13 to 15 and ≥98 for ages 16 to 18) (32). For those patients whose diastolic pressure remains in the range 90 to 100 mm Hg after 1 year of nonpharmacological management, drug treatment should be strongly considered.

Because of the psychological and social stresses associated with adolescence, the care of a chronic condition such as hypertension requires special considerations in this age group (see Chapter 5).

HYPERTENSION IN THE ELDERLY

Hypertension in the elderly is considered separately because the results of the major clinical trials described above cannot be applied to this group, which was under-represented in those trials. Information about hypertension in the elderly has been summarized in recent reviews (4, 16).

Epidemiology

Sustained hypertension is very common in older patients (Fig. 62.1). The risks associated with diastolic and/or systolic hypertension increase with each decade of life (Table 62.1). It is now known that treatment of diastolic hypertension in older patients reduces these risks somewhat. The impact of treatment on the risks of isolated systolic hypertension is still being evaluated.

Diastolic Hypertension. The placebo trial conducted by the European Working Party on Hypertension in the Elderly (EWPHE) has provided the most compelling information about risk reduction. This trial included men and women whose average age was 71 and whose average entering diastolic pressure was 101 mm Hg. Active treatment consisted of one or two pills daily of a diuretic (25 mg hydrochlorothiazide/50 mg triamterene), to which methyldopa could be added; 65% of patients reached the goal pressure (≤90 mm Hg) on just diuretic treatment. The summary findings were that cardiovascular, but not all-cause, mortality, was reduced and that cardiovascular morbidity was reduced modestly by active treatment (2). Subgroup analysis showed that there was no benefit in patients whose entering age was over 80 years (3).

Isolated Systolic Hypertension (ISH). The impact of drug treatment on morbidity and mortality due to ISH is being evaluated in a controlled trial, the Systolic Hypertension in the Elderly Program (SHEP), which will report its principal results in 1991 or 1992. The criteria for ISH in this trial is an average systolic pressure ≥160 mm Hg and diastolic pressure less than 90 mm Hg. During the initial phase of SHEP, it was found that low dose diuretic treatment reduced the blood pressure to the goal level (140 to 160 mm Hg) in most subjects (28).

Recommendations

The recommendations for older patients in the 1988 report of the Joint National Committee on Detection, Evaluation, and Treatment of Hypertension (JNC) are based on the findings from the EWPHE trial and other trials that included subgroups of older patients (32). For persons 65 or older with sustained diastolic pres-

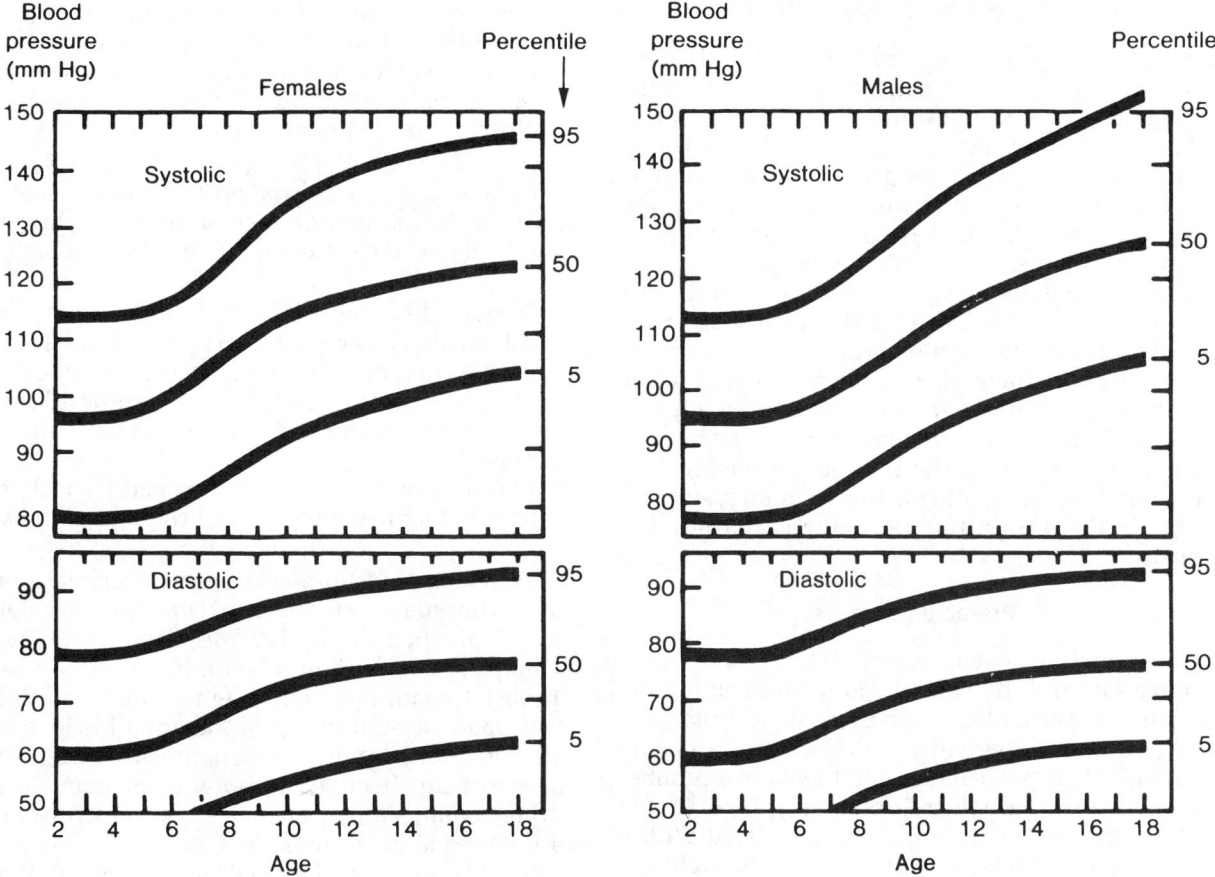

Figure 62.13. Percentiles of blood pressure measurement (right arm, seated) in children and adolescents. (From Report of the Task Force on Blood Pressure Control in Children. *Pediatrics* 59 (suppl):803, 1977.)

sures of 90 mm Hg or greater, reduction of the pressure to less than of 90 mm Hg is recommended and a trial of nonpharmacological measures (see above) before drugs is advocated in older patients with mild hypertension (diastolic pressure of 90 to 105 mm Hg). The JNC report recommends considering drugs for ISH if nonpharmacological measures do not help; but the report emphasizes that the benefit of treating ISH has not yet been demonstrated.

Because diuretics in small doses have been shown to lower blood pressure effectively in the majority of patients in the EWPHE and ISH trials, it is reasonable to select a diuretic for initial treatment of older persons with hypertension.

Caveats Regarding Drug Treatment

Several special characteristics of older persons should be considered in deciding how to treat their hypertension.

Orthostatic hypotension unrelated to drugs is fairly common in elderly persons (11). A combination of increase in sedentary activity and blunting of autonomic reflexes probably explains this. Thus, it is particularly important to obtain baseline and follow-up standing blood pressure (including standing after walking) in older patients taking antihypertensive drugs. When drug treatment is selected for an older person, it is prudent not to select the adrenergic inhibitor, prazosin, because of its tendency to produce marked orthostasis at low doses in some patients.

Other characteristics of older subjects that increase the risk of chronic antihypertensive drugs include the following:

1. Salt and fluid intake may vary significantly from week to week.
2. Concomitant large vessel atherosclerosis (kidneys, brain, heart) may increase the risk of ischemic damage resulting from accidental drug-induced hypotension.
3. Medication-taking errors may be increased.
4. Drug excretion rates are generally reduced as a function of aging.

Three precautions will minimize the risks of antihypertensive drugs in older patients: using the smallest recommended dose and increasing the dose very slowly; keeping the drug schedule simple; and promptly decreasing or discontinuing drugs if there are signs or symptoms of significant orthostatic hypotension or other annoying side effects.

HYPERTENSION IN PREGNANCY

Normally, the blood pressure falls during the first and second trimesters of pregnancy and reverts to the prepregnancy level in the third trimester. The maximal fall, on the average 15 mm Hg in the diastolic pressure, occurs during the second trimester. It is probably due to the general vasodilation that accompanies pregnancy. An increase in renin and aldosterone levels also occurs in normal pregnancy.

Based on previous records or history from the patient, it should be possible at the first prepartum visit to decide for most women whether they are usually normotensive or have chronic hypertension. This decision is very helpful in managing the two major patterns of hypertension that may be associated with pregnancy. These are gestational hypertension (hypertension developing during the pregnancy, during labor, or in the postpartum period) and chronic hypertension.

Pre-eclampsia

Pre-eclampsia is a syndrome in which the clinical data must be carefully considered before making the diagnosis, in particular to distinguish it from pre-existing chronic hypertension. Pre-eclampsia occurs in 5 to 10% of all pregnancies and there are a number of factors that increase the risk of developing it (Table 62.14). Untreated pre-eclampsia is associated with a high incidence of fetal mortality and with maternal morbidity, especially the convulsive syndrome known as eclampsia. The major pathophysiological derangements in pre-eclampsia are placental hypoperfusion, generalized vasospasm, and decreased glomerular filtration rate. The criteria for the diagnosis of pre-eclampsia are:

1. Development of new hypertension during the last half of pregnancy. The generally accepted criteria for hypertension in this instance are a baseline diastolic pressure below 90 mm Hg and a rise to 90 mm Hg or above, documented on 2 measurements at least 4 hours apart (15, 47).

   and

2. The development of new proteinuria during the last trimester (2 clean-catch specimens at least 4 hours apart that reveal 2+ proteinuria by dipstick).

   and

Table 62.14.
Risk Factors for Pre-eclampsia

Primagravida
Familial history of pre-eclampsia/eclampsia
Diabetes mellitus
Multiple gestation
Extremes of age
Pre-existing hypertensive vascular or renal disease
Hydatidiform mole
Fetal hydrops, but not isoimmunization *per se*
Previous history of pre-eclampsia/eclampsia

3. The development of new, generalized edema during the last trimester (dependent edema alone is not a predictor of pre-eclampsia; it is seen in approximately one-third of pregnant women whose blood pressure remains normal).

In the patient who does not have all three of these findings, the following considerations may help to decide whether to treat her as if she is pre-eclamptic:

1. Does she have one of the known risk factors for pre-eclampsia (Table 62.14)? The majority of affected women are primigravidas at the extremes of the childbearing age range. A primigravida whose mother or a sister had eclampsia is at particularly high risk.
2. Was the same degree of hypertension in fact present before the pregnancy (i.e., chronic hypertension)?

Fortunately most pre-eclampsia develops late in the third trimester when the fetus is mature and delivery can be planned promptly. The management for pre-eclampsia, which should be under the supervision of an obstetrician, is hospital admission, modified bed rest, frequent monitoring of maternal blood pressure and fetal status, and antihypertensive drugs. These measures are effective in resolving the manifestations of pre-eclampsia and ensuring a successful outcome of the pregnancy in most patients.

Pre-eclampsia resolves within 6 weeks of delivery. About 25% of primigravidas with pre-eclampsia will develop it during a future pregnancy. Epidemiological studies have shown, however, that women with a history of pre-eclampsia do not have an increased risk of developing chronic hypertension (13).

New Postpartum Hypertension

New hypertension is detected occasionally at the sixth week postpartum visit. At the end of 1 year, some of these patients remain hypertensive, wheras most revert to a normal blood pressure (53). When the hypertension is first detected at the sixth week visit, a urinalysis is critical in order to exclude the rare syndrome of postpartum nephrosclerosis. Women with diastolic blood pressures repeatedly 90 mm Hg or greater should be treated according to the treatment strategies discussed earlier in this chapter. For women with diastolic pressure always under 100 mm Hg and a normal urinalysis, nonpharmacological measures (see above) and regular follow-up are appropriate for the first 6 months to 1 year. A small proportion of these women remain hypertensive after this interval, and they should be treated for chronic hypertension.

Chronic Hypertension in Pregnancy

Chronic hypertension will be seen more commonly in pregnant women who are in their thirties because the prevalence of hypertension increases with age (Fig. 62.1). Because of the fall in blood pressure that occurs during the first two trimesters, a sustained diastolic pressure above 75 to 80 mm Hg is a generally accepted criterion for chronic hypertension during these trimesters, and a diastolic pressure above 85 to 90 mm Hg is regarded as hypertension in the last trimester (37).

There are two important questions to consider in patients with chronic hypertension:

1. *Should a woman with chronic hypertension avoid pregnancy?* In the woman with mild to moderate hypertension, there is a small increase in the risk to the mother or the infant. However, in women with evidence for end organ damage (cardiomegaly, renal impairment, or eye ground changes of accelerated hypertension), infant mortality is greatly increased; these women should be advised to avoid pregnancy.
2. *How should chronic hypertension be treated during pregnancy?* In general, a patient who becomes pregnant while taking antihypertensive medication should take her usual medication unless she becomes hypotensive during the pregnancy. In these patients, it is important to confirm that chronic hypertension was documented adequately before drug treatment. For patients not taking antihypertensives whose chronic hypertension is discovered during the first or second trimester, the hypertension should be treated. This recommendation is based on the finding of improved fetal survival in a controlled trial of methyldopa treatment (without diuretics) for women with chronic hypertension (46). Methyldopa, beta-blockers, and hydralazine have been found to be safe and effective during pregnancy; however, ACE inhibitors should be avoided because fetal abnormalities have been reported with this class of drugs (37).

Management of Hypertension during Lactation

Because there has been widespread recommendation for an increase in breast-feeding in the past decade, some women who need antihypertensive drugs will seek advice regarding the risks and benefits of breast-feeding. Most antihypertensive drugs appear in breast milk, and their impact upon suckling infants has not been well delineated. Based on what is known, the following guidelines have been suggested (64): The use of diuretics should be avoided during lactation because diuretics may significantly reduce milk volume. If a beta-blocking agent is indicated, propranolol should be used because it has the lowest ratio of milk to plasma concentration among beta-blockers; suckling infants of mothers taking propranolol, and other beta-blockers, have not had adverse effects. Because there is too little information about other adrenergic inhibitors, vasodilators, or calcium channel blockers, these drugs should probably be avoided when more potent drugs are needed. Captopril yields a very low concentration in milk relative to plasma, and it can

be recommended for a breast-feeding woman who needs a more potent antihypertensive drug.

ORAL CONTRACEPTIVES AND HYPERTENSION

Epidemiology

Longitudinal studies of women taking oral contraceptive pills (OCP) have shown the following:

1. A mild increase in blood pressure (systolic of 5 to 6 mm Hg and diastolic of 1 to 2 mm Hg) occurs shortly after initiating OCP in most women (62).
2. During the first 5 years of OCP use, there is a progressive rise in the blood pressure (mean of 14 mm Hg systolic and 8 mm Hg diastolic) (62).
3. The reported incidence of new hypertension has varied from 3 to 6/1000 OCP users after 3 years of use. These rates were 2 to 3 times higher than the rates in comparable nonusers (19).

Population studies have shown that OCP use does increase the risk of death from cerebrovascular and cardiovascular diseases. The absolute number of women affected is very small, but physicians must be aware of the potential hazards of this form of contraception.

The physiological basis for the modest increase in blood pressure accompanying OCP use may be volume expansion. After 3 weeks, it has been found that most individuals show a 100 to 200 mEq increase in total body sodium. In addition, increased renin and aldosterone activities are found. There is no difference in the degree of these changes between those women who remain normotensive and those who develop hypertension. A history of pre-eclampsia does not increase the risk of OCP-induced hypertension and is not a contraindication to OCP use. Furthermore, there are no contraindications to OCP use in the patient with well-controlled chronic hypertension who may wish to use this kind of contraception.

Approach to the Patient

The use of oral contraceptives has played a major role in the reduction of unwanted pregnancy during the past 20 years (see Chapter 93). Therefore, it is important to have an approach to the woman who develops hypertension while taking oral contraceptives. The following approach is recommended:

1. Assure that a baseline blood pressure is obtained before OCP use.
2. Dispense no more than a 6-month supply at one time.
3. Measure the blood pressure at least every 6 months. If the patient develops hypertension or if the blood pressure rises significantly (though remaining below 140/90), the patient should be advised to select another form of contraception, and when this has been done OCP should be discontinued.
4. Approximately one-half of women developing hy-

pertension during OCP use will revert to normal blood pressure within 3 months of discontinuation of OCP use. If the blood pressure does not revert to normal, the patient should be managed for chronic hypertension as described earlier in this chapter.

5. In the OCP user who develops hypertension and prefers to continue OCP after considering other options, treatment for sustained hypertension as outlined earlier is appropriate.

General References

Kaplan NM: *Clinical Hypertension*, 5th ed. Baltimore, Williams & Wilkins, 1990.

> Monograph covering in detail what the clinician needs to know about essential and secondary hypertension.

Kaplan NM:Nondrug treatment of hypertension. *Ann Intern Med* 102:359, 1985.

> Thoroughly referenced review of this subject.

The 1988 Report of the Joint National Committee on Detection, Evaluation, and Treatment of High Blood Pressure. *Arch Intern Med* 148:1023, 1988.

> Specific recommendations based on the consensus of a national panel of experts.

Specific References

1. Alderman MH, Budner N, Cohen H, et al: Prevalence of drug resistant hypertension. *Hypertension* 11(suppl II):II-71, 1988.
2. Amery A, Birkenheager W, Brixko P, et al: Mortality and morbidity results from the European Working Party on High Blood Pressure in the Elderly trial. *Lancet* 1:1349, 1985.
3. Amery A, Brixko R, Clement D, et al: Efficacy of antihypertensive drug treatment according to age, sex, blood pressure, and previous cardiovascular disease in patients over the age of 60. *Lancet*590, September 13, 1986.
4. Applegate WB: Hypertension in elderly patients. *Ann Intern Med* 110:901, 1989.
5. The Australian therapeutic trial in mild hypertension (editorial). *Lancet* 1:1261, 1980.
6. Health and Public Policy Committee, American College of Physicians; Philadelphia, Pa: Biofeedback for Hypertension. *Ann Intern Med* 102:709, 1985.
7. Birkenhager WH, Krauss XH, Schalekamp MADH, Kolsters G: Consecutive haemodynamic patterns in essential hypertension. *Lancet* 1:560, 1972.
8. Blood-pressure monitors How reliably can you take your pressure at home? We checked 36 devices for accuracy and ease of use. *Consumer Report*, May, 314, 1987.
9. Bravo EL, Gifford Jr. RW: Pheochromocytoma: diagnosis, localization and management. *N Engl J Med* 311:1298, 1984.
10. Brush Jr. JE, Cannon III RO, SchenkeW H, et al: Angina due to coronary microvascular disease in hypertensive patients without left ventricular hypertrophy. *N Engl J Med* 319:1302, 1988.
11. Caird FI, Andrews GR, Kennedy RD: Effect of posture on blood pressure in the elderly. *Br Heart J* 35:527, 1973.
12. Carey RM, Reid RA, Ayers CR, et al: The Charlottesville blood-pressure survey. Value of repeated blood-pressure measurements. *JAMA* 236:847, 1976.
13. Chesley LC, Annitto JE, Cosgrove RA: The remote prognosis of eclamptic women: sixth periodic report. *Obstetrics* 124:446, 1976.
14. Croog SH, Levine S, Testa MA, et al: The effects of antihypertensive therapy on the quality of life. *N Engl J Med* 314:1657, 1986.
15. Davey DA, MacGillivray I: The classification and definition of the hypertensive disorders of pregnancy. *Am J Obstet Gynecol* 158:892, 1988.
16. Davidson RA, Caranasos GJ: Should the elderly hypertensive be treated? *Arch Intern Med* 147:1933, 1987.
17. Detection, evaluation, and treatment of renovascular hypertension. Working Group on Renovascular Hypertension. *Arch Intern Med* 147:820, 1987.
18. England WL, Grim CE, Weinberger MH, Roberts SD: Cost effectiveness in the detection of renal artery stenosis. *J Gen Intern Med* 3:344, 1988.
19. Fisch IR, Frank J: Oral contraceptives and blood pressure. *JAMA* 237:2499, 1977.
20. Freestone S, Ramsay LE: Pressor effect of coffee and cigarette smoking in hypertensive patients. *Clin Sci* 63:403, 1982.
21. Frohlich ED, Grim C, Labarthe DR, et al: *Report of a Special Task Force appointed by the Steering Committee, American Heart Association. Recommendations for Human Blood Pressure Determination by Sphygomanometers.* Dallas, The American Heart Association, AHA publications no 70-1005 (SA)1987, pp. i.
22. Gifford Jr. RW: Resistant hypertension: introduction and definitions. *Hypertension* 11 (suppl II):II-65, 1988.
23. Goodwin FK, Bunney Jr. WE: Depression following reserpine: a reevaluation. *Semin Psychiatry* 3:435, 1971.
24. Haynes RB, Sackett DL, Taylor DW, et al: Increased absenteeism from work after detection and labeling of hypertensive patients. *N Engl J Med* 299:741, 1978.
25. Helgeland A: Treatment of mild hypertension: a five-year controlled drug trial. The Oslo study. *Am J Med* 69:725, 1980.
26. Hossmann V, Fitzgerald GA, Dollery CT: Influence of hospitalization and placebo therapy on blood pressure and sympathetic function in essential hypertension. *Hypertension* 3:113, 1981.
27. How far to lower blood pressure? *Lancet* 251, August 1, 1987.
28. Hulley SB, Furberg CD, Gurland B, et al: Systolic Hypertension in the Elderly Program (SHEP): antihypertensive efficacy of chlorthalidone. *Am J Cardiol* 56:913, 1985.
29. Hunt JC, Frohlich ED, Moser M, et al: Devices used for self-measurement of blood pressure: revised statement of the National High Blood Pressure Education Program. *Arch Intern Med* 145:2231, 1985.
30. Hypertension Detection and Follow-up Program Cooperative Group: Five-year findings of the hypertension detection and follow-up program. I. Reduction in mortality of persons with high blood pressure, including mild hypertension. *JAMA* 242:2562, 1979.
31. Hypertension Prevention Trial Research Group. The hypertension prevention trial: three-year effects of dietary changes of blood pressure. *Arch Intern Med* 150:153, 1990.
32. The Joint National Committee on Detection, Evaluation, and Treatment of High Blood Pressure. The 1988 Report of the Joint National Committee on Detection, Evaluation, and Treatment of High Blood Pressure. *Arch Intern Med* 148:1023, 1988.
33. Kaplan NM: Calcium entry blockers in the treatment of hypertension: current status and future prospects. *JAMA* 262:817, 1989.
34. Keane WF, Anderson S, Aurell M, et al: Angiotensin converting enzyme inhibitors and progressive renal insufficiency. *Ann Intern Med* 111:503, 1989.
35. Klein LE: Compliance and blood pressure control. *Hypertension* II (suppl II):II-61, 1988.
36. Kroenke K, Omori DM, Simmons JO, et al: The safety of phenylpropanolamine in patients with stable hypertension. *Ann Intern Med* 111:1043, 1989.
37. Lindheimer MD, Katz AI: Hypertension in pregnancy. *N Engl J Med* 313:675, 1985.
38. Medical Research Council Working Party. MRC trial of treatment of mild hypertension: principal results. *Br Med J* 291:97, 1985.
39. Memorandum from the WHO/ISH.1986 guidelines for the treatment of mild hypertension. *Hypertension* 8:957, 1986.
40. Messerli FH, Ventura HO, Amodeo C: Osler's Maneuver and pseudohypertension. *N Engl J Med* 312:1548, 1985.
41. Meyer JS, Leiderman H, Denny-Brown D: Electroencephalographic study of insufficiency of the basilar and carotid arteries in man. *Neurology (Minneapolis)* 6:455, 1956.

42. Mroczek WJ, Davidov M, Finnerty Jr. FA: Large dose furosemide therapy for hypertension: long-term use in 22 patients. *Cardiology* 33:546, 1974.
43. Multiple Risk Factor Intervention Trial Research Group: Multiple risk factor intervention trial: risk factor changes and mortality results. *JAMA* 248:1465, 1982.
44. Pentel P: Toxicity of over-the-counter stimulants. *JAMA* 252:1898, 1984.
45. Radack K, Deck C: Do nonsteroidal anti-inflammatory drugs interfere with blood pressure control in hypertensive patients? *J Gen Intern Med* 2:108, 1987.
46. Redman CWG, Beilin LJ, Bonnar J, Ounsted MK: Fetal outcome in trial of antihypertensive treatment in pregnancy. *Lancet* 2:753, 1976.
47. Redman CWG, Jefferies M: Revised definition of pre-eclampsia. *Lancet* 809, April 9, 1988.
48. Report of the second Task Force on Blood Pressure Control in Children—1987. *Pediatrics* 79:1, 1987.
49. Schulman SP, Weiss JL, Becker LC, et al: The effects of antihypertensive therapy on left ventricular mass in elderly patients. *N Engl J Med* 322:1350, 1990.
50. Shepherd RFJ, Zachariah PK, Shub C: Hypertension and left ventricular diastolic function. *Mayo Clin Proc* 64:1521, 1989.
51. Sheps SG, Jiang NS, Klee GG, van Heerden JA: Recent developments in the diagnosis and treatment of of pheochromocytoma. *Mayo Clin Proc* 65:88, 1990.
52. Stamler R, Grimm Jr. RH, Dyer AR, et al: Cardiac status after four years in a trial of nutritional therapy for high blood pressure. *Arch Intern Med* 149:661, 1989.
53. Stout ML: Hypertension six weeks postpartum in apparently normal patients. *Am J Obstet Gynecol* 27:730, 1934.
54. Svetkey LP, Himmelstein SI, Dunnick NR, et al: Prospective analysis of strategies for diagnosing renovascular hypertension. *Hypertension* 14:247, 1989.
55. Taguchi J, Freis ED: Partial reduction of blood pressure and prevention of complications in hypertension. *N Engl J Med* 291:329, 1974.
56. Tucker RM, Labarthe DR: Frequency of surgical treatment for hypertension in adults at the Mayo Clinic from 1973 through 1975. *Mayo Clin Proc* 52:549, 1977.
57. Tyroler HA, Heyden S, Sneiderman C, et al: *A 16-year follow-up of blood pressure in young adult residents of Evans County*. Pittsburgh, Medical Horizon Symposium: Hypertension in Childhood and Adolescents, September, 1976.
58. United States Public Health Service Hospitals Cooperative Study Group (Smith WM): Treatment of mild hypertension: results of a ten-year intervention trial. *Circ Res* 40 (suppl I):98, 1977.
59. Veterans Administration Cooperative Study Group on Antihypertensive Agents: Effects of treatment on morbidity in hypertension: results in patients with diastolic blood pressures averaging 115 through 129 mm Hg. *JAMA* 202:116, 1967.
60. Veterans Administration Cooperative Study Group on Antihypertensive Agents: II. Effects of treatment on morbidity in hypertension: results in patients with diastolic blood pressures averaging 90 through 114 mm Hg. *JAMA* 212:1143, 1970.
61. Weingarten KL, Zimmerman RD, Pinto RS, Whelan MA: Computed tomographic changes of hypertensive encephalopathy. *AJNR* 6:395, 1985.
62. Weir RJ, Briggs E, Mack A, et al: Blood pressure in women taking oral contraceptives. *Br Med J* 1:533, 1974.
63. Weiss NS: Relation of high blood pressure to headache, epistaxis, and selected other symptoms: the United States Health Examination Survey of Adults. *N Engl J Med* 287:631, 21972.
64. White WB: Management of hypertension during lactation. *Hypertension* 6:297, 1984.
65. Williams GH: Converting-enzyme inhibitors in the treatment of hypertension. *N Engl J Med* 319:1517, 1988.
66. Ying CY, Tifft CP, Gavras H, Chobanian AV: Renal revascularization in the azotemic hypertensive patient resistant to therapy. *N Engl J Med* 311:1070, 1984.

Musculoskeletal Problems

CHAPTER 63

Shoulder Pain

JOAN M. BATHON, M.D.

Shoulder pain is a common complaint in ambulatory practice. Often the general physician can, upon careful history-taking and examination of the patient, establish the correct diagnosis and direct appropriate therapy without orthopaedic or rheumatological consultation. This chapter will review the major causes of shoulder pain and provide a basis for diagnosis and treatment of these conditions.

ANATOMY, FUNCTION, AND EXAMINATION OF THE SHOULDER

To enable accurate diagnosis and treatment of disorders of the shoulder, an understanding of the *anatomy and function* of the shoulder structures is imperative (Fig. 63.1). Normal shoulder motion is dependent upon the smooth, integrated movement of the glenohumeral, acromioclavicular, and sternoclavicular joints and the scapulothoracic articulation.

The most superficial layer of the shoulder girdle is musculotendinous, consisting of the deltoid muscle (which abducts the shoulder and assists in both flexion and extension), the pectoralis major and minor muscles (which adduct the shoulder), and the trapezius muscle (which elevates and rotates the scapula). Superiorly, the roof of the shoulder girdle is composed of the deltoid muscle, the acromion, and the coracoacromial ligament. Deep to these structures is a bursa, variably referred to as the subacromial or subdeltoid bursa, which allows free movement of the underlying structures in relationship to the roof. Underlying the bursa is the rotator cuff, a group of short rotator muscle tendons, consisting of the supraspinatus superiorly, the infraspinatus and teres minor posteriorly, and the subscapularis anteriorly. The major function of the rotator cuff muscles is to stabilize the humeral head in the glenoid fossa. In addition, they assist in internal and external rotation and in abduction of the shoulder.

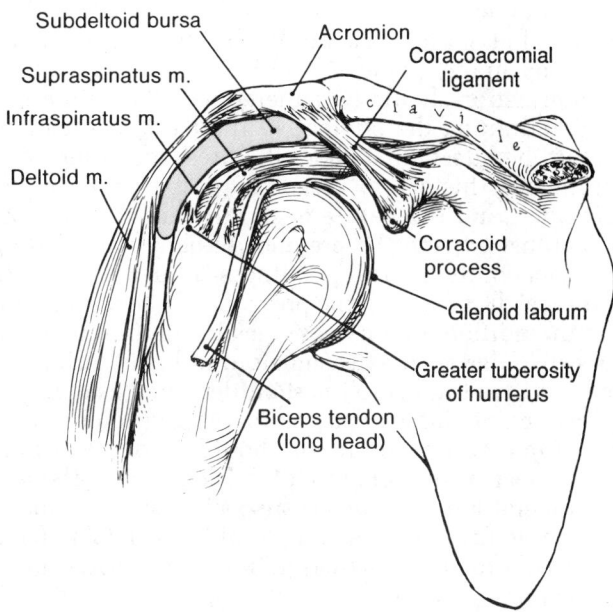

Figure 63.1. Coronal section of shoulder anatomy. Note the relationship of the subdeltoid bursa lying next to the supraspinatus tendon, but separate from the shoulder joint. Note the acromion, which is in a position to impinge the supraspinatus tendon on abduction of the arm.

Repetitive impingement of these structures between the acromion or coracoacromial ligament and the greater tuberosity of the humerus during abduction may lead to inflammatory and degenerative changes within the cuff. Deep to the rotator cuff and intimately attached to it is the ligamentous capsule of the glenohumeral joint. The capsule and rotator cuff are pierced anteriorly by the tendon of the long head of the biceps muscle. Deep to these structures is the glenohumeral joint. This joint is formed by the articulation of the humeral head with the shallow glenoid fossa of the scapula, the diameter and depth of which are significantly increased by the fibrocartilaginous glenoid labrum. The shallowness of the fossa enables nearly hemispheric motion of the arm, but this wide range of motion is achieved at the price of joint stability. Stability of the shoulder joint is dependent primarily, not upon bony structures, but upon the integrity of supporting soft tissue structures including the labrum, the capsule, and the rotator cuff.

Pain about the shoulder originates, generally, from one of three general sites: the glenohumeral joint; periarticular structures, such as the rotator cuff; and sites distant to the shoulder. A detailed *history* of the patient's complaint will facilitate the localization of disease to one of these three sites. The patient should be asked to identify the site of greatest pain or tenderness and to identify specific activities that exacerbate the pain. Periarticular disease, particularly rotator cuff tendinitis, is suggested by localization of pain to the acromion and by exacerbation of pain during abduction of the arm. In contrast, disorders of the glenohumeral joint present with poorly localized, diffuse aching of the shoulder that is exacerbated by movement of the joint in *any plane*. Pain that is referred to the shoulder from a distant site is also described as diffuse but is *not* exacerbated by movement of the shoulder in any plane.

Information should be gathered next that will assist in determining the etiology of the pain. The patient should be questioned about the presence of morning stiffness, a history of recent or past trauma to the shoulder, and the nature of the trauma, the occupational history, and the presence of pain and swelling in other joints. Morning stiffness of greater than 30 minutes' duration and the presence of pain and swelling in additional joints is suggestive of an inflammatory disorder such as rheumatoid arthritis. A history of repetitive trauma to the shoulder, such as that sustained in pitching a ball or in playing tennis, may result in chronic pain in the shoulder from tendinitis and/or tear of the rotator cuff. Dislocation of the glenohumeral joint should be suspected with traumatic injuries to the arm while the shoulder is abducted and externally rotated, whereas injury to, or separation of, the acromioclavicular joint usually results from a direct blow to the acromion.

Physical examination of the shoulder is performed next (Fig. 63.2). The shoulders should be compared visually while the patient's arms are resting at his sides. The general contours of the shoulders are examined for evidence of atrophy or displacement of bony landmarks. Physical findings of inflammation are rarely observed due to their obscuration by overlying musculature of the shoulder girdle. Palpation of the shoulder anteriorly, posteriorly, at the acromioclavicular and sternoclavicular joints, and over the bicipital groove is performed, noting areas of tenderness. Next, active motion is studied by having the patient perform a number of simple maneuvers. Internal rotation is assessed by the placement of the hands on the back inferiorly between the scapulae; external rotation, by placement of the hands on the back of the neck; adduction, by placement of the hands on the opposite shoulders; and forward flexion, by raising the arms with elbows extended so that both hands touch above the head.

Passive range of motion is then examined and compared with the active range. Internal and external rotation are best examined with the elbow flexed and the shoulder abducted to 90° in this manner, the total arc should measure approximately 180°. Passive abduction of the shoulder is assessed by pressing downward on the shoulder with one hand, thus immobilizing the scapula, and abducting the arm with the other hand. Abduction of the shoulder is a combination of glenohumeral motion and scapular abduction (approximately 2° of glenohumeral motion for each degree of scapulothoracic motion). Thus, by immobilizing the scapula, glenohumeral motion is isolated. In this situation the shoulder should be able to be abducted approximately 90°. If both active and passive ranges of motion of the shoulder are limited, a disorder of the glenohumeral joint or adhesive capsulitis should be suspected. In contrast, if passive range of motion exceeds the active range, it is likely that pain or mus-

cular weakness, such as that resulting from a rotator cuff tear, is the limiting factor. Finally, a neurological examination of the upper extremities should be performed, noting sensory or motor deficits in the affected arm. The spine and the remaining peripheral joints should also be examined for evidence of articular disease elsewhere in the body.

PERIARTICULAR DISORDERS

Impingement Syndrome

Most patients with shoulder pain have nonarticular disease caused, usually, by degenerative tendinitis of the rotator cuff. This condition is variably referred to by several names: *"impingement syndrome," supraspinatus tendinitis, subacromial bursitis, subdeltoid bursitis,* and *pericapsulitis.* The tendinous fibers of the rotator muscles undergo degenerative changes with advancing age. The tendons, particularly the supraspinatus that is the most superior, are thought to be worn down by attrition due to repetitive excursion between the greater tuberosity of the humerus and the acromion. Edema, hemorrhage, and inflammation associated with the attrition are thought to be the source of the acute pain that initially prompts the patient to seek medical attention. By the 6th decade, defects in the cuff are seen almost universally, and large ruptures or tears of the rotator cuff may then occur in the absence of significant precipitating trauma. In fact, acute tears resulting from trauma are rare and are reported almost exclusively in patients in their 20s and 30s. With aging, the biceps tendon, like the rotator cuff tendons, is also subject to inflammation, erosion, and rupture. Inflammation of the subacromial bursa may also occur in association with rotator cuff and/or bicipital tendinitis. As the overlying soft tissues are worn down, the greater tuberosity may then rub against the inferior surface of the acromion, and it too may erode.

The predominant presenting complaint in the impingement syndrome is pain, which is generally most severe over the anterolateral aspect of the acromion and which may radiate down the arm to the elbow. Examination of the patient for the *"impingement sign"* is helpful in the diagnosis of rotator cuff tendinitis. This test is performed by passively abducting the arm with the scapula immobilized. Subjects with the impingement syndrome will experience pain through 60 to 90° of abduction, when the greater tuberosity abuts the acromion. If the cuff is ruptured, active abduction cannot be sustained against resistance. *Rupture of the biceps tendon,* if present, will usually be evident as a mass of contracted muscle midway between the shoulder and elbow ("*Popeye*" sign). Radiographs in the early stages of degenerative tendinitis with impingement are normal. As the disease progresses, sclerosis and cysts may be observed in the greater tuberosity. Occasionally, calcific deposits will be apparent at the insertion of the supraspinatus tendon on the humerus ("*calcific tendinitis*").

Treatment for acute or "early" impingement syn-

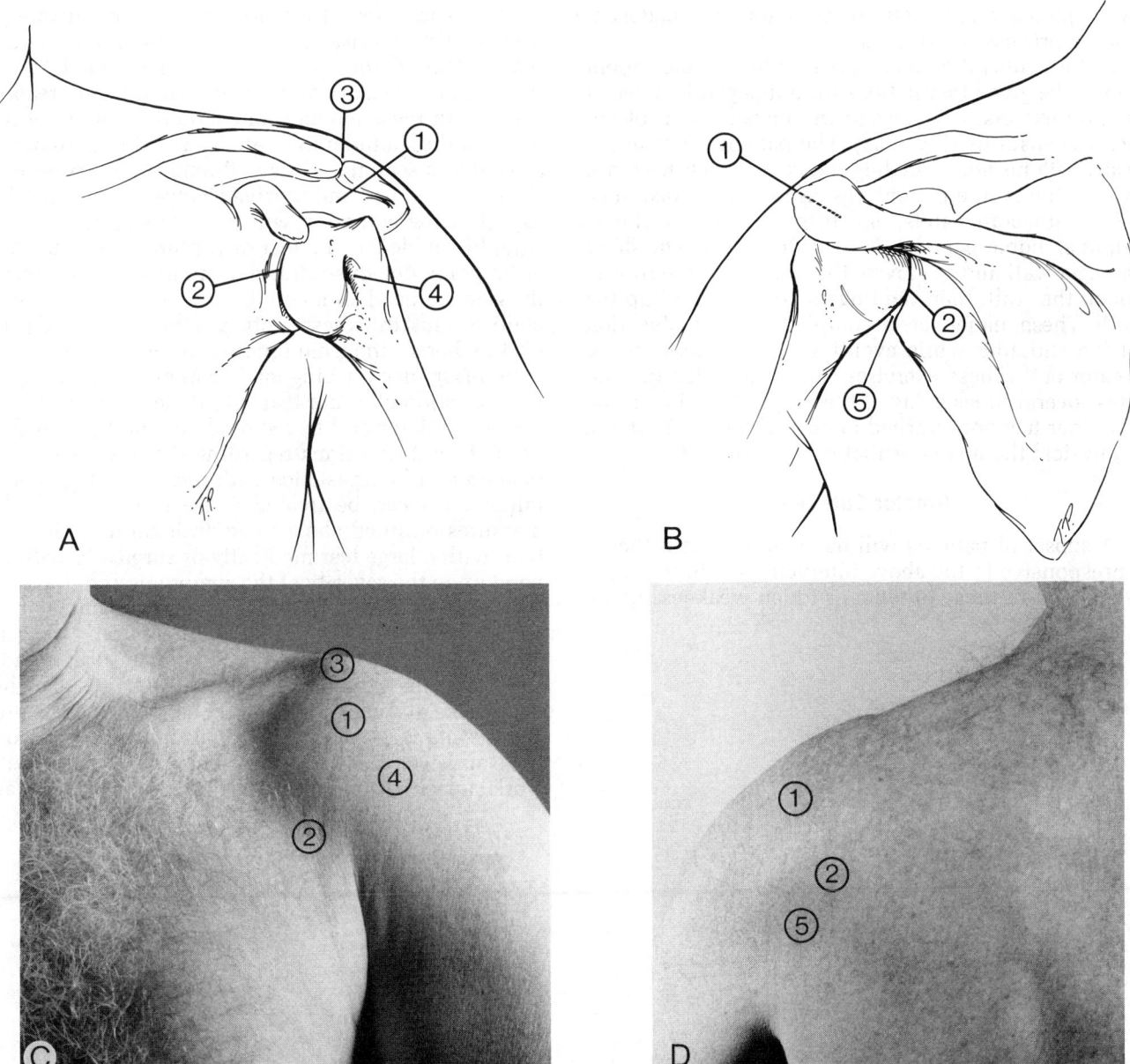

Figure 63.2. Topographical localization of pain and tenderness in specific shoulder disorders. *A* and *C*—anatomical and anterior views, *B* and *D*—posterior views. *1,* subacromial space (rotator cuff tendinitis/impingement syndrome, rotator cuff tear). *2,* Glenohumeral joint (glenohumeral arthritis, adhesive capsulitis, glenoid labral tears). *3,* Acromioclavicular joint (acromioclavicular arthritis, "shoulder sep- aration"). *4,* Bicipital groove (bicipital tendinitis, bicipital tendon rupture). *5,* Quadrilateral space (axillary nerve entrapment). Modified from Thornhill T: Shoulder Pain. In: Kelly WM, Harris ED, Ruddy S, Sledge CB (eds): Textbook of Rheumatology, 2nd ed. Philadelphia, WB Saunders, 1985, p. 492.

drome consists of a brief period (48 hours) of rest with the arm in a sling and a 2-week course of a nonsteroidal anti-inflammatory agent such as ibuprofen (e.g., Motrin), 800 mg three times a day (see also Chapter 70 for a full discussion of NSAIDs). Prolonged immobilization of the shoulder should be avoided since contracture of the shoulder capsule and periarticular structures may result. This entity is known as *adhesive capsulitis* or "frozen shoulder" (see below). An alternative initial approach, sometimes also beneficial in subjects in whom the conservative approach has failed, is the local injection of corticosteroids into the suba-

cromial space. A short-acting anesthetic (such as lidocaine) and a corticosteroid in a depot form (such as 20 mg of triamcinolone) are injected by an experienced generalist, orthopaedist, or rheumatologist. This approach frequently produces dramatic improvement in pain. The immediate alleviation of pain by the lidocaine also serves as diagnostic confirmation of the impingement syndrome. In addition, moist heat or ultrasound treatments may be beneficial in alleviating the acute pain, and, therefore, referral to a physical therapist in severe or persisting cases is appropriate. It is not unusual for patients to experience recurrence of the pain at a later date since the underlying degenerative process is still present.

As the acute inflammatory pain subsides, the patient should be given instructions for doing gentle range of motion exercises to prevent the development of adhesive capsulitis (Fig. 63.3). The patient bends at the waist with his arms dangling and circumducts his arms. Alternatively, the patient lies on his back, grasping a stick with both hands, and lifts the stick overhead. Another home exercise is to have the patient stand facing a wall and to elevate the arms until the fingers touch the wall; then the fingers are "walked" up the wall. These maneuvers accomplish forward elevation of the shoulder while avoiding undue stress on the rotator cuff. These exercises can be done for 10 minutes several times a day. If the range of motion of the shoulder has not returned to normal within 2 weeks, a physical therapy consultation is indicated.

Rotator Cuff Tear

A subset of patients will have chronic pain that is unresponsive to the above interventions. In these patients and in those in whom sudden weakness of ab-

duction and external rotation occur, more advanced degenerative disease of the rotator cuff and, in particular, a tear of the cuff should be suspected (1, 2). Radiographic examination of the shoulder is recommended in these patients and should include routine views of the shoulder in internal and external rotation, as well as a scapular Y view. Proximal subluxation of the humeral head and erosive changes in the anterior aspect of the acromion will provide suggestive radiographic evidence of a tear or rupture of the cuff. An arthrogram, demonstrating a communication between the glenohumeral joint and the subacromial space, will confirm a full thickness rupture of the rotator cuff (Fig. 63.4), whereas the techniques of ultrasound and magnetic resonance imaging may be more effective in the identification of minor tears (3). Patients suspected of having a rotator cuff tear should be seen by an orthopaedist for suggestions regarding the best diagnostic method and for assistance with treatment. In general, minor tears can be treated conservatively with the measures outlined above. The decision to treat a patient with a large tear medically or surgically will depend upon the severity of the symptoms and upon the functional demand of each individual patient. A joint decision between the patient and his family, his generalist, and the orthopaedist should be made. Indications for these surgical procedures remain somewhat controversial since the long-term benefits of these procedures are unclear. In individuals in whom shoulder pain and weakness may significantly interfere with work capacity, resection of the anterior acromion (ac-

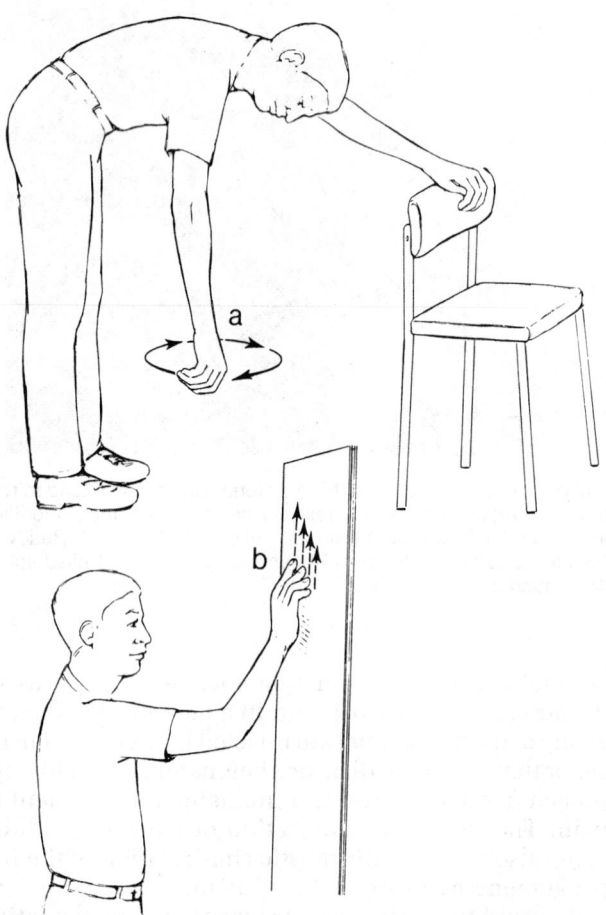

Figure 63.3. Range of motion exercises of the shoulder. Circumduction exercises of the shoulder (*a*) and the wall-climbing exercises for the shoulder (*b*) as described in the text.

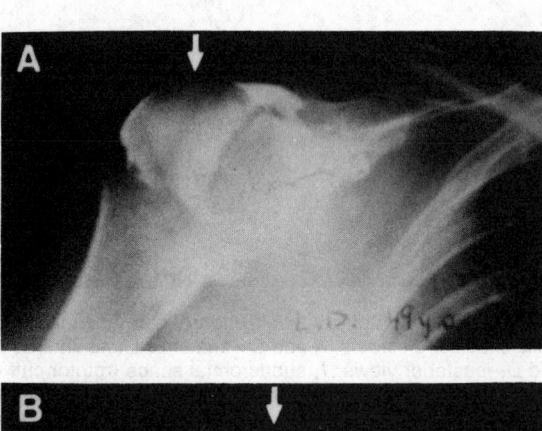

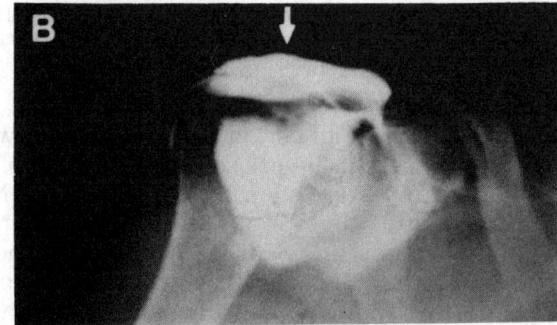

Figure 63.4. *A*, Normal shoulder arthrogram. The superior aspect of the joint should be smooth with a fine layer of contrast material. *B*, Rotator cuff tear. Note extravasation of the dye from the glenohumeral joint into the subdeltoid bursa, indicating a large tear of the rotator cuff tendon.

romioplasty) with repair of the rotator cuff may be performed. In individuals in whom pain and weakness do not create significant functional impairment, a conservative program with rest, analgesics, anti-inflammatory agents (see Chapter 70 for a full discussion of NSAIDs), and physiotherapy may suffice.

Acromioclavicular Arthritis

The acromioclavicular joint is formed by the articulation of the distal clavicle and the acromion. It contributes 20° of elevation to the full arc of motion of the shoulder. Osteoarthritis occurs commonly in this joint during middle age and later life and is usually seen in association with glenohumeral arthritis or chronic impingement syndrome. The patient's pain is poorly localized but is exacerbated by elevation of the arm above shoulder level. Direct tenderness over the joint is usually elicited. Plain radiographs may be helpful if degenerative changes are seen, but it should be noted that these changes are also frequently present in asymptomatic individuals. Alleviation of pain after an injection of a short-acting anesthetic, such as lidocaine, directly into the joint will confirm this site as the source of the pain. In patients in whom pain in this joint cannot be controlled with conservative measures such as nonsteroidal anti-inflammatory medication, referral to an orthopaedist should be made for consideration of resection of the distal clavicle. This is the procedure of choice since it provides good pain relief and is associated with minimal morbidity. Fusion of this joint is never performed since it results in painful restriction of motion of the shoulder.

Acute trauma, such as that sustained from a fall on, or a direct blow to, the shoulder, may result in subluxation or dislocation of the acromioclavicular joint. These injuries are also referred to as "shoulder separation" and are classified as follows: grade I—injury without subluxation; grade II—injury with partial subluxation; and grade III—injury with complete dislocation of the joint. In grade III separation, the physical examination may disclose a clavicle that is prominently displaced superiorly and posteriorly. Diagnosis of grade III and, occasionally, of grade II injuries is assisted by weight-bearing radiographs (anteroposterior view) of both acromioclavicular joints. Separation of this joint is only rarely associated with long-term disability, disfigurement, or pain. Several prospective studies of grade III injuries that have compared conservative management with strapping or a sling versus surgical repair of the coracoclavicular ligament have failed to demonstrate improved results from surgical treatment. Therefore, conservative treatment of shoulder separations of all grades is currently recommended (4). The patient is treated with an analgesic and the arm is rested in a sling until the acute pain subsides. Surgical repair of the coracoclavicular ligament may be considered only in the rare individual whose occupation is dependent upon continuous overhead arm activity (such as painters and some athletes) and in whom conservative treatment has failed to relieve pain.

GLENOHUMERAL DISORDERS

Disorders of the glenohumeral joint account for a minority of complaints of shoulder pain. In contrast to the impingement syndrome in which pain is localized to the distal acromion and is exacerbated by abduction, the pain associated with glenohumeral disease is diffuse, often associated with perceptible crepitus, and is exacerbated by active and positive motion in virtually any plane. The patient will attempt to reduce his pain, yet maintain some degree of motion in the shoulder, by increasing scapulothoracic motion and decreasing glenohumeral motion. This may result in contracture of soft tissues, thus further limiting range of motion of the shoulder. Disorders of the glenohumeral joint can be categorized by their inflammatory and noninflammatory etiologies (Table 63.1).

Inflammatory Arthropathies

The most common inflammatory disorder involving the shoulder joint is rheumatoid arthritis. Other disorders such as ankylosing spondylitis, Reiter's syndrome, and psoriatic arthritis can occasionally affect the shoulder. Shoulder pain in patients with an inflammatory arthropathy, however, usually occurs, not as an isolated complaint, but as part of a constellation of articular complaints and systemic symptoms. In a patient in whom shoulder pain of relatively new onset is the *only* presenting articular complaint, a septic or microcrystalline process (gout or pseudogout) should be considered. Synovial aspiration should be performed promptly to obtain fluid for culture for pathogens and for examination by polarization microscopy.

The patient with a *septic shoulder* should be hospitalized and treated with intravenous antibiotics and drainage by percutaneous or surgical means. The treatment of choice for the *aseptic, inflamed* shoulder is determined by the nature of the underlying condition; however, conservative treatment with a nonsteroidal anti-inflammatory drug is generally utilized first. Additional treatments such as gold therapy, intra-articular injection of corticosteroid preparations, and surgical intervention will generally require consultation with a rheumatologist since these decisions require an extensive assessment of the nature and the severity of the disease process in each individual.

Table 63.1.
Causes of Glenohumeral Disease

INFLAMMATORY
    Rheumatoid arthritis
    Ankylosing spondylitis
    Psoriatic arthritis
    Microcrystalline disease
    Infection

NONINFLAMMATORY
    Degenerative (osteoarthritis)
    Osteonecrosis
    Tears of the glenoid labrum

Noninflammatory Conditions

Shoulder pain originating from the glenohumeral joint may also be caused by noninflammatory conditions such as osteoarthritis, osteonecrosis (ischemic necrosis), and traumatic injuries. *Primary osteoarthritis* of this joint is rare. However, *secondary osteoarthritis* may occur as a result of recurrent glenohumeral dislocation, bone dysplasia, neuropathy due to syrinx or syphilis (Charcot joint), osteonecrosis, hemoglobinopathy, or inflammation. Osteoarthritis is confirmed radiographically by the presence of asymmetrical joint space narrowing, osteophytes, subchondral cysts, and sclerosis, and it is treated conservatively with nonsteroidal anti-inflammatory agents (see Chapter 70 for a full discussion of NSAIDs). In severe disease, total joint replacement may be indicated. Pain from *osteonecrosis* of the humeral head should be suspected in patients with a prior history of fracture of the shoulder, steroid treatment, hemoglobinopathy, or alcohol abuse. Plain radiographs are normal in early osteonecrosis and bone scan is required for diagnosis at this stage. *Tear of the glenoid labrum* is a rare cause of pain in the glenohumeral joint and usually occurs in individuals involved in throwing and racket sports. Consultation with an orthopaedist is indicated in a patient in whom a tear is suspected since arthrography or arthroscopy is usually necessary to diagnose this condition and since surgical excision or repair of the torn labral portion is usually necessary.

Adhesive Capsulitis

Adhesive capsulitis or "frozen shoulder" is a condition of unknown etiology in which progressive restriction of motion of the shoulder occurs (5). Frequently, an underlying painful condition of the shoulder, such as rotator cuff tendinitis or glenohumeral arthritis, precedes the development of adhesive capsulitis. However, this condition may also occur in association with chronic lung disease, coronary artery disease, cerebrovascular disease, and cervical radiculopathy. The common factor that appears to underlie these diverse conditions is prolonged immobility of the arm, and eventually the adhesive capsulitis may represent a greater disability than the initial cause of immobilization. At surgical exploration, thickening of the joint capsule and capsular adhesions to the underlying humeral head are observed. Inflammatory findings in the capsule or synovial lining of the joint have not been constant findings. It remains unclear, therefore, whether contracture of the shoulder capsule is a passive process related to lack of motion or an active process due to inflammation.

Adhesive capsulitis is more common in women than in men and generally occurs in the 5th decade or later. The patient characteristically complains of the insidious onset of diffuse shoulder pain and limitation of motion. In particular, the patient notes difficulty in the performance of tasks that require overhead arm motion, such as combing the hair and grasping objects from high shelves. Physical examination reveals pain at the extremes of motion and markedly reduced active and passive ranges of motion of the glenohumeral joint. Injection of an anesthetic agent into the glenohumeral joint may reduce the pain but does not result in an improved range of motion. The plain radiograph in adhesive capsulitis is generally normal.

The primary aims of treatment of adhesive capsulitis are pain relief, restoration of range of motion, and correction of the underlying cause. Analgesia is achieved by administration of a nonsteroidal anti-inflammatory (see Chapter 70 for a full discussion of NSAIDs) or, if necessary, a narcotic, medication for several days. In addition, ice packs may diminish the acute pain, whereas moist heat for several days is generally more efficacious in the relief of chronic pain. Ultrasound treatments may be beneficial in situations when the above measures have failed. As the acute pain resolves, a specific exercise program should be outlined by a physical therapist. This will be limited initially to passive range of motion exercises, and these can be performed in the home by a trained family member. With continued reduction in the patient's pain, exercises can be extended to include active range of motion without resistance, such as the circumduction and wall-climbing exercises described above (Fig. 63.3). Finally, active exercise with resistance is initiated and supervised by the therapist. It is important that the patient understand (a) that improvement is expected over the course of months, not days or weeks, and (b) that the range of motion achieved may not be entirely normal but will not, in most cases, significantly alter lifestyle. Manipulation of the shoulder under anesthesia to free capsular adhesions has been recommended in the past for patients in whom a functional range of motion is not attained, but the efficacy of this treatment has not been proven and is generally not recommended.

REFERRED PAIN

Not infrequently, pain in the shoulder area is referred from other regions of the body. Referred pain should be suspected: (a) when no localized tenderness in the shoulder girdle can be identified, and (b) when passive and active movements of the joint fail to elicit or exacerbate the pain. Conditions that may result in referred pain to the shoulder are numerous and diverse. Several of the more common of these conditions are discussed below, including compressive neuropathies, reflex sympathetic dystrophy, thoracic outlet syndrome, and visceral disorders (Table 63.2).

Compressive neuropathies that are manifested clinically by shoulder pain may originate at the level of the cervical spine, shoulder, and wrist. The pain is usually described as a dull ache, superimposed upon which may be a sharp or burning pain radiating down the arm. In addition to the pain, the patient may complain of paresthesias, numbness, and muscle weakness or atrophy. A careful neurological examination

Table 63.2.
Causes of Referred Shoulder Pain

COMPRESSIVE NEUROPATHIES
  Cervical nerve root compression
  Entrapment of axillary and suprascapular nerves
  Carpal tunnel syndrome
REFLEX SYMPATHETIC DYSTROPHY

THORACIC OUTLET SYNDROME

VISCERAL DISORDERS
  Diaphragmatic irritation—*e.g.*, subphrenic abscess, perforated
    viscera, pericardial disease
  Irritation of phrenic nerve—*e.g.*, carcinoma of lung
  Ischemic heart disease
  Apical (Pancoast) lung tumors
  Dissecting aortic aneurysms

will often delineate the nerve(s) or nerve root(s) affected:

1. *Cervical nerve root compression* characteristically occurs in middle-aged and elderly populations as a result of cervical disc disease or degenerative arthropathy. This subject is discussed in detail in Chapter 64. However, it is worthwhile noting here that neck pain usually accompanies the shoulder pain and that the pain in both areas is exacerbated by movement of the neck but not of the shoulder.
2. Compression of the median nerve in the carpal tunnel of the wrist (*carpal tunnel syndrome*) is sometimes associated with pain about the shoulder. Characteristically, pain originates within the wrist and radiates to the upper arm or shoulder. The patient generally complains of numbness or paresthesias in the fingers; these symptoms frequently awaken him from sleep and are relieved by rubbing or shaking the hand. Carpal tunnel syndrome is associated with inflammatory arthropathies involving the wrist, infiltrative processes such as

amyloidosis and myxedema, occupational trauma, and pregnancy; in 50% of patients no etiology can be found. Treatment of this condition is discussed in Chapter 81.

Reflex sympathetic dystrophy (also known by synonyms such as shoulder-hand syndrome and causalgia) is a poorly understood condition that is manifested in its acute stages by pain and swelling of the hand (or foot). Diagnosis and management are described in Chapter 83 but should be noted here as a cause of diffuse shoulder pain. The syndrome may occur in association with trauma to the involved extremity and with a number of nontraumatic conditions such as myocardial infarctions and cerebrovascular accidents.

Thoracic outlet syndrome is a rare condition but one in which pain in the shoulder is a frequent complaint. The thoracic outlet consists of a series of narrow, fixed passages within which the neurovascular supply of the upper extremity can become compressed as it exits the neck and thorax to enter the axilla (Fig. 63.5). Compression of the neural or vascular structures may result from conditions such as cervical rib, interscalene muscle compression, and anomalies of the first rib. The presenting complaints are dependent upon the predominant structure(s) being compressed. If neural in origin, the patient complains of a dull aching or burning sensation in the arm accompanied by paresthesias or numbness, usually in the distribution of the ulnar nerve. Muscle weakness and atrophy may be noted on physical examination. If vascular in origin, the patient may complain of an alteration in color or temperature, of swelling of the affected hand, or of a Raynaud-like phenomenon.

The physical examination may reveal a cool, cyanotic extremity as a result of arterial compression. Several tests can be performed that will aid in the diagnosis. The intensity of the patient's radial pulse

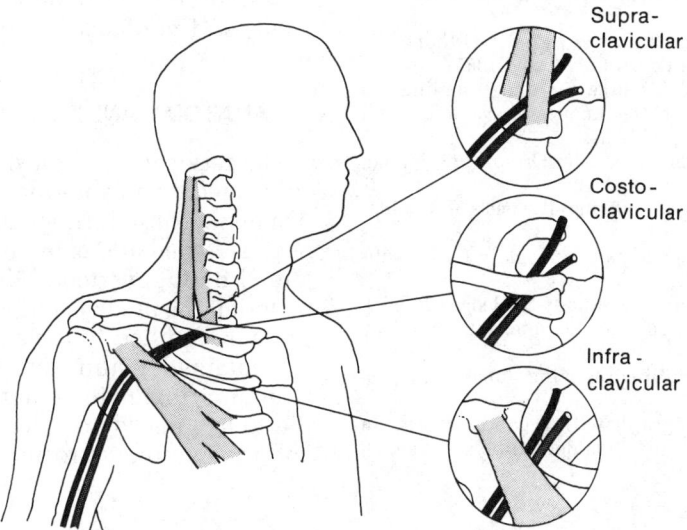

Figure 63.5. Points of neurovascular compression in the thoracic outlet syndrome. (From Ramamurti CP: *Orthopaedics in Primary Care.* Tinker RV (ed). Baltimore, Williams & Wilkins, 1979.)

is palpated during the following maneuvers: (a) the patient holds his breath in full inspiration while rotating the neck toward the side that is being examined (Adson maneuver); (b) the arm is abducted 180° in external rotation (hyperabduction maneuver); and (c) the patient assumes an exaggerated military posture with the shoulder braced posteriorly and inferiorly (costoclavicular maneuver). A "positive" test occurs when one or more of these maneuvers reproduces the patient's symptoms or results in dampening or obliteration of the patient's radial pulse. Noninvasive arterial Doppler studies of the extremity can then be performed at rest and during the maneuvers listed above. Arteriography may be performed for final confirmation of the syndrome, particularly if surgical intervention is being considered. Treatment of the thoracic outlet syndrome begins with conservative therapy with reassurance, education, and physical therapy to strengthen the musculature about the shoulder. In patients with severe or refractory disease, surgical intervention will then be necessary.

Pain may also be referred to the shoulder from disorders of the viscera, particularly those arising along the course of the phrenic nerve or from the diaphragm that it supplies (Table 63.2). Irritation of the nerve or diaphragm may arise from a variety of conditions involving the mediastinum, pericardium, liver, spleen and gall bladder. In addition, ischemic heart disease, apical (Pancoast) tumors of the lung, and dissecting aortic aneurysms may be causes of referred pain to the shoulder. Shoulder pain may, in fact, be the sole presenting symptom in these disorders. Disorders of visceral structures should be considered, therefore, when the clinical presentation suggests the shoulder pain to be referred and when no neural or vascular etiology can be identified.

General References

Calliett R: Shoulder Pain, 2nd ed. Philadelphia, FA Davis, 1981.
    A concise and well-illustrated manual with much practical information.
Halbach JW, Tank RT: In: Gould JA, Davies GJ (eds): Orthopaedic and Sports Physical Therapy. St Louis, CV Mosby, 1985.
    A well-illustrated, useful resource for understanding the mechanism of injury and the techniques of evaluation and rehabilitation of shoulder problems.
Post M (guest ed): The painful shoulder. Clin Orthop 173: March, 1983.
    A comprehensive monograph covering all aspects of shoulder pain problems.
Ramamurti CP, Tinker RV: Orthopaedics in Primary Care. Baltimore, Williams & Wilkins, 1979.
Thornhill TS: In: Kelley WM, Harris ED, Ruddy S, Sledge CB (eds): Textbook of Rheumatology, 2nd ed. Philadelphia, WB Saunders, 1985.
Wilgis EFS: Vascular Injuries and Diseases of the Upper Limb. Boston, Little, Brown, and Co, 1983.
    A well-illustrated monograph with a good chapter on compression syndromes of the shoulder, girdle and arm.

Specific References

1. Brems J: Rotator cuff tear: Evaluation and treatment. Orthopedics 11:69, 1988.
2. Colfield RH: Current concept review: rotator cuff disease of the shoulder. J Bone Joint Surg 67A:974, 1985.
3. Crass JR, Craig EV: Noninvasive imaging of the rotator cuff. Orthopedics 11:57, 1988.
4. Dias JJ, Steingold RF, Richardson RA, et al: The conservative treatment of acromioclavicular dislocation. J Bone Joing Surg 68B:719, 1987.
5. Lloyd JA, Lloyd HM: Adhesive capsulitis of the shoulder. South Med J 76:879, 1983.

C H A P T E R 64

Neck Pain*

NADIM E. AFEICHE, M.D.

Neck pain is a common problem. Nearly 50% of individuals over 50 years of age experience neck pain at some time. Because there are many structures in the neck that, when diseased, may cause pain, as well as multiple sources of referred pain, the physician must systematically evaluate patients who complain of neck pain that is new or persistent. This chapter provides a review of the skeletal structures of the neck, the method of evaluation for complaints of neck pain, a description of common problems and their treatment, and guidance for referral of selected patients with neck pain.

ANATOMY AND SOURCES OF PAIN (Fig. 64.1)

The cervical spine consists of seven vertebral bodies connected by an anterior and a posterior longitudinal ligament. These ligaments provide stability when the neck is flexed and extended. The vertebral bodies are joined by intervertebral discs composed of a gel-like material (the nucleus pulposus) that absorbs increased pressure applied to the spine. The nucleus pulposus is contained within an annulus fibrosus, a fibrous structure ringing the outer margin of the disc. During the fourth decade of life, both the nucleus pulposus and the annulus fibrosus undergo progressive degen-

---

*Drs. Noble M. Hansen and John R. Burton contributed to the first and second editions of this book.

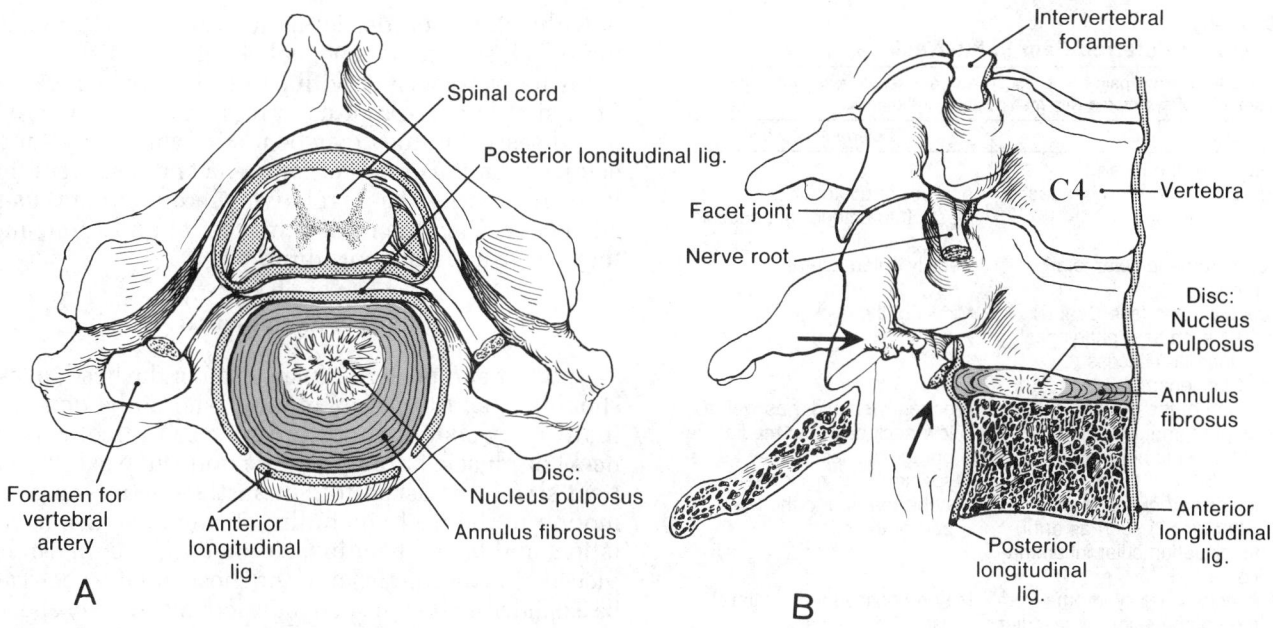

Figure 64.1. Anatomy of disc and ligaments of the cervical spine. *A.* Superior view. Note relationship of anterior and posterior longitudinal ligament to the intervertebral disc. *B.* Lateral view. Note relationship of intervertebral foramen to the intervertebral disc and facet joint. Bulg-ing of the intervertebral disc or bone spurs forming from the facet joint may cause compression of the nerve root within the intervertebral foramen (*arrows*).

eration, seen microscopically as a loss of the fibrous pattern and the collagen alignment. As a result, the ability of the disc to absorb shocks is reduced. There are facet joints found between vertebral elements posteriorly, one on each side of the spine; they are apophyseal (projecting) joints with a synovium-lined capsule. It is within these small joints in the posterior spine that osteoarthritis can occur, osteoarthritis being a breakdown of the articular cartilage within the joints. The intervertebral neural foramina, located laterally on either side of the vertebral bodies, are the canals through which the individual nerve roots emerge from the spinal canal. The spinal canal and the foramina can be encroached upon by a bulging intervertebral disc or an osseous proliferation (bony spur) originating in a vertebral body, by a facet joint, or from the bony margin of a neural foramen (Fig. 64.1). When the encroachment involves a nerve root, pain in the distribution of that root (radicular pain) may occur. The facet joint capsules and the intervertebral disc are innervated by fine unmyelinated nerves (called C fibers) that have simple nerve endings. When these nerve endings are stimulated by degenerative disease within the disc or joint capsules, the patient may experience pain, which is referred to the posterior aspect of the neck at any level. The pain felt in the neck may not be at the cervical level from which the nerve is arising. In addition, C fiber stimulation can cause pain to be referred to the interscapular area, superiorly and laterally over the shoulders, and in the lower arm and the hand. C fiber encroachment occasionally causes a decrease in sensation in the lower arm and in the hand.

Spasm of any of the many muscles of the neck region is also a common source of pain.

EVALUATION OF THE PATIENT

History

The date of onset of the patient's symptoms and any associated trauma should be ascertained. A history of recent trauma is an indication for a complete set of cervical spine X-rays (see below). Often, knowledge of the specific activity the patient was performing at the onset of pain will be quite helpful in establishing the cause of the pain. Prolonged extension of the neck, such as occurs in people doing overhead work, is a common occupational situation that can give rise to pain in the cervical region. Another common occupational cause of neck pain is prolonged sitting with the neck flexed in one position. This occurs commonly in computer operators or typists. The sustained position causes spasm of the neck muscles, which results in pain. Also, it is quite common that a patient sustains a minor twisting injury or trauma to the neck and does not experience neck pain within the first 24 hours, after which the patient's first pain may begin to appear and progress. Reproduction or increase of pain by neck motion is very helpful in localizing the problem to the cervical spine rather than to a referred source (Table 64.1). It is also important to know whether the pain is felt outside the neck as well, such as in the head, posteriorly between the scapulae, about the shoulder, down the arm, or in the hand. The patient should be

Table 64.1.
Sources of Referred Pain in the Neck

The clue to referred pain is the absence of any tenderness in the neck or of exacerbation of symptoms with manipulation of the neck,

Source	Referred Location
Disorders of the Head:	
Migraine or tension headache	Anterior or posterior
Sinus Infection	Most often anterior but occasionally posterior
Temporomandibular joint problem	Usually anterolateral
Oral problems (see Chapter 101) such as a pharyngeal or tonsillar abscess	Middle of the neck
Distant Lesions:	
Irritation of the surface of the diaphragm innervated by the phrenic nerve (C3, 4, and 5)	Frequently shoulder as well as low neck pain, but medial diaphragmatic lesion may be associated with neck pain
Shoulder problems (see Chapter 63) such as arthritis or periarticular inflammation	May be referred to the lateral part of the neck
Thoracic outlet syndrome from the compression of vascular and neural structures between the rib and the clavicle or between the scalene muscles	May be noticed in the lateral aspect of the neck
Lung problems such as superior sulcus tumor (Pancoast's tumor)	Initially may be located in the lateral aspect of the neck and shoulder
Cardiovascular problems such as a heart attack or an aneurysm of the thoracic aorta	May be localized to the base of the neck

asked about decreased *sensation* in his hands and, if possible, to say specifically which fingers are involved. If the pain and numbness are felt in a dermatome distribution, this indicates nerve compression (Table 64.2). Muscle weakness in the shoulder, arm, and hands should be elicited to help identify potential nerve compression (see Chapter 78). Pain associated with motion of the shoulder is not characteristic of cervical spine disease and suggests that the problem

is within the shoulder joint (see Chapter 63). Symptoms such as dizziness, visual changes, and ataxia are not usually associated with cervical problems arising from simple nerve root compression or degenerative disc disease, but they may be found when bony spurs encroach on the vertebral foramina and compress the vertebral arteries. These relatively rare symptoms usually occur when the neck is in a certain position, and they are usually of short duration.

Physical Examination

Anterior and posterior inspection of the head, neck, shoulders, and upper extremities should be done initially. Any abnormal posture such as torticollis (wry neck) or muscle atrophy will be noticed. Next the patient should be asked to demonstrate active range of motion of the neck, including flexion, extension, rotation, and lateral bending. Normally, the chin can be placed easily upon the anterior chest and the neck can be extended so that the patient is looking directly above. Normally, there is almost 90° of rotation of the neck to both sides. Simple hyperextension of the neck commonly exacerbates the pain caused by cervical disc degeneration. The patient should be asked to extend his neck and to maintain this position for a period of 30 seconds to determine whether the pain is made worse. Putting direct compression on top of the head also may produce or exacerbate pain in the patient with degenerative disc disease, especially if the head is compressed while the neck is extended. The posterior neck muscles are palpated for muscle spasm, which may be asymmetric and may give the patient the appearance of torticollis (wry neck). Next, the shoulder should be subjected to a range of motion to see whether this elicits pain within the shoulder itself.

Selected neurological tests (see Chapters 78 and 84) are important in the evaluation of the patient with neck pain whenever there is any suggestion of nerve root involvement or cord compression. These tests include reflex testing of the upper and lower extremities; muscle strength testing of the upper extremities; and

Table 64.2.
Characteristic Findings at Individual Cervical Nerve Root Levels

Nerve Root	Disc Level	History	Examination[a]
C3	(C2–3)	Pain into the back of the neck and around the mastoid process	No reflex changes
C4	(C3–4)	Pain into the back of the neck to the levator scapulae to anterior chest	No reflex changes
C5	(C4–5)	Pain into side of neck to the superior lateral shoulder, numbness over the deltoid muscle	Deltoid muscle atrophy and weakness of shoulder abduction
C6	(C5–6)	Pain to the lateral aspects of the arm and forearm and into the thumb and index finger with numbness of thumb and dorsum of hand	Weak biceps and brachioradial muscles and decreased biceps and brachioradial tendon reflexes
C7	(C6–7)	Pain into the midforearm to middle and ring fingers	Triceps muscle weakness with decreased triceps muscle reflex
C8	(C7–T1)	Pain to the medial aspect of the forearm into the ring and small fingers with numbness of the ulnar border and small finger	Triceps weakness with weakness of intrinsic muscles of the hand

[a] Sensory testing will usually show abnormalities in dermatome of the affected nerve root (see Fig. 78.2).

sensory testing of the upper extremities. The reflex testing should include the biceps, triceps, brachioradial, quadriceps, and gastrocnemius tendons, and the Babinski test. Muscle strength in the upper extremities should include the biceps (flexion of elbow), triceps (extension of elbow), wrist extensors and flexors, hand and finger flexors, and intrinsic muscles of the hand. The intrinsic muscles of the hand are tested by having the patient hold the fingers tightly together while the examiner tries to separate them. A sensory examination is then performed. An objective sensory deficit is one that conforms to a dermatome distribution (see Chapters 78 and 84).

Occasionally, cervical spine problems can cause cervical myelopathy when a bone spur forms posteriorly at the margin of an intervertebral disc and then impinges on the spinal cord, producing signs of cord compression: increased reflexes in the lower extremities with a positive Babinski sign. A spinal cord tumor at this level could give similar findings.

Laboratory Assessment

If the history reveals an episode of recent trauma or the neurological examination reveals abnormalities, a complete set of cervical spine X-rays should be obtained. These films should include an assessment of levels C1 through C7 with oblique and openmouth odontoid views. These X-rays will help the physician to rule out fracture or metastatic disease. There is not, however, a good correlation between clinical symptoms or signs and degenerative abnormalities on X-ray. In fact in asymptomatic individuals after the age of 40, cervical degenerative changes (spondylosis) are common and after the age of 50 are evident in over 90% of individuals (1). On the other hand, there may be serious cervical disease with minimal or no changes on X-ray. If there is no history of trauma and the neurological examination is normal, initial X-rays are not necessary but should be obtained if there is an inadequate response after 1 or 2 weeks of therapy.

Computerized tomography is also useful in the evaluation of problems of the upper cervical spine, especially after significant trauma when X-ray studies reveal no abnormality or if the positioning necessary for regular X-rays is difficult. Magnetic resonance imaging (MRI) is especially useful when evaluating patients who are suspected of having metastatic cancer or a primary disc problem. When MRI is available, it is best to consult with a radiologist, a neurosurgeon, or an orthopaedist to help decide whether a computed tomography (CT) scan or MRI should be done. Also, bone scans using radionuclides may be helpful when neoplastic disease is suspected; however, arthritis or positioning artifacts may confuse interpretation.

SELECTED SYNDROMES ASSOCIATED WITH NECK PAIN

Many problems of the neck may result in neck pain (Table 64.3). Because the most common problems—

Table 64.3.
Selected Problems of the Neck That May Result in Neck Pain

Problem	Comment
Arthritis	Especially rheumatoid (see Chapter 70) and degenerative joint disease (see the text and Chapter 68).
Disc disease	See the text.
Fibromyalgia	See Chapter 66.
Infection	Osteomyelitis or soft tissue infection—look for point tenderness.
Neoplasia	Myeloma or metastatic disease is associated with point tenderness and X-ray abnormalities.
Neuritis	Any nerve may be involved. A relatively common one is the spinal accessory nerve. Look for tenderness over the nerve—lateral aspect of upper one-third of sternomastoid muscle.
Platybasia	A congenital disorder that may not manifest symptoms before age 40 or from Paget's disease, X-rays show characteristic changes (i.e., invagination of the base of the skull).
Sprain	Whiplash (see the text).
Structures in neck	Any organ or structure located in the neck may become a source of neck pain. Careful examination will detect abnormalities such as thyroiditis, lymphadenitis, pharyngitis, sialadenitis, or tender carotid artery (carotodynia).
Tendinitis	Any tendon may be involved but occipital and sternomastoid are particularly common. Local tenderness is a clue.
Torticollis (wry neck)	Diagnosis is usually obvious by observation. An underlying structural problem could produce reflex muscle spasm; therefore, with an initial episode an underlying problem (such as tumor or infection) should be considered.
Trauma	Because of the danger of cord injury, trauma associated with neck pain should be carefully evaluated.
Vascular	Arteritis or dissection may cause neck pain.

cervical disc disease and cervical spondylosis (degenerative changes)—may have similar manifestations, they are discussed together based on the presence or absence of neurological findings (see below); and two other common problems—stiff neck and whiplash injury—are discussed separately.

Pain with Nerve Root Compression

Diagnosis

The objective signs of nerve root compression are muscle weakness, a decreased deep tendon reflex, and decreased sensation in a dermatome distribution.

Patients with nerve root compression present with the acute or gradual onset of posterior neck pain that radiates to the shoulder and down one arm into the lower arm and often into the hand itself. The pain will occasionally radiate into a finger that corresponds to the dermatome of the nerve root involved. The pain is made worse by movement of the neck and extreme neck positions. The patient may, in addition, complain of decreased sensation and paresthesias in the arm and hand. A patient may have nerve root compression from the cervical spine but have little or no neck and arm pain, and instead have arm weakness and loss of sensation. Nerve root compression can be caused by impingement of the nerve by a cervical disc—most common in younger individuals—or by osseous proliferation that can impinge upon the nerve as it exits through its foramen—most common in patients over 50. Also, the thoracic outlet syndrome may be confused with cervical disease associated with neurological findings, and this syndrome should be ruled out (see Chapter 63).

Management

Patients with neurological findings should be referred to an orthopaedist or to a neurosurgeon for more complete examination and follow-up. If muscle weakness and sensory impairment are of such a degree that they would be unacceptable if permanent, immediate surgical decompression may be considered. The orthopaedist or neurosurgeon will evaluate these patients further with CT, MRI, and/or myelography.

In mild cases of nerve root compression, treatment consists first of immobilization of the neck by use of a *soft cervical collar* that should allow slight flexion of the neck. If the collar forces the neck into extension, it may exacerbate the symptoms. A soft cervical collar, made of foam rubber and stockinette and fastened behind the neck, serves more as a reminder to a patient to restrict neck motion, as it will, based on clinical measurements, only restrict approximately 25% of flexion-extension and approximately 20 and 10% of rotational and lateral motion, respectively (2). These collars are well tolerated, inexpensive, and easily accessible (made in the office or available in pharmacies). Cervical collars that more fully restrict neck movements (such as the Philadelphia collar, Somibrace, four-poster brace, or cervicothoracic brace) are difficult to use, more expensive, and should be recommended only after consultation with an orthopaedist or neurosurgeon.

If the pain is severe, bed rest may be necessary. It is helpful to place a small pillow under the nape of the neck to provide proper positioning. If muscle spasm is present, moist or dry heat applied to the neck may give symptomatic relief. Analgesia using a nonsteroidal anti-inflammatory agent (NSAID) (see Chapter 70) or acetaminophen may help. If a stronger analgesic becomes necessary, codeine, 30 to 60 mg orally three or four times daily, may be added. Although not a first line agent, a muscle relaxant may be helpful (see Chapter 65, Low Back Pain) if symptoms persist after 3 or 4 days.

The acute phase usually lasts only 1 or 2 weeks. When symptoms become recurrent or chronic (lasting >2 to 3 weeks) *cervical traction* may provide relief and, although not studied in a controlled fashion, could be tried after the severe acute pain subsides. This is performed initially by a physical therapist. For a period of 30 minutes, 15 to 20 lb of chin halter traction are applied to the neck. The neck must be positioned in slight flexion; extension, which could worsen symptoms, must be avoided. After several sessions, the patient can be instructed in the use of a home cervical traction unit that can be applied for 30 minutes at a time, up to three times/day, for several months. Should the acute symptom not subside or if new signs develop, referral to an orthopaedist or a neurosurgeon is necessary for confirmation of the diagnosis and consideration of the use of a complex brace and possible surgery (usually discectomy and anterior interbody fusion).

Even when symptoms and signs subside there is a relatively high rate of recurrence of symptoms. It is therefore important to educate the patient in activities or positions that should be avoided and in exercises that may help to relieve muscle spasm (Figs. 64.2 and 64.3).

Pain without Nerve Root Compression

Diagnosis

The majority of patients who present with neck pain have no objective neurological findings. Changes in sensation in the lower arm or hand may occur from irritation of C fibers (i.e., those fibers innervating the discs, facet joint capsule, and the surrounding tissues) or from degeneration of the facet joints within the neck and, therefore, may be present without true nerve root compression. The patient may present either with an acute onset of pain (most of the time a disc herniation) or with a slowly progressive discomfort (most often from osteoarthritis) that has been building over several months. In the acute disc herniation syndrome, the patient presents with the rather sudden onset of neck pain that is associated with decreased range of motion of the cervical spine, bilateral muscle spasm, or occasionally asymmetric muscle spasm that produces torticollis (wry neck). The patient may have pain in the shoulder or arm but have no objective weakness or sensory findings on examination. X-rays of the cervical spine may be entirely normal.

Treatment

Initial treatment is basically the same as that outlined above for patients with nerve root compression. The neck is "immobilized" with a soft cervical collar; local heat and analgesics or NSAIDs (see Chapter 70) also may give symptomatic relief. Muscle relaxants (see Chapter 65) may be tried if symptoms persist after 3 or 4 days of initial treatment. In patients who have a chronic, more insidious onset of pain, it is helpful to examine the patient's occupational situation more closely to see if there are exacerbating circumstances. Any activity that creates a prolonged extension of the neck, such as overhead work (e.g., painting), or prolonged flexion of the neck, such as sitting at a computer or typewriter, may aggravate a preexisting

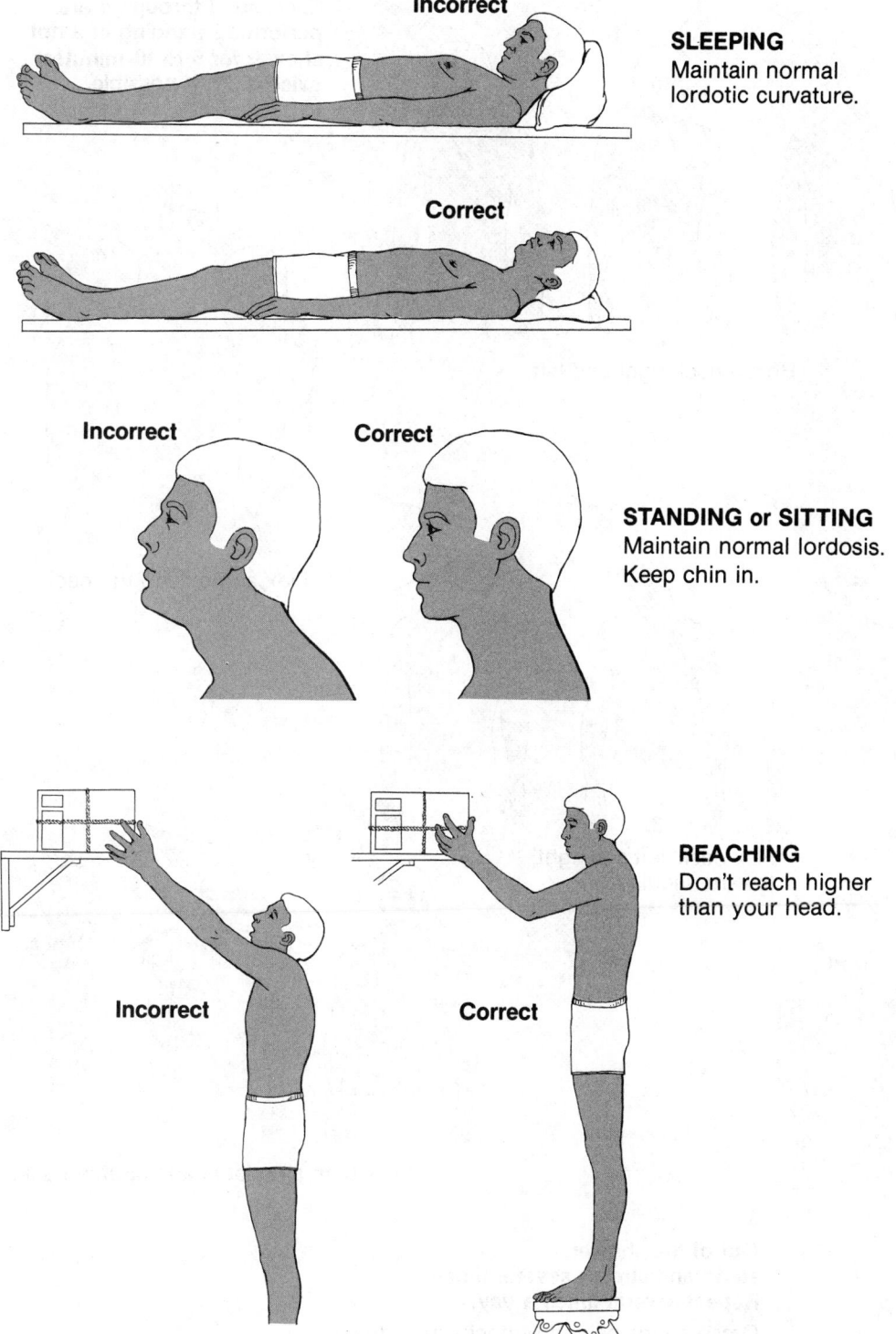

Figure 64.2. Position to prevent recurrence of neck pain.

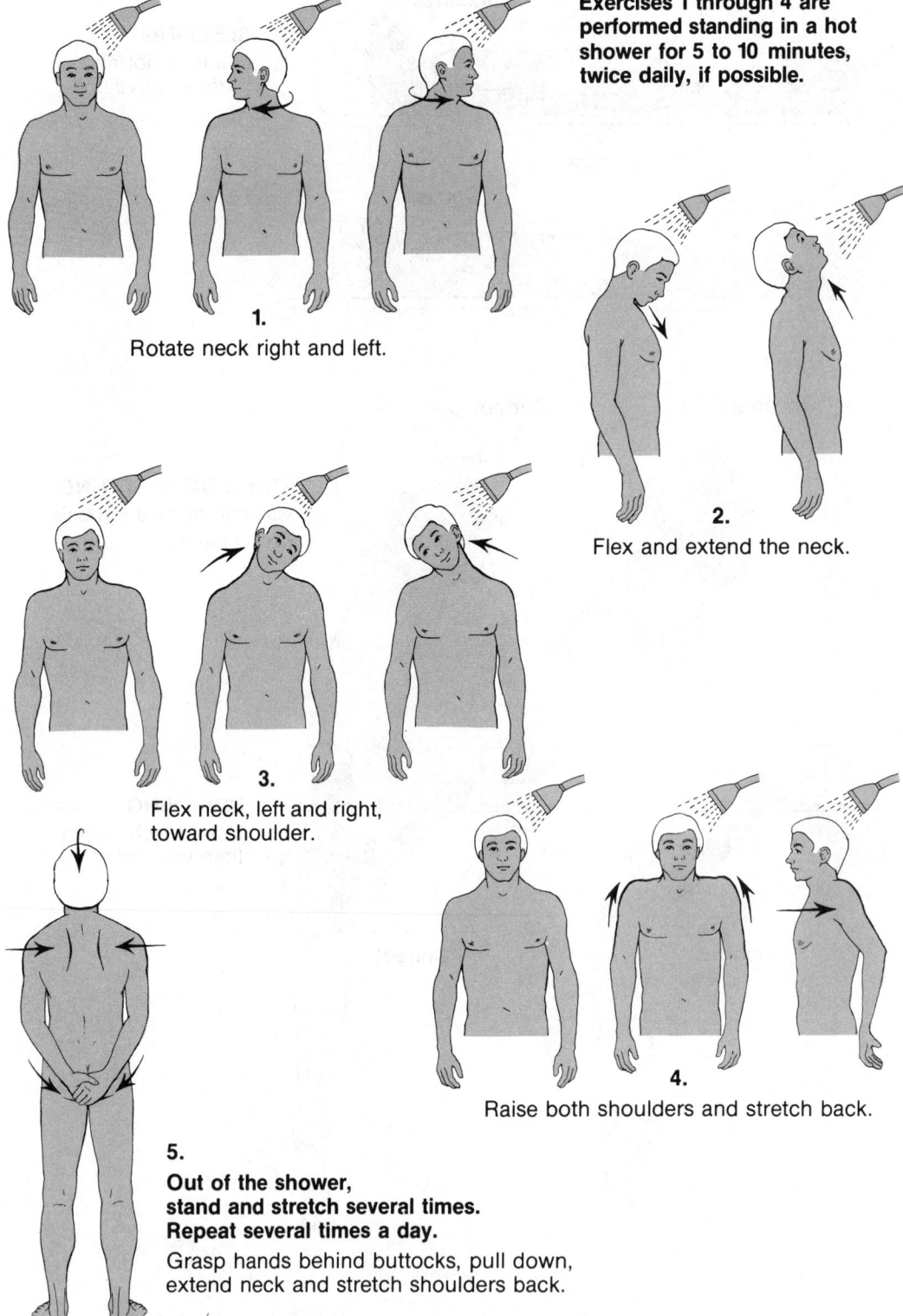

Exercises 1 through 4 are performed standing in a hot shower for 5 to 10 minutes, twice daily, if possible.

1.
Rotate neck right and left.

2.
Flex and extend the neck.

3.
Flex neck, left and right, toward shoulder.

4.
Raise both shoulders and stretch back.

5.
Out of the shower, stand and stretch several times. Repeat several times a day.

Grasp hands behind buttocks, pull down, extend neck and stretch shoulders back.

Figure 64.3. Exercises to rehabilitate the neck.

problem. If after initial treatment pain lasts more than 2 or 3 weeks, X-rays of the cervical spine should be obtained to look for a possible vertebral collapse, metastatic disease, or foraminal encroachment by bone. The treatment is based on the severity of the symptoms. An oral, rapidly acting anti-inflammatory agent, such as piroxicam (Feldene), 20 mg once a day, may be tried over a course of 2 or 3 weeks. (Alternative nonsteroidal anti-inflammatory agents, including aspirin, may be tried also; see Chapter 70.) When cost is a factor, aspirin is preferred; however, a daily dose of 3 to 6 g is needed for 7 to 10 days to achieve an anti-inflammatory effect. Shorter courses and lower doses of aspirin do provide analgesic benefit, however. The patient should be informed that his symptoms often may be chronic or recurrent, and he should be advised about how to avoid recurrences (Fig. 64.2).

If an acute severe episode of neck pain in this situation does not respond to treatment within the first week or 2, the patient should be referred. When the symptoms are more mild and chronic, a trial of treatment for several months would be reasonable before referral. Further evaluation by an orthopaedic surgeon or a neurosurgeon will include a complete cervical spine X-ray and a computerized cervical tomogram with or without a myelogram or MRI to identify the problem and its location. If a herniated disc is identified, consideration can be given to its removal, with anterior interbody fusion. This operation can give excellent relief of pain if the correct level of involvement has been identified.

Stiff Neck

Stiff neck is very common and is not a diagnosis, but rather a description of a symptom. Strain of the muscles or ligaments, strain of the neck, cold-induced muscular spasm, fibromyalgia, and neuritis are all possible causes. The problem is characterized by posterior cervical muscular spasm on one or both sides. The spasm usually lasts only a few days and is relieved by the application of heat and mild analgesics, such as acetaminophen or NSAIDs. The patient should receive advice about relieving muscle spasm and preventing recurrences (Figs. 64.2 and 64.3). Should the discomfort last beyond a week, an underlying disorder should be considered (e.g., disc disease), and an evaluation should be initiated.

Whiplash

Mechanism

Whiplash is a term given to acute injuries of the neck caused by sudden extension of the cervical spine. In this country, the most common cause is a rear end automobile collision. Patients with whiplash are frequently involved in litigation and compensation situations, which makes physicians skeptical of their complaints; it is, however, well documented experimentally that significant injury can occur by this mechanism. In cadaver studies, it has been shown that when the neck is suddenly and forcefully hyperextended, the muscles of the anterior aspect of the neck are stretched or torn, including the sternomastoid and longus coli muscles; a retropharyngeal hematoma can result; the anterior longitudinal ligament of the cervical spine may tear; and separation of the disc from the vertebral body can occur. Usually, however, the patient with whiplash injury sustains less intensive damage.

Diagnosis

It is not uncommon for the patient to be without discomfort initially. Pain usually begins several hours to 1 or 2 days after the injury. The patient experiences pain in the posterior and/or anterior region of the neck. It commonly radiates to the occipital aspect of the head, and it may radiate to the shoulders and down the upper lateral aspect of the arms. Occipital headaches often occur. Disc herniation and nerve root compression rarely occur from whiplash injury. X-rays after whiplash injuries are usually normal. However, there may be some loss of the normal cervical lordosis, which is an indication of muscle spasm and splinting of the neck.

Treatment

If muscle spasm or limitation of motion is present, the patient should be placed in a soft cervical collar (see above). Analgesics such as acetaminophen or NSAIDs (or occasionally for short periods, codeine), in adequate doses, should be given. The patient should be warned that extension of the neck will exacerbate the pain. Heat applied to the cervical spine, either moist or dry, may give symptomatic relief but does not speed healing. The patient should be encouraged to perform daily work and activities as much as possible. If the patient has severe pain and muscle spasm at the initial injury, the clinical course will probably last 4 to 6 weeks. When the patient's pain subsides and he has full range of motion without muscle spasm, the soft collar can be gradually discontinued, and the patient should also be advised of the methods of relieving muscle spasm and preventing recurrent symptoms (Fig. 64.2 and Fig. 64.3). If there are no symptoms of nerve root compression, the patient with persistent symptoms should be treated for a long period of time, perhaps a year, before consideration of further workup.

All patients with whiplash injury, especially those with nerve root signs, are probably best seen at least once by an orthopaedist or a neurosurgeon for confirmation of the diagnosis and for follow-up should the symptoms not resolve in a reasonable time.

General References

Bailey RW, Sherk HH, Dunn EJ, et al (eds): *The Cervical Spine. The Cervical Spine Research Society*. Philadelphia, J.B. Lippincott Co., 1983.
    A comprehensive textbook with in-depth and well-illustrated chapters on all problems of the cervical spine.
Cailliet R: *Neck and Arm Pain*. Philadelphia, FA Davis, 1981.

A very practical, concise, and well-illustrated manual covering the common causes of neck pain.

Nakano KK: Neck pain. In: Kelley WN, Harris ED, Ruddy S, Sledge CB (eds): *Textbook of Rheumatology*, 3rd ed, Philadelphia, WB Saunders, 1989.

An excellent discussion of the anatomy and biomechanisms and of the diagnosis, treatment, and differential diagnosis of common cervical spine problems.

Specific References

1. Elias F: Roentgen findings in the asymptomatic cervical spine. *NY J Med* 58:3300, 1958.
2. Johnson RM, Hart DL, Simmons EF, et al: Cervical orthoses. *J Bone Joint Surg* 59:332, 1977.

C H A P T E R   65

Low Back Pain

DAVID BORENSTEIN, M.D.

Second to the common cold, low back pain is the most common affliction of man. Between 70 and 80% of the population of the world experience back pain some time during their lives. The prevalence of back pain has ranged, in reports, from a low of 10% of adults during a 2-year period to a high of 20% of the population of a Western industrial society during a 2-week period (11, 21). Although as many as 30% of these individuals with back pain do not seek medical evaluation, the remainder eventually request medical advice (15). The outpatient office is the appropriate setting for the evaluation of these individuals. The vast majority of patients with low back pain have underlying conditions that can be diagnosed and treated in the ambulatory setting. Most patients do not require hospitalization or surgery. The task is to separate those few who require more aggressive therapy from those who will recover with conservative management.

ANATOMY AND BIOMECHANICS OF THE LUMBAR SPINE

The structure of the lumbosacral spine is complex. The lumbar spine is composed of five vertebrae with interposed intervertebral discs that consist of a gelatinous nucleus pulposus and a surrounding annulus fibrosus. The vertebrae and discs are supported by strong ligamentous structures and paraspinous muscles. The posterior aspects of the vertebrae surround the spinal canal, form the neural foramina, and interlock to form apophyseal joints whose main purpose is motion. The sacrum is the part of the spine that interdigitates with the iliac bones to form part of the pelvis.

An understanding of the nerve supply to the lumbosacral spine is essential in recognizing the patterns of pain associated with disease processes affecting individual anatomical components of the back (8). The sinuvertebral nerve (Fig. 65.1) is the major sensory nerve supplying structures in the lumbar spine. The nerve arises from the corresponding spinal nerve before it divides into anterior and posterior branches. The nerve enters the intervertebral foramen and divides into ascending, descending, and transverse branches that anastomose with the contralateral side and sensory nerves at adjacent levels, above and below. The sinuvertebral nerve supplies the posterior longitudinal ligament, superficial annulus fibrosus, epidural blood vessels, anterior dura mater, dural sleeve, and posterior vertebral periosteum. The posterior rami of the spinal nerves supply the apophyseal joints above and below the nerve and the paraspinous muscles at multiple levels. The complex innervation of lumbar spine structures helps explain the diffuse nature of pain associated with a wide variety of pathological disorders.

A number of organs are situated in the retroperitoneum, anterior to the lumbar spine. The kidneys, ureters, aorta, inferior vena cava, pancreas, and periaortic lymph nodes are retroperitoneal organs. Diseases that affect these organs may result in referred pain that is localized to the lumbar spine.

In the upright position with a normal curvature (lordosis), the ligamentous structures maintain the position of the spine with little need for contraction of the paraspinous muscles or weight-bearing by the apophyseal (facet) joints. However, if the normal curve is flattened or accentuated, the paraspinous muscles contract and the apophyseal (facet) joints become weight-bearing. This change in body mechanics results in pain.

The lumbar vertebrae are exposed to tremendous forces. This is due principally to the magnification of stresses that result from the lever effect of the arm in lifting and to vertical forces associated with the human

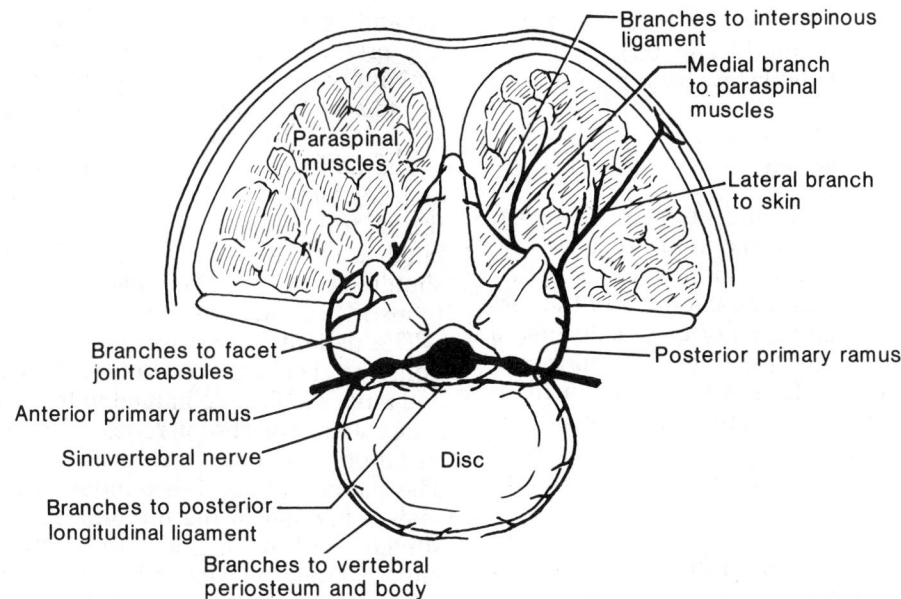

Figure 65.1. Cross-sectional view depicting nerve supply to the anterior (sinuvertebral) and posterior (posterior ramus) portions of the lumbar spine. Taken with permission from Borenstein DG, Wiesel SW. *Low Back Pain: Medical Diagnosis and Comprehensive Management.* WB Saunders, Co, Philadelphia, 1989, p. 14.

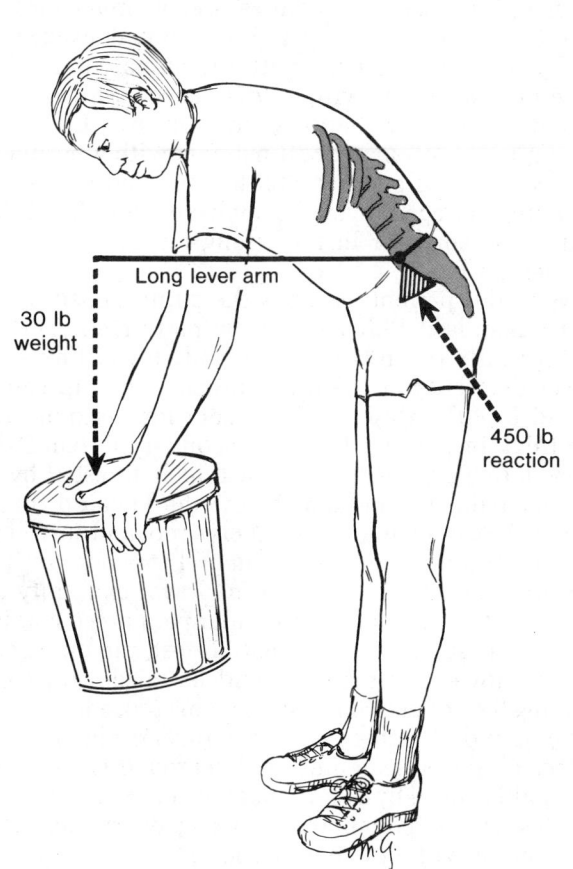

Figure 65.2. Forces in the lumbar area.

upright position. Figure 65.2 demonstrates how lifting an object away from the body introduces the lever magnification phenomenon, resulting in a marked increase in forces on the vertebral bodies and discs. Because each intervertebral disc is a fluid system, there is a hydraulic pressure created whenever a load is placed on the axial skeleton. This hydraulic pressure magnifies three to five times the force that occurs on the annulus fibrosus. This force is akin to the hoop stress that occurs in a barrel when pressure is applied to its liquid content. The ability of the annulus fibrosus to withstand stress decreases significantly with age, and by 60 years many individuals have only 50% of the strength in these fibers that they had at age 30.

The lumbar spine, however, is not just an isolated structure. Much support is obtained by the muscles and ligaments of the spine and by the muscles of the thoracic and abdominal cavities. These latter structures act as a sort of muscular cylinder that helps to decrease the load on the axial skeleton by as much as 30% in the lumbar area and 50% in the thoracic spine.

EVALUATION OF PATIENTS WITH LOW BACK PAIN

Certain facts pertaining to the etiology and natural history of back pain influence the evaluation and treatment of patients with this symptom. Back pain is most often associated with a mechanical etiology. Mechanical low back pain may be defined as pain secondary to overuse of a normal anatomical structure (muscle strain) or deformity of an anatomical structure (herniated nucleus pulposus). A majority of patients with mechanical back pain will not have an associated history of acute trauma, lifting, or strain (14). Most low back pain is self-limited. Of those individuals who are evaluated by their physician, 40 to 50% are better in 1 week, 51 to 86% in 1 month, and 92% within 2 months (7). Most patients with low back pain do not require surgery.

History

Questions about back pain concentrate on the onset, duration, frequency, location, radiation, time of day, quality, intensity, aggravating and alleviating factors along with the chronological development of the disorder. Historical evidence of motor or sensory nerve root irritation or of sphincter (bladder or rectal incontinence) or sexual dysfunction is important in identifying individuals with cauda equina compression (see below). Occupational history may reveal predisposing factors associated with recurrent episodes of back injury.

Patients are also questioned about systemic symptoms that are indicative of a nonmechanical cause of their back pain. Patients with fever, weight loss, pain with recumbency, extended morning stiffness, acute bone pain, or viscerogenic pain should be evaluated for a systemic illness. Patients who are over 60 years of age are also at greater risk of a nonmechanical cause for their pain.

Physical Examination

Physical Examination of the Lumbosacral Spine and Associated Musculoskeletal Areas

Abnormalities of the spine may be discovered while the spine is stationary or in motion. The patient is evaluated in an orderly fashion that tests the function of musculoskeletal and neurological structures of the lumbosacral spine (12).

Initially, the barefoot (or socks) patient is examined in a gown while he is *standing*. The spinal column is examined from all directions checking for excessive kyphosis, lordosis, or scoliosis. The presence of scoliosis is best determined by having the patient flex at the waist with arms extended in front. The asymmetry of the height of the shoulders can be appreciated. Any deviation of a spinous process from the midline is noted. Firm palpation of the paravertebral muscles and of each vertebral spine is performed. Isolated tenderness over a bone suggests a localized problem, such as tumor, infection, or compression fracture. Firm paraspinous muscles result from spasm secondary to local injury or referred pain.

Mobility of the spine is assessed by having the patient bend forward and attempt to touch his toes. Range of flexion can be determined by quantifying the expansion of a 10-cm line measured from the lumbosacral junction superiorly during maximal flexion (*Schober test,* see Chapter 71) or noting the distance of the fingertips from the floor. During this movement the normally smooth rhythm of the reversal of the lumbar lordosis is noted. If the rhythm is interrupted or hesitant, an abnormality of the apophyseal joints or paraspinous structures may be present. Lateral flex-

ion and extension are assessed. Lateral flexion is usually preserved in disc disease but may be limited in patients with a spondyloarthropathy. Increased discomfort with extension suggests disease of the apophyseal joints or spinal stenosis.

The patient is examined *bent forward* over the examining table. In this position, the inferior portion of the sacroiliac joints, ischial tuberosities, and sciatic notch are more easily palpated. The gait of the patient should be observed. Patients with back pain may walk in a stiff, guarded fashion.

The patient is next examined *sitting with his legs dangling.* The deep tendon reflexes of the knees (L4) and ankles (S1) are obtained to test the integrity of the reflex arcs. An absent reflex may signify nerve root irritation secondary to a herniated nucleus pulposus. The patient's knee is extended while the patient is seated. Flexion of the hip and extension of the knee stretch the lumbar nerve roots. Radicular pain that radiates from the back to below the knee is associated with nerve root irritation. The nerve root origin of the pain can be confirmed by lowering the leg just to the point where the pain disappears and then reproducing the pain by dorsiflexing the foot. This sign, if positive, suggests a herniated intervertebral disc, or less commonly, bony impingement of a nerve root caused by arthritis affecting the apophyseal joints, lumbar stenosis, or, rarely, a tumor of the spinal cord or surrounding structures. This "distracted" straight leg raising (SLR) test helps confirm the organic source of pain and identify those patients who may exaggerate their symptoms. Patients with functional complaints have no discomfort with a "distracted" SLR test but may describe excruciating pain with the SLR test in the supine position. Not all patients with a herniated disc will have a positive SLR test. An individual, especially over age 30 years, may have a herniated disc that is too small or in the wrong location to irritate the nerve roots.

Next, the patient assumes the *supine* position, so that a standard SLR test can be performed. The examiner fully extends the knee and slowly flexes the lower extremity at the hip. Normally the hip can be flexed to 80° without pain, except for discomfort in the thigh or behind the knee secondary to hamstring muscle tightness. A positive test is manifested by radicular pain that radiates below the knee on the affected side or bilaterally. The nerve root and surrounding dura do not move in the neural foramen until an elevation of 30° or greater of the lower extremity has been reached. Therefore, radicular pain present at less than 30° is suspect. After the SLR test, the unaffected or well lower extremity should be raised, thus performing the crossed SLR test (13). This procedure causes tension and stretch of the nerve roots of the opposite (affected) lower extremity and reproduces the radicular pain caused by SLR in that lower extremity. When this test is positive, there is a strong, but not absolute, correlation with disc herniation (24, 28).

Next, *sensory assessment* of the buttock, perineum, and lower extremities can be accomplished.

Figure 78.2 shows the relevant sensory dermatomes that can be evaluated by pinprick and touch. Abnormalities will help to localize a lesion and when present will help to decide on the need and urgency of an orthopaedic or neurosurgical consultation. An important component of the sensory assessment is the search for signs compatible with a *cauda equina syndrome* (compression of the lower portion of the nerve roots inferior to the spinal cord proper, often secondary to a central disc herniation). The signs of compression of the cauda equina include saddle anesthesia, loss of anal sphincter tone (assessed by rectal examination) bilateral sciatica, lower extremity motor weakness, as well as historical evidence of bowel, bladder, or sexual dysfunction. This syndrome, if present, is an indication for immediate referral to a neurosurgeon or orthopaedic surgeon for hospitalization as surgical decompression of the spinal cord is necessary.

A detailed assessment of *motor function* in the legs will also help to localize a lesion in the patient in whom neurological involvement is suspected (Table 84.7). This assessment can be done while the patient is supine, sitting, or standing. Muscles tested include the knee extensors (L3-L4), the dorsiflexors of the foot (L4-L5), the knee flexors (L5-S1), and the plantar flexors of the foot (S1-2) (Fig. 65.3). Subtle weakness may be elicited by having the patient walk on his toes (gastrocnemius muscle group—S1-2) and his heels (tibialis anterior muscles—L4-5).

While the patient is in the supine position, an assessment of the hip, sacroiliac, and knee joints is done. The hip and knee joints are assessed by moving these joints through a normal range of motion when they are unweighted. Pain with motion suggests an articular cause of leg pain. The sacroiliac joint is tested by the Patrick or "faber" (flexion, abduction, external rotation) test. The test is done by positioning the lateral malleolus of the tested leg on the patella of the opposite leg. Downward pressure is then placed on the medial aspect of the knee while stabilizing the pelvis by placing a hand on the contralateral anterior superior iliac spine. Pain associated with a quick pulse or downward pressure is usually localized to the lateral aspect of the lumbar spine and originates in the sacroiliac joint. Slow pressure may elicit groin pain indicative of hip joint dysfunction.

In the *lateral* position, the sacroiliac and hip abductors are tested. Pressure is applied to the iliac wing compressing the sacroiliac joints. Pain felt in the sacroiliac joint is suggestive of an intra-articular process or a strain of the posterior sacroiliac ligaments. Hip abduction (L5 function) is tested as the patient elevates the upper leg against downward pressure applied below the knee by the examiner.

In the *prone* position, the symmetry of the buttocks is assessed (gluteus maximus—L5, S1-S2). A femoral stretch test, i.e., extending the hip joint, elicits pain in the anterior thigh (L2-L3) or the medial aspect of the leg (L4) in patients with corresponding herniated intervertebral discs.

To evaluate patients suspected of *malingering* or of a psychiatric origin for their back pain, Waddell et al. identified five physical signs associated with functional disorders (25). First, over-reaction during examination was found to be the single most important nonorganic sign. Over-reaction may take the form of collapsing, sweating, tremor, muscle tension, bizarre facial expression, or disproportionate verbalization. Second, simulation testing may be used to elicit nonorganic pain. Two useful examples are axial loading and rotation. In the first test, with the patient standing, low back pain is reported in over-reactors on vertical loading by pressing down on the patient's head. Neck pain is common and does not constitute a positive sign. In the hip rotation test, the patient stands with feet together and arms fixed firmly to his sides at the hip level by the examiner's hands. In this manner the spine unit is passively rotated on the hips. Reports of low back pain constitute a positive nonorganic sign. However, in the presence of true radiculopathy, leg pain may be produced. Third is the use of distraction testing. This consists of observing the patient during the course of the examination for variable findings when the patient is unaware that he is being observed or tested. Specific tests include *distracted SLR* (see above). Fourth, superficial, nonanatomical or variable tenderness is also a nonorganic sign. A useful technique is *Magnuson's test* in which tender areas are subtly marked and later examined for reproducibility. Fifth, nonanatomical motor or sensory regional disturbances are important nonorganic signs. Sudden "giving away" or flaccidity of a muscle during strength testing and nonanatomical sensory changes often affect the same area and may be associated with regional tenderness. A finding of three or more of the five types of signs is clinically significant. Isolated positive signs are ignored.

Examination of Other Regions

Patients with constitutional symptoms or with viscerogenic symptoms associated with their back pain should undergo a general physical examination directed at those involved organ systems. The general

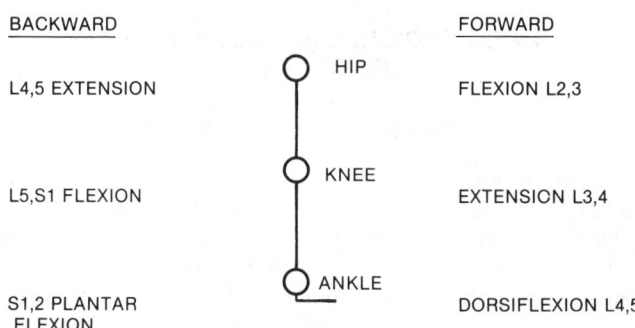

BACKWARD

L4,5 EXTENSION

L5,S1 FLEXION

S1,2 PLANTAR
FLEXION

HIP

KNEE

ANKLE

FORWARD

FLEXION L2,3

EXTENSION L3,4

DORSIFLEXION L4,5

Figure 65.3. Sequential pattern of muscle innervation of the lower extremity. Taken with permission from Borenstein DG, Wiesel SW: *Low Back Pain: Medical Diagnosis and Comprehensive Management.* Philadelphia, WB Saunders, Co, 1989.

physical examination is particularly important in individuals who describe new back pain and are 50 years of age or older.

Metastatic cancer of the spine is especially common from primary tumors of the breast, lung, prostate, thyroid, kidney, and rectum. These regions should therefore be examined carefully. Further, an abdominal examination, rectal examination, and, in women, a pelvic examination are necessary. Referred pain from cancer may also be felt in the back. For example, pancreatic lesions and posterior penetrating duodenal ulcers may cause pain to be referred to the high lumbar or low thoracic vertebral region. Bowel or urinary tract lesions may cause pain to be referred to the mid- or low lumbar region, and disease located in the pelvis may cause lower lumbar or sacral pain. Particular attention to the lymph nodes may provide a clue to the presence of an intra-abdominal lymphoma.

Important also is the assessment of the adequacy of the arteries emanating from the lower aorta. Abnormalities here may cause pain due to ischemia in the back, buttock, or lower extremities during exertion. In addition to diminished pulses and bruits over arteries, cutaneous signs of ischemia (ulcers, loss of hair or nails) should be sought in the legs or feet (see Chapter 87). Sudden change in a pain pattern associated with an abdominal aneurysm or episode of hypotension should alert one to the possibility of impending extension or rupture of the aneurysm.

Laboratory Evaluation

Radiographic Tests

A plain X-ray of the lumbar spine is not a necessary part of the initial evaluation of patients with back pain unless they have a history of recent major trauma or acute constitutional symptoms. Patients with back pain of a mechanical origin frequently have X-rays that are normal. In addition, many individuals with abnormal X-rays may be entirely asymptomatic (27). By age 50, 67% of normal individuals have evidence of "disc disease" characterized by narrowing of one or more disc spaces or disc calcifications; and an additional 20% of individuals have lumbar osteophytes. Only 13% of individuals this age have normal X-rays. Two-thirds of patients with roentgenographic evidence of lumbar disc degeneration are asymptomatic. Osteoarthritis of the apophyseal joints is not correlated with symptoms (18). In addition, plain films may not be sensitive enough to identify bony lesions unless 50% of the medullary portion of the bone has been destroyed (1). Therefore, plain X-rays of the lumbar spine should be obtained only in patients who have failed a course of conservative therapy, who persist with pain, who are 50 or older, who have reflex asymmetry, or who have point vertebral tenderness (10). Other radiographic techniques that are useful in the evaluation of patients with back pain include bone scan (infection, tumor, arthritis, fracture), computed tomography (disc, spinal stenosis, myeloma, retroperitoneal structures), and

magnetic resonance imaging (disc, intraspinal tumors). The technology of magnetic resonance imaging (MRI) has progressed to the point of replacing myelography as the imaging modality for herniated intervertebral discs (20). These more expensive imaging techniques are used to confirm the clinical diagnoses developed during the initial history and physical examination and continued evaluation of the patient with persistent back pain.

Other Laboratory Tests

The vast majority of individuals with low back pain do not require laboratory studies with their initial evaluation. Patients who are elderly, who have constitutional symptoms, or who have failed conservative therapy may benefit from a laboratory evaluation. The screening laboratory tests that are useful include complete blood count and erythrocyte sedimentation rate (inflammatory and neoplastic disorders), serum calcium concentration and alkaline phosphatase activity (diffuse bone disease), acid phosphatase activity (metastatic prostate cancer), urinalysis (renal disease), and occult blood in the stool (ulcers, gastrointestinal tumors). Other tests may be indicated based upon the diagnostic possibilities (e.g., serum immunoelectrophoresis—myeloma).

APPROACH TO DIAGNOSIS AND TREATMENT OF LOW BACK PAIN

Most patients with an acute onset of low back pain have a regional (mechanical) cause for their symptoms. Up to 90% of these patients respond to a course of conservative medical therapy. It is most important for the patients who receive conservative therapy to return for subsequent office evaluation. If on reassessment there are symptoms or signs of progression or of an incomplete response to treatment, evaluation for an alternative diagnosis is indicated. The follow-up contact should occur 3 to 4 weeks after the initial visit for all patients. The follow-up visit is also important for patients with resolved back pain so that they have an opportunity to be educated in regard to recurrent symptoms and for advice regarding prophylactic measures.

COMMON REGIONAL (MECHANICAL) BACK SYNDROMES

Lumbosacral Strain Syndrome

Lumbosacral strain is the most common cause of low back pain. The etiology of back strain is not always clear but may be related to muscular, ligamentous, or fascial strain secondary to either a specific traumatic episode or continuous mechanical stress. Individuals between the ages of 20 and 40 years are at greatest risk of developing muscle strain. Predisposing factors include obesity, chronic occupational strain requiring bending and lifting, abnormal forward pelvic tilt (accentuated lordosis), and leg length discrepancy (23).

Diagnosis

The patient complains of pain that may be severe in the back, buttock, or in one or both thighs. Usually symptoms follow a recent increase in physical activity for that individual, such as gardening, lifting, or an infrequently played sport. Usually the patient experiences no (or only minimal) discomfort during or immediately after the activity. Within the next 12 to 36 hours, as the soft tissues swell, pain develops and is associated with a feeling of muscular stiffness. The patient will complain of pain that is accentuated by standing and bending, and alleviated by lying (Table 65.1).

Examination of the back may show nonspecific signs of muscle spasm and loss of lumbar lordosis, but characteristically there is no evidence of nerve root irritation.

Management

The conservative therapy of low back pain and lumbosacral strain includes controlled physical activity, physical therapy, nonsteroidal anti-inflammatory drugs, and muscle relaxants. Back strain is improved with a decrease in physical activity (26). A period as short as 2 days has been shown to be effective at relieving back pain (4). Controlled physical activity allows injured tissues to rest, permitting a greater opportunity for healing without reinjury. To minimize back motion and provide support, the bed should be firm but comfortable. A bed board cut from 5/8-inch particle board or plywood (more expensive but will last for years) placed between the mattress and box spring is usually effective. The patient should be out of bed only for bathroom use. Physical therapy modalities, in the form of cold (ice massage) initially or heat subsequently, may decrease pain and diminish spasm. The application of dry heat by a heating pad for 20 to 30 minutes several times a day (on low or medium setting with a protective towel between skin and pad to prevent burns) is preferred by some patients. Others prefer moist heat, which is accomplished by using hot towels, or a heat pack, which produce sustained heat for up to 1/2 hour (available at pharmacies).

Non-narcotic analgesics in the form of nonsteroidal anti-inflammatory drugs are helpful in making patients comfortable while their injury heals. Nonsteroidal drugs with a rapid onset of action such as piroxicam (Feldene) or naproxen (Naprosyn or Anaprox) are most appropriate. Other nonsteroidals that are useful include aspirin, 600 mg four times a day, ibuprofen (Motrin) 600 to 800 mg four times a day, diflunisal (Dolobid), 500 mg twice a day, or naproxen sodium (Anaprox), 275 mg three times a day, or (Naprosyn) 500 mg twice a day. These drugs are useful adjuncts to bed rest for control of pain. The choice of any of these nonsteroidal drugs must be made in consideration of both patient and drug characteristics. For example, some patients prefer twice a day drug administration whereas others prefer more frequent dosing because of a perception of greater efficacy with a greater number of tablets. Nonsteroidal anti-inflammatory drug use is described in detail in Chapter 70. If added pain relief is necessary, acetaminophen may be used in conjunction with a nonsteroidal agent. Narcotic analgesics have too many side effects and potential toxicities to be given to the usual patient with low back pain. Muscle relaxants are not first line therapeutic agents but should be considered for the patient with significant muscle spasm on physical examination. Cyclobenzaprine (Flexeril) is more efficacious than placebo in the treatment of intractable pain syndromes with muscle spasm (3). Most patients will have a beneficial response to the drug at a dose of 10 mg once a day. The dose may be increased up to 10 mg three times a day, but this is associated with a greater frequency of drowsiness and dry mouth. Taking the drug 2 hours or more before bedtime may limit early morning drowsiness. This efficacy of cyclobenzaprine may be judged after a 7 to 10-day trial. Other muscle relaxants that may be useful, if cyclobenzapine is ineffective, include carisoprodol (Soma), 350 mg four times a day, chlorzoxazone (Parafon DSC), 500 mg four times a day, or orphenadrine citrate (Norflex), 100 mg twice a day (9). Diazepam (Valium) is no more effective than placebo in improving back spasm (2). This drug should not be used for patients with low back pain.

When improvement occurs after 3 to 4 days, the patient may increase his physical activities. Over a period of 1 to 2 weeks, ambulation is increased with a gradual decrease of the dose of drugs needed to con-

Table 65.1.
Mechanical Low Back Pain

	Lumbosacral Strain	Herniated Nucleus Pulposus	Osteoarthritis	Spinal Stenosis
Age (years)	20–40	30–50	>50	>60
Pain Characteristics				
Location	Back (unilateral)	Back, and leg (unilateral)	Back (bilateral)	Leg (bilateral)
Onset	Acute	Acute (prior episodes)	Insidious	Insidious
Standing[a]	+	–	+	+
Sitting[a]	–	+	–	–
Bending[a]	+	–	–	–
Straight leg	–	+	–	+ (stress)
Plain X-ray	–	–	+	+

[a](exacerbating +, alleviating –).
Adapted from Borenstein DG, Wiesel SW: *Low Back Pain: Medical Diagnosis and Comprehensive Management.* Philadelphia, WB Saunders Co, 1989.

trol symptoms. During this recovery period it is especially important to advise the patient to avoid activities that greatly increase the forces applied to the lower spine (e.g., lifting, pushing, force on outstretched upper extremity as in making beds or vacuuming, lurching, or bending). Should the patient fail to respond or should there be a recurrence of pain, the patient should be re-examined 3 to 4 weeks later to investigate the possibility of a systemic cause of back pain. If a mechanical cause remains the most likely diagnosis, a modification in drug therapy (prescribing an alternative nonsteroidal and, if needed, muscle relaxant drug) is indicated.

For the patient who is recovering satisfactorily, various exercise programs have been advocated. One simple but effective exercise program combines isometric gluteal and abdominal muscle contractions and pelvic tilt. These exercises, which are performed standing with the back against a wall (Fig. 65.4), should be recommended as soon as pain subsides. Additional exercises that stretch the lumbosacral muscles (Fig. 65.5) also provide comfort. The exercises should be performed for a few minutes four to six times a day. Exercises that are designed to strengthen the abdominal musculature, such as sit-ups with the knees flexed or straight leg raising, increase intradiscal pressure, may exacerbate symptoms, and are not recommended (however, see below for management of intercritical period).

Braces are reserved for patients who must remain active while healing continues. Lumbosacral supports theoretically help relieve back pain by increasing intra-abdominal pressure, which results in greater support of the vertebral column, allowing paraspinous muscles to relax. The lumbosacral support may be a cloth corset fitted with metal stays posteriorly or a smaller cloth brace with a molded plastic insert. The patient obtains a prescription for the corset or brace and is fitted by an orthotist or physical therapist. The patient should use the support while working and then remove the appliance. The use of a lumbosacral support weakens supporting back muscles, and, therefore, patients should be weaned gradually but steadily from the support. It is important for this group of patients to return gradually to full activity because an abrupt return may cause a recurrence of low back pain.

Herniated Intervertebral Disc

The intervertebral disc is composed of the annulus fibrosus and the nucleus pulposus. The annulus fibrosus maintains pressure on the contents of the nucleus pulposus allowing the intervertebral disc to perform as a cushion for the forces placed on the spine. Tears in the annulus fibrosus allow the contents of the nucleus pulposus to herniate beyond their normal confines. Tears in the annulus may be associated with transient episodes of low back pain. Herniation of the nucleus may result in sudden severe pain if neural elements are compressed and inflamed by the nuclear contents (Fig. 65.6). A sudden pressure placed on the

lumbar spine that may occur with flexion, e.g., bending over to lift a heavy object, lifting with the arms extended away from the body, a sudden lurch, or even a sneeze or cough, can precipitate the rupture. However, many patients who have a herniated disc will not give a history of injury or of a sudden increase in pressure. Lumbar disc disease is most common at the L4-L5 and L5-S1 levels and is less common between the other vertebral bodies.

Diagnosis

Patients with herniated intervertebral discs complain of sharp, lancinating pain. The pain radiates from the back down the leg in the anatomical distribution of the affected nerve root. The pain may be so severe that the patient resists examination and splints the back in an awkward position of lateral lumbar flexion and hip flexion. Patients with bilateral sciatica, progressive muscle weakness, or bladder or bowel incontinence should be evaluated for cauda equina compression (see page 817). The diagnosis of acute intervertebral disc herniation is most likely when physical examination reveals signs of nerve root irritation with either a loss of motor function, loss of deep tendon reflexes, and/or a localized sensory deficit. Specific disc herniations may result in well-defined motor, sensory, and reflex deficits that aid in their diagnosis (Table 65.2). Patients with progressive neurological deficits, particularly muscle weakness, should be referred to an orthopaedist or a neurosurgeon for close observation. These patients may benefit from early surgical intervention before a course of conservative therapy.

Documentation of the anatomical abnormality associated with radicular pain is necessary for those patients who have continued pain despite a 3 to 4 week course of conservative therapy. Electromyography (EMG) is useful for demonstrating the nerve root level associated with denervation of leg muscles. EMG may also be able to differentiate by the pattern of muscle involvement those patients with herniated disc and those with peripheral sciatic nerve abnormalities secondary to trauma (injection, radiation therapy, or blunt) or tumor. A number of radiographic techniques may be useful for demonstrating disc herniation. In the past computed tomography and myelography were the preferred techniques to identify herniated discs. Currently, magnetic resonance imaging readily identifies the location of herniated discs without the need for myelographic dye or radiation exposure (19). In many circumstances, MRI examination has replaced the myelogram as the preferred test for documenting disc herniation as it provides a better picture and is adequate for deciding on the need for surgery.

Management

The treatment for most patients with a herniated disc is nonoperative, since 80% of them will respond to conservative therapy when followed over a period of 5 years. In these patients whose pain and other

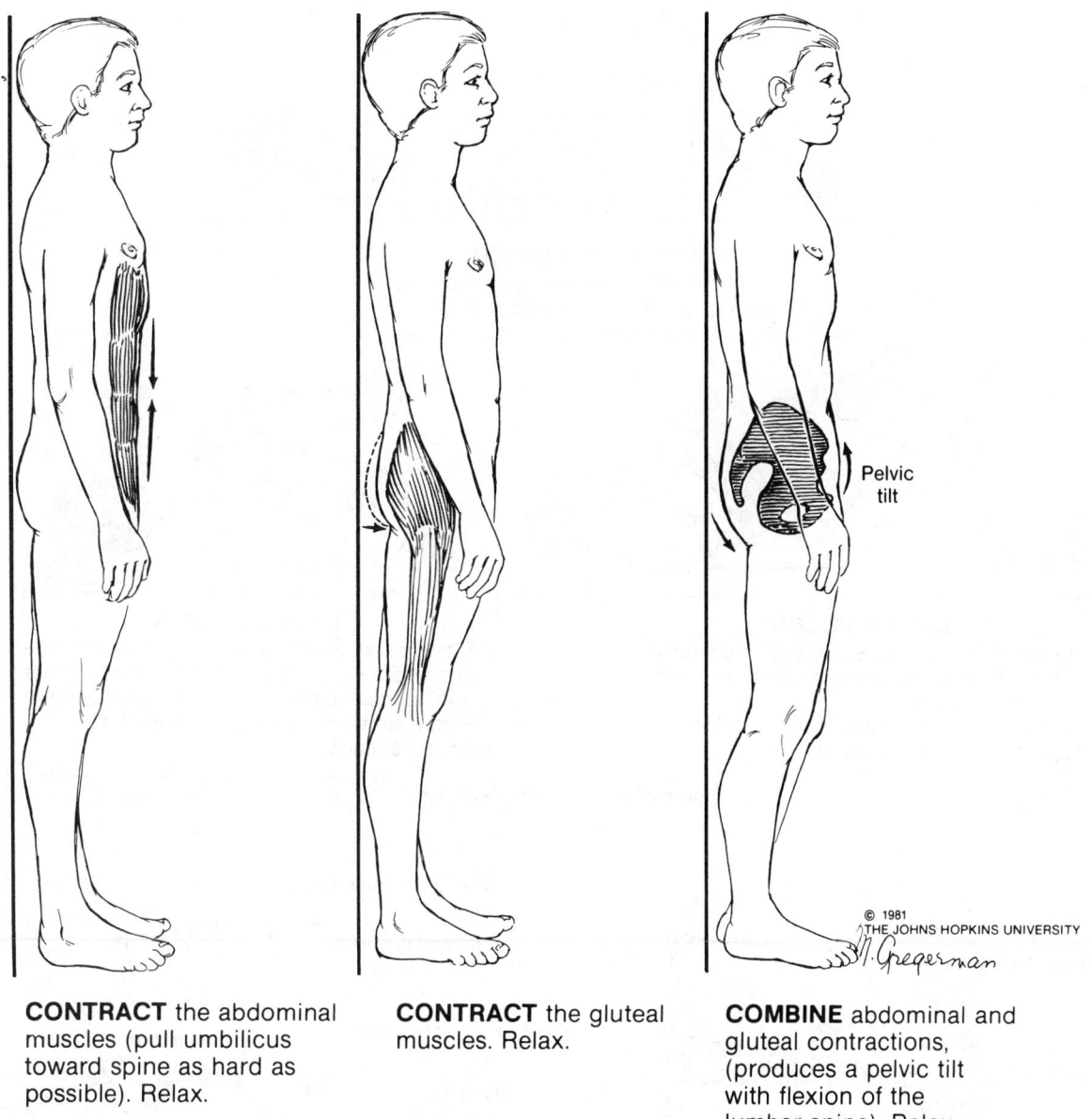

CONTRACT the abdominal muscles (pull umbilicus toward spine as hard as possible). Relax.

CONTRACT the gluteal muscles. Relax.

COMBINE abdominal and gluteal contractions, (produces a pelvic tilt with flexion of the lumbar spine). Relax.

© 1981
THE JOHNS HOPKINS UNIVERSITY

Figure 65.4. Exercises—abdominal muscles and pelvic tilt.

neurological abnormalities remit without surgical reduction of the disc, an adjustment of the annulus and posterior longitudinal ligament to the presence of the herniated disc fragment is the most likely reason for the diminution of edema, inflammation, back pain, and leg pain. Also desiccation of the fragment may play a role in resolution of symptoms.

Conservative therapy includes controlled physical activity with the patient at bed rest in the semi-Fowler's position (hips and knees flexed, supported by pillows). Drug therapy includes nonsteroidals and muscle relaxants, as described above, and narcotic analgesics if the pain is severe. Patients whose symptoms are so pronounced that narcotics are required should be hospitalized, and an orthopaedist or neurosurgeon should be consulted. Physical therapy is usually not necessary in managing patients with acute disc herniations. Active exercise programs may intensify symptoms and should be avoided. Therapy such as ultrasound, shortwave, diathermy, heat or cold packs may provide short-term pain relief but do not alter disc lesions or have any long-term effect on symptoms. Also, these therapies detract from compliance in regard to bed rest. Lumbar traction has not been shown to be more effective than bed rest in the treatment of lumbar disc disease (5). Patients should be prescribed a 3 to 4 week conservative regimen, and if they fail this, they may benefit from surgical decompression of the appropriate disc space, if a herniation has been demonstrated. For management of the intercritical period see "Management of the Intercritical Period," page 824.

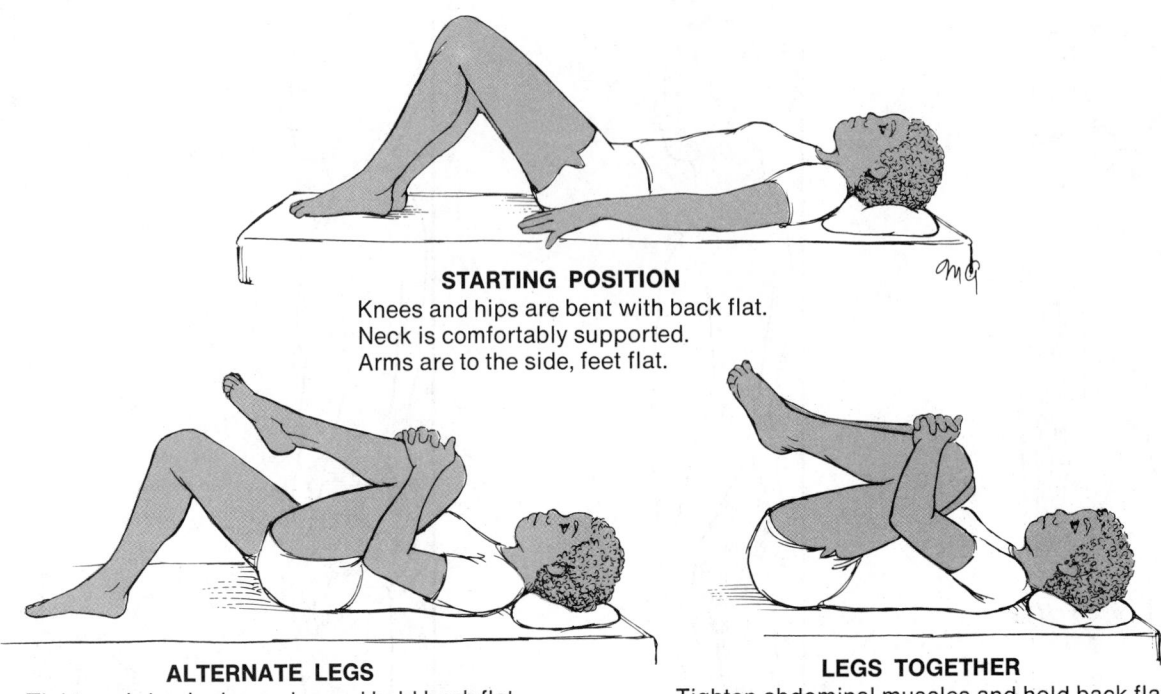

STARTING POSITION
Knees and hips are bent with back flat.
Neck is comfortably supported.
Arms are to the side, feet flat.

ALTERNATE LEGS
Tighten abdominal muscles and hold back flat.
With both hands on one knee, bring knee as
near chest as possible.
Return slowly to starting position. Relax.
Repeat, alternating legs, 10 times.

LEGS TOGETHER
Tighten abdominal muscles and hold back flat.
Bring both knees up to the chest, grasp knees
with hands and hold position for 30 seconds.
Return slowly to starting position. Relax.
Repeat 5 times.

Figure 65.5. Knee-chest exercises.

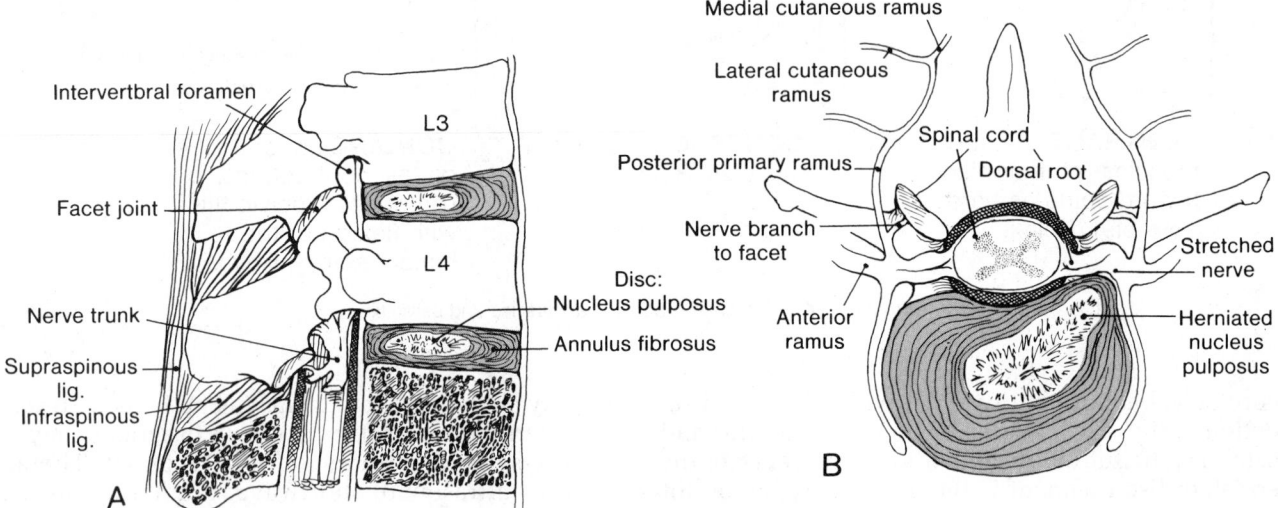

Figure 65.6. *A.* Normal disc. *B.* Herniated disc.

Osteoarthritis/Spinal Stenosis

The lumbar spine is one of the common locations for osteoarthritis, the most common form of arthritis. This noninflammatory joint disease is associated with joint pain, stiffness, deformity, and limitation of motion. Alterations over time secondary to osteoarthritis result in loss of disc volume, increased pressure on apophyseal joints, and hypertrophy of soft tissue and bony structures resulting in a decrease in the size of the spinal canal. Osteoarthritis is discussed fully in Chapter 68.

Diagnosis

Initially, patients may complain of pain after repeated episodes of hyperextension that traumatizes the apophyseal joints, resulting in a stretching or tear-

Table 65.2
Common Findings in Lumbar Disc Herniations[a]

Level of Disc Herniation	Nerve Root Compressed	Pain	Numbness (See Fig. 65.3)	Weakness	Reflexes (Decreased or Absent)
L3-L4	L4	Sacroiliac joint, hip, posterolateral thigh, anterior aspect of leg	L4 dermatome	Extension of knee (quadriceps)	Knee jerk
L4-L5	L5	Sacroiliac joint, hip	L5 dermatome (includes great toe)	Dorsiflexion of great toe (extensor hallucis longus)	
L5-S1	S1	Lateral aspect of leg and foot	S1 dermatome (includes lateral toes)	Unusual (plantar flexion of foot)	Ankle jerk
Massive midline lumbar disc herniation Cauda equina syndrome (usually L4 or L5)	Multiple roots in dural sac	Midline of back, posterior aspect of both thighs and legs	Perineum, posterior thighs, plantar aspect of feet	Paralysis of feet and sphincters	Absent ankle jerk

[a] Adapted from Vanden Briuk KD, Edmonson AS: The spine. In Edmonson AS, Crenshaw AH (eds): *Campbell's Operative Orthopaedics*. St Louis, CV Mosby, 1980.

ing of the ligamentous capsule of the apophyseal joint. Typically, back flexion (i.e., bending forward) relieves the pain whereas hyperextension exacerbates it. Patients may also experience back pain related to gradual degeneration of the intervertebral disc or the development of osteophytes either of which may impinge on a nerve root. Patients with lumbar osteoarthritis or degenerative disc disease describe back, buttock, or unilateral lower extremity pain. Examination usually reveals evidence of irritation of a specific nerve root resulting in loss of a localized motor or sensory neurological function or of an absent deep tendon reflex (L5-S1 disc, ankle; or L3-L4 disc, knee). The SLR may be positive. Many of these patients will respond to conservative therapy since the anti-inflammatory action of the nonsteroidal drugs is effective in diminishing the swelling of the soft tissues, which causes nerve impingement.

As patients grow older, particularly during the 5th to 7th decade, back symptoms become suggestive of irritation of multiple nerve roots at different levels on both sides of the spinal cord. Spinal stenosis occurs most commonly in men who complain of chronic low back pain with unilateral or bilateral lower extremity discomfort, exacerbated by extension of the spine (standing) who may develop frank hypesthesia or dysesthesias (see Table 65.1). There may be a history of prior disc surgery. In 30 to 40% of patients with lumbar spinal stenosis symptoms that suggest vascular insufficiency (e.g., buttock or lower extremity pain with walking), claudication may develop (16). These patients develop lower extremity pain while standing, walking, or hyperextension of the spine in the absence of any evidence of peripheral vascular disease. Painful paresthesias are present in the feet or legs and may radiate to the hip girdle or lower trunk. Patients may experience lower extremity numbness and weakness resulting in frequent falls. These symptoms are relieved by rest or flexion of the spine (the patient may report that he regularly gets relief by bending forward as if to tie his shoes). Physical examination may show no abnormalities until the patient is asked to walk. Abnormal motor sensory deficits may only be present during increased activity.

Plain X-rays show degenerative changes in the apophyseal joints and decreased anteroposterior canal diameter. Computed tomography (CT) is the best diagnostic radiographic technique for spinal stenosis. CT shows the narrowed canal and/or the impingement of osteophytes upon the intervertebral foramina.

Management

The majority of patients with spinal stenosis can be treated nonsurgically. Activities that bring on pain should be discouraged. Patients may respond to nonsteroidal anti-inflammatory drugs or a course of epidural corticosteroid injections (administered by a consulting rheumatologist or orthopaedist). Operative therapy for spinal stenosis is reserved for patients who are totally incapacitated by their condition.

MEDICAL BACK SYNDROMES

Spondyloarthropathies (see Chapter 71)

Patients with spondyloarthropathies (ankylosing spondylitis, Reiter's syndrome, psoriatic spondylitis, enteropathic spondylitis) frequently complain of low back, buttock, or leg pain. These patients have morning stiffness as a major component of their symptom complex. Although back pain is the first symptom in a number of young patients, it is frequently associated with other symptoms and signs of the specific disorder (iritis, conjunctivitis, skin rash, hematochezia). A clue to the presence of a spondyloarthropathy on physical examination is tenderness with percussion over the axial skeleton or sacroiliac joints. The sacroiliac joints may be painful when stressed while the patient is in the prone or supine position. Conditions affecting the axial skeleton and sacroiliac joints are discussed in Chapter 71.

Infections

Although rare, infections of the axial skeleton (osteomyelitis, discitis, or septic arthritis) must be considered in any patient with back pain. Osteomyelitis is an infection of the vertebral bodies. Discitis is an infection of the intervertebral disc (17). Septic arthritis of the back is an *infection of the sacroiliac joints*. These conditions are discussed in detail in Chapter 31.

Vertebral Fractures

Vertebral compression fractures are common and usually the result of a flexion injury when the spine is abruptly flexed as it is, for example, during jumping. The thoracic spine is most commonly involved. The force needed to compress a vertebral body in healthy bone is considerable. However, when the bone is diseased, e.g., as it is with osteoporosis, multiple myeloma, metastatic cancer, or hyperparathyroidism, the injury may be relatively insignificant. Pain is usually localized and immediate, although it may be delayed for several days after the fracture. Often tenderness over a single vertebra indicates the presence of a fracture, but an X-ray is necessary to confirm the diagnosis.

Other radiographic techniques are useful for identifying the locations of fractures that may not be detected by plain X-rays. A bone scan is often useful in demonstrating whether there are single or multiple fractures. CT, MRI, or myelography (the selection determined in consultation with an orthopaedist and radiologist) is indicated for patients with compression fractures who also have neurological deficits. These techniques are capable of localizing abnormalities associated with nerve impingement. Not all processes that weaken bone will be detected by bone scan (e.g., multiple myeloma). Blood chemistries, including the concentration of serum proteins, are helpful in identifying patients with myeloma.

With lumbar or thoracic vertebral compression fractures, management includes rest, adequate analgesia, and gradual ambulation when the patient is pain free. A lumbosacral support or, for the patient with a thoracic vertebral fracture, a chair-back or hyperextension brace may be helpful in alleviating pain. These may be obtained by prescription from an orthopaedic appliance shop.

Tumors

Tumors of the lumbar spine are unusual causes of back pain; however, these diseases are associated with the highest morbidity, mortality, and dysfunction of all. Patients with tumors of the lumbar spine usually have back pain as their initial complaint. Commonly, patients with tumor-associated pain have increased discomfort with recumbency. Physical examination demonstrates localized tenderness as well as neurological dysfunction if the spinal cord is compressed. Although laboratory evaluation frequently yields nonspecific data, radiographic evaluation is very useful in identifying the location and type of neoplastic lesion. In general, benign tumors are located in the posterior elements of vertebrae (spinous, transverse process), and malignant (both primary and metastatic)

tumors are located in the anterior components of vertebrae (body). The definitive diagnosis of a tumor must be derived from histological examination of biopsy material obtained from the lesion. The most effective therapy for both benign and malignant tumors is removal of the lesions that are accessible to surgical excision. When excision is not possible, partial resection, radiation therapy, corticosteroids, or chemotherapy may be indicated to control symptoms and compression of the spinal cord and nerve roots.

Referred Pain

Disease processes that affect organs in the retroperitoneum may not only cause pain locally but may refer pain in the distribution of the sensory nerve supplying the diseased tissue. Diseases of the vascular, genitourinary, and gastrointestinal systems may refer pain to the lumbar spine. Characteristically, referred pain is unaffected by the physical position of the patient. Patients usually have symptoms in the affected organ, which may serve as clues for the physician, raising the possibility of a viscerogenic cause other than the patient's back pain (Table 65.3).

MANAGEMENT OF THE INTERCRITICAL PERIOD

Although most patients with low back pain have a complete remission of symptoms within 3 to 4 weeks, many patients will experience a recurrence (7). Patients should return to the physician's office even if they have had a resolution of their pain. The purpose of these visits is to discuss ways to prevent recurrent attacks of back pain. Areas of discussion include posture, weight control, exercise, and work activities.

Figure 65.7 shows some correct and incorrect postures and practical advice that may be useful to give to patients who have experienced low back pain. Weight

Table 65.3.
Medical Causes of Low Back Pain

SYSTEMIC—constitutional symptoms, severe localized pain, morning stiffness are clues suggestive of generalized disorder
  Rheumatologic—Spondyloarthropathies, polymyalgia rheumatica, fibromyalgia
  Infectious—vertebral osteomyelitis, Pott's disease, discitis, septic arthritis, epidural abscess, herpes zoster
  Neoplastic—(Benign)—osteoid osteoma, osteochondroma, giant cell tumor,—(Malignant)—metastatic, multiple myeloma, chondrosarcoma, chordoma, lymphoma, retroperitoneal sarcoma, neural tumor
  Neurologic-Psychiatric—neuropathic (Charcot) joints, femoral neuropathy, depression, hysteria
  Miscellaneous—vertebral sarcoidosis, Paget's disease, retroperitoneal fibrosis

REFERRED PAIN—the absence of any tenderness, limitation of motion, or aggravation of pain or spasm during the physical examination is suggestive of referred pain
  Lower thoracic and upper lumbar pain—from an upper abdominal disease process (*e.g.*, pancreas)
  Low lumbar pain—from a lower abdominal disease process (*e.g.*, aortic aneurysm)
  Sacral pain—from a pelvic problem (*e.g.*, endometriosis, prostate cancer).

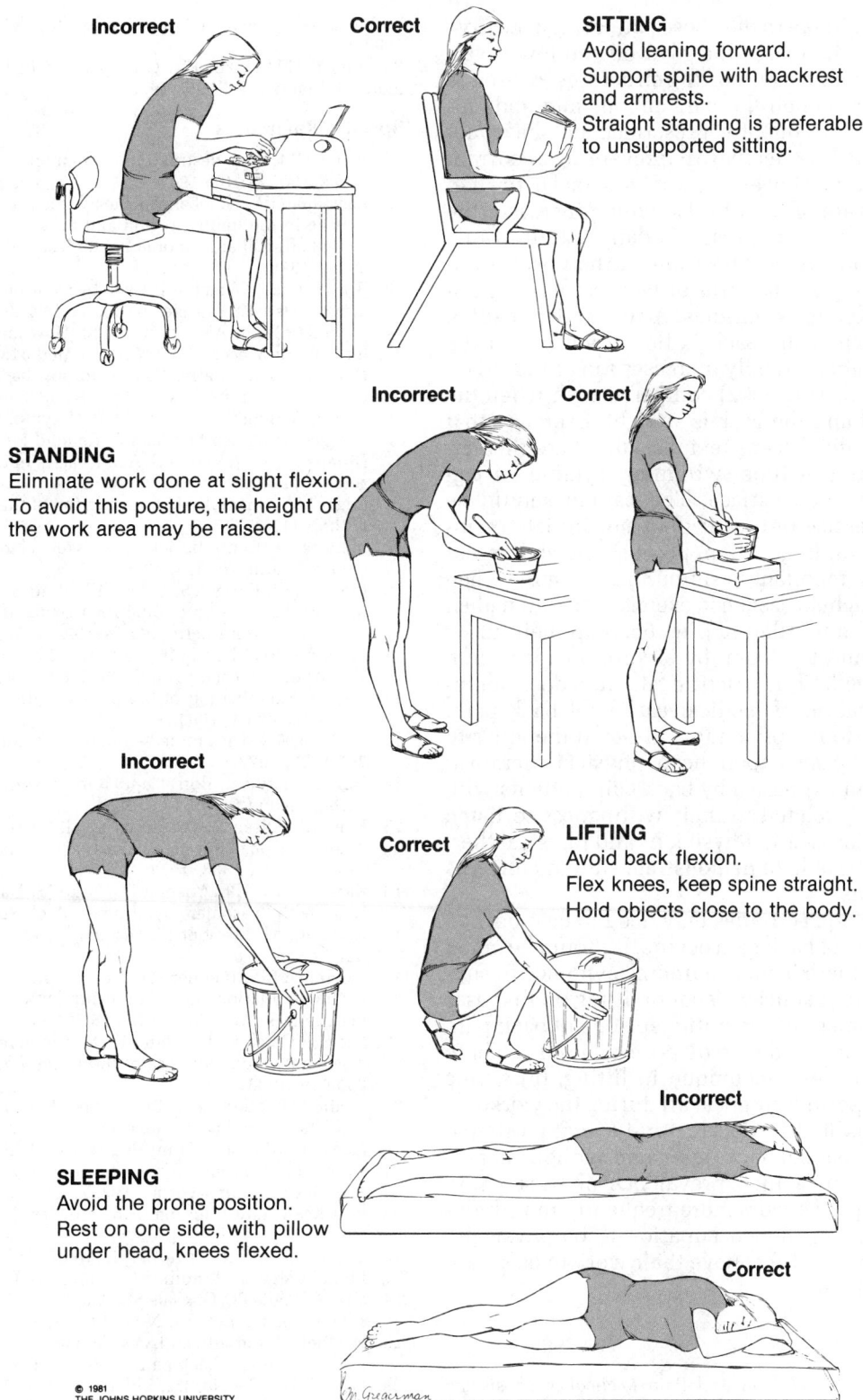

Incorrect **Correct**

SITTING
Avoid leaning forward.
Support spine with backrest
and armrests.
Straight standing is preferable
to unsupported sitting.

STANDING
Eliminate work done at slight flexion.
To avoid this posture, the height of
the work area may be raised.

Incorrect **Correct**

Incorrect

Correct **LIFTING**
Avoid back flexion.
Flex knees, keep spine straight.
Hold objects close to the body.

SLEEPING
Avoid the prone position.
Rest on one side, with pillow
under head, knees flexed.

Incorrect

Correct

© 1981
THE JOHNS HOPKINS UNIVERSITY

Figure 65.7. Postural attitudes—correct/incorrect.

reduction is desirable in the obese patient, as excessive weight directly increases the load on the lower vertebral column and its supporting structures. Exercises designed to strengthen the paraspinous and abdominal muscles are frequently prescribed but have not been shown to be effective in preventing recurrent episodes of pain. However, exercises make the patients more aware of their backs, which increases the likelihood that they will perform daily activities in a mechanically advantaged position for their back. Conservative therapy in the form of bed rest has the potential to weaken back muscles. Also, sudden loading of the spine when the back is flexed and when the knees are straight markedly increases forces placed on the lumbar spine (Fig. 65.2) compared with when the knees are bent and the back is straight. Exercises that strengthen the quadriceps (extend knees) are theoretically sound and include swimming, cycling, or jogging on a flat, even surface. The patient should be advised to exercise only if it does not initiate or increase back pain. In addition, because the abdominal musculature is important in supporting the spine when a weight is brought to bear on it, exercises that strengthen the abdominal musculature (Fig. 65.4) are helpful.

Evaluation and treatment by a chiropractor cannot be recommended. Chiropractic evaluation does not include investigation of medical causes of back pain. Chiropractors do not offer any additional therapies to those offered by an experienced physical therapist. The satisfaction expressed by back pain patients with chiropractors is related to their willingness to listen to patient concerns (15). Physicians and physical therapists should be able to demonstrate similar concerns to their patients.

Work or athletic activities may need to be modified once an episode of back pain occurs. It should be noted however, that there is no convincing evidence to support the concept that heavy labor or lifting predisposes to the development of the initial episode of back pain (22). Certain factors do predispose to injury. These include (a) improper technique in lifting, (b) sitting for prolonged periods or not at all during the workday, (c) sudden maximal physical activity (e.g., participation in an occasional vigorous game without conditioning results in a high prevalence of back pain). Further, back pain occurs more frequently in individuals who consider their occupation to be physically hard and in those who believe their work to be stressful to the spine (6).

General References

Borenstein DG, Wiesel SW: *Low Back Pain: Medical Diagnosis and Comprehensive Management.* Philadelphia, WB Saunders, 1989.
    A complete review of the diagnosis and management of mechanical and medical causes of low back pain.
Hall S, Bartleson JD, Onofrio BM, et al: Lumbarspinal stenosis. *Ann Intern Med* 103:271, 1985.
    A review of 68 patients with this condition.
Macnab I: *Backache.* Baltimore, Williams & Wilkins, 1977.

Rothman RH, Simeone FA: *The Spine.* Philadelphia, WB Saunders, 1982.
Ramamurti CP, Tinker RV: *Orthopaedics in Primary Care.* Baltimore, Williams & Wilkins, 1979.

Specific References

1. Ardan GM: Bone destruction not demonstrable by radiography. *Br J Radiol* 24:107, 1951.
2. Basmajian JV: Cyclobenzaprine hydrochloride effect on skeletal muscle in the lumbar region and neck: two double blind controlled clinical and laboratory studies. *Arch Phys Med Rehabil* 59:58, 1978.
3. Brown Jr BR, Womble J: Cyclobenzaprine in intractable pain syndromes with muscle spasm. *JAMA* 240:1151, 1978.
4. Deyo RA, Diehl AK, Rosenthal M: How many days of bed rest for acute low back pain? *N Engl J Med* 315:1064, 1986.
5. Deyo RA: Conservative therapy for low back pain. Distinguishing useful from useless therapy. *JAMA* 250:1057, 1983.
6. Dehlin O, Hedenrud B, Horal J: Back symptoms in nursing aides in a geriatric hospital. *Scand J Rehabil Med* 8:47, 1976.
7. Dillane JB, Fry J, Kalton G: Acute back syndrome—a study from general practice. *Br Med J* 3:82, 1966.
8. Edgar MA, Ghadially JA: Innervation of the lumbar spine. *Clin Orthop* 115:35, 1976.
9. Elenbaas JK: Centrally acting oral skeletal muscle relaxants. *Am J Hosp Pharm* 37:1313, 1980.
10. Frazier LM, Carey TS, Lyles MF, et al: Selective criteria may increase lumbarsacral spine roentgenogram use in acute low-back pain. *Arch Intern Med* 149:147, 1989.
11. Frymoyer JW, Pope MH, Costanza MC, et al: Epidemiologic studies of low back pain. *Spine* 5:419, 1980.
12. Hall H: Examination of the patient with low back pain. *Bull Rheum Dis* 33:1, 1983.
13. Hudgins WR: The crossed-straight leg-raising test. *N Engl J Med* 297:1127, 1977.
14. Hult L: Cervical, dorsal and lumbar spinal syndromes. *Acta Orthop Scand Suppl* 17:1, 1954.
15. Kane RL, Olsen D, Leymaster C, al: Manipulating the patient. A comparison of the effectiveness of physician and chiropractor care. *Lancet* 1:1333, 1974.
16. Karayannacos PE, Yashon D, Vasko JS: Narrow lumbar spinal canal with "vascular" syndromes. *Arch Surg* 111:803, 1976.
17. Kornberg M, Eismont FJ: Discitis: an elusive infection. *Infect Surg* 2:818, 1983.
18. Lawrence JS, Bremner JM, Bier F: Osteo-arthrosis. Prevalence in the population and relationship between symptoms and X-ray changes. *Ann Rheum Dis* 25:1, 1966.
19. Lee SH, Coleman PE, Hahn FJ: Magnetic resonance imaging of degenerative disk disease of the spine. *Radiol Clin North Am* 250:949, 1988.
20. Medic MT, Masaryk T, Boumphrey F, et al: Lumbar herniated disk disease and canal stenosis: prospective evaluation by surface coil MR, CT, and myelography. *AJNR* 7:709, 1986.
21. Nervill RLM, Turner JG: *Orthopaedic disorders in general practice.* Boston, Butterworths, 1985, p 35.
22. Rowe ML: Low back pain in industry. *J Occup Med* 11:161, 1969.
23. Turek SL: *Orthopaedics: Principles and Their Application.* Philadelphia, JB Lippincott, 1984, p. 1483.
24. Vaz M, Wadia RS, Gokhale SD: Another cause of positive crossed-straight-leg-raising-test. *N Engl J Med* 295:779, 1978.
25. Waddell G, McCulloch JA, Kummel E, et al: Nonorganic physical signs in low-back pain. *Spine* 5:117, 1980.
26. Wiesel SW, Cuckler JM, DeLuca F, et al: An objective analysis of conservative therapy. *Spine* 5:324, 1980.
27. Witt I, Vestergaard A, Rosenklint A: A comparative analysis of X-ray findings of the lumbar spine in patients with and without lumbar pain. *Spine* 9:298, 1984.
28. Woodhall B, Hayes GJ: The well-leg raising test of Fajersztajn in the diagnosis of ruptured lumbar intervertebral disc. *J Bone Joint Surg* 32A:786, 1950.

C H A P T E R   66

Nonarticular Rheumatic Disorders*

JOYCE KOPICKY-BURD, M.D.

BURSITIS

General Considerations

Definition

Bursitis, the inflammation of a bursal sac, is a very common problem. Bursal sacs are structures lined with synovial membrane that secretes and absorbs liquid. The bursae provide, thereby, a lubricating mechanism between structures such as bones, ligaments, tendons, muscles, and skin. Although usually isolated, occasionally they are in communication with a joint space. There are over 150 such structures in the body, but the number is not fixed and a new bursa may appear whenever there is friction between structures (1).

Most instances of bursitis can be diagnosed properly and treated in the office by the general physician; however, occasionally, because of the location of the bursa, the uncertainty of the diagnosis, or frequent recurrences of the problem, referral to an orthopaedist or rheumatologist may be necessary.

Etiology

The most common cause of bursitis is trauma; less often, a systemic process, such as rheumatoid arthritis or gout, causes the inflammation. Septic bursitis after trauma is especially a concern in patients with superficial bursitis (such as olecranon or prepatellar bursitis) (9). Basic calcium phosphate crystals are known to be associated with calcific periarthritis, tendonitis, and bursitis, but little is understood about the exact mechanism of calcium crystal deposition (7). Focal calcium deposits may be visible on X-ray.

---

*Drs. Raymond L. Malamet and Gregory B. Kelly contributed to this chapter in the second edition of this book.

Manifestations

Bursitis is particularly common in middle-aged and older individuals of either sex, but the reason for this age distribution is not known. Patients with acute bursitis usually describe the abrupt onset of localized pain and discomfort that is worsened by any movement of the structures adjacent to the bursa. Frequently, there is a history of trauma or of repetitively performed activity. Low grade fever is occasionally present.

When the inflamed bursa is superficial, an obvious swelling may be present that is often erythematous and tender. On the other hand, inflammation in deep bursae may be manifest only by regional tenderness and some limitation of motion. Computed tomography (CT) or magnetic resonance imaging (MRI) may be useful diagnostic studies if the diagnosis is unclear and involvement of a deeply situated bursa is suspected.

Aspiration of Bursae

When there is identifiable swelling that is fluctuant, especially accompanied by fever or evidence of surrounding cellulitis, it is important to aspirate fluid from the bursa. Examination of the fluid will differentiate between septic and nonseptic bursitis. Aspiration may be easily accomplished by the general physician when the bursa is superficial (Table 66.1). The appearance of the fluid varies, depending on the cause. It should be analyzed routinely (Table 66.1) in order to establish the diagnosis (Table 66.2). Septic bursal fluid manifests a significant leukocytosis with polymorphonuclear cell predominance (Table 66.2). Confirmation of sepsis occurs with culture proof of infection. The vast majority of septic bursae are caused by *Staphylococcus aureus*.

Therapy. If a septic bursitis is identified, the patient should be treated with antibiotics and by drainage of the bursal sac. The Gram stain of the bursal fluid should be a guide to the choice of antibiotics. If the Gram stain is negative or if Gram-positive cocci

---

Table 66.1.
Technique for Aspiration of Superficial Bursae (or Joints) and of Analysis of Bursal (or Synovial) Fluid

1. Determine by palpation the area of maximal tenderness and/or fluctuance and outline with indelible pen.
2. Clean the skin with iodine solution such as povidone (Betadine).
3. Anesthetize the skin with lidocaine in the area of planned aspiration.
4. Use an 18 gauge needle to aspirate.
5. Grossly inspect the fluid and analyze for the following:
   a. Cell count and differential—fluid needs to be in a tube containing heparin
   b. Glucose and total protein—fluid needs to be placed in a tube without anticoagulant
   c. Type of crystals (see Chapter 69)
   d. Gram stain and culture using transport media (even in the absence of a high white cell count)
   e. Mucin clot analysis
      (1) Add 1 to 2 drops of bursal fluid to 1 ml of 2–5% acetic acid in a test tube
      (2) Shake the mixture a few moments and observe the clot (good, if clot remains intact and this is normal or a noninflammatory state; poor, if clot disintegrates and this represents inflammatory disease states) (see Table 66.2)

Table 66.2.
Patterns of Bursal (or Joint) Fluid Findings in Common Problems

	Normal	Trauma	Sepsis	Rheumatoid Inflammation	Microcrystalline Inflammation
Color of fluid	Clear yellow	Bloody, xanthochromic	Yellow to cloudy	Clear yellow to cloudy	Clear yellow to cloudy
WBC/RBC	0–200/0	< 1200/many	10,000–200,000/few	1000–20,000[a]/few	1000–20,000[a]/few
Protein	Low	Low	Slightly increased	Slightly increased	Slightly increased
Glucose	Same as plasma	Normal	Decreased	Slightly decreased	Variable
Crystals	–	–	–	–	+[b]
Mucin clot	Good	Good to intermediate	Poor	Poor	Poor
Culture	–	–	+	–	–

[a] Cell count in noninfected inflammatory fluid may sometimes be as high as it is with sepsis; thus the need for culture.
[b] Gout: negatively birefringent sodium urate (see Chapter 69). Pseudogout: positively birefringent sodium pyrophosphate (see Chapter 69).

are found, then a penicillinase-resistant antistaphylococcal drug should be used. If Gram-negative organisms are found, blood cultures should be obtained and an extrabursal site of infection should be sought. Antibiotic choice should be based on the most likely organism causing the extrabursal infection. The need for hospitalization depends on the severity of the infection. Patients with high fever and chills, intense surrounding cellulitis, deep bursal involvement, extrabursal infection, or suspicion of an uncommon organism (especially if the host is immunocompromised) should be hospitalized for parenteral antibiotics (9). Patients who are less ill can be treated as outpatients with oral antibiotics and repeated bursal aspiration. The duration of therapy should be individualized according to culture results of serial bursal aspirations. Antibiotics should be continued for 5 additional days after achieving sterility of the bursal fluid (9).

Gout, pseudogout, or rheumatoid arthritis should be treated with anti-inflammatory agents (see Chapter 69).

Usually traumatic bursitis will resolve spontaneously if the area of inflammation is rested. The spontaneous resolution, however, requires several weeks and therapy shortens this period considerably. Therefore, if sepsis and gout are ruled out, the treatment outlined in Table 66.3 is indicated.

If there is no initial response to treatment with a nonsteroidal anti-inflammatory agent (see Chapter 70 for a description of NSAIDs), then the patient should be treated by an injection into the inflamed bursa of a mixture of lidocaine and depoglucocorticoid (Table 66.4). Immediate and dramatic, but transient, relief of pain secondary to lidocaine indicates that the proper

Table 66.3.
Treatment of Bursitis

1. Splint where feasible (especially effective in the hand and fingers).
2. Application of heat or cold may be of benefit in some patients.
3. Anti-inflammatory agents: A nonsteroidal anti-inflammatory agent with rapid onset of action is preferred (see Chapter 70 for a full discussion of NSAIDs).
4. Improvement is usual in several days, but the anti-inflammatory agent should be continued an additional 4–5 days to prevent recurrence.
5. If no significant response is noted in 5–7 days and if sepsis has been ruled out, the bursa may be injected with lidocaine and/or a steroid preparation (see Table 66.4).

Table 66.4.
Methods of Injection of Bursae or Joints with Lidocaine and/or Depoglucocorticoid Preparations[a]

1. Be certain sepsis has been ruled out (Tables 66.1 and 66.2).
2. Prepare the skin carefully with an iodine-containing solution such as povodine (Betadine).
3. Anesthetize the skin with intradermal 1–2% lidocaine.
4. Mix 2–3 ml of 1–2% lidocaine with 20–40 mg of a depoglucocorticoid (such as Celestone, Aristocort, or Kenalog) and inject the bursa with 1–3 ml of this mixture using a 20- to 22-gauge needle.

[a]Notes of caution: (a) injection into the skin will cause atrophy and thus should be avoided; the patient should understand that there is a possibility of this complication; and (b) injection into tendons themselves may cause degeneration and, in time, rupture and these structures should be avoided by careful palpation.

site has been injected. The anti-inflammatory effect of the steroid injection is seen in approximately 72 hours. If a satisfactory response has not occurred, the bursa may be reinjected in approximately 2 weeks. Waiting 2 weeks before reinjection provides ample time to rule out iatrogenic sepsis, which rarely occurs after a steroid injection. Depending on location, other modalities such as ultrasound, heat or cold application, and physical therapy may be used as adjuncts. If a bursitis does not respond to two steroid injections, rheumatological consultation to rule out associated systemic disease may be necessary. Rarely definitive treatment by surgical excision of the bursa may be necessary.

Specific Forms

Several forms of bursitis are particularly common; their unique aspects are described here.

Olecranon Bursitis

This common form of bursitis—also called student's or miner's elbow—is easily recognized by its location just behind the olecranon process of the ulna. Its special features are: (a) it is frequently associated with systemic disease, such as rheumatoid arthritis or gout; (b) symptoms frequently are chronic, in that they have been present for 2 or 3 weeks before a patient sees a physician; and (c) it is a common site for septic bursitis after trauma and may be associated with surrounding cellulitis (9). If rheumatoid arthritis or gout is present, it is important to realize that sepsis sometimes coexists. Traumatic olecranon bursitis is usually hemorrhagic, although xanthochromic fluid may be present.

Swelling in the area of the olecranon bursa should be aspirated if symptomatic (see Tables 66.1 and 66.2) and a stain, culture, white blood cell count, and crystal identification with polarizing microscopy should be obtained.

Therapy. Therapy depends on the characteristics of the fluid. If monosodium urate crystals are present, specific therapy for gout is indicated (see Chapter 69). Traumatic bursitis responds to simple removal of fluid; but if the fluid reaccumulates, a steroid injection (Table 66.4) should be given. If sepsis is identified, the patient should be treated with an antibiotic and bursal aspiration as outlined above. An X-ray of the elbow should be obtained to rule out osteomyelitis or a foreign body if the process has been present for more than 2 weeks.

Prepatellar Bursitis

Prepatellar bursitis (housemaid's or carpenter's knee) is a very common form of bursitis, easily recognized by its location overlying the inferior portion of the patella. It is particularly common in carpet layers, plumbers, and carpenters. It is most often caused by trauma from kneeling, but it may also be a site of sepsis, and the bursa, for this reason, should always be aspirated even if it feels dry (9).

Anserine Bursitis (11)

The anserine bursa is fan shaped and lies between the confluence of tendons and the tibia at the anterior medial aspect of the knee just below the joint space. Anserine bursitis is most often seen in individuals with arthritis, especially overweight middle-aged women with osteoarthritis of the knee, and is recognized by its location; the pain is typically produced when the knee is flexed and is particularly troublesome at night. The patient often seeks comfort by sleeping with a pillow between the thighs.

If there is surrounding erythema or if the patient is febrile, aspiration should be attempted because sepsis, although uncommon, may be present. Therapy depends on the findings (see Tables 66.2 and 66.3). When injection therapy is used, the solution should be injected in a fan-shaped pattern so that the entire bursa is treated.

Ischial Bursitis (17)

The ischial bursa is located over the ischial tuberosity, close to the sciatic nerve and the posterior femoral cutaneous nerve. When a person is sitting, the ischial bursae are covered only with subcutaneous tissue and skin; when a person is standing, the gluteus maximus also covers the bursa.

The most common reason for inflammation of this bursa is trauma, such as may occur in bicycling. It is rarely a site of sepsis.

Usually the inflammation results in an abrupt onset of pain, but occasionally the onset is more insidious. The patient often has exquisite pain when sitting or lying. Because of the close proximity of the sciatic

nerve to the bursa, there may be an associated neuritis resulting from pressure on the nerve, which causes pain to radiate into the leg. Direct pressure over the ischial tuberosity will cause sharp pain and the patient may hold the painful buttock elevated when sitting. In addition, the pain is intensified when the patient is supine and the hip is passively flexed. The patient will have difficulty standing on tip-toe on the affected side.

The differential diagnosis of symptoms suggestive of ischial bursitis includes lumbar spine disease, thrombophlebitis, and inflammatory back disease or sacroiliitis (see Chapter 71). Localization of the pain over the ischial tuberosity and the finding of induration near the ischial tuberosity on rectal examination establish the diagnosis of ischial bursitis.

Aspiration of the bursa, even when it is inflamed, is not recommended because it is often difficult to localize, and the surrounding structures, especially the sciatic nerve, may be injured. If aspiration is indicated because there is associated fever and, therefore, the possibility of septic bursitis, the patient should be referred to an orthopaedist for immediate evaluation.

Standard therapy (Table 66.3) with a nonsteroidal anti-inflammatory agent usually provides dramatic improvement within 2 to 3 days; but if there has been associated leg pain or weakness from sciatic nerve inflammation, those symptoms may persist for several months.

Ultrasound, administered by a physical therapist, may be effective and it should be considered if initial therapy has not relieved the symptoms within several days.

If the diagnosis is unclear, if there is a question of sepsis, and if the patient does not respond within a week to therapy, consultation with a rheumatologist or orthopaedist is recommended. If the diagnosis is confirmed, the consultant may aspirate the bursa and, if sepsis is ruled out, inject it with lidocaine and depoglucocorticoid, which often results in dramatic improvement.

Semimembranosus-Gastrocnemius Bursitis (Baker's Cyst) (5)

The semimembranosus-gastrocnemius bursa—commonly called a cyst—lies in the posterior medial aspect of the knee behind the femoral condyle and in 50% of individuals is continuous with the knee joint. Inflammation of this bursa is commonly associated with other knee problems such as internal derangements, rheumatoid arthritis, or degenerative arthritis. The bursa is rarely traumatized or infected. When the bursa is inflamed, pain is the major manifestation, especially during activities that require movement of the knee, such as repetitive squatting movements, and often it is relieved by rest. Contraction of the quadriceps (knee extension) compresses the suprapatellar bursa (which communicates often with the knee joint), causing fluid in the knee joint to flow directly into the semimembranosus-gastrocnemius bursa, thereby causing pain. A Baker's cyst can also be associated with calf swelling and tightness (the bursa descending several centimeters into the leg). Prolonged pressure from the cyst may lead to venous stasis resulting in true thrombophlebitis. Tenderness is present over the bursa, and often the patient complains of pain when the gastrocnemius muscle group is stretched—a positive Homans' sign. The location of the swelling may lead to confusion with a popliteal aneurysm. For this reason, careful examination, including palpation of the venous and arterial systems, is necessary. When there is any doubt about the diagnosis, special diagnostic studies and appropriate consultation as outlined in Chapters 70 (Rheumatoid Arthritis) and 87 (Peripheral Vascular Disease and Arterial Aneurysms), respectively, may be indicated. Diagnostic ultrasound is a useful screening examination (13). Occasionally a Baker's cyst ruptures spontaneously, resulting in swelling, heat, and diffuse tenderness of the calf. These features can mimic an acute deep vein thrombophlebitis (see Chapter 51). In those patients in whom the diagnosis is unclear, venography should be performed to exclude phlebitis.

Management of a patient with an uncomplicated Baker's cyst includes aspiration and instillation of a corticosteroid-anesthetic mixture. Usually this can be accomplished by aspirating and injecting the joint space. Rarely the cyst may need to be aspirated/injected from the posterior approach. Because of the important structures in the popliteal fossa (artery, nerve, and vein), aspiration of the bursa posteriorly should be done by an orthopaedist. Weight bearing should be minimized for several days. The response to this therapy is usually excellent. Management of a ruptured cyst consists of bed rest, heat, and elevation. Instillation of corticosteroids into the joint that has an effusion may be helpful. Nonsteroidal anti-inflammatory agents may also be of assistance; after symptoms have begun to abate, ambulation can slowly be increased.

Iliopectineal Bursitis

The iliopectineal bursa lies anterior to the hip joint, with which it communicates in approximately 15% of individuals. It lies between the inguinal ligament and the iliopsoas muscle just lateral to the femoral artery. Pain in the anterior pelvis, groin, and thigh is the most frequent manifestation of iliopectineal bursitis; swelling may result in a bulge resembling a femoral hernia (see Chapter 91) below the inguinal ligament. Bursitis may be present in conjunction with intrinsic inflammatory joint disease, such as rheumatoid arthritis. Extension of the hip (e.g., during walking) intensifies the pain so that the patient often limits the stride of the affected side. The anterior crural nerve (the largest branch of the lumbar plexus) lies just below the bursa and it may be irritated from bursal inflammation; resulting neuritis causes pain in the thigh, which often is also intensified by walking, and there may also be weakness of anterior muscles of the thigh. When a

bursa is quite enlarged it may compress the femoral vein, resulting in edema in the affected leg.

If a hernia can be ruled out (see Chapter 91), the bursa should be aspirated by an orthopaedist. Aspiration and injection with lidocaine and usually a corticosteroid result in lasting improvement.

Trochanteric Bursitis (16)

The trochanteric bursa lies in the lateral aspect of the thigh over the greater trochanter of the femur and is closely associated with tendons of the glutei muscles. The problem primarily affects older individuals. Most cases are of unknown etiology, although many are thought to result from osteoarthritis. Trauma accounts for approximately 20% of cases and sepsis is rare. The onset of pain may be abrupt, subacute, or chronic. There is frequently radiation to the knee or even to the groin. Discomfort is intensified by movement from the sitting to the standing position, going up and down stairs, or sleeping on the affected side.

On examination there is point tenderness over the bursa with reproduction of the pain. *Patrick's test* (external rotation of the hip combined with abduction) is often painful, whereas flexion and extension of the hip are usually pain free. An X-ray of this area is indicated, as frequently calcium is identified and its presence supports the diagnosis. Also, an X-ray may identify a problem in the hip joint or lower back that is causing referred pain that may simulate trochanteric bursitis.

Therapy, as outlined in Table 66.3, is usually quite effective. Additionally, it is important for the patient to sleep with a small pillow under the involved buttock to keep weight shifted off the bursa.

Subdeltoid Bursitis

This common condition is discussed in Chapter 63.

TENOSYNOVITIS

As with bursae there are many sites of potential tenosynovial inflammation. Tendinitis and tenosynovitis generally occur simultaneously. The synovial-lined tendon sheath is usually the site of maximal inflammation.

Inflammation of a sheath of a tendon is a relatively common problem. For the most part, only long tendons have sheaths. Tenosynovitis most often occurs from exercise, especially when a tendon has been used repetitively in an improperly conditioned individual (see Chapter 67). Tenosynovitis also may be part of a generalized inflammatory process. Sometimes tenosynovitis is the first manifestation of this process.

Tenosynovitis often affects the dorsal extensor tendons of the wrist. It is manifest most commonly by pain that is intensified with hand extension. In the acute stage, swelling and pain over the dorsal aspect of the wrist or over the dorsal radioulnar joint may occur. Occasionally, a friction rub is felt and/or heard when the appropriate muscle is contracted.

When tenosynovitis is identified in the absence of trauma, a systemic disease should be suspected. If present, specific therapy for that disease is obviously important. Gonorrhea should be suspected in sexually active individuals if inflammation involves the tendons of the ankle or wrist in the setting of a monoarthritis, fever, and skin rash. Using Transgrow media, culture of the endocervical canal and rectum in women and of the urethra in men is indicated (see Chapters 27 and 94).

If the tenosynovitis has developed because of trauma, such as exercise or overuse, or because of unknown reasons, nonspecific therapy initiated with a nonsteroidal anti-inflammatory agent, as for bursitis (Table 66.3), is appropriate. The fingers should be splinted in the position of function (see Fig. 67.2). If symptoms persist after 3 or 4 days of conservative therapy, the peritenon (loose tissue surrounding the tendon) should be injected with lidocaine and a corticosteroid (such as Aristocort or Kenalog) (Table 66.4). Occasionally, symptoms are recurrent, in which case referral to a rheumatologist or orthopaedist is indicated.

Tenosynovitis and tendinitis involving specific tendons are also discussed in Chapters 63 (Shoulder Pain), 67 (Exercise-Related Musculoskeletal Problems), and 102 (Common Problems of the Feet).

STENOSING TENOSYNOVITIS

Stenosing tenosynovitis is not a complication of tenosynovitis; rather, it occurs primarily when trauma is severe and localized. In stenosing tenosynovitis either a nodule forms on a tendon or an actual stenosis of a tendon sheath of a long tendon develops. This results in the affected part "sticking" in a fixed position that is sometimes also painful. When this affects the flexor tendons of the fingers, it is called *trigger finger*. The patient is unable to flex a digit fully or else, once it is flexed, the digit locks and literally must be straightened by external force until it suddenly snaps free. When stenosing tenosynovitis is present in the abductor or extensor tendon of the thumb, it is called *De Quervain's disease*, the most common form of stenosing tenosynovitis. Stenosing tenosynovitis is usually caused by repeated trauma (e.g., prolonged use of a screw driver), but it is occasionally seen in association with rheumatoid arthritis, amyloidosis, pregnancy, and myxedema.

The treatment is identical to that of bursitis as outlined in Tables 66.3 and 66.4. If the patient does not respond to several weeks of conservative therapy, surgical release may be necessary. When a nodule is palpable, it should be injected with a small amount of corticosteroid (such as 10 mg of Aristocort or Kenalog) and lidocaine. Frequently, it will resolve in several weeks (21).

DUPUYTREN'S CONTRACTURE

The palmar fascia may undergo nodular, hypertrophic fibroplasia of unknown cause. This results over many years in the development of a flexion contracture (Dupuytren's contracture). The process causes the skin to be fixed to the underlying fascia by adhesive bands, resulting in a fixed, puckered appearance. A Dupuytren's contracture is almost always painless but may result in significant functional disability. Although all digits may be involved, the 4th and 5th are affected most commonly. The condition primarily affects middle-aged or older men and, in nearly 40%, it is bilateral. It is more common in epileptics and alcoholics. Once the condition is present, passive extension of the fingers does not retard the process; in fact, it may accelerate it. If functional disability is present, the patient should be referred to an orthopaedic surgeon for consideration for surgery. Oral anti-inflammatory agents and local cortisone injections are not effective in retarding the process.

GANGLIONS

Ganglions, cystic swellings arising from the synovium of a joint or tendon sheath, are the most common benign tumor of the hand (18). They tend to occur more frequently in women from the teens through age 50. Onset may be sudden or gradual and the cyst may change over time, sometimes disappearing and then recurring. The swellings are usually smooth, tense, and fixed to the deep tissues. The most common site is the dorsum of the wrist between the extensor tendon of the thumb and the extensor tendon of the index finger. They may also occur on the volar aspect of the foot (the tarsal area) and ankle. There may be associated aching or weakness of the involved area. Nonoperative treatment in symptomatic patients, consisting of aspiration and/or cortisone injection, may be successful. Recurrences may need to be treated by operative excision.

FIBROMYALGIA

Fibromyalgia (commonly also referred to as *fibrositis*) is a form of nonarticular rheumatism characterized by chronic aches, pain, and stiffness in muscles, ligaments, tendon insertions, and subcutaneous tissues accompanied by increased tenderness at specific anatomical sites known as *tender points* (10, 20). It is a clinical and not a histological diagnosis. The recognition and management of fibromyalgia as a distinct entity is important because of its high prevalence (20 to 30% of patients referred to a rheumatologist) and because of the conditions with which it may be confused. The syndrome is considered primary when no known cause or associated disorder is present. *Secondary fibromyalgia* refers to instances in which another rheumatic disorder is an important concomitant illness.

Manifestations

The cardinal features of fibromyalgia are widespread soft tissue aching and stiffness, essentially daily, frequently involving the axial skeleton and the shoulder and pelvic girdles, of more than 3 months' duration (typically much longer). The condition is aggravated by fatigue, tension, excessive work activity, immobilization, and changes in the weather. Occasional spontaneous remission of several months' duration may occur. The long-term course is not fully known since the syndrome has only recently been defined. The condition primarily affects young and middle-aged women. The core feature of widespread pain and tenderness is essential for diagnosis (20). Specific locations termed tender points, which are painful when palpated (compared with control points) in patients with fibromyalgia, have been identified. Although some controversy exists regarding the exact number and location to examine, the eight paired tender points and four control points, illustrated in Figure 66.1, are a generally accepted core that is useful in clinical practice. Of these 16 points (eight paired points), most patients with fibromyalgia will have at least seven tender points. Approximately 85% of patients will also exhibit the characteristic features of nonrefreshed or disturbed sleep [actually a disturbance of non-rapid eye movement (REM) stage 4 deep sleep], fatigue, and morning stiffness (more diffuse stiffness than the specific joint pattern of morning stiffness seen in inflammatory arthritis) (10, 20). Patients often complain of swelling in the hands and fingers, although there is no objective evidence noted by the physician. Patients may also complain of numbness, usually in a nonradicular distribution and in the setting of a normal neurological examination. Other findings in these patients are headaches, symptoms of irritable bowel syndrome (see Chapter 40), and anxiety (see Chapter 13). Symptoms generally persist for years unless treatment is given (see below).

A thorough history and physical examination should be performed, as other conditions must be excluded before the diagnosis of fibromyalgia is made.

There are no specific laboratory abnormalities in fibromyalgia, and laboratory tests are generally done to exclude other diagnoses. Basic laboratory tests that should be performed include complete blood counts and measurement of erythrocyte sedimentation rate, serum proteins, muscle enzymes, and antinuclear and rheumatoid factor determinations. Other specific tests such as thyroid function tests may be appropriate depending on the patient's constellation of symptoms. By definition, all studies are normal in patients with fibromyalgia, and therefore any abnormalities should warrant a further search for an underlying disease.

The treatment of fibromyalgia is problematic and there is no good specific therapy (8). The nonsteroidal anti-inflammatory agents (NSAIDs) as well as corticosteroids have proven to be of little benefit. Many patients will have tried several NSAIDs without response. The only medications shown to be somewhat effective (approximately 1/3 of patients showing moderate to marked improvement) are the tricyclic antidepressant, amitriptyline (10 to 25 mg at bedtime), and cyclobenzaprine (5 to 30 mg at bedtime). Because of the lack of efficacy of most medications, appropriate treatment must include other modalities as well. These include patient education (emphasizing that fibromyalgia is not a prodrome of a more serious crippling disorder), physical therapy (relaxation, heat, massage), and a graded exercise program to maintain a good general level of aerobic fitness. Attempts should also be made to modify other aggravating factors such as mechanical/physical and psychological/emotional stress. Patients should be encouraged to be active participants in these aspects of the treatment program. "Doctor shopping," involvement in legal/disability cases, and the use of narcotic analgesics should be discouraged.

8 PAIRED TENDER POINTS (●)

1. Insertion of Nuchal Muscles into Occiput.
2. Upper Trapezius (mid portion).
3. Pectoralis Muscle-Just Lateral to Second Costo-Chondral Junction.
4. 2 cm Below Lateral Epicondyle.
5. Upper Gluteal Area.
6. 2 cm Posterior to Greater Trochanter.
7. Medial Knee in Area of Anserine Bursa.
8. Gastrocnemius-Achilles Tendon Junction.

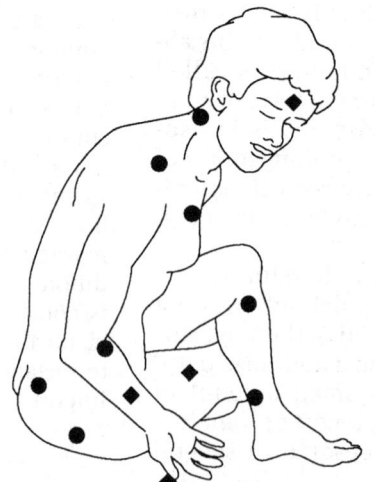

4 CONTROL POINTS (◆)

1. Middle of Forehead.
2. Volar Aspect of Mid-Forearm.
3. Thumbnail.
4. Muscles of Anterior Thigh.

Figure 66.1. The tender point locations in fibromyalgia are remarkably constant from patient to patient. Multiple locations have been described; the eight paired tender points shown represent frequently occurring points in a wide distribution. Most patients with fibrositis usually have seven or more tender points. Control points are not unduly tender; their examination should be interspersed with the tender points. Redrawn from Bennett RM: Fibrositis, In: Kelley WN, Harris ED, Rudy S, Sledge CB (eds): Textbook of Rheumatology, 3rd ed, Philadelphia, WB Saunders, 1989.

MYOFASCIAL PAIN SYNDROMES

Related problems, possibly distinct from fibromyalgia, are the myofascial pain syndromes (MPSs) (3). They are characterized by the presence of deep tender points also. However, in myofascial pain syndromes, the tender point is termed a *trigger point* because firm palpation of the point produces pain in a referred distribution. A second feature distinguishing MPS from fibromyalgia is the presence of just one or a regional clustering of points in MPS in contrast to the widespread distribution of symptoms and tender points in any given patient with fibromyalgia. A wide array of clinical syndromes in many different anatomical areas have been ascribed to MPS.

The pathogenesis of MPS is unknown. Patients with MPS may be helped by passive stretching of involved muscles after injection of the trigger point with a local anesthetic or use of a vapocoolant spray (e.g., ethylchloride). Attention should also be directed to elimination of any possible aggravating factors such as overuse or repetitive injury to involved muscle areas.

RAYNAUD'S PHENOMENON

Raynaud's phenomenon is a syndrome characterized by episodic vasospasm of the digital vessels in response to cold or emotional stress. Classically, a triphasic response occurs: first cutaneous pallor, extending from the fingertips to the midfingers; then mottling of the skin and cyanosis rapidly follow as a consequence of venous blood refluxing back into an empty cutaneous capillary bed (this pallor and/or cyanosis persists until rewarming of the digits); finally the recovery phase occurs over 15 to 20 minutes, resulting in intense hyperemia. Vasospasm is usually triggered by an abrupt change of environmental temperature, and, therefore, it may occur even in the summer months when a patient moves into air-conditioned or refrigerated areas. One or two digits may have more intense vasospasm, but generally the episodes are bilateral and symmetrical. Also, the feet and other acral parts (such as the ears or nose) may be involved. Patients often do not describe spontaneously the classical phases of Raynaud's phenomenon but do commonly note deep cyanosis associated with numbness, a pins and needles sensation, or frank pain on cold exposure.

Raynaud's phenomenon may occur secondary to a defined vascular abnormality or in association with a specific disease process (Table 66.5). It occurs most commonly in an idiopathic or primary form, Raynaud's disease, in which no underlying abnormality can be defined. Primary Raynaud's phenomenon is thought to be quite common, occurring principally in women aged 20 to 30 years. The true prevalence of Raynaud's phenomenon is unknown, but it has been estimated to be 2 to 6% of the general population and up to 20% of the selective population of young women (12). Patients with primary Raynaud's phenomenon

Table 66.5.
Classification of Raynaud's Phenomenon

A. Primary: Idiopathic Raynaud's, Raynaud's disease
B. Secondary: Disorders associated with Raynaud's phenomenon

1. *Connective tissue diseases*	*Percentage of Patients with Stated Disorder Who Also Have Raynaud's Phenomenon*
a. Systemic sclerosis	90
b. Systemic lupus erythematosus	20
c. "Mixed" connective tissue disease"	75
d. Dermatomyositis/polymyositis	20
e. Rheumatoid arthritis	10
2. *Neurovascular compression*	
a. Thoracic outlet syndrome (*e.g.,* cervical ribs, scalenus anticus syndrome)	
b. Carpal tunnel syndrome	
3. *Arterial disease*	
a. Arteriosclerosis	
b. Arteritis (thromboangitis obliterans)	
4. *Hematological Disorders*	
a. Paraproteinemia	
b. Cryoglobulinemia	
c. Polycythemia	
d. Hyperviscosity syndrome	Unknown
5. *Occupational*	
a. Vibratory tools (white finger syndrome)	
b. Polyvinyl chloride exposure	
6. *Drugs*	
a. Ergot-containing drugs (such as ergotamine)	
b. β-Adrenergic blockers	
c. Sympathomimetic agents (such as Actifed)	
d. Methysergide (Sansert)	
e. Chemotherapy (bleomycin, vinblastine)	
7. *Miscellaneous*	
a. Primary pulmonary hypertension	30
b. Migraine headache	10

are otherwise healthy, generally have relatively infrequent attacks (one to four episodes weekly), and rarely develop local cutaneous complications, such as digital pitting, ulcerations, or loss of hand function. Patients with primary Raynaud's phenomenon usually have an uncomplicated course with gradual decrease over a number of years in the frequency of episodes. Estimates suggest that 8 to 19% of patients believed initially to have the primary form will in time develop a defined secondary form (usually a connective tissue disease) (6, 19).

When patients present with Raynaud's phenomenon to a general physician, approximately 40% will have a defined secondary cause, the most common being a connective tissue disease (Table 66.5). Raynaud's phenomenon occurs in greater than 90% of patients with systemic sclerosis and may be the initial symptom, preceding the other features of the disease by years. Approximately 40% of patients with systemic lupus erythematosus and 10% of patients with rheumatoid arthritis may also have associated Raynaud's phenomenon. Raynaud's phenomenon may be a presenting feature in patients who have a systemic vasculitis. Disturbances of the axillary or cervical neurovascular bundle also can lead to Raynaud's phenomenon. Patients with neurovascular compression syndromes (cervical rib, scalenus anticus syndrome) and proximal vascular lesions (atherosclerosis) may present with unilateral Raynaud's phenomenon. Hematological abnormalities, such as cryoglobulinemia, paraproteinemia, or cold hemagglutinins, may present as typical Raynaud's phenomenon. Ergot-containing drugs, such as ergotamine, and β-blocking agents may be causative or potentiating agents. Occupational injury (vibration white finger syndrome) causing the syndrome occurs in a high proportion of workers operating vibratory tools (such as lumberjacks, shipyard workers, or meat cutters).

It may be difficult to determine whether a patient has a primary or secondary form of Raynaud's phenomenon when initially presenting to a physician; however, there are certain clues that should suggest a secondary form. Raynaud's phenomenon in children, men, or in women over age 30 is suggestive of a secondary form. Likewise, involvement limited to a single digit, vasospasm extending proximally to the proximal interphalangeal joint, and unilateral Raynaud's are more commonly associated with a secondary defined vascular occlusive lesion. Patients with signs or symptoms of another disease are likely to have a secondary form of Raynaud's phenomenon, especially if symptoms of a connective disease are present, such as myalgia, arthralgia, or unexplained fever.

Every patient presenting with Raynaud's phenomenon should have a complete history (including a drug review) and physical examination looking for underlying disease. An extension of the examination, evaluation of the nailbed with an ophthalmoscope, may reveal small telangiectasias or abnormal cutaneous capillary loops; these small vessel changes may be the earliest findings in an associated underlying connective tissue disease, primarily systemic sclerosis (6). The presence of ulcers on the digits should alert the physician that the Raynaud's is very severe and that the patient is very likely to have a secondary form of Raynaud's phenomenon. Patients with unilateral Raynaud's phenomenon should be carefully evaluated for a local vascular lesion, including bilateral blood pressure determination, auscultation over major vessels to determine the presence or absence or vascular bruits, and assessment of the peripheral pulses. Special testing for possible neurovascular compression syndrome (see Chapter 63) and consideration for chest X-ray and a noninvasive evaluation of the peripheral circulation (Doppler studies or digital plethysmography) are appropriate. Angiography may be necessary in cases in which a correctable occlusive vascular lesion is strongly suspected. Carpal tunnel syndrome has been implicated both in unilateral and bilateral Raynaud's phenomenon, and nerve conduction studies may be appropriate when a nerve compression syndrome is suspected (see Chapter 84).

Patients with typical symmetrical Raynaud's phenomenon should have, even in the absence of a suspicion of an underlying disorder, a complete blood count, Westergren sedimentation rate, urinalysis, antinuclear antibody (ANA) screen, cryoglobulins, and serum protein determination. Other studies may be initiated on an individual basis depending on the history, the physical findings, or the results of the screening studies (see above). Patients with a positive ANA are more likely to develop a clinically active connective tissue disease. The anticentrome antibody is the most frequent antinuclear antibody detected and may be useful in identifying a subgroup of patients with features suggestive of transition to the CREST (Calcinosis, Raynaud's, Esophageal Dysmotility, Sclerodactyly, Telangiectasis) variant of systemic sclerosis (15). Even when an associated illness is not identified, the patient should be followed carefully because an underlying illness might not manifest fully for several years (see above).

The principal mode of treatment in those cases in which a correctable cause cannot be found is avoidance of the cold. This includes protection of the hands and feet with mittens or gloves and avoiding a general chill of the body by wearing a hat and loose-fitting warm clothing in winter months. Smoking has been shown to aggravate Raynaud's phenomenon and should be stopped (4). Emotional stress should be assessed and controlled by appropriate measures (see Chapter 13). Patients with mild Raynaud's phenomenon often improve with education about the cause and nature of these episodes. Biofeedback therapy, usually offered by behavioral psychologists, is available in some communities and may provide partial benefit in patients with mild primary Raynaud's phenomenon. The nonpharmacological management of patients with Raynaud's phenomenon is summarized in Table 66.6. The majority of patients, particularly those with primary Raynaud's phenomenon, do not need and should not be treated with drugs. Rather, pharmacological

Table 66.6.
Management of Patients with Raynaud's Phenomenon

Education and reassurance
  Establish precipitating factors (such as refrigerator/freezer, air conditioning, emotional stress).
  Provide emotional support, *e.g.*, assurance of the mild nature of the disease in most patients may reduce some of stress that can precipitate attacks.
Avoidance of precipitating factors
  Wear gloves before reaching into refrigerator or freezer.
  Wear warm body clothing to avoid cold exposure when dressing.
  Keep head covered to avoid heat loss.
  Keep extremities warm and body well covered in cool weather or in air-conditioned environments.
  Be aware that stress can cause Raynaud's attacks.
Avoid certain drugs that precipitate attacks:
  β-Blockers (such as propranolol)
  Ergot-containing drugs (*i.e.*, ergotamine)
  Sympathomimetic agents (such as isoproterenol, Actifed, or other cold remedies)
  Nicotine (smoking)
  Oral contraceptives

treatment should be limited to patients with repeated attacks who limit their daily activities or who have significant loss of nutritional blood flow such that skin breakdown or ulceration may occur. There is no evidence that decreasing the number of episodes of Raynaud's phenomenon will alter the progressive changes that may occur in patients with scleroderma or another connective tissue disease.

A wide variety of vasoactive agents have been used in patients with Raynaud's phenomenon, but few agents have been proven of definite benefit. Many of these patients are young women who have the potential of childbearing; therefore, unproven treatment that may have a teratogenic effect should be avoided.

The calcium channel blockers, nifedipine and diltiazem, but not verapamil or nicardipine, have been demonstrated to be effective in several prospective, controlled, and double-blind studies (14). These agents relax smooth muscle, reduce peripheral vascular resistance, and increase peripheral blood flow. Patients with primary Raynaud's tend to respond better than patients with Raynaud's phenomenon secondary to a connective tissue disease, especially systemic sclerosis. The major side effects of these agents are secondary to their vasodilatory activity and include hypotension, dizziness, headache, and peripheral edema. Approximately 40 to 50% of patients will experience some lightheadedness and flushing on initiation of the calcium channel blockers; however, these side effects are usually transient, lasting 1 to 2 days, and do not require the discontinuation of the medication. Calcium channel blockers should never be used during pregnancy or in a patient planning to become pregnant because they have been shown in animal models to be teratogenic.

The calcium channel blocker that has been more extensively studied and the drug of first choice is nifedipine. The initial dose should be 10 mg orally given while the patient is in the physician's office. Sitting and standing blood pressures and pulse should be monitored in 15-minute intervals for 30 to 45 minutes. If the patient does not experience any significant adverse effects (a decrease in systolic pressure of 20 mm or greater below baseline, or a fall below 90 mm Hg), then nifedipine may be prescribed at a dose of 10 mg orally three times daily. The patient should be encouraged to assume usual activities and to keep a diary of the number and intensity of his Raynaud's phenomenon. The dose then may be increased every 3 to 4 days by 10 mg to a maximum of 30 mg three times daily or until good control is achieved. Once an effective dose has been achieved, monitoring every 2 to 4 months is important since the initial response may be transient and side effects, such as esophageal reflux, may limit the usefulness of the drug. If nifedipine fails or is not tolerated, diltiazem at a dose of 30 mg four times a day may be tried as an alternative calcium channel blocker. The dose may be advanced by 30 mg/day every 3 to 4 days until the symptoms improve or a maximum of 120 mg four times a day is reached. Patients generally have resolution or a dramatic re-

duction in the intensity and number of episodes of Raynaud's phenomenon in the summer months. For this reason, medication should be discontinued unless repeated cold exposure or active Raynaud's phenomenon is documented.

Other drugs that have been used for the treatment of Raynaud's are reserpine, phenoxybenzamine (Dibenzyline), and guanethidine (Ismelin). These agents have been generally disappointing with both unproven long-term control and intolerable side effects (orthostatic hypotension, reflex tachycardia, impotency, lassitude), and therefore they are not recommended. Prazosin (Minipress) has been studied in controlled trials and may occasionally be of benefit if tolerated (dose range of 2 to 8 mg daily in two or three divided doses). Topical nitroglycerin paste applied to the digits or a nitroglycerin patch have been used with some success, but their indications are not established and consultation with a rheumatologist is suggested before prescribing them. Research is now active in determining whether prostaglandins (PGE, prostacyclin) are helpful in the treatment of Raynaud's phenomenon.

Surgical sympathectomy was once popular for the treatment of Raynaud's phenomenon but is now infrequently performed, primarily because of the high relapse rate (40 to 50%) and frequency of significant postural hypotension (2). Selective digital sympathectomy may be done in centers where microsurgery is available; however, long-term controlled studies of this procedure are lacking. Sympathectomy should only be considered for short-term relief from an intractable course complicated by digital ulceration that has failed medical treatment. All patients who have had such a severe course or who have ulcers on their digits should be seen in consultation by a vascular surgeon and/or a rheumatologist. Local digital block performed by a vascular surgeon or rheumatologist has been used for temporary treatment of patients with significant digital tissue compromise; also a good response may predict which patient may have a good effect from digital or cervical sympathectomy. A patient who has severe disease with digital ulcers is susceptible to developing secondary soft tissue infection. Local debridement and antimicrobial treatment may be necessary if ischemic ulcerations become infected. Whirlpool treatment is the most effective method of ulcer debridement. In instances of secondary complications, consultation with a vascular surgeon and/or a rheumatologist is advised.

General References

Bennett RM: Fibrositis. In: Kelley WN, Harris ED, Ruddy S, Sledge CB (eds): *Textbook of Rheumatology*, 3rd ed, Philadelphia, WB Saunders, 1989.
Coffman J, Davies WT: Vasospastic disease: a review. *Prog Cardiovasc Dis* 18:123, 1975.
Owen Jr DS: Aspiration on injection of joint and soft tissues. In: Kelley WN, Harris ED, Ruddy S, Sledge CB (eds): *Textbook of Rheumatology*, 3rd ed, Philadelphia, WB Saunders, 1989.
Schumacher HR: Synovial fluid analysis and synovial biopsy. In: Kelley WN, Harris ED, Ruddy S, Sledge CB (eds): *Textbook of Rheumatology*, 3rd ed, Philadelphia, WB Saunders, 1989.

Spencer-Green G: Raynaud's phenomenon. *Bull Rheum Dis* 33:1, 1983.

Specific References

1. Bywaters EGL: Tendinitis and bursitis. *Clin Rheum Dis* 5:883, 1979.
2. Buddeley RM: The place of upper dorsal sympathectomy in the treatment of primary Raynaud's disease. *Br J Surg* 52:426, 1965.
3. Campbell SM: Regional myofascial pain syndromes. *Rheum Dis Clin North Am* 15:31, 1989.
4. Coffman JD: The attenuation by reserpine or guanethidine of the cutaneous vasoconstriction caused by tobacco smoking. *Am Heart J* 74:229, 1967.
5. Doppman JL: Baker's cyst and normal gastrocnemius-semimembranosus bursa. *AJR* 94:646, 1965.
6. Fitzgerald O, Hess EV, O'Connor GT, et al: Prospective study of the evaluation of Raynaud's phenomenon. *Am J Med* 84:718, 1988.
7. Halverson PB, McCarty DJ: Clinical aspects of basic calcium phosphate crystal deposition. *Rheum Dis Clin North Am* 14:427, 1988.
8. Goldenberg DL: Treatment of fibromyalgia syndrome. *Rheum Dis Clin North Am* 15:61, 1989.
9. Ho G, Mikolich DJ: Bacterial infection of the superficial subcutaneous bursae. *Clin Rheum Dis* 12:437, 1986.
10. Moldofsky H: Sleep and fibrositis syndrome. *Rheum Dis Clin North Am* 15:91, 1989.
11. Larsson L-G, Baum J: The syndromes of bursitis. *Bill Rheum Dis* 36:1, 1986.
12. Olsen N, Nielsen SL: Prevalence of primary Raynaud's phenomenon in young females. *Scan J Clin Lab Invest* 37:761, 1978.
13. Pathria MN, Zlatkin M, Sartoris DJ, et al: Ultrasonography of the popliteal fossa and lower extremities. *Radiol Clin North Am* 26:77, 1988.
14. Rodeheffer RJ, Rammer JA, Wigley F, Smith CR: Controlled double-blind trial of nifedipine in the treatment of Raynaud's phenomenon. *N Engl J Med* 303:880, 1983.
15. Sarkozi J, Bookman A AM, Lee P, et al: Significance of anticentromere antibody in idiopathic Raynaud's syndrome. *Am J Med* 83:893, 1987.
16. Spear IM, Lipscomb PR: Noninfectious trochanteric bursitis and peritendinitis. *Surg Clin North Am* 32:1217, 1952.
17. Swarbout R, Compere E: Ischiogluteal bursitis—the pain in the arse. *JAMA* 227:551, 1974.
18. Turek S: *The wrist in orthopedics*, 4th ed. Philadelphia, JB Lippincott Co., 1984.
19. Velogos E, Robinson H, Porcluncula F, Masi A: Clinical correlation analysis of 137 patients with Raynaud's phenomenon. *Am J Med Sci* 262:347, 1971.
20. Wolfe F: Fibromyalgia. The clinical syndrome. *Rheum Dis Clin North Am* 15:1, 1989.
21. Younghusland DZ, Black JD: De Quervain disease. *Can Med Assoc J* 89:508, 1963.

C H A P T E R 67

Exercise-Related Musculoskeletal Problems

RONALD P. BYANK, M.D.
DAVID F. MARTIN, M.D.

Activities such as jogging, marathon running, golf, tennis, softball, bowling, and many others are an integral part of the lives of millions of Americans.* Fitness has become a common goal, and health and exercise clubs are extremely popular. These can often place recreational athletes in a situation of overstress. Consequently, physicians are contacted frequently by patients with exercise-related problems. This chapter describes for a number of common exercise-related syndromes the mechanism of injury, the usual signs and symptoms, the treatment, the indications for referral, and the methods of preventing recurrences of the problem. Most of the injuries associated with exercise may also occur in nonexercising individuals who suffer mechanical stress due to falls, missteps into depressions, overactivity, or minor motor vehicle accidents. Evaluation and management are similar for exercising and nonexercising persons with these injuries.

---

*See Chapter 58 for a discussion of physical conditioning from the standpoint of the cardiovascular system.

PROBLEMS OF THE KNEE

Knee Structure and Function

The knee is the largest joint in the body. It has both hinge-like motion and rotatory motion (of the tibia on the femur) during flexion and extension. The principal components of the knee and their functions are the following (Fig. 67.1, *A* and *B*):

1. *Three articulations* that have a common articular cavity: the lateral and medial tibiofemoral articulations, each of which has an important cartilaginous buffer; the lateral and medial menisci; and the patellofemoral articulation. Weight-bearing stresses are seen in all three of these areas.
2. *The muscles* that control the motion of the knee: *flexors*—the hamstring muscles, which arise from the ischium, diverge to form tendons that insert into the tibia and the fibula; and the gastrocnemius muscle, which arises from the distal posterior femur and inserts on the calcaneus through the Achilles tendon. *Extensors*—the quadriceps muscles, which originate at the ilium and the femur and converge distally as the common quadriceps tendon, which attaches to the superior aspect of the patella, continuing on as the patellar tendon to insert into the tibia.
3. *The external tendons and ligaments*: the patellar tendon, a continuation of the common tendon of the quadriceps that joins the patella to the tibial tuberosity and makes possible extension of the knee joint; and the collateral ligaments, which give stability to the joint—the lateral connects the lateral femoral condyle to the fibula, and the medial connects the medial femoral condyle to the medial condyle and surface of the tibia.
4. *The cruciate ligaments*, which are located inside the joint and stabilize the joint in the anteroposterior plane: the anterior cruciate ligament, which is attached anteriorly to the intercondylar eminence of the tibia and posterosuperiorly to the lateral femoral condyle; and the posterior cruciate ligament, which is attached posteriorly to the posterior intercondylar fossa of the tibia and to the lateral meniscus and anterosuperiorly to the medial femoral condyle.
5. *The bursae of the knee*, which provide lubrication between the many dynamic components of the knee.

General Evaluation of Knee Injuries

Traumatic knee injury may be caused by a single event in which the knee is suddenly stressed or by chronic, repetitive stress. When there is no history of sudden trauma, two features are especially helpful in evaluating knee pain: (*a*) identification of any recently initiated physical activities or a sudden change in type or intensity of physical activities; and (*b*) identification of problems elsewhere in the lower extremity that may cause inappropriate stresses upon the structure of the knee (e.g., excessive pronation of the feet, see Chapter 102). When there is no clear-cut history of trauma and physical examination does not indicate injury to one or more anatomical structures, conditions that may cause spontaneous knee pain should be considered (see Chapter 66, Nonarticular Rheumatism; Chapter 68, Degenerative Joint Disease; Chapter 69, Crystal-Induced Arthritis; Chapter 70, Rheumatoid Arthritis).

Knee pain may be due to injury to any one of the structures described above. Except when there is a large effusion, the structure(s) responsible for the pain can usually be identified by systematic examination. Focal tenderness to palpation is present when pain is due to structural inflammation (e.g., bursitis) or to ligament, meniscus, or muscle injury. Specific tests for meniscal injury, ligament injury, and patellofemoral arthralgia are described below.

Examination for a small or moderate knee joint effusion is done in one of two ways:

1. *By inspection*, with the patient seated and both knees flexed 90°; if there is an effusion in the symptomatic knee, there will be a bulge on either side of the patellar ligament that is not seen in the normal knee.
2. *By ballottement* (Fig. 67.2), with the patient supine and the knee fully extended; the knee is compressed above and on either side of the patella, in order to localize any fluid under the patella, then the patella is compressed with an examining finger to determine whether it is ballotable.

Meniscal and Ligamentous Injuries

Definition and Mechanism of Injury

Tears of the medial or lateral meniscus (a disc-shaped fibrous cartilage) of the knee are common. When a rotary force is applied to the flexed knee joint, the meniscus can be trapped between the femur and the tibia; then when the knee is extended, the cartilage may be torn (11). Tears of the medial meniscus are about 10 times as common as those of the lateral meniscus. This problem is encountered, especially in individuals who play football, basketball, and lacrosse as well as in persons who are bowlers, golfers, or baseball players. A simple twisting motion can cause a meniscal injury and often a traumatic event is not identified.

Sprains or tears of the collateral ligaments and the cruciate ligaments are caused by a combination of angulating forces at the knee with rotational forces that cause rotation of the leg at the knee. Those forces that most frequently cause ligament injuries are forces that produce abduction of the leg at the knee (e.g., a direct blow to the lateral aspect of the leg with foot planted and fixed). In these injuries all four of the major stabilizers of the knee are at risk: medial collateral ligament, anterior cruciate ligament, posterior cruciate ligament, and lateral collateral ligament.

Superior View (tibial plateau)

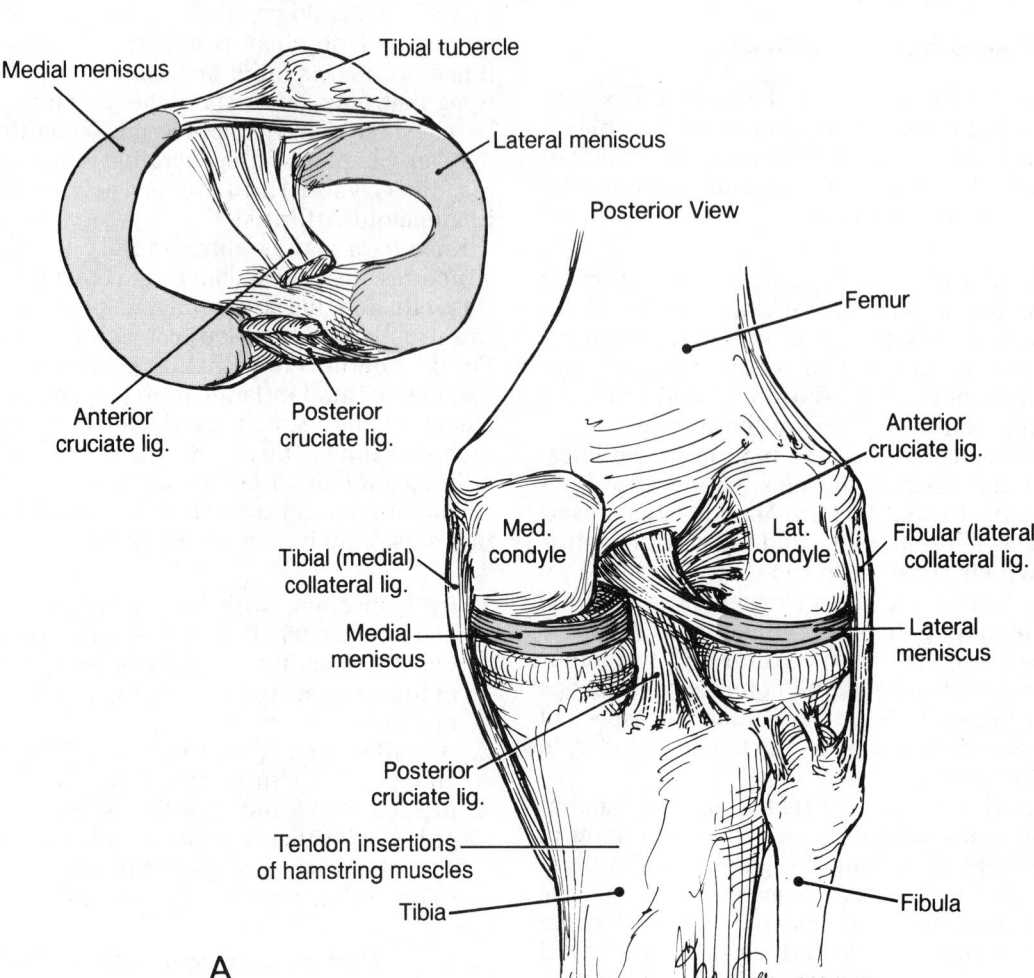

Figure 67.1. *A.* Important structures of the knee.

Symptoms and Signs

Meniscus Injury. The patient with a meniscus injury usually describes a twisting flexion injury of the knee followed by pain, and inability to flex the knee fully or to bear weight. Examination usually reveals knee joint effusion and tenderness over the joint line, either medially (medial meniscus injury) or laterally (lateral meniscus injury). Sometimes the onset is insidious and the patient notes episodes of knee effusion or of clicking or locking of the knee (which may last for several minutes or several hours). Examination of patients who suffer from this more chronic condition often reveals only minimal joint line tenderness. Quadriceps muscle wasting can be the only positive physical finding in this situation. Certain maneuvers are helpful in the diagnosis of meniscal injury; they are more likely to be diagnostic in patients with acute symptoms than in patients with chronic symptoms. The *McMurray test* is performed with the patient lying supine with the hip and knee fully flexed and the foot rotated outward to its full capacity to test the medial meniscus and inward to test the lateral meniscus (Fig.

67.3*A*). The knee is extended with the foot at first rotated out and again with it rotated in, and a painful click in the knee indicates a positive test. Not all meniscal tears will result in a positive test. The Apley or grinding test is performed by flexing the knee 90° when the patient is in the prone position, and then rotating the tibia internally and externally on the femur while compressing the leg against the femur (the direction of the rotation that produces pain does not accurately predict the meniscus that is injured), and then repeating the rotation while pulling the leg away from the femur (Fig. 67.3*B*). Pain during compression may be due to a tear of the lateral or medial menisci, and pain while pulling the leg is likely from a ligamentous injury.

Ligament Injuries. With a sprain of a ligament (usually the medial collateral ligament), the patient will describe pain at the time of injury and, in addition, there will be stiffness of the knee, tenderness, and often fullness over the ligament. Occasionally, there will be a serous joint effusion. (A strain, on the other hand, is a milder injury resulting in only stretching of a muscle.) Ligament sprains (see page 841) are clas-

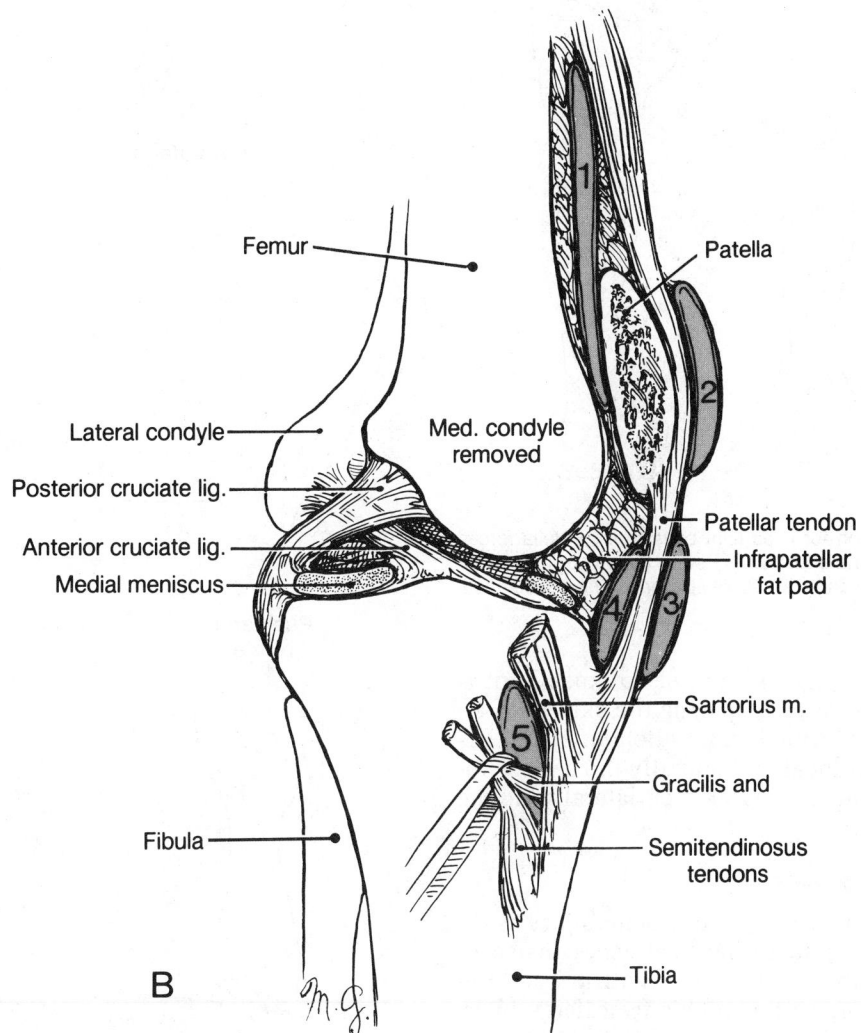

Figure 67.1. *B*. Five bursae of the knee: *1*, suprapatellar; *2*, prepatellar; *3*, superficial patellar tendon; *4*, retropatellar tendon; *5*, pes anserinus.

sified as grade I (stretching fibers without significant structural damage), grade II (partial disruption of fibers with increased laxity), and grade III (complete tearing of ligamentous tissues).

When injury to a ligament of the knee joint is suspected, the joint should be carefully evaluated for ligament instability, as illustrated in Figure 67.4. The laxity of ligaments varies tremendously between individuals; therefore, assessment of the uninjured knee first is important in evaluating an injured knee. The stability of the collateral ligaments should be tested with the patient supine and the knee in about 20° of flexion. Varus stress is applied to test the lateral collateral ligament, and valgus stress is applied to test the medial collateral ligament. If there is a grade I sprain, the affected ligament will be painful and tender, but there will not be instability as there would if the ligament had been ruptured. With grade II or III injuries, the lateral or medial joint space of the knee will widen when stress is applied to the leg with thigh fixed. The integrity of the anterior and posterior cruciate ligaments is tested with the knee at 15° and 90°

of flexion (see Lachman and Drawer tests, Fig. 67.4 A–C). Grasping the leg, the examiner exerts pressure posteriorly to test the posterior cruciate and then anteriorly to test the anterior cruciate. Instability in the direction of pressure indicates a tear of the cruciate ligament being tested. The most sensitive test of the anterior cruciate ligament is the *Lachman test* in which the knee is flexed to 15° and the tibia is pulled anteriorly on the femur. The test is defined as positive if there is anterior laxity.

Additional Evaluation. X-rays of the knee should always be obtained to exclude other problems, such as loose bodies within the knee, osteochrondritis dissecans, fractures, or arthritis. Radiographic evaluation should include anteroposterior, lateral, and sunrise patella views. If a large effusion is present, it should be aspirated for two reasons: first, removal of the fluid will result in relief of discomfort; and second, if a hemarthrosis is present, it may indicate a serious injury and the patient should be referred to an orthopaedist. If referral cannot be accomplished for several days, the knee should be splinted with a knee im-

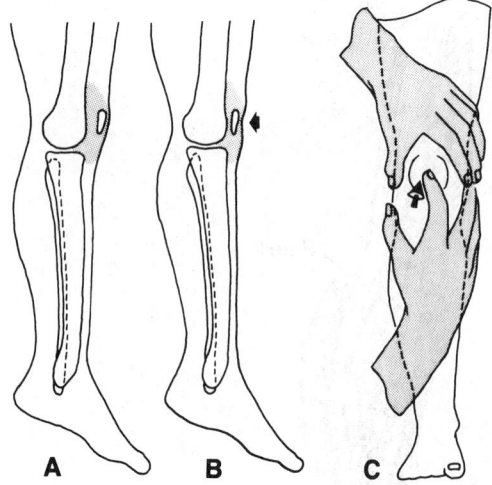

Figure 67.2. Examination for knee joint effusion. *A.* Patella forced away from the femur by the effusion. *B.* Patella forced downward into the femor ballottement maneuver. *C.* Illustration of the ballottement maneuver.

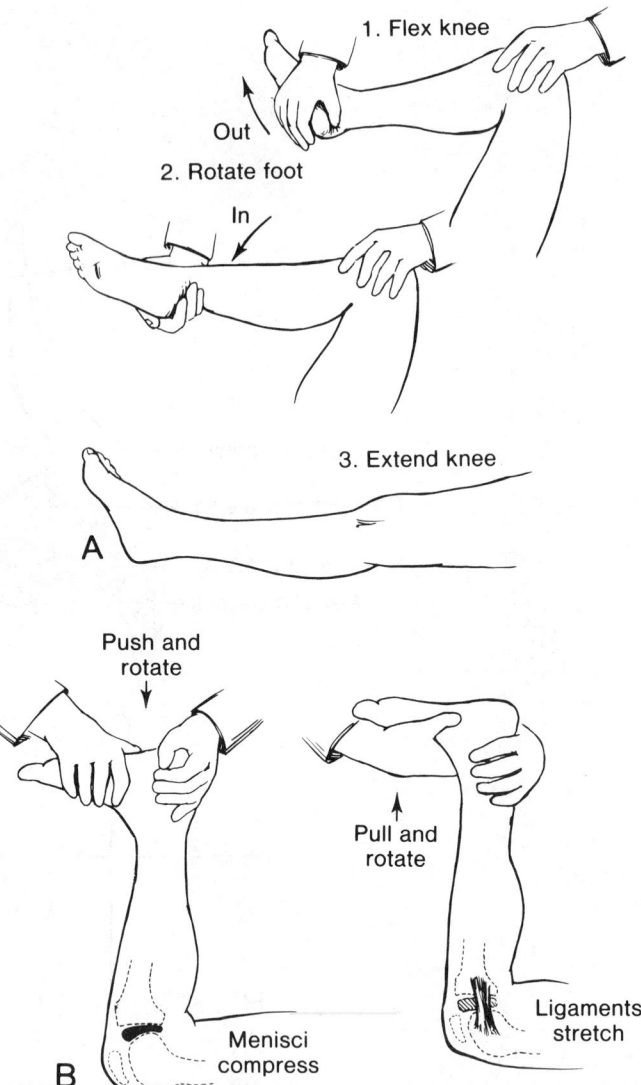

Figure 67.3. *A.* McMurray test. *B.* Apley test.

mobilizer (see below). Aspiration of the knee joint is easily accomplished after preparing the skin with an iodine-containing solution (such as Betadine) and anesthetizing it with lidocaine. Generally the easiest approach to aspiration is medially or laterally at the patellofemoral joint.

Treatment and Prognosis

Meniscus Injuries. When a meniscus injury is diagnosed or suspected, the initial treatment consists of immobilization of the injured knee with a knee immobilizer (a rigid support available from large pharmacies or orthopaedic appliance stores). An Ace bandage is not sufficient to provide stability, although it may help to diminish effusion. The patient should use crutches to keep his weight off the knee and should elevate the injured extremity when he lies down. Ice packs should be applied to the knee for 15 minutes several times a day to reduce swelling. Isometric quadriceps-strengthening exercises should be recommended as soon as the patient can do these comfortably (Fig. 67.5).

Most often symptoms subside within 14 days; if symptoms resolve, the prognosis is variable. In the instance of a small tear, complete healing may occur without subsequent symptoms. On the other hand, a larger tear may result in recurrent symptoms after initial improvement. Therefore, if symptoms persist beyond 2 weeks with conservative treatment or if they recur after return to normal activity, an orthopaedic referral is indicated for consideration of an arthrogram, magnetic resonance imaging (6), and/or arthroscopy to establish the diagnosis. *An arthrogram* is an X-ray of the joint and requires the injection of iodinated contrast material and air into the joint space. This is done by a radiologist or orthopaedist after administration of local anesthesia. After the procedure, which generally is well tolerated, crutches should be

used for 1 to 2 days, during which time usually only mild analgesics are needed. Magnetic resonance imaging (MRI) is a noninvasive procedure and is a good method of evaluating meniscal pathology. MRI scans are excellent for the evaluation of soft tissue structures about the knee. Sensitivity and specificity levels for meniscal tears are in the 90% range. Ligament imaging is less reliable. *Arthroscopy* is very valuable in evaluating and treating knee problems (see section below, Arthroscopy). If the diagnosis of meniscal tear is confirmed, surgical excision of the torn portion of the meniscus or of the entire meniscus may be necessary and may be performed either by arthroscopic surgery (an outpatient procedure) or through arthrotomy. With recent studies demonstrating the importance of the menisci to knee function, meniscal repair has also become an option.

After surgery for a torn meniscus, the patient is often able to return to light sports activity within 6 to 8 weeks, but it may be 3 months or longer before he can

A. Anterior Drawer Test

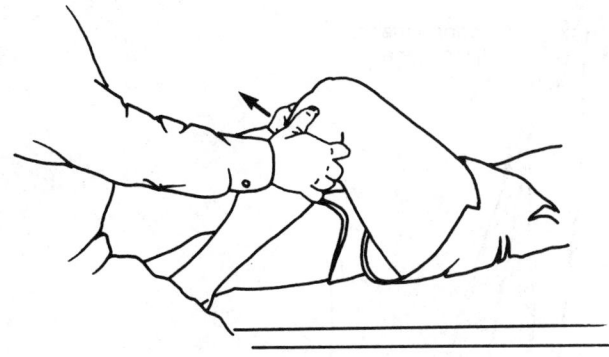

B. Lachman Test

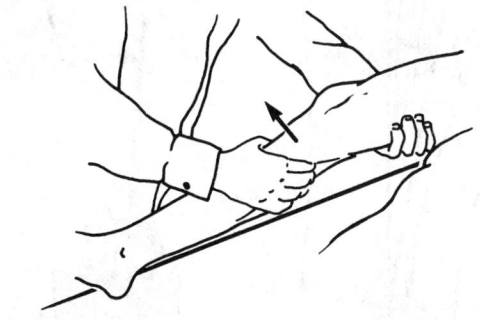

C. Posterior Drawer Test

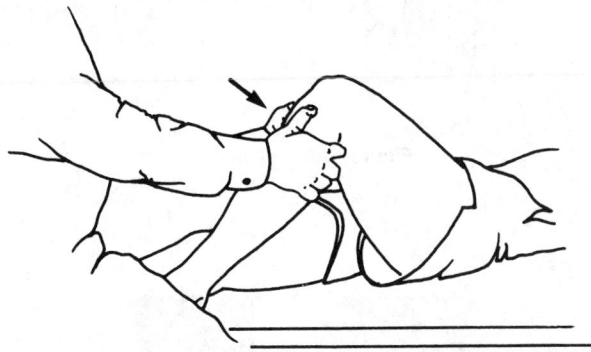

Figure 67.4. Examination for collateral and cruciate ligament injuries. *A.* Anterior drawer test. *B.* Lachman test. *C.* Posterior drawer test. Modified from Scott WN, Nisonson B, Nicholas JA (eds): *Principles of Sports Medicine.* Williams & Wilkins, Baltimore, 1984.

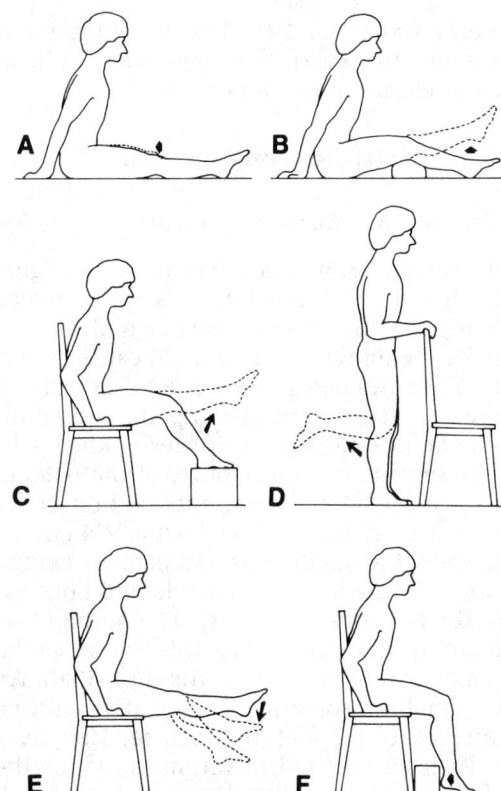

Figure 67.5. Restorative knee exercises. *A.* Isometric quadriceps exercise. *B* and *C.* Isotonic quadriceps exercises. *D,* Gravity-resisted isotonic flexion exercise. *E.* Gravity-assisted isotonic flexion exercise. *F.* Isometric flexion exercise.

resume such activities as running or tennis. A proper postoperative conditioning period of supervised physical therapy is important and will consist of strengthening the quadriceps and hamstring muscles (see Fig. 67.5) and of range of motion exercises to ensure normal mobility of the knee. Joint space narrowing and arthritic change almost always follow meniscectomy but may not limit a patient's activity significantly. The menisci are extremely valuable for knee stability, distribution of weight-bearing loads, and smooth range

of motion; therefore, it is imperative to aggressively treat meniscal tears to avoid further damage (1, 2).

Ligament Injuries. If a ruptured ligament is suspected, the patient's knee should be immobilized in a posterior splint or a rigid knee immobilizer, and the patient should be referred immediately to an orthopaedist.

If a grade I collateral ligament sprain (see page 838) is diagnosed, a patient with minor symptoms can be permitted to increase his activity gradually over the succeeding 1 to 2 weeks. For more pronounced symptoms, the knee should be immobilized with a knee immobilizer, and the patient should use crutches for 5 to 10 days. Ice packs and isometric quadriceps-tensing exercises should be recommended, as for meniscus injuries. When the knee brace is removed, the patient can progressively increase his activity and should begin isotonic quadriceps exercises (see Fig. 67.5) and range of motion exercises.

Prevention

Acute meniscus injury occurs by chance when a rotational force is applied to the knee when it is in the flexed position; it cannot be prevented by conditioning. Ligamentous injuries can be prevented to some degree by proper conditioning. Prophylactic braces (those placed on the normal knee to prevent ligamentous injury) are being used frequently, but their effectiveness is controversial (12). They may, in fact, preload the ligaments and make them more prone to injury and are therefore not recommended.

Patellofemoral Arthralgia

Definition and Mechanism of Injury

Patellofemoral arthralgia refers to pain originating from the patellofemoral joint. It is often associated with changes in the articular cartilage of the patella. *Anterior knee pain* can occur without cartilage changes as well. When the cartilage does become soft, it can break down, causing crepitus and pain. This condition is termed *chondromalacia* (5). Anterior knee pain can also occur secondary to instability of the patellofemoral joint—most often *lateral subluxation* or hypermobility of the patella. This can be due to an increased angle between the quadriceps and patellar tendon (Q-angle), by *patella alta* or by muscle and bony imbalances in the lower extremity (3). The normal Q-angle is up to 20°; if it is greater than this, increased lateral displacement of the patella results (Fig. 67.6). An abnormal Q-angle is sometimes associated with excessive pronation of the feet (flat feet, see Chapter 102). Patella alta is an anatomical variant in which the patella rides more proximally than usual, so that it becomes hypermobile. Patella alta can be identified on a lateral X-ray when the patellar tendon length exceeds the maximum length of the patella by more than 1 cm (Fig. 67.7). Normally, the lengths of these two structures are equal. Patients with a variation in hip joint anatomy that results in compensatory external tibial torsion (external rotation of lower leg in axial plane, slew foot) will also have lateral displacement of the patella and excess wear of the patellofemoral joint.

Anterior knee pain is a very common disorder, especially in adolescent athletes. This can be due to alignment problems, as discussed above, or overuse syndromes related to improper conditioning or stretching. Anterior knee pain can exist without changes in the anterior cartilage of the patella. The source of the pain may be the extensor mechanism (quadriceps muscle, quadriceps tendon, or patellar tendon) or in the patella itself. If stress on the articular cartridge is allowed to continue (whether secondary to subluxation or malalignment), cartilage breakdown may result. This is termed "chondromalacia." With appropriate treatment, this can be avoided in many cases (see below).

Symptoms and Signs

Pain, usually described as a soreness or aching around or under the patella, is the hallmark of this problem. The discomfort is aggravated by running up hills, climbing or descending stairs, kneeling, or hyperflexing the knee. Pain frequently disappears during activity only to recur just at the end of or after activity. The patient may also complain of the knee "locking"; however, upon careful questioning, this locking is found

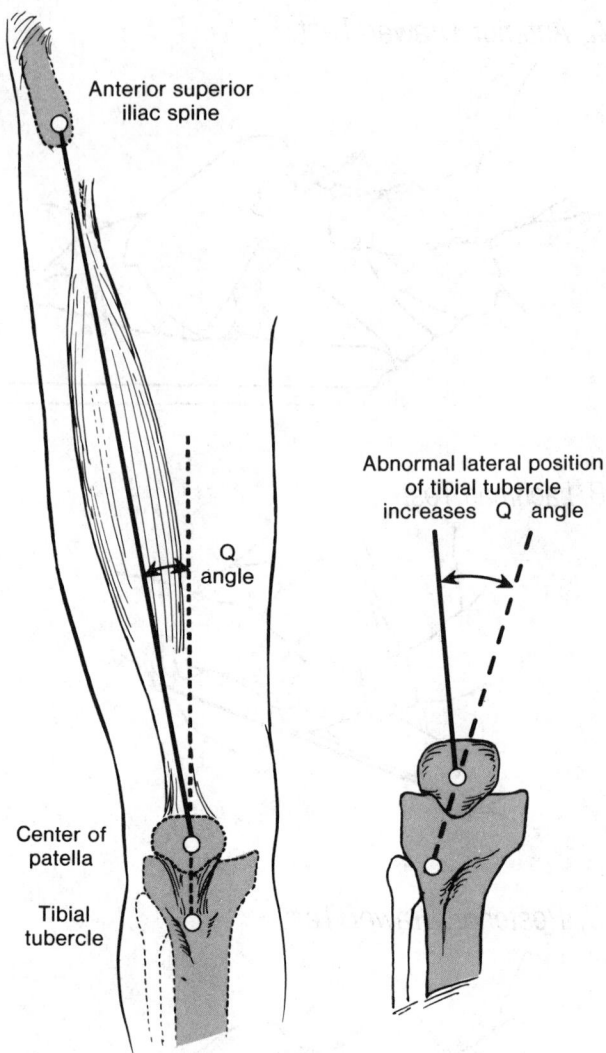

Figure 67.6. Q angle.

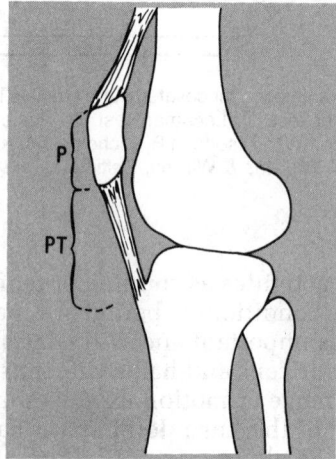

Figure 67.7. Patella alta. The ratio of PT to P is normally less than 1.2. In this case PT:P is 1.5 and therefore this is patella alta. *P*, patella; *PT*, patellar tendon.

to be only very transient and is not the true locking that is experienced in tears of the meniscus (see above).

Physical examination reveals any or all of the anatomical abnormalities described above. Patella alta and hypermobility of the patella are very frequent. Pain and/or crepitus with patellofemoral manipulation or palpation of the articular surface of the patella is usually present. Attempts to push the patella laterally may cause pain and involuntary contracture of the quadriceps, the so-called apprehension sign. If the patient extends his knee from 30° of flexion to full extension against resistance, pain will result. A knee effusion can be present.

Additional Evaluation

X-rays of the knees should be obtained routinely and should include a tangential or sunrise view to look for lateral subluxation of the patella, often with a hypoplastic lateral trochlear facet of the femoral sulcus.

Differential Diagnosis

Other problems that occasionally may be causes of anterior knee pain are prepatellar bursitis (Fig. 67.1B) (pain and tenderness localized to the prepatellar bursa, see Chapter 66), retropatellar (also called infrapatellar) tendon bursitis (Fig. 67.1B) (pain and tenderness localized to the area below the patella and behind the tendon), pes anserinus bursitis (Fig. 67.1B) (pain and tenderness in the bursa that lies deep to the combined insertion of the sartorius, gracilis, and semitendinosus tendons into the proximal medial tibial metaphysis), fat pad syndrome (trauma-related inflammation of the infrapatellar fat pad) (Fig. 67.1B), meniscal injury (see above), ligamentous instability of the knee (see above), arthritis, and osteochrondritis dissecans (necrosis within the condylar epiphysis characterized by insidious onset of knee ache at rest, worsened by weight bearing and confirmed by X-ray). Hip or pelvic disease is associated with referred pain from sciatic nerve root irritation. These problems can be differentiated by careful physical and radiological examination; if there is any doubt, referral to an orthopaedic surgeon is appropriate.

Treatment and Prognosis

Therapy is initiated as soon as possible after the appearance of symptoms. The use of crutches for up to 7 days to rest the knee is important; and the application of ice to the knee for approximately 15 minutes several times a day will help to decrease swelling. In addition, analgesic medications should be prescribed, such as enteric-coated aspirin, 600 mg four times a day, or Tylenol, 650 mg four times a day. Nonsteroidal anti-inflammatory agents also are very effective (see Chapter 70 for a full discussion of NSAIDs).

After the initial inflammation has subsided, the application of ice may be discontinued and heat may be applied for 15 to 20 minutes several times a day. The patient should avoid vigorous sports activities until symptoms subside, which often takes several weeks.

Progressive resistance exercises of the quadriceps should be supervised by a physical therapist (especially one experienced in sports medicine) to maximize quadriceps strength and stability (see Fig. 67.5). Stretching to increase flexibility is extremely important, especially in the hip flexors, quadriceps, and hamstring muscle groups (see below, Stretching Exercises). The course of patients with this problem is unpredictable. Orthopaedic referral is usually necessary if the patient has been forced to abandon his major sport for more than a few weeks, or if the problem recurs. Intra-articular corticosteroid injections by the orthopaedist may alleviate symptoms, but this treatment must be restricted, as it will increase cartilage deterioration if done to excess. Correction of the tracking problem in the patellofemoral joint may require the use of an orthotic to correct excess pronation of the foot (see Chapter 102) or the use of a cartilage knee brace (a heavy elastic brace containing a horseshoe-shaped pad to stabilize the patella—available from large pharmacies or orthopaedic appliance stores without prescription). Occasionally, if anterior knee pain progresses to cartilage damage, surgical treatment is necessary if conservative treatment fails. Surgery is designed to prevent subluxation of the patella and/or decrease stress in the patellofemoral articular cartilage. Results are variable depending on the extent of the problem and the type of surgery, but, occasionally, the patient may not be able to return to sports that place stress on the knee.

Prevention

Prevention of anterior knee pain and chondromalacia requires the use of proper foot gear (see Chapter 102), often including the use of orthotics, and "proper conditioning" of the athlete by gradually increasing his level of activity and by the performance of stretching exercises (see below).

PROBLEMS OF THE LEG

Apophysitis of the Tibial Tubercle (Osgood-Schlatter's Disease)

This is a relatively common cause of knee pain in adolescents. It is thought to be due to repetitive avulsions or stress fractures due to traction of the patellar tendon where it inserts into the growth plate of the tibial tubercle. This repetitive trauma causes inflammation and pain at the insertion point of the tendon.

The patient describes the insidious onset of pain of the tibial tubercle with activity. This condition is frequently bilateral. On examination there is enlargement and tenderness of the tubercle and adjacent tendon. There may be quadriceps atrophy from decreased activity, which frequently occurs because of use pain. There may also be tightness of the quadriceps and hamstrong muscle groups.

The adolescent with Osgood-Schlatter's disease should be instructed to avoid activities that entail resisted knee extension, such as climbing, running, and kicking, until pain has resolved (usually 6 to 8 weeks). Range of motion and stretching (see below, "Stretching Exercises") should be stressed early in the course of treatment. If pain persists after ossification is complete, surgical excision of heterotopic bone at the tibial tubercle and reattachment of the patellar tendon are sometimes necessary.

Shin Splints

Definition and Mechanism of Injury

Shin splints (10) are the occurrence of pain over the anteromedial aspect of the mid to distal portion of the lower leg (Fig. 67.8, *site A*). They are caused by overuse of the muscles of this region as may occur with running, jogging, or sustained walking. The pain is thought to result from tendinitis of the posterior tibial tendon and by periostitis from the pulling of this muscle from its bony attachment along the medial aspect of the tibia, the interosseous membrane, and the fibula.

Shin splints develop most often in individuals who (a) are not properly conditioned, (b) do not warm up properly, (c) run on hard or uneven surfaces, (d) wear improper foot gear, or (e) have anatomical abnormal-

ities such as variation in the anatomy of their hip joint with resultant excessive tibial torsion (external rotation of the tibia in the axial plane—slew feet) and hyperpronation of the feet (flat feet).

Symptoms and Signs

Shin splints are characterized by pain, usually gradual but occasionally abrupt in onset, which occurs during or just after exercise. Frequently, athletes continue to exercise in spite of the discomfort; but occasionally the pain is so severe that the exercise must be stopped. Examination reveals only the presence of tenderness along the medial aspect of the tibia.

Differential Diagnosis

If the area of tenderness is localized, a stress fracture may have occurred, although pain from a stress fracture is present immediately on starting activity. A compartment syndrome is similar to shin splints, but the location of pain and tenderness is different (see below). Occasionally fascial hernias, tenosynovitis, or tears of the interosseous membrane may produce symptoms suggesting shin splints; and, for this reason.

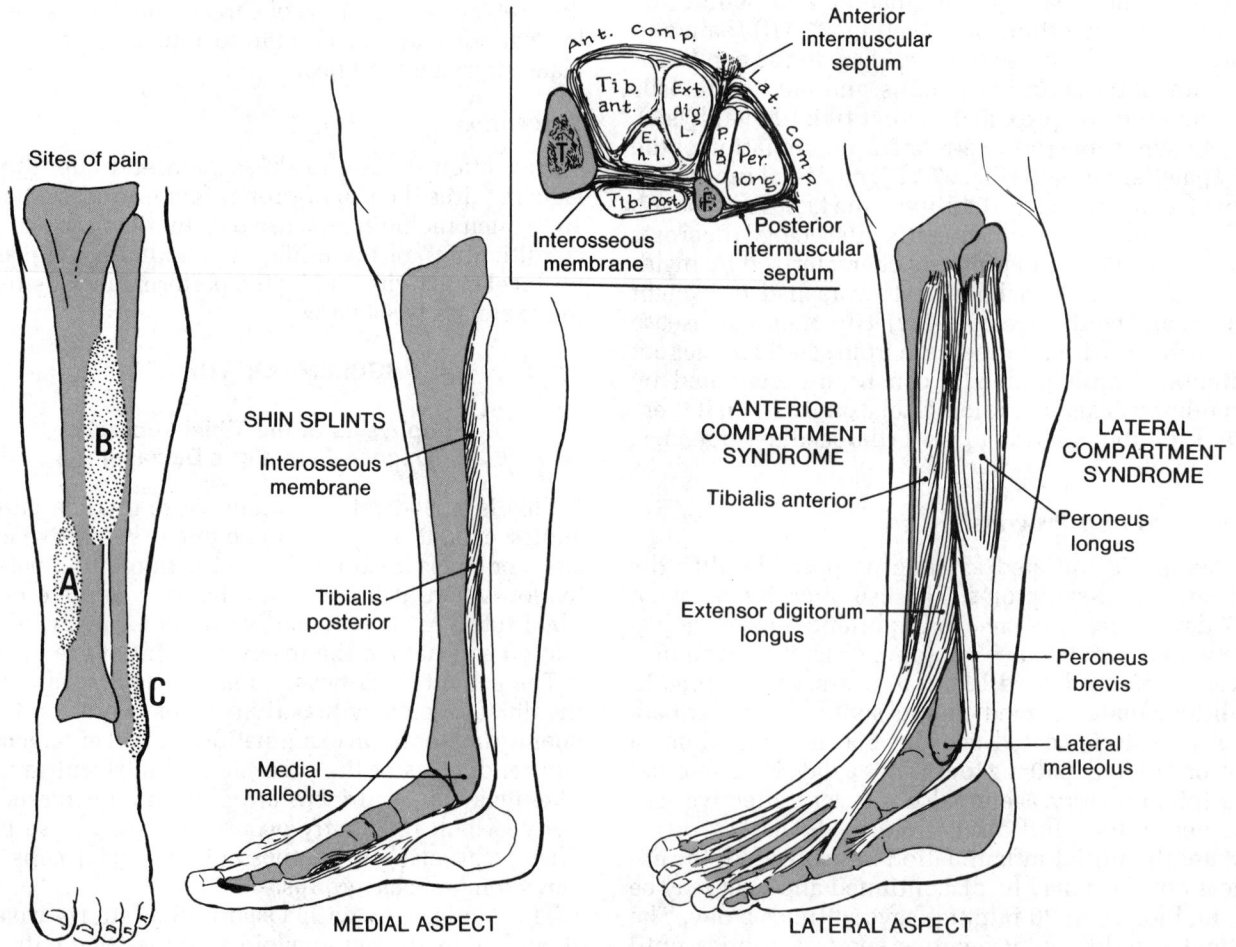

Figure 67.8. Sites of pain and relevant anatomy of (*A*) shin splints, (*B*) anterior compartment syndrome, and (*C*) lateral compartment syndrome.

an orthopaedic consultation should be requested if there is persistence of the symptoms after 3 weeks of therapy (see below) or if there is recurrence of symptoms. The orthopaedist will confirm the diagnosis and will look for anatomical abnormalities that predispose to this condition (see below). Also, an X-ray (indicated when symptoms are prolonged or recurrent) of the leg in the case of shin splints will occasionally show irregular bone formation of the tibia or fibula as a result of periostitis. A radionuclide bone scan is more sensitive than an X-ray in the diagnosis of shin splints and may be necessary if the diagnosis is uncertain. A positive bone scan shows increased uptake of radionuclide by the tibia, fibula, or interosseous membrane.

Treatment and Prognosis

Ice packs should be applied several times a day for 15 minutes at a time in order to reduce swelling and inflammation. In severe cases, the patient should avoid, for several weeks, the exercise that has precipitated the problem. The use of an elastic wrap on the lower leg provides some comfort, and the prescription of analgesic agents, such as enteric-coated aspirin, 650 mg four times a day, or Tylenol, 650 mg four times a day, will help to control the discomfort. Nonsteroidal anti-inflammatory agents also are very effective (see Chapter 70 for a full discussion of NSAIDs).

Acute shin splints should resolve with rest in 3 weeks; and, after this, conditioning is necessary before the patient can return to his sport. Stretching (see below, "Stretching Exercises") must be stressed in the therapy of this condition, and if symptoms persist, formal evaluation of foot and lower extremity biomechanics is indicated. The syndrome rarely recurs if conditioning has been correct.

Prevention

Prevention of this problem requires stretching exercises before physical activity (see below), running, or walking on soft level surfaces, and use of proper shoes (Chapter 102). An orthotic device may also be prescribed by an orthopaedist or podiatrist if hyperpronation of the feet or excessive tibial rotation is present. These also will be helpful in preventing recurrences.

Compartment Syndromes

Definition and Mechanism of Injury

There are two compartments in the leg that are prone to injury and subsequent swelling: the anterior (tibial) compartment and the lateral (peroneal) compartment. The anterior compartment syndrome is also called lateral shin splints and occurs when an athlete runs to excess on his toes or on a hill, or runs with shoes that have a sole that is too flexible. Activity can cause muscles to hypertrophy, and in addition repeated contraction can cause tissue edema. These factors lead to overswelling in the compartment, and blood supply to muscles and nerves can be compromised. This causes

the symptoms during exercise and can lead to permanent damage.

Compartment syndromes are usually seen in competitive runners, and they are much less common than shin splints.

Symptoms and Signs

Anterior Compartment Syndrome. The patient notices pain in the extensor muscles of the leg and in the lower leg, ankle, and foot. Discomfort usually occurs during or just after exercise. Examination reveals tenderness and often swelling of the anterior compartment, which is located over the midlateral aspect of the lower leg (Fig. 67.8, site B). Weakness of toe extensors and ankle dorsiflexors can also be seen.

Lateral Compartment Syndrome. In this situation the pain is located in the posterolateral aspect of the ankle above and behind the lateral malleolus (Fig. 67.8, site C); this is the area where the peroneal tendons are located. Frequently the patient feels as if his ankle has "given out." This syndrome is caused by excessive pronation of the foot (flat foot) and ankle (eversion) in runners with hypermobile ankles (weak ankles).

Treatment and Prognosis

Initially, ice should be applied for 15 minutes several times a day, and the patient must rest from exercise for 3 to 4 weeks. Anti-inflammatory agents are very helpful in controlling the inflammatory response. An anti-inflammatory agent with a rapid onset of action is suggested: naproxen (Naprosyn), 375 to 500 mg two times a day, or piroxicam (Feldene), 20 mg once a day, are both effective. If cost is a factor, enteric-coated aspirin is recommended, although it takes 7 to 10 days at a dose of 3 to 4 g/day to achieve an anti-inflammatory effect. Once symptoms subside, the patient should condition himself before returning to full exercise. This conditioning requires pre-exercise stretching (see below, "Stretching Exercises"), especially of the muscles that are involved, and then gradual return to running. The patient should have well-designed running shoes (see Chapter 102), should avoid toe running, and should always run on a level surface.

In the management of the lateral compartment syndrome an orthopaedist or podiatrist should be consulted to evaluate the use of an orthotic device or heel wedge to prevent hyperpronation, which predisposes to recurrence of the problem.

The prognosis for patients with either of these compartment syndromes is excellent provided the patient is properly conditioned. If symptoms persist, pressure elevation within the compartment can become a chronic and persistent problem and fasciotomy may be required.

Differential Diagnosis

Should symptoms not respond within a 7- to 10-day period, an X-ray of the area should be obtained to rule out other causes, such as a stress fracture or osteoid osteoma. A compartment syndrome also can be confused initially with thrombophlebitis, cellulitis, or vascular insufficiency, and these should all be investigated by means of serial observations and appropriate specific tests when indicated.

Prevention

Prevention of compartment syndromes requires stretching exercises (see below) before running, especially of the musculature involved in each of the compartments, and the use of good quality running gear, often including orthotics.

PROBLEMS OF THE ANKLE AND FOOT

Injuries of the Ankle Joints

Ankle Structure and Function

The ankle joint consists of articulations between the distal tibia and fibula, which form an arch, or mortice, and the talus, which fits into the mortice (see Fig. 67.9). The talus fits tightly into the mortice during dorsiflexion of the foot and is relatively mobile during plantar flexion. The stability of the ankle is provided by the various ligaments shown schematically in Figure 67.9.

Mechanism of Injury

Ankle injuries occur when there is sudden stress on one or more of the supporting ligaments. Such injuries

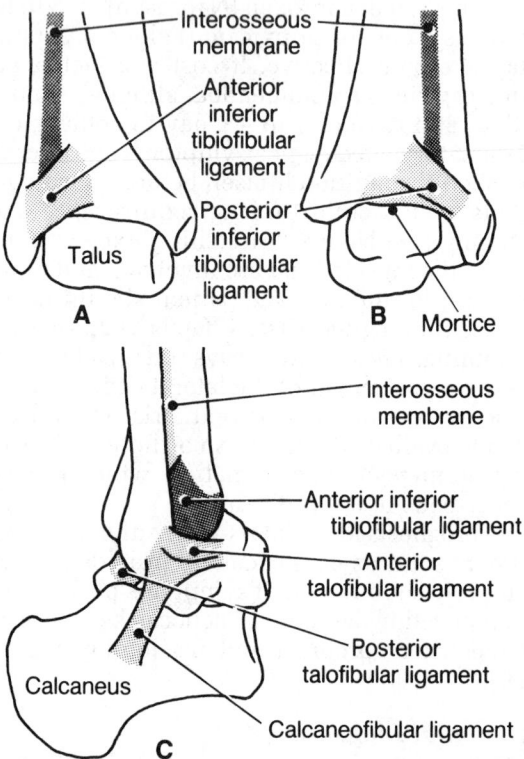

Figure 67.9. Distal tibiofibular joint and tibiotalar joint. *A.* Anterior view. *B.* Posterior view. *C.* Lateral view. (From Ramamurti CP, Tinker RV: *Orthopaedics in Primary Care.* Baltimore, Williams & Wilkins, 1979.)

may occur during vigorous activity or as a consequence of inadvertently stepping onto an uneven surface or off an unnoticed curb's edge, etc. Figures 67.10 and 67.11 illustrate schematically the spectrum of ankle ligament injuries and the stresses that cause them. The grades of ligament injury are discussed above (see "Problems of the Knee").

Signs and Symptoms

The patient usually can recall the position of the foot and whether there was a sensation or sound of tearing at the ankle. Immediate pain is noted, and if there has been a sprain, the patient will be aware of instability with weight bearing. Swelling over the injured ligament occurs within 1 hour of the injury, and it may be followed later by diffuse swelling of the foot and by an ecchymosis if there has been a significant ligament tear.

Examination of the strained or sprained ankle reveals marked tenderness over the injured ligament(s), made worse by replicating the stress that led to the injury (most commonly inversion of the foot). If there is not tense swelling, joint instability (e.g., obvious looseness or tilting of the talus with inversion of the foot) can be demonstrated when there has been a significant ligament tear. When the ankle cannot be easily manipulated to test for instability, a stress X-ray, under block anesthesia if needed, provides definitive diagnosis of severe sprain (see example, Fig. 67.12).

Treatment, Prognosis, and Prevention

Promptly after injury, the ankle should be immobilized (no walking, elastic bandage), ice packs (or ice water immersion) should be used for 10 to 15 minutes, and the leg should be elevated. If examination suggests that the injury represents a grade I (see above) or minor sprain (i.e., only modest pain, tenderness, and swelling, and no obvious instability), the ankle can be managed with an elastic bandage (used for 1 to 3 weeks), rest and elevation whenever possible, use of a cane for partial weight bearing, and gradual return to normal activities over 2 to 4 weeks. The technique and instructions for wrapping the ankle with an elastic bandage are shown in Figure 67.13.

If there is marked pain, swelling, or instability, it is likely that the patient has a significant (grade II or III) sprain (see above) of one or more ligaments, or, in the case of an eversion injury, an avulsion fracture (see Figs. 67.10 and Figs. 67.11). Referral to an emergency room or an orthopaedic surgeon's office for definitive diagnosis and management is indicated. For these patients, treatment consists of immobilization with a rigid ankle splint for 3 to 6 weeks and no weight bearing (i.e., use of a crutch) for 2 weeks, followed by progressive return to weight bearing. In order to assure optimal long-term outcome, convalescence from a significant ankle sprain should be planned and supervised by an orthopaedic surgeon. For severe injuries and for instability that does not improve with con-

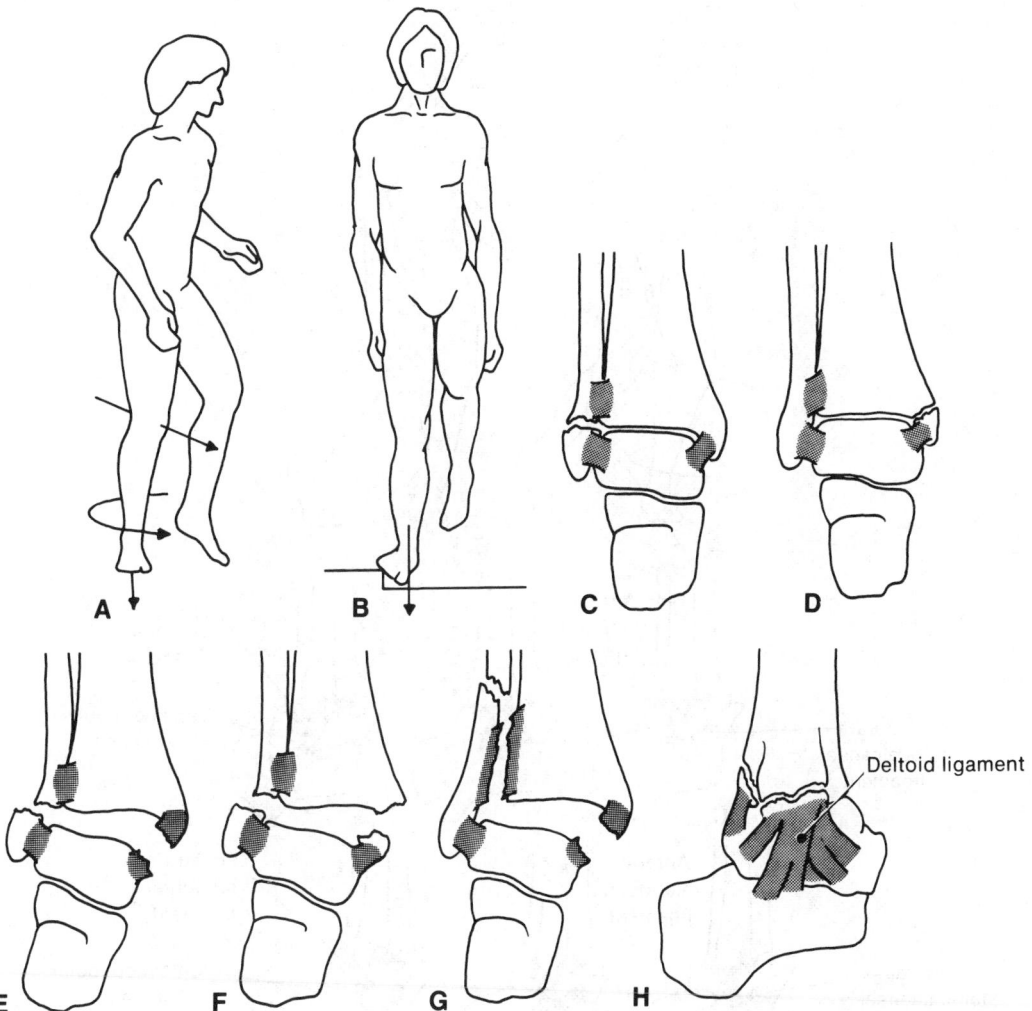

Figure 67.10. Pronation injuries of the ankle. *A* and *B*. Modes of injury. *A*. Extremity rotates internally on the fixed foot. *B*. The foot is forced into pronation by weight taken on the lateral aspect of the forefoot. *C* and *D*. Brief forces of lesser severity may fracture a mal- leoius without tearing a ligament. *E* through *G*. Forces of greater severity will destroy the mortice in one of three ways. *H*. When forward displacement of the tibia accompanies severe pronation forces, the posterior margin of the tibial articular surface may be fractured as well.

servative management, surgical realignment or repair may be necessary.

Prevention

Recurrent ankle sprain is common. Muscle rehabilitation and proprioceptive training are important for full return to function. Proprioceptive training can aid in regaining agility and in return of normal strength. Exercises consist of several positioning tasks for the foot: inversion and eversion resistance with surgical tubing and sliding on a teeter-totter are two examples. There are also commercially made teeter boards to improve ankle agility. Referral to a sports medicine physical therapist is appropriate for patients progressing slowly after ankle injuries. The optimal method for preventing recurrent injury, especially for an athlete with lax ankle joint(s), is to tape the ankle before engaging in exercise involving running. Alternatively, the patient can use a commercially available elastic ankle support whenever he exercises; these supports permit full range of motion but prevent the foot from falling into excessive inversion when it is not touching the ground (9).

Achilles Tendinitis

Definition and Mechanism of Injury

Achilles tendinitis is inflammation of the heel tendon and surrounding tissue and is due to overuse. The problem is most often caused by repetitive stretching of the tendon when the athlete is not properly conditioned. However, even with good conditioning it occurs in athletes who run on hills or who wear shoes with rigid soles. Furthermore, structural abnormalities such as tibia vara (bowlegged deformity), tight hamstring and calf muscles, a cavus foot (high arched foot often with claw toes), and a varus (inverted) heel deformity predispose to Achilles tendinitis. Initially, the peritendon (loose soft connective tissue surrounding the tendon) is inflamed, but in chronic cases the ten-

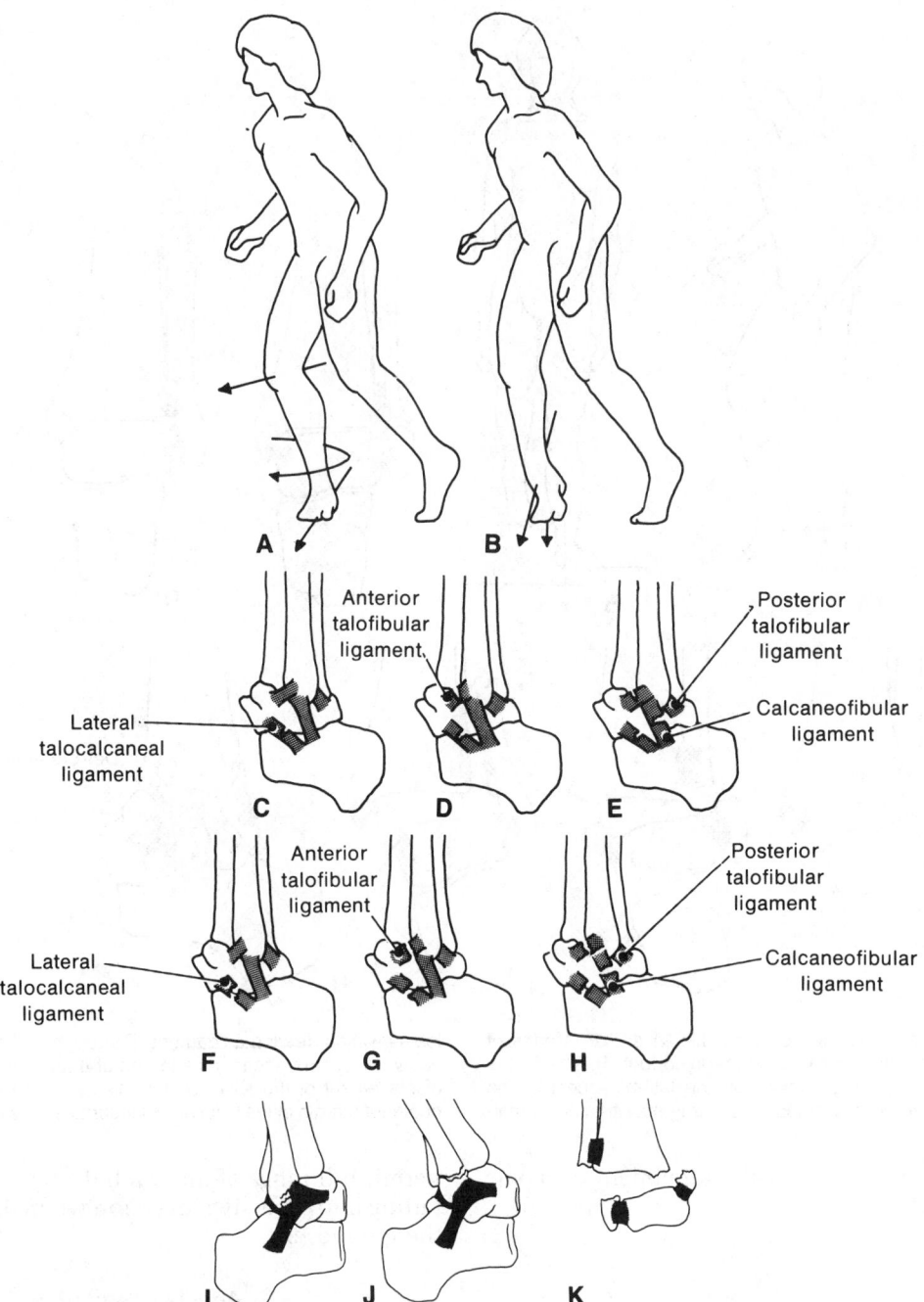

Figure 67.11. Supination injuries to the ankle. *A* and *B*. Modes of injury. *A*. Extremity rotates externally on the fixed foot. *B*. Plantarflexed foot is forced into supination. *C* through *E*. Sequence of injuries. Lateral talocalcaneal ligament (*C*) is injured before the anterior talofibular (*D*), which is injured before the calcaneofibular (*E*). *F* through *H*. When the injuring force is sufficient, the ligaments will tear completely and in the same sequence. *I* through *K*. Rather than tear the lateral ligaments, the injuring force may avulse a flake of fibula (*I*), or fracture off the end of the fibula (*J*), or fracture off both the end of the fibula and the medial malleolus (*K*).

don itself undergoes mucoid degeneration with the formation of longitudinal fissures and often nodule formation in the degenerate tendon.

This problem is commonly seen in recreational athletes, as well as in more serious runners.

Symptoms and Signs

The athlete with this problem notices a burning sensation in the heel, usually early during a run, which then lessens or disappears completely as running progresses. The discomfort often recurs upon completion of the run, in which case it is often more severe. Occasionally, a runner may note heel pain soon after awakening from sleep, which then subsides with daily activities.

On examination there is local or diffuse tenderness in the Achilles tendon; and, when the condition is chronic, there may be a tender nodule in the tendon, crepitus, and swelling.

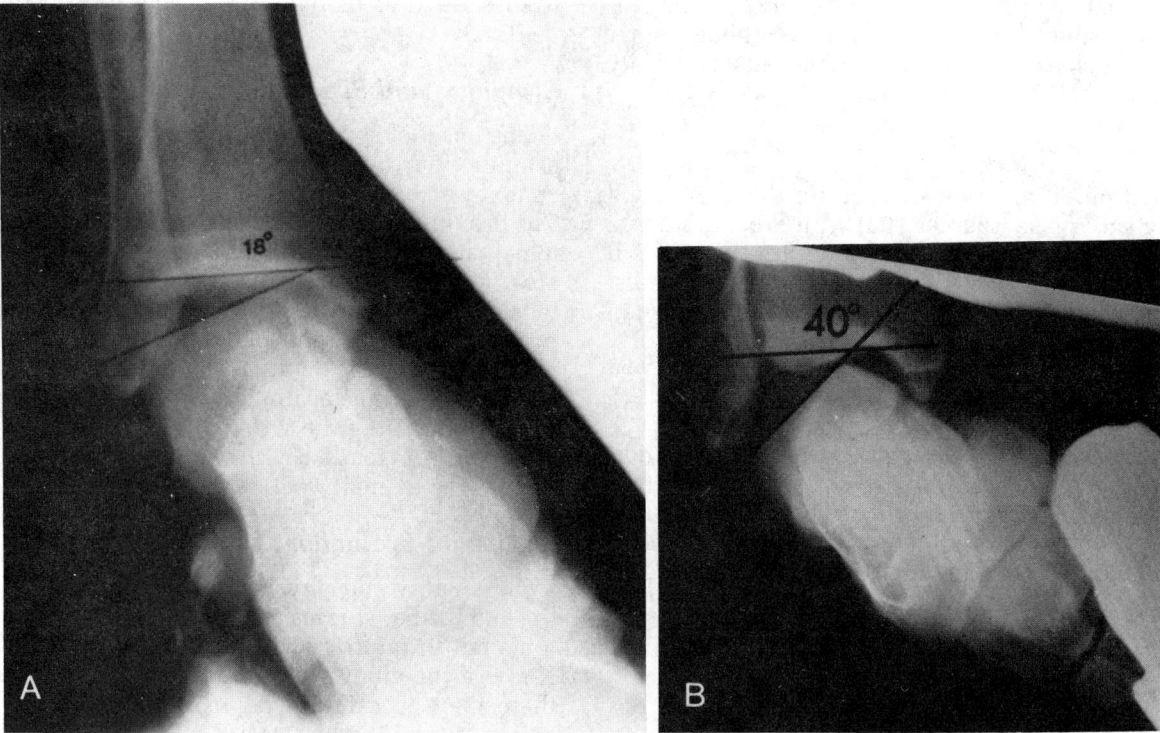

Figure 67.12. Examples of talar tilt. *A.* 15 to 20°. Complete single ligament tear with partial or complete injury to second ligament. *B.* Greater than 25°. Double ligament injury requiring more intensive treatment. (From Scott NW, Nicholas JA (eds): *Principles of Sports Medicine.* Baltimore, Williams & Wilkins, 1984.)

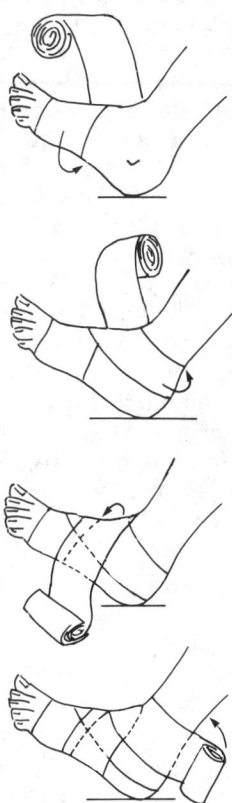

Figure 67.13. Technique for wrapping the ankle.

Treatment and Prognosis

The application of an ice pack to the area for 15 minutes several times a day will provide comfort and reduce swelling. Analgesic agents, such as enteric-coated aspirin, 650 mg four times a day, or acetaminophen, 650 mg four times a day, for several days will help to control the discomfort. Nonsteroidal anti-inflammatory drugs also are very effective (see Chapter 70 for a full discussion of NSAIDs). The runner should rest for several days, then reduce his running mileage and avoid hills until symptoms have been absent for 10 to 14 days. Exercises that gently stretch the tendon are important to condition the runner (see below) and to prevent recurrences. If symptoms persist, a rest from exercise for a period of 3 to 4 weeks or longer may be necessary to permit healing. Local injection of corticosteroids into the Achilles tendon must be avoided as this can weaken the tendon and cause a rupture. (Achilles tendinitis, if chronic, may lead to increased risk of rupture.)

In resistant cases, physical therapy, especially ultrasound, is helpful. In addition, when the syndrome is severe, splinting or casting of the ankle joint and the use of crutches are necessary to immobilize the Achilles tendon. In mild cases, with initial treatment and then proper conditioning, the prognosis is excellent. If the condition does not respond to therapy within 1 to 2 weeks, an orthopaedic consultation should be obtained since occasionally surgery is necessary. If surgery must be performed, it is unlikely that the athlete will be able to return to running, although other exercises, such as swimming or cycling, may be readily performed.

Prevention

Prevention of this problem requires the use of good running shoes (see Chapter 102) with flexible soles, a well-molded Achilles pad, and a rigid heel wedge. If the runner has a cavus foot (see above) an orthopaedist or a podiatrist should be consulted about the use of an orthotic device.

Plantar Fasciitis (Heel Spur)

Plantar fasciitis or "heel spur syndrome" is the most common cause of heel pain; it occurs most often in people who hike or run, but it may also occur in individuals who are not athletic. The name "heel spur syndrome" derives from the finding of a bone spur on X-ray of the calcaneus, but it is unlikely that this spur causes the symptoms in most patients. This problem is fully discussed in Chapter 102.

Retrocalcaneal Bursitis

Inflammation of the bursae that overlie the calcaneus (heel bone) may produce symptoms similar to those of Achilles tendinitis. Bursitis of the heel affects runners, but it may also occur at the upper border of the area just anterior to the Achilles tendon and just superior to the calcaneus, when tight-fitting shoes rub the heel with ordinary walking. On examination, there is focal tenderness confined to the calcaneus. Heel bursitis is managed with rest, properly fitted shoes, and, in runners, a heel pad (see Chapter 102).

PROBLEMS OF THE ELBOW

Lateral Epicondylitis (Tennis Elbow)

Definition and Mechanism of Injury

The term "tennis elbow" refers to inflammation in the region of the lateral epicondyle of the humerus at the origin of the common extensor muscles; it is a common exercise-related syndrome. It is caused by activities that combine excessive pronation and supination of the forearm with an extended wrist. Although the mechanism by which tennis elbow is produced is not known, the actual cause of pain may be due to radiohumeral synovitis or bursitis, tendinitis of the common extensor origin, traumatic epicondylitis or periostitis of the lateral epicondyle, or entrapment by scarring of a branch of the radial nerve in this region. Figure 67.14 identifies important structures of the elbow and provides an orientation to the common conditions seen there.

This problem is quite common in individuals performing activities such as tennis, badminton, and bowling, as well as with many non-sports-related activities, such as using a screwdriver or a wrench repetitively.

Symptoms and Signs

The onset of symptoms is usually gradual. Physical examination reveals tenderness over the lateral epicondyle or over the radiohumeral joint (Fig. 67.14). The proximal common extensor muscle is often tender to palpation and, on occasion, there is swelling in this area. The elbow usually has a normal flexion and extension, although the latter may sometimes be temporarily painful. Supination (palms up) and, especially, pronation (palms down) of the arm may be painful if they are performed against resistance. Pain can be elicited by stretching the wrist extensors by holding the elbow fully extended with the forearm pronated and the wrist maximally palmar flexed (Fig. 67.15).

Additional Evaluation

The history and physical examination are diagnostic, and further studies are not indicated unless symptoms fail to improve with treatment. In that case, an X-ray of the elbow should be obtained; on occasion, there may be calcium deposits noted at the lateral epicondyle of the humerus.

Treatment and Prognosis

The painful arm should initially be immobilized in a sling or, if symptoms are severe, immobilized in a long arm splint with the wrist held in dorsiflexion to rest the extensor tendons. Enteric-coated aspirin or acetaminophen or other analgesic agents will help to control symptoms. If mild analgesics are inadequate, a rapidly acting anti-inflammatory agent such as naproxen (Naprosyn) or piroxicam (Feldene) as described above (see also Chapter 70 for a full discussion of NSAIDs) may be prescribed. The injection of the area at the point of tenderness with a mixture of 3 ml of 1 to 2% lidocaine and 1 ml of glucocorticoid suspension (such as Aristocort or Kenalog) followed by the use of a sling for 1 or 2 weeks often provides dramatic relief of pain. A second injection may be repeated in approximately 3 weeks if symptoms fail to improve or if they recur during this period.

The prognosis is quite variable and depends to a large extent on the patient's activities. Tennis elbow may recur even in patients who are conscientious about their activity. If symptoms recur or if they fail to respond promptly to treatment, an orthopaedic consultation is indicated. Surgery may occasionally be required (7). The type of surgery depends on the problem, and occasionally a return to the vigorous activity that precipitated the problems may not be possible.

Prevention

Prevention of this problem requires conditioning of the muscle groups in the forearm and wrist through an exercise program. This program often needs to be specialized, and a physical therapist should be con-

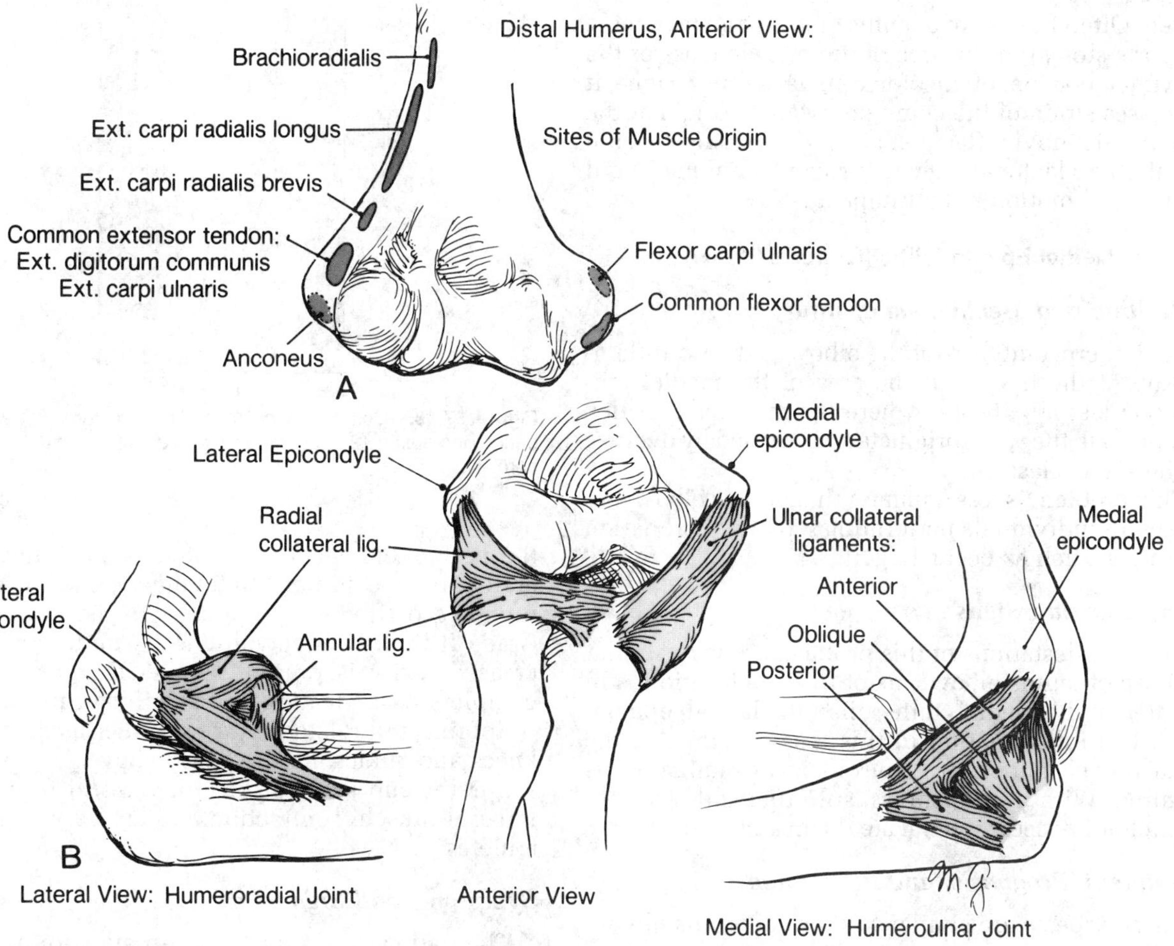

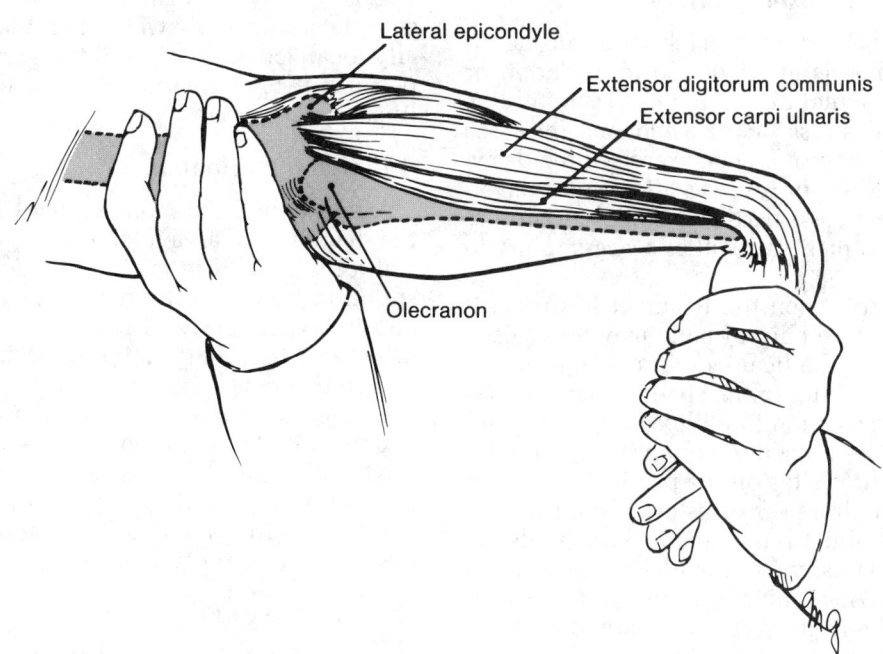

Brachioradialis

Ext. carpi radialis longus

Ext. carpi radialis brevis

Common extensor tendon:
Ext. digitorum communis
Ext. carpi ulnaris

Anconeus

Distal Humerus, Anterior View:

Sites of Muscle Origin

Flexor carpi ulnaris

Common flexor tendon

A

Lateral Epicondyle

Radial
collateral lig.

Lateral
epicondyle

Annular lig.

Medial
epicondyle

Ulnar collateral
ligaments:

Anterior

Oblique

Posterior

Medial
epicondyle

B

Lateral View: Humeroradial Joint

Anterior View

Medial View: Humeroulnar Joint

Figure 67.14. Important structures of the elbow.

Lateral epicondyle

Extensor digitorum communis

Extensor carpi ulnaris

Olecranon

Figure 67.15. Test for tennis elbow. The wrist is extended against resistance from a fully flexed position and the patient will notice pain at the lateral epicondyle. This usually mimics the patients symptoms if the diagnosis is correct.

sulted. Often the use of a tennis elbow strap (available at sports stores) in the area of the muscle mass of the proximal portion of the forearm is helpful since it decreases strain of the common extensor origin at the lateral epicondyle. Racquet size, weight, and tension can also be a factor along with proper technique (avoid using wrist motion at ball impact).

Medial Epicondylitis (Golfer's Elbow)

Definition and Mechanism of Injury

Medial epicondylitis of the elbow is due to inflammation of the tissues in the area of the medial epicondyle (see Fig. 67.14) where the muscles that flex and pronate the wrist originate. It is caused by overuse of these muscles.

This problem is less common than tennis elbow and is seen in individuals performing repetitive pronation exercises, such as occur in golf.

Symptoms and Signs

The manifestations of this problem are very similar to those of tennis elbow except that the location is in the area of the medial, rather than the lateral, epicondyle. The inflammation in this area can involve the ulnar nerve, so a careful neurological examination is required. With ulnar neuritis, splinting and rest with prompt orthopaedic referral are the treatment of choice.

Treatment, Prognosis, and Prevention

These aspects are similar to those of tennis elbow.

MISCELLANEOUS SPRAINS AND AVULSION FRACTURES

Definition and Mechanism of Injury

A *strain* is defined as overstretching a muscle although it sometimes is applied also to a tendon or ligament, without actual disruption of tissue. Strains occur during mild stress—e.g., when one overuses muscle groups that have not been exercised regularly. The pain of muscle strain resolves after 1 or 2 days.

A *sprain* is defined as a partial or complete rupture of the fibers of a ligament, as well as a stress injury to the joint capsule.

Avulsion fracture. When the ligament is strong, it does not rupture, but a chip of bone may be avulsed from the insertion of the ligament. These injuries are most common around the ankle, knee, elbow, and fingers. Violent muscle action in athletes, especially adolescents, may avulse a traction epiphysis (apophysis), usually at one of three sites on the pelvis: (*a*) anterior superior iliac spine from sartorius avulsion, (*b*) anterior inferior iliac spine from rectus femoris avulsion, and (*c*) ischial tuberosity from avulsion of the hamstring (Fig. 67.16). Also, injuries to the joint capsules and ligaments of the fingers are particularly common.

As described for ligament injuries above, strains and sprains are classified as grade I, grade II, or grade III depending on the amount of fiber involvement and

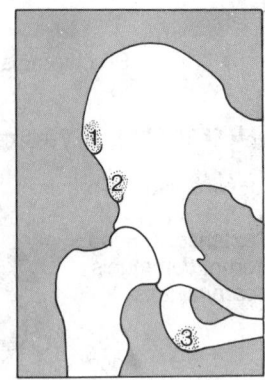

Figure 67.16. Common sites of avulsion fracture: (*1*) anterior superior iliac spine, (*2*) anterior inferior iliac spine, and (*3*) ischial tuberosity.

the amount of instability created. Grade I injuries generally involve minor stretching or tearing of small numbers of fibers. Symptoms are usually minimal. Grade II injuries involve more tissue tearing and increased laxity is present. Grade III injuries involve complete tissue tearing and significant instability.

Sprains and related injuries of the ligaments of the knees and ankles are discussed above.

Sprains and avulsion fractures result from sudden forceful muscle contraction and are very common in athletes.

Symptoms and Signs

The hallmark of a sprain or an avulsion fracture is pain in the area of the injury. Physical examination reveals swelling and stiffness of the involved joint with increased pain as the patient attempts to use it. The joint may be unstable if the ligament rupture is complete. Maximal swelling and tenderness are usually localized at the area of the sprain or fracture, especially if it is superficial as in the ankle, knee, or finger.

Additional Evaluation

X-rays of an injured area must be done to establish the diagnosis of an avulsion fracture.

If joint instability is found on examination, a consultation from an orthopaedic surgeon should be requested. Also, stress X-rays, especially of the ankle, knee, and finger, are often done by the orthopaedic surgeon under either local or general anesthesia to evaluate the degree of instability of the joints.

Surgical intervention by the orthopaedic surgeon to repair joint instability is occasionally necessary, especially in injuries in the area of the ankle and knee; even after surgery, an athlete will often not be able to return to the activity that resulted in the injury.

Treatment and Prognosis

The initial treatment of sprains and/or avulsion fractures consists of immobilization of the area with a splint, elevation, and application of ice for approximately 15 minutes several times a day to decrease swelling, and the prescription of analgesics such as aspirin or acetaminophen alone or in combination with codeine, 30 to 60 mg every 4 to 6 hours. If the injury is in the area of the ankle or knee, the patient must keep his weight off the injured joint by the use of crutches (see above). It is important to immobilize a finger for no more than 3 weeks and then only in the position of function, in order to avoid permanent stiffness of the joints (Fig. 67.17).

The prognosis for sprains and avulsion fractures is quite variable and depends to a large extent on the location of the injury; but with proper treatment and with subsequent conditioning of the patient, the outcome is generally good.

Prevention

The prevention of sprains and avulsion fractures requires proper conditioning, especially by the performance of stretching exercises (see below) before exertion and the use of proper foot gear and protective equipment.

STRESS FRACTURES

Definition and Mechanism of Injury

A stress fracture is a crack, which is sometimes minute, that can occur in almost any bone that has been repetitively subjected to impact. The most common sites of stress fractures are the metatarsal shafts, especially the second and third metatarsals, the distal fibula, the proximal tibia, and the symphysis pubis. Stress fractures may, however, occur in other bones, such as the lumbar vertebrae, the sacroiliac joint, the distal femur, the femoral neck (4), the tarsal navicula (13), the distal aspect of the tibia, the lateral malleolus, and the pubis ramus (8).

Stress fractures occur most commonly from walking or running, usually when an athlete has tried to do too much too fast, has used improper shoes, or has exercised on hard surfaces. Stress fractures occur in both poorly conditioned individuals and in highly conditioned athletes.

Symptoms and Signs

A patient who has sustained a stress fracture notices the gradual onset of aching of the affected bone during or just after exercising. Examination reveals localized tenderness and occasional swelling.

Additional Evaluation

The diagnosis depends on the symptoms and signs since X-rays of the affected area are usually normal at first; only after 2 to 4 weeks (sometimes longer) they may show bone resorption at the fracture site and/or the formation of callus (new bone). A radionuclide bone scan is positive, however, before the fracture can be identified on X-ray, and the scan may remain positive for up to 2 years after the injury. Therefore, a bone scan is indicated if symptoms persist for more than a few weeks and X-rays are negative.

Differential Diagnosis

Tibial stress fractures may be confused with pes anserinus bursitis, shin splints, and bone tumors, especially osteoid osteoma. If there is uncertainty about the correct diagnosis, a consultation should be requested from an orthopaedist.

Treatment and Prognosis

The treatment of stress fractures involves complete immobilization of the injured part in a splint. If the injury is in a lower extremity, the patient should not bear weight on it. The injured part should also be elevated, and ice should be applied initially for approximately 15 minutes several times a day until the swelling subsides, which usually occurs in 24 to 36 hours. After the swelling has subsided, heat may be applied for 15 minutes several times a day; but this should be discontinued if the discomfort is made more severe, which occasionally occurs. Pain should be controlled with aspirin or acetaminophen alone or combined with codeine, 30 to 60 mg every 4 to 6 hours as needed.

Metatarsal stress fractures should be treated initially with a cast, which should be left on 4 to 8 weeks. (If the physician is unfamiliar with the application of a short leg cast, referral to an orthopaedist is indicated.) Stress fractures of the tibia and fibula require more prolonged periods of immobilization and may require a cast for up to 12 weeks or longer. All patients with suspected stress fractures of the tibia or fibula should be seen by an orthopaedist. Patients who can bear weight without symptoms may be treated with rest of the injured extremity and avoidance of impact loading. The risk in stress fracture treatment is that the fracture will become a complete fracture and in areas such as the tibial shaft, femoral neck, and femoral shaft, these stress fractures can require surgical stabilization if they become complete.

With proper treatment and then appropriate conditioning, the prognosis is excellent and most patients will be able to return to normal sports activities. Occasionally bone grafting is required to obtain healing.

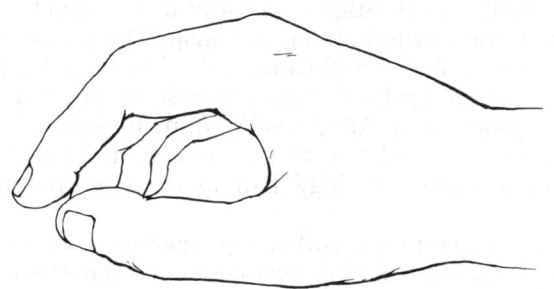

Figure 67.17. Position of function of fingers.

Prevention

Prevention of stress fractures requires proper conditioning with pre-exercise stretching exercises, proper footwear, and avoidance of hard surfaces and of too rapid an acceleration of physical activity.

STRETCHING EXERCISES

It has been pointed out that the occurrence (and recurrence) of some of the problems described in this chapter can be prevented by several measures—that is, selecting good shoes (see Chapter 102 for a description), not increasing the amount of stress on the musculoskeletal system too rapidly, and stretching the major muscle groups of the lower extremity before participating in sports. The four stretching exercises that should be practiced routinely are illustrated in Figure 67.18. Each exercise should be done for both sides for 15 to 30 seconds at a time for a few minutes before engaging in sports activities.

ARTHROSCOPY

Arthroscopic technique has progressed rapidly over the last 10 years and has greatly improved methods of diagnosis and treatment of joint problems.

Arthroscopic evaluation can now be carried out quite effectively in the knee, ankle, shoulder, elbow, and wrist. Surgical techniques through the arthroscope often enable the orthopaedist to avoid opening of the joint (arthrotomy). When arthrotomy is required, recovery time, rehabilitation, and complications are increased tremendously. To evaluate the interior of a joint, the arthroscope is fitted with fiberoptic light cables to illuminate and multiple lenses to identify and magnify all intra-articular structures.

The knee is the joint where arthroscopy has had its greatest advances, both diagnostically and therapeutically. Arthroscopy of the knee is indicated for diagnostic purposes in acute injury or in chronic knee pain where diagnosis has been difficult. The ligaments, articular cartilage, synovium, bony surfaces, and menisci can be accurately evaluated. Often meniscal injuries can be treated with partial meniscectomy or repair arthroscopically. Ligament reconstruction is performed with arthroscopic assistance to decrease morbidity.

Also, the hip can be viewed arthroscopically—loose body removal and synovial biopsy have been performed in the hip. The joint capsule in both the hip and wrist are small and somewhat tight, but as instrumentation advances arthroscopy is expected to have a larger role in evaluating and treating problems in these joints.

The ankle has long been a difficult joint in which to diagnose intra-articular pathology since the joint capsule is smaller and tighter. Nevertheless an experienced arthroscopic surgeon can adequately evaluate and treat various ankle problems. Chronic ankle pain has been treated effectively with arthroscopic synovectomy. Osteochondritis dessicans (transchondral talar

dome fractures), loose bodies, chondromalacia, rheumatological disorders, and infections have all been evaluated or treated in the ankle joint using arthroscopic methods. More recently, arthroscopic techniques have been applied to lateral instability and ankle fusions.

Arthroscopy has also been applied to the upper extremity in the shoulder, elbow, and wrist. In the shoulder joint, arthroscopy allows complete evaluation of the humeral head, glenoid, rotator cuff, anterior stabilizing structures, and subacromial space. Many athletes with vague shoulder complaints and nonspecific physical findings can be placed on proper rehabilitation or treatment programs after arthroscopic evaluation. Other areas where arthroscopy can be useful include the arthritides, dislocations, subluxations, loose bodies, rotator cuff lesions, labral tears, and frozen shoulders. Newer operative techniques have allowed subacromial decompression and anterior shoulder stabilization procedures to be performed arthroscopically. These procedures have reduced recovery time and postoperative rehabilitation dramatically since the musculature surrounding the shoulder (deltoid, pectoralis major, supraspinatus, infraspinatus) is not disrupted as it is with open techniques.

The elbow offers fewer diagnostic and therapeutic problems amenable to arthroscopic techniques. The ulnar, median, and radial nerves are in close proximity to the joint capsule, and anatomical knowledge is critical. The anterior and posterior compartments of the elbow can be evaluated with the arthroscope. The most common applications in the elbow are loose bodies or osteochondritic lesions or articular cartilage.

Arthroscopy of the wrist is also advancing, and patients with subtle carpal instabilities, chronic pain, and small chondral fractures have benefited from arthroscopic evaluation by skilled surgeons.

Arthroscopy is a surgical procedure and complications may occur. These complications include iatrogenic damage to intra- or extra-articular structures, hemarthrosis, thrombophlebitis, infection, synovial fistula, and instrument breakage (leaving intra-articular fragments).

There are many advantages to arthroscopic techniques, especially in the athlete. There is greatly reduced postoperative morbidity, and patients can often return to work or the field quickly. This is due to a decreased inflammatory response, smaller incisions, and decreased immobilization. Arthroscopy improves diagnostic capabilities, especially in the athlete with troublesome symptoms and a nonspecific physical examination. The complication rate, length of hospital stay, and even pain are often decreased compared with open procedures. Additionally, in many areas, the arthroscope provides a better view of intra-articular structures and pathology than open surgery provides.

Patient Experience. Arthroscopy may be accomplished using local, regional, or general anesthesia. The arthroscope is usually 3 to 5 mm in width and is inserted through a stab wound in the joint. A sterile solution is infused to irrigate

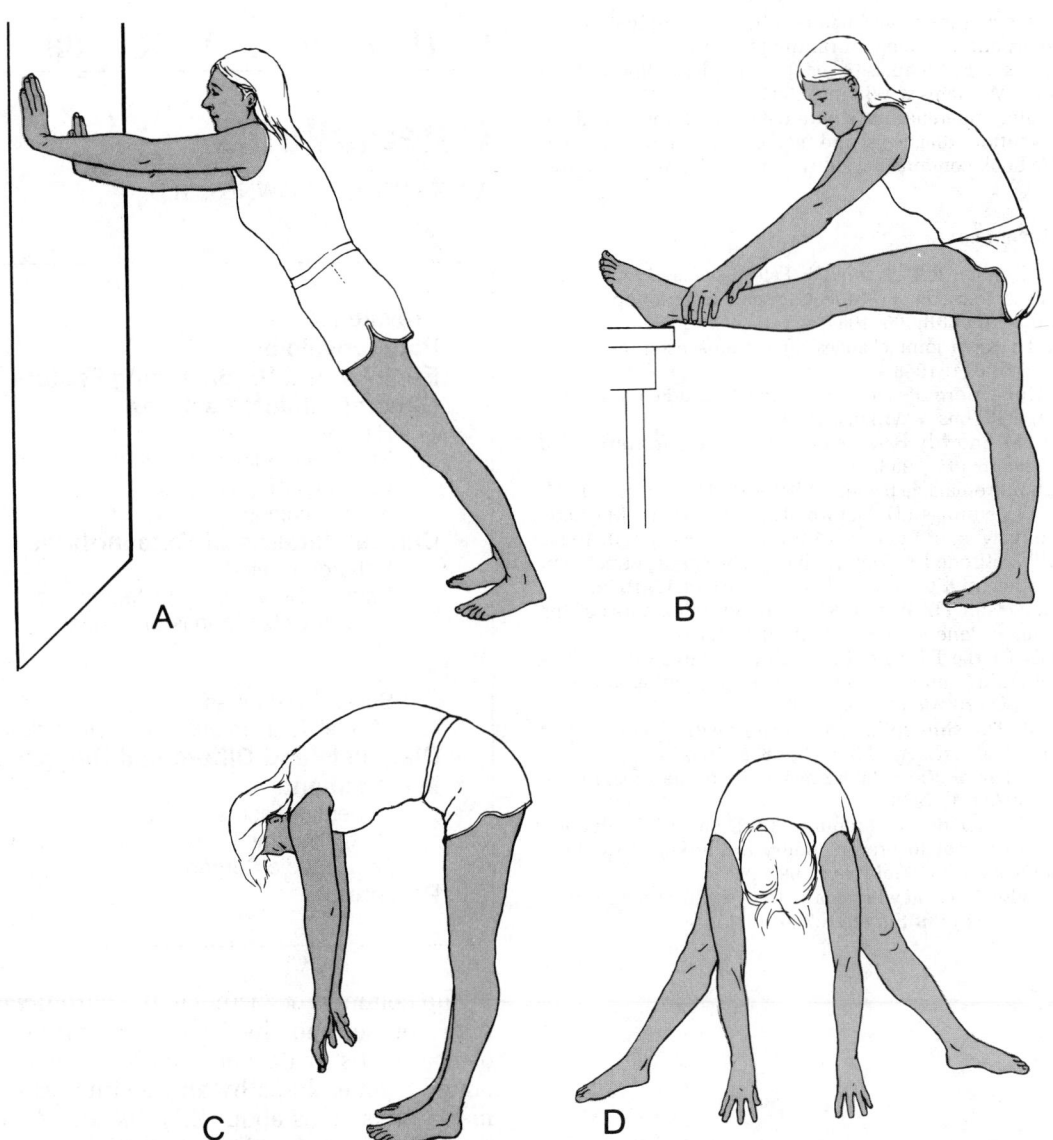

Figure 67.18. *A.* Stretch the Achilles tendon by leaning forward with the feet flat and placed at least 4 feet from the wall. *B.* Stretch the hamstring and gastrocnemius muscle groups by elevating the leg and bending forward as far as possible. *C.* Stretch the hamstring and back muscles by touching the toes slowly; bouncing should be avoided. *D.* Stretch the adductor muscle by gradually spreading the legs as far apart as possible; place the fingers on the floor for support.

and distend the joint. (Therefore in serious injury in which the joint capsule is disrupted, arthroscopy is difficult or even contraindicated because the fluid may dissect out of the joint into the tissue of the leg.) The procedure may be accomplished in 30 to 45 minutes. After the procedure the patient will need to rest the joint (and not bear weight) for 2 to 3 days. Mild analgesics for a few days are usually necessary to relieve discomfort.

General References

American Academy of Orthopaedic Surgeons: *Knee Braces—Seminar Report.* American Academy of Orthopaedic Surgeons, Chicago, 1985.

    A report that extensively reviews all types of knee braces—their indications, functions, and costs. Prepared by the Sports Medicine Committee of the AAOS.

Brody DM: Running injuries. *Ciba Clin Symp* 32:Nov 4, 1980.

    An excellent review of running injuries, including superb anatomical illustrations and a description of specific stretching exercises.

Crenshaw AH (ed): *Campbell's Operative Orthopaedics.* St Louis, CV Mosby, Co, 1987.

Fulkerson JP (ed): Patellofemoral Pain. *Orthoped Clin North Am* 17 (2):April 1985.

Hoppenfeld S: *Physical Examination of the Spine and Extremities.* New York, Appleton-Century-Crofts, 1976.

Hunter-Griffin, LY (ed): Overuse injuries. *Clin Sports Med* 6 (2): April 1987.

Minhoff J, Sherman OH (eds): Arthroscopy. *Clin Sports Med* 6(3):July 1987.

    A collection of review articles covering arthroscopic procedures in the knee, ankle, wrist, elbow, and shoulder.

Nicholas JA, Henshman EB (eds): *The Lower Extremity and Spine in Sports Medicine.* St Louis, CV Mosby, Co, 1986.

Paty JG: Diagnosis and treatment of musculoskeletal running injuries. *Semin Arth Rheum* 18 (1):August 1988.

Good review of the biomechanics, physical examination, injury types, and treatment of running injuries.

Scott WN, Nisonson B, Nicholas JA (eds): *Principles of Sports Medicine.* Baltimore, Williams & Wilkins, 1984.

An excellent reference book with detailed information about the prevention, diagnosis, and management of athletic injuries; the book contains a good section on the use of arthroscopy.

Specific References

1. Allen PR, Denhan RA, Swan AV: Late degenerative changes after meniscectomy. Factors affecting the knee after operation. *J Bone Joint Surg* 66B:666, 1984.
2. Fairbank TJ: Knee joint changes after meniscectomy. *J Bone Joint Surg* 30B:644, 1948.
3. Ficat RP, Hungerford DS: *Disorders of the Patello-Femoral Joint.* Baltimore, Williams & Wilkins, 1977.
4. Fullerton LR, Snowdy HA: Femoral neck stress fractures. *Am J Sports Med* 16:365, 1988.
5. Insall J: Chondromalacia patellae. *J Bone Joint Surg* 58A:1, 1976.
6. Jackson DW, Jennings LD, Maywood RM, Berger PE: Magnetic resonance imaging of the knee. *Am J Sports Med* 16:29, 1988.
7. Nirschl RP, Pettrone FA: Tennis elbow. The surgical treatment of lateral epicondylitis. *J Bone Joint Surg* 61A:832, 1979.
8. Pavlov H, Nelson TL, Warren RF, et al: Stress fractures of the pubic ramus. *J Bone Joint Surg* 64A:1020, 1982.
9. Rovene GD, Clarke TS, Yates CS, Burley K: Retrospective comparison of taping and ankle stabilizers in preventing ankle injuries. *Am J Sports Med* 16:228, 1988.
10. Slocum DB: The shin splint syndrome—medical aspects and differential diagnosis. *Am J Surg* 114:875, 1967.
11. Slocum DB, Larson RL: Rotatory instability of the knee. *J Bone Joint Surg* 50A:211, 1968.
12. Teitz CC, Henmarson BK, Krommal RA, Diehr PH: Evaluation of the use of braces to prevent injury to the knee in college football players. *J Bone Joint Surg* 69A:2, 1987.
13. Torg JS, Pavlov H, Cooley LH, et al: Stress fractures of the tarsal navicular. *J Bone Joint Surg* 64A:700, 1982.

C H A P T E R   68

Osteoarthritis

ALEXANDER S. TOWNES, M.D.

The common occurrence, the chronic and often benign course, and the lack of definitive treatment of osteoarthritis or degenerative joint disease have generated a general apathy and disinterest on the part of many physicians about this disease. A common attitude also among patients is that this form of arthritis is an inevitable consequence of aging and must be accepted as such. Advances in understanding of the pathophysiology of osteoarthritis, especially in the past decade, have accomplished a great deal in dispelling these undeserved attitudes. As a result a better perspective of the multiple etiological factors potentially involved in this disease and a better understanding of the clinical problems presented by patients with this disorder have developed.

Osteoarthritis is particularly important to the general physician who sees ambulatory adult patients. Estimates indicate that approximately half of all visits to physicians for joint disease are for this diagnosis. Osteoarthritis is the most common arthritis diagnosed in a general practice (22).

PREVALENCE

Prevalence of osteoarthritis increases with advancing age, beginning perhaps as early as the third decade of life and being almost ubiquitous as detected by radiography or by biochemical changes in articular cartilage in the seventh and eighth decades and beyond. It is fortunate and important, however, that clinical symptoms are not necessarily associated with structural changes, so that estimates of prevalence based on these findings exceed the magnitude of the clinical problem. Thus, symptoms and clinical findings of degenerative joint disease are not an inevitable accompaniment of aging. However, symptoms and findings are uncommon below age 35 and are more frequent above age 65, with perhaps as much as 30 to 40% of the population aged 65 and above having some symptoms related to this diagnosis. A recent survey of osteoarthritis of the knee in subjects aged 63 to 94 indicated an increasing prevalence of radiographic evidence of osteoarthritis with age to the level of 44% of subjects aged 80 or older and a higher proportion of symptomatic disease in women (11%) as compared with men (7%) (9).

PATHOPHYSIOLOGY

The pathogenesis of osteoarthritis is probably multifactorial (1); however, the final common pathway is believed to be injury to articular cartilage, which then undergoes a sequence of changes resulting eventually in loss of its proteoglycan matrix, cellular proliferation in attempted repair, release of enzymes with more destruction of all cartilage elements, and proliferation of subchondral bone (21). Changes are most severe in or may be confined entirely to areas of maximal stress on the articular cartilage, most striking in weight-bearing areas of the large joints. Although one hypothesis suggests a primary synovial lesion (12), most observers have concluded that the chronic synovitis that is found in more advanced cases of osteoarthritis is probably secondary to cartilage degeneration with secondary, usually mild inflammatory reaction to detritus shed into the joint cavity from this process (3, 28). A possible role for immune response to cartilage antigen has been suggested by the demonstration of antibodies to collagen in eluates of articular cartilage from patients with osteoarthritis (16). An important role of crystalline deposits of calcium pyrophosphate, hydroxyapatite, or basic calcium phosphates in the synovial inflammatory response or destructive arthropathy in certain patients, especially those with more advanced osteoarthritis, has been demonstrated (15) (see also Chapter 69). Remodeling and microfractures of subchondral bone with hardening and loss of ability to absorb stress as primary mechanisms in production of osteoarthritis have also been suggested (26).

Because there are no nerve fibers in articular cartilage, there are no symptoms due to early changes in the joints. There are multiple sources of pain, however, as the disease progresses. Periosteal irritation as a result of proliferating bone, denuded bone, compression of soft tissues by osteophytes in confined spaces, microfractures of subchondral bone, stress on ligaments as a result of loss of cartilage and joint incongruity, low grade synovitis, effusion, and spasm of surrounding muscles are all potential sources of pain in osteoarthritis.

ETIOLOGY AND PREDISPOSING FACTORS

The cause of osteoarthritis is not known. It is quite likely that there are multiple causes and many factors that may influence disease expression, some of which are listed in Table 68.1.

Because of multiple etiological mechanisms in the pathogenesis of osteoarthritis, the history should seek to determine specific factors that may be implicated in each patient. Heredity may be important, especially in development of Heberden's nodes (33) (see below). A family history may also draw attention of the patient to the benign occurrence of these bony enlargements in elderly family members and serve to reassure them about their course.

Obesity is perhaps an obvious factor, but its extent and duration are important in assessing potential damage to weight-bearing joints, especially the knees. Preceding trauma may be important in subsequent development of degenerative arthritis in a joint damaged by ligamentous instability, meniscal tear in the knee joint, etc. Traumatic episodes with sufficient damage to induce these abnormalities are likely to be severe enough to be recalled, for example, as severe "sprains" with swelling lasting several days or longer after a sports-related or other injury. Jogging is not known to predispose to osteoarthritis unless an injury has been sustained or pain, emanating from a joint, regularly results from the exercise (18, 19, 24). Prior

Table 68.1.
Factors Contributing to Development of Osteoarthritis

AGING
    Diminished proteoglycan aggregation
    Diminished resistance of cartilage to fatigue fracture
       (? defective collagen network)
    Decreased resiliency of soft tissues
    Loss of normal anatomical relationship (hip)
HEREDITY
    Heberden's nodes
    Primary generalized osteoarthritis
    Postural or developmental defects (e.g., scoliosis, slipped capital
       femoral epiphyses, Legg-Calvé-Perthes disease, etc.)
    Metabolic defects (ochronosis, Wilson's disease)
ABNORMAL DISTRIBUTION OF MECHANICAL STRESS
    Postural or developmental defects
    Joint instability or hypermobility
    Local incongruity of joint surfaces post-traumatic, after meniscec-
       tomy, prolonged immobilization
    Obesity (abnormal stress on knees due to adiposity)
EXCESSIVE REPETITIVE STRESS
    Occupational
    Sports related
    Associated with neuropathy
CRYSTALLINE DEPOSIT DISEASE
    Calcium pyrophosphate
    Hydroxyapatite
PREVIOUS INFLAMMATORY JOINT DISEASE
METABOLIC ABNORMALITIES
    Ochronosis
    Wilson's disease
    Acromegaly
    ? Diabetes mellitus

joint surgery with removal of a torn meniscus in the knee is also a predisposing factor to osteoarthritis of the knee. Repetitive stress of minor trauma may also predispose to development of osteoarthritis (e.g., in knees of basketball players) and may account for osteoarthritis in joints not commonly affected (e.g., elbows of baseball pitchers and elbows as well as shoulders of air hammer operators). Lifelong postural or mechanical defects also predispose to degenerative changes as the result of abnormal distribution of stress to the joint when force is applied. Because abnormalities such as varus or valgus deformities of the knees may also occur as a result of osteoarthritic damage to the joint, the history is important in determining which came first.

Osteoarthritis may also be associated with other disease states: preceding inflammatory arthritis; metabolic diseases, such as ochronosis, with deposition of metabolites in cartilage; diseases predisposing to chondrocalcinosis, such as hemochromatosis and hyperparathyroidism; and acromegaly. Diabetes mellitus may also predispose to osteoarthritis, although this association is less well documented.

GENERAL CLINICAL FEATURES

History

Characteristically there is involvement of only one or a few joints in osteoarthritis. Joints commonly affected and those usually spared are shown in Table 68.2. Because the presentations of patients may differ, depending upon the pattern of joints involved and predisposing factors, some of these presenting symptoms will be highlighted separately after a general discussion of the symptoms and findings in this disease.

Osteoarthritis usually begins insidiously and progresses slowly. Aching discomfort early in the course

characteristically increases in severity with use of the joint; therefore it tends to reach a peak after the activity of the day and is relieved by rest. Pain is often aching in character and may be difficult for the patient to localize precisely. It is usually felt in the areas surrounding the involved joint. However, it is important to remember that hip pain may be referred to the medial aspect of the thigh, the lateral portion of the buttock, or to the knee. Morning stiffness and stiffness after rest may be absent, or if present, last only 15 to 20 minutes or less, in contrast to a longer duration in inflammatory joint disease such as rheumatoid arthritis. However, in advanced disease stiffness may be more profound, and pain may occur at rest. When joint destruction is marked, the patient may be kept awake at night by the pain.

As the disease progresses, large pieces of degenerated cartilage may shed into the joint, producing loose bodies that may cause locking or giving away of the joint in addition to pain.

There are no systemic symptoms in osteoarthritis. This is an important negative feature of the history that helps to differentiate this disease from other forms of arthritis.

The influence of psychological factors on the level of pain and disability is an important consideration in evaluation and management of the patient with osteoarthritis. A recent study of patients with symptoms and objective clinical findings of osteoarthritis of the hip and knee demonstrated that psychological variables accounted for a far greater percentage of the variation observed both in functional impairment and in severity of pain than did objective estimates of disease severity (35). Thus in osteoarthritis as in other chronic diseases in which chronic pain may occur, it is essential in taking the history to learn as much as possible about the patient as an individual and about his environment in order to appropriately interpret findings and plan the most effective approach to treatment.

Physical Findings

Early in the disease there may be no physical findings. Most patients who present with symptoms will have some pain on passive motion of the involved joints or on motion against resistance. There is frequently a sense of crackling or crepitus as the joint is moved, probably due to joint surface incongruities and irregularities of opposing cartilaginous surfaces. Crepitus may be exaggerated by movement with weight bearing or by manual compression of the joint during movement (e.g., compression of the patella against the condyle of the femur when patellofemoral arthritis is present). In more advanced disease, joint motion may be limited and gross deformities may develop. Tenderness along the joint line is common but may be mild or absent. In contrast to most inflammatory joint diseases, soft tissue swelling is usually absent or minimal in osteoarthritis except in its most advanced stages. Bony enlargement and irregularity are common, especially in the hands at the distal interphalangeal joints

Table 68.2.
Distribution of Joint Involvement in Osteoarthritis

COMMONLY AFFECTED
  Hands:
    Distal interphalangeal (Heberden's nodes)
    Proximal interphalangeal (Bouchard's nodes)
    Carpometacarpal of the thumb (joints between first
      metacarpal and greater multangular and between greater multangular and navicular)
  Knees
  Hips
  Spine:
    Cervical
    Lumbar
    Thoracic
  Feet:
    Metatarsophalangeal (especially first)
USUALLY SPARED
  Ankles
  Hands:
    Metacarpophalangeal
    Carpometacarpal (except first)
  Wrists
  Elbows
  Shoulders

(Heberden's nodes) and less commonly in the proximal interphalangeal joints (Bouchard's nodes). Joint effusions are relatively infrequent compared with more inflammatory forms of joint disease. However, they may occur, especially in the knees. There is usually no detectable heat or redness over involved joints, although some warmth may be present as the disease progresses and chronic synovitis develops.

Physical examination of the patient with osteoarthritis should always include a careful evaluation of the neurological system and peripheral vascular system since disease in these systems may produce pain or limited motion in an extremity that may be erroneously attributed to osteoarthritis (see "Diagnosis and Differential Diagnosis").

Laboratory Findings

Osteoarthritis is characterized by normal laboratory tests unless it is associated with some other disease process. In particular acute phase reactants including the erythrocyte sedimentation rate (ESR) and the C-reactive protein are characteristically normal, in contrast to the inflammatory arthritides. Mild and transient elevation of ESR may occasionally be associated with the acute inflammatory events described below or may be due to intercurrent disease elsewhere.

Examination of synovial fluid is helpful when effusion is present in a large joint. Synovial fluid in osteoarthritis is usually of the noninflammatory type, i.e., with good viscosity, white blood cells <2000/mm^3, protein content <4 g/dl, glucose concentration approximately equal to a simultaneous serum glucose concentration, and a good mucin clot when mixed with acetic acid (see also Table 66.1). A more inflammatory fluid with elevated white cell count may occur especially when crystals of calcium pyrophosphate or hydroxyapatite are present (see Fig. 69.1 and Table 69.1).

X-ray Findings

Radiographic findings are important in the diagnosis and differential diagnosis of osteoarthritis since certain abnormalities are characteristic of this disorder. Therefore X-ray examination of the affected joints is indicated in the evaluation of most patients to confirm the diagnosis and to determine the extent of abnormalities present. However, it is important to point out that in early disease X-rays may be normal, and even with characteristic findings of joint narrowing and proliferation of subchondral bone with spur formation, symptoms may be absent. Hence, the importance of relating radiographic findings to the history and physical examination cannot be overemphasized. In general the more severe the radiographic changes, the more likely the patient is to have symptoms and findings of osteoarthritis. Radiographic findings from the earliest to the most advanced changes are listed in Table 68.3, and examples of X-rays are shown in Fig. 68.1.

Table 68.3.
X-Ray Findings in Osteoarthritis

EARLIEST
  No abnormality
EARLY
  Slight loss of articular cartilage thickness (narrowing of radiological joint space)
MODERATE
  Marginal osteophyte formation
LATE
  Loss of cartilage space (often focal in weight-bearing joints)
  Sclerosis of subchondral bone
  Subchondral cyst formation
  Loose bodies
  Subluxation or deformity

For evaluation of hands a single anteroposterior (AP) view of both hands is sufficient in most cases. Both hips can be visualized on a single AP film of the pelvis; more specific films may be required if an abnormality is detected or if findings do not correlate with the clinical picture. AP and lateral films are required for adequate evaluation of the knee joint. Special views of the patella ("skyline" view) may also be required to demonstrate the extent of patellofemoral arthritis. In evaluating the spine, AP, lateral, and oblique views are needed, the latter to visualize the neural foramina and the localization of nerve root compression by bony spurs.

In patients with degenerative disease of the spine, computerized tomography (CT) scans or magnetic resonance imaging (MRI) may demonstrate encroachment of osteophytes or of disc material on nerve roots. MRI is particularly useful in delineating soft tissue detail, e.g., in differentiation of the annulus fibrosus from the nucleus pulposus of the intervertebral disc. However, abnormal findings on CT scan and MRI in the absence of symptoms, or negative findings despite significant symptoms and signs, do occur. For example, in the cervical spine, false-positive and false-negative CT scan readings approximate 30% (6). Thus, as with plain radiographs, careful correlation of findings with clinical symptoms is imperative. In general, CT and MRI scans are reserved for patients in whom conservative management has failed and in whom surgery or alternative causes of pain or radiculopathy are being strongly considered. In general, it is advisable to consult with a rheumatologist or radiologist by telephone before deciding which of these procedures should be done when both are available.

CT and MRI scans can also demonstrate lesions in peripheral joints. The MRI is particularly helpful in demonstrating soft tissue structures including cartilages, which are not shown on conventional X-rays (34). On the other hand MRI may not show small calcific densities. Performance and interpretation of these procedures require experience and expertise, which are growing rapidly in tertiary centers but are still not widely available, and the full potential of application has not yet been realized. For this reason, and because of the expense of these procedures, they are best utilized by the rheumatologist or or-

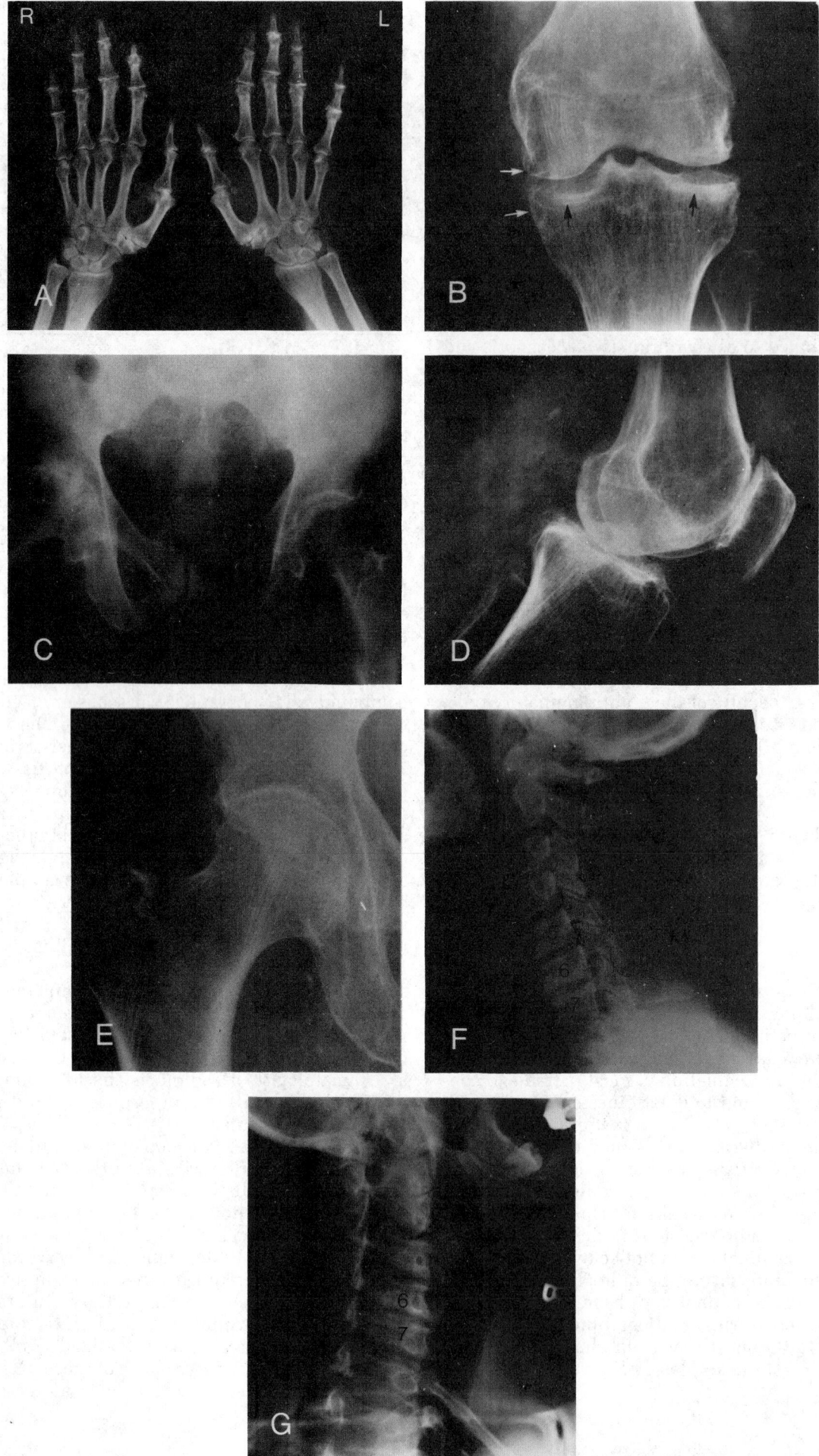

thopaedic consultant on patients referred because of uncertain diagnosis after careful evaluation, including standard radiographs.

CLINICAL PATTERNS OF OSTEOARTHRITIS

Heberden's Nodes

These bony enlargements of the distal interphalangeal joints are more frequent in women and commonly begin to appear in the fifth or sixth decade of life. They are often asymptomatic but a source of concern on the part of many patients who may view them as an outward sign of aging or as the beginning of a more serious and disabling arthritic disorder. This has been documented in a study of healthy elders in whom there was no correlation of osteoarthritis of the hands with objective measures of hand function, yet there was a definite correlation with subjective perception of functional limitation (2). Thus the physician must be aware of and be prepared to deal with the emotional investment of the patient that may focus concerns about declining functions (including menopause) upon an obvious change in physical appearance such as Heberden's nodes. With a curt dismissal, no explanation of the true significance of this abnormality, and no opportunity for the patient to ventilate personal concerns, the physician will miss an important therapeutic opportunity.

Primary Generalized Osteoarthritis

This term was applied by Kellgren and Moore (17) to a group of patients whom they characterized as having osteoarthritis involving the distal and proximal interphalangeal joints and the carpometacarpal joint of the thumb in addition to involvement of multiple other joints (hips, knees, metatarsophalangeal, and spine). The radiological appearance of the involved joints is similar to the usual changes of osteoarthritis, but the pattern suggests this syndrome. This pattern of osteoarthritis affects mostly middle-aged women who have a positive family history of a similar disorder of joint involvement. It is an uncommon pattern of osteoarthritis. Occasionally in early phases they will have had some inflammatory symptoms with an elevated ESR and an episodic course. It is suggested that these patients constitute a subgroup of patients with a heritable form of osteoarthritis that involves multiple joints and that perhaps has some distinctive radiological features. However, the nature of the proposed heritable factor has not been determined. It is important to recognize the syndrome clinically, primarily in order to differentiate it from rheumatoid arthritis and other polyarticular diseases (5).

Erosive Osteoarthritis of Hands

This term has been applied to patients with severe osteoarthritis of the hands [distal interphalangeal (DIP) and proximal interphalangeal (PIP) joints] in which extensive erosion of subchondral bone occurs with eventual deformity and significant limitation of motion of the finger joints (25). These patients also may have episodes of acute inflammation in these joints and their surrounding tissues. X-rays reveal the extensive bony erosion and subchondral cyst formation that may be interpreted incorrectly as rheumatoid or gouty erosions. The distribution of involvement in DIP and first carpometacarpal joints, sparing the metacarpophalangeal joints and wrists, should easily establish the true nature of the process. From the clinical point of view this syndrome is important because of the severity of symptoms and physical findings, which are not common in milder forms of osteoarthritis of the hands.

Hip

Hip involvement is potentially the most painful and disabling joint abnormality in osteoarthritis. It is more often unilateral. Developmental defects in the structure of the hip, including congenital hip dysplasia, slipped capital femoral epiphysis, or unrecognized avascular necrosis, may have gone undetected but have predisposed the patient to develop osteoarthritis; with age, disturbance of the normal anatomical relationship between femoral head and acetabulum may also predispose to osteoarthritis. In contrast to osteoarthritis of the knee, obesity is not a major causal factor in osteoarthritis of the hip.

Pain, which early in the disease is associated with weight bearing and movement, may become severe even at rest, and night pain is common in advanced disease. Patients may walk with a limp or with an abnormal gait. Pain and limitation of motion during internal rotation and extension are early physical signs, and subsequently all motions may be painful and re-

Figure 68.1. *A. Hands of patient* with degenerative joint disease. Note the following characteristics: soft tissue enlargement on right over the second distal interphalangeal joint (Heberden's node); the loss of joint space and bony proliferation of all distal interphalangeal joints, especially 2 and 3 in the right hand and 3 in the left hand; involvement of carpometacarpal joint of both thumbs with narrowing and increased density of subchondral bone; and normal metacarpophalangeal joints and wrist joints. *B. X-ray of knee* showing degenerative joint disease with loss of joint space (cartilage) especially in medial compartment, sclerotic subchondral bone, subchondral cysts, and early marginal spurs especially on lateral side. *C. Pelvic film* of a patient with advanced degenerative joint disease in the right hip. Notice the joint space narrowing and proliferation of subchondral bone. The left hip shows the minimal change of marginal sclerosis. *D. Lateral X-ray of same knee* (in *B*) illustrating involvement of patellofemoral joint with narrowing and spur formation superiorly. *E. X-ray of a hip* showing relatively early degenerative joint disease. Notice the narrowed joint space and spur formation of femoral head at upper margin of acetabulum. *F. X-ray of the lateral cervical spine* showing degenerative joint disease. Note narrowing of C5-6, and especially C6-7 interspace with anterior lipping and spur formation. *G. Oblique X-ray view of cervical spine* of same patient (*F*) showing osteophytes encroaching on neural foramina C5-6, C6-7.

stricted. Clear identification of pain on motion of the hip is important in differentiating hip disease from other causes of pelvic pain. Flexion and adduction contracture and shortening may occur as disability progresses. Most patients who are symptomatic will have characteristic changes of osteoarthritis on X-rays of the hip. CT scan or MRI may be useful to detect and differentiate early aseptic necrosis from osteoarthritis and a radiologist should be consulted regarding which procedure should be done when there is a question. Progression of disease is variable but perhaps more likely to occur rapidly in the hip than in other joints.

Knee

The knee is the most common symptomatic joint in osteoarthritis. There is a definite relationship to obesity, and the weight-bearing areas of the medial compartment are most often involved. Patellofemoral joint involvement is also common. The causative role of obesity in the development of osteoarthritis of the knee has been clearly shown in recent epidemiological studies. The association of obesity with knee osteoarthritis is stronger in women than in men (10), and the relative risk of knee osteoarthritis in obese black women is twice that of whites (1). In addition evidence indicates that knee osteoarthritis is a consequence of and not a risk factor for obesity (7).

Chondromalacia patellae (see also Chapter 67, Exercise-Related Musculoskeletal Problems) is a syndrome occurring usually in younger individuals (second, third, and fourth decades), probably resulting from trauma and shearing forces against the patella as it contacts the femur in midflexion. Knee effusion is frequently associated with this syndrome. In younger patients with knee effusion who do not respond to rest or palliative aspiration (see Chapter 66), arthroscopy may be indicated and will show characteristic changes. The relationship of this rather common syndrome to osteoarthritis is not entirely clear. Although a distinct etiological mechanism and pathology have been suggested, there are probably many contributing factors to this descriptive pathological condition.

Spinal Syndromes

Osteoarthritis can result in neck or back pain that may be acute or chronic (see Chapters 64 and 65). Particularly in cervical spine involvement, symptoms may be more related to referred pain than to neck pain. These syndromes can also result in pain without obvious nerve root compression or neurological abnormalities. Low cervical spine involvement can cause pain that is usually aching or burning in quality referred to the upper anterior chest, to the lower border of the scapula, and radiating down the arm to the elbow. Confusion with anginal pain may occur, but the history usually makes it clear that pain is localized to one side and occurs at rest, particu-

larly during the night or in the early morning after sleep (probably due to positioning of the head during sleep). Although it may also be exacerbated by activity during the day, pain related to cervical arthritis does not subside rapidly with rest and is not related to specific exertion. Physical examination usually can reproduce the pain on extremes of movement of the neck or with manual compression of the cervical segments in hyperextension, rotation, or lateral flexion. Degenerative arthritis of the thoracic spine can also cause radicular pain in the thoracic area, but this is surprisingly uncommon in contrast to frequent radiological findings of spur formation in the thoracic spine, probably because of the anterior position of most of these bony abnormalities.

Another spinal syndrome, the relationship of which to osteoarthritis is not clear, is *diffuse idiopathic skeletal hyperostosis* (DISH). Table 68.4 lists the radiological criteria for this diagnosis (27). Despite extensive hyperostosis and bony bridging between the vertebral bodies, in contrast to ankylosing spondylitis motion and function are usually relatively maintained since the apophyseal joints are usually spared. This syndrome is chiefly important because of its impressive radiographic appearance (Fig. 68.2), the diffuse bony changes with hyperostosis, and the importance of distinguishing it from ankylosing spondylitis (see Chapter 71).

"Acute" Exacerbations of Osteoarthritis

Patients with osteoarthritis may present occasionally with acute or subacute painful episodes with

Table 68.4.
X-Ray Abnormalities in Diffuse Idiopathic Skeletal Hyperostosis[a]

SPINAL

Laminated calcification and ossification along the anterior lateral aspect of at least four contiguous vertebral bodies continuing across the disc spaces and varying in thickness from 1 to 20 mm (see Fig. 68.2A, *arrows*) with relative preservation of the height of the disc space.

Bumpy spinal contour appearance from increased bone deposition located at the anterior disc space margins (see Fig. 68.2A)

Radiolucent disc extension (*i.e.*, L-, F-, or Y-shaped lucencies within the bone deposition along the anterior disc margin) (see Fig. 68.2B, *arrow*)

Radiolucency beneath deposited bone linearly located between the anterolateral calcification and the vertebral bodies (see Fig. 68.2A, *arrows*)

Absence of apophyseal joint anklyosis or of sacroiliac joint erosions

EXTRASPINAL

(Frequent and distinctive features that permit a diagnosis even without spinal X-rays)

Bony proliferation

Ligament calcification, ossification

Para-articular osteophytes

(These changes are always present in the pelvis and in approximately 75% of cases in the heel and foot and less commonly in the elbows, knees, shoulders, humerus, wrist, and hands.)

[a] Adapted from Resnick D, Shapiro RF, Wiesner KB, *et al.*: Diffuse idiopathic skeletal hyperostosis (DISH) (ankylosing hyperostosis of Forestier and Rotes-Querol). *Semin Arthritis Rheum* 7:153, 1978.

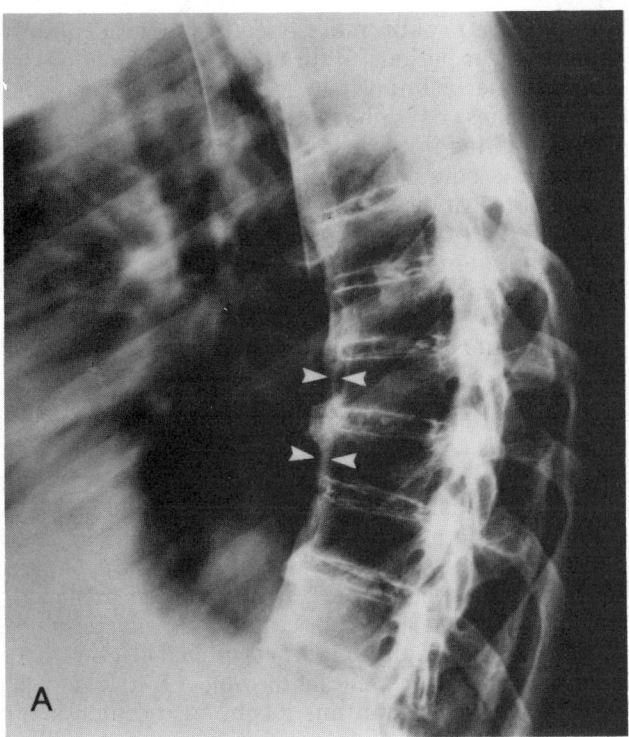
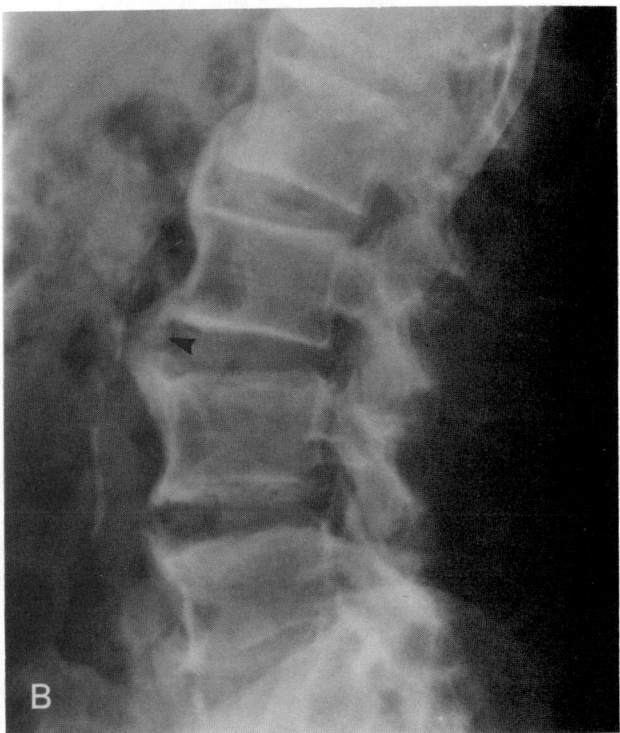

Figure 68.2. *A.* Lateral X-ray of thoracic spine of patient with diffuse idiopathic skeletal hyperostosis. *B.* Lateral X-ray of lumbar spine of patient with diffuse idiopathic skeletal hyperostosis. Prominent bony fusion and lipping anteriorly are seen.

swelling of the affected joint. These episodes are usually superimposed upon more typical preceding symptoms and signs of osteoarthritis, but they may be the event precipitating an initial visit to the physician. In these patients there may be evidence of inflammation with pain, swelling, warmth, and some erythema on occasion. When the knee is involved, there may be a joint effusion. The episodes, which may be precipitated by minor trauma, probably are caused by sudden release into the joint of large amounts of cartilaginous debris and/or microcrystalline deposits contained therein, and very rarely by complicating sepsis. In a study by Huskisson et al. (15) either calcium pyrophosphate or hydroxyapatite crystals or both were found in a high proportion of knee effusions of patients with such episodes, but, in addition, in a significant proportion of unselected patients with osteoarthritis of the knee with effusion. Thus the concurrence of crystalline deposit disease and osteoarthritis seems to be well established, although the relationship of cause and effect is not yet clear. From the clinical point of view, however, this interrelationship provides a better understanding of these acute inflammatory episodes that punctuate the course of otherwise typical osteoarthritis (see also Chapter 69, Crystal-Induced Arthritis). Sepsis may occasionally complicate an osteoarthritic joint, but it is a much less common event than occurs in a rheumatoid arthritic joint.

For these reasons a patient with established osteoar-

thritis who develops an acutely swollen, painful, hot joint should have the joint aspirated and the fluid analyzed because of the possibility of there being either a complicating microcrystalline-induced or a septic arthritis.

DIAGNOSIS AND DIFFERENTIAL DIAGNOSIS

The diagnosis of osteoarthritis is based upon the history and physical findings related to the joints, the absence of systemic signs, and typical radiological findings. Differentiation from other forms of arthritis is usually not difficult, with the possible exception of some of the more unusual diffuse or inflammatory patterns of involvement described above. Consideration of the age of the patient, the distribution of the joints involved, and the radiological findings will usually lead to the correct diagnosis.

The most common errors in differential diagnosis occur in attributing symptoms of pain or restricted movement to osteoarthritis when the problem is not the joints. This is a common mistake in the evaluation of shoulder pain particularly (see Chapter 63). Because X-rays may demonstrate changes of osteoarthritis in asymptomatic or mildly symptomatic patients, the physician must rely upon a careful history and physical examination to localize the disease to the joints. Table 68.5 lists other disorders, also common in older age groups, that often give rise to pain and to painful or restricted movement and that may be erroneously

Table 68.5.
Differential Diagnosis of Osteoarthritis:
Extra-articular Causes of Pain or Restricted Movement

BONE DISEASE
  Osteopenia or osteoporosis (see Chapter 74)
  Malignancy: myeloma, metastatic
  Paget's disease
  Osteomyelitis (see Chapter 31)
PERIARTICULAR SOFT TISSUE ABNORMALITIES
  Soft tissue contractures (Dupuytren's, postcerebrovascular acci-
    dent, or debilitating disease with disuse)
  Tendinitis or bursitis (see Chapters 63 and 66)
  Reflex sympathetic dystrophy
NEUROMUSCULAR DISEASES
  Neuropathy (diabetes, alcoholism, B_{12} deficiency) (see
    Chapter 84)
  Parkinsonism (see Chapter 82)
  Tardive dyskinesias (see Chapters 16 and 82)
  Senile dementia with rigidity (see Chapters 17 and 82)
VASCULAR DISEASES (see Chapter 87)
  Atherosclerosis
  Diabetes
  Vasculitis

attributed to osteoarthritis unless a careful examination is done.

MANAGEMENT

There is no cure for osteoarthritis and no therapy yet available that can be directed toward the specific pathophysiology of cartilage degeneration. However, much can be done to relieve symptoms, minimize disability, and perhaps delay progression of the disease. Certainly a nihilistic approach to therapy, e.g., "take aspirin and accept the fact you are getting older," which has been common advice in the past, is not justified. The criteria for the determination of medical disability under Social Security are listed in Chapter 9.

General Measures

Patient Education

Explaining to the patient the nature of the disease, that other joints are not likely to be involved, that progression of disease is slow, and that preservation of function is likely will reassure most patients. For the patient with Heberden's nodes or mild disease in other joints, this reassurance and understanding will be the most important therapeutic step in management. The physician should suggest some reading material for the patient such as *Learning to Live with Osteoarthritis* published in 1984 by Medicine in the Public Interest, Inc. (Suite 720, 600 New Hampshire Ave NW, Washington, DC 20037).

Rest

Pain and discomfort of osteoarthritis are frequently exacerbated by use, especially continuous use or weight bearing. Further, excessive use of joints already damaged by osteoarthritis may accelerate cartilage degeneration. Therefore, rest is an important modality of treatment for osteoarthritis. Short periods of rest through the day are usually more effective than are less frequent longer periods. With weight-bearing joints, rest is particularly important. Many patients, especially elderly ones, have the notion that use of a joint becomes limited if it is rested too much, so that needless overuse is common. When an understanding of the value of rest and reassurance about function are given, patients will often quickly learn to live within their own limitations without undue restrictions of activity and with improvement in symptoms.

Use of Canes, Crutches, and Walkers

In more severe disease, rest from weight bearing and stability when walking may be partially achieved by the use of a crutch, a cane, or a walker. The patient's attitude about the use of such assistive devices is an important consideration here since some will interpret their cane as a sign of infirmity and fail to use it, whereas others may carry it proudly as a badge of dependency even when it is not needed. Instruction in proper use of a cane, a crutch, or a walker should be given by the physician or a physical therapist. It should be remembered that the object is to take weight off the affected limb; thus a cane or a crutch should always be used on the opposite side and used simultaneously with the affected limb for weight bearing. Also, a cane should be held tightly and close to the body. Proper use is assured by pressing the handle against the good hip. A walker does not provide this type of unilateral support, but it may be needed in patients with bilateral knee pain or in patients whose instability requires more support than that provided by a cane or a crutch.

Correction of Postural or Mechanical Strain

This is an important consideration in patients with poor body mechanics. Thus the patient with pronated feet (see Chapter 102, Common Problems of the Feet) will have excessive stress on the knees and low back. Genu varus or valgum will stress the lateral or medial compartment excessively. Instruction in proper lifting and avoidance of unnecessary strain on certain joints or muscles by occupational or other activities may also need attention—for example, use of a cervical pillow in the patient with neck involvement (see also Chapters 64, Neck Pain, and 65, Low Back Pain).

Physical Therapy

Simple measures can be prescribed for home use without the need for referral to a physical therapist in patients with mild disease. However, the physician must be sure that the patient understands directions. Reinforcement on subsequent visits is also important to ensure compliance. Patients with more advanced disease should be referred to a physical or occupational therapist for more extensive instruction in an exercise program, joint protection maneuvers, use of assistive devices, gait training, and the like.

Heat. Application of heat often provides symptomatic relief of pain, reduces muscle spasm, and facilitates subsequent performance of an exercise program. Most patients prefer moist heat, which can be applied for 15 to 20 minutes via bathtub, hot towels, or commercially manufactured packs. Electric heating pads may also be used. Paraffin wax baths (available from large pharmacies) may be useful in patients with extensive hand involvement. With all modalities of heat therapy, temperatures that are very hot (above 110°F (43°C)) and prolonged or uninterrupted use should be avoided, to prevent skin damage. Use of diathermy, ultrasound, heat cabinets, and the like offers little advantage in most cases and requires a physical therapist.

Exercise. Goals of an exercise program are to maintain or improve function by preserving range of motion and improving muscle strength. The latter is important to help stabilize the joint and, by maintaining soft tissue cushioning of stress, to reduce the stress applied to the joint. Gradual conditioning is important so that muscle pain and soreness are not aggravated. Exercise should be graded according to the ability of the individual patient and carried out at least three times/day for optimal effect. In general, if muscle soreness or joint pain is worse after exercise, the intensity of the exercise should be reduced or progression halted until symptoms subside. Swimming is also a valuable means of exercise that does not involve weight-bearing stress. Bicycling also provides exercise with less weight-bearing stress than walking.

Maintenance of quadriceps strength is particularly important in osteoarthritis of the knee. This can be accomplished by beginning with slow full extension of the knee against gravity and then, as symptoms and progress allow, by extension with progressively increasing weight attached to the lower leg. (An old pocketbook or bag with a strap to which are added canned goods of specific weight from the pantry shelf will suffice.) In patients whose pain prevents active quadriceps strengthening, isometric exercises are useful. With the knee extended the patient is instructed to tighten the quadriceps maximally so that the patella becomes fixed, hold for 10 to 15 seconds by count, release, and repeat. The importance of maintaining muscle strength and conditioning is emphasized by studies measuring the energy expenditure of walking in patients with arthritis of the hip or knee (36). The markedly increased energy requirement results in excessive fatigue that discourages mobility and may begin a cycle of progressive functional impairment in the frail elderly patient.

Other Measures. For cervical spine disease gentle overhead traction may improve symptoms. This can be accomplished at home with a halter device and pulley and may be combined with the use of a soft cervical collar (see Chapter 64).

Many patients report remission of stiffness and pain and a sense of joint protection through the use of elastic supports around the joint. Such devices used at the knee, however, often obstruct venous circulation in the leg and cause edema, so that their use is not generally recommended. Wearing nylon stretch gloves (such as Iso-Toner gloves, available in department stores) may provide relief for some patients with extensive hand involvement (8).

Diet

Control of obesity (Chapter 76) is important in osteoarthritis of the knees, hips, and metatarsophalangeal joints. Otherwise there is no dietary imperative either to omit or to eat any specific foods, vitamins, or nutrients. Niacin, promoted by some as effective in controlling arthritis, has not been demonstrated scientifically to be beneficial in the treatment or prevention of osteoarthritis. Patients should be cautioned against food fads and unwarranted claims of relationship of diet and osteoarthritis.

Drug Therapy

Nonsteroidal Anti-inflammatory Drugs

Nonsteroidal anti-inflammatory drugs (NSAIDs) and analgesic agents are the mainstay of drug treatment of osteoarthritis. For patients with mild disease, pain is usually related to mechanical factors rather than to inflammation. Thus, analgesic doses are all that is required. Aspirin is an effective analgesic and usually is well tolerated in divided doses of 1.2 to 2.4 g/day. Acetaminophen is equally effective as an analgesic in patients unable to take aspirin.

Although mild by comparison with that of rheumatoid arthritis, the inflammatory component of osteoarthritis becomes more evident as the disease progresses and may warrant the use of anti-inflammatory doses of salicylates or other NSAIDs. The average dose of aspirin required may vary from 3.6 to 4.8 g/day for anti-inflammatory effect. At this dose gastrointestinal side effects of aspirin, including gastric ulceration and increased blood loss in the stool, are common. This may be largely obviated by the use of enteric coated aspirin, but erratic absorption in some patients requires a measure of blood salicylate level after several days of therapy to ensure an optimal level of 15 to 25 mg/dl. Other salicylate preparations such as choline salicylate (Arthropan liquid, 870 mg/5 ml, available without prescription), choline magnesium salicylate (Trilisate, 1500 mg), salicylsalicylic acid (Disalcid, 500 mg) and zorprin (all requiring a prescription) are also effective and have better gastrointestinal tolerance than aspirin, although they are also significantly more expensive—about equal in cost to other nonsteroidal anti-inflammatory drugs.

A large number of NSAIDs (32) in addition to salicylates are now available and more are being developed. It is probable that the efficacy and side effects of aspirin and the nonsteroidal anti-inflammatory agents are mediated, at least in part, through the ubiquitous prostaglandin system by inhibition of cyclo-oxygenase enzymes that are involved in the synthesis of prostaglandins from fatty acids of the cell membrane, principally arachidonic acid. The anti-inflammatory potency, duration of action, and side effects of each agent are somewhat variable because of the differences in tissue distribution and metabolism of the various drugs. Side effects are more prominent in the elderly and particular caution is necessary in this group of patients (see Chapter 70). For example, indomethacin (Indocin) is a potent NSAID which penetrates most tissues, including the central nervous system. Tolmetin (Tolectin) has a somewhat similar molecular structure and efficacy, but because it is largely excluded by the blood-brain barrier, has fewer central nervous system side effects, such as headache and psychic disturbances. Sulindac (Clinoril) is converted to an active metabolite after absorption so that it bypasses and does not inhibit the local gastroprotective effect of prostaglandins in the gastric mucosa. It also has little effect on renal function, perhaps because of tissue distribution of active metabolites in the kidney. Naproxen (Naprosyn) and piroxicam (Feldene) have a long half-life in the plasma, so that intervals between doses can be increased.

In controlled clinical trials none of the NSAIDs has been shown to differ significantly from aspirin in efficacy in the treatment of osteoarthritis or other forms of arthritis, although the frequency of side effects has been lower with some of these drugs than with regular aspirin. Also, any one agent may be unaccountably more effective than another, so that a serial trial approach is often warranted. NSAIDs have been shown to have variable effects on cartilage metabolism, including decrease of proteoglycan synthesis (23), and in experimental models of osteoarthritis may accelerate cartilage loss. These effects are more pronounced in osteoarthritic than in normal cartilage due to the enhanced uptake of NSAIDS with the depletion of matrix proteoglycans (4). Whether these observations are relevant to human disease or to the choice of a particular NSAID is not known. Adverse effects on progression of hip osteoarthritis by indomethacin have been suggested (30). However, until more specific therapy is available, NSAIDs will continue to be the principal drug treatment for symptomatic relief of osteoarthritis.

Although use of combinations of NSAIDs is fairly common practice, there is no convincing evidence that this practice is beneficial. Interference with absorption of indomethacin by aspirin, displacement from protein binding, and other potential interactions of NSAIDs would seem to indicate that the prudent choice is to use a single agent to its maximal effect. This may require increasing dosage over a period of 2 to 6 weeks until symptoms are relieved, side effects occur, or lack of efficacy is established before switching to an alternative agent.

Because many patients with osteoarthritis have other medical conditions for which they are receiving therapeutic drugs, one must be alert to problems of interactions with NSAIDs. For example, NSAIDs may mitigate the therapeutic effect of agents that depend on prostaglandins to mediate a response, such as the naturetic and antihypertensive effects of furosemide, thiazides, or captopril (29).

Some of the factors in choice of an NSAID include cost (32), frequency of administration required (a major factor in compliance), and side effects, which may be variably tolerated by different patients. These and other characteristics of NSAIDs are more fully discussed in Chapter 70.

Corticosteroids

Intra-articular injection of suspensions of corticosteroids (see Table 66.4) has been shown to be useful in the management of osteoarthritis when associated with effusions in large joints such as the knee (14). The removal of joint fluid (without corticosteroid injection) when an effusion is present in degenerative arthritis usually does not improve symptoms unless a microcrystalline arthritis is superimposed (see Chapter 69). If prolonged relief lasting several months is not achieved with one or two injections, this therapy should not be continued. The risk of serious side effects including enhanced destruction of the joint and infection may follow repeated injections, which should therefore be avoided.

There is absolutely no indication for systemic administration of corticosteroids in the management of osteoarthritis.

Orthopaedic Surgery

The orthopaedist should be consulted in management of patients with osteoarthritis who have a problem of malalignment or major instability in weight-bearing joints, for symptoms or findings of loose bodies in the joint, and for intractable pain with advanced disease of the hips or knees. Osteotomy may correct malalignment. Arthroplasty to improve instability and remove loose bodies, meniscal fragments, and perhaps large spurs may be useful in some patients. Arthroscopic lavage of the knee with gentle debridement is a much more tolerable procedure than open arthroplasty and may provide relief of pain for several months or longer before symptoms recur (11). It is useful particularly in knees that are not subject to undue stress in elderly patients (31). When pain or disability is refractory to treatment and joint destruction of a hip or a knee is advanced, consideration should be given to total joint replacement (13). Disabling pain is the principal indication for this procedure. Contraindications include neuromuscular or sensory deficits, severe peripheral vascular disease, marked obesity, dementia, and lack of motivation or inability to cooperate with a postoperative rehabilitation program. Results of joint replacement in osteoarthritis of the hip are generally excellent. Knee replacement has been somewhat less successful, but results have improved with new prostheses and in the hands of experienced surgeons; relief of pain approximates 90% but functional improvement is less certain. Arthrodesis (i.e., surgical fusion of the joint) is still useful in patients with unilateral, intractable, and severe knee involvement and may also be done when joint replacement has failed. Major complications of joint replacement are postoperative thrombophlebitis and infection. Elimination of potential foci of infection is important preoperatively, and prophylactic antibiotics are indicated after joint replacement surgery during dental or urinary tract procedures, which might produce bacteremia (20). Although the continued improvement in synthetic materials and surgical techniques has prolonged the durability of an artificial joint, still most rheumatologists do not refer patients with hip or knee arthritis for surgery until symptoms are pronounced and functional impairment is considerable.

PREVENTION

Because the etiology of osteoarthritis is uncertain, so is its prevention. However, recognition of predisposing factors and elucidation of normal physiology of articular cartilage suggest certain prudent steps that can be recommended.

Immobilization with avoidance of joint stress gives rise to biochemical changes in cartilage similar to early lesions in osteoarthritis. Thus normal stress and functioning of joints are important in maintenance of normal cartilage physiology. Perhaps one can abstract from this that a sedentary and inactive life is not good for the integrity of articular cartilage. Further, since strong periarticular muscles lend stability and help to absorb stress applied to joints, it seems logical that physical conditioning to maintain muscle strength and a lean habitus may be important in prevention of osteoarthritis. Soft tissues tend to lose mobility with advancing age and such changes have been shown to increase impact stress of joints. Physical activity may retard this loss of mobility and therefore should be encouraged in aging individuals.

At the same time it is evident that repetitive stress, especially when abnormally applied, is a strong predisposing factor to osteoarthritis. Thus correction of abnormal mechanical forces from developmental or postural defects, avoidance of unusual occupational stress, and avoidance of traumatic injury to joints are important in prevention of osteoarthritis.

General References

Brandt KD: Management of Osteoarthritis. In: Kelley WN, Harris CD, Ruddy S, Sledge CB (eds): *Textbook of Rheumatology*, 3rd ed. Philadelphia, WB Saunders, 1989.
Gardner PL: The nature and causes of osteoarthritis. Br Med J 286:418, 1985.
Mankin HJ Brandt KD: Pathogenesis of osteoarthritis. In: Kelley WN, Harris CD, Ruddy S, Sledge CB (eds): *Textbook of Rheumatology*, 3rd ed. Philadelphia, WB Saunders, 1989.
Hamerman D: The biology of osteoarthritis. N Engl J Med 320:1322, 1989.
Hough AJ, Sokoloff L: Pathology of Osteoarthritis. In: McCarty DJ (ed): *Arthritis and Allied Conditions*. Philadelphia, Lea and Febiger, 1989.
Moskowitz RW, Howell DS, Goldberg VM, Mankin HJ (eds): *Osteoarthritis, Diagnosis and Management*. Philadelphia, WB Saunders, 1984.
Radin EC: Chondromalacia of the patella. Bull Rheum Dis 34:1, 1982.

Specific References

1. Anderson JJ, Felson DT: Factors associated with osteoarthritis of the knee in the first national health and nutrition examination survey (Hanes I). Evidence for an association with overweight, race, and physical demands of work. Am J Epidemiol 128:179, 1988.
2. Baron M, Dutil E, Berkson L, et al: Hand function in the elderly: relation to osteoarthritis. J Rheumatol 14:815, 1987.
3. Boniface RJ, Cain PR, Evans CH: Articular responses to purified cartilage proteoglycans. Arthritis Rheum 31:258, 1988.
4. Brandt KD: Effects of non-steroidal anti-inflammatory drugs on chondrocyte metabolism in vitro and in vivo. Am J Med 83 (suppl 5A):29, 1987.
5. Buchanan WW, Park WM: Primary generalized osteoarthritis: definition and uniformity. J Rheumatol 10:4, 1983.
6. Daniels DC, Grogan JP, Johansen JG, et al: Cervical radiculopathy: computed tomography and myelography compared. Radiology 151:109, 1984.
7. Davis MA, Ettinger WH, Neuhaus JM, Hauck WC: Sex differences in osteoarthritis of the knee. The role of obesity. Am J Epidemiol 127:1019, 1988.
8. Ehrlich GE, DiPiero AM: Stretch gloves: nocturnal use to ameliorate morning stiffness in arthritic hands. Arch Phys Med Rehabil 52:479, 1971.
9. Felson DT, Naimark A, Anderson J, et al: The prevalence of knee osteoarthritis in the elderly. The Framingham osteoarthritis study. Arthritis Rheum 30:914, 1987.
10. Felson DT, Anderson JJ, Naimark A, et al: Obesity and knee osteoarthritis. The Framingham study. Ann Intern Med 109:18, 1988.
11. Friedman MJ, Berasi DO, Fox JM, et al: Preliminary results with abrasion arthroplasty in the osteoarthritis knee. Clin Orthop 182:200, 1984.
12. Glynn LE: Primary lesion in osteoarthritis. Lancet 1:574, 1977.
13. Harris WH: Total joint replacement. N Engl J Med 297:650, 1977.
14. Hollander JL: Treatment of osteoarthritis of the knees. Arthritis Rheum 3:564, 1960.
15. Huskisson EC, Dieppe PA, Tucker AK, Channel LB: Another look at osteoarthritis. Ann Rheum Dis 38:423, 1979.
16. Jasin HE: Autoantibody specificities of immune complexes sequestered in articular cartilage of patients with rheumatoid arthritis and osteoarthritis. Arthritis Rheum 28:241, 1985.
17. Kellgren JH, Moore R: Generalized osteoarthritis and Heberden's nodes. Br Med J 1:181, 1952.
18. Lane NE, Bloch DA, Wood PD, Fries JF: Aging, long distance running and the development of musculoskeletal disability. Am J Med 82:772, 1987.
19. Lane NE, Fries JF: Relationship of running to osteoarthritis and bone density. Compr Ther 14:7, 1988.
20. Liang MD, Cullen KE, Poss R: Primary total hip or knee replacement: evaluation of patients. Ann Intern Med 97:735, 1982.
21. Mankin HJ, Treadwell BV: Osteoarthritis: a 1987 update. Bull Rheum Dis 36, No. 5: 1986.
22. Marsland DW, Wood M, Mayo F: Content of family practice. I. Routine order of diagnosis by frequency. II. Diagnosis by disease category and age/sex distribution. J Fam Pract 8:37, 1976.
23. Palmoski MJ, Brandt KD: Effects of some nonsteroidal anti-inflammatory drugs on proteoglycan metabolism and organization in canine articular cartilage. Arthritis Rheum 23:1010, 1980.
24. Panush RS, Schmidt C, Caldwell JR, et al: Is running associated with degenerative joint disease? JAMA 255:1152, 1986.
25. Peter JB, Pearson CM, Marmnor L: Erosive osteoarthritis of the hands. Arthritis Rheum 9:365, 1966.
26. Radin EL, Parker HG, Pugh JW, et al: Response of joints to impact loading. III. Relationship between trabecular microfractures and cartilage degeneration. J Biomech 6:51, 1973.
27. Resnick D, Shapiro RF, Wiesner KB, et al: Diffuse idiopathic skeletal hyperostosis (DISH) (ankylosing hyperostosis of Forestier and Rotes-Querol). Semin Arthritis Rheum 7:153, 1978.
28. Revell PA, Mayston V, Lalor P, Mapp P: The synovial membrane in osteoarthritis: a histological study including the characterization of the cellular infiltrate present in inflammatory osteoar-

thritis using monoclonal antibodies. *Ann Rheum Dis* 47:300, 1988.

29. Rizack MA, Hillman CDM (eds): *The Medical Letter Handbook of Drug Interactions.* New Rochelle, NY, The Medical Letter, 1983.
30. Ronnigen H, Langeland N: Indomethacin treatment in osteoarthritis of the hip joint. *Acta Orthop Scand* 50:169, 1979.
31. Schonholtz GJ: Arthroscopic debridement of the knee joint. *Orthop Clin* 20:2:257, 1989.
32. Simon LS, Mills JA: Non-steroidal anti-inflammatory drugs. *N Engl J Med* 302:1179, 1237, 1980.
33. Stecker RM: Heberden's nodes, heredity in hypertrophic arthritis of the finger joints. *Am J Med Sci* 201:801, 1941.
34. Stoller DW, Genant HK: Magnetic resonance imaging of the joints. In: McCarty DJ (ed): *Arthritis and Allied Conditions.* Philadelphia, Lea Febiger, 1989.
35. Summers MN, Haley WE, Reveille JD, Alarcon GS: Radiologic assessment and psychologic variables as predictors of pain and functional impairment in osteoarthritis of the knee or hip. *Arthritis Rheum* 31:204, 1987.
36. Waters RL, Perry J, Conaty P, et al: The energy cost of walking with arthritis of the hip and knee. *Clin Orthop* 214:278, 1987.

C H A P T E R 69

Crystal-Induced Arthritis

ALEXANDER S. TOWNES, M.D.

Gout was the first form of arthritis that was recognized to be caused by the deposition of (urate) crystals in the joints and periarticular tissues. It is now known that other crystalline substances—most commonly calcium pyrophosphate dihydrate (CPPD) and hydroxyapatite—also are implicated in the pathogenesis of certain kinds of arthritic disease. Although disorders associated with these various crystals differ in etiology and in specific characteristics, they have in common the deposition of crystals in and around joints, the propensity to episodes of acute inflammatory arthritis, and sometimes the development of a destructive arthropathy. It is therefore appropriate to consider these varied clinical disorders together under the unifying concept of crystal-induced arthritis.

Mechanisms of Crystal-Induced Arthritis

Crystals such as monosodium urate and calcium pyrophosphate dihydrate when experimentally injected into joints produce an acute inflammatory response. The mechanisms involved in this response are complex but perhaps are as well studied as any of the stimuli that produce arthritis. By the nature of their electrostatic surface characteristics, crystals attract and bind many plasma proteins including fibronectin, IgG, C-reactive protein, and complement. Crystals are phagocytized by synovial lining cells probably as a result of binding of crystal-bound IgG, complement, or other proteins to membrane receptors. This initiates formation and/or release of prostaglandins, lysosomal enzymes, and other mediators that increase vascular permeability and promote the influx of polymorphonuclear neutrophils (PMN), which are essential for the inflammatory reaction to continue. Phagocytosis of crystals by PMNs is accompanied by the release of a potent chemotactic glycopeptide that further amplifies the PMN response. PMNs release lysosomal enzymes in the process of crystal phagocytosis and as a result of the membranolytic effect of urate crystals themselves on phagolysosomes after digestion of proteins from the crystal surface. In this process crystals are again released into the synovial fluid for further phagocytosis. Urate crystals also stimulate macrophages and synovial lining cells to produce interleukin-I, a potent pyrogen (7, 14).

Although the events that trigger acute inflammation in patients with crystal-induced arthritis are not entirely clear, it is likely that the precipitation of release of a sufficient volume of crystals from soft tissue deposits begins the cycle of crystal phagocytosis and inflammation. In patients with gout there is an association of acute attacks with rapid changes in serum urate concentration such as may occur with dietary indiscretion or initiation of therapy with drugs that lower serum urate. In CPPD deposit disease, release of crystals from tissue deposits in cartilage or soft tissues may result from trauma or from enzymatic digestion of matrix.

The invariable association between phagocytosis of crystals and the acute inflammatory response is important clinically since demonstration of crystals within leukocytes from synovial fluid constitutes a convenient method of making a definitive diagnosis in patients with acute inflammatory crystal-induced arthritis.

Although gouty arthritis and other crystal-induced diseases are usually characterized by symptoms and signs of acute inflammation, sometimes destructive arthropathy occurs with little evidence of inflammation. In these patients (preliminarily a few with CPPD and others with hydroxyapatite and other basic calcium phosphate crystals) for some reason the PMN response is markedly reduced, but protease and collagenase enzymes are released and activated resulting in destruction of synovial soft tissues and bone. This process then produces disruption of additional crystal deposits that are released into the joint, and the cycle continues (16, 18, 19).

Crystal Identification

The identification of crystals in synovial fluid or in periarticular tissue is fundamental to the diagnosis and management of patients with crystal-induced arthritis. Crystals of monosodium urate are best identified by placing a drop of aspirated tissue fluid directly on a glass slide and by examining the wet preparation through a microscope under polarized light (22); the crystals are difficult to see under nonpolarized light. Although specialized equipment is ideal, crystals can be demonstrated adequately in the physician's office by placing a plastic polarizing lens (made from an old pair of sunglasses, for example) between the light source and the microscopic stage, and by placing another lens in the body or in the eyepiece of the microscope. When one lens is rotated so that the field becomes dark, the negatively birefringent urate crystals (i.e., crystals capable of bending light rays in two planes; the notation of negativity is an arbitrary term used by physicists to describe the direction of bend), dimly seen in ordinary light, stand out brightly and can be identified within the cytoplasm of polymorphonuclear leukocytes. If a red plate compensator is placed between the light source and the stage of the microscope (one can be fabricated by wrapping a glass slide longitudinally with two layers of transparent (cellophane) tape (occasionally more layers of tape are required)) (6a), the crystals are even more easily identified since the field turns red and crystals parallel to the axis of the compensator will appear yellow, whereas those perpendicular to the axis will appear blue. Monosodium urate crystals are usually needle or rod shaped. The size varies, but some large crystals equal to or larger than the diameter of the leukocyte are usually seen. A wet slide of joint fluid prepared in this manner may be kept for a few hours at room temperature; however, once the cells die and lyse, evaluation is less valid. In the event the aspirated fluid cannot be examined immediately, it may be preserved overnight by refrigeration in a plain test tube.

Monosodium urate crystals (which are usually present in abundance) are pathognomonic of gout (see Table 69.1 and Fig. 69.1). Absence of crystals in an inflamed joint is strong evidence against the diagnosis, and, especially if leukocytosis is significant, infection or another diagnosis should be considered.

Table 69.1.
Identification of Crystals in Synovial Fluid

MONOSODIUM URATE
  Morphology
    Rod or needle shaped
    Length often approaches diameter of polymorphonuclear leukocyte (PMN)
  Polarized light
    Stand out brightly when field is dark
    Strongly negative birefringent
  Red plate compensator:
    Yellow crystals parallel and blue crystals perpendicular to axis
CALCIUM PYROPHOSPHATE DIHYDRATE
  Morphology
    Rhomboid, rod, or irregular rhomboid shape
    Length variable, often smaller than one lobe of a PMN nucleus
  Polarized light
    No increase in refractile appearance when field is dark
    Weakly positively birefringent
  Red plate compensator
    Blue crystals parallel and yellow crystals perpendicular to axis
HYDROXYAPATITE AND BASIC CALCIUM PHOSPHATES
  Not usually seen with ordinary or polarized light microscopy except as large aggregates that are not birefringent
  Stain nonspecifically with alizarin red S (available in histology laboratories) as clusters of crystalline material. Useful as a screening test.
  Requires electron microscopy, X-ray diffraction, or microprobe analysis for more definite identification.
CALCIUM OXALATE
  Morphology
    Polymorphic, irregular squares, short rods, bipyramidal. May appear in clumps.
  Polarized light
    Variable, most not birefringent, some strongly positively birefringent

Monosodium urate is usually easily distinguished from calcium pyrophosphate dihydrate (CPPD) on the basis of morphology and of characteristics of the crystals under polarized light (see Table 69.1 and Fig. 69.1). CPPD crystals vary much more in size and shape from rod-like to rhomboid and irregular forms, are usually much shorter, and are never needle-like. They are usually refractile without polarized light and do not increase appreciably in brilliance when the light is polarized. They are weakly positively birefringent and change color in the opposite direction to urate when the red plate compensator is placed between the polarizing lens (i.e., blue when parallel to the axis and yellow when perpendicular).

Because CPPD crystals are small and do not stand out in polarized light, they are overlooked more frequently by the occasional observer. Routine reports from unspecialized clinical laboratories are often falsely negative.

Other crystalline materials that may be seen include those from previously injected corticosteroids (which appear as crystals of varying and unusual configuration) and occasionally cholesterol crystals, which are easily distinguished from all of the above (resembling a folded envelope). Contaminating crystalline or refractile substances, such as ethylenediaminetetraacetic acid (EDTA) anticoagulant, talc, etc., can be avoided by use of careful technique.

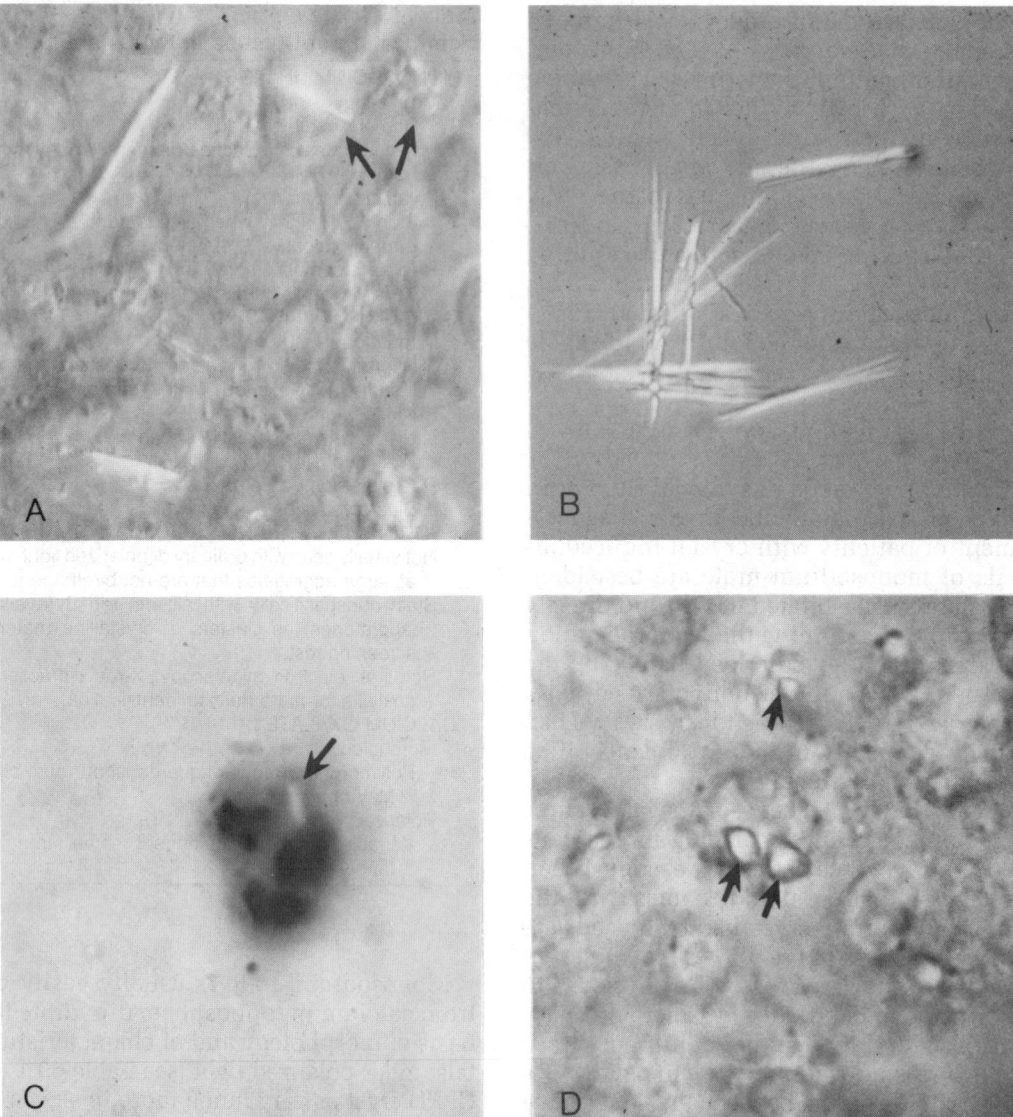

Figure 69.1. *A.* Urate crystals in synovial fluid examined by polarized light microscopy. Note the needle shape and variable size, but many have a larger diameter than white blood cells (oil immersion). *B.* Urate crystals from tophus examined by polarized light with red plate compensator (oil immersion). *C.* Calcium pyrophosphate dihydrate (CPPD) crystal in white blood cell found on Gram stain (oil immersion). Note the shape and size relative to nucleus and cytoplasm. Gram stain is not the usual method of demonstration, but it is occasionally useful. *D.* Wet preparation of synovial fluid demonstrating varied size and shape of CPPD crystal phagocytized by white blood cell (oil immersion lens, polarized light). Size and shape varies from squat rhomboid to rod shaped. Note several crystals in some cells.

GOUT

Pathophysiology

Gout is a syndrome that is caused by an alteration in purine metabolism, the end product of which is uric acid. This alteration results in hyperuricemia and in the deposition of urate crystals in various tissues. Periodic attacks of acute inflammatory arthritis, characteristic of gout, are due to the deposition of urate crystals in and about joints. Primary gout is caused by an inborn error in the production or excretion of uric acid. Secondary gout is caused by an increased breakdown of nucleic acids in association with one of a variety of acquired diseases or by impaired excretion of urate as a consequence of acquired renal disease (Table 69.2).

Most patients with gout (approximately 90%) have, usually for unknown reasons, an elevated renal threshold for the excretion of uric acid. The rest (approximately 10%) overproduce uric acid, although precise enzymatic defects in purine catabolism only rarely have been identified. Production and excretion of uric acid are best assessed by measurement of urate in a 24-hour sample of urine; normally less than 600 mg/day are excreted if the diet for 5 days has been free of foods that are rich in purines (fish, meat, and poultry—especially the solid organs of these food sources); although there is considerable dietary variation, an excretion of more than approximately 750 to 800 mg/

Table 69.2.
Causes of Hyperuricemia[a]

With Increased Urinary Uric Acid	With Normal or Low Urinary Uric Acid
10% of primary gout (defect unknown)	90% of primary gout (defect unknown)
Specific enzyme defects with primary gout	
Secondary causes:	Secondary causes:
Myeloproliferative disease	Renal insufficiency
Lymphoproliferative disease	Lead intoxication
Hemolytic anemias	Drugs:
Obesity	Salicylates (low dose, *i.e.*, < 2.4 g/ay)
Glycogen storage disease	Diuretics
Exercise	Pyrazinamide
Psoriasis	Ethambutol
	Nicotinic acid
	Alcohol
	Others
	Obesity
	Sarcoidosis
	Starvation

[a] Modified from Wyngaarden JB, Kelley WN: *Gout and Hyperuricemia.* New York, Grune & Stratton, 1976.

day while eating a nonrestricted diet may be considered indicative of overproduction in the absence of purine gluttony (8).

Normal levels of serum urate vary widely in the population, with a range of 3 to 8 mg/dl; also, there may be spontaneous variation within individuals. The upper limit of normal for serum urate measured by the uricase method usually is considered to be 7.0 mg/dl for adult males and 6.0 mg/dl for females. Ranges may be higher by 1 mg/dl or more if automated colorimetric methods, commonly used in multiphasic screening tests, are employed.

Serum "uric acid" concentration is primarily a measurement of urate. The concentrations of urate and uric acid are related to pH: at normal blood and interstitial fluid pH of 7.40, the ratio of urate to uric acid is approximately 45:1; as the pH falls—e.g., in the urinary tubule—the relative concentration of uric acid rises (e.g., at a pH of 4.50 the urate to uric acid ratio is approximately 0.06:1).

Epidemiology

Gout is estimated to occur at a lifetime frequency of 3/1000 population in the United States. It is 10 times more common in males in all of its forms and is rare in premenopausal females. Gout is infrequent below age 30 and increases in frequency to a plateau at about age 60. Age at onset is probably related to the duration and severity of preceding hyperuricemia. Gout is more common in obese or in hypertensive people, although the relationships are complex. The frequency of gout in hypertensive subjects, for example, is magnified if they are treated with thiazide diuretics (see below). Gout is also more common in patients with a chronically high alcohol intake, especially if they also are obese or have mildly impaired renal function. Associations of gout with hypertriglyceridemia has been

reported, but whether related to alcohol, diet, obesity, or genetic factors is unclear. Recent data from the Framingham population study has confirmed the long held clinical impression of an increased incidence of coronary heart disease (especially angina pectoris) in males with gout. A 60% excess prevalence of coronary heart disease was observed in men with gout as compared with men without gout in this population. Interestingly this was independent of other measured risk factors, and, as reported in other studies, there was no significant difference in the prevalence of diabetes mellitus or elevated serum cholesterol in the gouty men and in men without gout in the population studied over a 14-year period (1).

Clinical Features (Table 69.3)

Acute Arthritic Attack

The acute arthritic attack is the hallmark of gout. It is characterized by the onset of pain, swelling, and discomfort that progress rapidly to a peak level of intensity within 24 to 36 hours after onset. The pain is often severe enough to prevent use of the affected joint or even for the patient to bear the weight of bed clothing. The metatarsophalangeal joint of the great toe is the most commonly affected joint, followed by the forefoot, heel, ankle, knee, wrist, fingers, and elbow. The great toe is affected at some time during the course of perhaps 90% of gouty subjects. Usually a single joint is involved early in the course of the disease but pauciarticular arthritis (two or three joints) may occur; polyarticular (more than three joints) onset is rare. Polyarticular gout is more common in late disease associated with soft tissue tophi. Recurrent acute arthritis is more common in previously affected joints.

There are several events that may trigger an acute attack of gout: trauma, an acute illness such as an acute

Table 69.3.
Clinical Features of Gout

EPIDEMIOLOGY
  Sex: Males 10 to 1; Rare in premenopausal women
  Age: Usually middle age or older (peak age 60)
ACUTE GOUT
  History:
    Acute attacks, recurrent, with disease-free intervals
    Rapid progression to peak severity within 24 hours
  Physical findings:
    Usually monoarticular with swelling, tenderness, erythema, and intense inflammation
    Big toe metatarsophalangeal joint commonly involved (podagra)
    Forefeet, heels, ankles, knees, wrists, fingers, elbows, and other joints may be affected
    Occasionally polyarticular
    Fever may occur
  Laboratory: Joint aspiration with leukocytosis and identification of urate crystals is diagnostic
INTERCRITICAL GOUT
  No symptoms or findings except hyperuricemia
CHRONIC GOUT
  Often polyarticular
  Symptoms may persist between attacks
  Tophi are common (approximately 90–95%)
  Deformities may develop

myocardial infarction, dietary indiscretion, overuse of alcohol, starvation, and recent administration of drugs that lower serum urate concentration. Most of these events are associated with rapid changes in serum u-rate concentration, and it has been postulated that such changes cause dissolution of tissue deposits with discharge of crystalline material locally to induce the acute attack.

A family history of gout should be sought in patients with primary gout, and especially in those patients who excrete excess amounts of uric acid in whom a specific enzyme defect may be suspected. However, a positive family history is obtained in less than half of gouty subjects so that a negative history is of no differential diagnostic value.

On physical examination of the patient with acute gouty arthritis there is frequently erythema overlying or adjacent to the affected joints, especially when small joints are involved. The erythema often involves only a localized area rather than the entire joint. The intensity of the inflammatory reaction frequently results in a mistaken diagnosis of cellulitis, a diagnosis that may appear to be supported by a fever that may reach 101°F (38°C) or higher. Joint swelling usually is marked and joint effusion is also common. Tenderness on palpation or motion of the affected part also usually is marked.

The intensity and severity of these classical acute signs and symptoms may vary from one attack to another and may be less evident when a large joint such as the knee is involved, especially in elderly patients and in patients with polyarticular gout. However, the history will almost always indicate rapid progression to a peak intensity within 24 to 36 hours, an important feature in differential diagnosis.

Laboratory findings may include a mild leukocytosis and an elevated erythrocyte sedimentation rate. Serum uric acid almost always is elevated but is of limited diagnostic value because of the frequency of hyperuricemia in the absence of gout, and because the acute attack, which is related principally to the concentration of tissue urate, may occur at a time when the serum urate may be normal as a result of previous drug administration (such as high dose aspirin (>3.5 g/day) or another uricosuric agent) or of spontaneous variation. Examination of the synovial fluid provides diagnostic findings in almost all instances in which it can be obtained. There is a marked leukocytosis in the joint fluid with polymorphonuclear leukocytes that, when examined under polarized light, can be seen to contain phagocytized urate crystals (see section on crystal identification).

The acute attack is self-limited and even without treatment will subside in several days to weeks. Once the acute attack subsides or is treated, there are no residual joint symptoms—another important point in the differential diagnosis.

Recurrent acute attacks are usual: approximately 75% of patients will have a second gouty attack within 2 years of their first and most of these will have occurred within the first year; occasionally 10 years or more may elapse between attacks (32).

Intercritical Gout

Between acute attacks of gout, patients will be totally asymptomatic with no abnormal physical findings unless tophi are present or unless the disease has progressed to the chronic phase. If the patient's first visit to the physician is at this stage, a presumptive diagnosis can be made on the basis of a history of a typical prior attack, especially if there have been multiple attacks, and on the basis of hyperuricemia. Aspiration of the great toe during intercritical gout will demonstrate urate crystals in many (70%) patients with gout, but crystals may be occasionally found in patients with asymptomatic hyperuricemia or renal failure (28, 30, 31). Knee joint aspiration also yielded urate crystals in 58% of patients with intercritical non-tophaceous gout (4). Although reasonably specific for gout, the rather low sensitivity and the difficulty of obtaining synovial fluid in the absence of overt inflammation or effusion suggest that these procedures are not very useful in clinical practice.

Chronic Gout

This form of the disease is infrequent, especially since the advent of effective therapy to control hyperuricemia. Patients with chronic gout frequently have some persistent symptoms (such as morning stiffness) and manifest signs of synovial tissue thickening and some joint deformity. Acute exacerbations are still frequent and are often polyarticular. Tophi (soft tissue deposits of sodium urate) are present in 90 to 95% of patients. The rate of formation of tophi seems to be a direct function of the level and duration of hyperuricemia. Tophi are chalky or pinkish, gritty, usually superficial deposits that are palpable in joints or tendons, over pressure points, or in the pinnae of the ears. They are usually painless but after palpation they may be tender. Large tophi may look like bulbous swellings of the joints or, when they are located over the extensor surface of the forearm or in the ulnar bursa, may be mistaken for rheumatoid nodules. In such circumstances, aspiration or biopsy of tophi with demonstration of urate crystals will confirm the diagnosis of chronic gout. The actual concurrence of gout and rheumatoid arthritis is extremely rare.

Extra-articular Manifestations

It has long been known that primary gout may be associated with renal disease in three forms: *chronic gouty nephropathy, nephrolithiasis,* and *acute uric acid nephropathy.*

Chronic gouty nephropathy develops after many years of hyperuricemia and results from the deposition in the interstitial medullary tissue of sodium urate crystals that cause, ultimately, an interstitial nephritis. The frequency of this complication had, at one time, been assumed to be high. Controlled studies, however, have indicated that the incidence of renal insufficiency solely from gout and hyperuricemia is low and that renal dysfunction is usually mild; most often renal failure in patients with gout can be attributed to other causes such as vascular disease, or primary renal disease (3).

Renal failure from primary gout and hyperuricemia is usually silent and suspected only because of the identification of a mild abnormality of the concentration of blood urea nitrogen or of serum creatinine. Some patients will have slight proteinuria; only a few will be found to have peripheral tophi. It is not known whether secondary gout is associated with the development of chronic gouty nephropathy. The evaluation and management of patients who have renal failure are discussed in Chapter 48.

Uric acid nephrolithiasis accounts for only a small number of patients who have urinary calculi (see Chapter 47). However, approximately 20% of patients with gout develop calculi, although the stones may antedate acute gouty arthritis by years. From a different perspective, about 25% of patients with uric acid calculi have an abnormal serum urate concentration. The prevalence of uric acid calculi increases proportionately to the concentration of serum urate or to the excretion of uric acid whether or not gout is present. In one study, in which a cohort of men was followed for 12 years, serum levels of urate of 7 to 8 mg/dl, 8 to 9 mg/dl, and >9 mg/dl were associated with renal stones in 12.7, 22, and 40%, respectively (9). Also in gouty patients, urinary excretion rates of <300, 300 to 700, 700 to 1100, and >1100 mg/24 hours of uric acid were associated with an incidence of renal stones of 11, 21, 35, and 50%, respectively (33). The development of uric acid calculi is related not only to uric acid excretion but also to urinary pH and concentration. This subject is more fully discussed in Chapter 47.

Acute uric acid nephropathy is associated with a sudden increase in urate production and a marked rise in uric acid excretion, resulting in the formation of microcrystals in the renal tubules. This most often occurs in patients with lympho- or myeloproliferative disorders, especially during treatment. Acute uric acid nephropathy is rarely encountered in ambulatory practice.

Differential Diagnosis

During the acute attack gout must be differentiated principally from acute infectious arthritis, from bursitis related to a bunion (see Chapter 102), or from other forms of crystal-induced arthritis. It is important therefore to aspirate joint fluid for smear and culture (see Chapter 66 for technique and finding in the synovial fluid) as well as for crystal identification. Infectious arthritis is associated with a very low synovial fluid glucose, not found in gouty fluids. Rarely acute gout and infectious arthritis coexist (2).

X-rays (Fig. 69.2)

In the early course of gout, X-rays are normal except for acute soft tissue swelling. As the disease progresses, lucent areas of urate deposits may be seen in bone adjacent to the joints. These lesions may be mistaken for the erosions that are seen in rheumatoid or other arthritides but may be distinguished from them

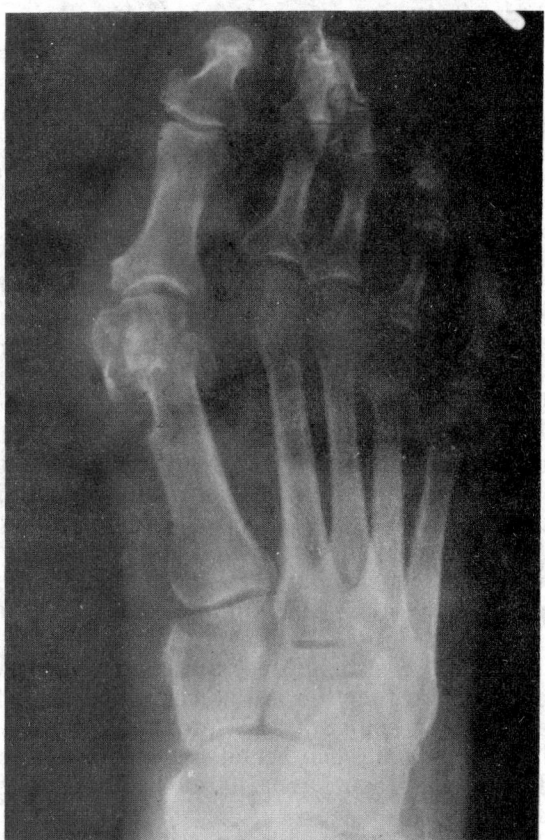

Figure 69.2. X-ray of the foot in patient with gout showing soft tissue swelling over first metatarsophalangeal joint and typical gouty erosion: away from joint margin, punched out with overhanging edge and no osteoporosis.

in that osteoporosis and bony sclerosis, which are common in other erosive diseases, are not present. Overhanging margins of bone are said to be characteristic of gouty erosions but are not frequently found.

X-rays of gouty joints are thus indicated mainly to evaluate the extent of possible tophaceous deposits in patients with gout of long duration, and only occasionally are X-rays indicated as an aid to diagnosis or differential diagnosis.

Management

If the diagnosis of gout can be established with certainty by the demonstration of urate crystals, the treatment is relatively simple and straightforward. Hospitalization is seldom required unless the diagnosis is in doubt; even the most severe case can be effectively managed on an ambulatory basis. The key elements in management are control of the pain of the acute attack and patient education to assure compliance with therapy administered to reduce serum urate concentration and to prevent recurrent attacks and progression to chronic tophaceous gout.

Management of the Acute Attack

If the diagnosis of acute gout is established or if gout has been diagnosed previously by the identification of urate crystals in the affected joints, rapid relief can be obtained in almost all cases by the administration of nonsteroidal anti-inflammatory drugs in appropriate doses. Indomethacin (Indocin), 50 mg (i.e., two 25-mg capsules), every 6 hours for six to eight doses is dramatically effective. There are few side effects if the dose is then quickly reduced to 25 mg every 6 hours after the initial response and maintained until the attack is completely resolved, usually no more than 5 to 7 days. Alternatively, other nonsteroidal anti-inflammatory drugs may be used (see Chapter 70 for a full discussion of NSAIDs). Phenylbutazone (Butazolidin), a potent anti-inflammatory agent, has been largely replaced by better tolerated and safer drugs. The plasma concentration and therapeutic effect of indomethacin (and of naproxen but apparently not of other nonsteroidal anti-inflammatory agents) are potentiated by an unknown mechanism by the simultaneous administration of probenecid (see below). Although the clinical significance of this interaction is unclear, especially with short course therapy, the manufacturer recommends that the dose of the nonsteroidal drug be reduced in patients who also are taking probenecid. Caution should also be used in elderly patients with impaired renal function or reduced renal blood flow due to cardiovascular disease since nonsteroidal anti-inflammatory drugs may acutely reduce renal function and precipitate acute renal failure or hyperkalemia (see Chapter 48).

Colchicine is the time-honored drug for treatment of acute gout; but its efficacy is limited by side effects that are almost invariable if an adequate dose is administered orally. The usual regimen is 0.6 mg every 1 to 2 hours up to 16 doses until relief is obtained or until side effects, usually diarrhea, nausea, or vomiting, develop. Dosage should be reduced in patients with impaired renal or hepatic function. It is no longer necessary to subject a patient to severe diarrhea when he already has a very painful joint, so that oral colchicine has largely been replaced by nonsteroidal anti-inflammatory agents. They are at least as effective and have fewer side effects (26). The exception is in the well-instructed patient who immediately after recognizing the onset of an acute attack of gout can institute oral colchicine and in doing so can abate the attack with a few doses and with minimal side effects.

Intravenous administration of colchicine rapidly provides a therapeutic plasma level of the drug and does not cause gastrointestinal side effects. It is useful in treatment of acute gout when the patient cannot take medication by mouth and in the patient with peptic ulcer disease, or with another contraindication to the use of nonsteroidal agents. Two milligrams of colchicine (available in ampules containing 1 mg in 2 ml) diluted with isotonic saline to 20 ml and given slowly (i.e., over 10 minutes) intravenously usually provide relief within 6 to 8 hours and, if necessary, may be followed by one or two doses of 1 mg in 20 ml of isotonic saline intravenously in 12 to 24 hours, not to exceed 4 mg in 24 hours. Reduced dosage is necessary in patients with impaired renal or hepatic function or in patients with neutropenia. Care must

be used to prevent extravasation of colchicine into the soft tissues since it may cause necrosis. Intravenous colchicine should not be used if the patient has recently received a course of oral colchicine.

A diagnostic therapeutic trial of colchicine has limited value since acute gout of several days' duration may not respond to colchicine and since pseudogout due to calcium pyrophosphate dihydrate-induced arthritis often shows a dramatic response as well. Because of its potential toxicity and even occasional deaths due to the inappropriate administration of intravenous colchicine, the therapeutic trail should be carefully considered. For example, acute podagra (acute arthritis of the metatarsophalangeal joint of the great toe) is highly characteristic of gout and uncommon in other arthritides.

Because diagnostic aspiration of this joint when acutely painful may cause marked discomfort for the patient, especially if undertaken by an inexperienced physician, a presumptive diagnosis of gout can be made on clinical grounds and the patient treated with nonsteroidal agents. A raised serum uric acid would further support the diagnosis of gout but is neither specific nor always present.

Corticosteroids provide another therapeutic alternative for acute gout in the patient who cannot take oral medications. Aspiration and intraarticular injection of corticosteroid is useful when a single large joint is involved. Intramuscular adrenocorticotropic hormone (ACTH), 40 to 80 units every 6 to 12 hours for up to 3 days, can also be used. Moderately high doses of oral corticosteroids are usually required (30 to 60 mg/day of prednisone) and its therapy is rarely indicated.

Drugs administered to lower serum urate have no place in the treatment of the acute gouty attack. In fact, these agents may cause exacerbation of acute attacks by the associated changes in plasma urate levels (see above).

Intercritical Gout

The efficacy of colchicine in doses of 0.6 mg one, two, or three times daily (dose frequency depends on control; most patients require two doses a day) in reducing the frequency of acute attacks of gout has been well established (21, 32). Thus, prophylactic colchicine should be given to all patients who have had more than one episode of acute gout to prevent recurrent attacks or to reduce the frequency of those attacks. Caution again is required in patients with impaired renal function. Reversible myopathy and neuropathy have been observed in some such patients even with two tablets per day (12). Infertility or azoospermia was also reported with the use of long-term prophylactic colchicine in four of 19 young men with familial Mediterranean fever (6). In patients without tophi (nontophaceous gout), with infrequent acute attacks and with mild hyperuricemia (i.e., <8 to 9 mg/dl), prophylactic colchicine may be all that is required. Some patients who have nontophaceous gout with infrequent attacks of arthritis (e.g., less than one or two a year) and who have relatively mild hyperuricemia (i.e., <8 to 9 mg/dl) may as an option elect not to take regular colchicine prophylaxis; in this instance, the episodic use of a nonsteroidal anti-inflammatory drug such as indomethacin (Indocin) (see above) is appropriate to control acute attacks. However, in most patients with gout and with persistent hyperuricemia of 9 mg/dl or higher, the serum urate concentration should be reduced to prevent recurrent gout and to reverse the accumulation of urate in the tissues. In this instance, colchicine prophylaxis should be continued until the patient has been free of attacks for at least 3 to 6 months after the concentration of serum urate has returned to normal.

Two classes of drugs that lower serum urate concentration are available: *uricosuric agents* promote urinary excretion of urate by blocking tubular urate resorption, and *allopurinol* (Xyloprim) decreases production of urate through inhibition of purine metabolism. Indications for the use of allopurinol are a history of urinary calculi or the presence of renal insufficiency, of chronic tophaceous gout, of excessive basal urinary uric acid excretion (i.e., >750 to 800 mg/24 hours), or of high levels of serum urate associated with secondary gout. Uricosuric agents are most effective in patients with nontophaceous gout with normal renal function and normal uric acid excretion (i.e., <750 to 800 mg/24 hours). Evaluation of urinary uric acid excretion is thus important not only as a clue to the mechanism of hyperuricemia (Table 69.2) but in the choice of therapy.

Probenecid (Benemid) is the uricosuric agent of choice because of its well-established safety and its relatively long duration of effect. An initial dose of 0.5 g twice daily should be increased to 1.5 g daily or to a maximum of 2 g/day (in two or three divided doses) to achieve a serum urate concentration consistently below 6.5 mg/dl, the level required to produce a urate gradient from tissue to plasma and to prevent further deposition of urate. In order to minimize the chance of precipitating a recurrent arthritic attack, the uricosuric agent should not be initiated until at least a week after an acute attack of gout has subsided and only after colchicine prophylaxis (see above) has been initiated for 3 or 4 days. The principal side effect of probenecid is gastrointestinal distress, but there is a risk of the formation of uric acid calculi in the renal tubules in the first week of therapy (the period of negative uric acid balance), especially when there is a large basal uric acid excretion (i.e., 600 to 800 mg/day); this risk can be eliminated if the patient drinks 2 to 3 liters of fluid/day and takes an alkalinizing agent such as sodium bicarbonate or citrate salt (Polycitrate), 0.5 to 1 mEq/kg of body weight in five or six doses a day, to keep the urine pH (measured from time to time with pH paper) above 6.0 to 6.5 for the first week of uricosuric therapy. Small doses of aspirin (2.4 g/day) block the effect of probenecid on renal excretion of urate and should be avoided.

Sulfinpyrazone (Anturane) is a more potent urico-

suric agent but must be given every 4 to 6 hours (400 to 600 mg/day) for maximal effect. This agent, which is an analogue of phenylbutazone, may cause gastric ulceration and platelet dysfunction. For these reasons, it should be used only when probenecid or allopurinol (see below) is not tolerated.

Allopurinol (Xyloprim) is a potent agent that reduces the concentration of serum urate. Because it blocks urate production, it is particularly useful in patients with renal dysfunction or with uric acid calculi. Serious side effects of rash, fever, leukopenia, hepatitis, and/or occasionally a generalized vasculitis occur in less than 2% of patients. These symptoms are most likely to occur within the first 2 months after initiation of therapy so that patients should be kept under close surveillance during this period. Toxicity seems to be enhanced when the drug is administered concomitantly with thiazide diuretics. Allopurinol (Xyloprim, available in 100- and 300-mg tablets) should be started at a dose of 200 mg daily and increased gradually (i.e., over 2 or 3 weeks) until the serum urate is consistently below 6.5 mg/dl; no more than 300 mg should be administered as a single dose. Prolonged use of doses in excess of 300 mg twice a day increases the risk of toxicity.

Concomitant use of allopurinol and probenecid has been advocated (29). These agents seem to have an additive effect in lowering serum uric acid. However, use of a single agent is preferable if possible.

Compliance is the major factor in the effective therapy of intercritical gout. Patients feel well between attacks, and continued compliance with medications requires reinforcement in patient education and in follow-up visits to ensure maintenance of normal serum levels of urate.

Dietary advice to patients with gout should be kept simple. Because of the complexity of urate metabolism and secretion, the role of ingestion of purine in gout is of importance only in extreme situations. Patients with an excretion of urate that is greater than 1100 mg/24 hours should be advised to decrease the use of purine-rich foods such as liver, kidney, and fish roe. Such foods are not, however, commonly used in excess. More important, dietary advice is to avoid alcohol (beer especially since it also adds to the purine load) and to avoid fasting beyond 24 hours as both these situations may be associated with an acute increase of serum urate concentration and this change may precipitate an attack of gout.

Chronic Gout

Compliance with appropriate therapy should eliminate this phase of gout except for a few patients with severe disease who are intolerant of one or more drugs used in treatment. Prolonged use of nonsteroidal anti-inflammatory agents (including aspirin in doses greater than 3.5 g/day—a uricosuric dose) may be required in some of these patients for adequate control of inflammation and chronic symptoms. Effective reduction in serum urate for months or years will result in dissolution of tophi and in general improvement. However, very large tophi may require surgical removal.

Asymptomatic Hyperuricemia

Asymptomatic hyperuricemia (>7 mg/dl in males and >6 mg/dl in females) should be evaluated first by assessment of urine uric acid excretion. If urinary uric acid excretion is significantly elevated (>600 mg/day on low purine diet or >750 to 800 mg/day in the absence of purine gluttony), a careful search for causes of hyperuricemia (see Table 69.2) should be made and consideration should be given to allopurinol therapy in order to prevent urinary stones and chronic renal insufficiency from interstitial deposition of urate. However, in the majority of such patients urine uric acid excretion will be normal or reduced despite hyperuricemia. In this situation, some of these patients may subsequently develop gouty arthritis, but the risk of urinary stones or renal disease is much less than if the urine uric acid excretion were elevated. The expense and potential toxicity of therapy to lower serum urate, therefore, are probably not warranted since therapy can be successfully initiated if gout develops and the risks of hyperuricemia are minimal (5, 13).

Hyperuricemia Secondary to Diuretics

The renal tubular handling of uric acid is complex: there is complete glomerular filtration followed by tubular resorption, tubular secretion, and further tubular resorption. The resorption of uric acid is in part modulated by the volume of extracellular fluid (expansion increases excretion and contraction decreases excretion). Diuretics modify the renal handling of uric acid by their effect on volume, and also some diuretics may directly affect urate transport. Thiazides regularly cause a dose-related rise of the serum urate level. This elevation is reversed upon withdrawal of the agent. The increase in concentration averages 1 to 2 mg/dl but occasionally may be 4 to 5 mg/dl. Furosemide also is frequently associated with a rise in concentration of serum urate; less commonly ethacrynic acid, acetazolamide, and rarely triamterene are associated with hyperuricemia. Spironolactone per se is not associated with hyperuricemia.

The incidence of gout after the initiation of a diuretic is a complex issue. Other factors that affect the incidence of gout—such as hypertension or obesity—are often present in patients treated with diuretics. Approximately 10% of hypertensive patients with hyperuricemia secondary to diuretic therapy actually develop gout. This risk increases in patients with known gout and those patients with diseases associated with elevation of serum urate, such as myeloproliferative disorders or psoriasis. Also in association with diuretic therapy, uric acid excretion is diminished and there is no increase in the incidence of urinary calculi. The risk of developing urate nephropathy is minimal (see above). For these reasons expectant management of patients with asymptomatic hyperuricemia secondary to diuretics is appropriate.

Should acute gout develop, treatment as described above may be initiated. Intercritical gout is managed similarly to primary gout, and uricosuric therapy with probenecid (if there is no renal failure) or therapy with allopurinol to decrease production of urate may be used. Stopping the diuretic is usually associated with a slight fall in the plasma urate concentration, but many patients will continue to have attacks of gout. Therefore, if a patient develops gout while taking diuretics, and the need for the diuretic continues, it is best to treat the gout as discussed above and to continue the use of the diuretic.

CALCIUM PYROPHOSPHATE DIHYDRATE (CPPD)-INDUCED ARTHRITIS

Pathophysiology

Pseudogout is a syndrome caused by the deposition of calcium pyrophosphate dihydrate in fibrocartilage (chondrocalcinosis) and joint tissue and in ligaments and tendons with an occasional resulting inflammatory response. It most often is idiopathic but may be associated with certain other diseases (see below).

Inorganic pyrophosphate is an important metabolite in many biosynthetic reactions where it is removed from macromolecules through the action of pyrophosphatases. It is adsorbed to hydroxyapatite and is probably involved in the regulation of mineralization, both in the accretion from amorphous calcium phosphate and in the dissolution of crystalline hydroxyapatite.

Epidemiology

Chondrocalcinosis increases in frequency with age; it is present in about 5% of the adult population at the time of autopsy and in 20 to 30% of people above age 80, most of whom are asymptomatic. The exact prevalence of CPPD disease is not known. In one series of consecutive patients with newly diagnosed crystal-induced arthritis, CPPD disease accounted for about one-third of the cases (15). Males are probably affected more than females with a ratio of males to females of 1.5:1 in the largest reported series (15).

Etiology

Familial cases with an autosomal dominant inheritance have been described (24) in which chondrocalcinosis appears at an earlier age. These families are uncommon, and many of these patients will remain asymptomatic for many years; the metabolic defect has not been identified, however. Most cases of CPPD disease are sporadic and idiopathic; a few are associated with one of a variety of metabolic diseases. Many of the diseases associated with deposits of CPPD involve metabolic abnormalities in connective tissues, but the precise mechanisms of CPPD crystallization are unknown. A list of these associated diseases is presented in Table 69.4.

Clinical Features (Table 69.5)

Patients are usually middle-aged to elderly at the time of onset of arthritic symptoms. There are several possible patterns of presentation: about one-quarter present with *self-limited acute gout-like attacks (pseudogout)* predominantly affecting the knees and wrists, but occasionally involving other joints, including rarely the first metatarsophalangeal joint. Monarticular attacks are the rule, but involvement of symmetrical joints and polyarthritis may occur rarely. Symptoms are often less intense than they are in gout, but the presentation is variable and some attacks may be quite severe. Systemic symptoms, including fever to 101°F (38°C) or more, may occur as in gout, and patients are frequently misdiagnosed as having infection. Attacks are often exacerbated by trauma and by acute illness. Long intervals (sometimes years) between attacks are common.

In about half the patients, and especially in women, the presentation *resembles osteoarthritis* with bilateral involvement, especially of the knees. The wrists, the metacarpophalangeal (MCP) joints, hips, shoulders, elbows, or ankles also may be affected. Acute exacerbations occur in about half of these patients with features that resemble osteoarthritis except that the disease is more progressive and destructive. Varus or valgus knee deformities are common, and extensive

Table 69.4.
Diseases Associated with Calcium Pyrophosphate Dihydrate (CPPD) Deposition Disease

Hemochromatosis—hemosiderosis
Gout
Hyperparathyroidism
Hypomagnesemia
Hereditary hypophosphatasia
Hypothyroidism
Neurogenic arthropathy

Table 69.5.
Clinical Features of Calcium Pyrophosphate Dihydrate (CPPD) Deposit Disease

EPIDEMIOLOGY
 Age: Middle aged or elderly
SITE
 Knee and wrist most common joints involved
 Metacarpophalangeal joints, hips, shoulders, elbows, ankles may be affected
 Arthritis usually monoarticular
PATTERN
 Acute gout-like attacks with symptom-free intervals in 25%
 Osteoarthritis-like disease in 50%, with superimposed acute attacks in half of these patients
 Rheumatoid-like polyarthritis in 5%
 Neuropathic-like arthritis without neurological damage (rare)
 Asymptomatic chondrocalcinosis in 20% (found on X-ray)
LABORATORY
 Synovial fluid shows leukocytosis and characteristic CPPD crystals

calcification around the patella may be seen on X-ray. Flexion contractures may occur also. The relationship to ordinary osteoarthritis is still unclear, except that the involvement of joints not usually affected in osteoarthritis (MCPs, wrists, shoulders, elbows) suggests a different pathogenesis (see also Chapter 68).

In a few patients persistent subacute inflammation with fatigue, morning stiffness, and synovial swelling in multiple joints lasting weeks or months resembles rheumatoid arthritis.

A few patients also have been reported with severely *destructive arthritis* resembling the Charcot joints of neuropathic arthropathy but associated with a normal neurological examination (19). CPPD disease may also be associated with a true neuropathic arthritis due to tabes dorsalis.

Laboratory Findings

Patients may have peripheral leukocytosis and an elevated erythrocyte sedimentation rate in association with acute or subacute attacks of arthritis. The synovial fluid will show polymorphonuclear leukocytosis that may exceed 50,000/mm³ in acute pseudogout but is more commonly in the range of 15,000 to 25,000. Crystal identification is the key to diagnosis (see above). In the absence of acute or subacute inflammation, leukocyte counts may be low (< 2000/mm³) and crystals may be largely extracellular.

Because of the occasional association with other disorders (Table 69.4), the patient's serum calcium, phosphorus, alkaline phosphatase, and uric acid concentrations should be measured, although they will usually be normal (17). Because pseudogout may be the presenting manifestation of hemochromatosis and because of the importance of early diagnosis in this disorder, measurement of serum ferritin is also indicated if there is any suspicion of this diagnosis.

X-ray Findings

The typical X-ray findings of CPPD deposit disease are punctate and linear calcifications (chondrocalcinosis) seen most frequently in the fibrocartilage of the menisci of the knee, usually bilaterally (Fig. 69.3). Other fibrocartilages may show similar changes, including the disc in the distal radioulnar joint, the symphysis pubis, the lip of the acetabulum, or the glenoid fossa or intervertebral discs. Hyaline cartilage may also be involved with similar punctate linear calcifications that may be identified as a dense line parallel to the subchondral bone. Calcification in the soft tissues of the joint capsule and occasionally in ligaments and tendons may also be seen but is less characteristic. In patients with the type of CPPD disease that resembles osteoarthritis, subchondral cyst formation with bony collapse may be prominent. Osteophyte formation is variable and inconsistent.

These radiographic findings may be helpful in suggesting or confirming the diagnosis of CPPD disease. However, it may not be possible to visualize the extent

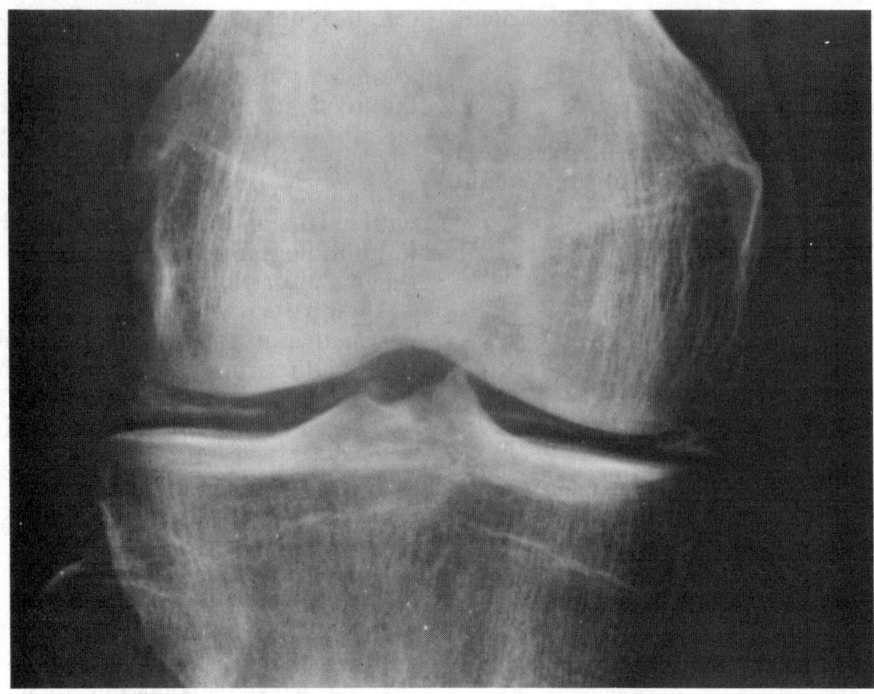

Figure 69.3. X-ray of knee of a patient with chondrocalcinosis. Stippled calcification of the medial and lateral menisci is easily identified.

of deposits radiographically, and their absence does not exclude the diagnosis if typical crystals can be demonstrated in synovial fluid or in biopsy material.

Management

There is no therapy that influences the deposition or resolution of tissue deposits of CPPD. In the acute episode diagnostic aspiration of synovial fluid with removal of crystals and leukocytes may provide significant clinical improvement. Local injection of depocorticosteroid is often effective and avoids potential side effects of systemic drug therapy (see Chapter 66, for technique). Efficacy of colchicine has been debated, and although it is sometimes effective, the use of indomethacin (Indocin) or other nonsteroidal anti-inflammatory agents is generally preferred as described above for acute gout (see above). Because many of these patients are elderly (and may therefore have an impaired glomerular filtration rate), caution regarding renal toxicity of these agents should be exercised (see Chapter 48). In patients with only recurrent acute attacks, no therapy is indicated between attacks, but early administration of anti-inflammatory agents on exacerbation may minimize or abort attacks. Therapy for patients with more subacute inflammation or for those with osteoarthritis-like disease is similar to that described for osteoarthritis (see Chapter 68), except that anti-inflammatory levels of drugs may be required for optimal symptomatic control.

HYDROXYAPATITE-INDUCED ARTHRITIS

The capacity of hydroxyapatite crystals to induce an inflammatory response was first appreciated in some patients with acute tendinitis (23). More recently hydroxyapatite crystals have been identified in patients with osteoarthritis, especially in association with acute inflammatory episodes (11) and in patients with destructive arthropathy of the shoulder joint (11). The latter, termed *Milwaukee shoulder*, is associated with painful limited shoulder motion, complete disruption of the rotator cuff, and extensive degenerative changes in the bone. In these conditions (see Chapter 63 for discussion) crystals of other basic calcium salts including octacalcium phosphate and tricalcium phosphate in addition to hydroxyapatite have sometimes been identified. This has prompted the use of the term *BCP (basic calcium phosphate) deposit disease* to describe these syndromes (10, 18). Calcium crystals may also be found in addition to BCP crystals in these syndromes in some cases. Alizarin red S dye (available from scientific supply houses) may be used to stain wet preparations of synovial fluid to screen for the presence of hydroxyapatite crystals, which appear with ordinary light microscopy as red-stained clumps of crystalline material (20). Because all other calcium-containing crystals and even noncrystalline calcium salts stain with this dye, specific identification of BCP crystals will require techniques not usually available, such as electron microscopy, microprobe analysis, or X-ray diffraction. Further definition of the role of hydroxyapatite in crystal-induced arthritis and of the spectrum of its clinical manifestations will be forthcoming as identification of crystals is applied more widely. At this time one need only be aware of the potential inflammatory properties of this crystalline material and consider its implication in the above clinical situations. The patient may be managed by the aspiration, from a joint or soft tissue, of the crystalline material and with the subsequent local injection of lidocaine/corticosteroids solution (see Chapter 66) or treatment using a nonsteroidal anti-inflammatory drug (see Chapter 70). These modalities should provide symptomatic relief in acute inflammatory arthritis or tendonitis associated with BCP crystal deposits. When symptoms become chronic or when extensive destructive arthropathy is present, rheumatological or orthopaedic referral is indicated.

ARTHRITIS ASSOCIATED WITH CALCIUM OXALATE

Another crystal-associated arthritis has been demonstrated in patients on long-term dialysis (usually hemodialysis but also seen with peritoneal dialysis) for end stage renal disease. Extensive deposits of calcium oxalate in soft tissues occurs in this setting, and these deposits may cause acute arthritis, destructive arthropathy, tenosynovitis, or bursitis (25, 27). These patients are difficult to manage because of the presence of extensive and continuing deposits and incomplete response to colchicine, nonsteroidal agents, and corticosteroids.

General References

Dieppe P, Doherty M, Macfarlane D (ed): Symposium on the crystal-related arthropathies. *Ann Rheum Dis* 42, London (Suppl 1), 1983.
    A collection of papers on this topic.
Kelley WN, Fox JH, Pallela TD: Gout and related disorders of purine metabolism. In: Kelley WN, Harris Jr ED, Ruddy S, Sledge CB (eds): *Textbook of Rheumatolgy.* 3rd ed. Philadelphia, WB Saunders, 1989.
Moskowitz RW: Diseases associated with the deposition of calcium pyrophosphate and hydroxyapatite. In: Kelley WN, Harris Jr ED, Ruddy S, Sledge CB (eds): *Textbook of Rheumatology.* 3rd ed. Philadelphia, WB Saunders, 1989.
    These two chapters in this comprehensive textbook provide an up-to-date review of all aspects of crystal-induced arthritis.
Steinbroker O, Neustadt PH: In: *Arthritis and Musculoskeletal Disorders.* Hagerstown, MD, Harper & Row, 1972.
    This is a very practical manual to aid the physician in the techniques of joint aspiration.

Specific References

1. Abbott RD, Brand FN, Kannel WB, Castelli W: Gout and coronary heart diesase. The Framingham Study. *J Clin Epidemiol* 41:237, 1988.
2. Baer PA, Tennenbaum J, Fain G, Little H: Coexistent septic and crystal arthritis. Report of four cases and literature review. *J Rheumatol* 13:604, 1986.
3. Berger L, Yu TF: Renal function in gout. *Am J Med* 59:605, 1975.
4. Bomalaski JS, Lluberas G, Schumacher JH Jr: Monosodium urate crystals in the knee joints of patients with nontophaceous gout. *Arthritis Rheum* 29:1480, 1986.
5. Campion EM, Glynn RJ, DeLabry LO: Asymptomatic hyperuricemia, risks and consequences in the normative aging study. *Am J Med* 82:421, 1987.
6. Ehrenfeld M, Levy M, Margolioth EJ, Eliakim M: The effects of long-term colchicine therapy on male fertility in patients with familial Mediterranean fever. *Andrologia* 4:420, 1986.
6a. Fagan TJ, Lidsky MD: Compensated polarized light microscopy using cellophane adhesive tape. *Arthritis Rheum* 17:256, 1974.
7. Gordon TP, Terkeltaub R: Gout: Crystal induced inflammation. In: Gallin JI, Goldstein IM, Synderman R (eds): *Inflammation.*
Basic Principles and Clinical Correlates. New York, Raven Press, 1988.
8. Gutman AB, Yu TF: Uric acid nephrolithiasis. *Am J Med* 45:756, 1968.
9. Hall AP, Barry PE, Dawber TR, et al: Epidemiology of gout and hyperuricemia. *Am J Med* 42:27, 1967.
10. Halverson PB, McCarty DJ, Cheung HS, Ryan LM: Milwaukee shoulder syndrome: Eleven additional cases with involvement of the knee in seven (basic calcium phosphate crystal deposition disease). *Semin Arth Rheum* 14:36, 1984.
11. Huskisson EC, Dreppe PA, Tucker AK, Cannell LB: Another look at osteoarthritis. *Ann Rheum Dis* 38:423, 1979.
12. Kuncl RW, Duncan G, Watson D, et al: Colchicine myopathy and neuropathy. *N Engl J Med* 316:1562, 1987.
13. Liang MH, Fries JF: Asymptomatic hyperuricemia: the case for conservative management. *Ann Intern Med* 88:666, 1978.
14. Malawista SE, Duff GW, Atkins E, et al: Crystal induced endogenous pyrogen production. A further look at gouty inflammation. *Arthritis Rheum* 28:1039, 1985.
15. McCarty DJ: Pseudogout and pyrophosphate metabolism. *Adv Intern Med* 25:363, 1980.
16. McCarty DJ, Halverson PB, Carrera GF, et al: "Milwaukee shoulder"—association of microspheroids containing hydroxy-apatite crystals, active collagenase and neutral protease with rotator cuff defects. I. Clinical aspects. *Arthritis Rheum* 24:464, 1981.
17. McCarty DJ, Silcox DC, Coe F, et al: Diseases associated with calcium pyrophosphate dihydrate crystal deposition. A controlled study. *Am J Med* 56:704, 1974.
18. McCarty DJ: Arthropathies associated with calcium containing crystals. *Hosp Pract* 21:109, 1986.
19. Menkes CJ, Simon F, Delrieu F, et al: Destructive arthropathy in chondrocalcinosis articulosis. *Arthritis Rheum* 19:329, 1976.
20. Paul H, Reginato AJ, Schumacher R: Alizarin red S staining as a screening test to detect calcium compounds in synovial fluid. *Arthritis Rheum* 26:191, 1983.
21. Paulus HE, Schlosstein LH, Godfrey RG, et al: Prophylactic colchicine therapy of intercritical gout. A placebo controlled study of probenecid-treated patients. *Arthritis Rheum* 17:609, 1974.
22. Phelps P, Steele AD, McCarty DJ Jr: Compensated polarized light microscopy. *JAMA* 203:508, 1968.
23. Pinals RS, Short CL: Calcific periarthritis involving multiple sites. *Arthritis Rheum* 7:359, 1964.
24. Reginato A, Valenzuela F, Martinez V, et al: Polyarticular and familial chondrocalcinosis. *Arthritis Rheum* 13:197, 1970.
25. Reginato AJ, Seonane JLF, Alvarez CB: Arthropathy and curtaneous calcinosis in hemodialysis oxalosis. *Arthritis Rheum* 29:1387, 1986.
26. Roberts WN, Liang MH, Stern SH: Colchicine in acute gout. Reassessment of risks and benefits. *JAMA* 257:1920, 1987.
27. Rosenthal A, Ryan LM, McCarty DJ: Arthritis associated with calcium oxalate crystals in an anephric patient treated with peritoneal dialysis. *JAMA* 260:1272, 1988.
28. Rouault T, Caldwell DS, Holmes EW: Aspiration of the asymptomatic metatarsophalangeal joint in gout patients and hyperuricemic controls. *Arthritis Rheum* 25:209, 1982.
29. Rundles RW, Metz EN, Silberman JR: Allopurinol in the treatment of gout. *Ann Intern Med* 64:229, 1966.
30. Wall B, Agudelo CA, Tesser JRP, et al: An autopsy study of the prevalence of monosodium urate and calcium pyrophosphate dihydrate crystal deposition in the first metatarsophalangeal joints. *Arthritis Rheum* 26:1522, 1983.
31. Weinberger A, Schumacher HR, Agudelo CA: Urate crystals in asymptomatic metatarsophalangeal joints. *Ann Intern Med* 91:56, 1979.
32. Yu TF, Gutman AB: Efficacy of colchicine prophylaxis in gout. Prevention of recurrent gouty arthritis over a mean period of five years in 208 gouty subjects. *Ann Intern Med* 55:179, 1961.
33. Yu TF, Gutman AB: Uric acid nephrolithiasis in gout. Predisposing factors. *Ann Intern Med* 67:1133, 1967.

C H A P T E R   70

Rheumatoid Arthritis

FREDRICK M. WIGLEY, M.D.

Rheumatoid arthritis is a chronic inflammatory systemic disease of unknown etiology that has a predilection for involvement of the joints. The articular inflammation has a variable course, but an additive (see below) symmetrical chronic polyarthritis associated with joint destruction, deformity, and loss of function is the primary clinical problem. Extra-articular features are recognized as an integral part of the disease and may antedate the onset of the inflammatory arthropathy by months.

In the past, patients with inflammatory arthritis were lumped under the diagnostic umbrella of either "rheumatoid arthritis" or "gout." In the last few decades it has been recognized that the spectrum of inflammatory arthritis can be separated into a number of individual disease processes. A clinician is now faced with an increasing complexity of diagnostic possibilities and, therefore, must develop a comprehensive approach that encompasses the history, physical examination, and appropriate laboratory studies.

EPIDEMIOLOGY

Population surveys have used somewhat different criteria for diagnosis of rheumatoid arthritis, but most have agreed that it has a worldwide distribution and, in white populations, a prevalence of definite classical disease of 1 to 2% (5). Important geographic and ethnic/racial variations exist. A high prevalence has been noted in North American Indians (3.5 to 5.3%) and a low prevalence has been reported in rural South African blacks and in Japanese (0.1%).

The prevalence increases with age, approaching 5% in women over age 55. The average annual incidence in the United States is about 70/100,000/year. Both incidence and prevalence of rheumatoid arthritis are two to three times greater in women than men. Although rheumatoid arthritis may present at any age, it most commonly affects patients in the third to sixth decades. Women tend to have a more severe articular disease, whereas extra-articular features are more common in men.

Seropositive rheumatoid arthritis (see below) aggregates in families, suggesting genetic and/or environmental influences on disease expression. The B cell alloantigen HLA-DR4 has been found in 70% of Caucasian seropositive patients compared with 25% of unaffected controls (17). DR4 associations have been confirmed in family studies in a variety of ethnic groups, thus defining an increased relative risk of four to five times in the DR4-positive individual.

PATHOGENESIS

Although the cause of rheumatoid arthritis is unknown, the infiltration of the synovia of affected joints by lymphocytes, plasma cells, and macrophages, associated with synovial lining cell proliferation (the so-called pannus), has suggested a cell-mediated immune process (10, 12). Local production of rheumatoid factor-containing immune complexes that are capable of activating complement and attracting inflammatory cells also has been shown. The inflammatory process is amplified by a variety of mediators including prostaglandins and a number of cytokines released by both synovial and infiltrating cells. The subsequent release of destructive enzymes and the altered cellular function cause destruction of cartilage and bone and subsequent loss of normal joint architecture.

HISTORY

The presentation of the disease (Table 70.1) varies from situations in which the diagnosis is obvious to ones in which the presentation is so atypical that it suggests other conditions. Diagnosis may be complicated further by the fact that rheumatoid arthritis may present with signs and symptoms that mimic other musculoskeletal disorders, such as gout or pseudogout (Chapter 69), polymyalgia rheumatica (Chapter 79), and fibrositis (Chapter 66).

The typical case of rheumatoid arthritis begins insidiously with the slowly progressive development of

Table 70.1.
Symptoms and Signs of Rheumatoid Arthritis

Symptoms		Signs	
Extra-articular	Articular[a]	Extra-articular	Articular
Fatigue	Morning stiffness	Rheumatoid nodules	Pain on passive motion
Depression	Pain and tenderness	Lymphadenopathy	Tenderness
Malaise	Swelling	Splenomegaly	Swelling
Anorexia		Ocular disease	Heat
		Entrapment neuropathies	Typical deformity

[a] Persistence (6 weeks or more) and symmetrical nature of signs and symptoms are important, but not invariable, diagnostic features.

symptoms and signs over a period of weeks to months. Occasionally, however, patients will experience an acute onset, usually polyarticular, within 24 to 48 hours; sometimes an acute presentation appears to be associated with either emotional or physical stress (for example, loss of a loved one or a recent injury).

Nonspecific systemic symptoms, primarily fatigue, malaise, and depression, are common but not invariable and may precede other symptoms of the disease by weeks to months. Usually the patient does not feel tired upon awakening but complains of rather severe fatigue 4 to 6 hours later. Fever occurs occasionally and is almost always low grade (37 to 38°C; 99 to 100°F); a higher fever suggests another illness, such as infection.

Arthritic symptoms (and signs) provide the definitive clues by which a specific diagnosis is made. Often the patient first notices stiffness (see below) in one or more joints, usually accompanied by pain on movement and by tenderness in the joint. Unlike a patient with gout (Chapter 69), a patient with rheumatoid arthritis can bear weight and can move the inflamed joint but has a persistent, deep, gnawing discomfort. In fact, severe pain in a patient with established rheumatoid arthritis should suggest a superimposed infection or an acute structural abnormality. The number of joints that are involved is highly variable, but almost always the process is eventually polyarticular (involvement of five or more joints). Rheumatoid arthritis is called an "additive" polyarthritis (there tends to be sequential involvement of joints) in contrast to the migratory or evanescent arthritis that can be seen in systemic lupus erythematosus or in the episodic arthritis of gout. The American Rheumatism Association, in its new revised criteria for the diagnosis of rheumatoid arthritis (1), has emphasized the importance of persistent swelling of the joints for greater than 6 weeks, stating that persistent soft tissue swelling of (or increased fluid in) a joint, followed by swelling of symmetrical joints, is characteristic of the disease. Any joints may be involved; but there is a predilection for peripheral joints with a relative sparing of the axial skeletal; the joints involved most often are the proximal interphalangeal (PIP) and metacarpophalangeal (MCP) joints of the hands, the wrists (particularly at the ulnar-styloid articulation), knees, elbows, temporomandibular joints, hips, ankles, and metatarsophalangeal (MTP) joints.

Morning stiffness may be a feature of any inflammatory arthritis but is especially characteristic of rheumatoid arthritis (almost all patients complain of it) and, in fact, is a useful gauge to measure the activity of the disease. The symptom is defined as stiffness, predominantly over joints, which persists at least for several hours (the average is 3 to 4 hours), thus distinguishing it from the transient gelation phenomenon of degenerative arthritis that lasts but a few minutes (see Chapter 68). Similar stiffness may, of course, occur after any prolonged period of inactivity.

It is typical of patients with rheumatoid arthritis that their symptoms wax and wane, especially at the beginning of the illness. Because of this and because objective signs may not be present at first, it is not unusual that the diagnosis is delayed for months. During this time the physician can best serve the patient by reassurance, careful interval history and periodic physical examination (see below), and, if appropriate, selected screening tests (see below). Symptomatic treatment with anti-inflammatory drugs may be instituted during this period (see below).

PHYSICAL EXAMINATION

A complete physical examination initially and then a limited examination every 3 to 6 months are important in patients with suspected rheumatoid arthritis, not only to make the diagnosis but to establish a baseline against which to assess the possible later development of both articular and extra-articular disease.

However, the primary focus of examinations in the physician's office will be the joints—repeated examinations and careful records of the status of affected joints, determined by history and previous examinations.

Joints

Swelling is the most measurable change that occurs in a joint that is affected by rheumatoid arthritis. The first change in involved joints is usually soft tissue swelling; eventually increased amounts of fluid within the joint space produce more readily recognizable (and, often, persistent) changes. In the hands, where the disease is often first manifest, typical fusiform swelling of the PIP joints commonly occurs (Fig. 70.1); the distal interphalangeal joints are less often involved. The MCP joints and the wrists are swollen even more

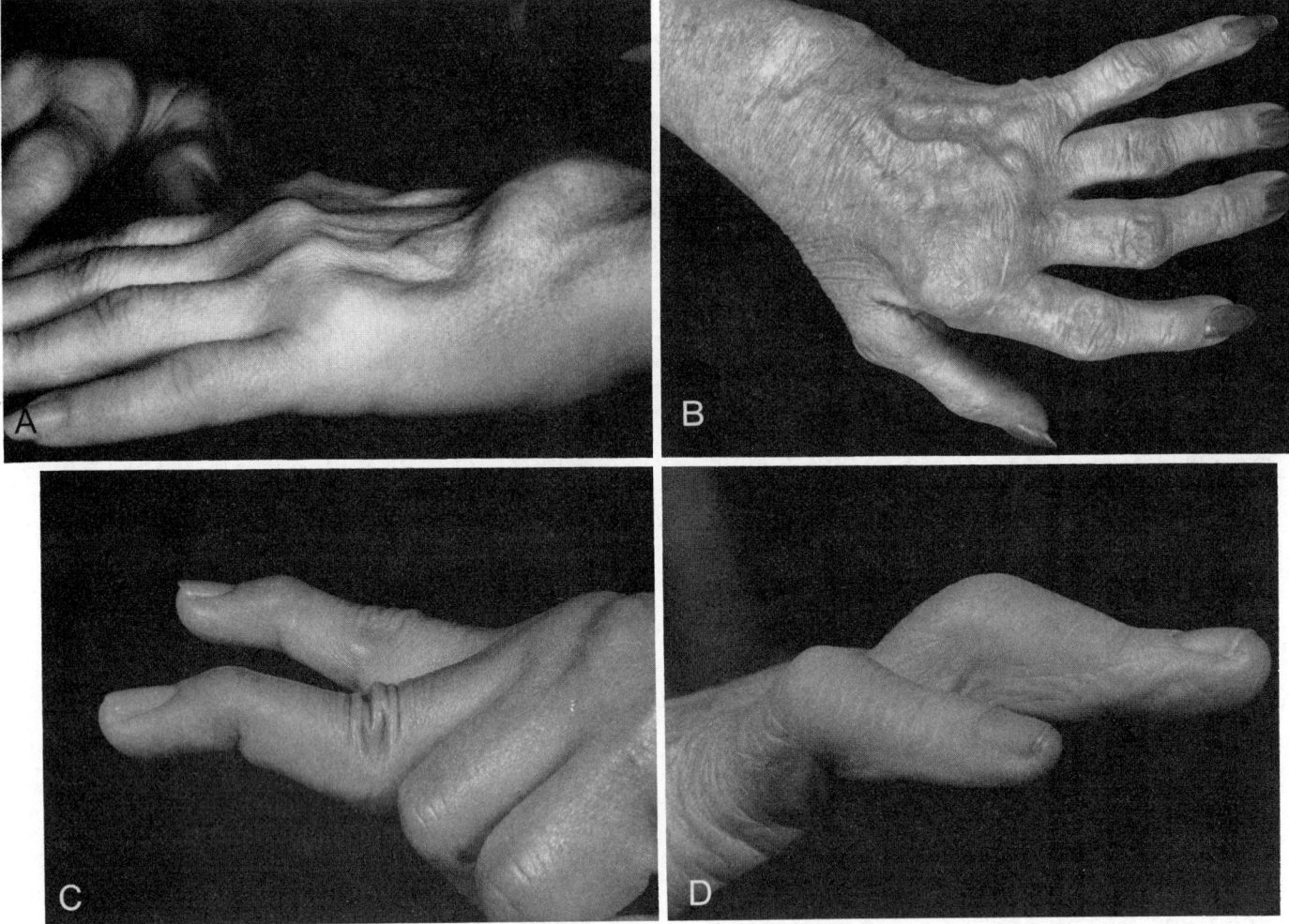

Figure 70.1. Hand deformities in rheumatoid arthritis. *A.* Typical fusiform swelling of the PIP joints; note also the synovial swelling of the wrist and MCP joints. *B.* Ulnar deviation of the fingers. *C.* Swan-neck deformity (hyperextension of PIP joint). *D.* Boutonnière deformity (flexion contracture of PIP joint).

often than are the PIP joints. The elbows, knees, ankles, and MTP joints are other common sites of disease where swelling may be readily apparent. Swelling of symmetrical joints, although not invariable, is characteristic of rheumatoid arthritis.

In contrast to gout (see Chapter 69) or to septic arthritis, redness of affected joints is not a prominent feature of rheumatoid arthritis.

Tenderness and pain on passive motion, although not specific for rheumatoid arthritis, are the most sensitive indices of inflammation of a joint. It is important to apply gentle but firm pressure when examining a joint so that tenderness due to inflammation will be elicited, but not so much pressure that a normal joint will be inappropriately symptomatic. Inflamed joints are also usually warmer than normal joints; the examiner may assess this best by feeling them with the back of his fingers.

The range of motion of the joint may be limited by inflammation and/or structural deformity, and it is important to determine which of these processes is play-

ing the major role in this regard so that appropriate therapy (see below) can be prescribed.

Weakness is a common feature of patients with rheumatoid arthritis; but, like range of motion, it is not easy to assess. The fatigue produced by the illness (see above) may contribute to an overall sense of weakness; but weakness of one or more limbs or parts of limbs may be caused by muscle atrophy, a result of joint deformity and of disuse. However, weakness may only seem to be present at times when, because of pain, the patient is unwilling to apply his full strength.

Permanent deformity may be an end stage of the inflammatory process that is first apparent as joint swelling. Persistent tenosynovitis and synovitis may lead to the formation of synovial cysts, which sometimes rupture (see below), to displaced tendons, and to compression by synovial fluid of the normal supporting structures of the joint (leading, for example, to muscle atrophy). These anatomical changes result in flexion contractures and subluxation (incomplete dislocation) of articulating bones. Typical visible changes (Fig. 70.1) include ulnar deviation of the fingers at the MCP joints, hyperextension or hyperflexion of the joints of the fingers, and, occasionally, ankylosis of the carpal and tarsal joints. Ankylosis of other joints is rare and may be a distinguishing feature when comparing rheumatoid arthritis with diseases that mimic it. Displaced toes ("cocked-up") with hallux valgus formation (angulation of the great toe laterally) are also common.

Synovial cysts are common in patients with rheumatoid arthritis and can be readily seen and palpated overlying the joints with which they communicate. Synovial cysts of the popliteal space (Baker's cysts) may develop in patients with a variety of disorders of the knee but seem to be especially prevalent in patients with rheumatoid disease. If popliteal cysts rupture, the signs and symptoms resemble closely those of acute thrombophlebitis (calf swelling and tenderness—even a positive Homans' sign). Proper therapy depends on the physician's ability to make the right diagnosis. An arthrogram (performed by injection of a radiopaque dye into the joint, followed by an X-ray of the knee) often will show the cyst and its connection with the joint space (Fig. 70.2). On occasion, venography may be necessary to rule out deep vein thrombosis. Decompression of the cyst by aspiration of synovial fluid from either the joint or the cyst and injection of a corticosteroid into the joint (see below)

usually effectively relieve the symptoms of the condition.

LABORATORY TESTS

Baseline diagnostic laboratory information in patients with suspected rheumatoid arthritis should include a hematocrit value, white blood cell count and differential count, erythrocyte sedimentation rate, urinalysis, and rheumatoid factor titer. The baseline determination of the concentration of electrolytes and creatinine and liver function tests are important to establish before initiating the use of drugs in the treatment of rheumatoid arthritis. In selected patients, synovial fluid analysis, additional serological studies, and appropriate X-rays may also be important (see below).

Hematology

A mild anemia with hematocrit values in the range of 30 to 34% occurs in approximately 25 to 35% of patients with rheumatoid arthritis. In most cases the reduced red cell mass is due to the so-called anemia of chronic disease (see Chapter 50) and is a normocytic-normochromic process characterized by a low concentration of serum iron, a low serum iron-binding capacity, and a normal or increased serum ferritin concentration. However, occasionally true iron deficiency

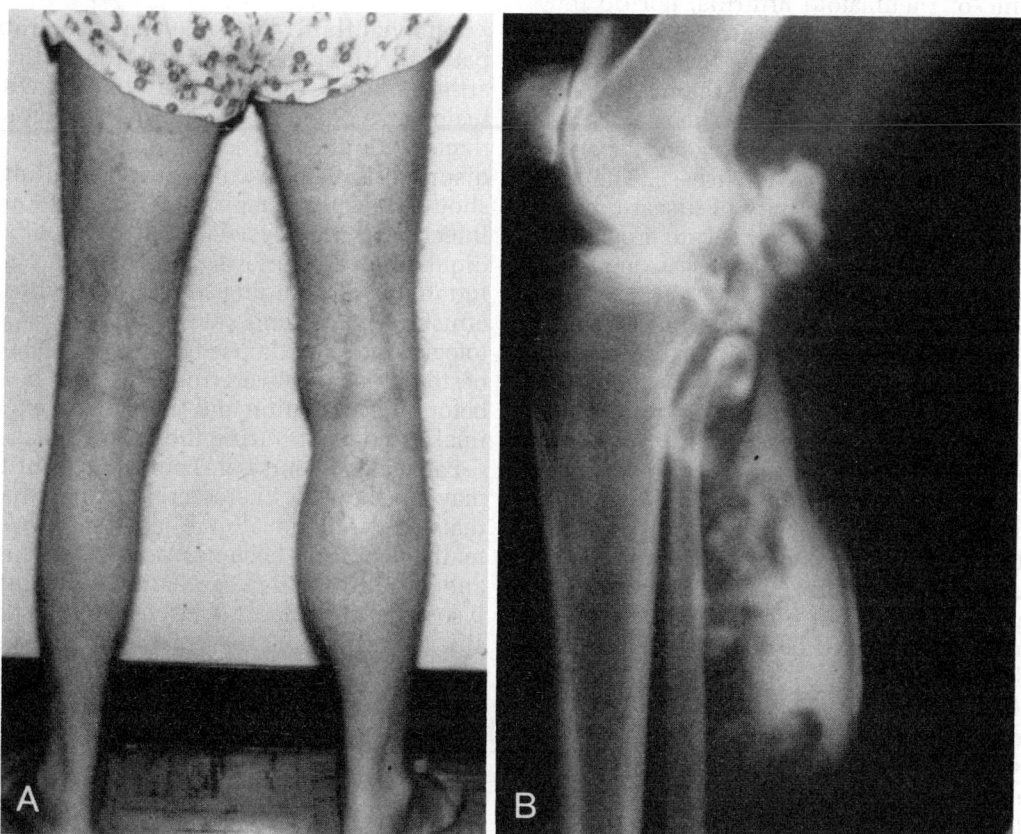

Figure 70.2. Baker's cyst. *A.* Swelling of the calf secondary to dissection of the cyst. *B.* Arthrogram of the knee, demonstrating the cyst.

anemia develops because of intercurrent stress ulceration and/or because of the irritative effects of nonsteroidal anti-inflammatory drugs (NSAIDs) (see below) on the gastric mucosa.

The white cell count is usually normal in patients with rheumatoid arthritis, but occasionally it is elevated in patients with a great deal of inflammatory disease and rarely is depressed (especially in association with Felty's syndrome, see below). Similarly the platelet count is usually normal but also may be elevated in association with the inflammatory process and may be reduced in patients with Felty's syndrome.

The erythrocyte sedimentation rate (ESR), most reliably measured by the Westergren method, is usually elevated in patients with rheumatoid arthritis and is a helpful adjunct in following the activity of the disease (see below).

Serology

Rheumatoid Factors

These are antibodies that react with the Fc fragment (a part of the molecule that can be produced in the laboratory by enzymatic cleavage of immunoglobulin G (IgG)). Although they may belong to any of the three major classes of immunoglobulins—IgG, IgM, and IgA—rheumatoid factors, as measured for clinical purposes, are IgM antibodies. The antibodies are by no means pathognomonic of rheumatoid arthritis, nor do they seem to be involved in its pathogenesis, but they are detectable in the serum of 70 to 80% of patients with the disease (16). A significant titer of rheumatoid factor is 1:80 or greater. In early disease the rheumatoid factor may be negative; it usually becomes positive within the first 6 months of active disease. The titer does not correlate with the activity of disease, but it does appear that patients with very severe erosive arthritis or with extensive extra-articular disease are likely to have relatively high titers.

Rheumatoid factor is also detectable in the serum of many patients without rheumatoid arthritis; most of these patients have had demonstrated or presumed chronic antigenic stimulation, such as prolonged infection (bacterial endocarditis, tuberculosis, viral hepatitis), collagen vascular disease, chronic lung disease (pulmonary fibrosis, asthma), and dysproteinemia (myeloma, macroglobulinemia, mixed cryoglobulinemia). Also, transient appearance of rheumatoid factor may occur in patients who have been recently vaccinated or who have had a self-limited viral infection. Finally, rheumatoid factor may be detected in the serum of apparently normal people, especially people over the age of 50, where its prevalence is anywhere from 10 to 25%, depending on the assay.

All of the clinical tests for rheumatoid factor depend on the agglutination, by serum that contains it, of particles (sheep red cells, latex, bentonite) coated with aggregated human or animal IgG. There is some variation in sensitivity of detection of rheumatoid factor according to which technique is used, so that the clinician should be familiar with the procedure used by his reference laboratory. The tests that employ latex or bentonite are more sensitive but less specific than tests that employ sheep red cells (2).

Antinuclear Antibodies

Antinuclear antibodies (ANAs), measured by immunofluorescent techniques, are present in approximately 20 to 30% of patients with rheumatoid arthritis. ANAs are more common in patients with extra-articular manifestations of disease and in patients with a high titer of rheumatoid factor. In comparison with systemic lupus erythematosus (SLE) the titer of antinuclear antibodies is ordinarily low in patients with rheumatoid disease, and antibodies to native DNA are unusual. The test is most useful as a predictor of extra-articular disease.

Serum Complement

Serum hemolytic complement (CH50), C_3 or C_4, is generally normal or increased in patients with rheumatoid arthritis; it may be low in an occasional patient with severe disease or with systemic vasculitis. The test is most useful in helping to distinguish the patient with early rheumatoid arthritis from patients with early SLE in whom it is often markedly decreased.

Synovial Fluid

Synovial fluid should be analyzed (Table 70.2) in a patient with monarticular arthritis, with polyarticular arthritis and fever, or in any patient with a joint effusion in whom the diagnosis is in doubt. Also patients with known rheumatoid arthritis who develop disproportionate discomfort and swelling of one joint should have fluid aspirated from that joint to rule out infection. If the physician is not familiar with the technique of arthrocentesis (see Table 66.1) or is uncomfortable about tapping the joint in which there is an effusion, the patient should be referred to a rheumatologist or to an orthopaedic surgeon. The patient should be told that the overlying skin will be anesthetized before the aspiration and that he will experience minimal discomfort during the procedure.

Early in the course of rheumatoid arthritis, joint fluid may not show the characteristic inflammatory changes that ultimately develop. Thereafter, however, the normally clear fluid becomes yellowish-white and turbid and, because of the degradation of hyaluronic acid by lysosomal enzymes, the viscosity of the fluid falls considerably and the so-called mucin clot becomes poor. [A simple method of testing the mucin clot is to add 1 ml of joint fluid to 4 ml of 2% acetic acid (Fig. 70.3).] Fluid aspirated from an inflamed joint also often clots spontaneously, another feature distinguishing it from normal. There is considerable variation in the total white cell count and the neutrophil count in synovial fluid of rheumatoid joints, but in general many more leukocytes (predominantly neutrophils) are present than are seen in the fluid of either normal joints or joints

Table 70.2.
Synovial Fluid Findings in Various Arthritidies

Synovial Fluid	Normal	Rheumatoid Arthritis	Noninflammatory Arthritis	Septic Arthritis
Color	Clear	Yellow	Clear-yellow	Variable
Clarity	Transparent	Turbid	Transparent	Opaque
Viscosity	High	Low	High	Low
Mucin clot	Good	Fair to poor	Fair to good	Poor
White cells (per mm³)	< 150	3,500–50,000	< 3000	50,000 → 100,000
Polymorphonuclear leukocytes (%)	< 25	> 70	< 25	> 75
Serum-synovial fluid glucose difference	0	≥ 30	≤ 5	≥ 30
Protein (g/dl)	1.8	4.2	3.0	4.9
CH50: protein[a]	> 2.5	< 2.5	> 2.5	Variable

[a] This ratio is low in synovial fluid of patients with arthritis associated with local immune complex formation (rheumatoid arthritis, SLE); it can be low in states associated with local consumption of complement (gout, infection), but it is frequently high or normal in other forms of arthritis.

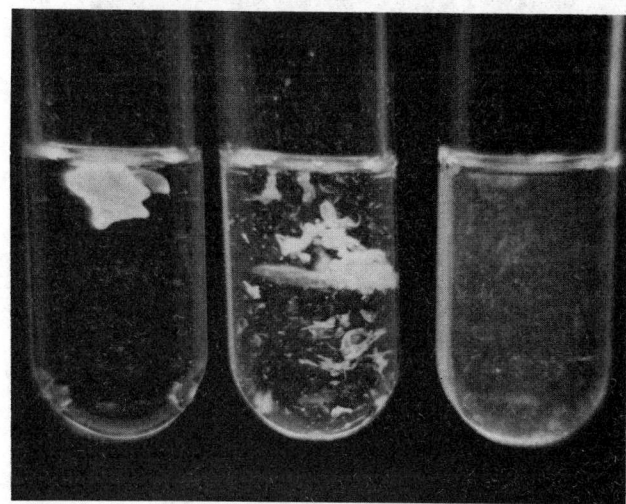

Figure 70.3. Mucin clot demonstrating (left to right) good, intermediate, and poor mucin clots.

that are arthritic but are not acutely inflamed. Cell counts can be done in the office with normal saline as a dilutent. At the same time, a smear can be made and stained for differential counting of white cells. If the physician is unable to perform these counts, the fluid should be transported to an appropriate laboratory, in which case the fluid should be added to a tube containing ethylenediaminetetraacetic (EDTA) acid to prevent clot formation. The cells will not lyse even if 4 to 6 hours pass before they are counted. However, rapid transport to the laboratory is essential so that an accurate glucose measurement can be made. The concentration of glucose in the fluid of inflamed joints, though usually normal, is occasionally moderately reduced; if it is less than half the serum glucose concentration, it suggests septic arthritis. The protein concentration in the synovial fluid is usually greater than 3 g/dl, typical of an exudative process.

A measurement of total hemolytic complement (CH50) in synovial fluid can be of diagnostic significance when the patient with rheumatoid arthritis has an atypical presentation. It need not be measured routinely, especially in patients in whom the diagnosis is known. If measured, CH50 in serum should be measured simultaneously. In nonrheumatoid inflammatory

arthritis, the titer of CH50 is the same in joint fluid and in serum. In seropositive rheumatoid arthritis there is a marked decrease in the titer of complement in synovial fluid (but not in serum). However, a similar decrease may be seen in microcrystalline arthritis and in septic arthritis. For complement determination the joint fluid and serum should be packed in ice and transported to the laboratory within hours of collection. If that is not possible, the specimens may be stored at −20°C (the usual temperature of a freezer in a refrigerator) for up to 1 week.

Radiology

Roentgenograms are rarely necessary in the diagnosis of rheumatoid arthritis but are useful in following the progression of the erosive process (Fig. 70.4). Furthermore, X-ray changes lag behind and require sufficient time (months) to evolve in a characteristic manner, limiting their usefulness early in the course of the disease.

Radiological findings vary in rheumatoid arthritis depending on the duration and severity of the illness. Early in the disease X-rays may show nothing other than soft tissue swelling. Thereafter periarticular osteoporosis may develop, and it is usually most noticeable in the small joints of the hands, wrists, and feet. With progression of the disease, narrowing of the joint space occurs due to loss of cartilage, and juxtaarticular erosions appear, generally at the point of attachment of the joint capsule. In end-stage disease, large cystic erosions of bone may be seen, bony proliferation may occur because of degenerative changes that follow inflammation, and the marked deformities that are visible to the naked eye (see above) are also visible radiologically. These changes are in contrast to the bony hypertrophy and fusion seen in patients with osteoarthritis (Chapter 68).

In general serial X-rays are not necessary in the management of patients with rheumatoid arthritis; they should be obtained if there is a suspicion of structural damage of a joint.

Special radiological studies are helpful in certain situations. *Arthrography* can be used to define possible internal joint derangement or injury to a supporting structure, such as a torn rotator cuff of the

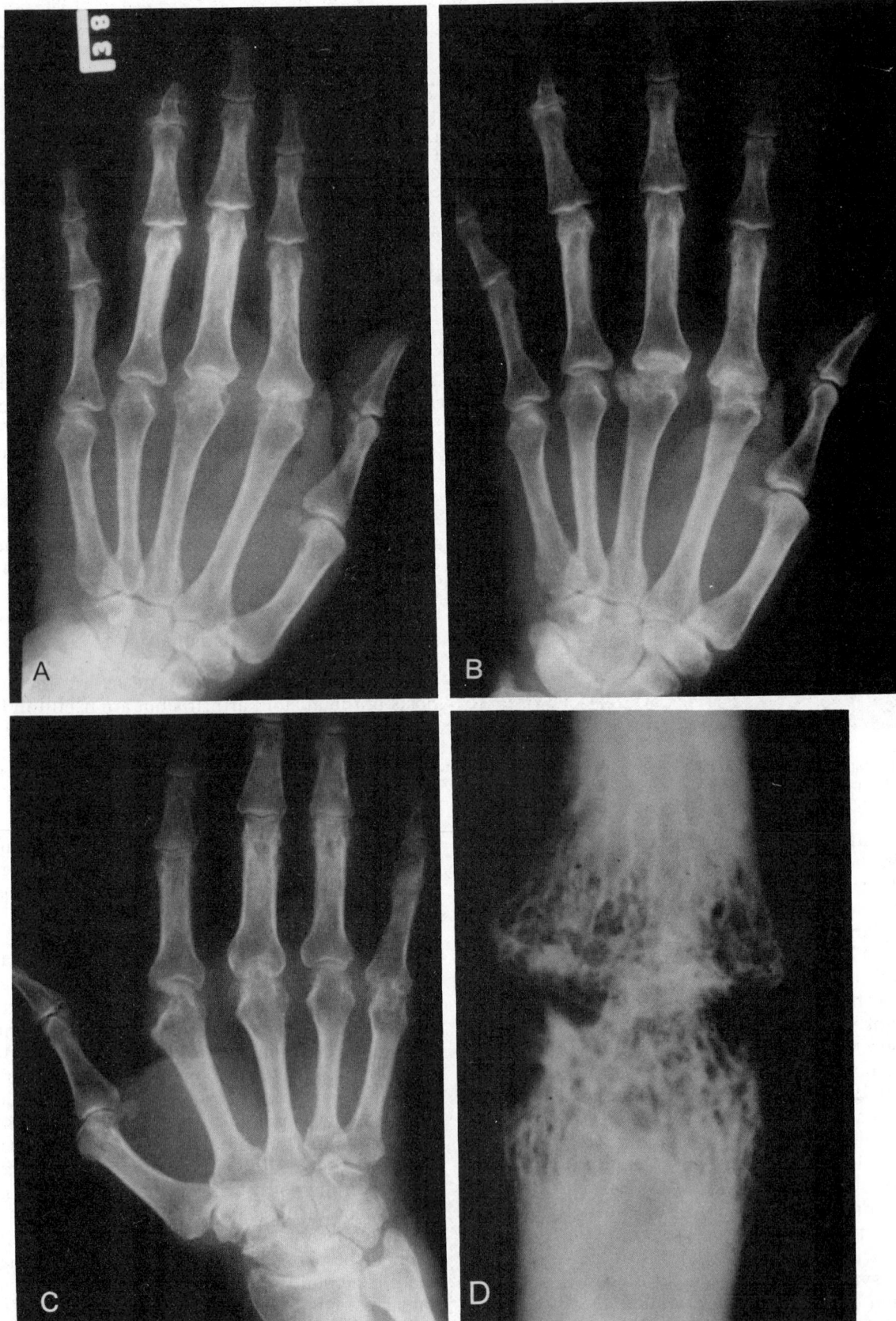

Figure 70.4. Radiological changes in rheumatoid arthritis. *A.* Early joint space narrowing in second and third MCP joints. *B.* Cystic changes, erosions, and further bony proliferation in second and third MCP joints. *C.* Periarticular osteoporosis, most noticeable in the interphalangeal joints, and numerous marginal erosions and cysts in the carpal bones and metacarpal heads. *D.* Juxta-articular erosions in a PIP joint.

shoulder; and bone scan can be helpful in establishing the diagnosis of aseptic necrosis. Computer tomography or magnetic resonance imaging may add important information in specific situations, particularly when evaluating cervical spine abnormalities.

Biopsies

Although the histology of rheumatoid arthritis is characteristic (see above), synovial biopsy is rarely necessary in the diagnosis of the disease. Similarly, biopsy of a nodule is only indicated to distinguish it from another process (e.g., a tumor); occasionally a nodule is excised because it is unsightly or because it has ulcerated or has eroded into an adjacent structure.

EXTRA-ARTICULAR DISEASE

Rheumatoid arthritis is a chronic inflammatory *systemic disease* (6). Although the joints are almost always the principal focus of the illness, other organ systems may also be involved, either because of rheumatoid granuloma formation or because of a generalized vasculitis. Usually, extra-articular manifestations of rheumatoid arthritis occur in patients with relatively more severe disease. In contrast to the predilection of classic rheumatoid arthritis for women, extra-articular manifestations of the disease (Table 70.3) are more common in men.

Rheumatoid Nodules

Although not specific for rheumatoid arthritis (similar nodules may be seen in patients with SLE or with rheumatic fever), the subcutaneous nodule is the most characteristic extra-articular lesion of the disease (Fig. 70.5). Nodules occur in 20 to 30% of cases, almost exclusively in seropositive patients. They vary in size from a few millimeters to several centimeters and may be either fixed to surrounding tissue or be freely movable beneath the skin. They are located most commonly on the extensor surfaces of the arms and elbows but are prone to develop also at pressure or contact points on the feet, the knees, and, rarely, the scapulae, the back of the head, the ischial tuberosities, and the base of the spine. Occasionally subcutaneous nodules may become painful, erode underlying bone, or ulcerate, but usually they are asymptomatic. Rheumatoid nodules may arise within tendons or ligaments and can result in joint dysfunction or tendon rupture. Rarely nodules may arise in visceral organs, such as the lungs, the heart, or the sclera of the eye. Wherever their location, nodules usually persist but occasionally regress when there is a remission of activity of the disease.

Pleuropulmonary Disease

There are several pulmonary manifestations of rheumatoid arthritis including pleurisy with or without effusion, intrapulmonary nodules, rheumatoid pneumoconiosis (Caplan's syndrome), diffuse interstitial

Table 70.3.
Systemic Manifestations of Rheumatoid Arthritis (Rheumatoid Disease)

I. General
    A. Fever
    B. Fatigue, malaise, diffuse stiffness
    C. Adenopathy
    D. Splenomegaly
II. Pulmonary
    A. Pleuritis (± effusion)
    B. Intrapulmonary nodules
    C. Interstitial pneumonitis
    D. Rheumatoid pneumoconiosis (Caplan's syndrome)
    E. Pulmonary fibrosis
    F. Arteritis (rare)
III. Cardiovascular
    (1) Heart
        A. Pericarditis, effusion, tamponade, constriction
        B. Myocarditis
        C. Endocarditis, including valvulitis
        D. Rheumatoid nodule (conduction defects)
    (2) Peripheral
        A. Vasculitis or arteritis
IV. Nervous system
    A. Peripheral neuropathy (mononeuritis multiplex) (sensory, motor, or both)
    B. Central nervous system
        1. Spinal cord lesion
            a. Vascular thrombosis
            b. Rheumatoid nodule
        2. Intracranial
            a. Arteritis (rare)
            b. Rheumatoid nodule (rare)
V. Ocular
    A. Keratoconjunctivitis (Sjögren's syndrome)
    B. Episcleritis (simple or nodular)
    C. Scleritis
        1. Diffuse
        2. Nodular (scleromalacia perforans)
        3. Necrotizing
VI. Hematological
    A. Anemia (chronic disease)
    B. Neutropenia (Felty's syndrome)
    C. Thrombocytosis
    D. Eosinophilia
VII. Skin
    A. Palmar erythema
    B. Nodules
    C. Vasculitic lesions
    D. Leg ulcers (Felty's syndrome)
VIII. Others
    A. Sjögren's syndrome
    B. Osteoporosis
    C. Hyperviscosity
    D. Lymphoma (Sjögren's syndrome)
    E. Secondary amyloidosis (controversial)

fibrosis, and, rarely, bronchiolitis obliterans, pneumothorax, or pulmonary arteritis (9). Severe lung involvement is more common in males and tends to occur in patients with high titer rheumatoid factor in the presence of other manifestations of rheumatoid arthritis. Commonly, there is a restrictive ventilatory defect with reduced lung volumes and a decreased diffusing capacity for carbon monoxide. Although the issue is controversial, most rheumatologists believe that rheumatoid arthritis does not cause intrathoracic obstructive airway disease. Extrathoracic airway obstruction may occur secondary to involvement of the cricoarytenoid joints of the larynx.

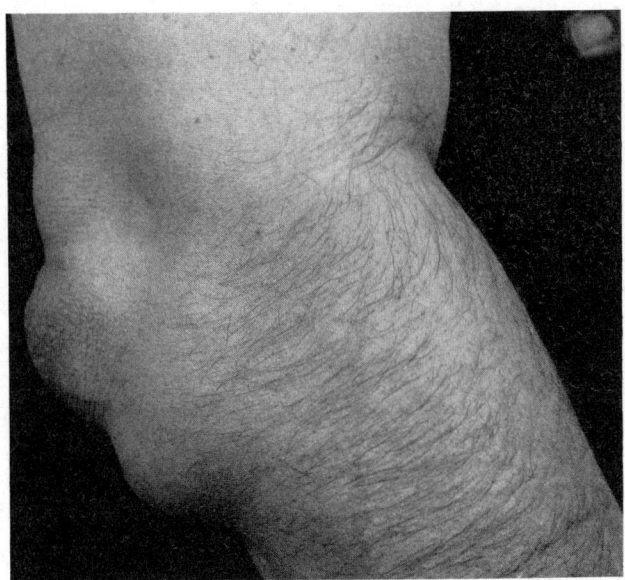

Figure 70.5. Rheumatoid nodules along the extensor surface of the forearm.

Pulmonary involvement may precede by months the onset of arthritis. Pleurisy, the most common problem, is clinically apparent in 5% of patients, but at autopsy is found 50% of the time, manifest by pleural thickening and inflammation. Pleural effusions, either unilateral or bilateral, are usually exudates (high lactate dehydrogenase activity and a protein concentration greater than 3 g/dl), but even in transudates the glucose concentration of the fluid is usually low (less than 30 mg/100 ml). A logical first approach to the management of a pleural effusion includes a diagnostic aspiration and/or pleural biopsy to exclude infection or malignancy.

Rheumatoid nodules in the lung are usually asymptomatic, but cavitation simulating cancer or infection may occur. Therefore, appropriate diagnostic steps should be taken to assure that an isolated pleural or pulmonary nodule is in fact rheumatoid in origin and not due to a complicating, intercurrent process.

Interstitial pneumonitis may precede a progressive pulmonary fibrosis, the most severe form of rheumatoid lung disease. This process is more common among patients who smoke.

To date no regression of rheumatoid lung disease has been shown with conventional modes of treatment. Patients with symptomatic pleural or pulmonary manifestations of rheumatoid arthritis should be followed in consultation with a rheumatologist and/or a pulmonologist.

Cardiac Disease (11)

Pericarditis is the most common cardiac manifestation of rheumatoid arthritis. Echocardiographic studies have demonstrated pericardial effusion in 55% of patients with subcutaneous nodules and in 15% of patients who do not have nodules. Symptomatic pericarditis usually presents with fever, chest pain, and a pericardial rub that resolve spontaneously. Recurrent or persistent pericardial disease, complicated by tamponade or constriction, is unusual. Myocarditis and conduction abnormalities secondary to nodule formation in the heart have been reported rarely. The treatment of patients with symptomatic cardiac disease should be planned in consultation with a rheumatologist.

Ocular Disease

The most common ocular manifestation of rheumatoid arthritis is the keratoconjunctivitis of Sjögren's syndrome (see below). *Episcleritis*, ordinarily a self-limited process of a few weeks' duration, occurs occasionally. It is manifest by discomfort, mild pain, and intense redness of the affected eye. Scleritis is a rarer but more serious problem. Unlike episcleritis it is a slowly progressive, frequently bilateral process; it is characterized by nodularity, intense redness, and often severe pain; and it may lead to perforation and/or loss of vision. The distinction between episcleritis and scleritis is difficult, and all patients with suspected scleritis should be referred to an ophthalmologist.

Neurological Disease

The most common neurological manifestation of rheumatoid arthritis is a mild, primarily sensory, *peripheral neuropathy*, usually more marked in the lower extremities. Entrapment neuropathies (for example, the carpal tunnel syndrome) sometimes occur in patients with rheumatoid arthritis because of compression of a peripheral nerve by inflamed edematous tissue. This problem is discussed in Chapter 84. Cervical myelopathy, secondary to arthritis of the cervical spine, is a particularly worrisome, although uncommon, complication; if caused by atlantoaxial subluxation, permanent—even fatal—neurological damage may ensue. Thirty percent of patients with rheumatoid arthritis have atlantoaxial subluxation without symptoms, and very few of them develop neurological dysfunction. However, neurosurgical consultation should be sought at the first sign of cord compression (radicular pain, difficulty voiding, focal weakness).

Lymphoid Hyperplasia

Lymphadenopathy, either local or generalized, occurs in 25% or more of patients with rheumatoid arthritis and is probably more common than that in seropositive patients. The nodes are nontender, firm, and freely movable; and, although the diagnosis of lymphoma sometimes is considered, the process almost always proves to be benign. When examined by biopsy, the nodes show a proliferation of normal plasma cells, consistent with the immunological reactivity of the disease. *Splenomegaly* occurs more rarely (5 to 10% of patients), usually in association with lymphadenopathy.

Felty's Syndrome

Felty's syndrome is characterized by rheumatoid arthritis, splenomegaly, and leukopenia—predominantly granulocytopenia (15). Patients with the syndrome usually are older, have a high titer of rheumatoid factor, and have relatively severe arthritis, often with other extra-articular manifestations of the disease. Recurrent bacterial infections and chronic refractory leg ulcers are the major complications, and splenectomy may benefit patients whose infections are severe.

Rheumatoid Vasculitis

Vascular inflammation is found in 10 to 25% of patients with rheumatoid arthritis on whom autopsies are performed. The most common clinical manifestations of vasculitis are small digital infarcts along the nailbeds. In a very small proportion of patients (less than 1%) a syndrome of accelerated vasculitis is seen, characterized by distal cutaneous ulcerations and gangrene, peripheral polyneuropathy, and visceral (intestinal, renal, cardiac, cerebral) ischemia. There does not appear to be a positive correlation, as was once thought, between the long-term administration of corticosteroids and the severity of this process. The syndrome ordinarily emerges after years of seropositive, persistently active, rheumatoid arthritis. Immediate consultation with a rheumatologist and, usually, hospitalization are indicated.

Sjögren's Syndrome

About 10 to 15% of patients with rheumatoid arthritis (most of them women) have Sjögren's syndrome, a chronic inflammatory disorder characterized by lymphocytic infiltration of lacrimal and salivary glands with impaired secretion of saliva and tears that results in the *sicca complex*, dry mouth (xerostomia), and dry eyes (keratoconjunctivitis sicca). Variably, other exocrine glands are affected as well. There is also commonly a lymphoproliferative reaction, characterized by lymphadenopathy and, sometimes, splenomegaly that may mimic or, rarely, actually transform into a malignant lymphoma. The syndrome may also be associated with a number of other systemic manifestations, including vasculitis, peripheral neuropathy, and thyroiditis, and with diffuse hypergammaglobulinemia (sometimes in association with renal tubular acidosis), cryoglobulinemia, an elevated titer of antinuclear antibodies, and a number of tissue-directed autoantibodies.

COURSE

Rheumatoid arthritis is a variable illness, and its course cannot be predicted precisely in a given patient. Several different patterns of activity can be described: *Spontaneous remission* may occur, particularly in the seronegative patient. *Recurrent explosive attacks* followed by periods of quiescence can be seen in the early phases, but activity usually is persistent and unpredictably waxes and wanes in intensity. Rarely, the inflammatory process is rapidly destructive, leading to early loss of function and to joint deformity. The degree of disability is probably directly proportionate to the severity and the duration of the inflammatory process. Although treatment can alter the course of the illness, complete remission is unlikely in people who have had symptomatic rheumatoid arthritis for a year or more. There is no clear-cut way to predict which patients will develop significant deformities (subluxation, ankylosis, etc., see above); most will not. On the other hand, one study showed that 60% of patients with rheumatoid arthritis are unable to work 10 years after onset of their illness (21). A minority of patients (approximately 25%) will have a course characterized by remissions and exacerbations—often with months or even years during which they are asymptomatic; a few have permanent remissions. Such patients often have an abrupt onset of their disease, which paradoxically may herald a better prognosis. Some patients who at first have episodic attacks of arthritis ultimately develop a more typical sustained progressive course. Patients who have a high titer of rheumatoid factor and nodules, particularly men, tend to have more severe disease and, conversely, seronegative patients are more likely to have spontaneous remissions and/or less severe disease.

Although significant morbidity from rheumatoid arthritis has been appreciated, only recently have studies demonstrated an increased risk for mortality. Patients at higher risk are those with systemic extra-articular involvement, low functional capacity, and lower social economic status.

DIFFERENTIAL DIAGNOSIS

The difficulty of diagnosing early rheumatoid arthritis emphasizes the importance of a systematic approach to patients with arthritis (Table 70.4). Epidemiological studies have clarified that the age, sex, and genetic matrix of the patient influence disease expression. Therefore, a clear definition of host features will form a framework to begin the evaluation of a patient with arthritis. Table 70.5 outlines examples of the differential diagnosis of polyarthritis based

Table 70.4.
Outline of Diagnostic Approach to Polyarthritis

A. Define the host features
 1. Age, sex, and ethnic background
 2. Genetic matrix
 3. Environmental factors
B. Describe the joint involvement
 1. Number
 2. Patterns
 3. Specific joints
 4. Intensity of pain
 5. Course
C. Characteristics of extra-articular features
D. Supporting laboratory studies
E. Response to therapeutic trial

Table 70.5.
Differential Diagnosis of Polyarthritis Based on Age and Sex

	Male	Both Sexes	Female
Childhood (1–15)	Juvenile ankylosing spondylitis (Chapter 71) Kawasaki's syndrome[a] Hemophilia (Chapter 51)	Juvenile rheumatoid arthritis—systemic onset (Still's disease)[a] Rheumatic fever[a] Leukemia[a]	Juvenile rheumatoid arthritis[a] Pauciarticular arthritis[a] Juvenile rheumatoid arthritis—polyarthritis onset[a]
Young adult (15–30)	Ankylosing spondylitis (Chapter 71) Reiter's syndrome (Chapter 71) "Reactive" arthritis[a] Behcet's syndrome[a]	Psoriatic arthritis (Chapter 100) Lyme disease[a] Inflammatory bowel disease (Chapter 39)	Systemic lupus erythematosus[a] Gonococcal arthritis (Chapter 27) Scleroderma[a]
Middle years (30–60)	Gout (Chapter 69) Palindromic rheumatism[a] Whipple's disease[a]	Seronegative polyarthritis (Chapter 70) Hypersensitivity reactions (Chapter 23) Vasculitic syndromes[a] Relapsing polychondritis[a]	Rheumatoid arthritis Sjögren's syndrome Sarcoidosis[a] Polymyositis[a] Erosive osteoarthritis (Chapter 68)
Elderly (60 +)	Diffuse idiopathic skeletal hyperostosis (DISH) (Chapter 68) Hypertrophic pulmonary osteoarthropathy (HPO)[a]	Pseudogout (Chapter 69) Tumor-related syndromes Secondary osteoarthritis (Chapter 68) Metabolic disorders	Primary generalized osteoarthritis (Chapter 68) Polymyalgia rheumatica (Chapter 79)

[a] These conditions are not discussed in this book. Information about them is contained in any of the general references at the end of this chapter.

on prevalence of disease expression defined by age and sex. Other important factors include the patient's occupation, habits, drug usage, and past medical history (Table 70.6). Finally, the characteristics of the arthritis itself provide important information in approaching the differential diagnosis (Tables 70.7 and 70.8).

Table 70.6.
Examples of Environmental Factors in Diagnosis of Arthritis

Occupation	Disease
Bartender, lead exposure	Gout (Chapter 69)
Health workers	Hepatitis (Chapter 43)
Sports	Secondary osteoarthritis (Chapter 68)
Outdoorsman	Lyme disease[a]
Gardener	Sporotrichosis[a]
Deep sea diver	Aseptic necrosis of bone[a]
Habits	
Alcohol abuse	Gout (Chapter 69), aseptic necrosis[a]
"Moonshine" ingestion	Saturnine gout (Chapter 69)
Smoking	Hypertrophic osteoarthropathy[a]
Intravenous drug abuse	Septic arthritis,[a] hepatitis, vasculitis
Sexual promiscuity	Gonococcal arthritis (Chapter 27), hepatitis (Chapter 43), Reiter's syndrome (Chapter 71)
Drugs	
Diuretics	Gout (Chapter 69)
Corticosteroids	Aseptic necrosis[a]
Hydralazine, procainamide	Systemic lupus erythematosus[a]
Any drug	Hypersensitivity reactions (Chapter 23)

[a]These conditions are not discussed in this book. Information about them is contained in any of the general references at the end of this chapter.

MANAGEMENT

General Principles

Rheumatoid arthritis is a chronic disorder for which there is no known cure. It therefore requires a comprehensive program that combines medical, social, and emotional support for the patient. An understanding of each patient's specific problems is essential. Serial observations (Table 70.9) and in-depth investigation of the impact of the disease on both the patient and his family provide the basis for effective management.

The major goals of treatment of the arthritis are (a) to reduce pain and discomfort, (b) to prevent deformities and loss of normal joint function, and (c) to maintain a productive and active life. To achieve these goals an understanding of the cause of pain is important. In rheumatoid arthritis pain and dysfunction are caused by (a) acute inflammation, (b) chronic proliferative synovitis, and (c) subsequent mechanical and structural abnormalities. Each of these processes warrants a different therapeutic approach. Often all three are present at once, although, depending on the stage of disease, one process may be predominant. Acute inflammation is always the major problem in early disease, and mechanical and structural abnormalities do not ordinarily develop until later in the course of the disease.

Management begins with effective communication between physician and patient. It is essential that the patient and his family be educated about the nature and course of the disease—the specific causes of the discomfort and the goals, problems, and expectations of treatment. Chronic arthritis is a major emotional, as well as physical, stress that often requires a major change in life-style. A misunderstanding about the disease and the setting of inappropriate goals will lead

Table 70.7.
Assessment of Joint Involvement

A. Number:

Monarthritis	Oligoarthritis (2–4)	Polyarthritis (>5)
Septic arthritis[a]	Reiter's syndrome	Rheumatoid arthritis
Gout	Inflammatory bowel disease	Systemic lupus erythematosus[a]
Pseudogout	Psoriatic arthritis	Serum sickness
Other crystals	Rheumatic fever[a]	Psoriatic arthritis
Local tumor[a]	Juvenile rheumatoid arthritis[a]	Tophaceous gout

B. Patterns:

Symmetrical	Asymmetrical
Rheumatoid arthritis	Psoriatic arthritis
Serum sickness	Reiter's syndrome
Systemic lupus erythematosus[a]	Gout, pseudogout

C. Intensity of pain:

Severe	Moderate
Septic arthritis[s]	All others including rheumatoid arthritis
Microcrystalline arthritis	

D. Course:

Acute	Infection, gout, pseudogout
Chronic	Psoriatic arthritis, rheumatoid arthritis, ankylosing spondylitis
Additive	Rheumatoid arthritis
Migratory	Rheumatic fever,[a] systemic lupus erythematosus[a]
Evanescent	Systemic lupus erythematosus,[a] viral[a]
Episodic	Gout, pseudogout, palindromic rheumatism[a]

[a]These conditions are not discussed in this book. Information about them is contained in any of the general references at the end of this chapter.

Table 70.8.
Diagnostic Clues Provided by Involvement of Specific Joints

First metatarsal (podagra)	Gout
Knee (acute, episodic)	Pseudogout
Distal interphalangeal	Psoriatic arthritis
	Osteoarthritis
Metacarpals, wrists, metatarsals	Rheumatoid arthritis
Sausaged digits	Reiter's syndrome
	Psoriatic arthritis
	Sarcoidosis
Sacroiliac	Ankylosing spondylitis
	Reiter's syndrome
	Psoriatric arthritis
	Inflammatory bowel disease
Sternoclavicular	Septic arthritis
	Polymyalgia rheumatica
Heel/ankle	Reiter's syndrome

Table 70.9.
Measurements to Be Made Serially in Patients with Rheumatoid Arthritis[a]

Duration of morning stiffness
Time of onset of fatigue
NSAID need/day
Grip strength
Number of joints that are tender or are painful on passive motion
Degree of swelling of affected joints
Erythrocyte sedimentation rate (Westergren)

[a]Adapted from McCarty DJ: Clinical assessment of arthritis. In McCarty DJ (ed): *Arthritis and Allied Conditions*, ed 9. Philadelphia, Lea & Febiger, 1979.

to frustration, depression, and withdrawal from social activity and from medical support.

A simple self-report questionnaire has been shown to be an effective, inexpensive method to assess the patient's status and response to treatment (Table 70.10) (13).

Treatment options include (a) reduction of joint stress, (b) physical and occupational therapy, (c) drug therapy, and (d) surgical intervention.

Reduction of joint stress is accomplished by a number of practical measures that do not depend on the use of drugs. Because of the stress of obesity on the musculoskeletal system, an ideal body weight should be maintained. Rest, in general, is an important feature of management; 8 to 9 hours' sleep at night and a 2-hour rest period in the middle of the day are reasonable recommendations for everyone with active disease. Also, vigorous activity (heavy work, brisk exercise) should be avoided because of the danger of intensifying joint inflammation. On the other hand, patients should be urged to maintain a modest level of activity to prevent joint laxity and muscular atrophy. Splinting of acutely inflamed joints, walking aids (canes, walkers), and specially designed furniture and household utensils are all effective means of reducing stress on specific joints; such aids are provided, on recommendation of the consultant rheumatologist, by an orthopaedist, a physiatrist or physical therapist, or an orthotics appliance store.

The *physical and the occupational therapist* should be consulted early in the course of treating a patient with rheumatoid arthritis. The therapist can effectively design a program of balanced rest and activity

Table 70.10.
Self-Report Questionnaire[a]

	Without Any Difficulty	With Some Difficulty	With Much Difficulty	Unable to Do
A. Dress yourself, including tying shoelaces and doing buttons?	_____	_____	_____	_____
B. Get in and out of bed?	_____	_____	_____	_____
C. Lift a full cup or glass to your mouth?	_____	_____	_____	_____
D. Walk outdoors on flat ground?	_____	_____	_____	_____
E. Wash and dry your entire body?	_____	_____	_____	_____
F. Bend down to pick up clothing from the floor?	_____	_____	_____	_____
G. Turn regular faucets on and off?	_____	_____	_____	_____
H. Get in and out of a car?	_____	_____	_____	_____

[a] Used to assess quantitatively the functional capacity of the patient to do the activities of daily living.

that is appropriate for the stage of the disease. Passive exercise (moving the joints through a full range of motion) is used when inflammation is active and poorly controlled; an active exercise program, when tolerated, can be designed to prevent contractures and muscular atrophy. Local heat, education in the use of various supporting aids and in joint protection, and maintenance of good joint function are all part of the therapist's role.

Either wet or dry local heat gives transient symptomatic relief of pain and stiffness, particularly to patients with chronic synovitis. A hot shower in the morning, coupled with passive "warming up" exercises, may relieve stiffness and help the patient to get the day started.

During periods when the inflammatory process is particularly intense, especially if they occur at the onset of the illness, hospitalization is helpful in removing the patient from the stresses of his everyday life, in beginning a structured rehabilitation program, and in evaluating the effect of drugs (see below) on the illness.

There is increased susceptibility of the rheumatoid joint to infection, usually by Gram-positive organisms. Whenever a single joint flares up or is accompanied by increased body temperature or follows a recent procedure (e.g., dental), infection should be ruled out by means of synovial fluid examination (see above).

Drug Treatment

A general discussion of the pharmacological approach to rheumatoid arthritis is followed by a description of the characteristics of individual drugs (7).

Anti-Inflammatory Drugs

In the presence of acute and/or chronic inflammation, it is appropriate first to prescribe aspirin or another nonsteroidal anti-inflammatory drug (NSAID). They should always be used in conjunction with the general modalities of rest, heat, etc. discussed above. The major effect of these agents is to reduce acute inflammation and thereby to decrease pain, improve function, and, it is hoped, prevent joint destruction. Recent studies have suggested that NSAIDs also may have more than an anti-inflammatory effect, i.e., they may alter cell function and, subsequently, the immune and/or inflammatory process, but the issue is controversial. All of these drugs also have mild to moderate analgesic properties independent of their anti-inflammatory effect.

Aspirin is a reasonable initial choice as drug treatment because compliance can be objectively measured and because of its low cost. However, many rheumatologists will initiate treatment with one of the newer NSAIDs. Aspirin is the generic name of acetylsalicylic acid. Several different preparations exist, including regular aspirin, aspirin buffered with antacids, and enteric coated aspirin (Table 70.11). Nonacetylated salicylates are mainly analgesic agents, but in clinical studies they have been shown to have anti-inflammatory activity. The main disadvantages of aspirin are the high incidence of gastrointestinal intolerance, the inconvenience of taking multiple doses, and the relatively long interval (4 to 7 days) before a full anti-inflammatory effect is reached. Gastrointestinal symptoms can be reduced by the use of various enteric

Table 70.11.
Salicylates

		Available Strength (mg)
Acetylated preparations		
Regular aspirin	Multiple brands	300–800
Buffered aspirin	Multiple brands	300–650
Enteric coated aspirin	Ecotrin, Encaprin	325–500
	Cosprin	325–650
	APF	500
	Easprin	950
Nonacetylated preparations		
Sodium salicylate	Pabalate	300
Salicylsalicyclic acid	Disalcid	500, 750
Choline-magnesium tris-alicylate	Trilisate	500, 750
Salicylate derivative		
Diflunisal	Dolobid	250–500

coated preparations. Therefore, when using aspirin an enteric coated aspirin is recommended. A trial of aspirin is usually continued for 4 to 6 weeks; if tolerated, 70 to 80% of patients can be expected to respond during this time. A lack of response may be due to noncompliance or to an inadequate dosage, so that a salicylate level should be measured before changing medications. The plasma salicylate level should be approximately 20 to 25 mg/dl (lower in the elderly) to ensure an effective trial (see below). If aspirin is not tolerated or if there is a lack of response at ideal drug levels (see details below), another NSAID should be prescribed.

There are now a large number of NSAIDs from which to choose (Table 70.12), but at full dosage all are potentially equally effective. In general, the NSAIDs have a more rapid onset of action, have a simpler dosage schedule, and are often better tolerated than aspirin and for those reasons are often used as initial therapy. However, there is a great deal of individual variation in patient tolerance and response to a particular NSAID. Therefore, a trial of approximately 4 weeks with one of these agents is indicated. Failure of response or intolerance can be followed by a new trial with another NSAID, usually of a different chemical class. (Combinations of two NSAIDs should be avoided.) If the second trial is also a failure, it is best to consider another approach.

Corticosteroids

Corticosteroids have both anti-inflammatory and immunoregulatory activity. Whether or not they can induce actual remission of rheumatoid arthritis is controversial. They can be taken systemically or can be injected intra-articularly depending on the clinical situation. If good control of active inflammation is not achieved with aspirin or another NSAID, a low dose of a corticosteroid (e.g., 5 to 15 mg of prednisone by mouth once a day) can be added as a "bridge" between the rapid acting NSAID and the slow acting remission-inducing agents (see below). It should be understood that, once started, corticosteroid therapy is very difficult to discontinue. Higher doses are rarely necessary unless there is a life-threatening systemic disease and, if used for prolonged periods, will lead to steroid toxicity. Although it is reasonable to initiate therapy with an every-other-day regimen, most patients will require corticosteroids daily. Repetitive short courses of high dose corticosteroids, intermittent intramuscular injections, adrenocorticotropic hormone injections, and the use of corticosteroids as the sole therapeutic agent are all to be avoided. The use of "pulse therapy" for management of very difficult cases is controversial and should be initiated only in conjunction with a rheumatologist. Clinical trials have found that high dose pulse (1 g of intravenous methylprednisolone) is not better than "low" dose (100 mg) pulse treatment.

Intra-articular corticosteroids (e.g., 40 mg of triamcinolone in a knee, 20 mg in a shoulder, or 2 mg in a finger) are an effective means of controlling a local flare in one or two joints without changing the overall drug regimen (see Chapter 66 for details about the technique of injection). Joint fluid should always be obtained, studied, and cultured at the time of injection to be certain that a complicating infection has not developed. The injection should be administered by a rheumatologist or an orthopaedist if the primary physician is inexperienced with the techniques. Many rheumatologists think that the same joint should not

Table 70.12.
Nonsteroidal Anti-inflammatory Drugs

		Available Strengths (mg)	Recommended Dosage	Maximal Daily Dosage (mg/day)
Propionic Acid Derivatives				
Ibuprofen	Motrin, Rufen	300, 400, 600, 800	600–800 mg 3 to 4 times a day	3200
	Nuprin, Advil	200	500 mg twice a day	1000
Naproxen	Naprosyn	250, 375, 500		
	Anaprox	275		
Fenoprofen	Nalfon, Fenopron	200, 300, 600	600 mg 3 times a day	2400
Ketoprofen	Orudis	50, 75	50 mg 3 to 4 times a day or 75 mg 3 times a day	300
Flurbiprofen	Ansaid	100	100 mg 2 to 3 times a day	300
Oxicams				
	Feldene	10, 20	10–20 mg a day	20
Acetic Acids				
Indomethacin	Indocin	25, 50 75 (slow release)	50 mg 3 to 4 times a day 1–2 times a day	150–200
Sulindac	Clinoril	150, 200	150–200 mg twice a day	400
Tolmetin	Tolectin	200, 400	400 mg 3 to 4 times a day	2000
Diclofenac	Voltaren	25, 50, 75	50 mg 2 to 3 times a day or 75 mg twice a day	150
Fenamates				
Meclofenamate	Meclomen	50, 100	50 to 100 mg 3 to 4 times a day	400
Pyrazoles				
Phenylbutazone	Butazolidin	100	100 mg 3 times a day	300 for no more than 7 days

be injected more than twice a year because of possible deterioration of intra-articular cartilage.

Remission-Inducing Agents (Agents with Delayed Onset of Action)

Although NSAIDs control the symptoms of active rheumatoid arthritis, remission-inducing agents theoretically alter the disease process itself—although that is still being debated. In any case they do have an effect upon rheumatoid arthritis that is different and more delayed in onset than is the effect of the anti-inflammatory drugs discussed above. Once persistent disease activity (chronic synovitis) is established, a remission-inducing agent should be considered. Persistent disease can be defined as either continued activity despite an optimal trial of an anti-inflammatory program (2 to 3 months) or the development of erosions on X-rays of the involved joints. High titer rheumatoid factor, the presence of nodules or of other extra-articular features of rheumatoid arthritis, or aggressive joint activity all predict progressive disease, and, therefore, a remission-inducing agent should be started early in such cases. The decision to use a remission-inducing agent is complicated by the time commitment, expense, and potential toxicity related to drugs of this class. The currently available drugs include antimalarials, sulfasalazine, gold, D-penicillamine, and cytotoxic agents.

Antimalarials or *gold compounds* (chrysotherapy) are the drugs of first choice. Antimalarials have the advantage of low toxicity. However, in general, they probably are better utilized in patients with relatively mild, although persistent, disease; gold is best used in patients with more active, aggressive disease. Consultation with a rheumatologist will be helpful in choosing the appropriate regimen. Approximately 60% of patients have some response to antimalarial drugs. The response to antimalarials is delayed, with increasing improvement noted up to 6 months; in patients who respond, continued use of the drugs dictates that the patient be examined by an ophthalmologist every 6 months so that early signs of ocular toxicity, the major side effect, can be detected (see below).

Sulfasalazine has its onset of action at approximately 2 to 4 months; two-thirds of patients will be intolerant of the drug and one-third will improve clinically. Its role in the treatment of rheumatoid arthritis is not yet firmly established. Fifty to seventy percent of patients improve after 2 to 4 months of chrysotherapy. If no response has occurred within 6 months or if toxicity is observed (see below), the drug is discontinued. If there is a good response, gold is given in a reduced dosage indefinitely.

If there is an inadequate or toxic response to gold, to antimalarial drugs, or to sulfasalazine, the next step in the treatment of rheumatoid arthritis is the use of *D-penicillamine*. In fact, some rheumatologists prefer methotrexate (see below) rather than D-penicillamine as the next step because of the high success rate and

the low prevalence of toxicity of methotrexate. Approximately 80% of patients will respond to D-penicillamine after it is given for 3 or 4 months. The use of D-penicillamine is often limited by its toxic effects (see below); and again, it should not be given without the advice of a rheumatologist. In patients who respond favorably, the drug can be administered indefinitely at a relatively low maintenance dose (see below).

Cytotoxic drugs other than methotrexate have a very limited role in the treatment of rheumatoid arthritis. They should be reserved for the relatively small number of patients with progressive, otherwise uncontrollable or life-threatening disease and should be used only in consultation with a rheumatologist and then only after the patient understands the risks of both short- and long-term toxicity (see below).

The traditional approach to the treatment of rheumatoid arthritis is being redesigned by many rheumatologists. It has been suggested that rather than moving from one drug to another in sequence that both rapid acting (NSAIDs and corticosteroids) and slow acting remitting agents should be started early and in combination. After control is established the corticosteroid and cytotoxic medication is eliminated and the dose of NSAID is lowered, to prevent progressive irreversible joint damage that can occur in the first several months. However, additional investigational studies are currently underway to address these important issues. This approach should be considered only after consultation with a rheumatologist.

Analgesic Drugs

Pain caused by inflammation is best treated with an anti-inflammatory drug (see above), although occasionally acetaminophen may be prescribed, together with an NSAID, for temporary analgesia. Narcotics should not be prescribed; dependency is a hazard in patients who have a chronic disease that may cause pain indefinitely. Mechanical pain secondary to structural changes, including joint space narrowing, subluxation, muscle atrophy, and weakness, is best approached through nonpharmacological modalities, such as splints, joint protection, surgery, etc.

Approach to Drug Treatment of Patients with Rheumatoid Arthritis

Figure 70.6 outlines a recommended sequence of therapeutic trials in the treatment of patients with rheumatoid arthritis.

Characteristics of Individual Drugs

Aspirin (acetylsalicylic acid)

MECHANISM. Aspirin inhibits the synthesis of prostaglandins, a family of potent mediators of inflammation that is derived from fatty acids within cell membranes. Although aspirin has other effects, inhibition of prostaglandin synthesis is thought to account for its major anti-inflammatory activity.

DOSAGE. The usual starting dose is 900 mg (three

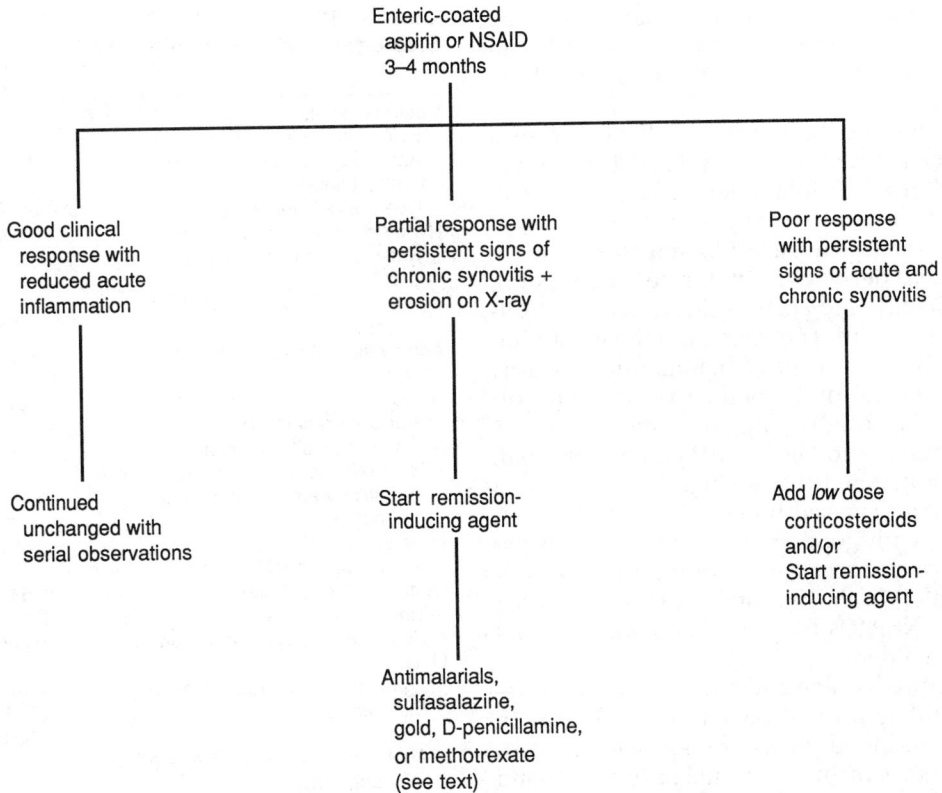

Figure 70.6. Suggested approach to anti-inflammatory drug treatment in rheumatoid arthritis.

USP aspirin tablets) four times a day. The drug should be an enteric coated preparation taken with meals and with a bedtime snack to minimize gastrointestinal side effects. If side effects do develop, dropping to a lower dosage (six tablets/day) and increasing by one tablet a day back to full dosage schedule may improve tolerance. Elderly patients are predictably less tolerant, and, therefore, a reduced dosage is advised at onset of treatment (eight to 10 tablets daily). A random serum salicylate level should be obtained approximately 7 to 10 days after beginning full dosage. A therapeutic level is 20 to 25 mg/dl, but elderly patients may be maintained between 15 to 20 mg/dl. If this level is not achieved on the initial schedule, and if the patient is believed to be compliant (see Chapter 4), the dose should be increased by one or two tablets a day until the desired anti-inflammatory level of salicylate is reached. There is a narrow margin between a good therapeutic level and toxicity. The earliest manifestation of toxicity is tinnitus or mild deafness. Should these symptoms occur, aspirin should be stopped until they abate and then restarted at a lower total dose that has been reduced by 1 or 2 tablets. After each change of dosage, it may take a week for a new steady state to be achieved. Younger patients can tolerate higher salicylate levels and do not usually have tinnitus or deafness until a level of 30 to 35 mg of salicylate/dl is reached.

USUAL TIME TO MAXIMAL EFFECT. The maximal anti-inflammatory effect of aspirin is achieved in 10 to 14 days if therapeutic levels are reached. Patients should be told of the importance of taking the medicine exactly as prescribed in order for the therapeutic effect to be achieved.

SIDE EFFECTS. Tinnitus (see above) and dyspepsia (nausea, heartburn, anorexia) are common side effects of aspirin therapy; both can be controlled: tinnitus, by reducing the dosage; dyspepsia, by taking the aspirin with food. Enteric coated aspirin reduces the incidence of dyspeptic symptoms, and, although absorption is somewhat reduced, an effective dosage can usually be achieved by appropriate monitoring of salicylate levels. Buffered aspirins are more expensive than, and have no clear-cut advantage over, the standard preparation.

The most troublesome side effects are gastrointestinal bleeding and peptic ulceration (see below). Because of the inhibition of platelet function by aspirin (see Chapter 52), it should never be prescribed to a patient with an underlying bleeding tendency (including patients taking anticoagulant drugs).

Nonsteroidal anti-inflammatory drugs (NSAIDs)

MECHANISM. Although chemically dissimilar, these agents, like aspirin, inhibit the synthesis of prostaglandins, currently their only well-defined anti-inflammatory effect.

DOSAGE. NSAIDs have an advantage over aspirin in that the dose schedule is simpler and analgesic and anti-inflammatory effects are achieved within hours of the first dose. Some preparations can be given once a day or twice a day, a schedule that maintains drug levels equivalent in effect to full doses of aspirin and that is particularly helpful in the treatment of elderly or less compliant patients.

If there is active inflammation, a full dosage of a NSAID should be prescribed (see Table 70.12); a lower dosage can be started if inflammation is mild, if mechanical pain is the major problem, if the patient is elderly, or if he is at added risk for toxicity (see below). The propionic acid derivatives (ibuprofen, naproxen), oxicams (piroxicam), and acetic acid derivatives (tolmetin, diclofenac sodium) are currently the most popular NSAIDs in the treatment of rheumatoid arthritis. If a particular preparation is ineffective or is not tolerated, then after resolution of symptoms of toxicity a trial for 4 weeks of another NSAID can be initiated. It has been demonstrated that a single dose (50 to 75 mg) of indomethacin at bedtime can be added to full doses of aspirin with good effect, particularly in patients with active disease who continue to have considerable discomfort in the morning (8). However, other combinations of NSAIDs have not been well studied and should be avoided.

There is an unpredictable and varied individual response in both tolerance and response to NSAIDs. In addition, assays of blood levels are not readily available, so that unlike aspirin, the clinician must depend on the clinical response to a trial of a given NSAID.

USUAL TIME TO MAXIMAL EFFECT. Although these agents have a maximal anti-inflammatory effect within hours, a reasonable trial period is 1 month.

SIDE EFFECTS (Table 70.13). The most common toxicity of NSAID is gastrointestinal disturbance (14). The term NSAID gastropathy has been suggested to describe a variety of gastric lesions including mucosal erythema, gastric erosions, and frank ulcerations. Life-threatening bleeding may occur and does so more commonly in the elderly patient. The gastropathy is caused by direct damage to the gastric mucosa and the blocking of locally produced protective prostaglandins. The patient should be carefully monitored every 3 months; a low dose should be used and chronic use of NSAID should be avoided when possible. At equivalent doses no one NSAID has been shown to be less toxic to the gastrointestinal (GI) tract. To prevent NSAID gastropathy the use of a "cytoprotective" agent may be helpful. The H₂ antagonists (e.g., cimetidine or ranitidine) have been less effective than sucralfate (1 g orally four times a day), or a new synthetic prostaglandin (PGE₁ analogue), misoprostol (100 or 200 μg orally four times a day). Misoprostol may cause diarrhea in 20 to 40% of patients and should not be used if pregnancy is planned. More studies will be needed to define the ideal use of cytoprotective agents in this setting.

A reasonable current practice is to use a cytoprotective agent when starting a NSAID in patients who have a high risk of developing a gastropathy. Such patients have a history of peptic ulcer disease or GI intolerance to a NSAID in the past, are anticoagulated, or are elderly (>70). If NSAID gastropathy develops, the NSAID should be stopped and, if the patient is not

Table 70.13.
Side Effects of Nonsteroidal Anti-inflammatory Drugs

	Approximate Prevalence
Gastrointestinal	10–20%
Epigastric pain, nausea	
Anorexia, dyspepsia, peptic ulceration	
Overt or occult bleeding	<1%
Hypersensitivity reactions	1–5%
Rashes, rarely Stevens-Johnson syndrome	
Very rarely, anaphylactoid reactions	
Aggravation of allergic rhinitis or asthma	10% of sufferers
Renal effects	>5%
Transient renal failure	
Water and salt retention	
Hypokalemia, inhibit diuretic action	
Interstitial nephritis, nephrotic syndrome	>1%
Hepatic effects	5–15%
Cholestatic hepatitis	
Central nervous system	>5%
Tinnitus/deafness	Primarily aspirin
Headache, vertigo, confusion	Higher with indomethacin
Others	
Agranulocytosis, aplastic anemia	<1% (pheylbutazone)
Diarrhea	10–15% (mefenamic acid, other fenamates)
Aggravation of congestive heart failure, angina	>1%
Parotitis	<1% (phenylbutazone)
Toxic amblyopia	<1% (ibuprofen)

already taking one, a cytoprotective agent(s) started before reinstituting new drug therapy. Evidence to date would suggest that misoprostol is the drug of choice, although diarrhea may limit its tolerance. It may be used alone or in combination with an H₂ antagonist, sucralfate, or antacids.

Because prostaglandins play a role in the regulation of renal blood flow, maintaining glomerular filtration and regulating salt, water, and renin metabolism, NSAIDs may impair renal function in high risk patients. The patients at highest risk are those with an imbalance in fluid status or compromise to renal function (e.g., heart failure, diuretic use, cirrhosis, dehydration, and renal insufficiency) (4). If NSAIDs are prescribed in such situations, renal function should be monitored by serial measurements of serum creatinine, and the drugs should be stopped if there is evidence of deterioration (increased edema or rise in concentration of serum creatinine).

Less than 5% of patients develop a hypersensitivity reaction, usually a rash, to an NSAID; the reaction is specific to a particular drug so that another NSAID can be substituted. Very rarely, an anaphylactoid reaction occurs (see Chapter 23) and, if so, subsequent exposure to all classes of nonsteroidal anti-inflammatory agents (including aspirin) is contraindicated.

Some side effects are more common for a particular NSAID. Phenylbutazone imposes an uncommon but important risk of producing aplastic anemia and, given the availability of many equally effective agents, should not be used in the treatment of rheumatoid arthritis. Indomethacin is more commonly associated than are other NSAIDs with gastrointestinal side effects and with neurological symptoms including severe frontal headache, dizziness, vertigo, lightheadedness, and mental confusion. Its long-term usefulness is therefore limited, particularly in elderly patients. The propionic acid derivatives (ibuprofen, naproxen, fenoprofen) are generally well tolerated (Table 70.13), although fenoprofen has been more frequently reported to cause acute interstitial nephritis than have other NSAIDs. Meclofenamate may cause diarrhea, and diclofenac sodium requires periodic monitoring of liver function test because of reversible elevation of serum transaminases.

Significant drug interactions can occur with any of the nonsteroidal anti-inflammatory drugs (Table 70.14) and must be anticipated.

Antimalarials. Antimalarials are rapidly absorbed, relatively safe, inexpensive, and often effective, remitting agents in the treatment of rheumatoid arthritis.

MECHANISM. The mechanism of action of antimalarials in the treatment of patients with rheumatoid arthritis is unknown.

DOSAGE. Hydroxychloroquine (Plaquenil) is the drug of choice among antimalarials. (Chloroquine is no longer recommended because of its greater ocular toxicity.) The daily dose should not exceed 400 mg/day (6 mg/kg); normally it is prescribed as a nighttime dosage to avoid gastrointestinal symptoms. The initial dosage of 6 mg/kg can be continued for 2 to 3 months,

or until a good clinical response is noted, and then lowered to a maintenance dose of 200 mg/day.

USUAL TIME TO MAXIMAL EFFECT. A period of 3 to 6 months is usual. A 6-month period without clinical effect should be considered as drug failure.

SIDE EFFECTS. The most important toxicities are ocular: loss of the corneal reflex, extraocular muscular weakness, loss of accommodation, and an irreversible retinopathy that may progress to visual loss. At the dosage recommended these toxicities are rare, but a baseline ophthalmological examination and a follow-up examination every 6 months are mandatory during the period of treatment. Gastrointestinal upset, pigmentation changes, leukopenia, and a variety of neurological side effects can rarely be seen also.

Gold. Gold is effective in the treatment of rheumatoid arthritis when it is given intramuscularly as a water-soluble thiosalt (gold sodium thiomalate (Myochrysine) or gold thioglucose (Solganal)). An oral gold compound (auranofin) is also available. Initial studies have demonstrated that it is as effective as intramuscular gold.

MECHANISM. A number of mechanisms have been postulated, but none has been proved to explain the effect of gold in patients with rheumatoid arthritis.

DOSAGE. Myochrysine or Solganal therapy should be initiated at 10 mg intramuscularly; if that is tolerated, 25 mg intramuscularly should be given the second week; and if that is tolerated, 50 mg intramuscularly should be given weekly until a response has occurred or until a total of 1 g has been given. If there is a favorable response, therapy should be maintained with 50 mg intramuscularly each month indefinitely.

Auranofin (oral gold) is now preferred by many rheumatologists because of ease of administration and, potentially, a lower incidence of serious toxicity. The dosage is either 6 mg once a day or 3 mg twice a day. Most believe auranofin is less toxic than intramuscular gold but less effective.

USUAL TIME TO MAXIMAL EFFECT. Maximal effect is achieved within 4 to 6 months or after administration of 1 g of gold.

SIDE EFFECTS. Chrysotherapy is associated commonly with side effects. Thirty percent of patients develop a rash, which can vary from a simple pruritic erythematous patch to a severe exfoliative dermatitis. Ulcerations and/or inflammation of the mouth, tongue, and pharynx occur occasionally as well. Up to 10% of patients have proteinuria, which is usually mild but rarely may be in the nephrotic range. Hematological reactions—immune thrombocytopenia, granulocytopenia, and aplastic anemia—occur rarely. Myochrysine, and less often Solganal, may produce a "nitritoid" reaction (flushing, dizziness, or fainting). Rarely, there is a paradoxical aggravation of musculoskeletal symptoms that requires discontinuation of treatment.

Patients receiving gold should have complete blood counts, including platelet counts, and have their urine tested for protein before each dose. Any evidence of hematological or renal toxicity warrants stopping treatment permanently. If a mild mucocutaneous

Table 70.14.
Nonsteroidal Anti-inflammatory Drugs: Drug Interactions

Antacids	Reduce rate and extent of absorption of NSAIDs; variable effect.
Anticoagulants	Phenylbutazone and oxyphenbutazone enhance the activity of warfarin. Aspirin, and potentially all NSAIDs, increases the risk of bleeding of an anticoagulant patient.
Oral Hypoglycemic Drugs	Aspirin, phenylbutazone, and oxyphenbutazone may potentiate the activity of sulphonylurea drugs. Other NSAIDs do not.
Digoxin	Aspirin or Ibuprofen may increase serum concentration.
Antihypertensive/Diuretics	NSAIDs may attenuate the effect of diuretics, beta-blockers, hydralazine, prazosin, angiotensin converting enzyme inhibitors.
Lithium	Elevation of plasma lithium level may occur particularly with indomethacin and diclofenac.
Methotrexate	Salicylate inhibits the renal clearance of methotrexate, and toxic levels may occur.
Phenytoin	Phenylbutazone inhibits the metabolism of phenytoin. Salicylates displace phenytoin from albumin and increase the concentration of free drug.
Probenecid	Inhibits renal clearance of several NSAIDs.
Combination of NSAIDs	Should be avoided.

eruption occurs, crysotherapy should be interrupted, but if the eruption abates, therapy may be restarted at a dose of 10 to 15 mg a week (and then increased by 5 to 10 mg every few weeks up to 50 mg a week again).

Oral gold is more likely to cause cutaneous eruptions or diarrhea than does intramuscular gold but is less likely to cause serious hematological or renal toxicity.

Sulfasalazine (Azulfidine en-tabs). Sulfasalazine has been reintroduced for the treatment of rheumatoid arthritis and offers an option for mild disease (18). Sulfapyridine has been linked to salicylic acid to create salicylazosulfapyridine, the currently used agent.

MECHANISM. The mode of action is unknown. Studies comparing sulfapyridine with 5-aminosalicylic acid have suggested that the active moiety in rheumatoid arthritis is the sulfonamide.

DOSAGE. There is an association with toxicity at the higher dose of sulfasalazine. The best results are found at a dosage of 40 mg/kg body weight. It is suggested to begin at 500 mg/day and increase dosage to 2 g/day over 1 month. The maximal dose of the enteric coated preparation is 2 to 3 g/day.

USUAL TIME TO MAXIMAL EFFECT. Clinical trials have shown improvement within 2 months of reaching full maintenance doses. A 4- to 6-month trial is suggested.

SIDE EFFECTS. There is a relatively high level of side effects (in the range of 20 to 60%.) These may be influenced by slow upward dosing (see above). The most common side effect is gastrointestinal upset including nausea, vomiting, anorexia, heartburn, and epigastric distress. These symptoms can be reduced by stopping medication and adjusting the dose downward. The enteric coated preparation is helpful in minimizing these side effects. GI symptoms are often accompanied by central nervous system symptoms including headache and dizziness. More serious side effects may occur in the first 3 months of treatment including bone marrow suppression, mucocutaneous reactions, and hepatotoxicity. Reversible infertility can occur secondary to oligospermia. Hypersensitivity reactions can be violent, and the drug should not be used in patients with sulfa allergy.

Monitoring should include full blood counts and liver function tests at 2 to 4 week intervals for 3 months, then every 6 to 12 weeks for 6 months and thereafter every 3 months.

D-Penicillamine. Dimethylcysteine, a product of hydrolysis of penicillin, is named penicillamine. It has remitting effects in the treatment of rheumatoid arthritis similar to those of gold.

MECHANISM. Penicillamine chelates metals, interferes with cross-linking of collagen fibrils, and disrupts sulfhydryl-disulfide bonds; but whether any of these actions explains the effects of the drug in patients with rheumatoid arthritis is unknown.

DOSAGE. Penicillamine (Cuprimine, Depen) is available in 125- and 250-mg capsules. Toxicity is reduced by starting at a low dosage (250 mg taken without other medications 1 to 1 1/2 hours after a meal once a day) and increasing the dose slowly (125 to

250 mg a day/every 3 months) until clinical benefit is observed or maximal dosage (750 to 1000 mg a day) is reached. Occasionally a slight reduction in dose (125 to 250 mg a day) may cause a dose-dependent side effect to abate (see below).

USUAL TIME TO MAXIMAL EFFECT. Maximal effect is noted within 4 to 6 months. The earliest response to therapy takes 8 to 12 weeks, and each time the dose is increased, another 8 to 12 weeks must pass before a response can be expected. If after 6 to 9 months of treatment, when the maximal dosage has been given for at least the last 8 to 12 weeks and a good clinical response has not been effected, the treatment should be stopped.

SIDE EFFECTS. Like gold, D-penicillamine treatment requires careful periodic monitoring of blood and urine, first on a weekly basis and then monthly once a stable dosage schedule is attained. The major early toxicities include skin rash, loss of taste, and gastrointestinal upset. These early side effects may be dose dependent and transient. After 3 to 4 months of treatment mouth ulcers, thrombocytopenia, renal toxicity (proteinuria, nephrotic syndrome), and skin eruptions are more likely to occur. Patients who have a history of gold-induced nephrotoxicity are more likely to have a nephrotoxic reaction to D-penicillamine. There is an increasing number of cases reported of unusual autoimmune syndromes secondary to penicillamine, including Goodpasture's syndrome, SLE, myasthenia gravis, polymyositis, and pemphigus. One or more of these side effects may occur in up to 30% of patients taking the drug, in which case treatment must be stopped.

Methotrexate. Methotrexate is a folic acid antagonist. It has been used at low doses in several trials, and many rheumatologists choose methotrexate rather than D-penicillamine after failure of antimalarial and gold therapy (3, 19). This drug should not be prescribed by the general physician without consultation from a rheumatologist.

MECHANISM OF ACTION. Immunosuppressive, cytotoxic, and anti-inflammatory effects have been described with methotrexate presumably secondary to inhibition of dihydrofolate reductase and, therefore, of normal cell metabolism.

DOSAGE. Methotrexate (available as a 2.5-mg tablet) is prescribed in an initial dosage of 7.5 mg once weekly (some prefer to use 2.5 mg every 12 hours for three doses). If no effect is noted in 6 to 8 weeks, then the dose can be increased to 15 mg once weekly (maximal dose of 25 mg weekly). Patients should be carefully selected not to have renal insufficiency, acute or chronic liver disease, alcohol abuse, leukopenia, thrombocytopenia, or untreated folate deficiency. Salicylates (and probably other NSAIDs) block the renal excretion of methotrexate and may lead to elevated serum levels and added toxicity and therefore should not be used simultaneously.

USUAL TIME TO MAXIMAL EFFECT. The onset of action is 3 to 6 weeks with 70% of of patients having some response. A trial of 3 to 6 months is suggested.

SIDE EFFECTS. The use of low dose weekly "pulse"

methotrexate therapy has proven effective and has reduced the toxicity (20). Hepatotoxicity has not been significant using this dose schedule if patients with pre-existing liver disease, alcohol abuse, or hepatic dysfunction are excluded from treatment. Elevated liver enzymes do not directly correlate with toxicity, but liver function tests and serum albumin should be monitored monthly along with the complete blood count. Gastrointestinal upset may occur (10%) but is usually mild in nature. Bone marrow suppression (3%), interstitial pneumonitis (<1%), stomatitis (6%), and alopecia (1%) can be seen. An increased occurrence of malignancy has not been found, nor have effects on sperm production or ovarian function. Women of childbearing potential must understand that methotrexate has potential for teratogenesis and should practice effective birth control.

Other Cytotoxic Agents.   The most commonly used drugs are azathioprine (Imuran) and cyclophosphamide (Cytoxan). Cyclophosphamide is not often used in the treatment of rheumatoid arthritis because of a somewhat higher incidence of toxic reactions. An increasing number of studies have shown the efficacy and relative safety of methotrexate, which is the preferred cytotoxic agent.

MECHANISM.   These drugs interfere with the synthesis of nucleic acids; one of the consequences of that interference is suppression of the immune response. The explanation for the effect of cytotoxic agents in patients with rheumatoid arthritis is unknown but presumably relates to these basic mechanisms.

DOSAGE.   Azathioprine (available as a 50-mg tablet) is used in a dosage of 1.0 to 2.5 mg/kg/day (100 to 200 mg), starting with the lower dosage and increasing it if necessary after 12 weeks of therapy.

USUAL TIME TO MAXIMAL EFFECT.   Maximal response to therapy is seen in 2 to 6 months.

SIDE EFFECTS.   Probably the most common side effect, in the first few months in this dose range, is a slowly falling blood cell count secondary to dose-related marrow depression; this effect is reversible if the drugs are withdrawn. The most serious side effect is the increased incidence, over a period of years, of malignant neoplasma (bladder cancer and lymphoproliferative and myeloproliferative neoplasms); however, this risk has been associated primarily with the use of cyclophosphamide. Less serious, but still important, complications of cytotoxic drugs are increased susceptibility to infection and dyspepsia (azathioprine). Thus, these agents should be strictly reserved for life-threatening complications of the rheumatoid process (e.g., vasculitis) or for patients with intolerable progressive disease despite conventional treatment, and they should only be prescribed in consultation with a rheumatologist.

Experimental Treatments

A number of experimental approaches to the treatment of rheumatoid arthritis have been devised but are not generally available. Levamisole is another new immunoregulatory drug that has been shown to be effective in rheumatoid arthritis, but it has unacceptable side effects. Plasmapheresis, lymphopheresis, and total nodal irradiation have all also been studied but are not recommended because of lack of controlled trials, unacceptable toxicity, and lack of long-term follow-up.

Surgery

Although rheumatoid arthritis is generally an inflammatory process of the synovium, structural or mechanical derangement is a frequent cause of pain or loss of joint function and may be improved by a surgical procedure. The patient, the primary physician, the rheumatologist, and the orthopaedist should participate in the consideration of such operations. The decision to have surgery is a complex one that must take into consideration the motivation and goals of the patient, his ability to undergo rehabilitation, and his general medical status.

Synovectomy is ordinarily not recommended to patients with rheumatoid arthritis, primarily because relief is only transient. However, synovectomy of the wrist is an exception and is recommended if intense synovitis is persistent despite medical treatment (6 to 12 months) in order to prevent extensor tendon sheath rupture.

Total joint arthroplasties, particularly of the knee, hip, wrist, and elbow, are highly successful. Arthroplasty of the MCP joints also can reduce pain and improve function. Other operations include release of nerve entrapments (e.g., carpal tunnel syndrome), ar-

Table 70.15.
Indications for Hospitalization of Patients with Rheumatoid Arthritis

Early in the course for assessment of the extent of the disease and for institution of a therapeutic regimen
At the time of acute painful flareups of arthritis
For assessment and treatment of severe manifestations of extra-articular disease

Table 70.16.
Indications for Referral of Patients with Rheumatoid Arthritis for Consultation

TO A RHEUMATOLOGIST:
1. If there is any question about the validity of the diagnosis.
2. If a arthrocentesis is indicated and the primary physician is not comfortable in performing the procedure (an orthopaedist can also do this procedure).
3. For advice about splinting (an orthopaedist can also provide this advice).
4. If the therapeutic regimen requires the use of remitting agents (see the text), at least telephone contact should be made.
5. If there is any consideration of corrective surgery (an orthopaedist can also provide this advice).
6. If there are severe manifestations of extra-articular disease.
TO AN ORTHOPAEDIST:
1. For advice about splinting.
2. If there is any consideration of corrective surgery.
TO A PHYSICAL THERAPIST:
1. Soon after diagnosis to advise and institute appropriate physical therapy.

throscopic procedures, and, occasionally, removal of a symptomatic rheumatoid nodule.

Summary of Indications for Hospitalization or Referral

The indications for hospitalization and for consultation are listed in Tables 70.15 and 70.16.

General References

Harris Jr ED: Rheumatoid Arthritis. Pathophysiology and Implications for Therapy. *N Engl J Med* 322:1277, 1990.
Kelly WN, Harris Jr ED, Ruddy S, Sledge CB (eds): *Textbook of Rheumatology*, 3rd ed, Philadelphia, WB Saunders, 1988.
McCarty DJ (ed): *Arthritis and Allied Conditions*, 11th ed, Philadelphia, Lea & Febiger, 1988.
Kippel JH, Schumacher HR, Robinson DR: *Primer on the Rheumatic Diseases*, 9th ed, Atlanta, Arthritis Foundation, 1988.
Tala N, Moutsopoulos HM, Kassan SS (eds): *Sjögren's Syndrome—Clinical Immunological Aspects*. Springer Verlag, 1987.

Specific References

1. Arnett FC, Edworthy SM, Bloch DA, et al: The American Rheumatism Association 1987 revised criteria for the classification of rheumatoid arthritis. *Arthritis Rheum* 31:315, 1988.
2. Cathcart ES: Rheumatoid factor B. Serologic techniques and in vitro assays of humoral and cellular immune function. In: Cohen AS (ed): *Laboratory Diagnostic Procedures in the Rheumatic Diseases*, 2nd ed, Boston, Little, Brown, and Co, 1975, p. 107.
3. Furst DE, Kremer JM: Methotrexate in Rheumatoid Arthritis. *Arthritis Rheum* 31:305, 1988.
4. Garella S, Matarese RA: Renal effects of prostaglandins and clinical adverse effects of nonsteroidal anti-inflammatory agents. *Medicine* (Baltimore) 63:165, 1984.
5. Hochberg MC: Adult and juvenile rheumatoid arthritis: current epidemiologic concepts. *Epidemiol Rev* 3:27, 1981.
6. Hund ER: Extraarticular manifestations of rheumatoid arthritis. *Semin Arthritis Rheum* 8:151, 1979.
7. Huskisson E: *Antirheumatic drugs in Clinical Pharmacology and Therapeutics Series*. New York, Praeger Scientific, 1983, vol 3.
8. Huskisson EC, Taylor RT, Burston D, et al: Evening indomethacin in the treatment of rheumatoid arthritis. *Ann Rheum Dis* 29:396, 1970.
9. Hyland RH, Gordon DA, Broden I, et al: A systematic controlled study of pulmonary abnormalities in rheumatoid arthritis. *J Rheum* 10:395, 1984.
10. Krane SM: Aspects of the cell biology of the rheumatoid synovial lesion. *Ann Rehum Dis* 40:433, 1981.
11. Lebowitz WB: The heart in rheumatoid arthritis (rheumatoid disease). A clinical and pathological study of sixty-two cases. *Ann Intern Med* 58:102, 1963.
12. McDermott M, McDevitt H: The immunogenetics of rheumatic disease. *Arthritis Found Bull* 39:1, 1989.
13. Pincus T, Callahan LF, Brooks RH, et al: Self-report questionnaire scores in rheumatoid arthritis compared with traditional physical, radiographic, and laboratory measures. *Ann Intern Med* 110:259, 1989.
14. Roth SH, Bennett RE: Nonsteroidal anti-inflammatory drug gastropathy. *Arch Intern Med* 147:2093, 1987.
15. Spivak JL: Felty's syndrome: an analytical review. *Johns Hopkins Med J* 141:156, 1977.
16. Stage DE, Mannik M: Rheumatoid factors in rheumatoid arthritis. *Bull Rheum Dis* 23:720, 1973.
17. Stastny P: Association of the B-cell alloantigen DRW4 with rheumatoid arthritis. *N Engl J Med* 298:869, 1978.
18. *The Medical Letter on Drugs and Therapeutics:* Drugs for Rheumatoid arthritis. 31:61, 1989.
19. Tugwell P, Bennett K, Bell M, Gent M: Methotrexate in rheumatoid arthritis. *Ann Intern Med* 110:581, 1989.
20. Weinblatt ME, Toxicity of low dose methotrexate in rheumatoid arthritis. *J Rheum* 12:35, 1985.
21. Yelin E, Meenan R, Nevitt M, Epstein W: Work disability in rheumatoid arthritis: effects of disease, social, and work factors. *Ann Intern Med* 93:551, 1980.

CHAPTER 71

Sacroiliitis, Ankylosing Spondylitis, and Reiter's Syndrome

FRANK C. ARNETT, JR., M.D.

SACROILIITIS

Chronic inflammation of the sacroiliac joints, *sacroiliitis*, may occur as an isolated clinical syndrome or as a component feature of several other chronic rheumatic disorders. Osteoarthritic changes in the sacroiliac joint do occur in older individuals, but this is a radiological change that is usually readily differentiated from sacroiliitis and is typically unassociated with symptoms. Sacroiliitis is considered the sine qua non for early *primary ankylosing spondylitis*; however, this latter diagnosis should only be applied when symptoms or signs indicate ascension of inflammation into additional segments of the axial skeleton. *Secondary forms of sacroiliitis* or spondylitis may complicate the clinical course in 10% of patients with inflammatory bowel disease (ulcerative colitis and Crohn's disease), 5 to 10% of those with psoriatic arthritis, and 20% of those with Reiter's syndrome. The dominant clinical problems that bring the patient with primary spondylitis to a physician and require careful management over many years relate to pain, limitation of motion, and deformity of the spine. In secondary spondylitis the same principles of diagnosis and management of the axial problem apply but must be accompanied by attention to the cutaneous, gastrointestinal, genitourinary, and peripheral articular manifestations of the primary disorders.

The pathogenesis of axial inflammation is unknown; however, there is a strong hereditary component marked by the histocompatibility antigen, HLA-B27. This genetic marker is strongly associated with sacroiliitis and spondylitis regardless of clinical setting (Table 71.1). Approximately 90% of patients with primary ankylosing spondylitis have HLA-B27. Conversely, if "normal" individuals with HLA-B27 are carefully assessed, clinical and/or radiographic evidence of disease can be found in only 2% (16). In addition to this genetic predisposition, certain environmental agents appear to be associated with these diseases in the B27-positive host. There is increasing evidence that *Klebsiella pneumoniae* in the gastrointestinal tract may be implicated in the pathogenesis of primary ankylosing spondylitis (10). A secondary spondylitis may occur in the setting of Reiter's syndrome that has been triggered by certain gastrointestinal, genitourinary, or other infections (see "Reiter's Syndrome").

ANKYLOSING SPONDYLITIS

Prevalence

The prevalence of spondylitis parallels the frequency of HLA-B27 in different populations in the United States and in other regions of the world. This tissue type occurs in 8 to 10% of Caucasian Americans, and the disease occurs in 0.1 to 0.2% of the white population (16) (Table 71.1). Black Americans have a much lower frequency of both disease and the HLA-B27 antigen (12). On the other hand, there is a high frequency of spondylitic disease and of HLA-B27 in American Indians. In other parts of the world, ankylosing spondylitis is common in Europeans and most Asian groups but is found rarely in African Blacks or in Japanese, again reflecting the relative frequency of the B27 marker.

Table 71.1.
Classification of Spondylitis and Frequency of HLA-B27[a]

Classification	HLA-B27 Positive
PRIMARY	
Isolated sacroiliitis[b]	70–90%
Ankylosing spondylitis	90%
SECONDARY	
Spondylitis of inflammatory bowel disease	50%
Psoriatic spondylitis	50%
Reiter's disease with spondylitis	90%
INFECTIOUS	
Sacroiliitis	Not increased
Discitis	Not increased
Osteomyelitis	Not increased
Degenerative spondylosis	Not increased

[a] Found in 8 to 10% of normal white and 2 to 4% of black Americans.
[b] May be the mildest form of ankylosing spondylitis.

Histopathology

The spondylitic diseases are characterized by chronic inflammation of *synovial* joints, especially those in the axial skeleton, *fibrous* joints such as sacroiliacs and symphysis pubis, and nonarticular bony areas where tendons and fascia have their insertions (*enthesopathy*). The chronic inflammatory infiltrates are nonspecific and histologically indistinguishable from those of rheumatoid arthritis. On the other hand, unlike the rheumatoid process in which there is cartilaginous and bony destruction, this inflammatory process tends to promote new bone formation across previous articulations. This ossification and calcification of the articular and ligamentous structures of the spine results in eventual fusion and gives rise to the characteristic radiographic findings.

History

The typical patient with sacroiliitis or ankylosing spondylitis is a young white man under the age of 40 years (Table 71.2). Occasionally the diagnosis of ankylosing spondylitis is made in older individuals but careful questioning will reveal that symptoms began years earlier. Women appear to be affected less often than men; however, this may be due to underrecognition of the disease in female cases. The initial symptoms of the disorder in women may be peripheral or cervical arthritis, and low back involvement may be absent or overshadowed by these complaints. Many are misdiagnosed and labeled seronegative rheumatoid arthritis (1) (see Chapter 70). Therefore, the physician must be mindful of these differences between men and women and must consider an emerging spondylitic process in young women who present with a seronegative arthritis. Similarly, children with ankylosing spondylitis are also more likely to develop a peripheral oligoarticular lower extremity arthropathy including severe hip disease, and symptoms in the axial skeleton may not develop for many years, if ever. Their illness is often inappropriately labeled juvenile rheumatoid arthritis (1).

The usual presenting symptoms of sacroiliitis or ankylosing spondylitis are pain and stiffness in the low back or buttocks. These symptoms begin insidiously, and the patient has usually noticed them for at least 3 months before seeking medical advice. Unlike mechanical low back syndromes, the pain and stiffness of inflammatory disease are usually worsened by rest and improved by exercise. The patient is unable to rest at night or sit for prolonged periods and must arise

Table 71.2.
Clues to Early Ankylosing Spondylitis

A young man
Pain/stiffness in buttocks, low back, chest wall
  Worse with rest
  Better with exercise
Sciatic-like pains
Family history of spondylitis
History of iritis

and walk in order to obtain relief. Like discogenic disease, however, symptoms of shooting pains into the buttocks and down the posterior or lateral thighs may mimic sciatica. These pains are usually transient and not associated with any demonstrable neurological deficits. Frequently, patients will already have been evaluated myelographically and/or treated conservatively or surgically for presumed disc disease.

With time the disease progresses into the lumbar and thoracic regions. Chest wall radicular pain occurs frequently and may mimic pleuritic, pericardial, or anginal pain syndromes. Progressive limitation of spinal movements ensues, and patients may note more difficulty in bending forward, the development of a stooped posture, and actual loss of height. Finally, the disease process reaches the cervical spine, and if appropriate preventive measures are not taken, the neck may become fused in a kyphotic position. Although other peripheral joints are uncommonly affected, the root joints (hips and shoulders) eventually become involved in 50% of patients. Occasionally fusion of the back may be entirely asymptomatic, and the patient will develop complaints only when the disease reaches the cervical spine, hips, or shoulders.

Additional important historical facts should be sought in the assessment of the patient. The family history will be positive for a first degree relative with spondylitis in 16% of patients (16). The past history should seek out prior episodes of peripheral arthritis, perhaps beginning in childhood, or even an episode of Reiter's syndrome. Acute anterior uveitis (iritis) may have been a harbinger of the articular syndrome, and at least 25% of patients will have iritis at sometime before or during their course of illness. The review of systems as well as the family history should seek out symptoms or diagnoses of psoriasis or inflammatory bowel disease in the patient or his family members. The patient with spondylitis may have relatives with psoriasis or inflammatory bowel disease but never manifest these disorders himself (5).

Physical Examination

A complete physical examination initially and every 4 to 6 months is important in patients with suspected inflammatory back disease. Although the primary focus of examinations will be the musculoskeletal system, especially the axial skeleton, shoulders, hips, and peripheral joints, additional attention must be directed toward the eyes, heart, skin, and gastrointestinal tract. This practice ensures the diagnosis and provides the baseline with which the physician can assess future articular or extra-articular complications or the superimposition of unrelated systemic or musculoskeletal disorders. It must be emphasized that ankylosing spondylitis is a disease in which the patient requires management over decades, and each new complaint cannot necessarily be ascribed to the basic disease process.

Articular Features (Table 71.3)

There are few measurable abnormalities in patients with early spondylitis. In fact the patient with sacroiliitis, despite significant symptoms of pain and stiffness in the low back region, may have an entirely normal physical examination. At most, there may be tenderness on direct palpation of these joints in the buttocks or upon compression of the pelvis. Stressing the sacroiliac joint to elicit pain (see Chapter 65, Low Back Pain) may also be useful.

Those abnormalities that eventually appear in the patient who has progressive disease relate to loss of range of motion and deformity in mobile structures. After evaluation of the sacroiliac regions the physician should next direct attention to the lumbar spine. The patient with lumbar involvement has often lost the normal lordosis, and there is flattening of that segment of the back. In addition, there is loss in range of motion when the patient attempts to bend forward and touch toes. It should be recalled that hip motion accounts for 90° of the flexion of the trunk on the lower extremities and that the lumbar spine provides the remaining stretch by reversing its lordosis and becoming kyphotic. It is important to obtain serial measurements of the distance between the patient's fingertips and the floor with maximal forward bending. Another objective measurement of lumbar motion is the *Schober test*. With the patient standing erect, a horizontal line is drawn at the L5-S1 region and another line 10 cm above that. With forward flexion the distance between these two points should increase to 15 cm in the normal lumbar spine. This test is best applied and interpreted in the young patient since lumbar motion normally decreases with age. Lateral bending of the lumbar spine should also be assessed at the same time.

Involvement of the *thoracic spine* is determined subjectively by the patient's complaints of pain or stiffness in that region and by demonstrable tenderness along the vertebral column and paravertebral muscles. Compression of the rib cage laterally and over the sternum may also elicit pain. Objective determination of fusion of the costovertebral joints is obtained by measuring the chest expansion. A tape measure is placed

Table 71.3.
Physical Examination in Ankylosing Spondylitis

SACROILIAC JOINTS	THORACIC SPINE
Tenderness	Increased kyphosis
Pain with compression/stress	Tenderness
LUMBAR SPINE	Pain with rib cage compression
Tenderness	sion
Paravertebral muscle spasm	Decreased chest expansion
Loss of lordosis	(< 3 cm)
Decreased flexion: Schober	CERVICAL SPINE
test (<5 cm) (see text)	Tenderness
Abnormal finger-floor	Pain on motion
Decreased lateral motion and	Muscle spasm
extension	Decreased motion
HIPS, SHOULDERS	Kyphosis, decreased lordosis
Pain on motion	Occiput to wall movement
Decreased range	(see text)

around the patient's chest wall at the nipple line or fourth intercostal space, and the change in circumference from full expiration to full inspiration is measured. Less than 3 cm is considered abnormal.

The range of motion of the cervical spine should be determined for extension, right and left rotation, lateral flexion, and forward flexion. Loss of extension is usually the earliest abnormality, and as the disease progresses there is a tendency for the patient to develop fixed deformity in the forward flexed position. Therefore, another rough estimate of developing cervical kyphosis is the occiput-to-wall measurement. This is obtained with the patient placing both heels against the base of the wall and attempting to extend the neck fully to touch the wall with the back of the head. This is normally readily accomplished.

Examination of the range of motion and elicitation of any pain on motion of both shoulders and hips is important since from one-third to one-half of patients will develop involvement of these joints at sometime during the course of the disease. Less often, peripheral joints become inflamed, but usually only transiently. The joints most commonly involved are the knees, ankles, and wrists. Approximately 10% of patients with ankylosing spondylitis will complain of pain in the heels either at the Achilles tendon insertion or over the attachment of the plantar aponeurosis in the sole of the foot. Swelling is usually not apparent in these areas, but tenderness to direct palpation is found.

Extra-articular Features (Table 71.4)

Cardiac abnormalities occur in less than 5% of patients with ankylosing spondylitis (3). The most common, first degree atrioventricular (AV) block, can be determined only electrocardiographically. A history of palpitations or syncope and the finding of a slow or irregular pulse on examination should alert the physician to higher degrees of AV block. At times a cardiac pacemaker is required for serious arrhythmias or complete AV dissociation. Aortic regurgitation due to inflammatory thickening of the aortic valve and root is another serious cardiac complication. Once the diastolic murmur becomes apparent there is usually cardiac decompensation requiring valve replacement in 1 to 2 years.

Table 71.4.
Extra-articular Manifestations and Complications of Ankylosing Spondylitis

CARDIAC	5%
First degree atrioventricular block	
Second and third degree atrioventricular block	
Aortic regurgitation	
OCULAR	25%
Acute iritis	
Chronic iritis	
NEUROLOGICAL	Rare
Cauda equina syndrome	
Cord injury due to fractures	
AMYLOIDOSIS	4%
PULMONARY FIBROSIS	Rare

Iritis occurs in approximately 25% of patients with ankylosing spondylitis and does not necessarily parallel the course of the articular disease. It may occasionally be the sentinel symptom. Its onset is usually abrupt and unilateral with intense pain, redness, and photophobia as the cardinal symptoms. Immediate ophthalmological attention is required to prevent serious damage to the anterior chamber of the eye. Local corticosteroids are usually successful in abating an acute episode; however, frequent slit-lamp examinations determine the response and help to dictate whether systemic steroids are required.

The *cauda equina syndrome* is a rare but serious neurological complication of spondylitis (see also Chapter 65). It is believed to be related to entrapment of exiting lumbar and sacral nerves through the inflamed spinal column; however, compressive inflammatory lesions within the spinal column may be found in some cases and are surgically remediable. Patients with ankylosing spondylitis should be questioned regularly about paresthesias and pain or weakness in the legs, as well as symptoms of bladder and/or bowel sphincter dysfunction. *Other neurological sequelae* of the disorder include injuries to the spinal cord from fracture dislocation of a rigid and brittle spine. The neck is especially prone to fracture, and paraplegia or quadriplegia may result (8).

Secondary amyloidosis can be found in approximately 4% of patients with ankylosing spondylitis, usually after many decades of persistent inflammatory disease. Proteinuria and nephrotic syndrome indicate renal involvement, which is usually the most serious manifestation of amyloid.

Apical pulmonary fibrosis, sometimes with cavity formation, is rare and usually of no clinical consequence. This radiographic abnormality may mimic tuberculosis, and vice versa.

Laboratory Tests

Radiographic evaluation of the sacroiliac joints provides the single most specific test for this disorder. Although a diagnosis of sacroiliitis/spondylitis can be suspected based on the history and physical examination, definitive diagnosis cannot be established without radiographic findings. A single anteroposterior view of the pelvis is usually adequate to define sacroiliitis; however, at times special views such as Ferguson's or oblique views are necessary to evaluate fully the integrity of the sacroiliac joints (15). The earliest radiographic change is usually bony sclerosis on both sides of the joint margins. Shortly thereafter bony erosions occur (Fig. 71.1). There is eventual fusion across the joint space with subsequent loss of the early sclerotic changes (Fig. 71.2). Sacroiliitis is not infrequently confused with the radiographic anomaly, *osteitis condensens ilii,* in which there is symmetrical sclerosis on the iliac side of each sacroiliac joint without any erosions. This finding is most common in young women who have borne children.

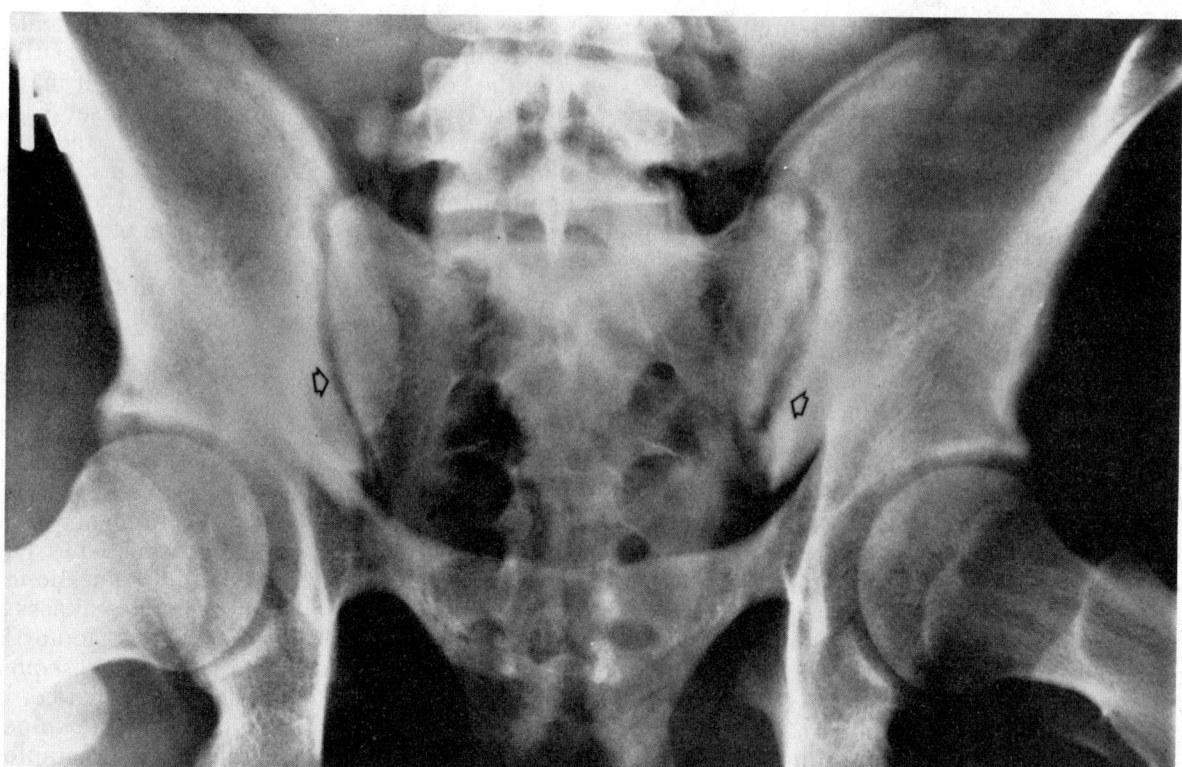

Figure 71.1. Relatively early X-ray changes of sacroiliitis showing bony sclerosis on both sides of the joint margins (see *arrows*). Joint space erosions, a later manifestation of the disease, are present on both sides also.

If the inflammatory disease has progressed beyond the pelvis, an early radiographic finding on lateral lumbar spine films is "squaring" of the vertebral bodies. This phenomenon may also be seen in the thoracic and cervical regions. The apophyseal joints of the spine become fused and, presumably due to immobility, diffuse osteoporosis ensues. Calcification and ossification of the ligamentous structures between vertebral bodies result in the characteristic syndesmophytes seen on X-ray, i.e., the bamboo spine (Fig. 71.2).

Radionuclide scanning (scintigraphy) of the sacroiliac joints is not useful if there is bilateral disease and is probably of most value in localizing pyogenic infections in the sacroiliac joints and other spinal structures (7). Computer tomography of the sacroiliac joints has been shown to be more sensitive than conventional X-rays in early disease (13).

Hematological studies are usually normal. In patients with severe disease, however, there may be a mild normocytic-normochromic anemia reflective of chronic disease. The white blood cell count is usually normal as is the platelet count, although again those with highly inflammatory disease may demonstrate mild thrombocytosis. The erythrocyte sedimentation rate is usually elevated. *Serological studies* are characteristically negative for rheumatoid factor and antinuclear antibodies, and serum complement levels are normal.

Tissue typing. HLA-B27 occurs in 90% of patients with sacroiliitis or spondylitis. This genetically de-

termined tissue type occurs in approximately 8% of the normal white American population. Recently, HLA typing by many commercial laboratories has become available to practicing physicians and when properly used may be a helpful diagnostic aid in the assessment of a patient with low back symptoms or seronegative peripheral arthritis (11). It must be emphasized, however, that indiscriminate HLA typing cannot be substituted for a thorough clinical and radiographic evaluation of the patient. In fact, determination of B27 is rarely needed in making the diagnosis of spondylitis. There are unusual circumstances, however, when the patient gives a strong history suggestive of inflammatory back disease but in whom the radiographs are not yet diagnostic of sacroiliitis. It is in such situations that HLA typing may be helpful, most especially for children and women with early or atypical disease. Even then a positive B27 does not confirm a diagnosis of sacroiliitis, but provides supporting data for the diagnosis when the most specific finding (radiographic sacroiliitis) is not present.

Many patients will already know their tissue type or wish to have the test performed because of the hereditary impact of disease on their family. In these circumstances the physician must offer proper genetic counseling. The facts should be simply presented to the patient as they are currently known. It should be emphasized that spondylitis is not usually a life-threatening or crippling disorder and that symptoms can be controlled medically in the ma-

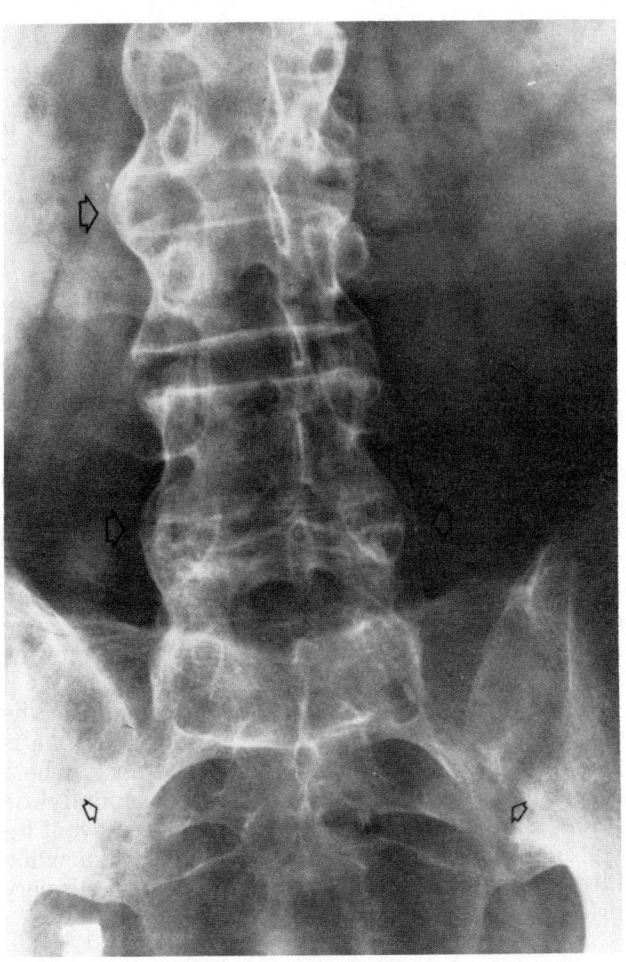

Figure 71.2. Late X-ray changes of sacroiliitis showing complete fusion of the joint space and loss of the early sclerotic change (*small arrows*). Bridging syndesmophytes are also present in the lumbar spine (*large arrows*).

Table 71.5.
New York Diagnostic Criteria for Ankylosing Spondylitis[a]

CLINICAL
1. Limitation of motion of the lumbar spine in all three planes—anterior flexion, lateral flexion, and extension.
2. History or presence of pain at the dorsolumbar junction *or* in the lumbar spine.
3. Limitation of chest expansion to 2.5 cm (1 inch) or less, measured at the level of the fourth intercostal space.

RADIOGRAPHIC
1. Sacroiliitis: grade 3 (sclerosis and erosions of the joint margins) or grade 4 (fusion across the joint).

[a] From Bennet PH, Burch TA: New York Symposium on population studies in the rheumatic diseases: new diagnostic criteria. *Bull Rheum Dis* 17:453, 1967. Definite ankylosing spondylitis = grade 3 or 4 bilateral sacroiliitis with at least one clinical criterion *or* unilateral grade 3 or 4 or bilateral grade 2 (sclerosis of joint margins) sacroiliitis with clinical criterion 1 *or* with both clinical criteria 2 and 3.

Table 71.6.
Principles of Management in Ankylosing Spondylitis

Ensure patient understanding of disease process and objectives in management
Alleviation of pain and stiffness with anti-inflammatory drugs
Physical measures to maintain posture and range of motion in affected areas

Course

It is impossible to predict the ultimate course of any patient presenting with sacroiliitis. The inflammatory process may remain confined to these isolated joints or it may progressively ascend into the lumbar, thoracic, and cervical spinal segments. Likewise, the duration of time from onset of symptoms to fusion of higher spinal segments is highly variable (4). Thus, each patient should understand the nature of this illness and the need for *continued medical surveillance*, as well as the principles of physical and pharmacological management of the disorder (Table 71.6).

Management

Pharmacological

Anti-inflammatory drugs are used to relieve the pain and stiffness of the disease and to promote the patient's ability to perform the physical exercises so important to maintaining a good posture. It is unclear whether these drugs actually affect the natural history of the disease since no long-term controlled studies are available. It seems likely, however, that they do alter and improve the overall functional capacity of the patient. Most often their use is required throughout the person's life; but, occasionally when symptoms completely remit, the anti-inflammatory agent may be tapered over several weeks and reinstituted if symptoms recur. Silent progress of the disease may occur; therefore, the physician should closely monitor these patients even when they are not taking medication.

Salicylates (aspirin) may be tried as the initial anti-inflammatory drug. An initial dose of 3 enteric-coated tablets four times/day is usually sufficient to attain

jority of patients. The likelihood that a family member will develop inflammatory back disease is low. Because HLA antigens, including B27, are inherited in a Mendelian dominant fashion, the risk of inheriting this tissue type would be 50% for each of a patient's children (this assumes that the opposite parent is negative for B27). Even if a child inherits this tissue type, his likelihood of developing arthritis is only 20% (16). Therefore, without any knowledge of HLA status, every child of a patient with B27-positive spondylitis has roughly a 10% (50% times 20%) chance of developing spondylitis.

The 90% probability of never developing this form of arthritis needs to be emphasized to patients concerned about this hereditary factor.

Diagnostic Criteria

The diagnostic criteria for ankylosing spondylitis are summarized in Table 71.5.

blood salicylate levels that are anti-inflammatory (15 to 25 mg/dl). Blood salicylate levels should be measured and the dosage adjusted to attain these levels. The majority of patients with ankylosing spondylitis will not have a dramatic response to salicylates; however, a trial of these inexpensive agents is often warranted before consideration is given to more potent and expensive nonsteroidal anti-inflammatory drugs (NSAIDs).

Indomethacin (Indocin) is especially effective therapy in many patients in dosages up to 75 to 150 mg/day. There are a number of side effects that are important to consider and these are discussed in detail in Chapter 70 (see page 896). Additional indole nonsteroidal anti-inflammatory agents such as tolmetin (Tolectin) and sulindac (Clinoril) are also useful in those intolerant of indomethacin. The reason that the indole NSAIDs seem more affective is unknown. In spite of this chemical impression, NSAIDs may be tried when the indoles are ineffective (see Chapter 70).

Phenylbutazone (Butazolidin, Azolid) appears to be the most effective agent in the majority of patients with spondylitic disease. Its long-term use is indicated in patients with very active disease unresponsive to other anti-inflammatory agents; however, because of its potential serious side effects its use is not recommended without a consultation with a rheumatologist.

Sulfasalazine (Azulfidine), a drug used for inflammatory bowel disease, has recently been found to be effective therapy for ankylosing spondylitis (14). Its mechanism of action is unknown but presumed to be anti-inflammatory. Its use should be reserved for patients unresponsive to nonsteroidal anti-inflammatory agents, and it may serve as an alternative to phenylbutazone. An enteric-coated preparation should be given starting at 500 mg twice daily for 1 week. Thereafter, doses of 2 to 3 grams per day (1 g 2 to 3 times a day) are recommended. Adverse reactions are common and include anorexia, headache, nausea, vomiting, gastric distress, and apparently reversible oligospermia in men. Serious blood dyscrasias (aplastic anemia, agranulocytosis, thrombocytopenia), hypersensitivity reactions, hepatic and/or renal damage, and central nervous system reactions occur occasionally, and complete blood counts and urinalyses should be monitored. Absorption of folic acid and digoxin are both reduced by sulfasalazine. Consultation with a rheumatologist should be obtained before using this agent.

Radiation therapy to the spine was once an effective means of relieving pain. This form of treatment is no longer recommended because of the risk of subsequent leukemia.

Physical Measures

While anti-inflammatory agents relieve the pain and stiffness of spondylitis, an equally important function is their promotion of the patient's ability to perform the physical therapy necessary to prevent spinal deformity and loss of motion in the joints. In fact, such a program usually cannot be instituted until symptoms have been brought under control. The natural history of the disease should be explained so that the patient understands the rationale for the exercise program that must be followed (and that the physician will need to reinforce) over many years. An erect posture when sitting or standing should be encouraged. The patient's bed should be quite firm or should be supported by a bed board. Use of a pillow should be avoided, or the smallest possible pillow should be used to prevent flexion of the neck. Sleeping in the prone position is most efficacious in promoting spinal extension, but the supine position is adequate if there is good support. The patient should refrain from sleeping on a side in a curled up posture.

An active exercise program, to promote extension of the back and increase range of motion of the axial and peripheral joints, as well as breathing exercises to maintain chest expansion should be instituted and executed two to three times/day. Referral to a physical therapist to provide specific instructions and determine that the patient is performing well is a good investment. Swimming is an excellent exercise for the patient with ankylosing spondylitis.

If spinal structures undergo complete ankylosis, the danger of spinal fracture after even minor trauma is increased. This is especially true in the neck, where whiplash types of injury occur. Thus, the spondylitic patient should take special precautions to prevent injury, including the use of a soft cervical collar when riding in an automobile or when walking on slippery surfaces.

Prognosis

The prognosis for patients with ankylosing spondylitis is excellent. The majority of patients can be managed successfully by pharmacological and physical means. Most continue to lead productive lives and change in vocational plans is usually not indicated (4). The morbidity from articular and extra-articular complications is low, and life span is not reduced significantly, if at all. In many instances pain in an affected area of the spine disappears after that segment has fused, and often disease halts at a particular segment and does not proceed to others. Although these facts should be optimistically presented to the patient, they are not cause for laxity in following the postural and exercise program and in maintaining close medical surveillance.

REITER'S SYNDROME

Definition

Reiter's syndrome is a reactive arthritis that occurs as an immunological response to several microbial agents at sites distant from the primary infection (9).

Unlike ankylosing spondylitis, Reiter's syndrome is primarily a peripheral arthritis. However, it shares with ankylosing spondylitis a predisposition to affect young white men and a tendency for sacroiliitis or spondylitis, inflammation of tendon and fascial attachments, uveitis, the same cardiac complications, and a strong association with HLA-B27 (75% positive). Although classically defined as the triad of nongonococcal urethritis, conjunctivitis, and arthritis, it has been found that the majority of patients do not express the classical triad, and that approximately 40% of patients will have arthritis as the only feature of the triad. This latter group has been termed "incomplete Reiter's syndrome," and diagnosis depends upon recognition of the typical pattern of arthritis, the presence of mucocutaneous lesions, and other features that are discriminating (2). Reiter's syndrome may, in fact, be the most common cause of arthritis in young men, even exceeding the prevalence of ankylosing spondylitis. Women are less often affected and comprise only 10 to 15% of most series. The diagnosis and management of the disease focus primarily on symptoms and signs referable to the joints and nonarticular musculoskeletal structures. The diagnosis is made on clinical grounds based upon a constellation of symptoms and signs. Typing for HLA-B27 may be a useful diagnostic aid in the incomplete or atypical case.

History and Examination

The principal clues to the diagnosis of Reiter's syndrome are summarized in Table 71.7. The patient presenting with Reiter's syndrome is usually a young white man between puberty and age 40. Rarely it occurs in older individuals. Blacks and Japanese (not other orientals) are affected far less commonly, presumably due to the relatively low frequency of HLA-B27 in these groups. The reason so few women are affected is unclear.

The disorder occurs in two main settings. First, the disease may follow an episode of diarrhea caused by *Shigella*, *Salmonella*, *Yersinia*, or *Campylobacter* (see Chapter 26). This postdysenteric form constitutes approximately 15% of most series in the United States. Second, the endemic form is believed to result from venereal exposure, and *Chlamydia trachomatis* (see Chapters 27 and 94) may be a causative agent. Recently, evidence of preceding *Borrelia burgdorferi* infection has been reported in 18% of cases from a region endemic for Lyme disease (17). Moreover, increasingly large numbers of cases are being seen in patients with acquired immune deficiency syndrome (AIDS) (18).

In the classical form, *urethritis*, usually painless

or with mild dysuria and a mucopurulent discharge, is usually the first symptom. Also, the prostate gland may be tender, although symptomatic prostatitis is not common. It generally lasts only 1 to 2 weeks. *Conjunctivitis* usually follows shortly. This is most often mild with redness, weeping, and morning crusting. Generally the conjunctivitis lasts only a few days. Photophobia is unusual, and its presence suggests uveitis (see below). Arthritis is usually the last feature of the triad to appear, usually from several days up to 1 month after the onset of urethritis. The arthritis is typically in the lower extremities, involving only one to four joints, most commonly the knees, ankles, and small joints of the feet. The patient notes pain, swelling, heat, and erythema over the joints in the majority of cases of this highly inflammatory disease. In addition to frank arthritis, over 50% of patients will have nonarticular musculoskeletal pain due to enthesopathy. Heel pain due to inflammation of the plantar aponeurosis or of the Achilles tendon insertion is one of the most prominent symptoms of the disease and may be one of the most disabling. Diffuse swelling of digits (sausaging), especially the toes, also occurs in over 50% of patients and is indicative of involvement not only of the joints but of tendons and periosteal structures.

The *mucocutaneous features* of Reiter's syndrome are often asymptomatic and must be sought on physical examination. These include (a) painless shallow oral ulcers, usually on the tongue and palate; (b) circinate balanitis (Fig. 71.3) manifested by shallow moist painless ulcers on the glans penis in uncircumcised men or a dry scaling eruption on the glans in the circumcised; and (c) keratodermablennorrhagia [hyperkeratosis and crumbling of nails (Fig. 71.4), a papulosquamous skin eruption usually beginning on the palms and soles (Fig. 71.5) that which closely resembles pustular psoriasis].

Additional features include fever in approximately one-third of patients, weight loss, and uveitis. The disease may begin abruptly and run a toxic course, or begin very insidiously and pursue an indolent one. Not infrequently heel pain (see Chapter 102) is the first symptom, and this complaint in a young man should raise the question of emerging Reiter's syndrome.

Laboratory Tests

Hematological studies will usually demonstrate a mild normocytic normochromic anemia characteristic of chronic disease. The hematocrit value rarely falls below 30%. A modest leukocytosis in the range of 10,000 to 15,000/mm^3 with a mild shift to the left occurs frequently in those with an acute toxic presentation. Thrombocytosis with platelet counts in the range of 400,000 to 600,000/mm^3 is found in approximately one-third. The erythrocyte sedimentation rate is usually elevated.

Serological studies for rheumatoid factor and anti-

Table 71.7.
Clues to the Diagnosis of Reiter's Sydrome

A young man with arthritis
Symptoms
    Preceding diarrhea, urethritis, or conjunctivitis
    Lower extremity oligoarthritis (knee, ankle, foot)
    Heel pain and/or sausaging of digits
    Rash on soles, penis; painless oral ulcers; dystrophic nails
    Fever, weight loss, leukocytosis
HLA-B27 antigen

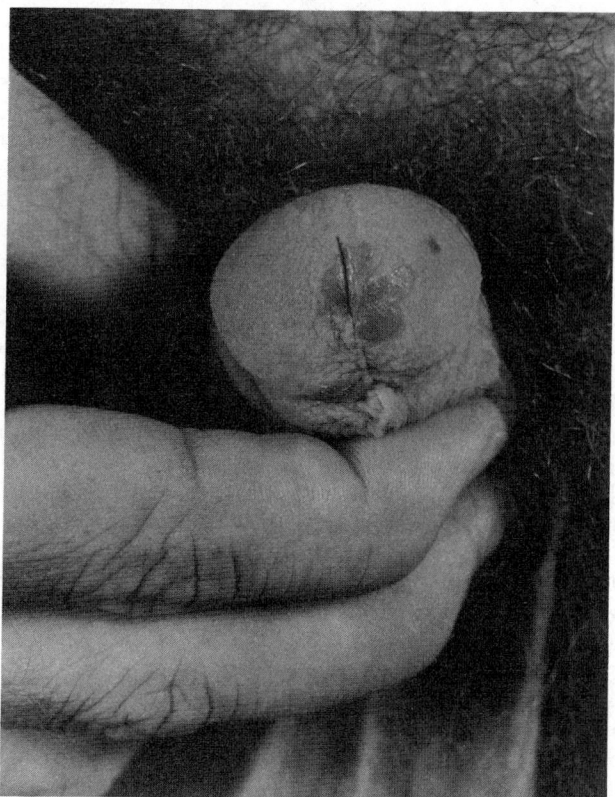

Figure 71.3. Moist, shallow circular lesions on the glans penis characteristic of circinate balanitis.

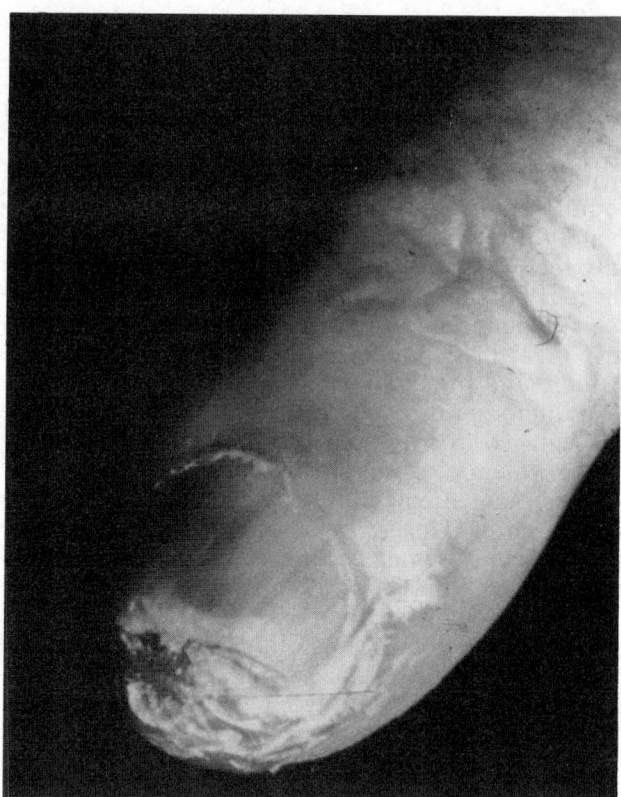

Figure 71.4. Opacification and onychodystrophy of fingernails in Reiter's syndrome. (Taken with permission from Arnett FC: Reiter's syndrome. In Fitzpatrick TB, Eisen AZ, Wolf K, *et al* (eds): *Dermatology in General Medicine,* ed 3. New York, McGraw-Hill, 1985.)

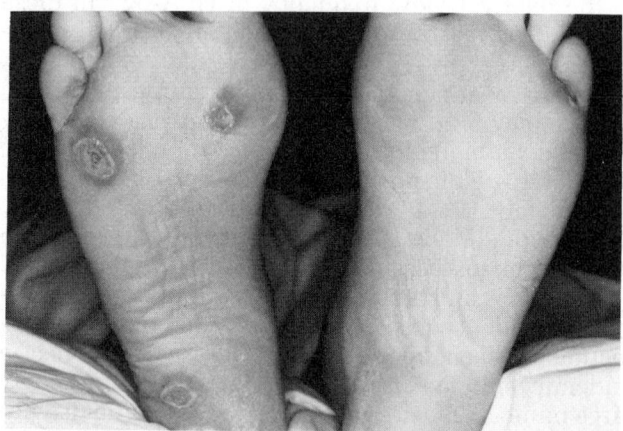

Figure 71.5. Typical keratoderma blennorrhagica involving the sole.

nuclear antibodies are negative. Serum complement is typically normal or elevated as an acute phase reactant. HLA typing will reveal the B27 antigen in 75% of cases but is rarely required in diagnosing the disease. *Radiographs* are typically normal early in the course of the disease; however, over time, periostitis may be seen involving the calcaneus or along the shafts of swollen digits. Should sacroiliitis appear (it does in about 20% of cases), it is more likely to be unilateral in this disease than in ankylosing spondylitis. This may be detected by examination (see above) and confirmed by X-ray if there is doubt. In severe disease cartilage may be lost in joint spaces, and bony ankylosis may ensue.

Synovial fluid has the characteristics of a moderate inflammatory process with a poor mucin clot, white blood cell counts ranging from 5,000 to 50,000/mm³, elevated protein, normal glucose, and a high complement (in contradistinction to the reduced complement in the synovial fluid of patients with rheumatoid arthritis). Culture shows that the synovial fluid is sterile. Synovial biopsy demonstrates an acute and chronic inflammatory process that is nonspecific and indistinguishable from that of many other inflammatory synovitides, and therefore it is not usually necessary. A urinalysis performed on the first voided specimen in the morning is a useful way to identify asymptomatic urethritis. *Urethral stains and cultures* are negative for gonococci in the majority, although the

concurrence of gonococcal urethritis with Reiter's syndrome has been documented. Therefore, this culture should not be overlooked. *Chlamydia trachomatis* infection by urethral cultures and/or serum antibodies can be found in 30 to 50% of cases (9).

It is now mandatory that underlying HIV and *B. burgdorferi* infections be considered and, when appropriate, excluded by serological testing (see Chapters 30 and 34).

Course and Prognosis

Reiter's syndrome follows a self-limited course and completely resolves in 3 months to 1 year in approximately one-third of patients. Another 30 to 40% of patients will have relapses after months or years of quiescence. It has been estimated that a patient with this disease has a 15% chance of having another episode each year for as long as 30 years. Less commonly, a chronic progressive course ensues, resulting in articular destruction and fusion of peripheral and usually axial skeletal joints. Disability results primarily from severe heel pain, deformities of the feet, visual loss due to uveitis, and, less commonly, cardiac complications. Approximately 10% of patients will become permanently disabled and unable to work (6).

Management

Treatment is directed toward suppressing the inflammatory process in joints and tendon insertions and preventing deformity of the peripheral and axial skeleton. Urethritis does not require specific therapy unless *C. trachomatis* (or gonococci) is identified, but the patient should be advised to use a condom during sexual intercourse since these or other transmittable infections are sometimes difficult to diagnose. Rarely an urgent circumcision is indicated if balanitis is extreme, but usually a protective dressing (e.g., petroleum gauze) is all that is needed to control discomfort. Conjunctivitis responds to compresses or astringent drops (see Chapter 99). Uveal tract involvement, if present, requires close follow-up and treatment by an ophthalmologist in order to prevent permanent visual loss. Indole NSAIDs [indomethacin or tolmetin (Tolectin), or sulindac (Clinoril)] are effective in the majority of cases of Reiter's syndrome. As in ankylosing spondylitis the indole NSAIDs seem more effective than other groups (see page 893 and Chapter 70). Sulfasalazine may be necessary occasionally for refractory arthritis or enthesopathy. Salicylates are helpful in a minority of patients but are worthy of trial because of their low cost. Dosage recommendations and adverse side effects are similar to those for ankylosing spondylitis. Systemic corticosteroids may be necessary to treat severe uveitis or inflamed joints that have been unresponsive to phenylbutazone or other nonsteroidal anti-inflammatory drugs, and in these instances consultation with a rheumatologist is suggested. At times, intra-articular corticosteroid injection (usually performed by a rheumatologist) may be useful when systemic therapy has not completely suppressed the inflammatory process. Only occasional patients with extensive cutaneous and articular disease will require more radical therapy (e.g., cytotoxic drugs), and consultation with a rheumatologist should be sought in these circumstances. Anti-inflammatory agents are generally continued for several months and then tapered in those whose symptoms are completely controlled. However, many patients will need continued, lifelong anti-inflammatory agents to suppress the inflammatory activity of the disease. Also, approximately 30 to 40% (see above) of those who have had symptomatic remissions will experience a relapse and require the reinstitution of anti-inflammatory medications. Tetracycline or erythromycin may be effective in treating chlamydia urethritis (see Chapters 27, 30 and 94); however, this therapy probably does not influence the subsequent emergence or course of the articular disease.

Physical measures are important adjuncts in the management of this disorder as in ankylosing spondylitis. There is a tendency for fusion of affected peripheral and axial joints. During acute inflammatory episodes, rest is important, and severely inflamed joints should be splinted to ensure comfort for the patient. As soon as inflammation can be brought under control with drugs, it is important that affected joints be exercised to maintain their ranges of motion. At first passive range of motion should be encouraged in all affected joints. Later, more active range of motion and strengthening exercises should be prescribed as the patient improves.

Painful feet, especially heels, may be helped by shoe inserts that shift weight bearing to nonaffected areas (see also Chapter 102).

General References

Arnett FC: Seronegative spondyloarthropathies. *Bull Rheum Dis* 37:1, 1987.
Calin A (ed): *Spondylarthropathies.* New York, Grune & Stratton, 1983.

Specific References

1. Arnett FC, Bias WB, Stevens MB: Juvenile-onset chronic arthritis: clinical and roentgenographic features of a unique HLA-B27 subset. *Am J Med* 69:369, 1980.
2. Arnett FC, McClusky OE, Schacter BZ, Lordon RE: Incomplete Reiter's syndrome: discriminating features and HL-A W27 in diagnosis. *Ann Intern Med* 84:8, 1976.
3. Bergfeldt L, Insulander D, Linbolm D, Möller E, Edhag O: HLA-B27: An important genetic risk factor for lone aortic regurgitation and severe conduction system abnormalities. *Am J Med* 85:12, 1988.
4. Carette S, Graham D, Little H, Rubenstein J, Rosen P: The natural disease course of ankylosing spondylitis. *Arthritis Rheum* 26:186, 1983.
5. Enlow RW, Bias WB, Arnett FC: The spondylitis of inflammatory bowel disease. *Arthritis Rheum* 23:1359, 1980.
6. Fox R, Calin A, Gerber RC, Gibson D: The chronicity of symptoms and disability in Reiter's syndrome. *Ann Intern Med* 91:190, 1979.
7. Gordon G, Kabins SA: Pyogenic sacroiliitis. *Am J Med* 69:50, 1980.
8. Hunter T, Dudo HI: Spinal fractures complicating ankylosing spondylitis. A long-term followup study. *Arthritis Rheum* 26:751, 1983.
9. Keat A: Reiter's syndrome and reactive arthritis in perspective. *N Engl J Med* 309:1606, 1983.
10. Keat A: Is spondylitis caused by *Klebsiella? Immunology Today* 7:144, 1986.
11. Khan MA: Clinical application of the HLA-B27 test in rheumatic disease. *Arch Intern Med* 140:177, 1980.
12. Khan MA, Braun WE, Kushner I, et al: HLA-B27 in ankylosing spondylitis: differences in frequency and relative risk in American blacks and Caucasians. *J Rheumatol* 3:39, 1977.

13. Kozin F, Carrerea GF, Ryan LM, Foley D, Lawson T: Computed tomography in the diagnosis of sacroiliitis. *Arthritis Rheum* 24:1479, 1981.

14. Nissila M, Lehtinen K, Leirisalo-Repo M, Luukkainen R, Mutru O, Yli-ker Hula U: Sulfasalazine in the treatment of ankylosing spondylitis. *Arthritis Rheum* 31:1111, 1988.

15. Ryan LM, Carrera GF, Lightfoot Jr RW, Hoffman RG, Kozin F: The radiographic diagnosis of sacroiliitis. A comparison of different views with computed tomograms of the sacroiliac joint. *Arthritis Rheum* 26:760, 1983.

16. Van der Linden S, Valkenburg HA, DeJongh BM, Cats A: The risk of developing ankylosing spondylitis in HLA-B27 positive individuals. A comparison of relatives of spondylitic patients with the general population. *Arthritis Rheum* 27:241, 1984.

17. Weyand C, Goronzy JJ: Immune responses to *Borrelia burgdorferi* in patients with reactive arthritis/Reiter's syndrome. *Arthritis Rheum* 32:1057, 1989.

18. Winchester R, Bernstein DH, Fisher HD, Enlow E, Solomon G: The co-occurrence of Reiter's syndrome and acquired immunodeficiency. *Ann Intern Med* 106:19, 1987.

Metabolic and Endocrinological Problems

C H A P T E R 72

Diabetes Mellitus

ROBERT I. GREGERMAN, M.D.

DEFINITION AND CLASSIFICATION

Diabetes mellitus is a condition characterized by an abnormality of glucose utilization and associated with elevation of blood glucose concentration. Approximately 10 million people in the United States are diabetic by this definition. Diabetes mellitus is not a single distinct disease entity. The commonest varieties of diabetes mellitus are known to be associated with abnormalities of insulin secretion and concentration, with cellular resistance to insulin action, and with vascular abnormalities such as basement membrane thickening. Nonetheless, diagnosis is based on the finding of persistently abnormal blood glucose concentrations at some time in life.

Until 10 years ago there was no general agreement on the classification of diabetes mellitus, based either on etiology or manifestations. The current classifications and terminology were proposed by the National Diabetes Data Group of the National Institutes of Health (27) and are followed in this chapter (Table 72.1).

Non-Insulin-Dependent Diabetes Mellitus (NIDDM: Type II)

This is the commonest form of diabetes mellitus and accounts for about 80 to 90% of patients presenting with an abnormality of glucose metabolism. About 9 to 10 million people in the United States are affected. Patients with NIDDM are neither absolutely dependent on treatment with insulin nor ketosis prone. Nonetheless, treatment with insulin may be necessary in the short term in order to control hyperglycemia, which leads to symptoms through osmotic diuresis or infection. Treatment with insulin may also be undertaken in an effort to prevent vascular complications, now believed by many to be a direct consequence of hyperglycemia. Furthermore, such patients do sometimes develop insulin dependence as the result of stress (severe infections, trauma). NIDDM is very likely a heterogeneous disorder. Although most patients are over age 40 at the time of diagnosis, this type of disease is also seen in young persons, and it is for this reason that older terms such as "maturity onset type diabetes" should be abandoned.

NIDDM has a much more obvious familial pattern of expression than does insulin-dependent diabetes mellitus (IDDM, see below). Glucose metabolism is commonly abnormal in the first-degree relatives of patients with NIDDM even when their oral glucose tol-

Table 72.1.
Classification and Clinical Characteristics of Diabetes Mellitus and Other States of Glucose Intolerance

Type of Diabetes	Former Terminology	Clinical Characteristics
INSULIN-DEPENDENT TYPE (IDDM, TYPE I)	Juvenile diabetes Juvenile onset type diabetes Ketosis-prone diabetes Brittle diabetes	Onset usually in youth but occurs at any age. Insulin deficiency requires exogenous insulin to prevent ketosis-acidosis. Non-insulin-dependent phases may occur during natural history. 10–12% of all cases.
NON-INSULIN-DEPENDENT TYPES (NIDDM, TYPE II): Nonobese NIDDM Obese NIDDM	Adult onset diabetes, maturity onset diabetes (MOD), stable diabetes, nonketosis-prone diabetes; in young people was called maturity onset diabetes of youth (MODY)	Onset generally after age 40, but may occur in young; not insulin dependent or ketosis prone, but may need insulin for control of persistent hyperglycemia; periods of ketosis-acidosis may occur during stress of illness; weight control of obese subtype may ameliorate disease. 80–90% of all cases.
OTHER TYPES: *Diabetes mellitus associated with* Pancreatic disease Hormone excess due to endocrine disease or hormone treatment (steroids of glucocorticoid type) Drug use Insulin receptor abnormalities	Secondary diabetes	Diagnosis demands usual abnormalities of glucose handling and documentation of associated condition.
Impaired glucose tolerance (IGT) Nonobese IGT Obese IGT IGT associated with certain conditions and syndromes Drug (chemical) induced Insulin receptor abnormalities Genetic syndromes	Asymptomatic diabetes; chemical diabetes; subclinical diabetes; borderline diabetes; latent diabetes	Diabetes is based on abnormality of glucose handling: may represent a stage of development of diabetes, although most remain in this class for years or revert to normal glucose tolerance.
Gestational diabetes mellitus (GDM)	Gestational diabetes	Glucose intolerance has *onset* during pregnancy; does not include diabetic who becomes pregnant: increased risk of perinatal complications and future diabetes.

erance is normal. Insulin resistance apparently develops first and is followed by a defect of first-phase insulin secretion resulting in impaired glucose tolerance. When there is further impairment of insulin secretion, i.e., defective second-phase secretion, overt NIDDM develops. Included in the group of NIDDM are patients who develop the disease before they reach adulthood (formerly known as "maturity onset diabetes of the young" or MODY). Behavioral and possibly environmental factors appear to be involved in the onset of NIDDM. Especially prominent is the role of excessive caloric intake and subsequent obesity in 60 to 90% of cases. In this type of diabetes, association with certain histocompatibility antigen (HLA) subtypes and with antibodies to islet cells has not been found. Blood insulin levels are variable and may be normal, subnormal, or even supranormal; insulin resistance is common. However, measurement of insulin concentration has no diagnostic usefulness.

Insulin-Dependent Diabetes Mellitus (IDDM: Type I)

This type of diabetes, which accounts for about 10 to 12% of cases, generally has its onset in childhood, often near puberty, hence the former name "juvenile onset diabetes mellitus." However, that designation was misleading, since this type of diabetes can occur during adulthood. In some reports a second peak of incidence occurs after age 40; in others, in the late 20s (21). Moreover, its essential characteristic is that insulin dependence is absolute; without insulin therapy, ketosis-acidosis usually ensues rapidly. Although the disease is probably heterogeneous, genetic determinants are important in most of these patients (see below). Rare cases may have a viral basis, but even in these, genetic predisposition may be important. Only 2% of siblings of patients with IDDM develop diabetes; when tested initially, these individuals may show only impaired glucose tolerance but eventually develop overt IDDM. Increased or decreased frequency of certain histocompatibility antigens, abnormal immune responses and autoimmunity, and antibodies to islet cells have been demonstrated in IDDM. None of these findings is currently useful in a diagnostic sense.

Recent studies have focused on IDDM as an autoimmune disease. When immunosuppressive therapy has been given within a few weeks after onset, remissions have been induced and up to one-half of patients may remain in remission at 1 year.

Inheritance and Genetic Counseling

The precise genetics of IDDM, however, are not clear, and prediction of the occurrence of diabetes in offspring of diabetic parents is not possible; even statistical estimates are crude (17). The prevalence of overt diabetes in offspring of conjugal diabetic parents is remarkably low, ranging from 3 to 12% in most reports. Contributing to the difficulty of prediction are the criteria for detection of diabetes (overt diabetes versus diabetes detected by glucose tolerance testing; see pages 917 to 919) and age of onset.

The conclusion that hereditary factors are more important in NIDDM than in IDDM comes from studies of twins. If expression of diabetes in IDDM were based entirely on genetic grounds, one would expect 100% concordance for diabetes in monozygotic twins; but this is not the case for patients diagnosed when young (before age 40). Both members of pairs become diabetic only about 50% of the time. Only in twins in whom diagnosis is made later in life is 100% concordance approached. Thus, environmental factors must be important in younger diabetics.

Studies of ethnic groups show distinctive patterns of diabetes and superimposed geographic (environmental) effects upon these patterns. The most easily apparent determinant is obesity. Certain American Indian tribes show a remarkably high prevalence of diabetes (Pima, Navajo); obesity appears to be the major factor in expression of the disease in these people. In terms of the patterns of disease, in South Africa, black and Indian populations have similar environments and diets, but only the black diabetics are ketosis prone. In contrast, the Indians have more frequent vascular disease. In non-Indian populations in the United States, no such distinctive ethnic or racial patterns have been recognized to date.

Parents who have an insulin-dependent diabetic child often wish to know the risk to future offspring. Prenatal HLA typing of fetal cells obtained at amniocentesis could be compared to that of the diabetic sibling; a fetus with the same HLA identity would increase the risk, but the accuracy of the prediction would still be only about 50%. The imprecise nature of this assessment is in contrast to the nearly 100% certainty of predicting Tay-Sachs disease or Down's syndrome. Thus, even with an accurate family history and pedigree, together with chemical assessment of diabetes (glucose tolerance testing), only crude predictions can be made for a couple who wish to know their own chances of developing diabetes and the risk for their offspring (17).

At this point, only a few generalities seem safe. Prospective parents should not be told to avoid procreation merely because one parent is diabetic. Even when both parents are diabetic, the risk seems relatively low. If avoidance of pregnancy is decided upon, a diabetic woman may be at increased risk from several commonly used contraceptive measures, although the evidence for this increased risk is not firm. High dose estrogen-based contraceptives may be unwise because of possibly increased risk in the diabetic of vascular thrombosis and hyperlipidemia. Low dose estrogen or progestogen alone would theoretically be safer. Intrauterine devices may possibly produce infection more often in a diabetic. Thus, mechanical means of con-traception such as the diaphragm or condom would seem to be the safest methods (see Chapter 93).

Other Types of Diabetes

Sometimes diabetes is associated with another condition or disease; usually the association is infrequent but more common than in the general population (Table 72.2). This heterogeneous group includes some disorders in which there is a clear relationship between the associated disease and the diabetes but many others in which an association has been noted but is not well understood. For example, in pancreatic insufficiency due to pancreatitis, insufficient insulin may be produced and insulin-dependent diabetes mellitus ensues. At the opposite extreme, an association between primary aldosteronism and diabetes mellitus has been observed, but the mechanism is not clear. Glucocorticoid excess, as in relatively rare Cushing's syndrome or very common steroid therapy, frequently produces diabetes mellitus. Rare cases of diabetes mellitus associated with insulin resistance and acanthosis nigricans have been described in which the insulin receptors show molecular abnormalities that impair their function.

Problems in Classification of Individual Patients

On occasion, classification may be difficult. For example, an adult presenting with ketoacidosis may be

Table 72.2.
Diseases Associated with Diabetes Mellitus or Abnormal Glucose Tolerance[a]

ENDOCRINE DISORDERS
Acromegaly
Aldosteronism
Glucocorticoid Excess (Cushing's syndrome; iatrogenic)
Pheochromocytoma
Thyrotoxicosis
Somatostatinoma/hypothalamic disorders
Insulin receptor abnormalities (lipodystrophy; virilization; acanthosis nigricans)
AUTOIMMUNE DISORDERS
Adrenal insufficiency (Addison's disease)
Hashimoto's disease
Hypoparathyroidism
Myasthenia gravis
Pernicious anemia
Polyglandular failure (adrenals/gonads/thyroid)
Primary hypothyroidism
Graves hyperthyroidism
OTHER DISORDERS INCLUDING GENETIC SYNDROMES
Amyloidosis
Hemochromatosis
Acute and chronic diseases of the pancreas
Cystic fibrosis
Malnutrition
Klinefelter's syndrome, Turner's syndrome, Werner's syndrome, optic-atrophy-diabetes mellitus, diabetes insipidus, Laurence-Moon-Biedl syndrome, Friedreich's ataxia, ataxia-telangiectasia, Refsum's disease, Down's syndrome, myotonic dystrophy

[a] Indicates relatively common disease or frequent association of disease with diabetes mellitus.

erroneously classified as IDDM when in fact the individual's diabetes is of the NIDDM type, with insulin dependence having been precipitated by the stress of infection. Similarly, the process of distinguishing between a patient with IDDM and a thin NIDDM patient for whom insulin has merely been prescribed may require discontinuation of the insulin therapy, a procedure that may be impractical. Diagnostic procedures necessary to exclude the possibility that the diabetes is one of the other types (e.g., Cùshing's syndrome, hemochromatosis, etc.) may not have been performed. In addition, for those patients in whom diagnosis was based on an abnormality of glucose tolerance, diagnostic criteria may not have been met or may have been equivocal (see page 917). In these situations, classification should be considered tentative.

CLINICAL PRESENTATION

Most diagnoses of diabetes mellitus are now made at an asymptomatic stage of the disease as a result of routine blood tests that reveal elevation of blood glucose concentration. In some institutions where the diagnosis is actively sought, glucose tolerance tests reveal many cases. Of those patients who are symptomatic at time of diagnosis, most will complain of increased frequency of urination (polyuria), excessive thirst with increased fluid intake (polydipsia), and, if the disease is very severe, increased appetite and increased food consumption (polyphagia) associated with weight loss. All of these symptoms are manifestations of excessive blood sugar and of secondary glucosuria. Other symptomatic manifestations include blurred vision, vaginitis (usually due to monilial infection), and skin infections. Furuncles and carbuncles, once common, are now rarely seen, but intertriginous candidiasis is common in the obese. Oral candidiasis is uncommon.

Usually, these symptoms are present for weeks or months before medical attention is sought. The onset of symptoms is often insidious and may be attributed by the patient, or even by the physician, to emotional factors or to a common problem such as a urinary tract infection. Indeed, the diagnosis may be missed for a time because the physician "knows" that the patient is not a diabetic on the basis of previous evaluation.

Some patients present with absent or minimal symptoms due to hyperglycemia and glucosuria but have already developed complications of the diabetic state such as neuropathy or, more commonly, vascular disease. However, only rarely will a patient be unaware of diabetes and yet present with severe complications of the disease such as diabetic retinopathy or nephropathy.

DIAGNOSIS

Elevation of blood sugar concentration is the hallmark of diabetes mellitus. Glucosuria alone is not a diagnostic finding, however, since rare individuals may have a renal tubular glucose "leak" (renal glucosuria) at normal concentrations of blood sugar. Only infrequently will individuals show diagnostically elevated blood sugar levels before glucosuria develops ("elevated renal threshold").

Criteria for Diagnosis of Diabetes Mellitus

Criteria have been suggested as follows (Tables 72.3 and 72.4) (27): (a) unequivocal elevation of plasma glucose (PG) concentrations associated with classic symptoms of diabetes mellitus, or (b) elevation of fasting plasma glucose (FPG) on more than one occasion, or (c) elevation of PG following an oral glucose challenge on more than one occasion. A single elevated

Table 72.3.
Normal Values for Plasma Glucose and for the Glucose Tolerance Test[a]

Fasting state (10–16 hours postprandial)	
Venous Plasma	< 115 mg/dl
Venous whole blood	< 100 mg/dl
Capillary whole blood	< 100 mg/dl
2-Hour oral glucose tolerance test (OGTT)	
Venous Plasma	< 140 mg/dl
Venous whole blood	< 120 mg/dl
Capillary whole blood	< 140 mg/dl

Values between those which are diagnostic (see Table 72.4) and those which are normal should be considered non-diagnostic. Impaired glucose tolerance (IGT) is considered present when three criteria are met: (a) fasting level is below diagnostic (b) 2-hour value is intermediate, and (c) some other value (½, 1, 1½) is elevated to:

Venous Plasma	> 200 mg/dl
Venous whole blood	> 180 mg/dl
Capillary whole blood	> 200 mg/dl

[a] To express values as millimoles per liter, multiply glucose in milligrams per deciliter x 0.056. Serum and plasma values are the same.

Table 72.4.
Diagnosis of Diabetes: Diagnostic Values of Glucose; and of the Glucose Tolerance Test[a]

Fasting state (10–16 hours postprandial)	
Venous plasma[a]	> 140 mg/dl
Venous whole blood	> 120 mg/dl
Capillary whole blood	> 140 mg/dl

Oral glucose tolerance test (OGTT) *preparation*: fasting 10–16 hours during which no caffeine-containing drinks or smoking is permitted.
  75-g glucose (40 g/m²)
    Use in nonpregnant adults: (1.75 g/kg for children. Up to 75 g maximum). Dosage form: flavored water, 25 g of glucose/100 dl. Drink over 5 minutes. Obtain blood samples at 0, ½, 1, 1½, 2 hours.
  Test positive for diabetes mellitus: *both* the 2-hour sample *and* at least one other sample must meet following criteria:

Venous plasma	> 200 mg/dl
Venous whole blood	> 180 mg/dl
Capillary whole blood	> 200 mg/dl

100-g glucose
  Use only in pregnant adults: obtain blood samples at 0, 1, 2, 3 hours.
Test positive for diabetes mellitus: *two* or more of the following values must be met or exceeded:

	Venous plasma (mg/dl)	Venous Whole Blood (mg/dl)	Capillary Whole Blood (mg/dl)
Fasting	105 mg/dl	90	90
1 hour	190	170	170
2 hours	165	145	145
3 hours	145	125	125

[a] Serum and plasma values are the same.

FPG or a single oral glucose tolerance test never establishes the diagnosis.

In most modern laboratories glucose is determined in plasma or serum. Plasma and serum values are identical, but both are 5 to 15% higher than are obtained using whole blood.

Impaired Glucose Tolerance (IGT) versus Diabetes Mellitus

The standards promulgated in Tables 72.3 and 72.4 are not arbitrary but have been derived from many studies and numerous considerations, including prospective studies conducted in the United States and Britain over the past 20 years. Although some disagreement will inevitably exist on all standards, perhaps the most important point is that no single value of fasting glucose or combination of values in glucose tolerance tests sharply divides diabetics from nondiabetics. Most populations exhibit a continuous unimodal distribution of values, usually skewed to the higher end. (An exception is the Pima Indian population in which bimodal distribution of both fasting and 2-hour postglucose values is seen (33).) The current criteria are derived from prospective observations of the fate of individuals whose glucose concentrations fall within certain ranges. The conclusions from such studies are as follows:

1. Individuals whose plasma glucose levels during the oral glucose tolerance test (OGTT) fall between normal (1 hour < 160 mg/dl; 2 hours < 140 mg/dl) and diabetic should be clearly classified into a group (impaired glucose tolerance, IGT) separate from those with overt glucose intolerance.
2. In this IGT group, one can expect 1 to 5%/year to develop symptomatic diabetes mellitus or diagnostically abnormal glucose tolerance. On the other hand, many such individuals eventually show normalization of glucose tolerance, and still others remain in the IGT range. The higher the blood sugar within the range of IGT, the greater the tendency for tolerance to deteriorate.

   Perhaps the most convincing evidence on IGT progression has come from a long-term study of Pima Indians (11, 27, 33). The risk of progression to overt diabetes in this group was clearly related to the level of glucose within the range of 160 to 200 mg at 2 hours (three times that of persons with lower values). In this group, however, the rate of decompensation to overt diabetes was still only 3%/year.
3. Treatment of the IGT group with oral antidiabetic (hypoglycemic) agents had no effect on the eventual development of diabetes.
4. Diabetic microvascular complications (retinopathy or nephropathy) do not develop in individuals with IGT. On the other hand, in the study of Pima Indians, values > 240 mg/dl were associated with such changes.

Significance of Impairment of Glucose Tolerance for Development of Cardiovascular Disease

Although morbidity and mortality from cardiovascular disease are unequivocally increased in patients with clinical diabetes mellitus, the issue of the impact of IGT on such events is unsettled. The National Diabetes Data Group Study concluded that morbidity and mortality from arteriosclerotic disease appeared to be significantly increased in patients with IGT, although to a lesser degree than the 2- to 3-fold increase seen in overt diabetes (27). On the other hand, no such conclusion could be drawn from later studies in 15 populations of the impact of IGT on development of coronary artery disease (35). In some of these studies, a strong relationship was found between IGT and coronary heart disease death rates, but in others no such relationship was evident. No satisfactory explanation is available to explain these discrepancies. At this time, IGT cannot be designated as an established risk factor for coronary heart disease or other cardiovascular diseases.

Fasting Plasma Glucose (FPG)

Elevation of FPG should be followed up by several repeated measurements of the FPG on different days. Because over 90% of individuals with repeated elevations of FPG will have an abnormal glucose tolerance test (OGTT), little is gained by proceeding directly to such a test. FPG may be elevated by stress and illness, but is actually less subject to this change than is the OGTT. When an illness results in elevation of FPG (or an abnormal OGTT) only to revert to normal with recovery, the question that arises is whether a "diabetic" state has been unmasked or whether the transient elevation is simply the result of disturbed carbohydrate metabolism associated with the illness. Only long-term follow-up may sometimes provide an answer. In the interim, the individual may be deemed to have IGT (see above). Such terms as subclinical, preclinical, chemical, latent, and borderline diabetes should be avoided, both because of their uncertain meaning and because of the psychological trauma and economic penalties (e.g., insurance ratings, job qualifications) that are often needlessly created.

The 2-Hour Postprandial Blood Sugar as a Screening Test

This procedure should be abandoned. Only infrequently will a gross elevation of postprandial sugar be seen when the FPG is normal. Initially nondiagnostic but abnormal elevations (e.g., 140 to 200 mg/dl) are often not observed on follow-up testing with an OGTT. Even a normal glucose concentration 2 hours postprandially has no established value for predicting that an OGTT would be normal. The 2-hour postprandial blood sugar with glucose added to the meal is similarly to be avoided.

Use of the Oral Glucose Tolerance Test

Diagnostic criteria for the OGTT are listed in Tables 72.3 and 72.4; Table 72.4 also shows how the test is performed. The OGTT is not necessary if there is unequivocal elevation of plasma glucose in a patient who has classic symptoms of diabetes or if the FPG is elevated on more than one occasion (see page 916). Indeed, in the absence of signs and symptoms of diabetes, relatively few clinical indications exist for attempted establishment of a diagnosis of diabetes mellitus solely by use of the OGTT.

Indications

The physician may wish to perform the test because of a positive family history. Occasionally, he may wish to prognosticate for a sibling of a diabetic. The OGTT does have a place in diagnosis during pregnancy (see below). The test is also sometimes performed in an individual who manifests premature atherosclerosis or has unexplained nephropathy, neuropathy, or retinopathy. However, under such conditions a positive OGTT is ordinarily, at most, no more than suggestive of a cause of the disorder at hand. For example, premature atherosclerosis certainly occurs in nondiabetics and in the face of normal glucose tolerance. Perhaps a greater constraint on the use of the OGTT for early diagnosis is the realization that, given the limitations of currently available therapeutic measures, the physician does not—except in obese individuals—undertake therapy directed at improvement of an abnormal OGTT. In many patients, therefore, no immediate therapeutic benefit is likely to result from uncovering an abnormal OGTT. Moreover, the "labeling effect" associated with an abnormal OGTT may create unnecessary morbidity in a previously healthy person.

Limitations

A number of other considerations impose limitations on the usefulness of the OGTT. A variety of illnesses, both acute and chronic, produce abnormalities of the OGTT. Infection, trauma, drugs, and even physical inactivity may produce a "diabetic" OGTT (Table 72.4). After myocardial infarction, many weeks may pass before normal glucose tolerance is again seen, and at least 2 weeks may elapse after a febrile illness. Testing with OGTT should certainly be postponed under these circumstances. Reduced food intake with less than 150 g of carbohydrate/day can also produce an abnormal test within a few days as can fasting beyond 16 hours. Even performance of the test in the afternoon rather than in the morning may produce elevated levels of blood sugar. Smoking immediately before or during the test can produce an abnormal result, as may the ingestion of caffeine-containing drinks (coffee, tea) in the period of fasting. If nausea, vomiting, or diaphoresis occurs during the test, the results are invalid and the test should be terminated. A repeated test may not necessarily provoke these symptoms. Beyond all of these caveats, great variability in any patient's OGTT response is well established, so that a diagnosis of diabetes cannot be established on the basis of a single abnormal test.

Drug Effects on Glucose Tolerance

Table 72.5 lists drugs and related substances that have been reported to be associated with decreased glucose tolerance and even with the development of symptomatic diabetes mellitus. The agents most often responsible are glucocorticoids (cortisone, prednisone, etc.) and the diuretics used in the long-term therapy of hypertension. Potassium depletion, which can be present even when serum potassium is normal, is one mechanism by which diuretics can produce glucose intolerance. Other drugs also affect glucose tolerance, but do so much less often. Despite their tendency to decrease glucose tolerance these drugs should not be withheld when their use is indicated. A common error is to fail to use a diuretic in a diabetic hypertensive patient for fear of exacerbating glucose intolerance. Although blood pressure control may be attempted by using nondiuretic agents (see Chapter 62), failure to achieve satisfactory blood pressure control should prompt the physician to proceed with use of a diuretic (see also below, page 940). If glucose tolerance worsens, therapy with the usual modalities for control of blood sugar should then be instituted. If the patient is already receiving insulin, an increase of insulin dose

Table 72.5.

Drugs Associated with Abnormal Glucose Tolerance or Diabetes Mellitus

HORMONES AND RELATED AGENTS ACTH
    Catecholamines (epinephrine, isoproterenol, levodopa)
    Dextrothyroxine
    Estrogens (oral contraceptives)
    Glucocorticoids (cortisone and derivatives)
    Thyroxine and triiodothyronine (toxic doses)
DIURETICS AND ANTIHYPERTENSIVE DRUGS
    Chlorthalidone (Hygroton, Combipres, Regroton)
    Clonidine (Catapres, Combipres)
    Ethacrynic acid (Edecrin)
    Furosemide (Lasix)
    Prazosin (Minipress)
    Propranolol (Inderal)
    Thiazides (Diuril, Hydrodiuril, etc.)
PSYCHOACTIVE AGENTS
    Chlorprothixene (Taractan)
    Haloperidol (Haldol)
    Lithium (Lithane, Eskalith)
    Phenothiazines (Thorazine, Trilafon, Etrafron, Triavil, etc.)
    Tricyclic antidepressants
        Amitriptyline (Elavil, Endep, Triavil, etc.)
        Desipramine (Norpramin, Pertofrane)
        Doxepin (Adapin, Sinequan)
        Imipramine (Presamine, Tofranil)
        Nortriptyline (Aventyl)
MISCELLANEOUS
    Antineoplastic drugs (L-asparaginase, streptozotocin)
    Dilantin (Phentoin)
    Indomethacin
    Isoniazid (INH)
    L-Dopa (Sinemet)
    Morphine; marijuana
    Nicotinic acid

may be all that is needed. Similar considerations pertain to the use of glucocorticoids. The course of diabetes provoked by the administration of corticosteroids or diuretics, once these agents have been discontinued, is variable.

Other Aspects of the Glucose Tolerance Test Including Effect of Age

Although age has no clinically significant effect on FPG, the values in the OGTT tend to increase with age. One method for dealing with this phenomenon was to report any given value as a percentile rank. Although this was a reasonable approach, the diagnostic criteria of the National Diabetes Data Group, as proposed above, take into account this effect of age (27). By this approach, aging merely results in IGT and is associated with the corollaries of this state, i.e., the possibility of higher risk for development of atherosclerotic disease and overt diabetes.

Gestational Diabetes

The term gestational diabetes (GDM) refers only to women who become overtly diabetic (Table 72.4) during pregnancy (see below, page 948). Women who are known to have diabetes and who become pregnant are not included. The majority of gestational diabetics return to a state of normal glucose tolerance postpartum. GDM occurs in some 1 to 2% of all pregnancies. Such patients are at increased risk (about 30%) for developing diabetes within 5 to 10 years after parturition.

Previous (PrevAGT) and Potential (PotAGT) Abnormalities of Glucose Tolerance

Persons with a normal OGTT who previously showed either IGT or overt diabetic hyperglycemia should be classified according to the presently accepted scheme as previous abnormality of glucose tolerance (PrevAGT). These individuals are not to be considered diabetic and should no longer be labeled with the terms prediabetic or latent diabetic. The economic and psychosocial stigmata of such labels are not justified.

The term potential abnormality of glucose tolerance (PotAGT) should never be used as a diagnostic label for any person. The term is useful only in research.

TREATMENT OF DIABETES MELLITUS

Education of the Patient

Of those chronic conditions that are common in ambulatory practice, diabetes stands apart because of the broad scope and the critical importance of patient education and long-term management. For all diabetics, the following factors are important: the impact of diet on diabetes; the implications of diabetes for ordinary activities; recognition of the signs of worsening diabetes; the importance of proper care of the feet; and the clarification of misconceptions about diabetes. For patients receiving insulin, the following additional factors are important: correct administration of insulin; the unique constraints that insulin therapy places on dietary management and changes of activity; the recognition of the symptoms of hypoglycemia; and the adjustment of insulin dose during intercurrent illness.

The patient's response to being informed of a diagnosis of diabetes varies widely. Many patients have already suspected the diagnosis as the result of previous observations of similar symptoms in family members. These individuals are often also aware of the complications of the disease (loss of vision, amputations) and the use of "the needle" (insulin, self-administration). Transient or even prolonged anxiety or depression occurs frequently and should be anticipated by the physician. Similar problems at this time are commonly seen in close relatives or friends of the patient. Management of these minor mood disturbances is described in Chapter 13.

Many patients are reluctant to accept the need for self-injection of insulin, and many physicians are unwilling to press the issue. The result is poor control, inappropriate use of oral hypoglycemic drugs, or both. Reluctance of both patient and physician may stem from unfamiliarity with the techniques. In point of fact, insulin injection is simple and almost without discomfort. A firm attitude on the part of the physician will overcome patient reluctance in almost all cases. The use of disposable syringes has eliminated the inconvenience of sterilization, and the modern thin, very sharp, plastic-hubbed or syringe-attached needles render the injections practically painless. Aspects of technique are described below (page 929).

A substantial proportion of "new" diabetics will quickly reveal a noncompliant pattern of handling their particular chronic illness. These patterns are usually difficult to alter. Perhaps the best way to prevent the development of poor compliance is to educate the patient and other members of the patient's household from the outset (see Chapters 3 and 4 for a detailed discussion of patient education and of compliance-promoting strategies).

Educational Process

The educational process should be as frank and as authoritative as possible, since much misinformation is apt to deluge the patient. Misconceptions should be explained and countered. The physician is not able to undertake and continue this process in the detail it deserves; therefore, a nurse or other trained individual should be available whenever possible to instruct the new diabetic and to continue the educational process as necessary. Excellent booklets are available from the American Diabetes Association and pharmaceutical manufacturers as adjuncts to personal instruction, as are a variety of teaching films and newsletters dealing with all aspects of diabetic care (14). In all aspects of management the need for reinforcement and continuing patient education must be stressed. Even the most intelligent patient often needs reiteration of treatment principles and procedures.

The goal of such instruction is correct patient self-care. Even such procedures as altering the dose of insulin to conform to changing needs should, whenever possible, be taught. Successful management is never possible without such education. On the other hand, all patients will need assistance from time to time. Telephone contact with the physician should be available and encouraged. Many problems of adjustment of insulin dosage, etc., can and should be handled by telephone in order to avoid excessive use of office time and unnecessary expense and loss of work time for the patient. Finally, the need for education of key members of the patient's family should not be forgotten. Alterations of diet and of eating patterns are not often made easily and may not be made at all if a spouse is unaware, for example, that punctual meals are essential for the patient receiving "conventional" insulin therapy. The distinctions between conventional, intensive conventional, and insulin therapy utilizing pumps are described below (page 929). The various programs impose different demands on the therapeutic process; conventional therapy is the most demanding in terms of the need for punctual meals.

Diet Therapy

Different diet strategies guide therapy for diabetes, depending on whether one is dealing with an obese, non-insulin-dependent (NIDDM) patient or an individual of appropriate weight who has insulin-dependent disease. For the obese NIDDM diabetic, the immediate and long-term goals are weight reduction, and almost any weight reduction scheme (diet plan) will suffice (see Chapter 76). Ideally, diet composition should approximate that shown in Table 72.6. Most obese diabetics are not symptomatic and do not require therapy with insulin or oral hypoglycemic agents for control of symptoms. The latter, if used, have the advantage that they do not complicate a low-calorie diet. Simultaneous institution of a weight reduction program and treatment with insulin, if prescribed, often lead to hypoglycemia and must be approached cautiously. The short-term goal of insulin therapy under these conditions is the relief of symptoms due to hyperglycemia. No attempt at "tight" control should be made at this time; such

efforts should be deferred until efforts at weight loss have ended.

The importance of *weight reduction* for the obese diabetic cannot be overstated. Population studies indicate that most diabetes is either made manifest by obesity in genetically predisposed persons or is actually caused by obesity. Hence, most overt diabetes in obese patients is potentially either preventable or "curable" by weight reduction provided that the diabetes has not been present for more than a few years. However, most patients are unable to achieve and/or maintain a weight that will reverse overt diabetes, even though they are made aware of the necessity for doing so. Chapter 76 on obesity, Chapter 3 on patient education, and Chapter 4 on compliance deal with this problem in greater detail.

Another goal of diet therapy is prevention of atherosclerotic disease. Atherosclerotic disease is both more prevalent and accelerated in diabetes and accounts for about 25% of deaths among IDDM diabetics with onset before age 20. Adults with NIDDM are two times as likely as those in the general population to die from coronary artery disease. A large portion of this excess mortality is undoubtedly due to the frequent abnormalities of lipids that are so common in diabetes mellitus. These do not appear to be genetically linked to diabetes, but poorly controlled hyperglycemia is accompanied by *secondary* disturbances of lipid metabolism. The evidence that this major problem of the diabetic may be preventable is to a large degree based on comparisons of the prevalence of atherosclerotic disease in different populations with widely varying diets (40, 41). The diabetics in this country who followed conventional high-fat, low-carbohydrate diabetic diets—at least until about 1970—had the highest rate of coronary disease seen anywhere in the world (three times the rate of the general population in this country). Because of this and the evidence from population studies, the American Diabetes Association (ADA) recommended in 1971 that its old standard diabetic diets be abandoned. From that time until a few years ago, the ADA avoided a firm recommendation regarding diets, suggesting only that diets should be individualized. The recent recommendations by the ADA are for diets high in carbohydrate (50% of calories) and low in fat (30%), diets similar to those recommended by the American Heart Asso-

Table 72.6.
Distribution of Major Nutrients in Typical, Traditional, Diabetic, and Current Diabetic Diets (United States)[a]

	Nutrients (Percentage of Total Calories)						
				Fat			
	Starch and other Complex Poly-saccharides	Sugars and Dextrins	Total Carbohydrates	Total	% Mono or Polyunsaturated	Protein	Alcohol
"Typical" Diet	25–35	20–30	45–50	35–45	30		1–10
Traditional diabetic diet	25–30	10–15	35–40	40–50	30	15–20	0
Current diabetic diets[b]	40[c]	10	50	30	20	20	—

[a] Modified from (40).
[b] The recommended diet of the American Diabetic Association provides additionally < 300 mg cholesterol and 28 g dietary fiber.
[c] Even higher levels of starch and lower levels of fat might be desirable, but are seldom possible in Western societies because they differ too much from the traditional diets of these cultures.

ciation for nondiabetics (Table 72.6). Although successfully used in diabetics studied on metabolic wards, the reported beneficial effects of such diets on blood lipids may be due to other factors: concomitant weight reduction, very low cholesterol content, high fiber content and absence of sucrose. One recent study in which patients with NIDDM received such diets resulted in unchanged low-density lipoprotein (LDL) cholesterol, lowered high-density lipoprotein (HDL) cholesterol and increased triglyceride levels (7). In contrast, another study used a high-monounsaturated-fat diet (50% of calories) relatively low in carbohydrate (35%). The result was improved plasma glucose, triglycerides, and HDL cholesterol compared with the ADA diet (16). The optimal diet for the control of blood lipids and glucose in the diabetic must still be considered unsettled.

Efforts to control hyperlipidemia in diabetics must include at least near normalization of blood glucose. At the present time no evidence is available that favors insulin or oral hypoglycemic drugs to achieve this goal, although a theoretical advantage for glipizide (see below) has been offered (36). Treatment of coexisting diseases that can cause hyperlipidemia is also necessary (e.g., hypothyroidism, obesity), but the presence of renal failure may preclude successful attempts to normalize blood lipids. If the nephrotic syndrome is present, gross hyperlipidemia will not be readily manageable, even with drugs.

In the approach to the typical NIDDM patient with mixed hypercholesterolemia and hypertriglyceridemia, normalization of blood sugar is attempted, along with initiation of the standard dietary program now recommended for nondiabetics (see above). The therapeutic goals for cholesterol and triglycerides are less than 200 and 150 mg percent, respectively. Drug therapy (see Chapter 75) is added after several months if diet is ineffective, but it is inappropriate and usually ineffective to introduce drug therapy if hyperglycemia is not controlled. Nicotinic acid, formerly thought to be inadvisable in diabetics, and gemfibrozil (Lopid) are current choices for combined hyperlipidemias. Lovostatin (Mevacor) may be effective when hypercholesterolemia is the only abnormality, but it is often inappropriately prescribed when hyperglycemia is not controlled and is contributing to a mixed hyperlipidemia. Weight reduction is an effective means of reducing hypercholesterolemia, but given the usual lack of success in achieving lasting weight loss, unrealistic expectations in this regard should not result in undue delay in initiation of the other lipid-lowering maneuvers.

A guiding principle for formulating diabetic diets should be the recognition that individual food preferences must be respected whenever possible. The dietician should obtain the patient's *preferred* dietary history and then attempt to construct the diet around these preferences. Such an approach is demanding for the dietician, but the issuance of a standardized "American" diet to a diabetic from an ethnic minority simply guarantees noncompliance.

In the past few years, diets containing large quantities of nonabsorbable plant fibers have been explored for use in diabetics. Fiber-rich foods decrease blood glucose after glucose loads or meals in both normal persons and in patients with NIDDM, whereas chronic ingestion of high-fiber, high-carbohydrate diets decreases fasting blood glucose and may permit decreased doses of oral hypoglycemic drugs or lower insulin requirements. The mechanisms of these effects are not fully understood. Although delayed carbohydrate absorption probably accounts for most of the acute effect, increased sensitivity to insulin seems also to be involved. Abnormalities of blood lipids often improve. However, a role for high-fiber diets in routine therapy has not been established. In many patients these diets produce a variety of unpleasant side effects, including increased frequency of stools, diarrhea, abdominal pain, and flatulence. The formulation of fiber-rich diets is difficult, and most patients do not accept the major alterations of diet that are necessary to produce the desired effects on blood glucose levels.

Estimation of Caloric Needs

Caloric requirements for maintenance of weight vary considerably from individual to individual and are influenced by activity level. Required calories are approximately 40 kcal/kg or 20 kcal/lb/day for an adult with "normal" activity. Thus an individual of 70 kg may require 2800 kcal, although some lean men performing ordinary activities may require as much as 3000 to 3500 kcal/day. Individuals who perform manual labor may need 4000 or more kcal, whereas sedentary persons may need only 2000 kcal or less.

In prescribing diets caloric requirements are often underestimated. Physicians commonly prescribe an 1800-kcal diet for maintenance even if it is grossly inadequate for a particular patient's caloric needs. Prescription of such a diet leads to frustration and noncompliance. Overzealous decreases of calories for weight reduction may be equally defeating. When maintenance of weight is the goal, a careful dietary history by a skilled dietician may give a good starting point for establishment of an individual's needs; the prescribed diet should then become simply a modification of that patient's ordinary pattern.

Diet during Conventional Insulin Therapy

Any patient receiving insulin faces a special problem. Unlike patients who are not receiving insulin—who require no special timing of meals and whose total intake can vary from day to day—the pattern of food intake for the individual receiving conventional therapy with insulin must be quite rigid; greater flexibility is possible with intensive conventional therapy (see page 931). Total caloric intake must be distributed among the meals of the day, which usually include midafternoon and bedtime snacks as well, so that insulin dose can be adjusted according to the patient's needs. The reverse procedure, selection of an insulin dose and adjustment of total caloric intake to this dose, is unphysiological and should never be used. Occasional patients strive to reduce insulin dosage by senseless starvation, incorrectly assuming that insulin dose has some relationship to "severity" of their disease. Needless to say, patients must be dissuaded from such practices.

The exact composition of the diet for the patient with IDDM is less important—from the point of view of blood sugar control—than is the constancy of distribution of the amount of food at each meal from day to day. Insulin effect (duration, intensity), even for a particular type of insulin, varies from patient to patient. Accordingly, avoidance of extremes of blood sugar concentration (hypo- and hyperglycemia) requires some adjustment of food apportionment for each individual. However, one should attempt to simulate as closely as possible the patient's usual and preferred pattern of food intake. The main modification is usually to add between-meal snacks. Once an acceptable food pattern has been established and insulin dose adjusted to that pattern, the patient must adhere to the program if extremes of blood sugar are to be avoided. Patients learn by trial and error how much latitude they can tolerate. Problems, not easily solved, are encountered in individuals who engage in strenuous sports or work that varies from day to day. Such persons may have to eat more on some days than others or make frequent adjustments of their insulin dose. Rigid control of blood sugar by use of conventional insulin therapy is not possible in such cases. Intensive conventional therapy (page 931) allows for better control of blood sugar and for greater variation in the level of physical activity.

The major adaptive problem with diet in patients treated with conventional insulin therapy (see page 929) is the need for most of them to eat in a programmed fashion, i.e., by the clock. No longer can the individual wait for hunger to prompt a meal; nor can he approach dining out at a restaurant with indifference to the time the meal will be served. To do so is to court a major hypoglycemic episode. However, delay of a meal may be unavoidable. In order to prevent hypoglycemia in this circumstance, about 10 g of carbohydrate/1/2 hour should be ingested. This can be provided by 4 to 6 oz (180 ml) of a sugar-containing soda ("soft drink") or 4 oz of orange juice, palatable premeal alternatives to glucose tablets, Life Savers, or a candy bar (see "Hypoglycemia during Insulin Therapy," page 935).

Exchange Lists and Special Foods

After a dietician estimates the constituents that will be acceptable to a patient, joint discussion should be held with the spouse or other involved family members. Cooperation and participation of a spouse in the process may be essential for successful adaptation, which, for practical reasons, may require that both partners participate in the diet modifications.

The intelligent use of diet exchange lists (food equivalents) is useful for many patients. Such lists are available from the American Diabetes Association, the American Dietetic Association, and most hospital dietetic units.

Special "diabetic" or "dietetic" foods are expensive and usually are unnecessary. Some such foods do contain less free sugar than is ordinarily the case, but the patient must read the labels carefully to avoid self-deception.

Exercise during insulin therapy. The pattern of glycemic response to exercise is quite variable. Some individuals may require an anticipatory reduction of insulin (e.g., 30%) in order to prevent hypoglycemia. Others may need additional food before moderate activity. In some individuals, especially those who exercise sporadically, prolonged exercise may result in severe hypoglycemia some 6 to 15 hours *after* cessation of exercise (23); again an anticipatory reduction of insulin dose and/or extra food may be needed. Modest exercise (walking at 3.5 miles in one hour) may utilize 350 extra calories; 10 to 20 g of carbohydrate, only a fraction of these extra calories, may be sufficient to prevent hypoglycemia. Similar considerations guide management of more vigorous exercise. The hypoglycemic effect of exercise may be greater if the insulin has been injected into an extremity being exercised. Many patients prefer to inject insulin into the thigh, but persons who engage in vigorous exercise (jogging, other sports, manual labor) may have to use abdominal or arm injection sites to avoid excessive insulin effect due to exercise-induced rapid absorption.

Effect of anorexia. When a patient with IDDM develops anorexia because of mild short-term illness ("cold," "flu," gastroenteritis), insulin should not be discontinued, but a reduction of the normal dose by one-third to one-half may be needed. More severe illness (e.g., a marked febrile state) may require continuation of the usual dose or even an increase in the dose. Every effort should be made to ensure intake of 50 g of carbohydrate in every 8-hour period to avoid both starvation ketosis and hypoglycemia. Careful monitoring of urine ketones (and glucose) during such periods and prompt adjustment of insulin dose if necessary may prevent a hospitalization for ketoacidosis.

Selection of Patients for Insulin Therapy or Oral Hypoglycemic Drugs

Non-Insulin-Dependent Diabetes (NIDDM)

A therapeutic approach to patients with NIDDM is shown in Table 72.7. As previously noted, the initial approach to the obese non-insulin-dependent patient is weight reduction. Such therapy—if followed—can be expected to reduce blood sugar within a few weeks. If FPG is less than 200 to 250 mg/dl, hyperglycemia and glucosuria will not ordinarily produce enough symptoms to be troublesome during this period and no additional drug therapy (oral hypoglycemics or insulin) is needed. Even a FPG of 300 may be tolerated. These patients are not ketosis prone; no urgency exists for instituting drug therapy. On the other hand, symp-

Table 72.7.
Therapeutic Approach to Patients With Non-Insulin-Dependent Diabetes Mellitus[a]

This table presents results of a poll involving specialists in diabetes. However, it does not represent the opinion of all experts. Treatment must be INDIVIDUALIZED for all patients. When two therapeutic approaches are listed, if both are capitalized, slight preference is given to the first one listed. If the second approach is in lower case letters, the first approach is strongly preferred. If both approaches are in lower case letters, no clear-cut preference can be stated.

Fasting Plasma Glucose (mg/dl)	Age of Patient (Yr)			
	20	40	60	80
	Obese Patient (Initial dietary treatment)			
5–139	DIET	DIET	DIET	diet or do nothing
140–199	ORAL AGENT or insulin	ORAL AGENT or insulin	ORAL AGENT	oral agent or diet
200	INSULIN or oral agent	INSULIN or ORAL AGENT	ORAL AGENT or insulin	oral agent or insulin or diet
Nonobese Patient (Initial dietary treatment)				
115–139	INSULIN or oral agent	ORAL AGENT or insulin	ORAL AGENT	oral agent or diet
140–199	INSULIN	INSULIN or ORAL AGENT	ORAL AGENT or INSULIN	ORAL AGENT or INSULIN
200	INSULIN	INSULIN or ORAL AGENT	INSULIN or oral agent	INSULIN or oral agent

[a] Modified from Amer. Diabetes Assoc. Physician's Guide to Non-Insulin Dependent (Type II) Diabetes. Diagnosis and Treatment, 2nd Ed. Alexandria, VA 1988.

tomatic hyperglycemia or glucosuria, persisting for weeks despite efforts at (or actual) weight loss, should not be ignored. In this case, drug therapy is indicated for symptomatic relief and can be discontinued if weight reduction is successful.

In the past, many patients with NIDDM and symptomatic disease have been treated with oral hypoglycemic drugs (see page 936). However, even asymptomatic patients have also been treated for only modest elevations of FGP or even for abnormal glucose tolerance. Such treatment may improve or normalize glucose tolerance. Extrapolation of results from patient surveys relating abnormalities of glucose tolerance to development of complications of diabetes would suggest that such treatment might be beneficial. However, no evidence exists to support this hypothesis.

The official recommendation of the American Diabetes Association, the AMA Council on Drugs, and the Food and Drug Administration is that sulfonylureas be limited to patients with symptomatic NIDDM who cannot be controlled by diet and in whom addition of insulin is impractical and/or unacceptable. This stand may be inappropriately conservative.

The indications for use of insulin in patients with *asymptomatic* NIDDM are unclear. Although evidence is accumulating that modest elevations of blood sugar do indeed relate to at least some of the complications of diabetes (11, 22), no prospective studies are available to demonstrate that insulin therapy of patients with asymptomatic hyperglycemia (FPG or OGTT) is beneficial. Insulin therapy is certainly indicated for control of symptomatic diabetes (see above, page 916) in NIDDM that cannot be controlled with diet or diet plus an oral agent.

Determination of hemoglobin A_{1c} in cases of modest elevation of blood sugar can serve as a guide (28) (see page 933). A normal value would deter a recommendation for drug or insulin therapy, whereas an elevated value would suggest that long-term benefit might outweigh the possible risks or inconvenience. Recommendations for or against therapy under these circumstances are presently determined not only by the clinical circumstances, but by the physician's convictions concerning the long-term deleterious effect of hyperglycemia (see "Normoglycemia as a Goal of Insulin Therapy," below).

Insulin-Dependent Diabetes

The IDDM patient should be started on insulin therapy as soon as insulin need is apparent. Ordinarily these patients have been hospitalized for treatment of ketoacidosis and have been switched from short-acting insulin, used in the treatment of the acute phase, to an intermediate or long-acting preparation. The insulin dependence has been established by the occurrence of the acute episode. Unless this acute event was precipitated by stress in an otherwise NIDDM patient, insulin dependence is usually absolute and permanent. Occasionally in adults (more often in children), insulin requirement may decrease or even disappear over several months; relapse is the rule in such cases.

Other Circumstances Requiring Insulin Therapy

Some patients who are not, strictly speaking, insulin dependent also need insulin therapy. Patients with NIDDM may be prescribed hypoglycemic drugs to control blood glucose but may be unresponsive with an initial attempt ("primary failures"). Others, adequately controlled by hypoglycemic drugs for a time, become unresponsive to these agents ("secondary failures"). Insulin therapy may become essential in such cases. Other patients with NIDDM develop grossly uncontrolled hyperglycemia during stress (trauma, infection, surgery). Whether ketosis ensues, the gross hyperglycemia may produce severe osmotic diuresis and its sequelae. Obviously, such patients require control of hyperglycemia with insulin therapy, which may be discontinued as soon as the situation warrants. Most young people of normal weight who develop diabetes will require insulin, even though they are not ketosis prone. The group of children or young adults termed MODY (see above) are also candidates for insulin, although many may be managed on diet alone.

Occasional adults, usually thin and not necessarily exhibiting much glucosuria, may exhibit unexplained weight loss and lack of well-being. Such patients may show dramatic improvement with insulin.

Some patients will be encountered who are receiving insulin therapy needlessly. Typically these are elderly individuals with NIDDM who have already developed an array of medical problems, usually cardiovascular. The degree of blood sugar control with large amounts of insulin (50 to 100 units) is poor. Although aggressive use of insulin will certainly normalize blood glucose, the development of hypoglycemia is risky in such persons. On the other hand, abrupt discontinuation of insulin in these patients often results in no worsening of diabetic control and reveals that, in fact, no significant insulin effect had been manifest at the prescribed dosage. Adherence to a proper diet and to weight reduction may suffice in such cases.

Exercise As Therapy

Although diabetics, like others, may derive benefits from regular exercise, the complexities of avoiding hypoglycemia during exercise make blanket recommendations tenuous (see above, "Exercise during Insulin Therapy"). In patients with NIDDM receiving sulfonylurea drugs the problem of hypoglycemia is not great, but obese patients on low-calorie weight-reduction diets who exercise at high intensity may be severely limited by lack of muscle glycogen unless they consume additional carbohydrate. Walking or cycling may be the least threatening form of exercise for these persons; attention to a period of adaptation is vital. Both types of patients must avoid exercise that will aggravate latent or existing problems, e.g., foot trauma that can lead to ulceration or exacerbation or retinopathy. It should be assumed that individuals with long-standing disease must be especially cautious when initiating an exercise program. The clearest rationale for exercise as therapy is as an adjunct to weight reduction programs. With weight loss, sensitivity to endogenous insulin may be restored in obese, insulin-resistant patients, and normoglycemia may ensue, sometimes obviating the need for oral agents or insulin. The blood sugar lowering effect of exercise often antecedes significant weight loss.

Normoglycemia As A Goal Of Therapy

The evidence for a relationship between the degree of blood sugar control and the development of microvascular complications remains uncertain (44). Studies in animals strongly suggest that microvascular complications of diabetes are a result of hyperglycemia. Maintaining euglycemia prevents or retards the development of retinopathy and nephropathy, whereas correction of hyperglycemia reverses early morphologic and functional abnormalities of nephropathy. Moreover, an initial period of hyperglycemia can initiate irreversible microvascular disease. Unfortunately, the studies in man are not nearly as convincing. However, in view of the growing evidence that control of hyperglycemia may prevent development of the microvascular complications of diabetes (11, 22), few would argue that normalization of blood sugar with insulin is undesirable, but this goal is not achievable using single dose or even two-dose insulin schemes without incurring unacceptable episodes of hypoglycemia. In which patients should the effort to achieve normoglycemia be vigorously promoted, and when in the history of the disease should such a program be undertaken?

Young patients with IDDM in the early years of their disease, at least in theory, stand to gain the most from normalization of blood sugar ("tight control"), since prevention of complications is the goal. Patients with IDDM who already have advanced complications of diabetes may not benefit at all, since no evidence is available that such complications are reversible or can even be stabilized. Nonetheless, the patient's hopes must be considered under these circumstances while the physician remains as supportive as possible.

For those patients with NIDDM, prevention or slowing the progression of vascular complications is also the most important rationale for tight control. Relatively young or even middle-aged patients with NIDDM may stand to gain as much as young patients with IDDM. In the elderly, whose life expectancy is limited by age, complications of diabetes, or concurrent disease, the problems associated with tight control should strongly influence the physician to avoid this approach, since the prevention of already present complications is not an issue, and slowing of their progression is likely to be impossible.

After an initial period of conventional therapy (see page 929) the issue of tight control should be considered and discussed with patients who are suitable candidates. In those to whom tight control is suggested, it is the physician's obligation to explain the current view that maintained normoglycemia may prevent the long-term complications of diabetes mellitus. The magnitude of the effort that is necessary to maintain normoglycemia must be explained, including the need for home blood glucose monitoring. One of the frequent-dose, intensified conventional insulin therapy schemes or its alternative, infusion pump delivery of insulin, must also be presented (see page 931). If the patient understands and accepts the problems and effort required, the physician may consider a program of tight control. However, serious consideration should be given to referral of the patient to an endocrinologist familiar with such a program since the process is difficult, very demanding of the physician's time, and usually requires a team approach utilizing a specially trained physician's assistant or nurse practitioner. The demands on the patient and the physician are greatest at onset of tight control therapy. The effort should always be made only when the schedules of all parties permit the undertaking.

Often therapy will be less than intensive. Such therapy attempts to achieve near normalization—as opposed to normalization—of blood sugar and is termed "minimal," "average," or "conventional" therapy (see page 929). Individuals with NIDDM tend to have relatively stable blood sugars and predictable responses to insulin, and an attempt to achieve near normalization can be made in such patients. In many, at least the fasting blood glucose can be normalized (see Table 72.3) without great difficulty using one or two doses of intermediate-acting insulin. Patients with IDDM are much more difficult to control, and even this degree of control is simply not possible using conventional therapy. Many physicians, failing to realize the limitation of one- or two-dose schedules, nonetheless still go through an agonizing trial of conventional therapy with such patients, only to have the effort end in failure and frustration for all involved. Usually several types and mixtures of insulin have been tried along with both single and two-dose schedules. At this point, a simplified treatment scheme that avoids excessive glucosuria with resultant symptoms and prevents development of ketoacidosis should be accepted. Reconsideration of institution of intensive conventional therapy may be appropriate at this stage.

Types of Insulin

Three major characteristics distinguish the various preparations of insulin: (a) onset and duration of action; (b) purity, important as it relates to cost and, rarely, to insulin allergy and resistance; and (c) species of origin, since this affects cost. A significant recent realization is that some human insulin preparations have a reduced duration of action.

Most of the preparations now in use are suspensions of insulin that have been modified to prolong their action after subcutaneous injection. The characteristics of these insulins are summarized below.

Regular Insulin (Crystalline Zinc Insulin; CZI)

This unmodified insulin is a completely dissolved ("clear") preparation, the main use of which is for acute therapy of ketoacidosis in hospitalized patients. In the treatment of ambulatory patients, regular insulin is not used alone but is used in mixtures with other insulins. The onset of action of subcutaneously injected regular insulin is 20 minutes; peak action is at 2 to 4 hours; and the duration of action is 4 to 6 hours. In occasional patients receiving one dose of intermediate-acting insulin daily, regular insulin may be given as the second dose. Special noncrystalizing solutions of human insulin are available for continuous subcutaneous injection with portable infusion pumps. Regular insulin is also increasingly used in combination with Ultralente insulin in tight control schemes; the long-acting preparation provides the equivalent of background activity provided by the basal infusion rate of a pump, whereas superimposed injections before meals are equal to bolus injections of the pump (see page 931) (Fig. 72.1).

Protamine Zinc Insulin (PZI)

This preparation, a loose chemical combination of insulin with the carrier protein, protamine, was the first long-acting insulin. At one time, PZI was amorphous material containing an excess of protamine, which precluded addition of regular insulin. However, all PZI now available is crystalline, contains no excess protamine, and can be mixed with regular insulin. Indeed, the commonly used NPH insulin approximates such a mixture (see below). PZI has a duration of action exceeding 24 hours.

PZI is rarely used by itself. Exceptions include diabetics who are not eating because of intercurrent acute or chronic illness. Other patients who may benefit from PZI are those who experience unacceptably frequent episodes of insulin-induced hypoglycemia when the "intermediate" insulins are used. When a long-acting form is to be used as sole therapy, most authorities have preferred—because of its allegedly more predictable effect—Ultralente insulin to PZI. For practical purposes, the two forms have identical uses and effects.

NPH (Neutral Protamine Hagedorn Insulin; Isophane Insulin)

This preparation is a standardized crystalline suspension prepared from regular insulin and protamine. Often termed "intermediate-acting," NPH in fact exhibits rather rapid onset of action and a duration of action up to 24 hours. Ideally, with a single injection of NPH, the short-acting component provides insulin effect during the day when meals are elevating the blood glucose, whereas the long-acting portion of PZI provides insulin effect through the night. For a few patients the achieved ratio of insulin effects is satisfactory. However, the duration of action of NPH is generally much less than 24 hours. Nonetheless, in the United States, many physicians continue to prescribe a single daily injection of NPH, a practice that has been discontinued in Europe where NPH is almost always given in two doses. NPH is the most commonly used intermediate-acting insulin in the United States. Mixtures of regular and NPH insulin are now available (see "Insulin Injection Technique").

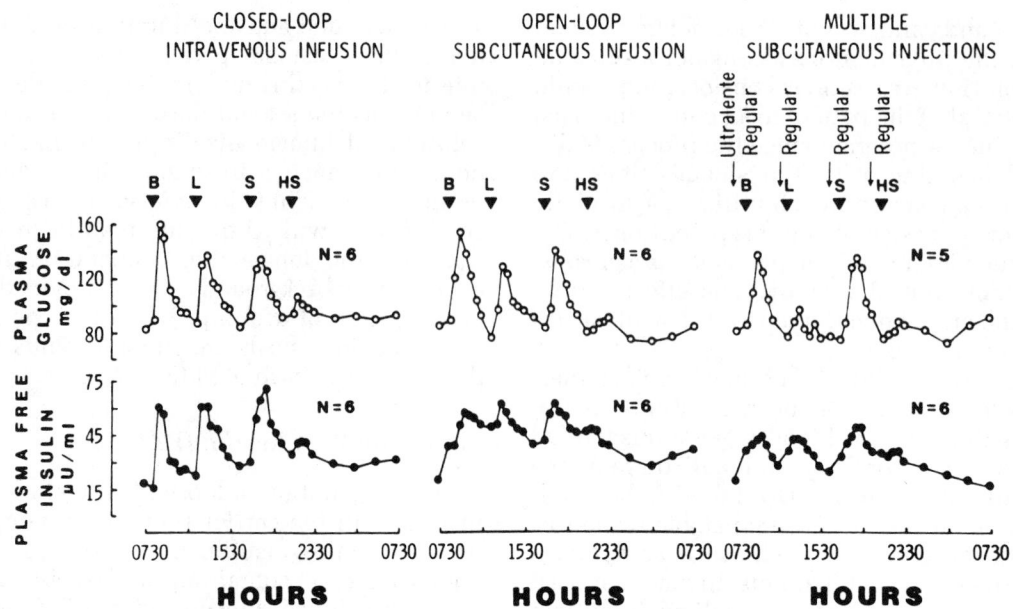

Figure 72.1. Plasma glucose and free insulin levels in patients with IDDM treated by three methods: closed-loop intravenous infusion (plasma glucose sensor controlled apparatus); open-loop subcutaneous infusion (insulin pump); and multiple subcutaneous injections (intensive conventional therapy). *B*, breakfast; *L*, lunch; *S*, supper; *HS*, bedtime snacks. Note that the results are essentially the same with all methods used.

(Modified from Rizza R, Gerich JE, Haymond MD et al: Control of blood sugar in insulin-dependent diabetes: comparison of an artificial endocrine pancreas, continuous subcutaneous insulin infusion, and intensified conventional insulin therapy. *N Engl J Med* 303:1313, 1980 and Schade DS, Santiago JV, Skyler JS, Rizza RA: Intensive Insulin Therapy. Garden City, NY, Medical Examination Publishing Co, 1983, p. 138).

The Lente Insulin Series

This group of insulins was devised at a time when PZI contained excess protamine, thus precluding the preparation of mixtures of short-acting regular with long-acting PZI. Controlled addition of zinc was used to prepare an amorphous, rapidly absorbed, and rapidly acting material (Semilente insulin) and another crystalline product with much slower absorption and longer action, Ultralente insulin. These insulins avoided the use of a foreign protein, protamine, and could be mixed in varying proportions. In some geographic areas, in both the United States and abroad, the Lente insulins are used almost exclusively.

Semilente insulin. This preparation is similar to regular insulin in onset and duration of action, although its effects are somewhat slower in onset and more prolonged. Semilente is always given subcutaneously. The chief use of Semilente is in mixtures with Ultralente or as a supplementary dose in conventional therapy schemes. Semilente is little used in the United States.

Ultralente insulin. This preparation has a duration of action exceeding 24 hours and is similar in action to PZI. Ultralente may, like PZI, occasionally be used alone (see PZI). However, the main use of Ultralente is as the long-acting component in the mixture that is known as Lente insulin. Ultralente insulin has recently become the backbone of "intensified conventional therapy." The prolonged effect of this preparation provides the background activity equivalent to the basal infusion rate of an insulin pump (see page 931).

Lente insulin is an intermediate-acting preparation.

It is a mixture of amorphous (Semilente) and crystalline (Ultralente) insulins. Although it is commonly thought to be equivalent to NPH, the duration of action of Lente insulin is significantly longer, usually exceeding 24 hours. If a single daily dose of insulin is the treatment goal, Lente is the insulin of choice.

Mixtures of Insulins

The usual goal of conventional insulin therapy is a single injection once daily. If this goal is to be reached, insulin effect must be prolonged sufficiently to produce normoglycemia in the morning and at the same time provide adequate daytime control of the increases of blood glucose that occur postprandially. However, the duration of action of NPH is usually too short for this goal and Lente, though a better choice, is often unsatisfactory as well. Either one of two scenarios is observed. In the first, the excessive daytime hyperglycemia and glucosuria dictates the need for additional rapidly acting insulin. Thus, regular insulin is added to NPH or Lente; or Semilente is added to Lente (see "Injection of Insulin", page 929). In the second, the single injection of NPH or Lente controls daytime hyperglycemia and glucosuria, but the total duration of action is inadequate, resulting in hyperglycemia at the beginning of the next day. Under these circumstances, additional long-acting component is needed. If Lente is used, Ultralente can be added, or a mixture of Semilente and Ultralente can be used with a ratio of 20:80 or 10:90. However, most diabetologists in the United States use NPH; their only option is to give an additional dose before dinner or at bedtime. This scheme has been called a "split-dose" program (see below, "Insulin Therapy").

Commercial Insulin Preparations

There are currently nearly 40 available commercial insulins in their various types, species of origin and, suppliers (Table 72.8). Clearly, no physician needs to memorize this changing list. However, even though most physicians write prescriptions for insulin without specifying the brand, it is important to be able to recognize the product that the pharmacist has dispensed. Not all preparations are available in a given region; pharmacies often supply the products of particular manufacturers according to local economic factors.

At the present time three companies market insulin within the United States: Lilly, Squibb/Novo, and Nordisk. All produce reliable, clinically comparable products within a particular category. Although no uniform terminology is established, these insulins can be grouped into grades, not to be confused with the various types of insulin already described (NPH, Lente, etc.) The principal determinant of which grade to prescribe is whether a clinical need exists for insulin more highly purified than standard grade material. The other major considerations are cost, which varies considerably between grades and use of animal-derived versus human insulin (obtained via recombinant technology or chemical modification of pork insulin).

Standard grades of insulin (Lilly; Squibb/Novo) are derived from the pancreases of pigs or beef cattle; Lil-

Table 72.8.
Insulins Currently Sold (11/89) in the United States[a]

Product	Manufacturer	Form	Strength
Rapid acting			
Humulin regular	Lilly	Human	U-100
Humulin BR (for external insulin pumps only)	Lilly	Human	U-100
Novolin R (regular; formerly Actrapid human)	Squibb-Novo	Human	U-100
Velosulin human (regular)	Nordisk-USA	Human	U-100
Iletin II regular	Lilly	Beef	U-100
Iletin II regular	Lilly	Pork	U-100, U-500
Purified pork R (regular Actrapid)	Squibb-Novo	Pork	U-100
Velosulin (regular)	Nordisk-USA	Pork	U-100
Purified pork S (Semilente; formerly Semitard)	Squibb-Novo	Pork	U-100
Iletin I regular	Lilly	Beef/Pork	U-40, U-100
Regular	Squibb-Novo	Pork	U-100
Iletin I Semilente	Lilly	Beef/Pork	U-40, U-100
Semilente	Squibb-Novo	Beef	U-100
Novolin R Penfill (regular)	Squibb-Novo	Human	U-100
Intermediate acting			
Humulin L	Lilly	Human	U-100
Humulin NPH	Lilly	Human	U-100
Insulatard human NPH	Nordisk-USA	Human	U-100
Novolin L (lente; formerly Monotard human)	Squibb-Novo	Human	U-100
Novolin N (NPH)	Squibb-Novo	Human	U-100
Novolin N Penfill	Squibb-Novo	Human	U-100
Iletin II Lente	Lilly	Beef	U-100
Iletin II NPH	Lilly	Beef	U-100
Iletin II Lente	Lilly	Pork	U-100
Iletin II NPH	Lilly	Pork	U-100
Insulatard NPH	Nordisk-USA	Pork	U-100
Purified pork lente (formerly Monotard)	Squibb-Novo	Pork	U-100
Purified pork N (NPH, formerly Protaphane)	Squibb-Novo	Pork	U-100
Iletin I Lente	Lilly	Beef/Pork	U-40, U-100
Iletin I NPH	Lilly	Beef/Pork	U-40, U-100
NPH	Squibb-Novo	Beef	U-100
Long acting			
Iletin II PZI	Lilly	Beef	U-100
Iletin II PZI	Lilly	Pork	U-100
Purified beef U (ultralente; formerly Ultratard)	Squibb-Novo	Beef	U-100
Iletin I PZI	Lilly	Beef/Pork	U-40, U-100
Iletin I Ultralente	Lilly	Beef/Pork	U-40, U-100
Ultralente	Squibb-Novo	Beef	U-100
Humulin U (Ultralente)	Lilly	Human	U-100
Mixtures			
Mixtard (30% regular, 70% NPH)	Nordisk-USA	Pork	U-100
Novolin 70/30	Squibb-Novo	Human	U-100
Novolin 70/30, Penfill			

[a]Modified from American Diabetes Association Physician's guide to Insulin-Dependent (type I) Diabetes. Diagnosis and Treatment, 2 ed., Alexandria, VA , 1988.

ly's material (Iletin I) is a variable mixture of the two species, mostly beef, whereas Squibb/Novo insulin is solely of beef origin. Standard animal insulins are the least expensive preparations and are satisfactory for use in almost all patients.

Purified animal insulins are of pig origin and are about as expensive as human insulin with which they are comparable in degree of purity. Human insulins are available in almost all types: regular, NPH, Lente, Ultralente, and PZI. Lilly's human insulin (Humulin) is of recombinant origin. Comparable human semi-synthetic insulins, prepared by chemical modification of pork insulin, are available from Squibb/Novo and Nordisk. The least expensive standard insulin costs about 50% of that of the most expensive human or purified pork insulin.

Although some physicians are inclined to use the most highly purified animal insulins or human insulin, standard insulin is nearly always satisfactory. Occasional patients receiving standard insulin who show allergy to this type (see below) should be switched to purified pork or human insulin. Insulin resistance is frequently ascribed to antibody formation, but little evidence exists to document significant immunogenic differences or improvement as the result of switching insulins. Human insulin is certainly immunogenic as is purified pork insulin. The various types of human insulin do differ from the products of animal origin by somewhat more rapid onset and peak of action and shorter duration of effect. Given the variability shown under clinical conditions (44), these differences may not be particularly important, especially in a split dose program. *However, it should be kept in mind that the intermediate (NPH; Lente) and long-acting human insulins (Ultralente) have a maximal duration of action in many individuals of less than 24 hours, making control impossible with a single dose.* Attempts to produce a satisfactory fasting (overnight) blood sugar with a single daily dose of human insulin could lead to excessive daytime or evening effect and to hypoglycemia. The insulins especially prepared for use in pumps must not be mixed with intermediate-acting insulins. Most of the problems due to impurities in insulin in the past disappeared with introduction of the relatively pure standard insulins nearly 2 decades ago. Allergic reactions and lipoatrophy were the two most troublesome events; both do appear to have been related to impurities and are now rarely seen.

Allergy to insulin is most commonly a local reaction at the site of injection. Local redness, swelling, heat, and itching occur within minutes to an hour after injection and persist for a few hours to a day, often with formation of an area of induration. Such reactions, no longer common, occur during the first few weeks of therapy and usually disappear as therapy is continued. Rarely, similar reactions develop many hours or up to a day after injection (delayed hypersensitivity). Local reactions may also be due to improper injection technique, the presence of preservatives in a particular brand, or even the injection of cold insulin.

Systemic allergic reactions, with or without a local reaction, are rare; they are manifest by urticaria, angioedema, and even anaphylactic shock (IgE mediated; see Chapter 23). Such reactions seem to occur most often in persons who have previously received insulin and appear during reinstitution of therapy after a lapse of months or years. Local reactions may progress to systemic ones; if this seems to be occurring, one should treat the patient before anaphylaxis occurs. The first maneuver involves a trial of highly purified insulin. If this approach fails, drugs such as antihistamines and glucocorticoids are helpful, but persistent insulin allergy is best treated by desensitization. With the patient receiving no antihistamines or steroids and no insulin in the preceding 12 to 24 hours, the procedure involves injection of 0.1-ml volumes of insulin that have been diluted 1:100 in 0.1% human serum albumin to prevent adsorption losses onto glass. An initial dose (0.001 unit) is given intradermally. Subsequent doses of 0.1 ml contain doubling amounts (units). After several intradermal injections at 30-minute intervals, the subcutaneous route is used. If a reaction occurs, epinephrine may be administered; the dose of insulin is reduced, but the process is continued. This procedure requires a series of solutions of insulin. These may be prepared by the physician or pharmacist but are also available by telephone request to Eli Lilly Co., Indianapolis, Indiana. Special kits and instructions for desensitizing patients who have delayed hypersensitivity reactions are also available from the same source.

Insulin lipoatrophy is now an uncommon event. Harmless but disfiguring localized atrophy of subcutaneous fatty tissue occurs around the site of insulin injections and is sometimes seen simultaneously with insulin allergy. The process may be related to impurities in insulin preparations rather than to insulin itself, since preparations of high purity are much less likely to produce this problem.

Insulin lipohypertrophy is even less common than insulin atrophy. This phenomenon is probably due to an intrinsic action of insulin and has not been improved by use of purer insulins. Repeated injections into the same area do appear to predispose to lipohypertrophy.

Trade Names, Unit Designations, and Syringes

All insulin (Table 72.8), regardless of type or source, is standardized at a specific concentration per milliliter. The symbol U refers to the insulin concentration in units per milliliter. All insulins are available at a concentration of 100 units per milliliter. Lilly still produces animal insulins at 40 units per milliliter, a useful concentration when doses are small, but a syringe for use with U-40 is necessary. Although long-term storage is best made under refrigeration, insulin is stable for weeks at room temperature, and vials need not be refrigerated after opening. When insulin is used during travel, extremes of temperature should be avoided, as in a sun-exposed automobile, next to a stove or heating element, etc.

Several sizes of syringe are available for use with

U-100. A 1-ml syringe can be used for all doses up to 100 units, but most accurate dispensing of less than 30 units is made when syringes of 0.5-ml (50-U) capacity are used. The bores of these syringes are smaller and the scales are consequently expanded. Alternatively, U-40 can be used with appropriate syringes designed to hold 40 units/1 ml. Occasional patients require more than 100 units/single injection. For such use 2-ml syringes (200-unit capacity) are manufactured, but these are in short supply and are difficult to obtain. A single insulin is available at 500 units/1-ml (Iletin II, regular).

The use of disposable plastic syringes with attached needles has greatly simplified use of insulin and is preferred by almost all patients (Becton-Dickinson: B-D, or equivalent). Many patients will reuse disposable syringes without obvious harm, but the practice should be discouraged. Reusable glass syringes requiring detachable needles are also available. Special syringes are available for use by patients with severe impairment of vision that prevents them from accurately measuring their insulin dose. However, a simple solution to this problem is often possible. Disposable syringes can be prefilled with ordinary sterile precautions by an able person (relative, friend) and safely stored in a refrigerator for at least a week.

Insulin Injection Technique

After initial instruction the patient should be observed during self-administration of insulin to be certain that the correct volume is being drawn into the syringe and that the technique of injection is proper. Sterilization of the skin with an alcohol wipe is not necessary, although the injection site should be clean. If the injection is made through skin that is wet with alcohol, unnecessary burning discomfort will be produced.

For use in ambulatory patients insulin preparations should always be given subcutaneously. Most needles in present use are 1/2 inch in length. Unless the individual is very thin, the best technique involves insertion of the needle at 90° to the skin surface. If the patient is very thin, or the needle is 5/8 inch in length, or the site is covered by thin skin, the needle may be inserted at approximately 45° to avoid intramuscular injection. After injection, the area should not be massaged, since that may accelerate absorption.

The choice of injection region is important, since the rate of insulin absorption—and hence the duration and magnitude of insulin effect—varies considerably between anatomical locations (44). Absorption is slowest from the thigh, fastest from the anterior abdominal wall, and intermediate from the arm. In addition, absorption from an exercising extremity is accelerated (page 922). The long-used technique of rotation of sites is unwise and may contribute to erratic control. On the other hand, the repeated use of precisely the same spot within a region should be avoided. Regular and NPH insulins can be mixed in the same syringe in all proportions without affecting the onset and duration of action of the separate components, although the net effects will be overlapping. In the United States 30/70 or 50/50 mixtures of regular and NPH are now sold; in Europe a series of such mixtures (10/90; 20/80, etc.) have long been available.

Regular and Lente insulins cannot be mixed and allowed to stand for more than a few minutes before injection; delay of injection will result in blunting of the action of the rapidly acting regular. Special regular insulins for use with pumps (Humulin-BR or Velosulin) cannot be mixed with Lente insulin without causing their precipitation.

Insulin Injection Devices

A variety of devices are of variable utility in facilitating injections of insulin. Button-like injection ports are devices that can be left in place, usually over the abdomen, all day and decrease the number of skin punctures when multiple injections are being given. Needleless injectors that use a high-pressure jet are used by some patients, but they are not always painless, and absorption may be more rapid than with ordinary injections. Fountain pen-shaped injectors use a cartridge-containing insulin; the needle need not be changed for several days. Delivery is with a push button or a preset dial. These devices are especially useful for diabetics taking more than one injection daily who are eating meals in a restaurant or are traveling (20).

Initiation of Insulin Therapy

Several levels of blood sugar can be established as goals of therapy.

Minimal Therapy

In this approach the goals are avoidance of the extremes of symptomatic hyperglycemia and hypoglycemia; use of the least amount of insulin in a single dose; minimal testing of blood or urine, usually urine; a blood $HgbA_{1c}$ that corresponds to an average blood sugar of 230 to 310 mg/dl, i.e., 9.5 to 12% (nondiabetic mean, 5%; range, 3.8 to 6.3). Diet is prudent (<30% as calories from fat; <10% from saturated fat; <300 mg cholesterol). Exercise is according to patient preference.

Average Therapy (Conventional Therapy; Near Normalization of Blood Sugar)

An attempt is made to approach a nearly normal fasting (prebreakfast) blood sugar, using one or two doses of intermediate insulin, usually mixed with added regular insulin. The prebreakfast blood sugar should range from 70 to 140 mg% and the mean glucose 160 to 230 mg%, corresponding to a $HgbA_{1c}$ of 7.5 to 9.5%. Self-monitoring of blood glucose will be necessary, usually daily, but sometimes up to three times a day.

Institution of insulin therapy coincides with or follows the establishment of a diet (see above). As pointed out earlier, relative constancy of food intake is essential. If such dietary compliance cannot be assured, the goal of insulin therapy should be modest, i.e., the avoidance of symptomatic hyperglycemia and ketoacidosis. Attempts to manipulate insulin dose while diet is varying widely will unquestionably result in hypoglycemic episodes. In any case, insulin therapy cannot possibly achieve even a near approach to normoglycemia when diet is varying.

First attempts at blood sugar control in almost all ambulatory patients treated by the conventional approach should be done with an intermediate-acting insulin (NPH or Lente). However, use of NPH will usually require two doses. A safe initial dose for a patient who has not received previous insulin therapy is 15 units for a nonobese individual and 25 units for an obese patient. Although initial doses are often expressed as units per kilogram, the range of requirements is so large that one might just as well begin with these doses, ignoring the weight. Many experts recommend addition of 5 to 10 units of regular insulin to the NPH or Lente to help normalize the postbreakfast blood sugar during the morning. Because of this common practice, several manufacturers are marketing mixtures of insulin (ratio of regular to NPH, 30:70).

Previously treated patients often require higher initial doses. Insulin-dependent patients will ordinarily have been started on insulin therapy while in the hospital, but the scheme below can be used for further adjustment of dose for both types of patient.

Continuing to Adjust Insulin Dosage. The dose of insulin can be increased by 5 units every 3 days until satisfactory control is approached. Usually, such a program will bring the patient under control within a few weeks. Increments of 10 units every 3 days are also safe as long as the patient is markedly symptomatic or if no effect is apparent within a week. During this time the patient should be monitoring urine or blood glucose (see "Monitoring Insulin Therapy"). A telephone call to the physician, nurse-practitioner, or physician's assistant can be made every week or more, but, at least when a single dose program is being established, the patient should be encouraged to proceed with the adjustments of dose as planned and should not require or expect a physician's instructions at every dose increment. Unnecessary dependence is thus discouraged, and the patient's involvement in management is enhanced.

When glucosuria begins to subside, almost always first apparent as decreased glucosuria or aglucosuria in the first A.M. specimen, the dose of insulin should be held constant until such time as fasting plasma glucose (FPG) can be obtained. Sometimes glucosuria first subsides during the day rather than in the A.M. If this pattern develops, the dose of insulin should be held constant until both FPG and the PG at the aglucosuric time are measured. At the time the PG is measured, a double-voided urine sample should be obtained and glucosuria should be measured simultaneously. A few such determinations allow an estimate of the patient's renal threshold; thereafter the physician can approximate elevations of the PG for that particular individual from the glucosuria. From the point of de-

velopment of aglucosuria during some portion of the day to eventual "control" requires continued adjustment of insulin dosage, almost always upward, and adjustment of the patient to the diet and the routine of monitoring. During this time the patient should be given reassurance that the period of close dependency on the physician will soon come to an end. Every effort must also be made to avoid rigidly scheduled visits to the physician's office or the clinical laboratory that interfere with the patient's livelihood or important personal affairs. Such intrusions will only discourage the patient and promote future noncompliance. On the other hand, achievement of reasonable control should not be prolonged and should be possible within a few weeks. When months pass and the patient's control remains irregular, seems to follow no pattern, or is marked by many hypoglycemic episodes, the problem is either noncompliance (see Chapter 4), usually dietary, or improper prescription of insulin. Noncompliance in the use of insulin can sometimes be ascertained by comparison of frequency of insulin purchase with the volume of insulin use predicted by prescribed therapy. For example, a 10-ml vial of U-100 insulin contains 1000 units; if the patient received 50 units daily, a vial should last 20 days (1000/50).

Evolution to a Two Dose Program. Many patients will not be controlled with a single dose of intermediate-acting insulin (NPH or Lente; see "Mixtures of Insulin" above). In these individuals hyperglycemia and glucosuria improve; the late A.M. or afternoon glucose measurements are the first to show a tendency to normalize. However, the long-acting component of the insulin preparation is insufficient to ensure normoglycemia in the fasting state, i.e., in the early morning. Two maneuvers can be tried. Usually, a predinner or bedtime dose of the same intermediate-acting insulin can be added, sometimes requiring a concomitant reduction of the A.M. dose. For example, if such a patient is receiving 60 units daily, up to 15 units may be given in the evening—usually before the dinner meal—and the A.M. dose can be reduced to 50 units. Additional increments of 5 units may then be made to either dose, depending on whether the fasting or postprandial glucose needs lowering. Patients using such a "split dose" schedule often receive 40 units or more daily with 50 to 70% of total daily dose in the A.M. and the remainder in the evening. A 2/3 A.M. versus 1/3 P.M. split is common.

To avoid a two-dose schedule the alternate approach of increasing the long-acting component can be instituted. In this case, the Lente insulins are best employed (see "Types of Insulin"). If the patient is already receiving NPH, a switch to the same dose of Lente is made. Ultralente insulin may then be mixed with Lente in increments of 5 to 10 units. Because Lente insulin is already a mixture of Semilente and Ultralente in a proportion of 30:70, addition of Ultralente merely alters this ratio in favor of the longer acting component, thus providing a greater likelihood that early A.M. PG will be controlled without producing midday hypoglycemia. To some extent, addition of a more long-acting component does, however, effect a lowering of glucose even during the day and may prompt a decrease of the A.M. dose. In any case, some patients can be controlled on a single dose of insulin in this way. For the patient who does not want a second daily injection, this approach is worthwhile.

Much effort can be expended in "fine tuning." Once the FPG is normalized (see above, page 930), efforts to attain normalization during the day with these approaches are only rarely successful and usually end in unacceptable hypoglycemic episodes. Because normalization of blood sugar is usually impossible by the schemes described, one should avoid machinations of this type. Normalization of blood sugar or "tight control" is simply unachievable in most diabetics treated with conventional therapy using one or two daily doses of insulin.

Intensive Insulin Therapy (IIT) with Multiple-Dose Insulin Programs or with Continuous Subcutaneous Insulin Infusion Pumps (Normalization of Blood Sugar)

This approach is an attempt to normalize blood sugar. It requires a maximal effort by the patient, the physician, and a team of support personnel (trained nurse or practitioner; dietician). An insulin pump or three or four daily doses of insulin are used. In the multiple-dose regimen, a long-acting form of insulin is required (Ultralente or PZI) to provide "background" insulin activity; boluses of regular insulin are given before meals to anticipate postmeal rises. Diet should provide less than 30% of calories as fat, 7% as saturated fat, and less than 200 mg of cholesterol, if possible. Preprandial sugars should be 70 to 120 mg/dl. Occasional postprandial blood sugars are obtained and should not exceed 180 mg. Weekly 3:00 A.M. levels should be determined to detect nocturnal hypoglycemia. The HgbA$_{1c}$ should not exceed 7.5%, corresponding to a mean glucose of 160 mg/dl. Diet must be optimized and home blood glucose monitoring practiced before initiating any program of intensive therapy with insulin.

Continuous subcutaneous insulin infusion (CSII) using a pump was first reported in 1978. In the past few years, many efforts attest to the efficacy and advantages of this approach and have defined the complications and risks of this method of therapy. Not as generally appreciated is the demonstration that identical success at normalization can be achieved by multiple dose programs that do not use a pump but do use a similar principle, delivery of insulin continuously from a subcutaneous depot site with additional doses of short-acting insulin given in bolus form (Table 72.9 and Fig. 72.1). Background insulin activity is provided not by the basal delivery rate of a pump but by absorption from the depot of long-acting insulin (usually Ultralente). The boluses are given before meals as individual injections of regular insulin. Approximately 50 to 60% of the total daily dose of insulin is given as a long-acting depot injection in the morning

Table 72.9.
Algorithm for Multidose Intensive Insulin Therapy

Target: Blood Glucose 70–140 mg/dl before meals, at bedtime, and not below 50 mg/dl at 3 AM

Insulin Regimen:

Insulin	Before		
	B	L	D
Regular	10	6	8
Ultralente	10	0	10

B = Breakfast; L = lunch; D = dinner

Algorithm:

Blood glucose before meals (mg/dl)	Inject Regular Insulin as below
60 mg/dl or less	2 units less
70–140 mg/dl	usual dose
141–200 mg/dl	2 units extra
201–250 mg/dl	4 units extra
251–300 mg/dl	6 units extra
Over 300 mg/dl	8 units extra

or before bed; the remainder is divided and given before meals as bolus injections of regular insulin. Regular insulin can be mixed with the long-acting form before breakfast, but two or three later injections are necessary.

If a physician decides to institute therapy with a pump, referral to a specialist familiar with one of these devices is usually necessary. Selection of a suitable current model of pump (cost of $1500 to $3000) and initiation of therapy are best made by a team active in this specialized field, although if necessary the continuation of therapy can thereafter be supervised by the general physician following the instructions available in published material (34).

Current pumps have fail-safe devices and alarms to guard against runaway pump action, power (battery) failure, empty insulin reservoir, and inadvertent turn-off. The insulin is administered through a 25-gauge scalp-vein needle attached to the pump via a piece of plastic tubing and inserted into the subcutaneous tissue of the abdomen. The needle is replaced every day or 2. Insulin reservoirs vary greatly in size and can accommodate one to several days' supply. Pumps must be worn almost continuously, being removed for only short periods (15 to 30 minutes) to allow showering, bathing, or swimming. Some patients need a respite from the pump, as for example in anticipation of sexual activity; in that case a dose of intermediate-acting insulin can be used at bedtime and the pump used during the day. Other physical activities, including sports, are performed with the pump in operation.

Initiation of therapy can be expected to take about 2 weeks, generally during a hospitalization in which the patient becomes familiar with pump operation as the dosage schedule is adjusted. Despite the apparent inconvenience of wearing the device, acceptance of the pump is remarkable. Many patients have continued pump therapy for 5 or more years. Patients, observing the improved blood glucose levels, are gratified by a sense of control of their destinies. In addition, they experience a normalization of activities by being freed from the tyranny of a clock-oriented existence, since meals no longer need be taken at fixed times but can be taken at will without great concern over the possible development of hypoglycemia. (However, hypoglycemia does occur even in the best managed cases.) The concentrations of lipids and lipoproteins, invariably abnormal in diabetics with even modest elevations of blood sugar, return to normal, in theory decreasing the increased risk of atherosclerosis of conventionally treated patients.

These forms of therapy that normalize blood sugar have been in use for only a few years, and it is not surprising that information on prevention of complications of diabetes is not yet available. Amelioration of minor degrees of proteinuria has been shown, possibly a result of membrane permeability changes, but renal insufficiency and major proteinuria are not reversed. Established retinopathy does not appear to be improved. Neuropathy is not clinically improved, although nerve conduction may improve.

A number of problems with pump therapy have become obvious. Pump failure, due to failure of the pump itself or to clogging of its infusion line, sometimes occurs. Diabetic ketoacidosis (DKA) rapidly ensues, often overnight, when the insulin infusion is interrupted. Local infection at the needle site also predisposes to ketoacidosis due to poor absorption of insulin, and it may be severe enough to require antibiotic therapy and hospitalization. The approximate frequency of DKA has been estimated at one episode/100 patient months; infection, at one/40 patient months; and severe hypoglycemia, at one/30 patient months.

Multidose intensive conventional insulin therapy has the advantage over the pump approach of lower cost and freedom from the hazards of DKA and local infection, but the disadvantage of requiring multiple injections. In crossover studies, an equal number of patients prefer one or the other form of therapy. Both forms of intensive therapy require extraordinary commitment by the patient, the family, and the physician's team.

Obstacles to Successful Intensive Therapy. Initial enthusiasm that diabetic complications could be prevented or stabilized often have given way to discouragement as patients and families realize the intense demands of such therapy. The logistics and mechanics of multiple blood sampling, wearing a pump, cost, and the constant reminder of the presence of chronic illness all serve to cause eventual abandonment of pump therapy by many patients. Moreover, in some individuals, blood sugars vary widely despite meticulous adherence to the rules of the program. Sometimes patients assume that they are at fault and stop reporting the truth about their control. Periodic monitoring with hemoglobin A_{1c} measurement is useful in defining the true state of control.

Monitoring Conventional Insulin Therapy

Efficacy of treatment in the conventionally treated ambulatory patient should be monitored by measuring FPG and urine glucose. Normalization of FPG—more reproducible than postprandial sugars—represents the basic or "coarse" adjustment of insulin dose, and postprandial normalization can be viewed as the "fine" adjustment. No useful purpose is served by attempts to adjust postprandial PG before normalization of the FPG is achieved; only thereafter should PG be monitored at midafternoon or before the evening meal.

Urine glucose monitoring before meals and before bedtime is also important and is too often neglected. Yet urine glucose monitoring remains simple and inexpensive and provides considerable information. As a sole technique for monitoring it is inadequate but much to be preferred to no monitoring or to inaccurately performed blood monitoring. One drawback is the variable renal threshold (normal range, 160 to 250 mg/dl). Inability to detect hypoglycemia is another disadvantage. Nevertheless, even two daily determinations of urine glucose can be a useful guide and complementary to blood monitoring.

Double voiding technique should be used whenever possible, especially for the first morning specimen, if the patient has not voided during the night. Although heavy daytime glucosuria is still present, no useful purpose is served by additional frequent monitoring of PG. On the other hand, when afternoon (before dinner) glucosuria has cleared, PG determination—like that of FPG—becomes essential to determine whether the PG has reached, or is approaching, hypoglycemic levels. The development of such episodes is, of course, an indication of need for adjustment of the treatment program.

In ketosis-prone patients, the urine should also be monitored for ketonuria. This can be accomplished using Acetest tablets or one of the combination "stix." Ordinarily, monitoring for ketones is not necessary as a routine procedure.

The optimal frequency of monitoring of FPG and/or of urinary glucose must be determined for each patient. During initiation of therapy, determination of glucosuria four times daily (first voided A.M. specimen, prelunch, predinner, and at bedtime) is essential if insulin is to be varied (increased) as described above. Typically, FPG must be determined every week or 2 while the insulin dose is being adjusted, and thereafter less often—perhaps only monthly or even every 2 to 3 months.

Monitoring Intensive Insulin Therapy

If "tight control" is the goal, and intensive insulin therapy is prescribed, self-monitoring of blood glucose (SMBG) is mandatory (see below). In the patient with NIDDM, complete absence of glucosuria can often be achieved without the need for frequent determinations of FPG, but this is not possible in patients with IDDM. The principal indication for SMBG is to permit normalization of blood glucose—tight control—by intensive insulin therapy or by insulin pump. However, other indications include patients with unusually low or high renal threshold for glucose, many patients with IDDM treated conventionally, all patients prone to hypoglycemic episodes, pregnant patients, and some patients with IDDM who, despite an inability to master effective therapy, seem to find SMBG more satisfying than the simpler and less expensive procedures of testing urine. The levels and ranges of blood glucose that indicate normoglycemia are fasting, 80 ± 20 mg%; 1 to 2 hours postprandial, 140 ± 0 mg%; and nocturnal (3 A.M.), not below 50 mg%.

The process of SMBG should be initiated as a prelude to tight control since, unless the patient shows an ability to master the technique and accept it as an ongoing necessity, the effort at tight control will fail. SMBG does not eliminate the need for dietary compliance. Recent studies indicate that, within the wide range of normal, neither intelligence, socioeconomic status, nor personality type has any predictive value for success with SMBG. Patients of limited financial means may drop out of such a program because of its high cost.

With programs of intensive therapy *initial* frequency of monitoring may be up to seven times daily: 1 hour before and after breakfast, lunch, and dinner, and before bedtime. Testing may be reduced to two to four times daily once a pattern of normalization is achieved. Patients who monitor less than four times daily are unlikely to maintain normalization of blood glucose.

The basis for all SMBG methods is a paper strip impregnated with an enzyme reagent (glucose oxidase) and suitable dyes. When placed in contact with a drop of capillary blood, the change of color intensity indicates the glucose concentration. Some strips are read only visually, others either visually or with a reflectance photometer. The characteristics of the commonly used strips are presented in Table 72.10. Accuracy of strips properly examined visually is excellent. For most patients a meter is not a necessity, but many feel more secure with machine readings.

In the United States two meters are in widest use. The Glucometer II (Ames) uses Glucostix; the Accu-Check II (Boehringer-Manheim) uses Chemstrips bG. All machines are reliable, portable, battery operated, and cost between $150 and $300. The retail cost of strips is approximately $0.70 each. If four are used daily the monthly cost is over $80.

Capillary blood is most commonly obtained from

Table 72.10.
Types of Reagent Strips for Self-monitoring of Blood Glucose by Visual Reading[a]

Name and Manufacturer	Instructions for Use
Chemstrip bG (Boehringer Mannheim)	Wipe after 1 minute, read; if > 240, wait an additional minute, read
Glucostix (Ames)	Blot for 30 seconds, wait 90 seconds, read
TrendStrips (Orange Medical Instruments)	Wipe after 1 minute, read; if over 240, wait an additional minute, read
Visidex II (Ames)	Blot after 30 seconds, wait 90 seconds, read

[a]Modified from American Diabetes Association Physician's guide to Insulin-Dependent (type I) Diabetes. Diagnosis and Treatment, 2nd ed, Alexandria, VA, 1988.

the tip of the finger, although some patients prefer the earlobe. The required drop of blood is obtained almost painlessly using a spring-triggered device such as the Autolet. Disposable Monolet lances are used to produce the puncture. At a current cost of $0.07 per Monolet, the monthly cost is approximately $10.

Blood flow from the finger can be enhanced before puncture by holding the hand in warm (not hot) water for 30 seconds. The skin should be quickly dried. Puncturing the thumb is least painful, but the ring finger has the best blood supply. Puncturing the lateral aspect of the fingertip (distal phalanx) is less painful than puncturing the ball. Pain is also less when sufficient pressure to produce erythema is applied to the palmar surface (ball) of the distal phalanx; an opposing digit of the same hand is used to apply the pressure. The first drop of blood produced suffices; the presence of extravascular fluid does not affect the result. An ideal puncture produces a $\pm/5$-mm drop. The finger is inverted and the drop is allowed to fall to the strip; timing is begun. The strip usually is blotted or wiped, following directions of the supplier, and the glucose level is read. If the earlobe is used, a second or third sample can subsequently be obtained on the same day without repuncture if the site is rubbed with an alcohol wipe, allowed to dry, and the earlobe is flipped with the finger. This procedure is preferred by some patients.

Glycosylated Hemoglobins

Long-term monitoring of overall blood sugar control by measurement of one of the chronic effects of hyperglycemia provides clinically useful information. Glucose reacts nonenzymatically in a concentration-dependent manner with the amino groups in proteins to produce glycosylated derivatives (5).

Chronic elevation of blood glucose results in an increase in the concentration of glycosylated hemoglobins, a major component of which is hemoglobin A_{1c} (Hgb A_{1c}). Determination of the level of either the total glycosylated hemoglobin A_1 or of Hgb A_{1c} gives essentially the same information, an integrated estimate of the degree of hyperglycemia over a period of weeks to months (Fig. 72.2). The normal range of Hgb A_{1c} is 3.8 to 6.3% of total hemoglobin and may rise to 15% with chronic hyperglycemia postprandially. Values of <7.5% suggest excellent control with fasting and 1 hour postprandial sugars in the range of 70 to 120 and 100 to 140, respectively. With 120 to 140 fasting and 141 to 160 postprandial, one might see Hgb A_{1c} at 7.5 to 9%. At 140 to 160 fasting and 160 to 200 postprandially; values of 9.1 to 11 are common, whereas minimal control gives values of greater than 11%. Glycosylated hemoglobin levels fall slowly with reduction of mean glucose, since circulating red blood cells containing high levels of glycosylated hemoglobin disappear normally in approximately 120 days. If euglycemia is established, glycosylated hemoglobins subsequently normalize in 4 to 6 weeks. Conversely, persistent hyperglycemia must be present for 1 to 4 weeks before elevated levels of glycosylated hemoglobins are seen. Short periods of hyperglycemia (6 to 24

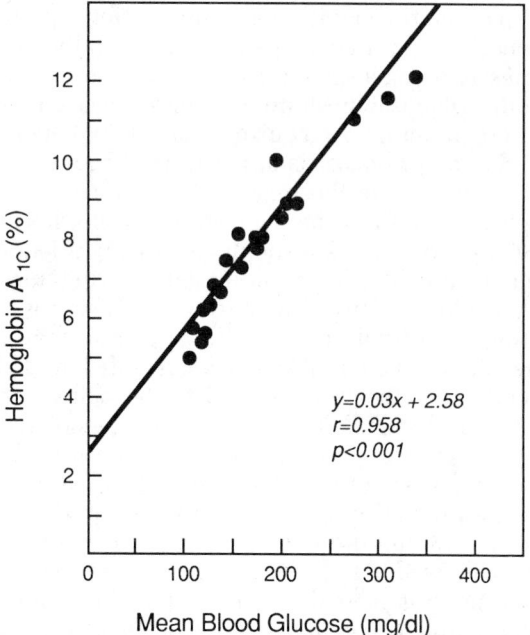

Figure 72.2. Relationship between hemoglobin A$_{1c}$ and mean blood glucose. Twenty-one subjects performed SMBG four to six times per day for 8 weeks. The arithmetic mean of those values was compared to the HgbA$_{1c}$ value determined at the end of the 8-week period. (From Nathan DM, Singer DE, Hurxthal K, et al: The clinical information value of the glycoslyated hemoglobin assay. *N Engl J Med* 310:341, 1984.)

hours' duration) may result in disproportionate elevations, since some methods include measurement of unstable glycosylated derivatives. Other conditions render interpretations of glycosylated hemoglobin values uncertain, including any in which red cell life span is low (bleeding; hemolysis) or in which hemoglobin F is increased (some hemoglobinopathies).

The measurement of glycosylated hemoglobins is a useful clinical adjunct in the assessment of the efficacy of control of hyperglycemia. However, proteins other than hemoglobin that also undergo glycosylation exist in nerve, ocular lens, kidney, cell membranes, and plasma. Of great importance is the realization that glucose is not an inert substance but one that can produce postsynthetic modification of many proteins. Some of these alterations may be harmful and provide a possible biochemical mechanism by which hyperglycemia, per se, may result in deleterious alterations of tissue structure and function and produce long-term complications of the diabetic state (28).

Factors Affecting Insulin Requirement

Insulin resistance. Classically, the term insulin resistance refers to a state in which the requirement for insulin exceeds 200 units daily. This extreme type of insulin resistance is usually due to the development of antibodies to insulin (see below). However, resistance to insulin occurs even in the absence of antibodies to insulin. This resistance—or decreased sensitivity to insulin—is most apparent in the diabetes that is associated with obesity and the state now termed non-insulin-dependent diabetes mellitus. Even non-

diabetic obese individuals who maintain normal levels of blood sugar do so by secreting supranormal amounts of insulin.

Although obese diabetics are insulin resistant in terms of their glucose homeostasis and certain aspects of lipoprotein metabolism, their metabolic state is not so deranged as to allow development of ketoacidosis. In the majority of insulin-resistant diabetics, weight reduction will reverse the insulin resistance. Glucose tolerance often improves to (or toward) normal, and the need for insulin to control hyperglycemia may decrease or disappear. In contrast, some nonobese patients with NIDDM have lower than normal levels of plasma insulin. Such patients comprise a spectrum of combinations of insulin resistance and insulin deficiency.

Current evidence suggests that sulfonylurea compounds, in addition to their action in facilitating insulin release, may act by returning insulin sensitivity toward normal, perhaps by increasing insulin receptors. The use of these drugs is dictated, however, by other considerations (see below).

Increases of insulin requirement. The stress of infection or trauma may increase insulin requirements quickly. Usually the site of any infection that is severe enough to produce this effect is obvious, or at least there is good evidence of an infectious process (fever, leukocytosis). Only rarely will a search for a hidden focus provide an explanation for changing insulin requirements or even for the development of ketoacidosis. Most episodes of ketoacidosis that are not related to stress are not caused by an increased insulin requirement. Rather, such episodes are usually related to noncompliance, although this may be unintentional, as when the patient mistakenly omits insulin because of intercurrent viral illness. Insulin requirement tends to increase after the end of the first trimester of pregnancy (see below).

A slow increase of insulin requirement (for the commonly used insulin of beef-pork origin) occurring over months may be related to development of insulin antibodies of the IgG type. Usually the patient may be stabilized at a new, higher dose level. Under these circumstances, the duration of action of short-acting insulin is often prolonged, whereas intermediate- or long-acting insulins may not carry a 24-hour effect. Insulin requirement may exceed 200 units/day and administration may become a problem. A switch to purified pork or human insulin may result in up to a 30% decrease in requirement. Occasionally, a short course of glucocorticoid therapy is necessary to effect a dose reduction. Prednisone (40 to 60 mg daily), rather than increase insulin requirement, will usually produce a dramatic fall in insulin requirement beginning at 7 to 10 days. Hospitalization should be considered after the first 5 days of such therapy in anticipation of rapid decrease of insulin requirement. When the decrease occurs, glucocorticoid therapy can be abruptly discontinued. Recurrence of the resistant state is infrequent and may not occur for months or years.

Decreases of insulin requirement. Vigorous exer-

cise reduces blood glucose and, in anticipation of such activity, the dose of insulin may need to be reduced (see page 922). *During pregnancy,* insulin requirement drops during the first trimester, rises and may double during the second and third trimesters, and falls suddenly at delivery (see below). Diabetics who develop *nephropathy* often show a decreased insulin requirement. A tendency to normoglycemia or even to hypoglycemia develops occasionally in patients previously requiring insulin who develop *chronic congestive heart failure.* Development of *adrenal or pituitary insufficiency* will also result in a decreased insulin requirement, but these are rare events and not specifically related to diabetes mellitus.

Hypoglycemia during Insulin Therapy: Recognition, Prevention, and Treatment

Hypoglycemia is an inevitable effect of an excessive insulin dose. Especially when severe, hypoglycemia causes central nervous system symptoms ranging from headache, subtle disturbances of mental function, confusion, and visual disturbances to personality change, seizures, unconsciousness, and transient hemiparesis. When hypoglycemia occurs during waking hours and is accompanied by the usual symptoms of epinephrine release (tremor, sweating, tachycardia, and palpitations), there is no problem in recognizing the condition. However, in some poorly controlled diabetics, as in some other persons, even mild reductions of blood glucose to levels (50 to 70 mg/100 ml) not clearly identifiable as hypoglycemia can sometimes produce epinephrine release with its resulting symptoms (see also Chapter 74). Under these circumstances, documentable hypoglycemia is not present and the clinical situation may be confusing.

By far the most frequent cause of hypoglycemia in the diabetic receiving insulin therapy is failure of the patient to eat at normal times. Despite repeated warnings many patients not only miss meals, but obfuscate the treatment program further by denying that they have done so. The physician must be ever on guard but tactful in constantly considering this possibility.

Diabetics may develop defects in mechanisms that normally counter-regulate hypoglycemia (8, 9, 10). This pathophysiological state may occur within a few years of onset of the disease. Deficiencies of glucagon secretion are common in IDDM and sometimes occur in NIDDM. Defective counter-regulation due to impaired secretion of epinephrine also becomes manifest in patients with autonomic (adrenergic) neuropathy late in the course of IDDM, although it occasionally develops within a year of onset of the disease. Other patients may have defective counter-regulation due to impairment of epinephrine action as a result of treatment with β-adrenergic blocking drugs, such as propranolol. In addition, such agents may mask many of the symptoms of epinephrine excess. Regardless of their precise mechanisms, these defective counter-regulatory responses undoubtedly contribute in many diabetics to their high risk of developing severe hypoglycemia during therapy with insulin, especially during intensive therapy (1, 8). In addition many intensively treated patients appear to develop tolerance to hypoglycemia and remain asymptomatic with markedly subnormal concentrations of glucose. Defective glucagon responsiveness to hypoglycemia in IDDM is not normalized (reversed) by establishment of tight control (1). In contrast, poorly controlled diabetics may develop *symptoms* of hypoglycemia at higher levels of glucose than do persons without diabetes (3).

Excessive insulin action often occurs during the night or early morning hours. The hypoglycemia-induced release of epinephrine and other counter-regulatory hormones (cortisol, growth hormone, glucagon) then causes rebound hyperglycemia, glucosuria, and ketonuria (Somogyi phenomenon). If the physician notes an elevated blood sugar and prescribes still more insulin, the result is further hypoglycemia, perpetuation of the cycle, and possible serious consequences. The physician is obliged to question the patient carefully for clues to the presence of nocturnal hypoglycemia leading to this sequence, such as nightmares, night sweats, and headache during the night or on arising, although these symptoms may not be present. Increasing intake of carbohydrate in the late evening and/or reduction of insulin dose by 10% in IDDM and up to 20 to 30% in NIDDM will often correct the situation. In the latter patients, such a brief and substantial reduction in insulin dose can be made with impunity. If the situation cannot be resolved by such maneuvers, frequent blood glucose monitoring including measurements during the night and early morning hours will be necessary (see page 932).

The classical Somogyi phenomenon must be distinguished from two other possibilities: (*a*) waning of insulin action; (*b*) the dawn phenomenon. Waning of insulin action occurs when the patient is receiving an insufficient amount of intermediate- or long-acting insulin; either a single A.M. dose is not carrying into the next day, or the second dose, given before dinner or at bedtime, is inadequate. The dawn phenomenon is an increase of blood sugar between 3 and 7 A.M. that occurs despite continuous subcutaneous infusion or background insulin action from Ultralente. An increased amount of insulin is necessary to overcome the action of growth hormone, which is secreted in pulsatile fashion during the night with considerable interindividual variation and, unfortunately, variation from day to day, as well. Because of this variation an amount of insulin that is sufficient one day may be quite inadequate the next. The point at which counter-regulatory hormones are secreted is quite variable; some diabetics trigger it at glucose concentrations as high as 50 mg/dl; others do not have counter-regulatory release until the blood sugar falls to as low as 30 to 40 mg/dl.

Obviously, waning insulin action and the dawn effect need more insulin, while the Somogyi effect requires that less be given. The simplest way to distinguish these is by self-monitoring of blood glucose (SMBG) with samples at 9 P.M., midnight, 3 A.M. and 7 A.M. Several nights and more frequent sampling may be needed. The differing patterns are shown in Figure 72.3. Constantly rising glucose indicates waning insulin. A plateau followed by a rise indicates the dawn phenomenon. A drop during the night to a clearly hypoglycemic level points to the Somogyi effect. If SMBG cannot be done, cautious reduction of the dose of (evening) insulin should be attempted. Although the existence of the Somogyi phenomenon has been repeatedly challenged (38), recent evidence convincingly points to its contribution to the problem of glucose regulation (29).

The immediate therapy of daytime hypoglycemia in a conscious patient is ingestion of food, preferably sugar. Patients should carry a ready carbohydrate source, such as candy, and must realize that a tiny piece of such material will not suffice. Five or six Lifesavers provide the necessary 10 g of carbohydrate, as will a piece of fruit. Glucose tablets are now available; at least four are recommended. If available, 4 to 6 ounces of sweetened juice or a soft drink are most satisfactory. A tablespoon of sugar may be added to fruit juice or merely dissolved in 1/2 cup of water. Relief should be obtained in 10 to 20 minutes. Family members or friends should be instructed in the treatment of such an emergency and should not waste time in attempting to reach medical assistance before administering sugar. Although no objection exists to seeking emergency medical care after sugar is given, the problem is usually resolved by the time medical assistance can be obtained. If no obvious cause is apparent for the episode of hypoglycemia—such as a missed meal that is subsequently eaten—the patient should be on guard for recurrence over the next few hours, during which time

repeated ingestion of sugar, at hourly intervals, may be advisable.

Most patients treated with less than intensive therapy will never require emergency medical assistance for treatment of hypoglycemia. However, occasional individuals will be prone to this problem and sometimes cannot be treated by the simple means described. Either because of a hypoglycemia-related alteration of mental status or because of unconsciousness, such persons will not be able to take oral sugar. A safe and effective emergency therapy is administration of 1 mg of glucagon subcutaneously by a person instructed in this technique. Glucagon is readily available in single dose form (1-mg vial) and should be kept available during initiation of insulin therapy and in hypoglycemia-prone persons. About 10 to 15 minutes are required for an obvious effect on sensorium. As soon as possible, oral sugar should then be given. An effort should always be made to identify the cause of the hypoglycemic episode and to reduce dosage or take other appropriate action to prevent recurrence.

Miscellaneous Factors Affecting Control

Although defects of counter-regulatory responses undoubtedly contribute to recurrent episodes of hypoglycemia in many patients, other factors in their daily lives also contribute (30). Noncompliance with diet may be deliberate or accidental: "small" snacks can be overlooked. Meals are often taken off schedule, upsetting the effort to adjust insulin dose to preferred time of meals, a scheme preferable to the opposite. Amounts of food, if greatly varied, will adversely affect insulin dosage. Emotional upset, difficult to evaluate as a cause of varying control, is nonetheless a significant factor in some circumstances. Injudicious use of alcohol is always a concern. Patients may have trouble measuring their insulin or may reverse the ratio of mixtures. Undocumented hypoglycemic reactions may be improperly treated and unreported. Techniques of urine or blood monitoring are often at fault. Patients misread directions or introduce variations that lead to errors of measurements.

Oral Hypoglycemic Drugs (Sulfonylureas)

Mechanism of Action

Within a few years after their introduction 35 years ago, these drugs came into wide use for the treatment of NIDDM. The acute hypoglycemic effects of the sulfonylureas appear to be mediated through insulin release. However, in chronic administration, during which blood glucose has been lowered, no increase of plasma insulin is apparent. Recent studies on the mechanisms of action of these drugs show both an increase in the number of insulin receptors and a potentiation of insulin action. Numerous effects other than the desired hypoglycemic action of the sulfonylureas have been studied in connection with drug-drug interactions of these compounds (see below).

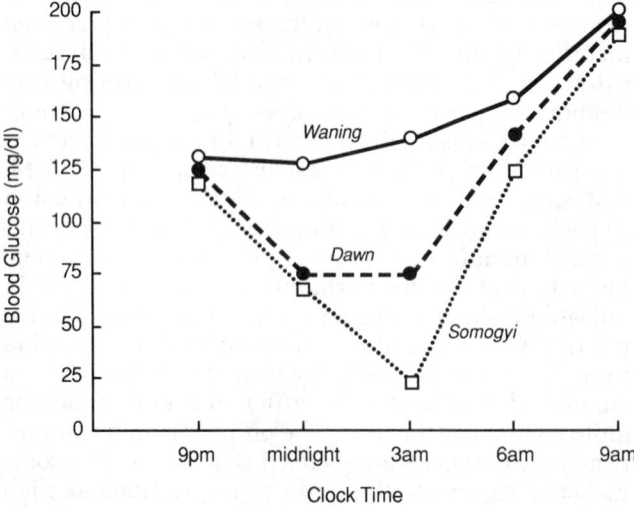

Figure 72.3. Idealized patterns of blood glucose concentrations during the night. The three patterns represent waning insulin action, the dawn phenomenon, and the classic Somogyi effect. All result in fasting hyperglycemia but are distinguished by the patterns of blood glucose concentration in the preceding hours.

Current Place in Therapy: University Group Diabetes Program (UGDP)

Although sometimes used to good purpose for treatment of symptomatic hyperglycemia, oral hypoglycemic drugs were often administered to patients with NIDDM who could have been treated with diet (i.e., by weight reduction). Many patients with minimal fasting or postprandial hyperglycemia or other abnormalities of glucose tolerance were also given these drugs.

A multicenter long-term cooperative study (UGDP) attempted to assess the usefulness of these agents in asymptomatic diabetics by comparing tolbutamide with diet and insulin treatment. The study began a vitriolic controversy in 1970 when it first reported that tolbutamide-treated patients fared no better than those given placebo and indeed had a higher cardiovascular (but not overall) death rate. Since that report, diabetologists have been divided concerning the usefulness (or dangers) of these agents. Although the harmfulness of these agents seems now, on reanalysis of the data, to be open to serious question, the long-term benefits in terms of prevention of complications of diabetes remain questionable. It is almost certain that the original UGDP study was too brief and involved an inadequate number of patients to have permitted answers to questions concerning prevention of complications. A number of other studies of this issue have now concluded that sulfonylureas do not result in harmful effects and the use of these drugs has therefore increased.

Therapeutic Effects versus Side Effects

No doubt exists that short-term symptomatic relief of hyperglycemia and its sequelae can be obtained in most NIDDM patients treated with sulfonylureas. This result can be most gratifying in properly selected patients. For example, patients who may have difficulty in self-administering insulin because of visual or other physical handicaps may benefit symptomatically from use of sulfonylureas. On the other hand, the use of sulfonylureas is not harmless, because of their intrinsic pharmacological action in lowering blood glucose and a number of toxic effects. Hypoglycemia can occur and may be both severe and protracted, especially in the elderly or in patients with decreased hepatic or renal function. Administration of certain of these agents to elderly patients, especially to patients with impaired cardiovascular function, may produce water retention and a syndrome identical to that of inappropriate secretion of antidiuretic hormone (SIADH) with severe hyponatremia and symptoms as profound as coma (39). The volume expansion that occurs may precipitate or worsen congestive heart failure. Chlorpropamide (Diabinese) is the classic offender in this regard, although tolbutamide (Orinase) has been rarely involved as well. The newer agents, glyburide and glipizide, are thought to be capable of producing this complication as well.

Candidates for Therapy with Sulfonylureas

Obese NIDDM patients who have not responded to a weight reduction diet or who, having started on a diet, need interim symptomatic relief from hyperglycemia that is producing osmotic diuresis (polyuria, polydipsia) may benefit. Typically these individuals are over age 40 and are more likely to respond if their diabetes has been present for only a few years. Other candidates are those who are unwilling to accept insulin therapy or in whom the risks of hypoglycemia seem unacceptable. The latter might include persons with occupations involving hazardous conditions (vehicle or dangerous equipment operators). Still others include nonobese individuals in whom insulin therapy is unacceptable, but for whom persistent hyperglycemia is believed by the physician to constitute a long-term risk factor for atherosclerotic and microvascular disease.

Although most physicians would currently be reluctant to change therapy to an oral agent for a patient who is managing well with insulin, such a change—if undertaken—is more likely to succeed if the diabetes has required less than about 40 units of insulin a day. Patients with a previous history of ketoacidosis are ordinarily not candidates for a transfer from insulin. A history of hyperosmolar nonketotic coma does not preclude a successful change from insulin. Patients with no tendency to ketosis, but whose diabetes is so severe that it has produced weight loss, may not respond to sulfonylureas given as initial therapy but may respond after hyperglycemia has been controlled for a short time with insulin.

Oral agents should not be prescribed for certain patients: individuals with a history of ketoacidosis, unless the latter has developed in relation to stress; patients with a history of severe toxic reaction to a sulfonylurea; and patients with severe hepatic or renal disease, although correct choice of an agent may make such therapy possible (Table 72.11).

Effectiveness. In optimally selected patients about one-half can be expected to experience normalization of fasting blood sugar while about one-third will not respond. In others, some drug effect will be evident, perhaps to a degree that permits symptomatic relief. Maximal drug effect can be expected within a few days to a week. Those who do not respond during initial therapy are considered to be "primary" sulfonylurea failures. In other cases, following a month or more of good response, the drug seems to become ineffective ("secondary" sulfonylurea failure). The frequency of this response has been estimated at 3 to 10%. Many secondary failures are due to noncompliance. Only occasionally in secondary failure will a switch from a maximal dose of one agent to another be successful.

Transfer from insulin or from one sulfonylurea to another sulfonylurea. NIDDM patients receiving insulin can be abruptly switched, provided that they do not need more than 40 units of insulin a day. A need for maximal doses of sulfonylurea can usually be an-

Table 72.11.
Characteristics of Hypoglycemic Drugs (Sulfonylureas)

Compound	Generic available	Trade Name	Tablet Size	Daily Dose Range	Duration of action (hr)	Doses/Day	Route of Inactivation
Tolbutamide	Yes	Orinase	0.5 g	1–3 g	12	2–3	100% in liver
Chlorpropamide	Yes	Diabinese	0.1 g 0.25 g	0.1–0.5 g	36+	1	100% excretion by kidney: as intact drug, 30%, plus less active metabolites, 70%
Acetohexamide		Dymelor	0.25 g	0.25–1.5 g	12–18	1–2	100% kidney excretion of active metabolites from liver plus unchanged drug
Tolazamide	Yes	Tolinase	0.1 g 0.25 g 0.5 g	0.25–1.0 g	12–24	1–2	Partial liver metabolism; partial excretion via kidney
Glyburide	No	Micronase Diabeta	1.25 mg 2.5 mg 5 mg	1.25–20 mg	16–24	1–2	100% metabolized to inactive compounds
Glipizide	No	Glucotrol	5 mg 10 mg	2.5–40 mg	12–24	1–2	100% metabolized to inactive compounds

ticipated in such cases. If the patient has manifested ketosis in the past, as for example during stress, but is otherwise thought to be a candidate for a switch to an oral agent, the dose of insulin may be cut in half as the drug is started. Subsequent monitoring over the next few days will show whether the oral agent can control hyperglycemia or must be abandoned. If a given sulfonylurea proves to be ineffective, it is unlikely that switching to another sulfonylurea will prove to be helpful, but occasionally a second generation agent (see below) will be effective when a first generation agent has failed.

Choice of drug. Tolbutamide is the only sulfonylurea studied in the UGDP. Although the admonitions of the Food and Drug Administration concerning other oral agents extrapolate from this study of tolbutamide, it may be useful to remember that the related available drugs might have fared better or worse. This caveat aside, for patients with normal hepatic and renal function, there is little to lead one to choose among the available agents (Table 72.11) except that the longer acting drugs need not be taken as often. The frequency of toxicity with tolbutamide is very low, probably lower than with the other agents, even at maximal doses. Chlorpropamide should never be used at a dose greater than 500 mg/day (above which hepatic toxicity is frequent). Because of the ability of chlorpropamide among the sulfonylureas to produce a syndrome of drug-induced water intoxication (SIADH) (see above), this drug should be avoided in the elderly in whom this effect has been seen almost exclusively. Acetohexamide is the least used agent, partly because it was introduced later than tolbutamide and chlorpropamide and partly because of lack of aggressive marketing. Tolazamide was introduced 20 years ago but has been marketed vigorously only within the past few years. Phenformin, a biguanide (not a sulfonylurea), was withdrawn from the market in 1977 as an "imminent hazard to the public health" after 18 years of general use. Fatal lactic acidosis, hypertension, and persistent

tachycardia were associated with its use. Metformin, a similar but apparently safer biguanide, is not yet available in the United States but is widely used in Europe, sometimes in combination with a sulfonylurea.

For many years, "second generation" sulfonylureas have been in wide use outside the United States. Glyburide (Micronase, Diabeta) and glipizide (Glucatrol) were introduced into use in the United States about 5 years ago and are being aggressively marketed. These drugs are safe agents but no long-term studies of the UGDP type are available with them. Although all sulfonylureas improve the second phase of insulin secretion, only glipizide in response to glucose stimulation improves both first and second phase responses and does not cause a rise of insulin levels in the fasting state. The latter characteristic has theoretical advantages over other oral agents, and possibly over insulin, for the prevention of atherosclerosis (36).

Comparative cost. At present, the approximate monthly retail cost of therapy with these drugs is from $4 to $80 depending on the dose and the agent used. Three of the drugs, tolbutamide, chlorpropamide, and tolazamide, are currently available in their generic forms at one-half to one-third the price of the trade name products. The cost of insulin therapy may be significantly less than that with the oral agents, depending on the dose and the grade of insulin that are used.

Instruction to the Patient on Use of Sulfonylureas

The sulfonylureas are most effective when administered about 30 minutes before breakfast and dinner.

The obese patient must be made to realize that diet, i.e., weight reduction, is the mainstay of therapy. In order to avoid unnecessary anxiety, the current status of the UGDP controversy should be discussed with the patient and the possible risks and goals of therapy clearly outlined. Although hypoglycemia is not common with the sulfonylureas, when it does occur, it is likely to be both severe and prolonged. Chlorpropamide and glyburide are the two drugs most likely to produce this problem. The symptoms of hypoglycemia should be clearly described to the patient, family, and/or friends and corrective measures outlined (see "Insulin Therapy"). The possibility of drug-drug interactions (see below) should be mentioned lest another physician prescribe a drug that potentiates or decreases the effectiveness of the sulfonylureas. Loading doses of sulfonylureas may have a place in patients under observation in the hospital but should not be used in ambulatory patients.

Monitoring Therapy with Sulfonylureas

Because patients receiving sulfonylurea drugs are not ketosis prone and have fairly stable diabetes, monitoring is relatively simple. Similar considerations apply to patients being treated with diet alone. No compelling indication exists for self-monitoring of blood glucose in most such patients (see page 932). Patients who have FPG in or near the normal range exhibit little or no fasting glucosuria but may show glucosuria in the postprandial state. Such patients can check their overnight (early A.M.) urine samples for glucose as infrequently as once a week or even every 2 weeks. More important they should understand that appearance of glucosuria where none had been evident or the worsening of glucosuria is an indication for contact with a physician. Similarly, these patients must be taught that, should they develop symptoms and signs of uncontrolled hyperglycemia (heavy glucosuria, polyuria, polydipsia, blurred vision), prompt advice from a physician is absolutely necessary. Routine testing for urinary acetone is not necessary unless the patient has new onset of persistent glucosuria or at some earlier time had an episode of ketoacidosis, perhaps during stress.

FPG should be determined every few months in most patients and is the best means of monitoring sulfonylurea-treated patients who respond to treatment with normalization of blood sugar. Determination of glycosylated hemoglobin is also useful (page 933). Development of hypoglycemia, which may be detected before symptoms develop, is an indication for downward adjustment of drug dosage.

Special Considerations in Treatment of the Geriatric Patient

Some elderly patients may best be treated with oral agents. These individuals may have special problems (e.g., poor vision or manipulative skills) that make self-administration of insulin more difficult than usual. Moreover, simple symptomatic therapy may be the foremost consideration in these individuals. On the other hand, many elderly persons can manage insulin therapy, especially of the type that is not excessively aggressive, and age alone should not deter the physician from appropriate institution of insulin therapy. As noted above (page 929), insulin syringes can be prefilled and stored in the refrigerator for 1 to 2 weeks; this plan is useful for the older person who cannot accurately draw up the correct amount of insulin. The elderly are especially likely to suffer from multiple diseases and to use multiple drugs. The risk of drug-drug interactions in this group is therefore greater than in younger individuals (see below). The elderly are also especially prone to development of severe and prolonged hypoglycemia with use of the sulfonylureas, which may be related, in part, to the decrease of renal function that normally accompanies aging and that may be worse in the diabetic. Decreased renal function (glomerular filtration rate, creatinine clearance) is frequently present in the elderly even when the serum creatinine is normal, since creatinine production decreases with age as muscle mass decreases. Thus, sulfonylureas that are disposed of exclusively by excretion (acetohexamide) or in part by this route (chlorpropamide, tolazamide) are more likely to produce hypoglycemia when renal function decreases. Chlorpropamide is also capable of inducing enhanced endogenous antidiuretic hormone action and of inducing a water intoxication syndrome, a phenomenon seen almost exclusively in elderly diabetics (39). Tolbutamide and tolazamide are probably the safest of the older sulfonylureas for use in the elderly; the initial dose should be low and increases should be made cautiously. Loading doses should not be used in the elderly.

Drug-Drug Interactions

Various drugs enhance the hypoglycemic action of sulfonylureas, and others decrease their effect. The magnitude of the effects varies with the different sulfonylureas. Several mechanisms are involved, some of which are known. Among the more commonly used drugs, salicylates, some sulfonamides, chloramphenicol, phenylbutazone and its derivatives, and bishydroxycoumarin all enhance the hypoglycemic action of the sulfonylureas either by displacement of binding to plasma proteins or by interfering with metabolic disposal. β-blockers may mask the hypoglycemia-induced release of epinephrine and thus prolong and intensify the hypoglycemic reactions. β-blockers, by blocking insulin release, may also precipitate hyperosmolar coma. Clonidine (Catapres) may, like β-blockers, mask the signs and symptoms of hypoglycemia. Acute ingestion of alcohol can enhance hypoglycemia; chronic alcohol use accelerates metabolic disposal of sulfonylureas and antagonizes their hypoglycemic action. Sulfonylureas, especially chlorpropamide, interfere with the metabolism of alcohol and may produce a disulfiram-like (Antabuse) effect (see Chapter 21). The thiazide diuretics, chlorthalidone, furosemide, and ethacrynic acid may produce hyperglycemia even in normal persons and antagonize the sulfonylureas. Another commonly used drug, the anticonvulsant phenytoin (Dilantin), also has an antagonist action. *Numerous other drugs may enhance or negate the effect of the sulfonylureas*; equally important, the sulfonylureas themselves produce numerous alterations of drug action. These problems should not be overstated, but the physician should be aware of these possibilities and interactions.

Treatment of "Other Types" of Diabetes Mellitus (Secondary Diabetes)

Drug-induced diabetes (e.g., thiazides) and diabetes associated with the use of glucocorticoids are usually not ketosis prone and ordinarily resemble that of NIDDM. Treatment with sulfonylureas may be tried, but insulin is often necessary. Withdrawal of the offending agent does not always ameliorate the diabetic state. The possibility of precipitating diabetes in patients with a strong family history should not deter the physician from the judicious use of diuretics or glucocorticoids when these agents are necessary. Similarly, a diabetic who is already receiving insulin should not be denied diuretic therapy (e.g., when hypertension develops) or glucocorticoids for fear of "aggravating" the diabetes. If such aggravation occurs, usually only an increase of insulin dose is necessary to reestablish the previous state of control.

Diabetes secondary to chronic pancreatitis or pancreatectomy should be treated with insulin. The insulin requirement is usually 20 to 40 units/day. The patients should be instructed to follow the dietary strategy outlined for insulin-dependent diabetes in Table 72.6. Alcoholic patients with this form of diabetes are particularly difficult to manage if they continue to drink heavily and to eat erratically.

COMPLICATIONS OF DIABETES MELLITUS

Diabetes mellitus is a leading cause of death in the United States today. Most of these deaths are due to the complications of the disease—primarily those complications associated with accelerated atherosclerosis and with chronic renal failure (Fig. 72.4). The risk of both atherosclerotic heart disease and of atherosclerotic peripheral vascular disease is increased approximately 3-fold in diabetics and is proportionate to the duration of disease (in patients with both NIDDM and IDDM). Atherosclerotic disorders are discussed in Section 8 and in Chapters 83 and 87; chronic renal failure is discussed in Chapter 48.

Hypertension and Its Therapy

Hypertension in diabetics requires aggressive therapy (see Chapter 62). Hypertension seems to accelerate diabetic retinopathy and diabetic renal disease and is a major risk factor for coronary atherosclerosis and probably other large vessel atherosclerotic disease. Indeed, control of hypertension is the only intervention that has been shown to slow the progression of renal disease. The choice of a specific antihypertensive drug or combination of drugs is influenced by the type of diabetes present and the stage of complications.

In uncomplicated IDDM and NIDDM, thiazides are

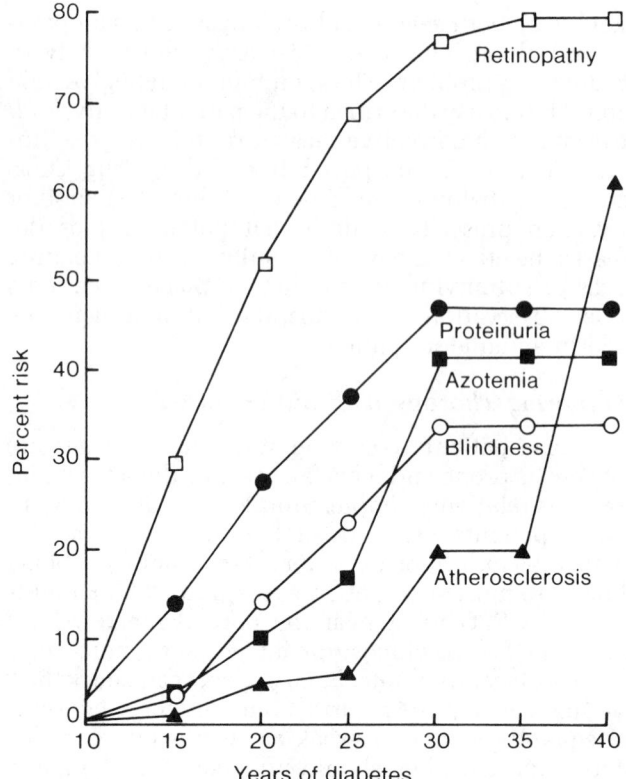

Figure 72.4. Complications of diabetes mellitus as a function of duration of the disease. (From Davidson MB: The continually changing "natural history" of diabetes mellitus. *J Chronic Dis* 34:5, 1981.)

still useful, although concern over their tendency to worsen glucose intolerance often deters their use. In NIDDM patients the dose of insulin can be increased slightly to compensate for this adverse effect. In contrast, a patient with NIDDM may show enough of a change of glucose tolerance to compromise what was acceptable therapy with an oral agent. Worsening hyperlipidemia is also a concern with these agents. Loop diuretics resemble the thiazides in their adverse action on glucose tolerance. Agents that promote orthostatic changes such as prazosin and methyldopa may be unacceptable in a diabetic who has autonomic dysfunction and already tends to have orthostatic changes. The β-adrenergic blocking agents are useful in many cases, despite some concerns. The nonselective β-blocking agents (propranolol, pindolol, nadolol, timolol) are best avoided because of possible worsening of glucose tolerance (inhibition of insulin release in NIDDM) and interference in recovery from hypoglycemia, masking of hypoglycemic symptoms, and occasional promotion of hyperkalemia. However, the selective β_1-blockers (atenolol, metoprolol) can be used since they are much less likely to produce these problems. Concern over aggravation of hyperlipidemia is unwarranted, since these drugs have only trivial effects on blood lipids. The so-called angiotensin-converting enzyme (ACE) inhibitors are also useful, especially in patients with nephropathy. Despite the occasional production of proteinuria in some patients,

ACE inhibitors may actually decrease proteinuria and slow progress of disease in diabetics with nephropathy. The calcium channel blockers, newly introduced for the treatment of hypertension, seem at this early point to be safe and effective for use in diabetics. Other problems with antihypertensives that may be especially troublesome in diabetics are impotence (diuretics, α or β adrenergic blockers), and hyperkalemia (triamterene, ACE inhibitors), presumably in relation to the hyporeninemic hypoaldosteronism often present in these patients.

Diabetic Peripheral Neuropathy

(See Chapter 84 for a general discussion of peripheral neuropathy.)

The prevalence of neurological deficits in diabetics is not known, although it is clear that in most patients the occurrence and severity of involvement are related to duration of the disease. The biomedical basis of functional change in diabetic neuropathy has been thought to involve excess formation of sorbitol and its sequelae, including altered tissue myoinositol (18). Microvascular insufficiency may also play a role (2, 6).

The most commonly appreciated abnormality is that which affects peripheral sensory nerves. Several types of sensation are involved (pain, proprioception, vibration, light touch) and can lead to unsteadiness, ataxic gait, and such uncommon but striking disorders as neuropathic arthropathy. Less well appreciated are the autonomic disorders that give rise to disturbances of cardiovascular function (postural hypotension, resting tachycardia), genitourinary function (impotence, bladder dysfunction), and gastrointestinal function (nocturnal diarrhea, fecal incontinence). Motor deficits are much less common but may occur with striking suddenness. Weakness is distal (neuropathic) rather than proximal (myopathic), although a specific type of myopathy also occurs in diabetics (see "Diabetic Myopathy" below). Some authors use the term *distal symmetrical sensorimotor polyneuropathy* to describe the commonest form of diabetic polyneuropathy.

Peripheral Sensory Neuropathy

Classically, the deficit is distal, with the lower extremities being first affected, followed by the upper extremities. The term "stocking-glove" distribution is appropriate. The disorder is a symmetric polyneuropathy with a proximal-distal gradient of dysfunction. In severe cases, even the sensory innervation of the trunk is involved; in this instance the most distal fibers are those of the anterior abdomen and lower thorax. Rarely, even the distal portions of the cranial nerves are affected (e.g., the distal sensory portion of the trigeminal nerve). The patterns of loss are not specific for diabetes mellitus and can be seen in such diverse states as amyloid neuropathy and toxic (e.g., lead) neuropathies. Whether the process represents a "dying back" of those nerves that are longest or is the cumulative result of randomly scattered lesions along the nerve trunks is not known.

The nerve damage may at first be asymptomatic but is revealed with careful questioning of the patient. Alternatively, the patient may first complain of hyperesthesia and dysesthesia, including tingling and burning sensations. Later, various symptoms are experienced including sensations of numbness or heaviness. Patients often complain that their feet feel "dead" or that they have a sensation of walking on a soft or nonexistent surface. Loss of ability to perceive temperature and firmness gives rise to these complaints. Severe, spontaneous, short-lived stabbing leg pains and cramps are common. Frequently these pains are most troublesome at night.

On neurological testing skin hypesthesia is the commonest finding (pinprick, two-point discrimination, light touch). The hypesthesia and loss of temperature perception lead to unappreciated skin trauma and predispose to infection. The sensory loss in the fingertips can prevent the blind diabetic from learning Braille letters. Deep tendon reflexes, especially that of the Achilles tendon, are lost, often in the early stages of the neuropathy.

Peripheral Motor Neuropathy

Much less common and less well recognized are the motor function abnormalities that occur as part of diabetic neuropathy. The intrinsic muscles of the feet are those most commonly involved. Interosseous atrophy produces inability to separate toes but, more important, allows the foot to assume abnormal positions. When claw or hammer toe develops, new pressure points appear at the tips of the toes and along the dorsal aspects; hyperkeratosis, callus formation, and ulceration follow. The interosseous atrophy that may affect the hands does not lead to total loss of function but does result in weakness of grip. Diffuse weakness of the legs and upper extremities may also occur.

Therapy of Painful Peripheral Neuropathies

Medical therapy is probably useless, except for analgesics as needed. Codeine or a similar agent is often necessary for relief of pain, and it may be required chronically. A number of drugs (phenytoin, amitriptyline, carbamazine, and diphenhydramine) have been recommended for treatment of pain in peripheral neuropathy, but there have been no controlled trials to test their efficacy (see Chapter 84 for additional details). Transcutaneous electrical nerve stimulation also has been said to be useful. Vitamin therapy is also frequently given but is almost certainly useless for this purpose. Aldose reductase inhibitors are promising, but still experimental, drugs.

Mononeuropathies

Mononeuropathy (mononeuritis simplex and multiplex) may occur in any superficial nerve (simplex) or asymmetric simultaneous combination (multiplex). The lower extremities are more commonly involved (femoral, lateral femoral cutaneous, sciatic, peroneal) than the upper (ulnar, radial, etc.). Onset is usually sudden with intense, often cramping and lancinating pain (see Tables 84.6 and 84.7). Typically, the pain is worse at night and, when the lower extremities are involved, may be relieved by pacing about. When the pain is radicular (trunk or abdomen) intrathoracic or intra-abdominal disease may be misdiagnosed.

At onset, diagnosis can only be surmised, although tenderness along a nerve trunk is very suggestive. Herpes zoster may be suspected, especially when hyperesthesia occurs, but when no vesicles appear and muscle weakness and atrophy are eventually evident, the diagnosis becomes obvious. The prognosis is quite good, with complete recovery within a few months the rule.

Cranial and oculomotor neuropathies. These monooneuropathies are distinguished from other mononeuropathies mainly by their location. Pain and headache may be present. The commonest nerves involved are III (palpebral ptosis, pupillary function undisturbed), VI (inward deviation of eye, diplopia), and IV (inward and upward deviations, diplopia). Recovery within 3 months is almost universal. When the facial nerve is involved, distinction from Bell's palsy is not possible (see Chapter 84), although the diabetic variety tends to be less severe and recovery is usually complete.

Neuropathic Foot Ulcers and Infections

Foot ulcers are common manifestations of diabetic neuropathy. Although the diabetic is certainly prone to vascular (arterial) insufficiency as well, and although the presence of large and small vessel disease often contributes, the origin of the problem is primarily the sensory deficit. Neuropathy often is asymptomatic until this late complication. Because the patient does not perceive pain normally, unappreciated trauma occurs, for example from poorly fitting shoes that produce pressure points that go unrelieved and end in penetrating abrasions. Wounds can also result from penetration by foreign materials or from self-trimming of nails. In addition to the sensory deficit, simultaneous motor weakness of extensor or flexor muscles together with proprioceptive defects can also contribute to anatomic deformity that in turn produces pressure points and ulceration.

Typically foot ulcers are plantar and occur at the point where weight bearing is greatest. Altered motor nerve function leads to muscle atrophy and tendon shortenings, which results in chronic toe flexion and finally hammer-toe deformity. This anatomic change shifts weight from the padded ball of the foot to the metatarsal heads where calluses form and contribute to the formation of new pressure points. The calluses themselves may develop fissures, which further promote ulceration.

The therapy of ulceration is primarily that of local foot care. Decreased weight bearing is usually essential. Infection is invariably present and is almost always a mixture of aerobic, facultatively anaerobic, and anaerobic organisms. Antibiotics of choice are a broad spectrum β-lactam or a combination of drugs that can be expected to be effective against all of these types of organisms (42). Because callus formation aggravates the tendency to increase local pressure and worsens ulceration, regular debridement is essential. Some patients can be taught debridement techniques, which may at least delay the intervals between visits for this purpose, but usually periodic professional assistance is essential. Such care is often best provided by podiatrists (see Chapter 102). Fitting of custom-made molded shoes is very helpful and is essential in some cases for prevention of ulceration. Remarkably, with proper treatment the ulcer may heal completely and not recur. However, recurrence is likely as long as the anatomic distortion or continued pressure is unchanged.

Autonomic Neuropathy

Abnormal Sweat Production

Almost always associated with other evidence of diabetic autonomic neuropathy, this complication in its typical form produces heat intolerance and increased sweating (hyperhydrosis) of the upper half of the body with decreased or absent sweating (anhydrosis) below the midtrunk. In other cases, anhydrosis is generalized and recognition of the complication may be difficult. In women the condition may be confused with menopausal sweats.

Affected patients have decreased thermoregulatory reserve and are predisposed to hyperthermia and heat stroke. Another consequence of impaired sweating includes failure to recognize hypoglycemia (see "Hypoglycemia Unawareness," page 935). This is a serious problem, since one of the warning signals of insulin reaction is lost. Many elderly patients, including those without diabetes mellitus, already have impaired sympathetic responses as a result of aging rather than of diabetes.

Cardiovascular Autonomic Neuropathies

In addition to abnormalities of innervation that result in abnormal cardiovascular reflexes (see below), diabetic cardiac denervation apparently accounts for the phenomenon of painless myocardial infarction, which is said to occur in more than 30% of diabetics who experience an acute event. Diagnosis is difficult unless acute electrocardiographic changes are present. Precipitation of unexplained ketoacidosis or myocardial failure may divert attention to these secondary events.

Resting Tachycardia. Heart rates of 90 to 100 beats/minute are common in patients with autonomic neuropathy; occasionally even higher rates are observed. Normal sleep-related bradycardia is absent. Parasympathetic damage is the apparent explanation; the sympathetics appear to be less affected. A β-blocker is useful if therapy is needed. In severe cases, the tachycardia subsides over the years as denervation becomes more complete and the sympathetics are also lost.

Several noninvasive tests are available to assess the presence of autonomic cardiovascular dysfunction. These include the Valsalva maneuver, beat-to-beat heart rate variation, and the lying-to-standing heart rate response. Such assessments are more subtle indicators of the presence of autonomic dysfunction than is postural hypotension. These tests are rarely of use clinically but do allow objective assessment. The consequences—or at least the associations—of these abnormal cardiovascular reflexes in diabetics are important. Once they have developed, there is a marked decrease of 5-year survival. Sudden death—not attributable to myocardial infarction—has been described in many such patients (13).

Postural Hypotension. The most readily recognized, and a most troublesome, cardiovascular abnormality is postural hypotension (see Chapter 84). The patient may complain merely of dizziness or faintness on standing, or the problem may be more severe, with visual disturbances and syncope. These symptoms may be confused with episodes of hypoglycemia. Remarkably, some patients with fairly marked postural hypotension are asymptomatic.

On initial examination, every diabetic patient should be checked for a postural decrease in blood pressure. In addition, a check for postural hypotension should be made whenever a potentially aggravating condition occurs. The onset or aggravation of postural hypotension is often associated with the beginning of therapy with a variety of drugs often used in diabetics such as antihypertensive drugs, including diuretics, vasodilators/antispasmodics such as nitroglycerin (glyceryl trinitrate), antidepressants (tricyclic), and phenothiazines. Occasional diabetic patients may be unable to tolerate effective doses of these drugs because of this problem.

The mechanism of this disorder is thought to reside in the efferent limb of the baroreceptor arc secondary to damaged sympathetic vasoconstrictor fibers in the splanchnic bed, muscles, and skin. Diminished plasma renin responses to postural change have been noted in such patients, as have abnormalities of plasma norepinephrine, but the role of these defects is not clear.

Various mechanical maneuvers, including the use of antigravity or "space" suits, have been recommended but are not useful. Drug therapy with vasopressors such as phenylephrine or combinations of tyramine or amine-containing cheeses and monoamine oxidase inhibitors have had their advocates. Clonidine has recently been advocated for this condition. For patients with severe postural hypotension, the most useful drug may be the mineralocorticoid, fludrocortisone (Florinef). In doses of 0.1 to 1.0 mg/day, the drug is often helpful, but since one of its actions is to expand fluid volume, it can precipitate cardiac failure or produce severe hypertension in the recumbent state. Refractoriness may eventually occur. In mild cases, the simple advice that the patient assume upright positions slowly by sitting on the edge of the bed after recumbency may help to avoid syncopal episodes, although continuing postural hypotension, though easily measured, may not be especially symptomatic (also see Chapter 84).

Digestive System Dysfunction

Most of the disorders of the gastrointestinal tract in diabetes are related to disturbances of motility. Esophageal motor dysfunction can be demonstrated on testing but is usually not a clinical problem.

Atony of the stomach (gastroparesis diabeticorum) is often asymptomatic but may be troublesome. Symptoms include anorexia, early satiety, postprandial fullness and bloating, and, occasionally, vomiting. Delayed and unpredictable emptying of the stomach may produce irregular diabetic control in already difficult to manage patients with IDDM. Diagnosis is apparent—sometimes as an incidental finding—on barium X-ray of the upper gastrointestinal tract. Metoclopramide (Reglan) 10 mg, three times daily, is helpful (see Chapter 37).

Small bowel dysfunction is common and symptomatic, leading to "diabetic diarrhea." Typically the diarrhea is nocturnal. Fecal incontinence, a result of impaired sensation of rectal distention, may occur and is very distressing. The disorder tends to be episodic, with attacks lasting from a few days to weeks or rarely months. Watery brown diarrhea, usually without steatorrhea, is typical. On barium X-ray studies of the small bowel the findings are those of disturbed motility. Despite the distressing symptoms, the patient appears well; weight loss is uncommon. When steatorrhea occurs, pancreatic exocrine insufficiency and sprue syndrome, more common in diabetics than in the general population, enter the differential. Fully developed sprue is associated with gross evidence of malabsorption. A trial of antibiotic therapy (e.g., tetracycline, 250 mg four times a day for 2 weeks) may improve the diarrhea and the malabsorption if the latter is due to small bowel stasis and bacterial colonization. Symptomatic treatment with antispasmodics (e.g., Lomotil) may be useful, especially when attacks of diarrhea are short lived.

Large bowel complaints, especially of constipation, are common in the elderly. It does not appear that diabetics are especially prone to any additional problems in this regard.

Patients with poorly controlled diabetes may develop fatty changes of the liver. Hepatomegaly and/or elevations of liver enzymes may occur. Effective control of blood sugar results in disappearance of these abnormalities.

Bladder Dysfunction (Neurogenic Bladder)

The symptoms of bladder dysfunction in diabetics are often overlooked (4). Onset is insidious and occurs over many years. Most patients (80%) will have clinical evidence of neuropathy affecting other systems. The first clinical manifestation of bladder dysfunction is an increase in the interval between voidings until urine is passed only twice or even once daily. A need to strain, slow stream, dribbling, and sensation of incomplete voiding may be present. These symptoms should be routinely solicited from diabetics, especially when there are symptoms or signs of peripheral neuropathy.

Demonstration of residual urine is the hallmark of clinically symptomatic cystopathy, but many diabetic patients, when studied by cystometric techniques, have objective evidence of a neurogenic involvement and a grossly enlarged bladder well before symptoms are evident (4). At this stage, residual urine is not present and other urinary tract abnormalities (recurrent infections) are not evident. If large volumes of residual urine do develop, patients become prone to infection (see Chapter 27) and incontinence (see Chapter 6).

Patients suspected to have cystopathy should be referred to a urologist for evaluation and for recommendations about treatment.

Sexual Dysfunction

The frequency of erectile impotence is high in diabetes, perhaps 50 to 60% overall. This complication, like many others in diabetes, is related to duration of disease. The problem is usually due to a type of autonomic neuropathy involving the pelvic parasympathetic nerves, put impaired blood flow is the cause in some cases.

Impotence is a common problem in nondiabetic men, and the problems leading to such impotence must be included in the differential diagnosis in the diabetic. Psychogenic factors probably account for the large majority of nondiabetic cases. Although no evidence suggests that psychogenic problems are any more common in diabetics, neither are diabetics immune to psychogenic disturbances. The onset of diabetic impotence is usually slow (6 months to several years), often associated with retrograde ejaculation; impotence eventually becomes complete. Despite this, libido is characteristically retained. Although patients with psychogenic impotence often report nocturnal erections and emissions and may retain masturbatory activity, all of these are absent in diabetic impotence.

An important point on clinical examination is that testicular sensitivity to pressure sufficient to cause pain is retained in men with psychogenic impotence but is often greatly diminished or lost in the diabetic in whom accompanying sensory neuropathy is common.

Endocrinological causes of impotence (see also Chapters 18 and 77) should be considered because they are potentially treatable, but it is rare to find an endocrine basis for impotence in the diabetic. Testosterone secretion, easily verified by plasma testosterone measurement, is invariably normal in diabetics; therefore, as one would expect, testosterone therapy is useless.

A variety of drugs, especially ones that are often used in diabetics, may cause impotence. The most common offenders are the nondiuretic antihypertensives (see Chapter 62).

Several studies report that, in contrast to the male, sexual function in diabetic women appears to be unaffected by the disease. Others have asserted that many diabetic women lose the ability to achieve orgasm (12).

The differential diagnosis and therapy of impotence are discussed in detail in Chapter 18. Considerable success has been achieved in diabetics by use of penile implants, including inflatable prosthetic devices. One of several vacuum devices can produce a functional erection (43). Intrapenile injections of papaverine plus phentolamine are effective in some cases (24).

Neuropathic Arthropathy (Charcot's Joint; Diabetic Charcot's Foot)

This complication of diabetes is frequently unrecognized or misdiagnosed. The disorder, preceded by a sensory neuropathy, is a progressive, degenerative change of the bony structure of the foot, most often involving the tarsal and tarsometatarsal joints (60%), but also the metatarsophalangeal joints (30%) and the ankle (10%). The prevalence has been estimated at one in 680 cases, but the disorder is probably more common. The patient presents with a swollen foot, often attributed to or associated with recent trauma. The foot may be painful or may be remarkably free of pain, considering the appearance. Examination shows moderate to gross deformity of the foot with "rocker-bottom" subluxation of the midtarsal region or subluxation of the metatarsophalangeal joints. Usually the foot is erythematous and warm to the touch. An infected neuropathic ulcer may be present. More often than not, the pulses are intact. Physicians unfamiliar with this presentation are likely to diagnose some other type of inflammatory arthritis or osteomyelitis, and their impression may be "verified" by the X-ray findings. In these early stages, the X-rays show severe osteoarthritis, but, as the disease progresses, there is complete destruction of the involved joints with resorption of the metatarsal heads and phalangeal diaphyses. Various other bony changes occur, including fractures, joint effusions, and subluxations. When these changes are at the maximal stage, i.e., when soft tissue involvement is most prominent, the diagnosis of osteomyelitis is frequently entertained, especially when there is an associated, often infected, ulcer. Synovial biopsy showing a thickened synovium containing osseous debris may provide the correct diagnosis and avoid the necessity of embarking on a prolonged and difficult course of antibiotic therapy for suspected osteomyelitis.

Diabetic Charcot's foot may also be confused with the changes associated with osteoarthritis and gouty, rheumatoid, and psoriatic arthritis. Consultation by an orthopaedic surgeon, rheumatologist, or podiatrist to confirm the diagnosis and to assist with therapy is almost always indicated.

Treatment is based on the cessation of further trauma

to the affected area, which is best accomplished by elimination of weight bearing. Hospitalization may be necessary for this purpose. Reduction of edema and signs of inflammation may take several weeks. Immobilization with a cast may be helpful but should not be undertaken in the acute stage and, if used, should be done with great care to ensure the integrity of the areas covered by the cast. Simpler boot-like devices may also be used. Crutches can be used at this point, followed eventually by a walking cast. Up to 4 months of treatment may be required. Thereafter, molded or contoured shoes are essential to proper long-term management. Surgical intervention is inadvisable, although occasionally a stabilization procedure may be required if conservative therapy fails. Amputation is not indicated unless osteomyelitis unequivocally coexists or the entire process fails to respond to prolonged conservative efforts. Despite the discouraging appearance of the foot at its worst stages, sufficient healing and stabilization to produce a useful foot can be anticipated.

Other foot problems in the diabetic. A number of common foot problems (e.g., bunions, calluses, corns, fungal infections, and ingrown toenails) can lead to devastating complications in diabetic patients. Prevention through proper foot care and early recognition and treatment are important considerations in the long-term care of every diabetic patient. These problems are discussed in detail in Chapter 102.

Neuropathic Cachexia

Another rare complication is known as neuropathic cachexia. Seen in both men and women, the typical case is a man in his 60s suffering from anorexia and profound weight loss. The extremities are painful and bilateral neuropathy is common. Spontaneous recovery in about 1 year can be expected in most cases.

Diabetic Myopathy (Amyotrophy or Proximal Asymmetric Motor Neuropathy)

This is a rare but devastating complication of diabetes mellitus that is thought by some to be a proximal motor neuropathy. Severe asymmetric proximal muscle weakness and pain usually affect the pelvic girdle and thigh muscles, although upper truncal musculature can also be involved. The typical patient is an elderly, NIDDM patient with mild disease. Men are more frequently affected than are women. Onset may be fairly rapid, and low grade fever and elevated erythrocyte sedimentation rate may be present. Cerebrospinal fluid protein may be very high. Muscle biopsy shows fiber degeneration. Prognosis for improvement is good, but significant residuals are common.

Diabetic Nephropathy

Progressive renal failure is another life-threatening complication of diabetes. The relationship between hyperglycemia (or insulin deficiency) and the development of microangiopathy with eventual nodular glomerulosclerosis (Kimmelsteil-Wilson disease) remains to be unequivocally established, but experimental evidence is accumulating in favor of such a relationship. Moreover, from observations in man, it now seems clear that the cause is either hyperglycemia, per se, or some other factor in the internal milieu of the diabetic that is responsible for the development of diabetic renal disease, since kidney transplants in diabetic patients often develop typical lesions of diabetes.

Diabetic patients with even minimal elevations of serum creatinine above 1.1 mg/dl, but not those with normal renal function, are at increased risk of acute renal failure from contrast media used in various radiographic procedures. Although the risk is only moderately increased (about 10 to 15% in the highest risk patients versus 5% in low risk patients and <2% in those with no renal disease and in normals), these procedures can often be replaced by others with less risk [magnetic resonance imaging (MRI); sonography]. If contrast media are to be used, the dose should be minimal and the patient well hydrated.

The clinical course of diabetic nephropathy and the impact of failing renal function on insulin requirement and the oral hypoglycemic drugs are discussed in Chapter 48.

Infections

Although it has never been established unequivocally that diabetics are more prone to infections than nondiabetics, most clinicians will encounter patients who have experienced repeated bacterial or fungal skin infections (carbuncles, furuncles, external otitis, moniliasis) or gastrointestinal moniliasis at some time before the diagnosis of diabetes was made or in association with uncontrolled hyperglycemia. Most authorities seem to agree that, once established, infections in the diabetic are difficult to treat and patients are prone to develop complications. Experimentally, hyperglycemia inhibits the phagocytic activity of granulocytes, a factor that may contribute to lowered host resistance. Control of blood sugar, therefore, should be part of any treatment program for an infection.

Urinary tract infections are an especially troublesome problem in diabetics. Although infections are not clearly increased in incidence, a greater prevalence of complications is obvious. Half of all cases of papillary necrosis occur in diabetics. Diabetic patients also seem prone to develop infections with unusual pathogens. However, no statistical case has been made for the desirability of suppression of asymptomatic bacteriuria in diabetics. Development of pyelonephritis is an indication for immediate hospitalization and vigorous antibiotic treatment; risk of renal carbuncle formation is a special hazard for the diabetic.

Skin infections due to *Candida* occur frequently in diabetics, especially those with NIDDM who are obese and require therapy with a local antifungal agent (see Chapter 100) as well as control of hyperglycemia.

Diabetic Retinopathy

This complication of diabetes mellitus has become one of the leading causes of blindness in the United States. In IDDM patients some degree of retinopathy can be detected by the most sensitive technique, angiography, after as little as 1 to 2 years in 10% of patients. By 10 years, retinopathy is evident in 50% of cases by ophthalmoscopy with a 70% prevalence by angiography. At 25 years nearly all patients can be shown to have some degree of retinopathy. By the time diabetes has been present for 15 to 20 years, about one-third of patients have severe disease and another one-half have obvious but lesser degrees of progressive retinal involvement. Remarkably, not all cases of early retinopathy are progressive.

Patients with NIDDM also develop retinopathy, apparently with less frequency (11), but when retinopathy does develop in this older group, the process seem to progress even more rapidly than it does in IDDM patients. Hyperglycemia, as indirectly measured by glycosylated hemoglobin, appears to predict the incidence and progression of diabetic retinopathy in NIDDM (22). However, attempts to normalize blood glucose in small numbers of patients have thus far not slowed the progression of retinopathy. The Diabetes Control and Complications Trial (DCCT) is underway. This prospective study of 1400 patients assigned to either intensive or conventional insulin treatment should provide more reliable information on the efficacy of therapeutic intervention.

Blindness in Diabetic Retinopathy

The visual loss in diabetic retinopathy is potentially even more severe than in blindness due to other causes. Many persons who are legally blind (defined as visual acuity less than 20/200 in both eyes) due to causes other than diabetes have slow onset of visual loss, thus allowing time for adaptation. In addition, they often retain reasonably full visual fields and visual acuity at or close to the legal limit. Such persons can see well enough to ambulate independently and to perform a variety of common activities (self-care, housework). With the aid of special devices they may even be able to read newsprint and to engage in some occupations. In contrast, the visual loss from diabetic retinopathy is often due to sudden hemorrhage or retinal detachment and frequently leaves the patient with only light perception. In addition, the diabetic frequently already has other complications of the disease when blindness develops.

Although total blindness afflicts only a minority of diabetic patients (11), a larger number suffer some degree of loss of visual acuity due to macular edema, the commonest cause of visual loss in diabetics (see below).

Ocular Symptoms

Diabetics who experience symptoms of visual disturbance need not be experiencing a catastrophic complication. Like others, diabetics develop changes of visual acuity such as a change in refractive error and astigmatism. In addition, they can experience decreased visual acuity as a result of marked changes in blood sugar, e.g., as the lens swells during acute normalization of blood sugar after prolonged hyperglycemia.

Persistent change of visual acuity requires examination by an ophthalmologist, especially when advanced retinal disease, proliferative diabetic retinopathy (PDR), is present. A common cause of visual loss in PDR, macular edema (see below), is not readily detectable by the direct ophthalmoscopy available to internists and requires stereoscopic examination by an ophthalmologist.

Sudden, painless loss of vision in PDR is often due to hemorrhage from proliferating new vessels or from retinal detachment. Lesser degrees of hemorrhage may cause "floaters" or "cobwebs." Another complication in PDR is outflow obstruction of the aqueous humor produced by fibrous scar tissue extending into the "angle" of the anterior chamber causing a marked rise in intraocular pressure and acute ("neovascular") glaucoma with severe pain. Loss of vision will occur unless emergency therapy is given.

Types of Retinal Disease in Diabetics

The current classification of diabetic retinal disease is nonproliferative (synonym, "background") (BDR), preproliferative (PPDR), and proliferative retinopathy (PDR). The latter, more advanced stage is the point at which sudden and massive visual loss becomes a problem.

Nonproliferative (BDR) and preproliferative (PPDR) retinopathy. The earliest lesions—readily visible with an ordinary ophthalmoscope—are in the region of the macula: microaneurysms, punctate retinal hemorrhages, hard exudates, soft exudates ("cotton wool"), and so-called intraretinal microvascular anomalies (IRMAs). Both microaneurysms and small "dot" intraretinal hemorrhages appear as red dots, and both tend to fade within months. Blot hemorrhages are larger. Distinction can best be made by fluorescein angiograms in which only microaneurysms "light up." This procedure, performed by an ophthalmologist, often identifies extensive intraretinal disease when only a few abnormalities are evident by ophthalmoscopy.

Hard exudates are glistening yellow or white lipid deposits located in the outer retinal layers. If they are greater than one disc diameter from the macula, they are not ominous. Soft exudates are areas of ischemia or infarction of the nerve fiber layer; they disappear within a few months. IRMAs are dilated, hypercellular vessels that are thought to represent either dilated capillaries or intraretinal vascular proliferation. These telangiectatic vessels are identifiable using the green filters of an ordinary ophthalmoscope but are best seen in the secondary phase of fluorescein angiograms during which they leak dye into the retina. IRMAs occur adjacent to areas of capillary closure. Their identification is not essential in the routine examination.

Whereas changes of background retinopathy indicate capillary damage and leakage, preproliferative changes [many soft exudates, extensive hemorrhages, IRMAs, and venous bleeding from enlarged dilated (beaded, sausage-link) retinal veins] indicate areas of intraretinal vascular occlusion with resulting nonperfusion. Decreased visual acuity at this stage requires an ophthalmologist's examination to determine with stereoscopic techniques whether macular edema is present. It is not usually appreciated by general physicians that *even without proliferative disease*, macular edema may result in visual loss as severe as the 20/200 level. Spontaneous improvement is not common but may occur. Visual acuity can also become poor due to lack of proper perfusion of the perifoveal capillaries. In this instance, visual acuity may be as low as 20/200 in the absence of macular edema. Fluorescein angiography will reveal the cause of poor visual acuity due to the lack of perfusion of the perifoveal capillaries. In the absence of accompanying proliferative disease, patients at this stage can usually ambulate freely and can engage in some occupations. Ability to read a newspaper, except with a vision aid, is unlikely, and the patient will have to relinquish driving a vehicle because driver's license vision requirements will no longer be met.

Eyes with retinal ischemia and moderate to severe preproliferative changes have a 50% chance of developing new vessel proliferation (neovascularization) within 1 year.

Proliferative retinopathy (PDR). At this stage of retinal disease, new vessels and accompanying fibrous tissue extend from the retinal substance and grow along the inner retinal surface and the posterior surface of the vitreous gel, often causing contraction of the gel and traction on the vessels and the retina. This process creates the conditions for retinal detachment and hemorrhage into the vitreous.

In addition, in advanced PDR, growth of new vessels and scar tissue into the "angle" of the eye may cause acute glaucoma (see "Ocular Symptoms"). When the new blood vessels grow into the optic nerve heads, they are termed *new vessels on the disc* (NVD); elsewhere in the retina, usually extending from large vessels, they are termed *new vessels elsewhere* (NVE).

The National Diabetic Retinopathy Study (DRS) not only established the efficacy of photocoagulation therapy (see below), but defined high risk characteristics as follows: (*a*) NVD greater than 25% of the optic disc area; (*b*) any NVD with preretinal or vitreous hemorrhage; or NVE equal to or exceeding 50% of the disc area with preretinal or vitreous hemorrhage. The presence of high risk characteristics increases the chance of blindness to 30 to 50% within 3 to 5 years unless appropriate photocoagulation therapy is given.

Treatment of Diabetic Retinopathy

Two forms of surgical therapy are now available for the treatment of proliferative retinopathy and its complications. Photocoagulation is of proven value in the prevention of visual loss due to proliferative disease, and vitrectomy restores and appears to stabilize vision after hemorrhage and/or retinal detachment.

Photocoagulation therapy. Argon *laser* therapy has been shown to reduce severe visual loss by nearly 60% over 5 years in patients with proliferative disease (31). Multiple (1200 to 1600 500-micrometer) burns are placed in the retinal periphery. The Early Treatment Diabetic Retinopathy Study (ETDRS) is currently evaluating panretinal photocoagulation (and laser photocoagulation using 450 to 650 widely spaced burns) to determine whether such therapy affects the course of disease in eyes with high risk characteristics or PPDR.

Diabetic macular edema is also treated with photocoagulation therapy. Leaking microaneurysms and other lesions in the macula are treated with 50- to 100-micrometer burns. ETDRS recently showed a reduction of visual loss due to macular edema of 50% over 3 years.

Patient experience. Photocoagulation therapy is an office procedure, usually performed in several sessions. Ordinarily only topical (corneal) anesthesia is necessary. Occasionally, some discomfort may be experienced, in which case a local anesthetic is injected into the retro-orbital tissues to allow a completed, pain-free procedure.

Vitrectomy for proliferative retinopathy. Hemorrhage into the vitreous is the usual indication for vitrectomy, a procedure that removes old blood and opaque vitreous and can be combined with cataract extraction. Retinal detachment resulting from traction bands that are formed in the vitreous is another indication for vitrectomy. Other repair procedures can be attempted. The results of vitrectomy can be dramatic in restoring sight after vitreous hemorrhage. Currently, however, vitrectomy is used only in severely diseased eyes. Recovery of near-normal vision is the exception rather than the rule.

Every effort should be made to control hypertension in an effort to prevent retinal hemorrhages. Lifting of heavy objects, jarring exercise, and exposures to high altitudes may also increase the risk of hemorrhages and should be avoided.

Role of the Internist versus Ophthalmologist; Indications for Referral

The internist or primary care physician should perform regular examinations of the eyegrounds of diabetic patients in order to ensure prompt and appropriate referral to an ophthalmologist (Table 72.12). Because most diabetic retinopathy occurs within several disc diameters of the macula, most lesions are visible by examination with the direct ophthalmoscope after dilation of the pupils. Nonophthalmologists frequently

Table 72.12.
Reasons for Referral of Patients with Diabetes Mellitus to an Ophthalmologist[a]

High Risk Patients
Neovascularization covering more than one-third of optic disk;
vitreous or preretinal hemorrhage with any neovascularization, particularly on optic disk; or
Macular edema (suspect from hard exudates in macula).

Symptomatic patients
Blurry vision persisting for more than 1 to 2 days or not associated with a change in blood glucose; suspect macular edema;
sudden loss of vision in one or both eyes; or
black spots, cobwebs, or flashing lights in field of vision.

Asymptomatic patients
Yearly examinations; (an optometrist can check pressures if no retinal changes or if only BDR is present);
hard exudates near macula;
any preproliferative or proliferative characteristics; or pregnancy.

[a]Modified from American Diabetes Association Physician's Guide to Non-insulin Dependent (Type II) Diabetes. Diagnosis and Treatment. 2nd Ed. Alexandria, VA. 1988.

defer this examination out of concern over precipitating acute angle-closure glaucoma. Such reluctance is not warranted, since this complication is rare at any age and is hardly ever seen before age 40. A drop of dilating solution (2.5% phenylephrine; 1% tropicanide) in each eye is sufficient and causes only sensitivity to bright light (requiring dark glasses) that lasts but a few hours. In addition to examining the retina, the physician should note the condition of the lens, since senile cataracts occur prematurely in diabetics and metabolic cataracts result from chronic elevation of blood glucose levels.

If only nonproliferative diabetic retinopathy is present, the patient need not be referred routinely provided that visual acuity is normal. Early preproliferative changes (see above) also do not warrant referral, but more extensive changes and proliferative changes should be followed by an ophthalmologist who is expert in photocoagulation. Periodic checks of intraocular pressure to detect glaucoma, especially important in diabetics, are, of course, part of routine health maintenance but can be made by an optometrist (see Chapter 98).

DIABETES DURING PREGNANCY

General

Pregnancy in the diabetic woman presents a major challenge to the physicians involved in the care of the mother and the fetus. Ideally, the medical team should include both an experienced internist/diabetologist and an obstetrician who cooperate actively in the management of the pregnancy. Others in the team may include an experienced teaching nurse and, ultimately, a pediatrician/neonatologist.

The course of the pregnancy in a diabetic woman and its impact on the fetus will depend on the type of diabetes and the stage of the disease at which the pregnancy occurs. Unless these are defined, it is not possible to address the issues of management and out-

come; generalizations tend to be meaningless. Thus, when pregnancy occurs in the IDDM diabetic without diabetic complications, who is already under close medical supervision and is practicing intensive insulin therapy, management of the diabetes consists of continuation of therapy with institution of even lower limits for blood glucose and special attention to avoidance of nocturnal hypoglycemia (see below). When pregnancy occurs in a diabetic woman with vascular disease, the mother is in danger of an adverse outcome. Nephropathy may worsen, at least temporarily, especially if hypertension is present. Premature delivery and smaller than normal infants occur with even modest increases of serum creatinine (greater than 1.5 mg/dl) and with proteinuria. Diabetic retinopathy, especially if already proliferative, or if hypertension is present, may progress rapidly and result in loss of visual acuity. Under these latter circumstances, various questions must be asked. Should an abortion be considered? Does the woman fully understand the risks of continuing the pregnancy?

Many experts are now convinced that modern *optimal* management of diabetes during pregnancy has reduced perinatal infant mortality to that of nondiabetic women. However, the treatment of most pregnant diabetic women is in fact less than optimal. It is the exceptional baby that is conceived in a mother whose diabetes is under rigorous control by intensive therapy, whose physical and emotional health is uncompromised by the diabetes, and whose physicians always provide unerring exemplary advice and care.

Implications for Pregnancy of GTT-Diagnosed Glucose Tolerance

A study of the effect of glucose intolerance, not overt diabetes, diagnosed by glucose tolerance test reported significant step-wise increases of macrosomia, congenital abnormalities, perinatal mortality, prematurity, toxemia, and cesarean section as the 2-hour plasma glucose increased from 100 to 164 mg/dl (37). These observations have been challenged (26). However, on the basis of this report and others, many obstetricians initiate therapy with insulin that is designed to maintain fasting and postprandial blood sugars that are normal *for pregnancy*. Such an approach demands self-monitoring of blood glucose (SMBG). Many physicians, especially internists, remain skeptical of this approach as overtly aggressive. Studies utilizing such intervention are not yet available. However, one can be certain that such therapy will be attended by many episodes of hypoglycemia. In numerous earlier studies the prognosis for the pregnant state and the perinatal morbidity of infants born of mothers with an abnormal OGTT but with essentially normal FPG did not differ from normal. This has led some to advocate diet therapy alone, so long as maternal fasting and postprandial glucose levels remain within the range of normal for the nonpregnant state. Nonetheless, the current authoritative view is that pregnant women with abnormalities of blood glucose should probably be vigorously treated (15).

Fetal Mortality and Congenital Malformations

The view that the more severe the diabetic state, the worse the perinatal survival has been definitively substantiated by a recent, large, multicenter study (25) that has shown that overtly diabetic women with nearly normal blood glucose levels are at no greater risk of having a spontaneous abortion than nondiabetic women (83% successful outcome). In contrast, those with elevated blood glucose and elevated glycosylated hemoglobin in the first trimester have additional risk, estimated to be increased by 3% for each standard deviation above the normal range. In contrast to earlier reports, patients classified according to White Class scale rating (severity of diabetes based on age at onset, duration of disease, presence of complications) showed no difference between groups (26). Ketoacidosis occurs in 2 to 10% of diabetic pregnancies and is associated in these cases with fetal losses of 80 to 100%.

The incidence of significant congenital abnormalities in nondiabetic women is about 2 to 3% but rises as much as 4-fold overall to 8 to 12% in infants born to type I diabetics and reaches 25% when control is poor, as evidenced by grossly elevated glycosylated hemoglobin. All authorities now agree that hyperglycemia during the early weeks of pregnancy (gestational weeks 3 to 7 when embryogenesis occurs) appears to account for the increased incidence of congenital malformations. Near normalization of blood sugar before conception and continued normalization through the critical first weeks has been reported to reduce this increased incidence to normal.

Maternal Mortality and Morbidity

Maternal mortality during pregnancy is definitely increased and at 0.5% is about 20 times that in nondiabetics. Most deaths are due to ketoacidosis or to hypoglycemia, the latter usually occurring in the first trimester or immediately postpartum, times at which insulin requirements often decrease. Obviously, optimal management could eliminate most or all of these deaths. Some deaths that may not be preventable include infections after cesarean section or hemorrhage after traumatic delivery of a large infant. Diabetics with overt heart disease (ischemic heart disease, congestive heart failure) have a very high mortality (75%) when allowed to go to term. Such patients should never become pregnant or should have an abortion if pregnancy occurs.

Maternal morbidity also increases during the diabetic pregnancy. Polyhydramnios occurs in 25% of pregnancies (10 times greater incidence than expected). Asymptomatic bacteriuria (20%) and frank pyelonephritis (7%) occur three times more often than in the general population. Pyelonephritis is said to occur in 25% of bacteriuric diabetics and is associated with a very high rate of fetal loss.

Diagnosis of Diabetes during Pregnancy

In 1985 the American Diabetes Association recommended that all pregnant women be screened for diabetes between the 24th and 28th weeks of pregnancy using a 50-g oral glucose load and a single blood sample 1 hour later. If the value exceeds 140 mg/dl, a glucose tolerance test is performed using 100 g of glucose. Criteria for diagnosis of diabetes are given in Table 72.4. The screening procedure identifies 80 to 90% of diabetics but has 15 to 20% "false-positives."

Management of Overt Diabetes during Pregnancy

Insulin Therapy; Monitoring Control

Patients with overt diabetes including gestational diabetes who are receiving insulin therapy should be monitored to establish optimal control of blood sugar. Although some obstetricians still favor hospitalization with frequent daytime blood sugar determinations ("glucose panel") as an aid to establishment of optimal control, the procedure is useless unless patient compliance can be foreseen after the hospitalization.

Several studies have reported that normalization of blood sugar ("tight control") is associated with reduction of fetal loss from 25% to 3 or 4%. On the basis of this information, the goal of insulin and diet therapy should be the closest approximation of normalization of blood sugar that is possible using self-monitoring of blood glucose (SMBG) while avoiding therapeutic heroics, i.e., multiple and prolonged hospitalizations solely for the purpose of blood sugar control. Normal fasting blood sugar (not exceeding 90 mg/dl), preprandial blood sugar less than 105 mg/dl, and 2-hour postprandial blood sugars that do not exceed 120 mg/dl are considered "tight control." However, some obstetricians using conventional therapy with insulin strive for blood sugar levels *averaging* 100 mg/dl, a goal probably impossible to achieve without prolonged hospitalizations and excessively frequent hypoglycemia. If normalization of blood sugar is attempted, either intensified conventional therapy or an insulin pump should be used in conjunction, of course, with SMBG (see page 932). Intensified therapy is probably to be preferred, since ketoacidosis and infection are significant risks with pump therapy; either complication could be lethal to the fetus.

Most patients managed with less than intensive therapy will require at least two doses of intermediate-acting insulin or mixtures of intermediate- and short-acting insulin. A few NIDDM patients may have satisfactory control on a single dose of insulin. It should be kept in mind that insulin requirements often decrease in the first trimester only to increase during the third trimester by up to 50% and to fall again after delivery. Patients on intensive therapy should monitor their glucose in the fasting (overnight) state, before each meal, and, possibly, 2 hours after meals. In addition, monitoring during the night (2 to 3 A.M.) may be necessary, since nocturnal hypoglycemia is common during pregnancy, especially in the first and third trimesters. Frequent monitoring of glucosuria and ketonuria remains an invaluable adjunct to ambulatory management, but only SMBG with frequent determinations can provide optimal management. Minor ketonuria due to carbohydrate lack is common but can usually be distinguished from ketoacidosis by rough quantitation of the ketonuria, minimal or absent glucosuria, and by measurement of the blood sugar at less than 200 mg/dl. Determination of plasma bicarbonate and plasma "ketones" (negative when ketonuria is due to carbohydrate lack) should be made if any doubt still exists. The development of ketoacidosis is an indication for immediate hospitalization.

Diet Therapy

Diet therapy is often modified slightly to include increased protein intake. Weight gain of about 25 lb (11.5 kg) is expected and acceptable in both normal and diabetic pregnancies. Severe weight control, previously advocated by some, has been abandoned.

Timing of Delivery

This issue is decided by the obstetrician (and neonatologist) and has been argued for decades, since it was recognized that the incidence of stillbirths in diabetics increases beyond the 36th week. However, attempts to deliver infants early (before 40 weeks) resulted in a high rate of cesarean section and a high rate of neonatal loss due to neonatal respiratory distress syndrome (RDS). Currently, if fetal surveillance is normal, delivery is delayed to term when it is induced if the cervix is favorable or if spontaneous labor occurs. However, if the pregnancy has been complicated by vascular disease, poor control of glucose, or if there are other adverse factors such as a prior stillbirth, delivery may be performed at 38 weeks in an effort to prevent late fetal death. Such early delivery is predicated upon finding suitable values for amniotic fluid phospholipids (lecithin:sphingomyelin (LS) ratio and the presence of phosphatidylglycerol), biochemical markers of fetal pulmonary maturation. RDS is highly unlikely if LS is greater than 2.0. Delivery despite fetal pulmonary immaturity may be necessary if the pregnant patient worsens (pre-eclampsia, renal failure) or there is other evidence of fetal distress.

Counseling the Diabetic Woman—Risks of Pregnancy

The issue of the complexity of diabetic management is not likely to deter pregnancy. On the other hand, the possibility of diabetes in the newborn or young child is often of great concern; this issue has already been discussed (see "Inheritance and Genetic Counseling"). Other questions concern maternal and fetal mortality. Although the diabetic mother without overt complications suffers little or no increased risk, the fetal issues must be presented with candor. Of special importance beyond that of infant survival is the problem of an increased risk of congenital abnormalities (see above) and long-term neurological abnormalities

in children of diabetic mothers (19). Therefore, preconception patient education and intensive therapy are extremely important for young diabetic women who plan to become pregnant.

Whether complications of diabetes are accelerated by pregnancy is not clear, although nephropathy and retinopathy may worsen, as discussed above. The long-term survival of the diabetic with microvascular disease is already significantly compromised and an honest prognosis in this regard may deter pregnancy, not necessarily because of concern over acceleration of the diabetic complications, but out of concern for the future welfare of a child born to a mother whose state of health may be poor and whose survival is threatened.

General References

American Diabetes Association: *Diabetes Care.*
>This journal contains reviews and practical articles.
Brody SA, Kent U (eds): *Endocrine disorders in pregnancy.* East Norwalk, CT, Appleton and Lange, 1989.
Davidson MB: *Diabetes mellitus. Diagnosis and treatment,* 2nd ed., New York, John Wiley & Sons, 1986.
>This text contains a wealth of practical information for treatment of the ambulatory patient: numerous references to literature available to patients, diet, sources of aids for the visually impaired, syringe magnifiers, etc.
DeGroot LJ, Besser GM, Cahill GF, et al (eds): *Endocrinology,* 2nd ed, 3 vols. Philadelphia, Saunders, 1989.
>The largest textbook of endocrinology, by outstanding authorities. Diabetes is covered in vol 2, pp. 803–1798.
Diabetes Self Management, PO Box 1186, Dover, NY, 07801.
>A periodical (6 issues per year), aimed at patients, devoted to a variety of practical subjects for patients. Publishes articles on ratings and prices of available equipment (glucose meters, etc.).
Hare JW (ed): *Diabetes complicating pregnancy: the Joslin Clinic Method.* New York, Alan R. Liss, 1989.
International Diabetes Center, Park Nicollet Medical Foundation, 500 W 39th St, Minneapolis, MN 55415.
>Booklets, slides, narrative cassettes for a variety of problems of interest to the diabetic ranging from diet exchange lists to impotence.
Lebovitz HE (ed): *Physician's Guide to Non-Insulin-Dependent (Type II) Diabetes. Diagnosis and Treatment,* 2nd ed. Alexandria, VA, American Diabetes Association, 1988. 63 pp. (paperback).
>This publication and the one edited by Sperling (below) are successful efforts to present to the practicing physician practical guidance in the care of diabetics. Carefully edited by outstanding authorities, they contain a wealth of up-to-date information in readable form. Highly recommended as an alternative to a larger textbook. Many references. May be ordered by mail ($22.45 per volume) from the American Diabetes Association, Alexandria, VA 22314.
National Diabetes Data Group: Classification and diagnosis of diabetes mellitus and other categories of glucose intolerance. *Diabetes* 28:1039, 1979.
>The latest criteria for diagnosis; a milestone in our concepts of the problem. Many references.
Practical Diabetology, Rapaport Publishing, Inc, 42-15 Crescent St, Long Island NY 11101.
>Short reviews of topics of interest to physicians treating diabetics.
Rifkin H, Porte Jr D (eds): *Diabetes Mellitus: Theory and Practice,* 4th ed. NY, NY, and Amsterdam, The Netherlands, Elsevier, 1990.
>This is the standard textbook on the subject.
Rizza RA, Green DA (eds): Diabetes Mellitus. *Med Clin North Am* 72:1271, 1988.
>A recent, up-to-date series of articles on all clinical aspects

of diabetes mellitus by a group of leading experts. A small minitextbook containing extensive bibliographies.

Schade DS, Santiago JV, Skyler JS, Rizza RA: *Intensive Insulin Therapy.* Garden City, NY, Medical Examination Publishing Co, 1983.

This book presents in great detail the art and practice of intensive therapy with various regimens including insulin pumps.

Sperling MA (ed): *Physician's Guide to Insulin Dependent (Type I): Diabetes. Diagnosis and Treatment.* Alexandria, VA, American Diabetes Association, 1988. 150 pp. (paperback).

See comment under Lebovitz, above.

Specific References

1. Amiel SA, Tamborlane WV, Simonson DC, Sherwin RS: Defective glucose counter-regulation after strict glycemic control of insulin-dependent diabetes mellitus. *N Engl J Med* 316:1376, 1987.
2. Asbury AK: Understanding diabetic neuropathy. Editorial. *N Engl J Med* 319:57, 1988.
3. Boyle PJ, Schwartz NS, Shah SD, et al: Plasma glucose concentrations at the onset of hypoglycemic symptoms in patients with poorly controlled diabetes and in nondiabetics. *N Engl J Med* 318:1487, 1988.
4. Bradley WE: Diagnosis of urinary bladder dysfunction in diabetes mellitus. *Ann Intern Med* 92 (part 2):323, 1980.
5. Brownlee M, Cerami A, Vlassara H: Advanced glycosylation end products in tissue and the biochemical basis of diabetic complications. *N Engl J Med* 318:1315, 1988.
6. Correspondence. *N Engl J Med* 320:57, 1989.
7. Coulston AM, Hollenbeck CB, Swislocki ALM, et al: Deleterious metabolic effects of high carbohydrate, sucrose containing diets in patients with non-insulin-dependent diabetes mellitus. *Am J Med* 82:213, 1987.
8. Cryer PE: The metabolic impact of autonomic neuropathy in insulin-dependent diabetes mellitus. (Editorial) *Arch Intern Med* 146:2127, 1986.
9. Cryer PE, Gerich JE: Glucose counter-regulation, hypoglycemia, and intensive insulin therapy in diabetes mellitus. *N Engl J Med* 313:232, 1985.
10. Cryer PE, White NH, Santiago JV: The relevance of glucose counter-regulatory systems to patients with insulin dependent diabetes mellitus. *Endocrine Rev* 7:131, 1986.
11. Davidson MB: The continually changing "natural history" of diabetes mellitus. *J Chronic Dis* 34:5, 1981.
12. Ellenberg M: Sexual dysfunction in diabetic patients. *Ann Intern Med* 92 (part 2):331, 1980.
13. Ewing DJ, Campbell IW, Clarke BF: Assessment of cardiovascular effects in diabetic autonomic neuropathy and prognostic implications. *Ann Intern Med* 92 (part 2):308, 1980.
14. FILMS: Millner, Fenwick, Inc: Diabetic Teaching Films. 2125 Greenspring Dr, Timonium, MD 21093. NEWSLETTERS: Diabetes in the News. 233 East Erie Str, Suite 712, Chicago, IL 60611 (no charge; junior high school level or above); Forecast. 600 5th Ave, New York, NY 10020 (about $15/year; high school level or above).
15. Gabbe S: Gestational diabetes mellitus. (Editorial) *N Engl J Med* 315:1025, 1988.
16. Garg AG, Bonanome A, Grundy SM, et al: Comparison of a high-carbohydrate diet with a high mono-unsaturated fat diet in patients with non-insulin-dependent diabetes mellitus. *N Engl J Med* 319:829, 1988.
17. Goldstein S, Podolsky S: Inheritance of diabetes and genetic counseling. In: Podolsky S (ed): *Clinical Diabetes: Modern Management.* New York, Appleton-Century-Crofts, 1980, ch. 1, p. 1.
18. Greene D: The pathogenesis and prevention of diabetic neuropathy and nephropathy. *Metabolism* 37:25, 1989.
19. Haworth JC, McRae KN, Dilling LA: Prognosis of infants of diabetic mothers in relation to neonatal hypoglycemia. *Dev Med Child Neurol* 18:471, 1976.
20. Jovanovic L: Insulin on the go. *Practical Diabetology* 7:10, 1988.
21. Karjalainen J, Salmela P, Ilonen J, et al: A comparison of childhood and adult type I diabetes mellitus. *N Engl J Med* 320:881, 1989.
22. Klein R, Klein BEK, Moss SE, et al: Glycosylated hemoglobin predicts the incidence and progression of diabetic retinopathy. *JAMA* 260:2864, 1988.
23. MacDonald MJ: Postexercise late-onset hypoglycemia in insulin-dependent diabetic patients. *Diabetes Care* 10:584, 1987.
24. Mandel E: Diabetes-related impotence and self-injection therapy. *Practical Diabetology* 7:1, 1988.
25. Miles JL, Simpson JL, Driscoll SG, et al: Incidence of spontaneous abortion among normal women and insulin-dependent diabetic women whose pregnancies were identified within 21 days of conception. *N Engl J Med* 319:1617, 1988.
26. Mills JL, Knopp RH, Simpson JL, et al: Lack of relation of increased malformation rates in infants of diabetic mothers to glycemic control during organogenesis. *N Engl J Med* 318:671, 1988; and Correspondence *N Engl J Med* 319:647, 1988.
27. National Diabetes Group: Classification and diagnosis of diabetes mellitus and other categories of glucose tolerance. *Diabetes* 28:1039, 1979.
28. Nathan DM, Singer DE, Hurxthal K, et al: The clinical information value of the glycosylated hemoglobin assay. *N Engl J Med* 310:341, 1984.
29. Perriello G, DeFeo P, Torlone E, et al: The effect of asymptomatic nocturnal hypoglycemia on glycemic control in diabetes mellitus. *N Engl J Med* 319:1233, 1988.
30. Polonsky K, Bergenstal R, Guillermo P, et al: Relation of counter-regulatory responses to hypoglycemia in Type I diabetics. *N Engl J Med* 307:1106, 1982.
31. Preliminary report on effects of photocoagulation therapy. *Am J Ophthalmol* 81:383, 1976.
32. Rizza R, Gerich JE, Haymond MD, et al: Control of blood sugar in insulin-dependent diabetes: comparison of an artificial endocrine pancreas, continuous subcutaneous insulin infusion and intensified conventional insulin therapy. *N Engl J Med* 303:1313, 1980.
33. Rushforth NB, Miller M, Bennett PH: Fasting and two-hour post-load glucose levels for the diagnosis of diabetes. *Diabetologia* 16:373, 1979.
34. Schade DS, Santiago JV, Skyler JS, Rizza RA: *Intensive Insulin Therapy.* Garden City, NY, Medical Examination Publishing Co, 1983. p. 138.
35. Stamler R, Stamler J (eds): Asymptomatic hyperglycemia and coronary heart disease. A series of papers by the International Collaborative Group, based on studies in fifteen populations. *J Chronic Dis* 32:683, 1979.
36. Stolar MW: Atherosclerosis in diabetes: the role of hyperinsulinemia. *Metabolism* 37(2) Suppl 1:1, 1988.
37. Tallarigo L, Giampietro O, Penno G, et al: Relation of glucose tolerance to complications of pregnancy in nondiabetic woman. *N Engl J Med* 315:389, 1986. and Correspondence, *N Engl J Med* 316:1343, 1987.
38. Tordjman KM, Havlin CE, Levandowski LA, et al: Failure of nocturnal hypoglycemia to cause fasting hyperglycemia in patients with insulin-dependent diabetes mellitus. *N Engl J Med* 317:1552, 1987.
39. Weissman PN, Shenkman L, Gregerman RI: Chlorpropamide hyponatremia. Drug-induced inappropriate antidiuretic-hormone activity. *N Engl J Med* 284:65, 1971.
40. West KM: Diet therapy of diabetes: an analysis of failure. *Ann Intern Med* 79:425, 1973.
41. West KM: Diet and diabetes. *Postgrad Med* 60:209, 1976.
42. Wheat LJ, Allen SD, Marietta M, et al: Diabetic foot infections. Bacteriologic analysis. *Arch Intern Med* 146:1935, 1986.
43. Zasler ND: Managing erectile dysfunction with external devices. *Practical Diabetology* 8:1, 1989.
44. Zinman B: The physiologic replacement of insulin. An elusive goal. *N Engl J Med* 321:363, 1986.

C H A P T E R 73

Thyroid Disorders

ROBERT I. GREGERMAN, M.D.

Disturbances of thyroid growth and function are among the most common endocrinological disorders encountered in ambulatory practice. Excessive production of the iodine-containing thyroid hormones, thyroxine (T_4) and triiodothyronine (Fig. 73.1), results in hyperthyroidism or thyrotoxicosis; decreased hormone production results in hypothyroidism. Generalized enlargement of the thyroid, regardless of cause, is termed goiter. Focal enlargement of the thyroid is termed a "nodule" and is usually benign. Either goiter or focal enlargement may be associated with abnormal thyroid function. Goiter can produce anatomical changes ranging from simply cosmetic to obstruction of contiguous structures such as the trachea and esophagus.

THYROID PHYSIOLOGY

Thyroid Regulatory Mechanisms

The principal regulatory mechanism of the thyroid is the hypothalamic-pituitary-thyroid negative feed-

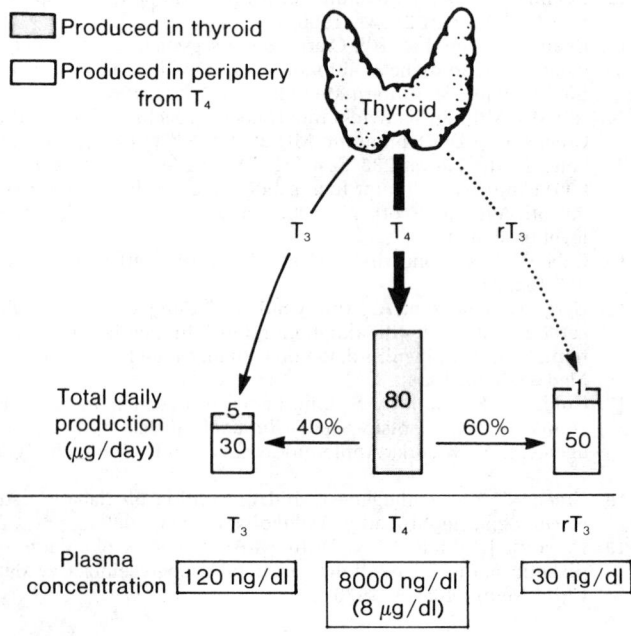

Figure 73.1. Production rates by the thyroid and in the periphery of thyroid hormones and their mean concentrations in the plasma.

back control system. The hypothalamus secretes thyrotropin-releasing hormone (TRH), which travels via the hypophyseal portal system to the pituitary, where it stimulates release of thyroid-stimulating hormone (TSH). TSH stimulates many aspects of thyroid activity, including hormone synthesis, thyroid growth, and the release of thyroid hormones. Secretion of TSH by the pituitary is inhibited by the thyroid hormones—thus the term "negative feedback loop."

Iodide from plasma is concentrated by an active process (iodide "pump") that can maintain a thyroid/plasma iodide ratio as high as 500 to 1. Iodide is thereafter converted through a series of enzymatic steps resulting in the formation of T_4 and T_3 within the thyroglobulin sequence. The iodide pump transports a number of anions other than iodide, a phenomenon that has been exploited diagnostically and therapeutically. For example, the pertechnetate anion, TcO_4^-, as the radioactive isotope ^{99m}Tc, has been widely used for thyroid imaging, although ^{123}I is now preferred.

The minimal daily requirement of iodide is only about 100 to 200 μg, an amount that is determined by obligatory loss, mainly through the kidney. The minimal daily requirement is enormously exceeded by dietary intake; for example, iodinated salt provides about 1000 μg in a normal 10-g daily intake. Thus, iodide deficiency is no longer seen in the United States; however, iodide deficiency is still a major problem in many parts of the world.

Any chemical substance that interferes with thyroid hormone function or release may lower blood hormone concentration and induce compensatory hypertrophy of the gland (goiter) via stimulation of TSH secretion. Certain substances are known to prevent iodide accumulation by impairment of the iodide "pump." Other substances interfere with hormone synthesis or inhibit hormone release. Clinically useful agents that have been employed for therapeutic effects in states of excess hormone production (hyperthyroidism) are known to act at one or another of these points. Perchlorate, no longer commonly used therapeutically, inhibits the iodide "pump." The thiocarbamide drugs interfere with hormone synthesis by blockade of incorporation of iodide into the tyrosines ("organification") and of the coupling reactions in iodothyronine formation, but have more effect on coupling than on organification. Lithium ion (currently in wide use for the treatment of affective disorders, Chapter 15), interferes with thyroglobulin proteolysis and hormone release and may result in goiter and, occasionally, hypothyroidism. Interestingly, lithium interferes with the action of TSH on the thyroid, and therefore some cases of hypothyroidism due to lithium are not associated with goiter. Iodide itself in pharmacological amounts interferes with hormone formation and release and in some individuals is a goitrogen.

Metabolic Effects of Thyroid Hormone

The thyroid hormones exert their actions through a variety of mechanisms. A classic thyroid hormone ef-

fect is on metabolic rate. Measurement of basal metabolic rate (BMR) was the basis for the first laboratory method for clinical assessment of thyroid status. The numerous known actions of thyroid hormone range from specific stimulation of mitochondrial oxidative metabolism to the nuclear regulation of protein synthesis. Thyroid hormones also exert specific regulatory effects on membrane physiology, e.g., potentiation of catecholamine effects. This action of thyroid hormones explains the signs of exaggerated sympathetic activity in hyperthyroidism and the effectiveness of the therapy of this condition by β-adrenergic blockade.

Hormone Transport

The thyroid hormones in the blood are T_4 and a much smaller quantity of T_3. Both hormones are tightly but reversibly bound to several plasma proteins, mainly thyroid hormone-binding globulin (TBG). In the normal person 65 to 70% of the thyroid hormones are bound to TBG, about 15% to the secondary carrier, thyroxine-binding prealbumin (TBPA), and about 15% to albumin. Variations of TBG occur in many clinical states and account for most of the changes in T_4 concentration in plasma that are seen in diseases other than hypo- and hyperthyroidism. Small quantities of T_4 (0.03%) and T_3 (0.3%) are not protein bound but are "free" and in rapid equilibrium with the protein-bound fraction.

The concentrations of free T_4 and T_3 in plasma are thought to reflect the amount of hormone exerting an effect on tissues. Clinical status in a number of conditions correlates with free T_4 rather than with total hormone in plasma. A good example of this correlation is the normal pregnant state in which total T_4 is high but in which there is no evidence of free thyroid hormone excess. The explanation is that plasma TBG is elevated, a consequence of the hyperestrogenism of pregnancy.

In some pathological states that affect the quantity of TBG in plasma (Table 73.1), and hence the total T_4,

Table 73.1.
Factors Affecting Thyroxine-Binding Globulin (TBG)

TBG INCREASED
  Estrogens:
    Oral contraceptives
    Pregnancy
  Hypothyroidism
  Acute hepatitis
  Cirrhosis
  Genetic TBG excess
  Acute intermittent porphyria
  Perphenazine (Trilafon)
TBG DECREASED
  Androgens
  Anabolic steroids
  Cirrhosis
  Glucocorticoids
  Nephrotic syndrome
  Severe chronic nonthyroidal illness
  Cushing's syndrome
  Genetic TBG deficiency

the absolute concentration of free T_4 may not adjust to a normal value. During a variety of nonthyroidal illnesses, factors other than the concentration of TBG and TBPA appear to determine the free hormone concentration, presumably by affecting the affinity of the TBG-T_4 interaction.

Metabolism and Interconversion of Thyroid Hormones

Practically all tissues metabolize and degrade the thyroid hormones, but the liver is quantitatively most important as a site at which regulation of hormone degradation occurs. T_4 metabolism is the major source (80%) of circulating T_3 in the normal individual. The normal thyroid secretes mainly T_4 and only a small amount of T_3 (Fig. 73.1). Only in hyperthyroidism, iodine deficiency, and certain other pathological circumstances is T_3 sometimes the predominantly secreted hormone.

Most of the T_4 secreted (about 85%) is ultimately deiodinated and further degraded. The physiologically most important pathway involves conversion of about 35% of the T_4 to metabolically active T_3, which is itself further deiodinated. About an equal amount of T_4 is converted to reverse T_3 (rT_3) (Fig. 73.1). Although not active in calorigenesis, rT_3 does antagonize a number of the effects of T_3 and thus may have some physiological importance. In a variety of pathological states the formation of T_3 is inhibited, whereas that of rT_3 is reciprocally enhanced. Measurement of rT_3 has some usefulness in the differential diagnosis of the "euthyroid sick syndrome" (see "Differential Diagnosis" under "Hypothyroidism").

LABORATORY TESTS OF THYROID FUNCTION AND OF THYROID DISEASE

Most thyroid "function" tests assess secretory activity of the thyroid gland only indirectly. Measurements of blood hormone concentrations, the most commonly used tests, cannot be equated directly with the rate of hormone production, although they reflect that rate when plasma binding of hormones is normal. However, various illnesses, drugs, and alterations of physiological state affect plasma binding. Accordingly, proper interpretation of plasma hormone concentrations demands concomitant assessment of plasma binding. Thyroid gland function can be assessed somewhat more directly by measurement of thyroidal iodide accumulation ("uptake"; RaIU) using isotopes of iodide (^{131}I, ^{123}I). These tests also must be properly interpreted, since uptake of tracer is only an approximation of the accumulation of stable iodide and of hormone synthesis.

Other laboratory tests are useful in the assessment of thyroid status and in the diagnosis of thyroid disease but are not, strictly speaking, tests of thyroid function. Such tests include measurements of the integrity of the physiological feedback control system (plasma TSH concentration before and after stimulation by ad-

ministered TRH), thyroid autoantibodies, and the immunoglobulins related to Graves' disease.

Measurements of Plasma Hormones: Plasma T_4 and T_3

The commonly used and important tests of thyroid function are measurements of the levels of T_4 and T_3, as determined by radioimmunoassay or other specific methods. Unlike the case with older techniques, no chemical interference is produced by drugs or iodine-containing substances, but it must be kept in mind that such agents may affect the actual level of thyroid hormones in blood. rT_3 is occasionally also used in differential diagnosis, especially of ill patients. The value of T_4 is certainly the single most important measurement in clinical evaluation of thyroid disease. However, interpretation of a given value (concentration) must take into account whether T_4 binding to plasma proteins is normal. Accordingly, T_4 must be measured in conjunction with assessment of hormone binding to plasma proteins or with determination of TBG. In practice this is done by determining the "free T_4" or the "free T_4 index" (see below). Normal values of the common tests are given in Table 73.2.

"Free T_4": Measurement of Non-Protein-Bound Thyroid Hormone in Plasma

The "free T_4" of plasma is estimated by separate measurements of the non-protein-bound T_4 (usually by equilibrium dialysis) and the total T_4; their arithmetic product equals the free T_4. The dialyzable (non-protein-bound) T_4 normally approximates only 0.03% of the total.

The free T_4 hypothesis (see page 953) has been helpful as a physiological concept. Determination of the free T_4 for clinical purposes is often useful, but the measurement has serious limitations. In some states, such as pregnancy or during estrogen therapy, both T_4 and TBG are elevated and thyroid status is accurately reflected by the free T_4. The dialyzable fraction is decreased, but since the T_4 is elevated, the free T_4 is normal. In hyperthyroidism, free T_4 reflects thyroid status better than total T_4, since the altered metabolic state itself lowers TBG; in some cases a normal or borderline elevation of T_4 is associated with an elevated free T_4. In hypothyroidism, TBG is often elevated and the free T_4 is decreased more than is the total T_4.

Problems of interpretation of the free T_4 arise in many seriously ill patients. A variety of nonthyroidal diseases ranging from acute infections to liver disease can result in elevation of the free T_4. In these situations, the patient is usually euthyroid with a normal T_4; the free T_4 is elevated only because the dialyzable fraction is increased. An explanation for this phenomenon is not readily available. Altered concentrations of neither TBG nor TBPA account for the increased free T_4. The appearance of a factor in plasma that interferes with protein binding of T_4 has been demon-

Table 73.2.
Thyroid Function Tests[a]

	Plasma T$_4$ (µg/dl)	Plasma T$_3$ (ng/dl)	T$_3$ Resin Uptake (T$_3$U) (%)	T$_3$ Resin Uptake Ratio (T$_3$UR)	TSH (µU/ml)	Free T$_4$ (FT$_4$) (ng/dl)	Free T$_4$ Index (FTI)[b]
Normal mean	8	120	30	1		1.5	8.0
Normal range	5–12	80–160	25–35	0.85–1.15	0.3–5	1.0–2.0	5.8–10.6
Confidence limits	±1	±20	±2	±0.05		±0.3	

[a] See the text for limitations of interpretation of normal ranges. Confidence limits (95%) of a single value are approximate and depend on both the laboratory and the level within the range.
[b] The FTI on any sample is calculated as T$_4$ × T$_3$UR, but the normal range for the FTI is determined empirically. The units of the FTI depend on whether the percentage T$_3$ resin uptake or the T$_3$ resin uptake ratio is multiplied times T$_4$.

strated. Thus, an elevated free T$_4$ is not a specific finding related solely to thyroid status. Moreover, the test is several times more expensive than the "free T$_4$ index," which is to be preferred as the "single" most effective screening test of thyroid function (see below).

Estimates of TBG: T$_3$ Resin Uptake and "Free T$_4$ Index" (FTI)

The T$_3$ uptake test (T$_3$U) is not to be confused with the concentration of T$_3$ in plasma. The T$_3$U is not a thyroid function test but merely provides an indirect estimate of the concentration of plasma TBG. To some extent, T$_3$U is also influenced by the quantity of T$_4$ in plasma, i.e., by the degree of saturation of the T$_4$ (and T$_3$) binding sites on TBG. The T$_3$U may eventually be replaced by direct quantitation of TBG. Technically the T$_3$U is measured by adding a tracer quantity of T$_3$ and a nonspecific T$_3$ binding absorbent (resin) to the sample of plasma to be tested. The tracer distributes itself between nonspecific binding sites on the resin and specific binding sites on TBG. Resin-bound tracer is therefore reciprocally related to the quantity of TBG in the plasma. The test result is expressed either as a percentage or as a ratio of the test sample to that of the laboratory's control plasma (T$_3$U ratio).

The usefulness of the T$_3$U is in interpreting a given level of T$_4$. A high (or low) T$_4$ can be interpreted as reflecting increased or decreased T$_4$ secretion only if the plasma binding of T$_4$ is normal, i.e., only if the TBG (T$_3$U) is normal. Otherwise, to reach a proper conclusion about thyroid function, disturbance of binding must be considered along with the high (or low) T$_4$. For convenience the T$_4$ and T$_3$U have been combined to give a so-called free T$_4$ index (FTI) by simply multiplying one number times the other (the index is sometimes designated the "T$_7$" or "T$_{12}$"). This widely used index "compensates" for the high or low T$_4$ value that results from abnormality of TBG concentration. In most, but not all, cases, FTI closely parallels free T$_4$.

In severely ill patients of the type more likely to be hospitalized than to be ambulatory, the FTI may be misleading. In such cases the resin uptake is elevated, not because TBG is low but as the result of the appearance in plasma of a nonspecific inhibitor of hormone binding that affects the distribution of tracer T$_3$ between sites in plasma and sites on the resin. Both the free T$_4$ and FTI tests must be interpreted with caution in any patient with severe nonthyroidal illness.

Tests of the Negative Feedback System

Thyroid-Stimulating Hormone

Plasma TSH is invariably elevated in primary hypothyroidism because of reduced feedback inhibition by the decreased concentrations of the thyroid hormones. The measurement of plasma TSH is important both in the diagnosis of primary hypothyroidism and in monitoring the adequacy of thyroid hormone replacement therapy (see below). Elevation of plasma TSH is the most sensitive indicator of hypothyroid status. Elevations of TSH were for many years reliably measured by radioimmunoassay, but the available assays were not sufficiently sensitive to detect suppression of TSH. Recently, new immunoradiometric assays have been introduced that quantitate the normal and subnormal range. As a result, the determination of TSH has become an important diagnostic measurement and alternative to measurement of TRH testing (see below) when blood levels of T$_4$ and T$_3$ are only borderline. Another use for the sensitive TSH assay is in assessing replacement therapy with thyroxine. Recent evidence indicates that suppression or modest elevation of TSH may accompany a variety of nonthyroidal illnesses, at least in hospitalized patients. Thus one should be cautious in interpreting these assays even in ambulatory patients.

Suppression Tests: Use of T$_4$ and T$_3$

In several thyroid diseases, gland function becomes independent of TSH, i.e., nonsuppressible by amounts of exogenous thyroid hormone that inhibit normal pituitary secretion of TSH. Nonsuppressibility is seen in hyperthyroidism due to any cause, in cases of hyperfunctioning adenoma ("hot nodule") with or without hyperthyroidism, and in 25% of cases of nontoxic nodular goiter. About one-half of patients with Graves' ophthalmopathy without hyperthyroidism have nonsuppressible thyroid function. Return of suppressibility in the course of Graves' disease indicates clinical remission, and the test is therefore a useful guide to therapy as well as to diagnosis. In the diagnosis of hyperthyroidism the test has been for the most part superseded by direct assay of plasma TSH (suppression) and by the TRH test (see below). Testing for suppressibility is done by administration of T_3 or T_4; a 50% decrease of radioiodide uptake is the end point. T_4 is given as a single 3-mg dose or 25 µg of T_3 are given every 8 hours. Radioiodide uptake is measured at 6 to 8 days (see below).

The TRH Test

Parenterally administered TRH produces release of TSH from the pituitary. Response to TRH is abnormal in several clinical circumstances and can be diagnostically useful. Until recently the most common use of the TRH test was in the diagnosis of suspected hyperthyroidism, but the advent of sensitive assays for TSH (see above) makes the TRH test obsolete, at least for this purpose.

The TRH test will remain useful for confirmation of a diagnosis of primary hypothyroidism. When the plasma TSH elevation is borderline, an exaggerated plasma TSH response to TRH is seen. The increment of TSH after TRH administration does not normally exceed 30 µU/ml, but elevations several times this amount may be seen in cases of borderline hypothyroidism.

The most common use of the test was as an alternative to the T_3 suppression test in the diagnosis of hyperthyroidism (see "Thyroid-Stimulating Hormone", above). Hypersecretion of thyroid hormones producing even minimal elevation of blood hormone levels blunts or abolishes the normal response to TRH. The TRH test is also useful in the differential diagnosis of severely ill patients with low plasma T_4 (see "Hypothyroidism versus Euthyroid Sick Syndrome"). The test is of limited use in the elderly in whom lack of TRH response can be normal.

The test is performed by injecting 500 µg of TRH intravenously. Plasma TSH is measured before injection and at 20 and 30 minutes. A significant response is an increase of more than 1 µU/ml. The general physician can easily perform the TRH test in the office. [The TRH (Thypinone) can be bought through any commercial pharmacy.]

Thyroidal Radioiodide Uptake (RaIU) Tests

The rate of tracer iodide accumulation (^{131}I, ^{123}I) in the thyroid can be measured by using times ranging from a few minutes to the plateau of accumulation (24 hours). These procedures, although still in wide use, have been rendered almost obsolete by the simpler and less expensive measurements of hormone concentrations in plasma. The diagnostic usefulness of the RaIU is also seriously limited by the "saturation" of Western diets with iodide. This has resulted in RaIU values that are too low to discriminate normal function from hypofunction, so that the test is now useless for the diagnosis of hypothyroidism. It is still of diagnostic usefulness in hyperthyroidism, although, since results are "normal" in up to 50% of cases of hyperthyroidism, a normal RaIU does not exclude the diagnosis. One important use of the test is in patients with hyperthyroidism associated with thyroiditis. If this condition is suspected, an RaIU is important; a low value deters inappropriate therapy. Determination of the RaIU is often part of the selection of dosages in RaI therapy. The RaIU is subject to interference by chemical agents and certain clinical states; both produce false-positive and false-negative results. The RaIU should no longer be used for the routine evaluation of thyroid function.

Immunological Tests

Assay of antibodies to thyroidal antigens (thyroglobulin, microsomes), so-called thyroid autoantibodies, is useful in determining the presence of autoimmune thyroiditis (see below, page 975, "Hashimoto's Thyroiditis"). Measurement of thyroid-stimulating immunoglobulin (TSI) (see "Graves' Disease") is not yet readily available. TSI measurements, when available, are useful in the pregnant patient, since high levels are associated with an increased likelihood of neonatal hyperthyroidism. A fall in TSI is a good indicator of remission in Graves' disease and will probably be useful for this purpose as the test becomes available. The long-acting thyroid stimulator (LATS) test, still available in some laboratories, is useless.

Other Tests: Imaging and Biopsies

Various scintiscan or imaging techniques are available to delineate the anatomy of the thyroid and to distinguish functional from nonfunctional tissue, a consideration in the differential diagnosis of thyroid neoplasms. Currently, ^{99m}Tc pertechnetate (TcO_4^-) is most widely used, but ^{123}I is the imaging agent of choice. (Some tumors will accumulate pertechnetate, thereby obscuring the diagnosis.)

Ultrasound imaging (sonography) is now a routine procedure for distinguishing cystic from solid nodules, an important point in differential diagnosis of these lesions. Moreover, ultrasound can accurately assess the size of nodules, providing an objective basis for evaluation of medical therapy.

Needle biopsy is a routine procedure in many centers. In proper hands, needle biopsy is a safe, outpatient procedure that gives a diagnosis in most cases. *Fine needle aspiration* with cytological examination is not as reliable as needle biopsy. Although both procedures may fail to distinguish benign adenomas from well-differentiated follicular carcinomas (15), an important limitation of the technique, the procedure may help avoid many operations and may provide much needed reassurance for the patient. Unfortunately, pathology reports that lack definitiveness or routinely end with ". . . cannot be excluded" or the like merely ensure that surgery *will* be done. Needle biopsy is performed ordinarily by an endocrinologist, surgeon, or radiologist who has been trained in the technique. The procedure, performed under local (cutaneous) anesthesia, is ordinarily painless. The only significant complication is local hemorrhage, but this is uncommon and usually of minor degree. Fine needle aspiration is without complications. Neither needle biopsy nor fine needle aspiration should be used unless the pathologist is specifically trained to interpret the biopsy material.

Nonspecificity of Thyroid Function Tests in Nonthyroidal Illness

Thyroid function tests may be nonspecifically altered in many nonthyroidal diseases, i.e., these tests are not specific when severe illness is present (Table 73.3). Moreover, a variety of drugs affect both thyroid function and the function tests (Tables 73.1 and 73.4). Some examples of these considerations are presented below; extensive discussions can be found elsewhere (3, 29, 30, and "General References").

Table 73.3.
Nonthyroidal Illness: Effects on T_4, Free T_4, and TBG in Plasma[a]

	Effects on T_4	Free T_4	TBG
LIVER DISEASE			
Active hepatitis	↑	↔↑	↑
Cirrhosis	↑↓	↔↑	↑↓
Cholangitis	↑	↔↑	↑
RENAL DISEASE			
Nephrotic syndrome	↔↓	↔	↔↓
Uremia, chronic	↔↓	↔↓	↔↓
INFECTIONS	↓	↑	↔
MALNUTRITION	↔↓	↔↑	↔↓

[a] Most illnesses and even such minor alterations of physiological state as decreased food intake will produce a decrease of plasma T_3.

Table 73.4.
Drug and Hormone Effects on Plasma T_4 and TBG

Gonadal Hormones	Effect on T_4	Free T_4	Effect on TBG
ESTROGENS	↑	↔↓	↑
Oral contraceptives			
Pregnancy			
ANDROGENS	↓	↔	
Testosterone		↑	
Anabolic steroids			
GLUCOCORTICOIDS	↓	↔	↓
Cushing's syndrome			
Pharmacological uses			
PSYCHOTROPIC DRUGS			
Perphenazine (Trilafon)	↑	↔	↑
Amphetamines	↑	↑	↔
ANTICONVULSANTS			
Phenytoin (Dilantin)	↓	↔↓	↔
HEPARIN	↔	↑	↔
ADRENERGIC BLOCKERS			
Propranolol (Inderal)	↔(↓T_3)	↔	↔
ANTIARRHYTHMIC DRUGS			
Amiodarone	↑	↑	↔
GALLBLADDER DYES	↑≲(↓T_3)	↔↑	↔
Iopanoic acid	↑↔(↓T_3)	↔↑	↔
Ipodate	↑↔(↓T_3)	↔↑	↔
OPIATES	↑		↑
MISCELLANEOUS			
Clofibrate	↑		↑
5-fluorouracil	↑		↑

Effects of Gonadal and Adrenal Hormones

Estrogens (pregnancy, contraceptives) raise, and androgens lower T_4 by altering plasma TBG. Glucocorticoids inhibit thyroid activity acutely by interfering with TSH secretion and affect the pituitary's responsiveness to TRH. The plasma T_4 is lowered during chronic glucocorticoid therapy, due mainly to a decrease of TBG. When dexamethasone is given acutely, the plasma T_4 decreases slightly and T_3 falls sharply.

Liver Diseases

Various alterations of thyroid function tests are produced by liver diseases. Early in infectious hepatitis, the T_4 is elevated secondary to an increase of TBG. Chronic liver disease produces many abnormalities in an unpredictable fashion. T_4 may be increased or decreased in parallel with TBG and the T_3U. Free T_4 is often elevated with no obvious relationship to the TBG. T_3 is usually low. A frequent and unexplained abnormality is elevation of TSH, although the response to TRH is not exaggerated as it is in hypothyroidism. RaIU is often elevated in acute alcoholic hepatitis with or without cirrhosis and in some cases of cholangitis. These changes have been attributed both to iodide depletion and to acceleration of T_4 metabolism.

Renal Diseases

The nephrotic syndrome is often associated with depressed T_4, but the decrease is not always explained by a lowering of the TBG. In chronic renal disease, the means of T_4, TBG, and the FTI are not significantly different from normal, but the range is greater and values may exceed the usual normal limits. Some patients with severe chronic renal failure receiving long-term dialysis show a progressive decrease of T_4. These patients and those with the nephrotic syndrome may represent examples of the recently recognized "euthyroid sick syndrome" (see "Hypothyroidism"). As one would expect in any chronic illness, the plasma T_3 is depressed.

Infections, Malnutrition, and Drugs

The T_4 may drop early in the course of acute infection and free T_4 may rise. Neither change is accounted for by an alteration of TBG. During starvation, plasma T_3 falls. Free T_4 is often increased without relation to the TBG. Plasma T_3 is often decreased in the elderly, a change that has been attributed to aging but is in fact due to diminished food intake and nonspecific illness. Closely correlated alterations of T_3U and plasma TBG have been reported in protein-calorie malnutrition. Some pharmacological agents affect the thyroid hormones of plasma (1). Phenytoin (Dilantin) lowers the T_4 and free T_4, often into the hypothyroid range. Although plasma TSH may be somewhat elevated, clinical hypothyroidism is not seen. Heparin acutely elevates the free T_4. The mechanisms of these changes are not known. Propranolol decreases plasma T_3 by inhibition of the normal T_4 deiodination route; rT_3 is increased. A similar decrease of T_3 through reduced hepatic metabolism of T_4 is produced by propylthiouracil, dexamethasone, the antiarrhythmic drug, amiodarone, and the radiopaque contrast media used for visualization of the gallbladder, iopanoic acid and ipodate. In the case of the latter agents, additional mechanisms are operative, since these compounds also elevate T_4 and TSH, an effect attributed to their inhibition of conversion of T_4 and T_3 in the pituitary as well as in the periphery. Amphetamine abuse may increase plasma T_4, presumably by central stimulation of TSH release (3).

Altered Plasma T₄ Due to Inherited Abnormalities of Protein Binding

In addition to those disease states in which T_4 levels are related to altered hormone binding to TBG, other situations that are explicable in terms of altered protein binding include inherited disorders of TBG excess, TBG deficiency, increases of concentration of TBPA, and increases of the number of T_4 binding sites on an albumin variant. The first two conditions are X-linked. The latter two conditions, inherited as autosomal dominants, are rare. Both can produce diagnostic difficulties, however, since neither is detected by the T_3 resin uptake; the free T_4 index is accordingly elevated in both situations, although the free T_4 is normal (3).

Alterations of Plasma T₄ in Nonthyroidal Illness Not Due to Abnormalities of Protein Binding

Elevations of T_4 that are unexplained by changes in thyroxine binding are quite common. These situations are most difficult to distinguish from hyperthyroidism. Included are the elevation of T_4 seen in acute nonthyroidal illness, in psychiatric disease, and as the effect of some drugs. The stress of serious illness may also lower T_4 and simulate hypothyroidism, but such severe illness is not ordinarily encountered in ambulatory patients. An exception may be seen in patients undergoing treatment by dialysis for chronic renal failure. Abnormal thyroid hormone levels in these situations and diseases that are regularly associated with such changes are described briefly below and reviewed in more detail elsewhere (3, 28, 29, and "General References").

Increase of Plasma T₄ during Nonspecific Illness. Although the phenomenon of decreased T_4 during severe illness is now widely recognized (see above), the frequent occurrence of increased T_4 (and FTI) due to illness is not generally appreciated. The increase of T_4 is modest and the T_4 generally does not exceed about 15 μg. This problem is commonly seen in severely ill elderly patients in whom it raises the issue of hyperthyroidism. Similar findings have been reported in hyperemesis gravidarum.

Acute Psychiatric Illness. Restlessness, hyperactivity, tachycardia, and tremor are often seen as part of severe, acute psychiatric illness. Clinical suspicion of hyperthyroidism leads to thyroid function tests and laboratory results consistent with this diagnosis. Such patients may have elevated T_4, FTI, and T_3. In some series up to one-third of acutely hospitalized psychiatric patients present with an elevated T_4. Although the phenomenon is documented only in hospitalized patients, it might be encountered in any severely disturbed individual. The T_4 returns to normal within 1 to 2 weeks of clinical improvement of the psychiatric disturbance.

Increased Plasma T₄ due to Resistance to Thyroid Hormones. A rare but well-recognized condition of increased T_4 unaccompanied by binding protein abnormalities is that of peripheral resistance to thyroid hormones. Originally described as a familial syndrome of increased T_4, goiter, deaf mutism, and some degree of hypothyroidism with delayed bone maturation and epiphyseal stippling, the most common situation is actually that of elevated T_4 in a phenotypically normal individual without evidence of hyperthyroidism. The abnormality occurs both sporadically and in familial form and is probably a heterogeneous group of disorders with variable inheritance (30).

Interpretation of Thyroid Function Tests: Statistical Considerations

No single numerical value divides normal from abnormal in any thyroid function test. The upper and lower limits of normal for plasma T_4, free T_4 index, and T_3 are set at ±2 standard deviations from the mean. By definition, therefore, 2.5% of normal persons will have abnormal values at each end of the distribution. To complicate the issue, a small number of hyperthyroid or hypothyroid persons have values that fall within the normal range. In addition to the statistical overlap, one must recall that both biological day-to-day variation and unavoidable analytical error further obscure the dividing line between normal and abnormal. For example, 95% confidence limits of a single T_4 test are ±1 μg/dl at the upper and lower limits of the normal range. For all of these reasons, and because of the occasional instance of laboratory or reporting error, a single determination can neither establish nor exclude a diagnosis with anything more than reasonable statistical certainty. Therefore, all abnormal values should be confirmed before therapy is undertaken, and borderline values should be repeated several times before drawing conclusions.

HYPERTHYROIDISM (THYROTOXICOSIS)

Hyperthyroidism, the clinical state resulting from an excess of thyroid hormone, is the most common functional disorder of the thyroid. Although essentially the same clinical picture results from any of several distinct pathological processes (Table 73.5), selection of proper therapy demands that the correct diagnosis be established. The most common variety of hyperthyroidism is Graves' disease, an autoimmune process also known as diffuse toxic goiter. Only slightly less common is hyperthyroidism due to a hyperfunc-

Table 73.5.
Causes of Hyperthyroidism[a]

COMMON
  Graves' disease
  Toxic nodular goiter
    Multinodular
    Uninodular
  Hyperthyroidism in association with thyroiditis
  Iodide induced (iodide, iodine-containing drugs and contrast media)
RARE TO VANISHINGLY RARE
  Thyrotoxicosis due to TSH or TSH-like stimulator
    Choriocarcinoma or hydatidiform mole
    Embryonal cell carcinoma of testis
    Pituitary tumor with TSH excess
    Idiopathic TSH excess
  Toxic thyroid carcinoma
  Hyperthyroidism due to exogenous thyroid hormone
    Factitia
    Medicamentosa (iatrogenic)
  Toxic struma ovarii

[a] Listed in approximate decreasing order of frequency.

tioning multinodular goiter (toxic nodular goiter). Occasionally hyperthyroidism is due to a solitary hyperfunctioning adenoma. Recently hyperthyroidism has been seen with increasing frequency as a transient phenomenon in the evolution of thyroiditis (10, 17). In addition, the induction of hyperthyroidism by iodide and iodide-containing drugs and contrast media has received considerable attention and should be kept in mind for those patients who have had such exposures (6). The other causes of hyperthyroidism listed in Table 73.5 are so rare that they are not usually encountered in ordinary practice.

Graves' Disease

Graves' disease is a complex disorder comprising toxic goiter, ophthalmopathy, and occasionally dermopathy. At any given time during the course of the disease, one of these manifestations may be an isolated finding. Graves' ophthalmopathy and Graves' dermopathy can occur independently of thyroid hormone excess. It is generally accepted that ophthalmopathy and dermopathy are closely related but separate and overlapping immunological disorders.

Various abnormal immunoglobulins are found in the plasma of patients with Graves' disease. Some of these immunoglobulins have TSH-like activity and are designated thyroid-stimulating immunoglobulins (TSI); they are antibodies to the normal receptor sites for TSH. The reasons for development of abnormal immunoglobulins in Graves' disease are not clearly understood. Recent thinking views Graves' disease as a failure of T cell surveillance rather than as a response to thyroid antigens released from thyroid damaged by unknown causes.

The plasma of some patients with Graves' ophthalmopathy contains a factor [exophthalmos-producing substance (EPS)] that produces exophthalmos and other abnormalities of orbital tissues in suitable test animals. In Graves' ophthalmopathy, the extraocular muscles show interstitial edema, increased connective tissue, fatty infiltration, and infiltration with lymphocytes. Eventually, gross degenerative changes such as fibrosis may occur (see "Ophthalmopathy of Graves' Disease," below).

Dermopathy, a unique, albeit unusual, finding in Graves' disease, consists of more or less circumscribed areas of mucopolysaccharide deposition, typically over the shins—hence the term "pretibial myxedema." This unfortunate designation unjustifiably suggests a relationship between the very different type of generalized mucopolysaccharide deposition in hypothyroidism and the localized deposition in Graves' disease. No relationship exists between these processes.

Clinical Presentation and Diagnosis of Hyperthyroidism

Historical Features

The presentation of the patient with hyperthyroidism is highly variable (Table 73.6). The severity of the thyrotoxic aspect is determined not only by the degree of hormone excess but also by its rapidity of onset, its duration, and by the age of the patient. The "typical" patient presents with one or more of the following spontaneous complaints: "nervousness," weight loss, palpitations (which at first may be intermittent), enlarging neck mass (goiter), change in appearance of eyes (Graves' disease), or symptoms of heart failure. These symptoms usually have been present anywhere from a few weeks to up to a year or longer.

As the disease progresses in severity, skeletal muscle wasting occurs, which tends to involve especially the limb girdle musculature, producing a proximal myopathy. This problem may result in weakness, expressed, for example, as great difficulty in climbing stairs or, on examination, in arising from a squatting position. Exertional dyspnea, without evidence of cardiac failure, is common and may be related to the myopathy.

The "nervousness" is typically irritability, inability to concentrate, restlessness, or overt emotional lability, but it is the tremor that most often leads the patient to express this complaint. Impairment of normal sleep pattern with frequent wakenings is common.

The weight loss classically occurs in the face of increased appetite, although frequently no obvious change in appetite is noticed or there may actually be anorexia, especially in elderly patients. The only prominent gastrointestinal symptom is increased frequency of bowel movements, but true diarrhea is not seen.

The "heat intolerance" of hyperthyroidism is often apparent only on questioning. Commonly the patient will admit to having reduced the number of covers used on the bed at night or to the development of new and unusual habits, such as sleeping in the nude or with feet extended from under the blankets. Sweating is increased but is not usually a spontaneous complaint.

Skin changes are hardly ever noticed by the patient and "silky skin" or hair is only occasionally seen on

Table 73.6.
Signs and Symptoms of Hyperthyroidism

Organ or System	Signs and Symptoms
ADRENERGIC MANIFESTATIONS	Excess sweating, heat intolerance, palpitations, tachycardia, tremor, lid lag, stare, nervousness, and excitability
HYPERMETABOLISM AND CATABOLISM	Increased appetite, weight loss
ONE SYSTEM PREDOMINANCE	
Eyes[a]	Periorbital edema, exophthalmos (proptosis), chemosis, ophthalmoplegia, papilledema
Cardiac	Arrhythmia, congestive heart failure
Muscle	Fatigue and weakness, muscle wasting, proximal myopathy, periodic paralysis
Gastrointestinal	Increased frequency of bowel movements, pernicious vomiting
Bone	Acropachy, osteoporosis, hypercalcemia
REPRODUCTIVE	Infertility, abortion, scanty menses, testicular atrophy, gynecomastia
MENTAL	Anxiety, irritability, psychosis, insomnia
SKIN	Onycholysis, "pretibial" myxedema, hyperpigmentation

[a] Graves' disease only.

examination. Hair loss is not infrequent, usually noticed as thinning of the scalp hair by women. Other skin changes include occasional cases in white persons of diffuse hyperpigmentation with darkening noted mostly over extensor surfaces of elbows, knees, and small joints. In black patients, darkening of skin is common.

Physical Findings

The thyroid is visibly or palpably enlarged in almost all young patients with hyperthyroidism, but in the elderly the thyroid may not be enlarged. Asymmetric enlargement is common, especially in patients with toxic nodular goiter. Extreme vascularity of the gland may result in palpable or audible blood flow, a bruit, usually heard over the enlarged lobes but occasionally best heard more rostrally over the superior thyroidal arteries. A bruit over the thyroid of a hyperthyroid patient is usually diagnostic of Graves' disease; this finding is not present in patients with toxic nodular goiter.

The *cardiovascular findings* include sinus tachycardia, systolic flow murmurs, and wide pulse pressure, commonly, and atrial fibrillation, occasionally. It is a common belief that most patients with hyperthyroidism have at least a tachycardia; but, in fact only 50% of patients, regardless of age, have an increased heart rate. The apex impulse is often prominent and forceful. Cardiac failure may develop in severe cases of long duration, especially in elderly persons.

The *eye findings* can be separated into those that occur as a result of thyroid hormone excess and those that are part of the ophthalmopathy of Graves' disease. Excessive thyroid hormone enhances sympathetic tone. The innervation of the eyelids is partially under sympathetic control. Lid retraction with increased scleral visibility above and below the iris, along with infrequent blinking, leads to the "stare" so commonly seen. Failure of the lid to follow promptly movements of the globe ("lid lag") is another manifestation of the same process. When Graves' ophthalmopathy is pres-

ent, there is forward protrusion of the globe. This process may be unilateral at first and is often asymmetrical. The protrusion represents true proptosis and contributes an additional component to the stare produced by increased sympathetic tone. Extraocular muscle weakness results in limitation of ability to converge and to perform extreme movements of gaze. Strabismus and diplopia are more severe manifestations. The most serious complications of Graves' ophthalmopathy are infiltrative (page 965).

The *dermopathy* of Graves' disease occurs most commonly on the legs ("pretibial myxedema") but also can be seen on the dorsum of the foot or on the back, the hands, or even the face. The plaque usually has a sharp, raised margin and may have an orange peel-like appearance. The affected areas are often intensely pruritic.

Clubbing of the fingers and toes is rare (thyroid acropachy) and distinguishable radiographically from that seen in pulmonary disease. A common sign is separation of the distal portion of one or more fingernails from their nailbed (onycholysis).

A postural tremor, usually of the hands, is a common physical finding (see Chapter 82).

Diagnosis

Recognition of Graves' disease in a typical case is not difficult, but, because of its frequently insidious onset, an absence of eye findings or of an overtly enlarged thyroid, or because of involvement of one or relatively few organ systems, the diagnosis may be missed for months or years.

The usual thyroid function tests will substantiate the diagnosis in most cases. If the results of the T_4 and free T_4 index are borderline or normal, the plasma T_3 must be measured, since hyperthyroidism may be due to elevation of T_3 alone. "T_3 toxicosis" (see page 966), however, occurs in less than 5% of cases. Occasionally, all of the tests of thyroid hormone levels are borderline. If the clinical suspicion of thyrotoxicosis is strong, every effort should be made to obtain laboratory confirmation by measurement of TSH, the response to TRH, or even the RaIU with suppression (see above). Clinical trials of antithyroid drugs should be avoided.

Differential Diagnosis

In some patients, particularly elderly ones, the clinical picture may not suggest hyperthyroidism. Such patients may present with only unexplained weight loss or weakness. Occult neoplasm may first be suspected, and the diagnosis of hyperthyroidism may be missed entirely or considered only after extensive evaluation fails to yield a diagnosis. These are the patients often labeled "apathetic hyperthyroidism." The term implies lethargy—which is, in fact, not often present—but should rather be used to denote that group of individuals who for unclear reasons lack the signs of sympathetic hyperactivity and hence do not exhibit tachycardia, lid retraction, tremor, etc.

Congestive heart failure or atrial fibrillation may be the presenting manifestation. So-called thyrocardiac patients have been incorrectly thought to be resistant to ordinary doses of digitalis. This is occasionally true, but a normal response to conventional therapy for cardiac failure or an arrhythmia should not be considered incompatible with a diagnosis of hyperthyroidism.

Some patients with anxiety may present with tachycardia, tremor, irritability, and weakness simulating hyperthyroidism. The "anxiety" of thyrotoxicosis is more likely to appear as irritability and hyperkinesis than as an expressed feeling of anxiety. Primary anxiety disorders are either related to identifiable stresses, coexist with symptoms of depression, or have distinctive characteristics that make them recognizable (see Chapters 12 and 13). In depression, weight loss is invariably accompanied by anorexia, a relatively unusual symptom of hyperthyroidism (see page 959).

The characteristic ophthalmopathy of Graves' disease may offer the first clue to the diagnosis. However, ophthalmopathy may not be accompanied by hyperthyroidism and may be unilateral. TSH measurement, the T_3 suppression test, or the TRH test will substantiate the diagnosis in most but not all cases of euthyroid Graves' ophthalmopathy. Without evidence of either thyroid hyperfunction, disturbance of the negative feedback system, or dermopathy, the diagnosis of Graves' ophthalmopathy cannot be made with absolute assurance. Indeed, other diseases of the orbit or retro-orbital space must be considered. Computerized axial tomography of the skull and the orbital contents and high resolution sonography are useful diagnostic tools. These procedures can visualize the enlarged extraocular muscles of Graves' ophthalmopathy, although such enlargement is also seen in pseudotumor. In many cases of Graves' ophthalmopathy, without hyperthyroidism, other aspects of Graves' disease eventually become apparent.

When hyperthyroidism is found in a patient without goiter or exophthalmos, suspicions of factitious hyperthyroidism may be warranted. An RaIU test and scan will establish whether the thyroid is functional, and scintiscan or sonogram will sometimes give evidence for enlargement that is not palpable. A very low uptake and a normal-sized gland on scintiscan or sonogram suggest ingestion of thyroid hormone or the presence of thyroiditis with hyperthyroidism (see below, page 965).

Therapy

Hyperthyroidism due to Graves' disease is frequently a self-limited process that terminates within a year or 2 in about one-half of patients. This natural history strongly influences selection of therapy. Other therapeutic considerations relate to the age of the patient and the presence or absence of complications.

Because there are currently no means of controlling the underlying cause of the disease, presumably TSI production, therapy is designed to interfere with thyroid hormone synthesis by drugs or by ablation of thyroid tissue by radioiodide or surgery. Opinions differ on approaches, but the views expressed here closely approximate those of conservative medical opinion in the United States. Each form of therapy has advantages and disadvantages; none provides a simple, definitive solution and none is truly curative. The objective of therapy is to assure minimal morbidity from both the therapy and the disease. The therapy of hyperthyroidism due to causes other than Graves' disease is discussed separately.

Thiocarbamide Antithyroid Drugs

These agents will predictably control excessive production of thyroid hormone in essentially all cases, although in only about one-half of cases will a permanent remission of the hyperthyroidism be seen. Of these latter cases, about one-half will become hypothyroid in the period between 15 to 20 years after successful treatment and onset of remission. Relapses may occur within 6 months to a year or even longer after apparent remission, but such relapses are uncommon except in postpartum patients.

Restoration of the clinically euthyroid state requires at least 4 to 8 weeks, although clinical improvement is usually seen much sooner. Antithyroid drugs are ordinarily the preferred initial treatment for children, some young adults without complications or other medical problems, and the pregnant patient. The antithyroid drugs are also routinely used as preliminary therapy in patients who are to be treated by surgery (see below, page 964). The objective in these cases is to ensure euthyroid status at the time of operation. Patients who are to be treated with radioiodide (see below, page 963) are also frequently treated with an antithyroid drug before and/or after ablation. Radioiodide is slow in producing its effect and may have to be given in multiple doses; use of an antithyroid drug before or after such therapy is therefore a temporary but useful adjunct.

In the United States, only two thiocarbamide drugs

are available, propylthiouracil and methimazole (Tapazole). Propylthiouracil may have an advantage when speed in restoration of euthyroid status is an urgent consideration. Propylthiouracil, unlike methimazole, in addition to its effects in inhibiting thyroid hormone synthesis, also inhibits conversion of T_4 to T_3 in peripheral tissues. Methimazole, on the other hand, is longer acting than propylthiouracil and may be given on a less frequent dosage schedule, thus facilitating compliance. In most adults with hyperthyroidism, 100 to 150 mg of propylthiouracil (available in 50-mg tablets) every 8 hours or 20 to 30 mg of methimazole (available in 5- and 10-mg tablets) every 12 hours will usually suffice as initial therapy, whereas maintenance is often possible with 50 to 100 mg of propylthiouracil twice daily or 5 to 10 mg of methimazole once or twice daily. The T_4 level should be measured after a month of treatment and every 2 to 3 months thereafter. If at these relatively low maintenance doses of antithyroid drug, the plasma T_4 falls below normal, efforts to "titrate" the dose further are frequently tedious and unsuccessful and should be avoided. A euthyroid state can be achieved under these circumstances by the addition of oral thyroxine, usually at somewhat less than full replacement dose. Another argument in favor of this approach is that higher doses of methimazole have been associated with higher rates of remission. A simple program is to initiate treatment with methimazole alone, and at a point when the T_4 has become normal, to institute maintenance with a single daily dose of 60 mg of methimazole plus 0.10 to 0.125 mg of thyroxine.

Although the recommended doses will control the disease in the vast majority of cases, some individuals clearly need higher doses. If the patient is severely ill, larger doses should be given from the beginning. The risk of an adverse drug effect may be increased, but this is not established and should not be a consideration under such circumstances. In order to achieve total blockade of hormone synthesis, as much as 200 mg of propylthiouracil every 4 hours may be necessary. Because methimazole has a longer duration of action, it need not be given so often, but 30 to 40 mg three times daily may be needed in some cases.

Duration of Therapy

A period of 12 to 24 months of therapy should elapse before consideration is given to discontinuation of the drug, although conflicting evidence suggests that lasting remission may not be related to duration of therapy beyond the point at which the patient becomes euthyroid. A few indicators are helpful in predicting success or failure of the outcome of a course of antithyroid drug therapy. Patients who have continued to require large doses of drug are almost certain not to have achieved remission. On the other hand, reduction of thyroid mass during therapy is often predictive of lasting clinical remission. Tests for restoration of the normal negative feedback system at the end of a period of drug therapy (thyroid suppressibility; see

above) are of little use in predicting long-term remission. For determination of short-term status the TRH test is of no use at all, but a suppression test using T_3 or T_4, although not accurately predictive of the long term, may nonetheless be helpful in establishing the clinical status at the time of discontinuation of drug therapy. To perform the test, the antithyroid drug is withheld through the period of the test. The patient is given 75 μg of T_3 (Cytomel) as a single dose daily for 7 days or one 3-mg dose of T_4. RaIU is then determined 1 week after initiation of T_3 administration (or after the single dose of T_4). Low postsuppression 24-hour uptake (<10%) indicates accurately that the patient is in remission at the time of the test. More significantly, an uptake above the normal range almost invariably indicates continuation of active disease. Intermediate values are not useful. If on clinical grounds, or as a result of testing, continued disease activity seems to be present, discontinuation of therapy is inadvisable and will almost certainly result in clinical relapse and needless morbidity. Measurement of titers of TSI may be useful in predicting relapse, but such measurements are not widely available and are also not accurate predictors.

If the clinical status indicates that remission may have been reached, antithyroid drug therapy is terminated and the patient is observed. Routine determination of plasma T_4 every 3 to 4 weeks for 3 to 6 months allows early recognition of return of thyroid overactivity. If the status is ambiguous, and especially if there is evidence of continued disease activity, antithyroid drug dosage may be reduced to one-half the maintenance level for 3 to 6 months in the expectation that, if recurrence occurs, it will be blunted. Prophylactic use of propranolol (see below) during withdrawal of antithyroid drugs is a useful maneuver that prevents emergence of symptoms of overt hyperthyroidism should relapse occur.

If the hyperthyroid state recurs, treatment with antithyroid drug may be reinitiated for another course (i.e., 1 year) or alternative therapy may be undertaken (^{131}I or surgery). A second course of antithyroid drug has a significant chance of inducing remission. In selected patients, prolonged or even indefinite drug therapy is reasonable, but with most patients such an approach is not desirable.

Minor side effects of drug therapy occur in 1 to 5% of patients. Skin rashes, the most common side effect, are usually seen in the first months of therapy and often disappear even if therapy is continued. Antihistamine drugs are useful in controlling these rashes and the sometimes associated urticaria and pruritus. Leukopenia is not uncommon but is usually not severe and is dose related. If the absolute number of polymorphonuclear leukocytes falls below 2000, the dose should be reduced or the drug discontinued. If the side effects are not tolerated, a switch to another agent will allow continuation of therapy in about half of the cases. Major complications of drug therapy occur in less than 0.1% of cases. Agranulocytosis is the most dreaded complication. Unlike leukopenia, thiocarbamide-induced agranulocytosis due to antileukocyte antibodies from thiocarbamides is not dose related and is of such sudden onset that routine blood counts are of no help in prevention. The patient should, however, be instructed to contact the physician promptly if severe sore mouth or sore throat and fever occur. Immediate hospitalization is indicated. Fortunately, most patients with agranulocytosis recover, albeit after a stormy course. Other toxic reactions include drug fever, arthralgias, and hepatitis. Elevations of alkaline phosphatase activity are commonly seen in patients receiving propylthiouracil. If other liver enzymes are normal, the drug may be continued, but persistent laboratory evidence of hepatocellular damage is an indication for discontinuation of therapy. White blood count should be monitored after several weeks of therapy and after increases of drug dose. Liver enzymes should be measured every 3 to 6 months.

Adjunctive Drug Therapy

Iodide. Iodide in the treatment of hyperthyroidism should be reserved for patients with severe illness. Occasionally, iodide therapy produces severe dermatitis. Use of iodide may preclude for many weeks the use of radioactive iodide, the uptake of which by the thyroid will be greatly diminished.

Iodide is the best agent available for inhibiting hormone release and is useful in patients who need rapid correction of the hyperthyroid state. Iodide also has a time-honored place in preoperative preparation (see below, page 964) for thyroidectomy, to reduce vascularity of the gland. When given after radioiodide therapy, iodide seems especially effective in accelerating restoration of euthyroid status.

The dose of iodide is one drop of a saturated solution of potassium iodide (40 mg) diluted in water or juice twice daily; larger doses are often given but are unnecessary. Lugol's solution is an obsolete pharmacological concoction containing iodine and iodide, which has no virtue over iodide alone.

Adrenergic antagonists. The symptoms and signs of thyrotoxicosis that are related to sensitization of the sympathetic nervous system are in large measure abolished by β-adrenergic blocking drugs. The current agent of choice is propranolol. Other newer, more selective β-adrenergic antagonists are probably equally effective, although no clear advantage has been demonstrated over propranolol. Some of these agents are partial adrenergic agonists (e.g., pindolol) and are inappropriate for use in hyperthyroidism. The indications for use of propranolol are severe tachycardia, tremor, sweating, and agitation. Propranolol is effective for relief of these manifestations of hyperthyroidism but does not appreciably affect excessive metabolic rate or reverse the catabolic state of severe cases. Propranolol has occasional undesirable side effects and is relatively contraindicated in some individuals (e.g., those with asthma). Concern is often expressed that patients with heart disease may be thrown into congestive heart failure or that heart failure, if present, may worsen.

On the other hand, some patients with congestive heart failure may respond well to the drug when excessive heart rate is a major contributing factor. Other uses for propranolol are in the prevention of symptoms during trial withdrawal of an antithyroid drug and while awaiting the effects of ^{131}I therapy. Most patients require propranolol in doses of *at least* 160 mg daily, but doses up to 720 mg may be necessary. The drug should be discontinued as soon as the patient is rendered euthyroid by other therapy.

Radioactive Iodide Therapy

Radioactive iodide (^{131}I) is uniformly effective therapy; it is simple to administer and inexpensive. It is the preferred form of therapy for most adults with Graves' disease and is much to be preferred over surgery.

The single disadvantage of radioactive iodide is that hypothyroidism is a frequent consequence. For many years, concern was expressed over the possibility of producing carcinoma of the thyroid, leukemia, or genetic damage in the future offspring of women in their childbearing years. All of these concerns have been shown to be groundless. Although low doses of external radiation do produce carcinoma of the thyroid, the higher doses used for treatment of hyperthyroidism do not. Long-term follow-up of treated patients over the past 30 years has failed to substantiate any such risk or any increased risk of leukemia. The amounts of radiation to the ovaries from therapeutic doses of radioiodide used for therapy of hyperthyroidism are lower than those delivered by diagnostic X-ray procedures and can be expected to produce no genetic effects. Thus, radioiodide therapy for hyperthyroidism can be considered for any adult patient, including women of childbearing age who plan to have children.

Hypothyroidism follows radioiodide therapy in the immediate few months after therapy in a more or less dose-related fashion. Large doses predictably eliminate hyperthyroidism with certainty but totally ablate the thyroid with great regularity. Small, single doses render the patient euthyroid with 50 to 70% likelihood but unavoidably still produce hypothyroidism within a year in about 10% of cases. Furthermore, of the patients rendered euthyroid, 3 to 4%/year develop hypothyroidism over the ensuing 20 years.

One may question whether the high frequency of post-treatment hypothyroidism constitutes a significant disadvantage of radioiodide therapy. The answer is that, for the majority of those who become hypothyroid, replacement therapy with thyroxine is a trivial inconvenience. For these patients, the advantages of radioiodide therapy far outweigh the one disadvantage. Unfortunately, a few patients, despite warnings to the contrary, discontinue their required lifelong replacement therapy, become lost to follow-up, and suffer all of the consequences of long-standing hypothyroidism and myxedema.

Some physicians advocate the use of deliberately ablative doses of ^{131}I. This approach to therapy certainly greatly simplifies patient management, accelerates restoration of the euthyroid state, and is reasonable in view of the high probability of post-therapy hypothyroidism regardless of dose. Nonetheless, most physicians do not advocate deliberate ablation unless the patient is elderly, has experienced a major complication of hyperthyroidism (e.g., severe heart disease), or has complicating medical problems that demand prompt control. In young patients who are tolerating their disease reasonably well, most physicians prefer to use small doses of ^{131}I, repeated if necessary, until the patient is euthyroid. Such an approach does not, of course, guarantee that hypothyroidism will be avoided.

As discussed below (page 966), larger (10 to 30 mCi) doses of ^{131}I are appropriate initially in the treatment of toxic nodular goiter.

In the past, elaborate schemes have been used to estimate the required dose of ^{131}I. Unfortunately, none of these has proven helpful, since the biological sensitivity to radiation effect, the most important variable, is not measurable. Currently, in a typical "low dose" treatment scheme patients with small glands are given 2 to 3 mCi, whereas those with moderately enlarged to large glands are given 5 to 10 mCi. Ablative doses approximate 15 mCi. Because of the unpredictable response with nonablative doses, antithyroid drugs are often used initially to render the patient euthyroid. Antithyroid therapy is then interrupted for 48 hours before the ^{131}I is given and reinstituted 24 hours afterward. Alternatively, an antithyroid drug can be initiated 24 to 48 hours after therapy with ^{131}I. Similar approaches combining antithyroid drug and ^{131}I are almost routinely used in patients with severe or complicated hyperthyroidism, e.g., thyrocardiac disease.

Radioactive iodide can be administered only by an appropriately licensed physician—usually an endocrinologist or a nuclear medicine physician. A few precautions are necessary. In women of childbearing age a negative test for pregnancy must be obtained by the therapist immediately before the therapy dose is given since exposure of a fetus to radiation is unacceptable. Women who have a young child at home are given no more than 8 mC and are instructed to avoid prolonged close contact (e.g., sharing a bed) for a week.

The undocumented notion has long persisted that radiation thyroiditis may produce excessive release of thyroid hormones 7 to 14 days after therapy, with the possibility of consequent worsening of the clinical state. This complication, if it occurs at all, must be rare. Nonetheless, prudence dictates a conservative approach in precarious patients, e.g., those in congestive heart failure, who are best brought to euthyroid status or who are at least significantly improved by antithyroid drug therapy before ablation with ^{131}I. At 3 months after ^{131}I therapy, when the short-term radiation effect becomes maximal, the antithyroid drug can be discontinued or tapered, provided, of course, that the laboratory and clinical evidence indicates return to euthyroid status. Adjunctive therapy with propranolol is useful at this point to ameliorate possible emerging

symptoms when the preceding dose of ^{131}I has been inadequate. If the laboratory evidence indicates continuing hyperthyroidism, another dose of ^{131}I will be required.

Therapy with ^{131}I is always successful if enough ^{131}I is given. "Failure" after one or more doses is never an indication for surgery or indeterminate therapy with antithyroid drug. Rather, additional ^{131}I should be given to complete the process.

Surgical Therapy

For many years surgical ablation of the thyroid, e.g., subtotal thyroidectomy, was the main therapy for hyperthyroidism. This procedure still has its advocates, especially for young adults and for children who cannot be successfully treated with antithyroid drugs. In the hands of experienced surgeons, subtotal thyroidectomy is certainly effective therapy, attended by minimal morbidity. However, complications include the small but real risk of anesthesia/operative mortality, recurrent laryngeal nerve damage with vocal cord paralysis, permanent hypoparathyroidism, and, most commonly, hypothyroidism. The latter two complications are, to a certain extent, unavoidable and are not merely the consequence of poor surgical technique. In addition to about a 10% occurrence of immediate postsurgical hypothyroidism, 2 to 3% of patients become hypothyroid each year after surgery, a figure only slightly lower than that after therapy with ^{131}I. A higher complication rate must be expected when the operation is performed by surgeons with limited experience in thyroid surgery. Surgery also is followed by a significant (5%) rate of recurrent hyperthyroidism, sometimes occurring many years later. In this case, even the most enthusiastic supporters of surgical treatment agree that recurrent hyperthyroidism should never be treated by a second operation, since the frequency of major complications rises to an unacceptable level.

Treatment of Hyperthyroidism during Pregnancy

Hyperthyroidism during pregnancy, almost invariably due to Graves' disease, should be treated with an antithyroid drug. Surgery has been used successfully during pregnancy but has no advantage and may be associated with increased fetal losses. Radioactive iodide is contraindicated. Therapy with antithyroid drugs during pregnancy is guided by two considerations. First, the antithyroid drugs freely cross the placenta and can, in large doses, produce goiter and hypothyroidism in the infant. Second, thyroid hormones do not cross the placenta from mother to fetus. The dose of antithyroid drugs should be the minimal amount adequate to control the hyperthyroidism. A dose of drug that totally blocks hormone synthesis along with a replacement amount of thyroxine is not appropriate during pregnancy. When ordinary doses of antithyroid drug are used, the fetus is usually born without goiter, but as a precaution the dose is often reduced, if possible, during the last month of pregnancy. Iodide should not be used during pregnancy, since the fetal thyroid is especially susceptible to the goitrogenic effect of iodide. Monitoring the plasma hormone level requires determination of free T_4 or the free T_4 index, since T_4 is normally elevated during pregnancy in association with the increased TBG.

TSIs (see page 959) of Graves' disease cross the placenta and enter the fetal circulation. Occasionally, the newborn infant is hyperthyroid as a result of this passive transfer of antibodies. The physician caring for the newborn should always be alerted to this possibility.

Ophthalmopathy of Graves' Disease

The exact frequency of ophthalmopathy in Graves' disease is not known, but most patients have either no obvious infiltrative eye involvement or show only minimal to moderate proptosis, which generally stabilizes at a tolerable level. Severe exophthalmos occurs in no more than a few percentages of cases of Graves' disease. Proptosis becomes more than a cosmetic concern, when the eyelids fail to close, setting the stage for exposure keratitis or corneal ulceration. Paresis of the extraocular muscles producing diplopia can also be troublesome and may require use of an eye patch or corrective surgery. The most disturbing and rarest eye involvement is chemosis or marked inflammation and edema of the conjunctivae and periorbital soft tissues. Ophthalmopathy of this severity is termed malignant or infiltrative exophthalmos. Rarely, optic neuritis leading to blindness occurs. The therapy of severe ophthalmopathy, which may include decompression of the orbit, is accomplished by an ophthalmologist with special competency in treating this condition.

Graves' ophthalmopathy follows a temporal course that may be totally dissociated from the hyperthyroidism, the treatment of which should be independent of and uninfluenced by the eye disease. Despite claims to the contrary, no form of treatment of hyperthyroidism has any advantage for control of the ophthalmopathy. The notion persists, however, that induction of hypothyroidism may aggravate exophthalmos. Development of clinical hypothyroidism should therefore be avoided, especially when exophthalmos is present.

Hyperthyroidism Associated with Thyroiditis (Lymphocytic Thyroiditis with Spontaneously Resolving Hyperthyroidism; Postpartum Thyroiditis with Hyperthyroidism; Silent Thyroiditis)

Classical subacute thyroiditis (see below, page 976) has long been known to be associated occasionally with short-lived, self-limited hyperthyroidism. The explanation for this phenomenon has been that the destructive inflammatory process causes release of preformed thyroid hormone. The hyperthyroidism invariably disappears within a few months.

Another apparently distinct variant of the thyroidi-

tis-hyperthyroidism syndrome has been recognized—lymphocytic thyroiditis. These patients present with a modestly enlarged thyroid gland that is nontender. No prior history of viral illness can be obtained. The radioiodide uptake is very low, as it is in subacute thyroiditis, whereas the T_4 and T_3 are high. About one-half of cases have significant elevations of thyroid antibodies, and about one-half of these high titers subside within a few months. A propensity of the condition to occur in the postpartum period has been noted, sometimes in successive pregnancies and sometimes followed by the development of hypothyroidism. On biopsy the changes seen differ from those of the peak phase of classical subacute thyroiditis, but the latter, in its late stages of evolution, may be indistinguishable from that of lymphocytic thyroiditis. Whether lymphocytic thyroiditis with spontaneously resulting hyperthyroidism (silent thyroiditis) is a new disease, as has been suggested by some, or is a newly recognized variant of subacute thyroiditis is a matter of debate (10, 17, 18).

It is important to obtain a radioiodide uptake measurement in all patients with hyperthyroidism who do not clearly have Graves' disease (i.e., who do not have associated eye findings) or toxic nodular goiter. A very low radioiodide uptake will establish the diagnosis of hyperthyroidism associated with thyroiditis and allow the physician to avoid inappropriate therapy (radioiodide or surgery). Treatment with an antithyroid drug may be useful; propranolol (see above, page 963) affords symptomatic relief and may be all of the treatment that is necessary.

Long-term follow-up studies on these patients show that about half persist in having some degree of thyroid abnormality; antithyroid antibodies or goiter, recurring bouts of hyperthyroidism, elevation of TSH ("decreased thyroid reserve"), and, occasionally, hypothyroidism (18).

Hyperthyroidism Associated with Multinodular Goiter (Toxic Nodular Goiter)

Toxic nodular goiter is usually seen in adults in midlife or in the elderly. Although the typical patient with Graves' disease usually relates symptoms extending over a few months to a year, the history in toxic nodular goiter is often much longer. Many years may pass before diagnosis. Because of the patient's age and the duration of illness, severe cardiac or musculoskeletal involvement is common.

Toxic nodular goiter appears to arise in the pathological evolution of some cases of nodular goiter. Most nodular goiters (see below, page 972) are initially TSH dependent, i.e., suppressible with exogenous thyroid hormone. Eventually, some of these goiters develop autonomous areas, with other regions of relatively decreased activity. Nodular goiters at this stage of evolution do not secrete enough hormone to produce clinical hyperthyroidism but in 20% of cases show nonsuppressible function. A few of these autonomously functioning goiters evolve to a stage in which excessive production of hormone and clinical hyperthyroidism ensue.

If the usual laboratory tests (T_4, free T_4 index) are borderline, special tests such as measurement of T_3, suppression of TSH (page 955), or TRH stimulation (page 956) should be considered. The suppression test can be undertaken cautiously in the elderly patient without overt heart disease but should not be used if heart disease is obvious. These tests are more helpful in excluding a diagnosis of hyperthyroidism than in establishing a state of hormone excess, since a significant number of cases of nontoxic nodular goiter are not suppressible. The TRH test is of limited value in the elderly. A normal response to TRH excludes a diagnosis of hyperthyroidism at any age, but failure to respond is a common occurrence in normal elderly persons.

Therapy of toxic nodular goiter is best accomplished with ^{131}I. Rather large doses, in the range of 10 to 30 mCi, are usually necessary. Hypothyroidism occurs much less frequently after ^{131}I therapy for nodular goiter than for Graves' disease. If the clinical situation demands prompt relief of the hyperthyroidism, an antithyroid drug can be used after the therapeutic dose of ^{131}I, since the response to radioiodide is often slow and multiple doses may be needed. Otherwise ^{131}I given alone is simple therapy, without side effects, and easily monitored by measurements of plasma T_4. Other therapeutic considerations including the use of adjunctive therapy follow those outlined for the therapy of Graves' disease with one exception. In hyperthyroidism due to toxic nodular goiter, antithyroid drugs alone cannot be expected to produce a lasting remission.

Hyperthyroidism Due to Excessive Secretion of T_3; "T_3 Toxicosis"

In most cases of hyperthyroidism, the thyroid secretes excessive quantities of both T_4 and T_3. However, in perhaps 5% of cases, T_3 is the predominant hormone secreted. T_3 toxicosis may occur in hyperthyroidism due to Graves' disease, toxic multinodular goiter, or autonomous adenoma. The patient who appears clinically hyperthyroid but whose T_4 is normal should have plasma T_3 measured. T_3 toxicosis sometimes occurs early in the course of hyperthyroidism due to Graves' disease and can develop during therapy with an antithyroid drug, in which case the dose should be increased. Continuing clinical findings of hyperthyroidism during such therapy—and despite a normal or low T_4—should raise the possibility that T_3 toxicosis is now present and that more, rather than less, antithyroid drug is needed. The treatment of T_3 toxicosis is the same as is that of other forms of hyperthyroidism.

Hyperthyroidism (and Hypothyroidism) Due to Iodide

Iodide from a variety of sources can induce hyperthyroidism (6). The agent currently most likely to produce hyperthyroidism is the antiarrhythmic drug, amiodarone (see Chapter 59). This drug contains nearly 40% iodine and can exert a number of effects on thyroid function. The drug inhibits conversion of T_4 to T_3; coincidentally an increase of serum T_4 and free T_4 occur. Although this circumstance, *per se*, does not cause thyroid dysfunction, amiodarone can cause either hyperthyroidism or hypothyroidism, the dominant dysfunction apparently depending on regional iodine intake. In Europe some 10% of patients receiving the drug develop hyperthyroidism whereas in the United States hypothyroidism is much more common, nearly 20% in one series. Most of the latter cases are presumably iodide induced in susceptible people with pre-existing Hashimoto's thyroiditis. The diagnosis of hyperthyroidism due to amiodarone depends on demonstration of an elevated T_3 and suppression of TSH. Treatment of hypothyroidism requires only ordinary replacement with T_4, but the hyperthyroidism cannot be treated with radioiodide (low thyroidal radioiodide uptake) and is often resistant to standard antithyroid drug therapy. The combination of propylthiouracil or methimazole plus perchlorate is quite effective.

Thyroid Storm (Thyrotoxic Crisis)

This dreaded complication of hyperthyroidism is now only rarely encountered. When thyroid storm does occur, it is usually in the setting of a severe medical or surgical stress imposed on a patient with uncontrolled or unrecognized hyperthyroidism. Clinical features of full blown thyroid storm include fever, sometimes to the level of extreme hyperpyrexia, marked tachycardia, great irritability, diarrhea, and hypotension. Thyroid storm often progresses rapidly to delirium and coma. Any such severe exacerbation of hyperthyroidism demands hospitalization and urgent consultation with an endocrinologist.

HYPOTHYROIDISM

Hypothyroidism, the metabolic state resulting from deficient thyroid hormones, is relatively common. Most cases can be diagnosed even when symptoms and signs are minimal, provided that the physician considers the diagnosis and seeks appropriate laboratory confirmation. The manifestations of hypothyroidism are varied and to a large measure age dependent. *Myxedema* is a severe form of hypothyroidism that results in deposition of mucopolysaccharides in the skin and other tissues, producing a characteristic appearance and a constellation of physical findings. The term myxedema is commonly but incorrectly used interchangeably with hypothyroidism. *Primary hypothyroidism* is a term used to indicate that the hormone deficiency results from a disease or other process within the thyroid gland. *Secondary hypothyroidism*, much less common, results from lack of thyrotropin (TSH) secretion, a result of pituitary or, rarely, hypothalamic disease. The thyroid is usually smaller than normal and not palpable. Plasma TSH, using new sensitive assays, may be low, but experience in this situation is limited. Almost invariably the hypothyroidism is part of a decrease in pituitary function involving tropic hormones in addition to TSH with consequent hypogonadism and/or adrenal insufficiency. Causes include postpartum necrosis, pituitary tumor, pituitary apoplexy, and granulomatous disease, or possibly part of an autoimmune process involving failure of other endocrine glands. Some cases occur without identifiable cause and are termed idiopathic (see also Chapter 74).

Etiology

Currently, the commonest cause of hypothyroidism is iatrogenic, i.e., the result of therapy of hyperthyroidism with radioiodide or by surgery. Spontaneous cases due to thyroid atrophy are also common. A clinical classification is given in Table 73.7.

Idiopathic hypothyroidism in most cases results from autoimmune destruction of the thyroid with subsequent thyroid atrophy. Some cases are the result of long-standing Hashimoto's thyroiditis. Both types occur frequently in association with other autoimmune diseases such as pernicious anemia. In both types, high titers of antibodies to thyroid antigens (thyroglobulin, microsomes) are seen in 90% of cases. As a clinically encountered thyroid abnormality, Hashimoto's thyroiditis is second in frequency only to nontoxic nodular goiter and is by far the most common cause of goitrous hypothyroidism. The clinical distinction between ordinary multinodular goiter and goiters due to Hashimoto's thyroiditis is made by measurement of thyroid autoantibodies.

Drug-Induced Hypothyroidism

A variety of drugs can produce hypothyroidism that is invariably associated with goiter formation. Only a few in current use have such an effect. Lithium, currently in wide use for the treatment of manic-depressive illness (see Chapter 15), is one such agent. If goiter occurs, lithium need not be stopped; addition of thyroxine relieves the hypothyroidism and causes regression of the goiter. Overtreatment of hyperthyroidism with an antithyroid drug will, of course, produce hypothyroidism. Iodide in pharmacological amounts is an antithyroid drug and will also occasionally produce goiter and hypothyroidism as in patients given long-term iodide therapy for asthma or another chronic lung disease. However, most adults who are susceptible to the antithyroid action of iodide have an underlying thyroid abnormality, such as Hashimoto's thyroiditis (see below, page 975) or radioiodide-treated Graves' disease. Amiodarone, an antiarrhythmic agent, contains iodine and can produce hypothyroidism in up to 20% of persons (see also "Hyperthyroidism Due to Iodide," page 966). One should also keep in mind the possibility of inapparent iodide administration during hospitalizations [contrast media, including those used in conjunction with computerized tomography (CT) scanning] with posthospitalization development of thyroid dysfunction.

Clinical Features

Hypothyroidism in the adult is highly variable in presentation. Usually, onset is insidious, often occurring over many years, with the result that the symptoms go unappreciated by patient and physician alike. The nonspecificity of the symptoms also contributes to the delayed diagnosis. No predictable progression of symptoms is apparent, but easy fatigability, lethargy, increased sleep requirement, cold intolerance, muscle aching, and stiffness are perhaps the commonest early symptoms. The skin is dry and scaling. Hair loss is frequent. The eyebrows become sparse, the face is "puffy," i.e., full, with edema of the periorbital areas. The voice often becomes low pitched and rough. Constipation is common and may be severe enough to produce megacolon; sometimes the diagnosis is suggested by the radiologist from the results of a barium enema. Diminished hearing, especially in old persons, is easily overlooked or attributed to "aging." Ordinarily, the affected individual becomes abnormally placid, but agitation or frank psychosis may occur. In the elderly, depression is the commonest psychiatric accompaniment of hypothyroidism. Dementia due to hypothyroidism is rare, but the association of the two processes in the elderly is not uncommon (9). Paresthesias of the hands due to carpal tunnel syndrome are common. Diminished sexual function is the rule. Women often experience menorrhagia. Rarely, galactorrhea may be seen in women of childbearing age. Fertility is diminished, but pregnancy may occur and normal delivery is possible. The newborn is euthyroid, unless the mother's hypothyroidism is drug related or the hypothyroidism is of the rare familial athyrotic variety.

Subclinical Hypothyroidism

The most common stage of hypothyroidism likely to be encountered in ambulatory patients is mild hypothyroidism, commonly termed subclinical hypothyroidism. This degree of hormone deficiency occurs

Table 73.7.
Clinical Classification of Hypothyroidism[a]

HYPOTHYROIDISM WITHOUT GOITER (DECREASE OF THYROID TISSUE MASS)
  Postablative for hyperthyroidism (radioiodide therapy or surgery)
  Idiopathic atrophy
  Developmental defect (congenital)
  Pituitary or hypothalamic disease
HYPOTHYROIDISM WITH GOITER
  Chronic thyroiditis (Hashimoto's disease, etc.)
  Drug induced (antithyroid drugs, iodide, lithium,[b] sulfonylureas, etc.)
  Iodide deficiency (remote geographic areas)
  Genetic biosynthetic defects

[a] Hypothyroidism in the United States is now most commonly the consequence of therapy for hyperthyroidism. Hypothyroidism due to idiopathic atrophy of the thyroid is second in frequency. Developmental defects (*e.g.*, lingual thyroid) are rare. Hypothyroidism with goiter is nearly always due to Hashimoto's thyroiditis, rarely to a drug. Genetic biosynthetic defects are rare and usually become manifest in childhood.
[b] Hypothyroidism due to chronic lithium therapy may occur without goiter.

with an overall prevalence of 2 to 7%. The condition is defined by a paucity of nonspecific but suggestive symptoms and few clinical findings, serum thyroid hormone levels that are within the normal range, but an elevation of thyrotropin (TSH). One study suggests that some of these patients are clinically improved after therapy with L-thyroxine (4).

Severe Hypothyroidism with Myxedema

In spontaneous cases of hypothyroidism, only with severe, long-standing disease does extensive deposition of mucopolysaccharide occur, producing the clinical state of myxedema. Rarely, myxedema may develop rapidly after radioiodide or after surgical ablation of the thyroid for hyperthyroidism.

In myxedema, a variety of manifestations can be appreciated on physical examination and, of course, they vary with the severity and duration of the disease. The skin, in addition to being dry and scaling, is typically cool. The scaling may be extensive so that large flakes are shed over the elbows and knees. The subcutaneous tissues may be infiltrated by mucopolysaccharides so that the skin appears to be "thickened" or "doughy." In the elderly, atrophy of the epidermis may occur simultaneously, producing a stiff, translucent, parchment-like appearance. Yellow-orange discoloration of the skin due to carotene may be evident, especially in the palms. The presence of edema is not obvious, since pitting is not noted except in extreme cases complicated by hypoproteinemia. An exception is the collection around the eyes of "bags of water." This finding is not, however, specific for hypothyroidism. The tongue is sometimes enlarged. The heart rate is usually slow (sinus bradycardia). The heart may appear enlarged, due either to dilation of the myocardium or to pericardial effusion. Pleural effusions and ascites may also be present, sometimes even in cases that are otherwise not clinically severe. Dilutional hyponatremia, clinically indistinguishable from the syndrome of inappropriate antidiuretic hormone excess, may be present. The deep tendon reflexes characteristically show a delay in their relaxation phase, the so-called "hung-up reflex." This is a highly suggestive finding but may be seen occasionally in other diseases. Mental functioning is slowed, as reflected in the characteristically slow speech. The reading speed may be greatly reduced. Hearing loss may be severe or of a degree apparent only on audiometric testing. Cerebellar dysfunction, if present, is usually evident only on extensive neurological testing, but in rare cases is grossly apparent as ataxia. These and other unusual aspects of hypothyroidism have been reviewed as has the clinical picture in the elderly (9, 13, 25).

Myxedema Coma

This severe, often fatal event is an infrequent complication of long-standing disease and is typically seen in the elderly patient. Myxedema coma is often associated with or precipitated by pneumonia, perito-nitis, or some other serious infection, the presence of which may not be immediately apparent. Severe respiratory failure is a major feature and can be due to a variety of factors ranging from upper airway obstruction to impaired chest wall mechanics.

Because elderly patients often become hypothermic on exposure to cold or during sepsis, the diagnosis of myxedema coma is more frequently considered than actually confirmed. Any of these events demands hospitalization.

Laboratory Findings

In primary hypothyroidism, the combination of low plasma T_4, free T_4 index (or free T_4), and high TSH is diagnostic. Difficulties in diagnosis are encountered only in occasional cases. The plasma T_3 is usually low, but since T_3 decreases in a variety of nonthyroidal illnesses ranging from malnutrition to liver disease, its measurement is not useful for diagnosis of hypothyroidism. Furthermore, it is normal in many patients with mild hypothyroidism. In hypothyroidism due to pituitary or hypothalamic disease the TSH should be low in the new sensitive assays. However, TSH may be low in severely ill persons with nonthyroidal illness also (see page 955). The TRH test is ordinarily not necessary for diagnosis of primary hypothyroidism but can be helpful when the T_4 and TSH are borderline. In this situation, an exaggerated response to TRH may be seen (TSH increment >30).

In addition to the definitive diagnostic tests, various other laboratory abnormalities are encountered, although they serve no useful diagnostic purpose. A common laboratory finding is elevation of plasma enzymes that originate in skeletal muscle: creatine kinase (CPK), serum aspartate aminotransferase (AST formerly SGOT), serum alanine aminotransferase (ALT formerly SGPT), and lactic dehydrogenase (LDH). Fractionation studies show that when these enzymes are elevated in hypothyroidism, they do not originate in cardiac muscle. Other abnormalities include electrocardiographic changes (such as flattened or inverted T waves, minor ST segment depressions, and low amplitude QRS complexes) and abnormalities of blood gas measurements due to hypoventilation. Anemia (see Chapter 50), usually normocytic and normochromic, may be present, as may macrocytic anemia of coexistent vitamin B_{12} deficiency (pernicious anemia). An abnormality of red cell shape (spiculation) also has been described in hypothyroidism.

Differential Diagnosis

The most difficult problem in diagnosis is the simple clinical appreciation of the possibility that the patient may be hypothyroid. Once suspected, the subsequent history, physical examination, and, particularly, laboratory findings will easily establish the diagnosis in all but a few cases. However, some special problems may be encountered. Any elderly patient who is sick, pale, and puffy faced becomes a suspect for the diagnosis, especially if an adequate history cannot be obtained. A patient with atypical chest pain, nonspecific electrocardiographic abnormalities, and elevated creatine kinase, ASP, or ALT is not infrequently labeled as having ischemic heart disease and myocardial infarction; the proper diagnosis may be hypothyroidism. A patient with the nephrotic syndrome might be mistaken for having hypothyroidism. However, although the plasma T_4 may be low (TBG is low in some nephrotic patients), the free T_4 index (or free T_4) is normal. More important, the patient with the nephrotic syndrome will have features characteristic of that disorder, i.e., massive proteinuria and hypoalbuminemia (see Chapter 44).

Diagnosis of Hypothyroidism in Patients Receiving Thyroid Hormone Therapy

Patients are frequently encountered who, having been diagnosed as hypothyroid at some time in the past, are receiving replacement therapy when first seen. Lack of documentation may lead one to question the original diagnosis. Alternatives include continuation of therapy despite an uncertain diagnosis, or discontinuation of therapy, a maneuver that will confirm or refute the need for continued treatment. In many instances, continuation of therapy may be simpler, less expensive, and more appropriate than an attempt to resolve the issue, but this can often be easily accomplished, even after many years of treatment, by abrupt discontinuation of hormone therapy. After 5 weeks, determination of plasma T_4 (and FTI) is made. If the value is normal, the patient is considered euthyroid and the original diagnosis is discarded. In contrast, a low T_4 (and a subsequently determined high TSH) verifies a diagnosis of hypothyroidism.

Occasional euthyroid patients who were inappropriately treated with thyroid hormone for long periods and most hypothyroid patients become symptomatic during the 5-week period of withdrawal. An occasional inappropriately treated patient can show a delay of several additional weeks in return of normal thyroid function. If the physician wishes to avoid the possibility of the development of symptoms as a result of withdrawal, a rapid but expensive way to determine thyroid status while the patient continues to receive full hormone replacement is to administer bovine TSH (10 units intramuscularly) followed 18 hours later by an RaIU test (page 956). A normal or elevated RaIU post-TSH injection indicates normal thyroid function and a previously inappropriate diagnosis of primary hypothyroidism.

Hypothyroidism versus "Euthyroid Sick Syndrome"

The diagnosis of hypothyroidism in severely ill patients presents special problems (28, 29). Patients with the simulating "euthyroid sick syndrome" are usually elderly and often have sepsis. The T_4 and T_4 indexes are low, TSH may be low, normal, or moderately elevated (up to 20μU/ml), depending on the stage of the illness, and response to TRH is normal or blunted. Plasma rT_3 is often elevated.

Although to date this "euthyroid sick syndrome" has been clearly recognized only in hospitalized, severely ill patients, it probably also occurs in less dramatic form in chronically ill, nonhospitalized individuals. Many patients with chronic renal failure undergoing hemodialysis appear to fall in this group. The mechanisms underlying this phenomenon appear to involve a combination of factors including accelerated T_4 metabolism, impairment of TSH secretion (29), and impairment of T_4 binding to plasma proteins.

Treatment

The best preparation for ordinary use is T_4 (levothyroxine, sodium l-thyroxine, Synthroid, Levothyroid). T_3 (liothyronine, Cytomel) is also effective and may possibly be more effective for treatment of goiter, but it has no special advantage for routine therapy of hypothyroidism and has the distinct disadvantage that one cannot monitor the plasma T_4 to determine adequacy of replacement. Combinations of T_4 and T_3 and desiccated thyroid should no longer be used.

Traditionally, initiation of thyroid hormone replacement therapy has been cautious and conservative and has utilized dosage schedules that ensure slow restoration of a normal metabolic state. Although the principle is rational, the practice is often faulty. Therapy should be adjusted to the individual case, with several points in mind. If the patient is not elderly and has never had overt cardiac disease, overcautious initiation of therapy will result only in needless prolongation of the hypothyroid state with its attendant morbidity. If the patient has evidence of pre-existing cardiac disease or is frail and elderly, therapy should be started at low dosage (see below), but unnecessary delay should be avoided. Only rarely will serious heart disease, such as angina pectoris, prevent at least partial therapy sufficient to eliminate myxedema, if not full correction of hypothyroidism.

The usual hypothyroid patient, without complicating medical problems, may be started on full daily replacement dosage. Even with this therapeutic schedule, the clinical response will be very slow. One can expect several months to pass before restoration of the normal metabolic state. If the patient is elderly or has known cardiovascular disease, a daily dose of 0.0125 to 0.025 mg of T_4 should be started, with 0.025-mg increases at 4-week intervals.

The objective of therapy is to restore the euthyroid state. Enough thyroxine is given daily to maintain the plasma T_4 at the mid- to upper range of normal, or, ideally, to the lowest level of T_4 at which the TSH is restored to normal. Most persons need about 0.125 mg/day; only rarely is as much as 0.2 mg necessary, and more is hardly ever needed. Elderly patients often require only 0.1 mg daily for maintenance; frequently as little as 0.05 or 0.075 mg may suffice (9). Once the patient is euthyroid, the T_4 need not be measured more than once a year.

Concern has been expressed over the bioavailability of hormone in certain generic preparations and even lack of standardization of certain brands of thyroxine, but clinically significant problems are not likely to be encountered with any of these preparations. Determination of plasma T_3 during therapy with T_4 is unnecessary.

Patients with grossly evident hypothyroidism who require surgery are poor risks until their thyroid status is at least partially corrected, a process that requires 3 to 4 weeks with ordinary oral therapy. Elective surgery is best delayed in such patients. In an urgent situation, an intravenous dose of T_4 is probably warranted to prepare the patient for surgery in a few days. The increased susceptibility of severely hypothyroid persons to respiratory depression by conventional doses of many central nervous system (CNS) active drugs should be borne in mind. This increased drug sensitivity has been responsible for precipitation of myxedema coma. On the other hand, recent studies indicate that patients with minimal hypothyroidism appear to tolerate ordinary surgical stress quite well.

POSTPARTUM THYROID DYSFUNCTION

Postpartum thyroid dysfunction is a common event, occurring in some 17% of women in one study (7). Both hyperthyroidism and hypothyroidism can occur; in some cases one state follows the other. The disease is usually transient, lasting 1 to 4 months and is most likely to occur in the first 8 months postpartum. However, in 30% of cases hypothyroidism is permanent. The majority of cases show antimicrosomal antibodies; antithyroglobulin antibodies are uncommon. In the United States, the hyperthyroid variety has been associated with postpartum lymphocytic thyroiditis (see "Hyperthyroidism Associated with Thyroiditis"). Postpartum hypothyroidism is often misdiagnosed as postpartum depression. Some women have repeated bouts of illness with successive pregnancies. The disorder is often familial.

GOITER

A goiter is an enlarged thyroid gland. The term implies nothing about the functional state of the gland. Goiter is the most common thyroid abnormality. *Diffuse goiter*, also called simple goiter, is a gland that is uniformly and symmetrically enlarged without apparent irregularities. (Some use the term *simple goiter* to denote any nontoxic or nonhyperfunctioning gland, regardless of its anatomy.)

In some areas of the world thyroid enlargement is so common as to be termed *endemic goiter*. Before the widespread introduction of iodized salt these areas were common, but this is no longer the case. Endemic goiter, for practical purposes synonymous with iodine deficiency goiter, is now found only in geographically isolated areas of the underdeveloped world. The term sporadic goiter refers to thyroid enlargement as now encountered in the United States and other developed areas. *Sporadic goiter* is seen in a small percentage of the population and increases in frequency with age. The cause is unknown.

Causes

Any process that prevents the synthesis of normal quantities of thyroid hormones may produce goiter. If impairment of hormone synthesis is severe enough, goiter formation is associated with reduction of blood hormone levels, eventually to be followed by clinical hypothyroidism. The mechanism of the thyroid enlargement in this situation is increased pituitary TSH secretion via activation of the feedback system. The resulting increased thyroid mass is a compensatory mechanism that may allow sufficient hormone synthesis to occur so that the patient remains euthyroid.

Drugs that interfere with thyroid hormone synthesis (thiocarbamides, lithium, iodides, etc.) can lead to goiter. Withdrawal of a goitrogenic drug results in regression of the goiter, as will administration of enough T_4 or T_3 to suppress endogenous TSH secretion.

Only one well-defined naturally occurring "goitrogen" is known, l-5-vinyl-2-thio-oxazolidone. This substance, with a mechanism of action much like that of the thiocarbamides, is in cabbage, turnips, soybeans, and several other vegetables. Other poorly characterized goiter-producing substances have been detected in the food and water supplies of some areas. No environmental factor has been incriminated, however, as a cause of sporadic goiter, the etiology of which remains obscure.

Recognition

A mass in the base of the neck is the usual mode of presentation of goiter. Occasionally, especially in the elderly, an enlarged thyroid is neither visible nor readily palpable but is incidentally found by X-ray of the chest or esophagus when either a retrosternal mass is noted or the trachea or esophagus is found to be deviated. Confirmation of the nature of a neck mass as an enlarged thyroid gland and precise determination of its size are now most economically and accurately performed by ultrasonic examination (sonography). Although radionuclide scintigraphy ("scanning") was previously used for this purpose, it is not as accurate and fails to show nodularity with comparable clarity. Computerized tomography is also quite accurate in delineating the anatomy of goiters and their relationship to contiguous structures but is not indicated on a routine basis.

Except in subacute thyroiditis, pain is not a usual symptom but can develop during cyst formation or hemorrhage, a fairly frequent event usually accompanied by rapid enlargement of a portion of the gland. Obstruction of the trachea or esophagus can be produced by goiter, but dysphagia should not be readily attributed to minor degrees of thyroid enlargement. Hoarseness may occur due to involvement of the recurrent laryngeal nerve, but this is rare in benign enlargement, and its occurrence suggests thyroid neoplasm.

Differential Diagnosis

Clinical and laboratory assessment of thyroid function should be made in all cases of goiter. The clinician must recognize that the functional state may change with time, sometimes rather rapidly, and hence the precise diagnosis may not be possible on a single examination. Goiter in association with hyperthyroidism suggests Graves' disease, toxic nodular goiter, or a hyperfunctioning ("hot") nodule. Hypofunction in association with goiter is likely to represent Hashimoto's thyroiditis (see "Hypothyroidism"), but other possibilities, such as drug ingestion, may have to be excluded. Rarities such as an infiltrative process (amyloid disease, metastatic neoplasm) and the inherited defects of hormone synthesis (organification or coupling defects) have to be kept in mind (Table 73.7).

If the clinical and laboratory assessments indicate normal thyroid function, the diagnosis of euthyroid goiter is made. Multinodular enlargement almost always indicates a process of many years' standing. Differentiation of diffuse enlargement from nodular enlargement may require ultrasonic examination since small nodules may be missed on physical examination, while ultrasound may detect nodules as small as 0.5 cm. If the ultrasound image is not helpful, an optimally performed scintiscan may show irregular ("patchy") uptake of tracer, but even the best technique can delineate nodules of only about 0.5 cm in size. A goiter composed of many such small nodules may appear to represent a non-nodular thyroid. Antithyroglobulin and antimicrosomal antibodies in serum are readily determined commercially and should be routinely sought in all cases of goiter. Such antibodies are elevated in the blood of 90% of patients with goiters due to Hashimoto's thyroiditis. A proper history will point to possible drug-related goiter. Rapidity of enlargement may help to differentiate benign from malignant lesions, and the presence or absence of pain will help in identifying inflammatory thyroiditis (see below, page 975).

Treatment

Although thyroid enlargement is idiopathic in sporadic goiter, the process is nevertheless dependent on the presence of TSH. Administration of a physiological quantity of thyroid hormone results in suppression of TSH release. When TSH secretion is chronically suppressed in this manner, the enlarged thyroid eventually regresses or at least ceases to enlarge. This suppression therapy may be accomplished with thyroxine (T_4, sodium l-thyroxine, Synthroid, Levothyroid) or triiodothyronine (T_3, liothyronine, Cytomel). The dose should not be excessive. T_4 at a dose of 0.125 ± 0.025 mg daily is usually ample. T_3 is given at a dose of 25 ± 5 μg daily. Some evidence suggests that T_3 may be effective in a greater proportion of cases.

Suppression therapy must be monitored by accurate determination of the plasma T_4, which should not exceed the upper limit of normal. One must be certain that the gland is suppressible, since 20% of nontoxic nodular goiters are autonomous. Other nonsuppressible goiters may represent inapparent euthyroid Graves' disease. These patients may, if not monitored, develop iatrogenic hyperthyroidism due to the exogenous thyroid hormone. Monitoring of therapy also assures that an adequate amount of hormone is being given. Although regression of goiter is evidence of adequacy of therapy, the physician should be certain that the dose is adequate in those cases that do not show obvious regression. In suppression therapy with T_3 the plasma T_4 falls to a level below normal if suppression is adequate. With either T_4 or T_3, adequacy of suppression can be determined by a low TSH in a sensitive assay. Subnormal but still detectable TSH in the morning indicates incomplete suppression of TSH secretion; in this circumstance, a nocturnal surge of TSH usually persists.

If the treated gland is diffusely enlarged, obvious regression by 6 months is to be expected in about one-half of cases. Nodular glands are less likely to respond, and any response that occurs is slower. Even if complete regression is not accomplished, prevention of further glandular enlargement can be expected. A baseline ultrasound examination—not necessary in every case—and follow-ups at 6-monthly or yearly intervals provide objective assessment of the therapeutic responses but are not always necessary.

Several years may be necessary to discern regression of a long-standing multinodular goiter, and during that time one or more nodules may become more easily palpable as the relatively normal portions of the gland regress. Some confusion may occur if the physician interprets this as a progression of the disease or as the appearance of a malignant area. Ultrasound examinations will help to avoid this error.

Suppression therapy is often properly performed for cosmetic reasons. Suppression therapy is also clearly indicated for individuals with many years of life expectancy during which time mechanical problems may develop. However, little is to be gained by treatment of patients whose glands are known not to have changed in size over many years and who are, therefore, unlikely to develop difficulties. A clear and unequivocal indication is found in the patient who has already had surgery for goiter. Recurrence of goiter is frequent in such persons but can predictably be prevented with suppression therapy.

Once started, suppression therapy is usually continued indefinitely but can be terminated or withdrawn if regression occurs. Some goiters do not recur; in those that do, therapy can be reinstituted. Suppression therapy does not lead to permanent loss of TSH secretion, even after decades of thyroid hormone administration, although rare individuals may manifest a brief period of hypothyroidism when prolonged therapy is withdrawn.

Goiter so large as to produce not merely a deviation

but significant tracheal compression, as assessed by plain X-ray views of the trachea, or to interfere with swallowing is now uncommon. In these cases, surgery, although attended by significant morbidity, should be considered, since suppression therapy is unlikely to be effective in significantly reducing the size of such large goiters. Radioiodide therapy can be considered in these cases, especially in the elderly or in individuals with other serious medical problems. Doses of 20 to 100 mC are necessary. Although the response is slow, useful reduction in the size of the goiter can be achieved (12).

The frequency of carcinoma in multinodular goiter has been debated for years. Unwarranted concern has resulted in countless unnecessary operations (see page 975).

THYROID NEOPLASMS

One of the most frequent abnormalities of the thyroid is a localized area of enlargement commonly known as a nodule. In evaluating a thyroid nodule, the possibility of malignancy is the main concern. About 90% are benign adenomas or cysts; the remaining ones are lesions of varying degrees of malignancy.

Benign Thyroid Neoplasms: the Solitary Nodule

Many solitary nodules are true adenomas and are encapsulated. Although most benign adenomas are relatively hypofunctioning, follicular adenomas may exhibit normal or greater than normal function, i.e., they take up iodine and elaborate thyroid hormone. The growth of most benign adenomas, hypofunctional though they may be, is dependent on endogenous TSH. Adenomas whose function is independent of TSH are termed *autonomous*.

Benign thyroid nodules are present in at least 5% of the population, but clinically aggressive thyroid carcinoma is rare. In a group of over 200 patients with thyroid nodules identified in the Framingham study (4% of 5000 patients examined, ages 30 to 60) and followed for 15 years, none developed clinically evident malignancy. In that population, new thyroid nodules continued to appear at a rate of about 1/1000 persons/year, about twice as frequently in women as in men (26).

Clinical Approach

The first point to be established is whether the patient really has only a single nodule. Palpation by an experienced examiner is essential. Frequently, the "solitary" nodule turns out to be one of several nodules in a nontoxic nodular goiter. A single nodule in a clearly enlarged thyroid has a similar connotation, since the enlarged gland is likely to be harboring many small, nondiscrete nodules. Although most patients with a nodule are euthyroid at presentation, T_4 index should be determined for confirmation. If any question about hyperthyroidism exists (see below), plasma T_3 should also be measured.

The next essential question is that of the functional state of the nodule relative to the remaining thyroid tissue, since the hyperfunctioning nodule is almost invariably benign. When scintiscanning is performed, accumulation of isotope in the nodule can approximate that of the surrounding gland ("warm" nodule), be greater ("hot" nodule), or be less ("cold" nodule). A hot nodule can be considered benign (99.8% with ^{123}I). "Warm" nodules are far more likely to be benign than not, but the statistics are not as unequivocal as they are for the hot nodule.

The Hot Nodule. Management of the hot nodule depends on whether an excessive amount of thyroid hormone is being produced. The autonomous hot nodule, if it produces an amount of hormone equal to or greater than that of normal gland output, suppresses TSH; the remaining normal tissue then becomes relatively inactive and may not be visible, or may be only poorly visible, by scintiscan. In cases in which the nodule is hyperactive but has not clearly suppressed the remaining thyroid tissue, demonstration of autonomous function may depend on a scintiscan after a period of suppression (see above, page 971) with administered thyroid hormone.

If the amount of hormone produced by the adenoma considerably exceeds normal, thyrotoxicosis should be clinically apparent. Usually T_4 and T_3 are produced in excess. However, hyperthyroidism due to T_3 alone (T_3 toxicosis) is fairly frequent with such hyperactive nodules (10).

The natural history of the hot nodule is variable. Over a 10-year interval about one-third will show little change, one-third will become frankly hyperactive, and the remainder will become cold, sometimes with obvious hemorrhagic infarction and cystic degeneration. Treatment of the hot nodule that is producing hyperthyroidism can be satisfactorily accomplished with radioactive iodine or surgery. Prophylactic ablative therapy is not indicated. Suppression therapy with thyroid hormone is, of course, not effective and will lead to iatrogenic hyperthyroidism.

The Cold Nodule. Most nodules are cold, i.e., functionally hypoactive relative to the remainder of the gland. The major concern with most nodules is, of course, malignancy. The diagnostic workup and therapeutic approach to these lesions should be determined by a number of clinical considerations, including the biological potential of the nodule and the age of the patient (11). In the elderly, even more than in the young, a conservative approach is necessary (9).

Most nodules—variously estimated at 75 to 90%—are benign lesions; most of these are adenomas, but 10 to 15% are cysts. Thus, the overall risk is small. The risk is smaller still when it is realized that the remaining lesions are almost always clinically relatively nonaggressive papillary or follicular carcinomas. These lesions are usually nonlethal (see below) and slow growing, so that a conservative course is always reasonable. Nonetheless, some patients—not to mention physicians—become extremely anxious when faced with the possibility of cancer. If reassurance fails and a conservative approach is insufficient, the patient or physician may wish to proceed with a definitive diagnostic procedure or even excision. However, immediate and indiscriminate excision of all thyroid nodules is irrational and cannot be justified.

Currently, some experts recommend needle biopsy of all nodules as the first diagnostic maneuver, bypassing scintiscanning and sonography. These authorities argue that this approach is more cost effective and helps to avoid unnecessary excisions (27). Cysts are immediately recognized by preliminary aspiration. Biopsy is by fine needle aspiration for cytological examination, or by aspiration or cutting needle for conventional histological examination. In experienced hands these procedures are safe, direct, and useful. It is probably possible under optimal conditions to make an accurate diagnosis in about 90% of cases examined by biopsy, although both procedures may fail to distinguish benign adenomas from well-differentiated follicular carcinomas (15), an important limitation of the technique. However, it must be strongly stressed that the most important consideration in the use of needle aspiration or biopsy is the expertise of the pathologist needed to examine the biopsy material. If a specifically trained pathologist is not available, needle biopsy, especially by fine needle aspiration, should be avoided. Similarly, if the patient is reluctant to undergo the procedure, a conservative approach using suppression therapy should be pursued.

The argument that needle biopsy helps to avoid unnecessary operations is correct if one considers that some physicians have long erroneously held that excision of all newly discovered nodules is indicated. However, when physicians have an initial approach that is conservative, universal institution of biopsy for a number of reasons probably adds to the number of unnecessary operative excisions. Reasons include indeterminate pathological diagnoses and discovery of papillary carcinomas that might have been adequately treated by suppression. The issue of whether to biopsy nodules or to treat them conservatively with initial suppression has received a detailed decision analysis and statistical treatment. The conclusion is that no "best approach" exists and that continued arguments over this issue will be futile. The decision to operate, suppress, or aspirate is thus a "toss-up," dependent in the individual case upon such subjective factors as psychological disability, relative cost, and attitudes toward operative risk and long-term medical therapy (16).

CONSERVATIVE APPROACH TO THERAPY OF COLD NODULES. Initiation of suppression therapy of nodules—with adequate monitoring—is reasonable even without antecedent biopsy, scintiscan, or sonogram, although most physicians prefer to obtain at least one or the other (16). A sonogram is preferred as the initial procedure. If a cystic lesion is identified, the need for scintiscan is obviated, since a cystic nodule is always "cold". Subsequent scintiscan of solid nodules is useful in identifying the occasionally en-

countered "hot" lesions. In neither of these two situations is biopsy necessary or helpful.

If a predominantly cystic nodule is identified on sonogram, aspiration and/or suppression therapy can be considered. Some cystic nodules require several aspirations, but most will eventually disappear with this approach. Suppression therapy is rational, since most cysts arise in benign adenomas, but its usefulness is not established. The sonogram provides an objective and accurate measurement of size of cold nodules so that regression or progression of the lesion can be followed during suppression therapy.

Regression of the nodule over a 6-month period indicates clinically benign disease; such patients can be followed indefinitely with continued suppression therapy. Some endocrinologists are satisfied that benign disease is present when a nodule at least does not grow larger during suppression therapy over the initial 6 months, after which suppression can continue. Regression of some nodules will occur, probably including an occasional papillary carcinoma. Physicians should not be dismayed by this statement, since suppression therapy is the mainstay of postoperative therapy of such lesions. A recent study has denied the efficacy of suppression therapy for single nodules, at least over a period of 6 months. However, the data presented actually indicate that some nodules do regress over this interval, perhaps spontaneously (8). Considering the probability that 90% of cases treated in this way represent benign disease in the first place and considering the low grade malignancy of almost all of the remaining cases, this approach is reasonable. However, close follow-up is necessary to ensure that appropriate therapy is instituted should the lesion enlarge further during suppression therapy or should lymph nodes become palpable.

Thyroid Carcinomas

General Considerations

About 95% of thyroid carcinomas are of the papillary or follicular variety; of these, 80 to 90% are papillary carcinomas. Anaplastic and medullary carcinomas probably account for no more than 5% of the total. The relative frequency of the various types of thyroid carcinomas is markedly age dependent (see page 974).

Occult thyroid carcinoma (defined as lesions with the histological appearance of carcinoma, but less than 1.5 cm in diameter) is found in 5 to 10% of United States and European populations and in 30% of Japanese samples at autopsy. Death from thyroid carcinoma is as rare in Japan as in the United States. Clearly, occult carcinoma behaves as a benign disease and does not warrant aggressive management.

In the United States, about 10,000 new cases of thyroid carcinoma are seen each year, but only about 1,000 persons die. Most of these deaths result from the aggressive forms of the disease, i.e., anaplastic lesions, the unusually aggressive follicular carcinomas, and a few from the very uncommon aggressive papillary lesions. Only rare deaths are attributable to medullary carcinoma.

Therapeutic Considerations in Thyroid Carcinoma

Papillary carcinoma. Enough information is now available to provide support for a middle-of-the-road approach, one that falls between that which advocated thyroid hormone suppression therapy without surgery and that which has employed radical surgery alone. Long-term observations have now also reasonably defined the role of radioiodide ablation therapy (14, 20).

Surgery for Papillary Carcinoma. Follow-up at 10 years indicates a recurrence rate of about 20% for subtotal resection versus 10% for total removal of the gland. Deaths due to carcinoma are 1.5 and 0.5%, respectively. This small difference is reported for one retrospective study to be statistically significant and currently strongly influences the surgical approach. However, the complication rate for total thyroidectomy (hypoparathyroidism, vocal cord paralysis) remains high. As a result, many surgeons have now adopted a modified or "near total" thyroidectomy. In this procedure the affected side is completely removed; most of the contralateral lobe is also removed but the posterior capsule is left, together with the tip of the upper pole. Whether this approach will succeed remains to be established. Meanwhile, conservative surgeons call anew for more limited surgery (2). Visibly involved lymph nodes are always removed, but radical neck dissection is not justified even in the presence of obviously involved nodes (14, 20).

The presence of cervical node metastases at operation or the extent of lymphadenectomy does not seem to influence either recurrence or death rate. The death rate in lesions under 2.5 cm without local invasion and without evident distant metastases at the time of surgery is less than 1% in 10 years and is 4 to 8% in the less favorable categories (14, 20).

Postoperative Therapy: TSH Suppression and Ablation with Radioiodide. Postoperative therapy with full replacement doses of thyroxine will suppress endogenous TSH and reduce recurrence, and is routine in all cases. In addition, postsurgical ablative therapy with radioactive iodide has a role, although not all cases of localized disease need such therapy. The patient with a minimal papillary lesion needs no such therapy, but the patient with a large, locally invasive lesion should receive ablative therapy with [131]I. In cases with an intermediate-sized lesion, without invasion of the thyroid capsule, and without lymph node metastases, the recurrence rate is greatly reduced by treatment with radioiodide, and deaths from recurrent disease may be completely abolished. The hesitation to use radioiodide routinely stems from the unwarranted fear of radiation-induced leukemia. Doses of ^{131}I smaller than those customarily recommended may be equally effective. In contrast to the constraints on radioiodide therapy of localized disease, known metastatic disease should always be treated vigorously.

Follicular Carcinoma. This tumor is somewhat more aggressive than papillary carcinoma, tends to be angioinvasive, and may metastasize to bones and lungs. The tumor may bypass regional lymph nodes, a marked difference from papillary disease. The most important prognostic feature is invasion, either through the tumor capsule or into blood vessels. Unlike papillary carcinoma, primary tumor size at presentation does not appear to influence prognosis (31).

The clinical presentation may be very different from that of papillary disease; the patient may present with metastatic disease involving lungs, bone, brain, or spinal cord. In these cases the primary tumor may be small and initially overlooked. Only rarely do the metastases produce sufficient thyroid hormones to cause thyrotoxicosis.

The surgical approach to follicular carcinoma should be that taken for papillary carcinoma. Suppression therapy with thyroid hormone replacement is routine. Postoperative ablative therapy with radioiodide appears warranted, especially for those patients with overtly invasive disease. However, the case for routine postoperative use of ^{131}I ablation therapy in the treatment of follicular carcinoma is not statistically established (31).

Anaplastic Carcinoma. This carcinoma is fortunately distinctly uncommon; its frequency depends on the age of the population. Anaplastic carcinoma is rare in children and in adults under the age of 35. By age 50, as many as 10% of cases of thyroid carcinoma are due to anaplastic disease, and by age 80, by which time the overall incidence of thyroid carcinoma has fallen markedly, nearly half of the cases that do occur are of this variety. The disease is locally invasive in a highly aggressive fashion and quickly produces pain, dysphagia, hemoptysis, and hoarseness. Death usually occurs within 6 to 12 months. Surgically resectable disease without evidence of metastases, even if it has extended outside the thyroid capsule, can be associated with long-term survival (20 to 30%). It is important to distinguish the small cell type from *lymphoma of the thyroid*. This rare disease, unlike anaplastic carcinoma, is radiosensitive and amenable to chemotherapy.

Medullary Carcinoma. Medullary carcinoma accounts for 1 to 2% of all thyroid cancers. The tumors arise from the parafollicular or C cells and produce thyrocalcitonin. Both sporadic and familial varieties are known. The sporadic case typically presents as a solitary nodule, whereas the familial variety is often multifocal and part of a multiple endocrine adenomatosis syndrome. Diarrhea occurs in some patients. Thyrocalcitonin in plasma is elevated in the basal state or after stimulation with calcium or pentagastrin infusion. When surgical excision is performed before regional nodes have become involved, 90% of patients survive for 10 years. Once the nodes are involved, only 40% survival can be expected. Medullary carcinoma does not appear to respond to suppression therapy with thyroid hormone.

The Question of Carcinoma in the Multinodular Thyroid

The risk of clinically significant carcinoma in a non-toxic nodular goiter is low. Occult carcinoma will be found in a significant proportion of such cases. However, the approach to such occult lesions is no different from that to occult carcinoma in the non-nodular gland. Demonstration of multinodularity by palpation or sonogram or its suggestion by scan leads some physicians, including the author, to a firm recommendation against surgical intervention. Suppression therapy is recommended, but only for prevention of further gland enlargement or to induce regression of symptomatic goiters and not out of concern for malignancy. Others feel that large nonfunctioning nodules within multinodular goiters should be treated with suppression therapy for a period of 6 months. Failure to regress is considered an indication for surgical excision. However, since most large nodules in multinodular goiters do not regress within such a period of time, while a significant number may actually become more prominent as less abnormal tissue regresses, this approach is certain to result in unnecessary surgery. Serial sonographic estimates of nodule size may prove useful in such cases.

Radiation-Associated Thyroid Carcinoma

Low-dose irradiation of the thyroid is a stimulus to thyroid carcinogenesis, with a latency period of 1 to several decades (23).

In recent years thyroid carcinomas have been reported to occur in increased incidence in patients who received radiation therapy some years earlier for enlarged tonsils, adenoids, or thymus; acne; cervical lymphadenopathy, etc. A distinction must be made between treatment with penetrating external radiation and local irradiation with point sources (radium rod and plaque treatment). Thyroid carcinoma has not been related to such limited exposure.

In a large, up to 40-year, follow-up study of over 4300 subjects irradiated with X-rays before age 15, 40% have developed nodules detectable by palpation or isotope scan of which one-third have been carcinomas. Thus, in this series, approximately 14% of irradiated persons have developed thyroid carcinomas, all of which were well differentiated (21, 22). Nodules continue to appear with no change in the ratio of benign to malignant. No relationship has been seen between radiation and the development of medullary or anaplastic carcinoma (21, 22).

Radiation-induced cancers appear to present more often with dissemination than those occurring spontaneously, an argument for early detection (21). Accordingly, high-resolution thyroid scans should be part of the follow-up, since nonpalpable lesions can be detected. The only blood test of value is determination of serum thyroglobulin, elevation of which predicts the development of nodules (24).

The approach to the patient with a history of irradiation to the head and neck is not currently stan-dardized. Examination of the patient at 2- to 3-year intervals should suffice. Routine isotope scintography or sonographic examination of the thyroid for patients with nonpalpable lesions is probably indicated. Many nonpalpable lesions (0.5 to 1.0 cm) can be detected by use of these methods. Although lesions too small to be palpable are clinically, if not pathologically, benign and should be managed conservatively, reports that carcinomas that are radiation induced may disseminate more readily than those occurring spontaneously should not be ignored. Thyroid suppression with thyroxine is recommended even for patients with nodules detected only by scintigraphy or sonography. If careful follow-up reveals an increase of nodule size despite suppression, surgery should be performed. A widespread, aggressive approach to nodules in these patients is <u>not</u> warranted.

Surgical therapy should involve the same approach as that for nonirradiated patients, i.e., near-total thyroidectomy, although a recent plea for a return to the earlier practice of lobectomy has been made (2). All patients who have had surgery for benign or malignant nodules should receive suppression therapy with thyroid hormone. Recurrence of benign nodules, but not malignant ones, is greatly reduced (5).

Radiation of the head and neck predisposes not only to thyroid cancer but to salivary gland tumors (parotids, others) with a ratio of benign to malignant lesions similar to that of thyroid. The incidence of benign neural tumors (neurilemomas; acoustic neuromas) and parathyroid adenomas is also increased.

THYROIDITIS

Pyogenic (Suppurative) Thyroiditis

Pyogenic or suppurative thyroiditis, also known as acute thyroiditis, is very rare, and most physicians will never encounter a case. The thyroid infection usually follows bacteremia but can occur as an isolated, primary event. The gland shows typical signs of an acute inflammatory process.

Riedel's Thyroiditis

Riedel's thyroiditis is another rare but indolent and painless form of thyroiditis. The intense induration associated with this process makes the clinical differentiation from infiltrating neoplasm difficult.

Hashimoto's Thyroiditis

This entity is common (see "Hypothyroidism," "Goiter," and Table 73.7). The process is painless and usually produces only modest enlargement of the thyroid. Nodularity is the rule. Distinction from nontoxic nodular goiter is made by the presence of high titers of thyroid autoantibodies in the serum of 80 to 90% of patients with Hashimoto's thyroiditis.

Subacute Thyroiditis

This entity, also known as granulomatous or de Quervain's thyroiditis, is common. Many mild cases are probably never diagnosed. The term subacute is often deceiving and sometimes inappropriate. Although the onset may be insidious, it is perhaps just as often acute over several days. Many patients give a history of recent antecedent upper respiratory tract infection.

The earliest symptoms may be referred pain, usually to the ear, but pain can appear to originate in the jaw or occiput. This phase may last a few hours or days before tenderness and discomfort in the thyroid area become apparent. Rarely, the patient is concerned only with the referred pain and is unaware of thyroidal tenderness until examination makes it apparent. When the onset is acute, the symptoms and signs are more likely to be severe. Initially, pain and swelling of the thyroid are often unilateral, but the process usually does not remain localized for more than a few days. Systemic symptoms include fever, especially in acute cases, and a sensation of intense fatigue and malaise. The course may be protracted with symptoms persisting for months, although usually they subside within a week or 2.

Erythrocyte sedimentation rate is elevated. Early in the disease, the thyroidal radioiodide uptake is depressed, and plasma T_4 may be elevated. Mild cases have no or only borderline abnormalities of the tests. Significant titers of thyroid autoantibodies are not common but can be seen. The radioiodide uptake test is not likely to be useful diagnostically, because in many normal persons the uptake is low (see page 956).

Clinical hyperthyroidism is occasionally seen with subacute thyroiditis (see above). Rarely hypothyroidism occurs and lasts several months. Permanent hypothyroidism is unusual. Recently a variant of this syndrome has been described in which neither hypo- nor hyperthyroidism is present but symptoms of severe systemic illness with fever and weight loss dominate (19). Blood tests of thyroid function are normal except for minimal elevation of free T_4 in a few. Thyroidal radioiodide uptake is low. Thyroid autoantibodies are not present. The thyroid is modestly enlarged and nontender in most cases, but even this clue is absent in some. Biopsies are typical of lymphocytic thyroiditis. Patients respond to anti-inflammatory therapy (see below).

Therapy

Therapy for subacute thyroiditis is symptomatic. The patient should be strongly reassured concerning the benign, self-limited character of the disorder. Thyroid tenderness often responds within several days to aspirin in doses sufficient to maintain therapeutic (anti-inflammatory) blood levels. Codeine should be added if neck discomfort is severe. In less than 10% of cases the process may be severe enough to require glucocorticoid therapy (30 to 60 mg of prednisone daily or equivalent). Glucocorticoid produces prompt relief of pain and tenderness but, if the disease is severe enough to require its use, will usually be necessary for weeks to several months. Relapse is common when therapy is discontinued, and retreatment may be necessary.

Lymphocytic Thyroiditis (Silent Thyroiditis)

This newly recognized process occurs in association with hyperthyroidism and is discussed on page 965.

General References

DeGroot LJ (ed): *The Thyroid and Its Diseases,* 5th ed. New York, John Wiley & Sons, 1984.
Ingbar SH, Braverman LE (eds): *The Thyroid,* 5th ed. Philadelphia, JB Lippincott, 1986.
    Comprehensive textbooks on all aspects of the subject.
Felig P, Baxter JD, Broadus AE, Frohman LA (eds): *Endocrinology and Metabolism,* 2nd ed. New York, McGraw-Hill, 1987.
Wilson JD, Foster DW (eds): *Textbook of Endocrinology,* 7th ed. Philadelphia, WB Saunders, 1985.
    Standard textbooks containing excellent chapters on the thyroid.

Specific References

1. Anonymous: Effects of drugs on thyroid function tests. *Med Lett* 23:30, 1981.
2. Baker RR, Hyland J: Papillary carcinoma of the thyroid gland. *Surg Gynecol Obstet* 161:546, 1985.
3. Borst GC, Eil C, Burman KD: Euthyroid hyperthyroxinemia. *Ann Intern Med* 98:366, 1983.
4. Cooper DS, Halpern R, Wood LC, et al: L-thyroxine therapy in subclinical hypothyroidism. A double-blind, placebo-controlled trial. *Ann Intern Med* 101:18, 1984.
5. Fogelfeld L, Wiviott MBT, Shore-Freedman E, et al: Recurrence of thyroid nodules after surgical removal in patients irradiated in childhood for benign conditions. *N Engl J Med* 320:835, 1989.
6. Fradkin JE, Wolff J: Iodide-induced thyrotoxicosis. *Medicine (Baltimore)* 62:1, 1983.
7. Fung HYM, Kologlu M, Collison K, et al: Postpartum thyroid dysfunction in Mid Glamorgan. *Br Med J* 296:241, 1988.
8. Gharib H, James EM, Charboneau J, et al: Suppressive therapy with levothyroxine for solitary thyroid nodules. A double-blind controlled clinical study. *N Engl J Med* 371:70, 1987.
9. Gregerman RI: Thyroid Diseases. In: Andres R, Bierman EL, Hazzard WR (ed): *Principles of Geriatric Medicine.* McGraw-Hill, New York, 1990.
10. Hamburger JI: Pitfalls in the laboratory diagnosis of atypical hyperthyroidism. *Arch Intern Med* 139:96, 1979.
11. Hamburger JI: The autonomously functioning thyroid nodule: Goetsch's Disease. *Endocr Rev* 8:439, 1987.
12. Kay TWH, d'Emden MC, Andrews JT, Martin FIR: Treatment of non-toxic multinodular goiter with radioactive iodine. *Am J Med* 84:19, 1988.
13. Klein I, Levey GS: Unusual manifestations of hypothyroidism. *Arch Intern Med* 144:123, 1984.
14. Mazzaferri EL, Young RL, Oertel JE, et al: Papillary thyroid carcinoma: the impact of therapy in 576 patients. *Medicine (Baltimore)* 56:171, 1977.
15. Miller JM, Hamburger MD, Kini S: Diagnosis of thyroid nodules. Use of fine needle aspiration and needle biopsy. *JAMA* 241:481, 1979.
16. Molitch ME, Beck JR, Dreisman M, et al: The cold thyroid nodule: an analysis of diagnostic and therapeutic options. *Endocr Rev* 5:185, 1984.
17. Nicolai TF, Brosseau J, Kettrick MA, et al: Lymphocytic thyroiditis with spontaneously resulting hyperthyroidism (silent thyroiditis). *Arch Intern Med* 140:478, 1980.
18. Nicolai TF, Coombs GJ, McKenzie AK: Lymphocytic thyroiditis

with spontaneously resolving hyperthyroidism and subacute thyroiditis. Long-term follow-up. *Arch Intern Med* 141:1455, 1981.

19. Rotenberg Z, Weinberger I, Fuchs J, et al: Euthyroid atypical subacute thyroiditis simulating systemic or malignant disease. *Arch Intern Med* 146:105, 1986.
20. Samaan NA, Maheshwari YK, Nader S, et al: Impact of therapy for differentiated carcinoma of the thyroid: an analysis of 706 cases. *J Clin Endocrinol Metab* 56:1131, 1983.
21. Samaan AN, Schultz PN, Ordonez NG, et al: A comparison of thyroid carcinoma in those who have and have not had head and neck irradiation in childhood. *J Clin Endocrinol Metab* 64:219, 1987.
22. Schneider AB: Thyroid nodules following childhood irradiation: A 1989 update. *Thyroid Today* 12:1, 1989.
23. Schneider AB, Recant W, Pinsky SM, et al: Radiation-induced thyroid carcinoma. Clinical course and results of therapy in 296 patients. *Ann Intern Med* 105:405, 1986.
24. Schneider AB, Shore-Freedman E, Ryo UY, et al: Prospective serum thyroglobulin measurements in assessing the risk of developing thyroid nodules in patients exposed to childhood neck irradiation. *J Clin Endocrinol Metab* 61:547, 1985.
25. Swanson JW, Kelly JJ, McConahey WM: Neurologic aspects of thyroid dysfunction. *Mayo Clinic Proc* 56:504, 1981.
26. Vander JB, Gaston EA, Dawber TR: The significance of nontoxic thyroid nodules. Final report of a 15-year study of the incidence of thyroid malignancy. *Ann Intern Med* 69:537, 1968.
27. Van Herle AJ, Rich P, Britt-Marie EL, et al: The thyroid nodule. *Ann Intern Med* 96:221, 1982.
28. Wartofsky L, Burman KD: Alterations in thyroid function in patients with systemic illness: "the euthyroid sick syndrome." *Endocr Rev* 3:164, 1982.
29. Wehmann RE, Gregerman RI, Burns WH, et al: Suppression of thyrotropin in the low-thyroxine state of severe nonthyroidal illness. *N Engl J Med* 312:546, 1985.
30. Wortsman J, Premachandra BN, Williams K, et al: Familial resistance to thyroid hormone associated with decreased transport across the plasma membrane. *Ann Intern Med* 98:904, 1983.
31. Young RL, Mazzaferri EL, Rahe AJ, Dorfman SG: Pure follicular carcinoma: impact of therapy in 214 patients. *J Nucl Med* 21:733, 1980.

C H A P T E R 74

Selected Endocrine Problems: Disorders of Pituitary, Adrenal, and Parathyroid Glands; Pharmacological Use of Steroids; Hypo- and Hypercalcemia; Osteoporosis; Water Metabolism; Hypoglycemia

ROBERT I. GREGERMAN, M.D.

PITUITARY DISEASES

Disorders of the pituitary gland are manifest by disturbance of function (hyper- or hyposecretion of trophic hormones), by anatomical encroachment on adjacent structures (enlargement of tumors), or by a combination of these processes. Many of the cases of hormone hypersecretion are due to benign tumors—often clinically inapparent microadenomas. Most commonly a small adenoma produces an excess of prolactin with resultant galactorrhea. Most cases of galactorrhea, however, are functional, in some cases idiopathic, and in others due to drugs.

When a pituitary tumor is large enough to produce increased pressure within the sella turcica, enlargement and erosion of the bony walls of that structure either produce no symptoms or may cause headache. Tumor enlargement superiorly—the direction of least resistance—leads to encroachment upon the adjacent optic chiasm and may produce visual field defects. Pituitary tumors large enough to be anatomically apparent are frequently associated with failure of hormone secretion (hypopituitarism), a process that results in end organ failure (hypoadrenalism, hypogonadism, and/or hypothyroidism). The pituitary may also be affected by a wide variety of systemic illnesses, including granulomatous, infectious, vascular, and neoplastic processes, but all are extremely uncommon causes of hypopituitarism.

A related problem is that of craniopharyngioma. This developmental abnormality may simulate pituitary tumor. The lesion is usually outside the pituitary and presents as a suprasellar mass lesion readily evident on computerized tomography. Most cases are manifest during childhood.

Clinical Presentations

When a patient presents with evidence of decreased endocrine function, routine evaluation must include consideration of whether the process is due to pituitary disease—i.e., "secondary" gland failure—or is "primary"—i.e., in the end organ. For example, in most patients with hypothyroidism thyroid-stimulating hormone (TSH) is elevated due to failure of normal inhibition of the negative feedback loop. However, if TSH is not elevated in the face of hypothyroidism, the possibility of hypopituitarism must then be further evaluated. Similarly, in patients with hypogonadism an easy differential diagnosis can be made, since levels of follicle-stimulating hormone (FSH) and luteinizing hormone (LH) invariably will be elevated if there is primary end organ failure. In patients with adrenal insufficiency, however, the plasma adrenocorticotropic hormone (ACTH) does not always clearly differentiate primary from secondary disease. In cases of endocrine hyperfunction, pituitary function may also be evaluated but not necessarily routinely (see "Hyperthyroidism," page 958; and "Adrenocortical Hyperfunction," page 983).

Not infrequently, the issue of pituitary disease is raised inadvertently. The patient's complaints lead to radiological examination of the skull because of headaches, suspected sinusitis, injury, or for some other reason. An enlarged or an abnormal sella turcica is noted. The issue then arises concerning further evaluation of what may be an incidental finding. Referral to an endocrinologist is appropriate at this point, but further evaluation by the nonspecialist is also possible.

Evaluation of an Abnormal Sella Turcica

The sella turcica as seen in ordinary X-rays of the skull may appear deceptively normal or may appear abnormal when it is not. Therefore, computerized tomography (CT) and magnetic resonance imaging (MRI) have almost totally replaced older techniques for evaluating the sella. In major medical centers MRI is used almost exclusively, even for initial examinations, but for this purpose CT is less expensive, more readily available, and completely satisfactory for the demonstration of 50 to 60% of lesions, most of which are intrasellar microadenomas. If a microadenoma cannot be demonstrated by CT, or if suprasellar extension proves to be present on CT, MRI should then be obtained; an additional 20% of microadenomas will be demonstrated. In a few centers venous sampling techniques for ACTH can lateralize many of the nonvisualizable adenomas that are the cause of Cushing's disease. In addition if suprasellar extension is present, the patient should be referred for ophthalmological examination of the visual fields, preferably with a red dot, the most sensitive technique for detection of field defects produced by suprasellar masses.

Empty Sella Syndrome

An enlarged sella does not always mean that a pituitary tumor is present. Not infrequently extensive evaluation leads to demonstration of an empty sella turcica. Such patients are often discovered during evaluation of skull X-rays obtained for reasons other than suspected hypopituitarism—usually headache—and, indeed, usually have no clinical endocrine disease. The cause of the empty sella syndrome is not known, but open communication of cerebrospinal fluid through a defect in the diaphragma sellae and/or a ruptured cyst have been postulated. In most cases, a rim of normal pituitary tissue remains and pituitary function, which should be routinely evaluated, is normal; in some there is minimal hypopituitarism and/or a visual field defect for reasons that are not clear but that could represent a previous cyst. The diagnosis can be suspected from CT that fails to show enhancement, but definitive diagnosis and differentiation from intrasellar tumor requires MRI, or if MRI cannot be done, use of radioopaque dye; pneumoencephagraphy for this purpose is now obsolete.

Chromophobe Adenomas

Chromophobe adenomas, the commonest of the pituitary tumors, account for about 85% of cases; most occur between ages 30 and 60, not infrequently in association with parathyroid or pancreatic islet cell adenomas and, sometimes, with the Zollinger-Ellison syndrome (see Chapter 37). These associations constitute the syndrome of multiple endocrine adenomatosis (MEA, type I). When the pituitary is not involved, but pheochromocytoma, medullary thyroid carcinoma, and—occasionally—parathyroid adenomata occur together, the syndrome is termed MEA, type II.

Chromophobe adenomas are usually noninvasive but may infiltrate local structures and on rare occasions even behave as locally malignant lesions. Long thought to be "functionless," many are now known to be prolactinomas. The term chromophobe adenoma belongs to the era in which pituitary tumors were classified by their histological staining characteristics (chromophobe, eosinophile, and basophile). A more precise classification can now be constructed that is based on the secretory product of the tumor (e.g., somatotrope tumor, growth hormone producing), but the old terms persist.

Pituitary function remains clinically normal until more than 75% of the normal pituitary has been destroyed by the adenoma. Hypogonadism is usually the earliest evidence of a hormone deficiency state (60 to 80% of cases), but hypothyroidism as an initial manifestation is almost as common. Adrenal insufficiency is usually the last problem to develop and is often inapparent except on laboratory testing. In about 10% of cases, diabetes insipidus develops.

Prolactin and Galactorrhea

Bilateral breast discharge may be the first clue to the presence of a prolactin-secreting chromophobe adenoma. In many cases discharge from the breast is minimal and may be apparent only on physical examination when a few drops of milk may be expressable. Breast enlargement may occur in the male, but prolactin excess is an uncommon cause of gynecomastia (Chapter 77). Prolactin secretion appears to inhibit the secretion of gonadotropins and hence may also be associated with evidence of hypogonadism, including impotence and amenorrhea (Chapter 77).

Most cases of galactorrhea are due not to tumor but to a functional disturbance of prolactin secretion, which in turn is either spontaneous or related to the use of certain drugs. In either case, the hallmark of galactorrhea is an increase of the concentration of prolactin in plasma. Radioimmunoassays for prolactin are widely available and present no special problems of interpretation except for the recent demonstration of a high molecular weight form of prolactin in some amenorrheic women. The significance of this material is unknown. The drugs most commonly incriminated in the production of galactorrhea are reserpine, phenothiazines, tricyclic antidepressants, α-methyldopa (Aldomet), and estrogens (oral contraceptives). If no drugs are involved, a functional disorder is still likely, but some cases will be due to chromophobe adenoma. Rarely, galactorrhea occurs secondary to hypothyroidism.

The degree of prolactin elevation is strongly suggestive of the cause of the disorder. Levels of prolactin greater than 200 ng/ml are essentially diagnostic of tumor, even in the absence of changes in the sella. Low levels of prolactin (less than 50 ng/ml) are much more likely to be due to a functional disorder, but in many cases differentiation is not possible by this means. Autopsy studies show that a significant proportion of the normal population harbors a nonsecreting microadenoma, and some normal persons may have minor abnormalities of the sella (CT or MRI). Such changes do not prove the presence of a functional microadenoma.

Many cases of galactorrhea, with or without microadenoma, can be successfully treated with the drug bromocriptine (Parlodel), which may lower the prolactin level, abolish the galactorrhea, and restore normal menses. Bromocriptine not only reduces prolactin secretion but in many cases causes the tumor to shrink so that even visual field defects can be reversed. A favorable response occurs in 80% of cases. The drug is now frequently given preoperatively, even when a large tumor is present, since surgical removal is thereby facilitated. Long-term drug therapy is also an alternative to surgery in some cases (18, 19). Treatment with bromocriptine can be undertaken by the nonspecialist provided that tumor is not likely. If prolactin levels are very high or if radiographic evidence of tumor is present, an endocrinologist should be consulted.

The indications for surgical intervention should be anatomical. Small tumors confined to the sella, or even those with some degree of suprasellar extension and associated with limited visual loss, are best treated by trans-sphenoidal surgery (see "Acromegaly"). Microadenomas can often be successfully removed and normal pituitary function restored. With marked suprasellar extension, a transfrontal surgical approach may be needed. This is a much more formidable procedure. In many cases a large tumor cannot be completely removed; postoperative radiation therapy will prevent clinical recurrence in these instances.

Acromegaly

Pituitary tumors that produce an excess of growth hormone result in the clinical state termed acromegaly. If the growth hormone excess occurs before cessation of growth, *gigantism* occurs. When growth hormone excess begins in the adult, the most common clinical feature suggesting the presence of acromegaly is insidious alteration of facial appearance over many years. Old photographs may be useful in helping to identify such changes. The various physical findings include enlargement (lengthening) of the mandible, sometimes with separation of the teeth; coarsening of facial features due both to overgrowth of frontal, malar, and nasal bones and soft tissue overgrowth producing widening of the nose and protrusion of the lips; enlargement of the hands and feet, often noted by increasing glove and shoe size; and dermatological changes that include skin thickening and sebaceous gland enlargement (hydradenitis). Very commonly, patients present with a nerve entrapment (carpal tunnel) syndrome. Osteoarthritis and diabetes mellitus, although frequently seen in this disorder, are too common to provide a clue to the presence of acromegaly. Tumors large enough to produce sellar enlargement may lead to headache; suprasellar extension may result in visual field defects.

The laboratory diagnosis is simple in overt cases but requires dynamic testing in mild cases. Elevation of serum growth hormone (GH) in the fasting, basal state to values consistently greater than 10 ng/ml is strongly suggestive of the diagnosis. However, stress and physical activity may also elevate the GH levels. Elevated values must therefore be confirmed with a test of the ability of glucose to suppress the GH. During a standard glucose tolerance test (Chapter 72), the GH—determined simultaneously with the glucose—should normally fall to a value less than 5 ng/ml. Most acromegalics show no fall of GH, and a few exhibit a "paradoxical" rise during the test. Laboratory evidence of elevated and nonsuppressible GH warrants referral to an endocrinologist, as does the presence of equivocal clinical or laboratory findings.

Treatment of Acromegaly

Treatment should be directed by an endocrinologist. Irradiation of the pituitary, usually by external high voltage techniques, has been standard treatment for years. Such therapy is effective but is usually extremely slow in its effect and may take several years to produce maximal suppression of hormone production. Surgery is indicated when there is a need for

rapid reduction of the elevated growth hormone (e.g., for cosmetic reasons in a young woman with early disease; visual field loss; or intractable headache). Trans-sphenoidal operation is now standard for most cases and should, if at all possible, include an attempt at selective removal of a microadenoma. The trans-sphenoidal operation involves minimal morbidity, a very low rate of complications, and essentially no mortality, but recurrences are common, leading some authorities to continue to advocate radiation therapy as the first approach for uncomplicated cases. Bromocriptine is effective in a minority of cases but can be useful occasionally in reducing the severity of headache.

Cushing's Disease

When evidence is obtained for overproduction of glucocorticoids and testing suggests the presence of adrenal hyperplasia (see "Adrenal Diseases"), X-ray evaluation of the sella turcica is in order. Only rarely will an abnormality be evident, even on CT. Most cases of Cushing's disease with adrenal hyperplasia are, nonetheless, due to a basophilic microadenoma of the pituitary (see page 984).

Other Secretory Pituitary Tumors

Although quite rare, pituitary tumors that secrete thyrotropin (TSH) and produce hyperthyroidism occur. Even rarer are cases of hypersecretion of TSH without demonstrable tumor. Patients with tumors have recently been successfully treated with a somatostatin analogue (19). Tumors producing excessive amounts of gonadotropins have not been described.

PITUITARY FAILURE (HYPOPITUITARISM)

Idiopathic Causes

Patients are occasionally encountered in whom pituitary failure occurs without evidence of pituitary tumor or of another anatomical defect demonstrable by current techniques. Some of these patients are eventually found to have infiltrative processes (sarcoidosis, histiocytosis, lymphoma). Hypopituitarism in these patients is diagnosed by the demonstation of end organ failure occurring in the absence of the expected elevation of trophic hormone. Isolated deficiencies of trophic hormones also occur but are rare. Among these, the most likely to be encountered is hypogonadotropic hypogonadism in the male, sometimes associated with anosmia (Kallmann's syndrome). In these patients, no anatomical basis is apparent.

Sheehan's Syndrome (Postpartum Pituitary Failure)

Massive uterine hemorrhage occurring at delivery occasionally results in pituitary infarction and panhypopituitarism. In this syndrome, failure of postpartum lactation and absence of menses are attended by debility and other evidences of end organ failure. Because of improvements in obstetrical care (prompt treatment of hemorrhage), such cases are now rare.

Pituitary Apoplexy

On rare occasions hemorrhagic infarction of a pituitary tumor may lead to severe headache and/or signs of a rapidly expanding intracranial abnormality. Radiographic examination of the sella turcica is abnormal. Another rare phenomenon is that of pituitary infarction ("apoplexy") occurring during the course of a febrile illness, presumably viral. Intense headache lasts for days and is usually but not always severe enough to require hospitalization. The acute febrile illness subsides with symptomatic therapy and without specific clinical or radiographic findings, only to be followed later by the development of hypopituitarism. Both men and women can be affected.

Hormone Replacement Therapy of Hypopituitarism

Pituitary insufficiency, regardless of the cause, is treated with thyroid hormone (thyroxine, see page 969) adrenal glucocorticoid (cortisol, see page 983), and gonadal hormone (testosterone, see Chapter 77, or an estrogen, see Chapter 77). At the present time, pituitary trophic hormones are not available for routine clinical use; furthermore, they are not necessary for maintenance of normal health and vigor. Occasionally, young women may be candidates for therapy with gonadotropins in order to produce ovulation and to restore fertility. Such therapy is possible but available at only a few centers. In men, normal libido and sexual performance can be assured with testosterone therapy. Restoration of fertility in the male is also possible with the use of a combination of gonadotropins, but such therapy is not generally available.

Disturbances of Pituitary Function Due to Nonendocrine Disease

Perhaps more common than decreased pituitary function resulting from intrinsic pituitary disease is altered gonadotropin secretion on a functional basis. Many illnesses can affect the functional integrity of the hypothalamic-pituitary-end organ axis. This phenomenon is most obvious as disturbance of menstruation in women (see Chapter 77). Any disease that results in malnutrition can produce decreased gonadotropins and (secondary) amenorrhea. Alcoholism is an outstanding example. Liver disease need not be present in alcoholism in order to produce amenorrhea, but various liver diseases are themselves associated with loss of menses. The common factor seems to be malnutrition.

The classical example of nonendocrine illness that simulates an endocrine disturbance is anorexia nervosa (see Chapter 5). In this psychiatric disturbance, which results in severe malnutrition with resultant weight loss, the most marked disturbance of endocrine function is cessation of menses resulting from a decrease of gonadotropins. Other trophic hormones are

not affected. Thyroid function is usually normal. Axillary and pubic hair are retained, giving important clinical evidence for the preservation of adrenal function. Although cortisol secretion is low (urinary steroid excretion is decreased), this results from slow metabolic disposal of cortisol rather than decreased ACTH secretion; plasma cortisol is normal. Growth hormone concentration may be elevated, a consequence of starvation due to any cause. The diagnosis of anorexia nervosa should be based on the association of psychiatric abnormalities and obvious decrease in food intake. The tests described will serve merely to support the diagnosis.

Other diseases may also result in secondary amenorrhea due to failure of gonadotropin secretion. These include such diverse conditions as severe emotional disturbances, marked obesity, poorly controlled diabetes mellitus, and severe chronic infections.

ADRENAL DISEASES

Adrenocortical Insufficiency (Addison's Disease)

In ambulatory patients the clinical presentation of adrenocortical insufficiency is related to a number of chronic complaints that are nonspecific in character. Although a high index of suspicion will certainly result in far more tests than positive diagnoses, detection of this relatively rare problem demands such an approach. The alternative is needless morbidity culminating in acute hospitalization for full blown disease, i.e., vascular collapse with Addisonian "crisis."

Etiology and Association with Other Autoimmune Diseases

Adrenocortical insufficiency is now most commonly due to "autoimmune" disease and is associated with the presence of antibodies to adrenal tissue. Most other cases are secondary to pituitary disease. Tuberculosis, once a common cause, now only rarely produces adrenocortical insufficiency, probably because of decreased frequency of tuberculosis and because of effective therapy. Many cases of autoimmune adrenocortical insufficiency are associated with autoimmune thyroiditis, although the two problems may develop years apart. The simultaneous occurrence of autoimmune thyroid and adrenal disease is termed Schmidt's syndrome. Rarely, autoimmune adrenocortical insufficiency, autoimmune hypothyroidism, and autoimmune gonadal failure occur in the syndrome of "polyglandular failure." There is also an association of autoimmune adrenocortical insufficiency with pernicious anemia and Sjögren's syndrome, and probably with systemic lupus erythematosus. Other rare causes of adrenocortical insufficiency include histoplasmosis and sarcoidosis.

Clinical Presentation

Chronic symptoms include anorexia, weight loss, weakness, and decreased physical endurance. Vomiting may occur, and abdominal pain, sometimes resembling that of peptic ulcer disease, can be a presenting feature. Other symptoms include mental sluggishness, irritability, and symptoms of either postural hypotension or of hypoglycemia. In primary adrenal insufficiency, increasing pigmentation (white patients) or further darkening of skin (black patients) may be noted. Loss of axillary and pubic hair—an important finding when present—may occur in women. Such hair loss is commonly overlooked on physical examination and is hardly ever volunteered as part of the history.

Physical examination often shows postural hypotension. Pigmentation is diffuse but in addition is especially evident in creases of the hands, the areolae, over pressure areas (knuckles, elbows), and in new scars. Pigmentation of buccal mucous membranes is a pathognomonic finding in white patients but is a normal finding in blacks. Lymphadenopathy is occasionally seen. When the adrenal insufficiency is secondary to pituitary disease, additional findings may relate to the manifestations of a pituitary tumor (headache, visual loss), to hypothyroidism (Chapter 73), or to hypogonadism (Chapter 77).

Laboratory Evaluation

Classically, hyponatremia associated with hyperkalemia and some degree of azotemia provided the clues to the diagnosis. These latter abnormalities are manifestations of severe disease and may be absent in the less severe cases that are likely to be encountered in an ambulatory practice. Various other nonspecific abnormalities occur, occasionally including anemia, lymphocytosis, and eosinophilia.

Laboratory diagnosis of adrenal insufficiency must be made or excluded by determination of plasma cortisol. Determinations of plasma cortisol made without prior adrenal stimulation by injected ACTH have many limitations. In this regard both the normal diurnal rhythm of cortisol and the high degree of variability of plasma cortisol in normal persons must be kept in mind. Plasma cortisol can be initially measured at any time of the day, and a normal value (15 to 25 μg/dl) will exclude the diagnosis. However, afternoon determinations may be "low" simply because of the normal P.M. drop, and even the fasting A.M. cortisol is highly variable. Values lower than 5 μg/dl at any time are highly likely to be due to adrenal insufficiency. Intermediate values (5 to 10 μg/dl) may be seen in less severe cases and may overlap those of normals. Thus, measurement of unstimulated plasma cortisol is useful, especially in excluding the diagnosis, but may fail to detect mild cases or may yield indeterminate values.

Plasma ACTH can be determined by immunoradiometric assay. An elevated level will be seen in primary adrenal insufficiency because of lack of inhibition of the negative feedback system. Plasma ACTH is an adjunct to diagnosis; its major usefulness is in establishing a diagnosis of secondary (pituitary) adrenocortical insufficiency.

Evaluation of the significance of low or borderline values of plasma cortisol should always be made by administering exogenous ACTH and then measuring plasma cortisol again—after the adrenal stimulation. The ease with which such testing is performed—and the frequent failure of unstimulated plasma cortisol values to give definitive information—provides a cogent argument for use of ACTH stimulation as the preferred screening procedure for adrenal insufficiency. Many variations of ACTH stimulation tests have been advocated. A simple and reliable procedure is the bolus intravenous injection of 0.25 mg of synthetic ACTH (Cortrosyn) (see below). Plasma cortisol obtained 2 to 3 hours after injection will normally increase 2 to 4 times over baseline and will be above the normal baseline range. Patients with adrenocortical insufficiency do not show a response. If the test is positive (no response), confirmation should be made with an 8-hour intravenous infusion of ACTH (Cortrosyn, 0.25 mg in 500 to 1000 ml of saline or glucose) and at least two plasma cortisols obtained between 6 and 8 hours. Expected increments of cortisol are somewhat greater in the latter test.

Synthetic ACTH (Cortrosyn) is readily available and has replaced the natural material in all of its forms. Rapid "1-hour" screening tests with ACTH should be avoided, since the increment of cortisol is less than when a longer period is used. The 1-hour test is therefore more difficult to interpret and less reliable. Intramuscular injections of ACTH can be given, but if there is no response, the test must be repeated by intravenous administration.

Tests of adrenal function based on urinary excretion of steroid metabolites [17-ketogenic (17-KGS) or 17-hydroxysteroids (17-OHS)] should be avoided as initial tests for adrenal insufficiency. These tests offer no advantage over plasma cortisol measurements and often yield artifactually low values due to incomplete collection of urine. After stimulation with ACTH, determinations of urinary steroids can, however, provide useful confirmation of the plasma cortisol response. The adrenal response to ACTH is slow in secondary adrenal insufficiency and requires stimulation for up to 3 days. However, other tests of pituitary function are available and serve better to identify the presence of adrenal insufficiency resulting from pituitary disease (see "Pituitary Diseases").

Although the adrenal mineralocorticoid, aldosterone, may be low in adrenal insufficiency, the hormone is secreted by the zona glomerulosa rather than the more central portion of the adrenal cortex and may be relatively unaffected by processes that destroy much of the adrenal. Therefore, measurements of plasma and urinary aldosterone have no place in routine diagnosis of adrenocortical insufficiency.

Treatment of Addison's Disease

The Addisonian patient should be made to realize the importance of taking hormone therapy regularly and of understanding self-care during situations of stress. Unless both patient and physician cooperate in this effort, the life of the Addisonian patient becomes a series of hospitalizations requiring emergency therapy for crises, most of which should be avoidable.

Steroid replacement therapy. Under normal circumstances patients are given 20 to 30 mg of cortisol (or equivalent) daily. Recommended dosage schemes vary. The simplest and least expensive therapy is 12.5 mg (1/2 of a 25-mg cortisone tablet) taken twice daily (morning and evening). In another scheme, 10 to 15 mg of cortisol (hydrocortisone) are used on the same schedule. Some authorities prefer to simulate the normal diurnal rhythm of cortisol secretion, although no evidence indicates that this scheme is of any benefit. In this approach, 10 to 15 mg of cortisol are given on arising and 5 to 10 mg in the evening. Equivalent doses of prednisone or another glucocorticoid (Table 74.2) may be used but have no advantage. Their use may, indeed, dictate a requirement for additional mineralocorticoid therapy, since glucocorticoids such as prednisone, dexamethasone, etc., have much less mineralocorticoid activity than does cortisol (or cortisone). Overtreatment with glucocorticoids should be avoided. Frequent increases of dose for treatment of nonspecific complaints are a common practice but are to be deplored, since iatrogenic Cushing's syndrome is a real hazard to the long-term well-being of patients with Addison's disease.

The requirement for glucocorticoids (cortisol) is, of course, increased during stress. In the ambulatory patient, minor stress can be handled by a properly instructed and motivated patient. Telephone contact with the physician is also useful—or even essential—on many such occasions, especially in the early months of therapy before the patient's ability to deal with these episodes has been demonstrated. The commonest stress for the ambulatory patient is a nonspecific, often viral, febrile illness. Ordinarily, a febrile response to approximately 101°F (38°C) that is unaccompanied by vomiting or diarrhea can be handled by simply increasing the cortisol dose to 50 to 75 mg daily in divided doses. A more severe episode (e.g., bronchitis) may require 100 mg. The occurrence of vomiting or significant diarrhea requires contact with a physician and may demand the use of parenteral glucocorticoids.

The need for hospitalization during stress must be determined by the physician and depends on the circumstances. It is obviously prudent to be cautious, but in this long-term chronic illness, frequent and precipitous hospitalizations should be avoided. Many minor events can be handled by judicious increase of steroid dosage. Preoperative management is described elsewhere (Chapter 86).

Although not all patients with fully developed adrenal insufficiency require mineralocorticoid therapy in addition to cortisol replacement, such therapy is usually started when the diagnosis is made. The initial dose is 0.1 mg of fludrocortisone daily (Florinef, 0.1-mg tablets). Aldosterone is not available for therapy of Addison's disease. Only rarely will patients require more than 0.1 mg of fludrocortisone. In the past doses as high as 0.2 mg daily were used, but hypertension and edema were common. Some individuals require as little as 0.05 mg every other day. Adequacy of therapy can be judged by determinations of serum sodium and potassium and clinical observations, including normalization of blood pressure without postural hypotension. When, during stress, the dose of cortisol is increased beyond 50 to 75 mg daily, fludrocortisone therapy becomes unnecessary, since the mineralocorticoid activity of cortisol is sufficient to maintain salt balance when taken in greater than baseline physiological amounts.

Patient education. The patient and members of the patient's household should be educated about the symptoms of Addisonian crisis and how to respond in emergencies. In addition, the patient should carry an identification document or wear an inscribed bracelet identifying the Addisonian state and instructing therapy. Appropriate information in addition to name, address, and telephone number should read approximately as follows:

I am a patient with adrenal insufficiency (Addison's disease). If I am seriously injured, found unconscious, or am vomiting, I should be given an injection of dexamethasone, as emergency treatment for Addisonian crisis. A filled syringe is with my belongings. Notify my physicians (name, telephone number) or other medical authority immediately.

Syringes containing dexamethasone phosphate (4 mg in 1 ml of water) are available for patients and can be conveniently carried.

All patients with Addison's disease should eat a diet that contains a liberal quantity of sodium (100 to 150 mEq/day), regardless of whether mineralocorticoids are used. In the event of intercurrent diarrhea or profuse sweating, additional salt should be consumed. Electrolytes should be checked periodically (every 3 to 4 months during the critical first year of therapy). Mineralocorticoid therapy should be cautiously reduced if edema, hypertension, or hypokalemia is noted, and salt and/or mineralocorticoid should be increased if postural hypotension, hyponatremia, or hyperkalemia appears. Overtreatment with glucocorticoids should be carefully avoided. Over the long-term, it should be borne in mind that, if the Addison's disease is idiopathic (i.e., autoimmune), related diseases and their own manifestations may appear at any time (hypothyroidism, hypoparathyroidism, hypogonadism).

Adrenocortical Hyperfunction; Cushing's Syndrome and Adrenal Androgen Excess

The adrenals produce several steroid products: glucocorticoids (chiefly cortisol), mineralocorticoids (chiefly aldosterone), and so-called adrenal androgens [a group of steroids collectively termed 17-ketosteroids (17-KS)]. Clinical disorders are known that affect predominantly the secretion of one or other of these hormones. Table 74.1 lists these disorders of adrenal hyperfunction. Most are rather uncommon or rare, but some essentially functional disorders are frequently

Table 74.1.
Adrenocortical Hyperfunction

GLUCOCORTICOID EXCESS PREDOMINATES
  Adrenal hyperplasia (60–70% of all cases):
    1. Pituitary microadenoma secreting ACTH (most cases of adrenal hyperplasia)
    2. Nonendocrine tumor secreting ACTH (rare)
  Adrenal neoplasm (30–40% of all cases):
    1. Adrenal adenoma
    2. Adrenal carcinoma   (about equal in frequency)
ADRENAL ANDROGEN EXCESS PREDOMINATES
(HIRSUTISM/VIRILISM)
  Some adrenal adenomas
  Some adrenal carcinomas
  Partial adrenogenital syndrome[a]
ALDOSTERONE EXCESS
  Primary aldosteronism:
    1. Adrenal adenoma
    2. Adrenal nodular hyperplasia
  Secondary aldosteronism:
    1. Salt and volume depletion, including diuretic use and various disease states causing increased production of renin
    2. Juxtaglomerular cell hyperplasia or tumor (rare)

[a] Complete enzymatic defects in steroid synthesis are rare and are invariably manifest early in life as adrenal insufficiency and abnormalities of genital development. In ambulatory adults, partial defects of synthesis of cortisol lead to compensatory adrenal hyperplasia with production of excessive quantities of adrenal steroids with weak androgenic activity. Hirsutism, with or without virilism, ensues (see Chapter 77).

encountered. The approach presented here is predominantly oriented to the recognition—or exclusion—and initial evaluation of these diseases in ambulatory patients. Once the practitioner is reasonably certain that a problem exists, detailed evaluation often requires consultation with an endocrinologist and sometimes hospitalization for special procedures. However, many relatively simple tests to define the situation can and should be performed on an ambulatory basis. It must be appreciated that details of diagnostic workups vary widely even among specialists and are in constant evolution as new hormone assays and tests emerge.

Cushing's Syndrome (Glucocorticoid Excess)

Etiology. In this syndrome a supraphysiological amount of glucocorticoid (cortisol) is secreted along with varying amounts of adrenal androgens. Most cases are due to hypersecretion of ACTH from the pituitary with resultant adrenal hyperplasia (Cushing's disease). In recent years it has become apparent that almost all of these cases are due to putuitary microadenomas that produce excessive amounts of ACTH (see "Pituitary Diseases"). A smaller number are due to adrenal adenoma or carcinoma. Cushing's syndrome may also occasionally be caused by ectopic production of ACTH by malignant tumors. Of these tumors, small cell carcinoma of the lung is most commonly involved. When a tumor causes Cushing's syndrome, the malignancy is usually obvious, although rarely a small neoplasm may be inapparent when the evidence of glucocorticoid excess first appears.

Clinical presentation. The severity of the signs and symptoms depends on the magnitude of the steroid excess, the rapidity with which it develops, and the

degree to which androgen production is increased. The signs and symptoms of glucocorticoid excess are familiar to all physicians who have seen the entire picture of this disease emerge as the result of long-term treatment of patients with prednisone and similar drugs. Glucocorticoid excess produces increased deposition of subcutaneous fat in the face ("moon facies"), and deposition of fat in the upper body produces "buffalo hump" and truncal obesity. Skin changes include telangiectasia over the face, atrophy and thinning of the skin with easy or spontaneous bruising, ecchymoses, and development of purplish abdominal striae. Hyperpigmentation is sometimes seen. Muscle weakness results from so-called steroid myopathy and is especially prominent in the shoulder and pelvic girdle areas. The extremities become thin as muscle wasting occurs. Eventually bone mineral loss occurs, producing osteoporosis with its resultant back pain. Crush fractures of the vertebrae are common and frequently spontaneous, and hip or wrist fractures may occur after minimal trauma. Hypertension and diabetes mellitus are common. Hypokalemia may occur. Probably less well recognized are the psychiatric disturbances that result from chronic glucocorticoid excess. Lability of mood, depression, mania, and frank psychoses may all be precipitated by glucocorticoid excess.

Androgenic effects occur from both the intrinsic properties of the glucocorticoids and the associated production of adrenal androgens. With glucocorticoid excess alone only mild signs are usually evident, i.e., hirsutism (facial, extremities, truncal) and acne. More profound androgen effects that include virilization suggest adrenal tumor. These signs include frontal baldness in women, oligomenorrhea, increase in muscle mass, and enlargement of the clitoris. Androgenic effects cannot, of course, be appreciated in men.

Differential Diagnosis

Obesity and Hirsutism. In women obesity is frequently associated with hirsutism, hypertension, and/or diabetes. When weight gain is rapid, striae may appear. These findings often raise the possibility of Cushing's syndrome and provoke laboratory screening for this disorder. Very few such patients will be found to have Cushing's syndrome.

One-half of obese persons have increased cortisol production, which is a phenomenon resulting from the obese state. In these individuals the urinary excretion of steroid metabolites is increased and falls into the range of that seen in Cushing's syndrome. However, in distinction from Cushing's syndrome, such obese individuals have plasma cortisol concentrations that are normal rather than elevated. Furthermore, the suppressibility of the pituitary-adrenal axis in obesity is also normal (see "Laboratory Diagnosis" below). The obesity-related increase of urinary steroid metabolite excretion is one of several reasons why such measurements are to be avoided for screening purposes.

Psychiatric Illness. Psychiatric symptoms are common in Cushing's syndrome. However, it has also been appreciated that depressive illness may be associated with markedly excessive production of glucocorticoids. These patients do not appear clinically to have full-blown Cushing's syndrome, but at least some clinical features suggest the diagnosis and lead to laboratory investigation. Differentiation from true Cushing's syndrome may be difficult at first, but the differential diagnosis eventually becomes clear, since remission of the psychiatric disturbance results in disappearance of the abnormal laboratory findings.

Laboratory Diagnosis

General. The tests of adrenal and pituitary function fall into two groups: (a) static measurements of blood or urine steroids or (b) dynamic testing of the pituitary-adrenal axis. Both procedures are useful and may be combined. With regard to the measurements themselves, in blood both plasma cortisol and ACTH can be assayed. In urine, assays are available for cortisol ("free cortisol"), two different groups of cortisol metabolites (17-OHCS and 17-KGS), and the adrenal androgens (17-KS), which also include some cortisol metabolites.

Screening for Suspected Cushing's Syndrome. Many patients with Cushing's syndrome have mild disease. Steroid production in such individuals is not greatly increased and there is considerable overlap with normal values. Accordingly, determination of plasma cortisol or urinary steroid excretion is not likely to be helpful. Screening can best be performed with an abbreviated suppression test with use of dexamethasone. A single oral dose of 1 mg is given between 11 P.M. and midnight, and the plasma cortisol is measured at 8 to 9 A.M. Normal patients will show suppression of cortisol to less than 5 µg/dl. If the test is abnormal, a more involved but more reliable suppression test is performed in which dexamethasone is given orally at a dose of 0.5 mg every 6 hours for 2 days. Plasma cortisol, urinary 17-OHCS, or both can be monitoried by this test. The plasma cortisol at the end of the suppression period should be suppressed to less than 3 µg/dl. Urinary 17-OHCS during the second 24 hours should not exceed 2.5 mg. Suppression is normal in obesity but may be abnormal in patients with psychiatric illness.

Other Screening Procedures. An alternative screening procedure is measurement of the 24-hour urinary excretion of cortisol (free cortisol). This test is relatively sensitive. Minimal elevations of plasma cortisol tend to result in marked increases of urinary cortisol. The test is not affected by obesity but may be altered in patients with psychiatric illness.

The normal diurnal rhythm of plasma cortisol tends to be obliterated in Cushing's syndrome. In normal individuals, the 4 P.M. cortisol is on an average 50% of that obtained in the early A.M. Although widely advocated for diagnosis, determination of this rhythm by measurement of A.M. and P.M. cortisol is not a reliable screening procedure.

*Interpreting tests and additional diagnostic maneu-*vers. Unfortunately, both false-positive and false-negative screening tests are occasionally seen. If the tests are equivocal and the clinical features strongly suggestive, referral to an endocrinologist is appropriate. In expert hands, a variety of maneuvers can usually establish or exclude the diagnosis and differentiate among the causes of Cushing's syndrome, but familiarity with the specialized test procedures is essential. Often a degree of laboratory precision is required that is not always achieved by ordinary commercial laboratories. Useful tests likely to be employed in such consultations, in addition to those described, include multiple samplings of plasma cortisol throughout the day and night ("integrated blood levels"), determinations of urinary excretion of steroids on multiple occasions, variations of the dexamethasone suppression test with the use of different doses of the steroid, and plasma ACTH measurements by special techniques.

Until strong laboratory evidence is at hand to indicate that steroid production is abnormal, procedures such as CT or MRI of the sella turcica and of the adrenal areas are not justified. These procedures are not useful in screening, although they are important in determining the locus and etiology of steroid excess once this phenomenon has been established.

Treatment of Cushing's syndrome. Surgery remains the treatment of Cushing's syndrome due to an adrenal adenoma. Although surgical removal of the adrenals (bilateral adrenalectomy) has been accepted for years as the most effective therapy for Cushing's disease (adrenocortical hyperplasia), this treatment is being rapidly abandoned. Induction of permanent adrenal insufficiency, the risk of development of an enlarging pituitary adenoma accompanied by hyperpigmentation (Nelson's syndrome), and significant operative mortality and morbidity are drawbacks of adrenalectomy for this condition. Over the past decade it has been appreciated that most cases of Cushing's disease can be treated by trans-sphenoidal surgical removal of a pituitary microadenoma, and this approach has become the preferred therapy (16, 21). However, a significant number (estimates range from 5 to 25%) treated in this manner recur within a relatively short time despite apparently successful removal of a microadenoma. Medical therapy with an inhibitor of adrenal steroid synthesis (mitotane; o,p-DDD), is effective, for these cases, either alone or preferably in combination with pituitary irradiation. Another inhibitor (e.g., metyropone, aminoglutethamide, and, most recently, ketoconazole) is also sometimes used instead of o,p-DDD (29). The selection of the therapeutic approach for the individual patient should be made by an endocrinologist.

Adrenal Androgen Excess

If evidence of Cushing's syndrome coexists with signs of androgen excess, the 24-hour excretion of 17-KS should be measured along with 17-OHCS or 17-KGS. The 17-KS measurement is, however, of no use in routine screening for Cushing's syndrome. Elevated values do occur, but do so less frequently than do the other indices of cortisol production. However, an argument can be made for including a single, 24-hour determination of urinary 17-KS in the initial screening workup for Cushing's syndrome, if there is clinical evidence of androgen excess. When adrenal tumor is present, measurement of urinary 17-KS may be the most abnormal test. Some adrenal tumors (benign adenomas or carcinomas) produce enormous amounts of 17-KS. In suspected cases of adrenal tumor, measurement of 17-KS is specifically indicated. Serum testosterone will also be elevated in women but not in men (see "Adrenal Mass Lesions" below).

Hirsutism. Hirsutism without virilism is extremely common (see Chapter 77). The combination of hirsutism plus virilism, which is exceedingly rare, is invariably associated with elevated 17-KS. When such a patient is encountered, referral to an endocrinologist is the most appropriate course. In adults, most cases will prove to be caused by adrenal tumors. Other causes, e.g., entities such as congenital adrenal hyperplasia (female pseudohermaphroditism, isosexual precocity in men, hypertension, and salt loss) all become apparent in childhood. Only a few cases (due to 21-hydroxylase deficiency) have ever been seen in adults.

Other Adrenal Diseases

Mineralocorticoid Excess

The classical condition resulting from mineralocorticoid excess is primary aldosteronism due to a benign adrenocortical adenoma (Conn's syndrome). Clinical features include hypertension and the manifestations of hypokalemia. A significant number of cases are due to bilateral adrenocortical nodular hyperplasia. The evaluation of this condition is described in Chapter 46.

Mineralocorticoid Deficiency

Aldosterone deficiency is part of classical adrenal insufficiency (Addison's disease) but may also occur as a selective, functional deficiency state in the syndrome of hyporeninemic hypoaldosteronism. The identifying feature is hyperkalemia. The syndrome is described in Chapter 48.

Pheochromocytoma

This rare catecholamine (epinephrine, norepinephrine)-producing tumor is usually considered in relationship to the evaluation of hypertension and is described in Chapter 62.

Adrenal Mass Lesions, Incidentally Identified

Adrenal masses were in the past occasionally discovered during intravenous pyelography, but such lesions are now commonly recognized during CT of the upper abdomen. When such a lesion is discovered, consideration should be given to the possible presence of Cushing's syndrome, of mineralocorticoid or cate-cholamine excess producing intermittent or sustained hypertension (pheochromocytoma, aldosteronism), of hirsutism and virilization, and of feminization. Biochemical testing should be initiated as appropriate.

Most of the lesions incidentally encountered during CT are benign, clinically silent adenomas, but a major concern is whether the mass represents a carcinoma. Three considerations are relevant in attempting to make this distinction: biochemical activity, size of the lesion, and the relative incidence rates. Most carcinomas produce biochemically measurable products, e.g., an excess of 17-KS; a few produce 17-KGS but have normal 17-KS; and rarely only testosterone or aldosterone levels are increased. Benign adenomas may also produce excess quantities of steroids. Nevertheless, in general, tumors producing biochemical products should be removed.

If no biochemical abnormality is demonstrable, the size of the lesion gives some indication of whether it is benign or malignant. When discovered, most adenomas are small (<6 cm diameter), and most carcinomas are large (>6 cm diameter). However, a conservative approach to all such biochemically silent lesions is warranted, because even with tumors over 6 cm, over 60 operations would be necessary to remove one carcinoma, while over 4000 operations would be needed to remove a single carcinoma, if one considers all lesions of diameter greater than 1.5 cm.

Occasionally the adrenal mass is cystic. Large cystic masses can be aspirated by needle puncture; clear fluid indicates a benign lesion, but bloody fluid is indeterminate, and cytology is not helpful. Similarly, needle aspiration biopsy is usually not useful in distinguishing benign from malignant cystic lesions.

In follow-up of biochemically silent adrenal masses, CT scans at 2, 6, and 18 months are indicated. Clear evidence of progressive enlargement is an indication for excision. Lesions that are stable at 18 months can be considered to be benign and should not be removed (9).

PHARMACOLOGICAL USES OF STEROIDS AS ANTI-INFLAMMATORY AND IMMUNOSUPPRESSIVE DRUGS

Most steroid (glucocorticoid) usage is related to treatment of diseases other than adrenal insufficiency. The doses used exceed those of physiological output and are best termed "supraphysiological" or, simply, pharmacological. The anti-inflammatory and immunosuppressive properties of these drugs constitute an invaluable part of the modern therapeutic armamentarium, but such uses, at least when prolonged, are invariably associated with side effects. Short-term uses are much safer, if not entirely innocuous. Although the glucocorticoid and mineralocorticoid actions of steroids have been chemically dissociated, no such separation has been possible for desired versus undesired effects. All available glucocorticoids share these properties to an equal degree, although potency (effectiveness per milligram) varies widely (Table 74.2). Despite this fact, certain glucocorticoid compounds

Table 74.2.
Commonly Used Glucocorticoids

Generic Name	Common Trade Name(s)	Equivalent Potency (mg)[a]	Sodium Retention Relative to Cortisol
FOR ORAL USE			
Cortisol (hydrocortisone)	Cortef	20	—
Cortisone[b]	—	25	1
Prednisone	Deltasone Meticorten Delta-Cortef	5	0.1
Prednisolone	Meticortelone Sterane	4	0.1
Methylprednisolone	Medrol	4	0
Triamcinolone	Aristocort, Kenacort	4	0
Dexamethasone[c]	Decadron	0.75	0
Betamethasone[c]	Celestone	0.6	0
FOR PARENTERAL USE			
Cortisol	Solu-Cortef		
Methylprednisolone	Solu-Medrol		
Triamcinolone	Aristocort		
Dexamethasone	Decadron		
Betamethasone	Celestone		
FOR TOPICAL USE			
Triamcinolone	Aristocort, Kenalog		
Fluocinolone	Synalar		
Betamethasone	Valisone		
FOR INHALATION			
Beclomethasone	Vanceril		

[a] Also equivalent to daily physiological replacement when given in divided doses.
[b] Cortisone acetate has long been given parenterally (intramuscular route) as well as orally; however, this compound is unpredictably absorbed from injection sites and cannot be relied upon to produce adequate blood levels.
[c] This compound has a relatively long duration of action and should not be used for alternate-day glucocorticoid therapy.

Most of the compounds listed are available in generic forms. All are marketed as ester derivatives or salts of esters, e.g., cortisol sodium hemisuccinate (Solu-Cortef). For practical purposes, only cortisol and cortisone have significant salt-retaining (mineralocorticoid) action.

Table 74.3.
Untoward Effects of Chronic Glucocorticoid Therapy

ACUTE
Fluid/electrolyte disturbances
  Sodium retention
  Fluid retention
  Potassium depletion
  Hypokalemic alkalosis
Gastrointestinal
  Peptic ulcer (hemorrhage, perforation)
  Ulcerative esophagitis
Endocrine
  Precipitation of diabetes mellitus
Ophthalmic
  Glaucoma
Neurological
  Mood swings
  Acute psychosis
  Convulsions
CHRONIC
Fluid/electrolyte disturbances
  See above, plus hypertension
Musculoskeletal
  Muscle weakness
  Muscle atrophy
  Steroid myopathy
  Osteoporosis/pathological fractures
  Aseptic necrosis of femoral or humeral heads
  Tendon rupture
Gastrointestinal
  Pancreatitis
Dermatological
  Impaired wound healing
  Atrophy of skin (fragility)
  Ecchymoses
  Increased sweating
Neurological
  Convulsions
  Increased intracranial pressure
  Insomnia
  Euphoria
  Depression
Endocrine
  Menstrual irregularities
  Carbohydrate intolerance/diabetes mellitus
  Adrenal atrophy/disruption of normal response to stress
    (iatrogenic Addison's disease)
Ophthalmic
  Cataracts
  Glaucoma
Hematological
  Thromboembolism
Other
  Weight gain
  Increased susceptibility to infections

have tended to become associated with the treatment of particular conditions, e.g., dexamethasone for treatment of cerebral edema. Often no secure pharmacological base supports such practices. On the other hand, legitimate pharmacological differences between available preparations do exist that include different rates of absorption, metabolic disposal, and solubility. Exploitation of such properties is seen in dermatological use. Triamcinolone and fluocinolone acetonides appear to be much more effective than hydrocortisone for cutaneous use, a phenomenon apparently related to properties of absorption (see Chapter 100). Another example is the use of beclomethasone (Vanceril) as an aerosol in the treatment of asthma (see Chapter 55) and allergic rhinitis (see Chapter 23).

Adverse Effects

Untoward effects of glucocorticoids are listed in Table 74.3. These problems are related to dose and—equally important—duration of therapy (12, 20). No contraindication ever exists to a single dose of glucocorticoid, regardless of the size of that dose. Thus, treatment of an allergic reaction with one or a few doses carries no risk. Chronic therapy, however, should be instituted only after consideration of the risk:benefit ratio. Therapy that is not intended as chronic may become so. For example, asthmatic patients may be so impressed by relief afforded by systemic steroids that other modalities are abandoned and the patient becomes totally dependent on glucocorticoids.

Side effects of steroids are closely related to desired effects. Anti-inflammatory effects are obviously desirable when treating a disease such as rheumatoid arthritis. However, many inflammatory responses are beneficial, as for example the inflammatory responses associated with bacterial infection. In this situation, glucocorticoids may inhibit a useful inflammatory response that otherwise would serve to localize the process. Thus, one ordinarily avoids pharmacological doses of glucocorticoids when infection requiring an antibiotic is necessary. Not infrequently, however, patients receiving glucocorticoids develop an infection. Ordinarily, steroid therapy is not discontinued; rather, vigorous antibiotic therapy is instituted and the dose of steroid is kept at as low a level as the clinical situation allows, thus preventing clinical evidence of adrenal insufficiency and the development of nonspecific but serious symptoms (see "Steroid Withdrawal Syndrome," page 989).

Adverse effects of steroids are related not only to duration of therapy but to dose used. Obviously, one should attempt to use a minimally effective dose. Nonetheless, some persons seem especially vulnerable to unwanted side effects. Poorly nourished, debilitated, and elderly patients are all more prone to the muscle-wasting effects of steroids. Postmenopausal women—already prone to develop osteoporosis—are especially vulnerable to the demineralization that accompanies steroid use. Genetically predisposed individuals may develop overt diabetes mellitus when given glucocorticoids. Peptic ulcer disease may be reactivated, and complications such as bleeding or perforation may be precipitated. Tuberculosis, clinically inapparent except for a positive tuberculin test, may become active. The role of isoniazid prophylaxis in this situation is described in Chapter 29.

Topical Therapy

Whenever steroids can be used locally, such use is preferred, especially when long-term treatment is involved. Although absorption may be complete from a local site, the amount of steroid required is often far less when use is local. One thus avoids—to some extent—systemic effects, side effects, and pituitary-adrenal suppression. In addition to dermatological use of topical steroids, treatments of some ophthalmological conditions, allergic rhinitis, asthma, and localized joint disease are examples of this principle.

Intermittent Therapy

Usually, severe disease requires initiation of steroid therapy given as multiple daily doses. When the disease intensity has waned (e.g., 1 to 2 weeks), conversion to alternate-day therapy can be made. Intermittent therapy of this type should always be considered whenever long-term use is contemplated. Such therapy is to be preferred because pituitary-adrenal suppression is not likely and the adverse effects of glucocorticoids are minimized (12, 20). When initiating intermittent therapy the daily divided dose is given as a single morning dose. After this dose has been shown to be tolerated for several days, the single daily dose may be doubled and given as a single dose every other day. Thereafter, the dose

given every other day can be reduced slowly, as clinically indicated. The "off" day, particularly when alternate-day therapy is first started, may result in the patient becoming symptomatic. To handle this situation small doses of glucocorticoid may be given on this day. Nonsteroidal anti-inflammatory agents may also be helpful in ameliorating symptoms at this time and in easing the transition.

Use of Adrenocorticotropic Hormone

The clinical indications for use of ACTH rather than a glucocorticoid are practically nonexistent. ACTH was available for clinical use even before cortisone. It is clear that in sufficient amounts (100 units) long-acting preparations (gel or zinc suspensions) given once daily are capable of stimulating adrenal secretion of up to 300 mg of cortisol daily. However, disadvantages are multiple: the route is parenteral; magnitude of response is unpredictable; mineralocorticoid effects (salt and fluid retention, potassium wasting) are considerable; response in patients previously treated with glucocorticoids is slow and unpredictable. The only advantage is that adrenal responsiveness is maintained during therapy. Combined ACTH-glucocorticoid therapy has been advocated for this reason, as has the occasional injection of ACTH to prevent adrenal atrophy. The advantage of such an approach over that of intermittent glucocorticoid therapy is not clear. Moreover, when ACTH is used alone in high doses for a prolonged period, pituitary suppression occurs even though adrenal suppression does not. Another disadvantage of ACTH therapy is failure to produce more than the equivalent of 300 mg of cortisol (60 mg of prednisone) despite maximal stimulation of the adrenals. Such a dose, although considerable, may be insufficient to produce the desired anti-inflammatory effect. The only current, fairly widespread use of ACTH is in the treatment of multiple sclerosis. It is not clear that such use is supported by anything more than anecdote.

Withdrawal from Chronic Glucocorticoid Therapy

Treatment with glucocorticoids (cortisone, hydrocortisone, prednisone, etc.) produces suppression of the hypothalamus-pituitary-adrenal axis; the output of ACTH falls, and there is subsequent adrenal atrophy and an inability to respond to stress with increased cortisol output. The time required for initial suppression is highly variable, but all patients receiving daily pharmacological doses of glucocorticoids for more than 1 week should be presumed to have a suppressed response to stress (30). If stressed by surgery, trauma, or severe infection, these patients should be treated with replacement glucocorticoids as if they had Addison's disease. On the other hand, glucocorticoids may be discontinued abruptly after 2 to 4 weeks of pharmacological steroid therapy provided that the patient is not under stress, since baseline—as opposed to stress-related—adrenal function will almost always be adequate. Patients who have been treated with alternate-day steroid therapy are not at risk, since pituitary-adrenal function seems well preserved in these individuals (12, 20).

When it becomes desirable to terminate glucocorticoid therapy, the question arises of how to accomplish this goal while avoiding adrenal insufficiency. In the presence of active underlying disease, for which the glucocorticoids may have been given in the first place, a dilemma quickly becomes apparent. The nonspecific symptoms of adrenal insufficiency may be similar or identical to those of the disease that was under treatment. In addition, the occurrence of the "steroid withdrawal syndrome" (see below) may further compound the issue.

Withdrawal Schedule

No single scheme can solve this difficult clinical problem although many have been proposed (4). However, a few general points can be made. First, even after prolonged therapy, in the absence of active underlying systemic disease, symptoms of adrenal insufficiency should not be expected until the daily dose of glucocorticoid drops below physiological replacement (30 mg of cortisol, 7.5 mg of prednisone, or equivalent; see Table 74.2). At this point most patients will tolerate a single 20- to 30-mg daily dose of cortisol (or 5 to 7.5 mg of prednisone). Continuation for 2 months at this level should ensure some degree of recovery of pituitary-adrenal function. Further withdrawal begins to re-establish the normal pituitary-adrenal relationship. Additional reductions of 5 mg of cortisol can be made every 2 to 3 weeks over the next 2 months or, alternatively, an every-other-day program can be tried over the same period; the glucocorticoid can then usually be stopped without producing symptoms. Assessment of the functional status of the patient's adrenals at this point is described elsewhere (see "Assessment of Recovery from Pituitary-Adrenal Suppression" below).

Steroid Withdrawal Syndrome

Abrupt withdrawal of pharmacological doses of glucocorticoids, even after months of therapy, does not always produce chemical evidence of adrenal insufficiency. Nonetheless, the patient may experience many of the symptoms of adrenal insufficiency, e.g., lethargy, malaise, anorexia, nausea, vomiting, myalgias, fever, and—in severe cases—desquamation of skin in a manner resembling exfoliative dermatitis. Such patients may be found to have normal or elevated levels of cortisol. This phenomenon is not simply adrenal insufficiency but rather is a pharmacological withdrawal syndrome. Symptoms subside promptly with reinstitution of glucocorticoid therapy (1).

Recovery from Pituitary-Adrenal Suppression

After long-term glucocorticoid therapy (pharmacological doses for a year or more), recovery of normal pituitary-adrenal responsiveness does not occur readily (14). At least several months must elapse, even if the patient receives no exogenous steroid therapy during that time. In the first month after withdrawal, both pituitary and adrenal function remain depressed (low plasma ACTH and low plasma cortisol). Over the following 4 months, pituitary function recovers (plasma ACTH is elevated), but adrenal function remains subnormal (plasma cortisol is lower than normal). Eventually, adrenal function recovers (plasma cortisol levels normalize) while elevated plasma ACTH returns to normal. The entire process may require up to 9 months. During this interval the patient may fare well, provided there is no stress, but replacement therapy with glucocorticoids may become necessary at any time. Accordingly, no patient should be considered to have normal pituitary-adrenal function unless at least 1 year has elapsed after complete withdrawal of chronic glucocorticoid therapy. Occasional patients seem never to recover normal responsiveness. Ideally, therefore, all patients with a history of chronic steroid therapy should be tested for normal responsiveness 1 year after withdrawal.

Assessment of a glucocorticoid-treated patient's adrenal function under baseline conditions is not difficult. Both plasma cortisol measurements and urinary excretion of steroid metabolites give a reasonable estimate of such baseline function. However, predicting the response to stress is more difficult. Because hypothalamic-pituitary function usually recovers first, followed by adrenal function, a normal response to exogenous ACTH usually indicates recovery of the entire axis (see page 982 for details of testing with ACTH). A more complete assessment of the integrity of the axis can be made by induction of hypoglycemia with insulin (insulin tolerance testing). Hypoglycemia triggers ACTH release and the cortisol secretory response of the adrenal. A normal insulin tolerance test assures that if the patient is subjected to stressful circumstances, replacement therapy with steroids will not be necessary. If neither an ACTH nor an insulin tolerance test has been done, clinical assessment, including perhaps plasma cortisol determinations or empirical treatment with glucocorticoids, becomes necessary. In the suppressed individual, testing with metyrapone (Metopirone), an adrenal 11-hydroxylase inhibitor sometimes used for evaluation of the integrity of the hypothalamic-pituitary-adrenal axis, may be misleadingly normal.

HYPOCALCEMIC STATES

Hypocalcemia is a relatively uncommon problem in ambulatory patients. The classic cause of hypocalcemia is idiopathic hypoparathyroidism, but most cases encountered are a consequence of inadvertent surgical ablation of the parathyroids during thyroidectomy or of a metabolic disturbance such as renal failure. The causes of hypocalcemia are listed in Table 74.4.

Clinical Manifestations of Hypocalcemia

The symptoms of hypocalcemia are primarily neuromuscular and are not usually evident until the serum calcium falls below about 8 mg/dl and often considerably lower. Mild symptoms are totally nonspecific and include psychological manifestations (irritability, mood changes, depression), paresthesias, and muscle cramps. More severe symptoms are delirium, psychosis, tetany (including laryngeal stridor), and seizures. Neuromuscular irritability can often be demonstrated by the twitching, which is induced by tapping over the facial nerve just anterior to the ear. A positive response is contraction of the facial muscles around the lip (Chvostek's sign). Another clinical maneuver is compression of the upper arm by a blood pressure cuff with the pressure elevated above the systolic pressure. A positive response is spasm of the hand induced within 3 minutes (Trousseau's sign). Signs of chronic hypocalcemia include patchy hair loss, scaling of skin, atrophy and brittleness of fingernails, and cataract formation. Candidiasis is common. Calcification of the basal ganglia may be seen on X-ray examination of the skull. Either osteosclerosis or osteopenia may occur depending on the etiology of the hypocalcemia.

Laboratory Findings

Hypocalcemia can be said to be present when the serum calcium falls below 8.5 mg/dl. However, since almost half of serum calcium is protein bound, reduction of serum protein by 1 g/dl lowers the serum calcium by about 0.8 mg/dl. The level of serum calcium must, therefore, always be evaluated in the context of the serum protein concentration; the serum magnesium concentration should also be evaluated at the same time (see below, "Other Causes of Hypocalcemia"). Plasma parathyroid hormone (PTH) levels are low or nondetectable in idiopathic or postablative hypoparathyroidism and in some cases of hypocalcemia due to magnesium deficiency, but they are elevated in pseudohypoparathyroidism, renal failure, malabsorption, and vitamin D deficiency. The interpretation and indications for determination of PTH levels are discussed below.

Idiopathic Hypoparathyroidism

This condition is rare. Although most patients are diagnosed in childhood, some do not exhibit the disease until adult life. Occasionally familial, the idiopathic disease is autoimmune, frequently associated with high titers of antibodies to parathyroid tissue, and may be seen in association with other autoimmune endocrine diseases (adrenal insufficiency, Hashimoto's thyroiditis) and pernicious anemia.

Post-thyroidectomy Hypoparathyroidism

Probably the most common cause of hypoparathyroidism, this condition is a complication of surgical thyroidectomy. The hypocalcemic state may become evident immediately after surgery but often takes many years to develop, presumably due to slowly progressive interference with the blood supply to the parathyroids. Routine screening of serum calcium in patients who have had thyroidectomy will reveal many asymptomatic patients. Most of these individuals will seem to need no therapy, but in view of the subtle neuromuscular changes that can result from hypocalcemia, careful consideration should always be given to this issue. Hypoparathyroidism is vanishingly rare after radioiodide therapy of thyroid disease. Only a very few cases have been reported.

Pseudohypoparathyroidism

This is a rare disorder of genetic origin (X-linked dominant trait). In addition to hypocalcemia and its manifestations, there are associated skeletal developmental defects that result in short stature, shortening of metacarpals and metatarsals, and round face. Clinical manifestations attributable to hypocalcemia may not appear until adult life. The biochemical basis of the hypocalcemia is end organ resistance to the action of PTH. The combination of hypocalcemia, elevated level of parathyroid hormone, and typical skeletal abnormalities is virtually diagnostic. In the absence of skeletal abnormalities, diagnosis depends on demonstration of resistance to administered PTH, a specialized procedure requiring referral to an endocrinologist.

Treatment of Hypoparathyroidism and Pseudohypoparathyroidism

The treatment of all forms of hypoparathyroidism is similar. A few patients with idiopathic or postablative PTH deficiency can be managed with calcium supplements alone. The dose is 1 to 2 g of calcium daily. Because calcium gluconate and lactate contain

Table 74.4.
Causes of Hypocalcemia[a]

HYPOCALCEMIA WITH HIGH SERUM PHOSPHATE
  Postablative hypoparathyroidism (post-thyroidectomy)
  Idiopathic hypoparathyroidism
  Pseudohypoparathyroidism
  Renal failure
HYPOCALCEMIA WITH LOW OR NORMAL SERUM PHOSPHATE
  Malabsorption (vitamin D deficiency)
  Magnesium deficiency (alcoholism)
  Renal rickets (renal tubular acidosis; phosphate diabetes; cystinosis; Fanconi's syndrome; vitamin D-resistant rickets)
  Medullary carcinoma of thyroid

[a] The serum alkaline phosphatase activity is elevated whenever severe metabolic bone disease is present. Parathyroid hormone levels are depressed in idiopathic hypoparathyroidism and may be depressed in magnesium deficiency. Parathyroid hormone levels are regularly elevated in renal failure and in pseudohypoparathyroidism. Urine calcium is depressed in most hypocalcemic states, except when the rare renal tubular calcium-wasting syndromes are responsible for the hypocalcemia.

only about 10% calcium, one must administer 10 to 20 g of these salts; the carbonate contains 40% calcium. Numerous tablets must be taken; patient compliance is a common problem. Every effort should be made to work out an acceptable, palatable, and economic program with a consistently available preparation for what is invariably lifelong therapy.

The second mainstay of therapy is vitamin D. The most commonly used preparation in the past has been ergocalciferol (vitamin D_2, Calciferol). The dose is usually 50,000 or 100,000 units daily, although higher doses may be necessary. The compound is available in 50,000-unit (1.25-mg) capsules. The sole advantage of ergocalciferol is cost; it is by far the least expensive form of vitamin D therapy. The disadvantage of ergocalciferol is somewhat unpredictable toxicity with resultant hypercalcemia and all of its manifestations (see page 993). Because vitamin D is fat soluble, toxicity may last for many weeks or even months after discontinuation of therapy. Glucocorticoids are effective therapy for hypercalcemia due to vitamin D toxicity.

A preferable vitamin D preparation is its synthetic analogue, dihydrotachysterol (DHT, Hytakerol). The dose varies from 0.2 to 2 mg daily. The compound is available as tablets and as a solution. The advantage of therapy with DHT is more rapid onset of action than D_2 and more rapid reversibility of toxicity upon withdrawal of the drug. The only disadvantage of DHT is its relatively high cost. Yet another effective compound is 1, 25-dihydroxyvitamin D_3 (calcitriol, Rocaltrol), the natural, active form of vitamin D. This compound is more rapid than DHT in onset and has a shorter duration of effect but has the disadvantage of even greater cost. The dose is 0.25 to 1.0 μg daily. Both 0.25- and 0.5-μg tablets are available.

The approach to chronic therapy of hypoparathyroidism is institution of a relatively fixed calcium intake at a total level of about 2 g, which is about 1 g over regular dietary intake. Thus, a patient whose normal daily calcium intake approximates 1 g needs an additional 1 g of calcium in the form of supplementary calcium salts (see above). Instruction of the patient by a dietician is essential. Vitamin D, in whatever form is selected, is given simultaneously, with adjustments of dose at weekly or biweekly intervals depending on the serum calcium level. The goal of therapy is a serum calcium concentration of 8.5 to 9.5 mg/dl. Hypercalcemia is to be avoided. Once a stable level of serum calcium is reached (1 to 2 months), the patient can be monitored at monthly intervals and eventually every 3 to 4 months. The possibility of toxicity due to hypercalcemia is always to be kept in mind. Even mild hypercalcemia predisposes to nephrocalcinosis and nephrolithiasis in these patients.

Hypocalcemia Due to Other Causes

When hypocalcemia is related to malabsorption, efforts to correct that situation should be undertaken, but simultaneous treatment with vitamin D and calcium may be indicated.

One relatively common cause of hypocalcemia is alcoholism with resultant magnesium deficiency. Overt malnutrition need not be present. The mechanisms by which alcohol abuse produces magnesium depletion include decreased dietary intake and alcohol-facilitated renal excretion of magnesium. Magnesium depletion results in both impaired secretion of PTH and impaired PTH action. Intramuscular magnesium therapy normalizes the serum calcium within hours.

Other diseases associated with hypocalcemia include osteomalacia (vitamin D and/or calcium deficiency) and variants of Fanconi's syndrome (a spectrum of renal tubular abnormalities). The hypocalcemia associated with renal failure is described in Chapter 48.

HYPERCALCEMIC STATES

In recent years routine, automated blood analyses have come to include determinations of serum calcium. This development has led to the detection of many cases of hypercalcemia (in most laboratories, serum calcium > 10.5 mg/dl), most of them mild and asymptomatic. The demonstration of hypercalcemia (in most laboratories, serum calcium > 10.5 mg/dl) always requires investigation.

Etiologies

In an ambulatory setting the most common cause of minimal, asymptomatic hypercalcemia may be that associated with use of thiazide diuretics, although the precise prevalence is really not known. The problem is fully reversible upon withdrawal of the drug. Once established as the cause of the hypercalcemia, thiazide therapy may be continued if otherwise clinically indicated, if the hypercalcemia is minimal, and if the patient is truly asymptomatic (see "The So-Called Asymptomatic Patient" below). When the serum calcium exceeds 11 mg/dl, one may switch to an alternative, nonthiazide diuretic.

Another common cause of benign hypercalcemia in ambulatory patients is hyperparathyroidism. In one of 1000 people who are screened, hypercalcemia is detected, due to a small, indolent parathyroid adenoma (15). The approach to such patients is described below (see page 992).

Some ambulatory patients who are found to have hypercalcemia will have weight loss, anorexia, etc. A calcium elevation in this setting is ominous. Because minimal elevations of calcium (less than 11.5 mg/dl) are ordinarily asymptomatic, the patient's symptoms of anorexia, weight loss, etc., are more likely attributable to the underlying disease, rather than to the incidental and associated but minimal hypercalcemia. The calcium elevation, however, is a finding that suggests a malignant process, e.g., carcinoma of the lung or breast. These patients are usually promptly hospitalized for diagnostic procedures and therapy of the underlying disease.

In the event that malignancy is not apparent, the differential diagnosis includes primary hyperparathyroidism (see below). At this point, determination of PTH concentration is useful in elucidating the cause of the hypercalcemic state. However, one should not rely on only a PTH assay to determine the cause of the hypercalcemia. A normal PTH level on repeated determinations excludes a diagnosis of hyperparathyroidism (see below), but an elevated PTH level does not necessarily indicate its presence. PTH assays do not always reliably differentiate between hypercalcemia due to hyperparathyroidism and that due to PTH-producing tumor. Elevations of PTH are often due to ectopic PTH production by tumors. Although tumor-produced PTH is not identical to normal PTH, the antibodies used to quantitate PTH often fail to distinguish between these substances. Improvements in PTH assays with more specific antibodies and radioimmunometric techniques have improved diagnostic accuracy to a high degree of specificity. Information concerning specificity should be available from the laboratory utilized.

Various other circumstances produce hypercalcemia. These are listed in Table 74.5.

Therapy of Hypercalcemia

The treatment of hypercalcemia due to hyperparathyroidism is discussed below (see "Primary Hyperparathyroidism").

Therapy to control hypercalcemia is not commonly

Table 74.5.
Causes of Hypercalcemia

Condition	Comment
COMMON CAUSES	
Thiazide drugs	Mild elevation (not > 12.5 mg/dl); requires 2 or more weeks to subside
Hyperparathyroidism	Frequently asymptomatic; commonly discovered on routine blood test
Malignancy (including myeloma)	Commonest cause in hospitalized patients; may lead to initial encounter in ambulatory patients
Spurious	Inappropriate technique while drawing blood (venous stasis produces hemoconcentration)
RARE CAUSES	
Milk alkali syndrome	Requires use (abuse) of both alkali (NaHCO$_3$) and large quantities of milk or calcium salts
Hypervitaminosis D	Usually 50,000 units or more daily
Thyrotoxicosis	Severe disease is evident
Paget's disease of bone	Immobilization is necessary
Immobilization	Body cast in adolescent males; patients with Paget's disease of bone; quadriplegia
Sarcoidosis	Hyperglobulinemia usually present
Chronic renal failure	Very uncommon; may exacerbate after transplantation or during hemodialysis
Adrenal insufficiency	Hemoconcentration present
Idiopathic elevation	Mild elevation in postmenopausal women; may revert to normal with physiological estrogen therapy

initiated in ambulatory patients. Most often the hypercalcemia or its underlying cause will have required initial therapy in a hospital. However, when the acute symptoms of hypercalcemia have been controlled during hospitalization, long-term palliative therapy may be needed for the ambulatory patient.

In malignancy, glucocorticoids (20 to 60 mg of prednisone daily) may control hypercalcemia, as may indomethacin (100 to 200 mg daily) in a small proportion of cases. Mithramycin is an effective agent for control of hypercalcemia of any cause, but this drug is ordinarily used only for the treatment of hypercalcemia due to tumor. Usually such therapy is given in a hospital, but ambulatory treatment is also feasible. The drug is given intravenously. At a dose of 25 μg/kg (15 μg/kg if hepatic disease is present or bone marrow function is impaired by disease or other drugs) side effects are not usually seen. Several days are often needed for a response to become apparent, but the effect often lasts for many days or even weeks. Calcitonin (Calcimar) is an effective calcium-lowering agent for many hypercalcemic states and can be self-administered. This hormone must be given subcutaneously on a daily or several times weekly schedule. The principal use of calcitonin is in the treatment of Paget's disease of bone. The major side effects are nausea and vomiting in a small percentage of cases. Glucocorticoids are often effective in lowering hypercalcemia due to sarcoidosis, vitamin D intoxication, and the milk-alkali syndrome. Mild hypercalcemia in elderly postmenopausal women may sometimes respond to physiological amounts of estrogen (8, 28). Treatment of hypercalcemia with phosphates administered orally is sometimes possible, especially in mild hyperparathyroidism (see below). Often partial control of hypercalcemia is sufficient to relieve symptoms; complete normalization of calcium level is often neither desirable nor necessary.

Primary Hyperparathyroidism

The term primary hyperparathyroidism refers to autonomous hyperfunction of one or more parathyroid glands. Hypercalcemia is the hallmark of this disorder. Secondary hyperparathyroidism, on the other hand, is a physiological or pathophysiological homeostatic response to situations that lower blood calcium.

The most common cause of primary hyperparathyroidism is a solitary benign adenoma (85% of patients). In a small proportion of patients more than one adenoma is present, and in the remainder the cause is idiopathic hyperplasia. Carcinoma of the parathyroid is rare (less than 1% of patients). Hyperparathyroidism may be familial and may occur as part of the syndrome of multiple endocrine adenomatosis (MEA, page 979).

Diagnosis

Most patients are now detected by routine automated analysis of blood electrolytes. The symptoms or sequelae of hypercalcemia may also alert the physician to the diagnosis (Table 74.6). Once the diagnosis is suspected, it is most important to establish beyond any doubt the presence of hypercalcemia. Multiple determinations of serum calcium should be made in a laboratory where a high degree of precision is assured. Because of spontaneous fluctuations of the serum calcium and because of analytical error, values that are only minimally elevated (10.5 to 11.5 mg/dl) must be repeated many times. The resulting mean level should be used for diagnostic purposes, not the last—sometimes normal—value obtained.

Once hypercalcemia is established as being present (greater than 10.5 mg/dl on multiple determinations), the next (or simultaneous) step is to determine the likelihood of the presence of other causes of hypercalcemia (see Table 74.5). Finally, assay of PTH in blood should be performed (see below).

Other routine laboratory studies may include low serum phosphorus concentration and, in severe cases with bone involvement, elevation of serum alkaline phosphatase activity. Other more elaborate indirect tests of PTH hyperfunction—none of which is useful for screening purposes—include the calculation of the tubular resorption of phosphate (TRP) and determination of urinary excretion of cyclic adenosine monophosphate (cyclic AMP). These tests, if they are to be used at all, are best performed by specialists. Other abnormalities in laboratory tests occur but are not useful for screening or in differential diagnosis, since they occur nonspecifically. Patients with hypercalcemia, regardless of cause, usually show hypercalciuria, but hypercalciuria may also occur without hypercalcemia. Increased excretion of hydroxyproline occurs, as it does in other bone diseases.

In severe cases of long duration, X-ray studies of various bones will reveal a variety of changes suggestive but not diagnostic of hyperparathyroidism. Demineralization (osteopenia) and subperiosteal resorption are most obvious in the clavicles and the hands, and the lamina dura of the teeth may be re-sorbed. Cystic changes occur in skull and long bones. None of these changes is likely to be seen in mild cases. X-ray studies are not useful for screening purposes.

Parathyroid hormone assays. Radioimmunoassays are quite useful but have several limitations. Specificity of the assay varies among laboratories, due to the use of different antibodies. Some laboratories offer several different PTH assays, each of which has its own advantages and limitations. The most commonly used procedure until recently, the so-called "C-terminal" assay, measures a peptide fragment derived from PTH. This assay, as performed on peripheral venous blood (plasma or serum), may be the most sensitive test for detecting hyperparathyroidism, but it is also elevated by impaired renal function, due in part to decreased peptide fragment excretion, and is frequently elevated in normal elderly persons, especially women over about age 65. The elevations seen in primary hyperparathyroidism are often only modest (e.g., 50% greater than the upper limits of normal). Accordingly, at least two or three assays should ordinarily be obtained. The assay also measures PTH-like materials produced by tumors.

Several other widely available assays measure "intact" hormone or N-terminal fragment(s). Interestingly, although these assays are more specific and less likely to be elevated in cases of ectopic (tumor) production of PTH, they are also less sensitive in detecting primary hyperparathyroidism, being normal in nearly half of cases. In patients with chronic renal failure, in whom secondary hyperparathyroidism is invariably present, the "intact hormone" assays are not artifactually raised by retention of PTH fragments, as are the C-terminal assays, and more or less reflect the degree of secondary hyperparathyroidism.

Recently introduced immunoradiometric assays for PTH (IRMAs) will probably soon replace the older radioimmunoassays. IRMAs have improved sensitivity and appear to be superior for detecting hyperparathyroidism. Moreover, they show a high degree of specificity and usually do not detect the PTH-like substances produced by tumors.

Steroid suppression test. Although most cases of hyperparathyroidism and of other hypercalcemic states can be diagnosed by the means described, the etiology of occasional cases of hypercalcemia remains in doubt. In these, a short course of prednisone therapy (30 to 40 mg daily for 10 to 14 days) may help diagnostically. The hypercalcemia of hyperparathyroidism does not respond to such therapy. Although only about one-half of cases of hypercalcemia due to malignancy respond, hypercalcemia due to diseases that are not always apparent—such as sarcoidosis, vitamin D intoxication, and milk-alkali syndrome—responds consistently. Daily determinations of blood calcium should always be obtained during such a test.

Further evaluation. Having established the presence of hypercalcemia and elevation of PTH, and having excluded by appropriate means malignancy, impaired renal function, and other conditions in Table 74.5, the diagnosis of hyperparathyroidism is reasonably well

Table 74.6.
Symptoms and Signs of Hypercalcemia

SHORT-TERM (READILY REVERSIBLE)
   General: weakness, anorexia, weight loss, fatigue
   Gastrointestinal: nausea, vomiting, constipation
   Genitourinary: polyuria, azotemia
   Musculoskeletal: bone aches
   Neurological: lethargy, sleepiness, difficulty concentrating, confusion, psychosis
   Cardiovascular: bradycardia, electrocardiographic abnormalities (short Q-T, arrhythmias, digitalis toxicity)
   Ophthalmological: difficulty focusing
   Dermatological: pruritis
LONG-TERM (IRREVERSIBLE OR SLOWLY REVERSIBLE)
   Gastrointestinal: peptic ulcer, pancreatitis
   Genitourinary: renal calculi (colic, hematuria); nephrocalcinosis; polyuria
   Skeletal: bone loss (osteopenia); subperiosteal resorption, bone cysts, pseudogout
   Neuromuscular: muscle atrophy
   Ophthalmological: band keratopathy; conjunctival calcifications (usually require slitlamp examination)

established. However, the urinary excretion of calcium should be determined at this point. Benign familial hypercalcemia due to parathyroid hyperplasia has been described. These patients—for reasons that are not understood—do not have hypercalciuria or other complications of minimal hypercalcemia and do not need surgical intervention. In most cases of hyperparathyroidism referral to an endocrinologist should be made if the diagnosis is in doubt or if surgery is contemplated.

The So-Called Asymptomatic Patient

A common dilemma in demonstrated hyperparathyroidism is the so-called asymptomatic patient with mild hypercalcemia. If the patient is truly asymptomatic, a conservative, expectant approach is appropriate given the nonspecific nature of the symptoms. The majority of cases of hyperparathyroidism are, in fact, however, associated with psychiatric and neuromuscular disturbances that are frequently not spontaneously articulated. Correlation with the degree of hypercalcemia is poor. The prominent symptoms include anxiety, "nervousness," indecision, daytime sleepiness, loss of energy, and typical manifestations of depression such as crying easily, excessive worrying, irritability, and lack of interest. Somatic symptoms are not increased. These psychiatric symptoms are reversible with relief of the hypercalcemia; indeed they may justify a decision in favor of surgery (17).

Therapy

In diagnosed patients the main question is whether surgical intervention is warranted. The rate of development of complications (urolithiasis, emotional disorders, bone disease, decreased renal function, peptic ulcer, pancreatitis) in patients with asymptomatic hypercalcemia is quite low. However, the decision for or against surgery will obviously be based not only on the presence of such problems, but on such factors as patient age, associated medical illness, the presence or absence of neuropsychiatric dysfunction, etc. (7, 15). In occasional patients, medical management of the hyperparathyroidism may be indicated (see below).

Surgical Therapy. If a decision is made to treat the patient surgically, referral to a surgeon experienced in parathyroid/thyroid exploration is warranted. In such experienced hands, an adenoma, if present, will be located and easily removed in 90 to 95% of cases. Parathyroid hyperplasia, which accounts for 10% of cases of hyperparathyroidism, is usually easily identified. In such cases, the surgeon should be prepared to perform a nearly total parathyroidectomy. Second neck explorations are technically difficult and may result in unnecessary morbidity (damage to the recurrent laryngeal nerve). Accordingly, any hyperplastic parathyroid tissue that is left behind should be identified with clips. As an alternative, many surgeons are now removing all parathyroid tissue from the neck and transplanting a portion of one hyperplastic gland

to an accessible location, usually a sternocleidomastoid muscle or into the forearm.

Failure to identify an adenoma and absence of hyperplasia may require partial thyroidectomy—the adenoma may be embedded in the thyroid—or exploration of the anterosuperior mediastinum. This procedure may be performed at the time of initial surgery or at some time later. Such "details" obviously involve the surgeon's preference and experience but should be considered and discussed before surgery. If the neck has already been explored unsuccessfully, a selective venous catheterization study with sampling of PTH levels is a useful procedure for preoperative localization of the tumor. Only a few major medical centers can perform this procedure. Such localization studies are not indicated before initial surgery.

Medical Therapy. The medical therapy of hyperparathyroidism with phosphate is ordinarily limited to those patients in whom surgery is not desirable but who require therapy. Although intravenous phosphate therapy carries the risk of soft tissue calcium deposition, no such problem attends the use of phosphate given orally. Sodium-potassium phosphate salts given orally (K-Phos, Neutra-Phos) may produce diarrhea. Dosage should be titrated upward as tolerated. A sodium-free preparation is also available (Neutra-Phos-K) for use in patients whose sodium intake should be restricted. Asymptomatic patients with mild hypercalcemia should probably not be treated with phosphate.

Estrogen has been recommended as an alternative to surgery for uncomplicated hyperparathyroidism. Because many patients with asymptomatic hyperparathyroidism are postmenopausal women, this approach has considerable appeal. Unfortunately, not all patients respond and even in those who do, some abnormalities of bone histopathology persist. Norethindrone, a progestogen, has a similar effect to that of estrogen in occasional patients (28).

OSTEOPOROSIS

Epidemiology and Manifestations

Primary osteoporosis is an age-related disorder characterized by a generalized decrease in bone mass (both the osteoid matrix and the inorganic macrocrystalline component) and increased risk of developing fractures in the absence of other known causes of bone loss. It is an important public health problem, affecting nearly 15 to 20 million persons in the United States (22). Approximately 1.2 million fractures related to osteoporosis occur annually in individuals beyond the age of 45. An estimated 32% of women and 17% of men who live to age 90 will experience a hip fracture. Among people so afflicted there is a 12 to 20% mortality within the first 3 to 4 months postfracture, and the physical, psychological, and socioeconomic toll on those who survive is formidable. In the United States alone, the annual cost of osteoporosis was estimated at 7 to 10 billion dollars in 1986 (24).

The proportions of the two major forms of bone, cortical (compact) bone and trabecular (medullary) bone, vary at different anatomical sites. Vertebral bodies contain mostly trabecular bone, and the proximal femur and radius contain mostly cortical bone. The two forms of bone differ in their response to mechanical forces, hormones, local regulatory factors, and their susceptibility to fracture. Peak bone mass is achieved at about age 35 for cortical bone and several years earlier for trabecular bone. Multiple factors including heredity, sex, race, nutritional status, level of physical activity, and general health influence peak bone mass. Bone mass is about 30% greater in men than in women and 10% greater in blacks than in whites. Throughout life, the normal process of bone remodeling exists as a dynamic equilibrium between bone formation and bone resorption. Women lose an average of 35% of their cortical and 50% of their trabecular bone over the course of their lives.

After reaching its peak in the 3rd decade, bone mass decreases steadily throughout adult life due to an imbalance in remodeling: The rate of mineral loss is variable but is greater in women (premenopause, about 1% per year) than in men. The two major etiologies of primary osteoporosis are estrogen deficiency (see Chapter 77 for details) and aging. Known risk factors for osteoporosis include a sedentary life style, prolonged bed rest, chronic cigarette smoking, nulliparity, diabetes mellitus, Caucasian race, and chronic glucocorticoid therapy. In women, bone mass decreases rapidly at 2 to 5% per year during the first 3 to 7 years after natural or surgical menopause or any other cause of estrogen deficiency. As a result, osteoporosis and fractures are more common in women than in men and in whites than in blacks. During the first 15 to 20 years after the menopause, vertebral fractures and Colles' fractures of the forearm predominate. The vertical fractures are of the "crush" type and tend to be deforming and painful. Loss of teeth is also common. This pattern of bone loss has been named type I or "postmenopausal" osteoporosis. In women over 70 and in men, fractures of the hip, proximal humerus, proximal tibia, pelvis, and distal radius are more common. Deformation of the spine occurs as trabecular thinning leads to vertical fractures of the "wedge" type and to dorsal kyphosis ("dowager's hump"). This type of bone loss has been named type II or "senile" osteoporosis. The mechanisms involved in the development of the two types have been postulated to differ. In type I the osteoporosis is caused by factors closely related to the menopause, one of which is decreased estrogen levels, whereas in type II the factors are thought to be related to aging (26).

Although age-related decreased production of 1,25-dihydroxyvitamin D and decreased calcium absorption may contribute to the development of osteoporosis, replacement therapy with neither agent has been shown to prevent bone loss or to increase bone mass in osteoporotic patients. Many workers in this area have concluded that factors other than those now recognized must contribute to the pathogenesis of osteoporosis. Recently, the focus has turned to growth factors acting and possibly produced locally (24, 25). Optimal, cost-effective use of radiological techniques (photon absorptiometry and CT scanning) for diagnosing early or established osteoporosis or for following progression of the process remains to be defined (11, 27). It is clear, however, that osteoporosis is quite advanced when it is detectable on plain X-rays.

Prevention of Osteoporosis

Patient management should emphasize the prevention of osteoporosis. The treatment of symptoms due to vertebral compression fractures is palliative (see Chapter 65, Low Back Pain).

Estrogen therapy begun at or within 5 to 6 years of the menopause is highly effective in preventing osteoporosis in women. Such treatment decreases bone resorption and postmenopausal bone loss and has been shown in case-controlled studies to reduce the incidence of hip and wrist fractures and vertebral fractures as well. Use of added progestin decreases or eliminates the risk of endometrial cancer. However, since the risks and acceptability of long-term therapy with estrogen and progestin in postmenopausal women have not been unequivocally defined (2, 3), a firm recommendation for such therapy should probably be reserved for women at high risk for developing osteoporosis, such as those with premature menopause. (Chapter 77 contains a detailed discussion of estrogen replacement in the menopause.)

Most adults consume diets deficient in calcium. In the absence of contraindications (e.g., history of hypercalcemia, kidney stones, or kidney failure), it is recommended that after the age of 40 calcium be taken in amounts sufficient to meet the daily nutritional calcium requirements of 1200 mg for premenopausal women and estrogen-treated postmenopausal women, or 1500 mg for non-estrogen-treated postmenopausal women and for men, especially Causasian men with risk factors for osteoporosis. In some early studies such calcium therapy was claimed to retard age-related bone loss greatly, whereas in recent reports calcium alone has had no beneficial effect. However, when postmenopausal women take calcium supplements in addition to estrogen replacement, the two modalities have a combined favorable impact and can be expected to reduce the rate of vertebral fractures by nearly one-half.

The major sources of calcium in the United States diet are milk and dairy products. Each 8-ounce glass (240 ml) of milk contains 275 to 300 mg of calcium. Skim or low fat milk is preferred to minimize fat intake. For those unable to take 1000 to 1500 mg of calcium by diet, supplementation with calcium tablets is recommended, with special attention to their elemental calcium content. Nonprescription oral calcium supplements, such as calcium carbonate, phosphate, lactate, or gluconate, can supplement a calcium-poor diet. The carbonate preparation has the highest percentage of calcium, containing 40% elemental calcium by weight; and calcium gluconate has the lowest percentage, only 9%. Patient compliance is greatest with the carbonate preparations, because fewer tablets are needed to achieve recommended calcium intake. However, the carbonate preparation can cause bloating, flatulence, and constipation, and some patients prefer calcium lactate or gluconate. Moreover, absorption of calcium from the carbonate form depends on the presence of gastric hydrochloric acid. Achlorhydria is common in older patients, so calcium carbonate may prove to be unsatisfactory for precisely those patients having the greatest need for calcium supplementation. Because the cost of calcium products varies greatly, patients should be told to take a recommended amount of elemental calcium and encouraged to shop for the least expensive preparation. Tables 74.7 and 74.8 list practical information about a number of calcium-containing foods and calcium supplements.

Other measures that may be important in preventing osteoporosis are modest weight-bearing exercise, such as walking; avoidance, if possible, of prolonged bed rest after acute illness; smoking cessation; avoidance of prolonged glucocorticoid treatment; and treatment of any coexisting conditions that are known to cause or accelerate osteoporosis.

DISORDERS OF WATER METABOLISM

The combination of excess thirst, increased intake of water, and increased output of urine is a common clinical presentation of a number of conditions (Table 74.9). In most of these, the symptoms are related to some event that results in excessive loss of fluid via the kidney. For example, hyperglycemia results in a large solute load (glucose) being presented to the renal tubules; an obligatory loss of water (osmotic diuresis) ensues. Hypercalcemia produces abnormalities of renal tubular function that result in impaired ability to concentrate urine. Lithium, widely used for treatment of bipolar affective disorders (manic-depressive illness), impairs the action of antidiuretic hormone and thereby produces water loss. Table 74.9 lists some of the conditions that cause polyuria.

A noteworthy disorder of water metabolism in ambulatory patients is that of *psychogenic water drinking*. In this disorder, the patient's psychiatric state alters normal behavior in such a way as to produce compulsive water drinking. Many of these patients have poorly defined psychiatric disorders, but some are overtly psychotic. Recent studies in these patients have identified unequivocal defects in urinary dilution, the osmoregulation of water intake, and in the secretion of vasopressin, but the precise causes of these abnormalities remain unexplained (13). Occasional individuals begin excessive water intake on receiving "health advice" from a lay source, i.e., the notion that

Table 74.7.
Calcium Content of Some Foods[a]

Food	Serving Size	Calcium Content (mg)
Sardines, canned in oil	8 medium	354
Spinach, frozen chopped, cooked	½ cup	113
Turnip greens, cooked	½ cup	246
Cheddar cheese (American)	1 ounce	211
Creamed cottage cheese	1 cup	211
Muenster cheese	1 ounce	203
Milk, whole	1 quart	1152
Milk, skim	1 quart	1212
Yogurt (lowfat, fruit flavored)	1 cup	345
Chocolate fudge	3½ ounces	100

[a] From Calcium for postmenopausal osteoporosis, *Med Lett* 24:105, 1982.

Table 74.8.
Commercially Available Calcium Supplements[a]

Drug	Tablet Size	Equivalent of 1 G of Calcium/Day
Calcium carbonate (40% calcium)		
Generic—Lilly	600 mg	4 tablets
—Rugby	600 mg	4 tablets
Alka-2—Miles	500 mg	5 tablets
Amitone—Norcliff Thayer	350 mg	7 tablets
Equilet—Mission	500 mg	5 tablets
Diacarbosil—Norcliff Thayer	500 mg	5 tablets
Mallamint—Mallard	420 mg	6 tablets
OsCal-500—Marion	1250 mg	2 tablets
TUMS—Norcliff Thayer	500 mg	5 tablets
Calcium gluconate (9% calcium) generic	600 mg	18.5 tablets
	1000 mg	11 tablets
	930 mg	12 tablets
Calcium lactate (13% calcium) generic	600 mg	12 tablets
Dibasic calcium phosphate (31% calcium) generic	500 mg	7 tablets
Chelated calcium (20% calcium)		
generic—Arco	750 mg	7 tablets
—Nature's Bounty	750 mg	7 tablets

[a] Adapted from Calcium for postmenopausal osteoporosis. *Med Lett* 24:105, 1982.

Table 74.9.
Causes of Polyuria[a]

Disorder	Mechanism
Glucosuria (diabetes mellitus)	Osmotic diuresis
Excessive intake of water	Psychogenic
Various drugs	Often due to anticholinergic effects producing dryness of mouth; possible central effects
Decreased antidiuretic hormone (ADH) effect	Deficiency of ADH secretion (idiopathic diabetes insipidus or due to pituitary-hypothalamic disease); nephrogenic diabetes insipidus
Renal disease, plus renal effects of potassium depletion, hypercalcemia, and lithium therapy	In all of these disorders, impairment of renal concentrating ability is present
Hyperthyroidism	Impairment of urinary concentrating ability; decreased salivary flow

[a] Disorders associated with increased urine volume.

drinking large quantities of water is healthful. Regardless of the cause, once such behavior is started, a compulsive behavior pattern tends to persist and is reinforced by a pathophysiological mechanism. Whatever the cause, large urine output, if it persists for a long time, produces a reversible impairment of urine-concentrating ability due to washout of renal medullary solutes. Thus, the behavior pattern, though basically of psychogenic origin, may become self-perpetuating. Attempts to have the patient restrict water intake when urinary concentrating ability is impaired under these conditions lead to continued water loss, and the resulting hyperosmolality leads to intense thirst. "Weaning" from excessive water intake may be very difficult.

A rare disorder of water metabolism in ambulatory patients is *diabetes insipidus,* a deficiency of antidiuretic hormone [ADH, arginine vasopressin (AVP)]. This condition is either idiopathic—in which case it is unassociated with other evidence of pituitary-hypothalamic disease—or, more commonly, is secondary to pituitary disease (tumor) or other disease in the hypothalamic-pituitary stalk-pituitary area (craniopharyngioma, aneurysm). Other rare causes include a variety of infiltrative diseases (sarcoidosis, tuberculosis), head trauma—especially with basal skull fracture or neurosurgical procedures—and central nervous system infections. The most common illness mimicking diabetes insipidus is the drug-related disorder that results from use of lithium for bipolar affective illness. Another very rare condition resembling lack of ADH results from an inherited renal tubular resistance to antidiuretic hormone, *nephrogenic diabetes insipidus.*

Approach to the Patient with Polydipsia and Polyuria

The history should be corroborated by family or friends if possible. Important historical points are rapidity of onset of symptoms, a preference for use of iced water, and nocturnal drinking habits. Sudden onset and preference for iced water are classical for diabetes insipidus. Numerous spontaneous awakenings at night in order to drink and urinate also strongly suggest this diagnosis, whereas absence of such events is in favor of functional disease. A careful psychiatric history is important. The use of drugs should be noted (10).

Initial laboratory workup should be simple. Urine glucose excretion should be measured. An A.M. serum sodium and/or osmolality determination along with serum potassium, calcium, urea nitrogen, and creatinine determinations should be made. The patient should collect all urine over one or two 24-hour periods. The sample should be examined to determine the volume, osmolality, and total creatinine excretion, the latter serving as a marker for completeness of the collection. Measurement of urine specific gravity is obsolete and should not be used.

These preliminaries will define the problem and provide an insight into the diagnosis. Unless considerable glucosuria is present, the patient's problem is not due to uncontrolled diabetes mellitus, even if blood glucose concentration is incidentally elevated. The presence of a normal serum sodium and/or osmolality indicates only that the process is not severe enough to have overwhelmed the ability to excrete water or the homeostatic (thirst) mechanism. Elevated serum osmolality strongly suggests diabetes insipidus; the opposite finding indicates psychogenic water drinking. The presence of normal serum calcium and potassium concentrations excludes several metabolic problems, whereas abnormalities of calcium, of potassium, or of renal function will make it clear that the problem is not primarily one of water metabolism (see Table 74.9).

At this point most patients will have normal findings in serum but a large volume of urine with low osmolality. Normal urine volume ranges up to 2500 ml; urine osmolality is decidedly low when the value is well below that of serum, i.e., less than 300 mOsm/kg (the urine is maximally dilute at 50 to 70 mOsm/kg). In both diabetes insipidus and psychogenic water drinking urine volume will usually exceed 4 liters daily. Values less than 5 to 6 liters daily do not distinguish between these possibilities but do indicate less than complete diabetes insipidus, in which urine volumes approach 10 to 12 liters daily, as they may in cases of severe psychogenic water drinking. If the serum sodium/osmolality is low and the urine volume is large with low osmolality, a diagnosis of psychogenic water drinking is likely.

Diabetes Insipidus versus Psychogenic Water Drinking

Having established the presence of a large urine volume of low osmolality together with normal serum electrolytes, additional testing is necessary to establish a diagnosis. Referral to an endocrinologist or nephrologist is appropriate at this juncture, although under optimal conditions further efforts to establish the diagnosis on the ambulatory patient may be undertaken before referral (see below). Hospitalization for testing under "metabolic" conditions is nearly always to be preferred in these cases; however, most ordinary hospital conditions are not appropriate for the gathering of definitive information on water handling.

The first additional test is that of water deprivation. Best performed during the day when monitoring is possible, the patient remains recumbent and refrains from fluid intake; all urine is collected in hourly batches for 6 hours. Volumes and osmolalities are determined on each sample. Body weight is determined hourly. When the urine volume and osmolality seem to have stabilized after several hours, antidiuretic hormone (ADH, Pitressin) is given (5 units, aqueous, subcutaneously). Urine osmolality and volume are then determined every 30 minutes for an additional 90 to 120 minutes. If at any point drop in body weight exceeds 3%, the ADH should be injected and the test terminated over the next 90 minutes.

In the normal individual, urine volume will fall and osmolality will rise over several hours. Urine osmolality will exceed 500 mOsm/kg. Administration of ADH produces an additional increase in urine osmolality, but the increase will be small if the level is already high. In the patient with partial diabetes insipidus, the plateau is at 300 mOsm/kg with an increase to at least 500 mOsm/kg after ADH; some patients will not respond maximally (osmolality 1000 mOsm/kg). Patients with nephrogenic diabetes insipidus will not respond to ADH. A prompt fall of urine volume and an increase of urine osmolality may not occur in some patients with psychogenic water drinking. These patients are often overhydrated and may not reach plateau levels for as long as 12 hours. If the diagnosis is still doubtful at this point, referral for consultation should be made. Further tests can be performed to provoke ADH release by infusion of hypertonic saline. Administration of intravenous ADH and other special maneuvers may be necessary. CT scans of the area of the sella turcica, although usually negative, are important in cases of diabetes insipidus to rule out space-occupying lesions. Anterior pituitary function must be assessed when diabetes insipidus is diagnosed.

Treatment

The treatment of psychogenic water drinking involves psychiatric counseling. These patients are difficult to manage, especially if they become severely hyponatremic. "Weaning" such patients from water may also be a slow process not only because of the profound nature of their psychiatric disturbance, but because of their acquired inability to concentrate urine, a process that is only slowly reversible.

The treatment of diabetes insipidus involves use of ADH in some form. Until the last few years Pitressin Tannate in oil was the preferred agent. This material is given intramuscularly. Great care must be taken to suspend the insoluble hormone before injection. The usual dose is 5 units every 24 to 72 hours, depending on the duration of effect in a particular individual. Antidiuretic hormone may also be administered as a nasal spray. Two forms are available; lysine vasopressin, with an effect that lasts only 4 to 6 hours, has been largely replaced by the synthetic analogue, desmopressin (DDAVP). This material acts for 12 hours or longer. DDAVP is a great advance in the therapy of diabetes insipidus. Nasal absorption may be impaired by rhinitis or respiratory tract infections, during which treatment with Pitressin Tannate may be necessary. Patients with partial diabetes insipidus can sometimes be managed with chlorpropamide (Diabinese, 250 to 500 mg daily), a drug that potentiates endogenous ADH. However, hypoglycemia is a significant hazard. Clofibrate (Atromid-S) is another drug that has been used to treat diabetes insipidus. Nephrogenic diabetes insipidus, both idiopathic and secondary to lithium, is partially responsive to thiazide diuretics (23).

Syndrome of Inappropriate Secretion of Antidiuretic Hormone (SIADH)

The clinical manifestations of this disorder are due to hyponatremia and the diagnosis is based on that finding. The causes are multiple. Classically, the disturbance was related to ectopic production of ADH by a neoplasm. The tumor most likely to produce this syndrome is a small cell (oat cell) carcinoma of the lung, but many other tumors have also been shown to produce the same syndrome. The presence of a tumor is usually obvious, but occasionally it may be clinically occult. In addition, a variety of acute and chronic diseases of the central nervous system can produce an identical syndrome. Drugs, acting centrally, may also produce ADH hypersecretion [morphine, barbiturates (23)]. The best described drug-related SIADH that is likely to be encountered in an ambulatory patient is that due to chlorpropamide (Diabinese) during the therapy of diabetes mellitus (Chapter 72). In this case, the disturbance is due to potentiation of ADH action, although increased ADH release may also be involved (23).

Treatment

The treatment of SIADH is usually that which is related to the underlying disease or involves withdrawal of drug therapy (e.g., chlorpropamide, Diabinese; see Chapter 72). Water restriction is effective but is difficult to maintain in an ambulatory setting. Lithium has been occasionally useful. Demeclocycline, a tetracycline analogue, is an ADH antagonist and is effective in some cases. An ADH peptide analogue that blocks ADH action has been developed and offers promise for therapy, but the agent is not yet available for clinical use.

HYPOGLYCEMIA

Because the symptoms of hypoglycemia are rather nonspecific, hypoglycemia is properly more often suspected than present. Chemical hypoglycemia, defined as a plasma sugar of less than 50 mg/dl, may not be symptomatic, although levels less than 30 mg/dl are nearly always associated with symptoms (see Chapter 72 for discussion of plasma versus blood glucose values).

Hypoglycemia produces symptoms by two mechanisms: (a) by triggering the release of epinephrine, one of several homeostatic responses that tend to normalize a low blood sugar; and (b) by deprivation of the nervous system of its essential energy source.

The causes of hypoglycemia are numerous, but by far the most common is a benign functional disturbance of insulin secretion that is temporally associated with absorption of food from the gastrointestinal tract. Most other hypoglycemic events are seen in diabetics being treated with insulin. A few other conditions producing hypoglycemia are associated with insulin overproduction, the rarest of which is an insulinoma. In most situations hypoglycemia is due not to insulin excess but to disturbances of glucose production, as in ethanol ingestion, or rarely to glucose overutilization, as in the presence of certain extrapancreatic tumors. The causes of hypoglycemia are listed in Table 74.10.

Clinical Diagnosis

Presentation of the Problem

In some patients the history will suggest to the physician that the patient is experiencing periodic hypoglycemia. Other patients will themselves suggest to their physician that hypoglycemia accounts for the symptoms. Much has been written in the lay literature about hypoglycemia, and many books attribute the entire range of human miseries to this disorder. Needless to say, the case has been overstated. The physician encountering such a patient may find mere reassurance ineffective, so convincing is some of the lay literature in this area and so obsessed are some patients. However, the physician inevitably embarks on a search, either to confirm or to refute the suspected diagnosis. Verification of the presence of hypoglycemia, or more precisely its exclusion, can be attempted by instructing the patient in the use of a glucose oxidase strip (e.g., Chemstrips bG). The strip can be brought or sent to the physician or laboratory within 1 week for confirmation of the reading. Unfortunately, failure to document the presence of hypoglycemia may not serve to dispose of the issue, and generation of dubious or equivocal laboratory results may merely serve to prolong the preoccupation, initiate useless diets, or even delay diagnosis of serious but unrelated disease.

Table 74.10.
Causes of Hypoglycemia in Ambulatory Adults

POSTPRANDIAL STATE
  Reactive (idiopathic)
  Early diabetes mellitus
  Ethanol ingestion
  Postgastrectomy state
FASTING STATE
  Insulin excess:
    1. Insulin injection
    2. Sulfonylurea ingestion[a]
    3. Miscellaneous drugs and poisons[b]
    4. Insulinoma
    5. Autoimmune hypoglycemia (very rare)
  Alcohol ingestion
  Hormonal deficiencies:
    1. Glucocorticoid
    2. Growth Hormone
  Prolonged fasting in normal women
  Malnutrition
  Liver disease
  Extrapancreatic tumors
  Renal failure (chronic end stage)
  Congestive heart failure

[a] Many drugs, including such diverse compounds as anti-inflammatory agents, antibiotics, and lipid-lowering agents, potentiate the effects of sulfonylureas and may cause hypoglycemia.
[b] Haloperidol, propoxyphene, salicylates, etc.

"Nonhypoglycemia"

The frequency with which self-diagnosis of hypoglycemia occurs depends on the population, but in one study from Los Angeles, the problem was very common. The condition has been termed "nonhypoglycemia" and extends the concept of "nondisease," as it originates from misattributes of the physician, such as misintepretation of laboratory values, to misattributes of the patient (31). Identification of such individuals is important, as is their re-education (5). The ready acceptance by patients of hypoglycemia as a diagnosis is perhaps related to its social acceptability, the comfort received from attributing vague symptoms (e.g., fatigue, mental "fogginess") to a "real" disease, the satisfaction of an escape into dietary rituals, and possibly relief from the anxiety that life-threatening or at least serious disease may be lurking.

The recognition of "nonhypoglycemia" requires a careful history that fails to demonstrate the legitimate symptoms of hypoglycemia as well as a clear demonstration that glucose metabolism is normal (see below). Exclusion of other organic disease is routine (Table 74.10). Distinction from the idiopathic postprandial syndrome must be made (see below). Finally, psychiatric disease must be considered, based on positive findings rather than merely on an exclusion of apparent organic illness.

If the evaluation fails to establish the presence of bona fide hypoglycemia, the issue of the therapy of "nonhypoglycemia" remains. This difficult problem includes at least three steps that have been termed (a) disattribution, (b) explanation and ventilation, and (c) reattribution (31). Disattribution involves confrontation of the patient with the results of the test procedure. For some patients the mechanics or ritual of the procedure itself are impressive and therefore helpful. If the patient clings to the diagnosis of hypoglycemia despite strong evidence to the contrary, the physician should attempt to explore the reason for the patient's need to do so. During this process, an effort should be made to have the patient fully explain his notions about hypoglycemia and verbalize what might happen if those notions are challenged. Finally, the physician must either provide an alternate explanation for the symptoms—reattribution—along with a treatment plan or be prepared to assist the patient in accepting an uncertain and ambiguous situation. Unless grossly apparent emotional problems become evident during this process, psychiatric referral should be made after considerable deliberation and only after an effort has been made by the internist to resolve the problem. (Chapters 10 and 11 describe in detail interviewing and psychotherapeutic techniques for working with patients such as these.)

Defining Hypoglycemic Symptoms

Because laboratory confirmation may be extremely difficult in some cases, an extraordinarily careful history is essential. The degree to which the history is convincing will determine the vigor with which a rather nebulous diagnosis is to be pursued. Two issues guide the process. First, what exactly are the symptoms? Second, do the symptoms occur postprandially or in the fasting state?

Adrenergic versus neuroglycopenic symptoms. Two groups of symptoms and signs are associated with hypoglycemia. Many of the symptoms of hypoglycemia relate to stimulation by low blood glucose of the release of epinephrine. These comprise the first group and are termed adrenergic or sympathetic. Usually these symptoms are of rapid onset and more than one is ordinarily present. Ordinarily they last only 15 to 30 minutes and include sweating, tremor ("shakiness"), a sensation of hunger, and anxiety. Irritability and palpitations are often mentioned but are rarely spontaneous or prominent complaints.

The second group of symptoms is related to glucose deprivation of the central and, to a lesser extent, peripheral nervous systems. These symptoms may be termed neuroglycopenic and when severe mimic those of central nervous system hypoxia. Minimal symptoms are headache, mental dullness, and sudden fatigue. Confusion and visual disturbances (blurring, dimming of vision) are associated with moderate to severe hypoglycemia, whereas unconsciousness and seizures are indications of very severe hypoglycemia.

Although adrenergic symptoms are mainly postprandial, neuroglycopenic symptoms, especially those of severe variety, are seen in association with fasting hypoglycemia. Minor neuroglycopenic symptoms may also be seen in the postabsorptive state, but symptoms severe enough to cause loss of consciousness are rare and should not be readily attributed to this cause. When severe symptoms do occur in the postprandial state, great difficulty in establishing a diagnosis may be encountered. The duration of this type of hypoglycemia is so short that, by the time the patient is seen by a physician and a blood sugar determination is obtained, the glucose concentration has often returned to normal.

Postprandial versus fasting hypoglycemia. An accurate history is essential in order to identify the hypoglycemia as either postprandial or fasting. The subsequent evaluation and the diagnostic possibilities segregate clearly once this distinction is made. If a distinction can be made based on the history, the alternate type of hypoglycemia should no longer be considered since the two types do not coexist.

Postprandial (reactive) hypoglycemia. In this situation the patient has no problem on arising and before breakfast. Similarly, no difficulty is experienced if the patient sleeps late. The symptoms usually develop 2 to 5 hours after a meal.

Inquiry concerning the patient's dietary habits may be revealing. Some patients restrict carbohydrate intake intermittently. When this is done and a large carbohydrate meal follows, hypoglycemia may be precipitated. A history of previous gastrointestinal surgery (gastrectomy) is also important. The amount of alcohol consumed should be noted, since ethanol ingestion may precipitate hypoglycemia, even in the nonfasting patient (see below). Often the patient may recall milder symptomatic episodes experienced over a long period, since the intensity of postprandial hypoglycemia tends to wax and wane over the years. A family history of diabetes mellitus should be sought. Postprandial hypoglycemia can be an early manifestation of diabetes mellitus of the non-insulin-dependent type (see Chapter 72). Although symptoms and signs of anxiety or depression may be present, they have no diagnostic usefulness.

General physical examination can be expected to be negative. Even when early diabetes mellitus is found by glucose tolerance testing to be the cause of the hypoglycemia, complications of diabetes that can be found on physical examination (retinopathy, neuropathy) will not be present.

Postprandial Hypoglycemia

Laboratory Evaluation

As noted under "Presentation of the Problem" (page 999), an attempt can be made to determine the presence or absence of hypoglycemia by instructing the patient in the use of a glucose measuring strip. However, unless such a simple maneuver eliminates the problem, an unlikely outcome, laboratory evaluation will be necessary. Although ordinary meals do not consist of carbohydrate alone, the only practical and standardized test for detection of postabsorptive hypoglycemia is the glucose tolerance test. For this purpose, the test as described for diagnosis of diabetes mellitus (Chapter 72) is modified to include more frequent sampling (30-minute intervals) and a longer period (5 hours). The patient is observed during the entire test. Correlation of blood sugar values with clinical symptoms is essential. If the patient develops hypoglycemia associated with typical adrenergic symptoms and signs that reproduce those ordinarily experienced, a diagnosis of postabsorptive hypoglycemia can be considered established. A more precise diagnosis depends on the type of curve observed (see below). If symptoms without signs occur in the absence of hypoglycemia, the diagnosis is psychiatric. If hypoglycemia is seen but no symptoms occur, the hypoglycemic response may simply not have been severe enough to have triggered symptoms. The diagnosis then remains presumptive. A repeated test may succeed in reproducing the clinical situation.

Criteria for Diagnosis of Hypoglycemia. Plasma glucose values are greater than 50 mg/dl during glucose tolerance testing in 75% of normal, asymptomatic persons. However, some normal individuals show values that fall to 50 mg/dl or somewhat lower and may exhibit hypoglycemic symptoms during the test, even though they never have such symptoms spontaneously. Thus, even a finding of hypoglycemia during testing should not be used to explain atypical symptoms. In addition, occasional normal individuals may reach levels below 35 mg/dl without any symptoms at all. The plasma epinephrine response during glucose tolerance testing has been proposed as a measure of "hypoglycemic" response, which exceeds the usually accepted glucose cut-off of 50 mg/dl. In individuals who develop typical adrenergic symptoms and signs, an increase of plasma epinephrine can be documented even though the glucose concentration never reaches a diagnostic level for hypoglycemia (6). This phenomenon appears to provide an objective criterion for what has been termed "idiopathic postprandial syndrome" (see below).

Determinations of plasma insulin, growth hormone, glucagon, and norepinephrine concentrations in connection with the glucose tolerance test are of no particular use in interpreting the results. Variability is very great and in no sense diagnostic.

Types of Hypoglycemic Response during Glucose Tolerance Testing

Early Diabetes Mellitus. The fasting glucose concentration is normal. In the first 2 hours, values diagnostic of diabetes mellitus are reached, although the highest values are usually between 200 and 250 mg/dl (Chapter 72). Thereafter, between 3 and 4 hours, the glucose concentration falls to its lowest value and below 50 mg/dl.

Postgastrectomy State. Plasma glucose concentration rises rapidly and may reach a peak over 300 mg/dl by 1 hour, after which a rapid decline occurs. The lowest value is seen at 2 to 3 hours.

Idiopathic. In this response the blood glucose values in the first 2 hours are normal, but at about 3 hours a fall to hypoglycemic levels occurs. Values usually return to baseline by 5 hours.

Management of Hypoglycemia

Early Diabetes Mellitus. If the patient is obese, weight reduction may normalize the glucose tolerance and abolish the hypoglycemic episodes. If the patient is not obese, dietary manipulation can be attempted, but no standardized approach is available. The diet most likely to succeed is one that simulates that now recommended for diabetes generally, i.e., a diet that contains a high proportion of complex carbohydrates rather than simple sugars (Chapter 72). Also important is the distribution of food intake into small meals—often as many as six. Alcohol may be an aggravating factor in producing hypoglycemia and should be restricted, at least on a trial basis. Caffeine (coffee, tea) need not be restricted. Sulfonylurea drugs are not useful.

Postgastrectomy State. As many as 75% of asymptomatic patients who have had a partial gastrectomy will show reactive hypoglycemia during a glucose tolerance test. The therapy of symptomatic patients is similar to that described above: frequent small meals and restriction of simple sugars. The anticholinergic drug propantheline (Pro-Banthine), 7.5 mg taken 30 minutes before meals, may be helpful. This drug inhibits gut motility and delays gastric emptying. At this dose, side effects (blurred vision, dry mouth) are minimal. Propranolol (Inderal) often blocks symptoms but does little to affect hypoglycemia and therefore may be hazardous.

Idiopathic Hypoglycemia. The course of this disorder is obscure. Some patients may present with anxiety and/or depression in association with onset of hypoglycemic symptoms. Although diet manipulation and/or propantheline therapy as described above may ameliorate the hypoglycemia, additional treatment may be needed for the psychological aspects. Recent introduction of high-protein, low-carbohydrate diets for weight reduction has also led to difficulties in some persons. Carbohydrate restriction followed by carbohydrate ingestion leads to the hypoglycemia in these individuals. Ethanol (doses of 3 ounces of gin or equivalent) may potentiate reactive hypoglycemia in normal subjects.

Idiopathic Postprandial Syndrome

In this situation patients complain of typical adrenergic symptoms and show objective signs, but during glucose tolerance testing (see below) never achieve diagnostic levels of hypoglycemia. This condition has been termed "idiopathic postprandial syndrome." Recently, plasma epinephrine has been shown to increase abnormally in such persons. In these individuals, or in some diabetics (see page 935), the release of epinephrine appears to be triggered at levels of blood glucose (50 to 70 mg/dl) not ordinarily considered to be in the "hypoglycemic" range. Determination of plasma epinephrine levels during the performance of the glucose tolerance test has been proposed as an objective criterion for this disorder (6). Whether release of epinephrine is caused by change of blood glucose concentration or some other mechanism is not clear. It should be stressed that affected individuals have typical adrenergic symptoms and signs; their complaints are not to be confused with the vague symptoms of "nonhypoglycemia" (see above).

Fasting Hypoglycemia

The classical entity associated with fasting hypoglycemia is the insulinoma, but such insulin-secreting tumors are very rare, and other causes of fasting hypoglycemia should be eliminated before embarking on the difficult task of establishing the presence of an insulinoma.

Fasting hypoglycemia in a well-nourished or obese individual suggests insulinoma, drug (sulfonylurea) ingestion, or insulin self-administration. Debilitation suggests hepatic disease (most often related to chronic alcohol abuse) or, rarely, extrapancreatic tumor. The history, physical examination, and routine laboratory studies will readily identify patients with chronic congestive heart failure or chronic renal disease, two other conditions occasionally associated with fasting hypoglycemia. Other aspects of these problems as well as endocrine deficiencies and alcohol abuse as causes of hypoglycemia are discussed below.

Laboratory Evaluation

As already noted (page 999) an attempt can be made to verify the presence or absence of hyperglycemia with the use of a reagent strip. However, if hypoglycemia remains a concern, determination of serum glucose concentration will need to be confirmed in a controlled setting.

When symptoms of hypoglycemia occur in the fasting state (usually overnight but in any case longer than 4 hours after a meal) a number of diagnostic possibilities more serious than those associated with postprandial hypoglycemia must be considered. However, the first step in evaluation of the problem is to establish the existence of hypoglycemia. Assuming that the symptoms are not so profound as to have caused coma, in which case hospitalization is mandatory, an overnight fast followed by determination of plasma glucose is the simplest screening procedure. This procedure may have to be repeated several times. If hypoglycemia cannot be documented in this way, the period of fasting may have to be extended to 24, 48, or even 72 hours. Hospitalization and close monitoring are necessary under these circumstances.

A sex difference in response to fasting is well established. Normal men may fast for up to 72 hours and will not show fasting plasma glucose (FPG) below 50 mg/dl. In contrast, women often exhibit a progressive fall in the concentration of plasma glucose during prolonged fasting. At 72 hours the majority of premenopausal women have a concentration of glucose less than 50 mg/dl and some as low as 25 mg/dl. Thus, prolonged fasting to establish the diagnosis of fasting hypoglycemia is not always useful, since so many normal women will become hypoglycemic.

Insulinoma

This tumor occurs with equal frequency in men and women and at any age. Symptoms of headache on arising, confusion before breakfast, or nocturnal or early A.M. seizures may be present for years before the diagnosis is suspected. Hyperinsulinism may produce abnormal hunger, weight gain, and obesity. Neuropsychiatric symptoms may lead to neurological or psychiatric evaluations or to hospitalizations. In some of these cases, permanent neurological deficits have been seen and are presumably related to long duration of symptomatic hypoglycemia before diagnosis.

Diagnosis. In addition to the demonstration of hypoglycemia, the determination of plasma insulin activity is important. During fasting in normal persons both glucose and insulin levels decline and the ratio of immunoreactive insulin (IRI) to glucose (G) is maintained at less than 0.3 (milliunits of IRI/milligrams of G/dl). In most patients with insulinoma an abnormally high IRI:G ratio is apparent after even overnight fasting. These determinations should be made repeatedly, since fasting hypoglycemia and an abnormal IRI:G ra-

tio often occur only intermittently even in patients with subsequently proven insulinomas. In addition, a single abnormal ratio never establishes the diagnosis. The physician should be very cautious in accepting the accuracy of IRI values obtained from commercial laboratories. Proinsulin levels are elevated in patients with insulinoma and can be a useful adjunct. A variety of other useful procedures should, if necessary, be conducted by an endocrinologist. If fasting fails to provoke hypoglycemia (see above), the patient should exercise as vigorously as tolerable. Up to 2 hours of exercise should be completed with sampling for glucose every 15 to 20 minutes before concluding that hypoglycemia does not develop. A bicycle exerciser, jogging, or vigorous calisthenics may be used. Exercise raises glucose levels in normal persons but lowers plasma concentration further in patients with insulinoma. Provocative tests of insulin secretion (tolbutamide, leucine, glucagon) can be utilized with appropriate caution. Suppression of endogenous insulin C-peptide is another useful procedure in difficult cases, but it requires induction of hypoglycemia by infusion of insulin under controlled conditions, a procedure that must be performed by an endocrinologist in a hospital. Computerized axial tomography and sonography can localize tumors of 2- to 3-cm size. Selective angiography can sometimes identify even smaller tumors. These procedures must not be used as alternatives to the tests described above but should be performed after demonstration of abnormal secretion of insulin. The definitive treatment of an insulinoma is surgical.

Insulin and Sulfonylurea Self-administration

Occasional nondiabetic patients, usually family members of diabetics or persons with medically related occupations (nurses, technicians), engage in surreptitious insulin administration. Examination may reveal needle marks. Other clues can be provided by the presence of antibodies to insulin, which are present only in persons given insulin of animal origin, or by the measurement of insulin C-peptide. In persons who are secreting insulin, C-peptide is also produced concomitantly, but C-peptide is not present in commercial insulin and will be very low or absent when hypoglycemia is induced by exogenous insulin.

Oral hypoglycemic drugs (sulfonylureas; see Chapter 72), like insulin, may occasionally be abused and cause fasting hypoglycemia. The drug can be detected by analysis of the blood, although only specialized laboratories perform these measurements.

Alcohol Abuse

This problem probably produces hypoglycemia more commonly than any other single cause. As stated above, ingestion of ethanol can produce postprandial hypoglycemia in normal, well-nourished persons who engage in "social" drinking. However, fasting hypoglycemia related to ethanol ingestion occurs in chronic alcohol abusers and especially in those who are malnourished. The situation most likely to provoke hypoglycemia is cessation of food intake and continued ingestion of ethanol over the ensuing 10 to 20 hours. Under these circumstances, ethanol intoxication, i.e., drunkenness, may mistakenly be thought to be responsible for the symptoms.

Liver Disease and Chronic Congestive Heart Failure

Although hypoglycemia can be seen in the course of severe, acute hepatitis or as a result of chronic passive congestion in long-standing congestive heart failure, liver disease does not usually produce hypoglycemia. Patients with severe cirrhosis may occasionally have fasting hypoglycemia, but the development of hypoglycemia in such a patient should suggest the presence of a hepatoma. In patients with well-differentiated hepatoma, hypoglycemia may be an early symptom.

Endocrine Disease

Glucocorticoids and growth hormone are important regulators of glucose metabolism. Thus, either pituitary insufficiency or adrenal insufficiency (primary or secondary to hypopituitarism) can result in hypoglycemia as a presenting manifestation. The diagnosis of these disorders is described elsewhere in this chapter.

Autoimmune Hypoglycemia

There are very rare conditions in which autoantibodies develop to insulin or its receptor. Patients have no history of insulin use. The hypoglycemia is often severe and refractory. These conditions are unlikely to be encountered in an ambulatory setting.

General References

DeGrott LJ, Besser GM, Cahill GF, et al (eds): Endocrinology, 2nd ed. Philadelphia, WB Saunders, 1989.
    A comprehensive, multivolume text.
Felig P, Baxter JD, Broadus AE, Frohman LA (eds): Endocrinology and Metabolism, 2nd ed. New York, McGraw-Hill, 1987.
    An authoritative textbook of manageable size.
Wilson JD, Foster DW (eds): Textbook of Endocrinology, 7th ed. Philadelphia, WB Saunders, 1985.
    The longtime standard textbook for the field, as authoritative as ever.

Specific References

1. Amatruda Jr TT, Hurst MM, D'esopo ND: Certain endocrine and metabolic facets of the steroid withdrawal syndrome. J Clin Endocrinol Metab 25:1207, 1965.
2. Barrett-Connor E: Postmenopausal estrogen replacement and breast cancer (editorial). N Engl J Med 321:319, 1989.
3. Bergvist L, Adami H-O, Perrson I, et al: The risk of breast cancer after estrogen and estrogen-progestin replacement. N Engl J Med 321:293, 1989.
4. Byyny RL: Withdrawal from glucocorticoid therapy. N Engl J Med 295:30, 1976.
5. Cahill GF, Soeldner JS: A noneditorial on nonhypoglycemia. N Engl J Med 291:905, 1974.
6. Chalew SA, McLaughlin JV, Mersey JH, et al: The use of the plasma epinephrine response in the diagnosis of idiopathic postprandial syndrome. JAMA 251:612, 1984.
7. Coe FL, Favus MJ: Does mild, asymptomatic hyperparathyroidism require surgery? N Engl J Med 302:224, 1980. (Editorial); and rebuttal (letters), Incidence of primary hyperparathyroidism. N Engl J Med 302:1312, 1980.
8. Coe FL, Favus MJ, Parks JH: Is estrogen preferable to surgery for postmenopausal women with primary hyperparathyroidism? N Engl J Med 314:1508, 1986.
9. Copeland PM: The incidentally discovered adrenal mass. Ann Intern Med 98:940, 1983.
10. Davis FB, Davis PJ: Water metabolism in diabetes mellitus. Am J Med 70:210, 1981.
11. Eastell R, Riggs BL: Diagnostic evaluation of osteoporosis. Endocrinol Metab Clin North Am 17:547, 1988.
12. Fauci AS, Dale DC, Balow JE: Glucocorticoid therapy: mechanisms of action and clinical considerations. Ann Intern Med 84:304, 1976.
13. Goldman MB, Luchins DJ, Robertson GL: Mechanisms of altered water metabolism in psychotic patients with polydipsia and hyponatremia. N Engl J Med 318:397, 1988.
14. Graber AL, Ney RL, Nicholson WE, et al: Natural history of pituitary-adrenal recovery following long-term suppression with corticosteroids. J Clin Endocrinol Metab 25:11, 1965.
15. Heath H III, Hodgson SF, Kennedy MA: Primary hyperparathyroidism. Incidence, morbidity, and potential economic impact in a community. N Engl J Med 302:189, 1980.
16. Jeffcoate WJ: Treating Cushing's Disease (editorial). Br Med J 296:227, 1988.
17. Joborn C, Hetta J, Lind L, et al: Self-rated psychiatric symptoms in patients operated on because of primary hyperparathyroidism and in patients with longstanding mild hypercalcemia. Surgery 105:72, 1989.
18. Johnston DG, Prescott RWG, Kendall-Taylor P, et al: Hyperprolactinemia. Long-term effect of bromocriptine. Am J Med 75:868, 1983.
19. Kohler PO: Treatment of pituitary adenomas (editorial). N Engl J Med 371:45, 1987.
20. Melby JC: Systemic corticosteroid therapy: pharmacology and endocrinologic considerations. Ann Intern Med 81:505, 1974.
21. Melby JC: Therapy of Cushing disease: A consensus for pituitary microsurgery (editorial). Ann Intern Med 109:445, 1988.
22. Melton, III LJ, Kan SH, Frye MA, et al: Epidemiology of vertebral fractures in women. Am J Epidemiol 129:1000, 1989.
23. Miller M, Moses AM: Drug-induced states of impaired water excretion. Kidney Int 10:96, 1976.
24. Peck WA, Riggs BL, Bell NH, et al: Research directions in osteoporosis. Am J Med 84:275, 1988.
25. Raisz LG: Local and systemic factors in the pathogenesis of osteoporosis. N Engl J Med 318:818, 1988.
26. Riggs BL, Melton LJ: Involutional osteoporosis. N Engl J Med 314:1676, 1986.
27. Riggs BL, Wahner HW: Bone densitometry and clinical decision-making in osteoporosis (editorial). Ann Intern Med 108:293, 1988.
28. Selby PL, Peacock M: Ethinyl estradiol and norethindrone in the treatment of primary hyperparathyroidism in postmenopausal women. N Engl J Med 314:1481, 1986.
29. Sonino N: The use of ketoconazole as an inhibitor of steroid production. N Engl J Med 317:812, 1987.
30. Spielgel RJ, Vigersky RA, Oliff AI, et al: Adrenal suppression after short-term corticosteroid therapy. Lancet 1:630, 1979.
31. Yager J, Young RT: Nonhypoglycemia is an epidemic condition. N Engl J Med 291:907, 1974.

C H A P T E R 75

Clinical Implications of Abnormal Lipoprotein Metabolism

MARC R. BLACKMAN, M.D.
DAVID E. KERN, M.D.

Interest in plasma lipids, lipoproteins, and apoproteins stems from their strong relationship to the development of atherosclerosis (3, 5). At a time when it is possible to reduce the frequency of premature death and disability from atherosclerotic disease, the physician should be knowledgeable about and capable of diagnosing and treating the major abnormalities of lipoprotein metabolism.

LIPOPROTEIN NOMENCLATURE AND COMPOSITION

Lipids are insoluble in the aqueous plasma medium. They circulate in plasma as component parts of macromolecules that consist of a nonpolar hydrophobic lipid core of cholesterol esters and triglycerides and a polar hydrophilic monolayer surface coat of protein, phospholipid, and unesterified cholesterol (Fig. 75.1). These macromolecules, which are made miscible in plasma by their surface coat, are called *lipoproteins*.

Lipoproteins have traditionally been classified as a family of molecules containing the same basic constituents, but in different proportions (Table 75.1). The major classes of lipoproteins can be separated from each other by differences in density (ultracentrifugation), net surface charge (electrophoresis), size, and composition. Ultracentrifugation, which provides the most useful means of classification, separates lipoproteins into five principal classes. From the least dense and largest to the most dense and smallest, these are the chylomicrons, very low density lipoproteins (VLDL), intermediate density lipoproteins (IDL), low density lipoproteins (LDL), and high density lipoproteins (HDL) (23).

Each lipoprotein contains characteristic proportions of lipids and type-specific apoproteins (apos) such that, with increasing lipoprotein density, the relative amount of lipid decreases and that of (apo) protein increases (Table 75.1). Thus, triglyceride is the major lipid component in chylomicrons and VLDL, whereas cholesterol is the major component of LDL. Intermediate density or remnant lipoproteins are catabolic products of chylomicrons and VLDL and contain similar amounts

A LIPOPROTEIN PARTICLE

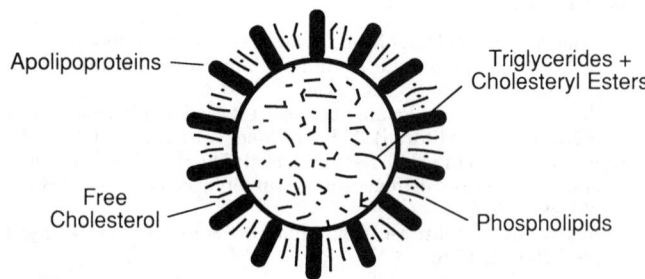

Apolipoproteins

Triglycerides + Cholesteryl Esters

Free Cholesterol

Phospholipids

Figure 75.1. Structure of the lipoprotein macromolecule with the nonpolar lipids, cholesterol ester and triglyceride, in the lipoprotein core surrounded by a monolayer composed of specific apolipoproteins and the polar lipids, unesterified cholesterol and phospholipid. (From: The Johns Hopkins Physicians Lipid Education Program, 2nd ed. The Johns Hopkins University, Baltimore, 1988, p. 11.)

Table 75.1.
Classification of Plasma Lipoproteins by Physical and Chemical Characteristics

Lipoprotein Fraction (Ultracentrifugation)	Density (g/ml)	Migration (Electrophoresis)	Composition as Percentage of Total Mass			
			Cholesterol	Triglyceride	Apoprotein	Phospholipid
Chylomicron	0.95	Origin	2– 7	80–90	2 (A, B-48, C, E)	3
Very low density (VLDL)	< 1.006	Pre-β	10–22	50–70	6 (B-100, C, E)	14
β-very low density (β-VLDL or VLDL$_2$)	< 1.006	β	30–40	45	12 (B-100, B-48, C, E)	15
Intermediate density or remnant (IDL)	1.006–1.019	Slow pre-β	30–40	40	18 (B, E)	22
Low density (LDL)	1.019–1.063	β	45–50	5–10	21 (B-100)	22
High density (HDL)	1.063–1.21	α	15–25	3–5	50 (A, C, E)	28

of both lipids and apos (see below, "Normal Physiology of Lipoprotein Transport"). The HDL are the densest lipoproteins; they contain the most apos and ordinarily consist of 15 to 25% cholesterol and a small amount of triglyceride in the core. HDL are further subdivided into HDL$_2$ and HDL$_3$. The former is more buoyant as reflected by its higher lipid to protein ratio and richer apo A-I and apo C and E content, relative to the more dense HDL$_3$, which has a lower lipid to protein ratio and a higher apo A-II than A-I composition. There is a strong inverse relationship of coronary risk to plasma concentrations of HDL$_2$ and apo A-I related to the heightened capacity of the latter molecules to transport cholesterol from cells (26) (see below).

PLASMA LIPOPROTEINS AS RISK FACTORS FOR ATHEROSCLEROSIS

The risk factor concept, which developed as an outgrowth of the Framingham study and other large epidemiological studies, is based upon the strong association between certain characteristics in people and the increased likelihood of developing cardiovascular disease (20). Among the risk factors for atherosclerotic vascular disease, the most clearly established ones are plasma total cholesterol levels (and plasma LDL and HDL content), hypertension, and cigarette smoking. Each has been clearly implicated and makes a sizable independent contribution to the overall risk of developing coronary artery disease (CAD).

Evidence from several large prospective and retrospective epidemiological studies among diverse populations has demonstrated that variations in plasma levels of certain lipids and lipoproteins are associated with an increased likelihood of developing or having CAD. *Hypercholesterolemia*, for example, is strongly associated with the subsequent development of CAD. The relationship is uniformly consistent, dose related, and independent of sex. The predictive value of the plasma level of total cholesterol is somewhat limited, however, by the fact that it reflects the opposing influences of LDL and HDL *cholesterol*. Levels of LDL correlate positively, whereas those of HDL are inversely related to CAD risk. The negative correlation between HDL levels and CAD depends mainly on its subfraction, HDL$_2$, which may provide, along with its major protein component, apo A-I, a better index of

risk than the total plasma level of HDL (26). Over the range of plasma levels of total cholesterol or of HDL cholesterol levels found in an average American population, the risk of CAD varies roughly 5-fold. Plasma levels of total cholesterol have less predictive value beyond the age of 50 or 60, but HDL cholesterol levels and the ratio of LDL to HDL cholesterol remain useful predictors in this age group. The relationships between plasma levels of total cholesterol, LDL cholesterol, and HDL cholesterol and CAD are independent ones, in that the associations remain significant even after statistical adjustment for the contributions of other risk factors (such as cigarette smoking, hypertension, obesity, impaired glucose tolerance, and other lipoprotein levels).

Elevated fasting levels of plasma *triglyceride* and its major lipoprotein transporter, VLDL, also correlate with an increased risk of atherosclerotic disease. In most large epidemiological studies, the association does not appear to be an independent one, but in the Framingham Heart Study, the plasma triglyceride level was found to be an independent risk factor for CAD (7). In certain subgroups of patients, such as those with familial combined hyperlipoproteinemia or familial dysbetalipoproteinemia, the hypertriglyceridemia may reflect altered lipoprotein and apoprotein composition and metabolism (33) and seems causally related to the development of premature atherosclerosis (5). In addition, hypertriglyceridemia may be prognostically important in patients with diabetes mellitus (36) or end-stage renal disease (13).

Not only do these lipoprotein and apoprotein abnormalities seem to increase one's predisposition to CAD, there is a parallel increased risk for cerebrovascular disease (17, 20) and peripheral vascular disease as well (17).

Plasma levels of other lipoproteins and apos also correlate with atherosclerotic disease. Elevated plasma concentrations of *LDL apo B* appear to discriminate between patients with and without atherosclerosis of the coronary and peripheral vasculature, even in the presence of normal plasma levels of total cholesterol and LDL cholesterol (5, 6, 33). The determination of plasma LDL apo B concentrations may prove useful in assessing risk in hypertriglyceridemic patients (5, 33). In familial dysbetalipoproteinemia, a genetic disorder characterized by elevated plasma levels of IDL and an abnormally migrating β-VLDL (27), there is an increased risk of both peripheral and coronary atherosclerotic disease. In contrast, fasting *chylomicronemia* is associated with recurrent episodes of abdominal pain and pancreatitis, but not with the early development of atherosclerosis.

In several epidemiological studies, plasma levels of total cholesterol below 180 to 195 mg/dl have been associated with an increased risk of cancer, especially cancer of the colon. The evidence does not, however, suggest a significant causal link, since (a) in most, but not all, studies the association was strongest in the first year of follow-up, then attenuated and disappeared in subsequent years, suggesting that preclinical cancer might have lowered levels of plasma cholesterol rather than vice versa; (b) studies comparing populations have shown a positive rather than a negative association between dietary fat intake and risk for major cancers, such as breast, prostate, and colon cancer; and (c) the relationship was generally weak, present in a minority of studies, and demonstrated no consistent relation between cholesterol level and cancer risk (22).

RATIONALE FOR DIAGNOSIS AND TREATMENT

The need for a preventive approach to the control of atherosclerotic disease becomes clear when one considers the following facts: Atherosclerotic disease constitutes the leading cause of death and disability in western industrialized societies. In the United States, approximately 725,000 individuals die annually from atherosclerotic disease, 550,000 of them from CAD. Many of the deaths occur suddenly and unexpectedly in otherwise apparently healthy people. Despite medical advances in the treatment of symptomatic disease, more than 40% of patients who sustain a myocardial infarction still die, with more than half of the deaths occurring outside the hospital before medical care is available. Complications and disability from atherosclerotic disease, once established, are seldom fully reversible. The economic costs are formidable, with more than $80 billion being spent annually in direct health care costs and lost wages and productivity.

The prevention, diagnosis, and treatment of plasma lipoprotein abnormalities constitute a major component of an overall effort to prevent atherosclerotic disease. The measurement of plasma concentrations of lipids and lipoproteins can identify asymptomatic individuals at high risk. A large and increasing body of data derived from pathological, genetic, metabolic, epidemiological, animal, and clinical studies has demonstrated that certain abnormalities in plasma lipoproteins (in particular elevated levels of total cholesterol and LDL cholesterol) actually promote or cause atherosclerosis. It is equally well established that both exogenous factors (such as imprudent diet, drugs, lack of exercise, and cigarette smoking) and endogenous metabolic factors (which are genetically determined and may be affected by various diseases) determine plasma levels of lipids and lipoproteins.

The "lipid (or "cholesterol") hypothesis," based upon the data described above, also postulates that favorable alterations of plasma lipoprotein levels by diet, drugs, or other therapy reduce the risk of atherosclerosis in humans. Although there had been much suggestive data based upon animal studies, clinical trials of diet and drug therapy, and observations of falling CAD mortality in the United States concurrent with widespread changes in dietary habits (as well as with the reduction of other risk factors), evidence supporting the lipid hypothesis was inconclusive until the completion of the Lipid Research Clinics Coronary Primary Prevention Trial (25). This trial was a prospective, randomized, double-blinded, multi-institutional trial of therapy with cholestyramine and diet versus placebo and diet in 3806 healthy hypercholesterolemic men aged 35 to 59 followed for an average of 7.4 years. During the study period, 155 of 1906 (8.1%) men in the cholestyramine group experienced definite CAD death and/or definite nonfatal myocardial infarction (the primary end points) as opposed to 187 of 1900 (9.8%) men in the placebo group. The resulting 19% reduction in the frequency of the primary end points in the treated group was accompanied by decreases in the development of new angina (by 20%), a positive exercise stress test (by 25%), and incidence of coronary bypass surgery (by 21%). There was a 2% reduction in overall CAD risk for each 1% reduction in plasma level of total cholesterol; thus in men compliant with the prescribed dose (24 g/day), a 25% decrease in total cholesterol level resulted in a 50% decrease in overall CAD risk. Another double-blinded, 5-year prospective, randomized study examined the effect of cholestyramine plus diet versus placebo plus diet on the angiographic progression of CAD in 116 hypercholesterolemic patients with prior angiographic evidence of CAD (1). The cholestyramine group evidenced a suggestive decrease in "definite" CAD progression and a significant decrease in "definite and probable" CAD progression. Favorable alterations in the ratios of plasma levels of total (or LDL) cholesterol to HDL cholesterol correlated significantly with a decrease in CAD progression, however defined.

More recently, a number of large-scale, randomized clinical trials have conclusively demonstrated that cholesterol-lowering drugs can decrease the incidence of both new and recurrent CAD events. One of the most influential of the recent reports is that of the Helsinki Heart Study (10), in which approximately 4000 asymptomatic, middle-aged men with elevated levels of total and LDL cholesterol were randomized and followed for 5 years on a regimen of either diet plus gemfibrozil therapy versus diet plus placebo. At the end of 5 years, the men receiving gemfibrozil exhibited average decreases in total and LDL cholesterol of 9%, an increase in HDL cholesterol levels of 8%, and a decrease in triglyceride levels of 35%. In addition, they experienced decreases in the frequencies of nonfatal myocardial infarctions of 37%, and of definite coronary deaths of 26%, for an overall reduction in the incidence of CAD end-points of 34%.

It should be noted that in neither the Lipid Research

Clinics Coronary Primary Prevention Trial (25) nor the Helsinki Heart Study (10) was hypocholesterolemic drug treatment associated with a significant decrease in all-cause mortality. Moreover, there was an excess of violent and accidental deaths in both studies that, although not statistically significant, remains unexplained and of sufficient potential concern to warrant attempts at confirmation in future trials of hypocholesterolemic drugs.

NORMAL PHYSIOLOGY OF LIPOPROTEIN TRANSPORT

Plasma lipoproteins arise from both exogenous dietary sources and from endogenous hepatic sources (Fig. 75.2). They carry lipids in three distinct but interacting pathways: The exogenous pathway consists primarily of chylomicrons; the endogenous pathway consists mostly of VLDL, IDL, and LDL; and the reverse cholesterol transport pathway consists mostly of HDL activity.

The exogenous pathway. After the ingestion of fat, dietary triglycerides are hydrolyzed in the gut and absorbed by intestinal enterocytes. Triglyceride-containing chylomicrons, formed in these cells, are secreted into lymphatic vessels and subsequently enter the venous system via the thoracic duct. Chylomicrons function as a system of high energy caloric transport, allowing the calories ingested in excess of the immediate needs of the body to be transferred to sites of storage between meals. Absorbed dietary cholesterol is also esterified and transported in chylomicrons.

Other triglyceride-rich lipoproteins are synthesized from endogenous sources by the liver and intestine. Cholesterol synthesis from acetate also occurs in the liver and is regulated by the enzyme hydroxymethylglutaryl (HMG) CoA reductase. Triglycerides synthesized in the liver combine with cholesterol ester and are enveloped in a lipoprotein monolayer before secretion into the hepatic venous outflow system as endogenous triglyceride-rich VLDL.

Chylomicrons and VLDL are transported to adipose tissue and muscle for storage and utilization. The uptake and storage of triglyceride are regulated by *lipoprotein lipase* (LPL). LPL is secreted by cells in virtually all parenchymal tissues and migrates to the endothelial cells of local capillary beds where it is activated by the apo C-II peptide normally found on chylomicrons, VLDL, and HDL. It hydrolyzes triglyceride and surface components from chylomicrons and VLDL to transform them into *remnant lipoproteins* (Fig. 75.2). The fatty acids released during this reaction migrate to muscle cells for combustion or to adipose cells for resynthesis and storage as triglyceride (28). The remnant lipoproteins are smaller, denser, and relatively enriched in cholesterol, apo B, and apo E compared with the chylomicrons and VLDL from which they derive. They are taken up by apo B-E (LDL) receptors in the liver. The chylomicron remnants are further degraded, and the VLDL remnants are processed into IDL and cholesterol-rich LDL (Fig. 75.2). Apo C-II and apo C-III, and the phospholipids and free cholesterol released during the LPL reaction, are transferred to HDL for utilization. The surface material generated by LPL-mediated removal of core triglyceride from VLDL and chylomicrons is the substrate (apo A-I is the cofactor) for the enzyme *lecithin-cholesterol acyl transferase* (LCAT), which converts nascent HDL to mature spherical HDL and plays a major role in reverse cholesterol transport (see below).

Hepatic triglyceride lipase, like LPL, is released into plasma by heparin administration, hence the term *postheparin lipolytic activity* (PHLA). Hepatic lipase and LPL differ in composition, yet both are involved in the regulation of the plasma concentration of HDL_2 and in the catabolism of triglyceride-rich lipoproteins. Hepatic lipase promotes the hepatic removal of phospholipids and cholesterol from HDL_2 to form either HDL_3 (which re-enters the circulation) or irreversible catabolic products of HDL.

The LDL are the principal carriers of cholesterol in plasma. Cholesterol is a major structural component

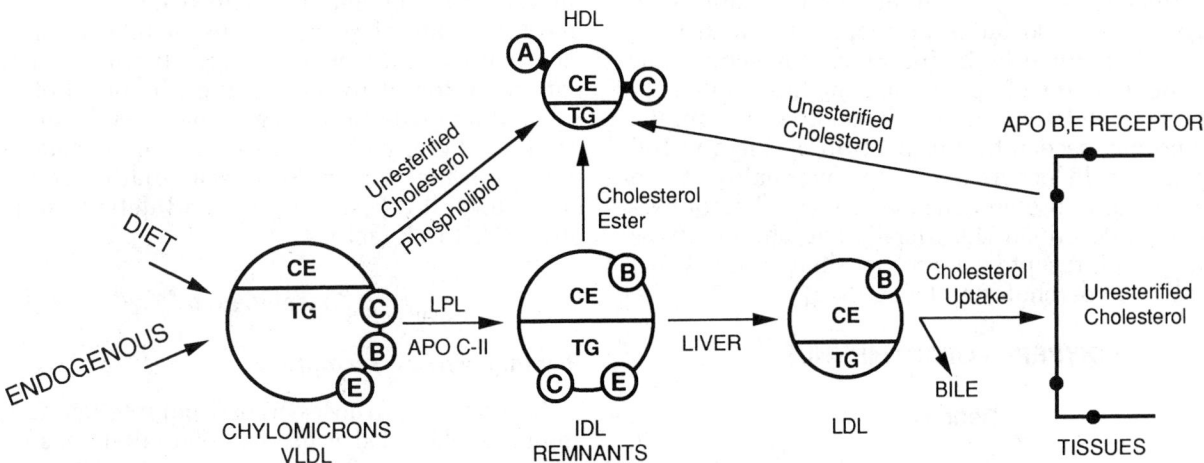

Figure 75.2.   The normal physiology of lipoprotein transport is illustrated schematically (see pages 1007 to 1008 for details).

of all cell membranes and is a precursor for steroid hormone synthesis by the adrenal glands and gonads. The LDL *cholesterol-rich particles* are derived mainly from VLDL and their catabolic remnants via the action of LPL and hepatic lipase. The principal removal of LDL occurs in the periphery by cells having a specific cell surface receptor (3) that recognizes all forms of apo B and is currently referred to as the apo B-E (LDL) receptor (Fig. 75.2). After specific cell receptor binding, LDL are internalized by receptor-mediated endocytosis and carried to lysosomes, where apo B is irreversibly degraded to amino acids and LDL cholesterol ester is hydrolyzed to free cholesterol. The free cholesterol is transported to an intracellular cholesterol pool where it regulates, by a cellular feedback pathway, the resynthesis of cholesterol, cholesterol ester, and apo B-E (LDL) receptors (19).

The cholesterol content of the cell is also regulated by a removal system involving HDL as a vehicle for cholesterol transport from peripheral to hepatic cells for catabolism and excretion into bile directly or after conversion to bile acid (19, 29). This reverse cholesterol transport system provides an efficient mechanism for the transfer of esterified cholesterol to LDL and VLDL, the absorption of free cholesterol from vascular endothelial cells, as well as the removal of cholesterol arising from cell membrane turnover and cell death.

Continued LDL catabolism in excess of that performed by hepatic and other parenchymal cells occurs in macrophages via a *scavenger pathway*. The latter is the predominant mechanism for LDL catabolism in persons with homozygous familial hypercholesterolemia (3).

An apparent antiatherogenic alteration in both the lipoprotein and apoprotein composition of HDL, the formation of HDL_c, occurs during high cholesterol feeding and represents one pathway by which the body can enhance its capacity to clear excess cholesterol from cells (19).

Apoproteins occupy specific domains on the three-dimensional structures of the individual lipoproteins. Alterations in lipid-protein interactions occur during the normal metabolism of lipoproteins, resulting in changes in the association of apoproteins with lipoproteins. Abnormalities in lipoprotein transport occur when the domains of apoproteins are altered by substitutions or deletions in amino acids. For example, the abnormal recognition of β-VLDL by the apo B-E receptor on cells occurs due to an abnormality in apo E in dysbetalipoproteinemia (see below, "Pathophysiology of Lipoprotein Disorders"), and abnormalities in the apo B-E receptors are responsible for the defect in familial hypercholesterolemia (3, 27).

HYPERLIPOPROTEINEMIA

Definition

Hyperlipoproteinemia is defined as the excessive accumulation in the blood of one or more of the lipoprotein classes of lipid-transporting macromolecules. The diagnosis of hyperlipoproteinemia is sometimes based upon plasma levels of lipids or lipoproteins above the 95th percentile of those found in a reference population. The distributions of plasma levels of total cholesterol, LDL cholesterol, total triglyceride, VLDL triglycerides, and HDL cholesterol among North American participants in the Lipid Research Clinics Prevalence Study have been published (24, 35). Although the participants in that study did not represent a random sample of the entire North American population, they did encompass a broad range of sociodemographic groups and thus provide the best available reference values for lipoproteins. Because lipoprotein values vary with age, sex, and race, these factors must be considered when assigning a range of normal or a percentile to an individual's lipid levels (Table 75.2).

Based upon the results of some treatment trials (25), the arbitrary use of a 95th percentile cut-off point in the diagnosis of hyperlipoproteinemia has some utility in suggesting the need for drug therapy in hypercholesterolemic patients. However, it should not be considered the dividing point between "diseased" and "healthy" individuals, since CAD risk increases continuously over a broad range of lipid values. Furthermore, lipid distributions vary between and within populations. For example, levels of total and LDL cholesterol (and the prevalence of CAD) are much higher in North American and Northern European populations than they are in the Japanese population. Many people diagnosed as normolipidemic in the United States would probably be classified as hyperlipidemic in Japan.

Decreased as well as increased plasma levels of certain lipoproteins can also pose a threat of atherosclerosis. Specifically, plasma levels of HDL cholesterol and apo A-I are inversely correlated with the risk for CAD, so that the 5th rather than 95th percentile can be used as the arbitrary cut-off point to distinguish those at greatest risk (Table 75.2).

More recently, the Adult Treatment Panel of the National Cholesterol Education Program (NCEP) has published a schema for categorizing patients by measurements of serum levels of total cholesterol (see below, "Indications for Evaluation"). Once a patient is found to have a high blood cholesterol concentration, decisions regarding possible diet, drug, or other therapy are made after a more detailed lipoprotein analysis, including calculation of the LDL cholesterol level (see below), and determination of other CAD risk factors.

Classification

Primary versus Secondary

For clinical purposes hyperlipoproteinemic states should be classified as primary (hereditary or sporadic genetic disorders of metabolism), secondary, or both. Secondary hyperlipoproteinemia is associated with an

Table 75.2.
Fasting Plasma Concentrations (mg/dl) of Lipoprotein Lipids in North Americans[a]

Caucasians[b]

Men

Age	TC[a] 5th%	TC Mean	TC 95th%	LDL-C 5th%	LDL-C Mean	LDL-C 95th%	TG 5th%	TG Mean	TG 95th%	HDL-C 5th%	HDL-C Mean	HDL-C 95th%
15–19	118	153	191	62	94	130	38	78	143	30	46	63
20–24	118	162	212	66	103	147	44	89	165	30	45	63
25–29	130	179	234	70	117	165	45	104	204	31	45	63
30–34	142	193	258	78	126	185	46	122	253	28	46	63
35–39	147	201	267	81	133	189	52	141	316	29	43	62
40–44	150	205	260	87	136	186	56	152	318	27	44	67
45–49	163	213	275	98	144	202	56	143	279	30	45	64
50–54	156	213	274	89	142	197	56	153	313	28	44	63
55–59	161	215	280	88	146	203	63	134	261	28	48	71
60–64	163	217	287	83	146	210	60	131	240	30	52	74
65–69	166	221	288	98	150	210	56	139	256	30	51	78
70+	144	210	265	88	143	186	54	133	239	31	51	75

Women

Age	TC[a] 5th%	TC Mean	TC 95th%	LDL-C 5th%	LDL-C Mean	LDL-C 95th%	TG 5th%	TG Mean	TG 95th%	HDL-C 5th%	HDL-C Mean	HDL-C 95th%
15–19		159	207	59	96	137	36	73	126	35	52	74
20–24		170	237	57	104	159	37	87	168	33	53	79
25–29		179	231	71	110	164	42	87	159	37	56	83
30–34		179	228	70	111	156	40	86	163	36	56	77
35–39		190	249	75	120	172	40	98	205	34	55	82
40–44		198	259	74	125	174	45	98	191	34	58	88
45–49		206	268	79	129	186	44	113	223	34	59	87
50–54		217	281	88	138	201	53	116	223	37	62	92
55–59		229	294	89	146	210	59	133	279	37	62	91
60–64		232	300	100	152	224	57	132	256	38	64	92
65–69		234	291	92	154	221	56	137	260	35	63	98
70+		225	280	96	149	206	60	128	289	33	61	92

Blacks

Men

Age	TC[c,d] 5th%	TC Mean	TC 95th%		Age	TG[d] 5th%	TG Mean	TG 95th%		Age	HDL-C[e] Mean ± SD
10–19	120	160	205		15–19	38	59	102		15–19	53 ± 11
20–29	—[e]	179	—		20–24	—	81	—		20–24	—
30–39	138	192	253		25–29	42	107	224		25–29	58 ± 15
40–49	148	207	—		30–34	52	126	294		30–34	54 ± 13
50–59	—	207	—		35–39	—	142	—		35–39	53 ± 16
60+	—	221	—		40–44	—	109	—		40–44	58 ± 20

Women

Age	TC[c,d] 5th%	TC Mean	TC 95th%		Age	TG[d] 5th%	TG Mean	TG 95th%		Age	HDL-C Mean ± SD
10–19	124	165	211		15–19	36	65	110		15–19	54 ± 11
20–29	124	177	235		20–24	38	77	137		20–24	—
30–39	132	185	243		25–29	38	80	150		25–29	57 ± 10
40–49	146	202	268		30–34	43	99	188		30–34	60 ± 13
50–59	—	217	—		35–39	—	104	—		35–39	59 ± 15
60+	—	234	—		40–44	—	120	—		40–44	62 ± 19

[a] 5th%, 5th percentile; 95th%, 95th percentile; TC, total cholesterol; LDL-C, low density lipoprotein cholesterol; HDL-C, high density lipoprotein cholesterol; TG, total triglycerides.
[b] Adapted from reference 31, visit 2.
[c] Levels determined routinely by clinical laboratories are often higher (up to 30 mg/dl or more) than those determined by a standard laboratory (e.g., Centers for Disease Control). Check how your laboratory is standardized.
[d] Adapted from reference 23, visit 1.
[e] Adapted from references 23 and 35.

identifiable disease or condition and is reversible with control or eradication of that disease or condition. The major causes of secondary hyperlipoproteinemia are listed in Table 75.3.

Phenotypic versus Genotypic and Pathophysiological

In the 1960s, it was popular to classify the various hyperlipidemic states *phenotypically,* based upon specific concentrations of lipids and lipoproteins and electrophoretic patterns (Table 75.4). Although the phenotypic classification describes in abbreviated fashion the plasma lipoproteins that are present in elevated or low concentrations, it does not reflect the genetic mechanisms or pathophysiology of the lipoprotein disorders (16). It is desirable to classify patients *pathophysiologically* and *genotypically* (Table 75.4) in order to diagnose and treat lipoprotein disorders accurately. Because apoproteins, enzymes, and cellular receptors are the major regulators of lipoprotein metabolism, it is appropriate to categorize lipoprotein disorders wherever possible in terms of pathophysiological defects in the structure, function, and metabolism of these molecules, rather than by using a rigidly fixed phenotypic classification. Often, the pathophysiological and genotypic classification can be surmised from a patient's phenotypic pattern, medical history, family history, and physical examination. Sometimes family members must be studied and/or more sophisticated laboratory analyses performed, necessitating referral to a specialist in endocrinology and metabolism.

Table 75.3.
Causes of Secondary Lipoprotein Disorders

Exogenous	Alcohol, oral contraceptives, estrogens, androgens, corticosteroids, diuretics (thiazides, chlorthalidone), β-adrenergic blocking agents, obesity, nutritional (diet high in cholesterol/saturated fat)
Endocrine-metabolic	Diabetes mellitus, hypothyroidism, Cushing's disease, Addison's disease, acromegaly, hypopituitarism
Hepatic	Obstructive or parenchymal disease, hepatoma
Renal	Nephrotic syndrome, chronic renal failure, hemodialysis
Acute stress situations	Acute myocardial infarction, sepsis, burns
Pregnancy	
Pancreatitis	
Dysgammaglobulinemias	Multiple myeloma, macroglobulinemia
Systemic lupus erythematosus	
Gout	
Viral infections	
Other	Glycogen storage disease, lipodystrophies, progeria, acute intermittent porphyria, anorexia nervosa, Klinefelter's syndrome

PATHOPHYSIOLOGY OF LIPOPROTEIN DISORDERS

The abnormal accumulation of lipoproteins in plasma results from their excessive production, defective removal, or both. Lipoprotein disorders may be primary (usually genetic), may be secondary to certain diseases (especially diabetes mellitus, chronic renal disease, hypothyroidism, dysglobulinemia) or drugs (corticosteroids, estrogens, thiazide diuretics), or may represent an interaction between primary and secondary factors. Abnormalities can occur in (a) triglyceride-rich lipoprotein synthesis, (b) lipoprotein lipase-mediated triglyceride catabolism, (c) remnant lipoprotein catabolism, (d) cholesterol-rich lipoprotein catabolism, and (e) cholesterol-rich lipoprotein (LDL cholesterol) synthesis and absorption.

Increased Triglyceride Synthesis

The majority of triglyceride input is from the diet in normal individuals. However, abnormalities in the regulation of the endogenous production of triglyceride-rich VLDL are fairly common and are the most frequent causes of hypertriglyceridemia. They are associated with an increase in plasma levels of VLDL (type IV) or VLDL plus chylomicrons (type V). The underlying metabolic cause for endogenous hypertriglyceridemia is usually related to hyperinsulinemia and insulin resistance, due most often to obesity, the ingestion of excessive calories or alcohol, or the use of estrogens or corticosteroids.

The primary forms of endogenous hypertriglyceridemia, familial hypertriglyceridemia, and primary familial combined hyperlipidemia also appear to be related to an increase in the synthesis of triglyceride-rich lipoproteins. *Familial hypertriglyceridemia* results in an increase in the endogenous synthesis of large triglyceride-rich VLDL. Many such patients are obese and exhibit mild glucose intolerance, hyperinsulinemia, and clinical evidence of diabetes mellitus, conditions that contribute to the excessive hepatic production of VLDL triglyceride.

In contrast, patients with *familial combined hyperlipidemia* (multiple lipoprotein-type hyperlipidemia) exhibit an increase in the production of apo B, which can appear in VLDL, LDL, or both. Various lipoprotein types (IIA, IIB, or IV) are found in patients with familial combined hyperlipidemia, and the presenting sign can be an increase in either VLDL triglyceride or LDL cholesterol, or both. The clinical expressions of this disorder vary among individual patients depending on diet, the degree of obesity, the level of physical activity, and the concomitant use of other drugs.

Familial hypertriglyceridemia and familial combined hyperlipidemia are inherited as separate autosomal dominant disorders, each occurring in approximately 1% of the general population. Familial hypertriglyceridemia is not associated with xanthomas unless hyperchylomicronemia supervenes. Basal concentrations (after a 12-hour fast) of total triglycerides and VLDL triglycerides are characteristically

Table 75.4.
Classification of Lipoprotein Disorders by Phenotypes and Genotypes and Corresponding Clinical Manifestations

Phenotype	Lipoprotein in Excess	Plasma Lipid Levels		Plasma Appearance[a]	Genotype	Age of Onset (Primary Form)	Xanthomas[b]	Other Clinical Manifestations
		Cholesterol	Triglyceride					
I	Chylomicrons	Normal or ↑	↑↑↑ lipemia	Clear plasma, creamy supernatant	Familial lipoprotein lipases deficiency, Apo C-II deficiency	Infancy or childhood	Eruptive, tuberoeruptive	Recurrent abdominal pain, other gastrointestinal symptoms, lipemia retinalis, hepatosplenomegaly
IIA	LDL	↑↑↑	normal	Clear	Familial hypercholesterolemia; Familial combined hyperlipidemia; Polygenic and sporadic hypercholesterolemia	Childhood for homozygous FHC,[c] late childhood to middle age for heterozygous FHC, adulthood for others	Tendinous, xanthelasma, tuberous; planar (homozygous)	Premature CAD,[c] arcus corneae, aortic stenosis (homozygous FHC), arthritic symptoms
IIB	LDL + VLDL	↑↑	↑	Clear	Familial combined hyperlipidemia; Familial hypercholesterolemia			
III	β-VLDL, IDL	↑↑	↑↑	Slightly turbid	Familial dysbetalipoproteinemia	Adulthood (occasionally late adolescence)	Planar (especially palmar), tuberous	Premature CAD and peripheral vascular disease, male > female, obesity, abnormal glucose tolerance, hyperuricemia, aggravated by hypothyroidism, good response to therapy
IV	VLDL	Normal or ↑[d]	↑↑	Turbid	Familial hypertriglyceridemia; Familial combined hyperlipidemia; Sporadic hypertriglyceridemia	Early to late adulthood	Usually none; rarely eruptive, or tuberoeruptive	CAD and peripheral vascular disease, obesity, abnormal glucose tolerance, hyperuricemia, arthritic symptoms, gallbladder disease
V	Chylomicrons + VLDL	Normal or ↑	↑↑↑	Turbid plasma, creamy supernatant	Homozygous familial hypertriglyceridemia	Childhood to middle age, usually adulthood	Eruptive, tuberoeruptive	Recurrent abdominal pain, other gastrointestinal symptoms, lipemia retinalis, hepatosplenomegaly, peripheral paresthesias, abnormal glucose tolerance, hyperuricemia

[a] Plasma obtained after 12 hours of fasting, left undisturbed in refrigerator overnight.
[b] Seen only in a minority of patients, but the frequency increases as plasma lipid levels rise.
[c] FHC, familial hypercholesterolemia; CAD, coronary artery disease.
[d] Cholesterol normal if triglycerides < 400 mg/dl.

elevated, but plasma levels of total and LDL cholesterol are normal or low unless levels of VLDL cholesterol are also increased. Familial hypertriglyceridemia is not associated with an increased incidence of premature CAD; however, patients with familial combined hyperlipidemia are at high risk, primarily due to their increased plasma levels of apo B and abnormalities in the composition of HDL, reduced levels of apo A-I and HDL₂ (5). Familial combined hyperlipidemia may be present in as many as 10% of the survivors of myocardial infarction under the age of 60 and thus represents a common and important risk for atherosclerosis.

The diagnosis of these disorders of lipoprotein metabolism and their exact definition can only be established by family studies. A strongly positive family history of atherosclerosis favors the diagnosis of familial combined hyperlipidemia in those hypertriglyceridemic patients in whom secondary causes for hyperlipidemia have been excluded. Differentiating between these two disorders of lipoprotein metabolism is important in the evaluation of a patient with hyperlipidemia, particularly with regard to deciding whether therapeutic intervention is warranted for the prevention of CAD and its complications.

Occasionally, patients present with marked *hypertriglyceridemia and hyperchylomicronemia* (triglyceride levels greater than 1000 mg/dl), pancreatitis, eruptive xanthomas, and lipemia retinalis. Coexistence of familial hypertriglyceridemia or familial combined hyperlipidemia with either obesity, uremia, untreated diabetes mellitus, chronic alcoholism, or the use of corticosteroids, thiazide diuretics, or estrogens can result in this syndrome. The chylomicronemia syndrome requires immediate treatment with elimination of dietary fat, nasogastric suction, and treatment of the secondary causes. Prevention is the primary means to avoid recurrences, and frequently patients with primary hypertriglyceridemia receive lipid-lowering agents prophylactically (19).

Decreased Lipoprotein Lipase-Mediated Triglyceride Catabolism

LPL is the rate-limiting enzyme for the uptake and storage of triglyceride by adipose tissue or muscle tissue and for the processing of triglyceride-rich lipoproteins to chylomicrons and VLDL remnants. In patients with the autosomal recessive trait of *apo C-II deficiency*, LPL activity is normal, but marked hypertriglyceridemia is present (19). In contrast, in the more frequently encountered (yet also rare) autosomal recessive syndrome of *familial LPL deficiency*, marked hypertriglyceridemia and chylomicronemia are both evident and LPL activity is absent. The type I phenotypic pattern is more likely to occur in patients with the familial form of LPL deficiency, rather than in those with apo C-II deficiency; yet both conditions manifest themselves in childhood with episodes of eruptive xanthomas and with the acute abdominal pain of pancreatitis. Most adult patients who have an ac-

quired impairment in LPL function usually have moderately severe diabetes mellitus, hypothyroidism, end-stage renal disease, or dysgammaglobulinemia, or are receiving corticosteroids or thiazide diuretics. The severity of the lipoprotein abnormality seems to be directly related to the decrease in LPL activity in postheparin plasma and adipose tissue.

The hypertriglyceridemia can be controlled by restriction of dietary fat and substitution of carbohydrates or medium chain triglycerides as energy sources. Effective treatment of diabetes mellitus with diet, insulin, or an oral sulfonylurea normalizes LPL activity and plasma triglyceride levels within 3 months. Similar changes are seen after appropriate therapy of hypothyroidism with thyroxine or of uremia with renal transplantation.

LPL also plays a role in the formation of HDL₂ (see "Normal Physiology of Lipoprotein Transport" above). This mechanism appears to mediate the increase in HDL₂ seen in endurance-trained athletes (8) and in patients with primary hypercholesterolemia treated with colestipol. Hence, diseases associated with abnormalities in LPL frequently have concomitant reductions in HDL cholesterol.

Defective Remnant Lipoprotein Catabolism and Dysbetalipoproteinemia

Excessive accumulation of lipoprotein remnants in plasma is usually caused by a defect in their removal due to an autosomal recessive derangement in the structure of apo E (27). Apo E3, the predominant form of apo E in the normal population, is absent in patients with the classic form of dysbetalipoproteinemia (type III hyperlipoproteinemia). The mutation causing this syndrome results in the occurrence of an abnormal form of apo E. Of the 1% of individuals homozygous for this condition, only 1 to 2% will exhibit hyperlipoproteinemia clinically.

Dysbetalipoproteinemia (remnant removal disease or broad β disease) has served as a prototype for the study of remnant lipoprotein metabolism. It appears that several defects in lipoprotein metabolism are required before excessive accumulation of IDL and of cholesterol-enriched β-VLDL can occur. The diagnosis is suggested by the initial findings of β (rather than pre-β)-VLDL and similarly elevated plasma concentrations of cholesterol and triglyceride. It is made more likely by the finding of an abnormally cholesterol-rich VLDL fraction (ratio of VLDL cholesterol to VLDL triglyceride of >0.42). The presence of tuberous and planar xanthomas (Fig. 75.3) is virtually pathognomonic for the disorder. Definitive diagnosis, however, requires analysis of VLDL to demonstrate the absence of apo E3. A strong association between this lipoprotein disorder and atherosclerosis of the coronary arteries and peripheral vessels has been reported and appears to diminish during treatment.

The accumulation of remnants in plasma is also found in certain patients with hypothyroidism, end-stage renal disease, and liver disease. The latter disorders are as-

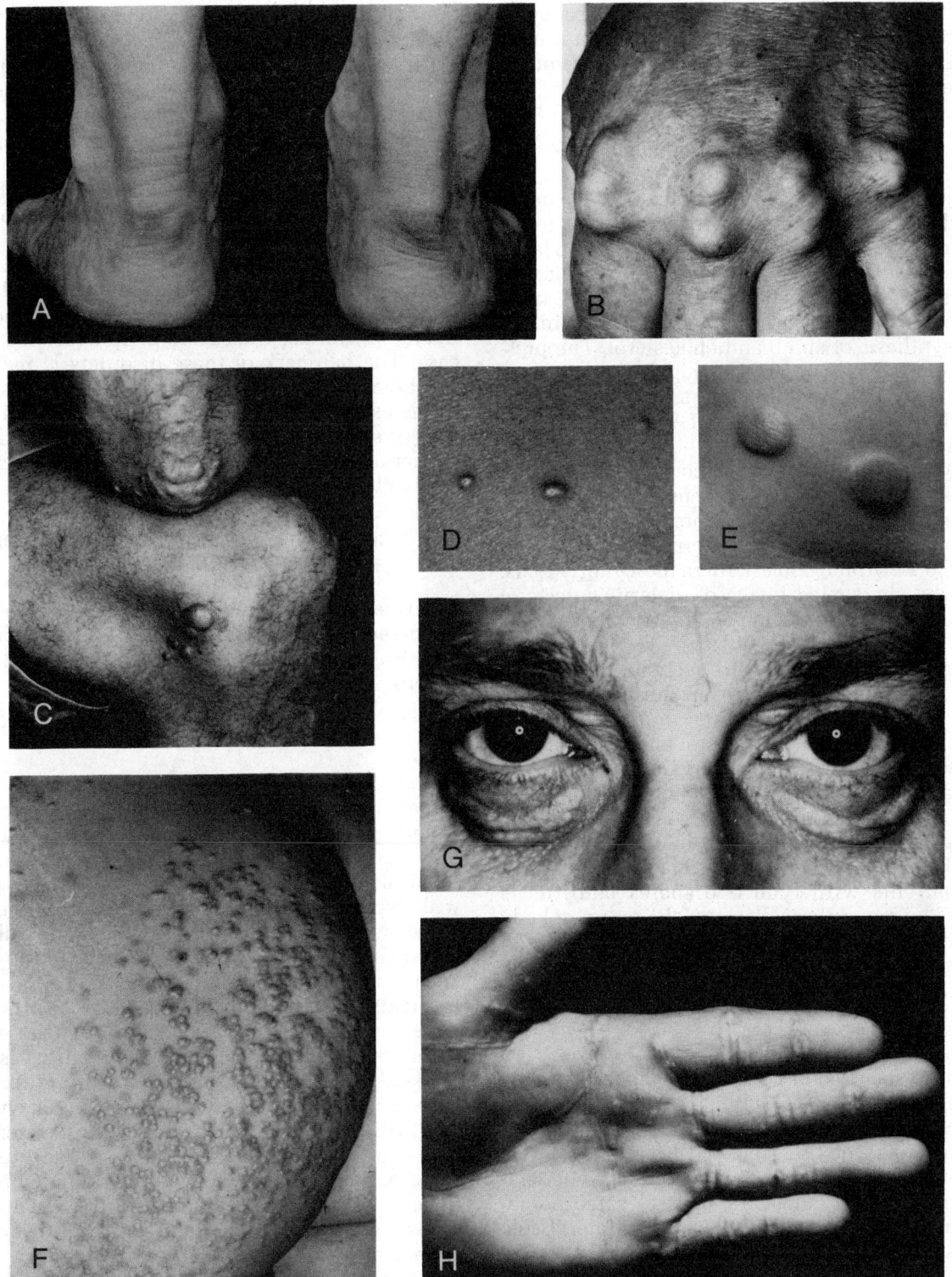

Figure 75.3. Dermatological manifestations of lipid disorders. *A.* Tendinous xanthomas. *B.* Tuberous xanthomas. *C.* Tuberous xanthomas. *D.* Eruptive xanthomas. *E.* Planar xanthomas. *F.* Eruptive xanthomas. *G.* Planar xanthomas on eyelids (xanthelasma). *H.* Planar xanthomas confined to palm creases (xanthoma striata palmaris).

sociated with an increase in the activity of the enzyme hepatic lipase, suggesting that a relationship may exist between this enzyme and the catabolism of remnant lipoproteins by the liver.

Increased Cholesterol Synthesis

The accumulation of cholesterol-rich LDL can occur as a result of an increased input of cholesterol into the plasma from dietary or endogenous sources. The latter occurs because of an increase in HMG CoA reductase activity and enhanced synthesis of cholesterol, or as a consequence of a primary genetic increase in the hepatic synthesis of apo B and cholesterol. The presence of apo B-enriched VLDL is highly suggestive of a genetic disorder of overproduction of apo B, as compared with the overproduction of VLDL triglyceride in familial hypertriglyceridemia.

The overproduction of apo B-containing LDL and VLDL leads to an increased propensity for the development of atherosclerosis (5). Moreover, the coexistence of obesity promotes the overproduction of apo B-enriched VLDL and cholesterol in these individuals. Finally, the augmented intake of dietary cholesterol usually contributes to the hypercholesterolemia characteristic of these patients.

Primary (sporadic) forms of hypercholesterolemia, with a genetic defect in the steps controlling the rate of hepatic synthesis of cholesterol from acetate, lead to an overproduction of cholesterol and resultant hypercholesterolemia. Usually dietary therapy involving an increase in polyunsaturated fat and a reduction in sucrose and simple carbohydrates is helpful in the treatment of these disorders; less often, drugs are required. Hypercholesterolemia in obese hyperinsulinemic patients with type II diabetes mellitus is decreased by hypocaloric diets and the return of body weight toward normal. In patients noncompliant with dietary measures, therapy with cholestyramine or nicotinic acid is usually effective in lowering plasma levels of cholesterol.

Defective Removal of Low Density Lipoproteins

Isolated primary elevations of plasma LDL or combined elevations of LDL and VLDL can be seen in affected members of families with familial hypercholesterolemia (3). Although the cells of some homozygous patients may be totally lacking in identifiable LDL (apo B-E) receptors, in other patients these receptors are present but functionally defective. Individuals heterozygous for familial hypercholesterolemia exhibit greater than a 50% reduction in LDL receptor number or a 50% defect in receptor-mediated catabolism; commonly their plasma levels of LDL cholesterol are elevated above 400 mg/dl regardless of their level of cholesterol synthesis. In patients who are homozygous, plasma levels of LDL cholesterol may reach 1000 mg/dl (19). Documentation of abnormal receptor binding in cultures of skin fibroblasts is necessary for the precise diagnosis of individuals with familial hypercholesterolemia.

Although primary causes (including familial combined hyperlipoproteinemia) predominate, secondary etiologies for increased concentrations of LDL cholesterol occur in patients with hypothyroidism, nephrotic syndrome, multiple myeloma, obstructive liver disease, and porphyria and in patients who have ingested excessive amounts of dietary cholesterol. Whatever the cause of the LDL accumulation in the plasma, the primary forms are associated with marked susceptibility to CAD and a high frequency of complications associated with early mortality, such as myocardial infarction, stroke, and severe peripheral vascular disease. The hallmark of these disorders is the tendon xanthomas that frequently affect the Achilles tendon or the extensor tendon of the forearm and hand (Fig. 75.3). Patients with secondary hypercholesterolemia appear not to develop atherosclerosis at as high a rate as people with the primary disorders.

COMMON SECONDARY DISORDERS OF LIPOPROTEIN METABOLISM

Several disease states are commonly associated with increased plasma levels of VLDL, elevated levels of both VLDL and LDL, or decreased levels of HDL cholesterol.

Diabetes Mellitus

Abnormalities in fat transport are frequently noted in patients with diabetes mellitus and are related to abnormalities in insulin action or insulin availability that lead to increased production and/or decreased removal of plasma lipoproteins. For example, patients with type II diabetes mellitus who are often obese, hyperinsulinemic, and insulin resistant exhibit both an enhanced production and reduced plasma clearance of triglycerides. These patients also have abnormalities in HDL cholesterol. In contrast, the hypertriglyceridemia that occurs in patients with insulin-dependent (type I) diabetes mellitus is due to markedly reduced levels of LPL activity, since insulin is required for normal synthesis of the enzyme (19). The diabetic lipemia syndrome is characterized by low or absent levels of LPL in the plasma and tissues of these patients. Although the underlying enzyme deficiency can be reversed after insulin repletion, normalization of the lipoprotein abnormalities can take as long as 3 months.

In the treated diabetic patient, variability in plasma levels of lipoprotein lipids is primarily related to dietary factors, body weight, physical activity, and the degree of glycemic control. If glucose tolerance deteriorates because of inadequate insulin administration or increased insulin resistance, severe hypertriglyceridemia may ensue and alter the concentrations of other classes of lipoproteins. In well-treated type I diabetic patients, plasma levels of HDL cholesterol are increased; in contrast, patients with type II diabetes usually have low plasma levels of HDL cholesterol. Regardless of the specific treatment or type of diabetes mellitus, women ordinarily exhibit higher plasma levels of VLDL triglyceride and LDL cholesterol, and lower levels of HDL cholesterol, than do diabetic men (36). This may explain the increased prevalence of atherosclerosis in diabetic women and the disappearance of the usual preponderance of atherosclerotic disease in men compared with premenopausal women (20).

Hypercholesterolemia, with increased plasma concentrations of LDL cholesterol and apo B, also can occur in patients with either type I or type II diabetes mellitus and is usually induced by diet. Intensive therapy with diet, exercise, and insulin usually normalizes lipoprotein levels unless a genetic lipoprotein disorder coexists.

Hyperlipidemia in the patient with diabetes mellitus increases the risk for the major complications of atherosclerosis, CAD, cerebrovascular disease, and peripheral vascular disease. The severity of peripheral vascular disease has been associated with the lipoprotein abnormalities in diabetic women. Whether treatment of the lipid abnormalities in diabetic patients will decrease their risk for CAD and other arteriosclerotic complications remains to be tested.

Chronic Uremia and Treatment with Dialysis

Many patients with chronic uremia have increased plasma levels of VLDL triglycerides and decreased levels of HDL cholesterol (13). These abnormalities persist during maintenance hemodialysis or peritoneal dialysis. The accelerated atherosclerosis observed in white versus black men undergoing chronic hemodialysis appears to be related to the abnormal composition of HDL$_2$ cholesterol in the plasmas of white men. A sedentary life style, obesity, high fat diets, or treatment with corticosteroids, β-blockers, or androgens worsens the lipoprotein profiles in these patients, whereas effective reversal of these secondary causes improves the lipid profile (13).

Hypothyroidism

Adequate levels of thyroid hormone appear to be necessary for the proper function of the lipoprotein cascade. Decreases in LDL receptor function, abnormalities in LPL and hepatic lipase-mediated metabolism of triglycerides and HDL, and reduced LCAT activity have been demonstrated in some patients with hypothyroidism. Consequently, increased plasma levels of VLDL, IDL, and LDL and reduced levels of HDL cholesterol have all been reported in patients with this disease. Treatment with thyroid hormone improves LDL receptor function, increases the activity and function of LPL and LCAT, and normalizes lipoprotein profiles.

Other Common Secondary Causes of Hyperlipidemia

Patients with the *nephrotic syndrome* frequently lose apo C-II in the urine, thus decreasing LPL-mediated triglyceride clearance. The hypoalbuminemia that accompanies the nephrotic syndrome increases hepatic VLDL synthesis, thereby elevating plasma levels of VLDL triglyceride and LDL cholesterol. Treatment of the primary disease causing the nephrotic syndrome usually corrects the lipoprotein abnormalities, but drug and diet (low fat) therapy may be required.

Hypercortisolemia of endogenous or exogenous origin increases hepatic synthesis of VLDL, LDL, or both. Kidney transplant recipients treated with high doses of corticosteroids frequently exhibit elevated plasma levels of both VLDL and LDL as well as reduced levels of HDL cholesterol. The atherosclerosis that develops in such patients is probably related to these lipid abnormalities, which should be treated accordingly.

Obesity, alcohol ingestion, and *androgen administration* tend to increase hepatic lipoprotein synthesis but have different effects on levels of HDL cholesterol and LDL cholesterol. In obese individuals, plasma levels of VLDL triglyceride and LDL cholesterol are increased, whereas those of HDL are decreased. Mild alcohol ingestion (up to 2 ounces/day) increases levels of VLDL triglyceride and HDL cholesterol but lowers levels of LDL cholesterol. Exogenous androgens raise levels of LDL cholesterol and lower HDL cholesterol levels. Diseases affecting the liver, such as hepatitis or cholelithiasis, alter lipoprotein metabolism. Diseases causing an obstruction in the hepatobiliary system tend to elevate plasma LDL, IDL, and remnant lipoproteins and cause abnormal lipoproteins (Lp X) to accumulate in plasma. Inflammatory processes usually lower levels of HDL and LDL cholesterol and raise VLDL depending on the nutritional state of the patient. Drugs used to treat hypertension, particularly thiazide diuretics and β-adrenergic blockers, raise levels of VLDL and LDL and lower levels of HDL cholesterol. Weight loss or the discontinuation of alcohol or these drugs usually normalizes lipoprotein profiles.

Hyperlipidemia occurs in patients with *systemic lupus erythematosus* or *dysgammaglobulinemia*. This may be related to interactions among amyloid protein, certain immunoglobulin fractions, and various steps in the lipoprotein cascade.

Table 75.3 lists common secondary causes for disordered lipoprotein metabolism. Table 75.5 lists the effect of several exogenous and endogenous factors on plasma levels of HDL cholesterol.

CLINICAL MANIFESTATIONS OF LIPOPROTEIN DISORDERS

Adverse clinical sequelae of the lipoprotein disorders most frequently manifest themselves as disorders of the vascular, dermatological, and gastrointestinal systems. The clinical manifestations associated with each of the major disorders of lipoprotein metabolism are outlined in Table 75.4.

Vascular

As discussed previously, elevated levels of total cholesterol, LDL cholesterol, and apo B-enriched lip-

Table 75.5.
Factors That Affect HDL Cholesterol Levels

Increase	Decrease
Exercise	Androgens (male sex, drugs)
Estrogens (female sex)	In males, puberty
Alcohol	In females, menopause
Familial (hyperalphalipo-	Obesity
proteinemia)	Hypertriglyceridemia
Leanness	Type II diabetes mellitus
Antihyperlipidemic drugs:	Familial hypoalphalipoproteinemia
Nicotinic acid, colestipol,	(Tangier's disease)
clofibrate, lovastatin	Cigarettes
gemfibrozil	Sedentary life style
Insulin	Probucol
IV Heparin	Uremia
	Vegetarian diet
	Progestogens

oproteins, and decreased levels of HDL cholesterol, HDL_2, and apo A-I, contribute to the development of atherosclerotic disease. The earlier the onset of symptomatic disease of the coronary, cerebral, or peripheral vasculature, the more likely it is that a lipoprotein abnormality and/or another major risk factor (cigarette smoking, hypertension, diabetes) is present (20). In the most severe form of hypercholesterolemia, homozygous familial hypercholesterolemia, plasma levels of total cholesterol vary from 600 to 1200 mg/dl, CAD generally develops in childhood, and very few patients survive past age 30. In heterozygotes, plasma levels of total cholesterol vary from about 270 to 550 mg/dl, and the time of onset of CAD varies between early adulthood and late middle age, with about 50% of men and women becoming symptomatic by age 50 and 60, respectively. Patients with monogenic familial combined hyperlipoproteinemia exhibit elevated levels of VLDL, LDL, or both, as well as abnormalities in HDL, apo A, and apo B; most patients manifest symptoms of CAD by age 60. Individuals with familial dysbetalipoproteinemia develop premature peripheral vascular disease and CAD at about equal rates, with the mean age of onset in both men and women of about 40. Such patients seem to be especially amenable to therapy. Individuals with monogenic familial hypertriglyceridemia or with fasting chylomicronemia do not appear to be at increased risk for CAD unless other risk factors for atherosclerosis are also present.

Dermatological

Xanthomas may occur in all of the hyperlipidemias; however, they are present in a minority of hyperlipidemic individuals. They occur with increasing frequency as the plasma lipid levels rise. They are present predominantly in the primary forms of hyperlipoproteinemia: familial hypercholesterolemia, familial dysbetalipoproteinemia, and familial LPL deficiency. Xanthomas are cutaneous and/or subcutaneous papules, plaques, or nodules characterized histopathologically by localized collections of lipid-laden histiocytes (foam cells). The presence or absence of xanthomas should always be noted. If present, their appearance (see below) can provide useful information about the nature of the underlying lipid disorder (Table 75.4). Unless tendons (especially the Achilles tendon) are palpated, tendon thickening characteristic of tendon xanthomas may be missed. Xanthomas are divided morphologically into several types:

1. *Tendinous* (Fig. 75.3 *A*)—firm subcutaneous masses that arise in tendons and occasionally in ligaments, fascia, or periosteum. They characteristically move in concert with the associated tendon and can appear as diffuse thickenings of the tendon. They most often occur on the Achilles tendons and the extensor tendons of the hands, knees, and elbows. The overlying skin is normal in color.
2. *Tuberous* (Fig. 75.3 *B and C*)—soft cutaneous and subcutaneous nodules that may harden with age and increasing fibrosis. Occasionally, they occur as superficial extensions of tendon xanthomas. They can also form from the confluence of eruptive xanthomas, an intermediate stage being called tuberoeruptive xanthomas. They occur most often on extensor surfaces and areas subjected to trauma, such as the elbows, knees, dorsa of the hands, heels, and buttocks. The overlying epidermis can be normal in color or have a yellow or orange hue.
3. *Eruptive* (Fig. 75.3 *D and F*)—small (1 to 4 mm) cutaneous papules, that tend to appear in crops, often coincident with an abrupt rise in plasma triglyceride levels. Compared with the other types of xanthomas, they contain more inflammatory cells, free fatty acids, and triglycerides and fewer foam cells and cholesterol esters. They most often occur over pressure areas, such as the buttocks, parts of the trunk, elbows, and knees. They often have a yellow center and red halo.
4. Planar (Fig. 75.3 *E, G, and H*)—flat, slightly elevated cutaneous lesions that occur most often in skin folds and scars but can be more widely distributed. When present on the eyelids, they are called *xanthelasma*. When located on the palms, they are called palmar xanthomas, and when confined to the palmar creases, *xanthoma striata palmaris*. They tend to be yellow or yellow-brown.

Hypercholesterolemia is associated with tendinous, planar, and tuberous xanthomas. Severe hypertriglyceridemia and chylomicronemia are associated with eruptive and occasionally tuberoeruptive or tuberous xanthomas. Palmar xanthomas are characteristic of familial dysbetalipoproteinemia and florid obstructive liver disease. Planar xanthomas on the body or palms in the presence of a type II lipid profile suggest homozygous monogenic familial hypercholesterolemia. The presence of tendinous or tuberous xanthomas or premature xanthelasma with a type II lipid profile suggests either heterozygous or homozygous monogenic familial hypercholesterolemia, as opposed to the polygenic or nongenetic forms. Tendon xanthomas are found in one-third to one-half of heterozygotes, whereas tuberous xanthomas are seen most often in patients with familial dysbetalipoproteinemia.

Occasionally, xanthomas appear in the absence of a hyperlipidemic state. For example, xanthelasma occur commonly in normolipidemic older individuals and in nonwhites, whereas planar xanthomas can occur in patients with lymphoma, leukemia, or myeloma. Studies in normolipidemic individuals with xanthelasma have revealed abnormalities in apo B and E suggestive of familial dysbetalipoproteinemia and/or elevated levels of LDL apo B, suggesting that these individuals may be at an increased risk of developing atherosclerosis.

Differences exist in the responses to treatment of the various hyperlipidemia-associated xanthomas. Thus, tendon xanthomas are the most resistant to treatment and, in practice, seldom disappear. In contrast, eruptive and planar xanthomas can disappear within a few weeks after return of plasma lipid levels toward normal.

Gastrointestinal

As many as 35 to 55% of patients with fasting chylomicronemia experience episodes of recurrent abdominal pain. Symptoms are ordinarily associated with marked elevations of plasma triglyceride levels (greater than 1000 to 2000 mg/dl). Abdominal pain may be so severe that it prompts unnecessary surgery, particularly if the lipid disorder is not suspected. The pain is often associated with pancreatitis, although the responsible pathogenetic mechanism is not well understood. It should be noted that routine serum amylase determinations are frequently subject to technical artifact when hyperlipidemia is present, due to the presence of an amylase-inhibiting factor that may or may not be triglyceride. In such cases, a more reliable estimate of the serum amylase value can be obtained by determining amylase levels on serial dilutions, until the value obtained no longer changes with further dilution. Another cause of abdominal pain may be rapid hepatic or splenic enlargement with capsular distension due to triglyceride deposition in reticuloendothelial cells. Often the cause is unclear. Gastrointestinal symptoms other than abdominal pain, such as nausea, vomiting, borborygmi, and diarrhea, also occur.

Other Clinical Associations

Other clinical concomitants of hyperlipidemia include the following: premature arcus corneae (grayish-white corneal ring due to lipid droplets) in hypercholesterolemia (elevated LDL); aortic stenosis in homozygous monogenic familial hypercholesterolemia; Achilles tendonitis in heterozygous monogenic familial hypercholesterolemia; obesity, glucose intolerance, hyperinsulinemia, hyperuricemia, and perhaps cholelithiasis in association with hypertriglyceridemia and elevated VLDL; recurrent polyarthralgias, arthritis, tenosynovitis, and sicca-like syndromes in hypertriglycer-

idemia (elevated VLDL) or hypercholesterolemia (elevated LDL); lipemia retinalis (cream-colored retinal vessels) in chylomicronemia (evident when plasma triglycerides rise above 3000 mg/dl; obvious when they exceed 10,000 mg/dl).

DIAGNOSIS

Indications for Evaluation

There is controversy about the optimal, cost-effective approach to the identification of hyperlipidemic persons at high risk for CAD (2, 11, 21). At present, the most widely used guidelines for case findings are those issued by the Adult Treatment Panel of the National Cholesterol Education Program (NCEP), which recommended that levels of total cholesterol should be measured in all adults 20 years of age or older at least once every 5 years, assuming blood cholesterol levels are below 200 mg/dl. The NCEP has published a schema for classifying individuals by measurements of serum levels of total and LDL cholesterol. In this classification, serum levels of total cholesterol less than 200 mg/dl are considered to represent a "desirable blood cholesterol"; levels from 200 to 239 mg/dl, to indicate a "borderline-high blood cholesterol"; and levels 240 mg/dl or above, to signify a "high blood cholesterol." Data from numerous epidemiological studies reveal that the relationships between serum levels of total (or LDL) cholesterol and CAD risk are continuous, and that CAD risk at a cholesterol value of 240 mg/dl is nearly double that at 200 mg/dl and rises rapidly at levels above 240 mg/dl. Total cholesterol levels of 240 mg/dl or more correspond to the uppermost 25% of cholesterol values in the entire population 20 years of age and older. Patients with levels of total serum cholesterol between 200 and 239 mg/dl and either known CAD or two or more known risk factors for CAD (see Table 75.6) are considered to have high blood cholesterol values.

Once a patient is found to have a high blood cholesterol level, or physical stigmata of hypercholesterolemia (e.g., dermatological signs), decisions regarding possible diet, drug, or other therapy are made after a more detailed lipoprotein analysis, including measurements of triglyceride and HDL levels on a blood

Table 75.6.
CAD RISK FACTORS AS DEFINED BY THE 1987 NCEP ADULT TREATMENT GUIDELINES[a]

Male gender
Family history of CAD before 55 years of age (parent or sibling)
Cigarette smoking
Hypertension
Diabetes mellitus
Definite cerebrovascular or peripheral vascular disease
Obesity ($\geq$30% overweight)
Known low HDL-C (<35 mg/dl)

[a] From The Johns Hopkins Physicians Lipid Education Program, 2nd ed. The Johns Hopkins University, Baltimore, 1988, p. 9.

specimen obtained after an overnight fast, calculation of the LDL cholesterol level (see below), and determination of other CAD risk factors. An LDL cholesterol level of 160 mg/dl or more is considered to represent a "high-risk LDL cholesterol," whereas levels of LDL cholesterol from 130 to 159 mg/dl signify "borderline high-risk" and LDL levels less than 130 mg/dl are considered to be "desirable." In patients with known CAD or two or more major CAD risk factors, LDL cholesterol levels from 130 to 159 mg/dl are considered to be "high-risk." Of additional note is that the NCEP considers an HDL level less than 35 mg/dl to be an independent risk factor for CAD. Thus, decisions regarding both the implementation and goals of therapy are based not on ratios of LDL (or total) cholesterol to HDL cholesterol but on absolute levels of LDL cholesterol. Such decisions are also influenced by the presence or absence of other CAD risk factors, one of which is an HDL level less than 35 mg/dl.

It is important to emphasize that assignment of risk levels using total and LDL cholesterol cut-off values, and the therapeutic actions that are based upon these values (see below), derive from studies in middle-aged men and have not yet been proved to be applicable to young and elderly men, or to women (2, 11, 21). Nonetheless, given the increasing evidence favoring the lipid (or cholesterol) hypothesis, most authorities believe it is appropriate to apply the diagnostic guidelines described above to all adult population groups.

Both the NCEP and the National Institutes of Health Consensus Development Conference on Treatment of Hypertriglyceridemia have considered fasting triglyceride levels greater than 500 mg/dl to represent "definite hypertriglyceridemia," levels from 250 to 500 mg/dl to signify "borderline hypertriglyceridemia," and levels less than 250 mg/dl to be normal. Some investigators, however, feel that fasting triglyceride levels between 150 to 249 mg/dl should be considered "borderline hypertriglyceridemia" and that only triglyceride levels less than 150 mg/dl are normal. As already noted, there is little evidence that hypertriglyceridemia per se is a risk factor for CAD in the absence of cholesterol abnormalities.

A more complete evaluation including measurement of plasma levels of total cholesterol, HDL cholesterol, and fasting triglyceride and calculation of the level of LDL cholesterol (see below) is desirable when (a) abnormalities are detected on screening; (b) there is a high suspicion of lipoprotein abnormalities (premature CAD, strong family history, xanthomata, etc.); or (c) conditions coexist that could cause secondary abnormalities in lipoprotein metabolism. Although the frequencies with which certain drugs (e.g., thiazide diuretics, antihypertensives, oral contraceptives) adversely affect lipoprotein metabolism are unknown, and direct causal interrelationships between such drug-associated lipid abnormalities and premature atherosclerosis are unproved, it seems prudent also to consider the more complete evaluation before therapy is initiated with these drugs.

Laboratory Evaluation

Serum levels of total cholesterol are not appreciably influenced by acute dietary intake and thus can be obtained from patients in the nonfasting state and at any time of the day. Cholesterol levels can also be measured in plasma, but the results should be multiplied by 1.03 to obtain the equivalent serum value. There is considerable biological variability in total cholesterol levels, with repeated measurements on the same person showing a standard deviation of as much as 18 mg/dl (37). Thus, the 95% confidence interval of a patient with a total cholesterol value of 220 mg/dl would be 184 to 256 mg/dl. In addition, both intra- and interlaboratory errors in measurement are common. Current estimates are that as many as one-half of all laboratory determinations of total cholesterol vary by 5% or more from the correct value, although several groups have proposed methods to reduce these errors in accuracy and precision to about 3% within the next several years. Thus, it remains important to obtain blood for cholesterol measurements from a non-stressed patient, to send the blood for measurement to a reliable laboratory, and to average the results of at least two to three measurements before final classification of the patient by total cholesterol level. Because measurements of HDL cholesterol are dependent upon the prevailing level of triglycerides, HDL cholesterol levels should be determined in patients after a standard 12- to 15-hour overnight fast.

Levels of total (and LDL) cholesterol fall during the first few days after myocardial infarction (14) so that cholesterol determinations should be made either within 24 hours of a severe acute myocardial infarction (when they are still valid) or postponed until 3 to 4 weeks after recovery. Fasting triglyceride (and VLDL) levels tend to rise slowly after a myocardial infarction, peaking at about 3 to 4 weeks and returning to baseline by 8 to 12 weeks. Triglyceride levels should, therefore, be obtained either within 24 hours of the acute event or delayed for 8 to 12 weeks.

The determination of HDL cholesterol is the measurement most subject to laboratory error. The precision of its measurement was inadequate in the majority of clinical laboratories surveyed by the Centers for Disease Control, Atlanta. It is, therefore, important for each physician periodically to assess the performance of an individual laboratory against one that is rigidly standardized. Repetition of the baseline measurement provides a further safeguard. Such measures to enhance validity are important, since there is a relatively narrow range of HDL cholesterol values within which even small differences are prognostically important. For example, a reduction in the level of HDL cholesterol of 5 mg/dl from 40 to 35 mg/dl increases the risk for CAD by about 25%. When triglyceride levels exceed 400 mg/dl, the standardized techniques for the precipitation of VLDL and LDL are ineffective and HDL cholesterol levels are unreliable. The plasma can be ultrafiltered to remove the interfering VLDL. If this is required, the physician should consult the laboratory. Despite these problems, the level of HDL cholesterol represents a potent index of CAD risk, an aid to diagnosis, and an important measure to follow during therapy. It also allows one to calculate LDL cholesterol (LDL-C) levels (provided triglyceride level is below 400 mg/dl) by the formula: $LDL\text{-}C = TC\text{-}(TG/5 + HDL\text{-}C)$, where TC is plasma level of total cholesterol, TG is fasting plasma triglyceride level, and HDL-C is the level of HDL cholesterol.

Observation of a fasting plasma sample, which has been left undisturbed overnight in a refrigerator at 4°C, is indicated in the presence of a significantly elevated fasting plasma triglyceride level. Elevated levels of total (or LDL) cholesterol do not affect the appearance of plasma, whereas hypertriglyceridemia associated with increased levels of VLDL imparts uniform turbidity to plasma, and hypertriglyceridemia associated with chylomicronemia is characterized by a creamy supernatant fraction that floats on the top of plasma.

A marked abnormality in serum lipid levels, especially marked hypertriglyceridemia (triglyceride >2000 mg/dl), can affect the validity of other laboratory tests. Marked hypertriglyceridemia has an inhibitory effect on the serum amylase assay, interferes with the measurement of liver enzymes (aspartate aminotransferase, alanine aminotransferase) and calcium by autoanalyzer, and causes artifactual reductions in the serum concentration of molecules restricted to the aqueous phase, such as sodium. Ultracentrifugation of plasma, with the removal of chylomicrons, permits these measurements to be performed accurately; but sometimes serial dilutions of the plasma are necessary, particularly for the measurement of amylase.

Clinical Evaluation

Clinical data contribute substantially to the diagnosis of specific lipoprotein disorders. History, physical examination, and indicated laboratory evaluation are required to rule out secondary causes of hyperlipidemia (Table 75.3). A positive family history, the presence of premature atherosclerotic disease, and the presence of specific dermatological manifestations may permit the diagnosis of a primary form of hyperlipoproteinemia (see Table 75.4).

Referral

When laboratory and clinical evaluations do not result in a clear-cut diagnosis of a lipoprotein disorder, referral to a specialist in endocrinology and metabolism is indicated. Such specialists can perform (or readily obtain) and interpret more sophisticated tests, such as ultracentrifugal quantification of lipoprotein levels, apoprotein measurement, receptor analysis, and determination of LPL activity. They may also assist in the evaluation of family members, so that the presence of a genetic disorder can be accurately diagnosed.

TREATMENT

General Considerations

The first step in the management of a lipoprotein disorder is accurate diagnosis. Secondary causes should be identified (Table 75.3) and treated. If the secondary cause is not reversible or a primary disorder exists, treatment may be required that is specifically directed at the abnormal lipoprotein pattern.

Such treatment should be part of the comprehensive management of other coexisting CAD risk factors (such as cigarette smoking, hypertension, diabetes mellitus, obesity, and inactivity). It will likely require behavioral change on the part of the patient and lifelong management, emphasizing the need for a positive patient-physician relationship, appropriate patient education, and skill on the part of the physician in using maneuvers to improve patient compliance (see Chapters 3 and 4). The long-term follow-up and monitoring of various parameters in such patients are necessary to enhance compliance, assess the effectiveness of therapy, and detect drug toxicity or the effect of concomitant therapy on plasma lipids (e.g., diuretics and other antihypertensive agents).

Patients classified as having a "desirable" total cholesterol level (<200 mg/dl) are usually instructed on the principles of a prudent diet and healthy life-style, educated about CAD risk factors (Table 75.6), and advised to have their total cholesterol levels rechecked at least once every 5 years. Patients with high total cholesterol levels (>240 mg/dl) undergo lipoprotein analysis and are advised about specific therapy depending upon their LDL cholesterol levels. Patients with "borderline-high" cholesterol values (200 to 239 mg/dl) who have neither CAD nor evidence of two CAD risk factors are advised to follow a Step 1 diet (see below) and to be re-evaluated yearly with repeated measurements of total cholesterol, as well as reassessment for CAD risk factors and dietary compliance. In contrast, those patients with borderline-high cholesterol values and either CAD or evidence of two or more CAD risk factors (male sex is considered to be one risk factor) are advised to undergo lipoprotein analysis, with treatment predicated on the levels of LDL cholesterol.

Treatment of hypercholesterolemia is based upon the results of lipoprotein analyses and determinations of LDL cholesterol levels. It is suggested that two or three measurements be performed 1 to 8 weeks apart, and that decisions about definitive therapy be based upon the average of these LDL cholesterol values. Patients with a "desirable" LDL cholesterol (<130 mg/dl) are treated as if the total blood cholesterol is also in the desirable range, and they are advised to follow a prudent diet and to repeat the LDL cholesterol measurement within 5 years. Patients with LDL cholesterol values between 130 and 159 mg/dl and neither CAD nor evidence of two or more CAD risk factors should be treated with the Step 1 diet and be re-evaluated yearly with total cholesterol measurements and reassessments of CAD risk factors and dietary compliance. Patients with LDL cholesterol values between 130 and 159 mg/dl and with CAD or two or more CAD risk factors and individuals with LDL cholesterol values greater than 160 mg/dl should be evaluated first for possible secondary causes of hypercholesterolemia before being advised about specific dietary or drug therapy. In addition, first-degree family relatives should be screened for hypercholesterolemia.

Management of hypertriglyceridemia must be individualized. When familial combined hyperlipidemia or familial dysbetalipoproteinemia is diagnosed, specific treatment is required. Patients with fasting triglyceride levels above 500 mg/dl sometimes accumulate chylomicrons and develop pancreatitis. The risk becomes substantial when triglyceride levels exceed 1000 mg/dl. The plasma triglyceride level should therefore be lowered in these patients. Individuals with familial hypertriglyceridemia or fasting triglyceride levels in the 250 to 500 mg/dl range in the absence of other CAD risk factors do not seem to be at increased risk of CAD or pancreatitis. Treatment is recommended only when risk factors coexist, such as (a) a family history of premature CAD; (b) abnormal levels of total (or LDL) cholesterol, HDL cholesterol, or apoproteins; (c) concomitant CAD, diabetes, end-stage renal disease, smoking, or obesity; and (d) young age. Isolated fasting triglyceride levels below 250 mg/dl do not require treatment.

Nonpharmacological Therapy

Diet (Tables 75.7 and 75.8)

It is now well established that plasma lipid levels can be altered by dietary manipulations. Under strictly controlled conditions (such as in a metabolic unit), elevated plasma levels of total (or LDL) cholesterol may be reduced by as much as 30% or more and levels of triglyceride or VLDL (in the presence of marked elevations) by as much as 80% or more. Fasting chylomicronemia can also be eliminated. Under ambu-

latory conditions, in which diets tend to be less restrictive and noncompliance more common, reductions in lipid levels are less dramatic. For example, among prospective studies of cholesterol-lowering diets, the decrease in plasma cholesterol averaged 15% (range, 8.5 to 22%).

Single diet approach (Table 75.7). It is now appreciated that one diet can be used to treat all of the common forms of hyperlipoproteinemia. As recommended by the NCEP, the diet consists of caloric restriction to attain ideal body weight (see Chapter 76), reduction of cholesterol intake to less than 300 mg/day, a decrease in total fat to less than 30% of total calories, and restriction of saturated fat to no more than 10% of calories, so that a polyunsaturated:saturated (P:S) fat ratio of 1:1 is achieved. There is a concomitant increase in the proportion of complex carbohydrate and fiber in the diet. Sodium intake is also reduced. Using the principle of "graduated regimen implementation" (see Chapter 4), the diet can be introduced in two steps, with the second step introducing further restrictions in dietary total fat, saturated fat, and cholesterol (Table 75.7). Step I represents the American Heart Association (AHA) "prudent diet," which is recommended for the entire American population. When severe chylomicronemia is present, more severe restriction of dietary fat is required (see below).

The AHA and other organizations publish useful booklets on this diet for the patient, physician, and nutritionist (see "General References"). Most patients with hyperlipoproteinemia will benefit from referral to a suitably trained dietitian.

The single diet actually incorporates several nutritional strategies, each of which tends to have a selective effect on plasma lipoprotein levels. It is helpful to consider each strategy separately.

Cholesterol reduction (Tables 75.7 and 75.8). The Step 1 diet to lower serum cholesterol levels is characterized by a restriction of dietary cholesterol to less than 300 mg/day, and reductions in daily total and saturated fat intake to less than 30 and 10% of caloric intake, respectively. The Step 2 diet further decreases cholesterol intake to less than 200 mg/day, and the intake of saturated fat to less than 7% of daily caloric intake. Caloric allowance is adjusted to ensure loss of excess weight or maintenance of ideal body weight (see Chapter 76). Restrictions in dietary cholesterol and saturated fats independently contribute to the reduction in plasma cholesterol levels. A modest increase in dietary polyunsaturated fat will result in further, though less marked, reduction in plasma cholesterol level.

The two major categories of polyunsaturated fatty acids are the omega-6 and omega-3 types. Linoleic acid is the principal omega-6 fatty acid and, when consumed in large amounts, can decrease levels of total cholesterol. Lecithin, a phospholipid derived from soybeans, is a widely publicized popular remedy for hypercholesterolemia, commonly sold in health food stores. Because it is not absorbed as such from the gastrointestinal tract, any hypocholesterolemic effect

Table 75.7.
Dietary Therapy of High Blood Cholesterol[a]

Nutrient	Recommended Intake	
	Step-One Diet	Step-Two Diet
Total Fat	Less than 30% of Total Calories	
Saturated Fatty Acids	Less than 10% of Total Calories	Less than 7% of Total Calories
Polyunsaturated Fatty Acids	Up to 10% of Total Calories	
Monounsaturated Fatty Acids	10 to 15% of Total Calories	
Carbohydrates	50 to 60% of Total Calories	
Protein	10 to 20% of Total Calories	
Cholesterol	Less than 300 mg/day	Less than 200 mg/day
Total Calories	To achieve and maintain desirable weight	

[a] From: The Expert Panel: Report of the National Cholesterol Education Program Expert Panel on Detection, Evaluation and Treatment of High Blood Cholesterol in Adults. *Arch Intern Med* 148:36, 1988.

Table 75.8.
Dietary Guidelines to Lower Blood Cholesterol[a]

Food	Recommended	Avoid or Use Sparingly
Fish, shellfish, poultry, shrimp, lean red meats Up to 6 to 7 oz are recommended per day (limit shrimp to 3 oz)	Fish; skinless chicken, turkey, Cornish hen; very lean cuts of beef, lamb, pork and veal; low-fat lunchmeats with 3 gm fat or less per oz. Dry beans or tofu may be used as a substitute for fish, poultry, and meat	Any fatty cuts of meat; lunchmeats; sausages; scrapple, bacon; hot dogs, caviar, fish roe; deep-fried meats, fish and poultry, organ meat, duck; goose
Fats and oils Up to 6 to 7 tsp may be used per day, including fat used in cooking	Unsaturated oils: safflower, sunflower, corn, soybean, sesame, olive, rapeseed (canola); margarine with first ingredient a liquid unsaturated oil listed above; 4 to 6 nuts or 3 olives count as 1 teaspoon of oil. Mayonnaise; salad dressing made with unsaturated oils listed above (2 teaspoons count as 1 teaspoon oil)	Butter; lard; palm kernel oil; meat fat; salt pork; bacon fat; coconut oil; palm oil; hydrogenated or solid shortenings; gravy; cream sauce; salad dressing made with cream, cheese, or sour cream
Milk and yogurt 2 or more cups recommended per day	Skim or 1% milk; including evaporated and powdered milk; buttermilk; nonfat and low-fat yogurt	Whole milk, including evaporated and condensed milk; eggnog; whole milk; yogurt; cream; sour cream; half and half; coconut milk
Cheese 1 oz of recommended cheese or 1/4 cup cottage cheese may be substituted for 1 oz of fish, poultry, or lean red meat	Low-fat cottage cheese; low-fat cheese with 4 gm of fat or less per oz	High fat cheeses containing more than 4 gm of fat per oz
Eggs Egg yolks should be limited to 2 per week including those used in cooking	Egg whites (2 egg whites will substitute for 1 whole egg in recipes); cholesterol-free egg substitutes	Egg yolks in excess of 2 per week
Vegetables and fruits 4 or more servings are recommended per day. Include at least 1 serving of citrus fruit or other source of vitamin C per day	Fresh, frozen, canned, or dried	Vegetables in cream, cheese, or butter sauces, deep-fried vegetables, french fries
Breads and cereals 4 or more servings recommended per day	Loaf bread and bagels (except egg); English muffins, pita bread; most sandwich and dinner rolls; Melba toast; water crackers; soda crackers; rice cakes; rye crisp; matzo, pretzels, breadsticks (made without cheese). All cereals except as noted. Pasta (except egg); all grains, including rice, barley, buckwheat, bulgur, corn, millet, rye, and oats	Croissants, biscuits, and other rich rolls; pastries; doughnuts; egg breads; commercial baked products; high-fat crackers; cereals with added oils and coconut, such as granola-type; egg pasta
Desserts and sweets Foods high in sugar are best used in small amounts. They should be used infrequently by persons with high triglycerides or excess weight	Fruit Sugar; jelly; cocoa powder, gelatin, Italian ice; frozen fruit bars; frozen low-fat yogurt; pudding made with skim milk; angel food cake; sherbet; sorbet; low-fat cookies; homemade baked products made with skim or low-fat milk, egg whites, and small amounts of unsaturated fat	Chocolate; ice cream; coconut; cream desserts; egg custard; commercial baked products
Miscellaneous	Bouillon; fat-free broths. Air-popped popcorn or popcorn made with small amounts of unsaturated oil; pretzels, chestnuts. Vinegar, spices, herbs, mustard, fat-free salad dressing	Cream or other fatty soups; High-fat snack foods, such as potato chips, corn chips, granola bars, microwave popcorn, nondairy creamers and whipped toppings made with coconut or palm oil

[a] From: The Johns Hopkins Physicians Lipid Education Program, 2nd ed. The Johns Hopkins University, Baltimore, 1988, p. 26.

probably derives from its high content of linoleic acid. Vegetable oils rich in linoleic acid, such as safflower oil, soybean oil, sunflower oil and corn oil, are the preferred dietary sources of the omega-6 fatty acids. The major sources of the omega-3 fatty acids are the fish oils. Taken as dietary supplements, high doses of fish oil lower elevated triglyceride levels but do not affect levels of total or LDL cholesterol. Recent evidence suggests that use of fish oil capsules may worsen hyperinsulinemia, insulin resistance, and glucose tolerance in patients with non-insulin-dependent diabetes mellitus (12, 32). Although epidemiological studies suggest both a lower incidence and prevalence of CAD in people who consume fish regularly, there is no evidence to date that this results from intake of omega-3 fatty acids. Thus, at present, the use of fish oil capsules containing omega-3 fatty acids is not recommended, particularly in patients with non-insulin-dependent diabetes mellitus.

The typical North American diet has a quite unfavorable P:S ratio of 0.4. On the other hand, there is no historical precedent that attests to the safety of diets very rich in polyunsaturated fats (e.g., P:S ratio ≥1.5). It does appear that the latter diets can promote formation of lithogenic bile and actually increase the incidence of symptomatic biliary tract disease. Although the data from at least one study suggested that such diets are associated with an increased risk of malignant disease, this finding was not supported when data from several trials were pooled (9). Another disadvantage to substantially increasing dietary intake of polyunsaturated fat is that the resultant high caloric intake might promote obesity. Finally, it should be noted that diets with very high P:S ratios (e.g. ≥3) may decrease HDL levels and lead to an unfavorable increase in the LDL:HDL ratio. For all of these reasons, a P:S ratio of about 1.0 is recommended in most hypocholesterolemic diets.

Recent evidence suggests that monounsaturated fatty acids, principally oleic acid, found in canola oil, olive oil, and certain forms of safflower and sunflower seed oil, lower levels of LDL cholesterol as effectively as do polyunsaturated fatty acids such as linoleic acid. Thus it is now recommended that both the Step 1 and Step 2 diets contain about 10 to 15% monounsaturated fatty acids, derived mainly from these vegetable oils.

The influence of dietary fiber on plasma cholesterol levels is complex, dependent on the type of fiber, and somewhat controversial. Guar, pectin, and unprocessed high fiber food, such as legumes and oats, lower plasma total cholesterol levels, whereas other fibers, such as wheat bran, do not. Effects on levels of HDL cholesterol and triglyceride are minimal. In the amounts consumed in a palatable diet, fiber plays a minor role compared to control of dietary fats and cholesterol.

The goals of dietary therapy are to reduce levels of LDL cholesterol to less than 160 mg/dl in patients who have neither CAD nor evidence of two or more CAD risk factors, and to less than 130 mg/dl in patients with CAD or two or more CAD risk factors. These are minimal goals of treatment, and even lower LDL cholesterol should be sought to further decrease CAD risk. The NCEP suggests that levels of LDL cholesterol be used for classification of patients and decisions regarding dietary (and drug) therapy, but that levels of total cholesterol be used for assessment of the efficacy of diet therapy. In patients with normal levels of HDL cholesterol and triglycerides, a total cholesterol of 240 mg/dl corresponds to an LDL cholesterol value of 160 mg/dl, whereas a total cholesterol of 200 mg/dl corresponds to an LDL cholesterol of 130 mg/dl. The level of LDL cholesterol should be monitored in patients with abnormal levels of HDL cholesterol or triglycerides to decide whether the goals of dietary therapy have been achieved, and on whether to pursue drug therapy.

Results of the Step 1 diet should be monitored after 4 to 6 weeks, and again at 3 months, when the effects should be maximal. In general, formal consultation with a dietitian is not required during implementation of the Step 1 diet, and the physician and other health care providers should serve as the primary sources of education and compliance monitoring of, and encouragement for, the patient. It is important to emphasize to all patients that diet therapy of hypercholesterolemia implies permanent, rather than temporary, changes in eating behavior. If the goals of diet therapy are not met after 3 months, it is recommended that the patient progress to a Step 2 diet, which leads to a reduction of saturated fatty acid intake from 10% to less than 7%, and of dietary cholesterol from less than 300 mg/day to less than 200 mg/day. Ordinarily, implementation of the Step 2 diet will require consultation with a registered dietitian. Decisions regarding the use of hypocholesterolemic drug therapy should not usually be made until the patient has undergone an adequate 6-month trial of diet therapy and has failed to meet the target LDL cholesterol goals. Dietary therapy alone is often sufficient in the approximately 85% of hypercholesterolemic patients with polygenic or nonhereditary forms of hypercholesterolemia. Adherence to a Step 1 diet in a diet-sensitive patient will often lower levels of total cholesterol by 30 to 40 mg/dl, whereas addition of the Step 2 diet will often reduce the total cholesterol level by another 15 mg/dl. Although diet usually reduces cholesterol levels in patients with monogenic hypercholesterolemia, concomitant drug therapy is almost always required. In elderly patients with hypercholesterolemia, the benefits of diet therapy should be weighed against the possibility of inadequate nutrition. For this reason, aged patients at high risk should generally be treated only with the Step 1 diet, and not with the more restrictive Step 2 diet.

Triglyceride reduction. Diets designed to reduce plasma triglyceride and VLDL levels emphasize the loss of excess weight by total caloric restriction. Plasma triglyceride levels usually fall, often to normal, after a few days of caloric restriction. The reduction is maintained as long as weight loss continues at a rate of 1 to 2 pounds (0.5 to 1 kg)/week. If normal weight is attained and maintained, further therapy may not be necessary. If hypertriglyceridemia persists or occurs in individuals of normal weight, a cholesterol-lowering diet, as outlined above, may be effective. Alcohol intake should be restricted since it can cause a striking rise in triglyceride levels in some patients with hypertriglyceridemia. Although extreme increases in the carbohydrate content of a diet can cause transient and, rarely, sustained hypertriglyceridemia, there is no firm evidence to suggest that total carbohydrate restriction is helpful in the treatment of hypertriglyceridemia. There are conflicting data regarding the effect on plasma triglyceride level of excessive intake of sucrose (common sugar) and simple sugars. In most studies, especially in patients who are already hypertriglyceridemic, they do raise plasma triglyceride levels and lower those of HDL cholesterol, but the effect is small. The rationale for dietary restriction of sugar is based more upon the need to avoid excessive caloric intake (and to prevent caries) than on its having a direct effect on plasma lipids. Like alcohol, sucrose provides "empty" calories in that it contains none of the valuable nutrients, such as protein, fiber, minerals, or vitamins. For this reason the substitution of complex (e.g., starches) for simple carbohydrates in the diet is recommended. A triglyceride-lowering diet should favorably affect plasma HDL cholesterol levels in most individuals, since obesity and triglyceride levels are inversely correlated with the levels of HDL cholesterol, and since plasma HDL levels usually rise during weight reduction. Plasma levels of total (and LDL) cholesterol often fall with loss of excess weight; when they rise, familial combined hyperlipoproteinemia may be present.

Chylomicron reduction. Treatment of fasting chylomicronemia (type I) involves the restriction of dietary fat intake to 5 to 20% of total calories (0.5 g of fat per kilogram of body weight is a reasonable starting point). The fat deficit should be corrected predominantly by substitution of complex carbohydrates. Because medium chain triglycerides (available as MCT oil) are transported directly from the intestine to the liver in the portal circulation without incorporation into chylomicrons, they may be added to the diet to provide calories. The recommended dose of MCT oil (available at most pharmacies) is 1 tablespoonful three to four times daily, mixed with foods. Five grams of vegetable fat rich in polyunsaturates should be included to prevent essential fatty acid deficiency.

Dietary fat is severely restricted until fasting chylomicronemia is eliminated and clinical symptoms are prevented or reduced in frequency; dietary fat is then chronically restricted to whatever degree is necessary to prevent fasting chylomicronemia. The efficacy of fat restriction in preventing recurrent abdominal pain is supported by clinical observations in individual patients.

When fasting chylomicronemia is accompanied by elevation of VLDL triglyceride levels, therapy is initiated with restriction of dietary fat intake and correction of coexistent secondary causes for the disorder. Once chylomicronemia has been eliminated, a tri-glyceride-requiring diet with a modest reduction in total fat intake (to approximately 30% of total calories) is all that is usually required to prevent recurrence. Total abstinence from alcohol is usually necessary.

Diets to raise levels of HDL. A dietary approach to the patient with an HDL cholesterol level below 35 mg/dl involves treatment of concomitant hyperlipoproteinemia and loss of excess weight. Although moderate alcohol consumption (2 to 3 ounces/day) is positively correlated with HDL cholesterol level and negatively correlated with CAD, it is not recommended for three reasons: (a) excessive use (greater than two or three drinks/day) increases the overall risk of morbidity and mortality, (b) its use may interfere with attempts to control obesity and hypertriglyceridemia, and (c) evidence is not conclusive that modest intake results in an overall health advantage.

Exercise

Evidence has accumulated over the past decade that regular isotonic exercise favorably affects plasma lipid levels. Most of the exercise programs that have been evaluated, including jogging, rapid walking, swimming, bicycling, cross-country skiing, and mountain climbing, have involved 30 minutes or more of continued effort at 70 to 85% of maximal heart rate at least three times weekly. In most studies, levels of HDL cholesterol have been shown to rise (approximately 20%) and triglyceride levels to fall (approximately 25%) with exercise (8). Although levels of LDL cholesterol usually do not fall in normal subjects, reductions of as much as 10% may occur in individuals with elevated levels of total and LDL cholesterol.

It has been demonstrated that individuals who exercise regularly are at a reduced risk for CAD in both cross-sectional and longitudinal epidemiological studies. Exercise also improves glucose metabolism, assists in weight reduction, and may reduce blood pressure (30).

Thus, exercise counseling (see Chapter 58) is an important part of the management of patients with abnormalities in lipoprotein metabolism.

Smoking Cessation

Plasma levels of HDL cholesterol have been found to be lower and levels of VLDL triglyceride higher in people who smoke cigarettes than in nonsmokers or ex-smokers. Moreover, an inverse relationship exists between the number of cigarettes smoked daily and the level of HDL cholesterol. Smoking cessation has been associated with a modest rise in plasma HDL level. It is not known what proportion of the increased risk of CAD associated with smoking is mediated through alteration in the plasma lipids or via other mechanisms. There is, however, substantial evidence that smoking cessation reduces CAD risk. There is also evidence that counseling of patients increases cessation rates. Therefore, all patients who smoke cigarettes should be counseled, regardless of their lipoprotein profile (see Chapter 20).

Drugs

In general, drug therapy is recommended only after an initial 3- to 6-month trial of nonpharmacological therapy (diet and exercise) has proved unsuccessful. Moreover, diet therapy should be continued during drug treatment since the effects of each are often additive. Information on drugs with which the general physician should be familiar is displayed in Tables 75.9 and 75.10.

Hypercholesterolemia

Patients whose LDL cholesterol levels fail to reach certain target goals, despite at least 6 months of adequate diet therapy, should be considered for drug therapy. The NCEP guidelines that suggest a need for drug therapy are an LDL cholesterol >190 mg/dl in patients without, or an LDL cholesterol >160 mg/dl in patients with, CAD or two or more known risk factors. Before considering drug therapy, however, one should be certain that the effects of other nonpharmacological interventions, such as a regular exercise program, weight control, and cessation of cigarette smoking, have been maximized. This is particularly important in patients who have failed to reach target LDL cholesterol levels on diet therapy but who do not meet criteria for drug treatment by the above guidelines. Patients with marked elevations of LDL cholesterol (>225 mg/dl), in whom dietary therapy alone is unlikely to normalize LDL cholesterol levels, should be considered for drug therapy after only 3 months of an adequate dietary trial. The minimal goals of drug treatment should be the same as those for dietary therapy, i.e., an LDL cholesterol level less than 160 mg/dl for patients without, and an LDL cholesterol level less than 130 mg/dl for patients with, CAD or two or more CAD risk factors. Some evidence exists that reducing LDL cholesterol levels to as low as 100 mg/dl leads to a further reduction in CAD risk, although it is unclear whether further therapeutic decreases in LDL cholesterol levels would be beneficial.

Cholesterol-lowering drugs can be categorized into three groups: (a) first-choice agents, such as bile acid sequestrants and nicotinic acid, which are effective in lowering total and LDL cholesterol levels, reduce CAD risk, and are generally safe for long-term use; (b) new drugs, such as lovastatin, which dramatically reduce total and LDL cholesterol levels, but whose efficacy in reducing CAD risk and long-term safety are unknown, and (c) other drugs, such as gemfibrozil and probucol, which lower LDL cholesterol levels.

Bile Acid Sequestering Resins

The bile acid-binding resins, *cholestyramine* and *colestipol*, remain the drugs of first choice for patients with primary hypercholesterolemia. They enhance LDL catabolism and excretion and prevent intestinal absorption by diverting cholesterol and bile acids into the feces. They also increase levels of triglycerides and

Table 75.9.
Commonly Used Lipid-Lowering Drugs

BILE ACID SEQUESTERING RESINS (Cholestyramine, Colestipol)

Mechanism: Anion exchange resins that bind bile acids, resulting in increased hepatic synthesis of cholesterol and bile acids, increased apo B catabolism, increased fecal excretion of cholesterol, increased LDL receptor activity, and usually a net reduction of plasma cholesterol levels.

Efficacy: Decreases total and LDL cholesterol up to 25–40% (onset 4–7 days, maximal effect within 1–3 weeks). In the LRC trial, mean reductions in experimental group of total and LDL cholesterol were 13.4 and 20.3%. Apo B level falls, while HDL level rises slightly. VLDL is unchanged or increased.

Pharmacokinetics: Not absorbed, but may bind other drugs (e.g., thiazides, digitalis preparations, anticoagulants, phenobarbital, thyroxine, phenylbutazone, propranolol, iron).

Side Effects: (a) Common—unpleasant sandy/gritty preparations, gastrointestinal (constipation in 10–20%, nausea, heartburn, abdominal discomfort, flatulence, etc., often resolve with continued therapy and/or treatment of constipation), lowered serum folate levels; (b) Uncommon—gastrointestinal (steatorrhea), hyperchloremic acidosis (small patients on high doses), fat-soluble vitamin deficiency; increased alkaline phosphatase and amino transferase (usually transient).

Administration: (a) Cholestyramine—12–32 g/day given twice daily to four times daily before or during meals; supplied as Questran 9-g packets each containing 4 g of active drug; (b) Colestipol—15–30 g/day, given twice daily to four times daily before or during meals; supplied as Colestid in 5-g packets or 500-g bottles.

Preparations should be taken in water or juice to prevent esophageal irritation or blockage. Other medicines should be taken 1 hour before or 4 hours after dosage. Monitor serum folate levels and consider supplemental multivitamins with folic acid.

Clinical Use: Drugs of first choice in the treatment of hypercholesterolemia, because of their relative safety and efficacy. Contraindications include marked hypertriglyceridemia and severe constipation.

NICOTINIC ACID (Niacin, and preparations such as Nicobid (time-released), 125, 250, or 500 mg, or Nicolar, 500 mg)

Mechanism: Diverse effects on lipid metabolism: decreases LDL and apo B synthesis by decreasing hepatic synthesis of VLDL, increases synthesis of HDL, inhibits lipolysis in adipose metabolized in liver and partially excreted unchanged in urine; plasma half-life is about 45 minutes.

Side Effects: (a) Common—cutaneous flushing and pruritis, which diminish after several weeks of therapy; gastrointestinal (nausea, diarrhea, abdominal pain, abnormal liver function); (b) Less common—dermatological disorders (e.g., increased pigmentation); activation of peptic ulcer; dysrhythmia; gout; urinary frequency and dysuria; glucose intolerance, etc.

Administration: (100, 250, 300, 400 and 500 mg tablets). Gradual increase over 1–3 weeks from 300 mg/day to 2–9 g/day; given in three times daily dosage; give with meals to diminish side effects. Flushing may be ameliorated by pretreatment with aspirin, one half to one 324 mg tablet 30 minutes before each dose. Generic form is inexpensive compared with time-release form (Nico-Bid); the latter may reduce the frequency of flushing, but increase the frequency of GI side effects. Administer with caution in presence of coronary artery disease.

Clinical Use: First-line (despite side effects) effective drug in the treatment of elevated LDL cholesterol or VLDL triglyceride. Contraindications include peptic ulcer disease, dysrhythmia, liver disease, diabetes mellitus, hyperuricemia, and gout.

HDL, particularly HDL_2. In doses of 20 to 24 g/day, a 20 to 30% reduction in LDL cholesterol may be achieved, but the expense is high ($50.00/month). Although these resins may be the safest of all of the hypolipidemic drugs, compliance is a problem because taste and gastrointestinal side effects prevent many patients from taking a full dose. Gradual increase of dose, contin-

Table 75.10.
Commonly Used Lipid-Lowering Drugs *(continued)*

HMG-COA REDUCTASE INHIBITORS (lovastatin = mevinolin)

Mechanism: Competitively inhibits HMG-CoA reductase, the rate-limiting enzyme in the synthesis of cholesterol, decreases production of LDL, increases LDL receptor activity in the liver and the rate of removal of LDL from the plasma.

Efficacy: Decreases total cholesterol (20–37%), LDL cholesterol (20–48%), LDL apo B (20–37%), VLDL cholesterol (27–40%), and triglycerides (7–27%). Provides variable and modest increases in HDL cholesterol (4–12%) and apo A-I and A-II.

Pharmacokinetics: Incompletely absorbed (average 30%); extensive first pass extraction by the liver with less than 5% reaching systemic circulation; inactive lovastatin converted to several active metabolites; peak plasma concentrations of active metabolites within 2 to 6 hours; steady state concentrations of total inhibitors achieved within 2 to 3 days; 83% of radiolabelled dose eliminated in feces (represents unabsorbed drug and active and inactive metabolites excreted in bile) and 10% in urine (as inactive metabolites).

Side Effects: (a) Generally well tolerated, discontinuation required in 1 to 2% of patients due to adverse effects; long term safety not yet established; (b) Occasional—headache (9% of patients), gastrointestinal (flatulence, abdominal pains or cramps, diarrhea, constipation, nausea, dyspepsia—usually mild and transient) (4–6%); elevation in liver aminotransferases and, uncommonly, alkaline phosphatases usually within 3 to 16 months (33 times increase in 2%), reverses over several weeks after discontinuation of drug; mild increase in creatinine kinase (11%); myalgias (3%); rash and pruritis (5%); (c) Uncommon—gastrointestinal (heartburn, dysgeusia), dizziness, insomnia, malaise, fatigue, myopathy (0.5%, but up to 30% in patients on immunosuppressant drugs), renal failure due to rhabdomyolysis; (d) Unknown—(?) cataracts.

Administration: Lovastatin (Mevacor, 20 mg, 40 mg)—20–80 mg/day once daily with evening meal or twice daily with meals (administration with food results in 50% higher plasma concentrations of total inhibitors, effectiveness greater when given as evening dose, perhaps because cholesterol synthesis occurs mainly at night). Obtain baseline liver function tests, then every 4–6 weeks for first 12–15 months, then every 3–4 months thereafter. Discontinue if aminotransferase rise ≥3 times normal. Because of the development of cataracts in animals on very high doses, baseline and yearly slit lamp examinations are currently recommended.

Clinical Use: Second-line (because of lack of data establishing long-term safety), very effective and well tolerated drug for the treatment of hypercholesterolemia. When response to a single drug is inadequate, lovastatin is effective in combination with a bile acid sequestering agent, nicotinic acid, or gemfibrozil. Each drug contributes separately to reductions in lipoprotein concentrations.

FIBRIC ACID DERIVATIVES (Clofibrate, Gemfibrozil, etc.)

Mechanism: Increases clearance of VLDL by enhancing lipolysis, may increase lipoprotein lipase activity, reduces hepatic cholesterol synthesis, and increases cholesterol excretion in the bile.

Efficacy: Clofibrate—decreases triglycerides/VLDL within 2–5 days (mean reduction 22% in Coronary Drug Project, up to 80% reduction in some patients), may decrease or increase LDL cholesterol (mean decrease in total cholesterol of 6% in Coronary Drug Project), reduces IDL in type III. Gemfibrozil lowers triglycerides to a greater extent, raises HDL more consistently and is less likely to raise LDL than clofibrate. In familial combined hyperlipoproteinemia, however, use of any fibric acid analog is likely to raise LDL cholesterol.

Pharmacokinetics: Completely absorbed, rapidly hydrolyzed to an active metabolite; peak concentration within 4 hours; metabolized in liver and excreted in urine; elimination divided into two kinetic phases, with half-lives of 1.7 and 15 hours. Gemfibrozil—completely absorbed; peak concentration within 2 hours; half-life 1.5 hours; undergoes enterohepatic circulation, metabolized in liver and excreted in urine. Both may enhance action of oral anticoagulants, phenytoin, and hypoglycemic agents, and of furosemide by displacing them from albumin-binding sites.

Side Effects: (a) Usually—well tolerated; (b) Occasional—(6-fold) increase in the incidence of cholelithiasis (may be less with gemfibrozil and newer analogs); other gastrointestinal (nausea, abdominal pain, diarrhea, weight gain); reduced libido, impotence; unusual flu-like syndrome; (c) Uncommon—rash, alopecia, breast tenderness, reversible abnormality in liver function, hepatomegaly, myositis, increased plasma glucose, etc.; (d) Unknown—(?)thromboembolism, (?)intermittent claudication, (?)dysrhythmia, (?)neoplasia.

Administration: Clofibrate (Atromid-S, 500 mg)—2 g/day in two or three divided doses. Gemfibrozil (Lopid, 300 mg and 600 mg)—600 mg twice daily (½ hour before meals). Some recommend periodic monitoring of asparate aminotransferase (formerly SGO-T), alanine aminotransferase (formerly SGP-T), and creatinine kinase (formerly CPK).

Clinical Use: Gemfibrozil is the drug of choice in the treatment of elevated VLDL triglyceride; it can also be used to lower total and LDL cholesterol and to raise HDL cholesterol, of particular utility in type III. Use with caution in the presence of hepatic or renal insufficiency.

uation of therapy, and concomitant symptomatic management of constipation may diminish side effects.

Nicotinic Acid

Nicotinic acid (3 to 6 g/day) significantly lowers plasma levels of LDL and VLDL while raising the level of HDL cholesterol. It is thus the drug of first choice for patients with concomitant elevations in LDL cholesterol and triglycerides. Its use is often limited, however, by unpleasant side effects and the frequent presence of coexisting contraindications. By starting at a very low dose of 100 to 200 mg daily and gradually increasing the dose of the drug and adding aspirin, increased tolerance often develops to the common side effects of cutaneous flushing, rashes, hives, and pruritis. Nicotinic acid is inexpensive, with monthly costs averaging $5.00 at a dose of 2 to 4 g daily. Nicobid, a slow release form of nicotinic acid, reduces some of the adverse effects, but the cost of the drug is high, averaging about $60.00/month.

HMG CoA Reductase Inhibitors

The new drug, lovastatin, and the related experimental drugs, simvastatin and pravastatin, are specific, potent competitive inhibitors of HMG CoA reductase, the rate-limiting enzyme in cholesterol biosynthesis. Lovastatin and related drugs increase hepatic LDL receptor activity and LDL clearance from the circulation and, in addition, decrease production of LDL (15). Lovastatin has been approved by the Food and Drug Administration for use in hypercholesterolemic patients and has been shown to reduce levels of total and LDL cholesterol by 20 to 50%, to decrease triglyceride levels slightly, and to increase the levels of HDL cholesterol in some patients (15, 34). It appears to be equally effective in individuals with familial and nonfamilial hypercholesterolemia. Although this novel class of hypercholesterolemic agent suggests great therapeutic promise, both its efficacy in decreasing CAD risk and its long-term safety remain to be established. At a dose of 40 mg/day, lovastatin costs about $75.00/month.

Gemfibrozil

Although gemfibrozil is approved for the treatment of hypertriglyceridemia, data from the Helsinki Heart Study (10) have revealed it to be effective as well in lowering LDL cholesterol, raising HDL cholesterol, and reducing the morbidity and mortality from CAD. Thus, gemfibrozil may soon be considered another first-line drug for the treatment of certain patients with hypercholesterolemia. It should be noted, however, that in patients with primary hypertriglyceridemia, gemfibrozil may increase LDL cholesterol levels, whereas in patients with elevations of both cholesterol and triglycerides, this drug can cause either an increase or a decrease in LDL cholesterol levels. A significant side effect of gemfibrozil is its tendency to increase bile lithogenicity. At a dose of 1.2 g/day, gemfibrozil costs about $30.00/month.

Probucol

Probucol has been used as a second-line drug for the treatment of hypercholesterolemia. It appears to lower LDL cholesterol levels by a receptor-independent mechanism and by an increase in LDL catabolism. In addition, it inhibits the oxidative metabolism and tissue deposition of LDL. Probucol use leads to a reduction in total and LDL cholesterol levels of 8 to 15%, and a concomitant reduction of HDL cholesterol levels of as much as 25%. The significance of the consequent reduction in the LDL:HDL ratio remains uncertain. To date, there are no reported studies of its efficacy in reducing CAD risk or of its long-term safety. The electrocardiogram (ECG) should be monitored in patients taking probucol, as the drug can cause prolongation of the QT interval (at which point the drug should be discontinued). At a dose of 1 mg/day, probucol costs about $30.00/month.

Combination Drug Therapy

When the response to one of the first-line drugs proves to be inadequate, combined therapy with two drugs should be considered. In general, one should choose drugs with complementary or synergistic mechanisms of action and should consult with a specialist in lipid disorders. The use of a bile acid sequestrant in combination with either nicotinic acid (4) or lovastatin (18) can lower levels of LDL cholesterol by 45 to 60% in patients with hypercholesterolemia and normal triglyceride levels. Probucol or gemfibrozil may also be used in combination with a bile acid sequestering resin, although these regimens are less effective. Lovastatin and nicotinic acid can be used together in patients with elevated levels of both LDL cholesterol and triglycerides, although there is rela-

tively little experience with this combination, particularly with regard to such adverse effects as hepatic toxicity. Patients with homozygous familial hypercholesterolemia may respond less well to treatment with drugs and diet than do patients with heterozygous monogenic, polygenic, or nonhereditary hypercholesterolemia.

Other Hypocholesterolemic Drugs

The use of *estrogen replacement therapy* (ERT) in postmenopausal women has a number of effects on cholesterol metabolism (Chapter 77). Treatment with oral estrogens usually lowers levels of LDL cholesterol and raises those of HDL cholesterol, but the doses required for these effects probably exceed those for "physiological replacement therapy." In contrast, administration of nonoral (e.g., transdermal) estrogens usually results in lower LDL cholesterol levels but unaltered levels of HDL cholesterol. Concomitant use of the progestin, medroxyprogesterone acetate (Provera), with either form of ERT appears not to influence either form of ERT adversely. *Neomycin* is effective in lowering cholesterol levels in hypercholesterolemic patients by enhancing the fecal excretion of neutral sterols. However, patients frequently develop diarrhea. Because neomycin is an aminoglycoside, renal function must be monitored during therapy. Treatment with *dextrothyroxine* should not be given because of its potential for inducing cardiac dysrhythmias.

Hypertriglyceridemia

Drugs that decrease hepatic production of VLDL and apo B, enhance VLDL clearance by stimulating LPL activity, or both are generally effective in treating hypertriglyceridemia. The fibric acid derivatives (clofibrate, gemfibrozil, bezafibrate, fenofibrate) and nicotinic acid do both.

Although nicotinic acid may be most efficacious, its use is limited by its side effects and the presence of coexisting contraindications. The fibric acid derivatives are, therefore, the drugs most commonly used. Gemfibrozil may be preferable to clofibrate, since it more consistently raises plasma levels of HDL, is less likely to raise the plasma LDL level, and may be less lithogenic. It is a relatively new agent, however, and long-term experience with it is limited. Although the fibric acid drugs are generally well tolerated, an acute myositis, which occasionally is associated with renal failure, may occur, particularly in patients with impaired renal clearance or hypoalbuminemia. These drugs either should not be used or their dose reduced by 70 to 90% in azotemic patients. Periodic monitoring of muscle enzymes (creatine kinase, aldolase) is required to avoid toxicity. When the level of LDL cholesterol rises in a patient taking a fibric acid drug, the diagnosis of familial combined hyperlipoproteinemia should be considered.

In compliant patients who remain hypertriglyceridemic with diet and a single drug, combined therapy with a fibric acid drug and nicotinic acid may be useful. Rarely, after consultation with a specialist in lipid disorders, the progestational agent, norethidrone acetate, or the androgenic anabolic steroid, oxandrolone, may be required to treat persistent hypertriglyceridemia plus chylomicronemia in women or men, respectively.

Dysbetablipoproteinemia

The decreased remnant catabolism characteristic of this clinically uncommon disorder can be corrected or improved by drug therapy. Clofibrate or gemfibrozil appears to normalize lipid levels and to enhance remnant clearance in patients with dysbetalipoproteinemia. They are the drugs of choice in this disorder. Furthermore, a reduction in the incidence of peripheral vascular disease has been demonstrated during clofibrate therapy. Ethinyl estradiol has a similar and even more dramatic effect, but in doses that greatly exceed those used for postmenopausal replacement therapy. Hence, its use requires careful monitoring for possible adverse estrogenic effects that would lead to discontinuation of the drug. Nicotinic acid is the drug of second choice.

Surgery and Other Therapies

More experimental forms of therapy (such as ileal bypass, portacaval shunt, plasma exchange, extracorporeal hemoperfusion, and liver transplantation) exist for the severely hypercholesterolemic patient who is resistant or only partially responsive to diet, exercise, and lipid-lowering drugs. These therapies should be implemented only in consultation with a specialist in lipid disorders.

Obtaining Consultation

The Lipid Metabolism Branch, National Heart, Lung and Blood Institute, National Institutes of Health, Bethesda, MD 20205, can provide the names of research centers in each geographic area where sophisticated evaluation of lipoprotein abnormalities, consultation services, and experimental forms of therapy are offered.

Additional information for the management of patients with hyperlipoproteinemia and other risk factors for CAD is available from both regional and national offices of the American Heart Association. This agency can provide information about diet, drugs, and exercise in the treatment of hyperlipidemia, hypertension, cigarette smoking, and obesity.

General References

Ad Hoc Committee to Design a Dietary Treatment of Hyperlipoproteinemia: Gotto AM, Bierman EL, Connor W, et al: Recommendations for treatment of hyperlipidemia in adults: a joint statement of the Nutrition Committee and the Council on Arteriosclerosis. *Circulation* 65:1067, 1984.

   Excellent detailed yet practical treatise on the management of patients with lipoprotein disorders.

American Heart Association Booklets

Eating for a Healthy Heart, Dietary Treatment for Hyperlipidemia.

   Booklet for patients on the American Heart Association (AHA) single diet approach to improving plasma lipoprotein levels.

Counseling the Patient with Hyperlipidemia.

   Short booklet for the physician or nutritionist on implementing the AHA diet.

Heart to Heart, Nutrition Counseling for the Reduction of Cardiovascular Disease Risk Factors.

   Detailed book for the physician or nutritionist on counseling patients regarding the AHA diet.

(All are available from your local chapter of the American Heart Association.)

Brunzell JD: Physiologic approach to hyperlipidemia. In: Schwartz TB (ed): *The Year Book of Endocrinology.* Chicago, Year Book Medical Publishers, 1984, p. 11.

   Well written, readily understandable, insightful physiological approach to lipoprotein metabolism and its relationship to atherosclerosis.

Kaplan NM, Stamler J: *Prevention of Coronary Heart Disease, Practical Management of the Risk Factors.* Philadelphia, WB Saunders, 1983.

   Excellent book that reviews numerous risk factors (including lipoprotein abnormalities, cigarette smoking, hypertension, physical inactivity, psychosocial factors, etc.) and their management in a thorough, yet concise and practical manner.

Lipid Research Clinics Program: *Lipid and Lipoprotein Analysis.* Manual of Laboratory Operations Vol 1: DHEW publ no. (NIH) 75-625, Washington, DC, US Government Printing Office, 1974.

   The methods book for lipoprotein analysis. A good reference to assist you in checking methodology and standardization of your local laboratory.

NIH Consensus Conference: Treatment of hypertriglyceridemia. *JAMA* 251:1196, 1984.

   Excellent discussion of when and how to treat the patient with hypertriglyceridemia.

The Expert Panel: Report of the National Cholesterol Education Program Expert Panel on Detection, Evaluation and Treatment of High Blood Cholesterol in Adults. *Arch Intern Med* 148:36, 1988.

   Major, highly influential report outlining an aggressive approach to the detection and management of elevated levels of total and LDL cholesterol in the adult population beyond 20 years of age.

The Johns Hopkins Physicians Lipid Education Program: *A Practical Approach to the Patient with a Lipid Disorder.* Baltimore, The Johns Hopkins University, 1988.

   An excellent compendium of useful information on the up-to-date management of patients with the major, common lipid disorders.

Specific References

1. Brensike JF, Levy RI, Kelsey SF, et al: Effects of therapy with cholestyramine on progression of coronary arteriosclerosis: results of the NHLBI type II coronary intervention study. *Circulation* 69:313, 1984.
2. Brett AS: Treating hypercholesterolemia: How should practicing physicians interpret the published data for patients: *N Engl J Med* 321:676, 1989.
3. Brown MS, Goldstein JL: How LDL receptors influence cholesterol and atherosclerosis. *Sci Am* 251:58, 1984.
4. Brown WV, Goldberg IJ, Ginsberg HN: Treatment of common lipoprotein disorders. *Prog Cardiovasc Dis* 27:1, 1984.
5. Brunzell JD, Sniderman AD, Albers JJ, Kwiterovich Jr PO: Apoproteins B and A-1 and coronary artery disease in humans. *Arteriosclerosis* 4:79, 1984.
6. Campeau L, Enjalbert J, Lesperance J, et al: The relationship of risk factors to the development of atherosclerosis in saphenous-vein bypass grafts and the progression of disease in the native circulation: a study 10 years after aortocoronary bypass surgery. *N Engl J Med* 311:1329, 1984.
7. Castelli WP: The triglyceride issue: A view from Framingham. *Am Heart J* 112:432, 1986.
8. Dufaux B, Assmann G, Hollman W: Plasma lipoproteins and physical activity: a review. *Int J Sports Med* 3:123, 1982.
9. Ederer F, Leren P, Turpeinin O, Frantz Jr ID: Cancer among men on cholesterol-lowering diets. *Lancet* 2:203, 1971.

10. Frick MH, Elo O, Haapa K, et al: Helsinki Heart Study: Primary prevention trial with gemfibrozil in middle-aged men with dyslipidemia. *N Engl J Med* 317:1237, 1987.

11. Garber AM: Where to draw the line against cholesterol. *Ann Intern Med* 111:625, 1989.

12. Glauber H, Wallace P, Griver K, et al: Adverse metabolic effect of omega-3 fatty acids in non-insulin-dependent diabetes mellitus. *Ann Intern Med* 108:663, 1988.

13. Goldberg AP: Lipid abnormalities in hemodialysis: prevalence, implications and treatment. *Perspect Lipid Disord* 2:17, 1984.

14. Gore JM, Goldberg RJ, Matsumoto AS, et al: Validity of serum total cholesterol level obtained within 24 hours of acute myocardial infarction. *Am J Cardiol* 54:722, 1984.

15. Grundy S: HMG-CoA Reductase inhibitors for treatment of hypercholesterolemia. *N Engl J Med* 319:24, 1988.

16. Havel RJ: Classification of the hyperlipidemias. *Annu Rev Med* 28:195, 1977.

17. Heiss G, Johnson NJ, Reiland S, et al: The epidemiology of plasma HDL cholesterol levels. The Lipid Research Clinics Prevalence Study. Summary *Circulation* 62(Suppl IV) IV:116, 1980.

18. Illingsworth DR: Mevinolin plus colestipol in therapy for severe heterozygous familial hypercholesterolemia. *Ann Intern Med* 101:598, 1984.

19. Havel RJ: (guest ed): Symposium on lipid disorders. *Med Clin North Am* 66:319, 1982.

20. Kannel WB, Schatzkin A: Risk factor analysis. *Prog Cardiovasc Dis* 26:309, 1983.

21. Leaf A: Management of hypercholesterolemia: Are preventive interventions advisable? *N Engl J Med* 321:680, 1989.

22. Levy RI: Consideration of cholesterol and nonvascular mortality. *Am Heart J* 104:324, 1982.

23. Lindgren FT, Jensen LC, Hatch FT: The isolation and quantitative analysis of serum lipoproteins. In: *Blood Lipids and Lipoproteins: Quantitation, Composition, and Metabolism.* New York, John Wiley & Sons, 1972, p. 181.

24. US Department of Health and Human Services, Public Health Service, National Institutes of Health: *Lipid Research Clinics Populations Studies Data Book, vol I. The Prevalence Study.* NIH publ no 80-1527, 1980.

25. Lipid Research Clinics Coronary Primary Prevention Trial Results: I. Reduction in incidence of coronary heart disease.; II. The relationship of reduction in incidence of coronary heart disease to cholesterol lowering. *JAMA* 251:351, 365, 1984.

26. Maciejko JJ, Holmes DR, Kottke BA, et al: Apolipoprotein A-I as a marker of angiographically assessed coronary artery disease. *N Engl J Med* 309:385, 1983.

27. Mahley RW, Angelin B: Type III hyperlipoproteinemia: recent insights into the genetic defect of familial dysbetalipoproteinemia. *Adv Intern Med* 29:385, 1984.

28. Nilsson-Ehle P: Regulation of lipoprotein lipase: triacylglycerol transport in plasma. In: Carlson LA, Pernow B (eds): *Metabolic Risk Factors in Ischemic Cardiovascular Disease.* New York, Raven Press, 1982, p. 49.

29. Oram JF, Brenton EA, Bierman EL: Regulation of high density lipoprotein activity in cultured human skin fibroblasts and human arterial smooth muscle cells. *J Clin Invest* 72:1611, 1983.

30. Paffenberger RS, Hyde RT, Wing AL, Steinmetz CH: A natural history of athleticism and cardiovascular health. *JAMA* 252:491, 1984.

31. Rifkind BM, Segal P: Lipid Research Clinics Program reference values for hyperlipidemia and hypolipidemia. *JAMA* 250:1869, 1983.

32. Schectman G, Kaul S, Cherayil GD, et al: Can the hypotriglyceridemic effect of fish oil concentrate be sustained? *Ann Intern Med* 110:346, 1989.

33. Sniderman AD, Wolfson C, Teng B, et al: Association of hyperbetalipoproteinemia with endogenous hypertriglyceridemia and atherosclerosis. *Ann Intern Med* 97:833, 1982.

34. The Lovastatin Study Group II: Therapeutic response to lovastatin in nonfamilial hypercholesterolemia. A multicenter trial. *JAMA* 256:2829, 1986.

35. Tyroler HA, Hess G, Schonfeld G, et al: Apoprotein A-I, A-II and C-II in black and white residents of Evans County. *Circulation* 62:249, 1980.

36. Walden CE, Knopp RH, Wahl PW, et al: Sex differences in the effect of diabetes mellitus and lipoprotein triglyceride and cholesterol concentrations. *N Engl J Med* 331:953, 1984.

37. Wyngaarden JB: Variability in individual cholesterol level clouds risk assessment. *JAMA* 260:759, 1988.

CHAPTER 76

Obesity

MARC R. BLACKMAN, M.D.

Obesity, defined as an excess of total body fat, is one of the most prevalent chronic medical disorders in the world. Moreover, its incidence and prevalence appear to be increasing, particularly in the highly industrialized nations (see below). Numerous complex, as yet ill understood, interactions among predisposing genetic and environmental factors influence the initiation, development, and persistence of excess adiposity. Although controversy exists about the exact health risks associated with mild obesity (3, 19, 34), in more obese patients, morbidity and mortality vary directly with the amount and topographical distribution of excess body fat, as well as with certain associated medical and behavioral abnormalities. Newer classification schemes need to be devised so that rational therapeutic interventions can be more specifically targeted toward those obesity syndromes associated with increased risk for morbidity and mortality. In so doing, perhaps both short- and long-term treatment results will improve substantially. In any event, there remains an urgent need to promote a variety of effective societal and individual approaches for prevention of excess adiposity.

DEFINITION

Obesity versus Overweight

Obesity must be distinguished from overweight, which refers to an increase in body weight due to increased bone, muscle, or fat. Although the two terms are often used synonymously, errors do occur in equating obesity with overweight, as for example in the muscular athlete with normal or decreased body fat. Because body composition and, in particular, body fat normally vary with age, sex, diet, physical activity, and population group, it is important to compare measurements of body fat in individual patients with those derived from appropriate control groups.

Methods for Quantifying Adiposity

Numerous methods exist for assessing and quantifying the amount and distribution of body fat. Although hydrostatic densitometry provides the most accurate estimates of total fat mass, the simplest, most common, and most reliable clinical approaches to date involve either determination of relative weight or measurement of skin-fold thickness. In the former approach, a patient's weight is expressed as a percentage or ratio of an "ideal," "desirable," or "acceptable" weight, such as that issued in the Metropolitan Life Insurance Company's Build and Blood Pressure Study of 1959 (35) and updated in the Metropolitan's Height and Weight Tables of 1983 (28). Of the various indices of weight and height tested, the body mass index (weight/height$_2$) has the highest correlation with other measures of body fat (Fig. 76.1). Although measurements of skin-fold thickness (using standardized calipers) are useful in assessing body fat in population studies, the technique is often less reliable in individual patients than are direct measurements of weight and height.

The topographical distribution of body fat is most conveniently and reliably ascertained by determining the waist-to-hip ratio (WHR), which is measured as the ratio of the minimal circumference at the waist to the maximal circumference at the hips with the patient in the standing position (see Fig. 76.2). Measurements of the WHR correspond very closely to more quantitative measures of central adiposity, such as quantitative computed tomography of the abdomen.

CLASSIFICATION

The heterogeneous nature and the many approaches to evaluation and management of the obesity syndromes have made classification schemes necessary but nonuniform. Thus, various classification systems might serve different purposes, as for example (a) to identify subpopulations of obese individuals at risk for increased morbidity and mortality, in whom therapeutic interventions might be beneficial; and (b) to distinguish among primarily genetic, environmental, and combined genetic plus environmental etiologies. With regard to the former, recent research suggests that

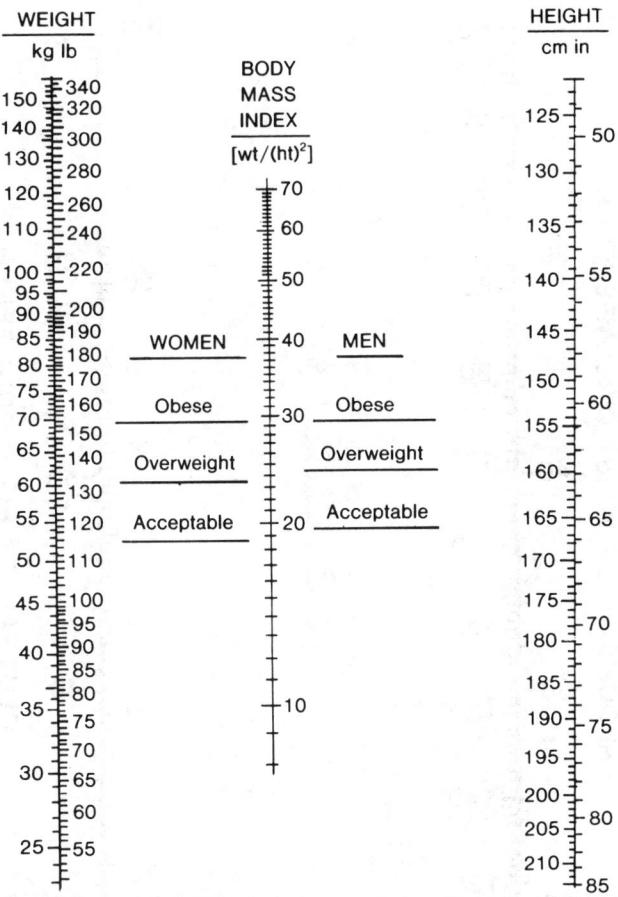

Figure 76.1. Nomogram for body mass index. (From Bray GA (ed): *Obesity in America*, DHEW publ no. (NIH) 79-359. Washington, DC, US Government Printing Office, 1979.)

patients with predominantly upper body obesity (i.e., increased fat in the back of the neck, shoulder areas and abdomen) exhibit an increased frequency of metabolic concomitants of obesity and an enhanced risk for developing diabetes mellitus, hyperlipidemia, and cardiovascular disease (12, 22, 25, 27, 29). In contrast, patients with predominantly lower body obesity (i.e., increased fat in the hips, thighs, and buttocks) are metabolically stable and are not at significantly enhanced risk for such diseases. Further research is necessary to discern whether therapeutic interventions should be targeted mostly toward patients with upper body obesity, and whether doing so will improve short- and long-term treatment results.

Although studies of adoptees and of monozygotic twins suggest an important genetic influence on some types of human obesity (36), genetic markers of the various obesity phenotypes remain to be identified. With regard to the latter classification scheme, categorization can be conveniently based upon anatomical/developmental and etiological criteria.

Anatomical/Developmental

It was once thought that the number of fat cells in healthy individuals increased steadily through the first few years of life, again increased slightly during the

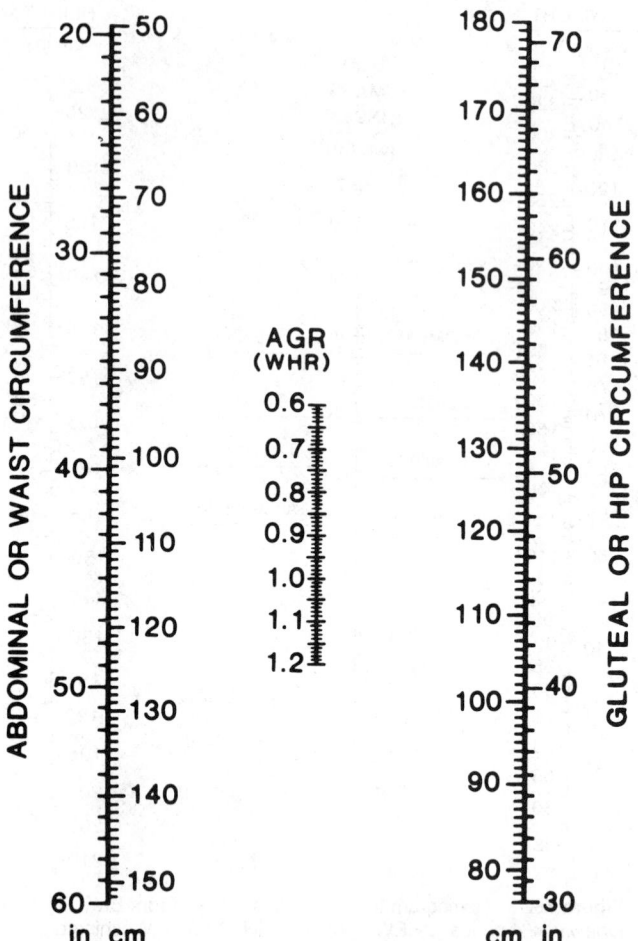

Figure 76.2. Nomogram for determining abdominal (waist) to gluteal (hips) ratio. Place a straight edge between the column for waist circumference and the column for hip circumference and read the ratio from the point where this straight edge crosses the AGR or WHR line. The waist or abdominal circumference is the smallest circumference below the rib cage and above the umbilicus, and the hips or gluteal circumference is taken as the largest circumference at the posterior extension of the buttocks. (From Bray GA: Classification and evaluation of the obesties. *Med Clin North Am* 73:161, 1989.)

peripubertal years, and remained fixed thereafter. Subsequent gains or losses of body fat in adulthood were considered to result solely from corresponding increases or decreases in fat cell size. Recognition that patients with *youth onset* (<15 to 20 years old) obesity more often had generalized obesity with both hyperplasia and hypertrophy of their adipocytes, whereas patients with *adult onset* (>15 to 20 years old) obesity more often had a centripetal distribution of excess fat and adipocyte hypertrophy without an increase in the number of fat cells (5, 18), tended to confirm this hypothesis.

With the increasing awareness of the considerable overlap between these two groups, the concept of hyperplastic versus hypertrophic obesity has undergone further revision. Thus, it is currently appreciated that, in any given individual, fat cell number can increase at any stage of life if a critical (presumably genetically determined) fat cell size has been surpassed. One fu-

ture therapeutic goal might be to identify and treat patients prior to their irreversible conversion from adipocyte hypertrophy to hyperplasia.

Other, much less common types of obesity fall within the anatomical classification. The *lipodystrophies* are localized accumulations of excess fat, most commonly single or multiple lipomas. The latter are inherited as an autosomal dominant trait. *Dercum's disease* (adiposis dolorosa) and *Weber-Christian disease* are two rare illnesses of unknown etiology characterized by focal (occasionally painful) distributions of single or multiple nodules of histologically normal fat.

Etiological

Various organic and environmental factors, none mutually exclusive, are included within the etiological classification of obesity.

Organic Factors

As already noted, even in patients with an apparently genetic predisposition to obesity, environmental influences seem to be important determinants of body weight (see below).

In both experimental animals and in man, certain *primary endocrine disorders* are important causes of obesity. These include hyperinsulinism, hypercortisolism, and deficiencies of growth hormone, thyroid hormone, or sex steroids.

Hyperinsulinemia can result from appropriate or surreptitious use of exogenous insulin, or from insulin hypersecretion by benign or malignant pancreatic neoplasms.

Hypercortisolism most often is iatrogenic, resulting from excess administration of exogenous glucocorticoids. Much less commonly, true Cushing's disease or syndrome is responsible.

Because *growth hormone* exerts an influence on conversion of fat stores into energy for body growth and protein deposition, its absence, either due to pituitary dysfunction or removal, leads to increased adiposity that is reversible by administration of the hormone.

Although *thyroid hormones* directly modulate the overall basal metabolic rate (BMR), hypothyroidism per se is most often associated with modest or no weight gain. Morbid obesity (defined below) due solely to hypothyroidism has not been documented, whereas moderate weight loss because of anorexia disproportionate to the decrease in BMR is occasionally seen.

The *polycystic ovary (Stein-Leventhal) syndromes*, a fairly common group of disorders in young women, is characterized by mild obesity, hirsutism, oligomenorrhea, and infertility in association with mild hypothalamic-pituitary-ovarian (and possibly adrenal) dysfunction. The obesity and the menstrual abnormalities are often ameliorated after ovarian wedge resection.

Hypothalamic obesity is a rare disorder associated most often with the presence of a craniopharyngioma or, less often, with other neoplastic or inflammatory diseases near the hypothalamic ventromedial nuclei, sites in the brain that appear to be involved in the control of normal feeding and satiety.

Of uncertain etiology, but increasingly recognized, are the *primary eating disorders* of bulimia (binge eating) and anorexia nervosa (self-induced starvation). Although the true incidence and prevalence of these conditions are unknown, bulimia is thought to occur in fewer than 5% of obese persons and in as many as 50% of patients with anorexia nervosa. It is generally refractory to most forms of medical and psychiatric management. In one study, phenytoin therapy was found to be helpful in controlling symptoms in about one-third of bulimics (40).

In addition to insulin and glucocorticoids, other pharmacological agents induce increases in food intake and body fat. The most commonly used are phenothiazines, oral contraceptives, and the antihistamine, cyproheptadine (Periactin). Weight gain associated with the latter drug probably results from its antiserotoninergic properties.

Most chronic cigarette smokers weigh less than age- and sex-matched nonsmokers but gain weight after they stop smoking. The weight gain frequently leads to resumption of smoking with its attendant risks for developing cardiovascular disease, emphysema, or cancer. Although the mechanisms responsible for weight loss during active cigarette smoking remain unknown, it has recently been shown that there is a strong positive correlation between the activity of the enzyme, adipose tissue lipoprotein lipase, in the fasting state and the amount of weight regained during the first 2 to 3 weeks after smoking cessation (10). Of additional note is the recent observation that cigarette smoking promotes an increase in the waist-to-hip ratio, despite its tendency to decrease body weight and BMI (33).

Environmental Factors

In view of the obvious imbalance between energy input and expenditure in obese individuals, it is not surprising to find numerous clinical studies that document the importance of nutritional habits and patterns of physical activity in the development of excess adiposity. The adverse effects of an absolute or relative excess in total caloric intake, of a maldistribution of foodstuffs (especially too much fat or carbohydrate), and of the general increase in sedentary life styles are particularly important.

In contemporary affluent societies, obesity is most frequently associated with behavioral and psychological determinants that affect both the circumstances and substance of food intake. Although numerous studies have sought to identify the obese persona, it appears that no such diagnostic personality profile exists. Nonetheless, a major distinction between youth and adult onset types of obesity may reside in the distorted perception of body image that is frequently associated with obesity in childhood and adolescence. Thus, in the latter group, affected individuals often

believe that their body habitus and weight are normal, a phenomenon rarely encountered in adult onset obesity. Moreover, in contrast to certain commonly held notions, it appears that obese individuals are often depressed, are unhappy about being fat, and are relieved by successful and sustained weight loss.

Socioeconomic factors exert strong influences on the development and persistence of obesity in individuals as well as in population groups. In the United States obesity is more common in (a) children and adults from the lower socioeconomic groups, (b) black versus white women, (c) white versus black men, and (d) first generation Americans versus their descendants. Interestingly, when body weights of women of similar ages were compared, those women born later in this century were less heavy than women born in the early 1900s; the opposite trend appeared true for men. The reason for this is unclear but may be related to the steadily increasing fashion consciousness and emphasis on exercise among American women, and to the generally more sedentary work habits and life styles of men.

Morbid Obesity

Morbid obesity defines a subset of patients who are 50 to 100%, or 100 lb (45.5 kg), above their "ideal," "desirable," or "acceptable" body weights. A predominantly genetic origin, with onset of disease in youth, a generally relentless progression through life, and a long-term cure rate of less than 5% are characteristic. In contrast, the onset and progression of the usual forms of mild to moderate adult onset obesity are influenced more by psychosocial factors. Whereas patients with youth onset morbid obesity often suffer from distorted perceptions of body image, this has not been true of patients with adult onset morbid obesity. The latter group, however, has been characterized as generally lacking in internal cues that control food intake, thus being more susceptible to external, environmental eating cues. This observation, confirmed in numerous psychological studies, has exerted a major influence upon the philosophy and design of behavior modification programs.

EPIDEMIOLOGY

Before the epidemiology of obesity in any population group can be ascertained, several general methodological concerns must be addressed. (a) A practical, standardized definition of obesity or overweight must be available and utilized. (b) The study population should be representative of the larger population group of which it is a part. (c) The presence and significance of coexistent morbid diseases or other conditions that may affect body weight must be known. (d) The effects of sex, age, socioeconomic, religious, ethnic, and other related factors must be considered. (e) The effects of confounding variables, such as cigarette smoking, should be analyzed. (f) Both cross-sectional and long-term longitudinal data should be collected. (g) Methods used for quantifying body fat in epidemiological studies, such as relative weight (e.g., body mass index), should be further refined to more closely approximate the most accurate known measures of adipose tissue mass. (h) The prevalence and significance of topographical variations in the distribution of body fat (i.e., upper versus lower body obesity) need to be assessed. Although many excellent, large scale demographic surveys have been reported, to date no single study has satisfied all of the above criteria.

Comparative data on weight and height derived from three major cross-sectional surveys of the United States population have been published by the National Center for Health Statistics and are in Table 76.1. Examination of the table reveals that for both men and women, weights and heights were greater in the periods from 1971 to 1974 and from 1976 to 1980 than they were from 1960 to 1962. These findings have been replicated in numerous studies, particularly in the Build Study of 1979 (9), a survey of 4.2 million generally healthy, middle class persons insured by 25 United States and Canadian insurance companies. Data from this latter study have been widely publicized by the Metropolitan Life Insurance Company as the 1983 Metropolitan Height and Weight Tables (28) and have led to upward revisions of the widely used "desirable" weights previously derived from the Build Study of 1959 (35). Because weights in these latter tables were not derived from a representative sample of the North American population, they should not be considered "desirable" and are therefore not labeled as such.

There is now widespread recognition that with advancing age, there are physiological alterations both in body weight (which increases gradually until the fifth to sixth decade, then tends to plateau) and body composition (with progressive loss of lean body mass and absolute or relative increase in total body fat). Table 76.2, originally reported by Andres (3), illus-

trates comparative weight for height data derived from the 1983 Metropolitan Height and Weight Tables (uncorrected for age) and from the Baltimore Longitudinal Study of Aging, conducted at the Gerontology Research Center of the National Institute on Aging. Perusal of these data reveals that, for most of the heights reported, the Metropolitan optimal weights for men and women are similar to those for the age-adjusted weights of individuals in their thirties and forties. Therefore, the Metropolitan tables overestimate the "norms" for younger adults but underestimate the corresponding "norms" for elderly people. In the age-adjusted data from the Gerontology Research Center, there is an increased weight allowance of about 10 lb/decade. More recent studies utilizing various anthropometric ratios (including WHR) have demonstrated an age-related increase in upper and central body adiposity. The ratios are independently influenced by BMI, and are higher in men than in women despite a postmenopausal acceleration in the trend in women (32).

In the United States Public Health Service Ten State Nutrition Survey of 1968 to 1970 (17), the prevalence of obesity in adolescents was determined by measurement of triceps skin-fold thickness. With use of the criterion of skin-fold thickness greater than the 85th percentile of adult values (18.6 mm in men and 25.1 mm in women), obesity in adolescents was found to vary with age from 11 to 39% for white males and from 9 to 19% for white females. White male adolescents were more obese than their black counterparts. In this study there were no consistent relationships between obesity and socioeconomic status. However, Stunkard et al. (38) have emphasized the importance of social factors in the prevalence of obesity or overweight in childhood. In one study overweight children from lower socioeconomic groups were identified by age 6, whereas overweight children from upper socioeconomic groups

Table 76.1.
Mean Weights and Heights by Age and Sex in Three Populations[a,b]

Age Group	Men		NHANES II	Women		NHANES II
	HES	NHANES I		HES	NHANES I	
Weight (kg)						
18–24 years	71.7	74.8	73.9	57.6	59.9	60.8
25–34 years	72.6	79.8	78.5	60.8	63.5	64.4
35–44 years	77.1	80.7	80.7	64.4	67.1	67.1
45–54 years	77.1	79.4	80.7	65.8	67.6	68.0
55–64 years	74.4	77.6	78.9	68.0	67.6	68.0
65–74 years	71.7	74.4	74.8	65.3	66.2	66.7
18–74 years	75.3	78.0	78.0	63.5	64.9	65.3
Height (m)						
18–24 years	1.74	1.77	1.77	1.62	1.63	1.63
25–34 years	1.76	1.77	1.77	1.62	1.63	1.63
35–44 years	1.74	1.76	1.76	1.61	1.63	1.63
45–54 years	1.73	1.75	1.75	1.60	1.62	1.61
55–64 years	1.71	1.73	1.74	1.58	1.60	1.60
65–74 years	1.70	1.71	1.71	1.56	1.58	1.58
18–74 years	1.73	1.75	1.76	1.60	1.62	1.62

[a] From Simopoulos AP, Van Itallie TBV: Body weight, health, and longevity. *Ann Intern Med* 100:285, 1984.
[b] The three populations are from the National Health Examination Survey (HES), 1960 to 1962 and the National Health and Nutrition Examination Survey (NHANES) I, 1971 to 1974, and II, 1976 to 1980. Two pounds were deducted from HES data to allow for weight of clothing; total weight of all clothing for NHANES I and II ranged from 0.1 to 0.3 kg and was not deducted from weights in table. Height was measured without shoes. Data are preliminary. Age-adjusted mean values and estimates of variation (standard error) about the mean estimates are not currently available.

Table 76.2.
Comparison of the Weight for Height Tables from Actuarial Data (*Build Study 1979*): Non-Age-Corrected Metropolitan Life Insurance Company and Age-Specific Gerontology Research Center Recommendations[a]

HEIGHT (Feet Inches)	Metropolitan 1983 Weights[b]		Gerontology Research Center[b]				
	Men	Women	Age-Specific Weight Range for Men and Women				
	25–59 yr		25 Yr	35 Yr	45 Yr	55 Yr	65 Yr
4 10		100–131	84–111	92–119	99–127	107–135	115–142
4 11		101–134	87–115	95–123	103–131	111–139	119–147
5 0		103–137	90–119	98–127	106–135	114–143	123–152
5 1	123–145	105–140	93–123	101–131	110–140	118–148	127–157
5 2	125–148	108–144	96–127	105–136	113–144	122–153	131–163
5 3	127–151	111–148	99–131	108–140	117–149	126–158	135–168
5 4	129–155	114–152	102–135	112–145	121–154	130–163	140–173
5 5	131–159	117–156	106–140	115–149	125–159	134–168	144–179
5 6	133–163	120–160	109–144	119–154	129–164	138–174	148–184
5 7	135–167	123–164	112–148	122–159	133–169	143–179	153–190
5 8	137–171	126–167	116–153	126–163	137–174	147–184	158–196
5 9	139–175	129–170	119–157	130–168	141–179	151–190	162–201
5 10	141–179	132–173	122–162	134–173	145–184	156–195	167–207
5 11	144–183	135–176	126–167	137–178	149–190	160–201	172–213
6 0	147–187		129–171	141–183	153–195	165–207	177–219
6 1	150–192		133–176	145–188	157–200	169–213	182–225
6 2	153–197		137–181	149–194	162–206	174–219	187–232
6 3	157–202		141–186	153–199	166–212	179–225	192–238
6 4			144–191	157–205	171–218	184–231	197–244

[a] From Andres R: Mortality and obesity. The rationale for age-specific height-weight tables. In Andres R, Hazzard WR, Bierman E (eds): *Principles of Geriatric Medicine*. New York, McGraw-Hill, 1985.
[b] Values in this table are for height without shoes and weight without clothes.

could not be identified until age 8, and there were fewer at later ages in childhood.

The Seven Country Study of Keys (21) (Table 76.3) provided comparative data on obesity and overweight, utilizing criteria of skin-fold thickness and relative weight; by either criterion men from the United States were among the most corpulent examined.

PATHOGENESIS

Energy Intake

In the United States the typical diet is composed of approximately 40 to 45% carbohydrate, 40% fat, and 15 to 20% protein. Energy intake that exceeds energy expenditure is the cardinal pathogenetic mechanism pro-

moting an increase in body fat. Although there is evidence to support the idea that, in healthy people, body weight is fairly closely regulated over long periods of time, body composition changes considerably with age, as noted previously. The numerous factors controlling normal food intake and distribution, storage, and expenditure of energy represent a complex, highly integrated series of events, as yet only partially understood.

Until recently, it was thought that normal control of hunger and satiety in man resided in certain nuclei of the lateral and medial hypothalamus, respectively, and that other neural, nutritional, endocrine-metabolic, gastrointestinal, and psychological factors exerted their influences by impinging upon these sites. Current evidence favors a more diffuse localization of feeding and satiety "centers" involving not only the perihypothalamic area but portions of the limbic system and cerebral cortex as well.

The application of contemporary techniques of cell, tissue, and organ culture has allowed for novel approaches to examine directly the basic cellular and molecular processes occurring in various tissues and cells (e.g., adipocytes, hepatocytes, etc.) known to be affected by metabolic derangements in obesity, in both humans and experimental animals. Data derived from such studies will undoubtedly provide important new information pertinent to understanding the pathophysiological derangements in cellular uptake, storage, and expenditure of energy in human obesity.

Table 76.3.
Prevalence of Overweight and Obesity in Groups of Men from Seven Countries[a]

Country	Percent of Sample	
	Overweight[b]	Obese[c]
Japan	2	2
Greece	11	11
Finland	15	14
Yugoslavia	19	29
Italy	33	28
Netherlands	13	32
United States	32	63

[a] Data adapted from Keys (21), from Bray GA: The obese patient. In Smith LH (ed): *Major Problems in Internal Medicine*, Philadelphia, WB Saunders, 1976, vol. 9.
[b] Overweight = men 10% or more over standard weight.
[c] Obesity = men with sum of triceps and subscapular skinfold > 28 mm.

Energy Expenditure

Even after adjustments for differences in age, sex, and body weight, energy expenditure varies considerably among normal adults. Under resting conditions, there are adaptations to the amount and type of food ingested that allow for increased or decreased utilization of, nutrients and that maintain a stable weight in most people. For example, after increased food intake above that required for maintenance of normal weight, healthy individuals exhibit an initial increase in weight followed by a new plateau of weight despite continued overeating, a phenomenon referred to as luxuskonsumption, or dietary-induced thermogenesis (DIT). Current evidence favors the hypothesis that DIT is an important factor in regulating body weight, and that the "missing energy" is burnt off in "brown fat," metabolically more active than the usual "white fat" (14).

In our sedentary society physical exercise plays a relatively minor role in energy expenditure. Nonetheless, evidence exists that energy expenditure differs in obese persons during exercise and during ingestion of food that contributes to the genesis of obesity. For example, recent studies in Southwestern American Indians suggest that a low rate of 24-hour energy expenditure contributes to the familial aggregation of obesity in that group (30). It should be noted that short-term vigorous exercise, such as weight lifting, competitive contact sports, etc., often leads to increases in dietary intake, utilization of muscle glycogen stores, and muscle mass. In contrast, frequent, sustained, moderate aerobic exercise, such as jogging, swimming, etc., mobilizes fat stores.

Despite the apparent long-term control of general energy balance and body weight in normal persons, there is no conclusive evidence of an endogenous set-point (e.g., glucostatic, lipostatic, or thermostatic) that modulates adipose tissue mass. However, Schwartz and Brunzell have reported that the activity of adipose tissue lipoprotein lipase (LPL), the rate-limiting enzyme in the uptake and storage of lipoprotein triglyceride in adipose tissue, is increased in obese Caucasians and that enzyme activity increases, rather than decreases, after weight loss (31). Moreover, there appear to be demographic/genetic differences in the occurrence of this phenomenon. These authors have proposed that adipose tissue LPL may exert a counter-regulatory role in preventing deviation from a set-point for fat cell size or mass, thus predisposing to return to the original obese state (31). As noted above (see page 1031), the correlation between baseline adipose tissue LPL activity and the amount of weight gained after cessation of cigarette smoking further supports this hypothesis.

Certain indices of cellular sodium potassium ATPase activity have been reported to be increased (6), decreased (11), or unchanged (4) in red blood cells or liver from obese subjects, as compared with controls. Further investigation is necessary to clarify whether alterations in the activity of this critical cellular enzyme contribute to the pathophysiological mechanisms by which cellular thermogenesis, and therefore the efficiency of energy expenditure, might be perturbed in human obesity.

The observation that most obesity in adult men is upper body in distribution, while that in most adult women is lower body in distribution, suggested that sex hormones might influence body fat topography and function. Increased androgenic activity has been reported in the blood of women with upper versus lower body obesity and has been shown to correlate with abnormalities in fat cell size and biochemical function (12). Moreover, abdominal adipocytes from patients with upper body obesity are metabolically active, whereas abdominal adipocytes from patients with lower body obesity, and thigh adipocytes from patients with upper or lower body obesity, are metabolically relatively stable.

NATURAL HISTORY

Much information has been adduced to show that obese infants and children become obese adults more often than do their lean counterparts. In addition, youth onset obesity tends to be more severe and persistent, and more resistant to treatment, than are the usually milder forms of later onset. This may be due to the fact that weight loss and decrease in adiposity per se result predominantly from a decrease in adipocyte size and not number, so that adipose hyperplasia (regardless of age of onset) (see page 1030) is ordinarily irreversible. In contrast, there is greater therapeutic promise for the more common adult onset obese population, who have a normal number of adipocytes.

Metabolic Concomitants

Although the exact roles of all organic and environmental factors in the pathogenesis of obesity remain to be elucidated, certain metabolic concomitants of excess adiposity have been characterized. Numerous studies document the close association between obesity and diabetes mellitus and suggest that obesity per se is diabetogenic. Obesity leads to increased pancreatic insulin production and hyperinsulinemia, both basally and after stimulation by ingestion of glucose, amino acids, etc. Evidence exists that the hyperinsulinemia and concurrent glucose intolerance are due to insulin resistance at the tissue level (e.g., liver, adipose tissue, and skeletal muscle) (23), caused in some individuals by a decrease in the number of cell surface receptors for insulin, and in others by aberrant, insulin-dependent intracellular glucose metabolism. Finally, it has been proposed that chronic hyperinsulinemia leads to a further decrease in the number of cell surface insulin receptors (i.e., "down-regulation"), the latter serving as an adipocyte response to prevent episodes of hypoglycemia.

There is a significant association between obesity and the presence of *hyperlipidemia*, especially hypertriglyceridemia. This latter relationship probably results, at least in some patients, from the hyperinsulinemia-induced increase in hepatic triglyceride synthesis and formation of triglyceride-rich very low density lipoproteins (VLDL), although this hypothesis requires further confirmation. Increased endogenous cholesterol synthesis is also more frequent in obese patients, leads to increased circulating concentrations of total cholesterol and low density lipoprotein (LDL) cholesterol and decreased concentrations of high density lipoprotein (HDL) cholesterol, and results in increased risk of coronary artery disease and, probably, cholesterol gallstones.

Many patients with adult onset upper body obesity appear cushingoid. Simple obesity is associated with an increased cortisol production rate leading to increased hepatic steroid metabolism and increased urinary excretion of certain steroid conjugates. Such patients typically have increased urinary 17-hydroxycorticoids; however, plasma cortisol, urinary-free cortisol, and overnight dexamethasone suppression tests are usually normal.

Salt and water retention is a common problem in obese patients, and it is in part mediated by increases in aldosterone secretion induced by dietary carbohydrate and, to a lesser extent, protein intake.

Onset of normal menarche does not occur until a critical body weight is reached (usually 40 to 45 kg), a finding that explains the earlier menarche in women with youth onset obesity. Menstrual abnormalities, such as dysfunctional uterine bleeding, amenorrhea, and infertility, are also more common in obese women and are often associated with aberrant cyclical reproductive hormone functional (subnormal levels of follicle-stimulating hormone (FSH) in the follicular phase, and of progesterone on the luteal phase).

Other important endocrinologic or metabolic sequelae of obesity, the mechanisms for which are unclear, are decreased growth hormone responses to provocative stimuli (including hypothalamic growth hormone-releasing hormone) and hyperuricemia. The former, by decreasing the availability of a lipolytic hormone, permits excess fat accumulation, and the latter is responsible for the increased prevalence of gout in obese individuals.

Risks

A large body of research and anecdotal data has suggested that obesity and overweight are graded phenomena, and that there is strong positive correlation between the degree of excess adiposity and increased morbidity and mortality, the latter particularly from cardiovascular and cerebrovascular diseases. It now appears that this hypothesis must be somewhat modified.

Critical analysis of data derived from retrospective life insurance studies suggested that there was no significant increase in mortality until body weight rose to values greater than 30% above ideal body weight. Data from a large number of prospective studies also suggest that severe to extreme, but not mild to moderate, obesity is associated with decreased longevity. More recent reanalyses of data from various large scale epidemiological studies have led several investigators to conclude that the "mortality for weight" curves are often "J-" or "U"-shaped, in that the highest mortality rates occur at both extremes of relative weight (e.g., body mass index), whereas the lowest mortality rates occur at intermediate weights (34). Andres has demonstrated that the body mass index associated with lowest mortality itself increases with advancing age, both in men and women, and has thus emphasized the need for age-specific weight-height tables (3). It is also evident, as noted above (page 1029), that the risks of obesity vary not only with the amount but with the topographical distribution of excess body fat. Finally, data published as part of a 26-year follow-up of subjects in the Framingham study (19) reveal that obesity per se is an independent risk factor for premature dying. Current evidence favors the view that hyperinsulinemia is the common pathogenetic mechanism by which upper body obesity influences known cardiac risk factors, such as hypertension, hyperlipidemia, and diabetes mellitus (20, 29). It seems likely that public health and other officials, as well as individual physicians, will become more cautious in their advice regarding evaluation and management of patients with mild to moderate obesity, particularly if it is lower body in distribution.

Medical Consequences

The major physiological and medical concomitants of moderate to extreme obesity are depicted in Table 76.4. Although a direct pathophysiological link between obesity and these conditions has not been unequivocally established, in each instance, the morbidity associated with the condition is proportional to the degree of excess adiposity and is partially or totally reversed after successful weight loss. In addition, obesity, particularly when severe, frequently exacerbates or complicates the course of a variety of other conditions—for example, by delaying surgical procedures, enhancing perioperative risks, prolonging convalescence from many illnesses, worsening pregnancy-associated problems, and exacerbating unstable behavioral patterns.

EVALUATION AND MANAGEMENT

Evaluation

The initial evaluation of the obese patient should include a medical and psychosocial history, physical examination, and appropriate laboratory and other studies. The history will usually indicate whether the patient has youth onset or adult onset obesity, and it will often provide important information regarding usual or unusual dietary practices, as well as patterns of physical activity. It is particularly important to identify any medical or psychological factors that may motivate the patient to lose weight or that militate for or against certain treatment plans. The physical examination should include an assessment of whether the patient has primarily upper or lower body obesity by measuring the ratio of the minimal circumference

Table 76.4.
Possible Medical Consequences of Obesity

ENDOCRINE-METABOLIC:
  Hyperglycemia, hyperinsulinemia, insulin resistance
  Hypertriglyceridemia, hypercholesterolemia ($\uparrow$ VLDL $\uparrow$ LDL $\downarrow$ HDL)
  $\uparrow$ Cortisol production but normal plasma cortisol, diurnal rhythm,
    urine free cortisol and overnight dexamethasone suppression
  Early menarche, menstrual abnormalities, hirsutism
  $\downarrow$ Growth hormone, basally and after provocative stimuli
  Hyperuricemia, gout
CARDIOVASCULAR:
  Hypertension
  Coronary artery disease
  Congestive heart failure
  Varicose veins
  Cerebrovascular disease
PULMONARY:
  Hypoventilation (*e.g.*, Pickwickian) syndromes
  Sleep apnea syndrome
  Chronic respiratory infections
GALLBLADDER:
  Cholelithiasis (cholesterol gallstones)
MUSCULOSKELETAL:
  Osteoarthritis
  Chronic orthopaedic problems
  $\downarrow$ Ambulation
RENAL:
  Nephrotic syndrome (normal or nonspecific biopsy)
ONCOLOGICAL:
  Endometrial, breast carcinoma (postmenopausal
    women), prostate, colon,
DERMATOLOGICIAL
  Acanthosis nigricans
  Chronic skin infections
PSYCHOSOCIAL:
  Depression, loss of self-esteem
  $\downarrow$ Employability
PREGNANCY:
  Worsen underlying hypertension, diabetes mellitus
  $\uparrow$ Maternal mortality
SURGERY (especially under general anesthesia)
  Increased perioperative morbidity and mortality

at the waist to the maximal circumference at the hips with the patient in the standing position. A waist to hip ratio (WHR) greater than 0.85 indicates definite upper body obesity, whereas a WHR less than 0.76 indicates lower body obesity.

Although secondary obesity is rare, its importance lies in its reversibility after identification and specific therapy of the underlying medical or pharmacological disorder. Special emphasis should therefore be placed on screening an obese patient for any contributing endocrine-metabolic process and on obtaining a history of medication use (see pages 1030–1031).

Evidence of glucose intolerance should be sought by obtaining fasting blood glucose levels with the patient on a regular (or, preferably, high carbohydrate) diet, and comparing the results with those from age- and sex-matched controls. The oral glucose tolerance test is not ordinarily necessary to make the diagnosis of adult onset diabetes mellitus. Hypercortisolemia should be suspected in any plethoric, hypertensive patient with upper body obesity, hypokalemia, and glucose intolerance. A normal overnight dexamethasone suppression test (i.e., 1.0 mg of oral dexamethasone at 11 P.M., followed by an 8 A.M. plasma cortisol

<5 μg/dl) or as a normal value for 24-hour urinary free cortisol excretion (<100 μg/24 hours) ordinarily eliminates the diagnosis of endogenous hypercortisolemia with a reasonable degree of certainty. Clinically significant hypothyroidism can usually be ruled out when the free thyroxine index (i.e., serum T_4 $\times$ resin T_3 uptake) is normal. On occasion, hyperthyroid patients "outeat" their increased BMR and complain to the physician of weight gain. The finding of menstrual irregularities, mild hirsutism (but not virilization), and obesity in a young woman prompts suspicion of the polycystic ovarian syndrome, a diagnosis made more likely by the additional findings of a mildly elevated serum testosterone level (60 to 100 ng/dl), flat basal body temperature curve (i.e., no ovulation), and palpable abnormalities on pelvic examination. Diseases of the hypothalamic-pituitary region should be considered in obese patients with otherwise unexplained neuroendocrine abnormalities. Certain rare syndromes, such as the Prader-Willi syndrome (obesity, short stature, hypogonadism, and mental retardation), are usually recognized in childhood by their characteristic clinical presentations.

In addition to the above, fasting blood samples should be sent for determinations of triglyceride, total cholesterol, HDL cholesterol, and uric acid levels. Most patients with hyperlipidemia have acquired (i.e., secondary), not genetic (i.e., primary), hyperlipidemias and will respond to appropriate diet regimens (see Chapter 75). Finally, in patients with clinically apparent or suspect hypoventilation syndromes or sleep-disordered breathing, pulmonary function should be tested.

A useful algorithm for the outpatient evaluation of the obese patient has been published by Bray and Teague (7). Initial experience with this algorithm, as applied to 234 obese women and 27 obese men, led to detection of the following significant abnormalities: hypertension (16%), hypertriglyceridemia (25%), glucose intolerance (25%), hypercholesterolemia (11%), and hyperuricemia (7%). In two of 57 patients studied, T_4 values were abnormal; one was high and one low.

Management of Mild to Moderate Obesity

Based upon the initial assessment of the patient, the type (adult onset versus childhood onset), topographical distribution, and degree of obesity should be ascertained, including the medical or psychological urgency for weight loss, the patient's motivation and readiness for weight loss, and the most suitable treatment plan. Because the usual form of simple adult onset, mild to moderate lower body obesity appears not to carry an increased risk of morbidity or mortality (see page 1035), it should probably not be treated at all. On the other hand, until the possible risks of mild to moderate upper body obesity are more clearly defined, it would seem prudent to treat it with a combination of moderate diet, regular exercise, and patient-motivated nutritional education and behavioral relearning. There is no justification for the use of anorexigenic drugs in the treatment of the problem. If the patient asks for them, the physician should explain that they are modestly effective, that they are of little or no help in maintaining long-term weight loss, and that many of them are potentially dangerous (see below, page 1039). Moreover, the patient should be cautioned against the purchase of patent medicines. It is now clear that several lay organizations for weight reduction [e.g., Weight Watchers, Take Off Pounds Sensibly (TOPS), Diet Center, and NutriSystem] are as capable as health professionals in effecting weight loss in this category of obese patient.

General nutritional guidelines for reducing the risk of diet-related chronic disorders, including obesity, have recently been published by the National Research Council (see Table 76.5). For most adults, a balanced diet containing 1500 to 1800 calories/day is necessary for maintenance of optimal body weight under conditions of basal activity. Thus, modest caloric restriction to 900 to 1200 calories/day for women and 1200 to 1500 calories/day for men is appropriate, with small increases proportionate to increases in levels of physical activity. It is often useful to advise patients who

Table 76.5.
Recommended Dietary Guidelines[a]

1. Reduce total fat intake to 30% or less of calories, saturated fatty acid intake to less than 10% of calories, and cholesterol intake to less than 300 mg daily. The intake of fat and cholesterol can be reduced by substituting fish, poultry without skin, lean meats and low- or nonfat dairy products for fatty meats and whole-milk dairy products; by choosing more vegetables, fruits, cereals and legumes; and by limiting oils, fats, egg yolks, and fried and other fatty foods.

2. Every day eat five or more servings of a combination of vegetables and fruits, especially green and yellow vegetables and citrus fruits. Also, increase intake of starches and other complex carbohydrates by eating six or more daily servings of a combination of breads, cereals and legumes. An average serving is equal to a half cup for most fresh or cooked vegetables, fruits, dry or cooked cereals or legumes, one medium piece of fresh fruit, one slice of bread, or one roll or muffin.

3. Maintain protein intake at moderate levels (less than 1.6 g/kg body weight for adults).

4. Balance food intake and physical activity to maintain appropriate body weight.

5. The committee does not recommend alcohol consumption. For those who drink alcoholic beverages, the committee recommends limiting consumption to the equivalent of less than 1 ounce of pure alcohol in a single day. This is the equivalent of two cans of beer, two small glasses of wine, or two average cocktails. Pregnant women should avoid alcoholic beverages.

6. Limit total daily intake of salt to 6 g or less. Limit the use of salt in cooking and avoid adding it to food at the table. Salty, highly processed salty, salt-preserved, and salt-pickled foods should be consumed sparingly.

7. Maintain adequate calcium balance. The potential benefits of calcium intakes above the RDAs (recommended daily allowances) to prevent osteoporosis or hypertension are not well documented and do not justify the use of calcium supplements.

8. Avoid taking dietary supplements in excess of the RDA in any one day.

9. Maintain an optimal intake of fluoride, particularly during the years of primary and secondary tooth formation and growth.

[a] Adapted from Diet and Health. Implications for reducing chronic disease risk. Committee on Diet and Health. Food and Nutrition Board. Commission on Life Sciences. National Research Council. Washington, DC National Academy Press, 1989.

are motivated to diet to purchase one of the readily available, inexpensive calorie counters and to use the information to limit their daily diet to a specific number of calories. In general, daily modest exercise programs should be tailored to the individual patient's ability and enjoyment. Regular physical conditioning will facilitate weight loss, as well as decrease or abolish obesity-associated hyperinsulinemia, insulin resistance, glucose intolerance, hypertriglyceridemia, hyperuricemia, and systolic and diastolic hypertension and will improve cardiovascular, respiratory, and musculoskeletal problems. A goal of a loss of 1 or 2 pounds (0.5 to 1 kg) a week is appropriate whenever a patient embarks on a weight reduction program.

Improved nutritional understanding often results from effective and practical dietary counseling. Diet sheets and booklets that set forth easy to understand and follow recommendations, particularly when attuned to the sociocultural and economic characteristics of the patient, are especially valuable. Improved patterns of eating behavior should be encouraged. Specific suggestions should include smaller, more frequent, or regular meals, eaten more slowly, in defined surroundings. Use of food diaries is especially helpful (Fig. 76.3), particularly in identifying abnormal behavioral patterns leading to excess food intake. For the patient who makes a significant effort, reinforcement of the improved eating behavior by his physician is important in maintenance of weight reduction. Usually, formal consultation with a professional behavioral therapist is not required.

Management of Morbid Obesity

Morbid obesity (see page 1031), particularly of the upper body variety, is associated with a measurably increased morbidity and mortality, as well as with a generally poor response to conventional methods of moderate caloric restriction. Although there are hazards associated with each of the more intensive forms of treatment, in many severely obese patients the risks and disadvantages of being overweight greatly exceed those of treatment. In some individuals, behavioral modification (see below), alone or in combination with other therapies, may offer an effective and safe management option.

Diet

Significant weight loss (up to 5 to 6 kg/week) can be achieved by prolonged (4 to 8 weeks) starvation of motivated, hospitalized morbidly obese patients. Within 1 to 2 years after such treatment, however, fewer than 25 to 30% of these patients have maintained their initial weight loss, and in the long-term, fewer than 5% attain and maintain their "ideal" body weight. A major hazard of such treatment is the extensive loss of lean body mass, and thus negative nitrogen balance, that occurs predictably within the first 1 or 2 weeks of starvation and continues at a somewhat lower rate thereafter. Other complications of this technique include orthostatic hypotension, ketoacidosis, electro-

FRANCIS SCOTT KEY MEDICAL CENTER
WEIGHT CONTROL PROGRAM

Name: _____ Date: _____

Day: Mon.   Tues.   Wed.   Thurs.   Fri.   Sat.   Sun.   (circle one)

Exercise or activity: A. Type_____   Minutes_____   B. Type_____   Minutes_____

Time	Minutes	Food Type	Amount	Meal/ Snacks	Hunger Yes No	Body Position	Activity while Eating	Location of Eating	Eating (with Whom)	Feeling

Time: starting time for a meal or snack; Meal/snack: indicate type of eating by the appropriate letter—M (meal) or S (snack). Hunger: check yes or no.

Figure 76.3. Food diary for identification of abnormal behavioral patterns leading to excess food intake.

lyte and vitamin deficiencies, weakness, decreased libido and impotence, menstrual irregularities, hyperuricemia and acute gout, renal uric acid calculi, emotional disturbances, and, rarely, sudden death. Despite these potential disadvantages, the need for hospitalization, and the high incidence of recidivism, total fasting appears to be a generally safe and efficacious technique for inducing significant short-term (e.g., presurgical) weight loss when supervised by physicians experienced in the technique.

Supplemented fasting is a technique that exploits in an ambulatory setting several of the advantages of total fasting, particularly those of significant short-term weight loss and high patient adherence. In general, patients consume 1 to 1.5 g of protein/kg of desirable body weight, enough to prevent loss of lean body mass, in a hypocaloric (e.g., 300 to 500 calories/day) diet supplemented by adequate hydration, potassium salts, and other vitamins and minerals. In one study of nearly 1200 patients who were followed clinically and biochemically at frequent intervals, approximately 75 to 80% of the patients lost more than 40 lb (18 kg) (15). Moreover, hypertension and glucose intolerance, as well as the need for appropriate medications, disappeared or diminished in the majority of affected patients; other benefits, such as improved exercise tolerance, ambulation, pulmonary function, psychosocial and employment status also became evident. The disadvantages of the technique are similar to, but of lesser magnitude than, those described above for total fasting; there have been, in addition, several sudden cardiac deaths in patients without known preexisting heart disease. A major problem with supplemented fasting is that the initial success rate drops to

about 25% on subsequent attempts at fasting after major weight regain.

A variant of the supplemented fast, the "liquid protein" diet, has been widely used in this country and consists of a very poor quality protein, collagen hydrolysate, supplemented with tryptophan. Because of the ready commercial availability of this diet, many obese patients have consumed it without appropriate vitamin or mineral supplementation or medical supervision. In one report (39), more than 60 sudden cardiac deaths were documented during or shortly after discontinuation of this diet. Although electrocardiograms often showed prolonged QT intervals, decreased QRS voltages, and refractory ventricular dysrhythmias, electrolyte abnormalities such as hypokalemia and hypocalcemia were not invariably present. Some autopsy studies have revealed a nonspecific cardiac muscle atrophy similar to that seen in protein-calorie malnutrition states in man and experimental animals. Also, transient, potentially life-threatening cardiac dysrhythmias were detected by 24-hour Holter monitoring, but not by standard 12-lead electrocardiograms, in three of six morbidly obese hospitalized patients followed for 40 days on a commercially available liquid protein diet (26). In none of the six patients was there an antecedent history of cardiac disease, and in all of the patients Holter monitoring was normal before and after the study diet. Except for mild hypokalemia in one of the affected patients, none of many routine chemical or metabolic parameters distinguished between patients with and without cardiac abnormalities. In a subsequent related study, six additional morbidly obese but otherwise healthy patients were hospitalized and fed for 40 days with a markedly hypocaloric (470 Kcal/day) experimental diet containing 60% high quality protein, 25% carbohydrate, and 15% fat and supplemented with the Recommended Daily Allowances or more of all essential minerals, trace elements, vitamins, and essential fatty acids (1). No dysrhythmias were detected on 24-hour Holter monitoring, nitrogen balance remained positive, and the previously noted electrolyte abnormalities were reversed or decreased. The results of the latter study suggested that appropriate supplementation of even a markedly hypocaloric diet was safer than the nutritionally inadequate liquid protein diet, and a model was thus provided for several popular diet programs, such as Optifast® and Medifast®. The Food and Drug Administration requires that warning labels be placed on all protein-supplemented diets and has suggested restricting such diets to certain individuals, all of whom should be aware of the potential hazards and should be followed by physicians experienced in using such diets. However, in view of the above observations, it appears prudent to discontinue use of liquid protein diets until the mechanisms of their cardiac toxicity are elucidated.

There are numerous palatable balanced and unbalanced low calorie diets in common use. Many patients find it easier to follow regimens that limit caloric intake by eliminating entire food groups, such as carbohydrates, or by providing nutritionally adequate food homogenates. Perhaps the benefits of these approaches derive both from a perception that they are more "medicinal" and from diminution in external feeding cues.

Diets that are very low in calories (fewer than 800 calories/day) and carbohydrates are usually ketogenic. They are particularly popular because of the commonly held ideas that (a) nutritional ketosis exerts an anorexic effect, (b) greater weight loss ensues than after a balanced diet containing an equal number of calories, and (c) such diets spare body protein better than do balanced diets. There are no unequivocal data to support the first two notions. Although low carbohydrate, low caloric diets do generally cause a more profound early (1- to 2-week) diuresis of salt and water than do balanced diets, the rate of fat loss is no greater. Moreover, hypocaloric, low carbohydrate diets, like fasting and supplemented fasting, are associated with weakness, dehydration, postural hypotension, and occasional hyperuricemia and acute gout.

The safest diets are balanced and contain more than 800 calories daily. Table 76.6 illustrates several popular fad diets that are nutritionally unbalanced and/or hypocaloric. Use of these and the numerous other related fad diets that are hypocaloric and unbalanced, particularly when medically unsupervised, should be avoided.

How effective are dietary attempts at long-term weight loss? Although quantitation of successful weight loss has been defined differently by various investigators, numerous studies confirm that at most only 10 to 20% of obese patients who initially lose significant amounts of weight on diets maintain or increase that weight loss several years later. Although all factors that promote such success or failure remain unknown, it has been shown that ability to continue in a diet program (nearly 25% of patients drop out within the first few weeks) and emotional stability are important. The appearance of pathological depression during or after dietary weight loss is well recognized and is more common in juvenile onset obese patients, in whom the baseline distortion of body image is often accompanied, paradoxically, by a perception of larger body size with progressive weight loss. It is to be hoped that improved classification schemes will better identify subpopulations of obese patients more amenable to specifically defined therapeutic programs.

Behavior Modification

The basis for behavior modification therapy in the management of obesity rests upon the finding that many obese patients, particularly those of adult onset, respond predominantly to external, rather than internal, feeding cues. Thus, the focus of treatment is to alter daily habits, such as eating behaviors and attitudes, social supports, exercise, nutrition, and other factors related to eating (8). Weight loss resulting from behavior modification, unlike that produced by dietary, pharmacological, or surgical therapy, has not been associated with serious adverse side effects. Although these techniques offer great therapeutic promise, particularly when used in conjunction with diet and exercise programs, not all obese individuals will respond, even in the short-term, to this form of therapy, a fact that underscores the need for improved categorization and prognostication of obesity subtypes.

The short- and long-term efficacy of group therapy for obesity has also been examined and appears to be similar to that of individual therapy, a finding that should prompt more effective use of trained therapists. Data published by two of the most popular lay self-help groups that advertise success at weight reduction, Weight Watchers and TOPS, confirm prior anecdotal impressions by experienced therapists that these groups achieve short-term results as good as, and long-term results as poor as, those in medically supervised programs.

Pharmacological Therapy

There is no known pharmacological agent for the treatment of obesity that is reliably effective, devoid of short- and long-term adverse side effects, inexpensive, and readily available. The anorexigenic derivatives of phenethylamine (Table 76.7), which include the amphetamines and fenfluramine, are the most commonly prescribed drugs. All possess certain pharmacological properties like those of epinephrine and norepinephrine; however, their various chemical modifications have led, to differing extents, to decreased cardiovascular and central nervous system toxicity and to preservation of anorexigenic properties. For the amphetamines, appetite suppression is probably mediated primarily by catecholaminergic

Table 76.6.
Characteristics of Several Widely Used Fad Diets

Diet	Composition	Deficiencies	Side Effects and Potential Hazards	Other Comments
HIGH PROTEIN/KETOGENIC DIETS Dr. Atkin's Revolutionary Diet The Drinking Man's Diet The Scarsdale Diet Dr. Stillman's Quick-Weight-Loss Diet	High protein Moderate to high fat Low carbohydrate Caloric intake varies from 1000–2000 calories	Likely deficiencies: Dietary fiber Calcium Riboflavin Folic acid Vitamins A, C Thiamine Iron	Potential exists for: Ketosis, anorexia, fatigue, dehydration, postural hypotension, hypokalemia/sodium loss, hyperlipidemia, hyperuricemia, constipation, halitosis	Long term maintenance unrealistic. NOT RECOMMENDED especially during pregnancy, in kidney disease, diabetes mellitus, lipid disorders. Can precipitate an acute attack of gout. Effectiveness due to high satiety values of foods consumed in diet. Large initial weight loss felt to be due to loss of body water. No greater actual fat loss than with balanced diet of equal calories.
PROTEIN-SPARING MODIFIED FAST (PSMF) Liquid Protein Diet The Last Chance Diet Cambridge Diet	Variation to total fast. Maximize fat loss but minimize lean body mass lost by adding 1.0 to 1.5 g of variable quality protein/kg of ideal body weight ~400 calories (300–700 calories) e.g., 330 calories/day 31 g of protein 44 g of CHO 2 g of fat and vitamin and mineral supplements	If poor biological quality protein, tryptophan deficiency. Likely deficiencies in poorly supplemented regimens: Potassium Phosphorus Calcium Magnesium Vitamin A Riboflavin	Ketosis Dehydration Hypokalemia Postural hypotension Cold intolerance Constipation Rarely—sudden death, felt to be secondary to cardiac arrhythmias	Unrealistic for long term maintenance. Not recommended for ambulatory management since needs careful medical monitoring. Tolerated more by morbidly obese than by mildly to moderately overweight individuals. Some programs do include instructions on nutrition, exercise, mental conditioning, life style modifications.
Pritiken Diet	80% complex CHP 10% fat 10% protein 650–1000 calories/day	Likely to be deficient in calcium, B$_{12}$, iron (slightly). Does not meet FDA's requirement for protein (especially high quality protein)	Dry skin, flatulence, gastric distress secondary to high fiber content	Long term compliance unlikely because of extreme change from average American diet. Exercise is encouraged.
Fasting	Fluid/electrolytes/vitamin and mineral supplementation	Extensive	Extensive	Inappropriate for ambulatory management. Needs to be done on metabolic ward only.

pathways, whereas for fenfluramine, these effects probably result from activation of serotonergic pathways. In a detailed analysis of the safety and efficacy of this group of drugs, the Food and Drug Administration has examined clinical data from nearly 10,000 patients reported in a large number of double-blind and two-drug comparison studies. At the end of 20 weeks, patients on either drug or placebo had equal dropout rates, whereas patients taking drugs averaged about 1/2 lb (0.25 kg)/week greater weight loss. There were no significant differences in weight loss when any drugs in this class were used. Intermittent therapy (2 to 4 weeks on, 1 to 2 weeks off) was often as effective as uninterrupted treatment, except with fenfluramine, which sometimes led to depression after the drug was stopped.

It should be noted that the above data from the Food and Drug Administration represent the analysis of pooled results of group performance, averaged over many weeks, using fixed dosages of drugs. It is evident, however, that individual patients exhibit considerable variations in short- and long-term responsivity to these drugs, and that patients often derive improved benefit, and avoid tolerance to the drug, after even small increases in their dosages. Thus, there seems to be a role for the judicious use of these anorexigenic agents in carefully selected patients followed in medically supervised, comprehensive, therapeutic programs that include diet, exercise, etc. However, exact guidelines for the optimal use of these drugs remain to be determined.

Although the most frequent side effects of the anorexigenic drugs are insomnia and dry mouth, and, for fenfluramine, depression and diarrhea, the major obstacle to their more widespread use is their potential for inducing physical and/or psychological dependence.

Table 76.8 lists other drugs, purported to promote

Table 76.7.
Appetite-Suppressing Drugs

Generic and Proprietary Names	Common Trade Names	Dosage (mg)	Administration[a] (mg)	Peak Blood Concentration (Hours after Oral Dose)	Half-Life in Blood (Hours)	Percentage Excreted Unchanged in Acidic Urine
Schedule IV						
Diethylpropion	Tenuate, Propion	25, 75	25 before meals (tid) 75 in morning	1–2	8–13	24
Fenfluramine	Pondimin	20	20–40 before meals	1	20	20
Mazindol	Sanorex, Mazanor	1, 2	1 before meals 2 in morning	2	13	22
Phentermine	Ionamin	15, 30	15 (tid) 30 in morning		Free 7–8	75
				1	20–24	
Schedule III[b]						
Phendimetrazine	Plegine, Obalan	35	35 before meals	—	4	??
Benzphetamine	Didrex	25, 50	25–50 before meals	1–2	2	??
Schedule II[b]						
Amphetamine	Dexedrine	5, 10, 15	5–10 before meals (tid)	1–2	5	55
Methamphetamine	Desoxyn	5, 10, 15	2.5 or 5 before meals (tid) 10 or 15 in morning	1–2	13	45
Phenmetrazine	Preludin	25, 50, 75	25 (bid or tid)	—	—	19

[a] tid = three times daily.
[b] The Federal Controlled Substance Act of 1970 places the prescription anorexiants into three of five schedule categories. Appetite suppressants in schedule II are most likely to be abused; those in schedule IV have little or no risk of abuse. The schedules of the Controlled Substance Act are numbered in order of decreasing potential for abuse; drugs in Schedule II (amphetamine, methamphetamine, and phenmetrazine) are the most restricted. (From Weintraub M, Bray, GA: Drug treatment of obesity. Med Clin North Am 73:237, 1989.)

Table 76.8.
Drugs of Unproved Efficacy or Safety in the Treatment of Obesity[a]

Human chorionic gonadotropin
Cholecystokinin
Glucagon
Indomethacin
Biguanides
Neomycin, cholestyramine
Diuretics, laxatives
Bulk fillers (methylcellulose)
L-Dopa
Hydroxycitrate
Amylase inhibitors
Thyroid hormones

[a] Adapted from Bray GA (ed): *Obesity in America.* DHEW publ no. (NIH) 79-359. Washington, DC, US Government Printing Office, 1979.

weight loss, which are of unproved efficacy or safety in humans and should not be used in the management of obesity.

Surgical Therapy

Because of the increased morbidity and mortality associated with extreme degrees of obesity, and the generally unsatisfactory results produced by more conservative therapies, several surgical techniques have been devised to effect substantial weight loss in massively obese patients. Although some controversy exists regarding optimal selection criteria, surgery should in general be reserved for psychologically stable, motivated patients with (a) massive obesity [usually 100 pounds (45 kg) or more above ideal body weight (28)] and repeated failures on strict diet and other therapies; (b) severe medical consequences of obesity (e.g., hypertension, diabetes mellitus, hyperlipidemia, ortho-

paedic problems) refractory to conventional therapy alone; and (c) unremitting, severe obesity-related despair and loss of self-esteem.

Until a few years ago, the most frequently used procedure was *jejunoileostomy*, performed by anastomosing the distal jejunum to the terminal ileum either as an end-to-side or end-to-end procedure; in the latter approach, the defunctionalized bowel was drained with an ileocolonic anastomosis. The major benefits from successful surgery were (a) permanent (if no reanastomosis) weight loss varying from 10 to 15 to 100 kg within 1 to 3 years postoperatively; this weight loss resulted primarily from a marked decrease in food intake (despite normal appetite), and only secondarily from an iatrogenic chronic malabsorption syndrome; (b) substantial improvement in blood pressure, hyperinsulinemia, and glucose intolerance, hyperlipidemia, etc.; and (c) dramatic improvement in sense of well-being and self-esteem.

Unfortunately, the list of adverse effects associated with the intra- or postoperative course of jejunoileostomy patients grew progressively more formidable. Even in large medical centers with experienced personnel, the overall mortality rate after surgery varied from 3 to 5%. Serious perioperative complications have included pulmonary embolus, renal failure, wound infection, gastrointestinal bleeding, and pancreatitis. Among the adverse long-term effects were chronic diarrhea and flatulence, malabsorption with electrolyte and vitamin imbalance, cholelithiasis, urinary tract stones (calcium oxalate), hyperuricemia, polyarthralgias, intestinal bacterial overgrowth (pseudo-obstructive megacolon and bypass enteropathy), and progressive hepatic dysfunction leading to hepatic failure. In one large series (16) 58% of patients experienced potentially life-threatening complications or major reoperations; 17% of patients required surgical reversal of reanastomosis, usually because of severe hepatic cirrhosis and failure.

Gastric bypass surgery and its variants (e.g., gastroplasty), currently more popular than jejunoileostomy (2, 24), induce significant weight loss by promoting decreased oral food intake while preserving normal gastrointestinal absorptive and digestive function. In the gastric bypass procedure, the proximal 10% of the stomach is fashioned into a 25- to 50-ml pouch by anastomosis to the jejunum through a 0.9- to 1.2-cm channel, thus producing rapid gastric filling, slow emptying, and prolonged satiety. One year postoperatively, weight loss in one review (24) of approximately 1500 reported patients averaged 30 to 35% of baseline weight, with one-third of patients losing 50 kg or more. Although carbohydrate and bile acids are absorbed normally after gastric bypass, glucose intolerance and hyperlipidemia (especially hypertriglyceridemia) are, nonetheless, substantially improved; in addition, liver function does not worsen and malabsorption, electrolyte and vitamin imbalance, and kidney stones do not occur. By taking frequent small feedings of high caloric foods, it is possible for patients to "outeat" the bypass. Within the first postoperative month, vomiting occurs two to three times weekly in nearly 65 to 70% of patients. However, this complication becomes progressively less frequent, so that by 2 years postoperatively, it occurs in less than 10% of patients. Other complications of the procedure include channel ulcers or obstruction, bile reflux, and the dumping syndrome. In centers with experienced personnel, the overall mortality rate has been reduced from 3 to 1% but remains as high as 8 to 10% in patients over 50 years old. Reoperation necessitated either by surgical complications or unsatisfactory weight loss appears to be uncommon, and "takedown" of the gastric bypass has been described in less than 1% of patients. The major variant of the gastric bypass, the gastroplasty (2), involves creation of a 0.9- to 1.2-cm stoma separating a 25- to 30-ml gastric pouch from the distal stomach. Thus, the distal 80 to 90% of the stomach is no longer excluded from the flow of nutrients, and gastrointestinal continuity is maintained.

Although more research is needed to determine the long-term efficacy and safety of gastric bypass surgery and its variants, it appears that these procedures may be of benefit in the treatment of selected morbidly obese patients. In contrast, the striking complication rates associated with jejunoileal bypass procedures militate strongly against use of this technique in all but the most extreme instances.

PREVENTION OF OBESITY

As is evident from the preceding discussion, psychological and sociocultural factors play prominent roles in the development and maintenance of nearly all types of obesity. Because the long-term results of therapy for both mild to moderate and morbid obesity are so unsatisfactory, much more attention should be paid to prevention of excess body fatness.

The finding that behavior modification techniques can benefit not only individual obese patients but also groups of such people, even in commercially run weight-reducing programs, is provocative and suggests that this approach to weight reduction may have much wider application. The ability to modulate community awareness of, and responsivity to, the need for maintenance of optimal weight has been proved in several large scale community studies, including that of the Stanford Heart Disease Prevention Program, which succeeded in a highly coordinated effort to decrease various risk factors of cardiovascular disease in three demographically matched communities (13).

Stunkard has suggested a variety of new, imaginative approaches to obesity prevention that could be initiated, singly or in combination (37). For example, organized industry, given the proper (financial) incentive, could (a) increase the number and availability of quality commercially run weight reduction programs and provide data regarding their short- and long-term efficacies; (b) develop new, more nutritious low calorie food products; (c) offer a wide variety of reasonably priced health foods throughout the general restaurant and food service (e.g., vending machines) industries; (d) increase, perhaps with aid from the sporting goods industry, the number of health and sports clubs; and (e) promote widespread improvement in general health habits by decreasing life insurance premiums for individuals who maintain normal body weight, blood pressure, etc. Analogous untapped potential for fostering good general health patterns, including the maintenance of optimal body weight, resides in other influential segments of our society, such as the media, education establishment, government, work site, and various volunteer agencies.

General References

Bray GA, (ed): Obesity. *Med Cl North Am* 79: No1, 1989.
    Excellent compendium of information on obesity-related research.
Bray GA, (ed): *Obesity in America.* DHEW publ no. (NIH) 79-359, Washington, DC, US Government Printing Office, 1979.
    Valuable resource, summary of NIH symposium.
Buchwald H (ed): Morbid obesity. *Surg Clin North Am* 59 (no. 6): 1979. Good account of a multidisciplinary approach to the extremely obese patient.
Diet and Health. Implications for Reducing Chronic Disease Risk. Committee on Diet and Health. Commission on Life Sciences. National Research Council. Washington, DC National Academy Press, 1989. Comprehensive, critical assessment of the roles of the major macro- and micronutrients as risk factors for diet-related chronic illnesses.
Greenwood MRC (ed): In: *Contemporary Issues in Clinical Nutrition.* New York, Churchill Livingstone, 1983. vol. 4.
    Excellent reviews of new directions in obesity-related research and treatment.

Stunkard AJ (ed): *Obesity*. Philadelphia, WB Saunders, 1980.
An important, comprehensive clinical text.

Specific References

1. Amatruda JM, Biddle TL, Patton ML, Lockwood DH: Vigorous supplementation of a hypocaloric diet prevents cardiac arrhythmias and mineral depletion. *Am J Med* 74:1016, 1983.
2. Andersen T, Backer OG, Stokholm KH, Quaade F: Randomized trial of diet and gastroplasty compared with diet alone in morbid obesity. *N Engl J Med* 310:352, 1984.
3. Andres R: Mortality and obesity. The rationale for age-specific height-weight tables. In: Andres R, Hazzard WR, Bierman E, Blass DA (ed): *Principles of Geriatric Medicine*. New York, McGraw-Hill, 1990.
4. Beutler E, Kuhl W, Sacks P: Sodium-potassium-ATPase activity is influenced by ethnic origin and not by obesity. *N Engl J Med* 309:756, 1983.
5. Bjorntorp P: Effects of age, sex and clinical conditions on adipose tissue cellularity in man. *Metabolism* 23:1091, 1974.
6. Bray GA, Kral JG, Bjorntorp P: Hepatic sodium-potassium-dependent ATPase in obesity. *N Engl J Med* 304:1580, 1981.
7. Bray GA, Teague RJ: An algorithm for the medical evaluation of obese patients. In: Stunkard AJ (ed): *Obesity*. Philadelphia, WB Saunders, 1980.
8. Brownell KD, Kramer FM: Behavioral management of obesity. *Med Clin North Am* 73:185, 1989.
9. *Build Study 1979*. Chicago, Society of Actuaries and Association of Life Insurance Medical Directors of America, 1980.
10. Carney RM, Goldberg AP: Weight gain after cessation of cigarette smoking: a possible role for adipose-tissue lipoprotein lipase. *N Engl J Med* 310:614, 1984.
11. DeLuise M, Blackburn GL, Flier JS: Reduced activity of the red-cell sodium-potassium pump in human obesity. *N Engl J Med* 303:1017, 1980.
12. Evans DJ, Hoffman RG, Kalkhoff RK, Kissebah AH: Relationship of androgenic activity to body fat topography, fat cell morphology and metabolic aberrations in premenopausal women. *J Clin Endocrinol Metab* 57:304, 1983.
13. Farquhar JW, Maccoby N, Wood PD, et al: Community education for cardiovascular health. *Lancet* 1:1192, 1977.
14. Garrow JS: Luxuskonsumption, brown fat and human obesity. *Br Med J* 286:1684, 1983.
15. Genuth SM, Castro JH, Vertes V: Weight reduction in obesity by outpatient semistarvation. *JAMA* 230:987, 1974.
16. Haverson JD, Wise L, Wazna MF, Ballinger WF: Jejunoileal bypass for morbid obesity. A critical appraisal. *Am J Med* 64:461, 1978.
17. Health Services and Mental Health Administration: *Ten State Nutrition Survey 1968–1970*. DHEW publ no. (HSM) 72-8130, Washington, DC, US Government Printing Office, 1972.
18. Hirsch J, Batchelor B: Adipose tissue cellularity in human obesity. *Clin Endocrinol Metab.* 5:299, 1976.
19. Hubert HB, Feinleib M, McNamara PM, Castelli WP: Obesity as an independent risk factor for cardiovascular disease: a 26 year follow-up of participants in the Framingham heart study. *Circulation* 67:968, 1983.
20. Kaplan NM: The deadly quartet. Upper body obesity, glucose intolerance, hypertriglyceridemia, and hypertension. *Arch Intern Med* 149:1514, 1989.
21. Keys A (ed): *Coronary Heart Disease in Seven Countries*. American Heart Association Monograph No. 29, 1970.
22. Kissebah AH, Vydelingum N, Murray R, et al: Relation of body fat distribution to metabolic complications of obesity. *J Clin Endocrinol Metab* 54:254, 1982.
23. Kolterman OG, Insel J, Saekow M, Olefsky J: Mechanisms of insulin resistance in human obesity: evidence for receptor and postreceptor defects. *J Clin Invest* 65:1272, 1980.
24. Kral JG: Surgical treatment of obesity. *Med Clin North Am* 73:251, 1989.
25. Krotkiewski M, Bjorntorp P, Sjostrom L, Smith U: Impact of obesity on metabolism in men and women—importance of regional adipose tissue distribution. *J Clin Invest* 72:1150, 1983.
26. Lantigua RA, Amatruda JM, Biddle TL, et al: Cardiac arrhythmias associated with a liquid protein diet for the treatment of obesity. *N Engl J Med* 303:735, 1980.
27. Larson B, Svardsudd K, Welin L, et al: Abdominal adipose tissue distribution, obesity, and risk of cardiovascular disease and death: 13 year follow-up of participants in the study of men born in 1913. *Br Med J* 288:1401, 1984.
28. Metropolitan Height and Weight Tables, 1983. *Stat Bull Metrop Life Found.* 64 (Jan–June): 2, 1983.
29. Peris AN, Sothmann MS, Hoffman RG, et al: Adiposity, fat distribution, and cardiovascular risk. *Ann Intern Med* 110:867, 1989.
30. Ravussin E, Lillioja S, Knowles WC, et al: Reduced rate of energy expenditure as a risk factor for body weight gain. *N Engl J Med* 318:467, 1988.
31. Schwartz RS, Brunzell JD: Increase of adipose tissue lipoprotein lipase activity with weight loss. *J Clin Invest* 67:1425, 1981.
32. Shimokata H, Tobin JD, Muller DC, et al: Studies in the distribution of body fat: I. Effects of age, sex, and obesity. *J Gerontol* 44:M66, 1989.
33. Shimokata H, Muller DC, Andres R: Studies in the distribution of body fat. III. Effects of cigarette smoking. *JAMA* 261:1169, 1989.
34. Simopoulos AP, Van Itallie TBV: Body weight, health, and longevity. *Ann Intern Med* 100:285, 1984.
35. Society of Actuaries: *Build and Blood Pressure Study*. Chicago, The Society, 1959, vol 1.
36. Stunkard AJ, Sorensen TIA, Hanis C, et al: An adoption study of human obesity. *N Engl J Med* 314:193, 1986.
37. Stunkard AJ: Obesity and the social environment: current status, future prospects. *Ann NY Acad Sci* 300:298, 1977.
38. Stunkard AJ, d'Aquili E, Fox S, Filion RDL: Influence of social class on obesity and thinness in children. *JAMA* 221:579, 1972.
39. Van Itallie TB: Liquid protein mayhem. *JAMA* 240:144, 1978.
40. Wermuth BM, Davis KL, Hollister LE, Stunkard AJ: Phenytoin treatment of the binge-eating syndrome. *Am J Psychiatry* 134:1249, 1977.

C H A P T E R 77

Common Problems in Reproductive Endocrinology

S. MITCHELL HARMAN, M.D., Ph.D.
MARC R. BLACKMAN, M.D.

Few general physicians feel comfortable dealing with their patients' sexual and reproductive problems. This is in part because medical school and postgraduate training have not generally included adequate exposure or specific education in these areas and in part because the subject of sex, although more openly dealt with in recent years, still may produce feelings of embarrassment in both patient and physician. In any case, most physicians view complaints involving the reproductive system as esoteric or rare, to be quickly referred to a specialist (i.e., endocrinologist, urologist, gynecologist, or psychiatrist). In fact, sexual and re-

productive dysfunctions are not rare. For example, nearly 50% of men will experience one or more periods of impotence between the ages of 20 and 50 (7); up to 10% of married couples have difficulty with conception; and approximately one in 400 males born will have Klinefelter's syndrome (two X and one Y chromosomes)(6).

Furthermore, the freedom with which sex and reproduction are now discussed both socially and in the popular media and the advent of scientific investigation of human sexuality have altered patient expectations. "Normal" sexual function is now an objective of many men and women, and dysfunction is legitimately viewed as a health problem. Thus, such problems are more likely to be brought to a physician than in former times. It is important, therefore, that the generalist be familiar with the major disorders of reproductive function and have adequate knowledge of the points of history, techniques of physical diagnosis, and modes of laboratory investigation to allow him to distinguish patients who require reassurance or can be treated simply in the office from those who should be referred to a specialist for more complex testing and therapy.

SEXUAL AND REPRODUCTIVE PHYSIOLOGY

Levels of Sexual Differentiation

The sexual differentiation of individuals can be viewed as a continuum proceeding in time from conception to adulthood and in biological "depth" from genetic to psychological and social as follows: (a) *Genetic sex* is determined at conception when the egg, bearing an X chromosome, is fertilized by a sperm bearing either a Y (XY = male) or X (XX = female) chromosome. The genetic sex determines (b) *Gonadal sex*—The development of an ovary or testis from the undifferentiated primitive gonad. (c) *Primary sex*—The embryonic testis secretes two important molecules, testosterone, the major male sex steroid, which causes the development of a penis and scrotum, and a peptide, müllerian inhibition factor (MIF), which causes the regression of the primitive müllerian duct structures. In the absence of MIF the müllerian ducts develop into a vagina, uterus, and fallopian tubes; without testosterone, female external genitalia (labia and clitoris) form; therefore, without testicular function the primary sex is female. Primary sex characteristics identify the individual's apparent sex at birth. (d) *Secondary sex* changes occur at puberty and are the result of greatly increased secretion by the gonads of sex steroid hormones. In males growth of body and pubic hair, beard growth, increase in muscle mass, deepening of voice, and onset of male libido with ejaculations and increased frequency of erections are characteristic effects of testosterone. In the female, rounding of body contours with breast growth and subcutaneous deposition of fat in the hips and buttocks, and also the onset of menses, are effects of cyclic estrogen secretion, and growth of pubic and axillary hair (and probably libido) are manifestations of adrenal androgen secretion. Both sexes experience a spurt of body growth at puberty, which is then followed by closure of epiphyses and cessation of growth of long bones. It is the hormone-dependent secondary sex characteristics that provide clues to adult sexual identity and that form the underpinning of (e) *Tertiary sex*, which is the way in which an individual identifies himself. There are few mammalian species whose level of sexual dimorphism is as extreme as that of humans. This is reflected by the fact that our identification as man or woman is crucial to balanced psychological and social function and is a critical component of self-image. The physician must bear in mind that any change that seems to alter a patient's masculinity or femininity is perceived as profoundly threatening and has power to harm well beyond its biological manifestations.

Male Reproductive Physiology

Activity of the male reproductive system is regulated by the hypothalamus, which produces, at irregular intervals of 60 to 120 minutes, secretory surges of a decapeptide, gonadotropin releasing hormone (GnRH), into capillaries of the median eminence, which drain into the pituitary portal veins that supply blood to the pituitary gland. GnRH stimulates pituitary gonadotropic cells to secrete pulses of the glycoprotein gonadotropic hormones, luteinizing hormone (LH), and follicle-stimulating hormone (FSH). FSH induces spermatogenesis in the seminiferous tubules whereas LH acts on the Leydig (interstitial) cells of the testis to stimulate testosterone secretion. Testosterone acts locally in the testis to promote spermatogenesis and is also the major circulating androgenic steroid. In plasma it is partially bound to a protein, sex hormone-binding globulin (SHBG), which decreases its clearance rate and also serves as a testosterone reservoir. The bound fraction of testosterone is not available to target cells so that the free fraction appears to correlate better than total plasma testosterone with peripheral androgenic effect. In most target cells testosterone is reduced to 5-α-dihydrotestosterone (DHT), which binds to specific cytoplasmic hormone receptor proteins and is translocated to the cell nucleus. Once in the nucleus the testosterone-receptor complex binds to regulatory elements on chromatin, activating downstream genes. This causes messenger RNA production, specific protein synthesis, and altered cell function. Testosterone is needed for growth of, and secretion by, the prostate and seminal vesicles. More general body effects include positive nitrogen and calcium balance (with increased muscle and bone formation) and augmented function of apocrine and sebaceous glands of the skin, which may result in comedones and acne. Another important effect of testosterone is to "feed back" to the hypothalamus and pituitary to inhibit secretion of gonadotropins. Thus, the reproductive hormones form a "closed loop" autoregulated system (Fig. 77.1).

Female Reproductive Physiology

The hypothalamic-pituitary relationship in the female is similar to that in males, except that complex modulation of hormone secretion in women results in a cyclic rather than tonic reproductive pattern. In women LH stimulates the interstitial-thecal tissue to make androgen and small amounts of estrogens (estradiol and estrone). Granulosa cells (the small cells surrounding the ovum to form a follicle) convert thecal androgens to estradiol, which, in concert with FSH, produces growth of a cohort of ovarian follicles by proliferation of their granulosa cells. A dominant (graafian) follicle emerges in each cycle as the major source of estradiol secretion, while adjacent follicles undergo atresia (degeneration). Rising estrogen secretion in this early or follicular phase of the cycle induces proliferation of the uterine endometrium and, by a "positive feedback" effect, a sudden surge of LH secretion around day 14 of the cycle. This LH surge results in ovulation. LH then induces the follicle to become a functioning corpus luteum producing both estradiol and progesterone during the latter half, or luteal phase, of the cycle. Progesterone acts on the uterus to produce a secretory endometrium, rich in glycogen and, in concert with estrogen, causes a neg-

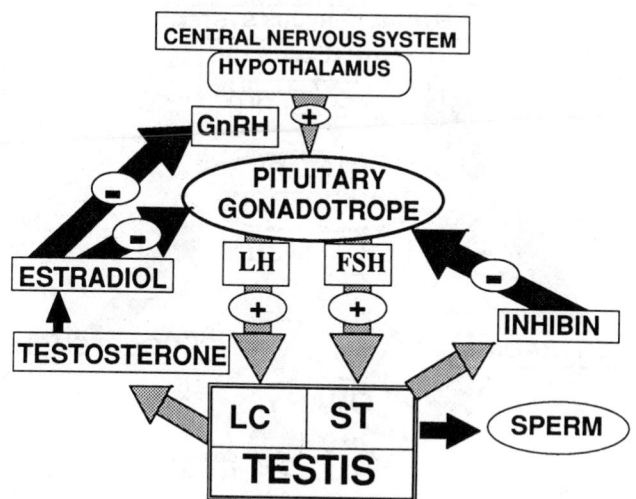

Figure 77.1. Reproductive endocrinology in the male. A variety of central nervous system inputs, from both exogenous (e.g., environmental stress) and endogenous (e.g., biorhythms) sources, act via neurotransmitters and neuropeptides to influence the amplitude and frequency of pulsatile hypothalamic neuronal output (secretion = light gray arrows) of gonadotropin-releasing hormone (GnRH) into the pituitary portal system. GnRH stimulates pituitary gonadotropic cells to release LH and FSH. LH induces the Leydig cell (LC) compartment of the testis to secrete testosterone (T). FSH and T act together to stimulate spermatogenesis in the seminiferous tubule compartment (ST). T acts via negative feedback (dark gray arrows) to inhibit gonadotropin and GnRH secretion, probably after aromatization locally to estradiol. Inhibin, produced by the ST in response to FSH also acts by negative feedback to decrease FSH release.

ative feedback effect that gradually reduces the secretion of LH and FSH. With loss of gonadotropic support, the corpus luteum involutes, steroid secretion diminishes, and the endometrium, left without estrogen and progesterone stimulation, sloughs off as the menstrual flow. At this point, with estradiol and progesterone at low levels, FSH and LH begin to rise and the stage is set for the next cycle. Ovarian estradiol is the major estrogen. Estrone, a weaker estrogen, is formed peripherally in fat, liver, kidney, and other tissues by conversion of adrenal and ovarian androgenic precursors. The secretion of these androgens also increases at puberty. Female reproductive hormone relationships are illustrated in Figure 77.2.

Male and Female Hormones and Libido

The reader is referred to Chapter 18 (Sexual Disorders) for a description of the stages of the sexual response that characterize sexual physiology in men and women. It is not clear in humans the extent to which sex hormones influence these events. There is no doubt that men who are completely deprived of testosterone (i.e., chemical or anatomical castration) experience a gradual loss (over 1 to 2 years) of interest in sex, reporting an absence of sensations of arousal in response to sexual cues (e.g., female nudity) and also less frequent erections and ejaculation. Many also report heightened emotional sensitivity, weepiness, and loss

of aggressive interest, ability to concentrate, or drive toward career goals, etc. Experimental evidence suggests that there is a direct effect of testosterone on the central nervous system to stimulate sexual behavior (4). In women, the relationship between libido and sex hormones is less obvious, but it has been reported that women are more likely to initiate sexual contact during phases of the menstrual cycle when androgen activity is highest (1) and that postmenopausal women, replaced with androgen as well as estrogen, have higher levels of sexual interest and activity. Clinicians also find that women with androgen-secreting tumors may report heightened sex drive and increased sexual content of dreams and fantasies. It has become apparent in recent years that the pituitary hormone, prolactin, which in women is responsible for lactation, is probably an "antisexual" hormone that reduces libido and potency in both sexes (3). In women, estrogens are necessary to maintain the vagina and the external genitalia in their mature reproductive states. In the absence of adequate estrogen, genital atrophy may result in pain on intercourse, with resultant loss of interest in sexual activity (see below).

SEXUAL AND REPRODUCTIVE DYSFUNCTION IN MEN

Hypogonadism

Etiologies

Failure of the testes to secrete adequate amounts of testosterone for development or maintenance of male secondary sex characteristics and libido results in the syndrome of male hypogonadism. In order to investigate and diagnose these patients it is helpful to classify the failure along each of the three axes shown in Figure 77.3. Criteria for classification are shown in Table 77.1.

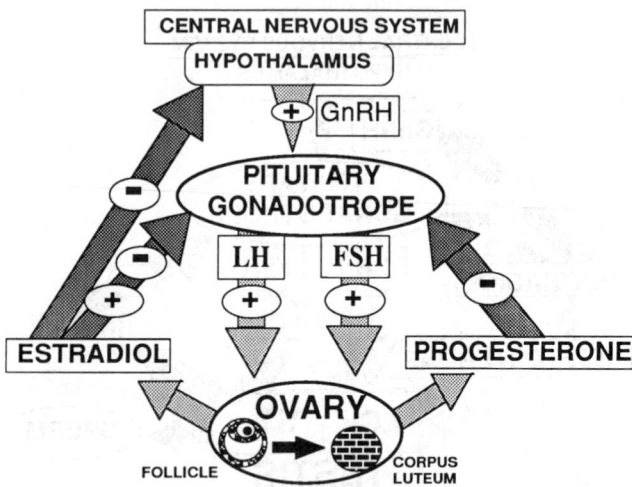

Figure 77.2. Reproductive endocrinology in the female. The central nervous system releases neurotransmitters and neuropeptides that influence the amplitude and frequency of pulsatile hypothalamic neuronal secretion (secretion = light gray arrows) of gonadotropin-releasing hormone *(GnRH)* into the pituitary portal system. GnRH stimulates pituitary gonadotropic cells to release LH and FSH. LH stimulates the thecal cells of the ovary to make androgens (e.g., androstenedione), which are converted into estrogens, mainly estradiol (E_2), by the follicular granulosa cells. Estradiol and FSH act together to promote follicular growth and maturation. At midcycle a sudden increase in secretion of LH induces ovulation and conversion of the follicle to a corpus luteum, which secretes both E_2 and progesterone (P). E_2 initially exerts positive feedback control on LH secretion leading to the ovulatory peak. Later in the cycle, E_2 and P act together to inhibit gonadotropin secretion.

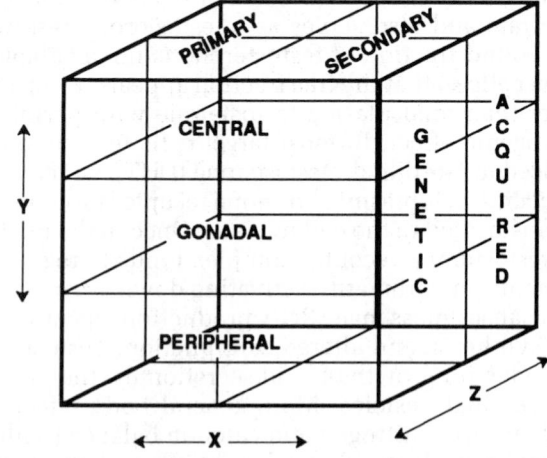

Figure 77.3. Each axis of the cube represents a different way of classifying hypogonadism. There are 12 possible categories and, hence, 12 "compartments" in the cube. The Y axis represents anatomical location (central, gonadal, peripheral); the Z axis etiology (genetic, acquired); and the X axis time of onset (primary, secondary).

Table 77.1.
Classification of Male Hypogonadism

Classification	Criteria
ACCORDING TO LOCATION OF LESION	
Central (hypothalamic or pituitary)	Gonadotropins ↓ or →
	Testosterone ↓
Gonadal (testis)	Gonadotropins ↑
	Testosterone ↓
Peripheral (failure of end organ response)	Gonadotropins ↑
	Testosterone ↑ or →
ACCORDING TO ETIOLOGY	
Genetic	History, (especially family history)
	Buccal smear, karyotype
Acquired	History, physical examination, radiology
	Evidence of infection, trauma, neoplasia, etc.
ACCORDING TO TIME OF ONSET	
Primary (failure of pubertal development)	History, physical examination
Secondary (loss of previously developed libido and secondary sex characteristics)	

Central. Central hypogonadism is characterized by low levels of gonadotropins and may be due to failure at the level of the pituitary or the hypothalamus. Common examples of different types of central hypogonadism follow. Kallmann's syndrome, which is characterized by hyposmia and is due to a defect in hypothalamic GnRH secretion, is a form of central, genetic, primary hypogonadism. Acquired hypothalamic failure may occur with diencephalic tumors. Pituitary hypogonadism is also central and usually acquired. The etiology may be infectious (e.g., tuberculosis or mycosis), traumatic, vascular (as in infarction with pituitary apoplexy), or, most commonly, neoplastic (usually either nonsecreting adenoma or craniopharyngioma). Central hypogonadism may also be associated with functioning pituitary tumors, such as those that secrete prolactin (prolactinoma) or growth hormone (acromegaly). Occasionally pituitary hypogonadism is congenital and idiopathic.

Gonadal. The most common cause of genetic, gonadal hypogonadism is Klinefelter's syndrome, which is due to chromosomal nondisjunction producing XXY genetic sex. These patients have very small, firm testes and gynecomastia. They usually enter puberty but fail to progress fully and present as phenotypic males with impotence, small phallus, and, often, gender confusion. Testosterone levels are generally in the low to low normal range in Klinefelter's patients (e.g., 200 to 350 ng/dl). Genetic gonadal hypogonadism may also occur if one or more critical enzymes in the steroid synthetic pathway leading to sex hormones is missing. Usually such defects involve enzymes common to the adrenal gland and testis and produce female primary sex in XY individuals. Acquired causes of gonadal hypogonadism include trauma and infection (usually

viral or granulomatous). Autoimmune damage to the testis may occur either alone or as part of a complex of multiple endocrine failure (Hashimoto's thyroiditis, idiopathic Addison's disease, adult onset diabetes mellitus, hypoparathyroidism, or pernicious anemia). Occasionally a varicocele will produce partial hypogonadism. Whether these entities result in secondary or primary hypogonadism depends on the time of life at which the damage occurs.

Peripheral. Peripheral hypogonadism is always genetic and is expressed as a continuum from complete androgen insensitivity or "testicular feminization" in which the phenotype is female (with normal estrogenization at puberty but lacking a uterus and, hence, menses), through varying degrees of partial androgen sensitivity, in which midline fusion of labioscrotal structures is highly variable (Reifenstein's syndrome), producing gender confusion, and ending with minor defects such as hypospadias and cryptorchidism, in which gender is clearly male. In all cases, the genetic sex is male (i.e., XY).

Approach to the Patient

The approach to the patient should be directed first at determining whether hypogonadism truly exists, then at its classification as discussed above, next at its specific etiology, and finally at providing appropriate therapy and/or referral for the condition diagnosed.

Patient presentations. Young patients are frequently brought to the attention of physicians by parents concerned with failure of pubertal onset or progression (see also Chapter 5). Primary hypogonadism may stem from almost any of the etiologies cited above and must be differentiated from so-called "constitutional delayed puberty," which is an idiopathic self-limited, familial condition. A strong family history of "late blooming" and beginning enlargement of the testicles are reassuring in this regard. A set of standards for pubertal development of adolescent boys is available (21) (see Table 5.5). In general, any boy reaching 17 years of age without signs of pubertal onset, or who begins but does not proceed through puberty, or who has other associated signs or symptoms (e.g., severe headaches) of a disease (e.g., pituitary tumor) that can produce hypogonadism deserves further investigation. Another presentation is genital intersexuality. A finding of hypospadias, cryptorchidism, or ambiguous genitalia in a patient with complaints suggesting hypogonadism should lead to further diagnostic procedures. The gradual loss of male secondary sex characteristics and libido is a third presentation of male hypogonadism. This may be so insidious as to be taken for "normal" by the patient, especially in a person progressing from middle toward old age, so that it is only noticed in association with the investigation of some related condition, such as hypothyroidism, adrenal failure, severe headaches, renal tuberculosis, etc. Finally, and probably most common, is the complaint of impotence, which may be the earliest manifestation of hypogonadism but is also seen in various other physical and psychological conditions. Impotence is discussed more completely below and also in Chapter 18.

History. A proper history should include a chronicle of pubertal progression, with time of onset of pubic hair, beard growth, voice change, growth spurts, erections, and ejaculations recorded as accurately as recollection allows. Of critical interest are loss or diminishment of libido and erections or ejaculations, slowing of beard growth, thinning of body and pubic hair, changes in the breast (i.e., swelling or tenderness), and loss of aggressive impulse or drive. The presence of headaches, double vision, or reduced peripheral vision may give clues to a pituitary tumor. Symptoms of hypothyroidism, adrenal failure, acromegaly, diabetes, anemia, pulmonary disease, and autoimmune disease should be sought. A history of urological problems, cryptorchidism, hypospadias, or episodes of orchitis is important. Finally, a family history of delayed puberty or of other endocrine abnormalities may be revealing.

Physical examination. The body habitus and facies should be examined first. Does the patient look mature or babyish, masculine or feminine? A lower body segment (femoral greater trochanter to floor) longer than the upper segment (femoral greater trochanter to crown) and arm span greater than height comprise "eunuchoid" proportions and suggest pubertal or prepubertal hypogonadism. Good muscle mass and axillary hair militate against long-standing hypogonadism. Male pattern baldness is an androgen-dependent process. The presence of comedones, especially in the tragus of the ear (a very common location), is a good sign of androgen activity. Complexion should be noted, since increased pigmentation suggests primary adrenal failure, and dry flaky skin, hypothyroidism. Vital signs should be taken and the presence of hypertension or of postural hypotension should be noted as possible indicators of adrenal enzyme defects or of Addison's disease. Special attention should be paid to the eyes for limitation of extraocular movements, papilledema, or restriction of visual fields, all suggestive of an intracranial tumor. Examination of the male breast should include careful palpation for the subareolar thickening and nodularity, which may be the only evidence of gynecomastia (see page 1049), and squeezing of the nipple to elicit galactorrhea, which, though rare in males, is pathognomonic of a prolactinoma. Careful attention should be paid to the genitals. Pubic hair pattern should extend up the linea alba to the umbilicus in a diamond shaped pattern (the so-called "male escutcheon"). Penis size and location of urethral meatus, scrotal rugation and pigmentation, and size and turgor of the testicles should be noted. The normal adult testis should be no less than 15 ml in volume (approximately 4.0 x 3.0 cm) and have the resistance to palpation of a firm ripe plum. An "overripe" softer feeling strongly suggests testicular atrophy. Careful palpation of the left side of the scrotum while the

patient performs a Valsalva maneuver may reveal the presence of a varicocele; significant varicoceles are always on the left, and approximately 5% of them are associated with reduced testosterone production from both testes (venous drainage from the left testis crosses over to the right). Rectal examination should assess prostate size, since the prostate shrinks with testosterone deficiency. Careful neurological examination should include testing of the sense of smell to detect Kallmann's syndrome.

Differential Diagnosis

The hormone tests that give the most information about suspected male hypogonadism are the serum testosterone and gonadotropin (LH and FSH) measurements. These are readily available from most commercial laboratories and are generally accurate within 20%. Normal adult males will have morning serum testosterone levels not less than 300 (and usually 450 to 700) ng/dl in most laboratories. Borderline values between 250 and 350 ng/dl are suspicious. It is important that testosterone levels be determined in the morning since the diurnal variation in testosterone can produce an afternoon and evening decrement in testosterone concentration of as much as 200 ng/dl. Abnormal or suspicious determinations should be repeated at least once for confirmation since there is considerable variability both in radioimmunoassay determination and from time to time within individuals. Serum LH usually varies from 2 to 30 mlU/ml and FSH from 2 to 16 mlU/ml, but different assays will have different ranges of normal. Low or normal LH and FSH in the presence of subnormal testosterone defines central hypogonadism. Elevated gonadotropins indicate gonadal failure. Central hypogonadism caused by prolactin (PRL)-secreting pituitary tumor will usually be accompanied by plasma PRL levels of 100 ng/ml or more (17). Impotence is an especially prominent symptom in hyperprolactinemic hypogonadism. Peripheral hypogonadism is characterized by elevated gonadotropin levels and normal or elevated testosterone levels. High gonadotropin and normal testosterone levels are also found in "compensated" gonadal hypogonadism. Table 77.1 shows the male hormonal patterns typical of central, gonadal, and peripheral hypogonadism.

Further investigation of patients with proven hypogonadism should probably be undertaken by a specialist in endocrinology. Table 77.2 lists various investigative procedures and types of patients for whom they are pertinent.

Referral to a urologist for testicular biopsy may be helpful in diagnosing traumatic or infectious damage. Biopsy also shows shrinkage and hyalinization of tubules in Klinefelter's syndrome. The procedure can often be done on an ambulatory basis under local anesthesia. However, it may cause hemorrhage and considerable pain, and about a week is required for full recovery. Therefore, it usually should be undertaken only after consultation with an endocrinologist.

Table 77.2.
Additional Investigations Useful in the Evaluation of Hypogonadism

Type of Failure	Radiological Procedure	Hormone Measurements	Other Tests
Central	Skull Film CT scan with contrast . Magnetic resonance scan Cerebral Angiogram	Prolactin Thyroxine TSH Cortisol (A.M.) Growth hormone (with GTT)	Visual Fields (formal) Clomiphene test LHRH test
Gonadal	Bone age (if primary)	Thyroxine Cortisol (A.M.)	Buccal smear Karyotyping Gonad Biopsy

Therapy

There are three aims of therapy in patients with central hypogonadism. The first is to suppress or remove any intracranial mass whose size or extent threatens vision or brain function. This may sometimes be accomplished by medical therapy (i.e., bromocriptine use in prolactinoma) but will usually require neurosurgery or radiation therapy, depending on the type and size of the lesion. The second aim is to suppress abnormal hormone secretion. In patients with prolactin-secreting adenomas treatment with bromocriptine (Parlodel), a synthetic dopamine agonist, given as 2.5 mg three times daily, by mouth, with meals and continued indefinitely, has proven effective, not only in lowering serum prolactin, increasing gonadotropins and testosterone, and restoring libido (4), but also in shrinking tumor mass. Unfortunately, bromocriptine has a high incidence of gastroenteric side effects, with dyspepsia, nausea, vomiting, cramping, and diarrhea in 10 to 12% of patients. In addition, in high doses, it has been associated with symptoms of depression and bizarre dreams or nightmares. The drug should be started at a dose of one 2.5-mg tablet/day (with food or antacid) and the dosage increased by one tablet/day each week up to a maximum of three/day to obtain the desired effect. The third aim, which is to replace deficient androgen, may be necessary in either central or gonadal hypogonadism. This is best accomplished by intramuscular injection of 200 to 300 mg of testosterone enanthate in oil (such as Delatestryl) every 2 to 4 weeks. The dose may be started at 200 mg every 4 weeks, after which the dose and interval can be adjusted depending on duration of the therapeutic (libido, sexual potency) effect. Oral androgen preparations are generally less effective. Interestingly, the mere replacement of testosterone by injection has not restored sexual competence in hyperprolactinemic patients. In central hypogonadism, three times weekly injections of 2000 to 4000 IU of human chorionic gonadotropin (hCG) (such as Pregnyl or Follutein) will normalize testosterone levels, generally within a month of initiation of therapy, and may also stimulate spermatogenesis. hCG is used because of its LH-like activity (human LH is unavailable). Because of the requirement for more frequent injections as compared with testosterone, hCG should replace testosterone only in those patients with central hypogonadism who are concerned about fertility. Follow-up of treated patients should include questions about sexual function, assessment of habitus, beard growth, and, in patients with failure of pubertal development, depth of voice. Libido and potency usually return within a few weeks of initiating treatment, whereas secondary sex characteristics improve gradually over 6 months to a year. Determination should be made as to whether gynecomastia or prostate enlargement with symptoms of urethral obstruction are occurring as a side effect of therapy. In older patients, it is a good idea to initiate therapy with an injection of a short-acting form of testosterone, such as aqueous testosterone propionate, 20 to 30 mg. Then, if prostate response leads to acute urethral outlet obstruction, the effect will be short-lived.

Gynecomastia

Importance

Significant enlargement of the male breast requires a physician's attention so that those cases with a serious hormonal and/or neoplastic etiology can be distinguished from the common benign idiopathic form.

Etiologies

Gynecomastia is common as sex steroids rise during early adolescence (occurring in up to 65% of boys age 14), but it regresses spontaneously (to less than 15%) by age 17. The prevalence increases again in the twenties, remains stable around 25%, and increases again to about 60% in the fifties. This idiopathic gynecomastia is nearly always less than 5 cm in diameter and causes no symptoms (25). Noticeable gynecomastia of >5 cm in diameter may be the first clue to the presence of an adrenal or testicular neoplasm or to a prolactinoma. In the case of adrenal tumors there is usually, but not always, an associated Cushing's syndrome. Various malignant tumors may secrete chorionic gonadotropin, which can overstimulate testicular steroid production and thus lead, indirectly, to gynecomastia. Hypo- and hyperthyroidism have been associated with breast enlargement. The taking of exogenous estrogen either purposely (by individuals with gender confusion or with prostate carcinoma) or incidentally because of estrogenic activity of various medications (e.g., diazepam, cimetidine, spironolactone, digitalis glycosides) should always be considered. Another iatrogenic cause is peripheral conversion to estrogens of excess androgens from testosterone or hCG therapy. Gynecomastia is also common in liver failure. Finally, true gynecomastia must be differentiation from the "gynecoid" breast seen in obesity and/or old age, which contains increased fatty tissue, but not glandular breast tissue, and also from carcinoma of the male breast. About 1% of all breast carcinoma occurs in men.

Approach to the Patient

History. The duration and age of onset of breast swelling is important. The presence of tenderness or discharge and the quality of the discharge (clear, turbid, bloody) should be noted. Any symptoms of hypogonadism (see above) should be elicited, as should symptoms of hypothyroidism (see Chapter 73) or Cushing's disease (see Chapter 74). Careful medication history and sexual history may reveal an exogenous etiology.

Physical examination. In general the examination should be the same as for hypogonadism (see above) with the addition that signs of Cushing's disease and thyroid disease should be emphasized (see Chapter 73). Deep palpation of the upper abdomen may reveal an adrenal tumor or downward displacement of the kidney by such a tumor. Careful bimanual palpation of the testicles may detect a secretory tumor (androblastoma). A useful formal system for staging breast development has been described by Marshall and Tanner (20). Briefly, at stage I there is minimal proliferation of glandular tissue just beneath the areola. At stage II a flat pad of glandular tissue spreads beyond the bounds of the areola (i.e., >5 cm). At stage III this pad rounds up, lifting the breast area forward from the chest wall in a cone shape with the nipple at the tip. At stage IV the areola spreads laterally as subareolar gland proliferation gives the breast a "double-contoured" appearance. Finally further maturation with increase in fatty tissue results in the mature single contour of stage V (see Fig. 5.2). Examination of the breast must also be directed at differentiation between presence of breast tissue (firm, slightly lobulated, and symmetrically distributed from the nipple outward with a limited boundary); fat (softer, diffusely distributed, and with no clear separation from surrounding subcutaneous adipose); and tumor (hard, nodular, frequently tender, often fixed to skin or underlying muscle, asymmetric with regard to the nipple). Milky nipple discharge on firm squeezing suggests prolactinoma; clear or bloody discharge suggests breast cancer. Unilateral breast enlargement should increase the suspicion of neoplasia, but asymmetry is not uncommon (10 to 15%) in patients with idiopathic gynecomastia. The decision whether further investigation is required depends on the age of the patient, the rapidity of enlargement of the breast, and the degree of such enlargement. Men between 18 and 45 years of age with recent onset of rapidly enlarging mammary glands, or glandular breast tissue diameter greater than 5 cm, or with symptoms or signs suggesting hypogonadism, hy-

pothyroidism, or Cushing's disease should receive further attention.

Diagnostic Procedures

Determinations of serum levels of estradiol, testosterone, and gonadotropins (LH and FSH) are indicated as are serum prolactin and specific determination of serum hCG. If the serum estradiol is greater than 50 pg/ml and if the testosterone:estradiol ratio is reduced to less than 100:1, the diagnosis of estrogen-secreting testicular tumor is strongly suggested. Elevation of 24-hour urinary 17-ketosteroids indicates an adrenal etiology in which case adrenal hyperfunction should be investigated with the diagnosis of adrenal neoplasm in mind (see Chapter 74). A low or low normal testosterone level with elevated FSH and LH suggests the diagnosis of Klinefelter's syndrome (XXY trisomy). Elevated serum hCG should prompt a search for occult malignancy with particular attention to gonads, lungs, and gastrointestinal tract. Elevated prolactin levels could be associated with taking certain medications (especially major tranquilizers, see Chapter 13) or with adenoma of the pituitary (see Chapter 74 and Table 77.2). The possibility of hypothyroidism should be evaluated by T_4, T_3, and TSH determinations. Finally, patients with firm, nodular, unilateral enlargement should be referred for mammography and/or surgical biopsy of the breast.

Therapy

Drug-induced gynecomastia remits gradually (several months) if the drug can be discontinued. Treatment of primary endocrine disease (e.g., prolactinoma, adrenal tumor, hCG-secreting carcinoma, etc.) should usually be undertaken by an appropriate specialist once the diagnosis is clear. When "idiopathic" gynecomastia is a cosmetic problem, plastic surgical excision of breast tissue is usually the therapeutic method of choice. It is important to bear in mind that breast development that has progressed beyond Tanner stage II (see Fig. 5.2) will never fully regress even if the proximate cause is corrected, and therefore it will require surgical intervention if complete cosmetic correction is desired.

Impotence

In this section, impotence and loss of libido will be considered only as they relate to physical disorders. For more general treatment of sexual dysfunction the reader is referred to Chapter 18. Briefly, impotence is the inability to achieve or maintain erection satisfactorily to effect penetration and ejaculation. Transient or occasional impotence is common and not necessarily evidence of a medical problem, but a pattern of repeated (>25% of opportunities) episodes over more than a month should be investigated. Impotence may or may not be accompanied by loss of sexual desire, depending on the etiology.

Etiologies

A disorder of any of the systems that maintain the sexual response and apparatus may lead to impotence. Etiologies may therefore be: (a) *psychological* (see Chapter 18); (b) *vascular*—This may be of the arterial type, with diminished blood supply to the corpora cavernosa (e.g., aorto-iliac atherosclerosis or disease of smaller peripheral vessels), or it may be venous incompetence, in which partial erections occur but blood drains off due to "venous leak" (12); (c) *neuropathic*—Damage to the peripheral pelvic autonomic nerves (e.g., neuropathy of diabetes mellitus or heavy metal poisoning or nerves severed by surgical trauma) or disease of the spinal cord or brain (e.g., tumor, trauma, or multiple sclerosis) may inhibit or obliterate the erectile response; (d) *toxic*—Substances of abuse, especially alcohol and opiates, can acutely and chronically diminish sexual ability; other medications affecting the autonomic and central nervous system, especially tranquilizers and sympatholytic antihypertensives, are often associated with impotence; (e) *debilitative*—Various severe and chronic medical illnesses (e.g., malignancy, renal failure) are commonly accompanied by loss of sex drive and/or impotence; and (f) *endocrine*—Hypogonadism and prolactinoma (see page 1047) have been discussed as causes of impotence. Other endocrine diseases, frequently producing sexual dysfunction, are hyper- and hypothyroidism, Cushing's syndrome, and acromegaly. In one series of patients referred to a major diagnostic center for persistent symptoms without apparent psychiatric etiology, 35% were found to have endocrine disorders (29).

Approach to the Patient

History. The duration of symptoms, the frequency with which intercourse is attempted, and the percentage of attempts ending in erectile failure should be recorded in order to determine whether the impotence is absolute or relative and whether it is progressing. Impotence unaccompanied by loss of libido suggests a neurological or vascular problem, whereas loss of interest in sexual activity is consistent with either hypogonadism or a psychological etiology. The history should include the patient's marital situation, whether there are sex partners other than the wife, the perceived level of partners' desire, and a social and work history to determine whether there is excessive stress. Situational impotence (i.e., with one partner but not another) is good evidence of a psychological problem. Normal men frequently awaken in the morning with an erection. This is a local response to a full bladder; detumescence follows urination. Preservation of morning erections is evidence against vascular or neuropathic disease; however, in the cited series (29) 14% of patients with an endocrine etiology still had morning erections. A history of medication use and substance abuse should be diligently sought. Heavy smoking is often associated with a peripheral vascular etiology of impotence. The physician should also ask about symptoms of hypo- or hyperthyroidism, Cushing's disease, and diabetes, peripheral neuropathy (paraesthesia, hyperesthesia, burning or shooting pains) or central nervous system disease, and vascular disease (claudication, angina, cold extremities, skin ulcers).

Physical examination. The physical examination should be conducted with particular attention to the manifestations of hypogonadism described above (page 1046), to signs of thyroid or adrenal disease (Chapter 73 and 74), and to signs of peripheral vascular disease (peripheral pulses, skin temperature, skin atrophy, or hair loss) (Chapter 87) and central or peripheral neuropathy (Chapter 84).

Diagnostic Procedures

Hormone determinations should be used to investigate for hypogonadism (page 1046) or prolactinoma (page 1047). If historical or physical findings lead to a suspicion of thyroid or adrenal disease, appropriate tests should be done (Chapters 73 and 74). A fasting blood sugar should always be obtained. Spontaneous erection during sleep (nocturnal penile tumescence) tends to be intact in psychogenic impotence but reduced when there is an organic cause. Nocturnal penile tumescence may be tested by the patient at home using a "snap gauge," but for definitive measurement studies should be conducted using quantitative instrumentation in a sleep laboratory (12). If peripheral neuropathy seems a likely etiology, this can often be confirmed by referral to a urologist for bladder manometrics and to a neurologist for nerve conduction velocity measurements (see also Chapter 84). Diagnosis of vascular causes may require Doppler estimation of penile blood flow and/or selective angiography; venous incompetence may be revealed by dynamic cavernosography.

Therapy

Therapeutic efforts should be directed at the specific entity underlying the impotence, whenever one can be found. Psychological impotence may respond to various therapeutic modalities (e.g., "sex therapy") depending on its severity and associated problems (see Chapter 18). Vascular causes may respond to surgical revascularization. Neuropathic impotence is occasionally reversible with removal of the inciting lesion (e.g., spinal cord tumor) but, if irreversible, may also be treated with an implantable penile prosthesis (see below), though results will vary depending on whether the spinal ejaculatory center or afferent pathways are damaged. Drug-induced impotence will usually be reversed by discontinuation of the offending agent. Therapy of hypogonadism has been discussed (see page 1049). If sexual function does not improve within 6 weeks after specific therapy for an organic cause has been instituted, consideration should be given to the possibility that the experience and expectation of sexual failure are inhibiting the response (so-called "performance anxiety") even though the primary etiology is no longer present. Such secondary psychological impotence may respond to psychological or behavioral therapy (see Chapter 18).

There are also nonspecific approaches to therapy that may succeed in restoring sexual function despite an irremediable (e.g., vascular or neuropathic) etiology. All of these therapies require urologic consultation. Implantable penile prostheses have been used extensively. These are of two types: those that are permanently stiff or semiflexible, and more complex devices that inflate by means of a pump and valve mechanism. A more recent approach is injection of papaverine or a mixture of papavarine and phentolamine directly into the corpus cavernosum, which produces erections lasting 30 minutes to several hours. Although highly effective, especially in neuropathic impotence of diabetes mellitus, this therapy should be supervised by a urologist familiar with its use since priapism is a potentially serious and fairly common (2 to 4%) complication. Another option is the use of a device that draws blood into the penis by negative pressure, then retains it there with an occlusive ring applied to the base of the penis. A number of different types of suction device are available, and this approach has given very satisfactory results in selected patients (33).

Aging

A series of early investigations found that men's testosterone levels declined with age and protein binding of testosterone to sex hormone-binding globulin increased with age, resulting in a profound decrease in mean free (bioavailable) testosterone. These changes were accompanied by an increase in circulating estrone and estradiol and in gonadotropins. More recent work, in which older men were carefully selected to match the younger men in terms of health, obesity, alcohol intake, social class, etc. revealed an increase in gonadotropins and minimal increase in SHBG, but little or no change in total and free sex steroids with age (11). Thus, a "male menopause" occurs infrequently, if at all, in healthy American men. Despite the relative stability with age of serum testosterone and other sex steroids, numerous studies in healthy men have revealed a steady decrease both in sexual appetite and ability with decreases in frequency of intercourse from an average of 2 to 3 events/week to less than 2/month by age 70 to 75 (22). This decrease cannot be blamed on hypogonadism but probably reflects changes in other (i.e., nervous and vascular) systems occurring with age. There are no scientific data to support a beneficial effect of administration of androgens to aging men whose testosterone levels are normal. Until and unless such data become available, this practice should be discouraged. Older men with abnormally low testosterone levels should be investigated in the same way as are other patients with suspected male hypogonadism (see page 1047) and treated appropriately.

SEXUAL AND REPRODUCTIVE DYSFUNCTION IN WOMEN

Hirsutism and Virilization

Growth of coarse dark hair (terminal hairs) in various body areas (besides the scalp and eyebrows) depends on the action of androgens. The pattern of hair growth reflects the relative sensitivity of different skin zones to androgen effect. Although pubic and axillary hair appear in both sexes, further hair growth diverges due to different androgen levels. Although male patterns vary, maximal expression of androgen effect includes terminal hair development over the face, limbs, chest, superior pubic triangle, linea alba, and back. In those carrying genes for "male pattern baldness," high levels of androgens are also associated with loss of scalp hair, first at the temporal hairline and later at the crown.

Most women (80%) develop some degree of dark hair growth over the legs and forearms but not much facial hair. About one-third have some hair on the chest and abdomen (extending along the linea alba). Abnormally high levels of plasma androgens can result in male distribution of hair growth, the state of "hirsutism." Very high levels of androgen production also lead, over time, to virilization, with increased muscle mass and decreased subcutaneous fat in hips and breasts ("male habitus"), clitoral enlargement (>2.0 cm), deepening of the voice, male pattern baldness, development of acne, and malodorous perspiration.

Excess body hair without signs of virilization is termed "simple" hirsutism. Hirsutism with virilization is rare and is almost always due to adrenal or ovarian tumor, congenital adrenal hyperplasia, male pseudohermaphroditism, or use of exogenous androgen (e.g., female athletes and body builders). Therefore, truly virilized patients should probably be referred directly to an endocrinologist.

Hirsutism without virilization. Although simple hirsutism may be an early manifestation of Cushing's syndrome or of an adrenal or ovarian neoplasm, most cases will fall into a group termed "idiopathic" or "constitutional." The prevalence of simple hirsutism has been estimated to be as high as 10% of adult North American women (23). It typically develops during the late teens, although progression may be so slow as not to produce troublesome amounts of hair for 10 or more years after onset of menses. In half to two-thirds of hirsute patients excessive ovarian production of androgens (testosterone and/or androstenedione) is demonstrable and is often associated with oligomenorrhea and decreased fertility. Ovarian structure may show hyperthecosis (overgrowth of interstitial tissue) or polycystic ovarian disease. The combination of hirsutism, obesity, acne, amenorrhea, and polycystic ovaries is known as the Stein-Leventhal syndrome. Women with this syndrome secrete excessive quantities of androgenic estrogen precursors (testosterone and Δ4-androstenedione) and normal quantities of estrogen. They usually have increased ratios of LH to FSH in plasma.

In perhaps half of all cases of simple hirsutism, elevated serum testosterone is not demonstrable; about one-half of patients with normal total testosterone have been shown to have increased plasma "free" (i.e., non-protein-bound) testosterone due to reduced sex hormone-binding globulin. Increased hair follicle conversion of testosterone to the more potent dihydrotestosterone has been demonstrated in some of the remaining cases, and other causes of increased sensitivity of hair follicles to androgens have been postulated.

Racial and ethnic factors are also important determinants of hair growth. Women of Asian ancestry and Caucasian women of northern European origins usually have relatively little terminal hair on face, torso, or extremities. In contrast, Caucasian women of Mediterranean origins frequently develop mustache, beard, or sideburn hair and have dark hair on legs and arms. Constitutional hirsutism and polycystic ovaries tend to run in families. Thus, a patient with moderate hirsutism who is of Mediterranean origin and has a mother with excessive facial hair is unlikely to have an identifiable disorder. The timing of onset is also important. Sudden development of hirsutism many years after onset of menses is more likely to be due to a tumor than to congenital causes.

Transitory hirsutism may occur during pregnancy and occasionally during menopause. A number of pharmacological agents can produce hirsutism, including glucocorticoids, phenytoin (Dilantin), minoxidil, diazoxide, and phenothiazines. Drug-induced hirsutism is characterized by the fact that increased hair growth is not limited to the androgen-sensitive areas of the skin. Rare cases include chronic local skin trauma and porphyria cutanea tarda.

Another major cause of adult onset simple hirsutism, sometimes with disturbance of menstrual pattern, is congenital adrenal hyperplasia (CAH). This group of diseases is caused by a deficiency of one of the several enzymes in the steroid synthetic pathway. Although such defects are usually manifest in childhood as ambiguous genitalia with salt loss (21-hydroxylase deficiency) or hypertensive (11-hydroxylase deficiency) syndromes, some patients with partial defects may manifest only hirsutism in adult life.

Approach to the Patient

A careful ethnic and family history is essential. The temporal evolution of the problem should be noted, including the menstrual history. On physical examination one should carefully note the distribution and density of terminal hairs in the sideburn and mustache areas, the periareolar and midsternal regions, and over the back and buttocks. Particular attention should be paid to the pattern of pubic hair. In the female the pubic hair forms an inverted triangle in the inferior pubic region only. The male escutcheon is a rhomboid space with terminal hairs filling the superior pubic triangle and extending up the linea alba to the umbilicus. A male-type escutcheon in a female is a good

presumptive sign of hyperandrogenism. Physical signs of virilization (see above) should be sought. Cases with virilism need referral to an endocrinologist, whereas those with severe ovarian dysfunction may require the attention of a gynecologist for therapy of abnormal menstruation or impaired fertility. Finally, signs of Cushing's syndrome (in which hirsutism may occasionally be more prominent than the classic changes) should also be sought.

The decision to proceed with laboratory testing depends on the severity of the hirsutism. Laboratory studies can be performed sequentially, if financial considerations are dominant, or simultaneously. Plasma testosterone, which is of ovarian and rarely adrenal origin, is measured first. Normal serum testosterone concentration suggests idiopathic hirsutism and excludes major ovarian disorders. Not excluded are mild cases of ovarian hyperthecosis with abnormal androstenedione production or decreased sex hormone binding globulin (increased "free" or bioavailable androgen). The uncovering of such borderline cases is usually not worthwhile since management would be unaffected. If the testosterone concentration is elevated to between 85 and 200 ng/dl, a diagnosis of ovarian hyperthecosis or polycystic ovaries (Stein-Leventhal syndrome) is most likely. These patients should have determinations of serum FSH and LH. Normal values suggest ovarian hyperthecosis, whereas increased LH and low normal or reduced FSH are highly suggestive of polycystic ovary disease. Levels of testosterone greater than 200 ng/dl suggest a diagnosis of ovarian neoplasm, and further diagnostic workup should be directed by specialists. This may include sonography, computerized axial tomography, laparoscopy with ovarian biopsy, or ovarian vein catheterization.

If testosterone levels are normal, excess production of weak androgens (e.g., androstenedione, dehydroepiandrosterone) by the adrenal remains a consideration and can be confirmed by appropriate plasma assays. In 21-hydroxylase deficiency, which is the most common type of CAH-producing adult hirsutism, plasma 17α-OH progesterone and urinary pregnanetriol may be elevated. Unfortunately, in about half of the patients with this syndrome these steroids will be significantly increased only after stimulation with exogenous adrenocorticotrophic hormone (ACTH). Therefore, if CAH is suspected, referral to an endocrinologist is appropriate. Large increases in serum dehydroepiandrosterone-sulfate or 24-hour urinary excretion of 17-ketosteroids suggests adrenal neoplasia (adenoma or carcinoma) and should also be evaluated by an endocrinologist.

Therapy. The therapy of simple hirsutism is usually local and essentially cosmetic, even when there is a hormonal abnormality, because medical reduction of androgen excess does not rapidly affect the presence of existing hair and is often incomplete.

Local measures include bleaching, wax stripping, shaving, plucking (tweezing), the use of hair removal creams (depilatories), and electrolysis. Contrary to popular belief, such measures do not accelerate the growth rate of hair. Plucking may cause local infection. Wax applications or hair removal creams are effective but may be irritating and must be used with care. All of these procedures must be repeated at intervals. Electrolysis and thermolysis are effective procedures for permanent removal of hair, but they are expensive and uncomfortable. Effectiveness and safety (avoidance of burns, scarring, and infection) are dependent on the technique of the operator. Referral of the patient requires that the physician be familiar with the electrologist's skill. Under the best of circumstances, electrolysis is generally successful in destroying about 50% of the follicles treated at one time. Thus, several repetitions are invariably required.

Patients given medical therapy should be cautioned not to expect rapid results, since dedifferentiation of androgenized follicles may require 6 to18 months, even when androgen excess is totally eliminated. The immediate benefit to be expected is prevention of progression of the hirsutism, with variable degrees of reversal occurring only as therapy is continued. Medical therapy is directed toward the suppression of androgen production, the blocking of peripheral androgen action, or both. Although such therapy appears more rational when androgen excess is demonstrable, patients with idiopathic hirsutism may occasionally respond. Adrenal suppression, although introduced on the erroneous assumption that adrenal androgens were responsible for most cases of hirsutism, is, nonetheless, effective in about one-third of cases. This seems to be due to an accompanying reduction of ovarian androgen secretion that is either directly dependent on ACTH or indirectly dependent via ovarian conversion of circulating adrenal steroids. Adrenal suppression is, of course, effective in cases of congenital adrenal hyperplasia. This form of therapy is simple and usually free from side effects. Dexamethasone can be given as a single dose of from 0.1 to 0.3 mg (as pediatric solution) orally at bedtime. At these low doses neither glucocorticoid excess (i.e., iatrogenic Cushing's syndrome) nor chronic adrenal suppression with adrenal insufficiency will occur. Side effects of dexamethasone therapy include occasional insomnia and appetite stimulation.

Another form of medical therapy is suppression of ovarian androgen production with a cyclically administered estrogen-progestin combination (oral contraceptive). This is effective in about one-half of cases. Estrogens also increase concentration of plasma sex hormone binding globulin, reducing the circulating free androgens. Because progestins have some intrinsic androgen-like activity on hair follicles, a combination that minimizes the content of progestational agent may be the most appropriate. Agents containing 2 mg or less of norethindrone or 0.5 mg or less of norgestrel are acceptable. When used, oral contraception should be given on the usual schedule recommended for fertility control for the particular preparation (see Chapter 93).

Disadvantages of oral contraceptives include their cardiovascular, thrombogenic, and other undesirable effects. The multiple disadvantages of administering these agents must be weighed carefully when they are to be prescribed for an essentially benign problem. Suppression of ovarian androgen production by oral contraceptives precludes pregnancy. Thus therapy must be interrupted when fertility is desired and the drug withheld until pregnancy is terminated. Hirsutism may recur during this time. Combined adrenal-ovarian suppression may be used if neither alone is effective.

Several other agents have been used successfully for the medical therapy of hirsutism. Medroxyprogesterone acetate (Provera), 100 mg intramuscularly every 2 weeks, or 30 to 40 mg orally, reduces testosterone production and interferes with testosterone action at the tissue level. A variety of side effects may be encountered and this mode of therapy is not recommended. Spironolactone (Aldactone), at a generally well-tolerated dose of 25 mg twice daily, also appears to suppress ovarian androgen production and may additionally antagonize androgen action at the hair follicle (27). Recently, experimental trials of local skin application of 4% spironolactone have shown good results, but no such product is available as yet. Cyproterone acetate and flutamide are competitive inhibitors of androgen action at the level of the hair follicle and have been used successfully outside the United States in the treatment of hirsutism. A new class of agents that inhibit conversion of testosterone to the active form, dihydrotestosterone, is also undergoing tests. Although none of the latter agents is currently approved in the United States for the treatment of hirsutism, a trial of oral spironolactone therapy may be justified in more severe cases of hirsutism, unresponsive to ovarian and adrenal suppression. Contraindications to spironolactone include concomitant taking of potassium supplements or renal insufficiency, either of which may predispose to hyperkalemia.

Dysmenorrhea

Dysmenorrhea (painful menstruation) is a very common problem. It is considered primary when it appears within a year or 2 of the menarche, a problem therefore beginning in the teenage years. When the painful menstruation appears for the first time or suddenly intensifies in a mature women, it is referred to as secondary dysmenorrhea and is nearly always a result of a specific pathological process, such as fibroids, endometriosis, pelvic inflammatory disease, or an intrauterine contraceptive device. Therefore, in secondary dysmenorrhea, the physician should seek an initiating cause. Patients with secondary dysmenorrhea should generally be referred to a gynecologist. Typical primary dysmenorrhea consists of the development within 1 or 2 days of the onset of menstruation of either crampy or sustained lower abdominal and pelvic pain that may radiate into the legs and that may be associated with nausea, vomiting, irritability, or abdominal distension. In a few patients, symptoms may be so severe that performance of usual daily activities is not possible. Usually the discomfort is most severe during the initial several hours of menstrual flow, fades gradually, and disappears within 2 or 3 days. The episodes tend to become less severe with increasing age and often disappear spontaneously within 5 or 10 years after the menarche or after the first pregnancy. The pathogenesis of primary dysmenorrhea is not completely understood, but it requires ovulation and it is believed to result from excessive myometrial contractions, possibly due to excess formation of uterine prostaglandins.

Mild forms of dysmenorrhea require only analgesic therapy, such as aspirin or acetaminophen, and reassurance from the physician. There are a number of preparations available without prescription that are marketed for menstrual cramps. Most are combination tablets and none has proven to be more effective than aspirin or acetaminophen alone. Examples of these combination tablets are: Femcaps (aspirin, phenacetin, citrate, ephedrine, and atropine) and Midol (aspirin, caffeine, and cinnamedrine). Analgesics work best when taken promptly at or slightly before the onset of menses and continued regularly (every 4 to 6 hours), rather than taken only when pain is perceived. When symptoms are more severe or incapacitating, therapy with nonsteroidal anti-inflammatory agents having antiprostaglandin activity greater than that of aspirin should be tried; they will be effective in approximately one-half of the patients. Ibuprofen (Motrin, 400 mg, four times/day, for 5 to 6 days), mefenamic acid (Ponstel, 250 mg, four times/day, for 5 to 6 days), and naproxen (Naprosyn, 500 mg, two times/day for five doses) have been approved by the Food and Drug Administration (FDA) for use in dysmenorrhea. More powerful nonsteroidal anti-inflammatory agents such as indomethacin (Indocin, 25 mg, four times/day for six doses) are effective in the treatment of dysmenorrhea but have not been approved for this purpose by the FDA. These drugs are most effective if given just before menstrual flow begins and continued for 2 to 3 days thereafter. However, because of the uncertainty of the effects of these agents in early pregnancy, it is suggested that their use be delayed until the beginning of menstrual flow in those patients who are sexually active and who are not using effective means of birth control. The patient should use one agent as a trial for three cycles and then this should be discontinued if there has been an inadequate response in controlling the symptoms. It is currently unknown whether one nonsteroidal anti-inflammatory agent might be effective when another has failed.

Oral contraceptive agents suppress ovulation and thereby dramatically control dysmenorrhea; these agents may occasionally be necessary for management of this problem when it is severe. The use of oral contraceptive agents is fully discussed in Chapter 93.

The unusual patient who does not respond to these therapies should be seen by a gynecologist for evaluation for an undetected problem causing secondary amenorrhea or to provide more experienced guidance in the drug therapy of primary amenorrhea.

Premenstrual Tension Syndrome

The premenstrual tension syndrome is an ill-defined complex of signs and symptoms that occurs to some degree in approximately 30% of women of reproductive age. Symptoms include irritability and increased aggressiveness, cravings for sweet or salty foods, nervousness, depression, tearfulness, mood swings, difficulty in concentrating, headaches, fullness and tenderness of the breasts, fatigue, and abdominal bloating. A significant minority of affected women find such symptoms severely disruptive to their lives. Any or all of the symptoms may be present, and the characteristic complaints vary from patient to patient, but the hallmark of the syndrome is that these problems appear during the latter half (luteal phase) of the menstrual cycle, disappear with the onset of menstruation, and are absent during the first part (follicular phase) of the cycle. Investigations of the etiology of this entity have not been very rewarding. No typical pattern of hormone or electrolyte changes has been found that sets symptomatic women apart from asymptomatic women. Nonetheless, it is clear that when ovarian function is suppressed (as by inhibition of pituitary function with a GnRH agonist), symptoms are abolished. It seems likely that the symptoms stem from an "abnormal" physical response to an essentially normal pattern of steroid hormone fluctuation during the menstrual cycle.

There is, at this time, no effective or accepted treatment for the premenstrual tension syndrome. Although progesterone supplementation, pyridoxine, minor tranquilizers, and thiazide diuretics have all been tried, their effectiveness has not been substantiated in clinical trials, nor is there a definite rationale for the use of any of these agents. Until such time as the pathophysiology of the syndrome has been better elucidated, it will remain a puzzling and frustrating clinical problem. The practitioner is advised to treat the most prominent symptoms empirically, while reassuring the patient that she is not mentally ill, but rather the victim of a common, hormonally mediated malady with no serious physical consequences.

Abnormal Vaginal Bleeding before Menopause

During the 35 to 40 years of menstruation nearly all women will have occasional variations in bleeding pattern. In women approaching the menopause, irregularity of the menstrual cycle is typical, as described below. In younger women, most changes in bleeding pattern will be of the type called dysfunctional uterine bleeding (DUB), which is defined as abnormal bleeding for which no anatomical source can be found. Most DUB is related to anovulation, generally as a manifestation of alterations in pituitary-gonadal physiology described as hypothalamic oligomenorrhea (see below). DUB may also be seen in the hirsutism-anovulation syndrome (e.g., Stein-Leventhal syndrome). A variety of physical and emotional stresses can precipitate DUB. In a few patients, abnormal vaginal bleeding will be related to unsuspected pregnancy or to anatomical problems.

Women frequently describe abnormal bleeding first to their general physician, and they will often be concerned about cancer. Therefore, it is important for the general physician to have a systematic approach to this problem. With careful history taking and a limited evaluation, a working diagnosis and plan can usually be developed in the office. Table 77.3 lists the various causes of abnormal vaginal bleeding in the premenopausal woman.

History. The patient should be asked how the abnormal bleeding differs from that which occurs during her normal cycle in terms of amount, timing, and quality, and when the normal pattern changed. Menorrhagia is present when menstruation occurs at the usual time or is extended by only a few days and blood loss is greater than usual (e.g., the patient has to change pads more frequently, pads contain more blood than usual). This characteristic is consistent with DUB, leiomyomata uteri, endometrial polyps, or an underlying medical problem (e.g., hypothyroidism). Metrorrhagia is present when the patient has vaginal bleeding (usually spotting) between otherwise normally spaced periods. This symptom may be found with leiomyomata, polyps, or local vulvar vaginal problems, but carcinoma of the endometrium or cervix and breakthrough bleeding related to oral contraceptives may also present this way. Menometrorrhagia indicates the presence of both menorrhagia and metrorrhagia. Polymenorrhea is present when menstruation occurs at intervals of less than 21 days. Oligomenorrhea is present when menstruation occurs at intervals of greater than 35 days. The latter two patterns are more commonly associated with alterations in hormone balance (i.e., DUB), often precipitated by physical or emotional stress.

The history can also provide evidence of ovulation.

Table 77.3.
Causes of Abnormal Vaginal Bleeding in the Premenopausal Woman

1. Dysfunctional uterine bleeding (hypothalamic idiopathic anovulation)
2. Perineal causes: bladder pathology, hemorrhoids
3. Vulvar causes: infection, laceration, tumor
4. Vaginal causes: infection, laceration, tumor, foreign body
5. Cervical causes: infection, erosion, polyp, carcinoma
6. Uterine causes: infection, polyp, leiomyomata, carcinoma, intrauterine device (IUD)
7. Ovarian causes: infection, polycystic ovary (Stein-Levinthal syndrome)
8. Pregnancy: threatened abortion, complete abortion, ectopic pregnancy
9. Oral contraceptive pills
10. Systemic medical conditions: bleeding diathesis (especially thrombocytopenia), thyroid disease, others

This may be very helpful since most DUB is associated with failure to ovulate. Features associated with ovulation include (*a*) mittelschmerz (mild or moderate pain in one iliac fossa at midcycle, indicating rupture of an ovarian follicle); (*b*) increased midcycle mucus (due to the secretory effect of progesterone); (*c*) premenstrual molimina (abnormal fullness, headaches, and irritability immediately preceding the onset of bleeding); (*d*) dysmenorrhea, and (*e*) a biphasic basal body temperature pattern; at time of ovulation, the temperature usually rises 1°F (½°C) and remains elevated until the onset of bleeding.

Sexually active women should be asked what type of contraception they are using and questioned regarding symptoms suggesting pregnancy. Breakthrough bleeding (metrorrhagia) is not uncommon in women using oral contraceptives, especially during the first year of use. Pregnancy-related bleeding is a problem in the first trimester, when it may be difficult to distinguish clinically whether the patient is pregnant. Almost always, the patient will have missed the most recent period, and she may have morning sickness, frequent urination, breast tenderness, and other early symptoms of pregnancy. Bleeding in the pregnant patient may be due to one of several conditions. Leakage of small amounts of blood from the cervical os is referred to as *threatened abortion.* This occurs in about 10% of pregnancies, but only half of these women will ultimately abort. Spontaneous abortion is characterized by intense cramping and bleeding with passage of clots. The abortion may be complete (the uterus is empty and no further management may be needed) or incomplete (partial loss of uterine contents and need for prompt attention by a gynecologist). Ectopic pregnancy is another cause of first trimester bleeding and is a life-threatening medical emergency. It is characterized by a missed period followed by bleeding that may range from spotting to frank hemorrhage. There is often associated unilateral pelvic pain.

In patients with menorrhagia, polymenorrhea or oligomenorrhea the history should include inquiry about abnormal vaginal discharge or other symptoms of pelvic infection or irritation (Chapter 94) because chronic pelvic infection may cause any of the abnormal bleeding patterns described above. The physician should also ask about certain medical conditions. Severe thrombocytopenia may cause menorrhagia. The patient with abnormal vaginal bleeding due to thrombocytopenia will usually have other manifestations of this problem (Chapter 51). Other coagulation abnormalities, including anticoagulant therapy, rarely cause abnormal vaginal bleeding. Hypothyroidism may cause menorrhagia whereas hyperthyroidism tends to be associated with oligomenorrhea (Chapter 73).

When dysfunctional uterine bleeding is suspected (absence of features of ovulation and lack of evidence for other causes), the patient should be asked about recent changes in her general health and in her daily activities. Among the factors that may precipitate DUB are diet change, weight gain or loss, emotional stress, jogging and other strenuous activities, sleep loss, mental strain, chronic medical conditions, and alcohol or illicit drug use.

Physical examination. All patients complaining of abnormal vaginal bleeding should have a pelvic examination to look for obvious anatomical causes of the bleeding. It is important not to defer the examination because of the bleeding. Hemorrhoids, vulvar conditions, vaginitis and cervicitis, cervical polyp or cervical erosion, and leiomyomata uteri are the principal anatomical problems that may be identified. Vulvovaginal and cervical sources of bleeding should be suspected especially in patients who describe metrorrhagia or postcoital bleeding. In an actively bleeding patient, orthostatic blood pressure and heart rate should be checked. The patient should also be examined for ecchymoses and petechiae, especially in the lower extremities, and for physical signs of thyroid disease.

Laboratory tests. A hemoglobin concentration or a hematocrit value should always be obtained. In addition, every woman with a change in her bleeding pattern should have a Pap smear evaluated (Chapter 95). Sexually active women should always have a pregnancy test. Pelvic sonography will nearly always reveal the presence of ectopic pregnancy and should be undertaken immediately whenever this diagnosis is suspected.

If the history or physical examination suggests the possibility of a bleeding diathesis, a platelet count, bleeding time, prothrombin time, and partial thromboplastin time should be obtained (Chapter 51). Thyroid function tests should be obtained if thyroid disease is suspected on clinical grounds.

Working diagnosis and management.

Anatomical Causes. The general evaluation described above is sufficient to identify most of the anatomical causes for abnormal bleeding in the premenopausal woman. A history of typical ovulatory symptoms increases the likelihood that the bleeding is due to an anatomical problem or a chronic medical condition. Because uterine problems (e.g., fibroid tumors, and, much less commonly, endometrial cancer) are more frequent in women over 35, these patients should be evaluated by a gynecologist if they develop any unexplained change that persists for more than two cycles. Except in the case of vaginitis or cervicitis, which may be treated by the general physician (Chapter 94), pelvic disease or pregnancy should be referred promptly to a gynecologist. The evaluation that a gynecologist will perform for possible gynecological cancer is described in Chapter 95. When a primary medical condition seems to explain the patient's problem, this condition should be managed appropriately (thrombocytopenia; see Chapter 51; thyroid disorders: see Chapter 73).

Dysfunctional Uterine Bleeding. For the large number of women in whom the working diagnosis is dysfunctional uterine bleeding, the general physician may elect to manage the problem himself or refer the patient to a gynecologist. The most common cause of DUB is anovulation. In this case no corpus luteum is formed so that a progesterone-primed endometrium is not produced. If levels of estrogen are fairly high, the endometrium will continue to proliferate, become hyperplastic, then break down irregularly and bleed. Two objective findings that help to confirm the absence of ovulation are the lack of a biphasic basal body temperature pattern described above and a failure of serum progesterone to rise during the patient's menstrual cycle. The two pieces of data should be obtained if possible before referral. In some women in whom these data indicate ovulation DUB may still be the correct diagnosis.

When dysfunctional bleeding has been a problem for a brief period (two or four cycles), appropriate management consists of explaining the problem to the patient and having her modify obvious precipitating factors whenever this is possible. If her menorrhagia is particularly heavy and is interfering with her usual activities, the problem can usually be controlled promptly by prescribing a 21-day package of a combination oral contraceptive such as Ovral-21. She should be given the following written instructions: Take the first three tablets immediately, then take one tablet twice daily for the next 9 days. Within 24 hours, the current bleeding will be suppressed, and she will then have withdrawal bleeding at the end of the 9-day course. Patients with persistent DUB, especially those in whom there is a problem of infertility, should be referred to a gynecologist or a reproductive endocrinologist. An endometrial biopsy will often be performed by the consulting gynecologist. This biopsy can confirm either the absence of ovulation (the endometrium will be proliferative, indicating only an estrogen effect) or the presence of ovulation (the endometrium will be secretory, reflecting a progesterone effect, or it may show a mixture of proliferative and secretory changes). Depending upon these findings and additional investigations, the gynecologist/endocrinologist will develop a management plan for the patient.

Oligomenorrhea and Hypogonadism

Gonadal dysfunction in women nearly always presents as alteration of the menstrual pattern, either irregular and infrequent menses (oligomenorrhea) or cessation of menses (amenorrhea). Oligo- or amenorrhea may be classified as primary or secondary; as juvenile, feminized, or masculinized; as central, gonadal, peripheral, or exogenous; and finally as congenital or acquired (see Table 77.4 for definitions of terms).

Primary. Primary central amenorrhea with maturational failure suggests idiopathic or genetic gonadotropin deficiency of pituitary or hypothalamic origin. A patient with primary gonadal failure is likely to have Turner's syndrome (XO sex chromosomes and no ovaries). Primary amenorrhea with normal maturation may be due to peripheral causes as simple as imperforate

Table 77.4.
Classification of Female Hypogonadism (i.e., Oligomenorrhea)

Classification	Criteria
ACCORDING TO TIME OF ONSET	
Primary (no onset of menses)	History
Secondary (cessation of established menses)	
ACCORDING TO SOMATOTYPE	
Maturation failure (juvenile)	Physical examination
Feminized (normal secondary sex)	
Masculinized (hirsute, deep voice, increased muscle mass, clitoromegaly)	
ACCORDING TO LOCATION OF LESION	
Central (hypothalamic or pituitary):	Gonadotropins ↓ or →
a. Without galactorrhea	
b. With galactorrhea	
Gonadal (ovarian failure)	Gonadotropins ↑
Exogeneous (disruption of menses by drugs, stress, or illness of other than reproductive organs)	History, physical examination, various laboratory and radiological tests
ACCORDING TO ETIOLOGY	
Genetic (chromosomal or familial)	History, buccal smear, karyotype
Acquired (infectious, neoplastic, traumatic, surgical, hemorrhage or infarction, autoimmune)	History, physical examination, radiology, other special procedures

hymen with obstruction of menses, or as serious as congenital uterine agenesis. A special case of this latter kind is testicular feminization (see page 1047).

Secondary. Feminized patients with central secondary amenorrhea may have brain tumors or anorexia nervosa but, most commonly, have hypothalamic amenorrhea. Although this may have an exogenous cause (see below), it is frequently idiopathic with no explanation even after thorough examination. Pituitary amenorrhea is usually acquired and is frequently accompanied by deficiencies in other hormone axes (adrenal, thyroid). Etiologies are the same as in the male (see above).

Gonadal secondary amenorrhea can be due to infection (e.g., tuberculosis), neoplasm (e.g., Krukenberg's tumor—metastasis of gastrointestinal neoplasm to ovary), trauma, surgery, or an autoimmune disorder. This latter category is often associated with a syndrome of polyglandular failures (see page 1047) and is the most common cause of "idiopathic premature menopause."

Exogenous. Exogenous amenorrhea may be caused by hyper- or hypothyroidism, liver failure, renal failure, or other nonendocrine illness. Hypothalamic (secondary, central, acquired) amenorrhea is also often exogenous in that there is a proximate cause such as weight loss, pathological obesity, vigorous exercise (e.g., runners or ballet dancers), or severe stress, as in grief or mental illness. Another form of exogenous interruption of menses may come from consumption of substances of abuse (opiates, alcohol) or prescribed medications (major tranquilizers, estrogens).

Galactorrhea

Galactorrhea (also see page 1059) is the production of milk (confirmed by demonstrating fat after staining the fluid with Sudan stain) in a woman who is not recently postpartum or nursing a baby. Secondary central amenorrhea is frequently (15%) accompanied by galactorrhea. In about 40% of cases galactorrhea-amenorrhea is due to a prolactin-secreting pituitary adenoma that may or may not be readily detectable (macro versus microadenoma) [18]. Other causes of galactorrhea amenorrhea include medication [isoniazid (INH), phenothiazines], recent pregnancy, hypothyroidism, and idiopathic hypothalamic dysfunction. It is not uncommon for a woman who has nursed to have mild persistent galactorrhea (without amenorrhea) for up to 5 years after weaning. In these cases prolactin levels are normal (<30 ng/ml).

Diagnosis of Female Reproductive Dysfunction

The diagnostic approach to female reproductive disturbances is aimed at classifying the kind of disorder (see above), identifying or eliminating specific disease entities that require medical or surgical treatment, and, having done this, determining to what extent the remaining symptoms represent a problem to the patient and treating these problems appropriately.

History

The physician should determine whether the problem is primary or secondary. A chronicle of pubertal events should be recorded including earliest budding of breast tissue (thelarche), pubic hair darkening and lengthening (pubarche), onset of menstrual flow (menarche), and time of growth spurt and its cessation. A menstrual history includes the average interval between menses, their regularity and when any irregularity developed, date of last period and previous period before that, the duration of flow and its magnitude, the presence of ovulatory pain (mittelschmerz), premenstrual tension, and dysmenorrhea (the latter three findings suggest ovulatory cycles). A pregnancy and nursing history (mature and premature deliveries, abortions, success with and duration of lactation, and living children's ages) and history of gynecological surgery (including dilation and curettage) are pertinent. A history of breast changes (swelling, tenderness, discharge) should be determined. The physician should ask whether the patient is troubled by growth of excessive hair, and, if so, the duration of symptoms, the location and severity of the problem, and the treatment used, if any. Also of interest are symptoms of masculinization: increased libido with greater sexual appetite or increased sexual dreaming and fantasies, voice deepening, and frontal hair loss. Symptoms of estrogen deficiency (hot flashes, vaginitis, dyspareunia, breast atrophy) are important. A careful history of medication and drug use, including oral contraceptive agents, may be helpful. A further general history should include weight gain or loss, dietary habits (especially rigorous dieting), strenuous exercise (e.g., running, ballet, gymnastics), symptoms of diabetes, adrenal or thyroid disease, and history of tuberculosis or hepatic, renal, or neurological problems. A family history should include ethnic origin and familial occurrence of reproductive and other endocrine dysfunctions (e.g., hirsutism, oligomenorrhea, hypothyroidism).

Physical Examination

On inspection the physician should note body habitus (obese or wasted, mature or child-like, masculine or feminine). The presence or absence of pubic and axillary hair, distribution of coarse dark hair on chest (periareolar, midsternal), abdomen, buttocks, and extremities, and the density of such hair must be noted. The quality of the patient's voice should be evaluated. Examination of breasts and pubic hair should include an estimate of their stage of maturity based on available standards (20) (see also Fig. 5.2 and Table 5.5). Nipples should be squeezed to look for galactorrhea. On pelvic examination it is important to look for clitoromegaly (>2.0 cm in length), state of the vaginal mucosa (dry versus moist, thick and rugated versus thin and atrophic), discharge, presence or absence and size and consistency of cervix and uterus. Bimanual examination should be done to attempt to estimate whether ovaries are enlarged (cystic) or not. In primary amenorrhea without maturation, signs of Turner's syndrome (wide set eyes, shield chest, wide set nipples, "webbing" of neck, short fourth metacarpal, and signs of aortic coarctation) should be sought. The remainder of the general physical examination (eyes, abdomen, etc.) should be as described in the evaluation of male hypogonadism (see page 1048), looking especially for signs of an intracranial mass lesion and thyroid or adrenal disease.

Diagnostic Procedures

All women with secondary amenorrhea should be considered pregnant until proven otherwise (even if sexual activity is not admitted, as, in adolescence, it may not be). Specific hCG assay is the most sensitive test for pregnancy (see Chapter 93). Further testing should be delayed until pregnancy is ruled out.

Serum estrogen radioimmunoassays have now improved to the point that one can generally distinguish low normal from definitely low (values less than 40 pg/ml are suspect and less than 25 pg/ml are low), but estrogen status may also be assessed by vaginal cytology and by the provocation of withdrawal bleeding. Cells for vaginal cytology should be obtained at the time of pelvic examination so that a maturational index can be estimated (see Chapter 94). A progesterone withdrawal test (7 days of 10 mg of medroxyprogesterone acetate (Provera) orally or a single 100-mg dose of progesterone in oil intramuscularly) will result in withdrawal bleeding within a few days (2 to 5 if oral

and 7 to 10 if intramuscular) if estrogen levels are adequate. If there is no bleeding, a 21-day course of estrogen [0.02 mg of ethinyl estradiol (Estinyl)/day] with 5 to 10 mg of medroxyprogesterone acetate (Provera) for the last 7 days should be administered. Absence of vaginal bleeding at this point indicates an absent or severely damaged endometrium, sometimes secondary to previous overvigorous dilation and curettage (Asherman's syndrome).

Serum or urinary gonadotropins are used to classify hypogonadism as gonadal (elevated) or central (low or normal). The investigation of central hypogonadism should include a serum prolactin level, especially if galactorrhea is present. Prolactin values between 30 and 100 ng/ml are elevated but may be consistent with prolactinoma or hypothalamic (idiopathic) galactorrhea. Values greater than 100 ng/ml nearly always mean that a prolactinoma is present (17). Further testing should be undertaken by appropriate specialists and is similar to that outlined for patients with male hypogonadism (Table 77.2). If hirsutism is present, the serum testosterone and urinary 17-ketosteroids should be measured (see page 1052).

Treatment of Women with the Oligomenorrhea Syndrome

Absence of Menses

The mere fact of amenorrhea is disturbing to some women, but not to others. Women with idiopathic oligomenorrhea who desire regular periods can be treated with low dose estradiol plus progestin regimens in cyclic fashion as outlined below. When fertility is an issue, appropriate referral should be made.

Galactorrhea (See Also Page 1058)

Women with hyperprolactinemia can be treated by transsphenoid removal of an adenoma (if present) or by suppression with bromocriptine (Parlodel), 2.5 mg, by mouth, two or three times a day, which treatment frequently also restores libido (see "Frigidity and Female Endocrine Dysfunction," below), suppresses lactation, and restores menses and fertility. Surgery is successful in restoring menses and reducing or eliminating galactorrhea in about 80% of cases. Risks of surgery include meningitis and cerebrospinal fluid (CSF) leakage into the sphenoid sinus, or permanent damage to the pituitary gland (hypogonadism about 5%, other axes, less than 2%), as well as the usual anesthetic and hemorrhagic risks of any surgical procedure. Risks of bromocriptine therapy have been described above (page 1049). When tolerated, this agent is 85 to 90% effective.

Intracranial Tumor

If vision or brain function is threatened, surgery or radiotherapy is indicated. Recent studies have shown that bromocriptine shrinks prolactin-secreting adenomas in size by reducing the volume (but not the number) of cells, so that it may be helpful, even in patients with suprasellar extension of tumor and visual symptoms, as emergency therapy prior to surgery. If only a microadenoma is present, it may be legitimate simply to follow visual fields and serial computed tomography (CT) scans at intervals of 6 months to 1 year and to treat hormone deficiency appropriately.

Estrogen Deficiency State

Estrogen deficiency is not a frequent occurrence in young women with central secondary amenorrhea but may occur in some women, especially those with hyperprolactinemia (18). It may be defined by a failure to develop withdrawal bleeding after progestin administration, by plasma estrogen levels less than 25 pg/ml, and/or by failure to ovulate and menstruate after being given clomiphene citrate (Clomid), 50 to 100 mg/day for 5 days. Estrogen deficiency is invariable in gonadal hypogonadism. Symptoms, complications, and therapy are discussed in the section on menopause(see below).

Female Sexual Dysfunction (Frigidity and Dyspareunia)

Definition

As in the male, female hyposexuality can be divided into reduced sexual interest or appetite (inhibition of desire), failure of arousal (inhibition of excitement), and anorgasmia (for a more complete discussion, see Chapter 18). Discussion below will be limited to physical and especially to endocrine etiologies.

Etiologies

Organic etiologies of female hyposexuality include diabetes mellitus with peripheral neuropathy, hyperprolactinemia, hypogonadism with estrogen deficiency, and organic disease of the vagina, uterus, fallopian tubes, or ovaries with resultant dyspareunia. Various endocrine (e.g., hyper- or hypothyroidism) and other systemic debilitating diseases can also cause loss of interest in sexual activity.

History

Questions should be the same as those asked of the woman with hypogonadism (see above). Additional questions should be asked about dyspareunia. If there is pain or discomfort on intercourse, it is important to know whether it occurs with attempts at penetration (local vaginal or vulvar problems) or only after deep penetration (pelvic disease, e.g., leiomyoma, endometriosis, salpingitis). The physician should determine whether there was a previous history of satisfactory sexual activity, and, if so, the time and circumstances of onset of its deterioration. Careful questioning should reveal to what extent the problem is one of loss of interest, excitation (lubrication and heightened pelvic blood flow), or orgasm. A history of symptoms of diabetes or peripheral neuropathy and of thyroid, adrenal, or other serious systemic disorders

should be obtained. Medication use (tranquilizers, oral contraceptives) and substance abuse (opiates, alcohol) are also pertinent.

Physical Examination

The physical examination should be conducted in the same way as for patients with female hypogonadism (see page 1059). Careful attention should be given to the genitalia, uterus, and adnexae for evidence of infection, atrophy, or neoplasia. Endometriosis, a frequent cause of dyspareunia, is sometimes detected on rectovaginal examination by palpation of nodules in the space between the rectum and vagina (pouch of Douglas). Neurologic examination should include testing of peripheral sensation and position sense and deep tendon reflexes.

Diagnostic Procedures

If evidence of hypogonadism exists, appropriate tests should be made (see page 1059). Measurement of serum prolactin level may be helpful even in patients without apparent galactorrhea or amenorrhea (see page 1059). Patients with pelvic disease should be referred to a gynecologist for further evaluation and therapy.

Therapy

Therapeutic efforts should be directed at the specific organic etiology whenever possible. Estrogen deficiency should be corrected (see below), and hyperprolactinemia should be treated surgically or medically (see above). When no organic cause is evident after careful examination, consideration of various modes of psychological diagnosis and treatment is appropriate (see Section 2, Psychiatric and Behavioral Problems).

PROBLEMS OF MENOPAUSE

Definition

Menopause is the irreversible cessation of the female reproductive cycle and menses that follows from a permanent loss of ovarian response to gonadotropins. This change generally occurs spontaneously between the ages of 45 and 55 in American women, with an average age of 50. Destruction or cessation of function of the ovary prior to age 40 is referred to as premature menopause. Hysterectomy terminates menstrual bleeding but not ovarian function and, hence, does not constitute a true menopause. In any year between 1990 and 2000, there will be approximately 30 million women of postmenopausal age (roughly one-third of the female population in the United States). Thus, an understanding of the medical problems of the menopausal period is important for all general physicians.

Physiology

The menopausal ovary is nearly depleted of primary follicles. The work of Sherman and Korenman (28) and others has shown that after age 35 to 40 there is a tendency for serum estradiol to decrease, probably reflecting a reduction in the responsive cohort of follicles at onset of a cycle. This results in less feedback inhibition, which in turn raises FSH levels and leads to a shortened follicular phase of the cycle (earlier ovulation), so that women in their late thirties may go from a regular 28- or 29-day menstrual interval to one of 25 to 27 days. In the early forties the luteal phase may also become inadequate with lower progesterone levels and early dissolution of the corpus luteum, resulting in further shortening of the cycle. Estradiol levels continue to decline. Next, anovulatory cycles and "missed" cycles, with long quiescent periods in which gonadotropins are high and estradiol very low, begin to occur. For a year or 2 menses are irregular and occur with reduced frequency, but occasional ovulatory cycles are seen. Finally cyclic bleeding ceases. FSH and LH levels become greatly elevated in serum and urine. Usually the FSH increase is greater. The ovary may still contain a few follicles, but these do not respond to gonadotropin. Estradiol levels become extremely low and adrenal estrone becomes the major estrogen.

Psychological Symptoms

The psychological response to the menopause may range from little or none to profound alteration of affect and personality, depending on the woman. Symptoms vary from minor irritability and emotional lability to severe depression and withdrawal from usual activities. Sexuality is also commonly affected, with some women reporting an increase in libido attendant on release from worries about conception, while other women have a reduction in sexual interest, usually associated with a perceived loss of attractiveness and femininity. Epidemiological and clinical studies have shown that there is no increase in mental illness attributable to menopause per se and that, in particular, women who develop depression during the menopausal years do not have a distinct syndrome but rather are characterized by a previous history of depressive illness or symptoms and/or the presence of situational factors (e.g., late life divorce, the empty nest, etc.) commonly associated with depressive episodes (32).

There are, however, many cultural misapprehensions about this period (e.g., expectations of loss of sexual interest and ability and expectations of an increased incidence of mental illness), and often these beliefs propagate feelings of inadequacy, somatic symptoms such as fatigue, and other complaints. Thus, some women who have previously been stable will still have psychological symptoms associated with the "change of life." For the most part, these will be minor and self-limited and will resolve with sympathetic support from the physician and the family. The organic changes of the menopause may reinforce these symptoms, and many women have had their symptoms worsened even further by the comment from a physician that the phenomenon is "an expected part of aging."

An attempt should be made to educate each patient about the menopause and evaluate her for any underlying psychological disturbances. In some cases a short course of a minor tranquilizer or an antidepressant may be justified. Women who develop significant psychological problems during the menopause should be managed appropriately, as described in the chapters in Section 2 of this book. In more severe cases psychiatric consultation is warranted.

Although there is little hard evidence that psychological symptoms accompanying menopause are due to estrogen deficiency, the value of estrogen replacement for relief of psychological symptoms in the menopausal transition remains controversial. A number of studies have suggested that significant relief of psychological symptoms and an overall increase in sense of well-being and ability to concentrate may occur when estrogen replacement is undertaken.

Estrogen Deficiency State

Ovarian estrogen production is minimal after the menopause. Ovarian interstitial and hilus cells still retain some secretory capacity but produce mainly small amounts of testosterone and androstenedione. Most estrogen is therefore formed from peripheral conversion of androgen, 75% of which comes from the adrenal. There is evidence that this rate of conversion is greater in obese women, who therefore tend to have higher estrogen levels postmenopausally. Estrogen deficiency results in various symptomatic manifestations in approximately 70% of postmenopausal women.

Hot flashes

Nearly 50% of menopausal women complain of a sudden sensation of flushing and extreme warmth, followed by profuse sweating and sometimes shaking or tremor. These episodes occur at irregular intervals from a few to many times a day and may awaken the patient at night. In about 15% of women they are severe enough to limit normal daily activities. It is important to remember that this, and other menopausal symptoms, may have their onset prior to actual cessation of the menses, since estrogen levels fall progressively in the premenopausal period. Investigations have shown that these episodes, objectively identifiable by altered skin and core temperature and skin resistance, are closely related temporally to episodic gonadotropin secretion by the pituitary gland. Hot flashes precede LH and FSH secretory rises by just a few minutes (30). LH and FSH secretory episodes are generally increased in amplitude, but not frequency, during the menopause, probably reflecting derepression of neurosecretory activity of the hypothalamus by loss of estrogen feedback. It is theorized that this exaggerated excitation of neurosecretory nuclei may spread to the adjacent thermoregulatory centers in the hypothalamus, setting off the "hot flash" (which is thus a sort of "hypothalamic seizure").

Genital and breast atrophy

The female reproductive organs undergo striking changes at the time of the menopause. Pubic hair becomes sparse and lank, and may turn gray. The labia majora lose their fullness as subcutaneous adipose is withdrawn from them and the mons veneris, thus exposing the labia minora. The skin and mucous membranes of the genitalia become thin and dry. The vaginal pH becomes more alkaline as glandular secretion of glycogen is lost. This change and the mucosal atrophy may result in a chronic vaginitis with itching, discharge, and local tenderness (see Chapter 94). Many women report decreased lubrication at intercourse and complain of dyspareunia. The cervix, uterus, and fallopian tubes also shrink. Estrogen deprivation is implicated in the relaxation of pelvic ligaments and muscles, which may result in uterine or bladder prolapse and contributes to the disturbing symptom of stress incontinence. At the same time glandular breast tissue atrophies, the breasts lose adipose and become shrunken and pendulous. There is a decrease in the erectile response of the nipple.

Osteoporosis (See Also Chapter 74, page 994)

Accelerated bone mineral loss occurs with any cause of estrogen deficiency, including the postmenopausal state (14). Replacement therapy prevents or greatly retards this process (see page 1063).

Atherosclerosis and Blood Lipids

Before the menopause, rates of myocardial infarction, angina, and sudden cardiac death are significantly lower in women than in men, even after accounting for known risk factors, such as blood pressure and cigarette smoking. These rates increase during the sixth through eighth decades to become equal to or slightly greater than those of age-matched men. Data from the Framingham population study (10) suggest that the level of coronary artery disease (CAD) risk is higher in postmenopausal women than in cycling women of the same age.

It is well established that plasma lipoprotein patterns predict risk of CAD (see Chapter 75). In particular, the greater the percentage of total cholesterol present in the high density lipid (HDL) fraction and the less cholesterol in the low density (LDL) fraction, the lower the risk of CAD. Cross-sectional measurements of HDL cholesterol in normal men and women (Fig. 77.4) have shown that mean levels are considerably higher in women than in men at every age and do not decrease in women at the age of the menopause. In contrast, although LDL levels (Fig. 77.4) are lower in young women than in age-matched men and increase gradually with age in both sexes, between ages 45 and 55 LDL cholesterol in women increases by a large increment and actually exceeds the LDL level in men after age 50. Thus, it would appear that HDL levels are higher in women, independent of endoge-

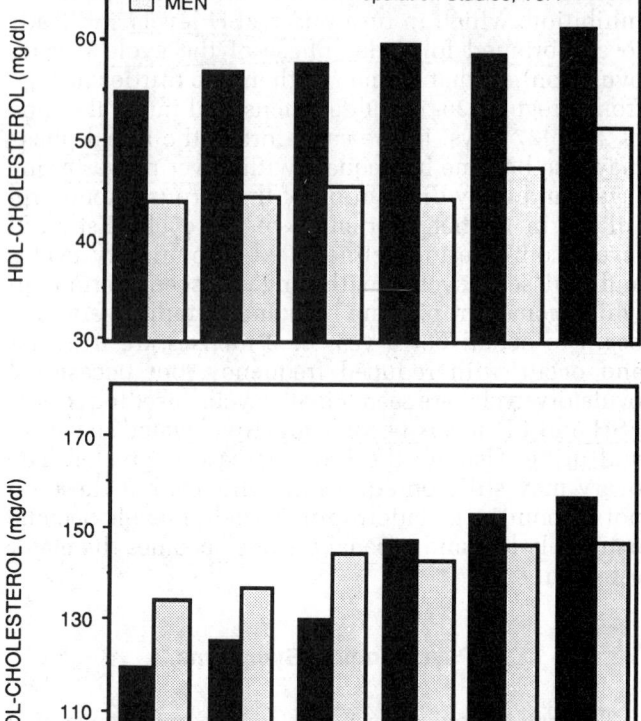

EFFECTS OF AGE ON CHOLESTEROL IN HDL AND LDL FRACTIONS IN MEN AND WOMEN

Figure 77.4. This figure, taken from data of the Lipid Research Clinics Population Study,[a] shows plasma levels of HDL cholesterol *(upper panel)* and LDL cholesterol *(lower panel)* in women (not using oral estrogens) and men by 5-year age intervals from 35 to 64. Menopause may be assumed to occur between ages 45 and 55. Note that during the perimenopausal period there is little change in HDL cholesterol but a relatively large increment in LDL cholesterol.

[a] The Lipid Research Clinics, Population Studies Data Book: Volume I, The Prevalence Study. United States Department of Health and Human Services, National Institutes of Health Publication No. 80-1527, 1980.

nous estrogen levels (and the menopause), and that LDL levels rise when estrogen is deficient.

The weight of available evidence favors the hypothesis that women are protected from coronary atherosclerosis by their endogenous estrogens and lose that protection at the menopause. Although there may be mechanisms for this protection that do not involve lipids, clearly, this effect is in part mediated by effects of endogenous estrogens on LDL but not HDL.

Endometrial Hyperplasia and Carcinoma

With loss of regular progesterone-induced maturation and subsequent shedding of the endometrium, the incidence of endometrial hyperplasia, due to the unopposed tonic effects of residual (adrenal) estrogen, begins to rise. This lesion is rarely seen in cycling premenopausal women but occurs frequently in those young women with a pattern of irregular anovulatory bleeding since these women also lack progesterone. Hyperplasia also appears to be more common in obese postmenopausal women, probably because of increased aromatization of androgens to estrogens in fatty tissue. Endometrial hyperplasia, especially the atypical adenomatous pattern characteristic of unopposed estrogens, appears to be a precursor of endometrial carcinoma. It is therefore not surprising that the carcinoma of the uterus is also more common in young anovulatory and postmenopausal obese women (16).

The incidence of endometrial carcinoma begins to rise at age 45, reaches a peak at about 0.08% (80/100, 000) at age 70, and falls off thereafter. It is usually suspected first by postmenopausal vaginal bleeding, is invasive (into myometrium and vessels) in only about 10% of cases, and has a relatively good prognosis if treated promptly by hysterectomy. It results in very few deaths, being relatively rare and frequently curable.

Estrogen Replacement Therapy

Benefits

Hot Flashes and Genital Atrophy. It is clear that the use of estrogen is highly effective, compared with placebo, in suppressing the symptoms of the "hot flash" (5). Even low doses (0.01 mg/day of ethinyl estradiol [Estinyl] or 0.625 mg/day of Premarin), which have no measurable effect on circulating serum gonadotropins, have been found effective. Such therapy is often given for 6 months to a year and then tapered; hot flashes recur in about 50% of cases, however. In this instance, a more prolonged course of low dose estrogens, or of cyclic or progestin-opposed estrogen therapy (see below), may be useful. Genital atrophy, vaginitis, and dyspareunia all are relieved by estrogen therapy, which may be systemic or local (by means of estrogen-containing cream). This latter form of therapy is not necessarily advantageous for preventing systemic effects of estrogen, since estrogens are taken up through the vaginal mucosa in unpredictable but significant amounts (26).

Bone Mineral Loss. Estrogen replacement has been shown to be effective not only in reducing bone mineral loss and maintaining bone density (13) but also in reducing the frequency of fractures in estrogen-deficient women (31). Thus, at present, prevention of osteoporosis is a persuasive indication for long-term postmenopausal estrogen replacement.

Coronary Artery Disease. Sex steroid hormones have specific and highly significant effects on lipoproteins (see below). In general, exogenous estrogens have beneficial effects, raising HDL (when taken orally) and lowering LDL cholesterol, whereas androgens do the opposite. A number of studies have found rates of CAD and cardiac death, as well as all-cause mortality, to be lower in women taking estrogens in the long term, although a few studies have shown no

apparent effect. If the former is true, prevention of CAD represents an even more compelling indication for estrogen replacement therapy than does osteoporosis prophylaxis, since CAD is an even more common cause of disability and death.

Risks

Cancer of the Uterus. The risk of estrogen therapy presently of greatest concern to physicians and patients is endometrial carcinoma (see above). A number of studies have demonstrated that postmenopausal estrogen therapy, as formerly practiced in the United States [i.e., 0.625 to 1.25 mg of oral conjugated estrogens (Premarin) given daily without interruption], is associated, after 2 or more years of therapy, with a 6- to 8-fold increase in the incidence of endometrial carcinoma (19). However, Hulka et al. (15) demonstrated that monthly interruption (see below) of therapy and/ or use of nonconjugated estrogen reduces the relative risk of invasive carcinoma to about 1.3 (not statistically significant). Furthermore, it is apparent from other studies that the use of an oral progestin for 7 to 10 days of the cycle to mature the endometrium does not produce any excess endometrial hyperplasia or endometrial carcinoma (9, 30). It is also of interest that women treated for up to 10 years with cycles of combined estrogen-progestin for birth control have not shown an increased rate of development of endometrial carcinoma, despite the high doses of estrogen employed. Thus, cyclic progestin-opposed estrogen therapy appears to be free of the risk of endometrial cancer and has now become the accepted practice in the United States. There is no reason why regular monthly bleeding in a 60-year-old should be confusing to the physician, trained to assume that postmenopausal bleeding indicates disease, if he is aware that the patient is receiving cyclic estrogen-progestogen therapy. As in a younger woman, it is intermenstrual spotting or unexpectedly heavy flow that should alert the physician to the necessity for investigation. Current gynecologic practice does <u>not</u> require <u>routine</u> endometrial biopsy when starting estrogen replacement therapy in healthy women without a history of abnormal intermenstrual bleeding, but this should be done if bleeding occurs at other than the expected withdrawal periods (see Chapter 95).

Risk Benefit Considerations

Although continued menstruation may be a small price to pay for protection from osteoporosis and CAD, prevention of genital atrophy, etc., some women find continuation or resumption of monthly vaginal bleeding unacceptable. For women who object to monthly bleeding, alternatives include cycling with progestogen at less frequent intervals (e.g., 90 days) or constant administration of estrogen and progestogen in a ratio that results in a quiescent endometrium. Although experience with these alternate modes of progestogen adminstration is too limited to produce data on actual risk of endometrial carcinoma, endometrial histology of women so treated gives reason to believe that protection will be obtained.

Carcinoma of the Breast. Although numerous investigations have been conducted, it remains uncertain whether estrogens used for postmenopausal replacement therapy are associated with an increased incidence of breast cancer. Moreover, a single study (8) suggested that the use of cyclic progestin in combination with estrogen by postmenopausal women may reduce the incidence of breast cancer. Recently, an epidemiologic study in Sweden found an increase of about 2-fold in the risk of breast cancer after 8 years in women using ethinyl estradiol but not in those using conjugated estrogens, and a 4-fold increased risk (after 6 years) in women receiving cyclic therapy with estrogen plus Provera (2). The type and dose of estrogen used in this study are different from those used in the United States so that the report should not affect current practice in this country.

Transdermal versus Oral Estrogen

The high doses of estrogen in oral contraceptives (OC) have a number of side effects, including increase in hypertension and thromboembolic disease (fully discussed in Chapter 93). These effects are due in part to portal absorption of orally administered steroid, which results in supra-physiologic levels in the liver on first pass and increased hepatic protein (e.g., renin substrate, clotting factors) synthesis. There is no dose of oral estrogen that will provide physiological replacement without increasing hepatic protein synthesis. Even though only one hepatic-related complication (gallbladder disease) has actually been shown to increase in women on estrogen replacement therapy (as opposed to those on OC), these effects are a legitimate consideration. Recently, dermal patches (Estraderm), which supply 50 or 100 μg of estradiol (E_2) per day, have become available. These devices provide slow constant release directly into the systemic circulation and, unlike oral estrogens, produce physiologic blood levels and ratios of E_2 and estrone (E_1). They do not cause elevations of hepatic proteins (TBG, SHBG, renin substrate) and presumably will not increase risks of hypertension, thromboembolic disease, or cholelithiasis. Results obtained to date suggest that transdermal estrogens have effects on calcium excretion and bone density comparable to those of oral estrogens, but no actual data relating their usage to fracture risk are yet available.

Recently it has become apparent that the route of steroid administration also influences the pattern of lipoprotein effects observed. When estrogens are given orally, there is a 10 to 30% increase in serum HDL cholesterol levels and a significant reduction in LDL cholesterol values. If estrogens are given by a nonoral route (e.g., by injection or transdermally), the HDL effect is not observed; however, prolonged (but not short-term) transdermal estrogen administration will lower LDL cholesterol. Thus, data suggest that use of nonoral exogenous estrogens produces a lipoprotein pattern resembling that seen before the menopause, whereas oral estrogen use has an added pharmacological effect to increase HDL beyond the high levels characteristic of women of any age. Because cycling women appear to be significantly protected from the risk of CAD, it is reasonable to suppose that transdermal estrogen confers a similar degree of protection; however, all currently available data showing decreased risk of CAD in estrogen-replaced women are derived from studies of oral therapy. Whether the greater HDL level produced by oral therapy leads to added benefit is not known, nor will it be until long-term studies comparing CAD rates in oral versus parenterally treated populations are completed.

The final consideration involves the use of progestogen. As noted above, cyclic progestogen appears to provide good protection against estrogen-induced endometrial hyperplasia and carcinoma. Progestogens, however, are weak androgens, antagonizing the beneficial effects of estrogens on LDL and HDL cholesterol, thus interfering with their cardioprotective action. Provera also has now been implicated in increasing the risk of breast cancer (see above). Thus, calculation of risk:benefit ratios for estrogen replacement therapy must factor in the route of estrogen administration, whether to use progestogen, and the type of progestogen to employ.

However, the current evidence still favors the use of estrogen replacement therapy continuously after the menopause, especially in women with premature loss of ovaries (under age 40) and in white women, especially those at high risk for osteoporosis (see above). Even if the mode of therapy used should result in some slight increase in the risk of endometrial carcinoma, comparison of incidences of morbidity and mortality shows that endometrial carcinoma is a relatively rare and infrequently fatal disease, whereas osteoporotic fractures and CAD are very common and often crippling or fatal. Estrogen replacement therapy is contraindicated in known cases of breast cancer or in women with a high risk of breast cancer (see Chapter 89) and in women who have suffered from stroke, phlebitis, or pulmonary emboli. The use of progestogen is not indicated in women who have had a hysterectomy.

Regimens and Costs

A regimen of 24 days of 1 or 2 mg of micronized estradiol (Estrace), 0.625 mg of conjugated estrogens (Premarin and others), or 50 or 100 μg of Estraderm by transdermal patch can be used. The routine addition of a progestogen (e.g., 10 mg of Provera) for the last 12 days must be considered controversial because of potential effects on plasma lipids and breast, but it does provide protection against endometrial cancer. Each cycle should be followed by 5 to 6 days without therapy before resumption of the cycle. Current cost for the oral regimen is approximately $10.00 per month and for transdermal patches $28.00 per month.

The addition of androgens to estrogen replacement therapy is not recommended. Increase in libido and other subjective beneficial effects of androgens have been described in some studies. Androgens also can produce virilization and may lead to a deterioration of the plasma lipoprotein pattern.

Alternatives to Estrogen Therapy

There is no good alternative to the use of estrogens for genital atrophy. As noted above, local estrogen cream produces unpredictable systemic estrogen absorption and thus has only illusory advantages over systemic therapy.

Because most older women consume calcium-deficient diets (400 to 600 mg/day), they are usually in a state of markedly negative calcium balance. As a result, some experts have recommended that postmenopausal women increase their daily dietary calcium intake to 1500 mg/day. There are no documented benefits of calcium intake above the recommended 1500 mg per day and the use of calcium supplements is therefore not justified if diet is adequate (24). Weight-bearing exercise (e.g., walking, but not swimming) has shown significant benefit in reducing bone loss and should be encouraged. Other aspects of the use of calcium in prevention of osteoporosis are discussed in Chapter 74.

Postmenopausal Bleeding

Postmenopausal bleeding is defined as any vaginal bleeding that occurs in a woman who has had no menstrual periods for 1 year (and is not on cyclic estrogen replacement therapy).

Postmenopausal bleeding must always be investigated because approximately 10% of women with such bleeding will be found to have a malignant process of some kind. The remainder have various problems such as endometrial hyperplasia, polyps, infections, traumatic lacerations, etc. It is important that patients be educated that any bleeding after one year of menopause is abnormal and needs to be reported to the physician.

History

The management of postmenopausal bleeding begins with a careful review of the history with respect to duration, frequency, and the characteristics of the bleeding in terms of color, amount, and flow. The presence or absence of hormone therapy is important. Even if cyclic hormones are being used, heavy bleeding or bleeding at unexpected times in the cycle should still be investigated.

Physical Examination

A careful physical examination should be undertaken. The abdomen must be evaluated for suprapubic masses and lower abdominal tenderness. The external genitalia must be inspected for neoplasia and/or atrophic changes. The vaginal mucosa should be inspected for atrophy or lacerations. The cervix must be visualized and a Pap smear obtained if needed. The size, shape, and position of the uterus must be noted and the adnexae evaluated for enlargement or tenderness. A rectal examination may reveal the presence of hemorrhoids and/or fissures. Samples of stool and of urine should be obtained for analysis for occult blood. These latter procedures may suggest the rectum or bladder rather than the uterus or genitals as the source of bleeding.

Diagnostic Procedures

Patients with obvious lesions of the vulva, vagina, or cervix should have a direct biopsy taken for histological evaluation. When there is no obvious lesion of the cervix, culposcopy (rather than biopsy) is indicated. Cervical biopsies are indicated only if the Pap smear is borderline or abnormal (see Chapter 95). Patients with significant adnexal disease should be further investigated by flat plate of the abdomen, intravenous pyelogram, barium enema, sonography, CAT, or magnetic resonance imaging (MRI) as appropriate. Bleeding from nonmalignant causes such as atrophic vaginitis, or traumatic lacerations secondary to intercourse, should not postpone the next and most important step, namely referral of the patient to a gynecologist.

The physician and patient should know that general anesthesia for a dilatation and curettage may be recommended by the gynecologist for patients who are obese, who have a low tolerance for pain, or who are new to the consultant. In those patients who have been seeing the physician for annual examinations over a number of years, a D and C under local anesthesia is usually a very satisfactory procedure and requires minimal hospital time.

General References

Blackman MR: Aging. In: DeGroot LJ, Besser GM, Cahill GF, et al (eds): *Endocrinology*, 2nd ed. Philadelphia, WB Saunders, 1989.
> Definitive review of effects of aging on hormone balance including male and female reproductive systems.

McLachan RI, Healy DL, Burger HG: The Ovary: Basic Principles and Concepts; B. Clinical. In: Felig P, Baxter JD, Broadus AE, Frohman LA (eds): *Endocrinology and Metabolism*, 2nd ed. New York, McGraw-Hill Book Co., 1987.
> Thorough exposition of diagnosis and management of disturbances of female reproductive system from puberty through menopause.

Santen RJ: The Testis. In: Felig P, Baxter JD, Broadus AE, Frohman LA (eds): *Endocrinology and Metabolis* 2nd ed. New York, McGraw-Hill Book Co., 1987.
> Excellent discussion of the physiology and pathology of the male reproductive system.

Upton V: The perimenopause: physiologic correlates and clinical manatgement. *J Reproductive Med* 27:1, 1982.
> Excellent summary of pertinent clinical issues and menopausal physiology.

Specific References

1. Adams DB, Gold AR, Burt AD: Rise in female-initiated sexual activity at ovulation and its suppression by oral contraceptives. *N Engl J Med* 299:1145, 1978.
2. Bergkvist L, Adami H-O, Persson I, et al: The risk of breast cancer after estrogen and estrogen-progestin replacement. *N Engl J Med* 321:293, 1989. and Editorial: Barrett-Connor E, Postmen-

opausal estrogen replacement and breast cancer. *N Engl J Med* 321:319, 1989.

3. Carter JN, Tyson JE, Tolis G, et al: Prolactin secreting tumors and hypogonadism in 22 men. *N Engl J Med* 299:847, 1978.
4. Davidson JM: Hormones and sexual behavior in the male. *Hosp Pract* 10:126, 1975.
5. DeFazio J, Speroff L: Estrogen replacement therapy: Current thinking and practice. *Geriatrics* 40:32, 1985.
6. Federman D: *Abnormal Sexual Development*. Philadelphia, WB Saunders, 1968,
7. Frank E, Anderson C, Rubinstein D: Frequency of sexual dysfunction in normal couples. *N Engl J Med* 299:111, 1978.
8. Gambrell RD, Maier RC, Sanders BI: Decreased incidence of breast cancer in postmenopausal estrogen-progesterone users. *Obstet Gynecol* 62:435, 1983.
9. Gambrell RD, Massey FM, Castaneda TA, et al: Reduced incidence of endometrial cancer among postmenopausal women treated with progestogens. *J Am Geriatr Soc* 27:389, 1979.
10. Gordon T, Kannel WB, Hjortland MC, McNamara PM: Menopause and coronary heart disease, The Framingham Study. *Ann Intern Med* 89:157, 1978.
11. Harman SM, Tsitouras PD: Reproductive hormones in aging men: I. Measurement of sex steroids basal luteinizing hormone and Leydig cell response to human chorionic gonadotropin. *J Clin Endocrinol Metab* 51:35, 1980.
12. Heller JE, Gleich PG: Erectile impotence: Evaluation and management. *J Fam Prac* 26:321, 1988.
13. Horsman A, Gallagher JC, Simpson M, Nordin BEC: Prospective trial of estrogen and calcium in postmenopausal women. *Br Med J* 2:789, 1977.
14. Horsman A, Jones M, Francis R, Nordin C: The effect of estrogen dose on postmenopausal bone loss. *N Engl J Med* 309:1406, 1983.
15. Hulka B, Kaufman DG, Fowler WC, et al: Predominance of early endometrial cancers after long-term estrogen use. *JAMA* 244:2419, 1980.
16. Judd HL, Lucas WE, Yen SSC: Serum 17β-estradiol and estrone levels in postmenopausal women with and without endometrial cancer. *J Clin Endocrinol Metab* 43:272, 1976.
17. Kleinberg DL, Noel GL, Frantz AG: Galactorrhea: a study of 235 cases, including 48 with pulmonary tumors. *N Engl J Med* 296:589, 1977.
18. Klibanski A, Neey RM, Beitins IZ, et al: Decreased bone density in hyperprolactinemic women. *N Engl J Med* 303:1511, 1980.
19. Mack TM, Pike MC, Henderson BE: Estrogen and endometrial cancer in a retirement community. *N Engl J Med* 294:1262, 1976.
20. Marshal WA, Tanner JM: Variations in pattern of pubertal changes in girls. *Arch Dis Child* 44:291, 1969.
21. Marshall WA, Tanner JM: Variations in pattern of pubertal changes in boys. *Arch Dis Child* 45:13, 1970.
22. Martin CE: Sexual activity in the aging male. In: Money J, Musaph N (eds): *Handbook of Sexology*. New York, Elsevier-North Holland, 1977, p. 813.
23. Muller SA: Hirsutism. *Am J Med* 46:803, 1969.
24. National Research Council Committee on diet and Health: *Diet and Health, Implications for reducing chronic disease risks.* Executive Summary, Washington, DC, National Academy Press, 1989.
25. Nutall FQ: Gynecomastia as a physical finding in normal men. *J Clin Endocrinol Metab* 48:338, 1979.
26. Schiff I, Tulchinsky D, Ryan KJ: Vaginal absorption of estrone and 17β-estradiol. *Fertil Steril* 28:1063, 1977.
27. Shapiro G, Evron S: A novel use of spironolactone: treatment of hirsutism. *J Clin Endocrinol Metab* 51:479, 1980.
28. Sherman BM, Korenman SG: Hormonal characteristics of the human menstrual cycle throughout reproductive life. *J Clin Invest* 55:699, 1975.
29. Spark RF, White RA, Connolly PB: Impotence is not always psychogenic. Newer insights into hypothalamic-pituitary-gonadal dysfunction. *JAMA* 243:750, 1980.
30. Tataryn IV, Meldrum DR, Lu KH, et al: LH, FSH, and skin temperature during the menopausal hot flash. *J Clin Endocrinol Metab* 49:152, 1979.
31. Weiss NS, Ure CL, Ballard JH, et al: Decreased risk of fractures of the hip and lower forearm with postmenopausal use of estrogen. *N Engl J Med* 303:1195, 1980.
32. Weissman MM: The myth of involutional melancholia. *JAMA* 242:742, 1979.
33. Witherington R: Suction device therapy in the management of impotence. *Urol Clin North Am* 15:123, 1988.

Neurological Problems

CHAPTER 78

Evaluation of the Patient with Neurological Symptoms*

MARGIT L. BLEECKER, M.D., Ph.D.
CONSTANCE J. MEYD, M.D.

This chapter describes approaches to history taking, physical examination, and laboratory evaluation that are most useful in ambulatory patients with neurological symptoms. One or more of these approaches is appropriate in patients with each of the neurological problems discussed in subsequent chapters (headache, seizures, dizziness, vertigo, syncope, tremor, Parkinson's disease, cerebrovascular disease, peripheral neuropathy).

NEUROLOGICAL HISTORY AND PHYSICAL EXAMINATION

General Principles

Four types of information should be obtained (or inferred) whenever there is a new neurological symptom: the temporal evolution of the symptom, any associated symptoms, the specific abnormality of neurological functions, and the anatomical localization of the problem. Figures 78.1 and 78.2 summarize

those facts that are most often needed for anatomical localization. Additional details regarding the anatomical relationships of peripheral nerves are shown in Figures 84.1 and 84.2.

It is important to remember that most individual neurological symptoms or signs are not specific for one functional or anatomical disturbance or for one etiology (e.g., loss of a reflex is not necessarily due to motor nerve damage, a hemiparesis is not necessarily due to cerebrovascular disease, and a resting tremor is not necessarily due to Parkinson's disease). The constellation of findings from the history and physical examination, however, is often quite specific. Therefore, a thorough history and physical examination are adequate for making a working diagnosis for most neurological problems encountered in office practice.

Depending on the circumstances, either a brief (but adequate) examination of each general neurological function may be required or only selected areas of the nervous system may need evaluation.

Brief Neurological History

Higher Functions and Consciousness

Handedness. Are you right-handed or left-handed?

Language. Have you had any problems with your thinking or with your speech? (Minor difficulty in finding words is very common in normal people, as are brief lapses of memory.)

Memory. How is your memory? What kind of things do you forget? (To the family: Have any problems with concentration, memory, or general abilities been noted?)

Acute cerebral dysfunction. Have you ever fainted, lost consciousness, felt dizzy, or had a seizure (fit, convulsion)? Do you have frequent or severe headaches? How often?

Mood. How are your spirits? Do you feel depressed? Are you worrying a great deal? How do you feel about the future? About yourself (confident, hopeless, helpless, guilty)?

Hallucinations/delusions. Have you seen or heard things that are unusual or that you think are not there? Does your imagination seem to play tricks on you? What do you feel is wrong? Is there anything or anybody controlling you?

Cranial Nerves

Nerve I (olfactory). Not tested in brief history and physical unless patient specifically mentions it, or has a history of head trauma with loss of consciousness.

Nerve II (optic nerve and vision). How is your vision? Do things seem blurred or are there patches where it is hard for you to see? Have you ever lost the vision in one eye or had trouble seeing out of one side or in one direction?

Nerves III, IV, and VI (extraocular motions). Have you ever had any double vision?

Nerve V (trigeminal nerve). Have you ever had any numbness over your face or difficulty chewing?

---

*Alfred C. Server, M.D., Ph.D., contributed to this chapter in the first and second editions of this book.

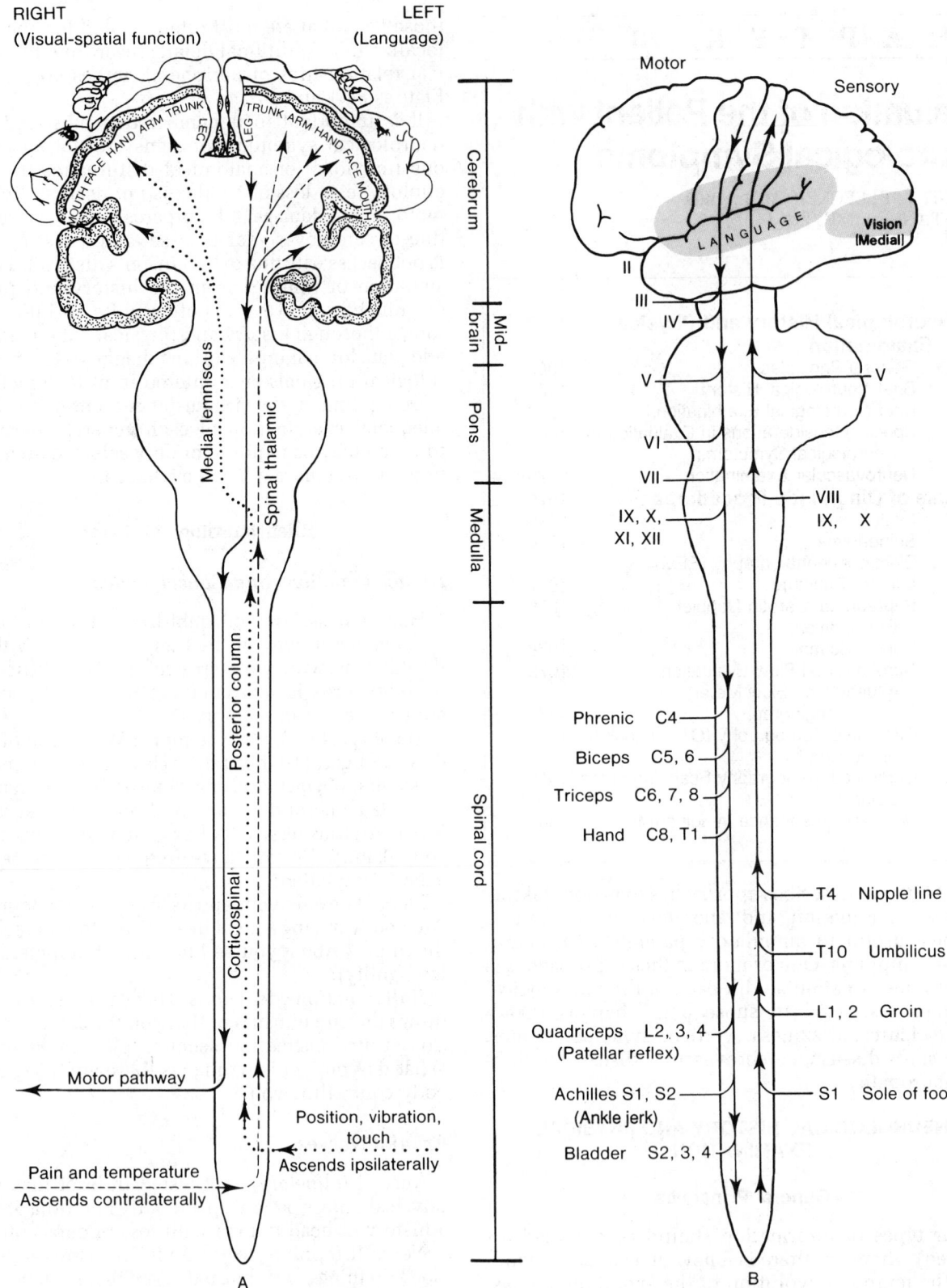

Figure 78.1. Schematic of neurological localization. Anterior (A) and lateral (B) schematics of central nervous system localization. Upper motor neuron signs and nonradicular sensory signs can only define the side of the lesion (A); in general, they do not reveal the level of the lesion. The presence or absence of other neurological signs or symptoms can help to specify the level of a localized neurological problem (B). (Courtesy of Barry Gordon, M.D. Ph.D.)

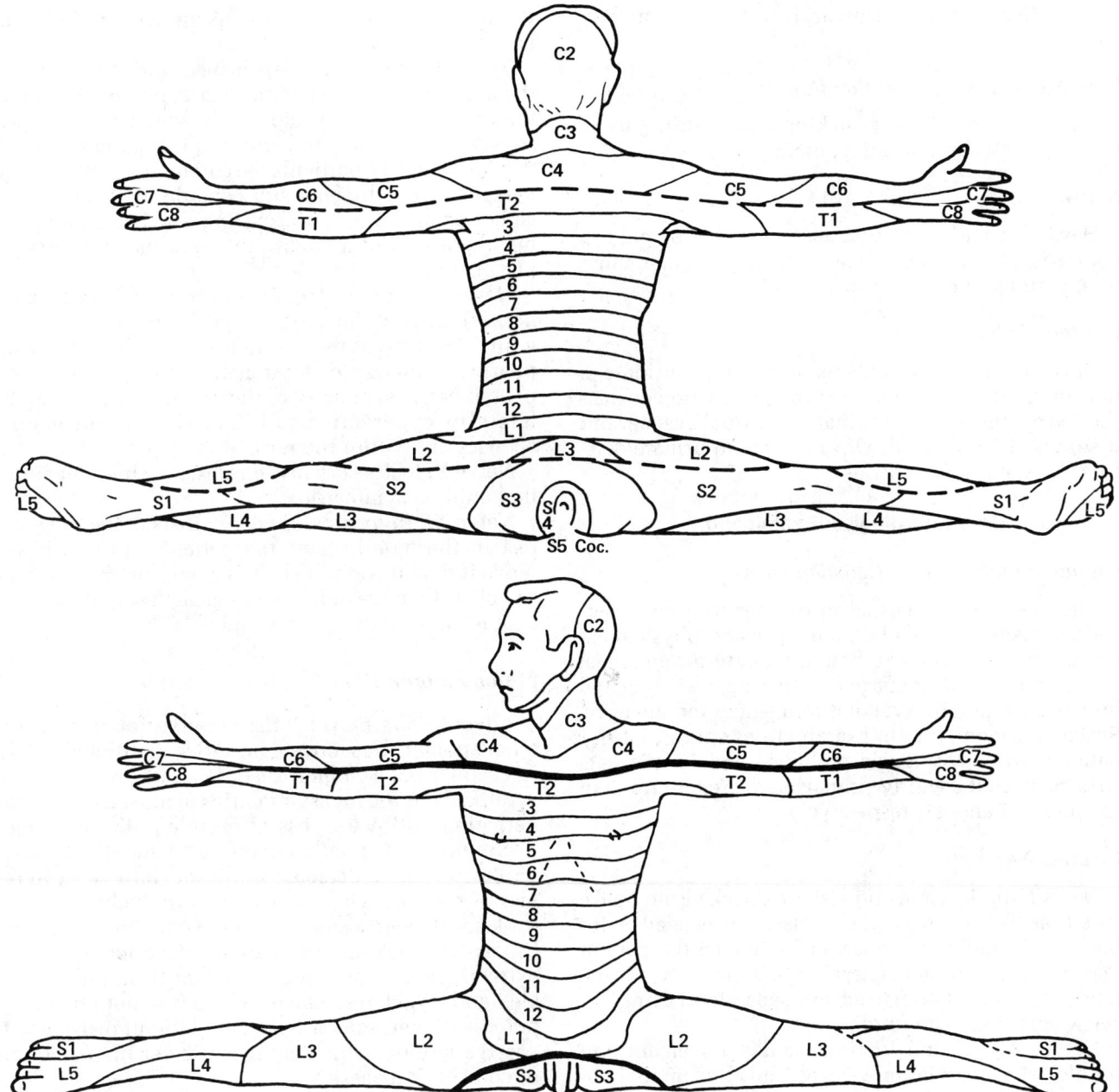

Figure 78.2. Cutaneous innervation areas of dermatomes. The numbers correspond to the spinal cord level of the dermatome. *C*, cervical; *T*, thoracic; *L*, lumbar; *S*, sacral. (From Haymaker W, Woodhall B: *Peripheral Nerve Injuries*, ed 2. Philadelphia, WB Saunders, 1962.)

Nerve VII (facial nerve). Have you ever had any weakness in your face or paralysis of your face?

Nerve VIII (auditory-vestibular nerve). How is your hearing? Have you had any ringing in your ears or difficulty hearing out of one side? Any loss of balance, spinning sensations, or dizziness?

Nerves IX, X, and XII (glossopharyngeal, vagal, and hypoglossal nerves). Have you had any problems chewing or swallowing your food? Does it seem to get caught anywhere? Where? What kinds of food do you have problems with? (Liquids are often the most difficult foods for patients with neurological problems.)

Motor

Have you noted any weakness in your arms or legs? Is it there all the time, or does it seem to come and go? Have you noted any twitching in your muscles? Where? How often? Any wasting of your muscles? Do you get any cramps in your legs? Under what circumstances?

Gait

Do you have any problems with walking? What kind? Where does it happen?—Climbing up stairs, walking certain distances, etc.? Do you feel unsteady on your feet?

Fine Motor and Cerebellar Function

Have you noticed any shaking or any difficulty in writing, drawing, buttoning, etc.?

Sensation

Have you had any numbness, tingling, or pain in your arms, legs, or feet? Where? Does position change or any other factor seem to bring it on?

Bladder/Bowel

Have you had any problems in starting to urinate or in urinating? Any difficulty with constipation or diarrhea? Any uncontrolled urination or stool evacuation? If so, was it associated with the urge to urinate/defecate, or was it spontaneous?

Brief Neurological Examination

Higher Functions and Consciousness

The questions suggested in the history plus observations made throughout the history and physical examination are usually sufficient for determining level of consciousness, language functioning, visual-spatial functioning, mood, level of intelligence, and memory. Systematic mental status examinations appropriate for patients with psychiatric problems and for patients with suspected cognitive impairment are described in Chapters 10 and 17, respectively.

Cranial Nerves

Nerve II (optic nerve and vision). Check vision (make sure that patients wear their glasses, if needed) with the use of the Snellen chart or by having the patient read from a newspaper, each eye separately. Check fields by confrontation (each eye separately) using finger wiggle. Examine fundi.

Nerves III, IV, and VI (extraocular movement and pupils). Have patient move eyes into all principal positions of gaze (horizontal, vertical, diagonal), observe for dysconjugate movements, and ask, while testing, about diplopia. Look for nystagmus and lid lag also. Look for ptosis and check pupils for size, symmetry, and reaction to light. (Normal pupil size for young adults is 3 to 5 mm. In the elderly, normal pupils are often 2 to 3 mm. A slight degree of pupillary asymmetry, 1 mm or less, is present in about 5% of the normal population; it usually varies from hour to hour and day to day, and it decreases in bright light.)

Nerve V (trigeminal nerve). Corneal reflexes should be tested at corresponding points on the cornea of each eye. Have the subject look up and away from the testing swab; use cotton as gauze is abrasive. With a pin, check for symmetry of perception over forehead, cheek, and chin. (There are wide variations in corneal sensitivity among normal individuals; some subjects, particularly those who have worn contact lenses, have virtually no response at all. Asymmetry is the most important clue to disease.)

Nerve VII (facial nerve). Inspect for asymmetry of the nasolabial folds when the face is not moving. Have the patient show teeth, close eyes, frown. (Normal persons may have a slight degree of resting asymmetry of the face; this is particularly common in edentulous persons. Normally both sides should move briskly together on showing teeth, smiling, etc. Lag on one side may be a sign of a slight 7th nerve palsy, central or peripheral.)

Nerves IX and X (glossopharyngeal and vagus nerves). Inspect the uvula for position and for motion with "Ahh." Test the gag reflex on both sides of the pharynx, looking for asymmetry of response. (Some people have asymmetry of the resting uvula. Also, bilaterally hyperactive to bilaterally absent gag responses are within the normal range.)

Nerve XI (accessory nerve). Observe shoulder shrug; it should be symmetric.

Nerve XII (hypoglossal nerve). Inspect the tongue at rest in the mouth; have the patient protrude it and move it to both sides. (The tongue normally has small twitches that are not pathological fasciculations; it should protrude in the midline.)

Motor Examination

Adventitious movements. Observe for tremor and other spontaneous movements. (See additional details in Chapter 82, Common Disorders of Movement.)

Bulk. Examine for asymmetries of muscle mass. (Denervation will cause loss of muscle bulk, reaching a maximum by 4 months; disuse over months to years will also cause a decrease in muscle bulk, e.g., in the legs of patients who are permanently bedridden.)

Muscle tone (resistance to passive motion). Test tone by passively flexing and extending the upper and lower extremities. Normal tone is a slight firmness of muscles and slight resistance to passive motion. In hypotonia, the muscles are flaccid, without resistance to passive motion. This may mean lower motor neuron or cerebellar disease.

There are several subtypes of *hypertonia*:

Rigidity is increased resistance to passive motion throughout the whole range of motion around a joint.

In *spasticity*, the initial passive motion is easy, but then there is a tightening of the muscle ("spastic catch") possibly followed by a sudden release ("clasp-knife effect"). Spasticity usually affects only one set of muscles around a joint (in the upper extremities, the biceps, forearm pronators, and finger flexors; in the lower extremities, the quadriceps, hamstrings, and plantar flexors).

In *gegenhalten* or *paratonia*, resistance is present in all directions but varies with the examiner's force and speed. It often seems to be voluntary ("fighting back"). Gegenhalten is seen normally in infants, but it appears pathologically in adults with dementias or frontal lobe disease.

Voluntary strength. Voluntary strength should be

sampled in several major muscle groups. Survey proximal and distal muscles in each extremity. An adequate screen is testing shoulder abduction, elbow extension and flexion, hand and finger extension, grip strength (with two fingers), hip flexion (with patient sitting), knee flexion, knee extension, and foot dorsiflexion. Also observe the patient's gait (see below).

For precise documentation, the following rating scale can be used:

0 = No movement
1 = Flicker
2 = Able to move with gravity eliminated (e.g., lateral motion of arm when recumbent);
3 = Able to move against gravity;
4 = Able to move against resistance;
5 = Normal strength

(In conversion reactions and malingering, strength on formal testing is usually jerky or "giving." With sudden passive motions in the opposite direction, the examiner may be able to demonstrate that the muscles can produce normal force. The examiner may note that the subject can do some voluntary activities, e.g., combing hair, reaching for objects, getting up or sitting down, etc., with muscles that the patients states are "too weak" to use for such motions on formal testing.)

Reflexes

The most important reflexes to test are the biceps (C5-6), triceps (C6-8), patellar (L2-4), Achilles tendon (S1-2), and plantar flexion ("Babinski"). Activity of the reflexes varies widely among patients and can vary in the same individual depending upon his emotional state and upon his ability to relax his muscles. As in the rest of the examination, asymmetries between two sides generally carry more weight than symmetric reflex changes; comparison must be made with the muscles relaxed to a similar degree and with the two extremities in identical positions. A decrease in the reflex or reflexes is generally due to disruption of the sensory or motor nerves (or both) of the reflex loop itself. Sometimes decreased reflexes are seen immediately after a cerebrovascular accident, in which case interpretation does not depend on the reflexes alone. Increased reflexes mean upper motor neuron (UMN) disease located anywhere from just above the anterior horn cell to the cerebral cortex. A Babinski response is dorsiflexion of the big toe, which may be associated with dorsiflexion and spreading of the other toes and dorsiflexion of the foot. The classic Babinski response is slow and deliberate. Nonspecific withdrawal may resemble the Babinski reflex, but it is usually rapid and the patient usually complains of subjective distress; a reliable Babinski sign can and should occur in the absence of any patient discomfort from the stimulus. A Babinski sign may be found as the sole indicator of upper motor neuron disease.

Sensation

The patient should be tested for symmetry and for differences in proximal and distal perception, in all four extremities. Sensitivity to pinprick (lateral spinothalamic tract) should be tested, as should both proprioception and vibratory sense (posterior column). There are normal differences in pinprick perception over different areas of the body—for example, it is decreased over the beard area—but patients generally ignore these differences. Particularly introspective or anxious patients can give very confusing responses and must be told to ignore small subjective differences. Repeated testing is often important to determine the reliability of a patient's response. Vibration sense should be tested with a 128-cycles/second (cps) tuning fork. Loss of vibration sense is often the earliest detectable abnormality in peripheral neuropathy. Mild distal loss of pin and vibration sense is very common in otherwise normal elderly patients.

Fine Motor and Cerebellar

The patient should be told to touch his thumb sequentially to each of the fingers of each hand separately and the speed, effort, and rhythm should be observed. Finger-to-nose-to-finger should be tested (subject has to touch examiner's moving finger, then touch his own nose, then touch the examiner's finger again, etc.) for speed, rhythm, intention tremor, and inaccuracy (dysmetria). The subject should be asked to tap each foot separately, and differences in speed, ease, and rhythm should be observed. In these tests, normal subjects show equal ability with either side or are slightly better on the side of their preferred hand. Slowness and subjective effort on repetitive movements, without a loss of rhythm, are characteristic of upper motor neuron lesions. Relatively preserved speed with erratic movements and loss of rhythm may be seen in cerebellar disease. Finger-nose-finger testing may be affected by tremor of various types as described in Chapter 82.

Station and Gait

Any tendency to list or any need for support while sitting, standing, or walking should be observed. The patient should be asked to walk normally and to walk on his heels and toes (tests strength and balance). A Romberg test should be performed (feet together in young patients, slightly apart in older patients).

In *cerebellar disease*, there is a wide base (legs widely separated), unsteadiness, and lateral reeling. (Lateral reeling can be evaluated by having the patient walk around a chair in both directions; he will tend to walk into the chair when it is on the affected side and to veer away from the chair when it is on the unaffected side.) Because of fundamental abnormality of motor coordination, the patient with cerebellar disease that affects the lower extremities cannot participate in a Romberg test, which requires standing with the two feet together; this is not an "abnormal Romberg test."

In *sensory ataxia* (loss of proprioception), there is uncertainty, slapping or stamping of the feet, and a "positive" Romberg test (the patient loses his balance with eyes closed but can avoid falling when his eyes are open because of visually mediated vestibular or cerebellar compensation).

In a *spastic gait* (in upper motor neuron disease), the leg does not flex but circumducts, and there is foot dragging (the toe of the sole of the patient's shoe becomes disproportionately worn); there is also loss of arm swinging on the spastic side.

In a *parkinsonian gait*, there is unilateral or bilateral loss of arm swinging; the patient is bent forward; and there is rigidity, shuffling, and festination (the upper part of the body advances ahead of the lower extremities; gait becomes faster as if to catch up).

In *lower motor neuron (LMN) paralysis* of the pretibial and peroneal muscles, there is drop-foot; hip flexion is preserved, and the patient lifts the foot very high, advances it by swinging it forward, then slaps it down.

In *frontal lobe disease*, gait may be wide based, shuffling, and slow, and turning is very slow, but there is no weakness or loss of sensation.

Special Considerations in Evaluation of Neurological Symptoms

The neurological symptoms seen in ambulatory patients are often less florid than are those of patients hospitalized for neurological disease, and many of these symptoms are related to prior acute neurological events. There are two important considerations in the evaluation of ambulatory patients with neurological symptoms: the variability in patient performance over time and the difference between the manifestations of upper motor neuron and lower motor neuron lesions.

Variability over Time

In dealing with abnormalities of the peripheral nerves, spinal cord, and brainstem, the physician can expect symptoms and signs to remain about the same after the basic problem has stabilized; subsequently, alterations of the findings usually reflect a change in the patient's disease. On the other hand, the performance of patients with ostensibly stabilized cerebral disease may vary greatly from minute to minute, hour to hour, or day to day. The variability affects the psychomotor domain, e.g., performance of everyday tasks, memory, speech and language, and mood. For example:

1. The patient may be able to dress, fix breakfast, and bring in the mail one morning; be incapable of these tasks the next morning; and perform them correctly on the third morning.
2. The patient may remember his wife's name in the morning but not in the evening of the same day.
3. The aphasic patient may be able to say something one minute and be unable to say it several minutes later.
4. The stroke survivor's affect may vary from depressed to euphoric from hour to hour and day to day.

As a result of this type of variability, members of the patient's family may become confused and, often, quite angry. They may frequently contact the physician to inquire whether a change in behavior means that the disease is getting worse, or they may conclude that the patient is capable of doing certain tasks but "just not trying" sometimes. When the pattern is clearly one of waxing and waning, the family should be reassured that, just as intact individuals have their "good days" and "bad days," brain-damaged subjects do also, but in exaggerated and different ways. The evaluation and management of behavioral changes of patients with cerebral damage are discussed in more detail in Chapters 17 (dementia) and 83 (stroke).

Difference between Upper Motor Neuron (UMN) and Lower Motor Neuron (LMN) Symptoms

The manifestations and the course of UMN and LMN damage differ fundamentally. UMN lesions affect the pathways bringing a command from the cortex to the anterior horn cell. UMN function depends upon integrity of the cortex and the corticospinal and corticobulbar tracts. LMN lesions affect the final common pathway for muscle movements. LMN function depends upon the integrity of the anterior horn cell in the spinal cord and its nerve fiber for carrying impulses to the muscle cell. A number of points are helpful in recognizing or distinguishing these common problems when they are less overt, which is often the situation in patients seen in office practice.

UMN Lesion Syndrome. If a UMN lesion is total, movements will be absent. However, there may be preservation of involuntary movements, such as those associated with yawning, laughing, crying, or anger.

When there is weakness (paresis) rather than paralysis due to UMN damage, the following patterns of weakness are seen.

In the face, the lower muscles are usually involved. There is variable but often some involvement of the orbicularis oculi (producing a widened palpebral fissure and weakness of eye closure), but the forehead is completely spared. This is in contrast to LMN (peripheral) 7th nerve damage in which usually both the upper and lower facial muscles are involved (although sometimes mild peripheral 7th nerve weakness— e.g., early Bell's palsy, an LMN lesion—can mimic a UMN pattern). One additional differential point is that the LMN lesion will produce the same amount of weakness with both a voluntary and an involuntary movement (e.g., laughing). A UMN 7th nerve paresis (from a stroke, for example) may not be apparent when the patient is laughing or crying involuntarily but may only be present when the patient is asked to smile voluntarily.

In the arm and leg, distal muscles are affected by UMN lesions much more than proximal muscles. In addition, some specific motor functions are affected more than others: in the arm, shoulder abduction and external rotation; in the forearm, extension and supination; in the wrist and finger, extension; in the hip, flexion; in the knee, flexion; and in the foot and toe, dorsiflexion.

Whether or not the muscles are weak in a UMN lesion,

voluntary movements are typically slowed and require greater effort than usual, and the ability of the affected limb's to make fine movements is lost. A patient with a very mild hemiparesis may be able to squeeze the examiner's hand with normal strength, but his movements are slower and clumsier than usual; he may be unable easily to use his fingers individually; also, when asked to extend both arms with his eyes closed, there may be downward and inward drift of the weak arm (pronator sign). In the lower extremity, a patient with such a mild defect may be able to dorsiflex his foot voluntarily. However, he may not be able to do this very rapidly (as revealed on attempted foot tapping), and the movement may not be automatically coordinated with walking, resulting in a "drop foot."

Typically (but not invariably), UMN lesions are accompanied by spasticity and hyperreflexia.

LMN Lesion Syndrome. Weakness resulting from a permanent LMN lesion is fixed and unchanging. Only those muscles served by the involved spinal cord segment or peripheral nerve are weak. There are none of the widespread effects characteristic of an UMN lesion. Atrophy is usually apparent within several weeks after a LMN lesion, in contrast to UMN lesions where atrophy is slight and late (many months). Pathological fasciculations may be present in affected muscle groups, distinguishable from benign occasional muscle twitching by the fact that they are frequent and occur only in the denervated muscles. Muscles are usually flaccid and hyporeflexic or areflexic. If a peripheral nerve has been involved, there may be associated hypesthesia or anesthesia.

Mixed UMN and LMN Lesions. In some situations, UMN and LMN lesions may occur together. For instance, spinal cord injury will typically give signs of a LMN lesion at the level of the injury, due to localized destruction of the anterior horn cells and their nerve roots; below the level of the injury, there may be a partial or complete UMN syndrome with spasticity, hyperreflexia, and preserved involuntary reflexes. Likewise, amyotrophic lateral sclerosis, an idiopathic degenerative disease, affects both pyramidal tract cells and anterior horn cells. Along with LMN type weakness, fasciculations, and wasting these patients have hyperreflexia and may have Babinski signs.

Neurovascular Examination

This section describes a systematic approach to the neurovascular examination. This examination is especially important in patients in whom cerebrovascular disease or an increased risk of cerebrovascular disease is the problem (see Chapter 83). The examination includes an assessment of the heart and peripheral vasculature with emphasis on the vessels of the head and neck.

Heart and Peripheral Vessels

The radial arteries should be simultaneously palpated at both wrists to determine any asymmetry in pulse amplitude or timing (pulse delay). The brachial arterial blood pressure should be measured in the su-

pine, sitting, and standing positions. Blood pressure should be measured in both arms to check for asymmetry. Unequal blood pressures in the two arms (≥ 20 mm Hg difference in systolic and greater than ≥ 10 mm Hg in diastolic pressure) are suggestive of a stenotic lesion of the subclavian or innominate artery on the side with the lower pressure. Orthostatic hypotension, defined as a fall in systolic pressure of greater than 15 mm Hg on moving from a supine to an upright position, may be important in explaining symptoms in patients with stenotic lesions of carotid or vertebral-basilar arteries.

A detailed cardiac examination can provide evidence of cardiomegaly, valvular disease, or an arrhythmia, each of which may predispose a patient to having a stroke. Finally, a complete assessment of the peripheral vasculature, for evidence of widespread atherosclerosis, should include palpation and auscultation of the femoral arteries and palpation of the arterial pulses in the feet.

Vessels of Head and Neck

The evaluation of the vessels of the head and neck should follow the time-honored format of inspection, palpation, and auscultation.

Inspection. Prominence of the superficial *temporal artery* with erythema, and, occasionally, ulceration of the overlying skin, in a patient with persistent malaise is suggestive of giant cell arteritis, an inflammatory process that can lead to retinal and/or cerebral infarction (see Chapter 79).

Dilation of the *episcleral arteries* of an eye can result from occlusion of the ipsilateral internal carotid artery (in this instance, the hemisphere on the side of the occlusion is being supplied in a retrograde fashion by the external carotid artery through enlarged ophthalmic arteries). The *funduscopic examination* allows direct visualization of the retinal vessels, and changes resulting from atherosclerosis, hypertension, or diabetes mellitus can be detected. Moreover, the absence of an expected change can be informative, as in the case of the hypertensive patient with normal retinal vessels on the side of a severely stenosed carotid artery. (In this instance, occlusive disease of the ipsilateral carotid artery protects the retina from the effects of chronic hypertension.) A detailed funduscopic examination may also demonstrate emboli, seen as white or refractile elements in the retinal arterioles (see Fig. 83.1). These emboli may be composed of cholesterol, platelets and fibrin, or calcium and are suggestive of atherosclerotic carotid occlusive disease or cardiac valve disease.

Palpation. The value of palpation of the carotid vessels has been the subject of debate. Reports of embolic stroke after firm palpation of a diseased carotid artery have left many clinicians with a sense of trepidation regarding manipulation of this vessel. The current consensus, however, is that gentle palpation of the carotid artery can be performed with limited risk and will occasionally provide useful information about the status of the vessel. Perhaps more valuable, and without risk, is palpation of the superficial temporal and facial arteries, which are branches of the external carotid artery. A weak or absent pulse in these arteries on one side of the head is suggestive of ipsilateral occlusive disease of the external or common carotid artery. In contrast, an increase in pulsation in these vessels may result from stenosis or occlusion of the ipsilateral internal carotid artery causing collateral flow through the external system. Finally, the finding of a tender superficial temporal artery with decreased pulsation may support other data consistent with the diagnosis of giant cell arteritis.

Auscultation. After auscultation of the heart to rule out the possibility of a transmitted cardiac murmur, the examiner should proceed to the following sites: the supraclavicular regions over the subclavian arteries; the carotid arteries up to their bifurcation at the angle of the jaw; the occipital, temporal, and parietal regions of the cranium; and the orbits. The finding of a cephalic bruit in an adult raises the possibility of an arteriovenous malformation; an orbital bruit suggests intracranial internal carotid artery disease; and a cervical bruit is suggestive, but not diagnostic, of atherosclerotic occlusive disease.

USE OF DIAGNOSTIC PROCEDURES

Patients may be referred for any of several diagnostic procedures in evaluating a neurological problem. For the majority of these procedures currently available for ambulatory application, the following information is provided here: definition, principal indications, limitations, and a description of what the patient experiences during the procedure. For nerve conduction tests and electromyography, this information is provided in Chapter 84.

Skull X-rays

Definition of Procedure

The term "routine skull X-rays" refers to a set of films that include three standard views: lateral, anteroposterior (AP), and inclined AP. Many other views are possible and may be indicated in specific conditions (e.g., basal skull views for a patient with atypical trigeminal neuralgia).

Principal Indications

1. Known or suspected significant head trauma.
2. Suspected pituitary tumor.
3. Suspected problems involving the bones—e.g., metastatic tumor (osteoblastic or osteolytic), myeloma, or Paget's disease.

Limitations

The skull X-ray has little value as a general screening test for intracranial disease. Relatively few neurological conditions are associated with bony changes; even when such changes are present, they can generally be evaluated better by procedures with greater sensitivity, specificity, and often nearly equivalent cost and risk, such as computed tomography (see below).

Patient experience. The patient should be informed that he will be asked to keep his head in several uncomfortable positions for short periods of time; accurate positioning might be impossible for patients who have neck problems or who are old.

Spine Films

Definition of Procedure

Standard spine films are usually AP and lateral views; oblique and flexion/extension views usually must be ordered specifically.

Principal Indications

1. Suspected cervical spondylitic radiculopathy—in this case, oblique films are necessary to examine the intervertebral foramina through which the roots pass.
2. Suspected cervical or lumbar stenosis or spondylolisthesis
3. Suspected vertebral fracture;
4. Suspected metastatic tumor;
5. To rule out other problems, such as tumor, fracture, and infection, in patients with suspected spondylosis or disc disease.

Limitations

Interpretation of "positive" findings: asymptomatic cervical spondylosis and interspace narrowing due to disc degeneration are so common after age 40 (see Chapter 64) that their presence has limited usefulness in the absence of more specific findings from the history and physical examination. Negative films provide good evidence against spondylosis as the cause of radicular symptoms.

X-rays are indirect studies; they do not show soft tissue or the actual status of the cord and nerve roots; these must be inferred. In patients with herniated intervertebral discs, films are usually normal or show only nonspecific intervertebral narrowing. However, patients with congenitally small bony canals (cervical or lumbar stenosis) are at high risk for these soft tissue problems occurring secondary to degenerative changes in the disc and ligaments; the radiologist should be specifically asked about these possibilities if they are clinically relevant.

Patient experience. The patient must cooperate for several views. Patients with neck problems or who are elderly may be unable to position themselves for adequate cervical spine films.

Electroencephalography (EEG)

Definition of Procedure

This is a record of the minute (1 to 50 μV) electrical rhythms of the brain.

Principal Indications

1. Known or suspected seizure disorders (see Chapter 80). (Recording during sleep or after sleep deprivation significantly increases the chances of a useful diagnostic examination; for complex partial seizures, nasopharyngeal leads record from the medial temporal regions where most of these seizures originate and, therefore, can increase the yield of the study.)
2. Confirmation of focal brain lesions in the absence of other evidence (e.g., in the diagnosis and localization of brain tumor, stroke, abscess, and other mass lesions);
3. Confirmation of diffuse brain disease, such as dementia, delirium, cerebral vasculitis, drug effect or withdrawal. (Because the general criteria for normal are broad, serial EEGs on the same subject are most helpful in these situations to confirm/disprove an abnormal condition.) The EEG is particularly useful in the differentiation of pseudodementia of depression from organic dementia.
4. Sleep disorders (see Chapter 85)—routine and special EEG recording techniques are often indicated.

Limitations

The EEG records cortical activity, and, although quite sensitive for processes affecting the cortex, is not useful for delineation of subcortical processes. This property, however, can be useful in investigating vascular lesions when a cortical versus subcortical lesion cannot be discerned by other criteria.

Negative EEG. A single negative EEG is not convincing evidence for the absence of a seizure disorder. For example, up to 50% of patients with known epilepsy have normal interictal records. Serial or repeated negative EEGs may be far more significant. A normal EEG in a patient with delirium suggests psychiatric illness.

"Mildly abnormal" EEG. Depending upon the reader and the classification scheme, some (5 to 30% or more) adult EEGs can be classified as minimally or mildly but nonspecifically abnormal. The relevance of these interpretations must be judged in the context of the patients' problems but should often not be given undue weight because of the broad range of normal. This is particularly true in infancy, childhood, adolescence, and old age. For instance, temporal slow activity (usually on the left, occasionally on the right or bilaterally) is a common finding after the age of 40 in as many as 30 to 40% of subjects; it may be confused with the slowing produced by a focal brain lesion.

Patient experience. Subjects are asked to lie down or recline while surface electrodes are attached with electrode paste (which tenaciously clings to hair, so that women should not get their hair done before coming for the study). The total procedure takes an average of about 40 to 60 minutes, with 20 to 30 minutes of actual recording time. For most of the actual recording, the patient will simply be asked to lie calmly with his eyes closed. Additional studies that most laboratories routinely perform include recording during hyperventilation (for 3 to 5 minutes) and photic simulation with a repetitive flash. (For many tracings, subjects will be encouraged to fall asleep. Some laboratories induce sleep with oral chloral hydrate if permitted by the referring physician.)

The EEG is extremely sensitive to patient movement, sweating, or muscle tension; any of these may make a tracing uninterpretable.

For sleep-deprived EEGs. The patient is generally asked to stay up the night before, and the EEG is done in the laboratory first thing in the morning.

Nasopharyngeal leads are generally applied through the nostrils after local anesthesia of the nasopharynx by spray; they may be annoying and they may interfere with nasal breathing, but they should not hurt.

Lumbar Puncture

Definition of Procedure

Lumbar puncture is performed to obtain cerebrospinal fluid for analysis and to measure intracranial pressure. A normal opening pressure does not exceed 200 mm of water. The opening pressure is dependent on the intracranial pressure, which can be elevated by measures that increase venous pressure such as straining and tightening of the abdominal musculature. An elevated opening pressure in a tense patient should be remeasured after encouraging the patient to relax prior to removing fluid. The closing pressure is dependent on the pressure/volume dynamics, which are influenced by the amount of fluid removed and the intracranial compliance. Normal cerebrospinal fluid is crystal clear and contains no more than five mononuclear cells; the normal glucose is two-thirds that of a simultaneously determined serum glucose, and the protein is less than 45 mg/dl. Xanthochromia is a yellowish discoloration of the spinal fluid present with red cell breakdown (indicating previous subarachnoid hemorrhage), hyperbilirubinemia, and extreme elevations of protein.

Principal Indications

The principal indications are:

1. Measurement of intracranial pressure: elevated pressure must be documented to diagnose pseudotumor cerebri (see Chapter 79). Low pressure syndromes can be documented by lumbar puncture but may be exacerbated by the procedure. Spurious elevations of pressure occur in tense patients.
2. Evaluation of patients with suspected demyelinat-

ing, or inflammatory disease such as multiple sclerosis, and inflammatory neuropathy (Guillain-Barre' Syndrome);
3. Evaluation of patients with suspected or known chronic infections such as syphilis, acquired immune deficiency syndrome (AIDS), Lyme disease, cryptococcus, tuberculosis;
4. Evaluation of patients with undiagnosed central nervous system disease.

Limitations

Abnormalities of cerebrospinal fluid are nonspecific; however, when interpreted in the context of the clinical presentation, diagnostic accuracy can be increased.

The procedure is completely safe if the following are ruled out: (a) infection of the skin overlying the puncture site, (b) an intracranial mass lesion, (c) bilateral supratentorial edema. Neurological consultation or a screening brain computed tomography (CT) or magnetic resonance imaging (MRI) study (see below) prior to the lumbar puncture will eliminate the potential for complications due to the latter two coexisting problems.

Patient experience. Patients are often reluctant to undergo lumbar puncture, based on widespread belief that it is dangerous and very painful. After neurological evaluation or an imaging study, the patient should be reassured that the procedure is safe. When performed with adequate local anesthesia, the discomfort is mild, certainly less than with upper endoscopy or colonoscopy, both widely accepted procedures. When done properly under aseptic conditions, the most common complication is a post-lumbar puncture (LP) headache (see Chapter 79). The probability of post-LP headache can be decreased by using the smallest gauge needle practical, a number twenty in most adults. Performing the tap with the patient in a sitting position also increases the likelihood of a first pass nontraumatic tap, however, the lateral decubitus position is necessary to obtain a precise opening pressure measurement. After the LP the patient is instructed to lie flat for about an hour and to drink copious amounts of fluid over the ensuing six hours. A minority of patients will complain of pain at the puncture site that may be treated with simple analgesics.

Supraorbital Carotid Doppler Examination

Definition of Procedure

The carotid Doppler examination is an ultrasonic study of blood flow in the supraorbital artery, with and without superficial temporal artery compression. The supraorbital artery is a branch of the internal carotid, with anastomotic connections with the external carotid system via the superficial temporal artery. With a patent internal carotid, flow through the supraorbital artery should be unaffected by compression of the temporal artery. (The direction of flow may transiently reverse as the internal carotid supply compensates.) However, with significant compromise of the internal carotid circulation, supraorbital artery flow becomes totally dependent upon the superficial temporal artery supply and will be abolished or markedly reduced by compressing it. This study is, therefore, dependent both upon a hemodynamically significant alteration of flow in the internal carotid and upon the "normal" pattern of vascular supply to the supraorbital artery.

Principal Indications

Suspected significant internal carotid artery stenosis (carotid bifurcation): a Doppler study has approximately 90% sensitivity and specificity as an indicator of significant (greater than 80%) carotid bifurcation stenosis.

Limitations

This procedure is useful for determining high grade internal carotid stenosis. It is normal if there is less than 80% occlusion. It does not reveal plaque ulceration or intracranial vascular disease in the middle cerebral artery. A negative Doppler study does not completely rule out significant stenotic disease; 10% of even highly stenotic lesions will be missed by the Doppler because of variations in collateral flow. It is never a substitute for thorough investigation of suspected cerebrovascular disease. It is not useful for the investigation of vertebral-basilar disease.

Patient experience. Subjects sit or recline with their eyes closed while an ultrasound-conducting gel is applied to the supraorbital region. An ultrasonic probe is then held over the artery for a few minutes while the temporal artery is being compressed and released. There is no discomfort or risk.

Duplex Scanning

Definition of Procedure

Duplex scanning combines B mode ultrasound scanning of the carotid bifucation with spectral analysis of a Doppler signal to assess plaque disease. The extent of plaque is classified into categories that vary with the laboratory, but generally approximate the following categories: 0 to 15%, 15 to 30%, 31 to 9%, 50 to 79%, 80 to 99%. Plaque characteristics such as calcification, hemorrhage, and ulceration can be determined. Plaque distribution in common, internal, and external carotid artery is delineated.

Principal Indications

This noninvasive screening technique may be used in the evaluation of patients with asymptomatic carotid bruits, transient ischemic attacks (TIAs), and stroke. With use of this procedure, stroke-prone patients may be better selected for hospital admission and arteriography.

Limitations

No more than 3 cm of the internal carotid artery can be imaged above the bifurcation. The distal common carotid is imaged for a variable distance, depending on its tortuosity. This technique cannot distinguish complete occlusion from a very high grade stenosis. No information about intracranial disease is obtained.

Patient experience. A comprehensive Duplex examination of the carotid arteries takes approximately 45 minutes. The transducer head is held over the carotid bifurcation at the angle of the mandible. There is no appreciable discomfort or risk.

Carotid Blood Flow Evaluation (Quantitated Flow Meter)

Definition of Procedure

While carotid Duplex scanning and angiography delineate anatomy, the quantitated carotid blood flow study measures actual blood flow in the common carotid artery in ml/second. An angle-independent A mode ultrasound probe is used to determine intima to intima vessel diameter and velocity, from which flow is calculated. This unique technique detects abnormalities of flow in the common carotid artery as well as "upstream" intracranial blood flow changes. When used in conjunction with an imaging technique (Duplex, angiography), the significance of stenotic lesions can be assessed.

Principal Indications

In patients with cerebrovascular disease (TIA, stroke, bruit) this technique is useful to evaluate the hemodynamic significance of stenotic lesions and in the detection of collateral flow patterns. Compensatory flow patterns in the carotid free of a high grade stenotic lesion may also be monitored. Bilateral abnormalities of flow are seen in dementia and in low cardiac output states.

Limitations

Carotid flow patterns remain normal in most patients until a 70 to 80% stenosis occurs; therefore, lower grade lesions cannot be followed serially.

Patient experience. The carotid blood flow study is similar to Duplex scanning except that the probe is held just cephalad to the clavicle. The study involves no discomfort or risk and takes about 20 minutes.

Cerebral Angiography

Definition of Procedure

Cerebral angiography provides imaging by intra-arterial or intravenous injection of a contrast agent. The major differences between the two routes are the superior resolution of the images and the visualization of intracranial arteries obtained with intra-arterial

studies. Duplex scanning (see above) provides information about the carotid bifurcation that is as accurate as that obtained with venous angiography, which it has widely replaced as a screening procedure for carotid artery stenosis. Intra-arterial studies may be accomplished using either *conventional angiography,* which usually requires hospitalization, or *digital subtraction angiography,* which can often be performed as an outpatient procedure because smaller catheters and lower doses of contrast agent are used.

A guidewire is placed in an artery, usually the femoral, and passed to the aortic arch where a catheter is advanced over the wire. The catheter is selectively advanced in the arteries of interest, including the common carotid and/or vertebral arteries, which are then injected with a contrast agent. Serial radiographs are taken.

Principal Indications

Cerebral angiography can be used in the delineation of a number of intracranial processes. Since the advent of CT and MR imaging, the principal indication for angiography has been the definitive diagnosis of cerebrovascular diseases including extra- and intracranial arterial stenosis, vascular malformations, aneurysms, and vasculitis.

Limitations

Adequate renal function is a prerequisite. Complications (about 1 to 2%) occur related to femoral puncture, manipulation of the catheter, and reactions to the contrast agent. Serious complications include femoral artery clot with embolization, strokes, and anaphylactoid reaction to the contrast agent. The ionic load of the contrast agent may precipitate heart failure in susceptible patients.

Patient experience. The patient lies on an X-ray table and a femoral puncture is made after local anesthesia with Xylocaine. The major discomfort is a burning sensation, which can be intense, felt with the injection of contrast. Less stressful is a metallic taste in the mouth, itching, and occasionally hives. Mild or severe bronchospasm, although less common, can occur. The patient must be able to lie still for the radiographs. After the procedure, patients are given instructions to drink a large amount of fluid, to limit activity, and to monitor for signs of bleeding or obstruction at or distal to the site of arterial puncture. Instructions usually include limiting ambulation, no lifting or other strenuous activity for 24 hours, and no bathing for at least 12 hours.

Computed Tomography (CT) Scanning of the Head

Definition of Procedure

Computed tomography uses narrow X-ray beams to exploit the differences in X-ray absorption between different kinds of intracranial tissues. Without contrast, the CT scanner can differentiate between the density of bone, calcified tissue, blood, gray matter, white matter, cerebrospinal fluid (CSF), and air. Its resolving power is proportional to the differences in the densities of these tissues; modern CT scanners can reveal hematomas only several millimeters wide, and infarcts of 1 to 1.5 cm wide. Although CT scan results are typically presented as horizontal slices through the brain, present technology allows slices to be reconstructed in the vertical or in any other plane to give a better perspective on abnormal findings.

Intravenous injection of contrast is used to enhance the X-ray contrast of vascular lesions; contrast material will diffuse into an area where the blood-brain barrier has broken down to increase the X- ray absorption density.

CT scanning is highly sensitive and often diagnostic; as such, it has a place in both screening and in specific investigation.

Principal Indications

Evaluation of patients with intracranial problems where structural alteration is known or suspected, e.g., tumor, ischemic cerebrovascular disease, hemorrhagic cerebrovascular disease, atrophic degenerative disease (Alzheimer's, Huntington's), hydrocephalus, subdural hematoma, or unexplained headache. Many conditions can be screened for without the use of radiographic contrast; this should be strongly considered in patients when the most common abnormalities do not require contrast for visualization (e.g., dementia, remote stroke) and in the elderly when the risks are somewhat greater.

Limitations

CT scanning is neither 100% sensitive nor infallible. For instance, a CT scan after a transient ischemic attack is often normal; this finding does not detract from the significance of the event and the need for further study. Furthermore, a negative CT scan does not exclude actual structural damage. The site of the lesion may not have been included in the slices done as part of a routine examination, or the damage may not have caused enough change in local absorption density to contrast with its surroundings. This is not uncommon in cerebral infarction a week or so after the initial insult, when the original edema has cleared, and new vessel formation (and phagocytosis) have not yet begun to affect brain density. A CT scan can also be negative because the damage is in an area of the brain that is poorly seen, such as the brainstem or spinal cord, or outside the brain tissue itself.

Patient experience. The patient is asked to lie down with his head inside what looks somewhat like a washing machine. In some scanners, a bag of water is pumped up around the head, but there is no direct contact. Straps will usually be applied over the forehead to prevent motion. (Patient motion will seriously impair the quality of the scanning and may make the scan uninterpretable). The procedure takes 5 to 20 minutes, depending on the scanner. Contrast material may be given intravenously, by single bolus, or by intravenous drip. When done without contrast injection, CT scan-

ning is essentially free of risk. When done with contrast, the risk is that of the contrast material itself—frequently, a warm flush in the face, nausea, and sometimes vomiting. In approximately one case in 100,000 there is the possibility of death from anaphylaxis. A serum creatinine should be done prior to infusion of contrast. If it is abnormal, the risks and precautions related to contrast media renal insult must be considered (see details, Chapter 48).

Computed Tomography Scanning of the Spine

Definition of Procedure

See "Computed Tomography Scanning of the Head."

Principal Indications

CT is an important diagnostic modality for studying the spine; it shows both the osseous and soft tissues of the spine better than conventional radiographic techniques, including myelography, without morbidity and without excess cost or exposure to radiation. Indications for primary CT of the spine include suspected disc herniation, spinal dysraphism, and facet joint pathology. Because 90% of herniated lumbar intervertebral discs occur at L4-L5 or L5-S1, a CT scan of these two levels can be performed quickly. In cases of spinal fractures it may demonstrate lesions missed by conventional tomography besides showing traumatic injuries of the spinal soft tissues. Spinal stenosis, narrowing of the spinal canal, or narrowing of the neural foramen and lateral recess may be most accurately diagnosed with CT. Other spinal lesions, including arteriovenous malformation, syringomyelia, spinal neoplasms, inflammatory processes, bone mineral analysis, and metabolic disease are accurately evaluated with CT.

Limitations

If the spinal region to be studied spans three or more vertebrae, myelography or MRI is more practical than is CT. Diagnostic accuracy of CT presupposes use of a localizer image for accurately selecting the plane and angle of the slice besides a relatively thin slice thickness and optimal resolution. CT diagnosis of a herniated disc may be inaccurate in patients with a previous laminectomy. If clinical criteria do not permit the selection of appropriate levels for scanning, CT may be a less satisfactory technique than myelography for examining the cervical spine.

Patient experience. See "Computed Tomography Scanning of the Head."

Magnetic Resonance Imaging (MRI)

Definition of Procedure

The basis of magnetic resonance imaging is the property of all nuclei with an odd number of protons, neutrons, or both to act as magnets. Hydrogen, because it is the most sensitive of the stable nuclei to a magnetic resonant effect, and because it is also the most abundant nucleus in the body, is ideally suited for MRI. Through the use of magnetic fields whose strength varies with their position, it is possible to define both the location and concentration of resonant nuclei, such as those of hydrogen, and to create thereby images that reflect the distribution of these nuclei in the tissues. Two concepts are particularly important to an understanding of MRI: (a) Because the radio waves emitted by nuclei in the magnetic fields commonly used in MRI are between 10 and 100 m in length, the images in this technique cannot be made through an optical process. (b) The intensity of the signal is not simply a reflection of the hydrogen density; rather, the observed intensity is actually the hydrogen density strongly modulated by local physical and chemical factors.

Principal Indications

MRI is a noninvasive imaging technique that gives better contrast and sensitivity for most central nervous system lesions than does X-ray CT. Many cranial abnormalities can be demonstrated with MRI, including intra- and extracranial tumors (especially posterior fossa), early cerebral infarctions, vascular malformations, hydrocephalus, sinusitis, white matter disease (multiple sclerosis), and spinal cord abnormalities.

In several aspects of brain imaging, MRI has already shown itself to be superior to CT. First, MRI provides better imaging of the posterior fossa than does CT because the surrounding bone causes no streak artifacts. Second, the soft tissue contrast with MRI is better than that with CT. As a result, gray matter and white matter are much better delineated in magnetic resonance images, and the extent of certain diseases is better appreciated with MRI. For example, MRI can reveal many more of the lesions of multiple sclerosis than can CT. Third, coronal and sagittal plane views can be made directly with MRI, rather than requiring the reformatting of serial transverse plane views, as required in CT. Fourth, major blood vessels can be identified with MRI without the need for contrast media because the flowing blood, as a result of its velocity, appears dark. The common carotid, internal carotid, external carotid, vertebral, and basilar arteries are easily seen. Aneurysms of the internal carotid artery have been detected and a thrombus in the lumen of the artery can be identified.

MRI will probably replace CT evaluation of the nervous system in many instances simply because of its ability to detect lesions not visible on the latter. For instance, in the evaluation of dementia, enlarged ventricles secondary to loss of parenchyma can be differentiated from enlarged ventricles secondary to increased pressure (normal pressure hydrocephalus) by the appreciation of increased transependymal fluid.

Limitations

MRI has high sensitivity for disease detection in the central nervous system, but it does not detect a signal from calcium deposits. Further, MRI does not have the sensitivity to describe glucose metabolic rate, neurotransmitter concentration, or amino acid transport with the spatial resolution of positron emission tomography, another novel technique.

The known hazards of MRI are due to the force and torque exerted by the field on ferromagnetic objects brought into the vicinity of the magnet and on patients' prostheses, such as surgical clips, pacemakers, and joint replacements. Cardiac pacemaker function can be disrupted and false signals produced, and ferromagnetic metal clips, such as those on cerebral aneurysms, may be dislodged.

Patient experience. The patient lies down on a table identical to the CT scanner, only the head holder consists of a plastic coil that passes very close to the nose of the patient. The entire table is then moved into a larger tunnel. The patient may experience claustrophobia and feel very warm. A knocking sound is heard during data collection, at which time the patient must remain absolutely still.

General References

Baker AB, Baker LH (eds): *Clinical Neurology*, (3 volumes). Hagerstown, Harper & Row, published since 1976, with yearly updates.
Although not the most comprehensive survey of neurological diagnosis and practice, many of its chapters are well recognized for their succinctness and clarity, and yearly updates of this loose-leaf book keep the information up to date. Some specific chapters of interest: Dejong RN: Case taking and the neurologic examination. O'Leary JL, Landau WM: Electroencephalography and electromyography. Short introduction to EEG and EMG.

Health and Public Policy Committee, American College of Physicians. Diagnostic evaluation of the carotid arteries. *Ann Intern Med* 835, November, 1988.
Specific recommendations for the use of tests in screening and diagnosis.

Heinz ER: *The Clinical Neurosciences*, vol 4 (Neuroradiology). Rosenberg RN, Grossman RG, Heinz ER, Willis WD (eds): New York, Churchill Livingstone, 1984.
Comprehensive description of neuroradiological procedures including all of the newer techniques covered in this chapter. Good background reading for a more thorough understanding of the technological advances made in this field.

Weinberger J (ed): *Noninvasive Imaging of Cerebrovascular Disease*. New York, Alan R. Liss, Inc., 1989.

CHAPTER 79

Headaches and Facial Pain*

MARGIT L. BLEECKER, M.D., Ph.D.
CONSTANCE J. MEYD, M.D.

EPIDEMIOLOGY

Although epidemiological surveys of headache are not always comparable or consistent with one another, all agree on the magnitude of the problem: 80 to 90% of the normal adult population reports recurrent headache, and in 30 to 50% of this population headaches are described as severe or disabling at times. Women suffer disproportionately from headaches, both in terms of numbers affected and in severity of headaches; the reported prevalence in women varies from slightly higher to as much as three times higher than in men (10, 17, 21). The majority of headache sufferers depend chiefly on self-care with over-the-counter remedies

*Barry Gordon, M.D., Ph.D., contributed to this chapter in the first and second editions of this book.

rather than on visits to their doctors to deal with their headache problems.

Findings from the National Ambulatory Medical Care Survey (NAMCS) provide a profile of that subset of headache sufferers who do go to a physician for headache. In this survey of office practice, headache was the seventh most frequent symptomatic reason for visits to all physicians; it accounted for approximately 2% of all visits to internists, general practitioners, and family practitioners. Table 79.1, adapted from the NAMCS, indicates the differences in visit rate for headache with respect to age group and sex of patients. Table 79.2 shows the distribution of headache duration reported by these patients; almost one-half of visits were for headache of less than 1 week's duration.

An important finding was the low frequency of recurrent headache in persons 65 and older. Fifty-seven percent of men and 43% of women in this age group report themselves as headache free, and only 18 to 30% report disabling or severe headaches. On the other hand, as indicated in Table 79.1, the frequency of vis-

Table 79.1.

Average Annual Rate of Office Visits for Headache, According to Sex and Age of Patient: United States 1977–1978[a]

Sex and Age (yr)	Average Annual Visit Rate/1000 Persons
BOTH SEXES	
All ages	43.2
Under 15	17.6
15–24	31.4
25–44	53.8
45–64	60.2
65 and over	63.9
FEMALE	
All ages	55.4
Under 15	15.8
15–24	40.8
25–44	67.0
45–64	82.0
65 and over	81.8
MALE	
All ages	30.3
Under 65	19.4
15–24	21.7
25–44	39.7
45–64	36.3
65 and over	38.4

[a] Adapted from Cypress BK: Headache as the reason for office visits, National Ambulatory Medical Care Survey: United States, 1977–1978. *Advance Data, Vital and Health Statistics of the National Center for Health Statistics.* Number 67, January 7, 1981.

Table 79.2.

Percentage of Office Visits with Headache as a New Problem with Respect to Sex of Patient and Time Since Onset of Complaint: United States, 1977–1978[a]

Time Since Onset of Complaint.	Female (%)	Male (%)
Less than 1 week	43.9	49.3
1–3 weeks	16.3	22.7
1–3 months	16.1	13.6
More than 3 months	20.5	13.7

[a] Adapted from Cypress BK: Headache as the reason for office visits, National Ambulatory Medical Care Survey: United States, 1977–1978. *Advance Data, Vital and Health Statistics of the National Center for Health Statistics.* Number 67, January 7, 1981.

its to physicians by those persons who do have headache increases with age.

Of all patients with headache, 80% or more will have what has been described as muscle contraction headache. Two to 7% will have migraine headaches. In practice, physicians see a disproportionate number of patients with migraine, since these individuals are much more likely to seek medical attention than are those with less severe or infrequent headache (11). In addition, physicians are likely to see a number of patients with nonmigrainous vascular headaches due to systemic infections with fever (2). Likewise, the relatively uncommon organic syndromes associated with significant headache (such as cluster headache, exertional headache, temporal arteritis, and sinusitis) are likely to be over-represented in a physician's office.

Life-threatening causes of headache are uncommon. In a study of a community hospital emergency department, 1% of patients complaining of acute headache had a subarachnoid hemorrhage or meningitis (2). In specialized headache clinics, which provide consultation for preselected patients, serious conditions (usually tumors, increased intracranial pressure, arteriovenous malformations, and the like) are found in about 5% of referrals. However, not surprisingly, such conditions (especially brain tumor) are often the major concerns of patients who come to a physician for evaluation of acute or chronic headaches.

GENERAL APPROACH TO THE PATIENT WITH HEADACHE

History

The history provides by far the most useful information for evaluating headache, particularly a careful account by the patient of the current or most recent episode. The most useful aspects of the history in determining etiology are the temporal profile, associated symptoms, and family history. The least specific is the character and location of the pain. Undue emphasis should not be placed on differentiating throbbing pain from pressure pain, etc. as the subjective interpretation of headache pain is so variable. The following questions are helpful in the differential diagnosis of headache (the interpretation of the patient's answers to these questions is discussed in detail in the sections on specific headache syndromes):

1. *Associated factors.* Is there any warning of the attack (prodromal feeling, focal numbness or weakness, or visual symptoms including the fortification hallucinations of classic migraine)? Is the patient aware of any factors that can bring on these headaches (alcohol ingestion, vasodilator use, psychosocial stresses, perimenstrual period, foods, drug use, position, sexual intercourse, exertion, tobacco)? What drugs is the patient taking for other conditions? To what does the patient attribute the headache? Does the patient fear a dreaded cause such as a tumor?

2. *Temporal features.* How does the headache begin— suddenly, or by building up slowly over a period of several hours or even days? When does the headache occur? Does it waken the patient from sleep or is it present on awakening? Does it recede after the patient is up for several hours? What is the frequency of headaches? (Have the patient recount the past month's and the past year's pattern.) How long do the headaches last (maximum, minimum, average)? Have there been intervals of weeks or months without the headache?

3. *Character and location of pain.* What kind of pain is the patient experiencing with the current headaches (band-like, squeezing, pressure, pounding, or throbbing)? Where is the pain located (one side of the head, all over the head, in the eyes, radiating up the back of the neck, etc.)? Does the pain radiate anywhere or seem to spread during the course of attack? How severe can the headaches be (on a scale of 1 to 10)? How does the patient rate this headache pain to the pain of other headaches or other situations (e.g., is it the "worst ever" or "the worst pain in my life")?

4. *Aggravating and alleviating factors.* Does anything make the headache pain worse (bending, standing up, sneezing, straining, coughing)? What factors seem to help the headache (lying down, pressing on the temples, avoidance of work, simple analgesics, narcotics, or other medications)? How is the patient currently treating the headache?

5. *Environmental exposures.* Does the headache occur predictably after exposure to an environment that may have elevated carbon monoxide levels (e.g., a closed room heated by a space heater)? Did the headache start after the patient began work (or activities at home) that entails exposure to fumes or dust containing lead? These and other environmental exposures that may cause headache are listed in Table 7.3.

6. *Associated neurological symptoms.* Does the patient have associated symptoms during the headaches such as spots before the eyes (very common in both tension and migraine headaches); inability to tolerate light, sound, touch or movement; nausea and/or vomiting; focal numbness or weakness; vertigo? Did the patient have motion sickness as a child? Does the patient note scalp tenderness?

7. *Prior evaluation.* Has the patient been evaluated for the headaches and what has he been told as a result of this evaluation? It is important to request previous records for all patients who give a history of severe, disabling headache, irrespective of the reported duration of the present headache problem or the nature of the previous evaluation; sometimes even just requesting the records reminds the patient of a 10- or 20-year history of severe headache and of multiple visits; sometimes the previous records confirm this despite a patient's poor recall. In either case, this information can be particularly valuable in evaluating a patient who describes recent onset of severe headaches.

8. *Functional impact.* How are the headaches currently affecting the patient (work and social relationships)?
9. *Family and household history.* Is there a history of headaches in the parents, siblings, children, or other people living in the patient's household? What type?

Physical and Laboratory Examination

In the majority of cases the history will usually suggest the probable basis for a patient's headache. Appropriate physical examination and laboratory examination are described under each type of headache below. The extent of the physical examination indicated may vary from no examination (e.g., in a patient with headache after vasodilator therapy), to an examination focused upon structures that may be the source of the headache (e.g., sinuses), to an extensive neurological and laboratory examination (e.g., the patient with new onset or marked change in prior headache pattern).

Principles of Initial Treatment

Most patients with headache can be treated presumptively for tension or migraine headache, as described below. A more extensive investigation should be carried out in patients who show either of the following situations after initial treatment: (*a*) Those patients who fail to respond to treatment of the presumed condition. Even in this situation, the extent of the evaluation should be tempered by the circumstances and the patient's expectations. For example, a middle-aged patient who fails a conservative treatment regimen for recent onset of what appear to be migraine headaches should have an earlier and more extensive evaluation than a middle-aged patient with 20 years of apparent tension headaches, and a repeatedly normal examination, who has not responded to the full spectrum of therapeutic options. (*b*) Those patients who show significant changes in complaints or physical findings that point to one of the less common causes of headache discussed below.

Treatment Expectations

When the issue of expectations of physicians and patients was studied, the majority of the physicians in this study expected that their patients would demand pain relief and not care very much about getting an explanation of their problem; in contrast, only 31% of the patients themselves stated that pain relief was most important, and 46% rated an explanation of their problem as their most important concern (12).

When treating the usual tension or migraine headache, the physician should neither expect always to achieve total relief of headache pain, nor should the patient be misled into thinking that this is always possible. The patient must be helped to understand the limitations of drug therapy and the potential for drug side effects that, in some cases, can be more distressing than the headaches. Selection of a treatment regimen is complicated by the high placebo response rate (20 to 40%) and by the variable natural history of headaches. Because of this variability, a detailed baseline history of the patient's headache problems is important for subsequent assessment of the patient's response to treatment.

SPECIFIC HEADACHE SYNDROMES

Tension (Muscle Contraction) Headache

Classification

In the absence of any rigorous criterion or physiological markers, the term "tension headache" has been applied to what is probably a heterogeneous group of headache syndromes.

There are two basic presentations, intermittent headache and continuous daily headache. Patients with intermittent headache that is not severe and that does not have the characteristics of migraine (see below) usually respond to simple over-the-counter analgesics. Most of these patients do not seek medical attention for their headaches but admit to headaches on review of systems. Patients with continuous daily headache of many months' or years' duration usually have depression and/or anxiety states. These patients describe constant headache that lacks any localizing characteristics and is refractory to analgesics and to migraine prophylaxis with the exception of the antidepressants.

Pathogenesis

The symptoms of this type of headache are presumed to be caused by contraction of scalp and neck muscles. The muscle contraction is thought to be a somatic consequence of coexisting psychosocial stress in the patient's life, although the stress cannot always be identified. Neither increased muscle tension nor precipitating stress is specific for tension headaches; both are also common in migraine, which is the prototype of vascular headache (see below). Table 79.3

Table 79.3.
Characteristics of Migrainous and Tension Headaches[a]

	Migraine (%)	Tension (%)
Age at onset		
<20 years	55	30
>20 years	45	70
Premonitory symptoms	60	10
Frequency		
Daily	3	50
<Weekly	60	15
Duration		
Constant, daily	0	20
1–3 days	35	10
Throbbing pain	80	30
Location		
Unilateral	80	10
Bilateral	20	90
Vomiting with attacks	50	10
Family history of headache	65	40

[a] Adapted from Raskin NH, Appenzeller O: *Headache.* Philadelphia, WB Saunders, 1980; as modified from Friedman AP, *et al*: *Neurology* 4:773, 1954.

summarizes the data on the frequency of several characteristics in a large number of patients and shows considerable overlap between tension and migraine headaches (3). Depressed mood is associated with chronic tension headache but the causal relationship between headache and depression is controversial, with some believing it to be the cause whereas others consider it to be secondary to headaches.

Presentation

The location and quality of the pain in tension headache is not diagnostic. Patients may describe bands, tightness, throbbing, shooting, or aching. The pain is usually bilateral, and the patient usually reports that recurring tension headaches are similar in quality and location. Patients frequently complain of spots before their eyes when the pain is intense, but these are not the true fortification hallucinations of migraine (see below). The duration of the headache varies from minutes to hours to days. Some patients complain of continuous headaches that have been unremitting for years; this kind of headache is almost always due to tension. Moreover, a history of increased psychosocial stress will often be associated with headache episodes. Finally, the patients may report some relief of pain with massage of their scalp.

Physical examination is unremarkable except for neck or scalp muscle tenderness, in some patients, and occasionally an exaggerated physiological tremor (see Chapter 82) due to anxiety.

Treatment

Nonpharmacological. It is usually helpful to explain to the patient the presumed pathogenesis of tension headache, i.e., scalp and neck muscle contraction or "tension." This information helps the patient to understand both the benign nature of his headache and its possible relationship to psychosocial stress. As explained elsewhere (Chapter 11), concerned listening to a patient's story often helps to reduce somatic symptoms due to stress. The physician can also help by encouraging any effort made by the patient to reduce stressful situations. For patients seeking nonpharmacological relief of symptoms, massage of the scalp and neck muscles by another person or use of relaxation techniques (see Chapter 13) can be recommended; in addition, any other procedure that the patient may have found helpful should be encouraged by the physician.

Pharmacological. Symptomatic treatment with drugs is an important adjunct to the general measures just described; for selected patients, prophylactic drug treatment can also be tried. Most patients will have used headache remedies containing aspirin or acetaminophen before consulting their physician about treatment. For mild to moderate headaches, however, an additional trial of these mild analgesics should be recommended if they have not been taken at the usual effective dose (625 mg every 4 to 6 hours). If these remedies fail to help, a trial of nonsteroidal anti-inflammatory medications other than aspirin is indicated.

A number of drugs are widely prescribed for patients with moderately severe intermittent headaches unresponsive to acetaminophen, aspirin, or other nonsteroidal agents. These drugs include codeine sulfate; propoxyphene (Darvon); and two products that contain combinations of analgesics, sedatives, and caffeine: Fiorinal (butalbital, caffeine, aspirin); and Percodan(oxycodone, aspirin). Each of these drugs can lead to habituation and dependency (see Chapter 22). Therefore, it is unwise to initiate treatment with these drugs unless it is clear that the patient can use them appropriately for limited periods.

Prophylaxis can also be tried for the occasional patient whose tension headaches are very severe or very frequent. The best results (60% improved versus 22% on placebo) have been obtained with the tricyclic antidepressant amitriptyline (Elavil), given in daily doses of 50 to 100 mg at bedtime (8). (A detailed discussion of the use of the tricyclics is found in Chapter 15). Somewhat less benefit has been obtained with prophylactic benzodiazepine anxiolytic drugs (diazepam and chlordiazepoxide) in the same study.

Migraine

Classification

The classification of migraine headache was revised in 1988 from classical and common migraine to *migraine with aura* and *migraine without aura* (5). Migraine with aura denotes a syndrome of headache with associated characteristic premonitory sensory, motor, or visual disturbances; and migraine without aura denotes a syndrome in which there is no neurological disturbance associated with the headache. Those headaches with aura are subdivided into typical, prolonged, familial hemiplegic, basilar, aura without headache, and acute onset aura. Further types of migraine include ophthalmoplegic, retinal, childhood periodic syndromes, complications of migraine (infarction, status migrainosis), and unclassified. Migraine is more common than generally appreciated, and many patients with recurrent moderate to severe migraine headaches are misdiagnosed as suffering from tension headache. Failure of analgesics in an emotionally healthy patient with recurring headaches is almost diagnostic of migraine.

Pathogenesis

For many years, the symptoms of a migraine headache have been attributed to sequential changes affecting intracranial and extracranial arteries. An initial stage of vasoconstriction, producing brain ischemia, is thought to be responsible for the fortification hallucinations (see below), transient hemiparesis or hemiparesthesias, confusion, vertigo, and other focal neurological manifestations that can be seen in migraine with aura. Although vasoconstriction presumably also occurs in migraine without aura, it is thought to be below the threshold necessary to produce obvious symptoms. Vasoconstriction is thought to last from 1/2 hour to several hours in a typical migraine attack. In the sequential theory, the initial vasoconstriction is thought to be followed by vasodilation of the affected vessels, resulting in typical "vascular headache" pain that throbs in unison with the pulse. Some patients report dilated, throbbing, aching vessels over one side of the scalp during an episode, tenderness of the scalp, and some relief during the attack by pressure on the temples, presumably decreasing blood flow to the dilated temporal arteries.

The vascular theory of migraine does not adequately account for many aspects of the migraine syndrome such as malaise, autonomic components (nausea, vomiting, diarrhea, bloating, fluid retention), and the postheadache elation or sense of well-being many patients describe. Other theories include electrical depression, an imbalance in sympathetic nervous system regulation, dysautonomia of the trigeminal nerve, and dysregulation of the ascending brain stem serotonergic system. Increasing evidence now makes it clear that migraine is an organic illness, not psychologically based.

Epidemiology and Natural History

The lack of a simple, specific test for migraine headache and variations in the definition of migraine headache make it difficult to determine the prevalence and natural course of this condition. Nevertheless, some characteristics are clear.

From 20 to 50% of migraine headache sufferers have a positive family history for migraine, usually in one parent. This seems to be particularly true with patients who have migraine with aura. Many patients report motion sickness and vertigo as a child with vertigo persisting into adulthood.

The onset of migraine is usually between the ages of 15 through 25 and the headaches are more common in women. Recurrence is a hallmark of migraine headache. The majority of migraine sufferers have several attacks each year, while some have one or more episodes per week and some have only rare episodes or even only a single typical episode in their lives. Migraine episodes usually become less frequent and less severe with age.

The perimenstrual period (particularly before the onset of bleeding, when levels of estradiol are falling), oral contraceptives (particularly off-days, presumably due to falling estrogen levels), and menopause are associated with migraine headaches. The following substances may initiate headaches in susceptible subjects: vasodilators (nitrates and antihypertensives); alcohol; chocolate; cheeses, wines, and other foods containing tryamine; and monosodium glutamate. Withdrawal of caffeine or of ergotamine can also cause headaches (presumably by rebound vasodilation). An unusual lengthy period of sleep, such as sleeping in on weekends, may provoke migraine. Attacks tend to occur also during a period of relaxation, such as weekends, holidays, and vacations. The patient should be asked about these associations and any others that he may have noted.

Diagnosis and Differential Diagnosis

The following are reasonably well-established criteria for the working diagnosis of a migraine headache:

1. Prodromal warning of some kind, ranging from vague malaise to focal neurological symptoms. So-called fortification hallucinations are almost specific for migraine; these are slowly enlarging scotomata that are surrounded by luminous angles and that slowly change shape and appear to move across the visual fields (Fig. 79.1). (Rarely occipital lobe tumors or arteriovenous malformations may produce the same effects.)
2. Unilateral head pain during any one attack. The pain usually increases gradually, reaching a peak in several hours and lasting for several hours to a day in typical cases. Attacks lasting 2 to 3 days are not uncommon, and some migraine attacks last for 1 to 2 weeks. The pain may be described as "pounding" or "throbbing," but the quality of the pain is variable and may be aching or stabbing. Although headaches are typically unilateral at the beginning of a single attack, they often generalize and most patients will have attacks on both sides of the head; however, in 20% of patients, headaches will always be on the same side.

Even these criteria are not broad enough to encompass all of the manifestations of migraine headache. Other frequent symptoms include photophobia, sonophobia, nausea, vomiting, and generalized malaise.

In the *differential diagnosis* of migraine, the most important considerations are transient ischemic attacks (TIAs) or other cerebrovascular events, partic-

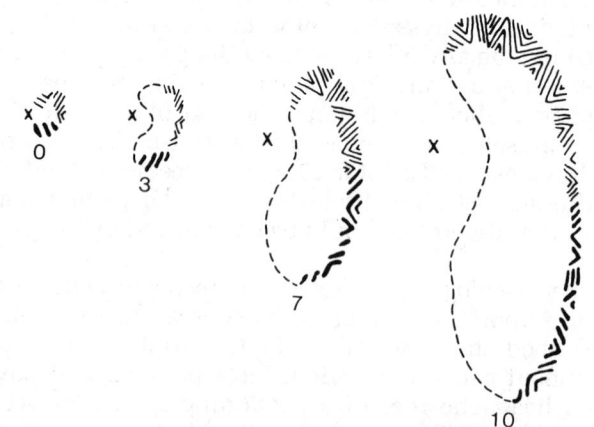

Figure 79.1. Lashley's maps of the progression of his own fortification spectra at varying time intervals after the onset of a migrainous attack. The X in each instance indicates the visual fixation point. The numbers represent minutes. (From Raskin NH, Appenzeller O: *Headache.* Philadephia, WB Saunders, 1980; as appeared in Lashley KS: *Arch Neurol Psychiatry* 46:331111941).

ularly in middle-aged and older patients (see Chapter 83 for details). Migrainous ischemia usually occurs in patients. with a prior history of similar attacks, often in young adulthood; the family history in these cases tends to be particularly strong. Symptoms of migrainous ischemia typically last 1/2 hour to several hours; TIAs usually last minutes to several hours. Headaches should be a prominent component of the migrainous ischemic event; although headache may occur in up to 25% of patients with transient ischemic events, it is usually relatively mild and transitory. Some patients with suspected migrainous ischemic events, particularly those with "migraine equivalents" (ischemic symptoms without headache), should be evaluated for TIA before their symptoms are attributed to migraine.

Treatment

The vast majority of migraine sufferers can be helped by treatment, principally pharmacological treatment.

Nonpharmacological. The most useful nonpharmacological treatment is elimination of avoidance of known trigger factors, when this is possible. Common drugs that may trigger an attack are nitrates, vasodilators, indomethacin, and oral contraceptives. Another common trigger factor, often less tractable, is psychological stress. Whenever possible such stress should be decreased, as discussed above under tension headache. Other trigger factors that can be eliminated are excess coffee use and irregular sleep habits. There are no consistently implicated dietary trigger factors; however, each patient should be encouraged to try eliminating any dietary component or other trigger factor that he can identify.

During an established attack, a patient usually feels better reclining in a dark cool room. This is the only practice other than drug treatment that appears to be helpful.

Pharmacological: mild attacks. Patients with mild migraine attacks often obtain relief from acetaminophen, aspirin, or another nonsteroidal anti-inflammatory agent, used as described above under tension headache.

Moderate and severe attacks. At the start of an attack in a patient with moderate to severe migraine, ergotamine tartrate is the agent of choice. Because of its relative specificity, ergotamine may be administered as a therapeutic trial to confirm a clinical suspicion of migraine headache. The action of ergotamine has traditionally been attributed to its vasoconstrictor property, but the reason for its effectiveness in aborting migraine symptoms is not understood clearly.

Ergotamine is available in preparations that permit administration by multiple routes (Table 79.4). The ideal route is one that is convenient, leads to prompt absorption of the drug, and is not affected by vomiting. Suppository, sublingual, and aerosol preparations meet these criteria. Ingested tablets may be vomited and are therefore less reliable. The traditional recommended schedules for ergotamine administration are summa-

rized in Table 79.5. The objective of these schedules is to attain a total dose that is effective but is below the dose that produces nausea and vomiting. Traditionally this has been accomplished by taking additional doses at 30 and 60 minutes if the first dose is ineffective. An alternative strategy may increase the likelihood of prompt attenuation of headaches: the patient should determine the dose that produces nausea for him (the nauseating dose), by following the traditional schedule on a headache-free day; the cumulative dose attained just prior to the nauseating dose is the appropriate total therapeutic dose (the subnauseating dose) for that patient to take (all at once) at the onset of future attacks.

A number of points are important in instructing a patient about the use of ergotamine. Above all, the patient should understand that ergotamine is not a "pain killer," but that it is used to interrupt the vascular events causing migraine pain. He should understand that for maximal benefit he must take ergotamine at the onset of prodromal symptoms or headache (waiting for the headache to become well established is a common problem in patients who report no benefit from ergotamine). In order to assure immediate access to their medicine, patients should be advised to carry some with them at all times. They should be informed that taking more than the recommended maximal daily dose (see Table 79.5) carries the risk of peripheral vasoconstriction in addition to nausea and vomiting. Because ergotamine preparations have a short shelf life, patients should obtain a new supply if they fail to obtain benefit from their medicine or if they have not used it for many months. Finally, patients should be warned not to use ergotamine more than twice in the same week.

Occasionally the patient has *side effects* from ergotamine even when taken at the subnauseating dose. These include abdominal cramps, vertigo, diarrhea, and distal paresthesia; less commonly, syncope, tremor, angina pectoris, and claudication may occur. Most patients, however, tolerate the drug well.

Serious adverse effects, including mental changes, edema, peripheral vascular occlusion, and distal gangrene, can occur if the daily dose of ergotamine exceeds 6 mg or the weekly dose exceeds 10 mg on a chronic basis.

The relative contraindications to ergotamine use are established angina and symptomatic peripheral arterial disease. Traditionally, hypertension has been named as a contraindication, but the risk has probably been overemphasized. Whenever there is concern about the effect of ergotamine on the blood pressure of an individual patient, the blood pressure response to ergotamine should be measured in the physician's office, following the protocol for determining the subnauseating dose of ergotamine outlined above.

Nonsteroidal anti-inflammatory agents may be of some benefit during an acute attack and should be used in full pharmacological doses (e.g., naproxen, 500 mg every 8 hours).

For an *established*, severe migraine headache, sim-

Table 79.4.
Ergot-Containing Drugs[a]

Brand and Generic Names	Route[b]	Ergot Alkaloid	Caffeine	Belladonna	Other
Bellergal	p.o.	Ergotamine 0.3 mg		0.1 mg	Phenobarbital 20 mg
Bellergal-S	p.o.	Ergotamine 0.6 mg		0.2 mg	Phenobarbital 40 mg
Cafergot	p.o.	Ergotamine 1 mg	100 mg		
Cafergot	p.r.	Ergotamine 2 mg	100 mg		
Cafergot-PB	p.o.	Ergotamine 1 mg	100 mg	0.125 mg	Phenobarbital 30 mg
Cafergot-PB	p.r.	Ergotamine 2 mg	100 mg	0.25 mg	Phenobarbital 60 mg
D.H.E. 45	i.m./i.v.	Dihydroergotamine mesylate 1 mg/ml			
Ergomar	s.l.	Ergotamine 2 mg			
Ergonovine	p.o.	Ergonovine 0.2 mg			
Ergostat	s.l.	Ergotamine 2 mg			
Ergotamine	s.c./i.m.	0.25 mg/0.5 ml or 0.5 mg/1 ml			
Ergotamine	Inhal.	0.36 mg/puff			
Ergotamine	p.o.	1 mg			
Ergotrate	p.o.	Ergonovine 0.2 mg			
Gynergen	p.o.	Ergotamine 1 mg			
Medihaler Ergotamine Aerosol	Inhal.	Ergotamine 0.36 mg/puff			
Migral	p.o.	Ergotamine 1 mg	50 mg		Cyclizine 25 mg
Wigraine	p.o.	Ergotamine 1 mg	100 mg	0.1 mg	Phenacetin 130 mg
Wigraine	p.r.	Ergotamine 1 mg	100 mg	0.1 mg	Phenacetin 130 mg

[a] Adapted from Raskin NH, Appenzeller O: *Headache.* Philadelphia, WB Saunders, 1980.
[b] p.o., by mouth; p.r., per rectum; i.m., intramuscular, i.v., intravenous; s.l., sublingual; s.c., subcutaneous; Inhal., inhalation.

Table 79.5.
Traditional Recommended Schedules of Ergotamine for Treating a Migraine Attack

Route	Strength per Dose	Initial Dose[a]
Sublingual (s.l.)	2 mg (tablet)	2 or 3 mg (1 or 1½ tablets)
Rectal (p.r.)	1 mg (suppository) 2 mg	1 or 2 mg
Oral (p.o.)	1 mg (tablet) 2 mg	1 or 2 mg
Aerosol (inhal.)	0.36 mg/puff (fine powder in cannister)	1 or 2 puffs

[a] Repeated at 30 and 60 minutes if necessary. This constitutes the maximal total dose for 1 day.

ple analgesics do not help. For this reason, reliable patients may be given small supplies of either codeine (60 mg) or oxycodone (5 mg) to be taken as needed if ergotamine and other measures have failed to abort an attack. This measure may save a patient many unnecessary trips to the physician's office or to an emergency department.

Prophylactic Therapy

Prophylactic therapy for migraine should be considered when the patient has two or more attacks/week or less frequent attacks that cannot be controlled with abortive therapy and that disrupt employment or social life.

The decision regarding prophylaxis must be the patient's, after the distinction between symptomatic and prophylactic therapy has been explained clearly. Even a patient who has not had adequate relief from routine measures may forego prophylactic treatment because of continuous drug therapy. Furthermore, for each of the drugs used prophylactically for migraine, a relatively long trial period (up to several months) may be necessary to assess effectiveness; and trials with a number of drugs may be necessary. These facts should also be explained to the patient. Finally, patients should understand that during the trial of prophylaxis they can continue the usual measures for treating their migraine attacks.

Those drugs that have been effective in migraine prophylaxis together with dose ranges and common side effects are listed in Table 79.6.

The following general conclusions can be drawn about migraine prophylaxis (14):

1. Fifty percent or more of patients report some improvement in their migraine syndrome during the first year, compared with a reported improvement in 25% of "control patients" (patients who choose not to take prophylaxis); during the second year of prophylaxis, the response rate may be lower.
2. Most of the improvement consists of a decrease in frequency or severity of headaches—freedom from headaches occurs in only a minority of patients.
3. Each of the drugs that has been tried (Table 79.6) gives similar results; failure of one drug does not predict response to another, so that a sequential trial of different drugs is reasonable.
4. Those drugs that are known best to the physician should be tried first for at least 2 to 3 months. (For the generalist, these are propranolol, amitriptyline, and calcium channel blockers.)
5. Failure to give an adequate dose is a common reason for failure of migraine prophylaxis.

Each patient who chooses prophylactic therapy

Table 79.6.
Propglactic Therapy of Migrainous Attacks—Prescribing Information

Drug	Tablet Size(s)	Daily Dose Range	Commonest Side Effects
Ergonovine	0.2 mg	0.4–2.0 mg	Nausea, abdominal pain, leg "tiredness"
Amitriptyline	10, 25, 50 mg	10–175 mg	Sedation, dry mouth
Propranolol	10, 20, 40, 80 mg	40–320 mg	Lethargy, insominia, constipation, light-headedness
Papaverine	150, 300 mg	300–900 mg	Nausea
Cyprohepatdine	4 mg	12–32 mg	Sedation, weight gain
Ergotamine-phenobarbital-belladonna	tabs	1–4 tablets	Nausea, sedation
Phenelzine	15 mg	15–75 mg	Insomnia, light-headedness, constipation
Methylsergide	2 mg	2–8 mg	Nausea, abdominal pain, muscle cramps, insomnia, weight gain, edema, peripheral vasconstriction, retroperitoneal fibrosis
Propranolol LA	80, 120, 160 mg	80–240 mg	Bradycardia, light-headedness, insomnia, nausea, short term memory loss
Verapamil[a]	80, 120 mg	240–640 mg	Hypotension, dizziness, constipation, skin rash
Nifedipine[a]	10 mg	20–60 mg	Hypotension, dizziness, flushing, nausea

[a]Not approved by the Food and Drug Administration for use in headache therapy.

should be asked to keep a log in which to record the frequency and severity of headaches and the nature of any associated factors.

The Patient with Intractable Migraine Headaches

A small number of migraine sufferers do not obtain relief from intractable and disabling headaches, even after prolonged and thorough attempts at therapy. For a complete assessment and an adequate trial of therapy, these patients should be referred to a neurologist. During particularly incapacitating episodes, hospital admission should be considered to provide adequate rest and treatment with potent analgesics.

Cluster Headache

Cluster headache is classified separately from migraine because of its distinct clinical characteristics and different therapy (8). It has previously been designated by a number of names, e.g., Horton's headache, histamine headache (a misnomer), and migrainous cranial neuralgia. Episodes of pain occur in clusters extending over days to weeks, thus giving the syndrome its name. Most episodes last from 4 to 6 weeks and are followed by long pain-free intervals. The intervals between episodes range from 3 months to 5 years, and occasionally longer; most patients, however, have one or two episodes/year. Eventually the problem ceases altogether.

Cluster headache is much less frequent than migraine in the population. It occurs predominantly in middle-aged men who are thin and smoke cigarettes. Onset usually occurs between the age of 20 and 50. There is no evidence for a familial basis for cluster headache.

Manifestations

In a typical attack, there is sudden stabbing or burning pain in the eye, orbit, and cheek on one side. The pain is usually excruciating. Unlike patients with migraine, patients with cluster headaches are usually agitated and they often pace the floor during the attack. Characteristically, the patient also describes ipsilateral lacrimation, rhinorrhea, and conjunctival injection. Ipsilateral ptosis and miosis may also occur; this is thought to be due to compression of the sympathetic plexus by the dilated carotid artery, which produces a partial Horner's syndrome. Usually the same side is involved during a cluster of attacks.

Attacks last from 30 minutes to 2 hours (mean, 45 minutes); occasional mild attacks may last only 10 minutes. The attacks range in frequency from six/day to one/week during a cluster; and they tend to occur at the same time each day, most commonly in the evening just after the patient has gone to bed. In some patients, alcohol may be a particularly potent trigger factor; nitrates and vasodilator drugs may also induce attacks. Therefore, there should be a full inquiry about the use of drugs in evaluating these patients.

These characteristics describe the typical syndrome of cluster headache. Some individuals have less well-defined episodes, whereas other patients may have almost daily attacks of pain for a number of years, a syndrome known as "chronic paroxysmal hemicrania" (13).

Except during an attack, when the unilateral findings described above are present, the physical examination in patients with cluster headache is unremarkable.

Differential diagnosis. Cluster headache must be distinguished from tic douloureux (see below); acute glaucoma (by the presence of miosis, normal tonometry, no lasting visual impairment); sinusitis (by lack of history of upper respiratory infection, lack of purulent rhinorrhea or sinus tenderness, and by negative X-rays); from peripheral dental abscess (by the absence of tenderness on tooth percussion); and from atypical facial neuralgia (see below).

Treatment

Because attacks may be short, lasting only 30 minutes, drug treatment may be ineffective in ameliorating an acute episode. The preferred method of aborting short attacks is 100% oxygen, administered for approximately 15 minutes at a 7 liters/minute flow rate (8). The therapeutic effect of oxygen may be secondary to its vasoconstrictor action. It will abort or diminish pain in about 75% of patients. Ergotamine, administered by inhaler or sublingually, may also be effective abortive therapy for cluster headaches. When administered by inhaler the dose is one puff every 5 minutes until a maximum of six puffs a day or 18 puffs a week is reached. A sublingual preparation of ergotamine containing 2 mg may be given at the beginning of the attack and repeated twice, at 30-minute intervals. No more than 6 mg should be taken in a 24-hour period, nor more than 10 mg/week.

The drug of choice for intervening after the onset of an episode of cluster headache is prednisone, 60 mg per day in divided doses, and tapered over 1 month (1). Prednisone shortens the duration of the episode and decreases the severity and frequency of the attacks. A maximal effect occurs within 2 or 3 days after initiation of therapy. Although side effects arising from a short course of prednisone are unusual, they do occur and include weight gain, salt retention, and emotional lability. Prednisone therapy should not be utilized in pregnant women or in patients with brittle diabetes mellitus, congestive heart failure, uncontrolled hypertension, or severe osteoporosis. (See additional information on prescribing and tapering of corticosteroids, Chapter 74.) There are reports of effective intervention and/or prophylaxis for cluster headache by treatment with propranolol, amitriptyline, verapamil, and cyproheptadine, in doses similar to those used in migraine (see Table 79.6).

For the patient who suffers from almost daily cluster headache (*chronic paroxysmal hemicrania*) lithium carbonate, 300 mg three times a day, has been used successfully. The use of this drug is described in detail in Chapter 15. Most patients with chronic cluster headache seem to be controlled at serum levels below 0.8 mEq/liter. Contraindications to lithium use include renal disease, congestive heart failure, dehydration, pregnancy, and concomitant diuretic administration. Major side effects relating to neurotoxicity include tremor, lethargy, and confusion. There must be a frequent check for polyuria, a symptom suggesting the onset of nephrogenic diabetes insipidus. Dermatological reactions include acne-like lesions and thinning of the hair. Lithium carbonate therapy is generally effective within 5 to 7 days. If lithium fails to control daily cluster headache, ergotamine tartrate may be added. Methysergide (see Table 79.6), either alone or with ergotamine, may be used if control still has not been achieved.

The patient for whom neither treatment nor prophylaxis with the above regimens helps should be referred to a neurologist or to an internist with wide experience in headache management.

Sinus Headache

The pain of *acute sinusitis* may be described by the patient as headache. The diagnosis is based upon the other manifestations of acute sinusitis and on the reproduction or exacerbation of the patient's "headache" by applying pressure to affected sinuses (see Chapter 28 for a full account).

Chronic sinusitis is often cited by patients as the reason for their headaches; it is actually a relatively uncommon cause for chronic intercurrent headache. Chronic sinusitis can present diagnostic difficulties, particularly when it involves the sphenoid sinus (causing a dull boring pain behind the eyes). The physician's suspicions should be aroused if there is a history of preceding acute sinusitis, especially if there is not a long history of headache. The diagnosis and management of chronic sinusitis are discussed in Chapter 28.

Acute Exertional Headache (Orgasmic, Cough, Sneeze)

The features of acute exertional headache are (a) that it is of sudden (or almost instantaneous) onset and (b) that it is directly related to exertion of some kind (orgasm, coughing, sneezing, straining, bending, running, lifting, etc.). It may last from minutes to 1/2 hour, rarely longer (15). In 90% of patients the headache is presumably due to intracranial-spinal pressure dissociations, and the course is benign. In 10% of patients significant organic disease has been found (Arnold-Chiari malformation, hydrocephalus, tumor, and subarachnoid hemorrhage).

Exertional headache must be differentiated chiefly from the headache of *subarachnoid hemorrhage*. The headache of major subarachnoid hemorrhage is usually far more persistent and is often associated with fever, stiff neck, progressive clouding of consciousness, and focal neurological signs. Exertional headaches may be quite severe, but they are brief and they recur with the trigger activity. Because it may be impossible to distinguish the first episode of exertional headache from a minor subarachnoid hemorrhage, and because of the 10% risk of another organic basis for the headache, computed tomography (CT), with and without contrast because of the possibility of tumor or arteriovenous malformation, or a magnetic resonance imaging (MRI) scan (see "Patient Experience," Chapter 78), should be considered when patients initially report the problem. If CT findings are normal, the benign nature of the condition should be explained to the patient. The patient will usually find ways to avoid some of the activities that produce headache. If desired, propranolol, 40 to 80 mg twice/day, or indomethacin, 25 mg three times daily, can be tried for prophylaxis when the patient plans to engage in a headache-provoking activity such as running.

Temporomandibular Joint Syndrome

On history and examination, some patients complaining of headache will have the stigmata of this common syndrome—pain brought on by motion of the jaw and tenderness of the temporomandibular joint. The epidemiology, course, and management of this syndrome are described in Chapter 101.

Headache Due to Drugs

Headache is an occasional side effect of many drugs. Among those commonly used drugs for which headache is more than an occasional side effect are indomethacin (Indocin), nalidixic acid (NegGram), trimethoprim-sulfamethoxazole (Bactrim, Septra), oral contraceptives, and vasodilators. Therefore, as noted earlier, it is important to ask the patient routinely about new drugs when evaluating a headache of recent onset.

A throbbing vascular-type headache frequently occurs shortly after initiation of treatment (or a dose increase) with a *vasodilator* drug. The most common offenders are the short- and long-acting nitrates, calcium channel blockers, and the vasodilators used to treat hypertension (hydralazine and minoxidil). The management of this problem depends upon the importance of the drug and the severity of the headache. Some patients, if informed in advance of the possibility of headache, will choose to take the drug anyway; this is particularly true of sublingual nitrates administered for angina. For the long-acting nitrates, dose reduction may effectively reduce headache for some patients, whereas alternate antianginal treatment will be needed for others (see Chapter 57). The headache associated with antihypertensive vasodilators can usually be prevented by treating the patient with a β-blocker before the vasodilator is added (see Chapter 62).

Headache in Acute Febrile Illnesses

Acute febrile illnesses may cause vascular-type throbbing headaches that remit when the illness resolves. A febrile patient in whom the headache is the major symptom and in whom nuchal rigidity or other manifestation of meningeal irritation is present requires a cerebrospinal fluid examination to exclude meningitis.

Giant Cell Arteritis and Polymyalgia Rheumatica

Giant cell arteritis (GCA) is a vasculitis that affects large arteries throughout the body. Clinical manifestations, however, are usually due to involvement of branches of the carotid artery and the most common syndrome is headache. GCA has also been called temporal arteritis (TA) because temporal headaches and a positive temporal artery biopsy are the findings that are most typical of the disease. The etiology of GCA is unknown.

Polymyalgia rheumatica (PR), a debilitating condition that presents with stiffness and aching of the neck and shoulder muscles, occurs in about 50% of patients with GCA (4). PR may also occur in patients who do not have GCA.

Epidemiology

GCA is almost exclusively a disease of persons over the age of 50; the average age of onset is 65. It is very uncommon in black individuals. It is somewhat more common in women than in men. In the single reported community study of GCA, it was found that the yearly incidence in persons over 50 was approximately 17/100,000 and the prevalence, 130/100,000 (6).

Manifestations

Giant cell arteritis. The headache of GCA does not have specific features that distinguish it clearly from other headaches. It is temporal in over one-half of patients; however, it may be frontal, occipital, parietal, or holocephalic. The patient usually reports that it involves the surface and is not intracranial. It may be made worse by hair brushing, resting the head on a pillow, and, at times, by exposure to cold. It is usually not described as throbbing. It is often described as being worse at night and building up gradually over a number of hours. Because these symptoms are not specific, the most important factors in suggesting the diagnosis of GCA are a number of associated findings, listed in Table 79.7. It is important to inquire specifically about pain (claudication) associated with chewing, swallowing, and arm or tongue motion, as these

Table 79.7.
Clinical Features of Giant Cell Arteritis[a]

Common Features (% of Patients with Feature at Initial Evaluation)		Less Common but Characteristic Features
Headache	(85)	Raynaud's phenomenon of
Temporal artery tenderness	(70)	limbs or tongue
Jaw claudication		Tender scalp nodules
Lingual, limb or swallowing	(65)	Thick, tender occipital arteries
claudication	(20)	Necrotic lesions of scalp,
Brachiocephalic bruits		tongue
Thickened or nodular temporal artery	(50)	Carotid artery tenderness
poral artery	(45)	Swelling of the hands
Pulseless temporal artery		Taste, smell disturbances
Visual symptoms	(40)	Distended, beaded retinal
Fixed blindness, partial or	(40)	veins
complete	(15)	Diminished or absent radial
Polymyalgia rheumatica		artery pulses
Weight loss >6 kg	(40)	Mononeuropathy—median,
Erythrocyte sedimentation rate	(35)	peroneal, cervical root
>50 mm/hour	(95)	
>100 mm/hour	(60)	
Fever(>37.7°C)	(20)	
Abnormal liver function	(50)	
Anemia (hematocrit <35%)	(50)	

[a]Adapted from Raskin NH, Appenzeller O: *Headache*. Philadelphia, WB Saunders, 1980.

symptoms are highly suggestive of GCA. The combination of one or more of the findings listed in Table 79.7 with a new headache in an older individual is sufficient to suspect GCA.

Polymyalgia rheumatica (PR). This condition is insidious in onset. The chief complaints are aching and stiffness of the shoulder girdle and, less commonly, of the thigh muscles. These symptoms may make it particularly hard for the patient to get up in the morning. Associated low grade fever, weight loss, and anorexia are common. On physical examination, there may be some tenderness of the shoulder and neck muscles, but there is no significant loss of muscle strength.

Diagnosis

Whenever GCA or PR is suspected, the erythrocyte sedimentation rate (ESR) measured by the Westergren method is the most useful screening test. The vast majority of patients will have a markedly elevated ESR (often 100 or greater). Because the upper limit of normal for persons over 60 may be as high as 40, an ESR of 40 to 60 is less informative than is a very high rate. *Definitive diagnosis of GCA* is made with a temporal artery biopsy. Because the typical histological changes (inflammatory cells, edema, and giant cells) are patchy in distribution, examination of serial sections of the resected segment of artery is essential; in occasional patients with GCA, even extensive sampling of one temporal artery does not yield a positive biopsy and the other artery must also be examined by biopsy.

Patient experience. A temporal artery biopsy can be done in an ambulatory surgery facility (by a general surgeon, vascular surgeon, plastic surgeon, or neurosurgeon). The scalp hair is shaved, the skin is anesthetized with Xylocaine, and the segment of artery (4 to 6 cm) is excised. The entire procedure requires about 1/2 hour. There are no serious sequelae.

The *diagnosis of polymyalgia rheumatica* is based on the combination of the typical symptoms, a high ESR, and exclusion of other explanations for the patient's symptoms. If a patient with typical PR has manifestations suggesting GCA (see Table 79.7), a temporal artery biopsy is indicated, since the recommended treatment for the two conditions is different.

Course and Treatment

Both GCA and PR are self-limited conditions, lasting up to 2 years. Treatment with corticosteroids produces dramatic symptomatic relief in patients with both conditions. More important, treatment appears to prevent almost entirely the most serious complication of GCA, blindness due to ischemic optic neuropathy. In untreated persons with GCA, unilateral or bilateral blindness occurs in 20 to 30% of patients.

If the diagnosis of GCA is strongly suspected, treatment should be initiated immediately and the temporal artery biopsy should be obtained within 3 to 4 days. The initial treatment is high dose prednisone (60 to 80 mg daily in four divided doses) for 4 to 6 weeks. During this time, symptoms usually remit entirely and there is a significant decrease in the ESR. After this initial period, the prednisone should be tapered weekly by about 10% until a dose of 10 to 15 mg daily has been reached. This dose should be continued for about 2 years, being discontinued by gradual tapering at the end of the second year (see Chapter 74 for details regarding long-term steroid therapy).

If the patient has isolated PR, the treatment is 10 to 15 mg of prednisone daily, from the outset. Treatment is also continued for approximately 2 years, with gradual discontinuation at the end of that time. The symptoms of PR, and the ESR, respond to this regimen within a few days to a week.

Although the symptoms of both GCA and PR may respond to aspirin and other nonsteroidal anti-inflammatory agents, these agents have not been shown to prevent the progressive vasculitis in GCA that may lead to blindness. The evidence for the efficacy of prednisone therapy in preventing blindness is based not upon controlled trials but upon the dramatic difference in the occurrence of blindness in untreated patients before prednisone was used (20 to 30% of patients) and in prednisone-treated patients (little or no occurrence of blindness).

The diagnosis and treatment of typical cases of GCA and PR can be accomplished readily by the generalist in the ambulatory setting. Whenever there is some question about the diagnosis or an unsatisfactory response to treatment, the opinion of a rheumatologist should be obtained.

Benign Intracranial Hypertension (Pseudotumor Cerebri)

Benign intracranial hypertension is a condition of unknown etiology characterized by headache, papilledema, and elevated intracranial pressure in the absence of a mass lesion or of venous sinus thrombosis (7). Headache in this condition is presumably due to stretching of the dura and perhaps the large vessels. Papilledema is a direct result of the increased pressure. The paucity of focal neurological symptoms and signs is due to the generalized nature of the pressure increase. Those focal signs that do appear (for example, 6th nerve palsies producing horizontal diplopia) are probably related to stretching of the involved structure.

This condition may occur *de novo* or may appear in association with a number of purported contributing factors (obesity, menstrual irregularity, steroid therapy or steroid withdrawal, oral contraceptives, nalidixic acid, vitamin A intoxication).

Manifestations

The prototypical patient is an obese young woman who develops progressively more severe headaches, nausea, vomiting, dizziness, and transiently blurred vision. In approximately one-half of patients, onset is abrupt, and the rest develop symptoms progressively over several weeks or months. The headache always precedes visual symptoms. It is usually generalized, constant, often more severe in the morning and aggravated by coughing, straining, or position change. The diagnosis is suggested strongly by these historical characteristics coupled with a physical examination that shows papilledema without focal neurological signs. Visual fields may be constricted and the blind spot enlarged. Rarely the papilledema involves the macular area, resulting in blindness (16).

The diagnosis of pseudotumor is always one of exclusion, as its name implies. The most important considerations in the *differential diagnosis* are intracranial mass lesion, hydrocephalus, hypertensive encephalopathy, and venous sinus thrombosis. To exclude an intracranial mass or hydrocephalus, a contrast CT scan or MRI scan (see "Patient Experience," Chapter 78) should be obtained. In pseudotumor, the scan may show small ventricles, but there will be no evidence of a mass lesion. After a negative scan, a lumbar puncture should be performed; in pseudotumor, the cerebrospinal fluid (CSF) pressure is high (200 to 400 mm H_2O or more), the content of CSF protein is normal or low, and the cell count is normal. The diagnosis of hypertensive encephalopathy should be made if the patient has the typical clinical features of pseudotumor, severe diastolic hypertension (equal to or greater than 120 mm Hg), and a negative CT scan. In a very obese woman, with a history of amenorrhea for many months, it is also important to consider pregnancy-induced hypertension (toxemia), which is ruled out by a negative pregnancy test (see Chapter 93).

For less clear-cut cases, such as a typical clinical presentation in an older male patient, referral to a neurologist is indicated.

Treatment and Course

Most patients recover completely from pseudotumor within several weeks or months; however, some patients require ongoing therapy to control headaches and prevent visual loss.

In a very obese patient, weight reduction is recommended although this may not directly affect the course of pseudotumor.

The goal of therapy is to reduce the intracranial pressure in order to reduce the risk of loss of vision. At the time of the initial lumbar puncture enough fluid should be removed to reduce the closing pressure to 100 mg H_2O or less (usually about 25 to 35 ml of CSF). Acetazolamide (Diamox), as 500-mg sustained release capsules, is then begun on a twice daily schedule with periodic check of serum electrolytes. If the patient remains asymptomatic and the papilledema clears, acetazolamide can be discontinued. For patients with continued headache, visual impairment, and papilledema, repeated lumbar punctures should be performed with removal of adequate volumes of CSF with each tap; and acetazolamide should be continued.

The use of corticosteroids to treat pseudotumor cerebri is controversial. Should the patient remain symptomatic after repeated LPs and acetazolamide, CSF shunting via a lumboperitoneal shunt or surgical incision of the optic nerve sheath should be considered. Management of these patients is difficult and requires the consultation of neurologists and neurosurgeons experienced in handling this disorder.

Post-traumatic (Postconcussive) Headache

Manifestations

Head trauma, which may or may not have been severe enough to cause loss of consciousness, may be followed by a number of symptoms that have been collectively entitled the postconcussive syndrome: headache, vertigo (often positional, see Chapter 81) lightheadedness or giddiness, poor concentration and memory, lack of energy, irritability, and anxiety. There is convincing evidence that these varied symptoms may be organic consequences of the injury, even though their exact causal mechanism is not understood. Raskin (see "General References") provide an excellent review of the syndrome, with the focus on headache.

Headache is the most frequent and often the most troubling manifestation of this syndrome. It typically begins within 24 hours of the trauma, as a dull, constant, generalized aching or cephalic discomfort that may wax and wane through the day or become concentrated at different points on the head (bifrontal or unilateral). During exacerbations, the pain typically has a throbbing quality. Headache may be worsened by sneezing, coughing, stooping, straining, or rapid head motions and changes in body position; it may be accompanied by nausea and vomiting.

Typically, these headaches worsen over days to weeks, then resolve over weeks or months; in some patients (roughly 15%) headache and other postconcussive symptoms continue for more than a year. It is now appreciated that minor head trauma in individuals with no prior headache history may lead to chronic recurrent headaches typical of migraine, with or without aura. Propranolol or amitriptyline used alone or in combination (see Table 79.6) has resulted in a dramatic reduction in frequency and severity of the headaches in some patients (20).

Differential Diagnosis

Subdural hematoma and other expanding mass lesions. Although postconcussive syndrome is a far more likely explanation of post-traumatic headache and ill-defined intellectual impairments than subdural hematoma, the seriousness of this possibility and the ease of ruling it out with CT scan make it an important consideration.

Post-traumatic dysautonomic cephalgia. Predominantly throbbing headache pain associated with sweating of one side of the face, pupillary dilation, and, sometimes, carotid bifurcation tenderness may represent a lesion of the carotid sympathetic plexus produced by whiplash-like injury (18). This condition may respond well to propranolol (see Table 79.6).

Pre-existing *migraine* or chronic *tension headaches* will have to be excluded by history; furthermore, post-traumatic headaches may make a pre-existing headache condition temporarily worse.

Cervical spine injury. See Chapter 64.

Objective Tests

In addition to the neurological history and examination, a number of currently available objective tests may be helpful for confirming the diagnosis of postconcussive syndrome: electroencephalography; vestibular function tests; electronystagmography; and auditory and visual evoked potentials. These tests, when positive, may be helpful medically and medicolegally. Because the abnormalities in these patients may be below the threshold of detectability, negative test results do not exclude an organic explanation of the patient's symptoms.

Treatment

For some patients with postconcussive headache, treatment similar to that used for migraine, with ergotamine and other agents, may occasionally be successful. In most patients, the course of the illness is self-limited even though fairly lengthy.

Low Pressure (Post-LP) Headache

Low pressure headache from persistent leakage of cerebrospinal fluid occurs most commonly after lumbar puncture (LP). Less commonly, it is due to a cerebrospinal fluid fistula caused by blunt trauma to any part of the neural axis (i.e., closed head or spine trauma); occasionally no causal event can be identified. The working diagnosis is based on the characteristic symptoms. The headache is markedly positional, relieved almost entirely by lying down. Nausea and dizziness are common nonspecific accompaniments. There are no focal neurological symptoms or signs, and the patient is afebrile.

The majority of postlumbar puncture and post-traumatic leaks close spontaneously, signified by resolution of the headache, within few days; occasionally the problem does not resolve for several weeks. Appropriate management is essential for rapid healing of the leak: the patient is instructed to remain recumbent for several days, after which usual activities can be resumed. The rare patient with persistent, typical post-LP headache should be referred to an anesthesiologist for epidural instillation of antologous blood; the blood will clot, forming a patch, at the site of the leak. Because of the risk of meningitis, any patient with a suspected persistent CSF fistula (i.e., a patient with a typical low pressure headache that persists after blunt trauma) should be referred to a neurologist or neurosurgeon for complete evaluation.

Characteristics of Headache Due to a Mass Lesion

For both the headache sufferer and the physician, concern about the possibility of a brain tumor often dominates the situation. The most important clue to the presence of an intracranial lesion in a headache sufferer is the simultaneous onset of headache and focal neurological signs/symptoms or a change in mental status. In a person over the age of 50, the onset of persistent headache for the first time is also very worrisome.

A number of other features, none of them specific, may be clues to the presence of an intracranial mass lesion:

1. Although the headache associated with a mass lesion can initially be intermittent, mild, and responsive to mild analgesics, typically it becomes more continuous and intense and, at the same time, less responsive to analgesics.
2. The headache may wake the patient from sleep or be present on waking every day, decreasing after the patient has been up for several hours. The value of these characteristics is somewhat diminished by the comparatively large number of patients with chronic tension headache, migraine, and cluster headache who are also awakened by or wake up with headache. True sinus headache may also be worse in the morning due to lack of postural drainage during the night.
3. Coughing, sneezing, and straining may aggravate a persistent headache due to a mass lesion, presumably by transiently increasing intracranial pressure and accentuating the stretching of pain-sensitive structures. Again, however, migraine headaches can have the same features.
4. Anorexia, nausea, and vomiting may accompany the headache, but these symptoms are not distinguishable from those caused by severe migraine headache. Projectile vomiting is rarely seen in adults with intracranial masses.

Except when there are focal neurological signs or symptoms, the decision to evaluate a patient for a mass lesion will usually be made after an initial period of observation and a trial of analgesics. A CT scan with contrast, or brain MRI (see "Patient Experience," Chapter 78), is the diagnostic procedure of choice when the decision is made to evaluate for a mass lesion. When the CT scan or MRI is positive for intracranial disease, the patient should be referred to a neurologist or a neurosurgeon for definitive care.

FACIAL PAIN SYNDROMES

Idiopathic Trigeminal Neuralgia (Tic Douloureux)

Manifestations

Trigeminal neuralgia is a problem seen almost exclusively in patients over the age of 40, most of them elderly. It has several distinguishing features: the pain is severe, paroxysmal, and lancinating; it lasts only a few seconds to a minute. The patient's face usually contorts with the pain, and the patient may find it impossible to control his emotional response. Between attacks the patient is usually pain free, although some patients may have a dull ache in the area. The interval between paroxysms is usually at least 2 or 3 minutes. The frequency of paroxysms is highly variable; some individuals have hundreds each day.

The pain is usually felt in those structures innervated by the second and third divisions of the trigeminal nerve (lips, gums, cheek, chin). There is a slightly greater tendency for tic to affect the right side of the face than the left. The pain is typically unilateral in a single attack, and in 95% of patients it remains unilateral. It is very uncommon for attacks to involve both sides of the face simultaneously.

The patient frequently can identify trigger points on the face or in the mouth that, when touched (even by contact with a gust of cold air) or moved, precipitate pain.

A few patients with idiopathic trigeminal neuralgia will have some areas of slightly decreased sensation that may be difficult to distinguish from normal; however, there is generally no objective decrease in sensation (in men, no more decrease than would normally be observed over the beard area).

Differential Diagnosis

A syndrome identical to or similar to idiopathic trigeminal neuralgia can be produced by a number of known conditions (secondary trigeminal neuralgia), e.g., multiple sclerosis, acoustic neurinoma, aneurysms, trigeminal neuromas, meningiomas, and others. These conditions should be considered, particularly if the patient is under 40 years, and has any of the following: pain predominantly in the upper division of the trigeminal nerve (forehead and eye); bilateral pain; or evidence of bilateral sensory loss or associated motor signs (e.g., weak jaw, facial weakness, swallowing difficulty).

In a patient with a typical clinical presentation, medical therapy (see below) can be initiated without further workup. If medical therapy is ineffective, or if there are any atypical features, referral to a neurologist is appropriate. He will usually request X-ray views helpful in evaluating the divisions of the trigeminal nerve that are clinically most involved (for the first division, the superior orbital fissure; for third division, the foramen ovale). A contrast CT or brain MRI scan (see "Patient Experience," Chapter 78) may also be obtained to check for a neuroma or a meningioma involving the trigeminal or other nerves.

Treatment

Advances in drug therapy have made the treatment of idiopathic trigeminal neuralgia relatively easy. The patient should initially be given carbamazepine (Tegretol, 200-mg tablets) 1/2 tablet (100 mg) twice daily, with meals, increasing every 2 to 3 days to a three times daily schedule and a total daily dose of 300 to 600 mg. An occasional patient may need doses as high as 1200 mg/day; in these cases, blood levels should be monitored to confirm the adequacy of the drug trial. Sixty to 70% of patients can expect excellent to satisfactory relief with carbamazepine. Benign side effects of the drug include nausea, vomiting, ataxia, vertigo, and transient leukopenia. The most serious side effects seem to be either allergic or idiosyncratic, including persistent leukopenia and aplastic anemia. Patients must be informed of these possible risks, the frequency of which is unknown but which appears to be quite low. Because of these risks, patients should have serial hemograms performed after 1 week, 6 weeks, 3 months, and on a periodic basis. Because trigeminal neuralgia may remit spontaneously after 6 months to a year, discontinuation drug therapy should be tried at periodic intervals (3 months).

If the patient fails to improve with carbamazepine or fails to tolerate the drug, two alternative medications can be tried: amitriptyline (several-week trial progressing from 25 mg to 150 mg at bedtime) or baclofen (several-week trial progressing from 10 mg twice daily to 40 mg twice daily). A patient whose symptoms cannot be controlled medically should be offered consultation with a neurosurgeon for possible percutaneous radiofrequency treatment of the trigeminal ganglion on the affected side.

Atypical Facial Pain

"Atypical facial pain" is a collective term for a variety of painful facial symptoms that do not meet the diagnostic criteria for any recognized entity (19). If untreated, most patients with this problem continue to complain of it for many years. The management of these patients involves excluding all reasonable possibilities; a one-time referral to a dentist and to an otolaryngologist should be part of this evaluation.

Most of these patients whose workup is negative have psychosocial problems and may improve with psychotherapy, provided either by the general physician or a psychiatrist. For additional details, see the discussion of the patient with chronic pain in Chapter 12.

General References

Delassio DJ (ed): *Wolff's Headache and Other Head Pain*, 5th ed. New York, Oxford University Press, 1987.
  The most recent edition of the classic reference work on headache.
Diamond S, Medina JL: Review article: current thoughts on migraine. *Headache* 20:208, 1980.
  A practical review.
Kumar KL, Cooney TG: Vascular headache. *J Gen Intern Med* 3(4):384, 1988.
  Up-to-date review, emphasizing management.
Raskin NH: *Headache*, 2nd ed., Philadelphia, WB Saunders, 1988.
  Extensively referenced book on selected headache syndromes (migraine, tension headache, cluster headache, post-traumatic headache, giant cell arteritis).

Specific References

1. Clinical Conferences at The Johns Hopkins Hospital: Cluster headache. *Johns Hopkins Med J* 150:246, 1982.
2. Dhopesh V, Anwar R, Herring C: A retrospective assessment of emergency department patients with complaint of headache. *Headache* 19:37, 1979.
3. Friedman AP, von Storch TJC, Merritt HH: Migraine and tension headaches: a clinical study of 2,000 cases. *Neurology* 4:773, 1954.
4. Hamilton Jr CR, Shelley WM, Tumulty PA: Giant cell arteritis: including temporal arteritis and polymyalgia rheumatica. *Medicine (Baltimore)* 50:1, 1971.
5. Headache Classification Committee of the International Headache Society: Classification and diagnostic criteria for headache disorders, cranial neuralgias and facial pain. *Cephalalgia* 8 (suppl 7):1, 1988.
6. Huston KA, Hunder GG, Lie JT, et al: Temporal arteritis: a 25-year epidemiologic, clinical and pathologic study. *Ann Intern Med* 88:162, 1978.
7. Johnston I, Patterson A: Benign intracranial hypertension. *Brain* 97:289, 1975.
8. Kudrow L: Response of cluster headache attacks to oxygen inhalation. *Headache* 21:1, 1981.
9. Lance JW, Curran DA, Anthony J: Investigations into the mechanism and treatment of chronic headache. *Med J Aust* 2:909, 1965.
10. Markush RE, Karp HR, Heyman A, O'Fallon WM: Epidemiologic study of migraine symptoms in young women. *Neurology* 25:430, 1975.
11. Monro J, Carini C, Brostoff J: Migraine is a food-allergic disease. *Lancet* 2:719, 1984.
12. Packard RC: What does the headache patient want? *Headache* 19:370, 1979.
13. Price RW, Posner JB: Chronic paroxysmal hemicrania; a disabling headache syndrome responding to indomethacin. *Ann Neurol* 3:183, 1978.
14. Raskin NH, Schwartz RK: Interval therapy of migraine: long-term results. *Headache* 20:336, 1980.
15. Rooke ED: Benign exertional headache. *Med Clin North Am* 52:801, 1968.
16. Rush JA: Pseudotumor cerebri, clinical profile visual outcome in 63 patients. *Mayo Clin Proc* 55:541, 1980.
17. Schnarch DM, Hunter JE: Migraine incidence in clinical versus nonclinical populations. *Psychosomatics* 21:314, 1980.
18. Vijayan N, Dreyfus PM: Post-traumatic dysautonomic cephalagia. *Arch Neurol* 32:649, 1975.
19. Weedington WW, Blazer D: Atypical facial pain and trigeminal neuralgia: a comparison study. *Psychosomatics* 20:348, 1979.
20. Weiss H, Stern BJ, Goldberg J: Chronic migraine after minor head trauma. *Ann Neurol* 16:113, 1984.
21. Ziegler DK, Hassasein RW, Cough JR: Characteristics of life headache histories in a nonclinic population. *Neurology* 27:265, 1977.

C H A P T E R 80

Seizure Disorders

ROBERT S. FISHER, M.D., Ph.D.

Approximately 2 million Americans are believed to have epilepsy. Many additional patients who do not carry the diagnosis of epilepsy present to their personal physicians or to emergency rooms for evaluation and management of seizures. Convulsive disorders are estimated to account for about 5% of visits to all physicians in private practice and for 20% of visits to neurologists (17).

DEFINITION AND CLASSIFICATION OF SEIZURES

The precise definition of a "seizure" is not easy, in part because no single behavior or laboratory result is pathognomonic. One approach is to define a seizure as an episode, with a clear start and finish, which affects motor control, sensation, speech, or consciousness and which is associated with certain characteristic electrical abnormalities of the brain. Most patients are relatively normal during the period between seizures (the interictal period), and their electroencephalograms (EEGs) may be normal as well.

The term "epilepsy" describes the condition of recurrent seizures due to primary (and persisting) nervous system disease. Therefore, single or even multiple seizures that occur as a result of temporally limited circumstances (such as high fever or alcohol withdrawal) should not be labeled as "epilepsy."

Although many predisposing factors are known, the basic mechanisms of seizures are still uncertain. Until a clear understanding of these mechanisms emerges, all classification schemes must be empirical. A widely accepted, clinically relevant scheme is shown in Table 80.1 (10). About 75% of all people with epilepsy can easily be classified according to this scheme. About 22% of classifiable patients over the age of 15 have generalized epilepsy and 78% have partial epilepsy. Complex partial seizures, labeled in the past "temporal lobe epilepsy," "psychomotor epilepsy," or "limbic epilepsy," are the most common form of seizures in adults. Specific causes of these different categories of seizures are considered below.

CLINICAL PRESENTATIONS OF SEIZURE DISORDERS

The clinical manifestations of a seizure depend upon several factors: the degree of maturity of the nervous system, the location of the initial abnormal electrical discharges, and the manner in which these discharges spread (8). A seizure focus in the motor cortex will produce jerking of those parts of the body normally governed by the region of the focus; a seizure in a "sensory region" of the brain will generate abnormal sensation; a seizure in the so-called areas of "higher function" leads to complex cognitive and behavioral manifestations (Fig. 80.1). Certain types of seizures

Table 80.1.
Classification of the Epilepsies[a]

PRIMARY GENERALIZED EPILEPSY
  Tonic-clonic (grand mal)
  Absence (petit mal)
  Myoclonic
  Atonic, others
PARTIAL (FOCAL) EPILEPSY
  With elementary symptomatology
    Focal motor
    Focal sensory
    Vegetative
    Psychic
    Mixed
  With complex symptomatology
    Partial complex (psychomotor)
SECONDARY GENERALIZED
UNCLASSIFIABLE

[a] Adapted from Dreifuss FE: Proposal for revised clinical and electroencephalographic classification of epileptic seizures. *Epilepsia* 22:489, 1981.

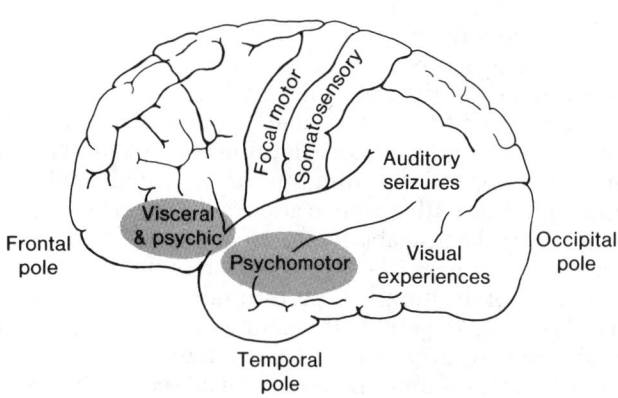

Figure 80.1. Relation of local seizure phenomena to brain topography.

present with sudden changes in consciousness rather than with focal motor or sensory signs of symptoms.

Generalized Tonic-Clonic (Grand Mal)

In patients with grand mal (now called "primary generalized tonic-clonic") epilepsy, seizure discharges present nearly synchronously in widespread regions of the cortex. The term "grand mal", should not be applied to seizures having focal onset and secondary generalization. These latter events should be called "generalized seizures" or "major motor seizures" instead of "grand mal," because the latter connotes initial generalization of seizure activity.

Grand mal seizures typically begin with an arrest of activity and sudden loss of consciousness, followed by trembling, tonic stiffening of the upper and lower extremities, then clonic rhythmical jerking of the limbs, followed by waxing and waning to a state of flaccidity. The usual duration of the sequence is 2 to 5 minutes. After a seizure, the patient may remain stuporous for minutes to hours. During the seizure, loss of consciousness is invariable; consequently, production of speech, purposeful eye movements, or subsequent recall for events during the seizure are features that rule out the diagnosis of grand mal epilepsy. Although a general sensation of unease may warn of an impending grand mal attack, a definite sensory, motor, or psychological aura should raise strong suspicion of a partial (focal) seizure that has become secondarily generalized. Common associated findings during both grand mal or secondary major motor seizures include incontinence, sweating, tachycardia, elevated blood pressure, and minor cardiac arrhythmias.

Grand mal seizures may first develop at any age, though onset is rare after about age 35. Frequency may range from one seizure in an entire lifetime to several seizures a day.

Generalized Absence (Petit Mal)

Petit mal (now designated "absence, typical") is another example of primary generalized epilepsy. It comprises about 10% of seizures, but it is primarily a disease of children, with onset usually between 4 and 12 years of age. The clinical presentation of petit mal seizures is quite distinct from grand mal. Petit mal is an entity in its own right and not a "little grand mal." Similarly, the use of the term "petit mal" to describe any brief lapse of consciousness or attention is a misnomer and an invitation to inappropriate therapy. Petit mal seizures present with absence attacks (i.e., lapses of consciousness) lasting about 3 to 30 seconds. There is no tonic-clonic phase nor loss of posture. Slight rhythmic twitching of the mouth or periorbital musculature may be observed. If petit mal seizures are atypical, with prolonged duration or notable automatism, the distinction from temporal lobe ("partial complex") seizures can be quite difficult. After a petit mal seizure, recovery of awareness occurs within seconds, but amnesia for events during the seizure is lasting. Petit mal seizures can occur over 100 times/day. Children who suffer such frequent seizures may be labeled daydreamers or slow learners, until a correct diagnosis is made.

The EEG during a petit mal seizure shows a characteristic 3/second spikewave pattern. Interictal EEGs in children with petit mal epilepsy are often normal. Sometimes hyperventilation or stimulation with regularly flashing lights may bring out abnormalities. Both clinical and EEG findings should be used to secure a diagnosis of petit mal epilepsy: neither alone is diagnostic.

About three of four children outgrow petit mal by age 20, but up to 50% (especially among those with atypical absence) may later develop grand mal seizures.

Myoclonic Seizures

Myoclonus consists of involuntary nonrhythmic jerking of limbs, trunk, or head, that is usually not fully synchronous (i.e., all parts do not move at the same time). When a series of frequent myoclonic jerks occurs for a few seconds, without alteration in the state of consciousness, the term "myoclonic seizures" is applied. Myoclonus is encountered by general physicians as a consequence of diffuse cortical injury from such causes as anoxia, hypoglycemia, severe renal or hepatic failure, or drug toxicity. In these conditions myoclonic seizures are often self-limited and resolve as the underlying illness stabilizes. Primary neurological disease, e.g., viral encephalitis, Jakob-Creutzfeldt disease, Huntington's chorea, or Wilson's disease, also may present in part with myoclonus.

Cases of familial myoclonus with associated neurological symptoms may be parceled into several different syndromes. These patients are generally managed in consultation with a neurologist.

Partial (Focal) Elementary Seizures

Focal motor or sensory seizures may present at any age. The clinical manifestations depend upon the site of the brain in which the seizure originates.

The motor cortex is the most common site of origin for focal seizures; as the seizure discharges spread across the motor strip, clonus (alternating contraction and relaxation) may "march" across the limb and face. Sensory seizures most often begin from a focus in the postcentral gyrus and are manifest by numbness in the face or fingers. Sensory seizures can also involve areas of special sensation. A focus in or near the visual cortex may cause perception of spots and lights, similar to the experience of patients suffering from classic migraine. Buzzing or ringing may be generated from a focus in the superior temporal lobe. Gustatory and olfactory sensations are components of partial complex (temporal lobe) seizures. Seizures dominated by vestibular symptoms are rare.

Retention of awareness is characteristic of focal seizures, so that patients may walk, talk, and think normally during a seizure—accomplishments that would be impossible during a generalized seizure. However, a large focus in the dominant hemisphere may generate seizures that blunt awareness.

After a focal motor seizure, there may be weakness of the body parts that have been involved. This so-called "Todd's paralysis" usually resolves within a few hours or, in unusual cases, after a few days. Distinction between cerebrovascular ischemic events with associated seizures and seizures with Todd's paralysis may be impossible without clues from the past history. Presence of a Todd's paralysis has localizing value and is good evidence that a seizure was focal.

Electroencephalography will not necessarily reveal a seizure focus, especially if it is small, particularly during the interictal stage.

Partial (Psychomotor) Complex Seizures

"Partial complex epilepsy" may be considered synonymous with "temporal lobe epilepsy," "psychomotor epilepsy," and "limbic epilepsy." This category of seizures is important for several reasons: the condition is common in the adult population; psychomotor seizures are often misdiagnosed; and correct diagnosis leads to a search for potentially correctable lesions and to effective therapy. Partial complex epilepsy is classified as a focal epilepsy because of clinical evidence linking these seizures with foci in or near the temporal lobe.

The presentation of partial complex epilepsy is more varied than that of the other forms of epilepsy and may include autonomic, psychic, visceral, sensory, or motor symptoms. Warning of an impending seizure may be signaled by an "aura." The classic aura of olfactory or gustatory hallucination is actually less common than is an aura of nondescript unpleasant visceral sensations or a sense of unease. There is, in general, no clear boundary between the aura and the seizure itself, particularly when seizures feature distorted visual or auditory sensations, or vertigo or general disequilibrium. Arrest of motor activity, rigid posturing of the head and eyes, and slow repetitive limb movements may occur and are easily distinguished in most cases from the tonic-clonic sequence of major motor attacks. Autonomic instability, including fluctuating heart rate or blood pressure, flushing, sweating, salivating, alterations in papillary reactions, or incontinence of urine or feces, has been described in patients with temporal lobe seizures. The term "psychomotor epilepsy" is derived from the frequent mental changes that characterize this form of epilepsy. Patients often say that they feel strange, in a "dream," or experience inappropriate emotions such as intense dread or strange serenity. During the seizure, consciousness is impaired to a variable extent; if they can talk, patients may portray what appears to be a primarily psychiatric illness. The distinction between partial complex epilepsy and psychosis may be obscured further in patients whose interictal personality is abnormal. Such individuals can easily be misdiagnosed as schizophrenic.

In a condition whose presentation may range from apparent appendicitis to apparent schizophrenia the physician must make special efforts to elicit a detailed history of a "spell" and, when possible, to observe one personally. Partial complex seizures should have a definite start and finish. Duration of seizure activity varies from 10 seconds to 5 minutes; most last from 30 seconds to 2 minutes. The seizures should be associated with some impairment in ability to register and process information during the seizure; and they should be relatively stereotyped from episode to episode. Observations of automatic behavior, such as repetitive mouth smacking, raising and lowering the arm, buttoning and unbuttoning a shirt, or pacing in circles, may secure the diagnosis of a partial complex seizure disorder, for such "automatisms" are common in psychomotor epilepsy and uncommon in other forms of seizures.

The standard EEG is abnormal in only about half of patients with partial complex seizures. The yield may be increased to 80 to 90% by recording EEGs during sleep and by using special electrodes positioned in the nasopharynx close to the undersurface of the temporal lobe.

Although partial complex seizures may begin at any age, the majority begin before age 20. Adult onset of temporal lobe epilepsy carries the same significance as does a new onset of any focal seizure; a significant structural lesion must be ruled out. Patients with onset of temporal lobe seizures, who come to surgery or to postmortem, may show either no histological abnormality of the brain or may have tumors, infarcts, granulomas, or infections, or more often a generalized gliosis of the mesial temporal lobe ("mesial temporal sclerosis"). It is not known whether gliosis causes temporal lobe seizures or follows from them.

Prognosis for spontaneous remission of complex partial seizures is not as favorable as it is for grand mal seizures.

Secondarily Generalized Seizures

Secondarily generalized seizures begin clinically as focal seizures (including those beginning as partial complex seizures) and then generalize to seizures in-

distinguishable from grand mal attacks. The focal onset can be as fleeting as a few tremors in an arm, numbness of the hand or one side of the face, or marked conjugate deviation of the eyes or head. Sensory or visceral auras are also evidence of focal onset, as is preservation of consciousness during the early part of a seizure.

Complex electrophysiological mechanisms govern whether seizure discharges remain in a local focus, spread along certain prescribed anatomical pathways, or generalize to much of the brain. A focal seizure may generalize when conditions of overall brain excitability are "right." Conversely, anticonvulsive therapy may convert a secondarily generalized seizure into a focal seizure. It is not known how often grand mal attacks are actually secondarily generalized seizures with occult primary origins.

Unclassifiable Seizures

With an adequate history, most seizures should be classifiable by the scheme given above. Unfortunately, the history is sometimes lacking, as when observers report "falling down and shaking," but cannot describe the full sequence of events. In these instances it is best to list the seizure as "unclassifiable" or to use nondescript terms such as "tonic-clonic" or an "absence attack" (if there was a brief lapse of consciousness), until the specific seizure type becomes evident.

EPIDEMIOLOGY

The reported yearly incidence of new onset epilepsy is approximately 20 to 50/100,000 population, and the prevalence is between 2 and 10/1,000 population (36). A 1981 review of multiple large series of referred adult patients with seizures show that 67% were partial in onset, 20% generalized, and 13% unclassified (32). Partial complex (previously designated "psychomotor") seizures were the most prevalent, at 41% of the entire seizure group; partial simple (focal motor or sensory) seizures were next, at 15%; primary generalized tonic-clonic (grand mal) and secondarily generalized each comprised about 11%; myoclonic seizures accounted for about 4%. Although these frequencies are based on groups of patients seen at seizure clinics, they probably parallel the frequencies seen in the community. At the younger end of the age spectrum, partial seizures are less frequent and generalized absence seizures more frequent than is represented by these crude percentages for all adults.

NATURAL HISTORY AND PROGNOSIS

The natural history of epilepsy is difficult to determine because all modern studies include heterogeneous mixes of treated and untreated patients (25). After a first unprovoked seizure the cumulative risk of recurrence has been estimated at between 30 and 70%. Until further data become available it is reasonable to estimate about a 50% risk for recurrence of a spontaneous tonic-clonic seizure in the few years after a first seizure. The role of treatment in reducing this risk is presently uncertain. If a person suffers a second, unprovoked seizure, then the risk for further seizures is high.

Once two spontaneous seizures have occurred, epilepsy is considered to exist, and the epidemiological focus switches to the possibility for remission. Before the development of anticonvulsant medication, the spontaneous remission rate for all types of seizures was about 10% to 32%. In one study (2) the remission rate, defined as 5 consecutive years seizure free (on or off therapy), was 70% 20 years after diagnosis of epilepsy. The role of treatment in the long-term outcome is unclear. It is useful to know that the probability of 5 years without seizures are 42% at 1 year and 51% at 2 years after diagnosis of epilepsy. The probability of being in remission at 20 years was 80 to 85% for patients with primary generalized epilepsies, but only 65% for those with partial complex epilepsies. Slightly less than half of the patient in this study remained on medication at 20 years. Another study (11) has shown the following to be poor prognostic factors in becoming seizure free for at least 2 years while on therapy: continuing seizures for the initial 2 years of treatment, presence of partial seizures, a high frequency of tonic-clonic seizures before treatment, a neuropsychiatric deficit, and positive family history for epilepsy.

It is generally possible to reassure a person with epilepsy that the long-term prognosis for remission is likely to be good; however, except for the primary generalized epilepsies in children, the remission can be expected to require many years.

Serious injury or death rarely occurs as a direct consequence of epilepsy, although anecdotal instances of sudden unexplained deaths in people with epilepsy have been reported.

ETIOLOGY OF SEIZURES

General Comments

Classification of seizures, as given above, depends upon clinical and EEG observation of the patient. A seizure represents a symptom: once the presence of a seizure has been established and the seizure classified, an etiology must be sought. How likely this search is to be successful is difficult to ascertain from the medical literature, because of serious biases in selecting populations for study.

Epilepsy secondary to identified causes is sometimes called "symptomatic" as opposed to "essential," "cryptogenic," or "idiopathic" epilepsy. It is agreed that most cases of primary generalized epilepsy are cryptogenic, so that a child presenting with typical petit mal or grand mal seizures, in the context of a normal examination, normal screening laboratory tests (see below), and a positive family history for similar seizures, would not warrant an extensive search for underlying causes. The yield is higher from investigation of partial or atypical generalized seizures.

Table 80.2 lists etiologies that should be considered for different types of seizures at various ages; the diagnoses are listed from top to bottom roughly in the order of their frequency (except that "idiopathic" is placed at the end of each list because it is a diagnosis of exclusion). It is worth emphasizing that all of the partial epilepsies can become secondarily generalized, and that the focal onset may be obscured. Therefore, focal etiologies should be considered even in apparently generalized seizures.

Special issues are raised by seizures that are manifest for the first time in the elderly. First, most seizure disorders have onset in the first three decades of life, and onset of the primary generalized forms of epilepsy almost never occurs after this age. Second, cerebrovascular disease accounts for 30 to 60% of all new seizures in the elderly population (28). Tumors, the major cause of focal seizures in middle-aged patients, cause 2 to 30% of seizures in elderly patients; however, brain tumors in this age group are very likely to be malignant. A cause is not found to explain seizures in half or more of this group. When an elderly patient presents with seizures, a special effort should be made to rule out treatable conditions such as carotid artery occlusions, cardiac arrhythmias, infection, and toxic-metabolic derangements.

Post-Traumatic Seizures

According to the National Head and Spinal Cord Injury Survey of the National Institutes of Health (1) 422,000 patients were hospitalized in 1974 for head injuries, 200/100,000 United States population. Four to 5 times that number of head injuries are sustained by people who are not hospitalized but who still have a significant risk of brain damage. New seizures usually partial in onset and often secondarily generalized may occur as a consequence of serious head injuries. The incidence of post-traumatic epilepsy depends upon several factors: the population under study, the severity of the injury, the duration of follow-up, and the criteria used to label a seizure as a manifestation of epilepsy. In patients with a mild injury (brief unconsciousness or amnesia) risk of later epilepsy is not increased significantly above baseline, whereas severe injuries (intracranial hematomas, focal neurological signs, unconsciousness for more than 24 hours) result in epilepsy in 7% of patients after 1 year and in 11.5% after 5 years (3). Moderately severe injuries (skull fractures or unconsciousness for 30 minutes to 24 hours) impose an intermediate risk. Injuries over the vertex are more epileptogenic.

The value of prophylactic therapy to prevent the onset of post-traumatic seizures has not been firmly established. Until more data become available, a reasonable approach includes the following elements: patients with minor scalp lacerations of brief loss of consciousness should not be considered to have a sig-

Table 80.2.
Etiological Factors for Seizures with Onset at Various Ages[a]

Adolescent (12–21 yr)	Adult (21–65 yr)	Elderly (65+ yr)
Common Causes		
Genetic (g)	Alcohol withdrawal (g)	Cerebrovascular (m)
Mesial temporal sclerosis (f)	Toxins or drugs (g)[c]	Thrombotic
Infection (m)	Drug withdrawal (g)	Embolic
Meningitis	Tumor (f)	Hemorrhagic
Viral encephalitis	Trauma (f)	Cardiac arrhythmia
Abscess	Scar	Trauma (f)
TORCHS[b]	Subdural hematoma	Scar
Parasites	Mesial temporal sclerosis (f)	Subdural hematoma
Psychogenic (m)	Genetic (g)	Tumor (f)
Toxins or drugs (g)[c]	Psychogenic (m)	Infection (m)
Drug withdrawal (g)	Infection (m)	Meningitis
	Meningitis	Viral encephalitis
	Viral encephalitis	Abscess
	Abscess	Syphilis
	Syphilis	Parasites
	Parasites	
Occasional Causes		
Metabolic (g)	Metabolic (g)	Alcohol withdrawal (g)
Hypoglycemia	Hypoglycemia	Toxins or drugs (g)[c]
Hyponatremia	Hyponatremia	Drug withdrawal (g)
Hypocalcemia	Hypocalcemia	Hypoxia (g)
Porphyria	Hypomagnesemia	Metabolic (g)
Trauma (f)	Hypoxia (g)	Hypoglycemia
Scar	Cerebrovascular (m)	Hyponatremia
Subdural hematoma	Thrombotic	Hypocalcemia
Tumor (f)	Embolic	
Arteriovenous malformation (f)	Hemorrhagic	
Subarachnoid hemorrhage (m)	Cardiac arrhythmia	
Eclampsia (m)	Renal failure (g)	
Renal failure (g)	Eclampsia (m)	
Rare Causes		
Collagen disease (m)	Collagen disease (m)	Hypertensive encephalopathy (m)
Hepatic failure (g)	Hypertensive encephalopathy (m)	Hyperosmolar (m)
Multiple sclerosis (f)	Hyperosmolar (m)	Renal failure (g)
	Multiple sclerosis (f)	Hepatic failure (g)
	Degenerative (m)	Degenerative (g)
		Factitious (m)
Idiopathic	Idiopathic	Idiopathic

[a] f, usually focal; g, usually generalized; m, often mixed.
[b] TORCHS, toxoplasmosis, rubella, cytomegalovirus, herpes, syphilis.
[c] See list of occupational exposures which may cause seizures, Table 7.3.

nificantly increased risk of epilepsy. A single seizure occurring during the first 2 weeks after head injury, or while the patient is still suffering from the acute effects of injury, should not be an indication for long-term therapy. A second seizure in this setting might be grounds for treatment. Some patients with brain injuries should be considered for a 2- to 4-year course of prophylactic phenytoin (unless there are particular contraindications to chronic medication), especially if there has been prolonged (greater than 24 hours) unconsciousness, penetrating injury to the brain, or if the vertex (topmost point of the vault of the skull) has been involved. If a patient has a "spontaneous" seizure more than 2 weeks after a head injury, he should be evaluated and treated as would any other patient with a new onset of a seizure disorder—the seizure should not be attributed to a recent or remote episode of head trauma until other treatable causes of seizures have been ruled out.

Alcohol-Related Seizures

Alcohol withdrawal is a very common cause of seizures (4); almost all of them occur within the first 48 hours of abstinence and most of them are generalized: In some series up to 25% of seizures have been focal, presumably because of a concomitant old cortical scar from trauma, infection, or vascular disease. If a known alcohol abuser has had a prior withdrawal seizure, presents a typical picture of a generalized seizure without focal features, has a normal examination and no complications, then investigations may be limited. More often, the history is imprecise and findings are equivocal, or the patient has a fever or an elevated leukocyte count. In these instances lumbar puncture, EEG, and continued observation are indicated. A computed tomography (CT) scan is likely to be of use when focal seizures, focal neurological deficits, or signs of acute head trauma are present.

Treatment of alcohol withdrawal is controversial, because the majority of patients (approximately 95%) in a state of withdrawal do not have seizures, or have them only once or twice. Many of the standard medications, such as chlordiazepoxide (Librium), which are used to treat the abstinence syndrome, have anticonvulsant properties as well. Nevertheless, the value of these medications (or of phenytoin) in the prevention of seizures is uncertain. Alcoholics with no prior seizure history should not be given prophylactic phenytoin during withdrawal. If a patient who is entering alcohol withdrawal gives a history of prior seizures, then a 5-day course of phenytoin (300 mg/day) may prevent the occasional seizure with its attendant risks of aspiration pneumonias and falls. Long-term therapy with anticonvulsants is not recommended.

Alcohol abusers are sometimes abusers of other drugs. Withdrawal from these, especially barbiturates or tranquilizers, at the same time as withdrawal from alcohol may cause fulminant seizures.

Recent work has suggested that seizures may also occur during the period of alcohol consumption, as distinct from the period of alcohol withdrawal (23).

For the alcohol abuser, ability to abstain is the principal determinant of seizure frequency. There is a strong relationship in this population between drinking and seizure frequency. On the other hand, nonalcoholic people with epilepsy can usually tolerate occasional alcohol and should be permitted to drink alcohol unless they clearly have seizures more often when they drink.

Seizures and Brain Tumors

Brain tumor is a relatively uncommon cause of epilepsy, but epilepsy is a common symptom of brain tumors. About one-third of intracranial and one-half of intrahemispheric tumors are associated with seizures. Slow growing tumors appear to be more epileptogenic: Seizures occur in 90% of patients with oligodendrogliomas, 69% of patients with astrocytomas, 34% of patients with glioblastomas, 37% of patients with meningiomas, and 41% of patients with metastases to the brain (24).

The prevalence of brain tumors among people with epilepsy varies from 2 to 12% (27) depending upon the population studied and on the type of seizures. Young and middle-aged adults with new onset of focal seizures have the greatest chance of harboring a tumor, with rates quoted at 35% (32). The following features suggest that seizures may be associated with a brain tumor: onset after 20 years of age, presence of focal neurological signs, signs of increased intracranial pressure, focal unilateral slow waves on the EEG, asymmetry of fast activity on the EEG, and inducibility by hyperventilation (34). If a tumor is suspected, a CT scan, with and without contrast, or an MRI are the tests of choice.

Seizures and Cerebrovascular Disease

Cerebrovascular disease is the most common, and epilepsy the second most common, of the serious neurological illnesses. The two conditions are found together fairly often. It is generally assumed in such patients that ischemia leaves a damaged area of brain, which then somehow "matures" into an epileptic focus. One series (15) reported an overall incidence of seizures of about 8% in patients with stroke, 4% in those with bland infarction, and 10% in those with hemorrhage. The seizures are more likely to be focal (60%) than generalized (40%). In 40% of the patients, seizures occur at the onset of the deficit or within the first 2 weeks; only a few of these patients later develop recurrent epilepsy. However, most patients who have seizures after the second week do develop epilepsy. Consequently, early seizures after stroke do not mandate the use of anticonvulsants, but late seizures should be treated as epilepsy.

As discussed above, seizures in the elderly should raise the suspicion of cerebrovascular disease and may be the first clue to the presence of transient ischemia or of impending stroke. In young patients, cerebral vascular disease is uncommon, but a seizure may lead to a diagnosis of an arteriovenous malformation, an aneurysm, collagen vascular disease, or a rare case of cortical thrombophlebitis.

Seizures and Infections

A seizure may be one of the first manifestations of bacterial meningitis, particularly in the very young and in the very old patient in whom the classic signs of meningitis may be lacking. Less fulminant forms of meningitis, such as cryptococcal or tuberculous meningitis, have been known to produce seizures that recur over weeks or months. Viral encephalitides, for example herpes simplex encephalitis, may also produce seizures. Human immunodeficiency virus (HIV) infection (see Chapter 34) is increasingly of concern as an etiology for neurological and systemic disease; most seizures in association with acquired immune deficiency syndrome (AIDS) result from opportunistic infections, such as cerebral toxoplasmosis, or from cnetral nervous system (CNS) lymphoma (20). Meningoencephalitis from any agent can scar the cortex, so that an epileptic focus is established that remains symptomatic years after the infection is eradicated.

For reasons that are poorly understood, systemic infections may trigger seizures in susceptible patients, even if the infection does not directly involve the central nervous system. However, when a patient presents with a seizure and signs of infection, especially if the seizure is focal or if focal signs are detected on neurological examination, the possibility of brain abscess must be explored.

EVALUATION OF A PATIENT WITH SEIZURES

When evaluating a patient for a possible seizure disorder, three questions must be answered: First, was the event a seizure? Second, if so, what type of seizure was it? Third, are there clues in the history, physical examination, or laboratory tests that point to an etiology of the seizure?

Differential Diagnosis of Seizure-Like Behavior

Determination of the nature of a seizure-like episode may be difficult (Table 80.3). Unless the physician has observed an attack, the patient and surrogate observers must specify whether or not it represented an episode "punched out in time" with specific signs of neurological dysfunction. The features that are most helpful in confirming that a seizure has occurred include tonic-clonic sequences, with or without tongue biting and incontinence; rhythmic jerking of a limb or of the face; and speech and motor arrest followed by automatisms. The differential diagnosis is dependent upon the character of the attack. Loss of consciousness raises the possibility of syncope (see Chapter 81); if a careful observer can specify sudden loss of consciousness and tone with no abnormal motor activity, syncope due to a cardiovascular problem is a much more likely diagnosis than is seizure. Transient numbness, weakness, speech or vision problems, or dizziness may occur as part of a cerebrovascular syndrome (see Chapter 83), including transient ischemic attacks, stroke, bleeding from an arteriovenous malformation or from an aneurysm, or migraine (see Chapter 79). Context may help to distinguish seizure from cerebrovascular disease, but particularly in the elderly, when the two conditions are linked, a firm diagnosis may have to be deferred.

Narcolepsy (see Chapter 85) is a relatively uncommon disorder in which people suddenly lapse into rapid eye movement (REM) sleep with associated inhibition of muscle tone ("cataplexy"). These patients can be aroused from their sleep, will often report that they dreamed during the attack, and will deny postictal confusion. Waxing and waning *delirium* (see Chapter 17) with occasional motor manifestations, such as might be produced by renal failure or by a drug

intoxication, may superficially resemble a seizure, but the episode will usually lack both the stereotypical aspects of a seizure and its clear start and finish.

Vertigo, from disease of the inner ear, can present paroxysmally and may be confused with epilepsy (see Chapter 81). Certain adults have tics that, unlike a true seizure, may be brought in part under voluntary control and often occur at predictable times.

In some patients, the major challenge is to decide whether episodes described as "seizures" are in fact *psychogenic symptoms*. Anxiety attacks can produce recurrent, fulminant, and moderately stereotyped symptomatology, all of which may be seen in patients with partial complex seizures. Because seizures may have emotional concomitants (for example, an aura of extreme fear) and may be triggered by stressful situations, it is evident how difficult the differential diagnosis may be. If a diagnosis of psychogenic illness can be supported on other grounds, if the attacks are strongly linked to preceding anxiety, and if automatisms are lacking, then a functional spell becomes a likely diagnosis.

Conversion disorder, presenting as "seizures," represent an extreme, but not uncommon, example of psychogenic seizure-like behavior. Unlike a malingerer, the patient with pseudoseizures due to a conversion disorder has no clear awareness of "faking" a spell. Observation of a generalized attack may reveal features unlikely to be part of physiological seizures— for example, retention of protective reflexes such as blink reflex, or the patient's making an effort to breath when the airway is briefly occluded, or talking, or showing directed eye movements. The motor activity may lack the organized tonic-clonic stages seen with grand mal epilepsy, unless the patient is sophisticated and has observed seizures before. (Unfortunately, this is often the case.) Psychogenic psychomotor spells may be the most difficult to diagnose. As a general rule, purposeful, goal-directed behavior, such as driving, shopping, talking in full sentences, or committing acts of specific violence, should not be considered to be part of the seizure unless there is strong supporting evidence. Positive features suggestive of conversion disorder—presence of secondary gain, "la belle indifference," inappropriate reactions to stress—may contribute to a correct diagnosis. Consultation among primary physician, neurologist, and psychiatrist may be required for proper diagnosis and management (see also Chapter 12, "Somatization").

Table 80.3.
Differential Diagnosis of Seizure-Like Behavior

Condition	See Chapter
Syncope	81
Cerebrovascular disease	83
Migraine	79
Narcolepsy	85
Fluctuating delirium	17
Paroxysmal vertigo	81
Breath-holding spells	
Episodic movement disorders	82
Functional episodes	12
Conversion Disorders	12

Classifying the Seizure

In actual practice, classifying a seizure (see above) goes hand in hand with establishing that a seizure has, in fact, occurred. Emphasis should be placed on a careful description of the start of the episode, because a fleeting focal onset or an aura may be the only indication that a seizure was a secondarily generalized rather than a grand mal seizure.

Establishing Etiology

The history usually supplies the main clues to the etiology of a seizure. Careful note should be taken of any birth trauma or perinatal illness, febrile convulsions, past head trauma, prior stroke or intracranial hemorrhage, previous encephalitis or meningitis, cancers, and any prior seizures. A family history of seizures is pertinent, because there is increased risk, particularly with primary generalized epilepsies, for seizures in relatives of people with epilepsy. Use of alcohol and/or barbiturates and of drugs that may provoke seizures, such as amphetamine, phenothiazines, tricyclic antidepressants, anticholinergics, or aminophylline, must be ascertained. Certain patients know of factors that precipitate their attack. For example, some will recognize as a precipitant the flashing-light effect that occurs in situations such as changing the channels on a television set, being in a setting where there are strobe lights, or driving rapidly past a row of trees. A small percentage of individuals with epilepsy have idiosyncratic precipitants, such as when certain regions of their skin are touched, loud sounds, or even such complex activities as reading, calculating, laughing, eating, or listening to music. These so-called "reflex seizures" may be aborted in some instances by avoiding the offending stimuli.

Physical examination will reveal whether a seizure patient is neurologically normal. Subtle asymmetries on the neurological examination may lead to diagnosis of a structural lesion that is generating the seizure. Furthermore, the general physical examination may give clues to an underlying cause (Table 80.4). One should be wary of findings that occur immediately after a seizure and should take the opportunity to recheck them in a few hours or a few days.

Laboratory Evaluation of a Patient with Seizures

Laboratory tests usually are not very helpful in determining whether a seizure has taken place, but they may be useful in establishing an etiology and in patient management.

Routine Laboratory Tests

The data base should include a hematocrit value, a white blood cell and differential count, a measurement of blood urea nitrogen or of serum creatinine, serum glucose, and serum electrolytes. Other tests (for example, measurements of blood gases and of liver function) should be ordered only if there is some suspicion that they may be abnormal. A number of striking abnormalities (metabolic acidosis, marked leukocytosis) may develop transiently immediately after an attack. A baseline electrocardiogram is useful, although immediately after a seizure it may show ST-T wave changes or arrhythmias that are transient and are results of, rather than causes of, seizure activity.

One test that may occasionally be helpful in seizure evaluation is measurement of serum prolactin. After tonic-clonic or complex partial seizures serum prolactin rises two to three times the upper limit of normal in more than 80% of cases that are not psychogenic seizures (16). Unfortunately, the rise in only present during the 10 to 60 minutes after a seizure. Positive findings are thus suggestive, but negative findings, especially measured remote in time from the episode, are inconclusive.

Table 80.4.
General Physical Signs Suggesting Causes of Epilepsy[a]

System	Signs	Disease
Skin and membrane	Petechiae	Subacute bacterial endocarditis (SBE), blood dyscrasias, leukemia, thrombocytopenic purpura, fat emboli
	Cyanosis	Cyanotic congenital heart disease, pulmonary disease
	Icterus	Liver disease, sickle cell disease, thrombotic thrombocytopenic purpura (Moschowitz)
	Malar skin rash	Systemic lupus erythematosus
	Facial port wine stain	Sturge-Weber-Dimitri disease
	Café au lait spots	Neurofibromatosis
	Depigmented spots	Tuberous sclerosis
Head	Head circumference ↑ or ↓	Hydrocephalus, macrocephaly, microcephaly
	Bruit	Arteriovenous malformation
Fundi	Papilledema	↑ intracranial pressure—brain tumor, hemorrhage
	Hemorrhage	Subarachnoid hemorrhage, hypertension, systemic bleeding tendency
	Exudate	SBE, diabetes mellitus, hypertension
	Retinal lesions	Intrauterine infections, tuberous sclerosis
Neck	Meningeal signs—stiff neck	Meningitis, subarachnoid hemorrhage, fractured odontoid, herniated cerebellar tonsils
	↓ Carotid pulses or bruit	Cerebrovascular disease
Circulation	Hypertension	Renal disease, cardiovascular disease, coarctation of aorta, collagen disease
	Arrhythmia	Cardiac disease—congenital, rheumatic, arteriosclerotic heart disease
Abdomen	Organomegaly	Liver disease, neoplasm, hematological disease
	Mass	Neoplasm
Bones and joints	Clubbing	Lung carcinoma, cyanotic congenital heart disease

[a] From Solomon GE, Plum F: *Clinical Management of Seizures.* Philadelphia, WB Saunders 1976.

Electroencephalography

The EEG is the most useful of the laboratory studies in the diagnosis of seizure disorders. An EEG may show generalized or focal epileptiform activity or, even in the absence of such activity, may demonstrate asymmetries of basic rhythms, focal slow waves, or diffuse slowing, all of which may give direction to further investigation. In general, the EEG should not be relied upon to make a diagnosis of a seizure but to confirm a clinical impression derived from the history. When history and EEG are at variance, primacy should go to the history. Patients should not be treated for epilepsy because of an abnormal EEG alone, since interictal epileptiform discharges may be seen in 0.4% of the healthy population, in 2.2% of patients with nonepileptic neurological disease, and in 3.5% of asymptomatic relatives of people with epilepsy (13). On the other hand, one should not be dissuaded from a clear impression of a seizure disorder because the EEG is negative. Interictal EEGs are usually normal in children with petit mal epilepsy, and they may be normal in from 10 to 50% of individuals with grand mal or partial elementary or partial complex seizures, depending upon the conditions of recording, the duration of recording, and the vagaries of any sampling process (24). When EEG confirmation of seizure activity is needed (for example, when the history is equivocal) repeated studies, 24-hour monitoring of tracings with concomitant observation of behavior, recordings after sleep deprivation, stimulatory techniques, such as hyperventilation or flash, or use of nasopharyngeal sphenopalatine leads may be indicated. Recently, epilepsy monitoring units have become available at centers specializing in diagnosis and treatment of epilepsy. Referral to such units is sometimes the most effective way to clarify the nature of spells not clarified by more routine maneuvers.

Epileptiform EEG discharges can usually be observed in the presence of anticonvulsant drugs, although some generalized discharges may be blunted. Medications should not be altered for the first EEG. If tracings are repeatedly negative and a suspicion of epilepsy remains, then admission to a hospital, rapid tapering of medicines in concert with EEGs, and direct observation off medicines may clarify the picture. Among patients with epilepsy, the pattern of generalized EEG slowing without seizure discharges is a fairly common finding, usually resulting from a postictal state or from intoxication due to a medication or other substance the patient has ingested.

Because EEGs can remain abnormal for a few weeks after a major seizure, any findings should be confirmed with repeated studies. An EEG is without risk, unless there are consequences from an injudicious interpretation. (See description of "Patient Experience," Chapter 78.)

Lumbar Puncture

Certain conditions that lead to seizures may require examination of cerebrospinal fluid to secure a diagnosis; chronic meningitis is an example. Data are not available from the medical literature on the yield of lumbar puncture in investigation of patients with various types of seizures; consequently, it is not possible to be dogmatic about whether this test is a requirement for all patients with seizures. The context of the seizure often resolves the issue. A normal child with classic petit mal epilepsy probably does not need a lumbar puncture. A patient in whom a mass lesion is strongly suspected should not have a routine spinal tap until other studies have given information on the risk of cerebral herniation. Most other patients, with focal or generalized seizures of uncertain etiology, should undergo spinal fluid analysis (see "Patient Experience," Chapter 78).

After prolonged generalized seizures the cerebrospinal fluid may show a pleocytosis of up to 100 cells, presumably from a transient breakdown of the blood brain barrier (26). Clearly, however, infection must be the diagnosis of first concern in this setting.

Imaging

Computerized tomographic scans (see "Patient Experience," Chapter 78) of patients with primary generalized seizures are abnormal (excluding nonspecific atrophy) in about 10% of instances. Scans of individuals with focal motor or secondarily generalized seizures show a focal abnormality about 65% of the time (21). Patients with partial complex seizures show abnormalities about 36% of the time. The most common findings are focal atrophy and evidence of old ischemia or hemorrhage; less commonly there is evidence of infection, tumor, or another abnormality. If the neurological examination reveals focal signs, the CT scan is especially likely to be positive. Magnetic resonance imaging (MRI), where available, is preferable to CT scanning in the evaluation of seizures, because the diagnostic yield is slightly higher than that of CT, at no added, or reduced (no contrast agent), risk (6).

The following recommendations seem reasonable: All patients with focal or secondarily generalized seizures or with an abnormal neurological examination should have an MRI or a CT scan with (unless there is a contraindication) contrast injection. In patients with a negative examination and in children the decision to perform a scan should be individualized. Lastly, imaging may be indicated when a stable pattern of seizures deteriorates.

Other Diagnostic Tests

"Traditional" neuroradiological studies—skull X-rays, radionuclide brain scan, pneumoencephalography, and arteriography—have to a great extent been supplanted by CT and MRI scanning in the initial evaluation of a seizure disorder, but each still has its own special indications that will be pointed out when appropriate by the consulting neurologist. Two techniques show promise for definition of seizure foci but are still considered experimental: imaging of brain metabolism and chemistry by positron emission tomographic (PET) scanning (19), and magnetoencephalographic recording of brain activity (30).

TREATMENT OF EPILEPSY

Except in unusual instances, epilepsy cannot be "cured." In about three of four patients it can, however, be controlled so that patients experience no seizures or only a very rare seizure. Most attention in the medical literature has been focused on details of pharmacological management for seizures, but the importance of a comprehensive approach cannot be overemphasized: an individual who is seizure free, but so toxic from medicines that employment is impossible, is at best a dubious success. Employment problems and other social aspects of managing epilepsy are considered below. Patient education, removal of precipitating factors for seizures, reduction of stress, provision for adequate amounts of rest, and attention to proper diet can all be important in control of epilepsy are also discussed below.

General Principles of Drug Therapy

It has been said that half of those patients who have generalized seizures monthly or more frequently are probably undertreated. In contrast, other patients are maintained on unnecessary or improper regimens of anticonvulsants. To achieve the ideal goal of seizure control without toxicity, the general principles listed in Table 80.5 should be followed.

In deciding *whether to treat a first seizure*, one should recall that a single seizure does not necessarily mandate a diagnosis of epilepsy nor a need for chronic therapy. As noted previously, early seizures after head trauma or stroke, or seizures in association with some clear precipitant such as alcohol withdrawal, should in general be treated conservatively. The more difficult decision involves the patient with a single "idiopathic" convulsion, because there is a 50% risk of having a second seizure (see above). Some patients are so frightened of the possibility of having another seizure, with potential repercussions for employment, social relations, and license to drive, that they are willing to accept the inconvenience of chronic medication. Other patients would prefer not to be medicated until they have another seizure. Clearly, the decision to treat after a first seizure must be individualized. After a second attack, most physicians would initiate therapy.

To select the appropriate anticonvulsant, it is important to know the type of seizure under consideration. Table 80.6 represents a general, but not unanimous, consensus on drugs of choice and alternates for the main forms of epilepsy. One large controlled trial has compared the effectiveness of four anticonvulsants—carbamazepine, phenobarbital, phenytoin, and valproic acid—for the treatment of partial and secondary generalized tonic-clonic seizures (18). Both carbamazepine and phenytoin were highly effective; both of these are recommended as drugs of first choice for these two common types of seizures. Valproic acid is generally recommended as the drug of first choice for primary generalized tonic-clonic (grand mal) seizures. Absence (petit mal) may be treated either with ethosuximide or valproic acid, although the former will not prevent concurrent tonic-clonic seizures. Myoclonic seizures are best treated with clonazepam (a benzodiazepine) or valproic acid. A certain percentage of generalized tonic-clonic seizures will respond to monotherapy with carbamazepine, and a certain percentage of partial seizures to valproate monotherapy. In several instances, more than one drug may be considered the "drug of choice" in terms of efficacy, in which case the selection can be made on the basis of personal familiarity with the drug, convenience of schedule, or the relative risk of side effects. There are several reviews comparing controlled trials of anticonvulsants that the reader may wish to consult (14, 31). Dosages, half-lives, serum levels, and main potential side effect of the drugs are given in Table 80.7.

Drugs should be initiated at one-quarter or one-half of the anticipated maintenance dosage (except for phenytoin and phenobarbital—see below), and the dosage should be advanced over several weeks, in order to avoid significant early toxicity that might discourage the patient from continuing with treatment. Because some of the medications remain in the blood for some time, it may take several days before the effects of a dosage adjustment are manifest.

There is a long and deplorable tradition of treating epilepsy with several drugs simultaneously, stemming

Table 80.5.
Principles of Drug Therapy

Decide whether to treat.
Select the proper drug for the particular form of epilepsy.
Start drugs slowly and build up levels gradually, to avoid toxicity.
Start with one drug, and use it to effect or toxicity before adding another.
Choose the simplest regimen possible.
Suspect compliance problems in treatment failures.
Monitor blood levels in problem cases.
Withdraw medications gradually.
Decide how long to treat.

Table 80.6.
Drugs of Choice

Seizure Category	Drugs of Choice	Alternatives
Primary generalized, tonic-clonic	Valproic acid Phenobarbital	Carbamazepine Phenytoin Primidone
Primary generalized, absence	Ethosuximide Valproic acid	Clonazepam
Primary myoclonic	Valproic acid Clonazepam	Phenytoin Phenobarbital
Partial simple and complex and secondarily generalized epilepsy	Carbamazepine Phenytoin	Valproic acid Phenobarbital Primidone
Mixed forms	Valproic acid Clonazepam	Carbamazepine Phenytoin Phenobarbital

Table 80.7.
Major Antiseizure Medications

Medication (Brand Name)	Available Strengths (mg)	Typical Adult Dose, Range, Schedule	Half-life (hr)	Levels (mg/liter[f])	Major Side Effects
Phenytoin (Dilantin)	100 capsules	300 mg 1 time daily[b] (200–500 mg)	22	10–20	Ataxia Cosmetic changes Rash Rare blood changes Osteomalacia
Phenobarbital (Luminal)	15, 30, 60, 100 tablets	100 mg 1 time daily	72	15–40	Sedation Hyperactivity Confusion Mood change
Primidone (Mysoline)	50, 250 scored tablets	250 mg 3 or 4 times daily (500–1500 mg)	3–12[c] 72[d]	6–12[c] 15–40[d]	Sedation Hyperactivity Mood change
Carbamazepine (Tegretol)	200 tablets (100 chewable)[e]	200 mg 3 or 4 times daily (400–2000 mg)	10–25	4–12	Gastrointestinal (GI) distress Ataxia Blurred vision Blood changes Hepatotoxicity
Ethosuximide (Zarontin)	250 capsules	250 mg 3 or 4 times daily (500–1500 mg)	30	50–100	GI distress Sedation Headache Dizziness
Valproic acid (Depakene)	250 capsules	250 mg 2 to 4 times daily (500–4000 mg)	8–12	50–100	GI distress Drowsiness Ataxia Alopecia Tremor Blood changes Rare liver toxicity Rare pancreatitis
Clonazepam (Klonopin)	0.5, 1, 2 tablets	2 mg 3 times daily (2–20 mg)	20–40	0.05–0.7	Drowsiness Ataxia Behavior change Dizziness

[a]These doses are usually attained gradually over days to weeks. The ranges are relatively rough guidelines; because absorption varies, serum levels are better guides to dosage.
[b]Only for Dilantin capsules (Kapseals).
[c]For primidone.
[d]For phenobarbital.
[e]Once daily slow-release form will probably be available in 1991.
[f]Lab may report same figures as micrograms per milliliter.

from times when most patients were started automatically on phenytoin, 100 mg, and phenobarbital, 32 mg, each three times a day. There is no evidence that two drugs in subtherapeutic doses are better tolerated or more effective than one drug in full dose. It has been pointed out that about 90% of new onset seizures can be controlled with one drug (phenytoin or carbamazepine), and that, when one drug is unsuccessful, addition of a second helps in only 36% of cases (29).

Compliance is a major factor in success of drug therapy for epilepsy (also see Chapter 4, Patient Compliance with Medical Advice). To promote compliance, every effort should be made to simplify the dosage regimen. Phenobarbital and certain formulations of phenytoin can be given in a once daily schedule. Therefore, medicines such as carbamazepine, primidone, and valproic acid, which must be given in divided doses, should be employed only when there is an identifiable advantage over phenytoin or phenobarbital. At each visit a patient (or the responsible person) should be asked to report on the exact medication regimen; all too often the answer indicates a need for better spoken, and written, communication with the patient. Familiarity with cost of medicines is important because patients may be hesitant to purchase an expensive medicine unless the need is clearly explained. Generic brands are less expensive; but, for several anticonvulsants, bioavailability of generic products has been quite variable. These are carbamazepine, primidone, phenytoin, and valproic acid. If generic brands of these are dispensed, especially brands from multiple manufacturers, drug levels may have to be checked more often to assure that the patient is getting adequate treatment.

The optimal dose of an anticonvulsant medication may vary several-fold among different patients. Determination of *serum levels* (Table 80.7) is a reliable way to measure how much medication is circulating, but such measurements should not be ordered indiscriminately. If a patient's seizures are controlled and there is no toxicity from a drug regimen, measurement of a serum level is wasteful and might even encourage one to alter a successful regimen. If control is not optimal, drug levels can document inadequate compliance or absorption, or highlight the occasional case when drug toxicity is manifest by increased seizures. The levels can also provide guidance for patients with symptoms that might or might not be due to drug intoxication. Ideally, levels to judge side effects should be taken at times of peak serum levels, and levels to judge anticonvulsant efficacy at times of trough serum levels. It is important to know that for some anticonvulsants, particularly phenytoin, drug dose and drug level are not linearly related: a saturation point is reached above which minor increments in daily dose (for example, increasing from 400 to 500 mg a day of phenytoin) may lead to major increases in serum level and in side effects. A level is most informative if measured in the "steady state" (see Table 80.7), which requires a stable dosage for about four or five half-lives of the medicine before measurement.

The determination of *how long to maintain treatment with anticonvulsants* is a difficult issue, because seizures remit over time, and thus freedom from seizures may or may not be due to the medicine. About one-half to two-thirds of patients will be entirely seizure free for 2 years with therapy. If an adult patient is seizure free for about 5 years on medication and stops treatment by gradual tapering, there is a 30 to 50% chance of relapse in the next 5 years (5, 12). About 90% of the relapses are registered within the first 2 years after discontinuing medication. As with the decision to initiate therapy, the decision to terminate anticonvulsant therapy must be individualized. A patient who was very difficult to control initially, who has an underlying structural lesion, or a persistently abnormal EEG may benefit from lifelong therapy. In contrast, a patient with idiopathic epilepsy who has been seizure free for 2 to 5 years and who is willing to accept an increased risk of having a seizure may be a candidate for drug withdrawal. If more than one drug has been prescribed, the medications should be tapered one at a time, each over a period of one or two months, and reinstated rapidly if seizures recur. An example of a cautious tapering schedule for a patient who has been taking carbamazepine 400 mg (two 200-mg tablets) three times daily would be a reduction by one pill per day every 2 weeks. During tapering and in the first few months after taper of all antiepileptic medications, it is prudent for the patient to refrain from driving.

INDIVIDUAL DRUGS

Phenytoin (Diphenylhydantoin, DPH, PHT, Dilantin)

Since its introduction in 1938, phenytoin has been one of the two major drugs used to treat seizures. It is most useful in grand mal epilepsy, partial simple epilepsy, and secondarily generalized epilepsy. Although it is also used for partial complex epilepsy, carba-

mazepine may have a better benefit:risk ratio in this seizure type. Phenytoin may make petit mal worse.

Phenytoin is absorbed from the gastrointestinal tract in 4 to 8 hours. Without a loading dose, a full week is required to reach therapeutic levels, but a load of three times the daily maintenance, given in the first day, will achieve immediate therapeutic levels. The mean half-life is 22 hours, with a range from 7 to 42 hours. Phenytoin is 90% protein bound, so that a low serum albumin level can lead to an increased concentration of the free agent and to increased toxicity. The drug is metabolized in the liver and is not excreted by the kidney. Therefore, dosage should only be lowered, by about 25%, in renal failure only when there is a decrease in serum albumin. In this situation, the total serum level may be low, but the free drug level will usually be adequate. Phenytoin is partially removed by hemodialysis.

The usual starting dose of phenytoin is 300 mg/day. This medication can be given once a day if it is given as Dilantin capsules, for this preparation is manufactured in slow release form. Other phenytoin preparations are fast release capsules. They are slightly less expensive but must be given in divided doses (i.e., 100 mg three times a day). The therapeutic level for phenytoin is generally between 10 and 20 mg/liter; the toxic range is usually over 20 mg/liter, but patients show fairly wide individual susceptibility to side effects. The lethal dose may range from 2 to 20 g.

Drug-drug interactions. Several drugs elevate phenytoin plasma levels: disulfiram and isoniazid, commonly; coumadin, chloramphenicol, methylphenidate, phenothiazines, benzodiazepines, and propoxyphene, less often. Other drugs may lead to increased phenytoin metabolism, resulting in decreased phenytoin levels: alcohol, folic acid, pyridoxine, theophylline, and occasionally carbamazepine, cimetidine, oral contraceptives, and sulfonamides. These potential drug interactions may be managed best by patient and physician awareness and by observation of serum drug levels during times of medication changes.

There are many potential *undesirable effects* of phenytoin. Dose- related acute effects include nystagmus (seen at therapeutic levels), ataxia (usually above 30 mg/liter), lethargy, paradoxical tendency to increased seizures at higher toxic levels (usually above 40 mg/liter), and allergic reactions. Chronic side effects of phenytoin are generally manifest after a few months to several years of daily ingestion. Chronically progressive cosmetic changes can be vexing in young women. Gum hypertrophy occurs in about 30%; it may be forestalled by good oral hygiene, but once established may regress only partially; hirsutism is seen in 5% overall, but in 30% of young women. Even more disconcerting are facial changes due to thickening of subcutaneous tissue about the nose and eyes, so-called "leonine faces." Cosmetic side effects can be avoided or even reversed by switching to a less well-known hydantoin, ethotoin (Peganone), given in doses of 500 to 1000 mg three times a day (up to 3 g total per day). Skin rash occurs in 2 to 10% of users of phenytoin, with a peak incidence about 2 weeks into the course. Stevens-Johnson syndrome occurs rarely. Lymphadenopathy develops in 2 to 5%, sometimes in association with fever, arthralgia, eosinophilia, and hepatosplenomegaly, presenting a picture of "pseudolymphoma" and, very rarely, true lymphoma. Hepatitis and a variety of blood dyscrasias have been reported. Megaloblastic anemia may occur, which responds to folate. Many patients develop measurable antinuclear antibodies in the serum; some will develop a lupus-like syndrome, characterized by arthralgias, that remits after discontinuing the drug; rarely a patient has progressed to irreversible systemic lupus erythematosus. Peripheral neuropathy with loss of deep tendon reflexes can be documented in about 20% of chronic users. Occasional pulmonary infiltrates and fibrosis have given rise to the term "Dilantin lung." Phenytoin can induce liver enzymes, thereby secondarily affecting metabolism of numerous hormones and drugs. Induced inactivation of vitamin D leads to radiological or biochemical evidence of bone disease in one of every three chronically treated patients. Teratogenic effects of phenytoin are strongly suspected (see below).

Phenobarbital

In past decades phenobarbital was a drug of choice for generalized tonic-clonic seizures. It is now a second-line agent for a variety of seizure types. Phenobarbital is particularly useful in the pediatric age group, where it may be better tolerated than phenytoin because it does not cause cosmetic side effects; it may, however, cause significant behavioral side effects (hyperactivity in up to 40% of children).

Phenobarbital is a long-lasting drug. The gastrointestinal absorption is slow so that levels reach a peak in 10 to 12 hours after an oral dose, compared with 20 minutes after an intravenous dose. The drug is detoxified by the liver and excreted by the kidney, but the dosage need be only slightly reduced in renal failure. The serum half-life is about 72 hours, ranging from 37 to 96 hours. Therapeutic levels are 15 to 40 mg/liter. Phenobarbital is a potent inducer of liver enzymes and leads to rapid tolerance, as well as to alteration of kinetics of numerous other medications. The dose of phenobarbital is 1 to 3 mg/kg/day, or about 100 mg/day for the average adult. Little justification, other than a patient's established pattern, can be made for giving it in divided doses.

The main acute side effect of phenobarbital in adults is sedation. After a few weeks, partial tolerance to the sedation usually develops. In elderly patients phenobarbital can cause confusion and respiratory depression. Subtle or overt personality changes due to phenobarbital probably occur more often than is generally recognized, especially in the elderly. Ataxia and nystagmus are common in all patients at high doses. Occasionally, there is idiosyncratic allergy, with accompanying dermatitis or gastrointestinal symptoms. Phenobarbital must not be administered to potential drug abusers or to unreliable patients who might precipitously discontinue their medicine.

Primidone (Mysoline)

Primidone is a barbiturate that is used for treatment of partial complex seizures (usually as a second choice after carbamazepine (see below). It has also been used in place of phenobarbital for treatment of grand mal or focal seizures, when the latter drug has failed, but it should not be a drug of first choice for these conditions. Primidone is excreted in part unchanged and is in part metabolized to phenobarbital and to phenylethylmalonic acid (PEMA). Primidone and PEMA are cleared in hours, whereas the phenobarbital persists for days. Serum levels of primidone and PEMA can be ascertained, but it often suffices just to confirm that a therapeutic steady state level of phenobarbital is present. In order to benefit from the short-lived primidone and PEMA, each of which has some anticonvulsant action, primidone must be given in three or four divided doses. A therapeutic dose is usually around 250 mg orally three or four times a day, but the initial doses should be much lower to avoid inducing extreme sedation. A test dose of 50 mg should be given to observe for idiosyncratic marked hypersomnolence. If none occurs, then it is reasonable to start with 125 to 250 mg daily, with increments each week, until therapeutic effect, therapeutic levels, unacceptable sedation, or the maximal dose of 2 g per day is reached. The dosage should be reduced by about half in patients with significant renal failure.

Side effects of primidone parallel those of phenobarbital, except that primidone tends to be more sedating.

Carbamazepine (Tegretol)

Carbamazepine is one of the newest of the major anticonvulsants used in the United States, but over two decades of use for seizures and for treatment of chronic neuropathic pains have proven it to be a safe and effective medicine. Carbamazepine is one of the drugs of choice in partial complex epilepsy. Studies comparing carbamazepine with other anticonvulsants for treatment of partial epilepsy have showed the highest rates of complete remission for patients taking carbamazepine (although mean seizure frequency was similar for patients taking carbamazepine, phenytoin, or phenobarbital) (18). Carbamazepine has efficacy probably equal to that of phenytoin in the treatment of partial simple and of generalized seizures. Therapeutic serum levels are 4 to 12 mg/liter. The adult dose is 400 to 2000 mg/day. Tablets come in 200-mg (or 100-mg chewable) sizes, and it is advisable to initiate therapy with no more than 200 to 400 mg/day, advancing to the full dose over a week or two. The half-life is about 10 to 25 hours, and dosage should be divided into three or four times a day regimens. If compliance is a problem, sometimes a twice daily dosage will suffice. A once daily slow-release form of carbamazepine may become available within the near future.

Because carbamazepine, in tablet form, may lose one-third or more of its effectiveness if stored in humid conditions, patients should be advised to keep their tablet containers in a dry location, away from the bathroom. Recently manufacturers have been asked by the Food and Drug Administration to package carbamazepine in moisture-proof containers.

The *side effects* of carbamazepine include fatigue, nystagmus, diplopia, dizziness, ataxia, dysarthria, rash (including rarely the Stevens-Johnson syndrome), inappropriate secretion of antidiuretic hormone, occasionally abnormal liver function tests, and an infrequent lupus-like syndrome. Gastrointestinal distress is the most common side effect, particularly if the medication is initiated too rapidly. Reversible leukopenia or thrombocytopenia is seen in 5 to 10% of patients, so that blood counts should be monitored weekly at the start of therapy and then every few months. This drug has had a reputation for causing aplastic anemia, based largely on six cases of this complication that were reported in the l960s (even though a causal relation to carbamazepine was not established). The actual incidence of aplastic anemia is not known, but it is thought to be very rare. The "black box" warning in the Physician's Desk Reference about carbamazepine and blood dyscrasias has recently been modified, to report a baseline population incidence of potentially fatal dyscrasia of 8 per million, and an incidence in a population that is taking carbamazepine of about 50 per million.

Ethosuximide (Zarontin)

Ethosuximide is the drug of choice for treatment of absence epilepsy in children. It has little efficacy in other types of seizures.

Valproic Acid (Sodium Valproate, Depakene, Depakote)

Valproic acid is a relatively recent addition to the list of major drugs used to treat seizures. Its effectiveness is quite broad, but it is thought to be particularly valuable for absence attacks in children, and for tonic-clonic and myoclonic epilepsy. Recent studies suggest some efficacy of valproate as a second-line agent for control of partial seizures (7).

Valproic acid is a fatty acid, structurally dissimilar from all other common anticonvulsants. It comes in 250-mg capsules (also as coated tablets purported by the manufacturer to cause less gastrointestinal upset) and as an elixir. Peak serum levels are reached in 1 to 4 hours after ingestion, and the half-life is about 8 to 12 hours. The drug is metabolized in the liver and excreted in the urine in modified form. Serum levels may be measured but at present have limited utility. The approximate therapeutic range is 50 to 100 mg/liter. The manufacturer suggests initiation of therapy with a dose of about 10 to 15 mg/kg/day, to be increased at weekly intervals by about 5 to 10 mg/kg/day to a

maximal dose of 60 mg/kg/day. A common final regimen is 250 to 500 mg orally, two to four times/day.

In studies on several thousand patients abroad, before the release of the drug in the United States in 1978, valproic acid proved to be quite safe. About one in five patients had significant side effects—commonly gastrointestinal upset, drowsiness, rash, reversible hair loss, weight loss or gain, ataxia, tremor, or hyperactivity. A limited number of studies suggest that valproic acid inhibits platelet aggregation and may prolong the bleeding time, but this effect is poorly documented. Less commonly, valproate may produce frank thrombocytopenia. The risk of valproate that has received the greatest attention in this country has been hepatic toxicity. Thirty-seven hepatic fatalities in association with valproic acid were reported in the United States over the period 1978 to 1984 (9). Among patients receiving valproate as monotherapy, the calculated rate of fatality from hepatic injury was 1 per 37,000. This rate was much higher for children less than 2 years old, and for children on polytherapy. These two risk factors together led to a hepatic fatality rate of 1 per 500 children. In contrast no hepatic fatalities were reported in patients over 10 years of age on monotherapy. Several patients have developed serious episodes of pancreatitis while taking valproic acid. Because of these recently discovered toxicities, and because of high cost, valproic acid has not yet replaced ethosuximide as the drug of choice for petit mal epilepsy unless there are concurrent atypical absence attacks or tonic-clonic seizures.

Clonazepam (Klonopin)

Clonazepam is a benzodiazepine drug, closely related to diazepam, that is used principally for treatment of myoclonus. It is not approved in the United States for treatment of partial seizures but has been used effectively for these conditions in Europe. Oral clonazepam has a serum half-life of 20 to 40 hours. Serum levels vary from .05 to .7 mg/liter and correlate only very roughly with clinical effect. Because of the sedative effect of clonazepam, therapy is usually initiated very gradually, beginning with 0.01 to 0.15 mg/kg, increased each third day to clinical effect or to maintenance at 0.1 to 0.2 mg/kg/day. In adults the daily maximal dose is 20 mg. Clonazepam commonly produces drowsiness, ataxia, and behavioral changes and can also cause dizziness and decreased muscle tone.

Other Anticonvulsants

No attempt has been made to catalog all of the agents used as anticonvulsants; only the major drugs of choice for the common types of seizures have been discussed. Ineffectiveness of the standard agents, when applied in accordance with the general therapeutic principles given previously, is certainly an indication for specialty referral and for possible trials of the more unusual therapies. Practitioners frequently use diazepam or chlordiazepoxide to treat seizures, and although these drugs do have some efficacy, this practice is not recommended except in special cases, such as in ethanol withdrawal or status epilepticus. Benzodiazepines, other than clonazepam, have drawbacks for chronic therapy; anticonvulsant effects tend to diminish as sedative effects accumulate.

REFERRAL TO A NEUROLOGIST

The use of a neurologist to help with diagnosis and evaluation of epilepsy depends upon the experience of the primary physician. Common management problems for which referral may be helpful are listed in Table 80.8.

HOSPITALIZATION

Few general statements can be made about the need for hospital admission of seizure patients, because availability of monitoring systems, emergency room "holding rooms," and availability of inpatient beds vary from locale to locale. A set of reasonable guidelines is shown in Table 80.8. Individuals brought to offices or emergency rooms after a first seizure are usually admitted in order to facilitate the diagnostic workup and to observe the patient in case a serious underlying cause, for example, meningitis or subdural hematoma, is present. This principle has exceptions. A young patient with a normal examination and a reliable family may be evaluated in an ambulatory setting. Any patient with new focal signs on examination should be admitted, as should obtunded patients, febrile patients, or those whose postictal lethargy persists for over 1/2 hour. A patient with a crescendo pattern of seizures, with several in one day, especially

Table 80.8.
When to Refer or to Hospitalize the Patient with Seizures

DIAGNOSTIC ISSUES
  Question about whether a seizure took place
  Abnormal physical examination
  Questionable focal findings
  Focal seizures
  Focality on the EEG
  Need for special diagnostics (e.g., lumbar puncture, CT or MRI scan)
  Uncertainty about etiology
THERAPEUTIC ISSUES
  Adjustment of an existing drug regimen that is complex
  Patient does not respond to a drug of choice
  Patient has significant medication side effects
  Patient wishes to become pregnant
  Patient wishes to taper off medication
  Significant change in the pattern of seizures
WHEN TO HOSPITALIZE
  Most new onset seizures
  New focal signs on examination
  Obtunded or prolonged "postical" patients
  Febrile patients
  Crescendo pattern of seizures
  All cases of status epilepticus
  Barbiturate withdrawal seizures
  Possibility of rapidly expanding mass lesion
  Seizures after recent head trauma
  Need for special inpatient studies
  Consideration for neurosurgery
  Monitoring of compliance

if tonic-clonic, should be admitted to a hospital immediately. Status epilepticus, when continuous or back-to-back seizures occur without intervening return of consciousness, is a true medical emergency and requires immediate hospitalization. Barbiturate withdrawal seizures may become fulminant; therefore, patients having seizures in this setting should be admitted. If the possibility exists of a rapidly expanding mass lesion, such as tumor, abscess, or possible hematoma after head trauma, then admission should not be delayed. Legitimate reasons for elective admissions include a need for special inpatient studies (arteriography, continuous monitoring), for evaluation for possible neurosurgical procedures for intractable epilepsy, and, lastly, for trials of supervised drug management to rule out noncompliance as a factor in treatment failure.

Admission is usually not needed for those patients who are known to have chronically recurrent seizures, whose pattern of seizures is stable, whose etiology is established or is thought to be idiopathic on the basis of a prior thorough workup, who have fully recovered from recent seizures, who have normal examinations (or static documented old deficits), and who are reliable enough to return for follow-up.

SOCIAL ISSUES AND PATIENT EDUCATION

Once a serious underlying etiology has been ruled out, the physician tends to view epilepsy as a benign disease. From the viewpoint of the patient, this is often far from the case. Seizures are distressing for every patient and for the patient's family. Fear of having a seizure can cause people with epilepsy to withdraw from society, and those who are willing to compete may be faced with nearly insurmountable discrimination.

The Commission for the Control of Epilepsy and Its Consequences (1977) found that the unemployment rate among those with epilepsy is twice the national average, and the underemployment rate is even higher. Suspension of a driver's license may make it nearly impossible to get to work. Children may be denied participation in sports or moved unnecessarily to "special sections" in school. People with epilepsy marry less often than matched cohorts; a significant fraction of the public believes that individuals with epilepsy are likely to be physically unattractive. Because of these and other social stigmata associated with epilepsy, it is important to focus on the patient's overall functioning, rather than simply on seizure control. The patient and family should be counseled regularly to help them to address those concerns that limit full participation in society.

Patients should be told that epilepsy is a medical illness, for too many carry notions, that it is a punishment for some past abuse. Whereas a single seizure should not be labeled as "epilepsy," definite epilepsy should not be mislabeled as something else, to avoid facing the correct diagnosis. The patient should know that individual seizures do not cause measurable brain damage and that the condition does not lead to mental deterioration. Numerous historical figures, including Julius Caesar, Emperor Charles V, Dostoevski, Flaubert, Napolean, Jonathan Swift, Handel and President William McKinley, achieved high stations while suffering from frequent seizures. The prognosis of epilepsy is good.

Restrictions of Activity

Patients often ask for guidelines about what they can and cannot do. Maximal activity consistent with avoidance of personal injury should be the goal. The specifics must be formulated by a physician familiar with the individual patient and his pattern of seizures. Patients with nocturnal seizures need not be restricted during the day. Contact sports are safe for people with infrequent seizures. Common sense dictates limits on activities when a seizure could be fatal, for example, flying, rock climbing, or scuba diving. Some potentially hazardous activities, such as swimming, are acceptable if provisions can be made for proper supervision. Seizures are not contraindications to strenuous activities, including sex. Alcohol consumption (in moderation) can be enjoyed by most with impunity.

Driving a Motor Vehicle

Overall, motor vehicle accident rates for people with epilepsy are about twice the rates in control subjects. The contribution to total traffic accidents by people with epilepsy is low, estimated at 1/10,000 accidents (33). By comparison, it is estimated that 6/10,000 of deaths at the wheel are from natural causes and that 5,000/10,000 are due to alcohol use. Approximately 12 to 20% of accidents in persons with epilepsy occur with the patient's first seizure. Despite these statistics, seizures at the wheel do occur and can represent both personal and public dangers. The key element of increased risk is blunting or loss of consciousness. Seizures without this element—for example, partial simple motor seizures—do not affect the risk of driving, and patients with this type of epilepsy are usually exempted from regulations.

Some states require that physicians directly report occurrence of seizures to the Department of Motor Vehicles; others require only documentation in the medical record that the patient has been informed of the risks for traffic accidents and has been instructed to contact the Motor Vehicle Department for a hearing. Patients and physicians should be honest in their communications; both are potentially liable for consequences of inaccurate or incomplete information. In general, the physician should address the medical facts of a case and leave the final determination of licensing to the state authorities. If an applicant has regular lapses of consciousness, the license will usually be suspended until a period of from 3 months to 2 years without seizures has elapsed (depending upon the state);

the recent trend in this country has been to consider shorter periods of suspension.

Employment

It is illegal to discriminate against handicapped individuals, including people with epilepsy, in the job marketplace. If an individual with seizures is unemployed or dissatisfied with work, the patient's physician should be quick to refer to a local rehabilitation agency for possible retraining, patient and employer education, or advice on legal action.

The Epilepsy Foundation of America (4351 Garden City Drive 406, Landover, Maryland, 20785, 301-459-3700) is a central nonprofit organization that can serve as a source for information and action on social aspects of epilepsy; at least one chapter exists in each state. Their training and placement service (TAPS) has been effective in training people with epilepsy for work and in finding them employment, either in the general work pool or in sheltered workshops. The same local organizations may further aid patients and physicians with regular group counseling for those who cannot live independently, or in providing for regular home visits by visiting nurses and other medical personnel.

Some patients with difficult to control seizures should be advised to apply for medical disability under Social Security (see criteria in Table 9.4).

Pregnancy

Special problems are raised by a woman with epilepsy who is, or wishes to become, pregnant (35). About 0.4% of all pregnancies occur in mothers with seizures. In women with epilepsy childbearing carries an above average risk for toxemia, vaginal hemorrhage, and complicated labor. The rate of premature births and perinatal deaths is elevated. Seizures become more difficult to control during pregnancy in about 50% of cases, easier to control in about 10%, and unchanged in the rest. Rarely, pregnancy can induce a new onset of recurring idiopathic seizures. Antiepileptic medications—phenytoin, carbamazepine, valproic acid, and to a lesser extent all of the other agents—are believed to be teratogenic. Studies suggest that the incidence of congenital abnormalities, particularly cleft lip, cleft palate, and cardiac defects, is two to six times more common in offspring of drug-treated mothers with epilepsy. Valproate has specifically been associated with about a 1% risk of neural tube closure defects.

Unfortunately, no study has delineated the relative contribution of medication and of epilepsy itself to this increased incidence of congenital abnormalities. Authorities agree that major motor seizures can produce anoxic, ischemic, or traumatic damage to a fetus and that this risk must be balanced against the teratogenic potential of medication. The best solution to the above dilemma is careful advance planning. Physicians should not only ask their patients to plan pregnancies, but to alert them to the plan months in advance. Prior to pregnancy special efforts can be made to taper medications or to switch to phenobarbital or carbamazepine, which may be less teratogenic than phenytoin or valproate. Brief psychomotor or absence seizures pose no known risk to a fetus, and a decision may be made by the patient to tolerate them during pregnancy. If pregnancy is unexpected, an ongoing successful regimen of anticonvulsants should probably be continued, to avoid the possibility of fulminant withdrawal seizures during a critical obstetrical stage. Ultimately, all of these relative risks must be discussed among primary and specialist physicians, patient, and husband, so that a mutually satisfactory plan can be chosen. The problems of childbearing are increased for mothers with epilepsy, but not greatly, and only the severely disabled epileptic woman should be flatly discouraged from having children.

Mothers taking anticonvulsants who wish to breast-feed may do so, because the amount of antiepileptic medications excreted in breast milk is low .

Potential parents wonder about the likelihood that their child will have epilepsy if they or one of their children have epilepsy. Although there are methodological problems in performing studies to answer this question, it can generally be said that there is about a 1 in 40 risk of transmitting primary tonic-clonic epilepsy (the risk is primarily from the mother, not the father) and that a positive family history increases the risk 2- to 4-fold (22). When seizures result from head trauma, tumor, drug withdrawal, or other identified causes, then the hereditary risk is not above baseline.

Family Counseling

Families must be told how to behave during a seizure; too often, frantic efforts to "treat" the seizure result in extreme anxiety and broken teeth. Seizures should be allowed to run their course; unless convulsions become nearly continuous (status epilepticus) they are not dangerous, and no first aid can shorten them. The mouth should not be forced open so that matchbooks, pencils, or other objects can be pushed in. The family should be informed that it is impossible to swallow the tongue. It is advisable to move the individual undergoing a seizure away from sharp corners and heights and to turn him on his side to decrease the risk of aspiration. Forcible restraint during a tonic-clonic phase is of no value, and during the automatisms of partial complex seizures restraints may increase agitation. There is little need to fear behavior during automatisms, because directed violence is extremely rare.

Concerned family members may be very helpful in promoting improved seizure control. They should be encouraged to discuss compliance, the cost of a medicine regimen, and how the seizures and/or drug toxicities affect school, work, and social relations. Patients may wish to keep a log of their seizures, medication times, side effects, and possible precipitating stresses. Perfect control of epilepsy with no toxicity is an ideal attained in only a minority of cases; in the remainder, patient, family, and physician can decide in concert how to balance the inconvenience of seizures against the unpleasant effects of medication and thereby achieve the best possible results.

General References

Engel Jr. E (ed): *Seizures and Epilepsy.* Philadelphia, FA Davis, 1989.
Hauser WA (ed): *Current Trends Epilepsy: A Self-Study Course for Physicians.* Landover, MD, Epilepsy Foundation of America, 1988.
Laidlaw J, Richens A: *A Textbook of Epilepsy.* New York, Churchill Livingston, 1982.
    A detailed general textbook about all aspects of clinical epileptology.
Penry JK, Newmark ME: The use of antiepileptic drugs. *Ann Intern Med* 90:207, 1979.
    A review of antiseizure medication, written for practicing physicians.
Solomon GE, Kutt H, Plum F: *Clinical Management of Seizures: A Guide for the Physician,* 3rd ed., Philadelphia, WB Saunders, 1983.
    Pithy summary of seizure therapeutics.
Temkin O: *The Falling Sickness: A History of Epilepsy from the Greeks to the Beginnings of Modern Neurology.* Baltimore, The Johns Hopkins Press, 1971.
    The definitive history of epilepsy from ancient to modern times.

Specific References

1. Anderson DW, McLawsin RL: The national head and spinal cord injury survey. *J Neurosurg* 53:51, 1980.
2. Annegers JF, Hauser WA, Elveback LR: Remission of seizures and relapse in patients with epilepsy. *Epilepsia* 20:729, 1979.
3. Annegers JF, Grabow JD, Grover RV, et al: Seizures after head trauma: a population study. *Neurology* 30:683, 1980.
4. Brennan FN, Lyttle JA: Alcohol and seizures: a review. *J Royal Soc Med* 80(9):571, 1987.
5. Callaghan N, Garrett A, Goggin T: Withdrawal of anticonvulsant drugs in patients free of seizures for two years. A prospective study. *N Engl J Med* 318(15):942, 1988.
6. Conlon P, Trimble MR, Rogers D, Callicott C: Magnetic resonance imaging in epilepsy: a controlled study. *Epilepsy Res* 2:37, 1988.
7. Dean JC, Penry JK: Valproate monotherapy in 30 patients with partial seizures. *Epilepsia* 29(2):140, 1988.
8. Delgado-Escueta AV: Epileptogenic paroxysms: modern approaches and clinical correlations. *Neurology* 29:1014, 1979.
9. Dreifuss FE, Santilli N, Langer DJ, et al: Valproic acid hepatic fatalities: a retrospective review. *Neurology* 37(3):379, 1987.
10. Dreifuss FE: Proposal for revised clinical and electroencephalographic classification of epileptic seizures. *Epilepsia* 22:489, 1981.
11. Elwes RDC, Johnson AL, Shorvon SD, Reynolds EH: The prognosis for seizure control in newly diagnosed epilepsy. *N Engl J Med* 311:944, 1984.
12. Emerson R, D'Souza BJ, Vining EP, et al: Stopping medication in children with epilepsy: predictors of outcome. *N Engl J Med* 304:1125, 1981.
13. Gastaut H, Tassinari CA: Epilepsies. In: Remand A (ed): *Handbook of EEG and Clinical Neurophysiology.* Amsterdam, Elsevier, 1975, Vol. 13, Part A.
14. Gram L, Bentsen KD, Parnas J, Flachs H: Controlled trials in epilepsy: a review. *Epilepsia* 23:491, 1982.
15. Louis S, McDowell F: Epileptic seizures in nonembolic cerebral infarction. *Arch Neurol* 17:414, 1967.
16. Luders WE, MacMilan JP, Gupta M: Serum prolactin levels after epileptic seizures. *Neurology* 34:1601, 1984.
17. Masland RL: Commission for the control of epilepsy. *Neurology* 28:861, 1978.
18. Mattson RH, Cramer JA, Collins JF, et al: Comparison of carbamazepine, phenobarbital, phenytoin, and primidone in partial and secondarily generalized tonic-clonic seizures. *N Engl J Med* 313:145, 1985.
19. Mazziotta JC, Engel Jr. J: The use and impact of positron com-

puted tomography scanning in epilepsy. *Epilepsia* 25(2):S86, 1984.

20. McArthur JC: Neurologic manifestations of AIDS. *Medicine (Baltimore)* 66:407, 1987.
21. McGahan JP, Dublin AB, Hill RP: The evaluation of seizure disorders by computerized tomography. *J Neurosurg* 50:328, 1979.
22. Newmark ME, Penry JK (eds): *Genetics of Epilepsy: A Review.* New York, Raven Press, 1980.
23. Ng SK, Hauser WA, Brust JC, Susser M: Alcohol consumption and withdrawal in new-onset seizures. *N Engl J Med* 319:666, 1988.
24. Niedermeyer E (ed): *Compendium of the Epilepsies.*Springfield, Illinois, Charles C Thomas, 1974.
25. Sander JW, Shorvon SD: Incidence and prevalence studies in epilepsy and their methodological problems: a review. *J Neurology, Neurosurg Psychiatry* 50:829, 1987.
26. Schmidley JW, Simon RP: Postictal pleocytosis. *Ann Neurol* 9:81, 1981.
27. Schmidt RP, Wilder BJ: *Epilepsy.*Philadelphia, FA Davis, 1968.
28. Schold C, Yarnell PR, Earnest MP: Origin of seizures in elderly patients. *JAMA* 238:1177, 1977.
29. Shorvon SD, Chadwick D, Galbraith AW, Reynolds EH: One drug for epilepsy. *Br Med J* 1:474, 1978.
30. Sutherling WW, Crandall PH, Engel Jr. J, et al: The magnetic field of complex partial seizures agrees with intracranial localizations. *Ann Neurology* 21:548, 1987.
31. Treiman DM: Efficacy and safety of antiepileptic drugs: a review of controlled trials. *Epilepsia* 28(3):S1, 1987.
32. Treiman DM: Seizure types and causes of epilepsy. *Semin Neurol* 1:65, 1981.
33. van der Lugt PJ: Traffic accidents caused by epilepsy. *Epilepsia* 16:747, 1975.
34. Vignaendra V, Ng KK, Lim CL, Loh TG: Clinical and electroencephalographic data indicative of brain tumors in a seizure population. *Postgrad Med J* 54:1, 1978.
35. Yerby MS: Problems and management of the pregnant woman with epilepsy. *Epilepsia* 3(28):S29, 1987.
36. Zielinsky JJ: Epidemiology. In: Laidlaw J, Richens A (eds):*A Textbook of Epilepsy.* New York, Churchill Livingstone, 1982, p 16.

C H A P T E R 81

Dizziness, Vertigo, Motion Sickness, Near Syncope, Syncope, and Disequilibrium

ERIC BASS, M.D.
HAMILTON MOSES, III, M.D.
WARREN ROTHMAN, M.D.

Dizziness is an extremely common symptom. Patients who complain of dizziness usually mean that they are uncertain of their position or their motion in relation to the environment—they are spatially disoriented. A large number of terms may be used by patients to describe this sensation Table 81.1). Sometimes patients who complain of "dizziness" are not

Table 81.1.
Terms That Patients May Use to Describe Spatial Disorientation

Dizziness	Vertigo	Fainting	Imbalance
Lightheaded	Spinning	Falling	Unsteadiness
Whoozy	Swaying	Blackout	Poor equilibrium
Haziness	Twisting	Pass out	Staggering
Weird feeling	Moving		Drunk feeling
Fuzzy-headed	Weaving		Bouncing
Floating	Rocking		Tilting
Swimming	Rolling		Listing
Blurred vision			

referring to spatial disorientation but to fatigue, dysphoric mood, or other subjective states. Proper diagnosis is usually possible when careful attention is paid to the history and when the patient is examined, with special attention to cardiovascular and neurological abnormalities. A limited number of diagnostic studies can aid the evaluation of selected patients, but these can only be interpreted properly in the light of information gained from the patient.

DELINEATING THE MECHANISM FOR A PATIENT'S DIZZINESS

Dizziness due to spatial disorientation may be classified according to one of the following *three mechanisms* : (*a*) the illusion that the patient or the environment is moving or rotating (vertigo), (*b*) a sensation of impending faint or actual loss of consciousness (near syncope, syncope), and (*c*) a sensation of impaired balance (disequilibrium) (7). Some patients have ill-defined "dizziness" that cannot be classified as vertigo, near syncope, or disequilibrium, and the basis for their complaint may be impossible to establish. Nevertheless, every attempt should be made to classify the mechanism of dizziness because the approach to specific diagnosis and management depends on the identified mechanism.

In taking a history from the patient with dizziness, the first objective should be to classify the probable mechanism for the complaint by determining the true character of the patient's symptoms. The patient should be asked to use words more specific than "dizziness," and should be asked to *describe a discrete recent episode*. Vertigo should be differentiated from near syncope, syncope, disequilibrium, and ill-defined lightheadedness. Questions about associated auditory symptoms, or neurological symptoms, may further help to classify the patient's problem more specifically (peripheral versus central vertigo, metabolic versus vascular presyncope, etc.). If the patient's brief account does not point to the probable mechanism, the following questions may help:

1. Is there actually the sensation of movement or rotation of your head or your body? (Positive response favors vertigo.)
2. Is it like the sensation you might get if you stand up too quickly after resting? A sensation as if you might black out? (Positive response favors presyncope.)
3. Is it a sensation of unsteadiness on your feet? A sensation that you are not sure where your hand or body is and that you cannot quite catch your balance and might fall? (Positive response favors disequilibrium.)

For a patient whose history does not establish the probable mechanism, asking *whether the patient can reproduce the symptoms* may be more efficient than exhaustive questioning.

The patient who claims to be dizzy "right now" while sitting before the physician should

1. Be checked for hypotension, first while seated, then recumbent and standing;
2. Be observed for hyperventilation (slow, hyperpneic breathing, not overt tachypnea);
3. Be examined for nystagmus (see below).

A patient who produces "dizziness" by turning his head should be asked to elaborate on the symptoms; vertigo (positional) and presyncope (due to compromise of cerebral blood flow) are the two problems most likely to be described.

If the patient reports typical dizziness on rising from a chair, orthostatic hypotension is likely; this can be confirmed by measuring supine and standing blood pressure. If the patient demonstrates gait ataxia (see Chapter 78) or reports dizziness upon turning while walking, the problem may be disequilibrium rather than vertigo.

As part of this preliminary inquiry, it is important to ask the patient whether dizziness has interfered with usual activities, especially driving a motor vehicle. This information will be important in management regardless of the mechanism of dizziness.

VERTIGO

Vertigo is defined as a hallucination of movement and may be described either as a sensation as if the external world were turning around the patient (objective vertigo) or as if the patient were turning in place (subjective vertigo). This sensation is similar to that experienced after being on a merry-go-round or after spinning in place for several minutes.

It has been estimated that somewhat less than a quarter of the patients who visit physicians for dizziness have vertigo (7). Most vertigo is due to conditions affecting labyrinthine structures or the vestibular nerve (peripheral vertigo) (see Fig. 96.1 anatomy of the ear and 8th cranial nerve); although these conditions are distressing and at times disabling, they are usually self-limited (26). In some patients, however, vertigo is a manifestation of progressive disease of the central nervous system (central vertigo) or is a secondary manifestation of a systemic condition. The major causes of vertigo in these three categories are listed in Table 81.2.

Vestibular Reflexes

In evaluating the patient with vertigo, it is helpful to have an understanding of the principal reflexes involved in vestibular function. The vestibular system functions through the vestibulospinal and vestibulo-ocular reflexes. The *vestibulospinal reflex* uses information from the sensory structures contained in the bony labyrinth (semicircular canals, utricle, and saccule) to determine the orientation of the head with respect to the ground and to promote appropriate postural adjustments to keep the body upright. The *vestibulo-ocular reflex* uses information from these sensory structures to detect rotational movements of the head and to generate appropriate

Table 81.2.
Major Causes of Vertigo[a]

PERIPHERAL CAUSES OF VERTIGO
  "Benign" positional vertigo
  Post-traumatic vertigo
  Peripheral vestibulopathy (labyrinthitis, vestibular neuronitis, acute and recurrent peripheral vestibulopathy)
  Vestibulotoxic drug-induced vertigo (aminoglycosides)
  Ménière's syndrome (endolymphatic hydrops)
  Inflammatory labyrinthitis (syphilis, vasculitis)
  Other focal peripheral disease (acute and chronic otitis media, cholesteatoma, tumor, fistula, genetic anomalies, rarely focal ischemia and others)
CENTRAL CAUSES OF VERTIGO
  Brainstem ischemia and infarction
  Cerebellopontine angle tumor (acoustic neurinoma, meningioma, metastatic tumor, etc)
  Demyelinating disease (multiple sclerosis, postinfectious demyelination, remote effect of carcinoma)
  Cranial neuropathy with focal involvement of 8th nerve
  Intrinsic brainstem lesions (tumor, arteriovenous malformation, trauma, etc)
  Other posterior fossa lesions (primarily intrinsic or extra-axial masses of the posterior fossa, such as meatoma, metastatic tumor, and cerebellar infarction)
  Seizure disorder (temporal lobe epilepsy)
  Migraine
  Heredofamilial disorders (spinocerebellar degenerations: Friedreich's ataxia, olivopontocerebellar atrophy, etc)
SYSTEMIC CAUSES OF VERTIGO AND DIZZINESS
  Drugs (anticonvulsants, hypnotics, antihypertensives, alcohol, analgesics, tranquilizers)
  Infectious disease (viral and bacterial meningitis, and systemic infection)
  Endocrine disease (diabetes and hypothyroidism particularly)
  Vasculitis (systemic lupus erythematosus, giant cell arteritis, and drug-induced vasculitis)
  Other systemic conditions (polycythemia, anemia, dysproteinemia, Paget's disease of the bone, sarcoidosis, granulomatous disease, and systemic toxins)

[a] Adapted from Troost BT: Dizziness and vertigo in vertebrobasilar disease. *Curr Concepts Cerebrovasc Dis* 14:21, 1979.

compensatory eye movements that are exactly equal and opposite to head movements. This reflex permits maintenance of ocular fixation during head movements. All reflex arcs between the vestibular sensory structures and the central nervous system utilize the vestibular branch of the 8th cranial nerve and the four vestibular nuclei of the brainstem.

In these reflex systems there is a tonic discharge from each vestibular sensory organ that elicits a perfectly balanced motor response in the central nervous system. When the head is moved in any direction, the labyrinthine output from one side increases while the output from the other side decreases; this temporary imbalance of sensory input elicits the compensatory motor commands for vestibulospinal and vestibulo-ocular reflexes. If the input from the labyrinths or its central processing becomes disordered, abnormal subjective states (i.e., vertigo) and motor responses (i.e., nystagmus and loss of balance) occur.

Approach to the Patient

Initial Office Evaluation

A systematic approach to the history and physical examination should be utilized for all patients with

vertigo. Even when a working diagnosis of a self-limited peripheral vertigo is made, follow-up is needed for confirmation, since there is significant overlap in the symptoms and signs produced by peripheral and central vertigo. The following information should be obtained in the initial office evaluation of the patient (the presentation and course of the major causes of vertigo are described on subsequent pages):

History

1. Was the onset gradual or sudden?
2. Are symptoms severe, moderate, or mild?
3. Are symptoms constant or episodic?
4. How long do symptoms last?
5. How frequently do symptoms occur?
6. Is there anything that brings on the attack (i.e., change in position, stress, etc.)?
7. Is there anything that makes symptoms worse or better?
8. Does the patient tend to fall, and to which side?
9. Is there associated nausea or vomiting?
10. Is this a first episode or a recurrent episode of illness?

Associated Auditory Symptoms

1. Is there a hearing impairment (unilateral or bilateral)?
2. Is tinnitus present (pulsatile or constant)?
3. Is there a history of prior ear infections or draining ears?
4. Is there a sensation of aural pressure?
5. Is there a history of prior head or neck trauma, recent barotrauma, or recent viral illness?
6. Has the patient been exposed to any ototoxic drugs?

Associated Neurological Symptoms

1. Are there changes in vision (diplopia, blurring of vision, flashing lights, etc.)?
2. Is there numbness of face or extremities?
3. Is there weakness in arms or legs (unilateral or bilateral)?
4. Is there clumsiness in the arms or legs?
5. Is there confusion or loss of consciousness?
6. Is there slurring of speech?
7. Is there difficulty with swallowing?

Examination

1. Inspection of external auditory canal and tympanic membrane (see Chapter 96).
2. Simple office assessment for hearing impairment (see Chapter 96).
3. Observation for spontaneous nystagmus (see below).
4. Tests for positional vertigo and positional nystagmus (see below).
5. Selective neurological and neurovascular examination (cranial nerves, particularly 5 and 7; cerebellar tests, gait testing, Romberg test; motor

testing—see Chapter 78 for recommended brief neurological and neurovascular examination).

Laboratory tests. If no clear cause of vertigo is identified from the initial history and physical examination, certain laboratory tests should be considered. Because luetic labyrinthitis and hypothyroidism can cause peripheral vertigo, a serological test for syphilis (FTA-ABS, since nontreponemal tests may be negative in tertiary syphilis; see Chapter 30) and a thyroid-stimulating hormone (TSH) level should be obtained on patients with peripheral vertigo. In addition, a hematocrit and a fasting blood sugar should be ordered to check for anemia and diabetes mellitus. There are no other routinely indicated laboratory tests in the initial office evaluation of vertigo. Several tests of vestibular function may be utilized by a consulting otolaryngologist (see below). Most of the systemic causes of vertigo listed in Table 81.2 will present with other symptoms in addition to the vertigo. Rarely, vertigo and decreased hearing may be the only symptoms described by a hypothyroid patient.

Evaluation of Nystagmus

Nystagmus is rhythmic movement of the eyes. When it is *pendular* (to-and-fro movements about equal in amplitude and speed), it is usually due to disturbance of central vision. *Jerk nystagmus* (having a slow and a quick component) is typically, but not exclusively, a sign of vestibular disease; every patient complaining of vertigo should be checked for this type of nystagmus. It is important to know how to recognize and test for jerk nystagmus since it is the only objective indicator of vestibular dysfunction.

Spontaneous Nystagmus. In patients with peripheral or central vestibular dysfunction, nystagmus may be present with the eyes in midposition or in any direction of gaze. The nystagmus may be detected even when the patient is not experiencing vertigo. During an episode of acute vertigo, there should usually be accompanying nystagmus if the vertigo is due to organic disease. Absence of nystagmus suggests that one of the other mechanisms for dizziness described above is present. Spontaneous nystagmus should be sought in five positions of gaze: straight ahead, right, left, up, and down. The patient should be instructed to turn the eyes only about 30° from midline, since extreme lateral gaze may produce end-position nystagmus in normal individuals. Visual fixation tends to suppress the spontaneous nystagmus of peripheral vestibular disease. Therefore, if spontaneous nystagmus is not observed, the patient should close his eyes (to eliminate visual fixation) and be observed for nystagmus through the eyelids, again in each of the five positions of gaze. Preferably, the patient can be examined with eyes open through Frenzel lenses (special 10-diopter lenses that distort the patient's view, making fixation impossible). If spontaneous nystagmus is present with the eyes open, the patient should be asked to fixate on a nearby object: *suppression of nystagmus with fixation favors peripheral vestibular disease,* whereas

persistence or enhancement of the nystagmus is typical of central disease.

Features that distinguish peripheral from central spontaneous nystagmus are summarized in Table 81.3.

Positional Nystagmus. Positional nystagmus (and vertigo) is produced by a sudden change in head or body position. The patient with positional vertigo usually gives a history of symptoms brought on by such changes as lying back in bed, turning the head while lying, arising from bed, bending over, or looking upward, but not when the head is stationary. The purposes of provocative testing are (a) to replicate the patient's symptoms, (b) to demonstrate nystagmus as objective evidence for vestibular impairment, and (c) to determine whether the nystagmus is fatigable.

The test utilized to detect positional vertigo was described by Bárány in 1921 (2) and is illustrated in Figure 81.1. The patient sits close enough to one end of the examining table so that his head would be over the edge if the patient were lying down. The patient is asked to keep the eyes open during the maneuver and to report any sensations (vertigo, nausea, etc.) that are experienced. Frenzel lenses are used, if available, to prevent suppression of the nystagmus. The patient is asked to turn his head 45° to one side. Then, while the examiner supports the head and shoulders, the patient is quickly brought to a reclining position with his head still rotated to one side and hanging over the end of the table. This position should be maintained for 20 seconds. In addition to listening to the patient's symptoms, the examiner should observe his eyes for nystagmus. If nystagmus appears, the examiner should note its time of onset (relative to the start of the maneuver), the direction of eye motion (horizontal, vertical, rotatory, or mixed), the nature of associated symptoms, the adaptability of nystagmus (does it disappear despite maintaining the same head position?), and its fatigability on repeated testing. The maneuver should then be repeated with the head turned in the opposite direction. In particular, if nystagmus was present in one position, the physician should pay careful attention to any change in its direction or amplitude when tested in the opposite direction.

Features that distinguish peripheral from central positional nystagmus are summarized in Table 81.4.

Peripheral Causes of Vertigo

Idiopathic Benign Positional Vertigo (BPV)

This is probably the most common type of vertigo seen in adult patients (1, 11). It occurs at all ages but is most common after the fourth decade and in persons with recent head trauma. The pathological basis for idiopathic BPV is not known. The differentiation of BPV from post-traumatic cervical vertigo, endolymphatic hydrops (Ménière's disease), and vertebral-basilar insufficiency is often the principal challenge for the physician.

Symptoms are first noted when the head is turned (a) as the patient is assuming a recumbent position, (b) when the patient is already recumbent, or (c) when

Table 81.3.
Features of Spontaneous Nystagmus

Feature	Peripheral	Central
Direction	Usually horizontal-rotatory Never purely vertical	Any direction May be purely vertical
Direction of fast component	Away from side with disease	Toward side with disease (or direction changing)
Effect of visual fixation	Suppressed	Not suppressed (may be enhanced)
Usual anatomical location of problem	Labyrinth or vestibular nerve	Brainstem or cerebellum

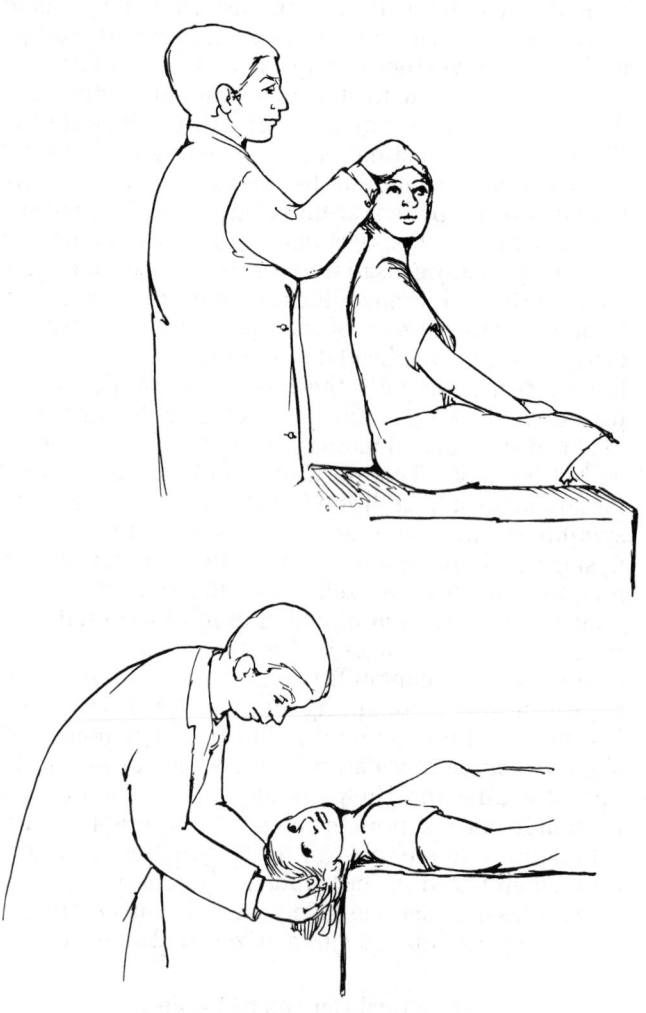

Figure 81.1. Bárány maneuever for testing a patient for positional vertigo and nystagmus.

the patient is rolling over in bed. The episodes of vertigo are brief (usually lasting less than 1 minute), and they are always brought on with a change in head position. If the vertigo is related to trauma (see below), it may begin immediately after the trauma or days to weeks later. Typically, patients with BPV do not complain of tinnitus or of hearing impairment. They may, however, have nausea during episodes of vertigo.

On examination, spontaneous nystagmus (see above) is *not* present. A positive positional test of the peripheral type (see Table 81.4) with the absence of other otological or neurological findings supports the working diagnosis of idiopathic BPV.

BPV is usually self-limited; however, symptoms may persist for weeks or months, and episodes may recur in later years. Because positional vertigo is observed in other conditions besides BPV, it is important to re-evaluate the patient serially, following the systematic approach utilized initially and looking for ancillary evidence for one of the other causes of vertigo listed in Table 81.2. Any patient whose course is atypical should be seen in consultation by an otolaryngologist or a neurologist.

BPV is usually treated with *positional exercises* (4, 21, 22). The patient should be instructed to do the following maneuvers, on a bed: assume the head position that will initiate symptoms and maintain this position until the vertigo disappears; then sit upright for a few seconds; then repeat the exercise multiple times (usually five times) until the exercise produces no symptoms. This should be done three or four times a day. Most patients report excellent relief of symptoms after performing these exercises for about 2 weeks (4). Younger patients tend to improve more rapidly than older ones.

Individuals with BPV who work at heights (repairmen, roofers, etc.) may have to curtail these activities until the symptoms have abated. Symptomatic treatment may be helpful, although this has never been confirmed in a controlled trial (see below).

Post-traumatic Vertigo

Vertigo is very common after both blunt head trauma and whiplash (flexion-extension) injury to the neck (12). The basis for the vertigo may be disruption of the utricular otolithic membrane (so-called "cupulolithiasis"), hemorrhage into the endolymph or into the eighth nerve, or fracture of the temporal bone, causing damage to the nerve. Clinically, it may be impossible to determine which of these mechanisms is responsible for a patient's symptoms. However, there are two typical patterns that are thought to suggest the dominant problem.

The first pattern is *immediate* post-traumatic vertigo, with associated spontaneous nystagmus (beating away from the side of injury), nausea and vomiting, positional nystagmus, and either conductive or sensorineural hearing loss. This pattern suggests temporal bone fracture and is typical of moderately severe trauma to the temporal bone or occiput. A history of brief

Table 81.4.
Features of Positional Nystagmus Elicited by the Bárány Maneuver

Feature	Peripheral	Central
Time to onset after quick position change (latency)	3–20 seconds	Immediate
Duration	Less than 1 minute (often only a few seconds)	Persists longer than 1 minute
Fatigability	Marked (may not be present on immediate repetition)	None
Subjective vertigo	Often marked	Often minimal or absent
Nystagmus direction	Fixed irrespective of head position	Changing with change in head position
Usual anatomical location of problem	Labyrinth or vestibular nerve	Brainstem or cerebellum

unconsciousness, the presence of Battle's sign (postauricular echymosis), and bleeding in the external auditory canal are other findings that suggest this diagnosis. Computerized tomographic scanning of the temporal bone is needed to detect the fracture. Because there is the possibility of finding surgically correctable damage, these patients should always be evaluated immediately by an otolaryngologist. Based upon this evaluation, an exploratory tympanotomy may be recommended. These patients must be carefully examined also for facial nerve paralysis. In general, immediate palsy requires immediate decompression, whereas delayed palsy may be followed conservatively, as in Bell's palsy (see Chapter 84).

In the majority of patients with immediate post-traumatic vertigo, the vestibular symptoms improve rapidly over the first few days and they are gone entirely within 6 to 12 weeks. Symptomatic treatment (see below) may be helpful.

The second common pattern is that of *delayed onset* (latent period of days to weeks) of post-traumatic vertigo, which presents in the same way as idiopathic BPV (see above). This pattern is more typical of minor head or whiplash injury and is thought to be due to cupulolithiasis. BPV, without spontaneous vertigo or nystagmus and without hearing deficit, is the typical finding on physical examination. The course and management are similar to those of idiopathic BPV.

Some patients with injuries of the cervical spine may experience *cervical vertigo*. This may be distinguished from benign positional vertigo by a modification of the Barany maneuver. To test for cervical vertigo the patient lies sideways with the affected ear down. Once again, the patient is placed sufficiently high on the table so that the head will clear the table. While lying sideways, the head is allowed to drop downward. If vertigo ensues, the patient has benign positional vertigo. If there is no vertigo, then the head is held in this position while the patient is allowed to lie supine. Should vertigo ensue, the diagnosis of cervical vertigo is established.

Some patients with post-traumatic vertigo may have a combination of the features of immediate and de-

layed vertigo. After systematic examination, these patients should be managed symptomatically (see below) since it is likely that their vertigo will be self-limited.

Peripheral Vestibulopathy (Acute Viral Labyrinthitis and Vestibular Neuronitis)

The collective term "peripheral vestibulopathy" has been suggested by Drachman and Hart (7) for a number of benign conditions for which the pathological basis is chiefly conjectural. Because these conditions often follow viral upper respiratory or gastrointestinal infections, they are thought to be due to inflammation of the vestibular end organ (labyrinthitis) or of the vestibular nerve (neuronitis). They are most common in the third to the fifth decade but may occur at any age. Occasionally, a cluster of cases occurs (epidemic vertigo). Like BPV, the working diagnosis of peripheral vestibulopathy is based on typical clinical features that are not pathognomonic; therefore, consideration of one of the progressive causes of central vertigo listed in Table 81.2 must be kept in mind in follow-up evaluation.

Typically, there is a sudden onset of moderate to severe spontaneous vertigo. Often there is accompanying nausea and vomiting, and symptoms are made worse by any change in position. The initial symptoms usually persist for several days, when they may be incapacitating. There is generally no complaint of hearing loss or tinnitus. There may be a tendency for the patient to fall when trying to walk.

On systematic examination spontaneous nystagmus with peripheral features (see above) is present. This is an important feature differentiating peripheral vestibulopathy from BPV in which spontaneous nystagmus is not present. Because involvement is usually unilateral, there may be a typical nystagmus pattern in which (a) the fast component is away from the side of the lesion when the subject is asked to look away from the lesion, and (b) the nystagmus may lessen or cease when the subject looks toward the side of the lesion. Caloric testing after recovery from the acute episode (see below) shows an absence or decreased response on the affected side, but this test is not needed routinely. Positional testing (if performed) may produce a positive response with peripheral characteristics (see Table 81.4). There is usually no hearing loss, and the neurological and neurovascular examinations are unremarkable.

The vertigo of peripheral vestibulopathy usually resolves within 6 weeks, although nystagmus may be demonstrated for several months, especially if electronystagmography (ENG) is performed (see below). In occasional patients, the vertigo may also persist for more than 6 weeks. Such patients should be systematically re-examined for evidence of a central cause of vertigo, in particular, acoustic neurinoma and brainstem or inferior cerebellar infarction (see below).

There is no specific treatment. Patients should be told that the worst symptoms will last only a few days, that all symptoms usually resolve within 4 to 6 weeks, and that they should adjust their usual activities according to how they feel (during the first few days, many patients will require strict bed rest for symptomatic relief). Antivertigo drugs may be helpful (see below). Diazepam (Valium), 5 mg three times daily, may also be useful in patients with peripheral vestibulopathy. An occasional patient may require hospital admission for intravenous hydration if nausea and vomiting are severe.

Vertigo Due to Vestibulotoxic Drugs

Ototoxicity is an occasional complication of aminoglycoside antibiotics, salicylates, and potent diuretics (ethacrynic acid and furosemide) (13). Most of these drugs are cochleotoxic and produce sensorineural hearing loss and tinnitus (see Chapter 96). Two aminoglycosides, streptomycin and gentamicin, are vestibulotoxic. The basis for aminoglycoside ototoxicity seems to be that these drugs are concentrated in the inner ear. Pathologically, there is destruction of the sensory hair cells of either the cochlea or the labyrinth. Ototoxicity due to an aminoglycoside can usually be prevented by avoiding serum concentrations above the therapeutic range and by limiting the duration of therapy.

In office practice, vestibular toxicity due to an aminoglycoside may appear shortly after the patient has been treated with an aminoglycoside drug while in the hospital. Because these drugs produce bilateral, symmetrical damage, the patient will usually not describe frank vertigo but will have unsteadiness and intolerance to motion and may describe difficulty walking in the dark. The pathological changes produced by aminoglycosides are permanent, and the symptoms usually persist indefinitely. Fortunately, most patients with vestibular toxicity are able to adjust to their problem, and hearing aids may help those with cochlear toxicity.

Mild vertigo or disequilibrium may occur as a side effect of a number of drugs (Table 81.2) that do not produce permanent pathological damage; these side effects remit promptly after stopping the drug.

Ménière's Syndrome (Endolymphatic Hydrops)

This condition is described in Chapter 96. Ménière's syndrome should always be considered in the differential diagnosis of a patient with the acute onset of severe vertigo with peripheral characteristics. The features that distinguish it from other causes of vertigo are the spontaneous onset of attacks, the limited duration of symptoms during each discrete attack (minutes to hours, not 1 or more days as seen with peripheral vestibulopathy), the associated tinnitus and sensorineural hearing loss (may vary in severity from day to day) found in most patients, recruitment on audiometric studies, and normal brainstem and cerebellar function. At times, Ménière's syndrome may present initially with only vertigo (isolated hydrops of the labyrinth) or only hearing loss (isolated hydrops of the cochlea). Serial observation is therefore important. In clinically suspected cases of isolated hydrops, a trial of diuretic treatment may be helpful.

Inflammatory Labyrinthitis

Labyrinthitis may occur, although rarely, as a manifestation of secondary or tertiary syphilis. It is always important to consider this etiology, as it may mimic other forms of peripheral vertigo and it requires antibiotic treatment. Typically, the patient has a combination of (a) sensorineural hearing loss, which may be unilateral or bilateral and fluctuating or sudden; (b) impaired ability to understand speech (loud enough but not clear); and (c) peripheral type vertigo, which is not positional. As noted earlier, this problem should be sought by sending a serological test for syphilis routinely (always including an FTA-ABS) in every patient with new peripheral type vertigo. If the test is positive, the patient should have a cerebrospinal fluid FTA-ABS determination and be treated according to the stage of the disease (see Chapter 30).

Systemic lupus erythematosus, polyarteritis nodosa, and other causes of vasculitis may present with vertigo or loss of hearing. Nearly always other manifestations of the disease will also be apparent simultaneously or will be evident from the history.

Central Causes of Vertigo

Table 81.2 lists the principal central causes of vertigo. Most are uncommon. The important clues to the presence of one of these conditions are the finding of associated neurological signs and symptoms, the presence of nystagmus with central characteristics (see Tables 81.3 and 81.4), or deviation of the patient's presentation and course from that expected for the common peripheral causes of vertigo. Whenever a central cause for vertigo is suspected, the patient should be referred for evaluation to a neurologist or an otolaryngologist. When the onset of symptoms is acute or there is evidence of rapidly progressive neurological symptoms, the patient should be hospitalized.

The principal manifestations of the two types of

central vertigo that a generalist is most likely to see (tumor and vascular disease) are described here.

Cerebellopontine (CP) Angle Tumor

Acoustic neurinoma, the commonest CP angle tumor, is described in Chapter 96. The usual manifestations of these tumors are due to compression of the auditory component of the 8th nerve (sensorineural hearing loss) and, much later, to compression of adjacent structures (the 5th and 7th cranial nerves in particular). Frank vertigo and nystagmus are present in a minority of patients. A vague complaint of unsteadiness, however, is present in almost half of the patients when they are first seen. Most patients complain of unilateral hearing loss and tinnitus. They generally have a great deal of difficulty in understanding speech in the affected ear. The electronystagmogram (see description below) usually shows a markedly decreased or absent response in the affected ear. The symptoms of CP angle tumor typically are insidious in onset (usually confined to sensorineural hearing loss for a prolonged interval), constant, and progressive. This time course distinguishes them from the periodic or severe symptoms typical of most peripheral vertigo and of the central vertigo of transient ischemia. Occasionally onset of vertigo may be acute, but even then hearing loss will have been apparent earlier.

As pointed out elsewhere (Chapter 96), consultation with an otolaryngologist is the most appropriate plan for a patient who may have a CP angle tumor. The consultant should determine which of a large variety of otoneurological tests is appropriate in pursuing this diagnosis (10).

Vertebrobasilar Arterial Disease

Cerebrovascular ischemia may cause vertigo. When this symptom is due to atherosclerosis, there are almost always symptoms or signs of other brainstem involvement, in particular clumsiness or weakness, loss of vision, diplopia, perioral numbness, ataxia, drop attack (sudden loss of motor tone in the lower extremities, without loss of consciousness), or dysarthria.

When these symptoms are transient, they may be due (a) to a transient ischemic attack (TIA) (see Chapter 83), (b) to mechanical compromise of the vertebrobasilar circulation (Fig. 81.2) brought on by rotation of the neck (detected either in the history or by having the patient replicate symptoms in the office), or (c) to diversion of blood from the brainstem to an arm during use of that arm—the subclavian steal syndrome (suspected on the basis of history and of the finding of a subclavian artery bruit or a decreased blood pressure in the symptom-provoking arm). When the symptoms are abrupt in onset and *persistent,* they may be due to infarction of the brainstem or cerebellum. Insidious onset of persistent symptoms would be more suggestive of tumor. Acute cerebellar infarction in the distal territory of the posterior inferior cerebellar artery (PICA), a relatively uncommon problem, may initially mimic

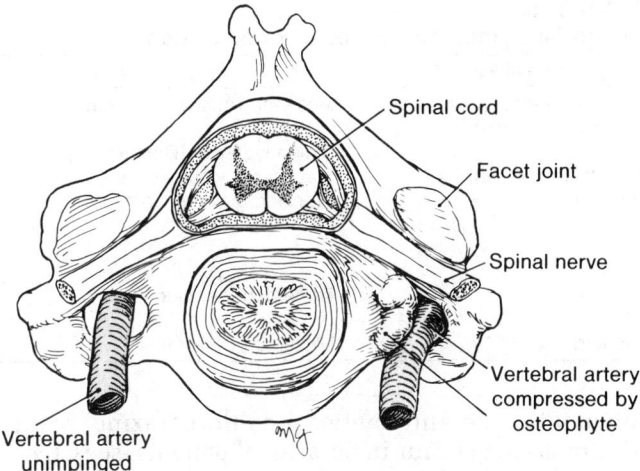

Figure 81.2. Anatomical relationship of the vertebral artery in a transverse foramen. The artery lies alongside the uncinate portion of the vertebra, the most common site of degenerative changes due to cervical spondylosis with osteophyte formation. (From Sheehan S, Bauer RB, Meyer JS: Vertebral artery compression in cervical spondylosis. *Neurology* 10:968, 1960.)

acute vestibulopathy, presenting as sudden marked vertigo, nausea, and vomiting. Usually infarction due to PICA occlusion will involve the brainstem, so that other neurological signs will be present (ipsilateral loss of pain and temperature sense of the face and contralateral loss of these sensations in the rest of the body, cerebellar ataxia, or ipsilateral Horner's syndrome).

Sudden vertigo and unilateral hearing loss may occur due to *selective occlusion of the internal auditory artery;* in such patients, a condition affecting small arteries (syphilitic arteritis or other vasculitides, or microembolism) is a more likely cause than atherosclerosis.

Symptomatic Treatment of Vertigo

When the working diagnosis is peripheral vertigo of any type, treatment with one of the "antivertigo" antihistamines may provide symptomatic relief (25). It is hypothesized that these agents work both by suppressing the vestibular end organ receptors and by inhibiting activation of vagal responses. Commonly recommended drugs in this group are listed in Table 81.5, with appropriate doses and schedules. Because peripheral vertigo from common causes is usually self-limited, the patient should be instructed to take an antivertigo agent only for a few weeks and then to try discontinuing the drug. The major side effects of these drugs are dry mouth and sedation.

When nausea and vomiting are pronounced, in either peripheral or central vertigo, an *antiemetic* can be tried. It is hypothesized that these agents work by suppressing central vestibular pathways that activate vagal responses. Commonly recommended antiemetic drugs are listed in Table 81.5. The major side effect occurring with short-term use is sedation; with the

Table 81.5.
Drugs for Symptomatic Treatment of Vertigo

Type of Action	Generic (Trade Name)	Available Preparation	Dose and Schedule
Labyrinthine suppressants (antihistamines)	Meclizine (Antivert, Bonine)	12.5 and 25-mg tablets	12.5–25 mg 3 or 4 times daily
	Dimenhydrinate (Dramamine)	50-mg tablets	50 mg 3 or 4 times daily
(anticholinergic)	Transderm scopolamine	1.5 mg disc	1 disc every 3 days
Antiemetics	Prochlorperazine (Compazine)	5- and 10-mg tablets	5–10 mg every 4 hours as needed
		10- and 25-mg suppositories	10 mg 4 times daily or 25 mg twice daily
	Trimethobenzamide (Tigan)	250-mg capsule	3 to 4 times daily
		200-mg suppository	3 to 4 times daily
Sedative	Diazepam (Valium)	5, 10 mg	3 times daily

phenothiazine antiemetic, prochlorperazine, acute dystonias may occur in occasional patients (see Chapter 16 for a full discussion of phenothiazine side effects).

Patients with persistent and disabling vertigo should be referred to an otolaryngologist for definitive evaluation and management. For permanent relief of symptoms, some persons will require surgery, which may consist of sectioning of the vestibular nerve, repair of an inner ear fistula, labyrinthectomy, or endolymphatic shunt. Several of these procedures produce unilateral deafness.

Tests Utilized in Evaluation of Vertigo

When a patient with vertigo that is difficult to diagnose is referred to a neurologist or an otolaryngologist, one or more of the studies listed in Table 81.6 will usually be conducted. A combination of results from several tests may support a specific diagnosis.

Audiometry

A number of audiological tests are usually performed in evaluating vertigo (i.e., puretone audiometry, speech audiometry, tone decay testing, acoustic reflex testing, and others) (23). Typically, there is no audiometric abnormality in the most common forms of peripheral vertigo (BPV and peripheral vestibulopathy), whereas there are typical patterns of hearing loss in Ménière's syndrome (low frequency hearing loss), acoustic neurinoma (high frequency hearing loss, with poor discrimination), and a variety of middle ear disorders (conductive hearing loss).

Patient experience.   These tests are performed in a small

Table 81.6.
Tests Used in the Evaluation of Vertigo

Audiometry (puretone, speech, tone decay, brainstem evoked potentials, *etc*)
Caloric tests
Electronystagmography
Skull X-rays
Mastoid X-rays
Polytomogram of temporal bone and internal auditory canal
CT scan and MRI
Air contrast myelogram, with CT scan

soundproof testing room. There is no significant discomfort for the patient. Complete testing may take up to 1 hour.

Caloric Stimulation

This is the only test that evaluates individually the vestibular end organs on each side of the head (16). The test is based upon the fact that the intact labyrinth responds to caloric stimulation with a typical pattern, i.e., warm water induces horizontal nystagmus with the rapid phase toward the stimulated ear, and cool water produces nystagmus in the opposite direction. Vertigo may be induced with both hot and cold stimulation. Under certain circumstances, electronystagmography is utilized (see below) in addition to direct observation during caloric stimulation. Ideally, the water temperatures are set at 30 and 44°C; these are equidistant from normal body temperature, constitute equal stimuli, and produce less distress than more extreme temperatures. Absence of the normal caloric response or deviation from the normal response may be helpful in diagnosis. Vestibular neuronitis and acoustic neurinoma are examples of conditions in which the normal response to caloric stimulation is absent or decreased on the involved side.

Patient experience.   The patient lies on one side with the head positioned comfortably at an angle of about 30°. Flowing water is introduced into the external auditory canal for 30 seconds. For optimal testing, there should be about a 30-minute wait between irrigations. During caloric stimulation, the patient will experience vertigo. An absent caloric response signifies vestibular disease.

Electronystagmography (ENG)

ENG records changes in the electrical potential between the cornea and the retina; when the eye moves, characteristic changes in electrical potential can be picked up (and recorded with a penwriter) in the skin adjacent to the eye (24). ENG has two advantages over direct inspection in detecting nystagmus. First, it is more sensitive than simple inspection and can confirm the presence of nystagmus when simple inspection is equivocal (often because the patient fixates, and suppresses nystagmus under these conditions). Second, it can provide serial tracings that permit comparison of a patient's nystagmus pattern over time. The disadvantages of ENG are that it requires considerable cooperation from the patient and skill from the operator both for correct conduction of the test and for proper interpretation. The principal value of ENG is in picking up subtle spontaneous nystagmus and in differentiating peripheral from central nystagmus, usually by caloric stimulation.

Patient experience. The patient is recumbent. Small electrodes are taped to the skin on either side of the eye. Nystagmus is measured under a number of conditions, including caloric stimulation (see above), optokinetic testing (the patient is asked to follow the stripes on a rotating drum), and others. The entire procedure may take up to 1 hour. The major discomfort is that associated with caloric stimulation (vertigo and occasionally mild otalgia).

MOTION SICKNESS

Motion sickness is experienced by most normal persons when they are exposed to conditions analogous to those of severe storm conditions at sea. About one-third of people experience some symptoms when exposed to the equivalent of moderate sea conditions such as may occur with automobile travel and air travel, as well as with boating. Normal vestibular function is necessary for an individual to experience motion sickness. Visual stimuli are contributory but not necessary for the experience of motion sickness (for example, looking out of the window of a vehicle on a curving or undulating road).

Manifestations

The symptoms of motion sickness vary from person to person, but an individual usually experiences the same symptoms each time. Malaise and nausea are always present, and vomiting is common. Other symptoms may include drowsiness, salivation, swallowing, hyperventilation, headache, flushing, and diaphoresis. There is a major psychological component in motion sickness; for example, some persons develop their typical symptoms in anticipation of an air flight or a boat ride. Vertigo is usually not present.

Most people adapt fairly rapidly to motion. After the first few days of a sea voyage, for example, they are able to tolerate the motion that made them ill at the beginning of the voyage.

Treatment

In tests simulating sea conditions, a number of drugs have been shown to be quite effective in preventing motion sickness (28). These drugs are much less effective if taken after the onset of symptoms. Because all drugs that prevent motion sickness are sedating, individuals should not operate cars, boats, planes, or potentially dangerous machines while taking these drugs.

Antihistamines

Either meclizine (Antivert, Bonine), 25 to 50 mg, or dimenhydrinate (Dramamine), 50 to 100 mg, can be used.

For persons who routinely get moderate or marked motion symptoms, taking one of these drugs about 1 hour before embarking in a car, plane, or boat may be very helpful. The protective effect from meclizine lasts from 12 to 24 hours, whereas that from dimenhydrinate lasts only 4 hours. The principal side effect is drowsiness; because this is more prominent with dimenhydrinate, meclizine is the better choice for persons who wish to remain alert during travel; others may prefer the greater sedating property of dimenhydrinate.

Scopolamine

The anticholinergic drug scopolamine prevents severe motion sickness in a high percentage of persons known to suffer from this problem. Scopolamine is available in tablet form and in the form of a plastic disc for continuous administration through the skin. A 0.4-mg tablet can be taken 1 hour before travel or boating. Alternatively, the button-sized disc (Transderm-SCOP) can be applied behind the ear. The disc works optimally when applied a number of hours before travel or boating. It is designed to deliver 0.5 mg of scopolamine over a period of 3 days. Dry mouth, sedation, and impaired visual accommodation may occur, probably more frequently with the oral preparation. Known closed angle glaucoma and benign prostatic hypertrophy are relative contraindications to the use of this and all anticholinergic drugs.

SYNCOPE AND NEAR SYNCOPE

Definitions and Normal Physiology

Syncope is defined as a sudden transient loss of consciousness, associated with an inability to maintain postural tone. Syncope must be distinguished from the following conditions that also lead to an alteration in the patient's state of consciousness: seizure disorder, vertigo, coma, shock, or delirium (17). Patients with syncope may be unconscious for a few seconds or minutes. Those who remain unconscious for many minutes or hours should be considered as experiencing stupor or coma, not syncope.

Near syncope refers to a transient sensation of imminent loss of consciousness. Many terms may be used by patients to describe this sensation (see Table 81.1). Although it may be difficult to distinguish between near syncope and nonspecific dizziness, the distinction is important because near syncope may be a prelude to frank syncope.

The physiological changes leading to syncope and near syncope depend on the underlying etiology. These changes are shorter in duration or less severe in the person who becomes dizzy without actually losing consciousness.

Unconsciousness implies that either both cerebral hemispheres have become impaired or that certain critical structures in the brainstem have failed. In general, unilateral diseases of the cerebral hemispheres do not lead to unconsciousness unless the brain becomes more generally affected.

Differential Diagnosis

Four classes of abnormalities should be considered in the differential diagnosis of syncope and near syncope: hypotension, cardiac disease, metabolic derangement, and intracranial conditions (Table 81.7).

Based on several series of patients with syncope, hypotension is the cause in 20 to 50% of patients, cardiac disease in 10 to 25%, metabolic disorders in less than 5%, and intracranial disease in less than 5% (6, 8, 17). In nearly 50% of patients, no cause can be clearly discerned on initial evaluation. For these patients with syncope of unknown origin, additional testing and prolonged follow-up may be necessary, but often a diagnosis is never established.

The single most common cause of syncope is the common faint or vasovagal episode. Orthostatic hypotension due to many causes is also very common. The commonest cardiac causes are arrhythmias. Hyperventilation is a very common cause of dizziness (through hypocapnea), but it rarely leads to frank syncope. Hypoglycemia rarely leads to syncope, although it frequently causes dizziness that is associated with other characteristic symptoms (palpitations, diaphoresis, hunger, etc.; see Chapter 72). Seizures and cerebrovascular events are the major neurological abnormalities that may be confused with syncope.

Because prognosis varies according to the underlying cause, optimal management depends on correct identification of the cause. The following discussion focuses chiefly upon the diagnostic evaluation of the patient. Appropriate management for the common causes of these problems is discussed elsewhere in the book, as indicated by cross-referencing.

General Approach to the Patient

Most patients who come to a physician after an episode of syncope or near syncope do so after their symptoms have resolved. The physician should obtain the history both from the patient and from anyone who observed the episode. The inquiry should focus upon

Table 81.7.
Differential Diagnosis of Syncope/Near Syncope[a]

HYPOTENSION	CARDIAC DISEASE
Simple faint (vasovagal syncope)	*Arrhythmia (heart block, brady- and tachyarrhythmias)*
Vasodilating drugs	*Outflow obstruction*
1. Angiotensin converting enzyme inhibitors	1. Aortic stenosis
2. Calcium channel blockers	2. Idiopathic hypertrophic subaortic stenosis
3. Nitroglycerine preparations	3. Aortic dissection
4. Vasodilator antihypertensives	4. Myxoma
Drugs affecting autonomic function	*Acute myocardial infarction*
1. Sympatholytic antihypertensives	*Mitral valve prolapse*
2. Neuroleptics	*Cyanotic congenital heart disease*
3. Tricyclics and monoamine oxidase (MAO) inhibitors	*Cardiac tamponade*
4. Levodopa	METABOLIC CONDITIONS
5. Cholinergic agents	*Hypoglycemia*
Autonomic neuropathy	1. Exogenous insulin
1. Peripheral neuropathy	2. Reactive
2. Postsympathectomy	3. Starvation (islet cell tumor)
3. Tabes dorsalis and diabetic pseudotabes	4. Dumping syndrome
4. Parkinsonism (Shy-Drager syndrome)	*Hypocapnia (hyperventilation)*
5. Idiopathic	*Hypoxia*
Decreased blood volume	1. Anemia
1. Hemorrhage	2. Airway obstruction
2. Salt and water deficit (diarrhea, vomiting, perspiration, diuretics, hyperglycemia)	3. Carbon monoxide
3. Fasting	*Hyperviscosity*
4. Adrenal insufficiency	*Electrolyte derangements (hyponatremia, hypokalemia, hypocalcemia, hyperglycemia)*
5. Hypoalbuminemia	*Drug overdose (sedatives and ethanol)*
Venous pooling	INTRACRANIAL CONDITIONS
1. Prolonged immobility while standing	*Seizure disorder*
2. Severe varicose veins	*Subarachnoid hemorrhage*
3. Late pregnancy	*Cerebral embolism or thrombosis*
4. After exercise	*Migraine*
Mobilization after bed rest	*Acutely increased intracranial pressure*
Orthostasis of aging	1. Tumor
Valsalva maneuver	2. Trauma
1. Tussive	3. Ventricular obstruction
2. Micturition	4. Hypertensive encephalopathy
3. Defecation (with straining)	*Brainstem compression*
4. Intermittent positive pressure breathing	1. Cervical or odontoid fractures
Compromise of cerebral blood flow due to cervical osteoarthritis or subclavian steal	2. Metastasis
Carotid sinus hypersensitivity	3. Cysts or anomalies of the posterior fossa
Pulmonary embolism	4. Platybasia

[a] Modified from Lee JE, Killip T, Plum F: Eopisodic unconsciousness. In Baron JA (ed): *Diagnostic Approaches to Presenting Syndromes*. Baltimore, Williams & Wilkins, 1971.

the events immediately preceding and following the attack; upon associated problems that may have been present for days to weeks before the episode; and upon evidence of significant trauma, neurological deficit, or aspiration complicating the current episode of syncope. The objectives of these initial steps are (a) to reach a working diagnosis or to decide what further evaluation is needed to do so and (b) to decide upon the appropriate initial management for the patient. Appropriate management may range from reassurance (e.g., the patient with vasovagal syncope) to volume expansion (e.g., the patient with a diarrheal illness) to hospital admission for observation, prompt diagnostic testing, and necessary treatment (e.g., the patient with a history suggesting recurrent life-threatening arrhythmias or the patient with a fracture or an aspiration pneumonia complicating syncope).

History

Current Episode. The patient should always be questioned about his position immediately before the attack. Syncope from most causes does not occur unless the patient is in the upright position. If the attack occurred when the patient first stood up, orthostatic hypotension due to venous pooling, loss of intravascular volume, or autonomic failure should be considered. If exercise preceded the attack, a number of cardiopulmonary abnormalities are possible, including aortic stenosis, hypertrophic cardiomyopathy, arrhythmia, or pulmonary hypertension. If syncope was associated with micturition, cough, or passing stool, this suggests diminished venous return due to a Valsalva maneuver. If there was psychological stress (e.g., an argument, fear associated with a medical or other procedure, etc.), vasovagal syncope is highly likely. In each case, the patient may recall feelings of dizziness, heaviness of the limbs, dimming of the vision just before loss of consciousness, or that surrounding events were distant or moving very slowly. Nausea, usually without vomiting, is quite characteristic of vasovagal syncope, syncope associated with bradyarrhythmias, and syncope associated with loss of intravascular volume.

Syncope that occurs when the patient is *seated or recumbent* should suggest hypoglycemia, carotid sinus hypersensitivity, cardiac arrhythmia, hyperventilation, a seizure, or hysteria. Syncope or dizziness occurring with position change while recumbent should always be distinguished from benign positional vertigo, which occurs most frequently in the recumbent position (see above).

Other manifestations just before syncope may suggest the diagnosis. Hunger may indicate hypoglycemia. Headache or characteristic visual disturbances may precede migrainous syncope. Hemiparesis, paraparesis, diplopia, dysarthria, or other neurological abnormalities may precede syncope/near syncope due to transient occlusion of the basilar artery or to vasospasm associated with migraine.

The physician should always take advantage of *observations made by others* who witnessed the period of unconsciousness. Particular attention should be paid to the duration of the spell, whether a convulsion occurred, if incontinence was noted, the sequence of events, and how the patient seemed during the period of recovery. In general, recovery of consciousness is swift. Slow recovery of clear consciousness (recovery after more than 5 minutes) should raise suspicion of a seizure, hypoglycemia, or an occluded intracranial vessel.

Associated Recent History. Information about the patient during the hours, days, or weeks preceding syncope/near syncope is often very helpful in the differential diagnosis.

A large proportion of patients will give a history of episodic near syncope. The patient will usually use the word "dizziness" or one of the other terms listed in Table 81.1. The circumstances surrounding these episodes may support a working diagnosis for a current episode of frank syncope. For example, the patient may have started, or increased the dose of, a drug known to cause orthostatic hypotension (see Table 81.7); or there may be a history of a problem leading to volume deficit, e.g., diarrhea, heat exposure, diuretic use, increased polyuria (in a diabetic), or melena. A patient convalescing from recent illness may relate the symptoms to being up and around after bed rest. An insulin-using diabetic or a patient with reactive or starvation hypoglycemia may describe episodic hypoglycemic symptoms, successfully aborted with carbohydrate intake, during the week(s) prior to frank syncope. In the absence of any relevant changes in the patient's circumstances, a history of recent near syncopal episodes is suggestive of arrhythmia, transient cerebral ischemia, or chronic idiopathic orthostatic hypotension.

A second group of patients will describe prior episodes of frank syncope, without prodromal near syncope. Most often, these will be patients with a history, often long-standing, of syncope due to vasovagal attack brought on by psychological or physical stress. A history of recurrent syncope without near syncopal episodes and without the features of vasovagal attacks warrants consideration of arrhythmia, transient cerebrovascular occlusion, or a seizure disorder.

Physical Examination

General Examination. The physical examination after an attack should include a systematic search for abnormalities in the blood pressure, heart and great vessels, abdomen, and central and peripheral nervous system. In particular, the blood pressure should be measured after the patient has been recumbent for several minutes, again after being seated, and finally while standing. The character, volume, and timing of the carotid pulses should be appraised, and any bruits should be noted. The pulse should be palpated for 1 to 2 minutes to look for irregularities. The heart should be carefully examined for murmurs, systolic clicks, or gallop rhythms. Abdominal examination may reveal a large bladder or signs of a visceral catastrophe. If unexplained orthostatic hypotension has been found, a rectal examination should be performed to check the stool for occult or gross blood.

Neurological Examination. A brief examination of the major components of the nervous system (see Chapter 78) may reveal evidence of either pre-existing neurological disease or of an acute insult related to the current episode of syncope/near syncope. Orientation, speech, memory for the event itself as well as for general information, and judgment should be noted. The fundi may reveal microemboli (see Fig. 83.1) or subhyaloid hemorrhages (a sign of subarachnoid hemorrhage). Nystagmus, ophthalmoplegia, or abnormalities of the pupils, facial movement and sensation, the corneal reflexes, speech, or movement of the palate or tongue indicate involvement of the midbrain, pons, or medulla. Weakness, sensory abnormalities, and pathological reflexes found in a general neurological examination may indicate a lesion elsewhere in the central nervous system. Any neurological abnormalities should raise the suspicion of cerebrovascular disease, a mass causing an epileptic focus, subarachnoid hemorrhage, or central nervous system infection. If trauma has occurred in the recent past or if a fall was sustained during the syncopal episode, subdural or epidural hemorrhage should be considered.

Significance of Seizures and Neurological Deficits. *Seizure activity* may occur after syncope due to any of the common causes, including the simple faint, hyperventilation, orthostatic hypotension, or venous pooling. This is not surprising since unconsciousness signifies a major disruption in normal brain function. A single tonic convulsion is the most common type of postsyncopal seizure; less often a focal seizure or a generalized convulsion may occur. In all three of these instances, the patient's evaluation should include routine tests for a seizure focus (see Chapter 80).

Minor neurological signs, such as slight focal weakness, reflex asymmetries, or pathological reflexes, may also occur after syncope from any cause. These findings may be present particularly if the patient is examined immediately after recovering consciousness, and they rarely persist for more than a few minutes. If such signs persist longer, are more profound, or occur in a constellation that suggests a particular anatomical lesion, they warrant further pursuit. However, one should not be surprised if a source is not found even after a thorough search is completed, since minor neurological signs are not uncommon after general ischemic or metabolic insults to the brain.

Laboratory Tests

No laboratory test is routinely indicated in the evaluation of syncope/near syncope, although an electrocardiogram generally should be performed if the cause of the patient's problem is not obvious. A carefully taken history with a screening physical examination, plus an electrocardiogram, will lead to the correct diagnosis in most patients. For the remaining patients, prolonged electrocardiogram (ECG) (Holter) monitor-

ing is usually recommended and has been found to reveal potentially important arrhythmias in 10 to 60% of cases (9, 17). In contrast, electroencephalography and head computerized tomography have less than a 1% yield in patients with a normal neurological examination and no symptoms suggestive of a seizure (8, 17).The indications for other laboratory tests are cited in the discussion of specific problems which follows.

Features of Common Causes of Syncope/Near Syncope

Hypotension

Because of autoregulation, cerebral blood flow is protected over a wide range of systemic blood pressure. In normal persons, a critical decrease in central nervous system (CNS) blood flow (clinically producing near syncope or syncope) does not occur until the mean blood pressure is below 50 mm Hg. Under a number of circumstances (e.g., sympatholytic drug treatment, cerebrovascular disease, aging), however, the minimal tolerated blood pressure may not be this low. Therefore, symptomatic failure of the systemic circulation may occur over a relatively wide range of blood pressures.

Simple Faint. The simple faint (vasovagal episode) has long been known to afflict young people; it is apt to occur in the setting of anxiety, tension, fatigue, or pain, and especially during venipuncture or other painful procedures. The simple faint is not just a disease of the young but can occur in older patients in identical settings. Early theories suggested that bradycardia due to vagal overactivity was the initial event; but it is now known that venous pooling due to peripheral arterial constriction with venous dilation occurs in the first phase, with a vagal phase (bradycardia) occurring only after the faint itself. Vasovagal attacks nearly always occur while the patient is upright, but they may occur while he is seated; and consciousness is nearly always regained promptly when the patient becomes recumbent. Typically there is a prodromal warning period, at times lasting up to 5 minutes, when the patient feels dizzy, light-headed, or flushed with mild nausea and occasionally palpitations or throat tightness. If the subject assumes a recumbent position during this stage, it may be possible to avoid loss of consciousness. An observer will note cold hands, pale skin, and tachycardia just before the patient loses consciousness. After the faint, when the patient is usually recumbent, a flush replaces the pallor and a bradycardia replaces the tachycardia. If the patient is unable to lie flat, recovery may be prolonged; and an occasional death has been noted, as in a faint occurring in a telephone booth or if the person is held upright during the spell. Bradycardia may persist for up to 1/2 hour after a simple faint. During this time the patient should remain in a recumbent position. The examination is otherwise normal unless there has been trauma or aspiration.

Autonomic Impairment. Syncope/near syncope due to autonomic impairment is always associated with orthostatic hypotension. To document this problem, blood pressure must be taken while the patient is supine, seated, and standing. In some patients, exercise while standing (walking for a few minutes, for example) may be required for a significant orthostatic drop (20 mm Hg systolic) to occur.

The most common cause of this problem is *antihypertensive drug use*; most syncope due to these drugs is preventable if these drugs are prescribed cautiously and the standing blood pressure, after exercise, is monitored routinely. Other drugs may also produce orthostatic symptoms (see Table 81.7). The initial management of drug-induced orthostasis is described in Chapter 62 (Hypertension); definitive management requires discontinuation or reduced dose of the offending drug.

Orthostatic hypotension can also be due to *autonomic neuropathy*. In patients suspected of having this problem, the integrity of the autonomic nervous system can be tested by noting the size and reaction of the pupils, the distribution of sweating, and the response to a Valsalva maneuver (14, 15). The Valsalva maneuver is performed by having the patient expire against a closed glottis for 20 to 30 seconds, then release air from the chest (Table 81.8). This maneuver creates a sudden reduction in cardiac output, stimulating vagal (afferent) and sympathetic (efferent) responses. Absence of the reflex tachycardia (phase II) and/or absence of the blood pressure overshoot and reflex bradycardia (phase IV) indicate autonomic impairment.

Sympathetic failure commonly occurs late in diabetic peripheral neuropathy (Chapter 72) but may be the presenting feature of amyloidosis or the neuropathy associated with various neoplasms. The Shy-Drager syndrome, which occurs in late life, is due to failure of certain central autonomic neurons and causes orthostatic hypotension, parkinsonism, and other autonomic symptoms in varying combinations. Sympa-

Table 81.8.
Four Phases of a Normal Valsalva Maneuver

ONSET (20–39 seconds) RELEASE	*Phase I:* A *sharp rise* in systolic pressure caused by an abrupt increase in intrathoracic pressure and emptying of the pulmonary bed during forced expiration against a closed glottis. *Phase II:* A *gradual fall* in systolic pressure and a concomitant narrowing of peripheral pulse pressures caused by decrease in pulmonic and systemic venous return. *Heart rate increases* during this phase. *Phase III:* A sudden *further drop* in blood pressure occurs. Pulse pressure may be very narrow for the few beats during refilling of pulmonary venous reservoir. *Phase IV* (overshoot): Cardiac output increases with the increase in ventricular filling. Within 30 seconds of release of intrathoracic pressure, blood pressure *rises above its original level* because of reflex vasoconstriction initiated by small pulse pressure during phase III. The pressoreceptor stimulation in phase IV results also in *transient bradycardia slowing*.

thectomy, particularly when done bilaterally or in the lumbar segments, may be followed immediately by orthostatic hypotension and syncope, though usually venous tone recovers several weeks after the operation. Tabes dorsalis and more commonly diabetic pseudotabes may present with lightning pains and autonomic failure. The management of orthostasis due to autonomic neuropathy is symptomatic; it is summarized in Chapter 84.

Decreased Intravascular Volume. Decreased intravascular volume due to hemorrhage or to salt and water loss (e.g., of gastroenteritis, heat exposure, diuretics, etc.) is recognized by the combination of orthostatic hypotension and an associated basis for the volume deficit. Hot weather and exercise predispose to volume depletion and thereby to syncope, particularly after vigorous exercise. Prolonged fasting, as in anorexia nervosa or with fad diets, also may produce syncope through volume depletion. Adrenal insufficiency due to pituitary or primary adrenal disease may produce syncope, due to the combination of chronic volume deficit and the loss of vascular tone; the syncope is often precipitated by an intercurrent illness that would not produce syncope in a healthy person. Hypoalbuminemia due to liver disease, enteropathies, or chronic disease can also lead to syncope/presyncope due to intravascular volume deficit. Volume expansion, either by increased salt and water ingestion or by intravenous fluids, is the initial treatment; the choice of ambulatory or hospital management and the planning of definitive treatment depends upon the severity and the primary cause for the volume deficit.

Venous Pooling. Venous pooling prevents return of blood to the heart, lowering cardiac output, at times sufficiently to produce near syncope or syncope. Symptoms may occur after prolonged standing in one position, particularly after exercise, as in recruits standing at attention. Severe dependent varicose veins or the compression of pelvic veins by a fetus or a large abdominal mass may produce symptoms due to a similar mechanism. Syncope 15 to 30 minutes after exercise has been attributed to dilation of the splanchnic circulation before blood flow to the skeletal muscles has completely returned to normal. Management of patients with these conditions is chiefly by avoidance of the precipitating circumstances after an initial episode. Supportive elastic stockings may be helpful for patients with marked pooling due to varicose veins (see Chapter 88).

Orthostatic Syncope/Near Syncope after Bed Rest. This problem is due to the combined effects of venous pooling, relative hypovolemia, and probably to some degree of lowered sensitivity of the baroreceptor system. It is a very common occurrence at all ages, but especially among the elderly, and should be anticipated in any person who has been at bed rest for more than a few days, in the hospital or at home; moreover, it may persist for 1 or 2 weeks, occasionally longer, after mobilization begins. Orthostatic symptoms may be minimized or prevented by having the patient gradually stand only after several minutes of sitting on the bed with the legs dependent. Practical exercises that may help convalescing patients in overcoming postural weakness and hypotension are illustrated in Figure 81.3. These patients should be encouraged to be out of bed for at least two hours a day, including morning, afternoon, and evening.

Orthostasis of Aging. Transient orthostatic symptoms are relatively common among older persons. An orthostatic fall of 30 mm Hg in systolic pressure is found in approximately 10% of healthy older persons (5). In addition, it has been shown that a significant fall in systolic blood pressure is common in elderly patients, in the sitting position, immediately after eating (20). This response may make elderly subjects especially susceptible to presyncope or syncope when getting up after a meal. The physiological basis for orthostatic blood pressure fall in the elderly is not established, although studies of small numbers of elderly persons have shown an impaired Valsalva response (15), indicating autonomic dysfunction. This often asymptomatic condition is important insofar as it increases the risk associated with drugs and conditions that may cause orthostatic hypotension. Clearly, older persons should have their standing blood pressure checked whenever they complain of even mild orthostatic symptoms, and they should be monitored similarly whenever a drug in one of the groups listed in Table 81.7 is prescribed. Those who are troubled by orthostatic symptoms should be advised to follow the steps recommended above for patients convalescing from bed rest.

Micturition Syncope. Micturition syncope, defined as syncope occurring at the beginning of, during, at the termination of, or immediately after urination (18), occurs typically in two types of subjects: (a) Young men who are otherwise healthy. Both the Valsalva mechanism and direct vagal stimulation have been hypothesized as the basis for this form of syncope. Alcohol, because it causes venous pooling, may be a predisposing factor in some patients. (b) Older men and women, many of whom have baseline orthostasis related to drugs or to aging. Persons with micturition syncope should be evaluated for orthostasis, and when this is found any factors contributing to it should be modified. In addition, all patients with recurrent micturition syncope should be advised to sit while urinating and to remain seated for a minute after urination.

Other Forms of Syncope Related to Systemic Circulation. *Tussive syncope* may follow a prolonged bout of coughing in otherwise normal individuals; in these persons, the syncope is thought to be due to the Valsalva mechanism (see above). Tussive syncope may also occur after only a slight cough in persons with obstructive airways disease; abnormalities of pulmonary and pleural vagal receptors in such individuals may aggravate their tendency to faint. Syncope during positive pressure breathing occurs by similar mechanisms.

Hypersensitivity of the carotid sinus is a controversial entity and probably an uncommon cause of syncope. Stimulation of the baroreceptors in the carotid sinus may provoke sympathetic relaxation and lead to hypotension with a normal heart rate; it may increase vagal activity leading to bradycardia without hypotension; or it may provoke abnormalities in the brainstem that lead to syncope without a change in circulatory dynamics. These mechanisms have been invoked in patients with long-standing and severe hypertension or with coronary or carotid arteriosclerosis. Older men wearing tight collars, women with cumbersome necklaces, or patients having large masses in the neck are predisposed to the problem. In some patients thought to have carotid sinus hypersensitivity, compression of the common or internal carotid arteries (or the external carotid, an important collateral in the case of a carotid occlusion) may lead to the symptoms of cerebral ischemia if the contralateral artery is not fully patent. Some authorities recommend provoking syncope by unilateral or bilateral carotid massage. This may be a dangerous maneuver, and it should be performed only in an emergency department or in the hospital, with intravenous fluid running, ECG monitoring, and atropine at hand, and only after checking the adequacy of the carotid pulses.

Sudden loss of consciousness may be the presenting manifestation in 10 to 15% of cases of pulmonary embolism (27). In such cases, unconsciousness may be brief (syncope) or prolonged (cardiac arrest), and may be accompanied by a small seizure or minor neurological abnormalities, even when paradoxical embolization has not occurred. The diagnosis of pulmonary embolism is suggested by the presence of dyspnea, hypotension, tachycardia, or acute cor pulmonale by ECG or physical examinations.

Cardiac Abnormalities

Rhythm Disturbances. Arrhythmias should always be considered in patients with syncope or near syncope who are older, have known heart disease, or have symptoms while seated or recumbent. Suspicion should also be raised in patients taking medications that may cause arrhythmias (e.g., quinidine, digoxin, tricyclic antidepressants, neuroleptics). Though premonitory warnings may be recalled (particularly grayouts, sweating, mild nausea, and fear), patients' reports regarding palpitations are notoriously unreliable and should not be used to substantiate or refute the diagnosis of an arrhythmia. Most patients with cerebral symptoms due to arrhythmias have normal resting ECGs. In general, at least 48 hours of ECG monitoring are necessary to identify all potentially important arrhythmias in patients with syncope that is not explained by the initial history, physical examination, and 12-lead ECG. Particular attention should be paid to ventricular tachycardia, paroxysmal sustained supraventricular tachycardia, profound bradycardia, high grade heart block, and spells of asystole. Definitive diagnosis is possible when recorded ECG abnormalities are accompanied by concurrent cerebral symptoms. In the absence of concurrent symptoms, definitive diagnosis may not be possible. However, asympto-

LEG EXERCISES

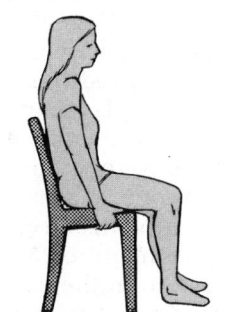 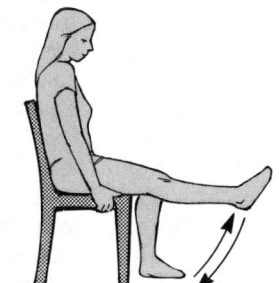 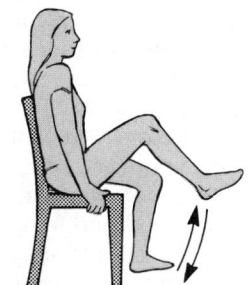

Starting position: Sitting in chair, exercise one leg at a time

Raise leg up and down. Repeat 10 times

Keeping knee bent, raise leg up and down

ARM EXERCISES: To increase effectiveness, hold a soup can in each hand for weight

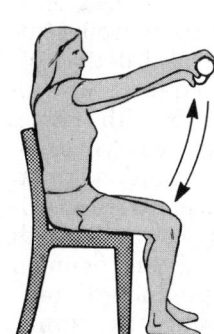 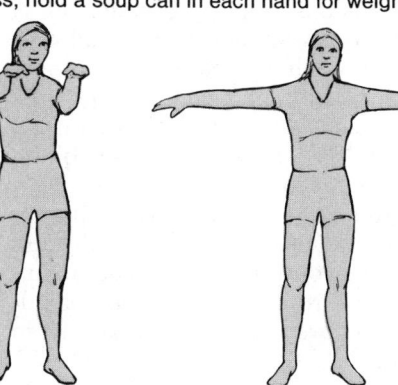

Start with arms straight out in front. Raise arms up and down, only to chin level. Repeat 10 times

Start with arms straight out in front. Swing arms out to sides and return to front. Repeat 10 times

RISING EXERCISE

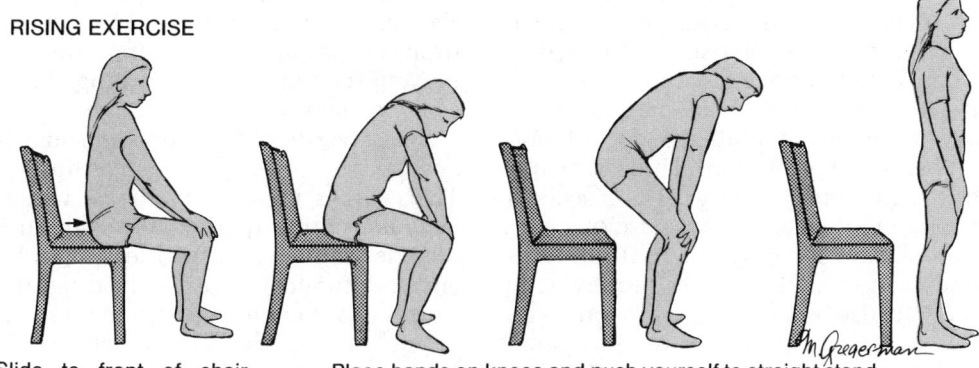

Slide to front of chair, keeping legs apart

Place hands on knees and push yourself to straight stand. Sit down, using hands on knees to help

Repeat 3–5 times using hands less and legs more each time. Repeat exercise without using hands to help

Figure 81.3. Exercise for weakness and orthostatic hypotension after prolonged bed rest. Patient must be out of bed 2 hours a day, morning, afternoon, and evening (for meals). Exercises are done three times a day. (Courtesy of Ms. Karen Ryder, Registered Occupational Therapist.)

matic abnormalities such as unsustained ventricular tachycardia, frequent ventricular ectopy, and sinus pauses are associated with an increased risk of sudden death that may warrant further evaluation (19). Details regarding the diagnosis and management of patients with these arrhythmias are found in Chapter 59.

Outflow Obstruction. An obstruction to ventricular outflow due to rheumatic or calcific *aortic stenosis* may lead to syncope. It nearly always follows exertion and is often associated with chest pain. Unconsciousness may be prolonged and may be followed by neurological abnormalities. Similarly, idiopathic *hypertrophic cardiomyopathy* in patients of any age may lead to syncope by outlet obstruction after exercise or by an arrhythmia at any time. The diagnostic approach to patients thought to have outflow obstruction from these causes is described in Chapter 60. A *left atrial myxoma* (very rare) may cause syncope by obstruction of blood flow when a patient leans over or undergoes exertion. *Cyanotic congenital heart disease* also leads to syncope after exercise or, rarely, during an airplane flight. Hypoxia and increased blood viscosity are contributing factors.

Myocardial Infarction. Acute myocardial infarction may present with syncope, which may result from an arrhythmia, low cardiac output, or severe pain. Embolization from a mural thrombus should be considered when syncope occurs during recovery from myocardial infarction.

Metabolic Abnormalities

Because some metabolic derangements (e.g., hypoglycemia or hypoxia) may lead to lasting damage, the physician should be very alert to the possibility of these problems in patients with syncope who have features or abnormalities characteristic of these derangements in their history or examination.

Hypoglycemia. Loss of consciousness due to hypoglycemia may occur in the adult when the blood glucose level is below 40 mg/100 ml. Hunger, palpitations, sweating, and anxiety nearly always occur 5 to 15 minutes before the patient loses consciousness. As the brain can survive for only about 10 minutes with a blood glucose of 20 mg/100 ml, the prophylactic administration of glucose is warranted in anyone who remains unconscious long enough for the physician to prepare the solution. Convulsions and incontinence commonly accompany hypoglycemic coma. The evaluation and management of hypoglycemia due to exogenous insulin are described in Chapter 72. *Reactive hypoglycemia and fasting* hypoglycemia (which may be due to insulinoma) may produce near syncope but not unconsciousness. These problems are described in Chapter 74. Mild hypoglycemic symptoms may also occur postprandially in patients who have had ulcer surgery, as part of the *dumping syndrome* (see Chapter 36).

Hypocapnia. Hypocapnia due to *hyperventilation* leads to syncope, near syncope, or ill-defined dizziness by decreasing cerebral blood flow through va-soconstriction of small arterioles throughout the brain. A pCO_2 of 25 mm Hg is sufficient to lower cerebral blood flow to levels at which symptoms may occur; such a value may be produced in some persons by a few very deep breaths. Athletes preparing to race, musicians playing wind instruments, or anyone who is fearful or anxious may develop transient symptoms in this way. Tetany or carpopedal spasm may or may not precede the cerebral symptoms. Recovery is prompt if ventilation is slowed. As many as 25% of patients with chronic dizziness have it on the basis of hyperventilation (7). The diagnosis and management of hyperventilation related to anxiety, the commonest cause of this problem, are described in Chapter 13.

Hypoxemia. Hypoxemia due to any primary cause may predispose to syncope/near syncope. *Severe anemia* (see Chapter 50) may sufficiently deprive the brain of oxygen to lead to syncope after exercise; it may also predispose to syncope from any other cause. Asphyxiation due to *obstruction of the upper airway* should be considered in small children, patients with bad teeth, or patients with masses in the neck. The "cafe coronary" due to laryngeal aspiration of food is usually betrayed by sudden collapse at the table. Patients with esophageal diverticula, however, may choke hours after a meal. Poisoning with *carbon monoxide* is suggested by a history of intentional or unintentional exposure to products of combustion (e.g., poorly ventilated space heaters, gas-burning engines in closed spaces). Manifestations may include prodromal headache and confusion plus bright pink color and prolonged unconsciousness.

Seizures are very common in patients with acute hypoxemia, and neurological sequelae are the rule after unconsciousness lasting more than 1 or 2 minutes. The management of hypoxemic syncope depends entirely on prompt and accurate diagnosis in order to prevent recurrence or worsening of the primary cause of hypoxemia.

Drug Overdose. Overdose of some drugs may cause syncope/near syncope due to orthostatic hypotension. These drugs include sedatives, which may produce venous pooling (particularly chloral hydrate, paraldehyde, and ethanol, and less often benzodiazepines and barbiturates) and all of the drugs listed as potential causes of autonomic impairment in Table 81.7. Stupor or coma due to the sedating effects of drug overdose is more common than are transient cerebral symptoms (syncope/near syncope) due to acute orthostatic hypotension.

Intracranial Abnormalities

Seizure. A seizure may occur with or without warning in any position and may be the primary event leading to loss of consciousness. The diagnosis and management of seizure disorders are described in detail in Chapter 80.

Subarachnoid Hemorrhage. A brief period of unconsciousness at the beginning of subarachnoid hemorrhage is the rule. This diagnosis is strongly suggested when the constellation of headache, confusion, and neck stiffness follows shortly after a syncopal episode. Any patient who is confused and who develops headache during initial evaluation demands more scrutiny, even if meningismus has not yet developed. Such patients should be admitted for observation and evaluation.

Embolism or Thrombosis. Cerebral embolism or thrombosis may cause brief (TIA) or prolonged (cardiovascular accident) unconsciousness if the basilar artery is affected. Rarely, a carotid occlusion may cause unconsciousness initially, even if the remaining vessels are patent. A carotid occlusion likewise may cause loss of consciousness if the contralateral carotid is already occluded; in this instance, the period of unconsciousness is usually prolonged and seizures may occur; neurological symptoms and signs nearly always are present. The ambulatory diagnosis and management of cerebrovascular disease are described in detail in Chapter 83.

Migraine. Migraine (see Chapter 79) may produce syncope/near syncope, due to spasm of the basilar artery or of the posterior cerebral arteries. Syncope that occurs with migraine is more often due to hyperventilation or to a vasovagal mechanism than to a central abnormality.

Increased Intracranial Pressure. Increased intracranial pressure, whether due to a brain tumor, trauma, or an obstruction to the ventricular system, may result in syncope when a Valsalva maneuver is performed such as during straining at stool or bending over. The hallmarks are pre-existing symptoms, papilledema, or neurological signs.

Brainstem Compression. Rarely, brainstem compression due to metastatic tumors, cystic anomalies, or a displaced fracture of C1 or of the odontoid process may lead to syncope with movement of the neck because of transient compression of critical structures of the brainstem. Patients with severe rheumatoid arthritis also may develop cervical instability leading to compression of the brainstem with neck motion. Associated neurological abnormalities are often present. The diagnosis and management of patients thought to have this problem require prompt hospital admission.

Overall Prognosis

The overall prognosis of syncope and near syncope depends ultimately on the underlying disorder and upon any trauma or other morbidity that may have occurred as a consequence of losing consciousness. The simple faint, hyperventilation, venous pooling, or syncope with a Valsalva maneuver may occur repeatedly when the patient is in the same circumstance and can be prevented by avoiding it. Drug-provoked syncope/near syncope can be eliminated by discontinuing or decreasing the dose of the offending drug; and syncope due to intravascular volume deficit is usually amenable to therapy. Although limiting exercise may prevent syncope due to cardiac outflow obstruction,

surgical therapy is usually needed (particularly for aortic stenosis), and the prognosis depends on the outcome of the surgery. Cerebral symptoms due to arrhythmias can be prevented by pacemaker or antiarrhythmic treatment. Similarly, most symptoms due to common metabolic or intracranial abnormalities are amenable to treatment. Patients with syncope of unknown origin have a relatively benign prognosis but may be troubled by recurrent syncope.

Selected Conditions That May Mimic Syncope

Hysterical Faint

Sudden, dramatic fainting was very common in the 19th century, especially in women. Today fainting preceded by hyperventilation is more common. Usually the fainting occurs in a manner to avoid injury, an important distinguishing feature from true syncope. The patient crumples to the ground with a limp body and shallow respirations. Recovery is usually immediate. Quite often, the faint may be embellished with movements that resemble seizures (referred to as pseudoseizures), but more often voluntary movements are the rule. Hyperventilation or coaxing may reproduce the spell. Chapter 12 provides additional detail regarding the evaluation and management of such patients, whose physical symptoms are often due to emotional factors.

Drop Attack

Older patients, especially men, may report sudden and unprovoked falls to the ground. Consciousness is not lost, and the patients can usually remember the entire episode. This maintenance of consciousness distinguishes drop attacks from syncope. Ischemia of the lower brainstem is thought to cause drop attacks, and occasionally patients will report other concurrent symptoms that suggest vertebrobasilar ischemia. Management is identical to that of TIAs occurring in the posterior circulation (see Chapter 83).

Cataplexy

Cataplexy is a special kind of drop attack, not due to ischemia, that occurs as part of the syndrome of narcolepsy (see Chapter 85). The patient falls suddenly to the ground because of a loss of extensor muscle tone but without loss of consciousness. These spells are usually provoked by a sudden startle, a joke, laughing, or sneezing. They may be effectively managed by tricyclic agents. *Sleep paralysis* (paralysis of the limbs for a minute or two upon awakening) and peculiar visual hallucinations on awakening or before falling asleep may also accompany narcolepsy. (See Chapter 85 for additional details.)

DISEQUILIBRIUM OF MISCELLANEOUS ORIGINS

Some patients with relatively persistent "dizziness" do not have manifestations that make it possible to classify their problem as vertigo or near syncope. Many of these persons have disequilibrium, or a sense of imbalance, that may be due to one of the following problems: cerebellar ataxia (see Chapter 78); multiple sensory deficits (3) (e.g., partial hearing, visual, and proprioceptive impairment); lower extremity weakness (e.g., from an old stroke or from disuse after a fracture or after a period of bed rest); pain in a weight-bearing joint; recently initiated drugs, especially sedatives; or the onset of a progressive central nervous system disease such as parkinsonism (see Chapter 82), normal pressure hydrocephalus (see Chapter 17), or CP angle tumor (see Chapter 96). These problems often occur in older persons, in debilitated persons (particularly chronic alcoholics), or in patients with long-standing diabetes. In these persons, cerebrovascular disease or autonomic neuropathy may cause periodic vertigo and near syncope to be superimposed on their day-to-day problem with imbalance.

The evaluation of persons describing imbalance consists chiefly of obtaining a history of the duration, progression, and day-to-day characteristics of the problem, focusing upon the limitations imposed upon their usual activities and upon any falls or near accidents that may have occurred. In the physical examination, it is important to determine which of the many problems listed above may be contributing to the patient's symptoms.

Depending upon the individual patient, management by the generalist may include (a) referring the patient for correction of deafness or cataract (see Chapters 96 and 97); (b) obtaining a consultant's opinion whenever unexplained progressive symptoms are found (for example, cerebellar ataxia in a relatively healthy person); (c) obtaining the help of a physical therapist if weakness or the need for selecting a cane or a walker is apparent; (d) discontinuing any drugs that may be contributing to the patient's symptoms and avoiding drugs that may worsen symptoms (see Tables 81.2 and 81.7).

CHRONIC DIZZINESS: GENERAL MEASURES IN MANAGEMENT

Patients with chronic dizziness, vertigo, syncope, or disequilibrium will have a far better prognosis if their physicians assure that their home environments are safe and that others in their households are aware of risks that should be avoided and of devices that may be helpful. A number of general measures to consider including the following: the use of night-lights, tacking down loose carpeting and floorboards, use of canes or walkers, installation of special railings in the bathroom, proper selection of footwear, and instruction on gradual assumption of an upright posture. These measures can be accomplished most effectively if the physician or a visiting nurse evaluates in his (the patient's) home.

General References

Baloh RW, Honrubia V: *Clinical Neurophysiology of the Vestibular System.* Philadelphia, FA Davis, 1982.

Excellent review of vertigo.
Lee JE, Killip T, Plum F: Episodic unconsciousness. In: Baron JA (ed): *Diagnostic Approaches to Presenting Syndromes.* Baltimore, Williams & Wilkins, 1971.
A detailed discussion of normal physiology and specific causes of syncope.
Wolfson RJ: Symposium on vertigo. *Otolaryngol Clin North Am* 6(1):1973.
Excellent coverage of all aspects of vertigo.

Specific References

1. Baloh RW, Honrubia V, Jacobson K: Benign positional vertigo: clinical and oculographic features in 240 cases. *Neurology* 37:371, 1987.
2. Bárány R: Diagnosis of disease of the otolith apparatus. *J Laryngol Otol* 36:229, 1921.
3. Brandt T, Daroff RB: The multisensory physiological and pathological vertigo syndromes. *Ann Neurol* 7:195, 1980.
4. Brandt T, Daroff RB: Physical therapy for benign paroxysmal positional vertigo. *Arch Otolaryngol* 106:484, 1980.
5. Caird FI, Andrews GR, Kennedy RD: Effect of posture on blood pressure in the elderly. *Br Heart J* 35:527, 1973.
6. Day SC, Cook EF, Funkenstein H, Goldman L: Evaluation and outcome of emergency room patients with transient loss of consciousness. *Am J Med* 73:15, 1982.
7. Drachman DA, Hart CW: An approach to the dizzy patient. *Neurology* 22:323, 1972.
8. Gendelman HE, Linzer M, Gabelman M, et al: Syncope in a general hospital patient population. Usefulness of the radionuclide brain scan, electroencephalogram, and 24-hour Holter monitor. *NY State J Med* 83:1161, 1983.
9. Gibson TC, Heitzman MR: Diagnostic efficacy of 24-hour electrocardiographic monitoring for syncope. *Am J Cardiol* 53:1013, 1984.
10. Glassock ME III, Hayes JW: Pitfalls in the diagnosis of acoustic and other cerebellopontine angle tumors. *Laryngoscope* 83:1038, 1973.
11. Harner SG: Peripheral labyrinthine causes of dizziness. *Postgrad Med* 81:251, 1987.
12. Hart CW: Evaluation of post-traumatic vertigo. *Otolaryngol Clin North Am* 6:157, 1973.
13. Hybels RL: Drug toxicity of the inner ear. *Med Clin North Am* 63:309, 1979.
14. Ibrahim MM: Localization of lesion in patients with idiopathic orthostatic hypotension. *Br Heart J* 37:868, 1975.
15. Johnson RJ, Smith AC, Spalding JMK, Wollner L: Effect of posture on blood-pressure in elderly patients. *Lancet* 1:731, 1965.
16. Jongkees LBW: The caloric test and its value in evaluation of the patient with vertigo. *Otolaryngol Clin North Am* 6:73, 1973.
17. Kapoor WN, Karpf M, Wieand S, et al: A prospective evaluation and follow-up of patients with syncope. *N Engl J Med* 309:197, 1983.
18. Kapoor WN, Peterson JR, Karpf M: Micturition syncope. *JAMA* 253:796, 1985.
19. Kapoor WN, Cha R, Peterson JR, et al: Prolonged electrocardiographic monitoring in patients with syncope. Importance of frequent or repetitive ventricular ectopy. *Am J Med* 82:20, 1987.
20. Lipsitz LA, Nyquist RP, Wei JY, Rowe JW: Postprandial reduction in blood pressure in the elderly. *N Engl J Med* 309:81, 1983.
21. Norre ME, Beckers AM: Vestibular habituation training. Specificity of adequate exercise. *Arch Otolaryngol* 114:883, 1988.
22. Norre ME, Beckers AM: Benign paroxysmal positional vertigo in the elderly. Treatment by habituation exercises. *J Am Geriatr Soc* 36:425, 1988.
23. Page JM: Audiologic tests in the differential diagnosis of vertigo. *Otolaryngol Clin North Am* 6:53, 1973.
24. Rubin W: Electronystagmography and its value in the diagnosis of vertigo. *Otolaryngol Clin North Am* 6:95, 1973.
25. Schmitt LG, Shaw JE: Alleviation of induced vertigo. Therapy with transdermal scopolamine and oral meclizine. *Arch Otolaryngol* 112:88, 1986.
26. Slater R: Vertigo. How serious are recurrent and single attacks? *Postgrad Med* 84:58, 1988.

27. Thames MD, Alpert JS, Dalen JE: Syncope in patients with pulmonary embolism. *JAMA* 238:2509, 1977.
28. Wood CD, Graybiel A: The antimotion sickness drugs. *Otolaryngol Clin North Am* 6:301, 1973.

C H A P T E R   82

Common Disorders of Movement: Tremor and Parkinson's Disease

STEPHEN G. REICH, M.D.
MAHLON R. DELONG, M.D.

TREMOR

Definition and Classification

Tremor is defined as the involuntary rhythmic or semi-rhythmic oscillation of a body part, resulting from alternating or simultaneous contractions of antagonistic muscle groups. Despite extensive clinical study, the pathophysiology of different tremor types is poorly understood and, as such, the differential diagnosis centers on clinical observation. Tremor is conveniently classified by its relation to the conditions of rest, postural maintenance, and movement. The three major clinical types of tremor are thus *resting*, *postural*, and *kinetic (intention)*. Accurate classification of temor type is important since each points to a group of specific underlying conditions (Table 82.1), each with specific therapy.

Table 82.1.

Conditions Associated with the Three Major Types of Tremor[a]

Resting Tremor

Parkinson's disease

Secondary parkinsonism: postencephalitic, toxic (phenothiazines, reserpine, carbon monoxide, manganese, carbon disulfide), tumor, trauma, vascular, metabolic (hypoparathyroidism, chronic hepatocerebral degeneration)

Heterogeneous disorders with parkinsonian features: striatonigral degeneration, olivopontocerebellar atrophy, progressive supranuclear palsy, Wilson's disease

Postural Tremor

Exaggerated physiological tremor
Anxiety, fright, fatigue, exercise
Endocrine: thyrotoxicosis, hypoglycemia, pheochromocytoma
Drugs: any sympathomimetics, caffeine, theophylline, levodopa, lithium, tricyclic antidepressants, phenothiazines, butyrophenones, thyroid hormone, hypoglycemic agents, withdrawal from alcohol and sedative-hypnotic drugs
Essential tremor
Familial (autosomal dominant)
Sporadic
Senile
With other neurological disorders: parkinsonism, torsion dystonia, spasmodic torticollis, neuropathy

Kinetic or Intention Tremor (Cerebellar Dysfunction)

Cerebellar degeneration, atrophy, infarction
Multiple sclerosis
Wilson's disease
Drugs and toxins: phenytoin, barbiturates, lithium, alcohol, mercury, 5-fluorouracil
Miscellaneous cerebellar and cerebellofugal lesions

[a] Adapted from:Jankovic J, Fahn S: Physiologic and pathologic tremors: diagnosis, mechanism, and management. *Ann Intern Med* 93:460, 1980.

Tremor can usually be distinguished from other hyperkinetic movement disorders by its rhythmicity and the presence or absence of other neurological signs. A brief review of the clinical phenomenology of other involuntary movement disorders will help to prevent diagnostic errors. *Chorea* consists of rapid, often distal, nonrhythmical, nonstereotyped movements that often coexist with the slower, writhing movements referred to as *athetosis*. In its extreme, when violent, flinging and more proximal choreoathetosis merges with *ballismus*. *Myoclonus* refers to rapid, brief muscle jerks that affect random body parts, are usually nonrhythmical, may persist during sleep (unlike tremors and other hyperkinetic movement disorders), and commonly occur in the setting of a metabolic or toxic encephalopathy. *Asterixis*, sometimes referred to as "negative myoclonus," consists of brief lapses of posture ("flapping") of the dorsiflexed hands due to inhibition of agonist muscle groups; like myoclonus, asterixis most often occurs in the setting of an encephalopathy. *Motor tics* can be distinguished from tremor by their lack of rhythmicity, erratic appearance in different body parts, complexity of the movement, onset in childhood or adolescence, and frequently associated vocalizations and behavioral disturbances. Tics are often preceded by a buildup of inner tension that subsides after the tic. Patients may be able to temporarily suppress a tic whereas most other abnormal movements lack such a degree of voluntary control. *Dystonia* refers to sustained, twisting movements usually lacking regular oscillations, although tremor-like movements of the head may occur in spasmodic torticollis, a form of dystonia.

EVALUATION OF THE PATIENT WITH TREMOR

The history and physical examination are fundamental in the diagnosis of tremors (Table 82.2). Important *historical* information includes the temporal onset of the tremor, associated neurological symptoms, whether it is suppressed by alcohol, family history, and a survey of medications and other medical illnesses. Almost all varieties of tremor increase in amplitude under stress, diminish with relaxation, and disappear during sleep. The impact of the tremor upon the patient determines whether treatment is indicated. Some patients do not find their tremor disabling and seek medical attention only for diagnostic purposes—young patients with essential tremor often just need reassurance that their tremor is benign and that they do not have Parkinson's disease or another degenerative disorder. However, the majority of patients find the tremor either physically or emotionally problematic.

Emphasis should be placed on the activities of daily living (ADLs; see Chapter 6 for definition). Patients with tremor typically have trouble with tasks requiring fine motor control such as buttoning, feeding, shaving, brushing their teeth, writing, and cooking. Embarrassment is often an unvoiced source of disability, and patients should be questioned about social isolation due to the tremor. The ADLs also provide objective parameters for judging the effectiveness of therapy.

The objectives of the *physical examination* are to determine the anatomical localization, frequency, and condition(s) of maximal activation of the tremor and to search for associated neurological signs. Patients should be examined with their hands resting on their lap, with their arms held outstretched, and while performing finger-to-nose and heel-to-shin maneuvers. Samples of handwriting and a drawing of a spiral should also be obtained. Observations while drinking from a cup or using a fork or spoon are also helpful in assessing functional impairment.

The *resting tremor* of parkinsonism typically consists of 4 to 6-Hertz (Hz, same as cycles per second) flexion-extension at the metacarpophalangeal joints, abduction-adduction of the thumb, and pronation-supination of the forearm; these produce the so-called "pill-rolling" tremor. Resting tremor is often brought out by having the patient walk or by distracting the patient with conversation or mental arithmetic. Early in its course, the parkinsonian tremor is often asymmetrical.

Postural tremor is characteristic of essential tremor and usually consists of 6 to 12-Hz symmetrical flexion-extension at the wrists and shoulders. It is brought on by having the patient assume an antigravity posture of the upper extremities (i.e., stretched-out arms), and it is not present when the arms are resting against the body or on a surface.

Kinetic tremor (also referred to as "intention tremor") is encountered most commonly in cerebellar disease and is characterized by 3 to 5-Hz irregular oscillations as the limb approaches a target. This type of tremor is often accompanied by inaccuracies in movement direction (dysmetria). In acquired cerebellar diseases, such as strokes and multiple sclerosis, kinetic tremors are often asymmetrical whereas heredofamilial and sporadic degenerative diseases involving the cerebellum produce bilateral, symmetrical tremor. Conditions that may mimic this aspect of cerebellar disease include marked postural tremor (which may impair purposeful movements) and proprioceptive loss. Care-

Table 82.2.
Principal Features of Different Tremor Types and Their Treatment

	Resting (Parkinsonian)	Postural (Essential)	Kinetic or Intention (Cerebellar)
History			
Age at onset	Middle age and beyond	All ages	All ages
Family history	Negative	Often positive (autosomal dominant)	Rarely positive
Response to alcohol	No effect	Often suppresses tremor	No effect
Physical Examination			
Frequency	4–5 Hz	6–12 Hz	3–5 Hz
Symmetry	Often begins asymmetrically	Symmetrically	Either symmetrical or asymmetrical
Body part(s) affected	Arms > legs	Hand>head >legs>jaw >tongue>trunk	Arms>legs>trunk/head
Associated Signs	Bradykinesia, rigidity, postural	None	Dysarthira, Nystagmus, broad-based gait
Treatment			
	Anticholinergics	Primidone	Stereotactic surgery
	Amantadine	Propranolol	
	Sinemet	Alprazolam	
	Bromocriptine	Stereotactic surgery	
	Pergolide		
	Stereotactic surgery		

ful assessment of all of the patient's signs and symptoms usually enables the physician to distinguish these conditions from true cerebellar dysfunction Table 82.3, which compares cerebellar and proprioceptive incoordination).

COMMON CONDITIONS PRESENTING WITH TREMOR

Parkinson's Disease

The typical resting tumor of Parkinson's disease is discussed below.

Physiological and Exaggerated Physiological Tremor

Most individuals have a barely perceptible postural tremor, so-called "physiological tremor," that may be best appreciated by placing a piece of paper over the outstretched hands. Although asymptomatic, this tremor may be *transiently* exacerbated during systemic illness, metabolic derangements, stress, and by the use or withdrawal of certain drugs or of alcohol (Table 82.1).

The most important step in management is identification and removal of the offending cause; resolution of the tremor confirms the diagnosis of exaggerated physiological tremor. Although discontinuation of tremorigenic drugs usually leads to prompt resolution of the tremor, it may take 1 to 2 weeks for the tremor to resolve after resolution of a systemic illness or a severe metabolic abnormality.

If the underlying condition cannot be eliminated (e.g., patients requiring lithium for manic-depressive illness), propranolol usually abolishes the tremor. For persons subject to situational anxiety, manifested by exaggerated physiological tremor, prophylactic treatment with propranolol (20 to 40 mg) 1 hour before an anxiety-producing situation (such as public speaking) may be helpful.

Essential Tremor

Essential tremor (ET), the most common form of postural tremor, affects over one million Americans (6, 9). Essential tremor is also called heredofamilial tremor, benign essential tremor, and "senile tremor." No neuropathological abnormalities have been identified in ETs but physiological evidence suggests that both the central and peripheral nervous systems are involved. The onset is insidious and may begin as early as childhood or appear for the first time in advanced age. Between 25 and 50% of patients have a positive family history, usually with autosomal dominant inheritance.

In its prototypical form, ET is characterized by a bilateral and symmetrical tremor of the hands, but it may also affect other body parts either in isolation or combined with a hand tremor. These include the head, chin, lips, tongue, lower extremities, or voice. At least half of patients with ET notice a beneficial effect from small amounts of alcohol (8). Although its regular use to suppress tremor should be discouraged, when used

sparingly, alcohol represents an effective treatment for ET particularly when exacerbated by situational stress. There does not seem to be an increased prevalence of alcoholism among patients with ET (17).

Treatment

When ET begins to interfere with the ADLs or causes significant embarrassment, treatment is indicated. Before starting medication, patients should be told that the goal of treatment is not to abolish the tremor, which is rarely possible, but instead, to reduce its severity. The patient's ADLs should be used as a gauge to determine the effectiveness of treatment.

The two medications most effective for ET are propranolol (Inderal or generic) and primidone (Mysoline). Neither has been shown to have consistent superiority, and the two drugs may be synergistic (19). Propranolol is started at 10 mg twice per day and gradually increased depending on the beneficial response and appearance of side effects to a maximum of 320 mg per day. Once a stable dose has been reached, patients can be converted to Inderal LA, as the once-daily administration is preferred by most patients (18).

Although other β-blockers have also been shown to be effective for ET, none is superior to propranolol (14, 21). Metoprolol has the theoretical advantage of being a β-1 selective blocker and therefore safer to use in patients with ET and asthma, but at higher doses, the β-1 selectivity is diminished. In general, β-blockers should be avoided in the presence of bronchospastic disease, second or third degree heart block, congestive heart failure, or insulin-dependent diabetes. Additional practical details about β-blockers are found in Chapter 62, Hypertension.

Primidone, an anticonvulsant, was found by serendipity to improve ET. The mechanism of action of primidone is unknown, but its effect does not appear to be due to either of its metabolites—(phenylethylmalonamide) or phenobarbital (20). Primidone is available as scored tablets in two (PEMA) strengths, 50 mg and 250 mg. The starting dose must be very low (e.g., 25 mg per day) since occasional patients, especially the elderly, develop severe side effects after even a single small dose—dizziness, lethargy, confusion, nausea, sedation, and ataxia, which usually diminish with continued use. The dose is initially given at bedtime and then gradually escalated to a maximum of 250 mg three times per day as tolerated. In general, if patients show no response to low doses (250 mg per day), it is rare for higher doses to be effective. If there is a beneficial but suboptimal response to either propranolol or primidone used alone, the two should be combined beginning at low doses and increasing in small increments, watching carefully for side effects, particularly in elderly patients.

The benzodiazepam, alprazolam (Xanax), has also shown to be effective in the treatment of ET. The maintenance dose is 0.75 to 3.0 mg per day, in a three times daily schedule. Its rapid onset of action and short half-life, in comparison with other benzodiazepines, allow for its intermittent use when situational stress temporarily exacerbates ET (11). Practical details regarding alprazolam are found in Chapter 13, TheAnxious Patient.

When ET is disabling and poorly controlled with optimal medical therapy, consideration should be given to referral to a neurosurgeon for stereotactic thalamotomy. When carried out at a center experienced in the procedure, there is a relatively high success rate with minimal morbidity (27).

Tremor Due to Cerebellar Dysfunction (Kinetic, or Intention, Tremor)

Tremor is rarely the sole presenting sign of cerebellar dysfunction and, most often, the underlying disease is already known or readily apparent—multiple sclerosis, stroke, or drug intoxication. Occasionally, severe essential tremor may be exacerbated with action giving the impression of cerebellar disease, but the faster frequency, prominent postural component, and lack of associated cerebellar signs usually suffice to distinguish the two.

With the exception of drug-induced cerebellar tremor (Table 82.1), which should be managed by discontinuation or reduction of the dose of the offending drug, a patient with newly diagnosed cerebellar tremor should be referred to a neurologist. Unless the underlying disease is amenable to treatment, there is little that can be done medically for cerebellar tremor. Adding weights to the affected limbs may offer a small amount of improvement but seldom enough to translate into a functional change. As is the case with severe essential tremor, stereotactic thalamotomy is a viable solution for disabling cerebellar tremor (27).

Miscellaneous Tremors

Two atypical types of tremor have been described recently: primary writing tremor (15) and primary orthostatic tremor (10).

Primary writing tremor is one variant of a group of "task specific" tremors. These are characterized by maximal activation during a specific act although there may be an associated mild postural tremor as well. Primary writing tremor occurs exclusively when patients attempt to write. It is not clear under which category of movement disorders primary writing tremor is best classified as it seems to lie somewhere along the spectrum between essential tremor and focal dystonia, i.e., writer's cramp (30). Writing tremor may respond either to drugs used to treat essential tremor or anticholinergics used to treat dystonia (see below).

Primary orthostatic tremor is characterized by rapid shaking of the legs only with standing and it may respond to clonazepam (0.5 to 3.0 mg per day).

PARKINSON'S DISEASE AND "PARKINSONISM"

History

In 1817 James Parkinson, a London general practitioner, published his *Essay on The Shaking Palsy* based on observations of six patients (28). Although much has subsequently been learned about the pathology, pathophysiology, and treatment of what later became known as "Parkinson's disease (PD)," little has been added to Parkinson's original clinical description of the movement disorder: "Involuntary tremulous motion, with lessened muscular power, in parts not in action and even when supported; with a propensity to bend the trunk forwards, and to pass from a walking to a running pace." Parkinson, however, did not appreciate the muscular rigidity or the relatively high frequency of depression and cognitive impairment associated with the disease.

Epidemiology

PD is one of the most frequently encountered neurological diseases in the ambulatory setting. Epidemiological studies have demonstrated varying incidence and prevalence rates among different geographical, socioeconomic, and racial groups but no one group has been found to be immune to PD. In the United States, the prevalence rate is approximately 100 per 100,000 for persons under 50 years of age and over 600 cases per 100,000 after age 70. The overall annual incidence rate is approximately 18 per 100,000 per year but, in the 70 to 79 age group, climbs to one to two cases per thousand. The average age of onset is 60 years with equal distribution between sexes.

Etiology

The cause of PD has remained elusive despite tremendous advances in understanding other aspects of the disease. Interest has focused on three main areas: infectious disease, genetics, and environmental toxins. A *viral* etiology for PD was suggested by the occurrence of a permanent parkinsonian syndrome after the epidemic of encephalitis lethargica (1918 to 1922) plus the appearance of transient parkinsonian features after other encephalitides. Attempts to identify either viral inclusions or serological markers of prior viral infection have been unsuccessful as have attempts to transmit PD to subhuman primates. The *genetic* hypothesis lost momentum after failure to demonstrate a higher prevalence of PD among first degree relatives of patients when compared with those of the spouse. Twin studies have also failed to demonstrate a higher-than-expected concordance rate.

More recently, enthusiasm has focused on the possibility of an *environmental toxin* after the discovery that 1-methyl-4-pheny-1, 2, 3, 6-tetrahydropyridine (MPTP), an impurity of "synthetic heroin," produced an outbreak of a severe, permanent parkinsonian syndrome in intravenous drug abusers (1, 22). Although neither MPTP nor its active metabolite MPP+ is known to occur naturally in the environment, the discovery that a toxin can selectively destroy the pigmented dopaminergic cells of the substantia nigra has not only opened new avenues of research but has also produced an animal model of PD. A current working hypothesis is that PD results from a subclinical toxic exposure leading to an acceleration of the "normal" aging process of the brain, which includes loss of nigral neurons and depletion of brain dopamine (2).

Diagnosis and Differential Diagnosis

The cardinal *signs* of PD include tremor at rest (often asymmetrical), bradykinesia, muscular rigidity, and postural instability. Common *symptoms* include impaired handwriting (micrographia), trouble walking, falling, poor coordination, trouble arising from a deep chair, couch, or the toilet, drooling, and trouble turning in bed. When the syndrome is fully developed, the diagnosis is straightforward. Errors in diagnosis are infrequent but are most often encountered when (a) the clinical picture is dominated by a severe tremor, in which case essential tremor may be mistakenly diagnosed; (b) tremor is absent in a patient presenting with unilateral rigidity and bradykinesia ("pseudohemiplegic PD") in which case diagnoses of upper or lower motor syndromes are entertained; and (c) patients are younger than 50, an age at which PD may not be considered in the differential diagnosis.

Although *idiopathic Parkinson's disease* is the most common diagnosis among patients presenting with parkinsonian signs, there are a number of other conditions that must be considered in the differential diagnosis (Table 82.3) (13). It has been estimated that as

Table 82.3.
Differential Diagnosis of Parkinsonism

Toxins
 Manganese
 Carbon monoxide
 Carbon disulfide Cyanide
 Methanol
 MPTP

Drug-Induced
 Neuroleptics
 Metoclopramide (Reglan)

Multisystem Degenerations
 Progressive supranuclear palsy
 Shy-Drager syndrome
 Olivopontocerebellar atrophy
 Striato-nigral degeneration
 ALS-PD-dementia complex of Guam

Primary Dementing Illnesses
 Alzheimer's disease
 Creutzfeldt-Jakob

Heredofamilial Diseases
 Wilson's disease
 Juvenile Huntington's disease
 Hallervorden-Spatz

Multi-Infarct State

Calcification of the Basal Ganglia
 Idiopathic
 Hypoparathyroidism

Postencephalitic

Trauma
 Dementia pugilistica

many as 20% of patients who carry the diagnosis of PD actually have another parkinsonian syndrome. In some of these cases typical signs of the patient's actual disease may appear late in the course but in other circumstances may not appear at all during life and only at postmortem examination is an alternative diagnosis discovered. The initial clue that a patient may have another parkinsonian syndrome is usually failure to respond to L-dopa. Other indicators include young age at onset or the appearance of cerebellar, corticospinal, lower motor neuron, autonomic, or ocular motor signs.

Although a discussion of each of the parkinsonian syndromes in Table 82.4 is beyond the scope of this chapter, three deserve special mention. *Neuroleptic-induced parkinsonism*, described in Chapter 16, may be clinically indistinguishable from idiopathic PD and can only be diagnosed retrospectively when parkinsonian signs resolve after discontinuation of the offending drug. In some patients signs may take as long as 1 year to completely resolve, emphasizing the need to periodically reassess antiparkinsonian therapy. In patients whose signs never resolve, it is likely that the neuroleptic simply uncovered a case of latent PD (34).

Progressive supranuclear palsy is the most common nonpharmacological mimicker of PD. It is distinguished by impaired vertical eye movements, although early in its course, ocular motility may be full with the only clinical clue being slow vertical saccades. Other signs include neck extension as opposed to the flexion seen in PD, early dysarthria and dysphagia, greater axial than appendicular rigidity ("axial dystonia"), progression to severe disability in 5 to 10 years, and limited response to antiparkinsonian medications (12).

Wilson's disease (hepatolenticular degeneration) is an autosomal recessive condition characterized by copper accumulation throughout the body. Parkinsonian features in a young patient should prompt an investigation for this condition. Liver disease may be present at the onset of neurological disease, but normal liver studies should not deter one from pursuing the diagnosis. The diagnosis is confirmed by demonstrating Kayser-Fleischer rings (green or golden deposits of copper in the Descemet's membrane of the cornea), low blood ceruloplasmin, and elevated urinary copper excretion (32).

Natural History of Parkinson's Disease

Although treatment ameliorates the manifestations of PD, and deprenyl (see below) has been shown to slow the progression of early PD, the condition remains a slowly progressive one. Nevertheless, patients can be reassured that the life span is rarely shortened in PD and that the majority of patients remain functional and relatively independent throughout the course of the illness. Table 82.5 summarizes the principal manifestations and the functional status of the patient in each of the stages that may occur in progressive PD.

Table 82.4.
Characteristics of Cerebellar and Sensory (Proprioceptive) Incoordination

Observation or Examination	Cerebellar	Sensory
Influence of vision	Elimination of visual aid (night, eyes closed) does not affect symptoms or signs	Symptoms and signs markedly increased by eliminating visual aid
Sensation	No necessary sensory problems (although may be superimposed, as in alcoholic cerebellar degeneration and sensory neuropathy)	Impaired position and vibration sense is *sine qua non* for diagnosis
Finger-nose-finger and/or toe-finger testing of coordination	Could be marked intention tremor and dysmetria (inaccuracy); affected limbs depend upon site of lesion(s)	Marked intention tremor and dysmetria (inaccuracy), usually most marked in legs
Gait	Wide based, asynchronous limb movements (depending upon nature of the lesion)	Wide based, high stepping, foot-slapping (steppage) gait (often due to foot drop from motor neuropathy)
Romberg testing	Patient equally unsteady with eyes open or closed	Patient can find a stable position with eyes open, but becomes markedly unsteady with eyes closed (positive Romberg)

Table 82.5.
Five Stages of Parkinson's Disease[a]

Stage	Principal Manifestations	Overall Functional Status
1	Unilateral involvement, blank facies, affected arm in semiflexed position with tremor and diminished swing, patient leans to affected side; gait slightly affected or normal	Patient can continue most activities as usual except those requiring quick motor responses (playing tennis, for example). Social embarrassment may be a problem.
2	(Usually within 1 to 2 years of stage 1.) Bilateral involvement with early postural changes (stooped); slow shuffling gait with decreased excursion of legs; executes turn slowly and deliberately	Patient usually must retire, if still working. High risk of becoming withdrawn (reactive depression) and abandoning valued social and recreational activities (although physical impairment may not prohibit them).
3	Pronounced gait disturbance with postural instability and tendency to fall	Patient begins to need assistance with some tasks because of slowness in accomplishing them (*e.g.*, dressing, packing a suitcase).
4	Significant disability; ambulation limited and only with assistance because of marked difficulty in standing and tendency to fall	Patient needs almost constant supervision and requires assistance in completing most activities of daily living.
5	Complete invalidism; confined to bed or chair; unable to stand or walk even with assistance; head becomes flexed on trunk; speech barely audible; face expressionless and blinking infrequent	Patient requires total care; death from aspiration or other form of infection related to immobolization.

[a] Adapted from Duvoisin R: Parkinsonism. In *Clinical Symposia*. Summit, NJ, CIBA Pharmaceutical Co, 1976, vol 28, no. 1.

Although some patients do reach the fifth stage (total disability), this is the exception rather than the rule.

Manifestations

Resting Tremor

Tremor is the presenting complaint in 70% of patients with PD. The tremor is maximal when the limb is at rest and has a frequency of 4 to 6 Hz. It consists of flexion-extension at the metacarpophalangeal joints, abduction-adduction of the thumb, and pronation-supination of the forearm producing the typical "pill-rolling" morphology. The tremor often affects the legs, feet, toes, and occasionally the lips, tongue, or chin, but it is relatively uncommon for it to involve the entire head. The tremor is accentuated by stress and distraction, diminishes with relaxation, and disappears during sleep. Although there may be an associated *postural* tremor in PD, typically, the resting tremor suppresses with posture and movement, which helps to distinguish it from essential tremor (see above).

Rigidity

Rigidity is defined as abnormal "plastic" resistance to passive movement. There is a "ratchety" quality throughout the entire range of motion producing the "cogwheel" phenomenon.

Patients rarely complain of "rigidity" per se and instead notice "stiffness" or often describe the abnormal tone as "weakness." Cogwheel rigidity is best felt at the elbow or wrist and may be demonstrated or increased as the patient performs a maneuver with the contralateral limb such as opening and closing the fist or drawing a figure in the air.

Bradykinesia and Akinesia

Patients with PD have difficulty initiating movements, and their movements are slow and performed with much greater conscious effort. Speech gradually becomes soft, slow, and monotonal. The blink rate is diminished as is facial expression producing the so-called "masked face." Because rigidity and akinesia can occur independently of each other, akinesia is not solely due to rigidity. This becomes apparent when treatment markedly decreases a patient's rigidity but has little or no effect on akinesia.

Gait and Postural Abnormalities

Patients with PD are flexed at multiple joints—neck, hips, knees, elbows, and fingers—producing the typical "stooped posture." Arising from a chair is often accomplished only with difficulty; patients may need to rock back and forth several times and eventually push off from arm rests. The gait is slow and shuffling with diminished associated movements. Turning is done "en bloc" with the entire body moving as the feet slowly rotate. There is a tendency to involuntarily progress from walking to running (festination) seemingly in an attempt to "catch up" with the body's center of gravity thrown forward by the flexed posture. Patients have difficulty maintaining balance and are often unable to correct for a rapid postural displacement, particularly backwards. The combination of the flexed posture, bradykinesia, freezing, festination, and impaired postural righting reflexes leads to one of the most difficult problems in the latter stages of PD—falling.

Other Associated Symptoms or Signs

Seborrhea and excessive perspiration are both common, and although often attributed to inadequate hygiene due to physical impairment, they are more likely an intrinsic part of the disease process.

Dysphagia is a common complaint in PD but is usually confined to the latter stages of the disease when it contributes significantly to morbidity and mortality due to inanition and aspiration pneumonia. Although not completely understood, swallowing abnormalities have been demonstrated at various levels: the voluntary muscles of the oral cavity plus the involuntary muscles of the pharynx and esophagus. Solids are usually more of a problem than liquids. If patients are unable to maintain sufficient caloric intake, consideration should be given to a feeding tube (see details in Chapter 6).

Sialorrhea is probably the result of decreased swallowing rather than overproduction of saliva; this can be treated with a low dose of an anticholinergic (see below).

Autonomic dysfunction may occur in PD itself and as a side effect of antiparkinsonian medication. When the clinical picture is dominated by severe dysautonomia, particularly when accompanied by cerebellar and lower motor neuron signs, with rapid progression, this is known as the Shy-Drager syndrome (33). Orthostatic hypotension and constipation are the most frequent autonomic signs in PD, but bladder dysfunction and impotence are also encountered. In each case, medications may be at fault and a thorough search for

other causes should be carried out before the defects are ascribed to PD.

Treatment

The treatment of PD can be divided into patient education and pharmacological treatment.

Patient Education

This consists of explaining to the patient the nature of PD, in particular, its very slow progression and the fact that with treatment, most patients can expect to remain functional and maintain a relatively normal lifestyle. Patient-oriented books (see "General References") and support groups are often helpful, sometimes as much to the caregiver as the patient, but these should be recommended with caution in the early stages of the disease as patients often concentrate only on the worst possible prognosis. Patients should know that their goals for social, professional, and physical activity will be utilized to guide decisions about when to initiate treatment and to make changes in the dosing regimen. Before starting treatment it should be emphasized to patients that the goal is not to eliminate all of the symptoms and signs of PD but rather to maintain an acceptable degree of functioning.

Physical activities should be encouraged, particularly walking. However, activities that can be dangerous if balance is impaired or motor response is delayed should be avoided (e.g., skiing, bicycling, driving in heavy traffic, using electric tools, etc.).

Weak or slow speech and poverty of facial expression can produce the impression of lack of interest during a conversation. Therefore, the patient should be advised tactfully to make a conscious effort to let others know that he is interested, despite his lack of facial expression. Having the patient practice speech by reading aloud and by recording and listening to his voice may help to overcome his reticence to speak.

Fear of falling is experienced by virtually all parkinsonian patients. Walking with hands clasped behind the back or using a standard walker or one on wheels (but not a cane) may improve stability. The patient's living environment should be free of obstacles that may cause him to stumble, and he should avoid walking in places where he is apt to encounter obstacles (rocky terrain, for example).

When the patient becomes progressively disabled, the assistance of others is necessary to avoid as much as possible the complications of bradykinesia and sedentary living. Such assistance includes periodic change in the patient's position to avoid skin breakdown, passive range of motion of the limbs and digits to avoid flexion contractures, and as much mobility, social, and intellectual stimulation as possible.

Pharmacological Treatment

General Principles. Pharmacological treatment is based on what is known of the neurotransmission in the basal ganglia. Two major neurotransmitters found in these regions are dopamine and acetylcholine. In PD, loss of the dopaminergic cells in the substantia nigra leads to depletion of dopamine in the striatum and a relative excess of acetylcholine. The two main classes of antiparkinsonian drugs currently available work by either increasing dopamine activity directly or indirectly (dopaminergic drugs), or by decreasing acetylcholine activity (anticholinergic drugs) (see details regarding available strengths, recommended doses, and schedules in (Table 82.6).

Step-wise Initiation and Adjustment of Medication. The treatment regimen for each patient must be individualized, but the general rule is to use the least amount of medication needed to achieve reasonable control of the symptoms and signs of PD. Early, when there is no significant impairment of ADLs or of occupational or social functioning, treatment is generally withheld unless the tremor or other signs cause embarrassment. Recently, it has been shown that deprenyl (see below), initiated at this point, may slow disease progression (35).

During the course of PD, it is necessary to follow a step-wise approach to prescribing, assessing, and adjusting antiparkinsonian medications. As the disease progresses, treatment should be initiated using either an anticholinergic or amantadine alone. Almost all patients will eventually require levodopa (L-dopa), but there is controversy about the optimal time to begin this drug. Proponents for early treatment cite studies indicating that this leads to decreased morbidity and mortality (4). However, there is also evidence that the length of time a patient is on L-dopa may be in itself a risk factor for later motor complications, leading some to advocate withholding treatment as long as possible (3, 5). A reasonable approach is to delay the use of L-dopa until the disease begins to compromise a pa-

tient's ability to function. At that point, L-dopa is added to the patient's initial regimen and the dose is gradually increased, using the patient's functional needs as a guide. Once the patient has responded to L-dopa, an attempt should be made to gradually reduce the dose of other antiparkinsonian medications or, if possible, discontinue them. Some patients will deteriorate as this is attempted, necessitating continued polypharmacy.

As the disease progresses and L-dopa alone is insufficient to control the symptoms and signs, a direct-acting dopamine receptor agonist such as bromocriptine or pergolide or the monoamine oxidase (MAO)-inhibitor deprenyl, which prevents catabolism of dopamine, should be added. Some recent evidence suggests that beginning with a combination of L-dopa and an agonist or beginning with an agonist alone is associated with a reduced incidence of later motor fluctuations including on-off and dyskinesias (see below).

Anticholinergics. Anticholinergics are helpful in the early stages of PD particularly when tremor is a predominant sign. Although there are a number of different preparations, none has clear superiority. They generally take 2 to 4 weeks before the maximal effect is observed. The common side effects include dry mouth (which may help sialorrhea), blurred vision, urinary retention, constipation, memory loss, and confusion. Narrow angle glaucoma is a contraindication to these agents. Anticholinergics should be avoided or used cautiously in very elderly or demented patients, who are often more sensitive to the side effects of these medications.

Amantadine (Symmetrel). Originally marketed as an anti-influenzal drug, amantadine was discovered by chance to help patients with PD. Its exact mechanism of action is not known but it has been shown to

Table 82.6.
Drugs Used for Parkinson's Disease

Drug	Available Preparation (mg)	Schedule	Starting Dose (mg)	Maintenance Dose (mg)
Anticholinergic Agents (representative examples)				
Trihexyphenidyl (Artane)	Scored tablets—2,5 Elixir—2 mg/5 ml	3–4 times daily	2	2–10
	Time-release capsules—5	Once daily	(May be substituted for regular Artane after maintenance dose is determined)	(May be substituted for regular Artane after maintenance dose is determined)
Benztropine mesylate (Cogentin)	Tablets—0.5, 1, 2	Once or twice daily	1	0.5–6
Dopaminergic Agents				
Carbidopa/levodopa (Sinemet)	Scored tablets 10/100, 25/100, 25/250	2–4 times daily	50/200 in 2 divided doses	400–500 levodopa
Bromocriptine (Parlodel)	Scored tablets—2.5 Capsules—5.0	2–3 times daily	1.25 qd	7.5–30
Pergolide (Permax)	Scored tablets—0.05, 0.25, 1.0	3 times daily	0.05 qd	1–3
Deprenyl (Eldepryl)	Tablets—5.0	2 times daily	5 qd	10
Amantadine (Symmetrel)	Capsule—100	2 times daily	200 qd	200

have both anticholinergic and dopaminergic activity. The full inpact of amantadine may not be seen for 2 weeks. Although helpful in the early stages of PD, the beneficial effect of amantadine is generally short-lived, approximately 6 months. Once L-dopa has been added, it is often possible to taper off amantadine without any clinical deterioration. Common side effects include pedal edema, confusion, hallucinations, and livedo reticularis. In the latter stages of PD, when the effect of L-dopa wanes or motor fluctuations appear, the addition of amantadine occasionally produces temporary improvement.

L-Dopa (as Sinemet). The hallmark of PD is depletion of dopamine in the striatum, and replacement of dopamine is the mainstay of treatment. Dopamine does not cross the blood brain barrier and is given instead in the form of its precursor, L-dopa. To avoid the extracerebral conversion of L-dopa to dopamine by peripheral dopa decarboxylase, L-dopa is usually combined with carbidopa, an enzyme inhibitor, in the form of Sinemet. Scored tablets combine 10 mg of carbidopa with 100 mg of L-dopa, or 25 mg of carbidopa with either 100 or 250 mg of L-dopa. Because at least 75 mg per day of carbidopa is required to inhibit dopa decarboxylase, the 25/100 preparation is best chosen to initiate treatment.

In the future, a controlled release preparation of Sinemet will be available combining 50 mg of carbidopa with 200 mg of L-dopa. This preparation was designed in an attempt to provide a more consistent blood level of L-dopa and reduce motor fluctuations (see below). Although it is helpful in some patients, the continual appearance of fluctuations in patients on the controlled release preparation underscores the fact that fluctuating peripheral L-dopa levels, as seen with standard Sinemet, is only one of many complex variables contributing to motor fluctuations.

The usual starting dose is one tablet (25/100) twice per day, but in the elderly it is best to begin with half tablets. Although Sinemet is absorbed best on an empty stomach, this also usually leads to an increased incidence of nausea and therefore Sinemet is initially prescribed with meals and, once tolerated, can be taken 1/2 hour earlier. Although some patients will have an immediate beneficial effect, it may take several weeks before a change is noticed. After that time, if there is no improvement, the dose is gradually increased every few days to a three to four times daily schedule, using full or half-tablet increments, until the patient has shown significant improvement or a total daily dose of 400 to 500 mg of L-dopa per day has been reached.

After about 5 years of treatment, the previously consistent response to Sinemet wanes and *fluctuations in motor functon* begin to appear in at least 50% of patients (25). These fluctuations follow a predictable pattern: the beneficial effect of a dose of Sinemet is noted within about 1/2 hour and lasts from 1 to 3 hours; then there is another 1/2- to 1-hour of loss of effect. This is referred to as "end-of-dose" wearing off. The initial treatment for decreasing effectiveness of Sinemet is to decrease the dosing interval, often using half-tablets

without increasing the total dose. Previously the total dose of L-dopa was advanced to at least 1 g per day, but a more recent approach has been to gradually increase the dose to no more than 400 to 500 mg and to start a dopamine agonist or deprenyl (see below) early. This approach is based on the observation that as the disease progresses, patients become more sensitive to the dyskinesias caused by L-dopa (see below).

Less predictable response fluctuations, referred to as "on-off," are manifested by frequent and often rapid changes in parkinsonian signs with freezing, hesitation when initiating movements, and akinesia. This class of fluctuations proves much more difficult to treat, but the addition of an agonist may help.

The reasons for fluctuations in response to Sinemet may include erratic gastric emptying and duodenal absorption, competition with dietary amino acids for transport across the intestine and blood brain barrier, inability of the remaining nigral dopaminergic neurons to metabolize and store dopamine, and alterations in the number and sensitivity of the remaining postsynaptic dopamine receptors. Fluctuations in motor response may diminish if *dietary protein* is limited during the day, to less than 7 g, and the balance is made up during the evening meal. This change eliminates the competition between large dietary amino acids and Sinemet for transport across the intestine and blood brain barrier. In a number of studies, the amount of time "off" has been found to diminish with this technique; but it has also been noted that dyskinesias may increase, necessitating a decrease in the dose of Sinemet (29). Improvement in resistant motor fluctuations has also been attained with delivery of a constant amount of levodopa directly into the duodenum with an infusion pump (31).

"Drug holidays" were once advocated when the effectiveness of Sinemet diminished. This method has fallen out of favor because of the frequent complications encountered as patients deteriorated while off treatment and because of the transient nature of the improvement when Sinemet was restarted.

Although most patients tolerate Sinemet well, *side effects* are not uncommon, particularly in the elderly or in patients with dementia (see below). These include confusion, hallucinations, hypersexuality, and fluid retention. Orthostatic hypotension is quite common; since this is often a finding in untreated PD, before starting Sinemet and after each dose increase, supine and standing blood pressure should be checked. All side effects resolve with reduction of the dose.

Drug-induced dyskinesias (choreiform movements of the limbs, face, or trunk) initially appear during peak dose, approximately 1 1/2 to 2 hours after Sinemet is taken. They can be reduced by decreasing the Sinemet dose and making up the difference with an agonist. Like "off" periods, dyskinesias may also occur unpredictably, and it is not uncommon in the late stages of the disease for patients to have a complex mix of "off" time, "on" time, and dyskinesias. When this mix of motor fluctuations begins to occur, consultation with a neurologist is suggested.

Direct Dopamine Receptor Agonists. These drugs have the theoretical advantage of acting directly on postsynaptic dopamine receptors and therefore bypassing the ineffective nigral dopaminergic neurons. As mentioned above, they are useful adjuncts to Sinemet, particularly when its effectiveness wanes and when there are motor fluctuations. When one of these drugs is added the Sinemet dose is maintained. In the United States, the available agonists include the ergot derivatives bromocriptine (Parlodel) and pergolide (Permax). Bromocriptine is available as scored 2.5-mg tablets and 5-mg capsules. The starting dose is 1.25 mg at night, and the dose is gradually increased, every 1 to 2 two weeks, in 1.25-mg increments, aiming for a maintenance dose of 7.5 to 30 mg per day in two or three divided doses. Pergolide is available as scored 0.05-, 0.25- and 1.0-mg tablets. It is started at 0.05 mg per day for 2 days and increased gradually (about every 3 days) to a maintenance dose of 1 to 3 mg per day, also in two or three divided doses. Although pergolide is at least 10 times more potent than bromocriptine, at present, there does not appear to be any compelling advantage of one over the other (23).

The side effects of bromocriptine and pergolide are similar to those of Sinemet, but there is a much lower incidence of drug-induced dyskinesias. Both drugs are tolerated poorly in the elderly and should be avoided in demented patients because of their propensity to cause confusion, hallucinations, and psychosis.

Deprenyl (Eldepryl, Seligiline). Deprenyl is a monoamine oxidase B inhibitor that prevents the catabolism and reuptake of dopamine. It has been shown to be an effective adjunct to Sinemet for patients with response fluctuations (24). Because only the "B" form of monoamine oxidase, which exists exclusively in the central nervous system, is inhibited, it is not necessary to restrict dietary tyramine to prevent systemic hypertension. Although dyskinesias may be exacerbated, necessitating a reduction in the Sinemet dose, deprenyl is otherwise relatively free of side effects. Reported side effects include nausea, dry mouth, dizziness, psychosis, and confusion. After a brief trial of 5 mg per day the patient should advance to a maintenance dose of 5 mg twice a day. As it may cause insomnia, both doses should be given early in the day.

It has been confirmed recently that deprenyl alone, in a dose of 5 mg twice per day, delays the need to initiate L-dopa therapy (35). The mechanism is believed to be blocking of the toxic transformation of unknown environmental substances such as MPTP (see above), which limits the death of nigral neurons.

Surgical Treatment

Stereotactic thalamotomy, when performed at a center specializing in the procedure, is a safe, effective treatment for patients with disabling tremor unresponsive to medical therapy. Thalamotomy also reduces rigidity and may improve mobility but does not relieve akinesia (16).

Initial findings of dramatic improvement in PD with implantation of autologous adrenal medullary tissue into the caudate nucleus were not substantiated in larger, better designed studies. More recently transplantation of nigral tissue obtained from aborted fetuses has been investigated. To date, tissue implantation has not been the panacea originally hoped for and should be a strictly experimental approach, appropriate only as part of a research protocol.

Dementia and Depression in Patients with PD

The estimated frequency of *dementia* in patients with PD varies widely based on the population studied, definition of dementia, and tools used to assess cognitive performance. A conservative estimate is that at least 15 to 20% of patients with PD will develop dementia (7). Although the incidence of dementia in PD is higher than in nonparkinsonian age-matched controls, it is crucial to appreciate that dementia is not an inevitable feature of PD and as such, must be approached with the same rigorous search for remediable causes used in nonparkinsonians (see Chapter 17). All of the medications used to treat PD have cognitive and behavioral side effects, particularly the anticholinergics; when cognitive abnormalities occur, an attempt should be made to reduce the doses of these drugs or, if possible, to discontinue them.

Dementia in patients with PD is occasionally complicated by bothersome hallucinations, agitation, psychosis, insomnia, or a reversal in the sleep-wake cycle. If these problems do not respond to reducing antiparkinsonian medications or the use of a mild sedative, a very low dose of a neuroleptic (see Chapter 16) may be required, recognizing that worsening of parkinsonian signs may result but the suppression of intolerable behavior usually leads to an overall improvement in the patient's condition and eases the burden of the caregiver.

Depression is common in PD, occurring in as many as 50% of patients (26). It is not clear to what extent it is the result of a intrinsic neurochemical defect or of a depressive reaction to the disability of the disease. Both PD patients and their physicians commonly fail to recognize depression and often mistakenly attribute a decline in motor function to PD when in reality it is the result of depression-induced psychomotor slowing; a rapid decline in a patient's functional status is often a clue to depression.

Depression in PD can be treated very effectively with tricyclic antidepressants. As depression resolves there is often concurrent improvement in many parkinsonian symptoms and signs. In severe cases—particularly when compounded by delusions, agitation, severe anxiety, or psychosis—tricyclics are either ineffective or not tolerated; in these patients electroconvulsive therapy is the treatment of choice. Chapter 15, Affective Disorders, contains details about three forms of treatment for depression.

General References

Tremor
Capildeo R, Findley LJ (eds): *Movement Disorders: Tremor.* London, Macmillan, 1984.

Jankovic J, Fahn S: Physiologic and pathologic tremors: diagnosis, mechanism, and management. *Ann Intern Med* 93:460, 1980.

Koller WC: Diagnosis and Treatment of Tremors. In: Jankovic J: *Neurologic Clinics* Vol 2 (3):Philadelphia, WB Saunders, 1984. pp. 449

Marsden CD, Fahn S: (eds): *Movement Disorders*. London, Butterworths, 1981.<RSH>Parkinson's Disease</RSH>

Duvoisin RC (ed): *Parkinson's Disease: A Guide for Patient and Family*, 2nd ed. New York, Raven Press, 1984.

Jankovic J, Tolosa E (eds): *Parkinson's Disease and Movement Disorders*. Baltimore, Urban & Schwarzenberg, 1988.

Koller WC (ed): *Handbook of Parkinson's Disease*. New York, Marcel Dekker, 1987.

Lieberman AN: Update on Parkinson's Disease. *NY State J Med* 87:147, 1987.

Marsden CD, Fahn S (eds): *Movement Disorders*. London, Butterworths, 1981.

Specific References

1. Burns RS, LeWitt PA, Ebert MH, et al: The clinical syndrome of striatal dopamine deficiency. *N Engl J Med* 312:1418, 1985.
2. Calne DM, Langston JW: Aetiology of Parkinson's disease. *Lancet* 2:1457, 1983.
3. de Jong GJ, Meerwaldt JD, Schmitz PIM: Factors that influence the occurrence of response variations in Parkinson's disease. *Ann Neurol* 22:4, 1987.
4. Diamond SG, Markham CH, Hoehn MM, et al: Multi-center study of Parkinson mortality with early versus late dopa treatment. *Ann Neurol* 22:8, 1987.
5. Duvoisin RC: To treat early or to treat late? *Ann Neurol* 22:2, 1987.
6. Findley LJ, Koller WC: Essential tremor: a review. *Neurology* 37:1194, 1987.
7. Gibb WRG: Dementia and Parkinson's Disease. *Br J Psychiatry* 154:596, 1989.
8. Growdon JH, Shahani BT, Young RR: The effect of alcohol on essential tremor. *Neurology* 25:259, 1975.
9. Haerer AF, Anderson DW, Schoenberg BS: Prevalence of essential tremor. *Arch Neurol* 39:750, 1982.
10. Heilman KM: Orthostatic tremor. *Arch Neurol* 41:880, 1984.
11. Huber SJ, Paulson GW: Efficacy of alprazolam for essential tremor. *Neurology* 38:241, 1988.
12. Jankovic J: Progressive supranuclear palsy: clinical and pharmacological update. In: Jankovic J (ed):*Neurologic Clinics*, Vol 2 (3). Philadelphia, WB Saunders, 1984.
13. Jankovic J: Parkinsonism-plus syndromes. *Movement Disorders* 4(suppl 1):S95, 1989.
14. Jefferson D, Jenner P, Marsden C: Beta-adrenoreceptor antagonists in essential tremor. *J Neurol Neurosurg Psychiatry* 42:904, 1979.
15. Kachi T, Rothwell JC, Cowan JMA, et al: Writing tremor: its relationship to benign essential tremor. *J Neurol Neurosurg Psychiatry* 48:545, 1985.
16. Kelly PJ, Ahlskog JE, Goerss SJ, et al: Computer assisted stereotactic ventralis lateralis thalamotomy with microelectrode recording control in patients with Parkinson's disease. *Mayo Clin Proc* 62:655, 1987.
17. Koller WC: Alcoholism in essential tremor. *Neurology* 33:1074, 1983.
18. Koller WC: Long-acting propranolol in essential tremor. *Neurology* 35:108, 1985.
19. Koller WC, Biary N, Cone S: Disability in essential tremor: effect of treatment. *Neurology* 36:1001, 1986.
20. Koller WC, Royce JL: Efficacy of primidone in essential tremor. *Neurology* 36:121, 1986.
21. Larson TA, Teravainen H: Beta-blockers in essential tremor. *Lancet* 2:533, 1981.
22. Langston JW, Ballard P, Tetrud JW, et al: Chronic parkinsonism in humans due to a product of meperidine-analog synthesis. *Science (Wash DC)* 219:9789, 1983.
23. Lewitt PA, Ward CD, Larsen TA, et al: Comparison of pergolide and bromocriptine therapy in parkinsonism. *Neurology* 33:1009, 1983.
24. Lieberman AN, Gopinathan G, Neophytides A: Deprenyl versus placebo in Parkinson's disease. *NY State J Med* 87:646, 1987.

25. Marsden CD, Parks JD: Success and problems of long term levodopa therapy in Parkinson's disease. *Lancet* 1:345, 1977.
26. Mayeux R: A current analysis of behavioral problems in patients with idiopathic Parkinson's disease. *Movement Disorders* 4 (Suppl 1):S48, 1989.
27. Narabayashi H: Surgical approach to tremor. In: Marsden CD, Fahn S (eds): *Movement Disorders* London, Butterworth, 1982.p. 292.
28. Parkinson J: *An Essay on the Shaking Palsy*. London, Wittingham and Rowland, 1817. (Reprint by) Chicago, American Medical Assn Press, 1959.
29. Riley D, Lang AE: Practical application of a low-protein diet for Parkinson's disease. *Neurology* 38:1026, 1988.
30. Rosenbaum F, Jankovic J: Focal task-specific tremor and dystonia: categorization of occupational movement disorders. *Neurology* 38:522, 1988.
31. Sage JI, Trooskin S, Sonsalla PK, et al: Long-term duodenal infusion of levodopa for motor fluctuations in parkinsonism. *Ann Neurol* 24:87, 1988.
32. Scheinberg IH, Sternlieb I: *Wilson's Disease*. Philadelphia, WB Saunders, 1984.
33. Shy GM, Drager GA: A neurological syndrome associated with orthostatic hypotension: a clinical—pathological study. *Arch Neurol* 2:511, 1968.
34. Stephen PJ, Williamson J: Drug Induced parkinsonism in the elderly. *Lancet* 2:1082, 1984.
35. The Parkinson Study Group: Effect of deprenyl on the progression of disability in early Parkinson's disease. *N Engl J Med* 321:1364, 1989.

CHAPTER 83

Cerebrovascular Disease

THOMAS J. PREZIOSI, M.D.

OVERVIEW

Epidemiology

Cerebrovascular disease is a major cause of disability and the third leading cause of death in the United States. The impact on society is far reaching with an estimated annual cost of greater than 7.3 billion dollars. According to a survey published in 1980 (35), the *annual incidence* of first stroke is 150 per 100,000 population; about 80% of strokes are due to thrombotic or embolic cerebral infarction, 12% to cerebral hemorrhage, and 8% to subarachnoid hemorrhage. As shown in Table 83.1, approximately 75% of strokes occur in individuals who are 65 or older. The *annual death rate* from stroke is 75/100,000 population, with a disproportionately greater number of early deaths among patients with hemorrhage as compared with patients with infarction. Data on *the prevalence of stroke* suggest that in a population of 100,000 there are approximately 500 stroke survivors at any point in time.

The incidence of stroke declined by more than 50% in one population (Rochester, Minnesota) during the 5-year period 1975 to 1979 compared with the 5-year period 1945 to 1949 (21). The decline was found for all age groups. Subsequent studies have shown that stroke incidence has decreased on a nationwide and indeed worldwide level (24, 50). Factors that may have contributed to the decline include more aggressive treatment of hypertension, more effective and early delivery of health care, and better management and recognition of the cardiogenic sources of cerebral embolization. Recent studies from the Rochester population have indicated a stabilization of decline; these studies also show a possible increase in stroke incidence, a finding that may be due to the earlier detection of stroke because of the introduction of new imaging techniques such as computed tomography (9).

Cerebrovascular disease presents *two major challenges in ambulatory practice* : first, the prevention of stroke in the large number of individuals with risk factors that make them stroke prone; and second, the optimal care of the many stroke survivors in each community.

Risk Factors

A major goal of patient evaluation in ambulatory practice is the identification of the individual with an increased risk of stroke. Patients who have previously suffered a stroke constitute an important subgroup of this high risk population. A community-based study of the natural history of stroke in Rochester, Minnesota, has shown that the first year recurrence rate among survivors of a first stroke was 10% and that the 5-year recurrence rate was 20% (39). In addition to a previous

Table 83.1.
Percentage Distribution of Stroke Occurrence by Age Group[a]

	Percentage of Total Persons in Each Age Group[b]							
	All ages	Under 35	35–44	45–54	55–64	65–74	75–84	84 +
US population	100.0	58.3	10.4	11.4	9.5	6.6	3.3	1.0
Stroke patients	100.0	1.2	2.0	6.8	15.6	28.3	33.4	12.7

[a] From National Survey of Stroke, US Department of Health, Education and Welfare, Public Health Service National Institutes of Health, NIH publ no. 80-2069; January 1980.
[b] Note that while the age group 65 years and older constitutes only 10.9% of the population, approximately three-fourths (74.4%) of all strokes occur in this age group.

history of stroke, other factors predispose a patient to stroke. Epidemiological data indicate that the incidence of stroke and the associated death rate increase markedly with age. Three other factors, all amenable to therapy, have also been found to correlate strongly with stroke occurrence: transient episodes of focal cerebral dysfunction of vascular origin called transient ischemic attacks (TIA), hypertension, and certain types of cardiac disorders.

Transient Ischemic Attacks (TIAs)

Approximately one-third of patients with a TIA subsequently develop a stroke, and the TIA provides a significant warning of impending infarction. The etiology, natural history, and treatment of TIA are discussed in detail later in this chapter.

Hypertension

Data accumulated during the Framingham study indicate that the risks of both nonhemorrhagic and hemorrhagic stroke are strongly related to hypertension. Atherothrombotic brain infarction occurred in hypertensive subjects (blood pressure greater than 160/95) four times more often than in normotensive subjects (33). Moreover, the available evidence suggests that stroke risk is significantly reduced by the treatment of hypertension in all patients including those with a history of cerebrovascular disease (6, 12, 48, 49). The evaluation and long-term management of hypertension is discussed in detail in Chapter 62.

Cardiac Impairment

Cardiac impairment clearly predisposes to stroke. It has long been known that the heart is often the source of emboli that lodge in cerebral vessels and lead to infarction. This type of stroke has more recently been found to account for 15 to 30% of all ischemic strokes and is highly associated with cardiac arrhythmias, particularly atrial fibrillation without valvular disease (25). Data from the Framingham study have identified cardiac impairment as a significant risk factor in the occurrence of the more frequently encountered nonembolic atherothrombotic brain infarction (ABI) (52). Subjects with electrocardiographic evidence of left ventricular hypertrophy (LVH) were nine times more likely to develop ABI than individuals without this abnormality. Patients with coronary artery disease (CAD) had five times the risk of ABI and those with radiographic evidence of cardiomegaly had three times the risk. When the contribution of concomitant hypertension was eliminated, LVH and CAD were each associated with a 3-fold increase in the risk of ABI; the contribution of cardiomegaly on X-ray was not found to be significant when other variables were controlled. On the basis of these findings it was concluded that cardiac impairment, especially if associated with hypertension, significantly heightens the risk of stroke occurrence. It is not clear that cardiac abnormalities, once established, can be modified so that the risk of subsequent stroke is reduced.

Other Factors

A number of other factors have been associated with an increased incidence of stroke: family history of vascular disease, elevated serum glucose concentration, elevated serum lipid levels, cigarette smoking, elevated blood hemoglobin and hematocrit levels, and the presence of a cervical bruit. To date, it is not known whether modification of any of these risk factors reduces the likelihood of stroke, and each requires some qualification. Data on *family history* are incomplete, although the available evidence suggests that in the family history of stroke patients there is a higher frequency of mortality from vascular disease. With regard to *diabetes mellitus*, prospective data from the Framingham study indicated an increased risk of cerebral infarction in subjects with even a modest abnormality of glucose tolerance (31). This study also demonstrated that *elevated serum lipid levels* were associated with increased stroke risk but only in subjects under the age of 50. The contribution of *cigarette smoking* to the risk of stroke occurrence remains controversial. However, in the Framingham study male cigarette smokers had a 3-fold greater risk of cerebral infarction than nonsmokers. The data on female smokers were too limited to draw a valid conclusion. *Elevated blood hemoglobin and hematocrit levels* have also been implicated as possible risk factors, but a cause and effect relationship has not been established (32, 47). *Oral contraceptive* use is associated with a 5- to 10-fold increase in risk of vascular diseases, including stroke (see details in Chapter 93). Finally, it is generally accepted that the presence of an *asymptomatic cervical bruit* correlates with an increased incidence of subsequent stroke, but there is controversy regarding the appropriate management of patients with this finding (see below).

CLASSIFICATION OF CEREBROVASCULAR EVENTS

Type of Event

Symptoms and signs of vascular origin are characterized by their relatively rapid onset. The following classification has been developed based upon their duration.

A *transient ischemic attack* is defined as a transient episode of focal cerebral dysfunction, rapid in onset (from no to maximal symptoms in less than 5 minutes) that usually lasts from 2 to 15 minutes but always resolves completely within 24 hours.

A *reversible ischemic neurological deficit* (RIND) is defined as an episode of focal cerebral dysfunction that lasts longer than 24 hours but resolves completely within 3 weeks.

A *completed stroke* is defined as an episode of focal cerebral dysfunction that has stabilized and may have improved but has not resolved completely after 3 weeks. The most characteristic pattern is the abrupt occurrence of a neurological deficit that improves or worsens, often repeatedly, over a period of minutes to hours to days and then becomes a fixed deficit. The term "stroke in evolution" is used to describe a vascular syndrome that is acute in onset and progressively worsens during the period of observation.

Vascular Territory

Cerebrovascular events are also classified on the basis of the vascular territory involved. Symptoms and signs referable to the two major vascular territories are listed in Table 83.2. There is some overlap in the symptom complexes, making the distinction between carotid and vertebrobasilar disease difficult at times. However, frequently the history alone provides the evidence necessary to diagnose a cerebrovascular episode and to identify the arterial territory involved.

Another group of ischemic events, presenting as *lacunar syndromes*, is due to occlusion of penetrating nonanastamosing branches of the major cerebral arteries. The pathology of the involved vessels has been characterized; occlusion is due either to miniature atherosclerotic plaques at the origin of vessels 400 to 1000 μ in diameter or, more commonly, to a degenerative process called lipohyalinosis affecting vessels 200 μ or less. These changes correlate strongly with the presence of hypertension. At least 20 clinical lacunar syndromes have been described (18); lacunar infarctions may also be silent, identified only by computed tomographic (CT) scan. The common syndromes are the following:

Pure motor hemiparesis (internal capsule or pons): hemiplegia or hemiparesis involving the face, arm, and leg without sensory deficit, dysphasia, or hemianopsia.

Pure sensory stroke (thalamus): numbness of the face, arm, and leg on one side without weakness or hemianopsia.

Homolateral ataxia and crural paresis (pons): cerebellar ataxia, weakness, and pyramidal signs involving the limbs on the same side, the lower extremity more than the arm.

The *dysarthria-clumsy hand syndrome* (pons): dysarthria, facial weakness, clumsiness of the hand with little or no weakness, a slight imbalance, and a Babinski sign on the affected side.

Multi-infarct dementia : a dementia syndrome char-

Table 83.2.
Clinical Features of Ischemia Involving the Major Vascular Territories

CAROTID ARTERIAL DISEASE
  Paresis (mono- or hemi-)
  Sensory loss or paresthesias (mono- or hemi-)
  Speech or language disturbances
  Loss of vision in one eye or part of one eye (amaurosis fugax)
  Homonymous hemianopsia
  Cognitive impairment
VERTEBROBASILAR ARTERIAL DISEASE
  Vertigo, diplopia, dysphagia, or dysarthria when two occur together
    or when one occurs with any of the following:
  Paresis (any combination of the extremities)
  Sensory loss or paresthesias (any combination of the extremities)
  Ataxia
  Homonymous hemianopsia (unilateral or bilateral)

acterized by stepwise progression (see description of dementia, Chapter 17).

COMPLETED STROKE

Any occlusive arterial disease may lead to a completed stroke. The vast majority of strokes are due to atherosclerosis, lipohyalinosis, or emboli from the heart. A number of conditions may produce a syndrome resembling a completed stroke, RIND, or TIA. These are summarized in the discussion of the differential diagnosis of TIA (see below).

Both the diagnostic evaluation and initial care of the patient with a new stroke should be accomplished in the hospital. This includes patients with lacunar syndromes, which vary in their etiology and their appropriate treatment (18). After hospital discharge, ambulatory or home care for the stroke survivor requires the collaboration of the patient, the family, the physician, and other professionals, as explained below.

Natural History

The major studies on the natural history of stroke differ with regard to two important variables: the type of stroke patient studied and the treatment available to the study population. The few studies that attempted to restrict the variables under consideration were performed before the advent of cerebral CT scanning and were therefore marred by a significant degree of diagnostic inaccuracy. Despite these criticisms, the extensive body of literature on the "natural history" of stroke provides useful information.

Early Prognosis

There is general agreement that age influences greatly the early prognosis for the patient who sustains a stroke, regardless of the type. The older the patient, the less likely he is to survive (Table 83.3). Studies that classify strokes on the basis of etiology indicate that the early prognosis is much better for thrombotic or embolic disease than for hemorrhage. During the interval 1955 to 1969, 82% of stroke patients from the Mayo Clinic with a clinical diagnosis of cerebral thrombosis and 67% of those with cerebral embolism were alive 30 days after the acute episode (39). These values compare favorably with the 1-month survival of 48% ob-

served for subarachnoid hemorrhage and 16% observed for intracerebral hemorrhage.

Morbidity in Stroke Survivors

A number of studies have evaluated stroke survivors on the basis of the degree of neurological, functional, and psychosocial impairment.

Table 83.4 shows the spectrum and frequency of *neurological impairments* found in stroke survivors in the Framingham study (23). Study subjects were living at home or in institutions at the time of functional evaluation. The interval between the stroke and the functional assessment ranged from 6 months to 33 years (mean, 7 years). It is notable that half of these individuals (63 of 123) had no motor deficit. These community-based data are probably representative of the situation in other communities.

In an extensive study of *overall function*, Katz et al (34) found that, of the patients who survive a stroke, approximately 50% are independent 2 years later and are able to ambulate and perform activities of daily living with minimal or no assistance. Spontaneous improvement is most rapid in the first few months after the stroke and is rarely noted after 2 years. Only a small percentage of stroke survivors remain bedridden and completely dependent. These findings are supported by results from the Mayo Clinic where only 4% of the survivors of a stroke required total care at 6 months; 36% had some degree of neurological deficit, yet were able to work; and 29% were functioning normally (39). On the basis of the authors' assessment, 54% of their patients may have benefited from rehabilitative care, including the 10% who were aphasic.

The Framingham study provided information on the equally important *social and psychological sequelae* of stroke (23). A significant decrease in the levels of vocational function and socialization outside the home was noted among stroke survivors as compared with age- and sex-matched controls (Table 83.5), and the decrease exceeded that anticipated based on the levels of neurological deficit. In a more recent study in Monroe County, New York, the social and psychological difficulties facing the stroke survivor were evaluated prospectively (17). Within the first 6 months after hospital discharge, 37% of the patients demonstrated moderate or severe depression, 32% anger and/or anxiety, 56% social isolation, 43% reduction in commu-

Table 83.3.
Percentage Distribution of Stroke Survivors by Age Group[a]

Age Group	Percentage Surviving									
		Days				Years				
	Onset	30	60	90	180	1	2	3	4	5
Under 65	100.0	73.7	71.1	69.4	65.9	63.2	57.6	57.6	52.0	49.2
65–74	100.0	75.6	69.5	65.2	63.1	59.4	52.9	46.1	42.7	34.5
75–84	100.0	68.1	62.1	57.6	52.4	45.7	37.2	30.0	23.1	21.9
85+	100.0	52.4	45.8	37.2	33.0	27.8	20.7	15.1	9.2	7.4

[a] From: National Survey of Stroke, US Department of Health, Education and Welfare, Public Health Service National Institutes of Health, NIH publ no. 80-2069, January 1980.

Table 83.4.
Prevalence of Neurological Deficits in the 123 Survivors of Completed Stroke, Framingham Study (1972 to 1974)[a]

Type of Peripheral Motor Deficit	Survivors	No. Surviving with:			
		Sensory deficit	Hemi-anopsia	Dys-arthria	Dys-phasia
No motor deficit	63	3	5	2	10
Left hemiparesis	28	13	6	3	2
Right hemiparesis	27	10	5	13	9
Bilateral motor deficit	4	4	3	2	1
No data	1	1	1	1	1
Total survivors	123	31	20	21	23

[a] From Gresham GE, Fitzpatrick TE, Wolf PA, *et al:* Residual disability in survivors of stroke—the Framingham study. *N Engl J Med* 293:954, 1975.

Table 83.5.
Prevalence of Four Types of Functional Disability in 119 Survivors of Completed Stroke and in 119 Controls, Framingham Study (1972 to 1974)[a]

Type of Disability	Survivors		Matched Controls[b]		P Value
	No.	%	No.	%	
All persons examined for functional disability	119	100	119	100	—
Dependent in activities of daily living	37	31	9	8	<0.0001
Dependent in mobility	24	20	6	5	<0.0001
Decrease in level of vocational function[c]	85	71	49	41	<0.0001
Decrease in socialization	74	62	37	31	<0.0001

[a] Gresham GE, Fitzpatrick TE, Wolf PA *et al*: Residual disability in survivors of stroke-the Framingham Study. *N Engl J Med* 293-954, 1975.
[b] Matched for age and sex.
[c] Either stopped working or incomplete resumption of homemaking activities.

nity involvement, 46% economic strain causing life style alteration, and 52% disruption of normal family functions. Additional studies have (a) confirmed the high incidence of moderate or severe depression in the first year after stroke; (b) shown that the risk of depression is particularly high in patients with damage in the left frontal hemisphere (42, 43). Longitudinal studies have shown that poststroke depression lasts up to two years. Recent studies suggest two types of depression: a major depressive syndrome and a minor or dysthymic depression. Patients with the major depressive syndrome respond well to tricyclic antidepressants, especially nortriptyline (44).

Recognition and treatment of the psychosocial problems of the stroke patient and his family are discussed in more detail below.

Mortality in Stroke Survivors

The death rate among stroke survivors is significantly greater than that expected for the general population matched for age and sex. The 5-year cumulative mortality is approximately 50 to 60%, with the greatest number of deaths occurring in the first year. With time, however, the mortality rate approaches that of the general population and in at least one study the accelerated rate of death after a stroke subsided completely after 24 to 30 months (34). There is evidence to suggest that the etiology of a stroke (occlusive versus hemorrhagic) is a less reliable predictor of late prognosis than early prognosis. Eisenberg et al (16) reported that although cerebral hemorrhage was more lethal acutely than cerebral thrombosis, those patients with cerebral hemorrhage who lived 1 month had a 5-year survival equal to or better than patients with cerebral thrombosis. The leading cause of death in stroke survivors is cardiovascular disease, with cardiac-related deaths exceeding deaths attributed to cerebrovascular disease by a factor of 2 to 1. Because cardiac disease is a major contributor to the etiology of the stroke, stroke recurrence, and the survival from stroke, a thorough evaluation and management of cardiac disease is of great importance in the care of stroke survivors.

Management

Management of the patient who has survived a stroke involves the evaluation and treatment of any physical and psychosocial sequelae and the selection of appropriate therapy to lessen the risk of recurrence. Once the patient has been discharged from the hospital, his personal physician plays a critical role in coordinating his care. Reduction in a patient's disability and dependency frequently requires the concerted efforts of the patient's family; physical, occupational, and speech therapists; and occasionally a psychiatrist. Stroke patients with significant deficits persisting for 3 months or longer may qualify for disability insurance under Social Security (see Table 9.3).

Role of the Family

At the time of discharge from the hospital, appropriate education is especially important for the stroke survivor and his family. It is during this period that the patient is confronted with the full extent of his functional loss and that the actions of well-meaning but uninformed family members can increase the patient's feeling of inadequacy. The patient's physician must dispel myths regarding stroke and supplant them with accurate and useful information. The American Heart Association (AHA) has produced a series of invaluable booklets that discuss stroke and its sequelae in lay terms and provide guidelines for the home management of the stroke patient. The titles of these publications are listed in Table 83.6.

Table 83.6.
Booklets Published by the American Heart Association[a]

Recovering from a Stroke—booklet written for the patient and the patient's family, on ways in which the patient can regain activities of daily living.
Stroke: Why Do They Behave That Way?—a detailed booklet providing recommendations for the care of the patient who has completed most of his spontaneous recovery of higher functions and has major residual deficits (see "Summary of Recommendations" in Table 83.7)
Aphasia and the Family—explains many of the problems in aphasia and suggests practical ways in which the family can help the aphasic patient

[a] Available without charge from local AHA chapters.

The following general suggestions can be helpful for the family of a stroke patient with residual disability:

Divide duties so that the full burden of care does not fall on one person.

Help the patient take responsibility for doing his exercises regularly.

Allow the patient to take on responsibilities for self-care and other activities gradually and by easy steps. It calls for fine judgment to encourage independence and still not to frustrate a patient with overdifficult tasks; to stimulate progress and still not to encourage unrealistic expectations.

Praise any successful efforts that he makes; don't be discouraged by failures. Recovery from a severe stroke is a slow process.

Have him participate in as many family activities and as much family planning as he can. Feeling useful is a tremendous morale builder.

Help him keep in contact with the world he has known. Don't relegate him to the side lines and leave him with only television and radio to occupy himself. Encourage him to develop a hobby. Spend time with him. . . . Encourage visitors if his condition warrants it. Make him feel wanted and a part of the social picture.

Get in touch with the doctor if things are not going as you think they should.

Role of Rehabilitation

Success in stroke rehabilitation is often dependent upon the extent of permanent central nervous system damage and the patient's ability to utilize alternative methods of function to compensate for fixed deficits. As noted above, spontaneous improvement in the stroke survivor may continue to occur for the first 6 to 12 months after the stroke, yet the mechanisms underlying such gains remain obscure. In studies to determine whether intensive rehabilitation results in functional gains after the period of spontaneous improvement, it has been found that even significantly impaired patients admitted to a rehabilitation program 12 months after a stroke may show marked improvement in dressing skills, bladder and bowel function, and walking (36). These findings form the basis for the conclusion that a program of rehabilitation does improve the outcome of the stroke survivor. It is estimated that the savings derived in returning a patient to his family or to independent living more than equals the costs of rehabilitation (36).

It is clear that not all patients in a rehabilitation program show significant functional improvement. A number of patient characteristics correlate with poor rehabilitation results, including bowel and bladder incontinence, low self-care status on admission, right hemispheric involvement, intellectual and perceptual deficits, heart failure, signs of generalized arteriosclerosis, and lower educational levels (7, 37). However, since none of these factors correlates strongly with poor outcome, the best approach is to offer rehabilitation services whenever possible to each stroke survivor with significant functional impairments.

It is generally agreed that, except for patients with

evidence of subarachnoid bleeding, for whom bed rest and mild sedation are indicated, a program of functional rehabilitation should begin as soon as possible after a stroke occurs. *There are several reasons for the early initiation of a program of rehabilitation.* First, it is generally accepted that patients who are provided with rehabilitation services early are likely to experience greater long-term functional improvement. Second, early transfer from bed to chair coupled with physical therapy reduces the complications that can develop in the immobile bedridden patient and that can subsequently limit the extent of functional recovery. Stretching of tight muscles, passive range of motion, and active or resistive exercises minimize the degree of muscle atrophy and prevent the development of contractures. In addition, even limited mobility of the patient will reduce the risk of circulatory complications such as thrombophlebitis, postural hypotension, and pressure sores. Third, early rehabilitation is of particular benefit to the patient who demonstrates an impaired ability to communicate due either to dysphasia or to dysarthria. Approximately one-third of stroke patients exhibit some form of communication disorder and many of these remain severely impaired beyond the period of spontaneous recovery (46). Such patients may feel desperately isolated because of their loss of ability to communicate. Therapists who specialize in speech and hearing are skilled in the evaluation and management of these problems and play an integral role in daily interactions with the patient and in recommending appropriate strategies to the patient's family and physician.

Everyone involved in the rehabilitation process must appreciate the significance of the functional losses sustained by the patient, and to do so, the losses must be viewed from the patient's perspective. This requires an *awareness of the patient's usual activities before the stroke;* this essential information should be obtained in conjunction with a social worker who can evaluate the patient's role at home prior to the stroke and can project how the stroke will alter that role when the patient returns to his home.

Ideally, the *rehabilitation initiated in the hospital is continued in the patient's home or in ambulatory care facilities.* Many communities have physical, occupational, and speech therapists available for both home and ambulatory follow-up (see Chapter 9 for details on home health services). The patient, his family, and the patient's personal physician should be acquainted with the goals and plans for rehabilitation before discharge to home or to a rehabilitation facility. The comprehensive text of Brandstater and Basmajian (see "General References") provides details about the many individualized approaches available for rehabilitation.

Management of Psychological and Behavioral Sequelae

The high incidence of psychological and behavioral problems among stroke survivors has been noted above. These problems often hinder rehabilitation efforts. Fear of a second stroke and depression due to loss of functional ability are readily understandable in the context of the patient's predicament. Appropriate counseling (as outlined above) of the patient and his family, coupled with participation in an active rehabilitation program, are the best ways to minimize these adverse psychological reactions to a stroke.

A number of stroke survivors experience *disturbances of mood that do not correlate with the level of functional disability*; and there is evidence that for many patients the mood disorder is a specific complication of cerebral damage rather than simply a reaction to functional loss (19, 42, 43). This mood disorder may augment the cognitive impairment of the patient or on occasion be expressed as an apparent cognitive impairment (pseudodementia of depression). Response in such patients to antidepressant treatment may be dramatic. Earlier observations have suggested that the type of mood disorder is dependent upon the side of the brain affected by the stroke (44). Gainotti (20) reported that behavior denoting a catastrophic reaction (see Chapter 17) and anxious depressive orientation of mood (anxiety reactions, bursts of tears, provocative utterances, depressed renouncements, or sharp refusals to go on with the examinations) are more frequent among patients with left (dominant) hemisphere damage. Symptoms denoting an opposite emotional reaction (denial of illness, minimization, indifference reactions, and tendency to joke) and expressions of hate toward the paralyzed limbs are more frequent among patients suffering from a lesion of the right (minor) hemisphere. Most authorities agree, however, that both psychological and physiological factors contribute to the development of mood disorders after strokes. Tricyclic antidepressants have been shown to benefit patients with poststroke depression (42, 43, 44). Practical information about these drugs is found in Chapter 15, Affective Disorders.

The AHA booklet *Stroke: Why Do They Behave That Way?* is particularly helpful for the family and for health care professionals caring for the patient who has survived a major stroke involving the cerebral cortex. Table 83.7 contains summaries of the recommendations for dealing with permanent behavioral problems in these patients.

Management of Late Complications

There are a number of late complications that may occur during the months to years after a stroke.

Shoulder Problems. The painful shoulder is one of the most disturbing complications encountered in the patient with a residual hemiparesis. Shoulder pain is frequently caused by increased traction on the shoulder capsule secondary to abnormal positioning of the paralyzed arm. The normal alignment of the joint can be restored through the use of a sling and proper positioning of the arm at night. Physical therapy, after initial symptomatic treatment with analgesics and the application of heat, can limit the extent of permanent structural damage (see Chapter 63, Shoulder Pain, for additional detail).

The *shoulder-hand syndrome*, also called reflex sympathetic dystrophy, occurs in approximately 5% of stroke patients. It is characterized by the occurrence of a painful shoulder associated with stiffness and swelling of the hand and fingers. Onset is acute or subacute (developing over a 3- to 6-month period) and may involve the hand and shoulder simultaneously or one followed by the other. Although a number of conditions can result in shoulder discomfort, the dystrophic changes in the hand are characteristic of the shoulder-hand syndrome. There is swelling below the wrist but no pitting edema, and the skin of the hand is warm and pink. With time, the intrinsic muscles of the hand atrophy and extension deformities in the metacarpophalangeal joints develop. At this stage radiographic examination of the hand often shows spotty demineralization of the carpal bones. The severe pain associated with this condition greatly hinders rehabilitation efforts. Therefore, early recognition and treatment are important. Ross and Chipman (45) offer the following plan for the management of this condition: Begin treatment with analgesics and with heat to the shoulder; then carefully initiate and gradually increase abduction and external rotation exercises of the arm (described in Chapter 63). If there is no significant improvement after 1 month, the patient should be referred to a neurosurgeon for stellate ganglion block, followed by a course of oral corticosteroids if symptoms persist.

Complications of Inactivity. The partially paralyzed stroke survivor often leads a sedentary existence. This life style is conducive to the development of vascular complications such as *thrombophlebitis* and *pressure sores*. Use of elastic stockings and frequent repositioning of the immobile patient by an informed family member will minimize these problems.

Neurological Complications. Prolonged pressure on a paralyzed limb may lead to a peripheral nerve lesion, which may be difficult to recognize when superimposed on brain damage resulting from the stroke. An awareness of this potential complication can expedite its recognition, and electrodiagnostic studies can confirm the lower motor neuron damage (see Chapter 84). Once a diagnosis is made, prompt initiation of physical therapy will limit the degree of functional loss resulting from this usually reversible lesion.

Approximately 2.5 to 5% of stroke survivors develop *focal or generalized recurrent seizures* (epilepsy) as a late complication. Patients with damage to their sensorimotor cortex are the most likely to develop epilepsy, with the first seizure usually occurring 6 to 12 months after the stroke (38, 41). Transient neurological dysfunction after a seizure in a stroke survivor is often attributed to a second stroke. The rapid resolution of symptoms and electroencephalographic (EEG) evidence of an epileptogenic focus point to seizure activity rather than ischemia as the cause. Recurrent seizures in the stroke survivor confirm the diagnosis of epilepsy. Seizure control can usually be achieved through the use of anticonvulsant medication (see Chapter 80).

Finally, *stroke-related deficits may transiently worsen*

Table 83.7.

Recommendations for Dealing with Behavioral Problems Associated with Permanent Loss of Higher Functions in Stroke Patients[a]

LEFT HEMISPHERE DAMAGE

Right hemiplegics will often have difficulties with speech and language. They also tend to be somewhat cautious, anxious, and disorganized when attempting a new task. Keep in mind the following suggestions:

1. Do not underestimate the patient's ability to learn and communicate even if he cannot use speech.
2. If he cannot use speech, try other forms of communication. Pantomime and demonstration are often useful.
3. Do not overestimate his understanding of speech and overload him with "static."
4. Do not shout. Keep messages simple and brief.
5. Do not use special voices.
6. Divide tasks into simple steps.
7. Give much feedback and many indications of progress.

RIGHT HEMISPHERE DAMAGE

If the patient is having difficulty with self-care activities, you can expect spatial-perceptual deficits. He will tend to talk better than he can actually perform. He may be impulsive or careless. Remember, when working with the patient who has significant spatial-perceptual deficits:

1. Do not overestimate his abilities. Spatial-perceptual difficulties are easy to miss.
2. Use verbal cues if he has difficulty with demonstration.
3. Break tasks into small steps and give much feedback.
4. Watch to see what he can do safely rather than taking his word for it.
5. Minimize clutter around him.
6. Avoid rapid movement around the patient.
7. Highlight visual reference points.

ONE-SIDED NEGLECT

One-sided neglect is a problem that involves more than a simple visual field cut or hearing loss. It can occur in both right and left hemiplegics but seems to be more common and more persistent among left hemiplegics. When dealing with a neglect problem, you should:

1. Keep the unimpaired side toward the action unless specifically working with neglected side.
2. Avoid trapping the patient in an unnecessarily confined environment.
3. Avoid nagging but give frequent cues to aid orientation.
4. Provide reminders of the neglected side.
5. Arrange the environment to maximize performance.

MEMORY PROBLEMS

Some memory problems can be expected in most stroke patients. When working with memory deficits, you can often increase the patient's ability to perform if you:

1. Establish a fixed routine whenever possible.
2. Keep messages short to fit his retention span.
3. Present new information one step at a time.
4. Allow the patient to finish one step before proceeding to the next.
5. Give frequent indications of effective progress; he may forget his past "successes."
6. Train in settings that resemble, as much as possible, the setting in which the behavior is to be practiced.
7. Use memory aids such as appointment books, written notes, and schedule cards whenever possible.
8. Use familiar objects and old associations when teching new tasks.

[a]Adapted from *Stroke: Why Do They Behave That Way?* American Heart Association.

when the patient develops a major intercurrent illness such as pneumonia or myocardial infarction. In this instance, neurological status returns to baseline after resolution of the intercurrent illness. (See discussion of upper motor neuron symptoms in Chapter 78.)

General Surgery. The approach to general surgery in the stroke patient is discussed in Chapter 86.

Prevention of Stroke Recurrence

The selection of appropriate therapy to lessen the risk of stroke recurrence is based on the pathophysiology of the initial stroke and upon the presence of any risk factors (see above) that can be modified. In this section only the most frequently advocated forms of preventive treatment are discussed.

Antihypertensive Therapy. In a prospective randomized clinical trial, Carter (12) assessed the efficacy of antihypertensive therapy in the treatment of hypertensive patients who had sustained a nonembolic ischemic stroke. He reported that 44% of the untreated patients, as compared with 20% of the treated patients, suffered another major stroke. At the end of a 2- to 5-year follow-up period 46% of the untreated patients and 26% of the treated patients had died. Although the number of recurrent strokes was too small to allow a valid comparison, the difference in mortality was statistically significant in favor of the treated group. Moreover, no treated patient sustained a major neurological complication as a result of a documented hypotensive episode.

Two subsequent studies of the effect of antihypertensive treatment on stroke recurrence included patients with hemorrhagic as well as ischemic strokes. Beevers et al (6) noted that the stroke recurrence rate varied inversely with success in controlling blood pressure. In patients with good, fair, and poor control of hypertension, the recurrence rates were 16, 32, and 55%, respectively. In contrast, the Hypertension-Stroke Cooperative Study Group (29) failed to demonstrate a significant reduction in stroke recurrence in treated as compared with control patients, although the incidence of congestive heart failure was reduced among the treated patients.

In summary, despite the differences in the studies cited above, critical assessment of the data yields the conclusions that antihypertensive medication can be safely administered to hypertensive stroke survivors and that it is indicated for these patients to reduce cerebrovascular and cardiovascular sequelae. (See Chapter 62 for details on the treatment of hypertension.)

Anticoagulant and Antiplatelet Agents. Anticoagulant and antiplatelet agents have been extensively evaluated for their efficacy in the prevention of stroke recurrence. There is evidence from noncontrolled studies that patients with ischemic infarcts due to emboli from the heart will benefit from long-term anticoagulation with Coumadin (14). However, for the large majority of stroke survivors, those with completed strokes due to atherothrombotic cerebrovascular disease, anticoagulation affords no benefits (22).

Data on the antiplatelet agents are somewhat more encouraging (8, 10). Chapter 52 ("Thromboembolic Disease") (a) summarizes the evidence regarding prophylaxis of atherosclerotic vascular disease with antiplatelet therapy and (b) provides practical guidelines for the use of antiplatelet (aspirin) therapy. These recommendations, based upon critical analysis of a vast literature, differ somewhat from approaches advocated in the past.

Carotid Artery Surgery. Based upon careful analysis of a number of studies, Kistler et al. (see "General References") concluded that carotid artery surgery may benefit a carefully selected group of patients with a completed stroke. According to these authors, carotid endarterectomy can be recommended to patients with a small infarct in the carotid system who have surgically correctable arterial lesions appropriate to the deficit (e.g., a large ulcerated plaque or stenosis of greater than 60%) and who are otherwise in good health and neurologically stable. Angiography and surgery should only be performed by a team of specialists with a record of documented success in the evaluation and treatment of occlusive cerebrovascular disease.

TRANSIENT ISCHEMIC ATTACK

As noted earlier, TIAs are defined as transient episodes of focal cerebral dysfunction, rapid in onset (no to maximal symptoms in less than 5 minutes), with symptoms referable to the carotid or vertebrobasilar arterial territory (see Table 83.2), which resolve completely within 24 hours.

Early studies on the pathophysiology of TIAs suggested that they are primarily caused by vasospasm or hypotension, but artery to artery emboli, resulting from atherosclerotic disease of intra- and extracranial cerebral vessels, are now thought to account for about 90% of TIAs (3).

Differential Diagnosis

Before the diagnosis of TIA is made, other conditions that can produce transient neurological dysfunction must be considered. *Epileptic seizures* (see Chapter 80) can result in transient neurological symptoms. A history of either a grand mal seizure with loss of consciousness, clonic movement of a subsequently weakened limb, or a rapid march of sensory symptoms will aid in reaching the correct diagnosis. *Migraine attacks* (see Chapter 79) are occasionally associated with sensory or motor symptoms that resemble TIAs. With migraine, however, the patients are usually younger, headache is almost invariably present, and the spread of symptoms often occurs with a characteristic march over minutes to hours. *Disorder of a vestibular end organ* (see Chapter 81) can lead to dizziness or vertigo suggestive of the brainstem ischemia of a vertebrobasilar TIA. However, as noted earlier, brainstem ischemia usually results in additional symptoms such as diplopia, dysphagia, dysarthria, weakness, sensory changes, ataxia, or loss of vision. A *mass lesion* such as a tumor or subdural hematoma will occasionally present with recurrent transient neurological symptoms. A careful examination of the patient may reveal mild persisting neurological signs that progress over time, and the lesion can often be de-

tected by CT scan (see "Patient Experience," Chapter 78). Occasionally an acute exacerbation of *multiple sclerosis* may mimic a transient ischemic attack. However, in such cases the patients are usually younger and have had previous and often multiple episodes of transient neurological dysfunction with multiple and different localization. *Hypoglycemia* can lead to transient neurological symptoms, which may be focal if the hypoglycemia is superimposed on existing occlusive cerebrovascular disease. Finally, transient neurological abnormalities may be present for a short interval *after syncope due to any cause* (see Chapter 81).

Natural History

The natural history of TIAs has long been debated (10).

Despite variability in the published reports, the available data indicate that TIAs represent a significant warning of impending stroke, with between 25 and 40% of patients experiencing a cerebral infarction within 5 years of their first TIA (40). The 15-year experience (1955 to 1969) of the Mayo Clinic perhaps provides the best information on natural history. During this period the average annual incidence of first TIA in Rochester, Minnesota, was 31/100,000 population with the rate increasing with age (51). Although long-term survival after the first TIA was not significantly different from that anticipated for the general population matched for age and sex, the risk of stroke occurrence was markedly increased. A large percentage of the strokes occurred in the first few months after the onset of TIAs indicating that this was a particularly high risk period. The risk was similar for TIAs in the carotid and vertebrobasilar territories.

Evaluation

Depending upon the history, initial evaluation of the patient with TIA may be in the hospital (for observation, in the patient who presents within hours or within a few days of the event) or in the ambulatory setting (the patient who describes a TIA that occurred days to weeks before). A detailed history is essential, to identify risk factors for cerebrovascular disease and to delineate and classify the focal symptoms (see Table 83.2). The physical examination should include assessment for hypotension, hypertension, cardiac disease, cerebrovascular and peripheral vascular disease, and any persisting neurological abnormality. The patient should also have a careful funduscopic evaluation to assess the status of the retinal vessels and to detect emboli (see example, Fig. 83.1) that suggest atherothrombotic carotid occlusive disease or cardiac valve disease. If there is clinical evidence of heart disease, in particular a murmur, atrial fibrillation, or left ventricular dysfunction, an echocardiogram should be obtained to look for an intracardiac source of arterial emboli. Patients with heart disease should also have Holter monitoring to check for cardiac arrhythmias.

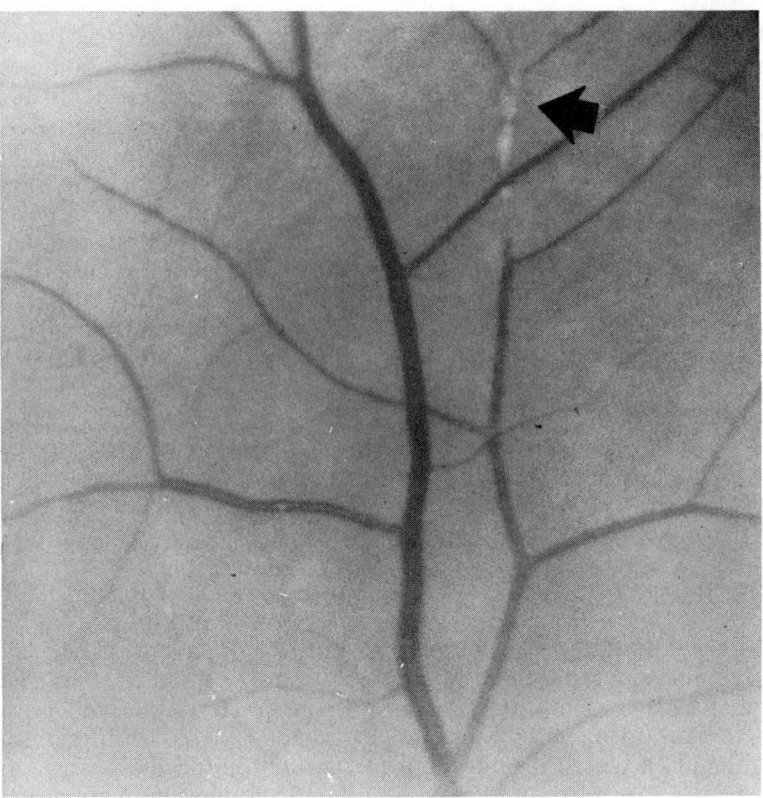

Figure 83.1. Atheromatous debris embolus lodged in retinal arteriole (*arrow*) in patient with recurrent hemisphere TIA and amaurosis fugax. These emboli persist for hours to weeks, and even permanently, while the platelet-fibrin emboli are fleeting and gone within a few minutes. (From Meyer JS, Shaw T: *Diagnosis and Management of Stroke and TIAs.* Baltimore, Williams & Wilkins, 1982.)

Screening tests, to check for specific causes of a TIA, should include a serum glucose measurement (hypoglycemia), a serological test for syphilis, a hemoglobin measurement (polycythemia), and an erythrocyte sedimentation rate (vasculitis).

Patients with carotid territory TIAs who are acceptable surgical candidates should have a *noninvasive carotid evaluation*, utilizing the available technique with the best performance characteristics. Decision analysis of the various available procedures has shown that the preferred noninvasive technique is duplex ultrasonography (1). If this is not available, carotid Doppler ultrasound combined with periorbital Doppler ultrasonography is an alternative approach with excellent performance characteristics. The characteristics and the patient experiences associated with these and other noninvasive diagnostic tests are described in Chapter 78.

Patients whose noninvasive studies show stenosis greater than 50% in a carotid artery, and who are candidates for surgery (see Chapter 86), should have carotid angiography (see description, Chapter 78). Planning of this preoperative evaluation should be coordinated by a consulting neurologist.

Management

Patients who have had a single TIA or multiple TIAs and are not surgical candidates should be placed on long-term *antiplatelet treatment* with aspirin (see details in Chapter 52).

Carotid endarterectomy, with or without long-term antiplatelet therapy, can be recommended to those patients whose diagnostic evaluation shows a significant arterial lesion that is at the carotid bifurcation and that could account for the patient's clinical symptoms. If stenotic disease is more severe in the intracranial carotid artery or the middle cerebral artery, then surgery of the carotid in the neck should not be recommended. If there is additional less severe disease in other extracranial or intracranial vessels, then, after surgery, long-term antiplatelet therapy is recommended.

A number of years ago, there was enthusiasm for *surgical revascularization*, utilizing an external to internal carotid bypass (2, 5), in patients with inoperable intracranial stenoses or total external occlusions. A controlled trial showed, however, that the incidence of strokes or recurrent TIAs was lower in the medically treated patients (4, 15).

In severe cases of *basilar vertebral insufficiency* with recurrent TIAs and/or strokes in the basilar vertebral territory and arteriographic evidence of bilateral vertebral compromise or high grade basilar artery stenosis, bypass procedures have been undertaken. The efficacy of these procedures has not yet been established, although they have been successfully completed with relatively low morbidity in small numbers of patients (13).

Because the guidelines for the management of patients with TIAs are still evolving, the advice of a neurologist who specializes in cerebrovascular disease should be sought liberally.

ASYMPTOMATIC CERVICAL BRUIT

The asymptomatic patient with a cervical bruit is encountered commonly in ambulatory practice. For example, 4.4% of subjects over the age of 45 had asymptomatic cervical bruits in a population-based study in Evans County, Georgia, and the majority of the bruits were heard anteriorly in the neck over the location of the carotid artery (27). Although atherosclerosis and/or arterial stenosis probably accounts for most of these bruits, a number of other mechanisms are possible (Table 83.8).

Natural History

Prospective studies of asymptomatic patients with an anterior cervical bruit have demonstrated an increased risk of cerebrovascular disease. There is disagreement, however, as to (a) whether the initial neurological deficit in the patient who becomes symptomatic is more likely to be transient or permanent and (b) whether the side of the bruit is of any value in predicting the location of the initial neurological event. At one extreme is the view that the initial deficit is often permanent and is most likely to occur in the vascular territory distal to the carotid artery with the bruit. At the other extreme is the belief that the initial event is almost invariably transient and can occur with equal frequency in the distribution of the affected or contralateral carotid artery.

Evaluation and Management

The evaluation and treatment of the asymptomatic patient with an anterior cervical bruit is controversial. Many authorities believe that there is no role for diagnostic evaluation and surgical intervention in the management of these patients (27), whereas others feel that for certain "high risk" patients these invasive procedures may be indicated (28). According to the latter view, a patient whose bruit is in the location of the carotid bifurcation (near the angle of the jaw) should have a careful funduscopic examination to look for emboli (see Fig. 83.1) as well as a noninvasive carotid evaluation similar to that for a carotid distribution TIA

Table 83.8.
Possible Causes of Cervical Bruit

Physiological murmur
Venous hum
Transmitted cardiac murmur
Atherosclerosis and stenosis of carotid, vertebral, subclavian, or innominate artery
Loops, kinks, inflammation, fibromuscular dysplasia of carotid artery
Arteriovenous fistula
Angiomatous malformation
Intracranial neoplasm
Paget's disease of the skull

(see above). A controlled trial is in progress to test the impact of surgery in such high-risk patients, when diagnostic studies show greater than 50% stenosis.

There is general agreement that patients should be followed closely for any change in the character of their bruit suggestive of progressive disease and for the occurrence of symptoms referable to an underlying arterial lesion. In patients who do undergo noninvasive study that shows carotid artery disease, it is reasonable to prescribe aspirin, although to date no study has assessed its role in this situation (see Chapter 52, "Thromboembolic Disease"). Preliminary data in small series of patients suggest that although antiplatelet therapy retards the rate of progressing carotid stenosis it does not prevent progression to eventual occlusion (26). Because serial angiographic studies have suggested that the rate of atheromatous change at the carotid bifurcation is directly related to hypertension (30), antihypertensive treatment is important in patients with asymptomatic bruits and high blood pressure; in these patients, it is particularly important to avoid the orthostatic hypotension that may accompany use of any antihypertensive drug.

General References

Benton AL (ed): *Behavioral Changes in Cerebrovascular Disease.* New York, Harper & Row, 1970.
  A detailed account of psychological problems complicating stroke.
Brandstater M, Basmajian J (eds): *Stroke Rehabilitation.* Baltimore, Williams & Wilkins, 1987.
  A detailed, well-illustrated, and extensively referenced resource on all aspects of the rehabilitation of stroke patients.
Feussner JR, Matchar DB: When and how to study the carotid arteries. *Ann Intern Med* 109:805, 1988.
  Detailed review of the literature and use of decision analysis to determine the relative value of diagnostic strategies.
Kistler JP, Ropper AH, Heros RC: Therapy of ischemic cerebral vascular disease due to atherothrombosis. *N Engl J Med* 311:27, 1984.
  Thorough review of the subject, extensively referenced.
Marler JR: Carotid endarterectomy clinical trials. *Mayo Clin Proc* 64:1026, 1989.
  Describes the three controlled trials of carotid endarterectomy that were in progress as of 1989, two for asymptomatic disease and one for symptomatic disease.
Sessler GJ: *Stroke—How to Prevent It/How to Survive It.* Englewood Cliffs, NJ, Prentice-Hall, 1982.
  A comprehensive discussion of stroke and its prevention for the physician and potential patient.

Specific References

1. American College of Physicians Health and Public Policy Committee. Diagnostic evaluation of the carotid arteries. *Ann Intern Med* 109:835, 1988.
2. Ausman J, Diaz F, DeLos RA, et al: Extracranial intracranial anastomoses in the posterior circulation. In: Berguer R, Bauer RD (eds): *Vertebrobasilar Occlusive Disease: Medical and Surgical Management.* New York, Raven Press, 1984, p 313.
3. Barnett HJM: The pathophysiology of transient cerebral ischemic attacks. Therapy with platelet antiaggregants. *Med Clin North Am* 63:649, 1979.
4. Barnett HJM, Peerless SJ: Collaborative EC/IC bypass study: the rationale and a progress report. In: Massey J, Reinmuth OM (eds): *Cerebrovascular Diseases.* New York, Raven Press, 1981, p 271.
5. Barnett HJM, Plum F, Walton JM: Carotid endarterectomy—an expression of concern. *Stroke* 15:941, 1984.
6. Beevers DG, Fairman MJ, Hamilton M, Harpur JE: Antihyper-

tensive treatment and the course of established cerebrovascular disease. *Lancet* 1:1407, 1973.

7. Bourestom NC: Predictors of long term recovery in cerebrovascular disease. *Arch Phys Med Rehabil* 48:415, 1967.

8. Bousser MG, Eschwege E, Haguenau M, et al: "AICLA" controlled trial of aspirin and dipyridamole in the secondary prevention of athero-thrombotic cerebral ischemia. *Stroke* 14:5, 1983.

9. Broderick JP, Phillips SJ, Whisnant JP, et al: Incidence rates of strokes in the eighties—the end of the decline in stroke? *Stroke* 20:577, 1989.

10. Brust JCM: Transient ischemic attacks: Natural history and anticoagulation. *Neurology* 27:701, 1977.

11. Canadian Cooperative Study Group: A randomized trial of aspirin and sulfinpyrazone in threatened stroke. *N Engl J Med* 299:53, 1978.

12. Carter AB: Hypertensive therapy in stroke survivors. *Lancet* 1:485, 1970.

13. Chambers BR, Norris JW: The case against surgery for asymptomatic carotid stenosis stroke. *Stroke* 15:964, 1984.

14. Easton JD, Sherman DG: Management of cerebral embolism of cardiac origin. *Stroke* 11:433, 1980.

15. EC/IC Bypass Study Group. Failure of the extracranial intracranial bypass to reduce the risk of ischemic stroke: results of an international randomized trial. *New Engl J Med* 313:1201, 1985.

16. Eisenberg H, Morrison JT, Sullivan P, Foote FM: Cerebrovascular accidents: incidence and survival rates in a defined population. Middlesex County, Connecticut. *JAMA* 189:883, 1964.

17. Feibel JH, Berk S, Joynt RJ: The unmet needs of stroke survivors. *Neurology* 29:592, 1979.

18. Fisher CM: Lacunar strokes and infarcts: a review. *Neurology* 32:871, 1982.

19. Folstein MF, Maiberger R, McHugh PR: Mood disorders as a specific complication of stroke. *J Neurol Neurosurg Psych* 40:1018, 1977.

20. Gainotti G: Emotional behavior and hemispheric side of the lesion. *Cortex* 8:41, 1972.

21. Garraway NW, Whisnant JP, Drury ID: The continuing decline in the incidence of stroke. *Mayo Clin Proc* 58:520, 1983.

22. Genton E, Barnett HJM, Fields, et al: XIV: Cerebral ischemia: the role of thrombosis and of antithrombotic therapy. *Stroke* 8:147, 1977.

23. Gresham GE, Fitzpatrick TE, Wolf PA, et al: Residual disability in survivors of stroke—the Framingham study. *N Engl J Med* 293:954, 1975.

24. Hachinski V: Decreased incidence and mortality of stroke. *Stroke* 15:376, 1984.

25. Halperin JL, Hart RG: Atrial fibrillation and stroke: new ideas, persisting dilemmas. *Stroke* 19:937, 1988.

26. Hemerci H, Heelshomer HB, et al: Spontaneous history of asymptomatic internal carotid occlusion. *Stroke* 17:718, 1986.

27. Heyman A, Wilkinson WE, Heyden S, et al: Risk of stroke in asymptomatic persons with cervical arterial bruits: a population study in Evans County, Georgia. *N Engl J Med* 302:838, 1980.

28. Hurst JW, Hopkins LC, Smith RB: Noises in the neck. *N Engl J Med* 302:862, 1980.

29. Hypertensive-Stroke Cooperative Study Group: Effects of antihypertensive treatment on stroke recurrence. *JAMA* 229:409, 1974.

30. Javid H, Ostermiller WE, Hengesh JW, et al: Natural history of carotid bifurcation atheroma. *Surgery* 67:80, 1970.

31. Kannel WB: Current status of the epidemiology of brain infarction associated with occlusive arterial disease. *Stroke* 2:295, 1971.

32. Kannel WB, Gordon T, Wolf PA, McNamara PM: Hemoglobin and the risk of cerebral infarction: the Framingham study. *Stroke* 3:409, 1972.

33. Kannel WB, Wolf PA, Verter J, McNamara PM: Epidemiologic assessment of the role of blood pressure in stroke. *JAMA* 214:301, 1970.

34. Katz S, Ford AB, Chinn AB, Newill VA: Prognosis after strokes. II. Long term course of 159 patients. *Medicine* (Baltimore) 45:236, 1966.

35. Kurtzke JF: Epidemiology of cerebrovascular disease. In: Siekert RG (ed): *Cerebrovascular Survey Report.* Rochester, Minnesota, Whiting Press, 1980.

36. Lehmann JF, DeLateur BJ, Fowler RS, et al: Stroke: does rehabilitation affect outcome? *Arch Phys Med Rehabil* 56:375, 1975.

37. Lehmann JF, Delateur BJ, Fowler RS, et al: Stroke rehabilitation: outcome and prediction. *Arch Phys Med Rehabil* 56:383, 1975.

38. Louis S, McDowell F: Epileptic seizures in nonembolic cerebral infarction. *Arch Neurol* 27:414, 1967.

39. Matsumoto N, Whisnant JP, Kurland LT, Okazaki H: Natural history of stroke in Rochester, Minnesota, 1955 through 1969: an extension of a previous study, 1945 through 1954. *Stroke* 4:20, 1973.

40. Millikan C: The transient ischemic attack. *Adv Neurol* 25:135, 1979.

41. Richardson Jr. EP, Dodge PR: Epilepsy in cerebral vascular disease: a study of the incidence and nature of seizures in 104 consecutive autopsy-proven cases of cerebral infarction and hemorrhage. *Epilepsy* 3:49, 1954.

42. Robinson RG, Starr LB, Kubos KL, Price TR: A two-year longitudinal study of post-stroke mood disorders: findings during the initial evaluation. *Stroke* 14:736, 1983.

43. Robinson RG, Starr LB, Lipsey JR, et al: A two-year longitudinal study of post-stroke mood disorders: dynamic changes in associated variables over the first six months of follow-up. *Stroke* 15:510, 1984.

44. Robinson RG, Balduc PL, Price TR: Two year longitudinal study of post stroke mood disorders: diagnosis and outcome at one and two years. *Stroke* 18:837, 1987.

45. Ross GS, Chipman M: The neuralgias. In: Baker AB, Baker LH (eds): *Clinical Neurology* Hagerstown, Harper & Row, 1974, vol 3.

46. Sarno MT: Disorders of communication in stroke. In: Licht S (ed): *Stroke and Its Rehabilitation* Baltimore, Williams & Wilkins, 1975.

47. Tohgi H, Yamanouchi H, Murakami M, et al: Importance of the hematocrit as a risk factor in cerebral infarction. *Stroke* 9:369, 1978.

48. Veterans Administration Cooperative Study Group on Antihypertensive Agents: Effects of treatment on morbidity in hypertension. Results in patients with diastolic blood pressures averaging 115 through 129 mm Hg. *JAMA* 202:1028, 1967.

49. Veterans Administration Cooperative Study Group on Antihypertensive Agents: Effects of treatment on morbidity in hypertension. II. Results in patients with diastolic blood pressure averaging 90 through 114 mm Hg. *JAMA* 213:1143, 1970.

50. Whisnant JP: The decline of stroke. *Stroke* 15:160, 1984.

51. Whisnant JP, Matsumoto N, Elveback LR: Transient cerebral ischemic attacks in a community. *Mayo Clin Proc* 48:194, 1973.

52. Wolf PA, Kannel WB, McNamara PM, Gordon T: The role of impaired cardiac function in atherothrombotic brain infarction: the Framingham study. *Am J Public Health* 63:52, 1973.

C H A P T E R   84

Peripheral Neuropathy

LORRAINE F. JOSIFEK, M.D.
MARGIT L. BLEECKER, M.D., PH.D.

DEFINITIONS AND PATHOPHYSIOLOGY

A peripheral nerve is a bundle of fibers called axons; the large and medium-sized axons are normally covered with a layer of myelin. Most peripheral nerves are mixed nerves carrying both incoming sensory information (afferent fibers) and outgoing motor and autonomic impulses (efferent fibers). Large diameter afferent fibers convey information about position and vibration; large diameter efferent fibers innervate the muscles themselves. Small diameter, often unmyelinated, fibers convey pain and temperature sensation, as well as autonomic information.

Peripheral neuropathies result from disease processes that involve nerve axons or their myelin encasements. Axonal neuropathies are the result of processes that primarily affect the cell body and axon, whereas demyelinating neuropathies result from processes that primarily affect the myelin sheath. Often, especially in chronic disorders such as diabetes mellitus, irrespective of the initial type of pathological process, the interdependence between axon and myelin produces secondary changes that, on biopsy, reveal a mixed pathological picture. The etiological diagnosis of peripheral neuropathies, therefore, usually depends upon their clinical features and on other supportive laboratory findings.

The three major patterns of peripheral nerve disease may be distinguished by clinical presentation: mononeuropathy, multifocal neuropathies (mononeuropathy multiplex), and polyneuropathy. *Mononeuropathies* are lesions of individual nerve roots or peripheral nerves; they usually are due to local causes such as trauma or entrapment (compression of a nerve by adjacent structures). *Multifocal neuropathy* (also called mononeuropathy multiplex) refers to involvement of two or more discrete nerves, usually asymmetrically and not contiguously, either at the same time or sequentially. This less common pattern is usually caused by systemic diseases such as polyarteritis nodosa or diabetes mellitus, which may affect several nerves focally. *Polyneuropathy* is the result of a generalized disease process affecting the peripheral nerves in a symmetrical distal distribution.

In both axonal and demyelinating diseases the longer and larger axons (nerves) are involved earlier and more severely than the shorter ones. In demyelinating neuropathies, this is because the longer axons have more potential sites for demyelination; in the axonal neuropathies, the longer axons require more metabolic support and are therefore more susceptible to curtailment of this support. Therefore, symptoms of both types of neuropathies tend to appear first in the feet and then in the hands. Most polyneuropathies indiscriminately affect both the sensory and the motor nerve fibers (mixed polyneuropathies or sensorimotor neuropathies); and some affect peripheral autonomic nerves. However, clinically (and occasionally pathologically), in some patients there will be a predilection for either the sensory nerves (sensory polyneuropathies) motor nerves (motor polyneuropathies), or autonomic nerves.

APPROACH TO THE PATIENT

History and Physical Examination

Symptoms of peripheral neuropathy include loss of sensation (sometimes accompanied by pain), weakness, and muscle cramps; and, if autonomic nerves are involved, impotence, urinary retention or overflow incontinence, constipation or diarrhea, and orthostatic hypotension. In patients with polyneuropathy, paresthesias (pins and needles) located in the feet are the most common presenting complaint. Many other sensory misperceptions occur and are difficult for the patient to describe. Frequently patients are bothered by non-noxious sensory stimuli (e.g., light touch perceived as burning), and they may report that symptoms are relieved by pacing the floor, by firm massage, or by cold (e.g., leaving the legs outside the covers at night). Complaints of heaviness or coldness of the extremities are also common.

The major *signs of peripheral neuropathy* are sensory loss, weakness, muscle atrophy, diminished or absent tendon reflexes, and trophic changes in the skin. The most common sensory modalities affected in polyneuropathy are pain and vibration, in a symmetrical stocking-glove distribution. Temperature is usually also affected, but this is harder to document in the clinical setting. In polyneuropathies the weakness is most often distal, affecting the intrinsic muscles of the feet, (e.g., inability to spread the toes and difficulty walking on uneven surfaces). In long-standing neuropathies the muscle imbalance causes high arched feet and hammer toes. Eventually the shin may appear prominent because of atrophy of the tibialis anterior muscle, and there may be striking wasting of the small muscles of the hand. The skin of the lower extremities may appear shiny, scaling, and atrophic. Marked loss of proprioception in the feet may be manifest as unsteadiness, ataxia, or a positive Romberg test (see Chapter 78 for additional details about neurological signs).

Etiologies and Distinctive Features

Whereas a limited number of conditions produce mononeuropathy and multifocal neuropathy (Table 84.1), there are many etiologies of polyneuropathy (Table 84.2). Diagnosis often depends on obtaining a thorough history (for example, of alcoholism or of occupational exposure to toxins) or on finding a relevant systemic condition (for example, diabetes mellitus). Table 84.3 lists the three features most useful in the differential diagnosis of a polyneuropathy (time course, selective functional involvement, distribution) and the etiologies associated with these features.

Time Course

Mononeuropathies are often acute in onset; that is, the patient remembers the time of onset. The most common of the acute polyneuropathies is the Guillain-Barré; syndrome, but other processes—metabolic, infectious, or toxic—may cause severe neurological dysfunction rapidly, sometimes within hours. Most toxic neuropathies (lead poisoning, for example) develop somewhat more slowly—within weeks—as do neuropathies associated with malnutrition (e.g., thiamine deficiency). The most common of the chronic neuro-

Table 84.1.
Common Causes of Mononeuropathy and Multifocal Neuropathy

MONONEUROPATHY
  Trauma—direct (occupational, recreational, e.g., ulnar or peroneal nerve), compression and entrapment (e.g., carpal tunnel, root compression, etc.)
  Infection—herpes zoster
  Toxins (e.g., penicillin injection into a sciatic nerve)
  Vascular—vasculitis, diabetes mellitus
  Neoplasm—lymphoma, neurofibroma
MULTIFOCAL NEUROPATHY (Mononeuropathy Multiplex)
  Diabetes mellitus
  Vasculitis
POLYNEUROPATHY
  Multiple etiologies (see Table 84.2)

Table 84.2.
Polyneuropathy: Etiology and Mode Of Predominant Involvement[a]

	Predominant Involvement[a]
METABOLIC	
Diabetes mellitus	S,SM,A
Polyneuropathy	
Mononeuropathy	SM
Lumbar plexopathy (diabetic amyotrophy)	M>S
Alcohol and vitamin deficiency	SM,A
Uremia	SM
Hypothyroidism	S>M
Porphyria	M>S
TOXIC (see Table 84.5)	
Lead	M
pyridoxine	S
Cis-platinum	S
Most others	SM
INFECTIOUS	
Diptheria	M
Leprosy	S
Lyme disease	SM
Human immunodeficiency virus	S>M
INFLAMMATORY	
Guillain-Barré	M
Recurrent inflammatory neuropathy	M
Noncarcinomatous sensory neuropathy	S
COLLAGEN VASCULAR	
Systemic lupus erythematosis	SM
Polyarteritis nodosa	SM
Sjögren's syndrome	SM
Rheumatoid arthritis	SM
NEOPLASTIC	
Carcinomatous	S,SM
Paraproteinemia, plasma cell dyscrasias	S,SM,A
Benign monoclonal gammopathy	S,SM
Waldenström's macroglobinemia	SM,M
Cryoglobinemia	SM
HEREDITARY	
Hereditary sensorimotor neuropathies	SM
Amyloidosis	S>M,A
Dysautonomia (Riley-Day)	S,A
Tomaculous neuropathy	SM
Tangier's (Bassen-Kornzweig)	S
Fabry's	S

[a] A = autonomic, M = motor, S = sensory.

pathies (gradual progression over months to years) are associated with diabetes mellitus (see Chapter 72) and with alcoholism (see below); and, in an unselected population, these are the most common of the polyneuropathies in general.

Patients with hereditary neuropathies sometimes may be unaware that they suffer from a long-standing progressive disorder. A history of a lack of athletic ability in school or difficulties with maneuvers in the military or of problems fitting shoes may be a useful clue in that regard. High arched feet and hammer toes reflect long-standing disease and may point to the diagnosis of one of these hereditary processes.

Patterns of Involvement

Mononeuropathy usually produces both motor and sensory involvement in the distribution of the affected

Table 84.3.
Polyneuropathy: Differential Diagnosis[a,b]

TIME COURSE	Predominately sensory:
Acute (days):	Global sensory loss:
Guillain-Barré syndrome	*Diabetes*
Porphyric neuropathy	Carcinomatous sensory neuropathy (ganglioradi-
Diphtheritic neuropathy	culitis)
Some toxins (triorthocresyl phosphate)	Paraproteinemic and cryoglobulinemic neuropathy
Subacute (weeks):	Tabes dorsalis
Many toxins	Dissociated loss of pain and thermal sensibility:
Nutritional neuropathies	Diabetes (small fiber type)
Carcinomatous neuropathies	Amyloidosis
Uremic neuropathy	Hereditary sensory neuropathies
Relapsing:	Lepromatous leprosy
Relapsing inflammatory neuropathy	Dissociated loss of joint position and vibration
Refsum's disease	sensibility:
Porphyria	Subacute combined degeneration
Chronic (many months or years):	Friedreich's ataxia
Diabetic motor-sensory neuropathy	Autonomic neuropathy:
Alcoholic neuropathy	*Diabetes*
Chronic inflammatory neuropathies	*Amyloid*
Very chronic (childhood onset):	Acute, chronic, and relapsing pandysautonomia
Heritable motor-sensory neuropathies (Charcot-Marie-Tooth	Dysautonomia (Riley-Day)
disease)	DISTRIBUTION[d]
SELECTIVE FUNCTIONAL INVOLVEMENT[c]	Proximal weakness:
Predominately motor:	Guillain-Barré
Guillain-Barré syndrome	Porphyria
Relapsing and chronic inflammatory neuropathy	Carcinomatous neuropathy with proximal weakness ("car-
Acute intermittent porphyria	cinomatous neuromyopathy")
Lead neuropathy	Spinal muscular atrophies
Heritable motor-sensory neuropathies (Charcot-Marie-Tooth)	Proximal sensory loss:
Diphtheritic neuropathy	Porphyria
	Tangier disease (analphalipoproteinemia)
	Temperature-related distribution:
	Lepromatous leprosy

[a] Adapted from Griffen JW: Peripheral neuropathies. In Harvey AM *et al* (eds): *Principles and Practice of Medicine*, ed 21. New York, Appleton-Century-Crofts, 1984.
[b] The most common etiologies are set in *italic*.
[c] Most polyneuropathies produce sensory and motor disturbances.
[d] Most polyneuropathies produce distal involvement.

nerve root or peripheral nerve (see below, Tables 84.6 and 84.7).

Most polyneuropathies produce both sensory and motor disturbances. Polyneuropathy with predominantly sensory involvement suggests diabetes mellitus, carcinoma, amyloidosis, dysproteinemia, and alcoholism. Occasionally, sensory losses are dissociated; that is, the patient has diminished appreciation of pain and temperature but preserved appreciation of light touch and joint position; this pattern is typical of small fiber neuropathies. When position and vibratory sense is lost but pain sense preserved, vitamin B_{12} deficiency (usually pernicious anemia) or, much more rarely, Friedreich's ataxia should be considered. In polyneuropathy, predominantly motor involvement suggests the Guillain-Barré; syndrome, hereditary neuropathies, lead intoxication, and acute intermittent porphyria. Predominantly autonomic involvement suggests diabetes mellitus, amyloidosis, alcoholism, dysautonomia, and dysproteinemia.

INVESTIGATIONS

Clinical Laboratory

It is important to identify the cause of a peripheral neuropathy because often neurological dysfunction will persist unless the underlying disease can be treated.

The common causes of polyneuropathy (shown in *italics* in Table 84.3) are usually obvious to the physician; but sometimes, even these require direct questioning (concerning alcoholism, for example) or specific laboratory tests (for example, measurement of blood glucose) before they are appreciated. If the cause of the neuropathy is not obvious, routine screening tests should include erythrocyte sedimentation rate, fasting blood glucose, serum creatinine, thyroxine (T_4), a complete blood count (CBC), a chest X-ray, and, in patients over the age of 40, a serum protein electrophoresis. There are many relatively unusual conditions that may be associated with neuropathy, but an extensive screening program to rule out all of these processes would be expensive and almost always unrewarding unless there is some clue in the history or physical examination to warrant a particular test (for example, measurement of blood lead in a patient with a history of occupational exposure). If, after evaluating a patient with neuropathy, no cause of the process has been identified, consultation with a neurologist should be considered.

Nerve Conduction Studies

The measurement of nerve conduction velocity is helpful in establishing the diagnosis, severity, and location of the neuropathy. A baseline measurement makes it possible to differentiate progression of the peripheral neuropathy from other clinical conditions at future points in time. Although there are laboratories that will perform nerve conduction studies upon demand, it is prudent to let a neurologist decide about the usefulness and the interpretation of the procedure.

Nerve conduction velocity measurements involve stimulating a nerve at one point and recording the response, either at the muscle (motor nerve), or at some distance along the nerve (sensory nerve). The results of nerve conduction studies usually include latency of response, conduction velocity, and amplitude of response. The latency of response refers to the time elapsed between the start of the stimulus and the muscle response (muscle fiber depolarization) or nerve response (sensory nerve action potential). The conduction velocity between two points along the nerve is always expressed in meters per second.

Conduction disturbances of the peripheral nerve may be localized, as in an entrapment syndrome, or may involve nerves more diffusely as in polyneuropathies. In general, early axonal degenerations are associated with normal conduction and the presence of denervation on electromyography (EM; see below), whereas demyelination is characterized by slowing of nerve conduction and normal EMG studies.

The procedure has several limitations. First, nerve conduction velocities (NCVs) only test directly that portion of the nerve between the two sites; they generally do not detect damage more distal than (e.g., muscle) or more proximal to (e.g., nerve root) the segment tested. F waves may detect proximal segment pathology but are not measured routinely. The standard test is therefore not directly applicable to such common situations as spondylosis or lumbar or cervical disc disease (see Chapters 64 and 65). Second, NCVs measure the speed of conduction in the largest and fastest conducting fibers of peripheral nerves. Therefore, nerve conduction studies are only sensitive to diseases that involve such fibers.

It is important for the clinician to be able to specify as precisely as possible the clinical problem and question to be addressed; stating only "numbness in the upper extremities" or "test nerves in lower extremities" without any specific guidance is unlikely to be productive.

Patient experience. With the patient comfortably positioned paste is applied over the sites to be tested and electrodes are taped over the appropriate muscles and nerves. The shocks may be mildly unpleasant. Usually the nerves on both sides of the body are compared. Testing takes approximately 20 to 60 minutes.

Electromyography (Table 84.4)

Electromyography (EMG) is not often helpful in patients with diffuse peripheral neuropathy. It may, however, detect the early denervation changes of axonal neuropathy before striking changes are recognized on nerve conduction studies. The principal use of EMG is to help define entrapment neuropathies (e.g., radial nerve entrapment) and differentiate these from more proximal radicular compression (e.g., carpal tunnel syndrome from C6 radiculopathy). The EMG can recognize denervation in muscles that are difficult to assess on physical examination.

EMG can also help differentiate the muscle wasting of neuropathic or myopathic disorders from disuse atrophy. Consultation with a neurologist will help define the clinical question for the EMG laboratory to answer.

EMG involves the insertion of needles into a muscle to record electrical activity directly. During complete rest, no electrical activity should be observed. *Spontaneous fibrillation* potentials are the action potentials of single fibers that are twitching spontaneously in the absence of innervation. Fibrillation potentials are usually, but not invariably, a good indication of primary denervation (they also occur in polymositis and more rarely in other myopathic processes). *Fasciculations* are the spontaneous firings of whole motor units (all of the muscle fibers innervated by a single nerve fiber). Fasciculations may be seen in normal individuals, although they are more frequent and likely to be more polyphasic in states of denervation. Therefore, the presence of fasciculations is only moderately useful in diagnosing denervation.

Muscle action potentials are examined individually by asking the patient to move only slightly. Large amplitude, long duration polyphasic potentials suggest a denervating process. Small amplitude, short duration polyphasic potentials are associated with myopathic processes.

The *interference pattern* is the pattern produced when the subject is asked to contract the muscle fully. A "full" interference pattern is normal. Anything less may indicate less than maximal effort (hysteria, malingering), poor conduction of nerve impulses to the muscle (denervation), or poor ability of the muscle to respond (myopathy).

The EMG electrodes damage and inflame the muscles into which they have been inserted (note—serum creatine phosphokinase activity is not altered by this procedure). Thus, if there is a possibility that a muscle biopsy will be required, the muscle that may be examined by biopsy should not be tested by EMG. The need for EMG for patients with bleeding tendencies or at risk from recurrent infection should be carefully reviewed with a neurologist.

Patient experience. There is usually discomfort with the initial insertion of the needles and also during movement of the muscles when the needles are in place. Because the needles are very thin and only penetrate skin and muscle, the risks of infection or hemorrhage are almost nil. The procedure takes 30 to 90 minutes.

Nerve Biopsy

Nerve biopsy should be reserved for those patients in whom a specific histological diagnosis is a possi-

Table 84.4.
Electromyography: Patterns Typical of Nerve and Muscle Disorders

Disorder	Insertional Activity	Complete Rest (Spontaneous Activity)	Action Potentials	Interference Pattern
Denervation[a]	Increased	Fibrillations, positive waves, fasciculations	High amplitude, long duration, polyphasic	Reduced or incomplete with fast firing rate
Myopathic				
Myopathy	Normal	Normal or rare fibrillations	Small amplitude, short duration polyphasic	Full, small amplitude
Myositis	Increased	Fibrillations, positive waves	Small amplitude, short duration polyphasic	Full, small amplitude

[a] Neuropathy, radiculopathy, disc disease.

bility (for example, amyloidosis or vasculitis). In general the procedure has limited usefulness, since the pathology is usually nonspecific; also the nerve tested by biopsy is usually a sensory nerve (the sural) and may not reflect a disease process that has affected the motor nerves. The biopsy may lead to painful sequelae in the distribution of the tested nerve (usually the sural distribution on the dorsolateral foot). If the nerve biopsy is done, the specimen must be specially processed for maximal information at centers that are familiar with nerve pathology. Consultation with a neurologist will be helpful in deciding whether a nerve biopsy is indicated.

COMMON PROBLEMS

Guillain-Barré; Syndrome

Most cases of the Guillain-Barré; syndrome (2) follow a mild viral illness (by 10 to 12 days); the syndrome also may be associated with pregnancy, the postoperative period, recent influenza immunization, and with human immunodeficiency virus (HIV) infection. There is rapid progression of symmetrical motor weakness (usually moving from the lower extremities to the upper extremities) accompanied by loss of deep tendon reflexes. Although acute pain or paresthesias in the back and posterior legs may be prominent early symptoms, objective evidence of sensory loss is minimal. Cranial nerve weakness may be present, with bilateral facial nerve palsy, in 40% of patients. NCVs may be abnormal, and the cerebrospinal fluid may show an increased protein concentration with normal cell counts (cytoalbumin dissociation). Because of rapid progression of the disease, patients suspected of having this disorder should be admitted to the hospital for close monitoring for potential respiratory distress and autonomic disturbances (hypotension, hypertension, cardiac arrhythmias, hyperpyrexia), which are often part of the course. There is some evidence that plasmapheresis early in the course shortens the period of disability. Recovery is complete in about half of the patients (although it may take 6 to 18 months); most of the remainder have only mild residual deficits; but 10% have severe permanent disability. The patients may remain at a plateau of function and then suddenly recover. Splints, to prevent contractures, and passive range of motion should be employed until the recovery

period is complete. The differential diagnosis includes diphtheria, botulism, and acute intermittent porphyria.

Diabetic Neuropathy

The prevalence of diabetic neuropathy (5, 19) is not known precisely, but it is clearly one of the more common neuropathies. The problem is discussed in detail in Chapter 72, Diabetes Mellitus.

Alcoholic Neuropathy

Neuropathies associated with alcoholism (3) and with associated vitamin deficiencies usually occur in the fourth to seventh decades, with a slow onset over a period of months. The presenting symptoms are varied, but they often reflect a distal, motor and sensory, symmetrical polyneuropathy with pain and paresthesias in the feet and legs. Autonomic features, including impotence, bladder dysfunction, and orthostatic hypotension, may also be seen. Malnutrition and vitamin deficiencies (particularly thiamine deficiency) probably make a major contribution to the neuropathy, although there is evidence that alcohol has a direct toxic effect on peripheral nerves.

Treatment is aimed toward improved nutrition and vitamin replacement as well as toward effective treatment for the alcoholism (see Chapter 21). The paresthesia of a mild neuropathy can be expected to improve with good nutrition and abstinence from alcohol. However, with moderate to severe sensorimotor and autonomic neuropathy, significant residual symptoms and findings will persist.

Carcinomatous Neuropathy

Carcinomatous neuropathy (11, 21) (excluding nerve damage from direct invasion of nerves by tumor) occurs most commonly in association with cancer of the lung, sometimes years before the tumor has been diagnosed.

Distal Sensorimotor Neuropathy

This is primarily an axonal process in which the sensory loss predominates in the lower extremities. It develops over weeks or months and often becomes stationary, or, if the underlying cancer responds to treatment, it may improve.

Carcinomatous Sensory Neuropathy

This has a distinctive pattern beginning subacutely, often with pain involving legs, arms, or face. Over many weeks a profound proprioceptive sensory loss develops accompanied by pseudoathetosis (seemingly purposeless movements that are due to loss of position sense). Areflexia is common. The patient may be unable to stand or walk unassisted. Nerve conduction studies may show normal motor potentials but reduced or unobtainable sensory potentials. The underlying tumor is most often oat-cell carcinoma of the lung, but breast, ovarian, uterine, and gastrointestinal tract tumors also occur. The neuropathy is usually progressive. A common chemotherapeutic agent for the treatment of ovarian cancer, cis-platinum, produces a similar picture.

Paraproteinemic Neuropathies

Peripheral neuropathy is commonly associated with paraproteinemic and dysglobulinemic disorders (12, 14). Often there are features of distal burning dysesthesias and autonomic dysfunction. Although the course is usually one of steady progression, improvement in the neuropathy may occur after the successful treatment of the underlying disease.

Toxic Neuropathy

Toxic neuropathies are becoming increasingly more frequent. They are important to recognize since they are potentially reversible if the toxin can be identified. The diagnosis may be made easily if there is a history of drug exposure (e.g., isoniazid, hydralazine, vincristine) or of industrial exposure (Table 84.5). Since these neuropathies have no distinguishing features on routine history or on physical examination, a detailed history of exposure to drugs and of the patient's occupation and recreational habits is important. Axonal involvement in the spinal cord may occur be masked by the toxic neuropathy. In these cases, a residual

Table 84.5.
Toxins Associated with Peripheral Neuropathies

INDUSTRIAL[a]
  Pesticides—organophosphates, dichorophenyoxyacetate (2, 4-D), Vacor rodenticide
  Metal work—lead, arsenic, mercury, thallium, methyl bromide
  Plastics, synthetic fabrics—*n*-hexane, methyl, *n*-butyl ketone, acrylamide, carbon disulfide, percholrethylene, trichlorethylene, dimethylaminoproprionitrile
  Gases—carbon monoxide, ethylene oxide
EUPHORIANTS
  Glue sniffing—*n*-hexane, solvents
  Nitrous oxide inhalation—whipped cream dispensers, dental offices
PHARMACOTHERAPEUTIC AGENTS
  Antimicrobial—isoniazid, nitrofurantoin, metronidazole
  Cardiovascular—hydralazine, procainamide, amiodarone
  Other—Phenytoin, disulfiram, pyridoxine, vincristine

[a] See also Chapter 7, Table 7.2.

spastic paraparesis becomes apparent when the peripheral neuropathy has resolved. Toxic neuropathies are classically associated with chronic low dose exposure (months to years), though they may appear within days to weeks with high level exposure. A delayed neuropathy associated with organophosphates develops 10 to 14 days after exposure whereas Vacor, a rodenticide, produces an acute toxic neuropathy within 2 to 3 days.

A recently recognized toxicity with megadose pyridoxine consumption produces a gradually progressive sensory ataxia and profound distal limb impairment of position and vibratory sense (18). General acceptance of vitamin B_6 therapy as safe and that "more might be better" by the public makes direct questioning about vitamin habits necessary. Because the original description, some patients have been reported who have ingested lower daily doses in the range of 0.5 to 1.0 g/day.

Multifocal Motor Neuropathy

Several acquired motor neuron syndromes (17) have recently been described. These syndromes, in which patients present with progressive asymmetrical motor weaknesses, have previously been considered to be variants of amyotrophic lateral scerlosis. Nerve conduction studies show multifocal motor nerve conduction block and high antibody titers to GM 1 ganglioside. Some patients with these syndromes have responded to immunosuppressive therapy.

HIV Infection

There are a number of peripheral nervous system manifestations of HIV infection (4).

A painful sensory neuropathy, usually confined to the feet, affects 30% of patients with the acquired immunodeficiency syndrome (AIDS). NCV studies show reduced or absent sensory potential and reduced motor nerve conductions. Primary HIV infection of the dorsal root ganglion has been proposed as the mechanism. Treatment is currently limited to symptomatic relief with tricyclic antidepressants such as amitriptyline (Elavil) and by carbamazapine (Tegretol), described below.

Multiple mononeuropathies have been described, most often in HIV-infected patients who have not yet developed AIDS. Some HIV-infected patients develop a chronic inflammatory demyelinating neuropathy. Treatment with plasmapheresis and prednisone has been tried.

Inflammatory demyelinating polyneuropathies (IDP) of both the Guillain-Barré; and chronic form have been seen, usually in the early stages of HIV infection, in otherwise asymptomatic seropositive individuals. Treatment has been tried with plasmapheresis as in seronegative cases of demyelinating neuropathy.

Chapter 34 provides a detailed account of the ambulatory care of patients with HIV infection.

Compression and Entrapment Neuropathies

When a peripheral neurological abnormality occurs in one upper or lower extremity, the abnormality is usually due to nerve entrapment or to compression caused by anatomical abnormalities or trauma, although polyneuropathy and mononeuropathy may present initially as a focal deficit in one extremity. With careful evaluation, it is usually possible to determine whether the patient's problem is due to nerve root damage or to damage to a peripheral nerve or one of its branches. Tables 84.6–84.8 and Figures 84.1 and 84.2 summarize the information needed to make this distinction, i.e., distribution of sensory, motor, and reflex deficits; common causative factors; and critical anatomical relationships.

Several commonly encountered compression and entrapment neuropathies are discussed here. Root compression symptoms due to cervical and lumbar spine disease are discussed in Chapters 64 (Neck Pain), 65 (Low Back Pain), and 68 (Osteoarthritis).

Median Nerve (Carpal Tunnel Syndrome)

Etiology. Carpal tunnel syndrome (CTS) is a very common pressure neuropathy in which median nerve injury results from compression by neighboring anatomical structures (see Fig. 84.1). The carpal canal or tunnel is formed by the concave arch of the carpal bones and is roofed by the transverse carpal ligament. These structures form a rigid compartment through which nine tendons and the median nerve must pass. Conditions that cause a decrease in the size of the carpal canal (e.g., Colles' fracture, rheumatoid arthritis, congenital carpal canal stenosis), enlargement of the median nerve (e.g., endoneural edema in diabetes mellitus, amyloid, neuroma), or increase in the volume of other structures within the canal (e.g., teno-synovitis, ganglion, lipoma, urate deposits in gout, hematoma, fluid retention in pregnancy) may all have one common result, namely, compression of the median nerve. Many cases previously classified as idiopathic are explained by occupational factors. CTS in the workplace is associated with occupations in which the wrist position deviates from the normal straight alignment and with occupations involving the use of greater hand force in all wrist positions (e.g., meat processing, fruit packing, upholstering, and waiting on tables). Median nerve compression can also be caused by tasks that require a sustained or repeated stress over the base of the palm, such as that caused by the use of screwdrivers, scrapers, paint brushes, and buffers. Vibration exposure (low frequency, 10 to 40 Hz), is another well-recognized risk factor for carpal tunnel syndrome (air-powered tools). Repetitive wrist and hand movements leading to CTS may also occur in activities such as knitting, crocheting, hooking rugs, playing a musical instrument, painting, woodworking, gardening, lifting weights, typing when the keyboard is too high.

Manifestations and Evaluation. Unless associated with direct trauma, the onset of symptoms of CTS is usually nocturnal and insidious. Symptoms in the hand may initially be described as episodic tingling and numbness with gradual progression to more severe symptoms referred to as burning, aching, pricking, or as a painful numbness in the fingers and deep in the palm. With the pain and tingling there is a subjective feeling of uselessness in the fingers, which are sometimes described as feeling swollen, even though, on inspection, little swelling is apparent. Many patients will have accompanying pain in the forearm, sometimes reaching the shoulder and described as a dull aching pain felt deeply in the limb.

Color changes in the fingers have been described, par-

Table 84.6.
Comparative Data on Root and Nerve Lesions in the Arm

Roots ⟶	C5	C6	C7	C8	T1
SENSORY LOSS[a,b]	Lateral upper arm	Dorsolateral forearm and thumb	Mid-dorsal forearm and middle finger	Medial forearm, ring and small fingers	Medial arm, axilla
MOTOR LOSS[b]	Deltoid, some biceps infra- and supras-pinatus	Biceps, brachioradialis, some deltoid	Triceps, wrist and finger extensors	Thenar eminence	Interossei of hand
TENDON REFLEX	Slight 1 biceps	Biceps, brachioradialis	Triceps	Finger jerk	None
CAUSATIVE LESION	Cervical spondylosis	Cervical spondylosis, disc disease	Disc disease, cervical spondylosis	Thoracic outlet syndrome, neoplastic disease at apex of lung or in cervical nodes	

PERIPHERAL NERVES ⟶	Axillary	Musculocutaneous	Radial	Median (Carpal Tunnel)	Ulnar (Cubital Tunnel)
SENSORY LOSS	Over deltoid	Radial forearm	Dorsal lateral hand	First 3½ digits	Small and ring finger
MOTOR LOSS	Deltoid	Biceps, brachialis	Triceps, wrist and finger extensors	Thenar, abductor pollicis brevis	Instrinsics of hand
TENDON REFLEX	None	Biceps	Triceps, brachio-radialis	Finger jerk	None
PAIN	Over deltoid	Lateral forearm	Dorsal lateral forearm and hand	Nocturnal lateral hand and fingers	Small and ring finger, tenderness at elbow

[a] See dermatomal pattern, Table 78.1.
[b] Pain distribution is usually from the neck along area of muscles supplied to the distal area of sensory loss.

Table 84.7.
Comparative Data on Root and Nerve Lesions in the Leg

Roots ⟶	L2	L3	L4	L5	S1
SENSORY LOSS[a]	Upper and medial thigh	Anterior thigh	Lateral thigh to medial thigh	Lateral leg to dorsum of foot	Posterior leg to plantar foot
MOTOR LOSS	Iliopsoas (hip flexion)	Quadriceps (knee extension), Adductor	Quadriceps, anterior tibial (dorsiflexion of foot)	Great toe extensor, anterior Tibial	Gastrocnemius, biceps femoris (flexion of knee), gluteus maximus (hip extension)
TENDON REFLEX	None	Adductor	Knee	Medial hamstring	Ankle
PREDOMINANT CAUSATIVE LESION	Neoplastic disease, neurofibroma	Neoplastic disease, rare disc disease	Disc lesions, neoplastic disease	Disc lesions, local metastatic	Disc lesion, local metastatic

PERIPHERAL NERVES ⟶	Obturator	Femoral	Lateral Femoral cutaneous (meralgia paresthetica)	Sciatic Peroneal Division	Sciatic Tibial Division (Tarsal Tunnel)
SENSORY LOSS PAIN AREA	Medial thigh	Anterior medial thigh	Upper lateral thigh usually 10–12 inches below the iliac crest	Dorsum of foot and lateral leg	Plantar foot (with burning pain), tips of toes
MOTOR LOSS	Adductor	Quadriceps (knee extension	None	Anterior tibial (dorsflexion of ankle), EDB (toe spreading)	Usually none detected
TENDON REFLEX	Adductor	Knee	None	None	Ankle

[a] See dermatomal pattern, Table 78.1.

ticularly with exposure to cold, but they are not related to the attacks of CTS sensory symptoms. Also, excessive sweating and mild degrees of edema are related to the vasomotor imbalance known to occur in CTS.

As CTS progresses, the nocturnal pain and tingling may begin to wake the patient after a few hours' sleep. Relief may be obtained by hanging the arm out of bed or shaking or rubbing the hand, but as symptoms increase, patients often get out of bed and walk about until the symptoms have eased. At this stage episodic tingling may develop during the day, but the associated pain in the arm occurs less often during the day than at night. In addition to sensory symptoms, there may be clumsiness and difficulty in performing certain tasks, such as unscrewing bottle tops, turning a key, or crocheting.

Objective changes in sensation and strength may appear in the hand, but some patients may suffer severe attacks of pain for many years without developing abnormal neurological signs. Sensory signs within the median nerve distribution (see Table 84.6) are best sought for in the fingertips, where impairment is, as a rule, more pronounced. Occasionally, instead of decreased sensation, there is an over-reaction to cutaneous stimuli in the median innervated lateral three and a half fingers. Isolated thenar wasting or sensory impairment in the distribution of one of the lateral three digital nerves may be the presenting feature of median nerve lesions at the wrist. Mild weakness of the abductor pollicis brevis (patient abducts thumb at right angle to palm, against resistance) or of the opponens pollicis muscle (patient touches base of little finger with thumb, against resistance) is frequently present with no visually apparent atrophy. Manual

pressure over the flexor aspect of the wrist or prolonged hyperextension or hyperflexion of this joint may reproduce sensory symptoms (Phalen's sign). Tinel's sign, consisting of shock-like pain and tingling elicited by percussion of the median nerve at the wrist, is a less common finding.

Although abnormalities of the nerve conduction studies (see above) are more likely to be found in the presence of a defect on clinical examination in CTS, a significant number of patients with typical symptoms have no abnormalities other than those detected on electrodiagnostic testing. Abnormalities of conduction in motor fibers of the median nerve in the carpal canal are frequent and are important findings in CTS, but abnormalities of sensory fibers occur with even greater frequency. Nearly 90% of patients have abnormalities on sensory nerve conduction studies from the index finger, and in some instances, this is the only objective evidence to support the clinical diagnosis. Needle-electrode examination of the thenar eminence is uncomfortable and less sensitive in CTS than are the routine nerve conduction studies.

Treatment. Immobilization of the wrist with a close-fitting anterior splint (extends from the upper part of the forearm to the metacarpophalangeal joints), which is worn by the patient at night or when resting, holds the wrist immobilized in a neutral position. This often will alleviate all symptoms, but if symptoms persist after a few weeks, additional therapy is indicated. Local corticosteroid injections or a trial of oral anti-inflammatory medication is frequently used but generally yields temporary relief at best.

Indications for *carpal tunnel release* include the failure of nonoperative treatment or clinical evi-

Table 84.8.
Entrapment Neuropathies: Common Causative Factors

Nerve, Location	Causative Factors
Median	
At wrist	Meat processing, upholstering, knitting, painting, weight lifting, using vibrating tools, pregnancy, musical instruments
At forearm	Repeated pronation, e.g., screwdriver, weight lifting
Ulnar	
At wrist	Bicycling, leaning on a walker, pliers, using palm as a hammer
At elbow	Injury to elbow, sitting in a wheelchair, chronic lying in bed, leaning on elbow on tables and desks
Radial	
At forearm	Lipoma, tennis, trauma
At arm	Saturday night palsy, bridegroom's palsy, crutches, pneumatic tourniquets
Axillary	Trauma to tip of shoulder, deep injections into deltoid muscle
Musculocutaneous	Weight lifting, shoulder dislocations
Tibial	
At knee	Chronic standing, poorly fitting shoes, ankle
At ankle	Trauma, weight gain, or edema
Peroneal	
At knee	Ankle sprains, crossed legs, after weight loss, squatting, kneeling
At ankle	Tight shoes, trauma
Femoral	Inguinal surgery, childbirth, psoas hemorrhage, dorsal lithotomy position
Lateral Femoral Cutaneous	Ascites, overweight, pregnancy, utility belts, blunt sports injury to anterior iliac spine
Obturator	Pelvic fracture, hip surgery, childbirth, retroperitoneal hematoma, and malignancy
Sciatic	Hip surgery, pelvic fracture, injections, endometriosis, retroperitoneal hematoma, lipoma

dence of thenar atrophy. A relative indication is constant sensory loss, especially if it is long standing. The surgical treatment for CTS is one of the most successful operations that can be performed on the hand. The operation demands care and skill by an orthopaedic, plastic, or neurological surgeon who is performing hand surgery regularly. Complications of the operation or poor results (i.e., reflex sympathetic dystrophy, severance of median nerve branches, hypertrophic scar, adherent flexor tendons) are almost always related to poor surgical technique. The usual postoperative recovery time is 6 to 8 weeks. An additional month may be needed for occupational rehabilitation. The majority of patients with ergonomically stressful jobs (jobs that involve repetitive wrist motion such as typing) are able to return to their preoperative activities after a work-hardening program.

Ulnar Nerve

Etiology. Ulnar nerve compression occurs most often at the elbow (see Fig. 84.1). The cubital tunnel refers to the area of entrapment of the ulnar nerve at the elbow as it runs beneath the aponeurosis of the flexor carpi ulnaris muscle just distal to the medial epicondyle. Minor pressure directly over the cubital tunnel during anesthesia, intoxication, stupor, coma, or by trauma may subsequently cause symptoms.

Cumulative trauma to the ulnar nerve at the elbow may occur with activities requiring repeated flexion and extension of the elbow. Hypermobility of the ulnar nerve in these cases results with hypesthesia in the fifth digit, often associated with elbow flexion.

Manifestations and Evaluation. Patients may awaken at night with elbow pain, shooting pain in the hand or fifth digit, and paresthesias and hypesthesias in the ulnar nerve distribution. These symptoms usually improve with elbow extension. The amount of pain and paresthesia varies, and for some the sensory loss is not bothersome. Patients usually see a physician when they experience motor dysfunction, such as weakness of grasp and pinch or loss of dexterity.

Ulnar sensory loss (see Table 84.6) is easiest to establish over the distal two phalanges of the little finger with two-point discrimination. Transition between the ulnar territory over the hypothenar eminence and the medial cutaneous nerve (branch from the brachial plexus) of the forearm is often detected at the skin crease at the wrist. Motor disability is manifested as decreased pinch strength, which is related to the degree of intrinsic atrophy of the involved muscles, and as impaired coordination and dexterity. Grasp may be decreased if the interossei and flexor digitorum profundus to the fourth and fifth digits are weak. One of the earliest signs of ulnar nerve entrapment is weakness of the third palmar interosseus manifested by an abducted posture of the fifth digit.

Ulnar neuropathy distal to the elbow occurs at the wrist or in the hand and must be considered if there is no weakness in the flexor digitorum profundus. This is most often caused by a ganglion, rheumatoid arthritis, or by trauma (such as long distance bicycling). Often lesions in the wrist or hand produce no paresthesias or sensory loss. Depending upon the level of entrapment at the wrist either all of the ulnar innervated muscles may be weak or there may be selective preservation of hypothenar function (i.e., abductor digiti quinti).

Focal slowing of the ulnar motor or sensory nerve conduction across the elbow is found with nerve conduction studies (see above) in one-third to one-half of patients, depending upon the severity. False-positive findings may be obtained and, therefore, close correlation with the clinical findings is mandatory. Increased distal latencies are found with entrapment at the wrist but must be correlated with EMG (see above) to determine the actual site of the lesion.

Treatment. Nonsurgical treatment is indicated for the patient with intermittent symptoms, acute or chronic mild neuropathy, or mild neuropathy associated with an occupational cause. For a mild ulnar neuropathy,

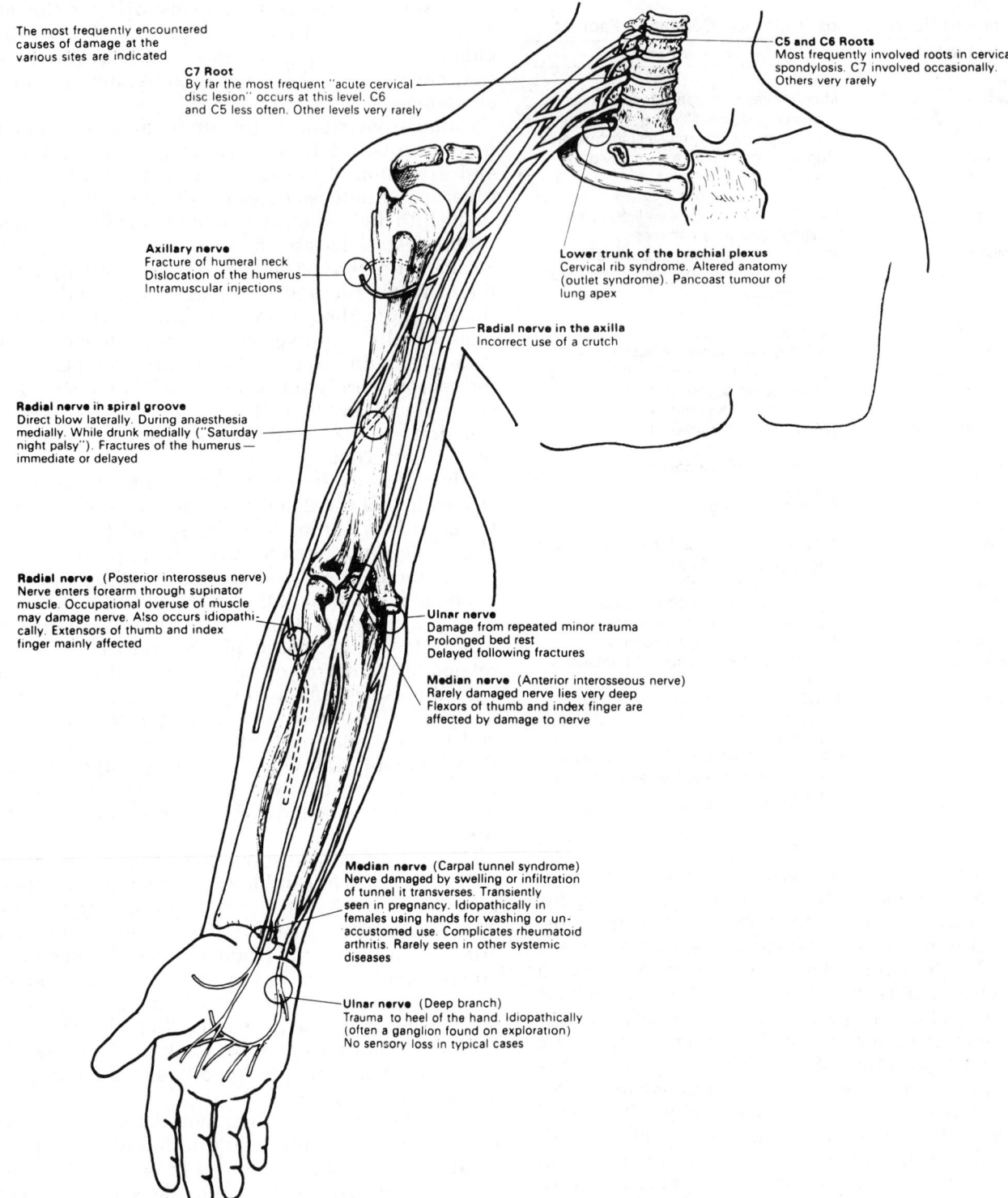

The most frequently encountered causes of damage at the various sites are indicated

C7 Root
By far the most frequent "acute cervical disc lesion" occurs at this level. C6 and C5 less often. Other levels very rarely

C5 and C6 Roots
Most frequently involved roots in cervical spondylosis. C7 involved occasionally. Others very rarely

Axillary nerve
Fracture of humeral neck
Dislocation of the humerus
Intramuscular injections

Lower trunk of the brachial plexus
Cervical rib syndrome. Altered anatomy (outlet syndrome). Pancoast tumour of lung apex

Radial nerve in the axilla
Incorrect use of a crutch

Radial nerve in spiral groove
Direct blow laterally. During anaesthesia medially. While drunk medially ("Saturday night palsy"). Fractures of the humerus — immediate or delayed

Radial nerve (Posterior interosseus nerve)
Nerve enters forearm through supinator muscle. Occupational overuse of muscle may damage nerve. Also occurs idiopathically. Extensors of thumb and index finger mainly affected

Ulnar nerve
Damage from repeated minor trauma
Prolonged bed rest
Delayed following fractures

Median nerve (Anterior interosseous nerve)
Rarely damaged nerve lies very deep
Flexors of thumb and index finger are affected by damage to nerve

Median nerve (Carpal tunnel syndrome)
Nerve damaged by swelling or infiltration of tunnel it transverses. Transiently seen in pregnancy. Idiopathically in females using hands for washing or un-accustomed use. Complicates rheumatoid arthritis. Rarely seen in other systemic diseases

Ulnar nerve (Deep branch)
Trauma to heel of the hand. Idiopathically (often a ganglion found on exploration) No sensory loss in typical cases

Figure 84.1. Anatomical relationships of nerves to the upper extremity. (From Patten J: *Neurological Differential Diagnosis*. New York, Springer-Verlag, 1977.)

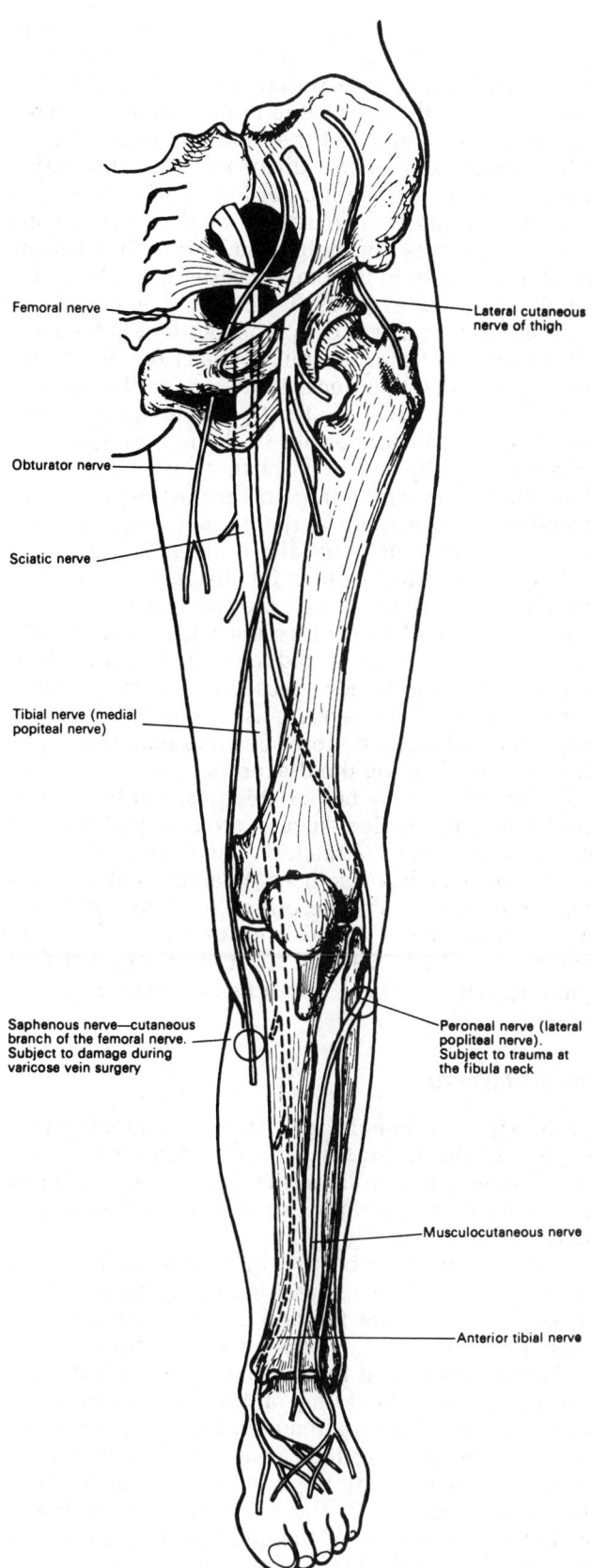

Figure 84.2. Anatomical relationships of nerves to the lower extremity. (From Patten J: *Neurological Differential Diagnosis*. New York, Springer-Verlag, 1977.)

splinting the elbow at night in an extended position may be helpful. An easy way to splint the elbow is to strap a pillow around it. Splinting should be continued for 2 to 3 months, especially if the symptoms are intermittent or show improvement. For ulnar compression at the wrist, whether due to a single traumatic event or to chronic trauma, conservative treatment with a splint is generally adequate. Surgical intervention is not necessary as long as symptoms do not progress and especially as long as there is no motor involvement or objective sensory loss. Surgical approaches to lesions of the ulnar nerve at the elbow depend on the etiology and the surgeon. These include simple release of the cubital tunnel, medial epicondylectomy, and anterior transplantation of the nerve. Complications from any of the surgical approaches include persistent or recurrent symptoms due to inadequate surgery or to recurrent scarring of the nerve.

Radial Nerve

Etiology. Radial nerve lesions are the least common of the major upper extremity nontraumatic compression neuropathies. Radial nerve entrapment or compression usually involves the radial nerve either at or proximal to the elbow (see Fig. 84.1).

Besides traumatic conditions such as humeral fractures, more proximal radial nerve injuries can occur when the arm has been held in a hyperabducted position that causes traction to the nerve. This may occur during surgery or sleep, and it may occur in patients who have been unconscious for a long time in abnormal positions ("Saturday night palsy"). Proximal nerve injury may also follow axillary pressure due to incorrect use of a crutch (central palsy).

Manifestations and Evaluation. Depending on the location of a high radial compression, the triceps function may or may not be affected. Elbow flexion and supination may be slightly weaker. The most obvious finding in a radial palsy is wrist drop and digital extensor paralysis.

The radial nerve is predominantly a motor nerve. High radial nerve lesions may produce sensory loss over the dorsum of the hand. Pain, tenderness, and a positive Tinel's sign (shock-like pain or tingling elicited by percussion of the nerve at the wrist) in the area of nerve damage may be present with radial nerve compression injuries. Nerve conduction studies (see above) can be helpful in localizing and quantifying radial nerve compression. For example, Saturday night palsy causes focal slowing of conduction at the site of pressure injury, but normal motor and sensory conduction below this lesion.

Treatment. The treatment of traumatic radial nerve compression is generally conservative. Cockup splint for the wrist joint should be accompanied by a spring-loaded extensor brace for the fingers if the weakness is long lasting. Individually constructed splints made by the occupational therapist are superior to those obtained from a surgical supply house. Treatment of compression of the posterior interosseus nerve (branch of radial nerve in the forearm) is surgical in most instances.

Peroneal Nerve

Etiology. The most common mechanism of damage to the peroneal nerve is compression at the head of the fibula (see Fig. 84.2), which may result from improperly applied plaster casts, tight stockings, bandages, and garters. Falling asleep with the side of the leg resting against a sharp or protruding object may occur in drug- or alcohol-induced stupor and even in the weakened bedridden patient. Occupations that require sitting, squatting, or kneeling may provoke peroneal compression. Entrapment may also occur in the fibular tunnel formed by the peroneus longus muscle.

Manifestations and Evaluation. Peroneal palsy produces foot drop due to weakness in the dorsiflexors of the foot, which may be accompanied by weakness of eversion. Symptoms usually consist of painless loss of motor power with partial sensory loss (over the lateral leg and dorsum of foot) when acute compressive lesions exist. Entrapment, however, does produce radiating pain with slowly progressive motor and sensory disturbances.

Nerve conduction studies can detect focal slowing across the fibular head as compared with the leg segment.

Treatment. Because the gait is quite unstable in the presence of foot drop, a rigid plastic splint worn in the shoe or a spring-loaded brace attached to the shoe is required. Compressive lesions of the peroneal nerve can be watched for several months before any consideration of a surgical approach is made. Entrapment presenting with pain and progressive motor and sensory loss is an indication for relatively early surgical exploration.

Tibial Nerve (Tarsal Tunnel Syndrome)

Etiology. The tarsal tunnel is located at the inferoposterior margin of the medial malleolus (see Fig. 84.2) and is formed by bones of the ankle and the flexor retinaculum (fibrous sheath from medial malleolus posteroinferior to the medial side of the calcaneus). In addition to the posterior tibial nerve the tunnel contains the posterior tibial artery and three long flexor tendons (8).

Enlarged tortuous veins within the tarsal tunnel, fracture or dislocation at the ankle, and nonspecific tenosynovitis may affect the other contents of the tarsal tunnel and lead to compression of the nerve trunk. Prolonged standing and walking often aggravate the pain, indicating that stasis or engorgement within the tunnel is likely to play some role. Also, sensory symptoms are made worse by the venous stasis and engorgement that occur at night during sleep. Except for a high prevalence in jockeys, no clear occupational factors have been identified.

Manifestations and Evaluation. The primary symptom of tarsal tunnel syndrome (TTS) is pain and dysesthesia in the sole of the foot. The burning pain

(description by patient may vary, e.g., walking on knives or pins, sole feels very thick) worsens with rest after a day of activity, and nocturnal pain is characteristic. Any or all of the three divisions (medial plantar, lateral plantar, and calcaneal) of the tibial nerve may be affected, resulting in sensory disturbance over the entire plantar surface or only one portion of it.

Specific points of the examination that help to confirm the diagnosis are the presence of a Tinel's sign, i.e., shooting pain to the plantar surface, produced by gentle percussion over the tarsal tunnel. Sensory loss, if present, is found over the plantar surface of the foot. It is easier to test sensory function over the tips of the toes (the sural and peroneal territories on the dorsum of the foot do not include the tips of the toes). Weakness in the intrinsic muscles of the foot may lead to a change in configuration of the foot and to instability of the phalanges, which impairs the pushing-off phase of walking. In contrast to carpal tunnel syndrome, tarsal tunnel syndrome is usually unilateral.

Nerve conduction studies for distal motor latency (see above) are done by stimulation proximal to the tarsal tunnel, and recordings are taken over the abductor pollicis brevis or abductor digiti quinti. Prolongation of motor latency or absence of motor potential may be recorded; however, sensory conduction studies appear to be much more sensitive than the motor studies in confirming the diagnosis.

Treatment. It may be possible to splint the foot or employ orthotic devices such as arch supports or heel wedges to reduce the stretch on the tibial nerve. Temporary response has also been obtained with corticosteroid injections. The definitive treatment of tarsal tunnel syndrome is surgical release of the flexor retinaculum, which can result in dramatic relief of symptoms if localized compression neuropathy is present.

Femoral Nerve

Etiology. The femoral nerve may be injured by stab wounds to the groin, hip, or pelvic fractures, by inguinal surgery (inguinal hernia, vascular repair, node resection), by angiography, or with retraction during pelvic surgery (see Fig. 84.2).

Stretch injuries can occur with prolonged lithotomy position or with hyperextention during gymnastics or dance. Pressure on the femoral nerve can be produced at the psoas muscle by hematoma or abscess.

Manifestations and Evaluation. The patient often complains about buckling of the knee (quadriceps weakness), and falls are frequent. The elderly may not recognize weakness as the cause of their falls. Pain in the groin radiating into the thigh may be severe. Sensory loss is present in the anteriomedial thigh and medial leg. Weakness of the quadriceps (knee extention) and loss of the knee reflex will be noted on examinations. Weakness of hip flexors indicates a more proximal lumbar plexus or root lesion. EMG tests help to differentiate these problems.

Femoral neuropathy is to be distinguished from diabetic lumbar plexopathy (diabetic amyotrophy). The latter disorder, seen in middle-aged mildly affected diabetics, begins abruptly with severe pain in the thigh and progresses over days to produce weakness, often most severe in the femoral nerve distribution. With EMG a wider distribution of involvement can be appreciated. Sensory signs are mild. The prognosis for recovery over 2 to 6 months is good (see Chapter 72, Diabetes Mellitus).

Treatment. Treatment depends on accurate diagnosis (e.g., discontinuation of anticoagulants when a psoas hematoma has been identified as the cause of the neuropathy). Physiotherapy may be required to maintain the mobility of the hip joint. The outcome and extent of rehabilitation measures will be determined by the etiology and extent of injury.

Saphenous Nerve

The saphenous nerve is one of three sensory branches of the femoral nerve (see Fig. 84.2). It is most often injured at Hunter's canal (10 cm proximal to the medial condyle of the femur). Vein stripping is a common cause. A small medial nerve branch can be injured by knee surgery. The patient has pain and numbness at the medial knee and leg. The pain may worsen with walking and climbing and be unaccompanied by sensory loss. Manual pressure over Hunter's canal produces pain that radiates. If the pain becomes chronic, local anesthetic can be injected to the area of injury.

Sciatic Nerve

Etiology. The sciatic nerve is often injured as a complication of trauma involving structures that the nerve traverses (see Fig. 84.2), including hip fractures, dislocations, and arthroplastic surgery. Compression of the nerve can occur in comatose or chronically bedridden patients, or after sitting on a hard edge. Hematoma, endometriosis, lipoma, and aneurysms of the gluteal artery are other causes of compression. Injections into the buttock are now less common causes of sciatic nerve injury. Benzylpenicillin and diazepam are particularly potent damaging agents. Injections usually cause immediate dysfunction with poor recovery.

Manifestations and Evaluation. Clinically, symptoms due to sciatic nerve compression may be confused with L5-S1 radiculopathy due to disc disease when the etiology is not readily apparent (see Chapter 65). The lateral trunk or peroneal division of the sciatic nerve is often affected more severely than the tibial division. Therefore, the distinction between a proximal sciatic injury and a more distal peroneal injury (e.g., after awakening from hip surgery) may be difficult. Careful strength testing of the short head of the biceps femoris (a lateral trunk, sciatic nerve innervated muscle) may help separate the two lesions; the patient lies on his back with hip flexed, then is asked to flex the leg at the knee against resistance. EMG studies may be particularly helpful in this clinical situation.

Lateral Femoral Cutaneous Nerve (Meralgia Paresthetica)

This nerve may be compressed or stretched at the anterior superior iliac spine at the lateral end of the inguinal canal (see lateral cutaneous nerve of the thigh, Fig. 84.2), causing burning pain, paresthesia, and decreased sensation over the lateral thigh. The sensory involvement is more lateral than that in femoral neuropathy, which causes sensory loss in the anterior-medial aspect of thigh, and there is *no motor involvement* or loss of patellar reflex. Point tenderness can usually be elicited at the passage of the nerve at the ipsilateral anterior iliac crest. Common causes include pelvic tilt, acute abdominal enlargement (ascites, pregnancy), external mechanical trauma (girdle, utility belt), and diabetes. The nerve compression may be relieved by weight loss or correction of the aggravating condition. Pain may respond to medical management (see below). If the pain is severe, local injection of an anesthetic may provide relief for long periods; sectioning of the ligament over the canal is only rarely needed. Paresthesias and pain usually disappear gradually, but an asymptomatic sensory loss in the lateral thigh may persist.

Bell's Palsy

Paralysis of the facial muscles due to inflammation and swelling of the 7th (the facial) cranial nerve (Bell's palsy) is seen occasionally in a general medical practice. One large series reported an incidence of 23 cases/100,000 population/year [10]. There is no predilection for a particular sex, age group, or race. In most patients, the cause of the condition is unknown. Two specific etiologies for 7th nerve neuropathy that have been recognized in recent years are Lyme disease [6, 9] Chapter 30) and HIV infection (Chapter 34). Although involvement of the facial nerve results in the predominant signs and symptoms of Bell's palsy, the process is actually a polyneuropathy that subclinically affects other cranial nerves as well. Usually patients will note the sudden onset, within hours, of a unilateral paralysis of a facial nerve: the eyebrow sags; The eye cannot be closed; the nasolabial fold disappears; and the mouth appears drawn to the unaffected side. Less commonly, there is loss of taste on the anterior two-thirds of the tongue, and there is hyperacusis (an accentuation of loud sounds) in the affected ear. There may be pain behind the ear. Most patients recover spontaneously within weeks to a few months; approximately 15% recover incompletely, but severe residual weakness is rare [10]. There is, in those who do not recover completely, a considerable risk of synkinesis, a contraction of all of the facial muscles on the affected side when the patient attempts to move just one or a few of them.

Corticosteroids appear to reduce the incidence of incomplete recovery [1, 22] of patients with Bell's palsy. When the palsy has been present less than four days, is moderately severe, and there is no strong contraindication to steroids (e.g., uncontrolled diabetes mellitus, hypertension, or active peptic ulcer disease), it is reasonable to begin a 10-day tapering course of prednisone beginning with 60 mg for three days and tapering by 10 mg each day thereafter. If pain behind the ear recurs during the tapering, the prednisone should be increased and a neurologist should be consulted. Some advocate early surgical decompression of the facial nerve in patients who demonstrate by EMG complete or nearly complete denervation, but most neurologists believe that the data do not support this radical approach.

THERAPEUTIC PRINCIPLES

General

Treatment of peripheral neuropathies first requires identifying and treating any underlying cause if possible. Efforts should be made also to prevent further damage; for example, patients with an underlying generalized polyneuropathy are more prone to pressure palsies, and it is important to educate them about habits that could be injurious (such as leaning on elbows or crossing legs). The daily administration of multivitamins is prudent in a patient whose nutrition may be poor.

For entrapment and compression neuropathies, eliminating pressure on the affected nerve is the primary mode of treatment, as discussed above. For deficits that are partial or recent in onset, recovery of function usually occurs within about 6 weeks after eliminating nerve entrapment or compression.

Symptomatic Treatment

Polyneuropathy is often irreversible and progressive. Symptomatic therapy and rehabilitative measures are, therefore, fundamental in helping these patients.

Motor

In most polyneuropathies, weakness usually affects dorsiflexion of the feet early (causing foot drop); ambulation can be greatly improved by a rigid plastic splint worn in the shoe or by a spring-loaded brace attached to the shoe obtained from a physical therapist. Fine motor weakness in the hands can be aided by special tools and other devices provided by occupational therapists.

Sensory

Anesthetic limbs are vulnerable to repeated, unrecognized trauma. The patient should always check the temperature of bath water, pot handles, etc. with parts of his body that have normal sensation. Small hard objects (keys, faucet handles) can be built up with soft materials. Occupational therapists can make useful suggestions in this regard. Meticulous care should be given to feet and toenails (see Chapter 102). Moisturizing cream for dry, insensitive skin

will reduce serious abrasions (see details, Chapter 100).

Pain associated with sensory neuropathies is usually chronic and difficult to treat. Simple analgesics (aspirin), whirlpool, and massage may help to relieve relatively mild pain. Narcotics should be avoided, because of the potential for addiction. Phenytoin (Dilantin), 300 to 500 mg/day to yield a serum level of 15 to 20 µg/ml, may provide relief of refractory pain and thus is worth a therapeutic trial. Details regarding the use of phenytoin are found in Chapter 80. If phenytoin has been maintained in the therapeutic range for 2 weeks and still proves unsuccessful, it should be discontinued and a trial of carbamazepine (Tegretol), 200 to 1000 mg/day in divided doses (two or three times a day), should be tried. This drug is started at 100 mg twice a day and is increased slowly (200 mg every 4 days in divided doses). Intolerance to carbamazepine (ataxia, drowsiness, and nausea) is especially likely in the older patient. Hematological values and liver function tests must be checked periodically (see details in Chapter 80). Tricyclic antidepressants (such as amitriptyline, 25 to 75 mg at bedtime) may also be tried (see details Chapter 15).

Autonomic

Autonomic dysfunctions should also be approached symptomatically (13). The *hypotonic bladder* may be treated by drugs that increase bladder tone (urecholine, 10 to 25 mg every 8 hours), by self-catheterization, or occasionally with surgery to decrease resistance to bladder emptying. Details regarding the evaluation and management of the hypotonic bladder are found in Chapter 6. *Sexual impotence* cannot be helped directly, although penile prostheses have been helpful for selected patients (see Chapter 18). The knowledge that sexual dysfunction has a neurological basis may relieve the anxiety that accompanies the problem. A check for medications that may be contributing to impotence is important (see Chapter 18). *Orthostatic hypotension* may be treated with salt supplementation and a volume-expanding mineralocorticoid (fludrocortisone, 0.1 to 0.2 mg daily) in patients without congestive heart failure or hypertension. Support stockings (e.g., Jobst) may be helpful to prevent venous pooling, but many patients do not tolerate these stockings well. Arising slowly from recumbent or sitting positions, maintaining active ambulation, and sleeping with the head of the bed on blocks (to stimulate renin release) are other measures that may help. Table 84.9 summarizes the practical ways to manage patients with this vexing problem.

OTHER PROBLEMS

Restless Legs Syndrome

This is a common syndrome, affecting perhaps 5% of the general population. It is an important cause of insomnia (see Chapter 85). Patients complain of an

Table 84.9.
Management of Patients with Orthostatic Hypotension Due to Autonomic Neuropathy

Avoid sudden changes in position
Avoid excessive intake of alcohol
Avoid diuresis
Correct hypovolemia
Discontinue or reduce the dosage of drugs known to cause orthostatic hypotension:
    Antihypertensive drugs
    Nitroglycerine
    Diuretics
    Neuroleptics
    Tricyclic antidepressants
    CNS depressants (opiates, alcohol)
    Levodopa
Prescribe mineralocorticoid (if no CHF or hypertension)
Supplement diet with salt
Tilt up the head of the bed (may stimulate renin release)
Use elastic support stockings

aching or painful crawling sensation "deep inside" the calf at rest, especially in the evening or in bed. Walking provides some relief over minutes but the dysesthesias often return quickly upon stopping (7, 20).

The exact pathophysiology has not been elucidated; both peripheral and central mechanisms have been proposed. The syndrome has been related in some patients to the peripheral neuropathies of diabetes and uremia. There has also been a relationship with iron and folate deficiency anemias, calcium and potassium deficiency, pregnancy, postgastric surgery state, excessive caffeine, sedative drug withdrawal, and exposure to neuroleptic medication. An idiopathic form is associated with periodic movements during sleep and a positive family history.

These patients should be evaluated for associated conditions for specific treatment. Simple analgesics (aspirin, acetaminophen) in the evening and at bedtime may often help early symptoms. In other patients nonsedating doses of clonazepam (Klonopin, 0.5 mg) or triazolam (Halcion, 0.125 mg) may relieve nocturnal symptoms. Tricyclic antidepressants have also been helpful.

Muscle Cramps

Cramps are localized involuntary painful contractions of skeletal muscles and produce a visible and palpable hard and bulging muscle. They must be distinguished from the sensation of cramp such as that described with intermittent claudication.

Ordinary muscle cramps are common and may be stopped by stretching the affected muscles. Cramps are associated with fatiguing exercises, salt depletion, dehydration, pregnancy, hypothyroidism, alcoholism, uremia, hypomagnesemia, myopathy, or denervation. Patients with frequent daytime cramps and no contributing factors should be referred to a neurologist for evaluation of the rare muscle enzymatic defects (e.g., phosphorylase, phosphofructokinase, or carnitine palmatyltransferase deficiency). If no associated condi-

tion exists, these patients may be given a therapeutic trial of phenytoin, carbamazepine, or amitriptyline (see above for dosages).

Nocturnal cramps occur in 15% of healthy young adults and are more common in the elderly. Two drugs have proved effective in a double-blind placebo trials: quinine sulfate, 200 mg at bedtime, and chloroquine phosphate, 250 mg a day (15, 16). Relief occurred in 1 to 3 weeks and often lasted several months after a several-week course of treatment ended. Even though cramps are more often associated with muscular dysfunction, nocturnal cramps (frequently in one leg) are a common presentation for entrapment of the tibial nerve (see above).

General References

Asbury A, Johnson P: *Pathology of Peripheral Nerves.* Philadelphia, WB Saunders, 1978. Dawson D, Hallett M, Millender L: *Entrapment Neuropathies.* Boston, Little, Brown, and Co, 1983. Dyck P, Thomas PK, Lambert EH, Bunge R (eds): *Peripheral Neuropathy,* 2nd ed. Philadelphia, WB Saunders, 1984.
    An excellent comprehensive review.
Harati Y: Diabetic peripheral neuropathies. *Ann Intern Med* 107:546, 1987.
    A thorough review of pathophysiological and clinical aspects.
Medical Research Council: *Aids to the Examination of the Peripheral Nervous System.* London, Her Majesty's Stationary Office, 1976.
    Well-illustrated guide to the physical examination for testing all peripheral nerves.
Schaumburg HH, Spencer PS, Thomas PK: *Disorders of Peripheral Nerves.* Philadelphia, FA Davis, 1983.
    A short work organized by disease processes that involve peripheral nerves.
Stewart JD: *Focal Peripheral Neuropathies.* New York, Elsevier, 1987.

Specific References

1. Adour KK, Wingerd J, Bell DN, et al: Prednisone treatment for idiopathic facial paralysis (Bell's palsy). *N Engl J Med* 287:1268, 1972.
2. Asbury AK, Arnason BG, Karp HR, McFarlin DE: Criteria for diagnosis of Guillian-Barré syndrome. *Ann Neurol* 3:565, 1978.
3. Behse F, Buchthal F: Alcoholic neuropathy: clinical, electrophysiological and biopsy findings. *Ann Neurol* 2:95, 1977.
4. Cornblatch D: Treatment of the neuromuscular complications of human immunodeficiency virus infection. *Ann Neurol* 2:S88, 1988.
5. Ewing DJ, Clarke BF: Diabetic autonomic neuropathy: present insights and future prospects. *Diabetic Care* 9:648, 1986.
6. Finkel M: Lyme Disease and its neurologic complications. *Arch Neurol* 45:99, 1988.
7. Gibb WRG, Lees AJ: The restless leg syndrome. *Postgraduate Med J* 62:329, 1986.
8. Goodgold J, Kopell HP, Spielholz NI: The tarsal tunnel syndrome. *N Engl J Med* 273:742, 1965.
9. Halperin JJ, Little BW, et al: Lyme Disease: cause of treatable peripheral neuropathy. *Neurology* 37:1, 700, 1987.
10. Hauser WA, Karnes WE, Annis J, Kurland LT: Incidence and prognosis of Bell's palsy in the population of Rochester, Minnesota. *Mayo Clin Proc* 46:258, 1971.
11. Horwich MS, Cho L, Porro RS, Posner JB: Subacute sensory neuropathy: a remote effect of cancer. *Ann Neurol* 2:7, 1977.
12. Kelly JJ: Peripheral neuropathies associated with monoclonal proteins: a clinical review. *Muscle and Nerve* 8:138, 1985.
13. McCleod JG, Tuck RR: Disorders of the autonomic nervous system II, investigation and treatment. *Ann Neurol* 21:519, 1987.
14. Meier C: Polyneuropathy in paraproteinaemia. *J Neurol* 232:204, 1985.
15. Moss HK, Herrman LG: Night cramps in human extremities. A

clinical study of the physiologic action of quinine and prostigmine upon the spontaneous contractions of resting muscles. *Am Heart J* 35:403, 1948.

16. Parrow A, Samuelsson SM: Use of choloroquine phosphate. A new treatment for spontaneous leg cramps. *Acta Med Scand* 181:237, 1967.

17. Pestronk A, Cornblath DR, et al: A treatable multifocal motor neuropathy with antibodies to GM 1 Ganglioside. *Ann Neurol* 24:73, 1988.

18. Schaumberg H, Kaplan J, Windebank A, et al: Sensory neuropathy from pyridoxine abuse new megavitamin syndrome. *N Engl J Med* 309:445, 1983.

19. Vinik A, Mitchell B: Clinical aspects of diabetic neuropathies. *Diabetes/Metabolism Reviews* 4:223, 1988.

20. Walters A, Hening W: Clinical presentation and neuropharmacology of restless legs syndrome. *Clin Pharmacol* 10:225, 1987.

21. Wilkinson M, Croft PB, Urich H: The remote effects of cancer on the nervous system. *Proc R Soc Med* 60:683, 1967.

22. Wolf SM, Wagner JH, Davidson S, Forsythe A: Treatment of Bell's palsy with prednisone: a prospective, randomized study. *Neurology* 28:158, 1978.

C H A P T E R 85

Sleep Disorders

RICHARD P. ALLEN, Ph.D.
PHILIP L. SMITH, M.D.
DAVID NEUBAUER, M.D.

EPIDEMIOLOGY

In a given year approximately one in three adults in some communities has a problem with sleep (19). Of these about one in five actually reports the problem to a physician. Moreover, 4% of adults report that they often use prescription medications for their sleep problems, and about 1% report habitual use of sleep medication on consecutive nights for two months or more (11, 18). Surveys also indicate that 4 to 8% of working adults complain of problems with excessive sleepiness that disrupt their normal daytime functioning (12); these problems of excessive sleepiness have been associated with the occurrence of industrial and automobile accidents.

The prevalence of serious sleep disturbances, and the association of these with mental illness, in adults was measured in a survey of several American communities from 1981 to 1985 (5). Overall 10% reported insomnia and 3% reported hypersomnia lasting at least two weeks. There were striking associations between sleep disturbances and mental illness: 40% of those reporting insomnia and 45% of those reporting hypersomnia had a psychiatric disorder; and the risk of developing new major depression was very high for those reporting insomnia at both the initial and the one-year follow-up interviews.

CLASSIFICATION OF SLEEP DISORDERS

The sleep-related problems described by patients should be regarded as symptoms rather than diagnoses per se. In recent years, a classification of sleep disorders has been developed to facilitate appropriate diagnosis and management of the sleep problems that patients describe (2). The four major categories in this classification are: (a) disorders of initiating and maintaining sleep—DIMS (the insomnias), (b) disorders of excessive somnolence—DOES (the hypersomnias), (c) disorders of the sleep-wake cycle, and (d) parasomnias (sleepwalking, sleep terrors, enuresis, etc.). A number of discrete entities have been identified within each of these categories.

PHYSIOLOGICAL PATTERNS OF NORMAL SLEEP

The fundamental sleep-wake cycle is maintained by at least two physiologically and neurologically distinct control mechanisms:

1. *Homeostatic mechanism* : establishes a balance between wake and sleep time over a period of 1 or 2 days (sleep-wake cycles). This balance varies greatly with species but for adult humans is set at about 30 to 40% sleep (7 to 9 hours/day). This balance works within a time frame of several days and accounts for sleepiness for a few days after significant sleep deprivation.
2. *Circadian oscillator* : establishes a sleep tendency variation over the normal 24-hour day. This oscillator also modulates core temperature and the activity levels of a large number of neurological hormonal functions (e.g., serotonin and cortisol levels). Without time cues, this circadian mechanism has a 25-hour cycle, and it therefore needs to be reset daily by 1 hour. Bright light and perhaps activity help to reset this clock.

These mechanisms each promote sleepiness or alertness and are usually in stable harmony (e.g., circadian oscillators and homeostatic mechanisms both increase sleepiness at the end of the day).

The normal sleep cycle is characterized by two physiologically different states: rapid eye movement (REM) sleep and nonrapid eye movement (NREM) sleep. Initially, sleep consists of the four successively "deeper" stages of NREM sleep. During each of these four stages, there is generally much less fluctuation in heart rate, blood pressure, and respiratory rate than that which occurs during REM sleep. The presleep wake stage and each sleep stage have additional distinctive clinical and electroencephalographic (EEG) characteristics.

Presleep wake (sleep latency period). As the patient begins to fall asleep, eye blinks, limb movements, and moderate tone in skeletal muscles are accompanied by either low voltage, mixed frequency EEG, or the characteristic alpha pattern (basic posterior rhythm).

Stage 1. This represents light sleep with slow rolling eye movements (pursuit eye movements). The alpha pattern disappears with lower frequency and usually higher voltage than the wake EEG. Sudden limb jerks may occur episodically, particularly during early stage 1 sleep.

Stage 2. Eye movements become infrequent or absent and muscle tone is usually reduced. The EEG shows characteristic occasional sleep spindle bursts, vertex sharp waves, K complexes, and some slow waveforms.

Stages 3 and 4. Slow wave sleep muscle tone is variable. EEG high voltage, slow wave activity predominates. Arousal is difficult from these deeper sleep stages.

At 1 to 2 hours after sleep onset, the first period of REM sleep occurs with a characteristic marked decrease in muscle tone and bursts of rapid eye movements. During REM sleep there is a paralysis of major skeletal muscles punctuated by occasional episodes of muscle twitches; hypercapneic and hypoxic respiratory drive are decreased; core body temperature fluctuates with ambient temperature; heart rate and blood pressure are extremely variable; and penile erections occur. Dreaming is also most closely related to REM sleep but may occur, usually less vividly, at other times.

On a typical night, a subject passes through three to five cycles of NREM and REM sleep. Typical sleep patterns for young healthy adults and for healthy elderly adults are shown in Figure 85.1. With aging there is a general decrease in slow wave sleep (stages 3 and 4), a shortening of the total sleep time, and more frequent awakenings during the night. The frequent awakenings and apparently decreased arousal threshold are the most prominent differences between sleep at age 50 and that at age 80. During the day, young adults require 10 to 15 minutes to fall asleep for a nap; older adults fall asleep more easily. As discussed later in this chapter, the recognition and deviations from the normal sleep cycles are helpful at times in establishing the correct diagnosis for a sleep disorder.

GENERAL OFFICE APPROACH TO DIAGNOSIS AND MANAGEMENT OF SLEEP DISORDERS

Although patients with significant sleep disorders or relatives of such patients will usually report the problem to the physician, it is important to inquire at least briefly about sleep in taking the medical history of any patient. Four questions will detect the presence of most significant sleep disorders:

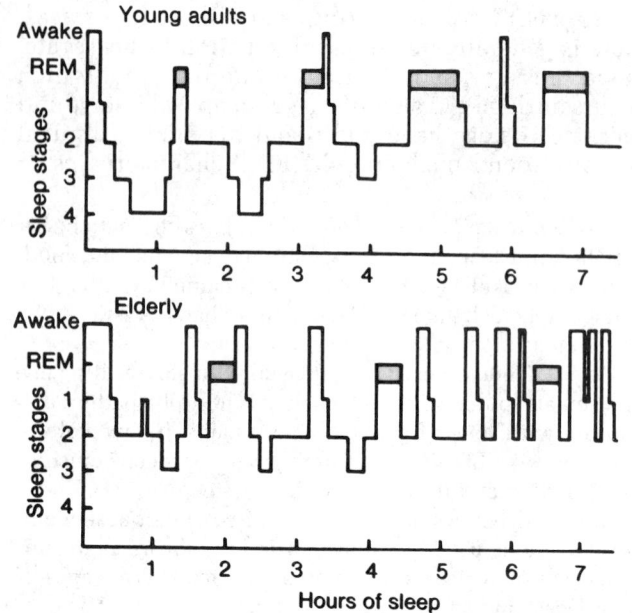

Figure 85.1. Normal sleep cycles in healthy young and elderly subjects. *Darkened area* indicates REM sleep. (Adapted from Kales A, Kales JD: Sleep disorders: recent findings in the diagnosis and treatment of disturbed sleep. *N Engl J Med* 290:487, 1974.)

1. Do you have trouble sleeping—either falling asleep, staying asleep, or getting enough sleep? (Positive response suggests a DIMS.)

2. Do you or others notice that you are disturbed by excessive sleepiness when engaged in your usual daytime activities? Do you tend to fall asleep in the day when you are sitting still or inactive? (Positive responses in a patient reporting no difficulty initiating or maintaining sleep suggests a DOES.)

3. Do you or your bed partner notice that you have any problem with unusual movement at night? (Positive response suggests a sleep disorder, especially if there is daytime sleepiness, insomnia, or parasomnia.)

4. Do you snore or note any abnormalities in breathing? (Positive response raises the possibility of a sleep-associated respiratory impairment and further questions should be asked, especially about excessive daytime sleepiness.)

It is very important at the outset to distinguish genuine sleepiness from other problems perceived by the patient as "sleepiness." Sleepiness by definition involves the need to fall asleep, and the patient usually reports some relief of the symptom after sleeping. Sleepiness is reported most often in situations with little activity; e.g., watching TV, riding in the car, reading, or studying. Muscle weakness, loss of interest in usual activities, exertional dyspnea, postural dizziness, and other symptoms may be referred to as sleepiness, tiredness, or fatigue. By having the patient describe concrete circumstances in which the symptom occurs, these problems can usually be distinguished from true sleepiness.

A number of strategies are helpful in assuring effective sleep for most people. These are summarized in Table 85.1. Counseling about the value of such strategies is often helpful for patients with a history of insomnia and poor sleep habits. In general, patients with excessive waketime sleepiness should be cautioned against driving a car, operating heavy machinery, and working in high places or other activities, where decreased attention or sleepiness could be dangerous.

The following sections describe the major sleep disorders by major presenting complaint—insomnia, excessive sleepiness, abnormal, sleep schedule, and abnormal behaviors in sleep.

DISORDERS OF INITIATING AND MAINTAINING SLEEP (DIMS)

An adequate evaluation of insomnia requires an inquiry to delineate the characteristics and duration of the sleep disturbance and to detect psychological, medical, pharmacological (including substance abuse), and environmental influences on the patient's sleep.

Transient Psychophysiological Insomnia

This is the most common sleep disorder in our society, even though the majority of affected persons do not seek medical help. By definition, transient psychophysiological insomnia lasts less than 3 weeks and,

Table 85.1.
Strategies That May Be Useful for Patients with Sleep Disorders

1. Sleep in the same room consistently, preferably not a room utilized for most wake time activities.
2. Develop a regular bedtime, with lights out or dimmed and a regular waking time, and avoid sleeping longer than usual except occasionally.
3. Adjust total sleep time to fit your needs—may be as little as 4 hours or as much as 10 hours.
4. Avoid routine daytime naps.
5. Plan regular daily exercise, preferably in the evenings and preferably exercising leg and arm muscles, no exercise for 30 minutes before bed.
6. Sleep in a cool room, avoiding temperature extremes.
7. Avoid heavy meals within 2 hours of bedtime; however, a light snack such as cheese and crackers at bedtime may be soporific.
8. Take no more than one alcoholic drink (equivalent of 2 ounces, 90 proof) after dinner; do not use alcohol to help you sleep, and do not drink alcohol within 3–4 hours of bed time.
9. Avoid stimulants, particularly within 8 hours of bedtime (e.g., no coffee, cola drinks, tea, cocoa, chocolates, etc.)
10. For poor sleep onset, do not stay awake in bed for more than 20 minutes. Instead, get out of bed, read, or engage in another productive activity. Try sleep again when you feel sleepy; if still unable to sleep, repeat this cycle.
11. For troublesome recurrent thoughts disturbing sleep onset, write them down with a possible plan of action. Try to start thinking about simpler, less troubling matters.
12. Accept an occasional night with sleeplessness; it is a normal healthy bodily adjustment to various conditions and provides extra time for hobbies, work, etc.
13. Use sleep medications only rarely and never for more than 4 days out of a week or for more than 2 consecutive weeks without consulting your doctor.
14. Unless you are unable to stay awake, do not alter your daily activities because you feel tired. You may think you are less alert than others do.

characteristically, has an abrupt onset related to an identifiable precipitating stressor (usually a domestic or occupational problem). These patients usually recover spontaneously, either because the stress subsides or the patient adapts to it. Prophylactic treatment may be useful when patients appear vulnerable to recurrence. Therapy includes short-term counseling (see Chapter 11), sleep hygiene advice (Table 85.1), and judicious use of hypnotic-sedative medications (see below). When frequent recurrent episodes of transient insomnia occur, a sleep cycle disturbance should be considered (see below). Personality or depressive disorders may also be present (see Chapters 14 and 15).

Another common cause of transient insomnia is periodic or permanent reduction or discontinuation of addictive substances, such as tobacco, alcohol, antianxiety drugs, or even sleeping medications. In mild cases, only transient insomnia occurs, but in more severe cases insomnia may become persistent and difficult to treat. These problems are discussed in Chapters 20–22.

Persistent Insomnia

By definition, patients with insomnia lasting more than 3 weeks have persistent insomnia. This problem may be seen in a number of situations, and more than one factor can contribute to the insomnia. The complaint of waketime fatigue and misery often seems excessive for the amount of sleep loss reported. After an interval of sleep loss, the patient may have mild improvement in sleep that is generally not sufficient to permit full recovery from the chronic sleep loss (1). These patients are usually evaluated after they have shown this mild improvement in their night sleep without improvement in waketime functioning.

Psychological and Psychiatric Disorders

These constitute the most common reasons for persistent insomnia. The sleep-related symptoms usually decrease as the primary disturbance improves.

Many patients with chronic difficulty initiating and/ or maintaining sleep have persistent psychophysiological insomnia. In presenting their history these individuals often recall a particular stress that occurred when the insomnia began, however, they note that the inability to sleep continued after the stress resolved.

These patients feel fatigued during the day but usually manage to function appropriately. They are tired in the evening when preparing for bed but then either remain in bed awake for several hours before falling asleep or they fall asleep quickly, only to awaken after just a few hours of sleep. In both cases there is considerable subjective distress about the continued problem. The harder they try to fall asleep, the more difficult it becomes. This process can be understood in psychological terms both because of the mental content of frustration and worry, and also because of the conditioned aspect of the sleeplessness. The nightly frustration and arousal are repeatedly associated with the nightly experience of going to bed. Whenever these individuals are sleepless in bed, they are reinforcing the association and increasing the probability of it occurring again.

Behavioral management is the most effective approach to this type of chronic insomnia; the use of hypnotic medications is not advisable because they do not alter the fundamental problem and use may lead to dependence. In addition to ensuring basic sleep hygiene (Table 85.1), two behavioral approaches may be recommended. In one approach, there is an attempt to separate the ongoing association of frustrated sleeplessness and the experience of going to bed. Patients are given a plan to follow, which includes getting out of bed and engaging in other activities (such as reading, watching television, doing household chores) until they are tired, then trying going to sleep again in bed. This may have to be repeated several times per night. Initially there may be a decrease in the total amount of sleep, however, in the long run this plan is often very helpful. A second behavioral approach attempts to consolidate sleep by restricting the amount of time the individual is permitted to be in bed. When the patient is able to sleep efficiently during the restricted period, the sleep time is progressively lengthened. The wake-up time is always kept constant, in order to reinforce the underlying circadian rhythm. With improved sleep the patient is allowed to go to bed at a slightly earlier time.

Affective disorders (see Chapter 15) often present initially with insomnia. Patients with unipolar depressions have less difficulty with sleep onset than with repeated awakenings and difficulty returning to sleep after awakening; depressed patients with bipolar disorder may commonly have episodic hypersomnia with complaints of awakening tired. In manic states, there is a profound inability to fall asleep, but even brief periods of sleep seem to restore wakefulness completely. Depression secondary to other medical or psychiatric conditions may also present with daytime sleepiness associated with premature arousals and sleep onset problems. A formal sleep study may occasionally be helpful in establishing the diagnosis of depression (6). Management of persistent insomnia includes appropriate treatment of the affective disorder as well as improvement in sleep habits (Table 85.1) and possible sleep cycle adjustment.

Patients with personality or anxiety disorders (see Chapters 13 and 14), particularly those with obsessive thoughts or phobias, frequently have insomnia associated with excessive ruminating thoughts at sleep onset. These patients may require psychotherapy. Hypnotics should be avoided because of their abuse potential, limited effectiveness in these patients, and possible masking of the the primary etiology. On the other hand, judicious use of 25 to 50 mg of amitriptyline (Elavil) may be effective (see below).

Chronic Sedative-Hypnotic Use

Protracted use of sedative-hypnotic medication paradoxically may cause poor sleep onset with repeated premature awakenings (10). This condition develops in patients with both transient and persistent insomnia who continue to use medication. The diagnosis is based on a history of prolonged sedative-hypnotic use with concomitant worsening insomnia. Treatment is usually difficult since drug withdrawal is mandatory in spite of the attendant transient worsening of symptoms. When withdrawal from medication is attempted, the patient must be told his sleep disorder will temporarily worsen and that overall improvement may not occur for several weeks, and in some cases months, after the drug has been stopped. The patient should be reassured that if his problem continues thereafter (i.e., it is not due solely to sedative abuse), the appropriate diagnosis and treatment can be accomplished after withdrawal. It is generally advised that the medication be stabilized for a fixed dosage and then gradually reduced, by one therapeutic dose per week. During withdrawal, frequent support and reassurance can be provided by brief contacts with the physician, either at weekly office visits or by telephone calls. More focused psychotherapy (Chapter 11) may be necessary in more difficult cases.

Sleep Apnea and Sleep-Induced Respiratory Impairment

This disturbance of respiration during sleep usually presents with hypersomnia and is discussed under DOES (page 1175). However, some patients with persistent insomnia, especially those with short sleep onset but frequent awakenings, may have this condition. As noted below, this condition will be exacerbated if treated with hypnotics, sometimes with serious complications (7).

Medical Conditions

Patients with most symptomatic medical conditions may describe persistent insomnia associated with their underlying condition, but only occasionally is insomnia a major presenting symptom (20). The sleep disturbance, although related to the pathophysiology of the disease in some conditions, may also be due to nonspecific psychological or physical distress in most situations. For example, patients with recurrent paroxysmal nocturnal dyspnea associated with either underlying congestive heart failure or obstructive pulmonary disease will note characteristic difficulties with recurrent arousals secondary to manifest shortness of breath. Similarly, patients who experience worsening daytime asthma will often note repeated awakenings at night and the need for bronchodilators before sleep can again be initiated. Chronic pain and arthritis are frequently associated with complaints of poor sleep. Insomnia in this clinical setting generally improves or worsens with the course of the associated medical condition. Sedative-hypnotic drugs (see below) are most helpful for patients whose insomnia is due to stress associated with their illness.

Periodic Leg Movements (Sleep-Related Myoclonus)

Periodic leg movements (also known as sleep-related myoclonus) are characterized by rhythmic, stereotyped leg movements or arm jerks occurring every 20 to 40 seconds for much of the sleeping time. Unlike other movement disorders, periodic leg movements begin after sleep onset, may appear in clusters for 15 to 30 minutes, or in severe cases persist throughout sleep. The movements typically involve flexion at the ankle and knee (occasionally also at the hip) with extension of the big toe. Arm movements are less common. The etiology, prevalence, and course of this condition are not well known. Prevalence is age related, occurring rarely before age 40 and most frequently after age 65. Once established, these movements persist with only rare spontaneous remission. This diagnosis should be suspected if the patient reports repeated nocturnal awakenings and very active sleep, or if a bed partner reports that the patient moves excessively in sleep, kicking his legs frequently. This condition may be exacerbated or even precipitated by renal failure or by the use of tricyclic antidepressants. For this reason, antidepressants should be avoided in the treatment of insomnia characterized by restless sleep.

Differential diagnosis includes normal twitches associated with REM sleep, sleep onset leg kicks, which cease after sleep is well established, and epileptic seizure activity during sleep. Diagnosis of periodic leg movement requires a nocturnal sleep study (13).

Treatment should be planned in consultation with a sleep disorders specialist. It usually involves moderate doses of short-acting benzodiazepines that suppress the associated arousal from sleep but do not reduce the frequency of leg movements. Low dose narcotic analgesics (propoxyphene or codeine) have proven effective for reducing both the number of leg movements and the number of arousals. These should generally be reserved for more severe cases because of the abuse potential for these medications. Clonazepam (Klonopin), oxazepam (Serax), or baclofen (Lioresal) before bed may also be effective, and tolerance is not a major problem.

"Restless legs" (see also Chapter 84) is a waketime disorder; almost all patients also have periodic leg movements during sleep (although most patients with periodic leg movements do not have daytime restless legs). The patient with restless legs reports deep, unpleasant leg muscle sensations that are resolved by moving the legs. Inactivity and tiredness exacerbate the problem. This condition often occurs in multiple members of the same family, and it generally becomes progressively worse with age. Treatment of the sleep-associated periodic leg movements is important in order to decrease waketime tiredness, but morning or waketime drowsiness may occur due to the medication used to treat the excessive movements. A small dose of Sinemet (carbidopa-L-Dopa, 25/100), taken before bed, may reduce the restlessness associated with severe cases of combined periodic leg movements in sleep and restless legs while trying to go to sleep. Despite promising results, the use of Sinemet in this condition is limited by the relatively short duration of the drug's action.

Sleep Disorders That Mimic DIMS

Disorders of excessive somnolence or DOES (see details below) may present commonly with disturbed nocturnal sleep and are occasionally misdiagnosed as DIMS. This problem is exacerbated by the patient's tendency to minimize waketime sleepiness and to emphasize disturbances of nighttime sleep. When there is a history of napping, particularly with an irresistible need to nap, DOES must be considered as the primary diagnosis.

Sleep-wake schedule disturbance (see details below) can also be confused with DIMS. Again, it is crucial that waketime functioning be carefully assessed. In patients who report marked drowsiness and impaired functioning in a particular part of the day associated with a delay in sleep onset or a premature awakening, a sleep-wake schedule disturbance should be considered.

Natural short sleepers, who are more commonly adult males, may also present with DIMS symptoms. Again, the significant information relates to waketime functioning. The amount of sleep needed by any person varies considerably; there are recorded examples of patients who sleep very little and appear to function without difficulty (9). A short sleeper awakens refreshed with little difficulty functioning during the day. Generally, sleep onset time is minimal and there are few awakenings during the night. Furthermore, the short total sleep time remains constant over weekends and holidays and will have been stable since late adolescence. The patient usually seeks consultation either because others have convinced him that his sleep is abnormal and might cause medical problems or because he has trouble using his waketime when others are asleep. Because his sleep restores wakefulness, he can be reassured that he has no sleep problem and can be advised to use his extra waketime constructively.

DISORDERS OF EXCESSIVE SOMNOLENCE (DOES)

Diagnostic Evaluation

Although insomnia complaints are more common, excessive daytime sleepiness usually has a more profound effect on the patient's life style and physical condition. A wide range of causal factors must be considered in evaluating this complaint. When a treatable cause such as substance abuse or medication side effects cannot be confirmed, sleep laboratory evaluation is generally indicated. This evaluation is needed to diagnose primary sleep disorders such as sleep apnea and narcolepsy (see below, "Sleep Center Evaluation").

Symptoms of hypersomnia, unlike symptoms of insomnia, are often difficult to elicit with certainty from the patient. Once reported, either by the patient or a reliable observer, the symptoms deserve attention for they may indicate the presence of life-threatening sleep apnea. The symptoms may range from tiredness throughout the day to a frank inability to stay awake during normal activities. Impairment in school or work performance and interference in valued social activities are common problems that will be uncovered in the evaluation of the patient. In severe cases, there may be a history of accidents that can be attributed to the excessive sleepiness. waketime activities that are associated with sleepiness in normal individuals result in marked sleepiness in patients with these disorders. These activities include watching television, riding in or driving a car, reading, sitting in a conference, waiting to be seen at a physician's office, and relaxing soon after a large meal.

Transient Hypersomnia

Excessive daytime somnolence lasting less than 3 weeks is usually due to a psychological response to stress. Onset is abrupt, symptoms consist of persistent fatigue and loss of energy, and behavior is characterized by long periods of time in bed, as a result of an identifiable precipitating event. In contrast to other patients with DOES, these patients spend excessive time in bed and generally do not express significant drive or effort to leave the bed. The condition should improve simultaneously with improvement in the psychological problem; however, if the patient's complaints persist, an alternate diagnosis should be considered. In particular, drug abusers may present with DOES symptoms in an effort to obtain stimulant medication; therefore, physicians must use judgment in treating patients complaining of hypersomnolence who are not well known to them.

Persistent Hypersomnia

By definition, persistent hypersomnia is present when symptoms last longer than 3 weeks. There may be a gradual increase in daytime sleepiness over months to years reflecting some developing disorder. Alternatively the hypersomnia may have been present since adolescence reflecting a more stable disorder.

Sleep Apnea and Sleep-Induced Respiratory Impairments

Definitions. These are by far the most serious disorders associated with sleep. They are characterized by breathing abnormalities that vary from reduction to complete cessation of airflow (hypopnea and apnea, respectively). The sleep apneas can be distinguished as central apnea (cessation of respiratory effort and, thus, no airflow) and obstructive apnea (occlusion of upper airway with continued respiratory effort). Isolated central apneas are usually associated with coexisting symptoms of insomnia, whereas obstructive apneas present typically with symptoms of excessive waketime somnolence. Importantly, all types of sleep-related apnea can be associated with hypoxemia and sleep fragmentation that lead to the systemic cardiovascular alterations and cognitive dysfunction noted in these individuals.

Epidemiology. The prevalence of sleep apnea is not well established; although it is suspected that as many as 1 to 2 million obese American men may have some degree of obstructive apnea. Recently, more young children and adolescents are being diagnosed with obstructive sleep apnea. The typical patient with obstructive sleep apnea is a middle-aged, mild to moderately obese man (male to female ratio of 20:1). Infrequently, this disorder is associated with specific abnormalities of the upper airway or of metabolic dysfunction (Table 85.2). By contrast, central sleep apnea occurs most commonly in either infants or normal individuals over 65. Frequently, central apnea may occur as a result of major cerebral disease, brainstem spinal disorder, or cardiovascular problem (Table 85.2).

Presentation. Characteristically, patients with obstructive apnea present with significant snoring or daytime hypersomnolence. The snoring is loud, intermittent, and often punctuated by respiratory efforts unaccompanied by obvious airflow. Arousals and twitching terminate the apneas, which cause demonstrable sleep fragmentation and subsequent daytime hypersomnolence. This sleepiness may range from subtle decreases in alertness toward the end of the day to the precipitous onset of sleep in the middle of a conversation. Because most patients are unaware of their breathing pattern and often underestimate the severity of daytime somnolence, a bed partner or other observer may provide useful information. Other clinical manifestations include choking or gasping episodes at night, systemic and pulmonary hypertension, and, in severe cases, cor pulmonale. By contrast, patients with central apnea will usually be observed to cease breathing with no associated respiratory efforts. In adults, there may be associated snoring, gasping for air, and arousal from sleep since often the central apnea occurs in combination with obstructive events; thus, it is often not possible clinically to distinguish the two forms of apnea.

The physical examination is usually not diagnostic in patients with obstructive apnea, although patients with narrowing of the upper airway are at significantly higher risk. In particular, children and adults who demonstrate a compatible history and marked tonsillar hypertrophy or retrognathia should be suspected of having this disorder. In elderly individuals with central apnea, the physical examination is normal, whereas patients with neurological or cardiovascular pathology will usually demonstrate obvious localizing neurologic signs (e.g., stroke) or cardiomegaly.

Course. The course of obstructive sleep apnea appears to be chronic, although not necessarily progressive if body weight remains stable. Some patients clearly develop progressive cardiopulmonary decompensation manifested by worsening hypercarbia and hypoxemia, which can be associated with cor pulmonale and life-threatening arrhythmias. Nevertheless, these complications are the exception and tend to occur in the more severely obese individuals after many years of disease. By contrast, the course of central apnea is determined by the underlying pathological process. Thus, if reversible central nervous system or cardiovascular disease exists, central apnea may resolve entirely. In normal elderly individuals with central apnea, the course and prognosis are unknown.

Diagnosis. A working diagnosis of sleep apnea can be made by direct observation of the patient during sleep, either at home or in a general hospital. However, even with ideal observation, clinically significant apnea may not be appreciated (8). Definitive diagnosis requires a sleep study (see below) that monitors the various parameters previously outlined. Other laboratory studies such as arterial blood gases and routine pulmonary function provide information about mechanical or gas exchange abnormalities useful in therapy but not diagnosis. Flow volume curves may demonstrate fluttering during expiration associated with evidence of variable extrathoracic obstruction in patients with obstructive apnea. This is a specific but not sensitive test; therefore, it is not recommended to screen patients. Although computerized tomography of the upper airway demonstrates narrowing of the upper airway in patients with obstructive sleep apnea, it is unclear at present how this information can be best utilized in the management of these patients.

Management. The treatment of obstructive sleep apnea continues to evolve. Management options for an individual patient will be recommended by the consultant who has evaluated the patient with a formal sleep study. Table 85.3 summarizes a number of the approaches that may be recommended. Initial man-

Table 85.2.
Disorders Associated with Sleep Apnea

OBSTRUCTIVE SLEEP APNEA
Narrowing of upper airway
Nasal abnormalities (deviation, polyps)
Oral abnormalities (tonsillar hypertrophy, acromegaly)
Bony abnormalities
Muscular abnormalities
Shy-Drager
Myotonic dystrophy
Hypothyroidism
CENTRAL SLEEP APNEA
Cerebral disorders (stroke)
Brainstem-spinal disorder (polio, infarction, neoplasia, surgery)
Cardiovascular disorders (increased circulation time)

Table 85.3.
Approaches to Management of Obstructive Sleep Apnea

GENERAL
Avoid CNS depressants
Weight loss
UPPER AIRWAY MEASURES
Constant positive airway pressure (CPAP)
Tracheostomy
Palatopharyngoplasty
MEDICATIONS
Medroxyprogesterone
Protriptyline
Oxygen

agement should emphasize correcting associated *medical conditions* such as hypothyroidism (14) or *anatomical factors* such as severe tonsillar hypertrophy, control of weight, and the avoidance of central nervous system (CNS) depressants. Although the mechanism is not known, it is clear that as little as 10% weight loss may markedly improve the severity of the apneas (17). Because most patients are 30 to 40% above ideal body weight, the minimal amount of weight reduction expected does not represent an unrealistic goal (see practical approaches in Chapter 76, Obesity).

Constant positive airway pressure (CPAP) has become the mainstay of therapy of patients with moderate to severe disease. The patient is fitted with a cup-like mask that entrains forced air, usually from a stationary unit in the bedroom, into the nasal airway. The pressure from the continuous airflow prevents upper airway collapse during sleep. Careful adjustment of pressure is important since patient compliance is dependent on elimination of the apneas at the lowest possible nasal pressure. Patients will note a pressure sensation in the upper airway and the ears when first using the mask. Drying of the mucosal membranes can be reduced by adding moisture to the forced air, and nasal congestion is improved by the addition of decongestants.

Selection of *surgical measures* to alter upper airway anatomy requires consultation with an otolaryngologist. Although tracheotomy was once employed regularly in the treatment of this syndrome, it is infrequently performed now because of the newer forms of medical therapy and the associated psychosocial adjustments and physical discomfort. Palatopharyngoplasty should be considered after medical therapy has been tried.

Medications such as medroxyprogesterone and protriptyline have been used to treat obstructive sleep apnea, but it is still unclear which patients will respond to pharmacological therapy (16). In general, protriptyline has been shown more consistently to reduce the snoring and severity of sleep apnea, while improving daytime hypersomnolence in people with mild to moderately severe obstructed apnea. The initial dosage is 5 to 10 mg given at bedtime or early in the morning if sleep onset is delayed as a result of the medication. In general, 30% of patients experience side effects that include dry mouth, difficulty initiating micturition in older men, and constipation. Because protriptyline is a mild appetite suppressant, it may facilitate weight reduction.

Presently, it is unclear which patients respond best to oxygen therapy; however, individuals with significant cor pulmonale appear to benefit the most. Patients usually will have evidence of hypoxemia both when awake and asleep; therefore, continuous 24-hour oxygen therapy will occasionally be required.

As a general rule, all forms of therapy discussed will reduce but not eliminate episodes of obstructive sleep apnea, except when the airway is either bypassed (tracheotomy) or opened (CPAP).

Presently, there are no therapies for central apnea

that consistently produce a reduction in frequency of events. Administration of oxygen will, however, almost always reverse any associated hypoxemia and bradyarrhythmias. CPAP and various respiratory stimulants have produced conflicting results, and there are too few studies evaluating diaphragmatic pacing.

Narcolepsy and Idiopathic Hypersomnolence

These are perhaps the best recognized primary disorders of excessive somnolence, even though they remain difficult to diagnose (21). Both narcolepsy and idiopathic hypersomnolence are characterized by the irresistible need for naps. The naps vary in duration from 30 seconds to 15 minutes and yet the subject awakens refreshed only to become somnolent within 2 to 3 hours. Most patients will report frequent near accidents and socially embarrassing situations related to their uncontrollable hypersomnolence. Narcolepsy also involves REM disturbances not seen in idiopathic hypersomnolence.

Narcolepsy. The prevalence of narcolepsy is approximately 4/10,000. It is equally common in men and women. Symptoms usually develop in the second decade of life and are relatively stable once the waketime sleepiness has developed fully. There is a probable genetic linkage with HLA-DR2 for at least narcolepsy with cataplexy. The pathogenesis involves abnormal control of REM sleep.

In narcolepsy, excessive waketime sleepiness is usually accompanied by one or more of the following symptoms: (a) *cataplexy* — a transitory sudden loss of postural muscle tone, sometimes causing collapse without loss of consciousness and often precipitated by an emotional response such as laughing, crying, or anger; (b) *sleep paralysis* — awakening with a transitory inability to move or speak, sometimes associated with dream-like hallucinations (this symptom is different from the sleep palsies experienced occasionally by most people—transient sensorimotor palsies of the ulnar, radial, and peroneal nerves that are subject to prolonged compression during deep sleep); (c) *hypnagogic hallucinations* — dream-like, usually visual, hallucinations occurring at the transition from wakefulness to sleep; and (d) *disturbed nocturnal sleep* — frequent brief awakening during a night's sleep. In some narcoleptic patients, these associated symptoms may occur before the development of waketime sleep attacks; in others they may never occur. Conditions that may be found in association with narcolepsy include sleep apnea (see above), sleep-related myoclonus (see above), and automatic behaviors, all of which occur more commonly in patients with narcolepsy than in the general population.

A working diagnosis of narcolepsy can be made on the basis of the history given by the patient and other observers. The definite diagnosis must be based upon characteristic findings in the napping tests performed in a sleep laboratory after other sleep disorders have been excluded by a nocturnal sleep study.

The *treatment of narcolepsy* utilizes both pharmacological and environmental measures to correct the two major symptoms, sleepiness and cataplexy. Before initiating treatment, the patient's usual pattern of daytime hypersomnolence should be documented to provide a baseline for assessing the response to therapy. Any of three stimulant drugs—magnesium pemoline (Cylert), methylphenidate (Ritalin), dextroamphetamine (Dexedrine)—and one tricyclic—protriptyline (Vivactil)—will provide relief from the waketime sleepiness. Tolerance is a major problem for all stimulants, and weekend drug "holidays" are advised. A minimally effective dose should be initiated with gradual increases in dosage every 1 to 2 weeks until symptom relief or side effects occur (Table 85.4). Medications that have sedating properties should be avoided if possible when treating patients with narcolepsy: hypnotics, anxiolytics, antihistamines, tricyclic antidepressants (other than those listed in Table 85.4), and trazadone, central-acting antihypertensives. Prazosin, a peripheral alpha-adrenergic inhibitor (and possibly other drugs with this property) can exacerbate cataplexy. Environmental management focuses on diet and planned waketime naps. Patients should avoid large meals and significant alcohol intake since both will exacerbate an underlying tendency for sleepiness. The cataplexy associated with narcolepsy is most effectively controlled by the tricyclics, imipramine (Tofranil) and protriptyline (Vivactil) (see Table 85.4). A regimen that was particularly effective in one large group of patients with sleep attacks plus cataplexy was treatment with imipramine, 25 mg, and methylphenidate, 5 to 10 mg three times daily (21). However, desipramine (Norpramin) and protriptyline (Vivactil) may be more effective than imipramine for reducing cataplexy with less sedation (see Chapter 15 for additional details about tricyclic antidepressants). New experimental treatments for cataplexy include the use of gamma-hydroxybuturate and yohimbine, an alpha-adrenergic inhibitor.

Idiopathic Hypersomnolence (IPH). Approximately 10% of patients presenting with excessive daytime hypersomnolence will be diagnosed as having idiopathic hypersomnolence. As opposed to narcolepsy, idiopathic hypersomnolence is not associated with inappropriate REM sleep during the daytime. These patients report a more pervasive sleepiness with less benefit from naps and less dreaming during naps than do narcoleptics; they also do not report

the other symptoms of narcolepsy—sleep paralysis, hypnogogic images, and cataplexy. Treatment includes use of stimulants, although the response is less consistent than in patients with narcolepsy.

In light of the difficult diagnosis, the variable response to treatment, and the significant risk of false reporting by individuals seeking stimulant medications, patients with suspected narcolepsy or idiopathic hypersomnolence should be evaluated in a sleep disorders center.

Medical and Environmental Causes

Causes for hypersomnia not due to a specific sleep disorder are varied and usually result in persistent wake time sleepiness. The more common medical conditions that should be considered are hypothyroidism (or apathetic hyperthyroidism in the elderly), hypoglycemia, anemia, uremia, hypercapnia, hypercalcemia, liver failure, and a number of neurological abnormalities (epilepsy, neurosyphilis, multiple sclerosis, delirium, brain tumors involving the brainstem and third ventricle, and progressive hydrocephalus from any cause). Progressive hydrocephalus may present initially as excessive somnolence without localizing findings; and sleepiness after head trauma may not develop until 6 to 18 months after the trauma.

Iatrogenic hypersomnia may accompany the use of a number of drugs with sedating side effects including centrally acting antihypertensives (reserpine, methyldopa, clonidine, β-blockers), antihistamines, anxiolytic agents, tricyclic antidepressants, neuroleptics, sedative-hypnotic drugs, and barbiturates.

Physical confinement and reduced environmental stimulation may lead to excessive somnolence. For example, in the elderly, there is a natural tendency toward waketime sleepiness, which in combination with some restrictions on activities, promotes excessive somnolence.

In each of these conditions, improvement in hypersomnolence depends largely upon improving the primary conditions. Thus, proper diagnosis, appropriate therapy, and discontinuation or adjustment of sedating medications will generally reduce but seldom completely reverse the sleepiness unless the

Table 85.4.
Drugs for Narcolepsy

Drug	Available Strengths (mg)	Minimum Effective Dose (mg)	Maximum Effective Dose (mg)	Time for Dose Effect
FOR HYPERSOMNOLENCE				
Dextroamphetamine (Dexedrine, generics)	5, 10, 15	5, every day	20, 3 times daily	3 days
Magnesium pemoline (Cylert)	18.75, 37.5	37.5, every day	112.5 every day	1 week
Methylphenidate (Ritalin, generics)	10, 20	10, twice daily	30, 3 and 4 times daily	3 days
FOR CATAPLEXY				
Protriptyline (Vivactil)[a,b]	5, 10	5, twice daily	10, 4 times daily	1 week
Imipramine (Tofranil, generics)[b]	25	25, twice daily	25, 4 times daily	1 week
Desipramine (Norpromin, Pertofrane)[b]	25, 50	25, twice daily	50, twice daily	1 week

[a] May also help reduce wake time sleepiness.
[b] For details on the use of tricyclics, see Chapter 15.

primary condition is resolved (e.g., hypothyroidism).

Psychosocial Conditions

Psychosocial stress, affective disorders, and schizophrenia may present with persistent waketime sleepiness. Recent community-based studies have shown that mental illness is present in almost half of those persons who report hypersomnolence (5). Patients whose hypersomnolence is due to mental illness will usually note precipitating stressful events or will demonstrate evidence of significant clinical depression; some may have hypersomnolence as a side effect of psychotropic drugs that have been prescribed for them. In these patients, the waketime status often involves a feeling of general fatigue and loss of energy, without need for sleep to restore wakefulness. These patients require management with a combination of psychotherapy and appropriate prescribing and adjustment of medications (see Chapters 12, 15, and 16).

Voluntary insufficient sleep occurs in our industrialized society, apparently related to social demands. For example, when college students are examined within the laboratory environment, they often demonstrate significant daytime hypersomnolence. With increased sleep time to approximately 9 or 10 hours, this sleepiness resolves. Thus, it is important to review the social and occupational circumstances under which the excessive daytime somnolence is occurring.

Other Sleep Disorders That Mimic DOES

Sleep-wake schedule disturbances (see below) may be incorrectly diagnosed as hypersomnia since these patients sleep late in the day and report an inability to stay awake for a large part of society's normal workday. In severe cases, the patient may have occasional reversal of the sleep-wake cycle with very long periods of sleep, short periods of wakefulness, and a complaint of never feeling very much awake. *Sleep-related myoclonus* (see above) often presents with waketime sleepiness and in extreme cases may be confused with narcolepsy. Minor symptoms generally associated with DIMS (insomnia) or DOES are present in waketime, e.g., morning malaise, minor irritations, diplopia, irritability, and multiple somatic complaints. Unlike DIMS, there is no problem initiating and maintaining sleep.

Natural long sleepers (usually adult females) also complain of excessive somnolence, sometimes because they have insufficient sleep owing to requirements of daily living, but more often because they feel they need too much sleep. The total sleep time required by a small subgroup of individuals (less than 2% of the adult population) is greater than 9 hours. When not under pressure, these individuals may sleep as much as 12 to 14 hours/day. This trend develops by early adolescence and remains stable throughout life. Therefore, when sleep time increases significantly later in life, it should not be attributed to this condition. Adequate protracted sleep, in one consolidated

sleep period each day, serves as both the diagnostic test and treatment for natural long sleepers. In difficult cases, sleep center referral should be considered to evaluate the patient for one of the causes of DOES.

DISORDERS OF THE SLEEP-WAKE SCHEDULE

Transient Problems

The homeostatic and circadian oscillation control of sleep and waking are usually well linked in a stable 24-hour pattern corresponding to social demands. Certain conditions may disrupt these relations leading to disorders of the sleep-wake cycle usually characterized by sleepiness at inappropriate times. Transient disturbances of the circadian cycle are well known to occur with transmeridian jet travel and with shiftwork. Recent understanding of these problems has led to improved techniques for reducing these types of sleep impairments.

For *jet travel*, short-acting sedative-hypnotics, such as triazolam (see "Sleep Medications" below), have been shown to permit sleep at the new time schedule and to facilitate wakefulness during the next day. Medication should be used for only 3 to 5 days. This treatment is useful for travel from east to west or west to east.

Shift workers demonstrate poor sleep during the daytime with subsequent sleepiness during the evening or night shift. The sleep-wake difficulties can be minimized by adjusting the sleep schedules with a forward rotation. In other words, an evening shift should be followed by a night shift followed by a day shift. In addition, adjustments to a new shift require 4 to 5 days; therefore, new changes in work shifts should be maintained for a minimum of 2 weeks before another change is initiated. In one study, this has clearly resulted in increased worker productivity with a concomitant decrease in accidents (4). Shift workers on night shift will generally do better sleeping in the afternoon than in the morning.

Persistent Problems

Persistent disruption of the normal sleep-wake cycle has only in recent years been recognized as a biologically based sleep disorder. This disorder may begin in childhood but usually develops in young adult life after some change in living schedule. The prevalence is unknown since the disorder has only been recognized recently.

Mechanism and Manifestations. The circadian biological rhythms of all species exert a major influence upon sleep. In an environment free of all time cues (e.g., prolonged living in a cave with constant light), the circadian rhythm for man runs slightly longer than 24 hours (about 24.5 to 25.5 hours). Under normal circumstances, the internal clock in each individual is reset every 24 hours in response to external cues. For reasons that are not clear, some people fail to entrain their internal cycle to the socially prescribed 24-hour clock. They either lose a stable cycle (progressive sleep cycle delay) or the cycle becomes fixed, out of phase with social demands. In the former case, the patient's sleep period changes rapidly, with occasional periods of prolonged sleepiness. In the latter case, the patient attempts sleep when he is physiologically most active and, therefore, finds sleep difficult to establish. Conversely, during the daytime, he must struggle to stay awake when he is physiologically ready for sleep. Under these circumstances, it is understandable why there are complaints about both insomnia and daytime sleepiness.

In contrast to most other sleep disorders, patients with sleep cycle disturbances report normal, good quality sleep when they are allowed to sleep for a few days on their own schedule, such as on nonworking days. Most report a nearly fixed delay in sleep onset (several hours after the expected bedtime), plus an ability to sleep late and to feel refreshed on the late awakening. Some report an advance in their cycle so that they are sleepy too early in the evening and unable to sleep in the early morning. Less commonly, the patients report the following cycle in their sleep disturbance: a period of insomnia with waketime sleepiness, followed by a period of premature sleepiness with premature awakenings. There is a brief period of normal sleep that ends in a repetition of the entire cycle beginning with insomnia with waketime sleepiness. Compared with the fixed sleep cycle delay, this progressive sleep cycle delay is an extremely unusual condition diagnosed by the characteristic history.

Diagnosis. A sleep-wake log and a temperature record assist in the diagnosis of a sleep-wake cycle problem. For 2 consecutive days, the patient is instructed to keep an oral temperature record for every 2 hours when not asleep. The temperature should not be taken within 10 minutes of consuming hot or cold beverages or food nor within 30 minutes after physical exercise. Body temperature fluctuates 1 to $2°$ F (about 0.5 to $1°$ C) during the day, reaching a peak during the time of greatest alertness and dropping off just before sleep onset (Figure 85.1). A temperature record showing no relative decrease before the planned bedtime supports the diagnosis.

Differential Diagnosis. A sleep-wake cycle disorder is commonly misdiagnosed as insomnia or as a problem of excessive somnolence. Both of these are excluded, if during extended sleep the patient sleeps well with good restoration of wakefulness. In some psychological disturbances, particularly manic type bipolar affective disorders and neurotic depression (see Chapter 15), sleep onset is delayed for a few hours. However, in these patients, the total sleep time is usually markedly reduced.

Schizophrenia may present with a sleep cycle disruption that resembles this disorder, but usually the underlying psychosis is diagnosed early. Some patients seen after chronic sedative-hypnotic (or stimulant) use may indeed have a primary disturbance in the sleep-wake cycle, a diagnosis that becomes apparent once the sleep-wake medication has been discontinued.

Treatment. Patients with the working diagnosis of fixed sleep-wake cycle delay can be placed on "light therapy." They need to be in bright lights in the early morning on awakening and to avoid seeing bright lights after about 4 P.M. This can usually be done by being in a sunlit area for about one hour in the morning and wearing dark sun glasses (such as mountaineer's glasses) whenever in sunlight after 4 P.M. When sunlight is not available, special very bright lights can be obtained that provide the needed 6,000 Lux when seated within 3 feet of the lights. Light therapy can reset the circadian rhythms within two weeks, but often patients with this condition need to continue the treatment to prevent relapse (15). Good sleep habits (Table 85.1) are then recommended to maintain the desired bedtime. Use of sedative-hypnotics or stimulants in this group of patients will not reset the sleep cycle and will complicate the treatment. Light therapy can also be used for patients with the progressive sleep cycle delay or sleep cycle advance, but the timing for the lights and dark glasses requires adjustment for each individual case. The best plan is referral to a sleep center for diagnosis and individualized environmental management.

DYSFUNCTIONS ASSOCIATED WITH SLEEP (PARASOMNIAS)

There are a number of miscellaneous problems associated with sleep, including three major disorders associated with incomplete arousal, usually from deep sleep (3). These incomplete arousals are increased by stress and tend to co-occur in the same person, who is often seen as a "deep" sleeper. There is a familial tendency for these disorders, and they occur most often in childhood. A fourth parasomnia involves abnormal behaviors during REM sleep.

Sleepwalking

Sleepwalking occurs in the first third of the sleep period with partial or total amnesia for the event on awakening. It is most common between ages 6 and 12, when it resolves. Occasionally, sleepwalking occurs in adults, although there is an antecedent history in childhood with complete remission until a recurrence in the late twenties or thirties when it may persist for several years. During sleepwalking, arousal from sleep can be difficult and the walking is complicated by associated clumsiness and accidents. Measures should, therefore, be taken to reduce the risks of accidents (e.g., ensure closed lower windows, restricted access to stairways, and cleared floor areas). Parents can be reassured that sleepwalking is otherwise of little concern, even though patients may report that it is worse during stress. In adults, however, there is usually an associated psychological problem requiring evaluation and appropriate psychotherapy. The possibility of sleep-induced seizures—particularly temporal lobe seizures in the REM stage of sleep—should be excluded (see Chapter 80). Sleepwalking in the elderly (over 65) is rare unless precipitated by sedative-hypnotic use.

Sleep Terrors

Sleep terrors occur in childhood as loud and uncontrollable screaming, usually during the first third of the sleep period, but occasionally repeating later in sleep. Throughout an episode, the child is generally uncontrollable until shortly before he returns to sleep. Fortunately, there is complete amnesia for the event, although the behavior is very disturbing to the family. Adults also experience sleep terrors characterized by sudden awakenings in the first third of the night accompanied by a profound sense of dread but not by the loud scream. Marked autonomic activity (tachycardia, diaphoresis) occurs in both children and adults. Sleep terrors occur in 1 to 4% of children beginning between ages 1 and 12 and ceasing by early adolescence. Adult onset is less common but does occur in the twenties or thirties but almost never after 40. Treatment of children includes reassurance of the family that the condition is benign. When the problem is very disrupting, a low dose anxiolytic agent, such as 2 to 5 mg of diazepam (Valium), at bedtime usually provides complete remission. Treatment for adults includes psychotherapy and a short course of treatment with a benzodiazepine agent. Bedtime doses of tricyclic antidepressants and neuroleptics should be avoided since exacerbation of the sleep terrors may result. The differential diagnosis includes sleep apnea, sleep-related epilepsy, and dream anxiety attacks. When sleep terrors persist in adults, sleep center referral (see above) should be considered to ensure correct diagnosis. For children, a referral should be considered if the condition is extreme and persistent.

Sleep-Related Enuresis

Persistent sleep-related enuresis is relatively common in childhood, occurring at age 5 in 15% of boys and 10% of girls. By puberty, the problem usually remits. Unless the sleep-related enuresis is associated with other problems, persists beyond puberty, or recurs after remission of several months, it can be considered benign. For adult onset or for recurring enuresis, the most important possibilities in the differential diagnosis are epilepsy, psychological disturbance, neurogenic bladder, dementia, and sleep apnea. Behavioral treatment for childhood enuresis is preferred to medication because it is more effective and safer.

REM Parasomnias

REM parasomnias or the REM behavior disorders are characterized by sudden usually aggressive or emotional behavior (hitting, crying out, swearing, diving off the bed in apparent fright) occurring during REM sleep. These events often occur without awakening, but the event may terminate when the patient is awakened by the discomfort caused by his behavior. Commonly one episode of a REM parasomnia will last for a few minutes with frequent repeated brief simple motor or verbal behavior stereotypic for the individual, repeated during the night and occurring on several nights during the week. The behaviors occur during REM periods and are commonly associated with dreamlike mentation that can be recalled by the patient if he is awakened during the event. The behaviors appear to be an acting out of some aspect of the dream accompanied by a breakdown in the usual skeletal muscle paralysis of REM sleep. On sleep studies these patients usually show frequent brief episodes of loss of muscle atonia during their REM sleep along with excessive muscle twitching during REM.

This disorder occurs almost exclusively in persons over 50 although a few cases have been reported for children and infants. In adults the disorder, once established, appears to be constant and not progressive. It is associated with other neurological disorders, particularly those related to brainstem pathology. Incidence of the disorder is not known. For this disorder, referral to a sleep disorder center is recommended both for diagnosis with a sleep study and for planning of treatment (usually use of a benzodiazepine hypnotic such as clonazepam).

SLEEP MEDICATIONS

Sedative-Hypnotic Drugs

As noted in previous sections, sedative-hypnotic drugs may be helpful for managing some sleep disorders and counter-productive when used for others. The benefits from these medications reported by patients may be very significant, even though the overall effects on sleep are a 10- to 30-minute reduction in sleep onset time and a 20- to 40-minute increase in total sleep time (18). The most important contraindication for sedative-hypnotic drug use is any symptom or sign of unexplained respiratory problems at night, including a history of heavy snoring or significant waketime sleepiness, as these may indicate sleep apnea (see above, page 1175).

Selection and Use

The sedative-hypnotics of first choice are the *benzodiazepines*. Table 85.5 summarizes available tablet sizes and recommended doses for sleep medications in this group. There is very little reason to select barbiturates or other sedative-hypnotics due to their significantly lower toxic to therapeutic ratio.

Because tolerance may develop to all sedative-hypnotics, the daily use of any of these drugs should be limited to 4 weeks. It is best to start at the minimal effective dose (see Table 85.5) and to permit an increase in dose, if necessary, every 3 to 4 days until the effective dose is found or the usual maximal dose is

Table 85.5.
Sedative-Hypnotic Benzodiazepine Drugs (in Order by Increasing Duration of Action)

Drug	Rate of Absorption or Appearance[d]	Half-life[e] (hr)	Available Strengths (mg)	Minimum Effective Dose (mg)	Maximum Recommended Dose (mg)
SHORT ACTING					
Midazolam (Versed)[a]	Rapid	1.5–3.5	7.5, 15	7.5	15
Triazolam (Halcion)[b]	Intermediate	1.5–5.0	0.125, 0.25, 0.5	0.125	0.5
Brotizolam[a]	Rapid	1–4	0.25, 0.5	0.25	0.5
INTERMEDIATE ACTING (half-lives usually 10–20 hours)					
Oxazepam (Serax)[c]	Slow	4–15	10, 15, 30	10	30
Lorazepam (Ativan)	Intermediate	10–20	0.5, 1, 2	0.5	4
Estazolam[a]	Intermediate	10–20	1, 2	1.0	2.0
Temazepam (Restoril)[c]	Slow	8–22	15, 30	15	30
Clonazepam (Klonopin)	Rapid	18–39	0.5, 1, 2	0.5	1.5
LONG ACTING					
Diazepam (Valium)	Rapid	40–120	2, 5, 10	2	15
Chlordiazepoxide (Librium)	Intermediate	36–200	5, 10, 25	5	25
Flurazepam (Dalmane)	Rapid	36–200	15, 30	15	30

[a] These medications were not available in the US market at the time this table was prepared.
[b] This medication commonly used at 0.125 mg starting dose for patients over 45, and 0.25 mg for younger patients.
[c] These medications have a somewhat delayed onset of action and should be taken about 1 hour before bedtime.
[d] Rate for most rapid significantly active compound in blood; correlates with onset of sedating action.
[e] Half-life for longest significantly active compound in blood.

reached. Most patients can titrate their own dose for symptom relief, but the dosage should not be increased once tolerance to an effective dose occurs. Even in the most unusual case, increasing doses more than twice is likely to create a new problem of drug dependence and does little to solve the patient's sleep problem.

In adjusting dosage, particular attention should be given to waketime function. Several of the popular benzodiazepines (flurazepam, diazepam, chlordiazepoxide) along with their active metabolites have long half-lives that may produce continuing daytime sedation even after one dose. When taken daily, the cumulative effects of these medications may lead to drowsiness during waking hours. Under these circumstances, the dose should be decreased. For the longer acting benzodiazepines, weekend drug-free intervals are recommended; alternatively, the shorter acting benzodiazepines, triazolam, oxazepam, lorazepam, and temazepam, may be considered. Very short-acting benzodiazepines, such as triazolam, cause little or no waketime sedation. They have, however, been reported to produce a "rebound insomnia" (insomnia after stopping the medication that is worse than that before treatment). Recent studies have indicated that one of two mechanisms may explain this problem: (a) oversedation on nights when the patient was taking medication (i.e., he may have reduced his sleep needs by attaining excess sleep on those nights); or (b) loss, in a hypnotic-using patient, of the self-correcting effects of insomnia (i.e., sleep deprivation from insomnia increases sleep need and results in compensatory sleep) (1). Rebound insomnia is usually mild and lasts only two days after stopping a hypnotic medication.

The *barbiturate sedative-hypnotics* have three distinct disadvantages in comparison with the benzodiazepines: the frequent occurrence of hangover after only one dose, the development of physiological dependence with the accompanying risk of a severe with-

drawal reaction, and the low toxic to therapeutic ratio. A number of *other sedative-hypnotics* (chloral hydrate, glutethimide, meprobamate, methaqualone, and methyprylon) have been shown to be effective but are associated with especially high potential for lethal respiratory depression with overdose. Therefore, there is little reason to select one of these agents or a barbiturate instead of a benzodiazepine. Of the entire group, chloral hydrate (500 to 1000 mg) is perhaps the safest if an alternative to the benzodiazepines is needed.

Information to Patients

When prescribing a sedative-hypnotic medication, it is recommended that sleeping medications be taken 10 to 60 minutes before bedtime, depending on the rate of absorption of the medication (see Table 85.5). The patient should be warned of the following: (a) the risk of tolerance and dependence with later withdrawal problems (especially with barbiturates and the short-acting benzodiazepines) and the risk of developing the "sleeping pill habit" and never adequately resolving the sleep problem; (b) potential problems of interaction with other drugs, particularly alcohol (alcohol abstinence, particularly after dinner, is essential and the patient should generally not take more than one sedating medication in the same day); (c) hangover effects and the possibility of becoming sleepy while driving, especially after the first few days on the longer acting benzodiazepines or barbiturates; and (d) the uncertain knowledge about effects on pregnancy.

Sedative-Hypnotic Withdrawal

For patients taking too much sleeping medication, the withdrawal must be gradual, particularly if the patient has been on a regimen for several months. These patients may report worsening insomnia due to chronic use of the medication (see above, page 1173) or develop physiological dependence and risk serious withdrawal symptoms. Nevertheless, withdrawal should be attempted and the patient should be informed that he will become temporarily worse before improving. The dosage of medication should be reduced by one therapeutic dose per week. If more than one medication is involved, one medication at a time should be reduced. Contact with the physician is essential in order to avoid relapses during this trying experience. Difficult but motivated patients may need assistance from persons who are expert in managing withdrawal from drugs (see Chapter 22).

Over-the-Counter Sleep Medications

Over-the-counter (OTC) sleep medications and antihistamines are effective for many patients with transient insomnia and may be as effective as low doses of the commonly prescribed sedative-hypnotics. The OTC medications contain small amounts of antihistamines (Table 85.6).

Antihistamines Requiring a Prescription

The prescription sedative-antihistamines include diphenhydramine (Benadryl), 50 mg strength, and hydroxyzine (Vistaril and Atarax), 25 and 50 mg. These drugs are more potent sedatives than the OTC sleeping medications. They may be particularly useful in patients with a history of drug or alcohol abuse.

Antidepressants

The most sedating of the tricyclic antidepressants, such as amitriptyline (Elavil), imipramine (Tofranil), and the nontricyclic agent, trazadone (Desyrel) are useful in low doses for the management of persistent insomnia associated with those psychological conditions in which there is a depressive or obsessive-compulsive component. These medications should be avoided when the patient reports restless sleep, excessive movement during sleep, or restless legs while awake.

Antidepressants are effective either when sleep onset is disturbed by anxiety or ruminating thoughts or when sleep is interrupted in the later part of the sleep period by dreams characterized by anxiety. Under these conditions, these agents are preferable to sedative-

hypnotics both because of better efficacy and less risk of dependence. Usual doses are 25 to 75 mg for the tricyclics and 50 to 150 mg for trazadone about 1 to 2 hours before bed. At this dose, the side effects are usually minimal. Additional information about antidepressants is found in Chapter 15.

SLEEP CENTER EVALUATION

For a number of the problems discussed in this chapter, referral for expert evaluation and management is recommended. Referral can be made to individual physicians who are expert in managing sleep disorders or to a sleep disorders center. Currently there are over 100 sleep disorder centers accredited by the American Sleep Disorders Association (ASDA). The ASDA can supply the locations of these centers (ASDA, 604 Second Street, S.W., Rochester, Minnesota, 55902). Access to these centers has become increasingly available; nevertheless, discussion about particular patients by telephone may be as useful prior to referral.

Patient experience. When a patient is evaluated at a sleep center, he undergoes a careful historical review of his sleep problem and a general physical examination. One or more all-night sleep studies (polysomnogram) may be scheduled in order to evaluate his sleep objectively. The polysomnogram is performed using noninvasive simultaneous measurements of a number of physiological activities during sleep: eye movements, brain activity by EEG, submental and anterior tibialis muscle activity, respiratory air flow and effort, cardiac rhythm, and continuous blood oxyhemoglobin saturation. Sometimes additional parameters are recorded such as rectal temperature, esophageal pH, and penile circumference.

A day test with 4 to 5 repeated 20-minute naps, spaced 2 hours apart, may also be scheduled. For this nap test (called a Multiple Sleep Latency Test or MSLT) the patient stays in his usual sleeping clothes and is asked to stay awake between the naps. A full sleep EEG is recorded as is done for the polysomnogram except the respiration and oxygen saturation measurements will usually either not be used or be used in a limited form, since the primary question addressed by this test is the degree of the patient's excessive sleepiness. The sleep latency (the time it takes the patient to fall asleep) for the naps provides the measure of the patient's sleepiness. The nap test is usually scheduled for the day after the night polysomnogram. A usual schedule for the patient in the sleep lab would be 9:30 P.M. to 8:00 A.M. for the polysomnogram and 8:00 A.M. to 4:30 P.M. for the nap tests.

Table 85.6.
Constituents of Commonly Used Over-the-Counter Sleep Remedies

Product Name	Constituent	
Miles Nervine[a] Sleep-Eze Sominex[c] Nytol	Pyrilamine maleate[b]	25 mg
Unisom Night-time Sleep Aid	Doxylamine succinate[d]	25 mg
Benadryl	Diphenhydramine	25 mg

[a] This product no longer contains bromine.
[b] Antihistamine of the ethylenediamine class.
[c] This product no longer contains scopolamine.
[d] Antihistamine of the ethanolamine class.

General References

Chase MH, Weitzman ED (eds):*Sleep Disorders: Basic and Clinical Research*, Vol 8, In: *Advances in Sleep Research.* Weitzman ED (Senior editor): New York, Spectrum, 1983.
    Very good technical but readable articles on the scientific basis for sleep disorders. Excellent section on hypnotics.
Coats TJ, Thoresen CE (eds): *How to Sleep Better: A Drug-Free Pro-*

gram for Overcoming Insomnia. Englewood Cliffs, NJ, Prentice- Hall, 1977.

> Useful self-help book emphasizing self-regulation techniques.

Feber R: *Solve Your Child's Sleep Problems.* New York, Simon and Schuster, 1985.

> A classic for pediatric sleep disorders—general guide, readable, suitable for many parents.

Guilleminault C (ed): *Sleeping and Waking Disorders: Indications and Techniques.* Menlo Park, CA, Addison-Wesley, 1982.

> Basic text on methodology and treatment.

Hauri P (ed): *The Sleep Disorders, Current Concepts.* Kalamazoo, MI, Upjohn, 1982.

> A useful general introductory work to sleep, sleep disorders, and their treatment. (The Upjohn Company provides copies of this small booklet.)

Kryger M, Roth T, Dement WC (eds): *Principles and Practice of Sleep Medicine.* Philadelphia, WB Saunders, 1988.

> The best available collection of solid secondary reference chapters covering both clinical and scientific basis for general sleep disorders. Some chapters are fairly technical.

Lamberg L (ed): *American Medical Association Guide to Better Sleep.* New York, Random House, 1984.

> Nontechnical introduction to sleep disorders written for the general public, but so well done it is useful as a secondary reference.

Phillipson DA, Bowes G: In: Fishman AP (ed): *Update: Pulmonary Diseases and Disorders,* 3rd ed., New York, McGraw-Hill, 1987.

> Excellent review of pathophysiology and diagnosis of obstructive sleep apnea.

Specific References

1. Allen RP, Mendels J, Nevins DB et al: Efficacy without tolerance or rebound insomnia for midazolam and temazepam after use for one to three months. *J Clin Pharm* 27:768, 1987.
2. Association of Sleep Disorders Centers: Diagnostic classification of sleep and arousal disorders. *Sleep* 2:1, 1979.
3. Broughton R: Sleep disorders: disorders of arousal? *Science (Wash DC)* 159:1070, 1978.
4. Czeisler CA, Moore-Ede C, Coleman RM: Rotating shift work schedules that disrupt sleep are improved by applying circadian principles. *Science (Wash DC)* 217:460, 1982.
5. Ford DE, Kamerow DB: Epidemiologic study of sleep disturbances and psychiatric disorders. An opportunity for prevention? *JAMA* 262:1479, 1989.
6. Gilin JC, Duncan W, Pettigew DK et al: Successful separation of depressed, normal and insomniac subjects by EEG sleep data. *Arch Gen Psychiatry* 36:85, 1979.
7. Guilleminault C, Eldridge FL, Dement WC: Insomnia with sleep apnea: a new syndrome. *Science (Wash DC)* 181:856, 1973.
8. Haponik E, Smith PL, Bleecker FR: Diagnosis of obstructive sleep apnea: is polysomnography necessary? *Chest* 84:354, 1983.
9. Jones H, Oswald I: Two cases of healthy insomnia. *Electroencephalogr Clin Neurophysiol* 24:378, 1968.
10. Kales A, Bixler EO, Tan TL, et al: Chronic hypnotic drug use: ineffectiveness, drug withdrawal insomnia and hypnotic drug dependence. *JAMA* 227:513, 1974.
11. Karacan I, Thornby JI, Williams R: A community survey. In: Guilleminault C, Lugaresi E (eds): *Sleep/Wake Disorders: Natural History, Epidemiology, and Long-Term Evolution.* New York, Raven Press, 1983.
12. Lavie P: Sleep habits and sleep disturbances in industry workers in Israel: main findings and some characteristics of workers complaining of excessive daytime sleepiness. *Sleep* 4:147, 1981.
13. Lugaresi E, Coccagna G, Gambi C, et al: Symond's nocturnal myoclonus. *Electroencephalogr Clin Neurophysiol* 23:289, 1967.
14. Rajagopal KR, Abbrecht PH, Derderian SS, et al: Obstructive sleep apnea in hypothyroidism. *Ann Intern Med* 101:491, 1984.
15. Rosenthal NE, Joseph-Vanderpool JR, Levendosky AA, et al: Phase shifting effects of bright morning light as treatment in delayed sleep phase syndrome. *Sleep* 13: 1990.
16. Smith PL, Haponik EF, Allen RP, Bleecker ER: The effects of protriptyline in sleep-disordered breathing. *Am Rev Respir Dis* 127:8, 1983.
17. Smith PL, Haponik EF, Gold AR, Bleecker ER: The effect of weight loss on sleep disordered breathing. *Am Rev Respir Dis* 129:A59, 1984.
18. Solomon F, White CC, Parron DL, Mendelson WB: Special report: sleeping pills, insomnia and medical practice, from the Institute of Medicine of the National Academy of Sciences. *N Engl J Med* 300:803, 1979.
19. Welstein L, Dement WC, Redington D et al: Insomnia in the San Francisco Bay area: a telephone survey. In: Guilleminault C, Lugaresi E (eds): *Sleep/Wake Disorders: Natural History, Epidemiology, and Long-Term Evolution.* New York, Raven Press, 1983.
20. Williams RL: Sleep disorders in various medical and surgical conditions. In: Williams RL, Karacan I (eds): *Sleep Disorders* New York, John Wiley & Sons, 1978.
21. Zarcone V: Narcolepsy. *N Engl J Med* 288:1156, 1973.

Selected General Surgical Problems

C H A P T E R 86

Preoperative Planning for Ambulatory Patients*

RICHARD J. GROSS, M.D.

---

* Everett Spees, M.D., contributed to this chapter in the first and second editions.

PREOPERATIVE PLANNING: OVERVIEW

The general physician often invests substantial effort in preoperative planning for a patient with a problem amenable to surgery. This includes scheduling tests to confirm the initial diagnosis, discussing the findings with the patient and the patient's family, proposing consultation with a surgeon, and consulting on the care of the patient's medical problems in the perioperative period.

Most preoperative planning should be done in the ambulatory setting. Increasingly, large proportions of operations are performed in ambulatory (same day) surgery units (Fig. 86.1). General guidelines on eligibility for same-day ambulatory surgery, based on the patient's medical status, are summarized in Table 86.1. These guidelines are derived from extensive experience with patients in all age groups during the past decade. In addition, many patients who will stay in the hospital after surgery (e.g., elective hysterectomy) are now admitted on the morning of surgery, increasing the need for preadmission medical evaluations (17). The principal reasons for office-based preoperative assessment in these two groups of patients are (a) that health care insurers now reimburse only for same day surgery for many procedures; (b) that this eliminates the costs and inconvenience associated with unanticipated cancellation of surgery, after the patient has been admitted; and (c) that better planning of care and higher patient satisfaction are often achieved.

In general, the surgeon expects the referring physician to have made an independent assessment of the need for surgery and of the patient's general fitness for surgery. Although the surgeon obtains the actual consent for the surgical procedure, the patient's ex-

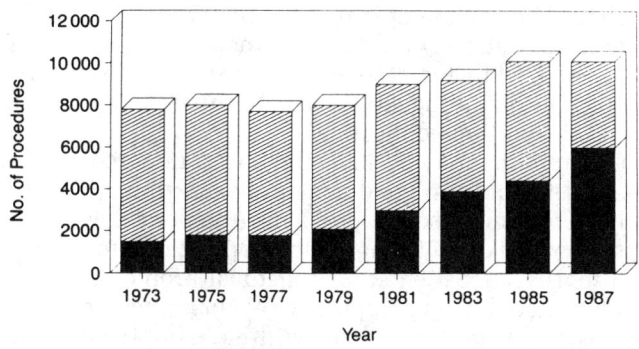

Figure 86.1. Numbers of ambulatory procedures (*black bars*) and surgical procedures (*hatched bars*) by year at Norwalk (Conn.) Community Hospital. Slightly modified from: Laffaye HA: The impact of an ambulatory surgical service in a community hospital. *Arch Surg* 124:601, 1989, copyright 1989, American Medical Association, with permission.

Table 86.1.
General Guidelines on Patient Eligibility for Ambulatory Surgery Based on Medical Condition (Not Considering Type of Surgery)[a]

1. American Society of Anesthesiologists Class 1-2 (some Class 3 for minor procedures).

   Class 1: There is no physiologic, biochemical, or psychiatric disturbance. The pathological process for which operation is to be performed is localized and not conducive to systemic disturbance. Examples: A fit patient with inguinal hernia; fibroid uterus in an otherwise healthy woman.

   Class 2: Mild to moderate systemic disturbance caused either by the condition to be treated surgically or by other pathophysiological processes. Examples: Presence of mild diabetes, essential hypertension, or anemia.

   Class 3: Rather severe systemic disturbance or pathology from whatever cause, even though it may not be possible to define the degree of disability with finality. Examples: Severe diabetes with vascular complications; moderate to severe degrees of pulmonary insufficiency; angina pectoris or healed myocardial infarction.

2. Stable medical problems, well controlled by medicines.

3. No recent myocardial infarction or unstable cardiac disease.

4. If diabetic, not taking insulin; if taking insulin, stable and patient capable of self-monitoring (insulin dependent diabetics should be operated upon early in the morning).

[a] Adapted from Kammerer WS, Gross RJ (eds): *Medical Consultation.* Baltimore, Williams & Wilkins, 1990.

pectations and assumptions are often based upon the counseling provided by his personal physician. The referral itself is usually understood by the patient and his family as an endorsement of a surgical opinion and of the consulting surgeon. For these reasons, it is important for referring physicians to know the place of surgery in the management of a broad array of conditions (10, 11).

In counseling the patient and his family, the patient's physician, as well as the consulting surgeon, should explain clearly the objective and the expected outcome of the operation. This is especially important for surgical procedures that are undertaken for asymptomatic conditions (such as elective cholecystectomy) and for procedures that may be disfiguring (such as mastectomy or amputation). Preoperative counseling should be documented in the patient's record, and this documentation should always include any special issues raised by the patient and how they were resolved (such as obtaining additional consultations or providing supportive counseling).

Approximately 50% of adults who undergo surgery are ostensibly in good general health; the other 50% have various medical problems (the percentages vary depending upon the age of the population). In perhaps 5 to 10% of patients, new medical problems will be identified during preoperative evaluation; a small proportion of these problems will have implications for the planning of surgery. Whenever surgery is planned, the patient's referring physician should complete an appropriate preoperative evaluation (see below), should assure that existing medical conditions that may affect the outcome of surgery are optimally controlled, and

should communicate specific recommendations to the surgeon regarding the care of the patient's medical problem(s) during the perioperative period. This chapter provides guidelines for these steps in the management of patients with a number of common medical problems.

GENERAL PREOPERATIVE EVALUATION

There is no consensus on the makeup of a general preoperative evaluation. For adult patients undergoing general or spinal anesthesia, most physicians currently perform a history and physical examination and order a number of routine laboratory tests (e.g., chest X-ray and electrocardiogram in patients over 40; and complete blood count, tests of hemostasis, electrolytes, glucose, measurement of blood urea nitrogen or creatinine, and urinalysis in all adults). This complete workup has been criticized for having a low yield and for being unnecessarily costly (17). The large number of factors that influence the preoperative evaluation make a consensus unlikely. The patient's age, the nature of the planned surgery (major or minor), the type of anesthesia to be used (general, spinal, regional, or local), and the interval since the patient's last comprehensive evaluation are relevant in the preoperative evaluation of every patient. In addition, one or more of the following considerations is often pertinent: estimating operative risk, establishing a baseline for expected postoperative changes or possible complications, avoiding harm to other patients or medical personnel [e.g., hepatitis, tuberculosis or human immunodeficiency virus (HIV) infection], documenting selected information for medicolegal reasons, determining drug dosage, and detecting rare but potentially catastrophic circumstances (e.g., thrombocytopenia in a patient scheduled for a craniotomy).

A practical approach for the individual patient is to select one of the two general types of preoperative evaluation as summarized in Table 86.2, i.e., *a limited or a comprehensive workup.* Guidelines for choosing between these alternatives are summarized in Table 86.3 Selected screening tests should be added to either workup in order to avoid potential catastrophes associated with certain high risk situations (Table 86.4). Routine HIV screening of preoperative patients is currently not recommended; instead the universal precautions described in Chapter 34 are recommended.

Frequently overlooked aspects of evaluation and planning in the assessment of the outpatient presurgical patient are listed in Table 86.5.

CURRENT MEDICATIONS AND KNOWN ALLERGIES

All drugs that a patient is taking and any known drug allergies should be specified at the time of referral for surgery. Planning should be initiated at that time, for the following reasons: to avoid possible interactions with anesthetic agents and possible complications during surgery, to manage the patient when an essential drug cannot be administered orally during

Table 86.2.
Two Types of General Preoperative Evaluation

Component of Workup	Limited Workup[a]	Comprehensive Workup[a]
History	HPI[b], past medical history, allergies, medications, heart, lungs, hemostasis, endocrine, family history of surgical/anesthesia problems and new symptoms (especially upper respiratory infection)	HPI[b], past medical history, social history, family history, allergies, medications, brief review of all systems
Physical examination	Vital signs, oral cavity, chest, heart, and abdomen	Complete physical examination
Laboratory[a]	Hematocrit, urinalysis, ECG (some cases >age 35), serum potassium (some cases), pregnancy test[c]	Chest X-ray, ECG (>age 35), complete blood count, blood urea nitrogen or serum creatinine, serum glucose, serum electrolytes, urinalysis, pregnancy test[c]

[a] Basic evaluation for screening and baseline data. Other tests may be added to evaluate known disease in a patient or to follow-up findings in the preoperative history and physical examination, see also Table 86.4.
[b] HPI = history of present illness.
[c] Women in childbearing age group.

Table 86.3.
Guidelines for Selecting the General Preoperative Evaluation

Limited Workup	Comprehensive Workup
Age <40	Age >40 (especially >60)
Recent comprehensive physical examination	No, old, or inadequate data base
Well patient	Patient with moderate-severe major organ disease
Local, regional, or spinal anesthesia	General anesthesia
Established patient; previously examined by physician	New patient, unknown to physician
Minor procedure	Major procedure (especially thoracic, abdominal, neurosurgical)

the perioperative period, and to avoid exposure to drugs to which the patient is allergic. The patient should be asked specifically about nonprescription drug use that, although very common, is often not mentioned spontaneously (particularly aspirin-containing compounds, which may potentiate postoperative bleeding; and sedatives, which may interact with anesthetic drugs); about prior allergic reactions to drugs for medical conditions (especially penicillin and other antibiotics that may be indicated postoperatively at a time when a patient is unable to provide information) and to local and general anesthetic agents (e.g., halothane); about use of corticosteroids within the past year (particularly patients with obstructive airways disease or seasonal allergy); about prior reactions to blood products; and about current use of recreational substances that may affect the patient's course during or after surgery (alcohol, tobacco, illicit drugs).

For patients taking one or more medications regularly, specific perioperative recommendations regarding those medications should be communicated to the surgeon (Table 86.6). Modification of chronic medications for surgery is best done before the patient is hospitalized rather than the night before surgery at the hospital, in order to allow time to detect unanticipated effects. Most medications have a duration of action between 6 and 12 hours, and omission of one or more doses may precipitate symptoms. For patients who are expected to be awake and to be able to take oral medications within this time span, it is appropriate to recommend giving a dose, with a small amount of water (1 ounce or less), in the morning before the induction of anesthesia and resuming the medication orally 6 to 12 hours later. When oral medications cannot be continued throughout the perioperative period, alternate

Table 86.4.
Additional Preoperative Screening Tests for Common High Risk Situations

High Risk Situation	Screening Tests
Patient undergoing neurosurgical, cardiac, vascular, or major abdominal procedure	Tests of hemostasis: platelet count, prothrombin time, partial thromboplastin time
Patient on diuretics, with vomiting/diarrhea, other abnormal fluid loss, cardiac disease, renal disease	Electrolytes
Patient with increased risk of active liver disease (e.g., alcoholism, drug addiction, homosexuality, dialysis patient, high risk medications) who is undergoing general or spinal anesthesia	Liver function tests: serum aminotransferases, alkaline phosphatase, bilirubin, hepatitis-associated antigen
Patient with increased risk of chronic pulmonary disease (e.g., smoker with ≥10 pack years) who is undergoing general anesthesia	Pulmonary function tests
Patient with increased risk of tuberculosis (e.g., known exposure, HIV positive, underprivileged population)	Chest X-ray, purified protein derivative skin test
Patient with increased risk of coronary artery disease (i.e., smoker, hypertensive, strong family history, diabetic, hyperlipidemia)	ECG
Malnourished patient or prolonged inability to eat	Nutritional assessment

Table 86.5.
Commonly Forgotten or Underestimated Items in the Office Evaluation and Management of the Surgery Patient[a]

A. Evaluation
  1. One disease (review the problem list).
  2. The generally sick patient.
  3. Inquiry about current medications (include aspirin and other, over-the-counter).
  4. Blood tests indicated by specific medical diseases or medications (e.g., drug levels, potassium for diuretics).
  5. Inquiry about abnormal bleeding or knowledge that one is a bleeder.
  6. Inquiry about prior history of transfusion or of transfusion reactions.
  7. Inquiry about previous problems with anesthesia.
  8. Inquiry about current use of alcohol or illicit drugs.
  9. Pregnancy test (serum qualitative HCG).
  10. Spirometry (smoker who may have unrecognized COPD).
  11. Echocardiogram (evaluation of murmur regarding SBE prophylaxis).
B. Management
  1. Tell patient to report even minor intercurrent illnesses between physical and day of surgery.
  2. Stop smoking, alcohol, illicit drugs, OTC medications (no new OTC medications).
  3. Medications—whether to take medications A.M. of surgery and when to restart postop. Discontinuing certain medications (such as aspirin, coumadin). Coverage for corticosteroids if indicated.
  4. SBE prophylaxis.
  5. Teach patient what to expect pre- and postoperatively; call if unexpected problems arise.
  6. Tell the patient about, and plan several weeks in advance, banking of one or more units of blood for autologous transfusion.

[a] Adapted from: Kammerer WS, Gross RJ (eds): *Medical Consultation*. Baltimore, Williams & Wilkins, 1990.

medications or routes of administration should be recommended.

SURGERY IN THE ELDERLY PATIENT

Size of the Risk

The mortality risk associated with anesthesia and surgery is increased in the elderly. However, the risk in elderly patients has fallen substantially over the past 10 to 20 years. The overall mortality risk for major surgery in patients under 65 is about 1%; the risk is about 5% between ages 65 and 80. Patients over age 80 have a 10% risk, although recently mortality as low as 6 to 8% has been reported (9, 18, 24).

A number of factors are more important than age itself in increasing surgical risk in older patients. These other factors are important because some that can be modified account for wide variations in surgical risks among patients of the same age. The most important factors are general overall health, nutrition, type of surgery (body cavity versus non-body cavity; elective versus emergency), type of anesthesia, and coexisting conditions [cardiac, infectious, renal, pulmonary, central nervous system (CNS)].

The conditions associated with very high surgical mortality in elderly patients are uncorrectable surgical lesions, such as infarcted bowel or ruptured aneurysm.

The next most important cause is cardiac disease, followed by infections (especially pneumonia), renal disease, and pulmonary disease. In the preoperative evaluation, attention should be focused on these problems, since they account for most perioperative deaths.

Certain common procedures can be performed at low risk in the elderly, often without general anesthesia. These low risk operations include cataract surgery, simple hernia repair, and transurethral prostate resection. The risks of some major surgical procedures in the elderly have fallen greatly over the past few years; examples include elective abdominal aortic aneurysm repair and repair of hip fractures.

Preoperative Planning

Office Evaluation. The elderly patient undergoing major surgery should have a comprehensive preoperative evaluation (see Table 86.2) because of the wide variety of coexisting, often unrecognized, medical conditions found in older individuals. The workup should be reviewed specifically for the risk factors listed above. Any major preoperative risks must be weighed against the benefits of the operation, with attention to the fact that quality of life may be as important as longevity in this age group. An accurate estimation of average future longevity for the patient's age group is important; this is often underestimated.

Preoperative cardiac evaluation is discussed below. Clues to occult infection (including simple upper respiratory infections) should be carefully sought, since classic signs may not be present in the elderly. Spirometry should be performed routinely in patients over age 65 if there is any suggestion of pulmonary disease, because of the increased incidence of pulmonary complications in older patients. It should be remembered that serum creatinine may be falsely low in elderly patients due to reduced muscle mass; therefore, a creatinine clearance should be obtained if the state of the patient's renal function is not certain, because of the importance in determining drug dosages. Finally, a baseline mental status examination (see Chapter 17) should be completed since postoperative changes in mental status occur frequently in the elderly. If there is hearing impairment due to cerumen impaction preoperatively, this problem should be corrected.

Recommendations to the surgeon. Elderly patients often have limitations of understanding because of memory deficits, hearing problems, and education. Because these are often known to the primary physician, communication to the surgeon of these limitations will improve the effectiveness of the surgeon's explanation of the procedure. Explanation of what to expect during hospitalization and surgery is even more important in the elderly, to avoid fear and confusion and because of outdated conceptions of the nature of surgery among the elderly.

Simple measures that can be planned before admission may help to reduce the high incidence of postoperative confusion in older patients. These measures include planning to allow family members to stay be-

Table 86.6.
Recommendations to the Surgeon Regarding the Patient's Regular Medications

Drug Class	Anticipated Problems	Recommendations to Surgeon for Perioperative Period
CARDIOVASCULAR		
Antihypertensives[b]	Interaction with anesthetics, hypotension	Inform anesthesiologist of use
	Inability to give orally	Plan postoperative regimen with alternative agents if needed
Antiarrhythmics[b]	Inability to give orally	ECG monitor in operating room and postoperatively, use alternative parenteral agents
β-Blockers	Myocardial depression, bradycardia	Continue intravenously, taper to lower dose, or discontinue depending on circumstances
Digitalis[b]	Toxicity	Obtain serum levels preoperatively
	Inability to give orally	Give 75% of daily oral dose of digoxin intravenously each day
Long acting oral nitrates[b]	Inability to give orally	Substitute transdermal nitroglycerine
GASTROINTESTINAL		
Antacids[b]	Inability to give orally	Intravenous H₂ blockers, nasogastric suction (if patient has active peptic ulcer disease)
ANTIBIOTICS		
Tetracycline	Risk of renal failure if given with methoxyflurane	Use alternative antibiotic or anesthetic
CORTICOSTEROIDS[b]	Adrenal insufficiency	Plan coverage (with intravenous corticosteroids) adequate for the stress of surgery
	Poor wound healing	Discuss with surgeon
NEUROLOGICAL		
Levodopa/Carbidopa[b]	Interaction with anesthetics (hypertension or hypotension), inability to give orally	Inform anesthesiologist of use; resume orally as soon as possible after surgery
Barbiturates	Increased CNS depression by anesthesia, inability to give orally	Inform anesthesiologist of use; give daily dose intramuscularly
Dilantin	Inability to give orally	Give daily dose slowly intravenously (or substitute phenobarbital before admitting patient for surgery)
BRONCHODILATORS		
Theophylline[b]	Inability to give orally	Switch to intravenous aminophylline
β₂-Sympathomimetics[b]	Inability to give orally	Switch to aerosolized or subcutaneous β₂-agent
PSYCHIATRIC		
Antidepressants[b]	Hypotension or hypertension, arrhythmias	Inform anesthesiologist of use; withhold monoamine oxidase inhibitors 2 weeks preoperatively; selectively withhold other agents 24 hours preoperatively.
Neuroleptics (i.e., phenothiazines and haloperidol)[b]	Arrhythmias, enhancement of neuromuscular blocking agents, hypotension	Inform anesthesiologist of use; withhold 24 hours preoperatively in some cases.
Benzodiazepines	Increased CNS depression by anesthesia	Inform anesthesiologist of use
Lithium[b]	Myocardial depression, hypernatremia	Inform anesthesiologist of use; determine blood levels; withhold 24 hours preoperatively; avoid diuretics and nonsteroidal anti-inflammatory agents; follow electrolytes closely
ANALGESICS		
Narcotics	Decreased cough reflex, increased CNS depression by anesthesia, hypotension	Inform anesthesiologist of use
Aspirin compounds[b]	Increased bleeding	Discontinue 1–2 weeks before surgery
ANTICOAGULANTS		
Warfarin[b]	Increased bleeding	Discontinue 48 hours before surgery, vitamin K₁ if needed, check prothrombin time before operation
DIURETICS	Electrolyte abnormalities, hypotension, inability to give orally	Obtain electrolytes and check blood pressure (lying, standing) within 24 hours preoperatively, use intravenous furosemide if needed
GOUT		
Benemid, allopurinol	Inability to give orally	Observe, treat acute gout with intravenous colchicine
DIABETES		
Oral hypoglycemics[b]	Inability to give orally	Switch to insulin preoperatively in selected patients
Insulin[b]	Risk of hyper- or hypoglycemia	Give one-third to one-half of usual dose preoperatively
THYROID THERAPY		
Thyroid hormone[b]	Inability to give orally	Usually can be discontinued for up to 7–10 days
Antithyroid drugs[b]	Inability to give orally	Use parenteral iodides or propranolol if necessary
TOPICAL DRUGS FOR GLAUCOMA		
Timolol	Systemic β-blockage	Notify anesthesiologist preoperatively
Phospholine iodide	Prolonged muscle relaxant activity	Discontinue 7–10 days preoperatively
RECREATIONAL DRUGS		
Alcohol	Affect drug metabolism, drug interactions, withdrawal syndrome, impaired respiratory function.	If possible, have patient discontinue use 1 or more weeks before admission for surgery; inform anesthesiologist and surgeon of recent use
Illicit drugs		
Tobacco[b]		

[a]If the patient will be able to take medication orally within 12 hours postoperatively, most maintenance drugs can be given at that time. If a shorter interval is crucial, a maintenance drug can be given with less than 1 ounce of water, several hours before anesthesia (e.g., 6 A.M.), and the drug can be resumed orally after surgery.
[b]See additional details in subsequent section of this chapter.

yond visiting hours, to return the patient to the same room postoperatively, to allow the presence of familiar objects, to leave a night light on, and to avoid unnecessary instrumentation. Tranquilizers, sedatives, hypnotics, and pain medications should be used in reduced doses and *for appropriate indications*, not routinely.

Postoperative mobilization of the elderly patient should be planned, and anticipated by the patient, preoperatively. In general, the patient should expect to resume ambulation as early as possible.

Surgery in the Pregnant Patient

Size of the Risk

Up to 2% of women require nonobstetric surgery during pregnancy. Risks posed to the mother and fetus include complications from the surgical problem, effects of anesthesia and medication (including teratogenicity), and precipitation of premature labor. Because of these problems, women of childbearing age who are not known to be pregnant should be screened for pregnancy before surgery. History, pelvic examination, and sensitive serum human chorionic gonadotropin pregnancy tests will usually suffice, but very early pregnancy may still be missed. If it is uncertain whether a woman is pregnant, nonurgent surgery should be postponed for 2 to 3 weeks until the situation is clarified; more urgent surgery requires judgment on an individual basis.

Physiological alterations in pregnancy that may complicate anesthetic-surgical management are listed in Table 86.7. Two common changes of pregnancy should be taken into account when evaluating the patient preoperatively: The "normal" serum creatinine is lower in pregnancy; and an S_3 gallop, a systolic murmur, or edema is commonly present in the pregnant patient without cardiac disease.

Fetal risks include teratogenicity of drugs and anesthetics, risk of diagnostic X-rays, premature labor, and fetal death. No definitive evidence exists that any one inhalational anesthetic is safer than another for the fetus.

Preoperative Planning

Preoperative planning for the pregnant surgical patient involves a number of complex issues. Considerations should include the following:

1. *Urgency of the surgery.* Can it be postponed until after delivery or is it urgent, e.g., acute appendicitis, when delay will increase fetal-maternal mortality? In general, emergency surgery should not be delayed because of pregnancy, and totally elective surgery should be postponed until the postpartum period. In intermediate situations, the duration and risk to the mother of waiting must be balanced against the risk of immediate surgery.
2. *Testing.* Tests should be carefully planned to allow a precise diagnosis with minimal risk, especially

risk from X-ray exposure. Whenever possible, other tests should be substituted for radiological procedures (e.g., a T_3 radioimmunoassay instead of I^{131} uptake in suspected hyperthyroidism or gallbladder sonogram instead of oral cholecystogram in suspected cholelithiasis). Routine X-rays, such as chest films or flat abdominal films, should be avoided. When these X-rays are unavoidable, use of lead screening, collimated equipment with minimal exposure, and few films can minimize fetal exposure. Avoidance of X-ray exposure should be remembered in the postoperative as well as the preoperative period.
3. *Medications.* Drugs required during the perioperative period should be anticipated. The potential effects on the fetus should be ascertained from obstetrical colleagues or available reference sources, and the least toxic alternative should be used. Routine drugs prescribed postoperatively should be avoided unless they are believed to be absolutely necessary.
4. *Anesthesia.* A decision on the type of anesthesia must be left to the anesthesiologist and obstetrician. Local or regional anesthesia would presumably be safer than general or spinal anesthesia, but no data exist to support this impression.
5. *Monitoring of fetal status* by the obstetrician should be planned throughout the perioperative period.

PROBLEMS AFTER DISCHARGE

Miscellaneous Problems

During the weeks and months after surgery, patients will often have questions about incisional pain, about various symptoms in the system that was operated on, and about restrictions of activity. These questions are best answered by the surgeon. In addition, patients who have major surgery will often complain of postoperative fatigue, a problem that can usually be handled by the patient's regular physician.

Postoperative Fatigue

Patients with postoperative fatigue may describe any of a number of symptoms: the need for increased sleep, weakness of the arms and legs when resuming usual activity, symptoms of orthostatic hypotension, and loss of interest in resuming usual activities (33). The physiological changes responsible for these symptoms have not been well defined.

Although the symptoms of postoperative fatigue often last for 1 or more months, it is important to evaluate each symptom carefully in order to identify drugs or underlying medical problems that may be contributing to the problem. Sleepiness may be related to sedatives, tranquilizers, or analgesics prescribed at the time of discharge and may improve with discontinuation of these drugs. The patient with orthostatic symptoms may have had a drug pre-

Table 86.7.
Physiological Alterations in Pregnancy and Their Relevance to the Surgical Patient[a]

System	Change	Clinical Implications
Cardiovascular	Uterine compression of vena cava and aorta in supine position	Decreased cardiac output and uterine perfusion; avoid supine recumbency; tilt hip 15° in perioperative period
	Decrease in blood pressure in early-mid gestation	Altered criteria for diagnosis of hypotension
	Presence of dyspnea, third heart sound and edema	No known increased risk, and such findings are not an indication for diuretic therapy or delay of surgery
Respiratory	Decreased arterial pO_2 when patient is in the supine position	Avoid supine recumbency
	Decreased pulmonary functional residual capacity and increased O_2 consumption	Increased risk of hypoxia perioperatively; avoid hypoventilation and increase inspired O_2 content prior to procedures inducing apnea (intubation or tracheal suctioning)
Arterial	Arterial pCO_2 and serum HCO_2 decrease to 30 mm Hg and 20 mmol/liter, respectively	Maternal and fetal acidosis may occur in patient ventilated to "normal," nonpregnant values of arterial pCO_2; normal values for pregnancy should be used to guide diagnosis and therapy of acid-base disturbances
Hematological	Decreased venous flow in legs and increased levels of clotting factors	Increased risk of thromboembolism; avoid supine position and consider use of support stlckings, pneumatic compression device, or prophylactic heparin
	Proximity of fetal and maternal circulations	Risk of isoimmunization; $Rh_0(D)$ immune globulin should be considered when urterine trauma is likely
Gastrointestinal	Decreased gastric motility and reduced competency of gastroesophageal sphincter	Increased risk of aspiration; preoperative antacids should be considered
Renal	Dilatation of urinary collecting system	Increased risk of urinary infection, and hence catheterization should be avoided when possible
	30 to 50% increase in glomerular filtration rate and renal plasma flow with a concomitant decrease in serum creatinine and urea nitrogen to 0.5 mg/dl and 9 mg/dl, respectively	Serum creatinine above 0.8 mg/dl may reflect impaired renal function; the clearance of many drugs is increased, and dosage schedules may require alteration

[a]From Barron WM: The pregnant surgical patient: medical evaluation and management. *Ann Intern Med* 101:683, 1984.

scribed that can produce this problem (diuretics, antihypertensives, long-acting nitrates, antidepressants); because bed rest alone may cause orthostasis, it is important to resume these drugs cautiously in a patient who has had recent major surgery and to try discontinuing the drug or reducing the dose whenever the patient complains of orthostatic symptoms. Loss of interest may also be secondary to drugs prescribed after surgery (see list of drugs that may cause a depressed mood, Chapter 15). Alternatively, this symptom may represent a minor mood disturbance in a patient who has had similar problems at previous times of stress (see Chapter 12); or it may represent a reactive depression, similar to a grief reaction (see Chapter 19), that is related to disfiguring surgery.

When evaluation of postoperative fatigue does not disclose contributing factors that can be treated, patients should be reassured that the problem will gradually resolve; and they should also be given a rough timetable for a return to regular activities that is realistic both in terms of the surgical procedure and of the fact that postoperative fatigue may take a number of months to resolve entirely. Simple exercises for patients convalescing from bed rest are illustrated in Chapter 81. For selected patients, these or similar exercises can be recommended during the period of recovery from postoperative fatigue.

THE PATIENT WITH CARDIOVASCULAR DISEASE

Overview

Most forms of general anesthesia may cause cardiovascular stresses (decreased myocardial contractility, peripheral vasodilatation, arrhythmias, hypotension); and spinal or epidural anesthesia may cause hypotension. These factors and the stresses associated with surgery itself probably account for the greatly increased risk of surgery for patients with underlying cardiovascular disease (19).

Ischemic Heart Disease

Size of the Risk

Ischemic heart disease poses two major risks perioperatively in the patient undergoing general anesthesia: myocardial infarction and death. These risks depend upon the patient's preoperative status. Overall, the risks for patients with arteriosclerotic heart disease are 2 or 3 times those of patients of the same age without cardiac disease.

The increased risk posed by ischemic heart disease is dependent on preoperative cardiac status (Table 86.8). *Stable angina pectoris* alone represents only a small increase in risk. The risk attending severe or unstable angina cannot be estimated accurately because of varying definitions and the small number of patients reported in the medical literature; but there is a significantly increased risk. A *myocardial infarction within 6 months* before surgery represents a very high risk, particularly in the first 3 months after infarction. Preliminary evidence (12, 31) suggests that aggressive perioperative management may significantly lower cardiovascular risk (e.g., reduce recurrent myocardial infarction risk from 30 to 4%); but this remains to be confirmed. Even 6 months after an infarction, the risk of a perioperative myocardial infarction is considerably larger than the risk in a control population.

In addition to a recent myocardial infarction, a number of factors contribute to the risk of perioperative cardiac complications or mortality. The most important of these factors are decompensated congestive heart failure, arrhythmias, and significant chronic obstructive lung disease. These and other factors have been incorporated into a *Cardiac Risk Index* (Tables 86.9 and 86.10) (7, 15, 16). This cardiac risk index has been validated in other studies (7), but it should not be used as an absolute classification. However, it provides helpful guidelines for assessing the significance of multiple risk factors.

Preoperative Planning

Office Evaluation. Patients with established ischemic heart disease should have a comprehensive preoperative evaluation (see Table 86.2). Noninvasive tests of cardiac function including echocardiography, nuclear scanning, and stress tests should generally be reserved for situations where the presence or severity of cardiovascular disease is questioned.

Based upon the preoperative evaluation, the risk of general anesthesia and surgery should be estimated for each patient. For patients with recent myocardial infarction (within less than 6 months), with unstable angina, or with less severe coronary artery disease and

Table 86.8.
Approximate Cardiovascular Risk in Relation to Preoperative Cardiac Status

Patient Preoperative Status	Approximate Risk of Postoperative Myocardial Infarction (%)	Approximate Mortality Risk (%)
No "cardiac" disease	0.2–2[a]	3[a]
"Cardiac disease" present	6	5
Angina (stable)	3	3–10
Postmyocardial infarction		
<3 months	30–35	25–40
<6 months	25	18–20
3–6 months	15–20	10–20
>6 months	5	No data

[a]Risk varies with age of population studied.

Table 86.9.
Cardiac Risk Index in Surgical Patients[a]

Risk Factors	Points for Cardiac Risk Index (see Table 86.7)
HISTORY	
Myocardial infarction in past 6 months	10
Age >70	5
PHYSICAL	
S_3 gallop or jugular venous distention	11
Significant aortic stenosis	3
ECG	
Rhythm other than sinus or premature atrial contractions on last preoperative ECG	7
>5 premature ventricular contractions/minute any time preoperatively	7
OTHER ORGAN SYSTEMS	
$pO_2 < 60$, $pCO_2 > 50$	
$K < 3.0$, $HCO_3 < 20$ mEq/dl	
BUN > 50	
CR > 3.0 mg/dl	
Signs of chronic liver disease or elevated aminotransferase	3 (each factor)
Bedridden from noncardiac causes	
OPERATION	
Intraperitoneal or intrathoracic	3
Emergency	4
TOTAL POSSIBLE	53

[a]Adapted from Goldman L, Caldera DL, Nussbaum SR, *et al*: Multifactorial index of cardiac risk in noncardiac surgical procedures. *N Engl J Med* 297:845, 1977.

Table 86.10.
Cardiac Risk Index (Based on a Prospective Study of Patients at the Massachusetts General Hospital)[a]

Class	Point Toal[b]	No or Moderate Complication (N = 943)[c] (%)	Life-Threatening Complication (N = 39)[d] (%)	Cardiac Deaths (N = 19)[e] (%)
I	0–5	99	0.7	0.2
II	6–12	93	5	2
III	13–25	86	11	2
IV	≥26	22	22	56

[a]Adapted from Goldman L, Caldera DL, Nussbaum SR, *et al*: Multifactorial index of cardiac risk in noncardiac surgical procedures. *N Engl J Med* 297:845, 1977.
[b]See Table 86.6.
[c]New or worsened heart failure without pulmonary edema, supraventricular tachyarrhythmia, or intraoperative or postoperative ischemia (as indicated by chest pain or ECG changes) without documented myocardial infarction.
[d]Documented intraoperative or postoperative myocardial infarction, pulmonary edema, or ventricular tachycardia without progression to cardiac death.
[e]Deaths due to arrhythmia or to low output heart failure.

multiple other risk factors (see Table 86.9), only urgent lifesaving surgery should be undertaken until the risk is lowered. Surgery may be done 3 months after infarction when the risk of waiting the additional 3 months is thought to be significant (e.g., recurrent cholecystitis). Patients with stable angina or uncomplicated recovery from myocardial infarction more than 6 months previously have an increased risk that does not decline further with time; thus, there is no need to postpone necessary operations.

Coronary artery bypass surgery should be considered before elective noncardiac surgery, in consultation with a cardiologist, in patients who have other indications for bypass surgery (see Chapter 57).

Recommendations to the Surgeon. A baseline electrocardiogram (ECG) should be obtained before surgery for all patients with known coronary artery disease and for all patients over age 35. Routine postoperative ECGs should be obtained only in high risk patients (e.g., all patients with known coronary artery disease and any adults who develop hypotension during surgery), since the yield of useful information from them is low.

For patients taking a long-acting oral nitrate for angina, the drug should be administered on the morning of surgery with a sip of water. Although the patient is unable to take medications orally, nitroglycerine paste or a transdermal patch should be substituted; because there is no simple way to determine the paste dose equivalent to an oral nitrate, an intermediate dose equivalent to 1 to 2 inches of nitral paste every 4 to 6 hours should be recommended.

For patients taking a beta-blocking agent for angina, intravenous small doses of propranolol (i.e., 1 to 2 mg every 6 hours or a continuous infusion of 1/2 to 3 mg/ hr*) should be substituted, given by a physician, while the patient is unable to take medications by mouth. This should protect the patient from the risk of acute cardiac ischemia, which occasionally follows abrupt cessation of beta-blocking agent. Patients able to resume oral intake within 12 to 24 hours usually can be observed without intravenous propranolol.

Calcium blocking agents should usually be given orally up to the morning of surgery. Another type of antianginal medication must be used postoperatively until the patient can resume oral intake.

Intensive intraoperative monitoring using Swan-Ganz and radial artery catheters should be planned for patients who are very sensitive to volume changes, such as those in congestive heart failure (see below), for operations when loss and replacement of large volumes of fluid are expected (e.g., aneurysm repair), and for patients with a recent myocardial infarction (< 6 months) or severe, unstable coronary disease.

Hypertension

Size of the Risk

Controversy still exists about whether mild to moderate hypertension (diastolic ≤110 mg Hg) increases anesthetic and surgical risks. The only prospective study showed no correlation between uncontrolled diastolic pressures in this range and the risk of perioperative cardiac, renal, or cerebrovascular events (14). Patients in this study often had other cardiac risk factors that did correlate with the incidence of perioperative cardiac morbidity (see Tables 86.9 and 86.11).

---

* This is not an United States Food and Drug Administration (FDA)-approved method of administration.

Too few patients have been studied to define adequately the risk for persons operated on when their diastolic pressure exceeds 110 mm Hg, but there is probably an increased risk (30). Likewise, control of hypertension may be more important in selected patients with severe cardiac, renal, or cerebrovascular disease.

Preoperative Planning

Office Evaluation. The basic preoperative evaluation in the hypertensive patient should establish whether there is end organ damage (renal: serum creatinine concentration and urinalysis; cerebrovascular: history, neurological and neurovascular examination; and cardiovascular: history, cardiac examination, chest X-ray, and ECG). Blood pressure and pulse measurements should be made with the patient lying or sitting and standing (after brief exercise, to identify the maximal orthostatic fall in patients taking antihypertensive drugs); the preoperative status of blood pressure control may then be classified as untreated, hypertensive despite therapy, or controlled.

Patients who are controlled, or patients who are partially controlled and have diastolic pressures ≤110 mm Hg, should be continued on their prescribed antihypertensive medication. Two exceptions to this rule are guanethidine and monoamine oxidase inhibitors. A patient taking either of these infrequently used drugs should be switched to a different drug as both of these drugs may cause markedly labile blood pressure during anesthesia.

Untreated patients with diastolic pressures ≤110 mm Hg may undergo surgery, with institution of antihypertensive therapy after convalescence from surgery.

Individual judgments must be made about patients with diastolic pressures ≥110 mm Hg, depending on the severity and duration of hypertension, the presence of end organ damage, and the extent of planned surgery. Most patients with diastolic ≥110 mm Hg should have their blood pressure at least partly controlled before admission for nonurgent surgery (30), although there are no studies proving that such control modifies risks. Attempts to control blood pressure too rapidly (for example, rapid increases in diuretic treatment over several days) may result in volume depletion, hypokalemia, or hypotension at the time of surgery. Therefore, these patients should have their blood pressure stabilized during 1 to 2 weeks before admission for surgery.

Recommendations to the Surgeon. For all hypertensive patients it is important to advise the surgeon to avoid significant intravascular volume expansion or contraction, as these conditions may either cause a significant rise in blood pressure (volume expansion) or fall in blood pressure (volume contraction, especially in the patient who is taking antihypertensive drugs).

Current antihypertensive medications should be

Table 86.11.
Risk of Perioperative Cardiac Complications in Patients with Mild to Moderate Hypertension[a]

Preoperative Characteristics	Mean Point Total[b] (± SEM)	Patients with No Cardiac Complication (%)	Patients with Minor Complications Only (%)	Patients with Major Nonfatal Complications (%)	Patients with Cardiac Death (%)
Normal blood pressure No history of hypertension	4.3 ± 0.3	89	9	2	0.2
Hypertension controlled Taking antihypertensive drug(s)	6.9 ± 0.6	76	15	8	1
Hypertensive Taking antihypertensive drug(s)	4.4 ± 0.5	93	8		1
Hypertensive Not taking antihypertensive drug(s)	5.5 ± 0.6	88	9	1	1

[a]Adapted from Goldman L, Caldera DL: Risks of general anesthesia and elective operation in the hypertensive patient. *Anesthesiology* 50:285, 1979.
[b]See Tables 86.10 and 86.11 for risk factor index.

continued through the morning of surgery and resumed postoperatively when the patient is stable and can take oral medications (diuretics are usually withheld the morning of surgery). Because of bed rest and inactivity during convalescence, some patients will require less antihypertensive medication postoperatively and during the first few weeks after major surgery.

In some patients, the diastolic pressure will exceed 110 mm Hg postoperatively, before oral medication can be resumed. For such patients, the surgeon should know that there are several regimens that will reliably control the blood pressure when carefully administered and adjusted. These regimens are (a) propranolol (1 to 2 mg intravenously every 4 to 6 hours or a continuous infusion of 1/2 to 3 mg/hour[†]) plus hydralazine (10 to 50 mg intravenously every 4 to 6 hours); (b) nifedipine (contents of a 10-mg capsule sublingually every 4 to 6 hours, not recommended as a first choice because of the possibility of excessive hypotension); and (c) transcutaneous clonidine (one or more patches, lasting up to 7 days), especially for patients who were taking clonidine before surgery and are at risk of rebound hypertension and tachycardia due to clonidine withdrawal. Further details about these drugs are found in Chapter 62.

Valvular Heart Disease

Size of the Risk

The risk of surgery in the patient with valvular heart disease varies with the valve affected (aortic versus mitral), the nature (stenosis versus insufficiency), and the severity of the lesion (16). The severity of valvular lesions as judged clinically by New York Heart Association (NYHA) classification (see Table 61.3A) provides a reasonable indication of surgical risk with the exception of aortic stenosis.

Valvular heart disease poses two major surgical risks: cardiac death and congestive heart failure. The presence of aortic stenosis of any degree of hemodynamic significance poses a high risk of surgical mortality. Mild to moderate mitral lesions or aortic insufficiency represent only slightly increased risks of cardiac death; however, hemodynamically severe valvular disease (i.e., NYHA class 3 or 4) due to these lesions creates major risks. In addition to increasing the risk of perioperative mortality, significant valvular disease poses an increased risk of decompensated heart failure.

Little specific information exists regarding the risks associated with prolapsed mitral valve or with hypertrophic cardiomyopathy. It is reasonable to assume that the risk in patients with prolapsed mitral valve depends upon the degree of mitral regurgitation. Patients with hypertrophic cardiomyopathy may be very sensitive to volume contraction and are probably best managed with a Swan-Ganz catheter in place during major procedures associated with rapid volume changes.

Patients with artificial heart valves, patients with any evidence of valvular heart disease (including mitral prolapse and hypertrophic cardiomyopathy), and patients with congenital structural defects (e.g., patent ductus arteriosus, ventricular septal defect) have a small but definite risk of acquiring bacterial endocarditis when they undergo procedures in the oral cavity and upper respiratory, gastrointestinal, or genitourinary tracts.

Preoperative Planning

Office Evaluation. The basic cardiac evaluation should delineate the nature and severity of the valvular disease and should identify any associated cardiac conditions. The uses of echocardiography and cardiac catheterization to evaluate valvular heart disease are described in Chapter 60. Patients with severe valvular disease should have corrective cardiac surgery followed by a period of convalescence before they undergo major noncardiac operations.

Recommendations to the Surgeon. Patients undergoing procedures attended by a risk of endocarditis should receive antimicrobial prophylaxis as summarized in Table 86.12.

[†]This is not an FDA-approved method of administration.

Table 86.12.
Prevention of Bacterial Endocarditis in Patients with Valvular Heart Disease, Prostatic Heart Valves, and Other Abnormalities of the Cardiovascular System[a]

ENDOCARDITIS PROPHYLAXIS[b]
Dosage for Adults

DENTAL AND UPPER RESPIRATORY PROCEDURES[c]

Oral[d]

Amoxicillin[e]	3 g 1 hour before procedure and 1.5 g 6 hours later

Penicillin allergy:

Erythromycin	1 g 2 hours before procedure and 500 mg 6 hours later

Parenteral[d,f]

Ampicillin	2 grams IM or IV 30 minutes before procedure
plus Gentamicin	1.5 mg/kg IM or IV 30 minutes before procedure

Penicillin allergy:

Vancomycin	1 g IV infused *slowly over 1 hour* beginning 1 hour before procedure

GASTROINTESTINAL AND GENITOURINARY PROCEDURES[c]

Oral[d]

Amoxicillin[e]	3 g 1 hour before procedure and 1.5 g 6 hours later

Parenteral[d,f]

Ampicillin	2 g IM or IV 30 minutes before procedure
plus Gentamicin	1.5 mg/kg IM or IV 30 minutes before procedure

Penicillin allergy:

Vancomycin	1 g IV infused *slowly over 1 hour* beginning 1 hour before procedure
plus Gentamicin	1.5 mg/kg IM or IV 30 minutes before procedure

[a] From *Med Lett* 31:112, 1989 (omits information for children).
[b] For patients with previous endocarditis, valvular heart disease, prosthetic heart valves, most forms of congenital heart disease (but uncomplicated secundum atrial septal defect), idiopathic hypertrophic subaortic stenosis, and mitral valve prolapse with regurgitation. Viridans streptococci are the most common cause of endocarditis after dental or upper respiratory procedures; enterococci are the most common cause of endocarditis after gastrointestinal or genitourinary procedures.
[c] For a review of the risk of bacteremia and endocarditis with various procedures, see D Durack in GL Mandell et al, eds., *Principles and Practice of Infectious Disease*, 3rd ed, New York: Churchill Livingstone, 1990, p. 716.
[d] Oral regimens are more convenient and safer. Parenteral regimens are more likely to be effective; they are recommended especially for patients with prosthetic heart valves, those who have had endocarditis previously, or those taking continuous oral penicillin for rheumatic fever prophylaxis.
[e] Amoxicillin is recommended because of its excellent bioavailability and good activity against streptococci and enterococci.
[f] A single dose of parenteral drugs is probably adequate, because bacteremia after most dental and diagnostic procedures is of short duration. An additional dose may be given 8 hours later in patients judged to be at higher risk.

The preoperative management of congestive heart failure, arrhythmia, or anticoagulant therapy (in patients with artificial valves) is described in subsequent sections of this chapter.

Congestive Heart Failure

Size of the Risk

Information on the risk of developing congestive heart failure (CHF) perioperatively is limited because of the few studies available. However, the best prospective studies (16) closely correspond to general clinical experience. The most significant risk factors for postoperative CHF are decompensated failure preoperatively and, to a lesser extent, prior CHF that is clinically stable preoperatively (Table 86.13). However, only 40% of patients who develop perioperative CHF have had prior failure. The best predictors for the other 60% of patients are age greater than 60, major surgery (especially abdominal aortic aneurysm repair or major abdominal surgery), and nonspecific electrocardiographic abnormalities.

Patients with postoperative pulmonary edema have a high total mortality (20 to 57%), most of which is cardiac. Patients who develop less severe postoperative CHF do not have an increased risk of postoperative cardiac death, although the overall mortality from all causes is increased. Most postoperative CHF occurs during or within several hours of surgery.

Preoperative Planning

Office Evaluation. Patients with compensated CHF should have a comprehensive preoperative evaluation (see Table 86.2). This evaluation should include an assessment of volume status (lying and standing blood pressures, inspection of neck veins, determination of whether edema is present) and examination for cardiac gallops and for rales. Laboratory data should include a digoxin level if that drug is being administered. Noninvasive methods for assessing left ventricular function (see Chapter 61) may be useful when the degree of cardiac dysfunction is uncertain.

Although there are no definitive studies in this regard, it is prudent to *digitalize* patients with a confirmed history of moderate or severe congestive cardiomyopathy, ideally during the week before admission. Most controversy about preoperative digitalization has concerned the patient who has a past history of no or minimal CHF yet has a "risk" of developing

Table 86.13.
Risks of Developing Congestive Failure (CHF) in Perioperative Period[a,b]

Patient Characteristics	Size of Risk	
	All CHF (%)	Pulmonary edema (%)
No prior CHF	4	2
Past CHF:		
All—now compensated	16	6
Past pulmonary edema (regardless of current status)	32	23
Decompensated CHF preoperatively	21	16
Preoperative physical findings:		
S₃ gallop	47	35
Jugular venous distention	35	30
New York Heart Association class preoperatively (see Table 61.3)		
1	5	3
2	7	7
3	18	6
4	31	25

[a] Adapted from Goldman L, Caldera DL, Southwick FS, *et al*: Cardiac risk factors and complications in non-cardiac surgery. *Medicine (Baltimore)* 57; 357, 1978.
[b] Based upon 1001 consecutive patients undergoing general surgery, orthopaedic surgery, or urological surgery (transurethral resection of the prostate omitted because of existing evidence of its safety even in elderly patients).

CHF because of an enlarged heart or because the surgery will involve major volume shifts. Although data are lacking, it is likely that digitalis does not help the latter type of patient and that the risk of digitalis toxicity is not warranted (8).

Patients with decompensated CHF should have all but lifesaving surgery postponed until the failure is controlled, either in the office or in the hospital.

Recommendations to the Surgeon. Patients with controlled CHF should be maintained on their usual oral regimen until midnight before surgery and maintained with intravenous diuretics and digoxin (75% of the oral dose) during the immediate postoperative period.

Arrhythmias

The arrhythmias that are encountered most frequently in ambulatory patients are described in detail in Chapter 59.

Size of the Risk

Patients with arrhythmias before surgery have significantly increased risks of cardiac morbidity and death. These risks have not been quantified for subgroups of patients with specific arrhythmias, except as indicated in the Cardiac Risk Index shown in Tables 86.9 and 86.10. Patients with complete heart block, Mobitz type II second degree block, and sick sinus syndrome have a significant risk of complications during anesthesia if a pacemaker is not inserted. On the other hand, there is little or no increased risk associated with bi- or trifascicular block on ECG in patients who are asymptomatic.

Arrhythmias do occur in approximately 20% or more of adult patients during general anesthesia; however, most of these patients do not have preoperative arrhythmias. Most intraoperative arrhythmias are supraventricular, transient, related to specific anesthetic or surgical manipulation, and do not require specific therapies. The number of arrhythmias that are detected clinically, without the use of continuous monitoring, is lower: Supraventricular arrhythmias are detected clinically in 4% of patients and other arrhythmias in 11% (13, 16).

Preoperative Planning

Office Evaluation. Patients with arrhythmias should have the comprehensive preoperative evaluation (Table 86.2) expanded in several ways. The probable etiology of the arrhythmia should be delineated (see Chapter 59). If the arrhythmia is intermittent or control is not certain, 24-hour Holter monitoring should be done. Drug levels of antiarrhythmic drugs that are being administered should be obtained. In general, this entire evaluation should be accomplished before admission for surgery.

Patients with *supraventricular arrhythmias* should have their ventricular rates controlled or should be converted to more stable rhythms. Except for atrial

fibrillation, this usually means conversion either to normal sinus rhythm or to atrial fibrillation, since other supraventricular arrhythmias are either hemodynamically unstable or give an unpredictable ventricular response even with appropriate drug therapy. Patients with atrial fibrillation should have their rates slowed but should be able to accelerate their heart rate under stress as indicated by their ability to raise their pulse rate more than 10 points by mild exercise.

Established indications for *preoperative digitalization* in patients with arrhythmias are control of rate in atrial fibrillation and prophylaxis of supraventricular arrhythmias in selected patients (e.g., patients with past histories of supraventricular arrhythmias, especially atrial fibrillation or flutter, who remain at high risk for recurrence; and patients with significant mitral stenosis).

Patients with ventricular premature beats (VPBs) or other ventricular arrhythmias should be treated according to the criteria outlined in Chapter 59.

Recommendations to the Surgeon. Antiarrhythmic drugs should be continued orally through the morning before surgery, after which the following intravenous treatment should be substituted until the patient is able to take oral medications again: intravenous digoxin (75% of the oral dose) for patients taking digoxin, and intravenous lidocaine or procainamide for patients taking quinidine or disopyramide for ventricular arrhythmias.

There is general agreement that patients undergoing general anesthesia should have a *prophylactic or therapeutic pacemaker* inserted for the following conditions:

1. Symptomatic or significant dysfunction of the sinoatrial node;
2. Idioventricular rhythm;
3. Current or past history of third degree or Mobitz type II second degree atrioventricular (AV) block;
4. Some instances of Mobitz type I second degree AV block;
5. Some patients with trifascicular block (right bundle branch block plus left anterior hemiblock plus first degree AV block; alternating left and right bundle branch block; or left bundle branch block and first degree AV block) especially in the presence of severe valvular disease, ischemic disease, or congestive failure;
6. A history of Stokes-Adams attacks.

Patients with a history suggesting bradyarrhythmias (especially a history of syncope or near syncope and an underlying ECG abnormality) probably should have a temporary pacemaker recommended if a full workup to evaluate the etiology of the symptoms cannot be performed preoperatively or is not revealing. Isolated conditions for which a pacemaker is more controversial, but generally not indicated, include bifascicular block, bundle branch block, first degree AV block, and sinus bradycardia that is asymptomatic.

THE PATIENT WITH PULMONARY DISEASE

Overview

Patients with significant pulmonary disease have an increased mortality and morbidity during surgery. The increased risks are due chiefly to the following physiological changes produced by the effects of anesthesia, sedatives, and analgesics: (a) abnormalities of pulmonary gas exchange, causing hypoxemia; (b) depression of the cough reflex and decrease in clearance of respiratory secretions; (c) respiratory depression; and (d) loss of sighing and normal lung inflation—each of which increases the risk of atelectasis and pneumonia. In addition, normal breathing and voluntary coughing are decreased after surgery because of pain and discomfort, especially after upper abdominal and thoracic surgery. Optimal preoperative treatment of pulmonary disease can reduce perioperative morbidity and mortality (27, 40).

Chronic Obstructive Pulmonary Disease (COPD)

Size of the Risk

The precise risk of perioperative death from pulmonary causes for patients with COPD is not known because of the lack of information regarding patients with mild lung disease. In patients with moderate to severe COPD, pulmonary deaths occur in about 4% (versus 0 to 2% of unselected patients) and pulmonary complications in 36% (versus 9% of unselected patients) (20).

The presence of a smoking history, dyspnea, cough, or abnormal spirometry increases the risk of minor postoperative pulmonary complications (i.e., atelectasis or infection without significant respiratory compromise). The risk of respiratory failure requiring vigorous postoperative respiratory therapy is increased in patients with an FEV_1 (forced expiratory volume in 1 second) less than 1.5 liters. A FEV_1 less than 1.0 liter or a pCO_2 greater than 45 mm Hg defines a high risk group with a marked increase in perioperative pulmonary mortality and in the incidence of postoperative respiratory failure requiring prolonged mechanical ventilation.

A number of nonpulmonary factors are helpful in predicting postoperative pulmonary complications in patients with COPD (Table 86.14). The greatest risks are in patients who are older than 60, who undergo upper abdominal and thoracic operations or operations under general anesthesia lasting more than 3 hours, or who have repeated operations within 1 year. A much lower risk is posed by operations on the extremities, back, breast, and central nervous system. Lower abdominal surgery represents an intermediate risk. Combining these factors with the pulmonary factors listed above increases the physician's ability to predict operative morbidity.

The type of anesthesia may affect the risk of pulmonary complications. Local anesthesia creates very little risk; if the patient is heavily sedated, however,

Table 86.14.
Nonpulmonary Factors that Increase Pulmonary Risks during General Surgery

MOST IMPORTANT
    Age over 60
    Upper abdominal or thoracic operation
    Repeat operations within 1 year
OTHER
    General anesthesia lasting more than 3 hours
    Obesity
    Abnormal ECG
    Poor patient effort/cooperation
    Narcotic analgesics
    Minor upper respiratory illness

there may be temporary deterioration in respiratory control and there may be a suppression of the cough reflex. Spinal anesthesia has been reported to be associated with a relatively low mortality rate in patients with COPD (37) in some studies. Because of the simultaneous use of sedatives and because the patient must ventilate in the supine position, spinal anesthesia creates a significant risk of intraoperative and postoperative respiratory complications; this is especially true of obese patients with chronic pulmonary disease. Because of these problems, general anesthesia, which permits control of ventilation and clearance of secretions, is often preferable to spinal anesthesia in patients with moderate or severe COPD.

Preoperative Planning

Office Evaluation. Patients with known COPD should have a comprehensive preoperative evaluation (see Table 86.2) and additional evaluation focused upon the status of their pulmonary disease (39). If they are taking aminophylline, they should have measurement of the serum aminophylline concentration and adjustment of the dose if it is above or below the therapeutic range. Any history of smoking, chronic or intermittent sputum production, recent upper respiratory infection, dyspnea on effort, or concomitant cardiovascular disease is particularly pertinent. Ideally smokers should stop smoking 2 weeks before admission for surgery to be performed under general or spinal anesthesia, and patients with upper respiratory infections should have surgery postponed at least 2 weeks, regardless of how minor the episode.

Table 86.15 summarizes for patients undergoing general or spinal anesthesia the principal indications for preadmission spirometry alone [forced vital capacity (FVC) and FEV_1] or for spirometry plus long volumes and arterial blood gases. Unfortunately, major operations are often performed without pulmonary function testing, despite the fact that even experienced clinicians sometimes misjudge the severity of obstructive lung disease. Spirometry will clarify the presence and severity of lung disease in questionable cases.

Pulmonary consultation should be obtained for patients whose FEV_1 is less than 1.0 liter and for patients with less severe pulmonary disease who are being evaluated for thoracic or upper abdominal surgery.

Table 86.15.
Indications for Pulmonary Function Test in Preoperative Patients with Pulmonary Disease

SPIROMETRY ONLY (FEV$_1$ and FVC)
  Smokers (>10 pack years)
  Any pulmonary symptoms (e.g., dyspnea, wheezing, cough, or sputum production)
  Upper abdominal surgery
  Age >60
  Repeat surgery within 1 year
  Multiple other risk factors (obesity, recent upper respiratory infections, narcotics abuse, abnormal ECG)
SPIROMETRY, LUNG VOLUMES, AND ARTERIAL BLOOD GASES
  Thoracic surgery
  Upper abdominal surgery and pulmonary disease
  Patients with restrictive lung disease
  Patients with chronic obstructive pulmonary disease with FEV$_1$ < 1.0 liter

Recommendations to the Surgeon. After admission to the hospital, the patient should be instructed preoperatively about coughing and deep breathing exercises, as well as the use of devices such as an incentive spirometer that will be used postoperatively. Patients already taking bronchodilators should continue their regimen through the morning of surgery; patients who have a history of intermittent airways obstruction should also be started on a theophylline compound before surgery. In order to prevent bronchospasm, especially in the immediate postoperative period, inhaled specific β$_2$-sympathomimetics and intravenous aminophylline should be administered, and the serum aminophylline level should be kept in the therapeutic range (10 to 20 mg/liter) during the time that the patient cannot take oral medications. Patients who have received corticosteroids for more than 2 weeks during the year before surgery should be appropriately covered for stress with parenteral steroids (see below). Patients with chronic purulent sputum production should receive a 5- to 7-day course of broad spectrum antibiotics (tetracycline, ampicillin, or trimethoprim-sulfamethoxazole) to decrease the quantity and purulence of secretions. Finally, arterial blood gases should be checked in all patients with moderate to severe COPD just before and just after surgery. There is some dispute about the efficacy of most of these individual measures. However, controlled trials have shown that the combination, preoperatively, of bronchodilators, antibiotics, lung expression, and mobilization of secretions decreases the number of perioperative complications (35, 37).

Lung Resection and COPD

Overall mortality rates for lung resection are about 5% for lobectomy and about 15% for total pneumonectomy. The mortality and morbidity rates for lung surgery vary widely depending upon patient factors (particularly age and pulmonary function), type of operation (pneumonectomy, lobectomy, segmental resection), and experience and skill of the surgical team.

Assessment of pulmonary function in the patient with COPD who has an indication for lung resection (usually a tumor) should be performed in the ambulatory setting. Use of the following criteria to select candidates for lung resection has reduced mortality for patients with COPD.

For *pneumonectomy*, the major criteria for operability are FEV$_1$ ⩾2 liters and FVC ⩾50% of predicted. Patients with an FEV$_1$ less than 2 liters should have quantitative perfusion lung scanning to determine the FEV$_1$ that can be expected after pneumonectomy (e.g., if 30% of perfusion and ventilation goes to the affected lung, the patient's pulmonary function will be decreased by approximately 30% postoperatively). Those with a predicted postoperative FEV$_1$ as low as 0.8 to 1 liter can undergo pneumonectomy, although their mortality risk is probably increased.

Patients not meeting the criteria for pneumonectomy may tolerate *lobectomy* or *segmental resection*. Most patients with a preoperative FEV$_1$ ⩾1.5 liters can tolerate a lobectomy. The patient may undergo resection of the segment or lobe if the predicted postoperative FEV$_1$ is greater than 0.8 to 1 liter.

Other measures in the preoperative planning for the patient with COPD undergoing pulmonary resection are similar to those described for such patients in the preceding section.

Asthma

Size of the Risk

Asthma affects approximately 3% of Americans, which makes it one of the most common pulmonary diseases (see Chapter 55). It is difficult to give a firm estimate of the operative risks posed by asthma because in most reports data on asthma are pooled with results for other types of obstructive airways disease. The most dangerous period for the asthmatic is not usually the period during general anesthesia, since the anesthetic may be an effective bronchodilator, but the immediate postoperative period. The major risks are severe bronchospasm and inspissation of thick secretions.

Preoperative Planning

Office Evaluation. The asthmatic patient should have a comprehensive evaluation (see Table 86.2) in the office before admission for surgery. This allows adequate time for changes in chronic management prior to admission. The patient should stop smoking 2 weeks before surgery.

Recommendations to the Surgeon. Spirometry (FEV$_1$ and FVC) should be performed in all asthmatic patients the day before the operation. Arterial blood gases should be measured in patients who are not in their stable baseline state or who have significant abnormalities in FEV$_1$. β$_2$-Sympathomimetics can be continued, as inhaled aerosols, until the induction of anesthesia and can be resumed in the recovery room. The serum concentration of aminophylline should be measured in all patients preoperatively because of the large number who have subtherapeutic or toxic levels on standard doses; planning for the immediate preoperative period should include continuation of oral bronchodilators through the morning of surgery and scheduling of surgery early in the day to avoid the need for preoperative intravenous aminophylline. In very severe asthmatics, a constant infusion of aminophylline should be recommended for the preoperative period and for the period when the patient is unable to take medicine by mouth; other patients are adequately managed by resuming aminophylline, intravenously, in the recovery room. Patients taking maintenance corticosteroids or who have been taking systemic corticosteroids for more than 2 weeks during the previous year should receive doses of parenteral steroids sufficient to cover the stress of surgery (see below) (29).

The Patient with Renal Disease

Size of the Risk

The size of the operative risk for patients with chronic renal disease depends upon the severity of their disease (see Chapter 47). Overall, the surgical mortality after major surgery in patients with severe renal disease (i.e., creatinine clearance less than 10 to 15 ml/minute including patients on dialysis) is about 2 to 4% when these patients are managed carefully. In patients not requiring dialysis, postoperative acute renal failure is the gravest complication, as it carries a high mortality (4, 5).

The major complications associated with surgery in the patient with moderate to severe renal disease are electrolyte disturbances (especially acidosis and hyperkalemia), volume contraction, volume overload, toxicity due to agents that are nephrotoxic or that are excreted by the kidneys, and bleeding. Volume contraction, with the risk of ischemic cerebral, cardiac, or renal damage, is a particular risk in patients with the nephrotic syndrome; these patients usually have a slightly contracted intravascular volume at baseline and are at risk of hypovolemia if an effort is made to decrease their edema with potent diuretics preoperatively. Toxic renal damage may follow the use of two agents that are frequently used in the perioperative period: radiocontrast agents and aminoglycoside antibiotics.

Preoperative Planning

Office Evaluation. Before admission for surgery, patients with chronic renal failure should have the comprehensive evaluation outlined in Table 86.2, and current volume status should be documented. Radiocontrast studies should be avoided, if at all possible, in the preoperative workup of patients with serum creatinine concentrations greater than 4.5 mg/100 ml or other risk factors, since the subsequent risk of acute renal failure is about 30% (4, 34).

Recommendations to the Surgeon. The most important consideration in perioperative management of patients who do not require dialysis is avoidance of

fluid imbalance. When the surgery carries a risk of significant volume shifts, Swan-Ganz catheterization should be considered to assure close monitoring of the intravascular volume. Administration of drugs such as antihypertensives should follow the guidelines stated elsewhere in this chapter. Adjustments in the doses of drugs should be appropriate for the patient's degree of renal insufficiency (2). The concentration of electrolytes and creatinine in the serum should be monitored carefully before and after surgery, to detect, particularly, hyperkalemia and deterioration of renal function. Patients with renal failure frequently have a metabolic acidosis compensated by hyperventilation; postoperatively continued appropriate hyperventilation will be necessary to avoid a potential precipitous fall in arterial pH. Preoperative prophylactic dialysis is not generally recommended in the patient not already on chronic dialysis. Furthermore, patients with a chronic anemia secondary to renal failure usually are well compensated and do not require preoperative transfusion unless they are symptomatic from the anemia or a large blood loss is expected during surgery.

In general, the nephrologist caring for patients on chronic dialysis should coordinate the medical management of these patients throughout the surgical episode. Although these patients have a very high postoperative complication rate (due to hyperkalemia, bleeding, arteriovenous fistula thrombosis, pneumonia, wound infection, and arrhythmias), their risk of dying due to surgery remains in the 2 to 4% range if they are carefully managed (3).

THE PATIENT WITH ENDOCRINE DISEASE

Diabetes Mellitus

Size of the Risk

Total surgical mortality for al diabetic patients is about 2 to 4%; less than 0.3% die as a result of poor control of their diabetes. About 14% of diabetics have postoperative complications that may be related to diabetes, particularly wound infection (41).

Preoperative Planning

Office Evaluation. Each diabetic patient should have the comprehensive preoperative evaluation outlined in Table 86.2. Patients controlled with diet alone or with oral agents may be handled as same day admissions if their diabetes is mild or if the planned procedure is minor. Otherwise they should be admitted one day before surgery, so that adequate time is allowed for switching to insulin. In general, insulin-dependent diabetics should be admitted 1 day before surgery in order to assure satisfactory preoperative control of their diabetes.

Recommendations to the Surgeon. Measurements of fasting blood sugars should be obtained on all diabetics on the day before and on the day of surgery, and their state of hydration should be evaluated to assure that they are not significantly volume contracted. Elective surgery should not be undertaken until diabetes is at least reasonably controlled (i.e., fasting blood sugar of 250 mg/100 ml or less).

The appropriate perioperative treatment of diabetes depends upon the type of surgical procedure planned and upon the preadmission regimen, as summarized in Table 86.16.

Diabetics who are controlled by diet can be monitored with daily fasting blood sugars throughout the operative episode and treated with insulin if unacceptable rises in glucose occur.

Management of *patients taking oral agents* varies because they represent a heterogeneous group. Patients with mild elevations of glucose who are undergoing minor procedures that will allow them to eat the same day can take their hypoglycemic drug on the day *before* surgery and resume it when they begin eating on the day of surgery. The exception is the patient taking chlorpropamide (Diabinese), which should be withheld 2 to 3 days before surgery because of its long half-life. If the patient is to undergo a major procedure, oral agents should be discontinued because they have long half-lives, control is less predictable, and the drugs cannot be given parenterally. Therefore, such a patient should be switched to management by diet only or to insulin. Human insulin is preferred for the patient who has not taken insulin previously.

For the patient who is *taking insulin before surgery*, one of several strategies is recommended for the preoperative period (see Table 86.16). Because of its simplicity and the small risk of hypoglycemia, the first regimen (giving one-half to two-thirds of the usual total daily dose of long-acting insulin preoperatively) is the preferred regimen. Postoperative management is easiest with a single morning dose of long-acting insulin, with the dose adjusted according to the metabolic status and calorie intake; supplemental regular insulin may be given as needed. Blood sugar measurement using a bedside technique is recommended; measurement of a fasting glucose and of electrolytes by the clinical laboratory should be obtained daily in the immediate postoperative period.

Adrenal Insufficiency and Chronic Steroid Therapy

Size of the Risk

It is generally agreed that patients who are currently taking a *pharmacological dose* of corticosteroids (i.e., more than the equivalent of 20 to 30 mg of hydrocortisone daily), who have taken corticosteroids at a pharmacological dose for 2 or more weeks in the past year, or who are receiving replacement doses for adrenal insufficiency are at risk of developing adrenal insufficiency because of the stress of surgery (41).

Patients in each of these groups should therefore receive extra corticosteroids in the perioperative period (see Chapter 74 for additional details).

Preoperative Planning

Office Evaluation. These patients should have a comprehensive evaluation before admission (see Table 86.2). For patients with adrenal insufficiency, the evaluation should include particular attention to factors that may reflect the adequacy of corticosteroid replacement (i.e., lying and standing blood pressure, concentration of serum urea nitrogen and/or serum creatinine, glucose, and electrolytes). Some authorities suggest adrenocorticotropic hormone (ACTH) stimulation or insulin-hypoglycemia testing to determine the need for steroid coverage in patients who are no longer receiving steroids but who have received large doses of steroids in the past; however, these tests cannot be recommended for routine use since adequate evidence that a normal response precludes the need for steroid coverage during surgery is lacking.

Recommendations to the Surgeon. The patient may receive his usual steroid dose by mouth the day before surgery. On the day of surgery, the patient should be given hydrocortisone, 100 mg intravenously, at 6:00 A.M.; a second 100-mg dose is infused continuously during surgery; then a 100-mg dose is given intravenously every 6 hours for the first 24 hours after surgery followed by 50 mg every 6 hours for the second 24 hours after surgery, and 25 mg every 6 hours for the

Table 86.16.
Management of Diabetes on Day of Surgery

Surgical Procedure	Treatment Required to Control Glucose Preoperatively		
	Diet Only	Oral Hypoglycemic Agent	Insulin
Minor	Observe	Withhold until after procedure	Withhold until after procedure or use "major" protocol
Major	Observe	Change to long acting insuling (achieve control with insulin before operation)	*Preferred regimen*: One-half to two-thirds of total long acting insulin dose preoperatively; regular insulin only if needed
			OR
			One-third of total long acting insulin dose preoperatively; one-third postoperatively; regular insulin only if needed
			OR
			Continuous low dose infusion of regular insulin
			OR
			Regular insulin in each liter of dextrose 5% in water (D$_5$W)

third 24-hour period. The patient may then return to his preoperative medical regimen.

There are two exceptions to these guidelines. First, the regimen is based on the assumption that there is no prolonged stress after surgery; if this occurs, higher doses of steroids must be continued for a longer time preoperatively. Second, for minor procedures, the patients may return to their usual dose within 24 to 48 hours postoperatively.

Hypothyroidism

Size of the Risk

The major potential complications of surgery in hypothyroid patients are increased sensitivity to and prolonged half-life of anesthetic agents, hypoventilation and respiratory arrest in the immediate postoperative period, hyponatremia due to decreased free water clearance, and myxedema coma. The risks of surgery in patients with mild to moderate hypothyroidism may be less than previously thought (25).

Preoperative Planning

Office Evaluation. Hypothyroid patients should be evaluated carefully before admission for surgery. The patient should have the comprehensive evaluation outlined in Table 86.2 and the thyroxine (T_4) level should be checked (unless a value from the past 2 months is available). The serum thyroid-stimulating hormone (TSH) concentration should be obtained in newly hypothyroid patients and in patients in whom there is a question about the adequacy of their replacement dose of thyroid hormone (see Chapter 73 for details).

Recommendations to the Surgeon. Specific recommendations for preoperative management depend upon the status of the patient's hypothyroidism. Patients with previously known and adequately treated hypothyroidism can undergo surgery. The half-life of administered thyroxine is about 7 days. Therefore, oral thyroxine can usually be discontinued before surgery and resumed when the patient is able to take oral medication. The stress of major surgery or of severe infection may accelerate the turnover of thyroxine, occasionally necessitating daily treatment with intravenous thyroxine (one-half the oral dose) in patients in either of these situations.

If the hypothyroidism has been effectively treated for a long period (as indicated by only minor symptoms or only a slightly decreased level of T_4), the patient can usually tolerate surgery and thyroid replacement can be adjusted postoperatively. For hypothyroid patients who have not been treated or who remain significantly hypothyroid because of inadequate replacement therapy, surgery should be postponed because of the risks listed above. Such patients should receive adequate thyroid replacement for a minimum of 1 to 2 months before elective surgery (4 to 6 months for patients with profound myxedema).

Surgery required before this period in mild to moderately hypothyroid patients may be considered, especially if minor surgery under local anesthesia is being performed, if the patient can be started on a total replacement dose immediately, and if there is prompt improvement in signs and symptoms of hypothyroidism (see Chapter 73 for additional details). Such patients should *not* be operated on as outpatients.

When a patient with previously undiagnosed hypothyroidism requires immediate major surgery, an endocrinologist should be consulted regarding perioperative treatment and monitoring.

Hyperthyroidism

Size of the Risk

The major risk of operation in patients with uncontrolled hyperthyroidism is thyroid storm. In one series, there were only 25 episodes of thyroid storm after 1,383 operations on thyrotoxic patients (26). However, surgery accounts for up to one-third of the cases of thyroid storm reported.

Preoperative Planning

Office Evaluation. The patient with known hyperthyroidism should be reassessed clinically and with thyroid function tests before admission for surgery. In previously undiagnosed patients, the usual approach should be used in evaluation and management (see Chapter 73).

Recommendations to the Surgeon. The treatment of the hyperthyroid patient during surgery depends on the patient's current thyroid status. Patients previously diagnosed and adequately treated should take their current treatment until midnight the night before surgery and should resume treatment when they can take substances by mouth again. Patients with new, known, or recurrent hyperthyroidism who are not euthyroid should be brought to a euthyroid state with thyroid blocking agents and/or iodides (see Chapter 73). Ideally, surgery should be postponed for several months in these patients until a consistent euthyroid state is attained.

An endocrinologist should be consulted regarding the treatment and monitoring of any patient with uncontrolled hyperthyroidism who requires urgent surgery.

The Obese Patient

Size of the Risk

Massive obesity significantly increases the mortality risk associated with surgery. In one study, for example, women undergoing surgery for adenocarcinoma of the uterus had a 20% operative mortality if they weighed more than 300 lb (136 kg), compared with a 1.5% mortality for obese women weighing between 200 and 240 lb (91 and 110 kg) (36). Less severe obesity probably does not increase mortality risks.

Moderate or massive obesity also increases the risk of a number of perioperative problems, including difficult intubation, difficulty in ventilating the patient during anesthesia, the need for a large amount of anesthesia during induction, potential delay in anesthesia washout because of slow release of anesthetic agents from adipose tissue, postoperative atelectasis and pneumonia, thromboembolism, difficult postoperative mobilization, nosocomial wound infection (particularly when there is increased moisture due to pannus adjacent to the surgical incision), wound dehiscence, and late incisional hernia.

Preoperative Planning

Office Evaluation. For massively obese persons, a program of gradual weight reduction (see Chapter 76) should be planned before any elective operation; this may require up to 6 months. When prompt surgery is needed, these patients should have a comprehensive evaluation (see Table 86.2). In particular these patients should be checked for uncontrolled diabetes mellitus and significant hypoventilation, two common complications of obesity that increase the risk of surgery. Either of these two problems should be managed preoperatively as discussed above.

Recommendations to the Surgeon. Massively obese patients should be given preoperative instruction in deep breathing and in the use of the incentive spirometer or of other devices designed to prevent pulmonary complications postoperatively. Other recommendations for perioperative management depend upon the obesity-associated conditions, such as diabetes, which the patient may have.

THE PATIENT WITH GASTROINTESTINAL DISEASE

Peptic Ulcer Disease

Size of the Risk

Data are lacking on the risk and the management of surgery in patients with active peptic ulcer disease.

Preoperative Planning

Office Evaluation. Patients with active ulcer disease should have elective nonulcer surgery postponed until the ulcer heals. The average time required for the healing of uncomplicated ulcers is 4 to 6 weeks for duodenal ulcer and 6 weeks for gastric ulcer (see Chapter 37). There is no consistent relationship between disappearance of ulcer symptoms, ulcer healing, and recurrence. Therefore, it is best to wait several weeks after all symptoms have disappeared and 2 to 3 months from the beginning of an episode before admission for elective nonulcer surgery. If surgery cannot be deferred this long or if ulcer recurrence is suspected, endoscopy should be performed preoperatively. Before admission, these patients should also have the comprehensive medical evaluation summarized in Table 86.2, and multiple stool samples should be checked to exclude active bleeding.

There are no empirical data to confirm these guidelines, nor to indicate whether surgery can be done safely as soon as an ulcer has healed (as shown by endoscopy). If abdominal surgery must be performed in a patient with active ulcer disease, consideration should be given to whether surgical treatment is needed for the ulcer as well (see detailed discussion of indications for and types of surgery, Chapter 37).

Recommendations to the Surgeon. Patients with remote or inactive ulcer disease require no special therapy preoperatively or postoperatively.

Patients with recently active ulcer disease should continue their current therapy until midnight the day before surgery. Because H_2 blockers (cimetidine, ranitidine, famotidine) can be given intravenously, one of these should be utilized throughout the period when the patient cannot take medications by mouth; nasogastric suctioning should also be recommended during this period.

Hepatitis

Size of the Risk

General anesthesia and surgery during acute hepatitis are associated with a high mortality and morbidity (21). The major problem accounting for these risks is postoperative hepatic encephalopathy and its complications. The catabolic effects of surgery, hypotension during anesthesia, and hepatic toxicity from anesthetic agents are the principal factors that may precipitate hepatic encephalopathy.

Preoperative Planning

Office Evaluation. Patients with a history of acute hepatitis should have a comprehensive evaluation (see Table 86.2), and liver function tests (serum transaminases, bilirubin, alkaline phosphatase, albumin, and prothrombin time) should be obtained before admission for surgery. Serological tests for hepatitis B antigen should also be performed (see Chapter 43).

Ideally, surgery should be postponed for a minimum of 6 to 12 months after all laboratory evidence of active liver disease has returned to normal. This cautious approach is advised because there is a risk of exacerbating hepatic injury if surgery is performed earlier. Only urgent, lifesaving surgery should be performed during the acute phase of hepatitis, whatever its etiology.

Recommendations to the Surgeon. Anticipation of postoperative complications (particularly bleeding and encephalopathy) is important in the patient with active hepatitis who must undergo surgery. For the patient with an abnormal prothrombin time (less than 50% of normal), fresh frozen plasma should be given throughout the immediate perioperative period. When immunological tests or epidemiological information indicates infectious hepatitis (see Chapter 43), the surgical team should be notified in order to minimize the risk of spreading infection.

Cirrhosis

Size of the Risk

Most of the quantitative data regarding the risks of surgery in the cirrhotic patient have been collected in trials of portal-systemic shunts; therefore, these data may not accurately reflect the risks of surgery unrelated to the liver. The most widely used measure of the mortality risk from shunt procedures is Child's index, which incorporates measurements of serum bilirubin, albumin, ascites, encephalopathy, and nutrition (see Table 86.17). The perioperative complications encountered in these patients are those associated with chronic cirrhosis: encephalopathy, jaundice, gastrointestinal hemorrhage, infection, and hepatorenal syndrome.

Regional and spinal anesthesia do not entirely eliminate the risks of complications in cirrhotic patients. For example, increased morbidity and mortality due to liver disease have been associated even with hernia repair under local anesthesia in some patients (1). The stress of the procedure itself, decreased hepatic blood flow, and complications such as hypotension and wound infection may worsen hepatic function, even in the absence of toxic general anesthetics.

Preoperative Planning

Office Evaluation. In addition to a comprehensive preoperative evaluation (see Table 86.2), patients with cirrhosis should have liver function tests (serum transaminase, bilirubin, alkaline phosphatase, albumin, and prothrombin time). Liver biopsy is indicated in selected patients to establish the presence of cirrhosis, to provide an additional indicator of the severity of liver damage, or to exclude active hepatitis. Liver scan is only occasionally needed to exclude other causes of hepatomegaly. In the history and physical examination, a careful search should be made for complications of cirrhosis, especially encephalopathy, bleeding, varices, and ascites.

The expected benefits of surgery must be weighed carefully against the risks in patients with cirrhosis. In general, risks are higher and only essential surgery should be performed. There are stable patients with mild cirrhosis, however, who have no ongoing injury (e.g., due to removal of a toxin or to discontinuation of alcohol) and in whom standards may be liberalized.

Table 86.17.
Child's Classification of Operative Risk in the Cirrhotic Patient[a]

	Group		
	"A" Minimal	"B" Moderate	"C" Advanced
Bilirubin (mg/100 ml)	<2.0	2.0–3.0	>3.0
Serum albumin (g/100 ml)	>3.5	3.0–3.5	<3.0
Ascites	None	Controlled	Poorly controlled
Encephalopathy	None	Minimal	Coma
Nutrition	Excellent	Good	Poor ("wasted")
Operative mortality	0%	9%	53%

[a]From Siefkin AD, Bolt RJ: Preoperative evaluation of the patient with gastrointestinal or liver disease. *Med Clin North Am* 63:1309, 1979.

Recommendations to the Surgeon. A number of precautions should be emphasized in the cirrhotic patient who does require surgery. Local (or, as a second choice, spinal) anesthesia may be safer than general anesthesia, although data are lacking. Therapy to prevent complications of liver disease, such as postoperative bleeding (fresh frozen plasma for the patient with an abnormal prothrombin time or partial thromboplastin time) and encephalopathy (see Chapter 43), should be established and maintained throughout the operative period, and the patient should be repeatedly checked for evidence of these two problems. The occasional patient who is taking chronic corticosteroid therapy for liver disease should have the steroid dose increased during the perioperative period as described above.

THE PATIENT WITH IATROGENIC IMPAIRMENT OF HEMOSTASIS

All anticoagulants increase the risk of intraoperative and postoperative bleeding and should be discontinued before any type of surgery. Patients receiving anticoagulants should have a comprehensive preoperative evaluation (see Table 86.2) before admission for surgery, and an appropriate plan for perioperative management of anticoagulation should be communicated to the surgeon.

Coumarin Derivatives

A reasonable protocol for discontinuing anticoagulation with coumarin derivatives is to stop treatment 48 hours preoperatively for most patients, including those with artificial heart valves (38). If there is less time or if the prothrombin time does not return rapidly enough to normal or near normal (less than 1.5 times normal), vitamin K_1 (Aquamephyton), 10 mg, can be given orally, subcutaneously, or intravenously over 10 to 15 minutes; the prothrombin time will usually return to normal within 24 to 36 hours. Where there is a particularly high risk of thromboembolic disease, such as in patients with artificial heart valves who have developed emboli in the past, anticoagulation can be stopped 24 to 36 hours before surgery, followed by intravenous vitamin K_1; when the prothrombin time becomes subtherapeutic (usually within 12 hours), full anticoagulation should be resumed with heparin and continued until 6 to 12 hours before surgery. In all of these situations, the prothrombin time (and if heparin is given, the partial thromboplastin time and platelet count) should be normal before surgery.

Warfarin (coumadin) ordinarily can be resumed 24 to 72 hours after surgery, at the preoperative dose if all surgical bleeding is controlled. Patients who have undergone intracranial, spinal, or ophthalmological operations probably should not be anticoagulated for 48 to 72 hours after surgery. For patients with a high risk of thromboembolism (artificial mitral valves, active venous thromboembolic disease), heparin can be reinstituted 12 to 24 hours postoperatively, if the surgeon is confident that hemostasis is assured, and continued until full anticoagulation with warfarin has been re-established. After the administration of vitamin K_1, the patient may be relatively refractory to the administration of warfarin for a week or more.

Aspirin

Aspirin prolongs the bleeding time and may increase blood loss during and after operation in some patients. Generally, if aspirin is not being used as a critical therapy, it should be discontinued 1 week preoperatively since aspirin continues to affect platelets for this period of time. Discontinuation of aspirin is particularly important prior to procedures when hemostasis is critical, such as neurosurgical operations.

THE PATIENT WITH CHRONIC BACTERIAL INFECTION

Two types of chronic bacterial infection pose risks to the patient and to others in the operating room and therefore require appropriate management before surgery—staphylococcal skin infections and pulmonary tuberculosis.

Skin Infections

Chronic bacterial skin infections (usually due to staphylococci) pose a high risk for wound sepsis and may be the source of infections in other patients (23). Therefore, they should be suppressed or eradicated prior to admission of the patient for an elective operation. Chapter 25 describes the antibiotic treatment of the various types of staphylococcal skin infection.

Tuberculosis

Active pulmonary tuberculosis poses a problem for the surgical patient because of the general debilitation it causes. It also creates the risk of infection for others in the operating room. Therefore, adult patients with a history of unexplained chronic cough or with a prior history of tuberculosis should be evaluated for active tuberculosis before admission for surgery. Patients with active pulmonary tuberculosis should be stable and have negative sputum cultures before admission for elective surgery. The ambulatory treatment of tuberculosis is described in Chapter 29.

THE PATIENT WITH NEUROPSYCHIATRIC DISEASE

Neuropsychiatric problems present ill-defined risks during surgery and the postsurgical period (42). The major concerns are worsening of mental status due to both metabolic changes and psychological stresses. The patient with psychiatric disease may decompensate postoperatively, making care difficult and jeopardizing wound healing.

Cerebrovascular Accident

Size of the Risk

Patients with recent strokes have a significant risk of worsening focal deficits during carotid artery surgery, but this cannot necessarily be extrapolated to other types of surgery. Patients with recent strokes (less than 6 weeks' duration) also have a risk of deterioration in their general mental status, regardless of the status of their focal deficits, if they undergo major surgery; but firm data are lacking on the size of this risk.

Preoperative Planning

Patients with recent strokes should have a comprehensive preoperative evaluation (see Table 86.2) emphasizing documentation of the preoperative neurological impairment. The data regarding the course of the patient's stroke should be reviewed, and additional testing (see Chapter 83) should be performed if necessary to exclude a treatable etiology.

No specific perioperative therapy for the patient with a stable completed stroke is needed. In general, it is prudent to delay elective, noncarotid surgery at least 6 weeks after a completed stroke, although no firm data are available to support this practice.

Asymptomatic Cervical Bruit

Size of the Risk

Cervical bruits are present in about 4% of persons over the age of 45 (22). These bruits may be due to a number of processes (see Chapter 83) including common or internal carotid stenosis. In the patient with an asymptomatic cervical bruit, there is slight or no increased risk of cerebrovascular accident during surgery (6, 32).

Preoperative Planning

Apart from a careful history and physical examination to exclude evidence of a prior stroke or a transient ischemic attack (TIA) related to the cervical bruit, there is no special approach needed for these patients. The value of duplex carotid ultrasound has not been established for estimating risk of postoperative stroke. Hypotension and excessive neck manipulation should be avoided in these patients during surgery. The patient with a history of symptoms possibly related to the bruit should be evaluated as described in Chapter 83.

Parkinson's Disease

Size of the Risk

The perioperative risks in patients with Parkinson's disease derive from the rigidity, which may impair voluntary postoperative ventilation, mobilization, and swallowing. The rigidity of patients taking antiparkinsonism medication may recur after the patient has missed several doses. Despite this potential problem, most patients with Parkinson's disease do tolerate anesthesia and temporary omission of medications (28).

Preoperative Planning

The patient should have a comprehensive preoperative evaluation (see Table 86.2), and the antiparkinsonian regimen should be tailored to provide the best possible relief of symptoms (see Chapter 82). For patients taking an anticholinergic agent, the drug may be continued until midnight before surgery and resumed when the patient is able to take oral medications. L-Dopa or Sinemet (L-dopa/carbidopa), should be continued up until induction of anesthesia, and the drug should be resumed as soon as possible after surgery. Postoperative physical therapy to maintain range of motion may help these patients until they are able to take oral medication.

Dementia and Organic Brain Syndrome

Size of the Risk

Patients with dementia have an increased risk of mortality and morbidity during surgery. The increase in mortality is largely due to lack of cooperation (e.g., with postoperative respiratory care). Much of the morbidity is related to worsening mental status due to anesthesia and surgical stress. Because surgery is always a difficult process for a demented patient and because the degree of increased risk is ill defined, the potential benefits of surgery should be carefully reviewed before the final decision to operate is made.

Preoperative Planning

The patient should have a comprehensive evaluation (see Table 86.2) before admission for surgery. A careful search for metabolic abnormalities that may worsen cerebral function should be made before admission, just before surgery, and throughout the postoperative period. Emphasis should be placed on detecting and correcting hypovolemia, electrolyte ab-

normalities, and hypoxia. Before major surgery it is advisable to document the patient's mental status formally (see Mini-Mental Status Examination, Table 17.1) so that mental states after surgery can be compared with baseline status.

For some patients undergoing major procedures, constant observation is recommended for the first 24 to 48 hours after surgery.

Other Psychiatric Problems

Size of the Risk

The major problems associated with general surgery in psychiatric patients are lack of cooperation with postoperative care, postoperative psychosis, and interactions between psychotropic medications and anesthetic agents (42). The degree of cooperation that can be expected postoperatively can generally but not always be predicted on the basis of the patient's past behavior and his preoperative mental status.

Preoperative Planning

Office Evaluation. A careful history of past psychiatric illness should be obtained. The patient's mental status should be documented preoperatively (see Chapter 10) so that it can be compared with postoperative changes. A psychiatric consultation should be obtained in all patients with psychosis or with other severe psychiatric problems. Additional issues that must be dealt with by the patient's personal physician and surgeon are the ability of the patient to give informed consent (see Chapter 10) and the effect of the patient's psychiatric state on the surgical evaluation (such as evaluating symptoms in a patient with one of the somatoform disorders, described in Chapter 12, or evaluating the need for cosmetic surgery).

Careful explanation of the operation is especially crucial to management of patients with psychiatric disorders or with anticipated stress reactions to surgery. The procedure should be explained in language the patient can understand. After the explanation, the patient should be asked to express any concerns that he has about the planned surgery, and the patient's comprehension of the planned surgery should be assessed. The need to ventilate about anxiety associated with disfiguring surgery (e.g., mastectomy, amputation, etc.) and with the fear of "not waking up" is particularly common in both anxiety-prone patients and in persons who are usually free of anxiety.

Patients with severe psychosis should be in a stable, manageable state before admission for elective surgery; this should be accomplished through close collaboration between the primary physician, the surgeon, and a psychiatrist.

Patients with mild to moderate anxiety or depression can be managed by supportive counseling, use of support by family members, selective use of antidepressants or minor tranquilizers, and careful explanation of the procedure to the patient. These interventions should be initiated before hospital admission, not at the last minute before surgery.

Recommendations to the Surgeon. The principal recommendation for the perioperative period is that the patient's use of psychotropic drugs should be communicated to the anesthesiologist.

Neuroleptics and tricyclic antidepressants can interact with anesthetics to cause increased sedation, hypo- or hypertension, and arrhythmias. Small to moderate doses of phenothiazines, haloperidol, and tricyclic antidepressants should be continued until about 12 hours before surgery. In the occasional patient taking very high doses of these agents, it is recommended that the drug be stopped about 24 hours before surgery, except in patients who have severely decompensated in the past when their medication has been changed.

The dose of benzodiazepines does not need to be changed unless it is very high.

Lithium carbonate can prolong the action of muscle relaxants and cause myocardial depression and hypernatremia. Lithium should be discontinued 24 hours preoperatively; however, the anesthesiologist should be aware that it has been administered recently. A blood lithium level and electrolyte measurements should be obtained before surgery as a guideline. Additional information about lithium is found in Chapter 15.

Monoamine oxidase (MAO) inhibitor antidepressants can lead to an enhancement of the effect of sympathomimetic agents, to enhanced sympathetic responses to anesthesia, and to a decrease in the rate of elimination of certain anesthetic agents. Because of these problems, MAO inhibitors should be discontinued at least 2 weeks before surgery, and the anesthesiologist must be informed of their recent administration.

General References

Barron WM: The pregnant surgical patient. Medical evaluation and management. *Ann Intern Med* 101:683, 1984.
    A comprehensive and up-to-date review of the subject.
Gross RJ, Kammerer WS: Medical consultation on surgical services: an annotated bibliography. *Ann Intern Med* 95:523, 1981.
Kammerer WS, Gross RJ (eds): *Medical Consultation: The Internist on Surgical, Obstetric, and Psychiatric Services*, 2nd ed. Baltimore, Williams & Wilkins, 1990.
    A comprehensive multicontributor book, extensively referenced.
Merli GJ, Weitz HH: Preoperative Consultation. *Med Clin North Am* 71:353, 1987. Smith NT, Miller RD, Carbascio AN (eds): *Drug Interactions in Anesthesia*, 2nd ed. Philadelphia, Lea & Febiger, 1986.
    Detailed account of interactions of commonly prescribed drugs with anesthetic agents.
Vandam LD (ed): *To Make the Patient Ready for Anesthesia: Medical Care of the Surgical Patient*, 2nd ed. Reading, MA, Addison-Wesley, 1987.
    Brief, practical recommendations for preoperative management of most common medical problems.

Specific References

1. Baron HC: Umbilical hernia secondary to cirrhosis of the liver. *N Engl J Med* 263:824, 1960.
2. Bennett WM, Muther RS, Parker RA, et al: Drug Therapy in renal failure; dosing guidelines for adults. Part 1 and Part 2. *Ann Intern Med* 93:62, 286, 1980.
3. Brenowitz JB, Williams CD, Edwards WS: Major surgery in patients with chronic renal failure. *Am J Surg* 134:765, 1977.
4. Briefel G, Turer P: Renal disease. In: Kammerer WS, Gross RJ (eds): *Medical Consultation*. Baltimore, Williams & Wilkins, 1990.
5. Burke GR, Gulyassy PF: Surgery in the patient with renal disease and related electrolyte disorders. *Med Clin North Am* 63:1191, 1979.
6. Corman LC: The preoperative patient with an asymptomatic cervical bruit. *Med Clin North Am* 63:1335, 1979.
7. Detsky AS, Abrams HB, McLaughlin JR, et al: Predicting cardiac complications in patients undergoing non-cardiac surgery. *J Gen Intern Med* 1:211, 1986.
8. Deutsch S, Daten JE: Indication for prophylactic digitalization. *Anesthesiology* 30:648, 1969.
9. Djokovic JL, Hedley-White J: Prediction of outcome of surgery and anesthesia in patients over 80. *JAMA* 242:2301, 1979.
10. Eisman B (ed): *Prognosis of Surgical Disease*. Philadelphia, WB Saunders, 1980.
11. Eisman B, Watkins RS (eds): *Surgical Decision Making*, 2nd ed. Philadelphia, WB Saunders, 1986.
12. Foster ED, Davis KB, Carpenter JA, et al: Risk of noncardiac operation in patients with defined coronary disease. *Ann Thoracic Surg* 41:42, 1986.
13. Goldman L: Supraventricular tachyarrhythmias in hospitalized adults after surgery. *Chest* 73:450, 1978.
14. Goldman L, Caldera DL: Risks of general anesthesia and elective operation in the hypertensive patient. *Anesthesiology* 50:285, 1979.
15. Goldman L, Caldera DL, Nussbaum SR, et al: Multifactorial index of cardiac risk in noncardiac surgical procedures. *N Engl J Med* 297:845, 1977.
16. Goldman L, Caldera DL, Southwick FS, et al: Cardiac risk factors and complications in non-cardiac surgery. *Medicine (Baltimore)* 57:357, 1978.
17. Gross RJ: Evaluation of the healthy patient and the ambulatory surgery patient. In: Kammerer WS, Gross RJ (eds): *Medical Consultation*. Baltimore, Williams & Wilkins, 1990.
18. Gross RJ, Kammerer WS: Special topics. In: Kammerer WS, Gross RJ (eds): *Medical Consultation*. Baltimore, Williams & Wilkins, 1990.
19. Gross R, Kern D: Cardiovascular disease. In: Kammerer WS, Gross RJ (eds): *Medical Consultation*. Baltimore, Williams & Wilkins, 1990.
20. Harman E, Lillington G: Pulmonary risk factors in surgery. *Med Clin North Am* 63:1289, 1979.
21. Harville DD, Summerskill WHJ: Surgery in acute hepatitis. *JAMA* 184:257, 1963.
22. Heyman A, Wilkinson WE, Heyden S, et al: Risk of stroke in asymptomatic persons with cervical arterial bruits: a population study in Evans County, Georgia. *N Engl J Med* 302:838, 1980.
23. Hiral D: Nasal Staphylococcus aureus and postoperative infection. *Am Surg* 46:310, 1980.
24. Hosking MP, Warner MA, Lobdell CM, et al: Outcomes of surgery in patients 90 years of age and older. *JAMA* 261:1909, 1989.
25. Ladenson PW, Levin AA, Ridgway EC, et al: Complications of surgery in hypothyroid patients. *Am J Med* 77:261, 1984.
26. McArthur JW, Rawson RW, Means JH, Cope O: Thyrotoxic crisis: an analysis of the thirty-six cases seen at the Massachusetts General Hospital during the past twenty-five years. *JAMA* 134:868, 1947.
27. Mohr DN, Jett JR: Preoperative evaluation of pulmonary risk factors. *J Gen Intern Med* 3:277, 1989.
28. Ngai SH: Medical intelligence: parkinsonism, levodopa, and anesthesia. *Anesthesiology* 37:344, 1972.
29. Oh SH, Patterson R: Surgery in corticosteroid-dependent asthmatics. *J Allergy Clin Immunol* 53:345, 1974.
30. Prys-Roberts C: Hypertension and anesthesia—fifty years on. *Anesthesiology* 50:281, 1979.

31. Rao Tadikonda LK, Jacobs K, El-Etr A: Reinfarction following anesthesia in patients with myocardial infarction. *Anesthesiology* 59:499, 1983.
32. Ropper AH, Wechsler LR, Wilson LS: Carotid bruit and the risk of stroke in elective surgery. *N Engl J Med* 307:1388, 1982.
33. Rose EA, King TC: Understanding postoperative fatigue. *Surg Gynecol Obstet* 147:97, 1978.
34. Schwab SJ, Hlatky MA, Pieper KS, et al: Contrast nephrotoxicity: a randomized, controlled trial of non-ionic and ionic radiographic contrast agents. *N Engl J Med* 320:149, 1989.
35. Stein M, Cassara EL: Preoperative pulmonary evaluation and therapy for surgery patients. *JAMA* 211:787, 1970.
36. Strauss RJ, Wise L: Operative risks of obesity. *Surg Gynecol Obstet* 146:286, 1978.
37. Tarhan S, Moffitt ED, Sessler AD, et al: Risk of anesthesia and surgery in patients with chronic bronchitis and chronic obstructive pulmonary disease. *Surgery* 74:720, 1973.
38. Tinker JH, Tanhan S: Discontinuing anticoagulant therapy in surgical patients with cardiac valve prostheses. *JAMA* 239:738, 1978.
39. Tisi GM: Preoperative evaluation of pulmonary function; validity, indications, and benefits. *Am Rev Respir Dir* 119:293, 1979.
40. Trautlein JJ: Preoperative pulmonary evaluation. In: Kammerer WS, Gross RJ (eds): *Medical Consultation*. Baltimore, Williams & Wilkins, 1990.
41. White VA, Kumager LF: Preoperative endocrine and metabolic considerations. *Med Clin North Am* 63:1321, 1979.
42. Woodcock J: Psychiatry. In: Kammerer WS, Gross RJ (eds): *Medical Consultation*. Baltimore, Williams & Wilkins, 1990.

C H A P T E R 87

Peripheral Vascular Disease and Arterial Aneurysms*

PETER J. GOLUEKE, M.D.

Most people, if they live long enough, develop atherosclerotic arterial disease. Each specific disease entity is only an isolated clinical manifestation of a generalized atherosclerotic process, and evaluation and management of specific problems of arterial disease must be viewed in this context. Quality and quantity of life may be improved by recognition, thorough evaluation, and appropriate therapy of peripheral arterial diseases. The purpose of this chapter is to provide guidelines for recognition and management of the more commonly encountered arterial problems: acute and chronic occlusive disease and abdominal and peripheral aneurysms.

ACUTE PERIPHERAL ARTERIAL OCCLUSION

Acute ischemia of the lower extremities demands immediate recognition and management since late recognition and treatment may eventuate in loss of limb or loss of life. If collateral circulation is not well developed, muscle necrosis and other irreversible changes may occur as early as 4 to 6 hours after acute arterial occlusion.

The two major causes of acute arterial occlusion are emboli and thromboses. Because surgical management

---

*Dr. Calvin B. Ernst contributed to this chapter in the first and second editions of this book.

of these two entities may be quite different, it is important to distinguish between them. Embolism demands immediate operation because pre-existing collaterals are scanty, and relief of ischemia can often be accomplished by a simple operation involving extraction of the clot using local anesthesia. Thrombosis usually can be managed under less emergent conditions than embolus because pre-existing collateral channels stimulated by chronic underlying occlusive arterial disease provide marginal but adequate blood flow. Furthermore, management of ischemia secondary to thrombosis often requires complex reconstructive surgical procedures that are best performed under elective conditions after adequate evaluation, which includes arteriographic study. However, faced with a nonviable extremity, immediate operation for thrombosis is mandatory.

Newer techniques utilizing thrombolytic therapy in appropriately selected patients, followed by angioplasty, atherectomy or endarterectomy, may salvage the thrombosed artery. These procedures can be performed on a semiurgent basis up to 1 to 2 weeks after thrombosis, but best results are obtained when they are performed soon after thrombosis.

Over 90% of the time, acute embolic occlusion may be distinguished from acute thrombotic occlusion on clinical grounds alone (see below). In instances in which doubt exists about the etiology, arteriography is essential to distinguish embolus from thrombosis (see below, "Laboratory and X-ray Studies").

Etiology

The majority of large arterial emboli originate in the heart. In a series of 338 patients, Fogarty and Buch (10) ascribed 94% of emboli to cardiac disease. Whereas years ago a preponderance of patients had rheumatic heart disease, in recent years peripheral embolization associated with the sequelae of arteriosclerotic cardiac disease has predominated. Arrhythmias secondary to coronary insufficiency, recent myocardial infarction with mural thrombosis, or old myocardial infarction with ventricular aneurysm are risk factors for embolization. Less common sources include proximal arterial lesions such as aortic aneurysms or large thromboulcerative mural aortic plaques. Such lesions cause arterioarterial emboli, which are often relatively small and which may cause the "blue toe syndrome" when they lodge in the most peripheral part of the circulation of the lower extremities (17). Left atrial myxomas, debris from prosthetic heart valves, paradoxical emboli (venous clots passing through a congenital cardiac defect into the arterial circulation), and foreign body emboli, although quite rare, all have been implicated in sudden arterial occlusion.

Although most acute arterial occlusions follow emboli, in situ thrombosis of an arteriosclerotic lesion accounts for approximately 25% of acute occlusive events. Such thrombotic complications are most likely to occur in segments of severe stenosis such as the aortic bifurcation, iliac bifurcation, common femoral bifurcation, and the superficial femoral artery just above the knee.

Upper extremity ischemia is usually secondary to arterial embolism. Acute thrombosis virtually never causes ischemia in the upper extremity, where chronic arteriosclerotic lesions are uncommon and collateralization is excellent. Thoracic outlet compression may give rise rarely to subclavian or axillary arterial thrombosis.

Concomitant problems such as hypovolemia from volume depletion or hemorrhage, congestive heart failure, polycythemia, or trauma all have profound influences on management.

Clinical Manifestations

Emboli lodge at arterial bifurcations (Fig. 87.1). The brachial artery in the antecubital fossa is the most common site of embolism in the upper body. Approximately 20% of upper body emboli go to the cerebral circulation. Multiple emboli result from a "shower discharge" of clots from the heart. Recurrent embolic episodes, during the same hospitalization, may affect 15% of patients. Therefore, although the legs are affected most often, there may be symptoms and signs of ischemia elsewhere.

Clinical manifestations vary depending on the adequacy of pre-existing collateral circulation and on the site of occlusion in the extremity. If pre-existing collateral vessels, stimulated by underlying occlusive arterial disease, are present, acute ischemic symptoms may be mild; however, total arterial occlusion of a previously normal arterial tree causes severe symptoms. Cardinal features include the six "Ps" of arterial occlusion: pulselessness, pallor, poikilothermia, pain, paralysis, and paresthesias. The latter three Ps reflect neurophysiological sequelae of ischemia, and the former three result from mechanical occlusion of an artery. Three-quarters of patients complain of pain, but 20% note numbness as the first manifestation of sudden arterial occlusion. Initially, pain may be mild; but as the ischemic process progresses, pain worsens only to subside late in the course of the disease as anesthesia and paralysis develop.

Additional findings other than the six Ps include poor capillary filling and collapsed or severely sunken veins on the dorsum of the foot. Pedal edema, if present, is not a result of arterial occlusion, but it may be secondary to heart failure or to pooling of blood in the extremities of patients who attempt to relieve ischemic pain by maintaining their legs in a dependent position for long periods of time.

Cardiac examination may reveal atrial fibrillation, a diastolic rumble or the opening snap of mitral stenosis, or a gallop associated with congestive failure. A recent history of chest pain or electrocardiographic evidence of myocardial infarction implicates a cardiac origin of acute leg ischemia.

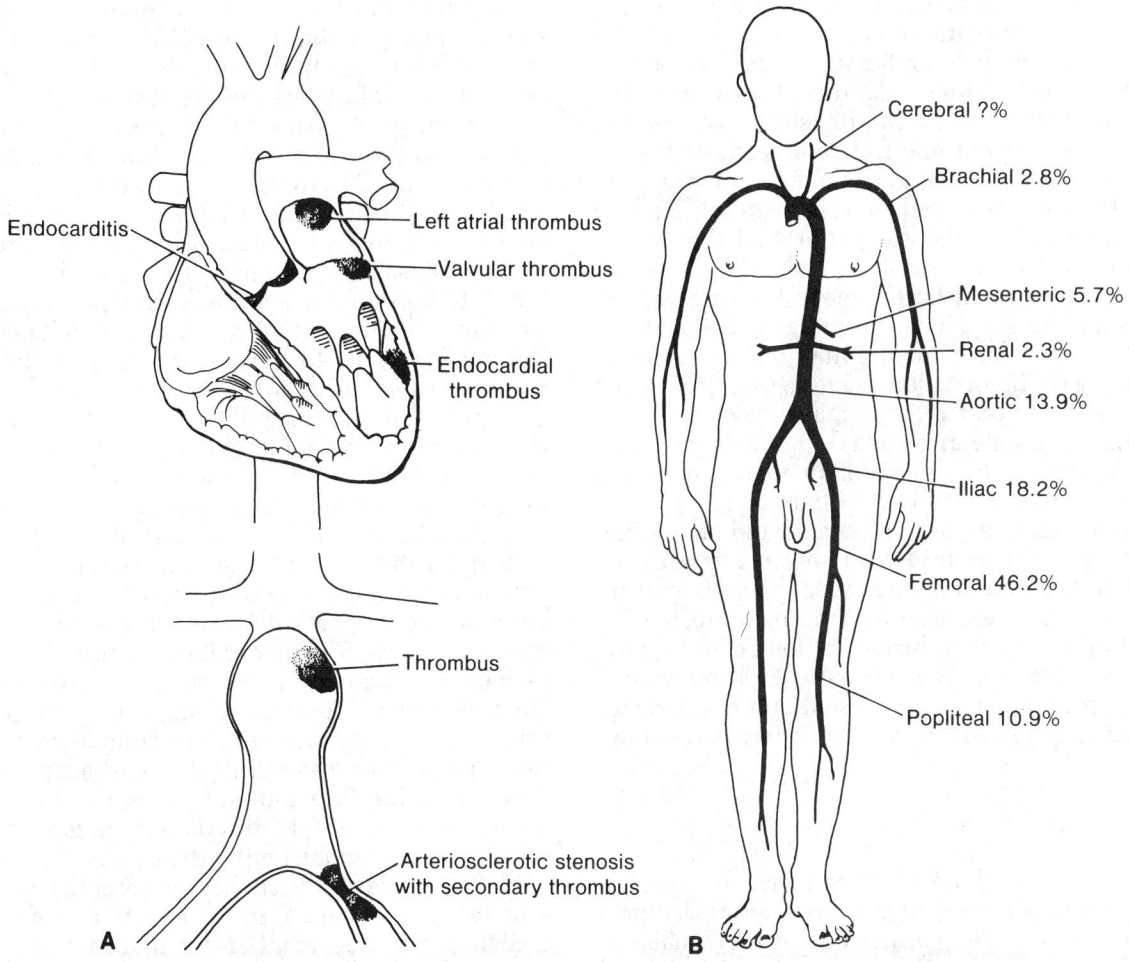

Figure 87.1. *A*. Source of arterial emboli in 338 patients. Over 90% originate in the heart. *B*. distribution of arterial emboli in the same group. Over 90% impact in the distal aorta or lower extremities. (Adapted from Rutherford RB (ed): *Vascular Surgery*, 2nd ed. Philadelphia, WB Saunders, 1984.)

Laboratory and X-ray Studies

Laboratory studies usually are not helpful in making the diagnosis of acute arterial ischemia of the lower extremities. Arterial blood gases and pH should be obtained to serve as baseline studies for subsequent comparative measurement as well as to identify metabolic acidosis from muscle ischemia, which might require correction prior to operation. Hyperkalemia may be manifest, particularly if advanced muscle ischemia has occurred. A roentgenogram of the chest may document cardiac enlargement or congestive heart failure. All of these studies should be obtained after the patient is hospitalized.

Arteriography is not routinely performed except, occasionally, in instances of modest ischemia when it is needed to distinguish between thrombosis and embolus (see below). Evidence of generalized and severe arteriosclerosis, tapered occlusions of arteries, and of well-developed collateral vessels indicates acute thrombotic occlusion. Normal-appearing arteries with scanty collateral circulation and an occlusion with an inverted meniscus configuration indicate embolic occlusion. However, embolization can occur in patients who also have chronic occlusive disease, and the diagnosis is occasionally still in question after angiography. In any case, the decision for immediate surgery is based on the clinical status of the extremity and not on the arteriogram.

Although noninvasive evaluation by Doppler ultrasonography or by plethysmography is often superfluous, the inability to obtain any arterial Doppler signal in the foot in a patient with an acute occlusion supports the decision for urgent revascularization.

Differential Diagnosis

The most important differential, because surgical management depends upon it, is to distinguish embolism from thrombosis. History is often quite helpful in separating these two entities. History of intermittent claudication or rest pain would implicate arterial thrombosis as the acute ischemic event. Complete lack of history of intermittent claudication usually indicates embolism. However, approximately 25% of patients who suffer acute superficial femoral arterial occlusion secondary to thrombosis have never had symptoms of intermittent claudication prior to the sudden occlusive event. On physical examination classic findings of chronic ischemia such as loss of hair on the toes and dorsum of the foot and the shin, along with nail, skin, and muscle atrophy, may be noted. Such findings also suggest arterial thrombosis rather than embolus. A pulsatile abdominal mass diagnostic of abdominal aortic aneurysm from which mural thrombus may have discharged to the distal arterial tree might be evident. Finally, if the acute ischemic episode involves only one leg, palpating the popliteal and femoral arteries may detect an aneurysm. If the contralateral vessel is vigorously pulsating and aneurysmal, a thrombosis of an aneurysm on the side of the ischemia may have occurred.

An acute dissection of the thoracic and abdominal aorta may present as unilateral lower extremity ischemia. Under these circumstances, patients will relate a history of severe, searing, ripping thoracic back pain and may provide a history of long-standing hypertension. Also, among such patients a murmur of aortic insufficiency may be present and chest roentgenograms may reveal a widened mediastinal silhouette.

Treatment

Evaluation and therapy must proceed simultaneously in the management of acute arterial ischemia of the extremities. The cornerstone of early management of acute arterial occlusions is administration of heparin sodium. When diagnosis of sudden arterial ischemia is first made, 100 to 150 units of heparin sodium/kg must be given intravenously. This injection should be given in the physician's office, if there are no major contraindications (see Chapter 52). Patients should then be hospitalized immediately and an urgent consultation obtained with a vascular surgeon.

Introduction of the balloon-tipped embolectomy catheter by Fogarty and his coworkers in 1963 revolutionized management of acute embolic occlusion (11). Adoption of the balloon-tipped catheter converted a previously complex undertaking to a simple operative procedure that invariably can be performed under local anesthesia. Consequently, since introduction of this device, improved survival and limb salvage rates have been reported from many centers. Practically any patient, no matter how ill, may be operated upon using this device.

The surgeon must be knowledgeable of vascular reconstructive techniques so that, should acute arterial thrombosis be encountered rather than acute arterial embolus, definitive treatment may be employed, which will usually require arterial reconstruction. In a critically ill patient in whom sufficient time has not been available for proper preoperative preparation, because the acutely ischemic limb mandates immediate management, aortofemoral bypass reconstruction may carry

prohibitive operative risks. Under such circumstances, extra-anatomical arterial reconstructive procedures such as axillofemoral, axillobifemoral, or femoral-femoral bypass may be warranted.

There may be a role for intra-arterial infusion of *fibrinolytic* agents directly into the site of the acute arterial occlusion (16, 28). A multiple purpose polyethylene catheter is imbedded into the occluding clot after the arteriographic study is performed. Urokinase (UK) is infused at a rate of 3000 to 4000 units/minute for 30 to 60 minutes and an arteriogram is repeated. Therapy is continued with UK at 1000 to 2000 units/kg/hour for 24 to 48 hours with clinical and angiographic re-evaluation at 8- to 12-hour intervals. Such therapy is contraindicated when the extremity may be in jeopardy, such as following an acute arterial embolus. The time required for lysis to occur may be longer than the safe ischemic interval, and amputation may then be necessary. It is generally accepted that clots older than 7 to 10 days are resistant to lysis. In patients with acute arterial thrombosis or with thrombosis of bypass grafts, however, this type of therapy may have merit. This is particularly true for high risk patients in whom operation may be contraindicated. Untoward bleeding is the major complication of fibrinolytic therapy and may compromise this form of treatment and lead to significant morbidity. Also, the duration of the infusion and the optimal dose to be administered to restore circulation are not yet firmly established. Therefore, until further experience is gained with this modality, it should be reserved for highly selected patients who are cared for in centers specializing in management of vascular disease.

After discharge from the hospital, patients are almost always maintained on therapeutic levels of oral anticoagulants for the rest of their lives (see Chapter 52). Furthermore, they must be evaluated several times a year in order to maintain optimal cardiac function and for continued evaluation of their peripheral circulation.

Results

In spite of improved diagnosis, preoperative care, operative management, and postoperative support, mortality from acute lower extremity ischemia continues to be discouraging. Prior to 1963 mortality after arterial embolectomy ranged between 34 and 63%. Mortality since 1963 has remained high and ranges between 10 and 40% (14, 22, 24). Virtually all deaths are related to complications of cardiovascular disease (12). Such findings reinforce the contention that recognition and correction of causes of embolism or thrombosis represent an important aspect in the management of such patients.

If the patient does not succumb to complications secondary to diffuse arteriosclerosis, limb salvage exceeds 95% in most series. Likelihood of successful limb salvage is directly related to time between arterial occlusion and restoration of blood flow. Therefore, it is improbable that a 100% limb salvage rate will ever be achieved.

CHRONIC ARTERIAL OCCLUSIVE DISEASE

In contrast to the management schema for acute arterial occlusion, which requires emergent or urgent treatment, chronic arterial occlusive disease, manifest by symptoms covering the spectrum from mild intermittent claudication to rest pain and gangrene, almost never requires emergent treatment. By virtue of development of collateral channels that bypass slowly developing atherosclerotic lesions, chronic arterial occlusive disease may be approached in an unhurried and organized fashion, often by nonoperative management. Thorough knowledge of the natural history of chronic arterial occlusive disease is key to proper management of patients suffering such problems. In an era of vascular surgery when practically any arterial circuit may be successfully reconstructed, and sophisticated diagnostic procedures offer objective data confirming clinical impressions and results of treatment, perspectives are occasionally distorted and operative management is enthusiastically overadopted.

Etiology and Pathophysiology

Atherosclerosis is the cause of chronic arterial occlusive disease in the vast majority of affected individuals. The symptoms and signs of the disease are unusual before the fifth decade. The disease process is influenced significantly and adversely by the presence of diabetes mellitus, hypertension, hyperlipoproteinemia, use of tobacco, factors affecting blood viscosity such as polycythemia, and by reduction in cardiac output. Furthermore, symptoms of arterial insufficiency of the legs are only regional manifestations of a generalized disease process. Chronic atherosclerotic disease rarely causes symptoms in the upper extremities.

Although atherosclerosis is a generalized disease, it has a remarkably segmental distribution. Arteriosclerosis is prone to develop at major arterial bifurcations, in areas of arterial fixation, and at points of marked arterial angulation such as the distal superficial femoral artery as it enters Hunter's canal, the bifurcation of the common femoral artery, the aorta distal to the renal arteries and, most commonly, at its bifurcation, and the common iliac bifurcations.

With gradual development of such lesions, the formation of collateral vessels compensates for segmental obstructive processes, and in many instances collaterals are sufficient to provide adequate blood flow even during moderate exercise. On the other hand, sudden occlusion of a previously unobstructed vessel may not be compensated by immediate collateral blood flow so that tissue necrosis and gangrene ensue. When collateral channels are adequate, no or only minimal symptoms may be present. However, as progressive main arterial involvement occurs, collateral channels may be progressively lost, and symptoms of severe exercise ischemia (intermittent claudication) occur that may progress to gradual development of rest pain and tissue necrosis. The spectrum, then, of symptomatic arterial occlusive disease of the legs extends from mild exercise ischemia to severe ischemic pain at rest to frank gangrene or nonhealing ulceration of the toes or foot (see Chapter 88).

Diabetes mellitus (see Chapter 72) has a unique influence on the pathogenesis of atherosclerosis. Diabetic patients manifest atherosclerosis of a more severe degree and at an earlier age than nondiabetic individuals. Furthermore, distribution of the atherosclerotic process in the lower extremity of a diabetic compared with a nondiabetic is different in that distal vessels such as popliteal, peroneal, and tibial arteries are more commonly involved than are aortoiliac and femoral segments. Microangiopathy also affects peripheral nerves as well as nutrient vessels to skin and muscle, which may result in insensitivity and progressive ischemia and in lack of natural protective mechanisms in the diabetic foot. Breakdown of skin and entry of bacteria with subsequent infection may cause extensive damage, since normal sensation is lost and significant symptoms may be obscured. Diabetic neuropathy (Chapter 72) also involves the sympathetic nervous system, and many of these patients have undergone autosympathectomy at the time they are initially seen by a clinician.

Buerger's disease, thromboangiitis obliterans, is a severe chronic panarteritis leading to fibrosis and obliteration of small vessels at the tibial and pedal levels. The arteries of the forearm and hand can be involved also, and superficial phlebitis may be seen as well. Buerger's disease is an infrequent cause of lower extremity arterial insufficiency in the United States. This entity affects young men in their twenties and thirties and is almost always associated with severe tobacco addiction. Successful management hinges on cessation of use of all forms of tobacco.

Natural History

Intermittent claudication reflects a relatively benign condition (2, 14, 15); approximately one-third of patients with claudication improve; one-third remain stable and tolerate their symptoms; and one-third deteriorate and require operation. Relentless deterioration of the lower extremity associated with intermittent claudication is unlikely in most nondiabetic patients, particularly if use of all tobacco products is discontinued. The chance of amputation occurring among individuals initially seen with intermittent claudication is approximately 1%/year. Patients with ischemic rest pain or gangrene, however, are at very high risk for amputation if surgical management is not employed.

The overall 5-year survival rate among individuals with intermittent claudication approximates 70%. The 10-year survival rate is approximately 40%. Of note is that of those individuals dying, three-quarters succumb to complications of coronary artery disease.

Clinical Manifestations

Symptoms among individuals suffering occlusive arterial disease to the legs range from mild muscular pain on exercise to severe rest pain, gangrene, or nonhealing ulceration. Such individuals should be carefully questioned for symptoms involving other arterial circuits such as transient cerebral ischemic attacks or angina. The distance a patient walks before developing claudication and the muscle groups involved (calf, thigh, buttock) should be documented. Men should be questioned specifically about impotence. Patients with ischemic rest pain will often note that they can alleviate their pain by dangling their legs over the side of a bed or a chair. Relief of pain with dependency suggests that blood flow is so marginal that the slight increase of flow with gravity can help to improve perfusion.

On *physical examination*, in the mildest form of the disease, only a diminution in intensity of peripheral pulses may be noted. Complete vascular examination should be performed noting locations of bruits, blood pressure measurements in both upper extremities, and the recording of all peripheral pulses. Among individuals with mild intermittent claudication, the skin of the feet may appear normal; there may be hair growth on toes; nails may appear normal; and there may even be faintly palpable dorsalis pedis and posterior tibial pulses. With progressive arterial involvement, however, trophic changes may involve the lower extremities with loss of hair on toes and anterior tibial areas. Poor skin nutrition is reflected by thin parchment-like skin. Lack of pulses below the inguinal ligaments, blanching and pallor with elevation of the extremity, and dependent rubor all indicate advanced ischemia. Gangrenous areas may be evident involving digits. The typical locations of ischemic ulcers are over the calcaneus, the lateral malleolus, and the dorsum of the foot (see Chapter 88).

Laboratory and X-ray Studies

The distribution and severity of peripheral arterial disease can be determined objectively by noninvasive Doppler flow studies. These studies are performed by the consulting vascular surgeon. A sphygmomanometer cuff is placed immediately above the malleoli, and the cuff is inflated to above systolic pressure. As it is slowly deflated, with the Doppler velocity detector placed over the dorsalis pedis or the posterior tibial artery, pulsatile sounds will occur at systolic opening pressure. The highest pressure recorded is utilized to compare with brachial arterial systolic pressure, and the ankle/arm pressure index is determined. Normal individuals have a mean index of over 1; for individuals suffering intermittent claudication the mean index is 0.59; for those with rest pain, 0.26; and patients suffering impending gangrene have a mean ankle/arm blood pressure index of 0.05 (30).

A Doppler study of lower extremity blood flow, although important, is not needed in evaluating all patients with lower extremity arterial occlusive disease. However, noninvasive testing is very helpful in distinguishing vascular insufficiency from other causes of leg pain (e.g., neurogenic claudication secondary to cauda equina compression from spinal stenosis). In the latter, Doppler ankle/arm indices are normal and, of particular note, remain normal after exercise. Noninvasive studies can also provide data that document objectively whether or not nonoperative therapy is effective in management or if deterioration of circulation is progressive. In addition, comparison of preoperative and postoperative noninvasive data is useful in documenting effectiveness of operative therapy.

The most important laboratory study, if it is determined the patient is a candidate for operation, is arteriography (see below). Although risks are very small in experienced hands, arteriography is utilized only when operation is indicated and agreed to by the patient.

Laboratory studies also may reveal hyperglycemia or hyperlipidemia that needs to be managed appropriately.

Treatment and Results

Treatment for arterial insufficiency of the legs may be either operative or nonoperative. Indications for operation are shown in Table 87.1. Patients should be managed by nonoperative therapy unless one of these indications is present. Knowing the natural history of the occlusive process aids significantly in determining whether or not the patient's symptoms warrant operative intervention in light of associated risk factors and life expectancy. Except for very poor surgical candidates, individuals with ischemic rest pain, nonhealing ulcers, pregangrenous changes, or gangrene always require operative intervention.

There are patients, however, who are not, and probably never will become, candidates for operation. This group includes individuals whose symptoms are not severe enough to warrant operation and those whose symptoms, although they may be severe, are of such recent onset that sufficient time has not elapsed to determine whether or not development of collateral circulation will cause symptoms to lessen or significantly abate.

General Measures

Much can be recommended to control or improve symptoms; and an itemized list of recommendations, written in layman's language, is often very helpful in managing such individuals. Such recommendations should first be reviewed with the patient, after which

Table 87.1.
Indications for Operation

Claudication that is intolerable in a good risk patient
Ischemic rest pain
Impending gangrene
Nonhealing ulceration

the patient should be given the list for ready reference (Table 87.2). Many of these recommendations pertain to protection of the feet. It should be emphasized that avoidance of trauma to the feet from ill-fitting shoes and avoidance of extremes of temperature are very important in the management program. If the patient finds that his feet are cold, particularly at night, he should be told not to use heating pads or hot water bottles since these may cause tissue breakdown and ulceration. A warm pair of socks or a muffler is advised. Patients should bathe their feet at least once a day in lukewarm water (tested by the hand) and thereafter apply lanolin or hand cream to the skin to keep it soft and pliable, thereby avoiding cracking and fissuring, particularly between the toes, which might lead to skin breakdown. Diabetic patients with peripheral occlusive disease are at very high risk of eventual foot amputation, and these protective measures are especially important for them. In addition, diabetic patients should be followed at least every 3 months by a podiatrist for trimming of callouses and nails and for close evaluation for early signs of infection or impending ulceration.

Other measures that significantly affect outcome include improving cardiac output, if congestive heart failure is present (see Chapter 61), and controlling diabetes mellitus. It is very important that the patient be advised to exercise to tolerance every day to stimulate collateral channel development. Exercise tolerance can be improved in up to two-thirds of individuals in this way. Also, it is most important to urge strongly the cessation of use of all tobacco products. It must be emphasized to patients that smoking accelerates atherogenesis, causes further hypoxia because of carbon monoxide poisoning, and causes vasospasm in the important collateral vascular bed that may last up to 1 hour after each cigarette. Patients must be admonished that nicotine in any form is absorbed through

Table 87.2.
Advice That Should be Given to Patients with Arterial Insufficiency

QUIT SMOKING—Use NO tobacco in ANY form[a].
If overweight, lose weight.
Exercise (walk) to the point of discomfort at least 2 miles a day.
Keep feet very clean. Bathe at least daily in LUKEWARM water.
Gently apply lanolin or mild hand cream to feet after bathing.
Use a night light to avoid hitting toes or shins.
Wear clean, preferably cotton, socks daily (cotton does not retain moisture).
Avoid injury to feet. Wear proper fitting shoes to prevent calluses, corns, blisters. Avoid shoes made of synthetic material that doesn't "breathe".
Place lamb's wool (available from pharmacies) between over-riding toes.
Avoid extremes of temperature. Do not put feet in hot water or use heating pads on lower extremities. In cold weather, wear socks to bed to warm feet. Do not get feet cold or wet.
If feet hurt at night, raise head of bed 6–10 inches (15–25 cm) on blocks.
For any sudden change in symptoms such as prolonged pain, numbness or tingling, or inability to move foot or leg, consult your physician *immediately*.

[a] See Chapter 20 for ways to help patients to stop smoking.

the buccal mucosa, be it pipe, or cigarette smoke, or tobacco juice.

Management of coexistent hypertension is sometimes challenging because among such patients, if blood pressure is too well controlled, symptoms may increase. Therefore, when managing hypertension in such individuals, one often may have to settle for less than ideal blood pressure control.

Pharmacological Management

There is little objective evidence to suggest that vasodilating drugs offer significant benefits to patients with symptomatic peripheral arterial insufficiency. Blood vessels in ischemic tissue beds are already maximally dilated as a local response to ischemia. When systemic vessels are dilated by these drugs, blood flow to the involved extremity may actually decrease and vasodilators may have the paradoxical effect of causing further ischemia. Therefore, vasodilator therapy should not be used in the treatment of patients with occlusive vascular disease.

Similarly, except for heparin anticoagulation in the hospital among patients who suffer acute deterioration of their peripheral circulation, long-term anticoagulation with oral agents has not been shown to have any beneficial effect on retardation of atherosclerosis or on improving symptoms. Oral anticoagulants in frail elderly, forgetful, or unreliable individuals may pose significant hazards from complications of anticoagulation therapy (see Chapter 52). Platelet-inhibiting agents have not been shown to be effective in management of lower extremity arterial occlusive disease (see Chapter 52).

Although drug therapy has been disappointing in the past, there has been recent enthusiasm for using drugs that improve blood flow through the microcirculation by a direct effect on the membrane of the red cell. It has been shown that erythrocytes from patients with obstructive arterial disease have a decrease in membrane flexibility and consequently may not deform adequately to squeeze through capillaries with a diameter of 4 to 5 μm. Pentoxifylline (Trental), a drug that returns erythrocyte deformability to almost normal, has been available for several years in the United States. It is a xanthine derivative whose precise mechanism of action is as yet undefined but probably is related to its inhibition of phosphodiesterase in red cells, thereby increasing intraerythrocyte cyclic adenosine monophosphate (AMP) (red cells depleted of cyclic AMP are more rigid). A randomized double-blind parallel group evaluation of the efficacy of pentoxifylline in the treatment of intermittent claudication documented that statistically significant improvement in claudication distance was found in individuals taking pentoxifylline (23). However, the degree of improvement was not enough to suggest that the drug would be effective by itself (i.e., if the patient continued to smoke and did not exercise appropriately).

Pentoxifylline is available in 400-mg tablets, usually prescribed in a dosage of one tablet three times a day with meals. A positive effect, if it occurs, will be seen in 1 to 2 months. The major side effects of the drug are nausea, dyspepsia, and dizziness, which often may be relieved by reducing the dose to one tablet twice a day.

Operative Intervention

It is only upon failure of nonoperative therapy or among individuals with clear indications for operation that arteriographic studies are obtained. It must be understood that arteriography serves as a guide for the vascular surgeon when reconstructing the vascular tree. There are no characteristic arteriographic findings that distinguish between patients with intermittent claudication, those with ischemic rest pain, and those suffering from gangrene and ulceration. As a generalization, however, patients who have intermittent claudication usually have hemodynamically significant proximal arterial occlusive lesions affecting the iliofemoral system or the femoral-popliteal-tibial system. Characteristically, such individuals have reasonably good outflow with two or more tibial vessels patent. Individuals with advanced ischemic changes will be found to have diffuse multisegment involvement and none or only one patent vessel in the lower leg or foot. However, overlap between various groups is wide, and no single arteriographic finding consistently characterizes any one symptom complex.

Rarely arteriography documents distribution of arterial involvement that is either too advanced or too peripheral to permit reconstruction. Advances in distal bypass surgery with the use of magnification lenses and nonreversed venous conduits almost always allows a reasonable chance of successful revascularization. However, there are times when an arteriographic pattern, with absence of any visible distal vessels, suggests that bypass is not possible. Under these circumstances, nonoperative therapy usually is recommended; but if ischemic rest pain and tissue necrosis are present, both patient and family are informed that when an operation is required, amputation is all that may be offered.

Indications for operation among patients with intermittent claudication relate mainly to the ability of the patient to tolerate the pain. Trivial claudication and even mild ischemic rest pain, controlled by non-narcotic analgesics, are not indications for operation, particularly in high risk individuals. A trial of conservative management is particularly important if other risk factors, such as recent myocardial infarction, are present (see Chapter 86, Preoperative Planning for Ambulatory Patients).

When it is determined that the condition of the patient warrants operative intervention and when arteriography documents repairable vessels, a number of options for arterial reconstruction are open to the vascular surgeon. Procedures employed include bypass reconstruction by use of an autogenous vein or prosthetic graft and endarterectomy. There is a definite preference for bypass reconstructive procedures over endarterectomy, an operation that is rarely used at the present time. Reconstructive procedures include aortofemoral bypass, femoral-popliteal bypass, and femoral-tibial bypass. Occasionally extra-anatomical reconstruction is done, bypassing the diseased aortoiliac arterial tree, particularly among individuals deemed to be at great risk from a major intra-abdominal procedure. Such extra-anatomical reconstructive procedures include axillounifemoral bypass, axillobifemoral bypass, and femoral-femoral bypass.

It is not appropriate to compare results between various surgical modalities and various patient populations because of variability among patient groups. As a generalization, however, operative mortality for aortofemoral bypass reconstruction is approximately 5%. The patency rate for aortofemoral bypass reconstruction is approximately 80 to 90% at 5 years. Operative mortality rates for extra-anatomical reconstruction are slightly less than for aortofemoral reconstruction, but graft patency rates are significantly worse.

Operative mortality for autogenous vein femoral-popliteal bypass procedures ranges from 0.5 to 1% depending on the general condition of the patient. Five-year patency rates for such procedures vary between 60 and 70%, but it should be emphasized that patency varies directly with the extent of the disease in the vessel being reconstructed.

In general, in contrast to arterial reconstruction for aneurysmal disease, arterial reconstruction for occlusive disease is at best palliative and does not significantly increase the patient's life expectancy because most individuals have significant coincident coronary artery disease. However, the quality of life is vastly improved, particularly among those individuals who would have undergone amputation if successful arterial reconstruction had not been feasible. Patients can often walk an unrestricted distance after successful arterial reconstruction.

Patients with aortofemoral arterial occlusive disease, but without coronary artery disease or diabetes mellitus, have survival rates that equal those of the normal age- and sex-adjusted population. Observed differences in life expectancy between "normal" populations and those undergoing arterial reconstructive procedures are usually due to the high prevalence of associated coronary artery disease and diabetes mellitus. It appears that the presence of coronary artery disease reduces life expectancy approximately 10 years, and the presence of diabetes mellitus reduces life expectancy by an additional 15 years (19).

Balloon Angioplasty and Laser and Mechanical Atherectomy

Since the mid-1970s percutaneous transluminal arterial dilation, as an alternative to surgical reconstruction, has been available for highly selected patients with arterial occlusive disease. Its advantages include low morbidity, low mortality, lower cost than arterial reconstruction, shorter hospital stay, repeatability, low complication rate, and patient acceptability. It must be understood that patients who are not candidates for arterial reconstruction, but may be candidates for percutaneous transluminal dilation, may also require operation for complications of transluminal dilation. Therefore, a cooperative team approach between the angiographer and the vascular surgeon is mandatory to provide optimal results and to minimize complications.

Most authors agree that the best results with percutaneous transluminal dilation are obtained in short stenoses in iliac arteries in which success rates at 1 year range from 76 to 93% and at 2 years range from 66 to 92%. The reported success rates for femoropopliteal disease range between 51 and 80% at 1 year and 46 to 75% at 2 years. There is general agreement that results are less satisfactory if the runoff, documented by arteriography, is poor. Recent evidence suggests that in the properly selected patient, the probability of early success of percutaneous transluminal dilation is high if the vessel is stenosed, the involved vessel is the iliac, and the runoff is good (18). Results are less satisfactory when multiple dilations are required.

Longer stenoses and occlusions have less favorable results but in very poor risk patients may be an alternative to reconstruction. Occlusions less than 5 cm long and stenoses less than 10 cm long appear to be the outer limits for successful percutaneous arterial dilation.

It is appealing to believe that percutaneous transluminal arterial dilation can be substituted for arterial reconstruction. However, the criteria for the use of this modality should be as rigid as those required for reconstructive surgery.

Recently, *laser atherectomy* has been introduced as an adjunct in the management of peripheral vascular disease (25). The laser is occasionally useful in developing a channel through an occlusion to allow passage of a balloon catheter for dilation (laser-assisted balloon angioplasty). At present the laser is not being used as sole therapy and its usefulness is actually somewhat limited since all stenoses and most short occlusions can be treated with angioplasty without the need for laser. In the case of long occlusions of the femoral artery, the laser may be better able to develop a channel for the balloon but the recurrent stenosis rate is very high in these cases (50% within 6 to 12 months).

Mechanical atherectomy devices, which use a cutting blade to remove rather than to dilate plaque, are currently under investigation and may further add to the armamentarium of the vascular surgeon for treating peripheral vascular disease.

Amputation

Occasionally the only form of therapy that can be offered is amputation. Debilitated patients with frank gangrene or continuous ischemic rest pain are not candidates for arterial reconstruction or arterial dilation, and amputation is the only feasible alternative. The object of amputation is to relieve the patient of disabling pain, remove nonviable and potentially infected tissue, and select a level that will provide the greatest chance of healing with maximal rehabilitation. Requirements that must be kept in mind when selecting amputation level are (a) the amputation must remove all necrotic and painful ischemic tissue, (b) the amputation stump must be able to be fitted with a functional and easily applied prosthesis, and (c) the blood supply to the skin at the level of the amputation must be adequate to permit primary skin healing.

If the gangrenous process is dry and does not involve the great toe, either autoamputation may be allowed to occur or formal surgical amputation may be performed. If pulses are palpable in the foot and the ischemic process affects the tips of the digits, primary healing will usually occur after toe amputation. In addition, neurotrophic (nonischemic) ulcers on the plantar aspects of the foot in diabetic patients will frequently heal if the head of the metatarsal is removed to relieve the pressure necrosis that occurs as a result of the diabetic neuropathy.

Mortality for amputation is directly related to the preoperative condition of the patient and to other complicating diseases. Mortality rates for amputations performed for occlusive arterial disease have been reported to be as high as 30% with the higher mortality rates recorded in the more proximal amputations.

After successful amputation, the most important aspect of therapy is rehabilitation. To this end, the more distal the amputation, the easier the rehabilitation. In addition, close cooperation between the surgeon and a rehabilitation center is essential to provide the greatest chance of functional ambulation with a minimum of delay. Although it is difficult to predict precisely which amputees will be able to use a prosthesis successfully, in general, patients who have had above-the-knee amputation, who are elderly, obese, or diabetic, adjust less well to attempts to restore ambulatory function.

ABDOMINAL AORTIC ANEURYSMS

Abdominal aortic aneurysm is the most commonly encountered aneurysm of the arterial tree. It is encountered two to three times more often than popliteal arterial aneurysm, the second most common aneurysm. Abdominal aortic aneurysms have been found in almost 2% of consecutive postmortem studies (3).

Men are affected by aneurysmal disease 10 times more often than women. The occurrence of abdominal aortic aneurysms increases with age.

Although it is not possible to implicate precisely a single etiology of abdominal aortic aneurysm, most are arteriosclerotic in origin. The infrarenal abdominal aorta is more susceptible to aneurysmal degeneration than are other arterial segments, although the reasons for this are unknown. Only about 5% of abdominal aortic aneurysms encroach upon visceral vessels, most commonly the renal arteries.

The *natural history* of untreated abdominal aortic aneurysms was unknown until the report of Estes (9) in 1950 that documented, for the first time, the grave consequences of this disease. Five-year survival of patients with untreated aneurysms approximates only 20%. Forty to 50% of patients with untreated abdominal aortic aneurysms die of rupture within 5 years; and 30% die of other causes, usually from complications of diffuse arteriosclerosis, most notably myocardial infarction. Multiple groups have presented corroborating data emphasizing the improved life expectancy after surgical treatment of this condition (5, 6, 13, 27) (see below).

Clinical Manifestations

History

The presentation of an abdominal aortic aneurysm depends upon whether complications have occurred. Over 50% of abdominal aortic aneurysms are asymptomatic when first discovered. Asymptomatic aneurysms may be noted during routine examination by a physician for another problem or may be found by the patient. Occasionally, patients complain of a "second heart" in the abdomen after they palpate a pulsatile epigastric mass.

The patient may complain of abdominal, flank, or back pain as the aneurysm expands and becomes symptomatic. Such symptoms are a harbinger of disaster because rupture may follow at an unpredictable time after onset of symptoms.

Rupture. Most aneurysms that rupture bleed into the retroperitoneal space, affording lifesaving tamponade after blood pressure falls sufficiently. Under these circumstances, the patient presents with a history of syncope, flank, or back pain, and in a hypovolemic-hypotensive state. Most patients suffering intraperitoneal rupture of abdominal aortic aneurysms are dead by the time they reach the hospital. However, a few do present for treatment; such individuals are profoundly hypotensive and require immediate operative intervention, in spite of seemingly lethal coincidental problems. Aneurysms may rupture also into an adjacent vein, causing a large arteriovenous fistula (such as an aortocaval or aortorenal fistula); or they may rupture into the gastrointestinal tract, usually duodenum, causing an aortoenteric fistula.

Other complications. If aneurysms are large enough, they may compress adjacent structures, such as ureter, duodenum, vena cava, or vertebral column, with production of appropriate symptoms (for example, symptoms of gastric outlet obstruction in patients with duodenal compression).

Dislodgement of laminated clots from the wall of the aneurysm may cause peripheral embolization to femoral, popliteal, or distal vessels. When emboli occur, patients may complain of symptoms of sudden leg ischemia as the first indication of an abdominal aortic aneurysm (see below). If embolic bits of debris are small and distal vessels are patent, patients may complain of small areas of tissue necrosis such as digital gangrene of the tip of a toe, or small punctate pretibial ischemic lesions.

Finally, aneurysms that suddenly thrombose may present with abrupt ischemia of a lower extremity that can be confused with the presentation resulting from cardiac or from arterial emboli.

Although the incidence of the various complications (other than rupture) is not known, they do underscore the pessimistic natural history of untreated abdominal aortic aneurysms. After seeking specific historical information regarding the aneurysm itself, it is important to question the patient regarding other symptoms of arteriosclerosis so that an estimate of the extent of involvement is obtained; this information will frequently influence recommendations for or against surgical therapy (see Chapter 86). Symptoms of transient cerebral ischemia or previous stroke, angina pectoris or previous myocardial infarction, or symptoms of cardiac decompensation such as significant severe shortness of breath, ankle edema, orthopnea, and paroxysmal nocturnal dyspnea all are especially important in determining the risks in this group of patients.

Physical Examination

Physical examination is the single most valuable source of information in the diagnosis of intrarenal abdominal aortic aneurysms and has been reported to be accurate in almost 90% of cases (9). Depending on the clinical presentation, either complicated or uncomplicated, physical examination will vary. As noted, most patients present with asymptomatic abdominal aortic aneurysms that are discovered on routine physical examination during evaluation for other problems. Under these circumstances, an epigastric pulsatile mass usually is felt. However, in obese individuals or in those with very small aneurysms, a mass may not be palpable. Among these individuals asymptomatic aneurysms may be discovered when X-rays are obtained for other intra-abdominal conditions such as peptic ulcer or renal or colonic disease.

It is important to palpate the epigastrium since the bifurcation of the abdominal aorta is at the level of the umbilicus. Only rarely when palpating inferior to the umbilicus will one identify an abdominal aortic aneurysm unless both common iliac arteries are also greatly aneurysmal. The laterally pulsatile nature of an abdominal aortic aneurysm is key to differentiating it from a mass that might feel pulsatile because it overlies the aorta. Lesions confused with abdominal aortic aneurysm include pancreatic neoplasms, pancreatic pseudocyst, horseshoe kidneys, neoplasms of the stomach or transverse colon, and retroperitoneal soft tissue tumors. Not uncommonly, a normal but prominently pulsatile abdominal aorta in a healthy individual is confused with an abdominal aortic aneurysm. Furthermore, in elderly patients an undilated but tortuous aorta may simulate an abdominal aortic aneurysm. In this circumstance, the pulsatile mass is felt to the left of the midline but not to the right. One should palpate the abdomen by approaching the midline both from the right and from the left to identify the laterally pulsatile characteristic of an aneurysm.

Risk of rupture correlates best with the size of the aneurysm (see below). Estimation of the size by physical examination alone, however, is so variable that it is completely unreliable.

One-quarter to one-third of patients have significant associated occlusive arterial disease as well as the abdominal aortic aneurysm; therefore, a systematic evaluation of all peripheral pulses should be performed. Systemic blood pressure in both arms should be measured because many patients with aortic aneurysms have hypertension. By listening with a stethoscope (the bell is most efficient) over the carotid bifurcations the physician may determine whether concomitant carotid arterial occlusive disease is present. When examining the lower extremities, particular attention should be directed to the character of the femoral, popliteal, and pedal pulses. In a small percentage of patients (probably less than 10%) there may be coexistent peripheral aneurysms involving the popliteal or femoral arteries.

Laboratory and X-ray Studies

It is particularly important that the suspicion, on physical examination, of an abdominal aortic aneurysm be confirmed by sonography. The accuracy of ultrasonic diagnosis of abdominal aortic aneurysm approaches 98% (21, 29). Anteroposterior and cross table lateral films of the abdomen will also document abdominal aortic aneurysms in 70 to 80% of cases because the aneurysm wall is frequently calcified (Fig. 87.2). Because the size of the aneurysm may affect therapy, particularly in asymptomatic and in very poor risk individuals, reliance on accurate ultrasonography or on X-ray assumes great importance. Although there are certain pitfalls in ultrasonography (e.g., the size of the aneurysm is often underestimated), it is an excellent technique, not only for detection of abdominal aortic aneurysms but for following patients who are not candidates for operation; repeated studies every 3 to 6 months are helpful in monitoring the size of the aneurysm.

Computed tomography (CT) is a useful means of assessing abdominal aortic aneurysms, which are seen on computed tomograms as areas of increased aortic diameter. An advantage of CT scanning is that it delineates both the lumen and the outer wall of the aneurysm with the intervening mural thrombus. Computed tomography also may document chronic aortic rupture with a contained hematoma as well as a very thin-walled aneurysm that may have a propensity for rupture.

It is useful, also, to have an objective measurement of peripheral pulses in the lower extremities to gauge the results of therapy or to follow the progression of coexistent occlusive arterial disease. This measure-

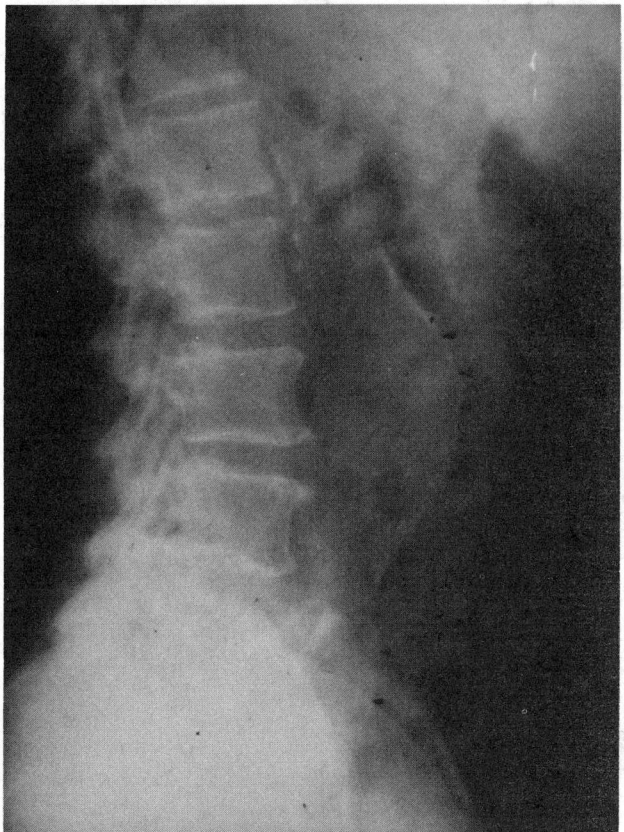

Figure 87.2. Cross table lateral abdominal X-ray documenting calcified abdominal aortic aneurysm.

ment is best made by the vascular surgeon by use of a Doppler blood velocity detection device.

Treatment and Results

Once the presence of an abdominal aortic aneurysm has been verified by either ultrasound or CT scan, a decision regarding therapy must be made. The risk of catastrophic rupture among patients with aneurysms greater than 6 cm in transverse diameter is so great that almost all such individuals must be considered candidates for operation (Fig. 87.3). Aneurysms between 4 and 6 cm impose an intermediate risk of rupture (10 to 30% within 2 to 3 years).

The natural history of abdominal aortic aneurysms dictates that even patients with small aneurysms should be treated surgically unless the risk is prohibitive. The classic study of Szilagyi et al. (27) comparing nonoperative with operative therapy is summarized in Fig. 87.3. Even with the worst operative mortality (13%), survival after surgical management of small aneurysms is better than nonsurgical management. As operative mortality declines, the disparity becomes greater. However, if patients have significant life-limiting concurrent disease and small asymptomatic abdominal aortic aneurysms, a close follow-up program can be instituted. Generally, aneurysms grow at an average

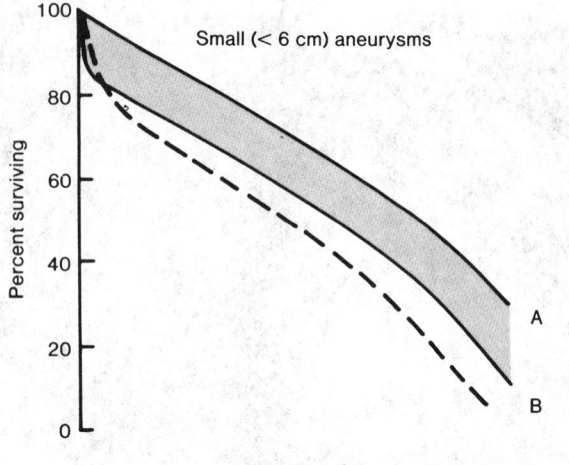

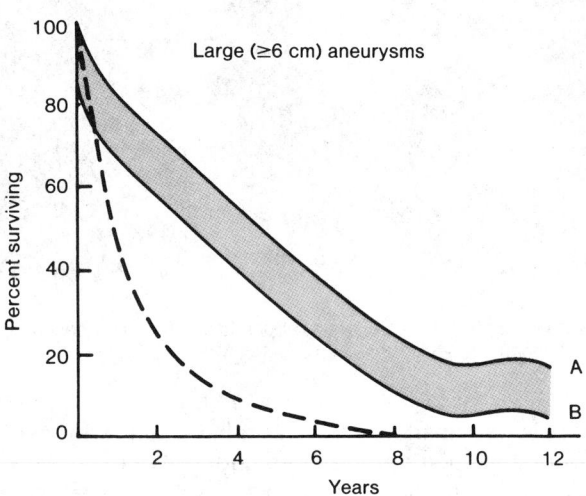

Figure 87.3. Survival curves for surgical and nonsurgical patients with large and small aortic aneurysms. The *dashed lines* represent survival rates in the nonsurgical groups; the bands, in the surgical groups (the top of the bands (*A*) assumed no operative mortality; the bottom (*B*), a 13% operative mortality). (Modified by Rutherford from data provided by Szilagyi). Even with 13% operative mortality, surgical treatment is better than nonsurgical treatment. (Adapted from Rutherford RB (ed): *Vascular Surgery* 2nd ed. Philadelphia, WB Saunders, 1984.)

rate of 0.4 cm/year (1), although one disputed (4) population-based study suggested a slower rate (20). There are no reported cases of spontaneous regression. When dealing with large aneurysms, even assuming an operative mortality rate of 13%, surgical therapy is clearly superior to nonsurgical therapy. Over the last two decades, operative mortality has declined to between 2 and 5% for elective aneurysmectomy (5, 8). Should operation be delayed until the aneurysm ruptures, operative mortality increases to a formidable 60 to 80%, particularly if the patient arrives at the hospital in hypovolemic shock. Even when such patients can be resuscitated adequately prior to operation, operative mortality remains approximately 50%.

Age in itself does not affect the risk of operation. Elective aneurysmectomy can be performed in a very elderly individual with an operative mortality rate comparable to a similar operation in younger individuals, provided the patient is a satisfactory operative candidate. Furthermore, as a group patients with major complications of their aneurysm (see above) do better with surgical therapy than they do without surgical therapy (26).

Therefore, it is generally advised that aneurysmectomy be performed in all individuals with a reasonable life expectancy who, in the judgment of the physician and surgeon, would tolerate the operative procedure with an operative mortality of less than 5%. Clearly, operation is mandatory for any individuals who have complications of their aneurysms (see above).

Controversy exists regarding routine use of preoperative aortography among patients with abdominal aortic aneurysms. Although some surgeons routinely recommend aortography, the majority employ aortographic studies selectively. One thing is clear—aortography should neither be used to confirm the diagnosis of an abdominal aortic aneurysm nor to make the diagnosis. Because of laminated clots within the aneurysmal sac, abdominal aortography may actually be misleading, giving an impression of an aneurysm that is actually smaller than it is or even giving the impression that an aneurysm is not present.

Under certain circumstances, abdominal aortographic studies are helpful and even mandatory. Indications for aortography include the possibility of the involvement of other blood vessels, either by the aneurysm itself encroaching upon the renal arteries or by concomitant occlusive arterial disease involving inferior mesenteric, superior mesenteric, or celiac vessels. It is important to determine the extent of reconstruction necessary so that these occlusive lesions do not go untreated and thereby jeopardize the overall result after aneurysmectomy. Drug-resistant hypertension, possibly on a renovascular basis, is another indication for aortography to document renal arterial involvement that might be correctable during abdominal aortic aneurysmectomy. Also, if aneurysmal disease is associated with extensive involvement of the iliac vessels, aortography is indicated. If there is suspicion of congenital arterial anomalies or other congenital defects such as horseshoe kidneys, abdominal aortography is helpful to delineate variances in blood supply associated with such abnormalities and to facilitate operative correction.

It is essential to inform the patient and family of various risks of operative versus nonoperative therapy. Equally important is explaining what complications may occur in the postoperative period. Although this is primarily the responsibility of the operating surgeon, it is appropriate for the primary physician to discuss with the patient what is likely to occur. The patient should know that a Dacron or Teflon prosthesis will be used to replace the abdominal aorta and that such arterial grafts are durable and, in general, never need to be replaced. Complications, fortunately, are very rare and in aggregate probably occur less than 2 to 3% of the time. Such complications include paraplegia from spinal cord ischemia, renal failure, loss of one or both legs (rare), graft infection, ischemic colitis, and aortoenteric fistula development. In addition, approximately one-quarter of male patients may develop impotence after abdominal aortic reconstruction. It should be stressed to the patient and family that postoperative complications of abdominal aortic aneurysmectomy are magnified by the urgency of the operative procedure.

If, for any reason, operation is not recommended or accepted, patients should be evaluated at 3- to 6-month intervals for progression of disease or for improvement of coincidental problems, either of which might mandate operation. Because abdominal aortic aneurysms do not dissect, symptoms mimicking dissecting thoracic aneurysms, such as pain shooting into the legs, do not occur. Most commonly, a patient with a rupturing or symptomatic aneurysm will complain of steady dull abdominal, flank, or back pain. If such pain occurs or if a change in existing symptoms is noted in a patient being followed with an abdominal aortic aneurysm, he and his family should be instructed to seek surgical attention promptly.

PERIPHERAL ARTERIAL ANEURYSMS

Peripheral arterial aneurysms may involve the carotid, subclavian, brachial, iliac, femoral, and popliteal arteries. Over 90% of peripheral aneurysms involve either popliteal or femoral arteries. Popliteal arterial aneurysms predominate. More commonly, tortuous vessels presenting as serpiginous pulsations under the skin are mistaken for peripheral aneurysms. The most noted example of this is a tortuous subclavian or common carotid artery in an elderly, hypertensive individual that may be confused with a carotid or subclavian artery aneurysm.

Most peripheral arterial aneurysms are arteriosclerotic in origin although mycotic, traumatic, and syphilitic aneurysms are seen occasionally. Peripheral arteriosclerotic aneurysms are localized manifestations of a generalized disease process. This is underscored by noting that, among patients who have femoral arterial aneurysms, 95% have another aneurysm elsewhere; and, more important, 92% have abdominal aortic aneurysms (7). Almost 60% of femoral arterial aneurysms are bilateral. Similarly, among individuals with popliteal arterial aneurysms, almost 80% have another aneurysm elsewhere; two-thirds have abdominal aortic aneurysms; and about half have another popliteal arterial aneurysm (7). Therefore, upon identifying a peripheral arterial aneurysm, the physician should routinely look for a potentially lethal abdominal aortic aneurysm.

Femoral and, particularly, popliteal arterial aneurysms are associated with a very high incidence of distal thromboembolism and of eventual limb loss. Untreated peripheral aneurysms may eventuate in limb loss approximately 75% of the time from either distal embolization or acute thrombosis. On the other hand, rupture with exsanguinating hemorrhage from femoral or popliteal arterial aneurysm is not a major risk.

Clinical Manifestations

Most patients presenting with peripheral arterial aneurysms are elderly, and many may be asymptomatic. Femoral arterial aneurysms usually are quite evident, particularly when they measure 4 or 5 cm in diameter. Similarly, popliteal arterial aneurysms, if they are large, are easily identified. However, popliteal arterial aneurysms may be overlooked because many clinicians do not routinely palpate the popliteal fossa during a physical examination.

Clinical manifestations depend upon whether or not complications are associated with peripheral aneurysms. Patients may present with sudden acute ischemia of an extremity because of thrombosis of the popliteal or femoral arterial aneurysm and manifest any of the six "Ps" of acute arterial ischemia: pallor, pulselessness, poikilothermia, pain, paresthesia, or paralysis. Among individuals in whom complications of peripheral aneurysms develop, successful limb salvage is significantly less likely than among patients in whom surgical therapy is offered before the development of such complications.

Similar to abdominal aortic aneurysms, lateral expansileness of a prominent femoral or popliteal pulse is characteristic of a femoral or popliteal aneurysm. A bruit may be associated with the aneurysm, but it is of no clinical significance. Diagnosis of femoral arterial aneurysm is easily made on clinical examination alone. The diagnosis of popliteal aneurysm may be more difficult. When palpating the popliteal fossa, it is helpful to have the patient relax his leg in a passively flexed position to allow the examiner's fingers access to the fossa. If an unusually prominent popliteal fossa is palpated and the examiner suspects aneurysm, the patient may be placed in the prone position and the lower leg supported by the examiner's arm to facilitate popliteal arterial palpation. If diagnosis of popliteal arterial aneurysm is in doubt, a sonogram or CT scan should be obtained. Occasionally, the only manifestations of a popliteal arterial aneurysm are small punctate necrotic areas of skin over the anterior tibial region or small gangrenous areas of the tips of toes. This "blue toe syndrome" is a result of microemboli from the aneurysm that have showered to the periphery.

Once the diagnosis of a peripheral arterial aneurysm is made, the patient should be referred to a vascular surgeon. Although arteriography is not required, but is highly recommended in management of abdominal aortic aneurysms (see above), arteriography is mandatory in management of peripheral aneurysms and, in particular, of popliteal arterial aneurysms. The arteriogram is used not so much to make the diagnosis but to document patency of arteries distal to the aneurysm, information that is critical to the vascular surgeon in planning arterial reconstruction.

Treatment and Results

Treatment of peripheral aneurysms is indicated in all instances in which it is the physician's estimate that the patient has a reasonable life expectancy. Because the natural history of peripheral aneurysms is one of eventual limb loss, it is important to offer surgical therapy to maintain or improve quality of life by avoiding amputation. If, however, patients have concurrent significant disease or are bedridden for other reasons, operation is not justified. Surgical correction includes replacement of femoral arterial aneurysms with Dacron grafts or with segments of reversed autogenous saphenous vein. Similarly, popliteal arterial aneurysms are managed by bypassing the diseased segment, preferably with autogenous saphenous vein but, if vein is not available, with any suitable prosthetic material.

Operative mortality for management of peripheral aneurysms approximates 1 to 3%. Limb salvage is obtained in over 90% of cases and is related to the degree of arterial involvement peripheral to the aneurysm. In almost all series reporting repair of popliteal arterial aneurysms, amputations in the postoperative period have been associated with severe occlusive arterial disease manifest by gangrene and rest pain preoperatively.

General References

Boyd AM: The natural course of arteriosclerosis of the lower extremities. *Angiology* 11:10, 1960.

> This study of 1440 patients with intermittent claudication, carefully evaluated and followed over an interval of 15 years, for the first time documented the natural history of intermittent claudication. This study provides the control data base against which results of surgical and nonsurgical therapy are judged.

Crawford ES, Saleh SA, Babb JW III, et al: Infrarenal abdominal aortic aneurysm; factors influencing survival after operation performed over a 25-year period. *Ann Surg* 193:699, 1981.

> Experience of an outstanding vascular surgeon evaluating 920 consecutive patients operated upon for abdominal aortic aneurysm. This paper is the "gold standard" against which the results of others are measured.

Dent TL, Lindenauer SM, Ernst CB, Fry WJ: Multiple arteriosclerotic arterial aneurysms. *Arch Surg* 105:338, 1972.

> Evaluation of 57 patients with peripheral aneurysms among 1488 having aneurysmal disease. Importance of coincidental multiple aneurysms when encountering patients with aneurysmal disease stresses need for thorough vascular evaluation.

Rutherford RB (ed): *Vascular Surgery*, 3rd ed, Philadelphia, WB Saunders, 1989.

> The first comprehensive text of vascular surgery. Specific disease entities are extensively discussed including nonoperative as well as operative aspects. Basic pathophysiological concepts are lucidly presented. This work should be in the library of all interested in vascular diseases.

Specific References

1. Bernstein EF, Dilley RB, Goldberger LE, et al: Growth rates of small abdominal aortic aneurysms. *Surgery* 80:765, 1976.
2. Boyd AM: The natural course of arteriosclerosis of the lower extremities. *Angiology* 11:10, 1960.
3. Carlsson J, Sternby NH: Aortic aneurysms. *Acta Chir Scand* 127:466, 1964.
4. Crawford ES, Hess KR: Abdominal aortic aneurysm. *N Engl J Med* 321:1040, 1989.
5. Crawford ES, Saleh SA, Babb JW III, et al: Infrarenal abdominal aortic aneurysm; factors influencing survival after operation performed over a 25-year period. *Ann Surg* 193:699, 1981.
6. DeBakey ME, Crawford ES, Cooley DA, Morris Jr GC: Aneurysm of the abdominal aorta; analysis of results of graft replacement therapy 1 to 11 years after operation. *Ann Surg* 160:622, 1964.
7. Dent TL, Lindenauer SM, Ernst CB, Fry WJ: Multiple arteriosclerotic arterial aneurysms. *Arch Surg* 105:338, 1972.
8. DeWeese JA, Blaisdell FW, Foster JH: Optimal resources for vascular surgery. *Arch Surg* 105:948, 1972.
9. Estes JE: Abdominal aortic aneurysm. A study of 102 cases. *Circulation* 2:258, 1950.
10. Fogarty TJ, Buch WS: The management of embolic and thrombotic arterial occlusion. In: Rutherford RB, (ed): *Vascular Surgery*. Philadelphia, WB Saunders, 1977, p. 423.
11. Fogarty TJ, Cranley JJ, Krause RT, et al: A method for extraction of arterial emboli and thrombi. *Surg Gynecol Obstet* 116:241, 1963.
12. Fogarty TJ, Daily PO, Shumway NE, Krippaehne W: Experience with balloon catherter technique for arterial embolectomy. *Am J Surg* 122:231, 1971.
13. Foster JH, Bolasny BL, Gobbel Jr WG, Scott HW Jr: Comparative study of elective resection and expectant treatment of abdominal aortic aneurysm. *Surg Gynecol Obstet* 129:1, 1969.
14. Imparato AM, Kim GE, Davidson T, Crowley JG: Intermittent claudication; its natural course. *Surgery* 78:795, 1975.
15. Juergens JC, Barker NW, Hines EA: Arteriosclerosis obliterans. Review of 520 cases with special reference to pathogenic and prognostic factors. *Circulation* 21:188, 1960.
16. Katzen BT, Edwards KC, Albert AS, VanBreda A: Low-dose direct fibrinolysis in peripheral vascular disease. *J Vasc Surg* 1:718, 1984.
17. Kempczinski RF: Lower extremity arterial emboli from ulcerating atherosclerotic plaques. *JAMA* 241:807, 1979.
18. Lally ME, Johnston KW, Andrews D: Percutaneous transluminal dilatation of peripheral arteries: an analysis of factors predicting early sucess. *J Vasc Surg* 1:704, 1984.
19. Malone JM, Moore WS, Goldstone J: Life expectancy following aortofemoral arterial grafting. *Surgery* 81:551, 1977.
20. Nevitt MP, Ballard DJ, Hallett Jr JW: Prognosis of abdominal aortic aneurysms: A population-based study. *N Engl J Med* 321:1009, 1989.
21. Nusbaum JW, Freimans AK, Thomford NR: Echography in the diagnosis of abdominal aortic aneurysm. *Arch Surg* 102:385, 1971.
22. Panetta T, Thompson J, Talkington C, et al: Arterial embolectomy: a 34-year experience with 400 cases. *Surg Clin North Am.* 66:339, 1986.
23. Porter SM, Baur EM: Pharmacologic treatment of intermittent claudication. *Surgery* 92:966, 1982.
24. Satiani B, Gross WS, Evans WE: Improved limb salvage after arterial embolectomy. *Ann Surg* 188:153, 1978.
25. Seeger JM, Abela GS, Silverman SH, et al: Initial results of laser recanalization in lower extremity arterial reconstruction. *J Vasc Surg* 9:10, 1989.
26. Szilagyi DE, Elliott JP, Smith RF: Clinical fate of the patient with asymptomatic abdominal aortic aneurysm and unfit for surgical treatment. *Arch Surg* 104:600, 1972.
27. Szilagyi DE, Smith R, DeRusso FJ, et al: Contribution of abdominal aortic aneurysmectomy to prolongation of life. *Ann Surg* 164:678, 1966.
28. Towne JB, Bandyk DF: Application of thrombolytic therapy in vascular occlusive disease. A surgical view. *Am J Surg* 154:548, 1987.
29. Winsberg G, Cole-Beuglet C, Mulder DS: Continuous ultrasound "B" scanning of abdominal aortic aneurysms. *AJR* 121:626, 1974.
30. Yao JST: Hemodynamic studies in peripheral arterial disease. *Br J Surg* 57:561, 1970.

CHAPTER 88

Lower Extremity Ulcers and Varicose Veins

ANDREW M. MUNSTER, M.D.
ROBERT J. SPENCE, M.D.

LEG ULCERS

Ulceration of a lower extremity is a common and important problem in ambulatory medical practice, most often caused by either macro- or microvascular disease. Accurate diagnosis is based mainly on history and physical examination and is essential for appropriate treatment. Often the management of various types of leg ulcers is completely different, one from the other. Inappropriate therapy can lead to the loss of a toe or even of a limb. Generally it is necessary to (a) give detailed instructions to the patient and (b) have a great deal of patience.

History

A complete general medical history is extremely important. Illnesses such as arteriosclerotic vascular disease and/or hypertension, diabetes mellitus, sickle cell disease, and collagen vascular disease may be associated with ulcers of the lower extremities. A history of steroid therapy may explain failure of ulcers to heal. A history of drug abuse or a psychiatric history may be pertinent in the explanation of factitious ulcers.

Specific attention should be paid to the following: duration of ulceration and previous attempts at therapy; symptoms of peripheral arteriosclerotic vascular disease, such as intermittent calf claudication, intermittent thigh or gluteal claudication, impotence, calf pain at rest, and feelings of coldness and tingling in the legs; a history of thrombophlebitis, ulceration, or injury to the lower extremities; a history of discomfort associated with footwear or of chronic swelling; and, if swelling has occurred, whether it has been alleviated by lying down.

Ischemic pain in the calf at rest is usually a symptom of advanced arteriosclerotic vascular disease, and it is characteristically alleviated if the patient dangles his feet over the edge of the bed, or sits in a chair, when awakened at night by ischemic pain. These symptoms must be differentiated from nocturnal leg cramps that occur in many individuals who have no evidence of peripheral vascular disease. Leg cramps are usually accompanied by palpable hardening of the calf muscles and by involuntary muscle contraction of the flexor muscles of the toes. The cramps usually are relieved if the patient gets out of bed and walks around. Examination of the extremities in these patients (see below) is usually normal.

Physical Examination

A thorough general physical examination of the patient should be undertaken in conjunction with the examination of the lower extremities. The general examination should search particularly for abdominal aneurysm and other intra-abdominal masses, lymphatic masses in the groin, as well as for signs of hypertension and of cardiac disease. Needle tracks and brawny indurated hands may indicate a history of drug abuse.

Examination of the Lower Extremities

Both lower extremities should be bared. Initial examination is performed while the patient is supine. Both legs are examined and compared. Particular points to be noted are: (a) the presence of either pitting or nonpitting edema. Pitting edema is a sign of chronic venous obstruction or of an acute inflammatory process. Nonpitting edema is a sign of lymphatic obstruction. If edema is present, it is important to note whether it is unilateral, and if it is bilateral, whether it is asymmetrical or symmetrical. Very firm, "brawny," edema suggests a very long-standing process; (b) the presence of hemosiderin deposited in the skin of the ankles (a sign of venous insufficiency); (c) the general appearance and quality of the skin, including hair growth (hair loss may signify arterial insufficiency); (d) evidence of fungal infection (scaling, apparently pruritic lesions); and (e) the status of the nails (deformity and hypertrophy are associated with arterial insufficiency).

After inspection of the feet and legs, a vascular examination of the lower extremities should be conducted. Femoral, popliteal, dorsalis pedis, and posterior tibial pulses should be palpated and graded. The capillary refill time after pressure on the toes with the legs elevated 45° should be observed (normally less than 5 seconds). Auscultation from the midabdomen down to the popliteal regions should be performed to detect bruits that are produced by narrowed atherosclerotic arteries. The temperature of the legs should be felt with the dorsum of the hand, both descending from the thigh to the foot and symmetrically comparing one side with the other. The patient is asked to sit up and to dangle his legs so that venous filling time and dependent rubor can be assessed. Evidence of varicose veins is best sought with the patient standing.

Inspection of Ulcer or Ulcers

Ulcerated areas on the legs are often very tender; and palpation, although necessary, should be done gently, with the gloved hand.

Site. An accurate description of the site of the ulcer, preferably with reference to some immovable anatomic landmark (e.g., the medial or the lateral malleolus) should be made, and the findings should be recorded.

Size. The size of the ulcer must be documented, and the vertical and horizontal diameter in centimeters should be noted in the patient's record. This measurement is particularly important for future reference when the progress of healing and the efficacy of treatment are assessed.

General Character. It should be noted whether the ulcer is regular or irregular in outline. The edges should be examined to determine whether they are raised, heaped, everted, or flat, and whether they are undermined or if there is any evidence of epithelial ingrowth from the edge of the ulcer toward the center, i.e., healing. The base should be examined to see whether it is clean or covered with exudate, and to see the type of tissue of which it is constituted (clean fascia, granulation tissue, dirty exudate, debris, etc.). Most importantly, the vascularity of the base is the most critical characteristic to be noted when considering the potential of the ulcer for healing.

Tenderness. If the ulcer is tender, it should be determined whether it is very tender, such as in acute inflammation or ischemia, or only mildly tender as in a neuropathy with loss of superficial sensation.

Changes in adjoining skin. It should be noted whether there are fluctuant areas of purulence near the ulcer, particularly on the sole of the foot; any callosities surrounding the ulcer; heavy deposition of pigment near the ulcer; or local edema.

When the examination of the ulcer(s) is completed, the patient should stand, preferably on a stool, and face the examiner. Edema should now be looked for as should the presence of varicose veins along the course of the (Fig. 88.1). In particular, the appearance of perforator varicosities (see page 1230) should be noted, usually above the medial malleolus, and the relationship of these perforators to ulcerated areas should be sought.

Types and Characteristics of Leg Ulcers

The principal characteristics of common ulcers are shown in Table 88.1.

Venous—Associated with Varicose Veins

Ulcers associated with varicose veins (see pages 1229-1232) characteristically occur in the presence of ad-

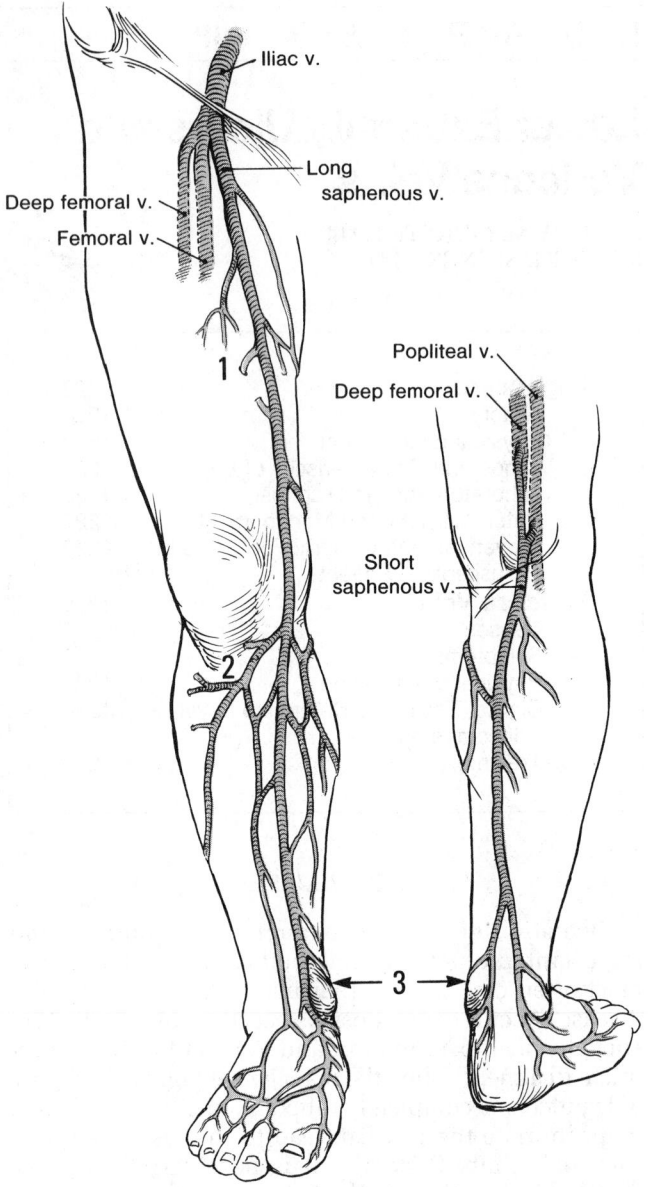

Figure 88.1. Venous circulation of the lower extremity. *1,* Hunter's canal perforator; *2,* anterior communicating vein of the leg; and *3,* ankle perforators.

vanced varicose veins, usually affecting the long saphenous system (Fig. 88.1). Such varicosities should be apparent when the patient has stood for a few minutes. Ulcerations associated with varicose veins occur where the deep perforators meet the long saphenous or the accessory long saphenous system just above, or 3 or 4 cm higher than, the medial malleolus. Edema and hemosiderin deposition are usually absent or minimal, and there are no signs of peripheral arterial insufficiency. The ulcers are characteristically fairly shallow, regular, and tender; they are usually initiated by minor trauma. They move with the skin and fascia over the underlying tissues. The edges are not undermined. There may be evidence of varicose veins on the unulcerated side of the extremity. The patient will

Table 88.1.
Characteristics of Common Leg Ulcers

Type of Ulcer	Usual Location	Edema	Pigmentation	Evidence of Arterial Insufficiency
Varicose	Medial leg	0 to +	0 to +	0
Stasis	Medial leg	+ + to + + + +	+ + +	0 to +
Arterial	Lateral leg, foot	0 to +	0	+ + + +
Dystropic	Sole, tip of toe	+ +	0	0
Traumatic	Midleg, toe	0	0	0 to + + + +
Diabetic	Toes, dorsum of foot	+ +	0	+ to + + +
Factitious	Anywhere	+	0	0

complain that the ulcer hurts and that he has a feeling of heaviness in the affected leg. Claudication and chronic edema are usually absent.

Venous—Associated with Chronic Venous Insufficiency ("Stasis Ulcers")

Chronic venous insufficiency is the most common cause of leg ulcers. The disorder probably follows deep venous thrombophlebitis with destruction of valves in the deep venous system and reversal of normal superficial-to-deep flow of blood in the perforating veins. The muscular action of the calf becomes ineffective, and blood flows to the superficial veins instead of in the usual centripetal direction through the deep venous system. Valves in the superficial (saphenous) system become incompetent, thereby raising the hydostatic venous pressure at the ankle. The old theory of stasis of venous blood with reduction of its oxygen content has long been disproven; therefore, the term stasis ulcer is technically a misnomer. The most recent research suggests that the venous hypertension distends the local capillary bed and widens the endothelial pores allowing large molecules to escape. The most important of these is fibrinogen, which polymerizes and forms a "fibrin cuff" around the capillary. This cuff forms a barrier to the passage of oxygen and other nutrients leading to cell death and ulceration (1). Extravasation of red cells also takes place; hemoglobin from these red cells is metabolized and the resultant hemosiderin is deposited in the tissues. The pigment acts as an irritant to the tissues, causing further collagen deposition (i.e., fibrosis), which results in strangulation of the nutrient arteriolar circulation to the skin. Both venous stasis and arterial capillary nutrient insufficiency, therefore, contribute to the formation of ulcers.

The patient usually gives a history of long-standing swelling of the affected leg. Often, there is a history of minor trauma at the site of the ulcer. The physical examination reveals edema, hemosiderin deposition, and ulceration, usually in line with the long saphenous vein, the short saphenous vein, or over a medial ankle perforator (Fig. 88.1). Arterial circulation in the leg may be entirely normal. Varicosities may or may not be present. The ulcer is usually fairly superficial and involves the skin, with irregular margins and with exudate covering the floor of the ulcer. The ulcer is usually movable with the skin and is tender. In grossly neglected cases, the ulceration may be massive and may involve most of the circumference of the leg. Occasionally, cellulitis may be evident, with erythema, tenderness, and fever secondary to superimposed bacterial infection (see Chapter 25).

Ulceration Associated with Arterial Insufficiency

Arterial insufficiency (see also Chapter 87) is the second most common cause of leg ulcers and, along with venous insufficiency, accounts for the great majority of leg ulcers. Ulcers associated with peripheral arterial occlusive disease usually begin with trauma and therefore appear at sites that are most subject to trauma—i.e., on toes, over the lateral or medial malleolus, at the base of the fifth metatarsal, at the head of the first metatarsal, on the heel or the ball of the foot, and in the distal pretibial region.

Ulcers secondary to occlusive arterial disease are characteristically quite painful, probably related to local inflammation and to ischemia. The foot may appear atrophic with shiny, fragile, transparent, hairless skin; the nails are often hypertrophied and deformed. Other hallmarks of arterial insufficiency—e.g., pulselessness and coolness—may be present. Because some patients are relieved of pain when they dangle the ulcerated leg, dependent edema may be present.

Dystrophic Ulcers

A neuropathic or dystrophic ulcer is usually associated with somatic or sympathetic neurological dysfunction. The precise pathogenesis of these ulcers is not known. Perhaps sympathetic dysfunction causes a reduction of arterial blood flow to local areas of skin that result in ulceration, or hypesthesia or anesthesia renders the patient more susceptible to trauma. Dystrophic ulcers are most commonly associated with peripheral neuropathies (see Chapter 84) and the neuropathies of congenital or acquired disease of the spinal cord, such as Friedreich's ataxia, syringomyelia, or multiple sclerosis. Peripheral neuropathies due to vitamin deficiency or to injuries may also result in ulcers. Ulceration almost always occurs in areas of pressure. The patient may complain of pain in the ulcer, but the ulcer is usually insensitive to light touch. There may be deformity in the foot associated with the neuropathy (talipes calcaneovalgus or equinus), or there may be a back deformity or a surgical scar as might occur in a patient with a meningomyelocele.

Usually, neurological examination of the lower extremity will be abnormal, revealing decreased proprioception, decreased cutaneous sensation, and perhaps impaired movement. The ulcer may be undermined and there may be subcutaneous tracking of infected material into adjacent tissues that, on pressure, will exude loculated pus from the undermined border of the ulcer. If the neuropathy is severe, the patient may be ambulating without pain, yet show quite advanced ulceration of the sole of the foot.

Post-traumatic Ulcers

Post-traumatic ulcers are common and usually are associated with impairment in nerve or vascular supply of the leg. Minor injury to the toe of a patient with arteriosclerotic occlusive vascular disease, or a leg injury in an individual with chronic venous insufficiency, may lead to ulceration. However, such ulcers may develop in the legs of otherwise healthy individuals, particularly after major injuries such as fractures, which involve areas where vascular supply is normally marginal. The most susceptible site is the junction of the middle and lower third of the subcutaneous surface of the tibia. In this situation, most traumatic ulcers, even in healthy youngsters, heal with some difficulty, and in older patients and in those with even minimal arterial insufficiency, injury at this site resolves with great difficulty. Post-traumatic ulcers may be accompanied by problems of chronic infection and present with tenderness and local cellulitis.

Diabetic Ulcers

Diabetic ulcers have features of dystrophic, traumatic, and arterial ulcers since all three factors contribute to their development. The characteristic location of such an ulcer is in an area of pressure, such as a corn or a callosity (see Chapter 102). The ulcer is fairly insensitive, often heavily infected, with undermined edges and tracks under the plantar fascia or proximally on the dorsum of the foot. Although usually patients are aware that they are diabetic, some are not, and a thorough evaluation upon suspicion of diabetes is mandatory since control of the ulcer will depend to a large extent on control of the diabetes. Radiological examination is important, for the bone underlying the ulcer may be the site of chronic osteomyelitis that will necessitate surgical intervention (see example, Fig. 31.1B).

Factitious Ulcers

Factitious ulcers commonly occur in the legs of addicts who inject drugs into slightly varicose leg veins. Perhaps the most common drug in this regard is pentazocine (Talwin), which, when either extravasated or injected in the suspension form, made by emptying the capsule into some water, is a strongly thrombogenic agent causing widespread skin necrosis. The distribution of these ulcers is usually bizarre. They may be multiple and bilateral; and if the history can be obtained, the diagnosis is easily made. Factitious ulcers may also occur in patients with poor hygiene, psychiatric disorders, or disorders associated with pruritis, such as scabies, which has led to excoriation. Any ulcer that fails to heal without a definite etiology in an apparently healthy environment should lead to the suspicion that it is factitious.

Neoplastic Ulcers

Neoplastic ulcers of the leg are rare; but when they do occur, they are usually either basal cell or squamous cell carcinomas and have the usual characteristics of these tumors (see Chapter 100). They have elevated or rolled edges, are anesthetic, and are usually attached to deeper tissue. Marjolin's ulcer, a rare form of squamous cell carcinoma that occurs in burn scars of long duration, may also be seen on the legs.

Hypertensive Ulcers

Another rare type of ulcer is associated with uncontrolled hypertension. It is thought that there is a progressive increase in the thickness of the arteriolar wall, decrease in the diameter of its lumen, progressive ischemia, and infarction of the skin (2). These ulcers are extremely painful and occur most frequently in women and on the posterolateral aspect of the leg and ankle.

Miscellaneous

Ulceration of the legs may occur in sickle cell disease, in polyarteritis nodosa and other collagen diseases, and in other systemic conditions (e.g., ulcerative colitis). In these instances, the diagnosis depends on making the diagnosis of the systemic disorder.

Corticosteroid therapy, particularly if it is long-standing, can lead to atrophy of the skin, increasing its fragility and susceptibility to injury. Furthermore, the impairment by corticosteroids of wound healing may prevent some ulcers from healing.

A toxic cause of skin ulceration is the brown recluse spider bite, common in the southeastern United States. The poison of the brown recluse spider contains a necrotizing enzyme that causes a rounded sloughing ulcer of approximately 3 to 4 cm with an indurated edge. The patient may not be aware of having been bitten by a spider. These ulcers are refractory to healing by use of conservative measures, and should be surgically excised and closed.

In the tropics, ulceration of the foot and leg may occur from local mycoses such as maduromycosis; these conditions should be kept in mind when an individual is returning from a tropical climate.

Laboratory Aids in Diagnosis

Bacteriology

Leg ulcers are often infected and almost invariably contaminated, usually with enteric organisms. Infections are particularly hazardous in the diabetic and in the patient with chronic arterial insufficiency. Cultures of the ulcer bed are useful, and cultures of obviously purulent ulcers are mandatory since antibiotic therapy is an important part of management, particularly when invasive infection is apparent (see Chapter 25). If fungal infection is suspected (unusual degree of scaling and of excoriation), unless the physician is experienced in the scraping of lesions and the microscopic identification of fungi, dermatological consultation is indicated.

Biopsy

Biopsy by a surgeon or a dermatologist is indicated if neoplastic or obscure fungal disease is suspected. Biopsy may be performed in the office under local anesthesia and should include a wedge-shaped section of the edge and floor of the ulcer. Any chronic ulcer that exists in a long-standing scar of any type should be biopsied to rule out squamous cell carcinoma. Sometimes only a biopsy of bone will make a definitive diagnosis of osteomyelitis that underlies a chronic ulcer.

Laboratory Tests for Systemic Disease

These tests are performed as dictated by the clinical diagnosis when the ulcer is suspected to be part of a systemic disorder—e.g., diabetes, polyarteritis nodosa, sickle cell disease, etc.

Noninvasive Vascular Testing

When ulceration is noted in a patient with occlusive arterial disease, he should be referred to a vascular laboratory for testing. This is more fully discussed in Chapter 87.

Natural History and Management (3)

Generally, chronic ulcers develop initially from skin trauma, which may be exceedingly minor. However, the insult is compounded by a milieu of macro- or microcirculatory disease or other unfavorable local or systemic factors. Once the wound becomes inflamed, the local metabolic rate increases the demand for oxygen and nutrients, which leads to compromise and death of tissue when the demands are not met. The tissue then may become infected, resulting in more inflammation and propagating the cycle, making the ulcer enlarge and then become chronic. Treatment of the ulcer requires the breaking of this cycle.

Chronic open wounds are all colonized by microorganisms to a greater or lesser extent. As long as an ulcer is an open wound, invasion by the organism is rare, and the threat of invasive infection and systemic toxicity is minimal. Furthermore, because the bacteria are on the surface of the wound rather than in the tissue and the tissue in the base of the ulcer is often poorly vascularized, systemic antibiotics do not affect the surface flora significantly. Topical antibiotics are generally more appropriate for open wounds, and systemic antibiotics are reserved for evidence of invasive infections.

Pus under pressure (i.e., an abscess) increases the risk of invasive infection greatly. When a collection of loculated pus exists, it must be drained adequately. Eschars that overlie ulcers may hide such loculated pus and should, therefore, generally be debrided.

Most ulcers of the lower extremities can be treated on an ambulatory basis. However, the presence of one or more of the following may be an indication for hospitalization:

1. the extent of the ulcer and the associated edema is so great that a period of absolute bedrest and elevation is required that is not possible outside the hospital;
2. the appearance of invasive infection heralded by cellulitis, lymphangitis, and systemic symptoms;
3. when there is serious concern about the etiology of the ulcer, particularly if arterial insufficiency may play a role.

Venous Ulcers Associated with Varicose Veins

These lesions will invariably heal with elevation and appropriate elastic compression to counteract the increased hydrostatic pressure in the varicose venous system. If the patient is at home, he should be at bed rest for a period of 2 weeks with only bathroom privileges. Smaller, clean ulcers may be treated by applying a nonadherent (e.g., Telfa gauze) or hydrocolloid dressing (e.g., Duoderm) to the ulcer and by carefully wrapping the leg with Ace bandages. Dressings that adhere to the ulcer on removal may damage the growing epithelium as the ulcer heals. Therefore, wet-to-dry dressings are discouraged and wet-to-wet dressings (see below, Ulceration of Chronic Venous Insufficiency) may be used cautiously. Alternatively the leg may be wrapped in gauze impregnated with a zinc-gelatin dressing (Unna boot or Unna bandaged). If an Unna boot is used (the impregnated gauze is commercially available), it is imperative that it not be wrapped tightly and that it be placed smoothly from the metacarpal-phalangeal joints to just below the tibial tuberosity, including the heel. This can be done best by keeping the bandage roll on the surface of the leg as the leg is wrapped. Wrinkles, failure to wrap the heel, and either too tight or too loose compression will result in treatment failure and, potentially, can result in further ulcerations. When first applied it should be removed within 48 hours to ascertain that the compression is adequate and no further problems are being created. The bandage may then be reapplied and changed weekly, and healing will usually result.

If the ulcer is grossly infected, a Unna boot should not be used. After adequate bacteriological cultures, it is best to treat an infected ulcer with a suitable topical antibacterial preparation such as silver-sulfadiazine cream and Ace bandage compression. A careful wet-to-wet dressing using a Chlorpactin, Dakin's, or other antibacterial solution is an alternative that has greater potential for removing exudate and necrotic debris without damaging the regenerating epithelium. It is important never to apply a Unna or Ace bandage to a leg when peripheral arteriosclerotic vascular disease is suspected or cannot be excluded.

The patient should be followed at twice weekly intervals in the physician's office. After healing of the ulcer, the patient should be referred for surgical opinion about whether stripping and ligation of the long saphenous vein and ligation of the incompetent perforators are indicated to prevent recurrence.

If surgery is not indicated, compression stockings will often counteract the hydrostatic pressure and prevent further ulceration. If the ulcerations do not heal in 2 to 3 weeks, hospitalization and surgical consultation are indicated.

Ulceration of Chronic Venous Insufficiency ("Stasis" Ulcer)

There is probably no other form of ulcer that taxes the patient or the physician as much as those associated with chronic venous insufficiency. The mainstays of therapy are elimination of infection, cleansing of the ulcer bed to facilitate healthy tissue growth, and reduction of edema by elevation and compression. The patient should be at bed rest, and the ulcer should be treated with dressings and with topical antibacterial agents, if infected (see Chapter 25).

The patient should be instructed to apply and change the dressing twice a day. One of the following approaches can be used: (a) Wet-to-dry dressing—a sterile gauze pad, moistened in normal saline (not soaking wet, as this can cause maceration), is secured over the ulcer (with a rolled bandage, not with an adhesive tape as this can damage the skin adjacent to an ulcer) and left to dry; necrotic tissue and other debris will be removed when the dry dressing is removed, gently, at the end of each dressing interval. This procedure is appropriate early in ulcer management when there is substantial exudate and debris to remove. (b) Wet-to-wet dressing—cleaner ulcers may have a similarly moistened dressing applied but moistened again before removing. This results in somewhat less vigorous debridement but protects the healing tissue of the ulcer. (c) Hydrocolloid dressing—When the ulcer is clean, or if it is quite shallow, a good alternative is a hydrocolloid dressing (e.g., Duoderm) under an elastic bandage. This dressing does not disrupt the growth of healing tissue and allows healing in a moist environment (4). This has the added advantage of not requiring change as frequently. This is similar to the Unna bandage described above, which can also be used in this setting. (d) In patients with particularly dirty or wet ulcers, the application of hydrophilic beads (e.g., Debrisan beads) every 12 hours (or more frequently if the beads change color, a sign that they are saturated) and the use of a whirlpool bath for a few days may be helpful.

Resolution of edema is important in the management of these ulcers. Leg elevation and elastic stockings should be used. Occasionally, diuretics may be helpful even when no element of cardiac or renal fail-

ure exists; but, to avoid the danger of volume depletion, elastic stockings should be tried first. If the edema can be controlled, the ulcers usually can be healed, although several weeks to months may be required. After the healing, the patient must be advised to keep the leg elevated, if possible, when sitting down and to wear some form of elastic compression permanently; preferably a made-to-measure elastic support garment such as a Jobst stocking.

If with these measures the ulcer still fails to heal, skin grafting may be required along with venous ligation and stripping. This will require surgical consultation and hospitalization.

Arterial Ulcers

Arterial ulcers are almost impossible to heal unless improvement of blood flow to the area can be achieved. Therefore, if there is any suspicion of arterial insufficiency, the patient should be referred for surgical evaluation. If the patient's lesion is unsuitable for surgical correction, or if the patient has already had an operation but ulceration persists, the ulcer can sometimes be healed with painstaking debridements every 2 or 3 days. This treatment, however, requires expertise; in case of doubt, surgical referral should be made.

A pair of sharp scissors or a scalpel is used to remove the dry eschar that covers the ulcer and to remove the necrotic edges of the ulcer carefully without causing bleeding. Wet-to-wet dressings are then applied, using a topical antibiotic solution such as Polymixin-Bacitracin 5% aqueous suspension to set the bandages. The patient is instructed to apply the bandage wet in the morning and to remove it in the evening after wetting it again. This has the effect of debriding the ulcer and allowing the delicate epithelial edges the best chance for ingrowth.

If there is a great deal of debris in the ulcer bed, twice daily application of a hydrophilic debriding agent (such as Debrisan beads) applied for a few days will usually help to clear the thick debris from the ulcer. Whirlpool therapy, if available, is an excellent adjunct to this therapy. Very tenacious necrotic debris may be removed with a short course of a proteolytic enzyme (e.g., Travase) applied 3 to 4 times a day, followed by the application of a wet-to-dry dressing. In conjunction with these measures, meticulously compulsive foot protection, soft footwear, elevation of the extremity, and avoidance of weight bearing are mandatory.

Dystrophic Ulcers

Dystrophic ulcers are a real threat to the limb because infection will often advance unnoticed by the patient until there is considerable spread of pus under the eschar or in the tissue around the ulcer. Treatment consists of bed rest, appropriate antibiotic therapy as indicated after culture (see Chapter 25), debridement of necrotic skin edges (which can be done without anesthesia in the office), and wet-to-wet dressings as described above. Dystrophic ulcers probably take the longest of all to heal, perhaps several months. If, despite office measures and adequate bed rest at home, no progress seems to be made, the patient should be hospitalized in a setting where debridement can be performed once or twice a day by a skilled individual.

Traumatic Ulcers

Traumatic ulcers will usually heal by avoidance of weight bearing, elevation, topical antibiotic therapy when the ulcer is infected, and protection of the ulcer by dressings. If no progress is made within 2 to 3 weeks, the patient should be seen by a surgeon for possible operative debridement and surgical closure of the wound.

Diabetic Ulcers

An ulcer in the diabetic foot imposes such serious risk of limb loss that the majority of these patients should be hospitalized.

In the hospital, diabetes can be more meticulously regulated; any pockets of suppuration can be drained, and treatment of osteomyelitis in the metatarsals and proper debridement can be carried out.

Factitious Ulcers

The key to the management of factitious ulcers is a high degree of suspicion, particularly in those ulcers that have no clear etiology and occur in what appears to be an otherwise healthy environment. These ulcers will usually heal if the cause can be found and controlled. An ulcer suspected of being a factitious ulcer can often be diagnosed and treated simultaneously by placing an occlusive dressing that prevents the patient from manipulating the ulcer.

These patients must be carefully followed to monitor the patient and to avoid the development of problems under the occlusive dressing.

Hypertensive Ulcers

Control of the patient's chronic hypertension and education of the patient regarding the importance of long-term control are the two keystones in the management of hypertensive ulcers. Otherwise the management follows the general principles applied to venous stasis ulcers.

Chronic Ulcers Associated with Corticosteroid Treatment

Systemic corticosteroids have an inhibitory effect on wound healing that can be partially reversed by vitamin A. Ulcers that fail to heal in patients being treated with corticosteroids may be given vitamin A, 25,000 U orally daily; and ointments containing vitamin A (e.g., A Ointment) may be used alone or in combination (with silver sulfadiazine cream for example) directly on the ulcer.

Neoplastic and Other Ulcers

Neoplastic and other unusual ulcers, such as that from the previously mentioned brown recluse spider bite, are a surgical problem; and these patients should be referred promptly for consultation.

Prevention and General Foot Care in Susceptible Patients (See also Chapter 102)

Foot and leg ulcers from any cause often recur after healing, since, with the exception of varicose veins, factitious ulcers, and occlusive arterial disease surgically corrected, the underlying disease is difficult to reverse. It is therefore mandatory to be familiar with the principles of foot care, and patients must understand and carry out instructions aimed at minimizing exposure to trauma. Patients with peripheral arterial disease or diabetes should wear very comfortable footwear, even if it is not fashionable. The front of the shoe should be broad so that the toes can spread. Areas of pressure caused by foot deformities should be corrected by orthopaedic shoes with appropriate fittings—e.g., insoles or metatarsal bars; patients with these problems should be referred to an orthopaedic surgeon or to a podiatrist. Patients should be instructed to keep their feet very clean—i.e., at least once-daily showers or footbaths in tepid water; nails should be very carefully trimmed, preferably with clippers; under no circumstances should sharp scissors be used to trim the sides of nails, as they may cause injury to the delicate nail fold and become a portal of entry for infection. Patients can protect their toes during walking by the insertion of small, fluffy pieces of cotton wool between them. Lanolin or other emollient creams are useful in preventing cracking of hardened areas of skin and in keeping the skin soft and supple. Patients should avoid extremes of temperature and should reduce exposure to trauma (e.g., a night light in the bedroom to avoid "stubbing" a toe). With attention to these small details, recurring trouble can often be prevented.

VARICOSE VEINS

Causes

Varicose veins of the lower extremities are common, affecting women more often than men, and usually becoming symptomatic between the ages of 20 and 40. The global epidemiology of varicose veins varies widely, ranging from a low incidence among women of lowland New Guinea of 0.1%, to a high among the women of South Wales at 50%. In the United States, varicose veins affect 19% of men and 36% of women.

Varicose veins are due to an incompetence of the valves of the long or short saphenous veins (see Fig. 88.1), permitting retrograde or downward flow of blood, or simply stagnation of the normal centripetal flow. In the perforator system, which is a system of veins communicating between the deep and the superficial veins, destruction of valves interferes with the unidirectional movement of blood from superficial to deep.

The disorder is aggravated, indeed may be caused, by conditions elevating intra-abdominal pressure, such as pregnancy, large intra-abdominal tumors, conditions causing chronic straining—e.g., prostatic obstruction, carcinoma of the sigmoid colon, and occasionally by mechanical interference with venous return in the venous system itself such as thrombosis of the pelvic veins.

Symptoms

The symptoms of uncomplicated varicose veins usually consist of heaviness and aching in the area of the veins or in the calves. The patient may complain of mild edema at the end of a long day's work. Occasionally, patients will complain of varicose veins for cosmetic reasons and desire treatment. Patients with uncomplicated varicose veins do not complain of intermittent claudication or severe pain; in the presence of these symptoms, other causes must be carefully sought. Occasionally, thrombophlebitis will supervene in a varicose vein and cause severe pain; the culpable vein is then palpable as an inflamed cord. After bed rest, elevation, application of local heat, and appropriate anti-inflammatory therapy (e.g., aspirin), the varix in the thrombosed vein will disappear.

Physical Examination

It is useful to have some idea of the anatomy of the venous system of the leg (Fig. 88.1). This will enable the clinician to judge the patient's symptoms on the basis of an anatomical abnormality detected by physical examination. There are several types of varicose veins that conform to the underlying anatomic arrangement of these veins.

Subcutaneous Varicose Veins ("Sunburst" Varices)

These are not, in the true sense of the word, varicose veins, but rather dilations of subcutaneous venous plexuses that have a spider-like arrangement and an unsightly purple color. These veins are quite frequently the object of cosmetic complaints by patients. Otherwise, they are essentially asymptomatic.

Varicosities of Long Saphenous System

These are the most common type of varicose veins. The long saphenous vein begins anterior to the medial malleolus at the ankle, courses superficially to the medial side of the knee, and then curves upward to enter the deep system just below the inguinal ligament medial to the femoral artery. The vein has several tributaries in the calf and in the thigh that are superficial, and it is also joined by several perforating veins from the deep venous system; the valves at these junctions can become incompetent and lead to focal varicosities (Fig. 88.1). There are three or four consistent perforators—three above the medial malleolus at a distance separated by approximately 3 cm, and a fourth just above the knee joint. If varicosities appear in this situation, the perforator system is almost certainly in-

competent. Varicosity of the long saphenous vein is clearly visible with the patient standing.

Varicosities of Short Saphenous System

The short saphenous vein arises behind the lateral malleolus and courses upward behind the calf to join the popliteal vein in the popliteal space (Fig. 88.1). Varicosities of this system are best seen with the patient standing with his back to the examiner.

Perforator Varicosities

As mentioned above, perforator incompetence is usually noticed in the long saphenous vein where the ankle perforators and the above-the-knee perforator join the vein; however, perforators join other superficial veins that, in turn, join the long and short saphenous system. Examination may reveal that there is no incompetence of the short or long saphenous veins, only of the perforators.

Clinical Testing to Determine Level of Incompetence

One or two easy clinical tests can be performed in the office that will aid in the determination of the severity of the problem and in the selection of appropriate treatment.

Trendelenburg's Test

The patient lies on his back and raises the affected leg to empty the veins. A venous tourniquet is applied just below the saphenous opening about 3 inches (7.7 cm) below the inguinal ligament and the patient then stands up. Constriction is released; if the saphenofemoral valve is incompetent, the veins will fill immediately from above; if not, the veins fill slowly from below. If the veins fill rapidly from above before the release of the tourniquet, this indicates an incompetent valve at the entry of the long saphenous vein into the femoral vein and signifies major long saphenous incompetence. This test is now repeated at successively lower levels in the leg; and thereby, the location of incompetence may be mapped.

Perthes' Test

This is a test for deep venous thrombosis in association with varicose veins. A tourniquet is lightly applied below the inguinal ligament as in Trendelenburg's test and the patient is instructed to walk in place. If varicose veins are accompanied by a thrombosed deep femoral system, the varicose veins will become very prominent after this exercise.

Noninvasive Vascular Testing

The advent of the modern vascular laboratory has revolutionized the evaluation of varicose veins, particularly with regard to competence of the venous valve at the junction of the long saphenous and femoral veins. Precise diagnosis is now possible. A determination of competency or incompetency of valves at the groin level is imperative before addressing methodologies of treatment. The full range of these tests is beyond the scope of discussion of this chapter, but they include Doppler ultrasonography, impedance plethysmography, and venography (see Chapter 52). Any patient who, by physical examination, is suspected of having venous incompetence at the saphenous femoral junction should be referred to a noninvasive vascular laboratory for evaluation before treatment is planned.

Treatment

Subcutaneous Varicosities Asymptomatic Except for Cosmetic Appearance

If the offending venous plexus is deemed large enough to accommodate a 25-gauge needle, a sclerosing solution may be injected. The technique is described below. Other treatments such as freezing with carbon dioxide snow, cautery under local anesthesia, and even laser therapy have been advocated, but their use requires a great deal of skill, and unnecessary skin scarring may result that is, in the end, more unsightly than the original vein. Probably the safest treatment of this kind of vein is the use of masking cosmetic creams, together with reassurance.

Localized Small Varicosities Not Accompanied by Major Long Saphenous or Short Saphenous Incompetence

These veins are suitable for treatment by a sclerosing injection and compression therapy. The procedure can easily be performed in the office by anyone skilled with a needle; however, the patient should be warned that several sittings may be required for complete elimination of the veins.

Technique. The patient stands with a tight tourniquet around the thigh, just enough to make the vein prominent. The area of the vein is lightly prepped with a suitable antiseptic, and 0.5 ml of sclerosing solution is injected by use of a 2-ml syringe, after initial aspiration to make sure the needle is in the vein. Immediately after the end of the injection, the needle is withdrawn; and the vein is gently compressed with a 2- × 2-inch gauze for 3 minutes, after which the tourniquet is released and compression continued for 2 minutes more. The patient now wears an Ace bandage on the area for approximately 4 hours. The sclerosant produces an inflammatory reaction in the intima, which obliterates the vein by phlebitis. Failure to use a tourniquet may release an unnecessarily large amount of sclerosant into the major veins of the leg and cause undesirable thrombosis at distant sites. The patient should be warned that extravasation of the sclerosant is a possibility and may cause a small skin slough. There are several commercially available sclerosant solutions, morrhuate sodium and sodium tetradecyl sulfate (Soltradecal), that are suitable for injection.

Major Long or Short Saphenous Varicosities, or Perforator Varicosities, in Symptomatic Patients

Symptomatic patients should be referred for surgical consultation. Attempts to inject and compress veins associated with clear-cut varicosities of the major superficial systems are doomed to failure without surgical intervention; nevertheless, injection or primary treatment of saphenous varicosities is preferred in some centers, mostly in Europe.

If an operation has been performed on either the long or short saphenous system or both, there are often residual varicosities of a minor degree requiring additional injection therapy that may be performed in the office. The recurrence rate of major varicosities after operation is 10 to 20% in most large series.

Varicose veins should not be treated in individuals who have an underlying cause associated with increased intra-abdominal pressure until the primary cause has been removed. The wearing of elastic stockings may, however, give comfort during this time. Such stockings may be advisable for support in any individual with varicose veins in whom other treatment is either undesirable or contraindicated. A further consideration in the selection of therapy is whether the patient has coronary artery disease; although veins that are severely varicose are not suitable for use in coronary bypass surgery, if patients have minimal varicose veins and may become candidates for a coronary artery bypass, these veins should be preserved, if at all possible, for potential use. Weight reduction in overweight patients is advisable for anyone with varicose veins, regardless of other modes of treatment.

Patient Experience. Outpatient surgery is often adequate for varicose vein operations on one leg, but hospitalization is recommended when both legs are to be operated. For minor varicose veins local anesthesia may suffice. For more extensive varicose veins, or those involving both legs, general or spinal anesthesia is necessary. The patient is instructed to shower or to bathe the legs and groin several times with surgical soap before operation to reduce the bacteria colonizing the skin. Usually the upper end of the vein is tied off in the groin to stop backflow of blood in the upper vein due to a defective valve. Next the lower end of the vein is identified and an incision is made in the skin. The vein is opened and a hard plastic or metal wire is inserted into the vein and passed all the way up to the groin. Next all enlarged branches of the varicose vein and all defective valve areas that have been marked before operation are opened and the smaller veins at these sites are tied off and removed, and the incisions are closed with sutures. Then, a ball is screwed onto the wire at the distal incision that allows the vein to be uprooted, the leg is elevated and wrapped with elastic dressings, and the vein stripper is slowly pulled upward, removing the varicose vein through the proximal incision. After varicose vein removal the legs are kept elevated for 6 to 8 hours. Walking is permitted with elastic wrapping of the legs. Elastic wraps or elastic stockings are used for at least 6 weeks after operation and the patient is instructed to elevate the legs periodically during the day. The patient is advised to avoid prolonged sitting or standing, but walking is encouraged. The patient can return to light work after a few days' convalescence but should not return to heavy lifting or hard manual labor for a month or so. Bleeding under the skin is the most frequent complication, but it is usually not serious. Infection occurs rarely and is treated with antibiotics and local application of heat. Damage to nerves can occur if the saphenous or sural nerves, located just under the skin, are injured during the process of making incisions or stripping the veins. This can cause pain or numbness over part of the lower leg, which usually resolves within a few weeks. About 10% of varicose veins will return after surgical treatment. These are usually the result of failure to tie off all of the communicating branches to varicose veins.

General References

Bailey JL: Leg ulcers. *Nurs Time* 72:1752, 1976.
    Primarily directed to nurses, it carries some practical suggestions on equipment and on dressing techniques for dealing with leg ulcers in the office.
Beninson J: Medical management of the peripheral vascular ulcer. *Angiology* 30:48, 1979.
    A simple, sensible description of management by a physician who has over 30 years' experience running a major leg ulcer clinic. Some very practical suggestions on basic advice to the patient with leg ulcers.
Kistner RL: Veins and lymphatics. In: Hardy JD (ed):*Textbook of Surgery*. Philadelphia, JB Lippincott & Co, 1988.
    A good discussion of modern noninvasive vascular testing, as well as a discussion of surgical techniques available for the treatment of varicose veins.
Litchfield R, Wolfson P, Haspel L, Dunlap S: Differential diagnosis of leg ulcers. *J Am Osteopath Assoc* 78:204, 1978.
    An excellent series of photographs showing various types of ulceration and a good description of the clinical features of the more common ulcers.
Ludbrook J: Primary great saphenous varicose veins revisited. *World Surgery* 10:954, 1986.
    An excellent overall review of the status of varicose vein therapy, and a discussion of theories of etiology.
Robson MC, Edstrom LE: Conservative management of the ulcerated diabetic foot. *Plast Reconstr Surg* 59:551, 1977.
    An article on a currently controversial subject, the management of diabetic ulcer. It points out the disastrous complications of mismanagement and the excellent results that can be obtained from meticulous conservative therapy.
Tremblay S, Lewis EW, Allen PT: Selecting a treatment for primary varicose veins. *Canad Med Assoc J* 133:20, 1985.
    A sensible discussion of options.
Young JR: Differential diagnosis of ulcers on legs of vascular cause. *J Dermatol Surg Oncol* 4:687, 1978.
    A useful discussion of vascular ulceration.

Specific References

1. Browse NL, Burnand KG: The cause of venous ulceration. *Lancet* 2:243, 1982.
2. Duncan HJ, Faris IB: Martorell's hypertensive ischemic leg ulcers are secondary to an increase in the local vascular resistance. *J Vasc Surg* 2:581, 1985.
3. Friedman SJ, Su WPD: Management of leg ulcers. *Am Fam Phys* 27:219, 1983.
4. van Rijswijk L, Brown D, Friedman S, et al: Multicenter clinical evaluation of a hydrocolloid dressing for leg ulcers. *Cutis* 35:173, 1985.

C H A P T E R 89

Diseases of the Breast

MICHAELPURTELL, M.D.
ROBERT M. QUINLAN, M.D.
LARRYWATERBURY, M.D

One of every 11 women in the United States will develop breast cancer. It is the second leading cause of cancer deaths among women, with 130,000 new cases seen each year and 40,000 deaths (45). Not surprisingly the fear of breast cancer is prominent in the patient who presents with breast-related complaints, although most of these are secondary to benign causes. The primary care physician must have a rational approach to the diagnosis and treatment of breast complaints and breast masses. He will carry out the screening program for cancer and supervise the patients' referral. If cancer is found, he will be the one to whom the patient initially will turn for information. A reassuring patient-doctor relationship is critical in dealing with this emotionally charged area of medicine.

NORMAL ANATOMY AND PHYSIOLOGY OF THE BREAST

The breast is a modified sweat gland. There is an extension of breast tissue reaching toward the axilla.

There are 12 to 20 acini arranged like a bunch of grapes with draining ducts emptying into openings on the nipple. These ducts are lined by two layers of epithelium, one of which serves as a basement membrane and source of epithelial cell reproduction. It is this "reverse layer" that can proliferate in certain pathological conditions. Surrounding each duct is a specialized periductal fibrous layer, which is under hormonal influence.

With each menstrual cycle, a fall in hormonal activity at the menses results in the desquamation of duct lining, which proliferates again at the cessation of menses. Increases in periductal vascularity and lymphocytic infiltration accompany this proliferation. During pregnancy the ducts and acini proliferate maximally, often never returning to normal in the postpartum period. In many parts of the breast the glandular hypertrophy will remain until it involutes at menopause. At that time there is a loss of parenchyma and an increase in fat, especially in the periductal region. The lobular anatomy slowly disappears. Variations in hormonal balance result in various benign pathological conditions occurring during the active menstrual childbearing years and at menopause. It is important to realize that anatomic changes associated with normal hormonal fluctuations during a menstrual cycle do not occur to the same degree in all areas of the breast. This accounts for the asymmetric palpatory findings in the normal breast, which is often very "lumpy."

SCREENING PROCEDURES

Physical examination (see page 1235) and mammography are useful screening procedures for the detection of breast masses (10, 14, 44, 48). Over the last several years, mammographic techniques have improved considerably and the radiation exposure per examination has dropped to very low levels so that the risk of inducing breast cancer from routine screening mammography is almost negligible. Routine screening mammography in women over the age of 50 (poorly studied over the age of 74) has been proven in controlled studies to decrease death from breast cancer (10, 48). The American Cancer Society recommends yearly screening in this age group, although other studies have shown similar effectiveness with screening intervals of 2 to 3 years (48). All physicians should encourage routine physical examination and screening mammography in woman over the age of 50. Although mammography is the more sensitive of the two screening procedures, physical examination is also important as up to 15% of palpable breast cancers are not visualized on mammography (28).

Routine screening mammography in women under the age of 50 remains controversial except for those women with increased risk by virtue of a previous breast cancer or a strong family history (4, 9, 10, 14, 16, 28, 50). The American Cancer Society recommends base line mammography between ages 35 and 40 and yearly or every other year mammography between ages

40 and 50. Other organizations disagree. Both American and Canadian Task Forces on the periodic health examination do not recommend routine screening mammography under the age of 50 (9, 50). There are several reasons for this controversy. Although mammography can certainly identify nonpalpable highly curable breast cancers in young woman, studies today have not demonstrated a convincing effect on survival in woman under age 50. Many of the tumors found in the young are in situ cancers that may not become invasive for years, if ever. Of major concern is the lack of test specificity in young women who frequently have a dense breast pattern on X-ray, complicating interpretation. This leads to a much higher benign:malignant biopsy ratio than in older women. In order to find cancer, lesions that are associated with cancer only 5% of the time or less are frequently biopsied (35). Thus, large numbers of normal woman must undergo physical and psychological trauma in order to find the occasional woman potentially benefited by the diagnosis of an early cancer. The recommendation for early follow-up of a suspicious lesion is potentially more harmful than biopsy. The impact of this frequent recommendation on a young woman (usually with no disease) is poorly studied but likely to be profound especially if she has problems with anxiety, depression, somatization, etc.

Whatever decision the primary physician makes about the usefulness of screening mammography in the young woman, it is important that he schedule an office interview for anyone contemplating screening. A woman needs to understand her likely experience when she goes for testing, particularly if it is her first mammogram. Patients should know that mammography may be uncomfortable because of the need for breast compression. The postmammography plan of communication should be worked out ahead of time to minimize the anxiety of waiting for a phone call. Young women in particular should understand the poor specificity of the test and the high likelihood of a recommendation for intervention (biopsy or early follow-up), especially with the first mammogram. The patient should know that if she receives that recommendation in most instances, the chance of benign or no disease far outweigh the chance of cancer.

CLINICAL CHARACTERISTICS OF COMMON DISEASES OF THE BREAST

Benign Tumors

Fibroadenoma

Fibroadenoma is the most common cause of a unilateral discrete mass in the 15- to 35-year-old age group. The peak incidence is from 20 to 25 years of age. In 10 to 15% of cases, there will be multiple tumors. Rapid growth seen during pregnancy, just prior to menopause, and in animals given estrogens, all suggest that fibroadenomas are under hormonal control. The natural history of a fibroadenoma is that of a tumor growing old with the patient, perhaps calcifying in the postmenopausal woman and rapidly growing in the pregnant patient.

A fibroadenoma has both fibrous and epithelial components. The tumor probably arises from terminal ducts and lobules, and the rare finding of lobular carcinoma rather than intraductal carcinoma within or in the vicinity of a fibroadenoma is consistent with such an origin.

The patient with a fibroadenoma usually complains only of the mass and denies pain, nipple discharge, or other breast changes. On physical examination, the lesion is usually firm, but not rock hard; it is smooth and well circumscribed, nontender, and easily movable. It often rolls about in the breast, mimicking a very large marble. In some adolescents giant fibroadenomas can be confused with virginal hypertrophy; however, they are usually more discrete than is diffuse hypertrophy. Mammography is frequently diagnostic, usually revealing a discrete, round, well-circumscribed lesion without associated calcium. However, because of the rare possibility of simultaneous lobular carcinoma or of progression to cystosarcoma phylloides and the inability to definitely exclude carcinoma (present in 2 to 3% of cases), excisional biopsy is usually recommended.

Cystosarcoma Phyllodes

Cystosarcoma phyllodes is a sarcomatous tumor of the breast that may arise from a fibroadenoma. The overgrowth of stroma mainly distinguishes it from a fibroadenoma. It has a malignancy rate of 20 to 30% with 2 to 3% of cases having already metastasized at diagnosis. Benign tumors are treated with wide excision and malignant tumors by modified radical mastectomy.

Intraductal Papilloma

Intraductal papillomas often present with serosanguinous, spontaneous, recurrent, or persistent nipple discharge from a single duct. These small tumors are not palpable, but their location can usually be determined by applying pressure on various quadrants of the areolocutaneous margin and noting which quadrant produces the discharge. An intraductal papillary cancer is a possibility that must be excluded by excising a small pie-shaped segment in the area producing the discharge.

Fibrocystic Disease

Fibrocystic changes of the breast are quite common and occur to some extent in most women. Because up to 90% of women will have some degree of cysts and epithelial hyperplasia on biopsy or at autopsy, it may be reasonable to consider fibrocystic disease as a normal variant rather than an actual pathological entity (31). The patient with fibrocystic change usually complains of dull, aching pain in the area of most pronounced nodularity, and this pain is often more prominent just before the onset of menses. It is possible that much of the pain related to fibrocystic change is due to cancer phobia, and it often lessens with a positive doctor-patient relationship. On physical examination the breast feels "lumpy" with bilateral, diffuse, tender, easily movable ill-defined masses, usually in the upper outer quadrant of the breasts. At times, especially with a discrete cystic lesion, it will be hard to distinguish cystic changes noted on examination or on a mammogram from cancer, making management of such patients difficult. Because of this uncertainty, many patients will undergo at least one biopsy to rule out cancer. The vast majority will be benign (15). Over 95% of the time the histology will be either normal (70%) or show only epithelial hyperplasia (25%). These findings are of little concern, and such patients are at low risk for developing breast cancer and do not require more vigilant follow-up than normal (15). In contrast, when hyperplasia with atypia is reported (3 to 4% of benign biopsies), this is significant, particularly if the mother or a sister of the patient has had breast cancer. In the absence of a positive family history the finding of atypia increases the risk of the patient developing breast cancer 4-fold, and in association with a positive family history this risk is increased nearly 11-fold (15). These patients do require careful follow-up with annual mammograms and biannual physical examinations, and in selected cases even prophylactic bilateral mastectomies may be considered.

Sometimes fibrocystic disease is associated with *duct ectasia*, usually heralded by spontaneous discharge of thick, gray-green fluid from multiple dilated ducts. At other times duct ectasia and discharge may be present in the absence of palpable fibrocystic lesions. In the first instance, a biopsy should be done to rule out carcinoma; in the second, the administration of estrogen may stop the discharge. If it does not, mammography should be performed and then a biopsy should be considered.

Premature Hyperplasia

A concentric unilateral swelling can occur beneath the nipple before puberty in girls. This commonly occurs during the ages 7 to 9. The lump can be 1 to 2 cm in diameter and is usually nontender. Within a year, a contralateral lump will appear and often both lumps remain static until puberty. A biopsy is *contraindicated* and would be equivalent to total mastectomy.

Gynecomastia

The main differential in male breast masses lies between gynecomastia (see Chapter 77) and male breast cancer. The latter is extremely rare, accounting for approximately 1% of all breast cancers. Although gynecomastia has many causes, its physical characteristics are usually unvaried. Gynecomastia presents as a breast mass beneath the areola, is usually slightly tender, and is easily movable. It is never associated with ulceration or nipple retraction. If gynecomastia is ruled out, a breast mass in a male should be examined by biopsy.

Cancer

The increased practice of routine screening for breast cancer by mammography, utilizing sensitive equipment, has resulted in a change in the presentation of breast cancer. A large percentage (15 to 20%) now are detected by mammography alone without an associated palpable mass (28). The remaining breast cancers are found by the patient or by the physician and 15% of these are clinically advanced. These advanced cases may be recognized by some of the following signs: skin changes (e.g., dimpling, peau d'orange, erythema), matted fixed axillary nodes, or a mass fixed to the chest wall. Less advanced cases may present with a painless, hard irregular mass, frequently (37%) located in the upper outer quadrant of the breast. These may be associated with subtle skin dimpling or nipple retraction. Palpable movable axillary lymph nodes less than 2 cm in diameter about half of the time on biopsy will only be reactive in patients with breast cancer, without tumor involvement.

EVALUATION OF A BREAST MASS

History: Risk Factors (Table 89.1) and Symptoms

The chance of a woman developing cancer increases with age (44, 45). The risk to age 50 is about 2.5% and to age 70 about 7% (and to age 110 about 10%). Many factors have been shown to alter these numbers. The *menstrual* and *reproductive* history is important (6). Early menarche and late menopause (i.e., prolonged duration of ovarian activity—greater than 40 years) have been associated with a slightly increased risk of developing breast cancer, whereas menopause before age 35 (normal and surgical) reduces the risk. The risk of breast cancer is increased in nulliparous women, while a full term pregnancy before age 18 offers some protective benefit. At this time it is still unclear whether the use of oral contraceptives changes a woman's risk for breast cancer. A family history of breast cancer is a major risk factor (2, 3, 41). The occurrence of breast cancer in a first degree relative (sister/mother) will increase a woman's probability of developing cancer by 2- to 4-fold. It is debatable whether and to what extent this increase in risk depends on the relative having been premenopausal when diagnosed and/or

Table 89.1.
Risk Factors for Carcinoma of the Breast

Factors	Relative Risk
Positive family history	1–5 (see the text)
Early menarche and late menopause (cyclic ovarian activity greater than 40 years)	slight
Nulliparity	3
Previous breast cancer	5
Benign disease of the breast	1–4 (see the text)
Radiation	Dependent on dose

having developed bilateral cancers. For instance some reports have estimated that the lifetime risk of developing breast cancer for a daughter or sister of a premenopausal woman with bilateral disease is 50%, but that the risk is not increased if the relative was postmenopausal with unilateral disease (3). Others have suggested that these estimates are too high on the one hand and too low on the other. It is important to assure patients that breast cancer in more distant relatives (e.g., aunts) has little or no effect on a woman's risk. The other major risk factor other than family history is a prior history of breast cancer, which increases the risk of contralateral breast cancer 5-fold (36, 39, 51).

The patient should be questioned about the presence of other symptoms (pain, discharge) related to a breast mass, the duration of those symptoms if present, and whether the discovery of the mass or onset of the other symptoms was associated with changes in the menses, injury to the breast, pregnancy, or to changes in medication.

After the presence of a mass, nipple discharge is the second most frequent sign of breast cancer. Nonlactational nipple discharge can be unilateral or bilateral, spontaneous or evoked only by pressure and massage, and persistent or recurrent. If the discharge is associated with a mass on physical examination, the mass should be the primary concern. Nipple discharge in women over 50 must be viewed with more suspicion than in younger women, regardless of its presentation. Discharge evoked only by trauma, massage, or pressure has no clinical importance. Spontaneous, recurrent, or persistent discharge from one or two ducts not associated with a mass requires surgical exploration of the duct to differentiate benign papilloma from intraductal papillary carcinoma. Both are possible without a presenting mass, and the character of the discharge is not helpful.

Physical Examination

The patient should be seated undressed to the waist on an examining table. Inspection and palpation of the nodal drainage areas (supraclavicular and axillary) should be performed. Inspection and palpation of the nipples, areolae, and breasts are done next. While the patient is sitting, her arm on the side being examined can be raised by the physician to allow palpation high into the axilla. The examination should then be repeated with the patient in the supine position with her arm raised over her head so that the breast flattens on the chest wall. If the clinician cannot appreciate a mass noted by the patient, it is critical to allow the patient sufficient time to find the lesion herself rather than to dismiss the complaint. If both the patient and the physician cannot locate the mass, the patient should be reassured that benign fibrous masses often disappear spontaneously as do menstrual-related cysts.

Initial Management

The three most common masses found in the breast are fibroadenoma, fibrocystic changes, and carcinoma.

Each of these common lesions has a peak incidence at different ages but there is considerable overlap. It is because of this overlap and the inability of the physician from history, physical examination, or radiographic studies to make a diagnosis with certainty that a biopsy usually is the only definitive test to rule out carcinoma.

Ages 15 to 30

An easily movable, nontender, smooth, marble-like mass in a woman less than 30 years of age is most likely a fibroadenoma. The mass should be electively excised. This can be delayed up to several months if the mass is not growing rapidly and if there are no major risk factors (significant family history or prior breast cancer). A mammogram should not be routinely obtained in the evaluation of a discrete mass in this age group. The tissue is too dense to allow useful interpretation, and the radiation may slightly increase the risk for developing a neoplasm. Perhaps a patient with large breasts that are hard to examine, persistent symptoms, or a strong family history deserves a mammogram.

Ages 30 to 50

A discrete mass noted during the reproductive years that feels cystic might be watched through one or two menstrual cycles. A sonogram can be useful in distinguishing a cystic from a solid mass. If the mass persists, then a surgical consultation will most likely be necessary to allow histologic examination of the mass. A mammogram can be obtained before the consultation, especially if the patient has never had one. It should be noted that a persistent mass that is not seen on mammogram should not be ignored. Ten to 15% of palpable breast cancers are not seen on mammography (28).

Ages 50 and Over

A patient with a suspicious mass should be referred for possible biopsy. A mammogram should be obtained to search for other areas suspicious for multicentric or contralateral disease that may also need to undergo biopsy.

All Ages

The usual evaluation of a persistent palpable discrete breast mass involves histologic examination even if the mammogram is not suspicious. An exception is a cystic mass that disappears after aspiration or menstruation. If the mass is larger than 2 cm, then an incisional biopsy is usually done; otherwise it should be removed in toto. A fine needle aspiration for cytology is frequently obtained first since it is easier and less traumatic than an open biopsy. Simultaneous biopsy, frozen section, histologic examination, and, if malignant, immediate mastectomy should be considered only in very special cases at the wish of the patient and only after detailed discussion. Waiting for permanent sections allows detailed examination of the pathology and certainty of the diagnosis. In addition, the treatment of primary breast cancer has undergone many changes in recent years with several treatment options now available to the patient. The one step approach deprives a patient of what is in some states her legal right to a second opinion in regard to treatment options for her breast cancer.

Needle Aspiration

In the past, aspiration was limited to nodules felt to be cystic with sonography used to help distinguish cystic from solid lesions. More recently aspiration by the surgeon of solid lesions to obtain material for cytological examination has allowed the diagnosis of carcinoma to be made in the office and perhaps can spare some patients a surgical biopsy. In the case of the cystic lesion, if the mass does not completely disappear, or if the fluid is bloody or if the mass rapidly reoccurs, an open biopsy will be necessary. (Cytologic examination of the fluid is usually of little use and need not be done routinely.) If the lesion disappears completely without recurrence, routine follow-up is sufficient. If the cytology of a needle aspiration of a solid lesion is negative, then formal biopsy usually will be required as false-negatives are common.

Surgical Biopsy

It is important not only for the referring physician to inform the patient of the need for surgical consultation, but also to explain clearly the reasons why this is needed and that a biopsy may be recommended by the surgeon. The patient should be encouraged to ask questions. The consultation is stressful and the patient is more likely to absorb information from her personal physician. In addition, the patient needs support from her personal physician and the reassurance that he will continue to be involved in her care should a biopsy reveal cancer.

Preparation. Most biopsies can be carried out as an outpatient in an ambulatory surgery unit. Either local (preferred) or general anesthesia can be used. The patient should not eat or drink after midnight on the night before the biopsy.

Operation. A 2.5- to 7.5-cm incision is used to allow an adequate biopsy to be made and to be cosmetically satisfactory. The incision site is selected very carefully to minimize the potential for disfigurement should cancer be found and breast-conserving therapy subsequently be chosen.

It should be explained to the patient that in addition to a possible residual mass, there is often a ridge of tissue secondary to sutures and scar remaining after the operation. Removal of a large mass might necessitate a small drain, which is withdrawn in the office 1 or 2 days after the biopsy. If a mass is palpable, then the tissue of concern is easily located and biopsied. As noted previously, increasingly biopsies are being obtained for a mammographic lesion found in the absence of a palpable mass. In these instances the procedure is more complicated. Under mammographic guidance, a radiologist will place thin needles or hooks into the breast, with the tips within a centimeter of the suspicious area on the mammogram. Methylene blue or some other color marker will then be injected into the breast to mark visually the abnormal area of the breast noted on the mammogram. The patient will then proceed to the ambulatory surgery unit where the surgeon will excise the stained area. If the mammographic abnormality contains microcalcifications, the biopsy specimen will be X-rayed to ensure that these have been removed with the biopsy. Several weeks after the biopsy the patient will need a mammogram to confirm that the suspicious area is no longer present.

Follow-up. Ecchymoses or hematoma (5% of the patients) and wound infection (1 to 2% of the patients) are main complications of breast biopsy. A large hematoma may require evacuation, but this usually can be done in the office. Exercise and strenuous activities should be avoided for 7 to 10 days after a breast biopsy to guard against late bleeding.

The long-term sequelae of breast biopsy are minimal; chronic scar formation may cause some difficulty with follow-up examinations and interpretation of mammograms. Detailed descriptions of the biopsy site should be noted in the chart by physicians on follow-up, and details of the biopsy should be conveyed to the radiologists reading future mammograms.

FOLLOW-UP MANAGEMENT OF A BENIGN BREAST MASS

Fibroadenoma

After excision of a fibroadenoma, the patient should have routine follow-up as defined by risk factors for carcinoma and age. The patient should be reassured that there is no increased risk of malignancy because of the fibroadenoma.

Fibrocystic Disease

If on pathology the epithelium is normal, then no special follow-up is necessary for the patient with a benign biopsy. Even if proliferative epithelial changes are noted, the increased risk is so minimal (less than 2-fold) that again the patient should be reassured and no special follow-up is warranted. Only the finding of atypia, especially in a patient with a history of breast cancer in a sibling or mother, requires special consideration. Without such a family history monthly self-examinations of the breasts, a physician examination *twice* yearly, and an annual mammogram should suffice. With a positive family history the patient may consider the 40% lifetime risk of developing breast cancer sufficient to consider bilateral prophylactic simple mastectomy with reconstruction (15). Subcutaneous mastectomy with implants should not be con-

sidered as a compromise. The 15 to 20% of the breast that will be left behind remains at risk.

As mentioned, the pain associated with fibrocystic changes is often ameliorated once a cancer has been excluded. If pain continues, the patient should be advised to wear a brassiere both day and night. A number of pharmacological and dietary strategies have been said to be effective in the management of patients with painful fibrocystic changes (e.g., avoidance of caffeine), usually without adequate supporting evidence (30, 42). However, danazol, a weak androgenic steroid, has been shown to decrease pain and nodularity in up to 70% of patients with fibrocystic changes when used in doses of 100 to 400 mg a day for 4 to 6 months (7, 32). Side effects are relatively minor, weight gain, acne, and amenorrhea being the most common. Tamoxifen, an antiestrogen, also has been reported to be useful (17).

CANCER

If the biopsy reveals carcinoma, then consultation with a medical oncologist and radiation oncologist should be considered. The treatment of breast cancer is complex and rapidly changing and involves the coordinated efforts of the surgeon, radiation oncologist, medical oncologist, and the primary physician. Whereas one would not expect the primary care physician to be knowledgeable in all of the details of treatment, he should be aware of the general concepts discussed below as it will be to him that the patient will look for support and clarification as she struggles with difficult treatment decisions.

Several clinical staging systems have been devised for breast cancer, but none facilitates the management of individual patients. It is perhaps simplest to divide tumors into three main groups: *resectable*: tumors not fixed to the chest wall and not associated with fixed matted axillary nodes; *locally advanced*, unresectable: tumors fixed to the chest wall or associated with the presence of matted axillary nodes, or inflammatory skin changes, but without signs of metastases; and *metastatic tumors*.

In the absence of symptoms or physical findings, patients with resectable tumors require minimal further studies consisting of a chest X-ray and measurement of serum alkaline-phosphatase activity and of calcium concentration and, if not done prior to the biopsy, a mammogram to look for contralateral disease or multicentric lesions. In addition, the patient's history should be retaken to ensure there are no musculoskeletal complaints consistent with bony metastases. If there are, scan and local X-rays of the symptomatic region should be obtained. In general, liver and bone scans should not be obtained routinely since in the absence of symptoms, physical findings, or abnormal serum chemistries, they are more likely to produce confusing false-positive results than to disclose unexpected metastases, especially with tumors less than 5 cm (11).

Surgery

Radical mastectomy, the standard for years, is no longer performed. The modified radical mastectomy (removal of the breast and the ipsilateral axillary lymph nodes), which preserves the pectoral muscles, is of equal efficacy but is less disfiguring, allows easier reconstruction, and rarely leads to clinically significant arm edema (21).

For patients with small (less than 2.5 cm) intraductal (noninvasive) carcinomas, local excision of the tumor (usually already accomplished by the biopsy) may ultimately prove to be sufficient treatment (29). Currently the National Surgical Adjuvant Breast Project (NSABP) is conducting a study comparing local excision for such patients with local excision combined with breast irradiation. This is an important study since with the increased use of mammography screening many more (up to 20%) of all new breast cancers found are intraductal lesions (43). However, until the results of this study are known, most experts do *not* recognize local excision alone as adequate treatment for these tumors.

A modified radical mastectomy requires general anesthesia, and hospitalization varies from 5 to 14 days. Most patients are ambulatory and eating normally within 24 hours of the operation and discharged within 1 week. Occasionally patients may be discharged with drains, which are removed at the time of follow-up. Serous fluid may accumulate under the skin flaps even after the drains are removed and may require aspiration in the office. In the early postoperative period the patient may be inconvenienced with arm and shoulder discomfort but usually can use the arm normally within 2 to 3 weeks. Some patients may experience shoulder and arm pain for a much more extensive period. It is important for these patients to continue arm exercises as prescribed by the surgeon. In 10% of the patients, after modified radical mastectomy, lymphedema of the ipsilateral upper extremity develops. Usually swelling is minimal in the morning and increases during the day. Typically, the degree of swelling gradually becomes worse over several years. Management includes the following:

1. Instruct the patient to sleep with the arm propped up on a pillow and to take special care not to sleep with the arm under the head.
2. Minimize the amount of time that the arm is allowed to hang down (e.g., while sitting).
3. Minimize trauma to the arm. This includes limiting the use of the affected arm for blood pressure determinations, for phlebotomy, and for insertion of intravenous catheters.
4. Aggressively treat any infection of the arm. Patients should be instructed to see their physician as soon as signs or symptoms (erythema, swelling, or pain) of infection are noted, no matter how minimal. (Cellulitis is the major complication of lymphedema.)
5. If the degree of swelling is unsightly or uncomfortable, the patient can be fitted with a Jobst sleeve (available at Jobst outlets in most cities) to be worn during waking hours. A trial with a lymphedema pump (a pneumatic sleeve, sold by medical supply houses, that applies intermittent compression to the affected arm) can be considered for severe, refractory cases.
6. The physician should be attentive to sudden changes in the rate of edema formation, especially when associated with new arm pain. This may indicate recurrence of tumor in the axilla.

It is most important to be sensitive to cosmetic and emotional needs of the patient for what most patients consider disfiguring surgery. Most hospitals have a representative from the American Cancer Society "Reach for Recovery" program or someone serving a similar role who can assist in this regard, and this person should make contact with the patient in the perioperative period to offer her help. Within 3 to 6 weeks of operation, most patients can be fitted with a breast form if skin healing is complete. These forms can be obtained in medical appliance stores.

Breast reconstruction should be discussed with the patient before the surgery to allow referral to a plastic surgeon *before* her scheduled mastectomy. The patient then can decide which of several reconstruction procedures she prefers and whether she would like reconstruction done simultaneously with the mastectomy or later. Breast reconstruction with implants, as opposed to using muscle flaps, is currently popular. There are no contraindications to this procedure other than inadequate chest wall tissue to allow a satisfactory result. Commonly, such reconstruction involves implantation of a balloon that is gradually inflated over several weeks to effect sufficient stretching of the chest tissues to allow the later insertion of the implant after removal of the balloon. Although flap reconstruction or balloon implantation can occur at the time of mastectomy, most advise a delay of 3 to 6 months to allow complete healing from the mastectomy.

Radiotherapy Combined with Surgery

Radiotherapy alone as treatment for primary breast cancer has not been systematically studied. The NSABP has established (for patients with resectable primary tumors 4 cm or less) that complete excision of the primary tumor ("lumpectomy," usually with removal of lymph nodes, unless the tumor is only intraductal— see below) followed by breast irradiation five times a week for 5 weeks is as curative as a modified radical mastectomy (22). For larger lesions, the information is not as well established, but a certain number of these women, especially those with tumors less than 5 cm, might also be considered for excision and radiotherapy. The main considerations are cosmetic. These include the relative sizes of the tumor and the remaining breast and how close to the nipple complex the tumor lies. The larger the ratio of tumor size to uninvolved breast the more likely a poor cosmetic result will occur, as a larger percentage of the normal breast will be exposed to radiation doses that will lead to·disfiguring fibrosis. Usually if tumors are close to or involve the nipple complex, a better cosmetic result is achieved after mastectomy and reconstruction than after lumpectomy and radiotherapy.

Patients should be warned that there is a significant incidence of recurrent breast cancer in the irradiated breast. In most reported series this ranges from 5 to 15% in contrast to 3% local recurrence rate after mastectomy (22, 38). (The results from the NSABP study are an exception with a very low rate of breast recurrences after radiation, perhaps because of patient selection and study design.) Even higher percentages (30%) of local relapses after lumpectomy and radiotherapy for invasive carcinoma have been reported if an extensive intraductal (noninvasive) carcinoma component is also present in the biopsy specimen (27). For this reason many physicians feel that patients with invasive breast cancer associated with a significant intraductal component should be treated with a modified mastectomy instead of lumpectomy and radiotherapy. This remains a controversial issue. Fortunately the occurrence of a local relapse after breast-conserving therapy does not appear to affect survival, unlike that that after a mastectomy (22, 38). Current data suggest that after a "salvage" simple mastectomy, these patients survive as long as those who had their tumor treated initially with a modified radical mastectomy. However, because of the prior radiotherapy, reconstruction in such patients will be more difficult than in those choosing a modified mastectomy initially.

For patients choosing lumpectomy and radiotherapy, over 80% are satisfied with the cosmetic results. The treatment is complicated with minimal, if any, postoperative lymphedema or impaired wound healing. The irradiated breast will atrophy over a number of months, and for some patients reduction mammoplasty of the opposite breast may need to be considered.

In summary, for most patients with tumors less than 5 cm that can be completely excised without affecting the nipple/areolar complex when there is sufficient remaining breast tissue, there exists a choice for the patient between mastectomy and breast-conserving radiotherapy. All patients should have the choices well outlined and be given information that clearly describes the benefits and disadvantages of both treatment options.

Multimodality Treatment

Those patients with locally advanced unresectable disease or with inflammatory disease should be considered for therapy with initial systemic chemotherapy followed by surgery if sufficient tumor reduction occurs and/or local irradiation with perhaps further chemotherapy (25). For a select group such an approach may allow long-term survival.

PROGNOSIS, FURTHER THERAPY, AND FOLLOW-UP

Prognosis

Currently estimates of survival are based mainly upon whether the tumor is wholly intraductal (noninvasive) or not and the results of the axillary node sampling. The cure rate with mastectomy approaches 100% for women whose tumor consists only of intraductal carcinoma. (Axillary node involvement occurs in less than 5% of these patients and so node resection gives little further information and can be omitted).

A special case is lobular carcinoma in situ (LCIS). This diagnosis should more accurately be classified as a premalignant lesion and not considered a neoplasm. It should be viewed as a risk factor in a manner similar to the finding of hyperplasia with atypia on a biopsy. Although there continues to be some disagreement between experts as to how significant a risk factor LCIS is, a reasonable estimate is that a woman with a finding of LCIS has between a 15 to 30% lifetime risk of developing invasive cancer or about 0.5 to 1% risk of cancer per year. It is important to realize that this risk applies to both breasts (just as does any other risk factor). Recommendations vary for LCIS, but most recommend close mammographic follow-up with prophylactic *bilateral* mastectomies reserved for those women psychologically unable to deal with the increased risk of breast cancer (26, 40).

For women with invasive cancer the status of the axillary lymph nodes is the best indicator of prognosis (Table 89.2) (5, 18, 21). Survival at 10 years is approximately 65% with no node involvement: 37% with one to three nodes: 13% with four or more nodes involved (5, 24). Within these subgroups patients whose tumor is estrogen receptor (and progesterone receptor) rich do better than those whose tumors lack significant receptor levels (8, 34, 46). Patients with tumors larger than 5 cm do somewhat worse, especially if there are positive nodes and patients with tumors smaller than 2 cm, and uninvolved nodes do better (1, 23). Adjuvant systemic therapy increases the overall survival by 5 to 15% (37). Unfortunately these figures apply to large groups and tell little about the survival estimate for the individual patient.

Recent advances may allow more accurate prognosis for specific subgroups and eventually for individual patients. For example, patients whose tumors appear

Table 89.2.
Survival of Patients with Breast Cancer Relative to Status of the Axillary Lymph Nodes[a]

Status of Nodes	Crude Survival (%)		5-Year Disease-Free Survival (%)
	5-Year	10-Year	
All Patients	63.5	45.9	60.3
Negative axillary lymph nodes	78.1	64.9	82.3
Positive axillary lymph nodes	46.5	24.9	34.9
1–3 positive axillary lymph nodes	62.2	37.5	50.0
≥4 positive axillary lymph nodes	32.0	13.4	21.1

[a] National Surgical Adjuvant Breast Project.

well differentiated to the pathologist may do significantly better than those tumors appearing poorly differentiated. Of greater interest is that tumors from individual patients are now being characterized by molecular biologic analysis to assist in estimates of prognosis. Patients whose tumors show aneuploidy or more than 6 to 7% of their cells in S-phase (synthesizing DNA) appear to do much worse than predicted by the current criteria of node status (12). DNA analysis of these parameters by flow cytometry is readily available through several commercial laboratories. Analysis for the increased presence and functioning of certain oncogenes (e.g., HER-2/Neu) in individual tumors is just beginning to show promise in predicting survival and may be available commercially in the near future (47). The need to determine more accurately the prognosis of individual patients is important, since prognostic category is the basis for patient selection for adjuvant therapy after the treatment of the primary tumor.

Adjuvant Therapy

For certain patients with poor prognoses, further treatment with radiation or chemotherapy will be recommended by the medical or radiation oncologist in an attempt to improve disease-free survival and cure. Currently patients are selected by the number of axillary nodes involved, their menopausal status, and the quantity of estrogen receptors their tumor contained (46). Systemic chemotherapy lasting 6 months is recommended to all premenopausal women with metastases to their axillary nodes. (For patients opting for lumpectomy/radiotherapy, the chemotherapy is usually sandwiched between the lumpectomy and the breast irradiation.) Similarly, use of an antiestrogen, tamoxifen, is recommended for postmenopausal women with axillary node involvement if their tumors contain significant estrogen receptors. In addition patients with four or more nodes involved with tumor might be candidates for postmastectomy chest wall irradiation, since they are more at risk for local recurrences (18). Long-term side effects of these therapies are infrequent but need to be recognized by both the patient and the primary care physician involved in the long-term follow-up. Chemotherapy may cause premature menopause and a slight increase in the incidence of second neoplasms, mainly hematologic. Radiotherapy may lead to darkened skin, pulmonary damage, or later solid neoplasms (but not breast cancer in the unaffected breast). Tamoxifen may cause bothersome hot flashes, and perhaps an increased incidence of endometrial carcinomas, but does not appear to have any cardiovascular adverse side effects or to affect the course of postmenopausal osteoporosis. Tamoxifen does seem to *decrease* the risk of developing cancer in the unaffected breast (19). The selection criteria for adjuvant systemic therapy are being re-examined constantly as new information is obtained. Based upon recent studies (19, 20, 33) of the beneficial effects of systemic therapy on node-negative patients, the National Cancer Institute is recommending that all premenopausal women with breast cancer receive adjuvant chemotherapy, independent of axillary node involvement (hence sparing patients who choose lumpectomy and radiotherapy an axillary dissection) and that all postmenopausal women whose tumors contain estrogen receptors be given tamoxifen for 5 or more years (13). These criteria are felt by many to be too broad and surely will be refined as the importance of the molecular biological characteristics as an independent prognosticator is better understood. One would hope that as the treatment of breast cancer evolves, only those patients who could benefit from adjuvant therapies will be offered them and that those patients cured by initial therapy will be spared further treatment.

Follow-Up

The patient with breast cancer is at a higher (5-fold) risk for development of cancer in the other breast (36, 39, 51). Consequently she should be screened with routine mammography and physical examinations as would any woman of moderately increased risk. Those patients choosing lumpectomy/radiotherapy should have a biannual mammogram and careful examination of the irradiated breast every 3 months looking for local, potentially curable recurrence. Patients who have had a mastectomy should have the scar examined at regular intervals since a small number (10%) of patients with recurrences in the scar may be cured with local resection followed by radiotherapy.

At present there is little evidence to support the concept that the asymptomatic patient is benefited by prompt diagnosis and initiation of treatment of recurrent systemic metastases (49). No studies have demonstrated that monitoring patients with X-rays, liver function tests, carcinoembryonic antigens (CEAs), or other tumor markers at regular intervals serve to improve survival. When these studies are normal, they serve to reassure the patient. However, when they are abnormal, many times they initiate a series of difficult management issues that mainly provoke uncertainty in the physician and anxiety in the patient without clear benefit to either. Thus follow-up plans can be individualized.

General References

DeVita Jr VT, Hellman S, Rosenberg SA (eds): *Cancer-Principles and Practice of Oncology*, 3rd ed. Philadelphia, JB Lippincott Co, 1989. p. 1197.
  In-depth chapter on breast cancer by the authors of *Breast Diseases*.
Fibrocystic "disease" of the breast: what's in a name? *Contemporary Surgery* 32:43, 1988.
  Concise review of the complaint of most women.
Harris JR, Berg J, Henderson IC, Kinne DW: *Breast Diseases*. Philadelphia, JB Lippincott Co., 1987.
  An excellent and extensive reference.

Specific References

1. Adair F, Berg J, Joubert L, Robbins GF: Long-term followup of breast cancer patients: the 30-year report. *Cancer* (Phila) 33:1145, 1974.

2. Adami H, Hansen J, Jung B, Rimsten A: Characteristics of familial breast cancer in Sweden: absence of relation to age and unilateral versus bilateral disease. *Cancer* (Phila) 48:1688, 1981.

3. Anderson DE, Badzioch MD: Risk of familial breast cancer. *Cancer* (Phila) 56:383, 1985.

4. Bailar JC: Mammography before age 50 years? *JAMA* 259:1548, 1988.

5. Bonadonna G, Rossi A, Tancini G, et al: Adjuvant chemotherapy in breast cancer. *Lancet* 1:1157, 1983.

6. Brinton LA, Hoover R, Fraumeni JF: Reproductive factors in the aetiology of breast cancer. *Br J Cancer* 47;757, 1983.

7. Brookshaw JD: Danazol treatment of benign breast disease: a survey of U.S.A. multicenter studies. *Postgrad Med J* 55:52, 1979.

8. Butler JA, Bretsky S, Mendez-Botet C, Kinne DW: Estrogen receptor protein of breast cancer as a predictor of recurrence. *Cancer* (Phila) 55:1178, 1985.

9. Canadian Task Force on the Periodic Health Examination. The periodic health examination: 2, 1985 update. *Can Med Am J* 134:724, 1986.

10. Chu KC, Smart CR, Tarone RE: Analysis of breast cancer mortality and stage distribution by age for the Health Insurance Plan Clinical Trial. *JNCI* 80:1125, 1988.

11. Caitto S, Pacini P, Azzini V, et al: Preoperative staging of primary breast cancer—a multicentric study. *Cancer* (Phila) 61:1038, 1988.

12. Clark GM, Dressler LG, Owens MA, et al: Prediction of relapse or survival in patients with node-negative breast cancer by DNA flow cytometry. *N Engl J Med* 320:627, 1989.

13. *Clinical Alert*. National Cancer Institute: May, 1988.

14. Council on Scientific Affairs: Mammographic screening in asymptomatic women aged 40 years and older. *JAMA* 261:2535, 1989.

15. Dupont WD, Page DL: Risk factors for breast cancer in women with proliferative breast disease. *N Engl J Med* 312:146, 1985.

16. Eddy DM, Hasselblad V, McGivney W, Hender W: The value of mammography screening in women under age 50 years. *JAMA* 259:1512, 1988.

17. Fentiman IS, Brame K, Caleffi M, et al: Double-blind controlled trial of tamoxifen therapy for mastalgia. *Lancet* 1:287, 1986.

18. Fisher B, Bauer M, Wickerham L, et al: Relationship of number of positive axillary nodes to the prognosis of patient with primary breast cancer-an NSABP update. *Cancer* (Phila) 52:1551, 1983.

19. Fisher B, Constantino J, Redmond C, et al: A randomized clinical trial evaluating tamoxifen in the treatment of patients with node-negative breast cancer who have estrogen-receptor-positive tumors. *N Engl J Med* 320:479, 1989.

20. Fisher B, Redmond C, Dimitrov NV, et al: A randomized clinical trial evaluating sequential methotrexate and fluorouracil in the treatment of pataients with node-negative breast cancer who have estrogen-receptor-negative tumors. *N Engl J Med* 320:473, 1989.

21. Fisher B, Redmond C, Fisher ER, et al: Ten-year results of a randomized clinical trial comparing radical mastectomy and total mastectomy with or without radiation. *N Engl J Med* 312:674, 1985.

22. Fisher B, Redmond C, Poisson MD, et al: Eight-year results of a randomized clinical trial comparing total mastectomy and lumpectomy with or without irradiation in the treatment of breast cancer. *N Engl J Med* 320:822, 1989.

23. Fisher B, Slack NH, Bross IDJ: Cancer of the breast: size of neoplasm and prognosis. *Cancer* (Phila) 24:1071, 1969.

24. Fisher B, Slack N, Katrych D, et al: Ten year follow-up results of patients with carcinoma of the breast in a cooperative clinical trial evaluating surgical adjuvant chemotherapy. *Surg Gynecol Obs* 140:528, 1975.

25. Griem KL, Henderson IC, Gelman R, et al: The 5-year results of a randomized trial of adjuvant radiation therapy after chemotherapy in breast cancer treated with mastectomy. *J Clin Oncol* 5:1546, 1987.

26. Haagensen C, Lane N, Lattes R, Bodian C: Lobular neoplasia (so called lobular carcinoma in situ) of the breast. *Cancer* (Phila) 42:737, 1978.

27. Harris JR, Connolly JL, Schnitt SUJ, et al: The use of pathologic features in selecting the extent of surgical resection necessary for breast cancer patients treated by primary radiation therapy. *Ann Surg* 301:164, 1985.

28. Health and Public Policy Committee. American College of Physicians: the use of diagnostic tests for screening and evaluating breast lesions. *Ann Intern Med* 103:143, 1985.

29. Lagios MD, Westdahl PR, Margolin FR, Rose MR: Duct carcinoma in situ: relationship of extent of noninvasive disease to the frequency of occult invasion, multicentricity, lymph node metastases, and short-term treatment failures. *Cancer* (Phila) 50:1309, 1982.

30. London RS, Sundaram GS, Goldstein PJ: Medical management of mammary dysplasia. *Obstet Gynecol* 59:519, 1982.

31. Love SM, Gelman SR, Silen W: Fibrocystic "Disease" of the breast—A nondisease? *N Engl J Med* 307:1010, 1982.

32. Mansel RE, Wisbey JR, Hughes LE: Controlled trial of the antigonadotrophin danazol in painful nodular benign breast disease. *Lancet* 1:928, 1982.

33. Mansour EG, Gray R, Shatila AH, et al: Efficacy of adjuvant chemotherapy in high-risk node-negative breast cancer. *N Engl J Med* 320:485, 1989.

34. McGuire WL, Clark GM, Dressler LG, Owens MA: Role of steroid hormone receptors as prognostic factors in primary breast cancer. *NCI Monogr* 1:19, 1986.

35. Moskowitz M: The predictive value of certain mammographic signs in screening for breast cancer. *Cancer* (Phila) 51:1007, 1983.

36. Nielsen M, Christensen L, Andersen J: Contralateral cancerous breast lesions in women with clinical invasive breast carcinoma. *Cancer* (Phila) 57:897, 1986.

37. NIH Consensus Panel: Adjuvant chemotherapy for breast cancer. *JAMA* 254:3461, 1985.

38. Recht A, Silver B, Schnitt S, et al: Breast relapse following primary radiation therapy for early breast cancer I: Classification, frequency, and salvage. *Int J Radiat Oncol Bio Phys* 11:1271, 1985.

39. Robbins GF, Berg JW: Bilateral primary breast cancers. *Cancer* (Phila) 17:1501, 1964.

40. Rosen P, Lieberman P, Braum D, et al: Lobular carcinoma in situ of the breast. *Am J Surg Pathol* 2:225, 1978.

41. Sattin RW, Rubin GL, Webster LA, et al: Family history and the risk of breast cancer. *JAMA* 253:1908, 1985.

42. Schairer C, Rubin GL, Webster LA, et al: Methylxanthines and benign breast disease. *Am J Epidemiol* 124:603, 1986.

43. Schnitt SJ, Silen W, Sadowsky NL, et al: Ductal carcinoma in situ (intraductal carcinoma) of the breast. *N Engl J Med* 318:898, 1988.

44. Seidman H, Gelb SK, Silverberg E, et al: Survival experience in the Breast Cancer Institution Demonstration Project. *Ca-A Cancer J for Clinicians* 37:258, 1987.

45. Seidman H, Mushinski MH, Gelb SK, et al: Probabilities eventually developing or dying of cancer: United States. Data from Surveillance, Epidemiology and End Results (SEERS) *Ca-A Cancer J for Clinicians* 35:36, 1985.

46. Singhakowinta A, Potter H, Bueokwe BB, et al: Estrogen receptor and natural course of breast cancer. *Ann Surg* 183:84, 1989.

47. Slamon J, Godolphin W, Jones LA, et al: Studies of the HER-2/neuproto-oncogene in human breast and ovarian cancer. *Science* (Wash DC) 244:707, 1989.

48. Tabor L, Gad A, Holmberg LH, et al: Reduction in mortality from breast cancer after mass screening with mammography: randomized trial from the Breast Cancer Screening Working Group of the Swedish National Board of Health and Welfare. *Lancet* 1:829, 1985.

49. Tomin R, Donegan WL: Screening for recurrent breast cancer—its effectiveness and prognostic value. *J Clin Oncol* 5:62, 1987.

50. U.S. Preventive Task Force. Recommendations for breast cancer screening. *JAMA* 257:2196, 1987.

51. Webber BL, Heise H, Neifeld JP, Costa J: Risk of subsequent contralateral breast carcinoma in a population of patients with in-situ carcinoma. *Cancer* (Phila) 47:2928, 1981.

C H A P T E R   90

Diseases of the Biliary Tract

ROBERT M. QUINLAN, M.D.
ESTEBAN MEZEY, M.D.

Diseases of the biliary tract are encountered commonly in ambulatory practice. Many patients will be discovered to have asymptomatic gallstones during the course of evaluation of another condition; others will be found to have symptomatic chronic cholecystitis. Less commonly, patients will present with an acute illness due to acute cholecystitis or to common bile duct obstruction. This chapter describes the cause, diagnosis, and treatment of these various conditions.

CHOLELITHIASIS

Epidemiology

Approximately 10% of the Unites States population has gallstones. In their lifetime only 50% will ever be symptomatic, with 80% of them having chronic symptoms, and 20% presenting with an acute illness. About 500,000 cholecystectomies are performed each year in the United States.

Ninety percent of gallstones found in patients in this country are cholesterol gallstones; 10% are pigment (bilirubinate) stones. The prevalence of gallstones is greater in women than in men and increases with age. In the United States 10% of men and 20% of women between the ages of 55 and 65 are affected (4). The prevalence of cholesterol gallstones is particularly high

in the Southwest Indians of the United States; for example, 70% of Pima women over age 25 have cholelithiasis (18).

Gallstone Formation

Bile is produced in the liver and excreted into the duodenum. Bile contains bile acids (primarily cholic, deoxycholic, and chenodeoxycholic acid), phospholipids (primarily lecithin), and cholesterol. The solubility of cholesterol depends on its incorporation with bile and phospholipids into a micelle. In the intestinal tract, bile salts are necessary for the absorption of dietary fats; they solubilize fatty acids and monoglycerides into micellar solutions. The fatty acids are absorbed in the jejunum, whereas the bile salts are absorbed in the ileum and enter the enterohepatic circulation.

There are three major types of gallstones that form in human bile: cholesterol stones (> 70% cholesterol), mixed stones (50 to 70% cholesterol), and pigment stones (12% cholesterol). These stones probably develop in three stages: first, the formation of a supersaturated bile; second, the crystallization or initiation of stone formation; and third, the growth of the stone to a certain detectable size before crystals in the bile are expelled into the intestine. It is likely, but not clearly established, that one of these stages is more important in the formation of certain types of stones than in others.

Cholesterol Stones

Recent studies have focused on the hypersecretion of biliary cholesterol as the real culprit in the pathogenesis of cholesterol stones and, although the Pima indian also has a documented deficiency in the bile salt pool, that might not be true for all cholesterol stone formers. Several mechanisms of increased cholesterol secretion have been identified (2). Cholesterol crystals form when the amount of cholesterol in bile exceeds the solubilizing properties of bile salts and phopholipid (supersaturated bile). The cholesterol crystals are caught in a film of mucin gel that lines the gallbladder and provides a nucleus for formation of gallstones. Growth of these stones occurs, especially in a dyskinetic gallbladder, one in which contraction is impaired, as in diabetes mellitus and pregnancy. The mucin gel itself might decrease gallbladder motility and emptying.

Pigment Stones

Formation of pigment stones is probably initiated by supersaturation of unconjugated bilirubin in the gallbladder and common bile duct. Unconjugated bilirubin, like cholesterol, is relatively insoluble in water. An increased concentration of unconjugated bilirubin in bile results either from formation of unconjugated bilirubin from conjugated bilirubin in the biliary tree through the action of a glucuronidase (perhaps of bacterial origin, in patients with infected bile, see below) or from increased production of unconjugated bilirubin by the liver (e.g., in patients with hemolytic anemia). A diseased gallbladder is probably not a factor in the formation of pigment stones.

Risk Factors

Because most patients with cholelithiasis are asymptomatic, it is difficult to evaluate risk factors precisely. Known risk factors for the development of cholesterol and pigment stones are listed in Table 90.1 (1).

Cholesterol Stones

The demography of cholesterol stones probably reflects, in part, a genetic predisposition and, in part, nongenetic ethnic characteristics. For example, it is known that obese people, and nonobese people who eat a high calorie diet, secrete relatively more cholesterol into their bile than does the average person. Therefore, populations in whom obesity is common (e.g., the Indians of the American Southwest) or who consume high calorie diets (occidental societies in general) are more susceptible to cholelithiasis.

The reasons for the increasing incidence of gallstones in middle-aged and elderly people are unknown but may be related to the time that elapses, first, between formation of supersaturated bile and formation of stones, and second, between formation of stones and recognition of them.

The influence of estrogens on the secretion of cholesterol in bile is reflected in the increased prevalence of gallstones in women (between puberty and menopause) compared with men (see above) and in women who take estrogenic preparations compared with women who do not (see Chapter 93).

Finally, there are a number of ways by which the concentration of bile acids in bile is reduced, favoring

the formation of gallstones: drugs utilized to treat hyperlipidemia, such as clofibrate, cholestyramine, and colestipol (see Chapter 75), decrease bile acid secretion; and certain disorders of the gastrointestinal tract (ileal resection, Crohn's disease of the ileum) reduce bile acid resorption.

Pigment Stones

The demography of pigment stones is entirely different from that of cholesterol stones. The propensity of orientals to develop pigment stones is not entirely understood, but it may be attributable to the higher prevalence of bacterial infection of the bile (usually *Escherichia coli* infections), and of *Ascaris* infestation, in the Orient compared to the Occident. In the United States, patients with pigment gallstones do not usually have infected or infested bile. The recognized risk factors in this country are hemolysis and alcoholic cirrhosis. Like cholesterol stones, pigment stones are more common with advancing age but unlike cholesterol stones, endogenous and exogenous estrogens or obesity have no influence on their development.

Natural History

Many attempts have been made to study the natural history of gallstones among the 2 to 3 million people in this country known to harbor them. Fifty percent of these people are asymptomatic, having had gallstones discovered incidentally on abdominal film (10 to 15% are radiopaque) or during celiotomy for treatment of another condition. The other 50% are symptomatic: i.e., gallstones are discovered during evaluation of the typical or atypical abdominal pain of cholecystitis (see below).

Approximately 18% of individuals with "silent" gallstones will develop symptoms in 15 to 20 years, and 3% will develop complications of biliary tract disease: acute cholecystitis, pancreatitis, or jaundice (7). The risk of developing complications is unrelated to the severity of symptoms but does increase with the length of time symptoms have been present. Most complications occur only among symptomatic patients. However, 20% of the time acute cholecystitis is the first indication of cholelithiasis. If complications occur, they usually occur within 5 years of the discovery of gallstones. Causes of death related to cholelithiasis among patients not having cholecystectomy are acute cholecystitis, cholangitis with liver abscess, necrotizing pancreatitis, gallbladder carcinoma, and gallstone ileus with mechanical small bowel obstruction. In Lund's study of the natural history of cholelithiasis, 2.7% of the deaths among patients not operated upon were attributed to gallbladder disease (12).

The Asymptomatic Patient

It cannot be predicted, on the basis of the size, number of stones, sex, or age of the patient, which asymptomatic patients are likely to become symptomatic (23). Whether asymptomatic patients should undergo elec-

Table 90.1.
Risk Factors for Gallstones[a]

CHOLESTEROL STONES
  Demography: Northern Europe, North and South America more than the Orient; American Indians; probably familial predisposition
  Obesity
  High caloric diet
  Drugs used in the treatment of hyperlipidemia: clofibrate, cholestyramine, and colestipol
  Gastrointestinal disorders involving major malabsorption of bile acids; ileal disease, resection or bypass; cystic fibrosis, with pancreatic insufficiency
  Female sex hormones: women more at risk than men, use of oral contraceptives and other estrogenic medications
  Age, especially among men
  Probable but not well established; pregnancy, diabetes mellitus, and polyunsaturated fats
PIGMENT STONES
  Demography; oriental more than occidental; rural more than urban
  Chronic hemolysis
  Alcoholic cirrhosis
  Biliary infection
  Age

[a] After Bennion LJ. Grundy SM Risk factors for the development of cholelithiasis in man. *N Engl J Med* 299:1161, 1978.

tive cholecystectomy, therefore, depends largely on the bias of the general physician and the consulting surgeon. About 18% of patients become symptomatic (see above), sometimes at a point in their lives when operation is more dangerous because of age, intercurrent illness, or the presence of acute cholecystitis. The risk of complications of cholelithiasis, other than acute cholecystitis, is negligible in the asymptomatic patient. Carcinoma of the gallbladder is more common among people with gallstones but the risk—0.3 to 1% over a lifetime—is approximately the same as is the operative mortality from cholecystectomy. If the gallbladder is calcified, risk of cancer is markedly increased, however, and cholecystectomy should be performed. Otherwise, the general consensus at this point is not to recommend elective cholecystectomy in the asymptomatic patient. Recently the legitimacy of this same approach in the diabetic patient has been documented (5).

CHOLECYSTITIS

The hallmark of cholecystitis is abdominal pain, often epigastric at onset, but localizing within a few hours to the right upper quadrant. The pain is characteristically, but not always, severe and unremitting with only slight variations in intensity. Use of the term "biliary colic," therefore, is not precise because colic is defined as pain that waxes and wanes. Some patients describe the pain as heavy and aching; some, as knife-like. Occasionally it radiates into the right side of the back or, less often, into other parts of the abdomen. The pain usually begins abruptly, within 1 to 3 hours of eating a meal. Patients may also complain of being awakened in the middle of the night. Pain is often accompanied by slight nausea. A typical attack subsides spontaneously within 2 to 3 hours. The frequency of such attacks is extremely variable, from every few days to once or twice a year.

A patient who presents this history is very likely to have gallstones. However, the degree of inflammation of the gallbladder often cannot be determined from the history. There may be gallstones without any inflammation at all; there may be acute inflammation; or there may be chronic inflammation with fibrosis. However, an attack lasting more than 6 hours generally heralds the onset of "acute cholecystitis," i.e., acute inflammation. The severity of the symptoms and the presence or absence of signs of inflammation and/or biliary obstruction determine the physician's response (see below).

Acute Cholecystitis

Pathophysiology

Acute cholecystitis is caused over 90% of the time by a gallstone that obstructs the cystic duct. Acalculous cholecystitis occurs primarily in patients who have sustained major trauma, including major operations, or in patients with emphysematous cholecystitis due to infection with gas-forming bacteria.

Inflammation of the gallbladder in early acute cholecystitis is probably due to irritation by concentrated static bile. In some cases, as the process progresses, infection may play a role; bile cultures are positive in only 20 to 30% of patients during the first few days of an attack but, by 7 to 10 days, almost 80% of biliary cultures are positive. In certain patients, e.g., diabetics, mural ischemia might also play a role.

The difference between the presentation of acute and chronic cholecystitis (see below) is probably due to the length of time the cystic duct has been totally obstructed and to the intensity of the inflammation.

Signs and Symptoms

The pain of classical acute cholecystitis is severe and persistent. It is usually accompanied by nausea and fever (99 to 102°F; 37 to 39°C) and less often, by vomiting. Unless treated, the symptoms are likely to persist for up to a week.

The severity and persistence of the pain will usually cause the patient to call or see his physician (see Chapter 36 for a general discussion of abdominal pain). On examination, the patient is restless. There is considerable right upper quadrant abdominal tenderness, associated with involuntary guarding of the abdominal wall. This guarding, indicative of early peritoneal inflammation, is particularly important to recognize. It is not a feature of less acute disease (see below). Murphy's sign, the sudden involuntary arrest of inspiration (because of pain), when the examiner palpates the right upper quadrant during inspiration, is caused by the abutment of the inflamed gallbladder against the examiner's fingers as it moves downward with expansion of the chest cavity. This sign is more often elicited after several days of inflammation. In one-third of the patients, the gallbladder is palpable during an attack of acute cholecystitis if the right upper quadrant is probed very gently. Occasionally patients are mildly jaundiced (see below).

Laboratory Tests

Leukocytosis (12,000 to 15,000 white blood cells/mm^3) due to a neutrophilic granulocytosis is common. Serum amylase activity may be increased, in the absence of other evidence of acute pancreatitis. Often, serum aminotransferases (aspartate aminotransferase and alanine aminotransferase) are increased as well. Twenty percent of patients have mild hyperbilirubinemia (< 4 mg/100 ml).

Biliary scintigraphy is the test of choice in the diagnosis of acute cholecystitis. The imaging compounds are ^{99m}Tc-labeled derivatives of iminodiacetic acid (TcHIDA, PIPIDA, or DISIDA), which are concentrated in bile. The study requires injection of isotope intravenously and evaluation of uptake of the isotope by the gallbladder. If the cystic duct is obstructed, because of acute inflammation or because of a stone, uptake does not occur.

The test is performed in the nuclear medicine department of a hospital and takes 1 to 4 hours to complete. A positive study shows isotope in the biliary tree and in the duodenum but not in the gallbladder. A negative study shows isotope in the gallbladder as well. If isotope is not excreted, the test is uninterpretable; but, if it is excreted, the sensitivity of the test is extremely high (essentially 100%). Specificity also is high (95%), but false-positive results may occur in patients with chronic cholecystitis or acute biliary obstruction due to pancreatitis.

Differential Diagnosis

The differential diagnosis must include those disorders that might cause severe right upper quadrant abdominal pain and, usually, leukocytosis and slightly abnormal hepatic function: acute pancreatitis, appendicitis, hepatitis, hepatic abscess, a perforated or penetrated peptic ulcer, acute pyelonephritis, myocardial infarction, and right lower lobe pneumonia or pleuritis. Because of the severity of the illness, these distinctions should be made in the hospital.

Treatment

The patient suspected of having acute cholecystitis should be hospitalized for observation, hydration, and further diagnostic procedures (see page 1246 and Chapter 36 for a discussion of these procedures as they pertain to ambulatory patients). If the pain is intolerable, the physician can administer meperidine parenterally while arranging admission. Because this drug may increase biliary pressure by causing spasm of the sphincter of Oddi, it is reasonable to administer 0.6 mg of atropine along with the narcotic to prevent that effect. The patient should be told that, in the hospital, he will be fed intravenously, rather than by mouth; that, if he is vomiting, a nasogastric tube will be passed; and that antibiotics will be administered. If the temperature, white blood count, and pulse rate increase further and if abdominal tenderness and guarding increase as well, emergency operation will be required to prevent acute gangrenous cholecystitis and perforation. This progression of signs and symptoms occurs in 30 to 40% of patients. On the other hand, if the patient improves and the diagnosis is confirmed, elective cholecystectomy may be performed within a few days. A randomized prospective study that compared early and delayed cholecystectomy for acute cholecystitis concluded that the duration of hospitalization and the duration of disability were significantly reduced by early operation (10). Because of an increased likelihood of rapid progression of the disease to gangrene and perforation in elderly or diabetic patients (14, 15), cholecystectomy should be performed in these patients as soon as they can be prepared for it (assuming that they are considered able to tolerate an operation). Similarly, the presence of emphysematous cholecystitis due to gas-forming bacterial infection dictates emergency operation (air bubbles in the right upper quadrant on a plain film of the abdomen indicate the diagnosis).

A discussion of surgery of the biliary tract and of the results and complications of operations is provided below (pages 1248–1249).

Chronic Cholecystitis

Pathophysiology

Symptomatic chronic cholecystitis is associated with gallstones over 95% of the time; the remaining cases are due to other diseases of the gallbladder, such as cholesterolosis (the appearance of macrophages laden with cholesterol crystals in the wall of the gallbladder—often without stones). Recurring attacks of relatively mild acute cholecystitis cause eventual fibrosis so that the gallbladder empties poorly. The symptoms of chronic disease, like those of acute cholecystitis, are due to obstruction by a gallstone of the cystic duct. In chronic recurrent cholecystitis obstruction of the cystic duct is relatively short (probably no more than a few hours) compared with the length of time of obstruction in acute cholecystitis, and therefore, inflammation is less intense. Chronicity of symptoms may also be related to gallbladder dyskinesia secondary to mural fibrosis.

Signs and Symptoms

Many patients who complain of biliary pain for the first time probably already have chronic gallbladder inflammation. The character and location of the pain are identical to those of acute cholecystitis. Pain is variably associated with nausea and, occasionally, vomiting. Unlike classical acute cholecystitis, fever is unusual with chronic disease. Typically, pain follows eating, beginning 1 to 6 hours after a meal (see above), and lasts for 2 to 3 hours. Nonspecific symptoms—vague postprandial pain, bloating, belching, flatulence, so-called fatty food intolerance—thought by many to suggest gallbladder disease, are extremely common in the general population and therefore are not helpful diagnostically.

The patient with chronic cholecystitis usually seeks the physician less urgently than does the patient with acute cholecystitis. On examination during the attack, although there is tenderness to deep palpation in the right upper quadrant of the abdomen, there is no muscle guarding as there is in patients with acute inflammation. Murphy's sign (see above) is absent, the gallbladder is rarely palpable, and jaundice usually is not present. Between attacks, there is no abdominal tenderness.

Laboratory Tests

The white blood count, serum amylase, serum aminotransferases, and serum bilirubin are usually normal.

Unlike patients with acute cholecystitis, patients with symptoms due to chronic cholecystitis can be evaluated further in an ambulatory setting but some will be hospitalized early in an attack because of an inability to distinguish it from an episode of acute cholecystitis. If a TcHIDA scan is obtained to help in making that distinction, it may be positive, even in patients with chronic cholecystitis, because of transient obstruction of the cystic duct.

Ultrasound. Ultrasound has replaced the oral cholecystogram as the principal test for the detection of gallstones. The advantages of ultrasound are that it exposes the patient to no radiation, it is much quicker (5 to 10 minutes), and it has no side effects. It is not influenced by associated gastrointestinal or hepatic disease. The detection rate for gallstones 3 mm or greater in diameter is between 89 and 96% by ultrasound with 93 to 97% specificity (3 to 7% false positive) (3).

Oral cholecystogram. The oral cholecystogram (OCG) documents whether the gallbladder is functioning and whether radiolucent stones are present. This information is needed when considering nonoperative treatments for chronic cholelithiasis (see below).

To perform the test, the patient is given 3 g of iopanoic acid (Telepaque) in the evening after dinner and is instructed not to eat overnight; films of the abdomen are taken the following morning. If the gallbladder fails to visualize, the patient is given another 3 g of Telepaque and X-rays are repeated the following day. The patient should be warned that he may experience mild diarrhea for up to a day after the ingestion of the Telepaque.

Approximately 75% of gallbladders are visible on the first dose and another 15% will become visible on the second dose. Although, as stated above, 10 to 15% of gallstones are radiopaque and can be seen on plain film, confirmation of their location in the gallbladder should be obtained by OCG. The OCG is reliable only if the Telepaque is ingested at the proper time, retained in the gastrointestinal tract, absorbed from the small bowel, transported to the liver, esterified to glucuronide, and excreted by the liver into the bile. Therefore, gastrointestinal or hepatic disease may cause a false-positive study. However, the specificity of the test is high (4% false positive) if either radiolucent stones are present in an opacified gallbladder or if the gallbladder fails to concentrate contrast material after the second Telepaque dose. The sensitivity of the test is lower (10% false negative) and therefore OCG should be followed by sonography if the gallbladder is visualized and no stones are seen.

CT scan. Computerized tomography (CT) accurately identifies gallstones 80% of the time. Currently, it has no advantages over OCG and ultrasonography in the diagnosis of gallbladder disease. CT scans might be useful occasionally, however, if both the oral choelcystogram and ultrasound are equivocal.

Upper gastrointestinal series (UGI). Many patients are evaluated with an UGI series in addition to an oral cholecystogram, especially if symptoms are atypical of biliary tract disease. Max and Polk (13) reported 250 patients who underwent cholecystectomy, 145 of whom had an UGI and 105 of whom did not. Of the 145 patients selectively chosen for UGI only 39 had positive findings. In only seven of these patients was an associated gastroduodenal operation done at the time of cholecystectomy. Of these seven only three patients had any new information added by UGI. Based on these data, Max and Polk suggested guidelines for selectively choosing patients who might benefit from an UGI (Table 90.2).

Treatment

The treatment of choice for symptomatic chronic cholecystitis is elective cholecystectomy in patients who can tolerate an operation. Patients who are not surgical candidates either because of coexisting medical conditions or because they refuse surgery may elect gallstone dissolution or shock-wave lithotripsy as possible alternatives. Risks of not treating, surgically or medically, patients with chronic cholecystitis include gangrene and perforation of the gallbladder, choledocholithiasis (see below), pancreatitis, and, rarely, gallstone ileus (the obstruction of the small bowel by a large gallstone passed through an acute fistula that has formed between the gallbladder and the duodenum).

Gallstone Dissolution

Oral. The two naturally occurring bile acids, chenodeoxycholic acid and ursodeoxycholic acid, have been documented to dissolve cholesterol gallstones in a limited number of carefully selected patients. In a large multicenter study, chenodeoxycholic acid therapy for two years resulted in complete or partial dissolution of stones in 11 and 30% of patients, respectively. Dissolution occurred more frequently in women, thin patients, and in patients with small or floating gallstones (17). At the end of 2 years, treatment was discontinued, even if stones had not totally dissolved, because the safety of a longer course of treatment was not established. More recently ursodeoxycholic acid (Actigall) has been approved for use. Ursodeoxycholic acid is rarely associated with the diarrhea and is not associated with the hepatoxicity occasionally seen with chenodiol and therefore has become the drug of choice for oral dissolution. Actigall is sold as a 300-mg tablet; the recommended dose is 8 to 10mg/kg/day or 300 mg twice a day. The cost of treatment is about $750/year. Before institution of treatment, baseline liver function tests should be obtained and repeated 4 to 6 weeks after initiation of treatment. Follow-up ultrasonogra-

Table 90.2.
Suggested Indications for Upper Gastrointestinal Series in Patients with Documented Biliary Tract Disease[a]

Older patients (>50 years)
Men
Previous gastroduodenal operations
Previously documented upper gastrointestinal disease
History of pancreatitis
History or presence of jaundice
Long atypical history

[a] After Max MH, Polk HC: Routine preoperative upper gastrointestinal series (UGIS) in patients with biliary tract disease; a plea for more selectivity. *Surgery* 82:334, 1977.

phy to document gallstone dissolution should be obtained every 6 months. Ursodeoxycholic acid is more effective than chenodeoxycholic acid in gallstone dissolution during the first year of therapy, but there is no difference by 2 years (6). About 40% of patients will be stone free in 2 years. As with chenodiol, the treatment is most effective in patients with a few small calculi in a functioning gallbladder. It is reasonable to expect the stones to reform with cessation of treatment (21) so that, in the absence of side-effects, indefinite treatment is warranted.

Percutaneous. Thistle et al. (19) have recently reported on 75 patients who underwent percutaneously administered methyl tert-butyl ether to dissolve gallbladder stones. This invasive technique resulted in a 96% dissolution rate; yet it is far from standard treatment because it requires skilled accurate percutaneous transhepatic placement of a catheter into the gallbladder and then requires careful monitoring of this highly flammable organic solvent. As experience accumulates, indications will probably be liberalized but currently this technique should be considered experimental.

Gallstone Lithotripsy. Extracorporeal shock-wave lithotripsy (ESWL) combined with oral bile acids is an alternate effective therapy reserved for patients with symptomatic radiolucent stones less than 3 cm in diameter (calcified or pigment stones are resistant to dissolution by this technique) and a functioning gallbladder visualized by oral cholecystography. The shock-wave fragmentation of the stones is carried out under sonographic monitoring with the patient partially submerged in water and is followed by long-term therapy with chenodeoxycholic acid and/or ursodeoxycholic acid. In one study from Germany of 175 patients, gallstones completely disappeared in 30% within 2 months of lithotripsy; in 63% at 4 to 8 months; and in 90% at 12 to 18 months (16). The success was highest in patients with solitary stones greater than 2 cm in diameter. Complications of the therapy are petechiae and, rarely, hematuria, or pancreatitis. However, one-third of the patients experience episodes of biliary colic before there is complete disappearance of the gallstones. Patients are monitored closely with follow-up ultrasonography. Recurrent stones are expected with ESWL therapy alone in 40 to 50% of patients at 5 years (9), but it is hoped that subsequent administration of oral bile acids will reduce this high recurrence rate. There are now several centers in the United States involved in a clinical trial of the efficacy of ESWL before FDA approval.

SYMPTOMATIC PATIENTS WHO HAVE NO DETECTABLE GALLSTONES

Biliary Dyskinesia

Some patients with symptoms suggestive of gallstones have a normal abdominal sonogram, a normal OCG and a normal abdominal CT scan. These patients may have *biliary dyskinesia*, a term used to denote abnormally decreased emptying of the gallbladder. The diagnosis is best made by cholecystokinin (Kinevac)-stimulated cholecystography with a ^{99m}Tc-iminodiacetic derivative (i.e., TcHIDA). Often, the patient's pain is reproduced after the Kinevac injection (it stimulates gallbladder contraction), and abnormally decreased emptying of the gallbladder can be documented as a markedly decreased ejection fraction (% of the isotope excreted) when compared with a group of normal subjects. Such patients, if severely symptomatic, should be offered elective cholecystectomy, after which symptoms usually abate.

Biliary Sludge

There is a group of symptomatic patients who have no gallstones detectable by the standard techniques whose gallbladders reflect, on ultrasonography, echoes now recognized to be characteristic of biliary sludge (2). Biliary sludge is a term applied to excessively viscous bile that contains cholesterol crystals, calcium bilirubinate granules and mucin. In such patients duodenal drainage, ordinarily done by a consulting gastroenterologist, may prove useful in identifying the cholesterol crystals or the bilirubinate granules.

The test is performed by having the patient swallow a plastic double-lumened tube, weighted at the end by a mercury-filled bag. There are holes in the tube above the bag. When the bag has passed into the second portion of the duodenum (documented by fluoroscopy), magnesium sulfate is injected into one lumen of the tube to stimulate contraction of the gallbladder. Duodenal contents are then aspirated and the sediment is separated by centrifugation and examined under a microscope. The patient's experience during this procedure is similar to that of patients undergoing upper endoscopy (see Chapter 36).

Biliary sludge may be a precursor of gallstones, but in a given patient the course is entirely unpredictable. Nevertheless, as with biliary dyskinesia, severely symptomatic patients with biliary sludge should be offered elective cholecystectomy.

CHOLEDOCHOLITHIASIS

Epidemiology

Common duct stones occur in approximately 15% of patients with chronic cholecystitis, either before or after cholecystectomy. The incidence increases with age and the length of time symptoms of gallbladder disease have been present. There are three categories of common duct stones: (a) concomitant gallbladder stones and common duct stones, (b) retained stones found in the common duct soon after cholecystectomy and/or common duct exploration, and (c) common duct stones identified long after cholecystectomy and/or common duct exploration. The incidence of common duct stones decreases exponentially in the first year after cholecystectomy only to rise again, reaching a peak at 3 years. In one study 26% of symptomatic common duct stones occurred 10 or more years after cholecystectomy (20). Also, patients with congenital agenesis of the gallbladder have a 20% incidence of common duct stones. These observations support the concept that common duct stones originate either in the gallbladder or in the intrahepatic or common bile duct.

Signs and Symptoms

Approximately 6% of patients with common duct stones are asymptomatic. More typically patients develop severe colicky right upper quadrant pain, often associated with jaundice, mild fever, and nausea and vomiting. The pain usually begins abruptly and lasts up to an hour. If nothing is done, attacks recur at variable periods of time. Eventually cholangitis will develop, manifest by persistent malaise and anorexia and intermittent fever, chills, and jaundice—associated with persistently high serum alkaline phosphatase activity. Suppurative ascending cholangitis characterized by right upper quadrant pain, high fever, shaking chills, and jaundice (Charcot's triad) is life threatening and constitutes a surgical emergency.

On physical examination, if the patient is asymptomatic, no abnormal signs are elicited. If the patient is symptomatic, right upper quadrant abdominal tenderness and muscle guarding are usually present—similar to the findings in patients with acute cholecystitis. The patient is usually mildly to moderately jaundiced.

Laboratory Tests

Because of the acute onset of symptoms and the severity of pain in patients with choledocholithiasis, laboratory studies in the ambulatory setting are usually not appropriate. If such studies are done, leukocytosis and increases in serum alkaline phosphatase activity, serum bilirubin, serum aminotransferase activity, and serum amylase activity are likely to be observed.

Treatment

If common duct stones are discovered during cholecystectomy, they are removed. If the patient presents to the physician with severe right upper quadrant pain, tenderness, guarding, and/or jaundice, he should be hospitalized for further diagnostic studies and treatment. If sonography or CT scan shows a dilated biliary tree with probable distal obstruction, then endoscopic retrograde cholangiopancreatography (ERCP) should be performed. Common duct stones must be removed, either by operation (see below) or, if possible, at the time of ERCP. (ERCP is performed only in the hospital, usually in the radiology department since fluoroscopy and X-rays of the cannulated duct are required. The patient experience during the procedure is essentially the same as it is during other kinds of upper endoscopy (see Chapter 36), except that ERCP usually lasts for 30 to 60 minutes and may be complicated 5 to 10% of the time by postendoscopic infection, especially if the common duct is manipulated, and by pancreatitis.) Lithotripsy (see above) is also being evaluated in the treatment of common duct stones.

Cholangitis

Bacterial infection of the biliary tree generally occurs in association with bile duct obstruction due to either choledocholithiasis, tumor, or biliary strictures. The principal symptoms are fever, chills, and abdominal pain. Jaundice is often but not invariably present. On examination, there is abdominal tenderness and often rebound tenderness. Abnormal laboratory tests include leukocytosis and elevations of the serum bilirubin and alkaline phosphatase. Serum aminotransferases may also be moderately elevated. Blood cultures are often positive. The patient may deteriorate rapidly and develop hypotension and changes in mental status. Hospitalization is mandatory for therapy with antibiotics, followed by appropriate relief of biliary obstruction either surgically, by endoscopic sphincterotomy, or by placement of a biliary stent.

Primary sclerosing cholangitis (11) is a chronic inflammation of unknown cause of intra- and extrahepatic bile ducts that leads ultimately to fibrosis and to cholestatic liver disease. The majority of patients are men. There is a very high correlation with concomitant inflammatory bowel disease, most commonly ulcerative colitis. The course of the cholangitis is unpredictable, but patients with advanced disease develop jaundice, right upper quadrant abdominal pain, fever, pruritis, and weight loss and ultimately die of hepatic failure. Diagnosis is made most easily by the demonstration of typical cholangiographic changes during ERCP. There is no treatment that influences the outcome of affected patients (including those of inflammatory bowel disease) with the exception of liver transplantation (see below).

BILIARY TRACT OPERATIONS

The general physician should be aware of the mechanics of biliary surgical procedures so that he can inform and reassure the patient who is to be referred to a surgeon.

Cholecystectomy

Elective cholecystectomy has a mortality rate of 0.5% or less. Urgent or emergency operation for acute cholecystitis associated with common duct stones in an elderly patient with cardiac and/or pulmonary disease has a mortality rate of 10%. The morbidity of cholecystectomy primarily relates to superficial wound infection (< 5 to 7%). Wound infection is more common if the operation lasts longer than 2 hours, if the patient is obese or diabetic, and if the patient has acute rather than chronic cholecystitis. Other possible but rare (< 1%) immediate complications of cholecystectomy are postoperative bleeding, postoperative bile leak, injury to biliary ducts (common hepatic or common bile duct), and overlooked common duct stones. A drain may be left in place for 24 to 48 hours after operation.

Cholecystostomy

This operation may be required in the patient who is critically ill from acute cholecystitis and who has associated severe cardiac, pulmonary, or renal disease that contraindicates the use of general anesthesia. Another less often cited indication for cholecystostomy is inability to detect normal biliary anatomy because of a severe inflammatory process near the main bile ducts. Rather than risk possible injury to structures in the porta hepatis, a cholecystostomy may be performed.

A cholecystostomy can be done through a small incision in the right upper quadrant under local anesthesia. A large drainage tube is inserted into the gallbladder through a stab wound in the fundus. The tube is brought through the abdominal wall and allowed to drain freely. An attempt should be made to empty the gallbladder of stones before placing the tube. If a stone is impacted at the cystic duct, future cholecystectomy will be necessary or a mucous fistula will persist after the tube is removed. If, however, all stones are removed, only 30 to 50% of patients will develop recurrent symptoms of cholelithiasis within 2 years after the tube is removed. The operative mortality is very high from cholecystostomy, not because of the operation, but because of the patient's critical condition.

Choledochotomy

Common duct exploration or choledochotomy, whether combined with a gallbladder operation or as an isolated operation, has a higher morbidity and mortality rate than does simple cholecystectomy. The operation takes longer than cholecystectomy and patients are generally older, two factors very important in determining morbidity and mortality. Generally the patient will be hospitalized 3 to 5 days longer for common duct exploration than for cholecystectomy alone (see below).

COURSE AFTER OPERATION

Normal Course

The patient is usually discharged 5 to 10 days after an uncomplicated biliary tract operation. Skin sutures will have been removed and the patient will be allowed to bathe. Usually patients are requested to avoid driving and sexual relations for 1 week from the day of discharge. Patients are also advised to avoid heavy [approximately 15 pounds (7 kg) or more] lifting for 6 weeks. The incidence of incisional hernia (see Chapter 91) is very low after a right subcostal oblique incision, slightly higher with a vertical midline incision, and highest with vertical paramedian incisions. The patient returns to the surgeon's office for evaluation at 3 to 6 weeks after operation. The drain site and wound should be healed unless there has been wound infection. The patient should have been able to resume an unrestricted regular diet within a few days of operation without difficulty. Stools should be at preoperative frequency and of normal color.

The patient should be expected to complain about pulling sensations in the area of the incision since the right rectus muscle has been divided and resutured. If the subcostal incision was made close to the costal margin, the patient will often complain also about discomfort on bending or sitting. The area just below a right subcostal incision is apt to be numb for several months because of interruption of a cutaneous sensory nerve to this area. Sensitivity does return, however, in the majority of cases. It is not surprising to find patients gaining weight after cholecystectomy, especially if they had lost weight preoperatively.

Postcholecystectomy Syndrome

About 90% of patients operated upon for symptomatic biliary tract disease become asymptomatic or have relatively trivial symptoms (occasional dyspepsia, for example). The other 10% may continue to be symptomatic either because they were treated for the wrong disease or because they have developed a postoperative complication. In the former category are patients who had gallstones but whose symptoms actually emanated from another disease (e.g., recurrent pancreatitis, peptic ulcer disease, angina, reflux esophagitis, or hiatus hernia).

Postoperative problems associated with the operation itself include retained common duct stones, an excessively long cystic duct remnant, and common duct injury with eventual bile duct stricture and recurrent pancreatitis. Sphincter-of-Oddi dysfunction is being recognized increasingly as one of the treatable causes of postcholecystectomy syndrome. The diagnosis is made by showing a decrease in the emptying of the biliary tree by cholecystokinin cholecystography with ^{99m}Tc-iminodiacetic derivatives (see above) and by demonstrating an elevated sphincter pressure by manometry during ERCP. Sphincterotomy in patients with elevated sphincter pressure results in relief of pain in over 90% of cases (8).

Tondelli et al. (22) have collated data from a number of series on the incidence and cause of the postcholecystectomy syndrome (PCS) (Table 90.3). Mild PCS refers to symptoms of dyspepsia, constipation, diarrhea, and intolerance to certain foods. Severe PCS refers to severe upper abdominal pain, cholangitis, or biliary fistula. Organic biliary etiologies include retained common duct stones, papillary stenosis, bile duct stricture, cystic duct remnant, chronic pancreatitis, or bile duct tumor. Organic extrabiliary etiologies include esophagitis, ulcer disease, pancreatitis, liver disease, heart disease, colon or urinary tract disease, and adhesions. Nonorganic disease includes irritable bowel syndrome and psychiatric or metabolic disease.

Table 90.3.
Frequency of Postcholecystectomy Syndrome (PCS) and Distribution of its Etiology[a]

	Bodvall and Oevergaard (1967)	Stefanini et al. (1974)	Hess (1977)	Brandstatter et al. (1976)
Number of patients with cholecystectomy	1930	800	919	—
PCS total	764(40%)	249(31%)	241(26%)	—
Mild PCS	660(35%)	317(27%)	—	—
Severe PCS	104(5%)	32(4%)	—	—
Etiology:				
Organic total	—	—	58%	66%
Organic biliary	9%	14%	4.5%	43%
Organic extrabiliary	—	—	53.5%	23%
Nonorganic total	—	—	42%	34%

[a] After Tondelli P, Gyr K, Stalder GA, Allgöwer M: The biliary tract. Part I. Cholescystectomy. *Clin Gastroentercl* 8:487, 1979.

General Reference

Sherlock SD: *Diseases of the Liver and Biliary System*, 8th ed. London, Blackwell Scientific Publishers, 1989.
A comprehensive readable current text.

Specific References

1. Bennion LJ, Grundy SM: Risk factors for the development of cholelithiasis in man. *N Engl J Med* 299:1161, 1978.
2. Carey MC, Cahalane MJ: Whither biliary sludge? *Gastroenterology* 95:508, 1988.
3. Ferruci T: Body ultrasonography. *N Engl J Med* 300:538, 590, 1979.
4. Friedman GD, Kannel WB, Dawber TR: The epidemiology of gallbladder disease; observations in the Framingham study. *J Chronic Dis* 19:273, 1966.
5. Friedman LS, Roberts MS, Brett AS, Marton KI: Management of asymptomatic gallstones in the diabetic patient. A decision analysis. *Ann Intern Med* 109:913, 1988.
6. Fromm H, Roat JW, Gonzales V, et al: Comparative efficacy and side effects of urosodeoxycholic and chenodeoxycholic acids in dissolving gallstones. A double-blind controlled study. *Gastroenterology* 85:1257, 1983.
7. Gracie WA, Ransohoff DF: The natural history of silent gallstones. The innocent gallstone is not a myth. *N Engl J Med* 307:798, 1982.
8. Greenen JE, Hogan WJ, Dodds WJ, et al: The efficacy of endoscopic sphincterotomy after cholecystectomy in patients with sphincter-of-Oddi dysfunction. *N Engl J Med* 320:82, 1989.
9. Heberer G, Paumgartner G, Sauerbruch T, et al: A retrospective analysis of 3 years experience of an interdisciplinary approach to gallstone disease including shock waves. *Ann Surg* 208:274, 1988.
10. Jarvinen HJ, Hastbacka J: Early cholecystectomy for acute cholecystitis; a prospective randomized study. *Ann Surg* 191:501, 1980.
11. LaRusso NF, Wiesner RH, Ludwig J, MacCarty RL: Primary sclerosing cholangitis. *New Engl J Med* 310:899, 1984.
12. Lund J: Surgical indications in cholelithiasis; prophylactic cholecystectomy elucidated on the basis of long-term followup on 526 nonoperated cases. *Ann Surg* 151:153, 1960.
13. Max MH, Polk HC: Routine preoperative upper gastrointestinal series (UGIS) in patients with biliary tract disease; a plea for more selectivity. *Surgery* 82:334, 1977.
14. Morrow DJ, Thompson J, Wilson SE: Acute cholecystitis in the elderly, a surgical emergency. *Arch Surg* 113:1149, 1978.
15. Mundth ED: Cholecystitis and diabetes mellitus. *N Engl J Med* 267:642, 1962.
16. Sackmann M, Delius M, Sauerbruch T, et al: Shock-wave lithotripsy of gallbladder stones. The first 175 patients. *N Engl J Med* 318:393, 1988.
17. Schoenfield LS, Lachin JL: The Steering Committee, The National Gallstone Study Group: Chenodiol (chenodeoxycholic acid) for dissolution of gallstones: The National Cooperative Gallstone Study: a controlled trial of efficacy and safety. *Ann Intern Med* 95:257, 1981.
18. Thistle JL, Schoenfield LJ: Lithogenic bile among young Indian women; lithogenic potential decreased with chenodeoxycholic acid. *N Engl J Med* 284:177, 1971.
19. Thistle JL, May GR, Bender CE, et al: Dissolution of cholesterol gallbladder stones by methyl-tert-butyl ether administered by percutaneous transhepatic catheter. *N Engl J Med* 320:633, 1989.
20. Thurston OG, McDougall RM: The effect of hepatic bile on retained common duct stones. *Surg Gynecol Obstet* 143:625, 1976.
21. Tint GS, Salen G, Colallilo A, et al: Urosodeoxy cholic acid: a safe and effective agent for dissolving cholesterol gallstones. *Ann Intern Med* 97:351, 1982.
22. Tondelli P, Gyr K, Stalder GA, Allgower M: The biliary tract. Part I. Cholecystectomy. *Clin Gastroenterol* 8:487, 1979.
23. Way LW, Sleisenger MH: Cholelithiasis: chronic and acute cholecystitis. In: Sleisenger MH, Fordtran JS (eds): *Gastrointestinal Disease. Pathophysiology, Diagnosis, Management*, 4th ed. Philadelphia, WB Saunders, 1989, p. 1691.

C H A P T E R   91

Abdominal Hernias

DILIP S. KITTUR, M.D., Sc.D.
GARDNER W. SMITH, M.D.

DEFINITIONS

A hernia is a protrusion of a viscus or part of a viscus from its normal location in the body. Clinically common hernias are protrusions of a part of an abdominal viscus through the abdominal wall. Depending on the site at which hernias occur, they are described as inguinal, femoral, umbilical, epigastric, etc. A hernia is termed *reducible* if its contents can be pushed back into the abdominal cavity, *irreducible* or *incarcerated* if they cannot be pushed back. The most feared complication of a hernia, *strangulation,* occurs when the blood supply to the herniated viscus is compromised. All strangulated hernias are also incarcerated but incarcerated hernias may not be strangulated.

This chapter describes the more common types of hernias and discusses the role of the general physician in their diagnosis and treatment.

HERNIAS OF THE GROIN

Inguinal Hernias

Inguinal hernias (Fig. 91.1, *A* and *B*) are classified either as direct or indirect; the great majority (over two-thirds) are indirect. Direct hernias are portions of the bowel and/or omentum that protrude directly through the floor of the inguinal canal to emerge at the external inguinal ring (Fig. 91.2). Indirect hernias enter the inguinal canal through its internal ring, lateral to the inferior epigastric vessels, traverse the canal, and emerge also at the external inguinal ring (Fig. 91.2). The indirect hernias, as they get larger, have a propensity to extend into the scrotum.

Epidemiology and Etiology

Inguinal hernia is a common problem in ambulatory practice: it accounts for approximately 75% of all abdominal wall hernias. Approximately 85% of inguinal hernias occur in men. At some time in their lives, about 5 to 10% of men in the United States will develop an inguinal hernia. Even in women, inguinal hernia accounts for more than half of the abdominal hernias. Although femoral hernias (see below) are much more common in women than in men, the most common groin hernia in women is an indirect inguinal hernia. Less than 10% of inguinal hernias in adults are bilateral when the patient is first seen, but there

is a significant possibility that a hernia may occur on the opposite side at some time in the future. The chance of developing a contralateral inguinal hernia is the same regardless of the side affected first.

All *indirect inguinal hernias* are due to a congenital defect in which the processus vaginalis remains patent. The processus vaginalis is a tract lined with peritoneum that extends from the peritoneal cavity into the scrotum. With time this tract may enlarge, and abdominal contents may herniate into it. Occasionally, however, only intra-abdominal fluid may gravitate into the scrotum, causing scrotal swelling when the patient is erect but draining back into the abdominal cavity when the patient is supine. Such a lesion is termed a *communicating hydrocele* and is more commonly seen in children than in adults. The severity of the combination of this congenital abnormality and a predisposing acquired condition that increases intra-abdominal pressure (such as obesity, chronic obstructive airway disease, ascites, chronic constipation with straining at stool, prostatism with straining at urination, and hard physical labor) determine when an inguinal hernia develops.

Direct inguinal hernias are acquired lesions and are not only influenced by changes in intra-abdominal pressure but also by progressive attenuation of the inguinal structures as part of the normal aging process. Rarely, inherited defects in collagen synthesis (e.g., Marfan's syndrome) provide an obvious explanation for accelerated weakening of these structures.

Direct hernias are for the most part problems of the middle-aged and elderly. Indirect hernias, since they are associated with a congenital defect, are more likely to develop in younger people, but these too increase in incidence with advancing age and are about four to five times more common after the age of 50 than before.

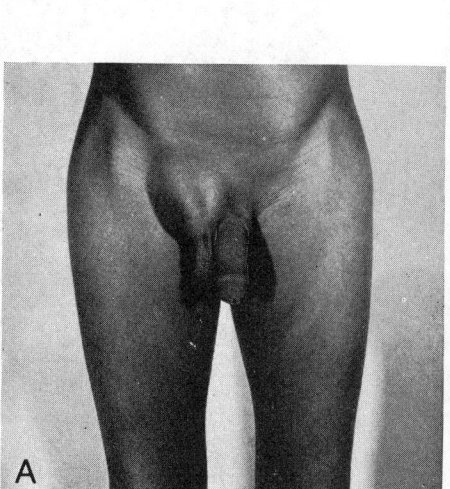 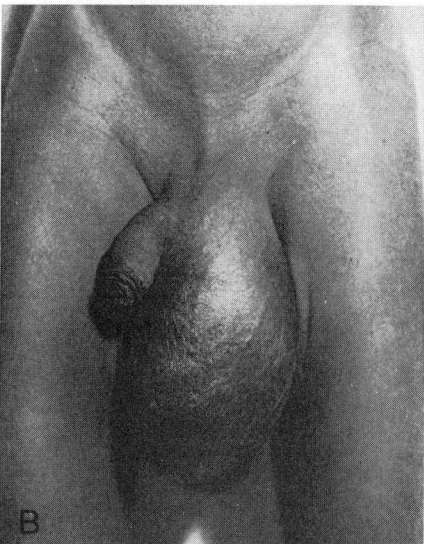

Figure 91.1. *A.* Right inguinal hernia in young adult male. *B.* Left scrotal hernia. (From Zimmerman LM, Anson BJ: *Anatomy and Surgery of Hernia,* 2nd ed. Baltimore, Williams & Wilkins, 1967, p. 152.)

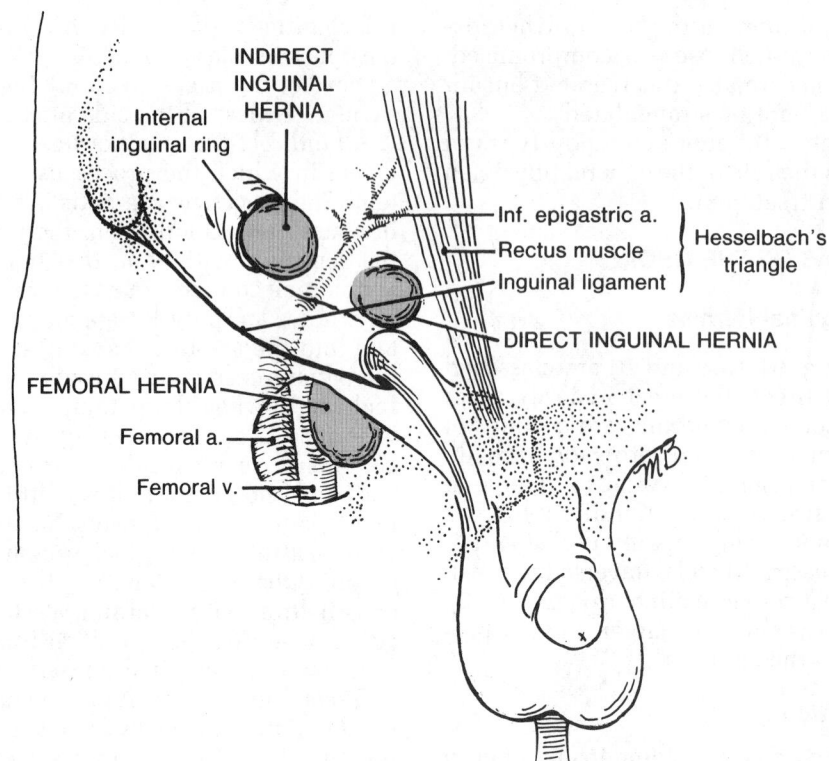

Figure 91.2. Artist's rendition of groin region illustrating femoral hernia and indirect and direct inguinal hernias. (Modified from Dunphy JE, Botsford TW: *Physical Examination of the Surgical Patient*, 3rd ed. Philadelphia, WB Saunders, 1964, p. 118.)

History

Most patients complain of a dull ache in the groin and of a bulge, either localized to the groin or extending into the scrotum (in women, the labia are the anatomical counterpart of the scrotum). Sometimes pain precedes discovery of the mass by some months (perhaps because, in early stages of herniation, the internal canal is stretched before omentum or bowel presents as a bulge at the external inguinal ring). Occasionally a patient will recall a short burning pain during straining, which represents the initial herniation. Often the patient, or the physician, notices the herniated mass, but no pain has been experienced. If the hernia becomes large enough, it may cause a dragging sensation when the patient walks. Small reducible indirect hernias may be noticed intermittently, at times of increased intra-abdominal pressure.

If a hernia incarcerates, it may become more painful, although many patients with chronically incarcerated hernias are pain free. Indirect hernias have an approximately 10% chance of incarcerating; direct hernias incarcerate only rarely. Strangulated hernias are always symptomatic: the hernia becomes extremely painful and tender; and nausea, vomiting, abdominal distention, constipation, and fever (with granulocytosis) are common.

Physical Examination

The patient should first be examined while he is standing. An indirect hernia sometimes can be distinguished from a direct hernia by inspection: an indirect hernia, once it has entered the inguinal canal, presents as an elliptical swelling descending toward or even into the scrotum (Fig. 91.3). A direct hernia presents as an isolated oval swelling near the pubis; it rarely is found in the scrotum (Fig. 91.4). If the hernia is visible, an attempt should be made to push it back into the abdominal cavity. If the hernia cannot be re-

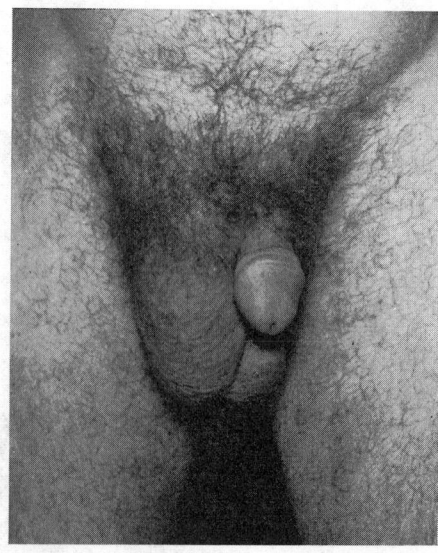

Figure 91.3. Indirect inguinal hernia. Swelling is oblique, cylindrical, and extends into scrotum. (From Zimmerman LM, Anson BJ: *Anatomy and Surgery of Hernia*, 2nd ed. Baltimore, Williams & Wilkins, 1967, p. 155.)

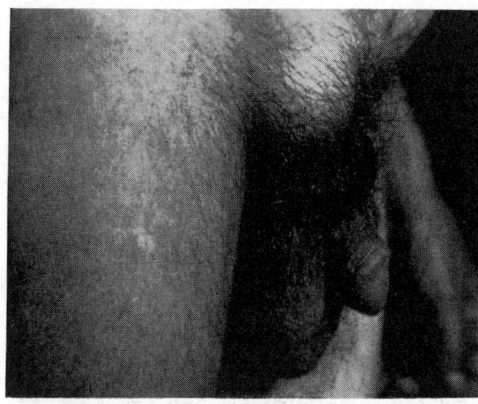

Figure 91.4. Direct inguinal hernia. Note medially situated globular swelling. (From Zimmerman LM, Anson BJ: *Anatomy and Surgery of Hernia*, 2nd ed. Baltimore, Williams & Wilkins, 1967, p. 154.)

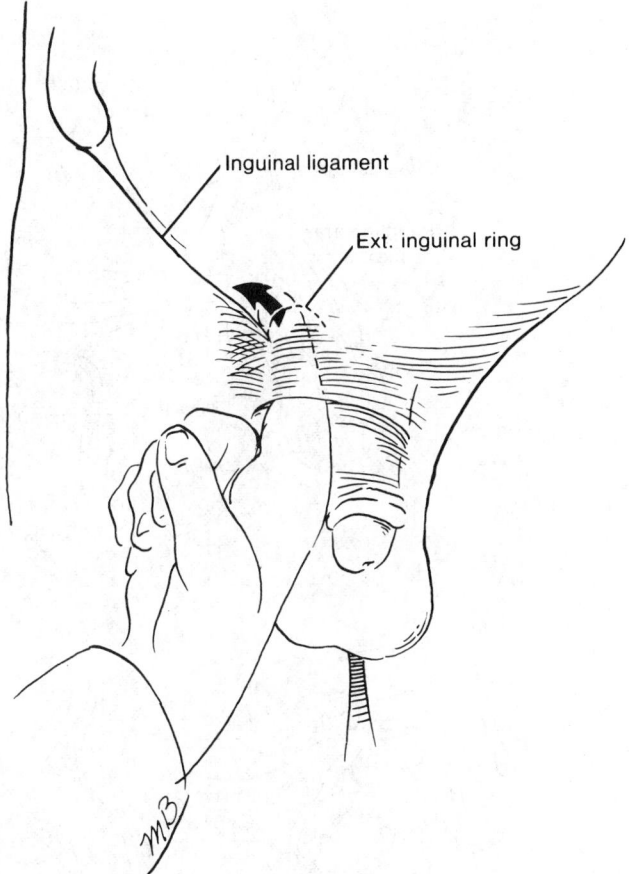

Figure 91.5. Examination of the inguinal canal. The examining finger gently invaginates the scrotum into the inguinal canal. (Modified from Dunphy JE, Botsford TW: *Physical Examination of the Surgical Patient*, 3rd ed. Philadelphia, WB Saunders, 1964, p. 116.)

duced, the patient should be asked to lie down and another attempt should be made to reduce it. Approximately 10% of inguinal hernias will be incarcerated when they are first diagnosed.

If the hernia is not visible, the physician's finger should be placed at the base of the scrotum and then gently advanced cephalad and laterally into the inguinal canal (Fig. 91.5). The external ring can be examined without causing the patient a great deal of discomfort. The size of the ring, in itself, does not predict the presence of a hernia or the propensity to develop one because the external ring is an opening in the aponeurosis of the external oblique muscle that does not contribute to the integrity of the floor of the inguinal canal. Further palpation will identify the crest of the pubic bone, the fibers of the external inguinal ring, the spermatic cord, and weakness in the posterior inguinal canal. When the examining finger has been directed through the external ring, having the patient increase intra-abdominal pressure by coughing or straining will cause a hernia to protrude and to be felt as an impulse or bulge at the tip of the examining finger.

Occasionally, contents of the hernia sac may be determined by physical examination: omentum may feel nodular and pliant; intestine, smooth and tense. Occasionally intestinal gas can be palpated as it moves through the bowel; also, a gas-filled loop of bowel may be tympanitic and on auscultation, bowel sounds may be heard within it. If one suspects a strangulated hernia, as when a patient presents with severe pain associated with a pre-existing hernia, an attempt should not be made to reduce the hernia forcefully since this maneuver has the risk of reducing gangrenous bowel, which has been the content of the hernia, into the general peritoneal cavity.

Differential Diagnosis

An incarcerated scrotal hernia must be distinguished from other scrotal lesions (Fig. 91.6). One of the most common of these is a *hydrocele*, a tense, slightly fluctuant mass that can be distinguished from a hernia and from a solid mass by transillumination. (The mass is made tense between examining fingers and, with the room darkened, a flashlight is pressed into the side of it; light passes through the hydrocele, but not through a solid mass.)

Another common scrotal mass is a *varicocele*, an enlarged venous plexus that on palpation feels soft and worm-like and that extends from the testicle up toward the spermatic cord. It does not transilluminate and, when the patient lies down, it collapses. If a varicocele is of recent onset in the adult, occurs on the left, and does not disappear in the supine position, one must suspect obstruction of the left spermatic vein (which enters the left renal vein) by retroperitoneal neoplasm.

A *spermatocele* is a localized but vaguely circumscribed mass that also does not transilluminate and that persists when the patient lies down.

Apart from distinguishing a hernia from another kind of scrotal mass, an important component of the physical examination is the examination of the testicle and its surrounding structures. In that way *epididymal cysts,* epididymitis, orchitis, testicular torsion, and testicu-

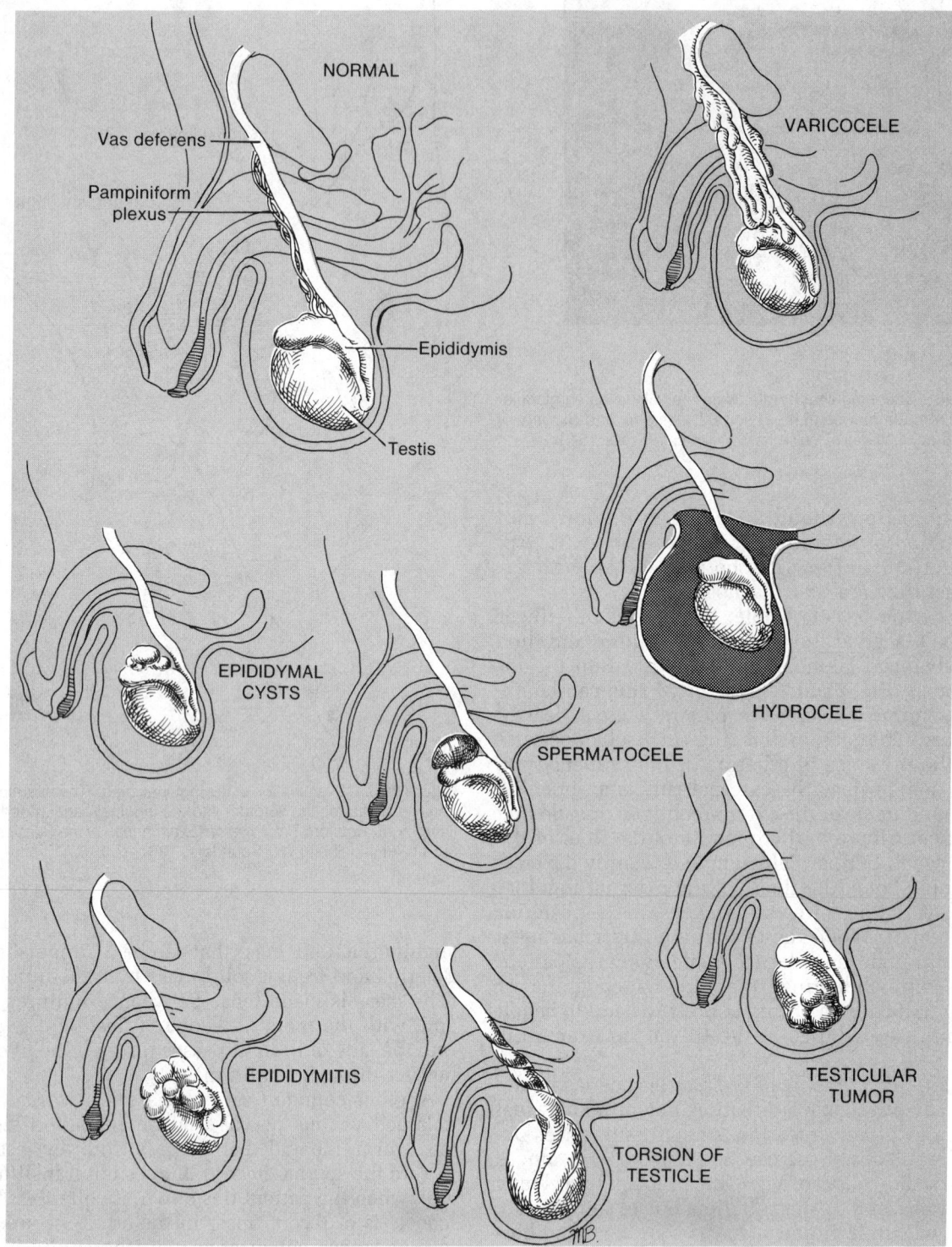

Figure 91.6. Lesions palpable in the scrotum. A correct diagnosis can usually be made if the normal anatomical relationships of the contents of the scrotum are borne in mind. (Modified from Dunphy JE, Botsford TW: *Physical Examination of the Surgical Patient*, 3rd ed. Philadelphia, WB Saunders, 1964, p. 111.)

lar tumors can be detected. *Epididymal cysts* may be in any portion of the epididymis and may be smooth or lobulated; some of them transilluminate; they are innocuous and require no treatment. *Epididymitis* presents as a tender, swollen epididymis. The inflammation, if untreated, may spread to the testicle (orchitis); see Chapter 27 for a discussion of this problem. Frequently, elevation and immobilization of the scrotum will relieve the pain associated with an inflammatory process. In contrast, the pain produced by *torsion of the testicle* is unremitting. Sudden onset of testicular pain in an otherwise healthy person is characteristic of this problem. On examination, the testicle is enlarged and exquisitely tender. The patient should be referred immediately to a general surgeon or to a urologist. *Testicular tumors* can involve the entire testicle or simply protrude as a small nodule from the testicular surface. These masses are more indurated than the common benign scrotal masses and usually lack the slight tenderness of the normal testicle. Patients with suspected tumors should be referred as soon as possible to a urologist.

Management and Course

Almost all inguinal hernias should be repaired. Severe coexistent illness is the only real contraindication to herniorrhaphy (see Chapter 86 for a discussion of anesthesia/surgery risks in patients with coexistent medical conditions). Although there is no sense of urgency associated with elective repair, it should be recognized that the risk of incarceration or of strangulation is much greater with indirect than with direct hernia. Accordingly the repair of a direct hernia may be more confidently deferred, or even declined, in the face of a significant medical illness. Nonoperative therapy should be discouraged; the wearing of a truss is potentially dangerous and does not guarantee that a hernia will remain reduced. Also, the pressure of the truss on the margin of a large defect will eventually lead to atrophy of the fascial and aponeurotic (broad tendinous) layers, causing the hernia to enlarge. Subsequent repair will be more difficult and, therefore, will carry a greater risk of recurrence.

Elective herniorrhaphy avoids acute incarceration (and strangulation) and the necessity to perform an emergency operation. If the hernia is chronically incarcerated and there are no symptoms of strangulation (strangulation is primarily a risk in acutely incarcerated, relatively small indirect hernias), repair may still be scheduled electively. If the hernia has incarcerated acutely, the patient must be hospitalized and attempts made to reduce the hernia before operation. Strangulated hernia is a true surgical emergency because delay in treatment can lead to gangrene of the intestine or omentum. Suspected strangulated hernias require immediate operative intervention.

Bilateral hernias may be repaired as staged procedures or at one operation, depending on their size, the type of repair required, the age of the patient, and coexistent problems. If the patient is elderly, and the hernias are large and require complex repair, herniorrhaphies should be staged, 4 to 6 weeks apart. Bilateral repairs of indirect inguinal hernias in children or young adults are routinely done at one operation.

Currently the majority of unilateral inguinal hernias are repaired under local anesthesia. The patient is rarely uncomfortable during the operation and can leave the hospital on the same day. This approach leads to fewer postoperative complications, such as atelectasis and acute urinary retention, and also reduces the cost of hospitalization. Spinal or general anesthesia is used in patients that cannot tolerate the procedure under local anesthesia, if the hernia is large requiring complex repair, and/or in obese patients in whom repair of the hernia under local anesthesia is technically difficult. Bilateral inguinal herniorrhaphy also requires spinal or general anesthesia. Repair of hernias in children is usually done under general anesthesia.

No matter which anesthesia is employed, certain *complications of herniorrhaphy* are possible (in about 7% of patients): recurrence (the most common complication, see below), urinary retention, wound infection, hydrocele formation, femoral neuritis, scrotal hematoma, and rarely, unilateral testicular atrophy. The general physician and the surgeon should discuss these complications with the patient before the operation and assure him that, except for recurrence of hernia, if they do occur, they are usually treatable or transient problems. Furthermore, the risk of wound infection, which greatly increases the likelihood of recurrence, can be reduced if the patient washes with an antiseptic soap for 1 week before operation.

When the patient is discharged from the hospital, he is ambulatory and usually requires no more than codeine for relief of pain. Patients are admitted to the hospital only if urinary retention or another complication such as bleeding or hypotension occurs. Patients with pre-existing medical illnesses such as heart disease or diabetes mellitus may be admitted to the hospital for observation. For the first week, the patient is advised to avoid lifting or straining and to use a stool softener and a mild laxative (see Chapter 39). The patient can return to light work (and light activity such as long walks) within another 2 weeks, but an occupation that requires heavy lifting or considerable exertion requires a total convalescence of about 6 weeks. Driving a car during the first 2 weeks should be discouraged, not because it is a form of strenuous activity, but because the patient, fearing pain or injury, may not step on the brake vigorously enough or soon enough in a crisis to avoid a collision. Sexual activity should be avoided for about 2 weeks. Resumption of normal recreational and work activities requires common sense. Most patients are fully rehabilitated and working less than 2 months after herniorrhaphy. Because recurrence may be related to premature untoward exertion, patients must be cautioned to avoid strenuous activity for 2 months. However, most episodes of recurrence are due to technical problems related to the hernia repair or to wound infections.

Approximately 1 to 7% of indirect and 4 to 10% of direct inguinal hernias recur. Over 50% of the recurrences will occur within 5 years of the initial repair. Unfortunately, the recurrence rate after repair of a recurrent hernia is very high, ranging from 5 to 35%. Apart from advising patients with a recurrent hernia that has been repaired to avoid straining and heavy lifting and to lose weight if they are obese, there is no special advice that these patients can be given.

Femoral Hernias

Epidemiology and Etiology

A femoral hernia is a protrusion of omentum and/or bowel through the femoral canal (Fig. 91.2). It is the second most common type of abdominal hernia, accounting for 10% of all abdominal hernias. It is much more common in women than in men; 33% of abdominal hernias in women, but only 3% of abdominal hernias in men, are femoral hernias. The incidence increases with increasing age, presumably again because of the degradation of collagen and attenuation of tissue that accompanies aging (see above, "Inguinal Hernia"). It is likely, however, that a contributing cause of a femoral hernia is a congenitally large femoral ring. Preperitoneal fat, forced through the large ring, enlarges it further. Increased pressure produced by straining or by pregnancy undoubtedly contributes to femoral herniation. Femoral hernias are bilateral in 15% or more of cases. The risk of incarceration, and particularly of strangulation, is especially high with this type of hernia.

History

The primary symptom of a femoral hernia is a bulge in the groin. A dull pain may be experienced, but less commonly than in patients with an inguinal hernia. About 20% of femoral hernias incarcerate (twice the rate of indirect inguinal hernias). The symptoms of incarceration and of strangulation are the same as they are in patients with inguinal hernias.

Physical Examination

A mass is often palpable, medial to the femoral vessels, and inferior to the inguinal ligament. The mass is usually reducible, and occasionally it is tender. Despite careful examination, the hernia frequently is difficult to detect, especially in obese women, even if it is incarcerated or strangulated. Therefore, women who present with signs and symptoms of unexplained intestinal obstruction should be examined carefully for evidence of a femoral hernia that has strangulated.

Differential Diagnosis

A femoral hernia must be distinguished from an enlarged lymph node, a lipoma, a saphenous varix, and a direct inguinal hernia. The first three of these possibilities are not reducible. A lymph node or lipoma may not transmit an impulse to the examiner's finger when the patient coughs. A saphenous varix may simulate a hernia impulse, however, since increased venous pressure induced by the Valsalva maneuver is transmitted to the varix. A lymph node or a lipoma is more movable than a hernia; and a varix can be collapsed by compression of the saphenous vein. The distinction between a femoral and other groin hernias sometimes can be made only at operation.

Management and Course

Femoral hernias should be repaired unless the patient is unable to tolerate an operation. The increased risk of incarceration and of strangulation adds to the urgency of the recommendation. The operative and postoperative considerations of inguinal hernia (see above) apply to femoral hernias as well except that for technical reasons, a larger proportion of these may have to be performed under spinal or general anesthesia. From 1 to 7% of femoral hernias recur; and, like inguinal hernias, 5 to 35% of repaired recurrent hernias also recur.

INCISIONAL HERNIAS

An incisional hernia is the protrusion of omentum and/or bowel through a surgical incision. Unlike the other types of abdominal hernia, a congenital weakness of the abdominal wall does not contribute to the development of the hernia. Any abdominal incision may be the site of a hernia. The major risk factors leading to the development of an incisional hernia are poor surgical technique, wound infection, and obesity. With the increasing use of chronic ambulatory peritoneal dialysis to treat patients in chronic renal failure (see Chapter 48), it has become apparent that incisional hernias (as well as inguinal hernias) are particularly common in this group of patients.

The hernia usually presents as a bulge through the incision that may enlarge if neglected (Fig. 91.7) and may even lead to intestinal obstruction. It should be repaired soon after the diagnosis is made to avoid the development of a larger defect that will complicate repair and will be more likely to recur. If repair must be delayed for some reason, the use of an abdominal binder will make the patient more comfortable and may retard progression of the size of the defect. If possible, an obese patient should lose weight before the operation (see Chapter 76).

UMBILICAL HERNIAS

An umbilical hernia is a protrusion of omentum and/or bowel through the umbilical ring. These hernias are probably due to congenital defects. Among adults, they appear most often in middle-aged multiparous women, in patients with cirrhosis of the liver and ascites, and in old, malnourished, chronically ill people. They are also common in infants, especially in Blacks.

Most umbilical hernias are obvious as an enlarge-

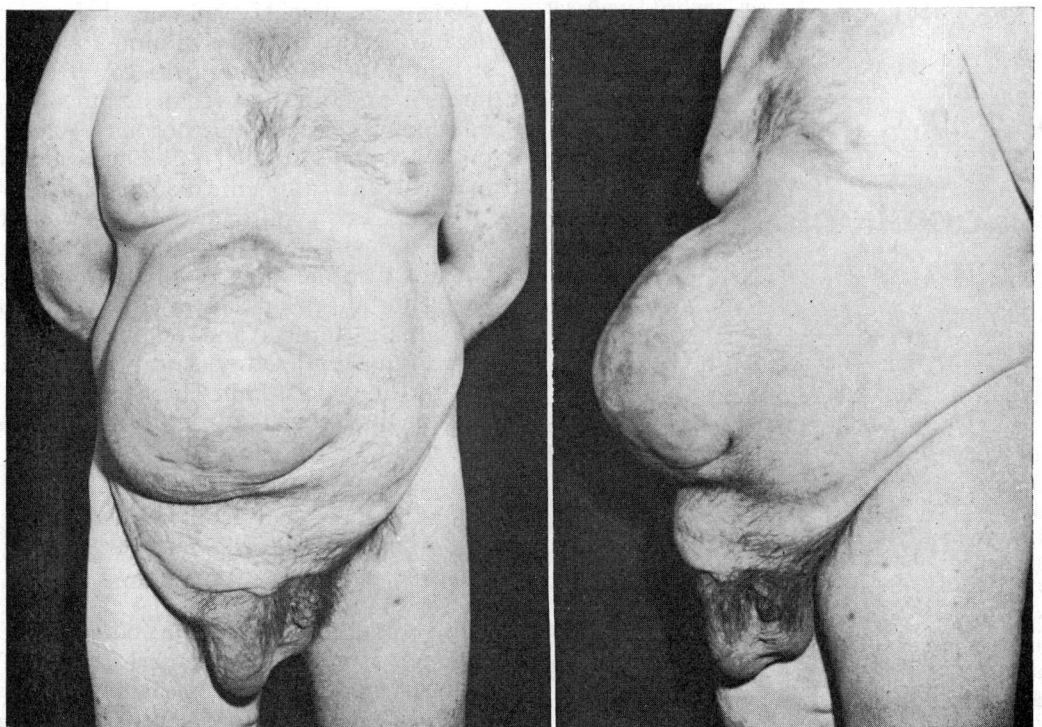

Figure 91.7. Large postoperative hernia after cholecystectomy. (From Zimmerman LM, Anson BJ: *Anatomy and Surgery of Hernia*, 2nd ed. Baltimore, Williams & Wilkins, 1967, p. 287.)

ment of the umbilical ring with protrusion of intraabdominal contents through it. However, a few patients complain only of vague intermittent pain and tenderness in the region of the umbilicus. On examination, a small defect is usually found that contains a small piece of omentum, preperitoneal fat, or a knuckle of bowel. If the patient is placed in the supine position and is asked to raise his head and cough, the hernia can be palpated.

The most common complication of umbilical hernia is incarceration with or without strangulation. For that reason, unless the patient simply cannot tolerate an operation, all umbilical hernias in adults should be repaired. Morbidity and mortality from such an operation are much lower if it can be done electively rather than in response to acute incarceration or strangulation. The only exception to this recommendation is umbilical hernias in infants. These tend to close spontaneously as the child gets older and repair should be deferred until school age.

EPIGASTRIC HERNIAS

An epigastric hernia is a protrusion of fat or omentum through the linea alba between the umbilicus and the xiphoid cartilage. These hernias almost never contain a viscus. A congenital defect in the linea alba is probably the major disposing factor. Epigastric hernias most commonly appear between the ages of 20 and 50 and are three times more common in men than in women.

Most patients complain of a small painless subcutaneous mass, most often just to the left of the midline. Usually the hernia consists of preperitoneal fat or of fat of the falciform ligament. Larger defects also contain omentum.

Complications are more common in patients with small hernias, because these are more likely to incarcerate. When this happens, there is usually local pain and tenderness and, less often, deep epigastric pain, abdominal distention, and nausea and vomiting.

Treatment must be individualized. Small asymptomatic hernias require no treatment; an asymptomatic hernia greater than 1.5 cm in diameter should be repaired. Incarceration of a small hernia is an indication for operation. The recurrence rate after epigastric herniorrhaphy is approximately 10% and usually can be attributed to failure to appreciate multiple defects in the linea alba at the time of the initial operation.

General References

Halverson K: Hernias. In: Goldsmith HS (ed-in-chief): Bryne JJ (ed General Surgery): *Practice of Surgery*, Vol 3. Philadelphia, Harper & Row, 1984. chap. 9.
    A succinct, well illustrated summary.
Nyhus LM (ed): Symposium on Hernias. *Surg Clin North Am.* 64 (2):183, 1984.
    Seventeen articles on different aspects of hernias.

Nyhus LM, Condon RE (eds): *Hernia.* Philadelphia, JB Lippincott, 1978.
A definitive text.

C H A P T E R   92

Benign Conditions of the Anus and Rectum

GARDNER W. SMITH, M.D.

Anorectal disorders are often encountered in ambulatory practice. This chapter describes five particularly common problems—pruritis ani, anal fissure, hemorrhoidal disease, perirectal abscess, and venereal diseases. Also included, because of their importance to the general physician, are somewhat less common problems such as proctalgia fugax and rectal prolapse. In addition to the more common venereal diseases, proctitis characterized by rectal pain, tenesmus, and often an anal discharge may also be caused by unusual organisms. In gay men, symptoms suggesting proctitis should raise suspicion of the *gay bowel syndrome,* a form of proctitis that results from the sexual transmission of a variety of pathogens (bacteria, helminths, protozoa, and viruses) (4, 5). Because of the difficulty in establishing a specific diagnosis, patients suspected of having this syndrome should be referred to a gastroenterologist or an infectious disease specialist. Cutaneous disorders that involve the perianal area and perineum are discussed in Chapter 94 (Benign Vulvovaginal Disorders) and Chapter 100 (Common Problems of the Skin). Other conditions that may affect the rectum are discussed in Chapters 26 (Acute Gastroenteritis and Associated Conditions) and 39 (Constipation and Diarrhea).

PRURITUS ANI

Definition

Pruritus ani, a distressing perianal itch, is a very common complaint, particularly in men. The intensity of the symptom is variable but is usually greatest at night. Often the itching abates spontaneously only to recur after widely variable asymptomatic periods.

Etiology

Although the cause of pruritis ani is often unknown (50 to 75% of the time), the symptoms may be a manifestation of many anorectal disorders (Table 92.1). Whatever the cause, the itching is frequently associated with fecal contamination of moist macerated skin, often complicated by excoriation and secondary infection.

Table 92.1.
Common Problems Associated with Pruritus Ani

DERMATOLOGICAL DISORDERS
  Psoriasis
  Atopic dermatitis
  Contact dermatitis
  Lichen planus
  Condylomata
  Venereal warts
  Herpes simplex
  Tumors
DIARRHEA
FISSURES
INFECTION
  Fungi and yeast (Especially in diabetic patients) (see Chapter 100, Common Problems of the Skin)
  Erythrasma
  Scabies (see Chapter 100, Common Problems of the Skin)
  Pinworm infestation—more common in children—*Enterobius vermicularis*
  Vaginal infections (see Chapter 94, Benign Vulvovaginal Disorders)
OBESITY
POOR ANAL HYGIENE
RECTAL PROLAPSE
PROLAPSED HEMORRHOIDS (most often hemorrhoids are not associated with pruritus and other causes should be sought)

Diagnosis

Whenever a patient complains of perianal itching, specific historical information should be obtained and several observations should be made to aid in establishing a diagnosis.

History

A limited dietary history is important since occasionally an excess intake of milk, coffee, tea, alcohol, cola, and spices may be associated with pruritus ani. It is important to review the drugs the patient is taking since medications, such as laxatives or colchicine, which cause gastrointestinal irritation, may be associated with perianal itching, as are certain oral antibiotics such as the tetracyclines.

General Examination

The patient should be examined for the presence of a dermatological problem such as psoriasis, scabies, or fungal infection (Table 92.1) that may be associated with pruritus ani. In addition, in women, a pelvic examination should be performed because of the occasional association of vaginal infection with pruritus ani (see Chapter 94).

With the patient in the lateral decubitus or the knee-chest position and with the buttocks separated, the perianal area should be inspected. During the inspection the patient should be asked to strain, a maneuver that may demonstrate prolapse or fecal or flatal incontinence.

If skin lesions are identified, appropriate evaluation (such as a KOH preparation) to establish a diagnosis (such as *Tinea* or *Candida*) should be done in order to initiate definitive therapy (see Chapter 100). If no lesions are visualized, or if only excoriated skin or hemorrhoids are seen, the evaluation should include a series of three to five cellophane tape preparations in an attempt to demonstrate the ova of pinworms (see below).

Rectal Examination

Digital rectal examination should always be accomplished using a well-lubricated gloved finger. Evaluation must be gentle in order to avoid spasm of the anal sphincter, which will preclude adequate examination. At initiation of the examination, the patient should be asked to bear down, which will minimize discomfort. Excessive pain or tenderness of one area should alert the physician to the presence of an anal fissure (see below). All structures of the anal canal within the limits of the reach of the finger should be assessed (the anus, the distal rectum, the prostate gland, the cervix).

Anoscopy

After rectal examination, and without laxative or enema preparation, an anoscopy (with the use of an instrument that permits a side or oblique view) should be performed. The usual disposable anoscope, although convenient, provides only a barely adequate side view. A well lubricated anoscope should be inserted gently, while the patient bears down to minimize discomfort. The instrument should be inserted slowly as deeply as possible. Then, after removal of the obturator, the rectum should be inspected using adequate light. Visualization is possible only through the side or oblique aspect of the instrument as it is withdrawn gradually. It is important to avoid rotation of the anoscope, which will be uncomfortable and which may actually tear the anal mucosa. For adequate inspection of all quadrants of the anal canal, the instrument must be reinserted and withdrawn three or four times.

Cellophane Tape Examination for Pinworms

This is easily accomplished by the patient at home or by the physician in the office. Swabs are commercially available (Pinworm Diagnostic Tapes, Parke-Davis), but they are also easily made by folding clear cellophane tape, sticky side out, over a tongue blade. At night pinworms migrate from the anal canal to the perianal area, where they deposit eggs. Therefore, the swab should be obtained upon arising, before a bowel movement, and before the perianal area is cleansed. The swab is placed at the anal verge and then the tape is mounted onto a glass microscopic slide. A specimen obtained in this way will keep for several days. The slides should be examined under the low power (×10) objective of the microscope searching for the typical ova of pinworm (Fig. 92.1).

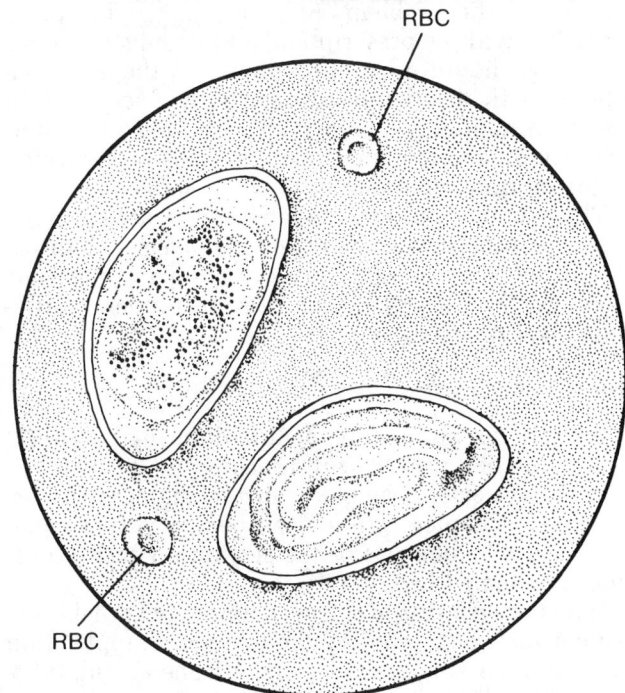

Figure 92.1. Appearance of the eggs of *Enterobius vermicularis* (pinworm). The egg is approximately 20 to 50 μm and typically has one relatively flattened side.

Treatment

General Measures

Most patients with pruritus ani can be diagnosed and treated adequately by the general physician. Even when the evaluation is inconclusive, except for the identification of excoriation, symptoms can be controlled by relatively simple measures:

Tepid sitz baths for 15 to 20 minutes provide excellent temporary relief (for example, at bedtime). If used several times daily at the outset of symptoms, sitz baths may be sufficient to control pruritus ani. However, often the patient will find frequent sitz baths impractical.

Anal cleanliness is mandatory; it should be thorough but gentle. After a bowel movement the anus should be cleaned with soft, white, nonperfumed toilet tissue (colored or perfumed tissue is potentially allergenic or irritative and should be avoided). If paper is too irritating, cotton swabs moistened with warm water or with glycerin may be used (cotton fiber is less irritating than paper fiber). Glycerin-witch hazel wipes (Tucks or generic, available without prescription) are helpful to cleanse the anal area. The patient should discontinue the use of these preparations if he notices intense burning and use plain glycerin (available without prescription) instead.

The anal area should be cleaned once or twice a day with plain soap, such as Ivory or Purpose, or plain shaving cream and should be kept dry between times by the application of plain talc (such as Johnson's Baby Powder); cornstarch is not a good substitute as it may promote the growth of microorganisms, which could compound the problem. At night, zinc oxide paste (available without prescription) may be substituted for talc. This should be applied thickly to the anal area where it will absorb moisture and provide comfort. In the morning it may be removed with soap and water, mineral oil, glycerin, or Tucks, or it may be reapplied in the morning and after each bowel movement.

The patient should use cotton underwear to provide better ventilation and should avoid polyester clothing. Prolonged sitting, especially on synthetic materials (such as vinyl seats), which prevent proper ventilation, should be avoided.

Specific Measures

If a specific problem is identified during the initial evaluation of a patient with pruritus ani (Table 92.1), it must be treated (see below or the chapters on dermatology (Chapter 100) and on benign vulvovaginal disorders (Chapter 94) or the section on gastrointestinal problems (Section 4).

When the pruritis is severe, commonly at night, the patient may gain relief by the temporary application of a minimal amount of hydrocortisone cream, 0.5% (available without prescription) or 1% (requires a prescription). Chronic use of fluorinated steroids should be avoided because of their tendency to cause atrophy and telangiectasias. Topical steroids will help the patient to avoid scratching the anal area, reducing trauma and subsequent injury.

The diet, when found to contain foods thought to be associated with pruritus ani (see above), may be modified, at least on a trial basis. If a food is incriminated, the patient may find that symptoms will not resolve for 1 or 2 weeks after the diet is appropriately modified. Moreover, the patient will note recurrence of symptoms, usually within 24 to 48 hours, after the reinstitution of an offending food.

Diarrhea and/or constipation should be controlled (see Chapter 39); stool softeners such as psyllium (Effersyllium or Metamucil), which are not irritating and which absorb mucus, a possible irritant to the sensitive perianal tissue, are preferred.

Occasionally these relatively simple measures do not provide adequate relief and it may be necessary to acidify the stool. There is evidence that in some patients with pruritus ani the stool pH is alkaline (pH 9 to 10) instead of slightly acid (pH 6 to 7) as it is normally. The stool pH may be measured in the office by using litmus paper or a urine dipstick after mixing some water with the stool specimen. If the pH is high, therapeutic acidification of the stool is indicated. Acidifiction may be accomplished with *Lactobacillus acidophilus* (such as Acidophilus, Bacid, or DoFus, all available without prescription), one to two capsules three times/day or with malt soup extract (Maltsupex), available without prescription in powder, liquid, or tablet form.

Occasionally antipruritic sedatives such as diphenhydramine (Benadryl), 25 to 15 mg, or trimeprazine (Temaril), 2.5 mg, taken before bed may be helpful in controlling nocturnal symptoms.

Referral. Should a patient with idiopathic pruritus ani not be responsive to these therapies, he should be referred to a gastroenterologist.

Enterobius Vermicularis (Pinworms). Because the infestation is passed via the fecal-oral route and because the ova may remain alive on bed clothing for up to 3 weeks, dissemination of the disorder within families readily occurs. Once the problem is identified, all members of the household should be evaluated with the cellophane tape test.

The drug of choice to eradicate this infestation is pyrantel pamoate (Antiminth). It is available as an oral suspension (50 mg/ml) and is given as a single oral dose (11 mg/kg, not to exceed a total dose of 1 g). An alternative drug, mebendazole (Vermox), 100 mg, is given as a single oral dose; it should not be used in infants or in pregnant women. These agents approach 100% effectiveness in killing the worms, and symptoms usually subside within 48 hours. The patient is no longer infective once the deposited eggs are removed from the perianal area and clothing by cleaning. Both drugs are well tolerated but may be occasionally associated with mild, transient gastrointestinal distress. Pyrantel pamoate may occasionally be associated with transient elevation of liver enzymes, and its use should be avoided in patients with known liver disease.

Patients who have been identified to have pinworm infection should launder their clothing and bed linens with detergent and hot water on the same day that they have received oral treatment. All infected members of the household should be treated simultaneously. Reinfection is common and re-evaluation is appropriate whenever symptoms recur. Retreatment is necessary with recurring infestation.

ANAL FISSURE

Definition

An anal fissure is a painful elliptical tear, usually located in the posterior portion of the anal canal where the mucosa is relatively fixed. The problem is very common and is observed with equal frequency in men and women. Fissures can extend to the pectinate line (Fig. 92.2) from their origin at the anal verge. A primary fissure represents a tear in the mucosa that occurs because of trauma associated with the passage of a large hard stool or with another similar insult.

Secondary fissures are much less common. They result from inflammatory bowel disease, infections, such as syphilis, gonorrhea, or tuberculosis, or an anatomical anal abnormality, such as scarring that may occur after a hemorrhoidectomy.

Presentation

An acute anal fissure presents with the sudden onset of sharp rectal pain that occurs during and immediately after defecation. This is often followed by a dull aching discomfort that may persist for several hours. A fissure may be associated with *spotty bleeding*, usually noticed as red staining of the toilet tissue or as blood on the surface of the stool. Occasionally, *pruritus ani* (see above) is the major symptom associated with a fissure, in which case a mucus discharge is

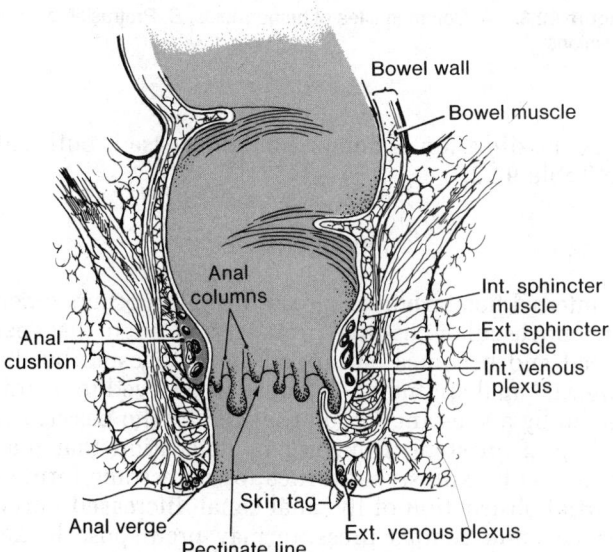

Figure 92.2. Important structures of the anal area.

almost always present. Enlargement and swelling of the associated "sentinel pile" may sometimes be perceived as a lump by the patient.

If the buttocks are gently retracted, thereby everting the anal mucosa, many anal fissures can be readily visualized, usually at the posterior margin of the anal verge. They are more likely to be seen if the patient is asked to strain. During this examination it is important to avoid inducing pain, which will result in spasm of the anal sphincter, increasing discomfort and masking the findings. If an anal fissure is identified by inspection, generally no attempt should be made to perform either a digital rectal examination or anoscopy until treatment has alleviated the symptoms.

If an anal fissure is identified or suspected, and if it is necessary to perform a rectal examination despite the presence of such a fissure (e.g., if a rectal cancer is suspected), a cotton pledget saturated with lidocaine gel may be placed over the fissure before the examination. During digital rectal examination the examining finger should be pressed away from the fissure. If anoscopy is required, abundant lidocaine gel should be used.

A chronic fissure, less common than an acute fissure, may be recognized by its indurated edges and especially by a collection of redundant tissue at the outer lip (the sentinel pile). If anal intercourse has been practiced, a venereal disease should be considered (see below).

Either acute or chronic fissures may be associated with development of a perianal abscess, readily recognized as an area of intense inflammation and fluctuation (see below).

Treatment

Many patients with an acute anal fissure can be made comfortable within a day or 2 and cured within 3 weeks by use of conservative therapy. Bulk laxatives such as Effersyllium or Metamucil should be taken as necessary to provide a soft stool. Irritant cathartics, such as Dulcolax, magnesia, and cascara, should be avoided as they exacerbate the problem. Once the fissure has healed, it is important for the patient to continue ingesting a high fiber diet and to continue using a stool softener as necessary. The use of bran cereals for breakfast and the consumption of at least eight glasses of water daily are important aspects of this regimen.

Anal discomfort may be relieved by the use of showers or sitz baths for 15 to 20 minutes two to three times/day, followed by the application of 0.5% hydrocortisone cream (available without prescription) or 1% hydrocortisone cream (requires a prescription) or by the use of topical anesthetics such as Nupercainal cream, ointment, or suppositories or Perifoam aerosol (both available without prescription). Two other excellent local agents are Anusol-HC cream (requires a prescription) and Balneol (nonprescription). Anesthetic agents may occasionally be associated with a contact allergy and should be immediately discontinued should the patient notice intensification of symptoms or a rash after their use. Topical corticosteriods and anesthetics should be used only on a temporary basis (i.e., 2 to 3 weeks).

If after 3 or 4 weeks of therapy the fissure has not improved or if initially the fissure appears to be chronic (see above), the patient should be referred to a surgeon, because in these instances conservative therapy is not likely to be successful.

If the problem is found to be primary, the surgeon may perform a lateral internal sphincterotomy. There is no need to excise the fissure, but a large sentinel pile may be removed. This procedure is usually done in an ambulatory surgery center, is well tolerated, and is quite successful. Although it can be done under local anesthesia, general anesthesia without a muscle relaxant is preferable. Postoperative complications are not common, but include anorectal abscess (less than 1%), temporary incontinence for flatus (6 to 10%) or for feces (1 to 2%) and prolapse of internal hemorrhoids (1%).

The results of this procedure are excellent. Postoperative discomfort is controlled with sitz baths and oral analgesics. Pain relief is usually noted within 48 hours; the incision heals in 6 days; and the fissure is healed in 3 to 4 weeks. Most patients return to work in 1 week or less. Complete and permanent healing of the fissure is achieved in 97% of cases.

HEMORRHOIDAL DISEASE

Definition

A precise characterization of hemorrhoidal disease is not possible since the pathogenesis has never been elucidated. To define a hemorrhoid as a varicosity of the rectal venous plexus is too simplistic.

Hemorrhoidal veins provide one of the normal communications between the systemic and portal venous systems. These veins have the tendency to dilate and to develop into a tortuous plexus. Anal cushions are part of the normal anatomy of the anal canal (Fig. 92.2). These cushions, which consist of hemorrhoidal venous and arterial plexuses, smooth muscle, and connective tissue, lie under the mucosa. The cushions apparently permit the passage of variable sized stools without disruption of the rectal mucosa. Hemorrhoidal disease is thought to be the result of displacement of these vascular anal cushions. The three cushions that are most likely to be involved are found in the right anterior, right posterior, and left lateral portions of the anal canal (Fig. 92.3). Venous drainage from these cushions is into the portal venous system.

Many physicians classify hemorrhoids as being external or internal; most of the time the diagnosis of external hemorrhoids is incorrect. Often the term is being used to describe redundant skin tags at the anal verge (Fig. 92.2). A small plexus of veins at the anal verge communicates with the systemic venous system. Dilation of these veins is uncommon and is usually associated with an internal hemorrhoid; however, isolated thrombosis may occur, and, while causing only minor discomfort, it may result in the development of a skin tag (Fig. 92.2).

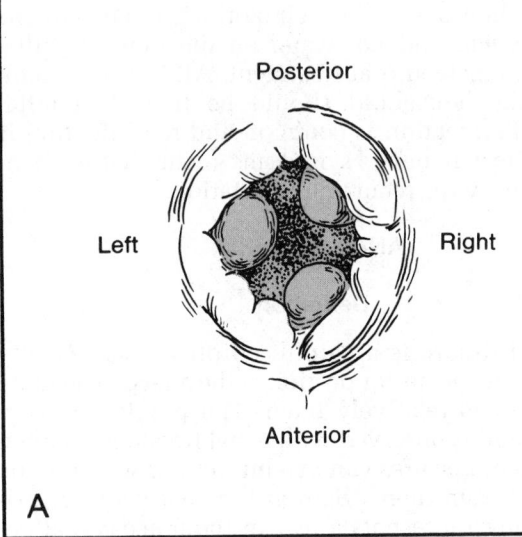

A

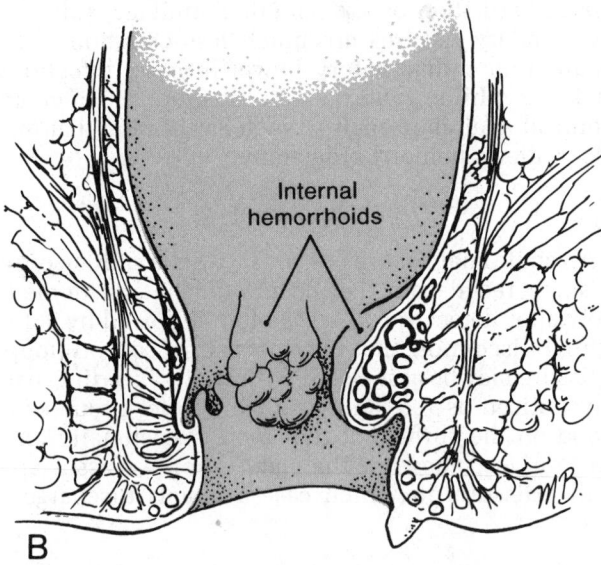

B

Figure 92.3. *A.* Common sites of hemorrhoids. *B.* Protrusion of anal cushions.

A classification of hemorrhoidal disease is outlined in Table 92.2.

Pathogenesis

Internal hemorrhoidal disease (or piles) occurs when an anovascular cushion prolapses through the anal canal and becomes entrapped and congested by the internal anal sphincter. Prolapse is believed to be initiated by a shearing force produced by the passage of a large firm stool, from urgent defecation that may occur with explosive diarrhea, or with some form of partial obstruction of the anal canal. Increased portal or systemic venous pressure may predispose to development of hemorrhoids. This increase in pressure might occur from congestive heart failure, pregnancy, portal hypertension, or pelvic inflammatory or neo-

Table 92.2.
Classification of Hemorrhoids

EXTERNAL SKIN TAGS: Small discrete skin tags arising from the anal verge

EXTERNAL HEMORRHOIDS: Hemorrhoids arising from the inferior hemorrhoidal plexus exterior to the anal verge, covered by pain-sensitive skin

INTERNAL HEMORRHOIDS: Hemorrhoids arising from the vascular cushions, normal structures, lying above the anal verge, covered by pain-insensitive mucosa. Internal hemorrhoids may be classified further:

   First degree: Hemorrhoids bulging into the lumen of the anal canal that produce bleeding

   Second degree: Hemorrhoids that prolapse during defecation but that reduce spontaneously

   Third degree: Prolapsed hemorrhoids that require manual reduction

   Fourth degree: Hemorrhoids that are irreducibly prolapsed

THROMBOSED HEMORRHOIDS: An internal hemorrhoid may prolapse and strangulate, which leads to thrombosis, an excruciating painful condition. If swelling progresses, gangrene of the hemorrhoids with ulceration, local infection, or pylephlebitis (septic phlebitis of the portal venous system) may result

---

plastic disease. Straining at micturition because of urethral or bladder outlet obstruction or straining that occurs with lifting or defecation has been implicated in causing hemorrhoids. Carcinoma of the rectum may be associated with hemorrhoidal development because of straining with bowel movements and local obstruction of venous outflow.

Epidemiology

Asymptomatic hemorrhoids are present in half of the population over age 50 but are uncommon in individuals under the age of 25 to 30 except in women who have been pregnant. A more precise definition of hemorrhoids—one in which symptoms are associated with these normal vascular plexuses—reduces the prevalence to approximately 5% of the population over age 50.

Presentation

Asymptomatic "hemorrhoids" noticed incidentally during an examination should not be considered a problem and should not be treated. Symptomatic hemorrhoids result in bleeding and prolapse. Symptoms that follow persistent prolapse, such as fecal soilage, mucus production, or pruritus ani, symptoms of localized infection, or rarely portal venous infection (pylephlebitis) may also occur. Severe pain is suggestive of a fissure (see above) rather than hemorrhoids. Thrombosis of an external hemorrhoid can cause significant discomfort. Pain is an uncommon symptom of internal hemorrhoids unless strangulation of a prolapsed hemorrhoid occurs. However, 80% of patients with symptomatic internal hemorrhoids will admit to some aching discomfort on occasion.

External Hemorrhoids

External hemorrhoids are covered by pain-sensitive skin. The most common manifestation, therefore, is pain, which results from thrombosis in the external venous plexus. Pain is perianal in location and can be

exacerbated by defecation. The patient may be aware of a tender perianal lump.

Internal Hemorrhoids

Internal hemorrhoids are covered by pain-insensitive mucosa, produce symptoms primarily from bleeding or prolapse, and are only painful in the event of thrombosis or strangulation (ischemia caused by constriction of a prolapsed hemorrhoid) with or without associated ulceration and infection.

Bleeding. Characteristically the bleeding from hemorrhoids is intermittent and bright red and spots toilet tissue or the surface of the stool. Occasionally it may be sustained and described as a dripping of blood. Rarely, massive hemorrhage may occur, particularly among patients with portal hypertension. Bleeding may also be occult; but because of their common occurrence, hemorrhoids should never be considered the cause of occult bleeding until other causes of gastrointestinal blood loss have been ruled out by appropriate evaluation. Gastrointestinal bleeding is fully discussed in Chapter 38.

Prolapse. Prolapse of internal hemorrhoids produces the sensation of fullness in the anal canal, especially after defecation. Usually prolapsed hemorrhoids will reduce spontaneously. Occasionally prolapse is more severe and manual reduction may be necessary. When reduction is not possible, prolapse may be associated with fecal soilage, mucus accumulation, and the development of pruritus ani (see above).

Pain. Pain from internal hemorrhoids suggests thrombosis or strangulation, and referral to a surgeon is necessary. Thrombosis and strangulation occur when prolapse of a hemorrhoid through the anal canal is followed by increasing congestion, created by spasm of the entrapping anal sphincter. If the hemorrhoid strangulates, it may ulcerate and cause infection, which is usually localized or which rarely may spread through the portal venous plexus, resulting in pylephlebitis.

Examination

Hemorrhoids can sometimes be visualized by observing the anal canal in good light after the patient gently retracts his buttocks and strains as if having a bowel movement. This maneuver produces slight eversion of the anal canal and may enable the examiner to see the internal hemorrhoidal plexus.

An *external hemorrhoid* will be seen as a mass just outside the anal verge. It is soft and painless unless thrombosed, in which case it is firm and tender with a bluish discoloration.

If the patient is in severe pain from thrombosis, strangulation, or ulceration, no further evaluation is necessary and urgent referral to a surgeon is appropriate (see below). In the usual case pain is not a problem and a more thorough evaluation of the anal canal should be accomplished by anoscopy (using a side view instrument, as described above, page 1259). It is important that this procedure be done carefully as described above. Anoscopy is the definitive diagnostic procedure for establishing the diagnosis of internal hemorrhoids.

Sigmoidoscopy should be performed in patients with recent onset of symptomatic hemorrhoidal disease because of the possibility that sigmoid or rectal carcinoma has caused the development of hemorrhoids. Currently this should be done with the flexible fiberoptic sigmoidoscope, a procedure that requires preliminary cleansing of the colon and rectum. The need for additional evaluation of the colon by barium enema, air contrast barium enema, or colonoscopy must be determined on an individual basis; it is mandatory if there has been significant or repeated bleeding (see Chapter 38).

Differential Diagnosis

Several problems may be confused with hemorrhoidal disease:

Hypertrophied anal papilla occurs along the pectinate line (Fig. 92.2) in association with an anal fissure (see above), Crohn's disease, or without obvious cause. These papillae usually are asymptomatic and require no therapy unless they have become particularly large, eroded, or infected, or unless they bleed. Hypertrophied anal papillae often have the appearance of a fibrous polyp and are easily differentiated from hemorrhoids by their location and by the absence of a vascular swelling.

Anal skin tags are very common. They appear as small projections of redundant skin external to the anal verge. They may be remnants of previously active external hemorrhoidal disease, associated with internal hemorrhoidal disease, or with Crohn's disease. One version is the sentinel pile seen in conjunction with an anal fissure (see above). They are of no consequence unless they are very large, bleed, or become infected or excoriated.

Prolapse of rectal mucosa is a problem that is much more common in the elderly. The pathogenesis may be similar to that of prolapsing internal hemorrhoids, except that the full thickness of the rectal wall may herniate. Prolapse is identified by the abnormal downward displacement of rectal mucosa without evidence of localized venous swelling (see below).

Protruding tumors such as rectal polyps, anal carcinoma, or, in women, endometriosis can be confused with hemorrhoids. If there is suspicion about the diagnosis, referral to a surgeon or a gastroenterologist for evaluation and biopsy is appropriate.

Course

Without treatment, symptoms due to hemorrhoids usually resolve spontaneously within several days to several weeks, even when thrombosis is present. Most patients, however, develop recurrent symptoms, although the intervals between symptoms may be long.

Treatment

The aim of treatment is to relieve symptoms while permitting spontaneous healing; treatment does not necessarily reduce venous bulges, although not infrequently they regress spontaneously. Most patients respond to conservative therapy:

Avoidance of direct pressure is essential in the relief of pain, especially due to thrombosed external hemorrhoids. The patient will usually find a position that gives him relief. For persons who must sit (doing desk work, for example) a donut-shaped inflatable ring is usually helpful in preventing pressure on a symptomatic hemorrhoid.

Sitz baths two to three times a day for 15 to 20 minutes on each occasion provide comfort. A moist, warm washcloth, firmly applied between the cheeks of the buttocks, may also provide good temporary relief of symptoms.

Stool softeners are mandatory, if stools are hard, to reduce straining with defecation and to prevent evacuation of hard stools that may prolapse the mucosa. Bran-containing breakfast cereal and/or whole wheat bread helps to maintain soft stools. An addition is the daily ingestion of a bulk laxative stool softener such as Effersyllium, Metamucil, Colace, or Peri-Colace (see also Chapter 39). Instructing the patient to increase fluid consumption, especially water, facilitates effectiveness of stool softeners. Use of stool softeners should continue, even after the resolution of the acute problem, as it may help to prevent recurrence.

Topical preparations may provide relief of pain or pruritis. *Hydrocortisone-containing rectal preparations*, such as Anusol-HC cream, Protofoam-HC aerosol, or Wyanoids-HC ointment (all require prescription), used three to four times a day, may provide symptomatic relief. Cream, foam, or ointment is preferred to suppositories, which tend to be expelled or drawn up in the rectum and, therefore, have less local effect. One-half percent (available without prescription) or 1% (requires a prescription) hydrocortisone cream (generic) is also useful.

Analgesic rectal preparations are also useful when pain is prominent, but they may occasionally result in contact allergy. Preparations such as Nupercainal (available without prescription) or lidocaine 2.5% ointment (requires a prescription) used three to four times a day may provide relief of rectal discomfort, particularly over the first several days when the discomfort tends to be most intense.

There is no acceptable evidence that Preparation H, which contains the antiseptic phenylmercuric nitrate, 3% shark liver oil, and "live yeast cell derivative," can shrink hemorrhoids, reduce inflammation, or heal injured tissue (6).

Systemic analgesics, such as meperidine (Demerol), 50 to 100 mg every 4 to 6 hours, may occasionally be necessary for pain associated with thrombosed hemorrhoids. However, such severe pain may be more effectively treated by a surgeon by thrombectomy (instant relief of pain) as compared with conservative therapy (4 to 5 days before pain is relieved). Systemic analgesics such as codeine or meperidine may be associated with constipation; therefore, they should be used in conjunction with laxatives.

Referral for Surgical Management

Patients should be referred to a surgeon for evaluation whenever there is doubt about the diagnosis (see above), if the patient does not respond within 1 or 2 weeks to conservative therapy, if pain is severe as may occur with thrombosis, or if there is evidence of strangulation, ulceration, or perianal infection. When uncomplicated hemorrhoids are recurrently symptomatic, the patient should be referred to a surgeon for definitive treatment.

The surgeon will evaluate the patient, confirm the diagnosis, and then consider several therapeutic options that are not normally provided by general physicians (7).

Injection of Sclerosing Agents

The submucosal injection of a symptomatic hemorrhoid with several milliliters of a sclerosing solution causes fibrosis and retraction of the hemorrhoid. This procedure is excellent therapy for small bleeding internal hemorrhoids (first or second degree) (see Table 92.2); it is simple, requires no anesthesia, and can easily be performed in the office (requires only a few minutes). There may be a period of several days when the patient experiences a sensation of anal fullness. This symptom is usually well tolerated or is easily controlled by the use of sitz baths three to four times/ day and by mild analgesics, such as acetaminophen or aspirin. After this procedure the patient usually requires no recovery period and can return to work immediately.

It is important that the physician performing this procedure be experienced with its use. If the solution is improperly injected, severe pain, necrosis, and rectal stenosis may occur. *Sclerotherapy* is rarely associated with the development of infection, an oleoma, or an oil embolus. Injection of sclerosing agents generally provides temporary relief, but it does not prevent the development of subsequent hemorrhoids. The procedure may be repeated several times. However, it produces an area of fibrosis and, if repetitively used, may result in rectal stenosis.

Rubberband Ligation

Rubberband ligation of hemorrhoids is a relatively simple office procedure that can be used for the treatment of symptomatic internal hemorrhoids of all degrees except the fourth (see (Table 92.2) (2, 3). The patient requires no special preparation, and usually the only discomfort results from anoscopy required during the procedure. No anesthesia is necessary. With use of an anoscope and a special instrument one or two rubberbands are applied near the base of one or two and occasionally three hemorrhoids, which are at

least 0.5 cm above the pectinate line. No more than two hemorrhoids should be treated at a single session. Constriction by the rubberband results in ischemic necrosis of the hemorrhoid, which eventually sloughs and is passed in the stool. Sloughing usually occurs between the 5th and 10th day after banding and is associated with passage of a small amount of blood. Rarely, bleeding may be massive, and urgent reassessment by the surgeon is necessary to control the bleeding by electrocautery or by ligation. Potentially fatal pelvic cellulitis has occurred on several occasions and, while exceptionally uncommon, must be promptly recognized and vigorously treated.

Usually, after rubberband ligation of hemorrhoids, the patient is not disabled and has only minimal discomfort characterized by a sensation of rectal fullness, a symptom that is usually well controlled by the use of sitz baths and/or mild oral analgesics, such as acetaminophen or aspirin. If the rubberband is improperly placed below the pectinate line, the patient may experience considerable pain, in which case reassessment by the surgeon is appropriate.

After rubberband ligation a bulk-forming stool softener such as Effersyllium or Metamucil should be prescribed to prevent straining. This will be necessary for several weeks and should be continued as long-term therapy to prevent straining, which may predispose to the subsequent development of new hemorrhoids.

Complete healing after this procedure occurs within 2 to 3 weeks, after which the patient may be treated with further rubberband ligations if there are other symptomatic hemorrhoids. Banding provides good relief of hemorrhoidal disease approximately 70 to 90% of the time. Symptoms may recur in 15 to 45% of patients after anywhere from 18 months to 5 years. In this circumstance, conservative measures may be employed (see above) or rubber band ligation may be repeated.

Manual Dilation of the Anus

This procedure is predicated on the belief that hemorrhoids result from partial obstruction of the anal canal necessitating increased pressure for evacuation of the bowel. The pressure is transmitted to the anal vascular cushion, resulting in the development of hemorrhoids. Despite the fact that some have considered dilatation to be an acceptable treatment alternative to hemorrhoidectomy (1), it is rarely used in the United States and is declining in popularity elsewhere. Initially promising reports of good results in 75 to 85% of patients are now being tempered by a 25% incidence of long-term partial sphincter incontinence, rectal prolapse, and the frequent recurrence of hemorrhoids. It is not an acceptable therapeutic alternative.

Partial Internal Sphincterotomy

This procedure is based on the same logic as manual anal dilation: that relief of partial obstruction of the anal sphincter, which leads to increased straining during defecation thus causing the development of hemorrhoids, will cure the hemorrhoids. Although it does not cause the severe long-term complications associated with anal dilatation, it is ineffective in the treatment of symptomatic hemorrhoids and is therefore not recommended.

Cryotherapy

This procedure is practiced in the United States by only a few surgeons. A freezing probe destroys the hemorrhoid, which in time sloughs. Usually the procedure is done in a surgeon's office without anesthesia. After the procedure there is often an uncomfortable, profuse, foul-smelling anal discharge that persists until the necrotic hemorrhoid sloughs, which usually occurs on about the 14th day. At this time bleeding may occur and is usually minor. However, in an occasional patient bleeding can be marked and will require re-evaluation with subsequent cauterization or ligation. After this procedure the patient is unable to return to his usual activities for a period of 2 to 3 weeks, primarily because of the anal discharge. Healing generally is complete by 6 weeks. Postoperatively, the patient is required only to take sitz baths and oral analgesics in addition to stool softeners. Because this procedure has no advantage over rubber band ligation and causes more postoperative discomfort, it has not become a popular alternative.

Laser Therapy and Infrared Photocoagulation

Both laser therapy and infrared photocoagulation are available as treatment modalities for first, second, and third degree hemorrhoids (see Table 92.2). The CO_2 laser has been most commonly employed and is effective. However, it requires expensive equipment and special expertise. The patient's experience and the results are similar to those achieved by cryosurgery.

Infrared photocoagulation is particularly efficacious in the control of bleeding from grade 1 and 2 hemorrhoids. When available, it may be particularly indicated in this situation.

Hemorrhoidectomy

Hemorrhoidectomy is indicated only for the treatment of large internal hemorrhoids and remains the only satisfactory approach to fourth degree hemorrhoids. It is probably the best emergency management for prolapsed thrombosed internal hemorrhoids. The procedure requires general or spinal anesthesia and the patient is usually hospitalized for 2 to 3 days, although good risk patients with less severe hemorrhoids may be able to have the surgery performed in an ambulatory center. The patient is prepared for the procedure by taking stool softeners for approximately a week before and is given a laxative the evening before the operation. The purpose of the operation is to remove hemorrhoidal tissue and to appose the skin and mucus membrane. The operation has a reputation for

severe postoperative pain. This problem can be greatly ameliorated, however, either by anal dilatation to four fingers prior to the resection of the hemorrhoids or by performing a lateral anal sphincterotomy in conjunction with the hemorrhoidectomy. The postoperative discomfort is then easily controlled by sitz baths, oral analgesics, and stool softeners. An uncommon but important postoperative complication is anorectal abscess (see below).

After hemorrhoidectomy there is a recovery period of 3 to 4 weeks before the patient is able to return to his usual activities.

When hemorrhoidectomy is performed by an experienced surgeon, the complications of infection, fistula formation, fissure development, significant bleeding, or acute thrombosis of an external hemorrhoid occur only rarely (less than 1%). Minor bleeding is more common but is usually present during the first 2 weeks. Acute urinary retention after hemorrhoidectomy occurs in about 10% of individuals and may require the short-term use of an indwelling catheter. Late complications of incontinence or of anal stenosis are quite rare. Skin tags are usually excised with the hemorrhoids, although small ones may develop after hemorrhoidectomy and are usually of no consequence (see above).

After hemorrhoidectomy the surgeon will usually evaluate the patient weekly for two to three visits until healing is complete and before the patient returns to work. The patient is seen 6 months after hemorrhoidectomy to be examined for the presence of additional hemorrhoids, stenosis, stricture, or skin tags.

Hemorrhoidectomy offers the best chance of long-term control with less than a 5% late recurrence rate. Its use has become increasingly limited because of the associated short-term morbidity and the observation that most symptomatic hemorrhoids can be eliminated by less traumatic procedures.

Special Considerations

Because of an increased rate of complications associated with operative procedures in individuals with severe congestive heart failure or debilitating disease, the treatment of hemorrhoids in these patients should be as conservative as possible. Patients who have portal hypertension present a special risk because of the frequent association of a coagulopathy and because operative hemorrhoidectomy in a few instances can diminish shunting between the portal and systemic systems and result in a rise in portal pressure that on occasion may be associated with esophageal or gastric variceal bleeding.

Hemorrhoids are very common in pregnancy and are best managed conservatively. They frequently resolve spontaneously after delivery. Occasionally, development of strangulated hemorrhoids requires surgical intervention during the pregnancy. Patients with inflammatory bowel disease and hemorrhoidal disease should be managed in consultation with a gastroenterologist and a surgeon.

ANORECTAL ABSCESSES AND ANORECTAL FISTULAS

Definition

An anorectal abscess is an abscess involving the perineum and perianal structures. Abscesses are classified by their anatomical location (Fig. 92.4). *Low intramuscular* or *perianal abscesses* are located in the subcutaneous tissue immediately surrounding the anus, which is the site of 50 to 75% of all anorectal abscesses. An *ischiorectal abscess* is located in the ischiorectal fossa, a fat-filled space between the levator ani (external anal sphincter) and the ischial tuberosity, and accounts for 20 to 40% of anorectal abscesses. *Intersphincteric, high intermuscular, pelvirectal,* and *submucosal abscesses* are far less common and account for about 10% of all abscesses. Anorectal abscesses are common, and the general physician should be familiar with presentation of such an abscess so that patients suspected of having this problem are promptly referred to a surgeon. Most anorectal abscesses are associated with anal fistulas. Occasionally, anorectal abscesses occur in association with other anal and perianal disorders (Table 92.3).

An *anorectal fistula* (fistula-in-ano) is a tract lined by granulation tissue having an internal opening in the anal canal and an external opening in the perianal skin. The internal opening is usually located in one of the anal crypts at the upper end of the anal canal just above the pectinate line (Fig. 92.2). If only one opening is identifiable, it is termed an *anorectal sinus*.

Etiology

Anorectal abscesses are more common in men. Most often they represent a primary bacterial infection of anal glands and ducts. Anal glands, thought to be diverticula of the anal canal mucosa, are located along the pectinate line. Many of these glands pass through the internal sphincter into the intersphincteric space. It is presumed that muscle tone in the internal sphincter prevents discharge from the glands causing stasis, dilation, and eventual infection. Bacterial cultures from the abscesses frequently isolate *Staphylococcus aureus, Escherichia coli, Bacteroides species, Proteus species, Streptococcus species,* or a mixed flora. Because anal glands in the adult are concentrated more in the anterior and posterior walls of the anus, abscesses and fistulas tend to occur in these areas. The majority of abscesses are located in the posterior rectal wall.

Most anorectal fistulas result from abscess formation in the anal glands and drainage through the perianal skin. Therefore, bacterial flora of fistulas are similar to those of anorectal abscesses. Some fistulas are not

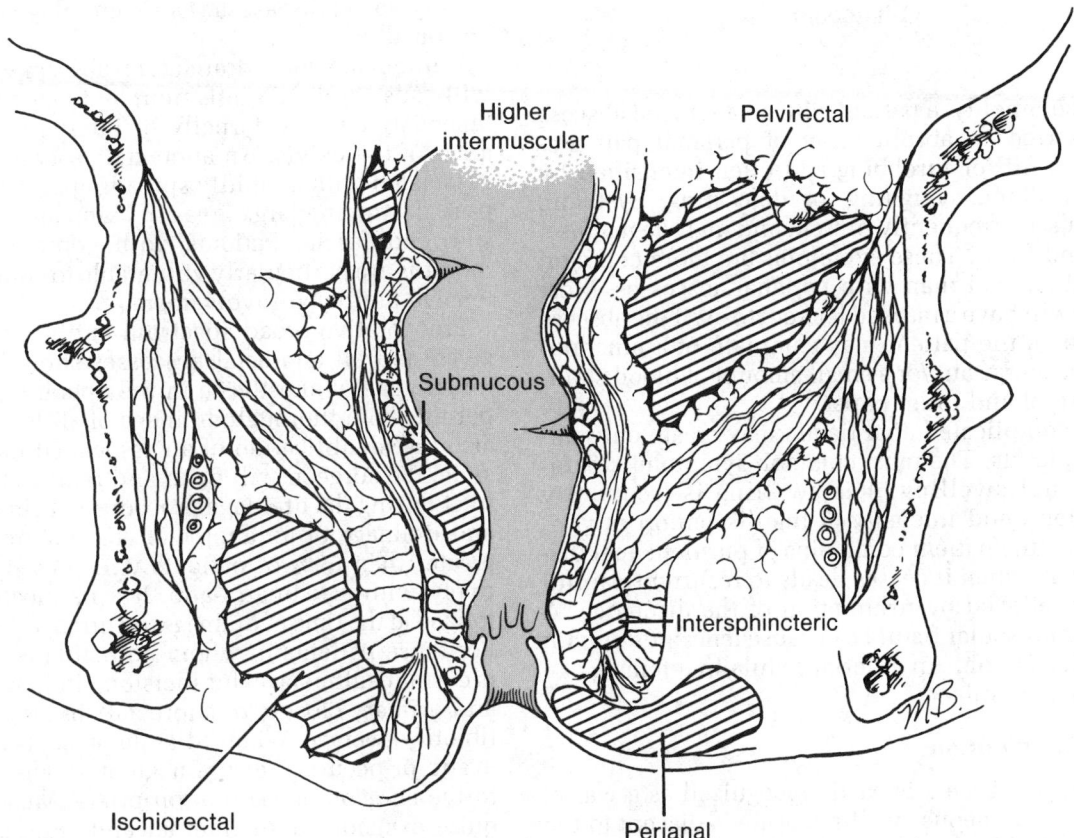

Figure 92.4. Anatomical classification of common anorectal abscesses.

Table 92.3.
Conditions That May Be Complicated by Anorectal Abscess and Fistula-in-Ano

INFLAMMATORY BOWEL DISEASE
CHRONIC INFECTIONS (uncommon)
    Actinomycosis
    Tuberculosis
    Lymphogranuloma venereum
    Schistosomiasis (rare)
    Amebiasis (rare)
INFECTION ANATOMICALLY ADJACENT TO THE RECTAL AREA AND PRESENTING AS ANORECTAL ABSCESS OR FISTULA-IN-ANO
   In women:
    Pelvic inflammatory disease
    Bartholin gland abscess
   In men:
    Infections of a Cowper gland (small periurethral glands)
    Pilonidal sinus (occasionally occurs in females)
FOREIGN BODY (e.g., an ingested bone or a penetrating wooden splinter)
TRAUMA
    Surgery (e.g., hemorrhoidectomy or prostatectomy)
    Radiation
    Laceration (e.g., from an enema)
ABNORMALITIES OF HOST DEFENSE (e.g., bone marrow aplasia, leukemia or lymphoma, diabetes mellitus)
CARCINOMA OF ANUS OR RECTUM

pyogenic in origin and are associated with inflammatory bowel disease or tuberculosis. Fistulas that do not originate in anal glands may result from diverticular disease, neoplastic disease, or trauma.

Diagnosis

History

Most commonly, a patient with an anorectal abscess will describe an abrupt onset of perianal pain described as full or throbbing and often intensified by sitting, walking, coughing, or defecating. Systemic symptoms are frequently present and include malaise, chills, and fever. These symptoms are more common with ischiorectal than with perianal abscesses. Most patients will have a marked leukocytosis. If the abscess has opened, the patient may complain of a mucopurulent discharge and/or a small amount of blood staining the stool and toilet paper.

An uncomplicated anal fistula may create only minor complaints. The most common symptom is painful perianal swelling. The swelling is frequently intermittent, and intensity of the discomfort is variable. Often the patient complains of purulent anal discharge that, when it ceases, leads to recurrent painful swelling relieved by resumption of the discharge. A high intramuscular fistula can cause tenesmus or pain during defecation. An anterior fistula in a female can cause dyspareunia.

Rectal Examination

A perianal abscess is easily recognized as a warm, tender, subcutaneous swelling located adjacent to the anus. An ischiorectal abscess may be identified by fluctuation in the ischiorectal fossa felt only on digital rectal examination. Often there is only tenderness detected by pressure to the skin overlying the ischiorectal fossa or the lateral wall of the anal canal during a rectal examination. Higher anorectal abscesses may present few or no findings on perianal examination. However, many of these individuals will complain of severe pain and pyrexia and exhibit a marked leukocytosis. Under such circumstances, digital examination of the anal canal usually reveals a high, exquisitely tender, posterior rectal wall mass.

The diagnosis of an anorectal fistula is established by inspection and palpation of the perianal area and performance of a digital rectal examination. Frequently the external opening of the fistula in the perianal area can be seen. Digital examination of the rectum may enable identification of the indurated tract of the fistula as it passes to its internal opening. Often the location of the internal opening is facilitated by the gentle passage of a probe. Anoscopy may also be helpful. Occasionally accurate localization must await surgical exploration. When perineal infection is present, the possibility of hidradenitis suppurativa must be considered (see Chapter 100, Common Problems of the Skin).

Treatment

Identification or suspicion of an anorectal abscess with or without a fistula-in-ano should lead to urgent referral to a surgeon. If there is a history of inflammatory bowel disease, a gastroenterologist should also be consulted.

Without adequate drainage an abscess will progress, will cause systemic infection, and can rupture spontaneously either externally or internally into deeper areas of the pelvis. An anorectal abscess may also be associated with a rapidly spreading necrotizing infection, destroying large areas of skin, subcutaneous tissue, and fascia. Patients with coincident diabetes mellitus are particularly vulnerable to complicated extensive perirectal involvement.

Preoperative broad spectrum antibiotics should be given and all anorectal abscesses should be drained under general anesthesia in the operating room. This permits both thorough drainage of all loculations and also the identification of an associated fistula. If possible, the surgeon will open and remove the fistulous tract during the drainage procedure. If simple incision and drainage of an anorectal abscess are performed, greater than 50% of patients will present postoperatively with a fistula-in-ano. If a fistulectomy is performed at the time of drainage, recurrence is uncommon. For those patients in whom no fistula is found, there is current enthusiasm for incision, drainage, curettage, and primary closure of anorectal abscesses under antibiotic coverage. When a fistula presents as a primary event, or occurs after drainage of an abscess, referral to the surgeon is again appropriate. Most fistulas require excision. Both internal and external openings must be excised, and the tract must be converted into an open wound and the granulation tissue excised or curetted. However, chronic fistulae can present very difficult technical problems and the wound can take 5 to 12 weeks to heal.

PROCTALGIA FUGAX

Occasionally healthy young adults develop the sudden onset of severe rectal pain, variably intermittent and generally lasting less than 30 minutes to 1 hour—proctalgia fugax. It frequently will awaken a patient at night. It is significantly more common in women than in men, and it can occur after sexual intercourse. The pain is described usually as a spasm or a cramp. The problem is not associated with systemic illness or with other gastrointestinal diseases such as the irritable bowel syndrome, and the etiology is uncertain. There is often an association with psychiatric disturbances. Proctalgia fugax is thought to result from spasm of a portion of the levator ani muscle. Patients with proctalgia fugax may obtain relief by taking a hot sitz bath or by applying pressure in the perianal area near the site of the discomfort. Occasionally if the attacks are severe and frequent, the patient may find relief by the use of sublingual or cutaneous nitrates. The problem usually persists for many years but then disappears in later life.

RECTAL PROLAPSE

Definition

Prolapse is a protrusion of the rectum through the anus. The protrusion may contain only mucosa, a mucosal prolapse, or it may contain all layers of the bowel wall, a full thickness prolapse (procidentia). There can also be an internal prolapse, or internal rectal intussusception, which produces typical symptoms without any external protrusion. This is often associated with the solitary rectal ulcer syndrome.

Etiology

Prolapse is more prevalent in women (approximately 80% of the cases) with a peak incidence between the ages of 60 and 80. In men the peak incidence occurs at about the age of 40. The exact pathogenic mechanism of this disease is not known. Factors that are associated with this disease are multiple. Weakening of fascial attachments of the rectum, attenuated muscles in the perirectal area and pelvic diaphragm, straining due to chronic constipation, and even congenital fascial defects all lead to the development of rectal prolapse. Prolapse is often observed after severe chronic diarrhea.

Diagnosis

History

Patients have variable symptoms, depending upon the degree of prolapse. Initially the protrusion occurs only with defecation, and the patient can easily reduce it manually. At this stage there may be no associated incontinence. The patient may complain of a sensation of displaced tissue at the time of a bowel movement, and there is often a feeling of incomplete evacuation. With progression of the problem, prolapse occurs with any straining and, eventually, simply with walking or even standing. At this stage incontinence is almost invariably a problem. With more profound prolapse the patient may complain of tenesmus and also develop a continuous mucous discharge. The prolapsed rectum may become excoriated and ulcerated, leading many patients to complain of bleeding. In instances of advanced degree of prolapse the patient may suffer urinary incontinence, and in the female there may be associated uterine prolapse. Patients with increasing degrees of prolapse suffer from considerable embarrassment and consequently will avoid social contact.

Examination

The physician will best recognize rectal prolapse by inspecting the anus when the patient strains in a squatting position or sitting on a commode. It is usually best to anticipate incontinence with this maneuver. If the prolapse is full thickness (procidentia), concentric folds of the rectal mucosa will be seen, whereas if there is only mucosal prolapse, only radial folds are seen. Digital examination will almost always reveal a patulous and relaxed anal sphincter that often will admit two to four fingers. Palpation of the protruding tissue between the examiner's finger will provide the sensation of only mucosa in mucosal prolapse and a double layer of bowel wall in full thickness prolapse. The rectal examination in patients with prolapse is usually associated with minimal if any discomfort.

Occasionally prolapsed hemorrhoids may be confused with rectal prolapse, but absence of concentric or radial folds of mucosa and the prominent location of prolapsed hemorrhoids in the left lateral or right anterior or right posterior edges of the anus suggest the proper diagnosis (Fig. 92.3). On occasion, a prolapse may be associated with a rectal tumor. For that reason a sigmoidoscopic examination should be performed on any patient with rectal prolapse. Other diagnostic studies are not usually required, but a defecatory videoproctogram (available in only a few centers) is very useful, especially for identifying either an associated rectocele or an internal prolapse.

Treatment

When the prolapse is small and limited to the mucosa, the patient may benefit from the use of stool softeners and by the use of an irritant rectal suppository (see Chapter 39) to initiate defecation and thereby avoid straining at stool. If prolapse progresses despite this treatment or if extensive mucosal prolapse is noted, it is appropriate to refer the patient to a surgeon. Redundant tissue may be treated either by rubberband ligation as for internal hemorrhoids or by sclerosis. Both procedures can usually be performed in the surgeon's office under local anesthesia and are usually successful in preventing progressive degrees of rectal mucosal prolapse.

When procidentia (full thickness prolapse) is present, only operative treatment will be effective. Several procedures are available for restoration of anal continence and reduction of prolapse. Virtually all of these operations require hospitalization and general anesthesia, although increasingly, in selected patients, ambulatory surgery is performed. All procedures are successful, with a recurrence rate of less than 4%. One important factor to consider before operation is whether incontinence will be improved. In some centers rectal manometric studies are advocated before surgical intervention. In instances when the gastroenterologist and surgeon believe that incontinence may not be improved, the alternative of providing the patient with a permanent diverting colostomy rather than doing an abdominal rectopexy must be considered. For elderly and/or very high risk patients with complete procidentia, a variety of perineal operations that do not require laparotomy are available. The results of these procedures are imperfect, but the situation is often made tolerable for a bedridden or inactive patient. All truly successful operative procedures for full thickness rectal prolapse require an abdominal proctopexy in which the rectum is secured to presacral fascia either by primary suture or by the use of synthetic mesh. This may or may not be accompanied by anterior resection of redundant sigmoid colon. Complications associated with surgical repair of prolapse are those of fecal impaction, presacral hemorrhage, stricture, infection, fistula formation, pelvic abscesses, and intestinal obstruction. The complication rate is less than 1 to 3%. Fecal impaction, however, can occur in up to 6 to 10% of the patients after operative repair. It is important to follow the patient carefully during this period so that this problem may be recognized early and treated appropriately. The long-term results are generally good, with recurrence rates in the range of 2 to 10%. However, for patients with preoperative fecal incontinence, 15 to 30% of them will continue to have some degree of postoperative incontinence.

VENEREAL DISEASE

Definition

The so-called "gay bowel syndrome" has become increasingly common as a consequence of the sexual practices of homosexual men (e.g., anal receptive intercourse, fist fornication, and anilingus). In fact, homosexuality is not, by itself, a risk factor for proctitis. However, the tendency toward promiscuity and the anonymity of the multiple contacts leads to a high likelihood of developing the syndrome.

Etiology

"Gay bowel syndrome" is a generic term that refers to numerous types of anal and rectal diseases seen in gay men (4, 5). Often the problem is a nonspecific

inflammation due to trauma or to unidentified minor infectious diseases. On the other hand, there are a number of specific causes of perianal disease and of proctitis in this population, the nature and prevalence of which are listed in Table 92.4. It should be noted that lymphogranuloma venereum (LGV) is caused by a specific immunotype of *Chlamydia trachomatis*.

Diagnosis

Perianal lesions are particularly seen in association with syphilis, condyloma acuminatum, and herpes simplex virus (HSV) infection. These lesions, when present in the absence of proctitis, are usually asymptomatic. In the case of syphilis and HSV infection, the symptoms of associated proctitis dominate the clinical presentation, whereas the venereal warts of condyloma acuminatum are usually asymptomatic. Perianal lesions in the form of abscesses, strictures, and fistulas are a late manifestation of both lymphogranuloma venereum and cryptococcosis.

A perianal chancre may suggest the diagnosis of syphilis, and the typical wart-like excrescence of a condyloma latum, while rare, is pathognomonic. The diagnosis must be confirmed by dark field examination for spirochetes. Condyloma acuminatum is recognized as a typical collection of venereal warts usually extending within the anal canal. There is no specific diagnostic test. HSV presents initially as perianal and/or anal canal vesicles, but these have usually ruptured and coalesced into ulcerations before the patient is seen. Diagnosis requires either a direct fluorescent monoclonal antibody technique or culture of the virus. Intranuclear inclusions on biopsy or a rising serum neutralizing antibody titer are suggestive, but not diagnostic.

The various kinds of proctitis in this population all have essentially similar and nonspecific symptoms of rectal discharge, pruritus, tenesmus, hematochezia, and constipation. Pain (odynochezia) is especially typical of HSV and may also accompany both LGV and syphilis. Amebiasis has a rather typical appearance of the associated proctitis on sigmoidoscopy, but the symptoms in this disease are those of colitis, not of proctitis. Constitutional symptoms also accompany HSV, LGV, and cryptococcosis. In the case of HSV, these symptoms consist of urinary retention, impotence, and unexplained but disabling dysesthesias of the peri-

Table 92.4.
Causes and Prevalence of Proctitis in Homosexual Men[a]

Gonorrhea	13–45%
Syphilis	5–10%
Lymphogranuloma venereum (LGV)	Uncommon
Non-LGV *Chlamydia trachomatis*	8–15%
Condyloma acuminatum	50%
Herpes simplex virus (HSV)[b]	6–30%
Amebiasis	20–30%
Cryptococcosis[b]	Rare

[a] From Peppercorn, MA Enteric infections in homosexual men with and without AIDS. *Contemp Gastroent* 2:23, 1989.
[b] Especially associated with acquired immunodeficiency syndrome (AIDS).

neum, buttocks, and posterior thighs. LGV causes fever and bloody diarrhea and is easily confused with inflammatory bowel disease, especially Crohn's colitis. Cryptococcosis is a disseminated disease with neurologic and skeletal manifestations. Inguinal adenopathy is a common finding in conjunction with syphilis, LGV, and HSV.

Diagnosis of all of these lesions requires anoscopy and sigmoidoscopy. Gonorrhea causes a nonspecific mucosal inflammation with erythema, friability, and an exudate. Gram stain of the exudate reveals Gram-negative intracellular diplococci, and a culture is confirmatory. Leutic proctitis is also nonspecific, and the diagnosis is made by dark field examination of the exudate and by serologic tests for syphilis. LGV, in addition to a nonspecific proctitis, causes linear and aphthous ulcers extending up from the rectum to the distal colon. Histologically as well as clinically these findings resemble Crohn's disease, and the diagnosis of LGV requires culture of the organism, preferably with immunotyping. Rising acute convalescent serum antibody titers to the L immunotypes of *C. trachomatis* are also confirmatory. Non-LGV *C. trachomatis* causes a mild proctitis that is nonspecific and is often localized to the anal crypts where it is hard to visualize and difficult to biopsy. Accordingly, it is commonly underdiagnosed unless serum for antibody titers is obtained. Although the warts of condyloma acuminatum usually present in the perianal area, anoscopy is necessary to look for involvement of the anal canal. HSV also causes predominantly perianal lesions, but anoscopy and sigmoidoscopy should be performed because the anal canal can contain vesicular lesions or ulcers and the distal rectum may reveal proctitis with or without ulcers as well. Amebiasis often presents a characteristic sigmoidoscopic appearance of punched out ulcers with a yellow base in addition to diffuse inflammation. Cryptococcal anal ulceration presents as a chronic perirectal abscess with fistula formation requiring anoscopic evaluation.

It should be emphasized that none of these lesions is likely to be recognized unless an appropriate history is obtained. These patients rarely volunteer information regarding their sexual practices, so the physician is obligated to ask the necessary questions or else the diagnosis will be missed.

Treatment

Surgical referral is rarely appropriate for these diseases, and, when surgery is required, evaluation by a gastroenterologist should precede any operative approach except in the case of condyloma acuminatum. Indeed for most of these lesions the differential diagnosis is sufficiently complex that gastroenterology consultation is usually appropriate. The exception is perhaps gonorrheal proctitis since the diagnosis, if

suspected, is easily made and treatment is usually successful (see Chapter 27). Luetic proctitis is also easily treated (see Chapter 30).

Chlamydia infections (see Chapter 27) respond to tetracycline, erythromycin, or a trimethoprim and sulfa combination. The duration and success of treatment depend first upon a correct diagnosis (Crohn's disease does not respond to antibiotics) and secondly upon the severity and duration of the infection. LGV may progress to abscess, fistula, and stricture formation and require surgical management, occasionally necessitating a colostomy.

Condyloma acuminatum, if the lesions are small, may respond to the topical application of podophyllin. Larger warts require surgical treatment by excision, fulguration, or, more recently, the CO_2 laser. Recurrence is likely, whatever method is used (see also Chapter 94, Benign Vulvovaginal Disorders).

Amebiasis is treated with metronidazole and, usually, with diiodohydroxyquin as well (see Chapter 26).

HSV may be and cryptococcosis is associated with the acquired immunodeficiency syndrome (AIDS). Accordingly, these patients need overall management of their disease in all of its manifestations (see Chapter 34). With respect to the specific treatment of HSV proctitis, mild cases may respond to a symptomatic approach with sitz baths and a topical cream containing lidocaine. More severe disease requires the use of topical, oral, or even parenteral acyclovir. Cryptococcal anal ulceration usually necessitates local surgical treatment. In addition, if it is a manifestation of systemic infection, as it usually is, parenteral amphotericin B should be used as well. Topical amphotericin B is ineffective.

General References

Goligher JC: *Surgery of the Anus, Rectum and Colon,* 4th ed. London, Bailliere Tindall, 1980.
Lieberman DA: Common anorectal disorders. *Ann Intern Med* 101:837, 1984.
Thompson JP, Nicholls RJ, Williams CB: *Colorectal Disease.* New York, Appleton-Century-Crofts, 1981.

Specific References

1. Lewis AAM, Rogers HS, Leighton M: Trial of maximal anal dilatation, cryotherapy and elastic band ligation as alternatives to haemorrhoidectomy in the treatment of large prolapsing haemorrhoids. *Br J Surg* 70:54, 1983.
2. Murie AJ, Sim AJW, Mackenzie I: Rubber band ligation versus haemorrhoidectomy for prolapsing haemorrhoids: a long term prospective clinical trial. *Br J Surg* 69:536, 1982.
3. Nivatvongs S, Goldberg SM: An improved technique of rubber band ligation of hemorrhoids. *Am J Surg* 144:379, 1982.
4. Peppercorn MA: Enteric infections in hemosexual men with and without AIDS. *Contemp Gastroenterol* 2:23, 1989.
5. Quinn TC: Gay bowel syndrome. The broadened spectrum of nongenital infection. *Postgrad Med* 76:197, 1984.
6. *Med Lett* vol 17:1975.
7. Thomson HJ: Rectal disease. Nonsurgical treatment of haemorrhoids. *Br J Hosp Med* 24:298, 1980.

Gynecological Problems

C H A P T E R 93

Birth Control*

GEORGE R. HUGGINS, M.D.

The avoidance of an unplanned or unwanted pregnancy is the decision of the patient and of her partner. In consultation with the physician, she (or they) acquires knowledge of the available contraceptive methods and then is helped in carrying out a satisfactory program.

There are many contraceptive methods (18). It is important for the physician to understand the limits and risks of all of them to be able to educate the patient fully about her options. The physician must be prepared to deal with patients who have varying knowledge and experience about contraception. Table 93.1 lists the current percentage distribution of use of contraceptive methods by married women in the United States.

Figure 93.1 shows the risks of using various methods of contraception. The figure displays the data that are provided in all oral contraceptive packages that are sold to patients. There is a low mortality rate associated with all methods in patients under 30 so that younger women have a wide choice. On the other hand, a patient who is over 35 years of age has a greater risk with oral contraceptives, and the physician must inform patients of these risks.

The theoretical and actual effectiveness of various

---

*Dr. J. Courtland Robinson contributed to this Chapter in the first and second editions of this book.

Table 93.1.
Contraceptive Use among Married Women at Risk[a, b]

Contraceptive Status	US Women Aged 15–44 (N = 6755)
TYPE USED	92
Oral contraceptive	27
IUD	6
Female sterilization	19
Male sterilization	13
Condom	12
Withdrawal	3
Diaphragm/cap	5
Rhythm	2
Other	5
NONE USED	8
TOTAL	100.0

[a] Adapted from Forrest JD, Henshaw SK: What US women think and do about contraception. *Fam Plan Perspect* 15:157, 1983.
[b] Percentage distribution of contraceptive use among married women at risk of pregnancy (including the contraceptively sterilized), arranged by method, United States, 1981.

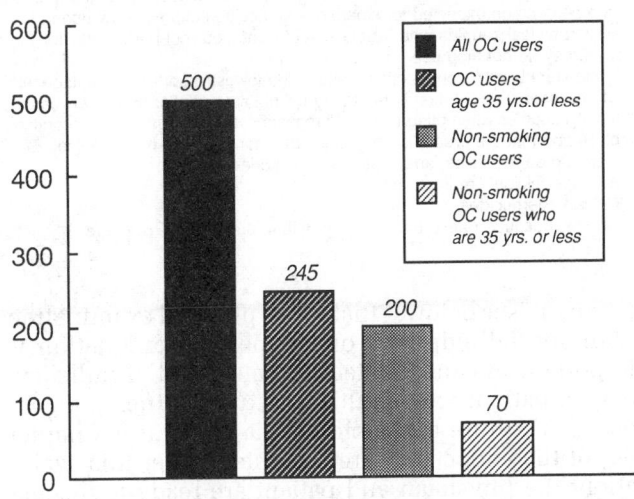

Estimated Number of Annual Deaths Among the Approximate 10 Million Oral Contraceptive Users in the United States

Figure 93.1. Adapted from Ory HW, Forrest JD, Lincoln R: *Making Choices: Evaluating the Health Risks and Benefits of Birth Control Methods.* New York: The Alan Guttmacher Institute, 1983.

methods of contraception is shown in Table 93.2. Theoretical effectiveness is determined in very carefully controlled studies in which a method is used exactly as it was designed to be used. Actual effectiveness is a measure of what is found when a method is used by large numbers of people in a less controlled manner. Clearly there is very little difference between the theoretical and actual effectiveness of some methods, whereas others show a considerable difference. This information should be used in helping to educate the patient.

Once it is established that fertility regulation is desired by the patient, a careful medical history should be obtained, including information about past pregnancies, menstruation, smoking, and family history that might suggest a contraindication to her getting

Table 93.2.
Lowest Expected Typical and Lowest Reported Failure Rates during the First Year of Use of a Method and First-Year Continuation Rates in the United States[a]

Method (1)	% of Women Experiencing an Accidental Pregnancy in the First Year of Use			% of Women Continuing Use at 1 Year[e]	
	Lowest Expected[b] (2)	Typical[c] (3)	Lowest Reported[d] (4)	Exc. Preg. (5)	Inc. Preg (6)
Chance	89	89			
Spermicides[f]	3	21	0	55	43
Periodic abstinence		20		84	67
Withdrawal	4	18	7[i]		
Cap[g]	5	18	8	77	63
Sponge	5 nullips	18 nullips	14 nullips	73	60
	> 8 parous	>28 parous	28 parous	73	<53
Diaphragm[g]	3	18	2	69	57
Condom[h]	2	12	4[i]	73	64
IUD		6		74	70
Medicated	1		0.5		
Non-medicated	2		3		
Pill		3		75	73
Combined	0.1		0		
Female sterilization	0.2	0.4	0		
Male sterilization	0.1	0.15	0		

[a] Adapted from the Population Council, from James Trussell and Kathryn Kost: Contraceptive failure in the United States: a critical review of the literature. Studies in Family Planning 18(5), September/October, 1987. Tables 1 and 2.
[b] Among couples who initiate use of a method (not necessarily for the first time) and who use it perfectly (both consistently and correctly), the authors' best guess of the percentage expected to experience an accidental pregnancy during the first year if they do not stop use for any other reason.
[c] Among typical couples who initiate use of a method (not necessarily for the first time), the percentage who experienced an accidental pregnancy during the first year if they do not stop use for any other reason.
[d] In the literature on contraceptive failure, the lowest reported percentage who experienced an accidental pregnancy during the first year following initiation of use (not necessarily for the first time) if they did not stop use for any other reason; however, see footnote [h].
[e] Among couples attempting to avoid pregnancy, the percentage who continue to use a method, under the alternative assumptions that no one becomes pregnant (col. 5) and that the proportion becoming pregnant is given by col. 2 (col. 6).
[f] Foams, creams, jellies, and vaginal suppositories.
[g] With spermicidal cream or jelly.
[h] Without spermicides.
[i] Too low, because rate is based on more than one year of exposure.

pregnant (see below, "Risks"). A physical examination with special emphasis on the pelvic examination is important. A cancer detection smear and, if indicated (e.g., a patient with multiple sexual partners), a gonococcus culture and a chlamydia smear (see Chapter 94) of the endocervix are suggested. After this evaluation, the physician and patient are ready to discuss the various contraceptive methods and to develop a satisfactory plan.

Although fertility declines with increasing age, protection is necessary until menopause (see Chapter 77). The uncertainty about pregnancy is further compounded by the increasing rate of abnormal menstrual cycles and, in particular, episodes of amenorrhea, as a woman gets older. Missing a period is very disturbing to a woman in the perimenopause unless a very reliable method of contraception is being used.

The postpartum patient needs help in getting back on a contraceptive program, and usually her obstetrician will have given her advice in this regard. In general, all methods are suitable for the healthy patient except for the breast-feeding mother, who should avoid the oral contraceptives. Also, the patient wishing to use an intrauterine device (IUD) will need to wait for involution of the uterus—which usually occurs 4 to 6 weeks postpartum—and, therefore, is at risk for pregnancy until the IUD is inserted.

THE ORAL CONTRACEPTIVE

Mechanism of Action

Oral contraceptives prevent ovulation by inhibition of gonadotropin-releasing factors in the hypothalamus. The principal effect of this inhibition appears to be suppression of the surge in activity of luteinizing hormone at midcycle, thereby removing a major stimulus to ovulation. In addition, oral contraceptives make cervical mucus more viscid and therefore less easily traversed by sperm. They also have a direct effect on endometrial development, making the uterus less receptive to implantation of the fertilized ovum (3).

Preparations and Dosage Schedules

The combined oral contraceptive was first introduced for use in the United States in 1960. In the ensuing years there have been significant changes made in steroid dosages. However, the hormones in the third generation oral contraceptives of today are the same found in the original pills introduced in 1960. Since 1970, all new oral contraceptives introduced in this country have contained ethinyl estradiol as their estrogen. Although there were more than 8 different progestins marketed commercially, today over 90% of currently used oral contraceptives contain either norethindrone or levo-norgestrel. Of the two, levo-norgestrel is by far the more potent.

There have been at least five different modes of administration:

1. The monophasic combined oral contraceptive, which contains the same dose of estrogen and progesterone for 21 days each cycle.
2. The now discontinued sequential oral contraceptives, which contained estrogen only for the first 2 weeks and a combination of estrogen and progestin for the last week of administration. These oral contraceptives were removed from the market in the early 1970s after reports of adenocarcinoma of the endometrium occurring in women under the age of 40 who took one particular brand of sequential pills.
3. The "mini-pill," which consists of daily continuous administration of progestin only. The progestin-only preparations do not consistently inhibit ovulation, and unwanted pregnancy is three to five times more likely than oral contraceptives that contain estrogen and progestogen. They should be prescribed, therefore, only for patients who cannot be given estrogen (e.g., those with a history of thromboembolism). Very few patients are taking these medications at present.
4. A biphasic regimen, which contains a low dose of estrogen for 21 days. The progestin dose in the first half of the cycle is essentially half the progestin dose in the second half.
5. The new triphasic oral contraceptives vary the progestin dose each week. Two of the three available preparations have a steady dose of ethinyl estradiol (35 µg). The third medication varies the estrogen dose from 30 to 40 µg.

Many of the currently available oral contraceptive preparations are listed in Table 93.3.

Absolute contraindications to oral contraceptives are listed in Table 93.4.

If oral contraception is selected, then the first choice should be a combination preparation containing 30 to 35 µg of estrogen and 1 mg or less of progestin. Occasionally it will be necessary to change to a higher dose of estrogen in order to control breakthrough bleeding (see below). However, preparations containing greater than 35 µg of an estrogen should be used only for a short period of time (e.g., two or three menstrual cycles). If higher doses seem necessary because there is no withdrawal bleeding or there continues to be breakthrough bleeding, consultation with an obstetrician-gynecologist is suggested.

In order to suppress ovulation and yet allow periodic bleeding the combination tablet is taken every day for 3 weeks. This cycle is accomplished by packaging the tablets for use during either a 21- or 28-day period and having the patient start the medication on the fifth day of her cycle, counting the first day of menstrual bleeding as day 1. An alternative is to start on the first Sunday after the onset of a menstrual period. This latter practice allows the packaging of the tablets to provide for the user a minicalendar, which minimizes missing a dose. The tablets are arranged in either circles or rows making it easier to use them regularly. The 21-day formulation and the 28-day formulation are packaging techniques to improve compliance. In all 28-day preparations the last seven tablets have no hormonal effect and are there only to keep the patient on schedule. The drop in hormone level after 21 days produces withdrawal bleeding just as it does in the normal menstrual cycle.

When a postpartum woman selects an oral contraceptive for contraception, it is initiated within a few days after parturition. Patients who have had a spontaneous or therapeutic abortion may start taking the drug on the first Sunday following the event. However, oral contraceptives are usually avoided in women who are breast feeding as the medication appears in the milk.

Benefits

In the past few years oral contraceptives have been found to be associated with a significant number of beneficial side effects. These involve a decreased risk of benign breast tumors, functional ovarian cysts, pelvic inflammatory disease, endometrial carcinoma, and carcinoma of the ovary. Table 93.5 depicts the estimated number of hospitalizations averted each year in the United States by oral contraceptive usage.

Taking into consideration the number of deaths averted by oral contraceptives because of the protective effect for ovarian and endometrial carcinoma, on balance, there are probably more deaths averted by oral contraceptive usage than caused by oral contraceptive use.

Recognition of these noncontraceptive benefits of oral contraceptives helps to place them in a much more positive perspective for patients and, indeed, puts the risk:benefit ratio of oral contraceptives in a more proper perspective.

Risks

Thromboembolic Disease

In the late 1960s the first epidemiological studies conducted in Great Britain and the United States showed an increased risk of thromboembolic disorders and myocardial infarction among oral contraceptive users. Very quickly it was determined that the risk of thrombophlebitis and other vascular accidents was related to the dose of estrogen, the age of the patient, and whether the patient was a smoker or nonsmoker (7, 14). Decreasing the estrogen dosage in the oral contraceptives from 80 to 50 µg achieved approximately a 30% reduction in incidence of thromboembolic disease. A further reduction from 50 µg into the range of 30 to 35 µg further decreased the risk of venous thrombosis and other serious vascular complications. In this country there are still substantial numbers of patients

Table 93.3.
Some Oral Contraceptives

Drug	Estrogen (mcg)	mcg per month	Progestin (mg)[a]	mg per month	Cost[b]
COMBINATION					
Loestrin 1/20 21, 28-Parke-Davis	Ethinyl estradiol (20)	420	Norethindrone acetate (1)	21	$15.47
Loestrin 1.5/30 21, 28-Parke-Davis	Ethinyl estradiol (30)	630	Norethindrone acetate (1.5)	31.5	15.47
Nordette 21 - Wyeth-Ayerst[c]	Ethinyl estradiol (30)	630	Levonorgestrel (0.15)	3.15	15.23
Levlen 21, 28 - Berlex	Ethinyl estradiol (30)	630	Levonorgestrel (0.15)	3.15	13.60
Lo/Ovral 21 - Wyeth-Ayerst[c]	Ethinyl estradiol (30)	630	Norgestrel (0.3)	6.3	15.94
Triphasil 21 - Wyeth-Ayerst[c]	Ethinyl estradiol (30,40)	680	Levonorgestrel (0.05, 0.075,0.125)	1.925	14.18
Tri-Levlen 21, 28 - Berlex	Ethinyl estradiol (30,40)	680	Levonorgestrel (0.05, 0.075,0.125)	1.925	12.98
Brevicon 21, 28 - Syntex	Ethinyl estradiol (35)	735	Norethindrone (0.5)	10.5	13.95
Modicon 21 - Ortho[c]	Ethinyl estradiol (35)	735	Norethindrone (0.5)	10.5	14.84
Genora 0.5/35 21, 28-Rugby	Ethinyl estradiol (35)	735	Norethindrone (0.5)	10.5	7.44
Nelova 0.5/35 21, 28-Watson	Ethinyl estradiol (35)	735	Norethindrone (0.5)	10.5	9.78
Norinyl 1 + 35 21, 28-Syntex	Ethinyl estradiol (35)	735	Norethindrone (1)	21	13.95
Norinyl 1/35 21, 28-Searle	Ethinyl estradiol (35)	735	Norethindrone (1)	21	8.15
Nelova 1/35 21, 28-Watson	Ethinyl estradiol (35)	735	Norethindrone (1)	21	9.78
Genora 1/35 21, 28-Rugby	Ethinyl estradiol (35)	735	Norethindrone (1)	21	11.00
Ortho-Novum 1/35 21-Ortho[c]	Ethinyl estradiol (35)	735	Norethindrone (1)	21	13.64
Tri-Norinyl 21, 28-Syntex	Ethinyl estradiol (35)	735	Norethindrone (0.5, 1.0)	15	13.95
Ortho-Novum 7/7/7 21-Ortho[c]	Ethinyl estradiol (35)	735	Norethindrone (0.5, 0.75, 1.0)	15.75	14.67
Ortho-Novum 10/11 21-Ortho[c]	Ethinyl estradiol (35)	735	Norethindrone (0.5, 1.0)	16	13.58
Nelova 10/11 21, 28-Watson	Ethinyl estradiol (35)	735	Norethindrone (05, 1.0)	16	9.78
Ovcon 35 21, 28 Mead Johnson	Ethinyl estradiol (35)	735	Norethindrone (0.4)	8.4	14.68
Demulen 1/35 21 - Searle[c]	Ethinyl estradiol (35)	735	Ethynodiol diacetate (1)	21	15.56
Norlestrin 1/50 21, 28-Parke-Davis	Ethinyl estradiol (50)	1050	Norethindrone acetate (1)	21	15.35
Ovcon 50 21, 28-Mead Johnson	Ethinyl estradiol (50)	1050	Norethindrone (1)	21	14.68
Genora 1/50 21, 28-Rugby	Ethinyl estradiol (50)	1050	Norethindrone (1)	21	11.00
Norlestrin 2.5/50 21, 28-Parke-Davis	Ethinyl estradiol (50)	1050	Norethindrone acetate (2.5)	52.5	15.80
Demulen 1/50 21-Searle[c]	Ethinyl estradiol (50)	1050	Ethynodiol diacetate (1)	21	17.32
Ovral 21-Wyeth-Ayerst[c]	Ethinyl estradiol (50)	1050	Norgestrel (0.5)	10.5	18.25
Norinyl 1 + 50 21, 28-Syntex	Mestranol (50)	1050	Norethindrone (1)	21	13.95
Ortho-Novum 1/50 21-Ortho[c]	Mestranol (50)	1050	Norethindrone (1)	21	13.64
Norethin 1/50 21, 28-Searle	Mestranol (50)	1050	Norethindrone (1)	21	8.15
Nelova 1/50 21, 28-Watson	Mestranol (50)	1050	Norethindrone (1)	21	9.78
PROGESTIN ONLY					
Ovrette-Wyeth-Ayerst	None		Norgestrel (0.075)	2.1	15.67
Nor-QD-Syntex	None		Norethindrone (0.35)	9.8	8.34
Micronor-Ortho	None		Norethindrone (0.35)	9.8	17.17

[a] Different progestins cannot be compared on a milligram basis.
[b] Cost to pharmacist for one month's use, based on manufacturer's listings in *Drug Topics Red Book, 1988,* and *October Update.*
[c] Also available in 28-day regimens at slightly higher cost.

Table 93.4.
Absolute Contraindications to Oral Contraceptives

Thrombophlebitis or thromboembolic disorders (current or remote)
Cerebral vascular or coronary artery disease (current or remote)
Known or suspected carcinoma of the breast
Known or suspected estrogen-dependent neoplasia
Undiagnosed, abnormal genital bleeding
Known or suspected pregnancy

who are taking medications with 50 μg or more of estrogen. Unfortunately, the group of patients using the greatest proportion of high dose estrogen preparations are those older than age 35.

Approximately 10 million women in the United States are current oral contraceptive users. Cardiovascular problems, heart attack, stroke, thrombophlebitis, and pulmonary emboli are the main causes of serious morbidity and death associated with oral contraceptive use. There are approximately 500 oral contraceptive-related deaths each year among this 10 million cohort of uses (11).

Age and smoking play a significant role in determining risk of serious cardiovascular events (see Fig. 93.1). An estimated 86% of deaths associated with oral contraceptive use result from a combination of smoking and pill use by women aged 35 and older. Because of the risk of thromboembolism oral contraceptives should be discontinued 30 days before major surgery. They need not be discontinued before minor surgery.

If all oral contraceptive users over the age of 35 were eliminated from studies, the estimated number of deaths could be cut by more than half, to approximately 245 per 10 million oral contraceptive users in the United States in a given year. Furthermore, if all smokers were eliminated from studies, the number of deaths could be reduced to approximately 240 deaths per year.

Most significantly, if there were no oral contraceptive takers who smoked or who were over the age of

Table 93.5.
Noncontraceptive Health Benefits of Oral Contraceptives

Rate of hospitalizations prevented and deaths averted annually by use of oral contraceptives, per 100,000 pill users, and estimated number of hospitalizations and deaths prevented annually, by specific disease in the United States[a]

Disease	Rate of Hospitalizations Prevented per 1,000,000 Pill Users	Number of Hospitalizations Prevented	Number of Deaths Averted
Benign breast disease	235	20,000	
Ovarian retention cysts	35	3,000	
Iron deficiency anemia[b]	320	27,000	
Pelvic inflammatory disease (first episodes)			
Total episodes[b]	600	51,000	100
Hospitalizations	156	13,300	
Ectopic pregnancy	117	9,900	10
Endometrial cancer[c]	5	2,000	100
Ovarian cancer[c]	4	1,700	1,000

Adapted from: Ory HW: The noncontraceptive health benefits from oral contraceptive use. *Family Plan Perspect* 14:182, 1982.
[a] Except where noted, figures refer to hospitalizations prevented among the estimated 8.5 million current users of oral contraceptives in the United States.
[b] Episodes prevented regardless of whether hospitalization occurred.
[c] Based on an estimated 39 million U.S. women who have ever used oral contraceptives.

35, the estimated number of deaths could be reduced from 500 to approximately 70 per 10 million oral contraceptive users in the United States in a given year. Clearly, for nonsmokers and women under 35 years, the oral contraceptives are safe medications.

Hypertension

With the older high dose oral contraceptives, the risk of developing high blood pressure was approximately 7%. With the new low dose preparations (under 50 μg of estrogen) evaluated in controlled studies, no significant hypertension resulting from the oral contraceptive has been identified. As such, if an oral contraceptive user develops hypertension, the hypertension should be promptly evaluated and not be ascribed to contraceptive usage. Women with pre-existing hypertension or with a family or personal history of hypertension are probably no more likely to develop high blood pressure when they take the new low dose oral contraceptive preparations.

Neoplasia

After 30 years of use the data concerning the relationship between oral contraceptive use and neoplasia are mostly reassuring (Table 93.6).

There is a relationship between the long-term use of oral contraceptives and the development of benign hepatic neoplasia (4). These lesions are extraordinarily rare and although the increased relative risk of developing one of these lesions in long-term users is high, the absolute incidence is very low. Long-term use of oral contraceptives has been associated with a significantly decreased incidence of both endometrial and ovarian cancer (15). This "protective effect" of oral contraceptives appears to be directly related to the length of usage, and the protective effect appears to persist for more than 5 years after discontinuing oral contraceptives.

There appears to be no relationship between oral contraceptive use and the development of either breast cancer or pituitary adenoma. The data are inconclusive for malignant melanoma and cervical neoplasia. With regard to the development of cervical neoplasia, there have been several recent studies that have shown a slightly increased risk directly related to the length of oral contraceptive use (1). Nevertheless, no firm conclusions can be drawn at this time.

The incidence of benign breast tumors and of fibrocystic disease is reduced by the administration of high progestin dose oral contraceptive hormones. Data on the newer low dose progestin contraceptive pills are inconclusive (9).

Altered Metabolism of Glucose or Lipids

With the oral contraceptives that contain greater than 50 μg of estrogen abnormal glucose tolerance tests could be seen after 3 months of use. This reduction in glucose tolerance is not, however, seen with the new low dose preparations. Also the new triphasic and low dose forms do not appear to alter the lipid profile even in long-term users whereas the high dose preparations (>50 μg of estrogen) adversely effect the lipid profile.

Gallbladder Disease

There is a 2-fold increase in the incidence of gallbladder disease requiring surgery within the first 1 to 2 years of oral contraceptive use. An estrogen-associated increase in the concentration of cholesterol in the bile has been demonstrated in patients taking oral

Table 93.6.
Oral Contraceptives and Neoplasia Risk

	Increased	No Effect	Decreased	Inconclusive Information
Hepatocellular adenoma	X			
Cervical neoplasia				X
Endometrial cancer			X	
Ovarian cancer			X	
Breast cancer		X		
Pituitary adenoma		X		
Malignant melanoma				X

contraceptives and may be the pathogenetic mechanism.

Headaches

Some patients with a history of migraine headaches will note a worsening of these headaches after oral contraceptive use. The development of severe recurrent headaches is a reason to recommend another contraceptive method.

Birth Defects

The relationship between hormonal ingestion during the first 3 months of pregnancy and the subsequent development of birth defects is uncertain. Initial epidemiological studies done in the 1960s and early 70s seem to favor an association with some cardiovascular and limb defects. More recent studies have tended to refute this association. There is no evidence that prior use of contraceptives has any effect on the development of any birth defect. Establishing a pregnancy within one to two cycles after discontinuation of oral contraceptives is not associated with a higher incidence of birth defects (8) and is therefore the recommended practice when pregnancy is desired.

Other Side Effects

In general, minor side effects occur early in the course of taking oral contraceptives and may be transient. Thorough education by the physician will increase the likelihood that the patient will tolerate these effects and will continue taking the medication.

Alopecia. Alopecia rarely is a reported side effect (see Chapter 100). Most often it is transient; but if hair loss is reported for greater than 3 months, the drug should be discontinued and the patient should use some other form of contraception.

Nausea. Nausea occurs in approximately 5% of patients but can almost always be eliminated by taking the contraceptive at bedtime.

Fatigue. Increased fatigability is occasionally described by patients but usually is of short duration.

Change in Menstrual Flow. The most typical pattern is a reduction in the amount and duration of menstrual flow. This is usually welcomed by the patient. On occasion, there will be no bleeding; and if the patient has taken the oral contraceptive regularly (so that pregnancy is not likely), she can be advised to continue it for another cycle. If she is again amenorrheic, a pregnancy test (see below) should be done. If pregnancy is ruled out, the patient can either select another contraceptive method or can be placed temporarily on a preparation with a slightly higher estrogen content, which results in more menstrual bleeding.

Breakthrough Bleeding. Breakthrough bleeding is most common in the early cycles after initiation of an oral contraceptive. It is of no concern as long as the patient has not missed a dose. Failure to take daily doses increases the chance of breakthrough bleeding, particularly in the early part of the cycle. If a dose or two has been forgotten early in the cycle, the patient should catch up and continue the normal regimen together with temporary use of a barrier form of protection. If breakthrough bleeding continues for several cycles, referral to a gynecologist is indicated to rule out an organic cause and to consider using a higher dose of estrogen.

Weight Gain. About 5% of patients will show some weight gain, sometimes associated with fluid retention.

Vaginitis. It has been difficult to document a close relationship between oral contraceptives and vaginitis. The hormones do alter the vaginal milieu, but vaginitis will develop in only a small proportion of patients. Standard diagnostic methods and subsequent therapy (see Chapter 94) will allow the vast majority of patients to continue to use the oral contraceptive.

Skin Changes. Some patients, especially dark-skinned individuals, will note chloasma (yellowish-brown discoloration of the skin) and a change in hair texture. Chloasma is unlikely to resolve with continued administration of the oral contraceptive and is, therefore, a reason to discontinue it if the cosmetic effect is unacceptable.

Emotional Changes. Some women have become depressed while taking oral contraceptives. Therefore, patients who have a history of depression should be followed especially carefully. If depression develops, the medication should be discontinued.

Effects on Laboratory Tests. Oral contraceptives can alter the results of a number of laboratory tests (16). The alterations reflect physiological changes in the patient in most instances but rarely signify clinically significant disease. Table 93.7 lists alteration in selected laboratory tests.

Drug Interactions. Oral contraceptives may alter the effectiveness of a number of other drugs; and, conversely, a number of other drugs may alter the effectiveness of oral contraceptives. Physicians should investigate the possibility of drug interaction before prescribing any other medication to a patient using an oral contraceptive preparation. Table 93.8 lists drugs that may interact with oral contraceptives.

Patient Follow-Up. A patient taking oral contraceptives should see a physician twice a year for an interim history (including a menstrual history) and any tests warranted by this evaluation. Any possible change in family planning should be discussed at that time. Once a year a pelvic examination should be done, which should include a cervical smear for cytology (at an appropriate interval, see Chapter 95). Sexually transmitted diseases (see Chapter 94) may need to be screened for if there are multiple sexual partners. Oral contraceptives may be discontinued at any time if pregnancy is desired or another method of contraception is planned. The first few menstrual periods after withdrawal may be heavier than during the time oral contraceptives were used. There is no change in fertility after a course of oral contraceptives.

Table 93.7.
Effects of Oral Contraceptives on Selected Laboratory Tests[a]

Laboratory Test	Effects	Probable Mechanism
SERUM, PLASMA, BLOOD		
Albumin	Slightly decreased	Decreased hepatic synthesis
Aldosterone	Increased	Activates renin-angiotensin system
Amylase	Slightly increased (common) Markedly increased (rare)	Pancreatitis
Antinuclear antibodies	Become detectable	Not established
Bilirubin	Increased (rare)	Reduced secretion into bile
Coagulation factors	Increased II, VII, IX, X	Increased synthesis
Cortisol	Increased	Increased cortisol-binding globulin Urinary free cortisol unchanged
Folate	Decreased or no change	Decreased folate absorption
Haptoglobin	Decreased	Decreased hepatic synthesis
High density lipoprotein cholesterol	Increased with estrogens and decreased with progestins	Not established
Iron-binding capacity	Increased	Increased transferrin levels
Magnesium	Decreased or no change	Decreased bone resorption
Phosphatase, alkaline	Increased (rare)	Altered secretion in bile
Platelets	Slightly increased	Not established
Prolactin	Increased	Not established
Renin activity	Increased	Increased synthesis of renin substrate
Thyroxine (total)	Increased	Increased thyroxine-binding globulin
Transaminases	Slightly increased	Not established
Triiodothyronine	Decreased	Increased thyroxine-binding globulin
Vitamin B$_{12}$	Decreased	Not established
URINE		
δ-Aminolevulinic acid	Increased	Increased hepatic synthesis
Calcium	Decreased	Decreased bone resorption
Porphyrins	Increased (may precipitate porphyria in susceptible patients)	Increased aminolevulinic acid synthetase
17-Hydroxycorticosteriods	Slightly decreased or no change	Increased binding proteins
17-Ketosteroids	Slightly decreased or no change	Increased binding proteins

[a] Adapted from *Med Lett Drugs Ther* 21:54, 1979.

INTRAUTERINE DEVICE

The intrauterine device (IUD) is one of the most effective methods of contraception, although its exact mode of action is unknown. Pregnancy rates range from one to three per 100 women per year. The first modern IUDs appeared in the early 1960s and were made of a biologically inert plastic. The second generation IUDs, copper- and progesterone-containing devices, have been available since the early 1970s (12).

During the late 1970s serious concerns were raised concerning the safety of all IUDs. Studies showed a strong relationship between IUD use and the development of pelvic inflammatory disease. The Dalkon Shield specifically was removed from the market because of its link to spontaneous septic abortions and pelvic inflammatory disease. The clearly increased risk for infection with this product has been attributed to the multifilament (versus monofilament on other IUDs) tail (the string that hangs into the vagina), which seemed to act as a wick for bacteria. Because of the publicity from the Dalkon Shield, distribution of other devices was discontinued by the manufacturers because of low sales volume or concern regarding litigation costs. The ongoing concern over the relationship between IUD use and the development of pelvic inflammatory disease with resultant tubal infertility is valid. However, epide-miological studies in the 1970s tended to overstate the risk of pelvic infection from IUD use. The reasons for this are:

1. In most early studies the control group included women who were using diaphragms and oral contraceptives. These are protective against pelvic inflammatory disease.
2. The risks for specific IUD devices were not analyzed separately. Dalkon Shield wearers, with substantially higher risk of infection, were included in most analyses.
3. Most studies did not analyze for factors that significantly affect risk of pelvic inflammatory disease, such as multiple sexual partners and previous history of pelvic infection.

Recent epidemiological studies have adjusted the relative risks of tubal infertility by type of IUD used and number of sexual partners. They have shown that women who had only one sexual partner in their lifetime had no significantly increased risk of tubal infertility. However, women who had more then one sexual partner had a three to four times higher risk (2). At present, IUD use is recommended only for women who desire no further pregnancies and who are in a mutually faithful monogamous relationship.

Table 93.8.
Selected Drugs That May Interact with Oral Contraceptive Preparations (OCPs)

Drugs that may decrease the effectiveness of OCPs resulting in breakthrough bleeding, pregnancy, or both:

A. Well-established, relatively commonly occurring drug reactions
  1. Anticonvulsants-barbiturates, phenytoin (Dilantin), or primidone (Mysoline)
  2. Antimicrobials-Rifampicin
B. Reported instances of possible drug interactions
  1. Antimicrobials
    a. (Breakthrough bleeding only)—Neomycin, Nitrofurantoin, phenoxymethylpenicillin (penicillin V)
    b. (Breakthrough bleeding and pregnancy)—Ampicillin, chloramphenicol, sulfamethoxypridaxine (Kynex, Midicel)
  2. Others—Chlordiazepoxide (Librium), meprobamate, Phenacetin, and phenylbutazone (Butazolidin)

Drugs whose effectiveness may be altered by OCPs:

A. Anticoagulants—The effect of anticoagulants may be reduced by the simultaneous administration of OCPs.
B. Clofibrate (Atromid-S)—Control of cholesterol and triglyceride levels may be lost when OCPs are simultaneously administered with clofibrate.
C. Thyroid hormone in patients without functioning thyroid gland—Mostly a theoretical concern; however, there may be a need for an increased dose of thyroid hormone in patients without a functioning thyroid gland.
D. Tricyclic antidepressants—Higher doses of estrogen may inhibit effect of antidepressants, and tricyclic toxicity may be increased.
E. Caffeine—There may be decreased metabolism of caffeine induced by OCPs. Patients who take large amounts of caffeine (e.g., 4–8 cups of coffee/day) should be cautioned regarding symptoms of caffeinism.

Types

There are two types of intrauterine devices available in the United States: The Progestasert and the ParaGard. The Progestasert is a plastic T-shaped device that contains a reservoir of 38 mg of progesterone in the vertical bar. This progesterone is released at a rate of 65 μg per day and exerts a local contraceptive effect. The progesterone reservoir is depleted after 12 months and the device must then be removed and replaced by a new one. A longer lasting levo-norgestrel-releasing IUD has been successfully tested but is not yet available. The ParaGard device has a body of polyethylene wound with copper wire and has a copper collar on each of its transverse arms (19). Clinical trials have shown that this device is effective for at least 5 years. Currently it is approved by the Food and Drug Administration (FDA) for 4 years of continuous use. This is a major benefit when compared with the Progestasert system, which is approved for only 1 year of continuous use.

Use and Insertion

If the physician is not experienced in IUD insertion, the patient should be referred to a gynecologist. The IUD is best inserted at the time of a menstrual period. The usual small amount of bleeding associated with insertion becomes a part of the normal menstrual flow; it is assurance that the patient is not pregnant, and it is easier to insert because the cervix is slightly dilated. The patient thereafter will usually notice some increased bleeding with her periods and possibly some increased cramping.

Patient Experience. Most often the patient experiences some cramps when the IUD is inserted. Nonsteroidal analgesics before the insertion (e.g., ibuprofen, 400 mg) affords some relief. These cramps usually subside in a few hours. Rarely they may be so severe as to necessitate removal of the device. If they persist beyond a few hours, this may be an indication that the device is not inserted properly and the device should be removed.

Risks

Contraindications to the use of an IUD are shown in Table 93.9. The most common serious side effect is the development of pelvic inflammatory disease. The patient must be instructed to report any fever, pelvic pain, or discomfort promptly. She must also report any missed menstrual periods since this mandates that she be evaluated for pregnancy. The patient who has missed a menstrual period must be evaluated also for ectopic pregnancy since the IUD prevents only intrauterine pregnancy. A patient who becomes pregnant with an IUD in place has a 5% risk of ectopic pregnancy and a 50% risk of spontaneous abortion. If the IUD strings are visible, the spontaneous abortion rate can be reduced to approximately 25% by removal of the IUD. Uterine perforation, a rare complication, is most likely to occur at the time of insertion. Finally, the use of the intrauterine device by a young nulliparous patient who has multiple sex partners is associated with a significantly increased incidence of uterine infection.

Table 93.9.
Contraindications

The IUD should not be inserted when one or more of the following conditions exist:

1. Pregnancy or suspicion of pregnancy.
2. Abnormalities of the uterus resulting in distortion of the uterine cavity.
3. Acute pelvic inflammatory disease or a history of pelvic inflammatory disease.
4. Postpartum endometritis or infected abortion in the past 3 months.
5. Known or suspected uterine or cervical malignancy, including unresolved, abnormal "Pap" smear.
6. Genital bleeding of unknown etiology.
7. Untreated acute cervicitis until infection is controlled.
8. Wilson's disease (copper-containing IUDs).
9. Known allergy to copper.
10. History of ectopic pregnancy.
11. Patient or her partner has multiple sexual partners.
12. Conditions associated with increased susceptibility to infections with micro-organisms. Such conditions include leukemia, diabetes, acquired immune deficiency syndrome (AIDS), and those requiring chronic corticosteroid therapy as examples.
13. Genital actinomycosis.
14. A previously inserted IUD that has not been removed.

Monitoring

There should be an annual follow-up at which time there should be a review of any problems, a pelvic examination including a cervical cancer smear, a gonorrhea culture and a chlamydia culture (if either is indicated), and detection of the device. The follow-up is best done by a gynecologist if the general physician is not experienced in managing patients with an IUD.

The IUD is easily removed by gentle traction on the string at or around the time of a menstrual period. Removal at this time allows the bleeding associated with removal to be part of the menstrual period. Also, it is easier to remove during menstruation than later in the cycle (see above).

As with oral contraceptives, if a patient terminates this form of contraception other than to attempt pregnancy, she will need help in choosing another form of contraception.

THE SPONGE

The sponge is a barrier contraceptive device. It is a small, donut-shaped, polyurethane plastic device filled with nonoxynol-9 (a spermicidal agent) that is placed high in the vagina before intercourse. Unlike the diaphragm (see below), it comes in one size. Studies have suggested that the pregnancy rate with the sponge is approximately that experienced with the diaphragm (15 to 18%). It should remain in the vagina no longer than 24 hours and should not be removed before 6 hours after intercourse. It is discarded after removal. If left in place longer than 24 hours, vaginal irritation may result. The chief advantages of the sponge are that it is available over the counter, it may be inserted well ahead of need, and intercourse may be repeated without further preparation. It is suggested for women having infrequent sexual intercourse, for postpartum patients, and for young women just starting to have intercourse for whom the diaphragm may be too complicated (6). Rare occurrence of toxic shock syndrome has been reported with the use of the sponge (see Chapter 94).

THE DIAPHRAGM

The diaphragm is a dome-shaped rubber device that is held open by a metallic band or spring. It is filled with a spermicidal cream or jelly before each use and placed in the vagina over the cervix to prevent sperm deposited during ejaculation from reaching the cervical os. As seen in Table 93.2, the theoretical effectiveness is much better than actual effectiveness, as is true of all barrier methods.

The diaphragm is fitted by a physician or an assistant. For better effectiveness, the patient should be asked to insert the diaphragm and have the physician or assistant check its placement. The device fits in the posterior fornix and tucks up behind the symphysis. The largest device that is comfortable is the proper one to use. Manufacturers of diaphragms have excellent booklets that are useful in helping a patient acquire the skill necessary for comfortable use of this form of contraception.

The patient will apply the spermicidal jelly to the inside of the dome and insert it in the vagina. She may insert it as long as 4 hours before intercourse. She should check for position with her finger and allow the device to remain in place for at least 6 to 8 hours after coitus. If repeated intercourse occurs within 6 to 8 hours, additional jelly should be first placed in the vagina without removal of the diaphragm.

With care a diaphragm should last 2 years. The patient will need a new fitting if she gains or loses significant weight, has a baby, or has pelvic surgery.

The cervical cap has recently been approved for use by the FDA (20).

The Prentif cap is a rubber device that fits snugly over the cervix. Initial fitting, which may be difficult, must be done by a specially trained health professional. Pregnancy rates are similar to those associated with the use of the diaphragm.

Benefits

The diaphragm is a low cost device that has no major risks other than the higher risk of unwanted pregnancy compared with oral contraceptives or the IUD.

Risks

Contraindications to the use of the diaphragm are sensitivity to the rubber or to the spermicidal material. Alterations in pelvic shape may also preclude the proper fitting of the different diaphragms available. It is not suited for individuals who will not or cannot touch their vagina as, for example, in patients who are very obese or who have a musculoskeletal disorder.

Some women may report discomfort during the time the diaphragm is in place. This discomfort is most often related to a wrong design or to improper fitting, and re-evaluation usually identifies the problem. A few patients will develop recurrent cystitis with frequent diaphragm use.

THE CONDOM

The condom is a latex rubber sheath that is placed over the erect penis. It is the only reversible effective "male method" of contraception except for coitus interruptus. Condoms properly used are an effective form of contraception and their failure rate with experienced and strongly motivated couples has been as low as 1 or 2 per 100 couple years of exposure. Failure rates during the first year of use or in less motivated couples may be considerably higher. Its effectiveness can be enhanced if it is combined with application of a spermicidal jelly or foam in the vagina. Some condoms are now being manufactured in containers with a spermicidal lubricant. The condom when used properly provides considerable protection against sexually transmitted diseases including: gonorrhea, herpes, chlamydia, and acquired immune deficiency syndrome (AIDS). Its only side effect is a rare instance of sensitivity to the lubricating material or skin irritation from friction.

VAGINAL SUPPOSITORIES, FOAM, OR JELLY

These methods all contain a spermicidal material combined with either cream, jelly, or aerosol (17). The material is inserted in the vagina at least 10 to 15 minutes before intercourse. The spermicidal material is dispersed in the vagina and over the cervix. This creates a barrier around the cervical os to prevent sperm from entering the intrauterine cavity. All of these forms of contraception may be obtained without prescription. They are especially useful when additional protection is desired at midcycle with the condom or to increase the effectiveness of the diaphragm when repeated intercourse occurs. The side effects are minor and are related to sensitivity or allergy to the spermicidal material.

RHYTHM

The human ovum probably is viable for only 12 to 24 hours after ovulation. Sperm probably do not retain the capability for successful fertilization for more than 48 hours. The development of a method of contraception that avoids intercourse at the fertile time is logical. Three methods have been developed:

1. The calendar method attempts to establish that portion of the cycle when intercourse is safe. The patient keeps a careful record of the duration of each cycle and then subtracts 18 days from the shortest cycle and 11 days from the longest cycle. This will then give her the beginning and the end of the fertile time. Obviously, the more regular she is, the shorter will be this interval and the better the protection. For example, if the shortest cycle is 27 days; and the longest is 33 days, then she is possibly fertile from day 9 until day 22, or an interval of 12 days. On the other hand, if she is very regular and bleeds every 28 days, her fertile period will be 7 days in duration.
2. The basal body temperature method takes advantage of the slight drop in body temperature associated with ovulation, followed by a rise in temperature of approximately 1°F (0.5°C). The woman takes her temperature each morning from day 3 of the cycle until it has remained elevated to approximately 98.6 to 99°F (36.8 to 37.2°C) for 72 hours. This indicates she is postovulatory and can resume coitus (the ovum must be fertilized within 24 or 48 hours).
3. The cervical mucus method requires the patient to learn, over a number of cycles, those changes that indicate ovulation. She is taught to examine her cervical mucus for clarity. She learns to identify abdominal discomfort associated with ovulation and then to use this information to avoid intercourse when conception is possible. This method requires

effort and regular cycles but has been used effectively by many women.

The rhythm method is the only method of birth control approved by the Roman Catholic Church and other religious organizations who oppose contraception. The risk of pregnancy in women who use this method of contraception is relatively high (Table 93.1).

STERILIZATION

Simple methods of permanent contraception are available to both men and women (5, 13). At present in the United States sterilization is the most popular method of contraception in persons over 30. The total number of sterilizations is rising, and at present the rate of elective sterilization is about equal for both sexes.

Patients considering sterilization need very careful education so that they understand its nature and risks. Informed consent is required for these procedures.

Vasectomy

Vasectomy when properly performed has a failure rate of only 1/200 to 1/500. The complication rate is approximately 4/1000; and, for the most part, complications are minor. They include infection, hematoma, epididymitis, and granuloma formation. Long-term serious side effects have not been reported among the very large numbers of men who have had the procedure performed. There was a transient concern, now known to be unwarranted (10), that antibodies to sperm that develop in some men after vasectomy predispose to atherosclerosis.

Patient experience. This procedure is done under local anesthesia in the urologist's office or outpatient surgical suite. There is minimal operative discomfort. Postoperatively mild discomfort is common but it is usually controlled with a mild analgesic, such as acetaminophen. Vigorous physical activity and sexual activity are restricted for 5 to 7 days until the wound has healed. Follow-up visits are necessary so that sperm counts can be performed. It usually requires 4 to 6 weeks for the ejaculate to become free of sperm.

Reanastomosis of the vas deferens may be accomplished surgically and results in patency in approximately 60% of patients. Vasectomy should, nevertheless, not be undertaken unless the patient genuinely wants permanent sterilization.

Tubal Ligation

The overall failure rate is approximately 2 to 3/1000. The major complication rate is approximately 4/1000. The complications are bleeding, infection, bowel, bladder, or uterine trauma.

Patient experience. Laparoscopy and/or minilaparotomy is usually performed using general anesthesia. Uncomplicated tubal ligation is generally performed as an outpatient procedure and is very well tolerated. Mild abdominal discomfort, when present, lasts usually only for a few days and rarely for a few weeks. Mild analgesics, such as acetaminophen, provide relief. The patient is usually able to return to her usual activities in 48 to 72 hours. Sterilization is immediate and intercourse is permitted as soon as the wound is no longer painful.

Tubal ligation is performed in the first half of the menstrual cycle before ovulation has occurred. This avoids the possibility of fertilization of an ovum occurring a day or 2 before the surgical procedure. If the woman is using effective contraception, tubal ligation may be performed at any time. Reanastomosis of the fallopian tubes can be accomplished surgically and results in a significant chance of fertility. The success of reanastomosis depends primarily upon the type and extent of the initial ligation and is not related to the time between ligation and anastomosis. Nevertheless, a woman should not undergo tubal ligation unless she genuinely desires permanent sterilization.

The existence of a post-tubal syndrome characterized by heavier menstrual bleeding, more pelvic pain, and more discomfort than found in the unsterilized populations has been questioned. The majority of patients following sterilization will notice no significant change in symptomatology associated with their menstrual periods.

DIAGNOSING PREGNANCY

Human chorionic gonadotropin is a glycoprotein hormone that is produced by the blastocyst and the placenta. Its secretion begins very early and can be detected in the maternal blood as early as 6 days after fertilization. In the past, there were a number of conditions that could give rise to a false-positive result such as the presence of foreign protein, cross-reaction with the luteinizing hormone (LH), follicular stimulating hormone (FSH), and thyroid stimulating hormone (TSH). The alpha subunit for human chorionic gonadotropin (HCG) is common to all of these hormones. The beta subunit for HCG is, however, unique, and the currently available pregnancy tests that utilize the monoclonal antibody methodology test only for the beta subunit. A false-positive reaction even with "home pregnancy detection kits" is extremely rare. There are four major types of pregnancy tests. The Icon is the most commonly used because of its simplicity, accuracy, and availability.

Radioimmunoassay (serum): Chorio Quant, Beta Tec, HCG Beta III

- Accurate (Close to 100% accuracy for positive result in normal pregnancy.) when used at least 7 days after conception;
- No LH cross-reaction;
- Specific for HCG (detects beta subunit);

- Used for assessing abnormal pregnancy (ectopic, molar, threatened abortion).

Enzyme-Linked Immunoassay (urine or serum): Icon, Confidot, Quest

- Accurate when used at least 12 days after conception;
- No LH cross-reaction;
- Specific for HCG (detects beta subunit).

Radioreceptorassay (serum): Biocept-G

- Accurate when used at least 14 days after conception;
- LH cross-reaction possible;
- Used for early confirmation of normal pregnancy.

Immunoassay (urine or serum): Neocept, Pregnosis

- Accurate when used at least 28 days after conception;
- LH cross-reaction possible;
- Used for routine pregnancy confirmation;
- Radioisotopes not required.

The biological half life of HCG is approximately 1.5 days. The serum HCG becomes negative approximately 10 days after delivery, artificial termination of pregnancy or spontaneous abortion, if all trophoblastic tissue is expelled.

The HCG test may remain positive for weeks to months if there are small foci of functioning trophoblastic tissue remaining. This could be seen after incomplete abortion, persistent hydatidiform mole, and choriocarcinoma. Every physician who cares for a patient who may be pregnant should have the capability to perform one of the new sensitive enzyme immunoassay tests. These may be done either on blood or urine.

General References

Hatcher RA, Guest F, Stewart F, et al: *Contraception Technology 1988–89*, 14th rev ed. New York, Irvington, 1988.
    A regularly updated text covering all aspects of contraception. It is highly recommended.
Mishell Jr DR: Contraception. *N Engl J Med* 320:777, 1989.
    A well-referenced review of all forms of contraception.

Specific References

1. Brinton LA, Huggins GR, Lehman HF, et al: Long term use of oral contraceptives and risk of invasive cervical cancer. *Int J Cancer* 38:339, 1986.
2. Burkman RT: The Woman's Health Study. Association between intrauterine device and pelvic inflammatory disease. *Obstet Gynecol* 57:269, 1981.
3. Durand JL, Bressler R: Clinical pharmacology of the steroidal oral contraceptives. *Adv Intern Med* 24:97, 1979.

4. Edmondson HA, Henderson B, Benton B: Liver-cell adenomas associated with use of oral contraceptives. *N Engl J Med* 294:470, 1976.

5. Hulka JF: Current status of elective sterilization in the United States. *Fertil Steril* 28:515, 1977.

6. Kafka D, Gold RB: Food and Drug Administration approves contraceptive sponge. *Fam Plan Pers* 15:146, 1983.

7. Layde PM, McCarthy PS, Lord JAH, Smith CFC: Incidence of arterial disease among oral contraceptive users: Royal College of General Practitioners Oral Contraceptive Study. *JR Coll Gen Pract* 33:75, 1983.

8. Linn S, Schoenbaum SC, Monson RR, et al: Lack of association between contraceptive usage and congenital malformation of offspring. *Am J Obstet Gynecol* 147:923, 1983.

9. LiVolsi VA, Stadel BV, Kelsey JL, et al: Fibrocystic breast disease in oral-contraceptive users. *N Engl J Med* 299:381, 1978.

10. Massey Jr FJ, Bernstein GS, O'Fallon WN, et al: Vasectomy and health. Results from a large cohort study. *JAMA* 252:1023, 1984.

11. Ory HW, Forrest JD, Lincoln R: *Making choices, evaluating health risks and benefits of birth control methods.* New York, The Alan Guttmacher Institute, 360 Park Ave, NY 10010, 1983.

12. Population Information Program.*Population Reports: Intrauterine Devices. IUDs—A New Look.* Johns Hopkins University, Series B, No. 5, Baltimore, MD, 1988.

13. Seiler JS: The evolution of tubal sterilization. *Obstet Gynecol Surv* 39:177, 1984.

14. Stadel BV: Oral contraceptives and cardiovascular disease (two parts). *N Engl J Med* 305:612, 672, 1981.

15. The Centers for Disease Control: Cancer and Steroid Hormone Study. Oral contraceptive use and ovarian cancer. *JAMA* 249:1596, 1983.

16. *The Medical Letter on Drugs and Therapeutics* 21:54, 1979.

17. *The Medical Letter on Drugs and Therapeutics* 22:86, 1980.

18. *The Medical Letter on Drugs and Therapeutics* 30:105, 1988.

19. *The Medical Letter on Drugs and Therapeutics* 30:25, 1988.

20. *The Medical Letter on Drugs and Therapeutics* 30:93, 1988.

C H A P T E R   94

Nonmalignant Vulvovaginal Disorders*

VANESSA CULLINS, M.D., M.P.H.
GEORGE R. HUGGINS, M.D.

Vulvovaginal symptoms comprise a significant proportion of problems presented to the primary physician. The diagnosis and treatment of these disorders can be both extremely satisfying and exasperating. Most diagnoses are readily made in one office visit. Treatment is usually easily rendered. Yet, the patient with recurrent or persistent symptoms presents special problems for the clinician. Appropriate evaluation and treatment of both the easily treated patient and the patient with persistent symptoms requires a knowledge of the anatomy, physiology and pathology, of the vulva and vagina.

---

*Drs J. Courtland Robinson and John R. Burton contributed to this chapter in the first and second editions of this book.

ANATOMY AND PHYSIOLOGY (See Fig. 94.1)

Vulva

The external genitalia of the female is denoted the "vulva." The vulva consists of the labia majora, labia minora, vestibule, clitoris, prepuce, and mons pubis.

The mons pubis (mons veneris) is a cushion of fat covered by stratified squamous skin and its appendages (hair follicles, sebaceous and apocrine sweat glands). The mons is located superior to the clitoris and encompasses the triangular-shaped hair-bearing tissue situated in front of the symphysis pubis. The labia majora are composed of longitudinal folds of fat and connective tissue corresponding to the dartos of the male scrotum. When the labia majora are parted, the vaginal vestibule is seen. The vestibule begins at the hymenal ring, extends outward to the labia minora, upward to the frenulum of the clitoris, and downward to include the posterior fourchette. The vaginal orifice (introitus) and urethral meatus open in the midline of the vestibule. Ducts of the Skene's glands (paraure-thral glands), Bartholin's glands (major vestibular glands), and the minor vestibular glands also open in the vestibule. The hymen, a firm, often crescentic-shaped membrane consisting of a double plate of stratified squamous epithelium, partially obscures the vaginal orifice (introitus) in virgins. Residual tags of the hymen, the "carunculae hymenalis," are often noted at the inferior edges of the introitus. The fourchette, the most posterior boundary of the vestibule, is formed by the fusion of the inferior aspects of the labia majora. The clitoris, homologue of the penis, is located in the midline at the most superior aspect of the vestibule. The labia minora bifurcate anteriorly forming the prepuce and frenulum of the clitoris.

Vulvar Glands

The major vestibular glands, or Bartholin's glands, are paired glands whose ducts exit at the introitus, above the fourchette at the 5 and 7 o'clock positions. The minor vestibular glands are numerous small glands whose ducts exit laterally to the hymenal ring. These

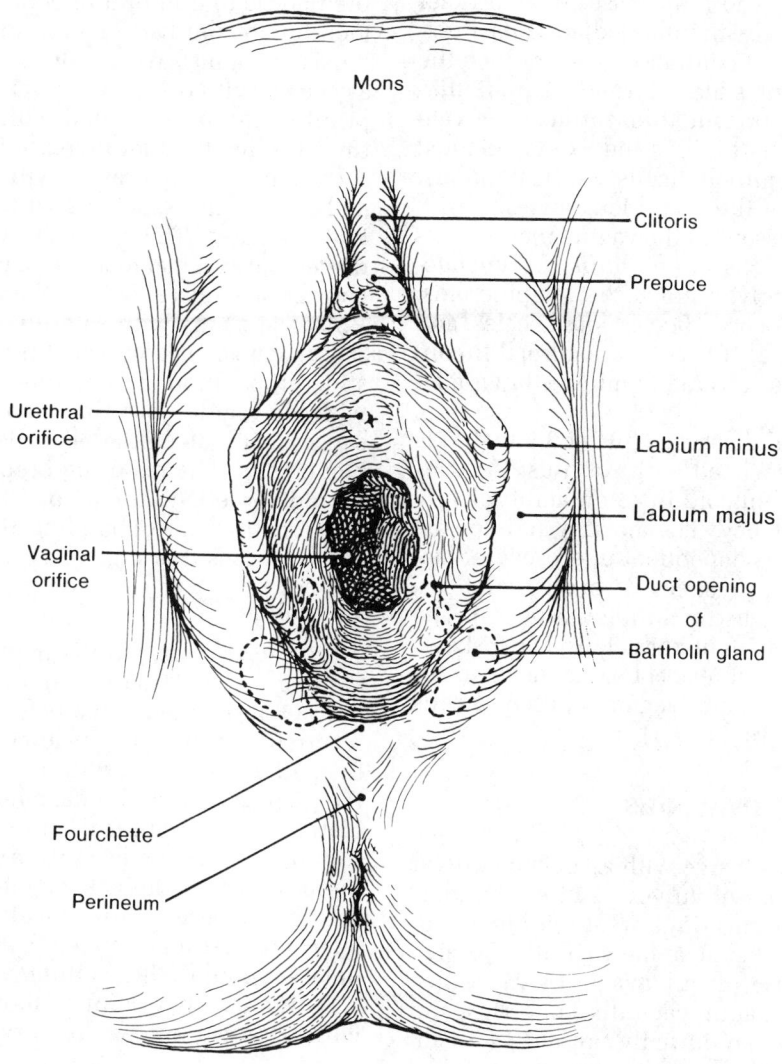

Figure 94.1. Anatomy of vulva.

small glands may extend superiorly to the region of the urethra. Ducts from the Skene's (paraurethral glands) open in the vestibule immediately beneath the urethral meatus.

Vagina

The vaginal canal extends from the vestibule to the uterine cervix. The vaginal wall consists of an outer fibrous layer, middle muscular layer, and inner epithelial layer composed of nonkeratinizing, stratified squamous cells. Glands are not present in the normal vagina.

When stimulated, the major nerve endings of the vagina cause the sensation of pain or light touch. Compared with the neural supply of the vulva, the vagina has few nerve endings. For this reason, vaginal infections are often asymptomatic until the discharge comes in contact with the vulva. The squamous epithelium of the vagina is hormone dependent. In the absence of estrogen, the vaginal epithelium is thin and fragile, and it consists of undifferentiated basal and parabasal cells. Progesterone leads to a decrease in superficial cells and a relative increase in intermediate cells. Pregnancy, lactation, and oral contraceptives produce the progesterone dominant state. Normal vaginal discharge is composed of transudation through the vaginal wall, secretions of Bartholin's and Skene's glands, desquamated vaginal epithelial cells, cervical mucus, endometrial fluid, tubal fluid, and leukocytes.

Bacteria normally present in the vagina include lactobacillus, *Staphylococcus epidermidis*, *Corynebacterium* species, nonhemolytic streptococci, diptheroids, peptococci, peptostreptococci, *Bacteroides* species, and *Eubacterium* species (12, 16). Yeast are normal inhabitants of the vagina in a substantial number of women (2, 15, 22).

Physiological vaginal discharge (pH of 3.5 to 4.1) is not malodorous or associated with pruritus. It varies in amount, is white or mucoid in color, and typically has a floccular consistency. The amount and consistency of the discharge is dependent upon several factors: hormonal profile, presence of menstrual flow, frequency of coitus, and use of antibiotics (8, 13). The *saline wet slide preparation* of normal discharge shows rare leukocytes, variable numbers of mononuclear cells, large Gram-positive rods, and vaginal epithelial cells with distinct borders (Table 94.1).

VULVOVAGINITIS

Abnormal vaginal discharge with associated vulvar irritation is the hallmark of vulvovaginitis. The most common vulvovaginal infections are: *Candida, Gardnerella, Trichomonas*, and atrophic vaginitis. Foreign bodies are a rare cause of vulvovaginitis in adults. Although not a cause of adult vaginitis, gonorrhea and chlamydial infections may initially present as an abnormal discharge and therefore be misinterpreted as a vulvovaginitis.

Candida

Candida (see Table 94.1) is an extremely common cause of adult vulvovaginitis. Approximately 40% of women with vulvovaginitis are infected with *Candida albicans*. *C. albicans* is a yeast that has no true mycelial form and for this reason infection should be referred to as *candidiasis* rather than moniliasis (a common term used in older literature), which implies infection by a mycelial form. The presence of *Candida* within the vagina is not sufficient for the diagnosis of the vulvovaginitis; up to 16% of nonpregnant, reproductive-aged women are normally colonized with the yeast (2, 15).

The change in *Candida* from normal flora to a pathogen occurs when the organisms proliferate to the point that the normal microbiological balance of the vagina is upset. Predisposing factors to infection include pregnancy, diabetes mellitus, immunosuppression, antibiotic or corticosteroid therapy, iron deficiency anemia, vaginal surgery, oral contraceptives, acquired immunodeficiency syndrome (AIDS), and AIDS related complex (ARC) (9, 14, 22). Skin conditions that predispose to *Candida* infection generally involve alterations of the barrier function of the skin through persistent moisture and development of maceration, as occurs with occlusive synthetic clothing. Candidal proliferation is associated with both an increased estrogen milieu and an increase in vaginal pH.

Patients usually present with intense vulvar itching and/or burning associated with a thick, curd-like vaginal discharge. The vulva and vagina are typically inflamed. The vaginal mucosa may exhibit adherent white patches of exudate similar in appearance to oral thrush. Vulvar erosions with satellite pustules may be seen. The diagnosis is confirmed through examination of a slide preparation of 10% potassium hydroxide mixed with the vaginal secretions. The potassium hydroxide causes lysis of epithelial cells, leukocytes, and red blood cells. The resulting preparation is thus not obscured by cells that may overlie the fungus and prevent identification of budding filaments, pseudohyphae, and/or spores (see Fig. 94.2).

Treatment

Candida vulvovaginitis may be treated either topically or orally. Usually the topical treatment is given first. Oral treatment (see below) is reserved for some recurrent infections (see below) or in situations in which the patient cannot or will not apply the topical agent. Fungicides include imidazole derivatives, gentian violet, and the antifungal antibiotic, nystatin. The imidazole derivatives and nystatin decrease the permeability of the cell membrane of fungi. This alteration of permeability results in the loss of the selective barrier function of the cell membrane such that potassium and other cellular constituents are lost.

Candida vulvovaginitis should be treated initially with a topical imidazole derivative such as:

1. Miconazole nitrate (Monistat)—One 200-mg sup-

Table 94.1.
Vaginal Discharge

	Physiological	Candida	Gardnerella	Trichomonas	Atrophic
Symptoms	None	Pruritis, Burning	± Pruritis, Burning	± Pruritis	+ ± Vulvar, vaginal dryness
Malodor	None	Yeast smell	Fishy or musty	Variable	Variable
Increased mucosal erythema	None	Yes	±	Yes	±
Consistency	Floccular	Thick, curd-like	Thin, creamy	Copious, frothy	Mucoid, blood tinged
pH	3.5–4.1	3.5–4.5	5.0–6.0	6.0–7.0	As high as 7.0
Wet Smear	Rare WBCs, large gram positive rods. Squamous epithelial cells	Budding filaments spores, Pseudohyphae	Clue cells	Copious WBCs Trichomonads	Copious WBCs parabasal and intermediate cells Paucity of superficial cells
KOH		Budding filaments, spores, Pseudohyphae	Fishy odor Musty odor		
Treatment of Choice	None	Imidazole derivative	Metronidazole	Metronidazole	Estrogen cream

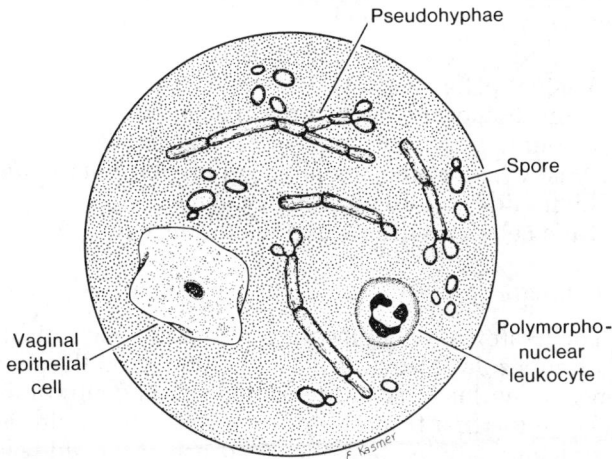

Figure 94.2. KOH preparation, showing yeast and pseudohyphi of candidiasis.

pository intravaginally at night for 3 days or 5 g of 2% cream intravaginally at bedtime for 7 days.
or
2. Butoconazole nitrate (Femstat)—One applicator full of 2% cream intravaginally at bedtime for 3 days.
or
3. Terconazole (Terazol)—One 80-mg suppository or 0.4% cream intravaginally at bedtime for 3 days.
or
4. Clotrimazole (Mycelex or Gyne-Lotrimin)—Two 100-mg tablets intravaginally for 3 days.

Most patients will feel much better in a day or 2 but they should complete the treatment course. The 7-day regimens described above are more effective during pregnancy when the infection can be more resistant.

Recurrent Candidiasis

Recurrent *Candida* infections of the vagina are of two types: *persistent* or *recurrent*. Persistent vulvovaginal candidiasis is a consequence of inadequate

treatment. Reinfection is due to reintroduction of the organism. The only method of distinguishing the two is by documenting eradication of the infection after a treatment course. This documentation in practice is not done commonly after an initial episode. However, when a second episode of *Candida* vulvovaginitis is experienced relatively soon, the physician should see the patient in follow-up within 1 to 2 weeks to re-examine the patient and determine by a KOH preparation (see above) if, in fact, the organism has been eradicated. Persistent infection should be treated with a 7-day course of a topical imidazole derivative as listed above for treatment of an initial infection. Recurrent infection requires more intensive treatment and an investigation for potential sources of the organism. In certain instances the inherent properties of *Candida* may be the cause of recurrent infection. *Candida* possesses the ability to change its surface antigens (18). A change in antigenicity alters susceptibility to antifungals. Because each imidazole derivative has a distinct spectrum of activity against the various species of *Candida*, switching to a different imidazole derivative may effect a cure. If these fail, referral to a gynecologist is appropriate for confirmation of the diagnosis and consideration of an alternative therapy such as gentian violet or nystatin.

Reinfection should trigger inquiry regarding the patient's sexual practices and sexual partner(s). Because the partner(s) may be colonized, he/she should be empirically treated with a fungicidal cream. For the male partner, the cream should be placed on the scrotum, penile glans, and shaft every night for 7 nights. *Candida* may also be transmitted during oral-genital contact. Therefore, if the patient's partner engages in cunnilingus, the partner should be treated with oral nystatin.

The gastrointestinal tract is a natural reservoir for *Candida*. Perineal contamination of the vulva through improper hygiene is thought to be another factor in the pathogenesis of recurrent infection. For this reason, patients with recurrent infections should be instructed to wipe from front to back when bathing and after urination or defecation. To decrease the intestinal candidal flora in patients with frequent reinfections, oral nystatin, 100,000 units three times a day for 1 week, will sometimes decrease the rate of reinfection. Such a course may be repeated from time to time if subsequent reinfections develop.

If recurrences are related to specific events, such as menses, prophylactic topical clotrimazole (Mycelex or Gyne-Lotrimin suppositories) used once a day for 3 days may be preventive. Sometimes recurrences are related to coitus, and for those women in whom coital events can be predicted, prophylactic therapy will be helpful.

Patients who continue to have recurrent infections despite the institution of these measures should be evaluated for diabetes mellitus (see Chapter 72) and human immunodeficiency virus (HIV) infection (see Chapter 34). If these are absent, a gynecologist should see the patient. Some of these recalcitrant patients may be found to have a primary deficiency of cell-mediated immunity to *Candida* that often is temporary.

Gardnerella Vaginitis (Bacterial Vaginosis)

Gardnerella vaginalis vulvovaginitis (bacterial vaginosis) (Table 94.1) is the second most common vulvovaginitis encountered in the United States. This entity was formerly referred to as "nonspecific vaginitis." The implicated organism, *Gardnerella* vaginalis, was previously known as *Haemophilus* or *Corynebacterium vaginale*.

Gardnerella vaginalis, like *Candida* albicans, may be found in the vaginas of females not experiencing signs or symptoms of vulvovaginitis. The concentration of *Gardnerella* is much lower in asymptomatic individuals. In addition to *Gardnerella*, an increased proportion of anaerobic bacteria such as *Bacteroides*, *Peptococcus* and *Eubacterium* are recovered from the vaginas of symptomatic women (5, 20, 21).

Patients with this infection usually complain of thin, creamy malodorous vaginal discharge with accompanying vulvar itching or burning. The vaginal mucosa and vulva may be mildly inflamed. The odor of this infection is usually described as "fishy" or "musty" and is commonly noted after coitus, when the alkaline seminal fluid has caused the release of volatile fatty acids and amines.

Diagnosis is confirmed through examination of the saline wet prep (see above), production of the characteristic odor, and determination of the vaginal pH. Using nitrazine paper, vaginal pH can be determined easily. Vaginal discharge of women infected with *Gardnerella* is typically between 5.0 and 6.0. The saline wet prep is significant for vaginal squamous cells covered with *Gardnerella* ("clue cells," see Fig. 94.3). Leukocytes are generally not abundant unless a mixed infection is present. The addition of a 10% potassium hydroxide solution to the discharge will cause the release of amines and volatile fatty acids that produce the "fishy" odor.

The diagnosis of *Gardnerella* vulvovaginitis is made

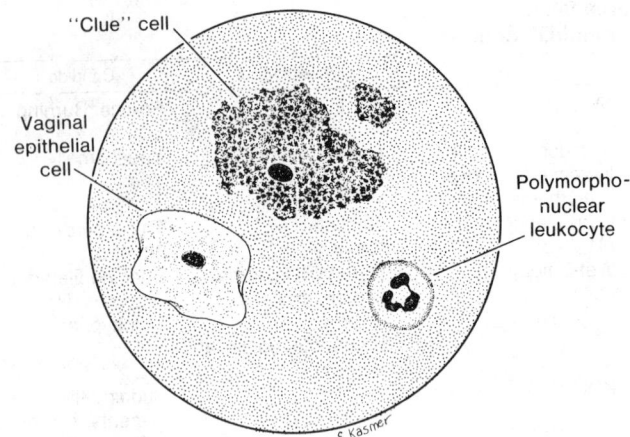

Figure 94.3. "Clue" cells.

when at least three of the four criteria listed below are met (1):

1. Vaginal pH above 4.5;
2. Thin, homogeneous vaginal discharge of variable amount;
3. "Fishy" odor after the addition of 10% potassium hydroxide solution to the discharge;
4. Clue cells on saline wet preparation.

Treatment

The treatment of choice for *Gardnerella* vaginitis is metronidazole (Flagyl, Protostat), 500 mg orally, two times a day for 7 days. Metronidazole is contraindicated in the first trimester of pregnancy. It should be used cautiously in alcoholics (because of the side effects that develop when the drug is taken with alcohol) or patients with severe hepatic disease. An alternative regimen that may be tried if metronidazole is contraindicated is:

Clindamycin, 300 mg, orally, two times a day for 7 days.

The role of sexual transmission in the acquisition of this vulvovaginitis has not been resolved completely. *Gardnerella* vaginalis can be recovered in the majority of male contacts of infected women; yet *Gardnerella* can be isolated from up to 1/3 of women who have never been sexually active. In addition, recurrence rates for the infection are the same for women whose partners harbor *Gardnerella* vaginalis as for those women whose partners do not have *Gardnerella* vaginalis (23). Because of the possible role of sexual transmission, condoms should be used during therapy. If the infection recurs, the patient's partner(s) should be treated.

Trichomonas

Trichomonas (see Table 94.1) is a common sexually transmitted disease. It is caused by the motile, unipolar flagellated protozoan, *Trichomonas* vaginalis. Aside from sexual transmission the organism can be acquired through close contact with contaminated water or clothing.

Patients generally present with a copious and often frothy vaginal discharge accompanied by vulvar pruritus. Additional symptoms include vaginal burning, vaginal spotting, and symptoms of urethral irritation—dysuria, frequency, and urgency. Pelvic discomfort may be experienced by some patients. Dyspareunia is very common. On physical examination, variable amounts of vulvovaginal erythema may be seen. Typically, there is less erythema than is seen in *Candida* vulvovaginitis. The vaginal mucosa and/or cervix may exhibit a characteristic "strawberry" appearance (reddish color with punctuation).

The diagnosis is established by assessing vaginal pH and examining the saline wet prep (see above). The vaginal pH is generally between 6 and 7. On saline prep (Fig. 94.4), a multitude of polymorphonuclear leukocytes will be seen. Among the white blood cells, trichomonads can be identified by the movement of their flagellae. It should be noted that cold saline or water will cause immobilization of the trichomonads. The solution should be at a comfortable room temperature. Atrophic vaginitis (see below) produces a discharge with a pH between 6 and 7 and copious white blood cells, but characteristically it does not contain mature squamous cells. Therefore, the presence of discharge-containing numerous white cells and *mature squamous epithelial cells*, with a pH between 6 and 7, is presumptive evidence of *Trichomonas* vulvovaginitis.

Treatment

Treatment consists of a single 2 g dose of oral metronidazole (Flagyl, Protostat). Patients who do not respond to this therapy may be treated with metronidazole, 500 mg two times per day for 7 days. Patients not responding to this regimen should be referred to a gynecologist for evaluation and treatment, which is likely to be difficult. Metronidazole is contraindicated in the first trimester of pregnancy and it should be

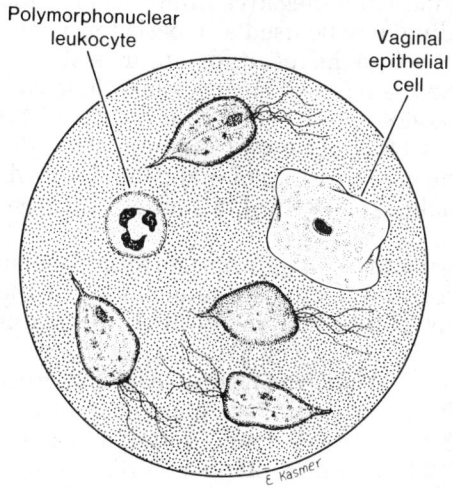

Figure 94.4. Saline preparation showing trichomonads.

used cautiously in patients with severe hepatic disease; when taken within 24 hours of alcohol consumption, metronidazole causes severe reactions similar to those when alcohol and disulfiram (Antabuse) are consumed together. In these situations or when there is an intolerance to metronidazole, clindamycin, 300 mg, orally, twice a day for seven days, may be used as an alternate. The sexual partner(s) should be similarly treated also, and it is usually pointless to attempt to recover the organism from the partner. Intercourse should be avoided or a condom used during treatment.

Atrophic Vaginitis

Atrophic vaginitis (see Table 94.1) is a common disorder of postmenopausal women. Caused by estrogen deficiency, it may be seen in women who are postoophorectomy, have premature ovarian failure, or are breastfeeding. Rarely, premenarchal (i.e., unestrogenized tissues) girls have atrophic vaginitis when an additional precipitant (e.g., occlusive clothing made of synthetic materials) occurs.

Estrogen deficiency results in thinning and fragility of the vaginal and vulvar epithelium. Instead of the glycogen rich superficial cells, the epithelium is composed primarily of parabasal and intermediate cells. This altered vaginal environment is associated with an elevation of pH to as high as 7.0. In this milieu, pathogenic bacteria may flourish. The patient may complain of a mucosal, blood-tinged vaginal discharge and vulvar and vaginal dryness. Some patients will also note urinary incontinence (see Chapter 6).

Visual examination of the normal atrophic vagina reveals a pale vaginal mucosa with decreased or absent rugal folds. Vulvar examination demonstrates thin, often shiny skin with decreased subcutaneous tissue and variable loss of hair. In atrophic vaginitis, erythema and petechial hemorrhages may be superimposed on these findings.

Saline wet prep examination (see above) of the discharge of women with atrophic vaginitis is significant for numerous leukocytes mixed with immature intermediate and parabasal epithelial cells. Microorganisms seen on the slide are generally secondary invaders of the inflamed mucosa. Often in the past a diagnostic smear of the vaginal wall maturation index was suggested; however, this test is no longer recommended since it has not proven reliable. Not all women with atrophy on vaginal examination have atrophic vaginitis. Treatment should be instituted only if symptoms are present.

Topical estrogen is the treatment of choice for atrophic vaginitis. Although oral estrogen may be used, the topical cream seems to be more effective. One-half to one applicator of estrogen cream every night for 1 to 2 weeks is followed by every other night application for 1 to 2 weeks. The medication can then generally be discontinued, and most patients will have only infrequent symptoms (e.g., every 3 to 6 months) such that an applicator full for 1 or 2 days when there are symptoms will provide adequate control. Absorption of estrogen to a level consistent with the early follicular phase of the female menstrual cycle may occur with topically applied preparations. Therefore, if prolonged administration (e.g., over 1 year) of a topical estrogen occurs, the patient will be at risk for complications of continuous estrogen therapy (see Chapter 77) including uterine cancer (see Chapter 95). Such patients should be followed concomitantly by a gynecologist so that appropriate screening for uterine cancer can be done or so that a progestin can be prescribed (see Chapter 77). The physician will need to be certain that none of the contraindications for estrogens (e.g., breast cancer) is present and that the same precautionary surveillance (e.g., for hypertension) is provided the patient using long-term topical estrogen preparations.

Some patients are unable or unwilling to use topical vaginal preparations. In this instance oral conjugated estrogen (Premarin) 0.625 mg daily may be prescribed for 1 month. Occasionally a repeated course of oral estrogens is necessary if symptoms persist. When retreatment courses become frequent, it is necessary to provide close surveillance for the complications of estrogen therapy (see above and Chapter 77). Generally a gynecologist should be consulted to participate in the care of a patient with frequently recurrent attacks of atrophic vaginitis.

Foreign Body

An occasional cause of vaginal discharge in adults is a foreign body. Lost tampons, forgotten diaphragms, and other smaller objects will be easily found by examination. Symptoms will improve after removal of the foreign body. Because secondary bacterial infection is also present, a triple sulfa cream (Sultrin), twice daily for 3 to 4 days, or a providone (Betadine or Femidine) douche, once daily for 3 to 4 days, may accelerate healing.

GONOCOCCAL AND CHLAMYDIAL INFECTIONS

Gonococcal and chlamydial infections are the most common upper genital tract sexually transmitted diseases in the United States. These infections may initially present as an abnormal discharge that is really the result of an associated cervicitis and not a vaginitis. The patient, however, will consider the discharge as a sign of a "vaginal infection." Although a purulent discharge is classically associated with gonorrhea, a mucopurulent discharge is seen with chlamydia. For both infections, most patients do not recognize signs or symptoms until the disease affects the upper genital tract.

Gonococcal Infection

In the United States, gonorrhea has always been considered the classic sexually transmitted disease. It is the entity with which other upper genital tract diseases are compared, and it is imperative, therefore, to understand this disease and its more common counterpart, chlamydia (see below).

Infected patients may have no symptoms, symptoms due to direct inoculation of organisms (cervical, rectal, or pharyngeal), or symptoms due to local or distant spread of infection. Transmission of gonorrhea from infected men to uninfected women or men is efficient and occurs in 90% of exposures; transmission from infected women to uninfected men or women is less efficient. Risk of infection from the latter mode of transmission is approximately 20% per exposure (4). The diagnosis and management of gonorrhea in male patients are discussed in Chapter 27.

Because the infection is initially asymptomatic, routine screening is important in women with multiple sexual partners, or with other sexually transmitted diseases. Symptoms generally occur once the organism has spread to the fallopian tubes and has initiated acute salpingitis and pelvic inflammatory disease (PID). Early consultation and prompt therapy will significantly reduce the serious sequelae of PID, i.e., ectopic pregnancy and infertility. A single mild episode of acute salpingitis will cause infertility in approximately 13% of patients (25). This figure rises to 75% after three or more bouts with PID (25). The clinical manifestations of uncomplicated gonococcal infection include vaginal symptoms (purulent vaginal discharge, vaginal itching, dyspareunia, dysuria, vague lower abdominal pain), anorectal symptoms (pruritus, painful defecation, rectal fullness), and pharyngeal symptoms. Pelvic inflammatory disease usually begins shortly after a menstrual period (which may itself be altered) and is characterized by fever, nausea, abdominal pain, and on examination marked tenderness of the pelvic organs to touch or motion. The adnexa may also be enlarged. The white blood cell count is usually elevated. The most common manifestation of disseminated gonorrhea is the *arthritis-dermatitis syndrome*. Symptoms and signs of this syndrome include polyarthralgia, tenosynovitis of elbows, wrists, or knees, purulent monoarthritis, and skin lesions. This syndrome usually develops 1 or more weeks after the initial infection.

Gram stain of the cervical material is diagnostic when intracellular Gram-negative diplococci are identified. This finding may be used as a basis for diagnosis and treatment before the results of culture (selective media that is chocolate based) are available. Gram stain alone, though, is not a very sensitive indicator of infections in females (4). Pharyngeal cultures are indicated in those who give a history of oral-genital sexual activity although the sensitivity of this procedure is only about 50%.

Management plans appropriate for the various forms of gonococcal infection are summarized in Table 94.2. Follow-up cultures to ensure that the treatment has been effective should be done 1 week after the therapy is completed. Women being treated for gonorrhea should either abstain from sexual intercourse or assure that their partner(s) uses a condom until a negative "proof of cure" culture is documented. Furthermore, the partner(s) must be treated for presumed infection (see Chapter 27 for treatment of male partners).

Table 94.2.
Management of Gonococcal and Chlamydia Infections

UNCOMPLICATED GONOCOCCAL INFECTION (asymptomatic, cervicovaginal, or anorectal symptoms; pharyngitis)
1. a. Ceftriaxone, 250 mg IM, once (or equivalent cephalosporin)
   or
   b. Spectinomycin, 2.0 g IM (once).
   or
   c. Ciprofloxacin, 500 mg, orally, once (contraindicated in pregnancy and in those age 16 and younger).
   or
   d. Norfloxacin, 800 mg, orally, once (contraindicated in pregnancy and in those age 16 or younger).
   or
   e. Amoxicillin, 3g orally with 1 g probenecid if infection known to have been acquired from a source proven not to have penicillin resistant gonorrhea.
2. Treat for chlamydia with doxycycline, tetracycline, or erythromycin (see below).
3. Treat partner(s).
4. Follow-up culture 1 week after completing treatment.
5. Report to local health department.

CHLAMYDIA CERVICITIS; POSSIBLE GONORRHEA/CHLAMYDIA INFECTION (a common situation with manifestations of infection present but without culture confirmation)
1. a. Doxycycline, 100 mg twice a day for 7 days.
   or
   b. Tetracycline 500 mg orally four times a day for 7 days.
   or
   c. Erythromycin 500 mg four times a day for 7 days.
2. Treat partner(s).
3. Follow-up culture for gonorrhea and *Chlamydia* (or assay for chlamydia) 1 week after completing treatment.

PELVIC INFLAMMATORY DISEASE (gonorrhea, *Chlamydia*, or both may be the cause)
1. Ambulatory treatment[a]
   a. Ceftriaxone 250 mg IM, one dose.
   or
   Cefoxitin (Mefoxin), 2 g IM, one dose
   plus
   Doxycycline, 100 mg orally twice a day for 10–14 days.
   or
   Tetracycline, 500 mg orally four times a day for 10–14 days.
   or
   Erythromycin 500 mg four times a day for 10–14 days.
   b. Contact or observation every 24–48 hours to assure improvement.
2. Indications for hospitalization
   a. Diagnosis uncertain (to exclude appendicitis, ectopic pregnancy, nongonoccal pelvic inflammatory disease, pelvic abscess).
   b. When an intrauterine device is present, in which case the addition of metronidazole (Flagyl) is recommended.
   c. Diagnosis is certain but patient is toxic or unable to follow ambulatory treatment reliably.
   d. Patient does not respond promptly to ambulatory treatment.
3. Inpatient Treatment
   a. Cefoxitin 2 g IV every 6 hours or cefotetan 2 g IV every 12 hours
   and
   Doxycycline 100 mg IV every 12 hours.
   or
   b. Gentamycin 2.0 mg/kg as an initial dose followed by 1.5 mg/kg every 8 hours
   and
   Clindamycin 900 mg IV every 8 hours.

GONOCOCCAL/ARTHRITIS-DERMATITIS SYNDROME (hospitalization is recommended)
1. a. Ceftriaxone 1.0 g, IM or IV daily.
   or
   Ceftizoxime 1g, IV every 8 hours.
   or
   Cefotaxime, 1 g, IV, every 8 hours.
   b. For patients allergic to β-lactim drugs, spectinomycin, 2 g, IM, every 8 hours should be given.
   c. Patients may be discharged in 48 hours with close follow-up, see 4 below.
2. When the infecting organism is proven to be penicillin sensitive, parenteral treatment may be switched to ampicillin 1 g every 6 hours.
3. Treat for potential coexistent chlamydial infection (see above).
4. The patient should complete 7 days of antibiotic therapy with either
   Cefuroxine axetil, 500 mg, orally, two times a day.
   or
   Amoxicillin, 500 mg with clavalanic acid, orally three times a day.
   or
   Ciprofloxacin 500 mg, orally, two times a day.

Note: In pregnant patients, use erythromycin instead of tetracycline or doxycycline.
   Ceftriaxone is effective against penicillinase-producing *Neisseria* gonorrhea.
[a] Adapted from *Morbidity and Mortality Weekly Report* 38(S-8), 1989 (see General References).

Whenever gonorrhea is confirmed, the patient should be reported to the local health department so that sexual contacts will receive appropriate evaluation and treatment.

Chlamydia Trachomatis Infection

In recent years the role of *Chlamydia trachomatis* in the production of genitourinary infections has been clarified (16, 17). Chlamydia is felt to be the etiological agent in a substantial number of cases of pelvic inflammatory disease. In the United States, chlamydial infections are more common than gonorrhea.

Chlamydial lower genital tract infection is more indolent than is gonorrhea, but symptoms are similar: lower abdominal pain, dysuria, mucopurulent discharge, and fever. On examination the cervix may be red, edematous, and friable. Typically, the cervical discharge is less profuse than it is in patients with gonorrhea.

Chlamydial infection is diagnosed with most certainty by culture, but the media are expensive and growth is slow. Therefore, culture is not ordinarily recommended. The fluorescent antibody staining technique and enzyme immunoassay are two relatively inexpensive and reliable methods (Microtrak and Chlamydiazyme), and one of these office tests is recommended to confirm chlamydia infection (24). For both the fluorescent antibody staining technique or enzyme immunoassay, a cotton swab impregnated with calcium gluconate is used to obtain a sample of endocervical discharge.

In addition to using the office tests in patients suspected of having chlamydia, the primary physician should screen any woman who has been diagnosed with another sexually transmitted disease.

When chlamydial infection is suspected, doxycycline or tetracycline is the drug of choice (see Table 94.2). Treatment should be initiated before the results of the diagnostic test are available. A negative test should alert the physician to an alternative diagnosis if the result is negative. In instances of uncomplicated pelvic inflammatory disease, when the initiating organism may not be recovered and secondary anaerobic infection is likely (6), the first line of treatment is a cephalosporin, such as cefoxitin or ceftriaxone, plus doxycycline (see Table 94.2). Erythromycin should be used in the pregnant patient because of the effect of tetracycline on fetal development and possible effect on maternal liver function. Because the male sexual partner is often infected as well, he should be treated also (see Chapter 27).

VULVAR ULCERATIONS

Herpes Simplex

The most common cause of vulvar ulceration is herpes simplex, an enveloped DNA-containing virus specific for humans. Although both herpes simplex types I and II may cause genital ulceration, type II is implicated in the majority of genital infections. This sexually transmitted disease is characterized by exacerbations and remissions that are independent of repeated exposure to the virus. The virus exists in latent form in pelvic nerve ganglia and within autonomic nerves along the uterosacral ligaments. Factors influencing recurrence of the infection are not well understood. It is known that recurrences are correlated with stress and the premenstrual period of the menstrual cycle. Fifty percent of individuals will develop a recurrence within 6 months of the initial infection (11).

When initially contracted, the patient may develop a prodromal illness characterized by fever, malaise, and lymphadenopathy. Rarely, meningitis or encephalitis can develop. Before lesions appear, paresthesias and burning may occur. The initial formation of vulvar vesicles may be asymptomatic. These vesicles typically measure from 1 to 10 mm in diameter. They are most commonly located on the labia minora, labia majora, and around the clitoris in a clustered, linear, or serpiginous arrangement (10) (see Fig. 94.5).

In the next stage of the process, the vesicles enlarge and rupture to form shallow painful ulcerations. The ulcerations generally coalesce and are surrounded by an erythematous border.

Clinical suspicion of this diagnosis should be confirmed through a viral culture (requires a special viral transport culture media) available through the local health department or with a cytological smear: *Pap Smear* or *Tzanck Preparation* (see Chapter 100). The

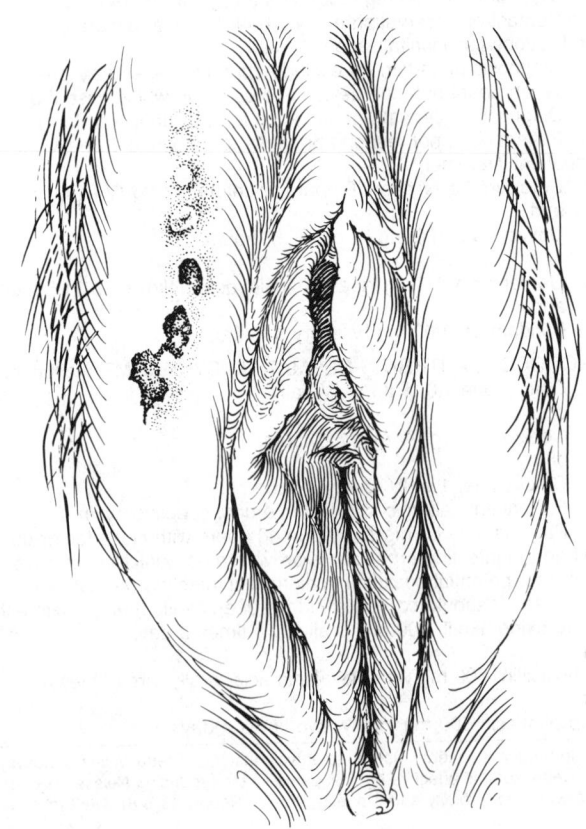

Figure 94.5. Herpes simplex.

culture or cytological smear should be prepared from fluid obtained from an unroofed vesicle or from the base of an ulcer. Viral identification via culture (usually positive in 48 hours but occasionally 7 days or longer is required) or smear is most likely during the first 3 days of infection. Therefore, a negative test obtained after this period is not a guarantee of the absence of herpes. The measurement of titers of serum antibodies to herpes virus is not generally helpful in the diagnosis of herpetic infection because of lack of specificity of the finding.

Ulcerations in close proximity to the urethra may result in dysuria or urinary retention. Although the cervix and vagina are involved in more than 50% of cases, cervical/vaginal ulcerations may be asymptomatic because of the lack of free nerve endings in the vagina or cervix. With extensive cervical involvement, though, cervical motion tenderness may be elicited. A honey-colored crust forms as the lesions heal. The ulcerations usually heal spontaneously in 1 to 3 weeks. Secondary bacterial invasion may prolong this healing process to 6 weeks or more. Usually, there is no permanent scarring.

The symptoms of recurrences are generally milder than the initial attack. Eighty-five percent of patients with recurrent infection experienced a prodrome of itching, tingling, burning, or tenderness.

Treatment

Therapy for herpes is aimed at palliation of symptoms. As yet, there is no means to eradicate the latent virus. Oral analgesics, topical anesthetics, compresses of 1:40 Burow's solution, witch hazel pads (e.g., Tucks or generic), and sitz baths may alleviate symptoms. Ten percent povidone iodine (e.g., Betadine) applied twice daily for several days inhibits secondary bacterial infection and promotes drying of the lesions. A patient who also has dysuria from the infection may benefit from phenazopyridine (Pyridium), 100 to 200 mg 3 to four 4 a day for three to four days.

The antiviral agent, acyclic purine analogue, acyclovir (Zovirax) may decrease the period of symptoms and viral shedding and it should be prescribed both topically and orally. Acyclovir therapy is effective for both primary and recurrent infections. Topical acyclovir, which when used alone (not recommended) is considered less effective than oral or intravenous therapy, may be placed on the lesions every 3 to 4 hours at the same time oral acyclovir is initiated. The combination of oral and topical therapy seems to result in quicker remission of symptoms. When applying acyclovir ointment, the patient should use a glove to prevent autoinoculation and transmission to others. The dosage of oral acyclovir is dependent upon whether the treatment is for an initial or for a recurrent attack or whether it is being prescribed for suppression. The initial attack should be treated with one 200-mg capsule of acyclovir five times per day *for 7 to 10 days.* Therapy for recurrences should be begun at the earliest sign. When the prodrome begins, one 200-mg capsule

every 4 hours for a total of five capsules daily *for 5 days* is administered. In patients with a history of severe recurrences (i.e., >6 a month), suppressive therapy should be prescribed. One 200-mg capsule three to five times daily for up to 6 months may be given. The dosage of acyclovir must be adjusted for patients with renal impairment.

Patients who experience a severe initial attack manifested by high fever, inability to void, meningitis, or encephalitis should be hospitalized for intravenous treatment with acyclovir. Intravenous acyclovir is also indicated in the treatment of initial and recurrent herpes simplex infections in immunocompromised patients. Vidarabine (Vira-A), another purine nucleoside analog, may be used in cases of herpetic encephalitis, or if intravenous acyclovir has been found to be ineffective.

Syphilis (Also See Chapter 30)

Vulvar ulcerations can be seen in all stages of syphilis. The primary chancre appears approximately 3 weeks after the infection has been contracted. It is a single, hard, painless lesion with an ulcerated central core. Frequently, multiple lesions occur that are painful and soft because of secondary bacterial invasion. Chancres are commonly found on the labia or introitus. Dark field examination of the base of the lesion will reveal spirochetes (*Treponema pallidum*). These initial lesions usually heal spontaneously in 1 to 6 weeks. Between 3 and 4 days after the appearance of the chancre, inguinal adenopathy develops. With time, these firm, nontender lymph nodes become bilateral.

Secondary syphilis develops 3 to 6 weeks after the chancre. Condyloma latum represent the classic vulvar, secondary syphilitic lesion. The plaques are multiple and commonly confluent. They are often grayish with a moist, necrotic appearance. The center of the lesion may be ulcerated. Other manifestations of secondary syphilis include malaise, flu-like syndrome, arthralgias, maculopapular rash, and lymphadenopathy.

Treatment

Primary, secondary, and latent syphilis of less than 1 year's duration should be treated with 2.4 million units of benzathine, penicillin G. (1.2 million units should be given in each buttock) (19). Alternative therapy for those allergic to penicillin is tetracycline, 500 mg orally four times a day for 14 days. A third choice is erythromycin, 500 mg orally four times a day for 14 days. Syphilis of more than 1 year's duration should be treated with 2.4 million units of benzathine penicillin G intramuscularly every week for 3 weeks for a total dose of 7.2 million units. Alternative therapy includes tetracycline, 500 mg orally four times a day for 30 days, or erythromycin, 500 mg orally four times a day for 30 days. Adequacy of treatment should be guided by the fall in Venereal Disease Research Laboratory (VDRL) titers (see Chapter 30). Pregnant women with syphilis should be referred to an obstetrician for therapy.

Other Causes of Vulvar Ulcerations

Less common causes of vulvar ulceration include granuloma inguinale, lymphogranuloma venereum, chancroid, hidradenitis suppurativa, Behcet's disease, Crohn's disease, and tuberculosis. A synopsis of common findings, diagnosis, and treatment of vulvar ulcerations is found in Table 94.3. Any patient with an ulcer that is nonhealing, recurrent, or not easily diagnosed should be referred to a gynecologist or dermatologist.

MISCELLANEOUS LESIONS (Tables 94.4 and 94.5)

Bartholin's Cyst/Abscess

Obstruction of the major duct of the Bartholin's gland (major vestibular gland) results in a Bartholin's cyst. Infection and obstruction of the duct will lead to a Bartholin's abscess. The majority of Bartholin's cysts occur because of mechanical blockage of the outflow of normal mucus secreted by the gland. If the cyst causes no symptoms and is only 1 to 2 cm in diameter, no treatment is necessary. Rapid enlargement, pain, hemorrhage, or secondary abscess formation requires the same therapy as a primary abscess; when a Bartholin's cyst/abscess is suspected to confirm the diagnosis and rule out carcinoma in an older woman and to initiate treatment, the gynecologist will create a fistula from the cyst or abscess to the vestibule by marsupialization, incision and drainage, or, rarely, excision. A Bartholin's abscess will harbor *Neisseria gonorrhoeae* in approximately 10% of cases. Therefore, culture for *Neisseria gonorrhoeae* is indicated. Adequate drainage usually obviates the need for systemic antibiotics. Sitz baths provide temporary symptomatic relief.

Condylomata Acuminata (Venereal Warts) (Anogenital Warts)

This common disorder is caused by a papovavirus and is transmitted sexually. This viral infection appears to be more prevalent now, and, importantly, it may be related to the subsequent development of cervical dysplasia (see Chapter 95). It occurs usually during the reproductive years and is most commonly seen in association with other vulvovaginal infections (including candidiasis, trichomoniasis, *Gardnerella* vaginalis infection, gonorrhea, or syphilis). It occurs more frequently in pregnancy and has a more active course in pregnant women.

The patient most often complains of a new growth on her vulva, perineum, or anus; and there is often associated itching and a vaginal discharge. These symptoms may be part of an associated vaginal infection or may represent infection in the crevices of the wart. Often there will be a history of warts on the penis of the sexual partner, who should also be evaluated.

The examination is characteristic and is almost always diagnostic. A wart of 1 to 2 cm usually first appears on the labia, frequently about the posterior introitus, but then spreads, with discrete or congruent lesions appearing on the perineum, anus, vagina, and cervix. They may coalesce into a cauliflower-like lesion that may become huge (Fig. 94.6).

Treatment

Treatment of the warts is best accomplished by painting them carefully with a 20% tincture of podophyllum. This solution is very irritating: it commonly causes transient discomfort and will burn normal skin if applied to it. If such contamination does occur, the skin should be washed promptly with alcohol and then with water. The podophyllum should be left on the warts for 8 to 12 hours and then removed with soap and water. During that time, the patient should not engage in sexual intercourse. The patient should be seen every 5 to 7 days for retreatment until healing occurs. If her sexual partner has warts, he should be treated also, and he should use a condom during intercourse until healing is complete.

Trichloroacetic acid (80–90%) is an alternative therapy. The trichloroacetic acid is applied to the warts at weekly intervals. The solution should be applied only to the warts. Plain talc or baking soda is useful

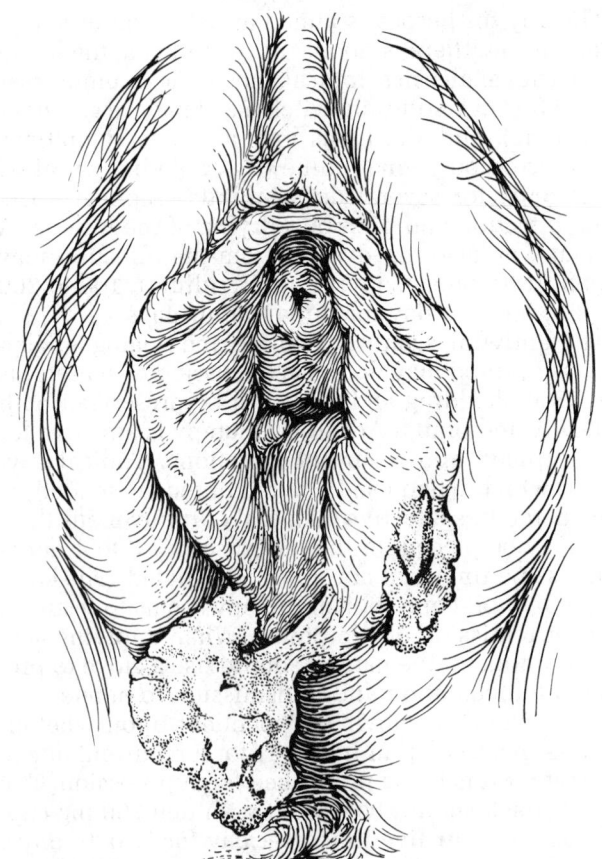

Figure 94.6. Condylomata acuminata.

to remove any excess solution. Neither Podophyllin nor trichloracetic acid is suitable for eradication of large warts (greater than 2 to 2.5 cm) on the cervix or vagina. Also, podophyllin has been reported to cause fetal abnormalities and should not be used during pregnancy. In these instances, referral to a dermatologist or a gynecologist is suggested for evaluation and for consideration of treatment using other modalities, such as cryosurgery, laser surgery, electrodesiccation, or simple surgical excision.

Sebaceous Cyst (Epidermal or Keratinous or Inclusion Cysts)

These conditions are discussed in Chapter 100.

Vulvar Papules

Folliculitis

Overgrowth of skin staphylococci and streptococci can result in vulvar folliculitis. Predisposing factors for this disorder include immunosuppressive therapy, local trauma, poor hygiene, or occlusive (synthetic) clothing. Infection of the hair follicle is identified by erythematous papules or pustules with a central hair shaft. Treatment consists of cleansing the area with a germicidal soap (e.g., Phisohex or Betadine). Warm sitz baths or compresses will help relieve the discomfort. Gentamicin or Neosporin ointment may be prescribed to accelerate healing. If the lesions do not heal within 1 week, systemic dicloxacillin or erythromycin should be prescribed.

Acrochordon

Acrochordons, commonly known as "skin tags," are sessile or pedunculated fibroephithelial polyps. Acrochordons are innocent and should only be removed if large, or annoying to the patient. A gynecologist should be consulted if removal is considered or if there is doubt regarding the diagnosis.

Molluscum Contagiosum

This benign lesion is caused by a pox virus and is transmitted by close contact, including sexual intercourse. However, sexual intercourse is not necessary for transmission as the disease may be spread via fomites or autoinoculation. Although trunk, face, and extremity lesions are common among school children, the lesions of adults are generally located on the genitalia. The adult patient characteristically sees a physician because of a painless new growth in the vulva, perineal area, or thighs. The lesions have a typical appearance permitting diagnosis by inspection, in most instances (Fig. 94.7). The individual lesions are wart-like papules varying from 1 to 10 mm in size. They have a smooth surface and a central umbilical depression containing keratin. There may be multiple separate lesions or one large coalesced lesion. If there is any doubt about the diagnosis, the central cheese-like core may be expressed onto a slide and examined un-

der a microscope using the low power objective. Characteristic large inclusion bodies, which occupy most of the cytoplasm of the cells, will be identified. Occasionally, the lesion resembles bacterial infection, such as folliculitis or furunculosis; but in these instances, the expression of pus versus a cheesy material from the lesion permits differentiation. If doubt remains regarding the diagnosis, the patient should be referred to a dermatologist or a gynecologist for confirmation or biopsy of the lesion.

Because spontaneous resolution may take from months to years, treatment should be given. Therapy consists of scraping open the papule (with a scalpel blade), evacuating its contents, and curetting or cauterizing the base. Large lesions may need to be anaesthetized with lidocaine injection before they are opened or curetted. The patient should be seen in approximately 1 week after the initial treatment for retreatment of any resistant or new lesions. Also the patient should be evaluated for the presence of another venereal disease that may have been acquired simultaneously. Even if another venereal disease is not found, a culture for gonococcal infection (see above) and a serological test for syphilis should be obtained. The patient's sexual partner should be evaluated for lesions of molluscum contagiosum or evidence of another sexually transmitted disease. A male sexual partner should use a condom until the patient's lesions have healed.

Hypo- and Hyperpigmented Lesions of the Vulva

Hypo- and hyperpigmented lesions of the vulva may range from nonmalignant to malignant disorders. Differentiation of the various processes is difficult by inspection alone. Biopsy must be performed to determine the diagnosis. For this reason, referral to a gynecologist or dermatologist is recommended when any such lesion is identified (see Chapter 95).

Intertrigo

This important and common disorder is discussed in Chapter 100.

Contact Dermatitis (Reactive Dermatitis)

This condition is discussed in Chapter 100.

Vestibular Adenitis/Vestibular Adenoma

Vestibular adenitis, inflammation or infection of the minor vestibular gland, results in chronic vulvar pain and dyspareunia. The lesions resulting from this infection are usually difficult to see on physical examination. However, careful inspection, using magnifying lenses if necessary, will usually reveal tiny, erythematous macules or papules lateral to the hymen, in the anatomical position of the minor vestibular glands (see above). Touching the reddened areas with a cotton-tipped applicator usually causes exquisite pain (26). Often the hymenal ring is constricted and/or the posterior aspect is rigid, edematous, and tender. Because

Table 94.3.
Causes of Vulvar Ulcerations

Disease Entity	Etiology	Appearance	Transmission	Symptoms; Other Manifestations	Diagnosis	Treatment
Herpes Simplex (see text)	Herpes simplex II Rarely herpes simplex I	Vulvar vesicle(s)	Sexual	Fever, malaise, lymphadenopathy, burning, paresthesia, dysuria, urinary retention, painful ulcer	Viral culture or Pap smear or Tzanck preparation	Oral acyclovir Topical acyclovir Palliative treatment of lesions
Herpes Zoster	Varicella zoster	Ulceration following the distribution of dermatome	Previous varicella zoster infection	Fever, malaise, lymphadenopathy, painful ulcer	Distribution of lesions Viral culture Pap smear or Tzanck preparation	Oral acyclovir Topical acyclovir Palliative treatment of symptoms
Syphilis (see text and Chapter 30	*Treponema pallidum*	*Primary:* Chancre—hard, painless lesions with central ulceration, lymphadenopathy *Secondary:* Condyloma latum—multiple flat plaques—often confluent. Rash—esp. palms and soles, lymphadenopathy *Tertiary:* Gummatous tumors or ulceration	Sexual	*Secondary:* Malaise, flu-like syndrome, arthralgias, lymphadenopathy *Tertiary:* CNS signs and symptoms	Positive FTA Rising VDRL titers	Benzathine penicillin G or Tetracycline or Erythromycin
Granuloma Inguinale	*Calymmatobacterium granulomatis*	Painless, erythematous nodule which ulcerates. Ulcers have irregular borders with a granulation ricine base. Lymphadenopathy latter stages—scarring and lymphedema	Sexual	Nonhealing ulcer that becomes painful after secondary bacterial infection	Donovan bodies (macrophages containing intracytoplasmic pleomorphic rods	Tetracycline Gentamicin Chloramphenicol Trimethoprim/Sulfumethoxzole (Bactrim Septra)

Disease	Etiology	Appearance	Transmission	Symptoms	Diagnosis	Treatment
Lymphogranuloma Venereum	Chlamydia Trachomatis Serotype L	Vulvar papule which ulcerates in 4–6 weeks. Hallmark inguinal adenitis—nodes are unilateral and edematous—Later bubo formation (enlarged matted nodes held together by inflammatory reaction) Fistula formation, vulvar fenestration	Sexual	Fever, malaise, initially painless	Titer of at least 1:64 on LGV complement fixation test	Aspiration of fluctuant bubos. Tetracycline Erythromycin Sulfamethoxazole Surgical reconstruction
Chancroid	Haemophilus ducreyi	Soft, painful, chancre-like ulcer	Sexual	Painful ulcer Inguinal adenopathy	(culturing the organism is difficult) Diagnosis of exclusion	Ceftriaxone Erythromycin Trimethoprim/Sulfamethoxazole
Hidradenitis suppurative (see Chapters 25 and 100)	Inflammation/infection of apocrine sweat glands	Vulvar abscess formation with draining sinuses, scarring and induration. Fistula formation	Nontransmittable	Pruritis, burning	Appearance	Surgical excision Occasionally—systemic antibiotics Rarely systemic or intralesional corticosteroids
Behçet's disease	? Autoimmune	Vulvar ulcerations with associated oral ulcerations and ocular inflammation	—	Arthritis, erthema nodosum, pyoderma, thrombophlebitis, acne, ulcerative colitis, neurologic symptoms	Diagnosis of exclusion	No definitive treatment High dose oral contraceptives Intralesional corticosteroids
Crohn's disease	Unknown	Linear ulcerations similar to a knife cut. Draining sinuses. Fistulous tracts	—	Oral ulcerations GI symptoms	Biopsy	Chlorambucil Corticosteroids Sulfones Metronidazole Surgical reconstruction
Tuberculosis (see Chapter 29)	Mycobacterium tuberculosis	Painless ulceration	Airborne Primary inoculation		Biopsy, acid fast cultures	Antituberculous therapy

Table 94.4.
Common Nonmalignant Vulvar Tumors

Disease Entity	Cause	Appearance	Symptoms	Complications	Diagnosis	Treatment	Other
Bartholin's Cyst	Obstruction of the duct of the gland	Discrete swelling of the inferior aspect of labium majus	None or vulvar irritation due to enlargement	Infection, hemorrhage into the cyst. Carcinoma, if ≥ age 40	Visual inspection	None, unless symptomatic, infected or hemorrhagic	
Bartholin's Abscess	Infection and obstruction of the duct of the gland	Discrete swelling of the inferior aspect of the labium majus	Pain	Hemorrhage	Visual inspection	Marsupialization Incision and Drainage Rarely, excision	Culture for gonorrhea
Condylomata Acuminata	Human papilloma virus	Single or multiple 2–3 mm diameter and 10–15 mm high, fine finger like projections or flat topped lesions. Lesions may become confluent	Itching, vaginal discharge	Secondary ulceration and infection	Visual inspection, biopsy	20–25% Podophyllum Trichloracetic Acid Liquid nitrogen or Nitrous oxide	5-Flourourucil for intravaginal lesions. Laser surgery, excision or electrosesiccation Treat partner
Sebaceous Cyst	?	Discrete swelling often, 1 cm in diameter. Firm, solid with a yellow color	Vulvar irritation due to enlargement. Pain, if infected	Infection	Visual appearance, biopsy	None Excision, if infected or bothersome	

Table 94.5.
Common Vulvar Papules

Disease Entity	Cause	Appearance	Symptoms	Diagnosis	Treatment
Folliculitis (see Chapter 25)	Staphylococcus and/or streptococcus	Erythematous papules or pustules with a central hair shaft	Asymptomatic Vulvar irritation or pain	Appearance	Germicidal soap, e.g., Phisohex Sitz baths or warm compresses Rarely, Gentamicin or Neosporin ointment Rarely, systemic dicloxacillin or erythromycin
Acrochordon	—	Soft, skin colored, sessile or pedunculated tags of skin	Asymptomatic unless infarcted	Appearance; Biopsy	No treatment or Excision, electrocautery, laser, or cryotherapy
Molluscum contagiosum	Pox virus possibly, sexually transmitted	Wart-like papules 1–10 mm in size with a central umbilical depression		Appearance; Biopsy	Scraping open the papule, evacuating the contents and cauterizing or curetting the base

this disorder is poorly recognized, patients with it frequently have been treated with numerous vaginal creams and/or topical steroids in the past. These measures are ineffective. The treatment of choice is a perineoplasty (a plastic repair of the perineum) (26). Because of the complexity in treating patients with this condition the patient should be referred to a gynecologist.

Adenomas of the vestibular gland may also develop (3). These tumors are generally 1 to 2 cm in size and are composed of the mucus secreting epithelium found in the vestibular glands. Patients typically describe dyspareunia and burning. Patients suspected of this condition should be referred to a gynecologist for definitive treatment.

Tampon-Related Ulceration/Toxic Shock Syndrome

Repetitive tampon use during periods of diminished or absent menstrual flow may result in vaginal ulceration. Typically, patients with this problem develop intermenstrual bleeding and/or abnormal vaginal discharge. The ulcers are usually located in one of the vaginal fornices. They are superficial, erythematous, and 1 or 2 mm in diameter (frequently they are mistaken for herpes). The ulcers will heal spontaneously in a few days if the tampon use is discontinued.

Toxic shock syndrome is caused by coagulase-positive Staphylococcus aureus. It is associated with fever greater than 102°F/39°C, severe headache, sore throat, vomiting, and diarrhea. Hypotension and shock may

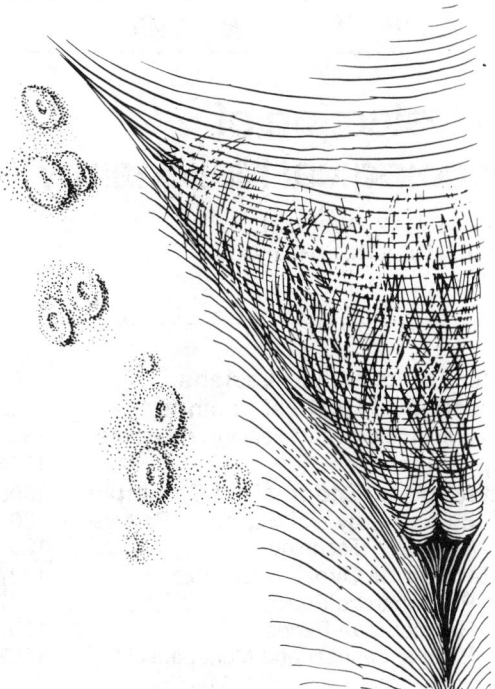

Figure 94.7. Molloscum contagiosum.

develop within 48 hours of the onset of the disorder. Other manifestations include palmar erythema, sunburn-like rash with skin desquamation, myalgias and conjunctivitis.

Pelvic examination typically reveals a purulent vaginal discharge. The vaginal walls are usually inflamed and may be ulcerated. Bimanual examination does not usually reveal any abnormal tenderness.

If a tampon is present at the time of the examination, it should be removed and cultured. A gonorrhea culture and chlamydial fluorescent antibody staining (Microtrak) test or the enzyme immunoassay (Chlamydiazyme) as described on page 1294 should be done to rule out either infection, which may be associated occasionally with symptoms that mimic the toxic shock syndrome.

After thorough cleansing of the vagina with Betadine, the patient should be hospitalized for intravenous therapy with a β-lactamase resistant penicillin and supportive care as needed.

Patients with toxic shock syndrome must be reported to the State Health Department as well as the Centers for Disease Control.

The patient should not use tampons for several subsequent menstrual cycles. In general all patients using tampons should be encouraged to change them every 8 hours at least and to avoid tampons made of superabsorbent material ("super" tampons).

Pubic Lice

This condition is discussed in Chapter 100.

Scabies

This condition is discussed in Chapter 100.

Urethral Syndrome

This condition is discussed in Chapter 27.

Psoriasis

This condition is discussed in Chapter 100.

However, the classic appearance of psoriasis is altered on the vulva. Because the vulva is moist, the psoriatic scale often is not present, and psoriasis may appear as a nonspecific dermatitis. It is rare for a patient to have psoriasis only on the vulva, and therefore a general dermatological examination should be performed. Patients suspected of psoriasis on the vulva should be referred to a dermatologist or gynecologist for confirmation of the diagnosis.

PSYCHOSEXUAL ASPECTS OF VULVOVAGINAL COMPLAINTS

A physician should not suggest treatment for an organic vulvovaginal disorder unless its diagnosis is confirmed. The vulvovaginal region is often the focus of symptoms of an emotional disorder. A psychiatric diagnosis should be considered when the patient seeks repeated appointments and the physician finds no organic cause of the symptom. The psychiatric section (Section 2) of this book deals in detail with diagnosis and management of specific sexual psychological disorders (see Chapter 18) and with other psychological disorders that may present with symptoms related to sexual function.

General References

Jones III HW, Wentz AC, Burnett LS (eds): *Novak's Textbook of Gynecology*, 11th ed. Baltimore, Williams & Wilkins, 1988.
> A comprehensive and authoratative text covering all aspects of gynecology.

Friedrich Jr EG: *Vulvar Disease*, 2nd ed. Philadelphia, WB Saunders, 1983.
> This text remains the classic reference for disorders of the vulva.

U.S. Department of Health and Human Services: 1989 sexually transmitted disease treatment guidelines. *Morbidity and Mortality Weekly Report* 38 (S-8):1989.
> The standard reference for the treatment of sexually transmitted diseases. Copies available at $3.00 each from Massachusetts Medical Scoiety, C.S.P.O. Box 9120, Waltham, MA 02254-9120.

Specific References

1. Amsel R, Totten PA, Spiegel CA, et al: Nonspecific vaginitis: Diagnostic criteria and microbial and epidemiologic associations. *Am J Med* 74:14, 1983.
2. Anyon CP, Desmond FB, Eastcott DF: A study of candida in one thousand and seven women. *NZ Med J* 73:9, 1971.
3. Axe S, Parmley T, Woodruff JD: Adenomas in minor vestibular glands. *Obstet Gynecol* 68:16, 1986.
4. Duncan NC: Gonorrhea 1983. *Derm Clinic* 1:43, 1083.
5. Erkkola R, Jarvomem H, Terho P, et al: Microbial flora in women showing symptoms of nonspecific vaginosis: Applicability of KOH test for diagnosis. *Scand J Infect Dis* 40:59, 1983.

6. Eschenbach DA, Buchanan TM, Pollock HM, et al: Polymicrobial etiology of acute pelvic inflammatory disease. *N Engl J Med* 293:166, 1975.
7. Deleted in editorial review.
8. Friedrich Jr. EG: Vaginitis. *Am J Obstet Gynecol* 152:247, 1985.
9. Galask'RP: Vaginal colonization by bacteria and yeast. *Am J Obstet Gynecol* 158:993, 1988.
10. Guinan ME, MacCalman J, Kern ER, et al: The course of untreated recurrent genital herpes simplex infection in 27 women. *N Engl J Med* 304:759, 1981.
11. Kaufman RH, Faro S: Herpes genitalis: clinical features and treatment. *Clin Obstet Gynecol* 28:152, 1985.
12. Larsen B, Galask RP: Vaginal microbial flora: practical and theoretic relevance. *Obstet Gynecol.* 55:1005, 1980.
13. Leppaluoto P: The coitus-induced dynamics of vaginal bacteriology. *J Reprod Med* 7:169, 1971.
14. McKay M: Cutaneous manifestations of candidiasis. *Am J Obstet Gynecol* 158:991, 1988.
15. Oriel JD, Partridge BM, Denny MJ, et al: Genital yeast infections. *Br Med J* 4:761, 1972.
16. Paavonen J: Physiology and ecology of the vagina. *Scand J Infect Dis Suppl* 40:31, 1983.
17. Schachter J: Chlamydia infections. *N Engl J Med* 298:428, 490, 540, 1978.
18. Soll DR: High-frequency switching in *Candida albicans* and its relations to vaginal candidiasis. *Am J Obstet Gynecol* 158:997, 1988.
19. Spence MR: The treatment of gonorrhea, syphilis, chancroid, lymphogranuloma renereum, and granuloma inguinale. *Clin Obstet and Gynecol* 31:453, 1988.
20. Spiegel CA, Amsel R, Eschenbach D, et al: Anaerobic bacteria in nonspecific vaginitis. *N Engl J Med* 303:601, 1980.
21. Spiegel CA, Davick P, Totten PA, et al: *Gardnerella* vaginalis and anaerobic bacteria in the etiology of bacterial (nonspecific) vaginosis. *Scand J Infect Dis, Suppl* 40:41, 1983.
22. Syverson RE, Buckley H, Gibian J, et al: Cellular and humoral immune status in women with chronic candida vaginitis. *Am J Obstet Gynecol* 134:624, 1979.
23. Vontver LA, Eschenbach DA: The role of *Gardnerella* vaginalis in nonspecific vaginitis. *Clin Obstet Gynecol* 24:439, 1981.
24. Watts DH, Eschenbach DA: Treatment of *Chlamydia, Mycoplasma,* and group B streptococcal infections. *Clin Obstet Gynecol* 31:435, 1988.
25. Westom L: Effect of acute pelvic inflammatory disease on fertility. *Am J Obstet Gynecol* 121:707, 1975.
26. Woodruff JD, Parmley TH: Infection of the minor vestibular gland. *Obstet Gynecol* 62:609, 1983.

C H A P T E R 95

Early Detection of Gynecological Malignancy*

PRESTON M. GAZAWAY, M.D.
GEORGE R. HUGGINS, M.D.

The female reproductive organs are common sites for the development of malignancy. Between 15 and 20% of cancers in women arise from the genital tract. Women who have gynecological cancers discovered while still confined to the site of origin can expect a 60 to 90% 5-year survival rate. In contrast, more extensive cancers involving distant spread have a 5-year survival of zero to 60% (8). If preinvasive lesions are detected and appropriate and punctual treatment is initiated, a 100% cure rate is expected. The vulva, vagina, and cervix all have well-characterized preinvasive lesions.

With the exception of the vulva and breast the patient is unable to perform a satisfactory gynecological self-screening examination. However, with the pelvic examination, all components of the genital system except the fallopian tubes may be inspected, palpated, and screened for cancer or its precursors.

DETECTION OF VULVAR LESIONS

The vulvar skin is subject to disease similar to that of the skin elsewhere, but the prevalence of various conditions is modified in that the vulva is unexposed to solar radiation. For example, squamous cell carcinoma comprises almost 85% of all vulvar cancers, followed by melanoma (5%), and sarcoma (2%). In contrast, basal cell cancer, common in sun-exposed skin, accounts for only 1.5% of vulvar malignancies (17).

Preinvasive lesions of the vulva are termed *vulvar intraepithelial neoplasia (VIN)*. VIN is the term now used to include diseases that were once called *Bowen's*

*J. Courtland Robinson, M.D., M.P.H., contributed to this chapter in the first and second editions of this book.

disease, erythroplasia of Queyrat, squamous cell carcinoma in situ, Paget's disease, and condyloma acuminata. The average age of women with preinvasive lesions is between 40 and 50. Most women with invasive vulvar cancer are in their 60s and 70s although it may occasionally develop in women less than 40. This age differential supports the hypothesis that progression from preinvasive lesions to cancer of the vulva is an indolent process taking several years.

The pathognomonic lesion of VIN is a papular or maculopapular lesion with a roughened surface; however, VIN may have many different guises and the lesions often appear to be well defined and innocent.

The lesions may vary from white to hyperpigmented. They may be sharply demarcated or generalized over the vulva and may even spread to adjacent regions. Some may resemble seborrheic keratoses, nevi, lentigo, intertrigo, condylomata acuminata, or condylomata lata. Because VIN and vulvar cancer can masquerade as many other disease entities, the diagnosis and definitive treatment are often delayed while treatment for an incorrectly diagnosed lesion is instituted.

Some women with vulvar cancer have noted symptoms for up to 16 months before seeking treatment. Furthermore, medical management was employed for up to 12 months before the definitive diagnosis was made (5).

One should be suspicious when any lesion is seen, especially if the lesions are chronic and not immediately responsive to topical treatment. The most common symptom of vulvar neoplasia is itching, which occurs in 70% of patients. Other symptoms include ulceration, bleeding, pain, or the presence of a mass.

Unfortunately, a vulvar equivalent of the cervical Pap smear is not available; therefore, the primary method of diagnosis of early lesions is the early recognition and prompt referral to a gynecologist for diagnosis by biopsy.

The treatment of VIN depends upon the extent of the lesion. If the vulvar lesions grossly appear to be condyloma acuminata and are not extensive, they may be treated empirically without biopsy (see Chapter 94 for details). If no decrement in size is apparent within 2 to 4 weeks, the suspected condylomata acuminata should be biopsied to confirm the diagnosis. The gynecologist and pathologist must be aware of prior treatment of the lesion because podophyllin and 5-fluorouracil (two common topical agents used in the treatment of condyloma acuminata) may cause abnormal mitoses and bizarre cells that cause an erroneous diagnosis to be made of advanced VIN or cancer.

Small lesions may be excised entirely. Laser vaporization, or skinning vulvectomy, is necessary for widespread disease.

Vulvar cancer may also masquerade as vulvar leukoplakia, lichen sclerosus et atrophicus, or kraurosis vulvae. Once these lesions are proven by biopsy they may be treated safely by a gynecologist by the twice weekly application of a topical androgen (usually 2% testosterone propionate ointment) made upon request by a pharmacist. When used only twice weekly, side effects are minimal.

Prevention of advanced disease requires that the patient be taught to examine her vulva periodically by use of a mirror, and to report any changes in the external genitalia. It is important that one examine the patient promptly if a change is noted and that a periodic examination be performed even when there are no complaints. Special sensitivity must be used in older women who are often reluctant to complain of a vagina or vulvar problem and who often are resistant to a screening vaginal examination.

DETECTION OF CERVICAL LESIONS

Epidemology and Etiological Factors

Invasive epidermoid carcinoma of the cervix is the second most common malignancy of the reproductive organs (endometrial cancer is the first) (14); 14,000 cases of cervical cancer (3% of all female cancers) were newly diagnosed in 1986. In that year there were 6,800 deaths from gynecological cancer (3.1% of all cancer deaths). Significant reduction in mortality and morbidity has been achieved by vigorous promotion and acceptance of the annual pelvic examination in combination with the cancer detection smear (Pap smear) (9). The incidence of cervical cancer has increased in younger women. In 1981, women less than 50 years old accounted for 21% of all cervical cancer deaths. By 1987 this figure had risen to 27% (2). This increase in cervical cancer in this population parallels the increasingly early onset of sexual activity among women. In 1971, 28% of 15- to 19-year-old women had had sexual relations; however, in 1982 42% of women in the same age group admitted to sexual activity (13).

The etiology of cervical cancer is still not settled, but the Human Papilloma Virus (HPV) is a significant etiological agent. The virus is transmitted sexually, by autoinoculation from condylomata elsewhere on the body, or from mother to neonate. Approximately 60 strains of HPV have been identified but only seven are tropic for the genital tract. HPV 6/11 is most often found in cervical condylomata and in low grade dysplasia. HPV 16 is found in about 55% of cervical cancers, HPV 18 in 15 to 20%, and HPV 33/33/35 are found occasionally (13). Women who become infected with HPV prior to 25 years of age are 40 times more likely to develop cervical cancer than those uninfected (4).

Infection with the herpes simplex virus, type 2, and the Epstein Barr virus both correlate with the incidence of cervical cancer. However, the question remains whether these viruses are promoters, cocarcinogens, or solely an index of past sexual behavior. Besides sexual activity at a young age and infection with HPV, early childbearing and multiple sexual partners are additional risk factors of cervical cancer.

PAP SMEAR

The mainstay of cervical cancer control is the performance of a regular Pap smear, with referral for colposcopy and biopsy whenever a significant abnormality is found. Colposcopy is an office procedure done during a pelvic examination that utilizes an instrument similar to a dissecting microscope that illuminates and magnifies 8- to 10-fold the cervix, vagina, and vulva. Also, if a patient is identified to be at high risk for cervical cancer (see above), then the use of barrier contraception until a mutually monogamous relationship is established may decrease the risk of transmission of potentially oncogenic agents.

The cancer detection smear, when properly obtained, is moderately effective in identifying a significant problem (9).

The efficacy of the Pap smear as a screening tool has never been tested in a prospective blinded study. The typical false-negative rate for a Pap smear in most laboratories is 20%, but reports have cited values from 3 to 60% (9). Despite this limitation the widespread use of the Pap smear has been accompanied by a significant decrease in the incidence of invasive carcinoma of the cervix. Likewise, there has been a corresponding increase in the detection of preinvasive lesions (Fig. 95.1). The success of cytologic screening of the cervix has led many physicians to place an inordinate amount of faith in the Pap smear. It should never be considered a perfect diagnostic test. Any visible cervical lesions of uncertain origin may represent an early cancer, and patients with such lesions should be referred to a gynecologist for evaluation.

A screening Pap smear should not be obtained if a woman has douched or used vaginal medication or a tampon in the previous 24 hours. These activities may alter or remove cells completely and yield an erroneous interpretation. Lubricants may also interfere with cytological interpretation. The speculum used in the examination should be unlubricated or, if necessary, lubricated only with water.

The most important area to be screened is the squamocolumnar junction, as most cervical neoplastic processes arise at this site. The anatomical relationship of this junction varies in the adolescent, the sexually active woman, and the postmenopausal women (Fig. 95.2). Once the cervix is visualized, the cervical spatula should be placed firmly against the cervix and rotated at least 360°, preferably 720°, in a continuous unidirectional sweep. A cotton swab moistened with normal saline should then be used to obtain an endocervical sample in all patients. Both specimens should then be smeared together onto a clean microscopic slide and immediately sprayed or immersed in fixative to prevent an air drying artifact. When because of narrowing of the cervical os a cotton swab cannot be introduced into the endocervical canal, a plastic brush (Cytobrush, Milex) may be used to obtain an adequate endocervical sample. An additional sample taken from the posterior vaginal fornix of perimenopausal or postmenopausal women may occasionally detect malignant cells that have exfoliated from the endometrium, fallopian tubes, or ovaries.

One should select a cytology laboratory that has satisfactory quality control, use the proper fixative techniques required by the laboratory, and learn the systems of reporting of the particular laboratory. Recently the National Cancer Institute Workshop has recommended a revision in the manner of reporting the results of the Pap smear (11). It is important to provide the laboratory the patient's age, the date of her last menstrual period, and to comment on the presence or absence of infection. The laboratory report should state whether the sample was satisfactory or unsatisfactory. An unsatisfactory slide must be repeated. The Pap smear is unsatisfactory if no endocervical cells are present in a specimen obtained from a premenopausal woman with an intact cervix (9).

The cytologist's report usually will describe the results as negative (with or without inflammation) or as showing atypia, dysplasia, or changes suggestive of cancer; these findings may be quantitated as mild, moderate, or severe. The presence of yeast or trichomonads may also be noted. However, the Pap smear is insufficiently specific to diagnose most organisms that cause vaginitis. If atypical cells are present in association with inflammatory cells, empirical treatment for chlamydia with doxycycline, 100 mg twice a day, or tetracycline, 500 mg four times a day for 10 to 14 days, should be instituted. Approximately 30% of women with atypia or mild dysplasia with inflammation may be infected with chlamydia. A few weeks after treatment, 90% of smears with atypia secondary to this infection revert to normal (10). When the Pap smear shows persistent atypia or inflammation, the

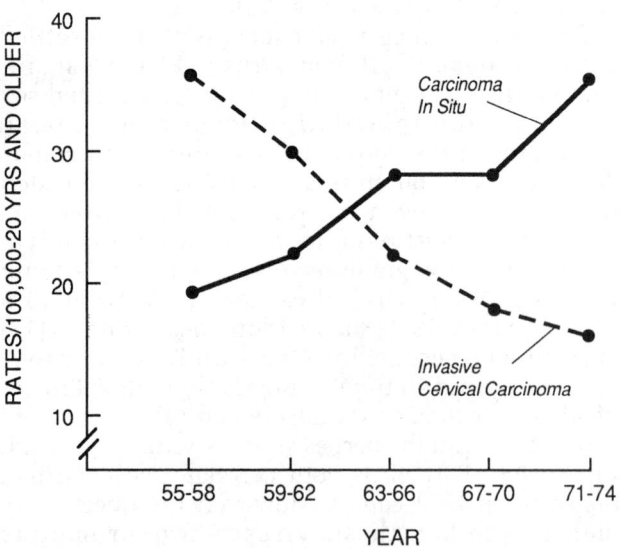

Figure 95.1. Average annual age-adjusted incidence rate trends for invasive carcinoma and carcinoma in situ of the cervix from the Toledo, Ohio area. (Redrawn from Kim K, Rigal RD, Patrick JR et al: The changing trends of uterine cancer and cytology; a study of morbidity and mortality trends over a twenty year period. Cancer 42:2439, 1978.)

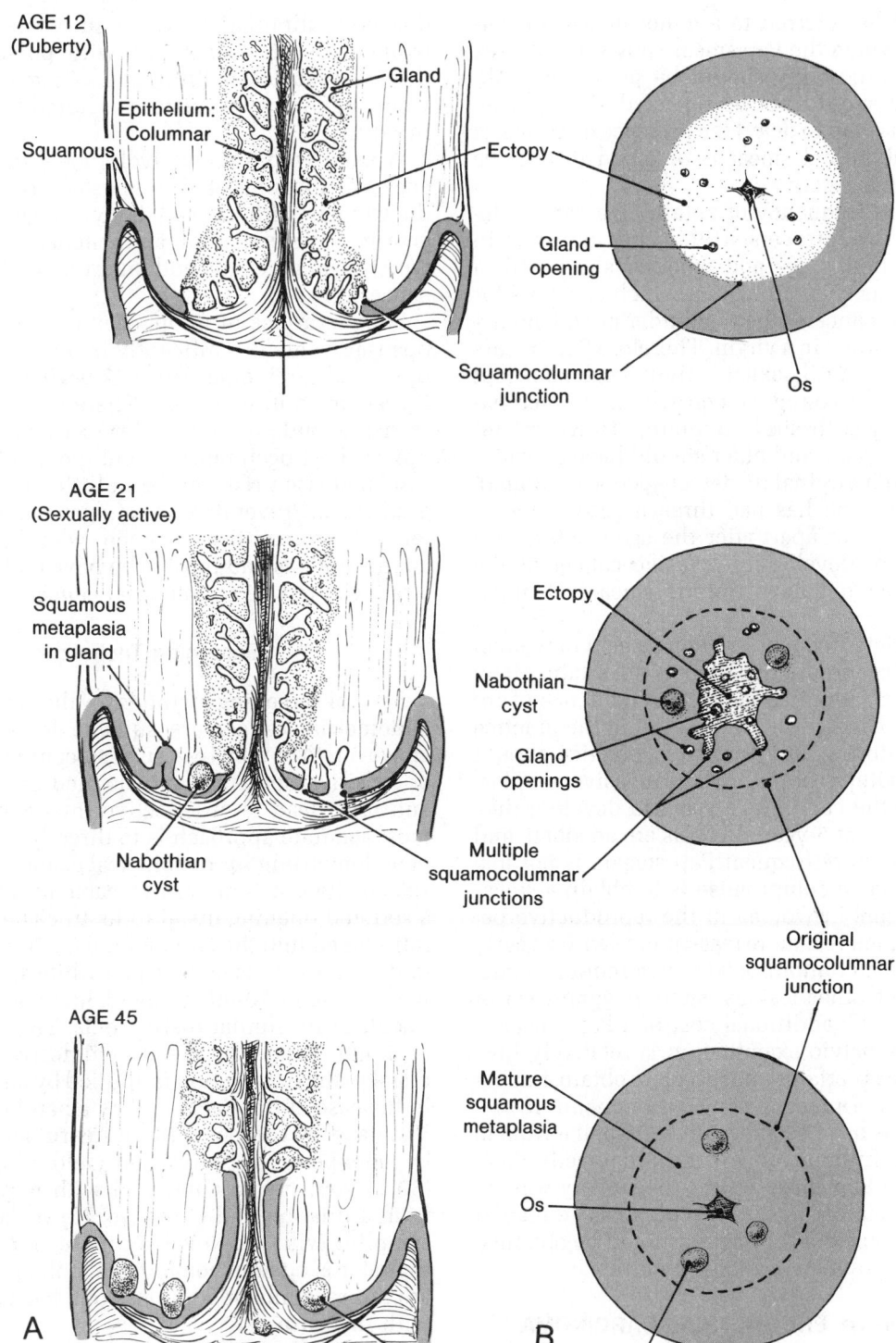

Figure 95.2.   The uterine cervix in women of various ages. *A*. Coronal section of the cervix and vaginal vault. *B*. Vaginal view of the cervix. (Redrawn from Briggs RM: Dysplasia and early neoplasia of the uterine cervix. A review. *Obstet Gynecol Surv* 34:70, 1980.)

patient should be referred to a gynecologist for colposcopy. Also when the Pap smear shows any degree of dysplasia, colposcopy should be performed. Abnormal smears should not be repeated since subsequent smears may fail to detect the presence of dysplasia (5). Once an abnormal smear is obtained it must be evaluated by colposcopy.

The suggested frequency of obtaining a cancer detection smear is controversial (9, 17); it depends in part on the patient's age and whether she is still a virgin. Squamous cell carcinoma, which accounts for 95% of cervical cancers (the remainder are adenocarcinoma), is unknown in a virgin. Therefore Pap smears are not necessary until sexual activity begins (except for adolescent and young women who have been exposed to diethylstilbestrol in utero). However, all women aged 18 years and older should have a regular Pap smear even if virginal (to detect adenocarcinoma). Also, a woman who has had three negative smears taken at least a year apart after the age of 60 is at a very low risk of developing invasive cancer of the cervix and need not have routine smears obtained thereafter.

The appropriate frequency of Pap smears in women who are in their reproductive years is uncertain. Many argue that the current decline in the incidence of invasive cervical cancer is a direct result of the practice of yearly monitoring, and that such practice should be continued. Others point out that invasive neoplastic changes in the cervix take years to develop; they argue that smears at 5-year intervals are adequate and that the cost of more frequent Pap smears is not justified. A reasonable compromise is to obtain a smear every 2 to 3 years in women in the reproductive period. Some women feel more reassurance with a yearly smear. Because an *annual pelvic examination* is suggested to detect other lesions, such as gonorrhea or ovarian cancer, the additional cost of a Pap smear at the time of the pelvic examination is relatively low. However, there is certainly no reason to obtain a smear every 6 months, a practice some recommend, if previous specimens have been negative. Also, if a woman has had a total hysterectomy (cervix removed), there is no need for a Pap smear unless the surgery was for cervical dysplasia or cancer, in which case a regular smear from the apex of the vagina should be obtained every year to evaluate for a local recurrence.

DETECTION OF ENDOMETRIAL CARCINOMA

Epidemiology and Etiological Factors

An estimated 36,000 cancers of the endometrium were detected in 1986. This cancer accounts for 8% of all cancers in women and almost 50% of all new gynecological cancers. Only 13% of cancer deaths resulted from endometrial carcinoma despite its high prevalence (14).

Unopposed estrogen stimulation has been firmly implicated in the genesis of this cancer, and there are several situations associated with such exposure: endogenous stimulation occurs in women who are anovulatory such as patients with polycystic ovarian disease, diabetes mellitus, and extreme obesity. These women often have a history of infrequent menses and infertility.

Women who are massively obese or who have diabetes mellitus metabolize sex steroids differently than do women with normal body weight. There is increased conversion of androstenedione to estrone, which stimulates the endometrium and perhaps even cancer.

Long-term use of unopposed estrogen in postmenopausal women significantly increases the risk of endometrial carcinoma. This risk begins to increase after 2 years of continuous use. There is a 14 fold increase in risk of endometrial cancer in women who use unopposed estrogen replacement therapy for 7 years (6). This increased risk can be nullified by adding a progestin (e.g., Provera) to the estrogen regimen (see Chapter 77). In contrast, women who have used oral contraceptives and those who have had children have a reduced risk of endometrial cancer.

Screening Techniques

Several screening methods for the early detection of endometrial cancer are suitable for office practice. However, to be effective, such screening methods must be sensitive, specific, well tolerated, safe, inexpensive, and must lead to an effective intervention (12). The most accurate approach is to directly obtain a sample of endometrium for histological examination. The Novak curette is a 4-mm resterilizable metal cylinder with a serrated opening distal to its tip. The instrument is introduced into the endometrial cavity and four quadrants of the uterus are scraped while applying suction with a 6-ml or 10-ml syringe. The Vabra aspirator and Vacutage are similar instruments. They consist of a 2- or 3-mm disposable metal cylinder with an opening distal to the tip. Suction is applied by an electric pump in the case of the Vabra and by a hand pump with the Vacutage. All three of these instruments when used by an experienced physician yield a high correlation (80 to 95%) when compared with material obtained from a dilation and curettage. However, endometrial sampling with the Novak's curette or a pump vacuum aspirator is often uncomfortable to the patient (5). They are not recommended unless one has had experience with their use.

The Pipelle Endometrial suction curette [available from United International Marketing Resources, 475 Danbury Road, Wilton, CT 06897, (800) 243-6608] is becoming very popular and is recommended for the general physician even though it has not been studied prospectively. It is a flexible plastic tube 1 mm in diameter with a small opening near the blunt tip. Suction is applied with an integral movable plastic plunger. Unfortunately, because of its flexibility, the Pipelle cannot always be inserted into a stenotic cervical os. This instrument produces minimal pain, and the specimen obtained is equivalent to the Novak's curette.

The Pap smear obtained without an additional specimen from the vaginal pool is unreliable for the detection of endometrial cancer. When a sample is obtained from the vaginal pool, the recovery of abnormal endometrial cells may be as high as 65%.

Patients who are at increased risk of endometrial cancer and all women who have postmenopausal bleeding should be referred to a gynecologist for suction endometrial aspiration if the general physician is not familiar with the technique.

DETECTION OF OVARIAN CANCER

Ovarian cancer is the most problematic of gynecological cancers. Most lesions are silent until they have reached a size large enough to produce symptoms from the pressure of the mass. By this time, they have usually metastasized. The cure rate for advanced lesions is low. In 1986 approximately 19,000 new cases of ovarian cancer were discovered among American women. They comprise 4% of all cancers and 26% of gynecological cancers. However, they account for 50% of deaths from gynecological cancers (14). The etiology of ovarian cancer is unknown, and little progress has been made in identifying the patient at risk, in early detection, or in improving the survival rate (15).

The symptoms of ovarian cancer are nonspecific and are often ignored by both patient and physician until the tumor is far advanced. Most commonly symptoms are referable to the gastrointestinal tract and consist of feelings of abdominal fullness, bloating, eructation, and pelvic pressure. Pain or constipation appears only very late. Abnormal uterine bleeding occurs only rarely in association with ovarian cancer.

The most common sign of ovarian cancer is an adnexal or abdominopelvic mass. The diagnostic evaluation of such a mass differs in each epoch of a woman's life.

Unfortunately neither ultrasound nor computed tomography (CT) of the abdomen and pelvis is able to indicate the malignant potential of ovarian masses. Nevertheless, these procedures are useful in determining the extent of the tumor. The determination of the concentration of tumor markers such as alpha-fetoprotein, human chorionic gonadotropin, and carcinoembryonic antigen may be helpful in the evaluation of an ovarian mass and in following the course of the patient after treatment.

Premenarche Period

About two-thirds of ovarian tumors are benign in this age group. The most common tumors are a *benign cystic teratoma (dermoid)*, a *benign simple cyst*, or a *cystadenoma*.

Malignant tumors in this age group arise from the germ cells or gonadal stromal cells in 80 to 90% cases (3). Generally no risk factors are elucidated. The most common presenting complaint is pain, which is caused by rapid tumor growth.

Reproductive Period

Most ovarian masses found during this period are functional cysts. The normal premenopausal ovary is 1.5 cm $\times$ 3 cm $\times$ 3.5 cm. If ovulation fails to occur, a unilocular cyst will be formed and may reach 10 cm in diameter. When ovulation does occur, a corpus luteum forms that may occasionally become enlarged because of internal hemorrhage. Both of these ovarian cysts are frequently detected because of the regular screening of women in this age group. These cysts usually resolve spontaneously within 2 to 4 weeks.

If the ovarian enlargement is demonstrated to be truly cystic by ultrasound, a period of observation is warranted. Oral contraceptive pills containing 35 to 50 micrograms of ethinyl estradiol (see Chapter 93) may be prescribed for 2 months to suppress gonadotropins. Estrogen blocks the pituitary gonadotrophins that are the stimulus for the formation and maintenance of ovarian cysts. When the ovarian cyst persists for longer than 60 days in spite of gonadotropin suppression, the diagnosis of ovarian neoplasia should be considered strongly and a gynecologist should be consulted.

Spanos found that 92% of persistent ovarian masses were neoplastic, and 6.8% were malignant (16). Ultrasound is the best method to diagnose and monitor ovarian cysts. Any ovarian tumor that is irregular, septated, semisolid, solid, or greater than 8 cm in diameter upon ultrasound evaluation should be strongly suspected to be malignant. For women with those lesions prompt arrangements for gynecological consultation should be made.

Perimenopausal and Menopausal Periods

During this era of a woman's life the incidence of ovarian cancer is highest. In the American population, the annual incidence increases from 15.7 per 100,000 for women aged 40 to 50 years to 35 per 100,000 after age 50. This dramatic increase in incidence has led some investigators to propose aggressive means to manage minimal ovarian enlargement.

In 1971, Barber proposed that any palpable ovary in a postmenopausal women was abnormal and required laparotomy. He termed this the *Palpable Postmenopausal Ovary Syndrome (PMPO)* (1). However, in recent years, experience has proven that a more conservative approach to the PMPO syndrome is warranted. Less than 10% of patients with the PMPO syndrome have ovarian malignancies (7).

The only available method today for screening for ovarian cancer is the periodic pelvic examination. All postmenopausal women should have an annual pelvic examination.

General References

Morow CP, Townsend DE: *Synopsis of Gynecologic Oncology.* New York, J. Wiley and Sons, 1987.
Jones III HW, Wentz AC, Burnett LS: *Novak's Textbook of Gynecology,* 11th ed. Baltimore, Williams & Wilkins, 1988.

Specific References

1. Barber HRK, Graber EA: The PMPO syndrome (postmenopausal palpable ovary syndrome). *Obstet Gynecol Surv* 28:357, 1973.
2. Booth M, Beral V: Cervical cancer deaths in young women. *Lancet* 1:616, 1989.
3. Breen JL, Marson WS: Ovarian tumors in children and adolescents. *Clin Obstet Gynecol* 20:607, 1977.
4. Butler EB, Stanbridge CM: Condylomatous lesions of the lower female genital tract. *Clin Obstet Gynecol* 11:171, 1984.
5. DiSilva PJ, Creasman WT (ed): *Clinical Gynecologic Oncology*. St. Louis, CV Mosby, 1989.
6. Ernster VI, Bush TL, Huggins GR, et al: Benefits and risks of menopausal estrogen and/or progestin hormone use. *J Prev Med* 17:201, 1988.
7. Goldstein SR, Sulramanyan B, Snyder JR, et al: The postmenopausal cystic adnexal mass: The potential role of ultrasound in conservative management. *Obstet Gynecol* 73:8, 1989.
8. Kennedy AW, Flagg JS, Webster FD: Gynecologic cancer in the very elderly. *Gynecol Oncol* 32:49, 1989.
9. Koss LG: The Papanicolaou test for cervical cancer: a triumph and a tragedy. *JAMA* 261:737, 1989.
10. Mecsei R, Haugen OA, Halvorsen LE, Dalen A: Genital *Chlamydia trachomatis* infections in patients with abnormal cervical smears: effect of tetracycline on cell changes. *Obstet Gynecol* 73:317, 1989.
11. National Cancer Institute Workshop. The 1988 Bethesda system for reporting cervical/vaginal cytologic diagnoses. *JAMA* 262:7, 1989.
12. Pritchard KI: Screening for endometrial cancer. Is it effective? *Ann Intern Med* 110:177, 1989.
13. Richard RM: Typing HPV DNA gains clues for therapy. *Contemp Ob/Gyn* 31:4, 1988.
14. Silverberg E, Lubera J: Cancer statistics. *CA* 36:16, 1986.
15. Smith LH, Oi RH: Detection of the patient at risk; clinical, radiological and cytological detection. *Clin Obstet Gynecol* 20:607, 1977.
16. Spanos WJ, Preoperative hormonal therapy of cystic adnexal masses. *Am J Obstet Gynecol* 116:551, 1973.
17. Walton RJ: Cervical cancer screening programs: summary of the 1982 task force report. *Can Med Assoc J* 127:581, 1982.

Problems of the Eyes and Ears

CHAPTER 96

Hearing Loss and Associated Ear Problems

WARREN ROTHMAN, M.D.

A 1971 report from the National Health Survey estimated that 13.2 million persons in the United States had significant bilateral hearing impairment. Of these, 5.5 million were over 65 years of age (2). The survey also indicated that a large proportion of symptomatic adults go directly to a hearing aid dealer rather than to a physician and/or audiologist for initial evaluation. This chapter provides an approach to hearing loss and associated ear problems when patients describe these problems to their physicians.

EAR STRUCTURE AND FUNCTION

Classification of the mechanism of hearing impairment (conductive or sensorineural), requires an understanding of the structure and function of the components of the ear (see Fig. 96.1).

The *external ear* is composed of the auricle, the auditory meatus, and the external auditory canal. The outer portion of the canal is cartilaginous and is covered by thick skin that contains hair follicles and the cerumen-secreting glands; cerumen protects the epithelium and captures foreign particles entering the canal. The inner portion of the canal is bony and is covered by squamous epithelium without hair follicles or cerumen glands.

The *middle ear* consists of the tympanic membrane, the air space behind it, and the three linked ossicles (malleus, incus, and stapes). The malleus is attached to the tympanic membrane, while the stapes makes contact with the inner ear via the bony stapes footplate at the oval window. The landmarks seen on inspection of the tympanic membrane are shown in Figure 96.2. The lining of the middle ear is a mucus-secreting epithelium similar to that which lines the nose. The middle ear communicates with the nose via the eustachian tube, which enters the lateral nasopharynx. Patency of the eustachian tube assures equal pressure on either side of the tympanic membrane, which facilitates the transmission of sound from the tympanic membrane to the oval window.

The *inner ear* is encased in very hard bone (the otic capsule) and is fluid filled. It consists of a sensory organ for hearing (cochlea) and the sensory organ for balance (vestibular labyrinth). Nerves from the cochlea and labyrinth unite to form the acoustic nerve (VIII), which runs through the bony internal auditory canal in the temporal bone to the brainstem.

The *conductive system* of the ear includes the external auditory canal, the tympanic membrane, the middle ear, and the ossicles. Hearing loss due to defects in this portion of the ear is termed conductive hearing loss. The *sensorineural system* of the ear consists of the cochlea, the auditory nerve, and the brainstem auditory pathways projecting to the auditory cortex. In these structures, sound waves delivered by the conductive system are transformed into nerve impulses. Hearing loss due to defects in this portion of the ear is termed *sensorineural hearing loss*, which may be localized as cochlear or retrocochlear.

DETERMINING SEVERITY AND MECHANISM OF HEARING LOSS

Office Testing

Regardless of the specific cause of hearing loss, the severity of the impairment and the probable mechanism (conductive or sensorineural) can be determined in the office. This determination can be made from a combination of the history, the patient's ability to hear

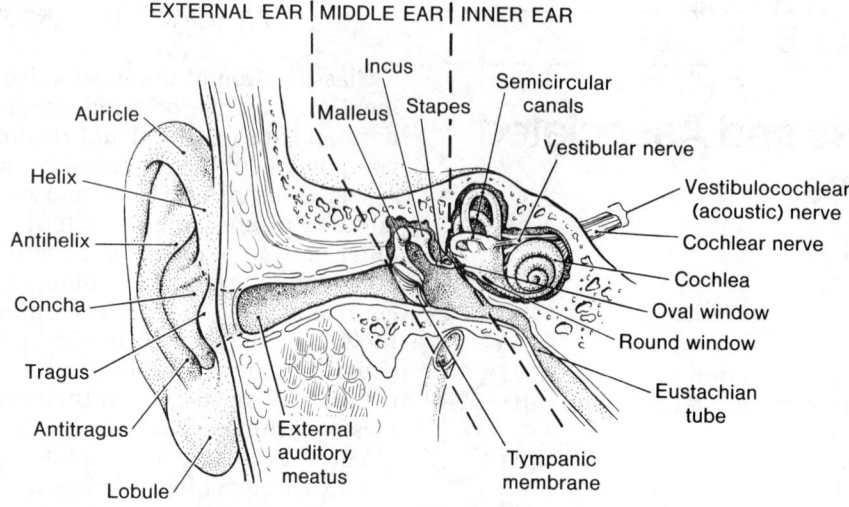

Figure 96.1.   Normal structures of the ear.

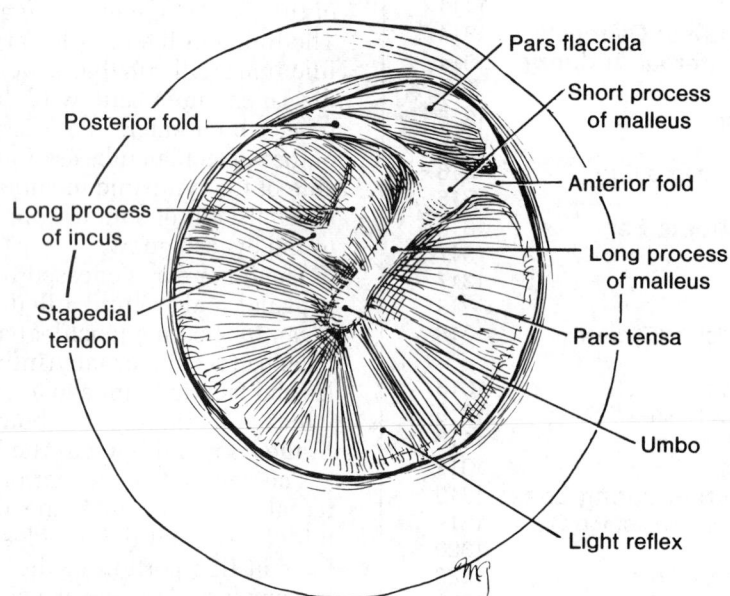

Figure 96.2.   Right tympanic membrane, showing important landmarks.

the spoken voice in the office, and testing with a tuning fork and a ticking watch.

A practical method for evaluating the *severity of hearing impairment* includes an estimate of the social problems that have occurred due to difficulty in hearing and an assessment of response to voice testing in the office; these two findings can be equated with various levels of abnormality in the audiogram (see Table 96.1). *Slight* impairment indicates difficulty in hearing long distance speech—for example, group meetings, social gatherings, or the theater. *Moderate* impairment includes some difficulty with short distance speech and conversation. *Severe* impairment indicates no understanding of the conversational voice but understanding of the amplified voice. Amplification may be achieved by raising the voice or elec-

tronically by use of a hearing aid (see below). *Profound* (or total) impairment indicates inability to hear and understand the spoken voice despite maximal amplification.

In the patient with significant hearing impairment, the *frequency range* that is involved can also be approximated in the office by testing recognition of words containing the sound "ah" (low frequency, vowel sound), such as apple, hot dog, airplane, and the sound "ss" (high frequency, consonant), such as ice cream, stairway, baseball, sunset, when these words are spoken about 2 feet behind the ear being tested, with the other ear covered. A ticking watch held 2 to 3 inches from the ear also tests hearing at high frequencies, whereas tuning forks test relatively low frequency hearing.

Table 96.1.
A Practical Method for Assessing Severity of Hearing Loss in the Office[a]

Severity of Hearing Loss	Social Difficulty	Office Voice Test	Puretone Audiogram
Normal hearing	None	18 ft or more using normal voice	No loss over 10 dB[b]
Slight hearing loss	Long distance speech	Not over 12 ft using normal voice	10–30 dB loss
Moderate hearing loss	Short distance speech	Not over 3 ft using normal voice	Up to 60 dB loss
Severe hearing loss	All unamplified voices	Raised voice at meatus	Over 60 dB loss
Profound hearing loss	Voices never heard	All speech and sound	Over 90 dB loss

[a]Adapted from Mawson SR: *Diseases of the Ear*. Baltimore, Williams & Wilkins, 1974.
[b]dB, decibel.

Tuning Fork Test

The mechanism of hearing impairment can be classified tentatively as conductive or sensorineural by the use of tuning fork tests (Rinne and Weber). A 256-Hertz (i.e., 256 cps) tuning fork should be used. The fork should be struck lightly for the Rinne test to avoid overtones. The interpretation of tuning fork tests is summarized in Table 96.2.

Rinne Test

This test is used to evaluate hearing loss in one ear. It is important to mask the hearing in the other ear by rubbing crumpled paper over that ear to create a rustling sound. The tuning fork is struck gently against a firm surface. It is then held against the mastoid bone until the patient no longer hears the sound; then it is held about 1 inch from the canal. The patient with normal hearing should hear the sound longer by air than by bone conduction. A modified Rinne is simply to have the patient compare the loudness of bone and air conduction. Air conduction should be louder than bone conduction in a patient with a normal ear.

Weber Test

This test is performed by placing the tuning fork on the forehead and asking the patient whether the sound is louder on one side. The reason for lateralization to the side with conductive loss is that environmental noise is masked on this side, increasing the efficiency of cochlear detection of sound transmitted by the vibrating mastoid bone.

Audiometry

When the patient is referred to an audiologist for evaluation of hearing loss, *puretone audiometry* is utilized to characterize the extent of impairment. Both air-conduction and bone-conduction measurements are made for sounds of varying intensity (decibels) and frequency (Hertz or cps). The usual frequencies tested are 250, 500, 1000, 2000, 3000, 4000, 6000, and 8000 Hertz. The results are plotted on a graph called an audiogram. The vertical axis shows hearing loss in decibels and the horizontal axis shows the frequency of the stimulus in Hertz. Examples of audiograms showing normal hearing, conductive hearing loss, and sensorineural hearing loss are reproduced in Figure 96.3. Speech audiometry, which measures the subject's ability to hear and understand the spoken voice, is also done as part of a formal hearing evaluation.

GENERAL APPROACH TO CHRONIC HEARING LOSS

Assessment and care for moderate or severe chronic hearing loss usually require the assistance of a consulting otolaryngologist. For many patients, little can be done to reverse the primary process, and care consists of compensating for existing hearing loss and preventing further loss.

Table 96.2.
Classification of Probable Mechanism of Hearing Loss Using Tuning Fork Tests

Classification	Rinne Test	Weber Test
NORMAL HEARING		
Both ears	AC > BC[a]	Midline
CONDUCTIVE LOSS[b]		
Right ear	Right ear—BC > AC Left ear—AC > BC	Lateralized to right ear
Left ear	Right ear—AC > BC Left ear—BC > AC	Lateralized to left ear
Both ears	Right ear—BC > AC Left ear—BC > AC	Lateralized to poorer ear
SENSORINEURAL LOSS		
Right ear	AC > BC bilaterally	Lateralized to left ear
Left ear	AC > BC bilaterally	Lateralized to right ear
Both ears	AC > BC bilaterally	Lateralized to better ear

[a]AC, air conduction; BC, bone conduction.
[b]Because sound transmission by air is much more efficient than by bone, air conduction may remain greater than bone conduction in early or minimal conductive hearing loss.

Communication

Counseling of the family and others who speak to the patient with moderate to severe hearing loss should emphasize two principles:

1. Facilitate communication by consistently using the following adjuncts to speech: face patients, obtain their attention before speaking, speak slowly, utilize gestures, and speak louder or move closer if the patient says that it helps.
2. Expect some difficulty in discriminating consonants (the high frequency hearing loss typical of most sensorineural deafness particularly affects this type of discrimination; for example, the word "yes" may be understood as "yet, get, less, mess," etc.).

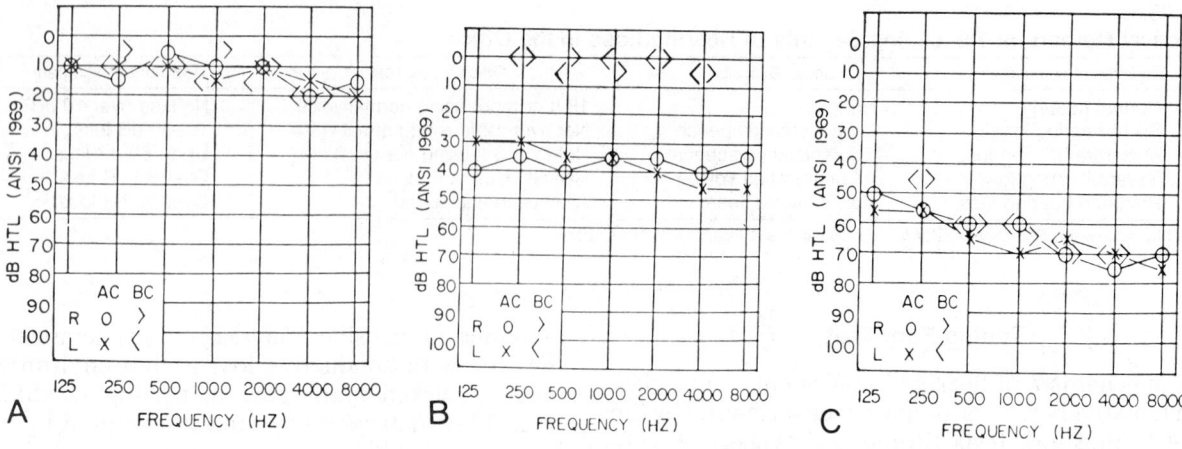

Figure 96.3. Examples of audiograms. *A*. Audiogram in a person with normal hearing. *B*. Bilateral conductive hearing loss (moderate). *C*. Bilateral sensorineural hearing loss (severe). (From Price L, Snider R: The geriatric patient: ear, nose and throat problems. In Reichel W (ed): *Clinical Aspects of Aging*. Baltimore, Williams & Wilkins, 1978, p. 489.)

For the patient with *profound or total hearing loss*, the principle governing all communication is that the message must be seen by the patient. Most patients will let the physician know the mode of communication they prefer: lipreading or writing. Whenever there is any question about the effectiveness of lipreading, written exchange of information should be utilized. This can be facilitated by assuring that paper and a pen or pencil are always available to the patient. In large communities, a translator who can communicate in American Sign Language may be available to assist patients who know sign language. Also various devices are now available that make it possible for totally deaf persons to receive telephone calls (messages are entered by the sender in code on a touch-tone unit and displayed visually for the deaf receiver) and to follow television programs.

Hearing Aids

Hearing aids (miniature, battery-powered microphone-amplifier-loudspeaker units) can assist the patient with sensorineural hearing loss (and some patients with irreversible conductive loss) (6, 7). Currently available aids vary from very small in-the-canal aids (costing up to $750, delicate, may be difficult to remove at night), aids fitted inobstrusively to the outer ear (also expensive; the choice of about 50% of users), behind-the-ear units (visible; has a tube that conducts sound to the ear; the choice of about 40% of users), and older devices incorporated into eye glasses or carried in a pocket with a wire connection to the ear mold. Hearing aids can increase the intensity of a sound by up to 70 dB. Thus, a sound of about 60 dB (the level of average conversational speech) passing through an aid may enter the ear at a level of 130 dB. This represents the maximal usable gain of an aid since sounds above this level become painful.

Federal law now prevents the sale of hearing aids to people who have not been evaluated first by a phy-

sician. Only trial and adjustment will determine whether an individual patient referred for a hearing aid will benefit. Medicare and other third party insurers do not pay for hearing aids. Most hearing aid dealers will allow a 30-day trial period during which the patient pays a rental fee; some states require this by law.

Patients may mention certain specific problems with the hearing aid to their personal physicians. There may be irritation of the conchal cartilage or even infection in the external canal. A poorly fitted hearing aid mold can cause pressure sores on the external ear (a particular hazard in the diabetic). Patients may also note an increase in cerumen accumulation in the aided ear. In each of these situations use of the aid should be discontinued until the process resolves. A better fitting mold will be needed to avoid recurrence in some patients. Others may do well by removing the aid periodically during the day.

For selected patients, implantable bone conduction aids (Audiant) and cochlear implants are now available (12, 22). The cochlear implant is used in patients who became profoundly deaf after first having normal hearing and normal speech development.

CAUSES OF HEARING LOSS: OVERVIEW

The major causes of hearing loss in adults are listed in Table 96.3. For each condition, the table indicates mechanism, onset (rapid or gradual), and whether the condition is unilateral or bilateral. The guidelines that follow will enable the general physician to reach a working diagnosis in most instances and to choose between primary treatment and referral for care by a specialist.

CONDITIONS OF THE EXTERNAL AUDITORY CANAL

A number of conditions may cause hearing impairment by blocking the external canal.

Table 96.3.
Causes of Hearing Loss in Adults

Causes	Mechanism[a]	Onset Rapid (Hours to Days) or Gradual (Months to Years)	Bilateral or Unilateral
EXTERNAL AUDITORY CANAL			
Cerumen impaction	C	Either	Usually unilateral
Foreign body	C	Rapid	Unilateral
Otitis externa	C	Rapid	Unilateral
New growth	C	Gradual	Unilateral
MIDDLE EAR			
Serous otitis media	C	Either	Either
Acute otitis media	C	Rapid	Unilateral
Barotrauma	C or SN	Rapid	Unilateral
Traumatic perforation of tympanic membrane	C	Rapid	Unilateral
Chronic otitis media	C	Gradual	Unilateral
Cholesteatoma	C or SN	Gradual	Either
Ossicular chain problems:			
Adhesive otitis media	C	Gradual	Unilateral
Tympanosclerosis	C	Gradual	Either
Traumatic injury	C or SN	Rapid	Unilateral
Otosclerosis	C and/or SN	Gradual	Bilateral
New growths	C or SN	Gradual	Unilateral
INNER EAR			
Presbycusis	SN	Gradual	Bilateral
Acoustic trauma	SN	Gradual	Bilateral
Drug-induced	SN	Either	Bilateral
Ménière's syndrome	SN	Rapid	Usually unilateral
Central nervous system infection:			
Meningitis	SN	Rapid	Either
Syphilis	SN	Either	Either
Tuberculosis	SN	Either	Either
Acoustic neuroma	SN	Gradual	Unilateral
Mumps (9)	SN	Rapid	Unilateral
ATRAUMATIC SUDDEN SENSORINEURAL HEARING LOSS	SN	Rapid	Unilateral

[a]C, conductive; SN, sensorineural.

Cerumen Impaction

The patient will usually complain of intermittent fullness and hearing impairment on the affected side and may give a history of prior episodes. These symptoms may increase after showering or swimming, as moisture may cause cerumen to swell. Diagnosis is made by otoscopy.

If the cerumen appears to be soft, it may be removed by irrigation with use of a rubber-bulb syringe and warm tap water (close to body temperature), directing the water upward and backward against the wall of the canal. If the cerumen is impacted and difficult to remove, a few drops of hydrogen peroxide (or carbamide peroxide, Debrox) should be instilled twice daily for 1 week before irrigation. Alternatively, a cerumenolytic agent (Cerumenex) may be utilized. In general, cerumenolytic agents should be used only in the office, as casual use by the patient at home increases the risk of allergic dermatitis (seen in about 1% of users). The following steps are taken: With the patient's head tilted laterally at 45° the ear is filled with cerumenolytic drops: a cotton plug is inserted for 15 to 20 minutes; the ear is then irrigated with lukewarm water and a soft rubber syringe. After irrigation, the tympanic membrane will usually show some injection around the handle of the malleus. In certain situations, cerumen removal should be done by an otolaryngologist:

(a) In the patient with a known tympanic membrane perforation or a history of mastoidectomy, irrigation is contraindicated because water may transport bacteria to the middle ear or mastoid and thereby initiate an infection; wax removal should be done by suction-tip aspiration; (b) in the occasional patient with an impaction that does not respond to the usual measures described above; in this instance, removal of cerumen is accomplished by aspiration or by the use of an operating microscope. Hearing impairment will usually be relieved immediately after removal of cerumen.

An impaction often follows vigorous efforts by the patient to remove wax with a cotton-tipped applicator. The patient should be reminded that ear wax is secreted to protect the lining of the canal and that the applicator should be used only to remove cerumen in the outer portion of the canal, for cosmetic purposes.

Patients who have had recurrent impactions, often due to excess secretion of cerumen, may prevent recurrences by gently syringing their ears once or twice per month, by using a soft rubber bulb and warm water. Also, instillation of baby oil drops weekly will help to keep the wax soft.

Foreign Body

Usually the history discloses accidental insertion of a foreign body or entrance of an insect, which is followed by fullness and hearing impairment. Foreign bodies can be removed by use of fine forceps or a wax spoon. Removal by irrigation should be avoided if the foreign body is a vegetable, as water will cause further swelling. Insects should first be killed by instillation of mineral oil. Hearing impairment resolves promptly after removal of a foreign body. Great care must be taken to avoid damage to the eardrum, especially in children and patients in whom the foreign body is deeply imbeded.

Otitis Externa (Swimmer's Ear)

This condition is most common in the summer months, when heat and humidity, plus moisture introduced by swimming or perspiration, promote swelling and maceration of the stratum corneum of the skin. In the external canal, this process may at first cause pruritus. The patient may give a history of having scratched the ear for a few days before the onset of drainage and pain. The pain is aggravated by movement of the external ear and sometimes the jaw. Hearing impairment will occur in those patients who present with swelling or debris that occludes the canal. The characteristics of the skin of the canal and of the exudate usually provide adequate clues to etiology, and cultures are needed only for patients who do not respond promptly to topical treatment. Copious or greenish exudate suggests *Pseudomonas*, the bacteria most frequently seen in otitis externa. Yellow crusting in the midst of a purulent exudate suggests *Staphylococcus aureus*. Canal skin that is scaling, cracked, and weeping indicates eczema (the history usually indicates that the condition is chronic). Fluffy material resembling bread mold, varying in color from white to black, suggests a fungal etiology (*Aspergillus* or *Candida*).

There are two general *principles* of *treatment* for all types of otitis externa: removal of all infected debris (with a cotton applicator with a tightly rolled fresh cotton bud and with a suction cannula if available) and instillation of an appropriate topical medication.

For *bacterial infections* the patient should instill an antimicrobial-corticosteroid combination, (e.g., Cortisporin Otic Suspension, containing polymyxin B-neomycin-hydrocortisone three or four times daily for 5 to 7 days).

For *fungal infections*, the canal should be thoroughly cleaned out and a light dusting of sulfanilamide powder should be applied, in the office. A dispenser containing sulfanilamide powder for this use can be obtained from any pharmacy. The fungal infection usually resolves after a single dusting with this powder. Clotrimazole (Lotrimin), 1% solution, three drops twice a day, is an effective alternative.

For *eczema* without superimposed infection, a topical steroid cream or solution is applied three to four times daily (e.g., triamcinolone, 0.1%).

In some patients, the canal may be so swollen that topical medication does not enter the canal efficiently.

In this case, a cylindrical cotton wick (or a commercially available sponge wick, such as Oto-wick), approximately the length of the ear canal (1 inch in adults), should be saturated with the desired medication and worked by gentle twisting into the canal until only the end is visible. The patient may then apply several drops of the medication to the wick three to four times daily, and the wick will carry it into the canal. The wick can usually be removed after 48 to 72 hours, and treatment can be completed as stated above.

Most episodes of otitis externa resolve completely after 5 to 7 days, and it is important to terminate topical treatment at this time. The ear canal cannot return to a normal state as long as topical medicine is constantly introduced into it; persistent treatment may lead to dermatitis medicamentosa. As a precaution against overtreatment, the prescription for eardrops should be nonrefillable, and only a small amount (10 ml) should be dispensed.

During treatment of otitis externa, moisture should be strictly avoided. During bathing, the ear should be plugged with cotton impregnated with petroleum jelly. To prevent recurrence, the patient should be warned against meddling with the ear (particularly frequent cleansing with cotton-tipped applicators, a common inciting cause).

Hearing impairment due to otitis externa should resolve promptly when swelling recedes.

In the following two situations, the patient with otitis externa requires prompt referral to an otolaryngologist: (*a*) patients whose findings suggest *mastoiditis* (slow response of the otitis externa to treatment plus tenderness over the mastoid process); and (*b*) patients with the findings of "*malignant otitis externa,*" usually diabetics or immunologically impaired individuals This process is actually an osteitis of the bone underlying the external auditory canal, caused by *Pseudomonas*. The distinguishing features are fever, excruciating pain, and the presence of friable granulation tissue in the area of apparent otitis externa. Because of the propensity for rapid spread to contiguous structures, this condition is an emergency, requiring hospital admission for debridement and intravenous antibiotics.

New Growth

Occasionally, unilateral, gradual onset hearing impairment may be due to a benign or malignant growth seen in the canal. Such patients must be referred for diagnosis and surgical excision of the growth.

CONDITIONS OF THE MIDDLE EAR

Most conductive hearing loss is due to conditions within the middle ear. In addition to history, evaluation of the middle ear includes assessment of eustachian tube function by air insufflation (pneumatic otoscopy), inspection for signs of acute inflammation (erythema, discharge, or bulging of the tympanic membrane), and inspection for changes in the tympanic membrane not due to acute inflammation (fluid level, retraction, scarring, distortion of normal structures, perforation) and cholesteatoma.

Serous Otitis Media

This problem is very common in childhood and relatively common in adults. The patient usually complains of fullness and decreased hearing in one or both ears with minimal or no pain. There is often a history of recent viral upper respiratory infection (see Chapter 28), exacerbation of allergic or vasomotor rhinitis (see Chapter 23), or recent acute otitis media (see below). Rarely, serous otitis media may be due to nasopharyngeal carcinoma. On physical examination the patient is afebrile, and there may be evidence of eustachian tube closure—retraction of the tympanic membrane, failure of the membrane to move on pneumatic otoscopy (a crude test of eustachian tube patency, not always abnormal in serous otitis), or an air-fluid level behind the membrane. Even when none of these signs is present, the presumptive diagnosis of serous otitis can be made in patients with typical symptoms and conductive hearing loss.

The objective of *medical treatment* is to relieve obstruction of the eustachian tube. This is accomplished by the use of topical decongestants. Systemic decongestants (e.g., pseudoephedrine) are not thought to be helpful (4, 5). Nasal sprays containing the decongestant phenylephrine (Neo-Synephrine Nasal Spray 0.25% or 0.50% or other over-the-counter preparations) are the simplest to use. The patient administers two puffs to each nostril followed 5 to 10 minutes later by two more puffs, four times daily. Alternatively, a phenylephrine-containing nasal solution (Neo-Synephrine, 0.25% or 0.50%, also over-the-counter) can be instilled by dropper four times daily. The head is hyperextended and three or four drops are instilled in each nostril to open the nasal passages; the head is then turned to the lateral position with the involved ear down, and three to four more drops are instilled into the nostril. After 3 or 4 days of topical treatment, rebound nasal mucosal hyperemia may occur. Therefore, the patient should be instructed explicitly to discontinue spray (or drops) after 3 days.

If a patient with serous otitis media has a history of allergic rhinitis, an antihistamine or specific treatment for their condition may be helpful (see Chapter 23). In addition to medications, patients should be instructed to promote eustachian tube patency by blowing the nose against closed nostrils with the mouth closed (Valsalva maneuver) every few hours during the day. This should not be recommended to the patient with a purulent nasal discharge.

All patients should be re-evaluated after 4 to 6 weeks. If conductive hearing loss persists beyond 6 weeks, the patient should be referred to an otolaryngologist who will confirm and quantify the conductive hearing loss and will check for other conditions that may be causing the hearing loss. Some patients with resistant serous otitis media will require myringotomy with aspiration of fluid from the middle ear and insertion of a ventilation tube to restore hearing.

Even with optimal treatment serous otitis media may recur in susceptible individuals. Sulfisoxazole (e.g., Gantrisin), 250 to 500 mg twice/day, or amoxicillin, 250 mg once daily, may be used for prophylaxis in infection-prone children (19).

Acute Otitis Media

All patients with this condition will complain of marked pain in the inner ear; most will give a history of a recent upper respiratory infection and fever, with or without drainage of purulent material from the ear (indicating tympanic membrane perforation); some will describe unilateral hearing impairment. On examination, there is injection and loss of luster of the tympanic membrane, grayish-pink coloration of the entire membrane, and, eventually, bulging of the membrane and loss of landmarks. Some patients will have a conductive hearing loss demonstrated by tuning fork tests (see above). There may be tenderness to palpation of the mastoid bone, since the mucosa lining the mastoid cells is continuous with that of the middle ear. Evidence of otitis externa is usually not present. The *most common* etiological agents are *Streptococcus pneumoniae* (pneumococcus), *Haemophilus influenzae, S. aureus,* and *β-hemolytic streptococcus.* Some cases are due to viral pathogens; since clinical distinction of these cases from those with bacterial infection is not possible, treatment should be the same for all patients with acute otitis media.

Medical treatment consists of systemic antimicrobials for 10 days.

Amoxicillin, 500 mg three times daily, is the best regimen. For penicillin-allergic persons, trimethoprim-sulfamethoxazole (Bactrim, Septra, generic), two tablets every 12 hours, is appropriate. Aspirin or acetaminophen every 4 to 6 hours should be recommended for pain. If needed, codeine, 30 mg, can be given with the aspirin.

If perforation with discharge occurs, Cortisporin otic suspension, four drops three times daily for 1 week, should be added to the treatment. If the tympanic membrane is bulging with pus and the patient describes severe pain or vertigo, myringotomy by an otolaryngologist is indicated.

Recovery from the pain of acute otitis media is usually prompt. Within 1 to 4 weeks, hearing impairment resolves, and the tympanic membrane returns to normal appearance. Serous otitis may be present after other signs or symptoms of acute otitis have resolved.

In the patient who is worse after several days of treatment or who is not well after 10 days, subacute mastoiditis may be present, and referral to an otolaryngologist is therefore indicated. Failure of serous otitis to resolve, persistence of a tympanic membrane perforation, and significant persistent hearing loss after 3 weeks are also indications for referral.

Barotrauma

Barotrauma refers to symptoms and signs produced by a sudden pressure differential between the middle ear and the surrounding atmosphere. The patient gives a history of fullness, pain, and decreased hearing in one or both ears. This problem is most commonly associated with flying or scuba diving. All patients with symptoms that are severe or that persist for more than a day should be examined. The findings on otoscopy vary from mild tympanic membrane retraction to hemotympanum with or without perforation. There may be conductive or neurosensory hearing loss. Any patient with moderate or severe unilateral hearing loss should be referred to an otolaryngologist because of the possibility of a surgically treatable fistula of the round or oval windows.

For patients with mild symptoms, treatment and outcome are similar to those described above for serous otitis media.

Prophylaxis against barotrauma consists of use of the Valsalva maneuver and swallowing or chewing of gum during descent in airplanes.

Traumatic Perforation of Tympanic Membrane

Traumatic rupture, affecting the pars tensa of the tympanic membrane (see Fig. 96.2), may be caused by solids (deliberate introduction of cotton-tipped applicator or other object for removing wax, foreign bodies entering during an accident, etc.); liquids (forcefully directed jet of water used in syringing the ear); and air (blast waves resulting from detonation of high explosives). Symptoms are decreased hearing, tinnitus, pain, and, at times, bleeding.

The *objective of treatment* is the prevention of infection. Most linear tears and small perforations of the membrane will heal spontaneously within 4 weeks without any residual loss of function. Large perforations may require fascia grafting by an otolaryngologist (myringoplasty). If there is a strong possibility that the middle ear has been contaminated at the time of injury (i.e., by syringing), antibiotics (ampicillin or erythromycin, 250 mg four times daily for 1 week) are indicated. In addition, it is essential to guard against the subsequent entry of organisms as long as the perforation persists. Thus the patient should prevent water or other contaminants from entering the ear. Before bathing, the patient should insert a petroleum jelly-covered cotton plug. Swimming should be avoided altogether. Patients whose perforation was self-inflicted should be warned against future syringing and probing to remove cerumen.

After spontaneous closure or myringoplasty, the hearing loss due to perforation usually resolves completely.

Chronic Otitis Media

Chronic otitis media implies discharge from the middle ear, either persistent or recurrent, with perforation of the tympanic membrane and usually some degree of conductive hearing loss. The management of this problem has two objectives: eradication of infection and restoration of hearing. When chronic otitis media is initially recognized, the patient should be referred to an otolaryngologist for evaluation.

Chronic otitis media can be divided into *two major subgroups*, *benign* and *dangerous*. The clinical characteristics of these two groups are summarized in Table 96.4. The fundamental difference in the dangerous subgroup is the presence of, or potential for, bone destruction due to invasion by squamous epithelium known as "cholesteatoma." Cholesteatoma occurs either when squamous epithelium of the auditory canal invades the middle ear through a pre-existing perforation (secondary acquired cholesteatoma) or when squamous epithelium spontaneously replaces the columnar epithelium of the middle ear, leading to perforation (primary acquired cholesteatoma). The cholesteatoma is the mass of whitish debris that accumulates at the site of invasion of squamous epithelium. As this mass enlarges, it has the potential to erode bone and promote chronic infection. Even a brain abscess may occasionally occur as a complication of active purulent cholesteatoma.

The commonly performed surgical procedures for chronic otitis media are the following:

Simple mastoidectomy. This procedure removes the mastoid cells and cholesteatoma, usually through a postauricular incision. The canal wall remains intact.

Modified radical mastoidectomy. In this operation, the mastoid cells are exteriorized so that they form a common cavity with the external auditory canal,

Table 96.4.
Chronic Otitis Media: Features Distinguishing Benign and Dangerous Forms

Feature	Benign	Dangerous (Cholesteatoma)
Discharge	Mucoid or mucopurulent	Purulent, foul
Location of pathology	Middle ear; eustachian tube	Middle ear, attic, antrum, any part of temporal bone
Tympanic membrane perforation	Pars tensa (central)[a]	Pars flaccida[a] or marginal
Middle ear mucosa	Mucous membrane	Stratified squamous epithelium
X-rays	Normal; clouding of mastoid cells	Underdevelopment of sclerosis of mastoid cells; bone destruction
Cholesteatoma formation	No	Yes
Bone erosion	No	Yes
Treatment of infection	Medical/surgical (surgery if the perforation fails to heal spontaneously)	Surgical

[a]See Figure 96.2.

draining and eradicating infection due to cholesteatoma.

Mastoid obliteration. After infection is eradicated by mastoidectomy, the cavity that has been created is obliterated with the use of muscle or other tissue graft. The purpose of this procedure is to restore normal anatomical contour and to avoid the aftercare that a mastoid cavity requires.

Myringoplasty. The tympanic membrane perforation is closed by use of a tissue graft.

Tympanoplasty. The conduction mechanism, including tympanic membrane perforation and ossicular disruptions, is repaired.

Complications of Otitis Media

Acute or chronic suppurative otitis media may become complicated by extension of infection beyond the confines of the middle ear into bone and other surrounding structures. These complicating infections are mastoiditis, facial nerve paralysis, petrositis (inflammation of petrous portion of the sphenoid with diplopia, pain around the eye, and persistent otorrhea), labyrinthitis, brain abscess, extradural abscess, subdural abscess, lateral sinus thrombophlebitis, meningitis, and otitic hydrocephalus. Symptoms not attributable to the typical course of acute or chronic otitis media may signify the presence of one of these complications. They are uncommon and usually occur in compromised hosts (diabetics, immunosuppressed patients, etc.) and in patients with untreated acute or chronic otitis media. All require immediate referral and hospitalization.

Ossicular Chain Problems

A number of chronic conditions affect the ossicular chain. These may be recognized by the combination of conductive hearing loss (usually chronic, either unilateral or bilateral), the absence of evidence for active otitis media, and, in some cases, typical findings on otoscopy. Each of these conditions requires referral to an otolaryngologist for accurate diagnosis and consideration of surgical management.

Adhesive Otitis Media

There is a history of prior ear infection, and the tympanic membrane is retracted and atrophic in areas of healed perforations. The eardrum is usually draped over the promontory and incudostapedial complex. Adhesive otitis media is usually a late complication seen in patients who have been inadequately followed up after treatment for repeated acute otitis or serous otitis and who have had persistent middle ear inflammation. Hearing loss is usually mild, though some patients may need a hearing aid. Surgical treatment is normally not necessary.

Tympanosclerosis

There is a history of prior infection, often bilateral. There is usually, but not always, a tympanic membrane perforation, and discrete plaques of whitish material consisting of dense collagen at times replaced with calcified hyaline may be seen in the middle ear. In selected patients, surgical removal of the plaques restores lost hearing. In others, ossicular reconstruction is necessary to improve hearing.

Traumatic Ossicular Injury

There is a history of external trauma (such as basal skull fracture and those causes of traumatic perforation listed above) followed by unilateral hearing loss, which may be conductive or mixed. A hemotympanum (blood behind the eardrum) is usually seen, although occasionally the tympanic membrane is normal. Hearing status after surgery depends upon the type of injury found at surgery.

Otosclerosis

This is a disease of the labyrinthine capsule in which a vascular type of spongy bone is laid down, causing fixation of the stapes and conductive hearing loss, usually bilateral. The history discloses slowly progressive hearing loss beginning in the second or third decade, usually bilateral, more commonly in females, and frequently accelerated after pregnancy. Also the use of oral contraceptive pills may induce or aggravate this disease. Examination of the tympanic membrane is usually normal. This is the most common cause of progressive conductive hearing loss in young adults. Because the results of surgery, consisting of stapedectomy or stapedotomy, and prosthetic replacement, are excellent, it is particularly important to detect and refer these patients. Sensorineural hearing loss is common as the disease progresses.

New Growths of Middle Ear

A number of benign and malignant growths may be seen on inspection of the tympanic membrane of patients with progressive unilateral conductive hearing loss. Malignant tumors most commonly present with a history of chronic discharge, occasionally bloody.

CHRONIC SENSORINEURAL HEARING LOSS

Presbycusis ("the Hearing of the Old")

A certain amount of hearing loss, beginning in the high frequency range, is virtually universal among elderly people. Approximately one in five people over 65 will develop moderate to severe hearing loss. The majority do not complain of deafness, and often a family member mentions the problem to the patient's physician. When hearing deficits are objectively evaluated in older persons, the deficits of the "complainers" and "noncomplainers" overlap considerably (20). Clearly, social and psychological factors are important in determining the seriousness of hearing loss reported by the individual patient.

Periodically the hearing status of every patient over 65 should be assessed (see Table 96.1). When an older patient is first found to have moderate hearing loss, the patient and his family should be counseled as outlined above, and the patient should be offered a referral for evaluation by an otolaryngologist (16).

Acoustic Trauma

This form of sensorineural hearing loss is found commonly in individuals employed in high noise industries or exposed to extremely loud, electrically amplified music (8). Like presbycusis, it is initially a high frequency hearing loss, eventually spreading to lower frequencies. Personal prevention by wearing earplugs in high noise settings and environmental prevention by reducing noise level are the best ways to prevent acoustic trauma. Established hearing loss due to noise is usually irreversible, but progressive hearing loss can be prevented. Acute hearing loss due to an acute episode of acoustic trauma, i.e., gunfire or cordless telephone ringer accidents, is frequently reversible; this is also referred to as "temporary threshold shift."

Drug-Induced Hearing Loss

A number of drugs may produce bilateral sensorineural hearing loss (Table 96.5), and the patient's personal physician will often be the first to learn of this problem. (Example: a patient will be seen in the office after hospitalization for an illness that was treated with aminoglycoside antibiotics or with intravenous diuretics and will complain of hearing loss.) For most of these drugs, ototoxicity is dose related; however, hearing impairment may occur even at therapeutic doses. One study showed that objective mild hearing loss (15 to 30 dB at high frequencies) occurs in as many as 10% of individuals whose serum levels of gentamycin and tobramycin are maintained within the therapeutic range (21).

The prognosis for drug-induced hearing loss varies according to the drug. Salicylates and quinine usually produce temporary, high frequency deafness; but permanent deafness has been reported in patients surviving salicylate poisoning and in infants of mothers who received quinine during pregnancy. Aminoglycoside ototoxicity may occur suddenly after a few doses, may be permanent, and may progress after discontinuation of the drug. Diuretic-induced ototoxicity may be seen after extremely high doses, usually in patients with renal insufficiency. Its onset may be sudden, after intravenous or (in a few reported cases) oral administration, and the hearing deficit may be permanent. This complication is rare with ethacrynic acid, very rare with furosemide, and may not occur at all with bumetanide.

Ménière's Syndrome

This benign but temporarily disabling condition will be seen one or more times per year in a typical practice. It may occur in any age group but is most common in the fourth to sixth decade. Symptoms are thought to be due to endolymphatic hydrops (excess fluid and pressure in the cochlea and the labyrinth).

The individual attack consists of a sudden temporary disturbance of vestibular function (vertigo) combined with fluctuating hearing loss, tinnitus, aural pressure, and nausea. An attack usually lasts for several hours. During the attack, spontaneous nystagmus will be present. The nystagmus will not be affected by position change. Between attacks, tinnitus and sensorineural hearing loss may persist. Symptoms are unilateral (3) in approximately 70% of cases. In about half of the cases vestibular and cochlear symptoms appear at the same time; in approximately 25%, deafness and/or tinnitus precedes the onset of vertigo; and in 25% vertigo precedes deafness (15). The vertigo is accompanied by nausea and vomiting, probably due to a spread of nervous impulses from the vestibular nerve to the vagal nuclei in the brainstem. In severe cases, other vagal symptoms may occur (abdominal pain, bradycardia, pallor, and sweating). Audiometry demonstrates sensorineural hearing loss, greater for lower frequencies in the early stage of the disease.

An attack may occur spontaneously at any time. Attacks may occur singly, with an interval of months or years between, or there may be a series of attacks over a period of weeks, followed by a long period of complete remission.

The *differential diagnosis* of Ménière's syndrome includes a number of conditions that may also present with hearing loss and vertigo unrelated to position change: viral labyrinthitis, acoustic neurinoma, syphilitic vertigo (14), labyrinthine fistula, vestibular granuloma, temporal bone fracture, or multiple sclerosis. Assessment of the patient with vertigo due to these and other causes is found in Chapter 81.

Treatment. Patients with suspected Ménière's syndrome should be referred promptly to an otolaryngologist to confirm the diagnosis and to initiate treatment. All patients will be treated with diuretics (25 to 50 mg of hydrochlorothiazide daily or its equivalent). Bed rest is recommended when the patient is having recurrent severe symptoms; bed rest does not prevent the periodic vertigo but prevents exacerbation due to position change. The antihistamine meclizine (as the prescription drug Antivert or nonprescription drug Bonine) can be tried in a dose of 25 mg three to four times daily. For nausea, the patient should take the antiemetic prochlorperazine (Compazine) either as a 5- or 10-mg capsule four times daily, or as a 25-mg suppository twice daily. After the acute attack has sub-

Table 96.5.
Drugs That May Cause Sensorineural Hearing Loss

ANTIBIOTICS	DIURETICS
Streptomycin	Ethacrynic acid
Neomycin	Furosemide
Gentamycin	
Tobramycin	OTHER DRUGS
Chloramphenicol	Salicylates
Vancomycin	Quinidine
	Quinine
	Cisplatin

sided, the patient should continue diuretic treatment; after 1 year without recurrence, diuretic treatment can be stopped. For the occasional patient with severe recurrent Ménière's syndrome refractory to medical treatment, one of a number of surgical procedures can be performed, selectively decompressing or destroying the vestibular labyrinth or sectioning the vestibular nerve.

Acoustic Neuroma

This uncommon, benign tumor usually arises from the vestibular fibers of the 8th cranial nerve. Rarely it may arise from the 7th cranial nerve. It grows slowly, expanding within the internal auditory meatus until large enough to extend into the posterior fossa and to cause damage to adjacent structures. Onset of symptoms is generally between the ages of 30 and 50. Essentially all patients will present with symptoms of 8th nerve impairment: unilateral hearing loss is found in the majority of patients and chronic, usually mild, positional vertigo or sense of imbalance occurs in many patients. Audiometry usually demonstrates significant sensorineural hearing loss with poor discrimination. Neurological examination shows involvement of the following neurological structures, in decreasing order of frequency: nerve VII, nerve V, nerve VI, and cerebellum (ataxia, with a tendency to fall toward the side of the lesion).

Referral to an otolaryngologist for evaluation is essential whenever unilateral sensorineural hearing loss is initially found. Diagnosis of acoustic neuroma is based on a characteristic audiogram and on computed tomography and/or magnetic resonance imaging (1). The results of surgical treatment generally permit the patient to resume his or her usual activity, but usually with permanent unilateral hearing loss (18). In a few patients with good hearing preoperatively it may be possible to preserve the hearing.

SUDDEN SENSORINEURAL HEARING LOSS

This condition, usually unilateral, is an otological emergency. The etiology is often difficult to ascertain and may include viral cochleitis, arterial occlusion (especially in patients with other evidence of arterial occlusive disease, such as embolic transient ischemic attacks), inner ear fistula, autoimmune factors (13), sudden expansion of a cerebellopontine angle tumor, temporal bone fracture, and noise trauma (gunshot, for example). The symptom, which occurs over a matter of minutes to hours, is either tinnitus or hearing loss. After prompt evaluation for conductive hearing loss (including simple cerumen impaction), these patients should be referred immediately for evaluation by an otolaryngologist. A number of empirical medical therapies have been tried. For patients with inner ear fistulas, surgical closure is possible.

The majority of patients will have permanent, severe unilateral hearing loss, and they and their families should be instructed regarding hearing safety (adequate noise protection for the other ear, preferential seating for optimal use of the good ear, precautions when driving in heavy traffic).

TINNITUS

Tinnitus ("ringing") refers to the perception of sounds in the absence of a normal external stimulus. Intermittent tinnitus is not uncommon in the general population. Persistent tinnitus may be due to a number of identifiable problems.

Subjective Tinnitus

The term *subjective tinnitus* is used when the subject complains of noises that cannot be heard by the observer. Subjective tinnitus may be subdivided into two types:

Tympanic. This usually arises as a result of a conductive lesion (all of the causes of conductive hearing loss). It is thought to be due to removal of the normal masking effect of ambient noise, with emergence of otherwise subaudible tympanic, vascular, and muscular noises. The patient will often describe the tinnitus as pulsating.

Petrous. This is due to conditions affecting the cochlea or 8th nerve (all of the conditions leading to sensorineural hearing loss). It is attributed to cerebral recognition of auditory stimuli produced by mechanical cochlear deformation or by hyperirritability of the acoustic nerve. It may be intermittent or continuous with varying intensity.

After the patient's primary otological problem has been defined, the most important requirement in dealing with tinnitus is reassurance (many patients believe that their tinnitus signifies the presence of a serious intracranial condition). Bedtime sedation to assure adequate sleep is important. Some patients will also find that the sound of a radio helps them to get to sleep by competing with the more distressing sound due to tinnitus. For patients with severe tinnitus, masking treatment by the consulting otolaryngologist may be helpful. Audiometry may be perfectly normal and the cause of the tinnitus unknown. Tinnitus clinics and support groups are now available in most large cities (10, 11, 17).

Objective Tinnitus

This is a noise audible to the examiner, sometimes inaudible to the patient, and originating from the region of the patient's ear. Causes include aneurysm of the internal carotid artery, temporomandibular joint problems, and myoclonus of palatal muscles. These patients should be referred to an otolaryngologist for a diagnostic workup.

VERTIGO

The problem of vertigo is discussed in depth in Chapter 81.

General References

Paparella MM, Shumrick DA: *Otolaryngology*, Vol 2. Philadelphia, WB Saunders, 1980.

Specific References

1. Armington WG, Harnsberger HR, Smoker WR, Osborn AG: Normal and diseased acoustic pathway: evaluation with MR imaging. *Radiology* 167(2):509, 1988.
2. Bailey Jr HAT, Pappas JJ, Graham S, Winston ME: Total hearing rehabilitation. *Arch Otolaryngol* 102:323, 1976.
3. Balkany TJ, Kires B, Arenberg IK: Bilateral aspects of Ménière's disease. *Otolaryngol Clin North Am* 31:4, 1980. (new edition due 1991)
4. Bluestone CD, Mandel EM, Cantekin EI, et al: Evaluation of decongestant antihistamine therapy for otitis media with effusion. *Ann Otol Rhinol Laryngol* 92 (6):35, 1983.
5. Cantekin EI, Mandel EM, Bluestone CD, et al: Lack of efficacy of a decongestant antihistamine combination for otitis media with effusion in children. *N Engl J Med* 308:297, 1983.
6. Corrado OJ: Hearing aids. *Br Med J [Clin Res]* 2;296(6614):33, 1988.
7. Department of Health, Education and Welfare: *A report on hearing aid health care.* Washington, DC, United States Government Printing Office, 1974.
8. Dobie RA: Noise-induced hearing loss: the family physician's role. *Am Fam Physician* 36(6):141, 1987.
9. Hall R, Richards H: Hearing loss due to mumps. *Arch Dis Child* 62(2):189, 1987.
10. Hawthorne MR, Britten SR, O'Connor S, Webber P: The management of a population of tinnitus sufferers in a specialized clinic: Part III. The evaluation of psychiatric intervention. *J Laryngol Otol* 101(8):795, 1987.
11. Hawthorne MR, O'Connor S, Britten SR, Webber P: The management of a population of tinnitus sufferers in a specialized clinic: Part I. Description of the clinic organization and the population seen. *J Laryngol Otol* 101(8):784, 1987.
12. Hough J, Himelick T, Johnson B: Implantable bone conduction hearing device: audiant bone conductor. Update on our experiences. *Ann Otol Rhinol Laryngol* 95(5):498, 1986.
13. Hughes GB, Barna BP, Kinney SE, Calabrese LH, Nalepa NJ: Clinical diagnosis of immune inner-ear disease. *Laryngoscope* 98(3):251, 1988.
14. Hughes GB, Rutherford I: Predictive value of serologic tests for syphilis in otology. *Ann Otol Rhinol Laryngol* 95(3 Pt 1):250, 1986.
15. Mawson ST: *Diseases of the Ear.* Baltimore, Williams & Wilkins, 1974.
16. Miller MH: Restoring hearing to the older patient: the physician's role. *Geriatrics* 41(12):75, 1986.
17. O'Connor S, Hawthorne M, Britten SR, Webber P: The management of a population of tinnitus sufferers in a specialized clinic: Part II. Identification of psychiatric morbidity in a population of tinnitus sufferers. *J Laryngol Otol* 101(8):791, 1987.
18. Ojemann RG, Montgomery WW, Weiss AD: Evaluation and surgical treatment of acoustic neuroma. *N Engl J Med* 287:895, 1972.
19. Paradise JL: Antimicrobial prophylaxis for recurrent acute otitis media. *Ann Otol Rhinol Laryngol* 90:53, 1984.
20. Price LL, Snider RM: The geriatric patient; ear, nose and throat problems. In: Reichel W (ed): *Clinical Aspects of Aging.* Williams & Wilkins, Baltimore, 1978, p. 489.
21. Smith CR, Lipsky JJ, Laskin OL, et al: Double-blind comparison of the nephrotoxicity and auditory toxicity of gentamicin and tobramycin. *N Engl J Med* 302:1106, 1980.
22. Youngblood J, Robinson S: Ineraid (Utah) multichannel cochlear implants. *Laryngoscope* 98(1):5, 1988.

C H A P T E R   97

Common Problems Associated with Impaired Vision: Cataracts and Age-Related Macular Degeneration*

ANDREW P. SCHACHAT, M.D.

CATARACTS

A cataract is an opacification of the lens of the eye. Ninety-six percent of individuals over 60 years of age will have some opacification of the lens, but most often these opacities are of no importance. A *significant cataract* results in interference with visual acuity. In the United States cataracts are a very common cause of diminished vision and may result in blindness. The incidence of diminished visual acuity from cataracts increases steadily after age 50, reaching nearly 50% of individuals over the age of 75. Cataracts are usually bilateral, and the progression is slow and may vary between eyes. The rate of progression is not individually predictable, and there is no treatment that will retard the progression. When the cataract is advanced, the only therapy is surgery.

Anatomy and Physiology

The lens is derived entirely from the evagination of surface ectoderm in the fetus. It is located immediately posterior to the iris and is suspended there by radially attached zonular fibers from the ciliary body (see Fig. 98.1, page 1330). It is a biconvex transparent structure with an elastic capsule whose shape may be altered

---

*Drs. Earl D.R. Kidwell, Jr., and John R. Burton contributed to this chapter in the first and second editions of this book.

by ciliary body contraction permitting images to be brought into sharp focus on the retina. The lens is acellular and avascular and lacks innervation. Nourishment is provided from the surrounding aqueous and vitreous humor, and metabolic by-products are removed by diffusion into the aqueous humor. The continued transparency of the lens requires the active metabolism of the elastic capsular epithelium so that any insult to the epithelium may result in lenticular opacities. New lenticular fibers are produced throughout life; and, since none are lost, increasing density of the fibers of the lens develops with age, which contributes to cataract formation as well.

Etiology

There are many causes of cataracts (Table 97.1). Although senescent cataracts—the result of the aging phenomena described above—account for the vast majority of cataracts, the general physician will occasionally see patients with congenital or traumatic lens opacities as well. The mechanism of opacification in all of these instances is thought to be due to interference with the metabolic activity of the capsular epithelium and with continued fiber production.

Many of these various types of cataracts have a distinctive appearance. The ophthalmologist may therefore suggest to the general physician the possibility of an underlying disorder such as myotonic dystrophy (iridescent spots) or Wilson's disease ("sunflower" cataract).

Symptoms and Examination

The primary symptom of cataract is impaired vision; usually patients describe a constant fog over the eye. They may also see rings or halos around lights and objects. The colors that objects appear change, particularly toward blue and yellow. Not infrequently, with

Table 97.1.
Etiology of Cataracts

CONGENITAL
  Autosomal dominant inheritance—25% of congenital cataracts
  Maternal malnutrition
  Maternal infections—e.g., rubella, syphilis
  Maternal metabolic disease—e.g., diabetes mellitus
  Maternal medication—corticosteroids
  Prematurity
TRAUMATIC
SENESCENT
SECONDARY
  Drug therapy—corticosteroids
  Degenerative eye disease—severe myopia
  Retinal dystrophy
  Essential iris atrophy
  Retinal detachment
  Glaucoma
  Intraocular neoplasia
  Ocular ischemia (e.g., Takayasu's disease)
ASSOCIATED WITH METABOLIC DISEASE
  Diabetes mellitus
  Wilson's disease
  Hypoparathyrodism

immature cataract formation, distant vision is impaired and near vision is preserved.

The location of the cataract within the lens determines the extent of the visual loss. Central opacities cause noticeable loss of vision and a distinct glare when the patient is in bright light. Bright light will constrict the pupil so that the dense portion of the lens occludes and diffuses light. For this reason the patient who has central opacities finds his vision is better in low light when his pupil is widely dilated. Peripheral opacities will cause noticeable loss of vision only late in the development of the cataract.

Cataracts are easily identified by illuminating the lens with a slitlamp, but most general physicians will find that they can see a cataract easily through the plus 4-10 lens of their direct ophthalmoscope. The lens appears cloudy. Similarly, a light from a small flashlight may be reflected off the opacity in the lens. Visual acuity should be tested in both eyes when cataracts are suspected. If the patient describes any visual symptoms or if the physician measures an impairment in visual acuity, the patient should be referred to an ophthalmologist. In adults, screening for cataracts is best done by a visual acuity examination with use of a *Snellen chart*. The Snellen chart is easy to use and the result is a ratio of the distance a patient stands from the chart to the distance that a subject with normal vision would stand to read the line of images in question. Therefore, 20/100 means the individual is seeing clearly at 20 feet an image that a person with normal vision would see at 100 feet. It is important to check separately the visual acuity of each eye with the other covered and with the patient using his glasses.

Cataract Surgery

Indications

Before surgery is indicated, optical manipulations such as mydriatics to help a patient see around a central cataract or new glasses for the progressive myopia associated with many nuclear cataracts may improve the vision of patients with cataracts. Also, visual aids, such as magnifying lenses and large print materials, may be helpful (see below, "Advice for the Visually Impaired"). The decision to remove a cataract, is determined by the visual needs of the patient, the degree of the cataract and the presence of any other ocular abnormalities. The ophthalmologist will perform a complete ocular assessment (see Chapter 98) before advising the patient about surgery.

Each patient must determine his own visual need based on his daily activities. The ability to read, drive, cross streets safely, and perform a daily routine are clearly of prime importance. For example, a patient usually requires visual acuity of at least 20/40 in the better eye to operate a motor vehicle safely or to continue moderately active daily life.

Surgery

Cataract surgery should not be performed without considerable deliberation as there are a number of complications that might occur (see below), and vision after cataract extraction may still be a major problem (see below). The general physician and the ophthalmologist should plan cataract surgery together. Cataract extraction is an elective procedure, and the patient should be in the best possible condition at the time of operation.

Approximately 600,000 cataract extractions are performed in the United States every year, and cataract surgery is the most commonly performed major surgical procedure performed in the elderly in this country. Surgery involves the removal of the opacified lens from the eye. The extraction may be intracapsular, involving complete removal of the lens, or extracapsular, leaving the posterior capsule of the lens intact. Microsurgical techniques have greatly improved the immediate outcome of surgery and have significantly shortened the period of disability. Extracapsular extraction is most commonly performed because it leaves the posterior capsule intact, permits easier lens implantation (see below), and is probably associated with fewer postoperative complications. Both eyes usually require operation, but normally only one lens is extracted at a time so that the patient will have vision in the nonoperated side when the eye that has been operated upon is covered by a patch for a few days after surgery. For patients with bilateral cataracts, the second procedure is usually performed a few months after the first.

Patient Experience. Cataract surgery is performed most often by use of local anesthesia supplemented with intravenous analgesia and sedation. Surgery is usually performed on an outpatient basis. The patient experiences moderate discomfort, but this lasts only a day or so and is controlled with analgesics. A hyperosmotic agent (such as glycerin or mannitol) may be employed to dehydrate and to soften the eye in preparation for surgery.

After discharge from the surgical unit a patient must restrict his activities for several weeks to minimize the frequency of complications. These restrictions are listed in Table 97.2. There are no permanent restrictions; however, caution with steps or when walking and working with machinery may be necessary if perception is seriously altered using aphakic spectacles (see below).

Table 97.2.
Temporary Restrictions After Cataract Surgery[a]

Wear eye shield during sleep and wear glasses at other times—shields are usually worn for 1 month and then discontinued.
Minimize bending or stooping for 3 or 4 weeks.
Do not sleep on side of operated eye for 3 or 4 weeks.
Do not wash hair for 2 weeks.
No showers for 2 weeks, although a bath is allowed (but with assistance to prevent a fall).
No strenuous or excessive physical activity for 4 weeks and then only after approval of the ophthalmologist.

[a]These are suggested to prevent inadvertent injury to the eye, diminish disruptive pressure on the wound, avoid sudden rise in ocular pressure, and diminish the chance of infection.

Complications

Complications occur in approximately 5% of patients who have had cataract extraction, and one of every 5000 eyes operated upon is lost because of complications. Knowledge of the possible complications after cataract surgery will aid the general physician in educating patients. Because of the potential for complications, the general physician must be sure that the patient keeps his scheduled postoperative appointments with the ophthalmologist.

Inflammation and Infection. All postoperative patients have some degree of traumatic intraocular inflammation. This is usually controlled effectively with topical corticosteroids. Bacterial endophthalmitis is a dangerous postoperative inflammation that must be recognized early before it devastates the eye. If a patient complains of decreased vision, pain, discharge, and redness, endophthalmitis may be present and the patient should be seen immediately by an ophthalmologist. Most infections occur within a few days of surgery; however, an operated eye is predisposed to infection from systemic infection, and therefore a patient with an acute red eye occurring at any time after eye surgery should be seen urgently by an ophthalmologist. Low grade chronic inflammation is common after cataract surgery and resultant macular edema is one of the most common causes of postoperative visual loss.

Hemorrhage. The sudden occurrence of hemorrhage in the uveal tract (the iris, the ciliary body, and the choroid) can adversely influence the final visual outcome. Although this complication is usually seen intraoperatively, rarely it may occur postoperatively. The event is characterized by a painless but precipitous change in visual acuity. Postoperative hemorrhage from the iris or from an inadequately closed corneoscleral wound is, however, more common than is vitreous hemorrhage. In all instances of hemorrhage, urgent referral to an ophthalmologist is indicated.

Retinal Detachment. The incidence of retinal detachment after cataract surgery is approximately 1 to 3%. Retinal detachment is characterized by suddenly decreased visual acuity, flashes of light, and the development of floaters, veils, and/or curtains in the visual field. Patients with symptoms of retinal detachment should be seen immediately by an ophthalmologist so that surgical reattachment of the retina may be accomplished. The success of reattachment is good provided that the procedure can be done expeditiously.

Glaucoma. This secondary form of glaucoma is due to several factors that lead to angle closure: the effect of the proteolytic agent, chymotrypsin, on the angular structures at the time of intracapsular operation (rare today); scarring due to postoperative inflammation; or the misdirection into and subsequent trapping of the aqueous in the vitreous gel see (Fig. 98.1, page 1330). Glaucoma may develop within a few days of surgery. Early glaucoma is usually transient, but it may become chronic. Glaucoma may appear as late as 1 to 2 years after surgery in 0.6 to 5% of patients depending on the type of surgery. The patient who has developed secondary glaucoma will usually complain of redness, tenderness, and pain in the eye. Further, if the patient has been fitted with a temporary spectacle, he will notice decreased visual acuity due to corneal edema. A postoperative patient suspected of having glaucoma should be seen by an ophthalmologist immediately.

Additional information related to glaucoma may be found in Chapter 98.

Delayed Opacification of the Posterior Capsule. The new technique of extracapsular extraction is most commonly performed since it is associated with fewer complications (as compared with intracapsular extraction). However, 20 to 50% of patients experience a gradual decrease in vision in the first few years after this technique due to opacification of the posterior lens capsule. This complication can now be treated highly effectively by a special laser instrument (YAG, yttrium aluminum garnet) that opens the posterior capsule without the need for intraocular surgery.

Optical Correction after Cataract Extraction

The removal of a cataract improves the transmission of light to the retina, but vision remains blurred without corrective lenses. Three types of lenses are used: aphakic spectacles, contact lenses, or intraocular lenses.

With aphakic spectacles there is a narrower field of vision, as well as considerable distortion of images, that appear rounded and three to five times larger than when the lens is present in the eye. Also, there are peripheral ring scotomata and loss of some depth perception. Even modern aphakic spectacles are heavy and thick so that a patient frequently will have considerable initial difficulty adjusting to them and will need support, understanding, and encouragement from family members. With experience, however, most patients will be able to function acceptably and perform all of their necessary daily activities.

A unilateral cataract extraction results in a pronounced disparity in image size if an aphakic spectacle is used postoperatively; therefore, unilateral surgery is generally not advised unless the patient will be able to use a contact lens or is a candidate for an intraocular lens implantation (see below). Under certain circumstances, however (such as when glaucoma or diabetic retinopathy is present in addition to cataract), monolenticular extraction may be indicated to permit the ophthalmologist to follow the course of these ocular diseases.

The use of contact lenses after cataract extraction provides considerable improvement over spectacles. There is, especially, reduction in distortion and expansion of the field of vision. The patient, however, must be motivated to use contact lenses, and this motivation must be considered before surgery is undertaken. Often elderly patients are concerned about being agile enough to insert contact lenses. The patient must also be fitted with a pair of spectacles with one lens missing so that he may see to place one contact lens.

A regular set of aphakic spectacles is also necessary as a backup to the contact lens.

Because of the visual handicap experienced after cataract extraction, plastic lenses are inserted at the time of surgery in nearly 85 to 95% of patients undergoing cataract extraction. Long-term survival of these inert prostheses is very good. The insertion of intraocular implants adds a few minutes to the operative time beyond that required for lens extraction. Utilizing this technique more than 90% of patients will experience an improvement in vision to 20/40 or better.

AGE-RELATED MACULAR DEGENERATION

Age-related macular degeneration is the leading cause of severe visual loss in people over age 50. The macula is the special central area of the retina used for fine focus such as reading. There is no universally agreed definition of the disease. It is characterized by the development of drusen, retinal pigment epithelial changes, and in some cases abnormal choroidal vessels and hemorrhage. Drusen are excrescences that develop along Bruch's membrane, which lies between the retina and choroid and appear, on ophthalmologic examination, as tiny discrete white or yellow deposits. They are at times difficult to visualize and the ophthalmoscope needs to be in sharp focus on the retina. The large majority of patients over age 50 have a few drusen and there is no consensus as to how many drusen and how extensive retinal pigment epithelial changes are required before a patient is labeled as having "macular degeneration." Drusen formation alone almost never reduces visual acuity.

Epidemiology

The Framingham Eye Study found that age-related macular degeneration was present in one or both eyes of almost 6% of individuals age 52 or older (3). The prevalence is strongly age related. Comparable rates were found in the Health and Nutrition Examination Survey (HANES) (2). Risk factors that have been identified in some series include hyperopia, decreased hand grip strength, light iris color, systemic hypertension, family history, cardiac hypertrophy, short height, history of previous lung infection, cigarette smoking, cardiovascular disease, chemical exposure, and sunlight exposure. The strength and validity of these associations are debated and at least two major epidemiological studies investigating risk factors are currently underway.

Clinical Features

There are two major forms of macular degeneration. The *atrophic form* is characterized simply by drusen formation and atrophic retinal pigment epithelial changes. It is the most common form of macular degeneration. The *exudative form* of macular degeneration, in which subretinal choroidal neovascularization occurs, can lead to subretinal hemorrhage and fluid accumulation and, eventually, extensive scarring. Although it is the rarer form of macular degeneration, it accounts for the majority of visual loss seen in patients with macular degeneration.

Drusen may vary in distribution, number, size, and shape. They may or may not have pigmentary alterations around them. Small drusen are difficult to see with the direct ophthalmoscope although larger or so-called "soft" drusen should be apparent (Figs. 97.1, 97.2). Atrophy associated with age-related macular degeneration may represent true atrophy of retinal pigment epithelium or may simply represent loss of pigment from within retinal pigment epithelial cells. Clinically, the distinction is impossible to make (Fig. 97.3). When atrophy involves the center of the retina (the "macula"), visual acuity is usually reduced.

Exudative macular degeneration is characterized by the accumulation of fluid, hemorrhage, or lipid beneath or within the retina (Fig. 97.4). Accumulation of fluid beneath the retinal pigment epithelium may lead to pigment epithelial detachment. Choroidal neo-

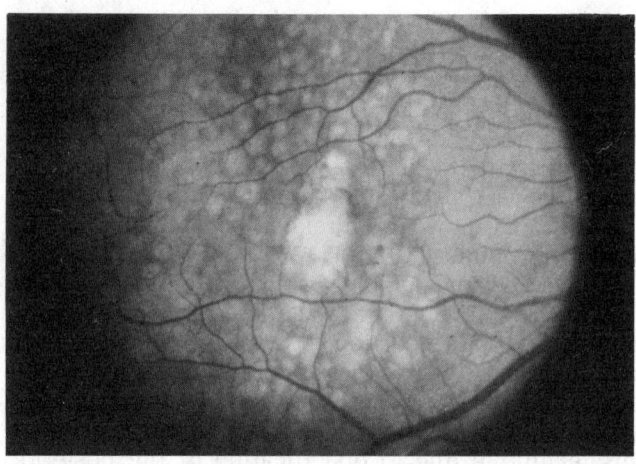

Figure 97.3. This patient with atrophic macular degeneration has hard and soft drusen. There is a zone of central atropy, and if the center of the macula is involved, vision is usually decreased.

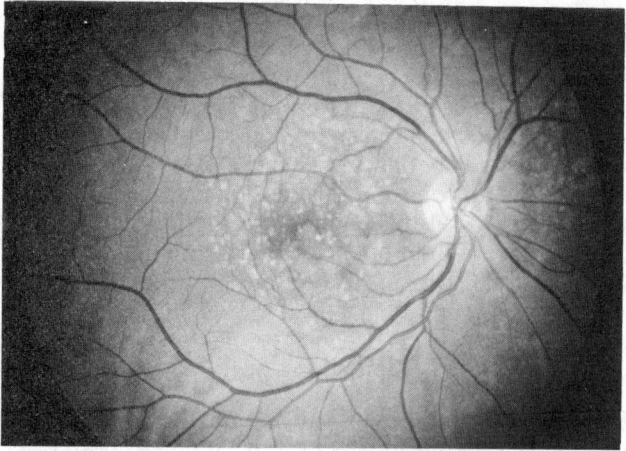

Figure 97.1. Hard drusen are the tiny dots in the central retina ("macular area"). They are minimally elevated and, when viewed in color, are yellow-white. The visual acuity is normal.

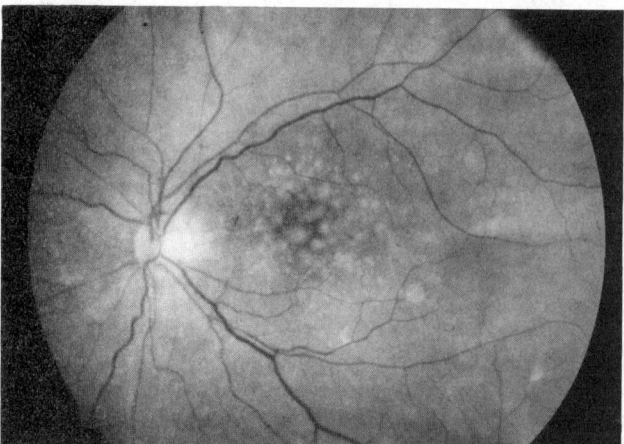

Figure 97.2. The larger blotches in the central retina are soft drusen. Patients with soft drusen are at increased risk of developing exudative macular degeneration. The visual acuity is normal.

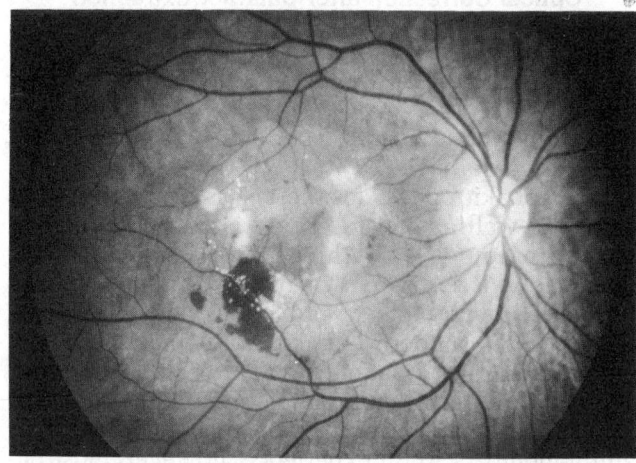

Figure 97.4. Exudative macular degeneration. There is subretinal blood and lipid. Subretinal fluid can be seen on stereoscopic photographs (not shown). This patient has choroidal neovascularization.

vascularization may grow through or actually cause breaks in Bruch's membrane. The new blood vessels beneath the retina are the cause of the hemorrhage and lipid accumulation (Fig. 97.5A). After the active phase, subretinal fibrosis or a so-called disciform scar is seen (Fig. 97.5B and C).

Although the subretinal new vessels are rarely directly visible, the technique of fluorescein angiography allows their diagnosis (Fig. 97.6). Intravenous fluorescein dye is injected in the antecubital fossa. Within 10 to 20 seconds, the dye can be photographed traversing vessels in the eye. The presence of increasing hyperfluorescence as the angiogram progresses is a marker for choroidal neovascularization. However, the interpretation of fluorescein angiograms is complex and use of the technique is beyond the scope of the nonophthalmologist.

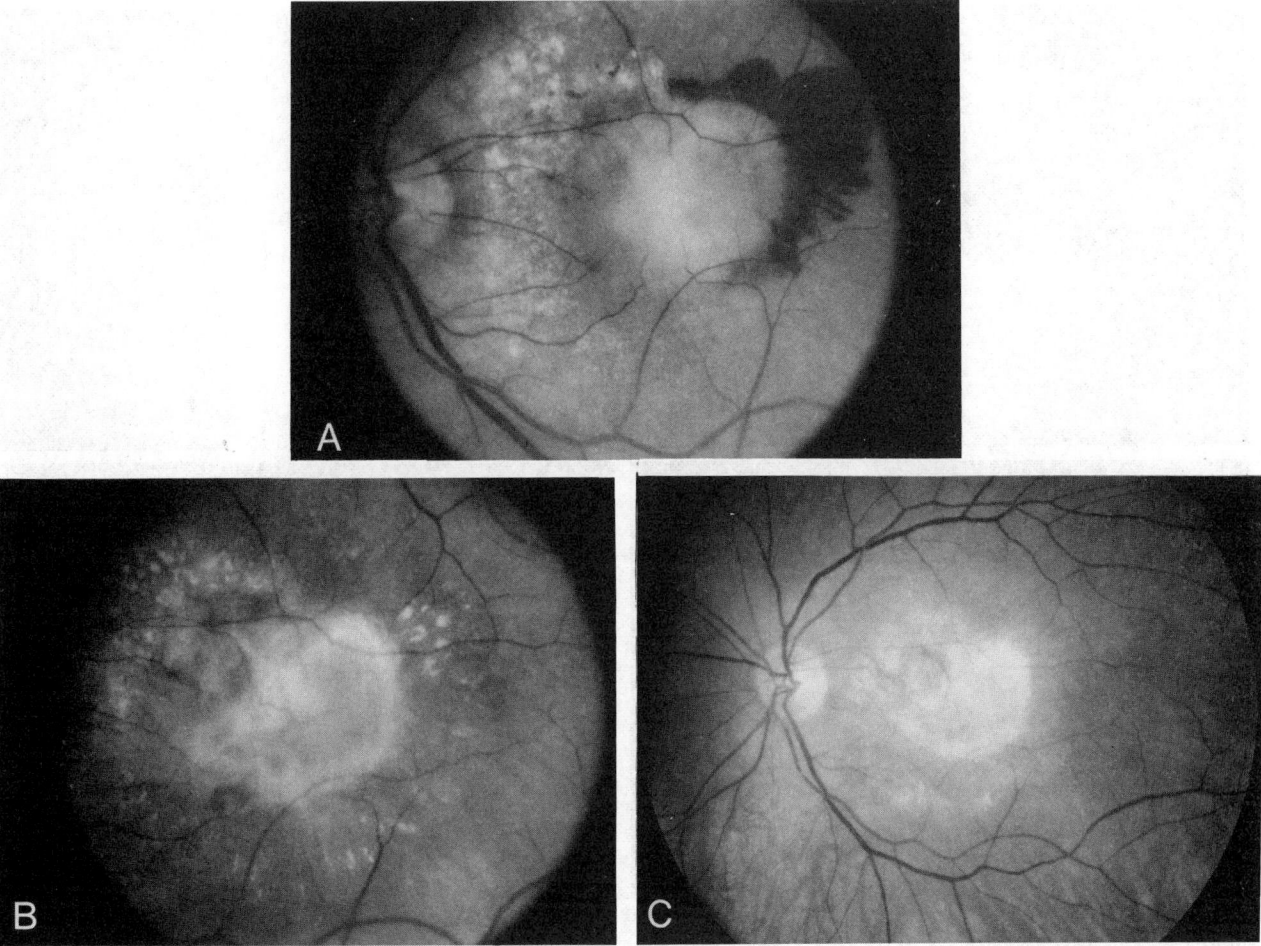

Figure 97.5. *A.* Exudative macular degeneration characterized by blood, lipid, and subretinal fluid accumulation, all sequelae of choroidal neovascularization. *B.* Six months later, the blood has resorbed, the lipid is less, and subretinal fibrosis is beginning. *C.* One year later, a "disciform scar" has formed.

Natural History and Treatment

The natural history of patients with bilateral drusen is uncertain. Patients who have exudative disease in one eye and drusen only in the second eye have a rate of between 4 and 15% per year of the development of exudative disease in the previously uninvolved eye. Patients with atrophic macular degeneration should be examined by an ophthalmologist at least annually.

Although numerous dietary and vitamin therapies have been recommended for patients with the atrophic form of the disease, there is no information available at this time that substantiates these recommendations. The one investigator who has reported a benefit for oral zinc supplementation for macular degeneration concluded that because of the pilot nature of the study and the possible toxic effects of the drug, widespread use of zinc in patients with macular degeneration is not now warranted (5). Because chronic light toxicity may play a role in the pathogenesis of macular degeneration, avoidance of sunlight has been considered. In a recent review (1), it was concluded that "no data exist (sic) to support the notion that any form of

sunglasses can reduce chronic photic insult and thereby reduce a putative factor in the development of age-related macular degeneration." Nevertheless, the use of sunglasses is relatively inexpensive and without side effects and, therefore, should not be "discouraged."

There is a treatment for a small subgroup of patients with exudative disease, but because the clinical features are subtle and the treatment is beyond the scope of the nonophthalmologist, referral to an ophthalmologist is indicated. The Macular Photocoagulation Study compared the value of laser photocoagulation with no treatment for patients with well-defined choroidal neovascularization outside the center of the macular area. After 3½ years follow-up, 62% of untreated patients had a loss of six or more lines of vision on a Snellen chart compared with 47% of treated patients. The difference is statistically significant (4).

ADVICE FOR THE VISUALLY IMPAIRED

When vision cannot be improved or maintained at an acceptable level, it is important for the physician

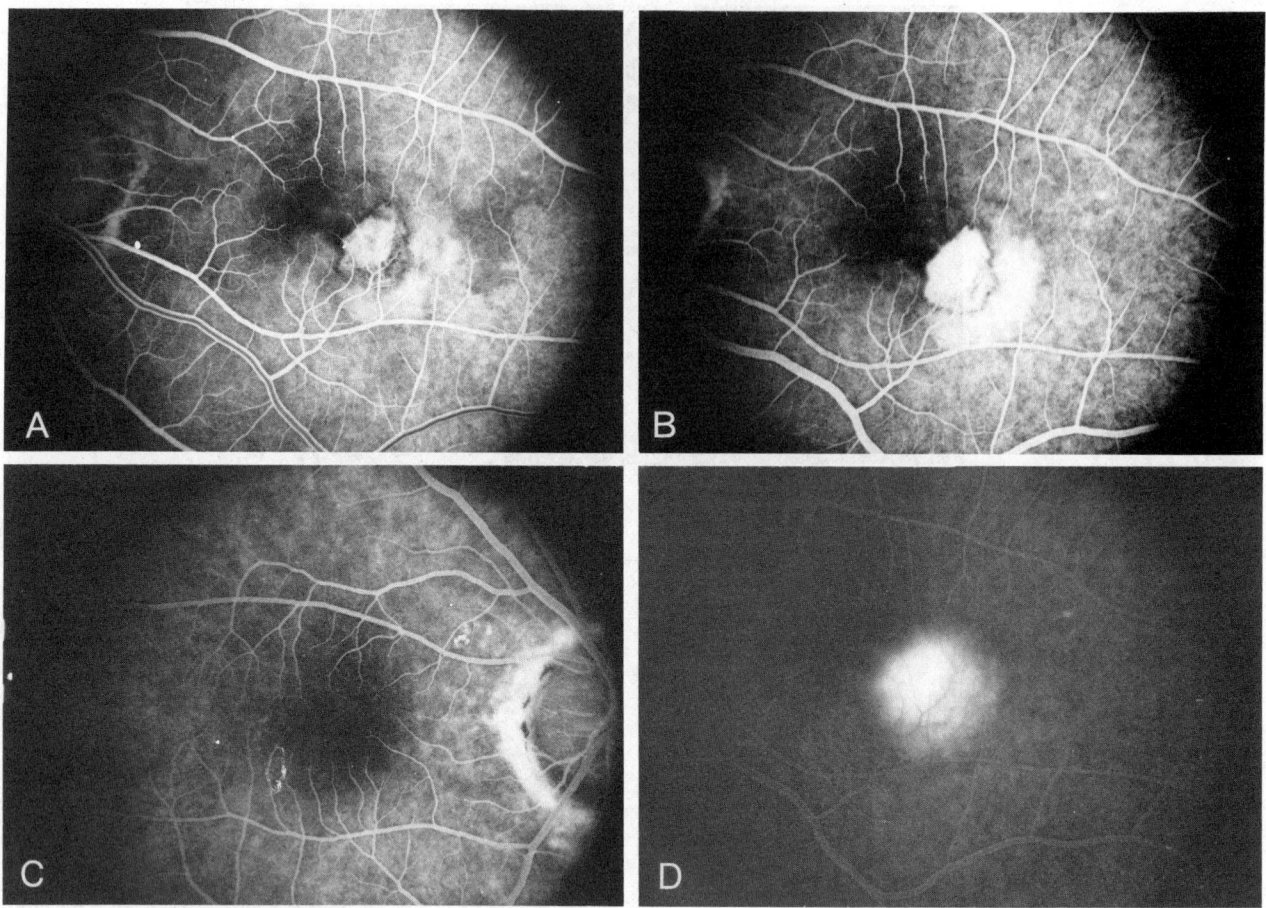

Figure 97.6. Fluorescein angiogram: choroidal neovascularization. *A.* In the early phase, 18 seconds after intravenous injection of dye, the fluorescein is seen filling retinal arteries and laminar venous filling is beginning. A zone of hyperfluorescence ("brightness") is seen at the inferotemporal aspect of the macula. This is caused by dye leaking form abnormal choroidal vessels ("choroidal neovascularization"). *B.* The leaking increases 10 seconds later. *C.* For comparison, a view of the normal fellow eye illustrates a normal angiographic pattern. *D.* A late frame, taken approximately 10 minutes after the injection, shows continued leaking of dye from the choroidal new vessels.

to aid the patient in finding resources that might provide some help in lessening the ever increasing isolation and loss of mobility resulting from blindness. Dr. DeWitt Stetten (see "General References") wrote an essay describing his experience with progressive blindness and outlined in that essay a number of useful aids that he identified. He described the increasingly available large print books, journals, and newsprint (e.g., *The New York Times*). There are also many books available on tape from the *Talking Books Program* of the Library of Congress. Most local libraries will be able to provide information on the availability of these tapes. Some journals may be obtained on tapes from *Recorded Periodicals* (919 Walnut St., Philadelphia, PA 19107). *Newsweek* magazine is available on disposable phonographic records (Newsweek, PO Box 6435, 1839 Frankfort Ave, Louisville, KY 40206). A variety of aids for the blind may be ordered from the catalog of SFB Products (Box 385, Wayne, PA 19087). A portable cassette tape recorder designed for the blind can be purchased through the American Printing House for the Blind, Inc. (General Office, PO Box 6085, Louisville, KY 40206). Talking clocks and Braille time pieces

may be very useful, and information concerning these and other aids are available from the National Institutes of Health (Volunteers for the Visually Handicapped, 4405 East-West Hwy, Bethesda, MD 20814). Several reading machines or magnifying devices are also available, although these are expensive (see Stetten, "General References").

Visual Foundation, Inc. (770 Center St., Newton, MA 02158) is a self-help organization that was developed by people losing their sight. They have published a handbook, *Coping with Sight Loss*, which provides information for the visually impaired on visual aids, devices, recreation, tax benefits, reading materials, and referral sources. The handbook is published in large print and on cassette tapes and will be a useful resource for the patient experiencing loss of vision as well as for physicians caring for these patients.

General References

Elman MJ, Fine SL: Exudative age-related macular degeneration. In: Ryan SJ (ed): *Retina.* St Louis, CV Mosby Co, 1989.
Liesegang TJ: Cataracts and cataract operations—two parts. *Mayo Clin Proc* 59:556, 622, 1984.

Sarks SH, Sharks JP: Age-related macular degeneration—atrophic form. In: Ryan SJ (ed): *Retina*. St Louis, CV Mosby Co, 1989.

Stark WJ, Woethen DM, Holladay JT, et al: The FDA report on intraocular lenses. *Ophthalmology* 90:311, 1983.

> The standard reference regarding intraocular lenses.

Stetten Jr D: Coping with blindness. *N Engl J Med* 305:458, 1981.

> A concise description of aids to help cope with blindness, written by Dr. Stetten as he experienced progressive loss of vision.

Straatsma BR, Foos RY, Horwitz J, et al: Aging-related cataract: laboratory investigation and clinical management. *Ann Intern Med* 102:82, 1985.

> This UCLA conference reviews all aspects of senescent cataracts and contains superb color photographs of a variety of common cataract patterns.

Weinstein G: Cataract surgery. In: Duane T, Jaeger E (eds): *Clinical Ophthalmology*, Vol. 5. Philadelphia, JB Lippincott, 1986. Chapter 7.

Specific References

1. Bressler NM, Bressler SB, Fine SL: Age-related macular Degeneration. *Surv Ophthalmol* 32:375, 1988.
2. Klein BE, Klein E: Cataracts and macular degeneration in older Americans. *Arch Ophthalmol* 100:571, 1982.
3. Leibowitz H, Krueger DE, Maudner LR, et al: The Framingham Eye Study Monograph. *Surv Ophthalmol* 24 (suppl):335, 1980.
4. Macular Photocoagulation Study Group: Argon laser photocoagulation for neovascular maculopathy: three year results from randomized clinical trials. *Arch Ophthalmol* 104:694, 1986.
5. Newsome DA, Swartz M, Leone NC, et al: Oral zinc in macular degeneration. *Arch Ophthalmol* 106:192, 1988.

C H A P T E R 98

Glaucoma*

ANDREW P. SCHACHAT, M.D.

Anatomy and Physiology	1329
Types of Glaucoma	1329
Primary Open-Angle Glaucoma	1329
Primary Angle-Closure Glaucoma	1333

Glaucoma is a common disorder characterized by an increase in intraocular pressure sufficient to cause damage to the optic nerve. The glaucomas are classified into primary and secondary groups (Table 98.1). The primary group accounts for 95% of all patients with glaucoma in the United States.

Patients with glaucoma will usually be followed by an ophthalmologist. However, the general physician will need to be familiar with the techniques of screening for and diagnosing glaucoma and with the long-term care of patients who are found to have glaucoma.

ANATOMY AND PHYSIOLOGY (Fig. 98.1)

The aqueous humor helps maintain the shape of the eye and the correct relationship among the refractile

*Dr. Earl D.R. Kidwell, Jr., contributed to this chapter in the first and second editions of this book.

Table 98.1.
Types of Glaucoma

PRIMARY
  Open-angle—90% of patients
  Angle-closure—5% of patients
  Congential—Infant and juvenile onset
SECONDARY
  Open-angle—Results from topical or systemic steroids, ocular inflammation, or obstructed venous return from the eye (e.g., carotid cavernous sinus fistula)
  Angle-closure—Results from trauma, neovascular change of the iris, ocular neoplasia, cataracts, and iris degenerations from various causes

elements of the eye; it also provides the nutrition of the avascular intraocular structures such as the lens. There is continuous production and removal of the aqueous humor. In most cases of glaucoma, an obstruction to the outflow of aqueous humor appears to be the basis for the increased intraocular pressure.

The aqueous humor is a clear ultrafiltrate of the blood and occupies part of the posterior and anterior chambers of the eye. It is produced by the ciliary epithelium of the ciliary body, which is a portion of the uveal tract of the eye. It appears most likely that the aqueous is formed partially by secretion and partially by a process of ultrafiltration. At least two enzymes have been implicated in aqueous formation: sodium/potassium-activated ATPase and carbonic anhydrase. Antagonists of these enzymes appear to reduce the rate of aqueous formation and thereby lower intraocular pressure; however, the precise mechanism of action of these drugs is uncertain. Acetazolamide (Diamox), a carbonic anhydrase inhibitor, has proved clinically important in the treatment of glaucoma. Once reproduced, the aqueous humor circulates from the posterior chamber into the anterior chamber of the eye. The trabecular meshwork, an intricate system of connective tissue fibers, is located in the periphery of the anterior chamber. The aqueous percolates through this meshwork to be reunited with the venous blood via Schlemm's canal.

TYPES OF GLAUCOMA

Table 98.1 outlines the major types and causes of glaucoma. However, only primary open-angle and primary angle-closure are discussed in this chapter since they are the only types of glaucoma likely to be seen with any frequency by the general physician. Open-angle glaucoma takes its name from the relatively normal appearing anterior chamber angle, a contrast to the narrow angle of angle-closure glaucoma as shown in Figure 98.2.

Primary Open-Angle Glaucoma

Prevalence and Risk Factors

Primary open-angle glaucoma is by far the most common cause of glaucoma in the United States; the prevalence increases after the age of 40 years and approaches 3% of individuals over 75 years of age.

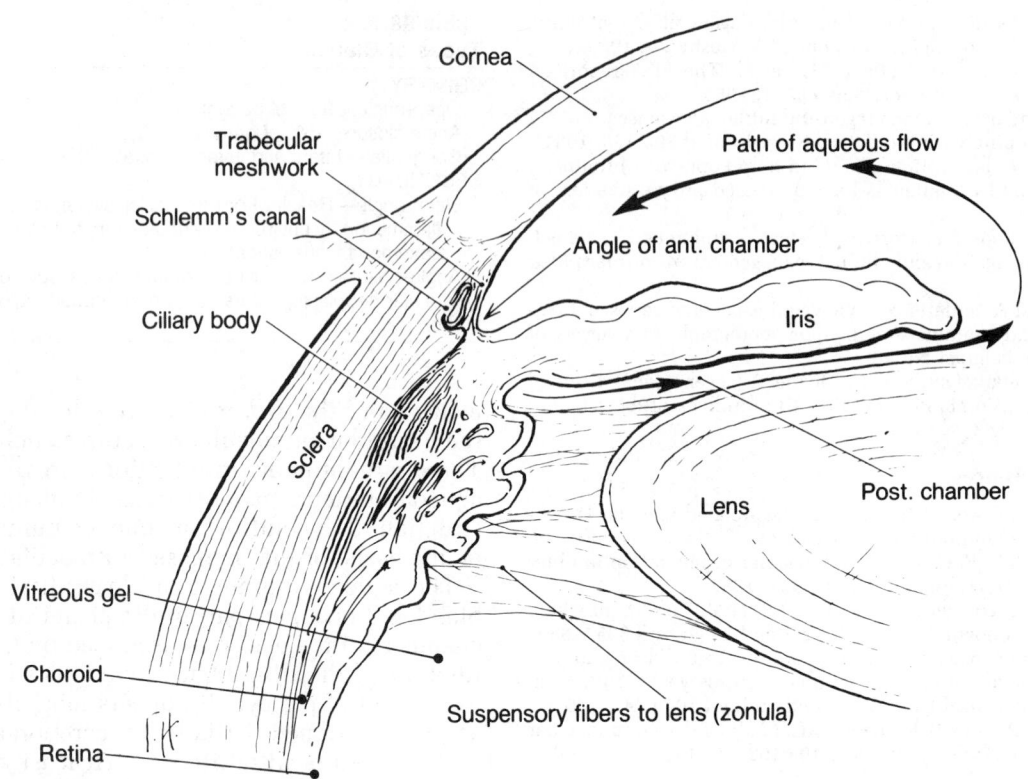

Figure 98.1.   Anatomy of the eye—cross section at the cornea. (From Basmajian JV: *Grant's Method of Anatomy*, 8th ed. Baltimore, Williams & Wilkins, 1971 p. 543).

Primary open-angle glaucoma causes 15 to 20% of all blindness in this country (see Chapter 97 for a discussion of blindness). Men and women are affected equally; but blacks are affected both at a higher frequency and at an earlier age, and open-angle glaucoma is the leading cause of blindness in black Americans. Open-angle glaucoma is familial, but the pattern of inheritance is not yet known with certainty. In patients who have a positive family history of glaucoma, there is an association between glaucoma and leukocyte antigen HLA B12. It has been proposed that there is an association between open-angle glaucoma and both diabetes mellitus and elevated blood pressure, but these hypotheses are controversial and more research will be necessary to define or negate such relationships. Patients who have high degrees of myopia (defective distant vision) are often said to have a higher risk of open-angle glaucoma, but there remains more controversy about this hypothesis as well.

Diagnosis

In primary open-angle glaucoma, ocular hypertension appears to result from resistance in the trabecular meshwork to aqueous outflow. The elevation of the intraocular pressure is roughly related to the degree of obstruction. The disease is asymptomatic in its early stages. When symptoms do occur, neural damage is present and may be substantial. Macular (central) vision and the ability to recognize forms on a vision test chart are preserved until very late. For this reason testing of visual acuity is not a reliable method to screen for glaucoma. Occasionally a patient with open-angle glaucoma may notice halos around lights and blurring of vision if there is a sudden rise in intraocular pressure such as might occur with rapid ingestion of a large quantity of fluid (e.g., 1 liter). Patients with this history should be referred to an ophthalmologist. Patients only rarely complain of headache that can be attributed to increased intraocular pressure. The ocular pressure may be elevated for years, however, before any change in the optic disc is noted. The change in the optic disc will be revealed by increasing excavation of the central physiological disc cup, visible on funduscopic examination (Fig. 98.3). This is most easily seen by use of the red filter of the direct ophthalmoscope. Over years the pink color of the disc fades and becomes pale, and vessels coursing over the disc show a sharp bend at the rim. Patients with an enlarged optic cup should be referred urgently to an ophthalmologist.

In evaluating the patient with increased intraocular pressure the opthalmologist will perform tonometry, gonioscopy (see below), funduscopy, and visual field examinations (see below). Characteristic visual field changes called "nerve fiber bundle defects" are seen in glaucoma.

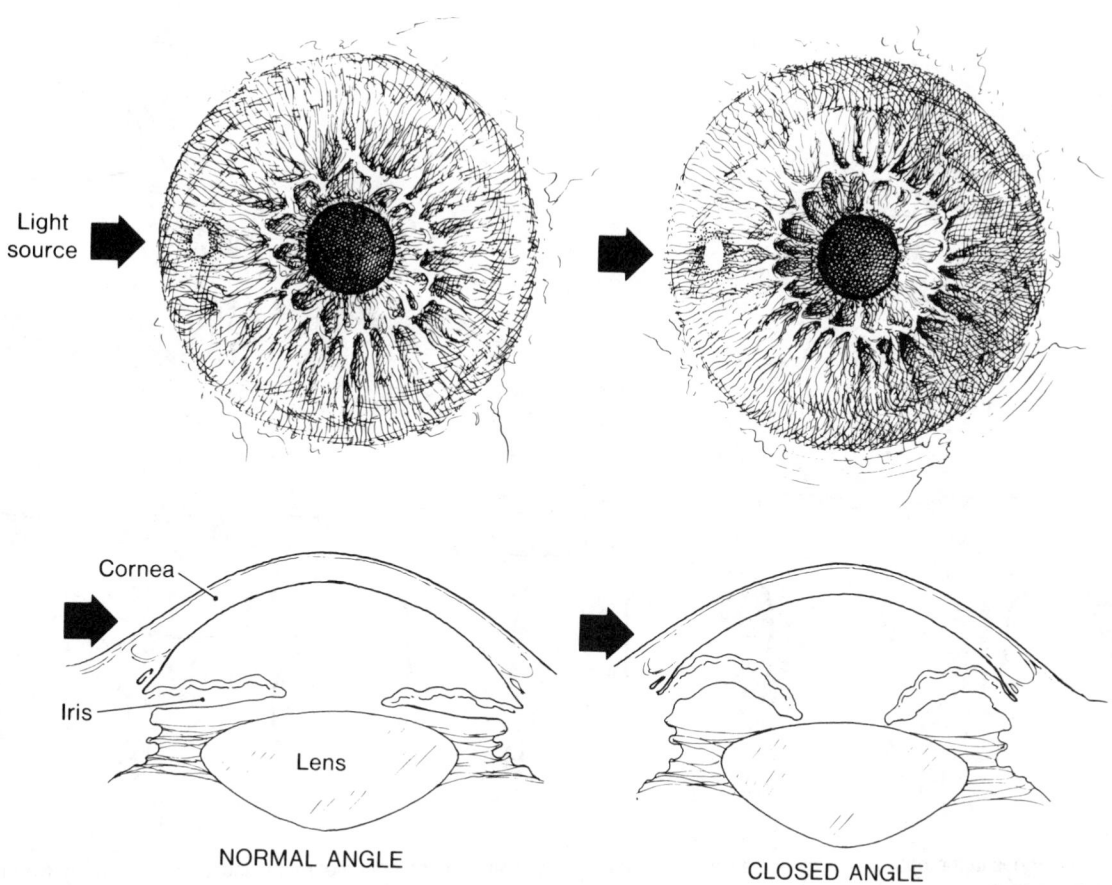

Figure 98.2. Illustration showing a shadow cast on the nasal side of the iris resultant from the bowed iris in angle-closure glaucoma. In open-angle glaucoma, the iris is not bowed and the shadow, therefore, is not cast.

Screening for Open-Angle Glaucoma

Screening for primary open-angle glaucoma is controversial, and high false-positive and false-negative detection rates are the norm. Nevertheless, screening seems reasonable because: (*a*) the disease is silent until permanent ocular damage has occurred; (*b*) screening is relatively simple in experienced hands and without significant risk; (*c*) treatment most likely can prevent eye damage; and (*d*) this form of glaucoma is common, especially in older individuals.

Screening in theory could be accomplished in one or more of three ways: tonometry, funduscopic assessment of the optic cup through the dilated pupil, and visual field assessment. For years it has been recommended that primary care physicians screen high risk patients for glaucoma by measuring eye pressure directly with a Schiotz tonometer. This screen done alone is now felt to be too insensitive and nonspecific to be of value. Rather, current thinking suggests that combinations of tests are needed to improve the sensitivity and specificity of glaucoma screening. Ophthalmologists generally do all three evaluations, but this is not practical for the general physician. For this reason, the report of the United States Preventive Service Task Force (see "General References") does not recommend the routine performance of tonometry by primary care physicians. Rather, primary care phy-

sicians are encouraged to advise patients aged 65 and older (those at high risk) to be referred to an eye specialist periodically for glaucoma screening.

Patients found by an eye specialist to have intraocular pressure equal to or greater than 20 mm Hg will generally have an evaluation consisting of several observations: confirmation of the intraocular pressure by applanation tonometry, by use of a complex piece of equipment, and requiring only a drop of topical anesthetic; funduscopic assessment of the optic disc and retina through the dilated pupil; formal visual field assessment; and gonioscopic examination, which permits the ophthalmologist to visualize the angle of the anterior chamber by using an instrument containing a contact lens and mirror. The patient usually experiences minimal or no discomfort during any of these procedures.

Approximately one-third of patients who on preliminary screening are found to have asymptomatic increased intraocular pressure will be found after thorough evaluation to have glaucoma. Approximately 30% may be found not to have elevated pressures on reassessment, and about 25% will have "ocular hypertension" without glaucoma. This latter group of patients with elevated intraocular pressure but with normal appearing optic discs and visual fields should be followed yearly by the ophthalmologist; about 1% of these

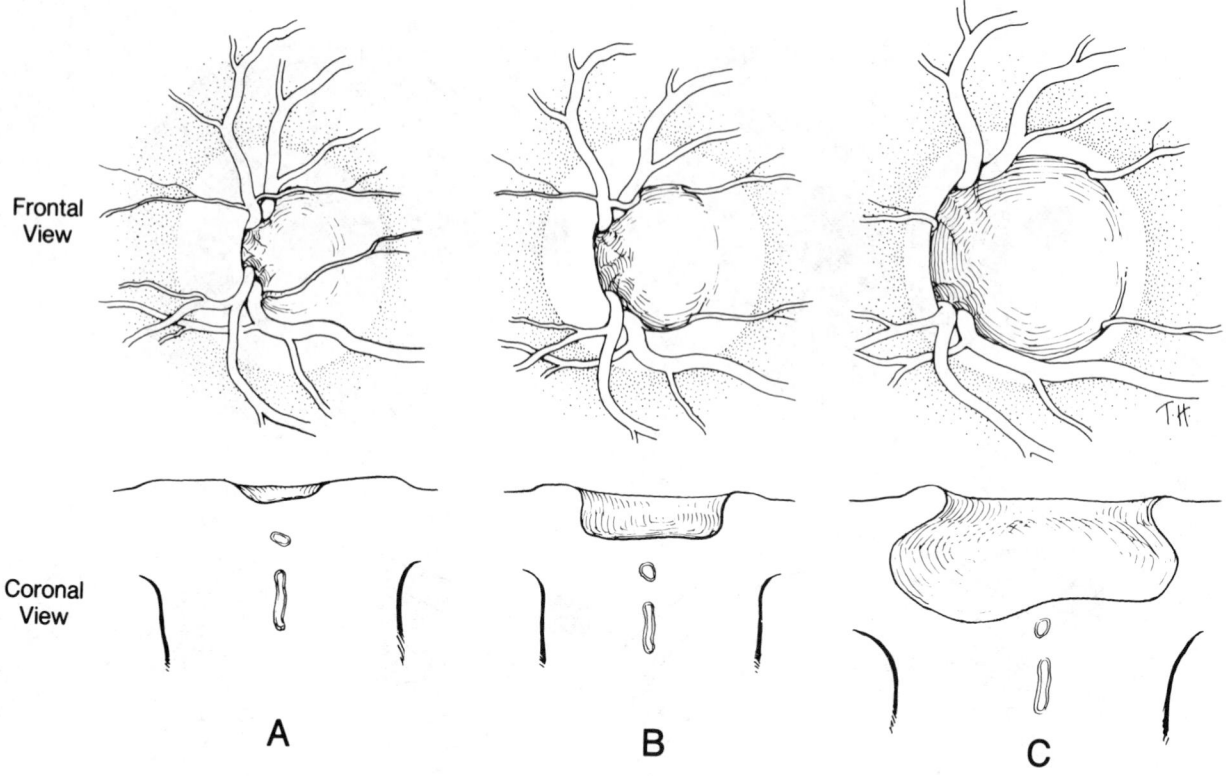

Frontal View

Coronal View

A   B   C

Figure 98.3.   Changes in the optic disc with increasing intraocular pressure showing on both the frontal and coronal views: *A.* Normal. *B.* Early change. *C.* Late change.

patients will develop glaucoma each year. The rate is higher for those with a positive family history of glaucoma and for those with higher pressure abnormalities.

Treatment

When the opthalmologist establishes the diagnosis of open-angle glaucoma, he will prescribe treatment based on the level of intraocular pressure, the degree of visual field loss, and the amount of optic nerve damage.

The treatment of open-angle glaucoma is largely medical, with use of agents that facilitate the outflow (e.g., miotics) or reduce the amount of production (e.g., β-blockers) of aqueous humor. The aim of therapy is to maintain the intraocular pressure at a level that does not lead to optic nerve damage. This target pressure is usually 20mm Hg. Patients are usually prescribed a topical β-blocker and sometimes a mild miotic, such as carbachol or pilocarpine. Other agents, such as carbonic anhydrase inhibitors and stronger miotics, are added or replace the milder agents as necessary. The β-adrenergic receptor blocking agent timolol maleate (e.g., Timoptic Ophthalmic Solution) will reduce ocular pressure and has the advantage of producing little or no effect on pupil size or visual acuity. For this reason decreased, blurred, or impaired night vision is

not the problem with timolol that it is with miotic agents. However, systemic effects of the β-blocker may occur. Newer more selective β-blocking agents such as levobunolol hydrochloride ophthalmic solution (Betagan) appear to have few systemic effects.

Frequently, early in the course, treatment may need to be changed by the ophthalmologist since drug tolerance is common and side effects may occur. Once the decreased ocular pressure has been attained, the ophthalmologist will usually examine the patient approximately three times/year for assessment of visual fields, measurement of intraocular pressure, funduscopic examination, and gonioscopy.

Argon laser trabeculoplasty may be used by the ophthalmologist to lower ocular pressure when medical therapy is unsatisfactory. This office procedure requires only topical anesthesia and can result in a significant reduction in ocular pressure in nearly two-thirds of patients. Most patients, however, will continue to require the continued use of medications. The mechanism by which laser trabeculoplasty exerts its beneficial effects is uncertain.

Surgery in primary open-angle glaucoma is designed to construct outflow channels for the aqueous humor or to freeze the ciliary body and destroy the site of aqueous production. Surgical procedures are reserved for patients in whom medical management fails. Medications may still be required after surgery.

Monitoring

The primary physician should ensure that the patient with open-angle glaucoma is receiving regular ophthalmological follow-up and should be alert to any side effects from the drugs prescribed by the ophthalmologist.

There has been particular concern about systemic medications that have anticholinergic (atropine-like), adrenergic, vasodilator, or corticosteroid properties and that may adversely affect ocular pressure. However, there are few data that would contraindicate the use of these agents in patients with open-angle glaucoma. Only if an anticholinergic drug paralyzes accommodation (noticeable as blurriness when the eyes are used for close work as in reading) should there be concern about it causing increased ocular pressure, in which situation the drug should be withdrawn; or if its use is mandatory, an ophthalmologist should be consulted. Systemic corticosteroids and, in particular, corticosteroids applied to the eye in the absence of intraocular inflammation may make the control of open-angle glaucoma more difficult. There is no evidence that vasodilator or adrenergic drugs affect the course of glaucoma.

Primary Angle-Closure Glaucoma

Although this form of glaucoma is far less common than open-angle glaucoma, it is important that the general physician be aware of it because an attack may be precipitated by the use of mydriatics; and if this occurs, urgent recognition and treatment are mandatory to prevent damage to the eye. Patients frequently have a positive family history and women are affected more than men.

The basic defect in primary angle-closure glaucoma is the inability of aqueous humor to reach the filtration apparatus. There is a blockage of the trabecular meshwork by the peripheral iris. When the pupil is mid-dilated, the iris is bowed forward, which blocks the outflow of aqueous humor (Fig. 98.2).

Individuals who have narrow anterior ocular chambers are predisposed to primary angle-closure glaucoma. Moreover, the lens may be of such size that there is encroachment of the aqueous-filtering trabecular meshwork. Individuals with these predispositions often have acute attacks of increased intraocular pressure when the eye is dilated, occluding aqueous outflow, as might occur in the dark or when a mydriatic is placed in the eye for funduscopic examination.

Diagnosis

Early diagnosis of this problem is critical because blindness may ensue and virtually every case is surgically curable if diagnosed early enough. Cure is increasingly less likely if repeated attacks have occurred and have resulted in scarring of the trabecular meshwork at the angle of the anterior chamber. The acute attack frequently is unilateral and often is precipitated by emotion (from associated pupillary dilation). The classical symptoms are episodes of ocular pain (usually located in the periocular or supraocular region), episodes of blurred vision, and seeing halos around lights at night. These symptoms occur because of corneal epithelial edema that has developed as a result of the increased intraocular pressure. Often patients find relief in well-lighted rooms or outdoors where daylight causes constriction of the pupil and opening of the angle of the anterior chamber.

Examination during an acute attack usually reveals marked elevation of intraocular pressure, to 60 to 90 mm Hg. However, chronic obstruction may compromise the circulation of the ciliary body and result in a fall in aqueous production and subsequently a reduction in ocular pressure. However, there is considerable individual tolerance of the vascular supply of the ciliary body to the increased pressure.

In patients predisposed to angle-closure glaucoma, the anterior chamber is shallow. This may be seen by illuminating the eye with a flashlight from the side and showing a shadow resulting from the bowed iris over the nasal portion of the eye (Fig. 98.2). Examination of the anterior chamber angle with a gonioscopic lens may reveal scarring of the trabecular meshwork—peripheral anterior synechia. Corneal edema will be present during an acute attack, and the anterior chamber may appear cloudy due to inflammation.

If the diagnosis of acute angle-closure glaucoma is suspected, immediate administration of acetazolamide (Diamox), 250 mg orally, and instillation of 2 drops of a miotic—such as pilocarpine (Pilocar), 4% every 15 minutes—are indicated, and the patient should be referred to an ophthalmologist immediately. In severe cases, the ingesting of hyperosmotic glycerol—1 ml/kg mixed as a 50% solution with chilled juice—almost always will interrupt an acute attack. Hyperosmotic agents such as glycerol or intravenous mannitol dehydrate the vitreous and lower eye pressure. Physicians who use mydriatics for funduscopic examination or patients who have narrow anterior ocular chambers and who do not have immediate access to an ophthalmologist should have an "angle-closure kit" consisting of pilocarpine (Pilocar, 4%), glycerol (glycerin—available as generic), and acetazolamide (Diamox) for use during an acute attack. Patients found to have a shallow anterior chamber even if they have not had a symptomatic attack of glaucoma should be referred to an ophthalmologist for evaluation, for education regarding specific manifestations of an acute attack, and for their initial treatment, usually prophylactic argon laser iridectomy.

Differential Diagnosis

The patient who has acute angle-closure glaucoma may come with an acute red eye to a general physician. Initially the physician will want to differentiate angle-closure glaucoma from acute iritis, acute conjunctivitis, and iridocyclitis. Chapter 99 discusses this differential diagnosis.

Course without Treatment

Severe attacks of angle-closure glaucoma may cause blindness in 2 to 3 days depending on the level of intraocular pressure and on the sensitivity of the ciliary body and optic nerve to ischemia. In some instances, ciliary ischemia stops aqueous production before blindness occurs; but repeated attacks are the rule, and these will eventually result in scarring of the trabecular meshwork. The frequency and rapidity of recurrences are unpredictable. An examination between attacks usually will reveal only a shallow anterior chamber (Fig. 98.2) and normal intraocular pressure. Peripheral anterior synechiae and segmental iris atrophy may be seen depending on the frequency and severity of previous attacks. A history of an acute attack, an actual acute attack, or the demonstration of a shallow anterior chamber should lead to prompt ophthalmological consultation.

Treatment

The treatment of primary angle-closure glaucoma is essentially surgical. If the diagnosis is made early enough in the course of the disease, a peripheral iridectomy can be done to prevent the attacks of increased intraocular pressure and the development of scarring. Argon or YAG laser peripheral iridectomy under topical anesthesia has little risk and results in cure in most cases. Surgical iridectomy may also be done by using a laser beam. The eye involved in an acute attack is operated upon as soon as the attack is controlled (see above). Generally, the other eye is operated upon prophylactically a week or so later. Follow-up care by the ophthalmologist after surgery is necessary. If pressure control has not been achieved, medical therapy (see above) may be necessary. This, however, is unusual if surgery is performed early.

When the physician is aware that a patient has a narrow anterior chamber or is under treatment for angle-closure glaucoma, there should be concern about the use of certain medications. Systemic anticholinergics or adrenegic drugs may rarely precipitate an acute attack by causing dilation of the pupils. Corticosteroids or vasodilating drugs are not contraindicated in patients with angle-closure glaucoma.

General References

Anderson DR: *Perimetry with and without automation*, 2nd ed. St. Louis, CV Mosby Co, 1987.
    Explains the details of visual field testing.
Editorial: Intraocular pressure control in glaucoma. *Lancet* 2:81, 1984.
    A brief overview of current therapy of elevated intraocular pressure with pertinent references.
Everitt DE, Avorn J: Systemic effects of medications used to treat glaucoma. *Ann Intern Med* 112:120, 1990.
    A brief review of the important systemic manifestations of topical and systemic drugs used to treat glaucoma.
Fraunfelder FT, Roy FN: *Current Ocular Therapy*, 2nd ed. Philadelphia, WB Saunders, 1985.
    This text provides a brief review of many common eye problems. It gives excellent therapeutic guidelines and has some pertinent references.
Havener WH: *Synopsis of Ophthalmology*, 6th ed. St Louis, CV Mosby, 1984.
Leske MC, Rosenthal J: Epidemiological aspects of open angle glaucoma. *Am J Epidemiol* 109:250, 1979.
Remis LL, Epstein DL: Treatment of glaucoma. *Annu Rev Med* 35:195, 1984.
Shields MB: *Textbook of Glaucoma*, 2nd ed. Baltimore, Williams & Wilkins, 1986.
U.S. Preventive Services Task Force: *Screening for Glaucoma.* Guide to Clinical Preventive Services, Baltimore, MD, Williams & Wilkins, Co., 1989, p. 124.

C H A P T E R   99

The Red Eye*

ANDREW P. SCHACHAT, M.D.

A patient who has developed a red eye is encountered frequently in an ambulatory practice. The problem is usually caused by an infection and most often is self-limited; however, there are serious considerations in the differential diagnosis that the general physician must recognize so that he can initiate urgent ophthalmological consultation if necessary. This chapter provides a framework for recognizing conditions that require consultation and provides a discussion of conditions that may be managed by the general physician. Figure 99.1 illustrates the important structures and landmarks of the external eye.

DIFFERENTIAL DIAGNOSIS (Table 99.1)

Conditions That Require Referral

The general physician can safely treat many conjunctival conditions that can cause a red eye. Keratitis (corneal inflammation), iritis or uveitis (inflammation of the uveal tract), and acute glaucoma are three im-

---

*Dr. Earl D.R. Kidwell, Jr., contributed to this chapter in the first and second editions of this book.

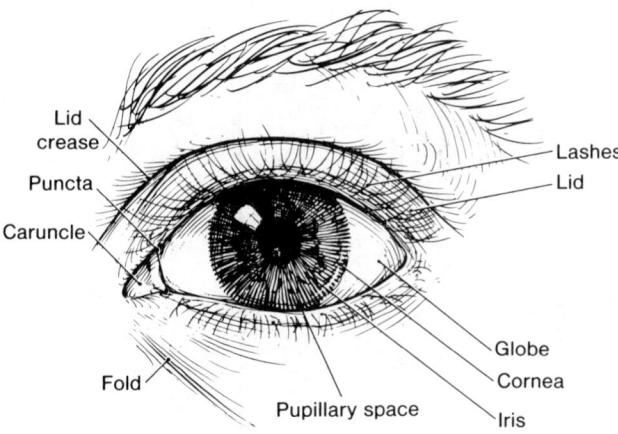

Figure 99.1. External landmarks of the eye.

Table 99.1.
Major Causes of a Red Eye

CONDITIONS THAT REQUIRE REFERRAL
  Acute Glaucoma
  Acute iritis
  Acute corneal tear or infection
  Acute scleritis and/or episcleritis
  Bacterial conjunctivitis—hyperacute

CONDITIONS THAT USUALLY CAN BE MANAGED BY THE
GENERAL PHYSICIAN
  Bacterial conjunctivitis—acute and chronic
  Viral conjunctivitis
  Inclusion conjunctivitis
  Allergic conjunctivitis
  Chemical conjunctivitis
  Foreign body
  Foreign body
  Subconjunctival hemorrhage

portant vision-threatening conditions that cause a red eye; and patients suspected of having one of these conditions should be referred to an ophthalmologist.

The conditions requiring urgent ophthalmological consultation can be recognized by the general physician who pays attention to several important features of the history and physical examination. Table 99.2 shows how this information may suggest a specific diagnosis. The patient should be asked specifically whether he has been treated for an ocular disorder or whether he has recently experienced pain in one or both of his eyes. He should be asked if there is visual loss or photophobia (light sensitivity). When the eyes are examined, it is essential to evaluate the following features: visual acuity, the nature of the discharge, the appearance of the cornea, the size and reactivity of the pupil, and the extent of the redness. When evaluating the extent of redness, an attempt should be made to determine whether there is simply conjunctival injection or ciliary injection. The ciliary vessels run in the sclera beneath the conjunctiva. Ciliary injection usually causes a purplish or violaceous zone of injection around the cornea. Unlike the conjunctival vessels, ciliary vessels do not constrict after the administration of a weak solution (e.g., 2.5 % solution)

of phenylephrine. The conjunctival vessels will move with the conjunctiva when the conjunctiva is touched with a cotton swab. Ciliary vessels do not. Glaucoma, keratitis, and scleritis will be characterized in most cases by ciliary injection. In selected patients special tests, such as measurement of ocular tension or inspection of the eye after fluorescein staining, are necessary.

Specific Conditions

Acute glaucoma is discussed in Chapter 98.

Iritis may be due to a specific problem such as trauma or infection, but often a specific etiology cannot be identified. In this condition failure to initiate proper treatment that usually includes a dilating agent and corticosteroids may result in permanent scarring that will affect pupillary movement and in some cases may lead to secondary glaucoma.

Iritis can usually be recognized by the general physician because it is a painful condition that characteristically is acute in onset and is associated with photophobia. Often vision is blurred as well. Occasionally, the pupil of the involved eye is small and fixed compared with the contralateral one. Typically the redness in iritis surrounds the cornea. Patients suspected of having iritis should see an ophthalmologist urgently so that the diagnosis can be confirmed, the cause found, and treatment initiated.

Corneal injury is usually recognized easily because of intense pain localized to the cornea after an injury and because of identification of a corneal lesion. If the injury is secondary to minor trauma (corneal abrasion) from a foreign body, the eye may be irrigated with a sterile eyewash (such as Collyrium) and a patch placed over it for 24 hours (see below, "Foreign Body"). If, on the other hand, an extensive epithelial defect (as revealed by fluorescein staining) is present, urgent ophthalmological referral is indicated.

Fluorescein staining is easily accomplished by moistening a sterile fluorescein strip in the lower conjunctival sac and waiting a moment for the fluorescein to diffuse into the tears. The eye is then gently irrigated with physiological saline or eyewash, and the epithelial defect will remain stained a brilliant green. A penlight with a cobalt blue filter (e.g., Blu-Spot No. 2015, available from medical supply companies) is inexpensive and will highlight fluorescein staining. A corneal ulcer will also stain with fluorescein, but staining will appear to be deeper, indicating subepithelial corneal involvement. Corneal ulceration can lead to blindness and patients with this condition should see an ophthalmologist urgently.

Scleritis usually is seen in association with a systemic disorder (such as rheumatoid arthritis). The deep vessels of the sclera are dilated; this may be demonstrated by the instillation of a drop of Neo-Synephrine 5 or 10%, which will constrict the superficial but not the deep vessels. This mydriatic should be avoided in patients with a history of narrow-angle glaucoma (Chapter 98). The patient usually complains of dis-

Table 99.2.
Important Observations in Evaluation of a Patient with a Red Eye

	Glaucoma	Iritis	Corneal Injury	Scleritis	Episcleritis	Bacterial Conjunctivitis	Inclusion Conjunctivitis	Viral Conjunctivitis
History of previous ocular disorder or condition predisposing to an ocular disorder	+/−	+/−	−	+	−	−	−	−
Pain	+	+ Photophobia	+	+	+	Mild discomfort or burning	Mild discomfort or burning	Mild discomfort or burning
Visual acuity	Dimished and blurred	Blurred	Usually diminished	Normal	Normal	Normal	Occasionally blurred, if chronic	Normal
Discharge	None	None	Usually some	None	None	Present: thick or thin	None or mucopurulent	Watery
Appearance of cornea	May be hazy	Normal	May be streaky	Normal	Normal	Normal	Normal except if late when superior dots or streaking may be seen	Normal
Pupil	Often dilated, mid-dilated, or fixed	Small and different from opposite side	Normal	Normal	Normal	Normal	Normal	Normal
Redness	Around cornea	Around cornea	Localized or diffuse	Localized or diffuse	Localized	Diffuse	Diffuse (variable)	Segmental or diffuse
Selected evaluations	Ocular pressure in eye is high (see Chapter 98)*	Normal	Fluorescein stain[b] shows epithelial defect as brilliant green	A drop of Neo-Synephrine 5 or 10% in conjunctiva will constrict superficial but not deep vessels (see the text)	None	None	None	None

[a] Should not be mesured if a discharge is present or if a corneal ulceration is seen.
[b] Use individually packaged sterile fluorescein strips.

comfort in the eye, and sometimes of severe pain, which is intensified if the eye is moved. Scleritis is often associated with iritis (see above). The treatment of scleritis is usually complicated and an ophthalmologist should be consulted urgently when scleritis is suspected.

Episcleritis is a relatively common problem characterized by pain caused by a sharply localized area of inflammation of the superficial layer of the sclera. The etiology is unknown, but it is occasionally associated with a systemic disorder such as rheumatoid arthritis or a specific infection such as herpes zoster or, rarely, tuberculosis. A few patients will have an associated iritis (see above) that is usually mild. The palpebral conjunctiva (i.e., that lining the eyelid) is not involved and there is no discharge; these two observations help to differentiate this problem from conjunctivitis. Episcleritis is short lived but is frequently recurrent; for this reason, ophthalmological consultation is indicated.

Hyperacute bacterial conjunctivitis (see below) is also a condition that should prompt urgent referral to an ophthalmologist.

Conditions That Usually Can Be Managed by the General Physician

The general physician can manage a number of ophthalmic conditions that present with a red eye. Before making the decision to treat, the physician should ask:

1. Has a thorough ocular examination been performed?
2. Is there impaired vision and, if so, has an explanation for impaired visual acuity been identified?
3. Is the natural history of the condition known or, if treatment is planned, is the usual response to treatment known?
4. Has the appropriate follow-up arrangement been made to confirm that the condition is self-limited, improving, and that referral to an ophthalmologist is not required?

Conjunctival infections, allergies, eyelid inflammation, and irritation are the commonest causes of red or irritated eyes and are discussed in detail below. Almost always a general physician can manage these problems without consulting with an ophthalmologist.

CONJUNCTIVITIS

General Considerations

The diagnosis and management of conjunctivitis can be confusing, considering the variety of ocular infections. Most cases are not absolute emergencies, and, frequently, they are self-limited. Conjunctivitis may, however, lead to serious complications such as corneal scarring, lid damage, or, in cases in which the patient has had antecedent intraocular surgery, endophthalmitis.

Conjunctival Flora

Under normal conditions the conjunctival sac has a bacterial flora composed of several species. The most commonly encountered organism is *Staphylococcus albus*, followed by corynebacteria, *Staphylococcus aureus*, and *Streptococcus* species. Some normal patients harbor *Pseudomonas* species as well as fungi. This complex flora complicates the establishment of a specific etiology in a patient with infectious conjunctivitis.

Presentation

Conjunctivitis is usually not painful, but often there is mild discomfort, burning, discharge, tearing, itching, and lid swelling. Vision is well preserved. Most often, infectious conjunctivitis is bilateral.

Laboratory Diagnosis

Whenever there is doubt about the diagnosis, a simple culture and/or staining of the conjunctival material will help in determining the cause and subsequent management of the condition. Most often, however, an adequate diagnosis can be made from the appearance of the conjunctiva, and a culture is not necessary. New immunological tests are available and permit immediate diagnosis of some causes of infectious conjunctivitis, especially chlamydia. The availability of these tests varies from community to community and over time. Therefore the general physician not familiar with their use should telephone an ophthalmologist for a recommendation.

Culture

Specimens for culture should be obtained with a sterile cotton swab by everting the eyelid and wiping the conjunctival sac. This material should be obtained without topical anesthesia because the preservatives in the anesthetic solution might inhibit the growth of organisms. The specimen must be transferred immediately into transport media or delivered immediately to the laboratory for culturing. Whenever a culture is considered necessary, both eyes should be cultured separately, even if there is only monocular involvement, so that the apparently uninfected eye will provide information about the nature of the normal flora.

Scraping

After culture, a topical anesthetic (such as Ophthaine) should be instilled, and scrapings of the conjunctiva, well away from the cornea, should be obtained. A sterile platinum spatula (available from medical supply stores) or the dull side of a sterile scalpel blade can be used to scrape the conjunctiva. The material obtained by this method is smeared on a glass slide and is stained with Gram stain and/or Giemsa stain.

The appearance of the cells found in these scrapings is helpful in determining the diagnosis and, therefore, scraping is recommended in the evaluation of patients with conjunctivitis when the diagnosis is uncertain. The differential findings are discussed below and listed in Table 99.3.

Specific Types

Hyperacute Bacterial Conjunctivitis

The name of this condition reflects its onset and the very thick exudate associated with it (Fig. 99.2). Typically, the discharge is so copious that it accumulates in the lashes or runs down the patient's cheek. One eye is usually involved before the other, but within several days the second eye becomes involved through autoinoculation. The infection quickly involves the surrounding structures and is associated with aching discomfort, swelling of the lid, and tenderness of the eye. Enlarged preauricular lymph nodes are often present. Early in the infection the cornea is not involved, but as the conjunctival swelling and reaction increase, a peripheral corneal ring ulcer may develop due to the compression of the peripheral corneal circulation.

Neisseria gonorrhoeae or *Neisseria meningitidis* is usually implicated in this infection. Inoculation is a result of fomite spread or through autoinoculation from infected genitalia. The gonococcus has the ability to penetrate the intact corneal epithelium so that central corneal ulceration and endophthalmitis also may occur. Meningococcal conjunctivitis is indistinguishable from gonococcal conjunctivitis, although the former occurs more frequently in younger individuals, may be bilateral at the onset, and can proceed to metastatic meningitis or meningococcemia.

Conjunctival scrapings reveal an overwhelming number of polymorphonuclear leukocytes and intracellular Gram-negative diplococci. Culture should be obtained on Thayer-Martin selective medium or be sent to the laboratory on Transgrow medium. The differentiation between gonococcus and meningococcus requires special bacteriological studies.

Therapy of hyperacute conjunctivitis must be prompt to avoid corneal damage or systemic spread and should include the administration of both systemic and topical antibiotics. Because of the seriousness of this condition an ophthalmologist should be consulted immediately. Institution of appropriate antibiotics

should result in the disappearance of the discharge within 24 to 48 hours, although lid swelling and conjunctival reaction do not abate for several days. If a corneal ulcer occurs, it is slow to heal; and if the cornea has been scarred, visual acuity may be affected. In rare cases endophthalmitis may occur and blindness is possible.

Acute Bacterial Conjunctivitis

This condition, like hyperacute bacterial conjunctivitis, has an abrupt onset but is characterized by a less thick, often mucopurulent, discharge. This form of conjunctivitis is often called catarrhal or pink eye (Fig. 99.3); it is seen at all ages and at any time of year. The most common cause of the condition is S. aureus infection. *Pneumococcus* and *Haemophilus* species also cause the problem, but infections with these organisms have a more restricted geographic distribution than do staphylococcal infections; pneumococcal infections occur primarily in the northern states during the colder months, and *Haemophilus* infections occur more commonly in the warmer regions of the United States throughout the year. Also, pneumococcal or *Haemophilus* conjunctivitis is more common in younger individuals than is staphylococcal conjunctivitis. Rarely, other bacteria, such as *Moraxella lacunata, Escherichia coli,* or *Proteus* species, cause this form of conjunctivitis.

Patients complain of eye irritation and watering, and typically the eyelids stick together after sleep. The infection starts unilaterally; but very often, because of autoinoculation, the contralateral eye becomes involved in 1 or 2 days. Examination reveals hyperemia of the palpebral conjunctiva (i.e., the eyelid); bulbar conjunctival petechiae, characteristic of *Haemophilus* infection, may be seen.

Acute bacterial conjunctivitis is usually self-limited and generally lasts 7 to 14 days, although *Haemophilus* infections may last somewhat longer.

The diagnosis is suspected by the examination; however, wherever there is doubt, diagnosis should be confirmed by examination of the scrapings of the conjunctiva and by culturing the exudate.

Topical treatment usually results in the resolution of symptoms in a day or 2. A number of topical antibiotics are available and one should be used for 5 to 6 days. Sodium sulfacetamide (Sulamyd-10%)—either the solution, 2 drops in the eye every 3 hours while awake, or the ointment, a small amount applied to the lower conjunctival sac four times a day and at bedtime—is generally satisfactory. If there is an allergy to sulfa drugs, a 1% chloramphenicol ointment (Chloromycetin ophthalmic ointment), four times a day and at bedtime, may be used. Also cool compresses several times a day may provide comfort and diminish matting.

Chronic Bacterial Conjunctivitis

S. aureus causes most cases of chronic bacterial conjunctivitis; but occasionally it is caused by other agents,

Table 99.3.
Diagnosis Based on Cells in Material Scraped from Conjunctiva

Cells	Significance
Polymorphonuclear leukocytes	Bacterial fungus, *Chlamydia* (inclusion conjunctivitis), trachoma, Stevens-Johnson syndrome
Mononuclear cells	Viral
Eosinophils	Allergy, ocular pemphigoid
Epithelial metaplasia (atypical, large cells)	*Chlamydia*, herpes simplex

(Fig. 99.7). Gram stain will not reveal these bodies but will show many polymorphonuclear leukocytes.

Therapy is effective but must be systemic. Oral tetracycline, 250 mg four times daily for 21 days, is the preferable regimen; but when tetracycline cannot be given, good results will be achieved with erythromycin, 250 mg four times a day for 21 days, or sulfamethoxazole-trimethoprim (e.g., Bactrim DS or Septra DS), 1 tablet twice a day for 21 days. It may take several months for the follicular hyperplasia to resolve, but the patient should experience symptomatic improvement within several days. The application of cool compresses for 20 minutes several times a day will also provide comfort in the first few days of treatment. Because this disease is difficult to diagnose, referral to an ophthalmologist is appropriate if there is any doubt.

Because the disease must be assumed to be sexually transmitted, the sexual partner should be similarly treated; other venereal diseases should be looked for, and the man should use a condom until therapy has been completed.

Allergic Conjunctivitis

This is a common and mild conjunctivitis frequently encountered in patients with allergic rhinitis (see Chapter 23). Often the patient describes a history of allergy to grasses and pollens as well as to other agents and usually complains of itching and tearing. Frequently, there is marked swelling of the conjunctiva (Fig. 99.8) and slight to moderate redness of the eye, and at times there is serous crusting in the morning.

Whenever there is doubt about the diagnosis, conjunctival scrapings may be examined. A finding of many eosinophils is diagnostic. When conjunctivitis is associated with allergic rhinitis, it usually parallels the rhinitis in severity and duration. When it occurs as an isolated problem, it is short lived and treatment is symptomatic. An over-the-counter topical astringent solution (such as Albalon, Naphcon-A, or Vasocon-A using 1 to 2 drops four times per day for a day or 2) and cool compresses as needed are very effective. Occasionally, symptoms are severe, and oral antihistamines may relieve itching.

Corticosteroid eyedrops (such as HMS Liquifilm or FMI Liquifilm) are very effective for this condition, but they must be used cautiously because their use is associated with corneal ulceration and perforation in the presence of herpes simplex infection, the development of fungal infection, and when used chronically, with the development in some individuals of open-angle glaucoma and, rarely, cataract formation. For these reasons, topical corticosteroids are not recommended without at least a telephone consultation with an ophthalmologist.

Chemical Conjunctivitis

Many agents may enter the conjunctiva and produce inflammation. Irritation from such agents as smoke, smog, sprays, chlorinated water, hair spray, makeup, or industrial dust occurs frequently. It is the history of the exposure that makes the diagnosis obvious. The patient should thoroughly rinse the conjunctival sac with water as soon as contamination with a chemical has occurred. The patient will also benefit from cool compresses for 15 to 20 minutes several times a day, and occasionally the use of an over-the-counter topical astringent solution (Albalon, Naphcon-A, or Vasocon-A) will be necessary.

In the case of an injury from an acid or alkali, serious permanent damage may occur and this problem is a true ophthalmological emergency. Patients should be advised to irrigate the conjunctival sac with copious amounts of water and to see an ophthalmologist immediately.

Foreign Body

Foreign bodies frequently lodge in the conjunctiva or cornea. Most often they can be visualized with the naked eye; but, if not, sterile fluorescein staining (see above) will outline the area of corneal epithelial damage. Foreign bodies may be removed by irrigation of the conjunctival sac with a sterile solution of physiological saline or eyewash. If they are not rinsed away, mechanical removal is indicated. This may be accomplished, when the object is in the cornea, by placing in the eye a drop of topical anesthetic (such as Ophthaine) and removing the foreign body with a sterile needle held carefully with the physician's arm braced. A cotton swab should not be used to remove a foreign body from the cornea since frequently it is very irritating to the structure and thus delays healing. If the foreign body is not on the cornea, removal is easier and usually does not require anesthesia. After removal, it is wise to instill a drop of antibiotic (such as Sulamyd or Bacitracin) and cover the eye with a patch for 24 hours. The eyepatch should be applied tightly enough to prevent the eyelids from moving. If the patch falls off before the 24-hour period is up, the patient should not try to reapply it, as often this may cause more irritation.

If the offending material is a piece of metal, rust rings surrounding the area of the epithelial defect may be observed. These rings are not harmful per se and only the foreign body should be removed.

In any instance when the foreign body is not easily removed, or if symptoms persist beyond a day after removal of a foreign body, an ophthalmologist should see the patient urgently.

Subconjunctival Hemorrhage

Subconjunctival hemorrhage is a common condition that very often is alarming to the patient. A small blood vessel ruptures in the conjunctival tissue after the patient coughs or strains and a painless wedge-shaped hemorrhage develops. Often the patient will have no memory of the coughing or straining, but incidentally notices the red eye. Occasionally, viral conjunctivitis may be manifest only by the appearance of a subconjunctival hemorrhage. Isolated subconjunctival hemorrhage requires no treatment and should resolve within several days. If the problem becomes recurrent and/or multiple, an abnormality of hemostasis should be considered.

EYELID CONDITIONS

Several conditions that affect the eyelid are commonly seen in ambulatory practice, and these may mimic a red eye. These conditions are usually readily diagnosed by their appearance and may be treated easily without an ophthalmological consultation.

Hordeolum

A hordeolum is a very common infection in the glands of the eyelid caused by *S.aureus*. It is characterized by the sudden onset of localized pain, swelling, redness, and often purulent discharge. The infected gland may be a meibomian gland just under the conjunctival side of the eyelid: an *internal hordeolum*. This infection may be quite large and may point to either the skin or conjunctival side of the lid. Also, a smaller gland associated with an eyelash follicle under the skin side of the lid may be infected: an *external hordeolum or sty*. A sty usually is smaller than an internal hordeolum and always points to the skin side of the lid.

Both types of hordeolum may be treated without obtaining a culture. Treatment is tripartite: hot compresses should be applied for 15 to 20 minutes several times a day and will provide comfort and establish drainage of the infected gland; the lid should be scrubbed with a neutral soap (e.g., Ivory) each morning; and every 3 to 4 hours for a few days a topical antimicrobial, such as a sulfonamide (e.g., Sulamyd-10%) or gentamicin (Garamycin), should be applied to prevent the development of an associated cellulitis or metastatic eye infection. If the hordeolum has not begun to respond to treatment in a day or 2, it may need to be incised; referral to an ophthalmologist is usually indicated.

Blepharitis

Marginal blepharitis is a very common chronic bilateral inflammation of the lid margins usually associated with seborrhea or a contact dermatitis, e.g., from mascara. Marginal blepharitis is discussed in Chapter 100, Common Problems of the Skin. Blepharitis also may be associated with chronic bacterial infection (see above, "Chronic Bacterial Conjunctivitis").

Chalazion

A chalazion is a lipogranulomatous inflammation of a meibomian gland secondary to chronic inflammation and it may follow a hordeolum. It presents as a swelling similar to an internal hordeolum (see above) except that it is chronic and usually does not manifest acute inflammation. The swelling may appear anywhere on the eyelid (although the upper lid is a more common location) and it usually points toward the conjunctival side. Usually a chalazion will not spontaneously resolve, and if the patient is symptomatic, referral to an ophthalmologist for excision is indicated.

General References

Fraunfelder FT: *Drug Induced Ocular Side Effects and Drug Interactions*, 3rd ed. Philadelphia, Lea & Febiger, 1988.
> A useful text that provides a resource for possible drug-induced eye problems, including conjunctivitis, iritis, cataracts, and many other problems.

Havener WH: *Synopsis of Ophthalmology*, 6th ed. St Louis, CV Mosby, 1984.
> A very well written short textbook that provides an overview of many eye problems, including the differential diagnosis of the red eye and of the different forms of conjunctivitis.

Schachat AP, Cruess AF: *Ophthalmology*. Baltimore, Williams & Wilkins, 1984.
> This short paperback text provides a useful overview and general approach to many common problems, including the red eye.

SECTION

15

Miscellaneous Problems

Most patients with a primary dermatological complaint consult a general physician or an internist rather than a dermatologist, according to a survey conducted by the American Academy of Dermatology (17).

This chapter provides assistance in diagnosing and managing common dermatological problems that are likely to be encountered in the general practice of internal medicine. In addition a thorough generic discussion of topical and intralesional therapy is provided.

ACANTHOSIS NIGRICANS

Acanthosis nigricans is a dermatological problem occasionally encountered in office practice. It gets its name from its velvety texture and brown to black color. Friction areas—axilla, neck, and groin—are the sites involved. Although most patients with the condition have the "benign" form associated with obesity or even an endocrinopathy such as diabetes mellitus, pituitary or adrenal adenomas, chronic hepatitis, or drugs, such as systemic corticosteroids, some patients have an underlying malignancy. This form, *malignant acanthosis nigraicans*, should be considered if the patient is thin, over 40 years old, and the eruption is recent in origin. The most commonly associated tumor is an abdominal adenocarcinoma, usually of the stomach. Therapy should be aimed at discovering the cause; local therapy is of little benefit.

ACNE

Definition

Acne vulgaris is a chronic disorder of the sebaceous glands, particularly those on the face, chest, and back, where the glands are the largest and most dense. Sebum from these glands reaches the surface by emptying into the hair follicle and flowing along the hair shaft, the two skin appendages forming the pilosebaceous unit. The earliest lesion of acne is the *comedone*, a plug formed by impaction of the opening of the pilosebaceous duct by horny material and dried sebum. The plugs are visible as closed comedones ("whiteheads") and, if the surface is darkened, open comedones ("blackheads"), black not due to dirt but to oxidation of melanin and sebum in the plugs. Comedones become inflamed as nonpathogenic bacteria, normal residents within the duct and gland, especially *Staphylococcus epidermidis* and an anaerobic diphtheroid, *Corynebacterium acnes*, proliferate within the obstructed glands and produce erythematous tender papules. As inflammation progresses, these papules may become pustular and, in severe cases, cystic. Cysts are presumed to be due to abscess formation deep in the dermis. Various manifestations of the disorder usually are present in the same patient.

Epidemiology

Acne occurs primarily in adolescents; there is an equal incidence in males and females, although the eruption often is worse in males. Almost all teenagers have acne to some degree, but only a minority require treatment. In most, the lesions resolve by age 20. Sometimes acne persists into adulthood or develops for the first time in adults, especially women, who use cosmetics (so-called acne cosmetica).

Acne can be produced or exacerbated by drugs, including corticosteroids, androgenic steroids, pheny-

toin, iodides, and lithium, and by external irritants, such as creosote, tar, and industrial cutting oils (chloracne). Pomade acne is acne near the hair line, especially common in blacks, caused by the use of hair pomades.

Pathogenesis

The underlying cause of acne is unclear, but several events contribute to its development. These include proliferation of sebaceous glands and increased production of sebum by sebaceous glands under the stimulation of androgens as puberty occurs and obstruction of the sebaceous glands with debris from the proliferation of bacteria, followed by inflammation. The precise reasons why some individuals develop severe disease whereas most have mild disease is not known, although severe acne often is hereditary.

Evaluation

The following information should be recorded before planning therapy:

1. *Topical medications* used, past and present, including prescription and nonprescription preparations. Many patients will have initiated therapy themselves, and the preparations they have used may be irritating. Response or failure to previously used antibiotics is particularly important information.
2. *Face care*, including soap used, scrubbing technique, use of skin machine, and cosmetics (brand and type). Information about the use of foundations, cold creams, and astringents also is important. These preparations or techniques may be irritating or actually acnegenic.
3. *Factors that improve or worsen the acne*, including menses, diet, and stress, should be explored. Diet is not an important factor, although patients who believe that certain foods lead to flare-ups may avoid those foods.
4. *Other medical conditions and current medications*, including oral contraceptive agents, corticosteroids, etc. (see above).

A chart should be entered into the patient's record for use in selecting and following therapy (Table 100.1). These data allow one to evaluate progress objectively.

Therapy

No single treatment is effective for all patients with acne. The overall goal is to reverse and prevent plugging of the sebaceous ducts as well as to reduce and prevent inflammation of the sebaceous glands and surrounding tissue (15). General instructions include STOP hard scrubbing, including the use of skin machines; STOP use of antibacterial soaps because nonpathogenic bacteria are reduced and replaced by pathogens; instead, substitute a plain soap such as Ivory, Camay, Purpose, or Basis; STOP use of oil-based cosmetics

Table 100.1.
Data to Be Recorded in Evaluation and Follow-up of Patients with Acne

	Face	Back	Chest
Comedones	( )	( )	( )
Papules	( )	( )	( )
Pustules	( )	( )	( )
Cysts	( )	( )	( )

```
0  = none
1+ = few
2+ = moderate
3+ = many
4+ = extensive
```

(ingredients of cosmetics are listed on the labels) as they obstruct the sebaceous duct. Water-based and oil-free makeup may be safe for some, but it is best to avoid all foundations. Blusher and eye shadow do not seem to aggravate acne. Improvement after exposure to large doses of summer sun does occur, probably from ultraviolet light entering the skin and damaging the sebaceous glands or ducts, but the improvement is temporary and the actinic damage is long term. There is no justification for artificial ultraviolet exposure in acne. Patients should be told that a delay of 4 to 8 weeks before obvious improvement is common with any treatment of acne. If there is no improvement after 2 to 3 months or if lesions are cystic or deep and inflammatory with scarring, referral to a dermatologist is appropriate.

Comedones

If only comedones are present, a desquamating agent such as 5% benzoyl peroxide lotion, gel, or cream (such as Desquam-X 5 Gel, Oxy-5 lotion, Persadox lotion or cream, Xerac BP5 gel) should be prescribed. Initially the agent should be applied only at bedtime as it may cause intense inflammation if used excessively. After a few weeks, if treatment is tolerated, the end point being slight erythema and dryness, the frequency of use may be increased to twice a day and then the concentration increased to 10% (such as Desquam-X 10 Gel, Oxy-10 lotion, Persadox HP cream or lotion, or Xerac BP10 gel). Some of these agents are available without prescription, such as Oxy-5, Oxy-10, Persadox, and Persadox HP.

Patients who do not respond to benzoyl peroxide within 4 to 8 weeks should be given topical vitamin A acid. The 0.01% gel (Retin-A gel, requires a prescription) seems to be least irritating and easiest to use. This agent appears to interfere with keratinization of the follicular duct, thereby decreasing the comedone plug. Because vitamin A acid is quite irritating, it too should be started at a low concentration at bedtime, applied to the entire face, increasing the dose to 0.025% gel gradually over 2 to 3 months. The patient need not experience discomfort and peeling for the drug to be effective. The drug should be avoided in blacks as it may darken their skin. Experiments in mice have shown an increased incidence of skin cancer when vitamin A acid was used with high doses of

ultraviolet light. Therefore, patients should be told to stop using the medication if they intend to be in the sun extensively.

Inflammatory Lesions (Papules or Pustules)

If inflammatory lesions are present, the initial therapy differs depending on the sex of the patient (5, 20).

Females. (a) Topical clindamycin (Cleocin-T) should be applied to the entire face morning and afternoon after washing with plain soap (such as Ivory, Camay, Purpose, or Basis). This should be continued for 2 months before alternative topical antibiotics, such as topical erythromycin (ATS), EryDerm, or Staticin, or a systemic antibiotic is prescribed. Oral tetracycline (see below) generally should be avoided in women because of the common complication of vaginitis. However, if the lesions are pustular or cystic, systemic antibiotics will be necessary, at least initially. The dose schedule given for males (see below) may be followed. Tetracycline must not be used after the second month of pregnancy because it may damage the bones and teeth of the fetus. (b) In addition to the antibiotic, a topical desquamating agent will be needed. Benzoyl peroxide or vitamin A acid should be used as for comedone acne (see above).

Males. (a) An oral tetracycline, 250 mg three times daily, should be prescribed. However, if the acne is severe, up to 2 g/day may be used. The medication should be taken 1 to 2 hours before or after meals to maximize absorption. The starting dose should be continued for 6 weeks or until there is clear improvement, then slowly decreased by one capsule daily each month. At the point that the acne recurs or flares up, the dose should be increased to the level that had maintained clearing and left at that level for several months. The lowest dose that is effective should be used. The usual maintenance level of tetracycline is 250 mg twice a day. Alternative antibiotics useful for acne include minocycline, 50 to 100 mg once a day (available in 50- and 100-mg dose), and erythromycin, 250 mg twice a day. (b) In addition to the antibiotics, a topical desquamating agent will be needed. Benzoyl peroxide or vitamin A acid should be used as for comedone acne (see above).

Both men and women should wash their hair frequently and should not apply oil to the scalp.

Cystic Acne

A new therapy, 13-cis-retinoic acid (isotretinoin, Accutane, 10, 20 and 40 mg, orally by prescription) cures or greatly improves nearly all cases of cystic acne (20). However, side effects are universal and include cheilitis, dry skin, and conjunctivitis, and, less commonly, musculoskeletal tenderness, hair thinning, and headache. It also is teratogenic, and women must use stringent birth control measures, have a negative pregnancy test, and be informed of the danger before starting the drug. Informed consent is required for its administration in women. Some patients develop elevated triglyceride levels but the significance of this is unknown. Nevertheless, it is suggested that a baseline triglyceride level be obtained before starting the drug and then repeated in 30 days (most who will develop elevated triglyceride levels from this drug will have done so in this time). Should the level become elevated, dietary counseling usually results in improvement (see also Chapter 75). The usual dosage is 1 to 2 mg/kg divided in two daily doses for 2 to 4 months. The medication is expensive, costing about $150/month, and has not been approved for use in milder forms of acne. Patients with cystic acne generally should be followed by a dermatologist.

Prognosis

Acne in the adolescent may require treatment until age 20 or so. Good results from the treatment outlined above can be anticipated in 80%. About 15% will require alternative therapies, such as high doses of alternative antibiotics or such specialized techniques as cryotherapy, intradermal corticosteroid injections, or acne surgery performed by a dermatologist. The remaining 5% will not respond well to any therapy. Dermabrasion, the superficial abrasion of the skin to reduce scars, may be useful for some patients, although most scars flatten and become less noticeable with time. Persistent acne in middle-aged women usually is due to excessive use of occlusive cosmetics and moisturizers. Clearing will not occur until use of such cosmetics is stopped.

ATOPIC DERMATITIS (ATOPIC ECZEMA)

Atopic dermatitis is a chronic, pruritic inflammation of the skin that has a characteristic course and pattern and that is usually associated with a personal and family history of allergy (11).

Etiology

Although still debated, the cause appears to be immunological with both cellular and humoral mechanisms playing a role (see Chapter 23). Patients with severe atopy often have an elevated serum IgE level and about 30% have a personal history of allergic rhinitis or asthma. In addition, 60% have a family history of atopy with cutaneous and/or respiratory symptoms. However, more than the immune system may be involved as signs of decreased production of eccrine sweat and increased vasoconstriction of small blood vessels are often evident also.

Presentation

Onset may be as early as the second month after birth but almost always before age 10 years. The major distress is due to the chronic and pruritic nature of the condition. Sleep is difficult; the discomfort may make the individual appear nervous and demanding. Other manifestations of atopy, or hypersensitivity, also may develop, including hay fever, rhinitis, or asthma. Early cataracts are a complication in a small percent-

age of severe cases, but general health is otherwise unaffected. A parent with atopic dermatitis may need to be told that the disorder is inherited and that about half of his or her children are likely to be affected to some degree.

Although the entire skin seems "dry" with fine flaky scaling, dermatitis, with eczematous lichenified plaque, tends to involve certain regions, and the distribution depends on age. During infancy, the disorder involves the extensor and exposed parts, and only later does it take on the adult distribution in flexural folds including the antecubital and popliteal, the wrists, and the sides of the neck (Fig. 100.1). Itching is generalized but worse in the lichenified plaques, which sometimes become superinfected. Many patients will have an extra crease below the margin of the lower eyelids (Dennie or Morgan fold).

Itching may be triggered by low humidity, high temperature, sweating, environmental allergens such as irritating or occlusive medications, wool clothing, greases, and detergents. Dietary factors may be important, and control sometimes can be partially achieved through manipulation of the diet (see below). Many cases improve during infancy and about half of the cases have cleared by puberty. Some will remain clear but in many the dermatitis will recur. Many atopic patients have exacerbations throughout life, often when under physical or emotional stress. In most cases itching improves during the summer although skin infections may be more common then.

A rare complication, but a serious one, is infection with herpes simplex, particularly at the site of active dermatitis. This is called *eczema herpeticum*. It is a fulminant illness with diffuse vesicles and fever. The

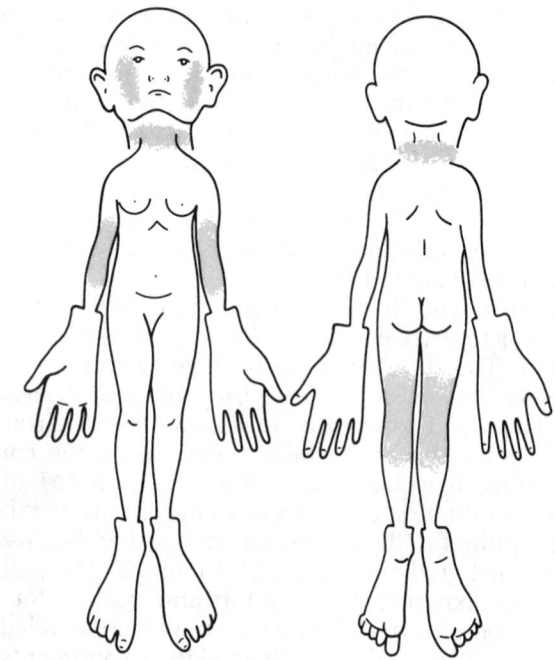

Figure 100.1.   Lichenified pruritic areas in flexural regions and on the face are typical locations for adult atopic dermatitis.

complication is life threatening. Hospitalization usually is required.

Differential Diagnosis

Seborrheic dermatitis, psoriasis, and contact dermatitis may be confused with atopic dermatitis (see below).

Therapy

Bathing and Lubrication

The patient should reduce the frequency of hot water bathing and the use of soap; both remove lipids and topical medications and increase water loss from the skin and result in itching. In general the patient should not bathe more than twice a week. The house should be humidified (see Chapter 23) during the winter. For additional details see "Bathing Instructions for Dry or Irritated Skin" (page 1376).

Topical Corticosteroids

Corticosteroids are the mainstay of topical therapy and will control most cases. The cream should be used when the eruption is subacute with oozing; however, the ointment is better absorbed than the cream and is less drying in chronic dermatitis. For the details of preparations, techniques of use, and complications, see "Corticosteroids," page 1377.

Because potent topical corticosteroids can induce vascular dilatation, which may become permanent, nothing stronger than 1% hydrocortisone cream should be used on the face.

Systemic

Recent studies have confirmed that some children are helped by elimination of certain foods from the diet, most commonly citrus fruits, wheat, eggs, and nuts. Two-week trials with elimination of different food groups may be worth attempting if the patient is sufficiently cooperative. Systemic antibiotics should be prescribed at the first sign of pyoderma—oozing, crusting, and odor. Erythromycin, 250 mg four times daily for 10 days for an adult, usually is sufficient. Dicloxacillin, 500 mg twice daily, may be used as an alternative. Cultures generally are not needed unless abscesses develop.

There is still a debate about whether antihistamines help beyond the side effect of sedation that normally accompanies their use. A trial for a week with 50 mg three times a day of diphenhydramine (Benadryl), 10 mg three times a day of hydroxyzine (Atarax, Cartrax, Vistrax), or an equivalent dose of other antihistamines (see Chapter 23) may be appropriate if the patient has marked pruritus and is restless. The use of sedating antihistamines is usually preferred to those that are less sedating in this distressing condition. The dose may be increased at bedtime to help with sleep.

Therapy for Resistant Cases. Systemic corticosteroids occasionally are necessary for severe flare-ups of atopic dermatitis. A suggested starting schedule in an adult is 40 mg of prednisone in a single daily morning dose, reduced by 5 to 10 mg a day as soon as improvement is seen and tapered off completely within 2 to 3 weeks. Patients may obtain so much relief from the systemic corticosteroids that the physician may not be able to persuade them to stop the drug; however, since atopic dermatitis may be lifelong, eventual difficulties from continuous systemic corticosteroids are bound to ensue.

CONTACT DERMATITIS

Definition

Contact dermatitis is a cutaneous reaction to an external substance and may be either an irritant or an allergic reaction. An irritant reaction affects most individuals exposed and generally produces discomfort immediately after exposure. Allergic contact dermatitis affects only individuals previously sensitized to the contactant. The reaction is delayed until the cascade of cellular immunity is completed, requiring up to several hours. Both in industry and in the home, irritant reactions are more frequent than are allergic reactions (8).

Irritant contact dermatitis is due to direct injury of the skin as, for example, that caused by detergents, solvents, or alkaline abrasives, including cement. If the irritant is a mild one, repeated or prolonged exposure, or exposure combined with abrasion, may be necessary to produce a reaction. In *allergic contact dermatitis*, lymphocytes, previously exposed to antigen that has been processed through the macrophage or Langerhans' cell system, react selectively to subsequent exposure with initiation of inflammation. Genetic predisposition, frequency of exposure to the antigen, and coexisting dermatitis are among the factors that affect the development of sensitization. Allergic sensitivity is usually a more difficult problem than irritation because sensitized individuals may respond to only minute quantities of the offending substance.

Characteristics

Diverse types of eruption with asymmetric or restricted distributions, such as a rash limited to the axillae or earlobes, or a rash only in exposed areas, such as the face, "V" of the neck, lower arms, and hands, probably are contact in origin. The deeper skinfolds protected from external contactants tend to remain clear, whereas an intrinsic dermatitis, such as seborrheic dermatitis, will involve the entire area, including the skinfolds. Involvement of the palms or soles or of the mucous membranes, ordinarily resistant to chemicals, is evidence against a contactant. Irritant and allergic dermatitides may be identical in appearance; distinction depends upon the history of exposure and the response to patch testing. The appearance of contact dermatitis varies from mild eruptions with itching and scaling to crusting, oozing, and even blistering lesions.

Allergic reactions to systemic medications are usually central and are worse on the trunk than on exposed peripheral parts. The major exceptions are reactions to drugs that induce *photosensitization* to ultraviolet light. Tetracycline, sulfonamides, phenothiazines, nalidixic acid, triptylines, sulfonylureas, and thiazides are known photosensitizers, leading to exaggerated sunburn reaction or eczematous dermatitis.

Common Contactants

Plant Dermatitis

Poison ivy, oak, and sumac, the most common of the plant contactants, produce eczematous or even blistering eruptions, usually restricted to exposed parts and often characterized by bizarrely shaped angular lesions, the result of contact with a plant resin (oleoresin). Contrary to popular belief, leakage of blister fluid does not "spread" the rash to other sites; however, lesions often are delayed in appearance because of the continuing unintentional exposure to the resin, which may persist on the patient's clothing, tools, or sports equipment or on the fur of the family pet. Sensitive individuals will continue to develop new lesions for up to the 3 weeks that is required for the resin to evaporate.

Metal Allergy

Nickel contact allergy is common, particularly in women, and it may be seen near hooks, zippers, or jewelry, such as on the earlobe and the wrist. Dermatitis under a gold ring could be due to metal allergy but is more often due to irritating soap residue. The eruption of metal allergy tends to be mild and chronic with scaling, pigmentation, and pruritus. A simple and convincing patch test can be performed to confirm the diagnosis of nickel allergy: a moistened 5-cent piece should be taped to the upper inner arm with an occlusive tape (such as Blenderm) and left on for 48 hours. The patient should remove the patch earlier if itching develops. Individuals allergic to nickel will develop dermatitis under the coin; the area should be examined by the patient for several days, as a reaction occasionally may be delayed.

Topical Medications

Allergy to topical medications is frequent, probably due to the loss of the protective barrier of dermatitic skin. Common culprits include neomycin, anesthetics (such as benzocaine or tetracaine), and preservatives, such as parabens and merthiolate. The original eruption may appear to persist, but the difficulty may be due to the imposition of a new contact allergy from the medication. The situation becomes even more confusing if corticosteroids are in the medication, thus partly masking the dermatitis.

Therapy

Plant Dermatitis

Immediately after exposure, the patient should wash the exposed parts thoroughly and wash or clean items that were in contact with the irritant or allergen. If the item is not washable, it should be isolated in a ventilated area for 3 weeks. The family pet should be bathed if it could have come into contact with suspect plants.

If acute dermatitis does develop, the patient should apply cooling compresses with saline (1 teaspoon of salt/pint of tap water) or Burow's solution (1 tablet or packet/pint of tap water) for 20 minutes every 2 or 3 hours. An antihistamine, such as diphenhydramine (Benadryl), 50 mg, or chlorpheniramine (Chlor-Trimeton), 4 mg every 4 to 6 hours (both are sedating), or terfenadine (Seldane), 60 mg twice a day (less sedating), as well as a topical lotion, such as calamine, or a corticosteroid cream, such as triamcinolone 0.1%, may be used. If the reaction is particularly extensive, or is located on the face and is acute with edema and blisters, or if the patient is known to have had severe reactions to the same antigen in the past, systemic corticosteroids are helpful. A substantial dose of prednisone is needed to suppress acute contact dermatitis; low doses are not effective. The average-sized adult patient should start with 60 mg each day in three divided doses until relief is produced and continue for a total of 2 or 3 weeks, decreasing the dosage as the condition subsides. It should be kept in mind that systemic corticosteroids will reduce the dermatitis only partially if the irritant or antigen remains in the environment. Secondary bacterial infection is uncommon but, if present, requires treatment with systemic antibiotics, such as erythromycin, 250 mg four times a day for a week. Currently available preparations for hyposensitization treatment of poison ivy, oak, or sumac cannot be recommended except in unusual situations (such as a sensitive forestry worker), and in these situations referral to a dermatologist or allergist is appropriate.

Other Contactants

To be effective, therapy must include the identification and elimination of the irritant or allergen. If the contactant cannot be eliminated from the environment, protection may suffice. For dermatitis of the hands, vinyl gloves, best worn with separate thin white cotton liners that can be removed and washed when needed, provide protection. Low grade exposure may be kept under control with topical corticosteroid ointments, such as triamcinolone, 0.1%, or fluocinonide (Lidex), while the source of antigen is being investigated.

In the case of jewelry (nickel) sensitivity, the patient may still be able to use the jewelry provided that it is painted with a clear acrylic paint or colorless nail polish to prevent the metal from coming into contact with the skin.

After the dermatitis has subsided and suspicious irritants and antigens have been removed from the patient's environment, it is important to prove that the patient did have a specific allergy or irritant so that the substance can be avoided in the future. The relationship is proven with patch tests. A kit to perform patch tests may be obtained from the American Academy of Dermatology (820 Davis Street, Evanston, IL 60201). However, patch testing is time consuming, and experience is needed to interpret the test results properly; therefore, patients are usually referred to a dermatologist or an allergist for this testing.

Cosmetics

Following Food and Drug Administration guidelines, ingredients of cosmetics are listed on the label. Manufacturers will make these substances available to the physician for patch testing. However, perhaps 40% of the reactions to cosmetics are caused by the perfume; the chemical composition of perfumes may not be known, even to the manufacturer. One should suggest discontinuing the cosmetic, a step the patient probably would have taken on her own. One percent hydrocortisone cream should be used sparingly until the reaction subsides. More potent topical corticosteroids are to be avoided on the face, since long use may lead to telangiectasis. The cosmetic should be discontinued for at least 2 weeks and during that time another brand should not be substituted; most cosmetics, used for the same purpose, have the same or similar ingredients. It should be recognized that cosmetic reactions may take weeks to regress. If after 2 weeks the eruption has not cleared or if it recurs when a different brand is started, referral to a dermatologist is appropriate since patch testing may be necessary to identify the allergen. Extensive investigation may be necessary before the cause can be determined; it is estimated that the average woman applies 13 cosmetic products, including deodorants and shampoos, to herself each day and that Americans are exposed to 30,000 chemicals during the year. Alternatively, another dermatitis, such as seborrheic dermatitis, may be present.

DRUG REACTIONS

Cutaneous eruptions from drugs take many forms ranging from a pink, evanescent, nonscaly rash to hives, blisters, pustules, erythema multiforme, purpura, or serum sickness.

The mechanism of drug eruptions may be allergic, toxic, or idiosyncratic. Allergic reactions may be IgE mediated or non-IgE mediated; IgE-mediated allergic drug reactions generally present with urticaria, angioedema, or anaphylaxis, whereas non-IgE reactions generally are macular, papular, petechial, or blistering. The only practical test for allergic reactions to an IgE-mediated sensitivity is the skin test to penicillin (Pre-Pen), but there are no laboratory tests to prove the cause of any of the non-IgE-mediated drug eruptions.

Drug eruptions usually improve or clear within 48 hours after the offending drug is discontinued, but occasionally they last for days or weeks, depending on the rate of clearance of the medication.

The drugs that are associated with the highest frequency of skin reactions are listed in Table 100.2.

When a cutaneous drug reaction is considered, elimination or change of all of the drugs suspected by causing the reaction is prudent; serious systemic reactions may develop if an attempt is made to suppress the reaction with antihistamines or systemic corticosteroids while continuing the drug. However, both of these agents relieve discomfort and help to speed resolution of an eruption once the offending agents have been stopped.

FOOT DERMATITIS

The most common dermatological disorders of the feet are: (a) tinea infection, (b) dyshidrosis, (c) contact allergy, (d) essential hyperhidrosis, and (e) erythrasma. The most important diagnostic clues are location (Fig. 100.2) and appearance; all of these disorders, except hyperhidrosis, are pruritic.

Tinea

Presentation

Tinea pedis, or superficial fungal infection of the feet, occurs in about 20% of the population, a problem related to the common use of closed shoes that retain generated heat and moisture, conditions perfect for

Table 100.2.
Drugs That Are Associated with the Highest Frequency of Skin Reaction[a]

Drug	Reaction/1000 Recipients
Amoxicillin	51
Trimethoprim-sulfamethoxazole	34
Ampicillin	33
Ipodate	28
Semisynthetic penicillin	21
Cephalosporins	21
Erythromycin	20
Dihydralazine HCl	19
Penicillin G	19
Cyancobalamin	18
Quinidine	13
Hyoscine butylbromide	13
Cimetidine	13
Phenylbutazone	12
Acetylcysteine	9
Phenazopyridine HCl	9
Hydralazine	8
Carbocysteine	7
Vincristine sulfate	6
Isoniazide	6
Cyclophosphamide	5
Gentamicin	5
Pentazocine HCl	5
Doxycycline	5
Barbiturates	4
Dipyrone	4
Metoclopramide HCl	3

[a] Modified from Bigby M, Jick S, Kick H, Arndt K: Drug-induced cutaneous reactions. A report from the Boston Collaborative Drug Surveillance Program in 15,438 consecutive inpatients, 1975-1982. *JAMA* 256:3358, 1986.

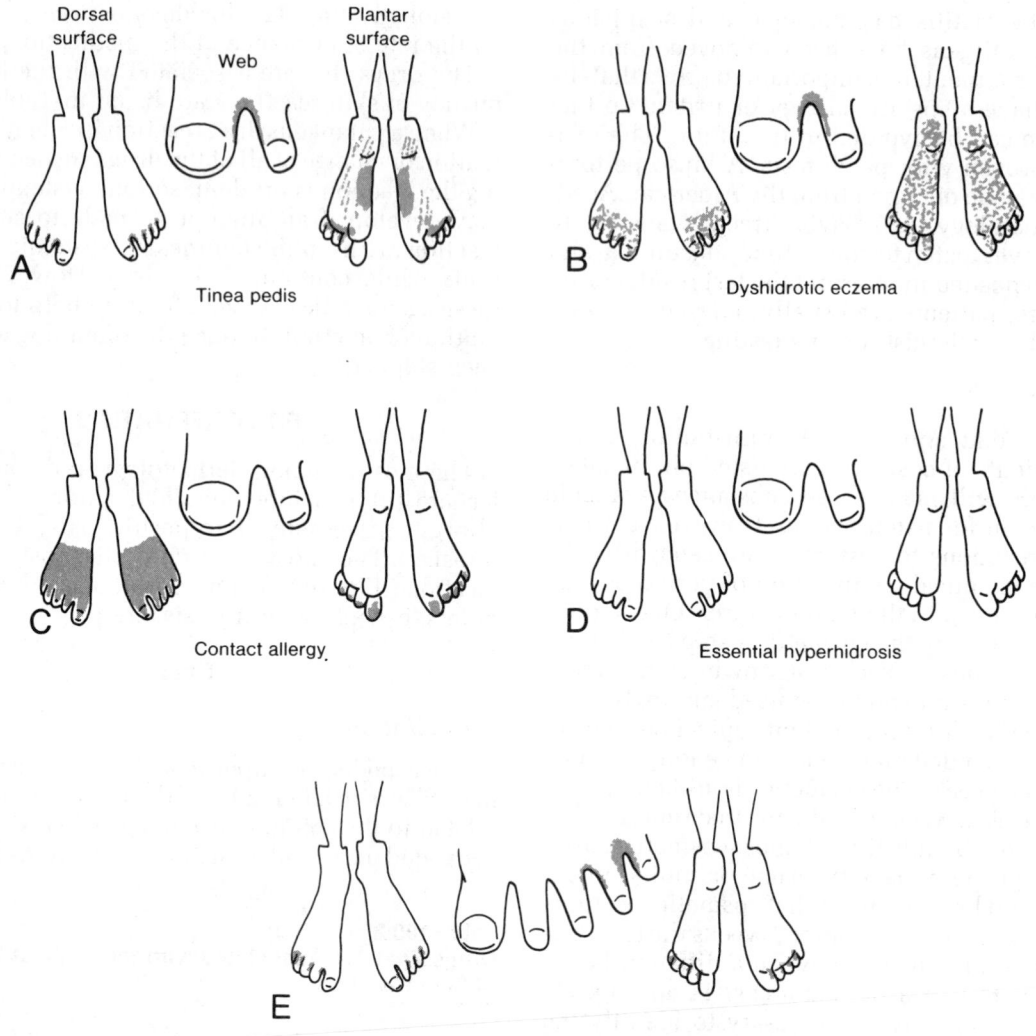

Figure 100.2. Distribution of lesions is useful to distinguish among causes of dermatitis of the feet. *A.* Tinea pedis—moisture, scale, and pruritus confined to the plantar surface (especially the instep) and between the toes. *B.* Dyshidrotic eczema—vesicles and severe pruritus on the dorsal as well as the plantar surface and between the toes. *C.* Contact allergy—the dorsum of the feet and underside of toes may be involved while the plantar surface and webs are clear. *D.* Essential hyperhidrosis—sodden soles but no dermatitis. *E.* Erythrasma—mild erythema and scale limited to the toe webs, especially the fourth to fifth.

fungal growth. Summer exacerbations are typical. This infection presents as scales, itching, and slight redness between the toes and on the soles. In acute stages, blistering can develop, usually involving the instep rather than the thick keratin on the balls of the feet. Secondary infection and lymphangitis may be superimposed in tinea pedis. Yellow crumbly toenails infected with fungi, onychomycosis, often are associated with chronic tinea pedis and serve as a source of continuing reinfection. A scraping of the scale or debris under the nail incubated on a slide with KOH for 10 minutes will reveal hyphae [see "Potassium Hydroxide (KOH) Preparation," page 1354]. Culture usually is not necessary.

Therapy

The patient should be instructed to dry the toe webs thoroughly after bathing and to use talc freely. Foot-

wear should be nonocclusive (ventilated leather shoes or sandals are best; vinyl footwear or sneakers should be avoided). The patient should use cotton socks (dark or light) and avoid wool and synthetic fibers that absorb moisture poorly. If the lesions are dry and pruritic, the physician should prescribe a topical antifungal agent such as miconazole cream (Monistat-Derm), haloprogin cream (Halotex), or clotrimazole cream (Lotrimin, Mycelex) to be applied to the feet sparingly each morning and evening. Antifungal powders seem to be less effective than creams and are not recommended. The patient should continue with the topical antifungals at bedtime until clear, then continue them for an additional month and reinstitute the therapy only upon recurrence. For additional details, see "Topical Antifungal Agents," page 1378. When the feet are particularly scaly and sweaty, a keratolytic in an insoluble ointment base (half-strength Whitfield's ointment, available without prescription) applied each morning, alternating with an antifungal cream at bedtime may be needed. If the lesions are moist and acute, they should be treated with compresses of Burow's solution for 3 days before starting topical antifungals. For additional details, see "Compresses," page 1376.

If initial therapy does not work, a 30-day course of griseofulvin, ultrafine (generic, by prescription), 250 mg three times a day with meals, usually will be effective (see page 1355 for a discussion of side effects). The topical antifungals should be continued after the griseofulvin is discontinued, to maintain clearing. If accompanied by hyperhidrosis (see below), 6% aluminum chloride in absolute ethanol (Xerac-AC, requires a prescription) applied to the feet each morning will induce dryness.

Onychomycosis of the toenails responds poorly to any therapy, including griseofulvin. See Chapter 102 for a more detailed discussion of the management by excision of the nail.

Dyshidrosis

Presentation

Dyshidrosis is the second most common dermatosis of the feet (although the feet are not involved by themselves, see below) and the most difficult of the common disorders to diagnose and treat. It affects both sexes with equal frequency. The cause of dyshidrosis is uncertain, but many patients have flare-ups after nonspecific irritation. One should inquire about causes, including contact allergens, especially from shoes, occupational sources, exposures to nonspecific irritants, and a history of atopy. The eruption also occurs on the hands where it is particularly common in persons whose hands frequently are wet—cooks, beauticians, and housewives. Dyshidrosis starts as minute, deep blisters on the sides of the palms and/or soles and between the fingers and/or toes. Scale and erythema accompanied by severe pruritus usually are present. Unlike tinea pedis, involvement of the dorsum of the foot is common. Dyshidrosis frequently is accompanied by hyperhidrosis (see below), but there is no disorder of the sweat glands, despite its name. The KOH examination will be negative. Scabies, although pruritic and often involving the feet and hands, typically involves the body (see below).

Therapy

Dyshidrosis is notoriously difficult to treat. During the blistering phase, the patient should compress for 20 minutes three times a day with Burow's solution (Domeboro, available without prescription), made with one packet or tablet dissolved in a pint of lukewarm water, followed by any high potency topical corticosteroid cream. For additional details, see "Corticosteroids," page 1377. At bedtime, in order to absorb serous fluid, a thick coating of zinc oxide paste, USP (available without prescription), should be applied and cotton socks used to keep the paste in place. In the morning, the patient should wipe off the paste with mineral oil on cotton balls and reap-

ply the steroid. During the acute phase, an antihistamine (such as Benadryl, 25 or 50 mg three to four times a day) for sedation will be useful. As the dermatitis becomes less acute, the compressing should be stopped and a corticosteroid ointment, instead of cream, used three times a day.

If initial therapy does not work within 2 weeks, a short course of systemic steroids may be necessary. Prednisone, 40 mg/day for the average adult, is prescribed, continued until relief is obtained, and then tapered by giving 20 mg/day for a week and then 10 mg/day for an additional 2 weeks, after which it is discontinued. Recurrences are typical. The dermatologist or allergist may help by performing contact allergy patch tests.

Contact Allergy

Presentation

Contact dermatitis of the feet is an allergic reaction to a footwear product, usually leather, tanning compounds, metals, dyes, adhesives, or foot medications (see also "Contact Dermatitis" above). It is less common than tinea pedis or dyshidrosis but should be considered when the dorsum of the feet and toes rather than the interdigital areas are involved with erythema, scale, and pruritus. If severe, even blisters may appear. Unlike tinea pedis, the toe webs, protected from direct exposure, and the soles, protected by thick keratin, do not become involved.

Therapy

Topical or even systemic corticosteroids do not fully suppress contact dermatitis if exposure to the antigen continues. If the dermatitis is severe, bed rest, compresses, and systemic antibiotics may be needed, while efforts to locate the source of the allergy are initiated. Referral to an allergist or dermatologist is suggested, as either will have access to specialized patch-testing materials as well as knowledge of sock and shoe components, and sources of less antigenic substitutes.

Hyperhidrosis

Presentation

This is a common disorder of excessive sweating of the soles, frequently accompanied by excess palmar sweating (9). It can be severe, with sweat dripping from the fingers and toes, interfering with the patient's occupation and social life. Pruritus or scale is not present. The increased moisture on the feet may lead to fissuring and infection and an objectionable odor.

Therapy

Six percent aluminum chloride solution (Xerac-AC or Drysol, requires a prescription), applied nightly until the condition has improved (usually by 48 hours) and then as needed, often is effective. It appears to work by causing the sweat duct to leak sweat back into the dermis rather than transporting it to the surface.

In severe cases, surgical sympathectomy has been used with success.

Erythrasma

Presentation

Erythrasma is a superficial skin infection with scale and erythema, particularly between the fourth and fifth toes. It is due to a bacterium, *Corynebacterium minutissimum*, which produces a porphyrin, recognized by a salmon-red fluorescence on exposure to Wood's light (see below). Although not a common cause of foot dermatitis, erythrasma should be considered when a scaly foot dermatitis does not respond to topical antifungal medications. A KOH examination (see below) will be negative.

Therapy

Erythrasma is successfully treated with erythromycin, 250 mg three times daily for 2 weeks, or with 2% erythromycin, topically for 2 weeks. Recurrences are frequent, but the infection generally is not passed among family members.

INTERTRIGINOUS DERMATITIS

General Considerations

Rashes in the groin, axilla, and submammery area are common, and most are due to one of four causes: candidiasis, tinea infections, intertrigo, and/or erythrasma. Less common causes of groin dermatitis are contact dermatitis, psoriasis, and seborrheic dermatitis. Rarely Bowen's disease and extramammary Paget's disease, forms of squamous cell carcinomas, must be considered, particularly if the lesions do not respond to topical therapy. Because of the moist environment, dermatitides of the intertriginous areas have some similarities in appearance regardless of cause. Most cases show erythema, scale, and oozing (if severe) and manifest some degree of pruritus. Table 100.3 provides criteria for the diagnosis of the four major causes of intertriginous dermatitis. The proper evaluation of groin dermatitis requires a KOH preparation and an inspection with use of a Wood's lamp; both are easily performed.

Table 100.3.
Diagnostic Criteria for Four Major Causes of Groin Dermatitis

	Moist	Sharp Border	Pustules at Edge	KOH[a]	Wood's Light[a]	More Pain Than Itch	More Itch Than Pain
Candidiasis	Yes	No	Yes	+	−	Yes	
Tinea cruris	No	Yes	No	+	−		Yes
Intertrigo	Yes	No	Maybe	−	−	Yes	
Erythrasma	No	Yes	No	−	+		Yes

[a] See the text for description.

Potassium Hydroxide (KOH) Preparation

The lesion should be scraped with a sterile no. 10 or 15 scalpel blade, and the scale should be transferred to a microscope slide. If the skin is moistened with a drop of water, the scales will adhere, which will make collection easier. A drop or two of 15% KOH should be placed on the slide with the scale, a coverslip applied, and the slide heated to dissolve epidermoid cells. KOH does not dissolve fungal hyphae. Boiling may "bubble" the scales off the slide and should be avoided. The preparation should be examined with the low power ($\times 10$) objective with the light turned low and the condenser racked down to increase contrast between hyphae and cell borders. Hyphae are thin, branching, double-walled filaments that can be distinguished from cell borders by their double-walled smooth appearance, often several cell diameters long (Fig. 100.3). The high dry ($\times 40$) objective can be used to confirm the observation.

Wood's Light Examination

An inexpensive "black light" can be obtained from physician supply stores or hobby shops. The examining room must be completely dark and the light placed close to the patient's skin since the light output is low. The physician should look for the coral red or salmon-colored fluorescence of erythrasma. The light also will be useful for examination of patients with tinea versicolor and vitiligo (see below).

Candidiasis

Presentation

Candidiasis is a yeast infection that is generally restricted to mucous surfaces and moist intertriginous areas of the skin. The eruption is moist, red, and often tender with a thin cheesy surface and frequent tiny pustules studding the indistinct margins.

Therapy

For inflammation with oozing and discomfort often associated with candidiasis, the patient should apply cool compresses of either saline (1 teaspoon of salt/pint of water) or Burow's solution (1 tablet or packet/pint of water) for 20 minutes three times daily. For details, see "Compresses," page 1376. The patient should, after compressing, thoroughly dry the area of dermatitis with a towel or fan and apply topical nystatin (Mycostatin, requires a prescription) cream or a broad spectrum antifungal agent, such as clotrimazole (Lotrimin or Mycelex, requires a prescription), Miconazole (Monistat-Derm, available without prescription) or ketoconazole (Nizoral, requires a prescription) cream. Antifungal powders are also useful in intertriginous rashes due to candidiasis. For additional detail, see Topical Antifungal Agents, page 1378.

In severe cases, where there is considerable oozing, the patient may layer zinc oxide paste (available with

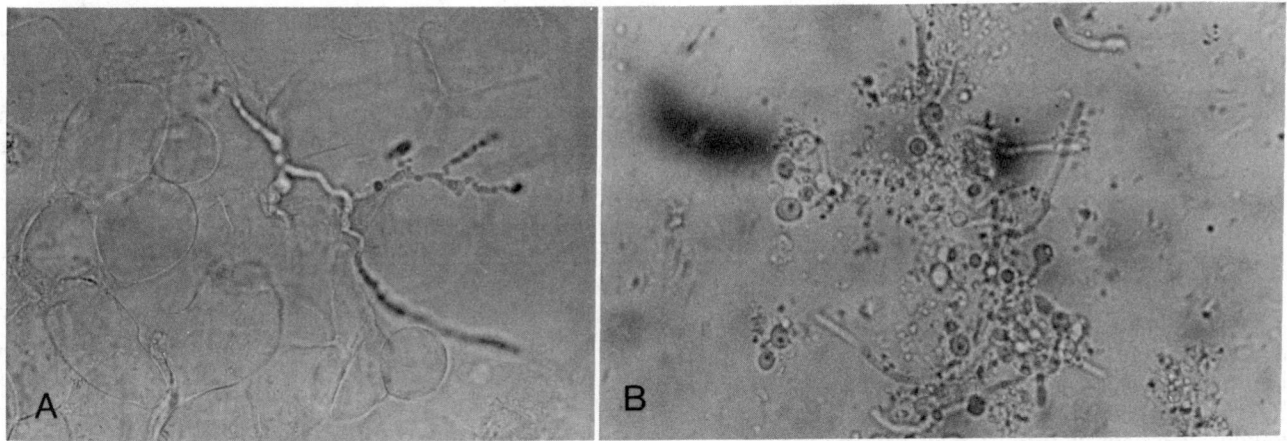

Figure 100.3. *A.* Hyphae of tinea (KOH preparation, × 400). *B.* Pseudohyphae of *Candida* (KOH preparation, × 400; photograph *B* courtesy of William G. Merz, Ph.D.).

out a prescription) thickly over the area at bedtime, to be removed with mineral oil-soaked cotton balls in the morning. Compresses usually are not needed for longer than 3 days. The antifungal agent, however, will need to be continued for 2 weeks. Distinct improvement should be apparent within 7 days of initiating therapy.

Evaluation and Therapy for Resistant Cases

A number of factors account for apparent clinical resistance, and these need to be considered if there has been no improvement within 7 days of initiating therapy (13). Local factors, such as polyester clothing that encourages sweat retention and maintains the infection, should be modified; loose, nonocclusive cotton clothes are preferred. Other skinfolds, such as the axilla, under the breasts, and about the neck and abdomen, should be examined for candidiasis. Candidiasis is likely to be present in the vagina and in the gut; organisms from these sites may be reinfecting the area (see Chapter 94). Reinfection is common, and the sexual partner should be examined for the presence of candidiasis. A KOH smear to search for pseudohyphae and spores is more practical than culture as results are immediate and are not invalidated by overgrowth of contaminants (Fig. 100.3B). Among the *Candida* species, only *Candida albicans* is a common pathogen.

Resistant cases in women should be treated with miconazole vaginal cream (Monostat 7), clotrimazole vaginal cream or tablets (Gyne-Lotrimin or Mycelex-G), or nystatin (Mycostatin) vaginal suppositories to be used daily for 2 weeks to control the vaginal candidiasis. Also for women with resistant cases, the gut may be the source of reinfection, and a 3-day course of oral nystatin suspension (100,000 units/ml) at a dose of 5 ml (1 teaspoon) four times a day should be prescribed. Furthermore, diabetes mellitus predisposes patients to candidiasis; however, if diabetes mellitus is a true causal factor, glycosuria will be present and

control of the glycosuria will help in the treatment of the candidiasis.

Tinea Cruris

Presentation

Tinea cruris, as the name denotes, is a fungal infection of the groin. Tinea cruris is common in males and uncommon in females and does not occur in childhood. It tends to recur during the summer months (13). It appears as most intertriginous dermatitides with erythema, scale, occasionally oozing and pruritis (see above).

Therapy

A topical antifungal agent (see "Topical Antifungal Agents," page 1378) (Monistat-Derm) should be applied to the rash sparingly twice a day for 3 weeks. The patient should try to decrease moisture in the area of the rash by using plain talc (such as Johnson's Baby Powder) and cotton underwear. If acute with oozing and discomfort, compresses for 2 or 3 days (see above) followed by the short-term application (e.g., 1 week) of a topical corticosteroid (such as triamcinolone cream, 0.1%) may be necessary before topical antifungal medications are begun.

If the lesions are extensive or involve other parts of the body as well, oral griseofulvin-UF (generic by prescription), 250 mg three times daily for 30 days taken with food, should be given. On occasion, griseofulvin may be the initial therapy with topical antifungal agents used to maintain the clearing. Griseofulvin generally is devoid of serious side effects; headaches and gastrointestinal distress develop when high doses are used and, rarely, photosensitivity can occur. Griseofulvin can reduce the effects of anticoagulants by increasing the rate of their metabolism by the liver.

Intertrigo

Presentation

Intertrigo is a moist, brightly erythematous and irritating dermatitis occurring in occluded body folds, generally in obese individuals. Excessive moisture, heat, and maceration produce conditions conducive to superficial infection with mixed bacterial flora.

Therapy

Therapy is directed at reducing heat and maceration by wearing light absorbent clothing (i.e., cotton rather than polyester), by frequent drying of the skin, and by the frequent use of plain talc (such as Johnson's Baby Powder). Cornstarch, which may encourage fungal and bacterial growth, should be avoided. After the drying measures, a corticosteroid-containing cream (such as 1 to 2 1/2% hydrocortisone cream) should be applied three times daily. Plain talc should be used over the cream during the day, and a thick layer of zinc oxide paste can be applied at bedtime, as with candidiasis, to absorb moisture. Improvement should be evident within a few days.

Treatment of obesity is important to prevent recurrences (see Chapter 76).

Erythrasma

Presentation

Erythrasma is a dry, slightly scaly, mildly inflammatory dermatitis in the intertriginous areas and can easily be mistaken for tinea infection (10). Moisture and maceration are frequent underlying conditions. It is due to an infection by a bacteria, *C. minutissimum*. The bacteria produce prophyrins, which fluoresce a salmon red color when exposed to a Wood's light (see above).

Therapy

Treatment with erythromycin, 250 mg three times daily for 2 weeks, or 2% erythromycin two times a day, topically for 2 weeks, generally is successful. Recurrences are frequent, but the disease generally is not transmissible.

HAIR

The social and sexual significance of hair is so great that the mention of hair loss should be received sympathetically and informed advice should be provided. Hair density varies considerably among individuals, and a substantial amount of hair, perhaps 20%, can be lost before the person notices the change; about 50% of the hair is lost before others notice thinning as well. Therefore the patient's estimate is more critical than the physician's assessment of hair loss.

Pathophysiology

The change from immature vellus hair of children to the coarse dark terminal hair of adults is induced by androgens, but is modified by genetic factors. Hair growth in humans is cyclical, not continuous. The period of active growth is called anagen; and the resting phase, telogen. Growing and resting hairs are intermingled and not synchronized so that, unlike molting in animals, no obvious thickening and thinning cycle occurs. At any one time about 80% of the scalp hairs are in anagen and 20% are in telogen. Once hairs have entered telogen, they do not restart their growth. Instead, as the hair follicle re-enters the growing phase, a new hair forms below the resting hair and eventually the resting hair is pushed up and out and is shed (much like the shedding of primary teeth). It takes about 3 months for hair to enter the resting phase and to be shed by newly formed hair from below. Shedding is quite normal and involves 25 to 100 hairs every day. A very high level of metabolic activity is maintained in anagen hair follicles. About 1 cm of hair emerges every month from a follicular base that is no thicker than this page.

Patterns of Hair Loss (Alopecia)

One must first decide whether the hair loss is diffuse or patchy (thinned in regions). For example, the usual male pattern balding is patchy. The second important observation that will be useful in the classification of alopecia is the appearance of the scalp (16).

Diffuse Alopecia with Normal-Appearing Scalp

It is important to determine whether the hair loss has been recent (weeks or months). If so, the cause was usually a precipitating event that took place within 3 months of the time hair began to fall out. Events associated with such hair loss include the use of many drugs (most frequently oral contraceptives, see below), pregnancy, or traumatic events, such as surgery, crash diets, severe accidents, a high fever, or severe illness. Hair follicles are susceptible to conversion from anagen to telogen from such events, and, when the hair follicle restarts its growth, the resting telogen hairs are shed in larger than normal numbers.

This hair loss is not seen at the time of the reversion from anagen to telogen but rather when growth resumes, generally 1 to 3 months later. This type of hair loss is called *telogen effluvium*. The hair eventually returns to its previous appearance. However, occasionally the thinned hair is not restored. In such individuals, mostly women, the hair loss apparently triggers a form of balding, female pattern baldness, that would have been delayed until a later age. Female pattern baldness is no more reversible than is male pattern baldness.

General debility due to any severe endocrine, nutritional, or other systemic disorder also can lead to hair loss, developing gradually over weeks, months, or even years. The mechanism of this loss is not talogen effluvium, however. The scalp usually does not appear abnormal or inflamed. If caused by a systemic medical disorder, the hair loss is usually a minor sign and the medical problem dominates the picture. However, either hypo- or hyperthyroidism and iron deficiency anemia may present as hair loss without obvious signs or symptoms; both should be ruled out by appropriate laboratory tests (see Chapters 50 and 73).

Drug-Induced Hair Loss. Hair thinning has been associated with numerous medications; the mechanism generally is that of telogen effluvium with excessive conversion of anagen hair follicles into telogen that persists until the drug is discontinued. Thinning of hair on the scalp is noticed anytime between about 3 months after beginning the drug and about 3 months after stopping it. Besides oral contraceptive preparations, other medications that may produce this effect include heparin, coumarin, high dose vitamin A, allopurinol, amphetamines, β-blockers, iodine, thiouracil, and trimethadione.

Cytotoxic medications cause another type of hair thinning that is usually more dramatic. The cytotoxic drugs have their greatest effect on rapidly growing cells; therefore, the disturbance is in the anagen rather than in the telogen phase follicle. It is easy to understand why the hair loss is dramatic—80% of hairs are in anagen and all of these may be damaged simultaneously. The result is a hair fall that is sudden and extensive. Fortunately, hair almost always regrows normally when treatment is concluded; in some patients hair grows back more profusely and darker than it was. The hair loss can be reduced in some instances by temporary reduction of the circulation to the scalp with a tight tourniquet about the head or cooling the scalp with icebags. This is practical only if perfusion of the scalp is not necessary for therapy and when the drug is given intravenously and has a short half-life in the circulation.

Intrinsic Hair Shaft Disorders. Intrinsic disorders of the hair shaft usually develop over months or years. These disorders can be congenital, with scalp hair never having grown normally, or, more commonly, can be acquired. Acquired forms are usually due to trauma, such as harsh chemicals or excessive brushing. The diagnosis may be evident on low power (× 10) microscopic examination of the hair shaft. The most common intrinsic hair shaft weakness developing in adulthood is *trichorrhexis nodosa*. In this disorder, the hair grows at a normal rate but breaks easily due to the development of clumps or nodes along the hair shaft, appearing as bristles under the microscope.

Diffuse Alopecia with Inflamed and/or Scaly Scalp

The most common dermatitic conditions of the scalp are psoriasis and seborrheic dermatitis, but these, by themselves, do not cause hair thinning. However, trauma from intense scratching or harsh "treatment" may break the hair and produce temporary and partial alopecia in the regions of the inflammation. Psoriasis tends to be restricted to the scalp, up to the margins, like a helmet, whereas seborrheic dermatitis tends to extend over the ears, forehead, and central part of the face. Seborrheic dermatitis and psoriasis of the scalp are best diagnosed by finding the condition elsewhere on the body (see pages 1366 and 1363). Psoriasis may be limited to the scalp, and in those cases the diagnosis is more difficult. Dermatologists distinguish between dandruff and seborrheic dermatitis; dandruff has scale and mild itching but lacks the inflamed and erythematous component of seborrheic dermatitis.

Treatment. One should follow the treatment outlined for psoriasis and seborrheic dermatitis of the scalp (see below). If unresponsive after 1 or 2 months of care, the patient should be referred to a dermatologist.

Patchy Alopecia with a Normal-Appearing Scalp

The usual cause is alopecia areata, particularly if the patches have appeared during the previous few days or weeks or have been recurrent. The patches of hair loss in alopecia areata are sharply demarcated from the surrounding normal scalp and are nearly or entirely devoid of hair. The patches may be single or multiple. A striking feature is the lack of inflammation; the scalp is not reddened or scaly. A history of severe emotional or physical trauma preceding the hair loss is common, but the underlying cause of alopecia areata is not known. Currently, the suspicion is that the fault is immunological since anti-epithelial and antithyroid antibodies have been found in many of the cases studied. Trichotillomania, compulsive hair pulling, is an important diagnostic alternative, but patches in this disorder are not completely bald; the patient cannot pull short hairs out until they regrow and are long enough to grab again.

Spontaneous resolution of alopecia areata is the rule. Most patients will have regrowth of all hair within several months and almost all will resolve within 2 years. Alopecia areata does not cause scarring, and the potential for hair regrowth always remains. One-third of the patients have recurrences. A severe course with recurrences is more likely if the patches appear at the nuchal hairline, if they are multiple, or if they began appearing in childhood.

Treatment. Moderate tugging of the hair at the margins of the patch with the fingertips is a useful test of activity of the process. If the hairs come out easily, the process is still active and the patch is going to continue to expand. Topical corticosteroids may slow or reverse progression. High potency topical steroids such as those used for acne keloid (see below) may be gently rubbed into the bald patch three times a day. Absorption can be increased by asking the patient to wear a plastic shower cap to bed. If hair does not appear in 1 month, intradermal injections of long-acting repository corticosteroids, such as triamcinolone acetonide, 10 mg/ml (Kenalog-10), may be tried. For details, see "Intralesional Corticosteroids," page 1378. Monthly repeated injections may be needed. In most cases, hair regrowth will be stimulated at the injection sites, although several weeks will pass before new hair growth becomes visible. The newly appearing hair often is light in color, but it will eventually darken to the patient's normal hair color. The hair produced by the injections usually is retained.

Patchy Alopecia with Sore, Inflamed, Scaly, and/ or Lumpy Scalp

This is most often caused by an infection, either fungal or bacterial.

Fungal Infection. Preadolescents with an infection of the scalp most frequently have a fungal ("ringworm") infection, due to either *Microsporum* or *Trichophyton* species. Although ringworm is a term commonly applied to these lesions, there are no distinct ring patterns in the scalp. Infections of scalp hair due to *Microsporum* species are not usually inflammatory or symptomatic and show a typical apple-green fluorescence when viewed with a Wood's lamp (see above). However, infections due to *Trichophyton* infections are now far more common. Hence, inflammation often is severe with pustulation and discomfort. If the inflammation becomes sufficiently severe, a boggy swelling, a kerion, will develop, which can lead to scarring of hair follicles and permanent hair loss. To diagnose a fungal infection, several hairs should be plucked, allowed to soak for 15 minutes in a drop of KOH on a microscope slide, and examined with the high dry objective to look for spores and hyphae in and on the hair shaft. Hair also should be submitted for fungal culture. Hair or scale should be submitted in a sterile tube without medium; fungi withstand transport well and the laboratory personnel can choose appropriate media depending upon the site and clinical diagnosis.

TREATMENT. If it seems likely that a fungal infection is present, ultrafine griseofulvin (generic by prescription) using 5 mg/kg/day in two or three divided doses (see page 1355 for a discussion of side effects), should be started, generally before the species has been identified by culture, which may take weeks. The drug is best absorbed when taken with food. It is best to treat *Microsporum* species for 3 weeks and *Trichophyton* species for 6 weeks and then to continue griseofulvin in both for 4 additional weeks after apparent cure.

Bacterial Infection. The scalp is generally resistant to bacterial infection because of its rich blood supply, but pyodermas, with pustules and bogginess of the scalp and with discomfort and adenopathy, can develop, usually secondary to an underlying dermatitis. It is important to look carefully for associated pediculosis capitis (head lice). The larvae and nits of *Pediculus humanus var. capitis* are sometimes difficult to find if bacterial superinfection has overshadowed the evidence of infestation (see full discussion, page 1362).

TREATMENT. As for other cutaneous pyodermas, erythromycin, 250 mg four times a day for a week, usually is sufficient. It is best to obtain a culture at the time the erythromycin is begun so that an alternative, such as dicloxacillin, can be chosen if insensitivity is found and if the scalp pyoderma proves unresponsive to erythromycin. The scalp should be cleansed by shampooing with a mild soap (such as Johnson's Baby Shampoo) up to four times a day.

Pediculosis should be treated with Kwell Shampoo, leaving the shampoo on for 5 minutes and then combing out the nits with a fine-toothed comb (see below). The shampoo treatment should be repeated 1 week later.

Acne Keloid. Acne keloid resembles a bacterial infection of the scalp with pustules and abscesses scattered among firm papules, but the condition is limited to the occipital part of the scalp and the back of the neck and is seen primarily in black males. It is a granulomatous and inflammatory foreign body reaction due to disordered and incurving ingrown hairs, perhaps first induced by barber clipping. Permanent hair loss can result from the scarring that develops.

TREATMENT. Therapy tends to be disappointing. However, partial relief may be achieved by courses of systemic antibiotics, such as tetracycline or erythromycin, 250 mg three times a day for 2 months; or topical high potency corticosteroids such as betamethasone cream (Diprolene), or fluocinonide cream (Lidex). Intradermal injections of long-acting steroids, such as triamcinolone acetonide (Kenalog-10), may be tried next if a satisfactory response has not been achieved. For details, see "Intralesional Corticosteroids," page 1378. The patient usually gets relief which may last for 1 or 2 months from this treatment.

Patchy Alopecia with Lumps and without Dermatitis

In this instance the hair loss is restricted to the scalp over the lumps. Nodules such as epidermal inclusion cysts, or tumors, benign or malignant, may lead to hair loss from either excessive underlying pressure or from infiltration of hair-bearing skin by tumor. These primary nodular conditions are described below.

Patchy "Pattern" Alopecia Progressive over Years without Dermatitis

The normal rate of scalp hair growth may slow and then stop due to androgen stimulation of hair follicles. The *thinning* and baldness usually accompanying aging is called *pattern baldness* because a stereotyped course and distribution are followed. If plugs of scalp containing viable hairs are transplanted into bald regions of the scalp, the newly planted hairs will follow the intrinsic growth pattern of the area the plugs came from rather than the bald area to which the plugs are placed. The hair follicles seem to have an intrinsic "clock." Underlying scalp vasculature has nothing to do with this clock; scalp massage cannot decrease baldness. Only the absence of hormones before puberty prevents the clock from being set, as in the case of male eunuchs castrated before puberty who never become bald. Graying of the hair also is dependent on this "clock," which, like balding, is modified by family inheritance patterns. The cause of graying is unknown.

The onset and rate of thinning vary with each individual due to complex genetic factors. It is often not appreciated that women as well as men develop thinning. The pattern in most women who develop thinning is not that seen in men but is rather a diffuse thinning over the crown. The balding process starts earlier in men than in women.

Treatment. The only medication that has been proven to induce hair is minoxidil, an effect first detected as a side effect of the systemic use of this antihypertensive. The topical form appears to be safe although the package insert suggests monitoring patients with underlying heart disease. This agent has only been approved for use in men. Perhaps only 10 to 20% of male users detect "acceptable" hair growth, but the majority report decreased hair loss. Topical minoxidil (Rogaine, 60 ml) is expensive ($50 to $70/month), and it usually takes 4 to 6 months to see a benefit. Also it appears that benefits diminish after 2 years and that retained hair is lost if minoxidil is discontinued. It also is important to treat underlying inflammatory scalp conditions (see below, "Psoriasis" and "Seborrheic Dermatitis").

The portion of the scalp at the back of the head is likely to retain hair into very old age. Surgical procedures that involve the transplantation of plugs or strips of hair from that region to bald areas do work and are of value; however, hundreds of plugs may be needed for good coverage and many months may be necessary for placement; the process is painful and expensive.

Implantation of artificial hair into the scalp should not be done; the technique simply does not work. The fibers act like foreign bodies and their rejection is accompanied by infection and pain.

HERPES SIMPLEX

General Considerations

Herpes simplex, caused by *Herpesvirus hominis*, is of two subtypes. One type appears in extragenital sites (most commonly about the mouth) and is caused by type 1 virus, whereas the type 2 strain causes most genital herpes infections. The initial or primary herpes simplex infection, due to type 1, usually occurs in childhood, whereas type 2 is spread by sexual contact, with most primary infections involving persons beyond the age of puberty. On occasion, type 1 virus causes genital herpes and type 2 causes extragenital infection usually due to sexual contact.

After primary infection, the virus remains latent within regional nerve root ganglia. Patients who suffer recurrent blisters do so because of periodic reactivation of the virus, which reaches the skin via nerve fibers and replicates.

Presentation

Cutaneous herpes simplex infection in the adult most commonly presents as a localized group of pinhead-to rice grain-sized blisters usually recurring at intervals and at the same site.

More frequent and quite troublesome are recurrent lesions, particularly if recurrences are frequent. Recurrent lesions usually are preceded by several hours to a day of a prodrome consisting of local burning or tingling. This is followed by the appearance of multiple small vesicles appearing at or near the site of previous episodes. The most common location for type 1 recurrences is about the mouth and is the usual cause of the "cold sore." The genitals and buttocks are the sites where type 2 infections appear.

The blisters last up to 7 days and are followed by dry crusting with complete healing in a total of 7 to 10 days. The episode may recur almost immediately or not for a year or more. However, recurrence every month to every few months is more typical. Eventually the tendency for recurrence diminishes. The lesions are not scarring. Recurrences are more likely to develop after febrile episodes, systemic illness, or local trauma, such as sunburn or intercourse (22).

Primary infection, particularly type 1, usually occurs in young children and is associated with severe systemic symptoms including fever, malaise, and localized tender adenopathy. The primary infection resolves in 1 to 3 weeks without a scar. Primary herpes simplex infections of neonates are serious and may be fatal; therefore, a pregnant woman with active vaginal or vulvar herpes should be delivered by cesarean section. Primary ophthalmic herpes simplex is quite painful and may lead to corneal ulcerations, scarring, and blindness. Patients should be urgently referred to an ophthalmologist for diagnosis and therapy.

Patients with atopic dermatitis may develop a generalized herpes infection, eczema herpeticum, with the worst lesions in the areas of pre-existing dermatitis. Patients who are immunosuppressed, either due to an inherited disorder or acquired due to malignancy or drug therapy, may become seriously ill from herpes simplex, and fatalities may occur.

The diagnosis of a herpes infection can be confirmed with a Tzanck smear, or the finding of rising levels of viral antibodies, or a positive viral culture, if the latter two specialized techniques are available.

Tzanck (Cytology) Smear

The purpose of a Tzanck smear is to identify multinucleated giant cells and intranuclear inclusion bodies that suggest herpes or varicella virus infection in cells obtained from the base of the blister. For the smear to be reliable, an early intact blister must be examined. The technique involves removing the blister roof with a scalpel or scissors and gently scraping the floor of the vesicle with a no. 10 or 15 surgical blade to obtain cells. The examiner should make a thin smear on a glass slide, immerse the slide in methanol or 95% ethanol for 1 minute, air dry, stain with Wright's or Giemsa as for blood smears, and examine for abnormal large multinucleated cells (Fig. 100.4).

Differential Diagnosis

Primary herpes simplex, particularly in an unusual location, may be misdiagnosed as cellulitis or acute contact dermatitis. Herpetic whitlow resembles bacterial paronychia but is a herpes infection of the fingertip, perhaps acquired by a nurse while providing mouth care to a patient. As herpes type 2 generally is acquired through sexual contact, other venereal diseases may have been transmitted at the same time and should be considered. A urethral or vaginal smear and culture for gonorrhea, a serological test for syphilis (STS), and a slide test for *Chlamydia* (see Chapter 27) at the initial examination, with the STS repeated 2 months later, are advisable.

The grouped vesicles seen in recurrent herpes zoster closely resemble those of herpes simplex, but the two conditions can usually be distinguished by the tendency for herpes zoster to involve a more extensive area and to follow a dermatomal distribution. Zoster is only rarely recurrent so that the history of repeated episodes of blisters, particularly if they are at the same site, also strongly favors a diagnosis of herpes simplex. The Tzanck smear will be useful to rule out other blistering disorders including impetigo, erythema multiforme, and pemphigus.

Erythema multiforme, an acute blistering eruption with target-like lesions and mucosal erosions, appears to be a hypersensitivity reaction and may resemble herpes simplex, particularly as patients frequently give a history of an antecedent "cold sore." Erythema multiforme often follows herpes simplex infections, although it also follows drug and bacterial or nonsimplex viral exposure (see also Chapter 101).

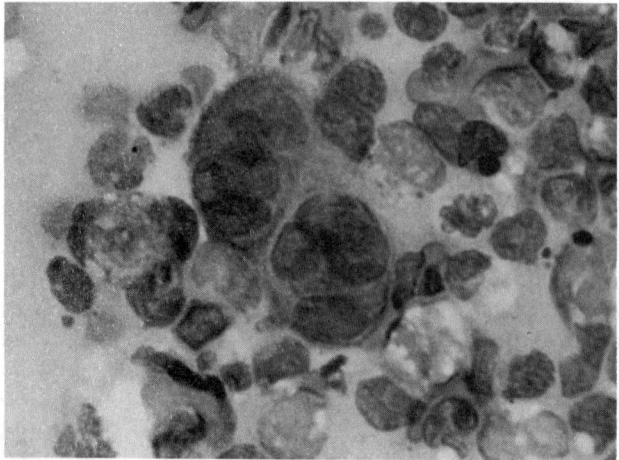

Figure 100.4. Tzanck smear: gentle scraping from the base of a vesicle and stained with Wright's or Giemsa stain. Multinucleated cells from herpes simplex are shown (×400).

Therapy

Therapy of the primary infection is aimed at relieving the discomfort by using anaglesia, both systemic, with salicylates or mild opiates, and topical anesthetics (Dyclone, Xylocaine), especially needed if mucosal surfaces are involved. The area should be kept cleansed. If oral lesions are extensive, the patient may need to be hospitalized for fluid replacement.

Some patients seem to have a decrease in the severity and length of recurrences with topical idoxuridine solution (Herplex, Stoxil), an analogue of thymidine available as an ophthalmic solution by prescription. A drop should be applied to the site hourly during the first 12 hours of a prodrome. There is no apparent benefit after vesicles have appeared.

Oral acyclovir decreases viral shedding and shortens healing time, and, in addition, reduces systemic symptoms and complications (22). For primary infection, one acyclovir (Zovirax, 200-mg capsules) given five times a day for 10 days. In the oral form it has virtually no side effects. Unfortunately it does not reduce the frequency or severity of subsequent recurrences. For treatment of infrequent recurrences, healing time is reduced if oral acyclovir is started at the time of the prodrome (five times a day for 5 days). Frequent (more than five times/year) and severe recurrences may be suppressed with continuous acyclovir (two to five times a day for up to 6 months, but the drug is expensive (about $50/month). Acyclovir ointment is not as effective as the oral form and is not recommended. A vaccine to prevent herpes simplex is not yet available.

Corticosteroids applied to the skin may decrease inflammation after vesicles have developed. Any full strength cream, such as triamcinolone 0.1%, may be used, four times a day, but the periorbital region should be avoided to prevent steroids from entering the eye. Secondary bacterial infection of herpes lesions is not common, and lesions heal at the same rate whether antibiotics are used or not.

The contagious nature of the infection must be stressed to the patient. Herpes simplex can be transmitted from either primary or recurrent lesions, and crusts as well as blister fluid contain infectious virus.

HERPES ZOSTER (SHINGLES)

General Considerations

Two weeks after primary infection with zoster-varicella virus, clinical lesions of chickenpox appear and, in most patients, clear without complication during the next 2 weeks. However, in many or perhaps all individuals who have had chickenpox, the virus continues to reside in a latent state within dorsal root or cranial nerve ganglia. Latent virus does not replicate and can only be identified with specialized culture or antibody techniques. The clinical signs of zoster are due to the reactivation of the virus and its emanation from the ganglia to peripheral nerve endings. In support of the premise that reactivation of virus rather than new infection is the cause of zoster, epidemiological studies have shown that patients with zoster have not been exposed to recent active cases of chickenpox and do not have an increased likelihood of acquiring zoster during epidemics of chickenpox.

Zoster is more likely to appear when mechanisms limiting reactivation of the virus are blunted. Conditions associated with reactivation include old age, acute systemic illness, injuries to or neoplasia of cranial nerves or the spinal column, and disorders associated with diminished immunocompetency, including lymphoma-leukemia and immunosuppressive therapy.

Presentation

A prodrome of 1 to 4 days, but occasionally up to 10 days, is characterized by tingling, tenderness, or itch restricted to the nerve segment involved. Patients with a severe prodrome may present with acute chest or abdominal pain or acute sciatica or joint pain. Before lesions are visible, hypesthesia, dysesthesia, or, more commonly, hyperesthesia will be evident in the dermatome so that a sensory neurological examination of the area may provide early confirmation of the diagnosis.

Very occasionally, zoster manifests only with localized pain, in which case establishing the diagnosis requires the demonstration of a rising antibody titer. Usually, however, there is a typical skin lesion: a patch of grouped vesicles on an erythematous base, each vesicle having a central dell. The eruption is almost always strikingly demarcated at the midline. However, the earliest lesions will present closest to the ganglia, and the dermatomal distribution may not be obvious. The lesion typically worsens for about a week then resolves over a second week. A Tzanck test may be performed (see above for technique) to confirm the presence of multinucleated giant cells and of intranuclear inclusions. Like herpes simplex and varicella, zoster can present a serious danger to immunosuppressed patients who may get severe chickenpox and varicella pneumonia; patients with zoster must be isolated from everyone who is immunosuppressed. The open crusted lesions are infectious and the isolation should continue until the crusts are completely healed.

Differential Diagnosis

Difficulties with diagnosis are more likely in the early stages before the blistering becomes evident. Patients may be considered to have cellulitis, contact dermatitis, neuralgia, arthritis, or a chest or abdominal disorder. Herpes simplex may present in a linear pattern but usually causes less local discomfort and dysesthesia than zoster.

There is no increased risk of subsequent cancer after the diagnosis of herpes zoster, whether the zoster is localized or disseminated.

Therapy

For most patients treatment is symptomatic. The pain may be excruciating and often requires mild opiates such as codeine at the dose of 30 to 60 mg every 3 or 4 hours as well as nighttime sedation such as with diphenhydramine (Benadryl), 50 to 100 mg. A thick coat of zinc oxide paste (available without prescription) or an antibacterial cream, 1% silver sulfadiazine (Silvadene, requires a prescription) one to two times a day, reduces the tendency of serum from the denuded blisters to stick to clothing and decreases discomfort by providing an air-tissue barrier. The zinc oxide may be removed with cotton balls moistened with mineral oil and reapplied morning and bedtime. Silvadene washes off with water. An alternative is to have the patient apply compresses (such as Domboros solution) several times a day.

Often severe, postherpetic neuralgia develops. It is a lancinating or persistent pain in the involved nerve root and dermatome that may continue for years and is particularly common in the elderly. Only a few patients, however, have pain persisting after a month or so. The mechanism of the pain probably is fibrosis and scarring of the nerve. Recent studies do not support the use of corticosteroids to prevent postherpetic neuralgia (6), but the use of large doses of oral acyclovir (800 mg five times a day for 5 days) appears to shorten the course and may reduce neuralgia (14).

If the eye is involved, urgent ophthalmological consultation is necessary. High risk patients, such as those with leukemia-lymphoma or who are immunosuppressed, and who have had an exposure to varicella or zoster within the previous 72 hours, should receive varicella-zoster-immune globulin, obtainable commercially through local blood blanks or the Red Cross. The place for acyclovir in zoster is being assessed in these situations. Varicella vaccines have been developed but are not yet available.

HIDRADENITIS SUPPURATIVA

Single occasional abscesses or inflamed cysts on the trunk or intertriginous areas are common. If, however, there are frequent recurrences in the axillae, groin, and/or perianal regions that heal leaving fibrotic scars, hidradenitis suppurativa should be considered. Patients with this disorder also may develop abscesses on the buttocks and, in women, about or under the breasts. Patients also tend to have active acne vulgaris or old acne scars and develop epidermal inclusion cysts.

Hidradenitis suppurativa, an infection of apocrine sweat glands, does not appear until apocrine glands develop at puberty. Although bacteria are not the underlying cause of hidradenitis, they participate in the process. The course is chronic, leading, if severe, to fistulae, lymphedema, and even restriction of arm or leg movement. The painful, draining abscesses and accompanying odor often produce considerable occupational and social disability. Figure 100.20 (page 1375) shows an example of hidradenitis suppurativa.

Therapy

Acute and fluctuant lesions may be incised and drained, just like any bacterial abscess. A bacterial culture for antibiotic sensitivities from a fresh, non-draining lesion should be obtained when the disorder flares. Systemic antibiotics, selected on the basis of sensitivity testing, help to resolve acute flares. Generally, erythromycin (250 mg four times a day) or dicloxacillin (125 mg every 6 hours) for 10 to 14 days generally is adequate. Long-term tetracycline (250 to 500 mg two to three times a day for months) may partially suppress the disorder. Between episodes, recurrences sometimes can be reduced with twice daily washing with hexachlorophene soap (PhisoHex, available with a prescription) or a quaternary iodine scrub (Betadine or Povidone, available without a prescription). Isotretinoin (Accutane) in doses used for acne (page 1347) sometimes is beneficial (4).

Permanent cure can be obtained by excision of the affected area, removing the apocrine glands, scars, and sinus tracts. This radical treatment is justified in severe cases. If the onset is recent and confined to one region, other causes of infection should be considered, such as tuberculosis, actinomycosis, cat-scratch disease, and, in the groin, granuloma inguinale.

MILIARIA (PRICKLY HEAT)

This common eruption is troublesome because of the prickling and itchy symptoms that accompany it. The eruption develops on occluded or rubbing skin surfaces such as flexoral areas when the skin temperature is abnormally hot. It usually consists of minute red papules, called *miliaria rubra*, but it sometimes presents as a myriad of pinhead-sized clear vesicles resembling water droplets, *miliaria crystallina*. The disorder is caused by occlusion of eccrine sweat ducts with rupture or leakage of the sweat into the surrounding tissue, with the specific type of miliaria depending on the depth of the obstruction within the duct.

Miliaria may develop in persons who work or exercise daily in a hot, humid environment as well as in patients who are wrapped with occlusive bandages, who are lying on plastic undersheets, or who have a high fever. The eruption clears when the skin is cooled and ventilated. Spending 8 hours in an air-conditioned sleeping room prevents the development of miliaria. Propylene glycol in water (50%) (available by prescription from most pharmacies), applied two times a day, may also help to clear the sweat duct blockage.

PEDICULOSIS CAPITIS (HEAD LICE)

Persistent itching of the scalp and crusting and oozing suggestive of a bacterial infection are the typical manifestations of pediculosis. Cervical lymph nodes frequently are enlarged and may be tender. The nits resemble grains of wild rice, in that they are brown and longer than they are wide (Fig. 100.5). They are attached to the scalp or loosely adherent in the hair. If the infestation has been prolonged, nits (egg cases) should be visible along the hair shaft as white granules, smaller than a pinhead. Because the eggs are deposited at scalp level, the duration of the infestation can be estimated by the distance of the nits from the scalp, each centimeter representing about 1 month of infestation.

Spread of pediculosis capitis requires close personal contact, such as may occur in children sleeping at one another's house or sharing the same towels and combs; ordinary contact between school children does not transfer the infestation.

Therapy

Treatment with lindane (Kwell, available by prescription) (this agent is also called gamma benzene hexachloride) shampoo is convenient and highly effective, but it is potentially neurotoxic and should not be used in pregnant or lactating women; pyrethrin with piperonyl butoxide (Rid, 60 and 120 ml) and permethrin (Nix, 60 ml), both available without prescription, appear to be safe for women in these groups and for children. One tablespoon of the medication or enough to saturate the hair is shampooed thoroughly into the hair for 10 minutes. Nits that may not be killed by the solutions should be removed with a fine-toothed comb and the shampooing repeated in 1 week if Rid is used, but one Nix treatment is sufficient. Combs and brushes should be submerged in boiling water, which quickly kills nits. Bed linens, towels, and clothing should be washed in hot water and dried at a high temperature or dry cleaned.

PITYRIASIS ROSEA

Pityriasis rosea (PR) is common, particularly during ages 15 to 35. Although the cause is not known, PR acts like an infectious disease as second episodes are uncommon and there are seasonal increases and min-iepidemics (3). Efforts to isolate an agent have been unsuccessful. There is no specific histopathology or blood test.

Presentation

The initial lesion, the "herald patch," is a 2- to 6-cm, round, scaly plaque that, in about half of the patients, appears on the trunk. Several days later, 1- to 2-cm, pale, red, round to oval macular and papular scaly lesions appear on the trunk and proximal parts of the extremities, forming a fern-like pattern (Fig. 100.6). The truncal lesions may clear at a time when new lesions are still appearing distally. The face is involved infrequently and less often in whites than in blacks. The eruption usually is pruritic and, at times, intensely so, but it may be asymptomatic. PR runs its course in 6 to 8 weeks.

The eruption mimics secondary syphilis; a serologic test for syphilis (STS) should be obtained in all sex-

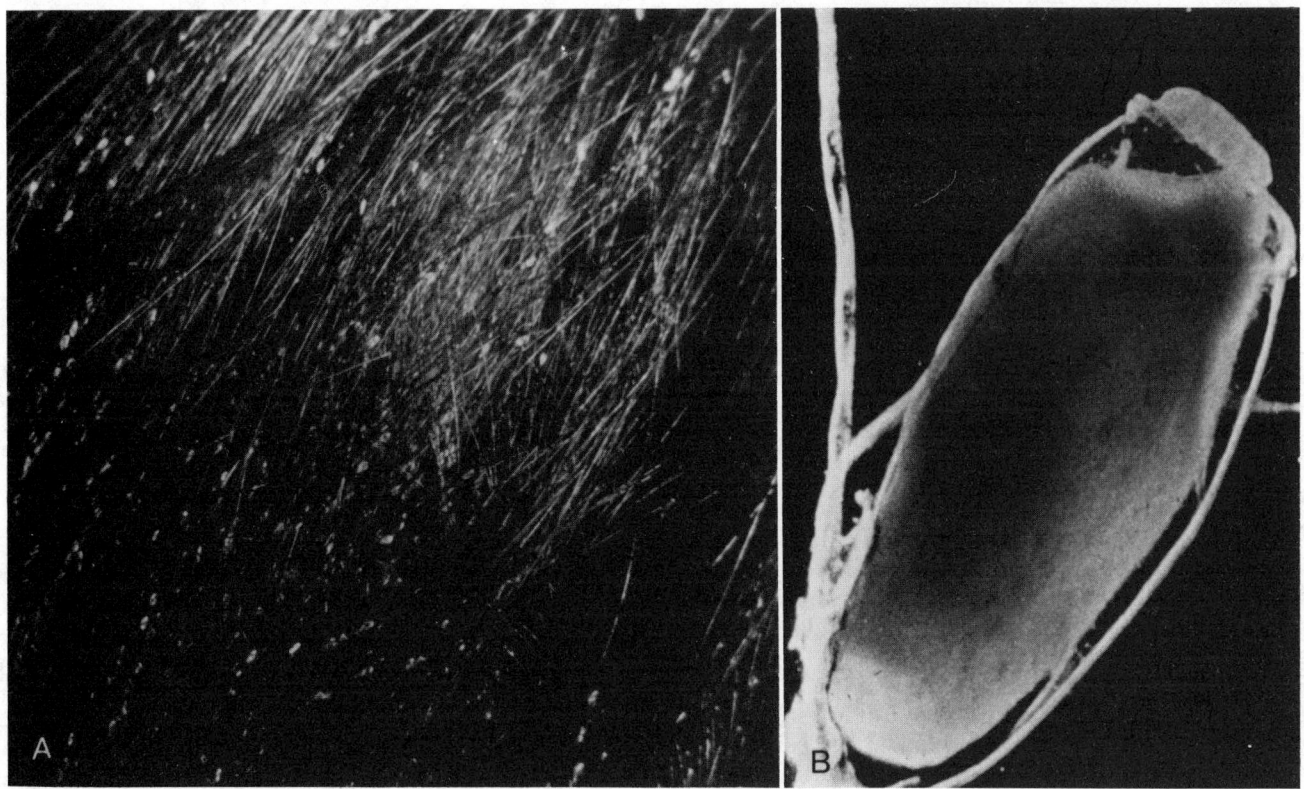

Figure 100.5. *Pediculus humanus var. capitis* (head louse). *A.* Gross appearance of nits on the hair shaft. *B.* Microscopic appearance (×100; photograph *B* courtesy of Reed and Carnrick, Kenilworth, NJ).

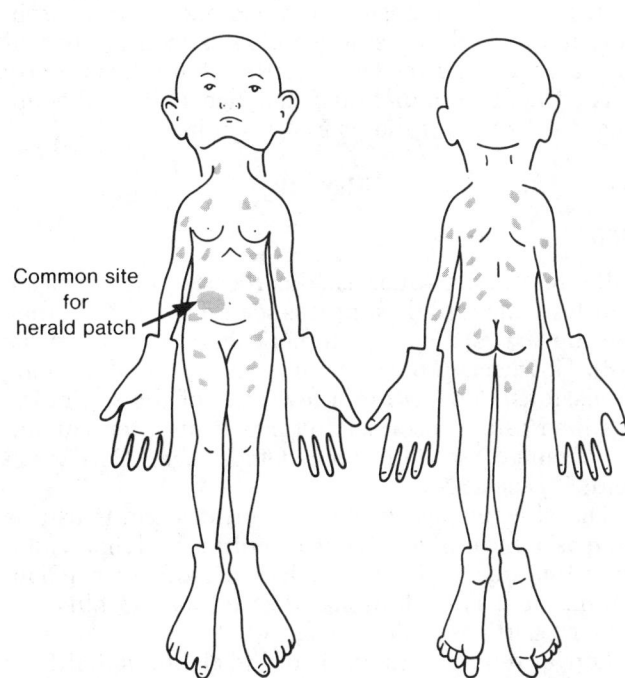

Common site for herald patch

Figure 100.6. Pityriasis rosea typically starts with a "herald patch" followed by oval patches in a fern-like pattern.

ually active patients suspected of having PR. The STS is always positive in secondary syphilis.

Therapy

If the lesions are not itchy, no treatment is needed. It is important, however, to explain the disease and to describe the anticipated course. If pruritus is mild, diphenhydramine (Benadryl), 25 to 50 mg three times a day, and a topical antipruritic suspension, such as calamine lotion with menthol or phenol added, may be prescribed.

Occasionally, pruritus is so severe that the patient cannot work or sleep. In that case, prednisone may be necessary to control the symptoms. Prednisone, 40 mg daily in four divided doses, should be prescribed until the patient is comfortable, usually a few days, then should be tapered over a 3-week period by prescribing one tablet less every third day. The patient does not require isolation and may attend school or work.

PSORIASIS

This probably genetic and usually lifelong disease affects 1 to 3% of the population. Psoriasis may first appear in childhood, especially in severe cases, but usually begins during the third decade. In most instances, it remains throughout adulthood, often improving in the summer and during pregnancies. The disease affects males and females equally. Most patients have only mild pruritus, but the scaly patches are unsightly and may interfere with work, social relationships, and self-image.

Certain histocompatibility antigens (HLA) are associated with the disorder and over one-third of patients have another family member with psoriasis, supporting the theory that psoriasis is inherited, but the underlying cause of the disease still is unknown. Vastly increased epidermal proliferation explains the histological alterations of elongation of epidermal ridges and increased numbers of mitotic cells; epidermal turnover rates may be increased up to 10-fold over normal. This epidermal proliferation is reflected clinically as overproduction of scale, the characteristic sign of the disease.

Presentation

The typical lesion is an erythematous, circumscribed plaque covered by loosely adherent, silvery scales appearing most often on the elbows, knees, and scalp; the external genitalia, the umbulicus, and the gluteal fold frequently are involved as well (Fig. 100.7). Peeling of the scale often produces minute bleeding points that reflect the proximity of underlying dilated capillaries (Auspitz sign). These dilated capillaries, rather than inflammation, are the cause of the plaque's redness. Nails may show pitting (Fig. 100.8) or, when more severely involved, a large volume of subungual keratotic debris leading to separation of the nail from the nail bed.

The diagnosis is not always obvious; the patient may present with severe "dandruff," with nail dystrophy, an apparent drug eruption, or arthritis and a rash. Se-

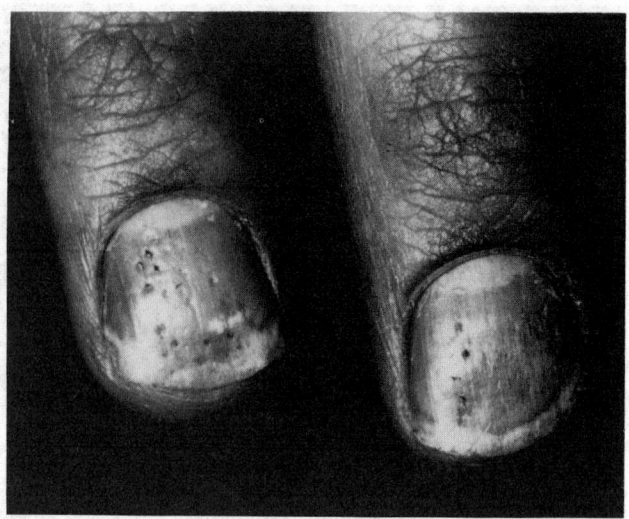

Figure 100.8.   Minute pits are commonly seen on the surface of nails in patients with psoriasis.

borrheic dermatitis (see below), fungal infection (see above), a psoriasiform drug eruption, or even a contact dermatitis to the therapy being used to treat the psoriasis must be considered.

There are several variants of psoriasis that are particularly virulent: *psoriatic erythroderma*, a generalized exfoliative dermatitis characterized by diffuse erythema and scaling and by systemic toxicity including chills and fever; and generalized *pustular psoriasis*, characterized by a diffuse pustular eruption and also by systemic toxicity.

The association between arthritis and psoriasis is still not precisely defined; some patients appear to have a typical seropositive rheumatoid arthritis, probably not related to the dermatological condition; others have a destructive arthritis, characteristically involving the terminal interphalangeal joints, that appears to be part of the psoriatic syndrome.

Therapy

Skin

Because topical fluorinated corticosteroids are clean, odorless, and rapidly suppress scale and pruritus, they are the first step in the topical therapy of psoriasis (18). However, topical steroids do not produce long remissions, and, within a few days of discontinuing the medication, psoriasis returns to its pretreatment appearance. For additional details, see "Corticosteroids," page 1377.

The effectiveness of topical corticosteroids can be increased by applying them at bedtime and then wrapping the area with any kitchen plastic wrap (Glad, Saran, etc.). For additional details, see "Occlusion" under "Corticosteroids," page 1377.

Longer relief for psoriasis of the glabrous (hairless) skin often can be achieved through the addition of tar preparations including Alphosyl, Estar Tar Gel, or Psorigel—all of which are available without prescription.

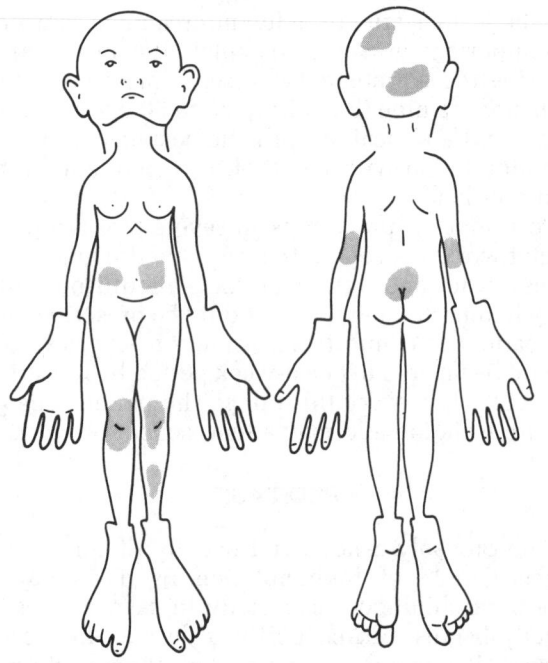

Figure 100.7.   Psoriasis tends to be found on extensor surfaces and areas of repeated trauma, such as the waistline.

Their use is empirical. All of these have a slight tar odor and tint; they should be applied sparingly, only to the patch, and generally only at bedtime. If corticosteroids with occlusion by wrapping are being used at bedtime (see above), the two therapies can be used on alternate nights.

Further benefits may result from the use at home of ultraviolet (UV) light. The patient should choose a floor model (if the unit is too small the patient will become frustrated by the long time that the therapy requires) with a timer (an absolute necessity) and can expect to pay approximately $150 for it. The patient should follow the instructions with the unit to determine the initial exposure, as this time will vary among models. Treatments should be every other day, with increasing exposure each time until slight redness is still visible 24 hours after the UV light exposure. The patient can increase the dose when the persistent erythema no longer develops. Tanning will deepen after several weeks of UV light. The morning after the nighttime application of a tar preparation is the best time to use UV light, but the tar appears to be effective if left on for as short a time as 2 hours prior to the light. The psoriasis-suppressing effect of natural sunlight appears to be more effective than artificial UV light and should be utilized when it is available. Little evidence for late developing skin cancers has ever appeared in psoriatics exposed to UV light and tars.

Scalp

The patient should shampoo every day or 2. Frequent shampooing may be all that is needed in mild cases. Although a number of shampoos containing tars (Ionil T, Sebutone, Zetar), selenium sulfate (Exsel, Iosel, Selsun), and zinc compounds (Danex, Head and Shoulders, Zincon) often are prescribed, very little medication will be left on the scalp after shampooing, so that medicated shampoos alone will help only those patients with minimal involvement.

If shampooing is not sufficient, a topical corticosteroid solution or lotion (Diprosone lotion, Lidex solution, Valisone lotion, Synalar solution) should be rubbed into the scaly plaques with the fingertips immediately after shampooing while the scalp is still moist. Ointments and creams are difficult to use in hairy parts. If scales are too thick to be loosened by shampoos alone, the patient may apply phenol/saline lotion (Bakers P + S liquid, available without prescription) to the scalp at bedtime before the morning shampooing. A stronger, but messier, preparation is a mixture of sulfur, salicylic acid, and tar (Pragmatar cream, available without prescription), which may be used if the phenol/saline lotion does not produce resolution of the thick scale within a month of use. Both preparations are used in the same way. Wearing a showercap at night may be advised to protect bed linens.

Nails

No consistently effective and easy treatment exists. On occasion, dermatologists inject nailfolds with ste-

roids, but the treatment is painful and relief is temporary.

Treatment used by a dermatologist for patients with extensive psoriasis include psoralen with long wave ultraviolet light (PUVA), etretinate (Tegison), systemic antimetabolites (methotrexate, hydroxyurea), or tar and UV light treatment, the Goeckerman regimen. Etretinate, the newest agent used in psoriasis, is a petinoid with substantial systemic side effects and should be prescribed only by physicians experienced in its use.

SCABIES

Presentation

Scabies is an infestation caused by a mite, *Sarcoptes scabiei var. hominis*. Scabies seems to run in cycles; there has been a dramatic upswing in cases since the 1970s, now apparently leveling off. Most of the signs and symptoms of scabies are due to sensitization to the mite and mite products rather than to the physical effects of the mite itself. Hence, there is delayed appearance of the rash until approximately 14 days after exposure, and there is delayed clearing after effective therapy. Because of the sensitization, symptoms start sooner with recurrent infection. Only a few mites usually are present, generally fewer than 10, even though the signs and symptoms can be extensive. The distribution of the mite does not correspond closely with the distribution of the rash (Fig. 100.9). Untreated scabies continues to progress; it is not self-healing.

The overwhelming symptom is severe itching, typically worse at night. The lesions appear as excoriated, inflamed, rice- to pea-sized papules, some with a burrow. Sites most involved are the finger webs, wrists,

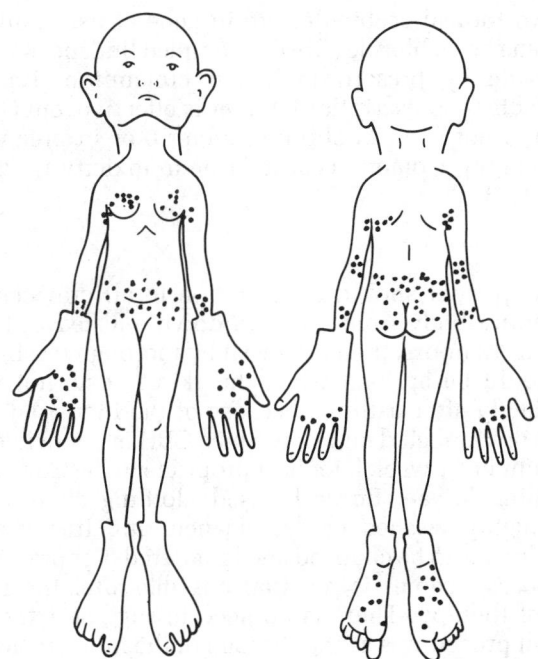

Figure 100.9. Pruritic papules are most prevalent about the waist, pelvis, elbows, and hands and feet in scabies.

antecubital fossae, elbows, areolae, umbilicus, lower abdomen, genitalia, and gluteal cleft. Superimposed excoriations and eczematous dermatitis are common. Findings may be minimal in scrupulously clean individuals. Family members and sexual partners almost invariably are involved and should be treated. Transmission requires close contact, such as sleeping in the same bed or living in the same house; scabies usually is not transmitted casually, as between schoolmates. If the patient is sexually active, it is important to look for other venereal diseases.

A diagnosis of scabies should be considered in any patient who has a pruritic eruption with excoriated papules, especially if family members or close friends also are experiencing itching. Scabies can be proven by finding the mite microscopically. This is accomplished by placing a drop of glycerol or mineral oil, preferably sterile, on the papule to keep the scales and scrapings in place, and scraping through the oil with a blade or syringe needle to the point of just drawing blood. The mite or its eggs must be sought using the ×10 microscope objective. The mite is an ugly, bristled ectoparasite about 0.4 mm long with four pairs of legs. It is hard to find; even experts may be unable to confirm the diagnosis. Therefore, it is appropriate to treat on strong clinical suspicion (7).

Scabies is sometimes difficult to diagnose and may be confused, even by the experienced clinician, with a variety of cutaneous disorders. Atypical presentations account for delayed treatment and provide opportunities for spread. Further confusion is often generated by the use of topical corticosteroids that can partially suppress the eruption.

Therapy

Two topical scabicides are in general use, gamma benzene hexachloride (GBH), also called lindane (Kwell, available by prescription), and crotamiton (Eurax, available by prescription). Either is effective, but GBH often is not used in children under 6 or in pregnant or lactating women because of neurotoxicity in children (17).

GBH

The patient should apply lotion to all crevices of the entire body from the chin down and leave it on for 8 to 12 hours, then remove it by thorough washing. It should be applied when the skin is dry, not immediately after bathing, because of the increased absorption through damp skin. Since GBH is not ovicidal, retreatment 1 week later is appropriate to destroy later hatching larvae. Recently used clothing should be thoroughly washed or dry cleaned, and linens and towels should be changed and laundered. For practical purposes, scabies is not transmissible after the first day of therapy. There is no need to suggest extermination procedures as the lifespan of the mite on clothing and bedding is short. All symptomatic family members should be treated at the same time. The physician should prescribe enough to apply 30 ml to each person for each of the two treatments and should not allow refills; extensive repeated use of GBH may cause irritation and pruritus, which may be confused with the original symptoms.

Crotamiton

Crotamiton is an alternative to GBH but is not as effective. It is applied from the chin down and to all body folds and creases in the same way as GBH, but it is reapplied 24 hours later. Clothing and linen should be changed the first morning after treatment. The medication should be left on for a total of 72 hours, after which patients should take a cleansing bath. Crotamiton is antipruritic and appears to be safe for use in children and pregnant women.

A safe and effective, but messy, alternative in small children is 6% sulfur in hydrophilic ointment, applied nightly for 3 nights and washed off each morning.

Follow-up

If the initial therapy did not appear to work, there are several points to consider. First it must be kept in mind that itching often persists for 1 to 3 weeks after effective scabicide treatment, as a result of slow subsiding of the hypersensitivity reaction to the mite and mite products. An antihistamine, such as diphenhydramine (Benadryl, a 25- or 50-mg capsule three or four times a day), a topical corticosteroid ointment, such as triamcinolone 0.1%, or, if severe, systemic corticosteroids, such as prednisone, 30 mg/day in three divided doses and tapered over 2 weeks, may be needed to provide relief. Second, if symptoms persist beyond 2 weeks or recur when the antipruritics are stopped, the patient should be re-examined for persistent infestation or reinfestation. If there are signs of secondary infection, a 7-day course of an antibiotic, such as erythromycin, 250 mg four times a day, is indicated. The pruritic papules that frequently accompany scabies may require weeks to clear. Animal scabies is different from human scabies; therefore, pets are not a reservoir and do not have to be treated in order to control human infestation.

SEBORRHEIC DERMATITIS

Presentation

Seborrheic dermatitis takes its name because it is found in regions where sebaceous glands are in greatest density, i.e., the scalp, eyebrows, ear canals, midface, and midchest area (Fig. 100.10). The main features are erythema and a yellow, greasy scaling in the regions of involvement. Itching is mild but troublesome. Typically, the severity fluctuates so that patients recall months of relative clearing and months of relative worsening.

Onset of seborrheic dermatitis is generally at puberty when it appears concomitantly with acne; the condition continues in its fluctuating course for years or decades without a decrease in old age. Both sexes

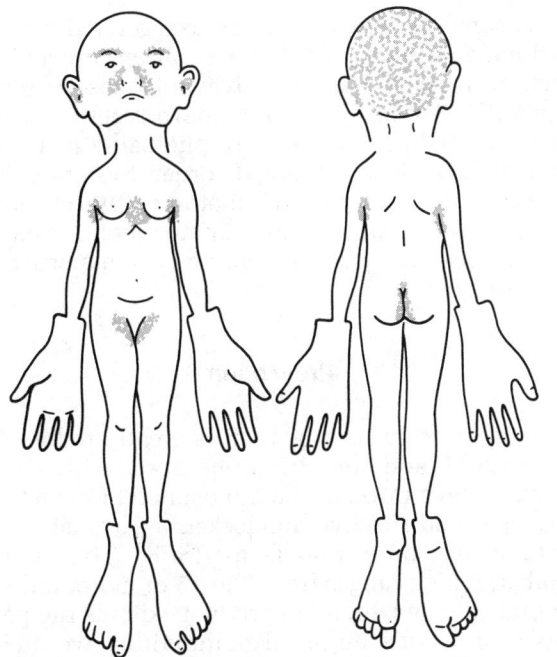

Figure 100.10. Usual location of erythema and scale in seborrheic dermatitis.

are equally affected. Seborrheic dermatitis is worsened in patients with Parkinson's disease, syringomyelia, emotional stress, and at the time of an acute stroke or myocardial infarction.

Occurring in regions of dense sebaceous glands, seborrheic dermatitis appears to to result from infection or sensitization to a common yeast, *Pityrosporon ovale* (21).

Differential Diagnosis

The common scalp condition, *dandruff*, is distinguished from seborrheic dermatitis by the absence of erythema and the lack of involvement in other regions. The most frequent confusion is with psoriasis, as both conditions are erythematous, scaly, and chronic. Psoriasis, however, tends to involve the extensor surfaces, particularly the elbows and knees; a search for such lesions in patients with severe scalp dermatitis may be helpful. Psoriasis of the scalp often stops at the hairline; seborrheic dermatitis does not. The differential diagnosis also includes contact dermatitis, a drug eruption, tinea corporis, and tinea versicolor. These alternative diagnostic possibilities should especially be considered when the response to therapy for seborrheic dermatitis is not satisfactory.

Therapy

Scalp

If mild, control with shampoos (see above, "Psoriasis") may be sufficient. Frequent, even daily, shampooing is not harmful and does not cause hair loss. If simple dandruff (see above) is the only problem, these

shampoos are usually sufficient for control of the problem.

If the condition is severe or is unresponsive to simple shampooing, a topical broad-spectrum antifungal solution, such as clotrimazole (Lotrimin, 20 to 60 ml) should be applied for a few weeks and then as needed to the scalp after shampooing. If there is severe itching or erythema, a topical steroid lotion (1 to 2 1/2% hydrocortisone lotion) can also be applied during the first week or two. If the condition proves resistant to this therapy, psoriasis is more likely to be the diagnosis than is seborrheic dermatitis.

Skin

The patient should apply a broad-spectrum antifungal cream, such as clotrimazole (Lotrimin, 30 g) or ketoconazole (Nizoral, 15 g) twice a day until clear, then once or twice a week for 4 weeks and then as needed to maintain clearing. Pruritis and erythema can be more promptly reduced if 1 to 2 1/2% hydrocortisone cream also is used during the first week or 2 of treatment.

If, after a 2-month trial, this therapy proves insufficient, oral ketoconazole (Nizoral), 200 mg daily for 2 weeks, may be tried. The course may have to be repeated occasionally as the yeast will slowly reappear as will the dermatitis. Oral ketoconazole has been associated with hepatitis in about one of 10,000 courses. Tetracycline, 250 mg twice daily, an hour before or 2 hours after meals, for up to 2 months may be tried and is often helpful, perhaps by altering the fatty acids on which the yeast subsists. The possibility of psoriasis should be considered if the dermatitis is resistant to treatment.

Eyelids

Seborrheic marginal blepharitis is chronic scaling at the lid margins without signs of conjunctivitis or globe discomfort. It can be controlled by gentle scrubbing each morning with baby shampoo, diluted one to one with water, using a cotton-tipped applicator to cleanse the lids. If not sufficiently controlled, a topical antifungal, as used above, or a mild topical corticosteroid such as 1% hydrocortisone cream twice daily may be used. However, long use of potent fluorinated topical corticosteroids can lead to glaucoma, is dangerous in the presence of herpes infection, and should not be used. Treatment should continue at this frequency only until the condition has cleared, after which the patient should decrease the frequency of application to two or three times a week for an additional 2 weeks and then should stop therapy. Like seborrheic dermatitis, the condition tends to recur; therapy can be restarted when needed.

Contact dermatitis to mascara or eye shadow can manifest as blepharitis, and both of these agents should be discontinued for at least a month to determine whether either is causal. The patient should be referred to an ophthalmologist if unresponsive or if the rash is accompanied by conjunctivitis and/or cornea or globe discomfort.

SUNBURN

Symptoms and Consequences

The redness, pain, and tenderness from excessive sun exposure are maximal in 12 to 24 hours. When burning is severe, the skin may blister or peel 1 to several days later. The skin attempts to protect itself from further injury by the induction of melanin; indeed tanning is a response to injury. Acute sunburn heals without scarring unless a secondary infection develops. Long-term, chronic excessive sun exposure, especially in light-complexioned persons, eventually leads to fine wrinkling and sometimes actinic keratoses, basal cell and squamous cell carcinomas; sun exposure is a risk factor for malignant melanoma as well.

Sun Exposure

Most of the energy from the sun that reaches the earth's surface on a sunny day is in the long wave, UVA spectrum, the so-called "tanning" portion. About 10% of the energy is at the short wave, UVB end of the ultraviolet spectrum. These are the so-called "burning" rays. The proportion of UVB decreases if the sunlight is filtered by clouds or when the sun is low on the horizon. Nonetheless, because UVB is about 1000 times more potent than UVA in evoking the burning reaction, it is UVB that causes most solar-induced damage. "Suntan parlors" often advertise that they provide primarily UVA or "safe" exposure, but even UVA in sustained high doses is potentially harmful.

Except for inducing vitamin D, now incidental because of the widespread use of fortified foods, the effects of ultraviolet light are destructive. There is no "safe" ultraviolet light exposure and tanning offers only partial protection. The nearly universal frequency of skin cancers in albinos and the much decreased wrinkling and frequency of skin cancers in blacks attests to the potential danger of the sun.

Therapy

A sunburn is like any other physical injury: the damage cannot be reversed and must be allowed to heal. Aspirin decreases the pain and perhaps lessens the inflammatory reaction by interfering with tissue prostaglandin metabolism. Large doses soon after exposure, 600 mg every 2 hours for six doses, seem beneficial. An extensive burn can be soothed with a 20-minute colloidal oatmeal bath, made by adding one-quarter cup of Aveeno Oatmeal, available without prescription, to lukewarm or cool bath water. If large blisters appear, they may be punctured with a sterile needle or surgical blade, but the roof should be left intact to serve as a pain-reducing biological dressing. Prophylactic antibiotics are not helpful.

Although the cause of sun exposure usually is obvious, some people develop an exaggerated response producing an unexpected "burn" or an unusual skin reaction, perhaps papules, hives, plaques, or a scaly dermatitis. An exaggerated sunburn reaction may be associated with a phototoxic or photoallergic drug reaction or a photosensitizing disorder. Systemic determination of the degree of photosensitivity and the separation of phototoxic and photoallergic responses require specialized equipment and the expertise of a dermatologist.

Prevention

Radiation from natural UVB is greatly reduced before 10 A.M. and after 2 P.M. because of filtration of the sun's rays through the atmosphere. Cosmetically acceptable and effective sunblockers are available, rated by their sun protection factor (SPF). The assigned number, which ranges from 3 to 15 or more, indicates the multiple by which the product extends the period of exposure. For example, if an individual would have developed a sunburn from a 30-minute exposure, a sunblock with SPF of 15 extends that time to 7.5 hours (0.5 hours × 15), obviously an effective level of protection for most purposes. Sunblocks should be applied 30 minutes prior to sun exposure. Most sunblocks are less effective in blocking UVA than UVB, and most are washed away by sweat or water; the directions for use of each product should be followed.

TINEA VERSICOLOR

Presentation

Tinea versicolor is a common superficial fungal infection caused by *Malassezia furfur*. It appears as desquamating macular patches found primarily on the trunk, between the chin and the waist. The rash may be mildly itchy. The varied colors of the rash, from red to pink to brown, gives the eruption its name. Tinea versicolor is most common in hot, humid environments.

The fungus interferes with normal pigmentation, so that the patches become more noticeable during the summer when the skin under the patches does not tan as well as the rest of the skin. This effect is seen in blacks as well as whites. The infection does not seem to be contagious; marital partners usually are not both affected. However, individuals who have had tinea versicolor seem prone to have recurrences.

An examination with KOH shows short hyphae and spores ("spaghetti and meatballs") (Fig. 100.11). The physician should search under the high dry objective (×40); the low power objective (×10) is too low to reveal the fungal structures. A Wood's light examination (see page 1354) is useful as it reveals the extent of the infection better than does room light. The organism cannot be cultured on usual office media.

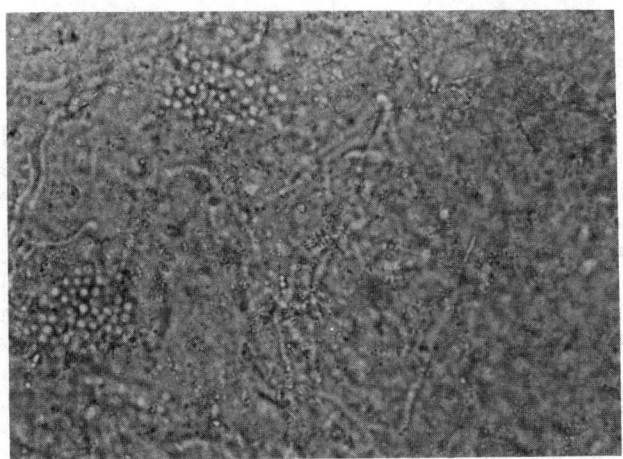

Figure 100.11. Short hyphae and spores of *Malassezia furfur* seen in tinea versicolor (KOH preparation, ×400).

Differential Diagnosis

Because of the pigment disruption, vitiligo must be considered. However, vitiligo is never scaly and a KOH examination will be negative. The pigment loss in tinea versicolor is partial; the pigment loss in vitiligo is complete. Other disorders to consider are seborrheic dermatitis (see above), pityriasis rosea (see above), and infection due to other tinea species. Seborrheic dermatitis most commonly involves the face and scalp, but tinea versicolor almost never goes above the chin; pityriasis rosea may be worse on the upper trunk but usually extends below the waist and the KOH examination will be negative; a KOH examination of the tinea that causes tinea cruris and corporis ("ringworm" of the groin and body) reveals long hyphae without spores, not short hyphae with spores.

Therapy

Numerous therapies work, but recurrences are common. An irritating soap applied at bedtime and showered off in the morning usually is sufficient. Selenium sulfide suspension (Exsel, 2.5%, requires a prescription; or Selsun Blue, 1%, available without prescription) or a peeling soap (Fostex cream, available without prescription) should be used for 4 consecutive nights or fewer if the skin shows irritation. The patient should apply the material from neck to wrists to waist, the areas most commonly affected. The use of 25% sodium thiosulfate (generic or Tinver, a prescription is required) twice a day for an additional 10 days assures resolution but should be used only after work and at bedtime as it has an unpleasant smell. Prescription antifungal agents, such as miconazole, clotrimazole, and haloprogin, are effective but too expensive to apply to the large surface area usually involved. Ketaconazol (Nizoral, 200-mg tablets, by prescription) is a newer, more convenient oral therapy and is effective in short courses (19). Some reports suggest daily use for 1 month, but a shorter course, such as 200 mg each day for 5 days, repeated with three tablets at 2 additional monthly intervals, also is effective. Nizoral probably is safe for short-term use, but hepatitis has been associated with the medication in about one of 10,000 courses.

After the initial therapy, the patient may expect the lesions to be cleared of fungi; a return visit is not needed. However, the patient must be warned that the lightened patches will remain until ultraviolet light-induced retanning occurs. Otherwise, the patient may consider the treatment to be a failure. Patients also should be told that recurrences are common and advised to repeat therapy if needed, generally in the following summer.

VITILIGO

Presentation

When melanocytes stop producing melanin and, later, completely disappear from the site, the skin turns nearly ivory in color, regardless of background racial coloration. The patches have sharp borders without erythema or inflammation. They are most frequent over bony prominences and around orifices such as the mouth and eyes (Fig. 100.12). The patches reflect light and appear bright white under a Wood's lamp (see page 1354), an examination that may be useful in revealing additional patches of vitiligo, especially if the patient is light complexioned. Vitiligo may be inherited, and its course is unpredictable.

Differential Diagnosis

The usual confusion is caused by postinflammatory hypopigmentation. In this case there is typically a his-

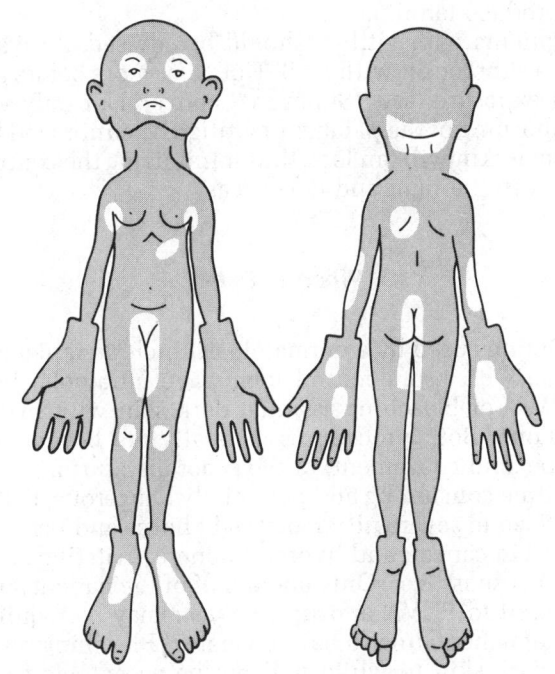

Figure 100.12. Depigmented macules of vitiligo occur most commonly at orifices, on extensor surfaces, and at areas of repeated trauma.

tory of a preceding inflammatory or traumatic condition as well as a persistence of at least some pigment, so that the patches are not ivory white as they are in vitiligo. Phenolic compounds, ingredients of some industrial janitorial products, may destroy melanocytes and lead to permanent depigmentation. The depigmentation may be indistinguishable from vitiligo, except by distribution, as the patches induced by phenol are restricted to the region of contact, notably the hands and arms.

Tinea versicolor also may be confused with vitiligo (see above). Vitiligo is more frequent in patients with thyroid disease, Addison's disease, pernicious anemia, and alopecia areata.

Therapy

There is no early medical therapy for vitiligo that will affect its course. Therefore, if new vitiliginous patches are appearing or extending, it is best to wait for the depigmentation to stabilize before beginning treatment. Several products are available that hide the lesions, with various degrees of success. They are either stains, including Dy-O-Derm and Vitadye, or cosmetics, such as Covermark, Dermablend, and Erase; all of these preparations are available without prescription at local department store or drug store cosmetic counters. The proper shading and use of Covermark needs to be taught; the Lydia O'Leary Co. (New York, NY 10022) will provide the names of local cosmetologists trained in the use of their products. One advantage of cosmetics over stains is that they provide a barrier to sunlight; the patches of vitiligo are easily sunburned since there are no melanocytes to produce tanning.

Patients with vitiligo should be advised always to use a sunblocker with an SPF of 15 or more before any sun exposure (see "Sunburn," above). Not only will sunburning of the patches of vitiligo be minimized but normal skin will tan less, thus minimizing the contrast between the light and dark areas.

When to Refer

Options used by a dermatologist include repigmentation with psoralen and long wave ultraviolet light (PUVA) or bleaching residual dark skin with hydroquinone. Both procedures generally are beyond the scope (and equipment) of the generalist; further, both are time consuming and potentially dangerous; PUVA can lead to severe ultraviolet light burns and perhaps, late skin cancer; and hydroquinone is irritating and a contact sensitizer. Only about half of the patients will respond to PUVA and up to a year may be required for repigmentation to be "adequate." Bleaching residual dark skin to white will not be acceptable to all patients.

WARTS

Presentation

There are several types of warts, generally classified on the basis of their location or their appearance. These clinical types were once thought to be caused by the same virus, but each is known now to be due to a DNA papilloma virus (papovavirus) of a different antigenic subtype (2). Warts are all mildly contagious, venereal warts more than the others, and have an incubation period, after inoculation, of 1 to several months. They are frequent in immunosuppressed individuals in whom they may be nearly impossible to eradicate. However, in normal individuals, spontaneous involution is common; half will clear in 1 year.

The major types of warts are vulgaris, plantar, flat, and venereal.

Verruca Vulgaris (Common Wart)

Presentation

Common warts start as minute papules and grow over many weeks or months to raised, rough, cauliflower-like papules. They are most common on the extremities but may be found on any part of the body in persons of all ages. One should consider that the patient may have become infected by a friend or family member. Should they be the source, they will need to be treated also.

Differential Diagnosis

It is important to consider molluscum contagiosum (scattered small pearly umbilicated papules in the skin and caused by a virus, also discussed in Chapter 94) in children and young adults, and seborrheic keratoses or cutaneous horns in the elderly.

Therapy

Numerous methods to treat warts are used, some easier than others (Table 100.4). A most convenient, painless, and usually effective office treatment is salicylic acid and lactic acid in flexible collodion (Duofilm or Occlusal HP, requires a prescription), which works by softening the keratin in which the wart is growing, thereby allowing the wart to be pared away. It is particularly useful for warts around the nail as the medication seeps under the nail. The patient should follow the directions in the package insert, which suggests soaking the wart, at bedtime, in warm water for 5 minutes and then applying a small drop of medi-

Table 100.4.
Treatment of Warts in Order of Ease of Use

1. Salicylic acid/lactic acid in collodion (Duofilm or Occlusal HP) (podophyllin for venereal warts)
2. Liquid nitrogen
3. Electrodesiccation and curettage
4. Surgical or laser excision

cation to the wart with the applicator or a toothpick; the surrounding skin should be avoided to reduce irritation. The solution dries quickly. The patient should reapply three more drops, allowing each to dry before applying the next one. Excess dead tissue should be pared using a pumice stone or razor blade (if the patient is able) the next morning. The therapy should be stopped for a day or 2 if the area becomes sore. The patient should continue treatment for 5 days, after which the wart usually is tender; at that time the patient should stop treatment to allow the inflammation to subside and should repeat the course every 2 weeks until clear.

A common alternative initial therapy is liquid nitrogen. If liquid nitrogen is available, each wart should be frozen for 20 seconds by using a thick cotton swab pulled to a narrow point. The aim is to get full freezing of the wart as well as 2 to 3 mm beyond. It is important to avoid the lateral sides of the fingers as the digital nerves are subject to damage. The digital nerve is located at the tip of the crease made when the finger is flexed. Liquid nitrogen freezing is painful; the area will hurt for several hours. A blister usually develops 2 to 3 days later. If the blister becomes inconveniently large, the patient can be allowed to puncture it with a sterile needle to drain the contents, but it need not be deroofed. An 80% cure rate is usual. The patient should return in 1 month for retreatment if not clear. A large number of patients with warts must be treated to justify the expense of the material. Storage vessels are available (costing approximately $500), and only monthly replenishment (from a gas-medical supplier, listed as such in the telephone directory, costs about $80) is needed.

If initial therapy did not work and if facilities are available, the next best alternative is electrodesiccation and curettage; referral to a dermatologist may be appropriate at this point. One should consider underlying immunosuppression, such as Hodgkin's disease, diabetes mellitus, or drug abuse, if the warts are extensive and resistant.

Plantar Warts (See Also Chapter 102)

Presentation

Plantar warts can be troublesome in that they tend to be persistent and painful. They are not raised from the surface like other warts but extend into the horny layer. They may be distinguished from corns and calluses by paring them down with a scalpel blade. Warts show a speckled surface due to blood in dilated capillaries, whereas a shiny smooth surface is typical of corns. Corns and calluses are likely to be bilateral and over pressure points, especially the metatarsal heads, whereas warts may develop at any site.

Therapy

The goal of treatment is to destroy the wart without producing a scar, as such scars may be permanently painful. The best way to avoid scars is to avoid the use of surgical or electrodesiccation techniques in therapy. Surgical procedures may be justified if the wart proves untreatable by chemical means, but surgery is not appropriate initially. X-ray therapy is infrequently used as it also produces late scarring.

For initial therapy, the patient may use salicylic acid and lactic acid in flexible collodion (Duofilm or Occlusal HP) in the same way as suggested for verruca vulgaris. A single drop covered by an occlusive tape, as described, seems to work better than does the open technique. Salicylic acid plaster (such as Duke—available in rolls from a physician supply store or pharmacy or Scholls—available in individual plasters; both available without prescription) also may be used at bedtime under occlusive tape, followed by paring each morning (see above).

Freezing with liquid nitrogen does not work as well on the sole as elsewhere because of the thickness of the plantar surface.

Treatment of plantar warts can be frustrating; the physician may wish to refer a patient to a dermatologist or podiatrist if the warts are extensive or prove resistant.

Flat Warts

Presentation

Flat warts remain smaller than verruca vulgaris, usually only 2 to 3 mm in size, and are barely raised above the surface. Although always superficial, flat warts are troublesome because they usually are numerous and affect exposed parts, such as the face, neck, or legs. Flat warts often are spread by nicking the skin during shaving, with implanting of the virus.

Therapy

For a small number of flat warts, liquid nitrogen, salicylic acid/lactic acid in flexible collodion (Duofilm—see above), or gentle electrodesiccation may be satisfactory. Aggressive procedures should be avoided in order to prevent scarring. If numerous, 0.025% vitamin A acid gel (Retin-A gel, requires a prescription) should be prescribed once or twice daily. An electric razor or depilatory may be used to decrease spreading of the warts through nicks and autoinoculation. Spread to other family members is unlikely.

Flat warts take a long time to cure, perhaps months. Patients with flat warts usually are referred to a dermatologist.

Venereal Warts

Presentation

Also called moist warts, acuminate warts, or condyloma acuminatum, these primarily affect the anogenital area and usually are acquired through sexual contact. They seem to be more contagious than other types of warts. Patients may not be aware of intraurethral, anal, or intravaginal warts and must be properly examined. The physician should suspect homosexuality in a male with anal or perianal warts. All patients with venereal warts should be examined for other venereal diseases that may have been contracted. Venereal warts are also discussed in Chapter 94.

Differential Diagnosis

Condylomata of secondary syphilis (an STS always is positive in secondary syphilis) and malignancies, such as Bowen's disease or extramammary Paget's disease, must be considered (see Chapter 95).

Therapy

The mainstay of treatment is 20 to 25% podophyllin, an extract of the mandrake plant, in tincture of benzoin. Podophyllin is a poison and should never be dispensed to the patient. It works only for the moist verrucous warts, less well on dry warts located on the shaft of the penis or on the scrotum. Podophyllin should be applied carefully with a wooden stick just to the wart; it is quite irritating to normal skin. The benzoin should dry for a few minutes before the patient is allowed to dress. The medication should be thoroughly washed off in 4 hours. If this initial treatment has not been too irritating, the medication may be left on longer after the next application. It is important not to apply podophyllin to large areas at one time if the warts are extensive because it is quite irritating. The patient should return weekly for retreatment.

After several treatments, a nubbin of the wart may remain. As the wart is now dry, it may not resolve further with podophyllin; liquid nitrogen or electrodesiccation may be needed for final cure. Usually at least four treatments are necessary. Podophyllin should not be used in pregnant women as it is potentially cytotoxic to the fetus.

If the warts are vaginal or urethral, referral to a gynecologist or urologist is appropriate. If cutaneous warts recur or prove recalcitrant to therapy, a biopsy or referral to a dermatologist for diagnosis and further therapy is warranted.

XEROSIS (DRY SKIN)

Presentation

"Dry," itchy, and scaly skin is common, increasing in frequency and degree in the elderly. Although usually generalized, xerosis is most frequent and severe on the legs. The cause is not fully understood, but there are diminished epidermal lipids, allowing loss of normally retained moisture from the stratum corneum. For that reason, dry skin is exacerbated by excessive soapy bathing and relieved somewhat by lubricating creams. Xerosis is worse in the winter when the humidity of warm air in the house is lowest.

Differential Diagnosis

A generalized itchy dermatitis, especially in the elderly, may be associated with underlying renal or hepatic insufficiency, diabetes mellitus, thyroid and other endocrine diseases, or lymphoma. Xerosis, to varying degrees, is present in all patients with atopic dermatitis. If present since an early age, the physician should consider congenital ichthyosis.

Therapy

The patient should reduce the frequency of hot water bathing generally to no more than twice a week and reduce the use of soap; both remove lipids and increase water loss and itching. For additional details, see "Bathing Instructions for Dry or Irritated Skin," page 1376.

Topical corticosteroids are not helpful. Antihistamines merely sedate and should be avoided for simple xerosis. The house or at least the sitting and sleeping rooms should be humidified. Successful treatment requires persistent care.

The patient should be much improved after the first course of treatment; if not relieved, the physician should consider underlying disease and obtain appropriate laboratory studies (see above).

BENIGN AND MALIGNANT GROWTHS

New growth on the skin are common, particularly in later life. It is important to be on the lookout for lesions during the physical examination and to distinguish benign from premalignant and/or malignant new growths. Two references provide resource information on skin tumors (1, 12).

Cysts

Epidermal inclusion cysts are the most common newly appearing nodules in the skin. Their size ranges from 3 to 30 mm. Their surface is normal in color, but they may have a central, horny punctum. Most cysts start as dermal inclusions of epidermis and expand as horny material and sebum are produced within the cyst. About 10% of cysts, most on the scalp, are pilar cysts, composed of the expanded outer root sheath of a hair follicle.

Cysts are asymptomatic, except that they are annoying and unsightly, unless ruptured. If the wall of a cyst ruptures, their contents of keratin, hair, and sebum leak into the skin, and a brisk foreign body inflammatory reaction ensues. The reaction eventually subsides or drains, causing the cyst to shrink or disappear. If the cyst persists or reappears, it will be more bound in place. Cysts are not premalignant.

If the cyst is unsightly or irritating it may be excised or, if large, may be drained through a small incision and the sac pulled out through the opening with a hemostat. An inflamed cyst resolves more quickly after being injected with 0.2 to 0.5 ml of undiluted triamcinolone acetonide (Kenalog, 10 mg/ml).

A *milium* is a superficial 1- to 2-mm epidermal inclusion cyst that looks like a grain of rice embedded in the skin. Milia develop in adulthood, most commonly on the face and more frequently in women than men. They persist but remain small. Milia can be removed by nicking the surface with a surgical blade and expressing the contents.

Fibroma

Any fleshy, skin-colored growth with a normal-appearing, noneroded surface extending out from the skin is almost certainly benign and is most likely a fibroma or an intradermal nevus. *Skin tags* are small fibromas that appear at sites of friction, especially the neck, axilla, and groin. Skin tags can be easily snipped off with a scissors, often without anesthesia.

Keloid or Hypertrophic Scar

A keloid is a hyperplastic mass of fibrous connective tissue occurring in the dermis and originating from a scar. A keloid extends beyond the edge of the scar and involves normal skin, whereas a hypertrophic scar is restricted to the scar line. Keloids alone tend to recur if excised, but both conditions may be unsightly, and tenderness in the firmer lesions can interfere with wearing of clothing. Keloids are most common in blacks.

Both keloids and hypertrophic scars can be made softer and less tender by injecting them with undiluted triamcinolone acetonide (Kenalog, 10 mg/ml). One should use a 1-ml tuberculin syringe with no finer than a 25-gauge needle, as high pressure often is needed to inject the suspension into the growth. The injections are repeated at monthly intervals for 2 to 3 months, using enough material to make the keloid bulge out. If the keloid is treated by excision, postoperative intralesional injections of triamcinolone acetonide diminish the likelihood of recurrences. An injection at the time of surgery and at 2- to 3-week intervals for two to three injections after surgery should be used. Because the corticosteroid delays wound healing, the wound must be protected from dehiscence by adhesive taping. The patient should be advised not to repierce an ear that has had a keloid. Pressure garments (require referral to a physical therapist) have been used for large keloids or hypertropic scars and can produce excellent results, but 4 to 6 months of use may be required. They also may be used to decrease recurrence after keloids or hypertrophic scars are surgically removed.

Lipoma

Lipomas are soft lumps ranging in size from a bean to a fist or larger, located deep within the subcutaneous fat. The overlying skin may be elevated, but there are not surface changes. Usually only one or two are present, but some patients have multiple lipomas. Single lipomas are more common in women than men and are sporadic, whereas the multiple type usually occurs only in men and is hereditary. Lipomas develop during adulthood and persist indefinitely. Lumps in the skin that become inflamed are more likely to be epidermal inclusion cysts. Malignant degeneration is rare; liposarcomas generally arise de novo, not in pre-existing lipomas.

Seborrheic Keratoses

These are common and practically universal, characterized by an irregular, rather than smooth, surface that feels waxy on being rubbed. These keratoses are superficial and they feel "stuck on" the skin rather than implanted or growing into the skin. They vary in color from beige or dark brown to black, occasionally resembling a malignant melanoma. Seborrheic keratoses never become malignant. Examples of seborrheic keratoses are shown in Figure 100.13.

The usual reason for their removal is bothersome irritation from clothing, belts, or straps or because their appearance is unacceptable to the patient. The simplest usually effective therapy for seborrheic keratoses is to paint them with trichloroacetic acid (obtainable from a pharmacy for office use but too caustic to be dispensed to the patient). The compound should be kept in the refrigerator. The keratoses should be lightly painted, taking care to avoid normal skin using a 50% solution on the face and 75% elsewhere. After about a minute the lesion will turn white and the patient will notice mild burning, which will subside shortly. A wet gauze sponge may be used to cool the skin and to remove excess acid. During the next week, the lesion will form a crust and fall away; however, thick lesions may require two or three monthly applications. One drop of trichloroacetic acid in the wrong place can cause great damage; therefore, the physician should take care not to hold the bottle or the applicator near the patient's eyes. If the lesions are thick or irritated, they may be lightly curetted after local anesthesia. Hemostasis may be obtained by fulguration or by application of Monsel's solution with a cotton-tipped applicator.

Cherry Angiomas

These common lesions are 1- to 3-mm bright red, cherry-colored, nonblanching, shiny papules usually located on the trunk (Fig. 100.14). These are not premalignant. Because of their small size and lack of bleeding tendencies, therapy is not warranted.

Nevi

A nevus, which is a new growth, typically is round, tan to dark brown in color, sharply outlined and present since early adulthood. Although nevi usually are benign, each must be examined with care. If the patient believes the lesion recently has changed, or if the lesion has been bleeding, has irregular or dark pigment, or is large, removal is justified. However, less than half of all malignant melanomas come from pre-existing nevi and the average adult has 20 pigmented nevi; prophylactic removal of all moles is practically impossible and certainly unjustified. If the primary reason for removal is cosmetic, without evidence of recent changes or suspicious signs, and if the mole is in a site visible to the patient, such as the face, the mole can be shaved with a scalpel blade to reduce it to the level of the skin surface. Hemostasis is achieved as with seborrheic keratosis removal (see above). The portion removed should be sent for histological examination. The cosmetic result of this "shave removal" is better than with excision, and removal does not increase the likelihood that the nevus will evolve into a melanoma. On the other hand, if there have been recent changes or suspicious signs, the lesion should be excised in its entirety and with adequate margins. Malignant melanoma is discussed below.

Actinic Keratoses

These appear as red, scaly, nonhealing crusty lesions, predominantly restricted to light-exposed areas such as the face, nape, and back of the hands (Fig. 100.15). These keratoses are most common in light-complexioned individuals who have spent a lot of time in the sun. These lesions have a low but real malignant potential and should be destroyed using any one of several methods, usually desiccation and curettage, with local anesthesia or freezing with liquid nitrogen. 5-Fluorouracil (Fluoroplex, Efudex, require prescription) is useful for patients with more than a dozen or so keratoses and has the advantage that early lesions will be destroyed as well. The medication is applied twice daily until irritation develops, normally in 2 weeks, and then continued for an additional 2 weeks. The patient should expect discomfort, redness, and peeling. A topical corticosteroid cream (such as triamcinolone, 0.1%) can be applied four times a day for a week once the reaction has reached its peak. The keratoses will be cleared, but new ones will appear again in about 2 years as the tendency for their development remains. Any lesion still present after the course of topical therapy should be examined by biopsy or removed.

Individuals with actinic keratoses should be examined for recurrence twice yearly. Such patients are most often treated and followed by dermatologists.

Cutaneous Horn

A cutaneous horn is a single, hard, keratotic growth, resembling a wart. Its elevated hard center gives the lesion its name. Although disordered keratin suggests disordered epidermis, most of these lesions are benign. However, they should be surgically removed for microscopic examination, since a few have a focus of squamous cell carcinoma at their base. Patients suspected of having this problem should be referred to a dermatologist or surgeon for removal.

Keratoacanthoma

A keratoacanthoma is a tumor that grows rapidly, usually within weeks, often becoming as large as a marble with a characteristic umbilicated hard keratotic center (Fig. 100.16). Most patients are over the age of 50. Because most of the tumors occur in men and appear on the arms and hands, an occupational etiology has been suggested. These tumors also are more frequent in immunosuppressed patients.

Although technically benign, keratoacanthomas resemble squamous cell carcinoma and act aggressively. Although it is safest to treat a keratoacanthoma by excision, wide excision is unnecessary. Left untreated, some have healed spontaneously in 4 to 12 months, generally leaving an unsightly scar. Although local surgery is curative, new tumors may appear elsewhere. Patients with a keratoacanthoma usually are referred to a dermatologist or surgeon.

Basal Cell Carcinoma

Basal cell carcinoma is a slowly spreading malignant growth that usually is single, shiny or pearly colored, with fine telangiectasias over the surface and a depressed center (Fig. 100.17). Most appear on light-exposed parts of the skin, particularly the face, neck, or forearms. Basal cell carcinomas account for about 80% of skin cancers. If left untreated, they can invade deeply, but they rarely spread distantly; fewer than 100 cases of metastatic basal cell cancer have been reported.

Sunlight is the most obvious environmental inducer of basal cell cancers. These cancers are rare in blacks. After confirmation of the diagnosis by biopsy, the lesion can be destroyed by either desiccation and curettage or excision, with about equal cure rates when performed by skilled practitioners. Because invasion tends to be deeper in the folds about the mouth, nose, and eyes, surgery in these areas needs to be more aggressive. Patients suspected of having a basal cell carcinoma should be referred to a dermatologist or surgeon.

Squamous Cell Carcinoma

A squamous cell carcinoma usually is firm and irregular with a scaly, keratotic, bleeding, and friable surface (Fig. 100.18). Like basal cell cancers, squamous cell cancers occur most often on sun-exposed parts, but they also appear on covered areas or adjacent to chronic trauma, such as leg ulcers, burn scars, or sites of radiation therapy. Squamous cell cancers arising in trauma sites have a higher potential to metastasize than do those that arise in an actinic keratosis. The lower lip is a frequent location because of both chronic sun exposure and chronic irritation from heat and tobacco tar in smokers. Squamous cell cancers account for about 20% of skin cancers.

Patients suspected of having squamous cell carcinoma should be referred to a dermatologist or surgeon. Primary treatment is surgical. Electrosurgery, radiation, and cryosurgery are less definitive alternative techniques.

ing and are useful for pruritic lesions, such as poison ivy dermatitis, sunburn, acute drug eruptions, viral exanthems, and urticaria. The most commonly used shake lotion is calamine lotion, a suspension of zinc oxide and iron oxide with glycerin and calcium hydroxide. Phenolated or mentholated calamine improves the antipruritic properties of the lotion and is available in most pharmacies. Diphenhydramine in calamine lotion, such as Caladryl, should not be used because of the risk of sensitization to the antihistamine.

Pastes

Zinc oxide, as either paste or ointment (available without prescription), is used to provide protection and adsorption of serous drainage in acute and subacute oozing dermatitis, such as diaper dermatitis, intertrigo, pruritus ani (see Chapter 92), and acute dyshidrotic eczema. The paste is applied thickly, like icing on a cake, twice daily, and is easily removed with cotton balls moistened with mineral oil.

Corticosteroids

Topical corticosteroids are the most common topical anti-inflammatory agents prescribed. At least 20 brands are marketed, and most are available in various vehicles and in different strengths. A weak formulation with up to 0.5% hydrocortisone is available under several brand names without a prescription. The range of potency of preparations available by prescription is given in Table 100.5. Although a more potent preparation is occasionally needed for a recalcitrant eruption, the main difference between products is a difference in the speed of onset of improvement, differing by a day or 2, rather than a difference in final outcome. The most common reason that a prescribed

Table 100.5.
Some Topical Corticosteroids Grouped by Potency (within Potency Groups, Arranged Alphabetically)

VERY HIGH POTENCY
  Temovate ointment
  Diprolene ointment
  Psorcon ointment
HIGH POTENCY
  Cyclocort ointment
  Diprosone cream and ointment
  Halog cream
  Lidex cream, ointment, and solution
  Topicort cream
  Valisone ointment
INTERMEDIATE POTENCY
  Cordran cream, lotion, and ointment
  Cyclocort cream
  Synalar cream, ointment, and solution
  Triamcinolone cream, gel, lotion, and ointment
  Valisone cream and lotion
  Westcort cream and ointment
LOW POTENCY
  Desonide cream (nonfluorinated)
  Locorten cream (nonfluorinated)
  Hydrocortisone, dexamethasone, flumethasone, prednisolone, and methylprednisolone

corticosteroid is ineffective is that it is given for the wrong diagnosis or in too small an amount.

All topical corticosteroids are expensive, generally $5 to $10 an ounce. It is common for insufficient amounts to be prescribed because of this expense and because physicians generally underestimate the amount needed. About an ounce of any topical preparation is needed to cover the entire body once. As an example of the amount needed, consider treatment of both thighs and legs three times a day for 3 weeks: Although only about a third of the total surface area is to be treated, about 1.5 pounds will be required (30 g $\times$ 0.33 $\times$ 3 times a day $\times$ 21 days = 630 g), which may cost $50 to $100. There are several ways to reduce the amount and costs of topical corticosteroid therapy. Creams can be spread further if applied when the skin is slightly damp, and the use of the corticosteroid should be limited to inflamed parts with only a moisturizer (see above) used elsewhere. Patients may use the steroid preparation for lubrication unless instructed otherwise. Also the corticosteroid may be used at bedtime with plastic wrap occlusion. The least expensive full strength topical corticosteroid is triamcinolone, which is available as a generic and in amounts up to 240 g.

Choice of Vehicle

Creams contain oils emulsified into water and appear white, whereas ointments are oils or oils into which water is emulsified and look and feel greasy, like petrolatum. Creams should be used for acute and subacute dermatitis where there is oozing because creams are miscible with serous fluids; ointments should be used for chronic dermatitis with scale and itching because they are better absorbed through intact skin. Corticosteroid solutions (Lidex or Synalar), lotions (Cordran or Valisone), or gels (triamcinolone, Benisone, or Lidex) are useful in hairy or intertriginous regions or in the ear canals.

Occlusion

Absorption and effectiveness are increased by covering a corticosteroid cream with plastic film, such as plastic gloves or kitchen wrap (e.g., Glad or Saran) held in place by cotton gloves or socks. The plastic holds the preparation in place, interferes with scratching away the steroid, and improves absorption by hydrating the horny layer. A cream should be used for occlusion treatment rather than an ointment, which is more likely to induce miliaria and folliculitis. A convenient occlusive treatment for small areas is an occlusive tape, Cordran tape, available in 60- and 200-cm lengths by prescription, in which a corticosteroid has been incorporated in the adhesive. The tape can be left on for up to 36 hours and removed for 12 hours to prevent maceration.

Warnings

Potent topical corticosteroids may mask underlying skin infections, contact allergies, and even suppress inflammatory reactions to cutaneous tumors and lymphoma. Discrete lesions should be examined by biopsy, and referral to a dermatologist should be considered for any eruption that is persistent.

Local complications may follow the use of any topical corticosteroid but are most common after the use of those in the high and intermediate potency groups. Complications include persistent erythema and telangiectasis, an acneform eruption, interference with healing, atrophic striae, and easy bruising. Glaucoma and cataracts may develop after months of use near the eyes. Systemic effects from absorbed corticosteroids in adults do not develop unless more than half the body is treated with high potency corticosteroids under plastic occlusion for several months. When systemic effects occur, they include hypertension, glucose intolerance, glaucoma, salt and water retention, and depressed pituitary-adrenal responsiveness. However, growth retardation and hypertension have been reported in small children after using potent topical corticosteroids without occlusion.

Intralesional Corticosteroids

Long-acting corticosteroids injected intralesionally often shrink epidermal inclusion cysts, inflammatory acne cysts, and hypertrophic scars and keloids. This therapy also may benefit other disorders, including lichen simplex chronicus, alopecia areata, granuloma annulare, psoriasis, and discoid lupus erythematosus. The most common preparation used is a suspension of triamcinolone acetonide (Kenalog, 10 mg/ml). The full strength concentration should be used only for scar reduction because that dose will induce skin atrophy. For general use, the preparation may be injected after diluting it to about 3 mg/ml, because this level usually does not cause atrophy. The dilution is made by first drawing up two volumes of saline and, after thorough shaking of the stock, one volume of corticosteroid suspension. The benefit usually occurs slowly over about a month when a second injection should be given if needed.

Warnings

Complications of intralesional corticosteroid injections include atrophy or dimpling, local increase or decrease in pigmentation, and, rarely, telangiectasis or local infection. Atrophic dimpling usually resolves in 6 to 12 months. Patients with disorders requiring intralesional steroid injections usually are referred to a dermatologist.

Topical Antimicrobials

Topical antibiotics have only limited use, because infections superficial enough to respond to topical antibiotics also respond to simple cleansing and compresses. However, they have proven useful in mild inflammatory acne vulgaris. All have the potential to induce sensitization and allergic contact dermatitis, suggested by the appearance of redness, scale, and itching. For example, contact dermatitis is a common development during therapy of chronic leg ulcers. The reaction may be against the active agent or against a preservative or fragrance.

Topical Antifungal Agents

Common superficial fungal infections are caused either by dermatophytes or by a yeast, almost always *Candida albicans*. Infections may involve any body surface but are most frequent in warm moist areas, such as the feet and groin.

Broad spectrum topical antifungal preparations (all require a prescription except as noted), effective against both dermatophytes and yeast, include ciclopirox (Loprox cream, 15/30 g), clotrimazole (Lotrimin cream, 15/30/45/90 g, and solution, 10/30 ml, and Mycelex cream, 15/30/45 g, and solution, 10/30 g), econazole (Spectazole, 15/30/85 g), ketoconazole (Nizoral cream, 15g) and miconazole (Monistat-Derm cream, 15/30/90 g, and lotion, 30/60 ml, available without prescription). Haloprogin (Halotex cream, 15/30 g, and solution, 10/30 ml) and tolnaftate (Tinactin cream, solution, and powder, available without prescription) are useful for dermatophytes but not *Candida*. Nystatin requires a prescription, (Mycostatim or generic cream, ointment, or powder) and is effective against candidal infections only. Nystatin oral preparations are poorly absorbed from the gastrointestinal tract and, therefore, have no effect on skin or systemic infections. However, oral nystatin may be needed if a groin infection recurs, as the gastrointestinal tract may be a reservoir for *Candida*. Oral nystatin is given as 1 teaspoon of the suspension (100,000 units/teaspoon) four times for 3 days for a total of 60 ml. Topical amphotericin B (Fungizone cream, 20 g, lotion, 30 ml, and ointment, 20 g) also is effective against candidiasis, but it is more expensive and may stain the skin.

Topical antifungal agents are used twice daily, on arising and before bedtime, except for yeast infections in the diaper area that should be retreated with each diaper change. In addition to the topical agent, local heat and moisture must be decreased. Measures that increase ventilation and maintain dryness include the use of cotton underclothing or socks, open and leather shoes rather than vinyl or rubber boots or sneakers, and the liberal use of talcum powder. Although topical antifungal agents are believed to be safe when used during pregnancy, there are no adequate studies, and, therefore, the drugs should be used in pregnant women only if necessary.

General References

Arndt KA: *Manual of Dermatologic Therapeutics*, 4th ed. Boston, Little, Brown, and Co, 1989.
  Handbook of therapy including details of usage, trade names, and prices.
Epstein E: *Common Skin Disorders*, 3rd ed. Oradell, NJ, Medical Economics Co, 1988.
  Practical advice including tear-sheets for the patient.
Fitzpatrick TB, Eisen AZ, Wolff K, et al: *Dermatology in General Medicine*, 3rd ed. New York, McGraw-Hill, 1987.
  Complete reference for the specialist. It includes an exclusive discussion of pathophysiology of skin disease.

Lamberg SI: *Dermatology in Primary Care*. Philadelphia, WB Saunders, 1986.

    A practical, problem-oriented guide to dermatology.

Specific References

1. Andrade R, Crumport S, Popkin L (eds): *Cancer of the Skin*. Philadelphia, WB Saunders, 1976.
2. Beutner KR: Human papilloma virus infection. *J Am Acad Dermatol* 20:114, 1989.
3. Bjornberg A, Hellgren I: Pityriasis rosea. *Acta Derm Venereol* 42:1, 1962.
4. Dicken CH, Powell ST, Spear KT: Evaluation of isotretinoin treatment of hidradenitis suppurativa. *J Am Acad Dermatol* 11:500, 1984.
5. Eady EA, Holland CT, Cunliffe WJ: The use of antibiotics in acne therapy. *J Antimicrob Chemother* 10:89, 1982.
6. Esman V, Geil JP, Kroon S, et al: Prednisone does not prevent post-herpetic neuralgia. *Lancet* 2(8551):126, 1987.
7. Estes SA: Diagnosis and management of scabies. *Med Clin North Am* 66:955, 1983.
8. Fisher AA: *Contact Dermatitis*, 3rd ed. Philadelphia, Lea & Febiger, 1986.
9. Grice K: Treatment of hyperhidrosis. *Clin Exp Dermatol* 7:183, 1982.
10. Habif TP: *Clinical Dermatology*. St. Louis, CV Mosby, Co., 1985. p. 214.
11. Hanifin JM: Atopic dermatitis. *J Am Acad Dermatol* 16:1, 1982.
12. Lever WF: Schaumburg-Lever G: *Histopathology of the Skin*, 6th ed. Philadelphia, Lippincott, 1983.
13. Jones HE: Therapy for superficial fungal infections. *Med Clin North Am* 66:871, 1982.
14. McKendrick MW, McGill JI, White JE, Wood MJ: Oral Acyclovir in acute herpes zoster. *Br Med J* 293:1529, 1986.
15. Melski JW, Arndt KA: Topical therapy for acne. *N Engl J Med* 302:503, 1980.
16. Muller SA: Alopecia: syndromes of genetic significance. *J Invest Dermatol* 60:475, 1973.
17. Odland GF, Kraning KK: Prevalence, morbidity and cost of dermatological diseases. *J Invest Dermatol* 73:395, 1979.
18. Roenigk Jr HH (eds): *Psoriasis*. New York, Marcel Dekker, Inc., 1985. p.667.
19. Savin RC: Systemic ketoconazole in tinea versicolor. *J Am Acad Dermatol* 10:824, 1984.
20. Shalita AR, Cunningham WJ, Leydin JJ: Isotretinoin treatment of acne and related disorders. *J Am Acad Dermatol* 9:629, 1983.
21. Shuster S: The etiology of dandruff and the mode of action of therapeutic agents. *Br J Dermatol* 111:235, 1984.
22. Strauss SE: Herpes simplex virus infection, biology, treatment and prevention. *Ann Intern Med* 103:404, 1985.

C H A P T E R 101

Common Problems of the Teeth and Oral Cavity

DOUGLAS K. MACLEOD, D.M.D.

    The purpose of this chapter is 2-fold: first, to provide guidelines for recognizing, treating, and referring patients with acute dental and oral problems properly; and second, to increase the physician's awareness of chronic dental and oral problems that may require referral and treatment. These types of problems are often neglected by the patient because of fear or ignorance about possible corrective treatment, because of anticipated pain from the procedure, or because of the anticipated cost of treatment.

ORAL EXAMINATION

    The oral cavity should be examined systematically. The examination should include lips, cheeks (buccal mucosa), hard and soft palate, salivary ducts (parotid duct orifice in the buccal mucosa opposite the upper second molars and submandibular duct orifice beside the lingual frenulum), tonsillar area, tongue, floor of the mouth, gingiva, and teeth, noting the normal structures and any deviations from normal.

    A dental examination includes an evaluation of the number (20 in the primary dentition and 32 in the permanent dentition—see Fig. 101.1), position, and

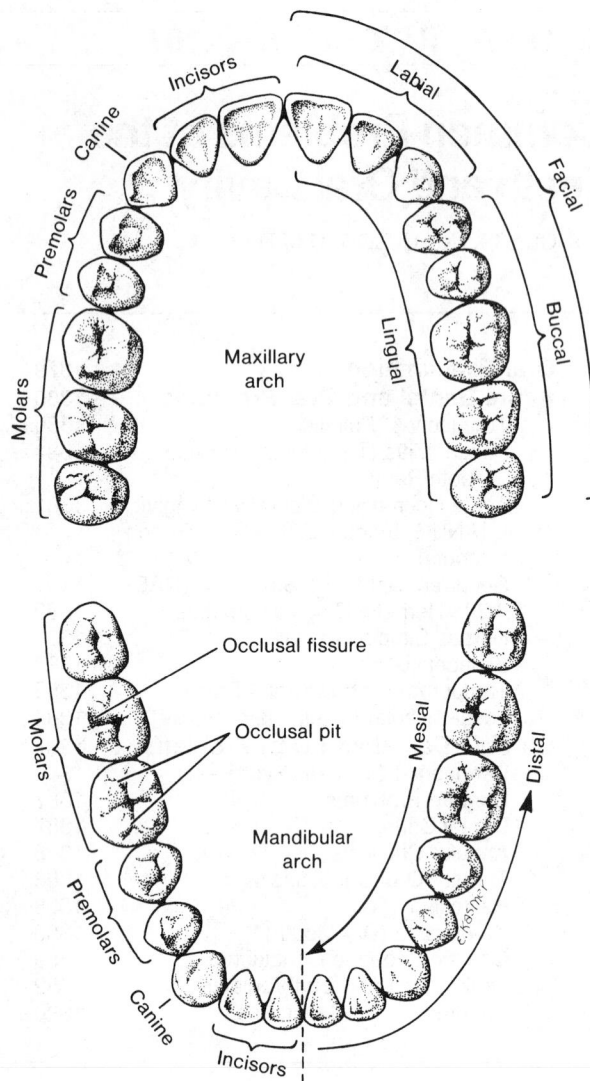

Figure 101.1. Permanent dentition.

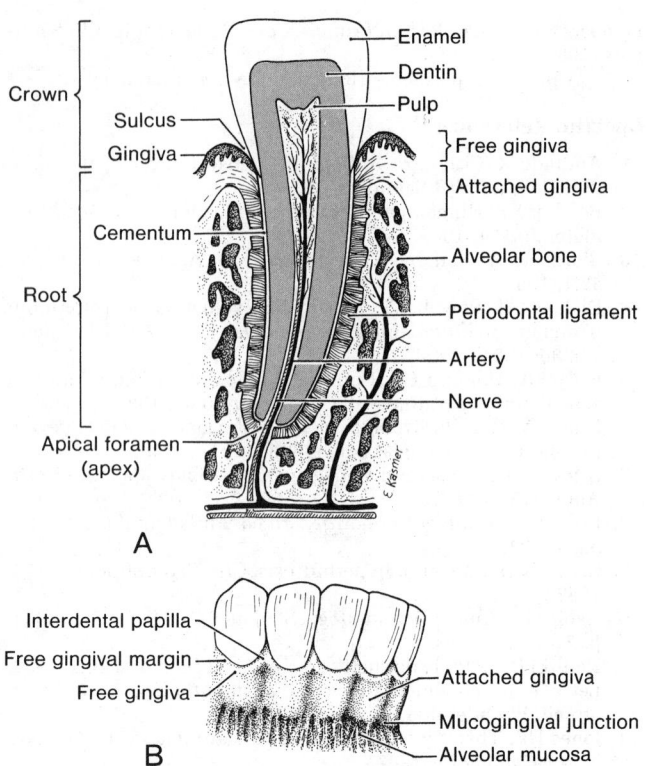

Figure 101.2. Structure of normal teeth and gingiva. *A.* A tooth and its parts. *B.* Teeth and gingiva.

arrangement of the teeth, and a check for caries (see below), erosions, abrasions, and fractures. It is important to examine the gingiva completely. The normal healthy gingiva is firm, pink, nontender, and does not bleed on palpation. The parts of a tooth and its adjacent structures are shown in Figure 101.2, A and B.

ACUTE DENTAL AND ORAL PROBLEMS

Toothaches (Pulpitis)

Presentation

Patients with toothache present with a large carious lesion (see "Dental Caries," page 1387), a large restoration (filling), or a combination of both. In the early stages, there is inflammation involving a portion of the pulp tissue (the central portion of the tooth, containing vital soft tissue—see Fig. 101.2A). There is relatively severe pain in response to thermal stimuli,

particularly to cold, and this pain persists for longer than 15 seconds after the stimulus is removed. As the area of inflammation increases, the pain becomes more severe; it may radiate to the suborbital area, to the side of the face, or to the ear. When total necrosis of the pulp occurs, sensitivity to thermal stimuli is lost. If at this point the inflammatory exudate cannot escape into the oral cavity, the pressure is released via the root apex; and there is exquisite sensitivity to percussion of the crown of the tooth. The signs and symptoms of pulpitis may be confused with pericoronitis (painful wisdom teeth, see below) or periodontitis (see below), and without further diagnostic aids (i.e., dental radiographs) it may be difficult to differentiate between these conditions.

If pulpitis is not treated, complications may occur, ranging from a localized alveolar abscess (an abscess of the bony supporting structure of the teeth) to facial cellulitis. The rate and type of complication depend upon the location of the affected tooth, host resistance, and the virulence of the bacteria present.

Treatment

Depending upon the situation when the patient is seen, one has three options. For patients who are afebrile and have no extraoral swelling (a swelling producing facial asymmetry) or intraoral swelling (swelling causing disruption of the supporting alveolar bone and soft tissue), analgesics (acetaminophen, 650 mg, and/

or codeine, 30 mg every 4 hours) and referral within 24 hours are indicated. When either slight extraoral or intraoral swelling or a low grade temperature elevation is present, antibiotics (penicillin V, 250 mg, or, for patients allergic to penicillin, erythromycin, 250 mg, every 6 hours) should be added, and the patient should be seen by a dentist within 12 to 24 hours. Patients with temperatures greater than 101°F (38.5°C) with intraoral and/or extraoral swelling causing facial asymmetry need immediate consultation and treatment by a dentist. Treatment of these types of problems varies from extraction of the affected tooth, root canal therapy (endodontics), or incision and drainage, to hospital admission for intravenous antibiotics for facial cellulitis.

Pericoronitis (Third Molar or Wisdom Tooth Pain)

Presentation

Pericoronitis is acute inflammation of the tissue around the crown of a partially erupted tooth. Patients presenting with pericoronitis are usually between the ages of 15 and 25 although the condition rarely can be seen in older individuals if they still have their third molars (see below) and they may give a history of previous subacute episodes of pain of the gingiva that partially covers the crown of an incompletely erupted tooth. The tooth most often affected is the mandibular third molar (wisdom tooth). The space between the crown of the tooth and the overlying gingival flap is an ideal area for the accumulation of food and bacteria; this leads to inflammation. The flap is traumatized by contact with the tooth in the opposing jaw, usually the maxillary third molar, and the inflammation is aggravated.

The patient describes pain that radiates to the ear, the throat, and the floor of the mouth. He complains of a foul taste, and there is swelling of the affected area so that he cannot close the jaw properly. In severe cases, pain spreading to the oropharynx and base of the tongue makes it difficult to swallow. The gingival tissue is markedly red, swollen, and tender (Fig. 101.3A). Occasionally, tender lymphadenopathy and systemic manifestations (fever, leukocytosis, and malaise) are present. Peritonsillar abscess, cellulitis, and Ludwig's angina (cellulitis of the floor of the mouth) are possible complications.

Treatment

In afebrile patients one needs only to make a dental referral and to prescribe analgesics. Febrile patients should be treated with antibiotics (penicillin V, 250 mg, or, for patients allergic to penicillin, erythromycin, 250 mg, every 6 hours) and moderate analgesics (acetaminophen, 650 mg, and/or codeine, 30 mg, every 4 to 6 hours). All patients should be seen by a dentist within 24 hours. Depending upon many factors, the dentist will either excise or debride the flap or remove the partially erupted lower tooth. The preferred treatment for third molars that are erupting in a position

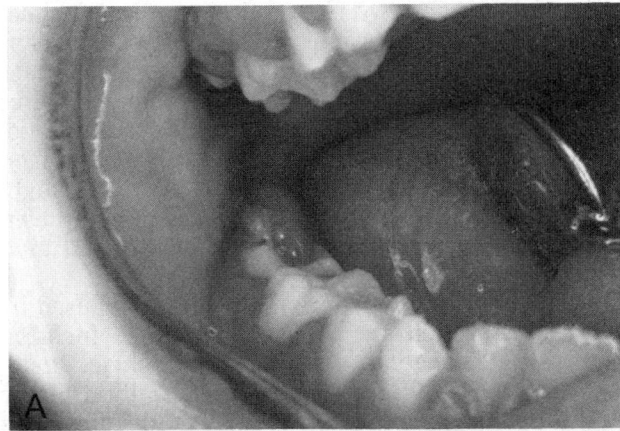
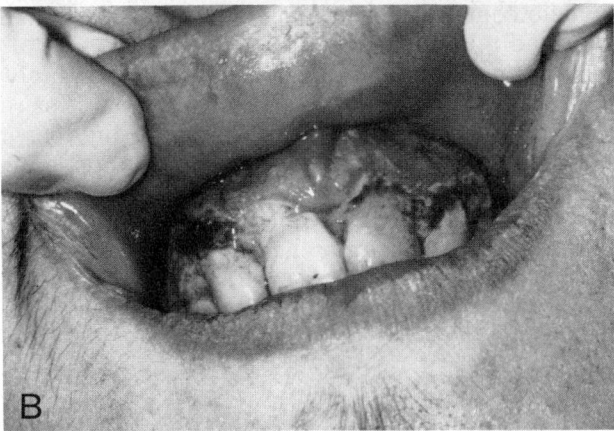

Figure 101.3. *A.* Pericoronitis of the mandibular third molar. *B.* Acute necrotizing ulcerative gingivitis.

that produces poor occlusion is to remove the traumatizing maxillary third molar tooth and to allow the infected flap to heal. The mandibular tooth is then removed 7 to 10 days later, after the acute infection has resolved. When pericoronitis involves eruption of third molars that are in good position for occlusion, the inflamed gingival flap is removed and the teeth are left in place.

Acute Necrotizing Ulcerative Gingivitis (ANUG, Vincent's Infection, Trench Mouth)

Acute necrotizing ulcerative gingivitis, or ANUG, may occur at any age, but is more common among young to middle-aged adults.

Presentation

ANUG has a sudden onset and is usually associated with a debilitating illness or an acute respiratory infection. Often there is a history of a change in the patient's life; for example, protracted work without rest or recent psychological stress. There is a fetid mouth odor and the patient describes a foul metallic taste, increased salivation, spontaneous gingival hemorrhage, and pronounced bleeding upon the slightest stimulation. The lesions are extremely sensitive to touch; pain is constant and gnawing and is intensified by hot or spicy foods. The oral findings are punched-out, crater-like depressions at the crest of the interdental papillae and/or marginal gingiva. The surface of the gingiva is covered by gray pseudomembranous slough that is demarcated from the gingiva by a pronounced linear erythema (Fig. 101.3B). Patients usually have submandibular lymphadenopathy and slight elevation in temperature; in severe cases, high fever, tachycardia, leukocytosis, loss of appetite, and malaise are seen.

Most investigators believe that ANUG is caused by two agents, which are normal oral flora, a fusiform bacillus, and *Borrelia vincentii*, a spirochete. Histologically, the stratified squamous epithelium of the gingiva is ulcerated and replaced by a thick fibrinous exudate containing many polymorphonuclear leukocytes and micro-organisms.

Complications include destruction of the gingiva and underlying supporting tissues, which after repeated episodes of ANUG can result in the loss of teeth. In rare cases, severe sequelae, such as noma (rapid spreading gangrene of oral and facial tissue, which occurs in the debilitated and nutritionally deficient patient), fusospirochetal meningitis, peritonitis, pneumonia, bacteremia, and brain abscess, have been reported.

Treatment

Patients with severe ANUG need immediate hospital admission, intravenous antibiotics, and supportive care (analgesics, hydrogen peroxide mouthwashes) until systemic symptoms subside. Patients with less severe ANUG need immediate attention by a dentist. At this visit, after treatment with a topical anesthetic, a cotton pellet and glyoxide (an oxygenating and foaming agent) are used to remove the pseudomembrane and the surface debris. Antimicrobials are usually prescribed for a few days by the dentist. After irrigating with warm water, the superficial calculus is removed. Patients are instructed to avoid tobacco and alcohol, to rinse with warm water and 3% hydrogen peroxide every 2 hours, and to confine toothbrushing to the removal of surface debris. When these instructions are followed after effective removal of all irritants by the dentist, a patient usually improves markedly within 5 days. If after the acute phase the patient does not continue periodic dental care, ANUG may recur and lead to eventual tooth loss.

Recurrent Aphthous Stomatitis (RAS)

Aphthous ulcers, also called *canker sores*, occur at some time in 20 to 50% of the adult population, are slightly more common in females, have familial tendencies, and occur most frequently during the winter and spring months (5). RAS was once thought to be a recurrent infection by the herpes simplex virus (HSV), but that is not the case; the cause of the condition is, in fact, still unknown.

Presentation

Aphthous stomatitis is characterized by superficial ulcerations on the mucous membranes of the lips, cheek, tongue, floor of the mouth, palate, and gingiva. This condition begins with a prodromal burning 1 to 48 hours before the appearance of discrete vesicles, which are approximately 2 to 5 mm in diameter and are painful. After 2 days, they rupture and form saucer-like ulcers that consist of a red or grayish red central portion and an elevated rim-like periphery. There may be a single lesion or multiple ulcers.

The lesions heal spontaneously within 7 to 10 days. As a rule the lesions are larger than those seen in acute herpetic gingivostomatitis (see below) and do not exhibit the diffuse gingival involvement or systemic symptoms seen in that condition.

RAS occurs in the following forms:

1. *Occasional aphthae* (a single lesion, at intervals from months to years, healing uneventfully).
2. *Acute multiple aphthae* (acute episode persisting for weeks, with lesions developing sequentially at different sites in the mouth, often associated with acute gastrointestinal disorders).
3. *Chronic recurrent aphthae* (one or more lesions always present for a period of years).

Treatment

Treatment of aphthae is symptomatic. A mouthwash containing equal parts of Benadryl suspension and Kaopectate (Benadryl, 5 mg/ml mixed with an equal amount of Kaopectate, prepared by a pharmacist) is helpful in reducing the pain as is viscous Xylocaine applied by cotton-tip applicator to painful lesions. Another useful agent is Zilactin (available without prescription), a 7% tannic acid suspension that is applied four times a day for a few days (usually a minimum of 2 days is necessary). In more severe cases, tetracycline has been successful in decreasing pain and duration of the ulcers; the patient should be instructed to empty a 250-mg capsule in 50 ml of water and to use this as a rinse, which is then swallowed, three or four times a day for 5 to 7 days. The patient should be encouraged to take sufficient amounts of nonirritating liquids or soft food to maintain hydration and nutrition. Intake may be facilitated by using a straw to prevent contact with the painful ulcers.

Acute Herpetic Gingivostomatitis

Acute herpetic gingivostomatitis occurs most frequently in infants and children below the age of 6 years, and it is observed with equal frequency in males and females. It is caused by the herpes simplex virus (HSV), and most oral infections are due to HSV type 1. It does, however, occur in older individuals including rarely the elderly. Most adults have developed immunity to herpes simplex virus as a result of childhood infection, usually inapparent. Although recurrent acute herpetic gingivostomatitis has been reported, it does not usually recur unless immunity has been altered by a debilitating systemic disease.

Presentation

Acute herpetic gingivostomatitis appears as a diffuse, erythematous, shiny involvement of the gingiva and the adjacent oral mucosa with varying degrees of edema and gingival bleeding. In the initial stage it is characterized by the presence of discrete spherical gray vesicles that may occur in the gingiva, the labial and buccal mucosa, the soft palate, the pharynx, the sublingual mucosa, and the tongue. Within 24 hours the vesicles rupture and form small painful ulcers with a red, elevated, halo-like margin and a depressed yellowish or grayish white central portion. Regional lymphadenopathy, fever as high as 105°F (40.5°C), and generalized malaise are common. The course is limited to 7 to 10 days and the ulcers heal without scarring. It is differentiated from RAS (see above) by the diffuse gingival involvement and the systemic symptoms.

Treatment

The management is exactly the same as that for recurrent aphthous stomatitis (see above). Antibacterial agents are not helpful, and corticosteroids are contraindicated. Idoxuridine has been used successfully in treating immunosuppressed patients with primary herpes infections, but because of toxicity its use should be limited to such patients, in consultation with a specialist in infectious disease. The role of oral acyclovir in herpetic gingivostomatitis is uncertain. Its use is probably warranted in the management of severe infection although this should be done in consultation with an infectious disease specialist or a dentist (see Chapter 94, for a discussion of acyclovir).

Herpes Simplex Labialis

Recurrent herpes simplex infections of the lips or perioral area occur in 20 to 40% of the adult population. Evidence suggests that recurrent herpes is not a reinfection but a reactivation of virus that remains latent in the nerve tissue.

Presentation

The natural history of this problem has been well delineated. Most affected subjects have several episodes during an average year. In approximately 60% of episodes, there is prodromal tingling for a number of hours before the appearance of the first vesicles. Pain is moderate to severe during the first 24 hours after appearance of vesicles and then rapidly diminishes. After 48 hours, vesicles are usually replaced by ulcer crusts. The process usually resolves after 7 to 9 days, but lesions may persist as long as 2 weeks.

The therapy of this condition is discussed in Chapter 100, Common Problems of the Skin.

Sialadenitis

Presentation

Sialadenitis is an inflammation of the salivary gland. Patients with sialadenitis present with pain and enlargement of the affected gland. In bacterial sialadenitis, the pain and swelling are not related to eating. The overlying skin may be red and tense, and the affected gland will yield a purulent discharge at the duct oriface. Bacterial sialadenitis is more common in children than in adults. Obstructive sialadenitis is more common than is bacterial infection of the salivary glands and is associated with salivary stones or a mucous plug. It occurs most frequently in middle-aged males. The involved gland is enlarged and painful, and the symptoms are more prominent before, during, and soon after eating. The submandibular gland is most often affected (75% of cases), whereas the parotid (20% of cases) and major sublingual glands (5% of cases) are less often involved. Mumps is more common in children but does occur in adults when it often is more severe. The parotid gland is swollen and tender and there is usually no redness, heat, or discharge. Most often both parotids are involved and, frequently, other salivary glands. Systemic symptoms are common.

Treatment

Treatment of bacterial sialadenitis consists of heat application (external moist heat packs to the affected gland for 15 to 20 minutes and intraoral warm rinses), analgesics (acetaminophen, 650 mg, and/or codeine, 30 mg, every 4 to 6 hours), antibiotics (penicillin V, 250 mg, or, for patients allergic to penicillin, erythromycin, 250 mg, every 6 hours for 10 days), and a liquid diet for the first 2 to 3 days.

The management of obstructive sialadenitis is more complex. When this diagnosis is suspected, the patient should be referred to a dentist or an otolaryngologist. In cases in which the stone is lodged in the duct, the acute phase is managed in the same manner as is bacterial sialadenitis, after which a sialagram is obtained to determine the extent of the problem. Surgical removal of the stone from the duct is eventually performed to prevent recurrence. In chronic obstructive sialadenitis, surgical excision of the gland is often necessary. The likelihood of recurrence after the first episode is unknown.

Temporomandibular Joint Pain

Several studies of healthy populations have shown that symptoms of temporomandibular joint (TMJ) disorders are present at some time in 25 to 50% of people but are not considered a serious problem by most patients (4). The vast majority (70 to 90%) of patients who present with these symptoms are women between the ages of 24 and 40. Multiple factors may lead to TMJ pain; there may be a history of emotional tension, bruxism (grinding of teeth), external blows to the jaws, or whiplash injury. TMJ pain may be present at some point in 20% of patients with rheumatoid arthritis. Patients with osteoarthritis of other joints may complain of TMJ clicking and snapping, but pain is usually absent.

Presentation

TMJ disorders are characterized by pain and tenderness in the muscles of mastication and in the TMJ, by crepitus when the joint is moved, and by a decrease in range of motion. In some severe cases there is a noticeable incoordination on the opening and closing of the jaw. This appears as a unilateral shift of the chin upon opening or closing the mouth. Examination may show malocclusion due to teeth that interfere with the normal movement of the mandible or to tenderness of the muscles of mastication.

Treatment

Patients with acute TMJ pain should be managed with moderate analgesics (acetaminophen, 650 mg, and/or codeine, 30 mg, every 4 to 6 hours) and referral to a dentist within 24 to 48 hours to begin therapy. The dentist's goal will be to make the patient aware of the etiology of his problem through education. Depending upon the severity of symptoms and the state of the patient's dentition, the dentist will prescribe one or a combination of the following: avoidance of excessive jaw motion; moist heat to affected muscles; soft diet; disengagement of upper and lower jaws with a night guard (a hard or soft appliance constructed by a dentist, used to separate the teeth); therapeutic exercises; and vapocoolant spray (ethyl chloride to decrease muscle pain). In atypical cases, trigger point injections of Xylocaine may be utilized to distinguish TMJ symptoms from trigeminal neuralgia (see Chapter 79). Once the acute episode has subsided (in about 7 to 14 days) the dentist can detect and eliminate any occlusal interferences and rule out any degenerative joint disease that may have predisposed the patient to TMJ symptoms. In the past, injections of sclerosing agents into the TMJ and condylectomy were tried, but with very poor success.

In a 10-year study, 97 of 100 patients treated conservatively improved. Of these, 83 had permanent improvement. Of the three patients who had intractable, severe symptoms, two required prolonged psychotherapy and one developed systemic arteritis (1).

Local Alveolar Osteitis (Dry Socket)

Local alveolar osteitis (dry socket) is the most common complication of tooth extraction. It occurs in approximately 5% of all tooth extractions, but it is more common after the removal of an impacted third molar. This problem results from the loss of the blood clot located at the site of the extraction. Most often this occurs when the extraction has been difficult and has resulted in considerable trauma to the socket and gum.

Patients with this problem will describe intense localized pain 2 or 3 days after an extraction. This pain is caused by irritation of the sensory nerves in the dry exposed bony socket. Also there is often a foul odor emanating from the socket, but no suppuration is present.

One should control the pain the patient is experiencing with codeine, 30 mg every 3 to 4 hours, and acetaminophen, 650 mg three to four times/day. The patient should be referred promptly to a dentist for irrigation and for the placement of a dressing. The dentist will need to see the patient every day or 2 for approximately 10 days until the socket becomes re-epithelialized. There are no long-term sequelae.

CHRONIC DENTAL AND ORAL PROBLEMS

Periodontal Disease (Pyorrhea) (Figs. 101.4 and 101.5)

Periodontal disease is a general term used to describe diseases that destroy the gingival and bony structures that support the teeth. Periodontal disease is usually subdivided into gingivitis and periodontitis. The major difference between the two is that in periodontitis there is loss of the supporting bony apparatus of the teeth.

Two-thirds of young adults, 80% of middle-aged adults, and 90% of people in the United States over 65 suffer from periodontal disease (7). Poor oral hygiene, which permits plaque to accumulate on the teeth, is the major etiological factor. Most periodontal disease, and therefore most loss of teeth, is preventable. Prevention consists of routine plaque control (see below).

Gingivitis

Presentation. Gingivitis is usually seen in one of four forms: *acute*, a painful condition that has a rapid onset and is of short duration; *subacute*, which is less severe than the acute condition; *recurrent*, which reappears after being eliminated by treatment or after disappearing spontaneously; and *chronic*, the most common form, which has a slow onset, is of a long duration, and is usually painless unless complicated by acute exacerbations (see Fig. 101.5).

The early signs of inflammation of the gingiva, which precede frank gingivitis, are increased gingival fluid secretion and bleeding from the gingival sulcus upon gentle probing. Healthy gingiva is usually "coral pink," whereas in gingivitis the gingiva becomes "bright red" secondary to increased vascularity and a decrease in keratinization. These changes start in the interdental papillae and free gingiva and spread to the attached gingiva. Both acute and chronic forms produce changes in the normally firm, resilient consistency of the gingiva. In acute gingivitis the gingiva has a diffuse edematous appearance, whereas in the chronic form the tissue has a fibrous appearance that pits on pressure.

The development of gingivitis is a consequence of supragingival and subgingival plaque formation (see Fig. 101.4). Plaque is a transparent deposit that is com-

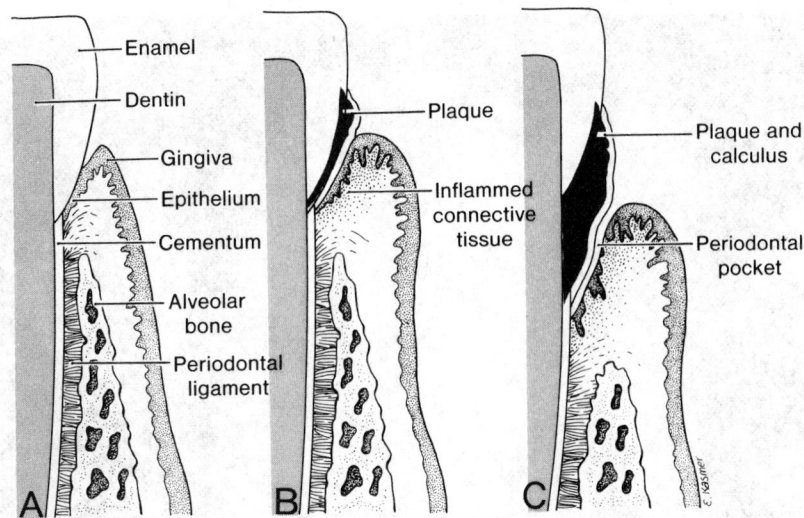

Figure 101.4. Dentogingival junction in health-plaque free (A), gingivitis resulting from plaque accumulation with inflammation of soft tissue (B), and periodontitis resulting from long-standing inflammation that has caused bone loss and tooth mobility (C).

posed primarily of bacteria and their by-products. Gram-positive filamentous rods, mainly *Actinomyces*, appear to be of major significance. Small amounts of plaque are not visible unless they are stained. As plaque accumulates, it becomes visible as a mass that varies in color from gray to yellowish gray to yellow. Measurable amounts of plaque may form within 1 hour after a thorough cleaning of the teeth with maximal accumulation in 30 days or less. Bacterial plaque, if left undisturbed, will mineralize and form calculus (tartar), as shown in Figure 101.4C. This process usually starts between the first and fourteenth day after plaque formation. Calculus is always covered by plaque. When calculus is present, the gingival tissues are unhealthy by definition.

The major complication of untreated gingivitis is periodontitis, that is, the extension of the inflammation to the supporting bony structures of the teeth (see below and Fig. 101.4C).

Treatment. Patients presenting with any one of the four forms of gingivitis usually require one to three dental visits (spread over a 4-week period) for treatment. The mechanical removal of plaque and calculus from the affected areas of the teeth and gingiva is achieved with the appropriate instruments. After all of the plaque and calculus have been removed by the dentist, the disease process is explained to the patient, who is then instructed in proper *plaque control measures*, i.e., effective toothbrushing (a soft bristled toothbrush that facilitates cleansing of the gingiva and the teeth without laceration should be recommended) and effective flossing (the floss should be rubbed vertically up and down three to five times in each interdental space, once daily). Maintenance of the disease-free state is only possible by continued effective plaque control measures by the patient and by professional cleaning every 6 to 12 months (to remove plaque and calculus that may be missed by brushing and flossing). In the last few years, mouth washes have been devel-

oped that are helpful in the treatment of gingivitis (3). Chlorhexidine gluconate, 0.12% (Peridex, available by prescription), has been shown to be microbicidal. Complications are frequent and include a brown stain of the teeth, possible taste alterations, and increase in calculus formation. For these reasons a patient should not use the material without consulting a dentist.

Factors that usually result in recurrence are (a) incomplete removal of plaque and calculus, (b) inadequate plaque control because of insufficient patient instruction, (c) premature dismissal of the patient before he demonstrates competence, and (d) lack of patient cooperation.

Periodontitis (See Fig. 101.4C)

Presentation. A patient with periodontitis has red and bleeding gums and an unpleasant taste in his mouth, but he is usually free of pain unless there is an acute infection superimposed upon the underlying chronic process. The principal physical findings are the signs of inflammation of the gingiva described above and periodontal pockets around the teeth from which pus may often be expressed upon gentle pressure. As periodontitis advances, the teeth loosen and spread apart, creating unattractive spaces and exposing the roots of the teeth as the bony support is lost. Mastication is impaired, and spontaneous pain and acute abscess may occur. The most important consequence of periodontitis is the destruction of the alveolar bone, which deprives the teeth of their support and is responsible for the loss of the teeth. The essential steps leading to destruction of bone are gingivitis, degeneration of collagen bundles of the periodontal ligament, and conversion of the shallow (<3 mm) physiological gingival sulcus to a deepened periodontal pocket (> 3 mm). As this pocket deepens, more debris accumulates in it. Inflammation progresses further inward, and the gums recede permanently. The apically progressing inflammation eventually reaches the alveolar crest, and

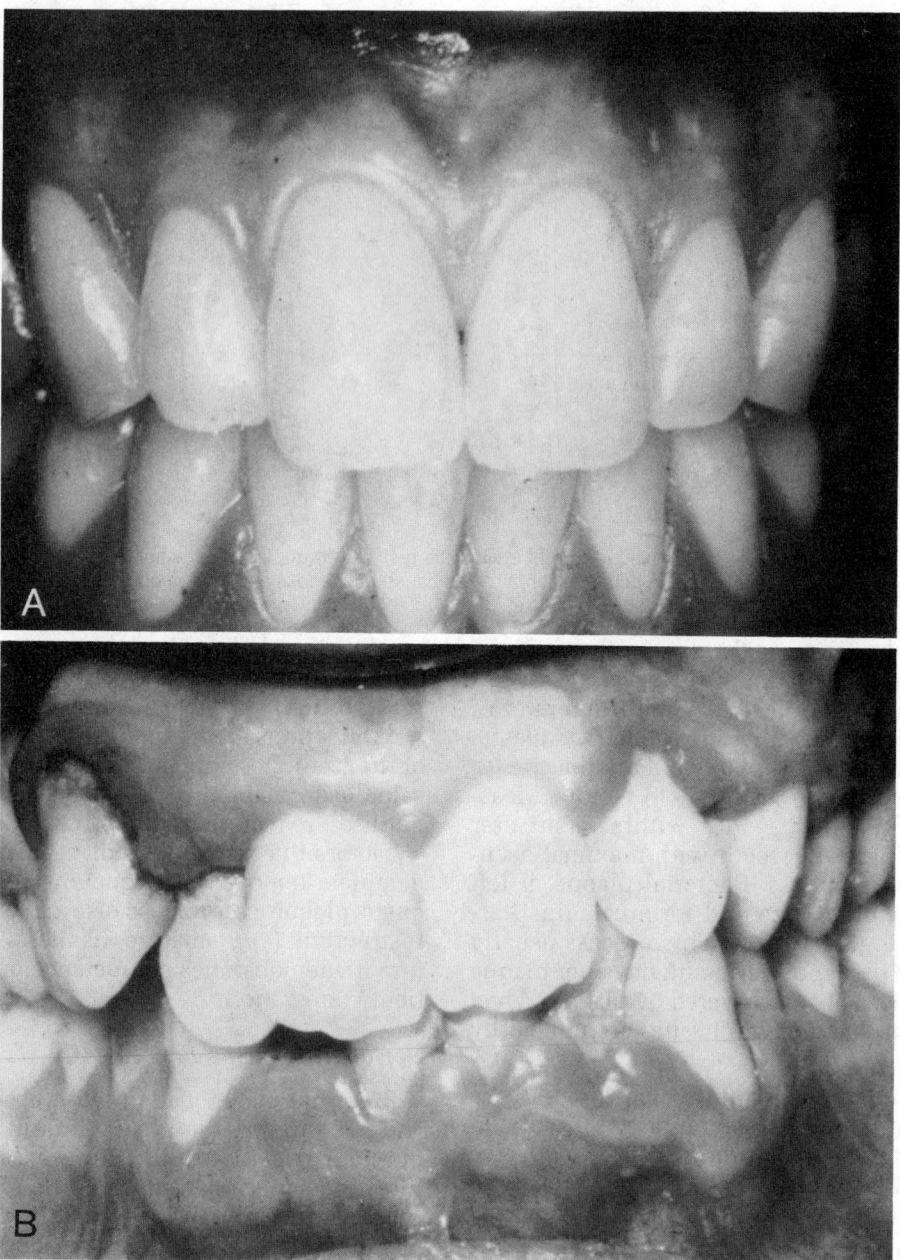

Figure 101.5. Normal gingiva (*A*) and chronic periodontal inflammation (*B*) showing swelling, blunting of interdental papillae, erythema, and bleeding.

bone resorption begins. This process continues, resulting in continued destruction of the alveolar bone.

Treatment. Most patients with periodontitis can be treated effectively, provided that the diagnosis is made before a significant amount of supporting alveolar bone is lost. The aims of treatment are to preserve the teeth by eliminating the disease, to restore effective function, and to prevent recurrence. When treated in the early stages, the major consequence of periodontitis (loss of bone support for the teeth) can be prevented. If proper treatment is postponed, there may be insufficient bone support once treatment is undertaken, and the natural teeth may eventually be lost. Some patients

are not concerned with this problem but are ultimately disappointed when their dentures do not function efficiently.

Treatment of periodontitis is divided into two phases. Phase I is similar to the treatment of gingivitis described above, i.e., removal of local irritant (plaque and calculus) and institution of effective plaque control (continual removal of the plaque). This treatment allows resolution of the inflammation. The success of this phase of therapy depends largely upon the patient's ability to maintain plaque-free teeth (see above under "Acute Necrotizing Ulcerative Gingivitis"). Phase II is the surgical phase in which the goal is to improve the gingival architecture that remains in spite of the disease. Experience has shown that patients have difficulty in preventing inflammation in periodontal pockets greater than 5 mm. Surgical treatment is therefore designed to decrease the depths of the pockets.

Denture Problems

Twenty million American adults are missing all of their teeth. Of these, many have obtained dentures. In addition, many of the edentulous population have managed well without teeth, are content to remain as they are, and, regardless of the quality of dentures constructed, are unwilling and/or unable to adapt to using dentures.

Presentation

Often the physician will be confronted with a patient who, although he has had dentures for years, upon specific questioning indicates that the dentures are not as satisfactory as the patient would wish. The most common denture problems are looseness and discomfort. If the patient is followed at least yearly by his dentist, the physician can generally assume the present situation is the best that can be achieved. On the other hand, if the patient has tolerated the same set of loose or uncomfortable dentures without seeking help for a number of years, he should be encouraged to seek care promptly. Failure to remove dentures at night is the reason for denture problems in some patients. This practice can cause (a) bony erosion with loss of conformity of the dentures to the supporting structures, (b) mucosal ulceration, and (c) oral candidiasis.

Treatment

Depending upon the condition of the patient's oral cavity, the present dentures, and the edentulous ridges, a number of treatment modalities are available, including rebasing or relining the existing dentures (5 to 7 days), making a new set of dentures (2 to 5 weeks), and preprosthetic correction of soft and hard tissue (4 to 6 weeks healing), followed by relining, rebasing, or remaking of dentures. In recent years, there have been marked improvements in dental implants for patients who have had trouble using dentures (especially lower dentures). The placement of implants is expensive ($700 to $800 per implant and usually five to six implants are used per arch) and time consuming (2 to 3 months) and requires that new dentures be made after placement of implants. The implants function as a replacement for the teeth roots that the patient had previously lost through dental caries, periodentitis, or trauma. Most conservative dentists reserve implants for the patient missing at least all posterior teeth or all natural teeth.

Dental Caries

Dental caries is a disease of the calcified tissues of the teeth characterized by demineralization of the in-

organic portion (enamel and dentin—see Fig. 101.2A of the tooth).

Dental caries is one of the most common diseases of man. It affects all persons regardless of race, location, or economic stratum, and it can occur at any age. Poor oral hygiene and a diet high in sugar promote caries, whereas routine oral hygiene and raw, coarse foods tend to reduce caries. Ingestion of fluorides in drinking water reduces susceptibility to caries. The form of the tooth affects caries, i.e., the deep pits and fissures on molars and premolars especially predispose these teeth to the disorder.

Presentation

Dental caries usually presents as a nonpainful, white, brown, or black spot on the enamel of a tooth. The most common location is the biting surface in conjunction with the pits and fissures of the tooth. Other locations include the smooth surfaces where the teeth come into contact with each other. Without the aid of special equipment (radiographs and hand instruments) and expertise of dental personnel, the best indicator of dental caries is the presence of brown or black spots in areas associated with lost portions of the tooth.

When a caries progresses rapidly to involve the pulp, as in children, the term acute caries is used. Slowly progressing caries seen in adults is referred to as chronic caries. Occasionally a carious lesion may cease to progress (arrested caries). This is due to breakage of enamel walls, thereby exposing the lesion to the cleaning action of the toothbrush, saliva, fluoride, and mastication. The term recurrent caries is used for carious lesions that begin around the margins of defective restorations.

A carious lesion usually develops after bacterial plaque (see above) forms on the tooth surface. The primary bacteria involved in this process are *Streptococcus mutans* and *Lactobacillus acidophilus*. These bacteria metabolize dietary fructose to produce lactic acid, which results in decalcification of the enamel. The rate of development of caries depends upon the susceptibility of the enamel.

Treatment

The treatment for most carious lesions is their removal, followed by a restoration (filling) that replaces the lost portions of the tooth. The goals are to remove the lesion, to protect the pulp from irritants, and to restore the tooth to function. In those cases when caries involves a tooth already significantly affected by periodontal disease, the tooth must be removed.

The major *complication* that results from delaying treatment is acute pulpitis and its complications (see above). In addition, delaying treatment may result in a more difficult restoration or possible loss of the involved tooth. In those cases in which the existing decay process is very close to the pulp, the heat generated by the rotary instruments used to prepare the restoration may result in a transient pulpal inflammation.

This inflammation results in a dull ache in the tooth for 2 to 3 days, which is usually relieved by aspirin. When the restoration process leaves only a paper-thin layer of dentin covering the pulp tissue, the transient pulpitis may be converted to acute pulpitis (irreversible), which then requires either tooth extraction or root canal therapy for relief of pain. Root canal therapy consists of three parts: the removal of the infected nerve tissue, the debridement and preparation of the nerve canal space, and obturation (filling) of the canal space with a biologically inert material.

Angular Cheilosis

Presentation

Angular cheilosis is characterized by a feeling of dryness and a burning sensation at the corners of the mouth. The epithelium at the commissures appears wrinkled and macerated. In time, the wrinkles deepen to fissures that appear ulcerated but do not bleed, although a crust may form. These lesions stop at the junction of the mucous membranes. They show a tendency for spontaneous improvement; only rarely do the lesions completely disappear.

There are several etiologies for cheilosis. A number of microorganisms may cause it in otherwise healthy people: *Candida albicans*, staphylococci, and streptococci. In addition, angular cheilosis due to overclosure of the jaws may be seen in edentulous patients. Overclosure causes a fold to be produced at the corners of the mouth in which saliva tends to collect, inviting the growth of micro-organisms. Angular cheilosis is also seen in riboflavin deficiency, which usually occurs in patients with multiple vitamin deficiencies. The lips show fissures, painful cracks, and scaling; these changes become severe at the corners of the mouth and are similar in appearance to angular cheilosis due to overclosure of the mandible.

Treatment

Edentulous patients troubled by angular cheilosis should be referred to a dentist who will evaluate them for mandibular overclosure, as correction of this problem (making or remaking of dentures) may lead to remission. Treatment is otherwise symptomatic and consists of applying petrolatum-containing ointment (e.g., Vaseline, Chapstick) to the scaling area to minimize discomfort.

Thrush (Oral Candidiasis)

Presentation

The typical lesions of oral candidiasis are white, curd-like plaques on an erythematous mucosa (Fig. 101.6). These plaques are loosely attached and may be scraped off the oral mucosa. They begin as pinpoint spots. Involvement may include the corners of the mouth, as noted in the previous section. The tongue is often reddened, and the patient describes a burning sensation.

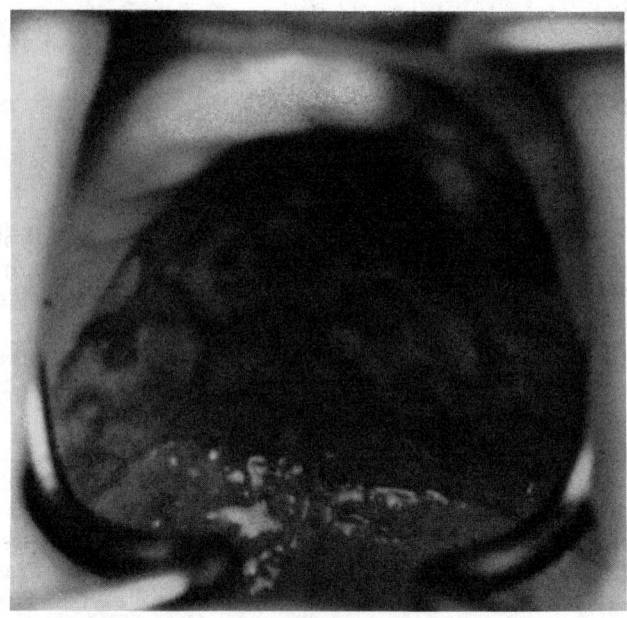

Figure 101.6. Candidiasis (thrush) of hard palate.

Thrush may occur chronically in patients with poor oral hygiene and poor nutrition. It may also be brought on or exacerbated by debilitating systemic illness, antibiotic therapy, impaired immune system, use of steroids or antimetabolites, or dental extraction. Thrush does not appear to be more common in diabetics. It is very common in patients with human immunodeficiency virus (HIV) infection (see Chapter 34).

The white plaques of thrush may suggest hyperkeratosis or leukoplakia. In these instances, a scraping will reveal hyphae and blastospores when the condition is candidiasis.

Treatment

The patient should be advised to practice good oral hygiene practices. Specific treatment consists of nystatin oral suspension, 4 to 6 ml held in the mouth for several minutes before swallowing, four times daily. Thrush usually resolves entirely after 1 to 2 weeks of treatment. Treatment should be continued for several days after visible lesions have disappeared. More intensive treatment is needed in patients with HIV infection (see Chapter 34).

Halitosis

Presentation

Halitosis is a foul or offensive odor emanating from the oral cavity. Mouth odors originate from local or remote sites. The local causes can be retention of odoriferous food particles on or between the teeth, ANUG (see page 1381), caries, chronic periodontal disease, dentures, tobacco smoking, and healing of surgical or extraction wounds. Extraoral causes of halitosis include infection in adjacent structures (rhinitis, sinusitis, tonsillitis), pulmonary infections, alcoholic breath, the acetone odor of the diabetic, or the uremic breath associated with renal failure.

Treatment

Local causes of this condition are treated by improvement in oral hygiene and by specific treatment of the underlying conditions by a dentist. If these measures are unsuccessful, pleasant-smelling mouthwashes or breath fresheners used frequently (every 2 to 4 hours) may greatly reduce the problem. Halitosis due to remote factors may be masked with mouthwashes and fresheners until the remote problem has been resolved.

Xerostomia (Dry Mouth)

Presentation

Xerostomia or dry mouth results from a partial or complete lack of saliva. This defect results in cracking of the lips, difficulty in swallowing, and/or changes in the tongue texture. The patient often increases liquid consumption in order to eliminate the dryness. Xerostomia may be a secondary complication of salivary gland disease (e.g., Sjögren's syndrome) or radiation treatment, but medication is the commonest cause. Anticholinergic, decongestant, and antihistamine drugs are the most common offenders.

The loss of saliva results in a loss of the protective coating of the mucous membranes of the oral cavity. Infections, severe dental caries, and problems with dentures very commonly result from the loss of saliva.

Treatment

Treatment of xerostomia is symptomatic. Patients should be referred to a dentist for a complete dental evaluation and to eliminate any caries and for instruction in the use of daily topical fluoride to help prevent recurrence of caries. The dryness may be lessened if the patient regularly irrigates his mouth with topical methylcellulose, glycerin, or a saliva substitute (Oralube, Xerolube, or MOI-STIR—all available without prescription). The saliva substitutes also decrease somewhat the risk of caries because they contain sodium fluoride.

Common Tongue Conditions

Geographic Tongue

Benign migratory glossitis or geographic tongue is an asymptomatic inflammatory condition consisting of multiple areas of desquamation of the filiform papillae of the tongue in an irregular pattern (Fig. 101.7A). The central portion of an affected area is usually denuded, and the border may be outlined by a thin, yellowish white line or band. The fungiform papillae persist in the desquamated area as small elevated red dots. The areas of desquamation remain for a short time in one location, then heal and reappear in other locations. The condition may persist for weeks or months and then regress, only to recur at a later date.

Women are affected twice as often as men and there is no racial difference. Because the etiology is unknown and the condition is benign, management consists of reassurance. Large doses of vitamins are not effective.

Hairy Tongue

Hairy tongue is a condition characterized by hypertrophy of the filiform papillae of the tongue due to the lack of normal desquamation of the keratin layer (Fig. 101.7B). This results in a thick, matted layer on the dorsum of the tongue. The color of the papillae varies from yellowish white to brown or even black depending upon their staining by extrinsic factors (tobacco, foods, or medications). The hypertrophied tissue may touch the palate and produce gagging in some patients. The majority of patients with hairy tongue are heavy smokers, but the etiology is unknown. Treatment of this benign condition is to brush the tongue with a tongue blade or toothbrush to promote desquamation and to remove debris.

Median Rhomboid Glossitis

Median rhomboid glossitis is a congenital abnormality of the tongue that appears clinically as an ovoid, diamond, or rhomboid-shaped reddish patch on the dorsal surface of the tongue. On examination, there is a slightly raised or flat area that is distinctive because there are no filiform papillae (Fig. 101.7C). Despite its name, this abnormality is not inflammatory; it is due to failure of the tuberculum impar to retract before fusion of the lateral halves of the tongue, so that a structure free of papillae is interposed. The prevalence of the abnormality is less than 1%, and there are no sex or racial differences. The only clinical significance of this innocuous condition is that it is occasionally mistaken for a carcinoma; differentiation from cancer is aided by a history of the presence of the lesion since childhood and by the fact that a carcinoma rarely develops on the dorsum of the tongue. If the physician is unsure of the diagnosis he should refer the patient to a dentist.

Leukoplakia and Erythroplakia

Presentation

Leukoplakia and erythroplakia are asymptomatic conditions of the oral mucosa that may become malignant.

Leukoplakia varies in appearance from a grayish white flattened scaly lesion to a thick, irregularly shaped plaque (Fig. 101.8). Histologically, there is hyperkeratosis, acanthosis, and some degree of dyskeratosis. It is commonly associated with underlying inflammation due to a chronic irritant (tobacco, alcohol, poorly constructed dentures). Leukoplakia may be found anywhere in the oral cavity, but most frequently it is found in the buccal mucosa, followed, in descending order, by the alveolar mucosa, tongue, lip, hard and soft palates, floor of the mouth, and gingiva.

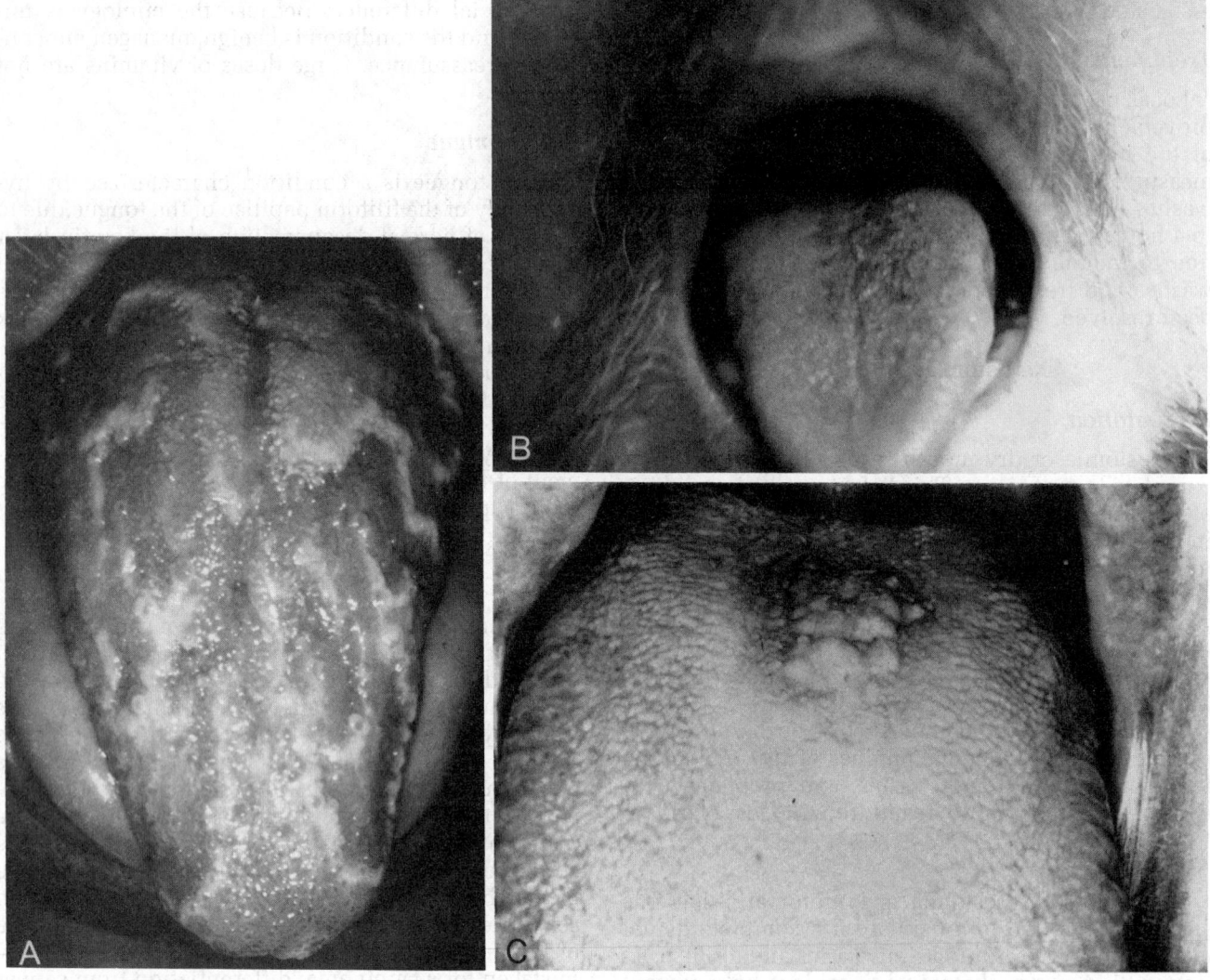

Figure 101.7. Common benign problems of the tongue. *A.* Geographic tongue. *B.* Hairy tongue. *C.* Median rhomboid glossitis.

Erythroplakia refers to a lesion that is velvety red in appearance, small (2 cm or less), and with or without a hyperkeratotic component. It is found in the floor of the mouth, soft palate, and ventrolateral border of the tongue.

The significance of these lesions has been delineated in a longitudinal study of mucosal lesions (6). Of 200 white lesions examined by biopsy, only four were malignant. In the same study, an erythroplastic component was present in 90% of the 158 asymptomatic squamous cell carcinomas that were found, suggesting, but not proving, that erythroplakia may be an important precursor of squamous cell cancer.

Treatment

It is impossible to determine which lesion showing leukoplakia or erythroplakia will undergo malignant transformation. Discontinuance of chronic irritants is recommended, followed by a 14-day observation period to allow inflammatory lesions to heal. If the lesion persists, referral to a dental surgeon for a biopsy and regular follow-up surveillance even if the lesion is benign is indicated. The biopsy procedure is as simple as having a restoration (filling) or a tooth extraction.

Other conditions that may resemble leukoplakia or erythroplakia are lichen planus, chemical burns, candidiasis (thrush), psoriasis, lupus erythematosus, and syphilitic mucous patches. Each of these has characteristic histological features.

Squamous Cell Carcinoma

Over 90% of all malignant tumors of the oral cavity are squamous cell carcinomas. They are four times more common in men than women and are most common after the fourth decade. In the United States oral cancer is the eighth most common form of cancer in men and the twelfth in women. Fifteen thousand new cases are found each year, and about 7500 patients die of this disease annually. Of lip carcinomas, 95% occur on the lower lip and appear as an ulcer, wart, sore, or

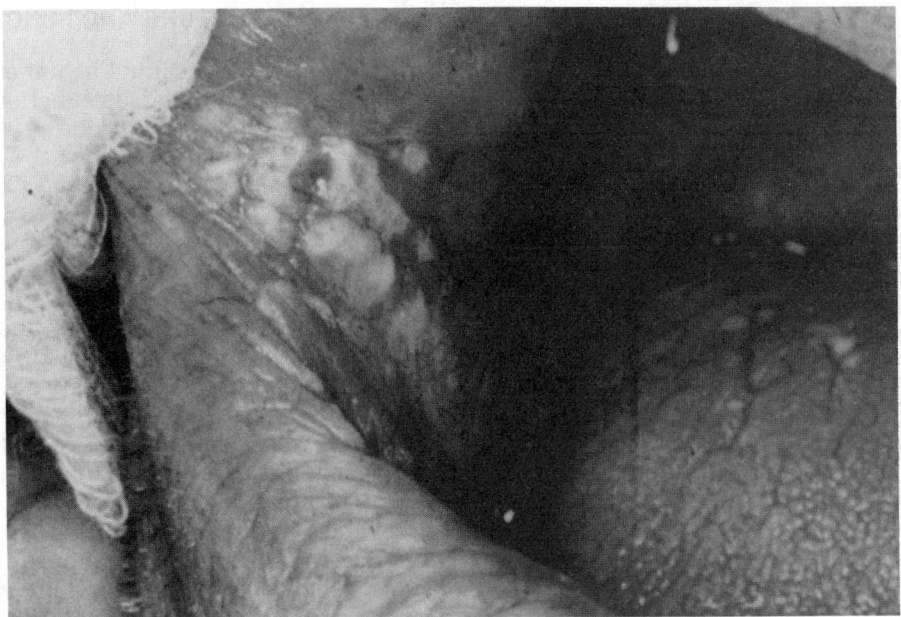

Figure 101.8. Leukoplakia showing early changes of epidermoid carcinoma.

scale (6). This lesion is more frequent in fair-skinned individuals. Of the intraoral carcinomas, 50% occur on the tongue (usually ventrolateral border, Fig. 101.9) and 16% on the floor of the mouth; the remaining 34% are equally distributed between the gingival mucosa, palate, and buccal mucosa. Sixty percent of intraoral carcinomas present as ulcers, 30% as growths, and the remaining 10% as white lesions or other abnormalities of the mucosa (2). Carcinoma of the tongue and floor of the mouth metastasizes early and carries a very poor prognosis.

The etiology of oral carcinoma is unknown. Ill-fitting dentures, actinic radiation, tobacco, jagged teeth, syphilitic glossitis, and alcoholism are believed to be risk factors.

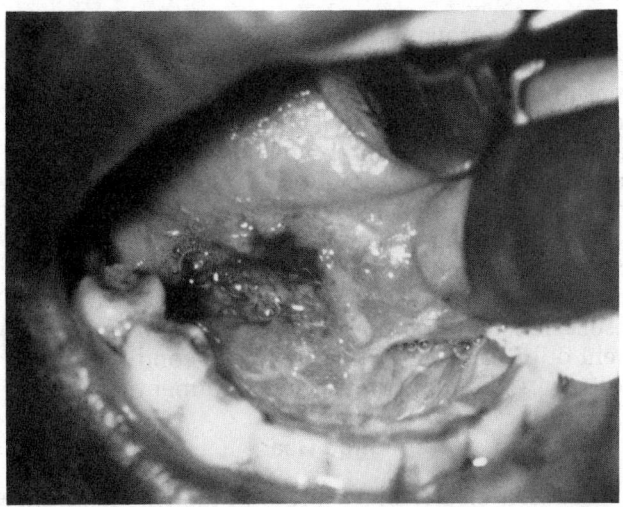

Figure 101.9. Squamous cell carcinoma of the floor of the mouth.

Presentation and Evaluation

Patients usually give a history of knowledge of the lesion for 6 to 18 months when they first present; for many reasons they have not sought evaluation. All patients with suspicious lesions should be referred promptly to a dental surgeon for biopsy. Biopsy is a simple procedure, not very different from having a restoration or tooth extraction; usually it is done under local anesthesia.

Treatment

Definitive surgery is a team effort between the otolaryngologist and the dentist. The dentist's role is to evaluate, for long-term prognosis, any of the teeth that are not to be removed in the surgical field and to remove any of these teeth that are affected with untreatable periodontitis; this is done to avoid osteoradionecrosis, a condition seen in the postradiation patient in whom the socket of an extracted tooth fails to heal as the result of diminished blood supply. Lip tumors have the highest success rate (10-year cure rate between 80 and 92%), whereas only one-fifth of patients with tongue cancer live longer than 5 years.

General References

Friedman MH, Weisberg J: *Temporomandibular Joint Disorders.* Lombard, IL, Quint Pub Co, 1985.
Lynch MA (ed): *Bunket's Oral Medicine, Diagnosis and Treatment,* 8th ed. Philadelphia, JB Lippincott, 1984.
Thaller SR, Montgomery WW (eds): *Guide to dental problems for physicians and surgeons.* Baltimore, Williams & Wilkins, 1988.
Williams RC: Periodontal Disease. *N Engl J Med* 322:373, 1990.
Wood NK, Goaz PW: *Differential Diagnosis of Oral Lesions,* 3rd ed. St Louis, CV Mosby, Co., 1985.

Specific References

1. Apfelberg DB, Lavey E, Janetos G, et al: Temporomandibular joint disease: results of a ten year study. *Postgrad Med* 65:167, 1979.
2. Bhaskar SN: *Synopsis of Oral Pathology*, 4th ed. St Louis, CV Mosby, 1973. p. 463.
3. Briner WW, Grossman E, Buckner RY, et al: Effect of Chlorohexidine glucenate mouth rinse on plaque bacteria. *J Periodent Res* 21 (suppl 16):44, 1986.
4. Franks AS: The social character of temporomandibular joint dysfunction. *Dent Pract Dent Rec* 15:94, 1964.
5. Graykowski EA, Barile MF, Lee WB, Stanley Jr HR: Recurrent aphthous stomatitis: clinical, therapeutic, histopathologic, and hypersensitivity aspects. *JAMA* 196:637, 1966.
6. Mashberg A, Morrissey JB, Garfinkel L: A study of the appearance of early asymptomatic oral squamous cell carcinoma. *Cancer* (Phila) 32:1436, 1973.
7. United States Department of Health, Education and Welfare, Public Health Service: *Research Explores Pyorrhea and Other Gum Diseases: Periodontal Disease*, (PHS Publication 1482). Washington, DC, United States Government Printing Office, 1970.

C H A P T E R   102

Common Problems of the Feet

BRUCE S. LEBOWITZ, D.P.M.

The general physician is often called upon to treat patients who complain of problems with their feet. Although disorders of the feet are not life threatening, they should not be taken lightly. Any patient with a painful foot will attest that his pain can and does take the joy out of living.

STRUCTURE AND FUNCTION

The abnormal foot cannot be understood unless the structure of the foot and its function during gait are understood.

Normal Gait (See Fig. 102.1, *A* and *B*)

The bones and joints of the feet facilitate walking and running in an upright position. The foot and leg function together to allow a smooth, even transfer of weight as one extremity moves ahead of the other. During gait, the foot first adjusts to a variable terrain and then acts to propel the body's weight forward.

In the *first stage of gait*, the heel strikes the ground and body weight begins to move distally over the lateral aspect of the foot. The foot is in a pronated position, meaning that the arch is relatively flattened. In effect, the foot resembles a "loose bag of bones" during this stage, permitting it to adapt to the terrain and to act as a shock absorber when body weight strikes the ground.

In the *second stage of gait*, as weight moves distally to the ball of the foot and the body is propelled forward, the foot must convert to a rigid lever. This conversion, or supination, takes place in the subtalar and midtarsal joints. Supination serves to heighten the arch, pushing the bones and joints of the foot together rigidly enough to propel body weight forward efficiently.

For the lower extremity to function normally, certain structural criteria must be met; if they are not met, compensation will occur. Ideally, the leg should be in a plane perpendicular to the foot and ground, as in a stick figure drawing. The forefoot should be in a plane parallel to the rearfoot; but various congenital factors may act to prevent this normal angulation. Varus (toward the midline or inverted) or valgus (away from the midline or everted) positions of the forefoot or hindfoot are the most common of these congenital factors.

Excessive Pronation

Excessive pronation (pronation extended through too much of the gait cycle) is the most common compensating mechanism when structural abnormalities are present. When the foot remains pronated during gait and does not resupinate in time, or at all, the condition known as "flatfoot" exists. The degree of this flatfoot position reflects the degree of pronation that is present. A number of problems may evolve from excessive pronation during gait—among them bunions, calluses, and hammertoes. As pointed out in the discussion of these conditions that follows, assessment of the mechanical basis for the condition is important in planning appropriate treatment for it.

Shoe Gear

Shoe gear clearly plays a role in the way feet function. Shoes protect feet from the elements, cushion the

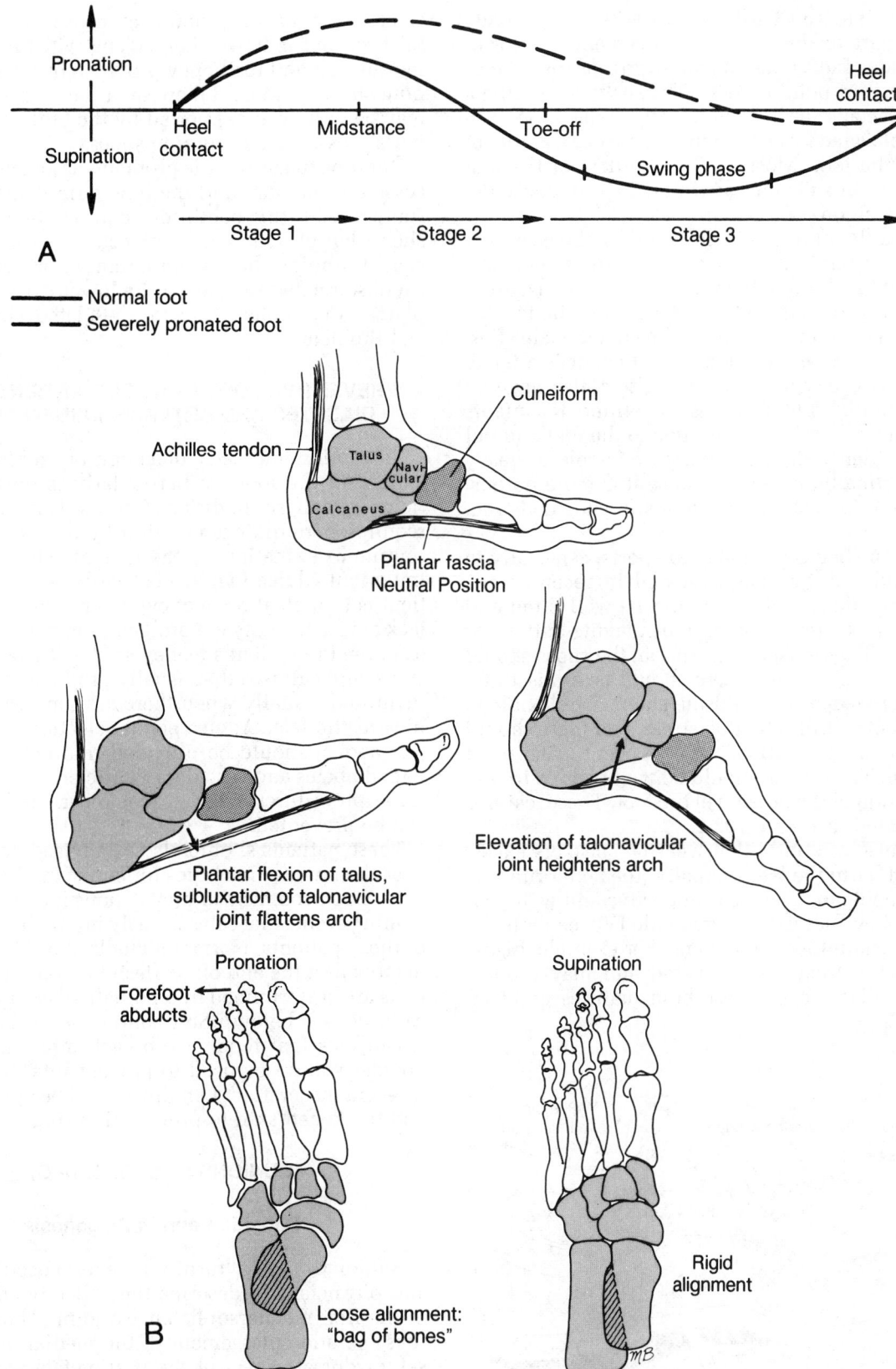

Figure 102.1. *A.* Schematic representation of the gait cycle for a normal foot and for a foot with excessive pronation. *B.* Schematic illustration of foot structure during pronation and supination.

effect of walking on hard, flat surfaces, and provide some support to the bones and ligaments. Unfortunately, many individuals favor short, narrow shoes, high heels, and pointed toes. Obviously, squeezing a basically rectangular foot into a triangular shoe with the heels elevated from 2 to 5 inches creates significant stress for the foot. Most of the disorders of the foot discussed in this chapter are intensified by these demands of fashion.

Most people, in fitting themselves for shoes, do not take into account the variations in their foot size throughout the day and the variation in shoe size from manufacturer to manufacturer. Therefore, the following advice is often helpful: buy shoes in the late afternoon when any swelling that might occur is already present; try to buy shoes in stores that also have an active trade in infant shoes, as shoe fitters for infants are experienced in fitting the shoe to the foot and not vice versa; lightweight shoes are preferable to heavy ones; and, finally, leather, because it is more porous, is preferable to synthetic materials in shoe construction.

Interest in shoe gear related to sports, especially to jogging and running, has escalated in recent years. Sneakers or running shoes should be well fitted and firm enough to prevent excessive splaying of the foot during activity. For shock absorption, the shoes should have studded soles; and there should be a raised, resilient heel wedge. The midsole should be flexible to help prevent Achilles tendon stress, and there should be a well-molded Achilles pad to prevent irritation of the tendon. The tongue should be well padded to prevent irritation of the dorsum of the foot. These features are illustrated in Figure 102.2.

It is a misconception that wearing sneakers excessively will harm the feet. Actually, the better running shoes available today are so supportive and well padded that they may be recommended to patients for numerous painful foot conditions. For example, highly arched feet (which are supinated and may pronate only slightly) lack shock-absorbing qualities; and con-

stant impact on the ground can cause severe metatarsal, heel, and arch pain. For patients with this condition, the support and resiliency provided by a modern running shoe are ideal. Likewise, a flat or pronated foot may be very well supported by the built-in arch supports of well-made running shoes.

Running magnifies the problems associated with excessive pronation, and the long-term management of runners with this condition requires the selection of shoes that provide good support. The use of well-designed running shoes is important in preventing most exercise-related injuries of the lower extremity as explained in Chapter 67, Exercise-Related Musculoskeletal Problems.

PREVENTIVE FOOT CARE FOR PATIENTS WITH DIABETES AND ARTERIAL INSUFFICIENCY

Prevention and early detection of problems on the surface of the foot are particularly important in patients with these conditions (see also Chapter 87). This requires periodic examination by the physician and routine examination by the patient. The single most important advice that can be impressed upon the patient is to look at his feet every day. When obesity or lack of visual acuity is a problem, someone else should examine the patient's feet every day. Irritations, abrasions, and calluses that usually produce pain must be identified visually when there are sensory abnormalities in the feet. Advice about selection of shoe gear (see above) should be provided routinely to patients with diabetes and vascular insufficiency. By following these procedures, serious foot ulcers and infections can be prevented.

These patients should also be advised not to utilize over-the-counter remedies for corns and ingrown toenails. Such commercial preparations include acids and tanning agents that can seriously injure the tender skin of these patients. Normal toenails should be allowed to grow past the end of the fleshy part of the toe; thick nails are best trimmed by a podiatrist, as are corns and calluses (see below). Soft cotton should be worn between toes that tend to rub each other, and talcum powder should be used to prevent interdigital moisture and maceration. Lanolin should be applied to dry and thickened skin to prevent fissuring.

BUNIONS (Fig. 102.3, *A–D*)

Definition and Pathogenesis

Bunion (literally "turnip") is a term used by laymen and physicians to describe the collective deformities of the first metatarsophalangeal joint. These deformities include enlargement of the medial, medial-dorsal, or dorsal aspect of the first metatarsophalangeal joint and lateral deviation of the great toe. The enlargement of the joint may consist of bone or soft tissue or a combination of the two.

For many years, tight-fitting shoes were mistakenly considered to be the cause of bunions. It is known

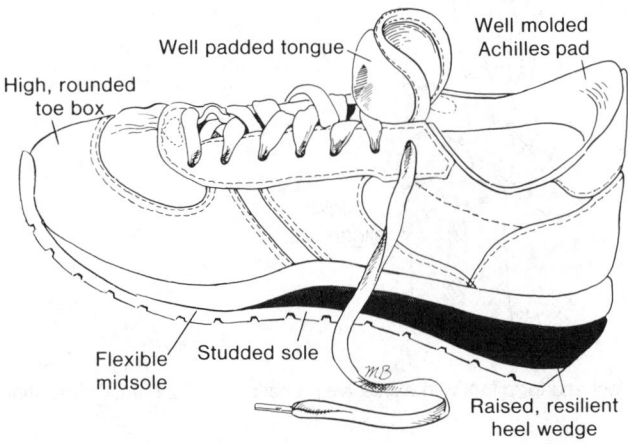

Figure 102.2.   Features of a well-designed running shoe.

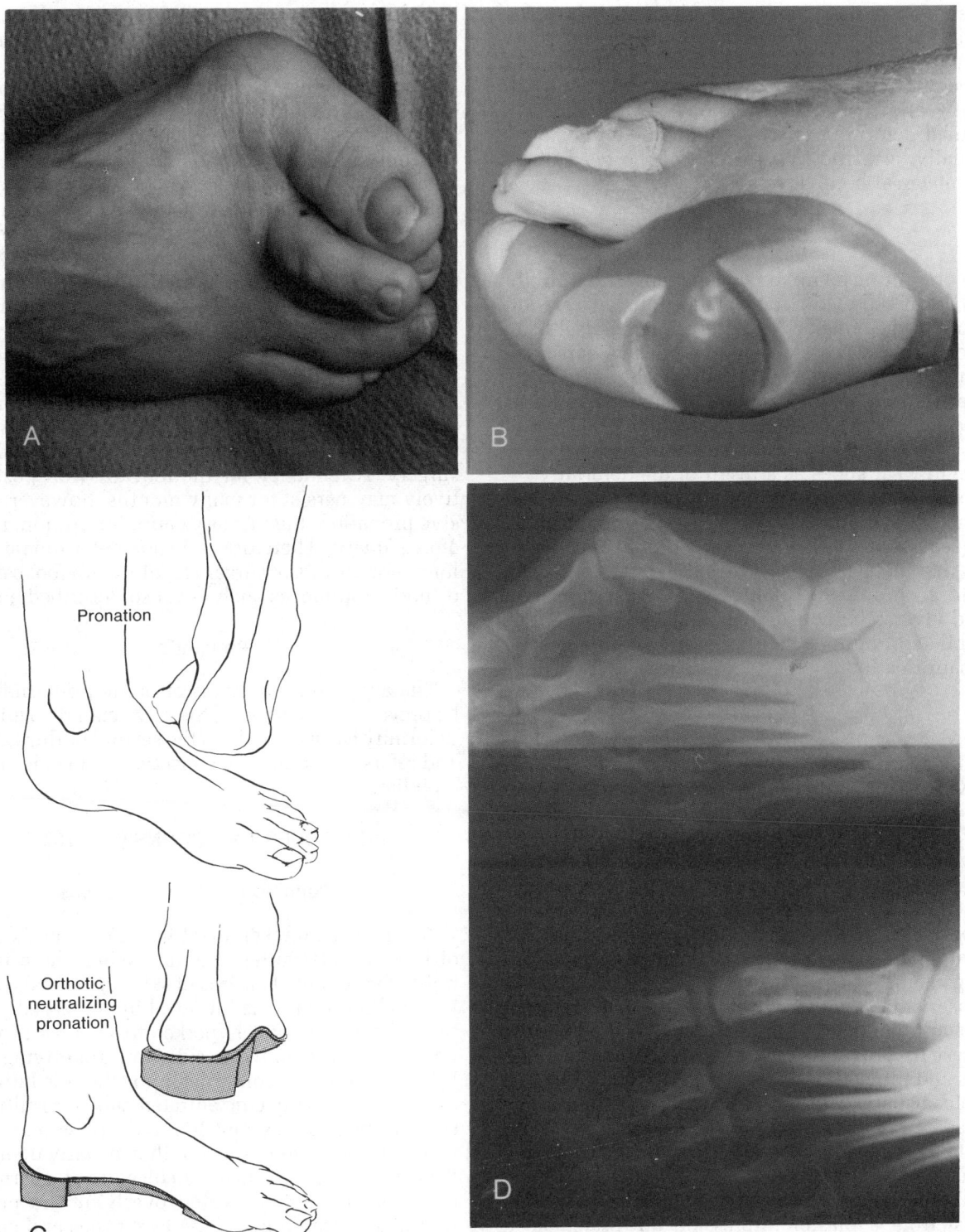

Figure 102.3. Bunions: appearance, orthotic compensation, and surgical repair. *A.* Bunion deformity. *B.* Bunion protected by latex shield. *C.* Leather orthotic arch support. *D.* Bunion deformity shown radiologically before and after surgical correction.

now that, although the pressure of tight shoes on an existing bunion can certainly result in pain that calls attention to the problem, bunions are not caused by poorly fitted shoes. The chief cause of the deformity is a hypermobile first metatarsal bone most often related to excessive pronation (see above). The first

metatarsal and great toe, which help to propel body weight forward, should be quite stable during the final stage of gait when a tight, rigid bony structure is needed. The intrinsic and extrinsic musculature should help to hold the metatarsal tight at this point. When there is excessive pronation, the entire foot remains loose and relatively unstable. One result of such laxity in this stage of gait is the hypermobility of the first metatarsal and the "buckling" of the first toe: intrinsic and extrinsic muscles cause the first metatarsal to deviate medially and the great toe to deviate laterally. The combined deformity is called hallux abducto valgus. Eventually, arthritic hypertrophy of the head of the first metatarsal bone develops.

Symptoms

The presenting complaint of a patient with a bunion is pain localized to the first metatarsophalangeal joint. Pressure of the shoe on the enlarged metatarsal head, with or without pressure on adventitious bursa, can cause pain that is severe and even disabling; pain can also result from the joint motion itself. Often, crepitus can be felt within the joint. Sometimes the patient seeks help, not because of pain, but because he is unable to wear shoes as a result of the deformity.

In evaluating a patient, the physician must be certain that the symptoms are a result of the bunion alone. Gout (see Chapter 69) may not only produce acute pain in the first metatarsophalangeal joint but may also aggravate a chronically painful joint. Therefore, gout should always be considered, especially in patients with bilateral bunion deformity and acute monarticular pain in a foot.

Management

Acute symptoms due to a bunion should be managed with rest, elimination of pressure on the bunion, soaks in warm water, and systemic anti-inflammatory medication such as naproxen (Naprosyn), 250 to 500 mg every 8 to 12 hours, or piroxicam (Feldene), 10 to 20 mg every 24 hours; aspirin, 600 mg every 4 to 6 hours, may also be used, but the onset of action is slower. After the acute symptoms have subsided, the patient should be started on a program of long-term management.

Conservative long-term management of a bunion involves accommodating the deformity and attempting to arrest its progress. This is achieved by the use of molds and protective shields (see Fig. 102.3, *B* and *C*). A mold, usually referred to as an arch support, may be made from various types of materials to accommodate the plantar aspect of the foot. Protective shields are made of latex rubber.

Full foot molds or protective shields made by a podiatrist from a plaster impression are preferable to commercially made devices found in pharmacies and shoe stores. Commercial devices are manufactured to fit average shoe and foot sizes and do not take into account the shape of the individual patient's foot. The mold should be in place during the fitting of all new shoes. Occasionally, if the mold makes conventional shoes too tight, a specially built shoe, called an extra depth-inlay shoe, may be used. These enlarged shoes have a removable insole, for which one may substitute the patient's mold. The mold and shoes should min-

imize pressures against the bunion. In addition, the mold acts to reduce excessive pronation, thereby reducing the deforming forces in the forefoot.

Patients whose bunion symptoms are not adequately controlled with conservative measures should be considered for surgery. The surgical management of a bunion must be individually planned for each patient and, in fact, for each foot, to correct the specific deformity. Correction might involve resection of the bony protuberance of the first metatarsal head only. In occasional patients with severe degenerative joint disease surgical management involves removal of all or part of the joint and insertion of a Silastic joint replacement (see Fig. 102.3*D*). Depending on locale, referral for surgical correction of a bunion may be made to a general, orthopaedic, or podiatric surgeon. A patient should expect to return to most of his preoperative activities within 6 to 8 weeks after bunion surgery; the interval may be somewhat longer after bilateral surgery. A tendency for the foot to swell postoperatively may persist for many months, however. Excessive pronation, the primary cause for bunion, persists after surgery. Therefore, a major determinant of the long-term results of surgery is follow-up foot care with orthotic appliances such as those described above.

Prevention

The annoying symptoms of bunion deformity may be prevented altogether if the physician recognizes the deformity early (usually in the second or third decade) and refers the patient for conservative management by a podiatrist.

CALLUSES AND CORNS (Fig. 102.4)

Definition and Pathogenesis

A callus is a thickening of the epidermis as a result of chronic intermittent trauma. When there is intermittent irritation of an area of skin, the initial response is vasodilation; this is followed by increased production of corneum and hyperkeratosis. This process is normal and protective to skin and underlying tissue. When the process continues until there is buildup of excessive or highly concentrated callus, resulting in a corn, problems may develop. Skin lines may remain visible in callused tissue, but they usually do not pass through the highly concentrated center of a corn. Corns are most frequently located overlying the proximal interphalangeal joints of the lesser toes and centrally within plantar calluses. A number of processes not related to chronic trauma can produce focal calluses as well, namely *verruca plantaris* (*plantar wart*), *foreign body granuloma*, and *porokeratosis plantaris discreta*. These lesions are discussed below.

The primary cause for most symptomatic calluses is excessive pronation (see above) and not restrictive shoes or walking on unyielding surfaces. During excessive pronation, the long flexor and extensor tendons pull on the distal phalanges, the toes appear to

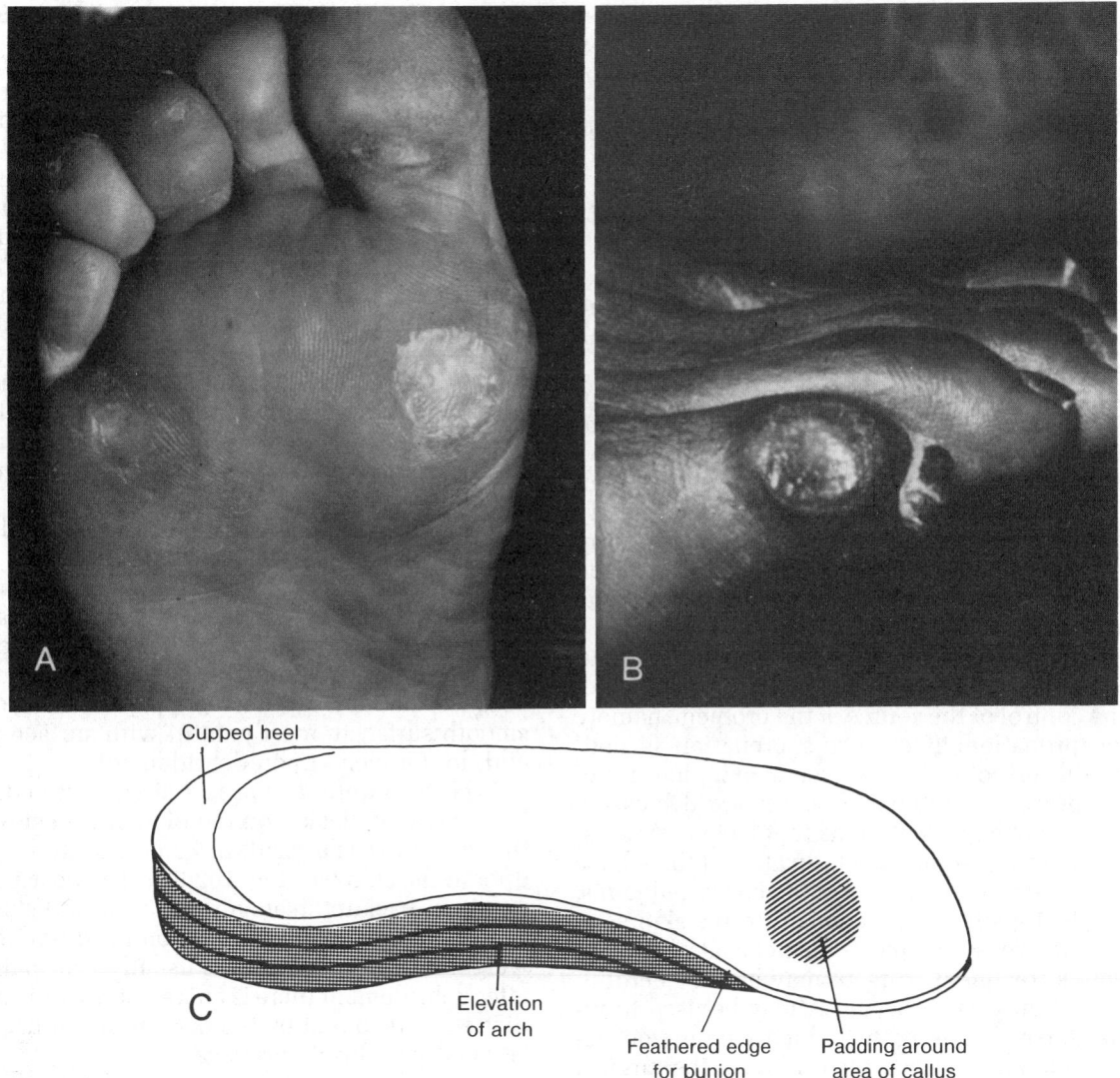

Figure 102.4. Calluses and corns. *A.* Typical plantar callus. *B.* Corn on the fifth digit. *C.* Orthotic device designed to shift weight from area of callus formation. (Photographs courtesy of Max Weisfeld, D.P.M.)

"hammer," and a retrograde force pushes down on the metatarsal heads, increasing pressure on the plantar skin. Other conditions that may promote this increased pressure are excessive supination (highly arched foot) and imbalance of the peroneal and tibial muscles due to weakness, arthritis, or other conditions affecting one or both legs.

Symptoms

Diffuse callus is usually asymptomatic and easily controlled by the patient with pumice stones and cleansing agents readily available in pharmacies. Both calluses and corns produce pain. Thick accumulation of callus tends to cause a burning sensation in the foot. A corn located within a plantar callus gives the sensation of walking on a sharp pebble. Corns that occur dorsolaterally on fifth toes (Fig. 102.4*B*) often cause exquisite pain, especially with tight-fitting shoes. Such

corns often have adventitious bursae associated with them and may produce symptoms due both to bursitis and to the discomfort of the corn pressing down on subcutaneous tissues.

Although corns and calluses can cause discomfort for the average person, they can cause serious morbidity in a diabetic patient. If hyperkeratotic lesions on an extremity are added to a diabetic's lowered resistance to infection, circulatory impairment, and decreased perception of pain, there is a clear potential for serious problems. A discrete lesion on the foot produces constant pressure on the underlying dermis. It is not unusual for this pressure, in a diabetic, to result in local breakdown of tissues, ulceration, and infection. Diabetics have the additional medical and mechanical problem of neurotrophic joints. In patients with the tendency to develop hammertoe and plantar-flexed metatarsal heads, these changes (and the calluses and corns that accompany them) may be accelerated by the loss of normal proprioception and pain sensation of a neurotrophic joint.

Corns and calluses can be a serious problem also for patients with conditions other than diabetes that impair arterial circulation to the lower extremities (see Chapter 87).

Treatment

Treatment of corns and calluses depends upon the location, severity, and type of lesion and upon the physical condition of the patient.

The physician will occasionally see patients who complain of severely painful corns and calluses. Dramatic relief may be obtained from the simple debridement of these very painful lesions, using a sterile no. 10 or no. 15 scalpel blade. If the blade is kept nearly parallel to the skin, injury to the underlying healthy dermis can be avoided. There is no need to debride the entire callus; any reduction in the thickness of the lesion will bring relief to the patient.

Conservative long-term management of corns and calluses in the feet of otherwise healthy people requires the control of the source of the problem, namely excessive pronation. If excessive pronation is neutralized with orthotic devices (see above), foot function is improved, pathological forces are decreased, and lesions may regress. Lesions that have been present for a year or longer usually indicate that there have already been structural changes in the bones and joints, as well as histopathological changes in the skin.

For patients whose symptoms are not controlled with conservative treatment, surgery may be very helpful. A number of surgical procedures may be used to realign metatarsal heads or to reduce hammertoe deformities. Often it is necessary to combine the surgical reconstruction of affected areas with control of pronation in order to achieve lasting resolution of symptoms. This may mean 6 to 8 weeks of convalescence (i.e., non-weight bearing for several days, then progression to partial, and then full weight bearing usually by 6 weeks) after foot surgery and the continued use of orthotics in shoes. The result, however, is greater foot health and comfort.

For the patient with diabetes or peripheral vascular disease, conservative treatment involves frequent debridement of the hyperkeratotic areas, padding for protection, and the fabrication of molds (by a podiatrist or orthopaedist) to shift weight away from problem areas and to accommodate deformities (see Fig. 102.4C). Extra depth shoes are often prescribed in conjunction with such appliances. When refractory infection or ulceration occurs despite conservative management, surgical procedures may be performed to eliminate a bony prominence. Surgery may return a bedridden patient to his feet or eliminate the need for future amputation. The management of this type of patient requires close collaboration between the patient's physician and the consultant.

OTHER HYPERKERATOTIC LESIONS

Other discrete hyperkeratotic lesions commonly found on the foot include verruca plantaris, porokeratosis plantaris discreta, and foreign body granuloma.

Verruca plantaris, or *plantar warts*, occur on the plantar aspect of the foot, usually on weight-bearing surfaces (Fig. 102.5A). They are discussed also in Chapter 100, Common Problems of the Skin, but a brief account is provided here because of the importance of differentiating them from corns, calluses, and other hyperkeratotic lesions. Plantar warts can by asymptomatic or extremely painful. They are caused by a papilloma virus for which there is no specific treatment or prevention. Because they are benign and often resolve spontaneously, aggressive or untried therapies should be avoided.

The appearance of a verrucous lesion is illustrated in Fig. 102.5A. They may vary in size from 1 mm to 1 cm. The lesions can be differentiated from hyperkeratotic corns in several ways: warts usually have rough surfaces, are painful with the application of both surface and lateral pressure, and bleed upon debriding because of their capillary supply; corns are usually smooth surfaced, most painful with surface pressure, and do not bleed upon debridement.

A *porokeratotic lesion* is a circumscribed, discrete hyperkeratotic lesion on the plantar aspect of the foot that develops as a result of keratin occluding a sweat duct in the skin (see Fig. 102.5B). The obstruction and resultant backup create a reaction in the skin similar to a deep, large corn. This lesion need not be under a weight-bearing surface. It is usually very painful, and after debridement there is characteristically even more distress. Treatment by the dermatologist or podiatrist is usually by local curettage.

Foreign bodies in the plantar surface of the foot can generate a local inflammatory reaction and thus create a hyperkeratotic lesion. One of the most common offending substances is hair (animal or human). For example, a dog hair, trapped in a carpet long enough to have dried out, can penetrate the skin rather easily. This lesion, although grossly resembling a simple callus, will, upon examination with a magnifying glass, have a small aperture (entry wound) near the center. The local reaction may or may not include infection. Treatment is simple excision of the foreign body.

NAIL CONDITIONS

There are only two nail conditions that are frequently brought to medical attention: onychomycosis (fungal infection) and ingrown toenails, with or without concomitant inflammation (paronychia).

Onychomycosis (Fig. 102.6)

Etiology and Findings

The typical fungal infection of a toenail begins distally at the tip of the toe and moves proximally,

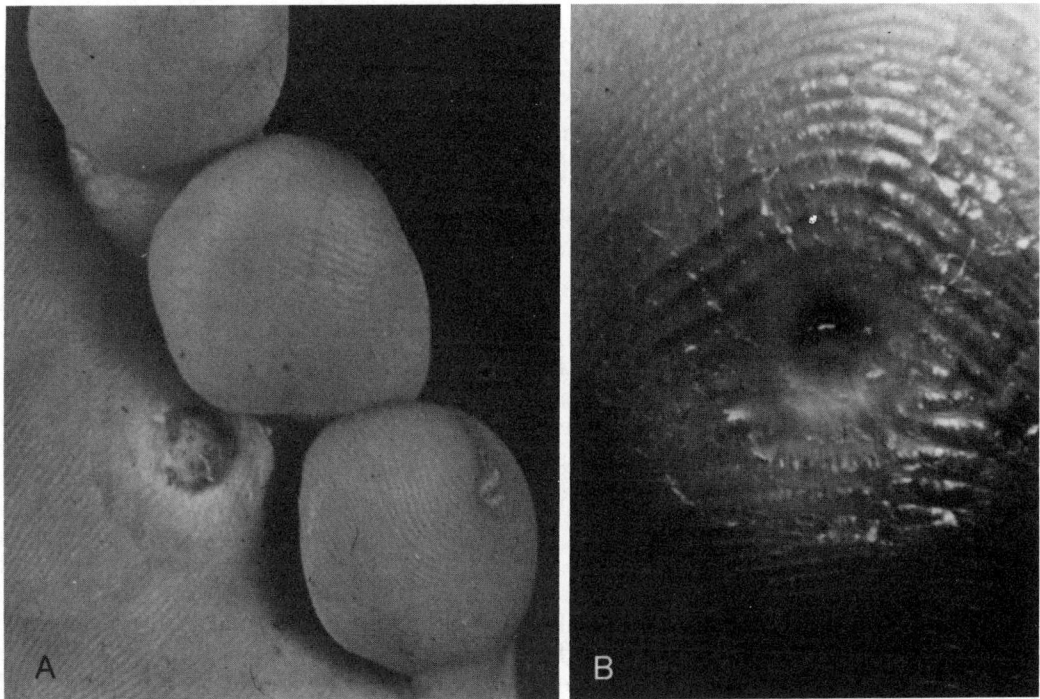

Figure 102.5. Hyperkeratotic lesions not due to chronic trauma. *A.* Plantar wart. *B.* Porokeratosis on plantar surface. (Photographs courtesy of Max Weisfeld, D.P.M.)

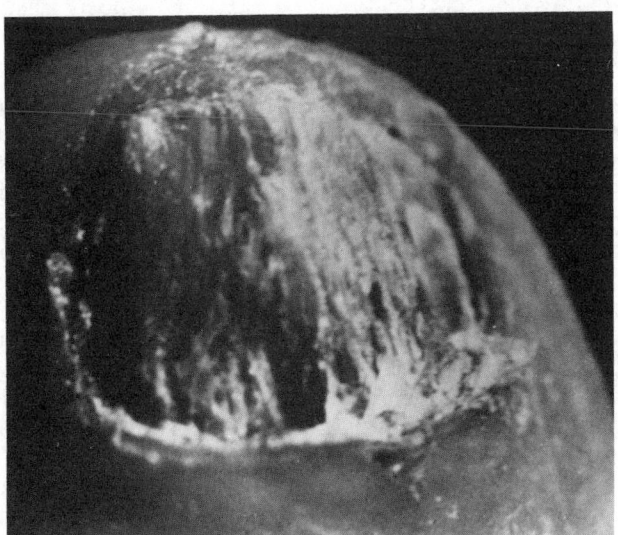

Figure 102.6. Mycotic toenail.

subungually, and through the nail plate itself. Etiological agents are *Trichophyton mentagrophytes, Trichophyton rubrum,* or *Candida albicans.* The fungus produces yellowish discoloration and longitudinal striations in the nails and in the epidermis; the accompanying local inflammatory reaction stimulates hyperkeratosis under the nail. This hyperkeratotic accumulation tends to lift the nail up from the epidermis, facilitating further progression of the fungus.

Eventually, the nail becomes brownish-yellow mottled, thickened, and powdery. Usually these infections are asymptomatic; patients are most concerned about the appearance of their nails, the possibility of spread of infection, and sometimes the inability to wear shoes when severe thickening of the nail plate is present.

Treatment

Fungus infections of toenails are difficult to eradicate medically. There are no topical medications that have been shown to be effective. Only the griseofulvin group of medications, taken orally, may eliminate the infection. Griseofulvin treatment is prolonged (1 to 2 years) and carries a small risk of bone marrow suppression. There is also the possibility that, after such a regimen, the infection will recur. Therefore, simple debridement or permanent removal of the nail is the treatment of choice for this problem.

When nail thickening is regarded as a problem by the patient, the process can be controlled by regular and thorough debridement. The debridement of mycotic or otherwise thickened toenails is a process generally performed by podiatrists. The debridement first involves soaking of the feet and cutting of the nails by heavy duty cutters. Finally, the nails are thoroughly filed down with an electrically powered, diamond-studded burr. These drills are fitted with vacuum extraction systems to protect the patient and podiatrist from breathing in the nail dust.

Another treatment is permanent removal of the nail,

including matrixectomy. Because toenails serve no useful function, their absence causes no functional impairment. Surgical correction should be reserved, however, for those patients whose nails are painful or for whom the appearance of the feet is a significant factor. The most frequent type of surgical correction of toenails performed by dermatologists, podiatrists, or surgeons is nail excision, followed by chemical destruction of matrix tissue and nailbed with 88% phenol. After a sterile dressing is applied to the toe, the patient may continue his normal routine. He needs only to change bandages and soak his feet daily until healing is complete in 2 to 3 weeks. Skin formerly below the nail plate thickens. Women can disguise the fact that their nails have been removed by applying nail polish to this thickened skin.

Ingrown Toenails (Fig. 102.7)

Etiology and Findings

Ingrown toenail, a painful condition in which the medial or lateral border of a toenail penetrates the flesh, is a common problem. Ingrown toenails have been attributed to factors such as improper trimming, heredity, bony pathology, improper shoe fit, tight socks, obesity, and trauma. However, there is no clear-cut etiology, and there are probably many contributing causes. The nail of a great toe is almost always involved, and the problem can be identified by inspection and by finding point tenderness upon pressing the margin of the toenail.

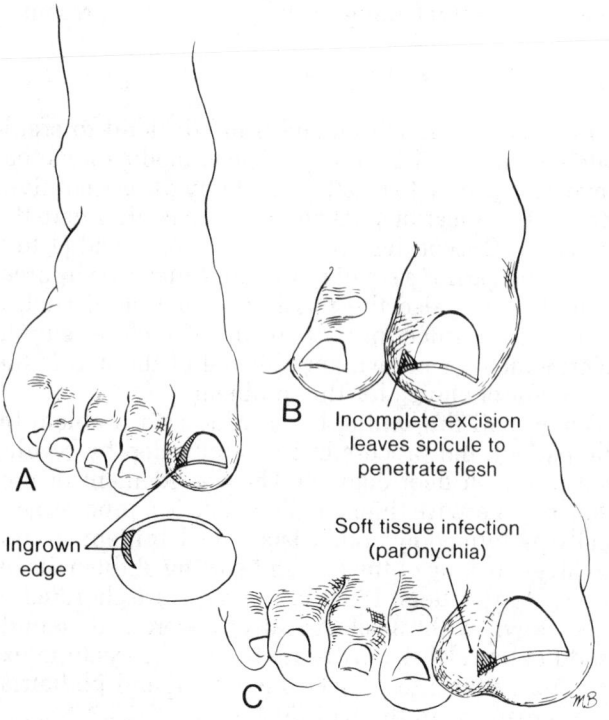

Figure 102.7. Schematic illustration of an ingrown toenail and complications that may occur.

Treatment

There is a popular misconception among many people that cutting a "V" in the center of a toenail will cause the lateral borders to grow toward the center, thereby relieving the ingrown condition. This belief has no basis in fact, since the nail plate is merely hornified keratin—nonliving, fixed tissue in which growth no longer occurs.

Initial treatment of ingrown toenail depends upon whether the patient's toe is infected (paronychia) or is chronically painful but not infected when the patient seeks care. The patient with an ingrown toenail will often seek help after attempting to excise the offending edge of toenail with whatever instruments are available; most of the nail edge may be removed in this way by the patient, but a small, sharp piece of nail usually remains that pierces the skin with each step and promotes infection: the toe becomes red, swollen, and exquisitely tender. The most vigorous soaking and the use of local and systemic antibiotics will not arrest such an infection as long as a nail spicule continues to penetrate the flesh. Therefore, the patient should be referred (to a dermatologist, podiatrist, or surgeon) for excision of the offending border of the nail; this procedure is done under local anesthesia and it is curative. However, approximately 10% of patients will have a recurrence, usually within 1 year. Systemic antimicrobials are rarely necessary. Definitive treatment of the ingrown nail itself varies according to the condition and needs of the patient.

For otherwise healthy patients, the procedure described above for removal of the entire toenail and for matrix destruction can also be utilized to eradicate permanently an ingrown border. After local anesthesia, the offending edge of toenail is excised; then phenol and alcohol are applied to cauterize the matrix tissue. This procedure, followed by 2 to 3 weeks for complete healing, will usually eliminate permanently this painful and sometimes dangerous condition.

Management of diabetics and patients with arterial insufficiency must be conservative, as wound healing may be poor after surgical removal of the nail. In these patients, frequent and thorough debridement of ingrown borders is effective and safe. Treatment by a podiatrist or other practitioner who is skilled in this procedure may be needed every 3 to 4 weeks to prevent complicating soft tissue infection.

HEEL PAIN

Heel pain is a common complaint. The most common pattern is pain that is localized to the medial plantar aspect of the heel. (Heel pain localized to the posterior aspect of the foot, the heel cord, is discussed in Chapter 67; and heel pain as a manifestation of the tarsal tunnel syndrome is discussed in Chapter 84.) Characteristically, the first step in the morning is particularly painful. After 5 to 10 minutes of walking the pain eases, but during the course of the day's activities it becomes progressively worse. The reason that these symptoms appear, disappear, and reappear is not understood.

Examination of the foot reveals a tender area of the heel approximately 4.5 cm from the posterior margin of the plantar surface, corresponding to the medial condyle of the calcaneus. X-rays frequently reveal a calcaneal exostosis or spur at the point of tenderness (Fig. 102.8). These spurs are commonly found on X-rays of asymptomatic heels, and they are not the cause of pain in symptomatic heels. Because the attachment of the plantar fascia coincides with the point of greatest tenderness, it is felt that pain is due to plantar fasciitis. One can picture the plantar fascia as an extension of the Achilles tendon, with the calcaneus acting as a fulcrum between fascia and tendon (Fig. 102.1B). Any condition that increases stress on the Achilles tendon may also stress the plantar fascia, e.g., overuse in running or jogging (especially with shoes having inflexible midsoles), excessive pronation (see above), or a sudden change to flat shoes after wearing high heels for prolonged periods. Heel pain may also be a manifestation of gout or Reiter's syndrome, and these diagnoses should always be considered when evaluating such a patient (see Chapters 69 and 71).

Treatment

Treatment should be aimed at both the local inflammatory process and the underlying mechanical problem. Initial treatment includes use of an oral anti-inflammatory medication (see Chapter 70), rest, and soaking in warm water. An injection of a corticosteroid and lidocaine (approximately 0.5 to 1 ml of suspension of a corticosteroid diluted with 1 to 2 ml of 1 to 2% lidocaine) into the tender area from the medial aspect of the heel will usually bring dramatic relief from pain that has not responded to other measures (see also Table 66.4).

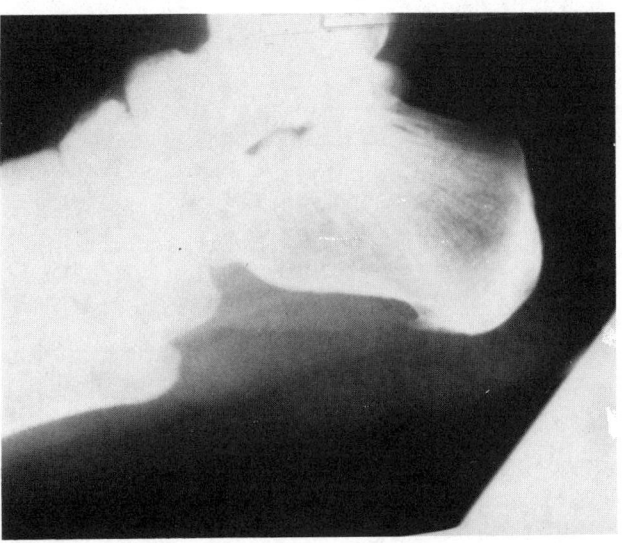

Figure 102.8. Radiological view of a calcaneal exostosis (spur). (Photograph courtesy of Max Weisfeld, D.P.M.)

Recurrent symptoms can be prevented by having the patient use a 1/4-inch felt heel pad. When this is inserted into the shoes, it decreases tension on the Achilles tendon, and, consequently, tension on the plantar fascia is also reduced. The increased angulation of the foot shifts weight away from the heel to the forefoot. Felt rather than foam, which is too compressible, is available from medical and surgical supply houses. When a simple heel pad is not sufficient, consultation with an orthopaedist or podiatrist is indicated. The consultant will fabricate an appropriate orthotic to minimize pronation, raise the heel, and protect the painful area. Rarely, a painful heel will require surgical fasciotomy and removal of the spur.

METATARSALGIA

Definition and Pathogenesis

Metatarsalgia refers to pain in the forefoot. The most common condition causing metatarsalgia is *Morton's neuroma*. This is a condition in which two interdigital plantar nerves between adjacent toes become compressed, inflamed, and ultimately painful. The compression of these nerves is enhanced by elevating the heel and compressing the forefoot. Therefore, women's fashionable highheeled, pointed toe shoes are associated with this condition. In fact, 80 to 90% of patients with neuroma are female.

Symptoms and Signs

The symptoms of neuroma are quite specific and consistent. Typically, the patient will describe a shooting, burning or cramping pain in the foot involving two adjacent toes. The third and fourth toes are involved most commonly. However, the second and third toes also are frequently affected. The patient will describe spontaneous pain during walking or running. Invariably, the patient will instinctively remove the shoe and massage the affected area, thereby relieving the pain. Presumably, the swollen nerve (neuroma) has been pinched by the metatarsal bones causing the pain that radiates to the toes. Stopping walking eliminates the trauma and massage may change the position of the neuroma. All of these measures result in alleviation of the pain. When foot pain is sudden, severe, and unremitting, metatarsalgia should be differentiated from a stress fracture by obtaining an X-ray (see Chapter 67).

Examination of the foot reveals that the neurovascular status will be normal unless another disease is present. Palpation between the metatarsal heads will reveal marked tenderness. If the forefoot is compressed while palpating the web space, the area may be exquisitely tender.

Treatment

The most effective treatment for metatarsalgia is the wearing of low, flat, wide, soft leather shoes. Corticosteroid (lidocaine) injections into the web space and reaching the plantar surface (0.5 ml of deposteroid with 1 ml of lidocaine) may provide temporary relief. Nonsteroidal anti-inflammatory drugs are not effective. Orthotics are helpful; however, if the patient is willing to wear wide enough shoes to accommodate them, the condition will usually resolve, even without the orthotic. Surgical excision is successful in 80 to 90% of cases and is indicated if symptoms persist. For those patients undergoing surgery, a recovery period of 4 to 6 weeks is necessary before they can return to full activity and wear their usual shoes.

Metatarsalgia not caused by neuroma is more difficult to characterize, evaluate, and treat. Nonneuritic metatarsal pain may occur anywhere in the forefoot with or without radiation and be exacerbated by high or, at times, low heeled shoes. Palpation often will reveal pain directly on a metatarsal head rather than between them. Rest, the application of ice, and elevation of the foot may help some patients but most require referral to a podiatrist for padding, orthotics, or other treatment.

General References

Lemont H: Common foot disorders. In: Berkow R (ed): *The Merck Manuel*, 15th ed. Rahway, NJ, Merck, Sharp and Dohme Research Laboratories, 1987.
Levin ME, O'Neal LW (ed): *The Diabetic Foot*, 4th ed. St Louis, CV Mosby, Co., 1988.
McClamy ED (ed): *Comprehensive Textbook of Foot Surgery*. Baltimore, Williams & Wilkins, 1987.
    This two-volume text covers all aspects of foot care including both medical and surgical treatments.
Williams PL: The painful heel. *Br J Hosp Med* 38:562, 1987.

INDEX

Page numbers followed by t and f indicate tables and figures, respectively.

eating disorders in, 53
hypertension in, 789–790
interview of, 60–61
physical development
common problems, 51–53
normal patterns and concerns, 51
physical examination of, 61–62
pregnant, 56
psychosocial development, 57–59
sexual development
common problems, 54–57
normal patterns and concerns, 53
sexual disorders in, 185
sexually transmitted disease in, 53, 55–56
suggested approach to, in office setting, 60–62
suicidal, 58–59
Adolescent athlete, examination of, 62, 62t–63t
Adrenal adenomas, 503, 986
Adrenal androgens
excess, 983, 984t, 985–986
secretion, 983
Adrenal diseases, 981–986
Adrenal function
of glucocorticoid-treated patient, 989
tests of, 982, 985
Adrenal hyperplasia, 980
bilateral, 503
Adrenal insufficiency, 978–979, 992t. See also Adrenocortical insufficiency
hypoglycemia in, 1003
laboratory diagnosis of, 982
mineralocorticoid therapy, 983
office evaluation, 1202
operative risk posed by, size of, 1202
preoperative planning with, 1202–1203
recommendations to surgeon, 1202–1203
secondary to pituitary disease, 982
Adrenal mass. See also Adrenal adenomas
biochemically silent, 986
carcinomas, 986
cystic, 986
incidentally identified, 986
α-Adrenergic agonists
central acting, for hypertension, 780–781
for stress incontinence, 76
β-Adrenergic agonists
antiallergic properties, 254, 254t
effect on serum potassium, 503
selective actions, 615
side effects of, 615
Adrenergic blocking agents. See also α-Blockers; β-Blockers; α-β-Blockers
as antiarrhythmics, 698
effect on thyroid function, 957t
for heart failure, 751
for hypertension, 779–783
pharmacological characteristics of, 778t
in treatment of hyperthyroidism, 963
Adrenergic drugs, and angle-closure glaucoma, 1334
Adrenocortical adenoma, benign, 986
Adrenocortical hyperfunction, 983–986, 984t
Adrenocortical insufficiency, 981–983. See also Addison's disease; Adrenal insufficiency

association with other autoimmune diseases, 981
clinical presentation, 981–982
etiology, 981
Adrenocorticotropic hormone
clinical use, 988
for gout, 874
plasma, 978
synthetic, 982
Adrenocorticotropic hormone-glucocorticoid therapy, 988
Adrenocorticotropic hormone stimulation tests, 982
Adson maneuver, 806
Adsorbents, 456
Adult children of alcoholics, 228
Adult children of dysfunctional families, 228
Adult respiratory distress syndrome, 307
Adult T cell leukemia, 583
Advance directives, from patients and families, 190
Adventitious movements, assessment of, in neurological exam, 1072
Adverse drug effects. See also specific agent
incidence of, with renal failure, 533
Advice, as counseling technique, 114
Advil. See Ibuprofen
Aerobic bacteria, lung abscesses, 345
Aeromonas hydrophilia, wound infections, 279t
Aerophagia, 459
Affect, 107
in schizophrenia, 159
Affective disorders, 147–158. See also Depression; Mania
bipolar, 137, 150, 157
counseling distressed family of patients with, 157
and hypersomnolence, 1179
with insomnia, 1173
major, 150–157
unipolar, 150
Affective symptoms, detection of patients with, 148
Afferent loop syndrome, 433t
Afterload, 737–738, 738f
adjusted, by use of drugs, 745
reduction therapy, in ambulatory setting, 752
Agency for Toxic Substances and Diseases Registries, 90
Aging. See also Elderly
and male sexual function, 1052
usual vs. successful, 77
Agnosia, 169
Agoraphobia, 131, 133–135
strategies adopted by patients with, to reduce anticipatory anxiety, 134t
without history of panic disorder, 134
Agranulocytosis
drug-induced, 163
thiocarbamide-induced, 962–963
AIDS. See Acquired immune deficiency syndrome
AIDS-associated retrovirus, 375
AIDS-related complex, 379
Air bronchogram, 597, 597f
Air-filtering devices, 258
Air pollution, 90–91
and obstructive pulmonary disease, 624
Airway hyperreactivity

in asthma, 608
after influenza, 306–307
in obstructive airways disease, 625
Airways. See also entries under Alveolar; entries under Bronchial; entries under Upper airway; Upper respiratory
collapse, 604. See also Lung(s), collapse
normal, morphology of, 607f
Airways obstruction. See also Obstructive airways disease
in infectious mononucleosis, 580
lower, chronic cough with, 588
measurement of, 605
mechanisms of, 605t
in asthma, 620
in rheumatoid arthritis, 887
risk factors, 623t
and syncope, 1130
upper, 594, 613, 1130
Akathisia, 163
Akinesia, with Parkinson's disease, 1138–1139
Al-Anon, 214, 218, 226, 228
process of, 227t
Alateen, 218, 226
Albalon, 261, 1340–1341
Albuterol, 615t
for asthma, 615
Alcohol. See also Blood alcohol level(s)
abuse/dependence, 18t, 149, 178, 205, 236
characteristics of, 236t
frequency, by sex and age, 106t
and hypoglycemia, 1002–1003
and acute gastritis, 425
addiction, 205
annual national consumption of, 206
effects of
on essential tremor, 1135
on sexual response, 176t
experimental use of, 232
and gout, 871
and hypertension, 770
interactions with sulfonylureas, 939
and lipoprotein metabolism, 1015
and management of heart failure, 745
metabolism, 205–207
and migraine, 1086
panic symptoms simulated by, 133
recommendations to surgeon for perioperative period, 1191t
social and recreational use of, 232
tolerance, 205, 207
and ulcer disease, 424
use
loss of control of, 210
prevalence of, 234
quantity or frequency of, 212–213
withdrawal
delirium caused by, 172
and hypertension, 787
seizures in, 1100
prevention of, 223
symptoms, 205, 221
treatment of, 1100
Alcohol amnestic disorder, 207–209
Alcohol–drug interactions, 219–220
Alcohol hallucination, 221
Alcoholic(s)
fever in, 272, 274
one-on-one confrontation of, 214–216

Ambiguous genitalia, 1047
Ambivalence, in schizophrenia, 159
Ambulatory medicine
  definition of, 4
  distinctive characteristics of, 3–12
  domain of, 3–6
  goals of, 7
  knowledge and skills important in,
    7–12
  longitudinal nature of, 5, 6t
  patient's expectations of, 7
    implications for practice, 7
  temporal dimension in, 5, 6t
Ambulatory (Holter) monitoring, 657, 693
Ambulatory patient(s), 4–5
  definition of, 3
  percentage distribution of diagnostic
    and therapeutic services
    ordered or provided for, 4, 5t
  principal diagnoses, 4, 4t
  problems of, 4
Ambulatory surgery
  guidelines on patient eligibility for,
    1187, 1188t
  numbers of procedures, 1187
Amebiasis, 358, 451, 454, 1271
  proctoscopy in, 450
  reporting, 21t
  treatment of, 288–289
Amenorrhea, 53, 178, 979, 1057
  exogenous, 1058
  hypothalamic, 1058
  primary, 1057–1058
  secondary, 981, 1058
    diagnostic procedures with, 1059
    treatment of women with, 1059
American Cancer Society, 92
American Heart Association, 1027
  information booklets, 753
  local affiliates of, 674
  prudent diet, 1020
American Medical Association, Council
    on Scientific Affairs, address,
    70
American Psychiatric Association,
    classification of personality
    disorders, 143–144
American Sleep Disorders Association,
    1183
Amiloride hydrochloride, 746
  characteristics of, 746t
  for hypertension, 779
    available strengths, 777t
    dose range, 777t
  for prevention of urinary calculi, 512
  for primary aldosteronism, 503
  in renal failure, 529, 530t
Aminoglycosides
  nephrotoxicity, 521t
  ototoxicity, 1120, 1320
  renal damage with, 1201
Aminophylline, 1199–1201
  for asthma, 616, 619
Aminotransferases, serum, 478
  elevated, 479–480
  in hepatitis, 473–474
  in hypothyroidism, 968
Amiodarone
  adverse effects of, 696t
  as antiarrhythmic, 698–700
  characteristics of, 695t
  doses, 698
  effect on thyroid function, 957t, 958
  hyperthyroidism with, 966

hypothyroidism with, 966–967
side effects of, 698
Amitriptyline
  for cluster headache, 1090
  doses, 152t
  effect on glucose tolerance, 918t
  for fibromyalgia, 832
  in migraine prophylaxis, 1089t
  prophylaxis for tension headaches,
    1085
  side effects, 152t
  as sleep medication, 1183
  strength of oral preparations, 152t
  therapeutic plasma level, 152t
  for trigeminal neuralgia, 1095
Amnesia, 121, 123
Amnestic syndrome, resembling alcohol
    amnestic disorder, 209
Amodiaquine, 364
Amoeba, diarrhea secondary to, 449
Amoebic colitis, 449
Amoxicillin
  for Lyme disease, 338–339
  for opportunistic infections in HIV-
    infected patients, 386t
  oral
    available strengths, 318t
    drug (and food) instructions, 318t
    for respiratory infections, 318t
    side effects, 318t
    usual adult dose and schedule, 318t
  for sinusitis, 310
  skin reaction to, 1351t
  for UTI, 294–295, 296t
Amoxicillin-clavulanate
  for acute bronchitis, 314
  oral
    available strengths, 318t
    drug (and food) instructions, 318t
    for respiratory infections, 318t
    side effects, 318t
    usual adult dose and schedule, 318t
    for recurrent pharyngitis and tonsillitis,
    309
  for sinusitis, 310
Amoxicillin rash, 267
Amoxil. *See* Amoxicillin
Amphetamines, 160
  abuse of, 238
    effect on thyroid function, 958
  chronic adverse effects of, 239
  effects of
    on sexual response, 176t
    on thyroid function, 957t
  fever due to, 271
  and hair loss, 1357
  usual effects of, 238–239
  for weight loss, 1039–1040, 1041t
Amphojel. *See* Aluminum hydroxide
Amphotericin B
  hypersensitivity, fever due to, 271, 271t
  for opportunistic infections in HIV-
    infected patients, 385t–386t
    available strengths, preparations,
    388t
    common adverse effects, 388t
    dosage change with renal/hepatic
     failure, 388t
    dosage/schedule/route, 388t
    drug interactions, 388t
    duration/maintenance, 388t
    organisms and syndromes, 388t
  topical, 1378
Ampicillin

for acute bronchitis, 314
diarrhea associated with, 455
oral
  available strengths, 318t
  drug (and food) instructions, 318t
  for respiratory infections, 318t
  side effects, 318t
  usual adult dose and schedule, 318t
for sinusitis, 310
skin reaction to, 1351t
for UTI, 296t
Ampicillin rash, 267
Amputation
  for arterial occlusive disease, 1217
  level, selecting, 1217
  mortality for, 1217
  rehabilitation after, 1217
  risk for, 1213
Amyloidosis, 444, 451, 653
  bleeding in, 565
  with chronic osteomyelitis, 344
  diagnosed by small bowel biopsy, 452
  esophageal motility disorder in, 407
  neuropathy of, 1157
  secondary, with ankylosing spondylitis,
    903
Amyotrophic lateral sclerosis, 1075, 1160
Amyotrophy, of diabetes mellitus, 945,
    1167
Anabolic steroids
  and cholestasis, 477
  effect on thyroid function, 957t
Anaerobic bacteria
  lung abscesses, 345
  osteomyelitis, 342
  sinusitis, 310
Anaerobic streptococci, lung abscesses,
    345
Ana-Kit, 267
Anal bleeding, spotty, 1261
Anal carcinoma, 1264
Anal cleanliness, to control pruritus ani,
    1260
Anal cushions, 1262
Anal fissure, 444, 1259
  treatment of, 1261–1262
Anal fistula, 1268
Analgesics
  dosage, in renal failure, 534
  for headache, 1085
  nephrotoxicity, 521t
  for pain associated with sensory
    neuropathies, 1168
  recommendations to surgeon for
    perioperative period, 1191t
Anal glands, 1267
Anal intercourse, and transmission of
    HIV, 376
Anal papilla, hypertrophied, 1264
Anal skin tags, 1264
Anal sphincters, examination, 444
Anaphylatoxin, 253
Anaphylaxis/anaphylactoid reactions,
    264
  definition of, 265–266
  management of, 266, 266t
  symptoms, 266
  therapeutic and diagnostic substances
    reported to have caused, 265t
Anaprox. *See* Naproxen
Androblastoma, 1050
Androgens. *See also* Adrenal androgens
  addition of, to estrogen replacement
    therapy, 1065

Dietary-induced thermogenesis, 1034
Diet exchange lists, 922
Diethylpropion, for weight loss, 1041t
Diethylstilbestrol, for metastatic prostatic
 cancer, 545
Diffuse esophageal spasm. *See*
 Esophageal spasm, diffuse
Diffuse idiopathic skeletal hyperostosis,
 862, 890t
 X-ray abnormalities in, 862t
Diffuse toxic goiter. *See* Graves' disease
Diffusion capacity, 594
 measurement of, 606
Diflunisal, for low back pain, 819
Digitalis, 271
 for arrhythmias, 694
 drug interactions, 748–749
 gastrointestinal side effects, 749
 indications for, 748
 therapy, 748–749
 use of
  general considerations in, 694
  recommendations for, 748–749
  recommendations to surgeon for
   perioperative period, 1191t
Digitalis toxicity, 703
 due to drug interactions, 749
 and hypokalemia, 497
 recognition of, 749
 treatment of, 749
Digitalization
 in ambulatory patient, 748
 in older patient, 748
 preoperative, 1197–1198
  in patients with arrhythmias, 1198
Digital subtraction angiography, 766,
 1079
 patient experience, 766
Digoxin, 1198
 dosage, 748
  in renal failure, 535
 drug interactions, 786
 effect on sexual response, 176t
 for prevention of recurrent attacks of
  supraventricular tachycardia,
  704–705
 radioimmunoassay, 749
 use of
  in elderly, 69
  recommendations for, 748–749
Dihydralazine HCl, skin reaction to, 1351t
Dihydrotachysterol, 532
 for therapy of hypoparathyroidism, 991
5-α-Dihydrotestosterone, 1045
1,25-Dihydroxyvitamin D, production of,
 age-related decrease, 995
1,25-Dihydroxyvitamin D₃, 516, 531–532
 for therapy of hypoparathyroidism, 991
Diiodohydroxyquin (Diodoquin), for
 amebic dysentery, 289
Dilantin. *See also* Phenytoin
 effect on glucose tolerance, 918t
 recommendations to surgeon for
  perioperative period, 1191t
Dilantin lung, 1109
Dilaudid. *See* Hydromorphone
Diltiazem
 adverse effects of, 696t
 for angina, 660, 662t, 664
 available strengths, 662t
 characteristics of, 695t, 751t
 contraindications to, 785
 duration of action, 662t
 for hypertension, 785–786

onset of action, 662t
 pharmacological characteristics of, 778t
 for Raynaud's phenomenon, 835
 usual maximum dose, 662t
 usual starting dose, 662t
Dimenhydrinate
 for motion sickness, 1123
 for symptomatic treatment of vertigo,
  1122t
Dimetane. *See* Brompheniramine
Dimetapp, 261t
Dimethylcysteine, 896
Di-methyltryptamine, 242
DIMS. *See* Disorders of initiating and
 maintaining sleep
Dioctyl sodium sulfosuccinate, 446
Diodoquin. *See* Diiodohydroxyquin
Diphenhydramine, 163
 for allergic rhinitis, 260t
 antipruritic effect, 1260
 for aphthous stomatitis, 1382
 for atopic dermatitis, 1349
 in calamine lotion, 1377
 in detoxification process, 222, 222t
 for herpes zoster, 1361
 intramuscular, 156
 in management of urticaria, 265
 for plant dermatitis, 1350
 for scabies, 1366
 as sleep medication, 1183
Diphenoxylate, 448
Diphenoxylate-atropine, 288, 456–457,
 463
 control schedule, 248t
 for diarrhea, 369
 prescribing patterns, 248t
 therapeutic use, 248t
Diphenylhydantoin. *See* Phenytoin
Diphtheria, 309
 annual incidence of, 354
 cutaneous, 279–280
 immunization, 354
  for travelers, 361
 reporting, 21t
Diphtheria antitoxin, 280
Diphtheria-pertussis-tetanus vaccine, 354
Diphtheria-tetanus toxoids, combined,
 354
Diphtheria toxoid, 354
Diphtheria vaccine, 352t
 history of, 17t
Diplopia, 1125
Diprolene. *See* Betamethasone, cream
Dipstick, urine, 491, 521
Dipyridamole, 576–577
 for angina, 665
Dipyrone, skin reaction to, 1351t
Direct fluorescent antibody for *T.
 pallidum* (DFA-TP) test, 329,
 331
Direct fluorescent microscopy, for
 syphilis, 331
Disability
 vs. malingering, 127
 Social Security definition of, 97
Disability insurance, 97–100
 appeal process, 98
 benefits, 97–98
 eligibility, 97
 process of disability determination, 98
 and return to work, 98–100
Disalcid. *See* Salicylsalicylic acid
Disc. *See* Intervertebral disc
Disciform scar, 1326, 1327f

Discitis, 823–824
Discoid lupus erythematosus, 1378
Disease
 ethnic concepts of, and compliance, 40
 of known or unknown etiology,
  reporting, 21t
 of known or unknown etiology that
  may be a danger to public
  health, reporting, 21t
 models of, and compliance, 40
 patient's previous experience of, and
  compliance, 40
Disequilibrium
 definition of, 1115
 of miscellaneous origins, 1131–1132
DISH. *See* Diffuse idiopathic skeletal
 hyperostosis
Disodium cromoglycate, antiallergic
 properties, 254, 254t
Disophrol, 261t
Disopyramide
 adverse effects of, 696t
 characteristics of, 695t
 dosage, in renal failure, 535
 effects of, 697
  on sexual response, 176t
 toxicity of, 697
Disorders of excessive somnolence, 1171,
 1175–1179
 diagnostic evaluation, 1175
 medical and environmental causes,
  1178
 psychosocial conditions, 1179
 sleep disorders that mimic, 1179
Disorders of initiating and maintaining
 sleep, 1171–1175
Displacement, 108
Disseminated intravascular coagulation,
 559, 569
Distal symmetrical sensorimotor
 polyneuropathy, 941
Disulfiram
 advantages of, 219
 contraindications to, 218–219
 effect on sexual response, 176t
 office prescribing of, 219
 to prevent drinking, 218
 side effects of, 218
 supervised use of, approach to, 219,
  219t
Disulfiram–alcohol interaction, 218
Ditropan. *See* Oxybutynin
Diucardin. *See* Hydroflumethiazide
Diulo. *See* Metolazone
Diuresis, 481
Diuretics, 1320. *See also* Loop diuretics;
 Potassium-sparing diuretics;
 specific agent; Thiazides
 abuse, 503
 characteristics of, 746t
 classes of, 746
 effect on sexual response, 176t
 for heart failure, 745–748
 hemodynamic effects of, 749
 for hypertension, 777–779
  available strengths, 777t
  dose range, 777t
  mechanism, 777
 hypokalemia caused by, 500
 mechanism of action, in heart failure,
  745
 metabolic alkalosis caused by, 500, 747
 nephrotoxicity, 521t
 ototoxicity, 1120

Dust allergy, 255
Dyazide, 777t. *See also* Triamterene
Dying. *See* Death and dying
Dyrenium. *See* Triamterene
Dysarthria, 1125
Dysarthria-clumsy hand syndrome, 1145
Dysautonomia, neuropathy of, 1157
Dysautonomic cephalgia, post-traumatic, 1093–1094
Dysbetalipoproteinemia, 1005, 1012
    drug therapy, 1027
Dysentery, 369
Dysfibrinogenemia, 572
Dysfunctional uterine bleeding, 1055–1057
    management, 1057
Dysgammaglobulinemia, liporprotein metabolism in, 1015
Dyshidrosis
    presentation, 1353
    therapy for, 1353
Dyshidrotic eczema, 1352f
Dysmenorrhea, 121, 1054–1056, 1058
Dysmetria, 1134
Dyspareunia, 120t, 174, 1060
    assessment, 183
    causes, 175t–176t
    diagnostic criteria for, 183
    estrogen therapy, 1063
    treatment of, 184
Dyspepsia, 895
    definition of, 434
    essential, 434
    nonulcer, 434
Dysphagia, 401–409
    causes of, 401, 402t
    clinical evaluation, 401–402
    esophageal, 401, 402t
    history, 401
    oropharyngeal, 401, 402t
    in Parkinson's disease, 1139
    postgastrectomy, 433t
    special studies with, 401–402
    with thyroid enlargement, 970
Dysphoric reaction, marijuana-induced, 240–241
Dyspnea, 120t, 591–595, 602, 722
    acute, 592–593
    acute intermittent, 604
    causes of, 592, 592t
    chronic, evaluation of, 593–594
    with chronic airways obstruction, 625, 632
    definition of, 591
    evaluation of, 592
    of heart failure, 740
    intermittent, 608
    with lung cancer, 638
    mechanisms of, 591
    postflu, 307
    progressive, 604
        evaluation of, 593–594
    psychogenic, 592
    at rest, 729
    treatment of, 595
        in renal failure, 537
Dysproteinemia
    bleeding in, 565
    neuropathy of, 1157
Dysthymic disorder, 137, 147–149
    diagnosis, 148–149
    diagnostic criteria for, 149t
    in elderly, 166
    epidemiology of, 148

frequency, by sex and age, 106t
    management, 149
    prognosis, 149
Dystonia, 1134
    axial, 1137
    drug-induced, 163
Dysuria-pyuria syndrome, 297–298

E

Ear(s). *See also* Inner ear; Middle ear
    conductive system of, 1311
    function, 1311
    pain, environmental causes, 84t
    problems, 1311–1321
    structure, 1311, 1312f
Eardrops, 1316
Eating disorders, 1031
    in adolescents and young adults, 53
    DSM-III-R criteria for, 53t
EBV. *See* Epstein-Barr virus
Echocardiography, 719–720
    with aortic regurgitation, 733
    with aortic stenosis, 722
    with atrial septal defect, 726
    clinical applications of, 720–721
    in heart failure, 743–744
    in hypertrophic cardiomyopathy, 725
    with mitral regurgitation, 727
    with mitral stenosis, 731
    M-mode, 720
    two-dimensional (2-D), 720
Eclampsia, 792
Econazole, 1378
ECT. *See* Electroconvulsive therapy
Ecthyma, 275
    antibiotic therapy for, 276t
    bacterial cultures of, 276
    prevention of, 276
    treatment of, 276
Ectopic pregnancy, 1056–1057
    and intrauterine device, 1282
Eczema
    atopic. *See* Dermatitis, atopic
    in external auditory canal, 1316
Eczema herpeticum, 1348–1349, 1359
Edecrin. *See* Ethacrynic acid
Edema
    dependent, 1225
    in heart failure, 741
    lower extremity, management, 1228
    nonpitting, 1223
    nontender periorbital, 310
    peripheral pitting, in heart failure, 742
    pitting, 1223
    therapy, 489
Edentulous population, 1387
Edrophonium, esophageal stimulation, 409
Educational diagnosis, 31
    case example, 31–34
EEG. *See* Electroencephalography
Ehlers-Danlos syndrome, 465, 729
    chronic aortic regurgitation with, 732
Eicosopentanoic acid, 577
Ejaculation, 174
Ejaculation, delayed, 120t
Ejection fraction, 737–738, 738f, 743
Ejection sounds, 718
    pulmonic, 718
    systolic, 763
Elavil. *See* Amitriptyline
Elbow
    arthroscopy of, 854
    exercise-related problems of, 850–852
    structures of, 851f

Eldepryl. *See* Deprenyl
Elder housing, 78
Elderly
    abominal pain in, 414
    abuse or neglect of, 69–70
    adjustment disorder with depressed mood in, 166
    alcoholism in, 166, 205
    anemia in, 562
    antipsychotic dosage in, 163
    cervical cancer in, 77
    clinical evaluation of patient, 65–67
    cognitive assessment of, 166
    delusions in, 168
    depression in, 166
    depressive symptoms in, 166
    diabetes in, special considerations in treatment of, 939
    disability in, rates of, 64–65
    drug use in, 68–69
        acetaminophen, 69
        acetohexamide, 939
        antihypertensives, precautions with, 791
        chlorpropamide, 939
        cold remedies, 69
        desipramine, 167
        digoxin, 69
        fluoxetine, 167
        haloperidol, 168
        major tranquilizers, 69
        neuroleptics, 167–169
        nonsteroidal anti-inflammatory drugs, 69
        nortriptyline, 167
        oral hypoglycemics, 69
        safety, 68–69
        sulfonylureas, 939
        tolazamide, 939
        tolbutamide, 939
        toxicities, 68–69
        tricyclic antidepressants, 167
        trifluoperazine, 168
    dysthymic disorder in, 166
    electroconvulsive therapy in, 167
    excessive somnolence in, 1178
    exercise in, 77
    exercise stress tests in, 77
    falls in, 70
    false-positive nontreponemal test reactions in, 332
    fever in, 272
    functional assessment of, 67–68
    glomerular filtration rate in, 68
    hallucinations in, 168
    hearing loss in, 1319–1320
    housing programs for, 78
    hypertension in, 758, 790–791
    hypochondriasis in, 167
    immunizations for, 77
    insulin therapy, 939
    limiting therapy for, decisions about, 67
    long-term care of, 65
    major affective disorders in, 167
    medical care for
        advance directives guiding, 77–78
        public policy about, 65
    mental distress complications of primary physical illness, 166
    mental illness in, 165–173
        importance of diagnosis, 165
    mental status in, postoperative changes in, 1190

Pneumonia, 315–319, 590, 592. *See also*
    Pneumocystis carinii
    pneumonia
  adenovirus, 317
  anaerobic, 316
  antimicrobial therapy, 318, 318t
  atypical, 316
    epidemiological clues to presumptive
      diagnosis of, 317t
  atypical vs. bacterial, 315
  bacterial, 315–316
  chlamydial, 316
  clinical presentation of, 315
  cold hemagglutinin-positive, 315
  cough, 588
  definition of, 315
  distinction from bronchitis, 315
  evaluation of, 316
  false-positive nontreponemal test
    reactions in, 332
  follow-up, 318–319
  Gram-negative, 316
  in HIV-infected patients, 319
  during influenza epidemics, 307
  influenza viral, 307
  laboratory examination in, 316
  with lung cancer, 639, 644
  management
    ambulatory, 318
    hospitalization, 317–318
  mycoplasmal, 315
  pain caused by, 596
  physical examination in, 316
  pneumococcal, 315–317
  prevention of, 319
  recurrent, 600
  serological diagnosis, 317
  slowly resolving, 599
  sputum in, 316–317
  staphylococcal, 316
  viral, 315
Pneumonitis
  environmental causes, 84t
  interstitial, 888
Pneumothorax, 602f, 602–603
  in asthma, 620
  iatrogenic, 602
  in rheumatoid arthritis, 887
  spontaneous, 592, 602, 623
    chest pain associated with, 596
  traumatic, 602
  types of, 602
Podagra, 871t
Podophyllin, 1303, 1372
Podophyllum, for venereal warts, 1296–
    1297
Poikilocytosis, 557
Point of maximal impulse, 742
Poison centers, 88
Poison ivy, 1350
Poison oak, 1350
Poison sumac, 1350
Polaramine. *See* Deschlorpheniramine
Polio, 17t, 358
  reporting, 21t
  vaccine, 352t
    for adults, 361
    for travelers, 360t, 360–361
Pollen(s)
  allergy to, 255
  seasonal occurrence of, 257f
Polyarteritis nodosa, vertigo in, 1120
Polyarthralgias, with hyperlipidemia,
    1017

Polyarthritis
  additive, 880–881
  diagnostic approach to, 889t
  differential diagnosis of, 890t
  seronegative, 890t
Polycystic kidney disease, 517–518, 520–
    522
  course, 525
Polycystic ovary disease, 1030, 1036,
    1052
Polycythemia vera, 569
Polydipsia
  approach to patient with, 997
  in diabetes, 916
Polyglandular failure, 981, 1058
Polymenorrhea, 1056
Polymorphonuclear neutrophilic
    leukocytes, vacuoles in, 273
Polymox, for urinary tract infections,
    294–295
Polymyalgia rheumatica, 890t–891t, 1092
Polymyositis, 403t, 890t
Polymyxin-bacteria-neomycin ointment,
    for cutaneous ulcers, 279
Polyneuropathy, 1155
  differential diagnosis, 1156, 1157t
  etiology, 1156, 1156t
  inflammatory demyelinating, in HIV
    infection, 1160
  mixed, 1155
  mode of predominant involvement,
    1156t
  motor, 1155
    symptomatic treatment, 1168
  sensory, 1155
    symptomatic therapy, 1168
  symptomatic treatment, 1168
  time course, 1156
  weakness in, 1156
Polypectomy, 438
  colonoscopic, 439
  intestinal, 422
Polyphagia, in diabetes, 916
Polyps
  with colon cancer, 441
  colonic, 439–440
    relationship of size, histological type,
      and risk of carcinoma, 439t
  hyperplastic, 439
  intestinal, 438
  juvenile, 440
  nasal, 256–257
    management of, 263
  rectal, 440
Polysomnogram, 1183
Polythiazide, for hypertension
  available strengths, 777t
  dose range, 777t
Polyunsaturated fatty acids, 1020
Polyuria, 541
  approach to patient with, 997
  causes of, 996t
  in diabetes, 916
Pomade acne, 1346
Pondimin. *See* Fenfluramine
Popeye sign, 800
Popliteal arterial aneurysm, 1221
Porokeratosis plantaris discreta, 1396,
    1398, 1399f
Positron emission tomographic scanning,
    of brain, 1106
Postcholecystectomy syndrome, 1249–
    1250
  cause of, 1249, 1250t

  incidence, 1249, 1250t
  symptoms of, 1249
Postconcussive syndrome, 1093
  objective tests for, 1094
Posterior inferior cerebellar artery,
    occlusion, cerebellar infarction
    due to, 1121
Posterior interosseus nerve, compression
    of, 1165–1166
Postextrasystolic potentiation, 693
Postgastrectomy syndromes, 432, 433t
Postheparin lipolytic activity, 1007
Postherpetic neuralgia, 1361
Postmyocardial infarction syndrome, 679
Postnasal drip, 311
  cough with, 588
Postpartum thyroid dysfunction, 970
Postpericardiotomy syndrome, 666–667
Postphlebitic syndrome, 576
Postrenal azotemia, 517
Post-traumatic stress disorder
  description, 136
  diagnostic criteria for, 137t
  epidemiology, 136–137
  origins, 136–137
  treatment, 137–138
Postural abnormalities, with Parkinson's
    disease, 1139
Postural attitudes, correct/incorrect, 825f
Postural drainage, 630
Postural hypotension, 497
  in adrenal insufficiency, 982
  in diabetes, 943
  with prazosin, 781
  with vasodilator therapy, 752
Postural tremor, in hyperthyroidism, 960
Postvagotomy syndrome, 456
Potassium
  deficiency, 495 (see also Hypokalemia)
    with cirrhosis, 481
  depletion
    consequences of, 496–497, 498t
    renal effects, 497
  dietary, and blood pressure control,
    770
  dietary deficiency, 501–502
  distribution of, between intracellular
    and extracellular spaces, 495
  maintenance therapy, indications for,
    500, 501t
  monitoring, in patients receiving
    diuretics, 500
  restriction, with chronic renal
    insufficiency, 529
  secretion, factors influencing, 495,
    496f
  serum, 495–496
  supplements, 501
  total body, 495
  urinary losses, excessive, 502
  wasting, renal, 502–503
Potassium balance, 496f
  external, 495
  internal, 495–496
    disordered, 503
  physiological background, 495–496
Potassium chloride
  to correct diuretic-induced
    hypokalemia, 501
  preparations, 501
Potassium-conserving diuretics, 770
Potassium current blockers, 698–700
Potassium hydroxide preparation, 1354
Potassium salts, 501t, 747